Osborn's Brain

IMAGING, PATHOLOGY, AND ANATOMY

SECOND EDITION

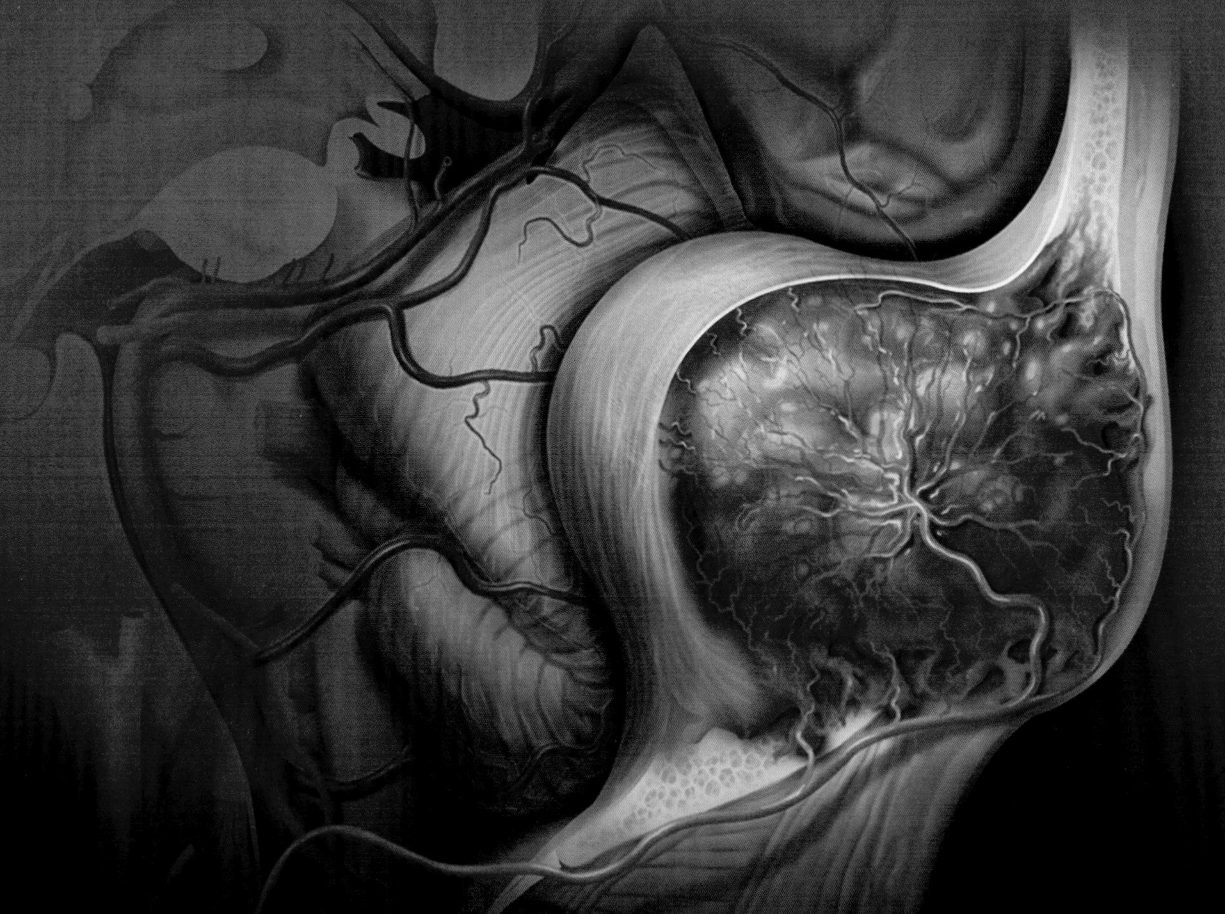

Anne G. Osborn

Hedlund | Salzman

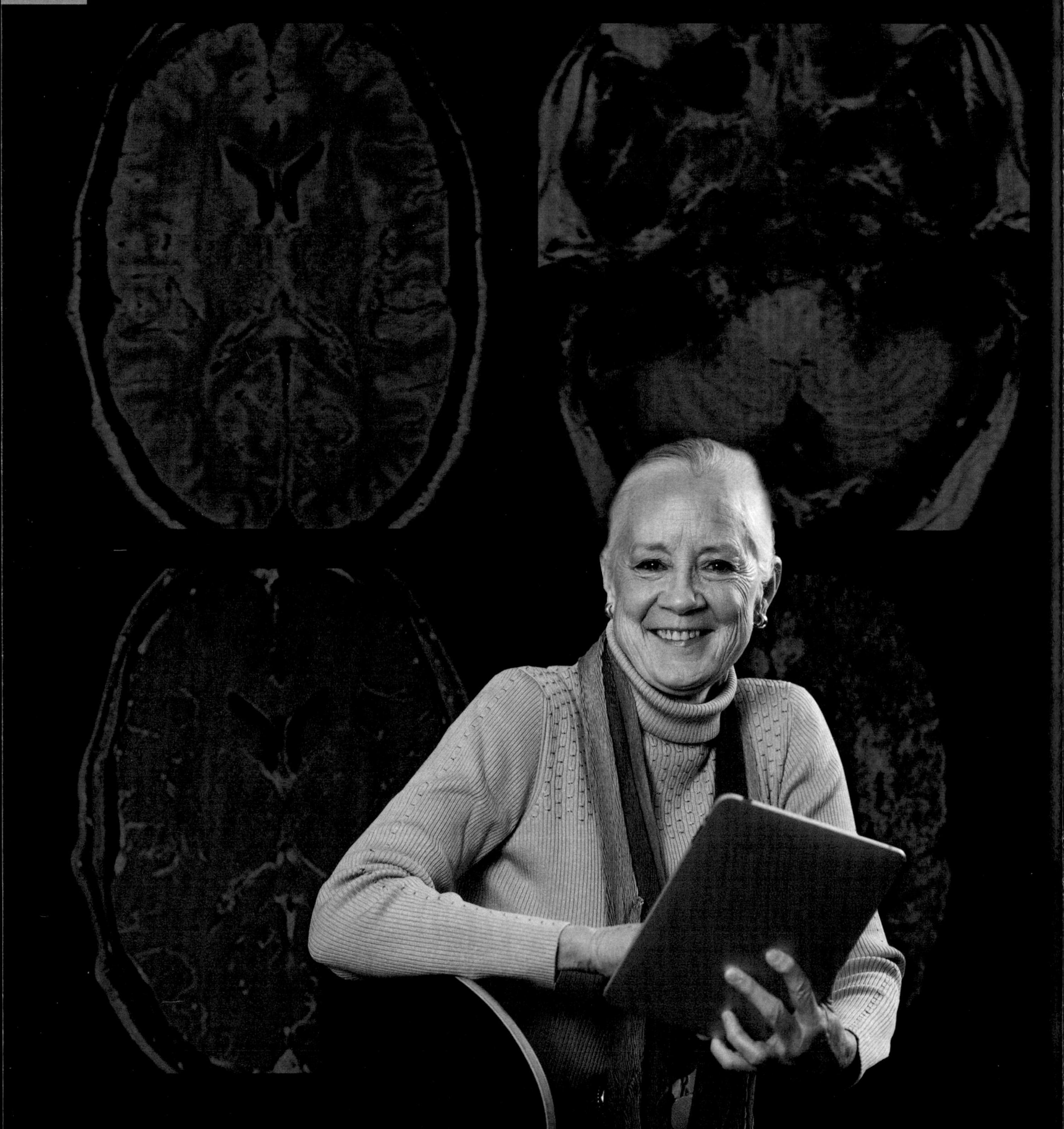

Osborn's Brain

IMAGING, PATHOLOGY, AND ANATOMY

SECOND EDITION

Anne G. Osborn, MD, FACR

University Distinguished Professor and Professor of Radiology and Imaging Sciences
William H. and Patricia W. Child Presidential Endowed Chair in Radiology
University of Utah School of Medicine
Salt Lake City, Utah

Gary L. Hedlund, DO

Pediatric Radiologist and Neuroradiologist
Primary Children's Hospital
Department of Medical Imaging
Intermountain Healthcare
Adjunct Professor of Radiology
University of Utah School of Medicine
Salt Lake City, Utah

Karen L. Salzman, MD

Professor of Radiology and Imaging Sciences
Neuroradiology Section Chief and Fellowship Director
Leslie W. Davis Endowed Chair in Neuroradiology
University of Utah School of Medicine
Salt Lake City, Utah

ELSEVIER

1600 John F. Kennedy Blvd.
Ste 1800
Philadelphia, PA 19103-2899

OSBORN'S BRAIN, SECOND EDITION

ISBN: 978-0-323-47776-5

Notices

Knowledge and best practice in this field are constantly changing. As new research and experience broaden our understanding, changes in research methods, professional practices, or medical treatment may become necessary.

Practitioners and researchers must always rely on their own experience and knowledge in evaluating and using any information, methods, compounds, or experiments described herein. In using such information or methods they should be mindful of their own safety and the safety of others, including parties for whom they have a professional responsibility.

With respect to any drug or pharmaceutical products identified, readers are advised to check the most current information provided (i) on procedures featured or (ii) by the manufacturer of each product to be administered, to verify the recommended dose or formula, the method and duration of administration, and contraindications. It is the responsibility of practitioners, relying on their own experience and knowledge of their patients, to make diagnoses, to determine dosages and the best treatment for each individual patient, and to take all appropriate safety precautions.

To the fullest extent of the law, neither the Publisher nor the authors, contributors, or editors, assume any liability for any injury and/or damage to persons or property as a matter of products liability, negligence or otherwise, or from any use or operation of any methods, products, instructions, or ideas contained in the material herein.

Publisher Cataloging-in-Publication Data

Names: Osborn, Anne G., 1943-
Title: Osborn's brain / [edited by] Anne G. Osborn.
Description: Second edition. | Salt Lake City, UT : Elsevier, Inc., [2017] | Includes bibliographical references and index.
Identifiers: ISBN 978-0-323-47776-5
Subjects: LCSH: Brain--Pathophysiology--Handbooks, manuals, etc. | Central nervous system--Diseases--Handbooks, manuals, etc. | Brain--Imaging--Handbooks, manuals, etc. | MESH: Brain--physiopathology--Atlases. | Central Nervous System--pathology--Atlases. | Neuroimaging--methods--Atlases.
Classification: LCC RC386.5.O83 2017 | NLM WL 301 | DDC 616.8--dc23

International Standard Book Number: 978-0-323-47776-5
Cover Designer: Tom M. Olson, BA
Cover Art: Lane R. Bennion, MS

Printed in Canada by Friesens, Altona, Manitoba, Canada

Last digit is the print number: 9 8 7 6 5 4 3 2 1

Dedications

FOR RON

Beloved sweetheart, eternal companion, and soulmate, you didn't live to see the first edition completed and then watch it become an international bestseller. The second edition is even better, and I hope it makes you even more proud. I love you beyond expression and devote every day of my life in the service of others and in honor of your memory.

AO

FOR DIANA, AARON, AND JAIME

For Diana, my beloved, my best friend.
Your unwavering support nourishes my creative spirit. Thank you, sweetheart.
For Aaron, you honor the integrity of relationship and honest work. This inspires me.
For Jaime, your whole-hearted humanity illuminates the sacredness of our work in the service of others.

GLH

FOR MY FRIENDS AND COLLEAGUES IN NEURORADIOLOGY

To those of you at the University of Utah and around the world, thank you for the wonderful collaborations over the years. I am fortunate to practice in a field with such talented experts. My work is elevated because of your knowledge and support, for which I am in a constant state of gratitude.

KLS

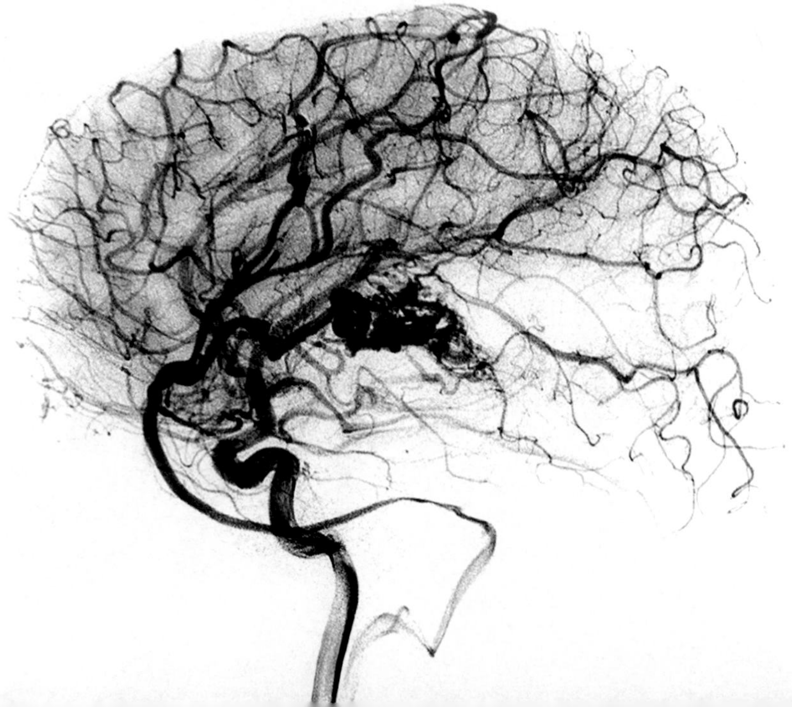

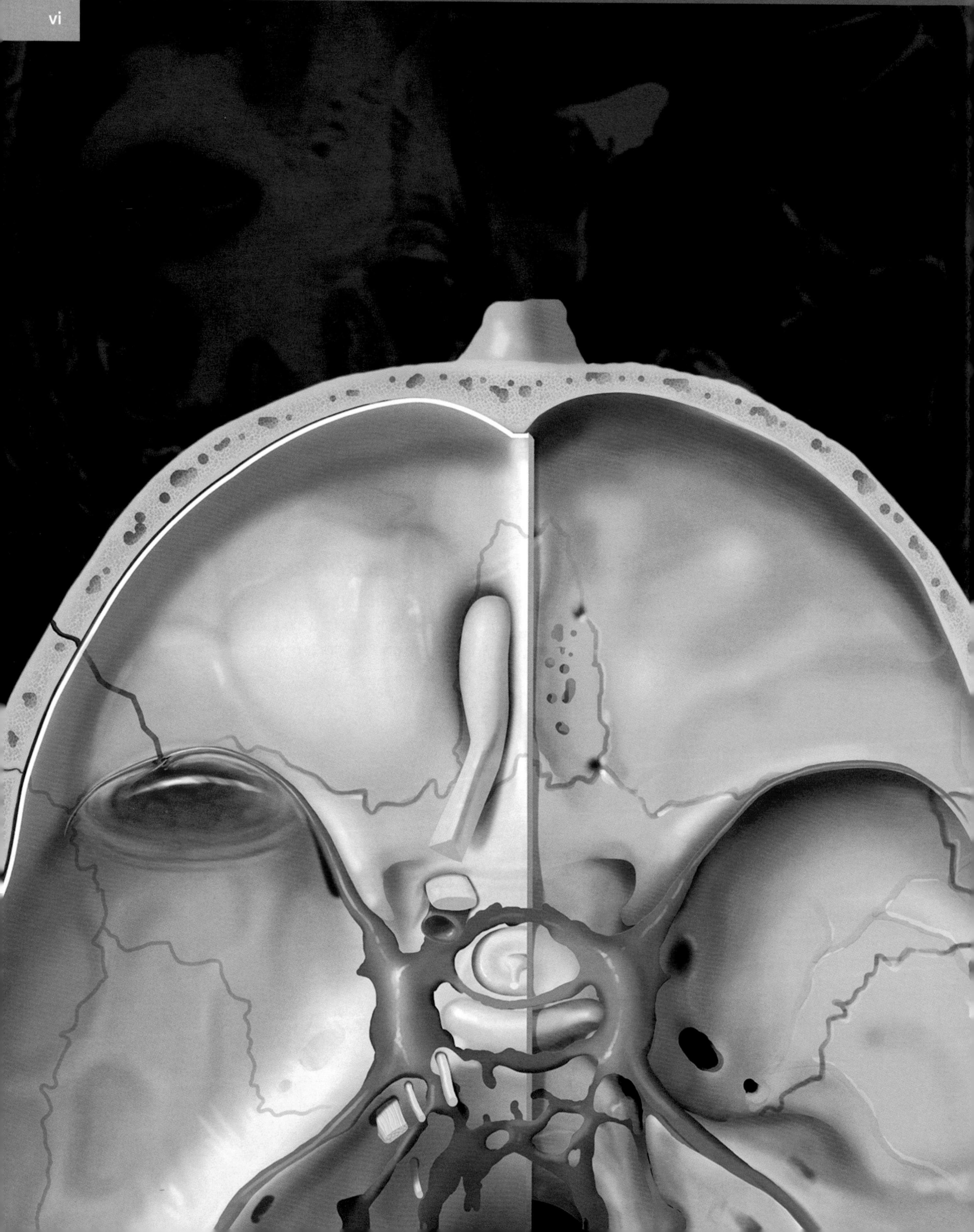

Preface

With *Osborn's Brain*, first edition, not only did I break a promise to myself that I would "never, EVER write another prose-based textbook," I would have been stunned to know I'd actually write a *second edition* of the book! But here we are, five years later, and I've done it. There have been so many changes in neuroradiology since the publication of the first edition that I wanted—and needed—to do a thorough update.

This edition is actually more than just an update; it is a major rewrite. Most of the 4,000+ images have been replaced with new, even better examples, and there are numerous new diagnoses that are presented. The Cancer Genome Atlas project has revolutionized our understanding of CNS neoplasms, and the exploding knowledge was reflected in the latest World Health Organization's *Classification of Tumours of the Central Nervous System*, published just a year ago. The "4-plus" WHO forms the basis of the completely rewritten neoplasms section of this edition.

For those of you who are new to *Osborn's Brain*, both the first and second editions are written as a curriculum in neuroradiology. The "must know—now!" topics such as brain trauma, stroke, and brain bleeds are covered in the first few chapters of the text. The book is meant to be read cover to cover, progressing through all the major areas of neuroimaging and neuropathology. While the basics are emphasized, there is a great deal of "advanced" information (read: fellow-and-beyond level stuff) that practicing neuroradiologists will find helpful and informative.

As with the first edition, this book is image-rich with hundreds of color graphics and gross pathology examples that inform the thousands of new, up-to-date images. I've expanded on my trademark summary "blue boxes" that are scattered throughout the text, allowing for a quick review of the essential facts.

Lastly, I invited two beloved colleagues, Drs. Gary Hedlund and Karen Salzman, to join me in authoring parts of the second edition. Gary is a revered pediatric neuroradiologist who is an international expert on (among other things) abusive head trauma. Karen's forte is tumor imaging, and her special focus is sella/parasellar disease. They are both highly respected members of our "Brain Team," and I have been privileged to work with them on this edition.

So as you start your journey through *Osborn's Brain*, second edition, best wishes and good reading to all of you! After all, you're why we write these things in the first place!

Anne G. Osborn, MD, FACR

University Distinguished Professor and Professor of Radiology and Imaging Sciences
William H. and Patricia W. Child Presidential Endowed Chair in Radiology
University of Utah School of Medicine
Salt Lake City, Utah

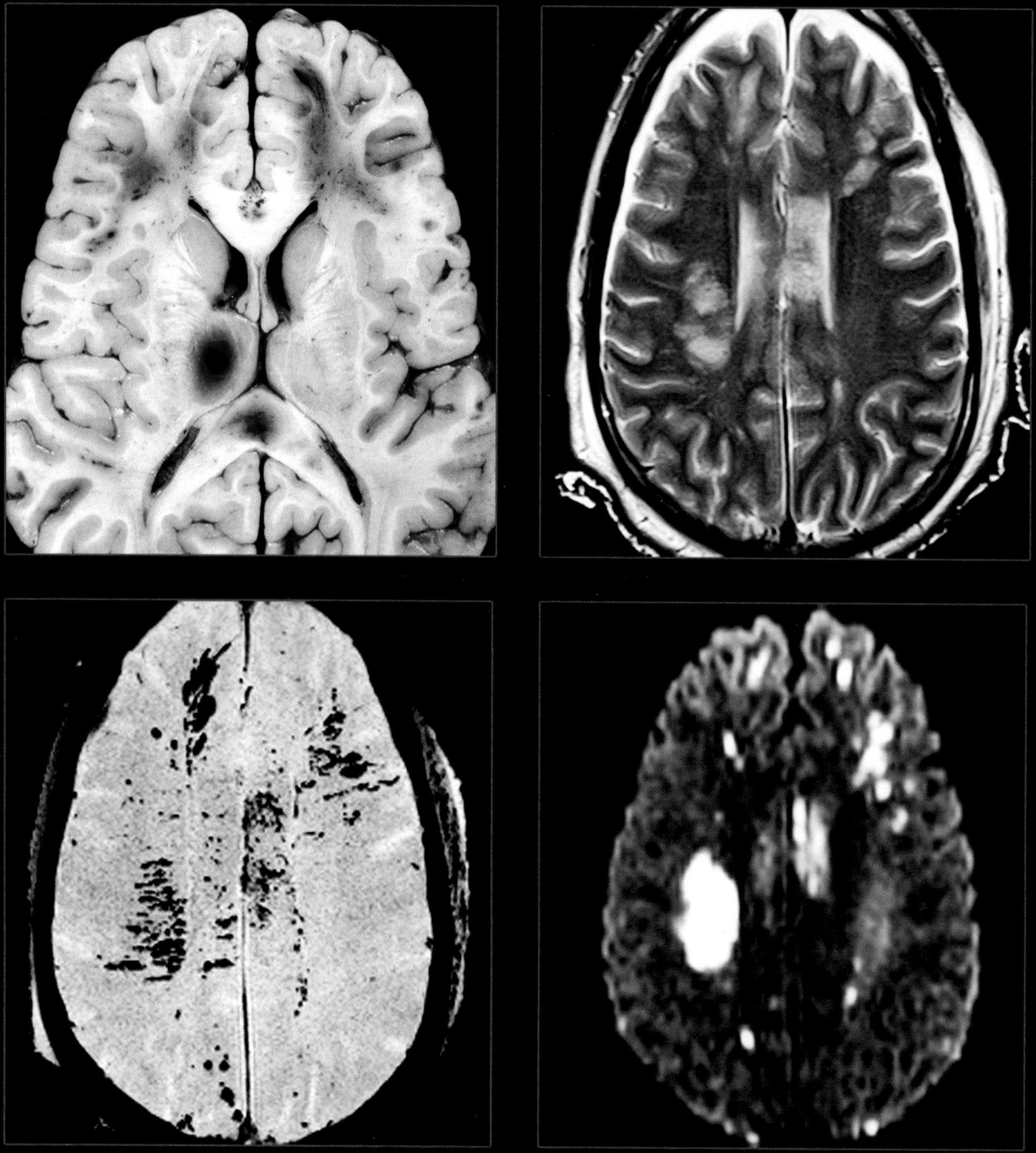

Image Contributors

AFIP Archives
D. P. Agamanolis, MD
N. Agarwal, MD
J. Ardyn, MD
M. Ayadi, MD
S. Aydin, MD
D. Bertholdo, MD
S. Blaser, MD
J. Boxerman, MD
M. Brant-Zawadski, MD
P. Burger, MD
S. Candy, MD
M. Castillo, MD
P. Chapman, MD
L. Chimelli, MD
S. Chung, MD
M. Colombo, MD
J. Comstock, MD
J. Curé, MD
B. Czerniak, MD
A. Datir, MD
B. N. Delman, MD
B. K. DeMasters, MD
K. Digre, MD
H. D. Dorfman, MD
M. Edwards-Brown, MD
D. Ellison, MD
H. Els, MD
A. Ersen, MD
W. Fang, MD
N. Foster, MD
C. E. Fuller, MD
S. Galetta, MD
C. Glastonbury, MBBS
S. Harder, MD
H. R. Harnsberger, MD
B. Hart, MD
E. T. Hedley-White, MD
G. Hedlund, DO
R. Hewlett, MD
P. Hildenbrand, MD
C. Y. Ho, MD
B. Horten, MD
C. Hsu, MD
M. Huckman, MD
P. Hudgins, MD
A. Illner, MD
B. Jones, MD
J. A. Junker, MD
E. C. Klatt, MD
D. Kremens, MD
W. Kucharczyk, MD
P. Lasjaunias, MD
S. Lincoff, MD
T. Markel, MD
M. Martin, MD
A. Maydell, MD
S. McNally, MD
T. Mentzel, MD
C. Merrow, MD
M. Michel, MD
K. Moore, MD
S. Nagi, MD
T. P. Naidich, MD
N. Nakase, MD
S. Narendra, MD
K. Nelson, MD
R. Nguyen, MD
G. P. Nielsen, MD
M. Nielsen, MS
K. K. Oguz, MD
J. P. O'Malley, MD
N. Omar, MD
J. Paltan, MD
G. Parker, MD
T. Poussaint, MD
R. Ramakantan, MD
C. Rambaud, MD
M. L. Rivera-Zengotita, MD
C. Robson, MBChB
F. J. Rodriguez, MD
P. Rodriguez, MD
A. Rosenberg, MD
E. Ross, MD
A. Rossi, MD
L. Rourke, MD
Rubinstein Collection, AFIP Archives
E. Rushing, MD
M. Sage, MD
B. Scheithauer, MD
P. Shannon, MD
A. Sillag, MD
E. T. Tali, MD
M. Thurnher, MD
T. Tihan, MD
K. Tong, MD
J. Townsend, MD
U. of Utah Dept. of Dermatology
S. van der Westhuizen, MD
M. Warmuth-Metz, MD
T. Winters, MD
A. T. Yachnis, MD
S. Yashar, MD

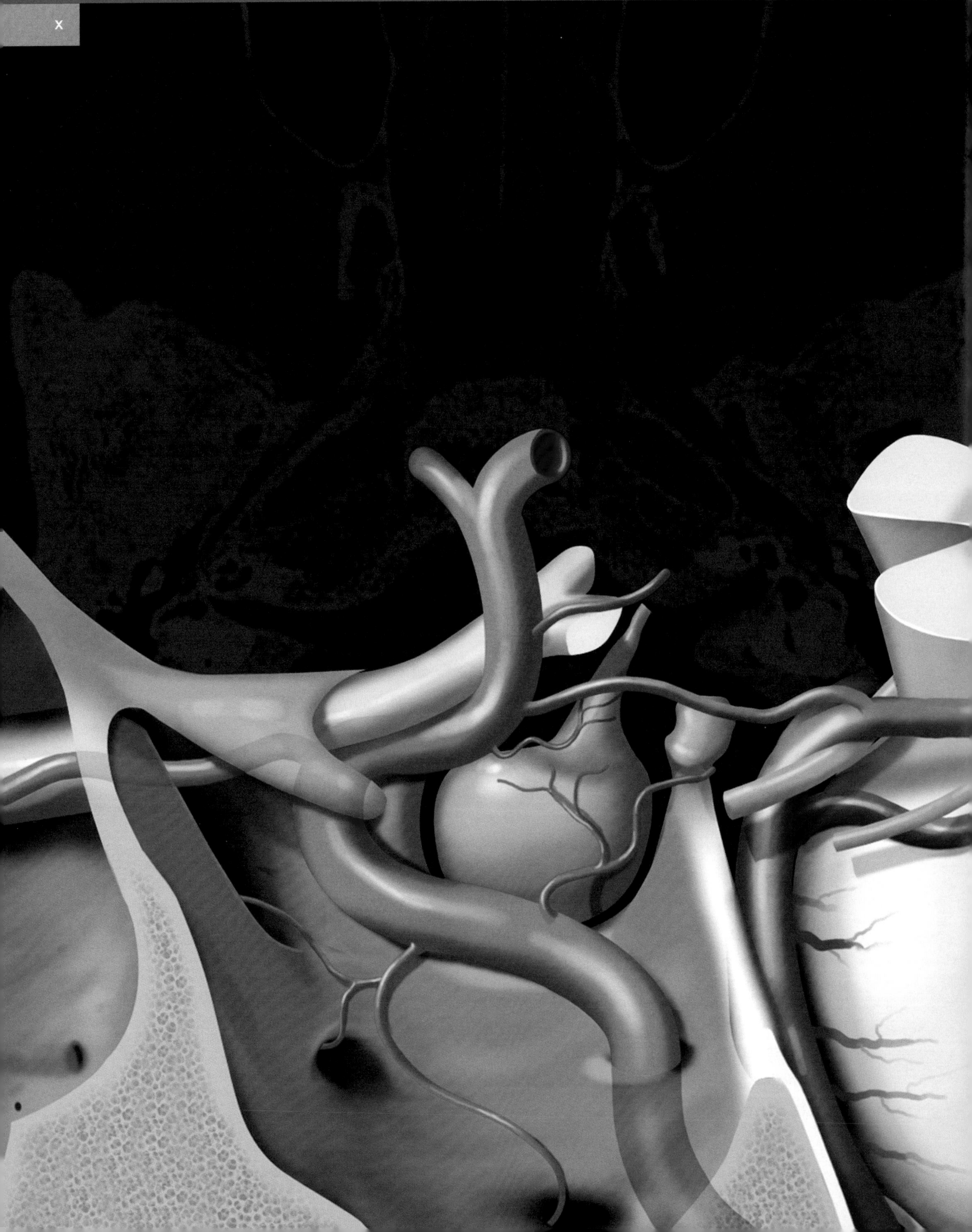

Acknowledgments

Editor in Chief

Karen E. Concannon, MA, PhD

Text Editors

Arthur G. Gelsinger, MA
Nina I. Bennett, BA
Terry W. Ferrell, MS
Lisa A. Gervais, BS
Matt W. Hoecherl, BS
Megg Morin, BA

Image Editors

Jeffrey J. Marmorstone, BS
Lisa A. M. Steadman, BS

Illustrations

Lane R. Bennion, MS
Richard Coombs, MS
Laura C. Wissler, MA
James A. Cooper, MD

Art Direction and Design

Tom M. Olson, BA
Laura C. Wissler, MA

Software Development and Support

Michael A. Hogenson, BS
Craig L. Moon, BS
Stephen Stephenson
Alma Miller

Production Coordinators

Rebecca L. Bluth, BA
Angela M. G. Terry, BA
Emily C. Fassett, BA

ELSEVIER

Table of Contents

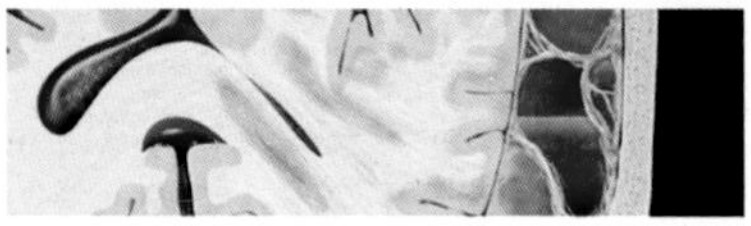

Section 1:

Trauma

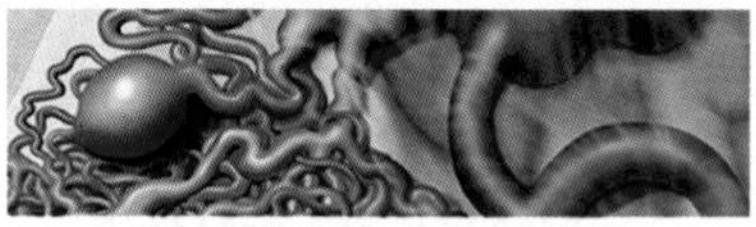

Section 2:

Nontraumatic Hemorrhage and Vascular Lesions

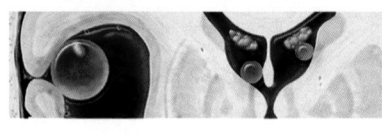

Section 3:

Infection, Inflammation, and Demyelinating Diseases

Table of Contents

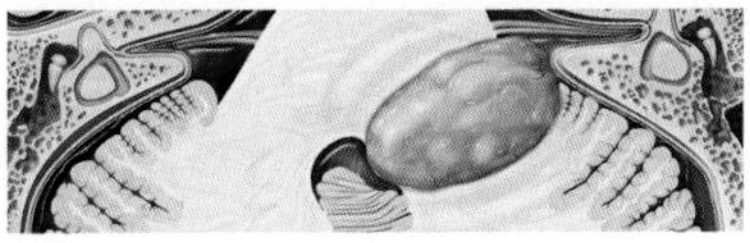

Section 4:

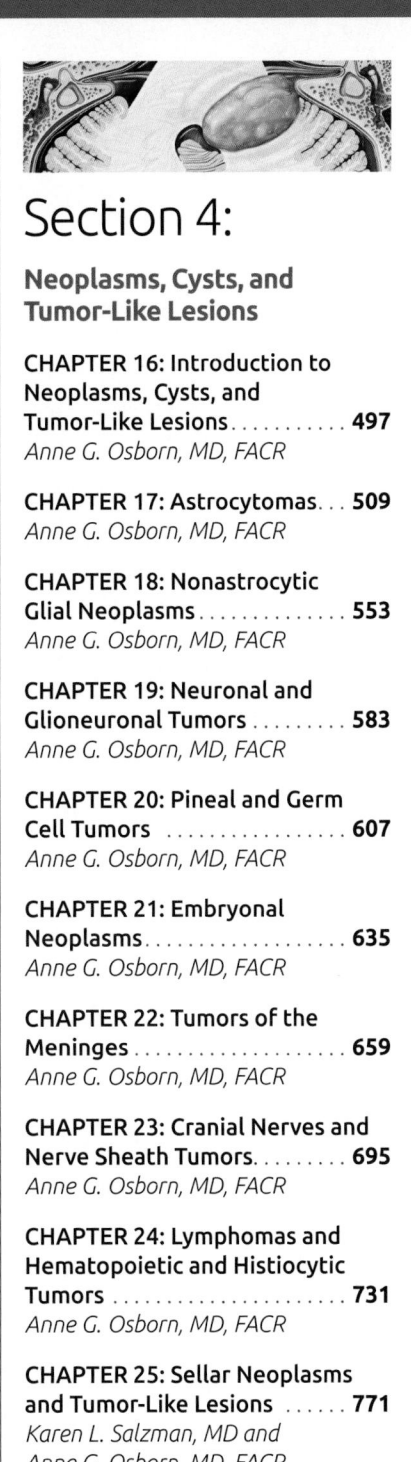

Neoplasms, Cysts, and Tumor-Like Lesions

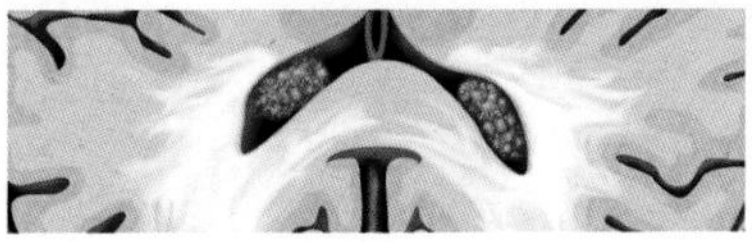

Section 5:

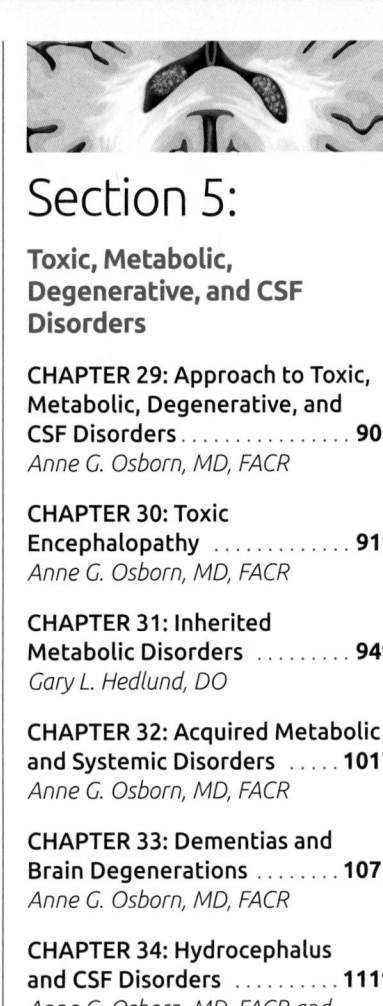

Toxic, Metabolic, Degenerative, and CSF Disorders

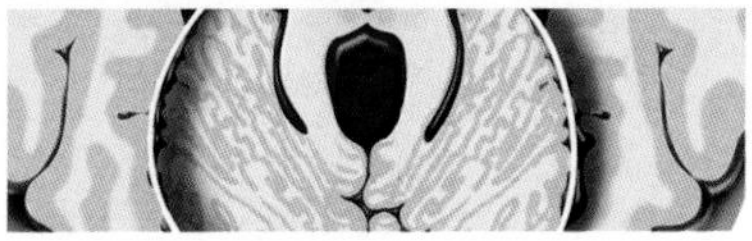

Section 6:

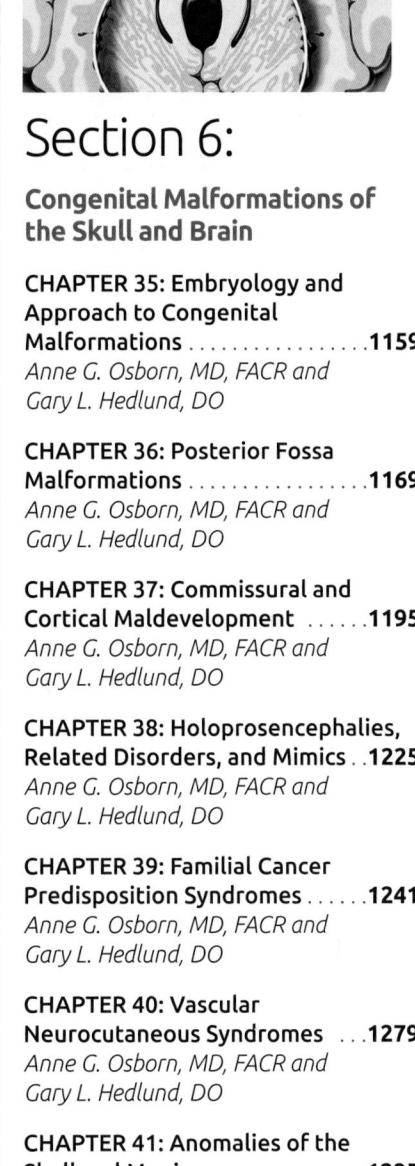

Congenital Malformations of the Skull and Brain

Osborn's Brain

IMAGING, PATHOLOGY, AND ANATOMY

SECOND EDITION

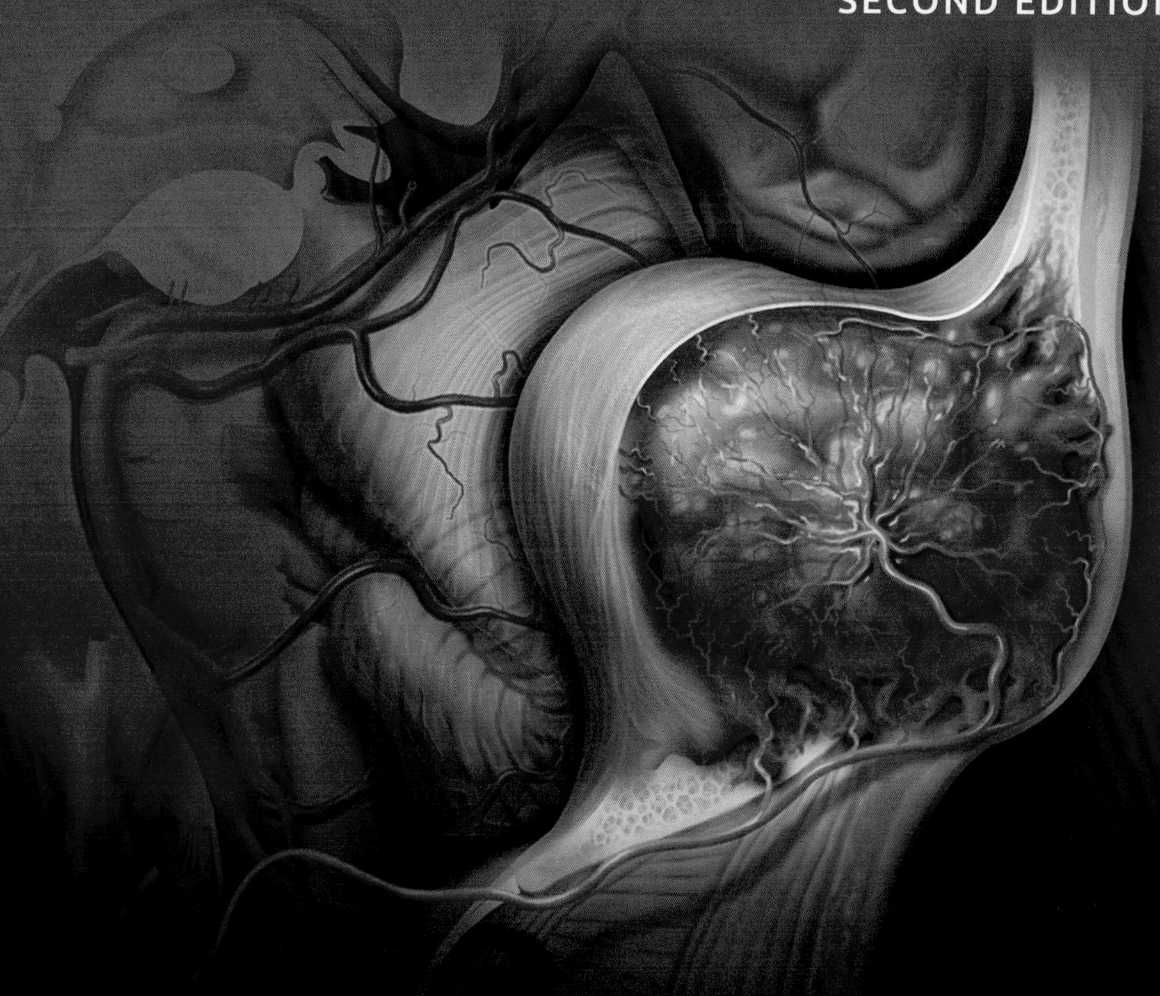

Anne G. Osborn

Hedlund | Salzman

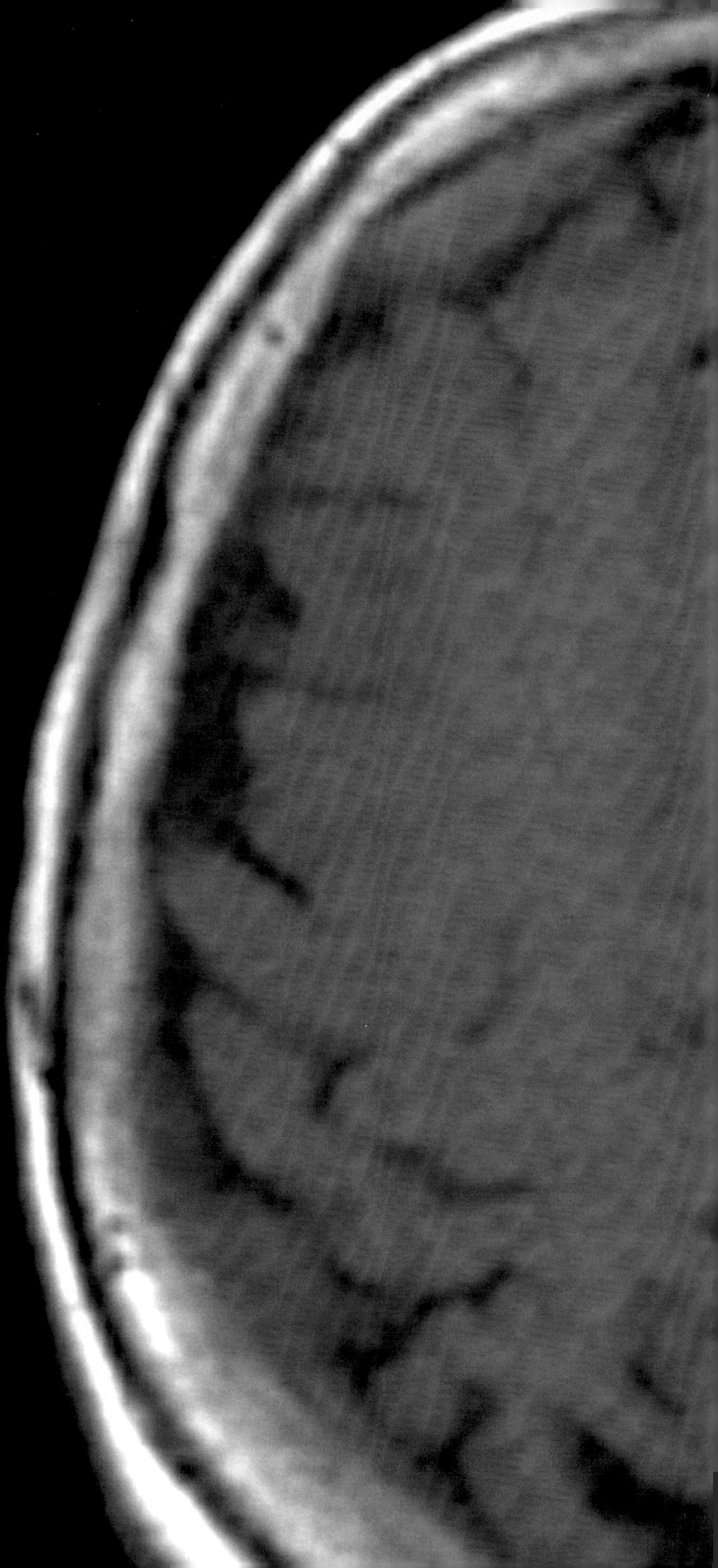

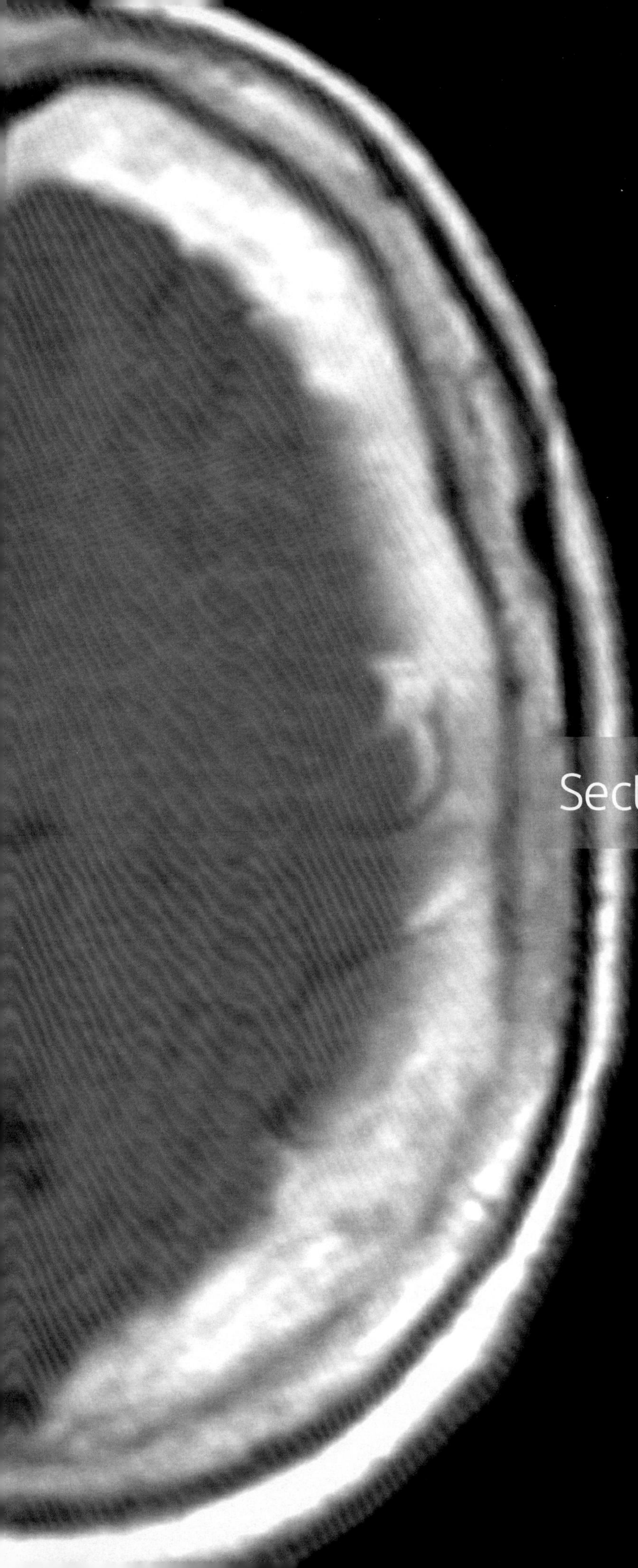

Section 1

Section 1

Trauma

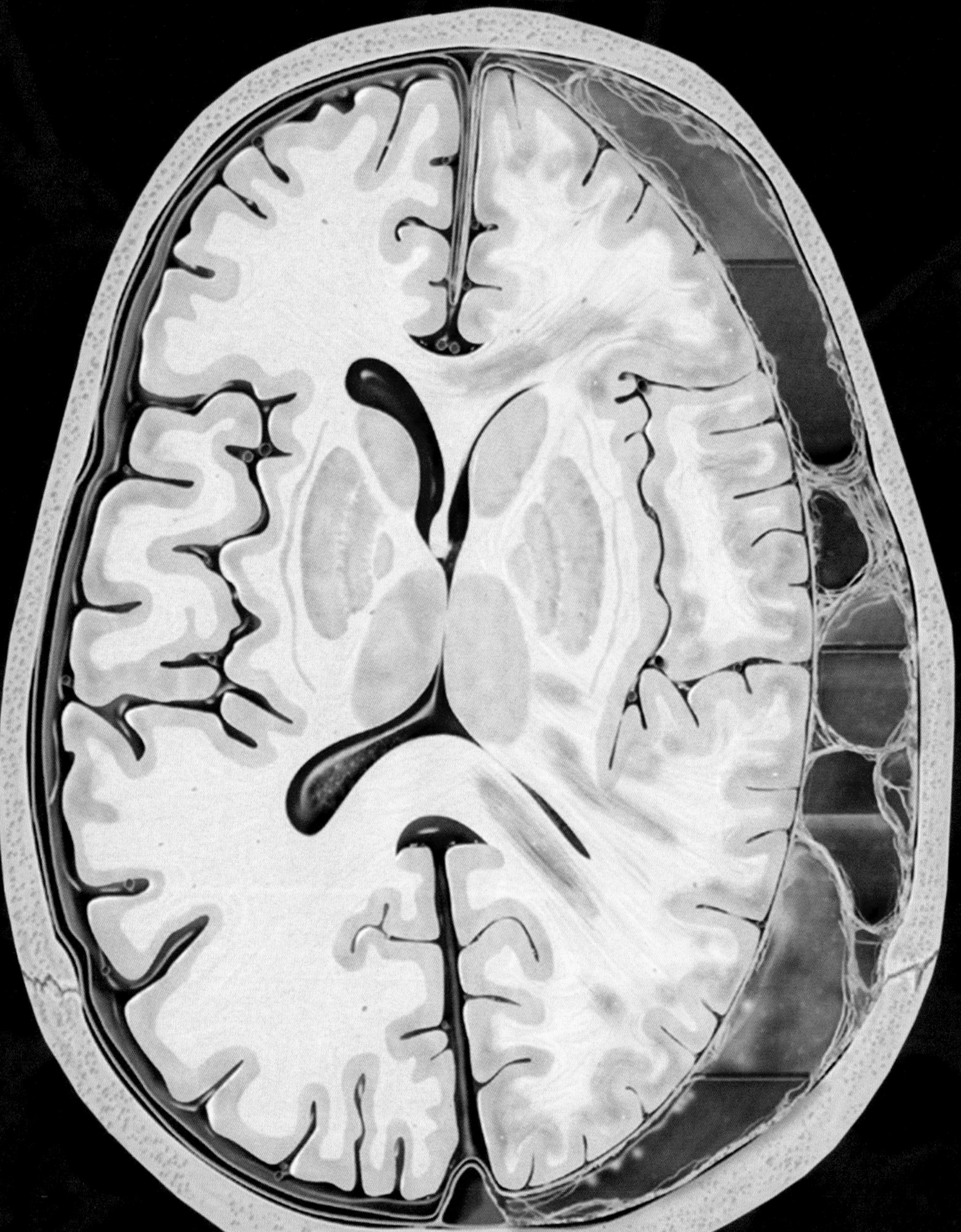

Trauma Overview

Trauma is one of the most frequent indications for emergent neuroimaging. Because imaging plays such a key role in patient triage and management, we begin this book by discussing skull and brain trauma.

We start with a brief consideration of epidemiology. Traumatic brain injury (TBI) is a critical public health and socio-economic problem throughout the world. The direct medical costs of caring for acutely traumatized patients are huge. The indirect costs of lost productivity and long-term care for TBI survivors are even larger than the short-term direct costs.

We then briefly discuss the etiology and mechanisms of head trauma. Understanding the different ways in which the skull and brain can be injured provides the context for understanding the spectrum of findings that can be identified on imaging studies.

Introduction

Epidemiology of Head Trauma

Trauma—sometimes called the "silent epidemic"—is the most common worldwide cause of death in children and young adults. Neurotrauma is responsible for the vast majority of these cases. At least 10 million people worldwide sustain TBI each year. In the USA alone, two million people annually suffer a TBI. Of these, 500,000 require hospital care.

Of all head-injured patients, approximately 10% sustain fatal brain injury. Lifelong disability is common in those who survive. Between 5-10% of TBI survivors have serious permanent neurologic deficits, and an additional 20-40% have moderate disability. Even more have subtle deficits ("minimal brain trauma").

Etiology and Mechanisms of Injury

Trauma can be caused by missile or nonmissile injury. Missile injury results from penetration of the skull, meninges, and/or brain by an external object, such as a bullet. Gunshot wounds are most common in adolescent and young adult male patients but relatively rare in other groups.

Nonmissile closed head injury (CHI) is a much more common cause of neurotrauma than missile injury. Falls have now surpassed road traffic incidents as the leading cause of TBI.

So-called "ground level falls" (GLFs) are a common indication for neuroimaging in young children and older adults. In such cases, brain injury can be significant. With a GLF, a six-foot tall adult's head impacts the ground at 20 mph. Anticoagulated older adults are especially at risk for intracranial hemorrhages, even with minor head trauma.

Motor vehicle collisions occurring at high speed exert significant acceleration/deceleration forces, causing the brain to move suddenly within the skull. Forcible impaction of the brain against the unyielding calvaria and hard, knife-like dura results in gyral contusion. Rotation and sudden changes in angular momentum may deform, stretch, and damage long vulnerable axons, resulting in axonal injury.

Classification of Head Trauma

The most widely used *clinical* classification of brain trauma, the Glasgow Coma Scale (GCS), depends on the assessment of three features: best eye, verbal, and motor responses. With the use of the GCS, TBI can be designated as a mild, moderate, or severe injury.

TBI can also be divided chronologically and *pathoetiologically* into primary and secondary injury, the system used in this text. **Primary injuries** occur at the time of initial trauma. Skull fractures, epi- and subdural hematomas, contusions, axonal injury, and brain lacerations are examples of primary injuries.

Secondary injuries occur later and include cerebral edema, perfusion alterations, brain herniations, and CSF leaks. Although vascular injury can be immediate (blunt impact) or secondary (vessel laceration from fractures, occlusion secondary to brain herniation), for purposes of discussion, it is included in the chapter on secondary injuries.

CLASSIFICATION OF HEAD TRAUMA

Primary Effects
- Scalp and skull injuries
- Extraaxial hemorrhage/hematomas
- Parenchymal injuries
- Miscellaneous injuries

Secondary Effects
- Herniation syndromes
- Cerebral edema
- Cerebral ischemia
- Vascular injury (can be primary or secondary)

Imaging Acute Head Trauma

Imaging is absolutely critical to the diagnosis and management of the patient with acute TBI. The goal of emergent neuroimaging is twofold: (1) identify treatable injuries, especially emergent ones, and (2) detect and delineate the presence of secondary injuries, such as herniation syndromes and vascular injury.

How To Image?

A broad spectrum of imaging modalities can be used to evaluate patients with TBI. These range from outdated, generally ineffective techniques (e.g., skull radiographs) to very sensitive but expensive studies (e.g., MR). Techniques that are still relatively new include CT and MR perfusion, diffusion tensor imaging (DTI), and functional MRI (fMRI).

Skull Radiography

For decades, skull radiography (whether called "plain film" or, more recently, "digital radiography") was the only noninvasive imaging technique available for the assessment of head injury.

Skull radiography is reasonably effective in identifying calvarial fractures. Yet skull x-rays cannot depict the far more important presence of extraaxial hemorrhages and parenchymal injuries.

Between one-quarter and one-third of autopsied patients with fatal brain injuries have no identifiable skull fracture! Therefore, skull radiography obtained solely for the purpose of identifying the presence of a skull fracture has no appropriate role in the current management of the head-injured patient. With rare exceptions, it's the brain that matters—not the skull!

NECT

Because of its wide availability and rapid detection of acute hemorrhage, CT is now accepted as the worldwide screening tool for imaging acute head trauma. Since its introduction almost 40 years ago, CT has gradually but completely replaced skull radiographs as the "workhorse" of brain trauma imaging. The reasons are simple: CT depicts both bone and soft tissue injuries. It is also widely accessible, fast, effective, and comparatively inexpensive.

Both standard and multidetector row CT (MDCT) are used in the initial imaging of patients with traumatic head injury. Identifying abnormalities that may require urgent treatment to limit secondary injuries, such as brain swelling and herniation syndromes, is essential.

Standard nonenhanced CT (NECT) scans (4 or 5 mm thick) from just below the foramen magnum through the vertex should be performed. Two sets of images should be obtained, one using brain and one with bone reconstruction algorithms. Viewing the brain images with a wider window width (150-200 HU, the so-called subdural window) should be performed on PACS (or film, if PACS is not available). The scout view should always be displayed as part of the study (see below).

MDCT is now in widespread use. Coronal and sagittal reformatted images using the axial source data are routinely performed in head trauma triage and improve the detection rate of acute traumatic subdural hematomas.

Three-dimensional shaded surface displays are helpful in depicting skull and facial fractures. If facial bone CT is also requested, a single MDCT acquisition can be obtained without overlapping radiation exposure to the eye and lower half of the brain.

Head trauma patients with acute intracranial lesions on CT have a higher risk for cervical spine fractures compared with patients with a CT-negative head injury. Because up to one-third of patients with moderate to severe head injury as determined by the GCS have concomitant spine injury, MDCT of the cervical spine is often obtained together with brain imaging. Soft tissue and bone algorithm reconstructions with multiplanar reformatted images of the cervical spine should be obtained.

As delayed development or enlargement of both extra- and intracranial hemorrhages may occur within 24-36 hours following the initial traumatic event, repeat CT should be obtained if there is sudden unexplained clinical deterioration, regardless of initial imaging findings.

CTA

CT angiography (CTA) is often obtained as part of a whole-body trauma CT protocol. Craniocervical CTA should also specifically be considered (1) in the setting of penetrating neck injury, (2) if a fractured foramen transversarium or facet subluxation is identified on cervical spine CT, or (3) if a skull base fracture traverses the carotid canal or a dural venous sinus. Arterial laceration or dissection, traumatic pseudoaneurysm, carotid-cavernous fistula, or dural venous sinus injury are nicely depicted on high-resolution CTA.

MR

Although MR can detect traumatic complications without radiation and is more sensitive for abnormalities such as contusions and axonal injuries, there is general agreement that NECT is the procedure of choice in the initial evaluation of brain trauma. Limitations of MR include acquisition time, access, patient monitoring and instability, motion degradation of images, and cost.

With one important exception—suspected child abuse—using MR as a routine screening procedure in the setting of *acute* brain trauma is uncommon. Standard MR together with susceptibility-weighted imaging and DTI is most useful in the subacute and chronic stages of TBI. Other modalities such as fMRI are playing an increasingly important role in detecting subtle abnormalities, especially in patients with mild cognitive deficits following minor TBI.

Who and When To Image?

Who to image and when to do it are paradoxically both well established and controversial. Patients with a GCS score indicating moderate (GCS = 9-12) or severe (GCS ≤ 8) neurologic impairment are invariably imaged. The real debate is about how best to manage patients with GCS scores of 13-15.

In an attempt to reduce CT overutilization in emergency departments, several organizations have developed evidence-based clinical criteria that help separate "high-risk" from "low-risk" patients. (Several of these are delineated in the boxes below.) Yet the impact on the emergency department physician ordering behavior has been inconsistent. In places with high malpractice rates, many emergency physicians routinely order NECT scans on every patient with head trauma regardless of GCS score or clinical findings.

Repeat head CT scans in trauma transfers from one hospital to another are common and add to both radiation dose exposure and cost. Inadequate data transfer from the referring hospital—not poor image quality—is the major reason for potentially preventable repeat head CT scans.

Whether—and when—to obtain follow-up imaging in trauma patients is controversial. In a large study of children with GCS scores of 14 or 15 and a normal initial CT scan, only 2% had follow-up CT or MR performed. Of these, only 0.05% had abnormal results on the follow-up study, and *none* required surgical intervention. The negative predictive value for neurosurgical intervention for a child with an initial GCS of 14 or 15 and normal CT was 100%. From this, the authors concluded that children with a GCS of 14 or 15 and a normal initial head CT are at very low risk for subsequent traumatic findings on neuroimaging and extremely low risk of needing neurosurgical intervention. Hospitalization for neurologic observation of children with minor head trauma after normal CT scan results was deemed unnecessary.

GLASGOW COMA SCALE

Best Eye Response (Maximum = 4)
- 1 = no eye opening
- 2 = eye opening to pain
- 3 = eyes open to verbal command
- 4 = eyes open spontaneously

Best Verbal Response (Maximum = 5)
- 1 = none
- 2 = incomprehensible sounds
- 3 = inappropriate words
- 4 = confused
- 5 = oriented

Best Motor Response (Maximum = 6)
- 1 = none
- 2 = extension to pain
- 3 = flexion to pain
- 4 = withdrawal to pain
- 5 = localizing to pain
- 6 = obedience to commands

Sum = "Coma Score" and Clinical Grading
- 13-15 = mild brain injury
- 9-12 = moderate brain injury
- ≤ 8 = severe brain injury

Appropriateness Criteria

Three major and widely used appropriateness criteria for imaging acute head trauma have been published: The American College of Radiology (ACR) Appropriateness Criteria, the New Orleans Criteria (NOC), and the Canadian Head CT Rule (CHCR).

ACR Criteria. Emergent NECT in mild/minor CHI with the presence of a focal neurologic deficit and/or other risk factors is deemed "very appropriate," as is imaging all traumatized children under 2 years of age. Although acknowledging that NECT in patients with mild/minor CHI (GCS ≥ 13) without risk

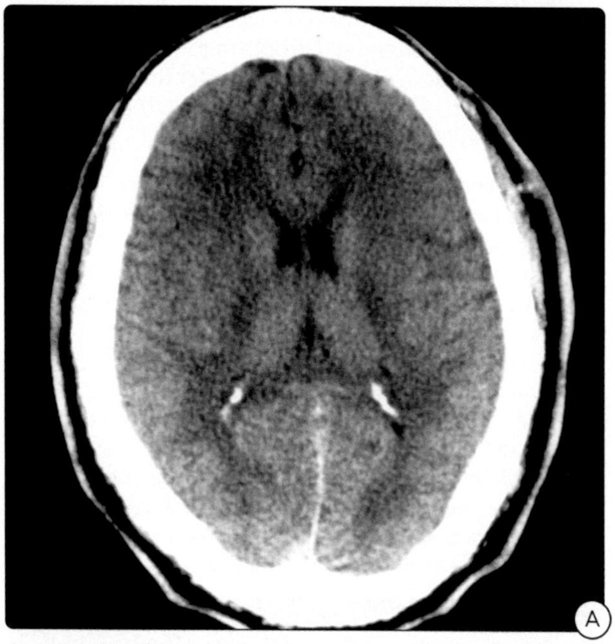

(1-1A) Axial NECT scan of a prisoner imaged for head trauma shows no gross abnormality. (Courtesy J. A. Junker, MD.)

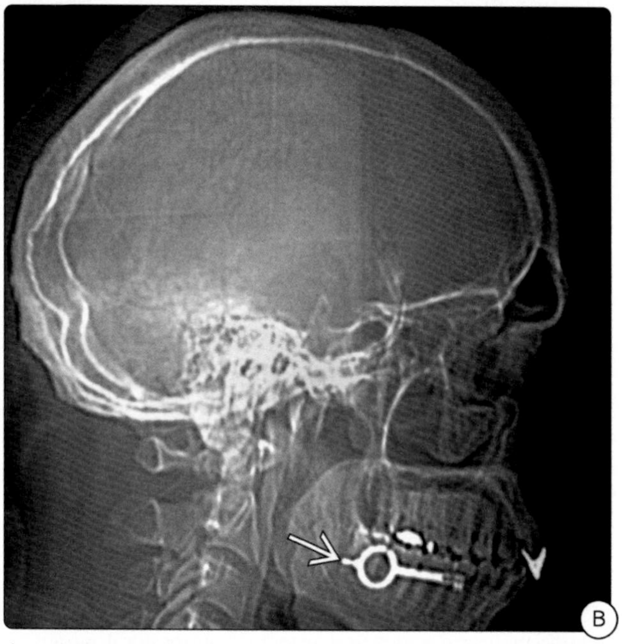

(1-1B) Scout view in the same case shows a foreign object → (a handcuff key!) in the prisoner's mouth. He faked the injury and was planning to escape, but the radiologist alerted the guards and thwarted the plan. (Courtesy J. A. Junker, MD.)

factors or focal neurologic deficit is "known to be low yield," the ACR still rates it as 7 out of 9 in appropriateness.

NOC and CHCR. Both the NOC and CHCR attempt to triage patients with minimal/mild head injuries in a cost-effective manner. A GCS score of 15 (i.e., normal) without any of the NOC indicators is a highly sensitive negative predictor of clinically important brain injury or need for surgical intervention.

NEW ORLEANS CRITERIA IN MINOR HEAD INJURY

CT indicated if GCS = 15 plus any of the following
- Headache
- Vomiting
- Patient > 60 years old
- Intoxication (drugs, alcohol)
- Short-term memory deficits (anterograde amnesia)
- Visible trauma above clavicles
- Seizure

Adapted from Stiell IG et al: Comparison of the Canadian CT head rule and the New Orleans criteria in patients with minor head injury. JAMA 294(12):1511-1518, 2005

According to the CHCR, patients with a GCS score of 13-15 and witnessed loss of consciousness (LOC), amnesia, or confusion are imaged, along with those deemed "high risk" for neurosurgical intervention or "medium risk" for brain injury.

Between 6-7% of patients with minor head injury have positive findings on head CT scans. Most of these patients also have headache, vomiting, drug or alcohol intoxication, seizure, short-term memory deficits, or physical evidence of trauma above the clavicles. CT should be used liberally in these cases, as well as in patients over 65 years of age, children under the age of two, anticoagulated patients, and patients with loss of consciousness or focal neurologic deficit.

Recent studies have also shown that compliance with established imaging guidelines such as the CHCR is poor, particularly in busy EDs that handle large trauma volumes. Despite efforts to educate urgent care physicians about limiting patient exposure to ionizing radiation and using clinically based risk stratification, nonenhanced head CTs remain one of the most frequently overutilized imaging studies.

CANADIAN HEAD CT RULE IN MINOR HEAD INJURY

CT if GCS = 13-15 and witnessed LOC, amnesia, or confusion

High risk for neurosurgical intervention
- GCS < 15 at 2 hours
- Suspected open/depressed skull fracture
- Clinical signs of skull base fracture
- ≥ 2 vomiting episodes
- Age ≥ 65 years

Medium risk for brain injury detected by head CT
- Antegrade amnesia ≥ 30 minutes
- "Dangerous mechanism" (i.e., auto-pedestrian, ejection from vehicle, etc.)

Adapted from Stiell IG et al: Comparison of the Canadian CT head rule and the New Orleans criteria in patients with minor head injury. JAMA 294(12):1511-1518, 2005

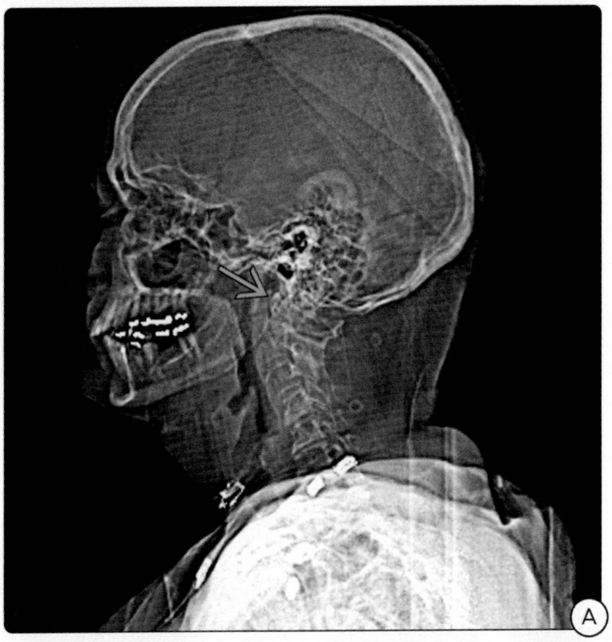

(1-2A) Scout view in a 66y woman with a CT head requested to evaluate ground level fall shows a posteriorly angulated C1-odontoid complex ⇨.

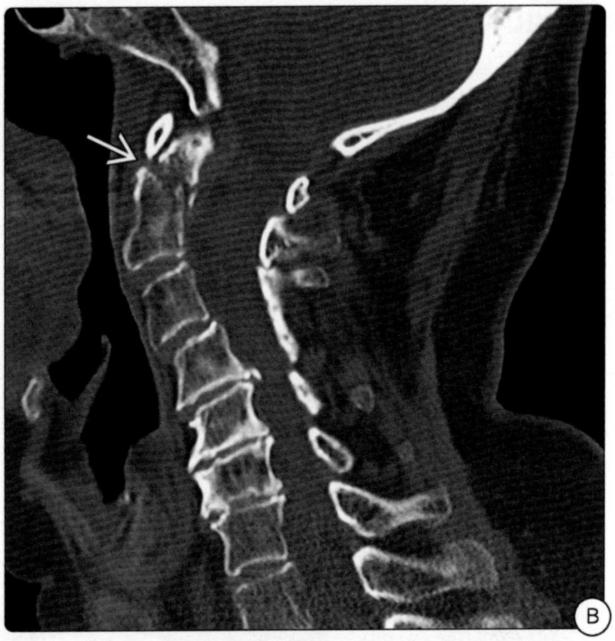

(1-2B) The head CT in the same case (not shown) was normal. Cervical spine CT was then performed. The sagittal image reformatted from the axial scan data shows a comminuted, posteriorly angulated dens fracture ➡.

Trauma Imaging: Keys to Analysis

Four components are essential to the accurate interpretation of CT scans in patients with head injury: the scout image plus brain, bone, and subdural views of the NECT dataset. Critical information may be present on just one of these four components.

Suggestions on how to analyze NECT images in patients with acute head injury are delineated below.

Scout Image

Before you look at the NECT scan, examine the digital scout image! Look for cervical spine abnormalities such as fractures or dislocations, jaw and/or facial trauma, and the presence of foreign objects **(1-1)**. If there is a suggestion of cervical spine fracture or malalignment, MDCT of the cervical spine should be performed before the patient is removed from the scanner **(1-2)**.

Brain Windows

Methodically and meticulously work your way from the outside in. First evaluate the soft tissue images, beginning with the scalp. Look for scalp swelling, which usually indicates the impact point. Carefully examine the periorbital soft tissues.

Next look for extraaxial blood. The most common extraaxial hemorrhage is traumatic subarachnoid hemorrhage (tSAH), followed by sub- and epidural hematomas. The prevalence of tSAH in moderate to severe TBI approaches 100%. tSAH is usually found in the sulci adjacent to cortical contusions, along the sylvian fissures, and around the anteroinferior frontal and temporal lobes. The best place to look for subtle tSAH is the interpeduncular cistern, where blood collects when the patient is supine.

Any hypodensity within an extraaxial collection should raise suspicion of rapid hemorrhage with accumulation of unclotted blood or (especially in alcoholics or older patients) an underlying coagulopathy. This is an urgent finding that mandates immediate notification of the responsible clinician.

Look for intracranial air ("pneumocephalus"). Intracranial air is always abnormal and indicates the presence of a fracture that traverses either the paranasal sinuses or mastoid.

Now move on to the brain itself. Carefully examine the cortex, especially the "high-yield" areas for cortical contusions (anteroinferior frontal and temporal lobes). If there is a scalp hematoma due to impact (a "coup" injury), look 180° in the opposite direction for a classic "contre-coup" injury. Hypodense areas around the hyperdense hemorrhagic foci indicate early edema and severe contusion.

Move inward from the cortex to the subcortical white and deep gray matter. Petechial hemorrhages often accompany axonal injury. If you see subcortical hemorrhages on the initial NECT scan, this is merely the "tip of the iceberg." There is usually *a lot* more damage than what is apparent on the first scan. A general rule: the deeper the lesion, the more severe the injury.

Finally, look inside the ventricles for blood-CSF levels and hemorrhage due to choroid plexus shearing injury.

Subdural Windows

Look at the soft tissue image with both narrow ("brain") and intermediate ("subdural") windows. Small subtle subdural hematomas can sometimes be overlooked on standard narrow window widths (75-100 HU) yet are readily apparent when wider windows (150-200 HU) are used.

Bone CT

Bone CT refers to bone algorithm reconstruction viewed with wide (bone) windows. If you can't do bone algorithm reconstruction from your dataset, widen the windows and use an edge-enhancement feature to sharpen the image. Three-dimensional shaded surface displays (3D SSDs) are especially helpful in depicting complex or subtle fractures **(1-3)**.

Even though standard head scans are 4-5 mm thick, it is often possible to detect fractures on bone CT. Look for basisphenoid fractures with involvement of the carotid canal, temporal bone fractures (with or without ossicular dislocation), mandibular dislocation ("empty" condylar fossa), and calvarial fractures. And remember: nondisplaced linear skull fractures that don't cross vascular structures (such as a dural venous sinus or middle meningeal artery) are in and of themselves basically meaningless. The brain and blood vessels are what matter!

The most difficult dilemma is deciding whether an observed lucency is a fracture or a normal structure (e.g., suture line or vascular channel). Keep in mind: it is virtually unheard of for a calvarial fracture to occur in the absence of overlying soft tissue injury. If there is no scalp "bump," it is unlikely that the lucency represents a nondisplaced linear fracture.

Bone CT images are also very helpful in distinguishing low density from air vs. fat. Although most PACS stations have a region of interest (ROI) function that can measure attenuation, fat fades away on bone CT images, and air remains very hypodense.

(1-3A) Axial NECT in an 18y man who fell off his skateboard shows a small right epidural hematoma that also contains air ➡. (1-3B) Two-millimeter bone algorithm reconstruction in the same case shows a nondisplaced linear fracture of the squamous temporal bone ➡ adjacent to the epidural blood and air ➡.

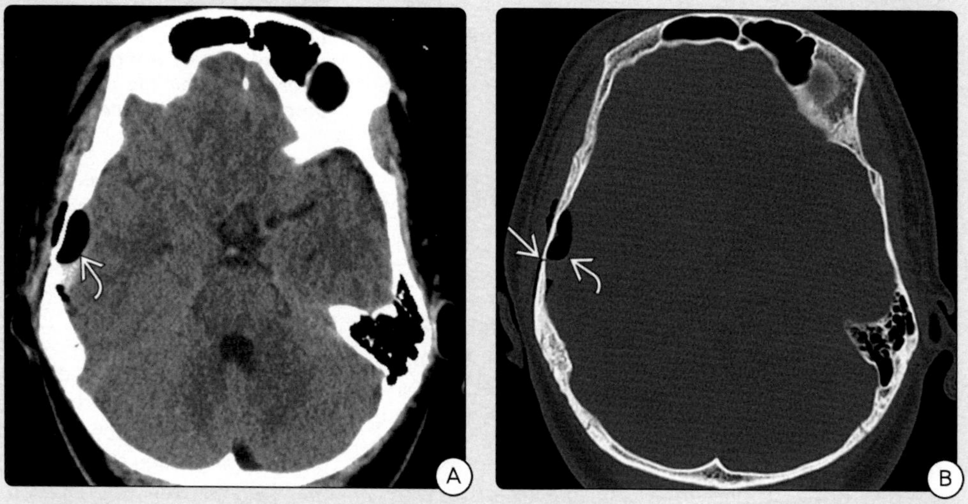

(1-3C) Coronal (left) and sagittal (right) bone CTs reconstructed from the axial source data show the temporal bone fracture ➡ is comminuted and crosses the mastoid ➡ and middle ear ➡. (1-3D) Bone CT with shaded surface display in the same case nicely shows the squamous ➡, mastoid ➡ aspects of the nondisplaced but comminuted fracture.

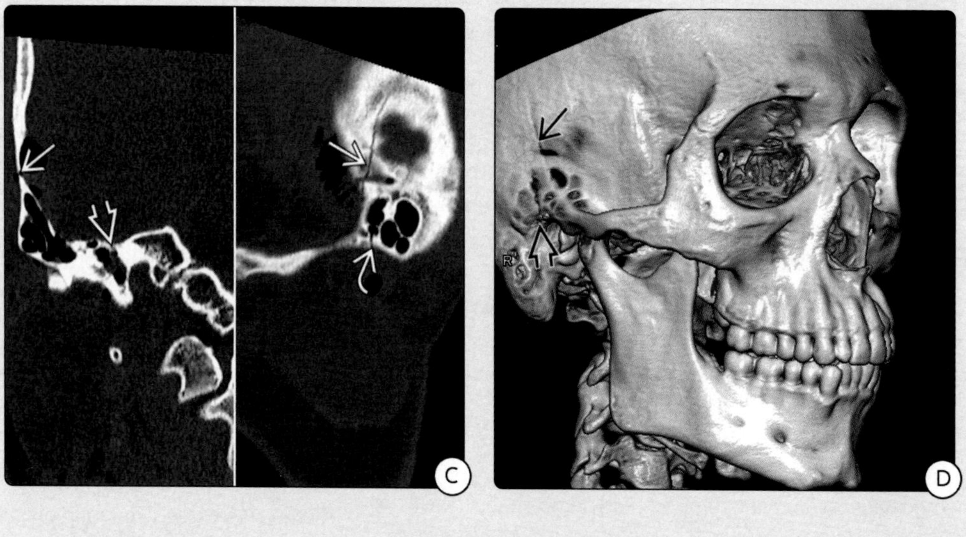

CTA

CTA is generally indicated if (1) basilar skull fractures cross the carotid canal or a dural venous sinus **(1-4)**; (2) if a cervical spine fracture-dislocation is present, especially if the transverse foramina are involved; or (3) if the patient has stroke-like symptoms or unexplained clinical deterioration. Both the cervical and intracranial vasculature should be visualized.

Although it is important to scrutinize both the arterial and venous sides of the circulation, a CTA is generally sufficient. Standard CTAs typically show both the arteries and the dural venous sinuses well, whereas a CT venogram (CTV) often misses the arterial phase.

Examine the source images as well as the multiplanar reconstructions and maximum-intensity projection (MIP) reformatted scans. Traumatic dissection, vessel lacerations, intimal flaps, pseudoaneurysms, carotid-cavernous fistulas, and dural sinus occlusions can generally be identified on CTA.

HEAD TRAUMA: CT CHECKLIST

Scout Image
- Evaluate for
  - Cervical spine fracture-dislocation
  - Jaw dislocation, facial fractures
  - Foreign object

Brain Windows
- Scalp swelling (impact point)
- Extraaxial blood (focal hypodensity in clot suggests rapid bleeding)
  - Epidural hematoma
  - Subdural hematoma (SDH)
  - Traumatic subarachnoid hemorrhage
- Pneumocephalus
- Cortical contusion
  - Anteroinferior frontal, temporal lobes
  - Opposite scalp laceration/skull fracture
- Hemorrhagic axonal injury
- Intraventricular hemorrhage

Subdural Windows
- 150-200 HU (for thin SDHs under skull)

Bone CT
- Bone algorithm reconstruction > bone windows
- Any fractures cross a vascular channel?

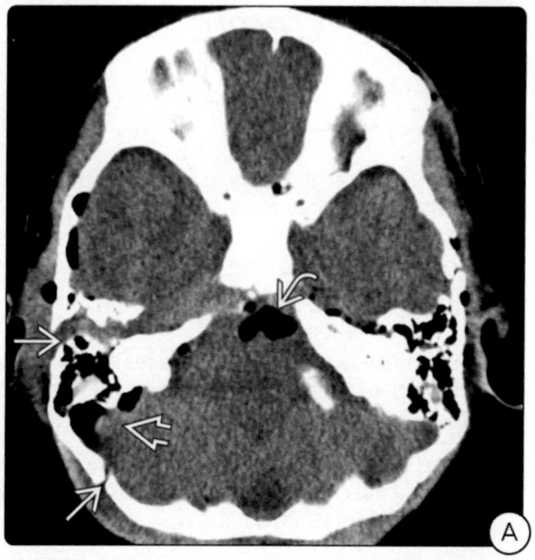

(1-4A) NECT shows pneumocephalus, base of skull fractures adjacent to air, which seems to outline a displaced sigmoid sinus.

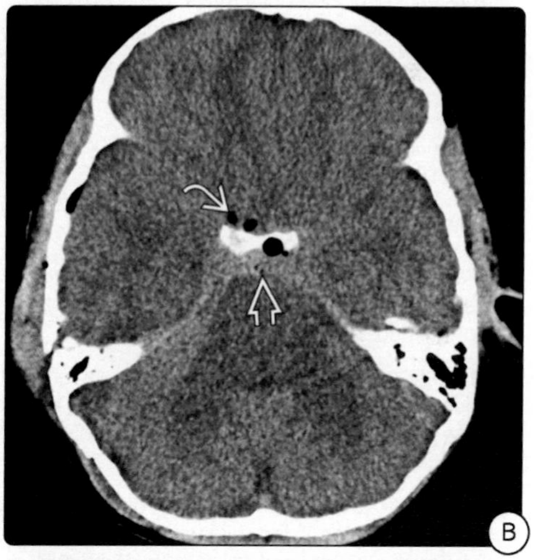

(1-4B) NECT in the same case shows diffuse brain swelling, pneumocephalus, and traumatic subarachnoid hemorrhage.

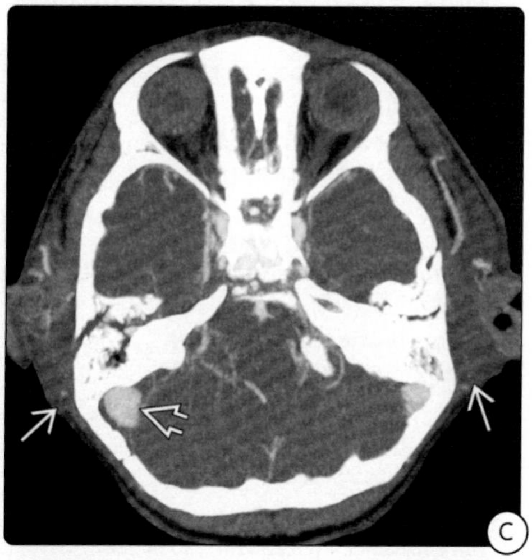

(1-4C) CTA in the same case shows the sigmoid sinus is intact but displaced medially. Note rapidly enlarging subgaleal hematoma.

Selected References

Introduction

Epidemiology of Head Trauma

Roozenbeek B et al: Changing patterns in the epidemiology of traumatic brain injury. Nat Rev Neurol. 9(4):231-6, 2013

Imaging Acute Head Trauma

How To Image?

Amrhein TJ et al: Reformatted images improve the detection rate of acute traumatic subdural hematomas on brain CT compared with axial images alone. Emerg Radiol. 24(1):39-45, 2017

Hinzpeter R et al: Repeated CT scans in trauma transfers: an analysis of indications, radiation dose exposure, and costs. Eur J Radiol. 88:135-140, 2017

Raja AS et al: "Choosing wisely" imaging recommendations: initial implementation in New England emergency departments. West J Emerg Med. 18(3):454-458, 2017

Thesleff T et al: Head injuries and the risk of concurrent cervical spine fractures. Acta Neurochir (Wien). 159(5):907-914, 2017

Lolli V et al: MDCT imaging of traumatic brain injury. Br J Radiol. 20150849, 2016

Bodanapally UK et al: Imaging of traumatic brain injury. Radiol Clin North Am. 53(4):695-715, viii, 2015

Who and When To Image?

Granata RT et al: Safety of deferred CT imaging of intoxicated patients presenting with possible traumatic brain injury. Am J Emerg Med. 35(1):51-54, 2017

Sharp AL et al: Computed tomography use for adults with head injury: describing likely avoidable emergency department imaging based on the Canadian CT head rule. Acad Emerg Med. 24(1):22-30, 2017

Atabaki SM et al: Comparison of prediction rules and clinician suspicion for identifying children with clinically important brain injuries after blunt head trauma. Acad Emerg Med. 23(5):566-75, 2016

Bharadwaj S et al: Minor head injury: limiting patient exposure to ionizing radiation, risk stratification, and concussion management. Curr Opin Pediatr. 28(1):121-31, 2016

Lolli V et al: MDCT imaging of traumatic brain injury. Br J Radiol. 20150849, 2016

Sadegh R et al: Head CT scan in Iranian minor head injury patients: evaluating current decision rules. Emerg Radiol. 23(1):9-16, 2016

Arab AF et al: Accuracy of Canadian CT head rule in predicting positive findings on CT of the head of patients after mild head injury in a large trauma centre in Saudi Arabia. Neuroradiol J. 28(6):591-7, 2015

Bodanapally UK et al: Imaging of traumatic brain injury. Radiol Clin North Am. 53(4):695-715, viii, 2015

Gunes Tatar I et al: Appropriateness of selection criteria for CT examinations performed at an emergency department. Emerg Radiol. 21(6):583-8, 2014

Ryan ME et al: ACR appropriateness criteria head trauma–child. J Am Coll Radiol. 11(10):939-47, 2014

Stiell IG et al: Comparison of the Canadian CT Head Rule and the New Orleans Criteria in patients with minor head injury. JAMA. 294(12):1511-8, 2005

Primary Effects of CNS Trauma

Primary head injuries are defined as those that occur at the time of initial trauma even though they may not be immediately apparent on initial evaluation.

Head injury can be caused by direct or indirect trauma. **Direct trauma** involves a blow to the head and is usually caused by automobile collisions, falls, or injury inflicted by an object such as a hammer or baseball bat. Scalp lacerations, hematomas, and skull fractures are common. Associated intracranial damage ranges from none to severe.

Significant forces of acceleration/deceleration, linear translation, and rotational loading can be applied to the brain *without* direct head blows. Such **indirect trauma** is caused by angular kinematics and typically occurs in high-speed motor vehicle collisions (MVCs). Here the brain undergoes rapid deformation and distortion. Depending on the site and direction of the force applied, significant injury to the cortex, axons, penetrating blood vessels, and deep gray nuclei may occur. Severe brain injury can occur in the absence of skull fractures or visible scalp lesions.

We begin our discussion with a consideration of scalp and skull lesions as we work our way from the outside to the inside of the skull. We then delineate the spectrum of intracranial trauma, starting with extraaxial hemorrhages. We conclude this chapter with a detailed discussion of injuries to the brain parenchyma (e.g., cortical contusion, diffuse axonal injury, and the serious deep subcortical injuries).

Scalp and Skull Injuries

Scalp and skull injuries are common manifestations of cranial trauma. Although brain injury is usually the most immediate concern in managing traumatized patients, superficial lesions such as scalp swelling and focal hematoma can be helpful in identifying the location of direct head trauma. On occasion, these initially innocent-appearing "lumps and bumps" can become life-threatening. Before turning our attention to intracranial traumatic lesions, we therefore briefly review scalp and skull injuries, delineating their typical imaging findings and clinical significance.

Scalp Injuries

Scalp injuries include lacerations and hematomas. Scalp **lacerations** can occur in both penetrating and closed head injuries. Lacerations may extend partially or entirely through all five layers of the scalp (skin, subcutaneous fibrofatty tissue, galea aponeurotica, loose areolar connective tissue, and periosteum) to the skull **(2-1)**.

Focal discontinuity, soft tissue swelling, and subcutaneous air are commonly identified in scalp lacerations. Scalp lacerations should be carefully evaluated

(2-1) Coronal graphic depicts normal layers of the scalp. Skin, subcutaneous fibrofatty tissue overlie the galea aponeurotica, loose areolar connective tissue. The pericranium is the periosteum of the skull and continues into and through sutures to merge with the periosteal layer of the dura. **(2-2)** NECT shows scalp laceration, hyperdense foreign bodies, and subgaleal air.

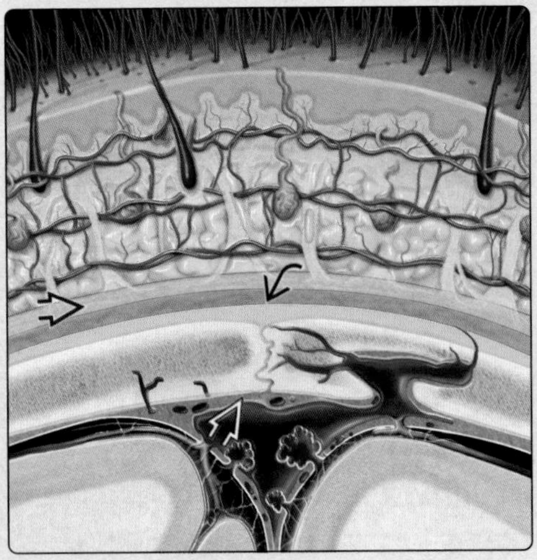

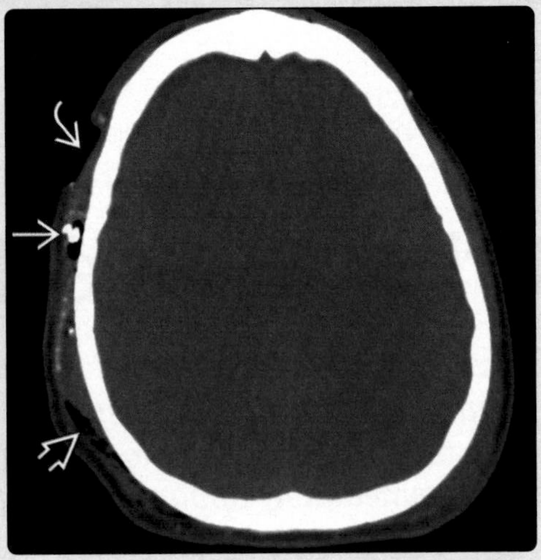

(2-3) Graphic shows the skull of a newborn, including the anterior fontanelle, coronal, metopic, sagittal sutures. Cephalohematoma is subperiosteal, limited by sutures. Subgaleal hematoma is under the scalp aponeurosis, not bounded by sutures. **(2-4A)** NECT scan in a newborn shows a small right and a large left parietal cephalohematoma. Neither crosses the sagittal suture.

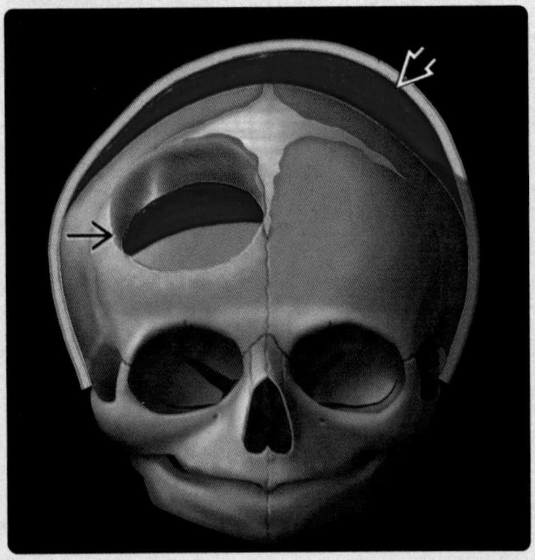

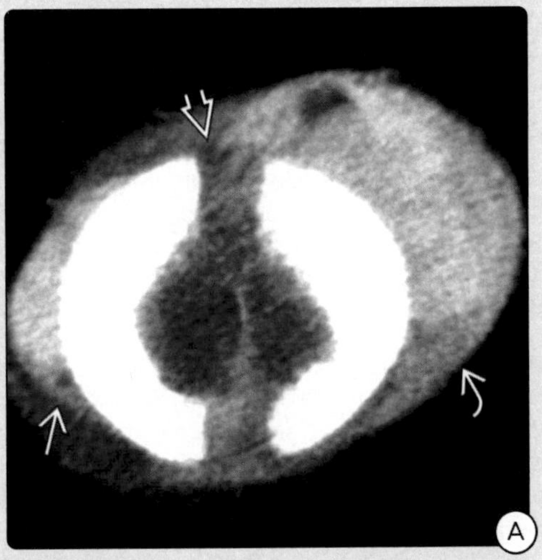

(2-4B) Coronal scan in the same case shows the small right, large left-sided cephalohematomas. The elevated periosteum clearly separates the two blood collections. **(2-4C)** Sagittal scan reformatted from the axial data shows that the left parietal cephalohematoma does not cross the coronal suture.

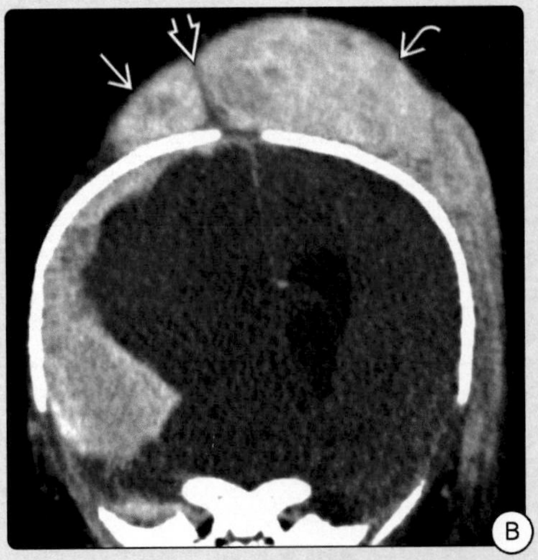

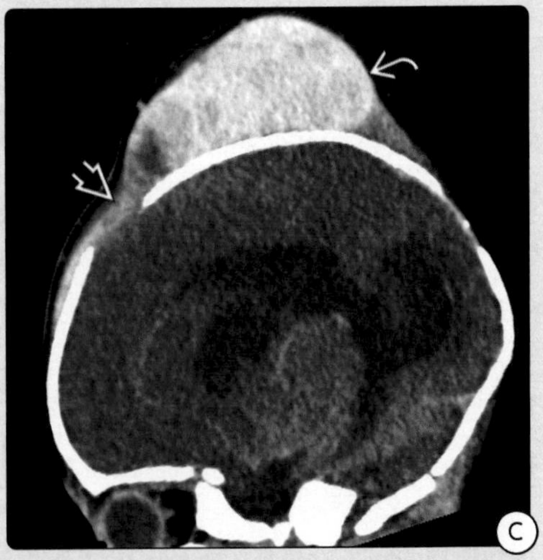

for the presence of any foreign bodies. If not removed during wound debridement, foreign bodies can be a potential source of substantial morbidity and are very important to identify on initial imaging studies. Wood fragments are often hypodense, whereas leaded glass, gravel, and metallic shards are variably hyperdense **(2-2)**.

Scalp lacerations may or may not be associated with scalp **hematomas**. There are two distinctly different types of scalp hematomas: cephalohematomas and subgaleal hematomas. The former are usually of no clinical significance, whereas the latter can cause hypovolemia and hypotension.

Cephalohematomas are *subperiosteal* blood collections that lie in the potential space between the outer surface of the calvarium and the pericranium, which serves as the periosteum of the skull **(2-3)**. The pericranium continues medially into cranial sutures and is anatomically contiguous with the outer (periosteal) layer of the dura.

Cephalohematomas are the extracranial equivalent of an intracranial epidural hematoma. Cephalohematomas do not cross suture lines and are typically unilateral. Because they are anatomically constrained by the tough fibrous periosteum and its insertions, cephalohematomas rarely attain large size.

Cephalohematomas occur in 1% of newborns and are more common following instrumented delivery. They are often diagnosed clinically but imaged only if they are unusually prominent or if intracranial injuries are suspected. NECT scans show a somewhat lens-shaped soft tissue mass that overlies a single bone (usually the parietal or occipital bone) **(2-4)**. If more than one bone is affected, the two collections are separated by the intervening suture lines.

Complications from cephalohematoma are rare, and most resolve spontaneously over a few days or weeks. Occasionally the elevated periosteum at the periphery of a chronic cephalohematoma undergoes dystrophic calcification, creating a firm palpable mass.

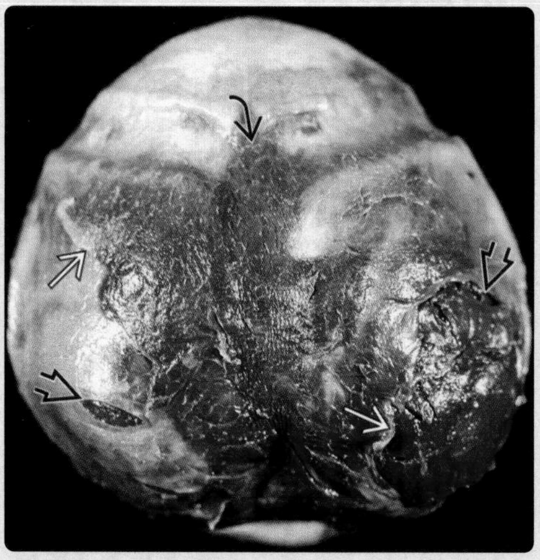

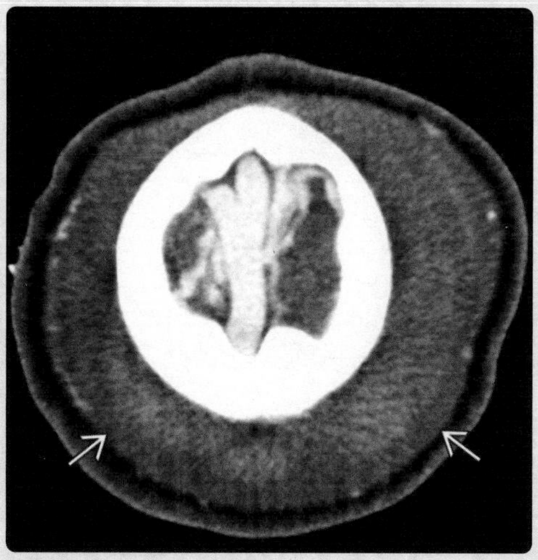

(2-5) Autopsy from a traumatized infant shows a massive biparietal subgaleal hematoma ➡. The galea aponeurotica has been partially opened ➡ to show large biparietal hematoma that crosses the sagittal suture ➡. (2-6) Axial CECT in 3y child shows massive subgaleal hematoma ➡ surrounding entire calvarium. Subgaleal hematomas cross sutures, can become life-threatening, while cephalohematomas are anatomically limited.

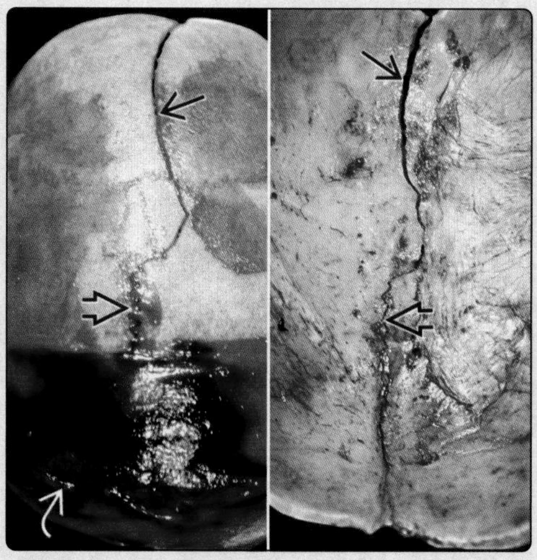

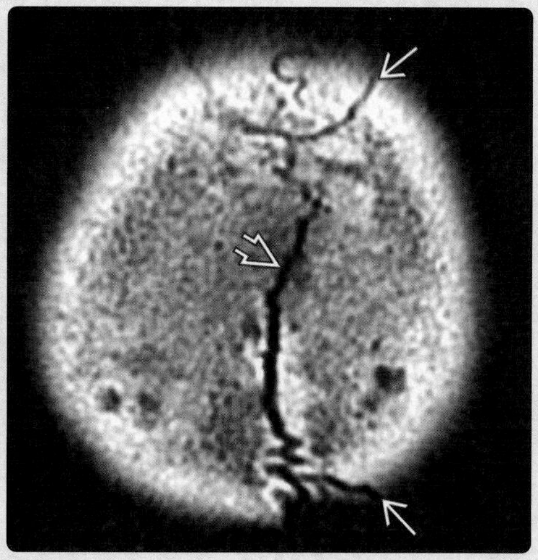

(2-7) Autopsied skull shows fatal trauma with exo- (L) and endocranial views (R). A linear fracture ➡ extends into the superior sagittal suture ➡, causing diastasis and a subgaleal hematoma ➡. (2-8) Bone CT through the top of the calvarium shows linear skull fractures ➡ extending into and widening the sagittal suture, causing a diastatic fracture ➡.

Subgaleal hematomas are *subaponeurotic* collections and are common findings in traumatized patients of all ages. Here blood collects under the aponeurosis (the "galea") of the occipitofrontalis muscle **(2-5)**. Because a subgaleal hematoma lies deep to the scalp muscles and galea aponeurotica but external to the periosteum, it is not anatomically limited by suture lines.

Bleeding into the subgaleal space can be very extensive. Subgaleal hematomas are usually bilateral lesions that often spread diffusely around the entire calvaria. NECT scans show a heterogeneously hyperdense crescentic scalp mass that crosses one or more suture lines **(2-6)**.

Most subgaleal hematomas resolve without treatment. In contrast to benign self-limited cephalohematomas, however, expanding subgaleal hematomas in infants and small children can cause significant blood loss.

Facial Injuries

Facial fractures are commonly overlooked on initial imaging (typically head CT scans). Important soft tissue markers can be identified that correlate with facial fractures and may merit a dedicated CT evaluation of the facial bones. These include periorbital contusions and subconjunctival hemorrhage as well as lacerations of the lips, mouth, and nose.

Holmgren et al. (2005) have proposed the mnemonic LIPS-N (**l**ip laceration, **i**ntraoral laceration, **p**eriorbital contusion, **s**ubconjunctival hemorrhage, and **n**asal laceration) be used in conjunction with physical examination. If any of these is present, a traumatized patient should have a dedicated facial CT in addition to the standard head CT.

Skull Fractures

Noticing a scalp "bump" or hematoma on initial imaging in head trauma is important, as calvarial fractures rarely—if

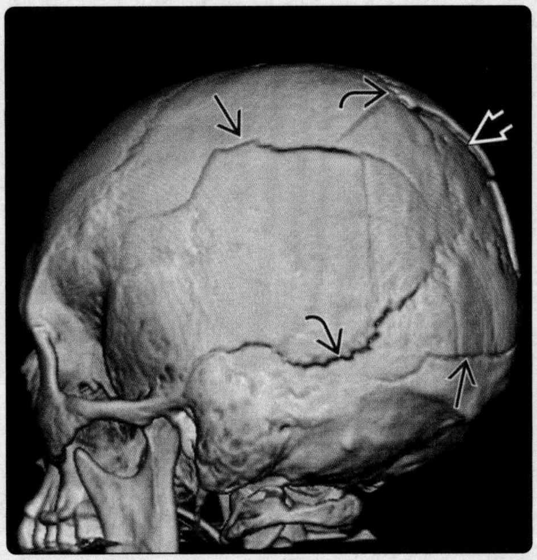

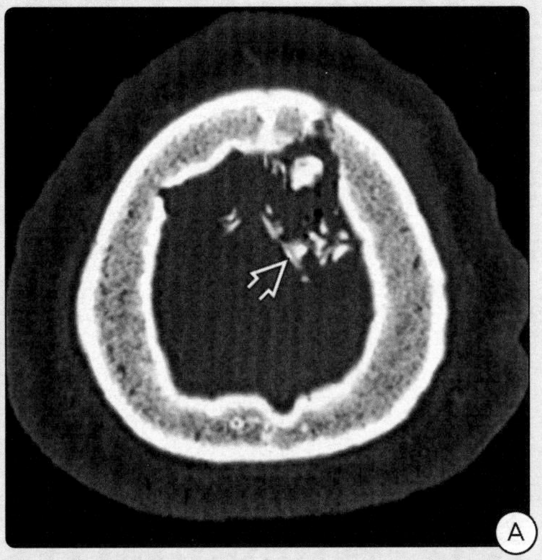

***(2-9)** 3D shaded surface display (SSD) in a patient with multiple linear ➔ and diastatic ➔ skull fractures shows utility of SSDs in depicting complex fracture anatomy. Note slight depression ➔ of the fractured parieto-occipital calvarium. **(2-10A)** Axial bone CT in a patient who was hit in the head with a falling ladder shows an extensively comminuted, depressed skull fracture ➔.*

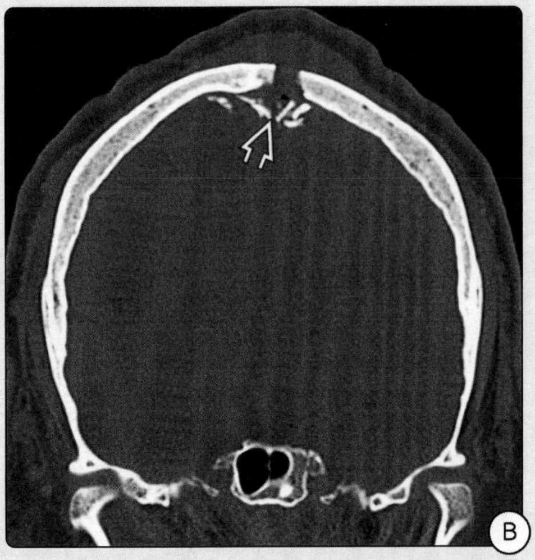

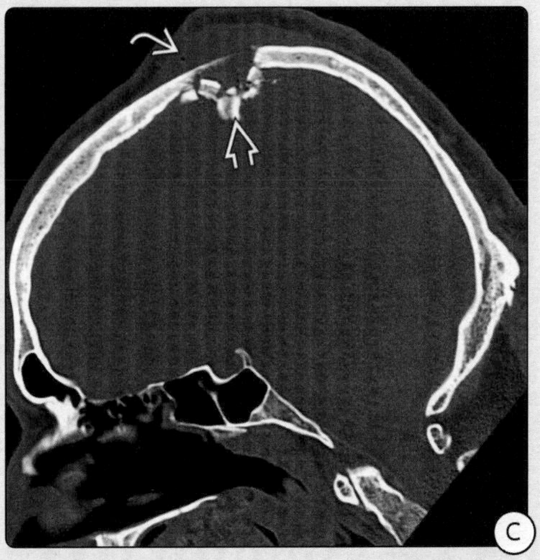

***(2-10B)** Coronal bone CT reformatted from the axial source data in the same case shows that the depressed skull fracture ➔ is near the midline, raising concern for superior sagittal sinus injury. **(2-10C)** Sagittal bone CT in the same case shows the depressed skull fracture ➔, associated with a focal scalp hematoma ➔. CTV (not shown) demonstrated SSS narrowing without occlusion or venous EDH.*

ever—occur in the absence of overlying soft tissue swelling or scalp laceration. Skull fractures are present on initial CT scans in about two-thirds of patients with moderate head injury, although 25-35% of severely injured patients have no identifiable fracture even with thin-section bone reconstructions.

Skull fractures can be simple or comminuted, closed or open. In open fractures, skin laceration results in communication between the external environment and intracranial cavity. Infection risk is high in this type of fracture, as it is with fractures that cross the mastoids and paranasal sinuses.

Several types of acute skull fracture can be identified on imaging studies: linear, depressed, elevated, and diastatic fractures **(2-7)**. Fractures can involve the calvaria, skull base, or both. Another type of skull fracture, a "growing" skull fracture, is a rare but important complication of skull trauma.

Linear Skull Fractures

A **linear skull fracture** is a sharply marginated linear defect that typically involves both the inner and outer tables of the calvaria **(2-8)**.

Most linear skull fractures are caused by relatively low-energy blunt trauma that is delivered over a relatively wide surface area. Linear skull fractures that extend into and widen a suture become diastatic fractures (see below). When multiple complex fractures are present, 3D shaded surface display (SSD) can be very helpful in depicting their anatomy and relationships to cranial sutures.

Patients with an isolated linear nondisplaced skull fracture (NDSF), no intracranial hemorrhage or pneumocephalus, normal neurologic examination, and absence of other injuries are at very low risk for delayed hemorrhage or other life-threatening complication. Hospitalization is not necessary for many children with NDSFs.

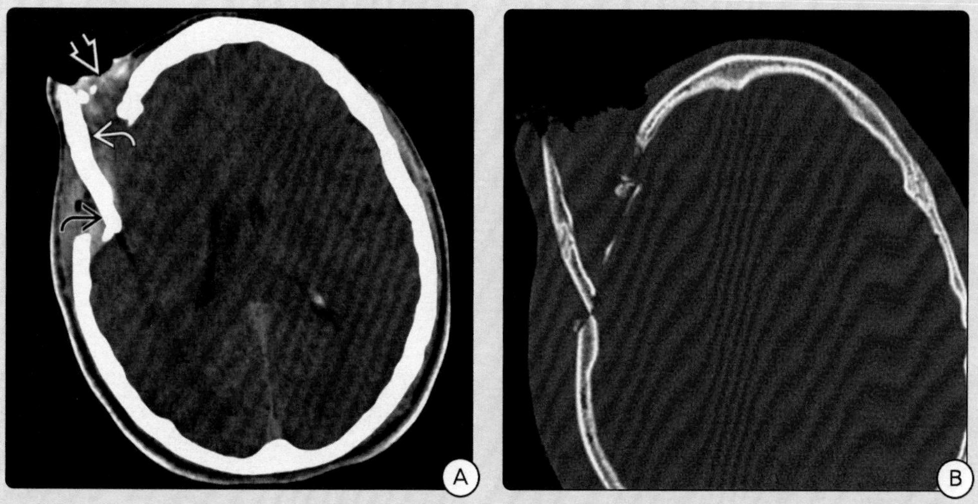

***(2-11A)** Axial NECT scan shows severe scalp laceration with a combination of elevated, depressed skull fractures. **(2-11B)** Bone CT in the same case shows that the elevated fracture is literally "hinged" away from the calvaria.*

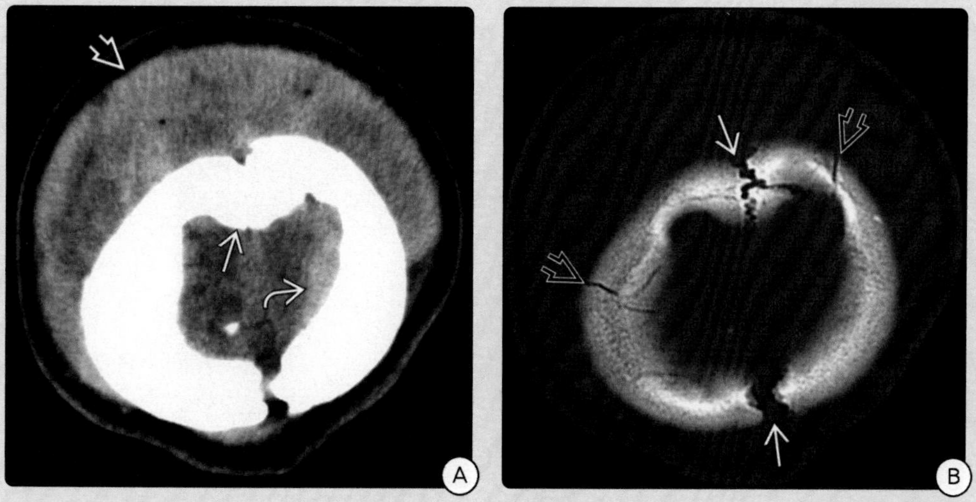

***(2-12A)** Axial NECT scan in a 20y man who had a tree fall on his head shows a massive subgaleal hematoma crossing the anterior aspect of the sagittal suture. A small extraaxial hematoma, most likely a venous epidural hematoma, is present. **(2-12B)** Bone CT in the same case shows a diastatic fracture of the sagittal suture. Nondisplaced linear fractures are also present.*

Depressed Skull Fractures

A **depressed skull fracture** is a fracture in which the fragments are displaced inward **(2-9)**. Comminution of the fracture fragments starts at the point of maximum impact and spreads centrifugally. Depressed fractures are most often caused by high-energy direct blows to a small surface with a blunt object (e.g., hammer, baseball bat, or metal pipe) **(2-10)**.

Depressed skull fractures typically tear the underlying dura and arachnoid and are associated with cortical contusions and potential leakage of CSF into the subdural space. Fractures extending to a dural sinus or the jugular bulb are associated with venous sinus thrombosis in 40% of cases.

Elevated Skull Fractures

An **elevated skull fracture**—often combined with depressed fragments—is uncommon. Elevated fractures are usually caused by a long, sharp object (such as a machete or propeller) that fractures the calvaria, simultaneously lifting and rotating the fracture fragment **(2-11)**.

Diastatic Skull Fractures

A **diastatic skull fracture** is a fracture that widens ("diastases" or "splits open") a suture or synchondrosis. Diastatic skull fractures usually occur in association with a linear skull fracture that extends into an adjacent suture **(2-12)**.

Traumatic diastasis of the sphenooccipital, petrooccipital, and/or occipitomastoid synchondroses is common in children with severely comminuted central skull base fractures. As it typically does not ossify completely until the mid teens, the sphenooccipital synchondrosis is the most common site.

"Growing" Skull Fractures

A **"growing" skull fracture** (GSF), also known as "posttraumatic leptomeningeal cyst" or "craniocerebral

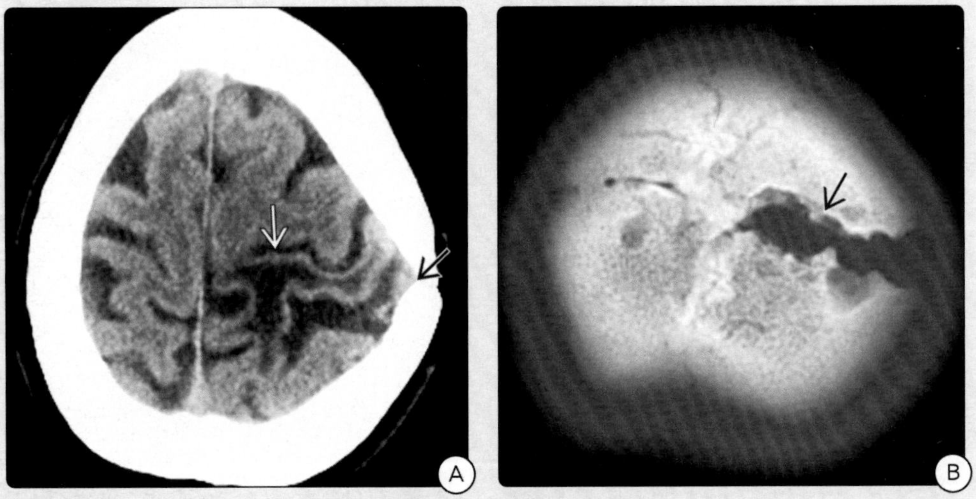

***(2-13A)** Axial NECT scan in a patient with progressive right hemiparesis following prior head trauma shows left parietal encephalomalacia ➡. The overlying skull appears focally deformed and thinned ⇨. **(2-13B)** Bone CT in the same patient shows a wide lucent skull lesion with rounded, scalloped margins ⇨.*

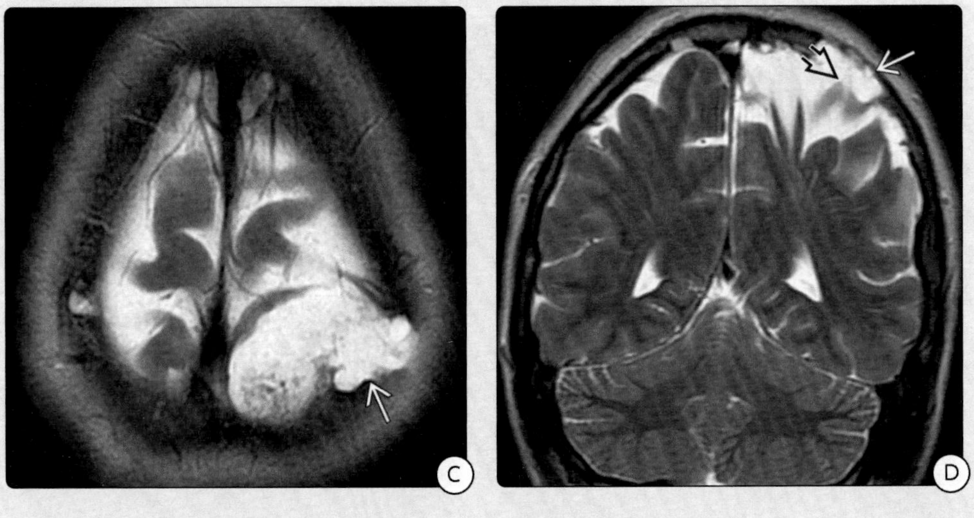

***(2-13C)** Axial T2WI in the same patient shows a lobulated CSF collection ➡ that extends into and almost completely through the calvarial vault. **(2-13D)** Coronal T2WI shows the intradiploic CSF collection ➡ with encephalomalacic brain stretched and tethered into the lesion ⇨. This is classic "growing" skull fracture (leptomeningeal cyst).*

erosion," is a rare lesion that occurs in just 0.3-0.5% of all skull fractures **(2-13)**. Most patients with GSF are under 3 years of age.

GSFs develop in stages and slowly widen over time. In the first "prephase," a skull fracture (typically a linear or comminuted fracture) lacerates the dura, and brain tissue or arachnoid membrane herniates through the torn dura. Stage I extends from the time of initial injury to just before the fracture enlarges. Early recognition and dural repair of stage I GSFs produce the best results.

Stage II is the early phase of GSF. Stage II lasts for approximately 2 months following initial fracture enlargement. At this stage, the bone defect is small, the skull deformity is relatively limited, and neurologic deficits are mild. Nevertheless, the entrapped tissue prevents normal fracture healing.

Stage III represents late-stage GSF and begins 2 months after the initial enlargement begins. During this stage, the bone defect becomes significantly larger. Brain tissue and CSF extend between the bony edges of the fracture through torn dura and arachnoid.

Patients with late-stage GSFs often present months or even years after head trauma. Stage III GSFs can cause pronounced skull deformities and progressive neurologic deficits if left untreated.

Imaging

General Features. Plain skull radiographs have no role in the modern evaluation of traumatic head injury. One-quarter of patients with fatal brain injuries have no skull fracture at autopsy. CT is fast, widely available, sensitive for both bone and brain injury, and the worldwide diagnostic standard of care for patients with head injuries. New generations of multislice CT scanners offer very short acquisition times with excellent spatial resolution.

Both bone and soft tissue reconstruction algorithms should be used when evaluating patients with head injuries. Soft tissue reconstructions should be viewed with both narrow ("brain") and intermediate ("subdural") windows. Coronal and sagittal reformatted images obtained using the axial source data are helpful additions.

Three-dimensional reconstruction and curved MIPs of the skull have been shown to improve fracture detection over the use of axial sections alone.

CT Findings. While fractures can involve any part of the calvaria or skull base, the middle cranial fossa is most susceptible because of its thin "squamous" bones and multiple foramina and fissures.

NECT scans demonstrate *linear* skull fractures as sharply marginated lucent lines. *Depressed* fractures are typically comminuted and show inward implosion of fracture fragments **(2-10)**. *Elevated* fractures show an elevated, rotated skull segment **(2-11)**. Diastatic fractures appear as widened sutures or synchondroses **(2-14)** **(2-15)** and are usually associated with linear skull fractures.

Stage I "*growing*" fractures are difficult to detect on initial NECT scans, as scalp and contused brain are similar in density. Identifying torn dura with herniated brain tissue is similarly difficult although cranial ultrasound can be more helpful.

Later-stage GSFs demonstrate a progressively widening and unhealing fracture. A lucent skull lesion with rounded, scalloped margins and beveled edges is typical **(2-13)**. CSF and soft tissue are entrapped within the expanding fracture. Most GSFs are directly adjacent to posttraumatic encephalomalacia, so the underlying brain often appears hypodense.

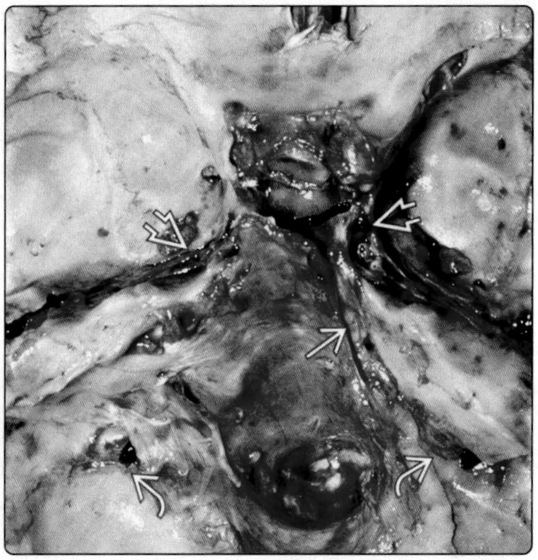

(2-14) Autopsy shows multiple skull base fractures involving clivus ➡, carotid canals ➡, jugular foramina ➡. (E. T. Hedley-White, MD.)

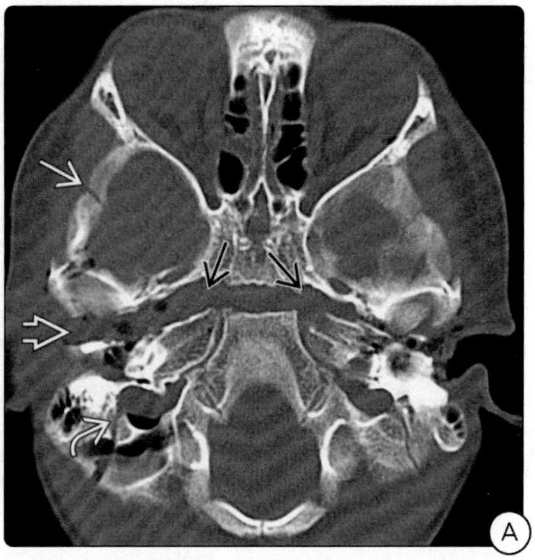

(2-15A) Linear ➡, diastatic ➡ fractures of the skull base are present crossing the jugular foramen ➡, both carotid canals ➡.

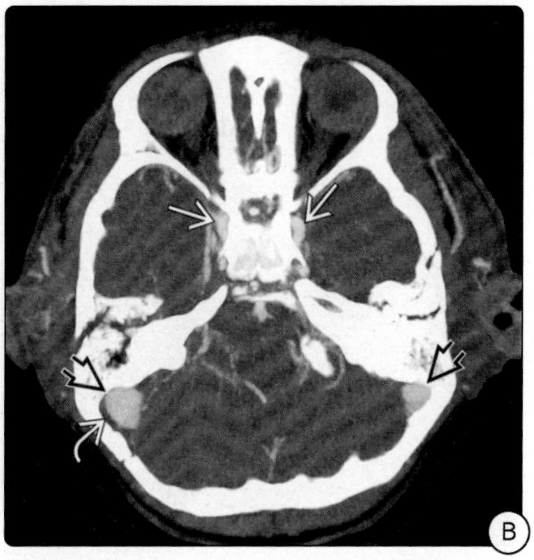

(2-15B) CT in the same case shows carotid arteries ➡, sigmoid sinuses ➡ are patent. A small right venous EDH ➡ is present.

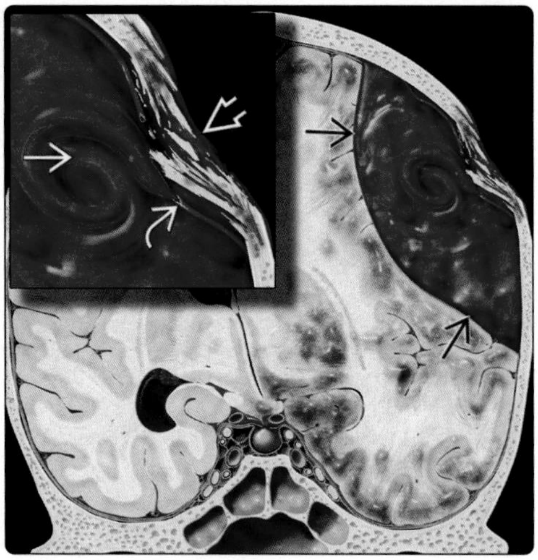

(2-16) Graphic shows EDH, depressed skull fracture lacerating middle meningeal artery. Inset shows rapid bleeding, "swirl" sign.

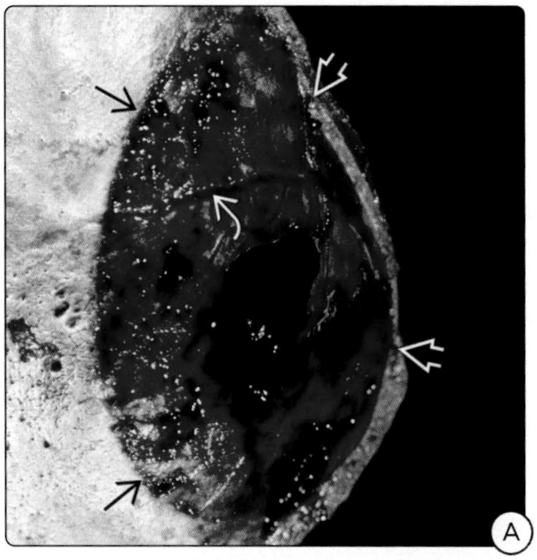

(2-17A) Endocranial view shows temporal bone fracture crossing the middle meningeal artery groove. Note biconvex margins of EDH.

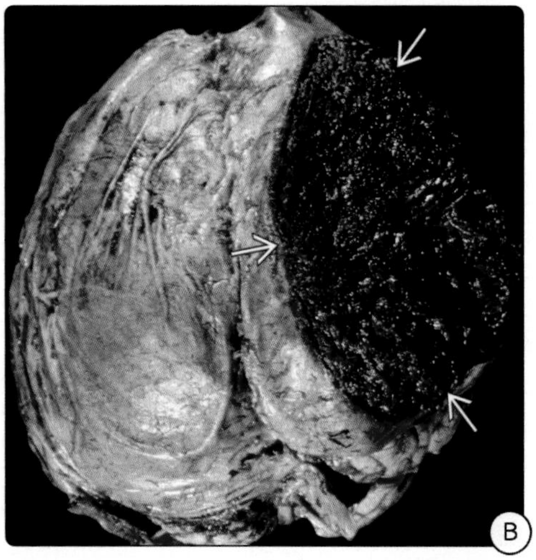

(2-17B) Dorsal view of the dura-covered brain shows the biconvex EDH on top of the dura. (Courtesy E. T. Hedley-Whyte, MD.)

MR Findings. MR is rarely used in the setting of acute head trauma because of high cost, limited availability, and lengthy time required. Compared with CT, bone detail is poor although parenchymal injuries are better seen. Adding T2* sequences, particularly SWI, is especially helpful in identifying hemorrhagic lesions.

In some cases, MR may be indicated for early detection of potentially treatable complications. A young child with neurologic deficits or seizures, a fracture larger than 4 millimeters, or a soft tissue mass extending through the fracture into the subgaleal space is at risk for developing a GSF. MR can demonstrate the dural tear and differentiate herniated brain from contused, edematous scalp.

Angiography. If a fracture crosses the site of a major vascular structure such as the carotid canal or a dural venous sinus **(2-14)**, CT angiography is recommended. Sagittal, coronal, and MIP reconstructions help delineate the site and extent of vascular injuries.

Clival and skull base fractures are strongly associated with neurovascular trauma, and CTA should always be obtained in these cases **(2-15)**. Cervical fracture dislocations, distraction injuries, and penetrating neck trauma also merit further investigation. Uncomplicated asymptomatic soft tissue injuries of the neck rarely result in significant vascular injury.

SCALP AND SKULL INJURIES

Scalp Injuries

- Lacerations
  - ± Foreign bodies
- Cephalohematoma
  - Usually infants
  - Subperiosteal
  - Small, unilateral (limited by sutures)
- Subgaleal hematoma
  - Between galea, periosteum of skull
  - Circumferential, not limited by sutures
  - Can be very large, life-threatening

Skull Fractures

- Linear
  - Sharp lucent line
  - Can be extensive and widespread
- Depressed
  - Focal
  - Inwardly displaced fragments
  - Often lacerates dura-arachnoid
- Elevated
  - Rare
  - Fragmented rotated outward
- Diastatic
  - Typically associated with severe trauma
  - Usually caused by linear fracture that extends into suture
  - Widens, spreads apart suture or synchondrosis
- "Growing"
  - Rare
  - Usually in young children
  - Fracture lacerates dura-arachnoid
  - Brain/arachnoid herniates through torn dura
  - Trapped tissue prevents bone healing
  - CT: Rounded edges, scalloped margins of skull
  - MR: CSF ± brain

Extraaxial Hemorrhages

Extraaxial hemorrhages and hematomas are common manifestations of head trauma. They can occur in any intracranial compartment, within any space (potential or actual), and between any layers of the cranial meninges. Only the subarachnoid spaces exist normally; all the other spaces are potential spaces and occur only under pathologic conditions.

Epidural hematomas arise between the inner table of the skull and outer (periosteal) layer of the dura. **Subdural hematomas** are located between the inner (meningeal) layer of the dura and the arachnoid. **Traumatic subarachnoid hemorrhage** is found within the sulci and subarachnoid cisterns, between the arachnoid and the pia.

To discuss extraaxial hemorrhages, we work our way from the outside to inside. We therefore begin this section with a discussion of epidural hematomas (both classic and variant), then move deeper inside the cranium to the more common subdural hematomas. We conclude with a consideration of traumatic subarachnoid hemorrhage.

Arterial Epidural Hematoma

Epidural hematomas (EDHs) are uncommon but potentially lethal complications of head trauma. If an EDH is promptly recognized and appropriately treated, mortality and morbidity can be minimized.

Terminology

An EDH is a collection of blood between the calvaria and outer (periosteal) layer of the dura.

Etiology

Most EDHs arise from direct trauma to the skull that lacerates an adjacent blood vessel **(2-16)**. The vast majority (90%) are caused by arterial injury, most commonly to the middle meningeal artery. Approximately 10% of EDHs are venous, usually secondary to a fracture that crosses a dural venous sinus (see below).

Pathology

Location. Over 90% of EDHs are unilateral and supratentorial. Between 90-95% are found directly adjacent to a skull fracture. The squamous portion of the temporal bone is the most common site.

Gross Pathology. EDHs are biconvex in shape **(2-17A)**. Adherence of the periosteal dura to the inner calvaria explains this typical configuration. As EDHs expand, they strip the dura away from the inner table of the skull, forming the classic lens-shaped hematoma **(2-17B)**. Because the dura is especially tightly attached to sutures, EDHs in adults rarely cross suture lines (10% of EDHs in children *do* cross sutures, especially if a fracture traverses the suture or sutural diastasis is present).

The typical gross or intraoperative appearance of an acute EDH is a dark purple ("currant jelly") lentiform clot.

Clinical Issues

Epidemiology. EDHs are much less common than either traumatic subarachnoid hemorrhage (tSAH) or subdural hematoma. Although EDHs represent up to 10% of fatal injuries in autopsy series, they are found in only 1-4% of patients imaged for craniocerebral trauma.

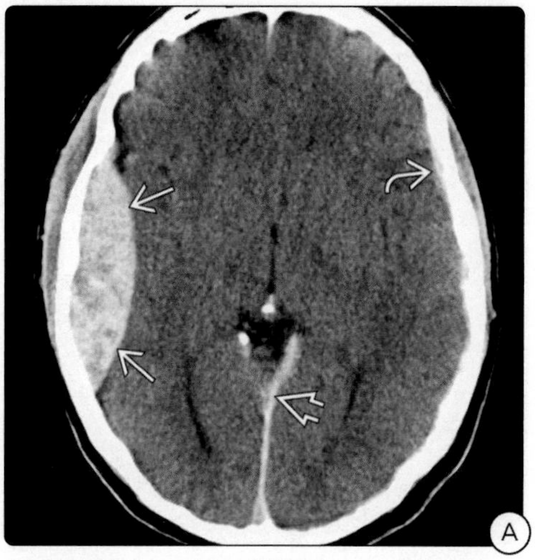

***(2-18A)** Biconvex aEDH is shown with a thin subdural blood collection along the tentorium, falx, and left hemisphere.*

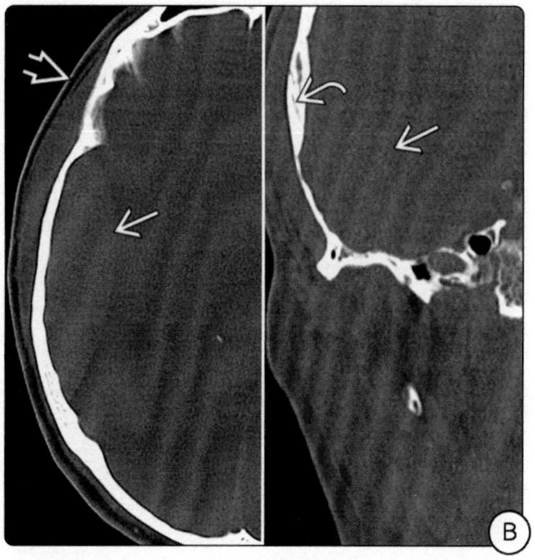

***(2-18B)** (L) Bone CT shows subgaleal hematoma, EDH. (R) Coronal bone CT demonstrates a subtle comminuted fracture.*

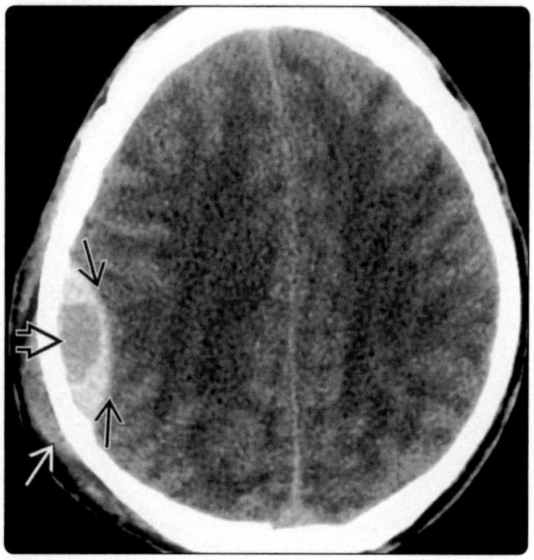

***(2-19)** Axial NECT shows an actively bleeding EDH with "swirl" sign, displaced cortex. A focal cephalohematoma is present.*

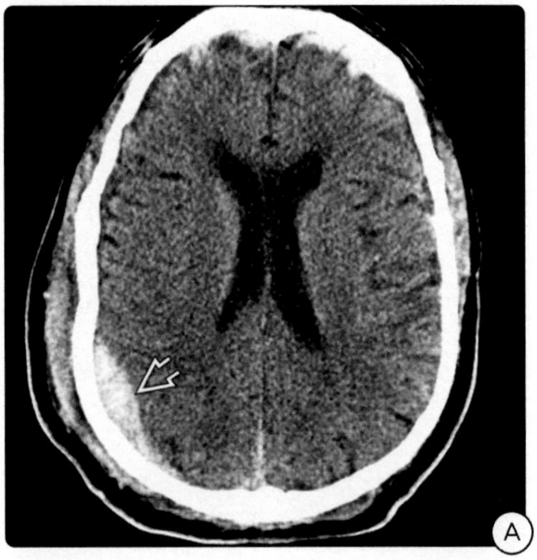

(2-20A) Serial imaging demonstrates temporal evolution of a small nonoperated EDH. Initial NECT scan shows a hyperdense biconvex EDH ➲.

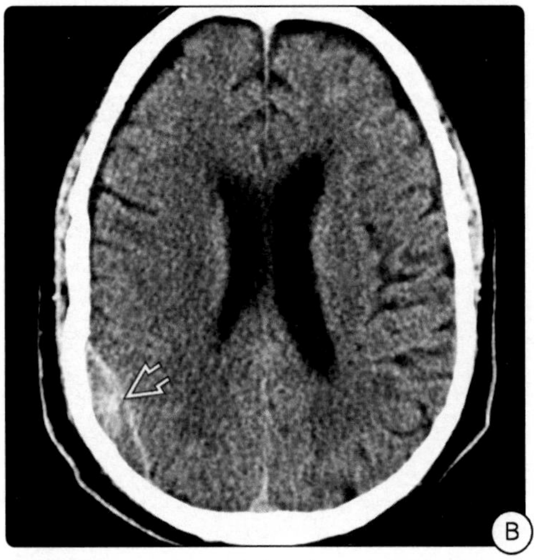

(2-20B) Repeat scan 10 days later reveals that density of the EDH ➲ has decreased significantly.

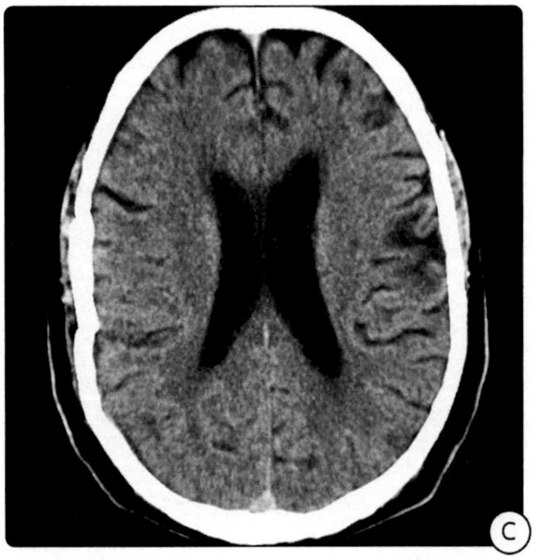

(2-20C) Repeat study 6 weeks after trauma reveals that the EDH has resolved completely.

Demographics. EDHs are uncommon in infants and the elderly. Most are found in older children and young adults. The M:F ratio is 4:1.

Presentation. The prototypical "lucid interval," during which a traumatized patient has an initial brief loss of consciousness followed by an asymptomatic period of various length prior to onset of coma and/or neurologic deficit, occurs in only 50% of EDH cases. Headache, nausea, vomiting, symptoms of intracranial mass effect (e.g., pupil-involving third cranial nerve palsy) followed by somnolence and coma are common.

Natural History. Outcome depends on size and location of the hematoma, whether the EDH is arterial or venous, and whether there is active bleeding (see below). In the absence of other associated traumatic brain injuries, overall mortality rate with prompt recognition and appropriate treatment is under 5%.

Delayed development or enlargement of an EDH occurs in 10-15% of cases, usually within 24-36 hours following trauma.

Treatment Options. Many EDHs are now treated conservatively. Most traumatic EDHs are not surgical lesions at initial presentation, and the rate of conversion to surgery is low. Most venous and small classic hyperdense EDHs that do not exhibit a "swirl" sign and have minimal or no mass effect are managed conservatively with close clinical observation and follow-up imaging **(2-20)**. Significant clinical predictors of EDH progression requiring conversion to surgical therapy are coagulopathy and younger age.

Imaging

General Features. EDHs, especially in adults, typically do not cross sutures unless a fracture with sutural diastasis is present. In children, 10% of EDHs cross suture lines, usually the coronal or sphenosquamous suture.

Look for other comorbid lesions such as "contre-coup" injuries, tSAH, and secondary brain herniations, all of which are common findings in patients with EDHs.

CT Findings. NECT scan is the procedure of choice for initial imaging in patients with head injury. Both soft tissue and bone reconstruction algorithms should be obtained. Multiplanar reconstructions are especially useful in identifying vertex EDHs, which may be difficult to detect if only axial images are obtained.

The classic imaging appearance of **classic (arterial) EDHs** is a hyperdense (60-90 HU) biconvex extraaxial collection **(2-18)**. Presence of a hypodense component ("swirl" sign) is seen in about one-third of cases and indicates active, rapid bleeding with unretracted clot **(2-16) (2-19)**.

EDHs compress the underlying subarachnoid space and displace the cortex medially, "buckling" the gray-white matter interface inward.

Air in an EDH occurs in approximately 20% of cases and is usually—but not invariably—associated with a sinus or mastoid fracture.

Patients with mixed-density EDHs tend to present earlier than patients with hyperdense hematomas and have lower Glasgow Coma Scores (GCSs), larger hematoma volumes, and poorer prognosis.

Imaging findings associated with adverse clinical outcome are thickness > 1.5 cm, volume > 30 mL, pterional (lateral aspect of the middle cranial fossa) location, midline shift > 5 mm, and presence of a "swirl sign" within the hematoma on imaging.

MR Findings. Acute EDHs are typically isointense with underlying brain, especially on T1WI. The displaced dura can be identified as a displaced "black line" between the hematoma and the brain.

Angiography. DSA may show a lacerated middle meningeal artery with "tram-track" fistulization of contrast from the middle meningeal artery into the paired middle meningeal veins. Mass effect with displaced cortical arteries and veins is seen.

CLASSIC ACUTE EPIDURAL HEMATOMA

Terminology
- EDH = blood between skull, dura

Etiology
- Associated skull fracture in 90-95%
- Arterial 90%
  - Most often middle meningeal artery
- Venous 10%

Pathology
- Unilateral, supratentorial (> 90%)
- Dura stripped away from skull → biconvex hematoma
- Usually does not cross sutures (exception = children, 10%)
- Does cross sites of dural attachment

Clinical
- Rare (1-4% of head trauma)
- Older children, young adults most common
- M:F = 4:1
- Classic "lucid interval" in only 50%
- Delayed deterioration common
- Low mortality if recognized, treated
- Small EDHs
  - If minimal mass, no "swirl sign" often managed conservatively

Imaging
- Hyperdense lens-shaped
- "Swirl sign" (hypodensity) = rapid bleeding

Venous Epidural Hematoma

Not all EDHs are the same!! **Venous EDHs** are often smaller, are under lower pressure, and develop more slowly than their arterial counterparts. Most venous EDHs are caused by a skull fracture that crosses a dural venous sinus and therefore occur in the posterior fossa near the skull base (transverse/sigmoid sinus) **(2-21)** or the vertex of the brain (superior sagittal sinus). In contrast to their arterial counterparts, venous EDHs can "straddle" intracranial compartments, crossing both sutures and lines of dural attachment **(2-22)** and compressing or occluding the adjacent venous sinuses.

Venous EDHs can be subtle and easily overlooked. Coronal and sagittal reformatted images are key to the diagnosis and delineation of these variant EDHs **(2-23)**. Several anatomic subtypes of venous EDHs, each with different treatment implications and prognosis, are recognized.

Vertex EDH

"Vertex" EDHs are rare. Usually caused by a linear or diastatic fracture that crosses the superior sagittal sinus, they often accumulate over hours or even days with slow, subtle onset of symptoms **(2-24)**. "Vertex" hematomas can be subtle and are easily overlooked unless coronal and sagittal reformatted images are obtained.

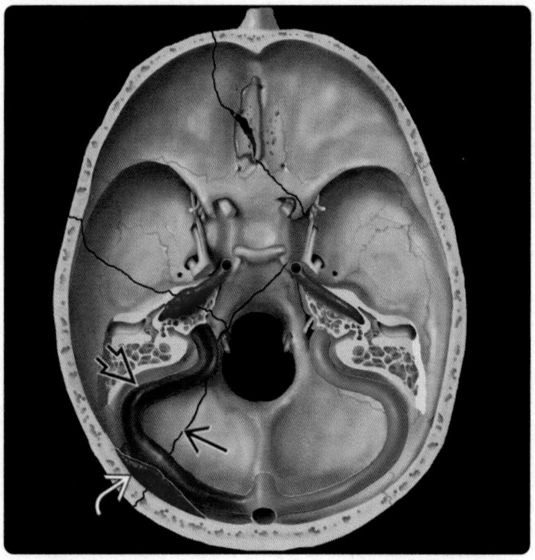

***(2-21)** Graphic shows basilar skull fracture ➡ with transverse sinus occlusion ➡ and posterior fossa venous EDH ➡.*

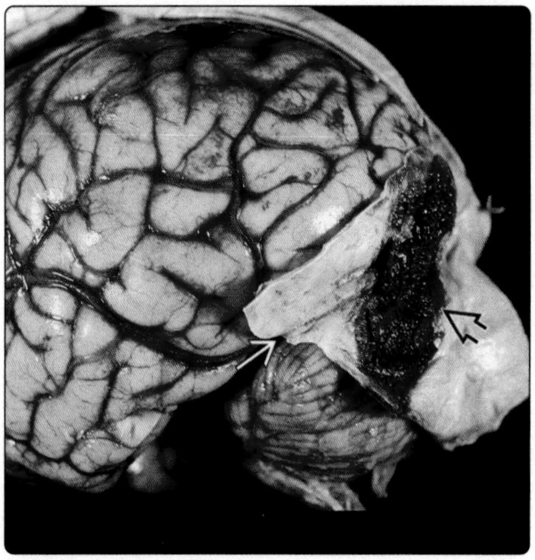

***(2-22)** Autopsy shows that venous EDH ➡ caused by transverse sinus injury "straddles" the tentorium ➡. (Courtesy R. Hewlett, MD.)*

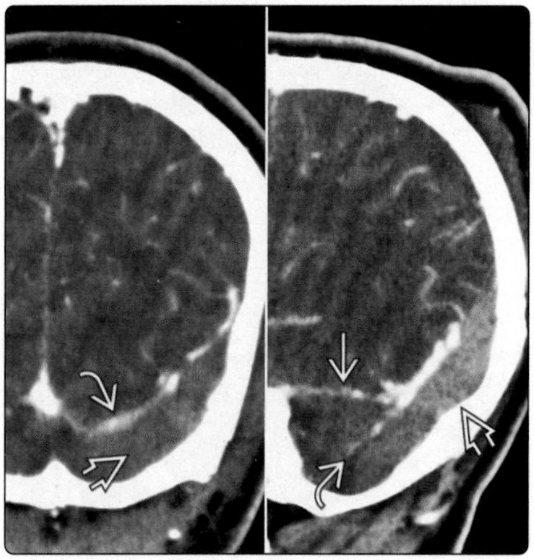

***(2-23)** (L) Coronal, (R) sagittal CTV shows venous EDH ➡ straddling the tentorium ➡, elevating the left transverse sinus ➡.*

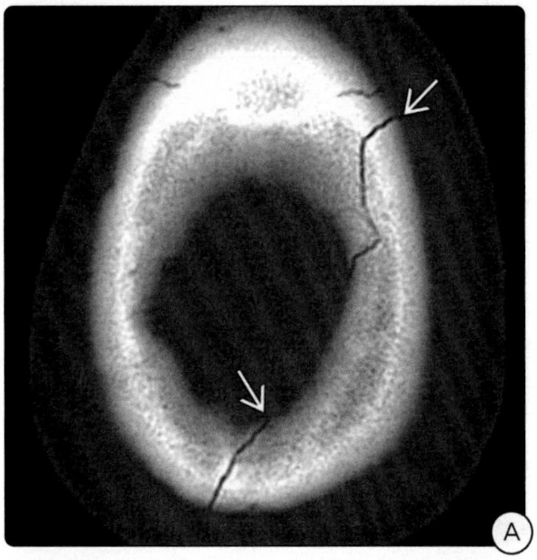

(2-24A) Bone CT in a 57y man shows a linear skull fracture that crosses the midline. No other abnormalities were present.

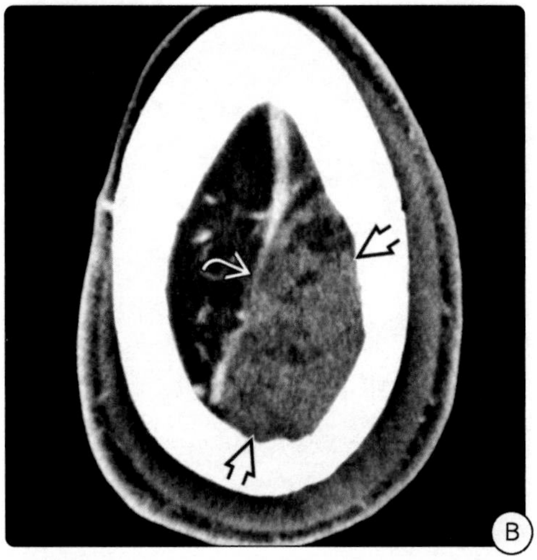

(2-24B) CT venogram after the patient deteriorated shows a large venous EDH. The middle SSS is compressed and thrombosed.

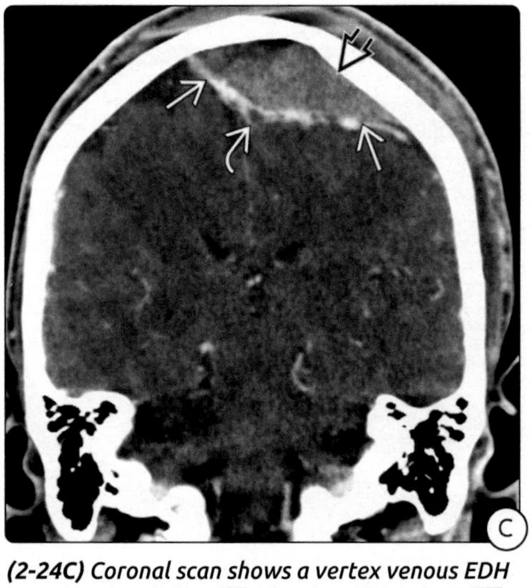

(2-24C) Coronal scan shows a vertex venous EDH crossing the midline. The thrombosed SSS, cortical veins are displaced inferiorly.

Anterior Temporal EDH

Anterior temporal EDHs are a unique subgroup of hematomas that occur in the anterior tip of the middle cranial fossa. Anterior temporal EDHs are caused either by an isolated fracture of the adjacent greater sphenoid wing or by an isolated zygomaticomaxillary complex ("tripod") facial fracture. The sphenoparietal dural venous sinus is injured as it curves medially along the undersurface of the lesser sphenoid wing, extravasating blood into the epidural space. Limited anatomically by the sphenotemporal suture laterally and the orbital fissure medially, anterior temporal EDHs remain stable in size and do not require surgical evacuation **(2-25)** **(2-26)**.

Clival EDH

Clival EDHs usually develop after a hyperflexion or hyperextension injury to the neck and are possibly caused by stripping of the tectorial membrane from attachments to the clivus. Less commonly, they have been associated with basilar skull fractures that lacerate the clival dural venous plexus.

Clival EDHs most often occur in children and present with multiple cranial neuropathies. The abducens nerve is the most commonly affected, followed by the glossopharyngeal and hypoglossal nerves. They are typically limited in size by the tight attachment of the dura to the basisphenoid and tectorial membrane **(2-27)**.

VENOUS EPIDURAL HEMATOMA

Not all EDHs are the same!
- Different etiologies in different anatomic locations
- Prognosis, treatment vary

Venous EDHs = 10% of all EDHs
- Skull fracture crosses dural venous sinus
  - Can cross sutures, dural attachments
- Often subtle, easily overlooked
  - Coronal, sagittal reformatted images key to diagnosis
- Usually accumulate slowly
- Can be limited in size; often treated conservatively

Subtypes
- Vertex EDH
  - Skull fracture crosses superior sagittal sinus (SSS)
  - SSS can be lacerated, compressed, thrombosed
  - Hematoma under low pressure, develops gradually
  - Slow onset of symptoms
  - May become large, cause significant mass effect
- Anterior temporal EDH
  - Sphenoid wing or zygomaticomaxillary fracture
  - Injures sphenoparietal venous sinus
  - Hematoma accumulates at anterior tip of middle cranial fossa
  - Limited anatomically (laterally by sphenotemporal suture, medially by orbital fissure)
  - Benign clinical course
- Clival EDH
  - Most common = child with neck injury
  - May cause multiple cranial neuropathies (CN VI most common)
  - Hyperdense collection under clival dura
  - Limited by tight attachment of dura to basisphenoid, tectorial membrane
  - Usually benign course, resolves spontaneously

Management of a clival EDH is dictated by severity and progression of the neurologic deficits and stability of the atlantoaxial joint. In patients with

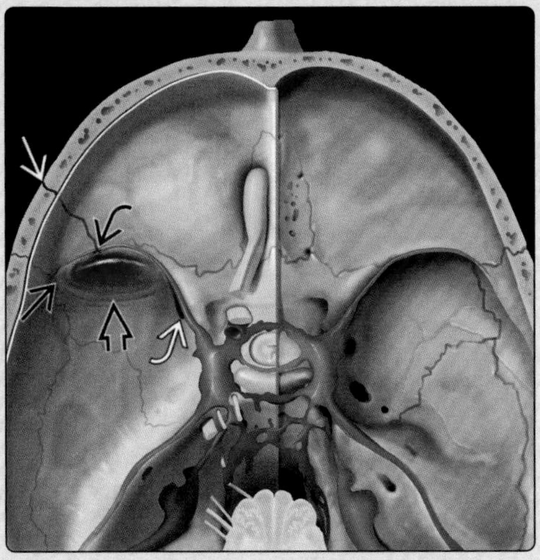

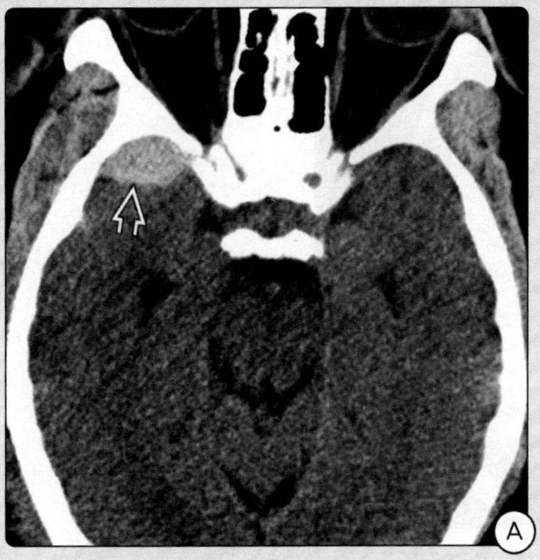

(2-25) Graphic depicts benign anterior temporal epidural hematoma. Fracture disrupts the sphenoparietal sinus. Low-pressure venous EDH is anatomically limited, medially by the orbital fissure and laterally by the sphenotemporal suture. (2-26A) Axial NECT in a 33y man with head trauma shows a biconvex anterior temporal acute epidural hematoma.

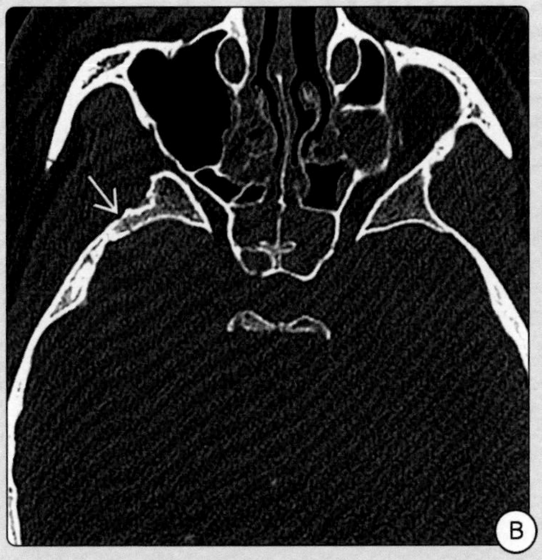

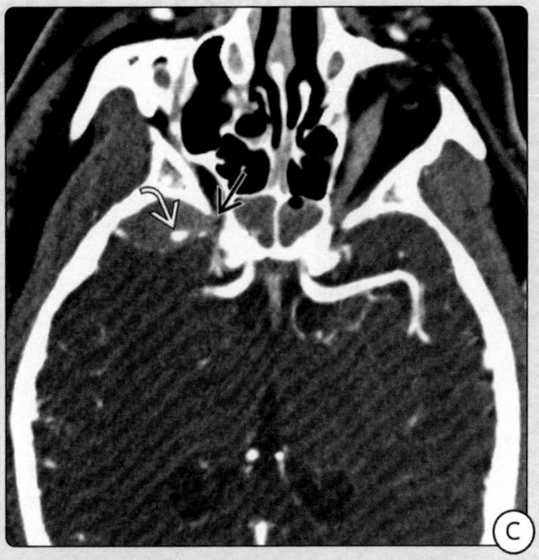

(2-26B) Axial bone CT in the same case shows a fracture through the right greater sphenoid wing. (2-26C) CT venogram in the same case shows a displaced, lacerated sphenoparietal sinus with contrast extravasation ("spot sign"). Note the EDH is limited medially by the orbital fissure. The patient was treated nonsurgically. The EDH showed no further enlargement and resolved completely.

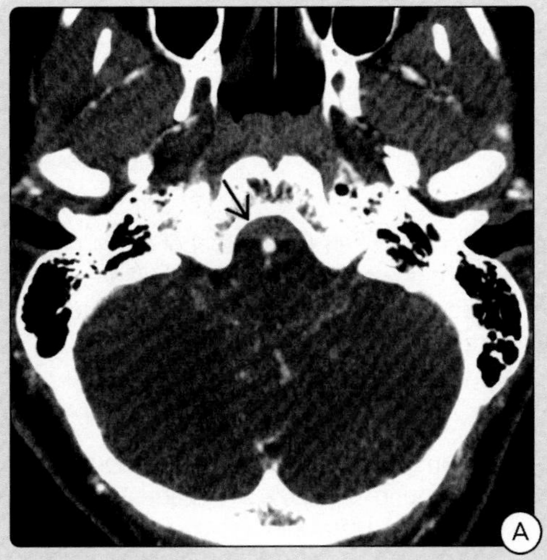

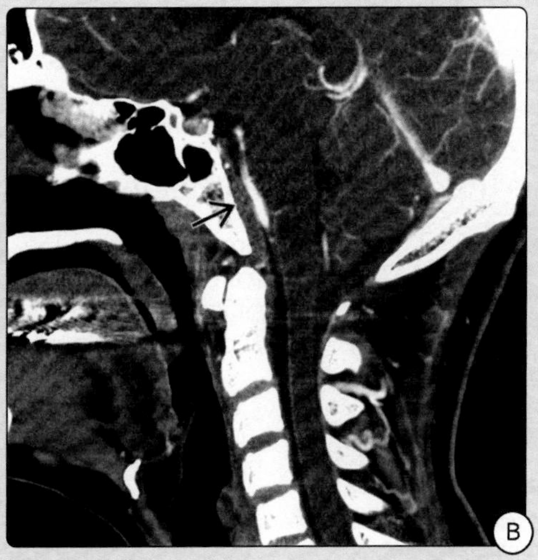

(2-27A) Axial CTA in a child with craniovertebral junction trauma shows a small clival EDH. There was no evidence for vascular injury. (2-27B) Sagittal CTA reformatted from the axial source date nicely demonstrates the clival epidural hematoma.

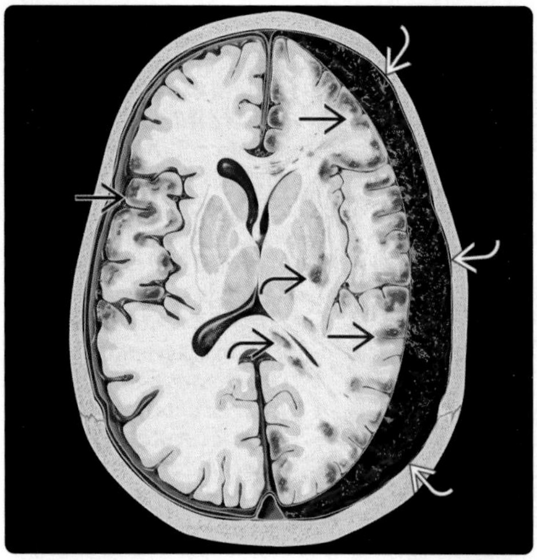

(2-28) Graphic depicts crescent-shaped acute SDH ➡ with contusions and "contre-coup" injuries ➡, diffuse axonal injuries ➡.

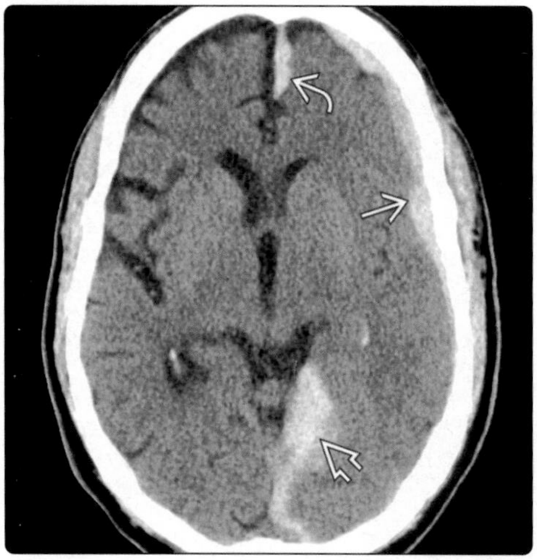

(2-29) Acute SDH spreads over left hemisphere ➡, along tentorium ➡, into interhemispheric fissure ➡ but does not cross midline.

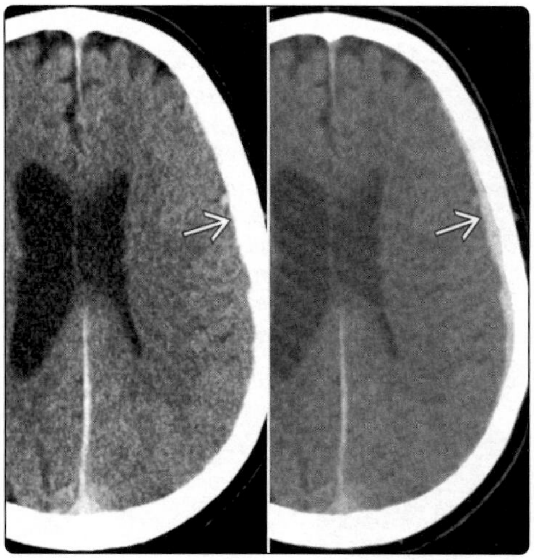

(2-30) NECT scan shows that small SDH ➡ is easier to see with wider (R) compared with standard (L) windows.

minor cranial nerve involvement, the clinical course is usually benign, and treatment with a cervical collar is typical.

NECT scans show a hyperdense collection between the clivus and tectorial membrane. Sagittal MR of the craniocervical junction shows the hematoma elevating the clival dura and extending inferiorly between the basisphenoid and tectorial membrane anterior to the medulla.

Acute Subdural Hematoma

Acute subdural hematomas (aSDHs) are one of the leading causes of death and disability in patients with severe traumatic brain injury. SDHs are much more common than EDHs. Most do not occur as isolated injuries; the vast majority of SDHs are associated with traumatic subarachnoid hemorrhage (tSAH) as well as significant parenchymal injuries such as cortical contusions, brain lacerations, and diffuse axonal injuries.

Terminology

An aSDH is a collection of acute blood products that lies in or between the inner border cell layer of the dura and the arachnoid **(2-28)**.

Etiology

Trauma is the most common cause of aSDH. Both direct blows to the head and nonimpact injuries may result in formation of an aSDH. Tearing of bridging cortical veins as they cross the subdural space to enter a dural venous sinus (usually the superior sagittal sinus) is the most common etiology. Cortical vein lacerations can occur with either a skull fracture or the sudden changes in velocity and brain rotation that occur during nonimpact closed head injury.

Blood from ruptured vessels spreads quickly through the potential space between the dura and the arachnoid. Large SDHs may spread over an entire hemisphere, extending into the interhemispheric fissure and along the tentorium.

Tearing of cortical arteries from a skull fracture may also give rise to an aSDH. The arachnoid itself may also tear, creating a pathway for leakage of CSF into the subdural space, resulting in admixture of both blood and CSF.

Less common causes of aSDH include aneurysm rupture, skull/dura-arachnoid metastases from vascular extracranial primary neoplasms, and spontaneous hemorrhage in patients with severe coagulopathy.

Rarely, an acute spontaneous SDH of arterial origin occurs in someone without any traumatic history or vascular anomaly. These patients usually have sudden serious disturbance of consciousness and have a poor outcome unless the aSDH is recognized and treated promptly.

Pathology

Gross Pathology. The gross appearance of an aSDH is that of a soft, purplish, "currant jelly" clot beneath a tense bulging dura. More than 95% are supratentorial. Most aSDHs spread diffusely over the affected hemisphere and are therefore typically crescent-shaped.

Clinical Issues

Epidemiology. An aSDH is the second most common extraaxial hematoma, exceeded only by tSAH. An aSDH is found in 10-20% of all patients with head injury and is observed in 30% of autopsied fatal injuries.

Demographics. An aSDH may occur at any age from infancy to the elderly. There is no sex predilection.

Presentation. Even relatively minor head trauma, especially in elderly patients who are often anticoagulated, may result in an aSDH. In such patients, a definite history of trauma may be lacking.

Clinical findings vary from none to loss of consciousness and coma. Most patients with aSDHs have low GCSs on admission. Delayed deterioration, especially in elderly anticoagulated patients, is common.

Natural History. An aSDH may remain stable, grow slowly, or rapidly increase in size, causing mass effect and secondary brain herniations. Prognosis varies with hematoma thickness, midline shift, and the presence of associated parenchymal injuries. An aSDH that is thicker than 2 centimeters correlates with poor outcome (35-90% mortality). An aSDH that occupies more than 10% of the total available intracranial volume is usually lethal.

Treatment Options. The majority of patients with small SDHs are initially treated conservatively with close clinical observation and follow-up imaging. Approximately 6-7% of these demonstrate an increase in SDH size over time and eventually require surgical intervention.

Patients with larger SDHs, a lesion located at the convexity, alcohol abuse, and repetitive falls are at the greatest risk for deterioration. Surveillance with follow-up CT scans is recommended until the SDH resolves or at least up to 5 weeks following the initial trauma.

Imaging

General Features. The classic finding of an aSDH is a supratentorial crescent-shaped extraaxial collection that displaces the gray-white matter interface medially. SDHs are typically more extensive than EDHs, easily spreading along the falx, tentorium, and around the anterior and middle fossa floors **(2-29)**. SDHs may cross suture lines but generally do not cross dural attachments. Bilateral SDHs occur in 15% of cases. "Contre-coup" injuries such as contusion of the contralateral hemisphere are common.

Both standard soft tissue and intermediate ("subdural") windows as well as bone algorithm reconstructions should be used in all trauma patients, as small, subtle aSDHs can be obscured by the density of the overlying calvaria **(2-30)**. Coronal and sagittal reformatted images using the axial source date are especially helpful in visualizing small ("smear") peritentorial and parafalcine aSDHs **(2-31)** **(2-32)**.

CT Findings

NECT. Approximately 60% of aSDHs are hyperdense on NECT scans **(2-29)**. Mixed-attenuation lesions are found in 40% of cases. Pockets of hypodensity within a larger hyperdense aSDH usually indicate rapid bleeding **(2-33)** **(2-34)**. "Dots" or "lines" of CSF trapped within compressed, displaced sulci are often seen underlying an aSDH.

Mass effect with an aSDH is common and expected. Subfalcine herniation should be proportionate to the size of the subdural collection. However, **if the difference between the midline shift and thickness of the hematoma is 3 mm or more, then mortality is very high.** This discrepancy occurs when underlying cerebral edema is triggered by the traumatic event. Early recognition and aggressive treatment for potentially catastrophic brain swelling are essential **(2-35)**.

In other cases, especially in patients with repeated head injury, severe brain swelling with unilateral hemisphere vascular engorgement occurs very

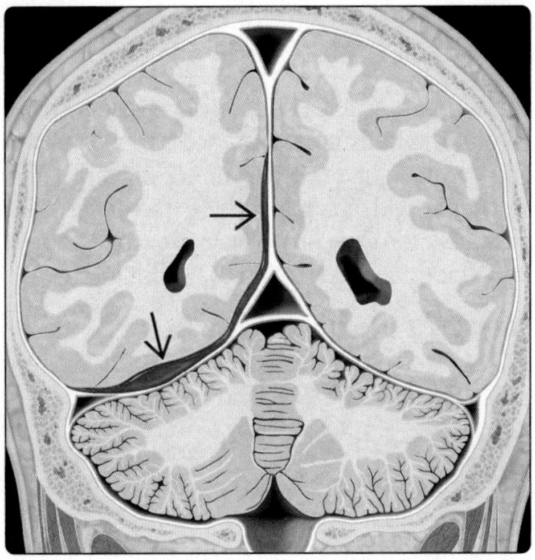

***(2-31)** Coronal graphic depicts thin aSDH layering along the tentorium and inferior falx cerebri* ⇨.

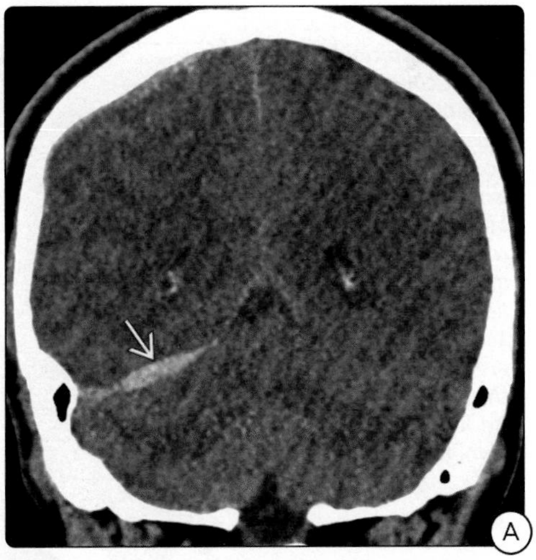

***(2-32A)** Reformatted coronal NECT scan using the axial source date shows a small right peritentorial aSDH* ➡.

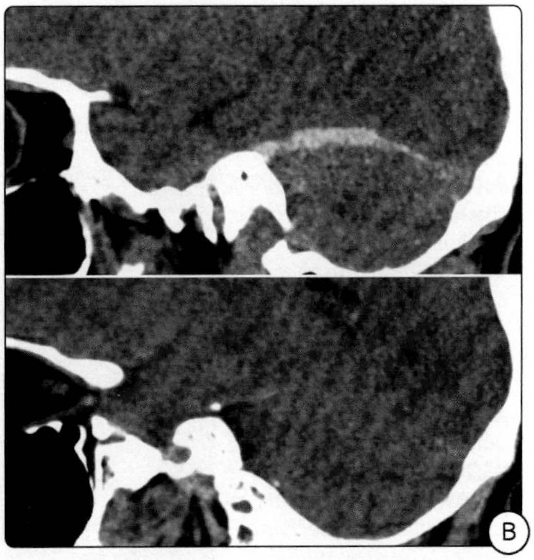

***(2-32B)** Sagittal scans in the same case show the right peritentorial aSDH (top) with normal left sagittal dura (bottom) for comparison.*

quickly. Here the mass effect is greatly disproportionate to the size of the SDH, which may be relatively small.

Occasionally, an aSDH is nearly isodense with the underlying cortex. This unusual appearance is found in extremely anemic patients (Hgb under 8-10 g/dL) **(2-36)** and sometimes occurs in patients with coagulopathy. In rare cases, CSF leakage through a torn arachnoid may mix with—and dilute—the acute blood that collects in the subdural space.

CECT. CECT scans are helpful in detecting small isodense aSDHs. The normally enhancing cortical veins are displaced inward by the extraaxial fluid collection.

Perfusion CT. CT or xenon perfusion scans may demonstrate decreased cerebral blood flow (CBF) and low perfusion pressure, which is one of the reasons for the high mortality rate of patients with aSDHs. The cortex underlying an evacuated aSDH may show hyperemic changes with elevated rCBF values. Persisting hyperemia has been associated with poor outcome.

MR Findings. MR scans are rarely obtained in acutely brain-injured patients. In such cases, aSDHs appear isointense on T1WI and hypointense on T2WI. Signal intensity on FLAIR scans is usually iso- to hyperintense compared with CSF but hypointense compared with the adjacent brain. aSDHs are hypointense on T2* scans.

DWI shows heterogeneous signal within the hematoma but may show patchy foci of restricted diffusion in the cortex underlying the aSDH.

Angiography. CTA may be useful in visualizing a cortical vessel that is actively bleeding into the subdural space.

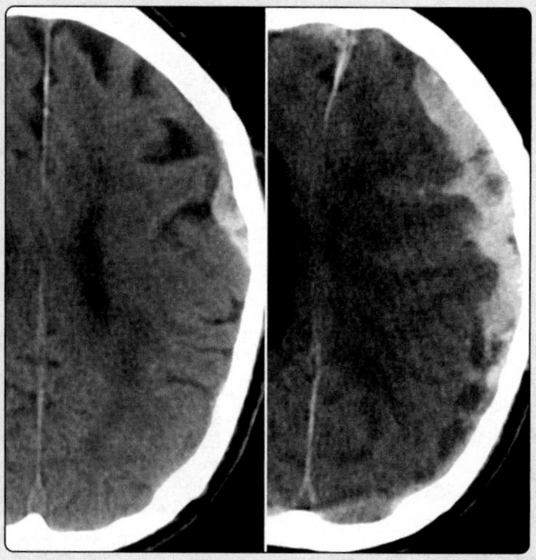

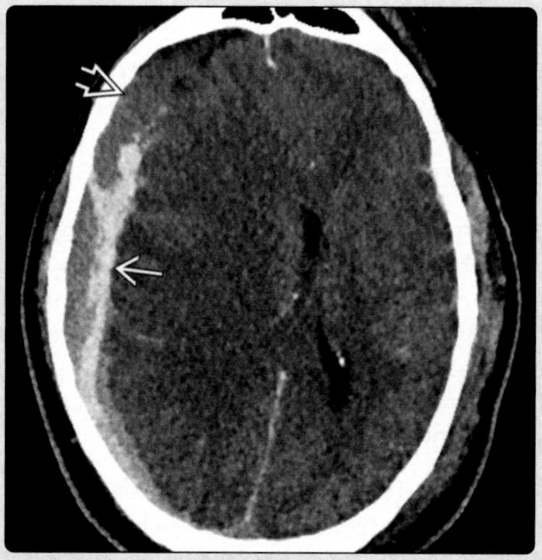

(2-33) (L) Initial NECT in an anticoagulated male patient shows a small mixed-density SDH. (R) Scan 6 hours later shows expanding, actively bleeding aSDH. (2-34) NECT scan shows a 55y man with an actively hemorrhaging aSDH. Some clotted blood is present ➡, but much of the hematoma consists of isodense unclotted hemorrhage ➡.

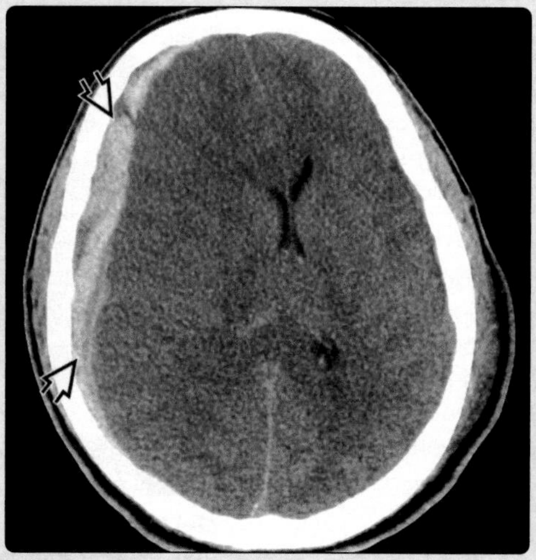

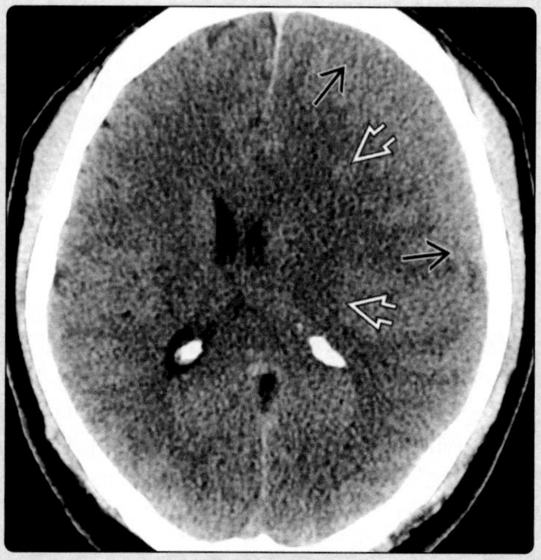

(2-35) NECT shows a mixed-density 12-mm aSDH ➡ with a disproportionately large subfalcine herniation of the lateral ventricles (17 mm), indicating that diffuse holohemispheric brain swelling is present. Subfalcine herniation ≥ 3 mm portends a poor prognosis. (2-36) NECT scan in a very anemic patient shows an isodense aSDH ➡. The aSDH is almost exactly the same density as the underlying cortex. The gray-white interface is displaced inward ➡.

Differential Diagnosis

In the setting of acute trauma, the major differential diagnosis is EDH. Shape is a helpful feature, as most aSDHs are crescentic, whereas EDHs are biconvex. EDHs are almost always associated with skull fracture; SDHs frequently occur in the absence of skull fracture. EDHs may cross sites of dural attachment; SDHs do not cross the falx or tentorium.

Subacute Subdural Hematoma

With time, subdural hematomas (SDHs) undergo organization, lysis, and neomembrane formation. Within 2-3 days, the initial soft, loosely organized clot of an acute SDH becomes organized. Breakdown of blood products and the formation of organizing granulation tissue change the imaging appearance of subacute and chronic SDHs.

Terminology

A subacute subdural hematoma (sSDH) is between several days and several weeks old.

Pathology

A collection of partially liquified clot with resorbing blood products is surrounded on both sides by a "membrane" of organizing granulation tissue **(2-37)**. The outermost membrane adheres to the dura and is typically thicker than the inner membrane, which abuts the thin, delicate arachnoid **(2-38)**.

In some cases, repetitive hemorrhages of different ages arising from the friable granulation tissue may be present. In others, liquefaction of the hematoma over time produces serous blood-tinged fluid.

Clinical Issues

Epidemiology and Demographics. SDHs are common findings at imaging and autopsy. In contrast to acute SDHs, sSDHs show a distinct bimodal distribution with children and the elderly as the most commonly affected age groups.

Presentation. Clinical symptoms vary from asymptomatic to loss of consciousness and hemiparesis caused by sudden rehemorrhage into an sSDH. Headache and seizure are other common presentations.

Natural History and Treatment Options. Many sSDHs resolve spontaneously. In some cases, repeated hemorrhages may cause sudden enlargement and mass effect. Surgical drainage may be indicated if the sSDH is enlarging or becomes symptomatic.

Imaging

General Features. Imaging findings are related to hematoma age and the presence of encasing membranes. Evolution of an untreated, uncomplicated SDH follows a very predictable pattern on CT. Density of an extraaxial hematoma decreases approximately 1-2 HU each day **(2-39)**. Therefore, an SDH will become nearly isodense with the underlying cerebral cortex within a few days following trauma.

CT Findings. sSDHs are typically crescent-shaped fluid collections that are iso- to slightly hypodense compared with the underlying cortex on NECT **(2-40)**. Medial displacement of the gray-white interface ("buckling") is often present, along with "dot-like" foci of CSF in the trapped, partially effaced sulci underlying the sSDH **(2-41)** **(2-42)**. Mixed-density hemorrhages are common.

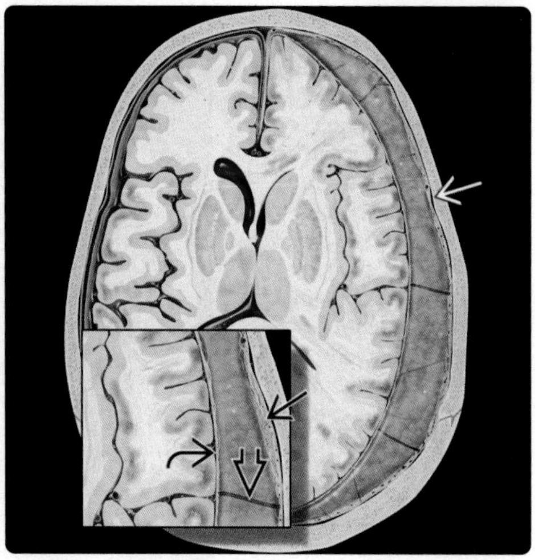

***(2-37)** Graphic depicts sSDH. Inset shows bridging vein and thin inner and thick outer membranes.*

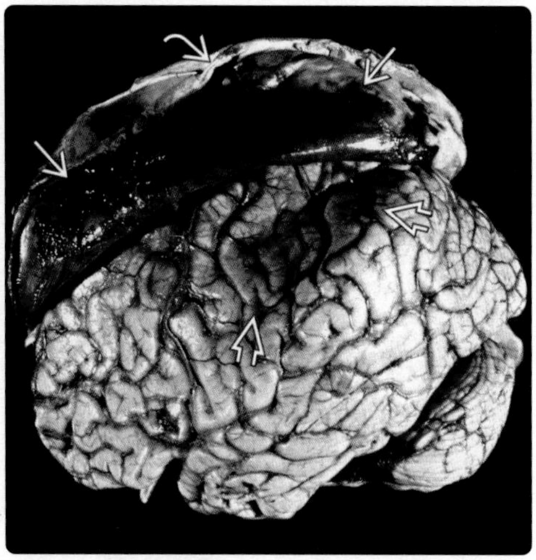

***(2-38)** Autopsy shows sSDH with organized hematoma, thick outer membrane, deformed brain. (Courtesy R. Hewlett, MD.)*

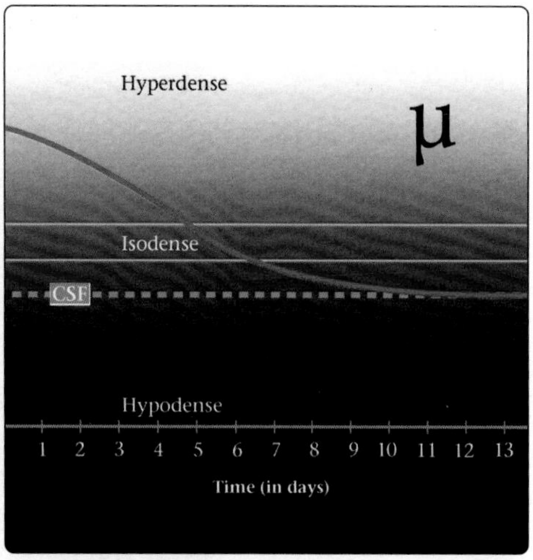

***(2-39)** SDHs decrease approximately 1.5 HU/day. By 7-10 days, blood in hematoma is isodense with cortex. By 10 days, it is hypodense.*

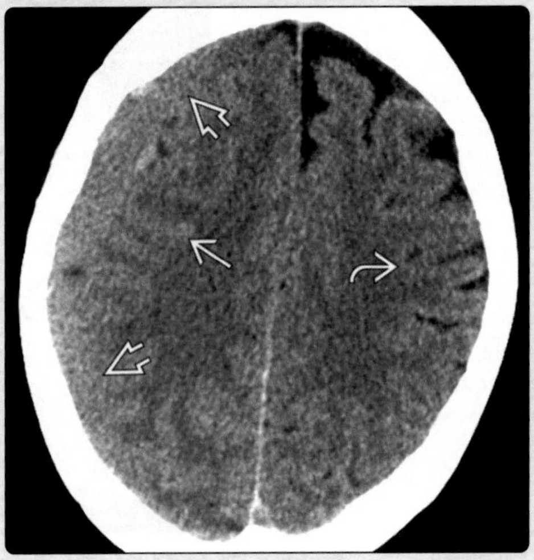

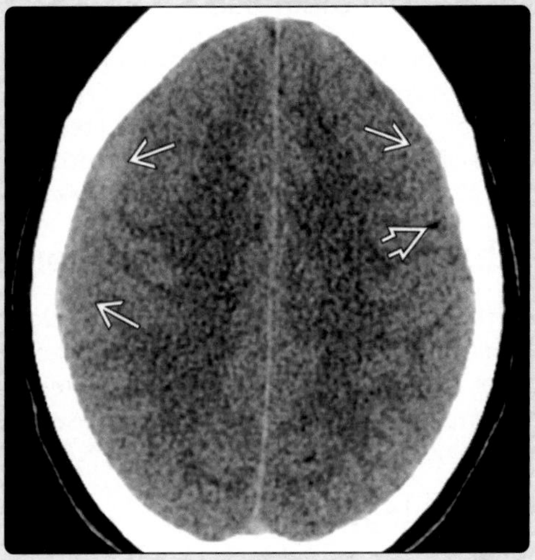

***(2-40)** Axial NECT scan shows right sSDH that is isodense with the underlying cortex. The right GM-WM interface is displaced and buckled medially compared with normal left side . **(2-41)** NECT scan in another patient shows bilateral "balanced" isodense subacute SDHs . Note that both GM-WM interfaces are inwardly displaced. A "dot" of CSF in the compressed subarachnoid space is seen under the left sSDH .*

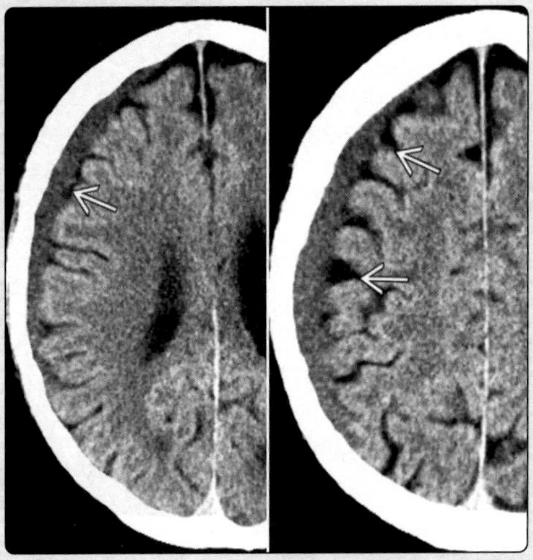

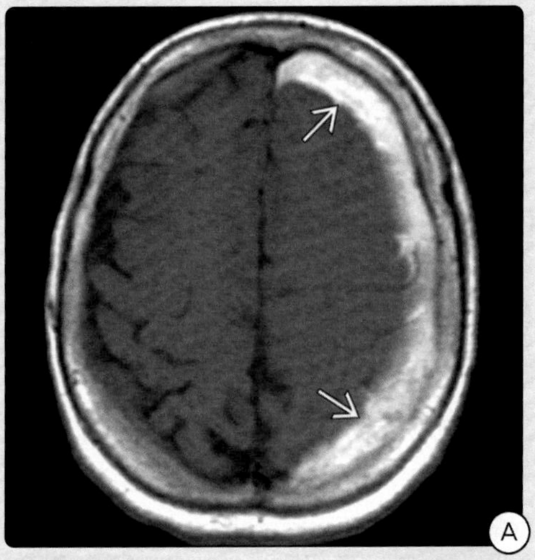

***(2-42)** NECT in elderly patient with sSDH, moderate cortical atrophy shows difference between nearly isodense SDH and CSF in underlying compressed subarachnoid space, sulci . **(2-43A)** Axial T1WI in patient with a late-stage aSDH shows crescent-shaped hyperintense collection extending over entire surface of left hemisphere, gyral compression with almost obliterated sulci compared with normal right hemisphere.*

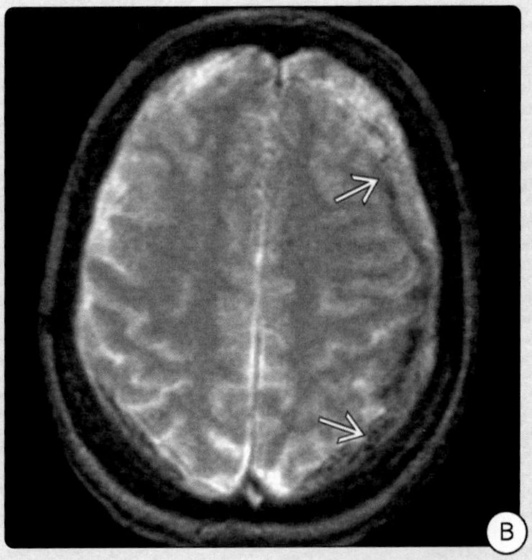

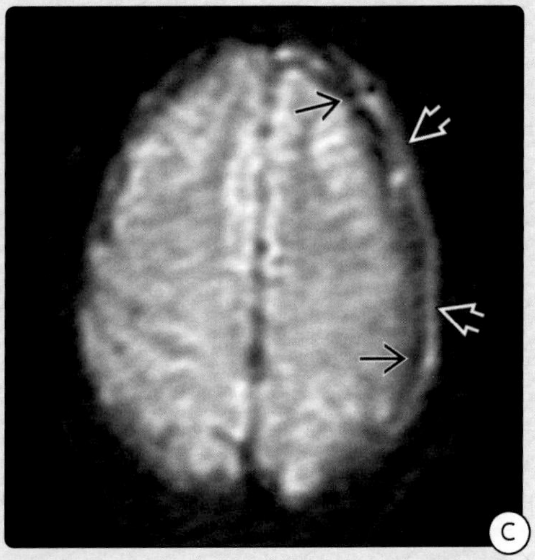

***(2-43B)** T2* GRE scan shows some "blooming" in the sSDH. **(2-43C)** DWI shows the classic "double layer" appearance of an sSDH with hypointense rim on the inside and mildly hyperintense rim on the outside of the clot.*

Bilateral sSDHs may be difficult to detect because of their "balanced" mass effect **(2-41)**. Sulcal effacement with displaced gray-white matter interfaces is the typical appearance.

CECT scans show that the enhanced cortical veins are displaced medially. The encasing membranes, especially the thicker superficial layer, may enhance.

MR Findings. MR can be very helpful in identifying sSDHs, especially small lesions that are virtually isodense with underlying brain on CT scans.

Signal intensity varies with hematoma age but is less predictable than on CT, making precise "aging" of subdural collections more problematic. In general, early subacute SDHs are isointense with cortex on T1WI and hypointense on T2WI but gradually become more hyperintense as extracellular methemoglobin increases **(2-43A)**. Most late-stage sSDHs are T1/T2 "bright-bright." A linear T2 hypointensity representing the encasing membranes that surround the SDH is sometimes present.

FLAIR is the most sensitive standard sequence for detecting sSDH, as the collection is typically hyperintense **(2-44)**. Because FLAIR signal intensity varies depending on the relative contribution of T1 and T2 effects, early sSDHs may initially appear hypointense due to their intrinsic T2 shortening.

T2* scans are also very sensitive, as sSDHs show distinct "blooming" **(2-43B)**.

Signal intensity on DWI also varies with hematoma age. DWI commonly shows a crescentic high-intensity area with a low-intensity rim closer to the brain surface ("double layer" appearance) **(2-43C)**. The low-intensity area corresponds to a mixture of resolved clot and CSF, whereas the high-intensity area correlates with solid clot.

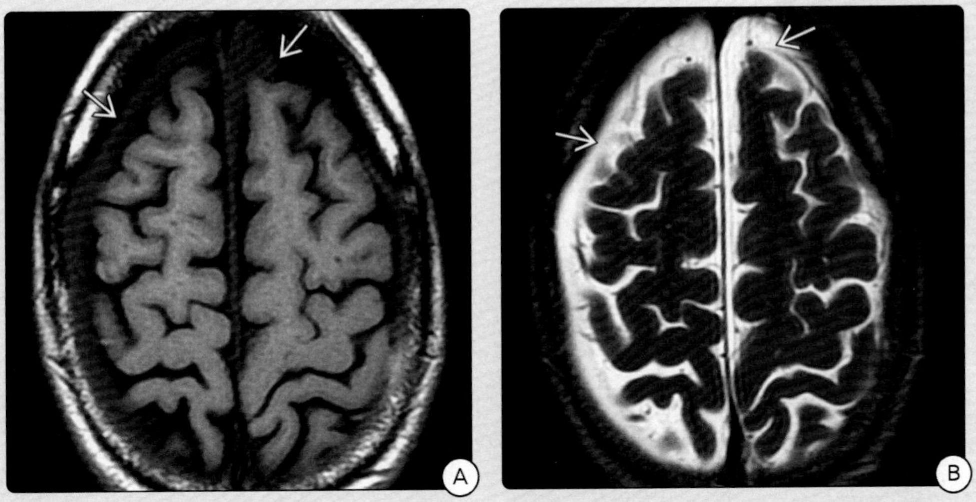

***(2-44A)** T1WI in a 59y man with seizures shows bilateral subdural collections ➡ that are slightly hyperintense to CSF. **(2-44B)** T2WI shows that both collections ➡ are isointense with CSF in the underlying subarachnoid cisterns.*

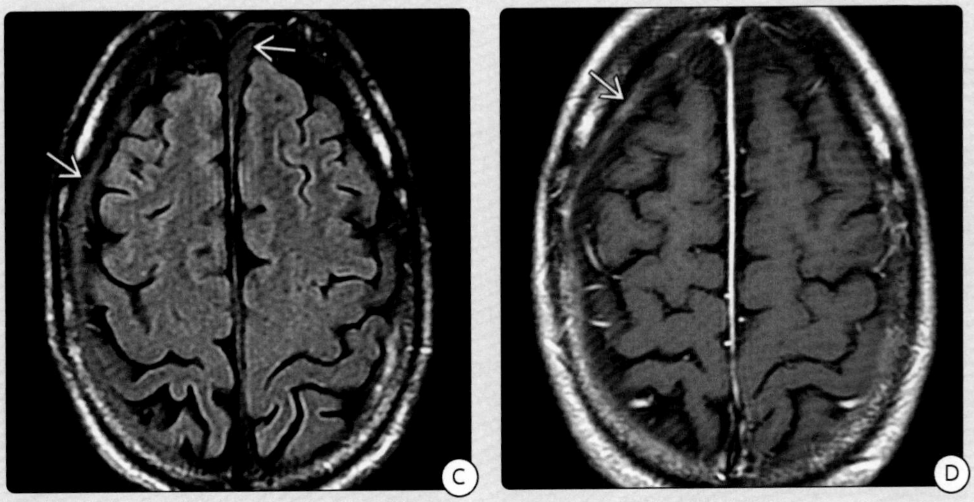

***(2-44C)** The fluid collections ➡ do not suppress on FLAIR and are hyperintense to CSF in the underlying cisterns. **(2-44D)** T1 C+ shows that the outer membrane of the SDH enhances ➡. Findings are consistent with late subacute/early chronic subdural hematomas.*

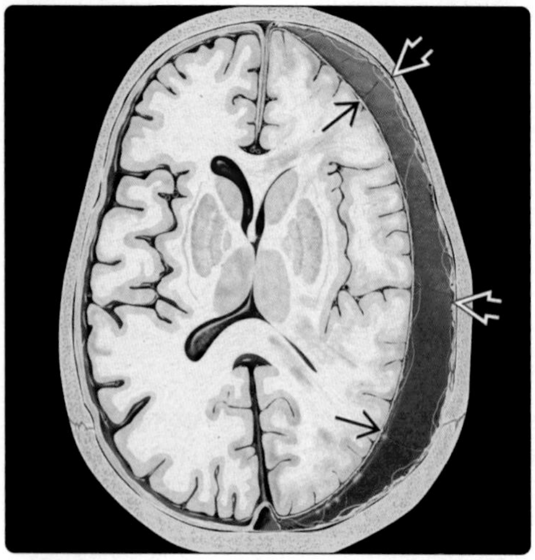

(2-45) Simple cSDHs contain serosanguineous fluid with hematocrit effect, thin inner ⇨, thick outer ➡ encapsulating membranes.

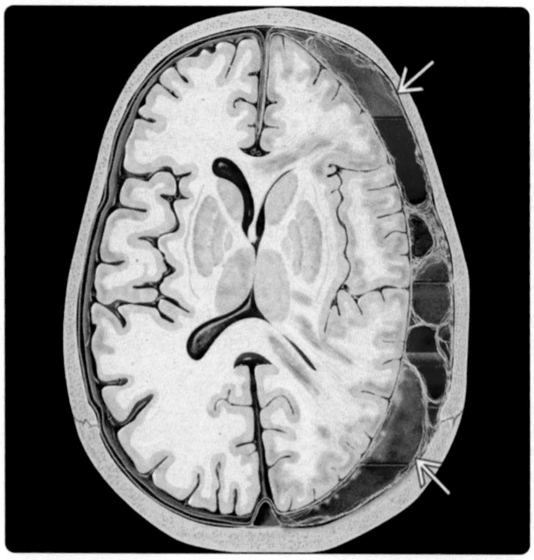

(2-46) Complicated cSDHs contain loculated pockets of old and new blood, seen as fluid-fluid levels ➡ within septated cavities.

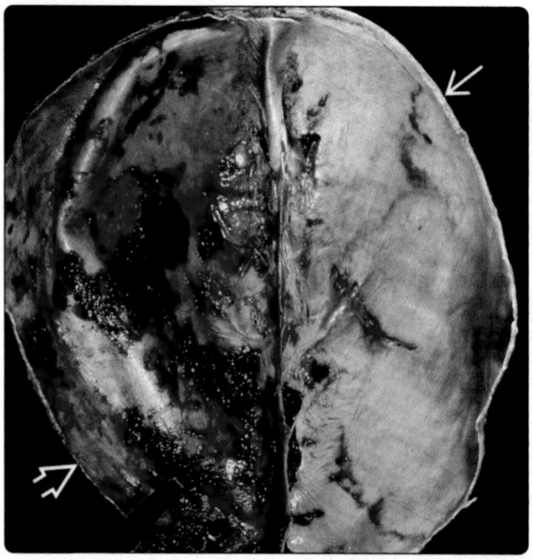

(2-47) cSDH autopsy has thickened dura 1 side ➡, mixed acute, subacute, chronic hemorrhages on other ➡. (From DP: Hospital Autopsy.)

T1 C+ scans demonstrate enhancing, thickened, encasing membranes **(2-44D)**. The membrane surrounding an sSDH is usually thicker on the dural side of the collection. Delayed scans may show gradual "filling in" and increasing hyperintensity of the sSDH.

Differential Diagnosis

The major differential diagnosis of an sSDH is an **isodense acute SDH**. These are typically seen only in an extremely anemic or anticoagulated patient. A **subdural effusion** that follows surgery or meningitis or that occurs as a component of intracranial hypotension can also mimic an sSDH. A **subdural hygroma** is typically isodense/isointense with CSF and does not demonstrate enhancing, encapsulating membranes.

Chronic/Mixed Subdural Hematoma

Terminology

A chronic subdural hematoma (cSDH) is an encapsulated collection of sanguineous or serosanguineous fluid confined within the subdural space. Recurrent hemorrhage(s) into a preexisting cSDH are common and produce a mixed-age or "acute on chronic" SDH (mSDH).

Etiology

With continued degradation of blood products, an SDH becomes progressively more liquified until it is largely serous fluid tinged with blood products **(2-45)**. Rehemorrhage, either from vascularized encapsulating membranes or rupture of stretched cortical veins crossing the expanded subdural space, occurs in 5-10% of cSDHs and is considered "acute-on-chronic" SDH **(2-46)**.

Pathology

Gross Pathology. Blood within the subdural space incites tissue reaction around its margins. Organization and resorption of the hematoma contained within the "membranes" of surrounding granulation tissue continue. These neomembranes have fragile, easily disrupted capillaries and easily rebleed, creating an mSDH. Multiple hemorrhages of different ages are common in mSDHs **(2-47)**.

Eventually, most of the liquified clot in a cSDH is resorbed. Only a thickened dura-arachnoid layer remains with a few scattered pockets of old blood trapped between the inner and outer membranes.

Clinical Issues

Epidemiology. Unoperated, uncomplicated subacute SDHs eventually evolve into cSDHs. Approximately 5-10% will rehemorrhage, causing multiloculated mixed-age SDHs.

Demographics. Chronic SDHs may occur at any age. Mixed-age SDHs are much more common in elderly patients.

Presentation. Presentation varies from no/mild symptoms (e.g., headache) to sudden neurologic deterioration if a preexisting cSDH rehemorrhages.

Natural History. In the absence of repeated hemorrhages, cSDHs gradually resorb and largely resolve, leaving a residue of thickened dura-arachnoid that may persist for months or even years. Older patients, especially those with brain atrophy, are subject to repeated hemorrhages.

Treatment Options. If follow-up imaging of a subacute SDH shows expected resorption and regression of the cSDH, no surgery may be required. Surgical drainage with evacuation of the cSDH and resection of its encapsulating membranes is performed if significant mass effect or repeated hemorrhages cause neurologic complications.

Imaging

General Features. cSDHs have a spectrum of imaging appearances. **Uncomplicated cSDHs** show relatively homogeneous density/signal intensity with slight gravity-dependent gradation of their contents ("hematocrit effect").

mSDHs with acute hemorrhage into a preexisting cSDH show a hematocrit level with distinct layering of the old (top) and new (bottom) hemorrhages. Sometimes, septated pockets that contain hemorrhages of different ages form. Dependent layering of blood within the loculated collections may appear quite bizarre.

Extremely old, **longstanding cSDHs** with virtually complete resorption of all liquid contents are seen as pachymeningopathies with diffuse dura-arachnoid thickening.

CT Findings

NECT. A hypodense crescentic fluid collection extending over the surface of one or both cerebral hemispheres is the classic finding in cSDH. Uncomplicated cSDHs approach CSF in density **(2-48)**. The hematocrit effect creates a slight gradation in density that increases from top to bottom.

Trabecular or loculated cSDHs show internal septations, often with evidence of repeated hemorrhages **(2-49)**. With age, the encapsulating membranes surrounding the cSDH become thickened and may appear moderately hyperdense. Eventually, some cSDHs show peripheral calcifications that persist for many years. In rare cases, a cSDH may densely calcify or even ossify, a condition aptly termed "armored brain" **(2-50)**.

CECT. The encapsulating membranes around a cSDH contain fragile neocapillaries that lack endothelial tight junctions. Therefore, the membranes show strong enhancement following contrast administration.

MR Findings. As with all intracranial hematomas, signal intensity of a cSDH or mSDH is quite variable and depends on age of the blood products. On T1 scans, uncomplicated cSDHs are typically iso- to slightly hyperintense compared with CSF **(2-51A)**. Depending on the stage of evolution, cSDHs are iso- to hypointense compared with CSF on T2 scans.

Most cSDHs are hyperintense on FLAIR **(2-51B)** and may show "blooming" on T2* scans if subacute-chronic blood clots are still present. In about one-quarter of all cases, superficial siderosis can be identified over the gyri underlying a cSDH.

The encapsulating membranes of a cSDH enhance following contrast administration. Typically, the outer layer is thicker than the inner layer **(2-51C) (2-51D) (2-52)**.

Uncomplicated cSDHs do not restrict on DWI. With cSDHs, a "double layer" effect—a crescent of hyperintensity medial to a nonrestricting fluid collection—indicates acute rehemorrhage.

Differential Diagnosis

An mSDH is difficult to mistake for anything else. In older patients, a small uncomplicated cSDH may be difficult to distinguish from simple **brain atrophy** with enlarged bifrontal CSF spaces. However, cSDHs exhibit mass effect; they flatten the underlying gyri, often extending around the entire

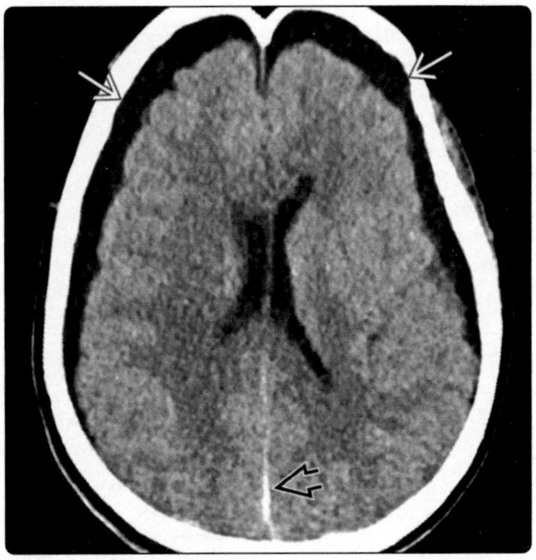

(2-48) NECT scan shows bilateral cSDHs ➡ causing mass effect on the underlying brain. A small left parafalcine aSDH is present ⇨.

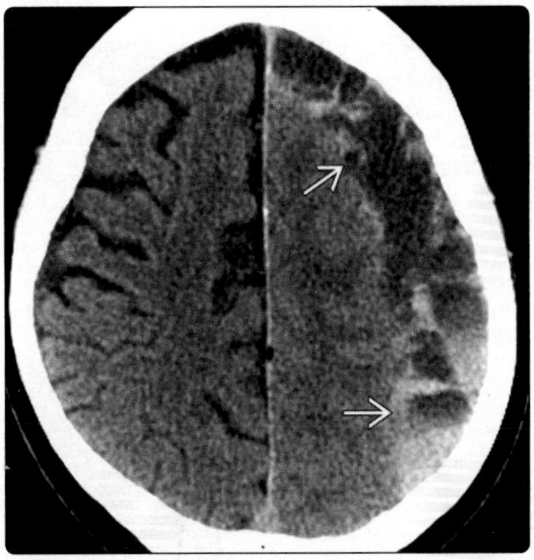

(2-49) NECT shows mixed cSDH ➡ that features multiple loculated pockets of blood with old blood layered on top of recent hemorrhages.

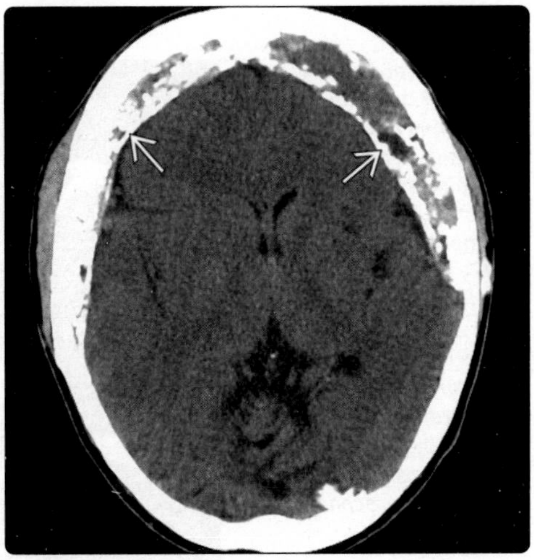

(2-50) NECT scan shows longstanding cSDHs, seen as densely calcified bifrontal subdural hematomas ➡, the "armored brain" appearance.

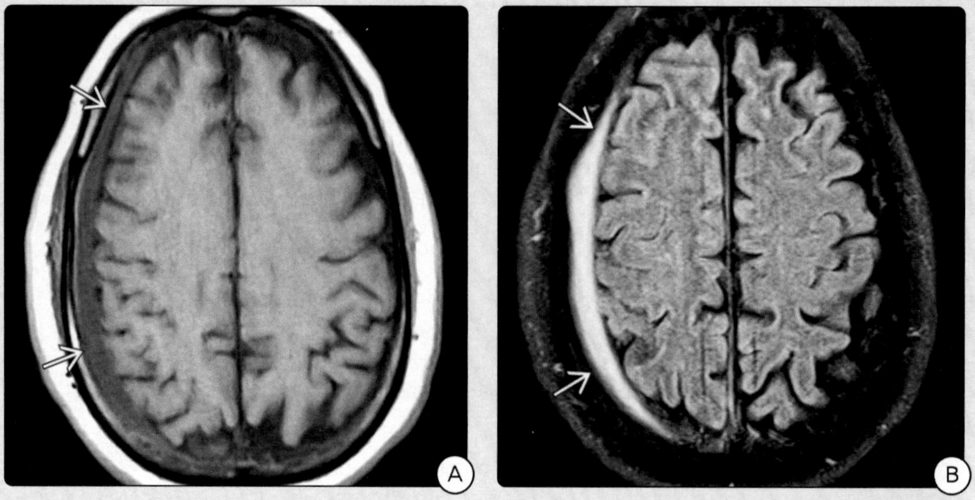

(2-51A) Axial T1WI shows a right-sided cSDH ➡. The collection is slightly hyperintense compared with CSF. (2-51B) Axial FLAIR in the same case shows that the cSDH ➡ is hyperintense relative to CSF.

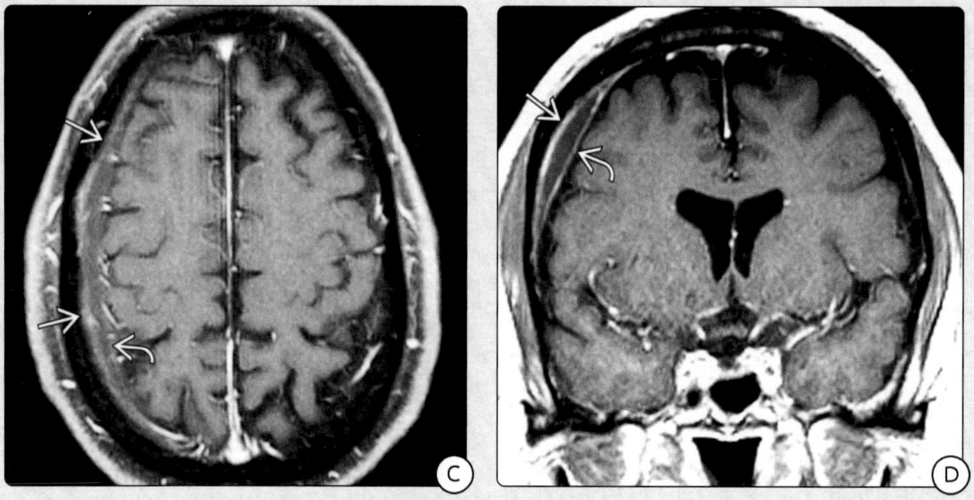

(2-51C) T1 C+ FS in the same case shows that the outer membrane is thick and enhances uniformly ➡. The inner membrane is thin, almost inapparent ↪. (2-51D) Coronal T1 C+ in the same case shows the thick outer ➡ and thin inner membrane of the cSDH ↪.

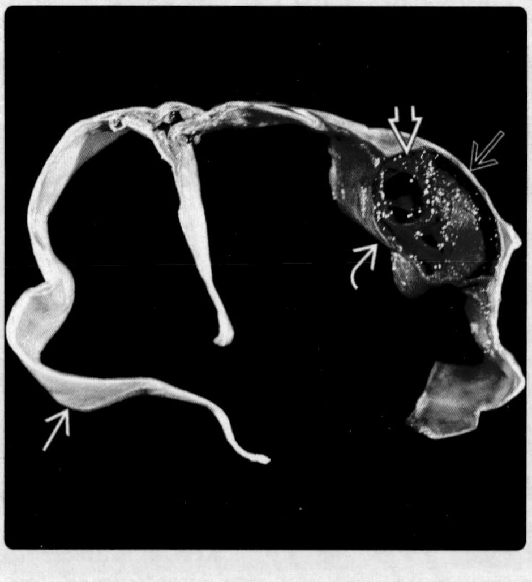

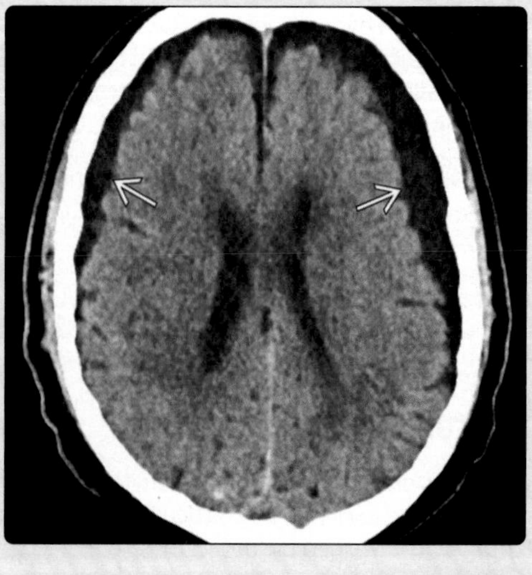

(2-52) Autopsy shows different aged cSDHs. Thickened dura-arachnoid ➡ residual clot ➡ is contained within a thin inner ↪, thick outer ⇨ membrane. (2-53) NECT in a 77y man with headaches 10 days following trauma shows bilateral hypodense collections ➡. These are measured CSF-like subdural hygromas, caused by CSF extravasating through a tear in the arachnoid.

hemisphere and into the interhemispheric fissure. The increased extraaxial spaces in patients with cerebral atrophy are predominantly frontal and temporal.

A traumatic **subdural hygroma** is an accumulation of CSF in the subdural space after head injury, probably secondary to an arachnoid tear. Subdural hygromas are sometimes detected within the first 24 hours after trauma; however, the mean time for appearance is 9 days after injury.

A classic uncomplicated subdural hygroma is a hypodense, CSF-like, crescentic extraaxial collection that consists purely of CSF, has no blood products, lacks encapsulating membranes, and shows no enhancement following contrast administration **(2-53)**. CSF leakage into the subdural space is also present in the vast majority of patients with cSDH. Therefore, many—if not most—cSDHs contain a mixture of *both* CSF and blood products.

A **subdural effusion** is an accumulation of clear fluid over the cerebral convexities or in the interhemispheric fissure. Subdural effusions are generally complications of meningitis; a history of prior infection, not trauma, is typical.

A **subdural empyema** (SDE) is a hypodense extraaxial fluid collection that contains pus. Most SDEs are secondary to sinusitis or mastoiditis, have strongly enhancing membranes, and often coexist with findings of meningitis. A typical SDE restricts strongly and uniformly on DWI.

Traumatic Subarachnoid Hemorrhage

Traumatic subarachnoid hemorrhage (tSAH) is found in virtually all cases of moderate to severe head trauma. Indeed, trauma—*not* ruptured saccular aneurysm—is the most common cause of intracranial SAH.

Etiology

tSAH can occur with both direct trauma to the skull and nonimpact closed head injury. Tearing of cortical arteries and veins, rupture of contusions and lacerations into the contiguous subarachnoid space, and choroid plexus bleeds with intraventricular hemorrhage may all result in blood collecting within the subarachnoid cisterns. Less commonly, tSAH arises from major vessel lacerations or dissections, with or without basilar skull fractures.

Although tSAH occasionally occurs in isolation, it is usually accompanied by other manifestations of brain injury. Subtle tSAH *may be the only clue* on initial imaging studies that *more serious injuries lurk beneath the surface.*

Pathology

Location. tSAHs are predominantly found in the perisylvian regions, in the anteroinferior frontal and temporal sulci, and over the hemispheric convexities **(2-54)**. In very severe cases, tSAH spreads over most of the brain. In mild cases, blood collects in a single sulcus or the dependent portion of the interpeduncular fossa. Rarely, Terson syndrome (intraocular hemorrhage) is associated with tSAH.

Gross Pathology. With the exception of location and associated parenchymal injuries, the gross appearance of tSAH is similar to that of aneurysmal SAH (aSAH). Curvilinear foci of bright red blood collect in cisterns and surface sulci **(2-55)**.

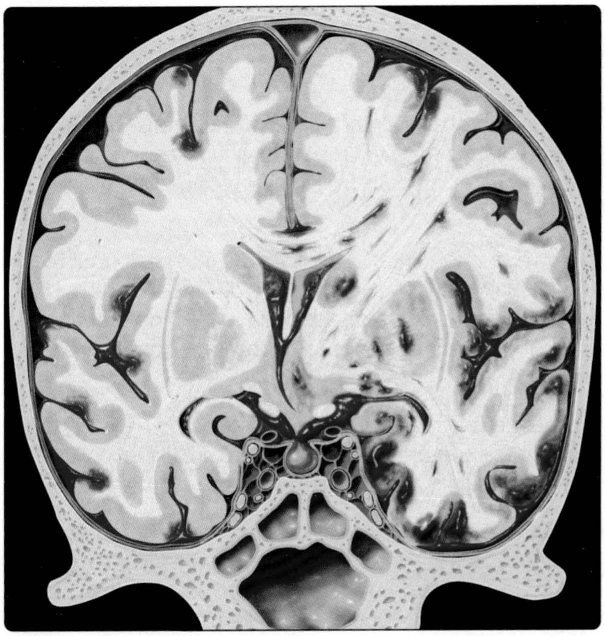

***(2-54)** Graphic depicts traumatic subarachnoid hemorrhage (tSAH). tSAH is most common around the sylvian fissures and in the sulci adjacent to contused gyri.*

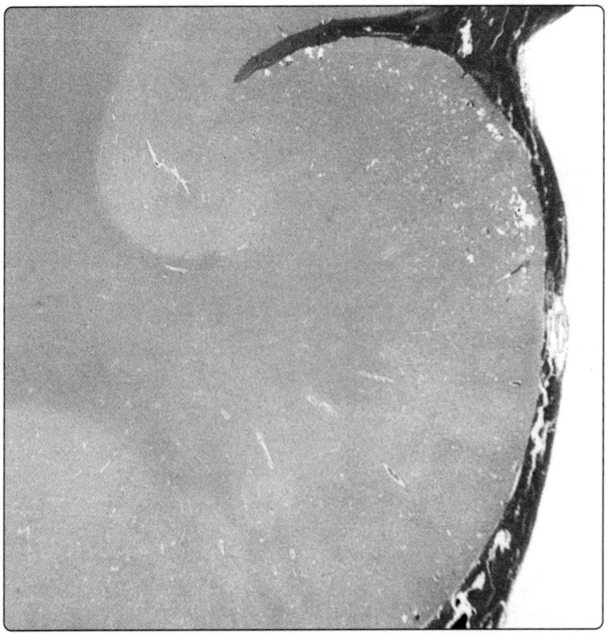

***(2-55)** Low-power photomicrograph shows an autopsied brain of a boxer who collapsed and expired after being knocked unconscious. Typical tSAH covers the gyri and extends into the sulci. (Courtesy J. Paltan, MD.)*

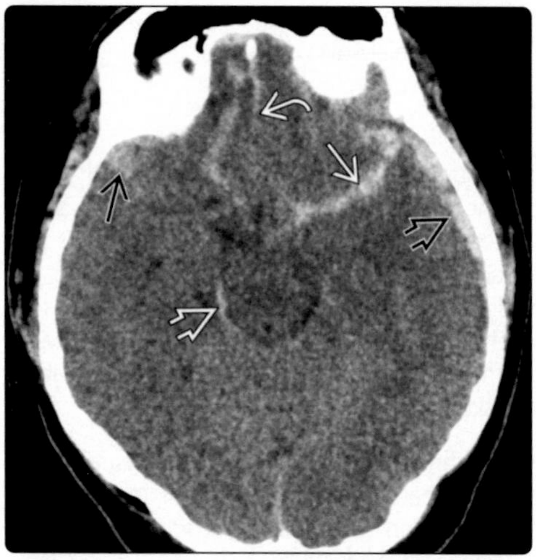

(2-56) NECT shows sylvian fissure ➡, inferior frontal ➡, perimesencephalic ➡ tSAH, contusions ➡, and small left aSDH ➡.

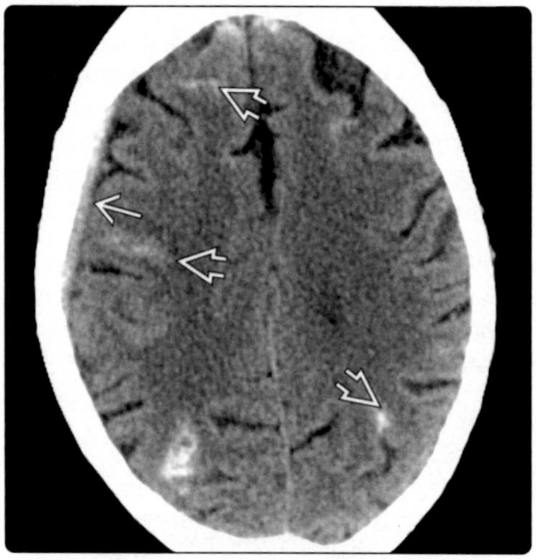

(2-57) NECT shows a small right SDH ➡ and multiple scattered foci of tSAH ➡ in the sulci over the convexities.

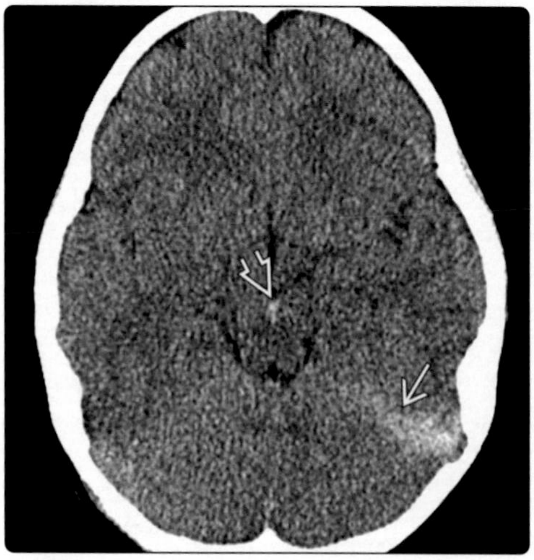

(2-58) Axial NECT shows a small peritentorial aSDH ➡ and a small amount of subarachnoid blood in the interpeduncular cistern ➡.

tSAH typically occurs adjacent to cortical contusions. tSAH is also commonly identified under acute epidural and subdural hematomas.

Clinical Issues

Epidemiology. tSAH is found in most cases of moderate trauma and is identified in virtually 100% of fatal brain injuries at autopsy.

Demographics. The prevalence of tSAH generally follows that of other traumatic brain injuries, i.e., it is bimodal and most commonly occurs in young adults (especially male patients) and the elderly.

Presentation. Clinical symptoms are primarily related to other traumatic injuries such as extraaxial hematoma, contusions, and axonal injury. In some cases, tSAH may cause delayed vasospasm and secondary ischemic symptoms.

Natural History. Breakdown and resorption of tSAH occurs gradually. Outcome is generally dictated by other injuries. Patients with isolated tSAH have very low rates of clinical or radiographic deterioration and typically do well.

Treatment Options. Supportive therapy is the primary treatment. In some cases, infusion of nimodipine or other calcium channel blockers such as verapamil may prevent vasospasm and its attendant complications.

Imaging

General Features. With the exception of location, the general imaging appearance of tSAH is similar to that of aSAH, i.e., sulcal-cisternal hyperdensity/hyperintensity **(2-56)**. tSAH is typically more focal or patchy than the diffuse subarachnoid blood indicative of aneurysmal hemorrhage **(2-57)**.

CT Findings. Acute tSAH is typically peripheral, appearing as linear hyperdensities in sulci adjacent to cortical contusions or under epi- or subdural hematomas. Occasionally, isolated tSAH is identified within the interpeduncular fossa **(2-58)**. Posttraumatic interpeduncular or ambient cistern hemorrhage is a good marker for possible brainstem lesions in patients with otherwise unexplained coma and may warrant further investigation.

Some cases of mild tSAH may have hemorrhage in a single convexity sulcus. In severe cases, tSAH spreads diffusely in the subarachnoid cisterns and layers over the tentorium. Chronic tSAH may appear as hypodense fluid that expands the affected sulci.

MR Findings. As acute blood is isointense with brain, it may be difficult to detect on T1WI. "Dirty" sulci with "smudging" of the perisylvian cisterns is typical. Subarachnoid blood is hyperintense to brain on T2WI and appears similar in signal intensity to cisternal CSF. FLAIR scans show hyperintensity in the affected sulci **(2-59)**.

"Blooming" with hypointensity can be identified on T2* scans, typically adjacent to areas of cortical contusion. tSAH is recognized on GRE or SWI sequences as hypointense signal intensity surrounded by hyperintense CSF.

tSAH also exhibits a unique morphology. Compared with smooth linear veins, SAH has a triangle shape with rough irregular boundaries and inhomogeneous signal intensity. Chronic tSAH causes focal superficial siderosis that appears as curvilinear hypointensity along gyral crests and sulci. DWI in tSAH may show foci of restricted diffusion in areas of frank ischemia or trauma-induced cytotoxic edema.

Angiography. Emergent CTA is usually unnecessary in cases with typical peripheral tSAH on NECT. Patients with suprasellar ("central") SAH may harbor a ruptured aneurysm and should be screened with CTA regardless of mechanism of injury.

DSA is rarely performed in acute brain trauma unless vascular injury such as dissection or pseudoaneurysm is suspected.

Differential Diagnosis

The major differential diagnosis of tSAH is **nontraumatic SAH** (ntSAH). Aneurysmal rupture causes 80-90% of all ntSAHs. In contrast to tSAH, aSAH is concentrated in the basal cisterns. CTA can identify a saccular aneurysm in most cases with aSAH.

Arteriovenous malformations account for 10-15% of ntSAHs and are easily identified on both CT and MR. Dissections and dissecting aneurysms, especially of the vertebrobasilar system, are less common but important causes of ntSAH.

SUBDURAL AND SUBARACHNOID HEMORRHAGE

Acute SDH (aSDH)
- Second most common traumatic extraaxial hemorrhage
  - Acute SDH > > epidural hematoma
- Crescentic collection of blood between dura, arachnoid
  - Supratentorial (95%), bilateral (15%)
  - SDHs cross sutures
  - SDHs do not cross dural attachments
- CT
  - Hyperdense (60%)
  - Mixed (40%)
  - Isodense acute SDH rare (anemia, coagulopathy, CSF mixture)

Subacute SDH (sSDH)
- Clot organizes, lyses, forms "neomembranes"
- CT
  - Density decreases 1-2 HU/day
  - Isodense with cortex in 7-10 days
  - Look for displaced "dots" of CSF under SDH
  - Gray-white interface "buckled" inward
  - Displaced cortical veins seen on CECT
- MR
  - Signal varies with clot age
  - T2* (GRE, SWI) shows "blooming"
  - T1 C+ shows clot inside enhancing membranes

Chronic/Mixed SDH (cSDH/mSDH)
- Serosanguineous fluid
  - Hypodense on NECT
  - Rehemorrhage (5-10%)
  - Loculated blood "pockets" with fluid-fluid levels common
- Differential diagnosis of uncomplicated cSDH
  - Subdural *hygroma* (arachnoid tear → subdural CSF)
  - Subdural *effusion* (clear fluid accumulates after meningitis)
  - Subdural *empyema* (pus)

Traumatic Subarachnoid Hemorrhage (tSAH)
- Most common traumatic extraaxial hemorrhage
- tSAH > > aneurysmal SAH
- Adjacent to cortical contusions
- Superficial sulci > basilar cisterns

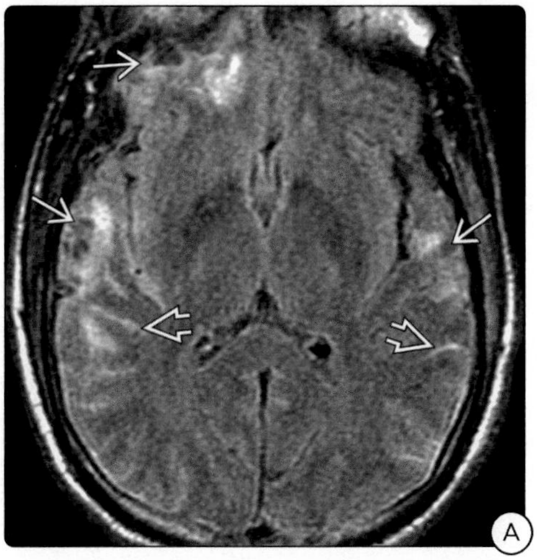

***(2-59A)** Axial FLAIR shows multifocal cortical contusions ➡ with traumatic SAH, seen as sulcal hyperintensities adjacent to the lesions ⇨.*

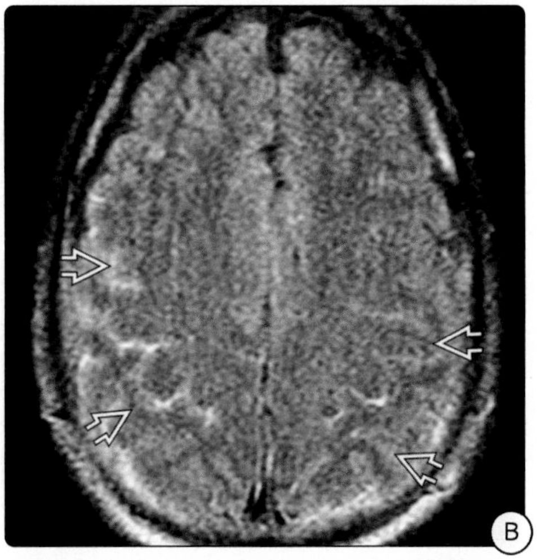

***(2-59B)** Artifactual sulcal hyperintensity ⇨ caused by incomplete water suppression is shown on FLAIR. Repeat scan (not shown) was normal.*

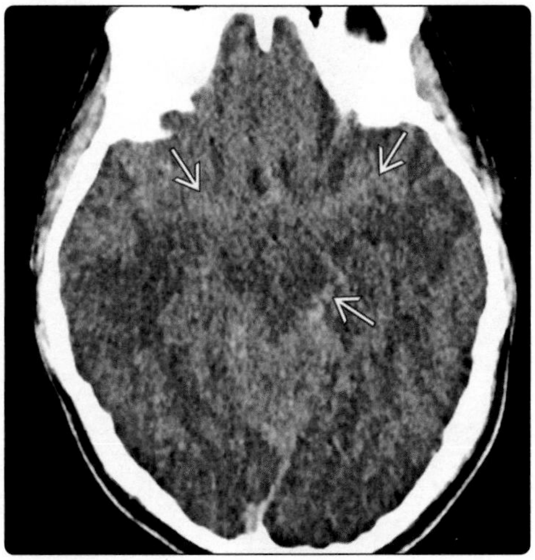

***(2-60)** Pseudosubarachnoid hemorrhage was caused by swollen low-density brain adjacent to normal blood vessels ➡.*

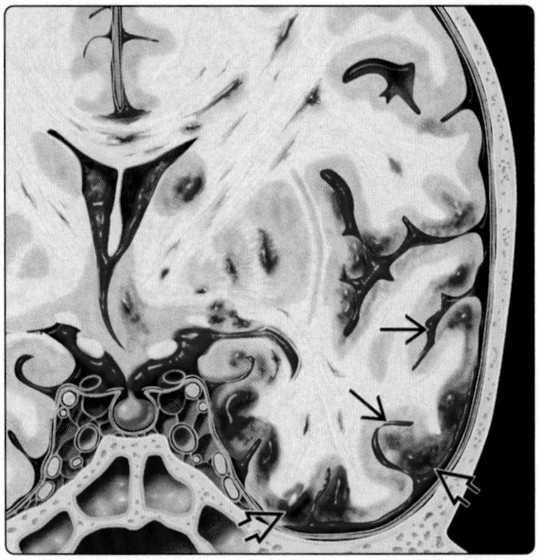

***(2-61)** Cortical contusions are located primarily along gyral crests ⇒, around a sylvian fissure. tSAH is common in adjacent sulci ⇒.*

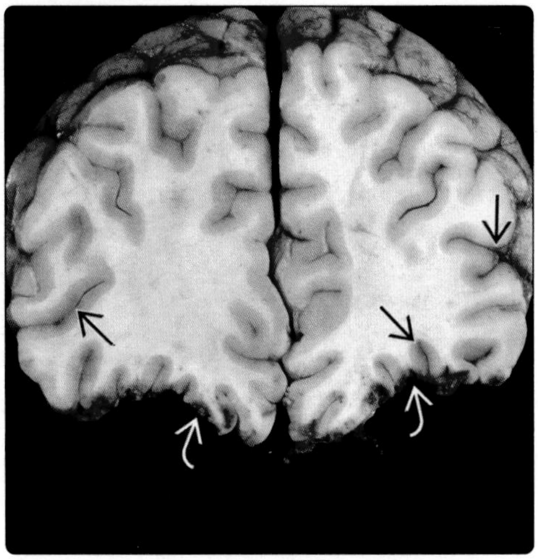

***(2-62)** Autopsied head trauma case shows bilateral inferofrontal cortical contusions ⇒, traumatic SAH ⇒. (From DP: Hospital Autopsy.)*

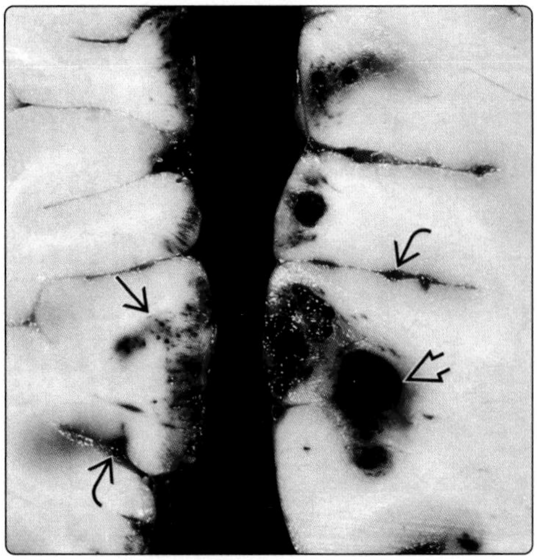

***(2-63)** Autopsy shows petechial ⇒ and larger confluent cortical contusions ⇒, tSAH in adjacent sulci ⇒. (Courtesy R. Hewlett, MD.)*

Sulcal-cisternal hyperintensity on FLAIR is nonspecific and can be caused by **meningitis, neoplasm, artifact** (incomplete CSF suppression), **contrast** leakage into the subarachnoid space (e.g., with renal failure), and **high inspired oxygen** during general anesthesia **(2-59B)**.

The term **pseudosubarachnoid hemorrhage** has been used to describe the CT appearance of a brain with severe cerebral edema. Hypodense brain makes circulating blood in arteries and veins look relatively hyperdense **(2-60)**. The hyperdensity seen here is smooth and conforms to the expected shape of the vessels, not the subarachnoid spaces, and should not be mistaken for either tSAH or ntSAH.

Parenchymal Injuries

Intraaxial traumatic injuries include cortical contusions and lacerations, diffuse axonal injury (DAI), subcortical injuries, and intraventricular hemorrhages. In this section, we again begin with the most peripheral injuries—cortical contusions—and work our way inward, ending with the deepest (subcortical) injuries. *In general, the deeper the abnormalities, the more serious the injury.*

Cerebral Contusions and Lacerations

Cerebral contusions are the most common of the intraaxial injuries. True brain lacerations are rare and typically occur only with severe (often fatal) head injury.

Terminology

Cerebral contusions are basically "brain bruises." They evolve with time and often are more apparent on delayed scans than at the time of initial imaging. Cerebral contusions are also called gyral "crest" injuries **(2-61)**. The term "gliding" contusion is sometimes used to describe parasagittal contusions.

Etiology

Most cerebral contusions result from nonmissile or blunt head injury. Closed head injury induces abrupt changes in angular momentum and deceleration. The brain is suddenly and forcibly impacted against an osseous ridge or the hard, knife-like edge of the falx cerebri and tentorium cerebelli. Less commonly, a depressed skull fracture directly damages the underlying brain.

Pathology

Location. Contusions are injuries of the brain surface that involve the gray matter and contiguous subcortical white matter **(2-61) (2-62) (2-63)**. They occur in very characteristic, highly predictable locations. Nearly half involve the temporal lobes. The temporal tips, as well as the lateral and inferior surfaces and the perisylvian gyri, are most commonly affected **(2-64)**. The inferior (orbital) surfaces of the frontal lobes are also frequently affected **(2-65)**.

Convexity gyri, the dorsal corpus callosum body, dorsolateral midbrain, and cerebellum are less common sites of cerebral contusions. The occipital poles are rarely involved, even with relatively severe closed head injury.

Size and Number. Cerebral contusions vary in size from tiny lesions to large confluent hematomas. They are almost always multiple and often bilateral **(2-66)**. Contusions that occur at 180° opposite the site of direct impact (the "coup") are common and are called "contre-coup" lesions.

Gross Pathology. Contusions range in appearance from small petechial to large confluent hemorrhages. Cortical contusions are usually associated with traumatic subarachnoid hemorrhage (tSAH) in the adjacent sulci **(2-63)**.

Microscopic Features. Perivascular microhemorrhages rapidly form and coalesce over time into more confluent hematomas. Edema surrounding the hemorrhages develops. Activation and proliferation of astrocytes together with macrophage infiltration ensue.

Necrosis with neuronal loss and astrogliosis as well as hemosiderin-laden macrophages are present in subacute and chronic lesions.

Clinical Issues

Epidemiology and Demographics. Cerebral contusions account for approximately half of all traumatic parenchymal lesions. They occur at all ages, from infants to the elderly. The peak age is from 15-24 years, and the M:F ratio is 3:1.

Presentation. Initial symptoms vary from none to confusion, seizure, or obtundation. Compared with diffuse axonal injuries (see below), cerebral contusions are less frequently associated with immediate loss of consciousness unless they are extensive or occur with other traumatic brain lesions (e.g., brainstem trauma or axonal injury).

Natural History. Neurologic deterioration is more common in older patients. Patients with large contusions, initial low Glasgow Coma Scores (GCS), coagulopathy, and presence of a coexisting subdural hematoma are prone to clinical deterioration. Those with small contusions, good initial GCS, and absence of clinical deterioration in the first 48 hours are unlikely to require surgery.

Hematoma expansion requiring surgical intervention occurs in approximately 20% of conservatively managed patients. Patients with unexplained clinical deterioration should have repeat imaging.

Treatment Options. Treatment options vary from observation with repeat imaging if the patient deteriorates to surgical evacuation of large focal hematomas. Craniectomy is performed in patients with severe brain swelling to prevent fatal brain herniation. Novel treatments such as Factor VII administration may prevent progressive hemorrhaging of brain contusions by protecting the microvessel endothelial cells.

Imaging

General Features. With time, cortical contusions become more apparent on imaging studies. Radiologic progression is the rule, not the exception. Nearly half of all patients show an increase in lesion size and number over the first 24-48 hours. In the absence of clinical deterioration, however, the relevance of documenting this progression is debatable.

CT Findings. Initial scans obtained soon after a closed head injury may be normal. The most frequent abnormality is the presence of petechial hemorrhages along gyral crests immediately adjacent to the calvaria. A mixture of petechial hemorrhages surrounded by patchy ill-defined hypodense areas of edema is common **(2-66)** **(2-67)**.

Lesion "blooming" over time is frequent and is seen with progressive increase in hemorrhage, edema, and mass effect **(2-68)**. Small lesions may coalesce, forming larger focal hematomas. Development of new lesions that were not present on initial imaging is also common.

MR Findings. MR is much more sensitive than CT in detecting cerebral contusions but is rarely obtained in the acute stage of traumatic brain injury

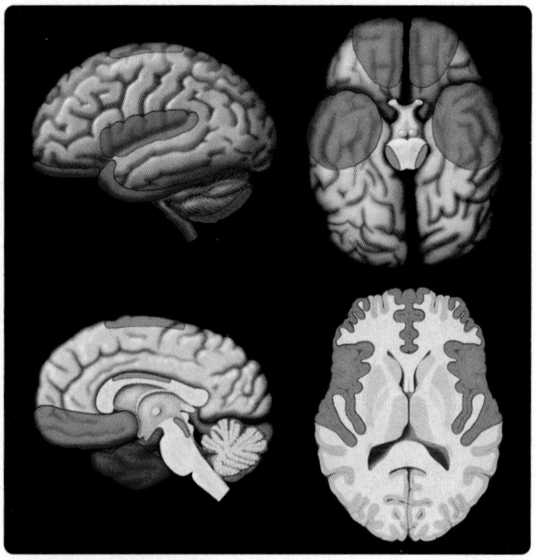

***(2-64)** Graphics depict the most common sites of cerebral contusions in red. Less common sites are shown in green.*

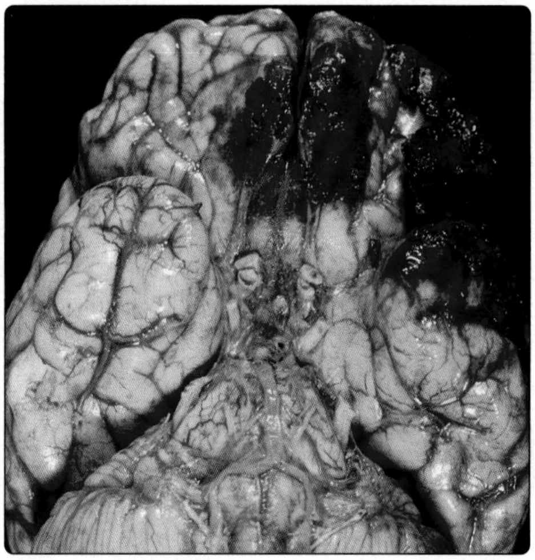

***(2-65)** Autopsied brain shows typical locations of contusions, i.e., the anteroinferior frontal and temporal lobes. (Courtesy R. Hewlett, MD.)*

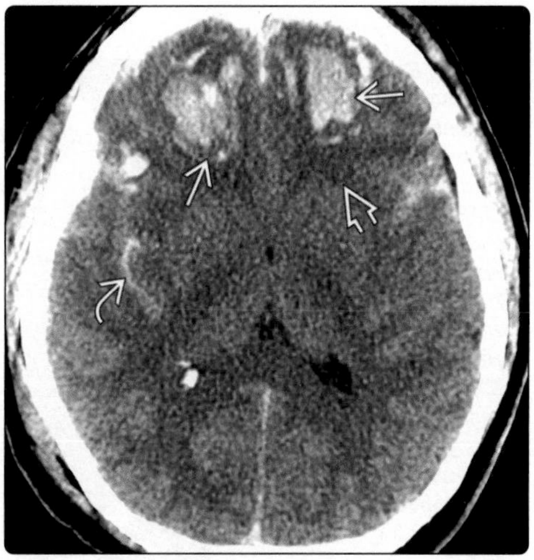

***(2-66)** NECT scan shows bilateral inferior frontal confluent contusions ➡, perilesional edema ➡, and traumatic SAH ➡.*

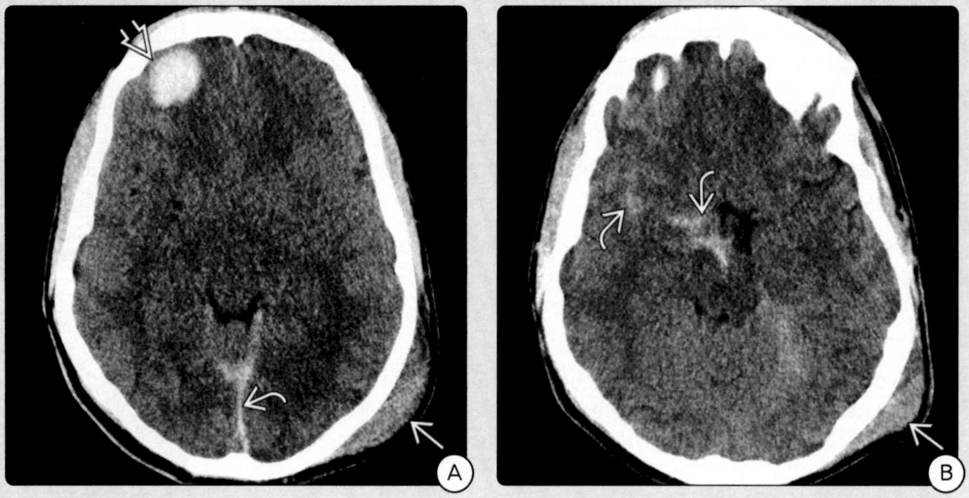

(2-67A) *Contusions are a common "countre-coup" injury. In this case, the initial trauma was to the left parieto-occipital region at the site of the scalp hematoma. A large right frontal contusion is seen directly opposite the impact site. Note small peritentorial aSDH.* ***(2-67B)*** *Lower scan in the same case shows the scalp hematoma and traumatic SAH, also opposite the impact site.*

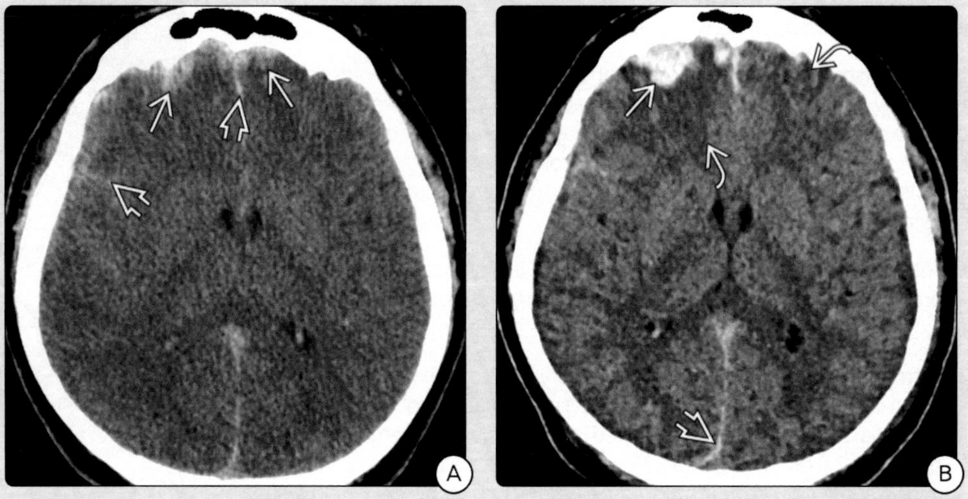

(2-68A) *Series of NECT scans demonstrates expected interval evolution of cortical contusions. Admission imaging shows bilateral inferior frontal contusions, some tSAH.* ***(2-68B)*** *Follow-up NECT 6 hours later shows that the contusions have enlarged and bifrontal hypodensities around the contusions have become apparent. Note small peritentorial aSDH.*

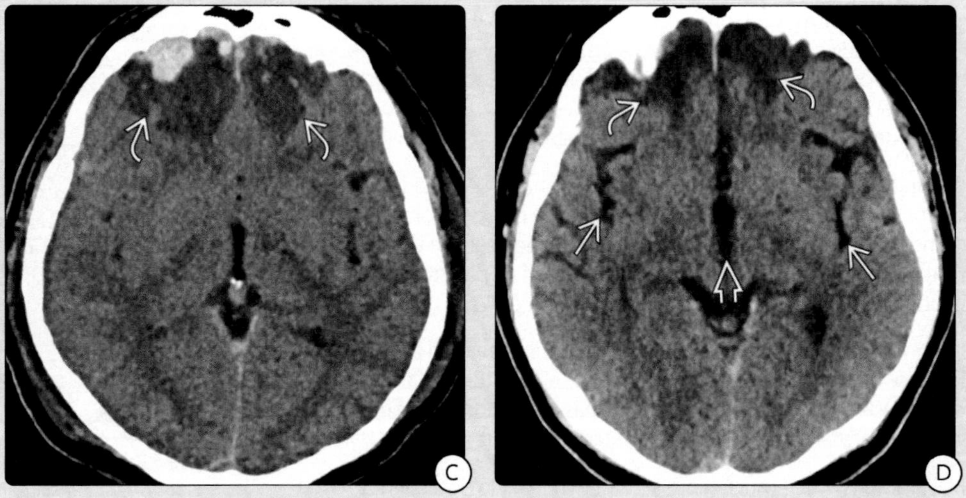

(2-68C) *Repeat NECT at 48 hours shows that the bifrontal hypodensities have consolidated around the hemorrhages. The tSAH and peritentorial aSDH have largely resolved.* ***(2-68D)*** *NECT at 2 months shows bifrontal encephalomalacia, enlarged sylvian fissures, and prominent third ventricle. These changes are common following moderately severe head trauma.*

(TBI). T1 scans may show only mild inhomogeneous isointensities and mass effect. T2 scans show patchy hyperintense areas (edema) surrounding hypointense foci of hemorrhage **(2-69A)**.

FLAIR scans are most sensitive for detecting cortical edema and associated tSAH, both of which appear as hyperintense foci on FLAIR. T2* (GRE, SWI) is the most sensitive sequence for imaging parenchymal hemorrhages. Significant "blooming" is typical in acute lesions **(2-69B)**.

Hemorrhagic contusions follow the expected evolution of parenchymal hematomas, with T1 shortening developing over time. Atrophy, demyelination, and microglial scarring are seen on FLAIR and T2WI. Parenchymal volume loss with ventricular enlargement and sulcal prominence is common.

DWI in patients with cortical contusion shows diffusion restriction in areas of cell death. DTI may disclose coexisting white matter damage in minor head trauma even when standard MR sequences are normal.

Differential Diagnosis

The major differential diagnosis of cortical contusion is **diffuse axonal injury** (DAI). Both cerebral contusions and DAI are often present in patients who have sustained moderate to severe head injury. Contusions tend to be superficial, located along gyral crests. DAI is most commonly found in the corona radiata and along compact white matter tracts such as the internal capsule and corpus callosum.

Severe cortical contusion with confluent hematomas may be difficult to distinguish from brain laceration on imaging studies. **Brain laceration** occurs when severe trauma disrupts the pia and literally tears the underlying brain apart. Parenchymal brain laceration in infants and young children is typically associated with abusive head trauma (see below).

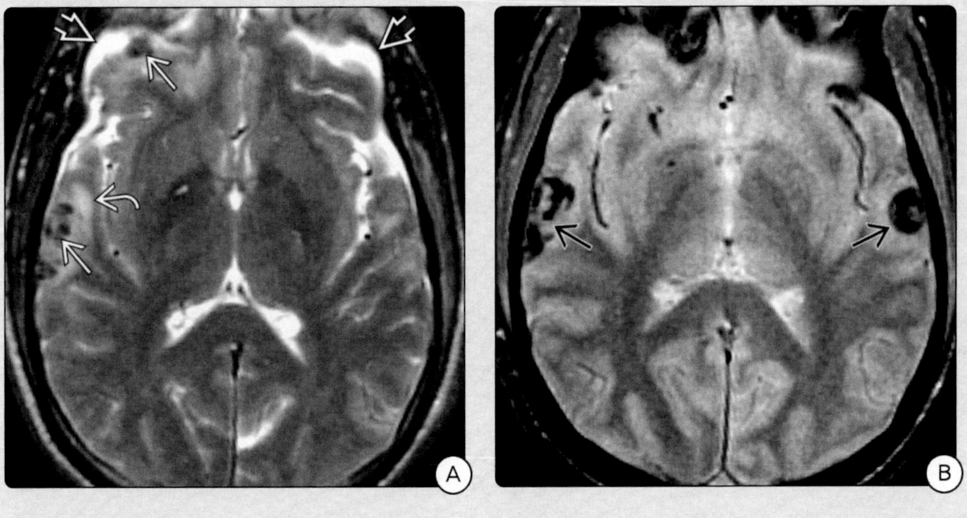

***(2-69A)** T2WI shows contusions ➡ with perilesional edema ➡ and bilateral subdural hygromas ➡. **(2-69B)** T2* GRE in the same case shows that the contusions bloom ➡.*

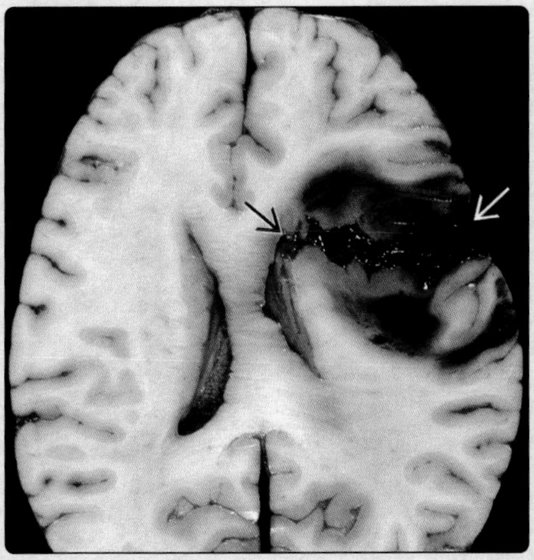

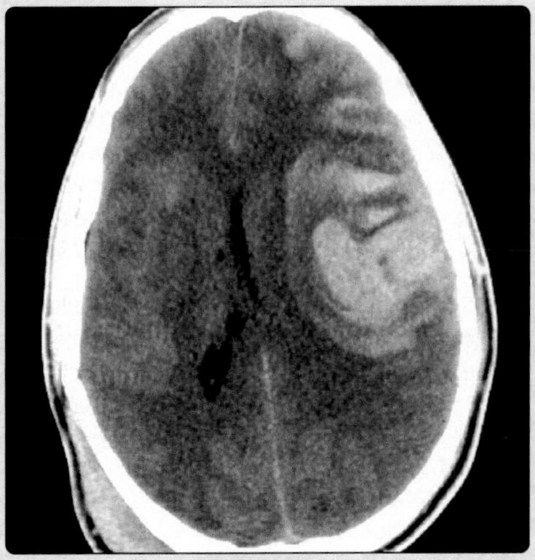

***(2-70)** Autopsy shows a "burst" lobe with a "full thickness" laceration extending from the pial surface ➡ to the ventricle ➡. (Courtesy R. Hewlett, MD.) **(2-71)** NECT scan shows a "burst" lobe with rapid parenchymal hemorrhage extending deep into the brain. The patient died shortly after this scan was obtained.*

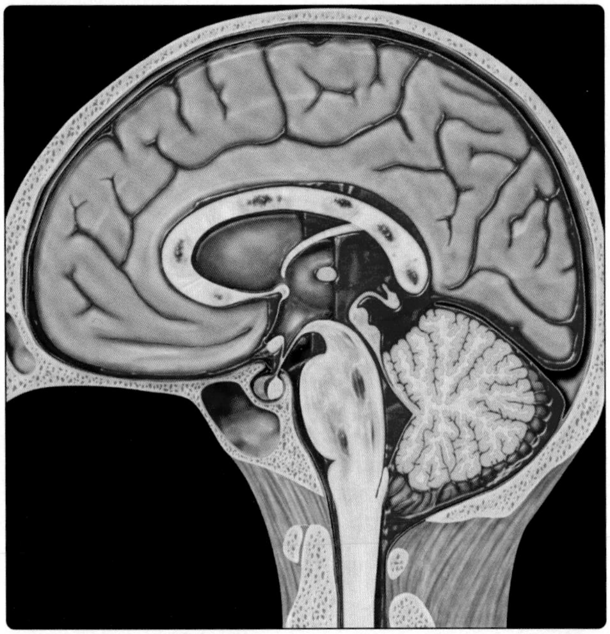

(2-72) Sagittal graphic depicts common sites of axonal injury in the corpus callosum and midbrain. Traumatic intraventricular and subarachnoid hemorrhage is present.

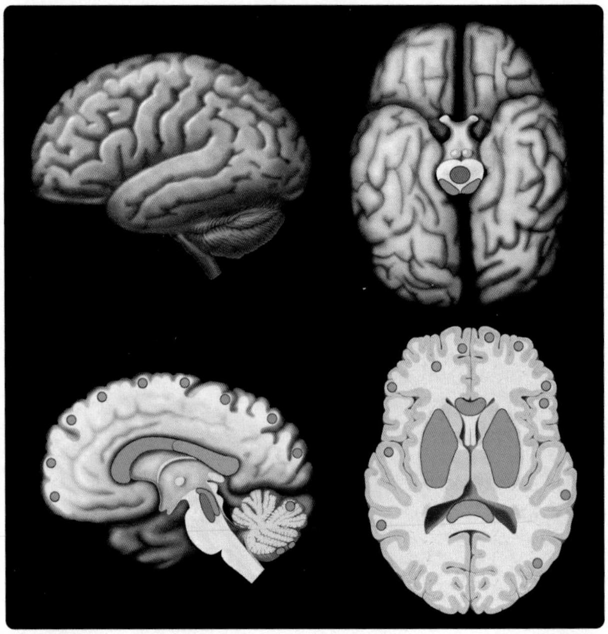

(2-73) Graphics depict the most common sites of axonal injury in red. Frequent but relatively less common locations are shown in green. Injury to the midbrain/upper pons (purple) is uncommon but often lethal.

A "burst lobe" is the most severe manifestation of frank brain laceration **(2-70)** **(2-71)**. Here the affected lobe is grossly disrupted, with large hematoma formation and adjacent tSAH. In some cases, especially those with depressed skull fracture, the arachnoid is also lacerated, and hemorrhage from the burst lobe extends to communicate directly with the subdural space, forming a coexisting subdural hematoma.

Diffuse Axonal Injury

DAI is the second most common parenchymal lesion seen in TBI, exceeded only by cortical contusions. Patients with DAI often exhibit an apparent discrepancy between clinical status (often moderately to severely impaired) and initial imaging findings (often normal or minimally abnormal).

Terminology

DAI is also known as traumatic axonal stretch injury. As most DAIs are stretch—not frank shearing—lesions, the term "shearing lesion" should be avoided. True "shearing" injury with frank axonal disconnection is uncommon and typically occurs only with very severe trauma.

Etiology

Direct head impact is not required to produce DAI. Most DAIs are not associated with skull fracture.

Most DAIs are caused by high-velocity motor vehicle collisions (MVCs) and are dynamic, deformative, nonimpact injuries resulting from the inertial forces of rotation generated by sudden changes in acceleration/deceleration. The cortex moves at a different speed relative to underlying deep brain structures (white matter, deep gray nuclei). This results in axonal stretching, especially where brain tissues of different density intersect, i.e., the gray-white matter interface.

The rapid deformation of white matter at the instant of trauma can lead to mechanical failure. A cascade of adverse events occurs, including calcium-dependent proteolysis of the axonal cytoskeleton in association with axonal transport interruption. Traumatic axonal stretching also causes depolarization, ion fluxes, and spreading depression. Amyloid precursor protein, excitatory amino acids, and proteolytic fragments of neurofilaments may be released. Cellular swelling with cytotoxic edema ensues, altering brain anisotropy. Significant and widespread alterations in brain perfusion may also occur as a result of TBI.

Pathology

Location. DAI occurs in highly predictable locations. The cortex is typically spared; it is the subcortical and deep white matter that is most commonly affected. Lesions in compact white matter tracts such as the corpus callosum, especially the genu and splenium, fornix, and internal capsule, are frequent. The midbrain and pons are less common sites of DAI **(2-72)** **(2-73)**.

Gross Pathology. The vast majority of DAIs are microscopic and nonhemorrhagic. Tears of penetrating vessels (diffuse vascular injury) may cause small round to ovoid or linear hemorrhages that sometimes are the only gross indications of underlying axonal injury **(2-74)**. These visible lesions are truly just the "tip of the iceberg."

Microscopic Features. Accumulation of transport products form axonal swellings or "retraction balls," leaving microscopic gaps in the white matter **(2-75)**. Neuronal apoptosis and microglial-mediated inflammatory changes ensue.

Staging, Grading, and Classification. The Adams and Gennarelli classification defines mild, moderate, and severe grades of TBI.

In mild TBI, lesions are seen in the frontotemporal gray-white matter interfaces. Injury is designated as moderate when the lobar white matter and corpus callosum are affected. In severe TBI, lesions are present in the dorsolateral midbrain and upper pons. More than half of all TBI cases with DAI are designated as moderate to severe.

Clinical Issues

Epidemiology and Demographics. DAI is present in virtually all fatal TBIs and is found in almost three-quarters of patients with moderate or severe injury who survive the acute stage.

DAI may occur at any age, but peak incidence is in young adults (15-24 years old). Male patients are at least twice as often afflicted with TBI as female patients.

Presentation. DAI typically causes much more significant impairment compared with extracerebral hematomas and cortical contusions. DAI often causes immediate loss of consciousness, which may be transient (in the case of mild TBI) or progress to coma (with moderate to severe injury).

Natural History. Mild TBI may result in persisting headaches, mild neurocognitive impairment, and memory difficulties. DAI is more common in moderate to severe injuries. Although DAI itself rarely causes death, severe DAI may result in a persistent vegetative state. Prognosis correlates with the number and severity of lesions as well as the presence of other abnormalities such as cortical contusions and herniation syndromes.

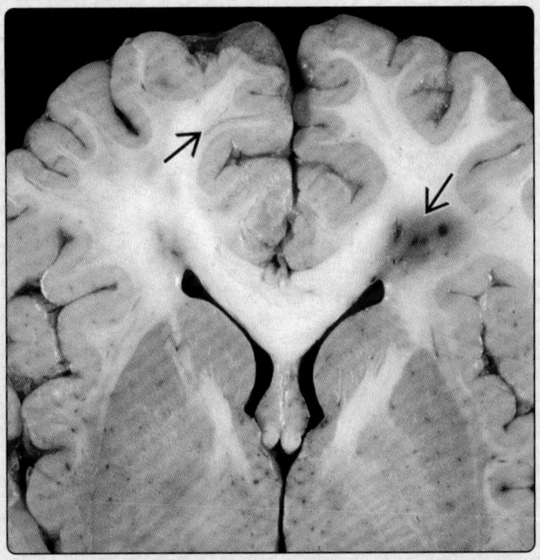
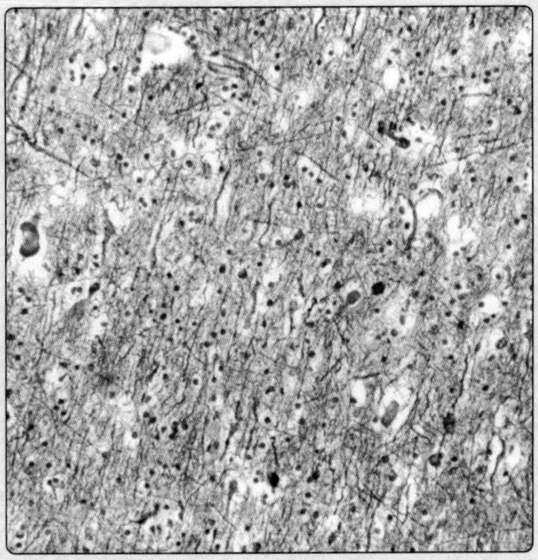

***(2-74)** Autopsy case shows typical findings of diffuse axonal injury with linear hemorrhages ⇨ in the subcortical and deep periventricular white matter. (Courtesy R. Hewlett, MD.) **(2-75)** H&E microscopy shows numerous white gaps or "bare" areas caused by axonal injury. (Courtesy R. Hewlett, MD.)*

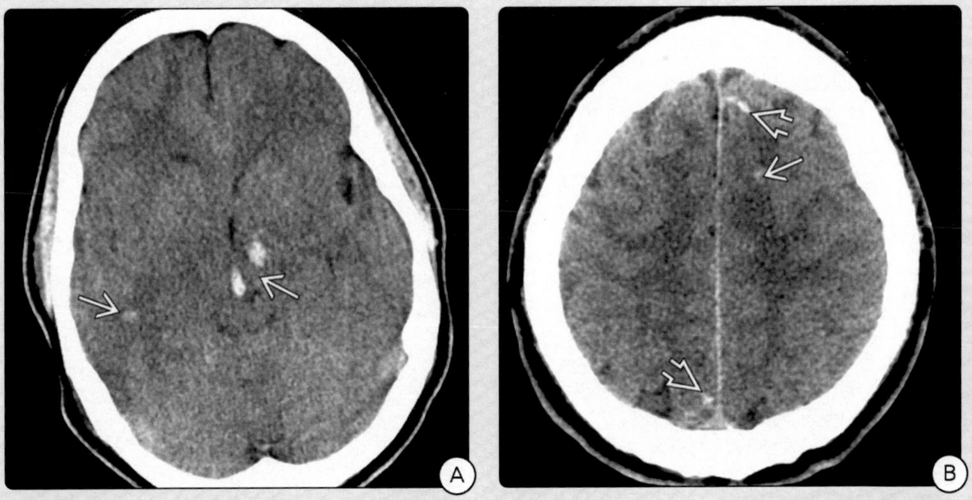

***(2-76A)** NECT in a patient with severe nonimpact head injury shows diffuse brain swelling with small ventricles, effaced sulci, and cisterns. DAI is present, seen as several punctate and linear hemorrhagic foci in the subcortical WM, midbrain, and left thalamus ➡. **(2-76B)** More cephalad scan in the same patient shows additional hemorrhagic foci in the corona radiata ➡ and subcortical WM ➡.*

Treatment Options. Management of intracranial pressure is the most serious issue. In some cases with impending herniation, craniectomy may be a last resort.

Imaging

General Features. One of the most striking features of DAI is the discrepancy between clinical symptoms and imaging findings. NECT scans are almost always the initial imaging study obtained in TBI **(2-76)**, although MR is much more sensitive in detecting changes of DAI. CT is very useful in detecting comorbid injuries such as extracerebral hemorrhage and parenchymal hematomas.

DAI typically evolves with time, so lesions are usually more apparent on follow-up scans. Between 10-20% evolve to gross hemorrhages with edema and mass effect.

CT Findings. Initial NECT is often normal or minimally abnormal **(2-77A)**. Mild diffuse brain swelling with sulcal effacement may be present. Gross hemorrhages are uncommon immediately following injury. A few small round or ovoid subcortical hemorrhages may be visible **(2-76)**, but the underlying damage is typically much more diffuse and much more severe than these relatively modest abnormalities would indicate.

MR Findings. As most DAIs are nonhemorrhagic, T1 scans are often normal, especially in the early stages of TBI. T2WI and FLAIR may show hyperintense foci in the subcortical white matter and corpus callosum. Multiple lesions are the rule, and a combination of DAI and contusions or hematomas is very common.

T2* scans are very sensitive to the microbleeds of DAI and typically show multifocal ovoid and linear hypointensities **(2-77B)**. SWI sequences typically demonstrate more lesions than GRE. Residua from DAI may persist for years following the traumatic episode.

***(2-77A)** NECT scan in a patient with closed head injury from high-speed motor vehicle collision shows no definite abnormalities. **(2-77B)** Because of the discrepancy between imaging findings and the patient's clinical status (GCS = 8), MR was obtained. T2* GRE scan shows multiple "blooming" foci in the subcortical/deep white matter and corpus callosum ➔, characteristic of hemorrhagic axonal injury.*

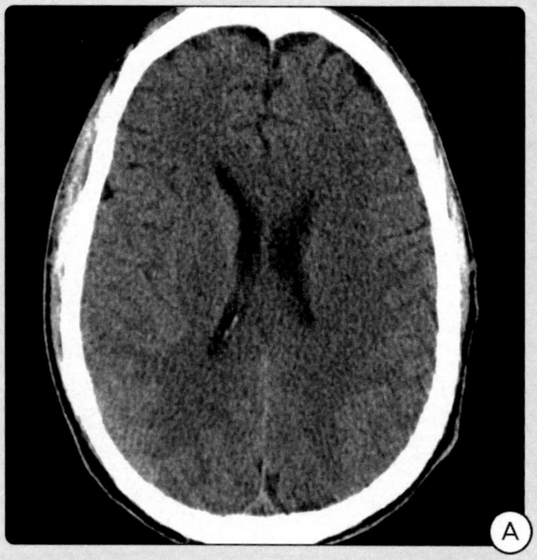

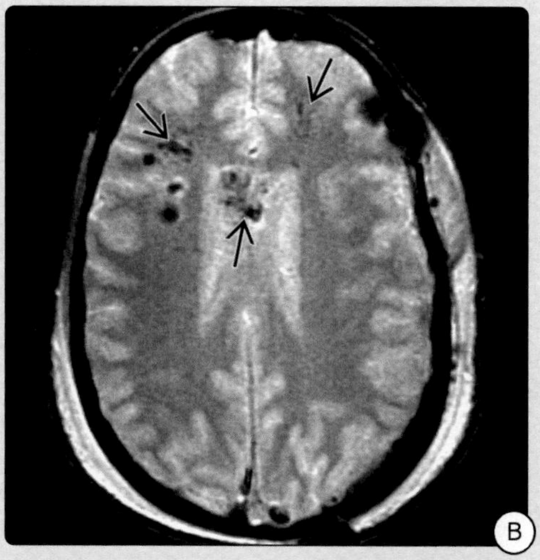

***(2-78A)** NECT scan in a head trauma patient with low GCS shows diffuse brain swelling with small ventricles, sulcal effacement. Hyperdense foci ➔ in the deep gray nuclei and fornix suggest axonal injury. **(2-78B)** DWI in the same patient shows restricted diffusion in the right fornix ➔ and corpus callosum ➔, characteristic of diffuse axonal injury.*

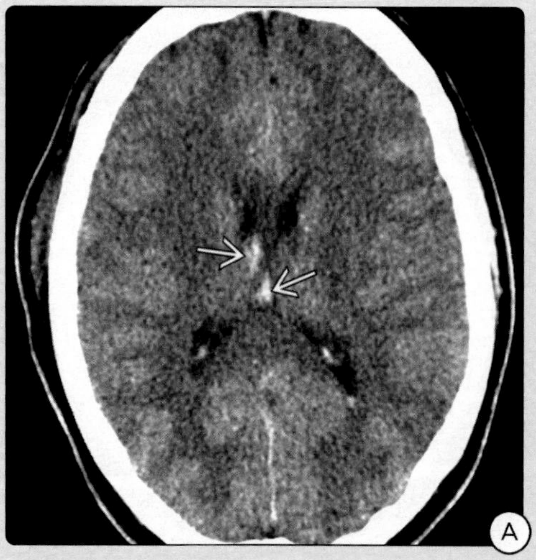

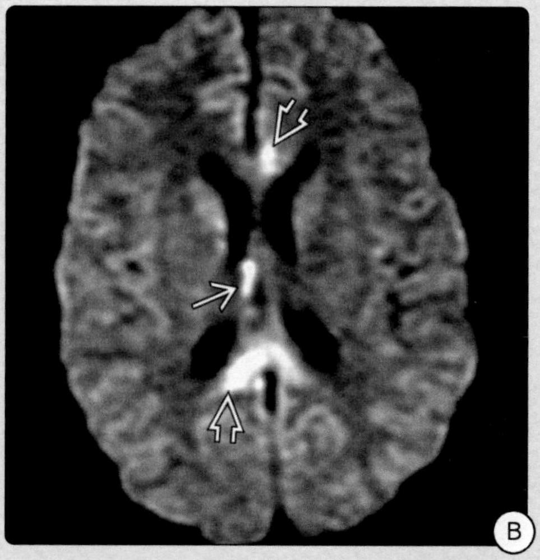

DWI may show restricted diffusion, particularly within the corpus callosum **(2-78)**. Whole-brain tractography may be useful in depicting white matter disruption. MRS shows widespread decrease of NAA with increased Cho.

Differential Diagnosis

Cortical contusions often coexist with DAI in moderate to severe TBI. Cortical contusions are typically superficial lesions, usually located along gyral crests.

Multifocal hemorrhages with "blooming" on T2* (GRE, SWI) scans can be seen in numerous pathologies, including DAI. **Diffuse vascular injury** (see below) appears as multifocal parenchymal "black dots." Pneumocephalus may cause multifocal "blooming" lesions in the subarachnoid spaces. Parenchymal lesions are rare.

Several nontraumatic lesions also appear as multifocal T2* parenchymal hypointensities. **Cerebral amyloid angiopathy** and **chronic hypertensive encephalopathy** are common in older patients. Zabramski type 4 cavernous malformations are also seen as "black dots" on T2* MR scans.

Diffuse Vascular Injury

Terminology

Diffuse vascular injury (DVI) probably represents the extreme end of the diffuse axonal injury continuum.

Etiology

DVI is caused by the extreme acceleration/rotational forces that are incurred in high-velocity MVCs. The brain microvasculature, particularly long penetrating subcortical and deep perforating vessels, is disrupted by high tensile forces. The result is numerous small punctate and linear parenchymal hemorrhages.

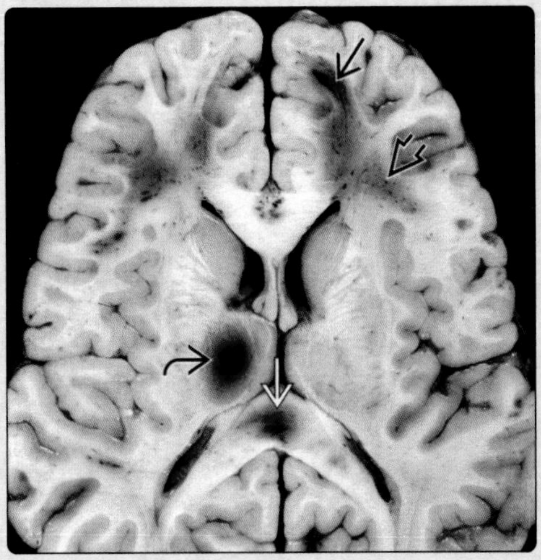

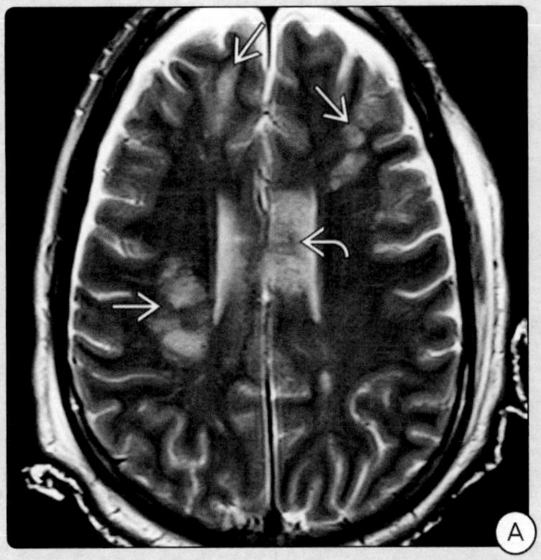

__(2-79)__ Autopsy case shows findings of diffuse vascular injury with multiple petechial ⇒ and linear ⇒ subcortical WM hemorrhages. Note subcortical injury to thalamus ⇒, corpus callosum splenium ➡. (Courtesy R. Hewlett, MD.) __(2-80A)__ 53y man was unconscious after MVA. GCS was 6; initial NECT was negative. T2WI from MRI 2 days later shows hyperintensities in subcortical/deep WM ➡ and corpus callosum ➡.

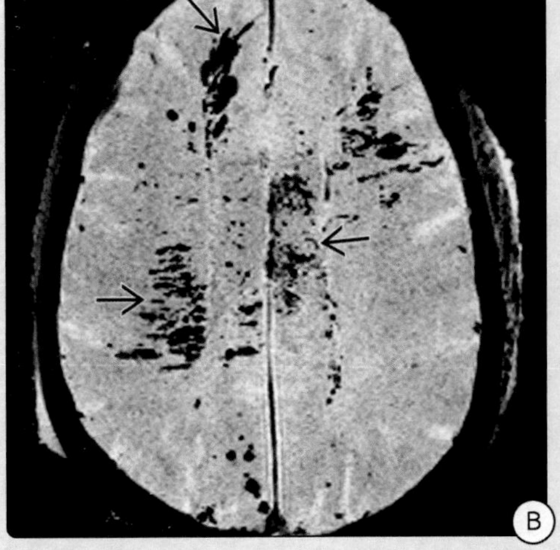

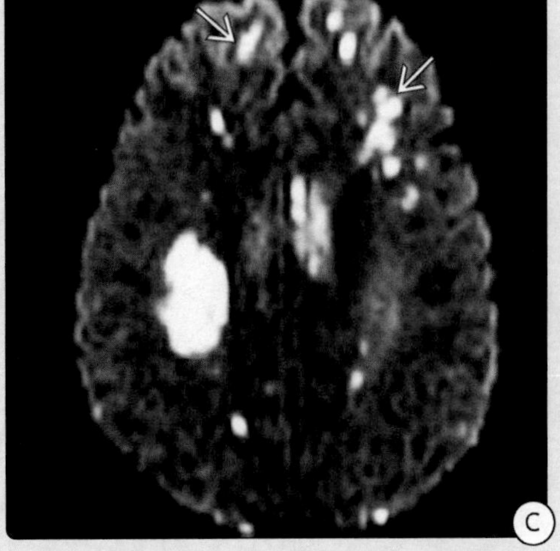

__(2-80B)__ SWI MIP in the same case shows innumerable punctate and linear blooming hypointensities ⇒ following the course of penetrating blood vessels, suggesting hemorrhagic axonal and vascular injury. __(2-80C)__ DWI in the same case shows multiple foci of restricted diffusion ➡.

Pathology

Gross Pathology. Autopsied brains of patients with DVI show numerous small hemorrhages in the subcortical and deep white matter as well as in the deep gray nuclei **(2-79)**.

Microscopic Features. Many more hemorrhages are detected on microscopic examination than are seen in the gross appearance of the brain. Blood is identified along periarterial, perivenous, and pericapillary spaces with focal hemorrhages in the adjacent parenchyma.

Clinical Issues

Epidemiology. Autopsy series suggest that DVI is present in 1-2% of fatal MVC victims and 15% of cases with diffuse brain injury.

Demographics. Although DVI can occur at any age, most occur in adults.

Presentation. Immediate coma from the moment of impact is typical. A very low GCS, often less than 6-8, is typical in patients who survive the initial impact.

Natural History. Death within minutes or a few hours following injury is typical although some long-term survivors have been reported.

Imaging

General Features. Many patients with DVI do not survive long enough for imaging. In those who do, the most striking feature is the dissociation between clinical severity and imaging findings.

CT Findings. NECT scans may show only diffuse brain swelling with effaced superficial sulci and small ventricles. A few small foci of hemorrhage in the white matter and basal ganglia can sometimes be identified. Bone CT shows multiple skull

(2-81) Autopsy specimen from a patient who died in a high-speed MVC shows a large hemorrhage → in the deep gray nuclei, characteristic of severe subcortical injury. (Courtesy R. Hewlett, MD.) (2-82) A 38y man was in an MVA. GCS at the scene was 8 and declined to 3 on arrival in the ER. NECT scan on admission (not shown) disclosed no abnormalities. Follow-up scan 8 hours later shows a large expanding basal ganglia hematoma →. He expired 2 days later.

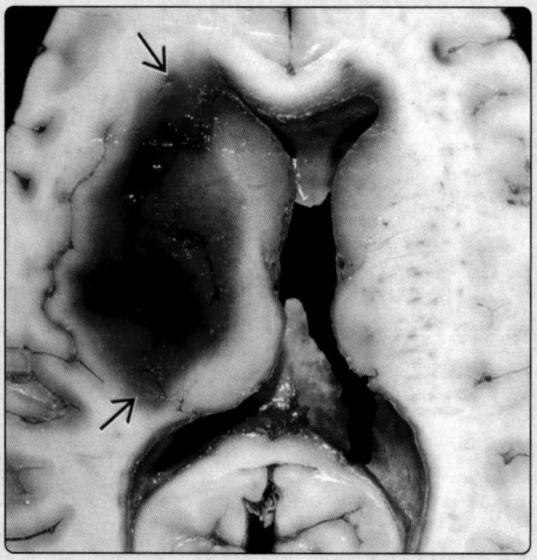

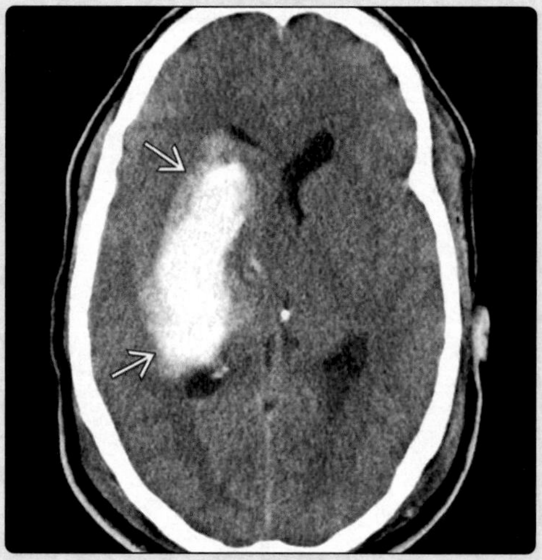

(2-83) Gross pathology shows deep parenchymal injuries with dorsolateral contusions →, traumatic tectal clefting →, and large focal hematoma surrounding the midbrain →. (Courtesy R. Hewlett, MD.) (2-84) NECT in a 52y woman after a moderate impact MVA shows hyperdensity in the left posterolateral midbrain → associated with focal tSAH →. Dorsolateral midbrain injury occurs when it is suddenly impacted against the tentorial incisura.

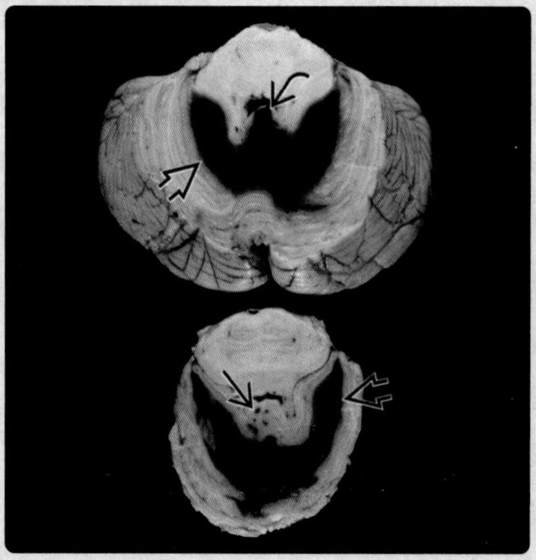

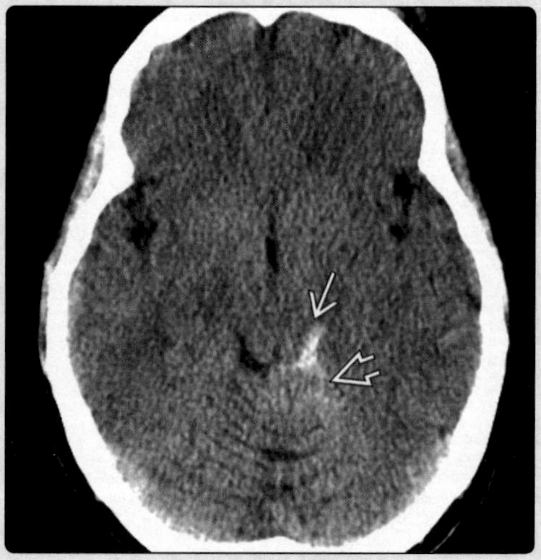

fractures in unrestrained passengers, but fractures are absent in one-third of individuals wearing seat belts.

MR Findings. T1WI shows only mild brain swelling. T2WI and FLAIR scans may demonstrate a few foci of hyperintensity in the white matter **(2-80A)**. Occasionally, scattered hypointensities can be identified within the hyperintensities, suggesting the presence of hemorrhage.

T2* scans, especially susceptibility-weighted sequences, are striking. Punctate and linear "blooming" hypointensities are seen oriented perpendicularly to the ventricles, predominantly in the subcortical and deep white matter, especially the corpus callosum **(2-80B)**. Additional lesions in the basal ganglia, thalami, brainstem, and cerebellum are often present.

DWI may demonstrate a few foci of restricted diffusion consistent with ischemia caused by the vascular injuries **(2-80C)**.

Differential Diagnosis

The major differential diagnosis is **diffuse axonal injury** (DAI). Although some lesions in DAI are hemorrhagic, the majority are not. DVI is characterized by the presence of innumerable petechial hemorrhages on T2* imaging. It is the number, severity, and extent of the hemorrhages that distinguishes DVI from DAI.

Subcortical (Deep Brain) Injury

Terminology

Subcortical injuries (SCIs) are traumatic lesions of deep brain structures such as the brainstem, basal ganglia, thalami, and ventricles. Most represent severe shear-strain injuries that disrupt axons, tear penetrating blood vessels, and damage the choroid plexus of the lateral ventricles.

Etiology

SCIs are caused by the violent acceleration/deceleration and brain rotation that occurs with severe, often fatal, motor vehicle collisions. Sudden craniocaudal displacement or lateral impaction of the midbrain against the tentorial incisura is common with these injuries.

Pathology

Gross Pathology. Manifestations of SCI include deep hemorrhagic contusions, nonhemorrhagic lacerations, intraventricular bleeds, and traumatic subarachnoid hemorrhage (tSAH) **(2-81)**. SCIs usually occur with other traumatic lesions such as cortical contusions and diffuse axonal injury (DAI).

Clinical Issues

Epidemiology. Between 5-10% of patients with moderate to severe brain trauma sustain subcortical injuries. SCIs are the third most common parenchymal brain injury, after cortical contusions and DAI.

Demographics. As with most traumatic brain injuries, SCIs are most common in male patients between the ages of 15 and 24 years.

Presentation. Immediate loss of consciousness with profound neurologic deficits is typical. Obtundation is the rule, not the exception. As with DAI, gross discrepancy between immediate imaging findings (often minimal) and GCS (low) is common.

Natural History. Prognosis is poor in these severely injured patients. Many do not survive; those who do typically have profound neurologic impairment with severe long-term disability.

Treatment Options. Controlling intracranial pressure is the most pressing issue. Craniectomy may be an option in exceptionally severe cases of brain swelling.

PARENCHYMAL BRAIN INJURIES

Cerebral Contusions
- Most common intraaxial injury
  - Brain impacts skull and/or dura
  - Causes "brain bruises" in gyral crests
  - Usually multiple, often bilateral
  - Anteroinferior frontal, temporal lobes most common sites
- Imaging
  - Superficial petechial, focal hemorrhage
  - Edema, hemorrhage more apparent with time
  - T2* (GRE, SWI) most sensitive imaging

Diffuse Axonal Injury (DAI)
- Second most common intraaxial injury
  - Spares cortex, involves subcortical/deep WM
- Imaging
  - GCS low; initial imaging often minimally abnormal
  - Subcortical, deep petechial hemorrhages ("tip of the iceberg")
  - T2* (GRE, SWI) most sensitive technique

Diffuse Vascular Injury
- Rare, usually fatal
- High-speed, high-impact MVCs
- May represent extreme end of DAI spectrum
- Imaging
  - CT shows diffuse brain swelling
  - T2 and FLAIR show a few scattered hyperintensities
  - SWI shows innumerable linear hypointensities

Subcortical Injury
- "The deeper the injury, the worse it is"
- Basal ganglia, thalami, midbrain, pons
  - Hemorrhages, axonal injury, brain tears
  - Gross intraventricular hemorrhage common

Imaging

General Features. Minimal abnormalities may be present on initial imaging but show dramatic increase on follow-up scans.

SCI typically exists with numerous comorbid injuries. Lesions ranging from subtle tSAH to gross parenchymal hemorrhage are common (2-82). Mass effect with cerebral herniation and gross disturbances in regional blood flow may develop.

CT Findings. NECT scans often show diffuse brain swelling with punctate and/or gross hemorrhage in the deep gray nuclei and midbrain **(2-83)** **(2-84)**. Intraventricular and choroid plexus hemorrhages are common and may form a "cast" of the lateral ventricles. Blood-fluid levels are common.

MR Findings. MR is much more sensitive than CT even though acute hemorrhage is isointense with brain on T1 scans. FLAIR and T2* are the most sensitive sequences. DWI may show foci of restricted diffusion. DTI mapping delineates the pattern of white matter tract disruption.

Differential Diagnosis

Secondary midbrain ("Duret") hemorrhage may occur with severe descending transtentorial herniation. These hemorrhages are typically centrally located within the midbrain, whereas contusional SCIs are dorsolateral.

Miscellaneous Injuries

A broad spectrum of miscellaneous primary injuries occurs in head trauma. Some such as pneumocephalus are relatively common. Other lesions are rare. We conclude this chapter with a consideration of these miscellaneous lesions, as well as the topics of child abuse and gunshot wounds.

Pneumocephalus

Terminology

Pneumocephalus simply means the presence of gas or air within the intracranial cavity; intracranial air does not exist under normal conditions. In pneumocephalus, air can be found

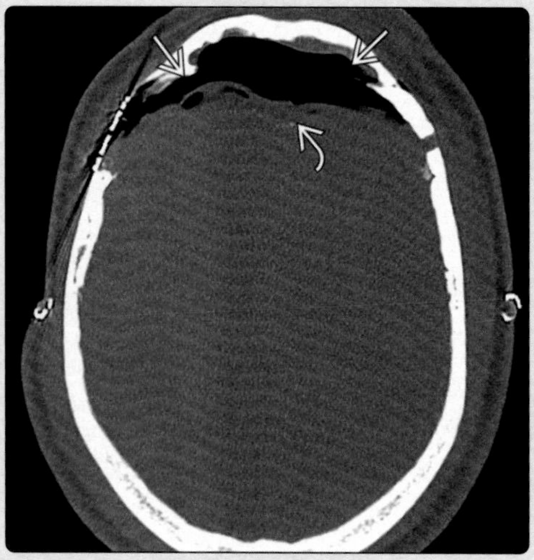

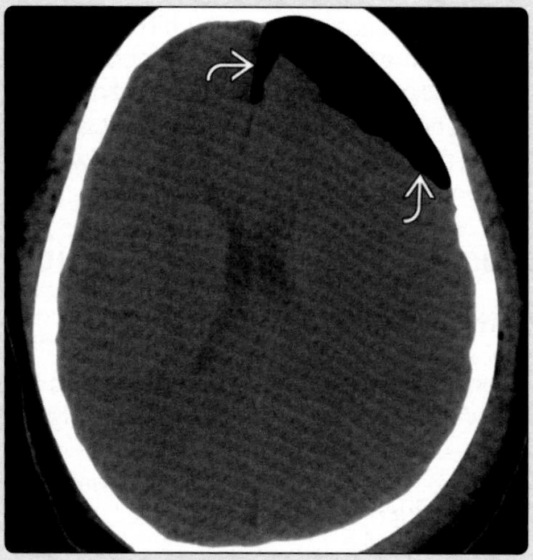

***(2-85)** Epidural air is seen in this immediate postoperative NECT following bifrontal craniotomy. The air collection → is continuous across the midline, and the fat packing and dura ↪ are displaced posteriorly, confirming epidural location of air. **(2-86)** Unilateral subdural air is an expected finding after supratentorial craniotomies. Subdural air ↪ forms a crescent-shaped collection over the hemisphere and does not cross the midline.*

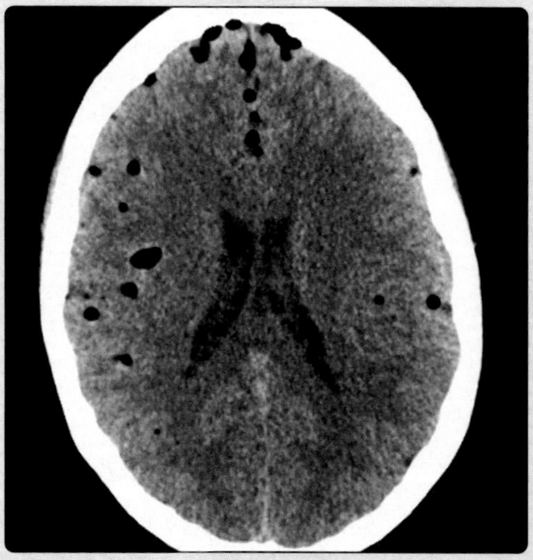

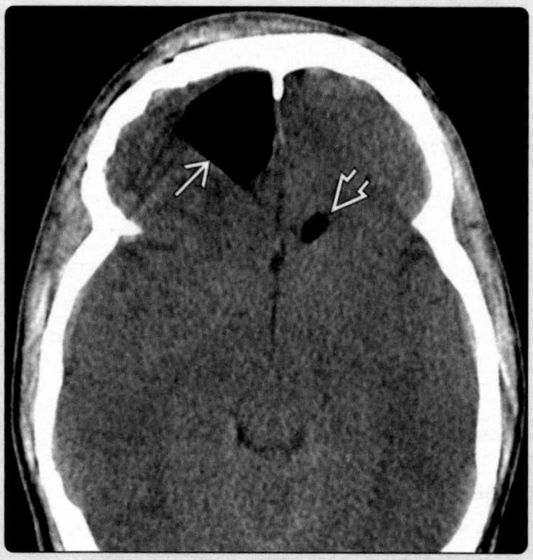

***(2-87)** Subarachnoid air appears as scattered, separate "spots" and dots" that collect in the sulci and cisterns. **(2-88)** NECT scan shows a focal pneumatocele in the right frontal lobe →. Some air is also present in the frontal horn of the left lateral ventricle ⇨.*

anywhere within the cranium, including blood vessels, and within any compartment. While intracranial air is never normal, it can be an expected and therefore routine finding (e.g., after surgery).

Tension pneumocephalus is a collection of intracranial air that is under pressure that causes mass effect on the brain and results in neurologic deterioration. Intracerebral pneumatocele or "aerocele" is a less commonly used term and refers specifically to a focal gas collection within the brain parenchyma.

Etiology

Intracranial air is most often associated with trauma and surgery. Infection by gas-forming organisms is a rare cause of pneumocephalus.

Any breach in integrity of the calvaria, central skull base, mastoid, or paranasal sinuses that also disrupts the dura and arachnoid can allow air to enter the cranium. A ball-valve mechanism may entrap the air, which can be exacerbated by forcible sneezing, coughing, straining, or Valsalva maneuver.

Intravascular air is usually secondary to intravenous catheterization, most commonly found in the cavernous sinus, and of no clinical importance. Intraarterial air is seen only with air embolism (transient) or brain death.

Clinical Issues

Epidemiology. Trauma is the most common cause of pneumocephalus. It is present in 3% of all patients with skull fractures and 8% of those with paranasal sinus fractures.

Virtually all patients who have supratentorial surgery have some degree of pneumocephalus on imaging studies obtained within the first 24-28 hours. **Tension pneumocephalus** is the accumulation of air under pressure leading to neurologic deterioration. Tension pneumocephalus is a relatively uncommon complication of surgery, usually seen after subdural hematoma evacuation.

Occasionally, **spontaneous pneumocephalus** can occur with primary defects in the temporal bone (**"otogenic pneumocephalus"**). Rarely, defects in or rupture of an enlarged paranasal sinus air cell ("pneumosinus dilatans") result in intracranial air.

Presentation. The most common presentation is nonspecific headache. Less commonly, neurologic deficit and disturbances of consciousness are observed.

Natural History and Treatment Options. Unless it is under tension, most intracranial air resolves spontaneously within a few days after trauma or surgery. Occasionally, air collections increase and may require evacuation with duraplasty.

Imaging

General Features. Intracranial air can exist in any compartment (epidural, subdural, subarachnoid, intraventricular, or intraparenchymal) and conforms to the shape of that compartment or potential compartment. The subdural space is the most frequent, and the most common site is frontal.

Epidural air is typically unilateral, solitary, and biconvex in configuration and does not move with changes in head position **(2-85)**.

Subdural air is confluent, crescentic, and often bilateral, frequently contains air-fluid levels, moves with changes in head position, and surrounds cortical veins that cross the subdural space **(2-86)**.

Subarachnoid air is typically seen as multifocal small "dots" or "droplets" of air within and around cerebral sulci **(2-87)**. **Intraventricular air** forms air-fluid levels, most often in the frontal horns of the lateral ventricles. Intraparenchymal air is uncommon, and such a collection is termed a **pneumatocele (2-88)**. **Intravascular air** conforms to the vascular structure(s) within which it resides.

PNEUMOCEPHALUS

Terminology
- Air in intracranial compartment
  - Always abnormal
  - Not always clinically significant
- Tension pneumocephalus
  - Air under pressure → neurologic deterioration

Etiology
- Surgery (most common)
  - Expected after craniotomy
- Trauma (8-10% of cases)
- "Spontaneous" (defect in temporal bone, sinus)

Location
- Epidural
  - Unilateral, biconvex
  - May cross midline
  - Does not move with change in position
- Subdural
  - Confluent, crescentic
  - Often bilateral ± air-fluid level
  - Shows crossing cortical veins
  - Changes with head position
  - Does not cross midline
- Subarachnoid
  - Discrete "spots" and "dots" in sulci, cisterns
- Intraventricular
  - Usually air-fluid levels, frontal horns
- Intraparenchymal
  - Confluent, well delineated

General Imaging Features
- CT
  - Extremely hypodense (-1000 HU)
  - Fat vs. air? Use wide windows!
- MR
  - Signal void
  - Prominent "blooming" on GRE
  - Alternating dark "holes" ± concentric bright rings
  - Chemical shift artifact in phase-encoding direction

(2-89) *NECT scan shows subdural air with "pointing" of the frontal lobes. This "Mount Fuji" sign is caused by cortical veins ➡ tethering the frontal lobes ➡, and it indicates tension pneumocephalus.* ***(2-90A)*** *Is this tension pneumocephalus or not? The frontal lobes appear moderately pointed ➡, suggesting the subdural air may be under pressure.*

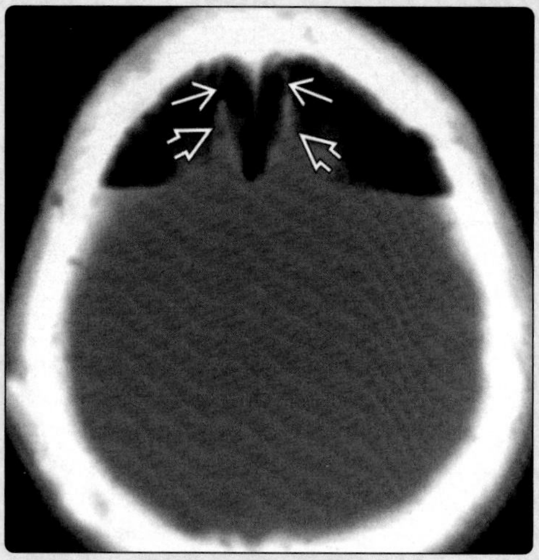

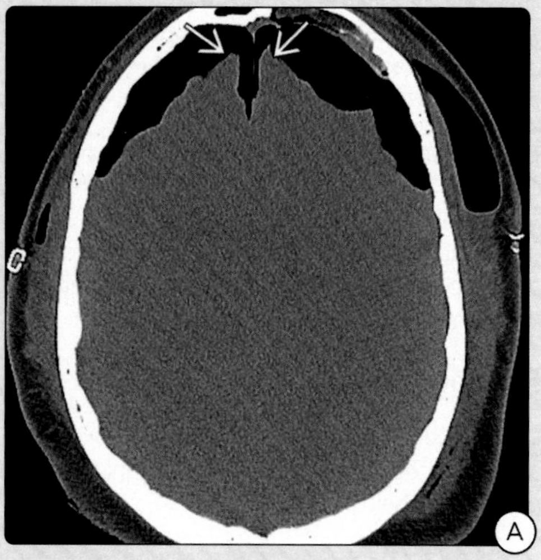

(2-90B) *Preoperative sagittal reformatted NECT in the same case shows normal position of the corpus callosum ➡ and anterior margin of the lateral ventricles ➡ relative to the limbus sphenoidale ➡.* ***(2-90C)*** *Sagittal postoperative NECT in the same case shows that subdural air has displaced the lateral ventricle ➡ posteriorly relative to the limbus sphenoidale ➡, indicating that the air is under tension.*

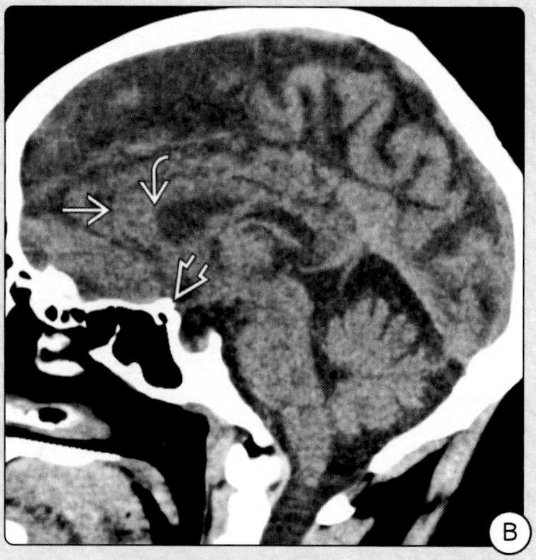

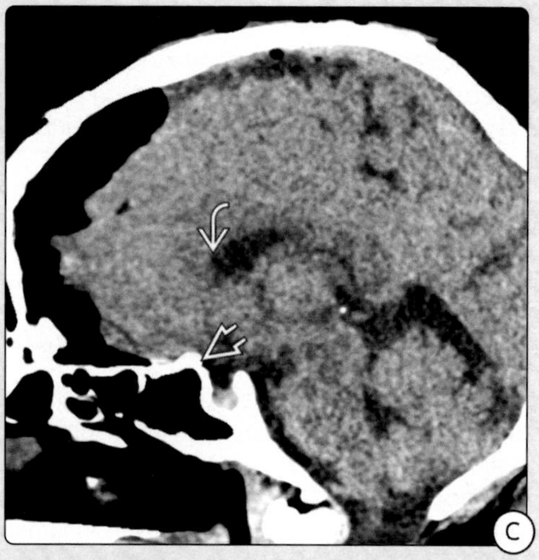

(2-91A) *Sagittal T1WI shows pneumocephalus after posterior fossa surgery. Some subdural air is present anterior to the frontal lobe, seen as a signal void ➡. "Spots" and "dots" of air with adjacent susceptibility artifact are present in the subarachnoid spaces ➡.* ***(2-91B)*** *T2* GRE scan in the same case shows multifocal blooming black dots ➡ representing air in the subarachnoid spaces.*

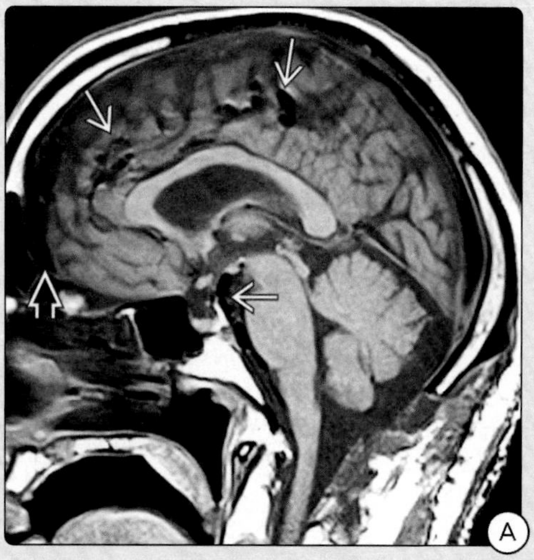

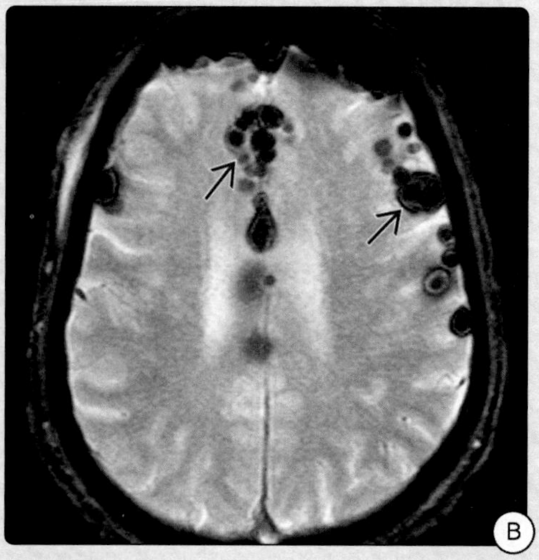

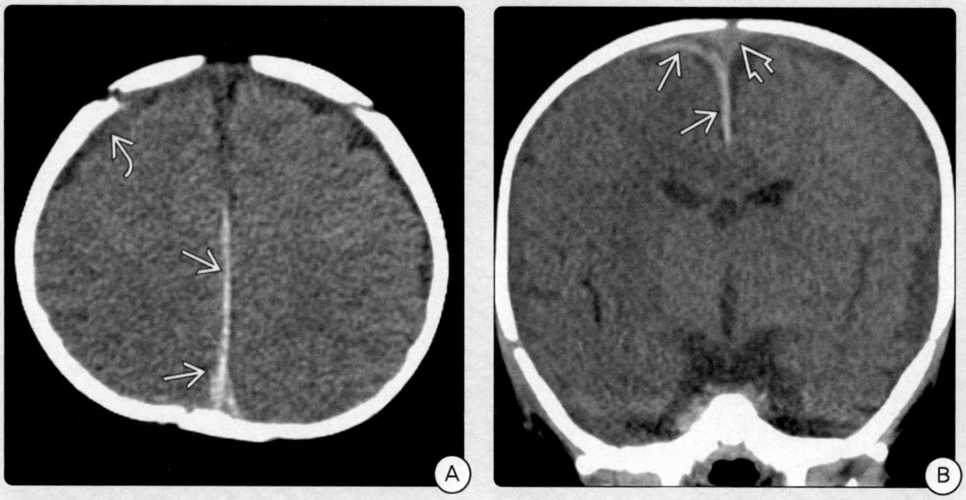

***(2-92A)** Axial NECT in a 3m boy shows acute parafalcine SDH ➡. There was no evidence of scalp or skull injury. Note the hypoattenuating right frontal subdural collection ⤻ that MR characterized as a chronic SDH. **(2-92B)** Coronal NECT, MPR shows an acute parafalcine and convexity SDH ➡. Note the triangular shape of the normal superior sagittal dural venous sinus ⇨. The falx cerebri limits the medial migration of the SDH.*

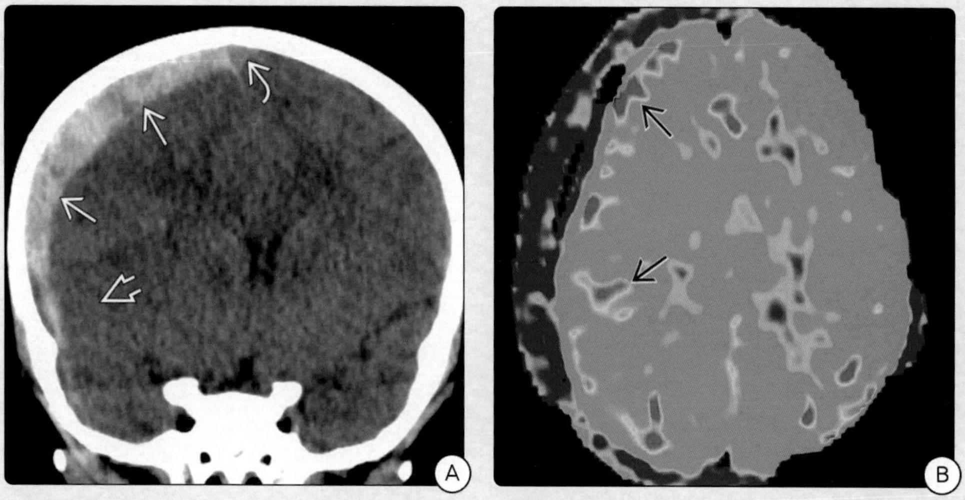

***(2-93A)** Coronal NECT in AHT shows mixed-attenuation SDH ➡ and subfalcine herniation ⤻. An acute hematoma was evacuated. Note the loss of GM-WM matter differentiation ⇨ representing cerebral edema. Extensive right hemispheric encephalomalacia followed. **(2-93B)** Arterial spin labeling (ASL) MR after SDH evacuation shows ↑ right cerebral hemispheric blood flow ➡ reflecting disordered autoregulation.*

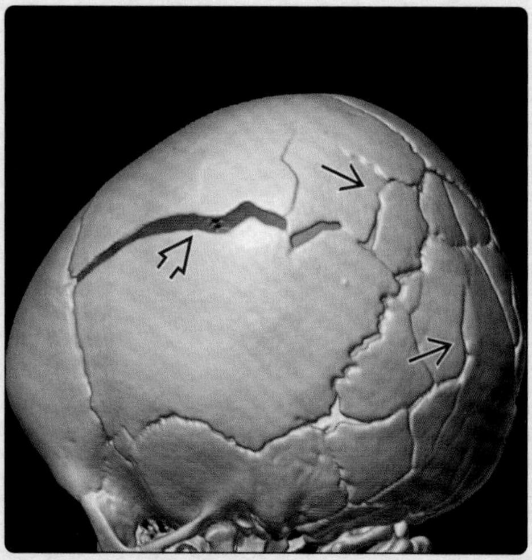

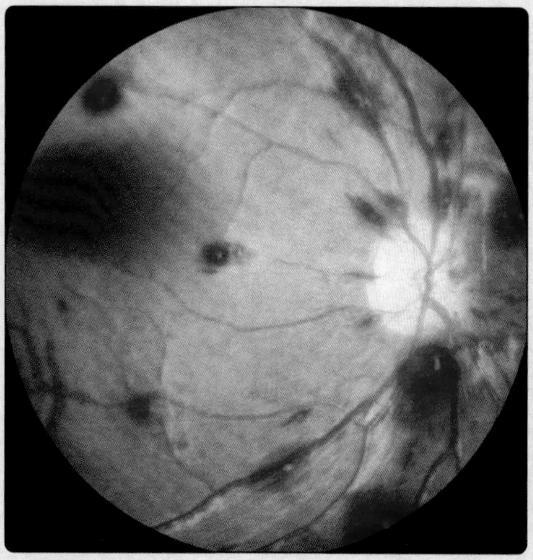

***(2-94)** 3D NECT in a 6m boy with scalp swelling is shown. There was no history of prior head trauma. Note the diastatic right parietal fracture ⇨ and innumerable occipital and parietal fractures ➡. Skull fractures are often absent in the setting of AHT. **(2-95)** Funduscopic exam in an infant victim of abusive head trauma (shaking) shows multiple retinal hemorrhages (RHs). RHs often accompany SDHs. (Courtesy K. Digre, MD.)*

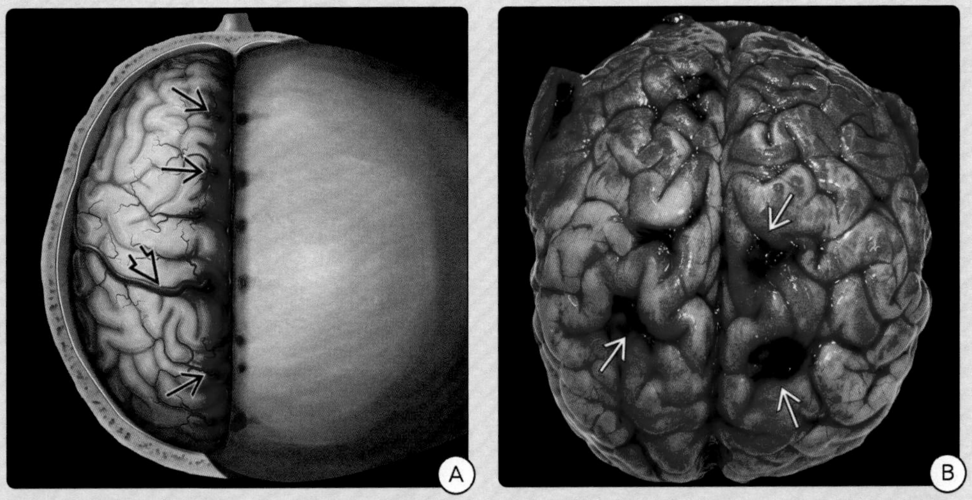

(2-96A) Convexity graphic demonstrates numerous torn bridging veins →. One torn bridging vein shows distention secondary to thrombosis ⇨. Bridging veins tear at the dural cuff where the vein penetrates the dura of the superior sagittal dural venous sinus. (2-96B) Autopsy photograph in an infant victim of fatal AHT shows numerous traumatically torn and thrombosed convexity bridging veins →. (Courtesy of C. Rambaud, MD.)

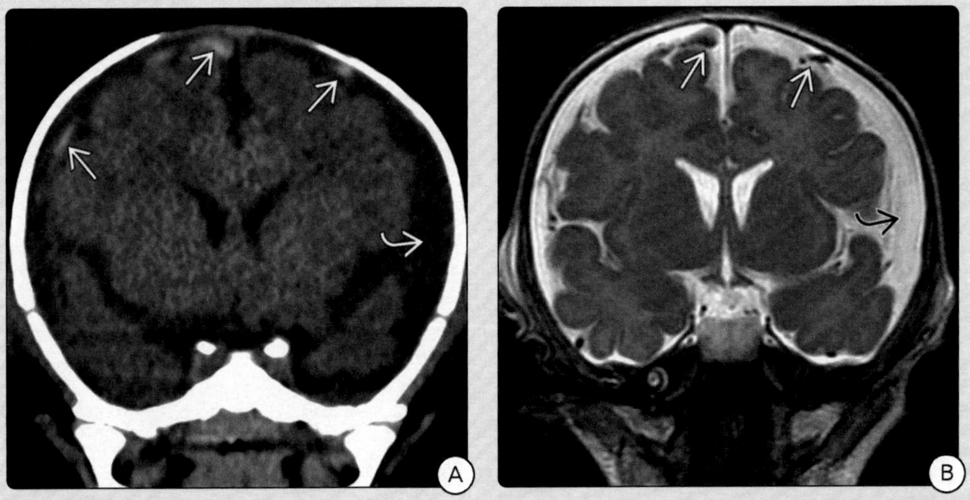

(2-97A) Coronal NECT in AHT shows confirmed infant shaking victim showing tubular and comma-shaped convexity hyperattenuating (torn and thrombosed) bridging veins →. Note CSF-like subdural collection ↪. MR showed features of hygroma (SDHy). (2-97B) Tubular hyperattenuating injured bridging veins from prior coronal NECT show on this T2WI corresponding T2 hypointensities →, with associated SDHy ↪.

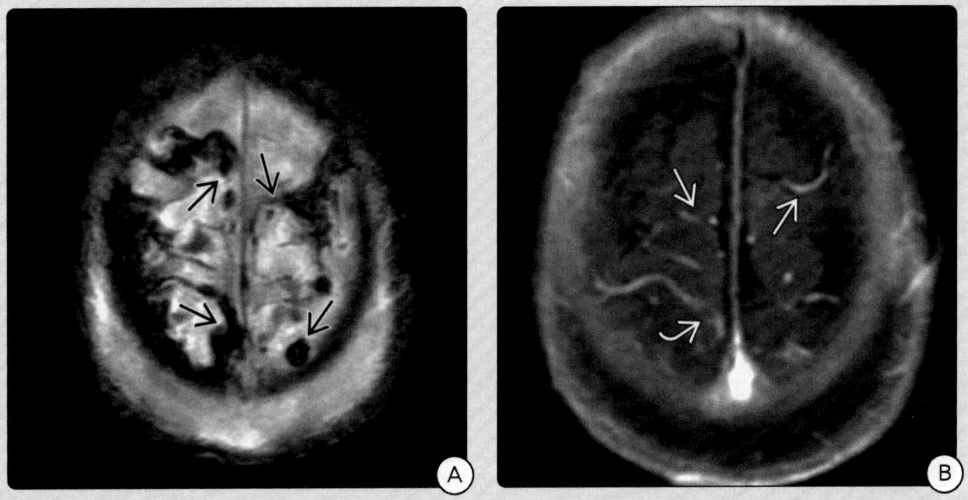

(2-98A) Axial SWI shows injured bridging veins in infant AHT victim with chaotic convexal tubular and rounded hypointensities → that at autopsy revealed torn and thrombosed bridging veins. Normal bridging veins converge and enter SSS. (2-98B) Axial T1 C+ MR shows the absence of normal bridging veins (normally 12-15/hemisphere). Thrombus is noted in a parietal bridging vein ↪. Note small cortical veins →.

CT Findings. Air is extremely hypodense on CT, measuring approximately -1,000 HU. The "Mount Fuji" sign of **tension pneumocephalus** is seen as bilateral subdural air collections that separate and compress the frontal lobes, widening the interhemispheric fissure **(2-89)**. The frontal lobes are displaced posteriorly by air under pressure and are typically pointed where they are tethered to the dura-arachnoid by cortical veins, mimicking the silhouette of Mount Fuji **(2-90)**.

Distinguishing air from fat on CT is extremely important. With typical narrow soft tissue windows, both appear similarly hypodense. Increasing window width or simply looking at bone CT algorithms (on which air is clearly distinct from the less hypodense fat) helps differentiate fat from air.

MR Findings. Air is seen as areas of completely absent signal intensity on all sequences. On T2* GRE, intracranial air "blooms" and appears as multifocal "black dots" **(2-91)**.

Differential Diagnosis

Air is air and shouldn't be mistaken for anything else. If wide windows are not used, a ruptured dermoid cyst with fat droplets in the CSF cisterns can mimic subarachnoid air.

Reminder!

With the exception of tension pneumocephalus, air itself generally isn't the problem; figure out what's causing it!

Abusive Head Trauma (Child Abuse)

Radiologists play a key role in the diagnosis of suspected child abuse. Imaging must be performed with care, interpreted with rigor, and precisely described. The final diagnosis of child abuse is typically made by a child abuse pediatrician, who leads a multidisciplinary team (in which the radiologist plays an important role). There is no rush to judgment. Thoughtful social, clinical, and scientific inquiry prevails.

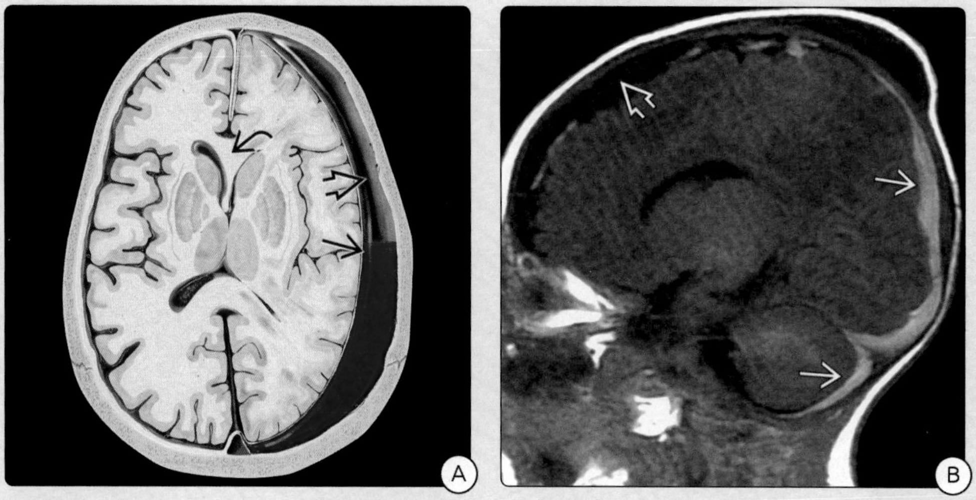

***(2-99A)** Graphic demonstrates hematohygroma and subfalcine shift. Dependent blood forms an interface with serum and CSF. To estimate hemorrhage age, assess the sediment! **(2-99B)** Parasagittal T1WI shows hematohygroma in a 4m victim of shaking. Dependent hyperintense acute hemorrhage (sediment) and CSF-like supernate are shown. The detection of hematohygroma in a child less than 2y old is a proxy for trauma.*

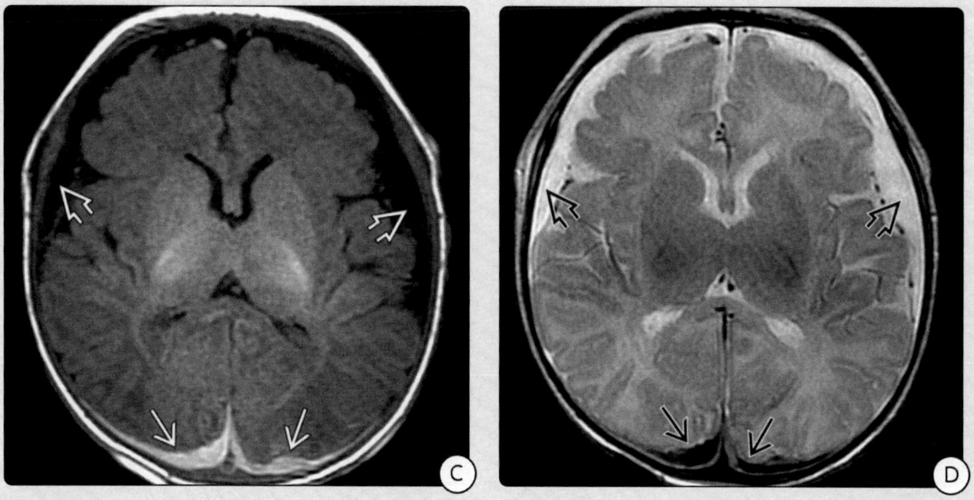

***(2-99C)** Axial T1WI is shown. Dating hematohygroma focuses on the sediment. Note the bilateral hygromas (supernate). Cortical veins hug the lateral cerebral fissures, confirming subdural location of hygroma. **(2-99D)** Axial T2WI shows hypointense acute SDH. This hematohygroma was assessed to reflect a single AHT event. Avoid defaulting to the diagnosis of new and old SDH in the setting of hematohygroma. Also note SDHy.*

Terminology

The term "nonaccidental trauma" (NAT), also known as nonaccidental injury (NAI) or shaken-baby syndrome (SBS), refers to intentionally inflicted injury. Our evolving understanding of the pathomorphologic underpinnings of inflicted injury influences our language. Currently, the American Academy of Pediatrics endorses the term, **abusive head trauma (AHT)**, which encompasses a spectrum of potential mechanisms of intracranial injury acting independently or in concert, including shaking with or without impact, impact alone, strangulation/suffocation, and hypoxic ischemic insult.

Etiology

AHT may involve linear translational forces with shaking and impact (impactive forces) or complex angular forces without impact (impulsive forces); AHT impulsive forces are commonly commotio forces with acceleration and deceleration often without impact. Resultant subdural and subarachnoid hemorrhages, cerebral edema, infarction, and brainstem or cervical cord injury may predispose the patient to respiratory arrest. Irreversible hypoxic ischemic injury may result. Death may follow.

Direct injuries are inflicted by blows to the head, impact of the cranium on an object such as a wall, or the brain impacting a rigid internal structure such as the pterion, rough floors of the anterior or middle cranial fossa, falx cerebri, or tentorium cerebelli. Direct impact may result in skull fractures, acute subdural hemorrhage (acute SDH), subarachnoid hemorrhage (SAH), contusions in the subjacent brain, parenchymal brain lacerations (PBLs) of the subcortical white matter in the young infant, and "contre-coup" injuries. **Importantly, victims of AHT commonly exhibit no skin, scalp, or calvarial evidence of trauma**, thus supporting shaking alone as the underpinning of intracranial hemorrhage and brain injury in AHT.

__(2-100A)__ Axial NECT in a 2m unresponsive boy shows SAH → and thin anterior, intermediate-attenuation subdural collections → (DDx being chronic SDH v. hematohygroma). Thin parafalcine convexal high-attenuation (acute) SDH was also detected (not shown). __(2-100B)__ Axial FLAIR MR performed 12 h after NECT shows enlarging SDHys →. These subdural collections followed CSF on all MR pulse sequences.

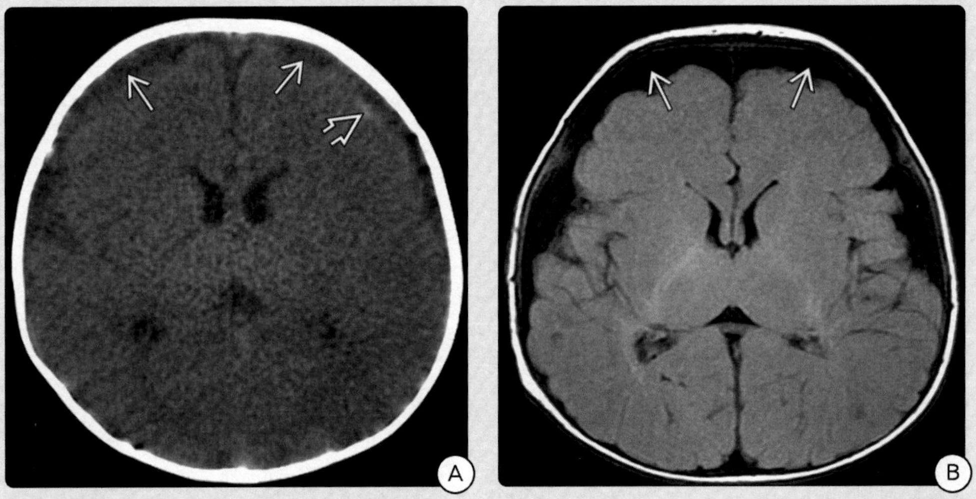

__(2-100C)__ Axial T2WI supports the CSF-like quality → of SDHy seen on prior FLAIR MR. Always consider trauma (accidental v. inflicted) as the etiology of SDHy in patients less than 2 y old. SDHy often enlarges quickly. __(2-100D)__ Coronal T2 GRE shows hypointense SAH → and thin bilateral peripheral SDHy →. SDHy follows CSF attenuation (CT) and intensity (MR). Note the small focus of ependymal → hemorrhage. Multiple acute rib fractures were detected.*

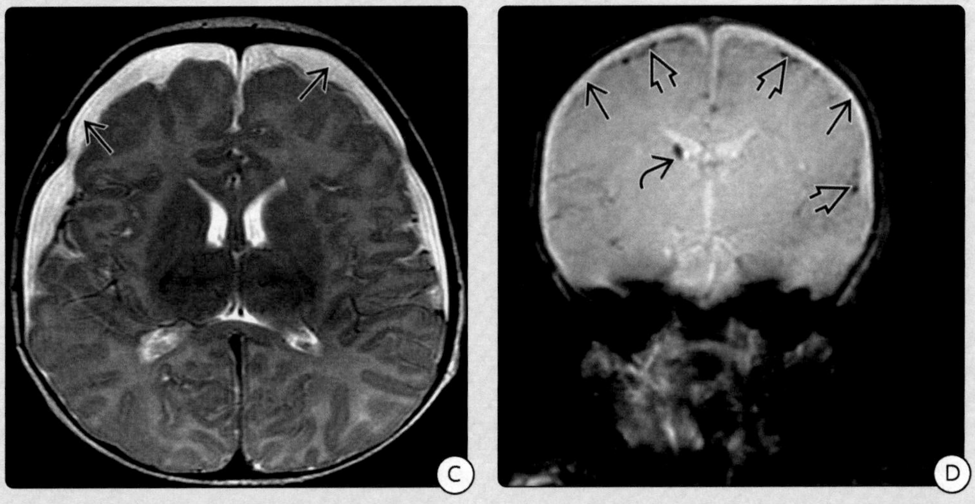

Indirect injuries of AHT lead to death and significant neurologic morbidity. The head of an infant or young child is relatively large compared with its body, cervical musculature is comparatively weak, and the incompletely myelinated cerebral white matter relatively fragile. Commotio motion alone (shaking) and potential for whiplash injury of the brainstem and upper cervical cord may lead to death. The most common result of shaking is diffusely distributed acute SDH. SAH is a common accompaniment of acute SDH. These extraaxial hemorrhages often represent proxies for underlying cerebral edema, early herniation, infarction, parenchymal contusions, subcortical laceration, and axonal shear injuries.

Pathology

SDH and subdural hygroma (SDHy) (CSF, CT attenuation, and MR signal intensity) detected in a child less than 2 years of age are strongly associated with trauma. SDH in a preambulatory infant (less than 1 year of age) or young child is highly suspicious for AHT. Subdural hematomas of differing ages support multiple traumatic insults and are common in AHT. SDH is the most common intracranial imaging finding in confirmed cases of AHT **(2-92A)**.

Clinical Issues

Epidemiology. In 2013, 678,932 cases of child abuse and neglect were reported in the United States. In that year, for infants, there were 23.1 victims per 1,000, and the estimated number of child abuse deaths was 1,520. Many more infants and children are left with permanent neurologic disability from abusive neurotrauma.

Although the magnitude of this health problem is sobering, the true prevalence of child abuse and neglect is unknown. Furthermore, the disruption of the family, community, and broader social fabric by this health blight and the psychosocial and economic impacts have yet to be fully illuminated.

Demographics. Trauma is the most common cause of death in childhood, and AHT is the most common cause of traumatic death and morbidity in infants (less than 1 year). Most abused children are less than 2 years of age. The peak age of inflicted injury is between 2 and 5 months. Although the majority of victims are male, in some cultures, female infants are more commonly injured.

No nationality or demographic group is exempt, and AHT can be found in all socioeconomic groups. Some predisposing factors include young age of the parents, single-parent households, domestic conflict, financial or emotional stress, and drug and alcohol abuse. Sadly, infants and young children with special needs are particularly at risk for inflicted injury.

Presentation. Clinical presentation of an abused child is variable. For the infant, nonspecific signs and symptoms may prevail, including lethargy, apnea, poor feeding, vomiting, irritability, unexplained weight loss, and macrocrania. More urgently, the infant or young child may present with seizure, respiratory distress, coma, and signs of cerebral herniation. There may be a lack of external signs of trauma. Retinal hemorrhages **(2-95)** are commonly detected in cases of AHT (80%). Discordance between stated history and severity of injury is common among victims of inflicted injury.

Patterned bruises, patches of torn hair, lip lacerations, and evidence of genital trauma raise the suspicion of inflicted injury and prompt appropriate imaging and consultation with the Child Protective Services team. It warrants repeating that the absence of external injuries (scalp, skull, skin, genitalia, and retinal hemorrhages) does not exclude AHT, nonneuro inflicted trauma, or neglect.

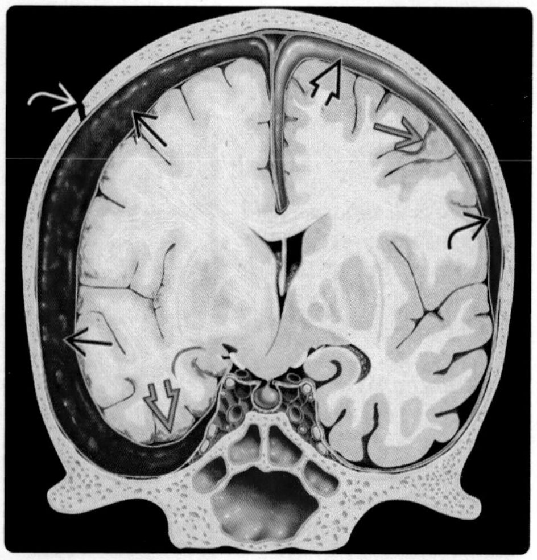

***(2-101)** Graphic shows aSDH ➡, subfalcine herniation, and cSDH ➡ with rebleed ➡. Note SAH ➡, cortical contusions ➡, and fracture ➡.*

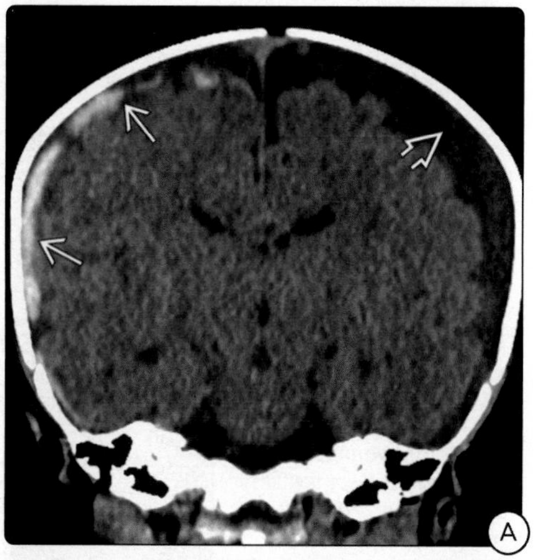

***(2-102A)** Coronal NECT in a battered infant girl shows aSDH ➡ and a large left holocranial low-attenuation subdural collection ➡.*

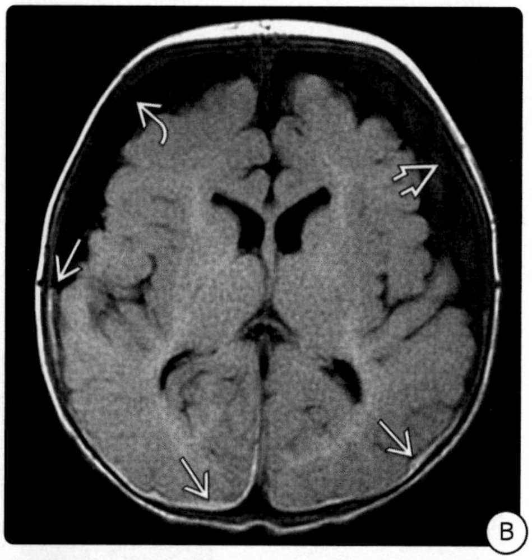

***(2-102B)** Axial FLAIR MR 24 h after NECT shows varied intensity subdural collections. Note hematocrit effect ➡, hygroma ➡, and cSDH ➡.*

(2-103) *Coronal NECT shows chronic SDH (cSDH) with bilateral intermediate-attenuation cSDHs. Thrombosed bridging vein and compressed subarachnoid spaces are seen. 3 days after this NECT, cSDHs were drained.* ***(2-104A)*** *Axial FLAIR of cSDH shows signal intensity greater than CSF. Membrane within the cSDH aids in dating the SDH as chronic. Compressed subarachnoid spaces and small rebleed are also seen.*

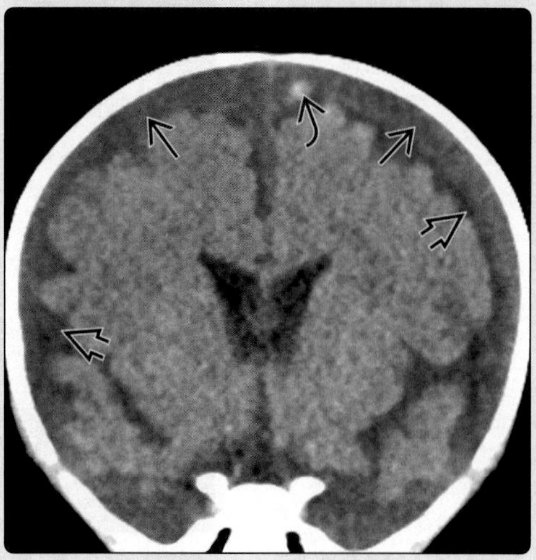

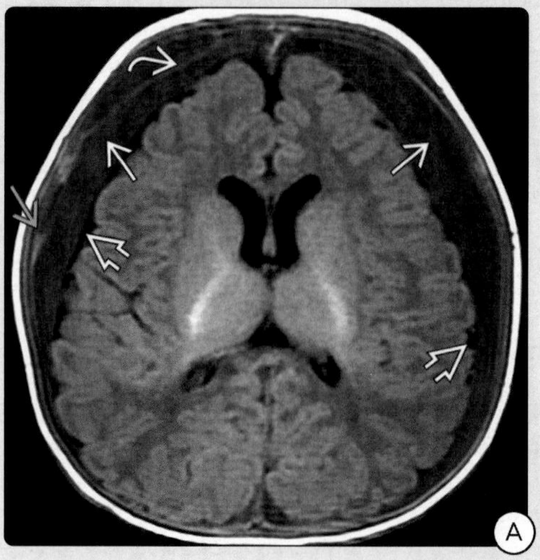

(2-104B) *T2WI shows large holocranial cSDHs slightly hypointense to CSF. Membranes are identified. Membranes represent a biomarker of cSDH and require 4-6 weeks to become macroscopically visible.* ***(2-104C)*** *Coronal FLAIR aids in depicting location of extraaxial fluid, fluid signal intensity, and membranes. Here, the cSDHs compress the subarachnoid spaces. Note the parafalcine membranes.*

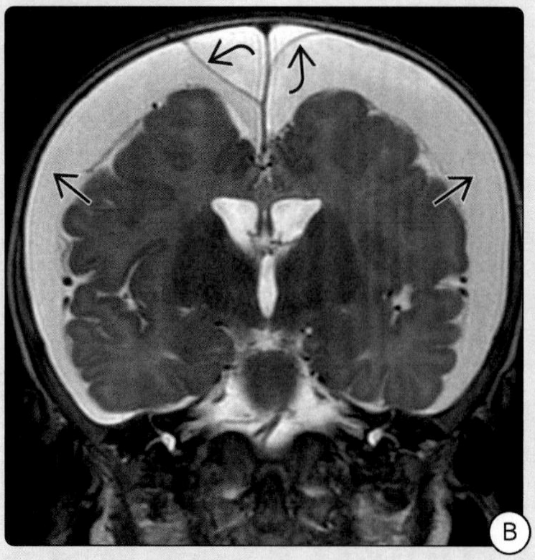

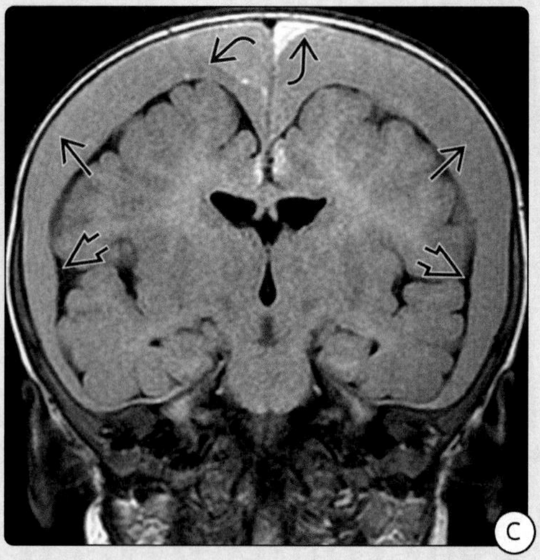

(2-104D) *Axial SWI reveals that cSDH on SWI and T2* GRE can look deceptively "simple," emphasizing the need to detect membranes when considering cSDHs. A small rebleed is seen here. Bilateral cSDHs were drained.* ***(2-104E)*** *Axial T1 C+ MR shows AHT and cSDH with enhancing membranes within the cSDHs. Also note the thick smooth bilateral enhancing endosteal dura.*

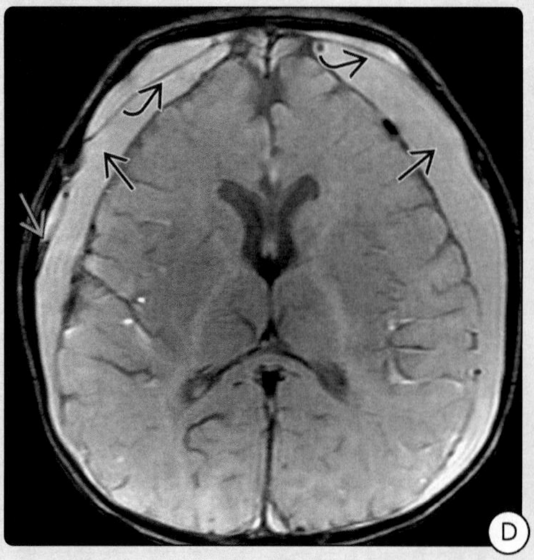

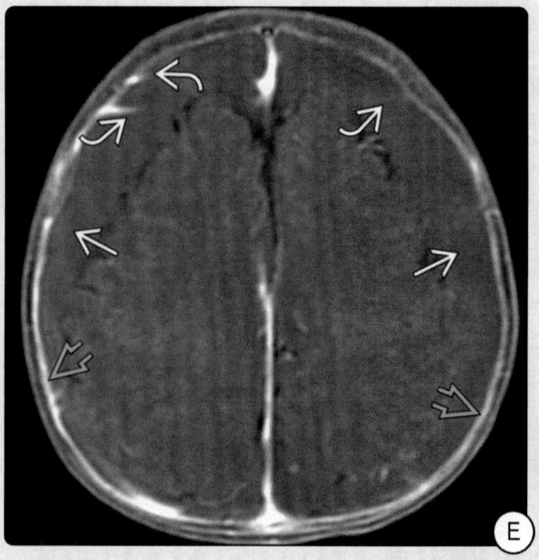

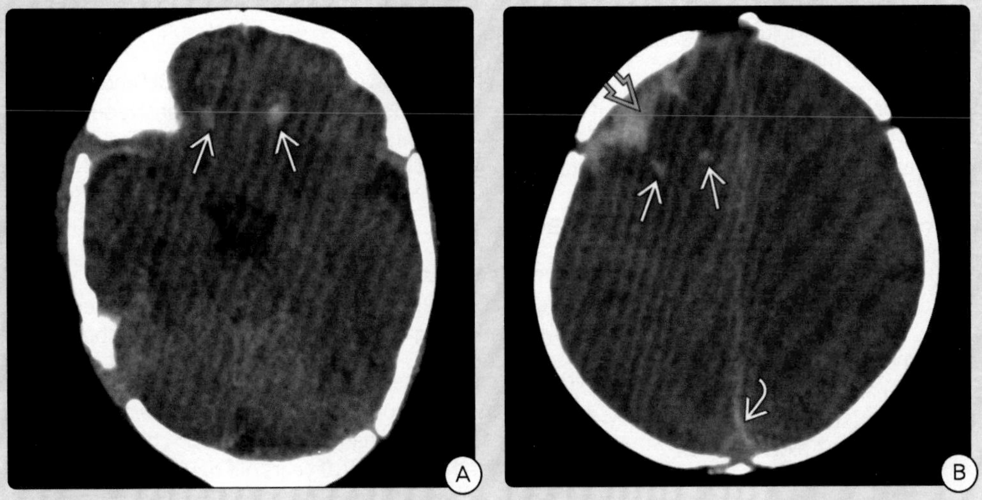

***(2-105A)** NECT shows bilateral parenchymal brain lacerations (PBLs) in a 3m male victim of confessed shaking injury. Note the inferior bilateral frontal subcortical parenchymal hemorrhages →. **(2-105B)** A more rostral NECT shows in this AHT victim combined right frontal PBLs → and frontal SDH and SAH →. Note the thin posterior parafalcine aSDH →. There was no evidence of blunt head trauma.*

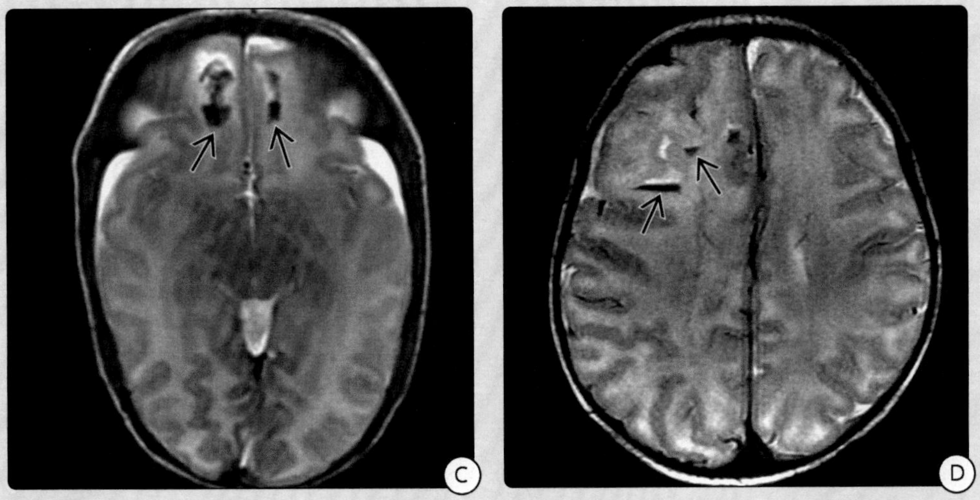

***(2-105C)** Axial T2WI shows frontal linear subcortical WM PBLs demonstrating hematocrit effect →. PBLs in the setting of AHT are most common in the first 6 mo of life. They represent a proxy for AHT. PBLs are uncommon in pediatric accidental head injury. **(2-105D)** Axial T2WI shows hematocrit levels within right frontal lobe PBLs →. PBLs in AHT involve the immature unmyelinated subcortical WM. The overlying cortex is intact.*

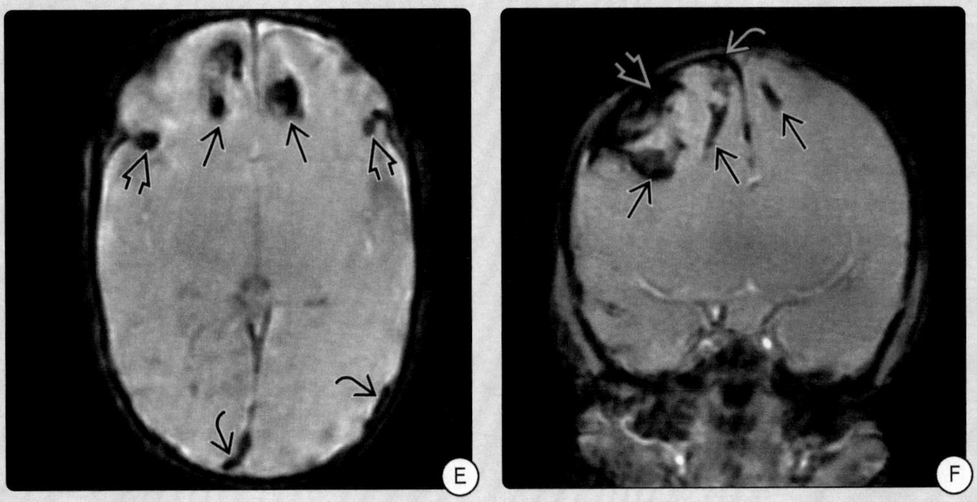

***(2-105E)** Axial SWI is a sensitive sequence to detect PBLs →. Also note the peri-pterional SAHs → and thin posterior SDHs →. PBLs occur in association with SDH and SAH. PBL injuries may appear remote from injury as subcortical WM clefts. **(2-105F)** Coronal SWI shows multiple WM lacerations (PBLs) → in association with right cerebral convexity subarachnoid and subdural hemorrhage →. Note the thin right frontal parafalcine SDH →.*

The main differential diagnosis is accidental injury, which is usually witnessed. Importantly, the intracranial injury patterns typical of AHT are not found in household falls < 3 feet.

Natural History. Early recognition of inflicted injury and intervention by Child Protective Services reduce mortality and morbidity. Finding evidence of repetitive violence indicates that the infant or child is at a higher risk for further injury and death. Mortality in AHT ranges from 15-60%, and morbidity is high. Posttraumatic brain damage with seizures and retardation are common, and the true prevalence is underestimated.

Treatment Options. The medical imperative is to protect the child. Radiologists are professionally mandated to clearly communicate any suspicion of abuse and the degree of certainty to appropriate clinicians. Notifying Child Protective Services of any suspected case of child abuse is legally required in many countries. All 50 states in the USA have statutes that mandate reporting cases of suspected child abuse or neglect.

The acute presentation of AHT with acute SDH and herniation will require emergent surgical drainage. Intensive supportive care is needed in the victim with seizures, encephalopathy, and acute cerebral injury.

Imaging

General Features. The Section on Radiology of the American Academy of Pediatrics recently updated its recommendations on diagnostic imaging in cases of suspected child abuse.

Initial imaging in cases of suspected child abuse should include a complete skeletal survey and NECT of the brain in the neurologically symptomatic infant or young child. MR is recommended for children 2 years old or younger. Ideally, we perform brain MR 3-5 days after admission to optimize the full appraisal of intracranial injury. MR detects thin-film SDHs over

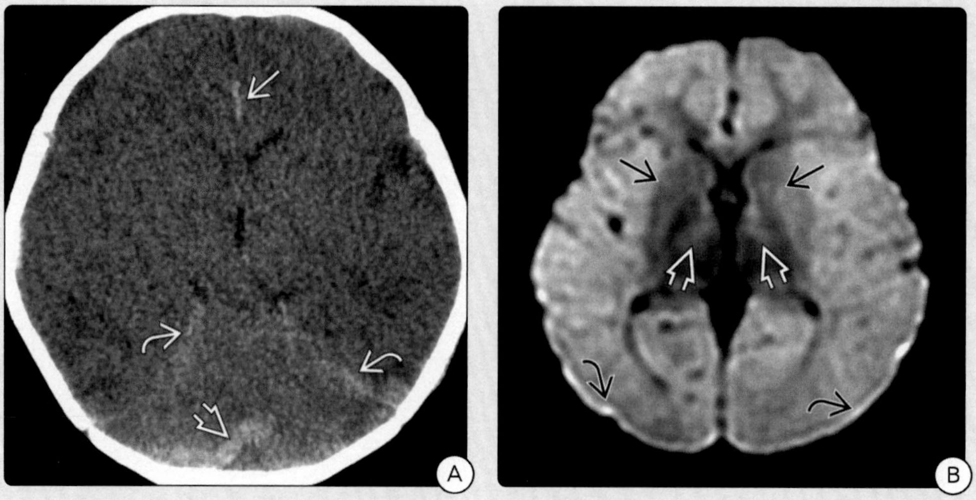

***(2-106A)** Axial NECT in AHT shows anterior parafalcine →, paratentorial →, and paratorcular → SDHs. Bilateral temporal lobe GM hypoattenuation > WM hypoattenuation (reversal sign). Cerebellum shows subtle increased attenuation (white cerebellum sign). **(2-106B)** Axial DWI shows diffuse cerebral hemispheric cortical and subcortical hyperintensity. Note focal hyperintensities within the BG → and thalami → and thin dependent SDHs →.*

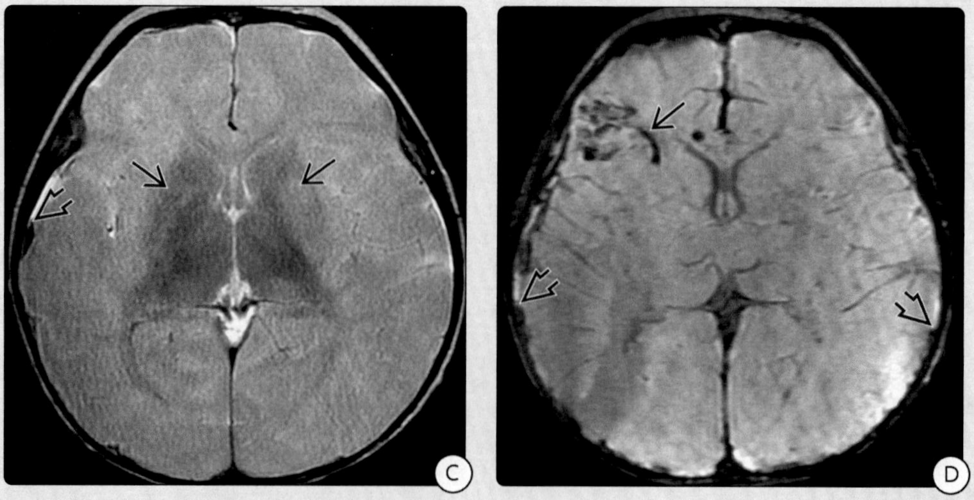

***(2-106C)** Axial T2WI shows diffuse cerebral hemispheric T2 prolongation and loss of normal GM-WM differentiation. Note the effaced cisterns, subarachnoid spaces, and lateral ventricles. Patchy BG hyperintensity is seen →. Note the thin lateral hematohygroma →. **(2-106D)** Axial SWI shows unexpected PBLs → in this 2m victim of shaking and strangulation. Bilateral hematohyromas are seen →. Patterned neck bruising was identified.*

the convexities and within the middle cranial fossa that were silent on NECT. MR contributes to the estimation of SDH age. Serial imaging (NECT and MR) plays an important role in dating AHT extraaxial hemorrhage and characterizing injury patterns.

Radiologists must resist strong dating language when reporting initial NECT findings in AHT. More precision in estimating hemorrhage age and magnitude of injury comes from serial imaging (NECT and MR). Experts emphasize that, although dating of both brain and skeletal injuries is imprecise, the more important goal is determining whether the pattern is that of "differing age" lesions regardless of location.

Birth related SDH is common, often asymptomatic, posteriorly located above and below the tentorium cerebelli, thin (< 3mm) and resolves by 1 month of age.

SDH discovered in the setting of Benign Expansion of the Subarachnoid Spaces (BESS) (a benign transient communicating form of hydrocephalus) in normally developing infants and young children are rare and warrant a thoughtful investigation by the child protective services team.

CT Findings. NECT including soft tissue and bone algorithms (including 3D surface-rendered modeling) with multiplanar reformatting is the minimum standard in the initial evaluation of AHT. Skull fractures are present in nearly half of all cases **(2-94)**, and scalp hematomas can be readily detected. Coronal **(2-92B)** and sagittal reformats detect small convexal SDHs. Sagittal reformations are particularly useful to detect peri-clival and cranial cervical junction hemorrhage that may reflect associated atlanto-occipital dissociation. When NECT is planned, omit skull radiographs from the skeletal series, thus reducing radiation exposure.

The identification and characterization of intracranial hemorrhage and detecting cerebral edema and herniation are critical. SDHs are shown in nearly 80% of all AHT cases **(2-92A)**. These are often thin film, parafalcine, and convexal in location. SAH accompanies SDH. Mixed-attenuation SDH is common in the acutely symptomatic AHT patient **(2-93A)**. Dependent SDH (hematohygroma and hematocrit effect) typically reflects a single event, not multiple bleeds **(2-99)**. SDHy (CSF-like on NECT) in children less than 2 years should be considered of traumatic etiology **(2-100)**. SDHy can enlarge rapidly. Epidural hematoma is rare in AHT. The presence of SDH and retinal hemorrhages increases the specificity of SDH as a proxy for AHT.

Causes of mixed-attenuation SDHs include the following: (1) acute SDH, (2) hyperacute + acute hemorrhage, (3) hematohygroma (SDH + CSF), and (4) old and new SDH **(2-102A)**. When there is associated underlying cerebral edema and herniation, invariably at the time of surgical drainage, the subdural collection is one of the first three considerations. Innocent rebleeding into a chronic SDH rarely leads to shift and cerebral edema.

The common origin of SDH and SAH in AHT are torn bridging veins (BVs) **(2-96A)**. On NECT, these appear as tubular or comma-shaped high-attenuation extraaxial collections over the parafalcine cerebral convexities. MR shows similarly shaped hypointensities on T2WI, GRE, and SWI. Underlying cerebral ischemia may be detected. These torn and thrombosed BVs represent a sign of trauma **(2-96)**.

Cortical contusions, PBLs **(2-105A)**, and occasionally diffuse axonal injuries may be detected with NECT, but MR more commonly identifies these abnormalities **(2-105C)**. Ischemic injury may also be present and varies from territorial infarcts to global hypoxic brain injury. Affected areas show NECT hypoattenuation.

Hemispheric or diffuse brain swelling occurs in some infants with acute subdural hematomas. This has been dubbed the "reversal sign" or "big black brain" for its striking low attenuation on NECT scans **(2-106A)**. Mortality is high in these cases. When "differing age" SDHs occur in the presence of severe hemisphere swelling, a "second-impact" type syndrome (see Chapter 3) from AHT should be considered.

MR Findings. SDHs of differing age on T1- and T2-weighted images showing mixed hyper-, hypo-, and isointense components are highly suggestive of AHT. FLAIR is helpful in compartmentalizing extraaxial collections and detecting small extraaxial collections (SDH, SDHy, and SAH) and white matter injury (PBLs) **(2-104C)**. SDH MR signal heterogeneity confounds estimates of blood dating. Use NECT and MR in conjunction for dating **(2-99)**.

Traumatic SDHy follows CSF on all MR pulse sequences **(2-100)**. Variance from this should invoke the radiologist to consider chronic SDH **(2-104)** vs. hematohygroma **(2-99)** in the differential diagnosis. Trauma, both accidental and inflicted, represents the most common causes of SDHy in a child less than 2 years of age.

T2* (GRE, SWI) scans are useful techniques for detecting blood products, particularly acute and subacute extraaxial and intraaxial hemorrhage, subtle petechial cortical contusions, PBLs, torn BVs, and hemorrhagic axonal injuries **(2-100D)** **(2-105F)**. Chronic convexity SDHs often lack susceptibility effect on T2* imaging (appearing deceptively as "simple fluid"); therefore, the radiologist must look for the presence of internal membrane structure within the SDH. DWI and ADC maps are essential for evaluating foci of ischemic injury **(2-104)**.

FLAIR, FSE T2, T2*, and post-IV contrast 3D T1-weighted imaging can detect membrane architecture within the SDH **(2-104)**. This is the best predictor of chronic SDH. Macroscopic subdural membrane formation within the SDH requires approximately 4-6 weeks to form. 3D post-IV contrast T1 imaging may display the traumatic disruption of BVs and the presence of traumatic cerebral sinovenous thrombosis **(2-98B)**.

DWI, ADC maps, DTI, FLAIR, and SWI provide insights into parenchymal injuries in AHT **(2-106B)**. Arterial spin labeling (ASL) pre- and postoperatively reflects alterations in cerebral blood flow following trauma **(2-93B)**. Altered cerebral vascular regulation is a pathophysiologic underpinning of the potentially catastrophic **second impact syndrome**.

Spine and spinal cord injuries are common in infants and children with shaking injuries. MR is the procedure of choice, as significant injuries can occur in the absence of fractures or subluxations. At our institution, MR of the cervical and thoracic spine is performed in conjunction with brain MR in the setting of suspected AHT.

Differential Diagnosis

Accidental traumatic brain injury is the most common differential diagnosis. Accidents are typically witnessed and more common after the child begins to ambulate. Household falls less than 3 feet do not result in imaging findings that mimic AHT. Accidental head trauma is more commonly impactive as opposed to the more common impulsive forces of AHT.

Other uncommon diagnoses such as **inborn error of metabolism** (e.g., glutaric aciduria and Menkes kinky hair syndrome) can cause retinal hemorrhages and bilateral SDHs.

Disorders of hemostasis can cause recurrent subdural hematomas. **Brain arteriovenous malformations** can cause intra- and extraaxial hemorrhage, and **metastatic neuroblastoma** with "raccoon eyes" can clinically mimic AHT. These uncommon "mimics" of AHT typically have compelling heritable, historical, clinical, and/or imaging features that sufficiently distinguish them from the imaging of inflicted injury and AHT. That being said, it is important to remember that infants and children with chronic illness and special needs are at higher risk for inflicted injury, including AHT.

Missile and Penetrating Injuries

The extent of tissue damage from a projectile depends on the type of bullet, its velocity and mass, and the physical characteristics of the affected tissues. Projectile craniocerebral injuries are qualitatively different from other traumatic brain injuries and from injuries in unconfined soft tissues with similar impact.

Although a detailed discussion of projectiles and their ballistics is beyond the scope of this text, we will briefly consider the ballistics of projectile injury and their craniocerebral consequences.

Readers interested in greater detail are referred to the definitive article by Jandial et al. 2008 (see Selected References). Much of the information on ballistics and tissue injury summarized below is derived from this excellent source.

Terminology

The high-velocity projectile brain injuries seen in noncombatant populations are predominantly gunshot wounds. Stabbing injuries inflicted by sharp objects such as a knife, screwdriver, or ice pick may also penetrate the calvaria and damage the underlying brain.

Etiology

The major factors that determine whether a projectile will penetrate the cranium are (1) its energy at impact on bone, (2) the contact area, and (3) the thickness of bone at the point of impact. Penetration by a ballistic projectile craters bone, punching it inward through the dura and into the brain.

The severity of tissue damage is proportional to the kinetic energy deposited in the tissue by the penetrating projectile *plus* a "rate effect" that is dependent on projectile size.

Pressure is very high at the tip of an advancing projectile. As a projectile penetrates the brain, it leaves a temporary cavity in

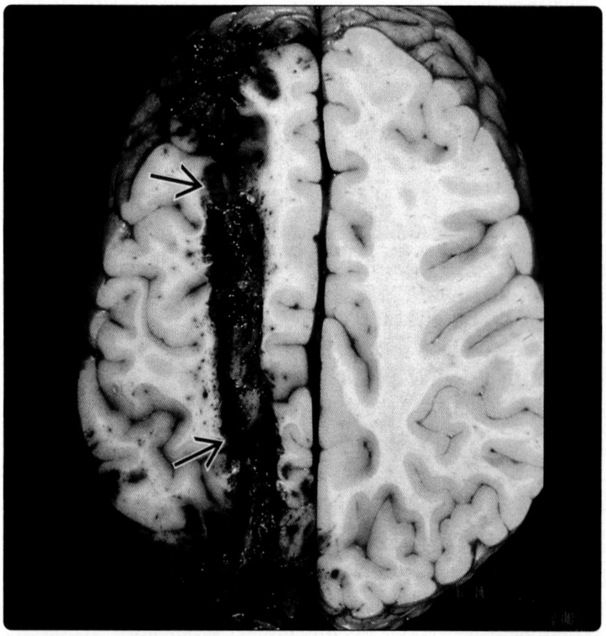

(2-107) Autopsy specimen from a patient with a gunshot wound from a 9-mm bullet shows the typical findings of a relatively high-velocity projectile, namely hemorrhage and disrupted macerated brain along the bullet path ⇨.

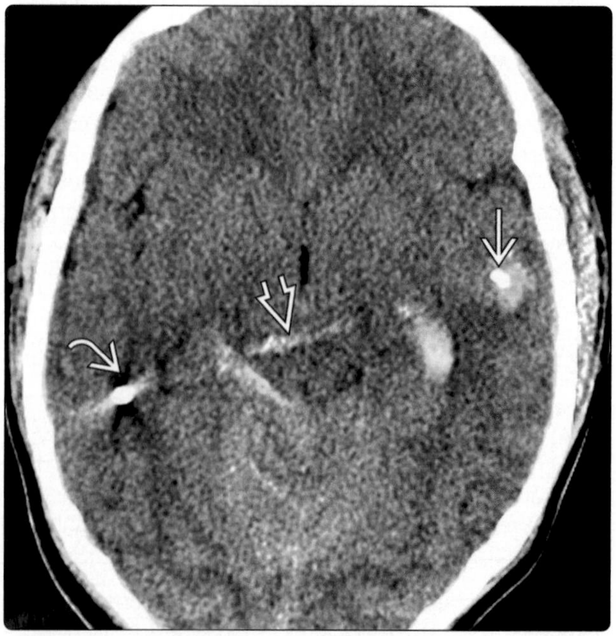

(2-108) NECT scan shows a low-velocity injury with a bullet fragment ➡, linear hemorrhage along a relatively narrow projectile path ➡, and a remaining fragment ➡ where the projectile slowed and then stopped.

its wake. It also causes outward radial stretching of adjacent tissue, depositing energy at very high strain rates.

As a bullet penetrates the brain, it yaws (not tumbles). This is why the entry wound is typically small and tissue damage expands as the bullet slows; the exit wound may be very large.

Projectiles with high kinetic energy may transfer enough energy to the skull to transform the bone fragments themselves into tiny secondary missiles. In the aggregate, these fragments can be just as lethal as through-and-through penetration by the projectile itself.

Pathology

The behavior of a projectile acting on tissue (the brain) that is anatomically constrained within a closed space (the skull) is different from injuries in unconfined soft tissue with similar impact.

Bullets passing through the firm brain tissue often take a slightly curved path between the entry point and final location. The trajectory is marked by macerated tissue, torn vessels, and disrupted axons **(2-107)**.

Clinical Issues

Presentation. Patients with gunshot wounds (GSWs) are overwhelmingly young males. Signs of brain swelling and herniation, including apnea and bradycardia, are common. The sudden increase in intracranial pressure caused by the cavitation and expansion of brain can cause coma or death, even if eloquent structures are not directly affected.

Patients with tangential GSWs commonly present with a fairly good GCS and no loss of consciousness. In these cases, the bullet typically does not breach the skull although the tangential GSWs may transfer considerable force to the brain and result in extraaxial hematoma, cortical contusion, and/or traumatic subarachnoid hemorrhage.

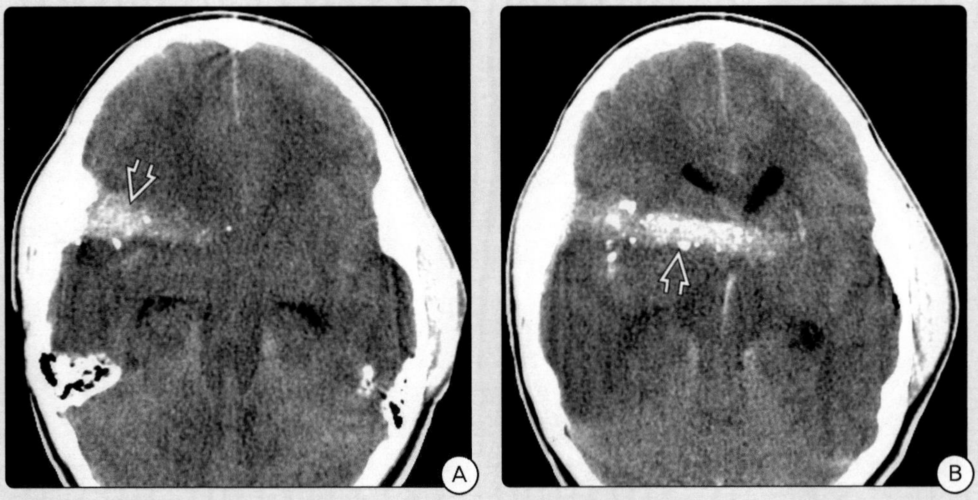

***(2-109A)** Series of NECTs depicts findings from a patient with a large-caliber, high-velocity gunshot wound. The entrance wound is through the squamous portion of the right temporal bone. Mass of blood, imploded bone, and a few bullet fragments ➪ are seen under the entrance wound. **(2-109B)** More cephalad scan shows the wide pathway ➪ formed by fragments that penetrated the brain at high velocity and high energy.*

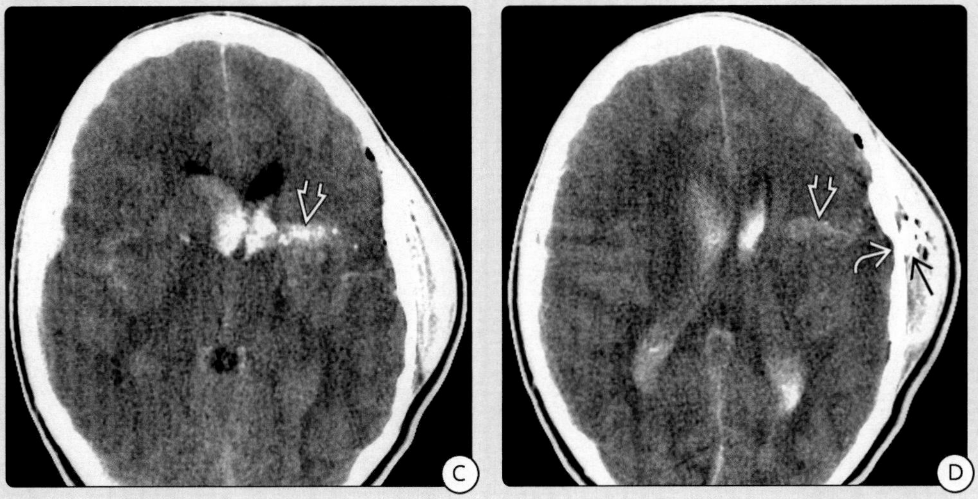

***(2-109C)** Scan through the frontal horns shows continuation of the pathway ➪ through the lateral ventricles. **(2-109D)** NECT through the upper lateral ventricles shows intraventricular hemorrhage. Blood is seen along the rest of the projectile pathway ➪. Enough kinetic energy was present to punch the remaining fragments through the left squamous temporal bone ➪, fracturing and exploding the skull outward ➔.*

Natural History. Prognosis is highly variable, ranging from death to full recovery. GSWs that have a central trajectory and are transventricular or bihemispheric have a high morbidity/mortality. Most fatalities occur within the first 24 hours after injury. Tangential GSWs with smaller-caliber, low-velocity bullets generally have a better outcome.

Imaging

The morphology of gunshot wounds is extremely variable. Injuries are most severe with large-caliber missiles traveling at high velocity that fragment early on entry into the cranium.

General Features. CT with both bone and soft tissue reconstruction is the diagnostic procedure of choice. The radiologist's report should identify the entry site, describe the missile path including bone fragmentation and ricochet paths **(2-110)**, and evaluate for exit wound. Possible damage to critical blood vessels should be noted along with secondary effects such as ischemia and herniation syndromes.

In general, a small-caliber, low-velocity projectile will have a relatively small linear track through the brain **(2-108)**. The track is larger with large-caliber, high-velocity bullets.

CT Findings. Entrance wounds are typically "punched-in" cones of bone. The bullet path is hyperdense and tends to curve slightly, broadening as the bullet yaws and slows. Bullet and bone fragments should be noted. The exit wound is typically either a ledge-shaped fracture or "punched-out" bone **(2-109)**. Pneumocephalus may be present.

Angiography. CTA with multiplanar reconstruction and MIP images is helpful in evaluating vascular injuries such as pseudoaneurysm, dissection, traumatic dural arteriovenous fistula, and venous injury or thrombosis.

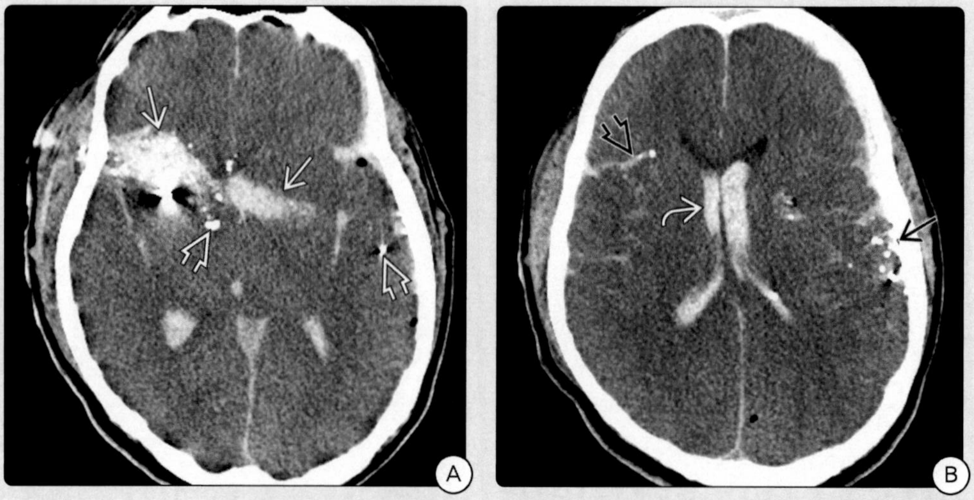

***(2-110A)** NECT in a 42y man who attempted suicide with a .22 pistol shows a cone-shaped track of hemorrhage ➡ and bullet fragments ➡. The brain exhibits diffuse low density without gray-white matter differentiation. The small lateral ventricles are filled with hemorrhage. **(2-110B)** Cephalad NECT shows intraventricular ➡ and subarachnoid ➡ blood. Small bullet fragments ➡ have lodged adjacent to the inner table of the skull.*

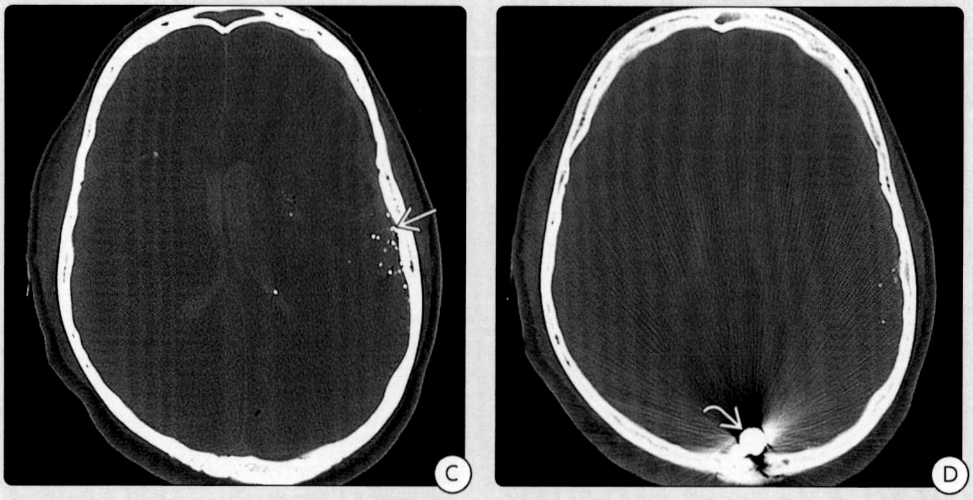

***(2-110C)** Bone CT shows numerous small bullet fragments ➡ adjacent to the inner table of the left parietooccipital bone. There is no overlying skull fracture. **(2-110D)** More cephalad bone CT shows that the low-caliber bullet ➡ has ricocheted from the inner table of the skull and lodged adjacent to the occipital bone without penetrating the skull.*

Selected References

Scalp and Skull Injuries

Leibu S et al: Clinical significance of long-term follow-up of children with posttraumatic skull base fracture. World Neurosurg. ePub, 2017

Rodà D et al: Epidemiology of fractures in children younger than 12 months. Pediatr Emerg Care. ePub, 2017

Sellin JN et al: Children presenting in delayed fashion after minor head trauma with scalp swelling: do they require further workup? Childs Nerv Syst. 33(4):647-652, 2017

Lolli V et al: MDCT imaging of traumatic brain injury. Br J Radiol. 89(1061):20150849, 2016

Fowler TR et al: Detecting foreign bodies in a head laceration. Case Rep Emerg Med. 2015:801676, 2015

Facial Injuries

Holmgren EP et al: Facial soft tissue injuries as an aid to ordering a combination head and facial computed tomography in trauma patients. J Oral Maxillofac Surg. 63(5):651-4, 2005

Skull Fractures

Arrey EN et al: Linear nondisplaced skull fractures in children: who should be observed or admitted? J Neurosurg Pediatr. 16(6):703-8, 2015

Orman G et al: Pediatric skull fracture diagnosis: should 3D CT reconstructions be added as routine imaging? J Neurosurg Pediatr. 16(4):426-31, 2015

Baugnon KL et al: Skull base fractures and their complications. Neuroimaging Clin N Am. 24(3):439-65, vii-viii, 2014

Extraaxial Hemorrhages

Arterial Epidural Hematoma

Peres CM et al: Endovascular management of acute epidural hematomas: clinical experience with 80 cases. J Neurosurg. 1-7, 2017

Basamh M et al: Epidural hematoma treated conservatively: when to expect the worst. Can J Neurol Sci. 43(1):74-81, 2016

Venous Epidural Hematoma

Singh S et al: Compression of the posterior fossa venous sinuses by epidural hemorrhage simulating venous sinus thrombosis: CT and MR findings. Pediatr Radiol. 46(1):67-72, 2016

Li J et al: Risk factors and early diagnosis of cerebral venous sinus occlusion secondary to traumatic brain injury. Neurol India. 63(6):881-8, 2015

Acute Subdural Hematoma

Al-Mufti F et al: Neurocritical care of acute subdural hemorrhage. Neurosurg Clin N Am. 28(2):267-278, 2017

Howard BM et al: Management and outcomes of isolated tentorial and parafalcine "smear" subdural hematomas at a level-1 trauma center: necessity of high acuity care. J Neurotrauma. 34(1):128-136, 2017

Vega RA et al: Natural history of acute subdural hematoma. Neurosurg Clin N Am. 28(2):247-255, 2017

Bajsarowicz P et al: Nonsurgical acute traumatic subdural hematoma: what is the risk? J Neurosurg. 1-8, 2015

Bartels RH et al: Midline shift in relation to thickness of traumatic acute subdural hematoma predicts mortality. BMC Neurol. 15:220, 2015

Cepeda S et al: Traumatic intracerebral hemorrhage: risk factors associated with progression. J Neurotrauma. 32(16):1246-53, 2015

Chronic/Mixed Subdural Hematoma

Castellani RJ et al: Symptomatic acute-on-chronic subdural hematoma: a clinicopathological study. Am J Forensic Med Pathol. 38(2):126-130, 2017

Rovlias A et al: Chronic subdural hematoma: surgical management and outcome in 986 cases: A classification and regression tree approach. Surg Neurol Int. 6:127, 2015

Traumatic Subarachnoid Hemorrhage

Balinger KJ et al: Selective computed tomographic angiography in traumatic subarachnoid hemorrhage: a pilot study. J Surg Res. 199(1):183-9, 2015

Parenchymal Injuries

Cerebral Contusions and Lacerations

Allison RZ et al: Derivation of a predictive score for hemorrhagic progression of cerebral contusions in moderate and severe traumatic brain injury. Neurocrit Care. 26(1):80-86, 2017

Yuan Q et al: FVIIa prevents the progressive hemorrhaging of a brain contusion by protecting microvessels via formation of the TF-FVIIa-FXa complex. Neuroscience. 348:114-125, 2017

Diffuse Axonal Injury

Abu Hamdeh S et al: Extended anatomical grading in diffuse axonal injury using MRI: hemorrhagic lesions in the substantia nigra and mesencephalic tegmentum indicate poor long-term outcome. J Neurotrauma. 34(2):341-352, 2017

Davceva N et al: Traumatic axonal injury, a clinical-pathological correlation. J Forensic Leg Med. 48:35-40, 2017

Izzy S et al: Revisiting grade 3 diffuse axonal injury: not all brainstem microbleeds are prognostically equal. Neurocrit Care. ePub, 2017

Zhao W et al: White matter injury susceptibility via fiber strain evaluation using whole-brain tractography. J Neurotrauma. 33(20):1834-1847, 2016

Miscellaneous Injuries

Pneumocephalus

Dabdoub CB et al: Review of the management of pneumocephalus. Surg Neurol Int. 6:155, 2015

Abusive Head Trauma (Child Abuse)

Expert Panel on Pediatric Imaging et al: ACR Appropriateness Criteria® suspected physical abuse-child. J Am Coll Radiol. 14(5S):S338-S349, 2017

Kralik SF et al: Radiologic head CT interpretation errors in pediatric abusive and non-abusive head trauma patients. Pediatr Radiol. ePub, 2017

Wright JN: CNS injuries in abusive head trauma. AJR Am J Roentgenol. 28:1-11, 2017

Zuccoli G et al: In vivo demonstration of traumatic rupture of the bridging veins in abusive head trauma. Pediatr Neurol. ePub, 2017

Girard N et al: Neuroimaging differential diagnoses to abusive head trauma. Pediatr Radiol. 46(5):603-14, 2016

Palifka LA et al: Parenchymal brain laceration as a predictor of abusive head trauma. AJNR Am J Neuroradiol. 37(1):163-8, 2016

Grant EP. Abusive head trauma: parenchymal injury. In: Diagnostic Imaging of Child Abuse, 3e, edited by Kleinman PK. Cambridge, UK: University of Cambridge Press, 2015, pp 453-486

Hedlund G. Abusive head trauma: extra-axial hemorrhage and nonhemic collections. In: Diagnostic Imaging of Child Abuse, 3e, edited by Kleinman PK. Cambridge, UK: University of Cambridge Press, 2015, pp 394-452

Hahnemann ML et al: Imaging of bridging vein thrombosis in infants with abusive head trauma: the "Tadpole Sign". Eur Radiol. 25(2):299-305, 2015

Li J et al: Risk factors and early diagnosis of cerebral venous sinus occlusion secondary to traumatic brain injury. Neurol India. 63(6):881-8, 2015

Wittschieber D et al: Subdural hygromas in abusive head trauma: pathogenesis, diagnosis, and forensic implications. AJNR Am J Neuroradiol. 36(3):432-9, 2015

Adamsbaum C et al: Dating the abusive head trauma episode and perpetrator statements: key points for imaging. Pediatr Radiol. 44 Suppl 4:S578-88, 2014

US Department of Health and Human Services and Children's Bureau, Administration on Children, Youth and Families. Child Maltreatment 2013.

Adamsbaum C et al: Abusive head trauma: don't overlook bridging vein thrombosis. Pediatr Radiol. 42(11):1298-300, 2012

Tung G. Imaging of abusive head trauma. In: Child Abuse and Neglect, edited by Jenny C. St. Louis, MO: Elsevier, 2011, pp 373-391

Missile and Penetrating Injuries

Feldman KA et al: Predictors of mortality in pediatric urban firearm injuries. Pediatr Surg Int. 33(1):53-58, 2017

DeCuypere M et al: Pediatric intracranial gunshot wounds: the Memphis experience. J Neurosurg Pediatr. 17(5):595-601, 2016

Jandial R et al: Ballistics for the neurosurgeon. Neurosurgery. 62(2):472-80; discussion 480, 2008

Secondary Effects and Sequelae of CNS Trauma

Traumatic brain injury (TBI) is not a single "one and done" event. TBI is an ongoing series of pathophysiologic reactions that extends from the moment of injury for days, months, or even years into the future. Acute TBI is just the initial triggering insult.

A veritable "cascade" of adverse pathophysiologic events continues to develop after the initial injury. Some—such as progressive hemorrhagic injury—occur within the first 24 hours after trauma. Others (e.g., brain swelling and herniation syndromes) may take a day or two to develop. Delayed complications such as CSF leaks and intracranial hypotension may develop weeks or months later. Finally, there is a broad spectrum of posttraumatic encephalopathic syndromes that may manifest years or even decades later.

Secondary effects of CNS trauma are defined as those that occur after the initial injury. These secondary effects are often more devastating than the initial injury itself and can become life-threatening. Whereas many of the primary effects of CNS trauma (e.g., cortical contusions and axonal injuries) are permanent injuries, some secondary effects are either preventable or treatable.

Many potentially serious secondary effects are at least partially reversible if recognized early and treated promptly. Emergent imaging assessment together with aggressive management of elevated intracranial pressure, perfusion alterations, and oxygenation deficits may help mitigate both the immediate and long-term effects of brain trauma.

Chapter 2 focused on the primary effects of TBI. In this chapter, we consider a broad spectrum of secondary effects that follow brain trauma, beginning with herniation syndromes.

Herniation Syndromes

Brain herniations occur when one or more structures is displaced from its normal or "native" compartment into an adjacent space. They are the most common secondary manifestation of *any* expanding intracranial mass, regardless of etiology.

In this section, we briefly discuss the relevant anatomy and physiology that explain the pathology underlying brain herniations. We then delineate the spectrum of brain herniations and their imaging findings, beginning with the most common types (subfalcine and descending transtentorial herniation). Posterior fossa herniations (ascending transtentorial and tonsillar herniations) are then considered. We conclude the discussion with a brief consideration of rare but important types of herniations, such as

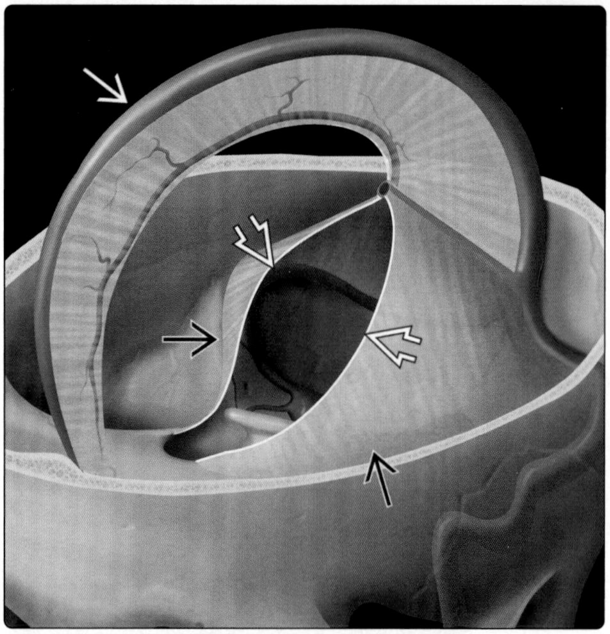

(3-1) Falx cerebri ➡ divides the supratentorial compartment into 2 halves. The tentorium ⇨ separates the supra- from the infratentorial compartment. Medial borders of the tentorium form a U-shaped opening ➡, the tentorial incisura.

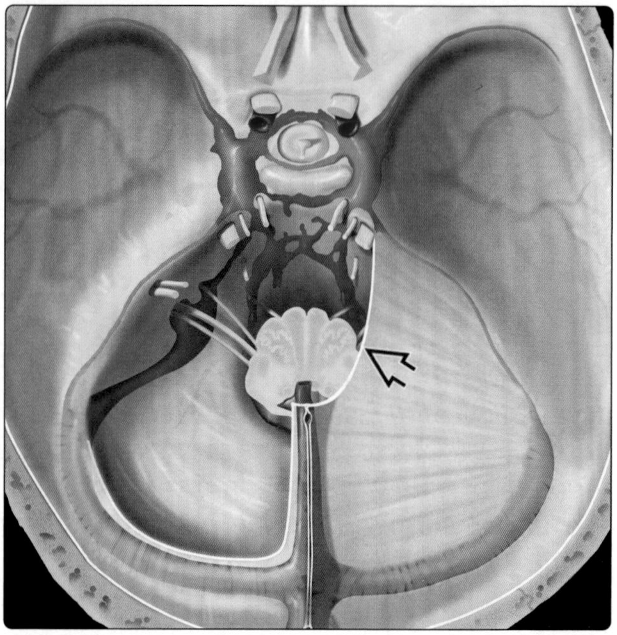

(3-2) The right half of the tentorium has been removed to show the posterior fossa. The left half is shown forming the edge of the tentorial incisura ⇨.

transdural/transcranial herniations and brain displacements that occur across the sphenoid wing.

Relevant Anatomy

Bony ridges and dural folds divide the intracranial cavity into three compartments: two supratentorial hemicrania (the right and left halves) and the posterior fossa **(3-1)**.

The dura mater consists of two layers, an outer (periosteal) and an inner (meningeal) layer. The periosteal layer is tightly applied to the inner surface of the calvaria, especially at suture lines. The meningeal layer folds inward to form two important fibrocollagenous sheets, the falx cerebri and tentorium cerebelli. The falx cerebri separates the right and left hemispheres from each other, whereas the tentorium cerebelli separates the supratentorial from the infratentorial compartment.

The **falx cerebri** is a broad, sickle-shaped dural fold that attaches superiorly to the inside of the skull on either side of the midline, where it contains the superior sagittal sinus (SSS). The falx descends vertically within the interhemispheric fissure. It is shorter in front, where it is attached to the crista galli, and gradually deepens as it extends posteriorly.

The concave inferior "free" margin of the falx contains the inferior sagittal sinus. As it courses posteriorly, the inferior margin of the falx forms a large open space above the corpus callosum and cingulate gyrus. This open space allows potential displacement of brain and blood vessels from one side toward the other. The opening is largest in the front and becomes progressively smaller, ending where the falx joins the tentorium cerebelli at its apex.

The **tentorium cerebelli** is a tent-shaped dural sheet that extends inferolaterally from its confluence with the falx, where their two merging dural folds contain the straight sinus. The straight sinus courses posteroinferiorly toward the sinus confluence with the SSS and transverse sinuses.

The tentorium is attached laterally to the petrous ridges, anteroinferiorly to the dorsum sellae, and posteriorly to the occipital bone. It has two concave medial edges that contain a large U-shaped opening called the **tentorial incisura (3-2)**. Displacement of brain structures and accompanying blood vessels from the supratentorial compartment or posterior fossa can occur in either direction—up or down—through the tentorial incisura.

Relevant Physiology

Once the sutures fuse and the fontanelles close, brain, CSF, and blood all coexist in a rigid, unyielding "bone box." The cerebral blood volume, perfusion, and CSF volume exist in a delicate balance within this closed box. Under normal conditions, pressures within the brain parenchyma and intracranial CSF spaces are equal.

The **Monro-Kellie hypothesis** states, "The sum of volumes of brain, CSF, and intracranial blood is constant in an intact skull. An increase in one should cause a decrease in one or both of the remaining two." Accordingly, any increase in intracranial volume from whatever source (blood, edema, tumor, etc.) requires a compensatory and equal decrease in the other contents.

When extra volume (blood, edema, tumor, etc.) is added to a cranial compartment, CSF in the sulci and subarachnoid cisterns is initially squeezed out. The ipsilateral ventricle becomes compressed and decreases in size. As intracranial volume continues to increase, the mass effect eventually exceeds the brain's compensatory capacity, and intracranial pressure (ICP) begins to rise.

If a mass becomes sufficiently large, brain, CSF spaces, and blood vessels are displaced from one intracranial compartment into an adjacent one, resulting in one or more cerebral herniations.

In turn, cerebral herniations may cause their own cascade of secondary effects. Parenchyma, cranial nerves, and/or blood vessels can become compressed against the adjacent unyielding bone and dura. Secondary ischemic changes, frank brain infarcts, cranial neuropathies, and focal neurologic deficits may develop.

If treatment is unavailable or unsuccessful, severe neurologic damage or even death is the result of what becomes, in essence, a brain "compartment syndrome."

Subfalcine Herniation

Terminology and Etiology

Subfalcine herniation (SFH) is the most common cerebral herniation and the easiest to understand. In a simple uncomplicated SFH, an enlarging supratentorial mass in one hemicranium causes the brain to begin shifting toward the opposite side. Herniation occurs as the affected hemisphere pushes across the midline under the inferior "free" margin of the falx, extending into the contralateral hemicranium **(3-3)** **(3-5)**.

Imaging

Mass effect displaces the brain from one side toward the other. The ipsilateral ventricle appears compressed and displaced across the midline, while the contralateral ventricle

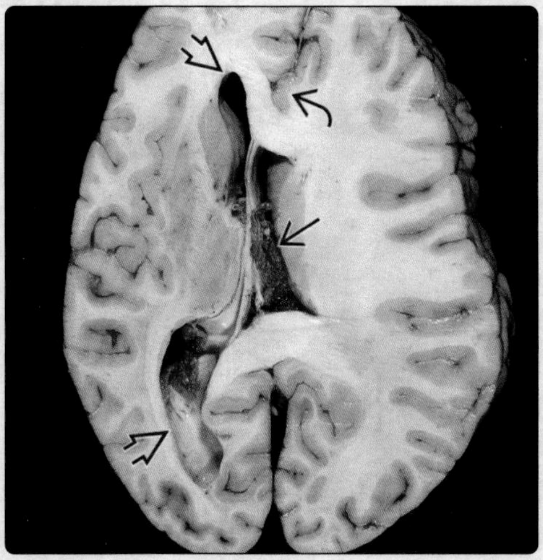

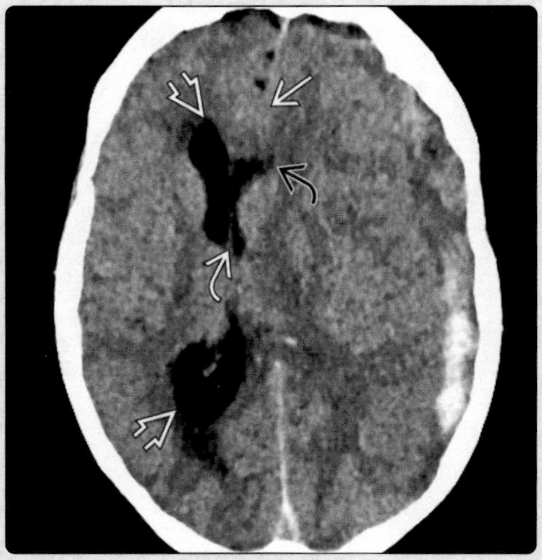

***(3-3)** Autopsy shows subfalcine herniation. Left lateral ventricle is compressed →, shifted across midline, as is cingulate gyrus →. Right lateral ventricle → is enlarged secondary to obstructed foramen of Monro. (Courtesy R. Hewlett, MD.) **(3-4)** NECT shows SDH with subfalcine herniation of cingulate gyrus →, compression of left lateral ventricle →, foramen of Monro obstruction →, and enlarged right lateral ventricle →.*

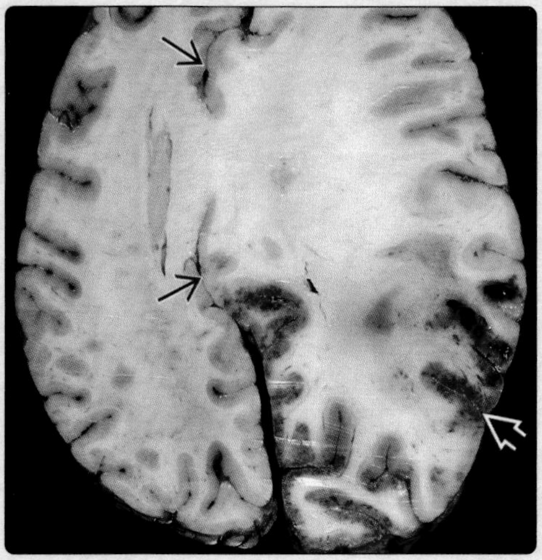

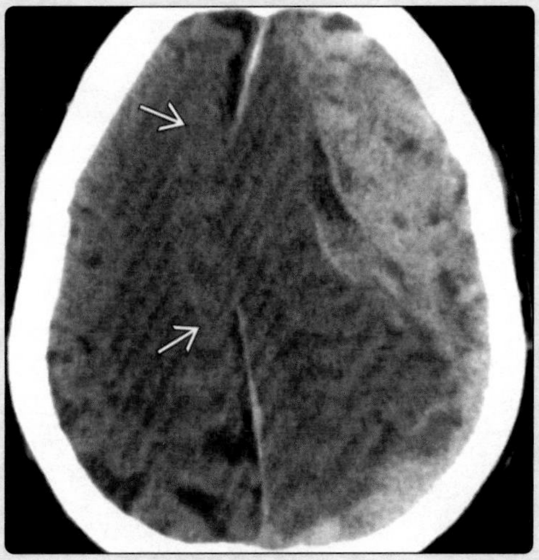

***(3-5)** Autopsy shows massive left hemisphere swelling with subfalcine herniation of cingulate gyrus →. Secondary left posterior cerebral artery hemorrhagic infarct → was caused by DTH. (Courtesy R. Hewlett, MD.) **(3-6)** An 80y anticoagulated man had a ground-level fall. NECT shows rapidly bleeding aSDH, subfalcine herniation of cingulate gyrus → under the falx cerebri, which is bowed by the mass effect.*

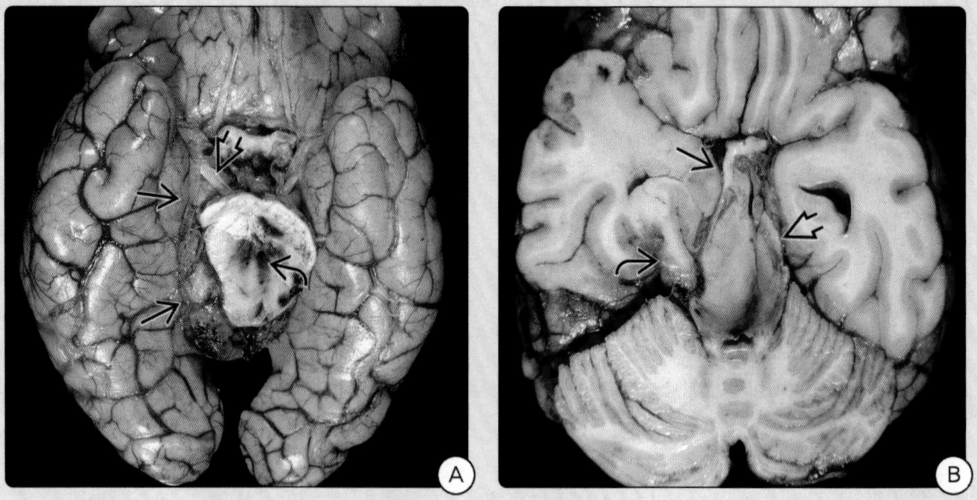

(3-7A) *Autopsy shows DTH. Right uncus and hippocampus are displaced medially and demonstrate "grooving" caused by impaction against tentorial incisura. CN III is compressed by herniating temporal lobe. Midbrain ("Duret") hemorrhage is present.* ***(3-7B)*** *Section shows uncal, hippocampal herniation compressing midbrain against the opposite edge of the tentorium ("Kernohan notch"). (Courtesy R. Hewlett, MD.)*

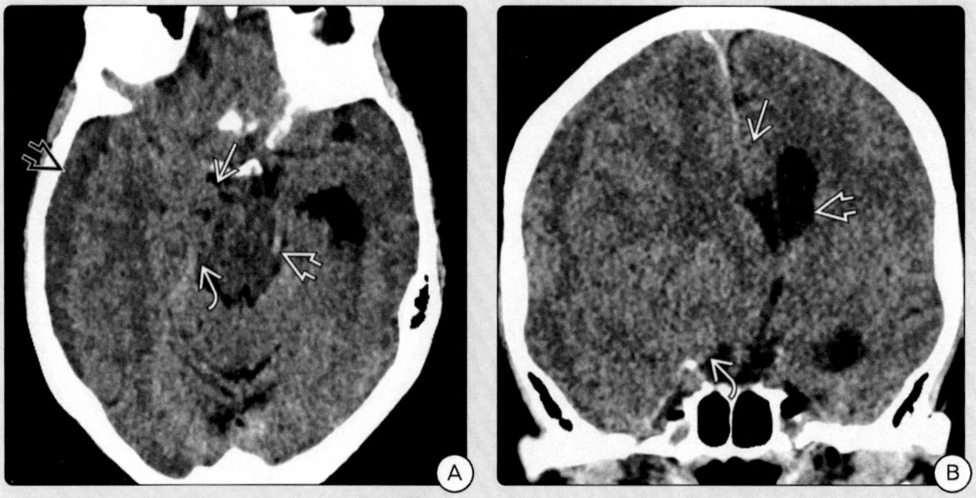

(3-8A) *Axial NECT shows a subacute SDH, descending transtentorial herniation of uncus, and hippocampus. The midbrain is compressed against the contralateral edge of the tentorial incisura.* ***(3-8B)*** *Coronal scan in the same case shows herniation of the cingulate gyrus under the falx cerebri, herniation of the uncus into the suprasellar cistern. The contralateral ventricle is obstructed, enlarged.*

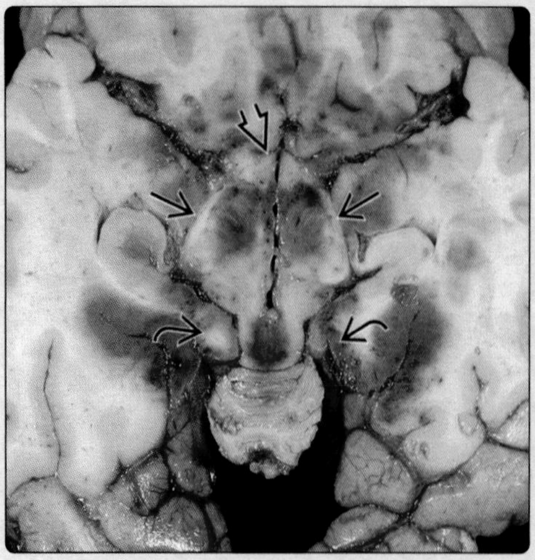

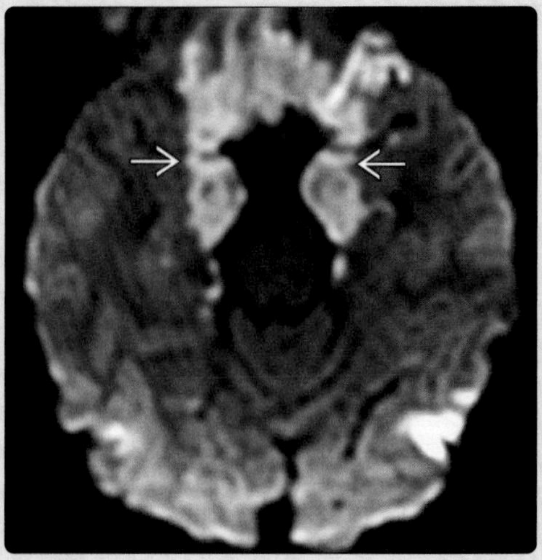

(3-9) *Autopsy of complete bilateral ("central") descending transtentorial herniation shows suprasellar cistern is obliterated by the inferiorly displaced hypothalamus. The uncus and hippocampus of both temporal lobes are herniated medially and inferiorly into the tentorial incisura. (Courtesy R. Hewlett, MD.)* ***(3-10)*** *DWI after central DTH shows restricted diffusion in the same areas.*

enlarges **(3-6)**. The cingulate gyrus and accompanying anterior cerebral arteries herniate under the falx **(3-6)**.

Complications

Early complications of SFH include unilateral hydrocephalus, seen on axial NECT as enlargement of the contralateral ventricle. As the mass effect increases, the lateral ventricles become progressively more displaced across the midline. This displacement initially just deforms, then kinks, and eventually occludes the foramen of Monro.

The choroid plexus in the contralateral ventricle continues to secrete CSF. Because the foramen of Monro is obstructed, CSF has no egress, causing the lateral ventricle to enlarge **(3-8)**. Severe unilateral obstructive hydrocephalus reduces drainage of extracellular fluid into the deep subependymal veins. Fluid accumulates in the periventricular white matter and is seen on NECT as periventricular hypodensity with "blurred" margins of the lateral ventricle.

If SFH becomes severe, the herniating anterior cerebral artery (ACA) can become pinned against the inferior "free" margin of the falx cerebri and then occluded, causing secondary infarction of the cingulate gyrus (see below).

SUBFALCINE HERNIATION

Etiology and Pathology
- Unilateral hemispheric mass effect
- Brain shifts across midline under falx cerebri

Epidemiology
- Most common cerebral herniation

Imaging
- Cingulate gyrus, ACA, internal cerebral veins displaced across midline
- Foramen of Monro kinked, obstructed
- Ipsilateral ventricle small, contralateral enlarged

Complications
- Obstructive hydrocephalus
- Secondary ACA infarction (severe cases)

Descending Transtentorial Herniation

Transtentorial herniations are brain displacements that occur through the tentorial incisura. Although these displacements can occur in both directions (from top down or bottom up), descending herniations from supratentorial masses are far more common than ascending herniations.

Terminology and Etiology

Descending transtentorial herniation (DTH) is the second most common type of intracranial herniation syndrome. DTH is caused by a hemispheric mass that initially produces side-to-side brain displacement (i.e., SFH). As the mass effect increases, the uncus of the temporal lobe is pushed medially and begins to encroach on the suprasellar cistern. The hippocampus soon follows and starts to efface the ipsilateral quadrigeminal cistern.

With progressively increasing mass effect, both the uncus and hippocampus herniate inferiorly through the tentorial incisura **(3-7)**.

DTH can be unilateral or bilateral. **Unilateral DTH** occurs when a hemispheric mass effect pushes the uncus and hippocampus of the ipsilateral temporal lobe over the edge of the tentorial incisura. In **bilateral DTH**, both temporal lobes are displaced medially.

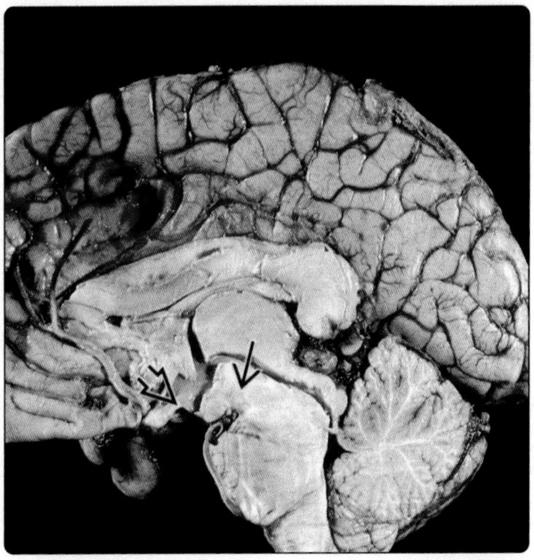

***(3-11)** Complete DTH shows midbrain is kinked inferiorly ➡, hypothalamus is smashed over dorsum sellae ➡. (Courtesy R. Hewlett, MD.)*

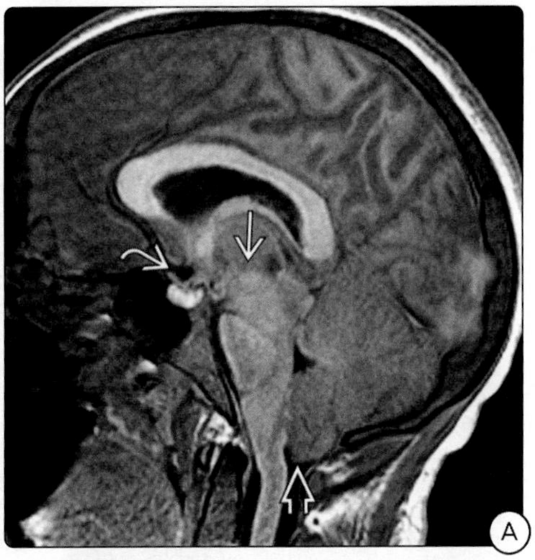

***(3-12A)** MP-RAGE shows complete DTH with obliterated suprasellar cistern ➡, downwardly displaced midbrain ➡, tonsillar herniation ➡.*

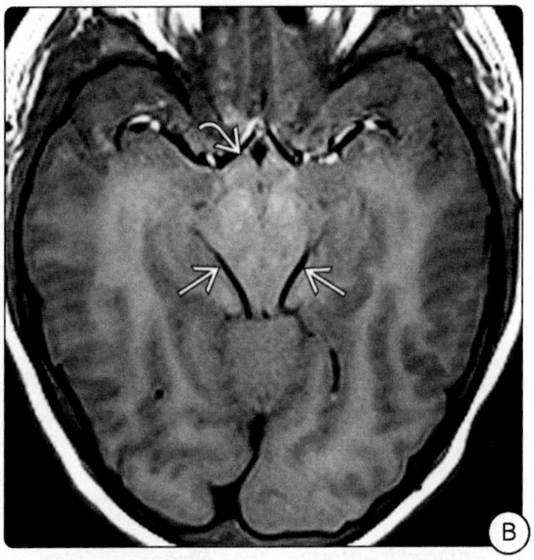

***(3-12B)** Axial T1WI in the same case shows obliterated suprasellar cistern ➡, herniating hippocampi causing midbrain compression ➡.*

"Complete" or **"central" descending herniation** occurs when the supratentorial mass effect becomes so severe that the hypothalamus and optic chiasm are flattened against the skull base, *both* temporal lobes are herniated, and the whole tentorial incisura is completely plugged with displaced tissue **(3-9)**.

Imaging

Axial CT scans in early **unilateral DTH** show that the uncus is displaced medially and the ipsilateral aspect of the suprasellar cistern is effaced **(3-8A)**. As DTH increases, the hippocampus also herniates medially over the edge of the tentorium, compressing the quadrigeminal cistern and pushing the midbrain toward the opposite side of the incisura **(3-8B)**. In severe cases, the temporal horn can even be displaced almost into the midline **(3-13A)**.

With **bilateral DTH**, both temporal lobes herniate medially into the tentorial hiatus. With **central descending herniation**, both hemispheres are so swollen that the whole central brain is flattened against the skull base. All the basal cisterns are obliterated as the hypothalamus and optic chiasm are crushed against the sella turcica, and the suprasellar and quadrigeminal cisterns are completely effaced **(3-9)** **(3-13B)**. The medial temporal and posterior frontal lobes become acutely ischemic **(3-10)**.

In complete (central) bilateral DTH, the midbrain is compressed and squeezed medially from both sides. It is also pushed inferiorly through the tentorial incisura, displacing the pons downward. The angle between the midbrain and pons is progressively reduced from nearly 90° to almost 0° **(3-11)** **(3-13B)**. In terminal central herniation, the pons eventually pushes the cerebellar tonsils inferiorly through the foramen magnum **(3-12)** **(3-14A)**.

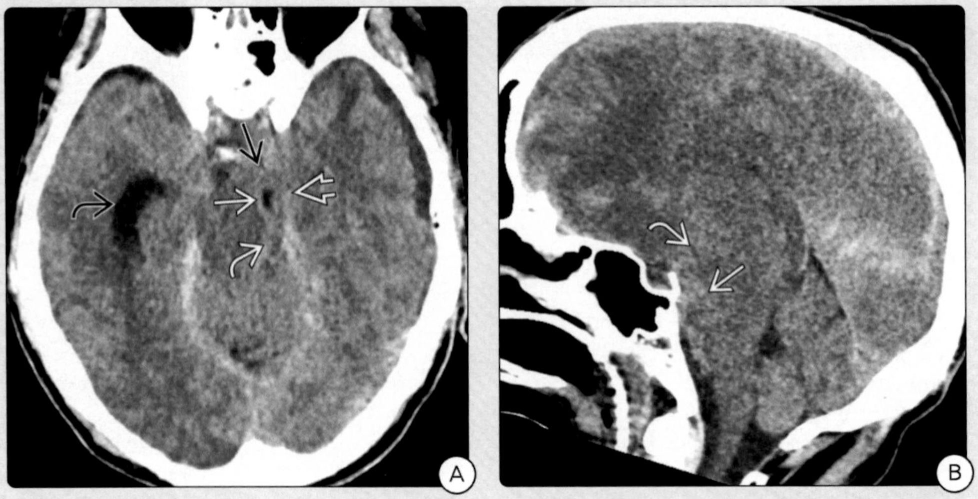

(3-13A) *NECT shows severe unilateral DTH. The uncus ➔ and hippocampus ➔ of the left temporal lobe are herniated medially over the edge of the tentorium ➔. The temporal horn ➔ of the compressed left lateral ventricle is almost in the midline. The contralateral temporal horn is enlarged ➔.* ***(3-13B)*** *Sagittal NECT shows that midbrain is displaced inferiorly ➔ and the midbrain-pons angle ➔ is obliterated.*

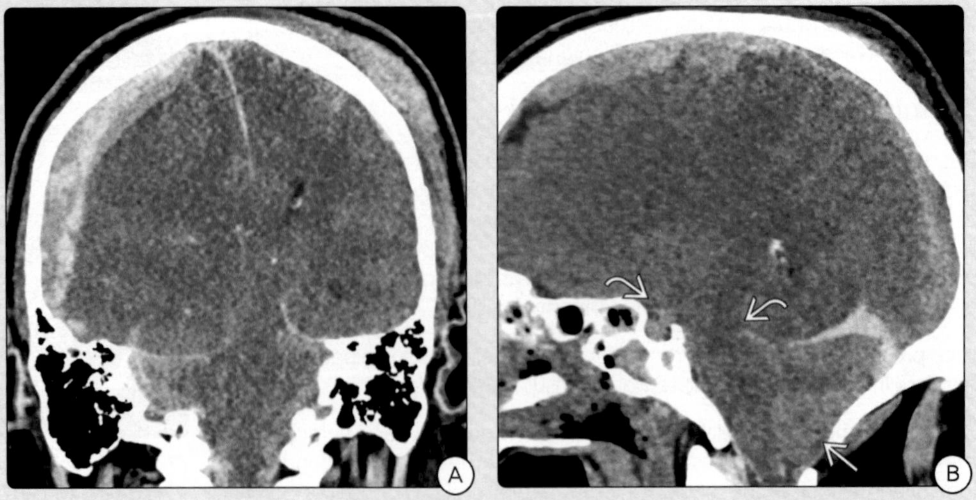

(3-14A) *Reformatted coronal NECT in the same case shows the severe subfalcine, descending herniations. Mass effect is so severe that the inferior falx is bowed and the tentorium displaced inward. The tentorial incisura is completely effaced by the herniating brain.* ***(3-14B)*** *Reformatted sagittal NECT in the same case shows complete DTH has effaced all basilar cisterns ➔. The tonsils are displaced inferiorly through the foramen magnum ➔.*

Complications

Even mild DTH can compress the third cranial (oculomotor) nerve as it exits from the interpeduncular fossa and courses anterolaterally toward the cavernous sinus **(3-7A)**. This may produce a **pupil-involving third nerve palsy (3-15)**.

Other more severe complications may occur with DTH. As the temporal lobe is displaced inferomedially, it pushes the posterior cerebral artery (PCA) below the tentorial incisura. The PCA can become kinked and eventually even occluded as it passes back up over the medial edge of the tentorium **(3-16)**, causing a **secondary PCA (occipital) infarct (3-17)**.

As the herniating temporal lobe pushes the midbrain toward the opposite side of the incisura, the contralateral cerebral peduncle is forced against the hard, knife-like edge of the tentorium, forming a **Kernohan notch (3-15)**. Pressure ischemia leads to an ipsilateral (not contralateral) hemiplegia, the "false localizing" sign.

Severe uni- or bilateral DTH may cause pressure necrosis of the uncus and hippocampus. "Top-down" mass effect displaces the midbrain inferiorly and closes the midbrain-pontine angle. Perforating arteries that arise from the top of the basilar artery are compressed and buckled inferiorly, eventually occluding and causing a secondary hemorrhagic midbrain infarct known as a **Duret hemorrhage (3-7A)**.

With complete bilateral DTH, perforating arteries that arise from the circle of Willis are compressed against the central skull base and also occlude, causing **hypothalamic and basal ganglia infarcts (3-32)**.

In a vicious cycle, the hemispheres become more edematous, and ICP soars. If the rising pressure exceeds intraarterial pressure, perfusion is drastically reduced and eventually ceases, causing **brain death (BD)** (see below).

DESCENDING TRANSTENTORIAL HERNIATION

Terminology and Pathology
- Unilateral DTH
  - Temporal lobe (uncus, hippocampus) pushed over tentorial incisura
- Severe bilateral DTH = "complete" or "central" herniation
  - Hypothalamus, chiasm flattened against sella

Epidemiology
- Second most common cerebral herniation

Imaging
- Unilateral DTH
  - Suprasellar cistern encroached, then obliterated
  - Herniating temporal lobe pushes midbrain to opposite side
- Bilateral DTH
  - Basal cisterns completely effaced
  - Midbrain pushed down, compressed on both sides

Complications
- CN III compression → pupil-involving third nerve palsy
- Secondary occipital (PCA) ± hypothalamus, basal infarcts
- Compression of contralateral cerebral peduncle ("Kernohan notch")
- Midbrain ("Duret") hemorrhage

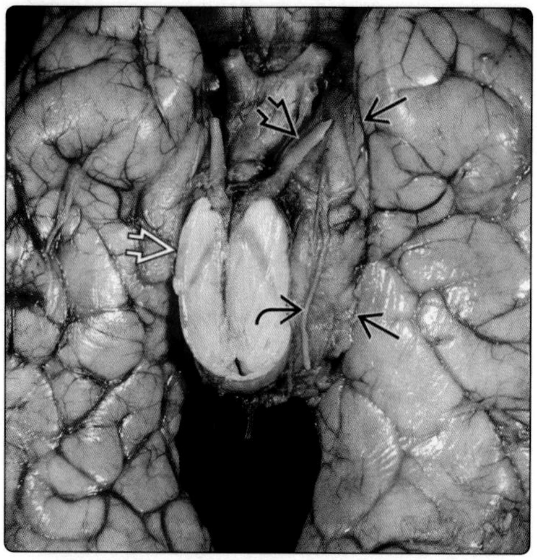

(3-15) Temporal lobe herniation by tentorium ⇨, compresses CN III ⇨, IV ⇨, midbrain Kernohan notch ➡. (E. T. Hedley-Whyte, MD.)

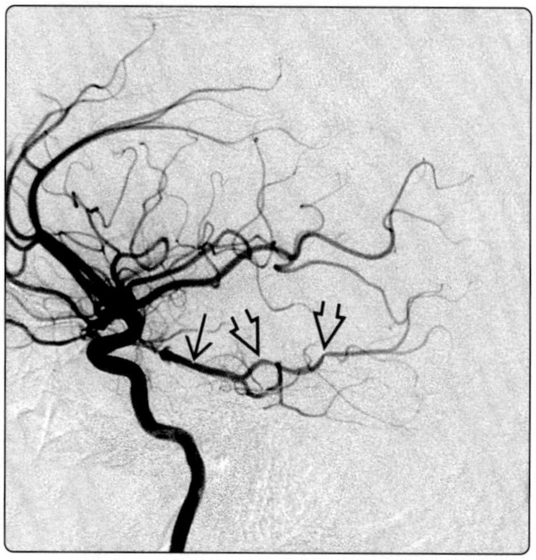

(3-16) In DTH proximal PCA ⇨ is displaced inferiorly through incisura, "kinked" ⇨, passes over tentorium edge. (Courtesy R. Hewlett, MD.)

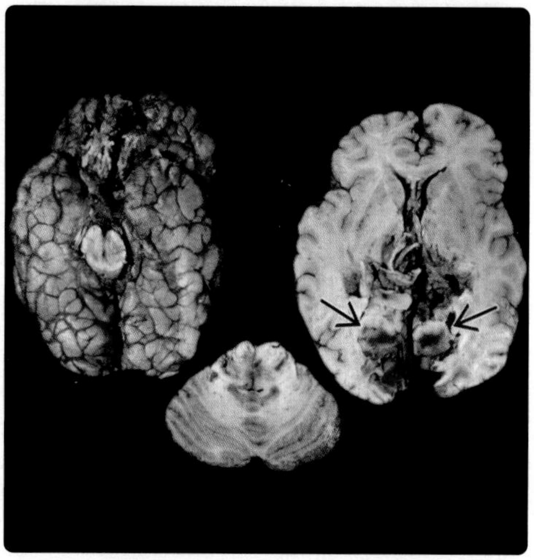

(3-17) Autopsy shows bilateral central DTH causing secondary PCA infarcts ⇨. (Courtesy R. Hewlett, MD.)

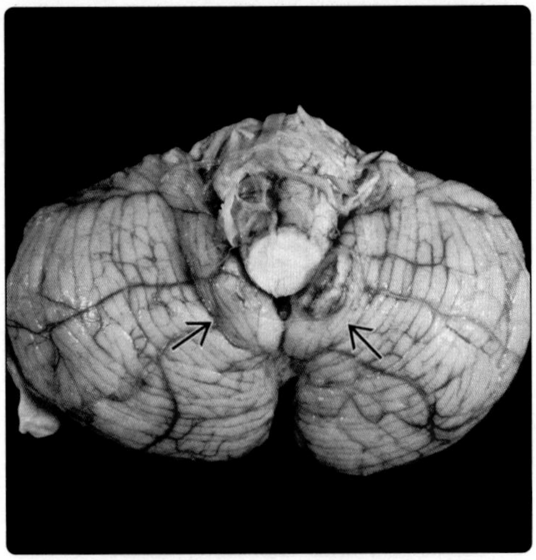

***(3-18)** Herniation shows tonsils are displaced inferiorly, "grooved" ➡ by bony margins of foramen magnum. (Courtesy R. Hewlett, MD.)*

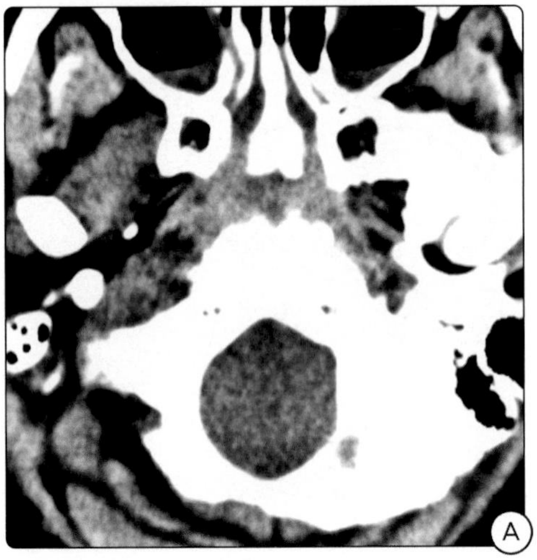

***(3-19A)** NECT in a patient with tonsillar herniation shows only effacement of CSF within the foramen magnum.*

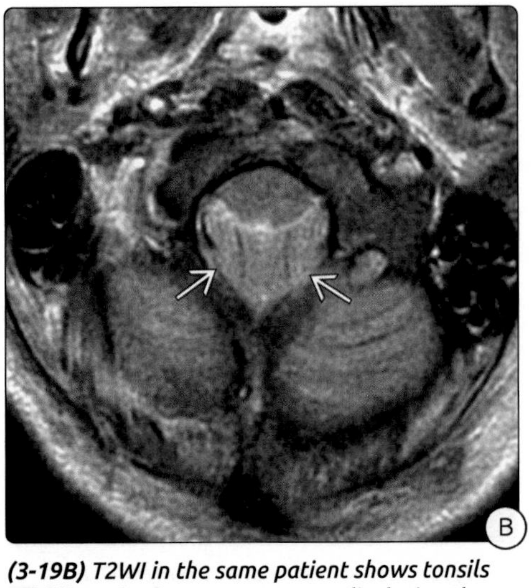

***(3-19B)** T2WI in the same patient shows tonsils ➡ filling the foramen magnum, displacing the medulla anteriorly.*

Tonsillar Herniation

Two types of herniations occur with posterior fossa masses: tonsillar herniation and ascending transtentorial herniation (ATH). Tonsillar herniation is the more common of these two herniations.

Terminology and Etiology

In tonsillar herniation, the cerebellar tonsils are displaced inferiorly and become impacted into the foramen magnum **(3-18)**. Tonsillar herniation can be congenital (e.g., Chiari 1 malformation) or acquired.

Acquired tonsillar herniation occurs in two different circumstances. The most common cause is an expanding posterior fossa mass *pushing* the tonsils downward into the foramen magnum.

Inferior tonsillar displacement also occurs with intracranial hypotension. Here the tonsils are *pulled* downward by abnormally low intraspinal CSF pressure (Chapter 34).

Imaging

Diagnosing tonsillar herniation on NECT scans may be problematic. The foramen magnum usually contains CSF that surrounds the medulla and cerebellar tonsils. Herniation of one or both tonsils into the foramen magnum obliterates most or all of the CSF in the cisterna magna **(3-19A)**.

Tonsillar herniation is much more easily diagnosed on MR. In the sagittal plane, the normally horizontal tonsillar folia become vertically oriented, and the inferior aspect of the tonsils becomes pointed. Tonsils more than 5 mm below the foramen magnum are generally abnormal, especially if they are peg-like or pointed (rather than rounded).

In the axial plane, T2 scans show that the tonsils are impacted into the foramen magnum, obliterating CSF in the cisterna magna and displacing the medulla anteriorly **(3-19B)**.

Complications

Complications of tonsillar herniation include obstructive hydrocephalus and tonsillar necrosis.

TONSILLAR HERNIATION

Etiology and Pathology
- Most common posterior fossa herniation
- Can be congenital (Chiari 1) or acquired
- Acquired
  - Most common = secondary to posterior fossa mass effect
  - Less common = intracranial hypotension
  - Rare = severe central DTH, brain death

Imaging Findings
- 1 or both tonsils > 5 mm below foramen magnum
- CSF in foramen magnum effaced
- Foramen magnum appears tissue-filled on axial NECT, T2WI
- Inferior "pointing" or peg-like configuration of tonsils on sagittal T1WI

Complications
- Obstructive hydrocephalus
- Tonsillar necrosis

Ascending Transtentorial Herniation

Terminology and Etiology

In ATH, the cerebellar vermis and hemispheres are pushed upward ("ascend") through the tentorial incisura into the supratentorial compartment. The superiorly herniating cerebellum first flattens and displaces, then effaces the quadrigeminal cistern and compresses the midbrain **(3-20)**.

ATH is much less common than descending herniation. ATH can be caused by any expanding posterior fossa mass although neoplasms are a more common cause than trauma.

Imaging

Axial NECT scans show that CSF in the superior vermian cistern and cerebellar sulci is effaced **(3-21)**. The quadrigeminal cistern is first compressed and then obliterated by the upwardly herniating cerebellum **(3-22)**. As the herniation progresses, the tectal plate becomes compressed and flattened. In severe cases, the dorsal midbrain may actually appear concave instead of convex **(3-20)**.

Eventually, the entire tentorial incisura becomes completely filled with soft tissue, and all normal anatomic landmarks disappear.

Complications

The most common complication of ATH is acute intraventricular obstructive hydrocephalus caused by compression of the cerebral aqueduct.

ASCENDING TRANSTENTORIAL HERNIATION

Relatively Rare
- Caused by expanding posterior fossa mass
- Neoplasm > trauma
- Cerebellum pushed upward through incisura
- Compresses, deforms midbrain

Imaging Findings
- Incisura filled with tissue, CSF spaces obliterated
- Quadrigeminal cistern, tectal plate compressed/flattened
  - Eventually appear obliterated

Complications
- Hydrocephalus (secondary to aqueduct obstruction)

Other Herniations

The vast majority of cerebral herniations are subfalcine, descending/ascending transtentorial, and tonsillar herniations. Other less common herniation syndromes are transalar and transdural/transcranial herniations.

Transalar Herniation

Transalar herniation occurs when the brain herniates across the greater sphenoid wing (GSW) or "ala." Transalar herniations can be either ascending (the most common) or descending.

Ascending transalar herniation is caused by a large *middle cranial fossa mass*. An intratemporal or large extraaxial mass displaces part of the temporal lobe together with the sylvian fissure and middle cerebral artery (MCA) up and over the GSW **(3-23)**.

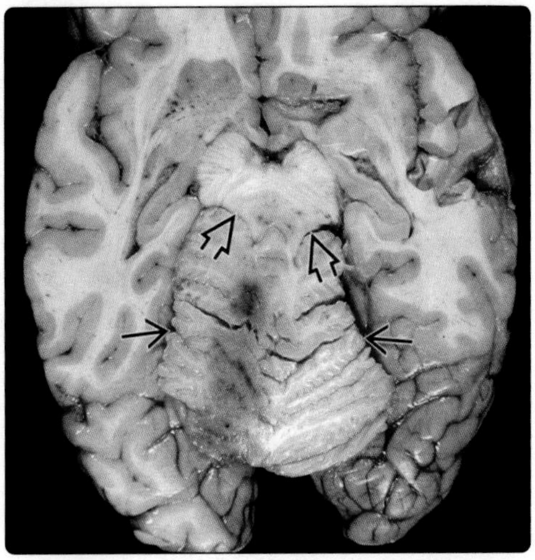

(3-20) Vermis, cerebellum ➩ push upward to tentorial incisura, compress midbrain/tectum ➩; ATH. (E. T. Hedley-Whyte, MD.)

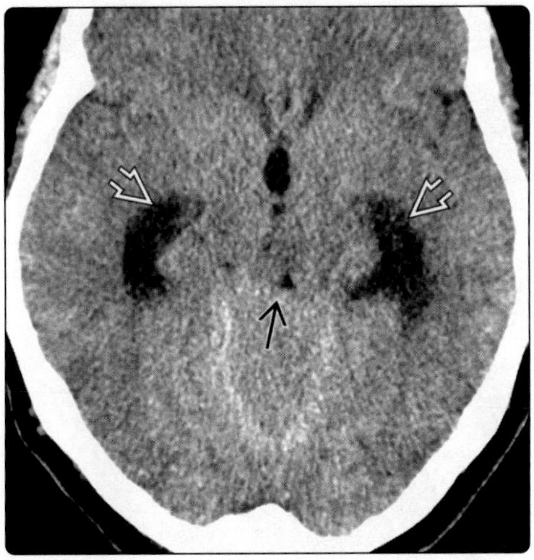

(3-21) NECT shows ATH with obliterated quadrigeminal cistern, compressed tectum ➩. Note severe obstructive hydrocephalus ➩.

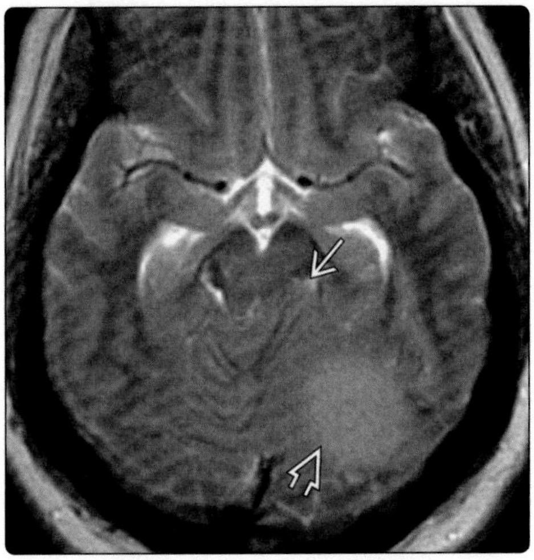

(3-22) T2WI shows unilateral ATH ➩ from a mass ➩ pushing the left cerebellar hemisphere superiorly through the tentorial incisura.

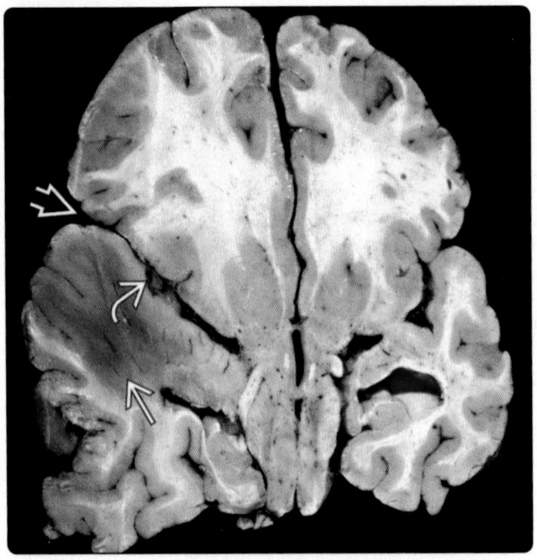

(3-23) Temporal lobe mass pushes sylvian fissure and MCA up/over the site of greater sphenoid wing . (E. T. Hedley-Whyte, MD.)

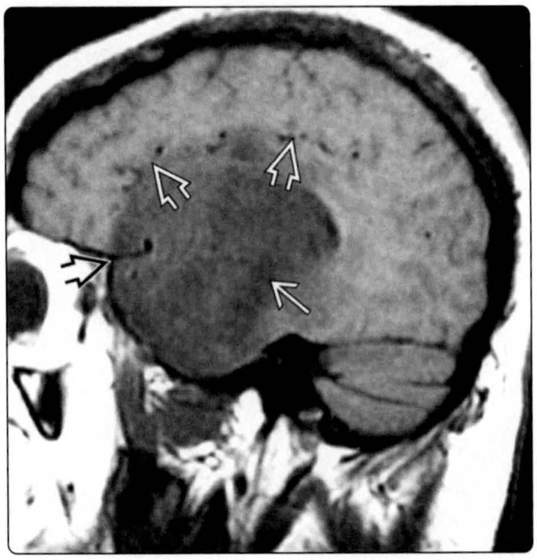

(3-24) Ascending transalar herniation shows mass elevates sylvian fissure, MCA , pushing temporal lobe up/over sphenoid wing .

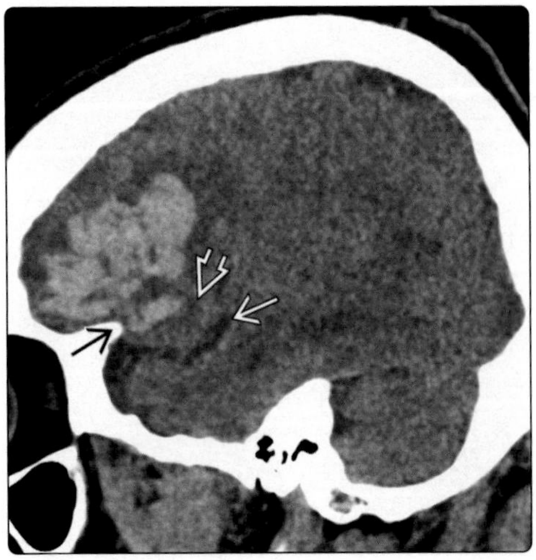

(3-25) Descending transalar herniation shows frontal lobe is pushed over the sphenoid wing displacing sylvian fissure posteroinferiorly.

Ascending transalar herniation is best depicted on off-midline sagittal MRs. The GSW is seen as the bony junction between the anterior and middle cranial fossae. The MCA branches and sylvian fissure are elevated, and the superior temporal gyrus is pushed above the GSW **(3-24)**.

Descending transalar herniation is caused by a large *anterior cranial fossa mass*. Here the gyrus rectus is forced posteroinferiorly over the GSW, displacing the sylvian fissure and shifting the MCA backward **(3-25)**.

Transdural/Transcranial Herniation

This rare type of cerebral herniation, sometimes called a "brain fungus" by neurosurgeons, can be life-threatening. For transdural/transcranial herniation to occur, the dura must be lacerated, a skull defect (fracture or craniotomy) must be present, and ICP must be elevated.

Traumatic transdural/transcranial herniations typically occur in infants or young children with a comminuted skull fracture that deforms inward with impact, lacerating the dura-arachnoid. When ICP increases, brain can herniate through the torn dura and across the skull fracture into the subgaleal space.

Iatrogenic transdural/transcranial herniations occur when a burr hole, craniotomy, or craniectomy is performed in a patient with severely elevated ICP. When the dura is opened, brain under pressure extrudes through the defect **(3-26)**.

MR best depicts these unusual herniations. The disrupted dura is seen as a discontinuous black line on T2WI. Brain tissue, together with accompanying blood vessels and variable amounts of CSF, is literally extruded through the dural and calvarial defects into the subgaleal space **(3-27)**.

OTHER HERNIATIONS

Ascending Transalar Herniation
- Most common transalar herniation
- Caused by middle fossa mass
- Sagittal imaging (best appreciated on off-midline images)
  - Sylvian fissure, MCA displaced up/over greater sphenoid ala
- Axial imaging
  - Sylvian fissure/MCA bowed forward
  - Temporal lobe bulges into anterior fossa

Descending Transalar Herniation
- Caused by anterior fossa mass
- Sagittal imaging
  - Sylvian fissure, MCA displaced posteroinferiorly
  - Frontal lobe pushed backward over greater sphenoid ala
- Axial imaging
  - Gyrus rectus pushed posteriorly
  - MCA curved backward

Transcranial/Transdural Herniation
- ↑ ICP + skull defect + dura-arachnoid tear
- Caused by:
  - Comminuted, often depressed skull fracture
  - Craniectomy
- Brain extruded through skull, under scalp aponeurosis
- Best appreciated on axial T2WI

Edema, Ischemia, and Vascular Injury

Traumatic brain injury (TBI) can unleash a cascade of physiologic responses that may adversely affect the brain more than the initial trauma. These responses include diffuse brain swelling, excitotoxic responses elicited by glutamatergic pathway activation, perfusion alterations, and a variety of ischemic events including territorial infarcts.

Posttraumatic Brain Swelling

Cerebral edema is a major contributor to TBI morbidity. Massive brain swelling with severe intracranial hypertension is among the most serious of all secondary traumatic lesions. Mortality approaches 50%, so early recognition and aggressive treatment of this complication are imperative.

Etiology and Epidemiology

Focal, regional, or diffuse brain swelling develops in 10-20% of patients with TBI **(3-28)**. Whether this is caused by increased tissue fluid (cerebral edema), or elevated blood volume (cerebral hyperemia) secondary to vascular dysautoregulation is unclear. In some cases, the trigeminal system may mediate brain swelling associated with subdural bleeding, providing the link between small-volume, thin subdural bleeds and swelling of the underlying brain.

Clinical Issues

Children, young adults, and individuals with repetitive concussive or subconcussive injuries are especially prone to developing posttraumatic brain swelling and are almost twice as likely as older adults to develop this complication. Although gross enlargement of one or both hemispheres occasionally develops rapidly after the initial event, delayed onset is more

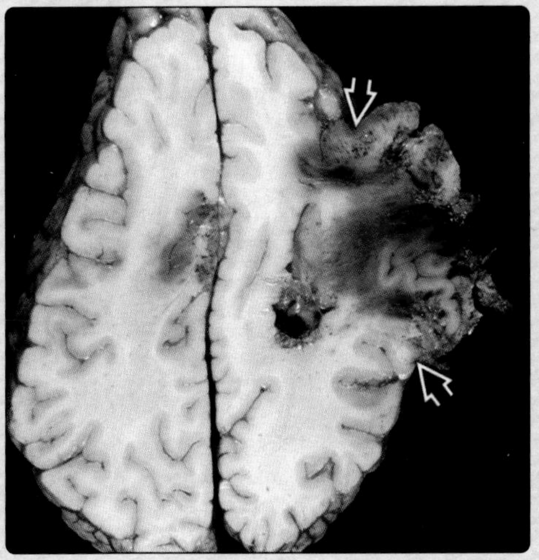
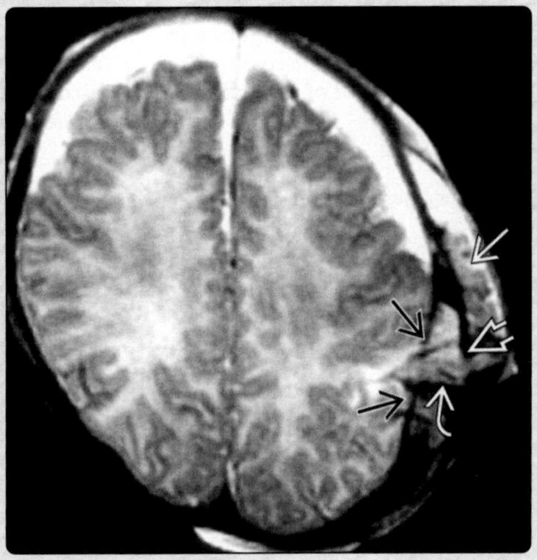

***(3-26)** Autopsy case shows transdural/transcranial herniation. Increased intracranial pressure caused brain extrusion through a large craniectomy defect ➡. (E. T. Hedley-Whyte, MD.) **(3-27)** Axial T2WI in an abused infant shows edges of torn dura ⇨ with brain ➡ extruding through the dura/arachnoid defect and extending under/over a comminuted skull fracture ➡. Extracranial macerated brain ➡ is seen under the scalp.*

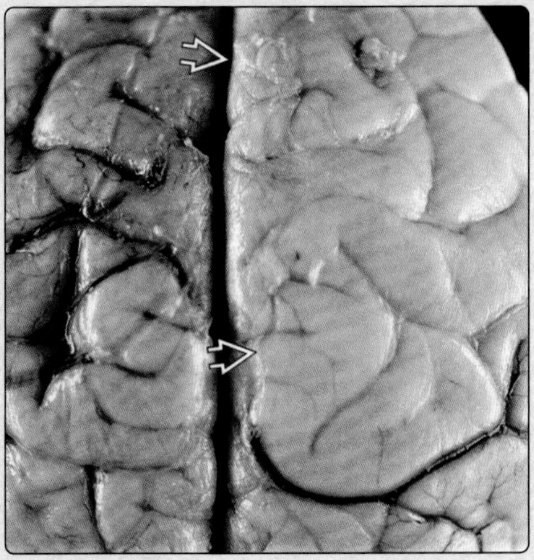
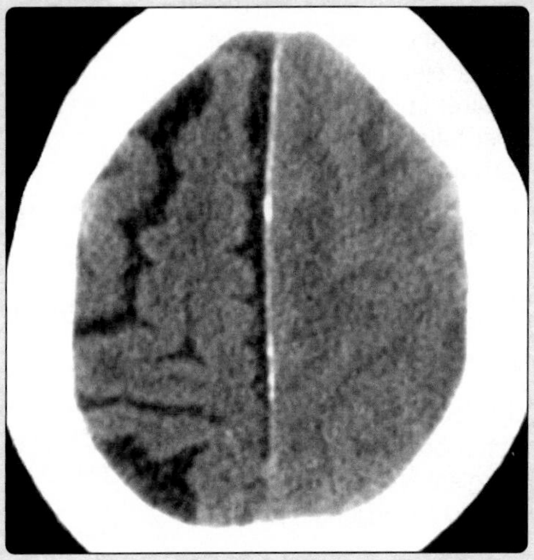

***(3-28)** Autopsy specimen shows unilateral hemispheric swelling ➡ that expands the gyri, compresses and obliterates the sulci. (Courtesy E. T. Hedley-Whyte, MD.) **(3-29)** Axial NECT scan shows normal right sulci and obliterated ("disappearing") convexity sulci over the swollen left hemisphere.*

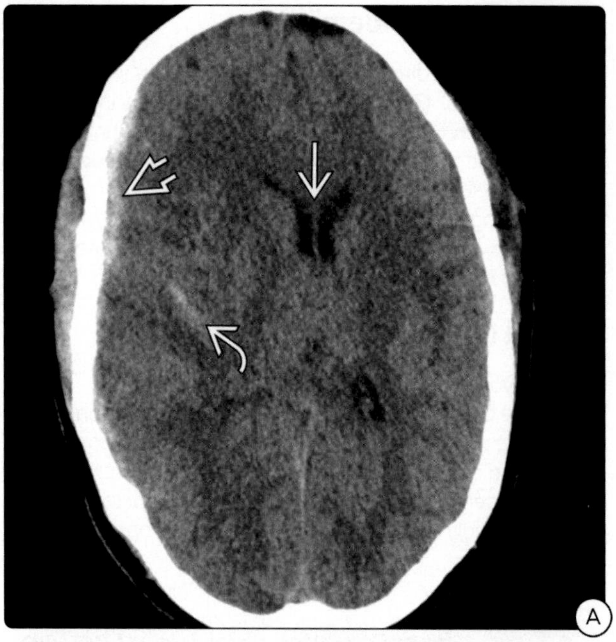

(3-30A) *A 35y man has a small right aSDH ➡ that measures only 6 mm in maximum diameter. Subfalcine herniation across the midline measured 15 mm ➡. Note small amount of tSAH ➡, preserved GM-WM interface.*

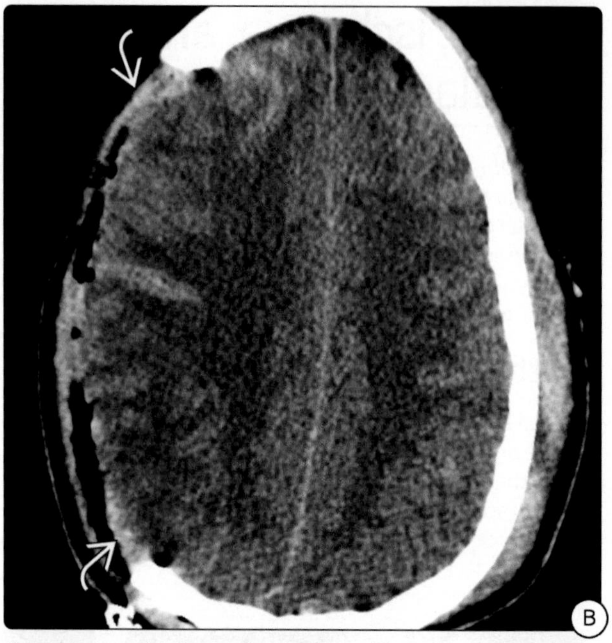

(3-30B) *Alerted to impending brain swelling, the neurosurgeons immediately evacuated the small aSDH. Because of severe intraoperative brain swelling, an emergency decompressive craniectomy ➡ had to be performed.*

typical. Severe cerebral edema generally takes between 24 and 48 hours to develop.

In some cases, aggressive measures for control of intracranial pressure (ICP) fail to restore cerebral metabolism and improve neurologic outcome. Decompressive craniectomy as a last resort is often performed, but evidence for reduced risk of death or dependence in severe TBI is lacking.

Imaging

The appearance of posttraumatic brain swelling evolves over time. Initially, mild hemispheric mass effect with sulcal/cisternal compression is seen on NECT scans **(3-29)**.

During the early stages of brain swelling, gray-white matter differentiation appears relatively preserved. Although the ipsilateral ventricle may be slightly compressed, subfalcine displacement is generally minimal. However, **if the mass effect is disproportionately greater (≥ 3 mm) than the maximum width of an extraaxial collection, such as a subdural hematoma (SDH), early and potentially catastrophic swelling of the underlying brain parenchyma should be suspected and treated proactively (3-30)**.

MR shows swollen gyri that are hypointense on T1WI and hyperintense on T2WI. Diffusion-weighted scans show restricted diffusion with low ADC values **(3-35)**.

As brain swelling progresses, the demarcation between the cortex and underlying white matter becomes indistinct and eventually disappears. The lateral ventricles appear smaller than normal, and the superficial sulci are no longer visible.

POSTTRAUMATIC BRAIN SWELLING

Epidemiology
- 10-20% of TBI
- Can be focal, regional, or diffuse
- Most common in children, young adults
- Potentially catastrophic

Imaging
- Earliest sign
  - SFH ≥ 3 mm than width of epidural or subdural hematoma
- Next
  - Sulcal effacement
- Later
  - Indistinct gray-white interfaces
- End-stage
  - One or both hemispheres uniformly low density
  - All sulci, cisterns obliterated
  - Small ventricles

Traumatic Cerebral Ischemia, Infarction, and Perfusion Abnormalities

Traumatic ischemia and infarction are uncommon but important complications of TBI. They have a variety of causes, including direct vascular compression, systemic hypoperfusion, vascular injury, vasospasm, and venous congestion. The most common cause of posttraumatic cerebral ischemia is mechanical vascular compression secondary to a brain herniation syndrome.

Posttraumatic Infarcts

The most common brain herniation that causes secondary cerebral infarction is descending transtentorial herniation (DTH). Severe unilateral DTH displaces the temporal lobe and accompanying posterior cerebral artery (PCA) inferiorly into the tentorial incisura. As the herniating PCA passes posterior to the midbrain, it courses superiorly and is forced against the hard, knife-like edge of the tentorial incisura. The P3 PCA segment occludes, resulting in occipital lobe infarction **(3-31) (3-32)**.

Less commonly, subfalcine herniation (SFH) presses the callosomarginal branch of the anterior cerebral artery (ACA) against the undersurface of the falx cerebri and causes cingulate gyrus infarction **(3-33)** **(3-34)**.

With complete bilateral ("central") DTH, penetrating arteries that arise from the circle of Willis are crushed against the skull base, resulting in multiple scattered basal ganglia and hypothalamus infarcts **(3-32)**. Pressure necrosis of the uncus and hippocampus can also occur as the herniated temporal lobes impact the free edge of the tentorial incisura **(3-10)**.

Traumatic Cerebral Ischemia

Focal, regional, and generalized perfusion alterations also occur with TBI. Extraaxial hematomas that exert significant focal mass effect on the underlying brain may cause reduced arterial perfusion and cortical ischemia. They may also compress the underlying cortical veins, causing venous ischemia **(3-35)**.

Global or generalized **cerebral ischemia** may result from hypoperfusion, hypoxia, membrane depolarization, or loss of cellular membrane integrity and ion homeostasis. Cellular energy failure may induce glutamate-mediated **acute excitotoxic brain injury**.

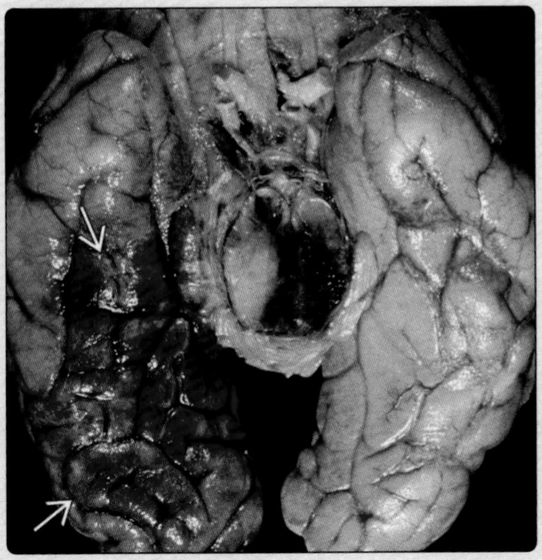

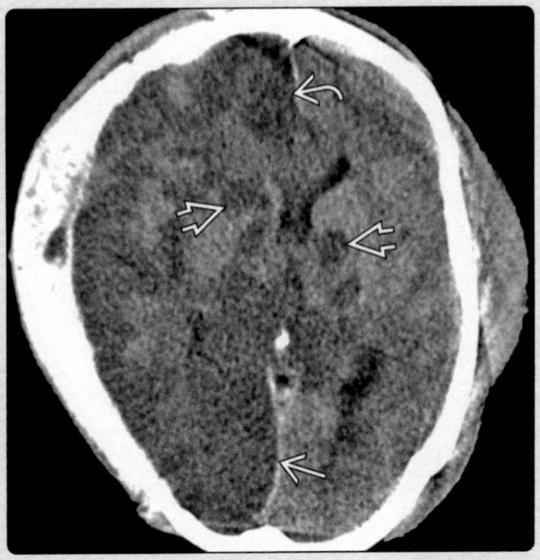

***(3-31)** DTH can occlude the PCA against the tentorial incisura, causing a secondary PCA territorial infarction ➡. (Courtesy R. Hewlett, MD.) **(3-32)** A severely traumatized patient is shown with diffuse brain swelling and right subfalcine herniation plus DTH. NECT obtained 5 days after the initial insult shows PCA ➡, anterior cerebral artery ➡, and multiple perforating artery ➡ infarcts.*

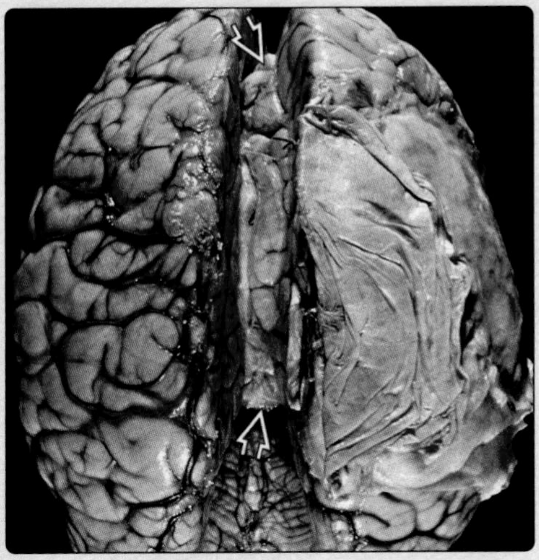

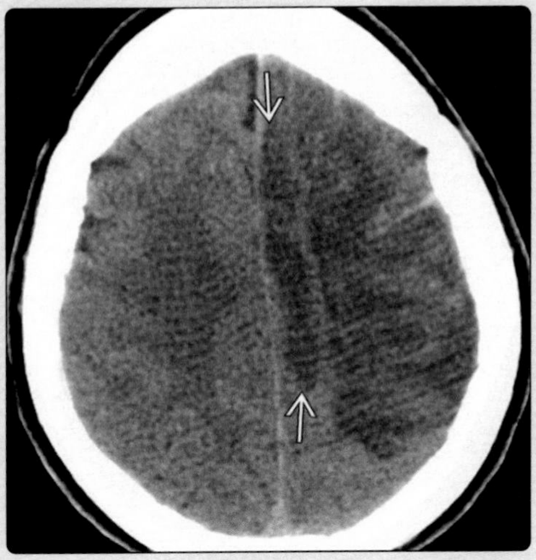

***(3-33)** Cephalad view of autopsied brain through the interhemispheric fissure shows subfalcine herniation of cingulate, callosomarginal gyri ➡. (Courtesy E. Ross, MD.) **(3-34)** NECT in a patient who survived a "malignant" MCA infarct shows secondary infarction of the left cingulate gyrus ➡. ACA was occluded when the acute, severe subfalcine herniation occurred.*

NECT scans show hypodensity with loss of gray-white differentiation in the affected parenchyma. CT perfusion may show decreased cerebral blood flow with prolonged time to drain. In cases of excitotoxic brain injury, MR shows swollen, hyperintense gyri on T2/FLAIR that do not correspond to defined vascular territories **(3-36)**.

Traumatic Cerebral Perfusion Alterations

In patients with acute SDHs, raised intracranial pressure typically leads to reduced cerebral perfusion pressure and impaired CBF. In contrast, patients with mixed or chronic SDHs may have significantly upregulated CBV and CBF in the cortex underlying the chronic SDH **(3-37)**. MTTs are often elevated.

Blunt Cerebrovascular Injuries

Blunt trauma cerebrovascular injuries (BCVIs) are associated with high morbidity and mortality. Patients with basilar skull fractures—regardless of whether fractures actually cross the carotid canal—and cervical spine fractures are at high risk for vascular complications and are typically screened with craniocervical CTA.

Posttraumatic **vasospasm** is seen as vascular irregularities without a clear dissection flap or intramural hematoma. Intracranial traumatic **dissection** is rare. The vertebral artery (usually between the skull base and C1) is the most commonly affected vessel. Anterior circulation dissections typically involve the supraclinoid internal carotid artery.

Vessel **tear/transection** is a very rare but potentially lethal complication of BCVI, causing rapidly expanding parenchymal hematomas or gross, widespread subarachnoid hemorrhage. CTA may show a "spot sign," indicating active bleeding **(3-38)**.

Traumatic **pseudoaneurysm** is rare. The vertebral artery and the distal ACA are the most common sites. Traumatic pseudoaneurysms are discussed in detail in Chapter 6.

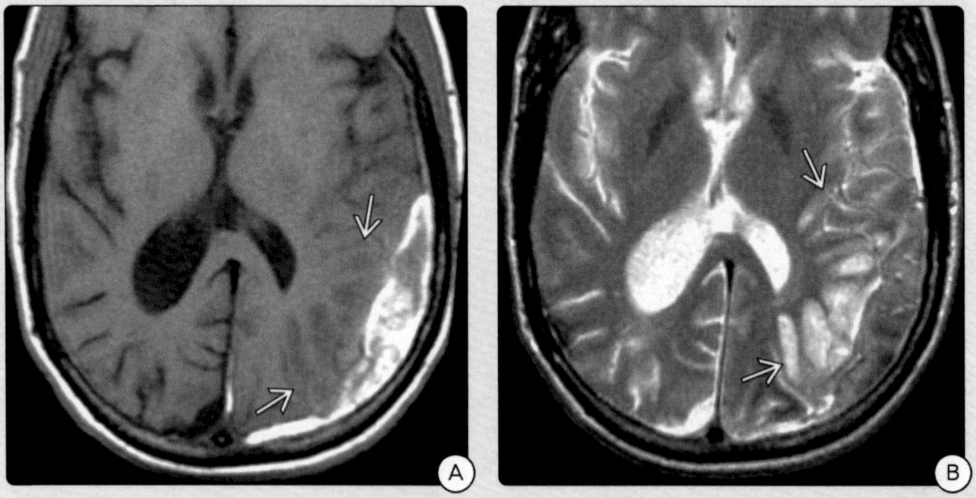

***(3-35A)** T1WI in a patient with an early subacute SDH shows sulcal effacement and gyral swelling in the underlying parietooccipital cortex ➡. **(3-35B)** T2WI in the same patient shows cortical edema ➡ under the SDH. Regional perfusion alterations are common under SDHs.*

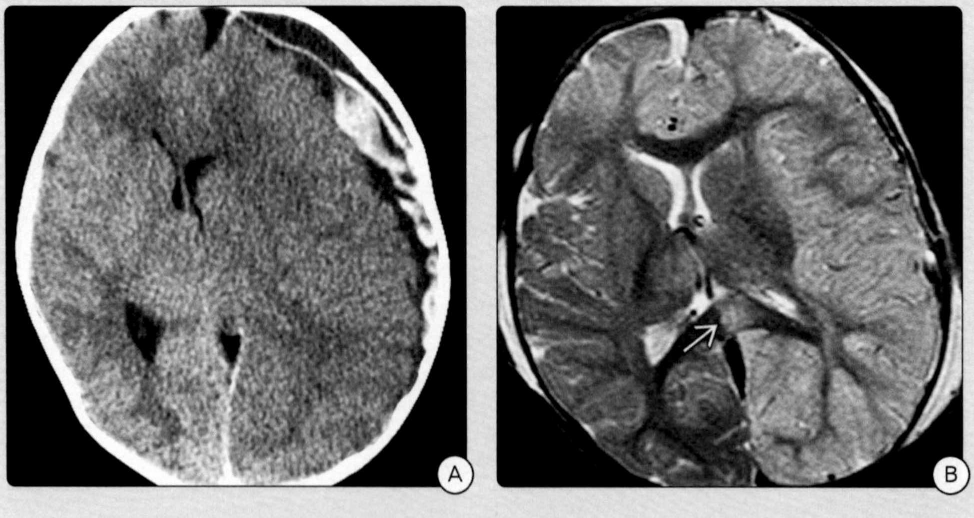

***(3-36A)** NECT scan shows mixed-density SDHs in an infant with inflicted (nonaccidental) trauma. Note the left hemisphere hypodensity ("big black brain"). The mass effect and subfalcine herniation are much larger than would be expected from the SDHs themselves. **(3-36B)** T2WI shows marked hemispheric edema, sparing only the basal ganglia. Hyperintensity in the corpus callosum ➡, right frontal lobe may represent excitotoxic injury.*

BLUNT CEREBROVASCULAR INJURIES
Vasospasm • Moderate/severe develops in 10% • Vessel irregularity without clear flap or intramural hematoma • Independent predictor of poor outcome

Intracranial Dissection
• Posterior circulation (vertebral artery) most common
  ○ Between skull base, C1 typical
  ○ Irregular wall, eccentric lumen ± flap or hematoma
  ○ 20% associated with posterior fossa traumatic subarachnoid hemorrhage (tSAH)
• Anterior circulation rare
  ○ Usually supraclinoid internal carotid artery

Transection
• Rare
• Can be life-threatening
  ○ Rapidly expanding parenchymal hematoma
  ○ Widespread tSAH
• Look for "spot" sign on CTA

Pseudoaneurysm • With or without dissection • Vertebral > > ACA

Brain Death

Terminology

Brain death (BD) is defined pathophysiologically as complete, irreversible cessation of brain function **(3-39)**. Some investigators distinguish between "whole brain death" (all intracranial structures above the foramen magnum), "cerebral death" (all supratentorial structures), and "higher brain death" (cortical structures).

The legal definition of brain death varies from country to country (e.g., the USA and the United Kingdom) and from state to state. Since adoption of the Uniform Determination of Death Act, all court rulings in the United States have upheld the medical practice of death determination using neurologic criteria according to state law.

Clinical Issues

BD is primarily a clinical diagnosis. Three clinical findings are necessary to confirm irreversible cessation of all functions of the entire brain, *including the brainstem*: (1) coma (with a known cause), (2) absence of brainstem reflexes, and (3) apnea.

Complex spontaneous motor movements and false-positive ventilator triggering may occur in patients who are brain dead, so expert assessment is crucial. Once reversible causes of coma (e.g., drug overdose, status epilepticus) are excluded, the clinical diagnosis of BD is highly reliable *if* the determination is made by experienced examiners using established, accepted criteria.

There are no published reports of recovery of neurologic function in adults after a diagnosis of BD using the updated 1995 American Academy of Neurology practice parameters.

Imaging

Imaging studies may be helpful in confirming BD but neither replace nor substitute for clinical diagnosis.

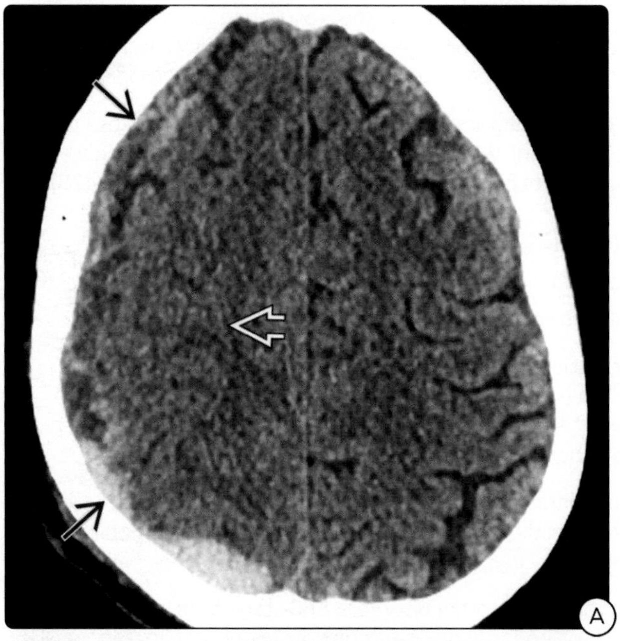

***(3-37A)** NECT in a patient with left hemiparesis shows a mixed-age right subdural hematoma → and cortical swelling ⇨ under the SDH.*

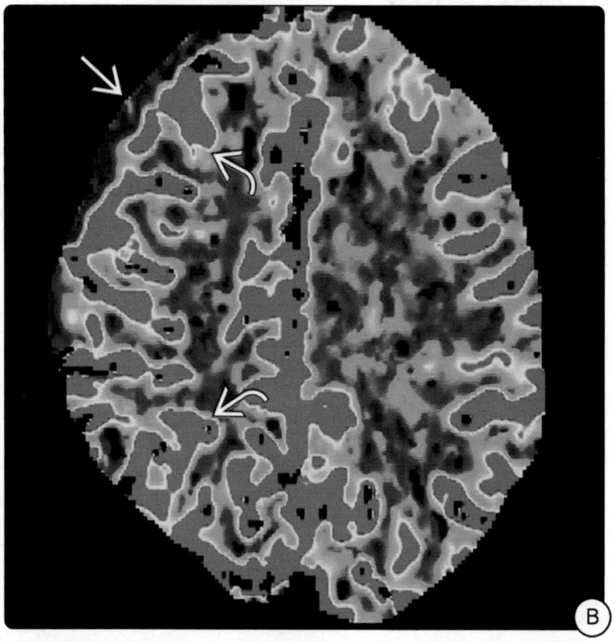

***(3-37B)** CT perfusion shows increased cerebral blood flow ↪ in the cortex under the SDH →. (Courtesy C. Hsu, MD.)*

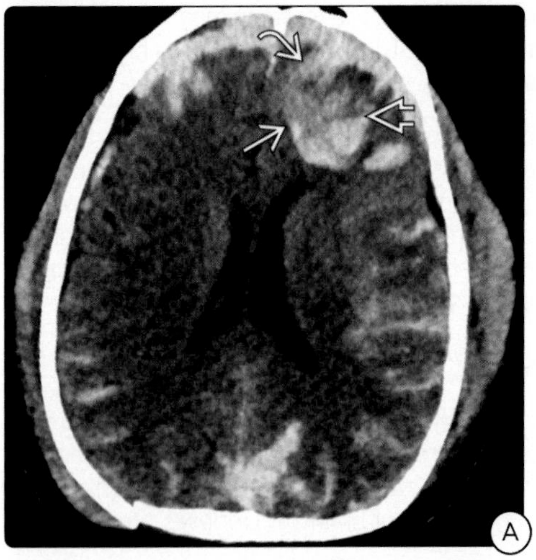

(3-38A) NECT shows extensive tSAH, left frontal hematoma ➡ with rapid bleeding, blood-fluid level ⇨, and probable brain laceration ↪.

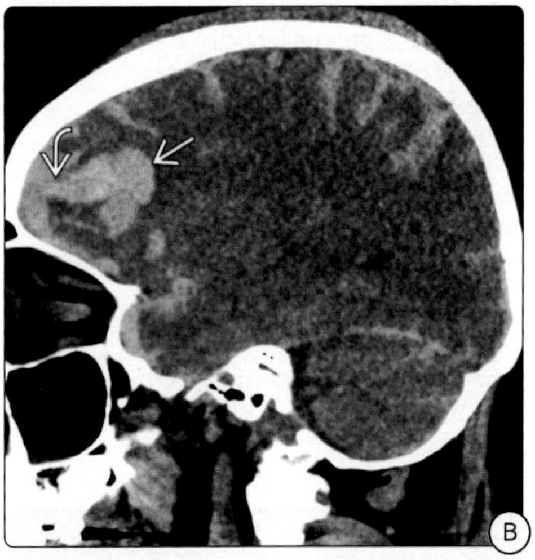

(3-38B) Sagittal scan reformatted from the axial source data shows the left frontal parenchymal hematoma ➡ and cortical tear ↪.

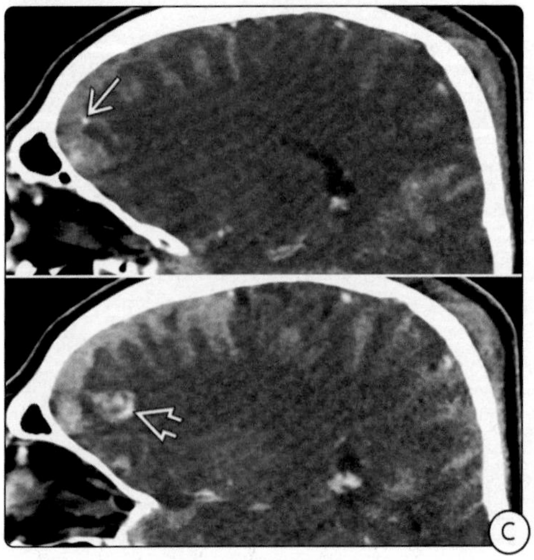

(3-38C) Reformatted sagittal CTA shows transected cortical artery ➡ and "spot" sign with contrast extravasation ⇨ into the hematoma.

CT Findings. NECT scans in BD show diffuse, severe cerebral edema. The superficial sulci, sylvian fissures, and basilar cisterns of both hemispheres are completely effaced **(3-40)**. The normal attenuation relationship between gray and white matter is inverted, with gray matter becoming iso- or even hypodense relative to the adjacent white matter (the **"reversal" sign**).

In striking contrast to the hypodense hemispheres, density of the cerebellum appears relatively normal (the **"white cerebellum" sign**). Density of the deep gray nuclei and brainstem may be initially maintained; however, all supratentorial structures eventually assume a featureless, uniform hypodensity.

MR Findings. Sagittal T1WI shows complete descending central brain herniation with the optic chiasm and hypothalamus compressed against the skull base and the midbrain "buckled" inferiorly through the tentorial incisura **(3-41) (3-42A)**. The hemispheres appear swollen and hypointense, with indistinct gray-white matter differentiation.

T2 scans show swollen gyri with hyperintense cortex. DWI in patients with brain death typically shows restricted diffusion with decreased ADC in both the cerebral cortex and white matter.

Angiography. Ancillary tests may be necessary to diagnose BD if clinical examination cannot be completed or confounding factors are present. Lack of cerebral circulation is an important confirmatory test in such cases. When ICP exceeds intraarterial perfusion pressure, brain blood flow ceases.

Conventional digital subtraction angiography (DSA) shows severe, prolonged contrast stasis with filling of the external carotid artery. Although most BD patients show no intracranial flow, almost 30% have some proximal opacification of intracranial arteries. The deep venous drainage remains unopacified throughout the examination.

CTA is emerging as an acceptable noninvasive alternative to DSA in many jurisdictions. Demonstrating lack of opacification in the middle cerebral artery (MCA) cortical segments and internal veins in CTA is an efficient and reliable method for confirming BD.

Ultrasound. Transcranial Doppler may show oscillating "to-and-fro" signal. Orbital Doppler shows absence or reversal of end-diastolic flow in central retinal arteries along with markedly increased arterial resistive indices.

Nuclear Medicine. Tc-99m scintigraphy shows scalp uptake but absent brain activity ("light bulb" sign). With increased extracranial activity ("hot nose" sign), these findings are both highly sensitive and specific for BD **(3-42B)**.

Differential Diagnosis

Potentially reversible causes of BD, such as deep coma due to **drug overdose** or **status epilepticus**, must be excluded clinically.

Technical difficulties with imaging studies that may mimic BD include a "missed bolus" on either CTA or nuclear medicine flow studies. Vascular lesions, such as arterial dissection and vasospasm, may also delay or even prevent opacification of intracranial vessels.

Massive cerebral infarction (especially "malignant MCA infarction") with severe edema can mimic BD but is typically territorial and does not involve the entire brain.

Brain death can also mimic other disorders. **End-stage brain swelling** from severe trauma or profound hypoxic encephalopathy (e.g., following cardiopulmonary arrest) makes the cranial arteries, dura, and dural venous sinuses all seem relatively hyperdense compared with the diffusely edematous low-density brain.

With very-low-density brain, comparatively high-density areas are seen along the basal cisterns, sylvian fissures, tentorium cerebelli, and sometimes even within the cortical sulci. This appearance is sometimes termed **pseudo-subarachnoid hemorrhage** (pseudo-SAH). Pseudo-SAH should not be mistaken for "real" SAH. The density of pseudo-SAH is significantly lower (between 30-40 HU) than the attenuation of "real" SAH (between 50-60 HU).

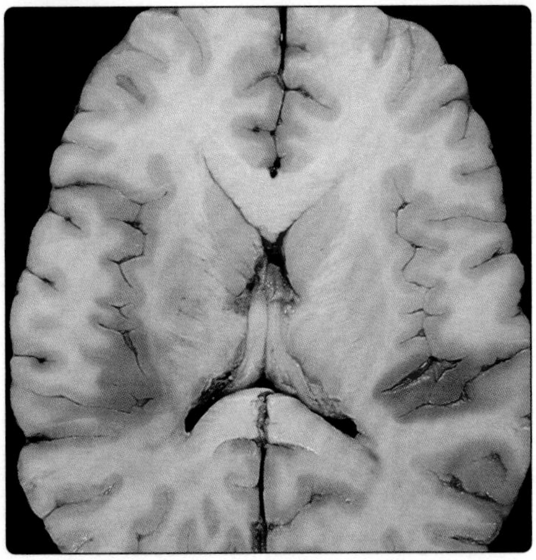

(3-39) Brain death shows diffuse swelling, poor GM-WM discrimination, small ventricles, and effaced surface sulci. (Courtesy R. Hewlett, MD.)

BRAIN DEATH

Terminology and Definition
- BD = Irreversible cessation of brain function
- Legal definition(s) vary with country, jurisdictions

Clinical Issues
- AAN 2010 checklist (BD in adults)
  - Coma (irreversible, known cause)
  - Neuroimaging explains coma
  - Neurologic examination, apnea testing performed

Ancillary Testing
- Only one needs to be performed
- Only if
  - Clinical examination cannot be fully performed OR
  - Apnea testing inconclusive/aborted
- Options
  - Cerebral angiogram (many jurisdictions accept DSA)
  - HMPAO SPECT
  - EEG
  - TCD

Imaging Findings
- DSA
  - Severe prolonged contrast stasis ICA
  - Most show no intracranial flow
  - 30% have some proximal opacification of intracranial arteries
- CTA, CTP
  - NO opacification of cortical MCAs and internal cerebral veins on CTA
  - Stasis filling on CTP
- HMPAO SPECT
  - No intracranial opacification of flow studies
  - Scalp uptake but no brain activity ("light bulb" sign)
  - Extracranial uptake ("hot nose" sign)

Differential Diagnosis
- Reversible causes of coma (e.g., drug OD, status epilepticus)
- Technical issues ("missed bolus")
- Severe brain swelling (other causes)
  - "Malignant" MCA infarct
  - Metabolic (e.g., hyperammonemia)

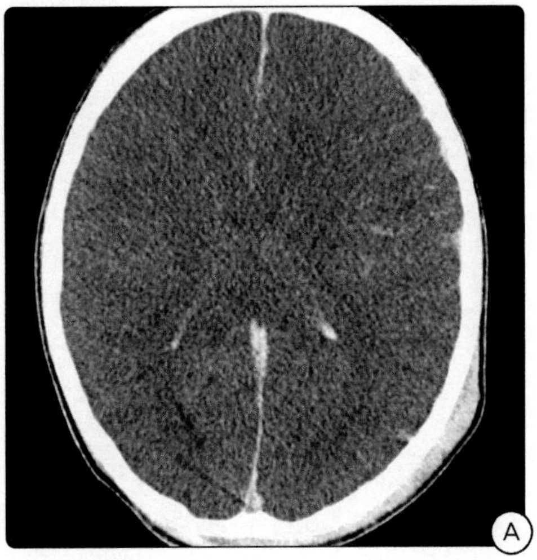

(3-40A) CECT obtained after near-drowning shows diffuse brain swelling with absent GM-WM interface. Lateral ventricles are almost invisible.

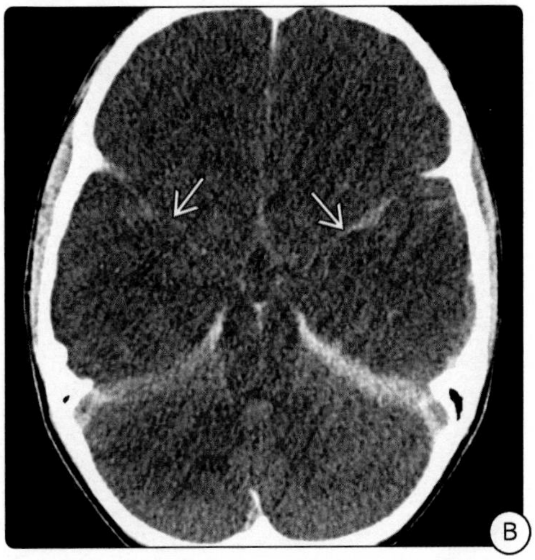

(3-40B) CECT in the same case shows severely attenuated MCAs ➡ and diffuse low-density brain. The patient expired shortly after the study.

Chronic Effects of CNS Trauma

Patients surviving traumatic brain injury (TBI) may have long-term sequelae, from mild cognitive disorders and neuropsychiatric effects to devastating neurologic deficits. Although a comprehensive discussion of all possible post-TBI effects is beyond the scope of this text, we will consider some of the more important sequelae of brain trauma in this section.

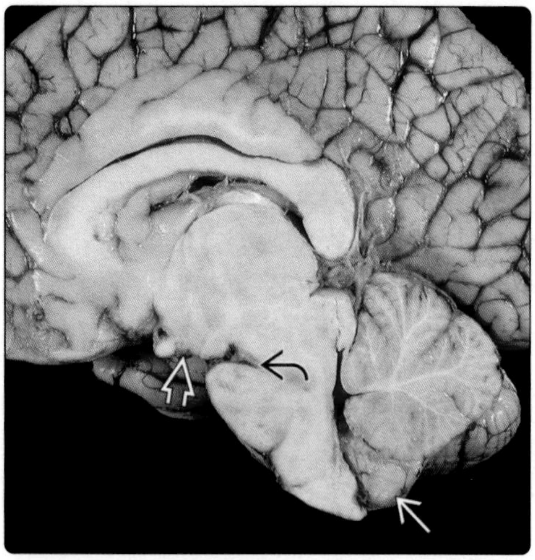

***(3-41)** Brain death autopsy shows severe brain swelling, complete central DTH ➡, inferiorly displaced midbrain ⇨, tonsillar herniation ➡.*

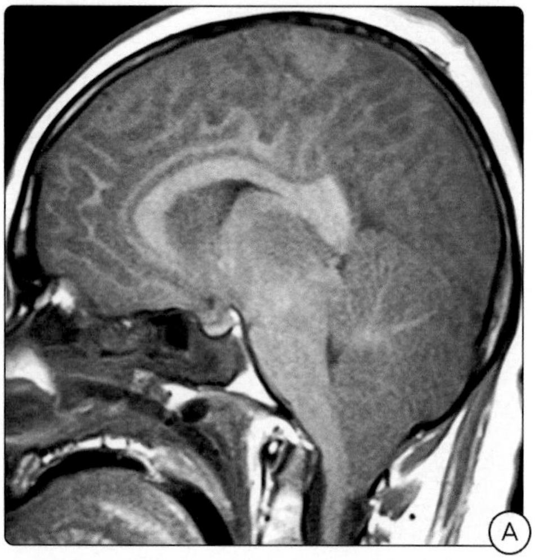

***(3-42A)** Antemortal sagittal T1WI for suspected brain death shows diffuse brain swelling and herniation similar to autopsy case shown above.*

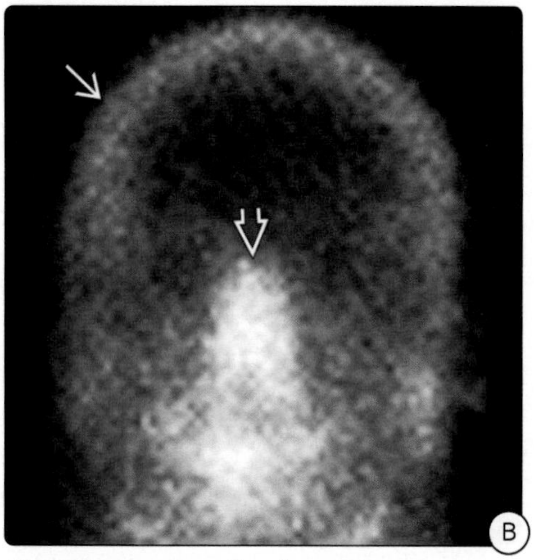

***(3-42B)** Tc99m Neurolite shows tracer accumulation in scalp ➡ ("light bulb" sign), nose ➡ ("hot nose" sign) consistent with brain death.*

Posttraumatic Encephalomalacia

Pathology

The pathologic residue of TBI varies from microscopic changes (e.g., axonal retraction balls and microglial clusters) to more extensive confluent areas of gross parenchymal loss and encephalomalacia. Focal areas of encephalomalacia are most commonly found in areas with a high incidence of cortical contusions, i.e., the anteroinferior frontal lobes and anterior temporal lobes **(3-43)**.

Imaging

Encephalomalacic changes generally appear as low-density foci on NECT. Hypointense areas on T1-weighted MR that appear hyperintense on T2WI and FLAIR are typical. T2* GRE scans may show hemorrhagic residua around the encephalomalacic foci. In patients with significant traumatic subarachnoid hemorrhage (tSAH), superficial siderosis can sometimes be seen as curvilinear hypointense foci along the pial surfaces of the brain **(3-44) (3-45)**.

Chronic moderate to severe TBI causes significant loss of gray and white matter volume with concomitant increase in CSF volume. These changes result in **generalized atrophy** and associated neurocognitive impairment. Whereas overall parenchymal volume loss with increased ventricular size and prominent sulci can be seen on standard imaging studies, subtle cases of regional or global atrophy may require quantitative MR (qMRI) studies for detection.

Reduced cerebellar volume can be seen in some patients following TBI, possibly reflecting the high vulnerability of the cerebellum and its related projection areas to fiber degeneration.

Advanced imaging studies can be helpful adjuncts in assessing residua of TBI. MR spectroscopy may demonstrate reduced neurometabolites following TBI. NAA levels may be low, even in a normal-appearing brain. FDG PET may show focal or more widespread areas of regional glucose hypometabolism.

Diffusion tensor imaging (DTI) demonstrates low FA and high ADC in the corpus callosum of some patients with persistent cognitive deficits following mild TBI.

Posttraumatic Demyelination

White matter tracts are particularly vulnerable to damage from impact-acceleration/deceleration forces. White matter injury after TBI involves both diffuse axonal injury and myelin pathology that evolves throughout the postinjury time course. Wallerian degeneration may occur as the axonal response to disconnection from initial mechanical forces and secondary insults. However, TBI can also cause demyelination of intact axons. In some cases, subacute demyelination causes striking restricted diffusion of the subcortical and deep white matter **(3-46)**.

Chronic Traumatic Encephalopathy

Terminology

Initially reported in boxers and called "dementia pugilistica," the term **chronic traumatic encephalopathy** (CTE) has been adopted to describe a wide spectrum of chronic neurobehavioral abnormalities that result from multiple blows to the head. Sports with concussions and repeated subconcussive injuries have been implicated in the etiology of CTE.

Etiology

CTE represents a cumulative process of repetitive head blows. There is some clinical and epidemiologic overlap of CTE with Alzheimer disease (AD). In addition, there is a close association of CTE and neurofibrillary tangle formation, suggesting a mixed pathology promoted by pathogenetic cascades that may result in both diseases. Both CTE and AD also have an overrepresentation of the *APOE*E3* allele.

Pathology

The gross findings in autopsied brains of deceased athletes suffering from CTE have been likened to that of an "octogenarian Alzheimer patient." Tearing of the septi pellucidi with frontotemporal volume loss, thalamic gliosis, substantia nigra degeneration, and cerebellar scarring are other common features.

Microscopic studies of CTE show variable histologic phenotypes predicated on the presence or absence of neurofibrillary tangles, neutrophil threads, amyloid plaques, and diffuse neuronal loss. In contrast to AD, the hippocampus is frequently spared in CTE.

Clinical Issues

Demographics. Between 15-40% of former professional boxers have symptoms of chronic brain injury. While most cases of CTE have been reported in male athletes playing high-impact sports (e.g., American football), they have also been reported in young female soccer players as well as battered women and abused children. Elderly patients with repeated falls may also be at risk for CTE. Anyone subjected to repetitive head injury from any etiology is at risk for developing CTE.

Presentation. Impairments in memory, language, information processing, and executive function as well as cerebellar, pyramidal, and extrapyramidal symptoms are characteristic of CTE. Progressive cognitive deterioration, recent memory loss, and mood and behavioral disorders such as paranoia, panic attacks, and major depression are common.

Imaging

CT Findings. In the largest series evaluating professional boxers with CTE, CT scans were normal in 93% and showed "borderline" atrophy in 6%. Increased prevalence of a cavum septi pellucidi was present in those boxers with atrophy.

MR Findings. Standard sequences in patients with CTE are often normal. Age-inappropriate volume loss and nonspecific white matter lesions are seen in 15% of cases **(3-47A)**. 3.0-T MR with susceptibility-weighted sequences (SWI) shows microhemorrhages in approximately 10% of patients with CTE **(3-47B)**.

Second-Impact Syndrome

Terminology

A more acute, potentially catastrophic complication of repetitive head injury has been recently recognized and dubbed **"second-impact syndrome"** (SIS) or **"dysautoregulation/second-impact syndrome."**

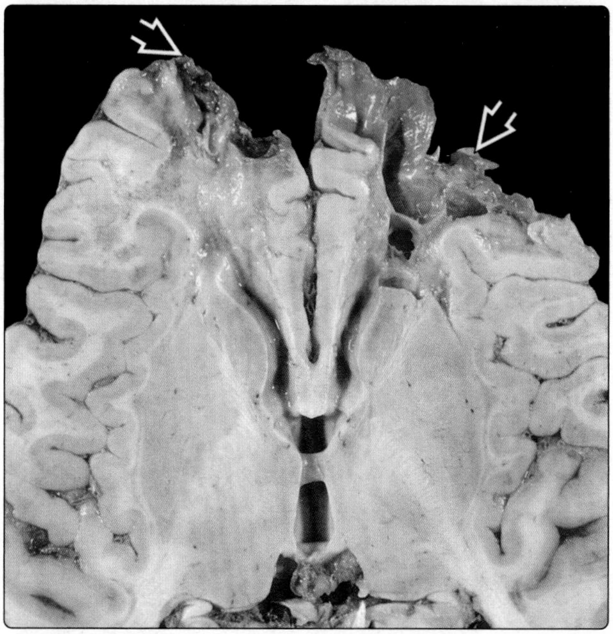

(3-43) Autopsy specimen shows effects of remote trauma with bifrontal encephalomalacia ➡. (Courtesy R. Hewlett, MD.)

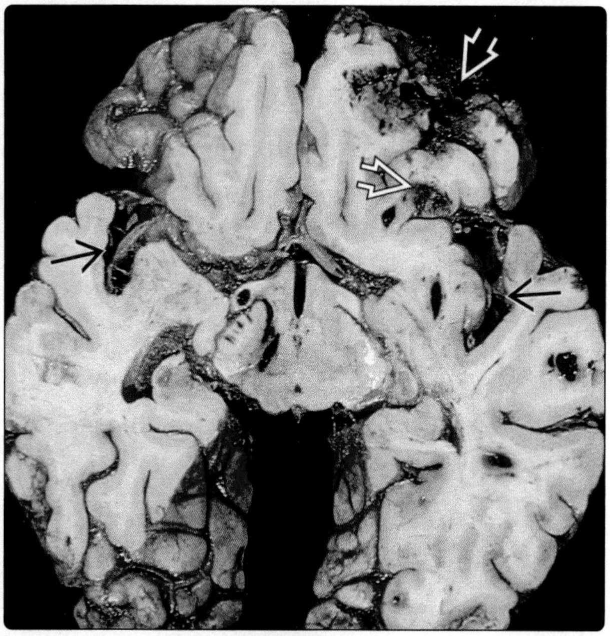

(3-44) Autopsy specimen from a patient with remote trauma shows contusions ➡ and extensive superficial siderosis ⇨. (Courtesy E. T. Hedley-Whyte, MD.)

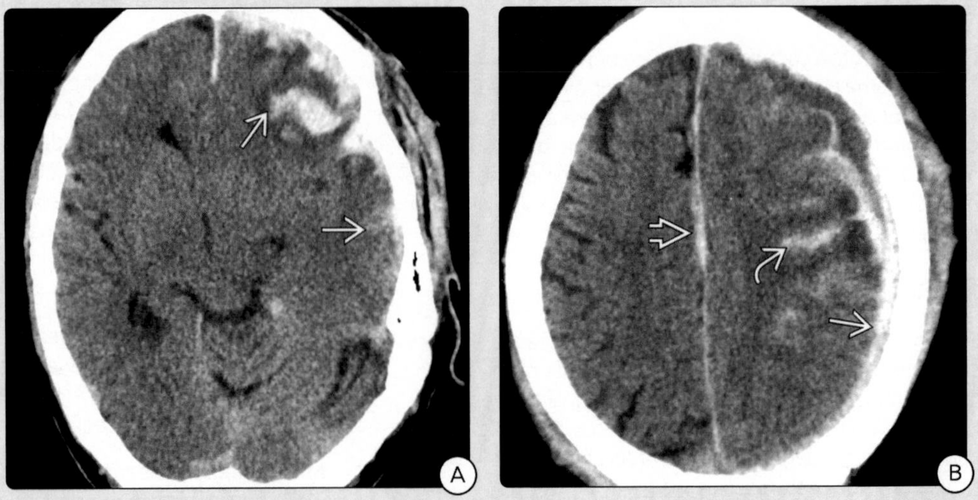

***(3-45A)** NECT scan in an elderly patient with moderately severe head trauma shows left frontotemporal contusions. **(3-45B)** More cephalad scan shows diffuse left hemisphere swelling with interhemispheric convexity SDHs. Several foci of tSAH are present within the compressed sulci.*

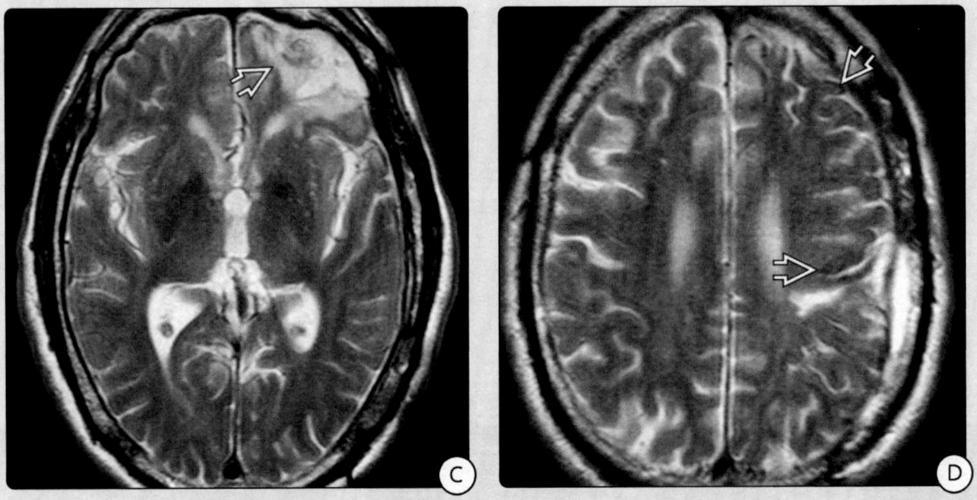

***(3-45C)** T2WI obtained 6 months later shows left frontal encephalomalacia. **(3-45D)** More cephalad T2WI shows several faint curvilinear hypointensities over some of the gyri and extending into the sulci.*

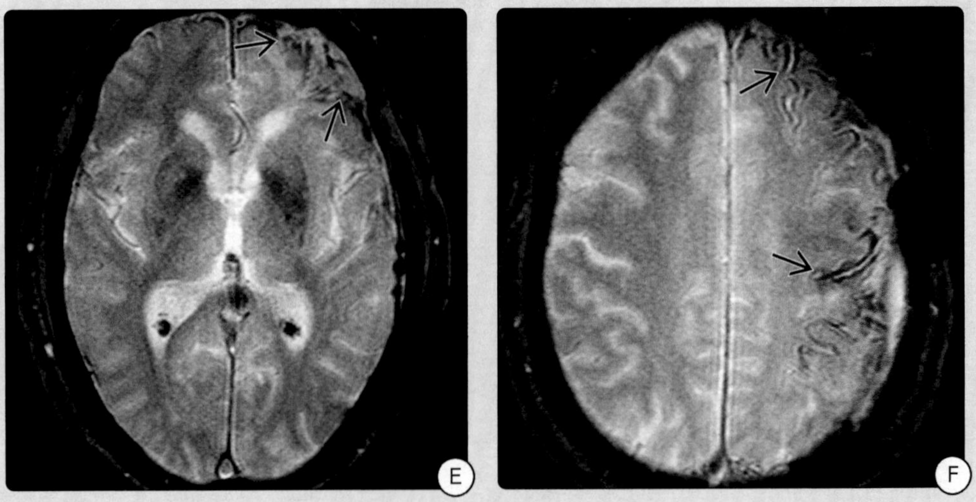

***(3-45E)** T2* GRE scan in the same patient shows "blooming" hemorrhagic residua around the left frontal encephalomalacia. **(3-45F)** More cephalad T2* GRE scan shows extensive posttraumatic superficial siderosis.*

Etiology

Clinical studies show that a single concussive brain injury opens a "temporal window" of metabolic abnormality that can be exacerbated by repeated trauma.

In SIS, individuals (often, but not exclusively, athletes) who are still symptomatic from a prior head injury suffer a second injury. In most cases, a small acute subdural hematoma (aSDH) is associated with disproportionately large brain swelling.

Brain swelling in SIS is probably due to dysautoregulation rather than simply the mass effect of the SDH on the underlying hemisphere. In SIS, loss of autoregulation of cerebral blood flow results in rapid cerebrovascular engorgement, increased intracranial pressure (ICP), and brain swelling.

Excitotoxic brain injury from either increased release and leakage or decreased reuptake of glutamate may also contribute to the unusually widespread cytotoxic edema seen in SIS patients.

Clinical Issues

Demographics. Most reported SIS cases are in young male athletes. Another group that may be susceptible to SIS is elderly patients with recurrent SDHs and repeat episodes of mild to moderate head trauma. Some investigators have also postulated that children with nonaccidental trauma and repetitive brain injury share common pathophysiologic features with athletes suffering from SIS.

Presentation. In SIS, the athlete is often suffering headaches and other symptoms from the initial concussion but returns to competition and sustains a second—often relatively minor—blow to the head. The athlete initially remains conscious but appears stunned and dazed ("got his bell rung") before collapsing and becoming semicomatose.

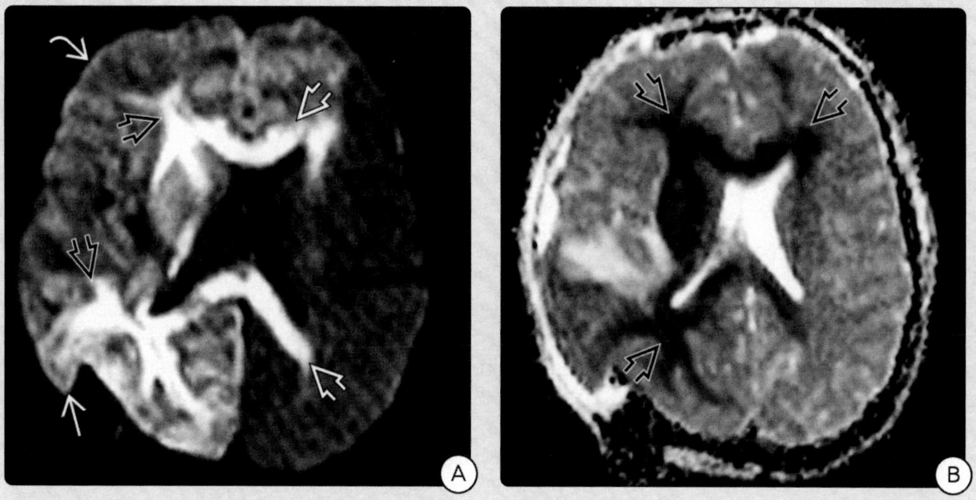

***(3-46A)** Axial DTI in a 22y woman 9 days following severe closed head injury requiring decompressive craniectomy shows residual brain herniation through the craniectomy site → and subacute traumatic cortical ischemia →. The subcortical/deep WM tracts → and corpus callosum → show striking acute diffusion restriction. **(3-46B)** DTI ADC map in the same case shows the striking restricted diffusion in the deep WM tracts →.*

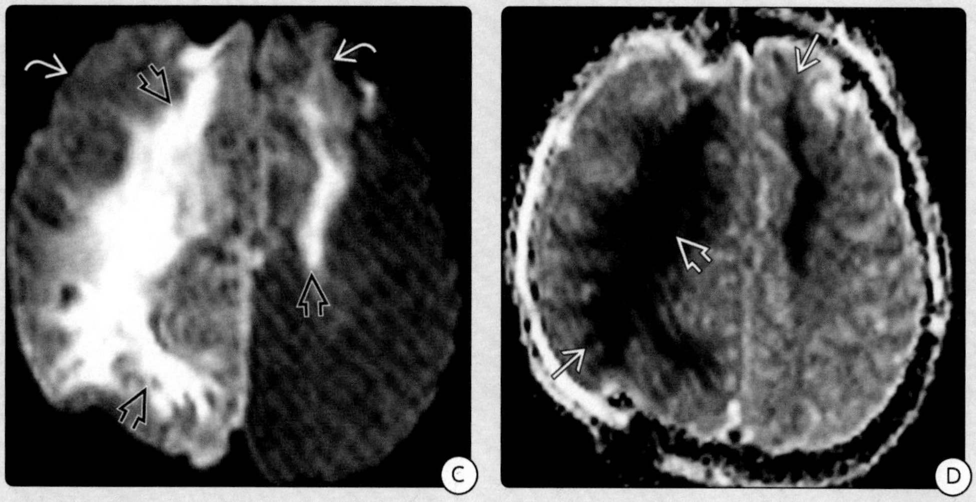

***(3-46C)** More cephalad DTI DWI shows the striking WM restricted diffusion → corresponds to tracts from the cortical infarcts →. **(3-46D)** More cephalad DTI ADC map in the same case confirms the striking acute restricted diffusion involves both the deep → and subcortical → WM tracts. In this case, it is unclear whether the striking posttraumatic WM changes reflect wallerian degeneration or damage to intact axons.*

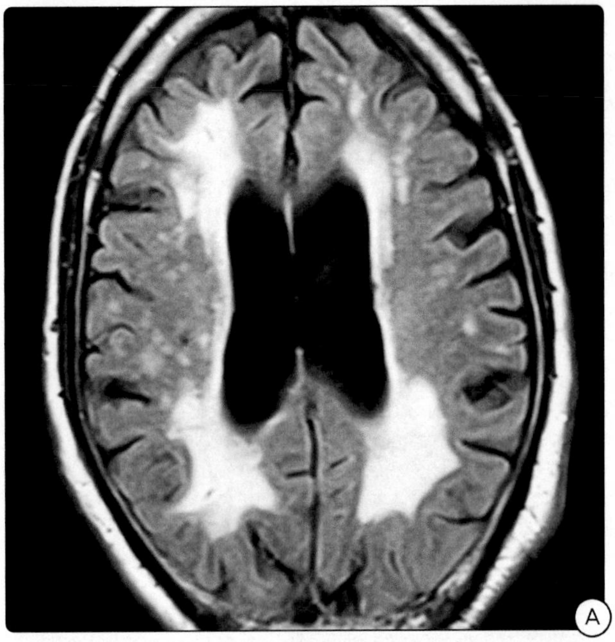

(3-47A) Axial FLAIR scan in a middle-aged former professional athlete with early-onset dementia shows diffuse bihemispheric volume loss, extensive confluent and punctate WM hyperintensities.

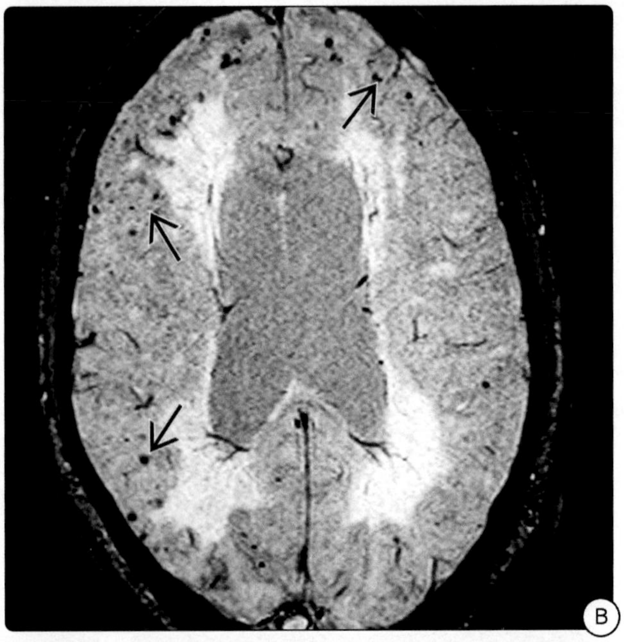

(3-47B) T2* SWI scan in the same patient shows numerous blooming microbleeds ➡. Imaging and clinical features are suggestive of chronic traumatic encephalopathy.

Recovery from a concussive event is nonlinear and does not coincide with the resolution of clinical symptoms.

Natural History. The clinical scenario of SIS is often catastrophic with rapid onset of coma and fixed, dilated pupils. Neurologic deterioration may occur within minutes. Mortality and morbidity are extremely high. Patients who survive, even with emergent decompressive craniectomy, often have multifocal ischemic infarcts with severe residual cognitive and neurologic deficits.

Imaging

NECT scans in patients with SIS show a small (usually < 0.5 cm) crescent-shaped, hyper- or mixed-density SDH overlying a swollen, hypodense cerebral hemisphere. The extent of the mass effect and midline shift is disproportionate to the relatively small size of the aSDH **(3-48)**.

Initially, the gray-white matter interface is preserved, but, as brain swelling progresses, the entire hemisphere becomes hypodense. The basal cisterns and cerebral sulci are totally effaced. Complete "central" descending herniation with brainstem compression ensues.

MR shows swollen T2/FLAIR hyperintense brain underlying a relatively small SDH. T2* (GRE, SWI) scans are usually negative for intraparenchymal hemorrhage. The swollen brain restricts strongly on DWI. MRS shows decreased NAA.

Posttraumatic Pituitary Dysfunction

Both anterior and posterior pituitary insufficiency, diabetes insipidus (DI), and inappropriate antidiuretic hormone secretion may occur following TBI. Posttraumatic DI is associated with high mortality, particularly when presenting very early following injury.

The diagnosis is based on clinical evaluation, laboratory testing, and neuroimaging. A spectrum of MR findings has been reported in posttraumatic pituitary dysfunction and includes hypothalamic and/or posterior pituitary hemorrhage, anterior pituitary lobe infarction, and stalk transection. Traumatic pituitary stalk interruption shows a partially empty sella with a very thin or transected stalk. Decreased vascularization on dynamic contrast-enhanced sequences may be present.

SECOND IMPACT SYNDROME

Etiology
- Concussion → "temporal window" of vulnerability
- Repeat injury before complete recovery → dysautoregulation
- Catastrophic brain swelling

Clinical Features
- Commonly affected
  - Young male athletes
  - Infants with abusive head trauma
  - Elderly patients with repeated falls

Imaging Findings
- Small aSDH
- Disproportionate mass effect
- Hemispheric edema

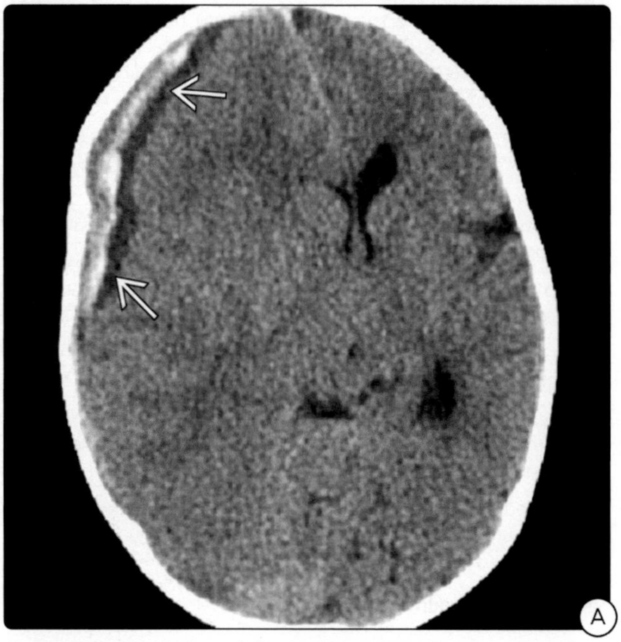

(3-48A) NECT scan in an infant with suspected nonaccidental trauma shows SDHs of 3 different ages ➡. Mass effect and subfalcine herniation are disproportionate to the size of the SDHs.

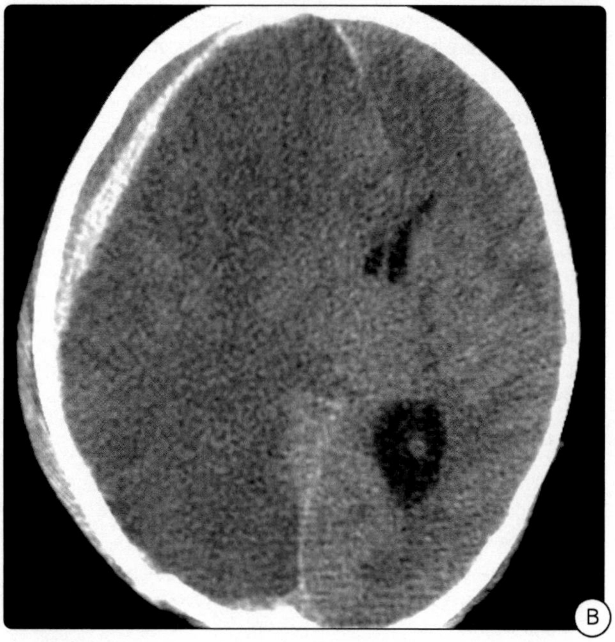

(3-48B) Repeat scan a few weeks later shows another mixed SDH with massive swelling, diffuse edema in the right hemisphere. This is probable second-impact syndrome following multiple concussive injuries.

Selected References

Herniation Syndromes

Mohseni M et al: Contralateral superior cerebellar artery syndrome: a consequence of brain herniation. J Korean Neurosurg Soc. 60(3):362-366, 2017

Smith J et al: Herniated gyrus rectus causing idiopathic compression of the optic chiasm. Clin Neurol Neurosurg. 153:79-81, 2017

Zhang CH et al: Kernohan-Woltman notch phenomenon: a review article. Br J Neurosurg. 31(2):159-166, 2017

Currie S et al: Imaging assessment of traumatic brain injury. Postgrad Med J. 92(1083):41-50, 2016

Wintermark M et al: Imaging evidence and recommendations for traumatic brain injury: conventional neuroimaging techniques. J Am Coll Radiol. 12(2):e1-14, 2015

McDougall CM et al: Angiographic demonstration of upward transtentorial herniation. Can J Neurol Sci. 41(1):82-3, 2014

Edema, Ischemia, and Vascular Injury

Posttraumatic Brain Swelling

Bruno A et al: A standardized method to measure brain shifts with decompressive hemicraniectomy. J Neurosci Methods. 280:11-15, 2017

Beuriat PA et al: Decompressive craniectomy in the treatment of post-traumatic intracranial hypertension in children: our philosophy and indications. J Neurosurg Sci. 59(4):405-28, 2015

Squier W et al: The pathophysiology of brain swelling associated with subdural hemorrhage: the role of the trigeminovascular system. Childs Nerv Syst. 28(12):2005-15, 2012

Ehrhart IC et al: Coronary vascular and myocardial responses to carotid body stimulation in the dog. Am J Physiol. 229(3):754-60, 1975

Traumatic Cerebral Ischemia, Infarction, and Perfusion Abnormalities

Kamp MA et al: Intraoperative indocyanine green (ICG)-based cortical perfusion assessment in patients suffering from severe traumatic brain injury. World Neurosurg. 101:431-443, 2017

Ogami K et al: Early and severe symptomatic cerebral vasospasm after mild traumatic brain injury. World Neurosurg. 813.e11-813.e14, 2017

Salehi A et al: Response of the cerebral vasculature following traumatic brain injury. J Cereb Blood Flow Metab. 271678X17701460, 2017

Kramer AH et al: Decompressive craniectomy in patients with traumatic brain injury: are the usual indications congruent with those evaluated in clinical trials? Neurocrit Care. 25(1):10-9, 2016

Malhotra A et al: Evaluation for blunt cerebrovascular injury: review of the literature and a cost-effectiveness analysis. AJNR Am J Neuroradiol. 37(2):330-5, 2016

Wang JW et al: Decompressive craniectomy in neurocritical care. J Clin Neurosci. 27:1-7, 2016

Bodanapally UK et al: Vascular complications of penetrating brain injury: comparison of helical CT angiography and conventional angiography. J Neurosurg. 121(5):1275-83, 2014

Wang WH et al: Risk factors for post-traumatic massive cerebral infarction secondary to space-occupying epidural hematoma. J Neurotrauma. 31(16):1444-50, 2014

Slotty PJ et al: Cerebral perfusion changes in chronic subdural hematoma. J Neurotrauma. 30(5):347-51, 2013

Ham HY et al: Post-traumatic cerebral infarction : outcome after decompressive hemicraniectomy for the treatment of traumatic brain injury. J Korean Neurosurg Soc. 50(4):370-6, 2011

Blunt Cerebrovascular Injuries

Jung SH et al: Surgical treatment of traumatic intracranial aneurysms: experiences at a single center over 30 years. World Neurosurg. 98:243-250, 2017

Nguyen H et al: Blunt traumatic brain injury patients: a role for CT angiography of the head to evaluate non-traumatic etiologies? World Neurosurg. 101:506-508, 2017

Kansagra AP et al: Current trends in endovascular management of traumatic cerebrovascular injury. J Neurointerv Surg. 6(1):47-50, 2014

Brain Death

Chakraborty S et al: Guidelines for use of computed tomography angiogram as an ancillary test for diagnosis of suspected brain death. Can Assoc Radiol J. 68(2):224-228, 2017

Garrett MP et al: Computed tomography angiography as a confirmatory test for the diagnosis of brain death. J Neurosurg. 1-6, 2017

Wang HH et al: Improving uniformity in brain death determination policies over time. Neurology. 88(6):562-568, 2017

Brasil S et al: Role of computed tomography angiography and perfusion tomography in diagnosing brain death: a systematic review. J Neuroradiol. 43(2):133-40, 2016

Greer DM et al: Variability of brain death policies in the United States. JAMA Neurol. 73(2):213-8, 2016

Smith M: Brain death: the United kingdom perspective. Semin Neurol. 35(2):145-51, 2015

Wijdicks EF: Brain death guidelines explained. Semin Neurol. 35(2):105-15, 2015

Chronic Effects of CNS Trauma

Armstrong RC et al: White matter involvement after TBI: clues to axon and myelin repair capacity. Exp Neurol. 275(3):328-33, 2016

Posttraumatic Encephalomalacia

Armstrong RC et al: Myelin and oligodendrocyte lineage cells in white matter pathology and plasticity after traumatic brain injury. Neuropharmacology. 110(Pt B):654-659, 2016

Konstantinou N et al: Assessing the relationship between neurocognitive performance and brain volume in chronic moderate-severe traumatic brain injury. Front Neurol. 7:29, 2016

Sundman M et al: Neuroimaging assessment of early and late neurobiological sequelae of traumatic brain injury: implications for CTE. Front Neurosci. 9:334, 2015

Posttraumatic Demyelination

Armstrong RC et al: White matter involvement after TBI: clues to axon and myelin repair capacity. Exp Neurol. 275(3):328-33, 2016

Lin M et al: Simulation of changes in diffusion related to different pathologies at cellular level after traumatic brain injury. Magn Reson Med. 76(1):290-300, 2016

Chronic Traumatic Encephalopathy

Frosch MP: Tau aggregates: where, when, why and what consequences? Neuropathol Appl Neurobiol. ePub, 2017

Gaetz M: The multi-factorial origins of chronic traumatic encephalopathy (CTE) symptomology in post-career athletes: the athlete post-career adjustment (AP-CA) model. Med Hypotheses. 102:130-143, 2017

Iacono D et al: Chronic traumatic encephalopathy: known causes, unknown effects. Phys Med Rehabil Clin N Am. 28(2):301-321, 2017

Manley GT et al: A systematic review of potential long-term effects of sport-related concussion. Br J Sports Med. 51(12):969-977, 2017

Perrine K et al: The current status of research on chronic traumatic encephalopathy. World Neurosurg. 102:533-544, 2017

Vile AR et al: Chronic traumatic encephalopathy: the cellular sequela to repetitive brain injury. J Clin Neurosci. 41:24-29, 2017

Hay J et al: Chronic traumatic encephalopathy: the neuropathological legacy of traumatic brain injury. Annu Rev Pathol. 11:21-45, 2016

Bramlett H et al: Long-term consequences of traumatic brain injury: current status of potential mechanisms of injury and neurologic outcomes. J Neurotrauma. 32(23):1834-48, 2015

Second-Impact Syndrome

Stovitz SD et al: What definition is used to describe second impact syndrome in sports? A systematic and critical review. Curr Sports Med Rep. 16(1):50-55, 2017

Cantu RC: Dysautoregulation/second-impact syndrome with recurrent athletic head injury. World Neurosurg. 95:601-602, 2016

Kamins J et al: Concussion-mild traumatic brain injury: recoverable injury with potential for serious sequelae. Neurosurg Clin N Am. 27(4):441-52, 2016

McLendon LA et al: The controversial second impact syndrome: a review of the literature. Pediatr Neurol. 62:9-17, 2016

Hebert O et al: The diagnostic credibility of second impact syndrome: a systematic literature review. J Sci Med Sport. 19(10):789-94, 2016

Guskiewicz KM et al: Acute sports-related traumatic brain injury and repetitive concussion. Handb Clin Neurol. 127:157-72, 2015

Cantu RC et al: Second-impact syndrome and a small subdural hematoma: an uncommon catastrophic result of repetitive head injury with a characteristic imaging appearance. J Neurotrauma. 27(9):1557-64, 2010

Posttraumatic Pituitary Dysfunction

Dalwadi PP et al: Pituitary dysfunction in traumatic brain injury: is evaluation in the acute phase worthwhile? Indian J Endocrinol Metab. 21(1):80-84, 2017

Alavi SA et al: Incidence of pituitary dysfunction following traumatic brain injury: a prospective study from a regional neurosurgical centre. Br J Neurosurg. 1-5, 2015

Capatina C et al: Diabetes insipidus after traumatic brain injury. J Clin Med. 4(7):1448-62, 2015

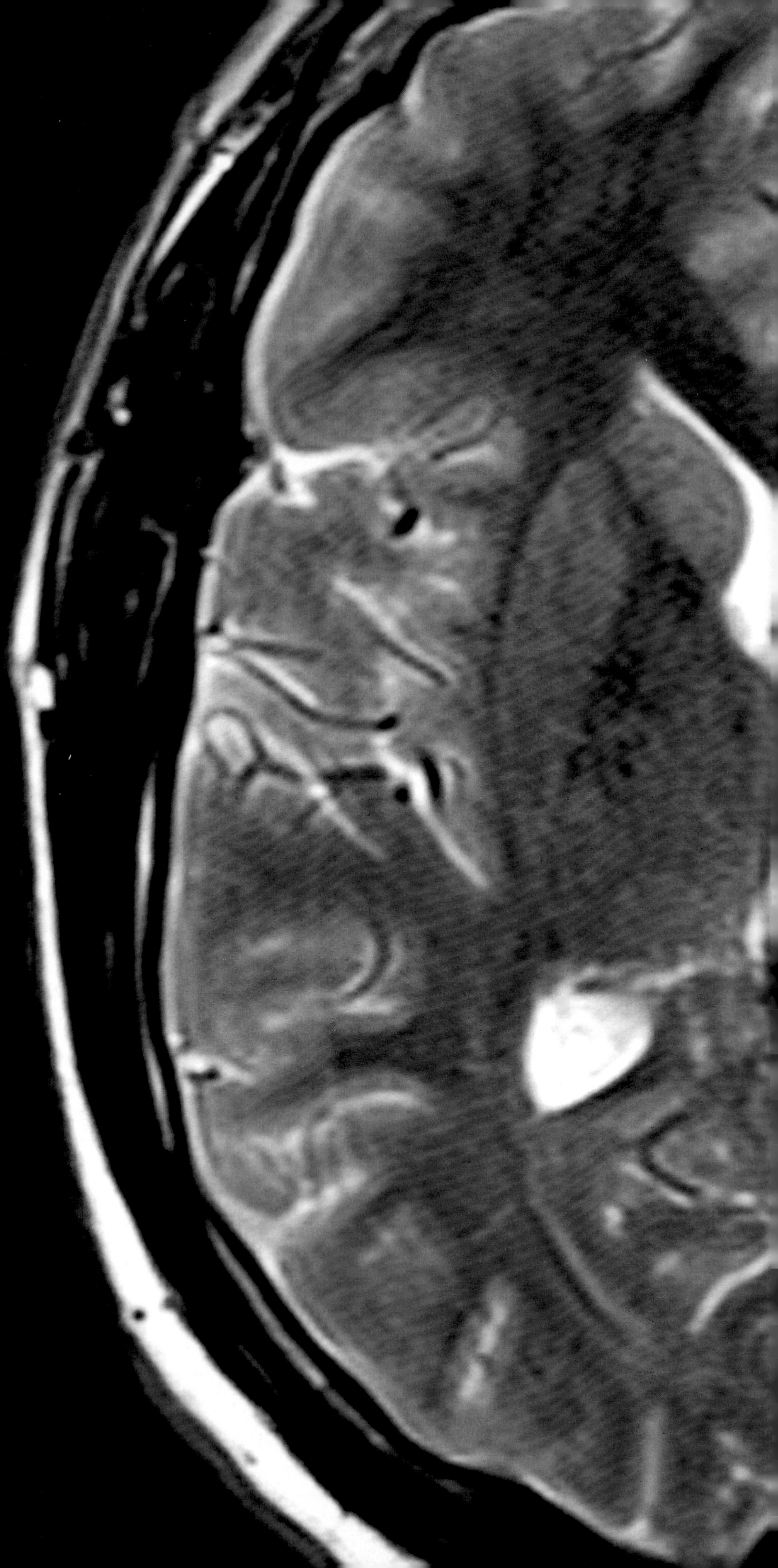

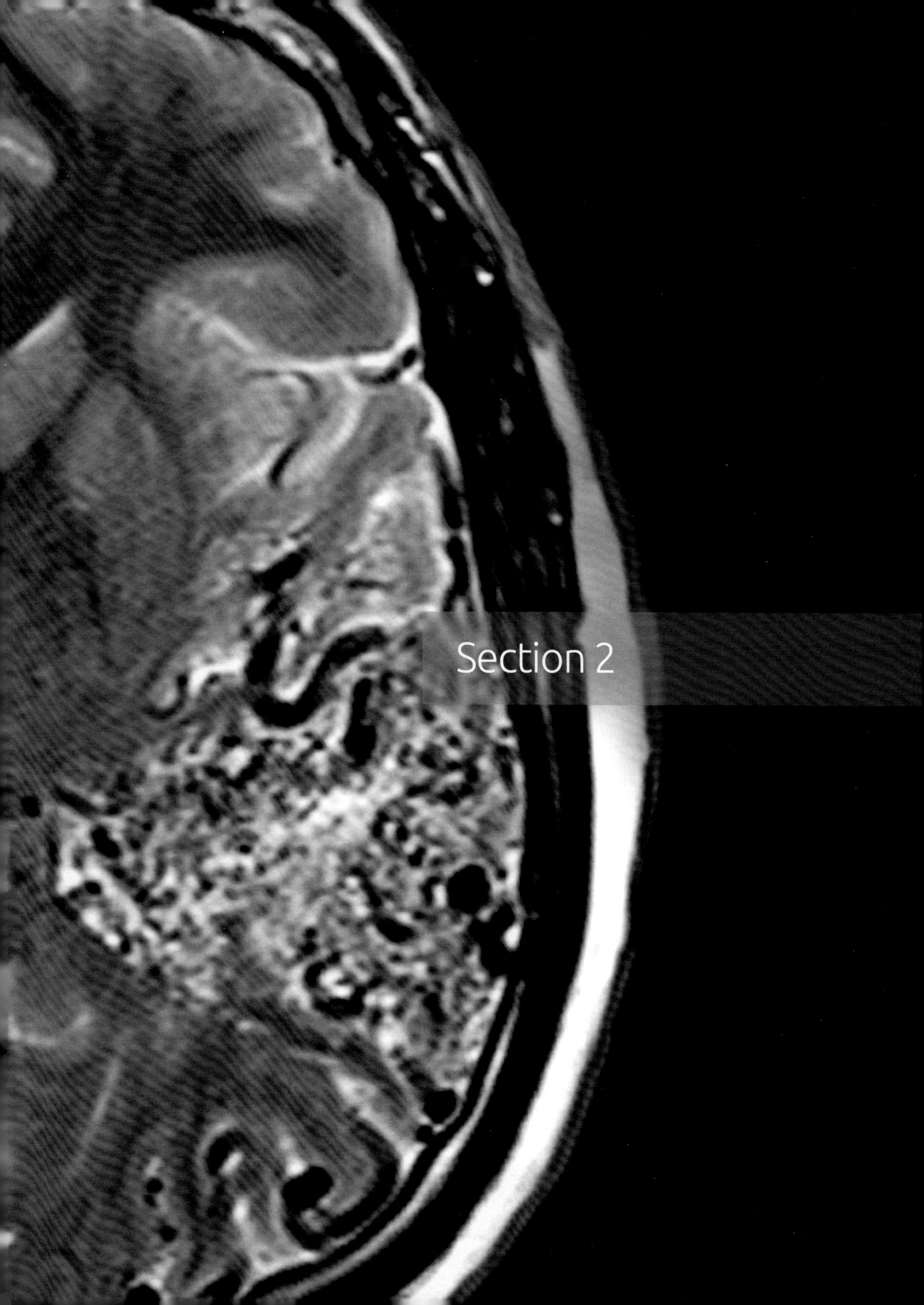
Section 2

Section 2

Nontraumatic Hemorrhage and Vascular Lesions

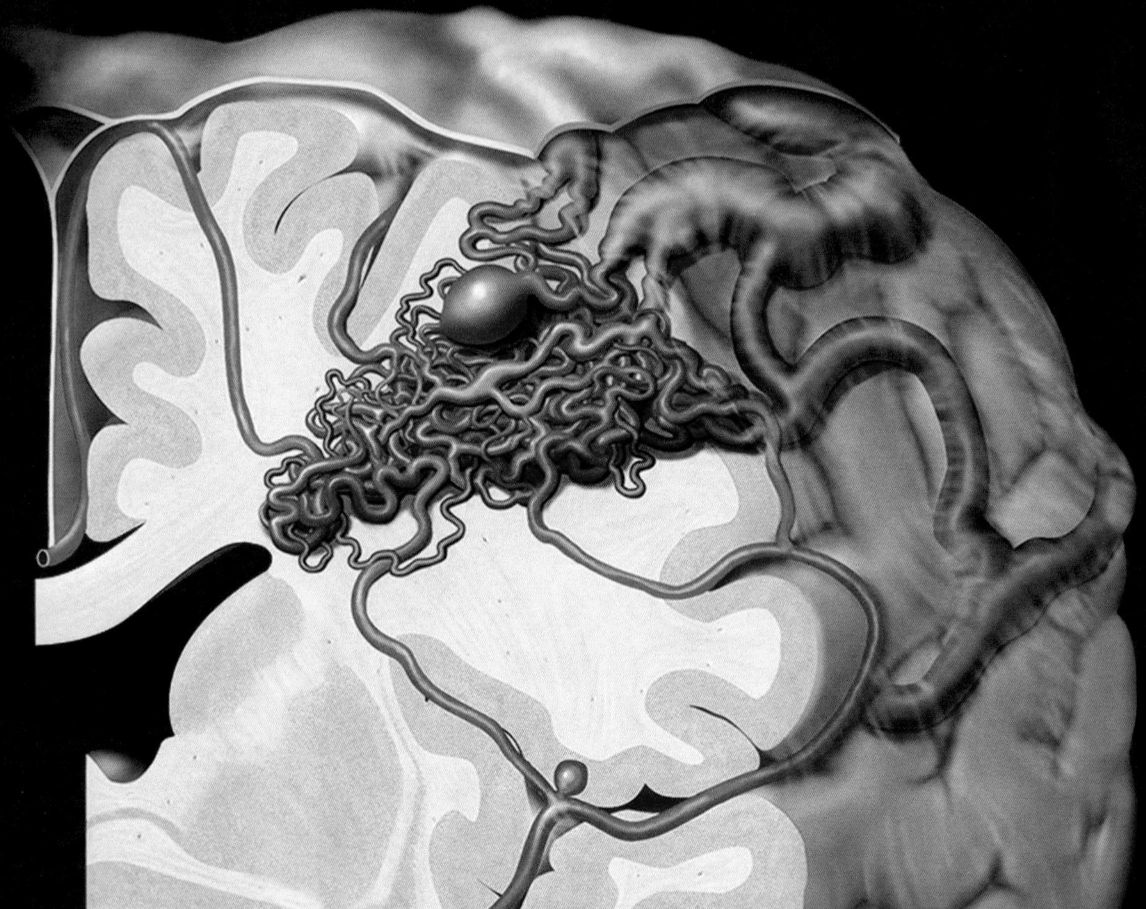

Approach to Nontraumatic Hemorrhage and Vascular Lesions

This part devoted to "spontaneous" (i.e., nontraumatic) hemorrhage and vascular lesions begins with a general discussion of brain bleeds. Subsequent chapters delineate a broad spectrum of vascular pathologies ranging from aneurysms/subarachnoid hemorrhage and vascular malformations to cerebral vasculopathy and strokes. Where appropriate, anatomic considerations and the pathophysiology of specific disorders are included.

Spontaneous (i.e., nontraumatic) intracranial hemorrhage (sICH) and vascular brain disorders are second only to trauma as neurologic causes of death and disability. Stroke or "brain attack"—defined as sudden onset of a neurologic event—is the third leading *overall* cause of death in industrialized countries and is the most common cause of neurologic disability in adults.

Imaging plays a crucial role in the management of stroke patients, both in establishing the diagnosis and stratifying patients for subsequent treatment.

Significant public health initiatives aimed at decreasing the prevalence of comorbid diseases, such as obesity, hypertension, and diabetes, have only marginally decreased the incidence of strokes and brain bleeds. Therefore, it will continue to be important to understand the pathoetiology of intracranial hemorrhages and the various stroke subtypes together with their imaging manifestations.

We start this chapter with a brief overview of nontraumatic ICH and vascular diseases of the CNS, beginning with a short discussion of who, why, when, and how to image these patients. We then develop an anatomy-based approach to evaluating nontraumatic ICH. We close the discussion with a pathology-based introduction to the broad spectrum of congenital and acquired vascular lesions that affect the brain.

Imaging Hemorrhage and Vascular Lesions

Who and Why To Image?

Because of its widespread availability and speed, an emergent NECT scan is generally the first-line imaging procedure of choice in patients with sudden onset of an unexplained neurologic deficit.

If the initial NECT scan is negative and no neurologic deficit is apparent, further imaging is usually unnecessary. However, if the history and clinical findings suggest a thromboembolic stroke or transient ischemic attack (TIA), additional imaging is indicated.

Emergent NECT imaging is also often obtained in patients with headache to screen for suspected subarachnoid hemorrhage (SAH), hydrocephalus, intracranial mass, or other unspecified abnormalities. The updated ACR Appropriateness Criteria indicate that most patients with uncomplicated nontraumatic primary headache do not require imaging. Several studies have confirmed the low yield of imaging procedures for these individuals with so-called "isolated" headache, i.e., headache unaccompanied by other neurologic findings.

In cases where history, physical, or neurologic examination elicits "red flags" or critical features of headache, imaging may be warranted to exclude a secondary cause (see boxes with brief summaries of ACR recommendations below; numerical ratings are 1-3, usually not appropriate; 4-6, may be appropriate; 7-9, usually appropriate).

For detailed explanation, including comments and anticipated exceptions, refer to the complete version at www.acr.org/ac.

ACR APPROPRIATENESS CRITERIA: CHRONIC HEADACHE

Chronic Headache (HA), No New Features, Normal Neurologic Examination

- NECT (3), CTA (2): Usually not appropriate
- MR (4): May be (minimally) appropriate

Chronic HA, New Feature or Neurologic Deficit

- Major concerns = mass lesion, brain bleed
- NECT (7), CTA (4): May be appropriate
- MR without/with contrast (8): Usually appropriate

Positional HA

- Major clinical concern = intracranial hypotension
- MR without/with contrast (8): Usually appropriate
- MR spine + MR myelography (7)

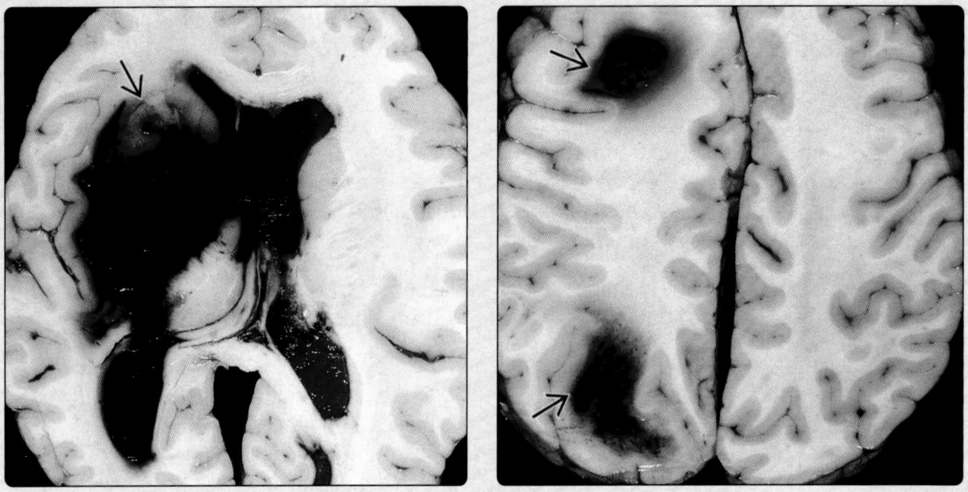

(4-1) Autopsy specimen from an elderly adult shows a parenchymal hematoma ⇨ centered in the striatocapsular region. The external capsule/putamen location is classic for hypertensive hemorrhage. (4-2) Autopsy case from a middle-aged patient with metastatic renal cell carcinoma shows 2 hemorrhagic metastases ⇨ at the gray-white matter interface, a typical location.

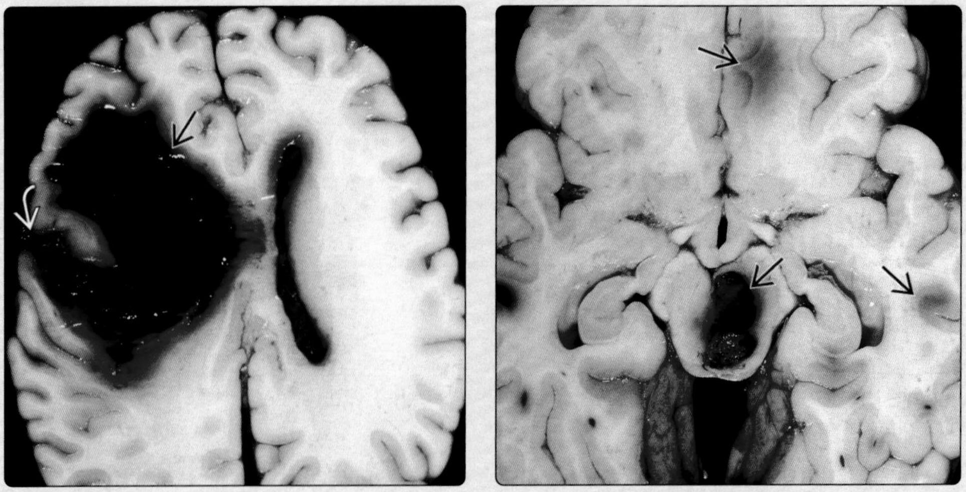

(4-3) Autopsy case is from a young patient with a large hematoma ⇨ centered in the hemispheric white matter with focal extension ➡ through the cortex. Underlying arteriovenous malformation (AVM) was the cause of this fatal intracranial hemorrhage. (4-4) Autopsy case is from a child with multifocal parenchymal hemorrhages ⇨ caused by leukemia. (All four cases courtesy R. Hewlett, MD.)

ACR APPROPRIATENESS CRITERIA: NEW HEADACHE

Sudden Severe HA ("Worst," "Thunderclap")
- Major concern = intracranial hemorrhage
- NECT (9), CTA (8): Highly appropriate
- MR (7), MRA (7): Usually appropriate

New HA in Pregnant Woman
- MR without contrast (8): Usually appropriate
- NECT (7): Usually appropriate

New HA, Suspected Meningitis
- MR without/with contrast (8): Usually appropriate

New HA, Immunosuppressed or Cancer
- MR without/with contrast (9): Highly appropriate

New HA, Focal Neurologic Deficit or Papilledema
- MR without/with contrast (8): Usually appropriate
- MR without contrast (7), NECT (7): Usually appropriate

When and How To Image?

Some of the most challenging questions arise when screening NECT discloses parenchymal hemorrhage. What are the potential causes? Should further emergent imaging be performed?

Many parenchymal "brain bleeds" carry high mortality and morbidity. Early deterioration secondary to rapid hematoma expansion and growth is common in the first few hours after onset. Imaging is crucial in further evaluating and managing these patients.

CTA is indicated in patients with sudden clinical deterioration and a mixed-density hematoma (indicating rapid bleeding or coagulopathy). A "spot" sign with active contrast extravasation caused by rupture of a lenticulostriate microaneurysm (Charcot-Bouchard aneurysm) can sometimes be identified. Contrast extravasation in spontaneous intracranial

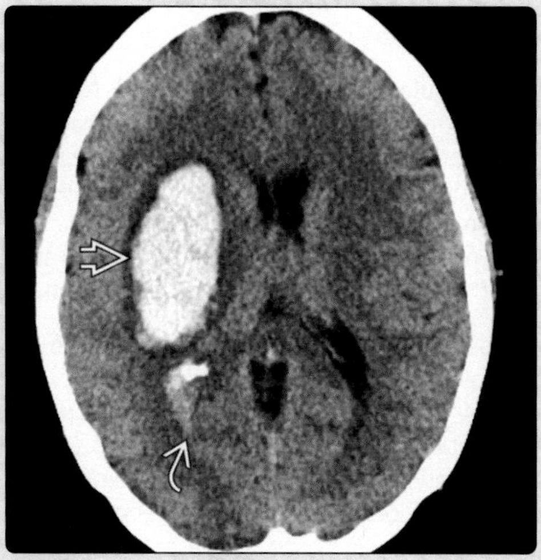

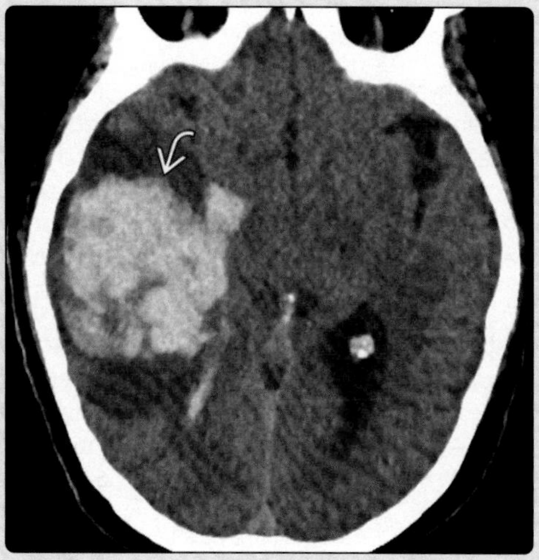

***(4-5)** NECT in a 60y woman with uncontrolled hypertension, sudden onset left-sided weakness shows classic putamen-external capsule hypertensive hemorrhage ➡. Note small amount of blood in the right occipital horn ➡. **(4-6)** NECT in a 59y normotensive man with headache, left-sided weakness, lethargy, and vomiting shows a right temporal lobar hemorrhage ➡. CTA was negative. Surgery disclosed glioblastoma.*

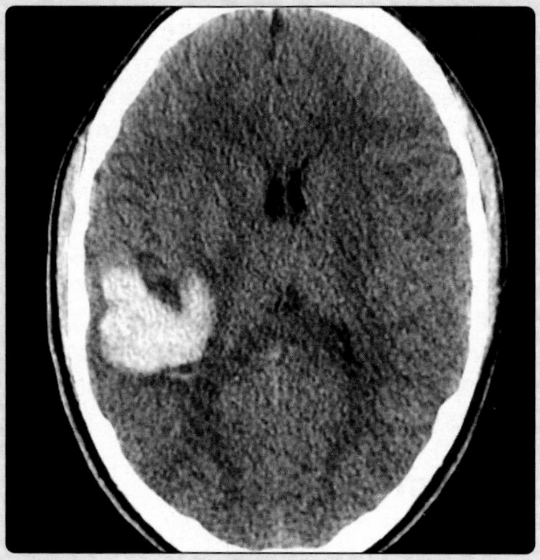

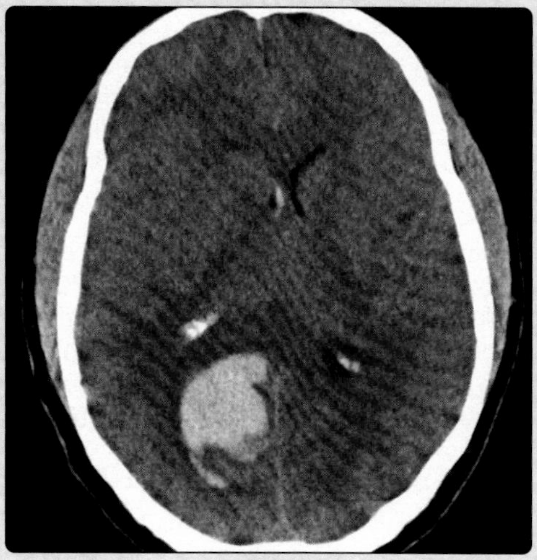

***(4-7)** NECT in a 15y boy with headache, mild left-sided weakness shows a right posterior temporal hematoma. DSA (not shown) disclosed a partially thrombosed AVM. **(4-8)** NECT in a 43y mildly hypertensive man who presented with a severe occipital headache shows a right occipital lobar hematoma. CTA and DSA (not shown) disclosed straight sinus thrombosis.*

hemorrhage (sICH) predicts hematoma expansion and poor clinical outcome.

CTA is also an appropriate next step in children and young/middle-aged adults with spontaneous (nontraumatic) ICH detected on screening NECT. In contrast to elderly patients—in whom hypertensive hemorrhage and amyloid angiopathy are the two most common etiologies of unexplained sICH—vascular malformation is the most common underlying etiology in younger age groups.

Emergency MR is rarely necessary if CTA is negative. However, follow-up MR without and with contrast enhancement can be very useful in patients with unexplained ICH. In addition to the standard sequences (i.e., T1WI, T2WI, FLAIR, DWI, and T1 C+), a T2* sequence—either (or both) GRE or susceptibility-weighted imaging (SWI)—should be obtained.

MR evidence for prior hemorrhage(s) and cerebral "microbleeds" can be very helpful in narrowing the differential diagnosis. Benign ICH typically follows an orderly, predictable evolution on MR scans. MR evidence of disordered or bizarre-looking hemorrhage should raise the possibility of neoplasm, underlying arteriovenous malformation, or coagulopathy.

If MR demonstrates multiple parenchymal hemorrhages of different ages, the underlying etiology varies with patient age. Multiple microbleeds in elderly patients are typically associated with chronic hypertension or amyloid angiopathy. Cavernous malformations or hematologic disorders are the most common causes in children and young adults.

Approach to Nontraumatic Hemorrhage

Hematoma location, age, and number (solitary or multiple) should be noted.

The differential diagnosis of spontaneous nontraumatic intracranial hemorrhage (sICH) varies widely with anatomic location. Because the brain parenchyma is the most common site, we begin with a discussion of intraaxial hemorrhages, then turn our attention to extraaxial bleeds.

Intraaxial Hemorrhage

Clinical Issues

Parenchymal hemorrhage is the most devastating type of stroke. Although recent advances have improved the treatment of ischemic strokes, few evidence-based treatments exist for ICH. Strategies are largely supportive, aimed at limiting further injury and preventing associated complications, such as hematoma expansion, elevated intracranial pressure, and intraventricular rupture with hydrocephalus.

Imaging

Parenchymal hematomas are easily recognized on NECT scans by their hyperdensity or, in the case of rapid bleeding or coagulopathy, mixed iso-/hyperdense appearance. Expansion of a parenchymal hematoma into the ventricular system is commonly encountered on initial imaging in patients with sICH and is associated with poor long-term outcome.

Hematomas typically expand the brain, displacing the cortex outward and producing mass effect on underlying structures such as the cerebral ventricles. The sulci are often compressed, and the overlying gyri appear expanded and flattened. The surrounding brain may appear grossly edematous.

Hematoma signal intensity on standard MR varies with clot age and imaging sequence. T2* (GRE, SWI) scans are especially important in evaluating patients with brain hemorrhage. They should be like your favorite credit cards: "Don't leave home without them!" Susceptibility-weighted imaging is particularly useful in identifying the presence and location of cerebral microbleeds.

Differential Diagnosis

Sublocation of an intraparenchymal clot is very important in establishing putative etiology.

If a classic **striatocapsular** or **thalamic** hematoma is found in a middle-aged or elderly patient, hypertensive hemorrhage is by far the most common etiology **(4-1)** **(4-7)**. Drug abuse should be suspected in a young adult with a similar-appearing lesion. Ruptured aneurysms rarely cause lateral basal ganglionic hemorrhage, and neoplasms with hemorrhagic necrosis are far less common than hypertensive bleeds in this location.

Lobar hemorrhages present a different challenge, as the differential diagnosis is much broader. In older patients, amyloid angiopathy, hypertension, and underlying neoplasm (primary or metastatic) are the most common causes **(4-2)** **(4-6)**. Vascular malformations **(4-3)** **(4-7)** and hematologic malignancies **(4-4)** are more common in younger patients. Dural sinus and/or cortical vein thrombosis are uncommon but occur in patients of all ages **(4-8)**.

Hemorrhages at the **gray-white matter interface** are typical of metastases **(4-2)**, septic emboli, and fungal infection.

Multifocal hemorrhages confined to the **white matter** are rare. When they are identified in a patient with a history of a febrile illness followed by sudden neurologic deterioration, they are most likely secondary to a hemorrhagic form of acute disseminated encephalomyelitis called acute hemorrhagic leukoencephalopathy (also known as Weston-Hurst disease).

Clot age can likewise be helpful in suggesting the etiology of an ICH. A hemosiderin-laden encephalomalacic cavity in the basal ganglia or thalamus of an older patient is typically due to an old hypertensive hemorrhage. The most common cause of a hyperacute parenchymal clot in a child is an underlying arteriovenous malformation.

Extraaxial Hemorrhage

Spontaneous extraaxial hemorrhages can occur in any of the three major anatomic compartments, i.e., the epidural space, subdural space, and the subarachnoid space. By far, the most common are subarachnoid hemorrhages (SAHs) **(4-9)** **(4-10)**. In contrast to traumatic hemorrhages, spontaneous bleeding into the epi- and subdural spaces is rare.

Subarachnoid Hemorrhage

Clinical Issues. Patients with nontraumatic SAH (ntSAH) usually present with sudden onset of severe headache ("worst headache of my life"). A "thunderclap" headache is very common.

Imaging. ntSAH is easily distinguished from a parenchymal hematoma by its location and configuration. Blood in the subarachnoid spaces has a feathery, curvilinear, or serpentine appearance as it fills the cisterns and surface sulci **(4-12)**. It follows brain surfaces and rarely causes a focal mass effect.

SAH is hyperdense on NECT scans. Bloody sulcal-cisternal CSF appears "dirty" on T1WI, hyperintense on FLAIR, and "blooms" on T2* sequences.

Differential Diagnosis. As with parenchymal bleeds, ntSAH sublocation is helpful in establishing an appropriate differential diagnosis. By far, the most common cause of ntSAH is **aneurysmal SAH** (aSAH). As most intracranial aneurysms arise from the circle of Willis and the middle cerebral bifurcation, aSAH tends to spread throughout the basal cisterns and extend into the sylvian fissures **(4-10)**.

Two special, easily recognizable subtypes of SAH are *not* associated with ruptured intracranial aneurysm. Blood localized to the subarachnoid spaces around the midbrain and anterior to the pons is called **perimesencephalic nonaneurysmal SAH** (pnSAH) **(4-11)**. This type of SAH is self-limited, rarely results in vasospasm, and is probably secondary to venous hemorrhage. CTA is a reliable technique to rule out a basilar tip aneurysm. DSA and noninvasive follow-up imaging have had no demonstrable increased diagnostic yield in such cases.

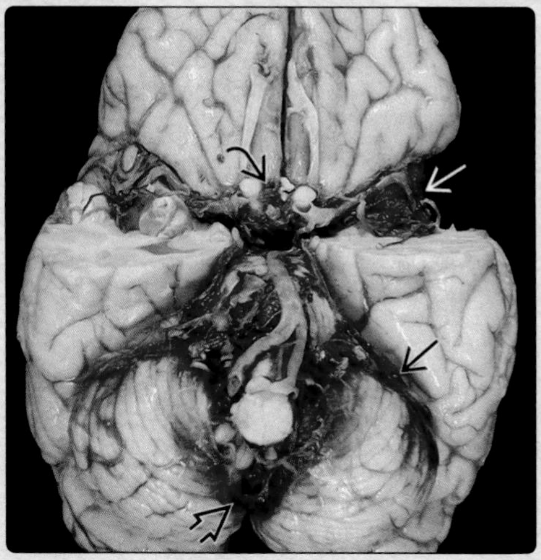

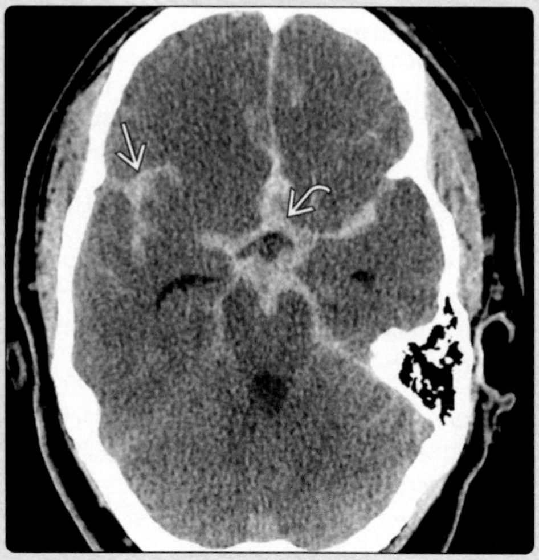

***(4-9)** Autopsy case demonstrates diffuse acute subarachnoid hemorrhage (SAH) in the basal cisterns. Blood fills the sylvian fissures, suprasellar cistern, and cisterna magna. Hemorrhage coats the surface of the pons and extends laterally into the cerebellopontine angle cisterns. **(4-10)** NECT scan shows a patient with aneurysmal SAH. Diffuse hemorrhage fills the suprasellar cistern and sylvian fissures.*

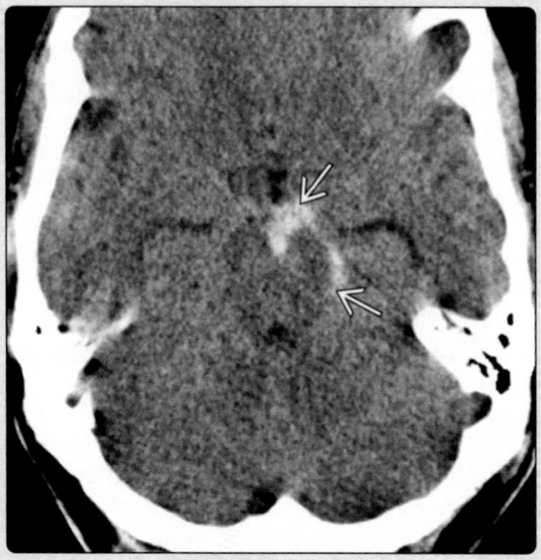

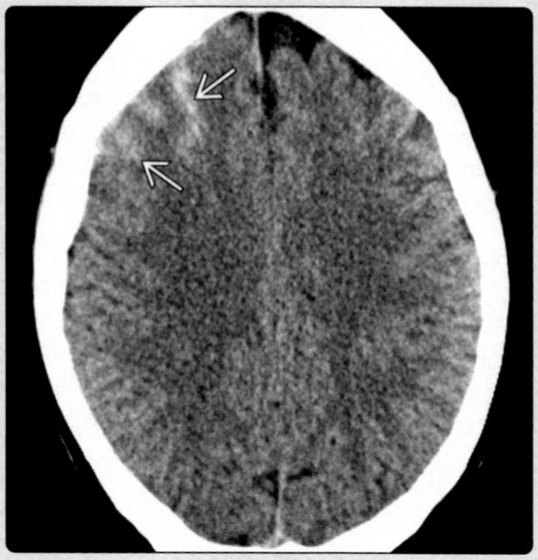

***(4-11)** NECT shows classic perimesencephalic nonaneurysmal SAH with subarachnoid blood localized around the midbrain, in the interpeduncular fossa, and in ambient cistern. CTA was negative. **(4-12)** NECT in a young woman with severe headache shows focal subarachnoid blood in right frontal convexity sulci. Basal cisterns (not shown) were normal. This is proven reversible cerebral vasoconstriction syndrome.*

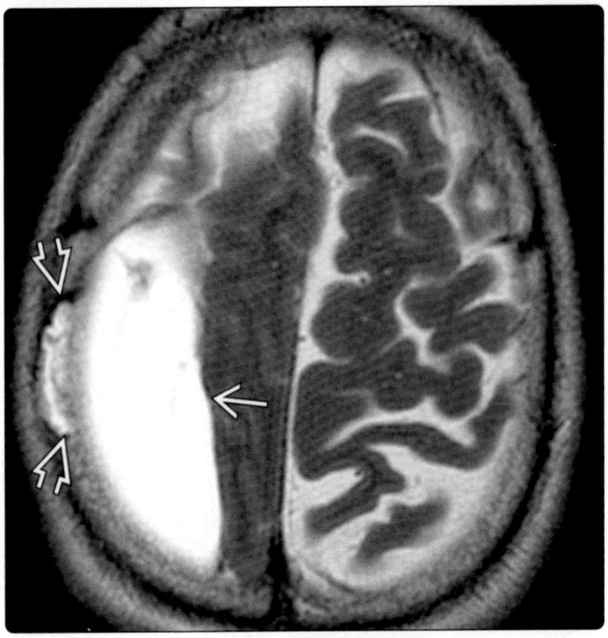

***(4-13)** T2WI shows a chronic epidural hematoma associated with a well-demarcated hyperintense lesion in the calvaria . Hemangioma was found at surgery.*

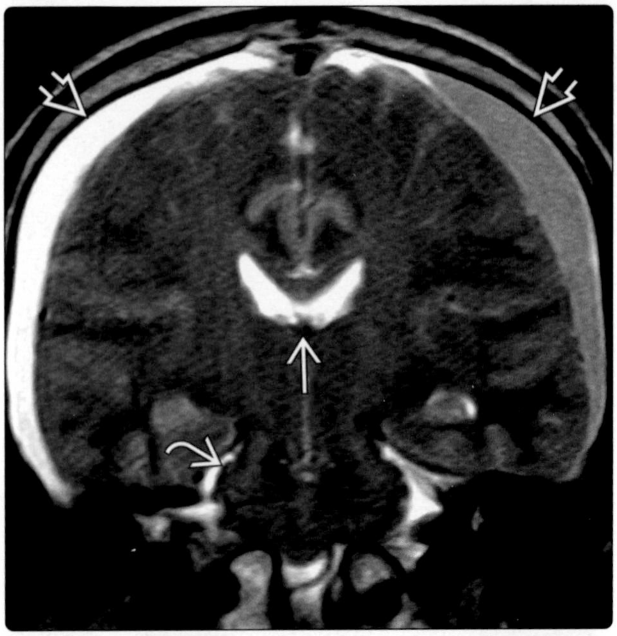

***(4-14)** Coronal T2WI in a patient with severe headaches and intracranial hypotension shows "fat pons" and lateral ventricles pulled inferiorly by brain sagging. Bilateral subdural hematomas of different ages are present .*

Blood in one or more sulci over the upper cerebral hemispheres is called **convexal SAH** **(4-12)**. This special subtype of SAH is associated with a number of diverse etiologies, including cortical vein thrombosis and amyloid angiopathy in older patients, as well as reversible cerebral vasoconstriction syndrome in younger individuals.

Despite extensive imaging evaluation, the origin of spontaneous ntSAH remains unidentified in 10-20% of patients. Hydrocephalus and delayed cerebral ischemia in these patients are infrequent, and long-term neurologic outcomes are generally good.

Epidural Hemorrhage

The pathogenesis of extradural hematomas is almost always traumatic and arises from lacerated meningeal arteries, fractures, or torn dural venous sinuses.

Most spontaneous epidural bleeds are found in the spinal—not the cranial—epidural space and are an emergent condition that may result in paraplegia, quadriplegia, and even death. Elderly anticoagulated patients are most at risk.

Intracranial spontaneous epidural hemorrhages are very rare. Most reported cases are associated with bleeding disorders, craniofacial infection (usually mastoiditis or sphenoid sinusitis), dural sinus thrombosis, bone infarction (e.g., in patients with sickle cell disease), or a vascular lesion of the calvaria (e.g., hemangioma, metastasis, or intradiploic epidermoid cyst) **(4-13)**.

Subdural Hemorrhage

Trauma also causes the vast majority of subdural hematomas (SDHs). Nontraumatic SDHs represent less than 5% of all cases.

Many nontraumatic SDHs occur with CSF volume depletion, i.e., dehydration or CSF hypovolemia. Both can become life-threatening if sufficiently severe.

Intracranial hypotension can be traumatic, iatrogenic, or spontaneous (see Chapter 34). Most cases of traumatic intracranial hypotension are secondary to CSF leak associated with spinal or dural injury. Iatrogenic intracranial hypotension occurs with dural tear following lumbar puncture, myelography, spinal anesthesia, or cranial surgery. Regardless of etiology, SDH is a common (but not invariable) association **(4-14)**.

Nontraumatic SDHs have been reported in association with a number of other conditions including hyponatremic dehydration, inherited or acquired coagulation disorders, dural venous sinus thrombosis, and meningitis.

A few cases of spontaneous SDH occur directly adjacent to a lobar peripheral hemorrhage and are associated with an underlying vasculopathy (such as cerebral amyloid disease with pseudoaneurysm formation) or vascular malformation. Others occur without an identifiable antecedent or predisposing condition.

Occasionally, a ruptured cortical artery or saccular aneurysm may result in a nontraumatic intracranial SDH. Dural hemangiomas have also been reported as causes of acute nontraumatic SDH. Elderly patients with intrinsic or iatrogenic

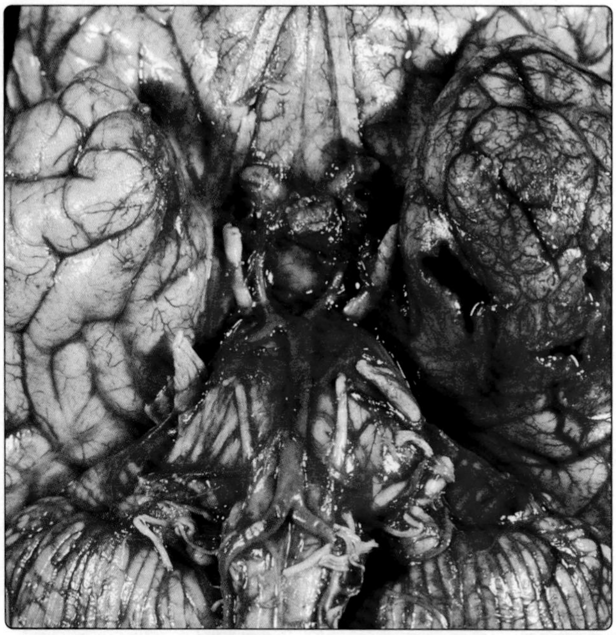

(4-15) Autopsied case shows extensive basilar SAH and vasospasm from a ruptured saccular aneurysm. (Courtesy R. Hewlett, MD.)

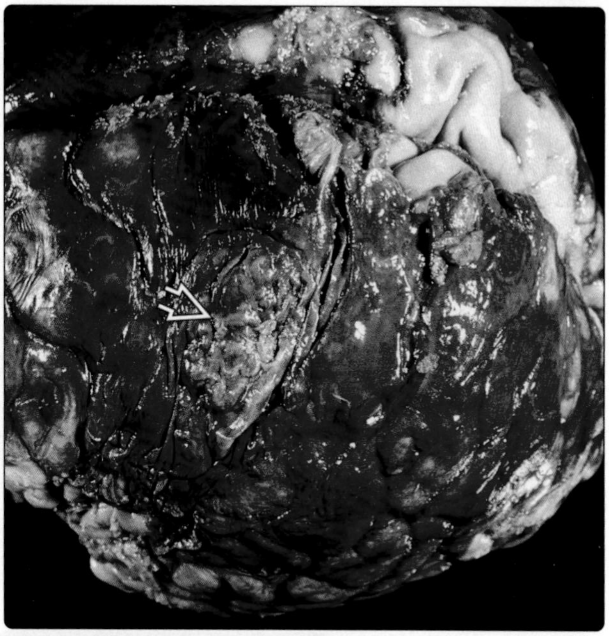

(4-16) Autopsy case shows an AVM causing massive intracranial hemorrhage. Note prominent draining veins ➡ over the surface of the hemisphere. (Courtesy R. Hewlett, MD.)

coagulopathy can present with an SDH and either minor or no definite evidence for head trauma.

Approach to Vascular Disorders of the CNS

Here we discuss a general approach to vascular disorders in the brain, briefly introducing the major chapters in this part. Details regarding pathoetiology, clinical features, imaging findings, and differential diagnosis are delineated in each individual chapter.

Subarachnoid Hemorrhage and Aneurysms

Trauma is—by far—the most common cause of subarachnoid hemorrhage (SAH). Traumatic SAH (tSAH) is found in 100% of patients with fatal severe head injuries and is common in those with moderate to severe nonfatal closed head trauma.

Chapter 6 focuses on *nontraumatic* "spontaneous" SAH, which causes between 3-5% of all acute strokes. Of these, nearly 80% are caused by rupture of a saccular aneurysm **(4-15)**. Aneurysmal SAH can generally be distinguished from nonaneurysmal SAH by its distribution on NECT scans (see above).

Classic saccular ("berry") aneurysms, as well as the less common dissecting aneurysms, pseudoaneurysms, fusiform aneurysms, and blood blister-like aneurysms, are discussed in this chapter.

Vascular Malformations

Cerebrovascular malformations (CVMs) are a fascinating, remarkably heterogeneous group of disorders with unique pathophysiology and imaging features. Chapter 7 discusses the four major types of vascular malformations, grouping them according to whether they shunt blood directly from the arterial to the venous side of the circulation without passing through a capillary bed.

CVMs that display arteriovenous (AV) shunting include AV malformations (AVMs) **(4-16)** and fistulas. Included in this discussion is the newly described entity called cerebral proliferative angiopathy. Cerebral proliferative angiopathy can mimic AVM on imaging studies but has unique features that may influence treatment decisions.

With few exceptions, most CVMs that lack AV shunting—i.e., developmental venous anomalies (venous "angiomas") along with cavernous malformations and capillary telangiectasias—rarely hemorrhage and are "leave me alone" lesions that are identified on imaging studies but generally do not require treatment.

Lastly, note that the topic of "occult" vascular malformation is not discussed. This is an outdated concept that originated in an era when angiography was the only available technique to diagnose brain vascular malformations prior to surgical exploration. Some vascular malformations such as cavernous angiomas and capillary telangiectasias are invisible (and therefore "occult") at angiography but are easily identified on MR.

Arterial Anatomy and Strokes

Chapter 8 begins with a discussion of normal intracranial arterial anatomy and vascular distributions, an essential foundation for understanding the imaging appearance of cerebral ischemia/infarction.

The major focus of the chapter is thromboembolic infarcts in major arterial territories, as they are by far the most common cause of acute strokes **(4-17)** **(4-18)**. Subacute and chronic infarcts are briefly discussed. Although typically not amenable to intravascular treatment, they are nevertheless seen on imaging studies and should be recognized as residua from a prior infarct **(4-19)** **(4-20)**.

The discussion of embolic infarcts includes cardiac and atheromatous emboli as well as lacunar infarcts and the distinct syndrome of fat emboli. The importance of recognizing calcified cerebral emboli on NECT scans is emphasized, as the risk of repeated stroke in these patients is very high.

The pathophysiology and imaging of watershed ("border zone") infarcts and global hypoxic-ischemic brain injury is also included. Miscellaneous strokes such as cerebral hyperperfusion syndrome are discussed.

The chapter concludes by illustrating strokes in unusual vascular distributions, including artery of Percheron and "top of the basilar" infarcts.

Venous Anatomy and Occlusions

The venous side of the cerebral circulation is—quite literally—"terra incognita" (an unknown land) to many physicians who deal with brain disorders. Although many could sketch the major arterial territories with relative ease, few could diagram the intracranial venous drainage territories.

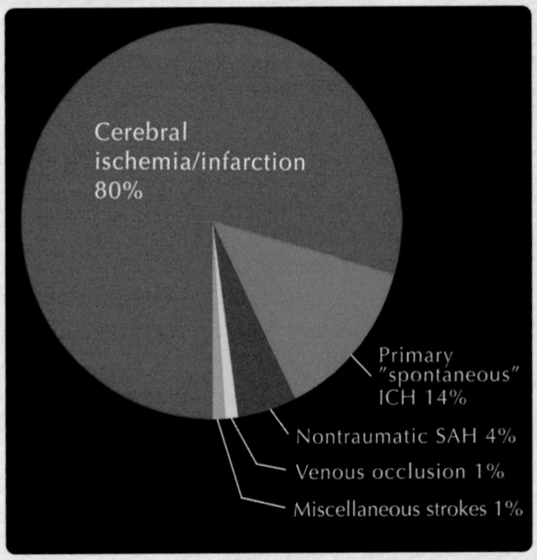

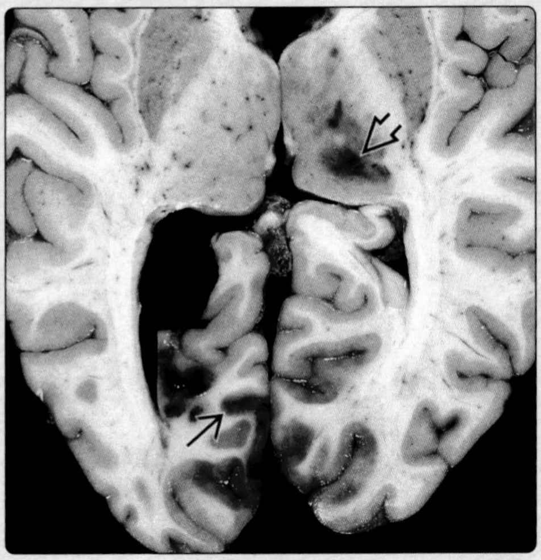

***(4-17)** Diagram shows cerebral ischemia-infarction represents vast majority of strokes. The second most common is primary intracranial hemorrhage (ICH), followed by nontraumatic SAH. **(4-18)** Autopsy shows subacute cerebral infarct, hemorrhagic transformation in occipital cortex ⇨, contralateral thalamus ⇨. Anatomic distribution is of posterior (vertebrobasilar) territorial infarct. (R. Hewlett, MD.)*

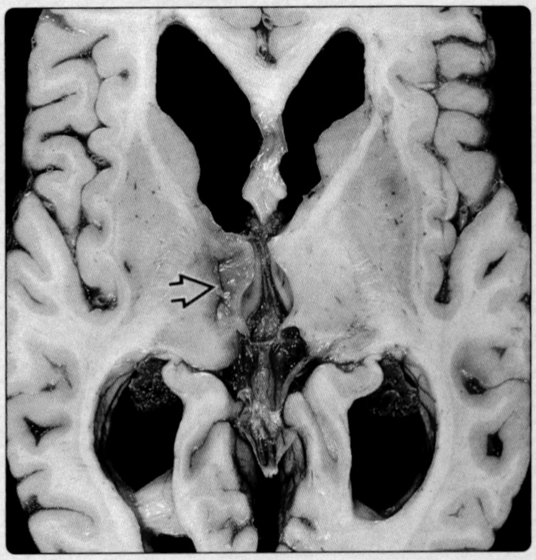

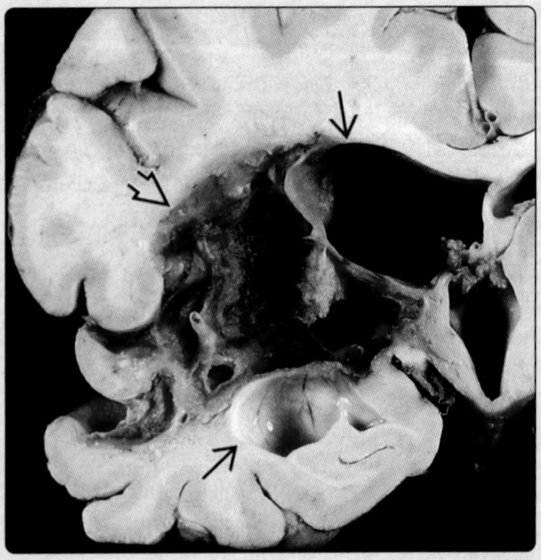

***(4-19)** Autopsied brain shows a chronic healed thalamic infarct ⇨. (Courtesy R. Hewlett, MD.) **(4-20)** Coronal autopsied brain shows encephalomalacic changes of an old middle cerebral artery (MCA) infarct ⇨. Note enlargement of the adjacent lateral ventricle ⇨. (From DP: Hospital Autopsy.)*

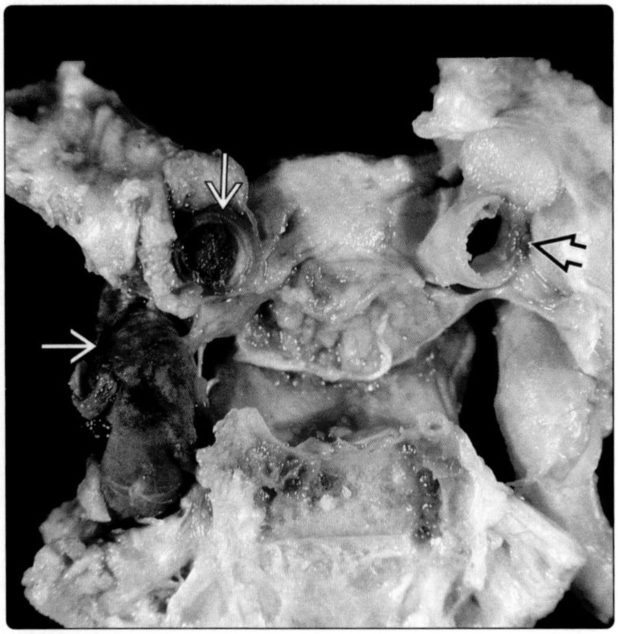

(4-21) Autopsy case shows thrombosis of 1 cavernous/supraclinoid internal carotid artery (ICA) ➡ and atherosclerosis ⇨ in the other ICA.

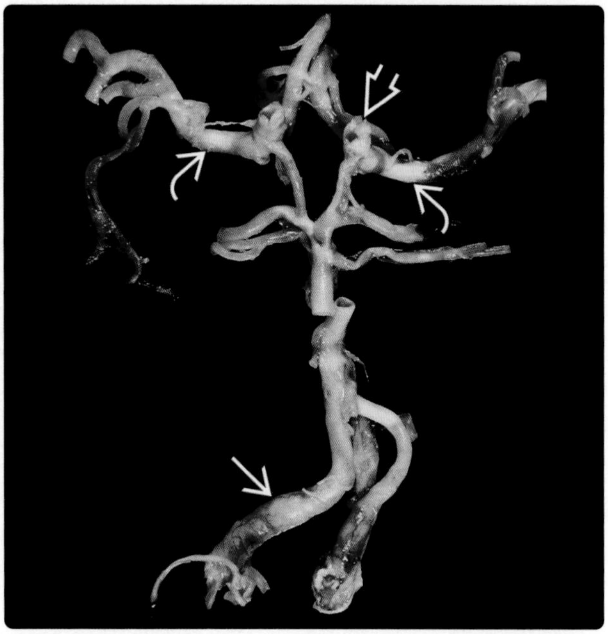

(4-22) Yellowish discoloration and ectasia from atherosclerotic vascular disease is most prominent in the posterior circulation ➡, but the ICAs ➡ and proximal MCAs ➡ are also affected.

The brain veins and sinuses are unlike those of the body. Systemic veins typically travel parallel to arteries and mirror their vascular territories. Not so in the brain. Systemic veins have valves, and flow is generally in one direction.

The cerebral veins and dural sinuses lack valves and may thus exhibit bidirectional flow. Systemic veins have numerous collateral pathways that can develop in the case of occlusion. Few such collaterals exist inside the calvaria.

Chapter 9 begins with a brief discussion of normal venous anatomy and drainage patterns before we consider the various manifestations of venous occlusion. Venous thrombosis causes just 1% of all strokes, and its clinical presentation is much less distinctive than that of major arterial occlusion. It is perhaps the type of stroke most frequently missed on imaging studies. Venous stroke can also mimic other disease (e.g., neoplasm), and in turn a number of disorders can mimic venous thrombosis.

Vasculopathy

Chapter 10, the final chapter in this part, is devoted to cerebral vasculopathy. This chapter begins with a review of normal extracranial arterial anatomy with special focus on the carotid arteries and their variants.

The bulk of the chapter is devoted to cerebral vasculopathy and is organized into two parts: atherosclerosis **(4-21)** and nonatherosclerotic disease. The concept of the "vulnerable" or "at-risk" atherosclerotic plaque is underscored. Indeed, although measuring the percentage of internal carotid artery stenosis has been emphasized since the 1990s as a major predictor of stroke risk and the basis for treatment-related decisions, identifying a rupture-prone plaque is at least as important as determining stenosis.

The relatively new but extremely important topic of high-resolution vessel wall imaging is introduced, and its role in distinguishing between different types of vasculopathy is emphasized.

The much-neglected but important topic of *intracranial* atherosclerosis is also discussed. Whereas major vessel and cardiac thromboemboli cause most arterial strokes, between 5-10% can be attributed to intracranial stenoocclusive disease **(4-21)** **(4-22)**. The topic of arteriolosclerosis (i.e., small vessel vascular disease) is also considered here and again in the subsequent section on metabolic disease.

Nonatheromatous diseases of the cerebral vasculature are much less common than atherosclerosis and its sequelae. However, a number of vasculopathies can have serious consequences and should be recognized on imaging studies. This heterogeneous group of disorders includes fibromuscular dysplasia, dissection, vasospasm, the unusual but important cerebral vasoconstriction syndromes, and the often-confusing topic of vasculitis.

The vasculopathy chapter concludes with the intriguing topic of nonatheromatous microvascular diseases, such as systemic lupus erythematosus, antiphospholipid syndrome, and amyloid angiopathy.

Selected References

Imaging Hemorrhage and Vascular Lesions

Expert Panel on Pediatric Imaging et al: ACR Appropriateness Criteria suspected physical abuse-child. J Am Coll Radiol. 14(5S):S338-S349, 2017

Flottemesch TJ et al: Age-related disparities in trauma center access for severe head injuries following the release of the updated field triage guidelines. Acad Emerg Med. 24(4):447-457, 2017

Hinzpeter R et al: Repeated CT scans in trauma transfers: an analysis of indications, radiation dose exposure, and costs. Eur J Radiol. 88:135-140, 2017

Klang E et al: Overuse of head CT examinations for the investigation of minor head trauma: analysis of contributing factors. J Am Coll Radiol. 14(2):171-176, 2017

Lambert L et al: Growing number of emergency cranial CTs in patients with head injury not justified by their clinical need. Wien Klin Wochenschr. 129(5-6):159-163, 2017

Nishijima DK et al: Out-of-hospital triage of older adults with head injury: a retrospective study of the effect of adding "anticoagulation or antiplatelet medication use" as a criterion. Ann Emerg Med. ePub, 2017

Raja AS et al: "Choosing wisely" imaging recommendations: initial implementation in New England emergency departments. West J Emerg Med. 18(3):454-458, 2017

Thesleff T et al: Head injuries and the risk of concurrent cervical spine fractures. Acta Neurochir (Wien). 159(5):907-914, 2017

Tranvinh E et al: Contemporary imaging of cerebral arteriovenous malformations. AJR Am J Roentgenol. 1-11, 2017

Alobeidi F et al: Emergency imaging of intracerebral haemorrhage. Front Neurol Neurosci. 37:13-26, 2015

Liu R et al: Modeling the pattern of contrast extravasation in acute intracerebral hemorrhage using dynamic contrast-enhanced MR. Neurocrit Care. 22(2):320-4, 2015

Douglas AC et al: ACR Appropriateness Criteria headache. J Am Coll Radiol. 11(7):657-67, 2014

Approach to Nontraumatic Hemorrhage

Intraaxial Hemorrhage

Nikoubashman O et al: MRI appearance of intracerebral iodinated contrast agents: is it possible to distinguish extravasated contrast agent from hemorrhage? AJNR Am J Neuroradiol. 37(8):1418-21, 2016

Witsch J et al: Intraventricular hemorrhage expansion in patients with spontaneous intracerebral hemorrhage. Neurology. 84(10):989-94, 2015

Yakushiji Y: Cerebral microbleeds: detection, associations and clinical Implications. Front Neurol Neurosci. 37:78-92, 2015

Extraaxial Hemorrhage

Weimer JM et al: Acute cytotoxic and vasogenic edema after subarachnoid hemorrhage: a quantitative MRI study. AJNR Am J Neuroradiol. 38(5):928-934, 2017

Elhadi AM et al: Spontaneous subarachnoid hemorrhage of unknown origin: hospital course and long-term clinical and angiographic follow-up. J Neurosurg. 122(3):663-70, 2015

Marder CP et al: Subarachnoid hemorrhage: beyond aneurysms. AJR Am J Roentgenol. 202(1):25-37, 2014

Approach to Vascular Disorders of the CNS

Vasculopathy

Takano K et al: Intracranial arterial wall enhancement using gadolinium-enhanced 3D black-blood T1-weighted imaging. Eur J Radiol. 86:13-19, 2017

Jung SC et al: Vessel and vessel wall imaging. Front Neurol Neurosci. 40:109-123, 2016

Lehman VT et al: Clinical interpretation of high-resolution vessel wall MRI of intracranial arterial diseases. Br J Radiol. 89(1067):20160496, 2016

Coutinho JM et al: High-Resolution vessel wall magnetic resonance imaging in angiogram-negative non-perimesencephalic subarachnoid hemorrhage. Clin Neuroradiol. 27(2):175-183, 2015

Spontaneous Parenchymal Hemorrhage

In the absence of trauma, abrupt onset of focal neurological symptoms is presumed to be vascular in origin until proven otherwise. Rapid neuroimaging to distinguish ischemic stroke from intracranial hemorrhage (ICH) is crucial to patient management.

Epidemiology of Primary ICH

Cerebral ischemia/infarction is responsible for almost 80% of all "strokes." Spontaneous (nontraumatic) primary ICH (pICH) causes 10-15% of first-time strokes and is a devastating subtype with unusually high mortality and morbidity. Death or dependent state is the outcome in > 70% of all patients.

Natural History of Primary (Spontaneous) ICH

Early deterioration with pICH is common. More than 20% of patients experience a decrease in Glasgow Coma Scale (GCS) score of two or more points between initial assessment by paramedics and presentation in the emergency department.

Active bleeding with hematoma expansion (HE) occurs in 25-40% of patients. Patients with large hematomas, history of anticoagulation, or hypertension are at particular risk for HE, which may occur several hours after symptom onset. HE is predictive of clinical deterioration and carries significantly increased morbidity and mortality. Therefore, swift diagnosis is needed to direct treatment.

The prognosis is grave, even with prompt intervention. Between 20-30% of all patients die within 48 hours after the initial hemorrhage. The 1-year mortality rate approaches 60%. Only 20% of patients who survive regain functional independence and recover without significant residual neurologic deficits.

Imaging Recommendations

The most recent American Heart Association/American Stroke Association (AHA/ASA) guidelines recommend emergent CT as the initial screening procedure to distinguish ischemic stroke from intracranial hemorrhage.

If a parenchymal hematoma is identified, determining its size and etiology becomes critically important in patient triage. CTA is easily obtained at the time of initial imaging and is now included in many institutions as an integral part of acute stroke protocols. If contrast or extravasation within the clot ("spot" sign) is present, these patients are at risk HE.

The management of unexplained brain bleeds also varies with patient age. If the patient is older than 45 years and has preexisting systemic hypertension, a putaminal, thalamic, or posterior fossa ICH is almost always hypertensive in origin. Vascular imaging may or may not be requested.

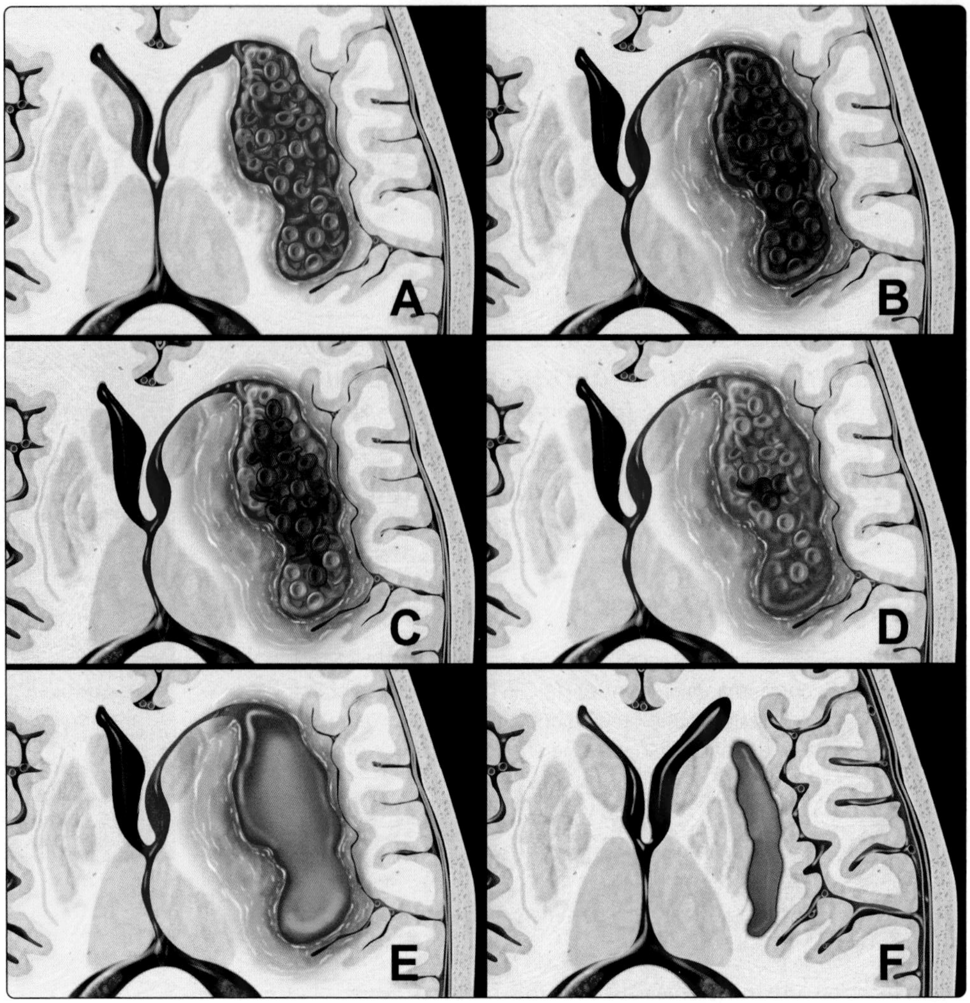

***(5-1)** Brain parenchymal hematomas have a fairly wide range of appearance depending on age of the clot, size of the hematoma, and oxygen tension in the environment. (A) Hyperacute hemorrhage is defined as less than 24 hours old. It consists of a water-rich clot that is 95-98% intracellular oxygenated hemoglobin (oxy-Hgb) (indicated by the intact red blood cells, RBCs, colored red). (B) Acute clots are between 1 and 3 days old. Here the hematoma consists mostly of RBCs (blue) containing intracellular deoxy-Hgb, with the conversion first appearing in the intensely hypoxic clot center. Early subacute clots between 3 (C) and 7 days (D) contain mostly RBCs with intracellular met-Hgb (yellow). (E) Late subacute clots (between 1 and 2 weeks) consist primarily of lysed RBCs with a liquid pool of extracellular met-Hgb. The mostly liquidized clot gradually shrinks with time until only a thin, slit-like yellowish residual fluid collection of extracellular met-Hgb surrounded by a hemosiderin rim remains (F).*

In contrast, lobar or deep brain bleeds in younger patients or normotensive adults—regardless of age—almost always require further investigation. Contrast-enhanced CT/MR with angiography and/or venography may be helpful in detecting underlying abnormalities, such as arteriovenous malformation, neoplasm, and cerebral sinovenous thrombosis.

In older patients with pICH, MR with T2* (GRE, SWI) is also helpful in detecting the presence of "surrogate markers" of small vessel disease such as brain microbleeds, white matter hyperintensities, and lacunar infarcts.

Overview of Primary ICH

We begin this chapter with a discussion of the pathophysiology of ICH. This provides the basis for considering how pICH looks on imaging studies and why its appearance changes over time. We then consider some major causes of spontaneous ICH, such as hypertension and amyloid angiopathy.

"UNEXPLAINED" ICH: WHAT YOU NEED TO KNOW AND DO

Key Clinical Information

- History (any predisposing conditions, e.g., hypertension)
- Medications, drugs (prescription, street)

Initial Imaging Survey = NECT ± CTA

Report

- Hematoma size
    - ABC/2 (width x length x height/2)
- Location
- Is there intraventricular hemorrhage, hydrocephalus?
- Edema, mass effect (herniations, etc)

Solitary lesions comprise the vast majority of pICHs. The presence of more than one simultaneous *macroscopic* brain bleed is actually quite uncommon, accounting for just 2-3% of all pICHs. Multifocal brain *microbleeds* are much more common. We therefore conclude this chapter with a discussion of multifocal brain microbleeds, their etiology, pathology, imaging appearance, and differential diagnosis.

Evolution of Intracranial Hemorrhage

Pathophysiology of Intracranial Hemorrhage

Clot Formation

Clot formation is a complex physiologic event that involves both cellular (mainly platelet) and soluble protein components. Platelets are activated by vascular injury and aggregate at the injured site. Soluble proteins are activated by both intrinsic and extrinsic arms that merge into a common coagulation pathway, resulting in a fibrin clot.

Hemoglobin Degradation

Hemoglobin (Hgb) is composed of four protein (globin) subunits. Each subunit contains a heme molecule with an iron atom surrounded by a porphyrin ring.

Hgb within red blood cells (RBCs) that are extravasating into a pICH rapidly desaturates. Fully oxygenated Hgb (oxy-Hgb) contains nonparamagnetic ferrous iron. In a hematoma, oxy-Hgb is initially converted to deoxyhemoglobin (deoxy-Hgb).

With time, deoxy-Hgb is metabolized to methemoglobin (met-Hgb), which contains ferric iron. As RBCs lyse, met-Hgb is released and eventually degraded and resorbed. Macrophages convert the ferric iron into hemosiderin and ferritin.

Ferritin is the major source of nonheme iron deposition in the human brain. Although iron is essential for normal brain function, iron overload may have devastating effects. Lipid peroxidation and free radical formation promote oxidative brain injury after intracranial hemorrhage (ICH) that may continue for weeks or months.

Stages of Intraparenchymal Hemorrhage

Five general stages in temporal evolution of hematomas are recognized: hyperacute, acute, early subacute, late subacute, and chronic. Each has its own features that depend on three key factors: (1) clot structure, (2) RBC integrity, and (3) Hgb oxygenation status. In turn, imaging findings depend on hematoma stage **(5-1)**.

Hematomas consist of two distinct regions: a central core and a peripheral rim or boundary. In general, Hgb degradation begins in the clot periphery and progresses centrally toward the core.

Hyperacute Hemorrhage. Hyperacute hemorrhage is minutes (or even seconds) to under 24 hours old. Most imaged hyperacute hemorrhages are generally between 4 and 6, but less than 24, hours old. Initially, a loose fibrin clot that contains plasma, platelets, and intact RBCs is formed. At this stage, diamagnetic intracellular oxyhemoglobin predominates in the hematoma.

In early clots, intact erythrocytes interdigitate with surrounding brain at the hematoma-tissue interface. Edema forms around the hematoma within hours after onset and is associated with mass effect, elevated intracranial pressure, and secondary brain injury.

Acute Hemorrhage. Acute ICH is defined as between 1 to 3 days old. Profound hypoxia within the center of the clot induces the transformation of oxy-Hgb to deoxy-Hgb. Iron in deoxy-Hgb is paramagnetic because it has four unpaired electrons.

Deoxyhemoglobin is paramagnetic, but, as long as it remains within intact red cells, it is shielded from direct dipole-dipole interactions with water protons in the extracellular plasma. At this stage, magnetic susceptibility is induced primarily because of differences between the microenvironments inside and outside of the RBCs.

Early Subacute Hemorrhage. Early subacute hemorrhage is defined as a clot that is from 3 days to 1 week old. Hgb remains contained within intact RBCs. Hgb at the hypoxic center of the clot persists as deoxy-Hgb. The periphery of the

Imaging the Stages of Intraparenchymal Hemorrhage

Stage	Time (Range)	Blood Products	CT	T1	T2	T2*	DWI	ADC
Hyperacute	< 24 hours	Oxy-Hgb	Hyperdense	Isointense	Bright	Rim "blooms"	Bright	Dark
Acute	1-3 days	Deoxy-Hgb	Hyperdense	Isointense	Dark	↑ "blooming"	Dark	Dark
Early subacute	> 3 days to 1 week	Intracellular met-Hgb	Isodense	Bright	Dark	Very dark	Dark	Dark
Late subacute	1 week to months	Extracellular met-Hgb	Hypodense	Bright	Bright	Dark rim, variable center	Bright	Dark
Chronic	> 14 days (≥ months)	Hemosiderin	Hypodense	Dark	Dark	Dark	Dark	Dark

(Table 5-1) *Deoxy-Hgb = deoxyhemoglobin; met-Hgb = methemoglobin; oxy-Hgb = oxygenated hemoglobin.*

clot ages more rapidly and therefore contains intracellular met-Hgb. Intracellular met-Hgb is highly paramagnetic, but the intact RBC membrane prevents direct dipole-dipole interactions.

A cellular perihematomal inflammatory response develops. Microglial activation occurs as immune cells infiltrate the parenchyma surrounding the clot.

Late Subacute Hemorrhage. Late subacute hemorrhage lasts from one to several weeks. As RBCs lyse, met-Hgb becomes extracellular. Met-Hgb is now exposed directly to plasma water, reducing T1 relaxation time and prolonging the T2 relaxation time.

Chronic Hemorrhage. Parenchymal hemorrhagic residua persist for months to years. Heme proteins are phagocytized and stored as ferritin in macrophages. If the capacity to store ferritin is exceeded, excess iron is stored as hemosiderin. Intracellular ferritin and hemosiderin induce strong magnetic susceptibility.

Chronic hemorrhage in the subarachnoid space typically coats the pial surface of the brain, a condition termed "superficial siderosis" (see Chapter 6). Superficial siderosis is sometimes seen adjacent to intraparenchymal hematomas, especially those associated with amyloid angiopathy (see Chapter 10).

Imaging of Intracranial Parenchymal Hemorrhage

The role of imaging in spontaneous ICH (sICH) is first to identify the presence and location of a clot (the easy part), to "age" the clot (harder), and then to detect other findings that may be clues to its etiology (the more difficult, demanding part).

The appearance of pICH on CT depends on just one factor, electron density. In turn, the electron density of a clot

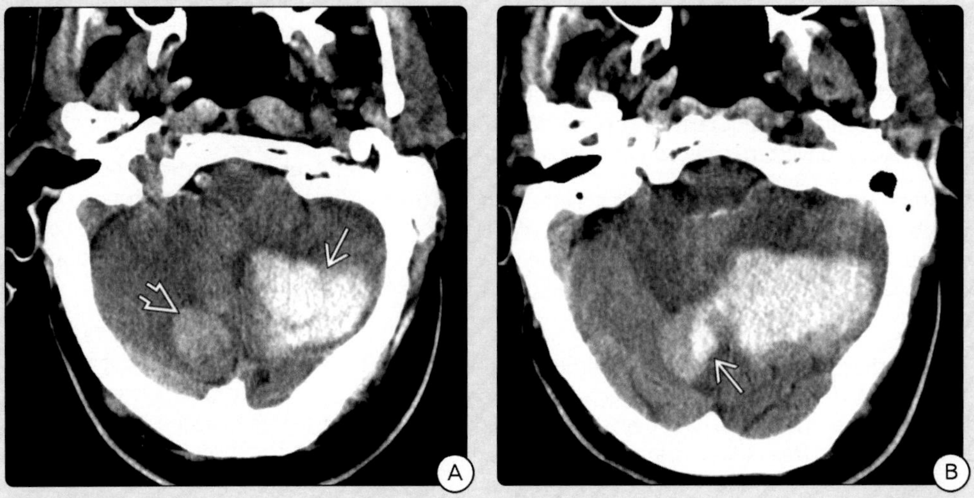

(5-2A) NECT in a hypertensive patient shows a large heterogeneous hematoma in the left cerebellar hemisphere ➡ and a smaller, much less hyperdense clot in the right cerebellum ➡. Findings are consistent with a hyperacute (loose, largely unretracted) clot. (5-2B) The patient suddenly deteriorated while still in the scanner. Repeat NECT scan now shows additional hemorrhage ➡. The patient died shortly after this scan was performed.

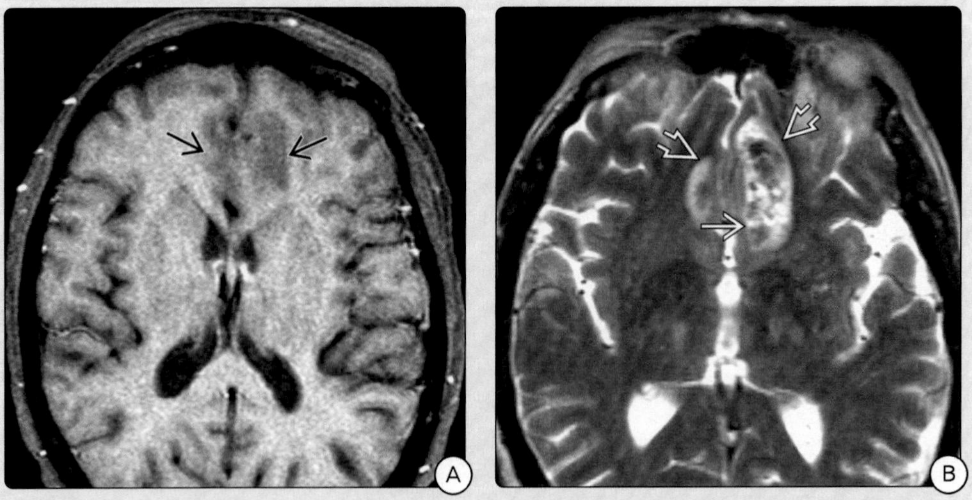

(5-3A) Patient is shown with acute myelogenous leukemia, acute visual symptoms. Emergent NECT scan showed no abnormalities. Sudden deterioration prompted MR. T1WI obtained within minutes shows an ill-defined bifrontal mass ➡ that appears isointense with gray matter. (5-3B) T2WI obtained 5 minutes later shows a mixed signal mass ➡ with fluid-fluid levels ➡. This is rapid hyperacute hemorrhage. (Courtesy M. Brant-Zawadzki, MD.)

depends almost entirely on its protein concentration, primarily the globin moiety of Hgb. Iron and other metals contribute less than 0.5% to total clot attenuation and so have no visible effect on hematoma density.

In contrast, the imaging appearance of ICH on MR is more complex and depends on a number of factors. Both intrinsic and extrinsic factors contribute to imaging appearance.

Intrinsic biologic factors that influence hematoma signal intensity are primarily related to macroscopic clot structure, RBC integrity, and Hgb oxygenation status. RBC concentration, tissue pH, arterial versus venous source of the bleed, intracellular protein concentration, and the presence and integrity of the blood-brain barrier also contribute to the imaging appearance of an ICH.

Extrinsic factors include pulse sequence, sequence parameters, receiver bandwidth, and field strength of the magnet. Of these, pulse sequence and field strength are the most important determinants. T1- and T2-weighted images are the most helpful in estimating lesion age. T2* (GRE, SWI) is the most sensitive sequence in detecting parenchymal hemorrhages (especially microhemorrhages).

Field strength also affects imaging appearance of ICH. The MR findings delineated below and in Table 5-1 are calculated for 1.5-T scanners. At 3.0 T, all parts of acute and early subacute clots have significantly increased hypointensity on FLAIR and T2WI.

Hyperacute Hemorrhage

CT. If ICH is imaged within a few minutes of the ictus, the clot is loose, poorly organized, and largely unretracted **(5-2)**. Water content is still high, so a hyperacute hematoma may appear isodense or occasionally even hypodense relative to adjacent brain. If active hemorrhage is present, the presence of both clotted and unclotted blood results in a mixed-density hematoma with hypodense and mildly hyperdense

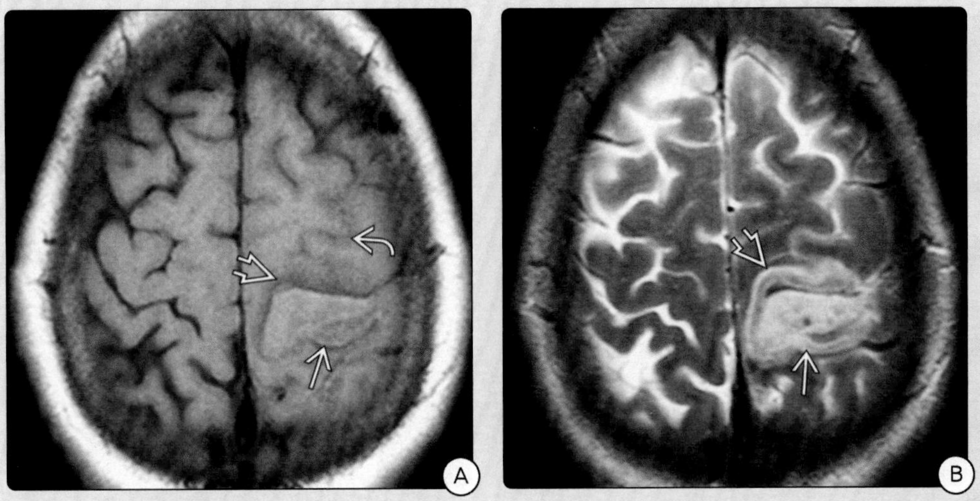

***(5-4A)** MR in normotensive patient with acute spontaneous intracranial hemorrhage (sICH) on NECT is shown. T1WI shows acute hematoma is intermediate in SI, surrounded by a rim of hypointense vasogenic edema. Adjacent sulcal effacement may be from subarachnoid hemorrhage (SAH). **(5-4B)** Clot is heterogeneously hyperintense on T2WI. Note vasogenic edema. "Dirty" CSF probably represents SAH.*

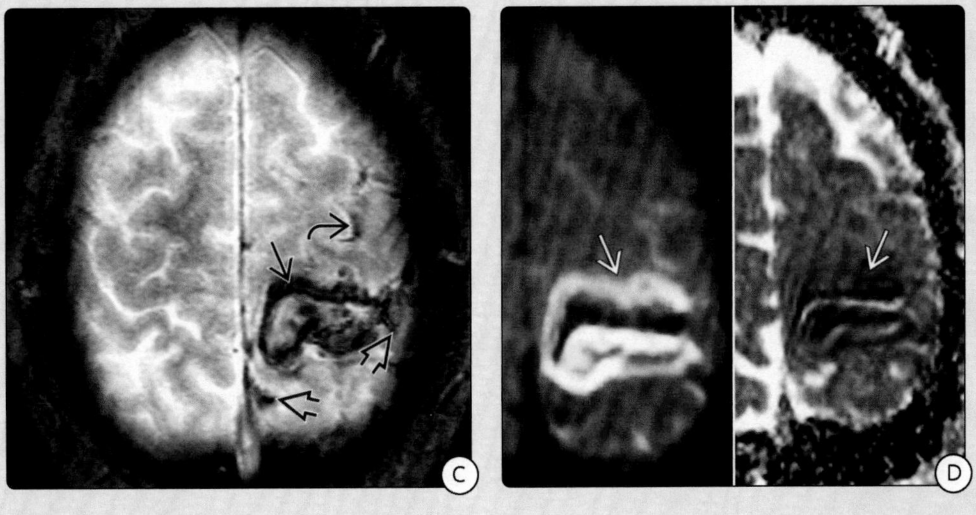

***(5-4C)** T2* GRE scan shows "blooming" around the periphery of the clot and in the sulci. Tubular hypointensity in adjacent cortical veins suggests venous thrombosis. **(5-4D)** DWI (L) and ADC map (R) in the same case show restricted diffusion in the layered, heterogeneous acute hematoma.*

components. Rapid bleeding and coagulopathy may result in fluid-fluid levels.

MR. Oxy-Hgb has no unpaired electrons and is diamagnetic. Therefore, signal intensity of a hyperacute clot depends mostly on its water content. Hyperacute clots are isointense to slightly hypointense to gray matter on T1WI **(5-3A)**. A hyperacute clot is generally hyperintense on T2 scans although they can appear quite heterogeneous **(5-3B)**.

Because the macroscopic structure of a hyperacute clot is so inhomogeneous, spin dephasing results in heterogeneous hypointensity ("blooming") on T2* sequences.

Acute Hemorrhage

CT. The hematocrit of a retracted clot approaches 90%. Therefore, an acute hematoma is usually hyperdense on NECT, typically measuring 60-80 HU. Exceptions to this general rule are found if hemorrhage occurs in extremely anemic patients with very low hematocrits or in patients with coagulopathies.

MR. Acute hematomas are low/intermediate signal intensity on T1WI **(5-4A)**. Significant vasogenic edema develops around the clot and is T1-hypointense and T2/FLAIR-hyperintense **(5-4B)**. As the clot retracts, water content diminishes. Intracellular deoxyhemoglobin predominates. Deoxyhemoglobin is paramagnetic with four unpaired electrons, and the hematoma becomes more profoundly hypointense on T2WI. Acute hematomas "bloom" on T2* (GRE, SWI) **(5-4C)**. Diffusion restriction is present on DWI and ADC although the presence of T2 and susceptibility effects can combine to produce a complex appearance in and around acute hematomas **(5-4D)**.

Early Subacute Hemorrhage

CT. Hematoma density gradually decreases with time, beginning with the periphery of the clot. Clot attenuation

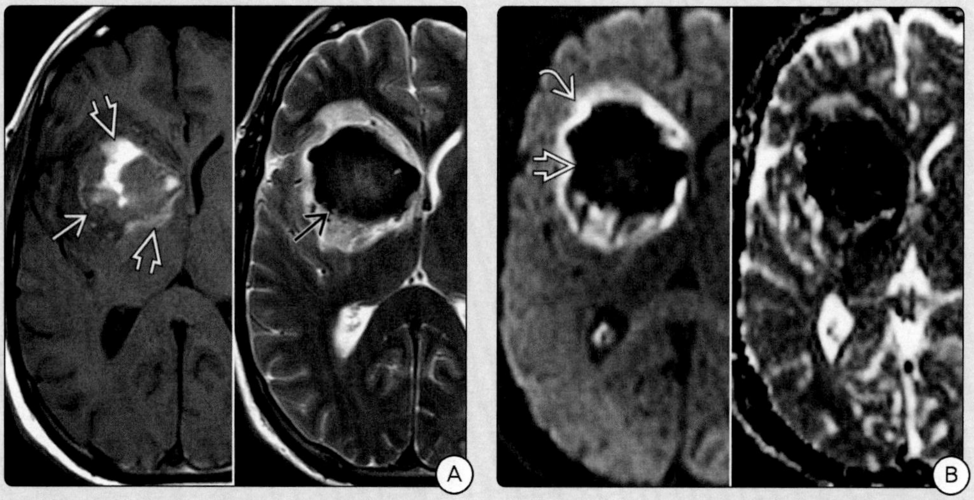

(5-5A) *Axial T1 (L) and T2WI (R) MRs in a patient with a 3-day-old left basal ganglionic hematoma. The clot is largely isointense with brain on T1WI and profoundly hypointense on T2WI. Some T1 shortening is beginning to appear in this late acute/early subacute hematoma.* ***(5-5B)*** *DTI DWI (L) and ADC (R) in the same case show "T2 blackout", which is surrounded by a hyperintense rim of "T2 shine-through".*

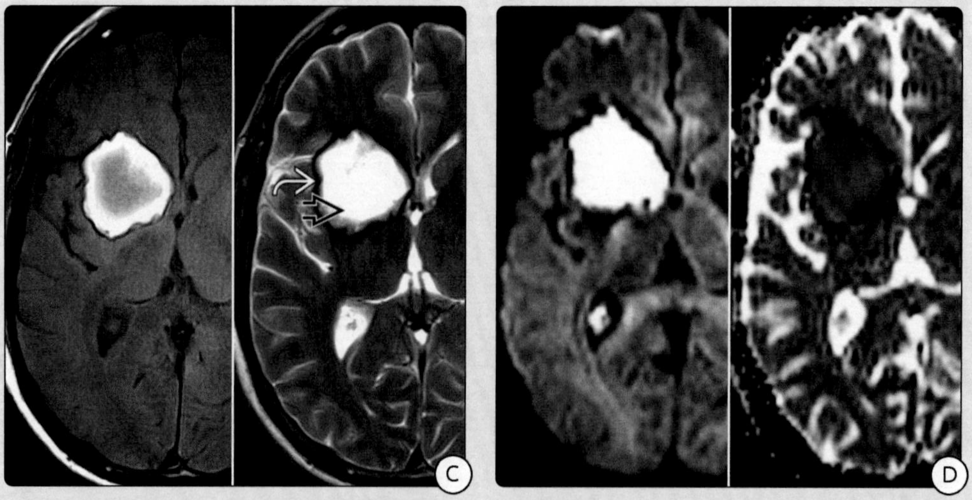

(5-5C) *Axial T1WI (L) and T2WI (R) 3 months later in the same case shows the hematoma is comprised mostly of "bright" extracellular dilute-free met-Hgb. Note hypointense rim (hemosiderin/ferritin) and some isointense clot remaining in the center of the hematoma.* ***(5-5D)*** *DWI (L), ADC map (R) show that the T2 effect dominates in the DWI, while the ADC is dark, indicating true diffusion restriction in the chronic hematoma.*

diminishes by an average of 1.5 HU per day **(5-6)**. At around 7-10 days, the outside of a pICH becomes isodense with the adjacent brain **(5-7B)**. The hyperdense center gradually shrinks, becoming less and less dense until the entire clot becomes hypodense. A subacute hematoma shows ring enhancement on CECT.

MR. Intracellular methemoglobin predominates around the clot periphery, whereas deoxyhemoglobin persists within the hematoma core. A rim of T1 shortening (hyperintensity) surrounding an isointense to slightly hypointense core is the typical appearance on T1WI **(5-7C)**. Paramagnetic methemoglobin is not very mobile and causes pronounced T2 shortening so early subacute clots are hypointense on T2WI. Profound hypointensity on T2* persists.

Clot appearance on diffusion-weighted imaging (DWI) varies. For many forms of hemorrhage, the T2/T2* effect comprises the dominant contribution to signal intensity and therefore appears markedly hypointense (T2 "blackout effect"). In acute and subacute hemorrhage, true restricted diffusion occurs with the intrinsically long T2 of these hematomas **(5-5D)**. The diffusion signal of hemorrhage at each stage of evolution is summarized in Table 5-1.

Late Subacute Hemorrhage

CT. With progressive aging, a pICH gradually becomes hypodense relative to adjacent brain on NECT scans. Ring enhancement may persist for weeks or up to 2 or 3 months.

MR. Once cell lysis occurs, mobile free dilute extracellular methemoglobin predominates in determining signal intensity. Clots develop hyperintensity around their rim on both T1WI and T2WI **(5-5C)**. Eventually the clot appears very hyperintense on both sequences. A rim of T2* blooming generally persists. With the exception of minor susceptibility artifacts, late subacute clots appear similar on both 1.5 T and 3.0 T.

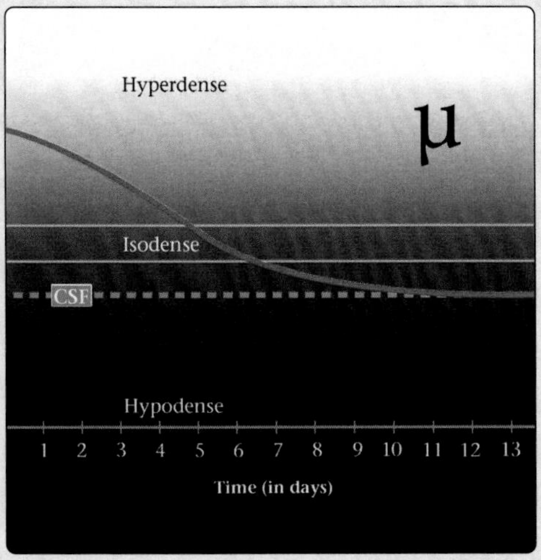

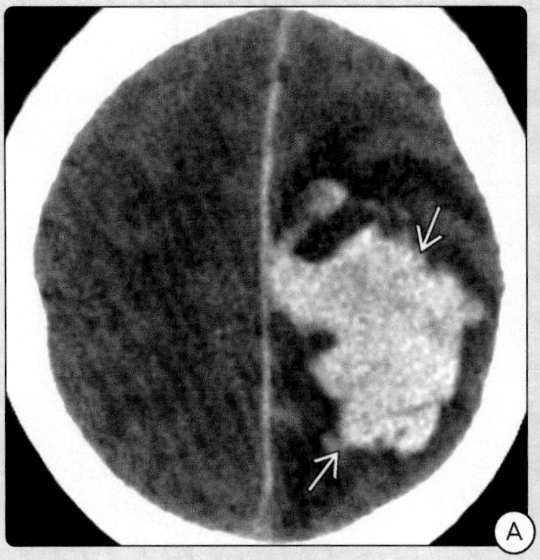

***(5-6)** Graphic depicts time-related progressive decrease in density of brain hematoma relative to parenchyma. Clots are initially hyperdense, become isodense between a few days to a week or so, then are hypodense. Eventually a resolving clot becomes nearly isodense with CSF. **(5-7A)** Axial NECT scan in a patient with an acute lobar hypertensive hemorrhage shows relatively uniform hyperdense clot in the left parietal lobe ➡.*

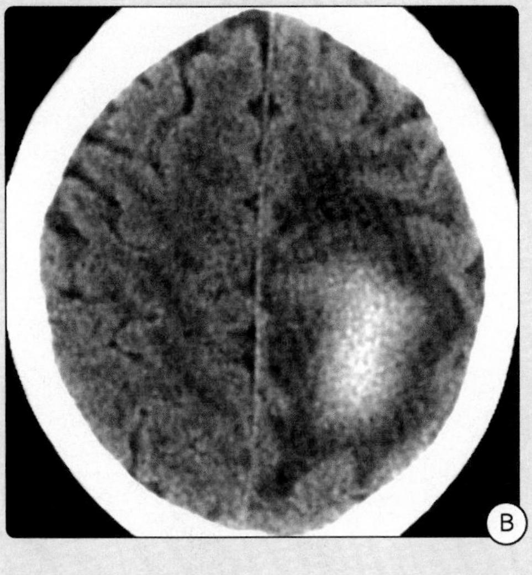

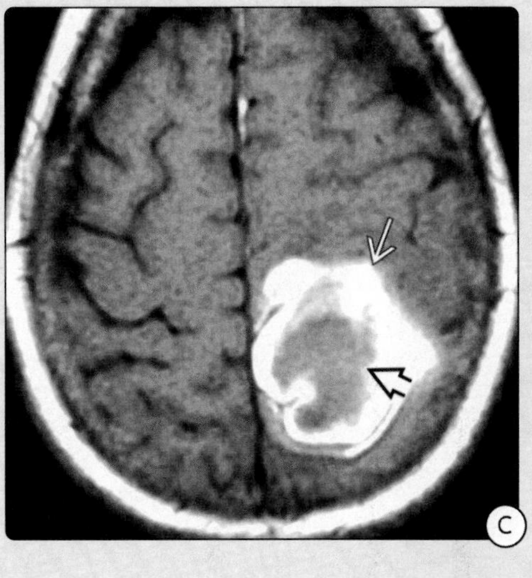

***(5-7B)** Follow-up NECT scan was obtained 1 week later. Clot density has decreased with a gradation from hyperdense in the center to isodense to hypodense at the periphery. **(5-7C)** MR scan was obtained immediately after the follow-up CT scan. T1WI shows that the subacute hematoma is hyperintense around the rim ➡, nearly isointense in the center ⇨.*

Chronic Hemorrhage

CT. A few very small healed hemorrhages may become invisible on NECT scan. From 35-40% of chronic hematomas appear as a round or ovoid hypodense focus. Another 25% of patients develop slit-like hypodensities. Between 10-15% of healed hematomas calcify.

MR. Intracellular ferritin and hemosiderin are hypointense on both T1WI and T2WI. A hyperintense cavity surrounded by a "blooming" rim on T2* may persist for months or even years **(5-9)**. Eventually, only a slit-like scar remains as evidence of a prior parenchymal hemorrhage **(5-8)**.

Etiology of Nontraumatic Parenchymal Hemorrhages

There are many causes of nontraumatic ("spontaneous") or unexplained ICH. The role of imaging in such cases is to localize the hematoma, estimate its age from its imaging features, and attempt to identify possible underlying causes.

The effect of age on the pathoetiology of sICH is profound. Knowing the patient's age is extremely important in establishing an appropriately narrowed differential diagnosis.

It can be difficult to discern enhancement within an already-hyperdense acute hematoma on CECT scans. Dual-energy CT (DECT) can display the presence of contrast enhancement, potentially helping distinguish between tumor bleeding and nonneoplastic ("pure") hemorrhage. Dual-energy CT can also help differentiate ICH from extravasated contrast material staining.

MR imaging with standard sequences as well as fat-saturated contrast-enhanced scans can be very helpful. A T2* sequence (GRE and/or SWI) should always be included, as the identification of other prior "silent" microhemorrhages affects both diagnosis and treatment decisions.

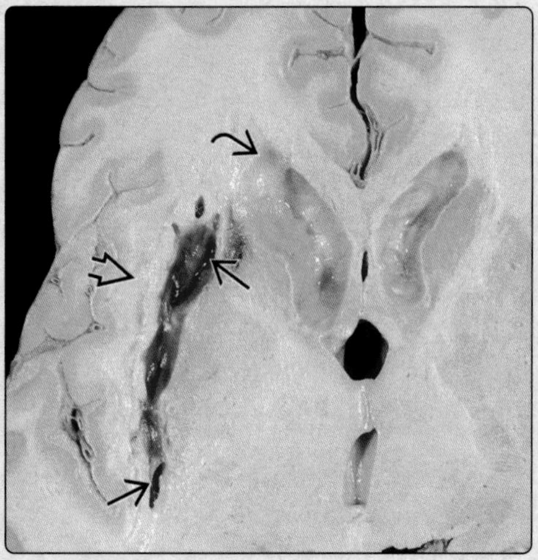

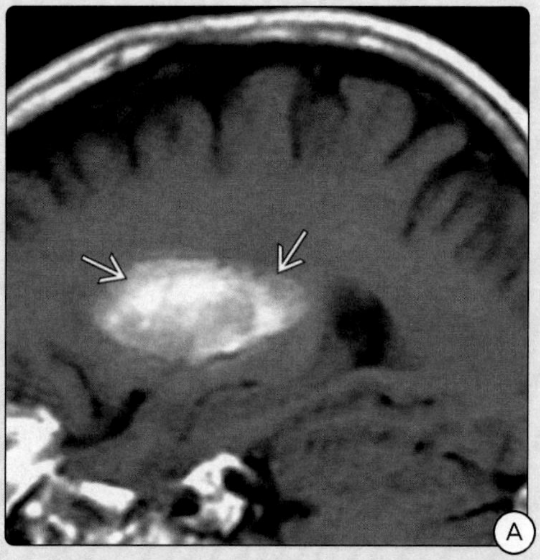

***(5-8)** Gross autopsy case shows residua of remote striatocapsular hemorrhage. A slit-like cavity with a small amount of yellowish fluid is surrounded by dark hemosiderin staining →. Note volume loss with enlarged right frontal horn ↷, gliotic brain ⇨ surrounding old hematoma. (Courtesy R. Hewlett, MD.) **(5-9A)** Sagittal T1WI in a patient 2 years following hypertensive hemorrhage shows ovoid hyperintense cavity ➡.*

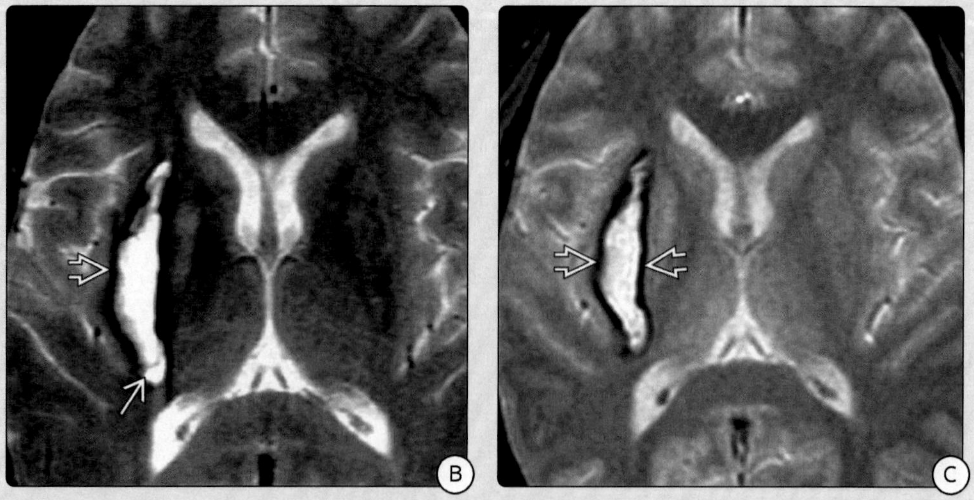

***(5-9B)** Axial standard (not FSE) T2WI shows that the cavity ➡ contains hyperintense fluid (dilute-free extracellular met-Hgb) and is surrounded by a hypointense rim of hemosiderin/ferritin ➡. **(5-9C)** T2* GRE shows "blooming" ➡ around the rim of the residual cavity. Findings are classic for chronic parenchymal hematoma.*

Newborns and Infants With sICH

ICH in the term newborn is most frequently associated with prolonged or precipitous delivery, traumatic instrumented delivery (e.g., forceps assistance or vacuum extraction), and primiparity. The most common cause of ICH in infants less than 34 gestational weeks is **germinal matrix hemorrhage (5-10) (5-11)**.

The germinal matrix is a highly vascular, developmentally dynamic structure in the brain subventricular zone. The germinal matrix contains multiple cell types, including premigratory/migratory neurons, glia, and neural stem cells. Rupture of the relatively fragile germinal matrix capillaries may occur in response to altered cerebral blood flow, increased venous pressure (e.g., with delivery), coagulopathy, or hypoxic-ischemic injury. Germinal matrix hemorrhage is discussed in greater detail later (Chapter 8).

Isolated choroid plexus and **isolated intraventricular hemorrhage (IVH)** do not involve the germinal matrix. **White matter injury of prematurity** generally does not show evidence of hemorrhage ("blooming") on T2* imaging.

The most common nontraumatic cause of spontaneous IVH in *neonates beyond 34 gestational weeks* is **dural venous sinus thrombosis** (DVST) **(5-12)**. In contrast to older children and adults in whom the transverse sinus is most commonly affected, the straight sinus (85%) and superior sagittal sinus (65%) are the most frequent locations in infants. Multisinus involvement is seen in 80% of cases. Thalamic and punctate white matter lesions are common in infants with DVST.

Children With sICH

The most common cause of sICH in children ages 1 to 18 years is an underlying **vascular malformation**. Vascular malformations are responsible for nearly half of spontaneous parenchymal hemorrhages in this age group **(5-13)**.

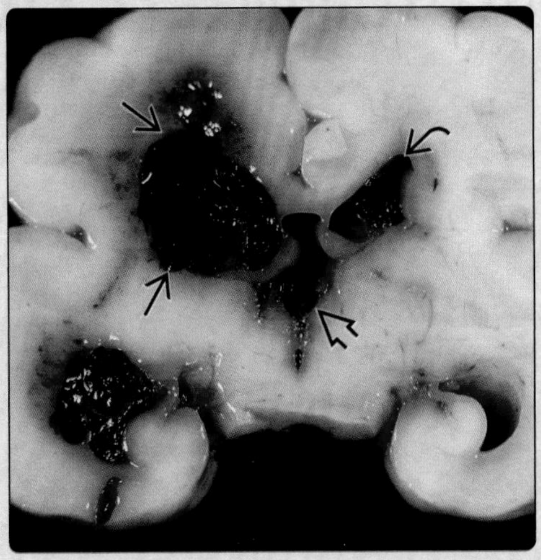

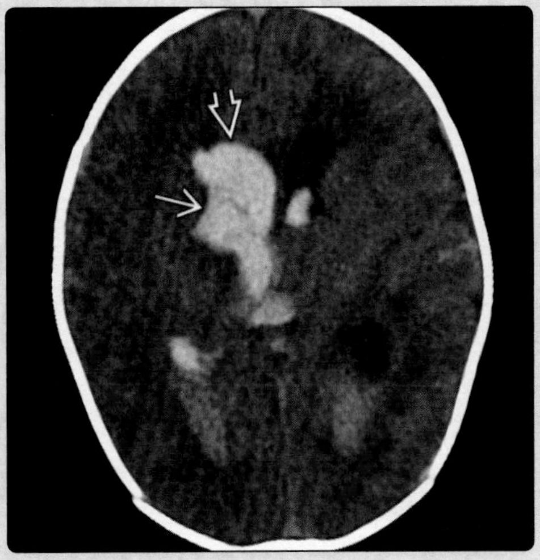

***(5-10)** Autopsied brain of a premature infant shows hemorrhage into the germinal matrix and the adjacent deep periventricular white matter. Blood is also present in both lateral and third ventricles. **(5-11)** NECT in a premature infant shows typical germinal matrix hemorrhage with dissection into the adjacent ventricles.*

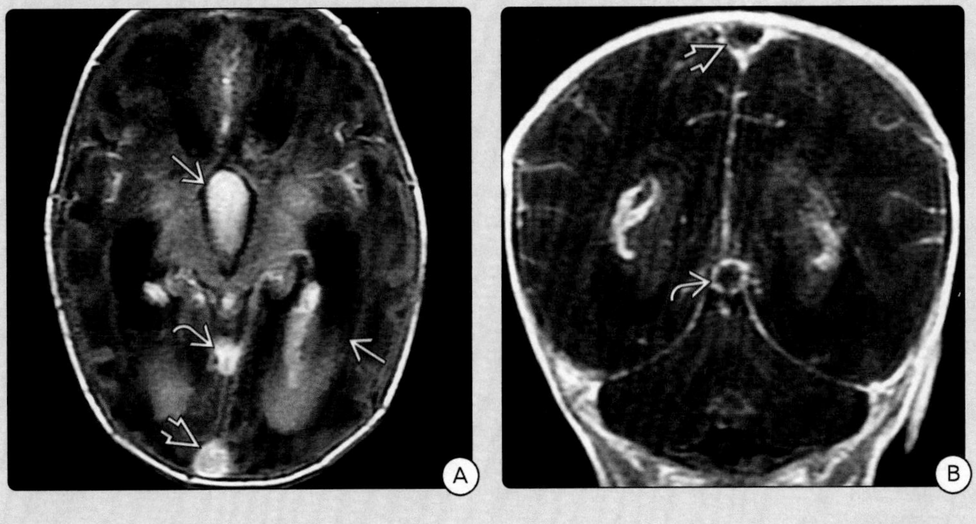

***(5-12A)** T1WI in a septic newborn infant shows blood in the third/lateral ventricles, thrombus in straight sinus, and torcular. **(5-12B)** Coronal T1 C+ in the same case shows thrombosis of superior sagittal, straight sinuses seen here as enhancing dura around nonenhancing clot ("empty delta" sign).*

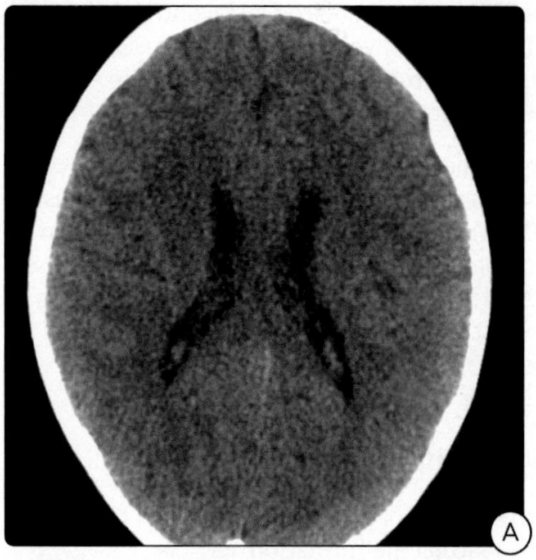

(5-13A) NECT in a child with headaches, family history of multiple cavernous malformations shows no abnormalities.

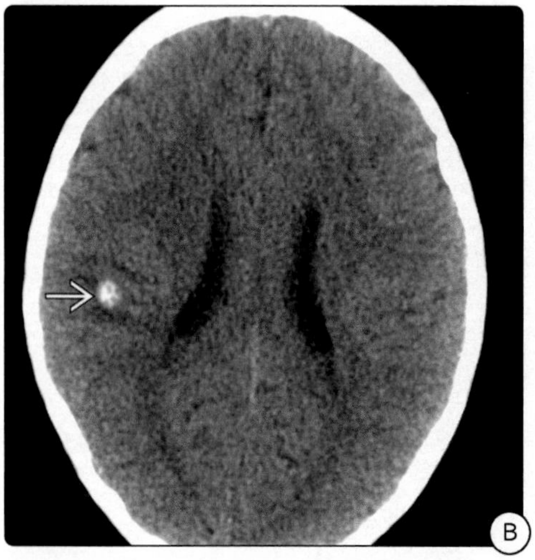

(5-13B) Follow-up scan 1 year later shows a small, solitary, calcified lesion in the right cerebral hemisphere ➡.

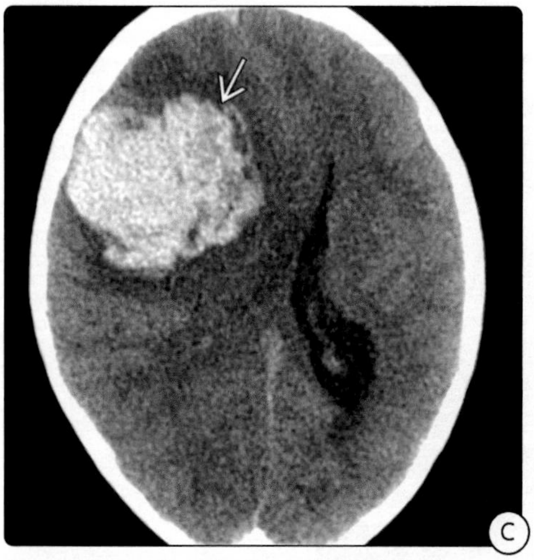

(5-13C) Several weeks later, the child had a severe headache, left-sided weakness, and bleeding into the cavernous malformation ➡.

At least 25% of all arteriovenous malformations hemorrhage by the age of 15 years. Cavernous malformations, especially familial cavernous malformations ("cavernomas"), are a less common but important cause of sICH in children.

Other less common but important causes of pediatric sICH include **hematologic disorders** and **malignancies**, **vasculopathy**, and **venous occlusion/infarction**.

Primary neoplasms are a relatively rare cause of sICH in children **(5-14)**. Infratentorial tumors are more common than supratentorial neoplasms.

Posterior fossa neoplasms that frequently hemorrhage include ependymoma and rosette-forming glioneuronal tumor. Patchy or petechial hemorrhage is more common than large intratumoral bleeds.

Supratentorial tumors with a propensity to bleed include ependymoma and the spectrum of primitive neuroectodermal tumors. Malignant astrocytomas with hemorrhage occur but are rare. In contrast to middle-aged and older adults, hemorrhagic metastases from extracranial primary cancers are *very* rare in children.

sICH IN INFANTS AND CHILDREN

Newborns and Infants

- Common
  - Germinal matrix hemorrhage (< 34 gestational weeks)
  - Dural venous sinus thrombosis (≥ 34 gestational weeks)
- Rare
  - Congenital prothrombotic disorder
  - Thrombocytopenia
  - Hemophilia
  - Vitamin K deficiency bleeding
  - Neoplasm

Children

- Common
  - Vascular malformation ≈ 50%
- Less common
  - Hematologic disorder
  - Vasculopathy
  - Dural venous sinus or cortical vein thrombosis
- Rare but important
  - Neoplasm (primary)
  - Drug abuse

Young Adults With sICH

An underlying **vascular malformation** is the most common cause of sICH in young adults as well **(5-15)**. **Drug abuse** is the second most common cause of unexplained hemorrhage **(5-16)**. Cocaine and methamphetamine may induce extreme systemic hypertension, resulting in a putaminal-external capsule bleed that looks identical to those seen in older hypertensive adults **(5-16)**.

Vasculitis and **reversible cerebral vasoconstriction syndrome** (RCVS) occasionally cause pICH in young adults **(5-17)**.

Venous occlusion/infarction with or without **dural sinus occlusion** is also relatively common in this age group, especially in young women taking oral contraceptives **(5-18)**. Severe **eclampsia/preeclampsia** with posterior reversible encephalopathy syndrome (PRES) may cause multifocal posterior

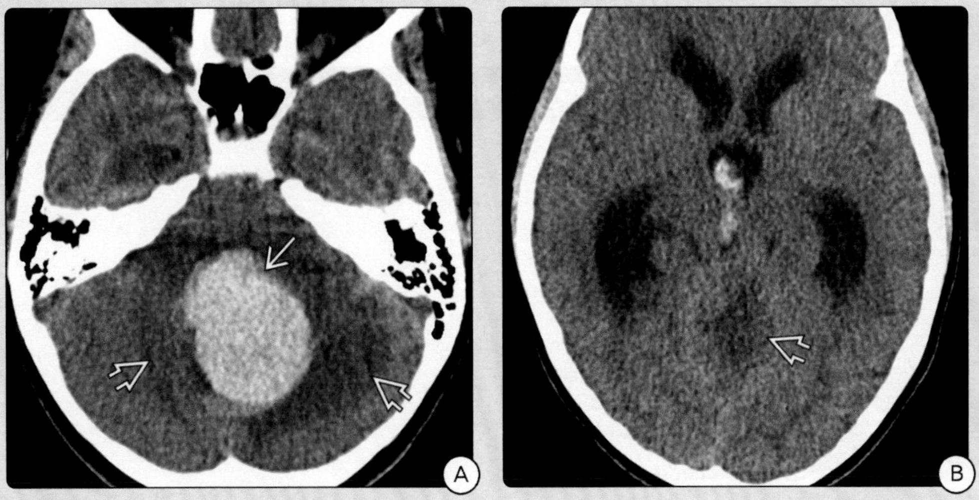

***(5-14A)** Axial NECT in a 10y child with morning nausea and vomiting, sudden onset of severe headache, shows a large posterior fossa midline hemorrhage → that involves the fourth ventricle/vermis. Edema is seen in both cerebellar hemispheres →. **(5-14B)** More cephalad scan shows upward herniation of the edematous cerebellum → and acute obstructive hydrocephalus. Hemorrhagic pilocytic astrocytoma was found at surgery.*

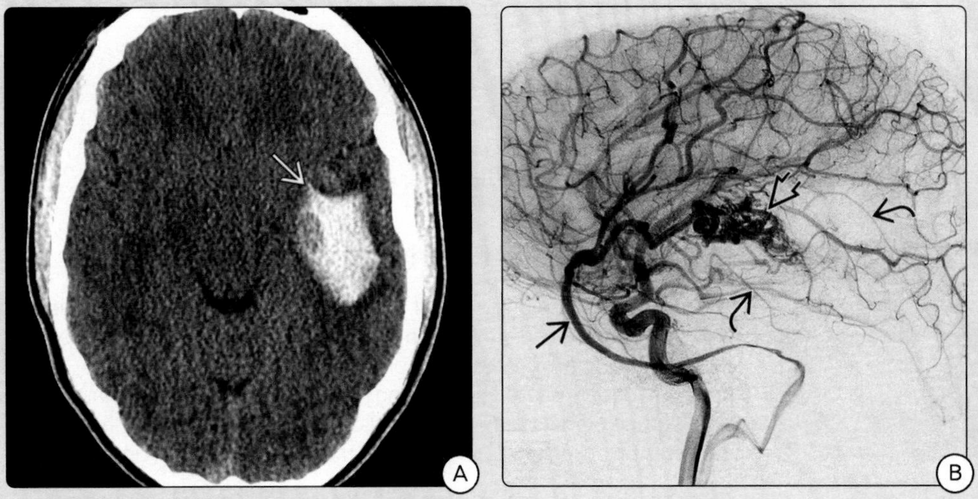

***(5-15A)** NECT in a 15y boy with sudden-onset severe headache, right-sided weakness shows an acute left anterior temporal hematoma →. **(5-15B)** Lateral view of the internal carotid angiogram in the same case shows a partially thrombosed arteriovenous malformation → with early draining superficial middle cerebral vein →. Most of the avascular mass effect → is from the hematoma.*

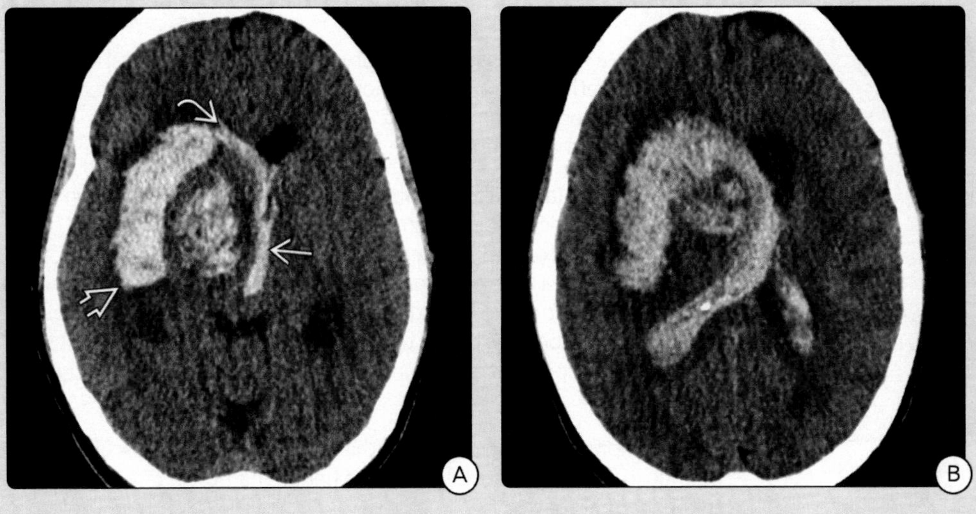

***(5-16A)** Axial NECT scan in a 22y male methamphetamine abuser with sudden-onset left-sided weakness shows a large right basal ganglionic hemorrhage → that has dissected into the right lateral → and third → ventricles. **(5-16B)** More cephalad scan in the same case shows the extent of the basal ganglia and intraventricular blood.*

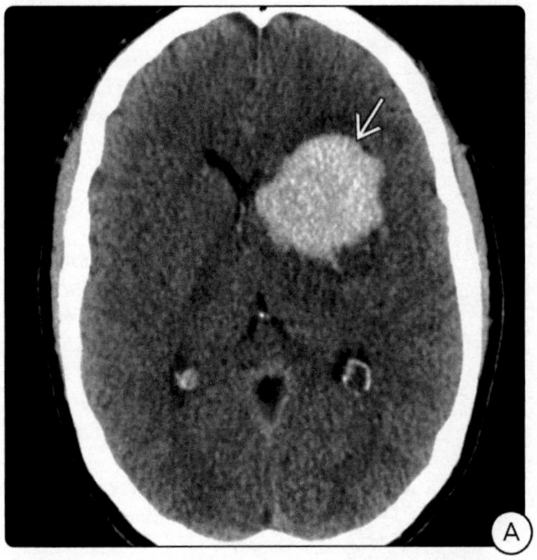

***(5-17A)** NECT in a 37y normotensive man with R-sided weakness shows a left basal ganglionic hemorrhage ➡. Drug screen was negative.*

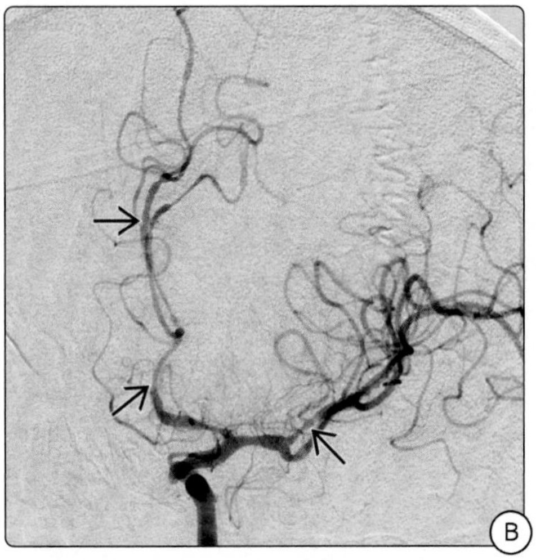

***(5-17B)** Oblique coronal DSA shows multiple areas of arterial dilatations, constrictions in the left ACA, MCA ➡. Initial diagnosis was vasculitis.*

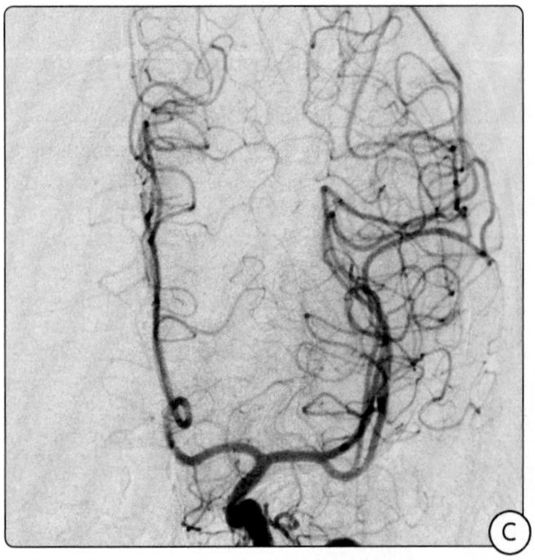

***(5-17C)** Repeat DSA 3 months later is normal. Final diagnosis was reversible cerebral vasoconstriction syndrome (RCVS).*

cortical and subcortical hemorrhages **(5-19)**. Hemorrhagic neoplasms (both primary and metastatic) are rare.

sICH IN YOUNG AND MIDDLE-AGED ADULTS

Young Adults
- Common
  - Vascular malformation
  - Drug abuse
- Less common
  - Venous occlusion
  - PRES
- Rare but important
  - Vasculitis
  - RCVS
  - Neoplasm

Middle-Aged Adults
- Common
  - Hypertension
  - Neoplasm (primary or metastatic)
- Less common
  - Dural sinus or cortical vein occlusion
  - Drug abuse
- Rare but important
  - Vascular malformation
  - Vasculitis
  - RCVS
  - Acute hemorrhagic leukoencephalopathy

Middle-Aged and Elderly Adults With sICH

The two most common causes of sICH in middle-aged and elderly patients are **hypertension** and **amyloid angiopathy**, both of which are discussed in detail below. Approximately 10% of spontaneous parenchymal hemorrhages are caused by bleeding into a brain **neoplasm**, generally either a high-grade primary tumor such as glioblastoma multiforme or hemorrhagic metastasis from an extracranial primary such as renal cell carcinoma **(5-20)**.

A less common but important cause of sICH in this age group is **venous infarct**. Venous infarcts are caused by cortical vein thrombosis, with or without dural sinus occlusion. Iatrogenic **coagulopathy** is also common in elderly patients, as many take maintenance doses of warfarin for atrial fibrillation.

Occasionally a ruptured **saccular aneurysm** presents with a focal lobar hemorrhage rather than a subarachnoid hemorrhage. The most common source is an anterior communicating artery aneurysm that projects superolaterally and ruptures into the frontal lobe.

Underlying **vascular malformation** is a relatively rare cause of sICH in older patients. With a 2-4% per year cumulative rupture risk, a first-time arteriovenous malformation bleed at this age can occur but is unusual. So is hemorrhage from a cavernous malformation. However, **dural arteriovenous fistulas (dAVFs)** *do* occur in middle-aged and elderly patients. Although dAVFs rarely hemorrhage unless they have cortical venous (not just dural sinus) drainage, spontaneous thrombosis of the outlet veins may result in sudden ICH.

Rare but important causes of sICH in this age group include **vasculitis** (more common in younger patients) and **acute hemorrhagic leukoencephalopathy**.

sICH IN OLDER ADULTS

Older Adults
• Common
  ○ Hypertension
  ○ Amyloid angiopathy
  ○ Neoplasm (primary or metastatic)
• Less common
  ○ Dural sinus or cortical vein occlusion
  ○ Coagulopathy
• Rare but important
  ○ Vascular malformation (usually dAVF)

Multiple sICHs

Solitary spontaneous parenchymal hemorrhages are much more common than multifocal bleeds. Etiology varies with patient age.

Multifocal brain bleeds that occur at all ages include venous thrombosis **(5-18)**, PRES **(5-19)**, vasculitis (especially fungal), septic emboli, thrombotic microangiopathy, and acute hemorrhagic leukoencephalopathy.

Multiple *nontraumatic* brain bleeds in children and young adults are most often caused by multiple cavernous malformations and hematologic disorders (e.g., leukemia, thrombocytopenia).

The most common causes of multiple ICHs in middle-aged and older adults are hypertension, amyloid angiopathy, hemorrhagic metastases, and impaired coagulation (either coagulopathy or anticoagulation).

MULTIPLE SPONTANEOUS ICHs

Children and Young Adults
• Multiple cavernous malformations
• Hematologic disorder/malignancy
Middle-Aged and Older Adults
• Common
  ○ Chronic hypertension
  ○ Amyloid angiopathy
• Less common
  ○ Hemorrhagic metastases
  ○ Coagulopathy, anticoagulation
All Ages
• Common
  ○ Dural sinus thrombosis
  ○ Cortical vein occlusion
• Less common
  ○ PRES
  ○ Vasculitis
  ○ Septic emboli
• Rare but important
  ○ Thrombotic microangiopathy
  ○ Acute hemorrhagic leukoencephalopathy

Macrohemorrhages

The top two causes of spontaneous (nontraumatic) intraparenchymal hemorrhage in middle-aged and elderly adults are hypertension (HTN) and amyloid angiopathy; they account for 78-88% of all nontraumatic ICHs.

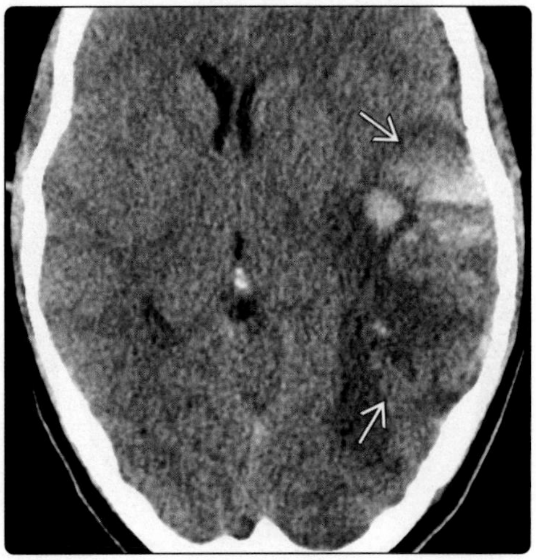

***(5-18)** NECT in a 23y woman with headaches shows left temporoparietal hemorrhage. CTV showed occluded TS, vein of Labbé.*

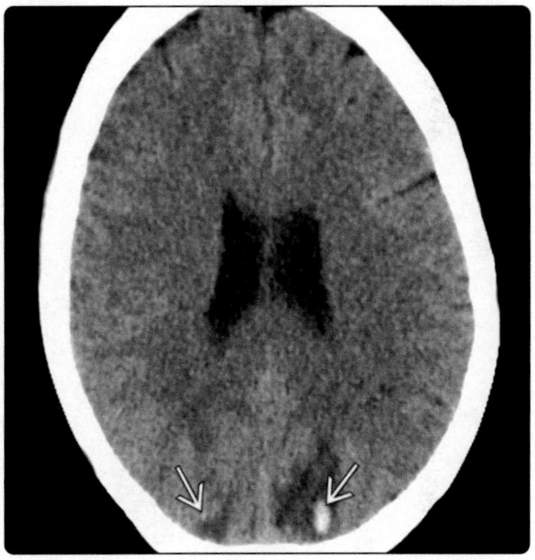

***(5-19)** A 22y eclamptic woman has occipital lesions with edema, hemorrhage; posterior reversible encephalopathy syndrome (PRES).*

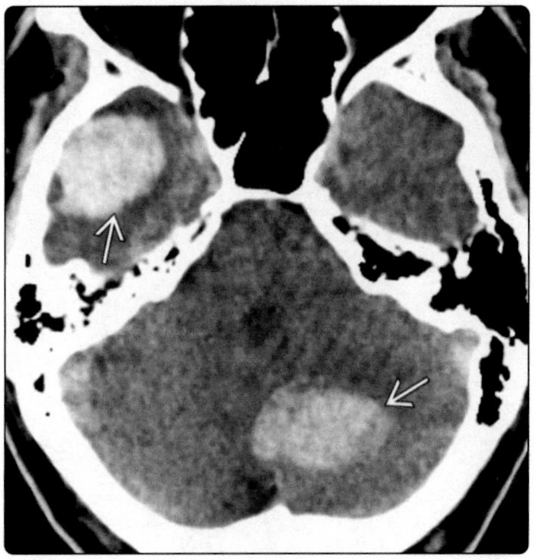

***(5-20)** Axial NECT scan in an elderly patient with known renal cell carcinoma shows multiple hemorrhagic metastases.*

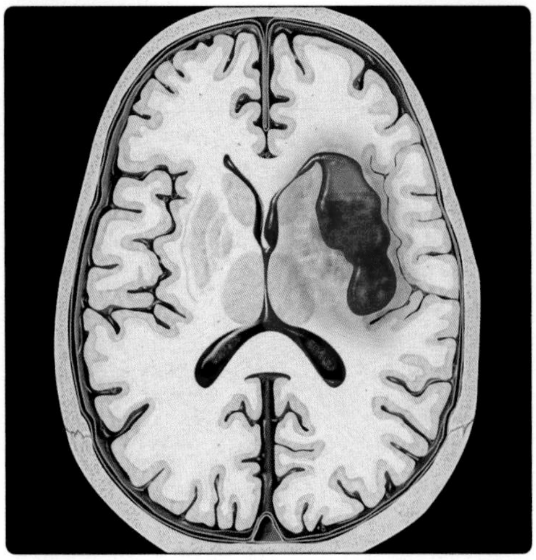

(5-21) Graphic depicts acute hypertensive striatocapsular hemorrhage with edema, dissection into the lateral and third ventricles.

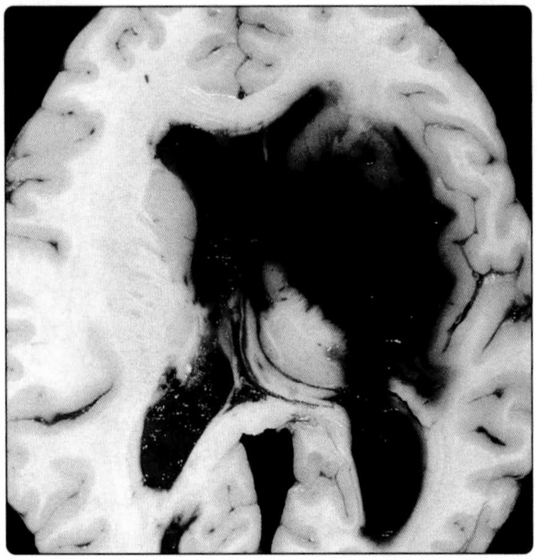

(5-22) Autopsy shows acute hypertensive ganglionic hemorrhage with intraventricular hemorrhage. (Courtesy R. Hewlett, MD.)

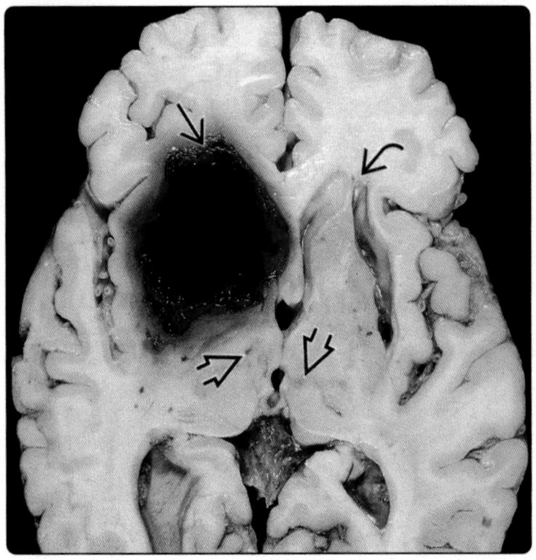

(5-23) Autopsy shows acute ⇨ and chronic ⇨ hICH, small remote thalamic microhemorrhages ⇨. (Courtesy R. Hewlett, MD.)

Although both can cause extensive nonhemorrhagic "microvascular" disease, their most common manifestations are gross lobar and multifocal microbleeds. We therefore discuss them here.

Hypertensive ICH

Terminology

Hypertensive intracranial hemorrhage (hICH) is the *acute* manifestation of nontraumatic ICH secondary to systemic HTN. *Chronic* hypertensive encephalopathy refers to the effects of longstanding HTN on the brain parenchyma and is mostly seen as subcortical white matter disease and/or multifocal microbleeds.

Etiology

HTN accelerates atherosclerosis with lipohyalinosis and fibrinoid necrosis. Penetrating branches of the proximal middle and anterior cerebral arteries, primarily the lenticulostriate arteries (LSAs), are most severely affected, possibly because of their branching angle from the parent vessels.

Progressive weakening and accelerated degeneration of the LSA wall permit formation of small pseudoaneurysms ("Charcot-Bouchard aneurysms" or "bleeding globes"). Ruptured LSA pseudoaneurysm is thought to be the genesis of most striatocapsular hypertensive hemorrhages.

Pathology

Location. The putamen/external capsule is the most common location **(5-21) (5-22)**. These so-called striatocapsular hemorrhages account for nearly two-thirds of all hICHs. The thalamus is the next most common site, responsible for 15-25% **(5-23)**. The pons and cerebellum are the third most common location and cause 10% of all hICHs. Lobar hemorrhages account for another 5-10%.

Multiple microbleeds are common in patients with chronic HTN. HTN-related microbleeds tend to cluster in the basal ganglia and cerebellum with fewer lesions in the cortex and subcortical white matter.

Size and Number. Size varies from tiny submillimeter microbleeds to large macroscopic lesions that measure several centimeters in diameter **(5-23)**. When T2* sequences are used, the majority of patients with hICH have multiple lesions.

Gross Pathology. The most common gross finding in hICH is a large ganglionic hematoma that often extends medially into the ventricles **(5-22)**. Hydrocephalus and mass effect with subfalcine herniation are common complications.

Microscopic Features. Generalized arteriosclerosis with lipohyalinosis and fibrinoid necrosis is common in patients with hICH. In some cases, small fibrosed pseudoaneurysms in the basal ganglia can be identified.

Clinical Issues

Epidemiology. Although the prevalence of hICH has declined significantly, HTN still accounts for 40-50% of spontaneous "primary" intraparenchymal hemorrhages in middle-aged and older adults. hICH is from five to ten times less common than cerebral ischemia-infarction, accounting for approximately 10-15% of all strokes.

Demographics. The overall risk of cardiovascular disease—including hICH—is significantly increased with systolic-diastolic HTN, isolated diastolic

HTN, and isolated systolic HTN. HTN increases the risk of ICH four times compared with normotensive patients.

Elderly male patients are the demographic group most at risk for hICH, with peak prevalence between 45-70 years. African Americans are the most commonly affected ethnic group in North America.

Presentation. Large hICHs present with sensorimotor deficits and impaired consciousness. Patients may—or may not—have a history of longstanding untreated systemic HTN.

Natural History. Neurologic deterioration after hICH is common. Hematoma expansion is frequent in the first few hours and is highly predictive of neurologic deterioration, poor functional outcome, and mortality. For each 10% increase in ICH size, there is a 5% increase in mortality and an additional 15% chance of poorer functional outcome.

Mortality rate approaches 80% in patients with large hemorrhages. Of hICH survivors, between one-third and one-half are moderately or severely disabled.

Treatment Options. Control of intracranial pressure and hydrocephalus are standard. Hematoma evacuation (whether open or stereotactic-guided) and craniectomy for brain swelling are controversial.

Imaging

CT Findings. NECT scans typically show a round or ovoid hyperdense mass centered in the lateral putamen/external capsule or thalamus **(5-24A)**. In the presence of active bleeding or coagulopathy, the hemorrhage may appear inhomogeneously hyperdense with lower density areas and even fluid-fluid levels. Intraventricular extension is common. Acute hICH does not enhance on CECT.

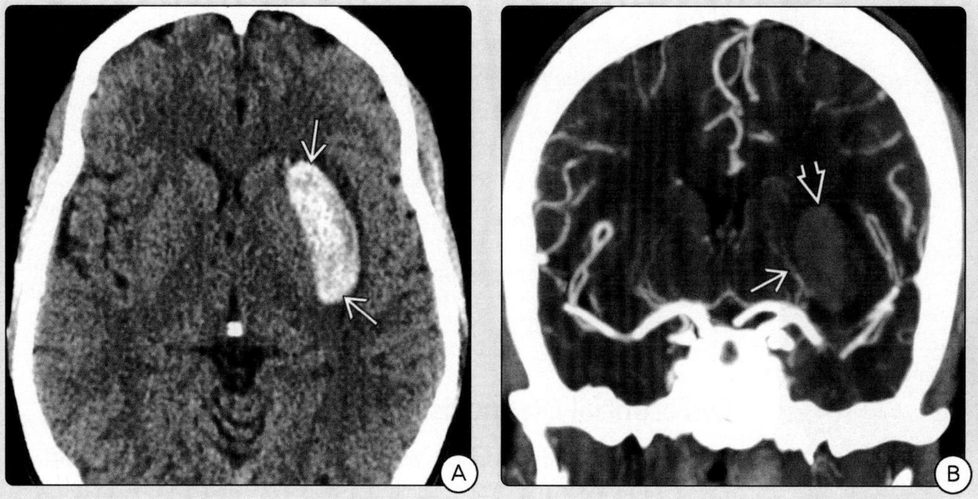

(5-24A) Axial NECT scan in a 57y hypertensive woman shows classic left striatocapsular hemorrhage ➡. (5-24B) Coronal MIP CTA shows that the left lenticulostriate arteries ➡ are displaced by the hematoma ⇨, but there is no evidence of contrast extravasation or "bleeding globe" to suggest increased risk of hematoma expansion.

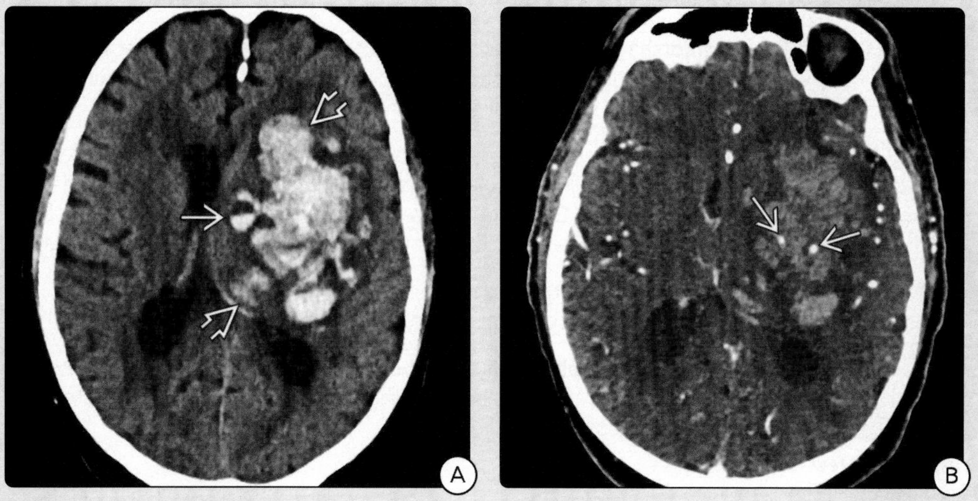

(5-25A) NECT in a 73y hypertensive man "found down" shows an acute left basal ganglionic hemorrhage ⇨ with mixed hyper-, hypodense foci, fluid-fluid levels ➡, suggesting rapid hemorrhage. (5-25B) CTA in the same case shows two "spot" signs with contrast extravasation ➡, indicating active bleeding into the expanding hematoma.

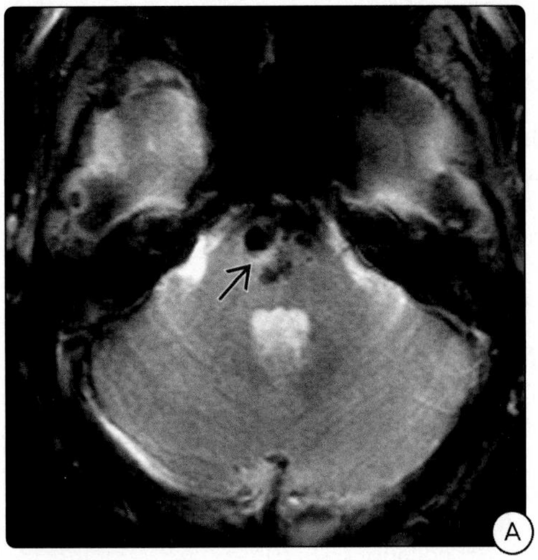

***(5-26A)** T2* GRE in a patient with chronic hypertension shows multiple blooming "microbleeds" in the pons ⇒.*

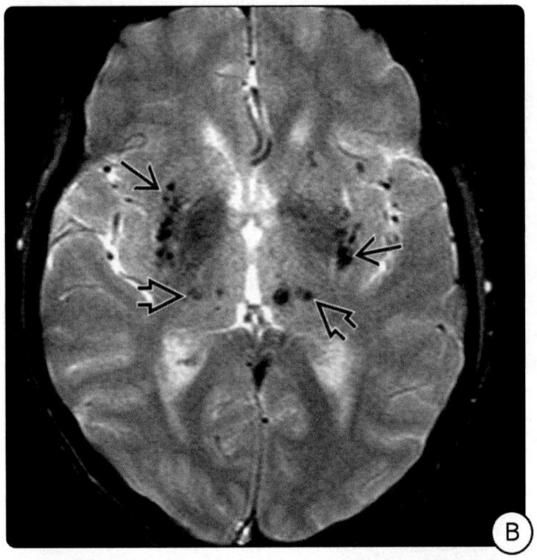

***(5-26B)** More cephalad T2* GRE shows multiple microbleeds in the putamina ⇒ and both thalami ⇒.*

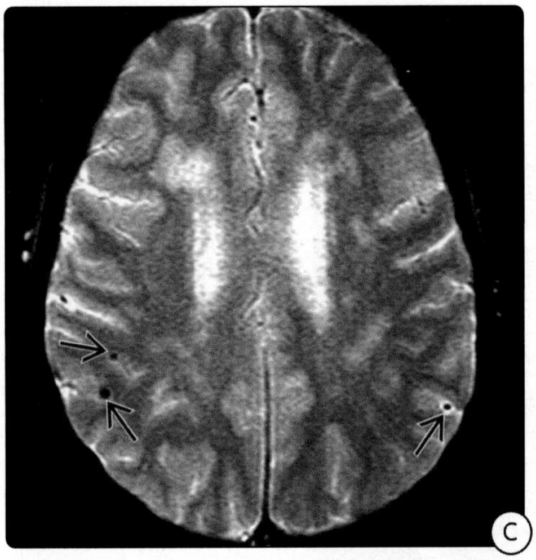

***(5-26C)** T2* GRE in the same case shows a few scattered cortical "blooming black dots" ⇒. This is chronic hypertension with microbleeds.*

MR Findings. Signal intensity on MR changes with clot age (see above) and varies from a large acute hematoma to a slit-like hemosiderin "scar." White matter hyperintensities on T2/FLAIR are common findings in patients with hICH. T2* sequences (GRE, SWI) frequently demonstrate multifocal "blooming black dots," especially in the basal ganglia and cerebellum **(5-26)**.

Angiography. Most hICHs are avascular on CTA **(5-24B)**. However, an enhancing "spot" sign with contrast extravasation can sometimes be identified in actively bleeding lesions **(5-25)**.

DSA in stroke patients with a classic striatocapsular hemorrhage and a history of hypertension is rarely required and usually does not contribute to patient management.

HYPERTENSIVE INTRACRANIAL HEMORRHAGE (hICH)

Location
- Putamen/basal ganglia (60-65%)
- Thalamus (15-25%)
- Pons/cerebellum (10%)
- Lobar hemispheric (5-10%)

Clinical Issues
- 10-15% of all "strokes"
- 40-50% of spontaneous hemorrhages in older adults
- Age, hematoma volume early predictors of death/disability

Imaging
- Classic = hyperdense clot in putamen/external capsule
- Look for old hemosiderin "scar," microbleeds on T2*

Differential Diagnosis
- Cerebral amyloid angiopathy
- Hemorrhagic neoplasm
- Internal cerebral vein thrombosis
- Drug abuse (e.g., cocaine use)

Differential Diagnosis

The major differential diagnosis for hICH is **cerebral amyloid angiopathy** (CAA). Patients with CAA are usually normotensive and have moderately impaired cognition. Although there is some overlap with hICH, the distribution of hemorrhages in CAA is typically lobar and peripheral more often than striatocapsular and central. Cerebellar hemorrhages are common in hICH but rare in CAA.

Hemorrhagic neoplasms (e.g., glioblastoma multiforme or metastasis) are more common in the white matter or gray matter-white matter junction and less common in the basal ganglia and cerebellum.

With the exception of dural arteriovenous fistula, first-time hemorrhage from an underlying **vascular malformation** is unusual in middle-aged and elderly patients. **Coagulopathy** can cause or exacerbate spontaneous ICH. Coagulation-related hemorrhages are typically lobar, not striatocapsular.

In younger patients, **drug abuse** (e.g., cocaine use) with extreme hypertension can cause putamen/external capsule hemorrhage.

Internal cerebral venous thrombosis can occur at all ages. These hemorrhages tend to be bilateral, thalamic, and more medially located than the striatocapsular bleeds of hICH.

Cerebral Amyloid Angiopathy

CAA is one of three morphologic varieties of cerebral amyloid deposition disease. Because CAA—also known as "congophilic angiopathy"—is a common cause of spontaneous lobar hemorrhage in elderly patients, we discuss it briefly here. The full spectrum of cerebral amyloid disease is discussed in greater detail in the chapter on vasculopathy (Chapter 10).

CAA causes approximately 1% of all strokes and 15-20% of primary intracranial bleeds in patients over the age of 60 years. Mean age at onset is 73 years. Patients with CAA are usually normotensive and moderately demented.

NECT may show one or more lobar hematomas, often in different ages of evolution. Some patients with CAA—especially those with "thunderclap" headache—may demonstrate vertex ("convexal") subarachnoid hemorrhage.

MR is the most sensitive study to detect CAA. Multifocal and confluent areas of white matter hyperintensity on T2/FLAIR scans are common. At least one-third have petechial microhemorrhages, seen as multifocal "blooming black dots" on T2* (GRE, SWI) sequences. Cortical superficial siderosis is also common and predictive of future lobar hemorrhages.

Remote Cerebellar Hemorrhage

Terminology and Etiology

Remote cerebellar hemorrhage (RCH) is a less well-recognized and often misdiagnosed cause of spontaneous posterior fossa parenchymal hemorrhage in postoperative patients. Most reported cases occur a few hours following supratentorial craniotomy. RCH also occurs as a rare complication of foramen magnum decompression or spinal surgery.

The etiology of RCH is most likely CSF hypovolemia, with inferior displacement or "sagging" of the cerebellar hemispheres. Tearing or occlusion of bridging tentorial veins is thought to result in superficial cerebellar hemorrhage, with or without hemorrhagic necrosis.

Clinical Issues

RCH is relatively rare, occurring in 0.1-0.6% of patients with supratentorial craniotomies, most often for aneurysm clipping, temporal lobe epilepsy, or tumor resection. There is a slight male predominance. Median age is 51 years.

Many—if not most—cases of RCH are asymptomatic and discovered incidentally at postoperative imaging. The most common symptoms are delayed awakening from anesthesia, decreasing consciousness, and seizures.

Prognosis is generally excellent. Treatment is generally conservative, as hematoma removal is rarely indicated.

Imaging

NECT demonstrates stripes of hyperdense blood layered over the cerebellar folia, the "zebra" sign. Hemorrhage can be uni- or bilateral, ipsi- or contralateral to the surgical site **(5-30)**.

MR findings are variable, depending on the age/stage of hematoma evolution. "Blooming" black stripes are seen on T2* (GRE, SWI) **(5-31)**.

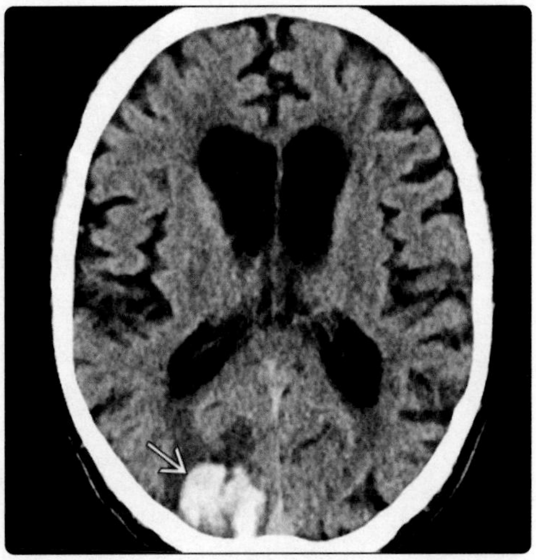

***(5-27)** NECT in an 82y normotensive man with sudden onset of left homonymous hemianopsia shows right occipital lobar hemorrhage ➡.*

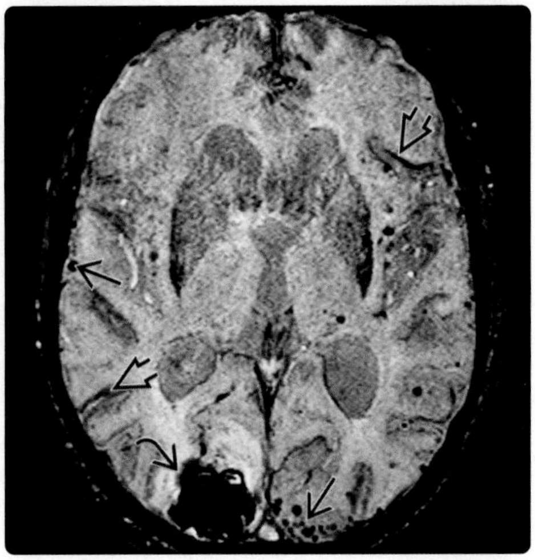

***(5-28)** T2* SWI MIP shows hematoma ⇨, multiple cortical microbleeds ⇨, and superficial siderosis ⇨. No basal ganglionic lesions are seen.*

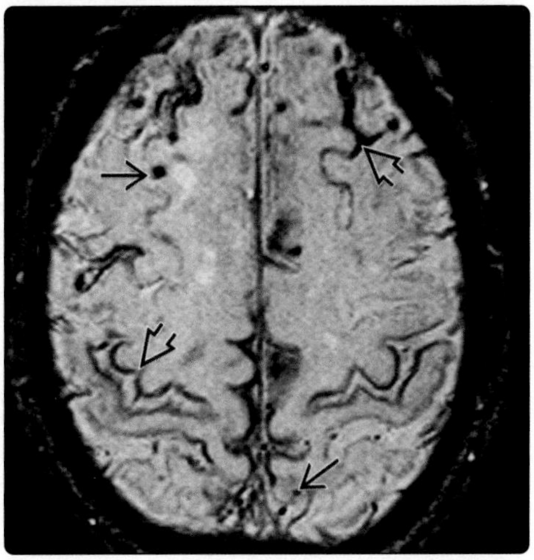

***(5-29)** More cephalad T2* SWI shows more microbleeds ⇨ and extensive cortical superficial siderosis ⇨. This is amyloid angiopathy.*

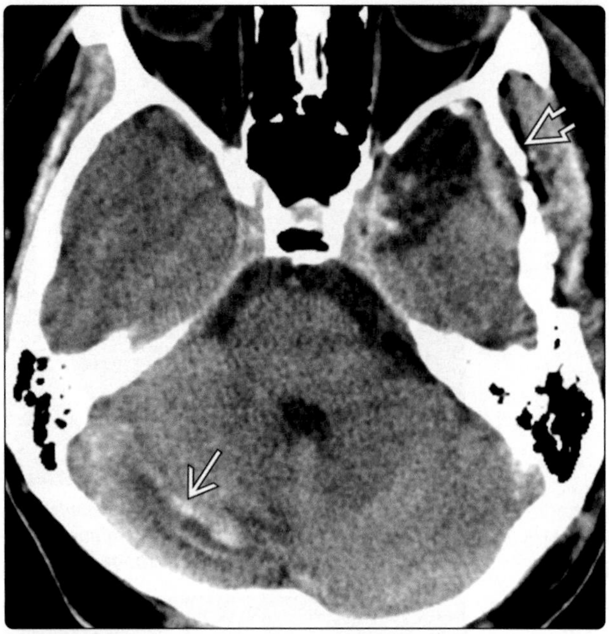

(5-30) NECT scan after supratentorial craniotomy ➡ shows linear "zebra stripes" ➡ of alternating hyperdensity (blood) and low density (edema) in the right cerebellum, consistent with remote cerebellar hemorrhage.

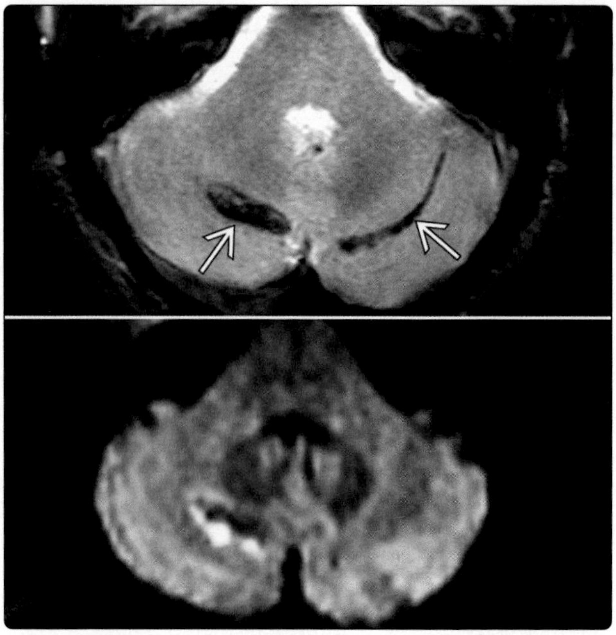

(5-31) Bilateral remote cerebellar hemorrhage is following resection of a supratentorial neoplasm. (Top) T2* GRE shows bilateral "blooming" lesions ➡. (Bottom) DWI shows some restriction in the right acute hemorrhage.

Microhemorrhages

For many years, pathologists have noted the presence of microhemorrhages in autopsied brains. While *macrohemorrhages* are easily detected on both CT and MR, until recently cerebral *microbleeds* (CMBs) were invisible. With the advent of T2* (GRE, SWI) imaging, microsusceptibility changes in the brain can now be detected with relative ease. More than 50% of patients with cerebral macrohemorrhages also have incident CMBs.

CMBs represent perivascular collections of hemosiderin-containing macrophages. They indicate prior bleeds from an underlying hemorrhage-prone microangiopathy. CMBs are almost always multiple and have many etiologies, ranging from trauma and infection to vasculopathy and metastases. Each is discussed in detail in the respective chapters that deal with the specific pathologic groupings.

In this section, we briefly summarize two distinct but related differential diagnoses: (1) entities that cause diffuse brain microbleeds and (2) the differential diagnosis of "black spots" or "blooming black dots" on T2* MR that often appear similar to but are *not* caused by microhemorrhages.

Multifocal Brain Microbleeds

A number of entities can cause diffuse brain microhemorrhages **(5-32)**, and the etiology of CMBs varies with age. Trauma with hemorrhagic axonal injury is the most common cause of CMBs in children and young adults. Corpus callosum-predominant CMBs have been described in middle-aged patients with critical illnesses such as DIC, respiratory failure, and viral infection. Chronic hypertension with arteriolar lipohyalinosis and amyloid angiopathy are the two most common pathologies responsible for CMBs in older adults.

"Blooming Black Dots"

In addition to CMBs **(5-33)**, many nonhemorrhagic entities cause appearance of multifocal "black dots" on T2* imaging.

Calcification has various signal intensities on conventional spin echo T1- and T2WIs. Calcifications are hypointense on T2* and appear as "blooming black dots" on GRE as well as SWI magnitude images. Blooming due to calcifications can be distinguished from hemorrhage by using phase imaging.

Pneumocephalus is common following neurosurgical procedures. Air has very low magnetic susceptibility, and small amounts of intracranial air can be difficult to detect on FSE T2WI. Air causes signal loss on T2* (GRE, SWI) sequences and makes the "blooming black dots" easy to identify **(5-35)**.

NONHEMORRHAGIC CAUSES OF "BLOOMING BLACK DOTS" ON T2*

Common
- Pneumocephalus

Less Common
- Multiple parenchymal calcifications
  - Neurocysticercosis
  - Tuberculomas

Rare But Important
- Extracorporeal membrane circulation
- Devices, complications
  - Metallic emboli (heart valves, etc.)

BRAIN MICROBLEEDS: ETIOLOGY, COMMON

Common
- Diffuse axonal/vascular injury
- Cerebral amyloid angiopathy
- Chronic hypertensive encephalopathy
- Hemorrhagic metastases

Less Common
- Multiple cavernous malformations
- Septicemia
- Hypoxemia, acute respiratory distress syndrome
- Fat emboli
- Vasculitis
  - Fungal
  - Sickle cell
- Coagulopathy

BRAIN MICROBLEEDS: ETIOLOGY, RARE

Rare But Important
- Acute hemorrhagic leukoencephalopathy
- Intravascular lymphoma
- Leukemia
- Radiation/chemotherapy
  - Radiation-induced telangiectasias
  - Mineralizing microangiopathy
  - SMART syndrome (**S**troke-like **M**igraine **A**fter **R**adiation **T**herapy)
- Thrombotic microangiopathy
  - Malignant hypertension
  - Disseminated intravascular coagulopathy
  - Hemolytic uremic syndrome (HUS), atypical HUS
  - Thrombotic thrombocytopenic purpura
- High-altitude cerebral edema

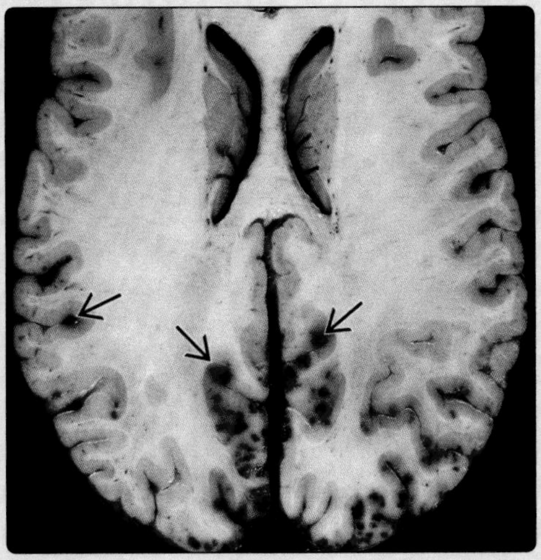
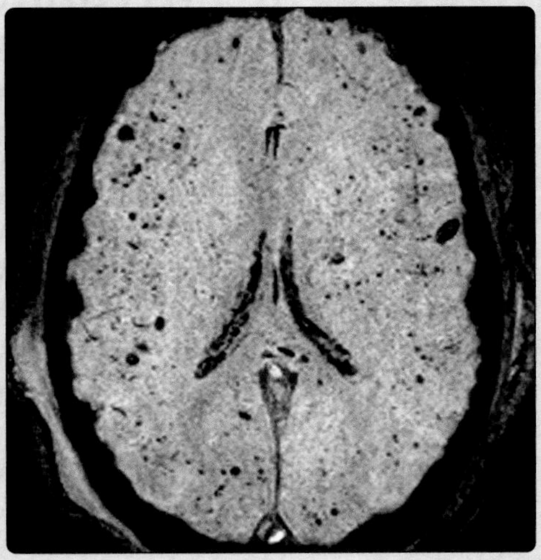

***(5-32)** Autopsy in a septic, immunocompromised patient shows multiple cortical microhemorrhages ➲. (Courtesy R. Hewlett, MD.) **(5-33)** T2* SWI in a 33y woman with meningococcemia, septic shock, purpura fulminans shows innumerable microbleeds scattered throughout both hemispheres.*

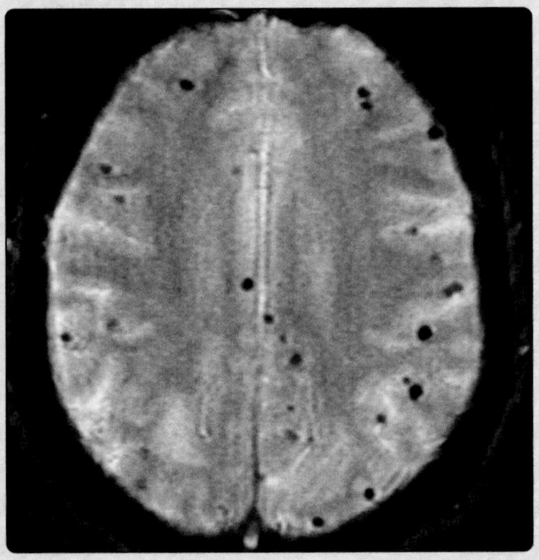
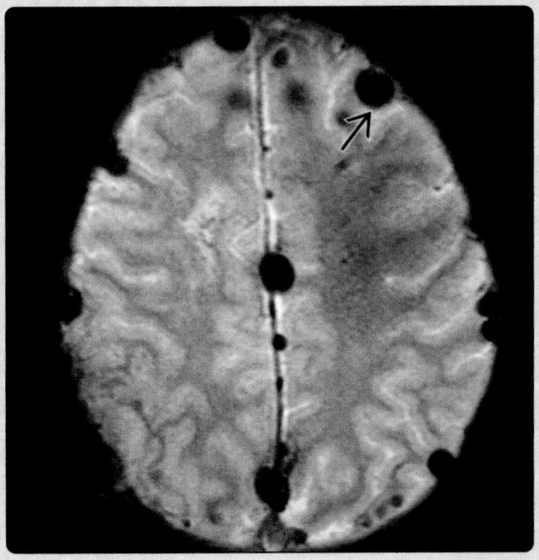

***(5-34)** T2* GRE shows a nonhemorrhagic cause of "blooming black dots." In this case, the patient had multiple calcified neurocysticercosis cysts. **(5-35)** Axial T2* GRE in a postoperative patient with pneumocephalus day 1 following surgery shows numerous "blooming black dots" ➲ caused by small bubbles of air in the subarachnoid spaces.*

Selected References

Evolution of Intracranial Hemorrhage

Imaging of Intracranial Parenchymal Hemorrhage

Demchuk AM et al: Comparing vessel imaging: noncontrast computed tomography/computed tomographic angiography should be the new minimum standard in acute disabling stroke. Stroke. 47(1):273-81, 2016

Morotti A et al: Diagnosis and management of acute intracerebral hemorrhage. Emerg Med Clin North Am. 34(4):883-899, 2016

Domingues R et al: Diagnostic evaluation for nontraumatic intracerebral hemorrhage. Neurol Clin. 33(2):315-328, 2015

Whang JS et al: Diffusion-weighted signal patterns of intracranial haemorrhage. Clin Radiol. 70(8):909-16, 2015

Wilson D et al: Investigating intracerebral haemorrhage. BMJ. 350:h2484, 2015

Macellari F et al: Neuroimaging in intracerebral hemorrhage. Stroke. 45(3):903-8, 2014

Etiology of Nontraumatic Parenchymal Hemorrhages

Cole L et al: Clinical characteristics, risk factors, and outcomes associated with neonatal hemorrhagic stroke: a population-based case-control study. JAMA Pediatr. 171(3):230-238, 2017

Joseph DM et al: Glioblastoma presenting as spontaneous intracranial haemorrhage: case report and review of the literature. J Clin Neurosci. 40:1-5, 2017

Fetcko KM et al: Atraumatic multifocal intracerebral hemorrhage. J Clin Neurosci. 31:213-6, 2016

Kranz PG et al: Spontaneous brain parenchymal hemorrhage: an approach to imaging for the emergency room radiologist. Emerg Radiol. 22(1):53-63, 2015

Kim SJ et al: Dual-energy CT in the evaluation of intracerebral hemorrhage of unknown origin: differentiation between tumor bleeding and pure hemorrhage. AJNR Am J Neuroradiol. 33(5):865-72, 2012

Macrohemorrhages

Hypertensive ICH

Nishiyama J et al: Occurrence of spot signs from hypodensity areas on precontrast CT in intracerebral hemorrhage. Neurol Res. 39(5):419-425, 2017

Chen G et al: Early prediction of death in acute hypertensive intracerebral hemorrhage. Exp Ther Med. 11(1):83-88, 2016

Cappellari M et al: The etiologic subtype of intracerebral hemorrhage may influence the risk of significant hematoma expansion. J Neurol Sci. 359(1-2):293-7, 2015

Cerebral Amyloid Angiopathy

Charidimou A et al: Cortical superficial siderosis and first-ever cerebral hemorrhage in cerebral amyloid angiopathy. Neurology. 88(17):1607-1614, 2017

Wollenweber FA et al: Cortical superficial siderosis in different types of cerebral small vessel disease. Stroke. 48(5):1404-1407, 2017

van Veluw SJ et al: Heterogeneous histopathology of cortical microbleeds in cerebral amyloid angiopathy. Neurology. 86(9):867-71, 2016

Remote Cerebellar Hemorrhage

Nagendran A et al: The zebra sign: an unknown known. Pract Neurol. 16(1):48-9, 2016

Sturiale CL et al: Remote cerebellar hemorrhage after supratentorial procedures (part 1): a systematic review. Neurosurg Rev. 39(4):565-73, 2016

Sturiale CL et al: Remote cerebellar hemorrhage after spinal procedures (part 2): a systematic review. Neurosurg Rev. 39(3):369-76, 2016

Microhemorrhages

Charidimou A et al: Cortical superficial siderosis and first-ever cerebral hemorrhage in cerebral amyloid angiopathy. Neurology. 88(17):1607-1614, 2017

Fanou EM et al: Critical illness-associated cerebral microbleeds. Stroke. 48(4):1085-1087, 2017

Wollenweber FA et al: Cortical superficial siderosis in different types of cerebral small vessel disease. Stroke. 48(5):1404-1407, 2017

Pasquini M et al: Incident cerebral microbleeds in a cohort of intracerebral hemorrhage. Stroke. 47(3):689-694, 2016

Linn J: Imaging of cerebral microbleeds. Clin Neuroradiol. 25 Suppl 2:167-75, 2015

Yakushiji Y: Cerebral microbleeds: detection, associations and clinical implications. Front Neurol Neurosci. 37:78-92, 2015

"Blooming Black Dots"

Salmela MB et al: All that bleeds is not black: susceptibility weighted imaging of intracranial hemorrhage and the effect of T1 signal. Clin Imaging. 41:69-72, 2017

Subarachnoid Hemorrhage and Aneurysms

Trauma is—by far—the most common cause of intracranial subarachnoid hemorrhage (SAH). Traumatic SAH occurs when blood from contused brain or lacerated vessels extends into adjacent sulci; it was discussed in connection with craniocerebral trauma (Chapter 2). This chapter focuses on nontraumatic SAH (ntSAH) and aneurysms.

We begin with an overview of the brain subarachnoid spaces, which provides the context for our discussion of ntSAH and aneurysms. We follow with detailed discussions of each topic.

Subarachnoid Space Overview

The subarachnoid spaces (SASs) are CSF-filled cavities that lie between the arachnoid and the pia. The SASs are crossed by numerous pia-covered trabeculae that extend between the brain and the inner surface of the arachnoid. It is the pia (*not* the arachnoid) that follows penetrating blood vessels into the brain parenchyma (see Chapter 34).

Prominent focal enlargements of the SASs, the cisterns, are found around the base of the brain, midbrain/pineal region, brainstem, and cerebellum. Most subarachnoid cisterns are named for their adjacent structures (e.g., suprasellar cistern, quadrigeminal cistern, cerebellopontine angle cistern). A few are named for their size (the great cistern or "cisterna magna"), shape, or sublocation.

The SASs are anatomically unique. They surround the entire brain, dipping into and out of the surface sulci and surrounding the cranial nerves. At some point, all major intracranial arteries and veins also pass through the SASs.

Nontraumatic Subarachnoid Hemorrhage

Spontaneous (i.e., nontraumatic) SAH (ntSAH) accounts for 3-5% of all acute "strokes." Approximately 80% of these are caused by a ruptured intracranial saccular aneurysm. Other identifiable causes of ntSAH include a variety of entities such as dissections, venous hemorrhage or thrombosis, vasculitis, amyloid angiopathy, and reversible cerebral vasoconstriction syndrome. No identifiable origin is found in 10-12% of patients presenting with ntSAH.

Hemorrhage into the SAS can be limited and quite focal. More often, blood is extravasated into the SAS, mixes easily with CSF, and spreads diffusely throughout the cisterns and sulci. Sometimes, blood in the SAS is refluxed into the cerebral ventricles, producing secondary intraventricular hemorrhage.

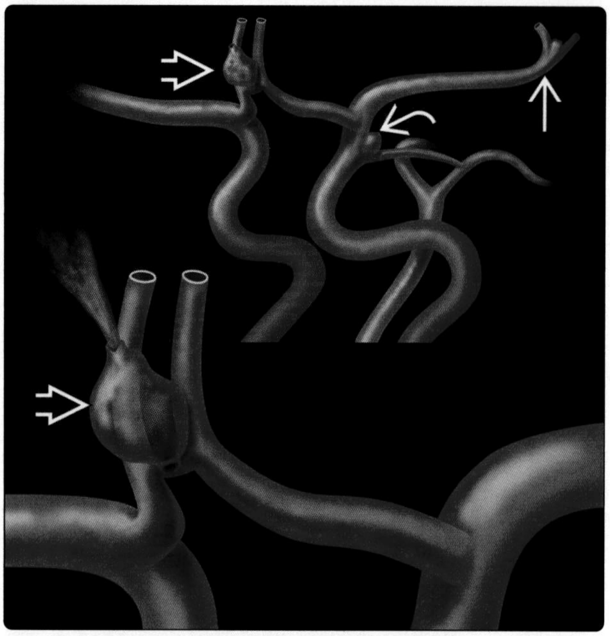

***(6-1)** Graphic shows a saccular aneurysm (SA) of the anterior communicating artery (ACoA) ➡ with active extravasation from a superiorly directed bleb ("teat"). Note additional posterior CoA (PCoA) SA ⇨, tiny bleb at the left MCA bifurcation ➡.*

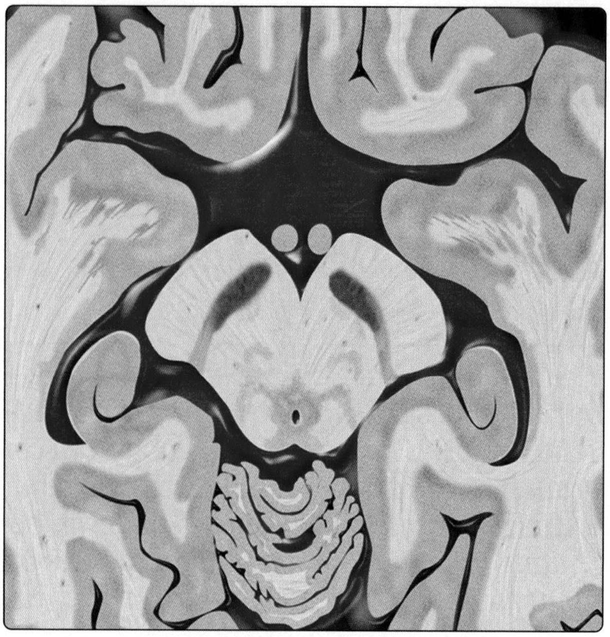

***(6-2)** Axial graphic through the midbrain shows subarachnoid hemorrhage (SAH) in red throughout the basal cisterns. With diffuse distribution of SAH without focal hematoma, statistically most likely location of the ruptured aneurysm is the ACoA.*

Aneurysms

The word "aneurysm" comes from the combination of two Greek words meaning "across" and "broad." Indeed, brain aneurysms literally are widenings or dilatations of intracranial arteries.

Intracranial aneurysms are classified by their gross appearance. **Saccular** or **"berry" aneurysms** are the most common type and typically arise eccentrically at vessel branch points **(6-1)**. **Pseudoaneurysms** often resemble "true" saccular aneurysms in shape but are contained by cavitated clot, not components of arterial walls.

Blood blister-like aneurysms are thin-walled hemispheric bulges that—as the name suggests—resemble cutaneous blood blisters in appearance.

Fusiform aneurysms are focal dilatations that involve the entire circumference of a vessel, extend for relatively limited distances, and do not arise at branch points. Fusiform aneurysms are most often secondary to atherosclerosis but can also occur with nonatherosclerotic vasculopathies.

Ectasias refer to generalized arterial enlargement without focal ("aneurysmal") dilatation. Although ectasias can affect any intracranial vessel, the most common site is the posterior circulation. Ectasias are not true aneurysms, so they are discussed in Chapter 10 on vasculopathy.

Subarachnoid Hemorrhage

Nontraumatic subarachnoid hemorrhage (ntSAH) can be aneurysmal or nonaneurysmal in origin and acute or chronic in presentation. We begin this discussion with aneurysmal SAH (aSAH) and its most devastating complications, vasospasm and secondary cerebral ischemia.

Proper classification of ntSAH subtype depends on early NECT (preferably within the first 24 hours following ictus), as subarachnoid blood rapidly redistributes and the initial pattern is quickly altered.

In this discussion, we review two special types of nontraumatic, nonaneurysmal SAH: **perimesencephalic SAH** and an unusual pattern of SAH called convexity or **convexal SAH**.

Lastly, in the first part of this chapter, we discuss chronic repeated SAH and its rare but important manifestation, **superficial siderosis**.

Aneurysmal Subarachnoid Hemorrhage

Terminology

aSAH is an extravasation of blood into the space between the arachnoid and pia. The typical location of aSAH (basal cisterns and sylvian and inferior interhemispheric fissures) usually helps distinguish it from other causes of ntSAH (*see* box, p. 125).

Etiology

aSAH is most often caused by rupture of a saccular ("berry") or (rarely) a blood blister-like aneurysm. Other less common causes of aSAH include intracranial dissections and dissecting aneurysms.

Subarachnoid Hemorrhage Grading

Grade	Hunt and Hess	WFNS	GCS	Modified Fisher CT
0	Unruptured/asymptomatic aneurysm	Unruptured aneurysm	Unruptured aneurysm	No visible SAH or IVH
1	Asymptomatic/minimal headache	GCS = 15	GCS = 15	≤ 1-mm SAH, no IVH
2	Moderate/severe headache + nuchal rigidity &/or cranial nerve palsy	GCS = 13-15, no neurologic deficit	GCS = 12-14	≤ 1-mm SAH + IVH
3	Drowsy, confused; mild neurologic deficit(s)	GCS = 13-15, focal neurologic deficit	GCS = 9-11	> 1-mm-thick SAH, no IVH
4	Stupor, moderate/severe hemiparesis, early decerebration	GCS = 7-12	GCS = 6-8	> 1-mm-thick SAH + IVH or parenchymal hemorrhage
5	Decerebrate, deeply comatose, moribund	GCS = 3-6	GCS = 3-5	N/A

(Table 6-1) *GCS = Glasgow Coma Score; IVH = intraventricular hemorrhage; SAH = subarachnoid hemorrhage; WFNS = World Federation of Neurological Societies.*

Pathology

Location. Because most saccular aneurysms arise from the circle of Willis or the middle cerebral artery (MCA) bifurcation, the most common locations for aSAH are the suprasellar cistern and sylvian fissures **(6-2)**.

Occasionally an aneurysm ruptures directly into the brain parenchyma rather than the subarachnoid space. This occurs most frequently when the apex of an anterior communicating artery (ACoA) aneurysm points upward and bursts into the frontal lobe.

Gross Pathology. The gross appearance of aSAH is typically characterized by blood-filled basal cisterns **(6-3)**. SAH may extend into the superficial sulci and ventricles. Varying degrees of arterial narrowing caused by vasospasm may be present (see below).

Clinical Issues

Epidemiology. The overall prevalence of aSAH is approximately 10-12 per 100,000 per year.

Demographics. The overall incidence of aSAH increases with age and peaks between the ages of 40 and 60 years. The M:F ratio is 1:2.

aSAH is rare in children. Regardless of their relative rarity, however, cerebral aneurysms cause the majority of spontaneous (nontraumatic) SAHs in children and account for approximately 10% of all childhood hemorrhagic "strokes."

Presentation. Nonspecific headache is a common presenting complaint in emergency departments, accounting for approximately 2% of all visits.

At least 75% of patients with aSAH present with sudden onset of the "worst headache of my life." The most severe form is a "thunderclap" headache, an extremely intense headache that comes on "like a boom of thunder" and typically peaks within minutes or even seconds. There are many causes of "thunderclap" headache. The most serious and life-threatening is aSAH although it accounts for just 4-12% of these severe headaches.

One-third of patients with aSAH complain of neck pain. Another third report vomiting. Between 10-25% experience a "sentinel headache" days or up to 2 weeks before the onset of overt SAH. These "sentinel headaches" are sudden, intense, persistent, and may represent minor bleeding prior to aneurysm rupture.

SCREENING FOR SUSPECTED ANEURYSMAL SAH

Clinical Issues
- Causes 3-5% of "strokes"
- "Thunderclap" headache (aSAH 4-12%)
- Peak age = 40-60 years, M:F = 1:2

NECT
- Sensitivity ≈ 100% if performed in first 6 hours
- Lumbar puncture unnecessary *if*
  - CT negative
  - Neurologic examination normal

CTA
- If NECT shows aSAH

Clinically Based Grading of SAH. Although a number of different scales have been proposed to grade aSAH, none has gained universal acceptance. The two most commonly used systems are the Hunt and Hess and the World Federation of Neurological Societies (WFNS) scales. Both are based on clinical findings.

The **Hunt and Hess scale** grades aSAH from 0 to 5. An unruptured, asymptomatic aneurysm is designated grade 0. Patients who are either asymptomatic or have minimal headache are grade 1. Grade 2 represents moderate to severe headache with nuchal rigidity and/or cranial nerve palsy. Grades 3-5 designate more serious aSAH. Drowsy or confused patients with mild focal neurologic deficits are grade 3. Grade 4 equates to stupor, moderate to severe hemiparesis, and an

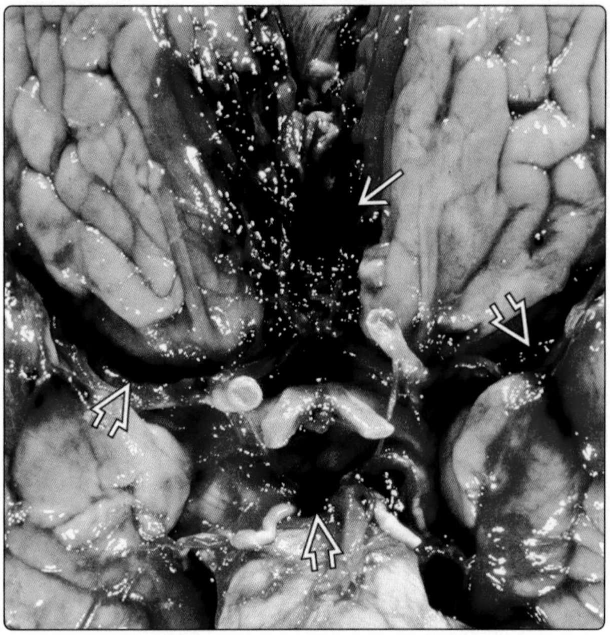

(6-3) Autopsy shows diffuse basilar SAH ➡ from a ruptured ACoA aneurysm. More focal clot is present in the interhemispheric fissure ➡. (Courtesy R. Hewlett, MD.)

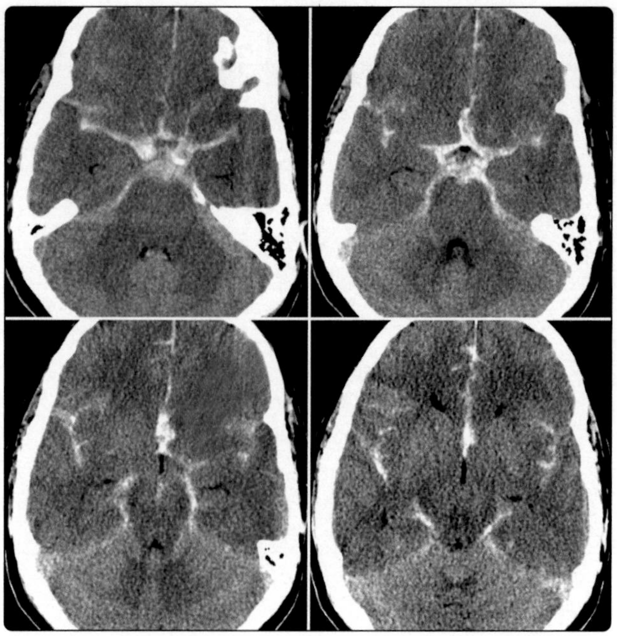

(6-4) Series of axial NECT scans shows the typical appearance of aneurysmal SAH. Hyperdensity in the basilar cisterns and sylvian fissures is typical.

early decerebrate state. Grade 5 patients are decerebrate, deeply comatose, and moribund.

The **WFNS scale** also recognizes six scales of aSAH but is primarily based on the **Glasgow Coma Score (GCS)**. Zero is an unruptured aneurysm. Grade 1 patients have a GCS of 15. Grade 2 patients have no neurologic deficits and a GCS of 13 or 14. Patients with GCS of 13-14 *with* a focal deficit are grade 3. GCS of 7-12 is grade 4. GCS scores of 3-6 are designated grade 5.

Recent studies have indicated that the best predictor of clinical outcome is based simply on the **GCS**. As with the other scales mentioned, an unruptured aneurysm is designated Grade 0. Grades 1-5 differ slightly from the WFNS system. Grade 1 is GCS of 15. Grade 2 is 12-14, 3 is 9-11, 4 is 6-8, and 5 is a GCS of 3-5. Its simplicity, reliability, predictive power, and wide familiarity among health care personnel make the GCS the most logical system for grading aSAH and guiding patient treatment.

A fourth schema, the modified **Fisher scale**, is based on CT appearance (not clinical findings) but is included on the summary table for comparison **(Table 6-1)**.

Natural History. Although aSAH causes just 3-5% of all "strokes," nearly one-third of all stroke-related years of potential life lost before age 65 are attributable to aSAH. The mean age at death in patients with aSAH is significantly lower than in patients with other types of strokes.

aSAH is fatal or disabling in more than two-thirds of patients. Massive SAH can cause coma and death within minutes. Approximately one-third of patients with aSAH die within 72 hours; another third survive but with disabling neurologic deficits.

Despite advances in diagnosis and treatment, in-hospital mortality continues to exceed 25%. Without treatment, ruptured saccular aneurysms have a rebleed rate of 20% within the first 2 weeks following the initial hemorrhage.

Unfavorable outcome is associated with several factors, including increasing age, worsening neurologic grade, aneurysm size, large amounts of SAH on initial NECT scan, parenchymal hematoma, intraventricular hemorrhage (IVH), and vascular risk factors such as hypertension and myocardial infarction.

Patients who survive aSAH also have an increased lifetime risk of developing new ("de novo") intracranial aneurysms and new episodes of SAH, estimated at 2% per year. They also carry an increased risk for other vascular diseases.

Treatment Options. The goals of aSAH treatment in patients who survive their initial bleed are (1) to obliterate the aneurysm (preventing potentially catastrophic rebleeding) and (2) to prevent or treat vasospasm (see below).

Imaging

General Features. NECT is an excellent screening examination for patients with thunderclap headache and suspected aSAH. Recent studies have shown that, in the first 6 hours after ictus, the sensitivity of modern CT scanners (16-slice or greater) for detecting aSAH approaches 100%. Lumbar puncture is now considered unnecessary if the NECT is negative and the neurologic examination is normal. Lumbar puncture-related complications are also more common than SAH diagnoses in patients with nontraumatic headache and a normal head CT.

The best imaging clue to aSAH is hyperdense cisterns and sulci on NECT. In some cases, subarachnoid blood surrounds and

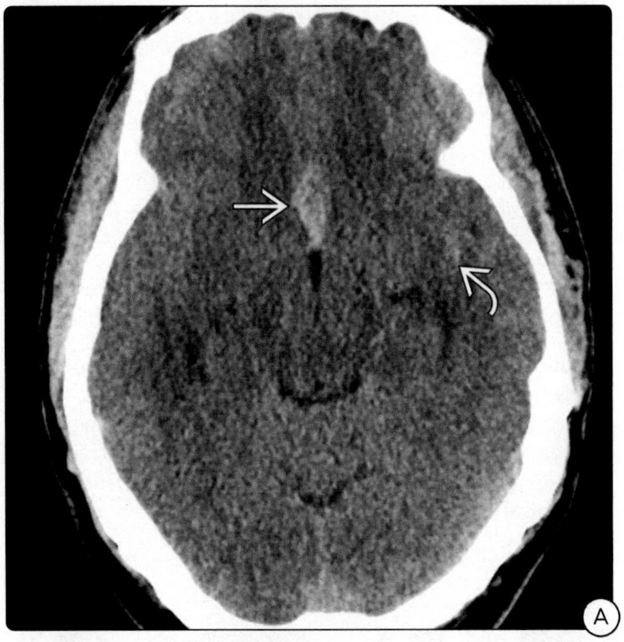

(6-5A) NECT in a 42y man with thunderclap headache shows a focal hematoma in the interhemispheric fissure ➡. A small amount of SAH is present in the left sylvian fissure ↶.

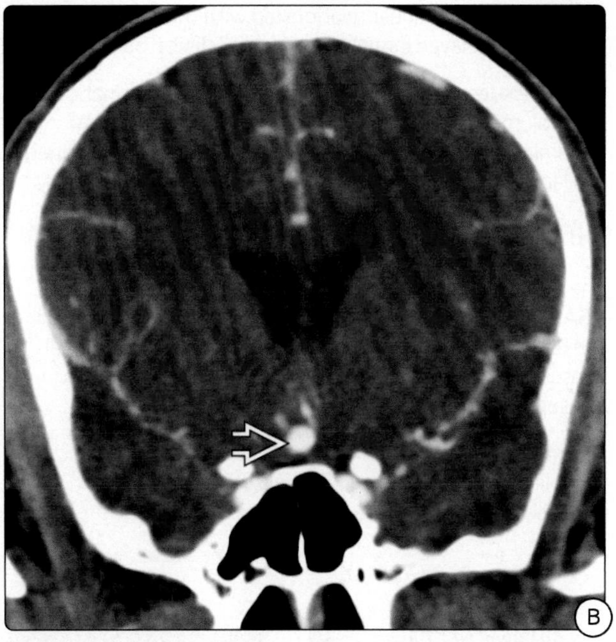

(6-5B) Coronal CTA in the same case demonstrates an 8-mm SA arising from the ACoA ➡. The aneurysm was successfully treated with endovascular coiling.

outlines the comparatively hypodense-appearing aneurysm sac.

CT Findings. The basal cisterns—especially the suprasellar cistern—are generally filled with blood **(6-4)**. Although SAH distribution generally depends on location of the "culprit" aneurysm, it is also somewhat variable and not absolutely predictive of aneurysm location.

ACoA aneurysms tend to rupture superiorly into the interhemispheric fissure **(6-5)**. MCA bifurcation aneurysms usually rupture into the sylvian fissure. Internal carotid-posterior communicating artery (ICA-PCoA) aneurysms generally rupture into the suprasellar cistern. Vertebrobasilar aneurysms often fill the fourth ventricle, prepontine cistern, and foramen magnum with blood.

IVH is present in nearly half of all patients with aSAH and is associated with a higher likelihood of in-hospital complications and poorer 3-month post-SAH outcome.

Focal parenchymal hemorrhage is uncommon but, if present, is generally predictive of aneurysm rupture site. Occasionally, a focal hematoma in the subarachnoid space forms. In most cases, it too is associated with bleeding from the "culprit" aneurysm.

MR Findings. Acute aSAH is isointense with brain on T1WI **(6-6B) (6-11)**. The CSF cisterns may appear smudged or "dirty." Because acute aSAH is hyperintense to brain on T2WI, it may be difficult to identify **(6-6C)**.

FLAIR is the best sequence to depict aSAH. Hyperintense CSF in the sulci and cisterns is present but nonspecific. Other causes of "bright" CSF on FLAIR include hyperoxygenation, meningitis, neoplasm, and artifact.

MR may also be a helpful additional examination when no structural cause for ntSAH is identified on screening NECT or CTA.

Angiography. CTA is positive in 95% of aSAH cases if the "culprit" aneurysm is 2 mm or larger **(6-5B)**. Although DSA is still considered the gold standard for detecting and delineating aneurysm angioarchitecture, many patients with aSAH and positive CTA undergo surgical clipping without DSA.

DSA identifies vascular pathology in 13% of patients with CTA-negative SAH, so such patients should be considered for DSA.

Standard DSA occasionally fails to demonstrate a "culprit" aneurysm. So-called angiogram-negative SAH is found in approximately 15% of cases. With the addition of 3D rotational angiography and 3D shaded surface displays, the rate of "angiogram-negative" SAH decreases to 4-5% of cases.

"Angiogram-negative" spontaneous SAH is not a benign entity, as there is a small but real risk of rehemorrhage and poor outcome. Repeat DSA following an initially negative DSA identifies aneurysms or pseudoaneurysms in an additional 4% of patients. Repeat DSA or CTA is recommended in patients with diffuse-type SAH if the initial DSA is negative.

Imaging-Based Grading of SAH. A simple scale based on NECT findings, the **modified Fisher scale**, has been proposed to grade aSAH. Grade 0 equates to no visible SAH or IVH. A focal or diffuse thin (less than 1 mm) layer of subarachnoid blood without IVH is designated grade 1. If IVH is present, it is a Fisher grade 2. Focal or diffuse thick (more than 1 mm) SAH without IVH is designated grade 3. The presence of intraventricular blood together with thick SAH is designated a grade 4 bleed. Stepwise increases in modified Fisher grade have a moderately linear relationship with the risk of vasospasm, delayed infarction, and poor clinical outcome.

Clinical Issues. Computerized quantitative determination of SAH volume is also a good predictor of delayed cerebral ischemia and functional outcome in aSAH but is not routinely available.

Differential Diagnosis

The major differential diagnosis of aSAH is **traumatic SAH (tSAH)**. aSAH is generally much more widespread, often filling the basal cisterns. tSAH typically occurs adjacent to cortical contusions or lacerations and is therefore most common in the superficial sulci.

Perimesencephalic nonaneurysmal SAH (pnSAH) is much more limited than aSAH and is localized to the interpeduncular, ambient, and prepontine cisterns. Occasionally, pnSAH spreads into the posterior aspect of the suprasellar cistern. It rarely extends into the sylvian fissures.

Convexal SAH (cSAH) is, as the name implies, localized to superficial sulci over the cerebral convexities. Often only a single sulcus is affected. Causes of cSAH are numerous and include cortical vein occlusion, amyloid angiopathy, vasculitis, and reversible cerebral vasoconstriction syndrome (RCVS).

Pseudo-SAH is caused by severe cerebral edema. The hypodensity of the brain makes blood in the cerebral arteries and veins appear dense, mimicking the appearance of SAH.

Sulcal-cisternal FLAIR hyperintensity on MR is a nonspecific imaging finding. It occurs with hemorrhage, meningitis, carcinomatosis, hyperoxygenation, stroke, and gadolinium contrast (blood-brain barrier leakage or chronic renal failure). FLAIR "bright" CSF can also result from flow disturbances and technical artifacts (e.g., incomplete CSF nulling).

(6-6A) Axial NECT in an 82y man with severe neck pain and suboccipital headache shows focal posterior fossa SAH ➡. (6-6B) Axial T1WI in the same case performed 48 h later shows "dirty" CSF with focal hematoma ⇨ surrounding the basilar artery ↷. Note relatively normal CSF in the left cerebellopontine angle (CPA) cistern ⇧. Blood in the right CPA cistern is beginning to show some T1 shortening ➡.

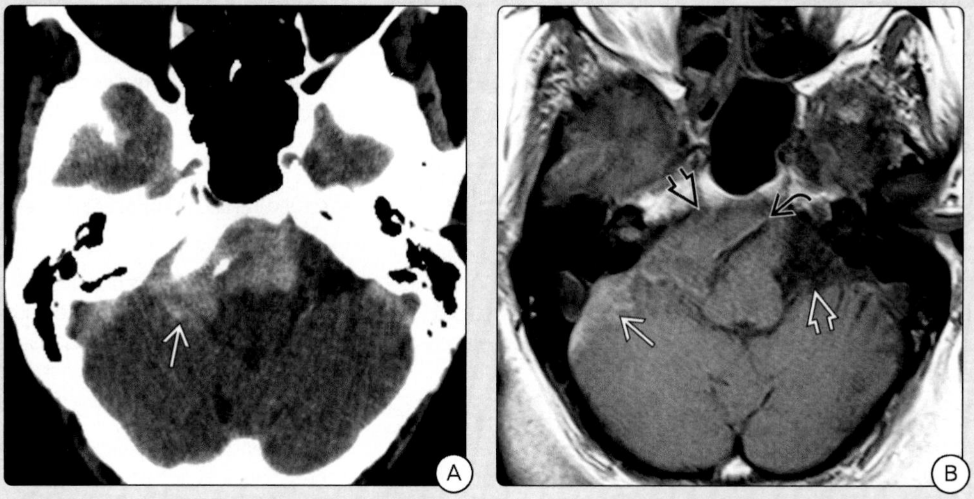

(6-6C) T2WI shows that the focal hematoma surrounding the basilar artery appears profoundly hypointense ⇨. CSF in the adjacent CPA looks "dirty" ➡, not as hyperintense as the relatively normal CSF in the left CPA ⇧. (6-6D) FLAIR scan shows the extraaxial hematoma is profoundly hypointense ⇨, while CSF in the adjacent sulci fails to suppress and appears hyperintense ➡. Nearly normal CSF in the left CPA cistern mostly suppresses ↷.

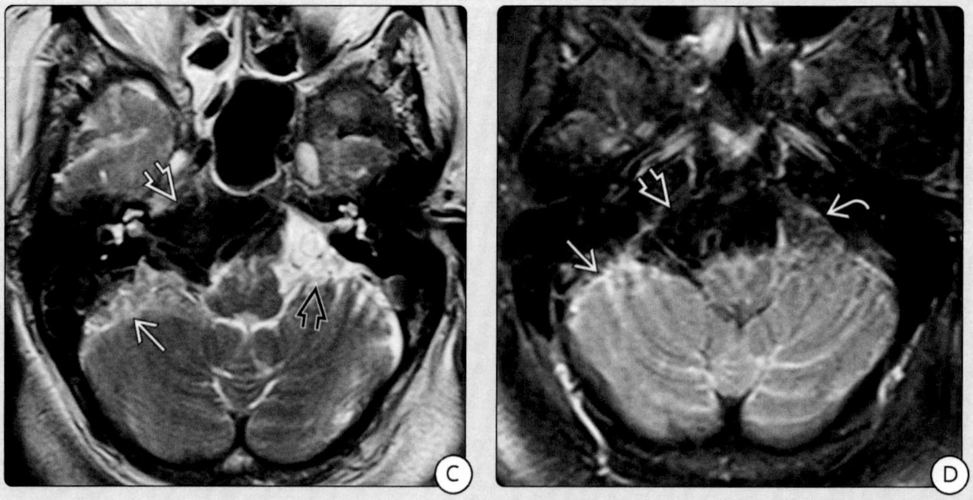

IMAGING OF ANEURYSMAL SAH

NECT
- Hyperdense basal cisterns, sulci
- Hydrocephalus common, onset often early

MR
- "Dirty" CSF on T1WI
- Hyperintense cisterns, sulci on FLAIR

Angiography
- CTA positive in 95% if aneurysm ≥ 2 mm
- DSA reserved for complex aneurysm, CTA negative
- "Angiogram-negative" SAH (15%; 5% if 3D used)
- Repeat "second look" DSA positive (5%)

Pyogenic meningitis, meningeal carcinomatosis, and high inspired oxygen concentration may also cause CSF hyperintensity on FLAIR. Prior administration of gadolinium chelates (with or without decreased renal clearance) can result in diffuse delayed CSF enhancement.

Other etiologies of sulcal-cisternal FLAIR hyperintensity include hyperintense vessels with slow flow (e.g., acute arterial strokes, pial collaterals developing after cerebral ischemia-infarction, Sturge-Weber syndrome, moyamoya, and RCVS).

Post-aSAH Cerebral Ischemia and Vasospasm

Cerebral ischemia is the major cause of morbidity and death in patients who survive their initial SAH. Two forms of ischemia occur: immediate/acute and delayed/subacute. Cerebral vasospasm (CVS) has traditionally been linked to delayed cerebral ischemia (DCI) and often used as a synonym for it. However, although both DCI and vasospasm occur in the same

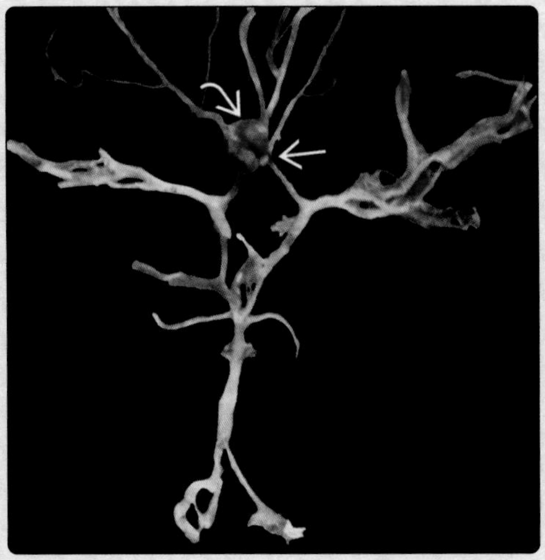

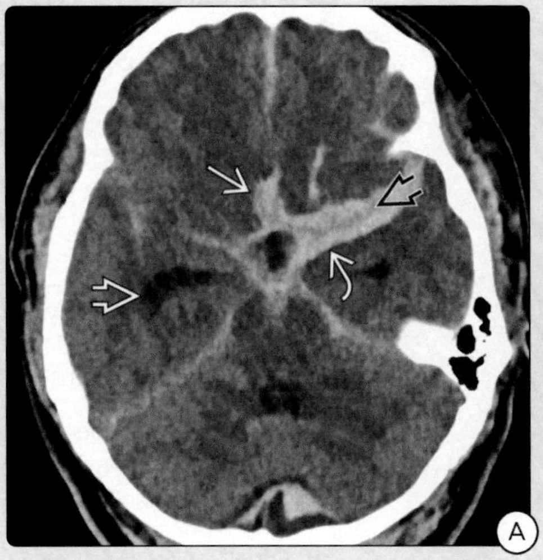

***(6-7)** Circle of Willis, proximal branches show bilobed ACoA aneurysm →, severe vasospasm →. (From DP: Hospital Autopsy.) **(6-8A)** NECT in 43y man with sudden, severe headache shows SAH filling basal cisterns. Blood is most prominent along the left sylvian →, inferior interhemispheric → fissures. The left MCA → is outlined by the SAH. Temporal horns → of the lateral ventricles are enlarged by early obstructive hydrocephalus.*

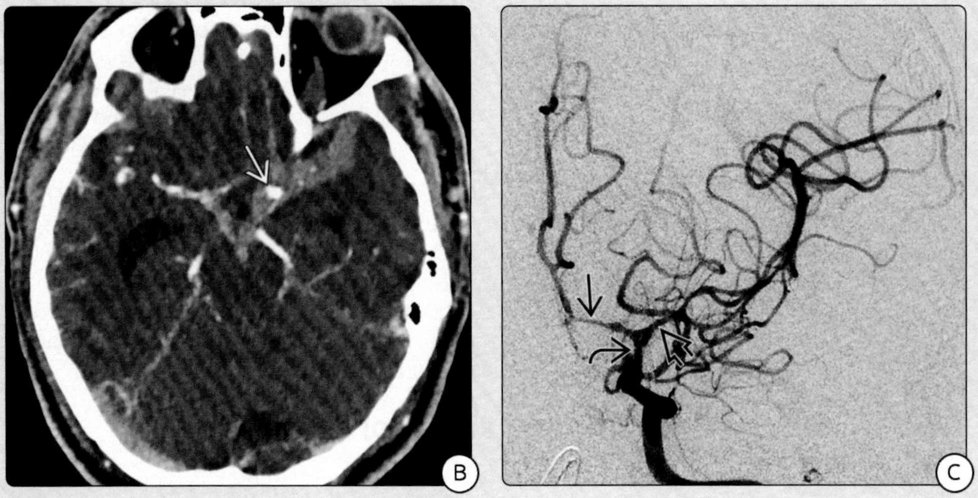

***(6-8B)** CTA shows an 8-mm bilobed aneurysm → at the left internal carotid artery (ICA) bifurcation. **(6-8C)** The aneurysm was clipped, but the patient deteriorated 4 days later. DSA shows moderate vasospasm involving the distal ICA →, proximal A1 →, and M1 → segments.*

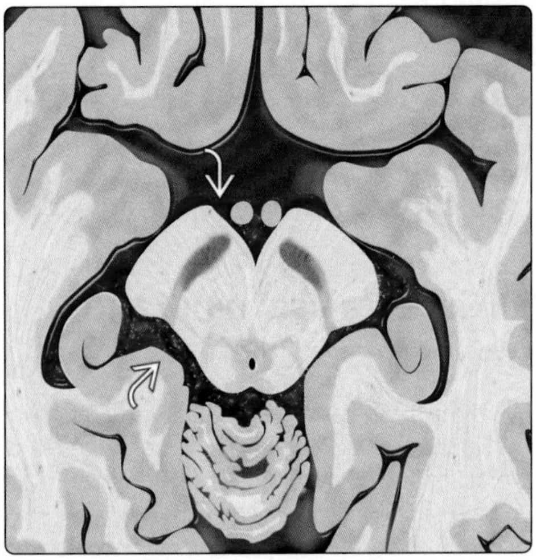

***(6-9)** In pnSAH, hemorrhage is confined to the interpeduncular fossa and ambient (perimesencephalic) cisterns ➡.*

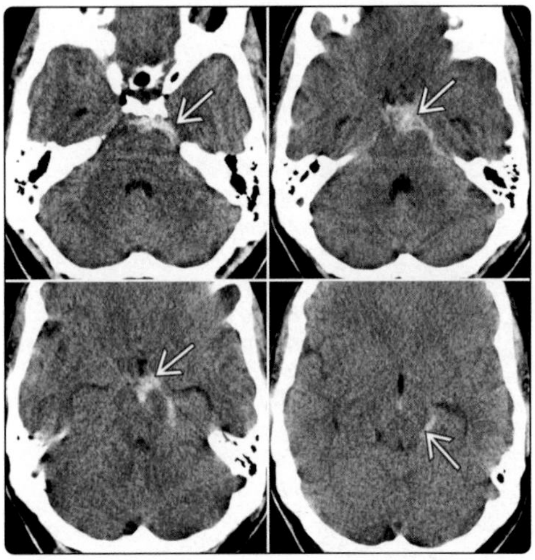

***(6-10)** NECT of pnSAH shows blood in prepontine, perimesencephalic cisterns ➡ but not anterior suprasellar cistern, sylvian fissures.*

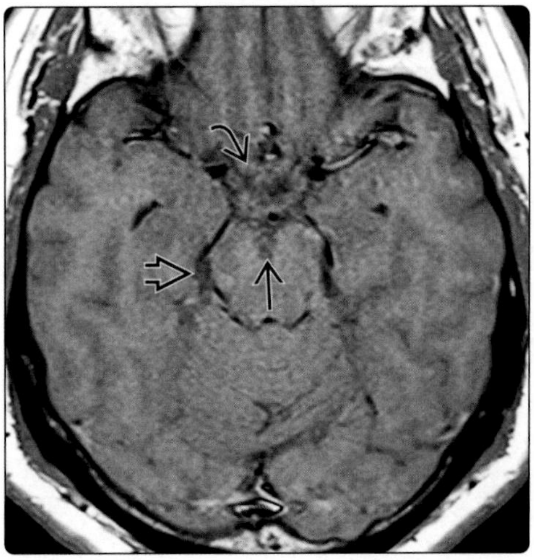

***(6-11)** T1WI shows pnSAH as "dirty" (isointense) CSF filling interpeduncular ➡, suprasellar ➡, perimesencephalic ➡ cisterns.*

time frame (usually 4-10 days after aSAH), not all patients with CVS develop DCI, and not all patients with DCI have vasospasm.

Immediate Cerebral Ischemia

Recent studies have stressed the importance of the *initial* ischemia that occurs immediately after aneurysmal rupture. Acute vasoconstriction can develop within minutes, and early ischemic changes can be detected in the majority of patients within the first 3 days following aSAH. Early ischemic changes are associated with higher death rates and poor outcome.

Many factors contribute to high mortality after SAH. Putative mechanisms involved in early brain injury include micro-thrombo-emboli, activation of inflammatory responses (e.g., cytokine production), oxidative stress (including lipid peroxidation), cortical spreading ischemia, and microvascular constriction.

Delayed Cerebral Ischemia

Vasospasm and *delayed* ischemia develop in two-thirds of all patients with aSAH. Approximately 30% become symptomatic. More than half develop delayed infarcts. Patients with large-volume SAH are at especially high risk for developing symptomatic vasospasm and DCI.

Imaging Post-aSAH Complications

Noninvasive methods to detect early-stage post-aSAH complications include color duplex ultrasound, transcranial Doppler ultrasound, CT angiography, and MR. MR with pMR is most sensitive for detecting early ischemic changes following aSAH.

CT perfusion (especially MTT and CBF) is a useful imaging surrogate for predicting DCI following aSAH. A CBF decrease of 7.6 mL/min/100 g or an MTT increase of 0.91 seconds at day 4 compared with day 0 predicts DCI with 100% and 84% sensitivity, respectively.

Many still consider DSA the gold standard for the diagnosis of CVS. Early angiographic vasospasm is demonstrable in 11% of patients within 72 hours of aSAH and is strongly correlated with delayed symptomatic vasospasm requiring endovascular intervention (intraarterial spasmolysis or angioplasty). Multiple segments of vascular constriction and irregularly narrowed vessels are typical findings **(6-8C)**.

Differential Diagnosis

The differential diagnosis of vasospasm within the context of existing SAH is limited. If the patient has a known aneurysm with recent SAH, the findings of multisegmental vascular narrowing indicate CVS. However, if the SAH is convexal (see below), the differential diagnosis includes **RCVS** and **vasculitis**.

Treatment of aSAH

Treating aSAH is aimed at preventing rebleeding (early aneurysm occlusion) and preventing DCI. Traditional treatment strategies have included "triple H" therapy (hypervolemia, hypertension, and hemodilution). More recent attempts to reduce the risk of DCI have included trials of antiinflammatory agents (e.g., statins), magnesium sulfate, and continuous lumbar drainage. To date, no statistically significant benefits have been demonstrated.

Other Complications of aSAH

DCI typically occurs 4-14 days after aSAH and is most commonly caused by vasospasm (see above).

Obstructive hydrocephalus commonly develops in patients with aSAH, sometimes within hours of the ictus, and may be exacerbated by the presence of IVH. Imaging studies show increased periventricular extracellular fluid with "blurred" lateral ventricle margins.

Neurodegeneration biomarkers (e.g., calpain-derived proteolytic fragments, hypophosphorylated neurofilament H, ubiquitin ligase, and neuron-specific enolase) increase after severe aSAH and may be early predictors of pathophysiologic complications and lasting brain dysfunction.

Terson syndrome (TS) is an intraocular hemorrhage that is found in 12-13% of patients with aSAH. TS is associated with more severe SAH grades and is probably caused by a rapid increase in intracranial pressure. The hemorrhage can be subhyaloid (most common), retinal, or vitreous.

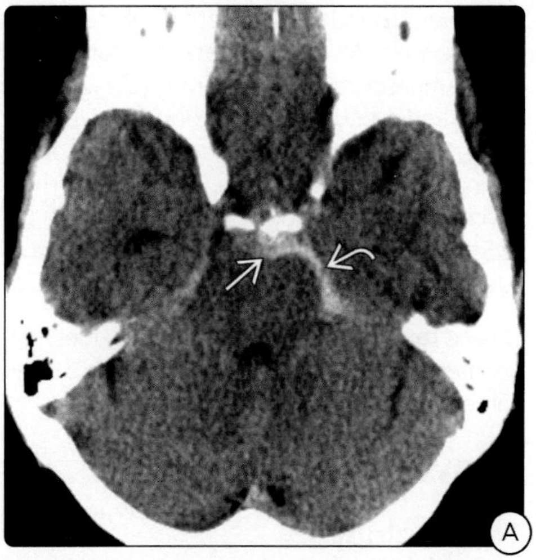

(6-12A) NECT in a 49y man with thunderclap headache shows prepontine → and perimesencephalic ↪ SAH.

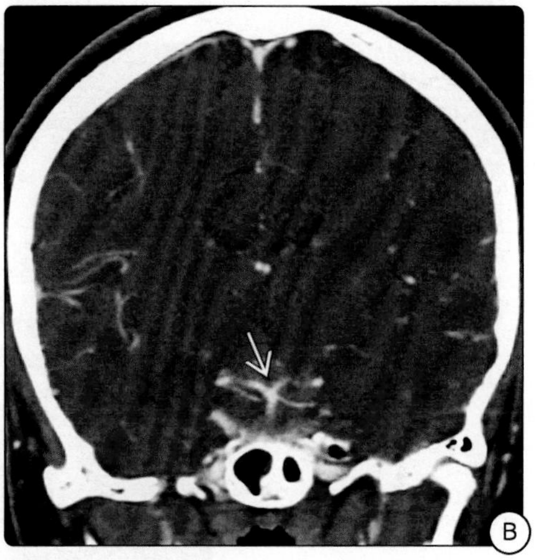

(6-12B) Coronal CTA shows that the basilar bifurcation → is normal.

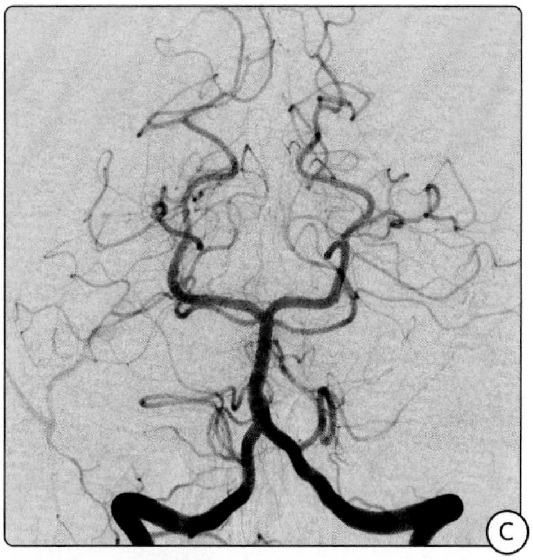

(6-12C) Anteroposterior DSA in the same case is completely normal. This is classic pnSAH.

Perimesencephalic Nonaneurysmal SAH

Terminology

pnSAH is also known as benign perimesencephalic SAH. pnSAH is a clinically benign SAH subtype that is anatomically confined to the perimesencephalic and prepontine cisterns **(6-9)**.

Etiology

The precise etiology of pnSAH is unknown, and the bleeding source in pnSAH is usually undetermined. Yet most investigators implicate venous—not aneurysmal—rupture as the most likely cause.

Clinical Issues

pnSAH is the most common cause of nontraumatic, nonaneurysmal SAH. The typical presentation is mild to moderate headache with Hunt and Hess grade 1-2. Occasionally patients experience severe "thunderclap" headache with meningismus.

The peak age of presentation in patients with pnSAH is between 40 and 60 years—identical to that of aSAH. There is no sex predilection.

Most cases of pnSAH follow a clinically benign and uneventful course. Rebleeding is uncommon (< 1%). In contrast to aSAH, vasospasm and delayed cerebral ischemia are rare.

Imaging

pnSAH has well-defined imaging features. NECT scans show focal accumulation of subarachnoid blood around the midbrain (in the interpeduncular and perimesencephalic cisterns) **(6-10)** and in front of the pons **(6-12A)**.

Although more than 90% of patients with pnSAH have negative DSAs, in 5-10% of cases, a ruptured posterior circulation aneurysm or vertebrobasilar dissection results in a pnSAH pattern of bleeding. Therefore, imaging the cranial circulation is generally recommended. High-resolution CTA is a reliable noninvasive alternative to catheter angiography in ruling out underlying aneurysm or dissection in such cases **(6-12B)**. If the initial CTA is negative, there is no significant additional diagnostic yield from DSA **(6-12C)** or MR.

Differential Diagnosis

The major differential diagnosis of pnSAH is **aSAH**. aSAH is significantly more extensive, spreading throughout the basal cisterns and often extending into the interhemispheric and sylvian fissures.

tSAH would be suggested both by history and imaging appearance. tSAH occurs adjacent to contused brain. It is usually more peripheral, lying primarily within the sylvian fissure and over the cerebral convexities. During closed head injury, the midbrain may be suddenly and forcibly impacted against the tentorial incisura. In such cases, the presence of perimesencephalic blood can mimic pnSAH. In contrast to pnSAH, interpeduncular and prepontine hemorrhage is usually absent.

cSAH is found over the cerebral convexities, not in the perimesencephalic cisterns. Blood within a single sulcus or immediately adjacent sulci is common.

Convexal SAH

Terminology

Isolated spontaneous ntSAH that involves the sulci over the brain vertex is called *convexal* or *convexity SAH* (cSAH). cSAH is a unique type of SAH with a very different imaging appearance from either aSAH or pnSAH: cSAH is restricted to the hemispheric convexities, sparing the basal and perimesencephalic cisterns **(6-13)**.

Etiology

A broad spectrum of vascular and even nonvascular pathologies can cause cSAH. These include dural sinus and cortical vein thrombosis (CoVT), arteriovenous malformations, dural arteriovenous fistulas, arterial dissection/stenosis/occlusion, mycotic aneurysm, vasculitides, amyloid angiopathy, coagulopathies, RCVS, and posterior reversible encephalopathy syndrome.

Clinical Issues

Although cSAH can occur at virtually any age, most patients are between the fourth and eighth decades. Peak age is 70 years.

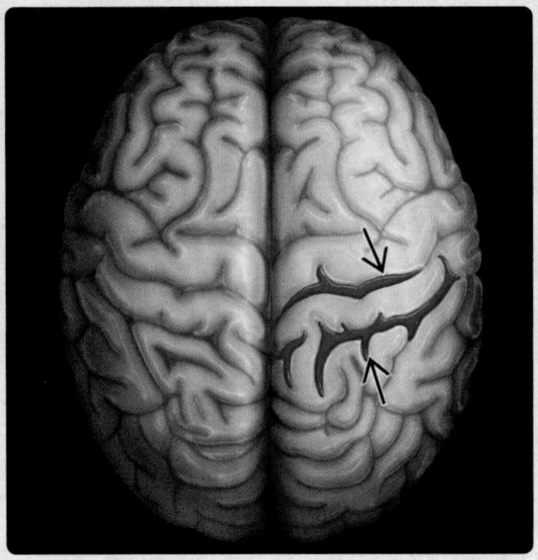

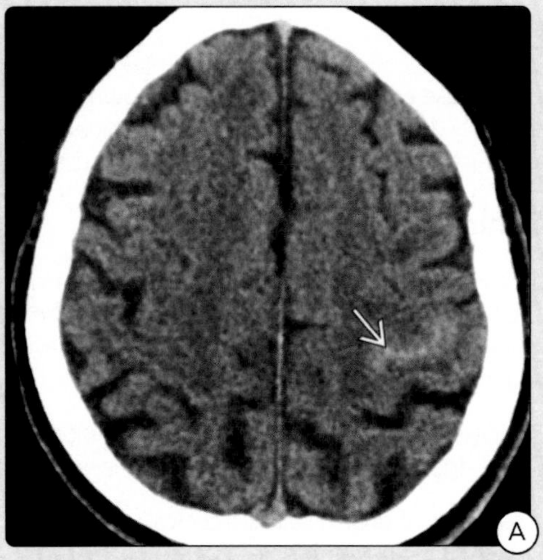

***(6-13)** Graphic depicts convexal SAH (cSAH) with focal subarachnoid blood ➡ in adjacent sulci along the vertex of the left hemisphere. **(6-14A)** NECT in a 78y man with headaches shows subarachnoid blood in a convexity sulcus ➡.*

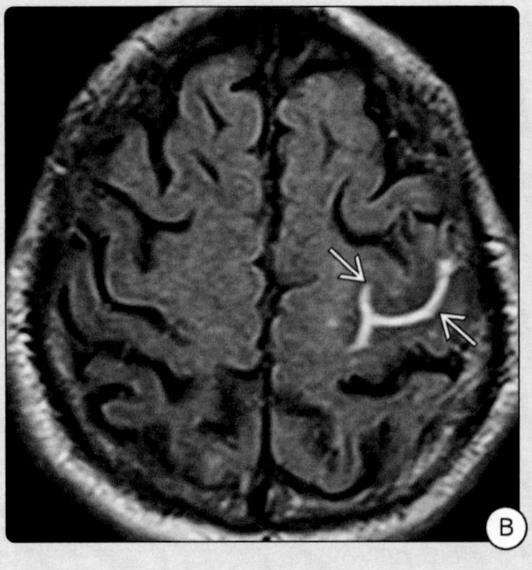

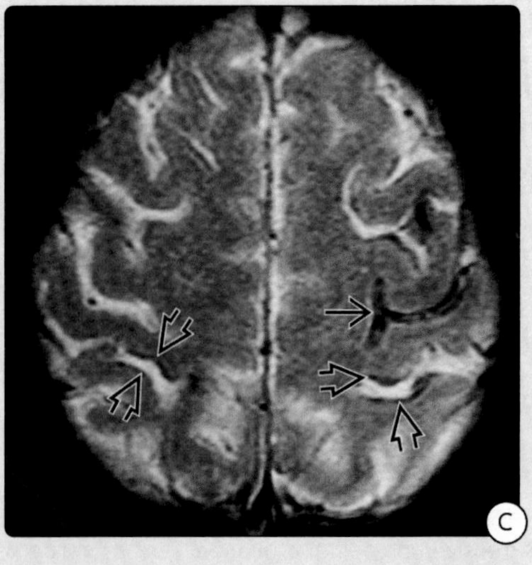

***(6-14B)** FLAIR MR in the same case shows hyperintensity in the convexity sulcus ➡. **(6-14C)** T2* GRE in the same case shows "blooming" of the hemorrhage filling the affected sulcus ➡. Also note subtle "track-like" hypointensities coating the pial surfaces of several other parallel sulci (cortical superficial siderosis) ➡. Final diagnosis was cSAH caused by cerebral amyloid angiopathy.*

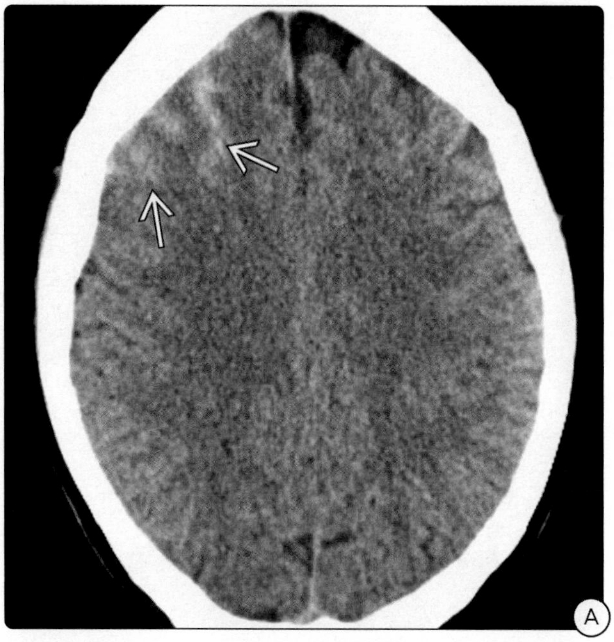

(6-15A) NECT in a 41y woman with thunderclap headache shows cSAH in several adjacent right frontal sulci ➡. The basilar cisterns (not shown) were normal, and there were no other foci of SAH identified.

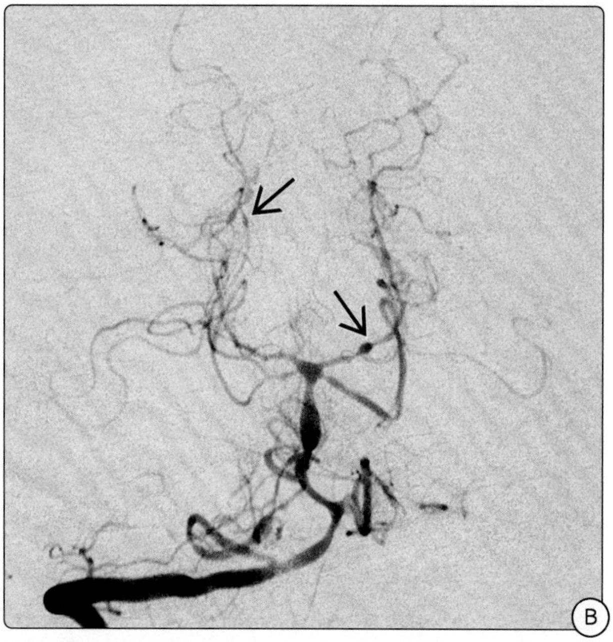

(6-15B) AP DSA in the same case shows multiple areas of alternating narrowing, dilatation in the posterior circulation ➡. Repeat angiogram several days later was normal. This is reversible cerebral vasoconstriction syndrome (RCVS).

The clinical presentation of cSAH varies with etiology but is quite different from that of aSAH. Most patients with cSAH have nonspecific headache without nuchal rigidity. Some present with focal or generalized seizures or neurologic deficits.

Patients with cSAH secondary to RCVS may present with a "thunderclap" headache. The vast majority are middle-aged women. cSAH caused by venous thrombosis or vasculitis may have milder symptoms with more insidious onset. Mean age of CoVT accompanied by cSAH is 33 years.

ETIOLOGY OF NONTRAUMATIC CONVEXAL SAH

Common
- Reversible cerebral vasoconstriction syndrome (RCVS)
  - Mean age ≈ 50 years
  - Typical presentation = thunderclap headache
- Cerebral amyloid angiopathy (CAA)
  - Mean age ≈ 70 years
  - Symptoms = confusion, dementia, sensorimotor dysfunction

Less Common
- Endocarditis
- Cortical vein thrombosis ± dural sinus occlusion

Rare
- Vasculitis

Cerebral amyloid angiopathy (CAA) is the major cause of cSAH in elderly patients. Worsening dementia and headache are the common presentations. cSAH in this age cohort is associated with cognitive impairment and CAA as well as APOE-ε4 overrepresentation compared with age-matched health controls. Between 40-45% experience recurrent cSAH and subsequent lobar hemorrhage (see Chapter 10).

The outcome of cSAH *itself* is generally benign and depends primarily on underlying etiology. Vasospasm and DCI are rare.

Imaging

CT Findings. Most cases of cSAH are unilateral, involving one **(6-14A)** or several dorsolateral convexity sulci. The basal cisterns are typically spared.

NONTRAUMATIC SAH: ANEURYSMAL VS. NONANEURYSMAL

Aneurysmal SAH
- Widespread; basal cisterns
- Arterial origin
- Complications (vasospasm, ischemia) common

Perimesencephalic Nonaneurysmal SAH
- Focal; perimesencephalic, prepontine cisterns
- Probably venous origin
- Clinically benign; complications, recurrence rare

Convexal SAH
- Superficial (convexity) sulci
- ≥ 60 years? Think cerebral amyloid angiopathy (CAA)!
- ≤ 60 years? Think RCVS!
- All ages: venous occlusions, vasculitis

MR Findings. Focal sulcal hyperintensity on FLAIR is typical in cSAH **(6-14B)**. T2* (GRE, SWI) shows "blooming" in the affected sulci **(6-14C)**. If the etiology of the cSAH is dural sinus or cortical vein occlusion, a hypointense "cord" sign may be present. Patients with CAA have multifocal cortical and pial

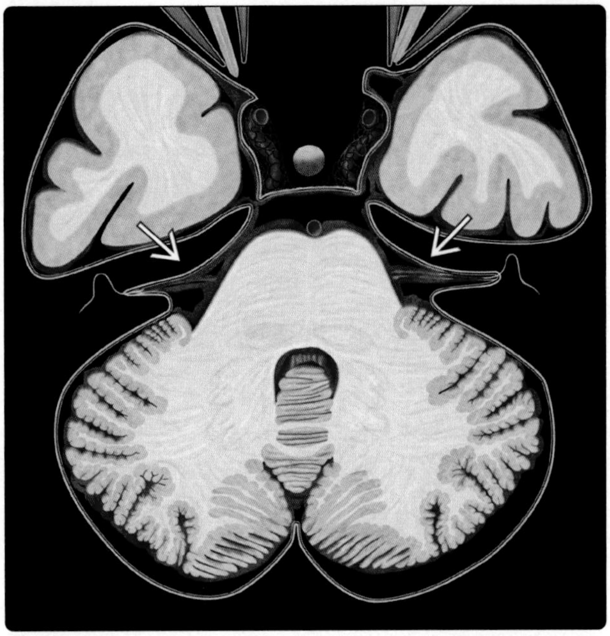

(6-16) Graphic of superficial siderosis shows darker brown hemosiderin staining on surfaces of the brain, meninges, cranial nerves. Notice that CNVII and VIII in the CPA-IAC ➡ are particularly affected.

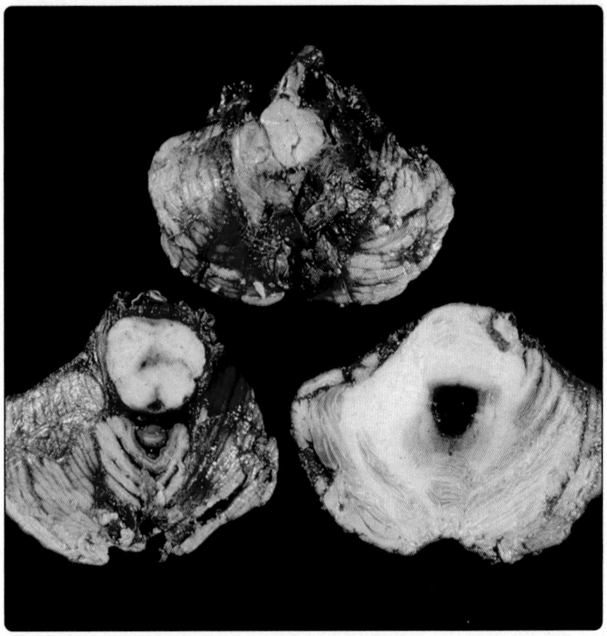

(6-17) Autopsy case shows classical superficial siderosis. The brainstem and cerebellum are covered with brown-staining hemosiderin deposits. (Courtesy E. T. Hedley-Whyte, MD.)

microbleeds ("blooming black dots") on T2*. They may also show evidence of siderosis and prior lobar hemorrhages of differing ages.

Angiography. CTA, MRA, or DSA can be helpful in evaluating patients with cSAH secondary to vasculitis, dural sinus and/or cortical vein occlusion, and RCVS **(6-15)**.

Superficial Siderosis

Terminology

Hemosiderin deposition along brain surfaces, cranial nerves, and/or the spinal cord defines the condition known as **superficial siderosis** (SS) **(6-16)**. Other terms for this condition include subarachnoid hemosiderosis and sulcal siderosis.

There are two types of siderosis, which differ in underlying pathologies and clinical presentation. "Classical" SS of the CNS primarily affects the infratentorial regions and spinal cord.

The term *cortical* SS describes a distinct pattern of iron-bearing blood-breakdown product deposition limited to cortical sulci over the convexities of the cerebral hemispheres. In cortical SS the brainstem, cerebellum, and spinal cord are spared.

Etiology

SS is a consequence of chronic intermittent or continuous minor hemorrhage into the subarachnoid space. Overall, trauma and surgery are the most common causes of classical SS. Other reported etiologies include hemorrhagic neoplasm, vascular malformations, and venous obstruction(s). SS due to repeated aSAH is relatively uncommon.

Cortical SS has many potential causes, but in older individuals cortical SS is most often associated with CAA.

Accelerated cerebellar ferritin synthesis and chronic intrathecal bleeding overload the ability of the microglia to biosynthesize ferritin, resulting in subpial iron excess. This facilitates free radical damage, lipid peroxidation, and neuronal degeneration.

Pathology

Location. Although it can occur anywhere in the CNS, *classical* SS has a predilection for the posterior fossa (cerebellar folia and vermis, CN VIII) and brainstem.

Cortical SS is seen in 60% of patients with CAA but is rare in non-CAA forms of intracerebral hemorrhages.

Gross Pathology. Brownish yellow and blackish gray encrustations cover the affected structures, layering along the sulci and encasing cranial nerves **(6-17)**.

Microscopic Features. Subpial hemosiderin depositions are the histologic hallmark of SS.

Clinical Issues

Patients with classical SS often present with slowly progressive gait ataxia, dysarthria, and bilateral sensorineural hearing loss. Some patients present with progressive myelopathy. Often decades pass between the putative event that causes SS and the development of overt symptoms.

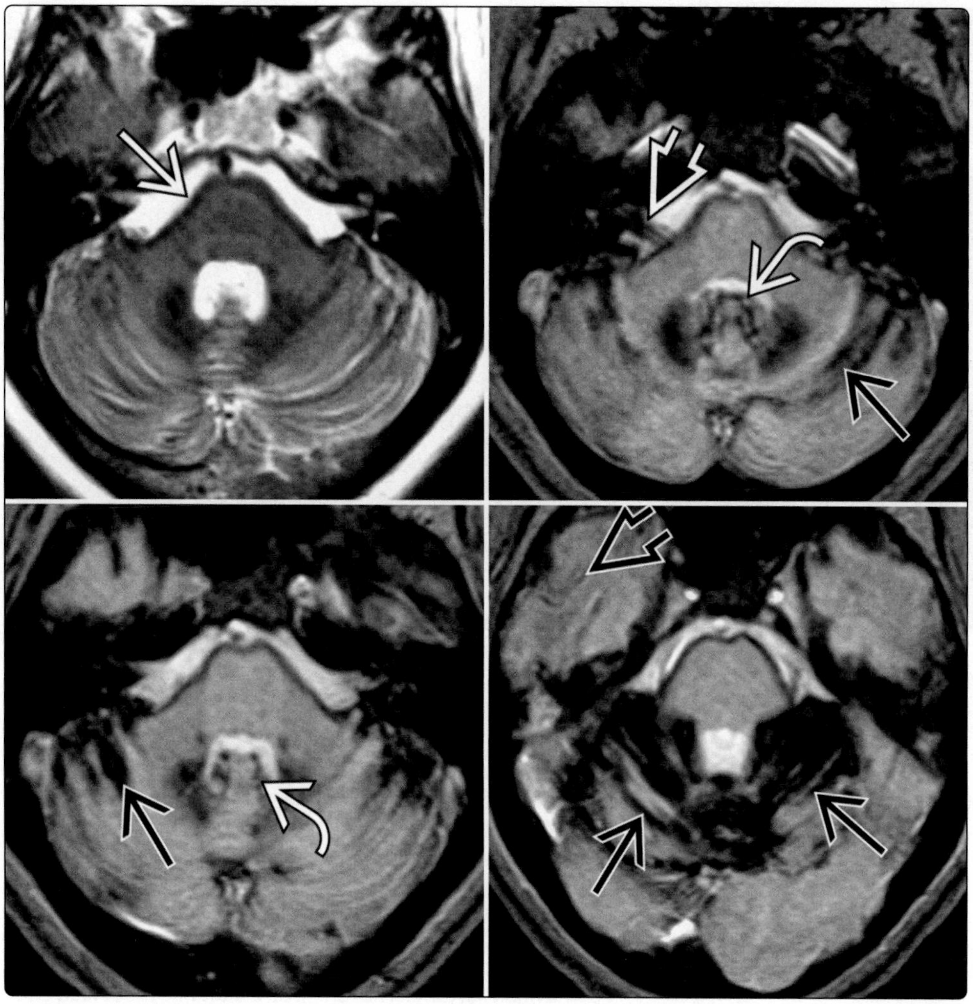

(6-18) Series of MR images shows typical findings of classic superficial siderosis in a patient with bilateral sensorineural hearing loss and progressive ataxia. (Upper Left) FSE T2WI shows linear hypointensity around the surfaces of the pons and cerebellum ➡. (Upper Right, Lower Left, Lower Right) T2 GRE scans show marked "blooming" covering the pons and cerebellar hemispheres, extending into and along the folia and great horizontal fissure ➡. Note siderosis along the right CN VII and CN VIII ➡. Hemosiderin deposition is also present in the choroid plexus of the fourth ventricle ➡. Other than minimal right temporal siderosis ➡, the supratentorial brain and subarachnoid spaces appeared normal. Despite detailed imaging of the entire neuraxis, no source for the chronic repeated SAHs was identified.*

Imaging

CT is usually normal in patients with SS. Occasionally, iron deposition is severe enough to cause hyperattenuation along brain surfaces.

SS on MR is best identified on T2* (GRE, SWI) imaging and is seen as a hypointense rim that follows along brain surfaces and coats the cranial nerves and/or spinal cord **(6-18)**. A characteristic bilinear "track-like" appearance is common with cortical SS.

Despite extensive neuroimaging, the source of the SS often remains occult. In 50% of classical SS, a hemorrhage source is never identified despite extensive investigation of the entire neuraxis.

Differential Diagnosis

The major imaging mimic of classic SS is **"bounce point" artifact**, which makes the posterior fossa surfaces appear artifactually dark.

Most cortical SS mimics contain deoxygenated blood or blood products. **Cerebral veins** appear markedly hypointense on SWI but do not run parallel to the convexity sulci. Slow flow in sulcal arteries (pial collaterals in stroke or moyamoya) can appear hypointense on SWI as well.

SUPERFICIAL SIDEROSIS (SS)

Classical SS
- Posterior fossa > > supratentorial
- Brain (typically cerebellum), cranial nerves coated with hemosiderin
- Chronic repeated SAH
- Cause undetermined in ≈ 50%
- Sensorineural hearing loss

Cortical SS
- Cortex over hemisphere convexities
- Most common etiology = CAA
- Transient focal neurologic episodes
- Parallel "track-like" hypointensities on T2*
- High risk of future intracerebral hemorrhage
- Lobar hemorrhages, microbleeds

In **Sturge-Weber syndrome**, hypointensity due to gyriform calcifications may be linear and cortical but can be easily identified on NECT. Rare causes of hypointensity over the brain surfaces include **hemorrhagic subarachnoid metastases**, **neurocutaneous melanosis** (hyperintense on

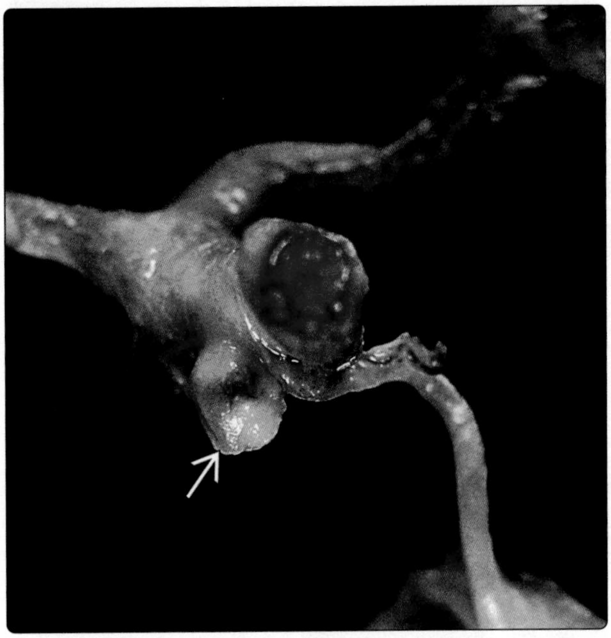

(6-19) Autopsy specimen shows an incidental unruptured SA ➡ at the ICA-PCoA junction. (Courtesy B. Horten, MD.)

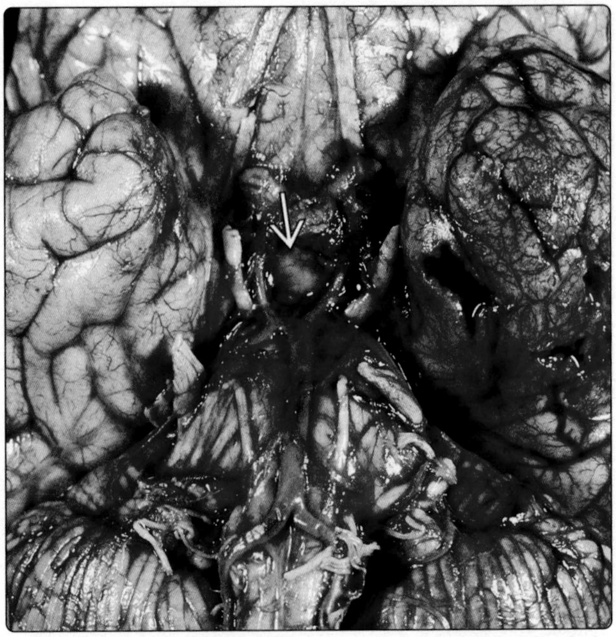

(6-20) Autopsy demonstrates a ruptured basilar bifurcation aneurysm ➡ with massive SAH extending throughout all the basilar cisterns. (Courtesy R. Hewlett, MD.)

T1WI), and **meningioangiomatosis** (thickened, enhancing, sometimes calcified and infiltrating proliferations of meningeal cells and blood vessels).

Aneurysms

Overview

Intracranial aneurysms are classified by their gross phenotypic appearance. The most common intracranial aneurysms are called **saccular** or **"berry" aneurysms** because of their striking sac- or berry-like configuration **(6-19)**. Saccular aneurysms (SAs) are acquired lesions that arise from branch points of major cerebral arteries in which hemodynamic stresses are maximal. SAs lack some of the arterial layers (usually the internal elastic lamina and media) found in normal vessels. More than 90% of SAs occur on the "anterior" (carotid) circulation.

Pseudoaneurysms (also sometimes called "false" aneurysms) are focal arterial dilatations that are not contained by any layers of the normal arterial wall. They are often irregularly shaped and typically consist of a paravascular, noncontained blood clot that cavitates and communicates with the parent vessel lumen. Extracranial pseudoaneurysms are more common than intracranial lesions. Intracranial pseudoaneurysms usually arise from mid-sized arteries distal to the circle of Willis. Trauma, drug abuse, infection, and tumor are the usual etiologies.

Blood blister-like aneurysms (BBAs) are a special type of aneurysm recently recognized in the neurosurgical literature. BBAs are eccentric hemispherical arterial outpouchings that are covered by only a thin layer of adventitia. These dangerous lesions are both difficult to detect and difficult to treat. They have a tendency to rupture at a much smaller size and relatively younger age compared with SAs. Although BBAs can be found anywhere, they have a distinct propensity to occur along the supraclinoid internal carotid artery.

Fusiform aneurysms (FAs) are *focal* dilatations that involve the entire circumference of a vessel and extend for relatively short distances. FAs are more common on the vertebrobasilar ("posterior") circulation. FAs can be atherosclerotic (more common) or nonatherosclerotic in origin. Nonatherosclerotic FAs are often associated with collagen-vascular disorders, such as Marfan or Ehlers-Danlos type IV.

Saccular Aneurysm

Terminology

Saccular ("berry") aneurysms (SAs) are sometimes called "true" aneurysms (to contrast them with pseudoaneurysms).

An SA is a pathologic outward bulge that affects only part of the parent artery circumference **(6-19)**. Most SAs lack two important structural components of normal intracranial arteries—the internal elastic lamina and the muscular layer ("media")—and often have a focally thinned wall that is prone to rupture.

Etiology

General Concepts. The development and subsequent rupture of intracranial SAs reflects several complex interactions. SAs are *acquired* lesions that develop from abnormal extracellular matrix (ECM) maintenance and excessive hemodynamic stress.

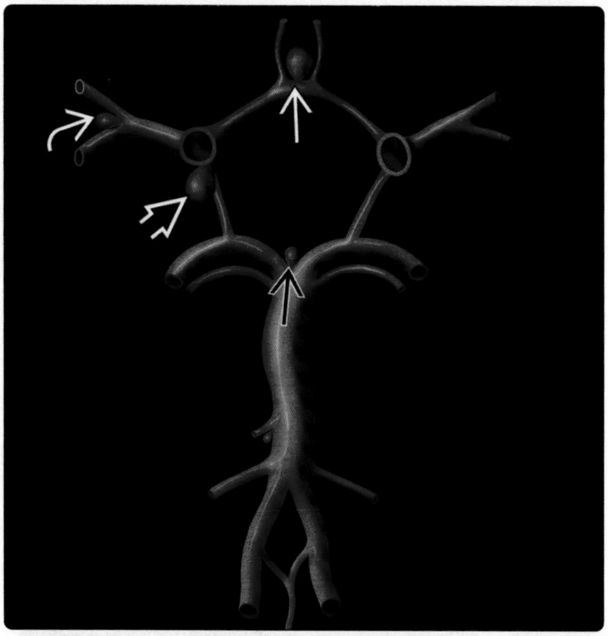

(6-21) The most common sites for SAs are the ACoA ➡ and the ICA-PCoA junction ➡. Other locations include the MCA bifurcation ➡ and the basilar tip ➡.

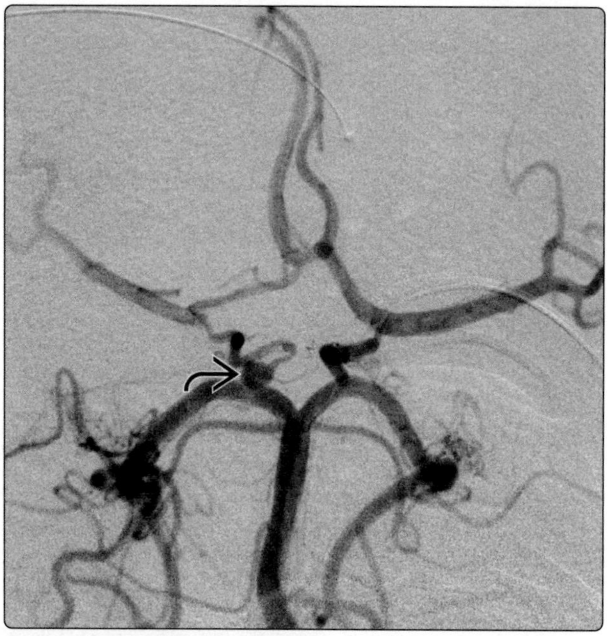

(6-22) Submentovertex view of DSA demonstrates entire circle of Willis. A small SA ➡ arises from the junction of the right PCoA and the P1 PCA segment.

Recent advances in molecular biology have revealed the common pathway of the initiation, progression, and rupture of SAs. SA formation begins with endothelial dysfunction followed by inflammatory cascades, pathologic remodeling, and degenerative changes in vessel walls.

Genetics. Very few SAs are congenital (i.e., present at birth). However, many studies have demonstrated a genetic component to aneurysm development and rupture.

Genome-wide association studies (GWAS) have identified some susceptible loci and genes related to cell cycle and endothelial function in SAs although no single disease-causing gene variant has been identified.

The 9p21 gene cluster plays an essential role in cellular proliferation and contains multiple genes that may be related to SA pathogenesis.

SOX17 mutation—a gene required for both endothelial formation and maintenance—has also been strongly implicated in most GWAS of SAs although it explains only a small fraction of the total genetic risk.

Inherited connective tissue disorders, anomalous blood vessels, familial predisposition, and "high-flow" states (i.e., vessels supplying an arteriovenous malformation) all increase the risk of SA development.

Demographic studies have also demonstrated that environmental factors such as systemic hypertension, smoking, and heavy alcohol consumption contribute significantly to the risk of developing SAs and may augment any underlying genetic propensities.

Anomalous Blood Vessels. A number of blood vessel asymmetries and some congenital vascular anomalies predispose to the development of an intracranial SA.

Bicuspid aortic valves, aortic coarctation, persistent trigeminal artery, and congenital anomalies of the anterior cerebral artery (i.e., A1 asymmetries or infraoptic course of the A1 segment) all carry an increased risk of SA. Whether arterial fenestrations (i.e., splitting and reuniting of a vessel such as the anterior communicating or basilar artery) are associated with an increased prevalence of SA is controversial.

SACCULAR ANEURYSM: ETIOLOGY

General Concepts
- Acquired, not congenital!
- Abnormal hemodynamics, shear stresses → weakened artery wall
- Underlying genetic alterations common

Increased Risk of SA
- Anomalous vessels
  - Persistent trigeminal artery
  - Fenestrated anterior communicating artery
- Vasculopathies, syndromes
  - Abnormal collagen (Marfan, Ehlers-Danlos)
  - Fibromuscular dysplasia
  - Autosomal-dominant polycystic kidney disease
- Familial intracranial aneurysm
  - 4-10x ↑ risk if first-order family member with aSAH

Inherited Vasculopathies and Syndromic Aneurysms. Some multiorgan heritable connective tissue disorders (such as **Marfan** and **Ehlers-Danlos II and IV** syndromes or **fibromuscular dysplasia**) are associated with increased risk of intracranial aneurysms. Arteriopathy is common in patients with **neurofibromatosis type 1** (NF1). Although the vascular changes in NF1 primarily affect the aorta and renal, coronary, and gastrointestinal arteries, some increased risk of developing intracranial aneurysms has been reported.

Autosomal-dominant polycystic kidney disease (ADPCKD) carries an increased lifetime risk (4-23%) of developing an SA. Patients with ADPCKD are also at increased risk for aneurysm rupture earlier in life (mean age 35-45 years) compared with the general population (mean age 50-54 years). Possibly because of the associated vascular defects due to mutations in the *PKD1* and *PKD2* genes, these patients are at increased risk of treatment complications.

Other, less common heritable conditions predisposing to SA development include pseudoxanthoma elasticum and multiple endocrine neoplasia type 1.

Familial Intracranial Aneurysms. A positive family history represents the strongest known risk factor for aneurysmal subarachnoid hemorrhage (aSAH) (4-10x general population). Up to 20% of patients with SAs have a family history of intracranial aneurysms. SAs in "clusters" of related individuals without any known heritable connective tissue disorder are termed **familial intracranial aneurysms** (FIAs). FIAs tend to occur in younger patients and rupture at a smaller size than sporadic SAs.

Pathology

Location. Most intracranial SAs occur at points of maximal hemodynamic stress. The vast majority arise from major blood vessel bifurcations or branches **(6-20)**. The circle of Willis plus the middle cerebral artery (MCA) bifurcations are the most common sites **(6-22)** **(6-23)**. Aneurysms beyond the circle of Willis are uncommon, as distal hemodynamic stresses are much lower. Many peripheral aneurysms are actually

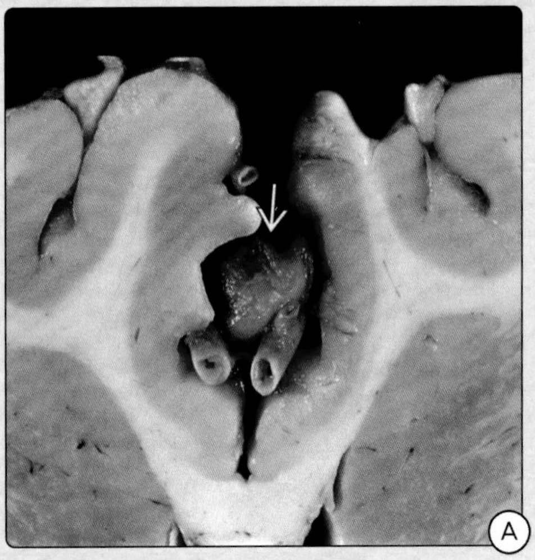

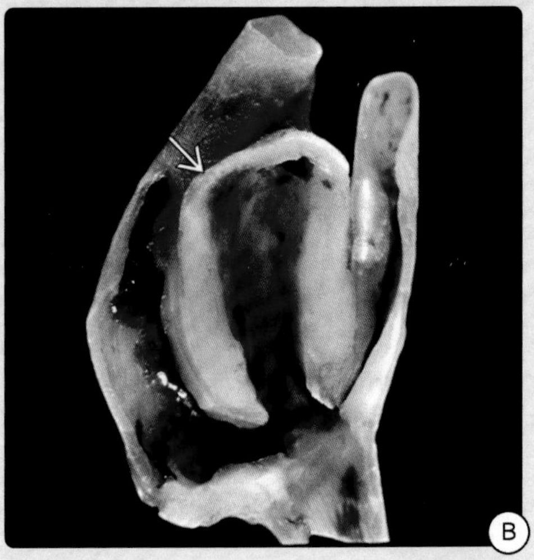

***(6-23A)** Autopsy shows an ACoA aneurysm projecting superiorly between the A2 segments of both anterior cerebral arteries. **(6-23B)** The aneurysm is dissected out and cut into a coronal section. Reactive changes thicken the base of the aneurysm, but the dome is relatively thin. (Courtesy J. Townsend, MD.)*

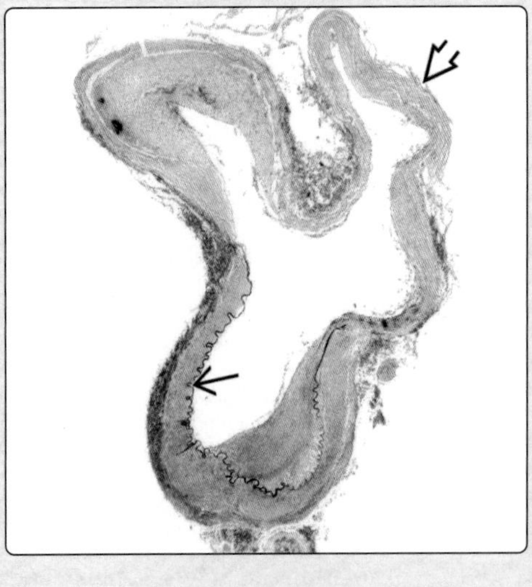

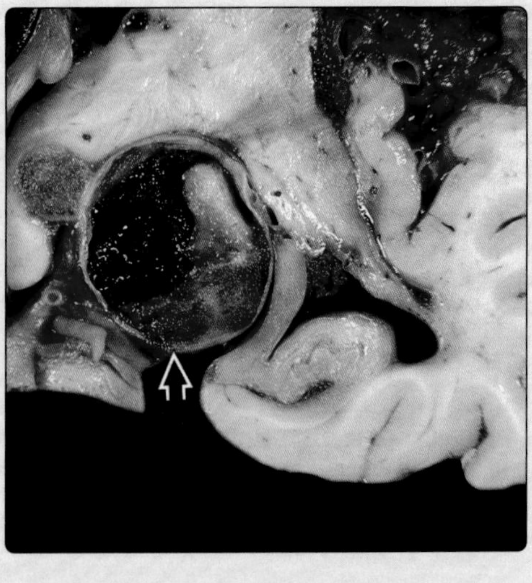

***(6-24)** Cross section of an aneurysm shows normal internal elastic lamina, muscular layer in the parent artery wall. The aneurysm sac lacks both these layers and is composed of only intima and adventitia. **(6-25)** Close-up view of a mostly thrombosed aneurysm demonstrates organizing clots of different ages. (Courtesy R. Hewlett, MD.)*

pseudoaneurysms secondary to trauma, infection, or tumor (see below).

Anterior circulation aneurysms. Ninety percent of SAs occur on the "anterior" circulation **(6-21)**. The anterior circulation consists of the internal carotid artery (ICA) and its terminal branches, the anterior cerebral artery (ACA), and MCA. The ophthalmic artery, anterior (ACoA) and posterior communicating (PCoA) arteries, anterior choroidal artery, and hypophyseal arteries are all considered part of the anterior circulation.

Approximately one-third of SAs occur on the ACoA with another third arising at the junction of the ICA and the PCoA. Approximately 20% of SAs occur at the MCA bi- or trifurcation.

Posterior circulation aneurysms. Ten percent of SAs are located on the vertebrobasilar ("posterior") circulation. The basilar artery bifurcation is the most common site, accounting for about 5% of all SAs **(6-20)**. The posterior inferior cerebellar artery is the second most common location.

Size and Number. SAs vary in size from tiny (2-3 mm) to large lesions over 1 cm **(6-23)**. SAs that are 2.5 cm or larger are called "giant" aneurysms.

Between 15-20% of aneurysms are multiple. About 75% of patients with multiple aneurysms have two SAs, 15% have three, and 10% have more than three SAs. Multiple SAs are significantly more common in female patients.

Gross Pathology. Intracranial SAs are dynamic—not static—lesions. Hemodynamic insults can elicit a pathologic vascular response that leads to self-sustained aneurysmal remodeling. Persistence of the original inciting hemodynamic factors is not necessary for continued pathologic progression.

The gross configuration of an SA changes with time as the arterial wall is remodeled in response to hemodynamic stresses. As it becomes progressively weakened, the wall begins to bulge outward, forming an SA.

The opening (ostium) of an SA can be narrow or broad based. Computational flow dynamics shows that intraaneurysmal flow patterns are complex and result in flow impinging on different parts of the aneurysm. Some impact the ostium, whereas others are most prominent at the dome. One or more lobules or an apical "tit" may develop as a result. Such outpouchings are usually the part of the aneurysm wall most vulnerable to rupture.

Microscopic Features. SAs demonstrate a disrupted or absent internal elastic lamina. The smooth muscle cell layer (media) is generally absent **(6-24)**. The delicate balance between the synthesis and degradation of the ECM—a dynamic network of proteins and proteoglycans—is disrupted. Therefore, the wall of an SA is usually quite fragile, consisting of intima and adventitia in a degraded ECM. Variable amounts of thrombus **(6-25)** and atherosclerotic changes may also be present, especially in larger "giant" SAs.

Inflammatory cell infiltration is a histologic hallmark of SAs. Macrophage infiltration is more prominent in ruptured SAs. Mast cells also seem to constitute an integral part of the inflammatory response in aneurysm development.

SACCULAR ANEURYSM: PATHOLOGY

Location
- 90% anterior circulation
  - Circle of Willis, MCA bifurcation
  - ACoA, ICA/PCoA junction most common
- 10% posterior circulation (basilar bifurcation)

Size, Number
- Tiny (1-2 mm) to giant (≥ 2 cm)
- 15-20% multiple (> 2 F:M = 10:1)

Gross, Microscopic Features of SA Walls
- SAs lack internal elastic lamina, media
- Variable thrombus
- Inflammatory changes common

Clinical Issues

Epidemiology. Unruptured intracranial aneurysms (UIAs) are found in 3% of the adult population and are increasingly detected due to more frequent cranial imaging. Asymptomatic unruptured SAs are at least 10 times more prevalent than ruptured SAs.

Demographics. Peak presentation is between 40 and 60 years of age. There is a definite female predominance, especially with multiple SAs.

SAs are rare in children, accounting for less than 2% of all cases, although they are the most common cause of spontaneous (nontraumatic) SAH in this age group.

Compared with adult aneurysms, pediatric aneurysms have a predilection for the posterior circulation. They also attain larger size and frequently develop a more complex shape. Childhood aneurysms exhibit a relative lack of female predominance and are more often associated with trauma or infection. Higher recurrence rates and de novo formation or growth are also common.

Presentation. Between 80-90% of all nontraumatic SAHs are caused by ruptured SAs. The most common presentation is sudden onset of severe, excruciating headache ("thunderclap" or "worst headache of my life").

Cranial neuropathy is a relatively uncommon presentation of SA. Of these, a pupil-involving CN III palsy from a PCoA aneurysm is the most common. Occasionally, patients with partially or completely thrombosed aneurysms present with a transient ischemic attack or stroke.

Natural History. The overall annual rupture rate of all SAs is 1-2%. However, the rupture risk varies according to size, location, and shape of the aneurysm.

Size and rupture risk. Aneurysms that are ≥ 5 mm are associated with a significantly increased risk of rupture compared with 2-4-mm aneurysms (unadjusted hazard ration 12.24). Demonstrable growth on surveillance imaging is also associated with an increased rupture risk.

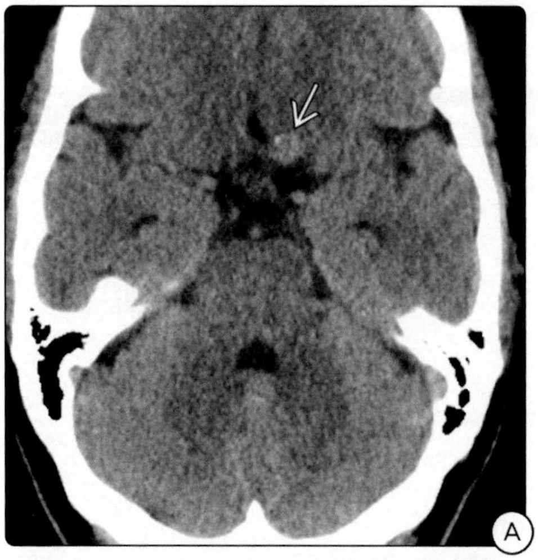

(6-26A) NECT in a 49y woman with headaches shows rounded hyperdense mass ➡ adjacent to the suprasellar cistern, with no evidence for SAH.

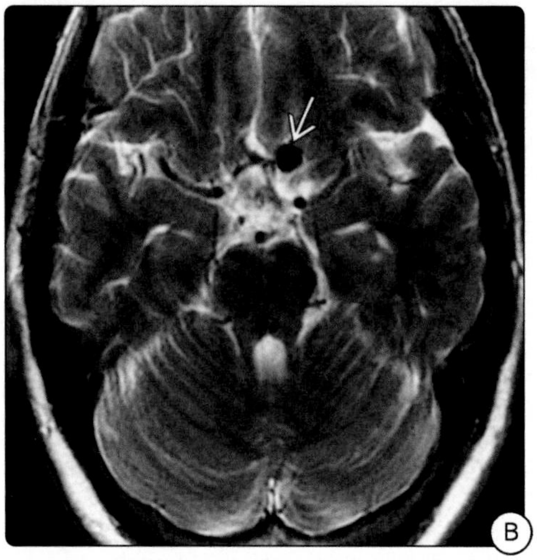

(6-26B) T2WI in the same case shows a very well-delineated "flow void" ➡ that appears to arise from the circle of Willis.

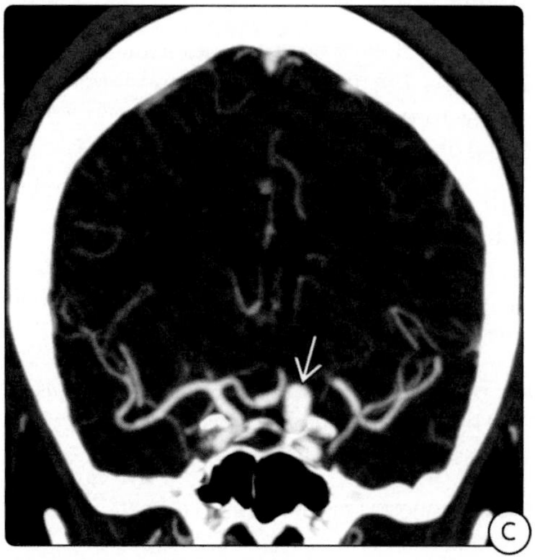

(6-26C) Coronal MIP of CTA in the same case shows that a lobulated SA ➡ arises from the distal ICA bifurcation.

Shape/configuration and rupture risk. In addition to size, shape and configuration also matter. Nonsaccular (nonspherical) shape increases rupture risk. The presence of a "daughter" sac (irregular wall protrusion) and increased aspect ratio (length compared with width) are independent predictors of rupture risk.

Location and rupture risk. Vertebrobasilar artery aneurysms have a significantly higher rupture risk, as do ICA-PCoA aneurysms. MCA and ACA aneurysms are associated with modest risk. Bifurcation aneurysms are more prone to growth than side-wall aneurysms.

Clinical history. Clinical history is important, as a prior history of SAH is a significant independent risk factor for aneurysm rupture. Female sex, hypertension, and smoking at baseline are other significant risk factors.

SACCULAR ANEURYSM: CLINICAL FEATURES

Epidemiology
- 3% of population; F > M
- Peak presentation 40-60 years (rare in children)

Presentation
- SAH with sudden severe "thunderclap" headache
- Mass effect (CN palsy) less common

Treatment Options. Treatment varies depending on whether the SA is ruptured or unruptured.

Ruptured SAs. Virtually all *ruptured* SAs are treated. Ideally, management should be tailored to the individual patient with all options considered for optimum outcome. Possible interventions include clipping, stenting, coiling, and flow diversion.

aSAH is a catastrophic event with high mortality and significant morbidity. Approximately one-third of patients die, and one-third survive with significant residual neurologic deficits. Only one-quarter to one-third of patients with aSAH recover with good functional outcome.

Patients who survive the initial SAH are typically treated as soon as possible. Rebleeding risk is highest in the first 24-48 hours after the initial hemorrhage. Approximately 20% of ruptured but untreated SAs rebleed within 2 weeks. Half rehemorrhage within 6 months.

Unruptured SAs. The management of *unruptured* SAs is controversial because of their unpredictable natural history. A new method of risk calculation, the PHASES score, was modeled on prospectively collected data from several cohort studies that provide absolute risks of rupture for the initial 5 years after aneurysm detection using six baseline characteristics such as age, aneurysm size and location, presence of hypertension, and previous SAH from a different aneurysm.

Recently, a multidisciplinary consensus developed a more complex treatment score (UIATS) that includes and quantifies key factors for clinical decision-making in the management of UIAs. These factors can then be used to score "in favor of UIA repair" (surgical or endovascular) and "in favor of UIA conservative management." The UIATS score models, not just morphologic UIA features, but also life expectancy, coexistent morbidities, family history, and modifiable or nonmodifiable risk factors.

NATURAL HISTORY OF SACCULAR ANEURYSMS

Most saccular aneurysms don't rupture!

What increases risk of rupture?

- **Size matters!**
  - Rupture risk increases with size
  - Aneurysms ≥ 5 mm greater risk than 2-4 mm (hazard ratio = 12)
  - However, no absolutely "safe" minimal size with zero risk
- **Shape, configuration matter!**
  - Nonround (nonsaccular shape) = ↑ rupture risk!
  - "Daughter" sac or "tit" = ↑ rupture risk!
- **Location affects rupture risk!**
  - Rupture risk of similarly sized aneurysms changes with location
  - Vertebrobasilar, ICA-PCoA location highest rupture risk
  - MCA, ACA moderate risk
  - Non-PCoA-ICA aneurysms lowest
- **Type**
  - Blood blister-like aneurysms rupture at smaller size

Imaging

General Features. SAs are round or lobulated arterial outpouchings that are most commonly found along the circle of Willis and at the MCA bifurcation. Imaging features depend on whether the aneurysm is unruptured or ruptured (with aSAH) and whether the aneurysm sac is patent or partially or completely thrombosed.

CT Findings. Very small unruptured SAs may be invisible on standard NECT scans. Larger lesions appear as well-delineated masses that are slightly hyperdense to brain **(6-26A)**. Rim **(6-28A)** or mural calcification **(6-29A)** may be present.

Acutely ruptured SAs present with aSAH, which is often the dominant imaging feature and frequently obscures the "culprit" aneurysm. Occasionally, an SA appears as a well-delineated, relatively hypodense filling defect within a pool of hyperdense subarachnoid blood.

A partially or completely thrombosed SA is typically hyperdense compared with the adjacent brain on NECT scans.

Patent SAs show strong, uniform enhancement of the aneurysm lumen. A partially thrombosed SA shows enhancement of the residual lumen. Completely thrombosed SAs do not enhance, although longstanding lesions may demonstrate rim enhancement secondary to reactive inflammatory changes.

MR Findings. MR findings vary with pulse sequence, flow dynamics, and the presence as well as the age of associated hemorrhage (either in the subarachnoid cisterns or within the aneurysm itself).

About half of all patent SAs demonstrate "flow voids" on T1- and T2WI **(6-26B)**. The other half exhibit heterogeneous signal intensity secondary to slow or turbulent flow, saturation effects, and phase dispersion. Propagation of pulsation artifacts in the phase-encoding direction is common. FLAIR scans may show hyperintensity in the subarachnoid cisterns secondary to aSAH.

If the aneurysm is partially or completely thrombosed, laminated clot with differing signal intensities is often present **(6-28)**. "Blooming" on susceptibility-weighted images (GRE, SWI) is common. Contrast-enhanced scans may show T1 shortening in intraaneurysmal slow-flow areas. High-resolution contrast-enhanced MR may demonstrate inflammatory changes in the aneurysm wall **(6-29C)** and adjacent brain **(6-28F)**.

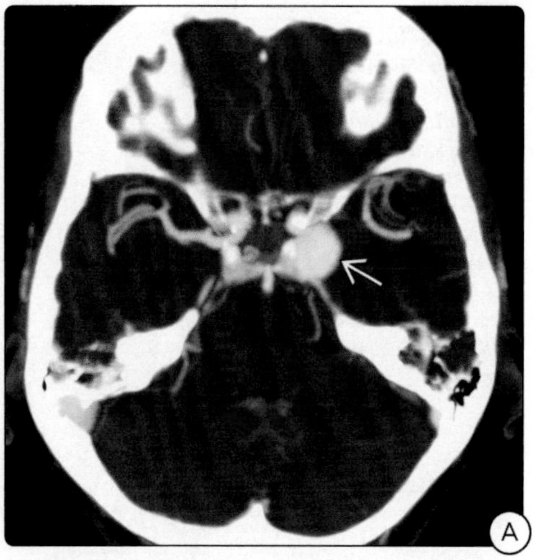

***(6-27A)** MIP of CTA in an 82y woman with diplopia shows a well-delineated, intensely enhancing mass ➡ in the left cavernous sinus.*

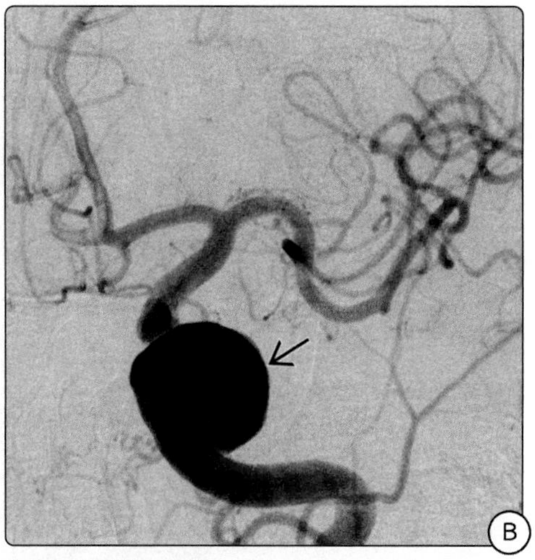

***(6-27B)** Oblique DSA of the left carotid angiogram shows a cavernous ICA aneurysm ➡, but details are difficult to appreciate.*

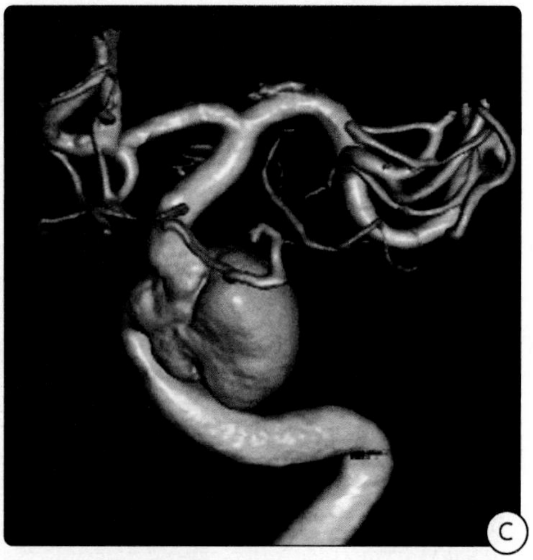

***(6-27C)** 3D rotational DSA with shaded surface display allowed full delineation of the aneurysm and its relationship to the parent vessel.*

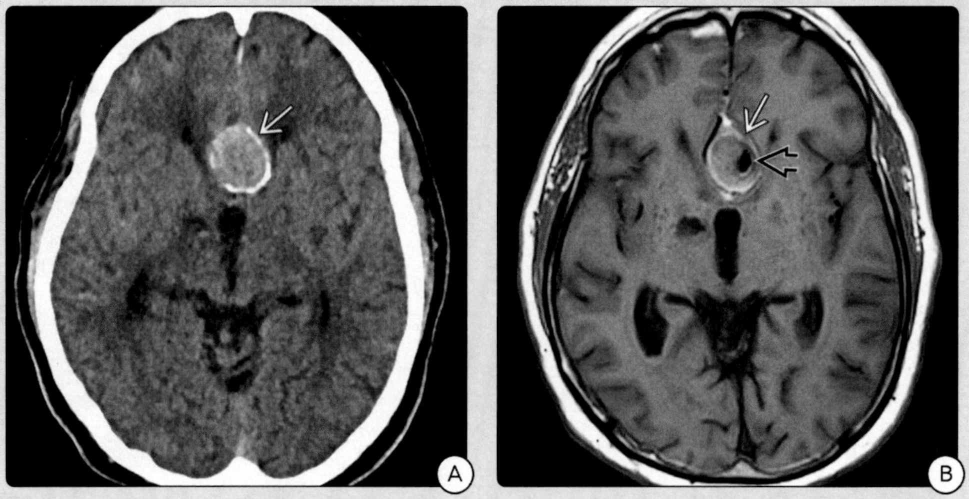

***(6-28A)** NECT shows a well-delineated hyperdense midline mass with peripheral calcification. The lesion is 2.5 cm in diameter. **(6-28B)** MR was obtained for further characterization. T1WI shows the lesion is hyperintense, with an eccentrically located oval flow void within the mass.*

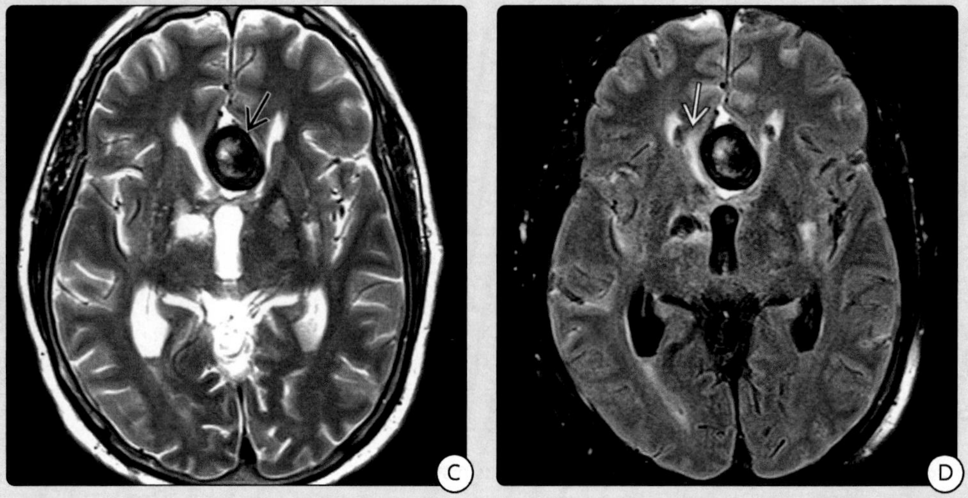

***(6-28C)** T2WI in the same case shows concentric hypointense layers of thrombus surrounding a mixed signal intensity core. **(6-28D)** FLAIR in the same case shows some hyperintensity in the adjacent brain.*

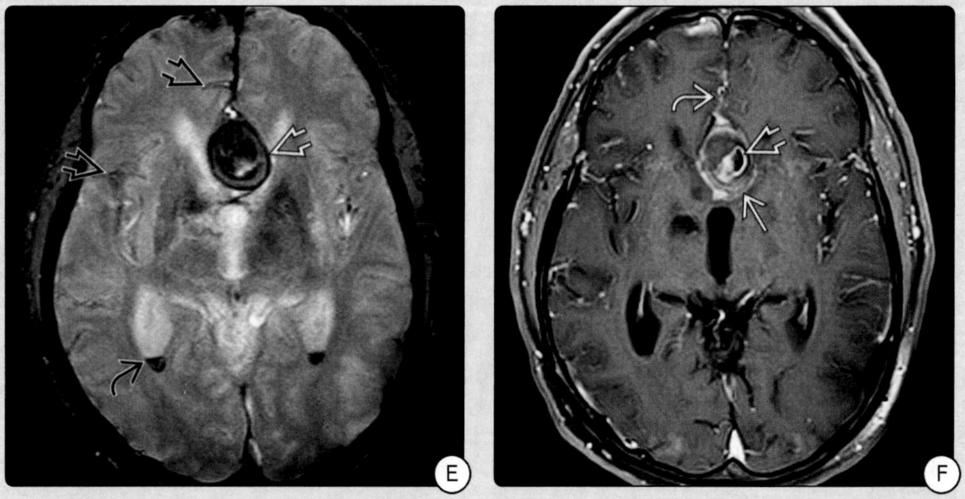

***(6-28E)** T2*GRE shows laminated thrombus of different ages. A small amount of intraventricular hemorrhage is present. Note associated superficial siderosis, indicating prior subarachnoid bleeds. **(6-28F)** T1 C+ FS shows enhancement around the mostly thrombosed aneurysm, along interhemispheric fissure, around residual lumen. This is a giant aneurysm with repeated SAH, perianeurysmal inflammatory changes.*

DWI sequences may show ischemic areas secondary to vasospasm or embolized thrombus.

Angiography. High-resolution multidetector CTA is a common screening procedure in patients with suspected aSAH. The sensitivity of CTA is more than 95% for aneurysms larger than 2 mm in diameter **(6-26C)**. The overall sensitivity of MRA is 90% for aneurysms larger than 2 mm in diameter.

Although many patients with aSAH and an SA that has been demonstrated on either CTA or MRA go directly to surgery, conventional DSA is still considered the gold standard for detecting intracranial SAs—especially if endovascular treatment is considered.

All four intracranial vessels as well as the complete circle of Willis must be demonstrated in multiple projections. Rotational 3D DSA with shaded surface displays is helpful in delineating the precise relationship between the aneurysm and its parent vessels and branches.

Multiple intracranial aneurysms are shown in 15-20% of cases. When more than one aneurysm is identified in aSAH patients, determining which aneurysm ruptured is essential for presurgical planning. Contrast extravasation is pathognomonic of rupture but rarely observed. Other angiographic features suggesting rupture include lobulation or presence of an apical "tit," size (the largest aneurysm is generally, though not always, the one that ruptured), and presence of focal perianeurysmal clot on CT or MR.

Computational analyses of intracranial aneurysms show that ruptured aneurysms are more likely to have complex and/or unstable flow patterns, concentrated inflows, and small impingement regions from the "jet" of blood entering the lesion. Volume variations with the cardiac cycle may also influence rupture risk.

Differential Diagnosis

The major differential diagnosis of intracranial SA is a **vessel loop**. Intracranial arteries curve and branch extensively. On 2D images (e.g., anteroposterior and lateral views of digital subtraction angiograms), overlapping or looping vessels may mimic the rounded sac of a small peripheral SA. Multiple projections and 3D shaded surface displays are helpful in sorting out overlapping or looping vessels from SA.

SACCULAR ANEURYSM: IMAGING AND DDx

Imaging
- Round/lobulated arterial outpouching
- CTA 95% sensitive if aneurysm > 2 mm
- DSA with 3D SSD best delineates architecture

Differential Diagnosis
- Vessel loop
- Arterial infundibulum
  - Conical
  - ≤ 2 mm
  - ICA-PCoA junction
- Blood blister-like aneurysm
  - Hemispherical bulge
  - Along superior surface of supraclinoid ICA
- Pseudoaneurysm
  - Usually distal to circle of Willis, MCA bifurcation
  - History of trauma, drugs, infection, neoplasm

The second most common differential diagnosis is an **arterial infundibulum**. An infundibulum is a focal, symmetric, conical dilatation at the origin of a

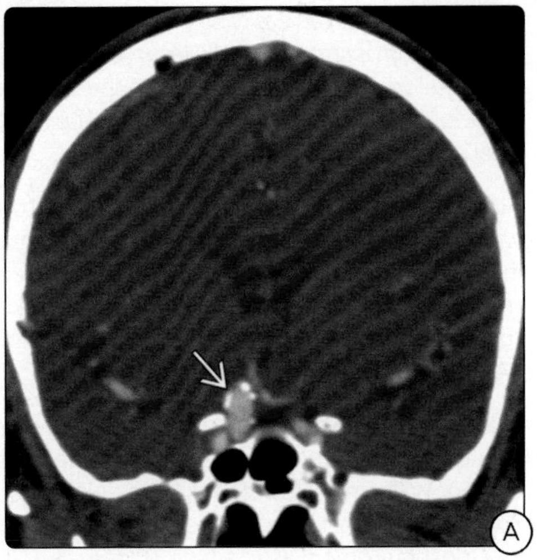

***(6-29A)** Coronal CTA in a 70y woman with headaches shows a partially calcified aneurysm of the distal right ICA ➡.*

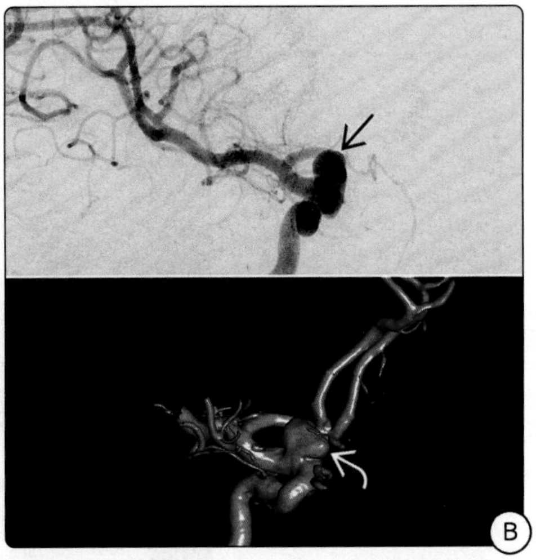

***(6-29B)** (Top) AP DSA in same case shows the aneurysm ➡. (Bottom) 3D SSA shows its detailed complex, multilobulated configuration ➡.*

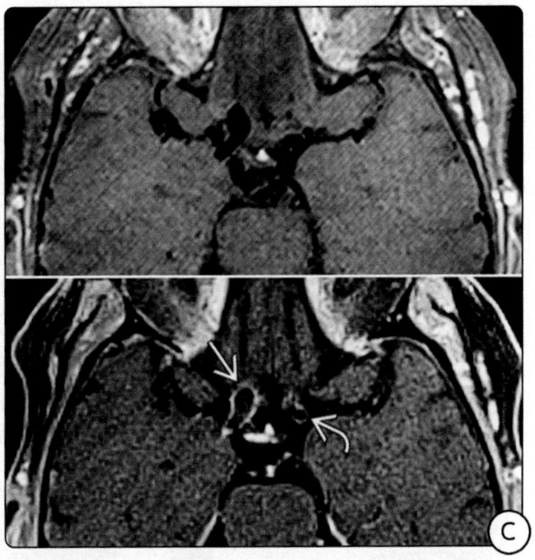

***(6-29C)** T1 C+ FS shows strong enhancement of the aneurysm wall ➡, normal enhancement of left distal ICA ➡. (Courtesy S. McNally, MD.)*

blood vessel that can easily be mistaken for a small SA. An infundibulum is small, typically less than 3 mm in diameter. The distal vessel typically arises from the apex—not the side—of the infundibulum. The PCoA is the most common location for an infundibulum.

Although most infundibula are incidental anatomical variants without pathogenetic significance, occasionally an arterial infundibulum ruptures or, over time, even develops into a frank aneurysm. When these rare "aneurysm-like infundibula" rupture and cause SAH, they are indistinguishable from classic SAs.

A **pseudoaneurysm** may be difficult to distinguish from an SA. Pseudoaneurysms are more common on vessels distal to the circle of Willis and are often fusiform or irregular in shape. Focal parenchymal hematomas often surround intracranial pseudoaneurysms.

Fusiform aneurysms (FAs) are generally easily distinguished from SAs by their shape. FAs are long-segment, sausage-shaped lesions that involve the entire circumference of a vessel, whereas SAs are round or lobulated lesions. Location is also a helpful feature in distinguishing an FA from an SA. FAs are more common in the vertebrobasilar ("posterior") circulation. SAs usually arise from terminal vessel bifurcations and are more common in the carotid ("anterior") circulation.

A **blood blister-like aneurysm** (BBA) may also be difficult to distinguish from a small, wide-necked SA. Although they can be found in virtually any part of the intracranial circulation, BBAs typically arise along the greater curvature of the supraclinoid ICA, not at its terminal bifurcation or PCoA origin.

An area of **signal loss** that mimics the "flow void" of an aneurysm on MR can be caused by an aerated anterior clinoid process or an aberrant supraorbital ethmoid or frontal sinus.

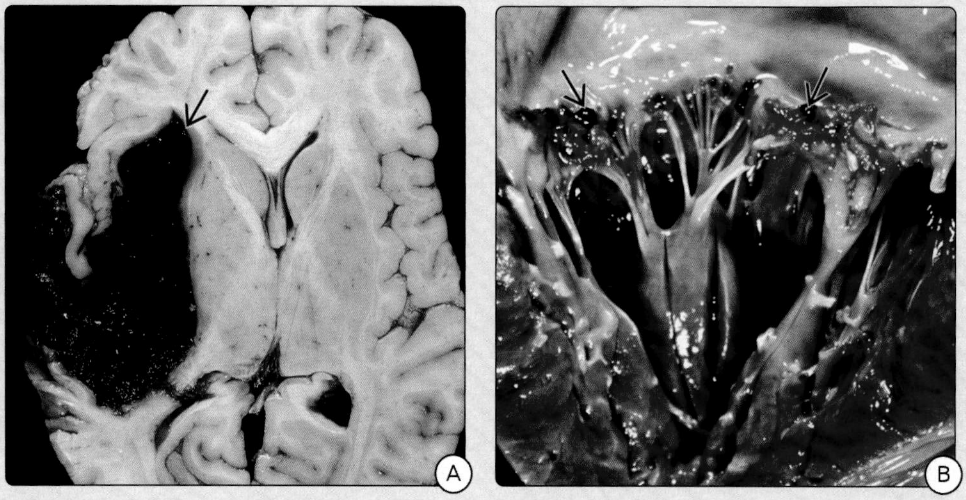

***(6-30A)** Axial autopsy section from a patient with bacterial endocarditis shows a large focal right temporal lobe hematoma → caused by a ruptured mycotic pseudoaneurysm of the MCA. **(6-30B)** Sectioned heart from the same patient shows extensive hemorrhagic vegetations → covering much of the mitral valve.*

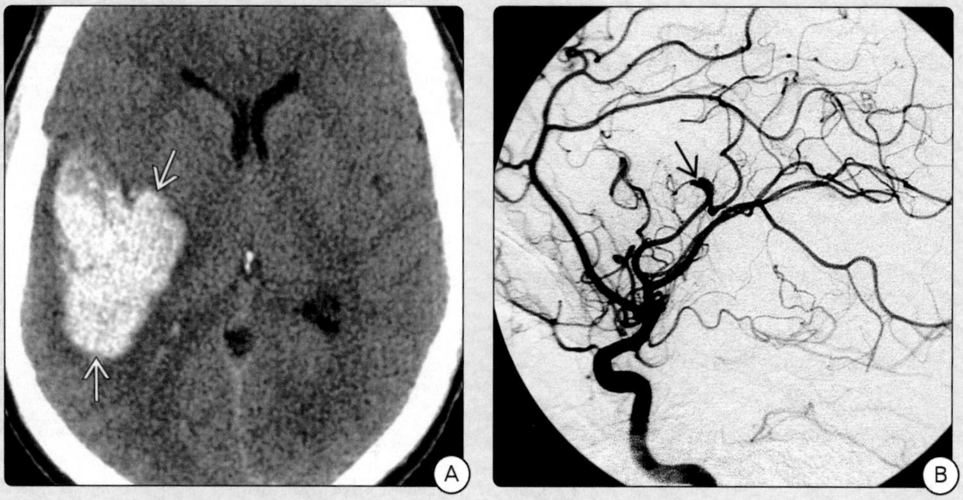

***(6-31A)** NECT shows spontaneous intracranial hemorrhage → in a patient with a history of bacterial endocarditis. The history raised suspicion for a mycotic pseudoaneurysm as the underlying etiology. **(6-31B)** Lateral DSA in the same patient demonstrates an irregular fusiform dilatation of an M2 MCA branch →. Mycotic pseudoaneurysm was confirmed during surgical evacuation of the hematoma.*

Pseudoaneurysm

Pseudoaneurysm is a rare but important underdiagnosed cause of intracranial hemorrhage, accounting for just 1-6% of all intracranial aneurysms. Delayed onset and continued deterioration of neurologic symptoms are common.

Terminology

Pseudoaneurysm—also sometimes called a "false" aneurysm to distinguish it from a "true" SA—is an arterial dilatation with complete disruption of the arterial wall.

Etiology

Pseudoaneurysms are usually caused by a specific inciting event—e.g., trauma, infection, drug abuse, neoplasm, or surgery—that initially weakens and then disrupts the normal arterial wall. When the weakened wall expands, a pseudoaneurysm is created.

Pseudoaneurysms are contained only by relatively fragile, friable cavitated clot and variable amounts of fibrous tissue. Necrosis and inflammatory or neoplastic infiltrates are additional features that may be present. As they lack normal vessel wall components, pseudoaneurysms are especially prone to hemorrhage **(6-30)**. Multiple hemorrhagic episodes, relapse, and complications such as distal embolic infarcts are common.

Pathology

Location. Approximately 80% of pseudoaneurysms affecting the carotid and vertebral arteries are extracranial, whereas 20% involve their intracranial segments.

Traumatic intracranial carotid pseudoaneurysms typically involve the proximal (cavernous or paraclinoid) ICA. Surgery and radiation therapy (typically for head and neck cancers) usually affect the extracranial carotid artery (carotid "blow-

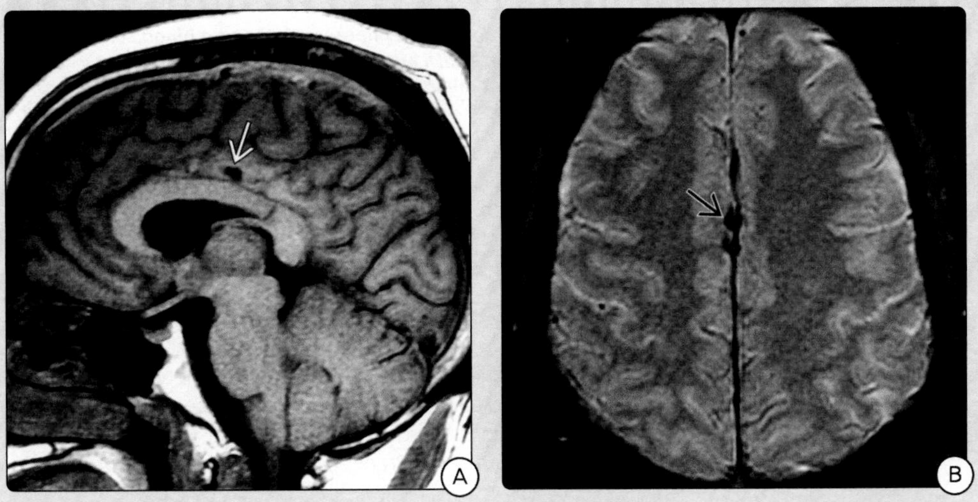

***(6-32A)** Sagittal T1WI in a 23y man with persistent headaches and a remote history of head trauma shows an unusual-appearing "flow void" ➔ above the corpus callosum. **(6-32B)** T2* GRE shows some hemosiderin staining along the falx cerebri ⇨.*

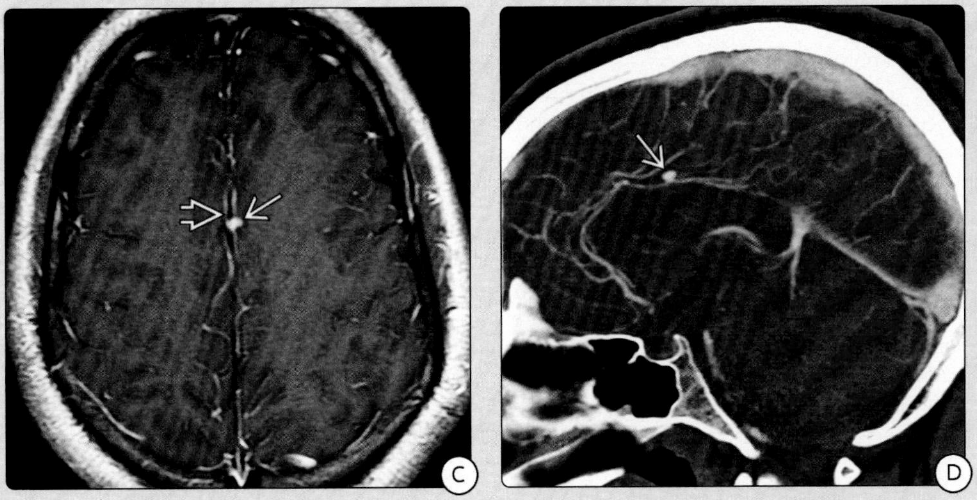

***(6-32C)** T1 C+ in the same case shows a bilobed aneurysm ➔ arising from the A3 anterior cerebral (pericallosal) artery (ACA) ➔. **(6-32D)** Sagittal CTA shows a pseudoaneurysm ➔ arising from the pericallosal artery. The pseudoaneurysm probably arose when the A3 ACA was forcibly impacted against the inferior margin of the falx cerebri during closed head injury.*

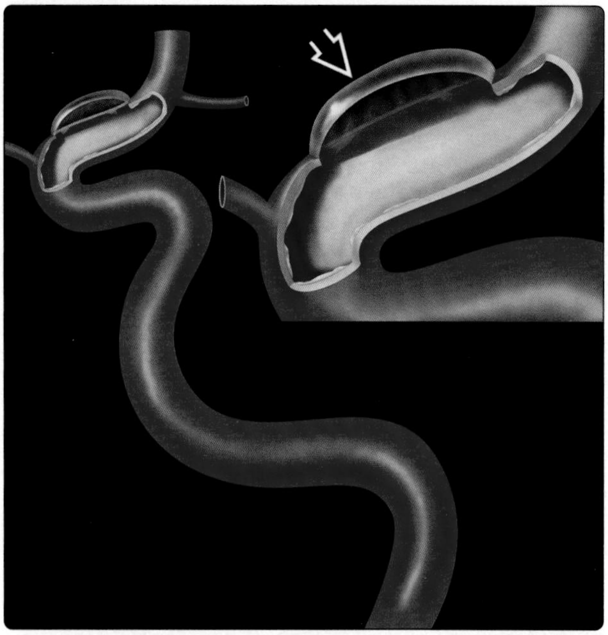

(6-33) Graphic depicts blood blister-like aneurysm, seen here as a broad-based hemispheric bulge covered with a tissue-paper-thin layer of adventitia ➡.

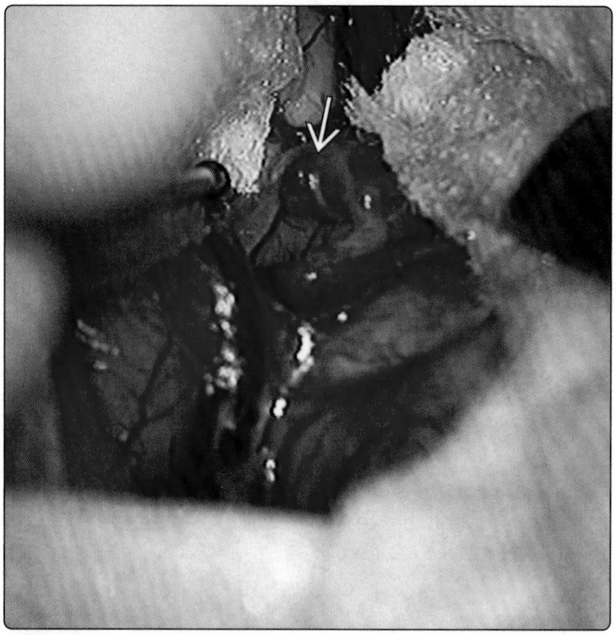

(6-34) Intraoperative photograph shows a blood blister-like aneurysm ➡ with blood swirling under the thin, nearly transparent aneurysm wall.

out" syndrome). Intracranial vertebral pseudoaneurysms typically affect the V4 segment.

Most pseudoaneurysms distal to the circle of Willis are infectious (mycotic), drug-related, neoplastic (oncotic), or traumatic. Traumatic pseudoaneurysms can form when the pericallosal artery is impacted against the inferior (free) margin of the falx cerebri during closed head injury **(6-32)**.

PSEUDOANEURYSM: PATHOLOGY

Pathology
- Arterial wall completely disrupted
- Often contained only by cavitated clot
- Inflammatory changes common

Etiology
- Rarely form spontaneously
- Trauma, infection, drugs or neoplasm

Location
- 80% extracranial
  - Cervical carotid, vertebral arteries
- 15-20% intracranial
  - Cavernous/paraclinoid ICA
  - Distal cortical branches

Gross Pathology. Pseudoaneurysms are purplish masses typically contained only by thinned, discontinuous adventitia and organized hematoma. Hematomas associated with pseudoaneurysms are often large and may contain clots of varying ages.

Microscopic Features. Wall disruption or necrosis is characteristic. Mycotic and oncotic pseudoaneurysms show extensive infiltration of the vessel wall by inflammatory or neoplastic cells, respectively. The parent vessel lumen is often occluded by thrombus, tumor, debris, or purulent exudate.

Clinical Issues

Patients with traumatic cavernous/paraclinoid ICA pseudoaneurysms often have skull base fractures. The interval between the initial injury and neurologic deterioration varies from a few days up to several months. The major clinical presentations include sudden headache, loss of consciousness, recurrent epistaxis, and cranial nerve palsies.

Patients with pseudoaneurysms distal to the circle of Willis often have a history of severe trauma (with or without skull fracture), systemic infection, or drug abuse.

Imaging

General Features. Findings suggestive of cerebral pseudoaneurysm include unexplained enlargement of an existing parenchymal hematoma. In the appropriate clinical setting, unusual or delayed evolution of hematoma also suggests the possibility of an underlying pseudoaneurysm.

CT Findings. NECT scans are generally normal or nonspecific. A parenchymal hematoma is common **(6-31)**. CTA sometimes shows a "spot" sign (focus of contrast enhancement) within a rapidly expanding hematoma. Because many pseudoaneurysms are small and nonsaccular, they may be difficult to diagnose on CTA.

MR Findings. Hematoma signal varies with clot age and sequence. A "flow void" representing the residual lumen may be present within the hematoma. Intravascular enhancement represents the slow, delayed filling and emptying often seen with pseudoaneurysms.

Angiography. Digital subtraction angiography shows a globular, fusiform, or irregularly shaped "neckless" aneurysm with delayed filling and emptying of contrast agent **(6-31B)**. Positional contrast stagnation is common.

Treatment. Endovascular occlusion with a flow-diverting stent is now the method of choice to treat most intracranial pseudoaneurysms. Surgical options include trapping or sacrificing the parent artery with or without bypass graft.

Differential Diagnosis

The major differential diagnosis of pseudoaneurysm is a "true" aneurysm or **SA**. Location is a helpful feature, as SAs typically occur along the circle of Willis and at the MCA bifurcation.

Dissecting aneurysm most frequently occurs in the posterior circulation, where the vertebral artery is the most common site. **Fusiform aneurysm** is also more common on the posterior circulation and typically involves the basilar artery.

PSEUDOANEURYSM: IMAGING AND DDx

Imaging Features
- Irregularly shaped outpouching
  - "Neck" usually absent
  - ± Surrounding avascular mass effect (cavitated hematoma)
- CTA
  - May show "spot" sign
  - Pseudoaneurysms often small, easily overlooked
  - DSA may be required if CTA is negative
- MR: Look for distal emboli

Differential Diagnosis
- Blood blister-like aneurysm
  - May be a form of pseudoaneurysm
- Saccular aneurysm
- Dissecting aneurysm
- Fusiform aneurysm

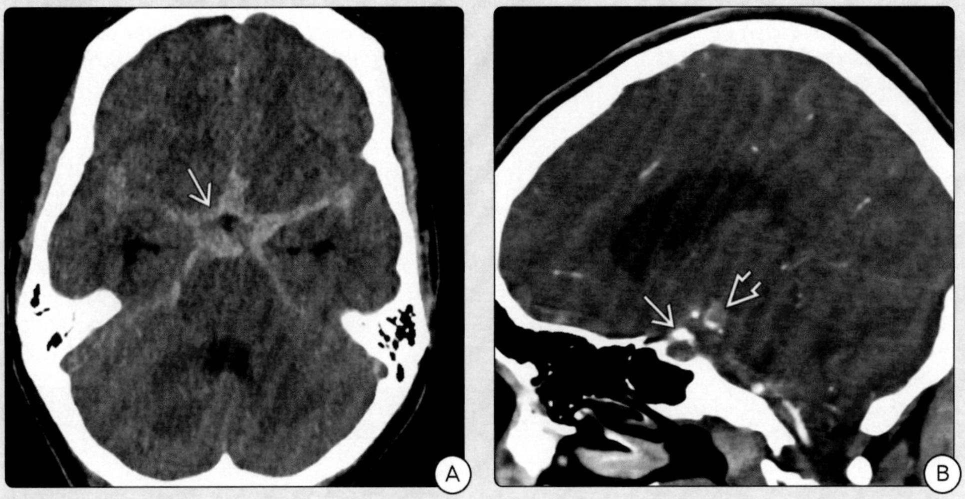

***(6-35A)** NECT in a 38y woman with sudden onset of "worst headache of my life" shows diffuse SAH throughout the basilar cisterns →, suggestive of aneurysmal SAH. **(6-35B)** Sagittal CTA shows the aneurysmal SAH →. The only suggestion of an abnormality is a slight hemispherical bulge along the left supraclinoid ICA →.*

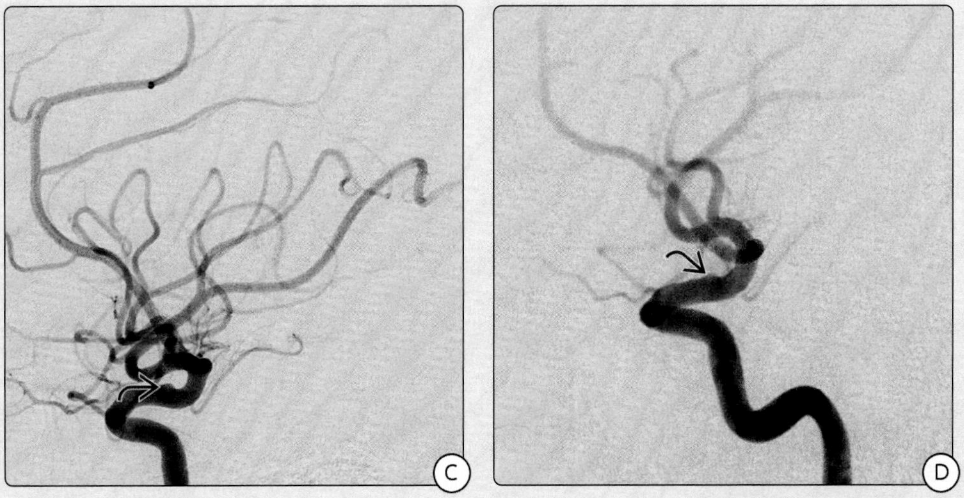

***(6-35C)** Lateral DSA in the same case shows that the hemispherical bulge along the supraclinoid ICA → is a blood blister-like aneurysm. **(6-35D)** Lateral oblique DSA confirms the presence of a blood blister-like aneurysm →.*

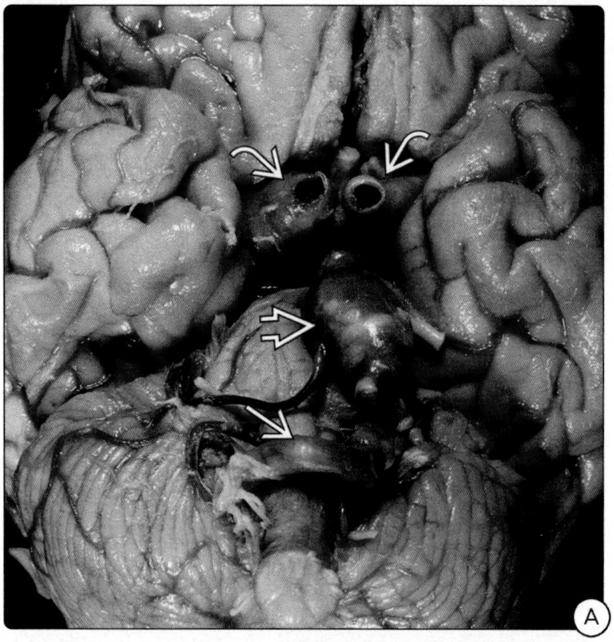

***(6-36A)** Autopsy case shows generalized atherosclerotic dolichoectasia of the vertebrobasilar system ➡ and both ICAs ➡. A fusiform aneurysm involving the distal basilar artery ➡ is present.*

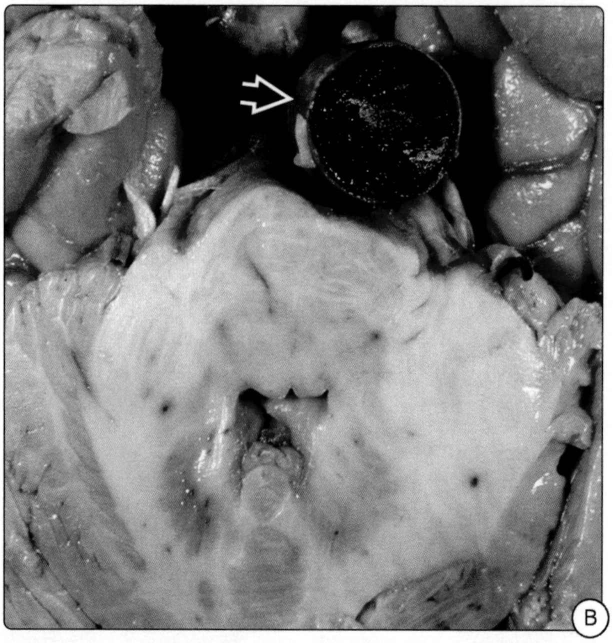

***(6-36B)** Close-up view of axial section through the posterior fossa shows the fusiform aneurysm ➡. (Courtesy R. Hewlett, MD.)*

Blood Blister-Like Aneurysm

Blood blister-like aneurysm (BBA), also known as blister or "dorsal variant blister" aneurysm, is an uncommon but potentially lethal subtype of intracranial pseudoaneurysm. BBAs can be difficult to diagnose and treacherous to treat. They represent approximately 1% of all intracranial aneurysms and 0.5-2.0% of all ruptured aneurysms.

BBAs are small, broad-based hemispheric bulges that typically arise at nonbranching sites of intracranial arteries (most commonly the supraclinoid ICA) **(6-33)**. BBAs have different clinical features and pose special diagnostic and treatment challenges compared with those of typical SAs. Preoperative recognition of a BBA is essential for proper management.

Etiology and Pathology

Hemodynamic stress and atherosclerosis seem to be the most important factors in formation of a BBA. BBAs are often covered with only a thin fragile fibrin layer or a friable cap of fibrous tissue **(6-34)**. Although BBAs can arise anywhere in the intracranial circulation, the anterosuperior (dorsal) wall of the supraclinoid ICA is the most common site.

Clinical Issues

BBAs exhibit more aggressive behavior compared with SAs. They tend to rupture at an earlier patient age and at significantly smaller size compared with typical SAs. They are also extremely fragile lesions that lack a definable neck and easily tear during surgical clipping. Intraprocedural rupture is common, occurring in nearly 50% of cases.

Coiling BBAs are rarely successful because of their wide necks and fragile walls. Multilayer flow-diverting devices have been tried with some success. If sufficient collateral circulation is present, trapping and occluding the parent vessel may be an option. If endovascular treatment is unsuccessful, wrapping and revascularization have been recommended as potential surgical options.

BLOOD BLISTER-LIKE ANEURYSM

Pathology
- Broad-based "blister" covered by thin friable tissue cap
- Usually solitary
- Can occur almost anywhere
- Dorsal wall of supraclinoid ICA most common site

Clinical Issues
- Easily rupture, may cause catastrophic aSAH
- Compared with saccular aneurysms
  - Rupture at earlier age
  - Rupture at smaller size

Imaging
- Small, easy to miss on CTA
- DSA with 3D shaded surface display best

Treatment
- Endovascular > surgical clipping
  - Flow-diverting stent
  - Stent-assisted coil embolization

Imaging

BBAs are small, often subtle lesions that are easily overlooked. A slight irregularity or small focal hemispherical bulge of the arterial wall may be the only finding **(6-35)**. 3D DSA with shaded surface display has been helpful in identifying these difficult, dangerous lesions.

Fusiform Aneurysm

FAs can be atherosclerotic (common) or nonatherosclerotic (rare). In contrast to SAs, FAs usually involve long, nonbranching vessel segments and are seen as focal circumferential outpouchings from a generally ectatic, elongated vessel.

Atherosclerotic FAs are typically seen in older adults. Nonatherosclerotic FAs can be seen at any age but are most common in children and younger adults.

Some investigators have recently noted that FAs—especially nonatherosclerotic lesions—are associated with aortic root dilatation and might be a form of neurocristopathy, as neural crest cells are the embryologic precursors of both the ascending aorta and intracranial arterial tree.

Atherosclerotic Fusiform Aneurysm

Terminology

Atherosclerotic fusiform aneurysms (ASVD FAs) are also called aneurysmal dolichoectasias, distinguishing them from the more generalized nonfocal vessel elongations seen as a common manifestation of intracranial atherosclerosis.

Pathology

Arteriectasis is common with advanced atherosclerosis of the cerebral arteries. Fusiform dilatation is a frequent complication. Generalized ASVD with a focally dilated fusiform enlargement is the typical gross manifestation of an ASVD FA **(6-36)**.

ASVD FAs are more common in the vertebrobasilar (posterior) circulation and usually affect the basilar artery. Plaques of foam cells with thickened but irregular intima and extensive

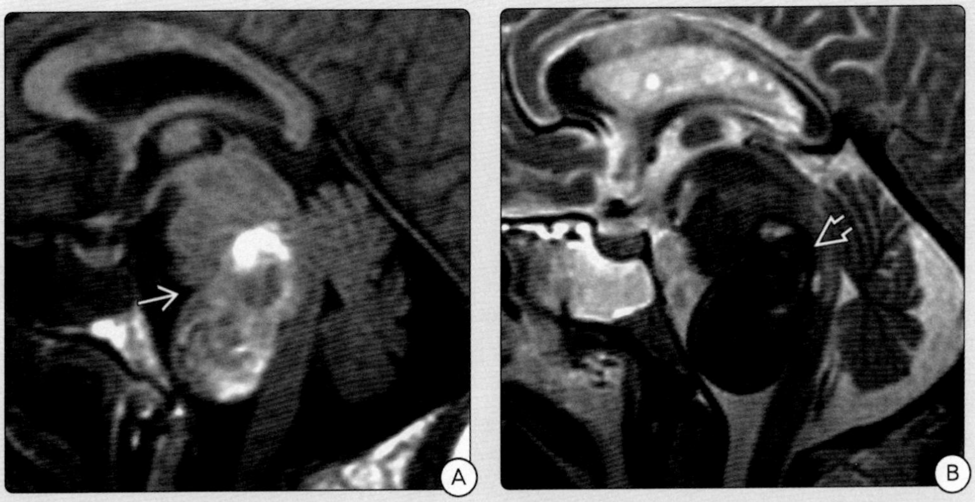

***(6-37A)** Sagittal T1WI in a 61y woman shows a huge, partially thrombosed atherosclerotic fusiform aneurysm of the basilar artery ➡. **(6-37B)** Sagittal T2WI in the same case shows that the aneurysm contains layered thrombus ➡ and indents and displaces the pons.*

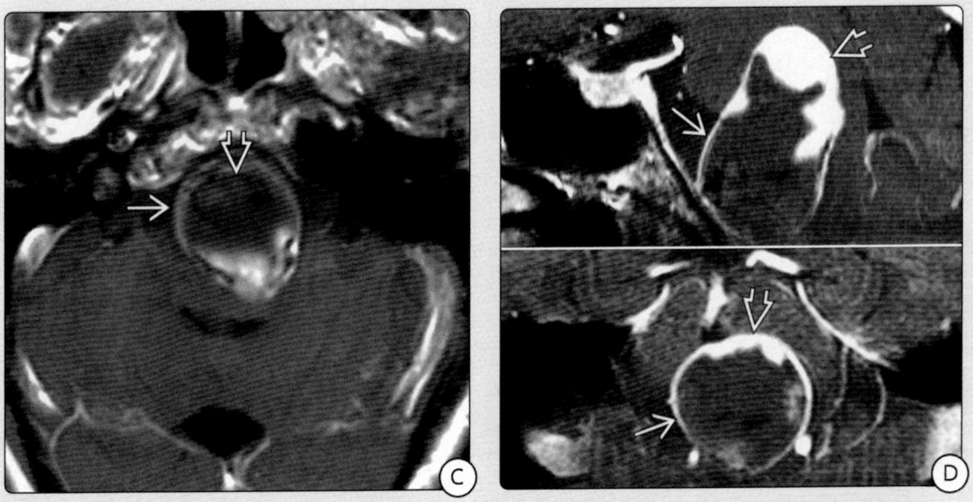

***(6-37C)** Axial T1 C+ MR in the same case shows that the atherosclerotic wall ➡ enhances, but most of the lumen is filled with nonenhancing clot ➡. **(6-37D)** Sagittal (top) and coronal (bottom) reformatted T1 C+ FS MRs show that the aneurysm wall ➡ and residual patent lumen ➡ enhance. This is a partially thrombosed atherosclerotic (ASVD) fusiform aneurysm.*

loss of elastica and media are present. Layers of organized thrombus surrounding a patent residual lumen are common.

Clinical Issues

Peak age of presentation is the seventh to eighth decade. Posterior circulation TIAs and stroke are the most common presentation. Cranial neuropathy is relatively uncommon.

Imaging

General Features. ASVD FAs are often large (more than 2.5 cm in diameter) fusiform or ovoid dilatations that are superimposed on generalized vascular dolichoectasias.

CT Findings. ASVD FAs are often partially thrombosed and frequently demonstrate mural calcification. Heterogeneously hyperdense clot is often present. The residual lumen enhances intensely following contrast enhancement.

MR Findings. Similar to SAs, the signal intensity of FAs also varies with pulse sequence, degree and direction of flow, and the presence and age of clot within the FA. Slow, turbulent flow in the residual lumen causes complex, sometimes bizarre signal **(6-37)**.

FAs often are very heterogeneous on T1WI and strikingly hypointense on T2WI. The residual lumen can be seen as a rounded "flow void" surrounded by complex thrombus that varies from hypointense to hyperintense. Intense enhancement of the residual lumen with prominent phase artifact is common following contrast administration.

Inflammatory changes are common in the walls of ASVD FAs. Vessel wall imaging may show variable enhancement. The enhancement is typically patchy, short segment, and discontinuous.

Angiography. CTA and DSA show generalized enlargement and ectasia of the parent vessel with a focal, round or

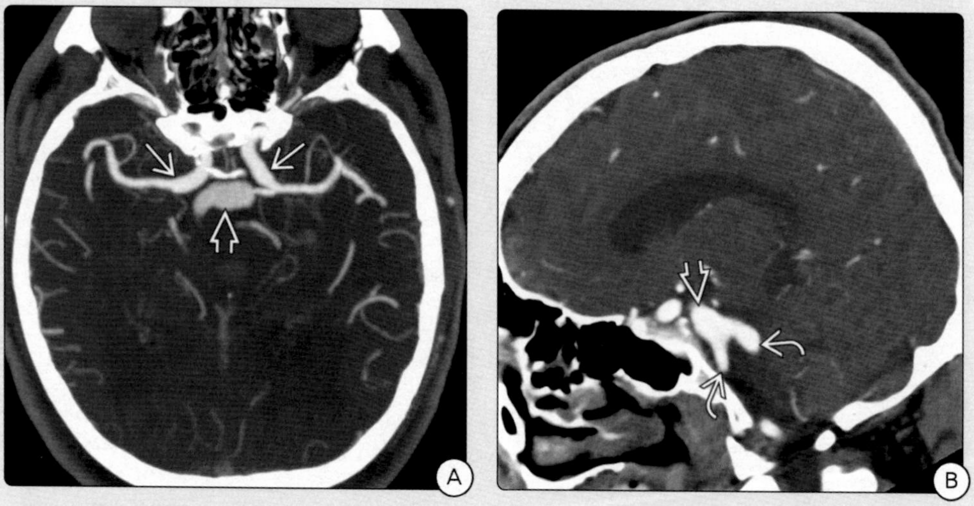

***(6-38A)** Axial MIP CTA in a 57y man with longstanding hypertension and coronary artery disease shows a fusiform aneurysm of the basilar artery ⇨ as well as fusiform vasculopathy of both supraclinoid ICAs ➡.* ***(6-38B)** Sagittal CTA in the same case shows the fusiform dilatation of the basilar artery ⇨ and enlarged ectatic distal vertebral arteries ↪.*

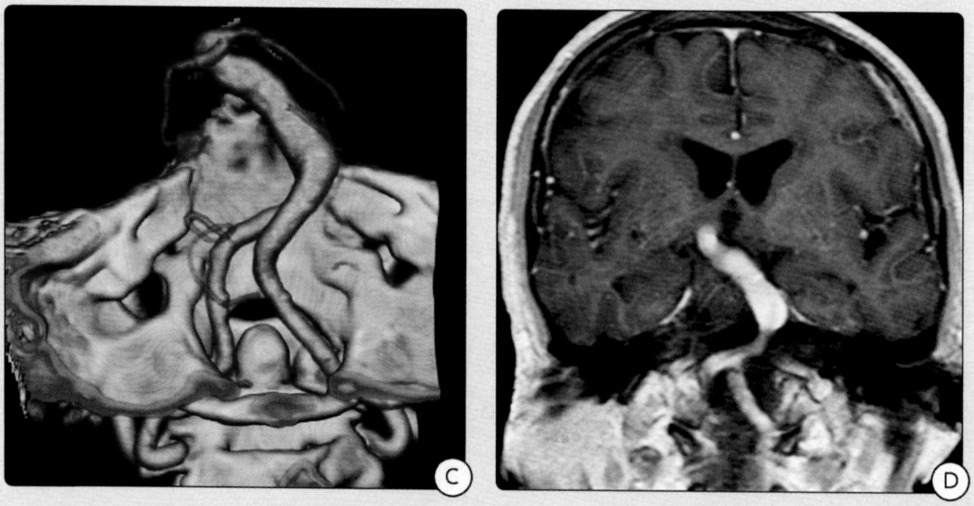

***(6-38C)** 3D SSD of the CTA shows that the fusiform aneurysm involves almost the entire basilar artery.* ***(6-38D)** Coronal T1 C+ MR in the same case shows almost the entire course of the fusiform ASVD basilar aneurysm. Because the flow is very slow, the entire vertebrobasilar system is opacified.*

fusiform, somewhat irregular contour **(6-38)**. In some cases, the residual lumen resides within a larger mass caused by mural thrombus.

Differential Diagnosis

The major differential diagnosis of an ASVD FA is **dolichoectasia**. Dolichoectasias are fusiform elongations of vessels—usually in the posterior circulation—without focal fusiform or saccular dilatations.

Nonatherosclerotic FAs are seen in younger patients who often have an inherited vasculopathy or immune deficiency (see below). Like ASVD FAs, intracranial **dissecting aneurysms** are most common on the vertebrobasilar (posterior) circulation. Findings of generalized ASVD are usually absent.

ATHEROSCLEROTIC FUSIFORM ANEURYSM

Terminology
- ASVD with a focally dilated fusiform enlargement
- Also called aneurysmal dolichoectasias

Pathology
- More common in vertebrobasilar artery
- Affects long nonbranching segment
- ASVD with irregular intima
- Extensive loss of elastica, media
- Layers of organized mural, intraluminal thrombus
  - Clot often much larger than residual lumen

Clinical Issues
- Middle-aged, older patients
  - Peak = 60-80 years
- Presentation
  - History of hypertension, systemic ASVD common
  - Symptoms vary with location
  - Posterior circulation TIAs, stroke
  - Less common = cranial neuropathies

Imaging
- CT, CTA
  - Generalized changes of ASVD present
  - Elongated vessel + fusiform or ovoid dilatation
  - Mural Ca++
  - Partial thrombosis common
- MR
  - Layered thrombus in wall, lumen
  - Signal intensity often complex
  - Clot surrounds variably-sized residual "flow void"

Differential Diagnosis
- Dolichoectasia
  - Elongated artery
  - No focal fusiform or saccular dilatation
- Dissection, dissecting aneurysm
  - Often younger patients
  - Also posterior circulation
  - ASVD changes minimal/absent
- Nonatherosclerotic fusiform aneurysm
  - Younger patient (including children)
  - Inherited vasculopathy (e.g., Marfan, Ehlers-Danlos type IV)
  - Vascular neurocutaneous syndrome (e.g., NF1)
  - Acquired immune deficiency

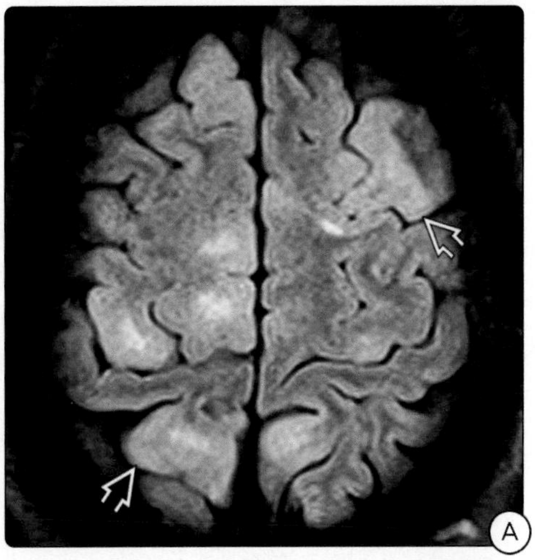

***(6-39A)** Axial FLAIR in a 22y man with tuberous sclerosis (TSC) shows multiple cortical tubers ➯.*

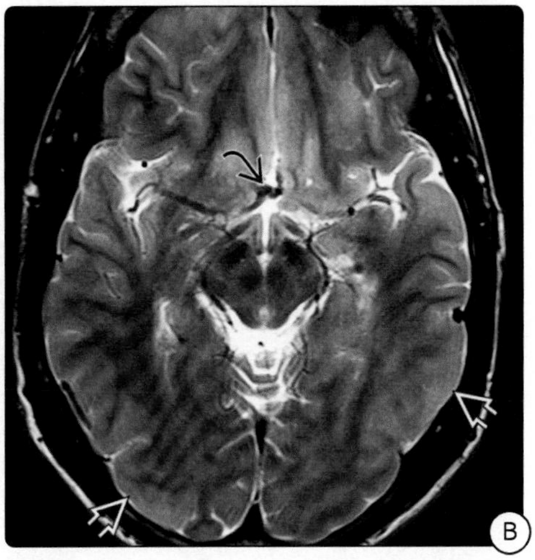

***(6-39B)** T2WI also shows several cortical tubers ➯. An unusual appearance of the ACoA was noticed ➯.*

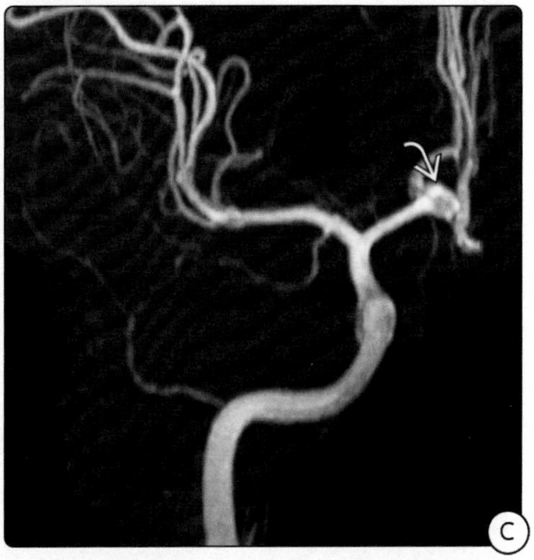

***(6-39C)** TOF MRA shows a fusiform aneurysm of the ACoA ➯. TSC is associated with both systemic and intracranial vasculopathies.*

Nonatherosclerotic Fusiform Aneurysm

Terminology

Nonatherosclerotic fusiform aneurysms (nASVD FAs) are fusiform elongations that occur in the absence of generalized intracranial ASVD.

nASVD FA is considered one manifestation of nonatherosclerotic large-vessel cerebrovascular arteriopathies.

Etiology

nASVD FAs occur with collagen vascular disorders (e.g., lupus), viral infections (varicella, HIV), and inherited vasculopathies (e.g., Marfan, Ehlers-Danlos) or vascular neurocutaneous syndrome (NF1, tuberous sclerosis) **(6-39)**.

Smooth muscle cells in the embryonic forebrain vessels are neural crest derivatives, which may explain the association of intracranial arteriopathy with neurocutaneous syndromes such as NF1 and tuberous sclerosis.

Pathology

nASVD FAs are focally dilated fusiform arterial ectasias that often involve nonbranching segments of intracranial arteries **(6-39)**. Multiple lesions are common. The carotid (anterior) and vertebrobasilar circulations are equally affected. Internal elastic lamina degeneration with myxoid changes and attenuation of the media are described findings at autopsy.

Clinical Issues

Patients tend to be younger than those with ASVD FAs. nASVD FAs are most common in children and young adults.

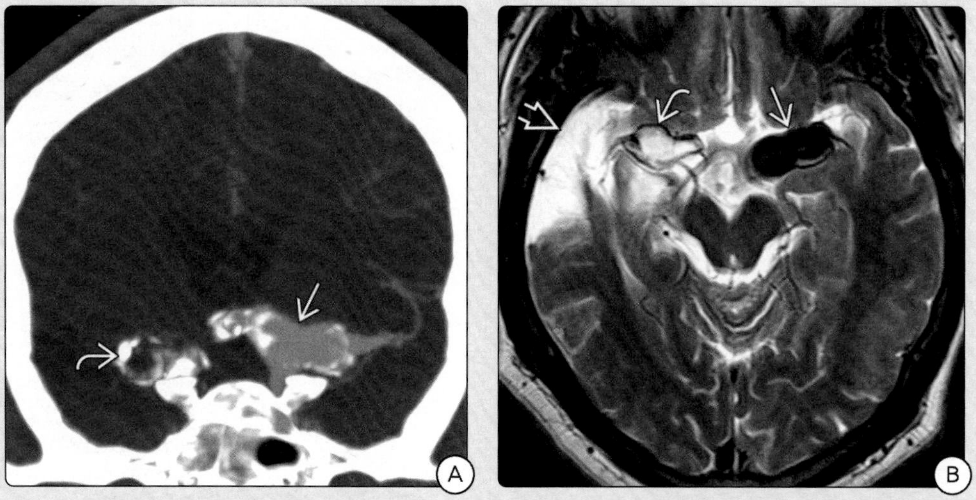

***(6-40A)** Coronal MIP CTA in a 25y HIV-positive man with a history of strokes shows striking fusiform aneurysms ➡ of both distal ICAs and their proximal branches. The right ICA fusiform aneurysm is thrombosed ↗. **(6-40B)** T2WI in the same case shows that the left fusiform aneurysm is patent ➡, but the right one is thrombosed ↗. Note the old right MCA territory infarct ⇨.*

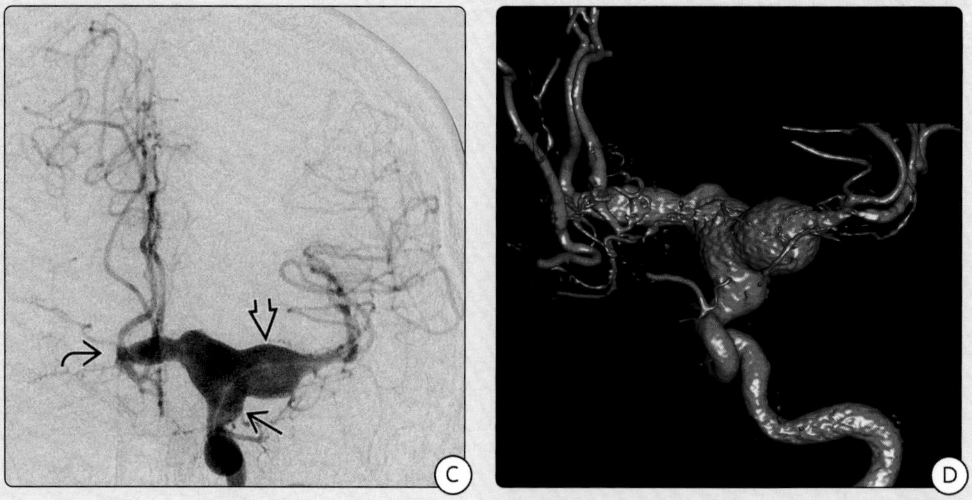

***(6-40C)** Anteroposterior view of the left carotid DSA in the same case shows that the fusiform aneurysm affects the distal ICA ➡ as well as the horizontal segments of both the ACA ↗ and MCA ⇩. **(6-40D)** 3D SSD of the left ICA shows the fusiform aneurysmal vasculopathy characteristic of HIV AIDS, once thought only to affect children.*

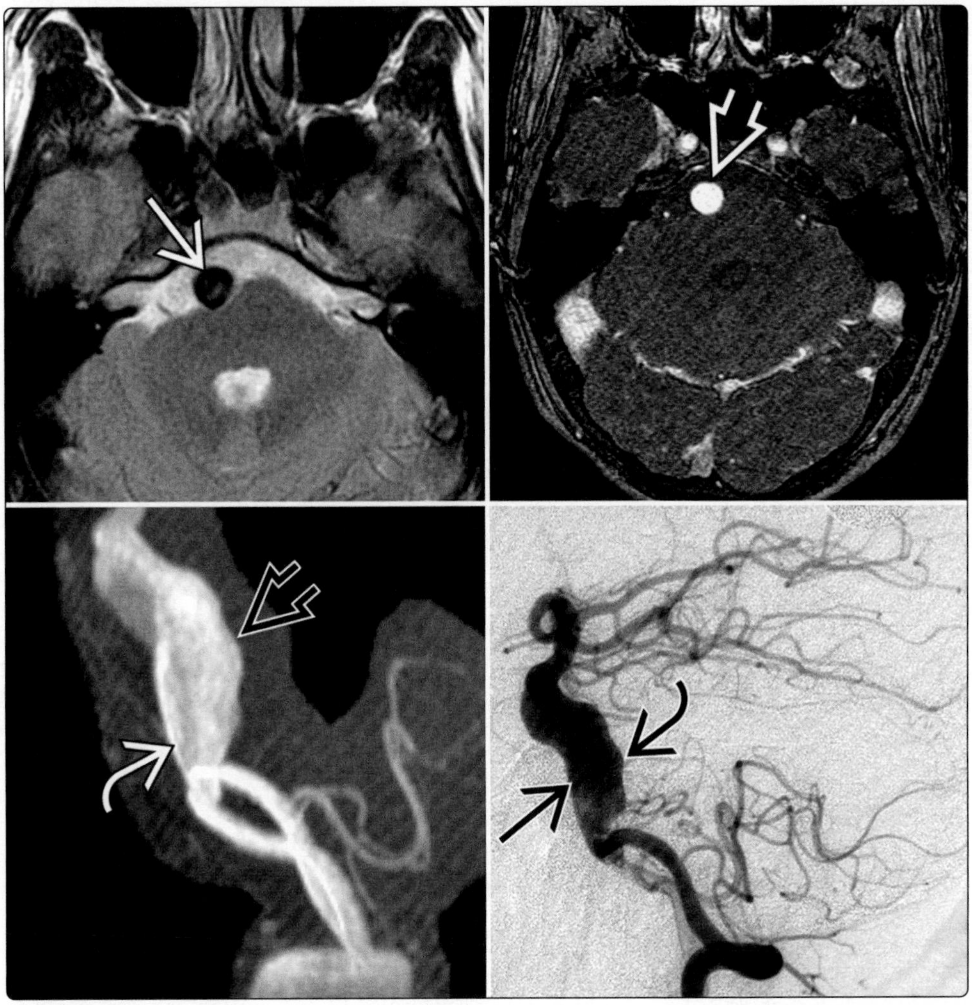

(6-41) (Upper left) T2WI in a 19y man with collagen vascular disease shows an enlarged basilar "flow void" . (Upper right) Source image from contrast-enhanced MRA shows the enlarged basilar artery . (Lower left) MIP view of MRA shows a fusiform aneurysm that involves almost the entire basilar artery . (Lower right) DSA shows the nonatherosclerotic fusiform aneurysm . The focal irregularities along the wall of the enlarged basilar artery seen here on both the MRA and CTA are due either to laminated thrombus in the aneurysm or defects in the microscopic structure of the vessel wall itself. Intimal lipid-laden plaques with true intraplaque hemorrhage are common in ASVD but absent in these inherited vasculopathies.

Nearly 40% of HIV-positive adults with dedicated neuroimaging of the intra- and extracranial cerebral vasculature have evidence of cerebral vasculopathy (vessel dolichoectasia and fusiform intracranial aneurysms) **(6-40)**. HIV-associated aneurysmal arteriopathy is linked with high morbidity; TIAs and stroke are common in these patients.

Imaging

Long segments of tubular, fusiform, or ovoid arterial dilatations are seen in the absence of generalized ASVD **(6-41)**. Circumferential involvement of the affected vessels is typical, as is extension into proximal branches.

Variable amounts of laminated thrombus may be present, complicating the imaging appearance of nASVD FAs. Differing ages of mural thrombus are also common. Calcification occurs but is less frequent than seen in ASVD FAs.

Differential Diagnosis

Fusiform intracranial dilatations in relatively young patients should suggest the possibility of nASVD vasculopathy and FA, with or without accompanying dissection. **Vertebrobasilar dolichoectasia** is seen in older patients with generalized changes of ASVD.

NONATHEROSCLEROTIC FUSIFORM ANEURYSM

Terminology
- Fusiform elongations without ASVD

Etiology
- Collagen-vascular disorders
- Viral infection (e.g., HIV)
- Inherited vasculopathies (Ehlers-Danlos, II and IV)

Pathology
- Long-segment fusiform dilatations of nonbranching segments
- ICA = vertebrobasilar

Clinical Issues
- Younger than ASVD FAs
- TIA, stroke, SAH

Imaging
- Long tubular, fusiform or ovoid dilatation
- No evidence for generalized ASVD
- Differential diagnosis
  - ASVD fusiform aneurysm
  - Dissecting aneurysm

Selected References

Subarachnoid Hemorrhage

Heit JJ et al: Cerebral angiography for evaluation of patients with CT angiogram-negative subarachnoid hemorrhage: an 11-year experience. AJNR Am J Neuroradiol. 37(2):297-304, 2016

Aneurysmal Subarachnoid Hemorrhage

Macdonald RL et al: Spontaneous subarachnoid haemorrhage. Lancet. 389(10069):655-666, 2017

Albertine P et al: The clinical significance of small subarachnoid hemorrhages. Emerg Radiol. 23(3):207-11, 2016

Dubosh NM et al: Sensitivity of early brain computed tomography to exclude aneurysmal subarachnoid hemorrhage: a systematic review and meta-analysis. Stroke. 47(3):750-5, 2016

Westafer LM et al: Hot off the press: an observational study of 2248 patients presenting with headache, suggestive of subarachnoid hemorrhage, that received a lumbar puncture following a normal CT head. Acad Emerg Med. 23(6):750-2, 2016

Post-aSAH Cerebral Ischemia and Vasospasm

Duan Y et al: Computed tomography perfusion deficits during the baseline period in aneurysmal subarachnoid hemorrhage are predictive of delayed cerebral ischemia. J Stroke Cerebrovasc Dis. 26(1):162-168, 2017

van der Kleij LA et al: Magnetic resonance imaging and cerebral ischemia after aneurysmal subarachnoid hemorrhage: a systematic review and meta-analysis. Stroke. 48(1):239-245, 2017

Weimer JM et al: Acute cytotoxic and vasogenic edema after subarachnoid hemorrhage: a quantitative MRI study. AJNR Am J Neuroradiol. 38(5):928-934, 2017

Jabbarli R et al: Early Vasospasm after aneurysmal subarachnoid hemorrhage predicts the occurrence and severity of symptomatic vasospasm and delayed cerebral ischemia. Cerebrovasc Dis. 41(5-6):265-272, 2016

Other Complications of aSAH

Oda S et al: Retrospective review of previous minor leak before major subarachnoid hemorrhage diagnosed by MRI as a predictor of occurrence of symptomatic delayed cerebral ischemia. J Neurosurg. 1-7, 2017

Perimesencephalic Nonaneurysmal SAH

Malhotra A et al: DSA of perimesencephalic hemorrhage. Radiology. 281(3):981-982, 2016

Potter CA et al: Perimesencephalic hemorrhage: yield of single versus multiple DSA examinations-a single-center study and meta-analysis. Radiology. 281(3):858-864, 2016

Convexal SAH

Graff-Radford J et al: Distinguishing clinical and radiological features of non-traumatic convexal subarachnoid hemorrhage. Eur J Neurol. 23(5):839-46, 2016

Superficial Siderosis

Charidimou A et al: Cortical superficial siderosis and first-ever cerebral hemorrhage in cerebral amyloid angiopathy. Neurology. 88(17):1607-1614, 2017

Wilson D et al: Infratentorial superficial siderosis: classification, diagnostic criteria, and rational investigation pathway. Ann Neurol. 81(3):333-343, 2017

Aneurysms

Saccular Aneurysm

Backes D et al: ELAPSS score for prediction of risk of growth of unruptured intracranial aneurysms. Neurology. 88(17):1600-1606, 2017

Björkman J et al: Irregular shape identifies ruptured intracranial aneurysm in subarachnoid hemorrhage patients with multiple aneurysms. Stroke. ePub, 2017

Choi HH et al: Growth of untreated unruptured small-sized aneurysms (7mm): incidence and related factors. Clin Neuroradiol. ePub, 2017

Kleinloog R et al: Risk factors for intracranial aneurysm rupture: a systematic review. Neurosurgery. ePub, 2017

Backes D et al: Patient- and aneurysm-specific risk factors for intracranial aneurysm growth: systematic review and meta-analysis. Stroke. 47(4):951-7, 2016

Blankena R et al: Thinner regions of intracranial aneurysm wall correlate with regions of higher wall shear stress: a 7T MRI study. AJNR Am J Neuroradiol. 37(7):1310-7, 2016

Mayer TE et al: The unruptured intracranial aneurysm treatment score: a multidisciplinary consensus. Neurology. 86(8):792-3, 2016

Pseudoaneurysm

Balik V et al: State-of-art surgical treatment of dissecting anterior circulation intracranial aneurysms. J Neurol Surg A Cent Eur Neurosurg. 78(1):67-77, 2017

deSouza RM et al: Subarachnoid haemorrhage secondary to traumatic intracranial aneurysm of the posterior cerebral circulation: case series and literature review. Acta Neurochir (Wien). 158(9):1731-40, 2016

Daou B et al: Dissecting pseudoaneurysms: predictors of symptom occurrence, enlargement, clinical outcome, and treatment. J Neurosurg. 1-7, 2016

Blood Blister-Like Aneurysm

Lozupone E et al: Flow diverter devices in ruptured intracranial aneurysms: a single-center experience. J Neurosurg. 1-7, 2017

Szmuda T et al: Towards a new treatment paradigm for ruptured blood blister-like aneurysms of the internal carotid artery? A rapid systematic review. J Neurointerv Surg. 8(5):488-94, 2016

Fusiform Aneurysm

Xu DS et al: Dolichoectatic aneurysms of the vertebrobasilar system: clinical and radiographic factors that predict poor outcomes. J Neurosurg. 1-7, 2017

Nonatherosclerotic Fusiform Aneurysm

Baeesa SS et al: Human immunodeficiency virus-associated cerebral aneurysmal vasculopathy: a systematic review. World Neurosurg. 87:220-9, 2016

Edwards NJ et al: Frequency and risk factors for cerebral arterial disease in a HIV/AIDS neuroimaging cohort. Cerebrovasc Dis. 41(3-4):170-176, 2016

Hammond CK et al: Cerebrovascular disease in children with HIV-1 infection. Dev Med Child Neurol. 58(5):452-60, 2016

Vascular Malformations

Brain vascular malformations, also known as cerebrovascular malformations (CVMs), are a heterogeneous group of disorders that exhibit a broad spectrum of biologic behaviors. Some CVMs (e.g., capillary malformations) are almost always clinically silent and are found incidentally on imaging studies. Others, such as arteriovenous malformations (AVMs) and cavernous angiomas, may hemorrhage unexpectedly and without warning.

In this chapter, we begin with an overview of CVMs, starting with a discussion of terminology, etiology, and classification. CVMs are grouped according to whether or not they exhibit arteriovenous shunting, and then each type is discussed individually.

Terminology

Two major groups of vascular anomalies are recognized: vascular *malformations* and vascular *hemangiomas*. All CVMs—the entities considered in this chapter—are malformative lesions and are thus designated as "malformations" or "angiomas." In contrast, vascular "hemangiomas" are true proliferating vasoformative neoplasms. Hemangiomas are classified as nonmeningothelial mesenchymal tumors and are discussed in Chapter 22 with meningiomas and other mesenchymal neoplasms.

Etiology

Most CVMs are congenital lesions and represent morphogenetic errors affecting arteries, capillaries, veins, or a combination of these elements.

Development of the human fetal vascular system occurs via two related processes: vasculogenesis and angiogenesis. In **vasculogenesis**, capillary-like tubes develop first and constitute the primary vascular plexus. This primary capillary network is subsequently remodeled into large-caliber vessels (arteries, veins) and small capillaries.

Angiogenesis is regulated by a number of intercell signaling and growth factors. Mutations in various components of the angiogenetic system have been implicated in the development of various CVMs.

Classification

CVMs have been traditionally classified by histopathology into four major types: (1) AVMs, (2) venous angiomas (developmental venous anomalies), (3) capillary telangiectasias (sometimes simply termed "telangiectasia" or "telangiectasis"), and (4) cavernous malformations.

Cerebrovascular Malformations

Type	Etiology	Pathology	Number	Location	Prevalence	Age	Hemorrhage Risk	Best Imaging Clues
CVMs With Arteriovenous Shunts								
AV malformations	Congenital (dysregulated angiogenesis)	Nidus + arterial feeders, draining veins; no capillary bed	Solitary (< 2% multiple)	Parenchyma (85%); supratentorial (15%); posterior fossa	0.04-0.50% of population; 85-90% of CVMs with AV shunting	Peak = 20-40 years (25% by age 15 years)	Very high (2-4% per year, cumulative)	"Bag of worms," "flow voids" on MR
Dural AV fistula	Acquired (trauma; dural sinus thrombosis)	Network of multiple AV microfistulas	Solitary	Skull base; dural sinus wall	10-15% of CVMs with AV shunting	Peak = 40-60 years	Varies with venous draining (increased if cortical veins involved)	Enlarged meningeal arteries with network of tiny vessels in wall of thrombosed dural venous sinus
Vein of Galen malformation	Congenital (fetal arterial fistula to primitive precursor of vein of Galen)	Large venous pouch	Solitary	Behind third ventricle	< 1% of CVMs with AV shunting	Newborn >> infant, older child	Low (but hydrocephalus brain damage common)	Large midline venous varix in neonate with high-output congestive heart failure
CVMs Without Arteriovenous Shunts								
Developmental venous anomaly	Congenital (arrested fetal medullary vein development)	Dilated WM veins; normal brain in between	Solitary (unless BRBNS)	Deep WM, usually near ventricle	Most common CVM (60% of all), between 2-9% of the population	Any age	Extremely low unless mixed with cavernous malformation	"Medusa head" of dilated WM veins converging on enlarged collector vein
Sinus pericranii	Congenital	Bluish blood-filled subcutaneous scalp mass	Solitary	Scalp	Rare	Any age (usually childhood)	Extremely low unless direct trauma	Vascular scalp mass connecting through skull defect to intracranial venous circulation
Cavernous malformation	Congenital (CCM, *KRIT1* gene mutations in familial autosomal-dominant syndrome; "de novo" lesions continue to form)	Collection of blood-filled "caverns" with no normal brain; complete hemosiderin rim	2/3 solitary (sporadic); 1/3 multiple (familial)	Throughout brain		Any age (peak = 40-60 years; younger in familial CCM syndrome)	High (0.25-0.75% per year; 1% per lesion per year in familial)	Varies; most common is solitary "popcorn ball" (locules with blood-fluid levels, hemosiderin rim); multifocal "black dots" in familial
Capillary telangiectasia	Congenital	Dilated capillaries; normal brain in between	Solitary >>> multiple	Anywhere but pons; medulla most common	15-20% of all CVMs	Any age (peak = 30-40 years)	Extremely low unless mixed with cavernous malformation	Faint brush-like enhancement, becomes hypointense on T2*

(Table 7-1) *AV = arteriovenous; BRBNS = blue rubber bleb nevus syndrome; CCM = cerebral cavernous malformation; CVM = cerebrovascular malformation; WM = white matter.*

Many interventional neuroradiologists and neurosurgeons group CVMs by function, not histopathology. In this functional classification, CVMs are divided into two basic categories: (1) CVMs that display arteriovenous shunting and (2) CVMs without arteriovenous shunting **(Table 7-1)**. The former are potentially amenable to endovascular intervention; the latter are either treated surgically or left alone.

In this book, we use a combination of functional and histologic classifications. We begin with a discussion of CVMs that display arteriovenous shunting, i.e., AVMs and arteriovenous fistulas. We then focus on CVMs that do not generally shunt blood from the arterial to the venous circulation. Nonshunting CVMs include developmental venous anomalies, capillary telangiectasias, and cavernous malformations.

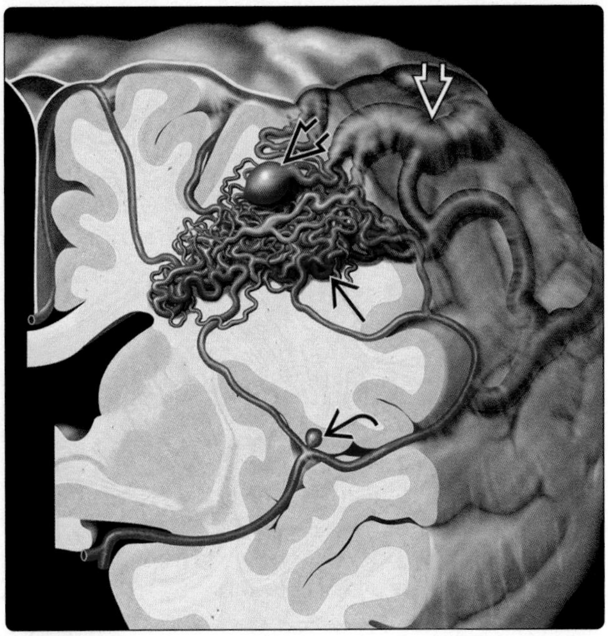

***(7-1)** Graphic depicts pyramidal-shaped AVM nidus ➡ with broad base toward the cortical surface. Intranidal aneurysm ➡, feeding artery ("pedicle") aneurysm ➡, and enlarged draining veins ➡ are shown.*

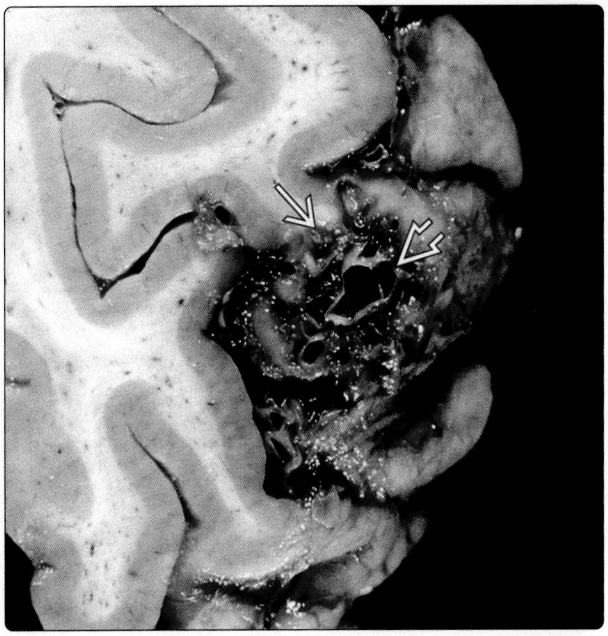

***(7-2)** Autopsy case demonstrates a classic AVM. The nidus ➡ contains no normal brain. An intranidal aneurysm ➡ is present. (Courtesy R. Hewlett, MD.)*

CVMs With Arteriovenous Shunting

Arteriovenous Malformation

Terminology

An arteriovenous malformation (AVM) is a tightly packed "snarl" or "tangle" of serpiginous, thin-walled vessels without an intervening capillary bed. Most brain AVMs (BAVMs) are parenchymal lesions and are also called "pial AVMs," although mixed pial-dural malformations do occur.

Etiology

General Concepts. AVMs are congenital defects of vascular development characterized by dysregulated angiogenesis. Endothelial cells in cerebral AVMs express GLUT1 (a protein in the embryonic microvasculature), matrix metalloproteinases, proangiogenic growth factors such as vascular endothelial growth factor (VEGF). This results in "downstream" derangements in vascular function and integrity.

Genetics. Most AVMs are solitary. The first genome-wide association study of sporadic (nonsyndromic) BAVMs found no common single nucleotide polymorphisms that contributed strongly to susceptibility. However, recent animal studies have demonstrated that endothelial Notch4-induced arteriovenous shunts arise from the enlargement of preexisting capillary-like vessels. Notch4 signaling in the microvasculature seems to be both sufficient and required for AVM formation.

Multiple AVMs are almost always syndromic. The genetic basis for several Mendelian syndromes with BAVM as part of the phenotype have been defined. These include **hereditary hemorrhagic telangiectasia** (HHT, also known as Rendu-Osler-Weber disease, OMIM #187300) and **capillary malformation-arteriovenous malformation** (CM-AVM, OMIM #608354).

HHT is a genetically mediated hereditary disorder characterized by epistaxis, mucocutaneous telangiectases, and visceral AVMs. HHT is caused by mutations in *ENG, ACVRL1, SMAD4,* and possibly *GDF2.* HHT is discussed in greater detail in connection with neurocutaneous syndromes (Chapter 39).

Segmental neurovascular syndromes called **cerebrofacial arteriovenous metameric syndrome** (CAMS) also have BAVMs as part of their phenotype. In CAMs, somatic mutations of the neural crest occur along predefined migration paths, resulting in specific combinations of facial and intracranial vascular malformations. **Wyburn-Mason syndrome**, in which AVMs are found in both the retina and brain, is one example of a CAMS.

Pathology

Location. Over 85% of AVMs are supratentorial, located in the cerebral hemispheres **(7-1)**. Only 15% are found in the posterior fossa.

Size. AVMs vary from tiny lesions to giant malformations that can occupy an entire cerebral lobe or hemisphere. Most are intermediate in size with a nidus ranging from 2-6 cm in diameter. Both the feeding arteries and draining veins are usually enlarged.

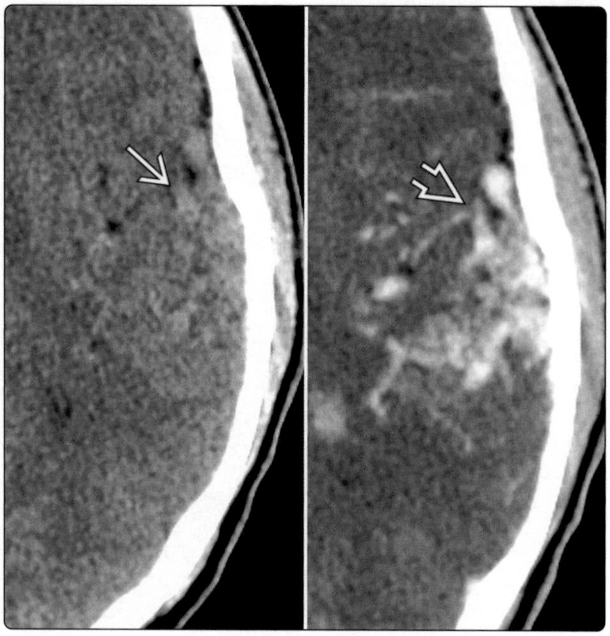

(7-3) (L) NECT shows serpentine hyperdensities ➡. (R) CECT shows strong uniform enhancement ➡. Wedge-shaped configuration is typical for AVM. Roughly 85% of AVMs are supratentorial.

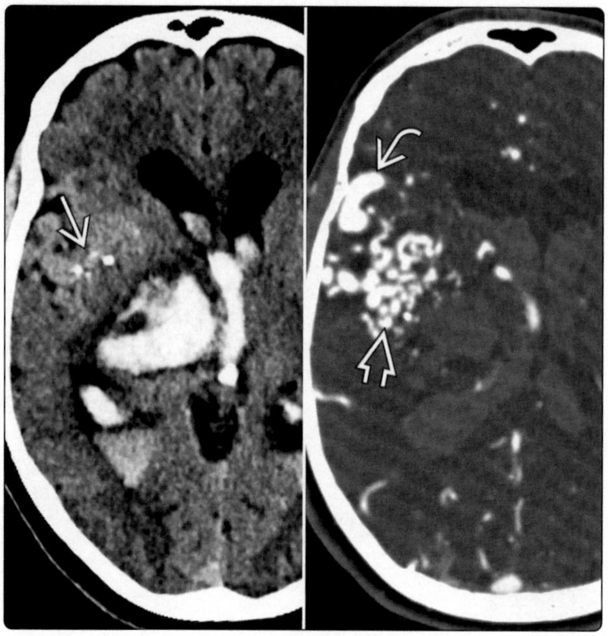

(7-4) (L) Axial NECT of a 58y woman with "stroke" shows right basal ganglionic spontaneous ICH with intravenous hemorrhage, calcifications (phleboliths) ➡. (R) CTA shows AVM with nidus ➡, dilated draining veins ➡.

"Micro"-AVMs have a nidus ≤ 1 cm; feeding arteries and draining veins are usually normal in size. Micro-AVMs are typically associated with HHT.

Number. Less than 2% of all brain AVMs are multiple. Almost all multiple AVMs are associated with vascular neurocutaneous syndromes (see above).

Gross Pathology. AVMs appear as a compact ovoid or wedge-shaped mass of tangled blood vessels **(7-2)**. Their broadest surface is at or near the cortex with the apex pointing toward the ventricles. Dilated draining veins are often found on the cortical surface overlying an AVM.

The brain surrounding an AVM often appears abnormal. Hemorrhagic residua such as gliosis and secondary ischemic changes are common, as are siderotic changes in the overlying pia. A "perinidal" capillary bed has been reported in some cases.

Microscopic Features. Vessels comprising the AVM nidus are of variable caliber and wall thickness. Some appear dysplastic and thin-walled without normal subendothelial support. Others exhibit intimal hyperplasia and fibrosis/hyalinization. Intranidal ectatic "arterialized" veins with thickened walls are common. Mural calcification and perivascular inflammatory changes may be present.

There are no capillaries and no normal brain parenchyma within an AVM nidus. Instead, varying amounts of laminated thrombus, dystrophic calcification, and hemorrhagic residua are often present. Small amounts of brain parenchyma within the nidus are occasionally identified but are typically gliotic and nonfunctional.

AVM: ETIOLOGY AND PATHOLOGY

Etiology

- Congenital defect
  - Abnormal vascular development
  - Dysregulated angiogenesis
- **Genetics**
  - Heritability studies suggest modest genetic contribution
  - To date GWAS have identified no responsible SNPs in sporadic BAVMs
  - Syndromic mutations (HHT, CM-AVM) known

Pathology

- Gross pathology
  - Ovoid or wedge-shaped with broad base toward cortex
  - 3 components: feeding arteries, nidus (center), draining veins
- Microscopic features
  - Dysplastic thin-walled vessels
  - Ectatic "arterialized" veins
  - Only nonfunctional gliotic brain in nidus

Clinical Issues

Epidemiology. Almost all AVMs are sporadic and solitary. With very rare exceptions ("de novo" AVMs), most are considered congenital lesions. Sporadic (nonsyndromic) AVMs are found in 0.15% of the general population.

Demographics. Prevalence is 10-18/100,000. Peak presentation occurs between 20-40 years of age, although

25% of patients harboring an AVM become symptomatic by age 15. There is no sex predilection.

Presentation. Headache with parenchymal hemorrhage is the most common presentation, occurring in about half of all patients. Seizure and focal neurologic deficits are the initial symptoms in 25% each. Small micro-AVMs in patients with vascular neurocutaneous syndromes such as HHT may be asymptomatic and only discovered when screening imaging studies are performed.

Natural History. The annual hemorrhage risk is approximately 3%, but, depending on the clinical and anatomical features of the AVM, the risk may be as low as 1% per year (in patients whose initial presentation was nonhemorrhagic) or as high as 33% in hemorrhagic lesions with deep brain or brainstem location and exclusively deep venous drainage. Other features associated with bleeding include feeding artery aneurysm and venous outflow restriction.

AVM: CLINICAL ISSUES

Demographics
- Peak 20-40 years (mean = 33 years)
- 25% symptomatic by 15 years

Presentation
- Headache with intracranial hemorrhage (ICH) 50-60%
- Seizure 25%, neurologic deficit 25%

Natural History
- Overall annual ICH risk 3% but wide variation

Several grading systems have been devised to characterize AVMs and estimate the risks of surgery. The most widely used is the **Spetzler-Martin scale**. Here AVMs are graded on a scale from 1-5 based on the sum of "scores" calculated from lesion size, location (eloquent vs. noneloquent brain), and venous drainage pattern (superficial vs. deep).

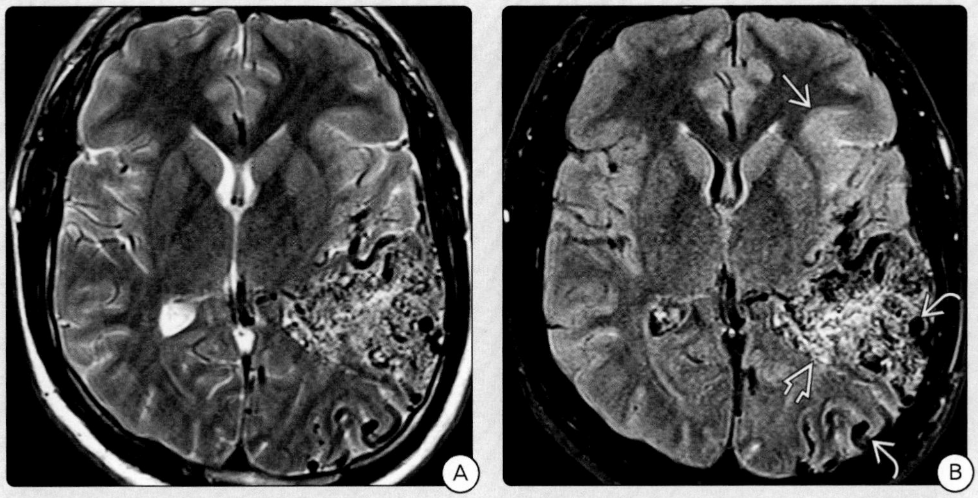

***(7-5A)** T2WI in a 29y man with a seizure shows a left parietal AVM with multiple "flow voids." Its "wedge" or pyramidal shape with broad base at the cortical surface is classic. **(7-5B)** FLAIR MR in the same case shows that the nidus contains some hyperintense gliotic brain. Note adjacent gyral swelling of the insula, left temporal lobe possibly related to vascular steal or postictal state. Dilated cortical veins along the cortex are present.*

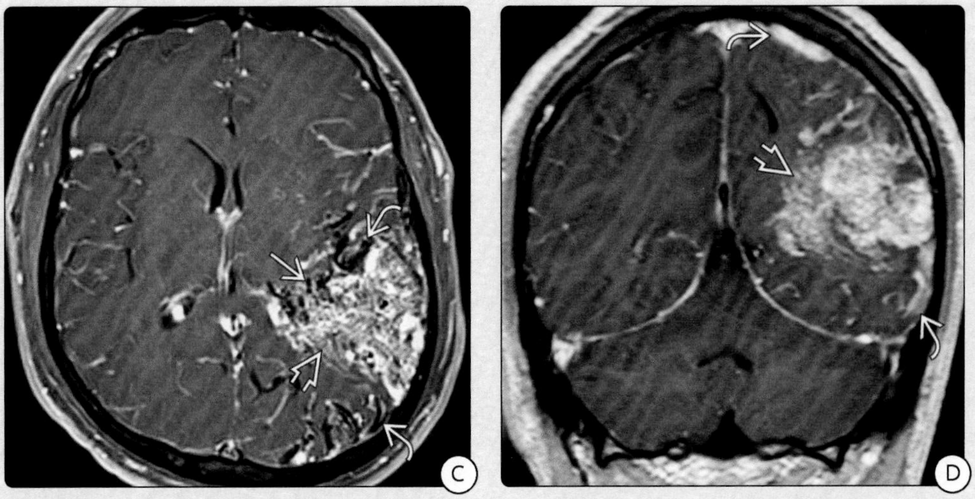

***(7-5C)** T1 C+ FS shows that the nidus enhances intensely. "Flow voids" around the nidus are dilated feeding arteries and prominent draining veins. **(7-5D)** Coronal T1 C+ MR demonstrates the wedge-shaped configuration of the AVM nidus especially well. The broad cortical surface of the lesion is apparent, as are enlarged draining cortical veins.*

Other imaging findings associated with hemorrhage risk include evidence of previous hemorrhage, presence of an intranidal aneurysm, and stenosis or thrombosis of one or more "outlet" draining veins.

Spontaneous regression of sporadic brain AVMs is rare (approximately 1% of cases). Most "obliterated" AVMs occur after a hemorrhagic episode and typically demonstrate venous stasis, thrombosis, and signs of elevated intracranial pressure. Rare nonhemorrhagic cases of spontaneous AVM regression have been reported.

Treatment Options. Embolization, surgery, stereotactic radiosurgery, or a combination of treatments are all current options in treating ruptured (i.e., hemorrhagic) BAVMs. The decision to treat asymptomatic AVMs and which treatment to use have been debated. Stereotactic radiosurgery in patients with small (mean = < 3 cm diameter) unruptured BAVMs achieves obliteration and avoids permanent complications in the majority of these cases.

SPETZLER-MARTIN AVM GRADING SCALE

Size
- Small (< 3 cm) = 1
- Medium (3-6 cm) = 2
- Large (> 6 cm) = 3

Location
- Noneloquent = 0
- Eloquent = 1

Venous Drainage
- Superficial only = 0
- Deep component = 1

Imaging

The imaging diagnosis of an uncomplicated AVM is relatively straightforward. However, the presence of hemorrhage or

__(7-6A)__ Lateral DSA in a 32y man with headache shows enlarged middle cerebral artery (MCA), anterior cerebral artery (ACA) feeding vessels with a tangle of smaller vessels in the wedge-shaped nidus. Faint opacification of the superior sagittal sinus (SSS) represents arteriovenous shunting of contrast. __(7-6B)__ Late arterial phase of the DSA shows the nidus and "early draining" veins emptying into the SSS.

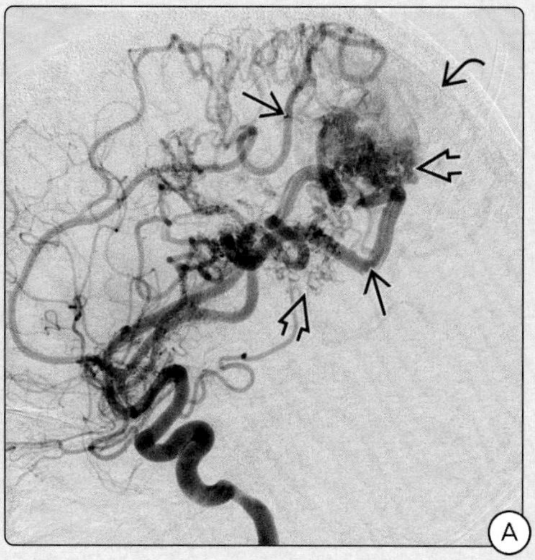

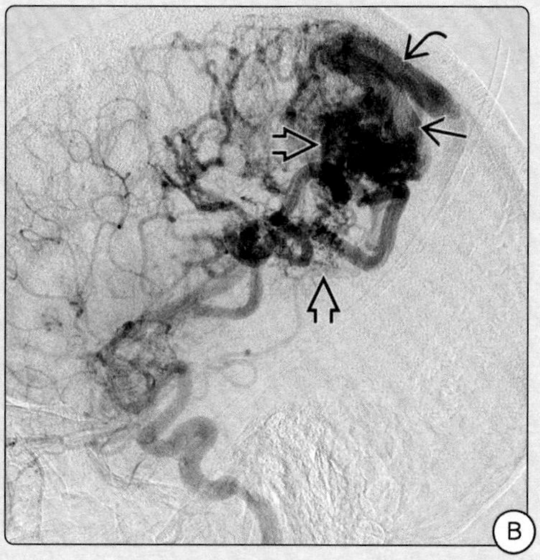

__(7-6C)__ Late capillary-early venous phase DSA in the same case shows some residual opacification of the nidus, multiple enlarged early draining cortical veins, including a huge superficial middle cerebral vein. No deep venous drainage was identified; it's Spetzler-Martin grade III AVM. __(7-6D)__ 3D MRA in the same case shows the nidus, multiple draining veins. Details of the angioarchitecture were best depicted by DSA.

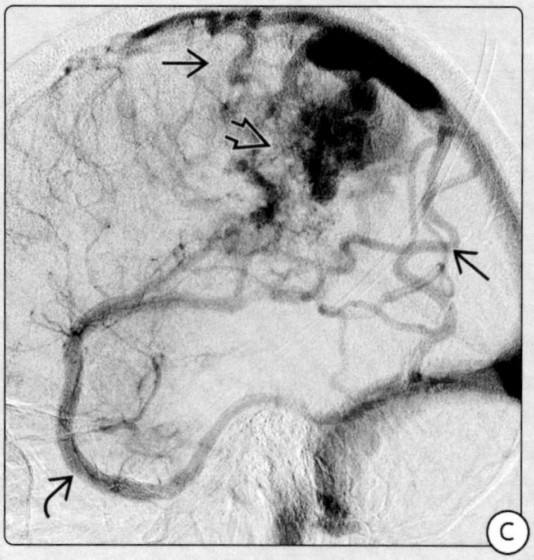

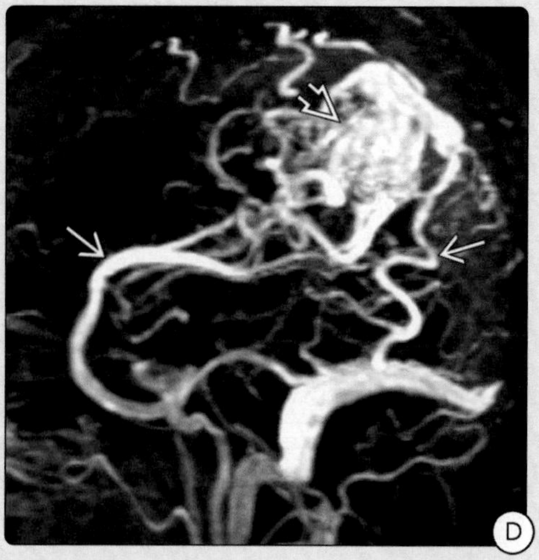

thrombosis can complicate its appearance. Acute hemorrhage may obliterate any typical findings of an AVM. Residua of previous hemorrhagic episodes such as dystrophic calcification, gliosis, and blood in different stages of degradation may also complicate its appearance.

General Features. AVMs are complex networks of abnormal vascular channels consisting of three distinct components: (1) feeding arteries, (2) a central nidus, and (3) draining veins **(7-1)**.

CT Findings. AVMs generally resemble a "bag of worms" formed by a tightly packed tangle of vessels with little or no mass effect on adjacent brain. NECT scans typically show numerous well-delineated, slightly hyperdense serpentine vessels **(7-3)**. Calcification is common **(7-4)**. Enhancement of all three AVM components (feeding arteries, nidus, draining veins) is typically intense and uniform on CECT scans.

CTA is commonly included as part of the initial evaluation in patients who present with nontraumatic "spontaneous" intracranial hemorrhage (sICH) and may be helpful in delineating the feeding arteries and draining veins of an underlying AVM **(7-4)**.

MR Findings. Findings vary with vascular hemodynamics, the presence (and age) of associated hemorrhage, and secondary changes in the surrounding brain.

Because most AVMs are high-flow lesions, spins rapidly pass through the lesion and do not receive a refocusing pulse. This produces the appearance of a tightly packed mass or a "honeycomb" of "flow voids" on both T1 and T2 scans **(7-5A)**.

Any brain parenchyma within an AVM is typically gliotic and hyperintense on T2WI and FLAIR **(7-5B)**. Contrast enhancement of AVMs is variable, depending on flow rate and direction. Draining veins typically enhance strongly and uniformly **(7-5C)**.

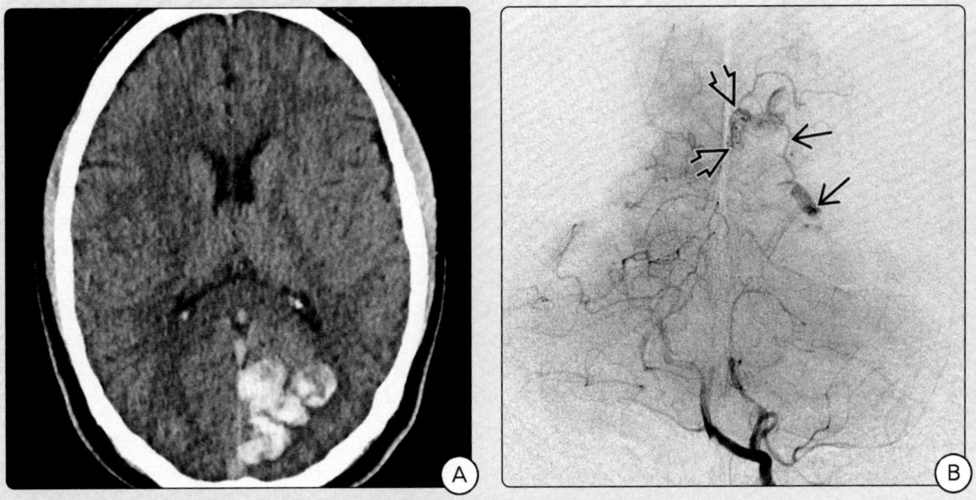

***(7-7A)** A 23y man had sudden onset of right homonymous hemianopsia. NECT shows an acute parenchymal hematoma in the left occipital lobe. **(7-7B)** Left vertebral DSA, anteroposterior view, late arterial/early capillary phase, shows stagnating contrast in the left posterior cerebral artery (PCA) ➡, prolonged vascular staining ⇨ in the calcarine cortex of the occipital lobe.*

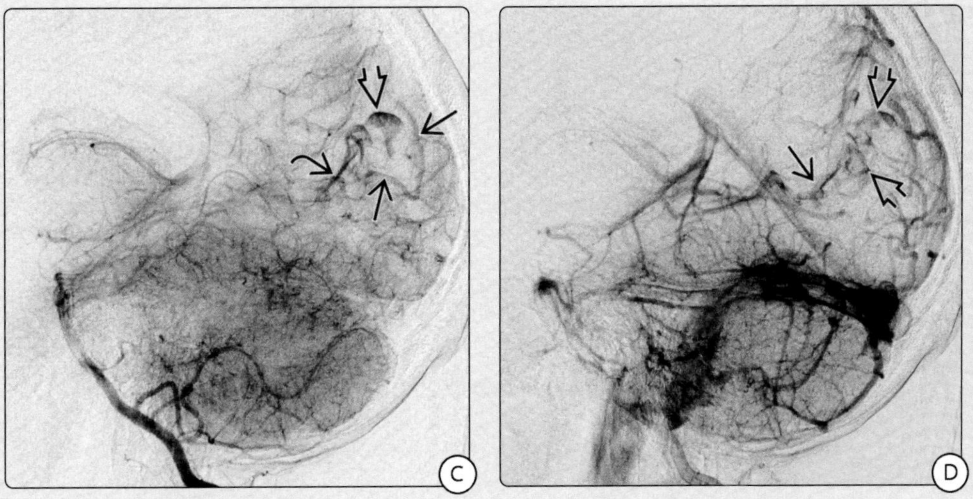

***(7-7C)** Left vertebral DSA, lateral view, capillary phase shows "stagnating" contrast in the distal PCA branches ➡, prolonged vascular "blush" ⇨. A vein draining the vascular blush is irregular and sharply tapered ↷. **(7-7D)** Venous phase of the vertebral angiogram shows thrombus in the draining vein ➡, persistent contrast staining in the lesion ⇨. DSA 6 months later showed no residual of the thrombosed AVM.*

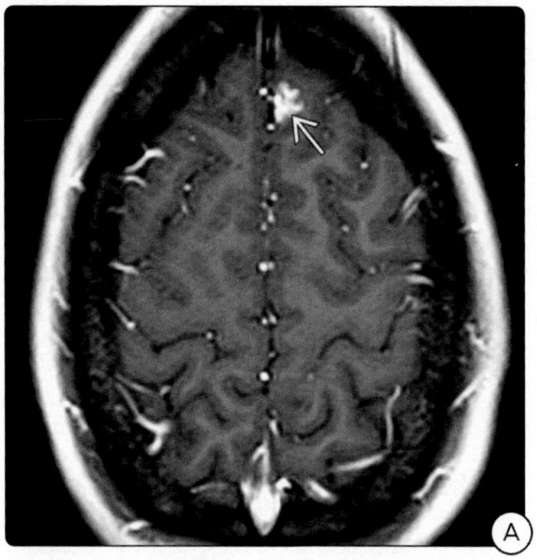

(7-8A) T1 C+ FS MR in an 18y man with family history of hereditary hemorrhagic telangiectasia shows enhancing left frontal lesion ➡.

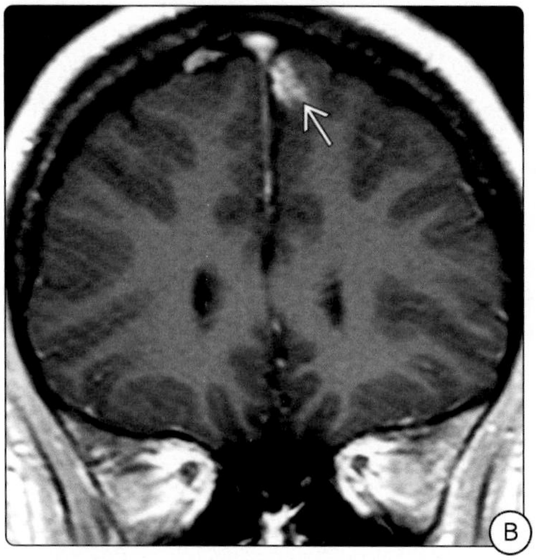

(7-8B) Coronal T1 C+ MR in the same case shows that the lesion has irregular, somewhat spiculated enhancement ➡.

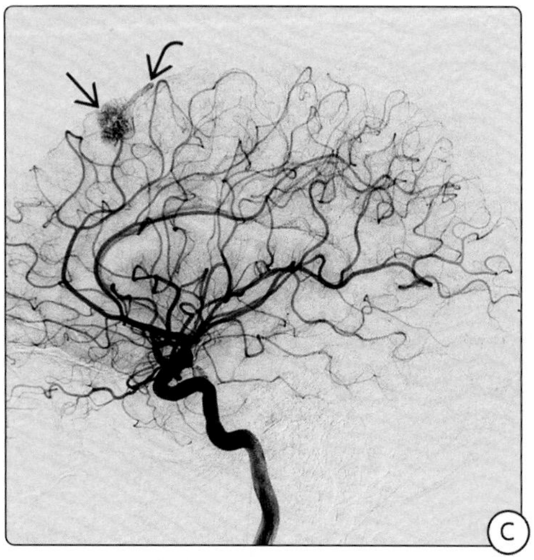

(7-8C) Lateral left internal carotid DSA shows that the lesion ➡ is a "micro-AVM" with an early draining vein ➡.

Hemorrhagic residua are common. T2* sequences often show foci of "blooming" both within and around AVMs as well as siderosis in the adjacent pia.

Angiography. DSA is needed to evaluate and diagnose macrovascular causes of sICH undetected by CTA or MR/MRA. Although ultra-high-field (i.e., 7 T) TOF MRA has been touted as comparable to DSA, most institutions still depend on DSA to delineate the detailed angioarchitecture of BAVMs.

All three AVM components (feeding arteries, nidus, venous drainage) must be thoroughly evaluated. The pial **feeding arteries** that supply an AVM are often enlarged and tortuous **(7-6A)**. Flow-related angiopathy may be present, ranging from simple dilatation to endothelial thickening, stenosis, and occasionally even thrombosis and occlusion. A flow-induced **"pedicle" aneurysm** is seen in 10-15% of cases.

Approximately 25% of superficially located, large, or diffuse AVMs have some transdural arterial contributions, so thorough evaluation of the dural vasculature should also be part of the complete angiographic delineation of AVM arterial supply.

The **nidus**, the core of the AVM, is a tightly packed tangle of abnormal arteries and veins without an intervening capillary bed **(7-6B)**. Up to 50% contain at least one aneurysmally dilated vessel (**"intranidal aneurysm"**). The nidus contains little or no brain parenchyma and hence causes no significant mass effect on the adjacent brain. Displacement of angiographic midline markers (e.g., the anterior cerebral arteries and internal cerebral veins) is therefore usually absent unless an acute hematoma is present.

As there is no intervening capillary bed between the arterial feeders and draining veins of an AVM, direct arteriovenous shunting within the nidus occurs **(7-6C)**. **Draining veins** typically opacify in the mid to late arterial phase ("early draining" veins) **(7-6B)** **(7-6C)**. Veins draining AVMs are typically enlarged and tortuous and may become so prominent that they form varices and exert local mass effect on the adjacent cortex. Stenosis of one or more "outlet" draining veins may elevate intranidal pressure and contribute to AVM hemorrhage **(7-7)**.

The internal angioarchitecture of an AVM is optimally delineated by high-resolution DSA **(7-8)**. Superselective injection of all feeding arteries delineates the nidus and helps define the presence of an intranidal aneurysm. Three-dimensional reconstructions with shaded surface display or 3D-printing models may be very helpful in surgical planning and endovascular treatment.

Differential Diagnosis

Occasionally a highly vascular neoplasm such as **glioblastoma multiforme** (GBM) displays such striking neoangiogenesis that it can mimic an AVM. Most GBMs, even extremely vascular lesions, enhance intensely and contain significant amounts of neoplasm interposed between the enlarged vessels. Sometimes **densely calcified neoplasms** such as oligodendroglioma can mimic the "flow voids" of an AVM.

A hemorrhagic AVM that is completely obliterated may be indistinguishable from other vascular malformations (such as **cavernous malformation**) or hemorrhagic neoplasm.

Cerebral proliferative angiopathy (CPA) is a large, diffuse malformation that has innumerable small feeding vessels, no definable nidus, and normal brain interposed between the proliferating vascular channels (see below). CPA is frequently misdiagnosed as a BAVM.

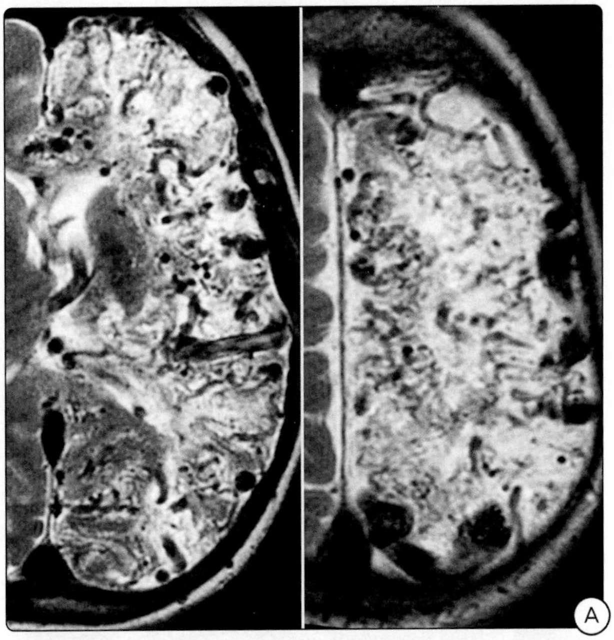

(7-9A) *Axial T2WI through the lateral ventricle (L) and upper corona radiata (R) shows almost complete replacement of the left hemisphere by a mass of dilated tortuous arteries and enlarged draining veins.*

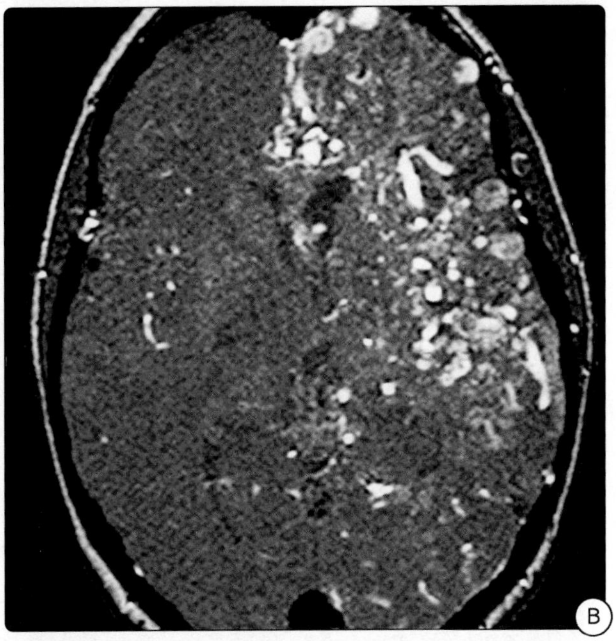

(7-9B) *Contrast-enhanced MRA shows innumerable enlarged vessels scattered throughout the left hemisphere with normal brain in between. This is cerebral proliferative angiopathy. (Courtesy P. Chapman, MD.)*

AVM: IMAGING

General Features
- Arteriovenous shunting
- 3 components
  - Feeding arteries
  - Nidus
  - Draining veins
- No intervening capillaries

NECT
- Slightly hyperdense "bag of worms"
- Tightly packed
- Little/no mass effect

CECT
- Strong serpentine enhancement

MR
- "Honeycomb" of "flow voids"
- No normal brain inside

Differential Diagnosis
- Highly vascular neoplasm (e.g., glioblastoma multiforme)
- Cerebral proliferative angiopathy

Cerebral Proliferative Angiopathy

Terminology

Cerebral proliferative angiopathy (CPA), formerly considered a variant of AVM known as "holohemispheric giant cerebral AVM" or "diffuse AVM," is now recognized as a separate entity with distinct imaging features and different natural history.

CPA consists of multiple small arterial feeders and numerous draining veins with no dominant feeders or nidus. **Unlike AVMs, CPAs contain normal brain tissue interspersed between the abnormal vessels.** Therefore, its treatment is very different from AVMs.

Pathology

Grossly, CPAs are large lesions that occupy most of a lobe or sometimes even an entire cerebral hemisphere. Their histopathologic features and angioarchitecture are unlike those of classic BAVMs: CPAs have brain parenchyma interspersed between the proliferative vascular channels.

Clinical Issues

The clinical profile and natural history of CPA are quite different from those of classic brain AVMs. Although it is a progressive disorder, CPA generally behaves less aggressively. Most patients present with seizure (45%) or severe headache (40%). In contrast to AVMs, neurologic deficits with TIAs or a hemorrhagic event are the presenting features in only 12-15% of CPA cases.

Mean age at symptom onset is 22 years. There is a 2:1 female predominance.

Long-term prognosis in CPA is poor. Unlike classic AVMs, CPA is characterized by ongoing angiogenesis and progressive hypervascular shunting. Over time, CPA may demonstrate progressive lesion enlargement with extension into previously uninvolved normal brain parenchyma.

Treatment

There is no definitive treatment for CPA. When misdiagnosed as an AVM, permanent neurologic damage to the normal interspersed brain parenchyma may occur if aggressive surgery or stereotaxic radiosurgery to devascularize a putative AVM is performed. Limited embolization of transdural arteries contributing to the CPA has been performed in some patients with uncontrollable seizures or headaches, although the risk of devascularizing normal brain in such cases is high.

Revascularization surgery with encephalo-duro-arterio-synangiosis to increase cortical blood supply by recruiting additional dural arteries has been performed with some improvement reported in a few patients. Bevacizumab, an antiangiogenesis monoclonal antibody that binds to VEGF, has been used in a few patients with inconclusive results.

Gamma knife radiosurgery has also been reported to improve headache but not the associated neurologic deficits.

Imaging

CPA is seen on MR as a large (usually more than 6 cm), diffusely dispersed network of innumerable dilated vascular spaces intermingled with normal brain parenchyma **(7-9A)**. Dense enhancement following contrast is typical **(7-9B)**. pCT and pMR show hypoperfusion ("steal") extending far beyond the morphologic abnormalities.

DSA shows numerous small feeding arteries, usually with no dominant arterial supply **(7-10)**. Recruitment of dural and even transosseous feeders is common. There with no discernible nidus. A dense, prolonged diffuse vascular "staining" of the affected parenchyma is common. Residual islands of brain parenchyma can usually be discerned in between the arterial network.

In contrast to AVMs, the veins draining CPA are only moderately enlarged relative to the large extent of the vascular abnormality. Venous varices are rare.

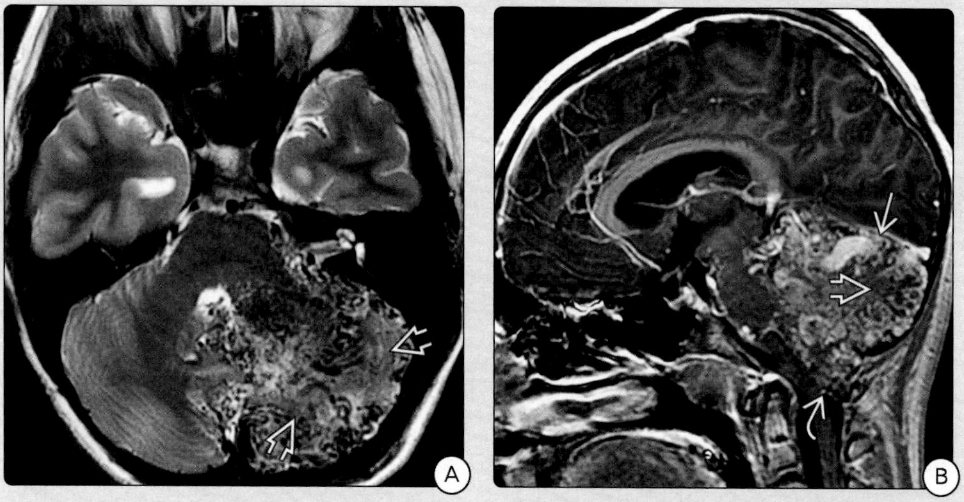

***(7-10A)** Axial T2WI in a 10y girl with ataxia shows innumerable tortuous, serpentine vessels occupying most of the left cerebellar hemisphere and vermis. Note islands of normal brain in between the "flow voids". **(7-10B)** Sagittal T1 C+ in the same case shows that the enhancing tortuous vessels fill almost all of the left cerebellum, including the tonsil. Note some areas of nonenhancing brain.*

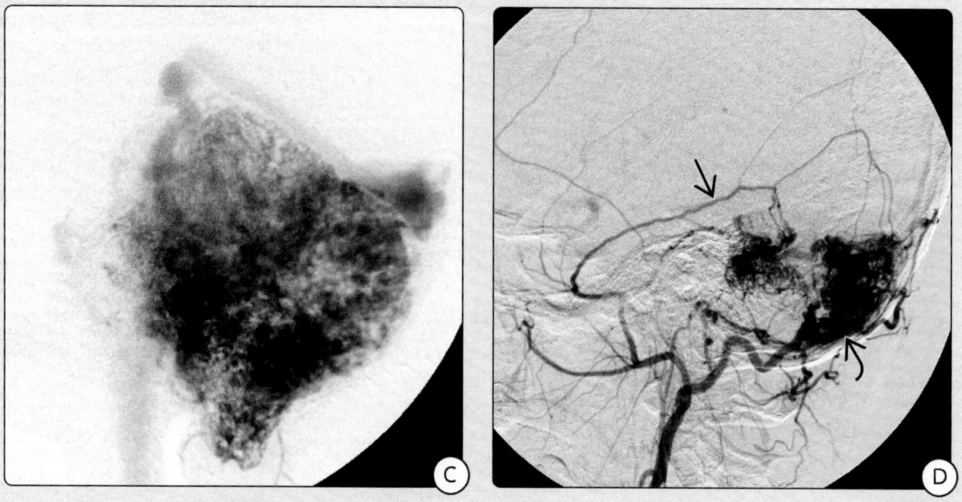

***(7-10C)** Lateral view of left vertebral DSA, late capillary phase, shows that many contrast-filled vessels occupy almost the entire cerebellum. **(7-10D)** Left external carotid DSA shows some contribution from the middle meningeal artery and the occipital artery. Initially diagnosed as an AVM, the child worsened after multiple embolizations before the correct diagnosis of cerebral proliferative angiopathy was made.*

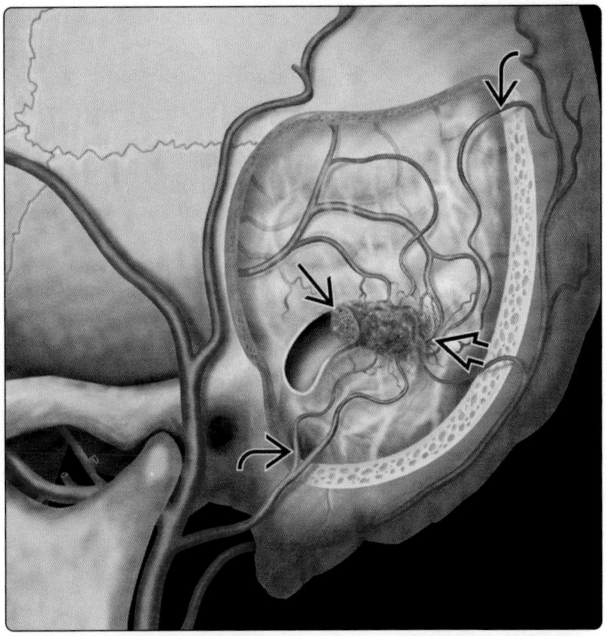

(7-11) Graphic depicts dural arteriovenous fistula (dAVF) with thrombosed transverse sinus ⇨ with multiple tiny arteriovenous vessels in the dural wall ⇨. Lesion is mostly supplied by transosseous feeders ⇨ from the external carotid artery (ECA).

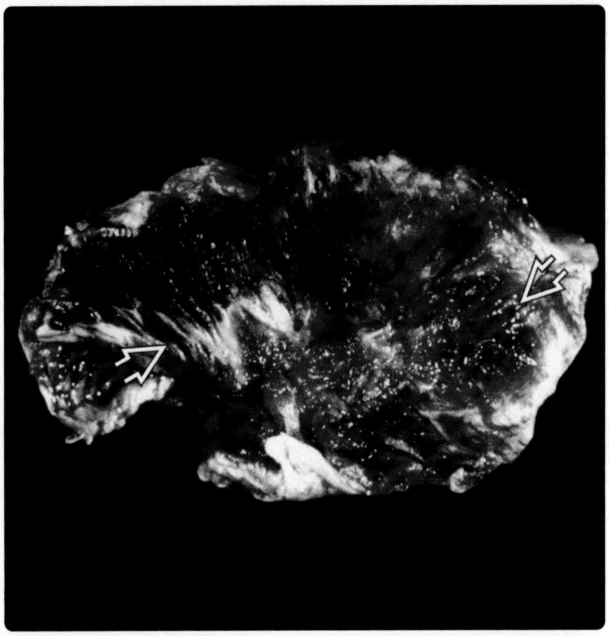

(7-12) Mass-like surgical specimen from a resected dAVF in the transverse sinus wall shows innumerable crack-like vessels ⇨. (Courtesy R. Hewlett, MD.)

CEREBRAL PROLIFERATIVE ANGIOPATHY

Clinical Issues

- Seizures, headache, neurologic deficits > > hemorrhage
- Progressive course, new areas of abnormal vascularity

Imaging

- Large, diffusely dispersed network of dilated vessels
- Numerous arterial feeders including dural
- **No nidus; normal brain in between!**

Dural AV Fistula

Dural arteriovenous fistula (dAVF) is the second major type of cerebrovascular malformation that exhibits arteriovenous shunting. Much less common than AVMs, they exhibit a spectrum of biologic behavior that ranges from relatively benign to catastrophic ICH. In this section, we consider typical dAVFs.

A special type of dAVF, carotid-cavernous fistula (CCF), has its own classification schema, distinctive clinical findings, and unique imaging features that differ from dAVFs elsewhere. CCF is discussed separately below.

Terminology

A dAVF, also known as a dural arteriovenous shunt, is a network of tiny, crack-like vessels that shunt blood between meningeal arteries and small venules within the wall of a dural venous sinus.

Etiology

Unlike parenchymal AVMs, adult dAVFs are usually acquired (not congenital). Although the precise etiology is controversial, local hypoperfusion in a thrombosed dural venous sinus that results in elevated intrasinus pressure is the most commonly cited mechanism. Upregulated angiogenesis within the dural sinus wall occurs after thrombosis and is considered the most likely etiology. Budding/proliferation of microvascular networks connects to a plexus of thin-walled venous channels, creating microfistulas.

Pathology

Location. Although dAVFs can involve any dural venous sinus, the most common locations in adults are the transverse, sigmoid, and cavernous sinuses (CSs). The superior sagittal sinus is a more common site in children.

Size and Number. Multiple lesions in anatomically separated dural sinuses are uncommon, accounting for slightly less than 8% of dAVFs. Multiple dAVFs can be synchronous (simultaneous multiplicity) or metachronous (sequential development of multiplicity).

Size varies from tiny single vessel shunts to massive complex lesions with multiple feeders and arteriovenous shunts in the sinus wall.

Gross Pathology. Multiple enlarged dural feeders converge in the wall of a thrombosed dural venous sinus **(7-11)**. A network of innumerable microfistulas connects these vessels directly to arterialized draining veins. These crack-like vessels may form a focal mass within the occluded sinus **(7-12)**.

Microscopic Features. Vessels within a dAVF often exhibit irregular intimal thickening with variable loss of the internal elastic lamina.

Clinical Issues

Epidemiology. dAVFs account for 10-15% of all intracranial vascular malformations with arteriovenous shunting. AVMs are approximately 10 times as common as dAVFs.

Demographics. Most dAVFs are found in adults. The peak age is 40-60 years, roughly 20 years older than the peak age for AVMs. There is no sex predilection.

Presentation. Clinical presentation varies with location and venous drainage pattern. Uncomplicated dAVFs in the transverse/sigmoid sinus region typically present with either bruit and/or tinnitus. dAVFs in the CS cause pulsatile proptosis, chemosis, retroorbital pain, bruit, and ophthalmoplegia.

"Malignant" dAVFs, lesions with cortical venous drainage, may cause seizures and progressive dementia in addition to focal neurologic deficits. Venous hypertension with dAVFs that drain into the vein of Galen may cause bithalamic edema with rapidly progressive dementia.

Patients who present with ICH or nonhemorrhagic neurologic deficits also have a higher risk of new adverse events than those with an asymptomatic fistula.

Natural History. The natural history of a dAVF remains poorly understood. Some lesions demonstrate angiographic progression, whereas others remain relatively stable. Progression of a dAVF from low to high grade occurs but is relatively uncommon.

Prognosis depends on location and venous drainage pattern. Almost 98% of lesions without cortical venous drainage will follow a benign clinical course. Hemorrhage is rare in such cases (approximately 1.5% per year). In contrast, "malignant"

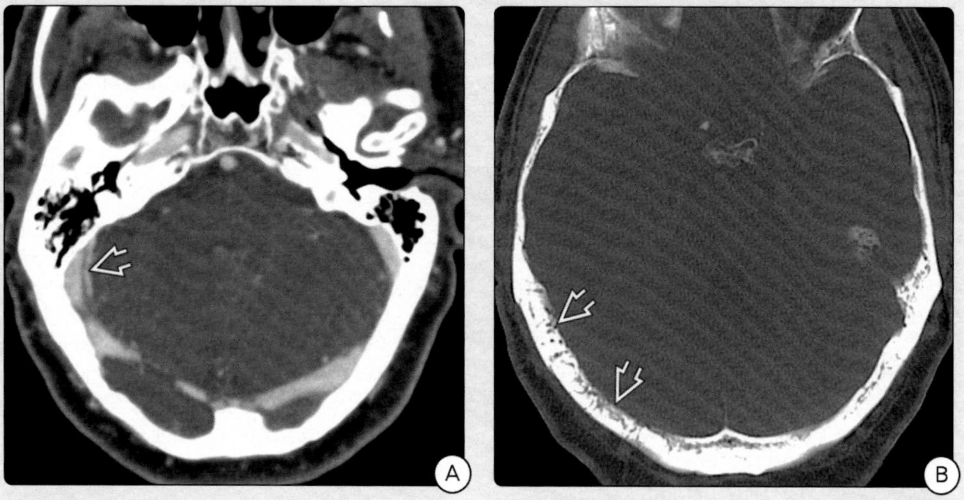

***(7-13A)** CTA source image in a patient with right-sided tinnitus shows no obvious abnormality, although the right sigmoid sinus ➡ looks peculiar. **(7-13B)** Bone CT in the same patient shows multiple enlarged transosseous vascular channels ➡ in the squama of the right occipital bone.*

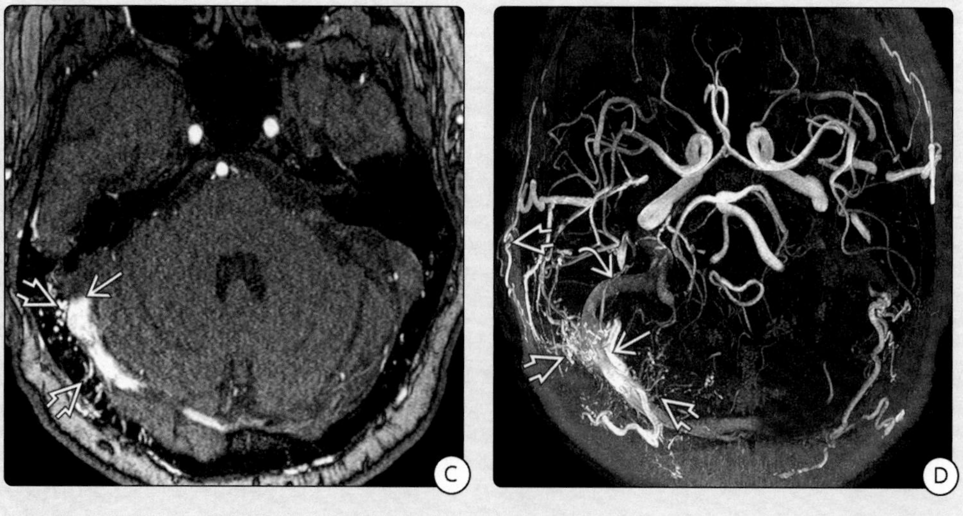

***(7-13C)** Contrast-enhanced MRA source image shows dural sinus thrombosis ➡, multiple enhancing vascular channels ➡ characteristic of posterior fossa dAVF. **(7-13D)** MRA in the same patient shows innumerable tiny feeding arteries ➡ supplying a dAVF at the transverse-sigmoid sinus junction. The sinus has partially recanalized ➡, and the distal sigmoid sinus ➡ and jugular bulb are partially opacified.*

dAVFs often have an aggressive clinical course, with hemorrhage (annual risk approximately 7.5% per year) and neurologic symptoms as common complications.

Multiple dAVFs are associated with angiographic progression and poor clinical prognosis, requiring an aggressive treatment and management strategy.

Treatment Options. Clinical observation may be appropriate in some patients who have minimal or no symptoms and dAVFs that demonstrate no cortical venous reflux.

Preventing the occurrence of ICH or nonhemorrhagic neurologic deficits is the goal of treating symptomatic dAVFs. Surgical or endovascular occlusion of the fistula or fistulous nidus is the ideal result. At a minimum, disconnection of the feeding vessels and draining veins is performed.

Endovascular treatment with embolization of arterial feeders using particulate or liquid agents with or without coil embolization of the recipient venous pouch/sinus may be performed. Surgical resection of the involved dural sinus wall or stereotactic radiosurgery are other options, used either alone or in combination with endovascular treatment.

Approximately 15% of endovascularly "cured" intracranial dAVFs recur.

Imaging

General Features. Most dAVFs are found in the posterior fossa and skull base. Although they can involve any dural venous sinus, the most common site is the transverse/sigmoid sinus junction. Between one-third and one-half of all dAVFs are found here. Less common sites are the CS and superior petrosal sinus. dAVFs involving the superior sagittal sinus are relatively uncommon.

Cross-sectional imaging alone may be insufficient to demonstrate a dAVF. CTA, MRA, and DSA may be required

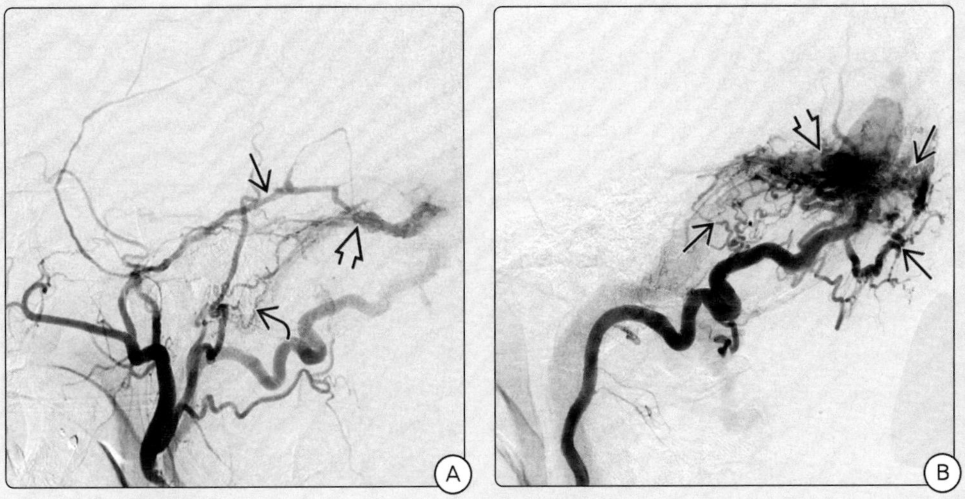

***(7-14A)** Lateral DSA of the ECA in a patient with pulsatile tinnitus shows a dAVF to a partial recanalized transverse sinus →. Numerous ECA branches including the posterior auricular → and middle meningeal arteries → supply the fistula. **(7-14B)** Superselective DSA of the occipital artery shows that it is the major contributor to the dAVF in the wall of the transverse sinus → through innumerable transosseous perforating branches →.*

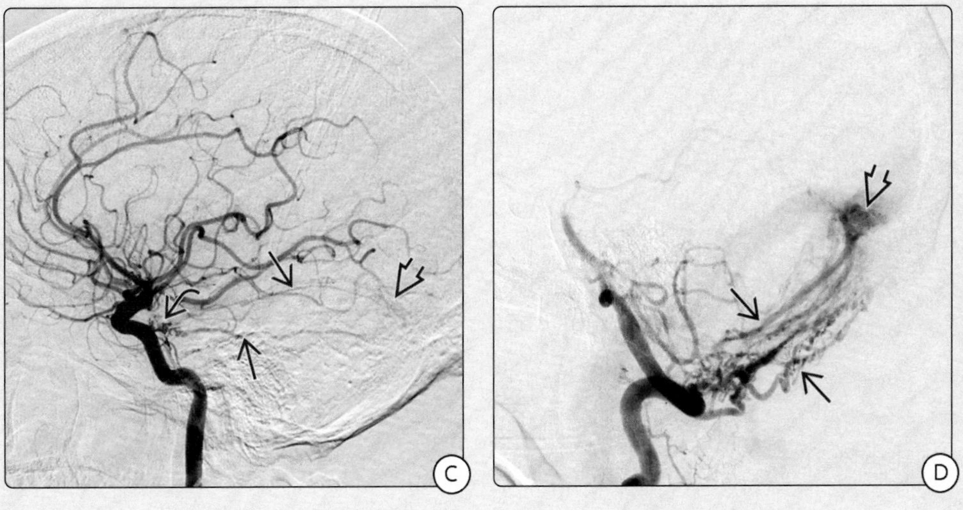

***(7-14C)** Lateral DSA of the left internal carotid artery (ICA) shows a markedly enlarged meningohypophyseal trunk → with several marginal tentorial branches → supplying the dAVF →. **(7-14D)** Lateral DSA of the left vertebral injection shows numerous enlarged posterior meningeal branches → that arise from the V3 segment and supply the dAVF →.*

both to identify a dAVF and to delineate its detailed angioarchitecture.

CT Findings. CT findings vary from none to striking. Hemorrhage is uncommon in the absence of cortical venous drainage or dysplastic venous dilatation. An enlarged dural sinus or draining vein can sometimes be identified on NECT scans. CCFs may demonstrate an enlarged superior ophthalmic vein. Dilated transcalvarial channels from enlarged transosseous feeding arteries can occasionally be seen on bone CT images and should be sought for all patients with pulsatile tinnitus **(7-13A)** **(7-13B)**.

Contrast-enhanced scans may demonstrate enlarged feeding arteries and draining veins. The involved dural venous sinus is often thrombosed or stenotic.

MR Findings. As with CT, MR findings on standard sequences vary from normal to striking. The presence of dilated cortical veins without an identifiable nidus adjacent to normal-appearing brain may suggest the presence of a dAVF. The most common finding of a dAVF itself is a thrombosed dural venous sinus containing vascular-appearing "flow voids" **(7-13C)** **(7-13D)** **(7-15B)**. Thrombus is typically isointense with brain on T1 and T2 scans and "blooms" on T2* sequences. Chronically thrombosed sinuses may enhance **(7-15B)**.

Parenchymal hyperintensity on T2WI and FLAIR indicates venous congestion or ischemia, usually secondary to retrograde cortical venous drainage.

Preoperative functional MRI (fMRI) and diffusion tensor imaging (DTI) are increasingly utilized to map eloquent brain and improve outcome in patients with motor cortical AVMs.

Angiography. While CTA/CTV with 3D shaded surface display may be useful in depicting static arterial supply and venous drainage patterns, time-resolved (so-called four-dimensional CTA) CTA acquires consecutive volumetric scans and can demonstrate flow dynamics in vascular malformations.

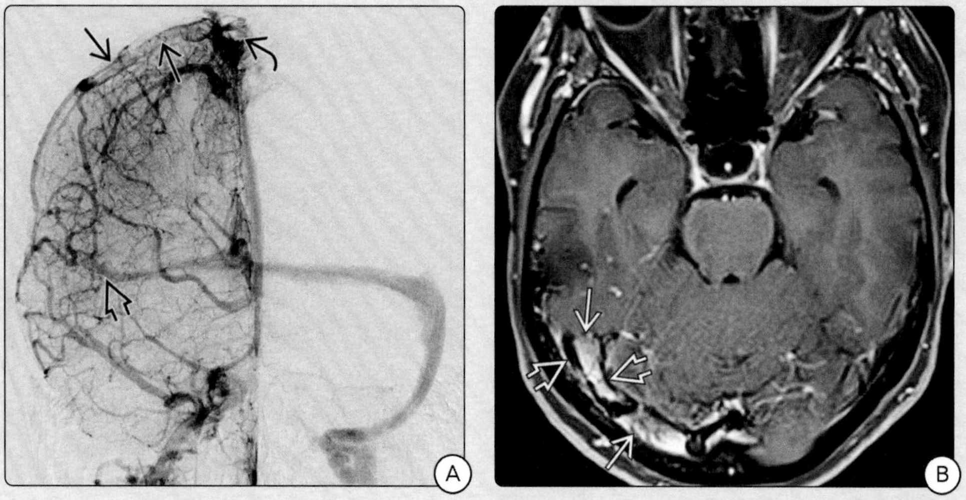

***(7-15A)** AP DSA in a 62y man with headaches shows thrombosis of the right transverse sinus and superior sagittal sinus. Note clot in vein of Trolard outlined by contrast. **(7-15B)** Two years later the patient developed pulsatile tinnitus. T1 C+ FS MR shows enhancing chronically thrombosed right transverse sinus and partially recanalized venous channels.*

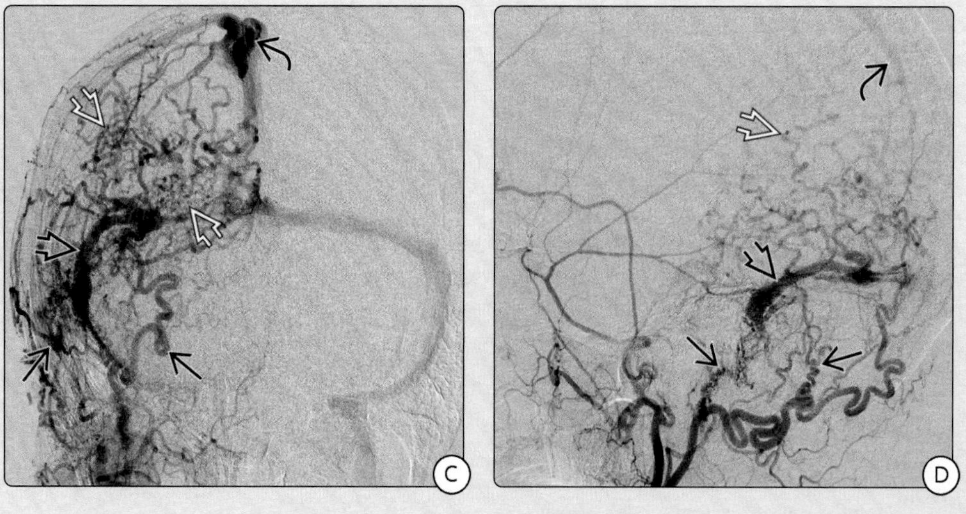

***(7-15C)** AP DSA shows the partially recanalized right transverse sinus with enlarged fistulous arterial feeders arising from the external carotid artery. Innumerable "pseudophlebitic" tortuous veins drain into the SSS, which is now patent. **(7-15D)** Lateral DSA shows the partially recanalized TS with transosseous branches from the ECA that supply a dAVF in its wall. Tortuous enlarged "pseudophlebitic" veins drain into the SSS.*

DSA is still regarded as the "gold standard" in evaluating AVFs. The arterial supply to the dura is rich, complex, and is derived from both the internal and external carotid systems. Complete visualization of all carotid and vertebral branches, often in combination with superselective catheterization of dural and transosseous feeders, is usually required to identify all arterial feeders, define the exact fistula site, delineate venous drainage, and identify pedicle aneurysms (found in 20% of cases).

As most dAVFs arise adjacent to the skull base, multiple enlarged dural and transosseous branches arising from the external carotid artery (ECA) are usually present **(7-14A)**. Dural branches may also arise from the internal carotid and vertebral arteries **(7-14D)**. An enlarged tentorial branch of the meningohypophyseal trunk commonly contributes to dAVFs at the transverse/sigmoid sinus junction **(7-14C)**.

The presence of dural sinus thrombosis, flow reversal with drainage into cortical (leptomeningeal) veins, and tortuous engorged pial veins (a "pseudophlebitic" pattern) should be identified and are more common in patients with progressive brain disease **(7-15)**.

High-flow venopathy associated with a dAVF may result in progressive stenosis, occlusion, and subsequent hemorrhage. Dysplastic venous "pouches" may cause focal mass effect. Risk of associated ICH rises significantly with the presence of leptomeningeal drainage and dysplastic venous dilatations.

Angiographic classification of dAVFs helps stratify risk of dAVF rupture and predict the clinical course of these lesions. The Cognard and Borden classifications are the most commonly used systems.

In either classification, *the presence of cortical venous drainage (CVD) puts a dAVF into a higher risk category* **(7-16)**. Subdividing lesions with CVD into symptomatic and asymptomatic types may help improve risk stratification. dAVFs are dynamic lesions and may spontaneously regress or

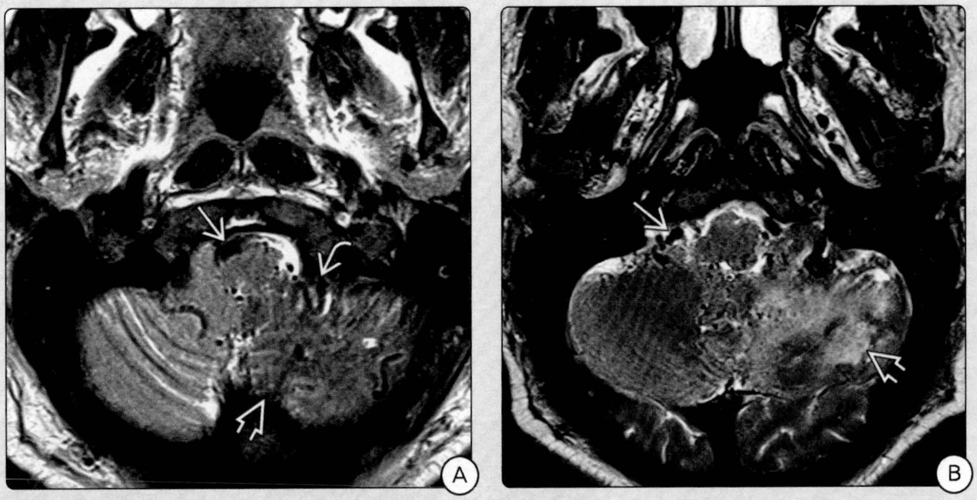

***(7-16A)** Axial T2WI in a 59y man with headaches, weakness, increasing lethargy, and rapidly declining mental status shows numerous vascular "flow voids" around the cervicomedullary junction ➡ and cerebellum ➡. The left cerebellar hemisphere is generally hypointense ➡, reflecting venous stasis. **(7-16B)** More cephalad T2WI shows numerous additional "flow voids" ➡ and edema in the left cerebellum ➡.*

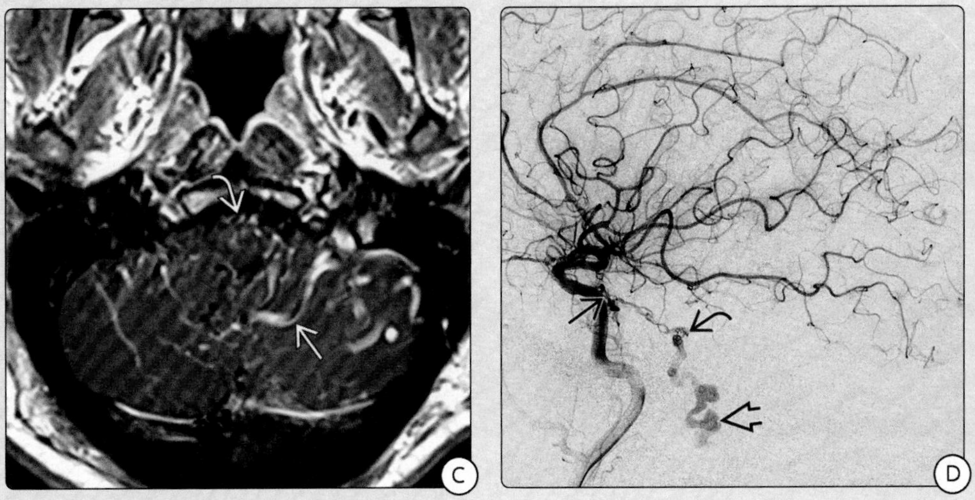

***(7-16C)** T1 C+ MR in the same case shows enhancement of numerous vessels in the cerebellar folia ➡ and around the cervicomedullary junction ➡. **(7-16D)** Lateral view of the DSA obtained in this case demonstrates a dAVF ➡ supplied by branches from the meningohypophyseal trunk ➡. Note slow flow into dilated variceal posterior fossa veins ➡. Venous drainage continued inferiorly into perimedullary veins. This is Cognard type V dAVF.*

progress. The risk of a low-grade lesion converting to a high-grade type is relatively low, but change in symptoms should prompt imaging reevaluation.

Differential Diagnosis

The most common mimic of dAVF is **acute dural venous sinus thrombosis** with prominent collateral venous drainage creating a "pseudophlebitic" pattern on MR and DSA.

Chronic dural venous sinus thrombosis can pose a difficult diagnostic challenge. There may be little or no evidence for residual clot, and the fibrotic thrombosed sinus enhances strongly, mimicking normal venous filling. If the proximal thrombosed sinus segment recanalizes while the distal outflow remains obstructed, collateral venous drainage through prominent tortuous medullary veins can mimic CPA, AVM, or a dAVF.

A **pseudolesion of the jugular bulb**, caused by slow or asymmetric flow, may create inhomogeneous signal within the jugular foramen. No thrombus is seen on T2*, and neither abnormal arterial feeders nor enlarged venous collaterals are present.

A **pial AVM** or **fistula** is rare and represents a direct arteriovenous shunt between a brain parenchymal ("pial") artery and a dilated cortical draining vein. These occur along the brain surface or within the brain itself, not within a dural venous sinus (see below).

Rarely, a dAVF adjacent to the brainstem can incite T2/FLAIR hyperintensity, mimicking an **infiltrating glioma**. Contrast-enhanced images should be carefully evaluated for abnormal perimedullary vascular enhancement.

COGNARD CLASSIFICATION OF dAVFs

Grade 1: In sinus wall; normal antegrade venous drainage (low risk; benign clinical course)

Grade 2A: In sinus; reflux to sinus, not cortical veins

Grade 2B: Reflux (retrograde drainage) into cortical veins (10-20% hemorrhage)

Grade 3: Direct cortical venous drainage; no venous ectasia (40% hemorrhage)

Grade 4: Direct cortical venous drainage + venous ectasia (65% hemorrhage)

Grade 5: Spinal perimedullary venous drainage

BORDEN CLASSIFICATION OF dAVFs

Type I
- Dural arterial supply with antegrade drainage into venous sinus
  - **Type Ia**: Simple dAVF with single meningeal arterial supply
  - **Type Ib**: Complex dAVF with multiple meningeal arteries

Type II
- Dural supply + ↑ intrasinus pressure → antegrade sinus, retrograde cortical venous drainage

Type III
- Dural arteries drain into cortical veins

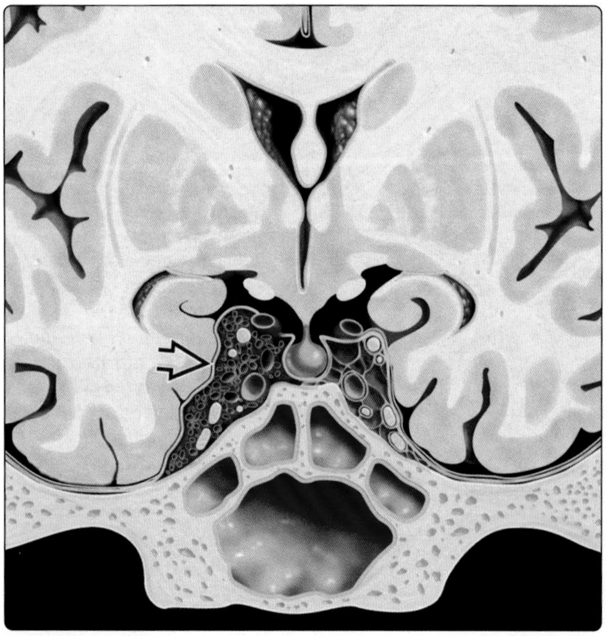

(7-17) Coronal graphic depicts a carotid-cavernous fistula (CCF). The right cavernous sinus (CS) ⇒ is enlarged by numerous dilated arterial and venous channels.

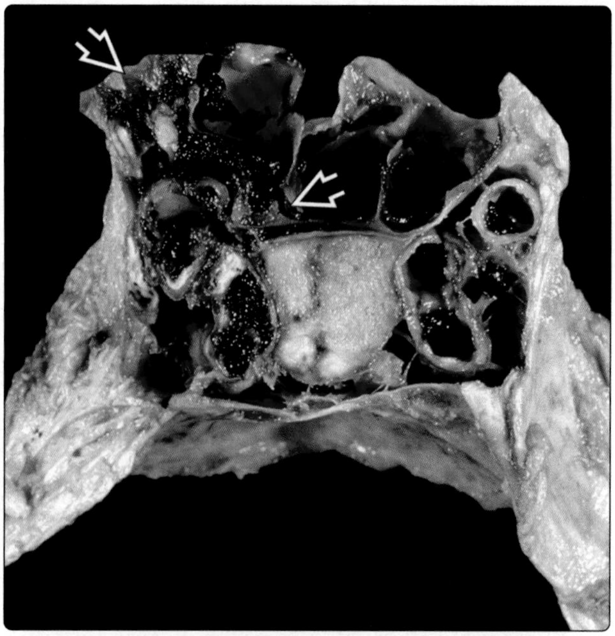

(7-18) Autopsy case of direct CCF with dissection of the CS and adjacent structures shows that the right CS is enlarged ⇒ by numerous dilated vascular channels. (Courtesy B. Horten, MD.)

Carotid-Cavernous Fistula

Terminology

Carotid-cavernous fistulas (CCFs) are a special type of arteriovenous shunt that develops within the CS **(7-17) (7-18)**. CCFs are divided into two subgroups, direct and indirect fistulas.

"Direct" CCFs are typically *high-flow* lesions that result from rupture of the cavernous internal carotid artery (ICA) directly into the CS, with or without a preexisting ICA aneurysm. **"Indirect" CCFs** are usually *slow-flow, low-pressure* lesions that represent an AVF between dural branches of the cavernous ICA and the CS.

Etiology

CCFs are almost always acquired lesions and can be traumatic or nontraumatic in origin. Most *direct* CCFs are traumatic, usually secondary to central skull base fractures. Either stretch injury to the ICA or direct puncture from a bony fracture fragment may occur. A single-hole laceration/transection of the cavernous ICA with direct fistulization into the CS is the typical finding. Spontaneous (i.e., nontraumatic) rupture of a preexisting cavernous ICA aneurysm is a less common etiology.

Indirect CCFs are nontraumatic lesions and are thought to be degenerative in origin. In contrast to dAVFs elsewhere, indirect CCFs rarely occur as sequelae of dural sinus thrombosis. Most indirect CCFs are found in the dural wall of the CS and supplied via intracavernous branches of the ICA and deep (maxillary) branches of the ECA.

Pathology

Gross Pathology. In a direct CCF, arterialized flow causes dilatation of the CS with venous hypertension and retrograde flow into the superior and inferior ophthalmic veins. Indirect

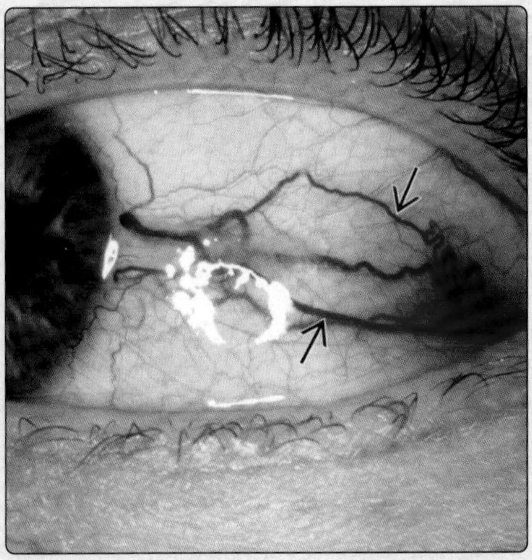

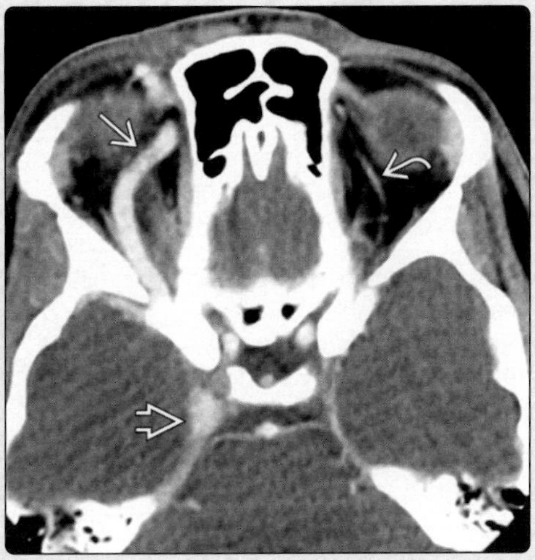

***(7-19)** Clinical photograph of a patient with a CCF shows numerous enlarged scleral vessels →. **(7-20)** CECT scan shows classic findings of CCF. The right CS is enlarged ➡, and the ipsilateral superior ophthalmic vein ➡ is more than four times the size of the left superior ophthalmic vein ➡.*

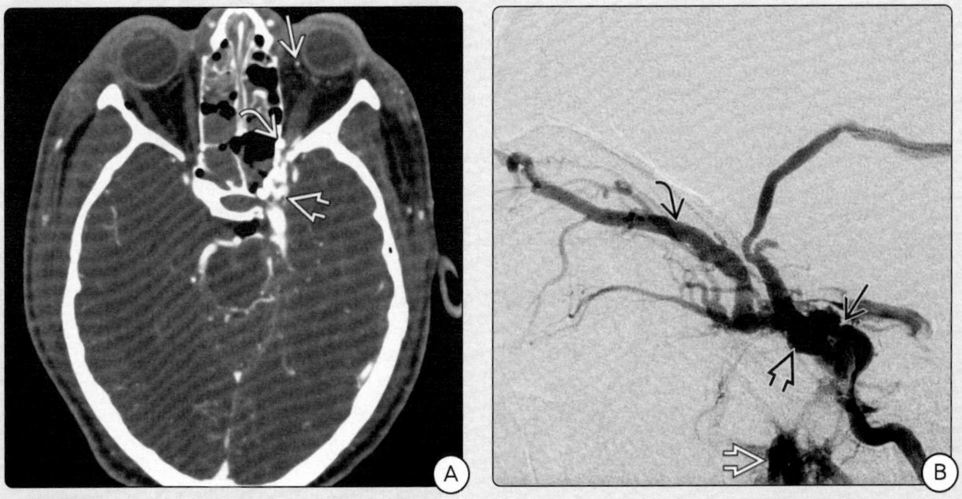

***(7-21A)** A 21y man developed left proptosis following severe trauma with multiple skull base fractures. CTA shows enlarged vessels around the left globe ➡, at the orbital apex ➡ and within the CS ➡. **(7-21B)** DSA shows a direct CCF at the C4-C5 segment →. The enlarged CS → drains anteriorly into the superior ophthalmic vein →, inferiorly into the pterygoid venous plexus ➡.*

CCFs demonstrate enlarged crack-like vessels within the CS that resemble those seen in typical dAVFs elsewhere.

Staging, Grading, and Classification. CCFs are a subtype of dAVF. A specific classification for CCFs, the Barrow classification, is based on the arterial supply.

BARROW CLASSIFICATION OF CAROTID-CAVERNOUS FISTULAS
Type A: Direct ICA-CS high-flow shunt
Type B: Dural ICA branches-CS shunt
Type C: Dural ECA-CS shunt
Type D: Both ICA/ECA dural branches shunt to CS

Clinical Issues

Clinical presentation, natural history, demographics, and epidemiology vary with whether the CCF is traumatic or spontaneous.

Epidemiology. An indirect CCF is the second most common site of intracranial dAVF, following the transverse/sigmoid sinus junction. Direct high-flow CCFs are much less common.

Demographics. As direct CCFs typically occur with trauma, they are found in both sexes and at all ages. Indirect CCFs are most frequent in women 40-60 years of age.

Presentation. Direct CCFs may present within hours to days or even weeks following trauma. Bruit, pulsatile exophthalmos, orbital edema, decreasing vision, glaucoma, and headache are typical **(7-19)**. In severe cases, vision loss may be rapid and severe. Cranial neuropathy may occur but is less common. In rare cases, rupture of an intracavernous ICA aneurysm may cause life-threatening epistaxis.

Indirect CCFs typically cause painless proptosis with variable vision changes.

Natural History. In severe cases with torrential ICA-CS shunting, hemispheric ischemia may result. If retrograde intracranial venous drainage is present, catastrophic subarachnoid hemorrhage from ruptured ectatic cortical veins can occur.

Treatment Options. The primary goal in treating a direct CCF is fistula closure, typically by transarterial-transfistula detachable balloon embolization. Transvenous embolization via the internal jugular vein and inferior petrosal sinus is another option. If the ICA is torn, covered stent placement may be effective. Less commonly, trapping the fistula and sacrificing the parent ICA with coils or balloons may be considered. This is an option only if the patient passes the balloon "test" occlusion or has sufficient collateral circulation to compensate for lack of antegrade ICA flow.

Indirect CCFs may be treated conservatively or with superselective embolization.

Imaging

General Features. The general imaging features of CCF reflect the presence of arteriovenous shunting within the CS. Depending on the degree of the shunt, findings can vary from subtle to striking.

CT Findings. NECT scans may demonstrate mild or striking proptosis, a prominent CS with enlarged superior ophthalmic vein (SOV), and enlarged extraocular muscles. "Dirty" fat secondary to edema and venous engorgement may be present. Occasionally, subarachnoid hemorrhage from trauma or ruptured cortical veins can be identified.

CECT scans often nicely demonstrate an enlarged SOV and CS **(7-20)**. Inferior drainage into a prominent pterygoid venous plexus and posterior drainage into the clival venous plexus are sometimes present.

CTA shows engorgement of the ophthalmic vein and CS **(7-21)**. Dehiscence of the intracavernous ICA is characteristic for direct CCF.

MR Findings. T1 scans may show a prominent "bulging" CS and SOV as well as "dirty" orbital fat. T2-weighted images may show asymmetric flow-related signal loss in the affected veins. Too many "flow voids" in the CS are a common finding with CCFs.

Strong, uniform enhancement of the CS and SOV is typical. Enlarged, tortuous intracranial veins may occur with high-flow, high-pressure shunts.

Rare cases of high-flow, aggressive direct CCFs with prominent pontomesencephalic and perimedullary venous drainage causing progressive myelopathy have been reported.

Angiography. DSA is required for definitive diagnosis and treatment. Complete delineation of the arterial supply and venous drainage pattern is the goal. *Direct* CCFs typically demonstrate rapid flow with very early opacification of the CS. Selective ICA injection with very rapid image acquisition is often necessary to localize the fistula site precisely. A single-hole fistula is usually present, typically between the C4 and C5 ICA segments.

Occasionally, injection into the vertebrobasilar system with manual compression of the ipsilateral carotid artery is necessary to determine the fistula site. Venous drainage via the superior and inferior ophthalmic veins, contralateral CS, clival, pterygoid, and sphenoparietal sinuses, and intracranial cortical veins should be delineated.

Indirect CCFs often have multiple dural feeders from cavernous branches of the ICA (meningohypophyseal and inferolateral trunks) as well as deep branches of the ECA (middle meningeal and distal maxillary branches). Anastomoses between ICA and ECA feeders, such as the artery of the foramen rotundum, are common and must be delineated completely prior to embolization.

Ultrasound. The normal flow in the SOV is from extra- to intracranial (i.e., from orbit into CS). Flow reversal (intra- to extracranial) within an enlarged SOV can be demonstrated noninvasively using Doppler US.

Differential Diagnosis

The major differential diagnosis with CCFs is **cavernous sinus thrombosis** (CST). Both CCF and CST may cause proptosis, intraorbital edema, enlarged extraocular muscles, and the appearance of "dirty" fat. In CST, the CS may appear enlarged, but prominent filling defects are present on T1 C+ MR.

Pial AV Fistula

Intracranial pial arteriovenous fistulas (pAVFs) are rare, accounting for less than 2% of all intracranial AVMs. Most occur in children but can occur in the elderly.

pAVFs usually consist of a single dilated pial artery connecting directly to an enlarged cortical draining vein **(7-22)**. No intervening capillary bed or nidus is present although a dilated venous pouch is common.

80% of pAVFs are supratentorial. They typically lie on or just within the brain surface or adjacent to the ventricular ependyma. Supratentorial pAVFs are supplied by the anterior, middle, or posterior cerebral arteries and are usually associated with a venous varix **(7-23)** **(7-24)**.

PIAL ARTERIOVENOUS FISTULA

Epidemiology and Clinical Issues
- 1-2% of all intracranial arteriovenous malformations
- Children > > elderly

Imaging
- 80% supratentorial; 20% infratentorial
- Pial artery connects directly to cortical vein
- Venous pouch common

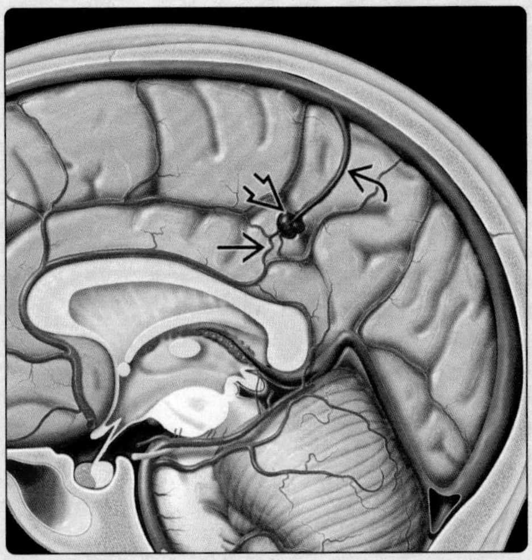

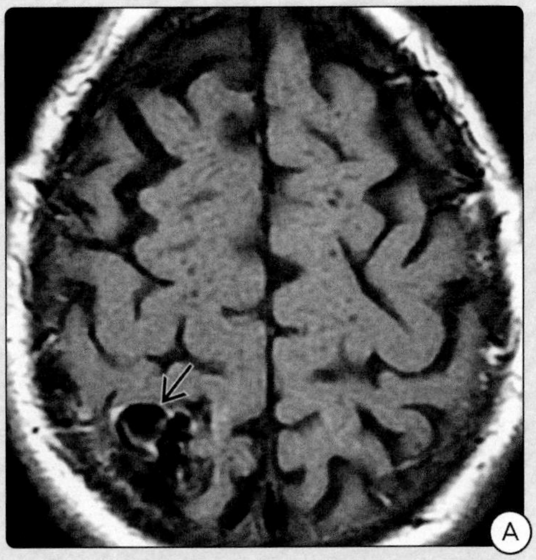

***(7-22)** Graphic depicts pial AVF with slightly enlarged ACA branches connecting to a venous varix, dilated cortical draining vein. **(7-23A)** Axial T1 MR in a 75y man with headache shows an unusual extraaxial "flow void" in the left parietal lobe.*

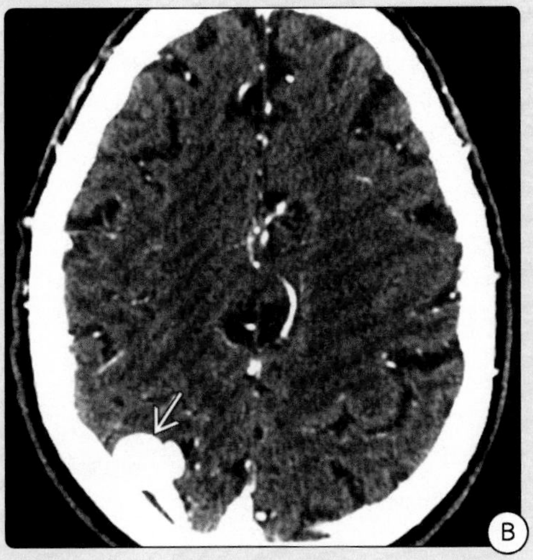

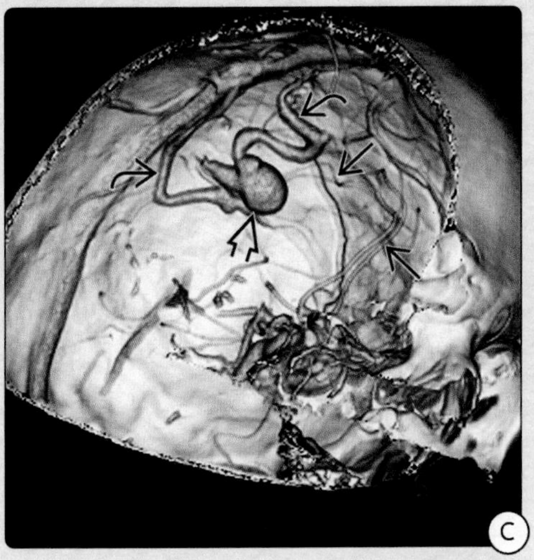

***(7-23B)** CTA in the same case shows that the well-demarcated lobulated lesion enhances intensely. **(7-23C)** 3D shaded surface display (SSD) of the CTA shows that the lesion consists of a venous pouch that drains into dilated superficial cortical veins and communicates directly with distal branches of the posterior cerebral artery. This is pial AVF.*

Vein of Galen Aneurysmal Malformation

Different types of vascular malformations share a dilated vein of Galen as a common feature, but only one of these is a true vein of Galen aneurysmal malformation (VGAM). A VGAM is the most common extracardiac cause of high-output cardiac failure in newborns and comprises 30% of pediatric vascular anomalies.

Terminology

VGAM is essentially a direct AVF between deep choroidal arteries and a persistent embryonic precursor of the vein of Galen, the median prosencephalic vein (MPV) of Markowski **(7-25)**. The presence of these arteriovenous shunts keeps the MPV patent and causes flow-related aneurysmal dilatation of this primitive vein, forming a large midline venous pouch that lies behind the third ventricle.

Etiology

General Concepts. At 6-10 gestational weeks, the developing telencephalon is supplied by multiple choroidal arteries that drain via a single transient midline vein in the roof of the diencephalon, the MPV of Markowski. Normally, the developing internal cerebral veins annex drainage of the fetal choroid plexus, and the MPV—the precursor of the vein of Galen—regresses. In a VGAM, a high-flow fistula prevents formation of the definitive vein of Galen.

Genetics. VGAMs are sporadic lesions with no known genetic predisposition.

Pathology

Gross Pathology. Enlarged arteries drain directly into a dilated MPV. Aneurysmal dilatation of the persistent MPV forms a large venous pouch behind the third ventricle that often drains into a markedly enlarged superior sagittal sinus

(7-24A) Axial T2WI in a 2-month-old infant shows a large venous pouch in the right choroidal fissure surrounded by numerous "flow voids." Note massively enlarged transverse sinuses. (7-24B) A markedly enlarged right PCA is identified as the likely primary feeder to the venous pouch.

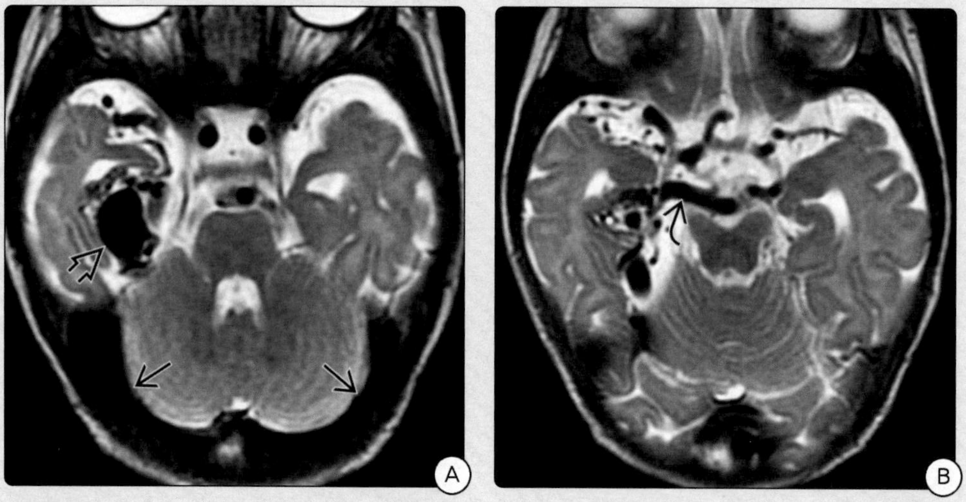

(7-24C) Coronal T2WI shows an enlarged artery that appears to connect with a tangle of abnormal vessels in the right medial temporal lobe. (7-24D) Left vertebral angiogram, anteroposterior view, early arterial phase shows an enlarged, tortuous PCA with a jet of contrast directly filling a markedly dilated draining vein. This is pial AVF.

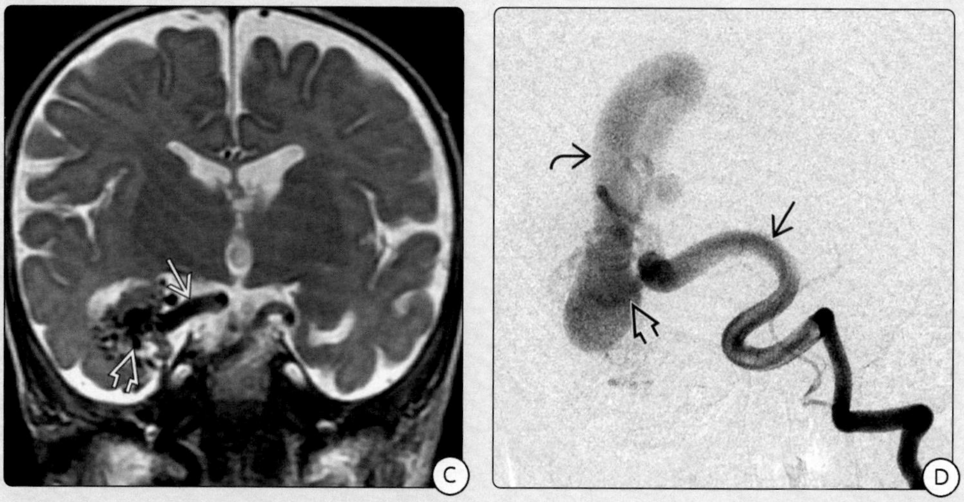

via an embryonic falcine sinus **(7-25) (7-26)**. The ventricles are often markedly dilated. The brain is frequently atrophic. Ischemic changes are common.

Microscopic Features. The wall of the venous pouch may become significantly thickened and dysplastic.

Clinical Issues

Epidemiology. VGAMs are rare, representing less than 1% of all cerebral vascular malformations. However, they account for 30% of symptomatic vascular malformations in children.

Demographics. Neonatal VGAMs are more common than those presenting in infancy or childhood. Adult presentation is rare. There is a definite male predominance (M:F = 2:1).

Presentation. Signs and symptoms vary with age of onset. In neonates, high-output congestive heart failure and a loud cranial bruit are typical. Older infants may present with macrocrania and hydrocephalus, with or without heart failure.

VGAMs in older children are often associated with developmental delay and seizures. VGAMs in young adults typically present with headache with or without hemorrhage and hydrocephalus.

Natural History. Prognosis is related to size of the arteriovenous shunt. Large VGAMs cause cerebral ischemia and dystrophic changes in the fetal brain. Left untreated, neonates with VGAMs typically die from progressive brain damage and intractable heart failure.

Treatment Options. Anatomic cure of the VGAM is not the main goal of treatment; rather, the ultimate goal is sufficient control of the malformation to allow normal brain maturation and development. Staged arterial embolization, ideally at 4 or

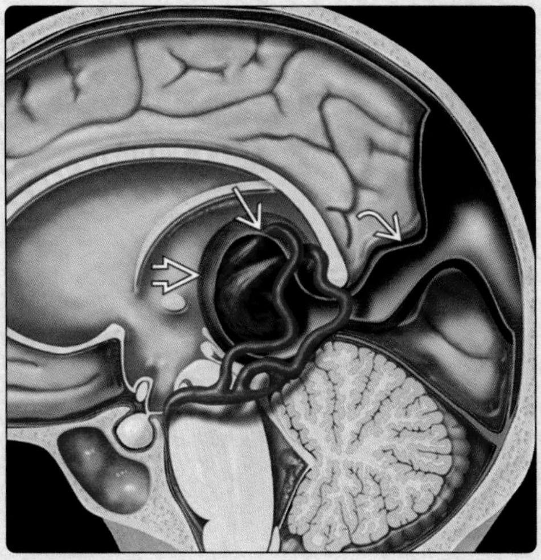
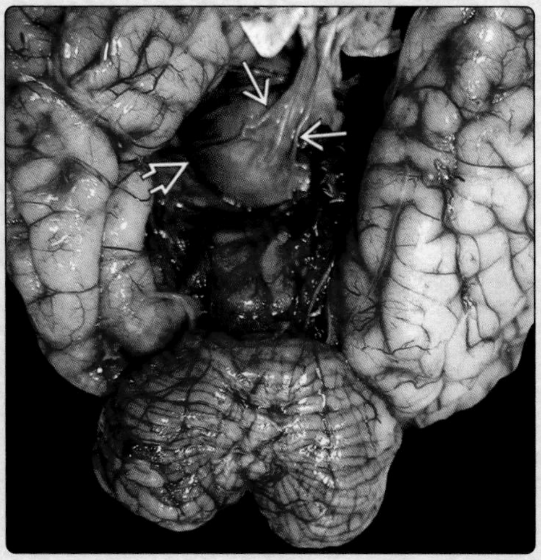

***(7-25)** Graphic illustrates vein of Galen malformation. Enlarged choroid arteries drain directly into dilated median prosencephalic vein, falcine sinus. Torcular herophili (venous sinus confluence) is massively enlarged. **(7-26)** Autopsied brain of infant with vein of Galen aneurysmal malformation (VGAM) shows large venous sac of malformation with several dilated arterial feeders emptying directly into sac. (From DP: Neuropathology, 2e.)*

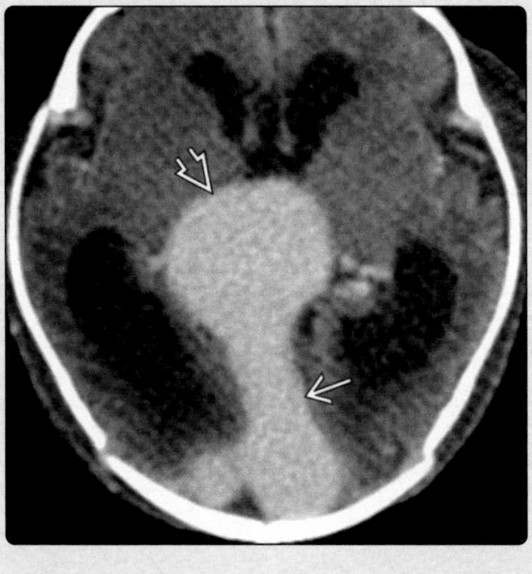
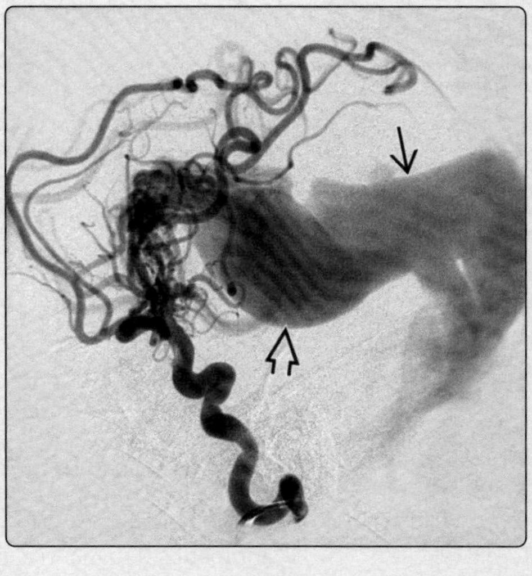

***(7-27)** CECT scan in a newborn demonstrates a massive VGAM draining into an enlarged falcine sinus, causing obstructive hydrocephalus. **(7-28)** Internal carotid angiogram, early arterial phase, lateral view, shows a VGAM draining into a massively enlarged falcine sinus. (Courtesy S. Blaser, MD.)*

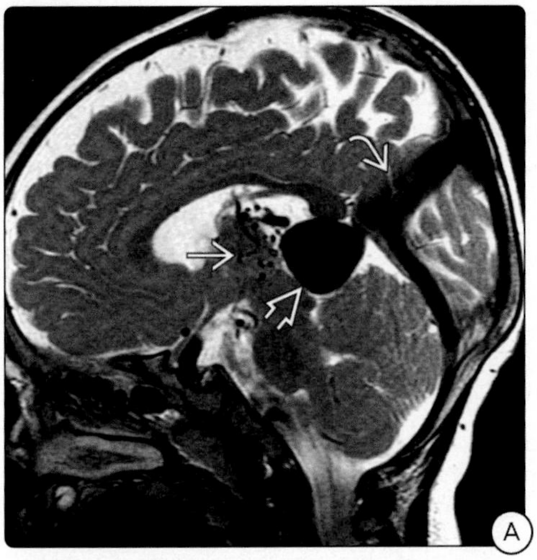

***(7-29A)** Sagittal T2WI in an 8m infant shows a classic VGAM with multiple dilated choroidal feeders, falcine sinus.*

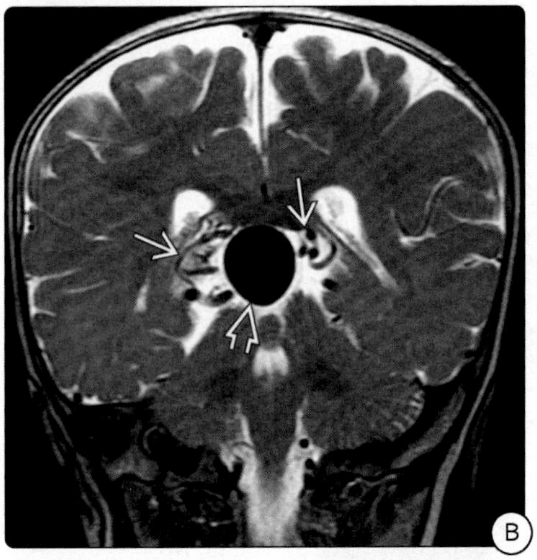

***(7-29B)** Coronal T2WI shows the midline venous pouch and enlarged choroidal feeders draining directly into the VGAM.*

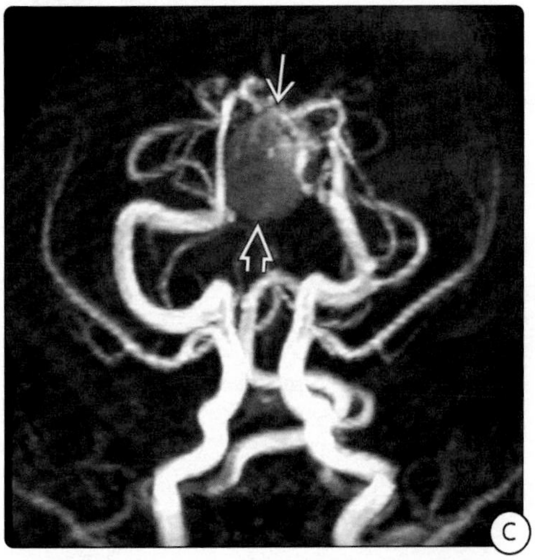

***(7-29C)** TOF MRA shows the VGAM with arterial feeders draining directly into the venous pouch.*

5 months of age, is the preferred treatment. The transvenous approach carries significant morbidity and mortality and is generally contraindicated.

Imaging

General Features. A large, rounded venous pouch drains into a persistent falcine sinus or prominent straight sinus. The venous sinus confluence is often markedly enlarged.

CT Findings. NECT scans show an enlarged, well-delineated, mildly hyperdense mass at the tentorial apex, usually compressing the third ventricle and causing severe obstructive hydrocephalus. Variable encephalomalacia, hemorrhage, and/or dystrophic calcification in the brain parenchyma are often present. CECT scans show strong uniform enhancement **(7-27)**.

MR Findings. Rapid but turbulent flow in the VGAM causes inhomogeneous signal loss and phase artifact (signal misregistration in the phase-encoding direction). Enlarged arterial feeders are usually seen as serpentine "flow voids" adjacent to the lesion **(7-29A)**. Thrombus of varying ages may be present lining the VGAM.

Fetal MR can identify important secondary complications of VGAM, such as hemispheric white matter injuries and progressive heart failure with development of fetal hydrops.

Angiography. Two forms of VGAM are recognized based on their specific angioarchitecture: choroidal and mural. In the **"choroidal"** form, multiple branches from the pericallosal, choroidal, and thalamoperforating arteries drain directly into an enlarged, aneurysmally dilated midline venous sac. In the **"mural"** form, a single or a few enlarged branches from collicular or posterior choroidal arteries drain into the sinus wall. Giant venous sacs are more commonly associated with mural-type VGAMs.

In more than 50% of all VGAMs, the straight sinus is hypoplastic or absent, and venous drainage is into a persistent embryonic **"falcine sinus."** The falcine sinus is easily identified, as it angles posterosuperiorly toward the superior sagittal sinus **(7-28)**.

Ultrasound. Many VGAMs are now diagnosed antenatally. A hypoechoic to mildly echogenic midline mass behind the third ventricle is typical. Color Doppler shows bidirectional turbulent flow within the VGAM.

Differential Diagnosis

Typical imaging findings in a neonate with high-output congestive heart failure are virtually pathognomonic of VGAM. A thalamic AVM with deep venous drainage may cause secondary enlargement of the vein of Galen. **Vein of Galen aneurysmal dilatation associated with an AVM** rarely presents in the neonatal period. A high-flow **giant childhood dAVF** may present in infancy and clinically resemble a VGAM. Involvement of the dural venous sinuses rather than the vein of Galen or MPV is typical.

CVMs Without Arteriovenous Shunting

Developmental Venous Anomaly

With the advent of contrast-enhanced MR, **developmental venous anomalies (DVAs)** have become the most frequently diagnosed intracranial vascular malformation. Once thought to be rare lesions with substantial risk of hemorrhage, the vast majority of venous "angiomas" are now recognized as asymptomatic and incidental imaging findings. Neurologic complications of these common lesions are rare.

Terminology

DVA, also called **venous "angioma"** or "venous malformation," is an umbrella-shaped congenital cerebral vascular malformation composed of angiogenically mature venous elements. Dilated, thin-walled venous channels lie within (and are separated by) normal brain parenchyma.

Very rarely, a dilated or tortuous venous pouch without discernible arterial or venous tributaries occurs. In these unusual cases, the term **isolated venous varix** is appropriate.

Etiology

General Concepts. The precise etiology of DVAs is unknown. Most investigators believe it is arrested medullary vein development between 8 and 11 gestational weeks that results in DVAs. In this model, the persistence of primitive medullary veins with recruitment of transparenchymal anastomotic drainage pathways eventually matures into a classic DVA. Others believe DVAs represent an extreme variant of otherwise normal venous drainage. Unlike many other cerebrovascular malformations (CVMs), DVAs do not express growth factors.

Genetics

Solitary DVA. Whereas genetic linkage studies have implicated a region on chromosome 9p in hereditary cutaneomucosal venous malformations, no genetic predisposition for the formation of isolated, sporadic brain DVAs has been identified.

An association of DVA and solitary (but not familial) cerebral cavernous malformations (CCMs) has been recently reported, suggesting that these vascular malformations probably have a different developmental mechanism. Solitary DVAs lack the *KRIT1* gene associated with familial CCMs.

Multiple DVAs. Between 6-7% of patients with a DVA have two lesions; multiple DVAs occur in 1%. Multiple DVAs have been reported in **blue rubber bleb nevus syndrome** (BRBNS) and other superficial craniofacial venous and venolymphatic malformations.

Pathology

Location and Size. Approximately 70% of DVAs are found in the deep white matter, adjacent to the frontal horn of the lateral ventricle **(7-30)**. The second most common location is next to the fourth ventricle (15-30%).

DVA depth is defined as where the medullary venous radicles converge into the collector vein. Three depths are recognized: juxtacortical, subcortical, and periventricular **(7-32)**. Some larger DVAs can have dual or even triple convergence sites.

DVA size varies from tiny, almost imperceptible lesions to giant venous malformations that involve most of the hemispheric white matter.

Gross Pathology. DVAs consist of two elements: a cluster of variably sized prominent medullary (white matter) veins (the so-called "caput medusa") that converges on an enlarged stem or single "collector vein." Medullary veins in the caput medusa have lost their normal connections to the brain surface or ependyma and depend on the collector vein. A DVA is embedded within and drains grossly normal-appearing brain parenchyma, forming its primary or sole venous drainage pathway **(7-31)**.

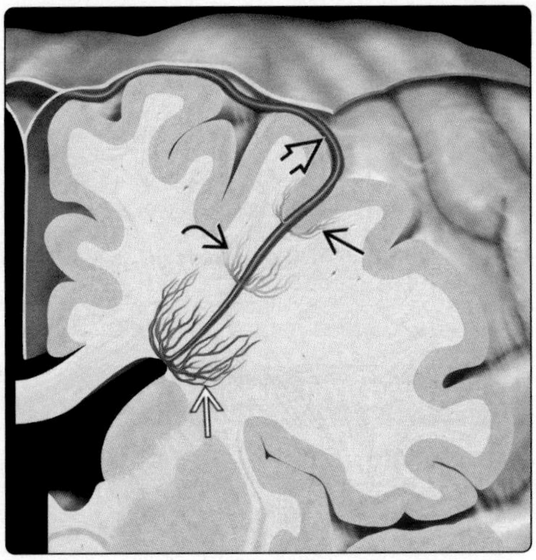

***(7-30)** DVA with enlarged juxtacortical →, subcortical →, periventricular → medullary veins drains into a single transmantle collector vein →.*

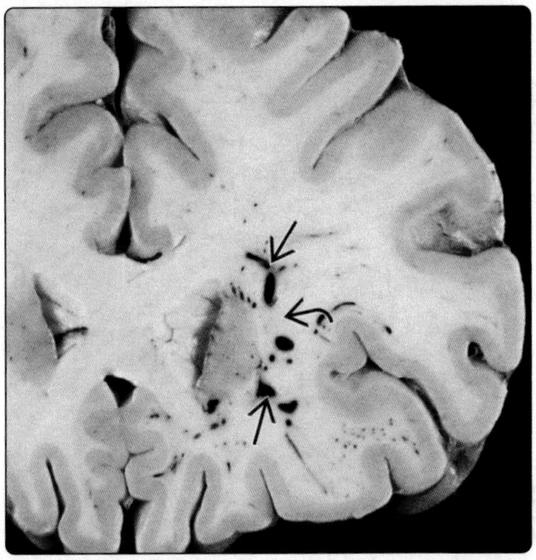

***(7-31)** Coronal autopsy shows a DVA →. Note normal brain → in between the enlarged medullary veins. (Courtesy P. Burger, MD.)*

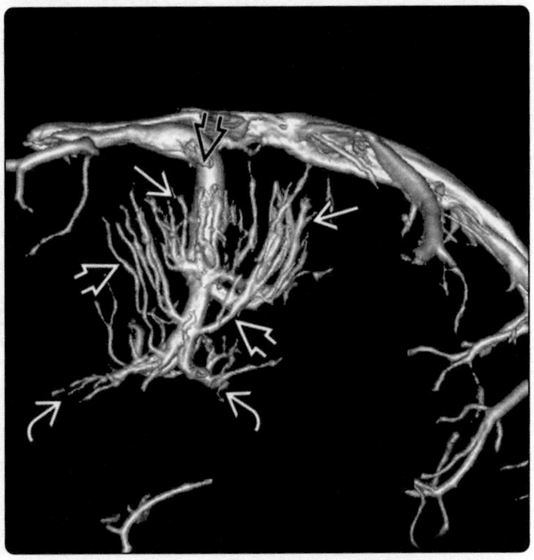

***(7-32)** 3D DSA shows DVA with juxta- → and subcortical →, periventricular → medullary veins, collector vein →. (P. Lasjaunias, MD.)*

Hemorrhage and calcification are uncommon unless the DVA is associated with a CCM or the collecting vein becomes thrombosed.

Microscopic Features. Thin-walled, somewhat dilated venous channels are interspersed in normal-appearing white matter. Occasionally, the vessel walls are thickened and hyalinized.

Varying degrees of focal parenchymal atrophy, white matter gliosis, neuronal degeneration, and demyelination have been reported within the venous drainage territory of some DVAs.

DEVELOPMENTAL VENOUS ANOMALY

Terminology
- DVA; also known as venous "angioma"

Pathology
- Solitary > > multiple; small > large
- Enlarged white matter veins interspersed with normal brain
- Usually found adjacent to lateral or fourth ventricle

Clinical Issues
- Epidemiology and demographics
  - Most common cerebrovascular malformation (60%)
  - Prevalence on T1 C+ MR = 2-9%
  - All ages, no sex predilection

Natural History
- Usually benign, nonprogressive
- May hemorrhage if mixed with cavernous malformation or collector vein thromboses

Clinical Issues

Epidemiology. DVA is the most common intracranial vascular malformation, accounting for 60% of all CVMs. Estimated prevalence on contrast-enhanced MR scans ranges from 2.5-9.0%.

Demographics. DVAs are found in patients of all ages without sex predilection.

Presentation. Most DVAs are discovered incidentally at autopsy or on imaging studies. A recent metaanalysis showed that 98% of all isolated DVAs are asymptomatic. Two percent present with hemorrhage or infarct, probably caused by stenosis or spontaneous thrombosis of the outlet collector vein.

DVAs may coexist with other vascular lesions that cause symptomatic intracranial hemorrhage. The most common "histologically mixed" CVM is a cavernous-venous malformation, found in 10-15% of patients with a DVA and is especially common in the posterior fossa. Occasionally a "triad" malformation that consists of cavernous, venous, and capillary components is identified.

DVAs may coexist with a **sinus pericranii**. Sinus pericranii is typically the cutaneous sign of an underlying venous anomaly. DVAs are also associated with hereditary hemorrhagic telangiectasia (HHT) (4% of cases) and **periorbital lymphatic/lymphaticovenous malformations**. Other reported associations include malformations of cortical development.

Natural History. Most DVAs remain asymptomatic. Longitudinal studies have demonstrated that incidentally

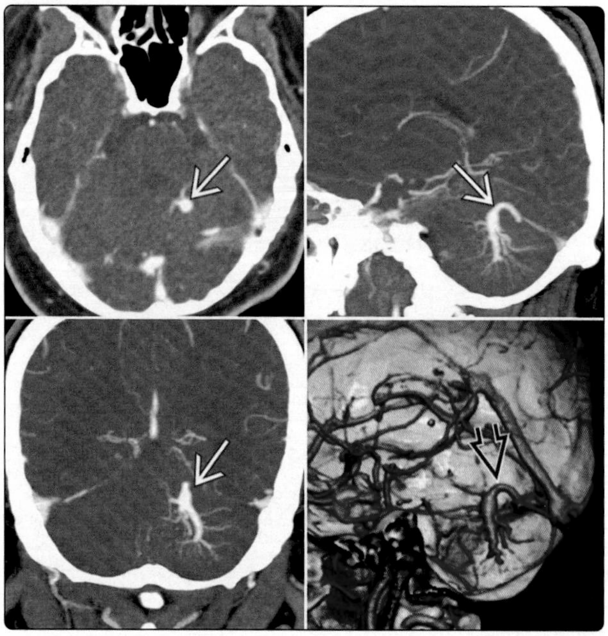

***(7-33)** Axial (upper left), sagittal (upper right), and coronal (lower left) CTA depict classic DVA in the left cerebellar hemisphere ➡. 3D rendering shows DVA ➩ and its relationship to other posterior fossa venous structures.*

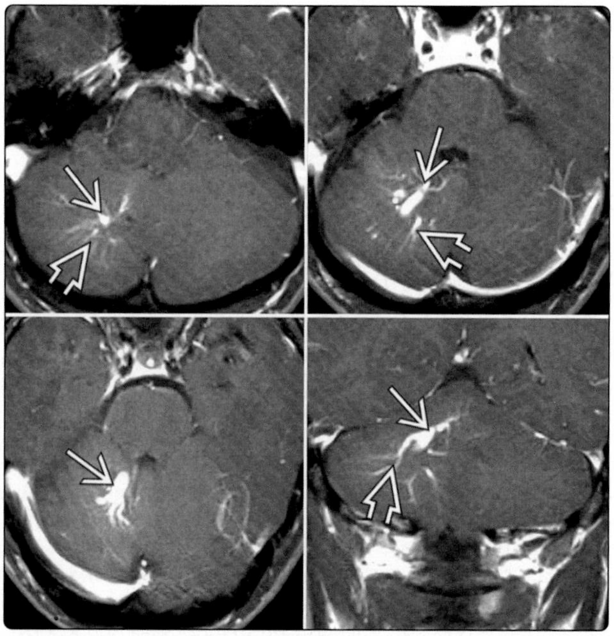

***(7-34)** T1 C+ MR scans show classic findings of DVA with enlarged white matter veins ➡ draining into a large collector vein ➩. This was an incidental finding in an asymptomatic patient.*

discovered DVAs had zero symptomatic hemorrhages or infarcts in nearly 500 person-years of follow-up.

Approximately 6% of DVAs present with symptomatic hemorrhage. Most are mixed with a lesion that has an intrinsic tendency to hemorrhage (such as cavernous malformation).

Treatment Options. No treatment is required or recommended for solitary DVAs (they are "leave me alone!" lesions). If a DVA is histologically mixed, treatment is determined by the coexisting lesion. Preoperative identification of such mixed malformations is important, as ligating the collector vein or removing its tributaries may result in venous infarction.

Imaging

General Features. DVAs are composed of radially arranged medullary veins that converge on a transcortical or subependymal large collector vein. The classic appearance is that of a "Medusa head" or upside-down umbrella **(7-32)**.

CT Findings

NECT. NECT scans are usually normal unless the DVA is very large and a prominent draining vein is present. Unilateral basal ganglia calcification has been reported in the drainage territory of some deep DVAs.

CECT. CECT scans show numerous linear and/or punctate enhancing foci that converge on a well-delineated tubular collector vein **(7-33)**. In larger DVAs, perfusion CT may show a venous congestion pattern with increased CBV, CBF, and MTT in the adjacent brain parenchyma.

MR Findings. If the DVA is small, it may be undetectable unless contrast-enhanced scans or susceptibility-weighted sequences are obtained.

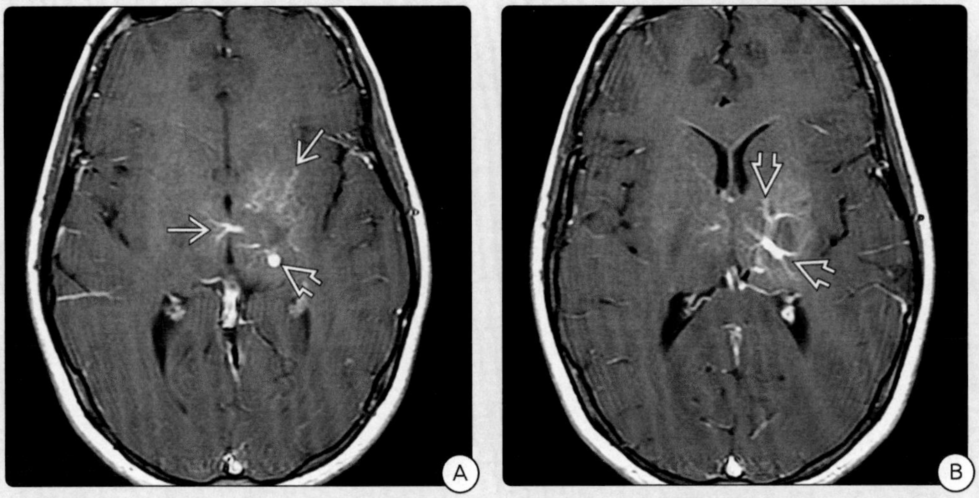

(7-35A) T1 C+ FS in a 30y woman with headaches shows a very large DVA ➡ in the left thalamus with a numerous dilated deep veins ➡ emptying into a collector vein. (7-35B) More cephalad T1 C+ FS scan shows that the large DVA consists of several larger "collector veins" ➡ that drain most of the thalamus. This was an incidental finding; the patient's neurologic examination was normal.

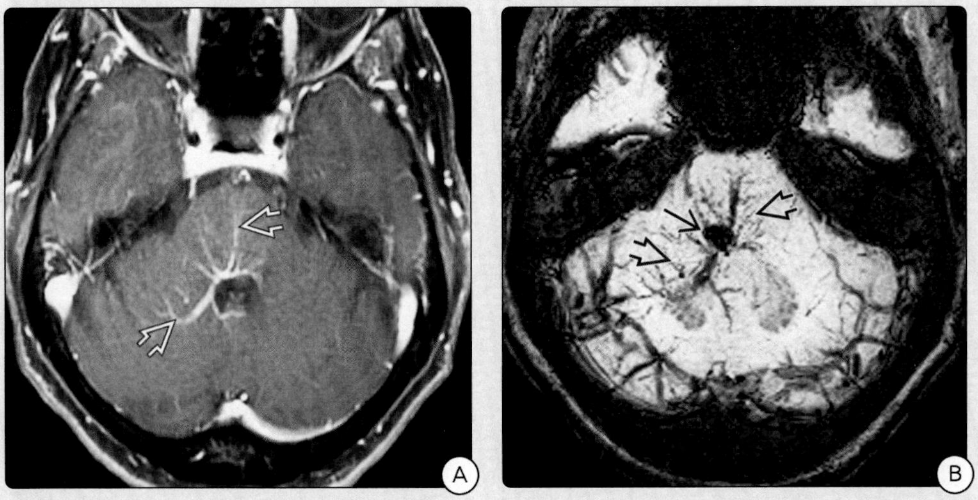

(7-36A) T1 C+ FS MR in a 55y man with sudden onset of right CN VI, CN VII palsies shows a classic DVA ➡ adjacent to the fourth ventricle. (7-36B) T2* SWI shows the hypointense DVA ⇨. In addition, a small focal hematoma ⇨ from a cavernous malformation in the floor of the fourth ventricle is identified; the hematoma is probably responsible for the patient's symptoms.

(7-37A) Axial NECT in a 30y man with sudden-onset left-sided weakness shows a hyperdense lesion with a fluid-fluid level surrounded by peripheral edema. (7-37B) T1WI in the same case shows multiple locules with mixed signal intensity, subacute hemorrhage with fluid-fluid levels.

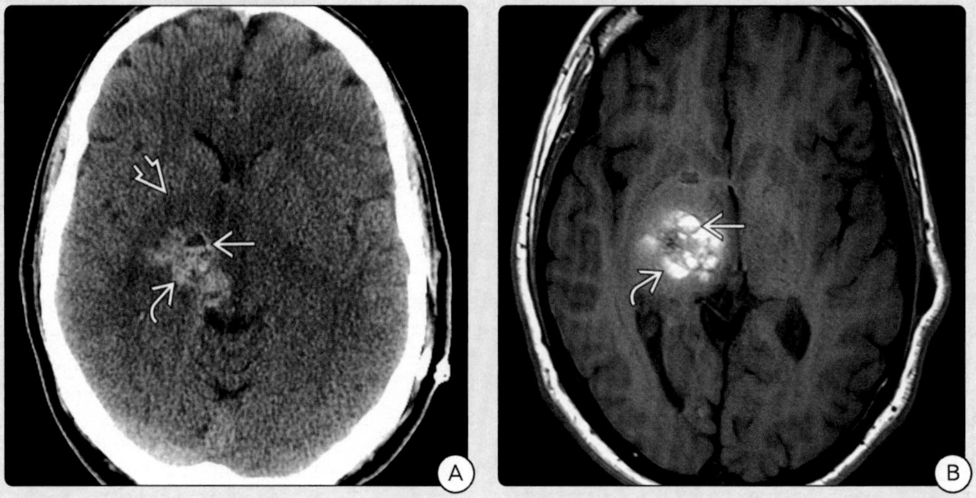

(7-37C) T2WI in the same case shows rings of dark hemosiderin staining around the locules, which contain fluid-fluid levels. A second subtle lesion is present in the right occipital lobe. (7-37D) T1 C+ FS in the same case shows some enhancement around the loculated mass. In addition, multiple enlarged venous channels are present.

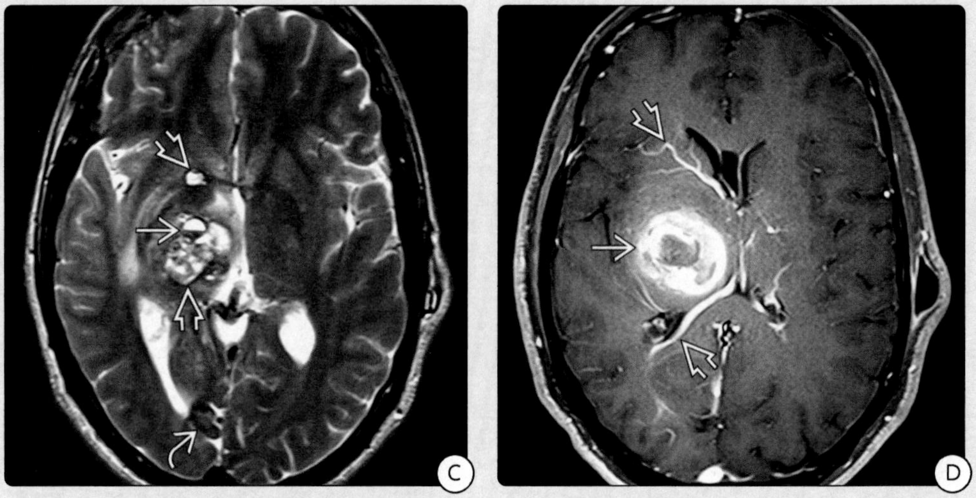

(7-37E) T2 SWI in the same case shows the mass with subacute hemorrhage blooms. The enlarged venous channels associated with the mass contain deoxygenated blood. In addition, a separate mass is present in the right occipital pole. (7-37F) Lateral DSA shows multiple "Medusa heads". These are multiple giant DVAs associated with cavernous malformations.*

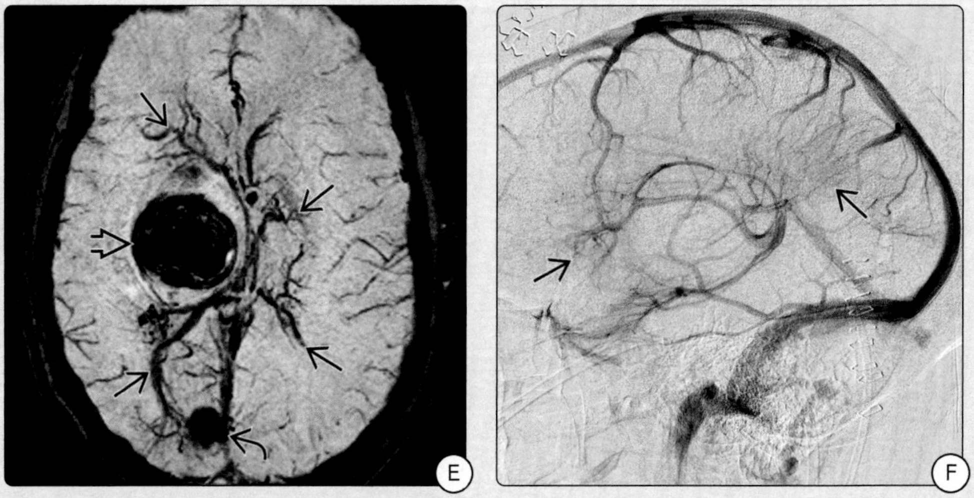

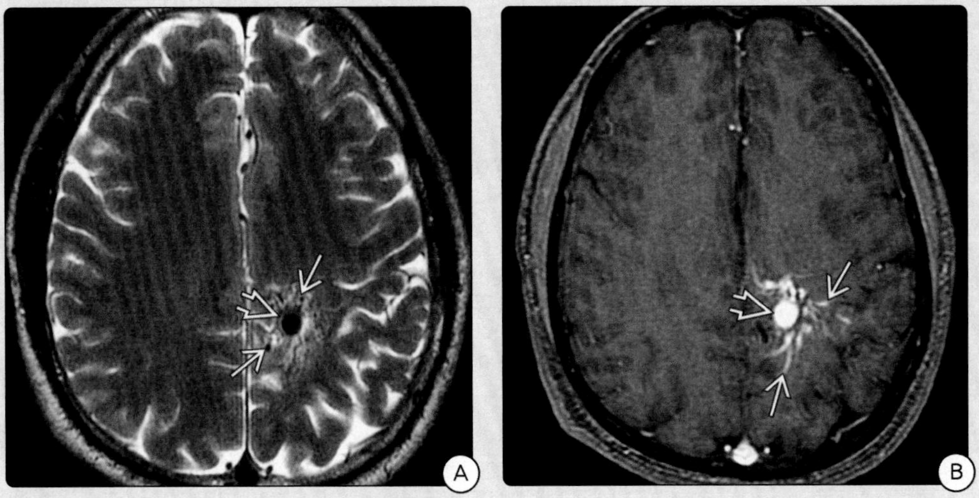

***(7-38A)** Series of images illustrates complex DVA in a 34y man. Here an axial T2WI shows a large "flow void" in the middle of many smaller, more tortuous-appearing vessels. **(7-38B)** T1 C+ FS shows an intensely enhancing, well-delineated central vessel surrounded by a cluster of linear enhancing foci.*

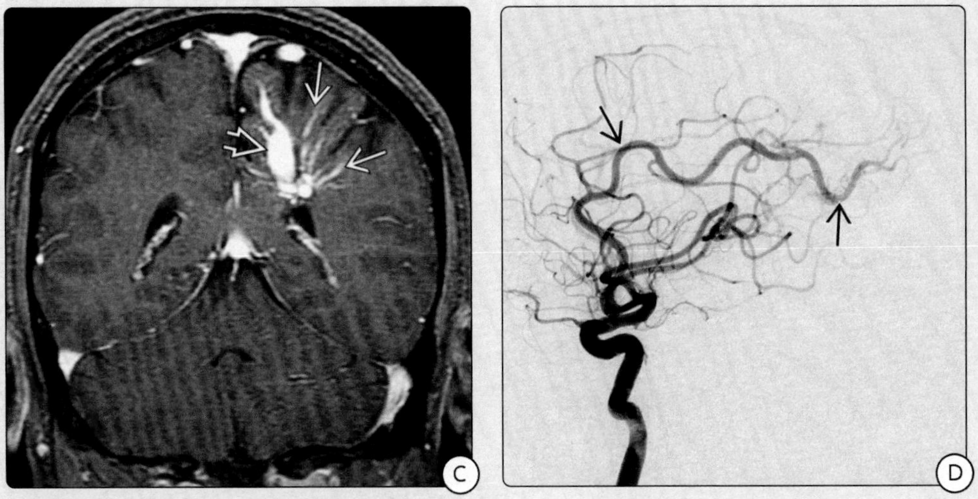

***(7-38C)** Coronal T1 C+ FS shows a "Medusa head" of enlarged white matter veins draining into a large "collector" vein. **(7-38D)** Lateral DSA, early arterial phase, shows a markedly enlarged pericallosal branch of the left anterior cerebral artery.*

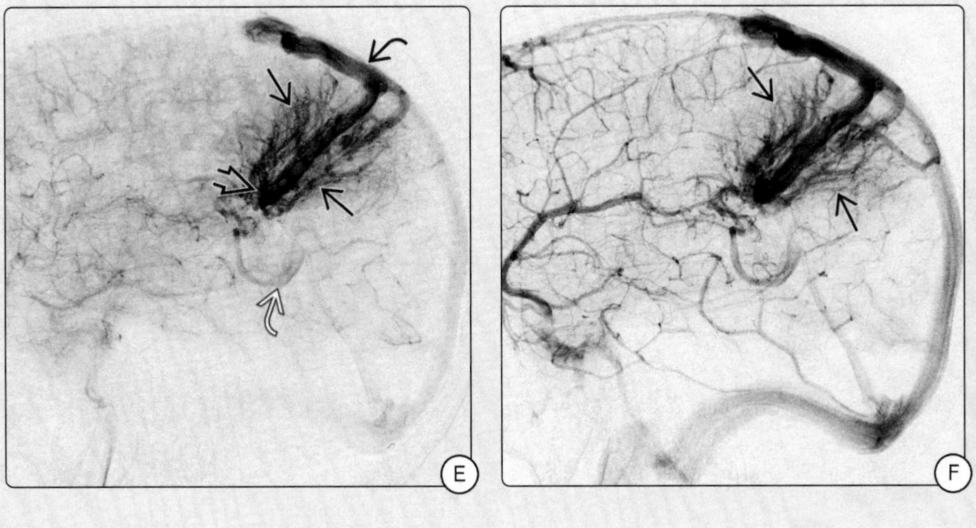

***(7-38E)** Lateral DSA, late arterial phase, shows a giant "Medusa head" blush of enlarged medullary veins draining into a dilated transmantle collector vein. Note A-V shunting with early draining vein of Galen and SSS. **(7-38F)** Venous phase of the DSA shows the giant DVA. This is a "complex DVA" with enlarged arterial feeders and A-V shunting with early draining veins. There is no "nidus" to suggest AVM.*

T2/FLAIR. Large DVAs can exhibit a "flow void" on T2WI. Venous radicles of the caput medusa are often hyperintense on FLAIR. T2/FLAIR parenchymal abnormalities are present in up to 11% of children and 25% of adults with DVAs **(7-39)**. The etiology of such associated hyperintensities is unknown but could represent gliosis, venous congestion or ischemia, demyelination or hypomyelination.

T2* (GRE, SWI). Because flow in the venous radicles of a DVA is typically slow, blood deoxygenates and T2* scans (GRE, SWI) show striking linear hypointensities **(7-36)**.

If a DVA is mixed with a cavernous malformation, blood products in various stages of degradation may be present and "bloom" on T2* sequences **(7-37)**. Discrete hypointense foci on 3T SWI are seen in the majority of cases, especially in DVAs that are associated with parenchymal hyperintensities on FLAIR. Venous congestion in a DVA may result in microhemorrhages or possibly promote the formation of small cavernous malformations.

T1 C+. T1 C+ sequences show a stellate collection of linear enhancing structures converging on the transparenchymal or subependymal collector vein **(7-35)** **(7-36)** **(7-39)**. The collector vein may show variable high-velocity signal loss.

pMR. DSC pMR is usually normal in small DVAs. Elevated CBV and CBF with mildly increased MTT are common within larger DVAs. Capillary perfusion as measured with arterial spin labeling is usually normal.

Angiography. The arterial phase is normal. The venous phase shows the typical hair-like collection ("Medusa head") of dilated medullary veins within the white matter **(7-37F)**. A faint, prolonged "blush" or capillary "stain" may be present in some cases.

Transitional forms of venous-arteriovenous malformation with enlarged feeders and a caput medusa that blushes during the arterial phase and AV shunting ("early draining" vein) have

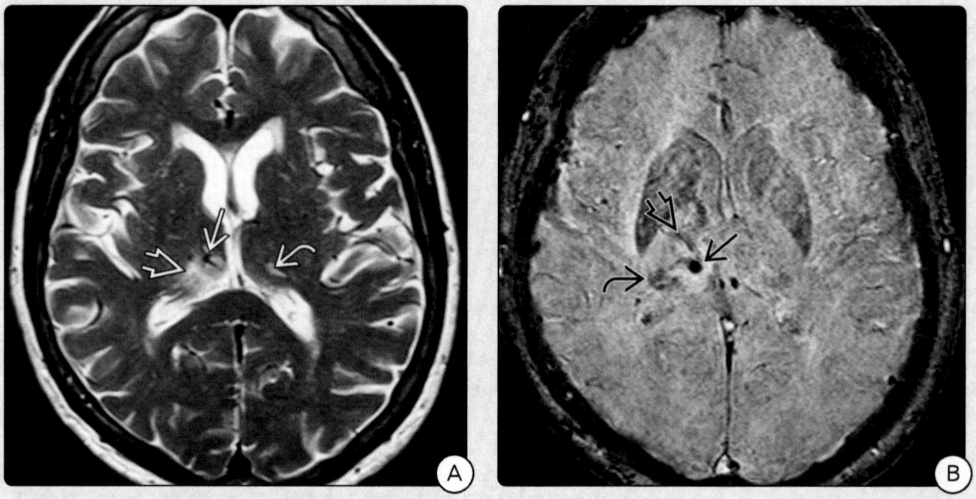

(7-39A) Axial T2WI in an 82y woman with a history of systemic atherosclerotic disease and cerebral lacunar infarcts shows a confluent hyperintensity in the pulvinar of the right thalamus. A branching "flow void" is present in the medial aspect of the lesion. (7-39B) T2* SWI in the same case shows a prominent "flow void" in the center of the hyperintensity. Ill-defined patchy and linear hypointensities are present in the lesion.

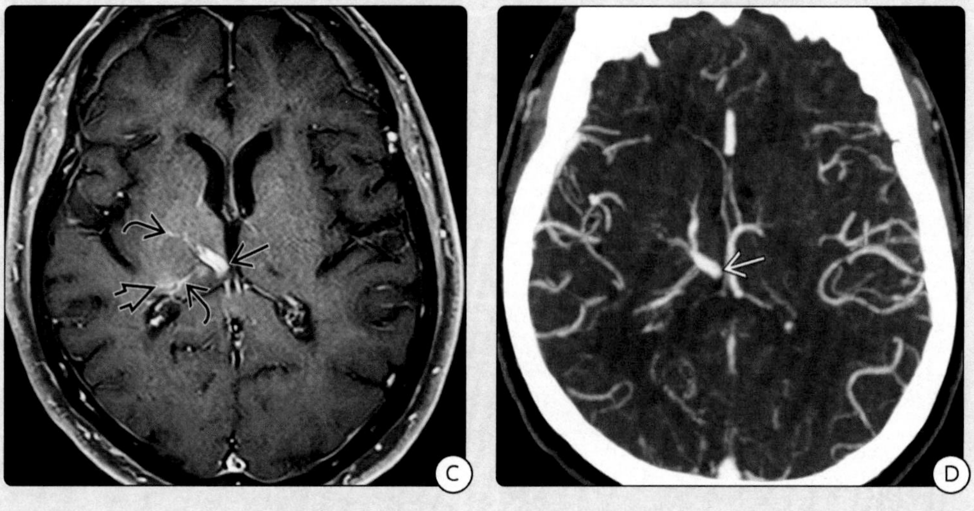

(7-39C) T1 C+ FS in the same case shows a large tubular enhancing structure in the medial thalamus. Linear and "brush-like" areas of enhancement drain into the dilated vessel. (7-39D) MIP of CTA in the same case shows the underlying vascular lesion is a large, complex thalamic DVA . Areas of T2/FLAIR hyperintensity may be due to venous congestion/ischemia.

been described but are uncommon **(7-38A)**. Rarely, a true venous varix or sinus pericranii may occur with a DVA.

Nuclear Medicine Studies. More than three-quarters of DVAs are associated with hypometabolism in the adjacent brain parenchyma on FDG-PET studies, often in the absence of any other structural abnormalities. There is a strong association between the degree of DVA-associated hypometabolism and increasing age, suggesting that DVAs may result in cumulative brain parenchymal injury. Rarely, DVAs exhibit increased uptake on 11C-methionine PET-CT, mimicking neoplasm.

Differential Diagnosis

A histologically-mixed vascular malformation in which the DVA provides prominent venous drainage is common. The most common combination is a mixed cavernous-venous malformation. Unusually large ("giant") **capillary telangiectasias** often have a dominant central collector vein and may therefore resemble a DVA.

DEVELOPMENTAL VENOUS ANOMALY: IMAGING

MR
- T2/FLAIR
  - Collector vein = flow void on T2WI
  - Radicles of "Medusa head" hyperintense on FLAIR
  - 10-25% have T2/FLAIR parenchymal hyperintensities
- T2* (GRE/SWI)
  - Linear hypointensities in radicles, collector vein
  - Blooming foci if mixed with CCM
  - 3T SWI may show microbleeds
- T1 C+
  - "Umbrella" of tubular radicles → collector vein
- pMR
  - ↑ CBV/CBF, increased MTT

DSA
- Classic "Medusa head" in venous phase

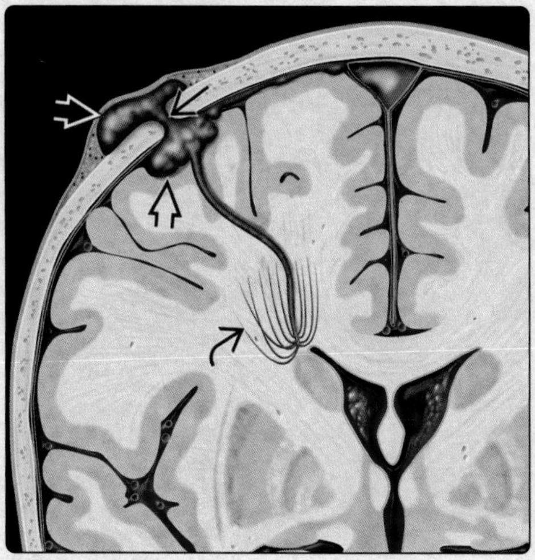

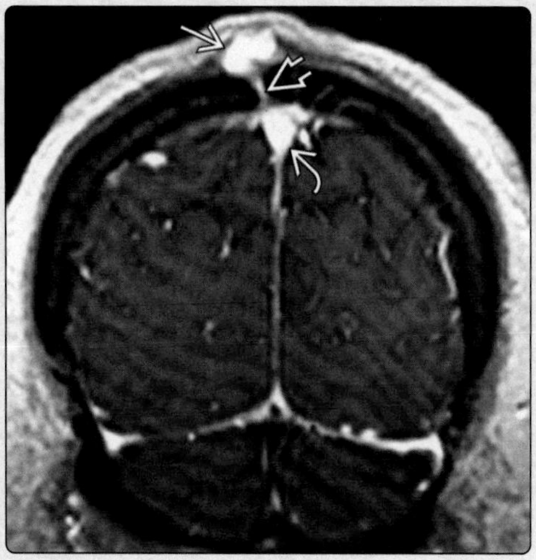

(7-40) Coronal graphic depicts a classic sinus pericranii (SP) with an expanded venous pouch under the scalp connecting to the intracranial venous system through a transcalvarial channel. Some SPs are associated with a DVA. (7-41) Coronal T1 C+ SPGR study shows classic SP. An extracranial venous pouch connects with the SSS via a transosseous vein.

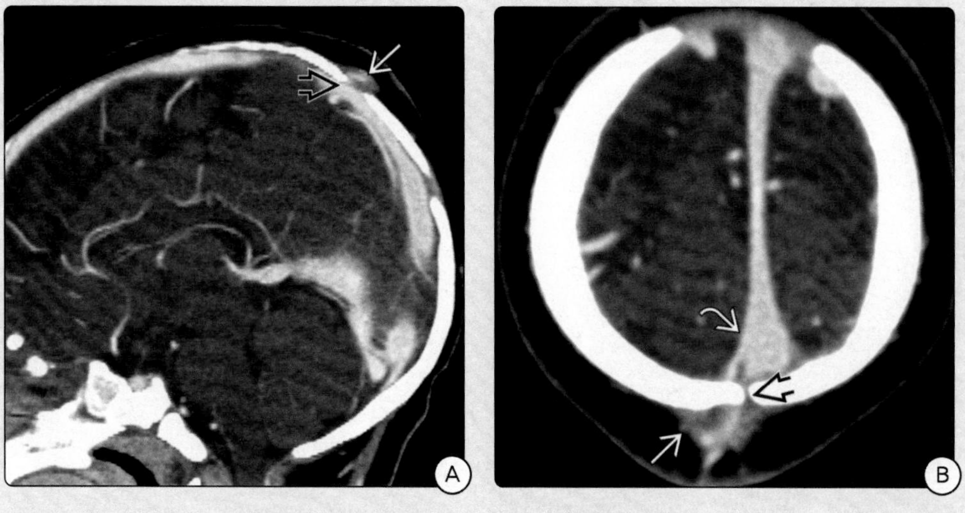

(7-42A) Sagittal CTV shows a small SP connecting to the SSS through an adjacent skull defect. (7-42B) Axial CT venogram in the same case shows that an enhancing extracranial scalp mass connects to the SSS via a channel passing through the skull defect.

Sinus Pericranii

Terminology

Sinus pericranii (SP) is a rare benign venous anomaly that consists of an emissary intradiploic vein that connects an intracranial dural venous sinus with an extracranial venous varix **(7-40)**. The dilated venous pouch hugs the external table of the skull. Some investigators consider SP the cutaneous manifestation of an intracranial developmental venous anomaly (DVA), as the two lesions are often—but not invariably—associated.

Etiology

SPs can be congenital or acquired, posttraumatic or spontaneous. A congenital origin of most SPs is likely, given their frequent association with DVAs and congenital mucocutaneous malformations, such as blue rubber bleb nevus syndrome **(BRBNS)**.

Other possible etiologies include incomplete sutural fusion over prominent abundant diploic or emissary veins, allowing aberrant communications between the epicranial and intracranial dural venous systems to develop.

Scalp laceration and skull fracture that disrupts emissary veins at the outer table of the calvaria may result in development of an acquired SP.

Pathology

A bluish sac beneath or just above the periosteum of the calvaria is typical. The dilated, blood-filled sac connects through an enlarged emissary vein with the intracranial circulation **(7-40)**. The frontal lobe is the most common site, followed by the parietal and occipital lobes. SPs in the middle and posterior cranial fossae are rare.

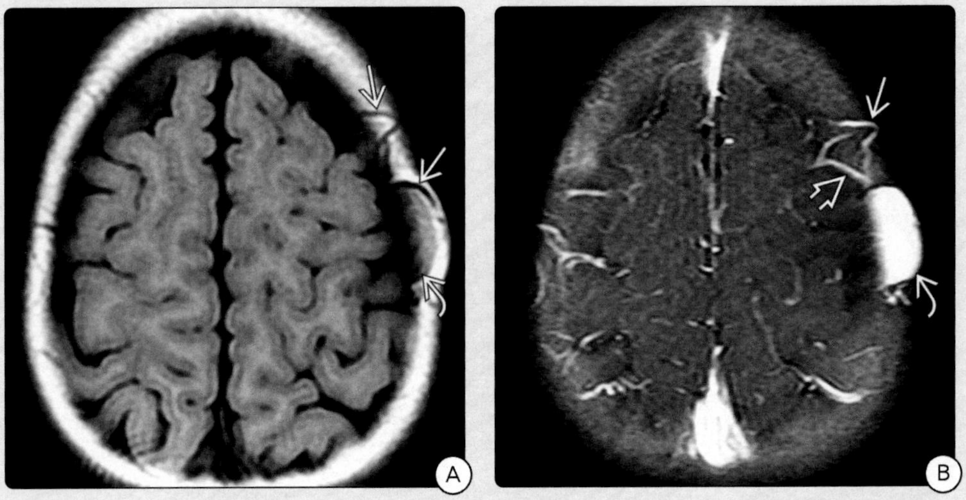

***(7-43A)** T1WI in a child with a soft scalp mass shows a well-delineated left posterior frontal subcutaneous mass ➡ associated with prominent scalp vessels ➡. **(7-43B)** T1 C+ FS in the same case shows the mass ➡ enhances intensely, uniformly. The adjacent scalp vessels ➡ communicate through the skull with intracranial cortical veins ➡.*

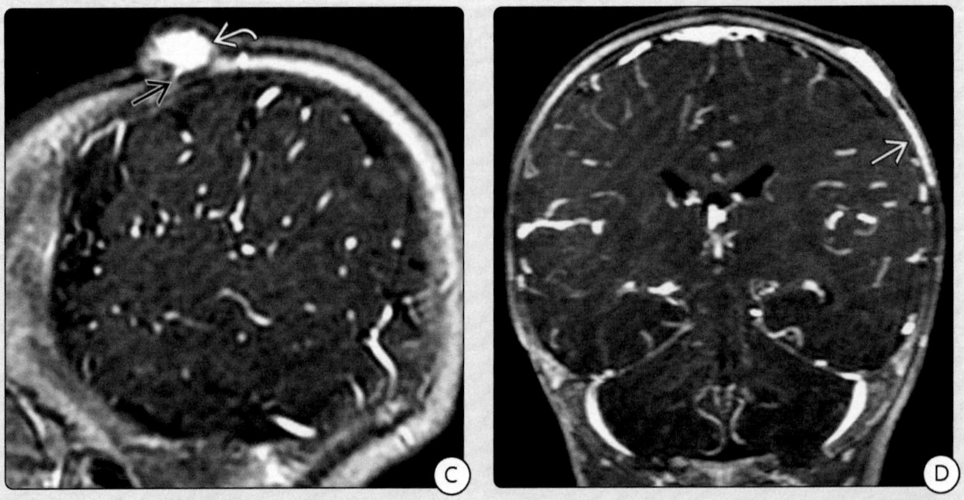

***(7-43C)** Sagittal contrast-enhanced SPGR shows that the enhancing subcutaneous vascular mass ➡ abuts the skull and communicates with the intracranial vasculature via a transosseous venous channel ➡. **(7-43D)** Coronal SPGR shows that prominent intradiploic venous channels ➡ also communicate with the vascular mass. This is SP.*

SP may be associated with single or multiple intracranial DVAs. Other reported associations include craniosynostosis and dural sinus hypoplasia. SP with multiple DVAs is associated with BRBNS.

Clinical Issues

Epidemiology. SPs are rare lesions, found in less than 10% of patients who present for treatment of craniofacial vascular malformations and 4% of patients with palpable scalp/cranial vault lesions.

Demographics. Although SPs can occur at any age, most are found in children or young adults. There is no sex predilection.

Presentation. A nontender, nonpulsatile somewhat bluish compressible scalp mass that increases with Valsalva maneuver and reduces in the upright position is typical. A history of "forgotten trauma" is not uncommon. Other than their cosmetic effect, most SPs are asymptomatic.

Natural History. If left alone, most SPs behave benignly and remain stable in size. There is a very small lifetime risk of air embolism or hemorrhage from direct trauma to the SP.

Treatment Options. Patients with SP may be referred to dermatologists because of discoloration in the scalp or forehead. Surgical removal of the extracranial component with cranioplasty is occasionally performed for cosmetic purposes. Surgery without adequate imaging may result in potentially lethal complications including hemorrhage, venous infarction (if the SP is associated with a DVA), and air embolism.

Imaging

General Features. A vascular or subperiosteal scalp mass overlies a well-defined bone defect. The mass communicates directly with the intracranial venous system through the bony defect **(7-41)**.

CT Findings. An SP is iso- or hyperdense on NECT and shows strong uniform enhancement after contrast administration **(7-42)**. The underlying calvarial defect varies in size but is typically well demarcated. Occasionally, an SP may contain calcifications (phleboliths) or thrombi.

In some cases, multiple anastomotic venous connections can course within the diploic space for several centimeters, causing extensive skull erosion.

MR Findings. Most SPs are isointense on T1WI **(7-43A)** and hyperintense to brain on T2WI. "Puddling" of contrast within the SP on T1 C+ is typical unless the lesion is unusually large and flow is rapid **(7-43)**. MRV is helpful in delineating both the intra- and extracranial components.

Angiography. The arterial and capillary phases are normal. Most SPs are visualized only on the very late venous phase. They are seen as well-defined rounded pools of contrast that slowly accumulate within and adjacent to the skull defect containing the transcalvarial vein.

Flow in SPs is variable. DSA is crucial in distinguishing between two basic patterns, each with different management implications. Dominant or "drainer" SP is present if the SP is used to drain the brain into the venous pouch and adjacent pericranial scalp veins, bypassing the usual venous outlets. If only a small part of the venous outflow occurs through the extradiploic vessels, the SP has an accessory drainage pattern. Whereas an accessory-type SP can generally be treated safely, incidental or iatrogenic closure of a dominant-type SP can result in intracranial hypertension, cerebral hemorrhage, and even death.

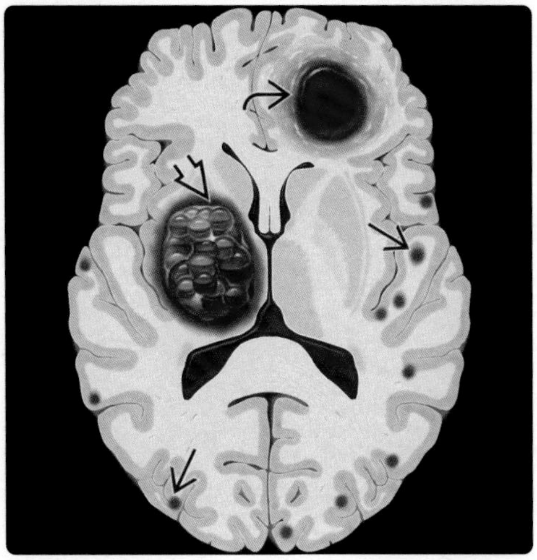

***(7-44)** Note subacute ➲, classic "popcorn ball" ➲ appearances of CCMs. Microhemorrhages are seen as multifocal "blooming black dots" ➲.*

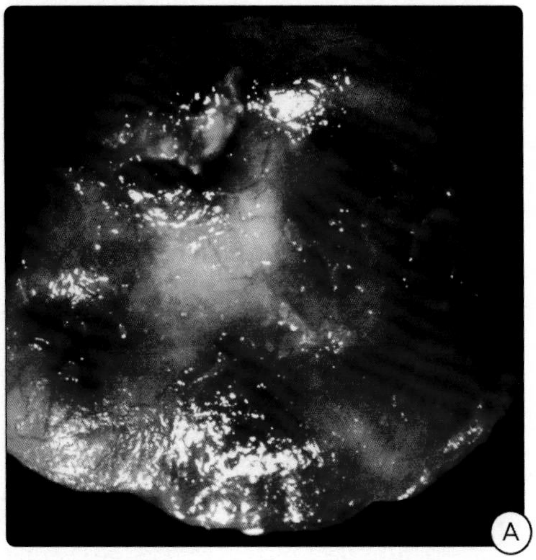

***(7-45A)** Resected surgical specimen of CCM shows the typical well-circumscribed, lobulated, berry-like appearance.*

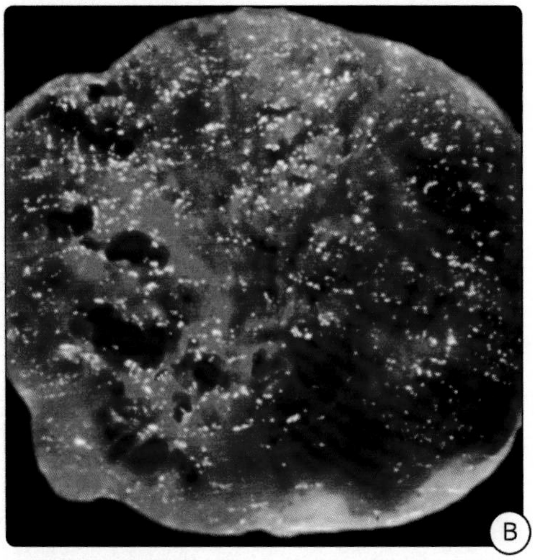

***(7-45B)** Cut section shows multiple locules of blood in various stages of evolution.*

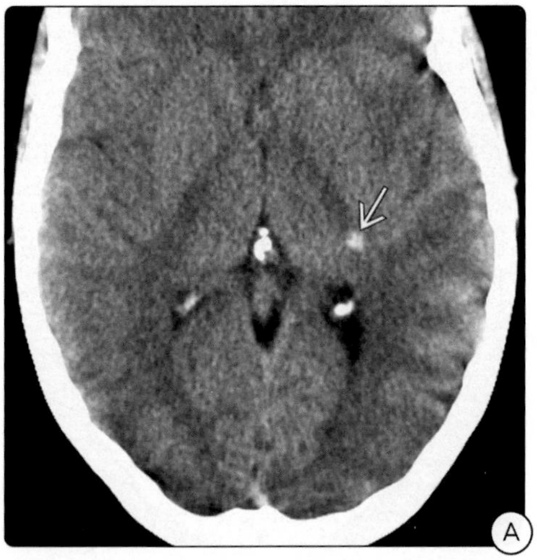

(7-46A) NECT in a patient with family history of CCM shows punctate hyperdense lesion in the posterior limb of the left internal capsule ➡.

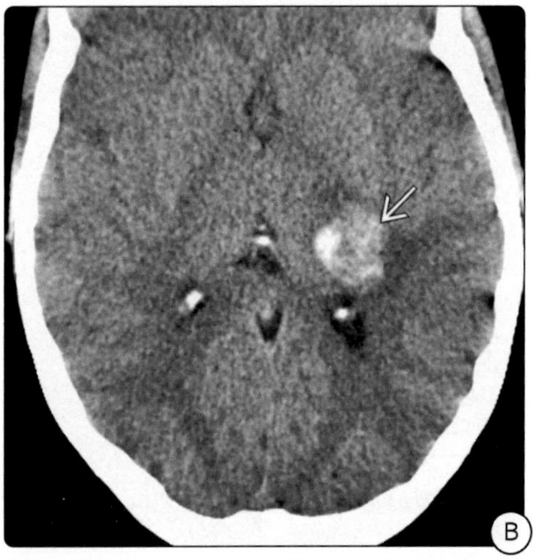

(7-46B) NECT scan obtained 6 years later when the patient developed acute right hemiparesis shows that the lesion ➡ has markedly enlarged.

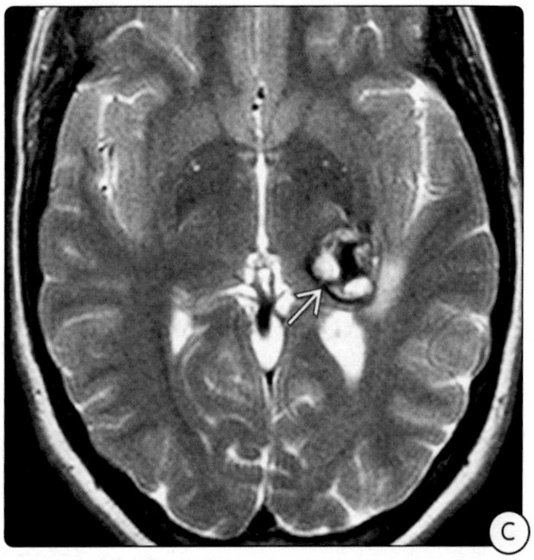

(7-46C) T2WI shows "popcorn ball" appearance of type II CCM. Blood locules in different stages are surrounded by hemosiderin rim ➡.

Ultrasound. Color Doppler may delineate the extracranial component and define flow direction. US does not define the intracranial component of an SP.

Differential Diagnosis

The imaging findings of SP are diagnostic. Other scalp and calvarial masses of infancy and childhood include **cephalocele**, **dermoid cyst**, **hemangioma**, **histiocytosis**,and **metastasis (neuroblastoma)**. In middle-aged and older adults, the most common scalp mass is a **sebaceous (trichilemmal) cyst**.

Cerebral Cavernous Malformation

Cerebral cavernous malformations (CCMs) are a distinct type of intracranial vascular malformation characterized by repeated "intralesional" hemorrhages into thin-walled, angiogenically immature, blood-filled locules called "caverns." CCMs are discrete, well-marginated lesions that do not contain normal brain parenchyma. Most are surrounded by a complete hemosiderin rim **(7-44)**.

Prior to the advent of CT and MR, cavernous malformations were sometimes called "occult" vascular malformations ("occult" to angiography, as they are extremely low-flow lesions that do not exhibit arteriovenous shunting). These lesions are now easily identified on MR and hence are no longer "occult" to imaging. Cavernous malformations exhibit a wide range of dynamic behaviors. They are a relatively common cause of spontaneous nontraumatic intracranial hemorrhage in young and middle-aged adults, although they can occur at any age.

Terminology

CCMs are also known as cavernous "angiomas" or "cavernomas." They are benign malformative vascular hamartomas. CCMs are sometimes erroneously referred to as "cavernous hemangiomas." Hemangiomas are benign vascular neoplasms, not malformations.

Etiology

General Concepts. CCMs are angiogenically immature lesions with endothelial proliferation and increased neoangiogenesis.

CCMs can be inherited or acquired. Acquired CCMs are rare and usually associated with prior radiation therapy (XRT). Approximately 3.5% of children who have whole-brain XRT develop multiple CCMs, with a mean latency interval of approximately 3 years (3-102 months).

Genetics. CCMs can be solitary and sporadic (80% of cases) or multiple and familial (20%). Familial CCMs are inherited as an autosomal-dominant disease with variable penetrance.

Three independent genes have been identified in familial CCMs: *CCM1* (KRIT1), *CCM2* (OSM), and *CCM3* (PDCD10). Endothelium-specific loss-of-function mutations in these genes account for 70-80% of all familial cases. Between 5-15% of familial CCM cases remain genetically unexplained.

CCM1 is a pivotal inhibitor of sprouting angiogenesis and is necessary to keep vascular endothelium quiescent. Biallelic loss of a CCM gene allowing uncontrolled sprouting angiogenesis may explain the chaotic vascular architecture and dynamic progression of CCMs.

Upregulation of *KLF4* (a transcription factor of the Kruppel-like factor Family) has been identified as the key initial event in CCM lesion formation. *KLF4* regulates different vascular functions such as angiogenesis and vascular permeability and is a master regulator of endothelial to mesenchymal transition, a key factor in the development and progression of both familial and sporadic CCM lesions.

Associated Abnormalities. CCMs are the most common component in mixed vascular malformations. Cavernous-venous and cavernous-capillary are the two most frequent combinations.

Pathology

Location and Size. CCMs can occur anywhere in the CNS and range in size from tiny, near-microscopic lesions to giant malformations that can occupy an entire lobe or most of the cerebral hemisphere.

Gross Pathology. A compact, spongy collection of reddish-purple blood-filled "caverns" devoid of intervening neural elements is typical **(7-45)**. Most CCMs are surrounded by a rust-colored rim of gliotic, indurated brain.

Microscopic Features. CCMs consist of tightly packed epithelium-lined vascular channels ("caverns") in a collagenous stroma. These endothelial cells are undergoing endothelial to mesenchymal transition, a key factor in the development of cavernous malformations.

Vessels within the caverns typically lack elastic tissue and usually have thin walls but may become thickened and hyalinized. Some channels are partly or completely thrombosed and contain hemorrhage in different stages of evolution. A gliotic, hemosiderin-stained rim surrounds the lesion.

CCMs do not contain brain parenchyma, but the surrounding brain often shows reactive changes and hemosiderin deposition. Dystrophic calcifications are common within CCMs.

Staging, Grading, and Classification. The most commonly used classification of CCMs, the Zabramski classification, is

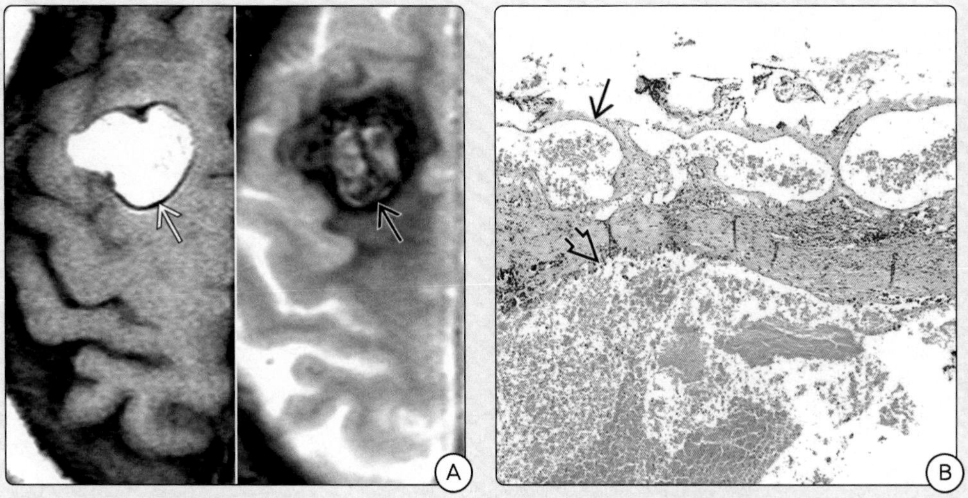

***(7-47A)** Zabramski type I CCM is illustrated. (L) T1WI shows that the lesion is hyperintense and surrounded by a hypointense hemosiderin rim ➡. (R) T2* GRE scan shows "blooming" hypointensity both around ➡ and within the lesion. **(7-47B)** Microscopic section from the resected specimen in the same case shows a blood-filled cavity ➡ surrounded by thin endothelium-lined vascular channels ➡. (Courtesy R. Hewlett, MD.)*

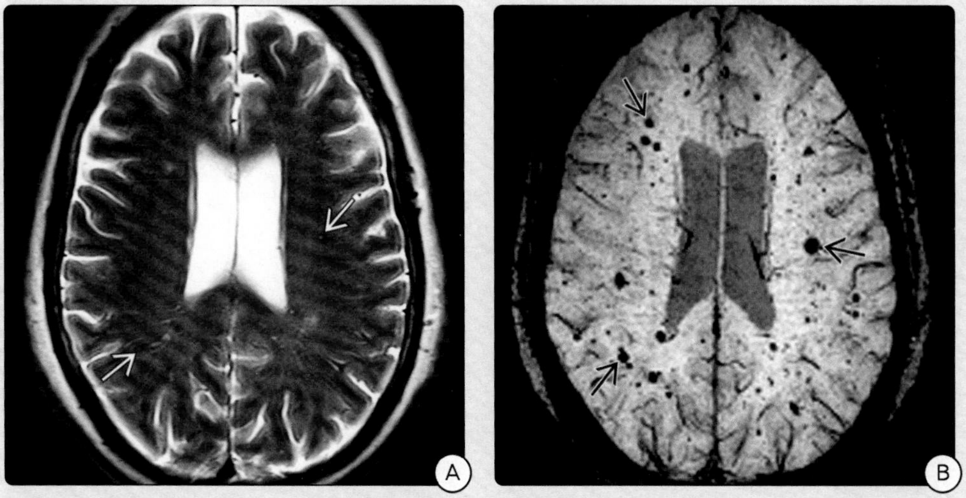

***(7-48A)** Axial FSE T2WI in a 70y Hispanic woman shows a few scattered faint hypointensities ➡ in the coronal radiata. **(7-48B)** MIP of T2* SWI in the same case shows innumerable blooming hypointensities ➡. These are Zabramski type IV CCMs.*

based on imaging appearance, not histologic findings (see shaded box on page 190).

Clinical Issues

Epidemiology. CCMs are the third most common cerebral vascular malformation (after DVA and capillary telangiectasia) and are found in approximately 0.5% of the population. Two-thirds occur as a solitary, sporadic lesion; approximately one-third are multiple.

Demographics. CCMs may occur at any age; they cause 10% of spontaneous brain hemorrhages in children. The imaging prevalence of CCMs increases with advancing age. Peak presentation is 40-60 years (younger in the familial multiple cavernous malformation syndrome). There is no sex predilection.

Multiple CCM syndrome is more common in Hispanic-Americans of Mexican descent. Over 90% of individuals with a positive family history have a *KRIT1* mutation and will develop one or more CCMs.

Presentation. Half of all patients with CCMs present with seizures. Headache and focal neurologic deficits are also common. Small lesions, especially microhemorrhages, may be asymptomatic.

Natural History. CCMs have a broad range of dynamic behavior, and the clinical course of individual lesions is both highly variable and unpredictable. Repeated spontaneous intralesional hemorrhages are typical. There is a distinct propensity for lesion growth in all patients. Patients with multiple CCM syndrome typically continue to develop de novo lesions throughout their lives.

Hemorrhage risk with solitary lesions is estimated at 0.25-0.75% per year, cumulative, and is greater for women. In the familial multiple CCM form, hemorrhage risk is much higher, approaching 1-5% cumulative risk per lesion per year.

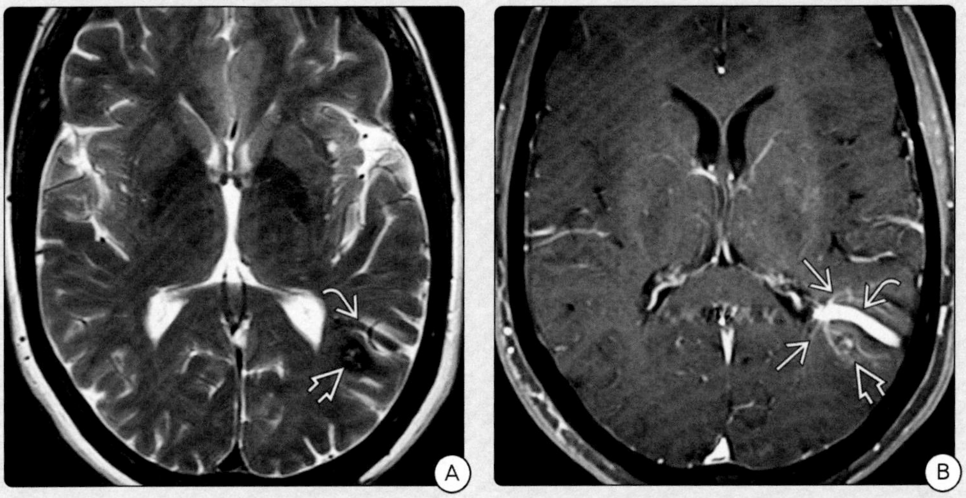

***(7-49A)** Axial T2WI in a 50y woman with seizures shows a mixed-intensity left parietal mass surrounded by a complete hemosiderin rim. A large tubular structure is seen in the adjacent sulcus. **(7-49B)** T1 C+ FS in the same case shows mild central stippled enhancement in the lesion. The tubular structure enhances strongly and has several well-defined linear tributaries that drain into it.*

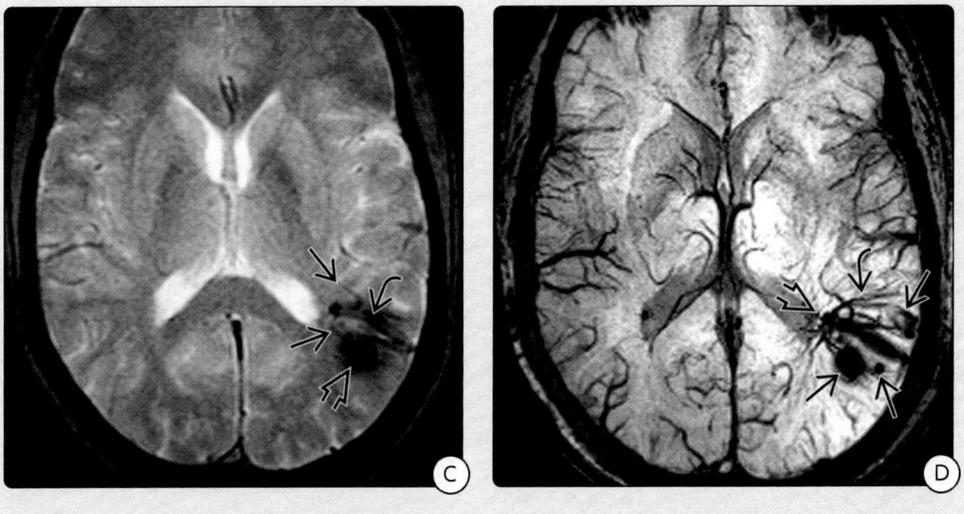

***(7-49C)** T2* GRE scan in the same case shows "blooming" around the area of hemosiderin staining. The tubular structure and its tributaries appear hypointense. **(7-49D)** MIP of T2* SWI in the same case shows three separate foci of blooming hypointensity. The DVA with its collector vein and dilated venous tributaries is well seen. This is a cavernous-venous vascular malformation, the most common mixed combination in the CNS.*

Hemorrhage rates also vary with imaging appearance based on the Zabramski classification (see below). Zabramski type I and II CCMs have a significantly higher hemorrhage rate than types III and IV.

The presence of acute or subacute blood-degradation products on MR (Zabramski I, II) is the strongest indicator for an increased risk of hemorrhage (mean annual hemorrhage rate of 20-25% vs. 3-4% without signs of acute or subacute blood). "Dot-sized" CCMs on T2* (GRE or SWI) that are invisible or barely visible on T1WIs and T2WIs (Zabramski type IV) have the lowest mean annual hemorrhage rate (1%).

Treatment Options. The management of deep-seated CCMs in critical locations is controversial. At present, total surgical removal via microsurgical resection is the treatment of choice for symptomatic lesions with recurrent hemorrhages. Stereotactic radiosurgery has been used with some success in patients with CCMs in critical locations such as the brainstem that are not amenable to microsurgery.

CEREBRAL CAVERNOUS MALFORMATIONS

Etiology
- *CCM1*, *CCM2*, or *CCM3* mutations in familial CCM
- Negative inhibition of sprouting angiogenesis lost

Pathology
- Occur throughout CNS
- Solitary (2/3), multiple (1/3, familial)
- Multiple thin-walled blood-filled locules ("caverns")
- No normal brain inside; hemosiderin rim outside

Clinical Issues
- Can present at any age; peak = 40-60 years
- Course variable, unpredictable
  - Repeated intralesional hemorrhages typical
  - Hemorrhage risk = 0.25-0.75% per lesion per year
  - Higher risk, de novo lesions in familial CCM

Imaging

General Features. CCMs occur throughout the CNS. The brain parenchyma is the most common site. A well-circumscribed mixed density/signal intensity mass surrounded by a complete hemosiderin rim ("popcorn ball") is the classic finding. CCMs can vary from microscopic to giant (more than 6 cm) lesions. In rare circumstances, a CCM (often mixed with venous malformations) may occupy an entire lobe of the brain.

CT Findings. NECT scans are often normal, as many CCMs are too small to be detected. Larger lesions appear hyperdense **(7-46A)** with or without scattered intralesional calcifications. Most CCMs are well delineated and do not exhibit mass effect unless there is recent hemorrhage **(7-46B)**. Adrenal calcifications are common in patients with familial CCM and may be a clinically silent manifestation of disease.

MR Findings. Findings are variable, depending on the stage of evolution and pulse sequence utilized. CCMs have been divided into four types based on imaging appearance (Zabramski classification).

The classic CCM (Zabramski type II) is a discrete reticulated or "popcorn ball" lesion caused by blood products contained within variably sized "caverns" or "locules." Fluid-fluid levels of differing signal intensities are common **(7-46C)**. The mixed signal core is surrounded by a complete hemosiderin rim on T2WI that "blooms" on T2* sequences. CCMs with subacute hemorrhage

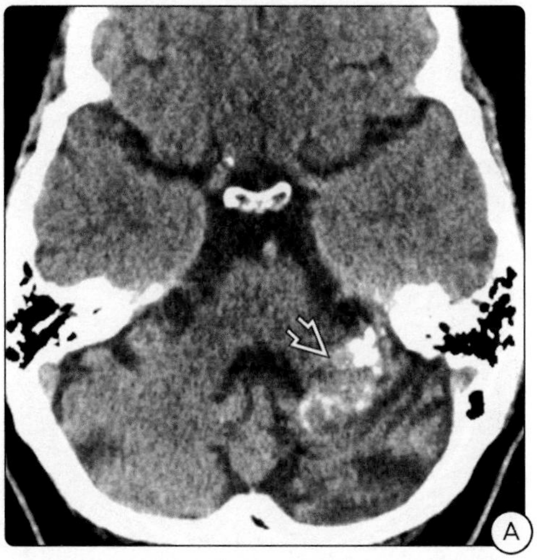

***(7-50A)** NECT scan shows a hyperdense, partially calcified mass ➡ in a moderately atrophic left cerebellar hemisphere.*

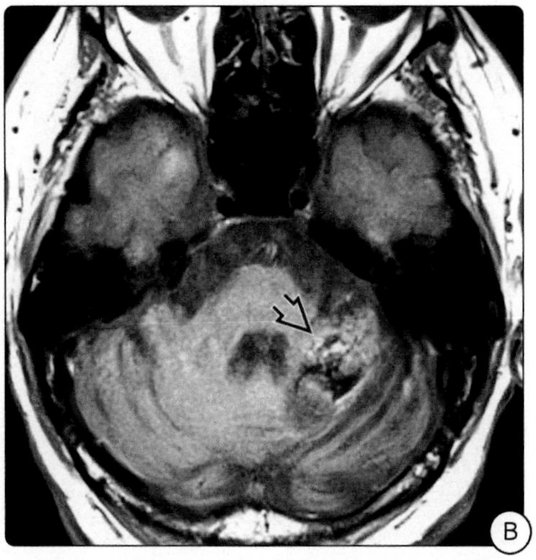

***(7-50B)** Axial T1WI in the same case shows mixed hyperdense and isodense signal within the mass ➡.*

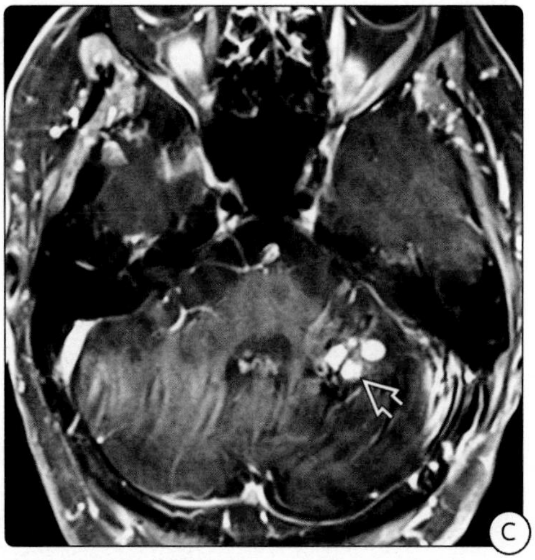

***(7-50C)** T1 C+ FS in the same case shows strong enhancement ➡ within the internal caverns of this variant CCM.*

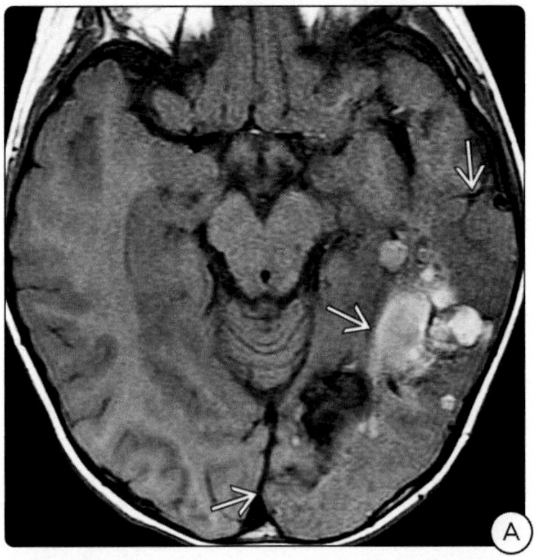

(7-51A) *Axial T1WI shows mixed signal-intensity lesion occupying most of the posterior temporal/occipital lobes.*

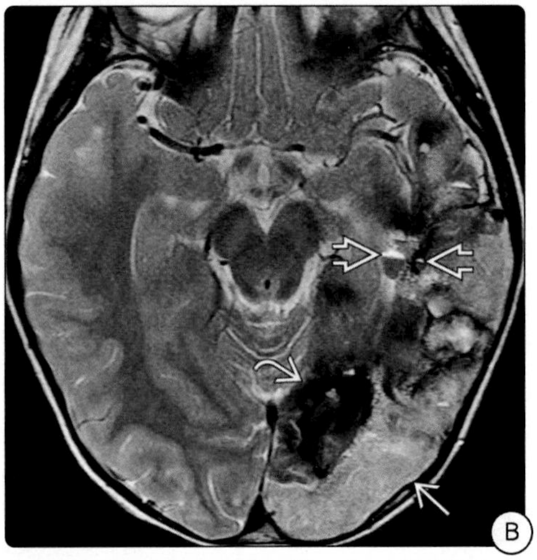

(7-51B) *T2WI shows several locules with fluid-fluid levels and areas of parenchymal hyper- and hypointensity.*

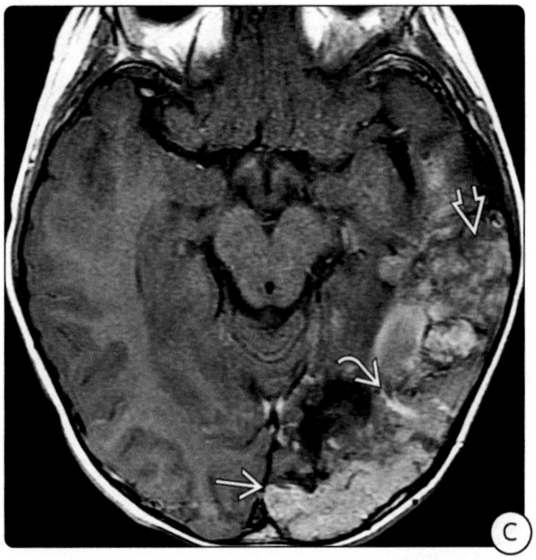

(7-51C) *T1 C+ shows diffuse, patchy enhancement, large vein; giant capillary-cavernous venous malformation. (W. Fang, MD.)*

(Zabramski type I) are hyperintense on T1WI and mixed hyper-/hypointense on T2WI **(7-47)**.

T2* scans (GRE, SWI) should always be performed to look for additional lesions. Punctate microhemorrhages are seen as multifocal "blooming black dots" (Zabramski type IV) in many cases with familial CCM **(7-48)**.

Enhancement following contrast administration varies from none (the usual finding) to mild or moderate **(7-50)**. If a CCM coexists with a DVA, the venous "angioma" may show strong enhancement **(7-49)**. If such a histologically "mixed" vascular malformation is resected, the venous drainage must be preserved to avoid postoperative venous infarction.

Some studies have demonstrated a higher prevalence of abnormal white matter hyperintensities in familial *CCM1* carriers that are spatially distinct from the cavernous malformations, suggesting an additional manifestation of endothelial abnormalities in this population.

Angiography. CCMs have no identifiable feeding arteries or draining veins. DSA, CTA, and MRA are usually negative unless the CCM is mixed with another vascular malformation (most commonly a DVA). If acute hemorrhage has occurred, an avascular mass effect may be present. Rarely, venous pooling with contrast accumulation in one or more of the "caverns" can be identified.

Differential Diagnosis

The most common differential diagnosis is a **mixed vascular malformation** in which a CCM is the dominant component **(7-51)**. Occasionally, a **hemorrhagic** or **densely calcified neoplasm** (such as a glioblastoma or oligodendroglioma, respectively) can mimic a CCM.

Multifocal "black dots" on T2* scans can be seen in a number of lesions besides type IV CCMs. Chronic hypertensive encephalopathy, amyloid angiopathy, axonal stretch injury, and cortical contusions may have similar appearances.

Hemangiomas are true benign vasoformative neoplasms and should not be mistaken for CCMs. Most are found in the skin and soft tissues of the head and neck. Hemangiomas within the CNS are rare and most commonly found in dural venous sinuses and cranial meninges, not the brain parenchyma.

CEREBRAL CAVERNOUS MALFORMATIONS: IMAGING

CT
- NECT
  - Hyperdense ± scattered Ca++
  - Variable hemorrhage
- DSA

MR (Zabramski Classification)
- Type I: Subacute hemorrhage
  - Hyperintense on T1
  - Hyper-/hypointense on T2
- Type II: Differently aged hemorrhages
  - Mixed signal with hyper/hypointensity on both T1 and T2
  - Classic = "popcorn ball"
  - Look for blood-filled locules with fluid-fluid levels
- Type III: Chronic hemorrhage
- Type IV: Punctate microhemorrhages
  - "Blooming black dots" on T2* (GRE, SWI)

DSA
- Usually negative (unless mixed with DVA)

Capillary Telangiectasia

Terminology

A brain capillary telangiectasia (BCT) is a collection of enlarged, thin-walled vessels resembling capillaries. The vessels are surrounded and separated by normal brain parenchyma.

Etiology

General Concepts. Although their exact pathogenesis is unknown, capillary telangiectasias are probably congenital lesions. BCTs have been reported with hereditary hemorrhagic telangiectasia (HHT).

Cranial irradiation may cause vascular endothelial damage and induce development of multiple cavernous or telangiectatic-like lesions in the brain parenchyma. Patients with radiation-induced capillary telangiectasias typically present with seizures several years after whole-brain XRT. Mean age of onset is 11-12 years, and mean latency period is nearly 9 years.

Genetics. No known genetic mutations have been identified for solitary BCTs. BCTs are the most common vascular malformation in HHT, occurring in 60% of patients. No specific correlation has been observed between genotype and phenotype of brain vascular malformation.

Pathology

Location and Size. BCTs can occur anywhere in the CNS. The pons, cerebellum, and spinal cord are the most common sites **(7-52)**. Solitary lesions are much more common than multiple BCTs. Although "giant" capillary telangiectasias do occur, the vast majority of BCTs are small, typically less than 1 cm in diameter.

Gross Pathology. Most BCTs are often invisible to gross inspection. Only 5-10% of BCTs are larger than 1 cm in diameter. Occasionally lesions up to 2 cm occur. These can be seen as areas of poorly delineated pink or brownish discoloration in the parenchyma **(7-53)**.

Microscopic Features. A cluster of dilated, somewhat ectatic but otherwise normal-appearing capillaries interspersed within the brain parenchyma is characteristic **(7-55)**. Unless mixed with other malformations (such as cavernous angioma), BCTs do not hemorrhage and do not calcify. Gliosis and hemosiderin deposition are absent.

Clinical Issues

Epidemiology. Capillary telangiectasias are the second most common cerebral vascular malformation, representing between 10-20% of all brain vascular malformations. Skin and mucosal capillary telangiectasias are even more common than brain telangiectasias.

Demographics. BCTs may occur at any age, but peak presentation is between 30-40 years. There is no sex predilection.

Presentation. Most BCTs are asymptomatic and discovered incidentally. A few cases with headache, vertigo, and tinnitus have been reported.

Natural History. Sporadic BCTs are quiescent lesions that do not hemorrhage. BCTs in patients with HHT also have a benign natural history.

Treatment Options. Isolated BCTs do not require treatment. Treatment of mixed lesions is dictated by the associated lesion.

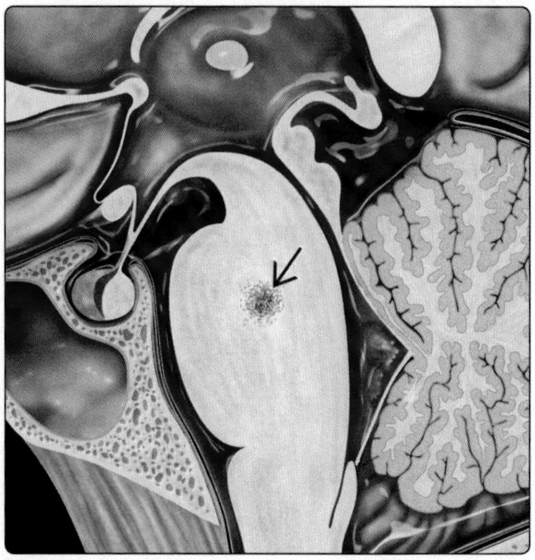

***(7-52)** Graphic depicts pontine capillary telangiectasia ⇒ with tiny dilated capillaries interspersed with normal brain.*

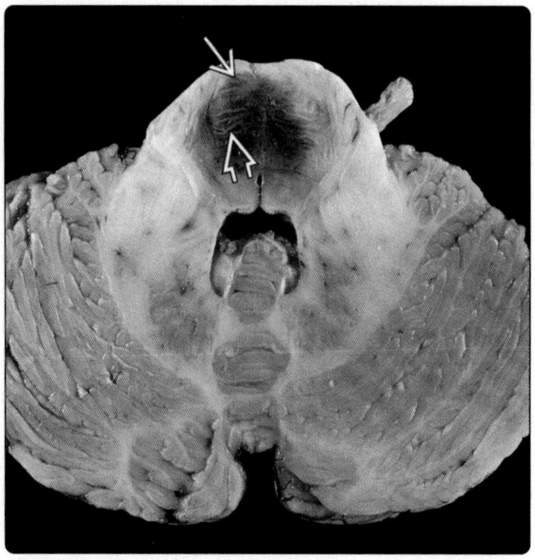

***(7-53)** Autopsy shows large pontine capillary telangiectasia ➡ with pontine fibers ➡ passing through the lesion. (Courtesy B. Horten, MD.)*

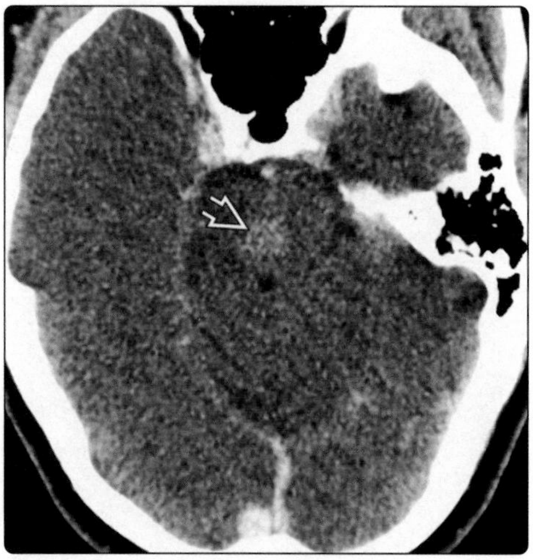

***(7-54)** Axial CECT of the cervical soft tissues shows incidental, asymptomatic large capillary telangiectasia ➡ in the upper pons.*

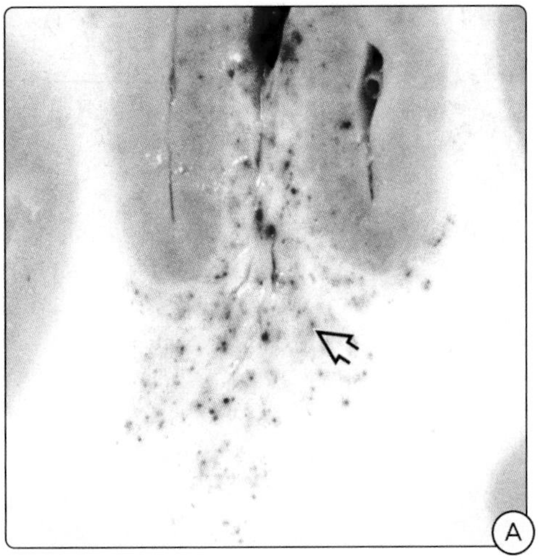

(7-55A) Subcortical capillary telangiectasia shows innumerable enlarged pink foci ➡ in the subcortical WM produced by enlarged capillaries.

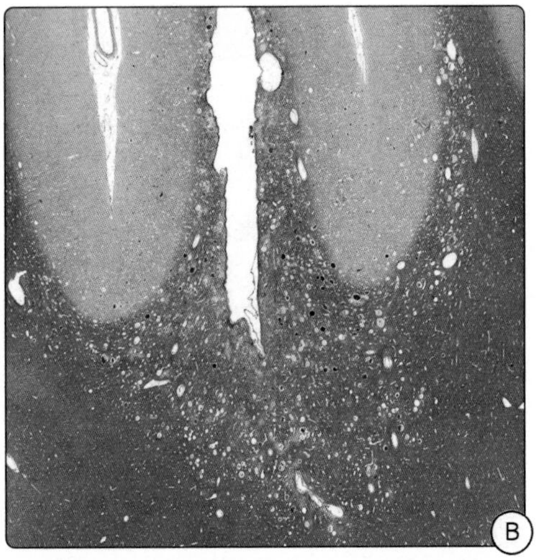

(7-55B) Blue myelin stain shows enlarged capillaries. in subcortical WM with normal blue-staining WM between the vessels.

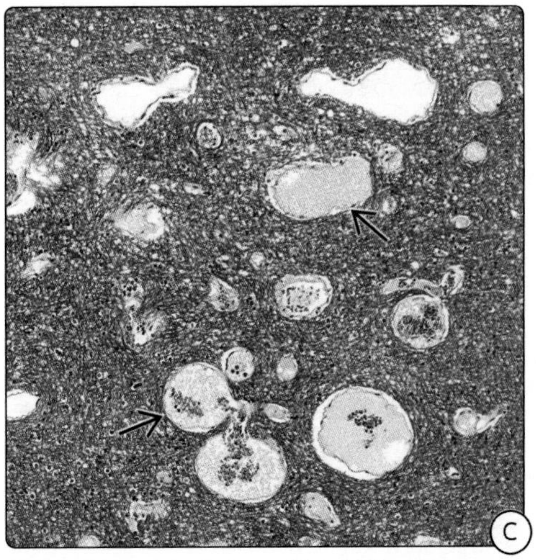

(7-55C) Micrograph shows blood-filled, thin-walled enlarged capillaries ➡, the hallmark of capillary telangiectasia. (Courtesy P. Burger, MD.)

Imaging

General Features. Because normal brain is interspersed between the dilated capillaries of a BCT, no mass effect is present. Unless they are histologically mixed with other CVMs (such as a cavernous malformation), BCTs lack edema, do not incite surrounding gliosis, and neither hemorrhage nor calcify.

CT Findings. Both NECT and CECT scans are usually normal unless the telangiectasia is unusually large **(7-54)**.

MR Findings. BCTs are inconspicuous on conventional precontrast MRs **(7-56A)**. T1 scans are typically normal. Large BCTs may show faint stippled hyperintensity on T2WI **(7-57A)** or FLAIR, but small lesions are generally invisible.

T2* (GRE, SWI) is the best sequence for demonstrating a BCT **(7-57)**. As blood flow within the dilated capillaries is quite sluggish, oxyhemoglobin is converted to deoxyhemoglobin and is visible as an area of poorly delineated grayish hypointensity.

BCTs typically show faint stippled or poorly delineated brush-like enhancement on T1 C+ **(7-56B)**. Larger lesions may demonstrate a linear focus of strong enhancement within the lesion, representing a draining collector vein **(7-57C)**.

As BCTs are interspersed with normal white matter tracts, DTI shows no displacement or disruption and no alteration of fractional anisotropy.

Differential Diagnosis

Because they show mild enhancement on T1 C+, BCTs are often mistaken for **neoplasms**. Yet they do not exhibit mass effect or surrounding edema. Signal intensity loss on T2* and focal brush-like enhancement in a lesion that is otherwise unremarkable on standard sequences easily distinguish BCT from neoplasm.

Radiation-induced vascular malformations are seen as multifocal "blooming black dots" on T2* (GRE, SWI) sequences. Most are cavernous malformations with microhemorrhages, not capillary telangiectasias.

CAPILLARY TELANGIECTASIAS

Pathology
- Cluster of thin-walled, dilated capillaries
  - Normal brain between vascular channels
- Location
  - Pons, cerebellum, spinal cord most common sites
  - BUT can be found anywhere

Clinical Issues
- 10-20% of all cerebrovascular malformations
- All ages
  - Peak = 30-40 years
- Rarely symptomatic
  - Most discovered incidentally at imaging

Imaging
- MR
  - T1/T2 usually normal unless unusually large
  - T2* key sequence (dark gray hypointensity on GRE)
  - May become very hypointense on SWI
  - "Brush-like" enhancement on T1 C+
  - ± Prominent central draining vein

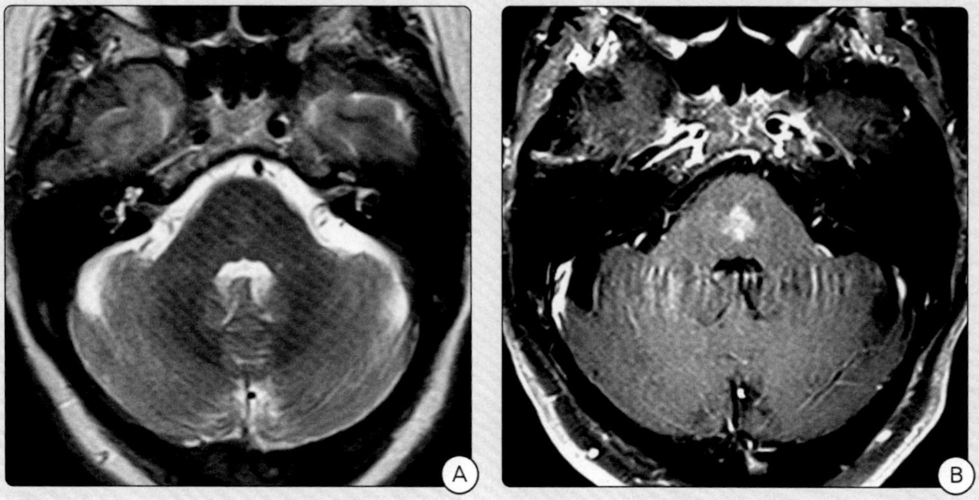

***(7-56A)** Axial T2WI in a neurologically intact 52y woman is normal. The faint hyperintensities in the cerebellar peduncles are artifactual. **(7-56B)** T1 C+ FS in the same case shows moderate brush-like enhancement in the lesion. The features of normal T2/FLAIR, mild to moderate hypointensity on T2* GRE and the brush-like enhancement pattern, are classic for capillary telangiectasia. The pons is the most common CNS location for capillary telangiectasias.*

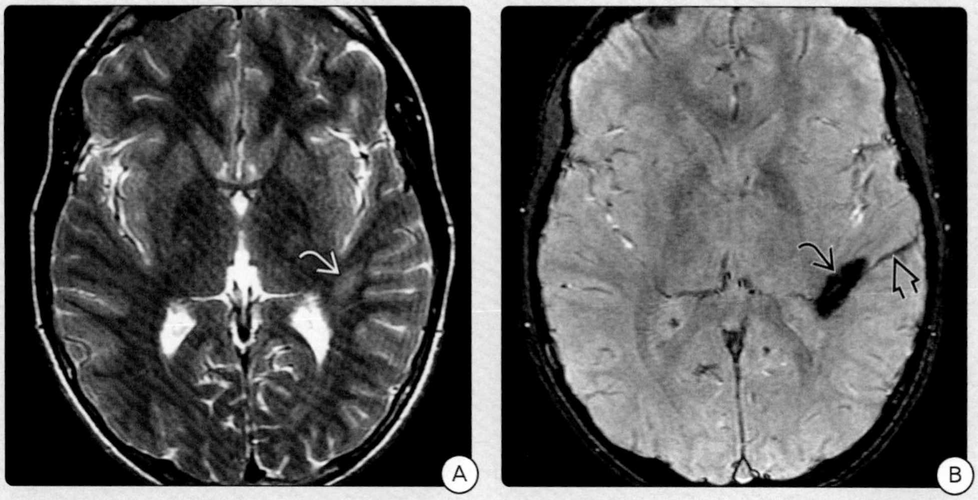

***(7-57A)** Axial T2WI in a 16y boy with headaches shows a faint, ill-defined hyperintensity in the left parietal white matter. **(7-57B)** T2* SWI in the same case shows blooming hypointensity in the lesion, prominent draining vein.*

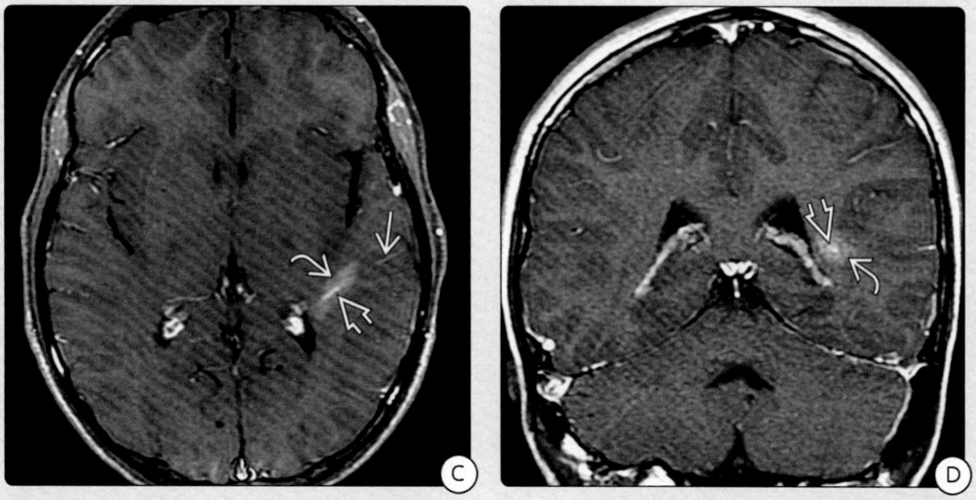

***(7-57C)** T1 C+ FS shows brush-like area of enhancement surrounding a prominent central draining vein. A superficial cortical vein also drains the lesion. **(7-57D)** Coronal T1 C+ shows the brush-like enhancement of a giant capillary telangiectasia with prominent central draining vein.*

Selected References

CVMs With Arteriovenous Shunting

Arteriovenous Malformation

Jiao Y et al: A supplementary grading scale combining lesion-to-eloquence distance for predicting surgical outcomes of patients with brain arteriovenous malformations. J Neurosurg. 1-11, 2017

Jimenez JE et al: Role of follow-up imaging after resection of brain arteriovenous malformations in pediatric patients: a systematic review of the literature. J Neurosurg Pediatr. 19(2):149-156, 2017

Solomon RA et al: Arteriovenous malformations of the brain. N Engl J Med. 376(19):1859-1866, 2017

Ding D et al: Radiosurgery for cerebral arteriovenous malformations in a randomized trial of unruptured brain arteriovenous malformations (ARUBA)-eligible patients: a multicenter study. Stroke. 47(2):342-9, 2016

Koo HW et al: Clinical features of superficially located brain arteriovenous malformations with transdural arterial communication. Cerebrovasc Dis. 41(3-4):204-210, 2016

Liakos F et al: Towards a revised Spetzler-Martin arteriovenous malformations grading scale. Redefining the "eloquent brain areas". J Neurosurg Sci. ePub, 2016

Weinsheimer S et al: Genome-wide association study of sporadic brain arteriovenous malformations. J Neurol Neurosurg Psychiatry. 87(9):916-23, 2016

Wrede KH et al: Non-enhanced MR imaging of cerebral arteriovenous malformations at 7 Tesla. Eur Radiol. 26(3):829-39, 2016

van Asch CJ et al: Diagnostic yield and accuracy of CT angiography, MR angiography, and digital subtraction angiography for detection of macrovascular causes of intracerebral haemorrhage: prospective, multicentre cohort study. BMJ. 351:h5762, 2015

Cerebral Proliferative Angiopathy

Karian V et al: Cerebral proliferative angiopathy. Pediatr Neurol. 66:115-116, 2017

Liu P et al: Cerebral proliferative angiopathy: clinical, angiographic features and literature review. Interv Neuroradiol. 22(1):101-7, 2016

Lopci E et al: Cerebral proliferative angiopathy (CPA): imaging findings and response to therapy. Clin Nucl Med. 41(12):e527-e529, 2016

Rohit et al: Diffuse proliferative cerebral angiopathy: a case report and review of the literature. J Radiol Case Rep. 9(9):1-10, 2015

Dural AV Fistula

Anand P et al: Venous hypertensive encephalopathy secondary to venous sinus thrombosis and dural arteriovenous fistula. Pract Neurol. ePub, 2017

Jermakowicz WJ et al: Cognard Type V intracranial dural arteriovenous fistula presenting in a pediatric patient with rapid, progressive myelopathy. J Neurosurg Pediatr. 1-6, 2017

Reynolds MR et al: Intracranial dural arteriovenous fistulae. Stroke. 48(5):1424-1431, 2017

Tsai LK et al: Diagnosis and management of intracranial dural arteriovenous fistulas. Expert Rev Neurother. 16(3):307-18, 2016

Ambekar S et al: Long-term angiographic results of endovascularly "cured" intracranial dural arteriovenous fistulas. J Neurosurg. 1-5, 2015

Bhogal P et al: Normal pio-dural arterial connections. Interv Neuroradiol. 21(6):750-8, 2015

Biswas S et al: Accuracy of four-dimensional CT angiography in detection and characterisation of arteriovenous malformations and dural arteriovenous fistulas. Neuroradiol J. 28(4):376-84, 2015

Hetts SW et al: Progressive versus nonprogressive intracranial dural arteriovenous fistulas: characteristics and outcomes. AJNR Am J Neuroradiol. 36(10):1912-9, 2015

Holekamp TF et al: Dural arteriovenous fistula-induced thalamic dementia: report of 4 cases. J Neurosurg. 1-14, 2015

Kanai R et al: Infratentorial pial arteriovenous fistula in the elderly. J Stroke Cerebrovasc Dis. 24(10):e307-9, 2015

Le Guennec L et al: Dural arteriovenous fistula mimicking a brainstem glioma. J Neuroimaging. 25(6):1053-5, 2015

Li C et al: Clinical and angioarchitectural risk factors associated with intracranial hemorrhage in dural arteriovenous fistulas: a single-center retrospective study. PLoS One. 10(6):e0131235, 2015

Carotid-Cavernous Fistula

Adam CR et al: Dilated superior ophthalmic vein: clinical and radiographic features of 113 cases. Ophthal Plast Reconstr Surg. ePub, 2017

Castaño C et al: Treatment of Barrow type 'B' carotid cavernous fistulas with flow diverter stent (Pipeline). Neuroradiol J. 1971400917695319, 2017

Park SH et al: Stereotactic radiosurgery for dural carotid cavernous sinus fistulas. World Neurosurg. ePub, 2017

Lee JY et al: Multidetector CT angiography in the diagnosis and classification of carotid-cavernous fistula. Clin Radiol. 71(1):e64-71, 2016

Lin TC et al: Systematic analysis of the risk factors affecting the recurrence of traumatic carotid-cavernous sinus fistula. World Neurosurg. 90:539-545.e1, 2016

Pial AV Fistula

Martínez-Payo C et al: Nongalenic pial arteriovenous fistula: prenatal diagnosis. J Clin Ultrasound. ePub, 2017

Satow T et al: Spontaneous resolution of cerebral pial arteriovenous fistula following angiography: report of two cases. World Neurosurg. ePub, 2017

Alurkar A et al: Intracranial pial arteriovenous fistulae: diagnosis and treatment techniques in pediatric patients with review of literature. J Clin Imaging Sci. 6:2, 2016

Yu J et al: Intracranial non-galenic pial arteriovenous fistula: a review of the literature. Interv Neuroradiol. 22(5):557-68, 2016

Bhogal P et al: Normal pio-dural arterial connections. Interv Neuroradiol. 21(6):750-8, 2015

Kanai R et al: Infratentorial pial arteriovenous fistula in the elderly. J Stroke Cerebrovasc Dis. 24(10):e307-9, 2015

Requejo F et al: Intracranial pial fistulas in pediatric population. Clinical features and treatment modalities. Childs Nerv Syst. 31(9):1509-14, 2015

Vein of Galen Aneurysmal Malformation

Agarwal H et al: Vein of Galen aneurysmal malformation-clinical and angiographic spectrum with management perspective: an institutional experience. J Neurointerv Surg. 9(2):159-164, 2017

Cohen JE et al: Clinical and angioarchitectural factors influencing the endovascular approach to galenic dural arteriovenous fistulas in adults: case series and review of the literature. Acta Neurochir (Wien). 159(5):845-853, 2017

Joo W et al: Vein of Galen malformation treated with the Micro Vascular Plug system: case report. J Neurosurg Pediatr. 1-5, 2017

Madhuban A et al: Vein of Galen aneurysmal malformation in neonates presenting with congestive heart failure. Child Neurol Open. 3:2329048X15624704, 2016

Zhou LX et al: Diagnosis of vein of Galen aneurysmal malformation using fetal MRI. J Magn Reson Imaging. ePub, 2016

Wagner MW et al: Vein of galen aneurysmal malformation: prognostic markers depicted on fetal MRI. Neuroradiol J. 28(1):72-5, 2015

CVMs Without Arteriovenous Shunting

Developmental Venous Anomaly

Harreld JH et al: Developmental venous anomalies mimicking neoplasm on 11C-methionine PET and DSC perfusion MRI. Clin Nucl Med. 42(5):e275-e276, 2017

Aoki R et al: Developmental venous anomaly: benign or not benign. Neurol Med Chir (Tokyo). 56(9):534-43, 2016

Linscott LL et al: Developmental venous anomalies of the brain in children - imaging spectrum and update. Pediatr Radiol. 46(3):394-406, 2016

Nabavizadeh SA et al: The many faces of cerebral developmental venous anomaly and its mimicks: spectrum of imaging findings. J Neuroimaging. 26(5):463-72, 2016

Larvie M et al: Brain metabolic abnormalities associated with developmental venous anomalies. AJNR Am J Neuroradiol. 36(3):475-80, 2015

Iv M et al: Association of developmental venous anomalies with perfusion abnormalities on arterial spin labeling and bolus perfusion-weighted imaging. J Neuroimaging. 25(2):243-50, 2014

Linscott LL et al: Brain parenchymal signal abnormalities associated with developmental venous anomalies in children and young adults. AJNR Am J Neuroradiol. 35(8):1600-7, 2014

Meng G et al: The association between cerebral developmental venous anomaly and concomitant cavernous malformation: an observational study using magnetic resonance imaging. BMC Neurol. 14:50, 2014

Sinus Pericranii

Simonin A et al: Three-dimensional printing of a sinus pericranii model: technical note. Childs Nerv Syst. 33(3):499-502, 2017

Pavanello M et al: Sinus pericranii: diagnosis and management in 21 pediatric patients. J Neurosurg Pediatr. 15(1):60-70, 2015

Cerebral Cavernous Malformation

Akers A et al: Synopsis of guidelines for the clinical management of cerebral cavernous malformations: consensus recommendations based on systematic literature review by the angioma alliance scientific advisory board clinical experts panel. Neurosurgery. 80(5):665-680, 2017

de Vos IJ et al: Review of familial cerebral cavernous malformations and report of seven additional families. Am J Med Genet A. 173(2):338-351, 2017

Flemming KD et al: Population-based prevalence of cerebral cavernous malformations in older adults: Mayo Clinic Study of Aging. JAMA Neurol. ePub, 2017

Strickland CD et al: Familial cerebral cavernous malformations are associated with adrenal calcifications on CT scans: an imaging biomarker for a hereditary cerebrovascular condition. Radiology. ePub, 2017

Takada S et al: Contribution of endothelial-to-mesenchymal transition to the pathogenesis of human cerebral and orbital cavernous malformations. Neurosurgery. ePub, 2017

Wetzel-Strong SE et al: The pathobiology of vascular malformations: insights from human and model organism genetics. J Pathol. 241(2):281-293, 2017

Zou X et al: Automated algorithm for counting microbleeds in patients with familial cerebral cavernous malformations. Neuroradiology. ePub, 2017

Bravi L et al: Endothelial cells lining sporadic cerebral cavernous malformation cavernomas undergo endothelial-to-mesenchymal transition. Stroke. 47(3):886-90, 2016

Dammann P et al: Correlation of the venous angioarchitecture of multiple cerebral cavernous malformations with familial or sporadic disease: a susceptibility-weighted imaging study with 7-Tesla MRI. J Neurosurg. 1-9, 2016

Ghali MG et al: Pediatric cerebral cavernous malformations: genetics, pathogenesis, and management. Surg Neurol Int. 7(Suppl 44):S1127-S1134, 2016

Kim J: Introduction to cerebral cavernous malformation: a brief review. BMB Rep. 49(5):255-62, 2016

Tan H et al: Quantitative susceptibility mapping in cerebral cavernous malformations: clinical correlations. AJNR Am J Neuroradiol. 37(7):1209-15, 2016

Taslimi S et al: Natural history of cavernous malformation: systematic review and meta-analysis of 25 studies. Neurology. 86(21):1984-91, 2016

Cha YJ et al: Pathological evaluation of radiation-induced vascular lesions of the brain: distinct from de novo cavernous hemangioma. Yonsei Med J. 56(6):1714-20, 2015

Cuttano R et al: KLF4 is a key determinant in the development and progression of cerebral cavernous malformations. EMBO Mol Med. 8(1):6-24, 2015

Golden MJ et al: Increased number of white matter lesions in patients with familial cerebral cavernous malformations. AJNR Am J Neuroradiol. 36(5):899-903, 2015

Nikoubashman O et al: Prospective hemorrhage rates of cerebral cavernous malformations in children and adolescents based on MRI appearance. AJNR Am J Neuroradiol. 36(11):2177-83, 2015

Capillary Telangiectasia

Brinjikji W et al: Natural history of brain capillary vascular malformations in hereditary hemorrhagic telangiectasia patients. J Neurointerv Surg. 9(1):26-28, 2017

Brinjikji W et al: Neurovascular manifestations of hereditary hemorrhagic telangiectasia: a consecutive series of 376 patients during 15 years. AJNR Am J Neuroradiol. 37(8):1479-86, 2016

Orgun LT et al: Symptomatic capillary telangiectasia of the pons: three pediatric cases diagnosed by suspectibility-weighted imaging. Childs Nerv Syst. 32(11):2261-2264, 2016

Yu T et al: Symptomatic large or giant capillary telangiectasias: management and outcome in 5 cases. J Neurosurg. 1-7, 2015

Arterial Anatomy and Strokes

"Stroke" is a generic term that describes a clinical event characterized by sudden onset of a neurologic deficit. However, not all strokes are the same! Stroke syndromes have significant clinical and pathophysiological heterogeneity that is reflected in their underlying gross pathologic and imaging appearances. Arterial ischemia/infarction—the major focus of this chapter—is by far the most common cause of stroke, accounting for 80% of all cases.

The remaining 20% of strokes are mostly hemorrhagic, divided between primary "spontaneous" intracranial hemorrhage (sICH), nontraumatic subarachnoid hemorrhage (SAH), and venous occlusions. Both sICH and SAH were discussed extensively in preceding chapters, and venous occlusions will be discussed in the following chapter.

We begin by briefly reviewing the normal intracranial arteries. With this solid anatomic foundation, we then turn our attention to the etiology, pathology, and imaging manifestations of arterial strokes.

Normal Arterial Anatomy and Vascular Distributions

Clinicians frequently discuss the intracranial vasculature in two parts, the "anterior circulation" and the "posterior circulation." The **anterior circulation** consists of the intradural internal carotid artery (ICA) and its branches plus its two terminations, the anterior cerebral artery (ACA) and middle cerebral artery (MCA). Both the anterior communicating arteries (ACoAs) and the posterior communicating arteries (PCoAs) are also considered part of the anterior circulation.

The **posterior circulation** is composed of the vertebrobasilar trunk and its branches, including its terminal bifurcation into the two posterior cerebral arteries (PCAs).

We begin our discussion with the anterior circulation. We briefly consider the ICA and its segments, branches, important variants, and anomalies and then delineate the anatomy of the circle of Willis. The three major cerebral arteries (i.e., anterior, middle, posterior) are next discussed, along with their branches, variants, and vascular distributions. We conclude this section with the normal anatomy of the vertebrobasilar system.

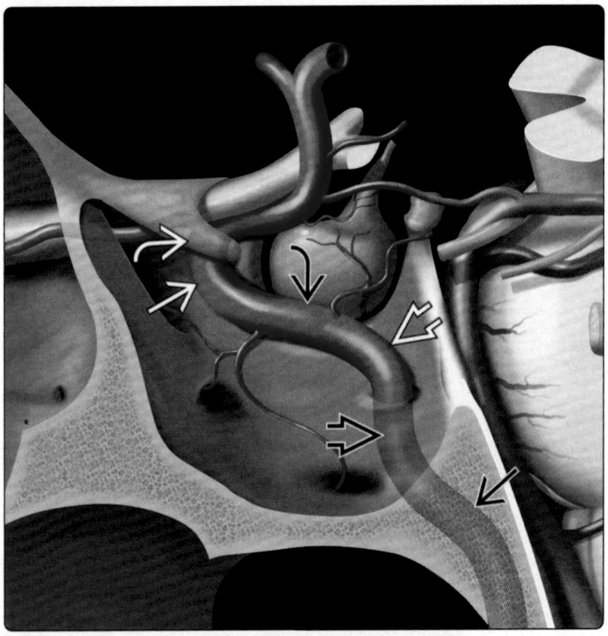

***(8-1)** Intracranial ICA, branches are shown; C2 (petrous) segment ➡ is long and L-shaped. C3 ➡ is a short segment between C2 and cavernous ICA (C4) ➡. C5 ➡ is last extradural segment. Posterior ➡, anterior ➡ genua of C4 are shown.*

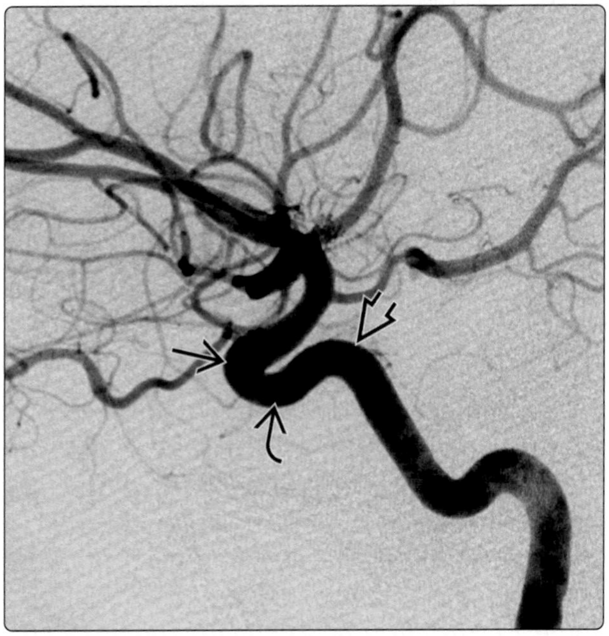

***(8-2)** Lateral DSA shows all ICA segments. The C4 (cavernous) segment ➡ has both a posterior ➡ and an anterior ➡ genu. Together, they form the angio-DSA carotid "siphon."*

Intracranial Internal Carotid Artery

The intracranial ICAs follow a complex course with six straight vertical or horizontal segments that are connected by three curved genua. The ICAs are divided into numbered segments. By convention, the extracranial ICA—which normally has *no* named branches in the neck—is designated the **C1 (cervical) segment**. The cervical ICA is discussed in detail along with the other extracranial cephalocervical arteries (Chapter 10).

Normal Anatomy

C2 (Petrous) ICA Segment. The C2 (petrous) segment is contained within the carotid canal of the temporal bone and is L-shaped **(8-1)**. As it enters the skull at the exocranial opening of the carotid canal, the ICA lies just in front of the internal jugular vein. At this point, the ICA goes from being relatively mobile (in the neck) to relatively fixed (in the bone), where it is more vulnerable to traumatic shearing forces and dissection injury.

The C2 ICA has a short vertical segment, then a genu or "knee" where it turns anteromedially in front of the cochlea, and a longer horizontal segment. The ICA exits the carotid canal at the petrous apex.

The C2 segment has two small but important branches. The **vidian artery**, also known as the artery of the pterygoid canal, anastomoses with branches of the external carotid artery (ECA). The **caroticotympanic artery** is a small ICA branch that supplies the middle ear.

C3 (Lacerum) ICA Segment. The C3 (lacerum) segment is a short segment that lies just above the foramen lacerum and extends from the petrous apex to the cavernous sinus (CS).

The C3 segment is covered by the **trigeminal ganglion** of CN V and has no branches.

C4 (Cavernous) ICA Segment. The C4 (cavernous) segment is one of the most important and complex of all the ICA segments. The C4 ICA has three subsegments connected by two genua **(8-2)**. In order, these are (1) a short posterior ascending (vertical) segment, (2) the posterior genu, (3) a longer horizontal segment, (4) an anterior genu, and (5) an anterior vertical ascending (subclinoid) segment. As the cavernous ICA courses anteriorly, it also courses medially. Therefore, on anteroposterior or coronal views, the posterior genu is lateral to the anterior genu.

The **abducens nerve** (CN VI) is inferolateral to the ICA and is the only cranial nerve that lies *inside* the CS itself (the others are in the lateral dural wall).

The C4 ICA segment has two important branches **(8-1)**. The **meningohypophyseal trunk** arises from the posterior genu, supplying the pituitary gland, tentorium, and clival dura. The **inferolateral trunk** (ILT) arises from the lateral aspect of the intracavernous ICA and supplies cranial nerves and CS dura. Via branches that pass through the adjacent basilar foramina, the ILT anastomoses freely with branches from the ECA that arise in the pterygopalatine fossa. This important connection between the external and internal carotid circulations may provide a source of collateral blood flow in the case of ICA occlusion.

C5 (Clinoid) ICA Segment. The C5 (clinoid) segment is a short interdural segment that lies between the proximal and distal dural rings of the CS. The C5 segment terminates as the ICA exits the CS and enters the cranial cavity adjacent to the anterior clinoid process. The C5 segment has no important branches unless the ophthalmic artery originates within the CS and not in the proximal intracranial (C6) segment.

C6 (Ophthalmic) ICA Segment. The C6 (ophthalmic) segment is the first ICA segment that lies wholly within the subarachnoid space. This segment extends from the distal dural ring to just below the posterior communicating artery (PCoA) origin.

The C6 segment has two important branches. The **ophthalmic artery** (OA) arises from the anterosuperior aspect of the ICA, then passes anteriorly through the optic canal together with CN II. The OA has extensive anastomoses with ECA branches in and around the orbit and lacrimal gland. The **superior hypophyseal artery** arises from the posterior aspect of the C6 ICA segment and supplies the anterior pituitary lobe (adenohypophysis) and infundibular stalk as well as the optic chiasm.

C7 (Communicating) ICA Segment. The C7 (communicating) segment is the last ICA segment and extends from just below the PCoA origin to the terminal ICA bifurcation into the ACA and MCA. As it courses posterosuperiorly, the ICA passes between the optic and oculomotor nerves.

The most distal ICA segment has two important branches. The **PCoA** joins the anterior to the posterior circulation. A number of perforating arteries arise from the PCoA to supply the basal brain structures including the hypothalamus.

The **anterior choroidal artery** (AChA) arises 1 or 2 mm above the PCoA and initially courses posteromedially, then turns laterally in the suprasellar cistern to enter the choroidal fissure of the temporal horn. The AChA territory is reciprocal with that of the posterolateral and posteromedial choroidal arteries (both are branches of the PCA) but usually includes the medial temporal lobe, basal ganglia, and intralenticular limb of the internal capsule.

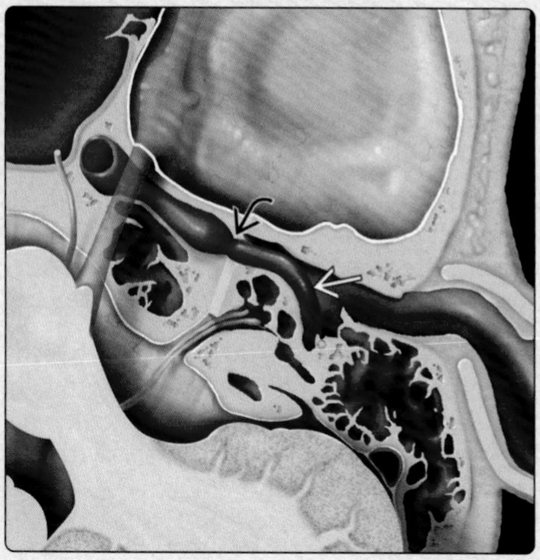

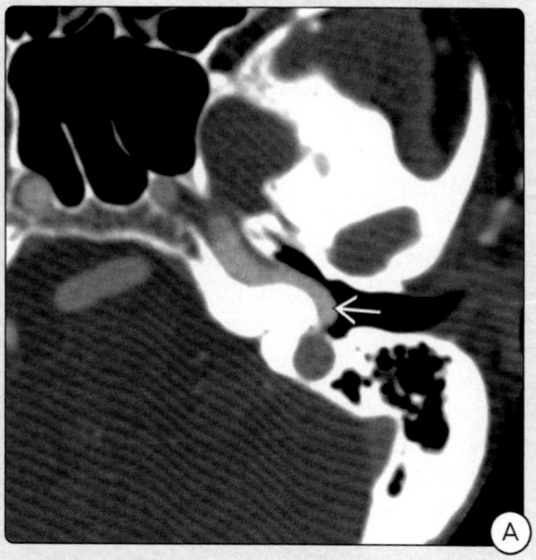

(8-3) Axial graphic illustrates a classic aberrant ICA ➡ arising along the posterior cochlear promontory and crossing along the middle ear to rejoin the horizontal petrous ICA. A stenosis ⇨ is often present at the reconnection site. (8-4A) Axial CTA source image through the middle ear shows an aberrant ICA (AbICA) ➡ looping over the cochlear promontory.

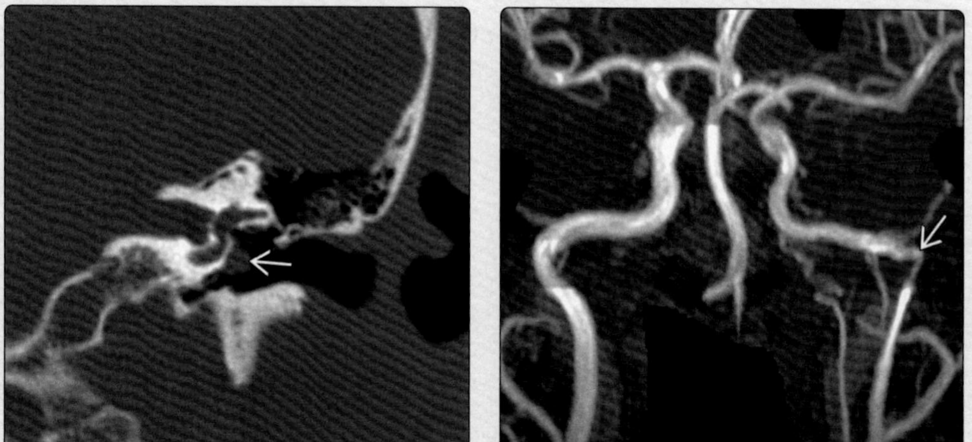

(8-4B) Coronal temporal bone CT at the oval window level shows an AbICA ➡ as a well-delineated soft tissue "mass" located on the cochlear promontory, mimicking a glomus tympanicum paraganglioma. (8-4C) Coronal MRA shows a normal right ICA. An aberrant left ICA passes more laterally with a characteristic, sharply angled shape that resembles a "7" ➡.

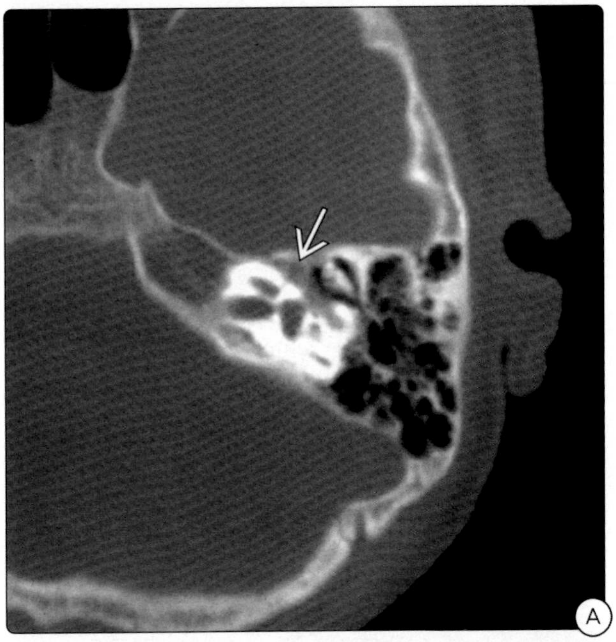

(8-5A) Characteristic findings of a persistent stapedial artery (PSA) are illustrated. Axial temporal bone CT demonstrates an enlarged anterior tympanic segment of the facial nerve canal .

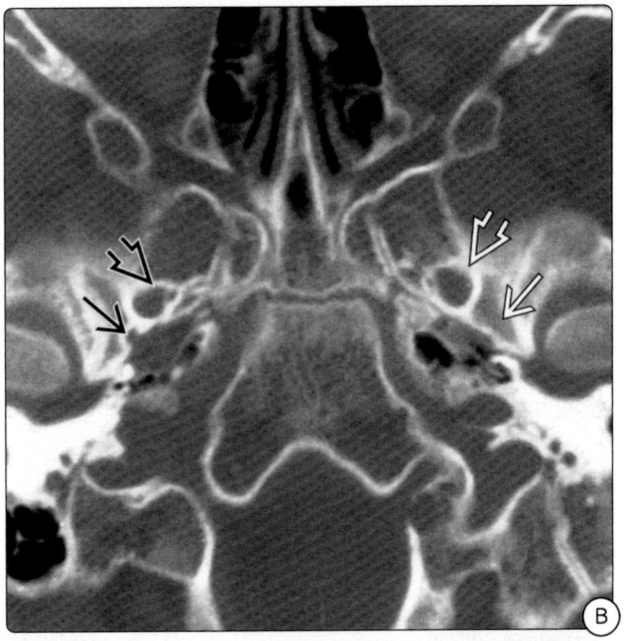

(8-5B) Bone CT in the same patient shows normal left foramen ovale , absence of left foramen spinosum (FS) . The right foramen ovale , FS are normal. Absent FS and enlarged anterior CN VII segment are pathognomonic for PSA.

Variants and Anomalies

Three important ICA vascular anomalies must be recognized on imaging studies: an aberrant ICA (AbICA), a persistent stapedial artery, and an embryonic carotid-basilar anastomosis.

Aberrant ICA. An AbICA is a congenital vascular anomaly that enters the posterior middle ear cavity from below and hugs the cochlear promontory as it crosses the middle ear cavity **(8-3)**. The ICA finally resumes its normal, expected course as it joins the posterior lateral margin of the horizontal petrous ICA.

Patients with an AbICA typically present with pulsatile tinnitus. An AbICA is identified on otoscopic examination as a vascular-appearing retrotympanic mass lying in the anteroinferior mesotympanum. An AbICA mimics the clinical appearance of paraganglioma (glomus tympanicum, glomus jugulare). Biopsy may result in stroke or fatal hemorrhage, so this anomaly *must* be recognized by the radiologist *and* communicated to the referring clinician.

The appearance of an AbICA on CT is pathognomonic. Axial bone CT shows a tubular lesion that crosses the middle ear cavity from posterior to anterior **(8-4A)**. Coronal images show a round, well-delineated soft tissue density lying on the cochlear promontory **(8-4B)**.

Angiography (DSA, CTA, MRA) shows that the AbICA has a more posterolateral course than normal. A distinct angulation that resembles a 7 is often present, together with a change in contour and caliber (pinched appearance) before the segment resumes its normal course **(8-4C)**.

Persistent Stapedial Artery. A persistent stapedial artery (PSA) is a rare congenital vascular anomaly in which the embryonic stapedial artery persists postnatally. Most PSA cases are discovered incidentally at imaging or at surgery.

A PSA arises from the C2 (petrous) ICA at the genu between the vertical and horizontal segments. The PSA passes through the stapes footplate and doubles the size of the anterior (tympanic) facial nerve segment **(8-5A)**. Intracranially, the PSA becomes the middle meningeal artery (MMA).

Pathognomonic imaging findings are (1) the absence of the foramen spinosum (because the MMA arises from the PSA, not the ECA) **(8-5B)** and (2) an enlarged tympanic segment of the facial nerve. A PSA is often—but not invariably—associated with an AbICA.

Embryonic Carotid-Basilar Anastomoses. Early in embryonic development, connections form between the primitive carotid artery and the two longitudinal neural arteries (the fetal precursors of the basilar artery). With the exception of the PCoA, all these primitive arterial connections regress and then disappear when the definitive cerebral circulation forms. If they fail to regress, a postnatal **persistent** ("primitive" or "embryonic") **carotid-basilar anastomosis** (PCBA) remains.

There are four types of PCBA. Each is recognized and named according to its anatomic relationship with specific cranial or spinal nerves. From superior to inferior, these are a persistent trigeminal artery (CN V), persistent otic artery (CN VIII), persistent hypoglossal artery (CN XII), and proatlantal intersegmental artery (C1-3) **(8-6)**.

Persistent Trigeminal Artery. A persistent trigeminal artery (PTA) is the most common of the persistent embryonic carotid-basilar anastomoses and is identified in 0.1-0.2% of

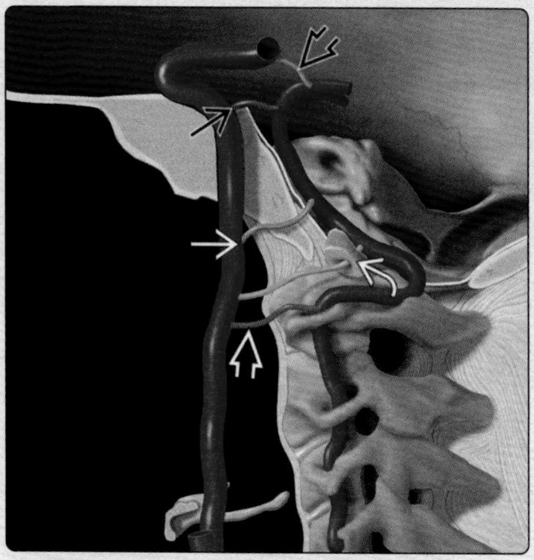

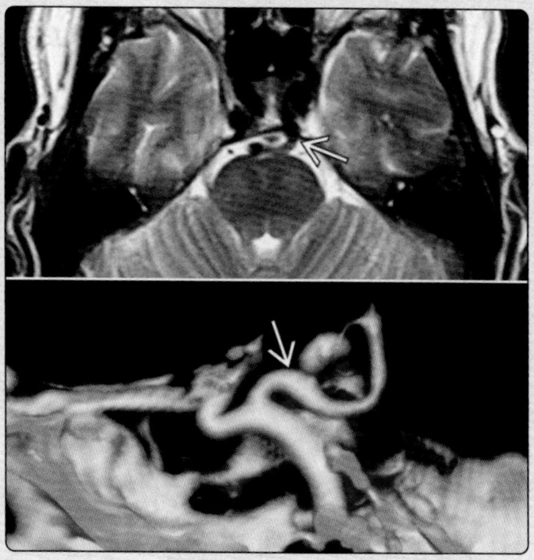

***(8-6)** Graphic shows anastomoses between the ICA, VA. PCoA is a normal connection. The PTA connects the cavernous ICA, BA. The POA connects the petrous ICA to the BA through the IAC. The PHA connects the cervical ICA, VA through the hypoglossal canal. The proatlantal artery connects the cervical ICA, VA. **(8-7)** T2WI (top), 3D CTA (bottom) show a PTA coursing posteriorly through dorsum sellae from ICA to BA.*

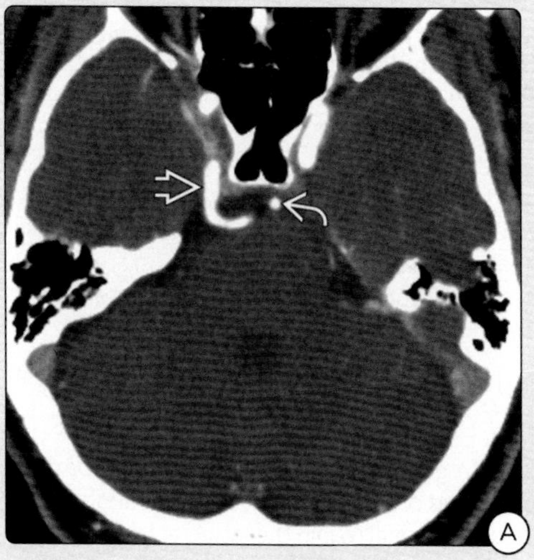

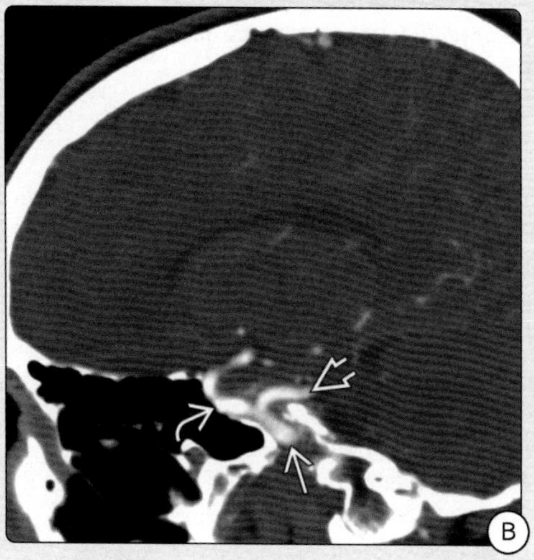

***(8-8A)** CTA shows a classic right PTA passing posterolaterally around the sella toward the basilar artery. **(8-8B)** Sagittal CTA in the same case reformatted from the axial source data shows the classic "Neptune's trident" appearance of a PTA. The "trident" is formed by the ascending and horizontal segments of the cavernous ICA and the PTA.*

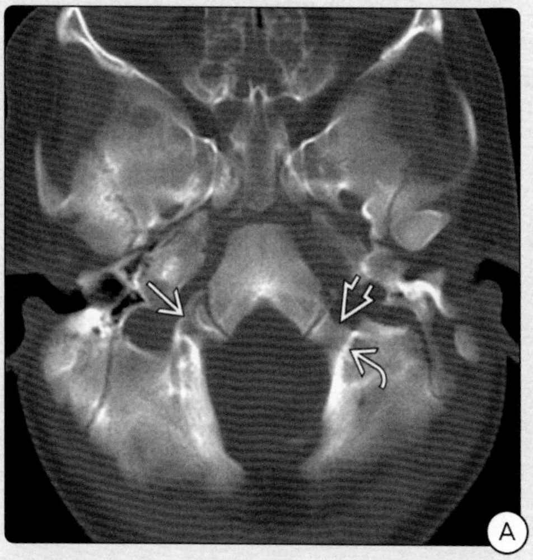

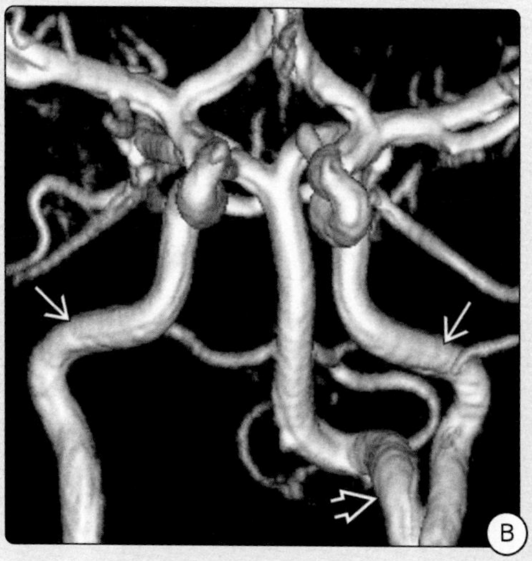

***(8-9A)** Axial bone CT shows a normal right hypoglossal canal. The left hypoglossal canal is almost twice its size. The cortical margins of the enlarged hypoglossal canal appear intact. **(8-9B)** Coronal 3D MIP MRA in the same patient shows normal right and left carotid arteries. The entire posterior circulation is supplied by a persistent hypoglossal artery, which accompanies the left CN XII through the enlarged hypoglossal canal.*

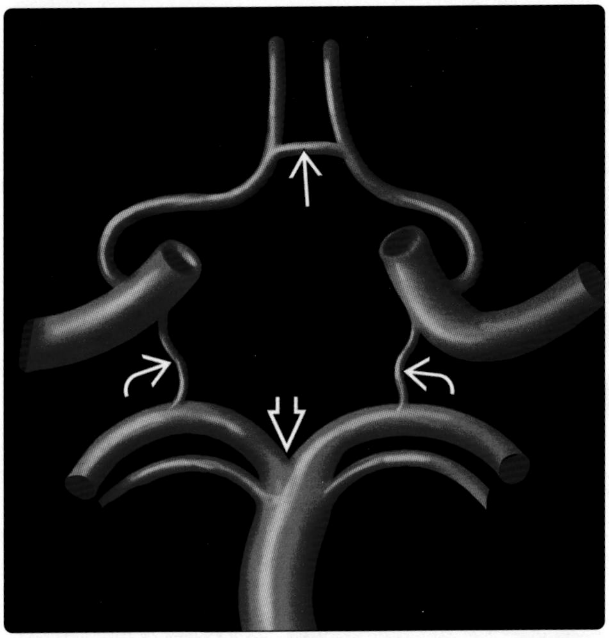

(8-10) Graphic depicts the circle of Willis with the ACoA ➡ and PCoAs ➡ connecting the anterior (carotid) circulation to the posterior (vertebrobasilar) circulation ➡.

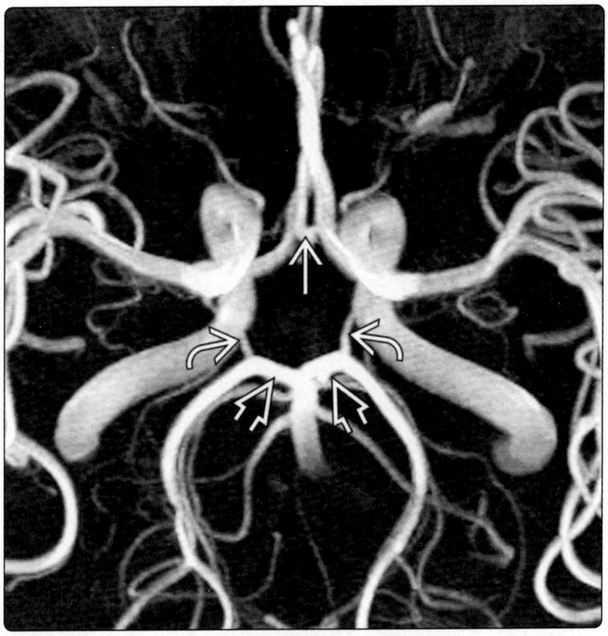

(8-11) Submentovertex view of normal MRA shows the ACoA ➡, small PCoAs ➡, and basilar bifurcation with large P1 PCA segments ➡ forming a "balanced" circle of Willis.

cases. Two types of PTA are recognized. In Saltzman type 1, the PTA supplies the distal basilar artery (BA), PCoAs are usually absent, and the proximal BA is hypoplastic. In Saltzman type 2, the PTA fills the superior cerebellar arteries, while the PCAs are supplied via patent PCoAs.

As they pass posteriorly, PTAs can course either lateral or medial to the sella turcica. In the latter instance, the PTA courses posteromedially, compressing the pituitary gland and penetrating the dorsum sellae before it anastomoses with the BA. This variant is important to recognize prior to transsphenoidal surgery for pituitary adenoma.

Imaging findings of a PTA show a large vessel that connects the cavernous ICA with the BA. In 60% of cases, the PTA courses posteromedially, running through the dorsum sellae to join the BA **(8-7)**. In 40% of cases, the PTA runs posterolaterally along the trigeminal nerve, curving around (not through) the dorsum sellae **(8-8A)**.

Sagittal CTA and MRA show a "Neptune's trident" configuration **(8-7)** **(8-8B)**. Nearly one-quarter of all PTAs have associated vascular abnormalities, such as saccular aneurysm, moyamoya, aortic coarctation, and arterial fenestrations.

Persistent Otic Artery. Postnatally, the incidence of PCBAs is inversely related to their order of disappearance. The primitive otic artery is the first of the fetal carotid-basilar anastomoses to regress and is therefore the rarest of these uncommon anomalies. Only a few cases of persistent otic artery have been convincingly demonstrated.

Persistent Hypoglossal Artery. A persistent hypoglossal artery (PHA) is the second most common type of PCBA, with an estimated prevalence of 0.03-0.09%. A PHA arises from the posterior aspect of the cervical ICA, generally at the C1-2 level, and courses along CN XII through the hypoglossal canal to anastomose with the basilar artery **(8-6)**. The ipsilateral vertebral artery and PCoA are hypoplastic. The posterior ICA arises from the PHA in 50% of cases.

A PHA has the highest incidence of associated aneurysms of any PCBA.

Imaging shows a large vessel that arises posteriorly from the distal cervical ICA and curves posteromedially through an enlarged hypoglossal canal to join the intracranial BA just above the foramen magnum **(8-9)**.

Proatlantal (Intersegmental) Artery. A proatlantal artery, also called a proatlantal intersegmental artery (PIA), is the most caudal of the PCBAs **(8-6)**. Two types are recognized. A type 1 PIA arises from the cervical ICA at the C2-3 (or lower) level, then runs posterosuperiorly and joins the suboccipital vertebral artery before coursing upward through the foramen magnum. A type 2 PIA follows a similar course but arises from the ECA.

Circle of Willis

The circle of Willis (COW) is the great arterial anastomotic ring that surrounds the basal brain structures and connects the anterior and posterior circulations with each other. In the event of arterial occlusion, the COW is the most important source of potential collateral blood flow to the occluded territory.

Normal Anatomy

The COW has 10 components: two ICAs, two proximal or horizontal (A1) anterior cerebral artery (ACA) segments, the anterior communicating artery (ACoA), two posterior communicating arteries (PCoAs), the basilar artery (BA), and two proximal or horizontal (P1) segments of the posterior cerebral arteries (PCAs) **(8-10)** **(8-11)**. The middle cerebral artery (MCA) is *not* part of the COW.

Vascular Territory

Important perforating branches arise from all parts of the COW and supply most of the basilar brain structures. Those that arise from the ACoA and PCoA are discussed below. Perforating branches from the ACAs, MCAs, PCAs, and BA are also described along with the anatomy of their parent arteries.

The ACoA has perforating arteries that pass superiorly to supply the anterior hypothalamus and optic chiasm, corpus callosum genu, cingulate gyrus, and pillars of the fornix. Occasionally a large, dominant perforating artery arises from the ACoA and is called the median artery of the corpus callosum. The PCoA gives origin to several perforating branches (anterior thalamoperforating arteries) that supply the thalamus.

Variants and Anomalies

COW *variants* are the rule, not the exception. One or more components of the COW is hypoplastic or absent in the majority of cases. A1 and P1 variants are described below. A hypoplastic or absent PCoA is the most common COW variant and occurs in one-quarter to one-third of all cases. An absent, duplicated, or multichanneled ACoA is seen in 10-15% of cases. Anatomic variants in the COW may cause significant flow asymmetries between the right and left ICAs or decreased volume in the BA on MRA and pMR studies; they should not be misinterpreted as vascular disease.

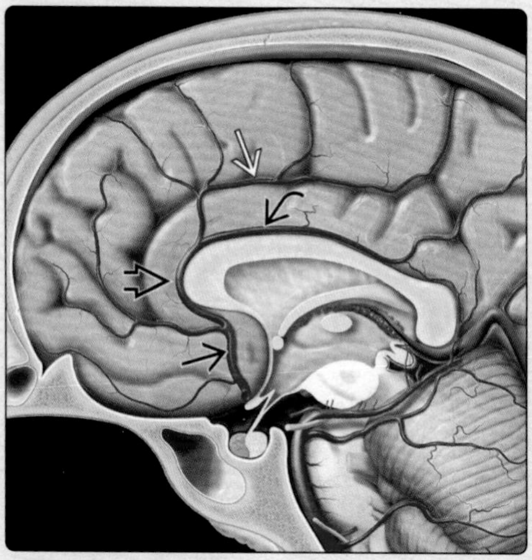

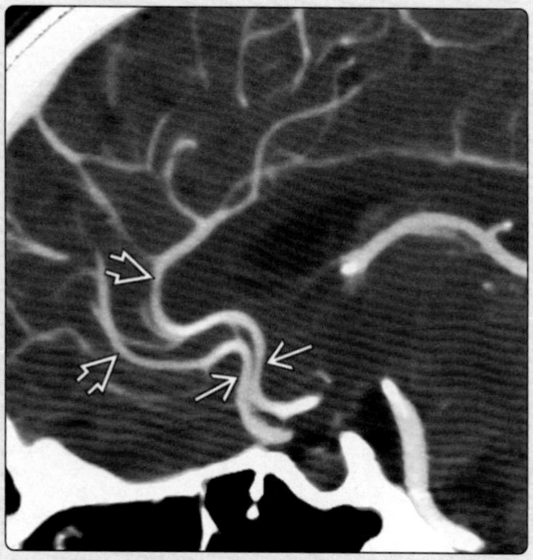

***(8-12)** Graphic shows relationship of ACA to underlying brain. A2 segment ascends in front of 3rd ventricle. A3 curves around corpus callosum genu. Pericallosal, callosomarginal arteries are major terminal ACA branches.* ***(8-13)** Sagittal MIP of CTA shows A2 segments of both ACAs ascending in interhemispheric fissure in front of 3rd ventricle, A3 segments curving around corpus callosum genu.*

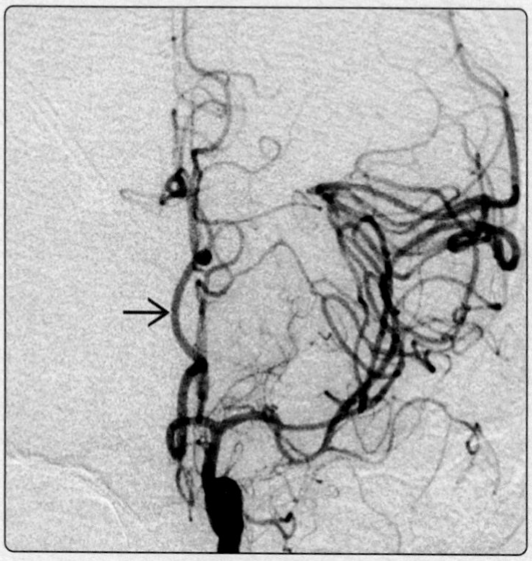

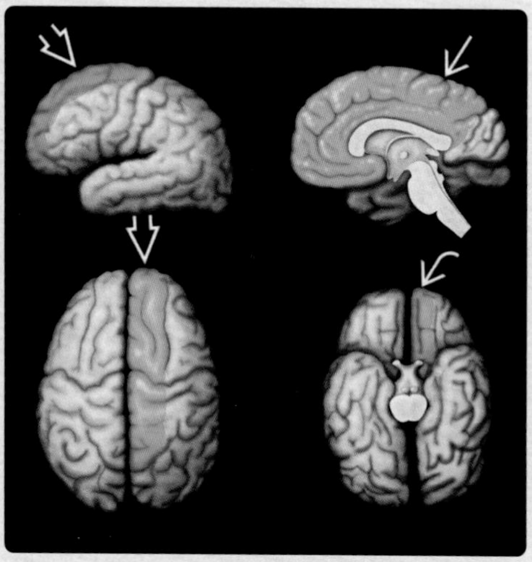

***(8-14)** AP view of a normal left internal carotid DSA shows the ACA "wandering" gently from side to side across the midline in the interhemispheric fissure.* ***(8-15)** ACA vascular territory (green) includes the anterior two-thirds of the medial surface of the hemisphere, a thin strip of cortex over the top of the hemisphere vertex, and a small wedge along the inferomedial frontal lobe.*

In contrast to normal variants, which are common, true COW *anomalies* are rare. When present, they are associated with a high prevalence of saccular aneurysms.

Anterior Cerebral Artery

The anterior cerebral artery (ACA) is the smaller, more medial terminal branch of the supraclinoid ICA. The ACA runs mostly in the interhemispheric fissure and has three defined segments **(8-12)**.

Normal Anatomy

A1 (Horizontal) ACA Segment. The first ACA segment, also termed the horizontal or A1 segment, extends medially over the optic chiasm and nerves to the midline, where it is joined to the contralateral ACA by the ACoA. Two important groups of branches arise from the A1 segment. The **medial lenticulostriate arteries** pass superiorly through the anterior perforated substance to supply the medial basal ganglia. The **recurrent artery of Heubner** arises from the distal A1 or proximal A2 ACA segment and curves backward above the horizontal ACA, then joins the medial lenticulostriate arteries to supply the inferomedial basal ganglia and anterior limb of the internal capsule.

A2 (Vertical) Segment. The A2 or vertical ACA segment courses superiorly in the interhemispheric fissure, extending from the A1-ACoA junction to the corpus callosum rostrum **(8-13)** **(8-14)**. The A2 segment has two cortical branches, the orbitofrontal and frontopolar arteries, that supply the undersurface and inferomedial aspect of the frontal lobe.

A3 (Callosal) Segment. The A3 ACA segment curves anteriorly around the corpus callosum genu, then divides into the two terminal ACA branches, the pericallosal and callosomarginal arteries. The pericallosal artery is the larger of the two terminal branches, running posteriorly between the dorsal surface of the corpus callosum and cingulate gyrus. The

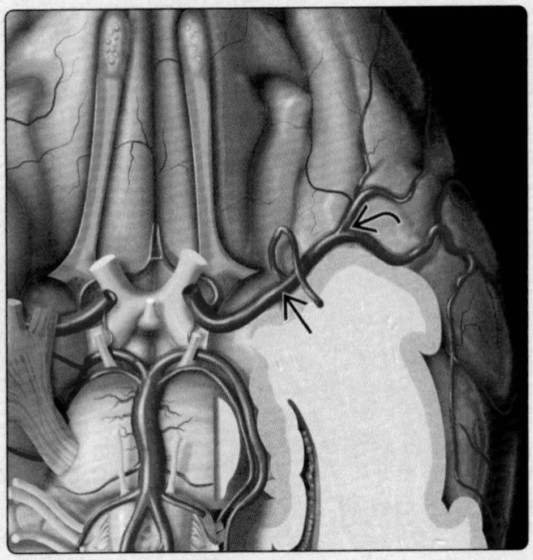

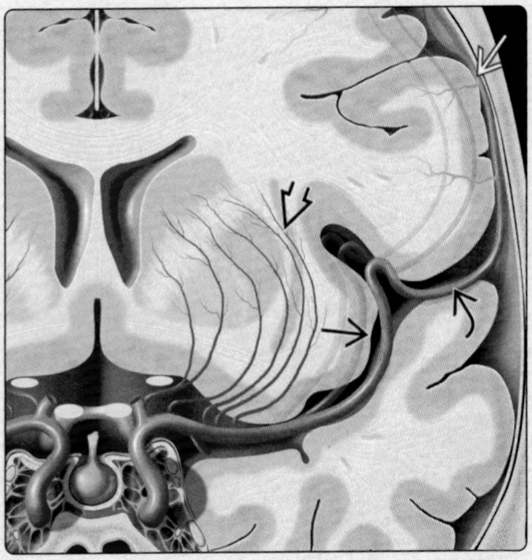

***(8-16)** Submentovertex graphic depicts the MCA and its relationship to adjacent structures. Note the horizontal (M1) segment and the genu with bifurcation into M2 branches. **(8-17)** Coronal graphic shows the lateral lenticulostriate arteries, M2 segments over the insula, M3 segments running laterally in the sylvian fissure, and M4 (cortical) branches coursing over the lateral surface of the hemisphere.*

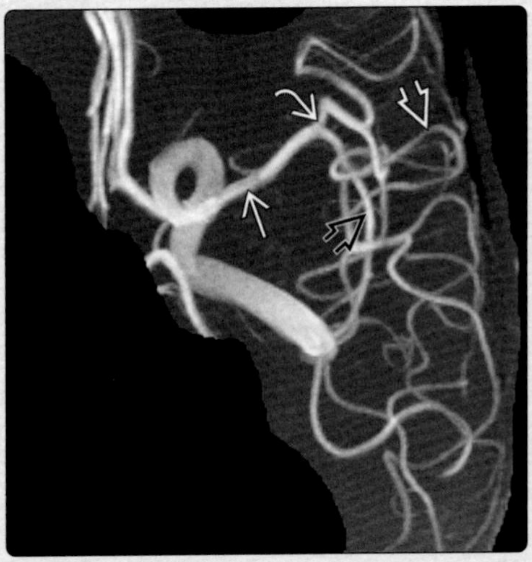

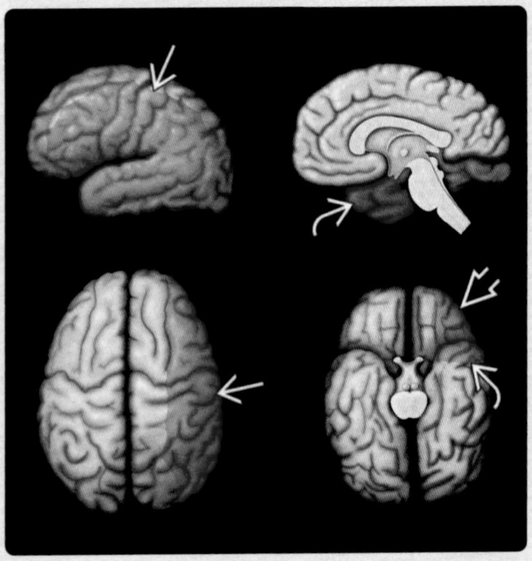

***(8-18)** Submentovertex view of MRA shows M1, genu and bifurcation, M2 segments coursing over insula, and M3 segments turning laterally to exit the sylvian fissure and course over the lateral surface of the hemisphere. **(8-19)** Vascular MCA territory (red) supplies most of the lateral surface of the hemisphere, the anterior tip of the temporal lobe, and the inferolateral frontal lobe.*

callosomarginal artery courses over the cingulate gyrus within the cingulate sulcus **(8-12)**.

Vascular Territory

The cortical ACA branches supply the anterior two-thirds of the *medial* hemispheres and corpus callosum, the inferomedial surface of the frontal lobe, and the anterior two-thirds of the cerebral convexity adjacent to the interhemispheric fissure **(8-15)**.

The penetrating ACA branches (mainly the medial lenticulostriate arteries) supply the medial basal ganglia, corpus callosum genu, and anterior limb of the internal capsule.

Variants and Anomalies

A rare variant is a **persistent primitive olfactory artery** (PPOA), which is a true ACA anomaly rather than a persistent carotid-basilar anastomosis (PCBA). In PPOA, a hypoplastic proximal ACA takes a very long anterior and inferomedial course along the ipsilateral olfactory tract just above the cribriform plate. It then makes a tight posterosuperior "hairpin" turn to continue as the normal distal ACA. PPOAs are frequently associated with saccular aneurysm, usually at the "hairpin" turn.

Two uncommon but important ACA anomalies are an infraoptic A1 and an azygous ACA. An **infraoptic A1** occurs when the horizontal segment passes below (not above) the optic nerve. An infraoptic A1 is associated with a high prevalence (40%) of aneurysms. A single midline or **azygous ACA** is seen with the holoprosencephaly spectrum.

Middle Cerebral Artery

The middle cerebral artery (MCA) is the larger, more lateral terminal branch of the supraclinoid ICA. The MCA has four defined segments.

Normal Anatomy

M1 (Horizontal) Segment. The M1 MCA segment extends laterally from the ICA bifurcation toward the sylvian (lateral cerebral) fissure. The MCA typically bi- or trifurcates just before it enters the sylvian fissure **(8-16)**.

The most important branches that arise from the M1 segment are the lateral lenticulostriate group of arteries and the anterior temporal artery. The **lateral lenticulostriate arteries** supply the lateral putamen, caudate nucleus, and external capsule **(8-17)**. The **anterior temporal artery** supplies the tip of the temporal lobe.

M2 (Insular) Segments. The postbifurcation MCA trunks turn posterosuperiorly in the sylvian fissure, following a gentle curve (the genu or "knee" of the MCA). Several branches—the M2 or insular MCA segments—arise from the postbifurcation trunks and sweep upward over the surface of the insula **(8-17)**.

M3 (Opercular) Segments. The MCA branches loop at or near the top of the sylvian fissure, then course laterally under the parts ("opercula") of the frontal, parietal, and temporal lobes that hang over and enclose the sylvian fissure. These are the M3 or opercular segments **(8-18)**.

M4 (Cortical) Segments. The MCA branches become the M4 segments when they exit the sylvian fissure and ramify over the lateral surface of the cerebral hemisphere **(8-19)**. There is considerable variation in the cortical MCA branching patterns.

Vascular Territory

The MCA has the largest vascular territory of any of the major cerebral arteries. The MCA supplies most of the *lateral* surface of the cerebral hemisphere with the exception of a thin strip at the vertex (supplied by the ACA) and the occipital and posteroinferior parietal lobes (supplied by the PCA) **(8-19)**. Its penetrating branches supply most of the lateral basal brain structures.

Variants and Anomalies

There is wide variability in the branching pattern of the cortical MCA vessels but few true anomalies. In contrast to the ACA/ACoA complex, MCA hypoplasia and aplasia are rare.

Duplicate origin of the MCA is rare. Here two MCA branches arise separately from the terminal segment of the ICA and then fuse to form an arterial ring. Fenestrated and accessory MCAs have been described.

Posterior Cerebral Artery

The two posterior cerebral arteries (PCAs) are the major terminal branches of the distal basilar artery. Each PCA has four defined segments **(8-20)**.

Normal Anatomy

P1 (Precommunicating) Segment. The P1 PCA segment extends laterally from the basilar artery (BA) bifurcation to the junction with the posterior communicating artery (PCoA). The P1 segment lies above the oculomotor nerve (CN III) and has perforating branches (the **posterior thalamoperforating arteries**) that course posterosuperiorly in the interpeduncular fossa to enter the undersurface of the midbrain.

P2 (Ambient) Segment. The P2 segment extends from the P1-PCoA junction, running in the ambient (perimesencephalic) cistern as it sweeps posterolaterally around the midbrain. The P2 segment lies above the tentorium and the cisternal segment of the trochlear nerve (CN IV). Two major cortical branches—the **anterior and posterior temporal arteries**—arise from the P2 PCA segment and pass laterally toward the inferior surface of the temporal lobe **(8-20)**.

Several smaller but important branches also arise from the P2 PCA segment. **Thalamogeniculate arteries** and **peduncular perforating arteries** arise from the proximal P2 and pass directly superiorly into the midbrain **(8-21)**.

The **medial posterior choroidal artery** (PChA) and the **lateral PChA** also arise from the P2 segment. The medial PChA curves around the brainstem and courses superomedially to enter the tela choroidea and roof of the third ventricle. The lateral

PChA enters the lateral ventricle and travels with the choroid plexus, curving around the pulvinar of the thalamus. The lateral PChA shares a reciprocal relationship with the AChA, a branch from the ICA.

P3 (Quadrigeminal) Segment. The P3 PCA is a short segment that lies entirely within the quadrigeminal cistern. It begins behind the midbrain and ends where the PCA enters the calcarine fissure of the occipital lobe **(8-22)**.

P4 (Calcarine) Segment. The P4 segment terminates within the calcarine fissure, where it divides into two terminal PCA trunks **(8-22)**. The medial trunk gives off the medial occipital artery, **parietooccipital artery, calcarine artery**, and **posterior splenial arteries**, whereas the lateral trunk gives rise to the **lateral occipital artery**.

Vascular Territory

The PCA supplies most of the *inferior* surface of the cerebral hemisphere, with the exception of the temporal tip and frontal lobe. It also supplies the occipital lobe, posterior one-third of the medial hemisphere and corpus callosum, and most of the choroid plexus **(8-23)**. Penetrating PCA branches are the major vascular supply to the midbrain and posterior thalami.

Variants and Anomalies

A common normal variant is the **"fetal" origin of the PCA.** Here the proximal PCA arises from the ICA instead of from the basilar bifurcation. "Fetal" PCA origin is seen in 10-30% of cases. This variant is easily recognized on CTA, MRA, and DSA.

Vascular transit time in the PCA territory decreases with increasing contribution of the anterior circulation relative to that of the posterior circulation. If a large PCoA or "fetal" PCA

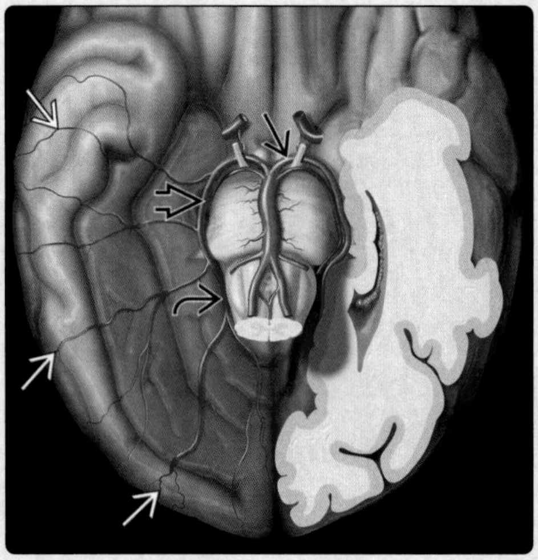

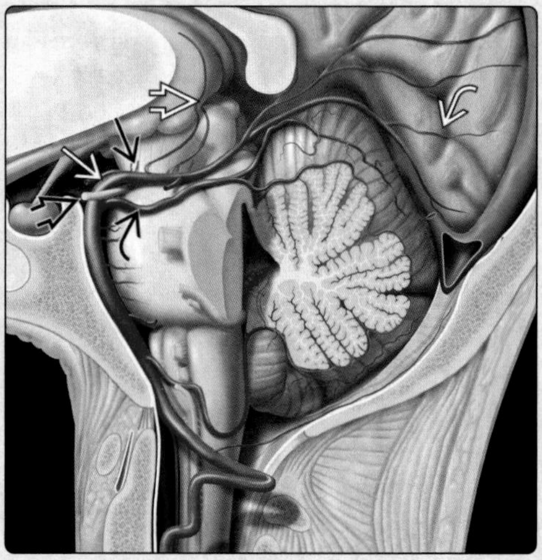

***(8-20)** Submentovertex graphic shows the PCA segments and their relationship to the midbrain. P1, P2, and P3 segments are shown. P4 segments (cortical branches) ramify over the occipital and inferior temporal lobes. **(8-21)** Lateral graphic depicts the PCA above and the superior cerebellar artery below the oculomotor nerve. Perforating, choroidal, and cortical PCA branches are also shown.*

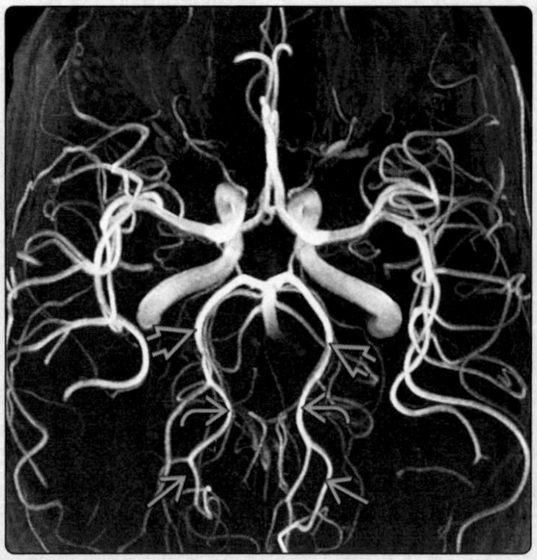

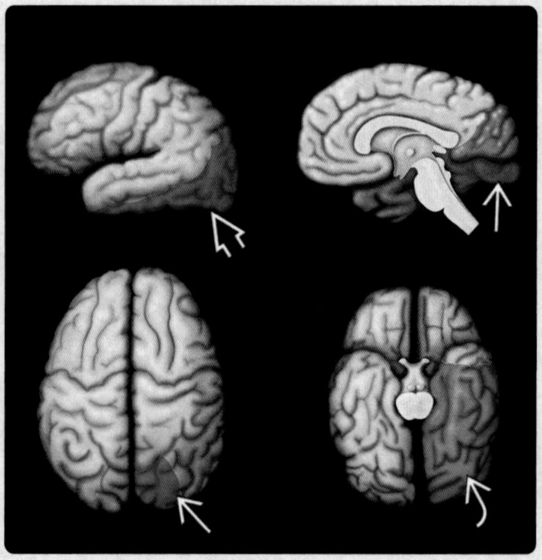

***(8-22)** Submentovertex MRA shows the posterosubmentovertex sweep of the P2 PCAs and the medial course of the P3 segments as they pass behind the midbrain. Calcarine and P4 cortical branches are shown. **(8-23)** The PCA territory (purple) includes the occipital lobe and posterior third of the medial and the posterolateral surfaces of the hemisphere, as well as almost the entire inferior surface of the temporal lobe.*

is present on one side, this can produce substantial left-right asymmetry on perfusion imaging. Knowledge of this common normal variant is essential, as such asymmetry can mimic cerebrovascular pathology.

A rare but important PCA variant is an **artery of Percheron** (AOP). Here a single dominant thalamoperforating artery arises from the P1 segment and supplies the rostral midbrain and bilateral medial thalami **(8-88)**.

With the exception of persistent carotid-basilar anastomoses (see above), true PCA anomalies are uncommon. Early bifurcation, duplication, and fenestration of the precommunicating (P1) PCA segment have been described.

Vertebrobasilar System

The vertebrobasilar system consists of the two vertebral arteries (VAs), the basilar artery (BA), and their branches. Four VA segments are identified. Only one—the V4 segment—is intracranial.

Normal Anatomy

V1 (Extraosseous) Segment. Each VA arises from the ipsilateral subclavian artery and courses posterosuperiorly to enter the C6 transverse foramen. Unnamed **segmental branches** arise from V1 to supply the cervical musculature and lower cervical spinal cord.

V2 (Foraminal) Segment. The V2 segment courses superiorly through the C6-C3 transverse foramina until it reaches C2, where it first turns superolaterally through the "inverted L" of the transverse foramen and then turns upward to pass through the C1 transverse foramen **(8-24)**. An **anterior meningeal artery** and additional unnamed segmental branches arise from V2.

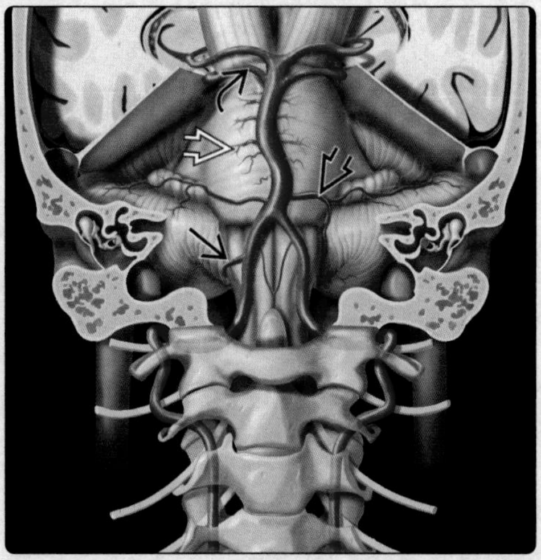

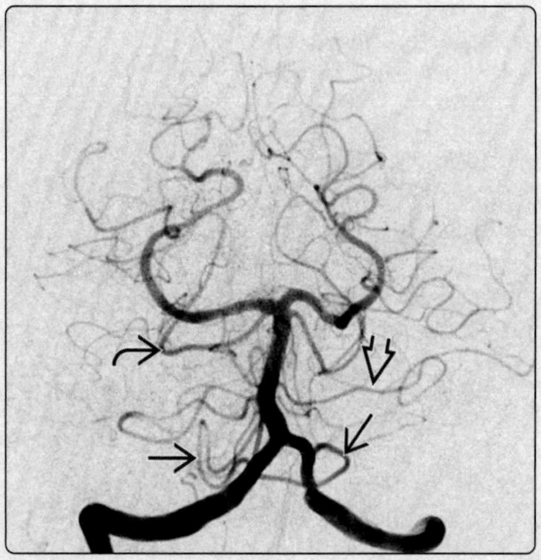

***(8-24)** AP graphic depicts the vertebrobasilar system. PICAs ⇨ arise from the VAs before the basilar junction and curve posteriorly around the medulla. AICAs ⇨ course laterally to the CPAs. Two or more SCAs ⇨ arise from the BA just below the tentorium. Perforating BA branches ➡ supply most of the pons. **(8-25)** AP DSA shows PICAs ⇨, AICAs ⇨, and SCAs ⇨. The SCAs and PICAs both curve posterolaterally around the midbrain.*

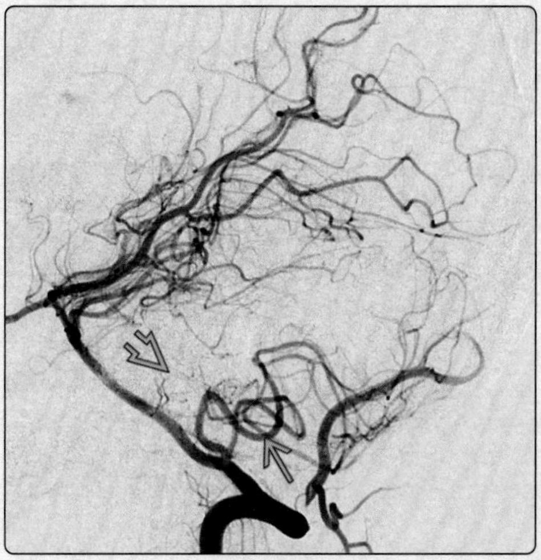

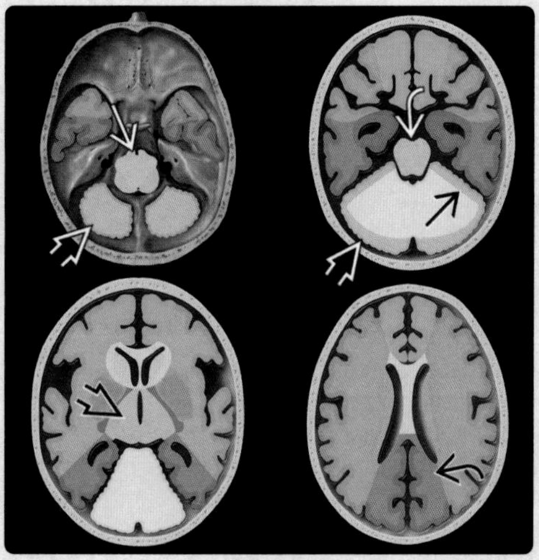

***(8-26)** Lateral DSA shows large PICAs ⇨ and small AICAs ⇨. **(8-27)** Graphic shows the posterior circulation vascular territories of PICAs (tan ➡), AICAs (blue-green ⇨), SCAs (yellow), medullary perforating branches of the VA ➡, and pontine perforating branches of the BA ➡. Thalamic perforating branches ⇨ arise from the top of the BA and PCoAs. PCA territory is shown in purple ⇨.*

V3 (Extraspinal) Segment. The V3 segment begins after the VA exits the C1 transverse foramen. It lies on top of the C1 ring, curving posteromedially around the atlantooccipital joint before making a sharp anterosuperior turn to pierce the dura at the foramen magnum. The only major V3 branch is the **posterior meningeal artery**.

V4 (Intradural) Segment. Once the VA becomes intradural, it courses superomedially behind the clivus and in front of the medulla. It gives off small **anterior and posterior spinal arteries** and **medullary perforating branches**. The **posterior inferior cerebellar artery (PICA)** arises from the distal VA, curves around/over the tonsil, and gives off the perforating medullary, choroid, tonsillar, and inferior cerebellar branches **(8-24)** **(8-25)**.

Basilar Artery. The two VAs unite at or near the pontomedullary junction to form the BA. The BA courses superiorly in the prepontine cistern, lying between the clivus in front and the pons behind. It terminates in the interpeduncular fossa by dividing into the two **posterior cerebral arteries**.

Numerous small but critical **basilar perforating arteries** arise from the entire dorsal surface of the BA to supply the pons and midbrain.

The first major named BA branch is the **anterior inferior cerebellar artery (AICA)** **(8-26)**. The AICA arises from the proximal BA and courses ventromedially to CNs VII and VIII, frequently looping into the internal auditory meatus. It supplies both nerves as well as a relatively thin strip of the cerebellar hemisphere that lies directly behind the petrous temporal bone.

One or more (usually two to four) **superior cerebellar arteries** (SCAs) originate from each side of the distal BA, course laterally below CN III, then curve posterolaterally around the midbrain just below the tentorium **(8-25)**. SCA branches ramify over the surface of the superior cerebellum and upper vermis, curving into the great horizontal fissure.

Vascular Territory

The vertebrobasilar system normally supplies all of the posterior fossa structures as well as the midbrain, posterior thalami, occipital lobes, most of the inferior and posterolateral surfaces of the temporal lobe, and upper cervical spinal cord **(8-27)**.

Variants and Anomalies

The vertebrobasilar system has several normal variants. The two vertebral arteries vary in size, with the left VA dominant in 50% of cases, both equal size in 25%, and the right VA dominant in 25%. The left VA originates directly from the aortic arch (instead of the left subclavian artery) in 5% of cases. A small VA that ends in the PICA without connecting to the BA is another common normal variant.

The BA commonly varies in course and branching patterns. The BA and VAs can be fenestrated or partially duplicated.

Arterial Infarcts

We first focus on the pathology and imaging of major arterial ischemia-infarction, starting with acute lesions. Subacute and chronic infarcts are then discussed, followed by a brief consideration of lacunar infarcts. Lastly, we discuss watershed and hypotensive infarcts.

Acute Cerebral Ischemia-Infarction

As the clinical diagnosis of acute "stroke" is inaccurate in 15-20% of cases, imaging has become *the* basis of rapid stroke triage. When and how to image patients with suspected acute stroke varies somewhat from institution to institution. Because of speed and accessibility, NECT and CTA (with or without CT perfusion) are the most commonly used modalities.

Acute stroke protocols are based on elapsed time since symptom onset, availability of emergent imaging with appropriate software reconstructions, clinician and radiologist preferences, and availability of neurointervention.

Because imaging has become so critical to patient management, we will focus in detail on hyperacute/acute stroke imaging. There are four "must know" questions in acute stroke triage that need to be answered rapidly and accurately. (1) Is intracranial hemorrhage or a stroke "mimic" present? (2) Is a large vessel occluded? (3) Is part of the brain irreversibly injured (i.e., is there a core of critically ischemic, irreversibly infarcted tissue)? (4) Is there a *clinically relevant* "penumbra" of ischemic but potentially salvageable tissue?

THE FOUR "MUST KNOW" ACUTE STROKE QUESTIONS

- Is there intracranial hemorrhage (or a stroke "mimic")?
- Is a large vessel occluded?
- Is part of the brain irreversibly injured?
- Is an ischemic "penumbra" present?

Terminology

Stroke—a generic term meaning sudden onset of a neurologic event—is also referred to as a cerebrovascular accident (CVA) or "brain attack."

The distinction between cerebral ischemia and cerebral infarction is subtle but important. In cerebral *ischemia*, the affected tissue remains viable although blood flow is inadequate to sustain normal cellular function. In cerebral *infarction*, frank cell death occurs with loss of neurons, glia, or both.

Timing is important in patient triage. *Hyperacute* stroke designates events within the first 6 hours following symptom onset. In hyperacute stroke, cell death has not yet occurred, so the combined term *acute cerebral ischemia-infarction* is often used. *Acute* strokes are those 6-48 hours from onset.

Etiology

Ischemic stroke is a heterogeneous disease with different etiologies and several subtypes. Etiology varies with stroke subtype, and stroke subtypes also vary by racial and ethnic groups. Recent genome-wide association studies (GWAS) have identified specific loci for a number of stroke subtypes.

Stroke Subtypes. Several systems have been used to classify major arterial stroke subtypes. These include the NINDS stroke data bank subtype, the Lausanne Stroke Registry, and the TOAST (Trial of Org 10172 in Acute Stroke Treatment).

One of the simplest classifications is the **ASCO** phenotypic system, which divides strokes into four subtypes: **a**therosclerotic, **s**mall vessel disease, **c**ardioembolic, and **o**ther.

Atherosclerotic (ASVD) strokes are the most common type of acute arterial ischemia/infarction, representing approximately 40-45% of cases. The relative distribution of intracranial, extracranial, and coronary ASVD varies with race and ethnicity. Intracranial atherosclerosis causes 30-50% of strokes in Asians but only 8-10% in North America.

Most large artery territorial infarcts are embolic, arising from thrombi that develop at the site of an "at risk" ASVD plaque. The most common site of ASVD in the craniocervical vasculature is the carotid bifurcation (see Chapter 10), followed by the cavernous internal carotid artery (ICA) segment. The most frequently occluded intracranial vessel is the middle cerebral artery (MCA).

Large artery atherosclerosis stroke susceptibility has a locus identified near TSPAN2. Genome-wide analysis has also identified a strong overlap between large artery stroke and migraine headaches, especially those without aura.

Small vessel disease represents 15-30% of all strokes. Small artery occlusions, also called **lacunar infarcts**, are defined as lesions measuring less than 15 mm in diameter. Many are clinically silent although a strategically located lesion (e.g., in the internal capsule) can cause significant neurologic impairment.

Lacunar infarcts can be embolic, atheromatous, or thrombotic. Most involve penetrating arteries in the basal ganglia/thalami, internal capsule, pons, and deep cerebral white matter. Small artery strokes have been associated with the 12q24 locus near ALDH2. The homocysteine levels-associated genetic variant *MTHFR* C677T is associated with lacunar stroke and cerebral small vessel disease (white matter hyperintensities) but not large artery or cardioembolic stroke.

Cardioembolic disease accounts for another 15-25% of major strokes. Common risk factors include myocardial infarction, arrhythmia (most often atrial fibrillation), and valvular heart disease. Cardioembolic stroke is associated with the locus ZFHX3.

Other is a heterogeneous group that combines strokes with miscellaneous but known etiologies together with strokes of undetermined etiology ("cryptogenic stroke").

Pathophysiology. An estimated two million neurons are lost each minute when a major vessel such as the MCA is suddenly occluded. Cerebral blood flow (CBF) falls precipitously. The center of the affected brain parenchyma—the densely **ischemic core**—typically has a CBF < 6-8 cm^3/100 g/min. Oxygen is rapidly depleted, cellular energy production fails, and ion homeostasis is lost.

Neuronal death with irreversible loss of function occurs in the core of an acute stroke. A relatively less **ischemic penumbra** surrounding the central core is present in about half of all patients. CBF in the penumbra is significantly reduced, falling from a normal of 60 cm^3/100 g/min to 10-20 cm^3/100 g/min. This ischemic but not-yet-doomed-to-infarct tissue represents physiologically "at risk" but potentially salvageable tissue.

There is a well-defined *histologic "hierarchy of sensitivity"* to ischemic damage among the different cell types that constitute the neuropil. Neurons are the most vulnerable. They are followed (in descending order of susceptibility) by astrocytes, oligodendroglia, microglia, and endothelial cells.

There is also a *geographic "hierarchy of sensitivity"* to ischemic damage among the neurons themselves. Neurons in the CA1 area of the hippocampus, neocortex layers III, V, and VI, and the neostriatum are more vulnerable than other regions (e.g., the brainstem).

Predisposing Factors and Genetics. Ischemic stroke is a multifactorial disease. Hypertension, diabetes, smoking, metabolic syndrome, and elevated triglycerides are significant known predisposing factors. However, all these factors together account for just part of stroke risk. Now with widespread availability of GWAS data, an ever-increasing percentage of overall stroke risk can be attributed to various genetic factors.

Pathology

Location. The MCA is the most common site of large artery thromboembolic occlusion **(8-28)**, followed by the PCA and vertebrobasilar circulation. The ACA is the least commonly occluded major intracranial vessel.

Size and Number. Acute infarcts can be solitary or multiple and vary in size from tiny lacunar to large territorial lesions that can involve much of the cerebral hemisphere.

Gross Pathology. An acutely thrombosed artery is filled with soft purplish clot that may involve the entire vessel or just a short segment **(8-29A)**. Clot extension into secondary branches with or without distal emboli into smaller, more peripheral vessels is common. Longer and larger thrombi are also associated with reduced probability of reperfusion after intravenous thrombolysis, so thrombectomy may be necessary to maximize the probability and speed of recanalization.

Gross parenchymal changes are minimal or absent in the first 6-8 hours, after which edema in the affected vascular territory causes the brain to appear pale and swollen. The gray-white matter (GM-WM) boundaries become less distinct and more

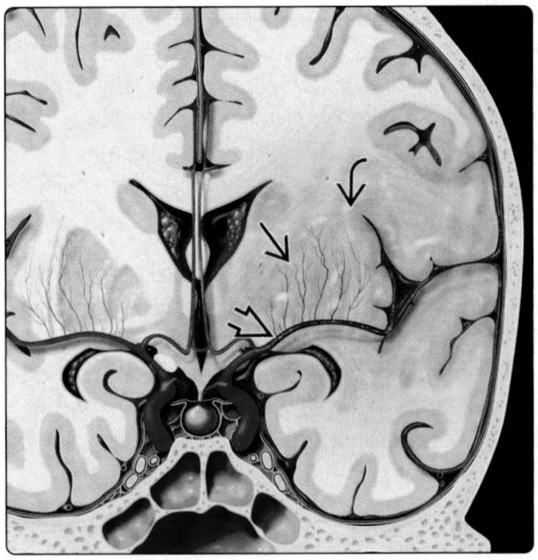

(8-28) Graphic shows M1 occlusion. Acute ischemia is seen as subtle loss of gray-white interfaces and "blurred" basal ganglia.

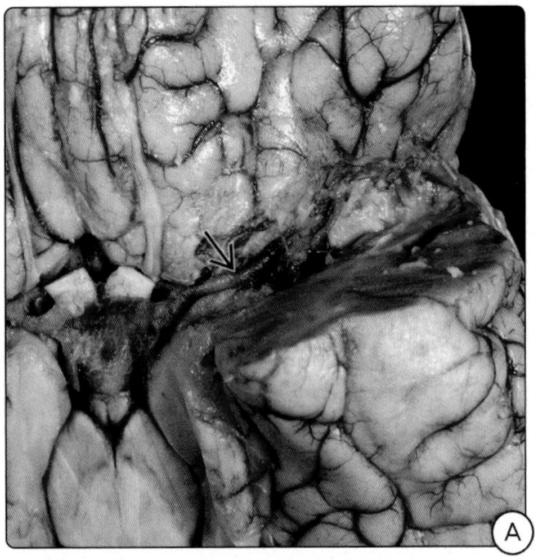

(8-29A) Autopsy specimen shows acute thrombus in the proximal MCA. (Courtesy R. Hewlett, MD.)

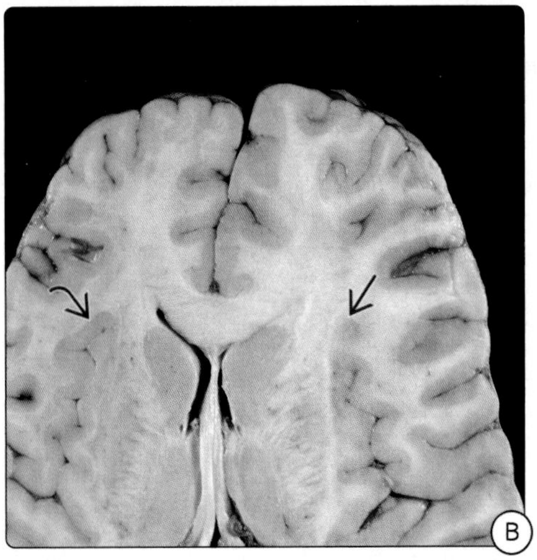

(8-29B) The same case shows swollen, "blurred" insular cortex compared with the opposite normal side. (Courtesy R. Hewlett, MD.)

"blurred." As the gyri expand, the adjacent sulci are compressed, and the sulcal-cisternal CSF space is effaced **(8-29B)**.

Microscopic Features. Frank cerebral infarction is characterized by irreversible damage to all cells within the infarcted zone. Microscopically, neurons appear histologically normal in the first 8-12 hours. Within 12-24 hours, acutely ischemic neurons classically appear "red and dead" with hypereosinophilic cytoplasm, early karyolysis, and pyknotic nuclei. Acute infarcts are pale and often vacuolized, especially near the junction with intact brain. Astrocytic swelling without cell death predominates in the penumbral zone.

Clinical Issues

Epidemiology and Demographics. Stroke is the third leading cause of death in many industrialized countries and is the major worldwide cause of adult neurologic disability. The age-adjusted incidence rate is about 180 per 100,000 per year.

Strokes affect patients of all ages—including newborns and neonates—although most occur in middle-aged or older adults. Children with strokes often have an underlying disorder such as right-to-left cardiac shunt, sickle cell disease, or inherited hypercoagulable syndrome. Strokes in young adults are often caused by dissection (spontaneous or traumatic) or drug abuse.

Presentation. Stroke symptoms vary widely, depending on the vascular territory affected as well as the presence and adequacy of collateral flow. Sudden onset of a focal neurologic deficit such as facial droop, slurred speech, paresis, or decreased consciousness is the most common presentation.

Natural History. Stroke outcome varies widely. Between 20-25% of strokes are considered "major" occlusions and cause 80% of adverse outcomes. Six months after stroke, 20-30% of all patients are dead, and a similar number are severely disabled.

Prognosis in individual patients depends on a number of contributing factors, i.e., which vessel is occluded, the presence or absence of robust collateral blood flow, and whether there is a significant ischemic penumbra. Nearly half of all strokes have inadequate collateral blood flow and no significant penumbra. Most patients with major vessel occlusions—even those with a significant ischemic penumbra—will do poorly unless blood flow can be restored and the brain reperfused.

Uncontrolled brain swelling with herniation and death can result from so-called malignant MCA infarction. In such cases, emergent craniectomy may be the only treatment option.

Treatment Options. Speed is essential, with the goal of a "door to needle" time (i.e., from arrival in the emergency department to intervention) under 60 minutes. Transporting stroke patients by EMS directly to the imaging suite can reduce the door-to-needle time to under 30 minutes. Prehospital notification, alerting and clearing the CT/MR scanner, acquiring history en route, and neurologic examination with intravenous tPA delivery on the table are key elements in implementing such ultrafast stroke triage.

Stroke treatment options and inclusion/exclusion criteria are continually evolving. The single most important factor in successful intervention is patient selection, with the two most important considerations being (1) elapsed time from symptom onset and (2) imaging findings on the screening NECT scan.

The clinically accepted therapeutic window for *intravenous* recombinant tissue plasminogen activator (rTPA) is less than 3 hours from ictus (the "golden hours"). *Intraarterial* thrombolysis is typically restricted to less than 6 hours. Exceptions to this general rule include basilar artery thrombosis and patients outside the 6-hour window who have a persistent significant perfusion-diffusion mismatch.

Endovascular thrombectomy benefits most patients with acute ischemic stroke caused by occlusion of the proximal anterior circulation and offers an alternative, potentially synergistic method to thrombolysis. Its advantages include delivering site-specific therapy and tailored thrombolytic dosage. Early studies have shown improved recanalization rates and 90-day outcomes. Mechanical thrombectomy may also be suitable in patients beyond the therapeutic window or in whom thrombolytic therapy is contraindicated.

Imaging

"Brain Attack" Protocols. The primary goals of emergent stroke imaging are (1) to distinguish "bland" or ischemic stroke from intracranial hemorrhage and (2) to select/triage patients for possible reperfusion therapies.

Most protocols begin with emergent NECT to answer the *first* "must know" question in stroke imaging: Is intracranial hemorrhage or a stroke "mimic" (such as subdural hematoma or neoplasm) present? If a typical hypertensive hemorrhage is identified on the screening NECT and the patient has a history of systemic hypertension, no further imaging is generally required. CTA is sometimes requested to evaluate for active bleeding ("spot sign").

Once intracranial hemorrhage is excluded, the *second* critical issue is determining whether a major cerebral vessel is occluded. CT angiography (CTA) can be obtained immediately following the NECT scan and is the noninvasive procedure of

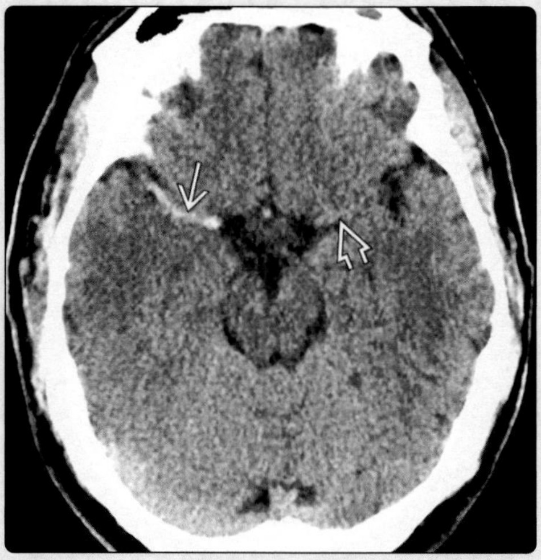

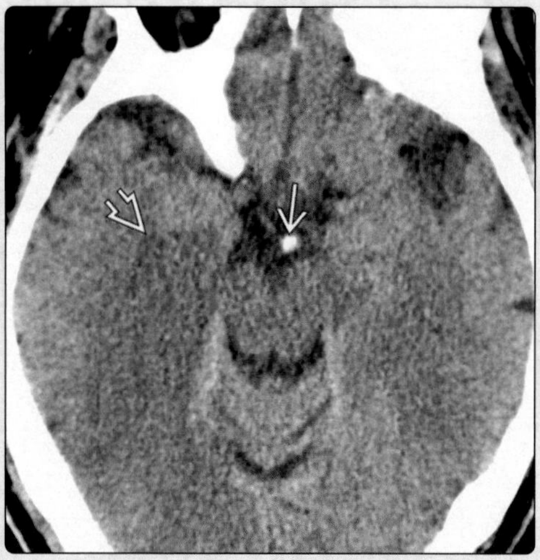

***(8-30)** NECT scan shows a classic "hyperdense MCA" sign with acute thrombus in the right MCA. Compare its striking hyperdensity with the normal, mild hyperdensity of the left MCA. **(8-31)** NECT scan shows "dense" artery sign in acute thrombosis of the basilar trunk. Note the hypodensity of the right occipital, inferomedial temporal lobes.*

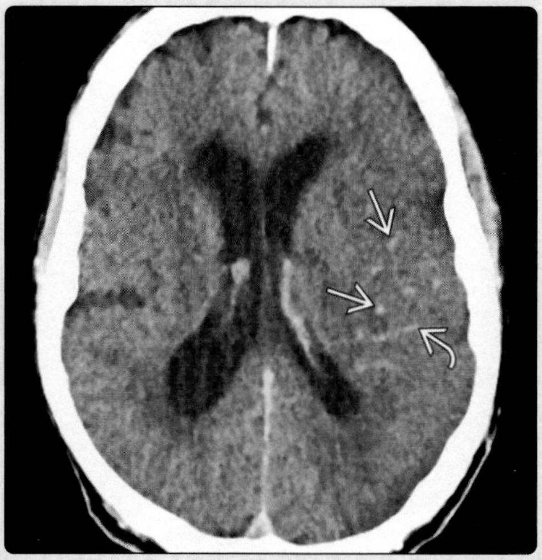

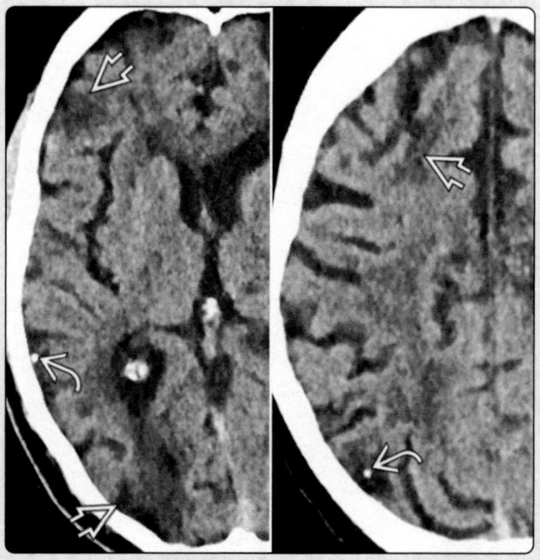

***(8-32)** NECT in a 75y man with acute onset of right hemiparesis shows hyperdense thrombus in the left M2 ("dot sign") and M3 MCA branches. **(8-33)** Axial NECTs in a 77y man with history of multiple strokes show old right-sided cortical infarcts and two calcified emboli. Patients with one or more calcified emboli are at high risk for repeated strokes.*

choice for depicting potentially treatable major vessel occlusions. MR angiography (MRA) is more susceptible to motion artifact, which is accentuated in uncooperative patients. DSA is typically reserved for patients undergoing intraarterial thrombolysis or mechanical thrombectomy.

The *third* and *fourth* questions can be answered with either CT or MR perfusion (pCT, pMR) studies. Both can depict what part of the brain is irreversibly damaged (i.e., the unsalvageable core infarct) and determine whether there is a clinically relevant ischemic penumbra (potentially salvageable brain).

CT Findings. A complete multimodal acute stroke CT protocol includes nonenhanced head CT, an arch-to-vertex CTA, and dynamic first-pass perfusion CT (pCT). With helical acquisition, the entire protocol can be completed within 15 minutes as a single examination with separate contrast boluses. Recent studies have demonstrated that CTA with or without CTP improves diagnostic accuracy compared with NECT alone and does not delay IV tPA or endovascular therapy.

NECT. Initial NECT scans—even those obtained in the first 6 hours—are abnormal in 50-60% of acute ischemic strokes if viewed with narrow window width.

The most specific but least sensitive sign is a hyperattenuating vessel filled with acute thrombus. A **"dense MCA" sign** is seen in 30% of cases with documented M1 occlusion **(8-30)**. Less common sites for a hyperdense vessel sign are the intracranial internal carotid artery, basilar artery **(8-31)**, and MCA branches in the sylvian fissure ("dot" sign) **(8-32)**.

Uncommon but important NECT findings that indicate vascular occlusion include a calcified embolus **(8-33)**, most likely from an "at-risk" ulcerated atherosclerotic plaque in the cervical or cavernous ICA. It is critically important to identify calcified cerebral emboli, as they carry a near 50% risk of repeat ischemic stroke.

Blurring and indistinctness of gray-white matter (GM-WM) interfaces can be seen in 50-70% of cases within the first 3

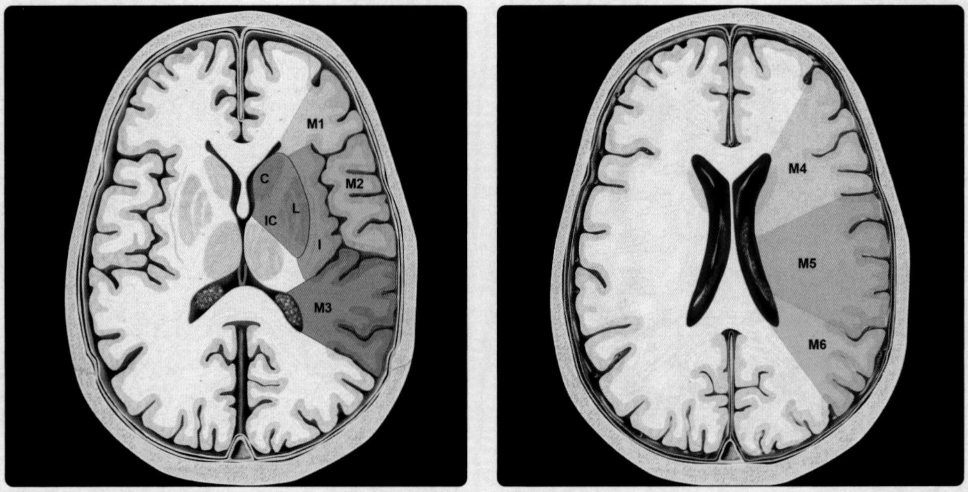

***(8-34)** Anatomic regions for calculating ASPECTS score are illustrated. M1-3 represent the middle cerebral artery cortex with each area allotted one point. The insular cortex (I), lentiform nuclei (L), caudate head (C), and internal capsule are scored with one point each. **(8-35)** More cephalad graphic shows the superior three MCA territories. ASPECTS score is calculated by subtracting 1 point for each affected area from 10 (normal total score).*

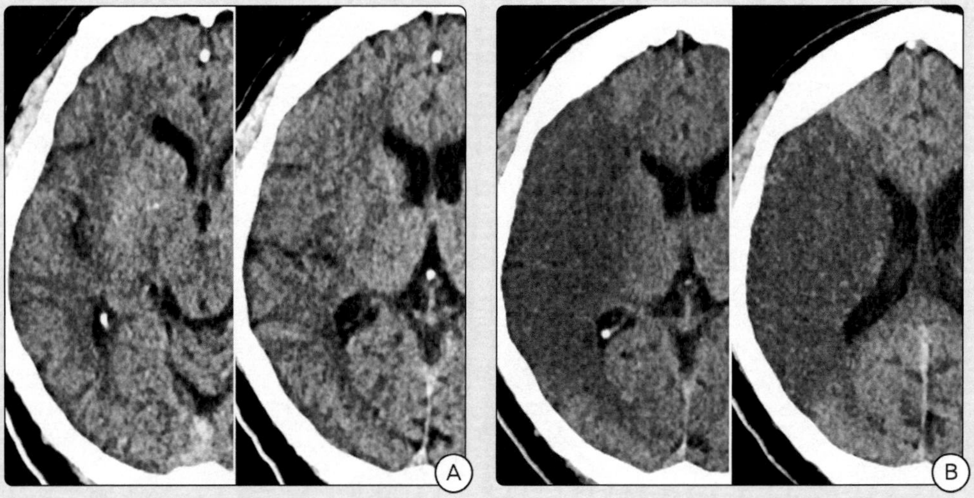

***(8-36A)** Axial NECTs in a 60y man with acute stroke symptoms show (L) hypodensity in the right insular cortex, M1, M2, and and M3 cortical areas. The caudate, lentiform nucleus, and internal capsule are spared. (R) More cephalad NECT shows hypodensity in the M4 to M6 cortical regions. ASPECTS score is 3. **(8-36B)** At 24 h the wedge-shaped infarction is sharply delineated. ASPECTS score of 3 has a poor prognosis.*

hours following occlusion **(8-36A)**. Loss of the insular cortex (**"insular ribbon" sign**) **(8-38A)** and decreased density of the basal ganglia (**"disappearing basal ganglia" sign**) are the most common findings **(8-37A)**.

Wedge-shaped parenchymal hypodensity with indistinct GM-WM borders and **cortical sulcal effacement** develops in large territorial occlusions. If more than one-third of the MCA territory is initially involved, the likelihood of a "malignant" MCA infarct with severe brain swelling rises, as does the risk of hemorrhagic transformation with attempted revascularization.

The **A**lberta **S**troke **P**rogram **E**arly **C**omputed **T**omographic **S**core (ASPECTS) is a straightforward, quick, and reproducible measure of early ischemic change **(8-34)** **(8-35)**. Originally described using NECT, the scoring system can be applied to both CT and MR. ASPECTS score is calculated by subtracting one point for each of 10 regions affected. The MCA cortex and insular ribbon are allotted seven points, and subcortical structures are allotted three points. An ASPECTS score ≤ 7 equates to more than one-third of the MCA territory and is associated with increased risk of hemorrhage and poor outcome **(8-36)**.

CECT. Standard CECT scans are rarely performed as part of most "brain attack" protocols. CECT may show enhancing vessels if slow antegrade flow or retrograde filling via collaterals over the vascular watershed zone is present. Cortical gyriform enhancement is rare in early arterial occlusion but may occur in late acute/early subacute infarction.

CTA. Multidetector row CT angiography (CTA) of both the intra- and extracranial circulation is used to visualize the craniocervical vasculature from the aortic arch to the cortex and is now standard practice in acute stroke imaging.

CTA (with or without CT perfusion) quickly answers the *second* "must know" stroke question **(8-38)**, i.e., is a major vessel

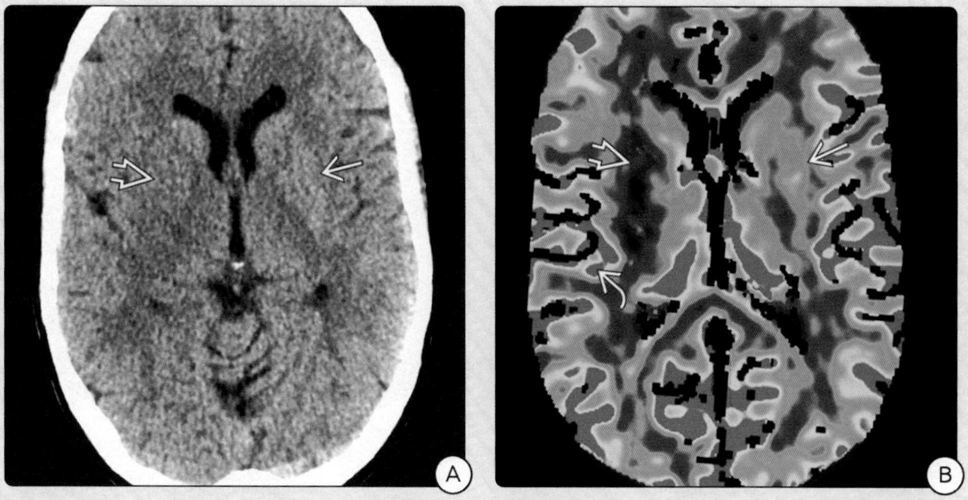

***(8-37A)** NECT scan 3 hours after stroke onset shows hypodensity of the right basal ganglia compared with the normal left side ("disappearing basal ganglia" sign). **(8-37B)** pCT was performed. Cerebral blood volume (CBV) shows markedly reduced blood volume in the right basal ganglia compared with the normal left side. CBV in the cortex overlying the basal ganglia infarct appears relatively normal.*

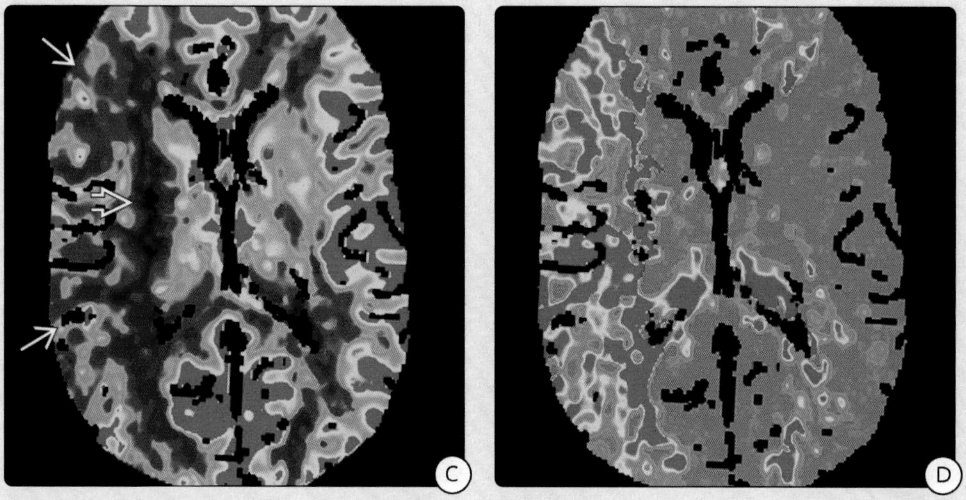

***(8-37C)** Cerebral blood flow (CBF) in the same patient shows markedly reduced blood flow to the entire right MCA distribution with the most profound deficit in the right basal ganglia. The CBV/CBF "mismatch" in the cortex represents a large ischemic penumbra surrounding the densely ischemic basal ganglia. **(8-37D)** MTT shows that blood flow to the right MCA distribution is slow with markedly prolonged transit time.*

occlusion with a "retrievable" intravascular thrombus present? CTA localizes and defines the extent of the intravascular thrombus, assesses collateral blood flow, and also characterizes atherosclerotic disease.

pCT. The *third* and *fourth* "must know" questions can be answered with whole-brain CT perfusion (pCT). Findings on pCT correlate well with those of DWI and pMR (see below).

pCT depicts the effect of vessel occlusion on the brain parenchyma itself, offering a time-sensitive and practical assessment of cerebral hemodynamics and parenchymal viability that is key to acute stroke management **(8-37)**. Baseline pCT can be used to estimate the extent of ischemic core and operational penumbra although correlation with final infarct volume is less unreliable. pCT is also less reliable in identifying those patients who will not benefit from intraarterial therapy.

Perfusion CT is obtained by monitoring the first pass of an iodinated contrast bolus through the cerebral circulation. As contrast passes through the brain, it causes transient hyperattenuation that is directly proportional to the amount of contrast in the vessels and blood in the brain.

pCT has three major parameters: cerebral blood volume (**CBV**), cerebral blood flow (**CBF**), and mean transit time (**MTT**). CBV is defined as the volume of flowing blood in a given volume of brain. CBF is the volume of flowing blood moving through a given volume of brain in a specified amount of time. MTT is the average time it takes blood to transit through a given volume of brain.

All three pCT parameters can be depicted either visually—on a color scale—or numerically, using selected regions of interest. Color-coded perfusion maps can be visually assessed quickly and accurately.

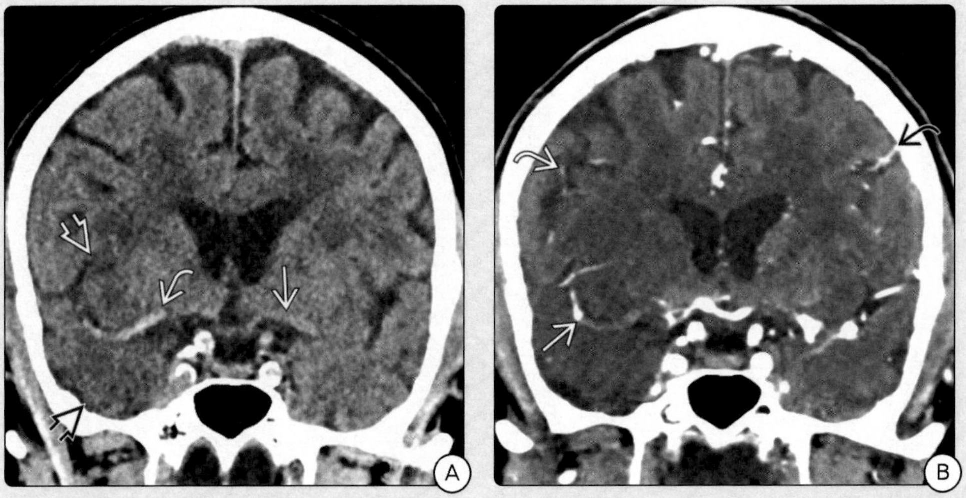

(8-38A) *Coronal NECT scan in an 82y woman with sudden onset of left-sided weakness shows a dense MCA sign. Thrombus ➡ extends through the right M1 segment from its origin to the bifurcation. Compare with normal left MCA ➡. Note hypodensity of the right temporal lobe ⇨, insular cortex ➡ ("insular ribbon sign").* ***(8-38B)*** *Coronal CTA shows right MCA occlusion ➡. Note poor opacification of M3, M4 branches ➡ compared with normal left side ⇨.*

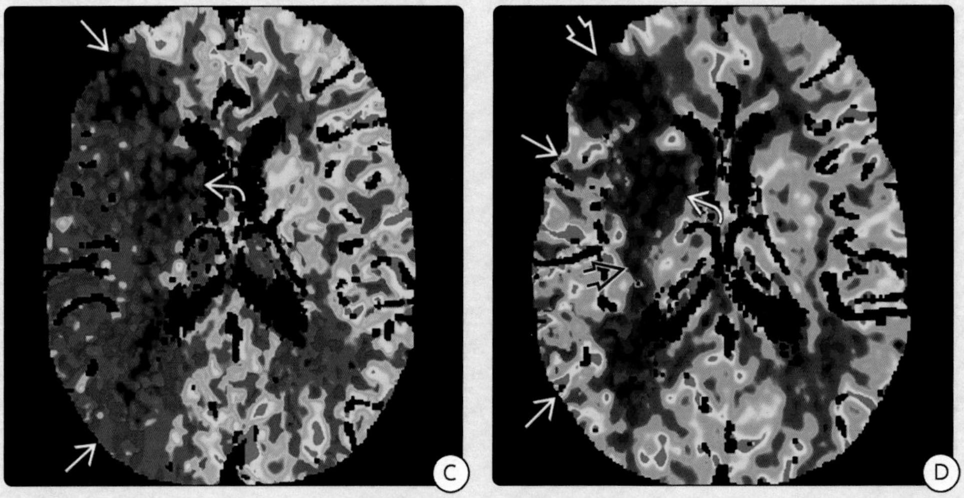

(8-38C) *Axial pCT in the same case shows wedge-shaped area of markedly reduced cerebral blood flow to the entire right MCA territory ➡, including the basal ganglia ➡.* ***(8-38D)*** *Cerebral blood volume in the same case shows much of the cortex is ischemic penumbra ➡, maintained by pial collaterals. The core infarct includes the right frontal lobe ➡, basal ganglia ➡, and deep/periventricular white matter ⇨.*

The standard color scale is graduated from shades of red and yellow to blue and violet. With CBV and CBF, perfusion is portrayed in red/yellow/green (highest) to blue/purple/black (lowest). In normal brain, there is bilaterally symmetric perfusion in the cerebral hemispheres with higher CBF and CBV in gray matter (cortex, basal ganglia) compared with white matter. Well-perfused gray matter appears red/yellow, white matter appears blue, and ischemic brain is blue/purple. Totally nonperfused areas (i.e., the ventricles and densely ischemic central core of a major infarct) are black **(8-38)**.

Of the three standard parameters, MTT shows the most prominent regional abnormalities. Here the color scales are reversed to emphasize the abnormally prolonged transit time in the ischemic brain. With MTT, the slower the transit time, the closer to the red end of the scale. Brain with normal transit time appears blue. Parameters similar to MTT that are often used in pCT include time to peak (TTP) and time to drain (TTD).

The densely ischemic **infarct core**—the irreversibly injured brain—shows matched reduction in *both* CBV and CBF. The infarct core is seen as a dark blue/purple or black area that contrasts with the normally perfused red/yellow brain **(8-37B)**. Prolonged MTT is seen as a red area, in contrast to the blue brain, in which transit time is normal **(8-37D)**. An MCA territory infarct core volume of 70-100 mL is highly specific for poor clinical outcome, independent of associated penumbra and regardless of subsequent recanalization.

An **ischemic penumbra** with potentially salvageable tissue is seen as a "mismatch" between markedly reduced CBV in the infarcted core **(8-37B)** and a surrounding area (penumbra) characterized by decreased CBF with normal or even transiently increased CBV **(8-37C)**. Thus the potentially salvageable brain tissue is equivalent to CBV minus CBF. Prolonged MTT over 145% that extends beyond the core infarct area (so-called CBV/MTT mismatch) also characterizes the ischemic penumbra.

An important ancillary finding in patients with large MCA infarcts is reduced perfusion in the opposite cerebellar hemisphere. Between 15-20% of large MCA infarcts cause hypoperfusion with reduced CBF in the contralateral cerebellum, a phenomenon called **crossed cerebellar diaschisis** (see below) **(8-40)**.

Ischemia-induced vascular damage predisposes to two highly morbid and potentially fatal **postischemic complications**, i.e., hemorrhagic transformation (HT) and malignant cerebral edema (MCE). pCT with blood-brain-barrier permeability techniques can quantify microvascular contrast extravasation, which correlates with subsequent development of HT and MCE.

MR Findings. Although CT/CTA/pCT is often preferred because of accessibility and speed, "expedited" rapid stroke protocols with only fast FLAIR, T2*, DWI, and pMR can be used **(8-39)**. MR is superior to CT in detecting small vessel and brainstem ischemia. MR is also helpful in delineating an ischemic penumbra when there is a discrepancy between CT/CTA and clinical stroke severity.

T1WI. T1WI is usually normal within the first 3-6 hours. Subtle gyral swelling and hypointensity begin to develop within 12-24 hours and are seen as blurring of the GM-WM interfaces. With large vessel occlusions, loss of the expected "flow void" in the affected artery can sometimes be identified.

T2/FLAIR. Only 30-50% of acute strokes show cortical swelling and hyperintensity on FLAIR scans within the first 4 hours. Nearly all strokes are FLAIR positive by 7 hours following symptom onset. T2 scans become positive slightly later, generally within 12-24 hours. Intraarterial hyperintensity on FLAIR is an early sign of stroke and indicates slow flow (not thrombosis), either from delayed antegrade flow or—more commonly—retrograde collateral filling across the cortical watershed **(8-41A)**. FLAIR-DWI "mismatch" (negative FLAIR, positive DWI) has been suggested as a quick indicator of viable ischemic penumbra and eligibility for thrombolysis.

T2* GRE. Intraarterial thrombus can sometimes be detected as "blooming" hypointensity on T2* (GRE, SWI) studies **(8-39C)**. Also look carefully for the presence of multifocal parenchymal microbleeds in older patients. In this age group, "blooming black dots" are most commonly caused by chronic hypertension or amyloid angiopathy. The presence of cerebral microbleeds may be an independent risk factor for subsequent anticoagulation-related hemorrhage.

T1 C+. Postcontrast T1 scans show intravascular enhancement. Parenchymal enhancement is uncommon in acute/hyperacute ischemia **(8-41E)**.

DWI and DTI. Cellular swelling begins to develop within minutes following an ischemic insult. ADC values decrease, producing high signal intensity on DWI images **(8-41C)**. Although most investigators posit cytotoxic edema as the basis for decreased ADC, part of the decrease is due to reduced water diffusibility caused by decreased levels of astrocytic aquaporin-4 (AQP4). Aquaporins are transmembrane proteins—water channels—that facilitate bidirectional selective water transport in and out of the cell.

Around 95% of hyperacute infarcts show diffusion restriction on DWI, with hyperintensity on DWI and corresponding hypointensity on ADC **(8-41C)**. DTI is even more sensitive than DWI, especially for pontine and medullary lesions.

A negative DWI does not exclude the diagnosis of stroke. Between 2-7% of patients with a final diagnosis of stroke are initially DWI negative. Very small (lacunar) infarcts, brainstem lesions, clot lysis with recanalization, and moderately reduced or fluctuating hypoperfusion that is not severe enough to restrict water movement have all been cited as possible reasons for DWI-negative acute strokes.

pMR. Restriction on DWI generally reflects the densely ischemic core of the infarct, whereas pMR depicts the surrounding "at-risk" penumbra. A **DWI-PWI mismatch** is one of the criteria used in determining suitability for intraarterial thrombolysis.

Angiography. As the diagnosis of acute cerebral ischemia-infarction with large vessel occlusion is already established using CTA or MRA, DSA is generally obtained only as a prelude

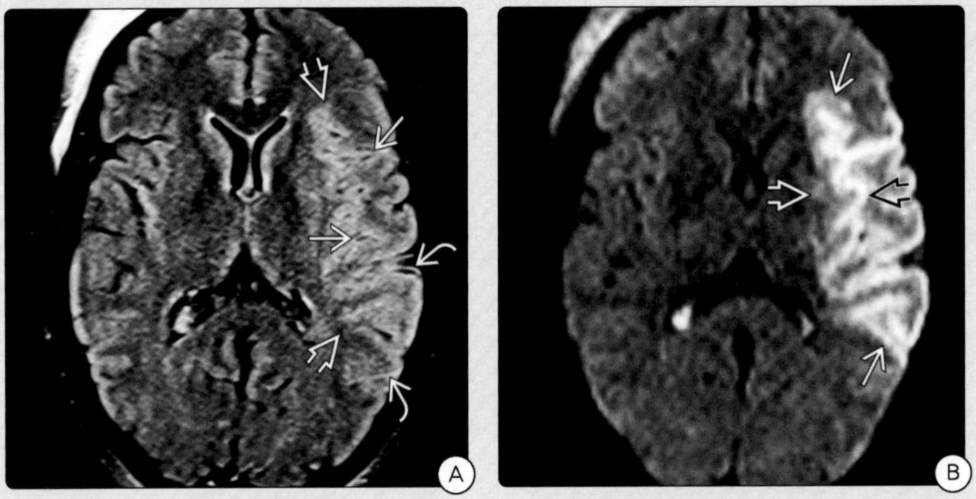

(8-39A) *Series of images depicts rapid MR stroke evaluation in a 51y woman with sudden onset of speech difficulties, right-sided weakness. ASPECTS score on NECT was 6. Fast FLAIR shows left MCA cortical hyperintensity with intravascular signal in the M3, M4 branches.* ***(8-39B)*** *DWI shows that restricted diffusion extends into the insular cortex and external capsule with minimal involvement of the lateral putamen.*

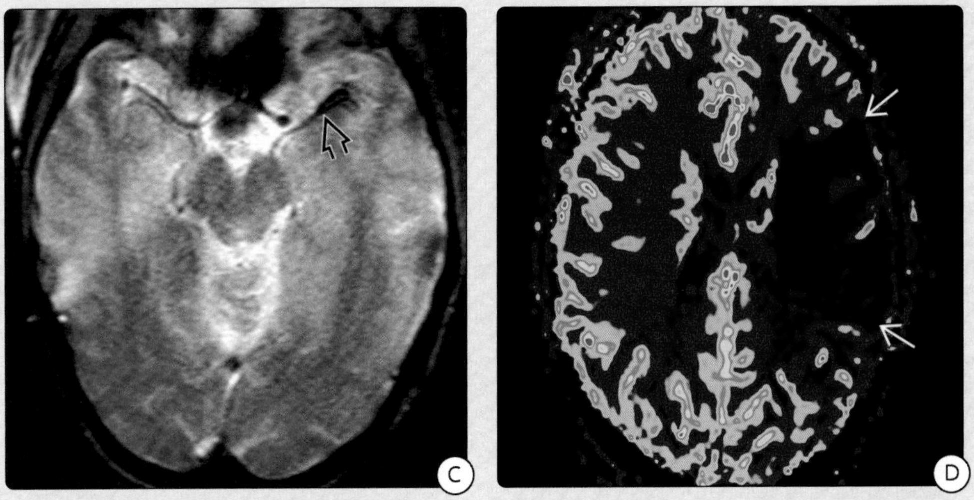

(8-39C) *T2* GRE in the same case shows "blooming" thrombus in the left M1 segment and bifurcation.* ***(8-39D)*** *pMR shows markedly reduced cerebral blood flow in the densely ischemic core infarct, which appears smaller than the corresponding DWI and FLAIR abnormality.*

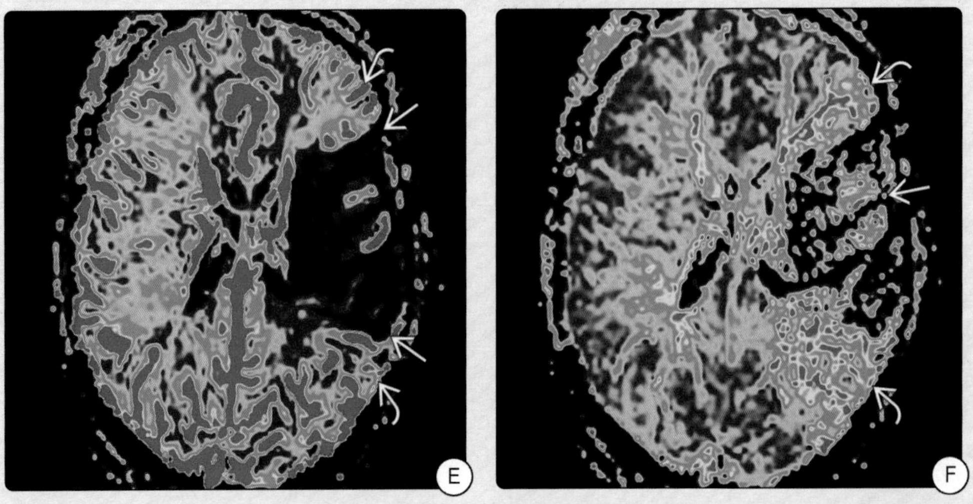

(8-39E) *CBV is markedly reduced in the densely ischemic core infarct, but this image shows a penumbra of well-maintained CBV in the adjacent brain.* ***(8-39F)*** *MTT shows the prolonged transit time in the large ischemic penumbra as well as some islands of slowed but still-perfused brain within the core infarct. Thrombectomy with clot retrieval was successfully performed within 3 hours of admission to the ER.*

to intraarterial thrombolysis or mechanical thrombectomy. Clot location and length can be precisely determined and collateral circulation delineated.

Major vessel occlusion is identified on DSA as interruption of the intraarterial contrast column. Frequent findings include an abrupt vessel "cut-off" **(8-42A)**, "meniscus" sign, tapered or "rat-tail" narrowing, or "tram-track" appearance with a trickle of contrast around the intraluminal thrombus.

Other common angiographic findings include a "bare" or "naked" area of nonperfused brain **(8-42B)** **(8-42C)**, slow antegrade filling with delayed washout of distal branches (seen as intraarterial contrast persisting into the capillary or venous phase), and pial collaterals with retrograde filling across the cortical watershed **(8-42D)** **(8-42E)** **(8-42F)**.

Less common signs are hyperemia with a vascular "blush" around the infarcted zone (so-called luxury perfusion) **(8-42F)** and "early draining" veins (arteriovenous shunting with contrast appearing in veins draining the infarct while the remainder of the circulation is still in the late arterial or early capillary phase).

Mass effect is rare in hyperacute stroke but very common in the acute/late acute stages.

Differential Diagnosis

Normal circulating blood is always slightly hyperdense compared with brain on NECT. A "hyperdense vessel" sign can be simulated by **elevated hematocrit** (all the vessels appear dense, not just the arteries), arterial wall **microcalcifications**, and **hypodense brain** parenchyma (e.g., diffuse cerebral edema).

Stroke "mimics" with restricted DWI include **infection, status epilepticus**, and acute **hypoglycemia**. Status epilepticus typically affects cortex in a nonvascular distribution while sparing the underlying subcortical WM **(8-43)**.

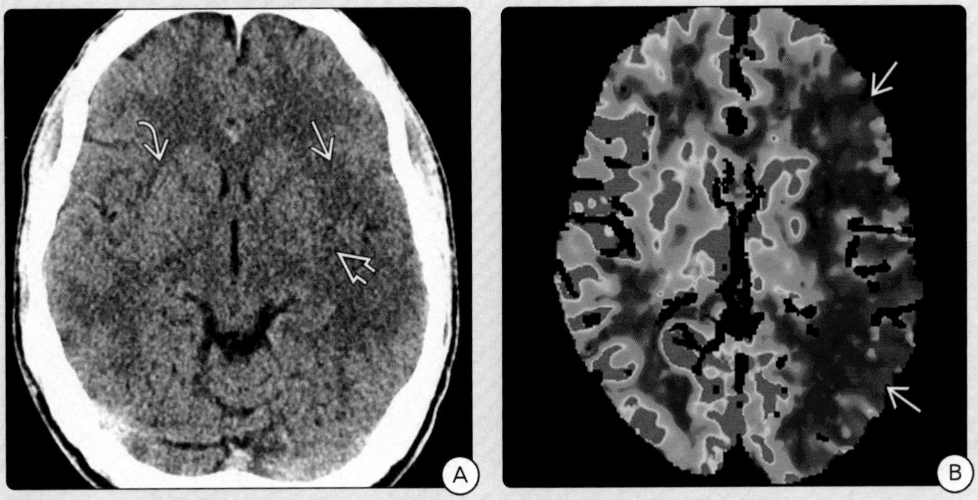

***(8-40A)** Axial NECT scan 5 hours after sudden onset of right hemiparesis shows left "insular ribbon" sign with hypodensity affecting the insular cortex ➡ and lateral aspect of the putamen ➡ ("disappearing basal ganglia" sign). Compare to the normal right insular cortex, external capsule, putamen ➡. **(8-40B)** CT perfusion with cerebral blood flow image shows markedly reduced CBF in the left MCA distribution ➡.*

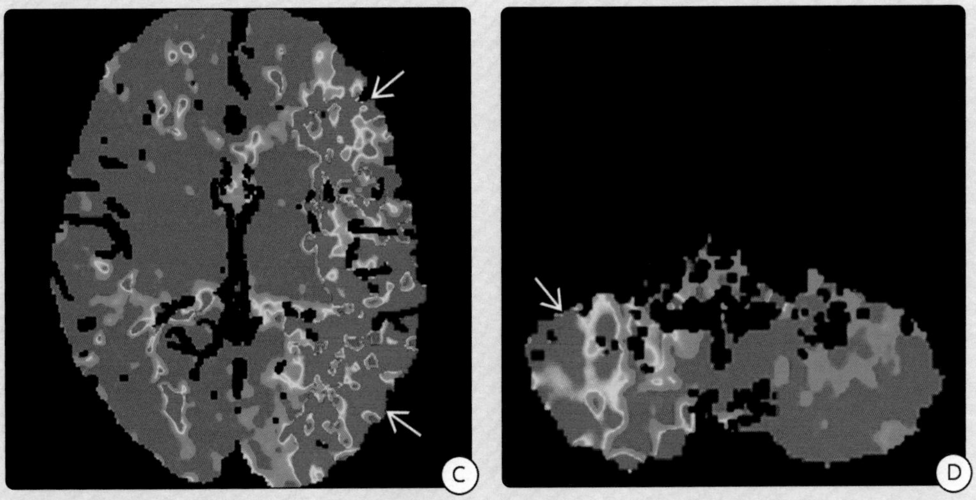

***(8-40C)** TTP image in the same patient demonstrates markedly prolonged time to peak in the same area ➡. **(8-40D)** TTP image through the posterior fossa demonstrates prolonged time to peak in the right cerebellar hemisphere ➡, indicating acute crossed cerebellar diaschisis.*

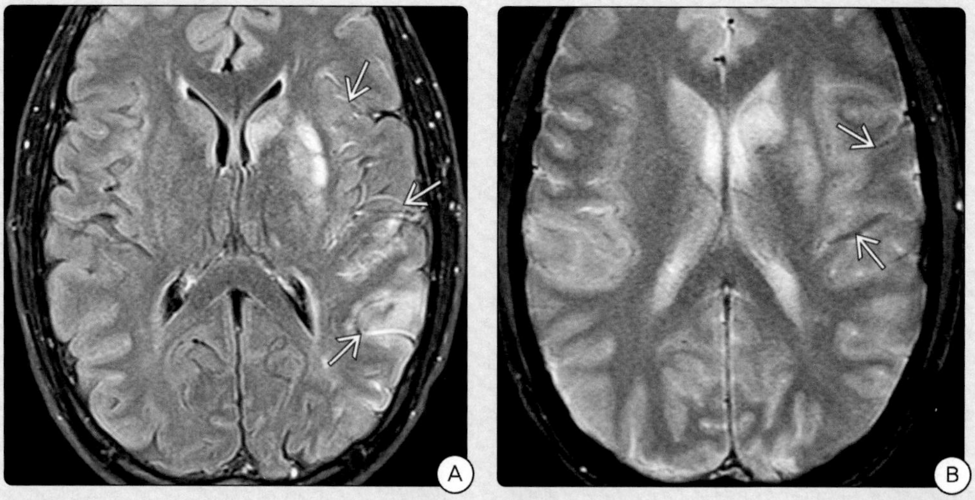

(8-41A) *Acute stroke in a 47y man shows patchy hyperintensity in left caudate nucleus, lateral putamen, and parietal cortex. Note multiple linear foci of intravascular hyperintensity ➡, consistent with slow flow in the MCA distribution.* ***(8-41B)*** *T2* GRE shows several linear hypointensities ➡ in the affected MCA branches, consistent with hemoglobin deoxygenation caused by slow, stagnating arterial blood flow.*

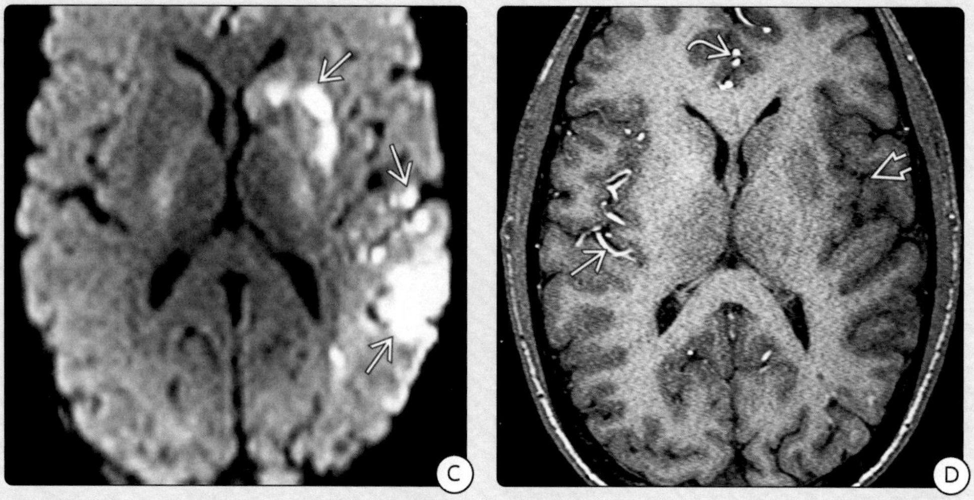

(8-41C) *DWI in the same patient shows multiple patchy foci of diffusion restriction ➡, consistent with acute cerebral infarct.* ***(8-41D)*** *Axial source image from 2D TOF MRA shows normal signal intensity in the right MCA ➡ and both ACA branches ➡ but no flow in the left MCA vessels ➡.*

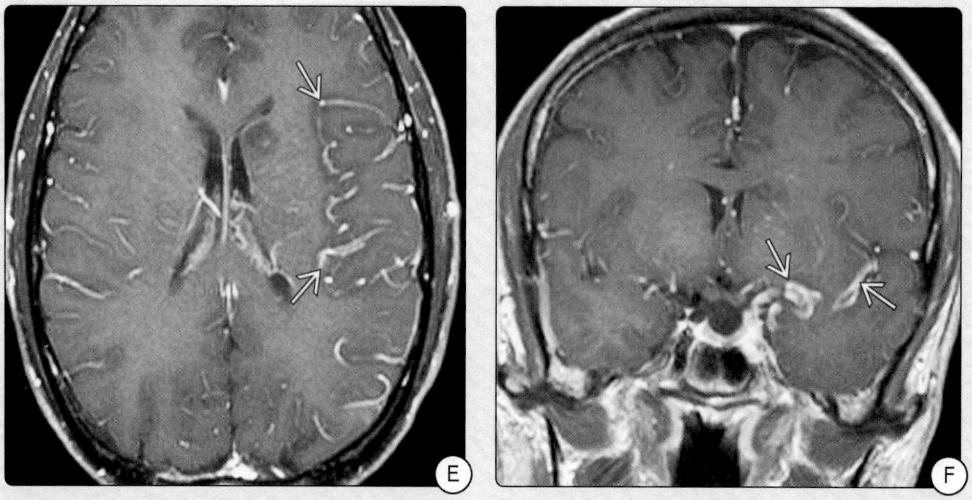

(8-41E) *Axial T1 C+ FS scan shows striking intravascular enhancement in the left MCA branches ➡, consistent with slow flow in patent (nonthrombosed) vessels.* ***(8-41F)*** *Coronal T1 C+ scan shows prominent intravascular enhancement in the left MCA ➡.*

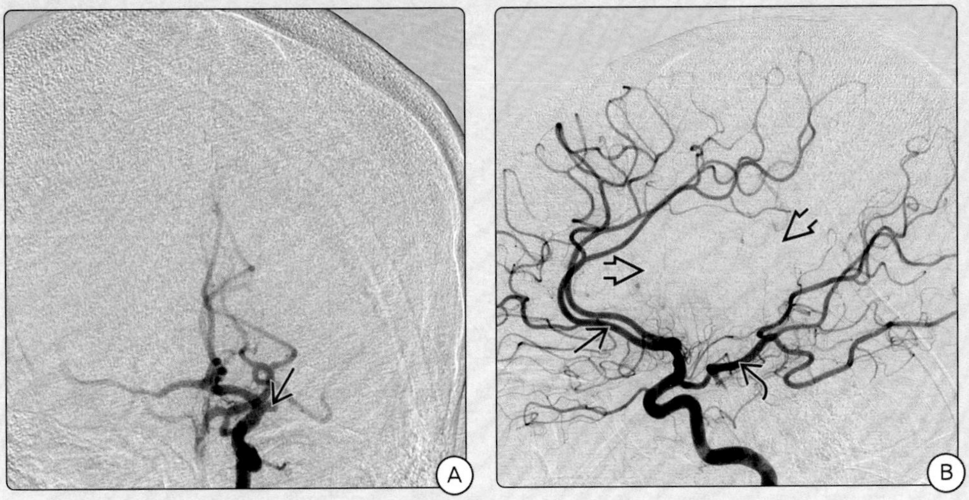

(8-42A) *Series of DSA images demonstrates classic angiographic findings of acute thromboembolic occlusion. Left internal carotid angiogram, early arterial phase, AP view, shows abrupt "cut-off" of the MCA →.* ***(8-42B)*** *Lateral view, early arterial phase, shows normal filling of both ACAs → and the ipsilateral PCA → via a large PCoA. The MCA distribution is not opacified, leaving a large "bare area" → of devascularized brain.*

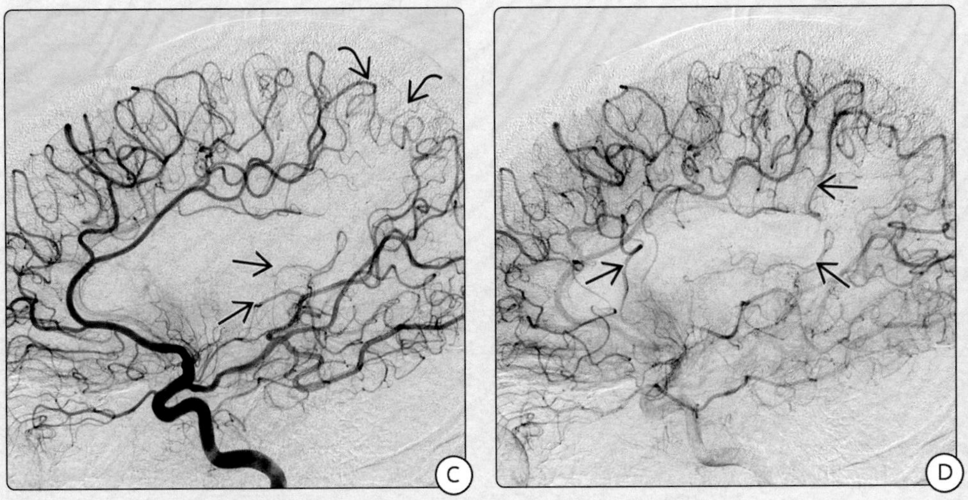

(8-42C) *Later image shows that the large "bare area" remains unopacified. Cortical branches are seen high over the left parietal convexity with early retrograde filling of the distal MCA branches → via pial collaterals from the ACA and PCA. Collateral flow is also seen from the posterior temporal PCA branches → into the MCA territory.* ***(8-42D)*** *Later image shows slow retrograde filling → into the MCA territory from ACA and PCA collaterals.*

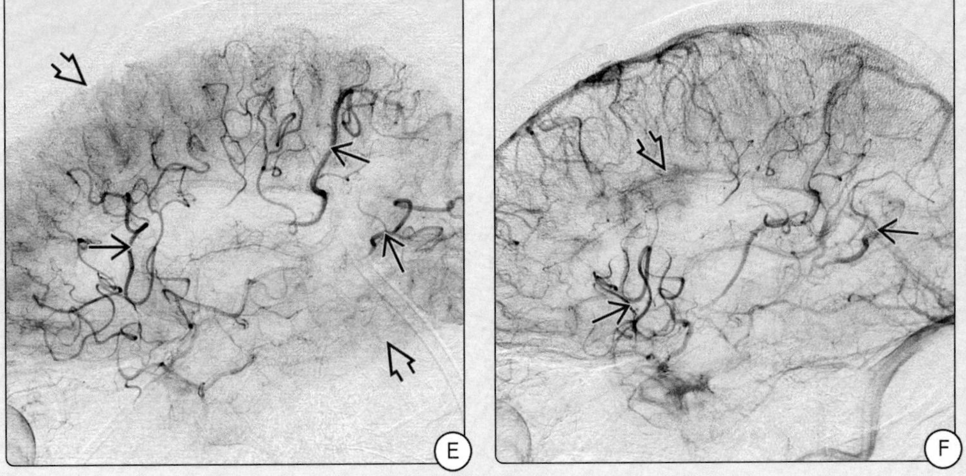

(8-42E) *Capillary phase shows diffuse brain "blush" → in ACA/PCA territories; contrast with "bare area" normally supplied by the MCA. Some MCA branches → are filling slowly via retrograde flow from ACA/PCA pial collaterals.* ***(8-42F)*** *Venous phase shows persisting contrast → in some MCA branches that have filled in retrograde fashion via pial collaterals and are slowly emptying. Note "blush" → at border of "bare area" caused by "luxury perfusion."*

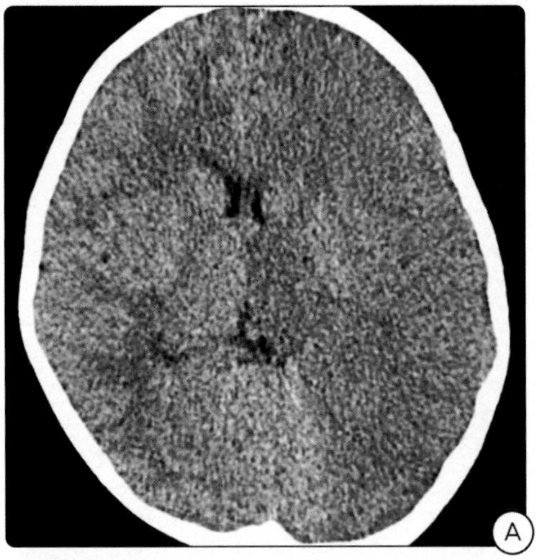

***(8-43A)** NECT in a 3y child in the ER with right-sided weakness shows that the left hemisphere appears strikingly hypodense.*

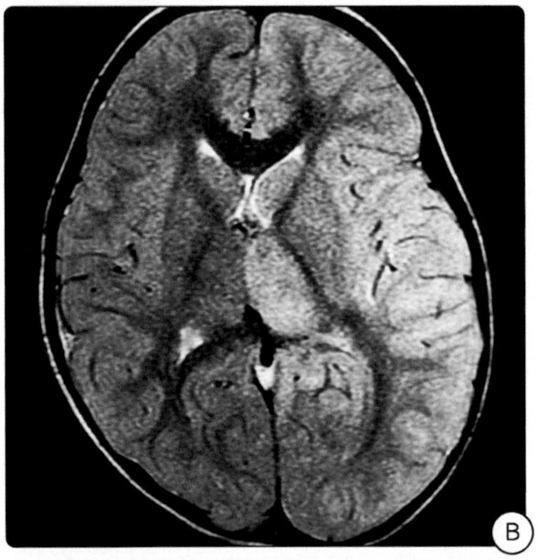

***(8-43B)** T2WI in the same case shows that the left hemisphere cortex and thalamus are hyperintense, but the underlying WM is spared.*

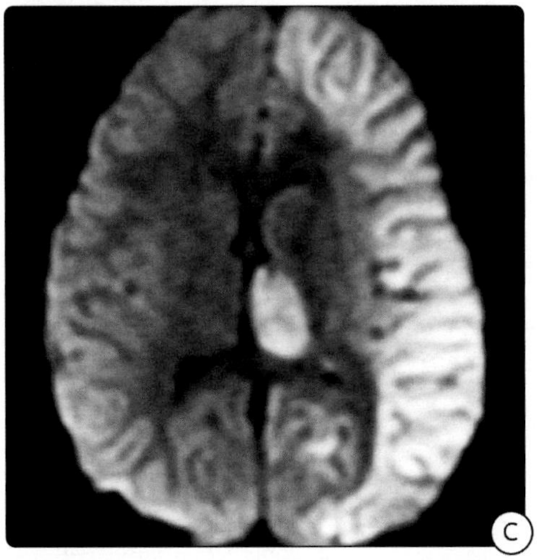

***(8-43C)** DWI shows cortical, thalamic restricted diffusion in a nonvascular distribution. Hyperemia is secondary to status epilepticus.*

ACUTE STROKE IMAGING

NECT
- Hyperdense vessel ± "dot" sign
- "Blurred," effaced GM-WM borders
  - "Insular ribbon" sign
  - "Disappearing" basal ganglia
- Wedge-shaped hypodensity
  - Involves both cortex, WM
- Look for Ca++ emboli (≈ 50% risk future stroke)

CECT
- ± Enhancing vessels (slow flow, collaterals)

CTA
- Shows site, length of major vessel thrombus
- ASVD
  - Extracranial: aorta, carotid bifurcation
  - Intracranial: cavernous ICA, circle of Willis + branches

pCT
- Infarct core (irreversibly damaged brain)
  - Matched perfusion (CBV, CBF both ↓)
  - ↑ MTT
- Ischemic penumbra
  - Perfusion "mismatch" (↓ CBF but normal CBV)

T1WI
- Usually normal in first 4-6 hours
- ± Loss of expected "flow void"

T2WI
- Usually normal in first 4-6 hours

FLAIR (use narrow windows)
- 50% positive in first 4-6 hours
  - Cortical swelling, gyral hyperintensity
  - Intraarterial hyperintensity (usually slow flow, not thrombus)

T2* (GRE, SWI)
- Thrombus may "bloom"
- Large infarcts may show prominent hypointense medullary veins
- Microbleeds (chronic hypertension, amyloid)

DWI and DTI
- > 95% restriction within minutes
  - Hyperintense on DWI
  - Hypointense on ADC map
- "Diffusion-negative" acute strokes
  - Small (lacunar) infarcts
  - Brainstem lesions
  - Rapid clot lysis/recanalization
  - Transient/fluctuating hypoperfusion

pMR
- DWI-PWI "mismatch" estimates penumbra
- CBV-CBF, DWI-FLAIR mismatches estimate penumbra

DSA
- Vessel "cut-off," "meniscus" sign, tapered/"rat-tail" narrowing
- "Bare" area of unperfused brain
- Slow antegrade or retrograde filling
- Delayed intraarterial contrast washout
- Luxury perfusion
  - "Blush" around "bare area"
  - "Early draining" veins

Subacute Cerebral Infarcts

Terminology

Strokes evolve pathophysiologically with corresponding changes reflected on imaging studies. Although there are no firm divisions that demarcate the various stages of stroke evolution, most neurologists designate infarcts as acute, subacute, and chronic.

"Subacute" cerebral ischemia/infarction generally refers to strokes that are between 48 hours and 2 weeks following the initial ischemic event.

Pathology

Edema and **increasing mass effect** caused by cytotoxic edema become maximal within 3-4 days following stroke onset. Frank tissue necrosis with progressive influx of microglia and macrophages around vessels ensues with reactive astrocytosis around the perimeter of the stroke. Brain softening and then cavitation proceeds over the next 2 weeks.

Most thromboembolic strokes are initially "bland," i.e., nonhemorrhagic. **Hemorrhagic transformation** (HT) of a previously ischemic infarct occurs in 20-25% of cases between 2 days and a week after ictus **(8-44)**. Ischemia-damaged vascular endothelium becomes "leaky," and blood-brain barrier permeability increases. When reperfusion is established—either spontaneously or following treatment with tissue plasminogen activator—exudation of red blood cells through the damaged blood vessel walls causes parenchymal hemorrhages. Petechial hemorrhages are more common than lobar bleeds and are most common in the basal ganglia and cortex.

Clinical Issues

HT itself generally does not cause clinical deterioration. HT is actually related to favorable outcome, probably reflecting early vessel recanalization and better tissue reperfusion.

Imaging

General Features. There are significant variations within the subacute time period. Early subacute strokes have significant mass effect and often exhibit HT, whereas edema and mass effect have mostly subsided by the late subacute period.

CT Findings. On NECT, the wedge-shaped area of decreased attenuation seen on initial scans becomes more sharply defined. Mass effect initially increases, then begins to decrease by 7-10 days following stroke onset. HT develops in 15-20% of cases and is seen as gyriform cortical or basal ganglia hyperdensity **(8-45A)**.

CECT follows a "2-2-2" rule. Patchy or gyriform enhancement appears as early as 2 days after stroke onset, peaks at 2 weeks, and generally disappears by 2 months.

MR Findings. Signal intensity in subacute stroke varies depending on (1) time since ictus and (2) the presence or absence of hemorrhagic transformation.

T1WI. Nonhemorrhagic subacute infarcts are hypointense on T1WI and demonstrate moderate mass effect with sulcal effacement. Strokes with HT are initially isointense with cortex and then become hyperintense **(8-46)**.

T2WI. Subacute infarcts are initially hyperintense compared with nonischemic brain. Signal intensity decreases with time, reaching isointensity at 1-2 weeks (the T2 "fogging effect") **(8-47)**. Early wallerian degeneration

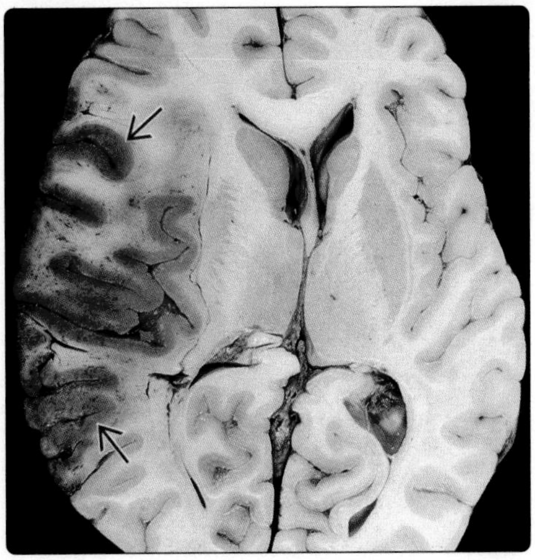

***(8-44)** Subacute stroke is shown with mass effect, gyriform hemorrhagic transformation. (Courtesy R. Hewlett, MD.)*

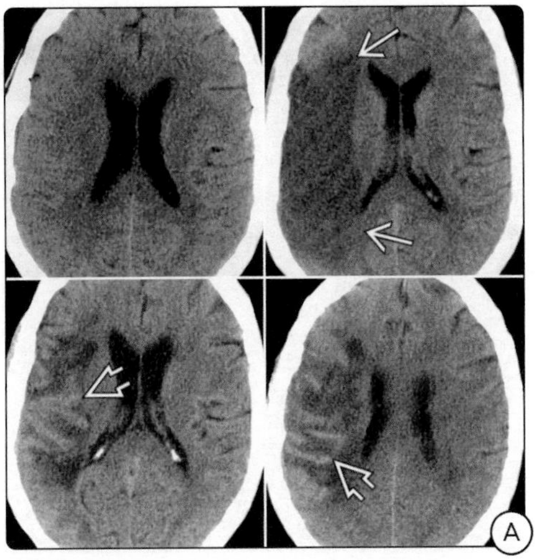

***(8-45A)** (Top) NECT at 2 h shows mild sulcal effacement. At 48 h, wedge-shaped hypodensity involves GM, WM. (Bottom) HT at 1 week.*

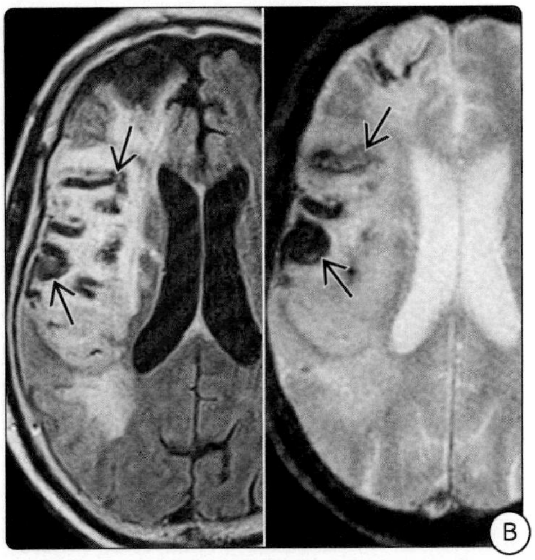

***(8-45B)** FLAIR (L) and GRE (R) in the same case show hemorrhagic transformation in this example of subacute stroke.*

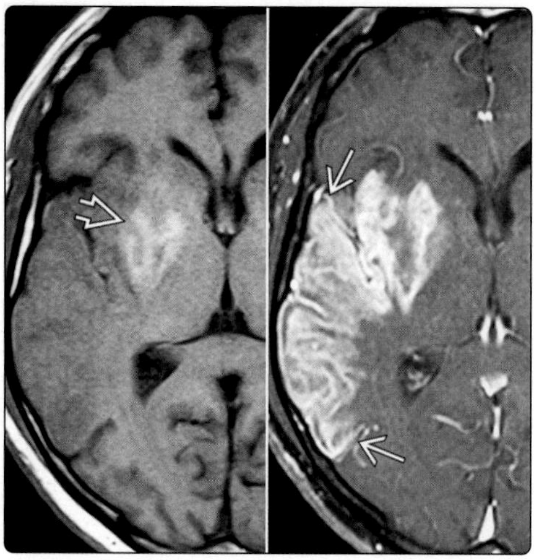

***(8-46)** MR 2 weeks after right MCA stroke shows HT ➡ (L) and the intense enhancement ➡ characteristic of subacute infarction (R).*

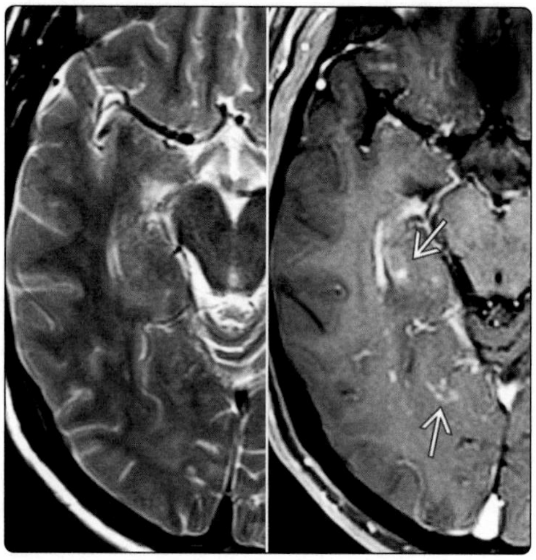

***(8-47)** T2 "fogging effect" 2 weeks after stroke. (L) T2WI appears normal. (R) T1 C+ FS shows patchy enhancement ➡ in PCA infarct.*

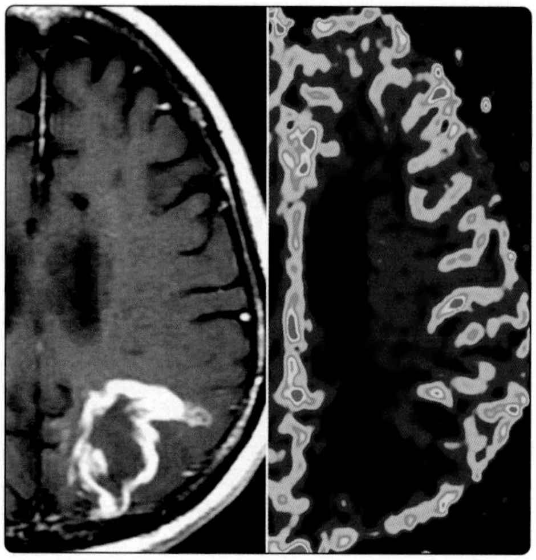

***(8-48)** (L) Subacute infarct with ring enhancement mimics neoplasm. (R) pMR shows "cold" lesion with profoundly decreased rCBV.*

can sometimes be identified as a well-delineated hyperintense band that extends inferiorly from the infarcted cortex along the corticospinal tract.

FLAIR. Subacute infarcts are hyperintense on FLAIR **(8-45B)**. By 1 week after ictus, "final" infarct volume corresponds to the FLAIR-defined abnormality.

T2* (GRE, SWI). Petechial or gyriform "blooming" foci are present if HT has occurred in the infarcted cortex **(8-45B)**. Basal ganglia hemorrhages can be confluent or petechial.

Prominent ipsilateral medullary veins on SWI in MCA territory strokes within 3-7 days of ictus are a significant predictive biomarker of poor clinical outcome. Prominent medullary veins in the contralateral (normal) hemisphere may indirectly reflect increased CBF and are associated with good clinical outcome.

T1 C+. The intravascular enhancement often seen in the first 48 hours following thromboembolic occlusion disappears within 3 or 4 days and is replaced by leptomeningeal enhancement caused by persisting pial collateral blood flow. Patchy or gyriform parenchymal enhancement can occur as early as 2 or 3 days after infarction **(8-46)** and may persist for 2-3 months, in some cases mimicking neoplasm **(8-48)**.

DWI and pMR. Restricted diffusion with hyperintensity on DWI and hypointensity on ADC persists for the first several days following stroke onset, then gradually reverses to become hypointense on DWI and hyperintense with T2 "shine-through" on ADC. pMR with arterial spin-labeling shows crossed cerebellar diaschisis in 50% of patients with subacute ischemic strokes.

SUBACUTE STROKE

Pathology
- Edema, mass effect initially increase
- Vessel damage → hemorrhagic transformation 25%

CT
- Hypodensity sharply defined
- Gyriform enhancement 2 days to several weeks

MR
- T1WI
  - Iso- to hypointense
  - May see T1 shortening (cortex, basal ganglia)
- T2WI
  - "Fogging effect" (isointensity)
  - ± Early wallerian degeneration
- FLAIR
  - Hyperintensity corresponds to final infarct
- T2*
  - "Blooming" HT
  - Prominent medullary veins
- DWI
  - Pseudonormalization
  - T2 "shine-through"
- T1 C+
  - Enhances (gyriform, even ring-like)

Differential Diagnosis
- Neoplasm
- Infection
  - Cerebritis
  - Encephalitis

Chronic Cerebral Infarcts

Terminology

Chronic cerebral infarcts are the end result of ischemic territorial strokes and are also called postinfarction encephalomalacia.

Pathology

The pathologic hallmark of chronic cerebral infarcts is volume loss with gliosis in an anatomic vascular distribution. A cavitated, encephalomalacic brain with strands of residual glial tissue and traversing blood vessels is the usual gross appearance of an old infarct **(8-49A)**.

Imaging

NECT scans show a sharply delineated wedge-shaped hypodense area that involves both gray matter (GM) and white matter (WM) and conforms to the vascular territory of a cerebral artery. The adjacent sulci and ipsilateral ventricle enlarge secondary to volume loss in the affected hemisphere **(8-49A)**. Dystrophic calcification occurs but is uncommon **(8-50)**.

Wallerian degeneration with an ipsilateral small, shrunken cerebral peduncle is often present with large MCA infarcts. Look for atrophy of the contralateral cerebellum secondary to crossed cerebellar diaschisis.

Chronic infarcts older than 2-3 months typically do not enhance on CECT.

MR scans show cystic encephalomalacia with CSF-equivalent signal intensity on all sequences. Marginal gliosis or spongiosis around the old cavitated stroke is hyperintense on FLAIR **(8-49B)**. DWI shows increased diffusivity (hyperintense on ADC).

Multiple Embolic Infarcts

Brain emboli are less common but important causes of stroke. Most consist of clots containing fibrin, platelets, and RBCs. Less common emboli include air, fat, calcium, tumor, and foreign bodies (e.g., debris from metallic heart valves).

Cardiac and Atheromatous Emboli

Pathoetiology. Simultaneous small acute infarcts in multiple different vascular distributions are the hallmark of embolic cerebral infarcts **(8-51)**. The heart is the most common source; cardiac emboli can be septic or aseptic. Peripheral signs of emboli such as splinter hemorrhages are sometimes present. Echocardiography may demonstrate valvular vegetations, intracardiac filling defect, or atrial or ventricular septal defect.

Ipsilateral hemispheric emboli are most commonly due to atheromatous internal carotid artery plaques. Many are clinically silent but convey a high risk for subsequent overt stroke.

Imaging. In contrast to large artery territorial strokes, embolic infarcts tend to involve terminal cortical branches. The GM-WM interface is most commonly affected.

NECT scans show low-attenuation foci, often in a wedge-shaped distribution. Atherosclerotic emboli occasionally demonstrate calcification **(8-33)**. Septic emboli are often hemorrhagic. CECT scans may demonstrate multiple punctate or ring-enhancing lesions.

MR scans show multifocal peripheral T2/FLAIR hyperintensities. Hemorrhagic emboli cause "blooming" on T2* sequences. The most sensitive sequence is

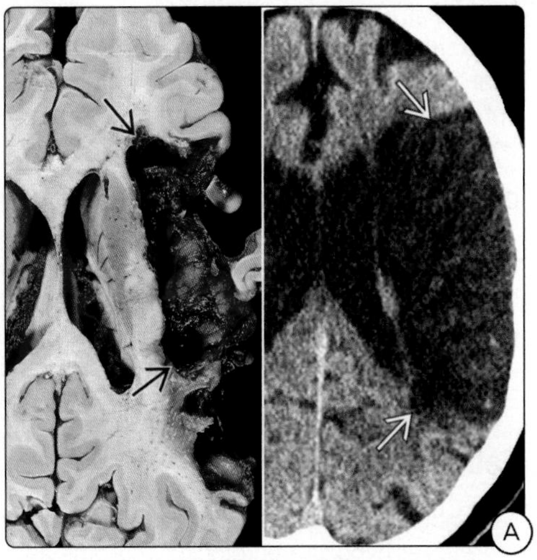

***(8-49A)** (L) Old MCA infarct with hemorrhagic transformation ⇨. (R. Hewlett, MD.). (R) NECT shows encephalomalacia, old MCA infarct ➡.*

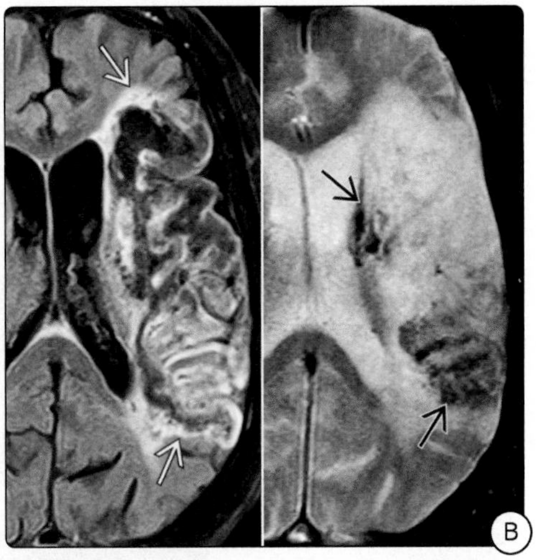

***(8-49B)** FLAIR (L) shows hyperintensity ➡ around the cavitated, encephalomalacic area, whereas T2* GRE (R) shows some HT ⇨.*

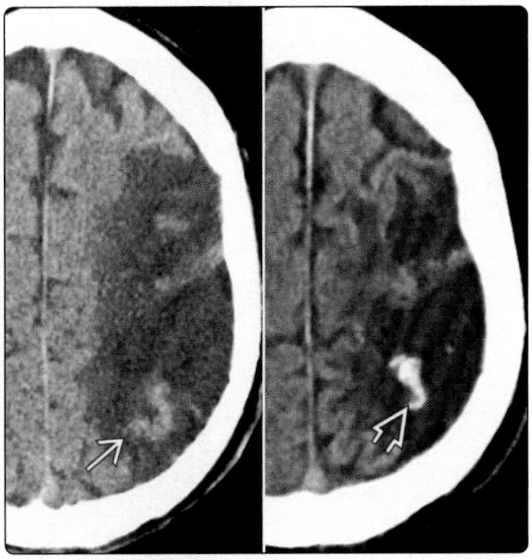

***(8-50)** (L) NECT of late subacute MCA infarct shows small focus of HT ➡. (R) Gyriform Ca++ ➡ is present in the same area 3 years later.*

DWI. Small peripheral foci of diffusion restriction in several different vascular distributions are typical of multiple embolic infarcts **(8-52)**. T1 C+ imaging may show multiple punctate enhancing foci. Septic emboli often demonstrate ring enhancement, resembling microabscesses.

Differential Diagnosis. The major differential diagnosis of multiple embolic infarcts is **hypotensive cerebral infarction** (see below). Hypotensive infarcts are usually caused by hemodynamic compromise and tend to involve the deep internal watershed zones. **Parenchymal metastases** have a predilection for the GM-WM interface, as do embolic infarcts, but generally do not restrict on DWI.

Fat Emboli

Fat embolism syndrome (FES) is an uncommon disorder that presents as hypoxia, neurologic symptoms, and/or a petechial rash in the setting of severely displaced lower extremity long bone fractures. The term "cerebral fat emboli" (CFE) refers to the neurologic manifestations of FES.

Pathoetiology. Two mechanisms have been proposed to explain the effects of FES: (1) small vessel occlusions from fat particles and (2) inflammatory changes in surrounding tissue initiated by breakdown of fat into free fatty acids and other metabolic byproducts.

The pathologic hallmark of CFE is arteriolar fat emboli with perivascular microhemorrhages **(8-53)**.

Epidemiology and Clinical Issues. The overall incidence of FES in patients with long bone fractures—most commonly the femoral neck—is 1-2%. FES also occurs with pelvic fractures, elective orthopedic procedures (e.g., total hip arthroplasty), anesthesia, and systemic illness (e.g., pancreatitis). FES in patients with bone marrow necrosis secondary to sickle cell crisis has also been reported.

(8-51) Autopsy specimen shows multiple old healed infarcts at the gray-white matter junctions ➾. (Courtesy R. Hewlett, MD.) (8-52A) A 70y man with decreasing cognitive function for one month became acutely worse. Emergent MR with axial FLAIR shows multifocal bilateral cortical ➦ and basal ganglionic ➡ hyperintensities.

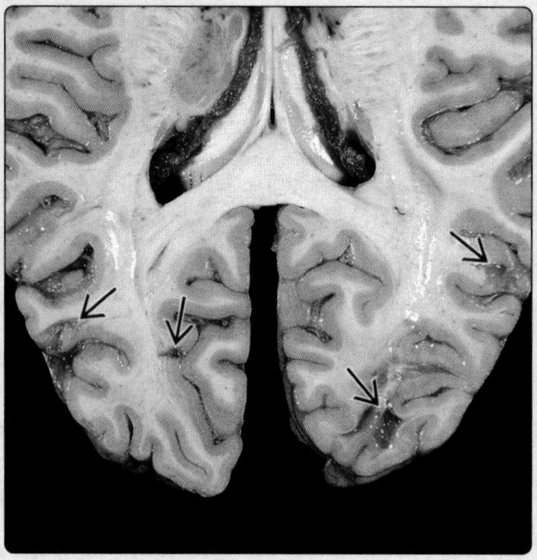

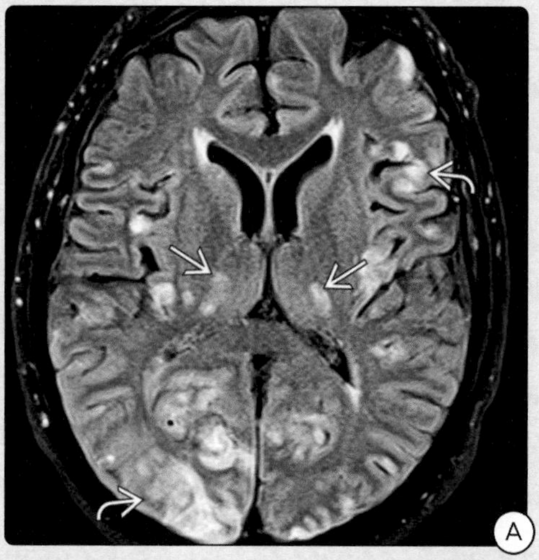

(8-52B) T2 GRE shows some of the cortical lesions ➦ exhibit blooming, consistent with petechial hemorrhages. (8-52C) DWI shows restricted diffusion in the lesions. Multiple septic and hemorrhagic embolic infarcts are seen.*

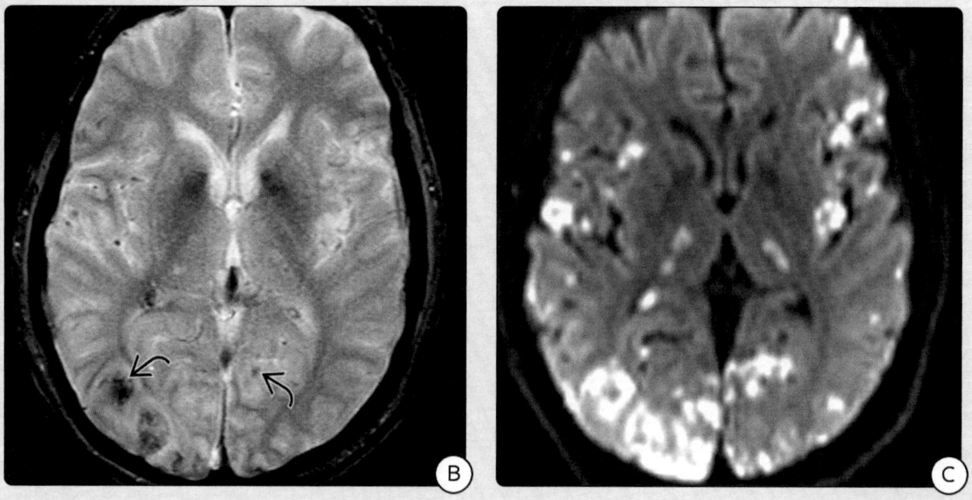

CFE occurs in up to 80% of patients with FES. Signs and symptoms vary in severity and include petechial rash, headache, seizure, drowsiness, altered mental status, and coma. Focal neurologic deficits are less common. Onset is from 2 hours up to 2 days after trauma or surgery, with a mean of 29 hours.

Imaging. Imaging findings reflect the *effect* of the fat emboli (i.e., multifocal tiny strokes and microhemorrhages) on brain tissue, not the fat itself. NECT scans are therefore usually normal.

MR shows numerous (average = 50) punctate or confluent hyperintensities in the cerebellum, basal ganglia, periventricular WM, and GM-WM junctions on T2/FLAIR **(8-54A)**. DWI shows innumerable tiny punctate foci of diffusion restriction in multiple vascular distributions, the "star field" pattern **(8-54B)**. The deep watershed border zones are commonly involved.

Solitary or multiple small hypointense "blooming" foci can be identified in up to one-third of all FES cases on T2* GRE. SWI discloses innumerable (> 200) tiny "black dots" in the majority of patients **(8-54C)**.

Differential Diagnosis. The major differential diagnosis of cerebral fat embolism syndrome is **multiple embolic infarcts**. Multiple cardiac or atheromatous embolic infarcts rarely produce the dozens or even hundreds of lesions seen with CFE. Lesions tend to involve the basal ganglia and corticomedullary junctions more than the white matter.

Multifocal "blooming" hypointensities on T2* can be seen with severe **diffuse axonal injury (DAI)** or **diffuse vascular injury (DVI)**. As patients with CFE often have polytrauma, the distinction may be difficult on the basis of imaging studies alone. DAI and DVI tend to cause linear as well as punctate microbleeds.

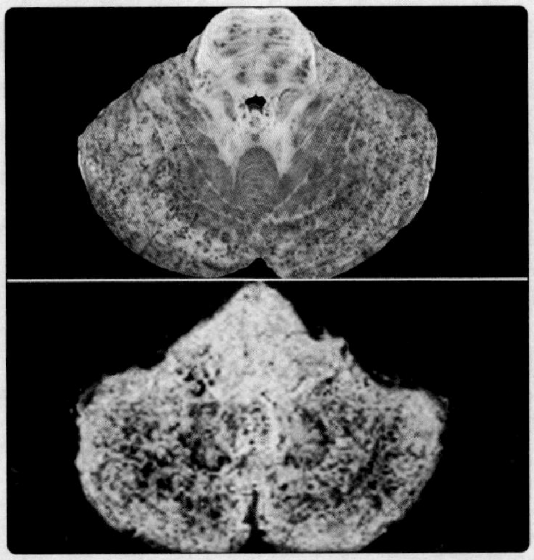

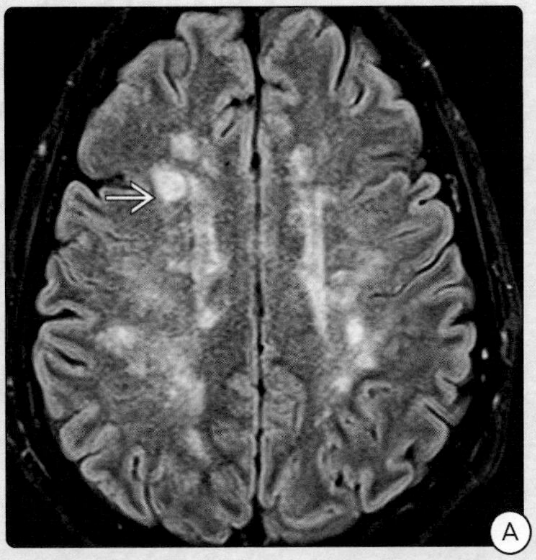

***(8-53)** (Top) Autopsy case of fat embolism shows innumerable small microbleeds throughout the pons and cerebellum (Courtesy Klatt, Robbins, and Coltran, Atlas of Neuropathology, 2015). (Bottom) MIP SWI in fat embolism shows multiple "blooming black dots."* ***(8-54A)** Axial FLAIR scan in a 62y woman with altered mental status following hip surgery shows multiple confluent hyperintense foci ➡ in the deep white matter of both hemispheres.*

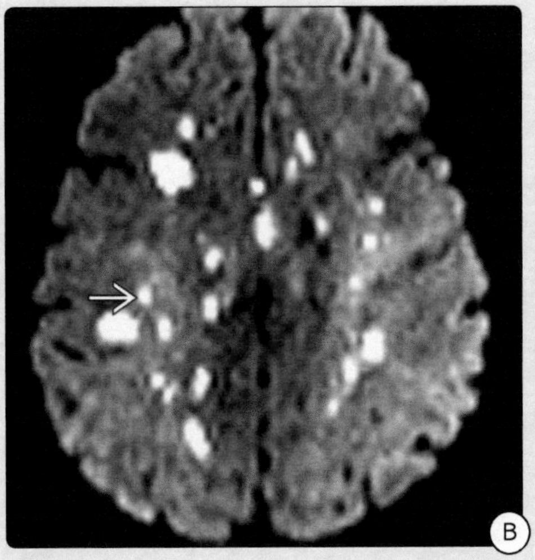

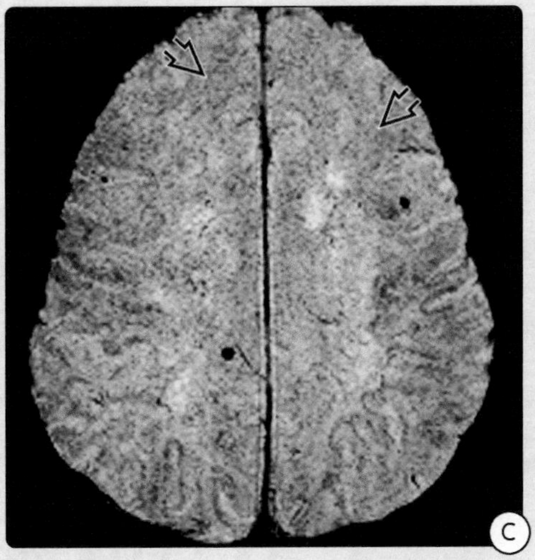

***(8-54B)** DWI in the same case shows innumerable tiny foci of diffusion restriction in the deep cerebral white matter ➡, the so-called "star field" pattern characteristic of cerebral fat embolism syndrome.* ***(8-54C)** T2* SWI in the same case shows literally thousands of tiny blooming hypointense foci throughout the hemispheric WM ⇨ characteristic of microbleeds secondary to cerebral fat embolism syndrome.*

Cerebral Gas Embolism

Pathoetiology. Minor amounts of air in the intracranial venous systems is usually iatrogenic, introduced during intravenous catheter placement.

Massive cerebral gas embolism (CGE) is a potentially catastrophic complication of central venous catheter (CVC) manipulation/disconnection and has been reported with cardiac procedures.

Other etiologies of arterial or venous air embolism include lung biopsy, craniotomy in the sitting position, and angiography. Penetrating trauma, decompression sickness, and hydrogen peroxide ingestion are other causes of gas embolism.

Clinical. Small amounts of CGE may be asymptomatic or mild and transient. In more severe cases, focal neurologic deficit, coma, seizures, and encephalopathy may ensue. Reported mortality of CGE associated with CVCs approaches 20%.

Imaging. Asymptomatic air following intravenous catheter placement is most commonly observed as an incidental finding, typically as dots of air in the cavernous sinus.

Intracranial air bubbles can be identified in 70% of symptomatic CGE cases, appearing on NECT as transient small intravascular rounded or curvilinear hypodensities, typically located at the depths of sulci **(8-55A)**. Intraparenchymal air is loss common.

Air is quickly absorbed and can rapidly disappear **(8-56)**. If massive air embolism occurs, cerebral ischemia or diffuse brain swelling typically ensues **(8-56)**.

(8-55A) 55y woman experienced left hemiparesis after esophageal dilatation. (L) Axial NECT of cerebral gas embolism shows multiple "dots" of air in the brain ➡. (R) FLAIR shows a much more extensive area of diffuse cortical/subcortical WM hyperintensity ➡. (8-55B) (L) DWI shows restricted diffusion ➡ in the cortex. (R) T1 C+ shows extensive patchy, linear enhancement ➡ in the cortex and subcortical WM. (Courtesy P. Hildenbrand, MD.)

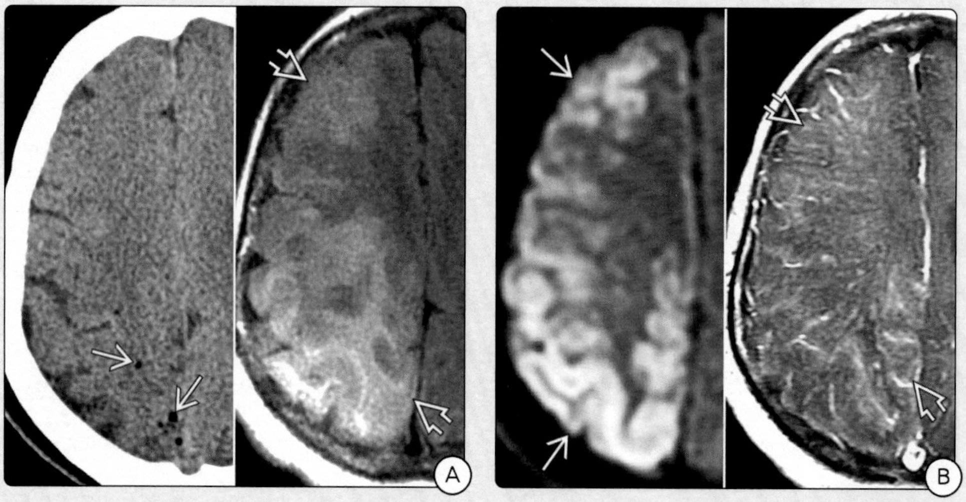

(8-56A) Axial NECT scan in a 69y man immediately after cardiac ablation shows massive cerebral gas embolism. (8-56B) NECT scan in the same case 1 hour later shows that most of the air has been resorbed with only two small parenchymal dots of air ⇨ remaining. Severe diffuse cerebral edema is now present.

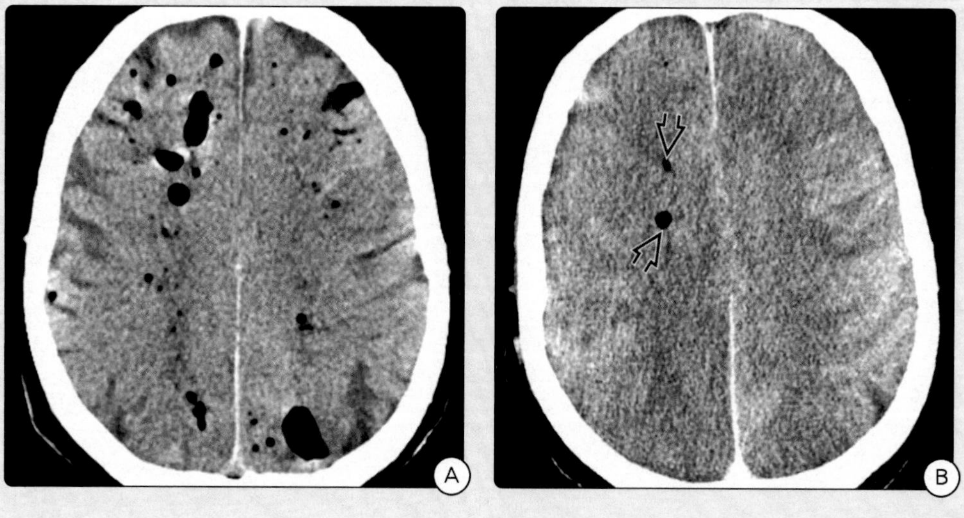

EMBOLIC INFARCTS

Cardiac and Atheromatous Emboli

- Small, simultaneous, multiple lesions
- Bilateral, multiple vascular distributions
- Typically involve cortex, GM-WM interfaces
- May be Ca++
- ± Punctate/ring enhancement
- Usually not hemorrhagic unless septic

Fat Emboli

- 12-72 h after long bone trauma, surgery
- Less commonly from bone marrow necrosis (e.g., sickle cell crisis)
- Arteriolar/capillary fat emboli
- Cause multiple tiny microbleeds
- Multiple foci of restricted diffusion in "star field" pattern (bright spots on dark background)
- Microbleeds best seen on T2* SWI > > GRE
- Deep WM > cortex

Cerebral Gas Embolism

- Usually iatrogenic (procedural) or traumatic
- Can occur with hydrogen peroxide ingestion
- NECT may show transient round or curvilinear air densities in sulcal vessels
- Quickly absorbed, disappear
- If massive, lethal brain swelling ensues rapidly

Lacunar Infarcts

Terminology

The terms "lacuna," "lacunar infarct," and "lacunar stroke" are often used interchangeably. **Lacunae** are 3- to 15-mm CSF-filled cavities or "holes" that most often occur in the basal ganglia or cerebral white matter **(8-57)**. They are often observed coincidentally on imaging studies in older patients but are not clearly associated with discrete neurologic symptoms, i.e., they are subclinical strokes. Lacunae are sometimes called "silent" strokes, a misnomer as subtle neuropsychologic impairment is common in these patients.

Lacunar stroke means a clinically evident stroke syndrome attributed to a small subcortical or brainstem lesion that may or may not be evident on brain imaging. The term "état lacunaire" or **lacunar state** designates multiple lacunar infarcts.

Epidemiology and Etiology

Approximately 25% of all ischemic strokes are lacunar-type infarcts. Lacunae are considered macroscopic markers of cerebral small vessel ("microvascular") disease. There are two major vascular pathologies involving small penetrating arteries and arterioles: (1) thickening of the arterial media by lipohyalinosis, fibrinoid necrosis, and atherosclerosis causing luminal narrowing and (2) obstruction of penetrating arteries at their origin by large intimal plaques in the parent arteries.

The *MTHFR* C677T genotype is correlated with lacunar stroke.

Pathology

Location. Penetrating branches that arise from the circle of Willis and peripheral cortical arteries are small end-arteries with few collaterals, so lacunar infarcts are most common in the basal ganglia (putamen, globus

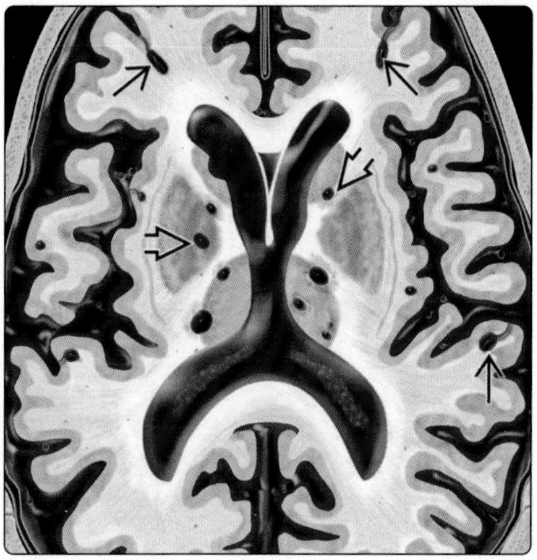

***(8-57)** Graphic shows lacunar infarctions in thalami, basal ganglia ⇨. Note also prominent perivascular (Virchow-Robin) spaces →.*

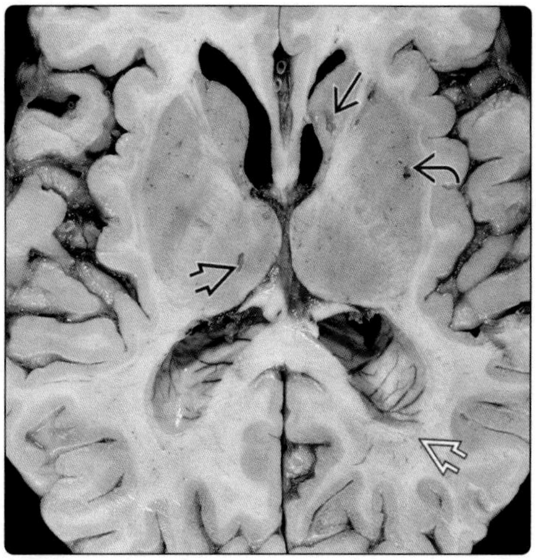

***(8-58)** Old lacunar infarcts are in the caudate →, putamen ⇨, thalamus ⇨, periatrial WM rarefaction ⇨. (Courtesy R. Hewlett, MD.)*

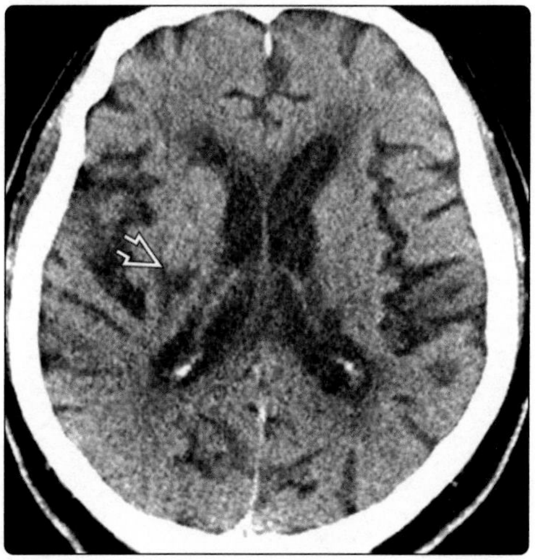

***(8-59)** NECT shows typical old thalamic lacunar infarct as hypodense, slightly irregular lesion ⇨.*

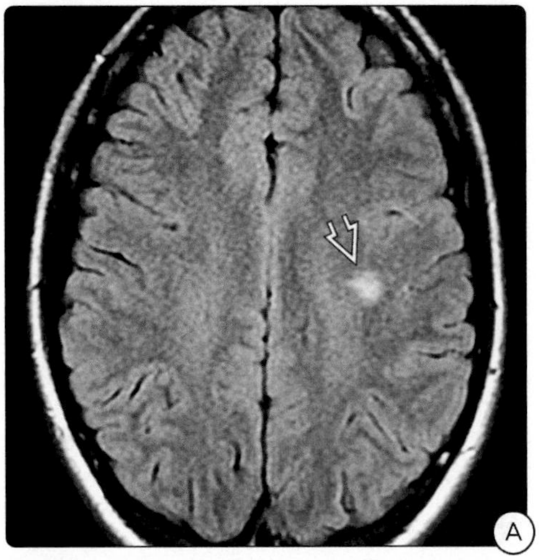

(8-60A) Axial FLAIR shows focus of irregular hyperintensity in left hemisphere WM ➯.

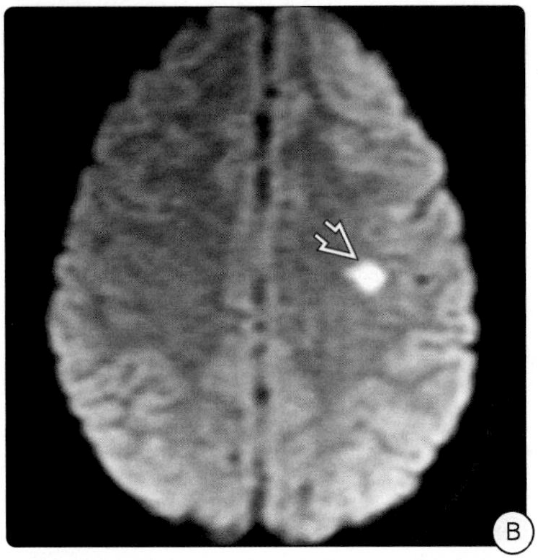

(8-60B) DWI in the same case shows solitary focus of restricted diffusion ➯.

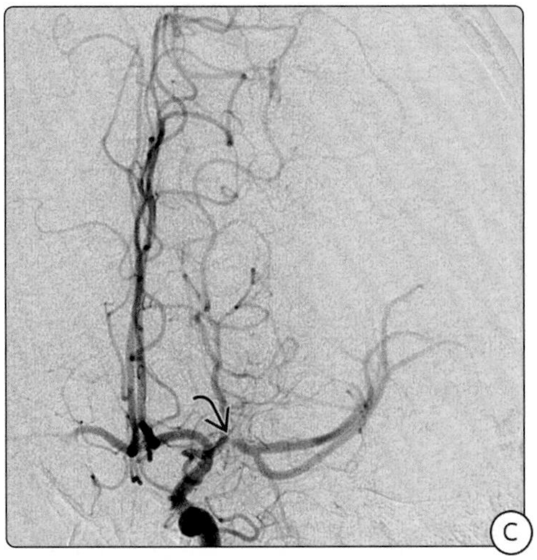

(8-60C) AP DSA in the same case shows high-grade stenosis of the proximal left MCA ➯ causing acute lacunar infarct.

pallidus, caudate nucleus), thalami, internal capsule, deep cerebral white matter, and pons.

Size and Number. Lacunae are, by definition, 15 mm or less in diameter. Multiple lesions are common. Between 13-15% of patients have multiple simultaneous acute lacunar infarcts.

Gross and Microscopic Appearance. Grossly, lacunae appear as small, pale, irregular but relatively well-delineated cystic cavities **(8-58)**. Brown-staining siderotic discoloration can be seen in old hemorrhagic lacunae. Microscopically, ischemic lacunar infarcts demonstrate tissue rarefaction with neuronal loss, peripheral macrophage infiltration, and gliosis.

Clinical Issues

Independent risk factors for lacunar infarcts include age, hypertension, and diabetes. Other contributing factors include smoking and atrial fibrillation.

Outcome of lacunar stroke is highly variable. Although most lacunae are asymptomatic, "little strokes" can mean "big trouble." A single subclinical stroke—often a lacuna—is associated with increased likelihood of having additional "little strokes" as well as developing overt clinical stroke and/or dementia. Nearly 20% of patients over 65 with white matter hyperintensities (WMHs) on T2/FLAIR MR will develop new lacunae within 3 years.

Between 20-30% of patients with lacunar stroke experience neurologic deterioration hours or even days after the initial event. The pathophysiology of "progressive lacunar stroke" is incompletely understood, and no treatment has been proven to prevent or halt progression.

Imaging

Imaging findings vary with whether the lacuna is acute or chronic.

Acute Lacunar Infarcts. Most acute lacunar infarcts are invisible on NECT scans. Acute lacunar infarcts are hyperintense on T2/FLAIR **(8-60A)** and may be difficult to distinguish from foci of coexisting chronic microvascular disease **(8-61)**. Acute and early subacute lacunae restrict on DWI **(8-60B)** **(8-61C)** and also usually enhance on T1 C+.

DWI overestimates the eventual size of lacunar infarcts. Cavitation and lesion shrinkage are seen in more than 95% of deep symptomatic lacunar infarcts on follow-up imaging.

Chronic Lacunar Infarcts. Old lacunae appear as well-defined but often somewhat irregular CSF-like "holes" in the brain parenchyma on NECT scans **(8-59)**.

Chronic lacunar infarcts are hypointense on T1WI and hyperintense on T2WI. The fluid in the cavity suppresses on FLAIR, whereas the gliotic periphery remains hyperintense. Multifocal white matter disease, seen as WMHs, is also common in patients with frank lacunar infarcts.

Most lacunae are nonhemorrhagic and do not "bloom" on T2* sequences. However, parenchymal microbleeds—multifocal "blooming black dots" on T2* (GRE, SWI)—are common comorbidities in patients with lacunar infarcts and chronic hypertension.

Differential Diagnosis

The major differential diagnosis of lacunar infarct is **prominent perivascular spaces** (PVSs). Also known as Virchow-Robin spaces, prominent PVSs are pia-lined, interstitial fluid-filled spaces. Prominent PVSs can be found in virtually all locations and in patients of all ages although they tend to increase in size and frequency with age. The most common locations for PVSs are the inferior third of the basal ganglia (clustered around the anterior commissure), subcortical white matter (including the external capsule), and the midbrain (see Chapter 28).

PVSs are sharply marginated and ovoid, linear, or round; lacunae tend to be more irregularly shaped. PVSs faithfully follow CSF signal intensity on all MR sequences and suppress completely on FLAIR. The adjacent brain is typically normal although a thin rim of FLAIR hyperintensity around the PVSs is present in 25% of cases.

Embolic infarcts are typically peripheral (cortical/subcortical) rather than the usual central and deep location of typical lacunae.

Watershed or **"border zone" infarcts** grossly resemble lacunar infarcts on imaging studies. However, "border zone" infarcts occur in specific locations—along the cortical and subcortical white matter watershed zones—whereas lacunae are more randomly scattered lesions that primarily affect the basal ganglia, thalami, and deep periventricular white matter.

The WMHs associated with **microvascular disease** (primarily lipohyalinosis and arteriolosclerosis) are less well defined and usually more patchy or confluent than the small (< 15 mm) lesions that represent true lacunar infarcts. WMHs tend to cluster around the occipital horns and periventricular white matter, not the basal ganglia and thalami.

A few scattered T2/FLAIR hyperintensities are common in the **normal aging brain**. A general guideline is "one white spot per decade" until the age of 50, after which the number and size of WMHs increase at accelerated rates.

LACUNAR INFARCTS

Etiology and Pathology
- Macroscopic markers of "small vessel disease"
- Atherosclerosis, lipohyalinosis
- Along small penetrating arteries (few collaterals)
- Most common in basal ganglia, deep WM

Imaging
- Acute lacunae often invisible on NECT
- T2/FLAIR hyperintense
- Use DWI to distinguish from WMHs of chronic microvascular disease
- Chronic lacunae irregular, CSF-like
- May be surrounded by gliotic rim

Watershed ("Border Zone") Infarcts

Terminology and Epidemiology

Watershed (WS) infarcts, also known as "border zone" infarcts, are ischemic lesions that occur in the junction between two nonanastomosing distal arterial distributions. WS infarcts are more common than generally recognized, constituting 10-12% of all brain infarcts.

Anatomy of the Cerebral "Border Zones"

Watershed zones are defined as the "border" or junction where two or more major arterial territories meet. Two distinct types of vascular border zones are recognized: an external (cortical) WS zone and an internal (deep) WS zone **(8-62)**.

The two major **external WS zones** lie in the frontal cortex (between the ACA and MCA) and parietooccipital cortex (between the MCA and PCA). A strip of

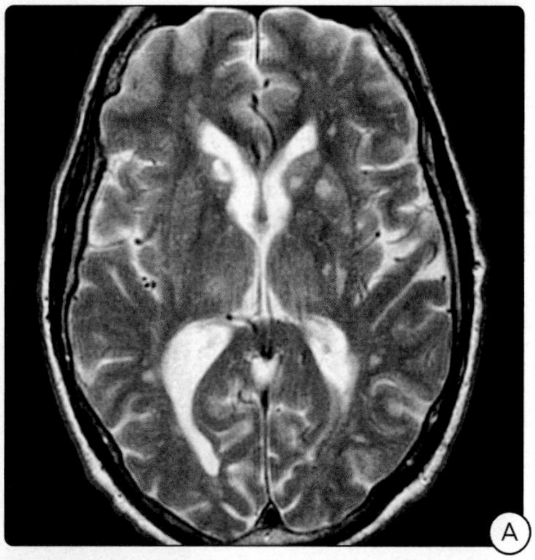

***(8-61A)** Axial T2WI shows multiple bilateral rounded and irregular hyperintensities in the basal ganglia and deep cerebral white matter.*

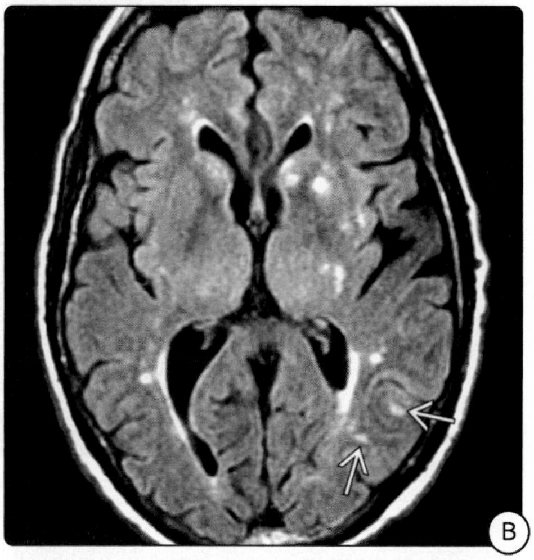

***(8-61B)** FLAIR MR (same case) shows multiple hyperintensities in both hemispheres. Some small subcortical lesions ➡ are also present.*

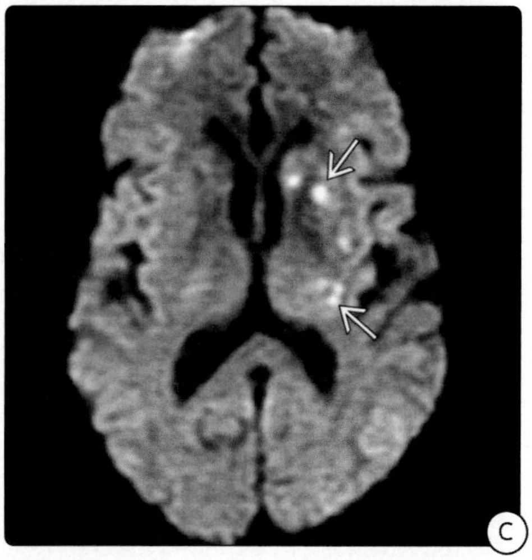

***(8-61C)** Some lesions demonstrate acute restriction ➡. DWI is helpful in distinguishing acute from chronic lacunar infarcts.*

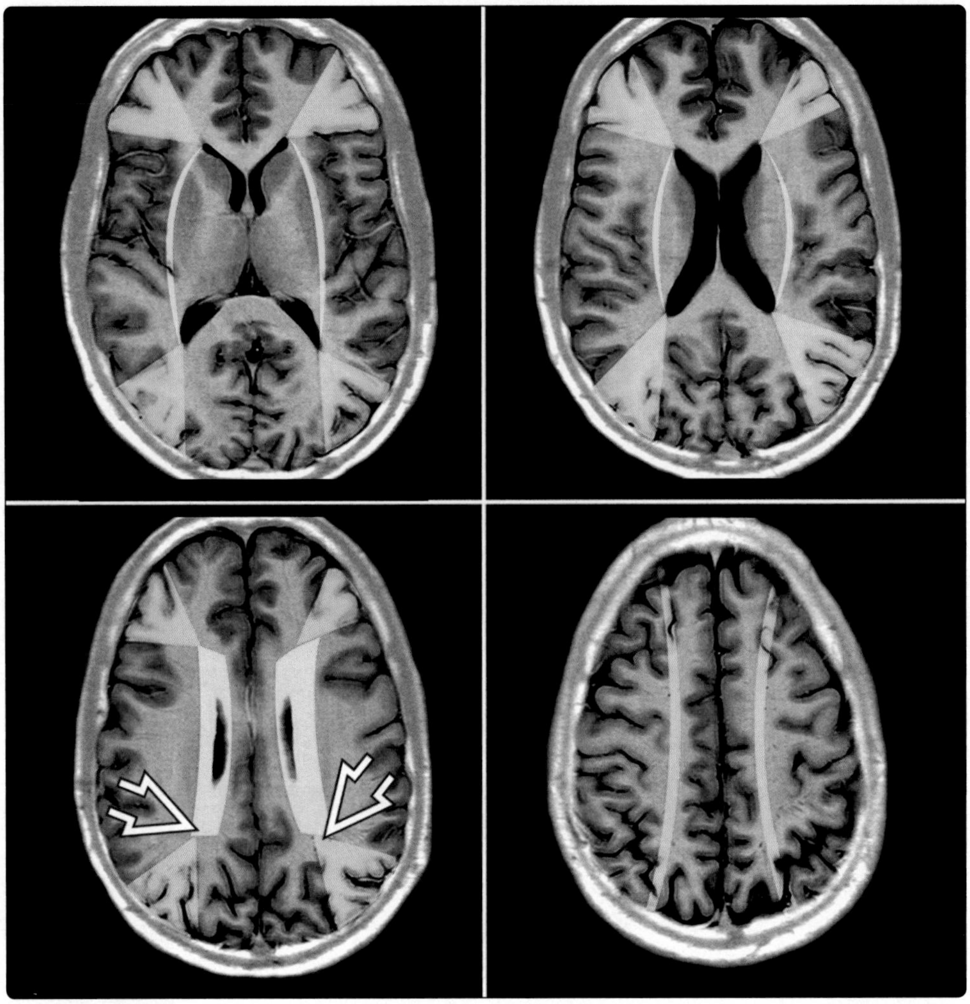

***(8-62)** T1-weighted images show two vascular watershed (WS) zones with external (cortical) WS zones in turquoise. Wedge-shaped areas between the ACAs, MCAs, and PCAs represent "border zones" between the three major terminal vascular distributions. Curved blue lines (lower right) represent subcortical WS. The triple "border zones" ➲ represent confluence of all three major vessels. Yellow lines indicate the internal (deep WM) WS zone between perforating arteries and major territorial vessels.*

paramedian subcortical white matter near the vertex of the cerebral hemispheres is also considered part of the external WS.

The **internal WS zones** represent the junctions between penetrating branches (e.g., lenticulostriate arteries, medullary white matter perforating arteries, and anterior choroidal branches) and the major cerebral vessels (MCA , ACA, and PCA).

Etiology

Two distinct hypotheses—hemodynamic compromise and microembolism—have been proposed as the etiology of hemispheric watershed infarcts. Both are likely contributing factors.

Terminal vascular distributions normally have lower perfusion pressure than main arterial trunks. Maximal vulnerability to hypoperfusion is greatest where two distal arterial fields meet together. *Hypotension with or without severe arterial stenosis or occlusion can result in hemodynamic compromise.* Flow in the affected WS zone can be critically lowered, resulting in ischemia or frank infarction. The most susceptible "border zone" is the "triple watershed" where the ACA, MCA, and PCA all converge.

External WS infarcts are the more common type. Most external WS infarcts are *embolic*. Anterior cortical WS embolic infarcts often occur in concert with internal carotid atherosclerosis. External WS infarcts in all three "border zones" are less common and usually reflect *global hypoperfusion*.

Internal WS infarcts are rarely embolic. They represent 35-40% of all WS infarcts and are most often caused by *regional hypoperfusion* secondary to hemodynamic compromise (e.g., ipsilateral carotid stenosis).

Pathology

Location. Distribution territories of the ACA, MCA, and PCA all vary considerably from individual to individual. WS infarcts likewise demonstrate moderate variability in location.

Internal WS infarcts tend to "line up" in the white matter, parallel to and slightly above the lateral ventricles **(8-63)**. Cerebellar WS infarcts occur at the borders between the posterior inferior, anterior inferior, and superior cerebellar arteries.

External (cortical) WS infarcts show a bimodal spatial distribution. Anteriorly, they center in the posterior frontal lobe near the junction of the frontal sulcus with the precentral sulcus. Posterior WS infarcts center in the superior parietal lobule posterolateral to the postcentral sulcus. The prevalence of WS infarcts decreases between these two areas. WS infarcts spare the medial cortex **(8-64)**.

Size and Number. WS infarcts vary in size from tiny lesions to large wedge-shaped ischemic areas. Multiple lesions are common and can be uni- or bilateral. Bilateral lesions are often related to global reduction in perfusion pressure, usually an acute hypotensive event.

Imaging

Imaging findings vary with WS infarct type. The main goals of neuroimaging in patients with WS infarcts are (1) to determine whether hemodynamic impairment (i.e., vascular stenosis) is present and, if present, (2) to assess its severity.

Internal WS Infarcts. Internal "border zone" infarcts can be confluent or partial. Confluent infarcts are large, cigar-shaped lesions that lie alongside or just above the lateral ventricles. Partial infarcts are more discrete, rosary-like lesions. They resemble a line of beads extending from front to back in the deep white matter **(8-63B)**.

Stenosis or occlusion of the ipsilateral internal carotid artery or MCA is common with unilateral lesions **(8-63D)**. The presence and degree of hemodynamic impairment can be determined using a number of methods, including pCT, pMR, SPECT, and PET.

External (Cortical) WS Infarcts. Cortical (external) WS infarcts are wedge- or gyriform-shaped **(8-65)**.

Differential Diagnosis

The major differential diagnosis of WS infarction is **lacunar infarcts**. Lacunar infarcts typically involve the basal ganglia,

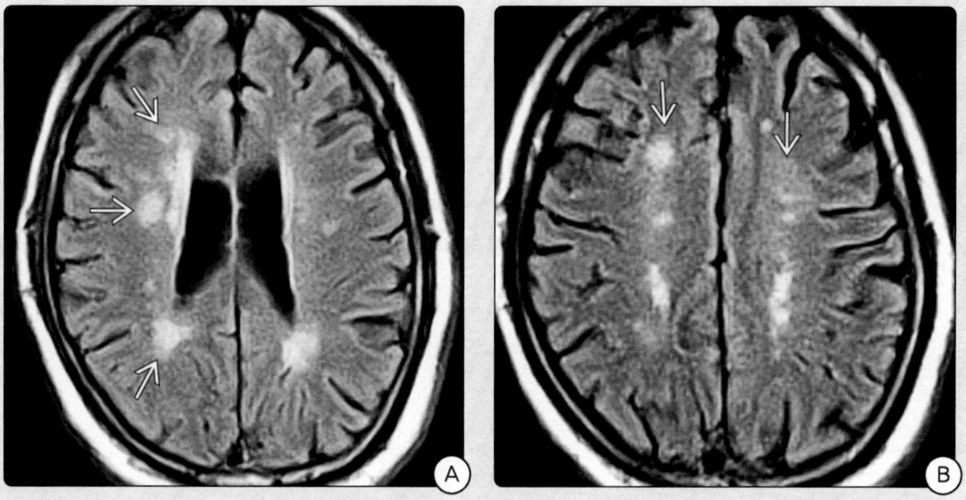

***(8-63A)** Axial FLAIR in a 69y woman with TIAs shows hyperintensities ➡ in the deep WM adjacent to the right lateral ventricle. **(8-63B)** More cephalad FLAIR in the same case shows bilateral WM hyperintensities lined up from front to back ➡ just above the level of the lateral ventricles.*

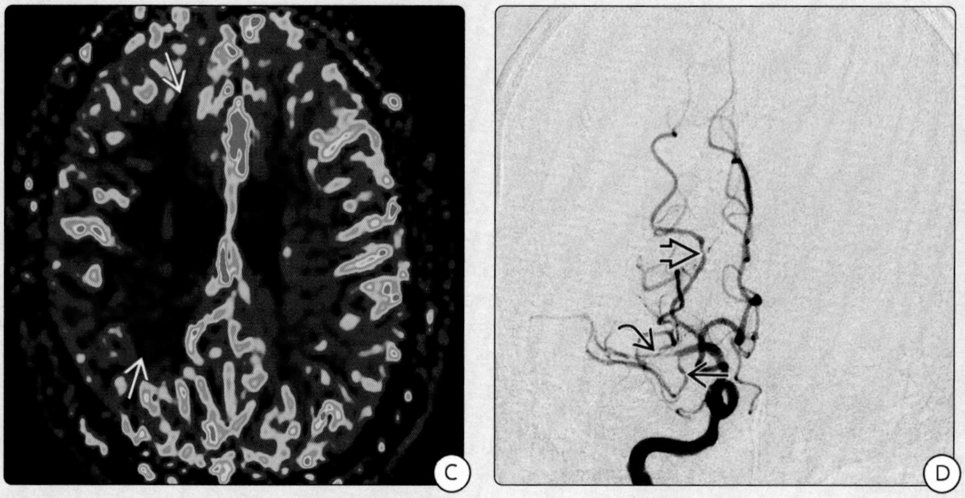

***(8-63C)** pMR in the same case shows reduced flow to the right hemisphere, with profoundly decreased perfusion of the deep WM ➡. **(8-63D)** AP view of DSA shows very high-grade stenosis of the right MCA ⇨ causing the deep watershed zone ischemia. Note changes of ASVD in the right posterior cerebral ⇨ and anterior temporal ⇨ arteries.*

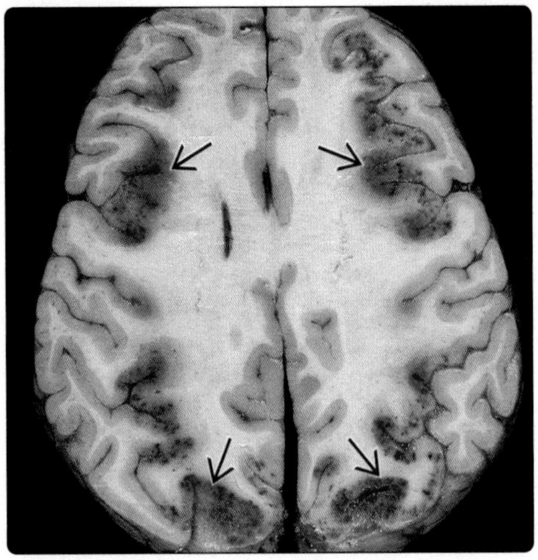

(8-64) *Autopsy case shows classic external (cortical) watershed infarcts ⇒.*

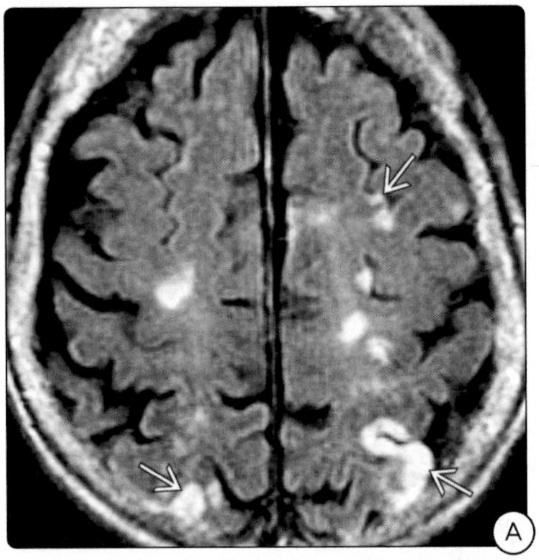

(8-65A) *Axial FLAIR scan demonstrates typical findings of bilateral external (cortical) watershed infarcts ➡.*

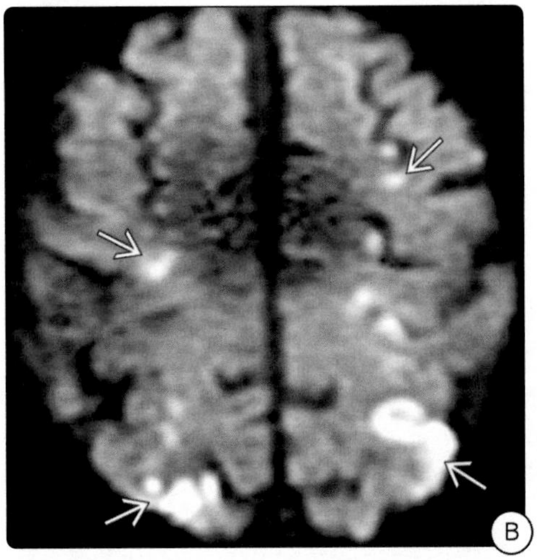

(8-65B) *DWI shows multiple cortical punctate, gyriform foci of restricted diffusion ➡, hypotension with transient global hypoperfusion.*

thalami, and pons and appear randomly scattered. Multiple **embolic infarcts** can also closely resemble WS infarcts. Emboli are often bilateral and multiterritorial but can also occur at vascular "border zones."

Posterior reversible encephalopathy syndrome (PRES) typically occurs in the setting of acute hypertension. The cortex/subcortical white matter in the PCA distribution is most commonly affected although PRES can also involve "border zones" and the basal ganglia. PRES rarely restricts on DWI (vasogenic edema), whereas "border zone" infarcts with cytotoxic edema show acute restriction.

WATERSHED ("BORDER ZONE") INFARCTS

Anatomy and Etiology

- 2 types of vascular "border zones"
  - External (cortical): between ACA, MCA, PCA
  - Internal (deep WM): between perforating branches, major arteries
- Etiology
  - Emboli (cortical more common)
  - Regional hypoperfusion (deep WM common)
  - Global hypoperfusion (all 3 cortical WS zones)

Imaging

- External: wedge or gyriform
- Internal: rosary-like line of WMHs

Perinatal Hypoxic-Ischemic Injury (HII)

PERINATAL HYPOXIC-ISCHEMIC INJURY

Global

- Hypoxic-ischemic injury (HII) in term newborns
  - Profound or central pattern
  - Watershed infarction
  - Diffuse or total pattern
- HII in preterm newborns
  - Profound or central pattern
  - Perinatal white matter damage (periventricular leukomalacia)
  - Germinal matrix-intraventricular hemorrhage
  - Periventricular hemorrhagic infarction
  - Cerebellar injury

Focal

- Perinatal stroke: arterial
  - Solitary
  - Multifocal
- Perinatal stroke: venous
  - Superficial
  - Deep

Hypoxic-ischemic injury (HII) is one of the most devastating of all neonatal brain insults. The acute clinical manifestation of HII in the newborn is termed **hypoxic ischemic encephalopathy**. Death or severe lifelong neurologic deficits, including motor impairment, cognitive deficiency, and developmental delay, are common. This section will emphasize the role of ischemia and hypoxia in perinatal brain injury and acknowledge that inflammatory factors (e.g., chorioamnionitis), metabolic conditions (e.g., hypoglycemia), and heritable predispositions (e.g., *COL4A1* gene mutations) play comorbid roles in **HII**.

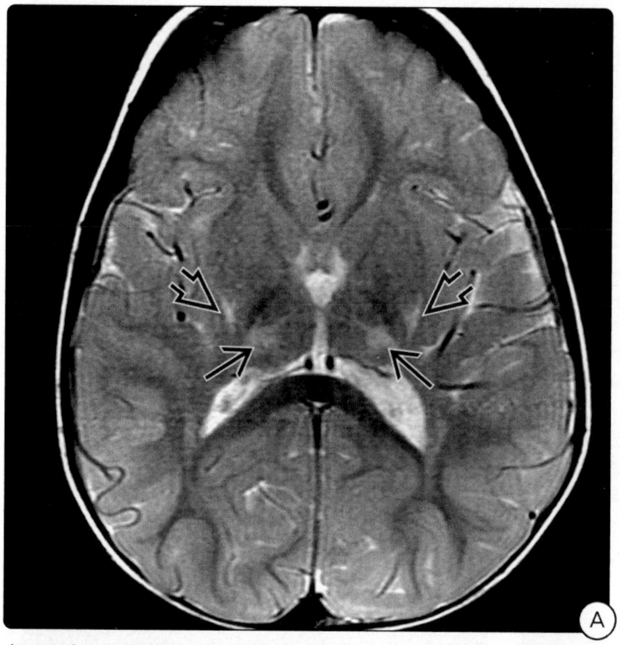

(8-66A) Axial T2WI in a 6m infant who was a preterm newborn shows thalamic ➡ and posterior putaminal ➡ atrophy and T2 prolongation (gliosis) from remote central HII. This shows perinatal preterm central pattern of HII.

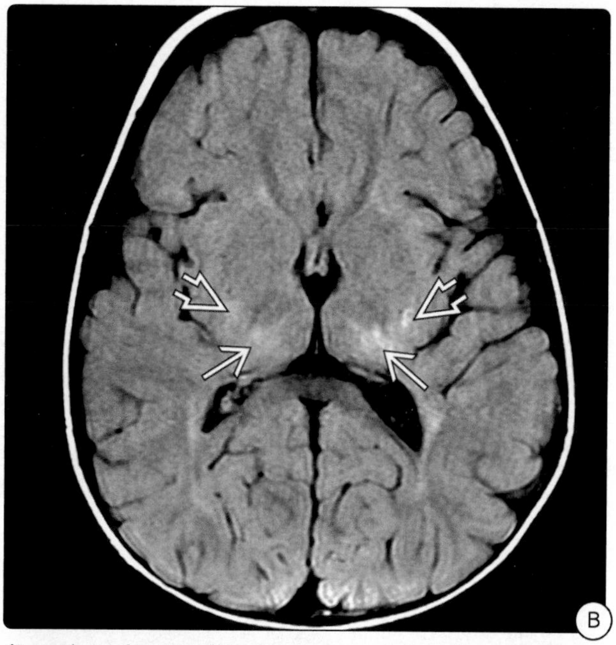

(8-66B) Axial FLAIR of the same preterm infant shows thalamic ➡ and posterior putaminal ➡ atrophy and hyperintensity (gliosis) from remote central HII. This shows the perinatal preterm central pattern of HII.

HII encompasses injuries that may be global or diffuse localized arterial infarction or localized infarction due to cerebral sinovenous thrombosis. All may have identical acute clinical presentations in the newborn. Perinatal HII imaging patterns are often distinctive compared with similarly mediated injuries among older children, adolescents, and adults.

The pathophysiology of HII in the perinatal period is recognizably complex. Cerebral ischemia is simply diminished blood flow. Ischemia can be focal or global. **Focal ischemia** refers to decreased or absent perfusion in a particular vascular territory. Focal patterns of ischemic injury are further subdivided into arterial (e.g., stenosis or occlusion) (solitary or multifocal) **(8-82A)** and venous (superficial or deep) **(8-84)**. Ischemia may or may not proceed to infarction (i.e., tissue death).

Global ischemia occurs when overall cerebral perfusion drops below the level required to maintain normal brain function (e.g., placental abruption). In addition to ischemia and hypoxia, hypoglycemia and inflammatory substances (e.g., circulating cytokines) play an important supporting role in HII. From the middle of the third trimester of pregnancy through the 40th postconceptional week, the dorsal brainstem, thalami, basal ganglia, and perirolandic cortex exhibit high metabolic activity. It is not until the 44th postconceptional week that the geniculocalcarine tracts (optic radiations) show increased metabolic/myelinating activity. As a rule, in the setting of mild to moderate HII, blood is shunted to preserve flow to the basal ganglia, thalami, brainstem, and cerebellum. Damage is reflected in the interarterial (watershed) boundary or border zones and cerebral cortex **(8-79A)**.

In severe or profound HII, the injury pattern is global with injury to the deep nuclei (thalami and globi pallidi) **(8-66)**, posterior brainstem, hippocampi, superior cerebellar vermis, and sensorimotor regions of the cerebral cortex. In the 2nd trimester (gestational age of 14-26 weeks), ischemic injury leads to liquefaction **(8-80F)**; in the third trimester (27-40 weeks), ischemic injury leads to astrogliosis.

Hypoxia or **hypoxemia** refers to reduced blood oxygenation. Asphyxia indicates the altered exchange between oxygen and CO_2 resulting in diminished blood oxygen (hypoxia). In contrast to ischemia, cerebral hypoxia is almost always global. In the initial stages of hypoxia, cardiac output and cerebral blood flow (CBF) may be maintained normally, but blood oxygenation is deficient (e.g., carbon monoxide poisoning).

Prolonged systemic hypoxemia results in cardiac hypoxia, which in turn diminishes cardiac output. Depressed cardiac output causes global brain hypoperfusion and ischemia. Interestingly, the presence of alternate energy metabolites (e.g., glucose and ketone bodies) confers on the newborn a resistance to hypoxia as long as normal cerebral perfusion is maintained.

The term **global HII** or *total injury* describes the pathologic and imaging findings (peripheral and central) of CNS ischemia and hypoxia acting in concert.

Secondary Energy Failure and HII

For the radiologist tasked with interpreting MR studies in newborns with HII, understanding the concept of *secondary energy failure* is critical in the timing of MR studies and to avoid false negative MR interpretations. HII leads to diffusion

__(8-67A)__ Coronal US of grade I germinal matrix hemorrhage (GMH) in a 33-week preterm newborn at 5 days of age shows an expansile hyperechoic germinal matrix hemorrhage at the left caudothalamic groove →. __(8-67B)__ Sagittal US shows grade I GMH. Focal hemorrhage is demonstrated at the caudothalamic groove →, which represents the location of the greatest aggregation of germinal matrix tissue.

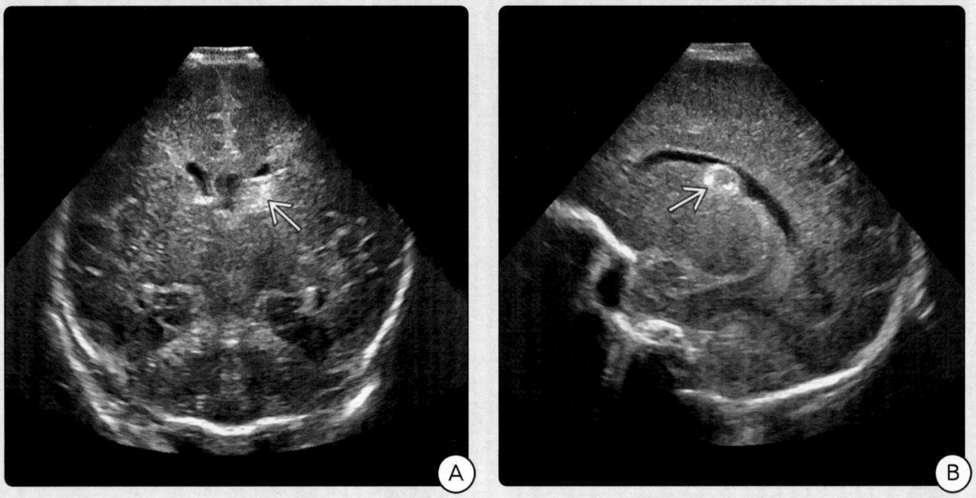

__(8-68A)__ Coronal US shows grade II GMH. Linear accumulations of intraventricular hemorrhage are demonstrated within the frontal horns →. Hemorrhage is also seen within the temporal horns ↪. __(8-68B)__ Sagittal US shows grade II GMH. Clot is identified within the lateral ventricle →. Intraventricular hemorrhage abuts the choroid plexus within the trigone ↪. Color Doppler US can discriminate choroid from clot.

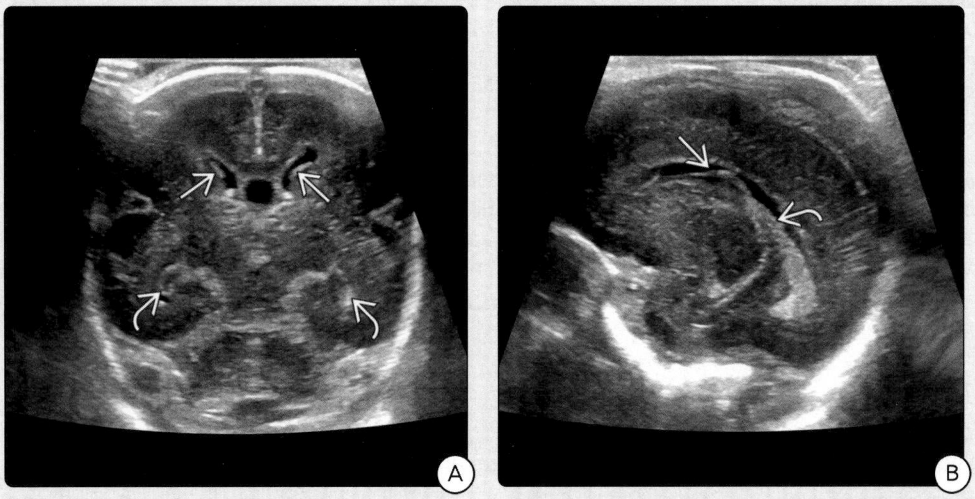

__(8-69A)__ Coronal US shows grade III GMH. Clot fills, distends the lateral ventricles →. Evaluate the periventricular tissue for hyperechoic changes of PVHI. __(8-69B)__ Sagittal US shows grade III GMH. Posterior fontanelle US shows distending clot within lateral ventricle →. Clot is encompassing the choroid plexus within the trigone ⇨. The posterior fontanelle approach to US allows clear visualization of the lateral ventricle and trigonal regions.

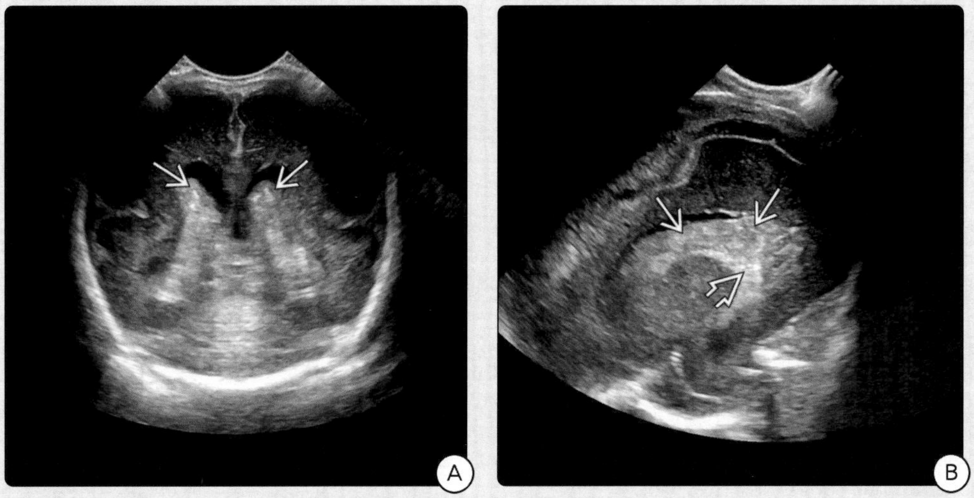

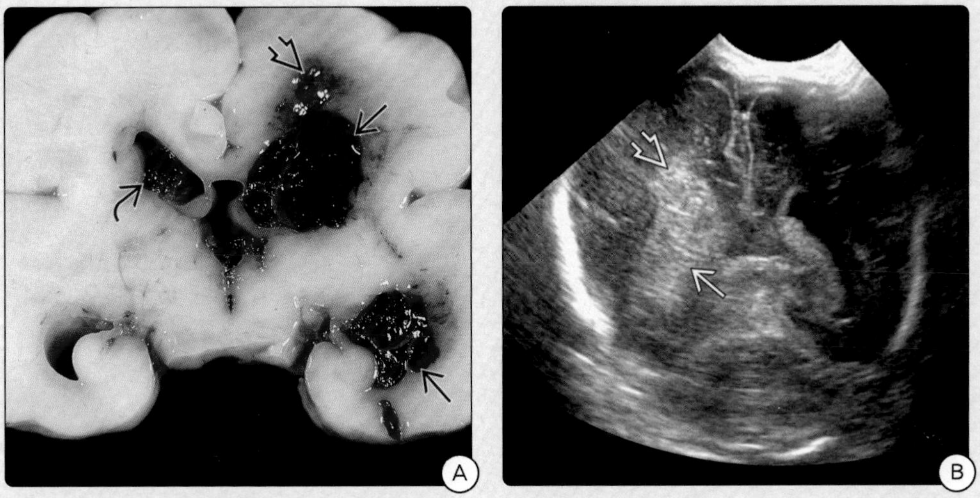

***(8-70A)** Coronal autopsy specimen shows expansile clot within the left lateral ventricle. There is left perifrontal periventricular hemorrhagic infarction (PVHI). There is hemorrhage within the right lateral ventricle. **(8-70B)** Coronal US at 72 h of age in a 28-week preterm newborn shows distending clot within the right lateral ventricle. Note the parenchymal hyperechogenicity of PVHI.*

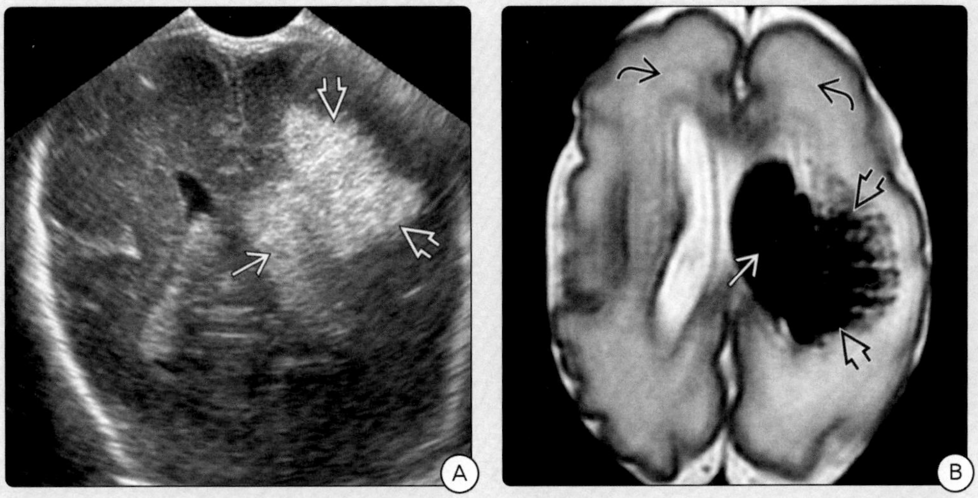

***(8-71A)** Coronal US in a 26-week preterm newborn shows distending ventricular hemorrhage and hyperechoic PHVI. **(8-71B)** Axial T2WI in the same newborn shows PVHI and ventricular clot. Note the bihemispheric hypointense halos, representing neurons migrating outward from the germinal matrix.*

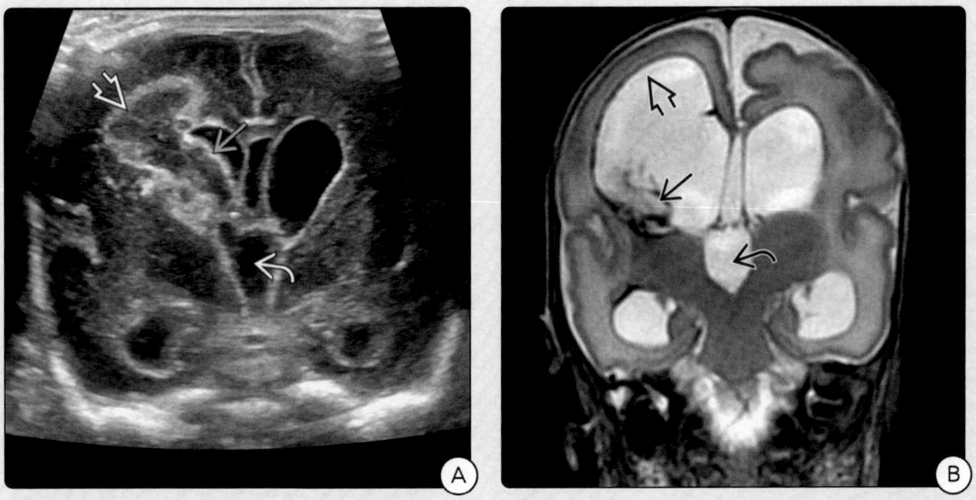

***(8-72A)** Coronal US at 15 days shows evolving PVHI. At 72 h of life, US showed distending clot within the right lateral ventricle. Posthemorrhagic ventriculitis and hydrocephalus are also noted. **(8-72B)** Coronal T2WI in the same patient with PVHI shows clot and infarcted brain debris. Porencephaly of the frontal lobe and posthemorrhagic hydrocephalus are noted.*

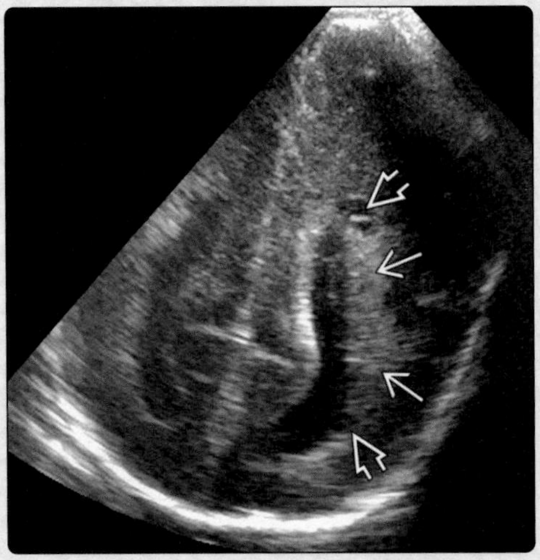

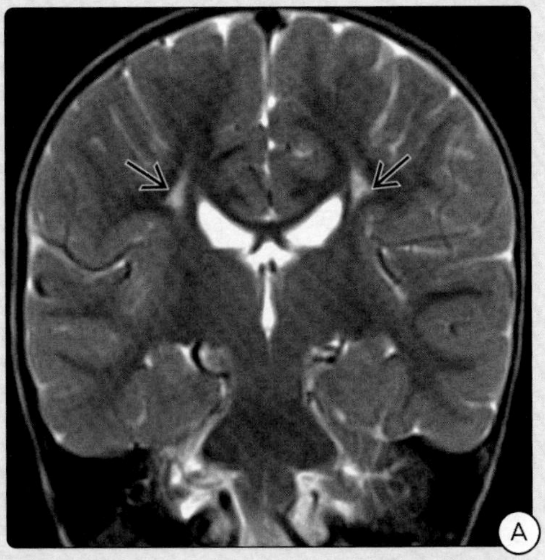

***(8-73)** Oblique coronal US in a preterm neonate at 2 weeks of age shows pathologic periventricular hyperechoic "flair" →. Note focal periventricular hypoechoic cysts →. **(8-74A)** Coronal T2WI in the same patient at 12m shows symmetric periventricular T2 prolongation consistent with gliosis [perinatal WM damage (PWMD), periventricular leukomalacia (PVL)] →. Note passive frontal horn dilation.*

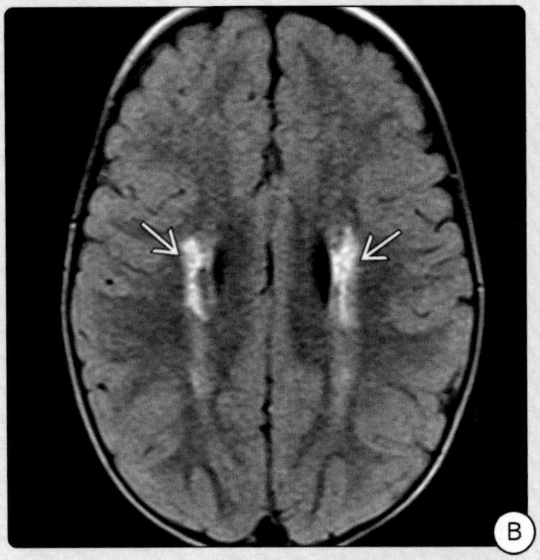

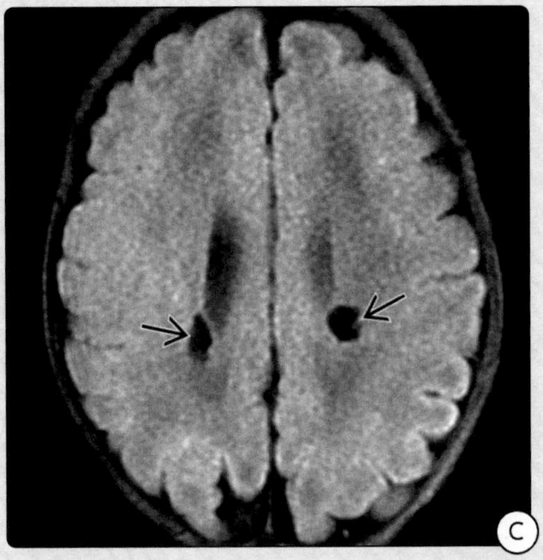

***(8-74B)** Axial FLAIR in the same patient shows periventricular hyperintensity representing gliosis from remote PWMD →. T2 FLAIR becomes more sensitive to detect WM injury after 8 months of age. **(8-74C)** Axial FLAIR in a 2m, 32-week preterm infant demonstrates cystic PWMD →. Note the limitation of T2 FLAIR in revealing gliosis (PVL) at this age.*

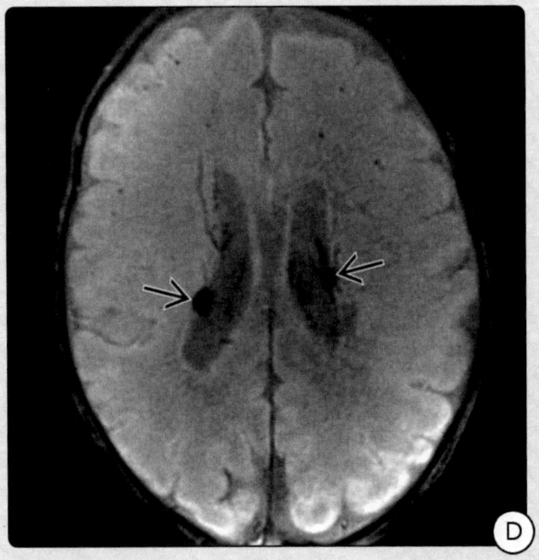

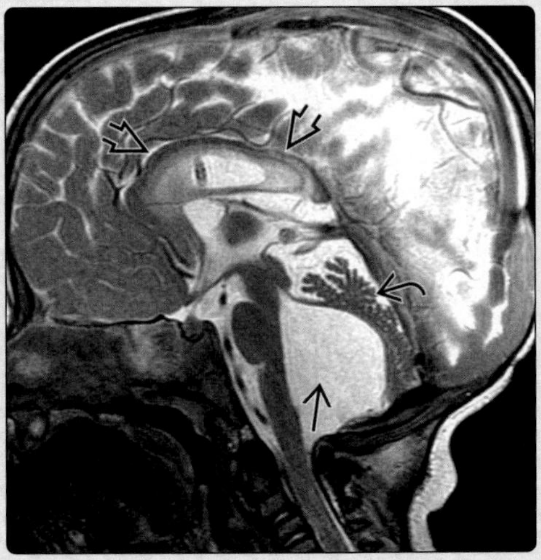

***(8-74D)** Axial SWI in the same patient shows focal periventricular hypointense "blooming" → consistent with hemorrhagic PWMD (PVL). **(8-75)** Sagittal T2* MR shows an 8m, 28-week preemie with remote grade III GMHs and PWMD. The image shows marked thinning of the corpus callosum → from PVL, cerebellar atrophy →, and trapped fourth ventricle → from remote IVH.*

restriction (DWI and ADC) **(8-78C)** and lactate elevation (MRS) **(8-80E)** within the first few hours following the ischemic-hypoxic insult.

During the period of *early recovery* (6-18 hours after insult), lactate and diffusivity abnormalities may transiently "*normalize*," only to revert to abnormality after 24 hours. The HII-driven cascade of damage including the disruption of molecular intracellular structures responsible for oxidative and phosphorylative cellular activities will progress, peaking at approximately 5 days. Therefore, we make every effort to time MR brain imaging in the setting of HII at **day 5**. This just so happens to complement the current brain cooling protocols that typically conclude on day 4.

Pressure-Passive Flow and HII

Cerebral vascular regulation in the newborn and particularly the preterm neonate differs from adults. Normally, blood vessels of the brain constrict when blood pressure increases and dilate when blood pressure decreases. The absence of this autoregulatory function leads to pressure-passive flow. In preterm neonates, pressure passive flow is normally present. In the term newborn, hypoxia and hypercarbia lead to the loss of cerebral vascular autoregulation. Therefore, in the setting of HII, varied patterns of hypoperfusion injury may occur in the preterm and term newborn.

Overview of Imaging Modalities and HII

MR is the modality of choice for the investigation of neonatal HII. It offers the greatest sensitivity and specificity. Physiologic monitoring is required, and sedation is often needed to control motion. *MR* is expensive and access may be limited.

Cranial sonography is well suited for germinal matrix and intraventricular hemorrhage detection, and follow-up, is low cost, requires no sedation, is portable to the bedside, and uses no ionizing radiation **(8-67A)**.

Ultrasound lacks sensitivity and specificity for detecting white matter damage and has a limited FOV.

CT rapidly screens for hemorrhage, calcifications, and clinical mimics of HII such as congenital brain tumors. CT lacks sensitivity for detecting the global and focal signs of HII and involves ionizing radiation.

From a practical standpoint, the **preterm** newborn is typically initially imaged with cranial US. Other organ system requirements (e.g., ventilator support for respiratory failure and need to maintain body temperature) often delay MR to the time of estimated term gestational age or planned time of discharge. For the **term** neonate in whom the timing of HII is known with greater precision, *US* is recommended immediately after birth, and *MR* is planned 5 days after delivery.

Perinatal HII

There is increasing evidence that some injury patterns that we have historically described as neonatal HII, particularly white matter damage of prematurity, have their onset in utero (prenatal). As an example, maternal chorioamnionitis leading to preterm birth at 30 weeks (third trimester of pregnancy) with the subsequent discovery of periventricular white matter damage likely represents a perinatal injury, not necessarily a neonatal injury.

This nuance of understanding has practical implications for our neuroimaging reports due to possible obstetrical and fetal maternal medicine legal consequences. The perinatal time frame is defined as the period beginning at 20-28 weeks of gestation prior to birth and extending 1-4 weeks after birth.

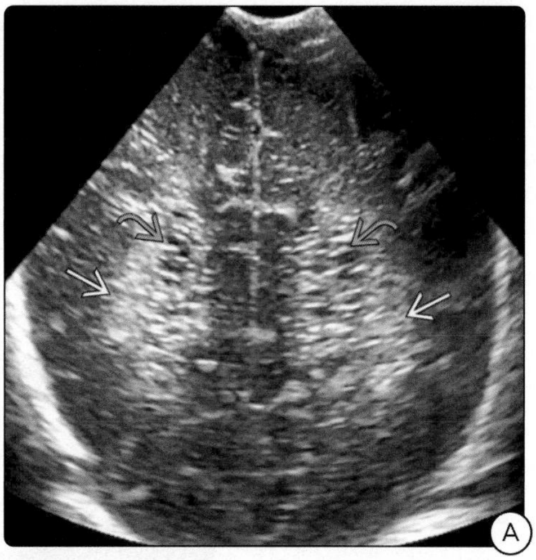

***(8-76A)** Coronal US at 17 days in 34-week preemie shows cystic and diffuse PWMD. Cystic PVL is an uncommon form of PWMD.*

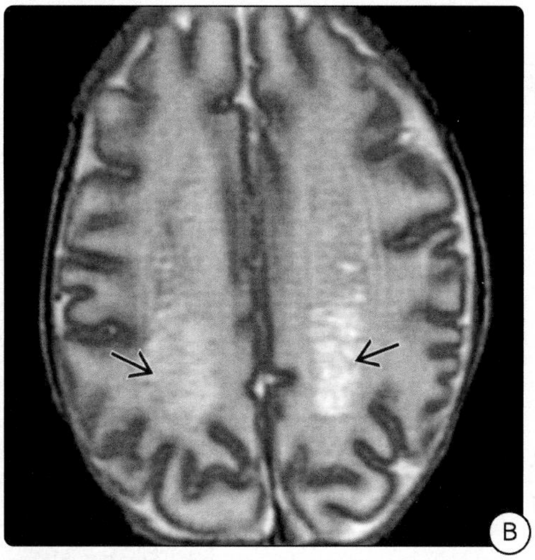

***(8-76B)** Axial T2WI in the same infant shows cavitating cysts of PWMD. Diffuse noncavitary form of PWMD is the most common type.*

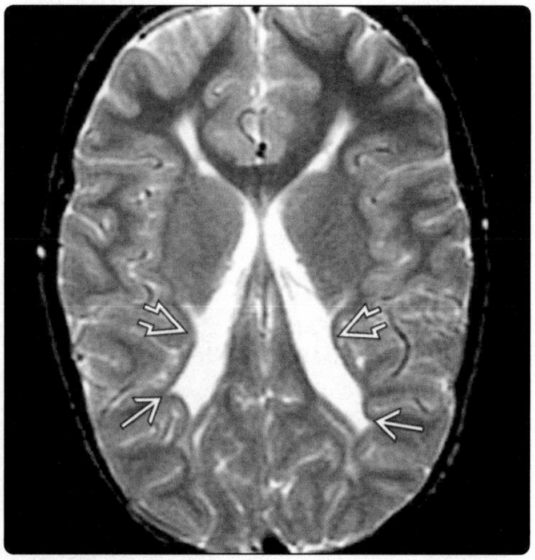

***(8-77)** Axial T2WI shows end-stage PWMD (PVL). Central WM loss allows the cortex to touch and "scallop" the ventricular margins.*

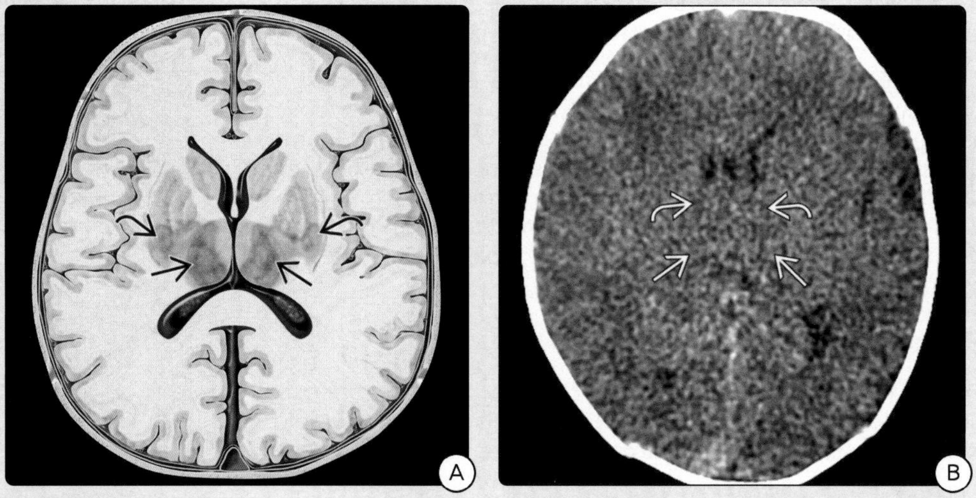

(8-78A) *Axial graphic depicts profound, severe, or central HII in a term infant with preferential involvement of the posterior putamina and ventrolateral thalami.* ***(8-78B)*** *Axial NECT in acute profound HII demonstrates loss of the normal GM attenuation of basal ganglia and thalami. This image shows diffuse loss of GM/WM discrimination and ventricular and sulcal effacement from cerebral edema.*

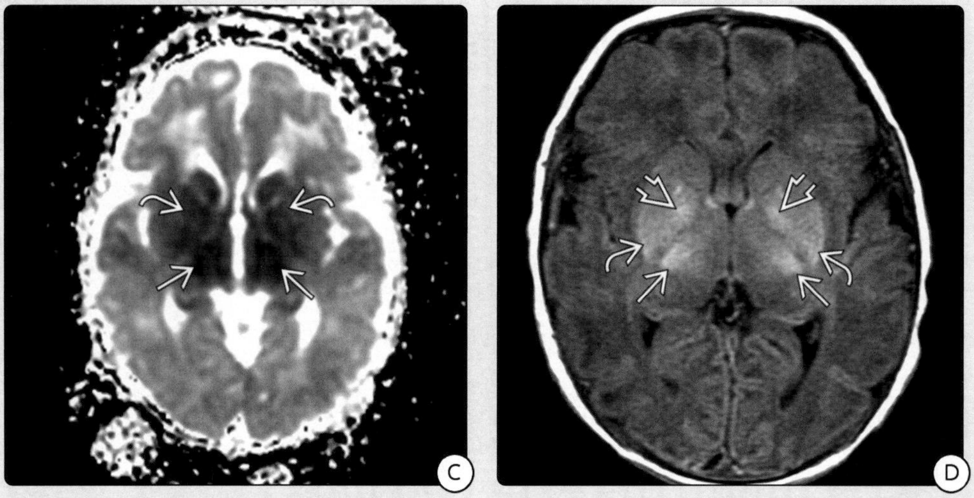

(8-78C) *Axial ADC map shows an acute central or profound pattern of HII in the term newborn primarily involving the striatum and thalami.* ***(8-78D)*** *Axial T1WI shows a term newborn with profound HII and pathologic T1 shortening within the thalami, putamen, and globi pallidi. Note the absence of expected T1 shortening (myelination) within the posterior limbs of internal capsule.*

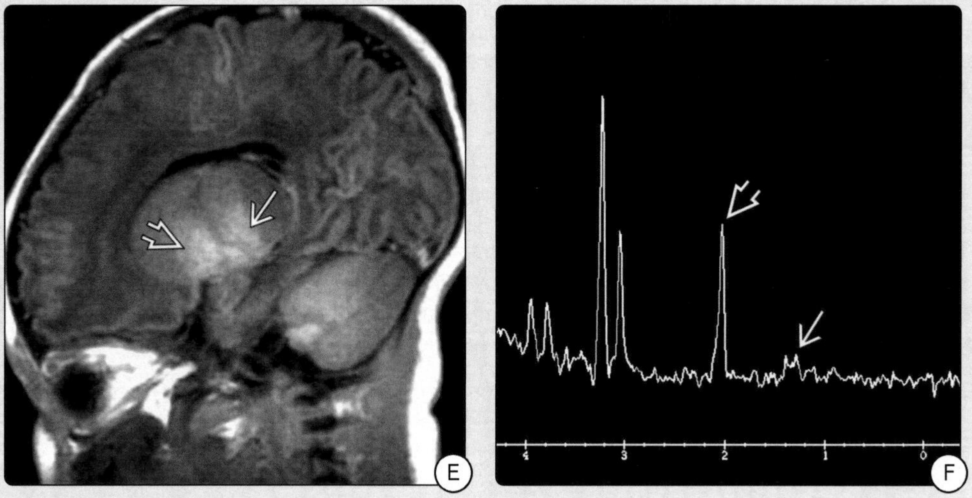

(8-78E) *Parasagittal T1WI in the same patient shows pathologic T1 hyperintensity within thalami and globi pallidi. Ca++, manganese, and lipids within injured tissue may contribute to T1 shortening.* ***(8-78F)*** *Long-TE (288 ms) proton spectroscopy sampling of the left basal ganglia at day 6 shows persistent lactate doublet at 1.3 ppm. This is a poor prognosticator for tissue recovery. There is decline of NAA.*

Imaging findings in perinatal HII vary with *maturation of the brain* at the time of injury, *severity of insult*, *duration of insult*, and *existing comorbidities* (e.g., inflammatory milieu, hypoglycemia, and genetic mutations). The spectrum of brain injury in the preterm and term neonate is surprisingly broad with distinctive qualities and points of overlap. The full appraisal of injury depends on the timing of imaging and the imaging modality selected.

In the preterm newborn suspected of HII, the radiologist must be familiar with central or profound injury, perinatal white matter damage, germinal matrix hemorrhage, intraventricular hemorrhage, periventricular hemorrhagic infarction, and cerebellar injury.

HII in Preterm Infants. Preterm newborns are born before 37 weeks of gestation and typically weigh less than 1,500 g. In the USA in the year 2000, 11% of all live births were preterm and of low birth weight. Perinatal HII is more common in preterm neonates, and, based on MR data, 50% of these newborns will exhibit some degree of white matter injury. For those that survive prematurity, 90% will manifest neurologic deficits, including cerebral palsy and cognitive, behavioral, and attention deficit disorders. The prevalence and severity of neurologic sequelae increase with the extremes of prematurity.

In this subgroup, the type of injuries that result from **severe or profound HII** reflect the state of brain maturation (areas of active myelination), metabolic demands of key anatomic structures, associated comorbidities (e.g., hypoglycemia, fetal-maternal inflammation), and the state of maturity of cerebral glutamate receptors. In aggregate, these interrelated factors affect the pattern of vulnerability to HII.

The pattern of severe HII in the preterm is similar to the profound or central pattern of HII in term newborns with a few notable exceptions. The superior cerebellar vermis, posterior limb of the internal capsule, and perirolandic cortex are uninvolved in preterm severe HII, as these structures

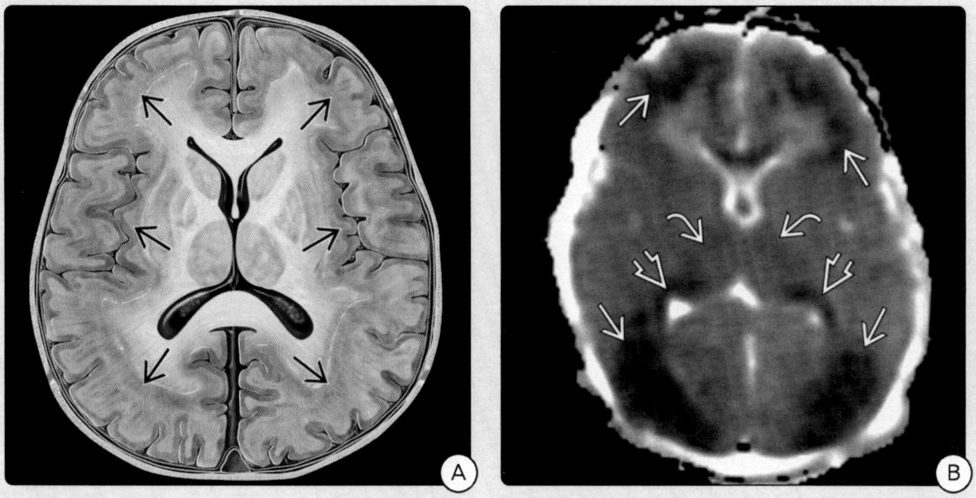

***(8-79A)** Graphic shows less severe HII, which generally spares the deep basal ganglia but involves the cortex and subcortical WM, especially in the interarterial watershed "border zones" →. **(8-79B)** Axial ADC map in "less severe," prolonged protracted HII shows predominant restricted diffusion in the watershed zones →. Also, note low ADC values in the optic radiations →, genu of the corpus callosum, and thalami →.*

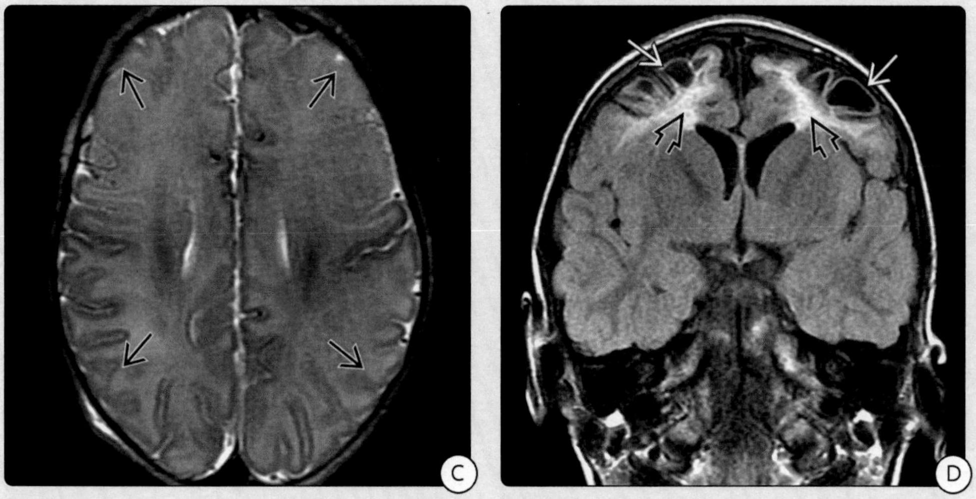

***(8-79C)** Axial T2WI in the same patient demonstrates loss of normal hypointense cortical GM → signal ("reversal sign"), representing cortical and subcortical edema. **(8-79D)** Coronal FLAIR in the same patient 8 months later shows cystic encephalomalacia → and subcortical gliosis →. Note the "mushroom shape" of the affected gyri (ulegyria).*

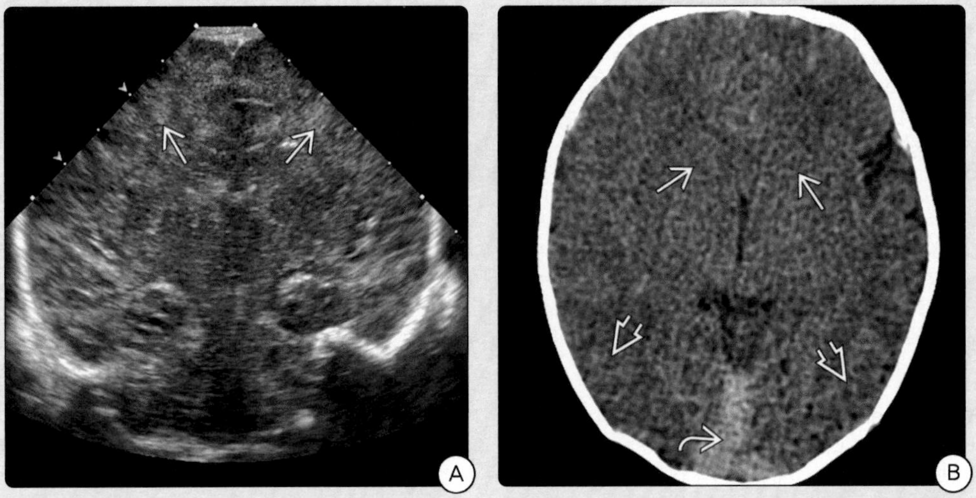

(8-80A) *Coronal cranial US in acutely asphyxiated term newborn shows diffuse "salt and pepper" pattern of heterogeneous echogenicity and lateral ventricular compression secondary to diffuse cerebral edema.* ***(8-80B)*** *NECT shows term neonate with total or diffuse pattern of HII and loss of central and peripheral GM/WM differentiation. Lateral ventricles are compressed, prominent normal torcula due to surrounding edema.*

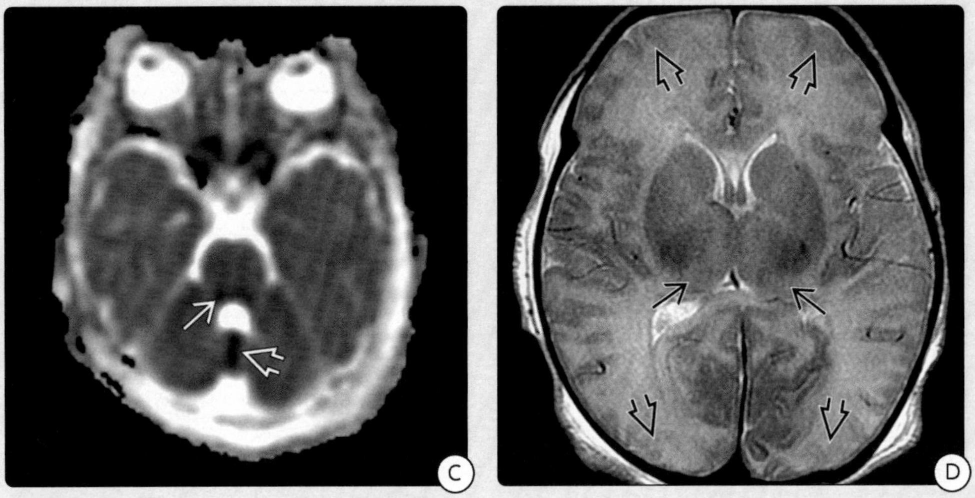

(8-80C) *Axial ADC map shows total or diffuse HII. Diffusion restriction is within the corticospinal tracts and superior cerebellar vermis.* ***(8-80D)*** *Axial T2WI in a term newborn with total or diffuse HII shows peripheral edema (reversal sign) and patchy thalamic edema. T2WI underestimates HII changes.*

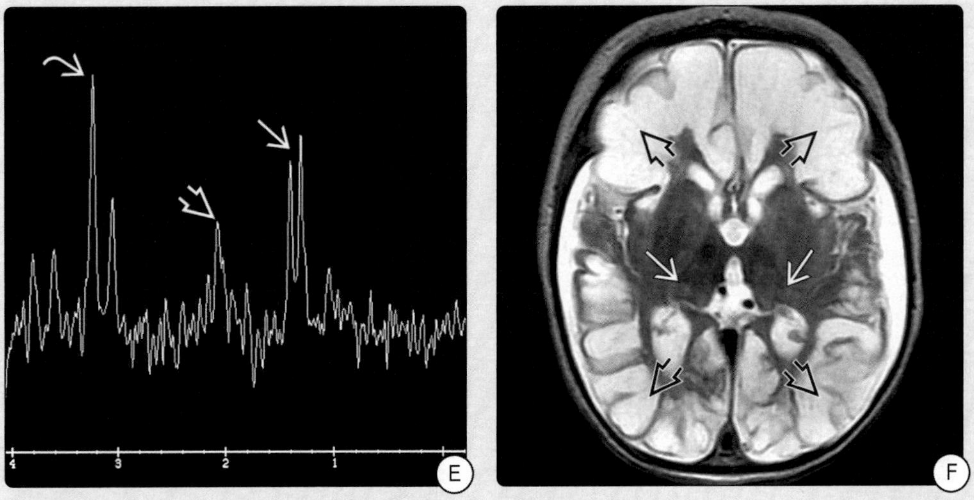

(8-80E) *Proton spectroscopy (short TE, 35 ms) from parietal WM of the prior patient, 5 days after birth asphyxia, shows large lactate doublet, reduced NAA, and elevation of choline.* ***(8-80F)*** *Axial T2WI shows the same patient, 6 months following diffuse or total HII event. Multicystic encephalomalacia and patchy thalamic hyperintensity are shown.*

normally myelinate at or near term. **Severe or profound HII** in preterm neonates preferentially affects the early myelinating and metabolically active structures, including the thalami, basal ganglia (particularly posterior putamin), and dorsal brainstem, with relative cortex sparing except for the pre- and postcentral gyri.

Imaging in the acute and subacute time frame when **severe or profound HII** is suspected is practically first accomplished with cranial US, which may show hyperechogenicity in the thalami often within 24 hours.

If MR is performed in the first week of life (often not feasible due to fragility of the preemie), it would show reduced diffusivity (e.g., DWI hyperintensity, ADC hypointensity) and MRS abnormalities (e.g., elevated lactate) in affected areas, including the thalami, dorsal brainstem, lentiform nuclei, and perirolandic gyri. T2 prolongation is often seen in affected areas in the first few days after injury, and T1 shortening may be detected after 3 to 4 days.

GERMINAL MATRIX-IVH IN PRETERM INFANTS

Grade I
- Subependymal GMH
  - Typically at caudothalamic groove
- No/minimal intraventricular extension

Grade II
- GMH + IVH (filling < 50% of ventricular area)
- No/minimal ventriculomegaly

Grade III
- GMH + IVH [near complete filling (> 50%) and distention of ventricle]

Periventricular Hemorrhagic Infarction (PVHI) (Grade IV)
- Periventricular parenchymal hemorrhagic infarction
- Secondary to hemorrhagic ventricular distention, venous ischemia, and hemorrhagic venous infarct
- *Unlike grade I-III bleeds, not true GMH*

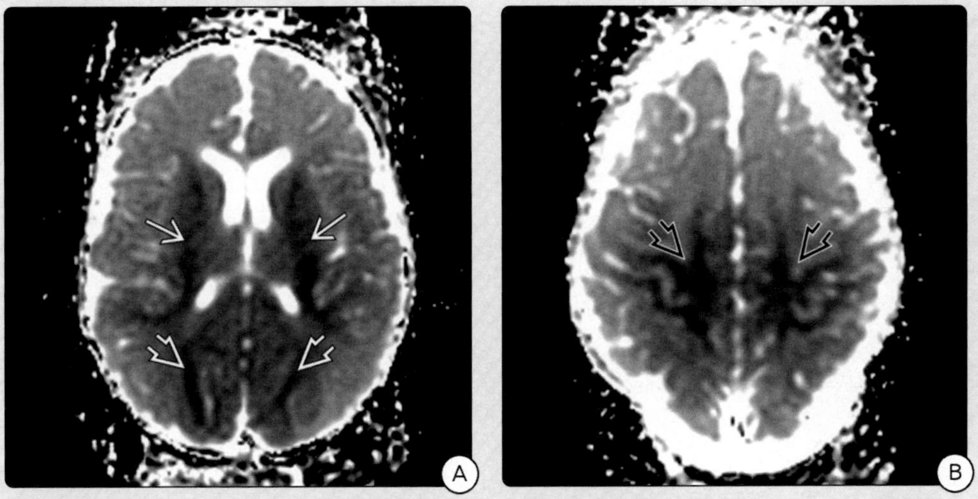

***(8-81A)** Axial ADC map shows a term newborn at 5 days of life with a mixed HII pattern. Note the deep nuclear ➡ and parietal occipital WM ➡ diffusion restriction. **(8-81B)** Axial ADC map in the same patient shows extensive cerebral hemispheric WM diffusion restriction ➡. Diffuse WM injury following HII may be delayed (up to a week after HII event).*

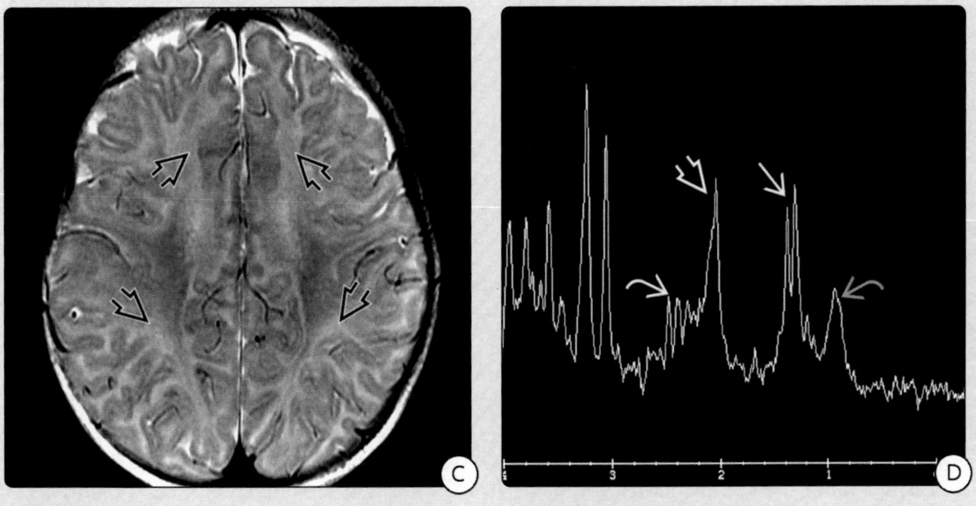

***(8-81C)** Axial T2WI in the same patient demonstrates nonspecific subcortical WM T2 prolongation ➡. T2WI has limited sensitivity in detecting injury in neonatal HII. **(8-81D)** Proton spectroscopy (MRS) of the basal ganglia in the same patient (mixed pattern of HII) shows lactate doublet ➡, NAA decline ➡, elevation of excitatory neurotransmitters ➡ (injury markers), and a broad lipid peak ➡.*

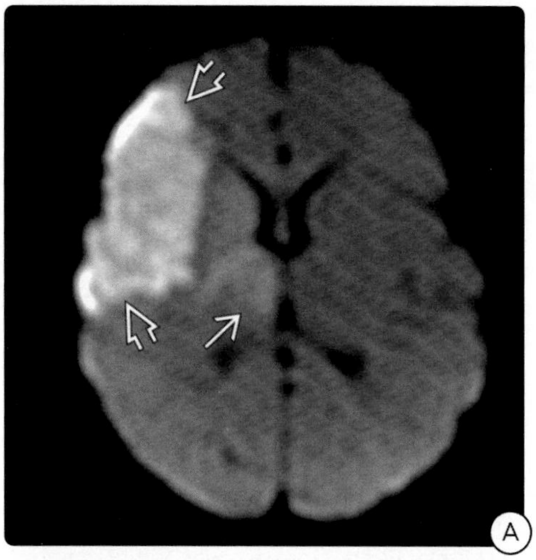

***(8-82A)** DWI in term newborn with seizures shows focal arterial distribution infarction and deep nuclear diffusion hyperintensity.*

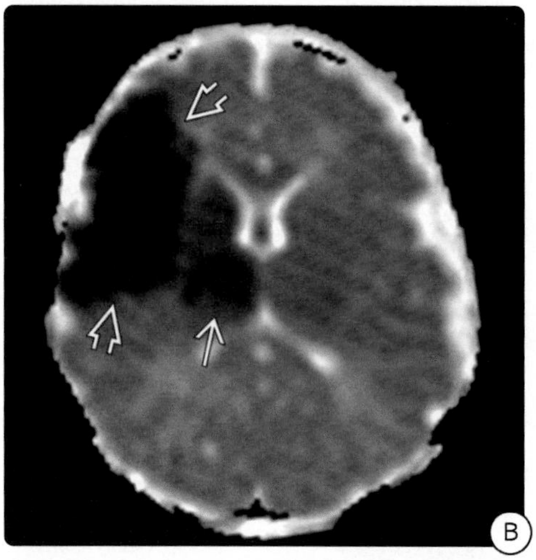

***(8-82B)** Axial ADC map in the same patient shows diffusion restriction in a peripheral and deep arterial distribution.*

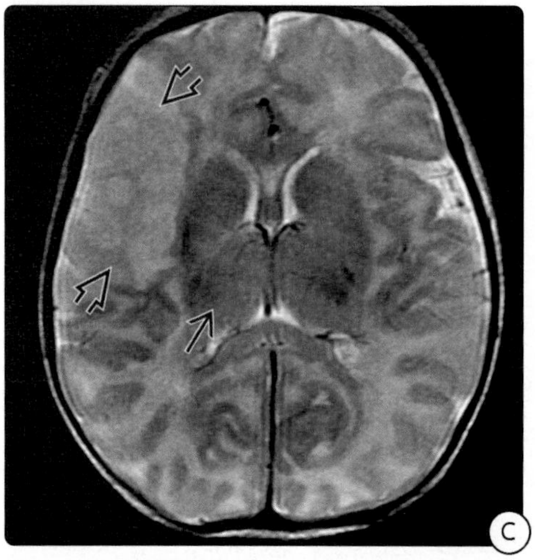

***(8-82C)** Axial T2WI in the same newborn shows peripheral T2 prolongation. Also note subtle thalamic T2 hyperintensity.*

When MR is delayed (> 2 weeks after delivery), injured tissues show volume loss (atrophy), T1 and T2 shortening, pseudonormalized DWI, and diminished NAA on MRS **(8-66)**.

Mild to moderate HII can manifest in one of three general patterns: (1) hemorrhagic: germinal matrix hemorrhage (GMH), intraventricular hemorrhage (IVH)/periventricular hemorrhagic infarction (PVHI); (2) perinatal white matter damage (PWMD) **(8-70A)**; (3) cerebellar injury. These patterns can occur independently or synchronously.

The germinal matrix (GM) forms the neuronal precursor cell zone. The largest aggregates of vascularized GM tissue are found at the caudothalamic grooves (ganglionic eminence), roof of the fourth ventricle, superior margins of the frontal horns, and the granular cell layer of the cerebellum.

The prevalence of GMH-IVH in preterm neonates is inversely related to gestational age and birth weight. The prevalence of GMH in preterm neonates under 2,000 g is approximately 25%. Ninety percent of GMHs occur within the first 4 days of life, and these bleeds become less frequent after 34 weeks of gestation. GMH-IVH is generally evaluated with cranial US and is divided into three grades that reflect hemorrhage location and degree of ventriculomegaly **(8-67)** **(8-68)** **(8-69)**.

PVHI (formally called Grade IV GMH) occurs with a prevalence of 15% in newborns with IVH. Eighty-ninety percent of neonates with PVHI manifest the injury in the first 96 hours of life. The US in cases of PVHI demonstrates hemorrhage casting and distending the lateral ventricle and ipsilateral periventricular parenchymal hyperechogenicity (e.g., region of hemorrhagic infarction).

Delayed MR (particularly T2* GRE and SWI) shows hemorrhagic debris within the periventricular infarction, the ipsilateral ventricle system, and subarachnoid spaces (siderosis). In cases of bilateral PVHI, consider heritable microangiopathy due to mutations in the gene *COL4A1* on Ch 13q34.

Perinatal White Matter Damage. PWMD is also known as periventricular leukomalacia (PVL). Prevalence is inversely related to gestational age at birth. Mild to moderate HII in the preterm newborn alone or in conjunction with maternal-fetal infectious/inflammatory conditions may lead to damage of the premyelinating oligodendrocytes in the periventricular WM and injury to neurons of the subplate (a transient deep layer of the cortex). Given the diffuse cerebral injury (neurons and axons) beyond just white matter, a more accurate encompassing but less commonly used description is **encephalopathy of prematurity**.

WM injury is most common adjacent to the foramen of Monro and lateral ventricle trigones. Three PWMD patterns have been described: diffuse, focal/multifocal-noncavitary, and focal/multifocal-cavitary. Cavitary PWMD is the least common. Motor and visual (geniculocalcarine) pathways course through the periventricular WM. Lower extremity axons run medial to upper extremity axons in the periventricular WM. Therefore, lower extremity axons are more frequently injured, often leading to the clinical presentation of spastic diplegia (e.g., cerebral palsy).

Cranial US, although the initial imaging modality of choice, is an insensitive method of diagnosing PWMD. When abnormal, the early findings are regions of periventricular hyperechoic "flares" that disrupt the normal echo striations of the periventricular WM **(8-73)**. Periventricular cysts do not commonly develop. When cavitation does occur and cysts develop (14-21 days) **(8-76)**, the cysts will ultimately over weeks to months contract and, through the process of astrogliosis, leave reduced WM volume in the periventricular regions **(8-77)**. If no cysts are detected by US, the only sonographic hint to the diagnosis of PWMD may be the unexplained ventricular dilation. Interestingly, in autopsy studies of preterm infants that show PWMD in 50%, their serial cranial US examinations suggested PWMD in no more than 10%.

MR of PWMD in the first week of life is expected to show decreased diffusivity and FA and increased radial diffusivity. Reduced FA at "corrected term" age is a poor prognosticator for normal motor and neurocognitive development. Spin-magnitude MR shows periventricular T1 hyperintensities (e.g., coagulative necrosis) and T2 hyperintensity **(8-76B)**. Hemorrhagic components of PWMD are more common in the extremes of prematurity, showing "blooming" on T2* GRE and SWI. MRS in the first week shows elevated lactate and delayed MRS (> 2 weeks) and demonstrates decreased NAA and lactate washout **(8-74)**.

End-stage PVL shows reduced WM volume and thinning of the corpus callosum **(8-75)**. The regions of PWMD show T2 and T2 FLAIR hyperintensity. In affected areas, the cortex nearly touches the lateral ventricles, which are enlarged and have irregular ("scalloped") margins **(8-77)**.

Cerebellar injury in the preterm newborn is underappreciated. Reduced cerebellar volume in preterm newborns is common and may reflect transsynaptic degeneration of cerebellar tracts and neurons resulting from supratentorial brain damage and/or disturbed signaling between the overlying leptomeninges and the underlying developing cerebellum.

HII IN PRETERM INFANTS

Clinical Issues

- < 37 wk gestational age
- HII causes 50% of all cerebral palsy (CP) cases
  - 5% < 32 wk develop CP; 15-20% < 28 wk develop CP

Imaging

- Severe HII affects mostly thalami; less severe HII causes GMH, IVH, PVL, and cerebellar injury
- Perinatal WM damage
  - Oligodendrocyte precursor cells vulnerable; periventricular, near trigones and frontal horns
  - 2/3 have coexisting hemorrhages (GMH-IVH)
  - Early on US: periventricular hyperechoic "flares"
  - Subacute: ± cysts, then resolve → gliosis, ventricular dilation

HII in Term Infants. Term newborns are those of a gestational age 37 weeks or greater. The prevalence of moderate to severe HII is estimated at 1.3/1,000 live births. Imaging findings of asphyxia in term infants vary with severity of insult, timing of imaging, and chosen modality. Although ultrasound is often used as the initial imaging study, MR with the adjuncts of DWI, DTI, and MRS is most sensitive for assessing the presence and magnitude of HII. As with the preterm brain, those regions with high metabolic demands (e.g., great glucose needs, richly perfused, and actively myelinating) are the first to exhibit vulnerability in HII.

Severe HII with profound perinatal hypotension or cardiocirculatory arrest in term neonates preferentially affects actively myelinating areas where NMDA receptors are highly concentrated. The deep gray matter (e.g., posterior putamina, ventrolateral thalami), hippocampi, dorsal brainstem, superior vermis, optic radiations, and perirolandic cortical regions are most severely affected **(8-78)**. Other at-risk regions include subthalamic nuclei, corticospinal tracts, and lateral geniculate nuclei. Severe HII in term infants may also preferentially lead to deep white matter injury and parasagittal and other interarterial watershed infarcts **(8-80) (8-81A)**.

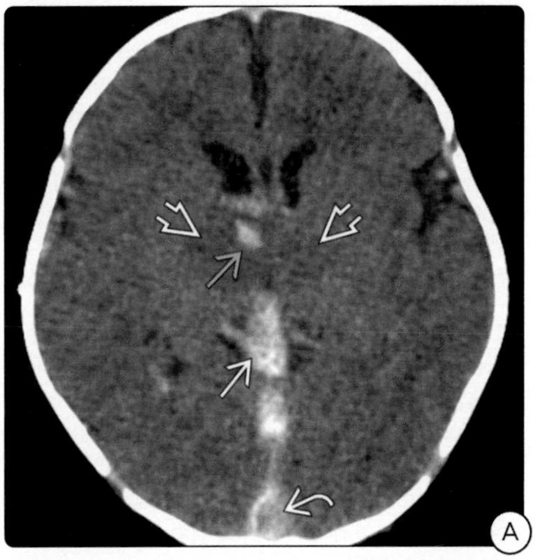

***(8-83A)** NECT in iron-deficient newborn with CSVT shows clot in vein of Galen ➡ and torcula ➡, deep BG edema ➡, focal hemorrhage ➡.*

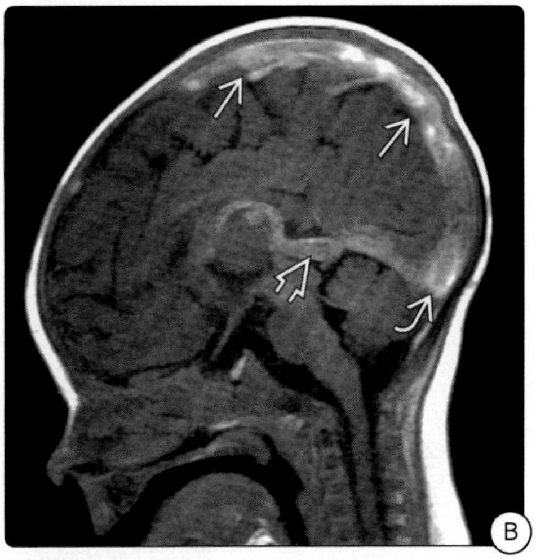

***(8-83B)** Sagittal T1 MR in same patient shows hyperintense clot within the superior sagittal sinus ➡, vein of Galen ➡, and torcula ➡.*

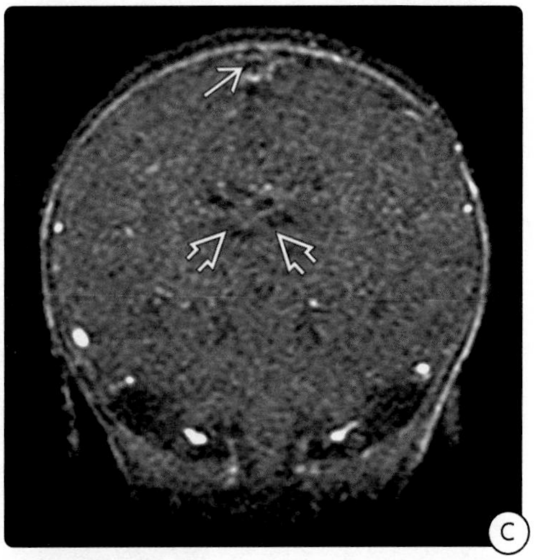

***(8-83C)** MR venogram MIP image in the same patient shows absent flow within the superior sagittal sinus ➡ and internal cerebral veins ➡.*

Immediate postparturition cranial US is recommended in the setting of HII. Sensitivity is recognizably lacking; however, if abnormalities are observed within the first 12 hours after birth [e.g., hyperechogenicity within the thalami and basal ganglia, poor GM/WM differentiation (e.g., salt and pepper hemispheric hyperechogenicity indicating diffuse edema), and ventricular compression], these ultrasound findings provide strong evidence for HII having begun prior to delivery, which is of clinical, forensic, and medical legal importance.

CT lacks sensitivity in detecting HII and exposes the newborn to ionizing radiation. However, if performed in the acute setting of suspected profound HII, look for diminished attenuation of the basal ganglia and thalami (normally of greater attenuation than WM), cortical attenuation less than WM (reversal sign), effacement of the cisterns, and compression of the ventricles (indicating diffuse cerebral edema) **(8-80B)**.

Spin-echo MR in HII is often normal in the first 8-10 hours. At 2-3 days of life, T1 shortening (e.g., hyperintensity) within the thalami and basal ganglia and absent or decreased T1 shortening in the normally myelinated posterior limb of the internal capsule (e.g., normally myelinated > 37 weeks) represent markers of profound HII. T1 shortening within the posterolateral putamina greater than T1 shortening within the posterior limb of internal capsule is a poor prognosticator. The pathologic T1 shortening likely represents accumulating Ca++, released myelin lipids, and manganese within infarcted tissue. T1 shortening may persist for a month(s). T2 hyperintensity begins within 24 hours and lasts for 3-4 days and then transitions to T2 hypointensity, which is seen by day 7 and persists for up to a month(s) **(8-78)**.

DWI is the most sensitive sequence in the first 24 hours, showing restricted diffusion and reduced ADC values in the basal ganglia and thalami. Remember to carefully review the ADC maps due to the fact that the long T2 values of the

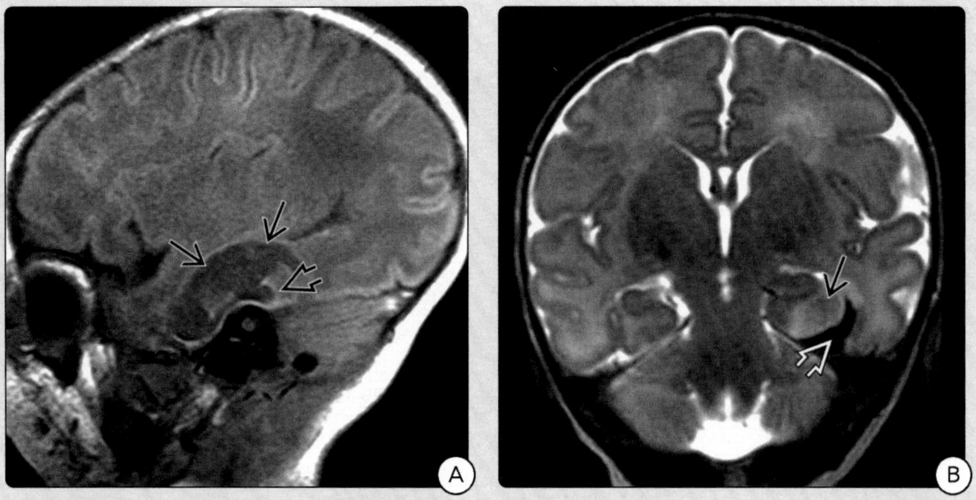

***(8-84A)** Parasagittal T1WI in a seizing term newborn with focal venous infarction shows edema of the temporal lobe →. T1 hyperintense SAH is also noted →. **(8-84B)** Coronal T2WI in the same patient shows edema of the temporal lobe → and sulcal distending hypointense SAH →.*

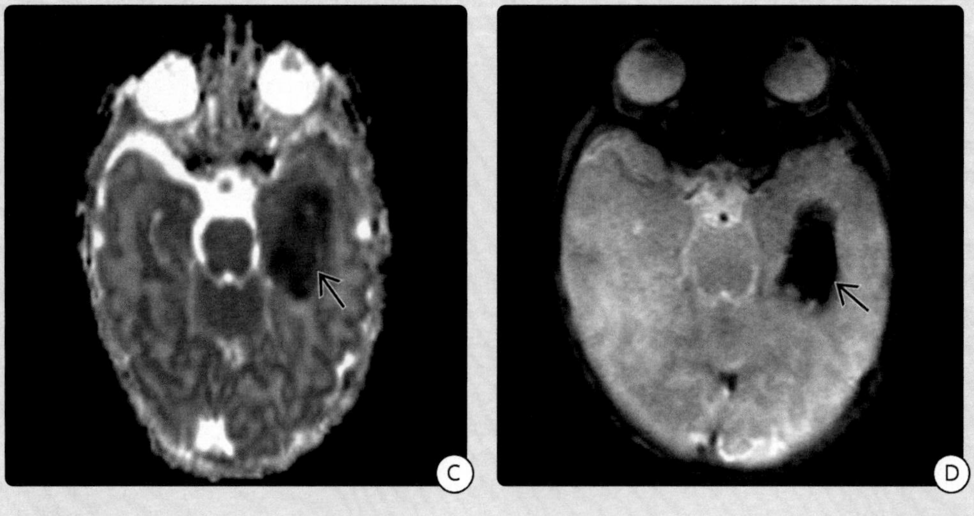

***(8-84C)** Axial ADC map in the same patient with venous infarction shows temporal lobe diffusion restriction →. **(8-84D)** Axial SWI in the same newborn shows hemorrhage within the temporal lobe venous infarction →. Venous infarcts are often hemorrhagic.*

neonatal brain may result in a "near normal" appearance on DWI in the setting of HII. Diffusion abnormalities peak near 5 days and then "pseudonormalize" by the end of the first postnatal week. "**NORMAL DWI**" does not exclude HII (e.g., early recovery period 6-18 hours after insult and pseudonormalization). It remains imperative to carefully review spin-echo images, particularly T1WI.

MRS shows elevated lactate at 1.3 ppm, which may be elevated as early as 4-8 hours after HII event. A lactate:NAA ratio > 0.5 portends serious neurologic injury. Elevation of glutamine-glutamate peak resonating at 2.3 ppm reflects acute brain injury. MRS voxel placement should include "targets" showing abnormal DWI/ADC findings. Avoid the sampling ventricular fluid, as lactate is present in the CSF of normal newborns. Be aware of the doublet resonance (lactate mimic) at 1.15 ppm from methyl protons of propane-1,2, diol (vehicle of the sedation agent phenobarbital). NAA begins to decline after day 3.

Atrophy and accompanying T2 and T2 FLAIR hyperintensity of the injured structures eventually ensue in the areas acutely showing restricted diffusion, T1 shortening, and elevated lactate. **Ulegyria**—shrunken cortex with flattened, mushroom-shaped gyri, representing a footprint of HII—is often found in the parietooccipital area. Cystic encephalomalacia represents end-stage findings.

Therapeutic hypothermia (TH) has become a mainstay of treating HII in term newborns. TH decreases cerebral metabolism, stabilizes the blood-brain barrier, decreases inflammatory mediators and excitatory amino acids, and suppresses apoptosis. TH prolongs the time to pseudonormalization and appears to reduce MR abnormalities in mild to moderate HII. The impact of TH in the setting of profound HII is uncertain.

Less severe HII with only partial asphyxia generally spares the brainstem, cerebellum, and deep gray nuclei. Prolonged partial asphyxia causes hypoperfusion in the watershed (e.g., interarterial border) zones **(8-79A)**. The parasagittal cortex and subcortical WM are most severely affected. T1 and T2 scans are initially normal, but wedge-shaped areas of diffusion restriction in the watershed zones can be seen on DWI **(8-79B)**. Late findings include multicystic "border zone" cystic encephalomalacia **(8-79D)**.

Potential Imaging Mimics of Perinatal HII. Infection (e.g., type II herpes encephalopathy), hypoglycemia, abusive head trauma (AHT), maple syrup urine disease, and nonketotic hyperglycinemia each have health history and distinctive imaging findings that aid in the differentiation from HII.

Focal Perinatal Hypoxic-Ischemic Injury

Perinatal Stroke: Arterial. Arterial strokes are underestimated in the pediatric population and represent a significant cause of neurologic morbidity and mortality. Thrombus can arise within an intracranial vessel, heart, or from the placenta. The MCA territory is the most commonly affected region. Multifocal ischemic injuries may arise from extracranial embolic sources. The estimated prevalence is 1:2,300-5,000 live births. Twenty-five percent of pediatric arterial strokes occur in neonates. Fifty percent occur in the first year. Symptoms vary with anatomic region involved and size of infarction. Fifty percent are idiopathic.

Known risk contributors include obstetrical factors, congenital heart disease, anemia, thrombotic/coagulation disorders, polycythemia, metabolic derangement (e.g., tetrahydrofolate reductase mutation), homocysteinemia, chorioamnionitis, and autoimmune disorders. *COL4A1* gene mutation has been associated with early arterial infarctions. Early US demonstrates hyperechogenicity of the involved area. NECT shows geographic hypoattenuation within 12-24 hours of the infarction, and MR demonstrates restricted diffusion almost immediately, with other spin-echo series (e.g., T1, T2, FLAIR) taking hours to reveal signal alteration. SWI has great sensitivity in detecting the paramagnetic effect of parenchymal hemorrhage. For vessel imaging, TOF MRA is recommended.

Perinatal Stroke: Venous. Focal venous infarctions are less frequent than arterial infarctions in the neonate. The estimated prevalence of cerebral sinovenous thrombosis (CSVT) in newborns is 0.67/100,000 cases per year. Up to 40% of these CSVT patients suffer venous infarctions, and 70% of are hemorrhagic. Risk factors for neonatal CSVT include sepsis, coagulation disorders (acquired and inherited), iron deficiency anemia, dehydration, and CNS infection **(8-83)**. Suspect venous infarctions when unexpected intracranial hemorrhage is detected (e.g., unexplained ventricular hemorrhage) and infarction does not fit an arterial distribution (e.g., thalamic, anterior temporal, frontal, parietal with sparing of the caudate nucleus). Venous infarctions tend to show a mixed pattern of vasogenic and cytotoxic edema. MR and IV contrasted 3D-MRV are recommended. CSVT in neonates tends to resolve without aggressive interventions **(8-84)**.

HII in Postnatal Infants and Young Children. *Mild to moderate anoxic events* in older infants and young children generally cause watershed zone injury, with wedge-shaped hypoattenuation regions on NECT and areas of restricted diffusion involving the interarterial "border zones" between the major cerebral artery territories.

Severe asphyxia (usually from drowning, choking, or nonaccidental trauma) in children younger than 1 year of age damages the basal ganglia, lateral thalami, dorsal midbrain, and cortex. A novel pattern of diffuse central and peripheral WM damage (restricted diffusion and T2 prolongation) and eventual WM volume loss is occasionally seen.

In infants between 1 and 2 years of age, the basal ganglia, hippocampi, and anterior frontal/parietooccipital cortex are involved, whereas the thalami and perirolandic cortex are relatively spared. On NECT, the cortex appears hypointense relative to the WM (the "reversal" sign). In severe HII, diffuse cerebral edema makes the difference between the extremely hypoattenuated hemispheres and normally perfused cerebellum and brainstem especially striking ("white cerebellum" sign).

HII in Older Children and Adults

Mild to moderate global HII typically results in watershed zone infarcts (see above).

Severe HII in older children and adults selectively affects the deep gray nuclei, cortex, hippocampi, and cerebellum. NECT shows diffuse cerebral edema with loss of normal gray-white matter differentiation and "disappearing" basal ganglia.

MR shows hyperintensity in the cortex, hippocampi, globi pallidi, and sometimes the cerebellum on T2/FLAIR **(8-85)**. DWI and ADC maps demonstrate restricted diffusion in the same areas. These diffusion abnormalities typically "pseudonormalize" within 1 week. In some cases of severe HII—especially those associated with drowning, hanging, and carbon monoxide poisoning—delayed WM injury develops sometimes up to a week following the initial insult.

In chronic HII, T1WI may show gyriform hyperintensity (caused by **cortical laminar necrosis**, not hemorrhage or calcification).

HII IN POSTTERM INFANTS, CHILDREN, AND ADULTS

Postnatal Infants and Young Children

- Severe
  - Basal ganglia, lateral thalami, dorsal midbrain, cortex
- Mild-moderate = cortical watershed zones

Older Children and Adults

- Severe
  - Deep gray nuclei, cortex, hippocampi, cerebellum
  - Later = gyriform T1 shortening (laminar necrosis)
- Mild-moderate = cortical watershed zones

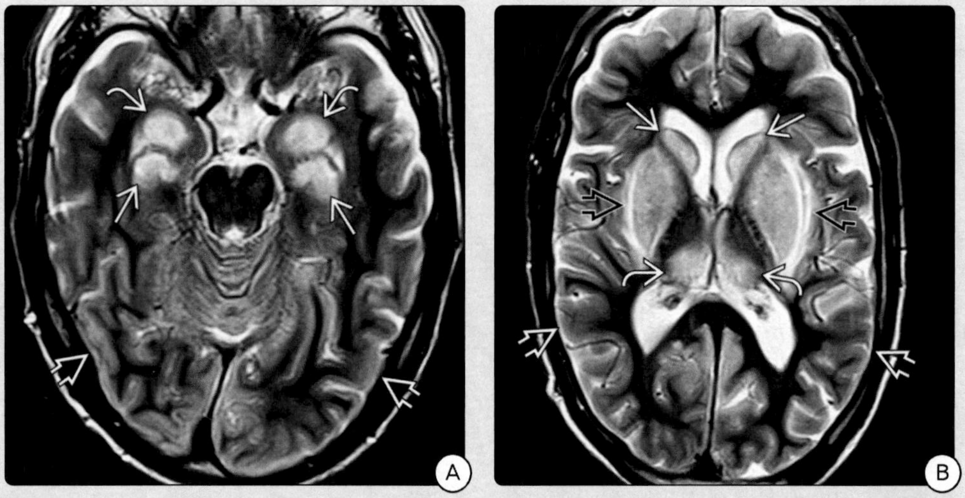

***(8-85A)** Axial T2WI in a 53y man after cardiac arrest and prolonged resuscitation shows diffuse cortical swelling and hyperintensity, as well as focal hyperintensity in both hippocampi and amygdalae. **(8-85B)** More cephalad T2WI in the same case shows more diffuse cortical hyperintensity as well as symmetric hyperintensity in the basal ganglia/external capsules, thalami, and caudate nuclei.*

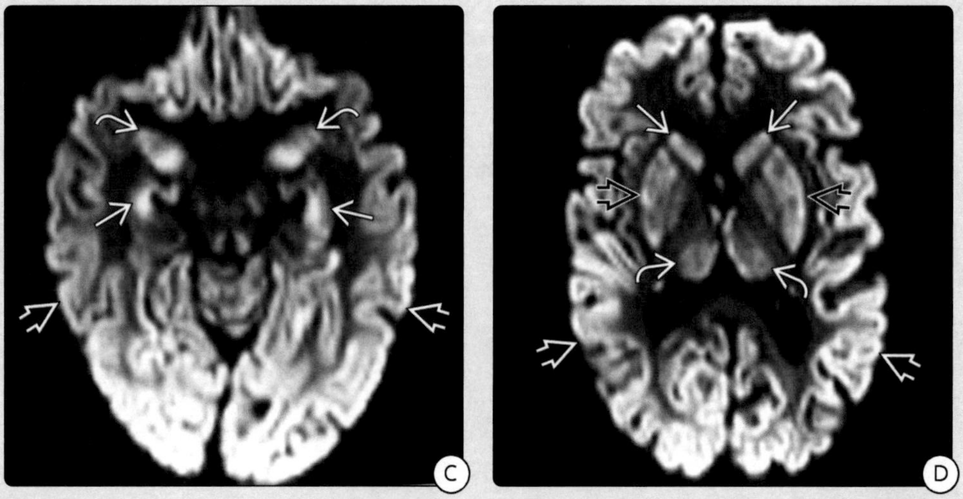

***(8-85C)** DWI in the same case shows symmetric restricted diffusion in the entire cortex plus hippocampi and amygdalae. **(8-85D)** More cephalad DWI shows the symmetric cortical restricted diffusion as well as involvement of the thalami, lentiform nuclei, and caudate heads.*

Miscellaneous Strokes

Cerebral Hyperperfusion Syndrome

Terminology

Cerebral hyperperfusion syndrome (CHS) is a rare but potentially devastating disorder. CHS is sometimes called luxury perfusion or postcarotid endarterectomy hyperperfusion and is defined as a major increase in cerebral blood flow well above normal metabolic demands.

Etiology

CHS most often occurs as a complication of carotid reperfusion procedures (i.e., endarterectomy, angioplasty, stenting, or thrombolysis). CHS has also been reported after STA-MCA anastomosis in moyamoya disease. Less common causes include status epilepticus, MELAS, and hypercapnia.

Critical carotid stenosis with chronic cerebral ischemia causes endothelial dysfunction and impaired arterial autoregulation. Loss of normal vasoconstriction results in chronic dilatation of the brain "resistance" vessels. When normal perfusion is restored, this can result in rapidly increased cerebral blood flow (CBF) in the previously underperfused hemisphere.

Comorbid clinical risk factors include age, hypertension (especially post procedure), bilateral lesions, hemodynamically significant disease in the contralateral carotid artery, poor collateral blood flow, and diminished cerebral vascular reserve.

Clinical Issues

Epidemiology and Presentation. Symptomatic CHS occurs in 1-3% of carotid reperfusion procedures, although 5-10% of

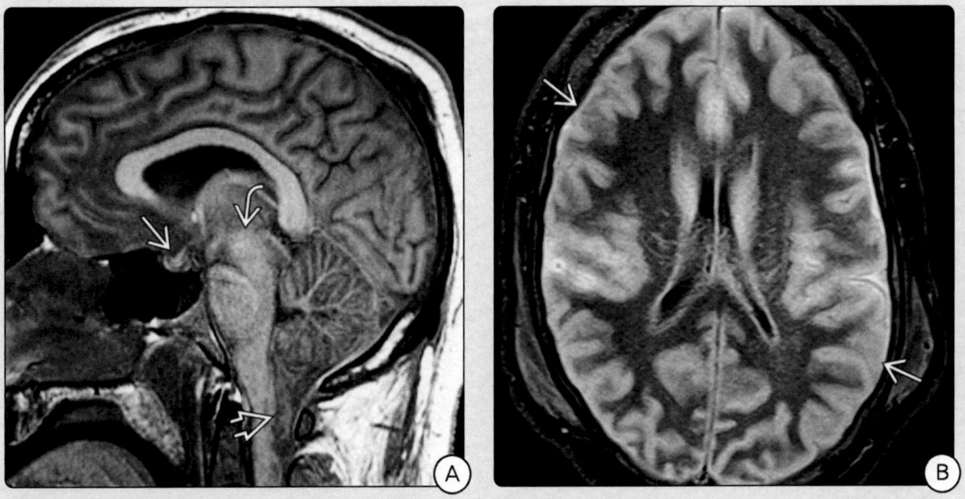

***(8-86A)** Sagittal MPORAGE in a 43y male drug abuser found down shows diffuse brain swelling with severe descending transtentorial herniation. The suprasellar cistern is obliterated, the midbrain is displaced inferiorly, and the cerebellar tonsils are herniated downward through the foramen magnum. **(8-86B)** FLAIR shows small ventricles, obliterated sulci, and diffuse gyral swelling.*

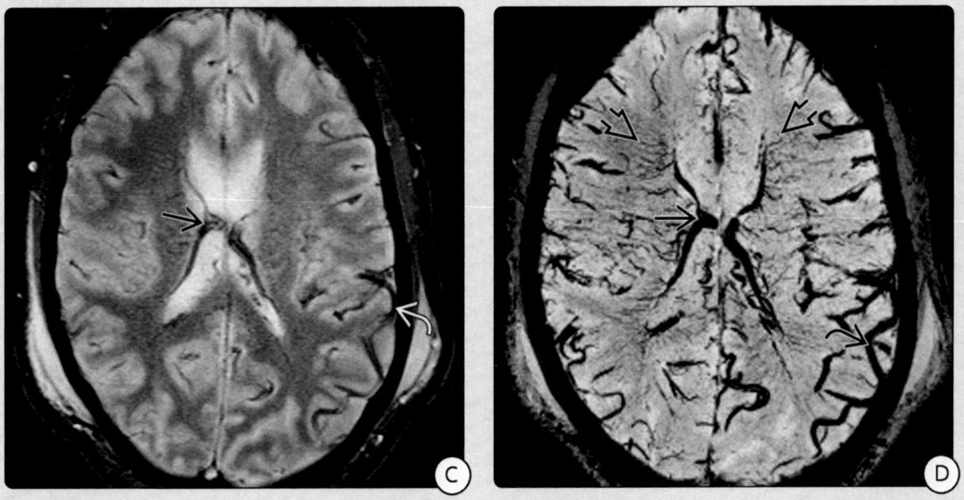

***(8-86C)** T2* GRE shows no evidence for parenchymal hemorrhage. The deep cerebral and superficial cortical veins appear unusually prominent. **(8-86D)** MIP of the T2* SWI in the same case shows near complete venous stasis with enlarged, hypointense deep cerebral and superficial cortical veins. Note unusually prominent medullary veins. This is end-stage HII. The patient expired shortly after the scan was obtained.*

patients develop mild, generally asymptomatic CHS. Patients typically present within a few hours following carotid endarterectomy (CEA), usually with unilateral headache, face or eye pain, cognitive impairment, and variable neurologic deficits.

Imaging

CT Findings. NECT scans may show only mild gyral swelling. CTA/pCT show congested, dilated vessels with elevated blood flow and decreased MTT/TTP **(8-87A) (8-87B) (8-87C)**.

MR Findings. T2/FLAIR scans show gyral swelling, hyperintensity, and sulcal effacement in the internal carotid distribution **(8-87D)**. T1 C+ scans may be normal or show mildly increased intravascular enhancement. DWI is typically negative, as the edema is vasogenic rather than cytotoxic. pMR shows elevated CBF and cerebral blood volume with decreased (shortened) MTT.

Postprocedure CHS on TOF-MRA is seen as an increase in the change ratio of signal intensity more than 1.5x the preoperative level.

Nuclear Medicine Findings. Single-photon emission computed tomography (SPECT) has demonstrated focal hyperperfusion at the revascularization site in STA-MCA anastomosis for moyamoya disease.

Differential Diagnosis

The major differential diagnosis of post-CEA CHS is **acute cerebral ischemia-infarction**. Here the MTT is prolonged (not decreased), and DWI typically shows restricted diffusion.

Acute hypertensive encephalopathy (PRES) is a dysautoregulatory disorder with a predilection for the posterior circulation. Lesions are typically bilateral, not unilateral as with post-CEA CHS.

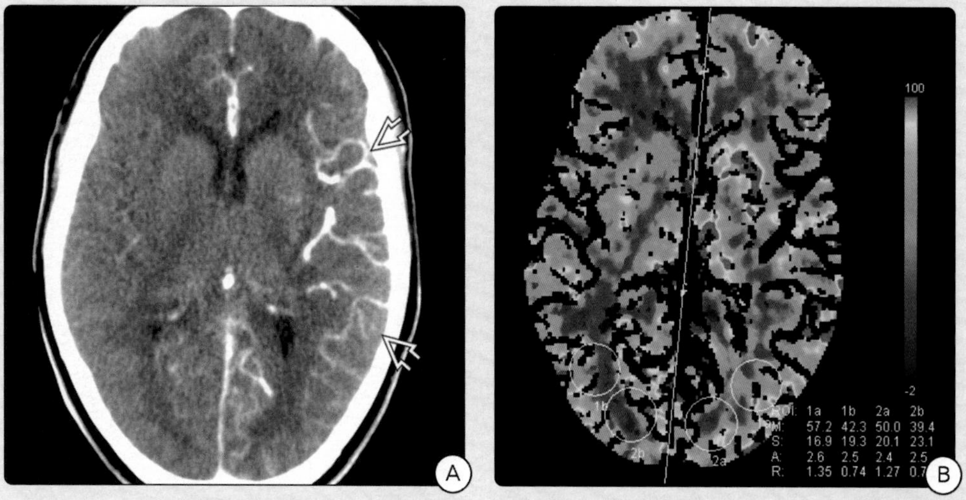

***(8-87A)** A 56y man with > 70% stenosis of his left cervical ICA underwent carotid endarterectomy. A few hours after surgery, he became acutely confused and developed right-sided weakness. CTA source image shows markedly increased vasculature in the left hemisphere ➡. **(8-87B)** CTA with CBF appears relatively normal, but blood flow on the left (2a, 2b ROIs) is increased compared with the right side.*

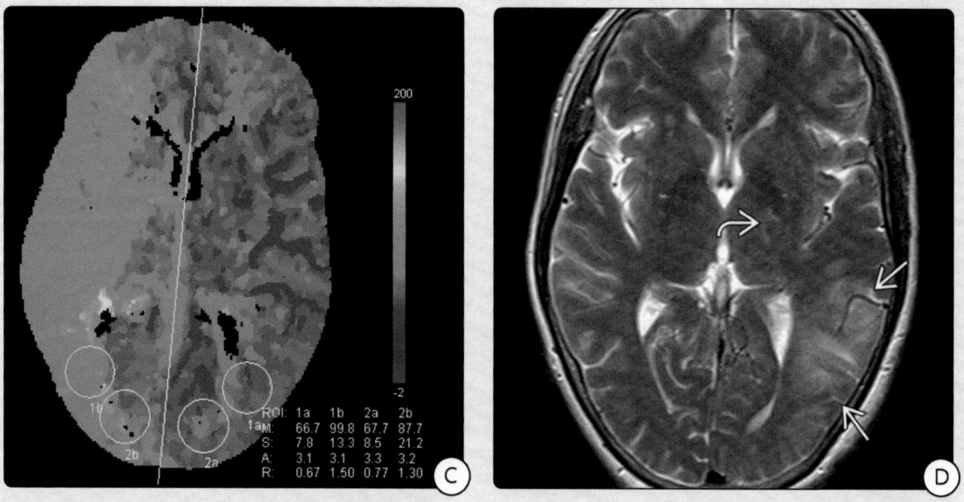

***(8-87C)** TTP study is even more striking. The abnormal side is NOT the right MCA distribution (green) but is the left side (blue), where the TTP is markedly shortened. **(8-87D)** T2WI shows gyral swelling, sulcal effacement, and hyperintensity in the left temporal and parietooccipital cortex/subcortical white matter ➡, basal ganglia ↪. DWI (not shown) was normal. This was post-carotid endarterectomy hyperperfusion syndrome.*

Status epilepticus can also result in hyperperfusion. The cortex is usually more selectively involved than the white matter. The stroke-like episodes in **MELAS** are related to vasogenic edema, hyperperfusion, and neuronal damage. Cortical hyperintensity on T2/FLAIR can resemble CHS, but MRS in "normal-appearing" brain shows a characteristically elevated lactate peak.

Strokes in Unusual Vascular Distributions

The vast majority of arterial strokes are easily recognizable, as they conform to the expected vascular territories of major cerebral arteries such as the ACA/MCA/PCA and posterior inferior cerebellar artery. Two unusual but important arterial occlusions are the artery of Percheron infarcts and the top of the basilar syndrome. Each is briefly discussed here.

Artery of Percheron Infarction

The artery of Percheron (AOP) is a vascular variant in which a single large midbrain perforating artery arises from the P1 PCA segment to supply the midbrain and medial thalami **(8-88)**. AOP occlusion can cause obtundation, oculomotor and pupillary deficits, vertical gaze palsy, ptosis, and lid retraction.

NECT scans in early acute AOP occlusion are usually normal. Hypodense areas in both thalami extending into the central midbrain may develop later.

MR with DWI is the procedure of choice. T2/FLAIR scans show round or ovoid hyperintensities in the medial thalami, just lateral to the third ventricle **(8-89A)**. In slightly more than half of all cases, a V-shaped hyperintensity involves the medial surfaces of the cerebral peduncles and rostral midbrain **(8-89B)**. DWI shows diffusion restriction in the affected areas.

The major differential diagnosis of AOP occlusion is **"top of the basilar" infarct**. "Top of the basilar" infarcts are much more extensive, involving part or all of the rostral midbrain, occipital lobes, superior vermis, and thalami.

Deep cerebral (galenic) venous occlusions involve the basal ganglia, posterior limb of internal capsules, and typically the entire thalami. T2* (GRE, SWI) scans demonstrate "blooming" clots in the internal cerebral vein, vein of Galen, and straight sinus (see Chapter 9).

"Top of the Basilar" Infarction

"Top of the basilar" infarct is a clinically recognizable syndrome characterized by visual, oculomotor, and behavioral abnormalities caused by thrombosis of the distal basilar artery. "Locked-in" syndrome is a rare but devastating manifestation of top of the basilar thrombosis.

Thrombus typically occludes both proximal PCAs as well as distal perforators that supply the rostral midbrain and thalami. Both occipital lobes are usually infarcted. Depending on the inferior extent of the clot, pontine perforators and one or more superior cerebellar artery territories may also be affected.

NECT scans show a dense basilar artery sign. Hypodensity in the occipital lobes and/or thalami may be apparent **(8-92)**.

MR findings vary depending on thrombus extent and vascular supply to the distal PCAs. T2/FLAIR hyperintensity and diffusion restriction in the midbrain, thalami, upper pons, and superior cerebellar hemispheres are common **(8-92)**.

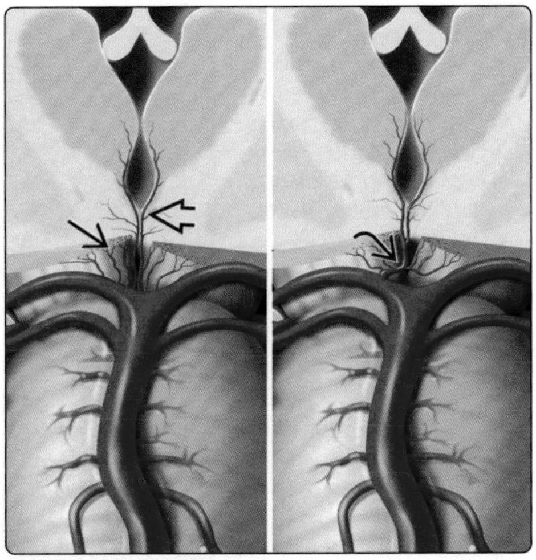

(8-88) (L) Normal BA, small perforating arteries supply midbrain ⇨, medial thalami ⇨. (R) AOP has single dominant trunk ⇨.

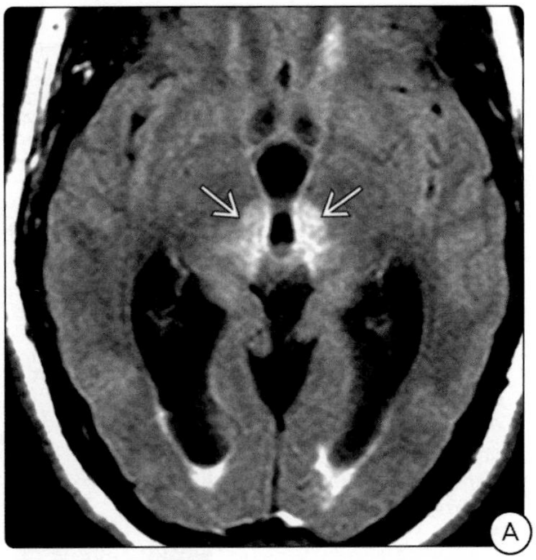

(8-89A) FLAIR scan in a patient with artery of Percheron infarct shows both medial thalami infarcts ➡.

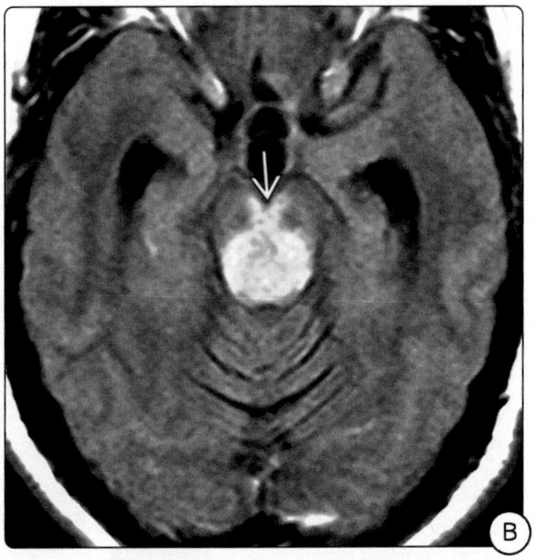

(8-89B) FLAIR in the same patient shows midbrain, peduncular "V" hyperintensity ➡.

*(**8-90A**) Autopsy case shows basilar artery thrombosis. The vertebrobasilar system is very ectatic and atherosclerotic. Bluish purple thrombus fills the distal vertebral and basilar arteries →. (**8-90B**) Inferior view of the same autopsied brain shows thrombus filling the basilar artery →. Both occipital lobes appear swollen and discolored.*

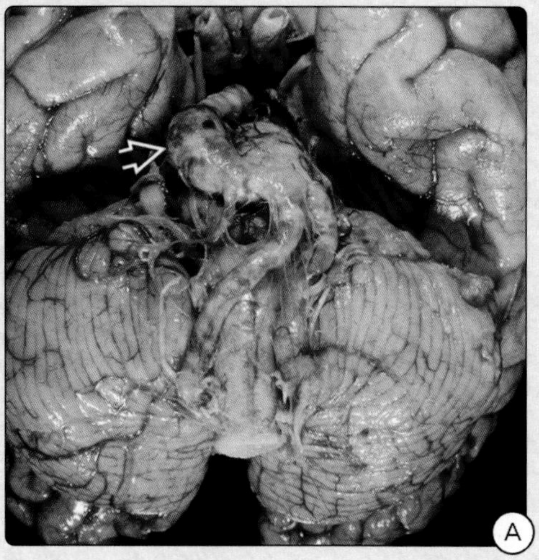

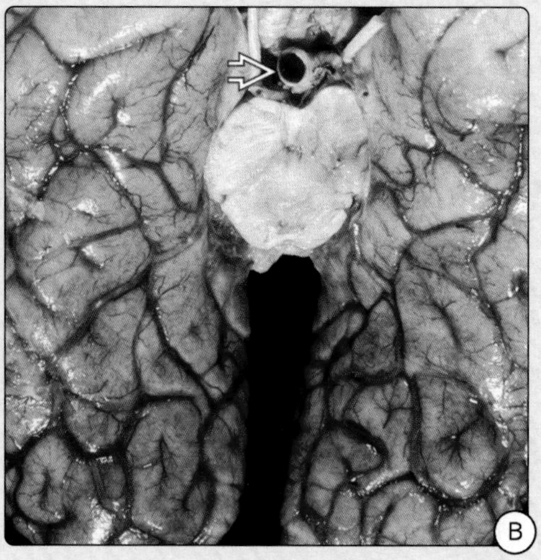

*(**8-90C**) Axial cut section shows thrombus extending into the P1 segment of one of the posterior cerebral arteries →. Bioccipital infarcts → with some hemorrhagic transformation in the cortex are present. (Courtesy R. Hewlett, MD.) (**8-91A**) NECT shows classic "dense basilar artery sign" with the top of the BA significantly more hyperdense → than either of the distal internal carotid arteries →.*

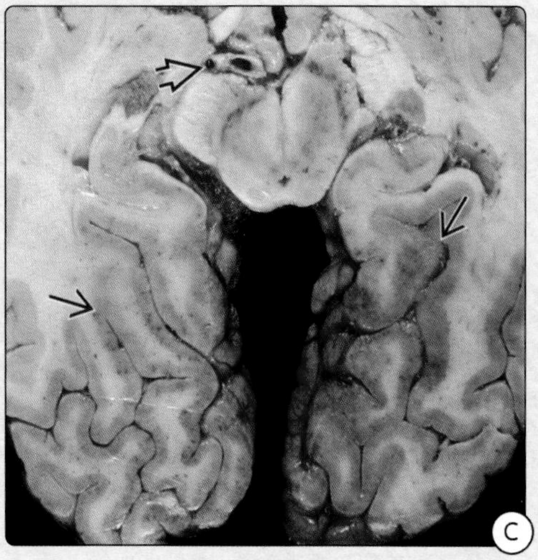

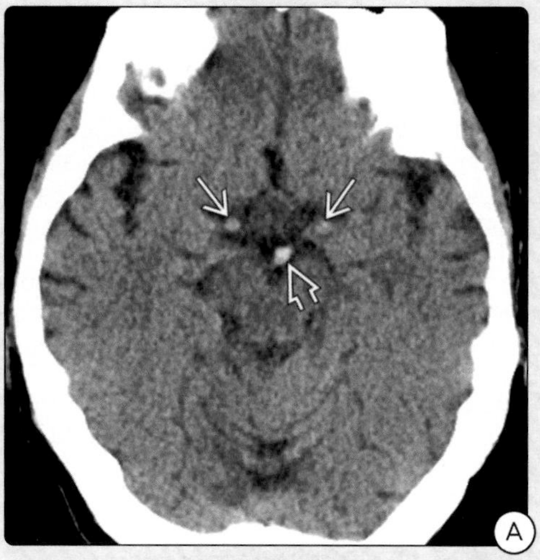

*(**8-91B**) Axial CTA in the same case shows nonopacification of the basilar artery →. (**8-91C**) Sagittal reformatted CTA in the same case shows that almost the entire length of the basilar artery is filled with thrombus →. The vertebral artery and proximal PCA are opacified →. Note absence of contrast in vessels supplying the pons and upper vermis. The patient expired 12 hours after imaging was performed.*

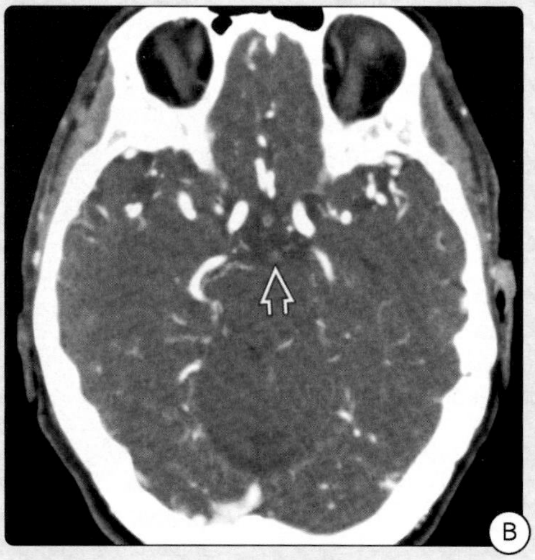

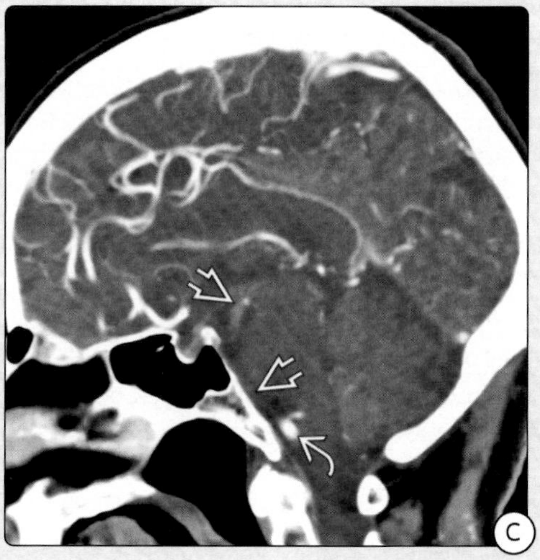

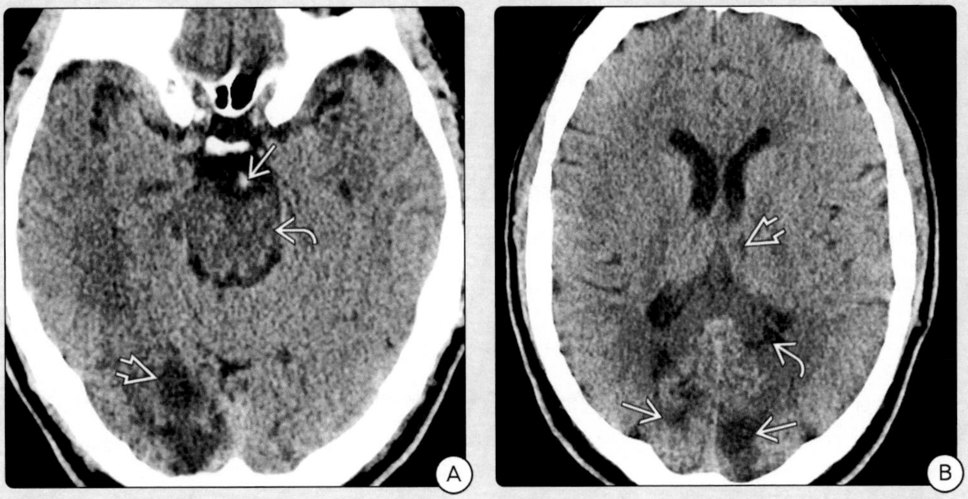

***(8-92A)** More extensive BA thrombosis is illustrated by a series of images in a 63y man. NECT scan through the midbrain shows dense BA ➡, hypodense midbrain ➡, and right medial occipital lobe hypodensity ➡. **(8-92B)** More cephalad scan shows hypodensity in the left thalamus ➡, corpus callosum ➡, and both occipital lobes ➡.*

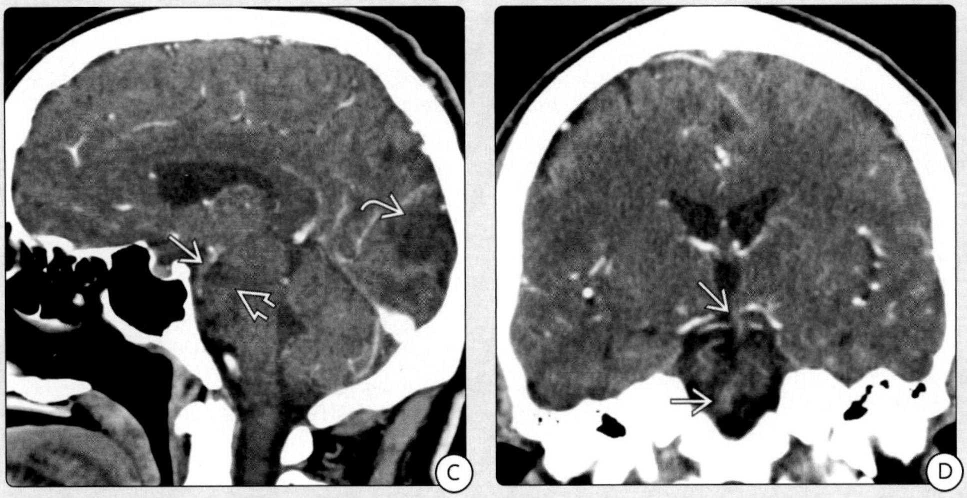

***(8-92C)** Sagittal CTA shows basilar artery thrombus ➡ with nonopacified distal basilar artery. Multiple patchy hypodensities are present in the pons ➡ and occipital lobe ➡. **(8-92D)** Coronal CTA shows extensive thrombus in the BA ➡.*

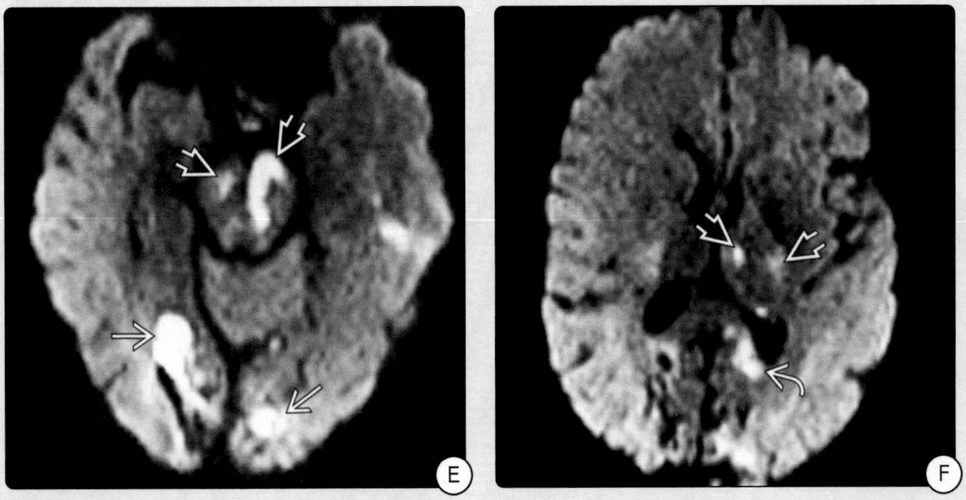

***(8-92E)** DWI in the same patient shows a bilateral midbrain perforating artery ➡ and occipital infarcts ➡. **(8-92F)** More cephalad DWI in the same patient shows infarcts in the left thalamus ➡ and corpus callosum splenium ➡. Both areas are supplied by perforating branches of the distal basilar artery.*

Selected References

Normal Arterial Anatomy and Vascular Distributions

Intracranial Internal Carotid Artery

Kirkland JD et al: The transclival artery: a variant persistent carotid-basilar arterial anastomosis not previously reported. J Neurointerv Surg. 9(3):e11, 2017

Arráez-Aybar LA et al: Persistent trigeminal artery: a cross-sectional study based on over 3 years conventional angiography, CT angiography and MR angiography images. Surg Radiol Anat. 38(4):445-53, 2016

Circle of Willis

Mahakkanukrauh P et al: Circle of Willis of the brain: anatomical variations and their importance. Anat Sci Int. 91(2):215, 2016

Vrselja Z et al: Penetrating arteries of the cerebral white matter: the importance of vascular territories of delivering arteries and completeness of circle of Willis. Int J Stroke. 11(3):NP36-7, 2016

Anterior Cerebral Artery

Cilliers K et al: Description of the anterior cerebral artery and its cortical branches: variation in presence, origin, and size. Clin Neurol Neurosurg. 152:78-83, 2017

Middle Cerebral Artery

Uchiyama N: Anomalies of the middle cerebral artery. Neurol Med Chir (Tokyo). 57(6):261-266, 2017

Posterior Cerebral Artery

Gunnal SA et al: Study of posterior cerebral artery in human cadaveric brain. Anat Res Int. 2015:681903, 2015

Vertebrobasilar System

Stojanović B et al: Variation of some arteries of the vertebrobasilar system: case report. Surg Radiol Anat. 39(6):689-692, 2017

Arterial Infarcts

Acute Cerebral Ischemia-Infarction

Hui FK et al: ASPECTS discrepancies between CT and MR imaging: analysis and implications for triage protocols in acute ischemic stroke. J Neurointerv Surg. 9(3):240-243, 2017

Kang DW et al: Prediction of stroke subtype and recanalization using susceptibility vessel sign on susceptibility-weighted magnetic resonance imaging. Stroke. 48(6):1554-1559, 2017

Leigh R et al: Imaging the physiological evolution of the ischemic penumbra in acute ischemic stroke. J Cereb Blood Flow Metab. ePub, 2017

Lin L et al: Whole-brain CT perfusion to quantify acute ischemic penumbra and core. Radiology. 279(3):876-87, 2016

Subacute Cerebral Infarcts

Yu X et al: Prominence of medullary veins on susceptibility-weighted images provides prognostic information in patients with subacute stroke. AJNR Am J Neuroradiol. 37(3):423-9, 2016

Multiple Embolic Infarcts

Novotny V et al: Acute cerebral infarcts in multiple arterial territories associated with cardioembolism. Acta Neurol Scand. 135(3):346-351, 2017

Zakhari N et al: Unusual cerebral emboli. Neuroimaging Clin N Am. 26(1):147-63, 2016

Lacunar Infarcts

Arvanitakis Z et al: The relationship of cerebral vessel pathology to brain microinfarcts. Brain Pathol. 27(1):77-85, 2017

Watershed ("Border Zone") Infarcts

Shi J et al: Cerebral watershed infarcts may be induced by hemodynamic changes in blood flow. Neurol Res. 39(6):538-544, 2017

Mangla R et al: Border zone infarcts: pathophysiologic and imaging characteristics. Radiographics. 31(5):1201-14, 2011

Perinatal Hypoxic-Ischemic Injury (HII)

Krishnan P et al: Neuroimaging in neonatal hypoxic ischemic encephalopathy. Indian J Pediatr. 83(9):995-1002, 2016

Veenith TV et al: Pathophysiologic mechanisms of cerebral ischemia and diffusion hypoxia in traumatic brain injury. JAMA Neurol. 73(5):542-50, 2016

Greer DM: Cardiac arrest and postanoxic encephalopathy. Continuum (Minneap Minn). 21(5 Neurocritical Care):1384-96, 2015

Kuban KC et al: Systemic inflammation and cerebral palsy risk in extremely preterm infants. J Child Neurol. 29(12):1692-8, 2014

Badve CA et al: Neonatal ischemic brain injury: what every radiologist needs to know. Pediatr Radiol. 42(5):606-19, 2012

Schwartz ES and Barkovich AJ: Brain and spine injuries in infants and childhood. In: Pediatric Neuroimaging, 5th ed, edited by Barkovich AJ. Philadelphia, PA: Lippincott, Williams, and Wilkins, 2012, pp. 240-366

Heinz ER et al: Imaging findings in neonatal hypoxia: a practical review. AJR Am J Roentgenol. 192(1):41-7, 2009

Khwaja O et al: Pathogenesis of cerebral white matter injury of prematurity. Arch Dis Child Fetal Neonatal Ed. 93(2):F153-61, 2008

Miscellaneous Strokes

Cerebral Hyperperfusion Syndrome

Andereggen L et al: Quantitative magnetic resonance angiography as a potential predictor for cerebral hyperperfusion syndrome: a preliminary study. J Neurosurg. 1-9, 2017

Newman JE et al: Post-carotid endarterectomy hypertension. Part 1: association with pre-operative clinical, imaging, and physiological parameters. Eur J Vasc Endovasc Surg. ePub, 2017

Strokes in Unusual Vascular Distributions

Vinod KV et al: Artery of Percheron infarction. Ann Neurosci. 23(2):124-6, 2016

Suthar PP et al: Top of basilar artery syndrome. J Clin Diagn Res. 9(7):TJ01, 2015

Venous Anatomy and Occlusions

Dural venous sinus and cerebral vein occlusions are relatively rare, accounting for only 1% of all strokes. They are notoriously difficult to diagnose clinically and are frequently overlooked on imaging studies, as attention is focused on the arterial side of the cerebral circulation.

The risk of venous "strokes" is increased by a number of different predisposing conditions. Dehydration, pregnancy, trauma, infection, collagen-vascular disease, coagulopathies, and a spectrum of inherited disorders all enhance the likelihood of developing sinovenous occlusion.

Familiarity with both normal venous anatomy and drainage patterns is essential for understanding the imaging appearance of sinovenous occlusive disease. Therefore, in this chapter, we first briefly review the normal gross and imaging anatomy of the cerebral venous system. Because about half of all venous occlusions result in parenchymal infarcts, we also discuss their drainage territories.

Once we have laid the anatomic foundation for understanding the cranial venous system, we turn to the fascinating topic of sinovenous occlusive disease—venous "strokes"—and their mimics.

Normal Venous Anatomy and Drainage Patterns

The intracranial venous system is unlike its systemic counterparts. Brain veins and sinuses lack valves and can have bidirectional flow. In the body, veins typically accompany arteries, and their vascular territories are relatively comparable. Not so in the brain. The dural sinuses and the cerebral veins travel separately, so their drainage territories do not mirror arterial distributions. Therefore, a venous "stroke" looks and behaves quite differently from a major arterial occlusion.

The intracranial venous system has two major components, the **dural venous sinuses** and the **cerebral veins**. We begin our discussion with the dural sinuses and then turn our attention to the cerebral veins. We conclude by delineating the drainage territories of the major dural sinuses and cerebral veins.

Dural Venous Sinuses

The dural venous sinuses are subdivided into an anteroinferior group and a posterosuperior group. The posterosuperior group is the more prominent and consists of the superior sagittal sinus (SSS), inferior sagittal sinus (ISS),

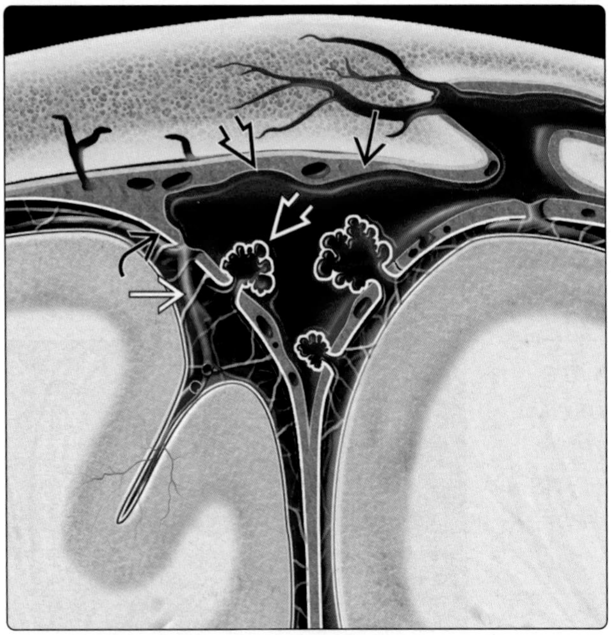

(9-1) Superior sagittal sinus (SSS) ⇨ is between the outer ⇨ and inner ⇨ dural layers. CSF-containing projections (arachnoid granulations) ➡ extend from the subarachnoid space (SAS) into the SSS. Cortical veins ➡ also enter the SSS.

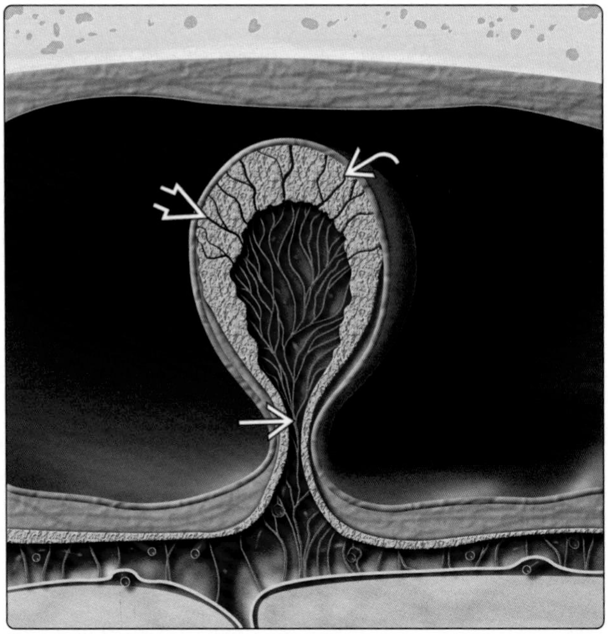

(9-2) Graphic depicts an arachnoid granulation (AG) projecting into a venous sinus. CSF ➡ extends from the SAS into the AG and is covered by a cap of arachnoid cells ➡. Channels in the cap ➡ drain CSF into the sinus.

straight sinus (SS), sinus confluence (torcular herophili), transverse sinuses (TSs), sigmoid sinuses, and jugular bulbs.

The anteroinferior group consists of the cavernous sinus (CS), superior and inferior petrosal sinuses (SPSs, IPSs), clival venous plexus (CVP), and sphenoparietal sinus (SphPS).

General Considerations

Dural sinuses and venous plexuses are endothelium-lined channels that are contained between the outer (periosteal) and inner (meningeal) dural layers. Dural sinuses and plexuses—especially the CS and clival plexus—are often fenestrated and multichanneled. At least one intrasinus septation or fibrous band is present in 30% of autopsy cases.

The dural sinuses frequently contain **arachnoid granulations** (AGs), also known as pacchionian granulations. AGs are CSF-containing projections that extend from the subarachnoid space (SAS) into dural venous sinuses **(9-1)**. A central core of CSF extends from the SAS into the granulation, which in turn is covered by an apical cap of arachnoid cells. Multiple small channels extend through the full thickness of the cap to the sinus endothelium and drain CSF into the venous circulation **(9-2)**.

Although AGs can occur in all dural venous sinuses, the most common locations are the TS and SSS. The CS is a relatively uncommon site.

Superior Sagittal Sinus

The SSS is a large, curvilinear sinus that parallels the inner calvarial vault. It originates from ascending frontal veins anteriorly and runs in the midline at the junction of the falx cerebri with the calvaria **(9-3)**. The SSS increases in diameter as it courses posteriorly, collecting a number of unnamed, small, superficial cortical veins and the larger anastomotic vein of Trolard.

Emissary and bridging veins connect the extracranial scalp veins with the SSS. A number of so-called "venous lakes" in the diploic space of the calvaria also drain into the SSS.

On coronal imaging, the SSS appears as a triangular vascular channel contained between the dural leaves of the falx cerebri. On sagittal DSA/CTA/MRA, the SSS is seen as a sickle-shaped structure that hugs the inner table of the skull. Filling defects—AGs and fibrous septa—within the SSS are common findings on imaging studies.

Normal SSS variants include absence of its anterior segment and off-midline position. When its anterior segment is hypoplastic or absent, the SSS begins more posteriorly near the coronal suture, where it receives prominent frontal veins. The SSS usually remains in the midline throughout its course. As it descends toward its termination in the venous sinus confluence, however, it may gradually course off midline.

Inferior Sagittal Sinus

Compared with the SSS, the ISS is a much smaller and more inconstant curvilinear channel that lies in the bottom of the falx cerebri.

The ISS lies above the corpus callosum and cingulate gyrus, collecting small tributaries as it curves posteriorly along the inferior "free" margin of the falx. The ISS terminates at the falcotentorial junction, where it joins with the great cerebral vein of Galen (VofG) to form the SS.

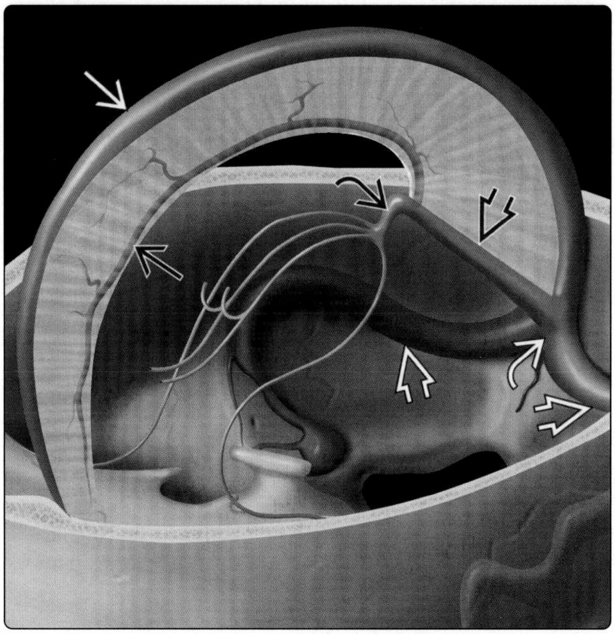

(9-3) Falx cerebri extends from the crista galli to the falcotentorial junction and holds the SSS ➡ and the ISS ➡. VofG ➡ receives the ICVs and basal vein of Rosenthal. Straight sinus ➡, sinus confluence ➡, transverse sinuses (TSs) ➡ are shown.

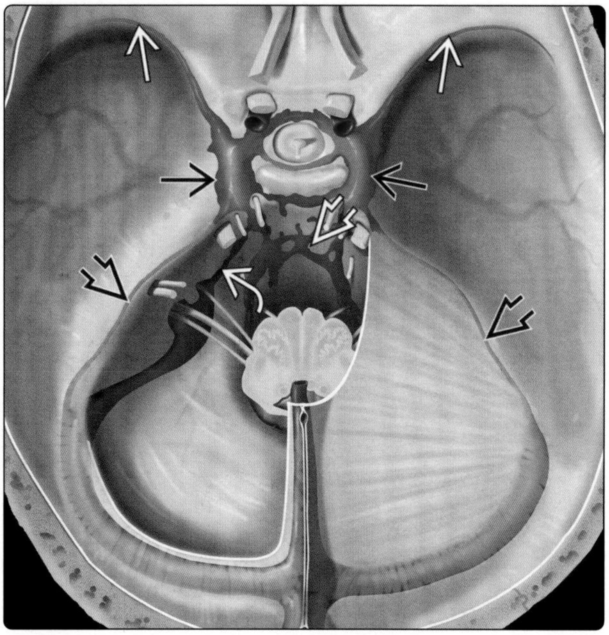

(9-4) Graphic shows the numerous interconnections among the cavernous sinuses (CSs) ➡, clival venous plexus ➡, sphenoparietal sinuses ➡, and the superior ➡ and inferior ➡ petrosal sinuses.

The ISS is often small or inapparent and is inconsistently visualized on imaging studies.

Straight Sinus

The SS is formed by the junction of the ISS and VofG. It runs posteroinferiorly from its origin at the falcotentorial apex. Along its course, the SS receives numerous small tributaries from the falx cerebri, tentorium cerebelli, and adjacent brain.

SS variants are relatively uncommon. A **persistent falcine sinus** is an unusual variant that is identified on 2% of normal CTAs. Here a midline venous structure—the persistent falcine sinus—connects the ISS or VofG directly with the SSS. Two-thirds of patients with a persistent falcine sinus have absent/rudimentary SSs.

Sinus Confluence and Transverse Sinuses

The SS terminates by joining the SSS and TSs to form the **venous sinus confluence** (torcular herophili). The venous sinus confluence is often asymmetric, with septations and intersinus channels connecting the TSs.

The TSs, also known as lateral sinuses, are contained between attachments of the tentorium cerebelli to the inner table of the skull. The TSs curve laterally from the torcular to the posterior border of the petrous temporal bone, where they turn inferiorly and become the sigmoid sinuses.

Anatomic variations in the TSs are almost the rule rather than the exception. The two TSs are frequently asymmetric, with the right side typically larger than the left. Hypoplastic or stenotic segments are present in one-third of the general population. Filling defects caused by arachnoid granulations and fibrous septa are also common.

Sigmoid Sinuses and Jugular Bulbs

The sigmoid sinuses are basically the inferior continuations of the two TSs. They follow a gentle S-shaped curve, descending behind the petrous temporal bone to terminate by becoming the internal jugular veins (IJVs). Side-to-side asymmetry of the sigmoid sinuses is common and normal.

The jugular bulbs are focal venous dilatations at the skull base between the sigmoid sinuses and IJVs. The IJVs provide the main venous outflow system of the brain. Alternative nonjugular venous (NJV) pathways exist normally and may become important routes of collateral drainage in sinus thrombosis or intracranial hypertension. The two major NJVs are the **vertebral plexus** and the **pterygopalatine plexus**.

The IJVs, TSs, and sigmoid sinuses are often asymmetric, and there is concomitant variation in size of the jugular bulbs and their osseous foramina. Jugular bulb pseudolesions with flow asymmetry are common and should not be mistaken for "real" masses (e.g., schwannoma or paraganglioma). Bone CT shows that the jugular spine and cortex around the jugular foramen are intact, not eroded or remodeled.

Cavernous Sinus

The CSs are irregularly shaped, heavily trabeculated/compartmentalized venous sinuses that lie along the sides of the sella turcica, extending from the superior orbital fissures anteriorly to the clivus and petrous apex posteriorly **(9-4)**.

Formed by a prominent lateral and much thinner—often almost inapparent—medial dural wall, the CSs contain the two cavernous internal carotid arteries (ICAs) and abducens (CN VI)

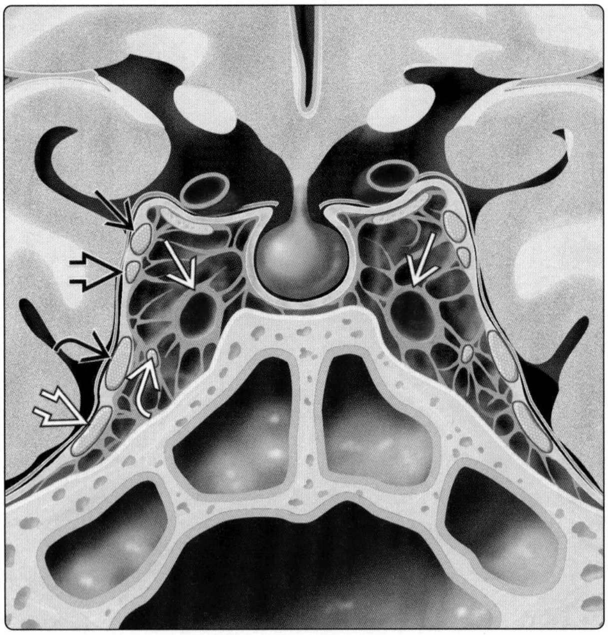

(9-5) Coronal graphic shows the CSs and their contents. The CSs are fenestrated, septated, and multichanneled. Internal carotid arteries and CN VI are inside the CSs. CN III, IV, V_1, and V_2 lie in the lateral dural wall.

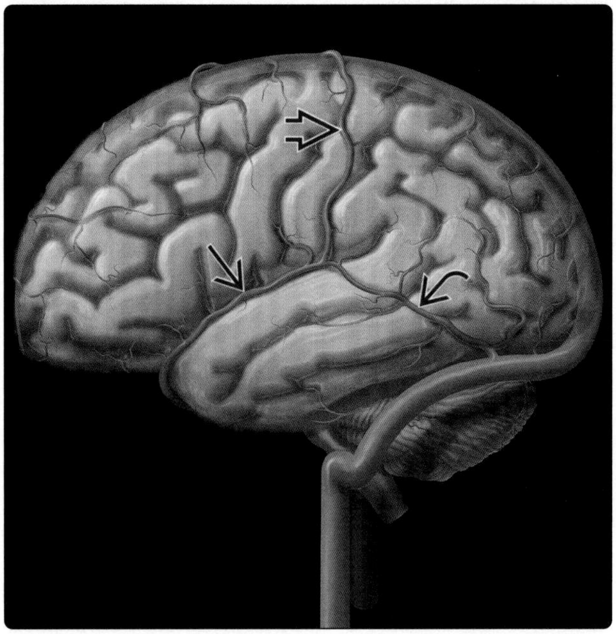

(9-6) Lateral graphic depicts the superficial cortical veins. The three named anastomotic veins—Trolard, Labbé, and the superficial middle cerebral vein—are depicted. One or two of the superficial cortical veins are usually dominant.

nerves. CN III, CN IV, CN V_1, and CN V_2 are actually *within* the lateral dural wall, not inside the CS proper **(9-5)**.

The major tributaries draining into the CSs are the superior/inferior ophthalmic veins and the SphPSs **(9-4)**. The two CSs communicate extensively with each other via intercavernous venous plexuses. The CSs drain inferiorly through the foramen ovale into the pterygoid venous plexuses and posteriorly into the CVP as well as the SPS and IPS.

Although the intercavernous septations and compartments are quite variable, the size and configuration of the CSs are relatively constant on imaging studies. The lateral walls normally appear straight or concave (not convex), and the venous blood enhances quite uniformly.

Superior and Inferior Petrosal Sinuses

The SPS courses posterolaterally along the top of the petrous temporal bone, extending from the CS to the sigmoid sinus. The IPS courses just above the petrooccipital fissure from the inferior aspect of the CVP to the jugular bulb **(9-4)**.

Clival Venous Plexus

The CVP is a network of interconnected venous channels that extends along the clivus from the dorsum sellae superiorly to the foramen magnum **(9-4)**. The CVP connects the CS and petrosal sinuses with each other and with the suboccipital veins around the foramen magnum.

Sphenoparietal Sinus

The SphPS courses around the lesser sphenoid wing at the rim of the middle cranial fossa. The SphPS receives superficial veins from the anterior temporal lobe and drains into the CS or IPS.

Cerebral Veins

The cerebral veins are subdivided into three groups: (1) superficial ("cortical" or "external") veins, (2) deep cerebral ("internal") veins, and (3) brainstem/posterior fossa veins.

Superficial Cortical Veins

The superficial cortical veins consist of a superior group, a middle group, and an inferior group.

Superior Cortical Veins. Between eight and twelve unnamed superficial veins course over the upper surfaces of the cerebral hemispheres, generally following convexity sulci.

The superior cortical veins cross the subarachnoid space, pierce the arachnoid membrane and inner (meningeal) layer of the dura, and drain directly into the SSS **(9-1)**.

In many cases, a dominant anastomotic superior cortical vein, the **vein of Trolard**, receives the superficial middle cerebral vein and courses upward from the sylvian fissure to join the SSS **(9-6)**. The vein of Trolard is typically located in a precentral, central, or postcentral location.

On lateral CTV, MRV, or venous-phase DSA, the superior cortical veins are arranged in a spoke-like pattern, coursing centripetally toward the SSS and entering it at right angles.

Middle Cortical Veins. The most prominent vein in this group is the **superficial middle cerebral vein** (SMCV). The SMCV begins over the sylvian fissure and collects numerous small tributaries from the temporal, frontal, and parietal opercula that overhang the lateral cerebral fissure.

On lateral CTV, MRV, or venous-phase DSA, the SMCV courses anteroinferiorly, paralleling the sylvian fissure, and curves around the temporal tip to terminate in the CS or SphPS.

Inferior Cortical Veins. The inferior cortical veins drain most of the inferior frontal lobes and temporal poles. The **deep middle cerebral vein** (DMCV) collects tributaries from the insula, basal ganglia, and parahippocampal gyrus, then anastomoses with the **basal vein of Rosenthal** (BVR).

After receiving the DMCV, the BVR courses posterosuperiorly in the ambient cistern, curving laterally around the midbrain to drain into the VofG.

A prominent posterior anastomotic vein, the **vein of Labbé**, courses inferolaterally over the temporal lobe to drain into the TS **(9-6)**.

All three named superficial anastomotic veins—the vein of Trolard, vein of Labbé, and SMCV—vary in size, maintaining a reciprocal relationship with each other. If one or two are dominant, the third anastomotic vein is usually hypoplastic or absent.

Deep Cerebral Veins

The deep cerebral ("internal") veins are themselves subdivided into three groups: (1) medullary veins, (2) subependymal veins, and (3) deep paramedian veins **(9-7)**.

Medullary Veins. Innumerable small, unnamed veins originate between 1 and 2 cm below the cortex and course straight through the white matter toward the ventricles, where they terminate in the subependymal veins **(9-8)**. These veins are generally inapparent on imaging studies throughout most of their course until they converge near the ventricles. DSA and contrast-enhanced MR may show faint linear stripes of contrast parallel to the ventricles **(9-9)**. T2* susceptibility-

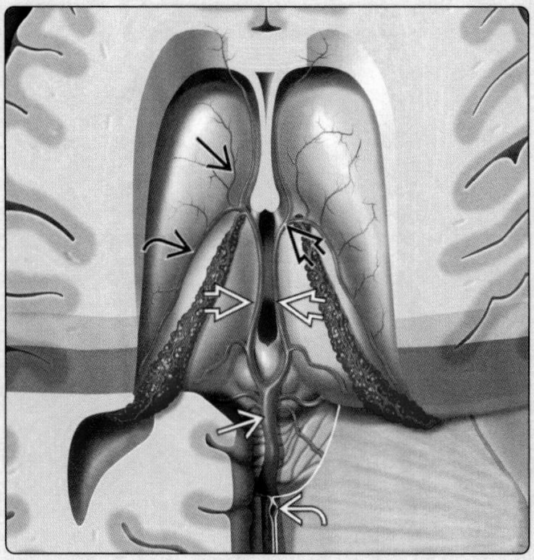

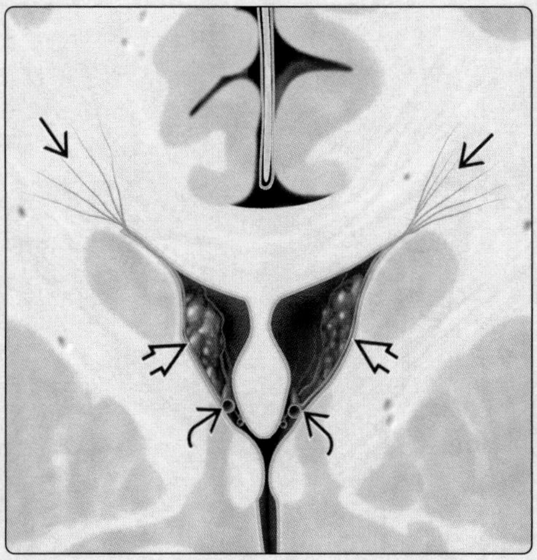

***(9-7)** Deep cerebral and subependymal venous drainage is seen from the top down. Caudate ⇒ and terminal veins ⇒ form the thalamostriate veins ⇒, which drain into the internal cerebral veins (ICVs) ⇒, VofG ⇒, and straight sinus ⇒. **(9-8)** Graphic through coronal ventricles shows medullary (deep WM) veins ⇒ converging at ventricular margins to drain into subependymal ⇒ and thalamostriate ⇒ veins. From there, they drain into the ICVs.*

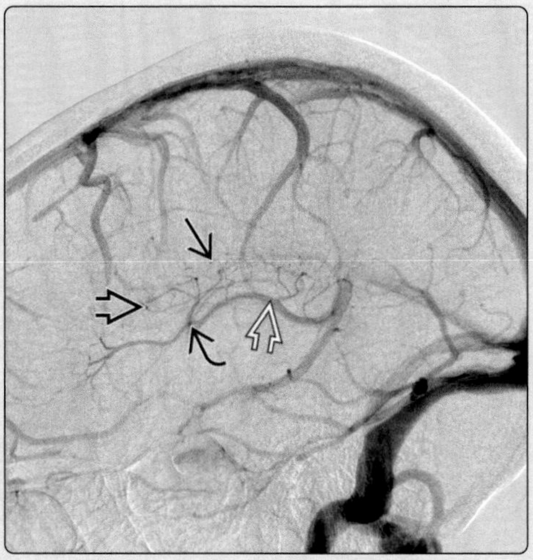

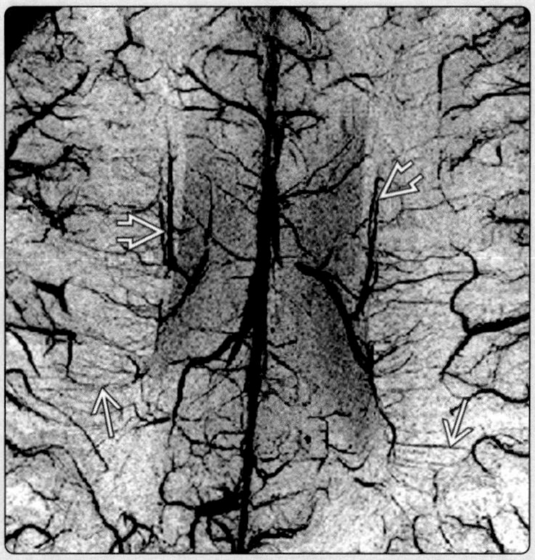

***(9-9)** Venous-phase DSA shows tiny medullary veins ⇒ draining into subependymal veins, seen here as "dots" on the end ⇒. The septal and thalamostriate veins converge near the foramen of Monro ⇒ to form the ICV ⇒. **(9-10)** Close-up axial view of 3.0-T T2* SWI scan shows deoxyhemoglobin in innumerable small medullary veins ⇒ draining into the subependymal veins ⇒.*

weighted imaging (SWI) best depicts the medullary veins because the deoxygenated blood is paramagnetic **(9-10)**.

Subependymal Veins. The subependymal veins course under the ventricular ependyma, collecting blood from the basal ganglia and deep white matter (via the medullary veins) **(9-8)**.

The most important named subependymal veins are the septal veins and the thalamostriate veins. The **septal veins** curve around the frontal horns of the lateral ventricles, then course posteriorly along the septi pellucidi. The **thalamostriate veins** receive tributaries from the caudate nuclei and thalami, curving medially to unite with the septal veins near the foramen of Monro to form the two internal cerebral veins (ICVs) **(9-8)**.

Deep Paramedian Veins. The **ICVs** and **VofG** provide drainage for most of the deep brain structures. The ICVs are paired paramedian veins that course posteriorly in the cavum velum interpositum, the thin invagination of subarachnoid space that lies between the third ventricle and the fornices. The ICVs terminate in the rostral quadrigeminal cistern by uniting with each other and the BVR to form the VofG **(9-8)**.

The VofG (great cerebral vein) curves posterosuperiorly under the corpus callosum splenium, uniting with the ISS to form the SS.

Brainstem/Posterior Fossa Veins

The veins that drain the midbrain and posterior fossa structures are likewise divided into three groups: (1) a superior ("galenic") group, (2) an anterior (petrosal) group, and (3) a posterior group.

Superior (Galenic) Group. As the name implies, these veins drain superiorly into the VofG. Major named veins in this group are the precentral cerebellar vein (PCV), the superior vermian vein, and the anterior pontomesencephalic vein (APMV) **(9-11)**.

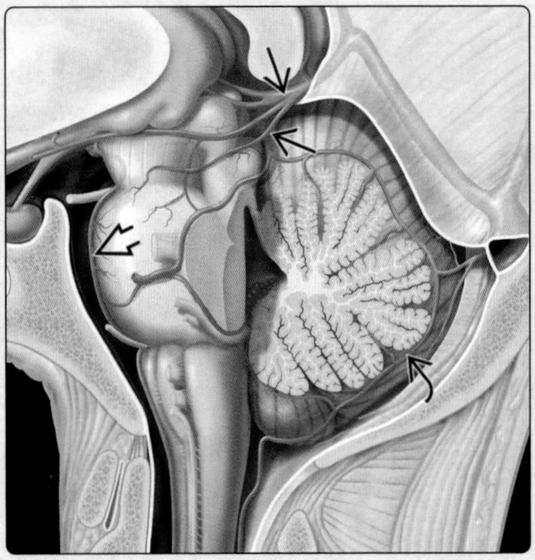

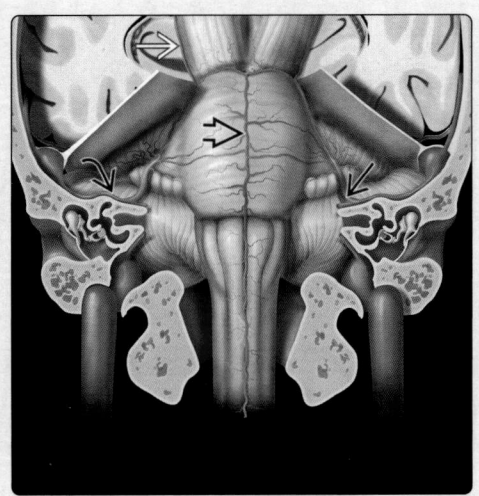

***(9-11)** Sagittal graphic through the vermis shows the superior (galenic) group of veins, the anterior group with the pontomesencephalic vein, and the posterior group. **(9-12)** Anterior pontomesencephalic and the petrosal venous plexuses drain the pons, anterior cerebellum, and cerebellopontine angle cistern. Note anastomoses with the superior petrosal sinuses and mesencephalic veins.*

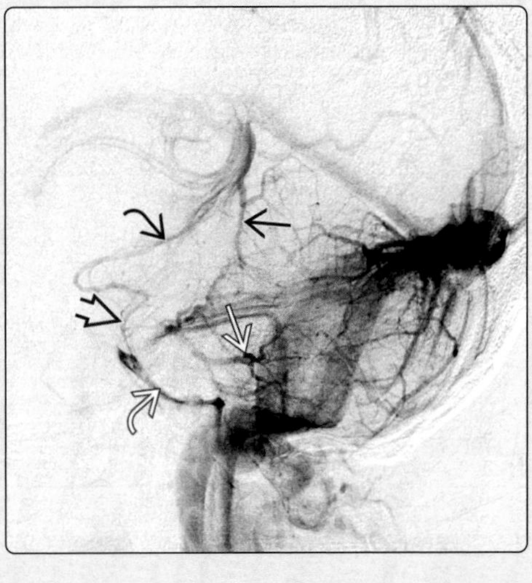

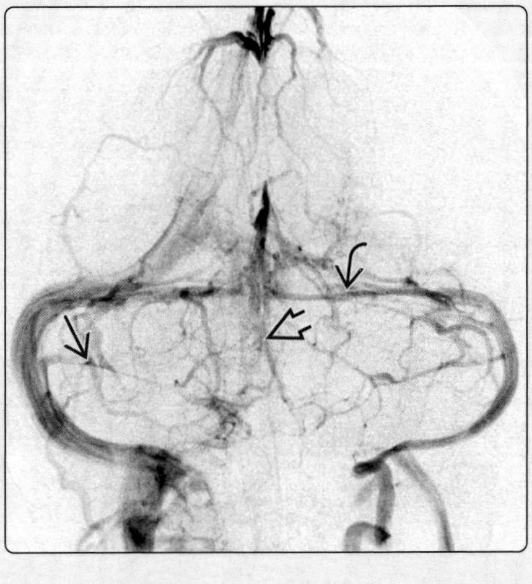

***(9-13)** Venous-phase vertebrobasilar DSA shows pontomesencephalic venous plexus and galenic group with precentral cerebellar vein, basal vein of Rosenthal. Note "star" of petrosal veins. Clival plexus drains into the inferior petrosal sinus. **(9-14)** AP view shows petrosal "star" and midline vermian veins. Note hypoplastic left TS segment, a common normal variant.*

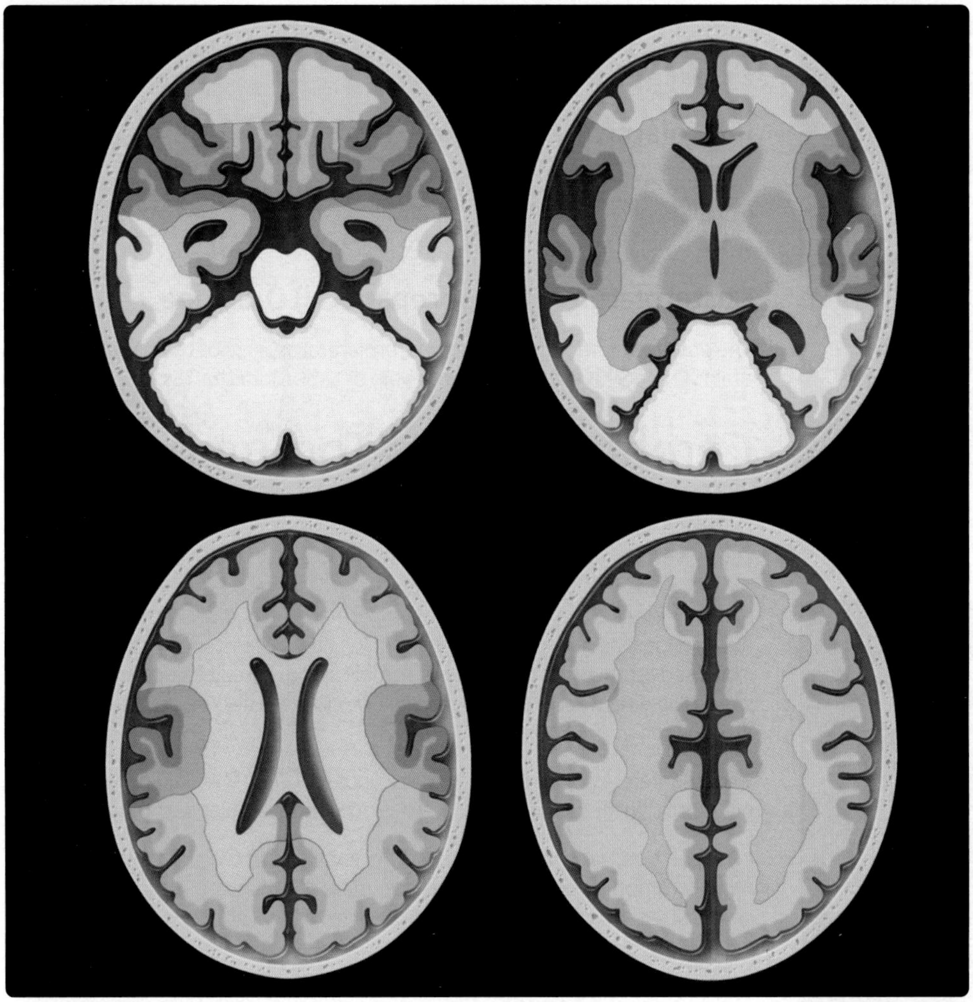

(9-15) Color-coded anatomic diagram depicting brain venous drainage territories is depicted at four representative levels: the base of the brain (upper left), basal ganglia and internal capsules (upper right), middle of the lateral ventricles (lower left), and upper corona radiata above the level of the corpus callosum (lower right). Superficial parts of the brain (cortex, subcortical white matter) are drained by cortical veins (including the vein of Trolard) and superior sagittal sinus (shown in green). Central core brain structures (basal ganglia, thalami, internal capsules, lateral and third ventricles) and most of the corona radiata are drained by the deep venous system (internal cerebral veins, vein of Galen, straight sinus) (red). The veins of Labbé and the transverse sinuses drain the posterior temporal, inferior parietal lobes (yellow). The sphenoparietal and cavernous sinuses drain the area around the sylvian fissures (purple).

The **precentral cerebellar vein** (PCV) is a single midline vein that lies between the lingula and the central lobule of the vermis. It terminates behind the inferior colliculi by draining into the VofG. The **superior vermian vein** runs over the top of the vermis, joining the PCV and draining into the VofG **(9-11)**.

The **anterior pontomesencephalic vein** (APMV) is actually an interconnected venous plexus, not a single dominant vein. The APMV covers the cerebral peduncles and extends over the anterior surface of the pons **(9-12)** **(9-13)**.

Anterior (Petrosal) Group. The **petrosal vein** (PV) is a large venous trunk that lies in the cerebellopontine angle cistern, collecting numerous tributaries from the cerebellum, pons, and medulla. The PV and its tributaries form a prominent star-shaped vascular collection seen on AP DSA or coronal CTV **(9-14)**.

Posterior (Tentorial) Group. The most prominent veins in this group are the **inferior vermian veins**, paired paramedian structures that curve under the vermis. The inferior vermian veins collect tributaries from the inferior surface of the cerebellum and drain into unnamed tentorial sinuses near the torcular.

Venous Drainage Territories

The cerebral venous drainage territories are both less familiar and somewhat more variable than the major arterial distributions. These drainage patterns follow four basic patterns: a peripheral (brain surface) pattern, a deep (central) pattern, an inferolateral (perisylvian) pattern, and a posterolateral (temporoparietal) pattern **(9-15)**. Accurately diagnosing and delineating venous occlusions depends on understanding these specific venous drainage territories.

Peripheral (Surface) Brain Drainage

Brain surface drainage generally follows a radial pattern. Most of the mid and upper surfaces of the cerebral hemispheres together with their subjacent white matter drain centrifugally (outward) via cortical veins into the SSS.

Deep (Central) Brain Drainage

The basal ganglia, thalami, and most of the hemispheric white matter all drain centripetally (inward) into the deep cerebral veins. The ICVs, VofG, and SS together drain virtually the entire central core of the brain.

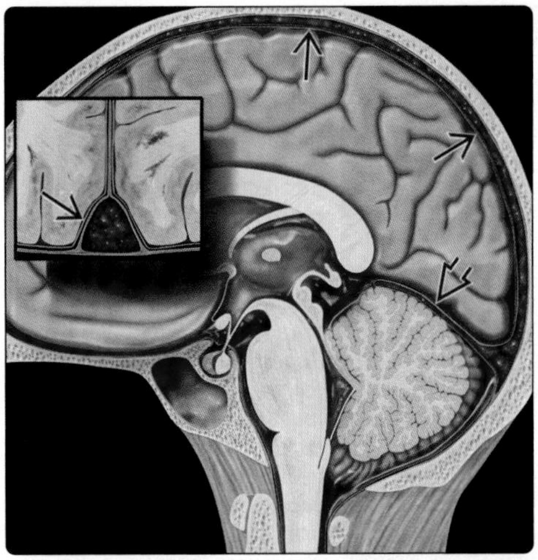

***(9-16)** Sagittal graphic shows SSS, straight sinus thrombosis. Insert shows pathologic basis of "empty delta" sign.*

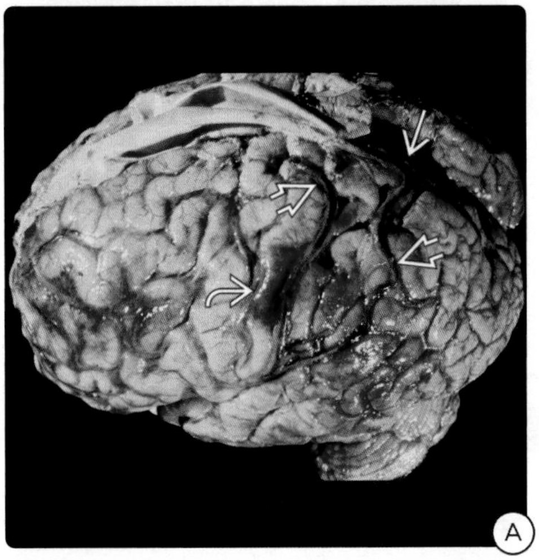

***(9-17A)** Autopsy case demonstrates acute SSS, cortical vein thrombosis, and venous infarcts.*

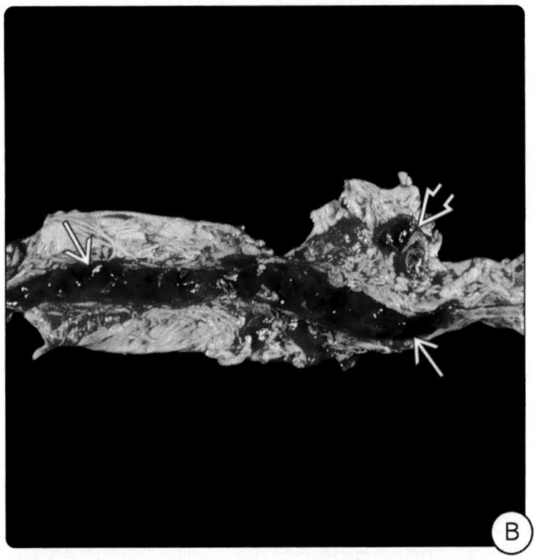

***(9-17B)** Gross photograph from the same case shows "currant jelly" clot in the SSS, cortical veins. (Courtesy E. T. Hedley-Whyte, MD.)*

The most medial aspects of the temporal lobes, primarily the uncus and the anteromedial hippocampus, also drain into the galenic system via the DMCVs and BVR.

Inferolateral (Perisylvian) Drainage

Parenchyma surrounding the sylvian (lateral cerebral) fissure consists of the frontal, parietal, and temporal opercula plus the insula. This perisylvian part of the brain drains via the SMCV into the SphPS and CS.

Posterolateral (Temporoparietal) Drainage

The posterior temporal lobes and inferolateral aspects of the parietal lobes drain via the SPSs and anastomotic vein of Labbé into the TSs.

Cerebral Venous Thrombosis

Dural venous sinus, superficial (cortical) vein, and deep vein occlusions are collectively termed cerebral venous thrombosis (CVT). CVT is an elusive diagnosis with a great diversity of causes and clinical presentations; it is also easily overlooked on imaging studies. Normal dura and circulating blood are mildly hyperdense compared with brain on NECT scans, so the subtle increased attenuation of venous thrombi can be difficult to detect. Venous sinuses lie directly adjacent to the skull, so clots can also be obscured by attenuation artifacts.

Venous infarcts can be relatively innocuous or lethal. They can mimic neoplasm, encephalitis, and numerous other nonvascular pathologies.

In this section, we consider several different types of CVT. We begin with the most common intracranial venous occlusion, dural sinus thrombosis. We next discuss superficial vein thrombosis and follow with deep cerebral occlusions.

We conclude the discussion with a consideration of cavernous sinus (CS) thrombosis/thrombophlebitis. Because of its anatomic proximity to the nose and paranasal sinuses, the CS is especially vulnerable to retrograde infection. The combination of infection and thrombosis means the clinical presentation and imaging findings of CS thrombosis have some special features not shared with other venous occlusions.

Dural Sinus Thrombosis

Terminology

Cerebral dural sinus thrombosis (DST) is defined as thrombotic occlusion of one or more intracranial venous sinuses **(9-16)**. DST can occur either in isolation or in combination with cortical and/or deep venous occlusions.

Etiology

Wide varieties of both inherited and acquired conditions are associated with increased risk of all CVTs. A predisposing comorbidity can be identified in the majority of cases, and many affected patients have more than one predisposing factor.

The most common acquired causes of CVT are oral contraceptive use and pregnancy/puerperium. Other conditions include—but are not limited to—trauma, infection, inflammation, hypercoagulable states, elevated hemoglobin levels, dehydration, collagen-vascular disorders (such as antiphospholipid syndrome), vasculitis (such as Behçet syndrome), drugs, and Crohn disease.

Between 20-35% of all patients with CVT have an inherited or acquired prothrombotic condition. Predisposing genetic factors are common and include antithrombin III, protein C, and protein S deficiency, as well as resistance to activated protein C caused by factor V Leiden gene mutation.

Pathology

When thrombus forms in a dural sinus, venous outflow is restricted. This results in venous congestion, elevated venous pressure, and hydrostatic displacement of fluid from capillaries into the extracellular spaces of the brain. The result is blood-brain barrier breakdown with vasogenic edema. If a frank venous infarct develops, cytotoxic edema ensues.

CEREBRAL VENOUS THROMBOSIS: CAUSES

Common
- Oral contraceptives
- Prothrombotic conditions
    - Deficiency of proteins C, S, or antithrombin III
    - Resistance to activated protein C (V Leiden)
    - Prothrombin gene mutations
    - Antiphospholipid, anticardiolipin antibodies
    - Hyperhomocysteinemia
- Puerperium, pregnancy
- Metabolic (dehydration, thyrotoxicosis, etc.)

Less Common
- Infection
    - Mastoiditis, sinusitis
    - Meningitis
- Trauma
- Neoplasm-related causes

Rare But Important
- Collagen-vascular disorders (e.g., antiphospholipid antibody syndrome)
- Hematologic disorders (e.g., polycythemia)
- Inflammatory bowel disease
- Vasculitis (e.g., Behçet disease)

Location. The transverse sinus is the most commonly thrombosed dural venous sinus, followed by the superior sagittal sinus (SSS).

Gross Pathology. In acute DST, the affected dural sinus appears distended by a soft, purplish clot that can be isolated to the sinus or may extend into adjacent cortical veins **(9-17)**. In chronic DST, firm proliferative fibrous tissue fills the sinus and thickens the dura-arachnoid.

The spectrum of associated brain injury in DST varies from venous congestion to ischemia to petechial hemorrhages and frank hemorrhagic infarcts **(9-18)**.

Clinical Issues

Epidemiology. CVTs represent between 1-2% of all acute strokes. Although CVT can occur at any age (from neonates to the elderly), it is most commonly seen in young individuals. Nearly 80% of patients are younger than 50 years of age. The estimated annual incidence is five cases per million adults.

Demographics. CVT predominantly affects women (F:M = 3:1). A sex-specific risk factor (oral contraceptives, pregnancy, puerperium, and hormone replacement therapy) is present in nearly two-thirds of all women with CVT. Because of these sex-specific risk factors, mean age at presentation is nearly a decade younger in women compared with men (34 years vs. 42 years).

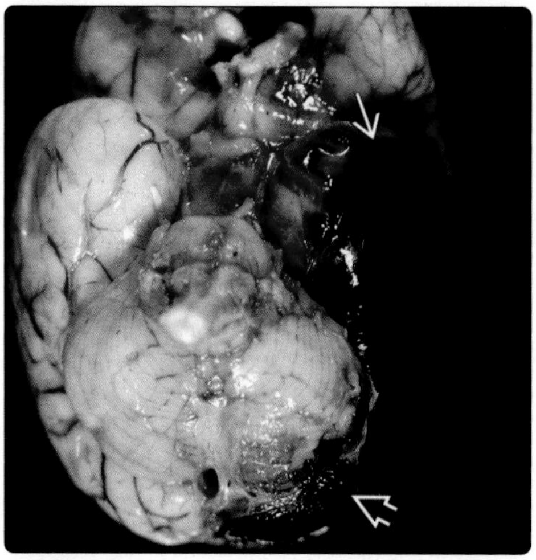

***(9-18)** Autopsy shows acutely thrombosed TS that caused a large temporal lobe hemorrhagic infarct. (R. Hewlett, MD.)*

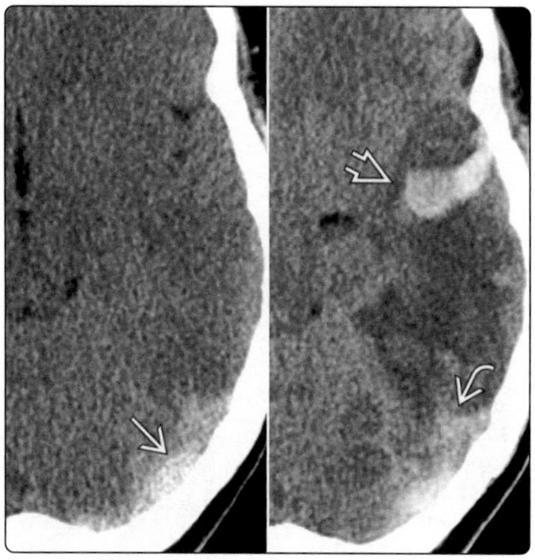

***(9-19)** 23y woman (migraine) NECT is "normal," hyperdense thrombus in left TS. CT in 24 h has VofL thrombosis, hemorrhagic infarct.*

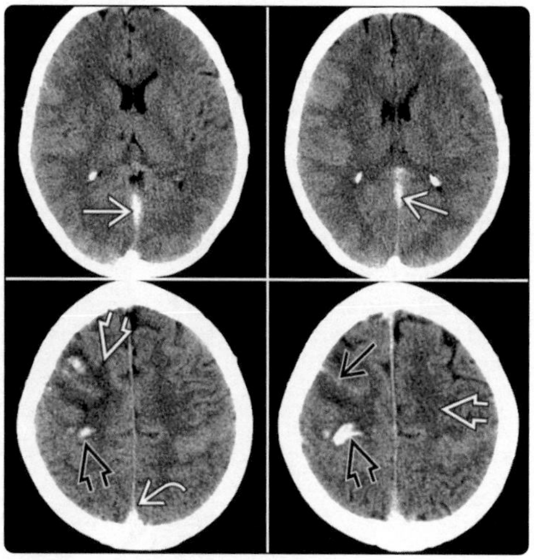

***(9-20)** NECT shows hyperdense thrombus in the SS, SSS with bilateral edema, parenchymal hemorrhages, convexal SAH.*

Presentation. The clinical manifestations of CVT are varied, often nonspecific, and may be subtle—especially in neonates, children, and the elderly.

Headache is the most common symptom, occurring in nearly 90% of cases. The headache is usually nonfocal, often slowly increasing in severity over several days to weeks. Nearly 25% of patients present without focal neurologic findings, making the clinical diagnosis even more difficult.

Natural History. The natural history of CVTs varies widely, as does outcome. Many DSTs recanalize spontaneously without long-term sequelae. In some cases, a thrombosed or partially recanalized venous sinus forms an arteriovenous fistula in the adjacent dural wall.

Prompt recognition of DST has a significant impact on clinical outcome. Diagnostic delay—averaging 7 days in large series—is associated with increased death and disability.

Imaging

Keys to the early neuroradiologic diagnosis of DST are (1) a high index of suspicion, (2) careful evaluation of dural sinus density/signal intensity and configuration, and (3) knowledge of normal venous drainage patterns.

CT Findings. *NECT is normal in up to 25-30% of CVT cases, so a normal NECT scan does* **not** *exclude the diagnosis of CVT!* Early signs are often subtle. Slight hyperdensity compared with the carotid arteries is seen in 50-60% of cases and may be the only hint of sinus or venous occlusion **(9-19)**. When present, a hyperattenuating vein ("cord" sign) **(9-21B)** or dural venous sinus sign **(9-21A)** **(9-22A)** is both a sensitive and specific sign of cerebral venous occlusive disease. Parenchymal edema with or without petechial hemorrhage in the territory drained by the thrombosed sinus is a helpful but indirect sign of DST **(9-20)**.

(9-21A) NECT in a 22y woman with "thunderclap" headache was obtained to evaluate for subarachnoid hemorrhage. Note hyperdensity of straight sinus ➡, torcular (venous confluence) ➡. The left thalamus also appears hypodense ➡. (9-21B) More cephalad NECT shows hyperdense thrombus filling and expanding the SSS ➡. Note hyperdensity in an adjacent superficial cortical vein ("cord" sign) ➡.

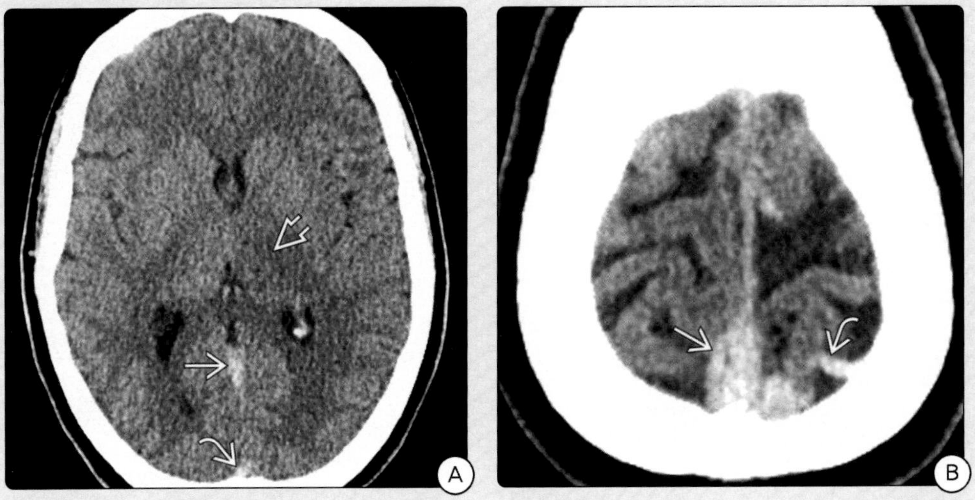

(9-21C) CECT in the same case shows classic "empty delta" sign ➡ formed by enhancing dura around nonenhancing thrombus. (9-21D) Sagittal CTA shows extensive thrombus filling the SSS ➡, straight sinus ➡, vein of Galen ➡, and torcular (sinus confluence) ➡.

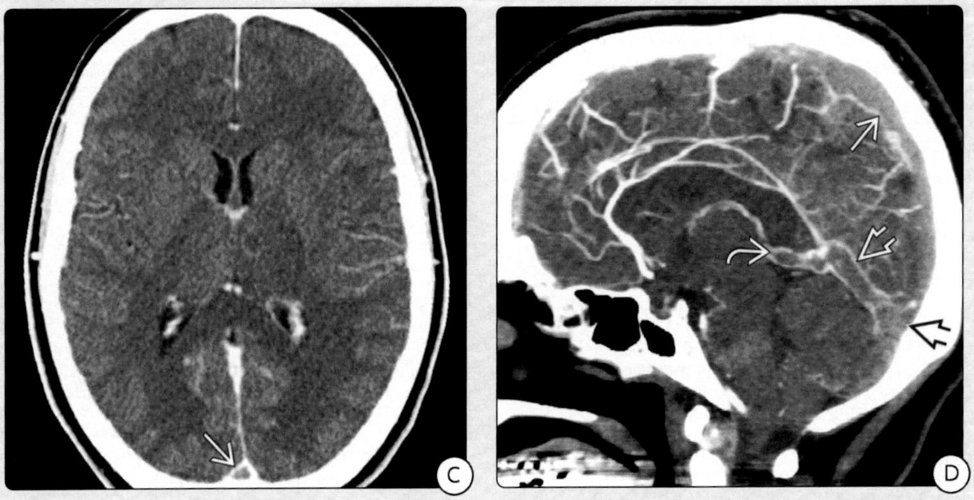

In 70% of cases, CECT scans show an **"empty delta" sign** caused by enhancing dura surrounding nonenhancing thrombus **(9-21C)**. "Shaggy," enlarged, or irregular veins suggest collateral venous drainage.

CTA/CTV has fewer artifacts than MRV and is therefore the best noninvasive method for delineating dural sinus filling defects. CTA/CTV readily demonstrates the thrombus within the intensely enhancing dura **(9-21D)**.

MR Findings. Diagnosing CVT on MR can be challenging because thrombus and normal venous flow can have similar signal intensities. The imaging appearance of DST also varies significantly with imaging sequence. Whereas normal dural venous sinuses have *opposite* signal intensities on FLAIR and T2*, in DST these sequences generally demonstrate the *same* signal intensity regardless of clot age.

Acute, subacute, and chronic occlusions have different findings on MR and are discussed separately below.

Acute DST. An acutely thrombosed sinus often appears moderately enlarged ("fat sinus" sign) and displays abnormally convex—not straight or concave—margins **(9-22C)**. The "flow void" of rapidly moving blood typically seen in large venous sinuses disappears **(9-22B)**. Acute DST appears *isointense* with the underlying cortex on **T1WI (9-22C)**.

As hemoglobin in blood clots rapidly desaturates to deoxyhemoglobin, it becomes very *hypointense* relative to brain on **T2WI** and **FLAIR (9-22D)**. Therefore the acute T2 "dark" DVT mimics normal intrasinus "flow void" **(9-32C)**. If venous congestion and edema develop secondary to obstructed outflow, they cause gyral swelling and parenchymal hyperintensity on T2/FLAIR.

Similar to parenchymal hematomas, acute venous clots "*bloom*" on **T2* (GRE, SWI) (9-32D)**. SWI shows the profoundly hypointense clot and slow flow with deoxygenated blood in dilated cortical veins. The appearance

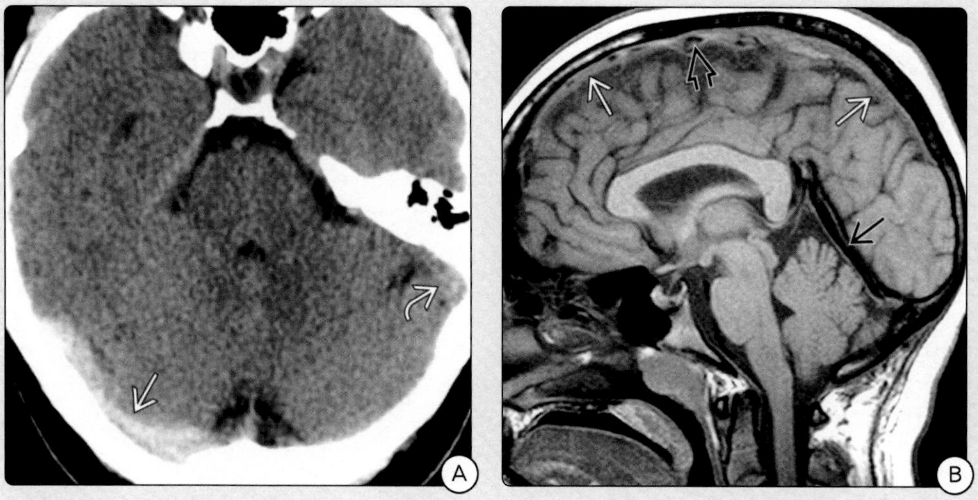

(9-22A) Axial NECT scan in a 29y pregnant woman with headaches, papilledema shows hyperdense right TS compared with the left sigmoid sinus. (9-22B) Sagittal T1WI in the same patient shows a normal "flow void" in the straight sinus. The SSS shows an absent "flow void" and—except for the CSF-filled arachnoid granulations—appears filled with clot that is almost isointense with brain.

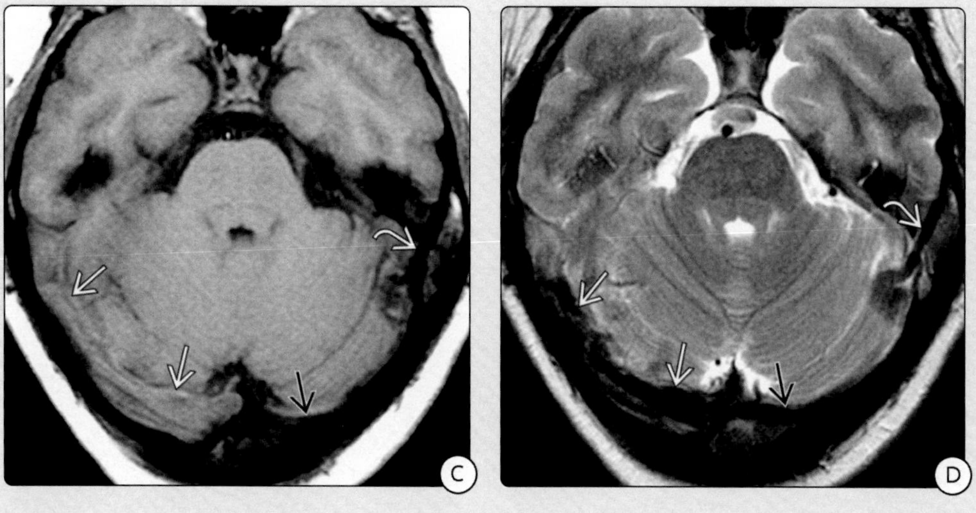

(9-22C) Axial T1WI in the same patient shows an enlarged right TS that appears filled with isointense clot. Compare with the normal "flow void" in the left vein of Labbé and TS. (9-22D) Axial T2WI in the same patient shows that the thrombosed right TS appears very hypointense and mimics the "flow voids" of the patent left TS and vein of Labbé; acute dural sinus thrombosis (DST).

may nonetheless be confusing, as normal-flowing but deoxygenated venous blood also appears hypointense.

Extensive acute (or longstanding chronic) DST may result in collateral venous drainage through the medullary (white matter) veins into the deep subependymal veins. The medullary veins enlarge and contain desaturated hemoglobin; thus, they are seen on T2* sequences as prominent linear hypointensities entering the subependymal veins at right angles **(9-36C)**.

When seen in cross section, **T1 C+** scans demonstrate an "*empty delta*" sign, similar to the appearance on CECT and CTA/CTV. Intrasinus thrombi usually appear as elongated *cigar-shaped* nonenhancing filling defects on axial T1 C+ **(9-24D)**.

DWI has low sensitivity for the visualization of acute clots but can be helpful in demonstrating areas of parenchymal venous ischemia.

Coronal 2D unenhanced TOF **MRV** may demonstrate *absent flow*, especially if the thrombus is in the SSS. As the transverse sinuses often have hypoplastic segments, a "flow gap" must be interpreted with caution (see below). **Contrast-enhanced MRV** has the highest sensitivity of all sequences for visualizing acute DST.

Late Acute DST. As the intrasinus thrombus organizes, the clot begins to exhibit T1 shortening and becomes progressively hyperintense.

With T2 prolongation, a thrombosed sinus progresses from appearing very hypointense to iso- and then hyperintense with brain on both T2WI and FLAIR **(9-23)**. T2* can be misleading, as clot signal gradually approaches that of normal sinuses. Late acute DST continues to exhibit an "empty delta" sign on T1 C+.

Subacute DST. Subacute thrombus is hyperintense on all sequences (T1, T2, FLAIR, T2*) **(9-24)** **(9-25)**.

(9-23A) Sagittal T1WI in a 56y man with electrolyte disturbance 4 days before imaging shows changes of pontine myelinolysis ➡ and late acute DST. Signal intensity in the thrombosed SSS and sinus confluence is beginning to demonstrate some foci of patchy T1 shortening ➡. (9-23B) Axial T1WI in the same case shows the right TS is enlarged ➡, slightly hyperintense relative to the adjacent cerebellum.

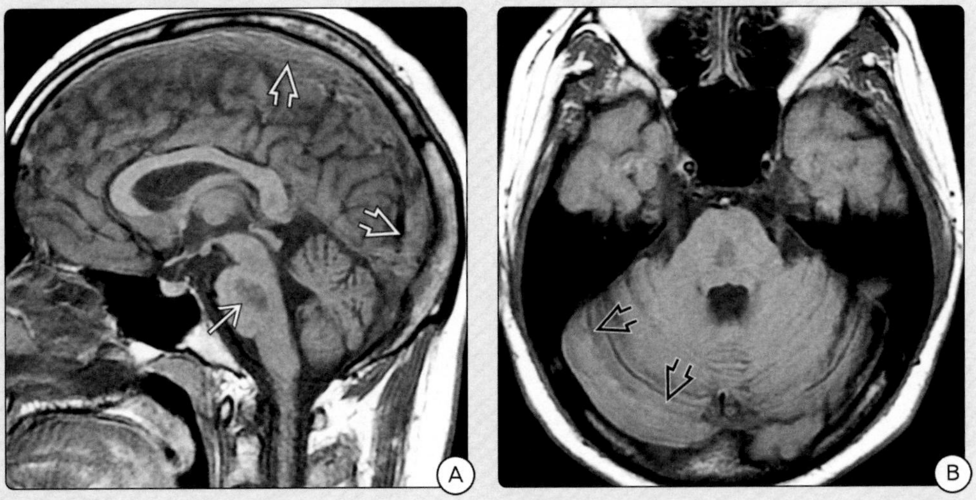

(9-23C) T2WI shows the pontine myelinolysis ➡. Thrombus in the enlarged right TS is mildly hypointense with some foci now appearing nearly isointense ➡ with the adjacent cerebellum. (9-23D) T2 GRE shows "blooming" hypointensity in most of the thrombus ➡. Note area of less prominent blooming ➡ that is now approaching signal intensity of the white matter. This is late acute DST.*

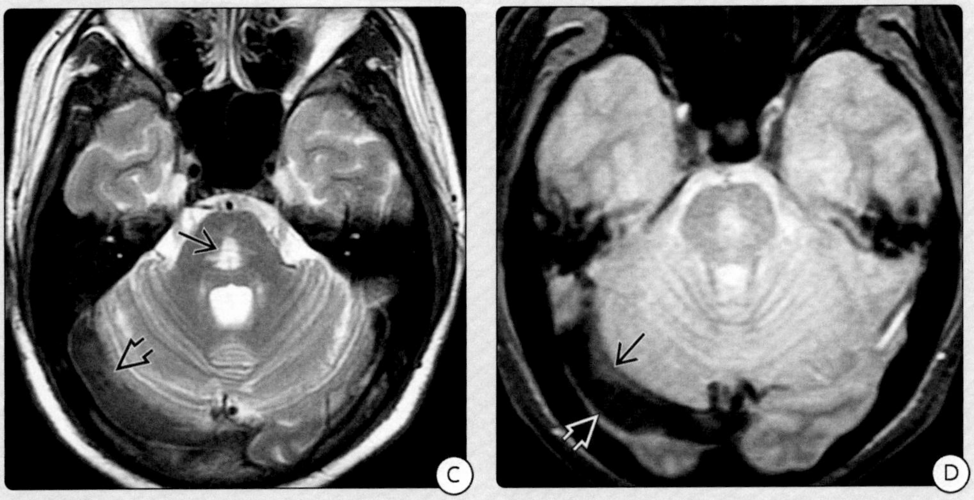

Chronic DST. Clot signal in chronic DST is very variable and depends on the degree of clot organization. Chronic organized, fibrotic thrombus eventually becomes isointense with brain on T1WI and remains isointense to moderately hyperintense on T2WI **(9-27A)**. As blood has resorbed and largely disappeared, there is little or no T2* "blooming."

Longstanding cerebral venous sinus thrombosis may develop significant collateral drainage through the medullary veins. This is seen as tortuous, "squiggly" intraparenchymal "flow voids" on T2WI that enhance on T1 C+ scans, sometimes becoming so prominent that they mimic an arteriovenous malformation on SWI and DSA **(9-27)**.

Dura-arachnoid thickening is also common in longstanding chronic DST. In some cases, the dural thickening becomes so pronounced that it appears very hypointense on T2WI **(9-26)**. Any residual clot may be reduced to a thin, almost inapparent isointense collection within the thick, strongly enhancing dura-arachnoid.

Angiography. Typical findings of DST on DSA are those of an occluded (nonfilling) sinus. Slow flow with or without clot in the adjacent cortical veins is common. Delayed emptying often makes the cortical veins appear as if they are "hanging in space" **(9-27D)**.

Differential Diagnosis

Asymmetry of the transverse sinuses is common. A **hypoplastic segment** is seen in one-quarter to one-third of imaged cases and may mimic DST. The presence of enlarged collateral venous channels is suggestive of DST.

A **"high-splitting" torcular** can mimic an "empty delta" sign on CECT.

Giant arachnoid granulations are focal round or ovoid CSF-like filling defects in the sinuses, whereas clots tend to be elongated, cigar-shaped lesions (see Venous Occlusion Mimics later in the chapter).

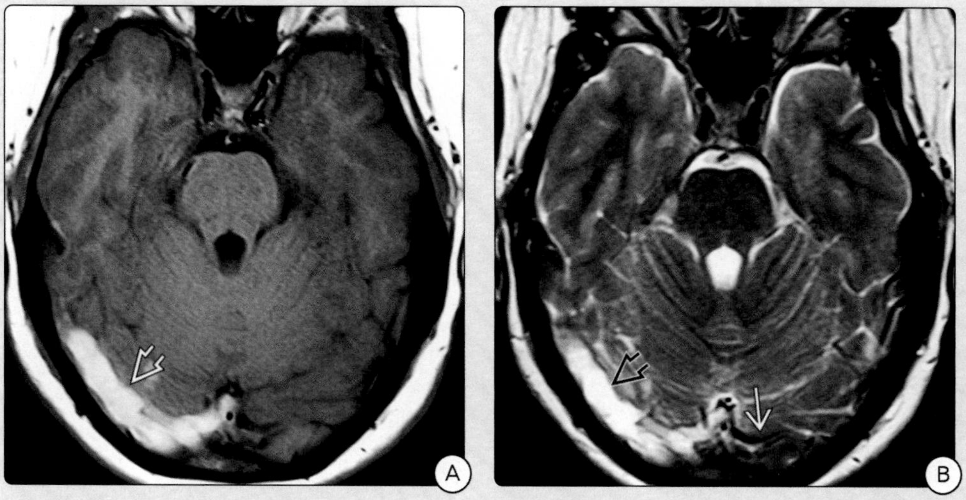

(9-24A) A 21y woman presented to the ER with 2 weeks of severe headache, papilledema on neurologic examination. Axial T1WI shows classic early subacute hyperintense thrombus ➾ in the occluded right TS. (9-24B) T2WI in the same case shows that the subacute thrombus is very hyperintense ➾. Contrast with normal "flow void" in the hypoplastic left TS ➡. The clot was hyperintense on FLAIR (not shown).

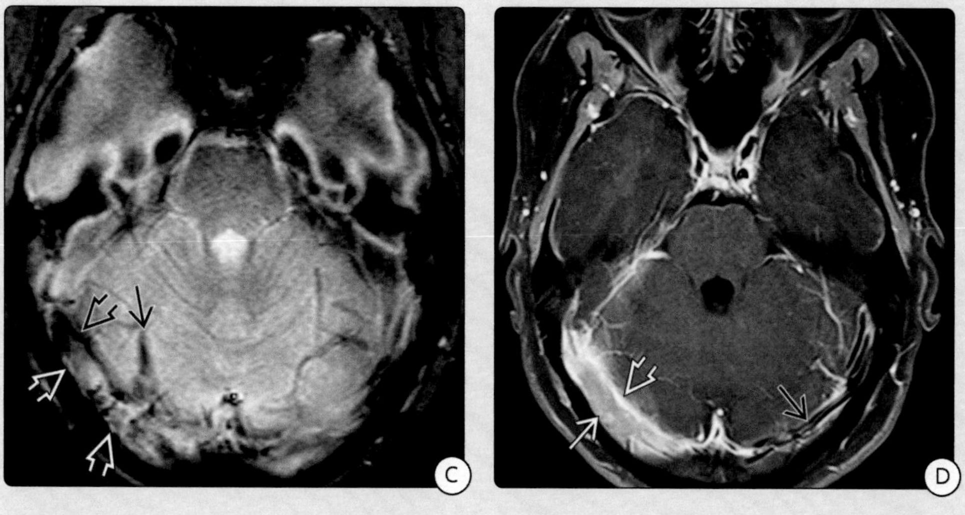

(9-24C) T2* GRE shows that the thrombus is mostly hyperintense ➾ with only some residual "blooming" in the right TS ➾ and in several tentorial tributary veins ➡. (9-24D) T1 C+ FS shows the intensely enhancing dura ➾ surrounding the nonenhancing, slightly less hyperintense subacute thrombus ➾. The left TS is hypoplastic but patent with a normal "flow void" ➡. This is subacute DST.

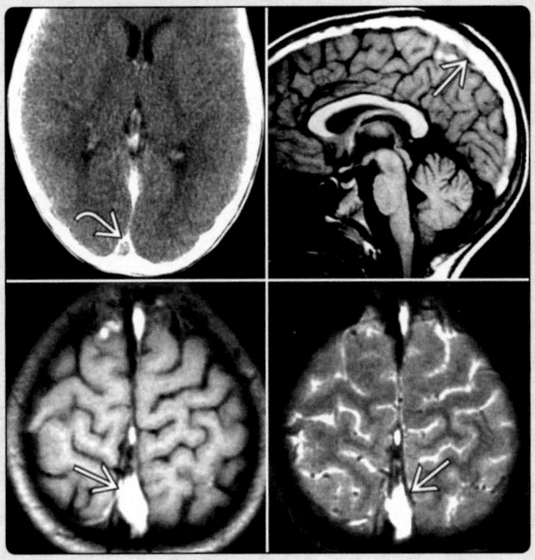

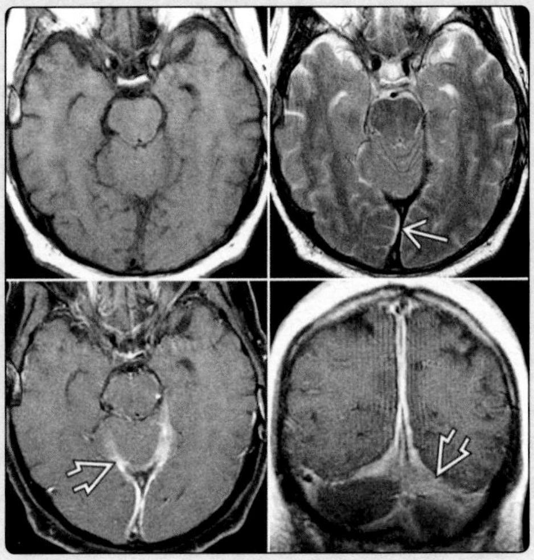

(9-25) *Late subacute SSS thrombosis shows "empty delta" sign on CECT and hyperintense thrombus on both T1WI and T2WI.* ***(9-26)*** *Longstanding chronic SSS thrombosis shows hypointense thick enhancing dura. (Courtesy M. Castillo, MD.)*

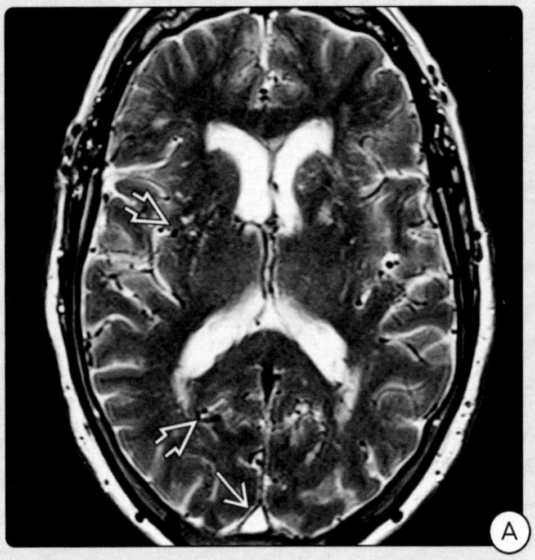

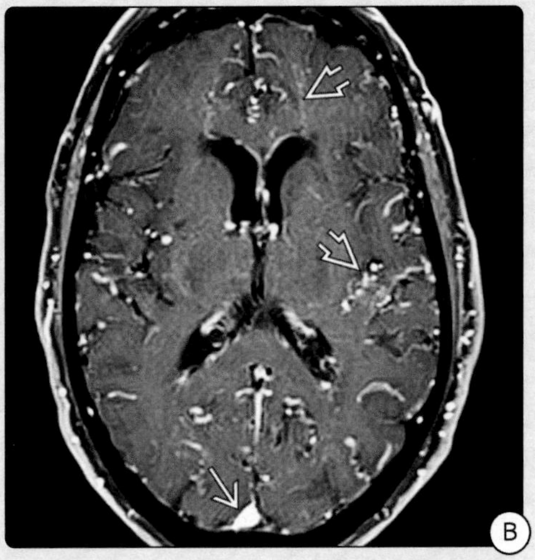

(9-27A) *T2WI in an 82y man with multiple episodes of confusion, falls, and altered mental status shows uniformly hyperintense SSS and unusually prominent, tortuous "flow voids" in the sulci, parenchyma.* ***(9-27B)*** *T1 C+ FS in the same case shows that the SSS enhances intensely and uniformly. Numerous tortuous, corkscrew vessels in the parenchyma and sulci also enhance intensely.*

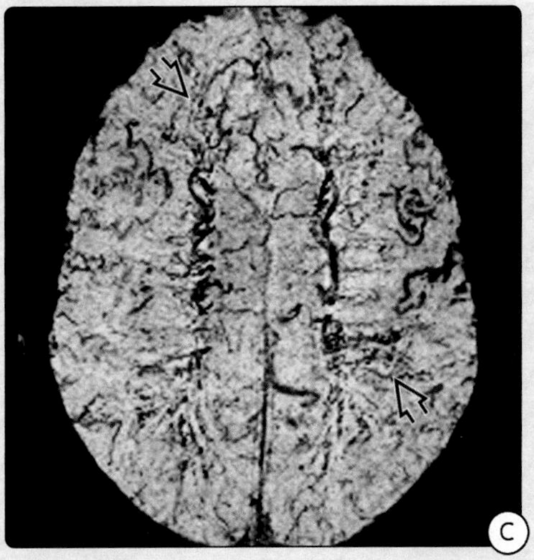

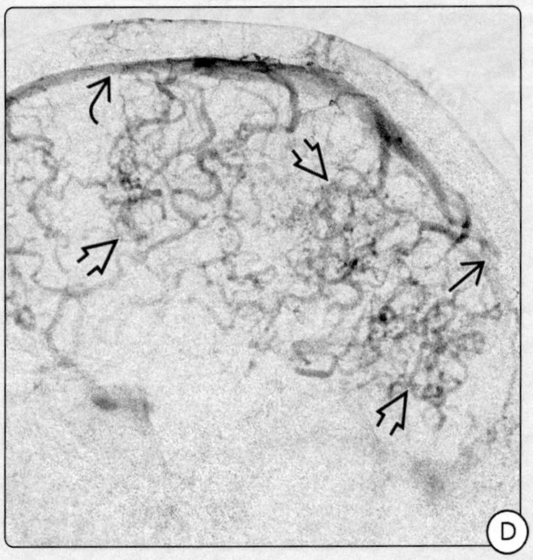

(9-27C) *T2* SWI shows innumerable prominent tortuous, corkscrew "squiggly" medullary veins throughout both cerebral hemispheres.* ***(9-27D)*** *Venous DSA shows that the distal SSS is occluded, while its proximal and middle segments are patent. Numerous enlarged "corkscrew" medullary veins appear to "hang in space." This is chronic SSS occlusion with medullary collateral venous ("pseudophlebitic") drainage.*

DURAL SINUS THROMBOSIS: MR

Acute
- "Fat" sinus with bulging convex walls
- T1 isointense, T2 profoundly hypointense
- T2* "blooms," T1 C+ shows "empty delta"

Late Acute
- T1 mixed isointense, mildly hyperintense
- T2/FLAIR mildly hypointense/isointense
- T2* "blooms"

Subacute
- T1 hyperintense, T2/FLAIR hyperintense
- T2* hyperintense

Chronic
- T1 isointense, T2/FLAIR moderately hyperintense
- T2*, T1 C+ show "squiggly" parenchymal enhancement
- T1 C+ shows thick, enhancing dura

Superficial Cerebral Vein Thrombosis

Superficial cerebral vein thrombosis (SCVT) can occur without or with DST **(9-28)**. When it occurs without accompanying DST, SCVT is termed isolated cortical vein thrombosis.

Superficial Vein Thrombosis *Without* DST

Isolated SCVT (iSVCT) without DST is rare, representing only 5% of all sinovenous occlusions. The clinical outcome of iSVCT is generally good.

iSCVT usually presents with a nonspecific headache. Approximately 10% of patients report sudden onset of a "thunderclap" headache that clinically mimics aneurysmal subarachnoid hemorrhage.

Symptoms such as focal neurologic deficits, seizures, and impaired consciousness are less common than with dural sinus or deep vein thrombosis.

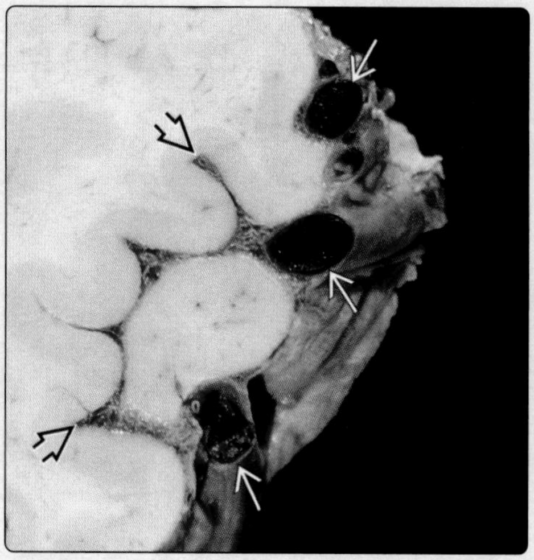

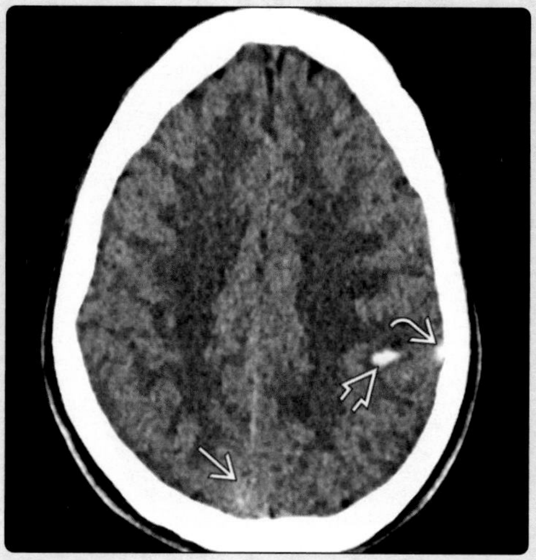

***(9-28)** Autopsy case shows thrombus in several cortical veins ("cord" sign), adjacent convexal subarachnoid hemorrhage. (Courtesy E. T. Hedley-Whyte, MD.) **(9-29)** NECT in a 29y woman with thunderclap headache shows small parenchymal hemorrhage, "cord" sign of thrombosed cortical vein. Contrast with normal density of the SSS, which is patent and uninvolved. This is isolated cortical vein thrombosis.*

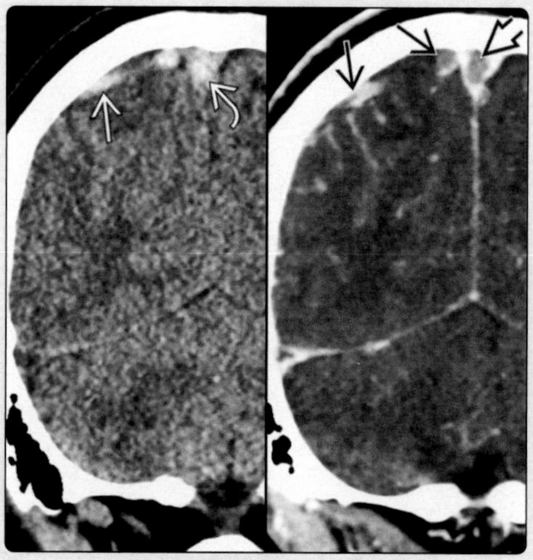

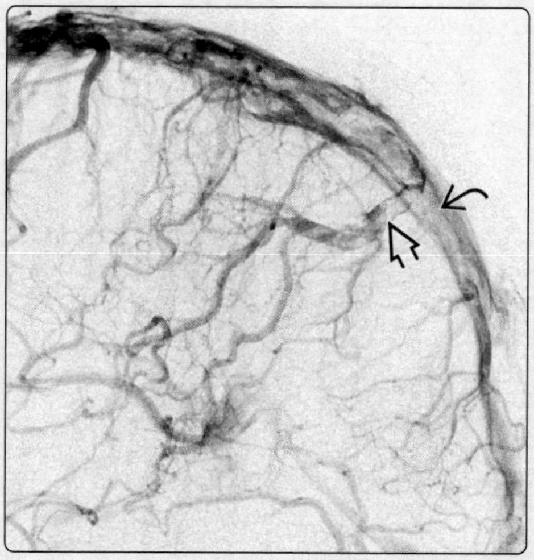

***(9-30)** Cortical vein occlusion is shown with dural sinus thrombosis. (L) Coronal NECT in a 62y woman with headache, left-sided weakness shows a hyperdense SSS and thrombus in the adjacent vein of Trolard. (R) CTV shows "empty delta" sign in the SSS, filling defects in the vein of Trolard. **(9-31)** Close-up view of lateral DSA in the same case shows thrombus in SSS and vein of Trolard.*

The imaging diagnosis of iSCVT can be problematic. NECT is usually negative although some cases may demonstrate focal **convexal subarachnoid hemorrhage** or a **"cord" sign**, representing a hyperdense thrombosed vein **(9-29)**.

CTA/CTV or DSA may show a thin round or tubular layer of contrast surrounding the thrombus.

The MR diagnosis of SCVT—whether with or without dural sinus involvement—is difficult to establish using only standard T1- and T2-weighted sequences. Acute thrombi are isointense with brain on T1WI and hypointense on T2WI, making them difficult to distinguish from normal "flow voids" **(9-32C)**.

FLAIR may demonstrate focal convexal subarachnoid hemorrhage, seen as hyperintense sulcal CSF. Cortical-subcortical hyperintensities consistent with vasogenic edema are common associated findings.

Intraluminal thrombus can sometimes be seen as a linear hyperintensity on FLAIR or DWI. Venous ischemia may result in transient diffusion restriction.

T2* (GRE, SWI) sequences are key to the noninvasive diagnosis of SCVT **(9-32)**. With a sensitivity of more than 95%, they are by far the best imaging sequences for detecting thrombosed cortical veins. A well-delineated tubular hypointensity with "blooming" of hemoglobin degradation products within the clot is observed at all stages of evolution, persisting for weeks. Patchy or petechial hemorrhages in the underlying cortex and subcortical white matter are common, as is associated convexal subarachnoid hemorrhage.

Superficial Vein Thrombosis *With* DST

Two general types of SCVT with DST are recognized: DST that involves one or more small cortical draining veins and DST that affects one of the great anastomotic veins (Trolard or Labbé).

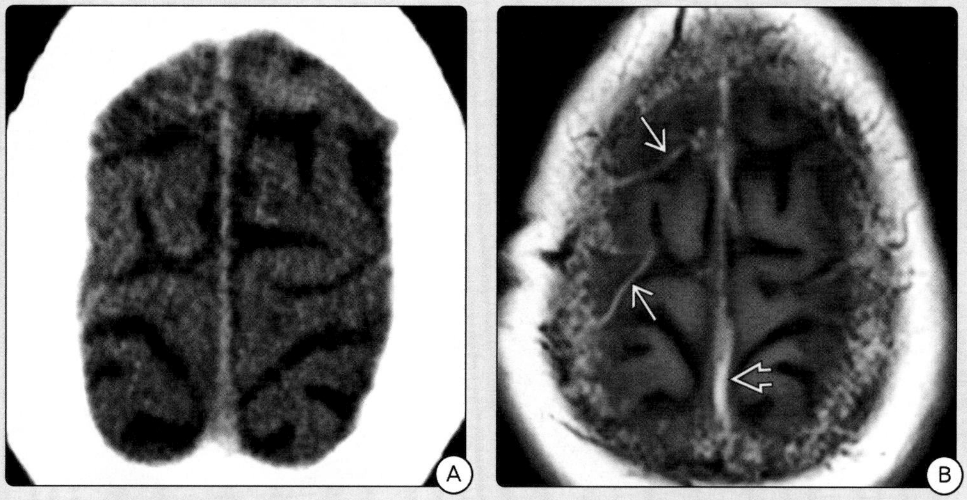

***(9-32A)** A 68y man presents with 3 days of headache. "Rule out vasculitis" shows no abnormality on NECT. **(9-32B)** T1WI in the same case shows slight T1 shortening in the SSS ➡ and right cortical veins ➡.*

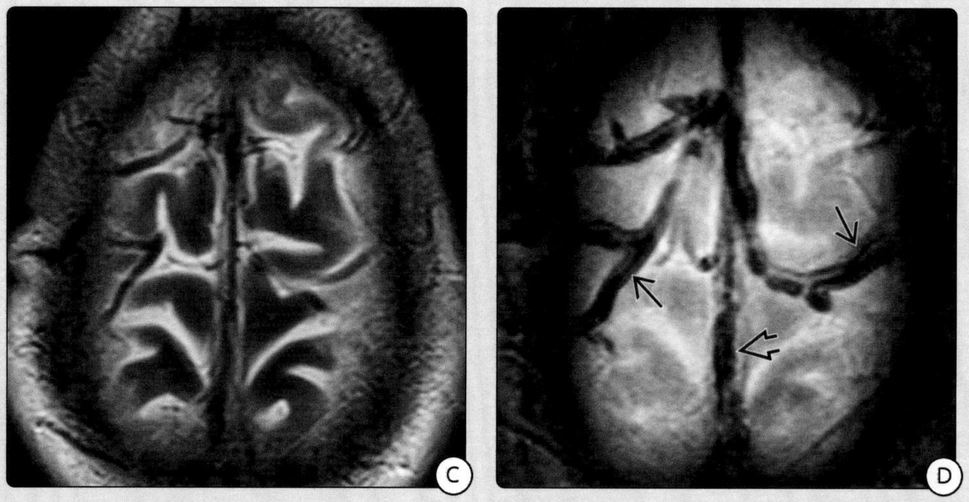

***(9-32C)** T2WI requested to "rule out vasculitis or stroke" in a 68y man with headache appears normal. **(9-32D)** T2* GRE in the same case shows multiple thrombosed cortical veins, seen as curvilinear hypointensities ➡. The adjacent SSS is also occluded ➡. The cortical vein and dural sinus thrombosis are late acute stage, with hypointense thrombus on T2WI mimicking normal "flow voids" (see image, left).*

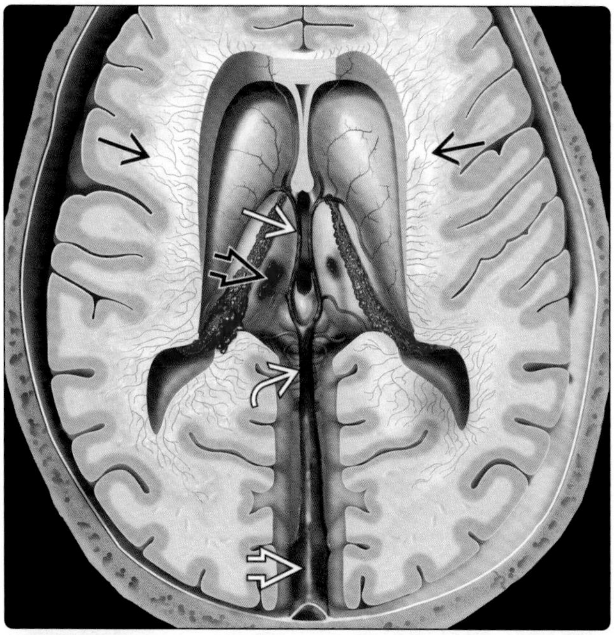

(9-33) Axial graphic depicts deep venous occlusion with thrombosis of both ICVs ➡, VofG ➡, and SS ➡ with hemorrhage in both thalami ➡. Note venous congestion with edema, and engorgement of white matter medullary veins ➡.

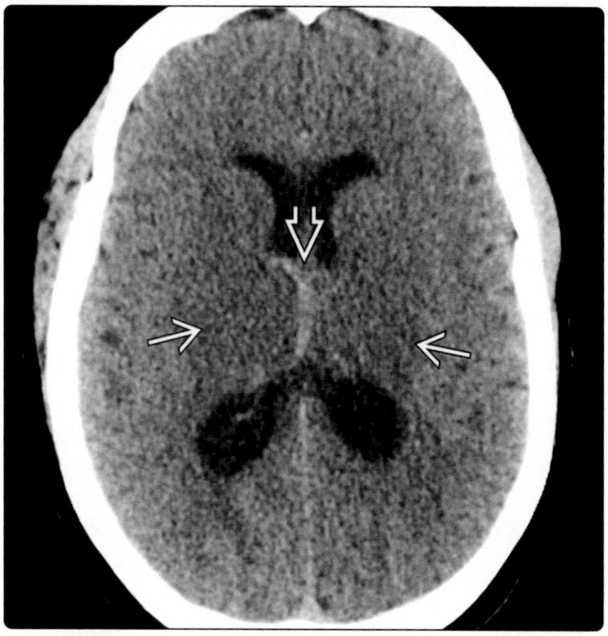

(9-34) Axial NECT scan in a 32y woman with severe headaches shows classic findings of deep cerebral vein thrombosis. Both ICVs are hyperdense ➡, and the thalami ➡ are hypodense ("disappearing" thalami).

Imaging findings of SCVT with accompanying DST are similar to those of DST alone. In addition to clot in the sinus, thrombus extends into one or more cortical veins **(9-17)**. SSS occlusion with SCVT may affect the superolateral surfaces of the hemispheres, with variable amounts of edema and petechial hemorrhage involving the cortex and subcortical white matter **(9-17A)**. If the anastomotic vein of Trolard is dominant, its occlusion may result in lobar hemorrhage.

Transverse sinus occlusion that extends into a dominant vein of Labbé often causes extensive posterior temporal and anterior parietal hemorrhage **(9-18)** **(9-19)**.

SUPERFICIAL CORTICAL VEIN THROMBOSIS

Superficial Thrombosis With DST
- DST extends into adjacent veins
- Edema, hemorrhage in cortex, adjacent white matter
- Can be extensive if vein of Trolard or Labbé occluded

Superficial Thrombosis Without DST
- Rare (5% of all CVTs)
- May cause convexal subarachnoid hemorrhage
- May see "cord" sign
- Deoxygenated thrombus can mimic normal "flow voids" on T2WI
- T2* (GRE, SWI) key to diagnosis
  - "Blooming" thrombus in vein(s)

Deep Cerebral Venous Thrombosis

Deep cerebral venous thrombosis (DCVT) is a potentially life-threatening disorder with a combined mortality/disability rate of 25%.

Etiology and Pathology

The deep cerebral venous system [the internal cerebral veins (ICVs) and basal vein of Rosenthal, together with their tributaries, the vein of Galen, and straight sinus] is involved in approximately 15% of all patients with cerebral venoocclusive disease **(9-33)**.

DCVT can occur either alone or in combination with other sinovenous occlusions. Isolated DCVT is present in 25-30% of cases. DCVT is almost always bilateral and results in symmetric venous congestion/infarction of the basal ganglia and thalami **(9-34)**.

Clinical Issues

Initial symptoms of DCVT are variable and nonspecific, making diagnosis difficult. Most patients present with headache (80%) followed by rapid neurologic deterioration and impaired consciousness (70%). Focal neurologic findings are frequently absent.

Imaging

Early NECT findings may be subtle. Hyperdense ICVs and straight sinuses resemble a contrast-enhanced scan **(9-35)**. Hypodense "fading" or "disappearing" thalami with effacement of the border between the deep gray nuclei and internal capsule are key but nonspecific findings of DCVT **(9-34)**.

MR is the imaging modality of choice. Acute thrombus is isointense on T1WI **(9-36A)** and hypointense on T2WI (pseudo-"flow void"). Venous congestion causes hyperintensity with swelling of the thalami and basal ganglia on T2/FLAIR in 70% of cases.

The most sensitive sequence is T2* GRE, on which acute clots show distinct "blooming" **(9-36B)**. Venous congestion in the medullary and subependymal veins is also hypointense due to slow flow and hemoglobin deoxygenation **(9-36C)**.

CTA/CTV and DSA show absent opacification in deep venous drainage system **(9-35D)**, and MRV shows absence of flow.

Differential Diagnosis

Extensive DCVT may make the NECT scan resemble a normal **contrast-enhanced CT (9-35A)**.

Differential diagnosis of DCVT includes other lesions with bithalamic abnormalities. **Arterial strokes** caused by artery of Percheron thrombosis or "top of the basilar" occlusion often affect both thalami. **Bithalamic gliomas** and **metabolic abnormalities** such as Wernicke encephalopathy are among many disorders that can affect medial thalami.

DEEP VENOUS THROMBOSIS

Pathology
- Uncommon (15% of CVTs)
- Usually both ICVs ± VofG, SS involved

Imaging
- Hyperdense ICVs (may look like CECT scan)
- Bithalamic edema common
- Variable hemorrhage
- CTV shows nonopacification of deep (Galenic) veins
- DSA shows absent visualization of ICVs ± VofG, SS
- Differential diagnosis
  - Neoplasm (bithalamic glioma)
  - Top of basilar, artery of Percheron thrombosis
  - Wernicke encephalopathy

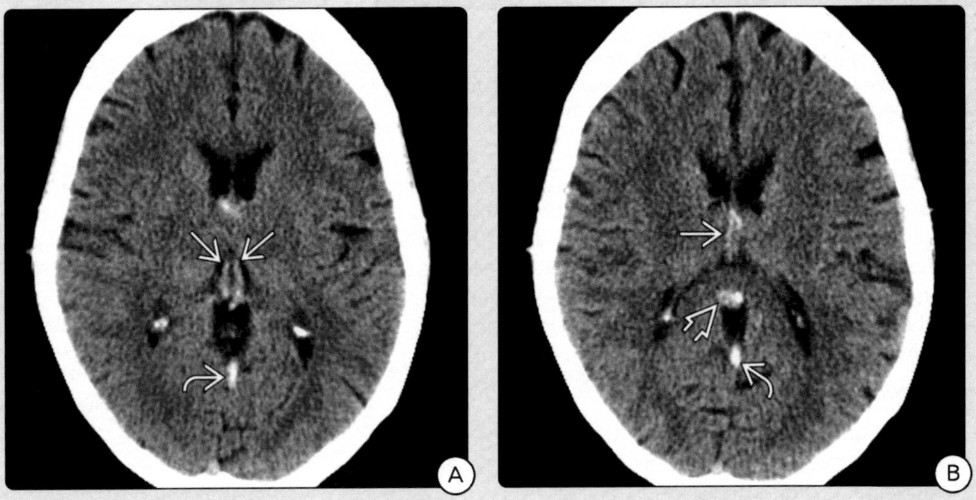

***(9-35A)** NECT in a 25y man with headache, dysmetria shows such uniform hyperdensity in both ICVs and straight sinus that the study looks like a contrast-enhanced scan. **(9-35B)** More cephalad scan shows that the hyperdensity in the ICVs also involves the vein of Galen as well as the straight sinus.*

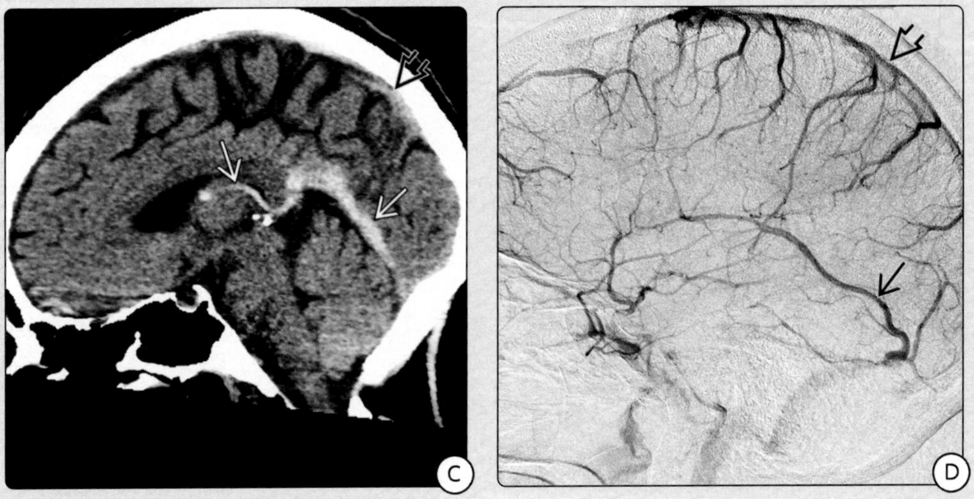

***(9-35C)** Sagittal NECT reformatted from the axial source data shows dense thrombus extending throughout the entire deep venous (Galenic) system. The SSS appears normal. **(9-35D)** Venous phase of the lateral carotid DSA in the same case shows normal cortical veins and SSS, vein of Trolard. The ependymal veins, ICVs, vein of Galen, and straight sinus are unopacified because they are completely filled with thrombus.*

Cavernous Sinus Thrombosis/Thrombophlebitis

Cavernous thrombosis/thrombophlebitis is the most common form of septic cerebral venous sinus thrombosis, a rare but potentially lethal condition with significant morbidity and high mortality.

Terminology

Cavernous sinus thrombosis (CST) is a blood clot in the cavernous sinus (CS). If it occurs in conjunction with sinus infection, it is termed cavernous sinus thrombophlebitis **(9-37)**.

Etiology and Pathology

The CS is composed of numerous heavily trabeculated venous spaces that have numerous valveless communications with veins in the orbit, face, and neck. Infection can thus spread easily through these venous conduits into the CS.

CST usually occurs as a complication of sinusitis or other midface infection. *S. aureus* is the most frequent pathogen. Other less common agents include anaerobes and angioinvasive fungal infections.

Otomastoiditis, odontogenic disease, trauma, and neoplasm are less frequent causes of CST.

Clinical Issues

Epidemiology. CS thrombosis without trauma, infection, or multiple other dural venous sinus occlusions is extremely rare.

Presentation. Headache, especially in the CN V_1 and CN V_2 distributions, and fever are usually the earliest symptoms. Orbital pain with edema, chemosis, proptosis,

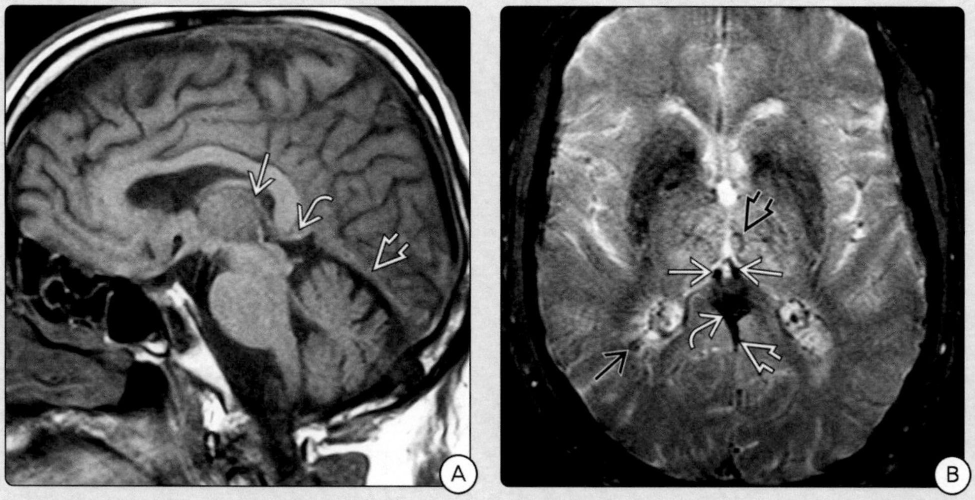

(9-36A) Sagittal T1WI in a patient with deep venous occlusion shows lack of normal "flow voids" with isointense clot present in the ICVs, vein of Galen, and straight sinus. (9-36B) Axial T2 GRE scan in the same case shows clot with "blooming" hypointensity in the ICVs, vein of Galen, and straight sinus. Note hypointensity caused by venous congestion with slow flow in the medial thalamic and deep WM medullary veins.*

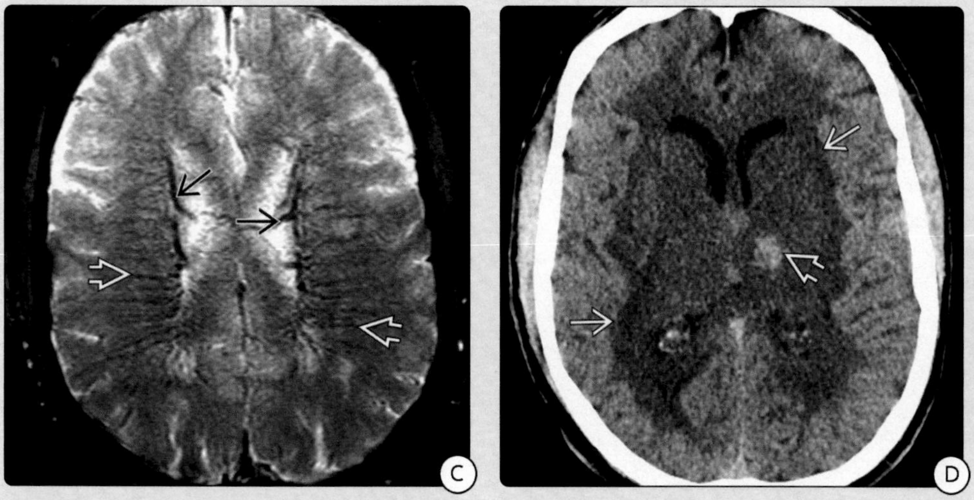

(9-36C) T2 GRE shows hypointensity from slow flow with deoxyhemoglobin in engorged subependymal and deep WM medullary veins. (9-36D) NECT scan 2 days later shows extensive confluent hypodensity in the entire central brain with a hemorrhagic focus in the left thalamus. The hypodensity represents infarction in the deep venous drainage territory (compare with Figure 9-15). The patient died shortly afterward.*

ophthalmoplegia, and visual loss is present in 80-100% of cases.

Natural History. Untreated CST can be fatal. Even with antibiotics, the mortality rate of CS thrombophlebitis is 25-30%.

Imaging

CT Findings. CS thrombophlebitis causes proptosis, "dirty" orbital fat, periorbital edema, sinusitis, and lateral bulging of the CS walls and may demonstrate a thrombosed superior ophthalmic vein (SOV) on NECT. CECT scans demonstrate multiple irregular filling defects in the expanded CS and SOVs **(9-37)**.

MR Findings. MR scans show enlarged CSs with convex lateral margins. Acute thrombus is isointense with brain on T1WI and demonstrates variable hypointensity on T2WI **(9-38A)**. Nonenhancing filling defects within the enhancing dural walls of the CS and thrombosed orbital veins on T1 C+ are the definitive imaging findings in CST **(9-38C)**.

Look for the normal intracavernous carotid artery "flow void," as CS thrombophlebitis can lead to thrombosis or pseudoaneurysm formation **(9-37C)**.

Angiography. Nonvisualization of the CS on DSA can be a normal finding and does not indicate the presence of CS thrombosis **(9-37D)**.

Differential Diagnosis

The differential diagnosis of CST includes neoplasm, carotid-cavernous fistula, and inflammatory disorders. **Neoplasms** (e.g., lymphoma, metastases) enhance uniformly. **Carotid-cavernous fistula** causes "flow voids," and **inflammatory disorders** (e.g., sarcoid, inflammatory pseudotumors) enhance strongly and uniformly.

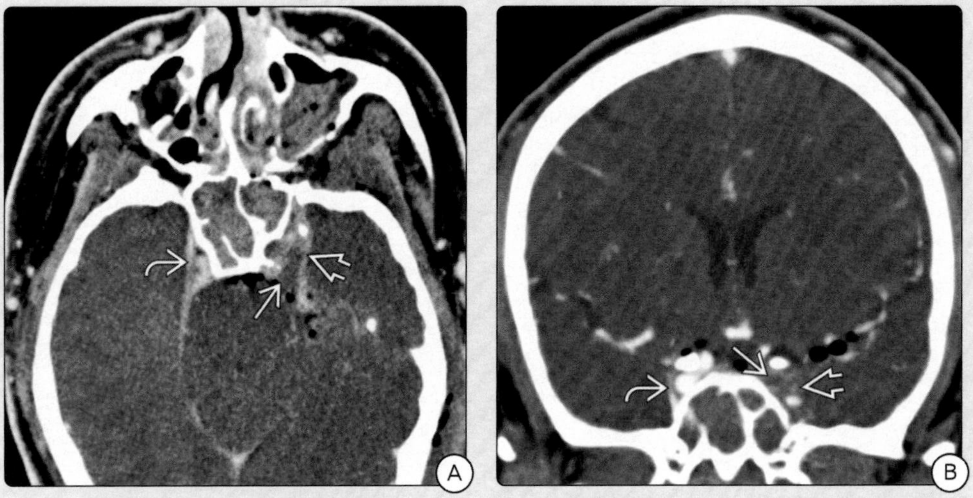

***(9-37A)** CECT source image from CTA in a 28y man with polytrauma shows filling defects in the left CS ➡. The affected CS has a lightly convex lateral margin ➡ compared with the normal right CS ➡. **(9-37B)** Coronal CTA in the same patient shows occlusion of the left cavernous internal carotid artery (ICA) ➡. The left CS remains unopacified because it is filled with thrombus ➡. Compare this to the normal right CS ➡.*

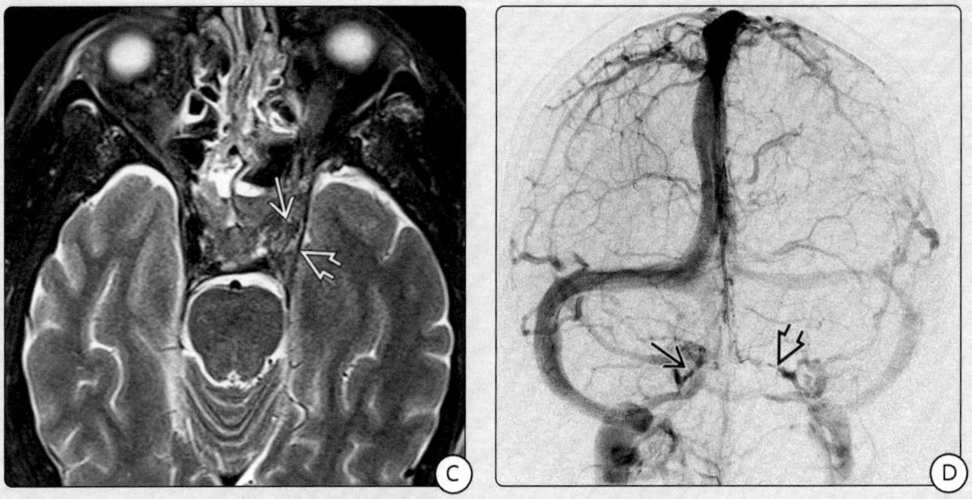

***(9-37C)** Axial T2WI in the same case shows left ICA occlusion, seen as an absent "flow void" ➡. The left CS is filled with iso-/hypointense clot ➡. **(9-37D)** Venous phase of right ICA angiogram demonstrates the difficulty in diagnosing CST on DSA. The right CS ➡ is opacified, draining inferiorly into the pterygoid venous plexus. Left CS is not visualized, and subtle thrombus ➡ is present, seen here as a filling defect.*

CAVERNOUS SINUS THROMBOSIS/THROMBOPHLEBITIS

Pathoetiology

- Numerous valveless communications between CS, orbit, face
- CS thrombosis secondary to sinusitis, dental disease > trauma, neoplasm
- Spontaneous, isolated CS thrombosis rare

Clinical Issues

- Headache, cranial neuropathy
- Proptosis, chemosis common

Imaging

- NECT may be normal early
  - Look for sinusitis, "dirty" orbit fat
  - Lateral bulging of CS walls
- CECT/CTV
  - Nonenhancing filling defects on CECT
  - Nonopacification on early-phase CTV
- MR
  - T1WI isointense, laterally bulging walls
  - T2 iso-/hypointense
  - Look for cavernous carotid thrombosis (loss of "flow void")
  - T1 C+ shows nonenhancing filling defects

Venous Occlusion Mimics

We conclude this chapter on venous anatomy and occlusions with a brief discussion of conditions that can mimic—or obscure—venous thrombosis.

Sinus Variants

The major differential diagnosis of cerebral venous thrombosis is a **congenital anatomic variation**. The right transverse sinus (TS) is usually the dominant venous sinus and is often significantly larger than the left side. A **hypoplastic TS** segment is present in one-quarter to one-third of all imaged cases and is *especially* common in the nondominant sinus (usually the left TS) **(9-39A)**. In such instances, the ipsilateral jugular bulb is typically small **(9-39C)**. Correlation with bone CT can also be helpful in demonstrating a small bony jugular foramen or sigmoid sinus groove. A hypoplastic TS or sigmoid sinus is also often—but not invariably—associated with alternative venous outflow pathways, such as a persistent occipital sinus or prominent mastoid emissary veins.

Variations in the torcular herophili (sinus confluence) are also common. A **high-splitting**, **segmented**,or **multichanneled sinus confluence** can have a central nonopacified area that mimics dural sinus thrombosis (DST).

The absence of occluded draining veins, enlarged venous collateral channels, or abnormally thick dural enhancement supports the diagnosis of TS sinus hypoplasia or anatomic variant vs. true cerebral venous sinus thrombosis.

Flow Artifacts

A **"flow gap"** on 2D TOF MRV can result from a number of factors including slow intravascular or in-plane flow or complex blood flow patterns. Flow parallel to the plane of acquisition (in-plane flow) can cause signal loss on MR venography and is most prominent in vertically oriented structures such as the distal sigmoid sinus. Use of inferior saturation pulses with axial 2D TOF MRV can saturate flow in parts of the curving superior sagittal sinus (SSS) but can be avoided by imaging in the coronal plane.

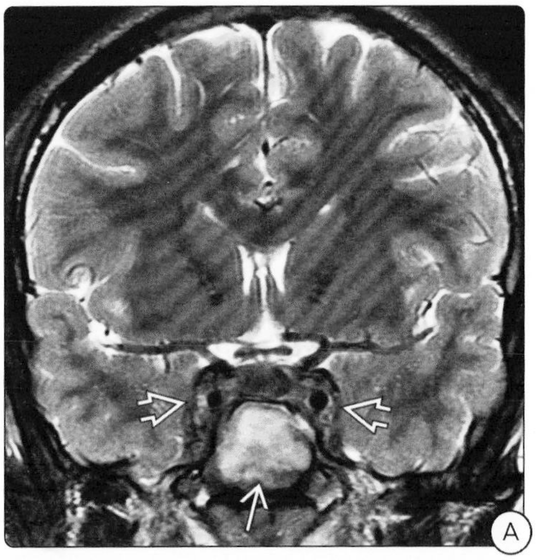

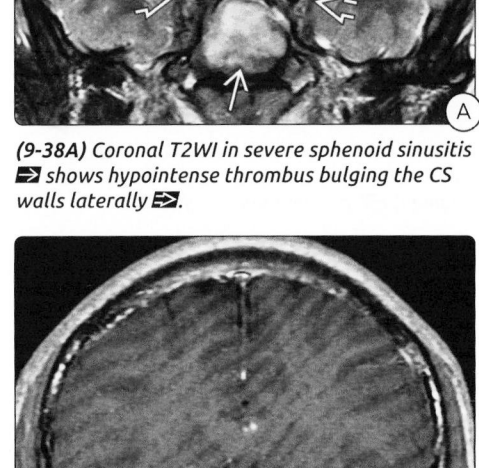

***(9-38A)** Coronal T2WI in severe sphenoid sinusitis shows hypointense thrombus bulging the CS walls laterally.*

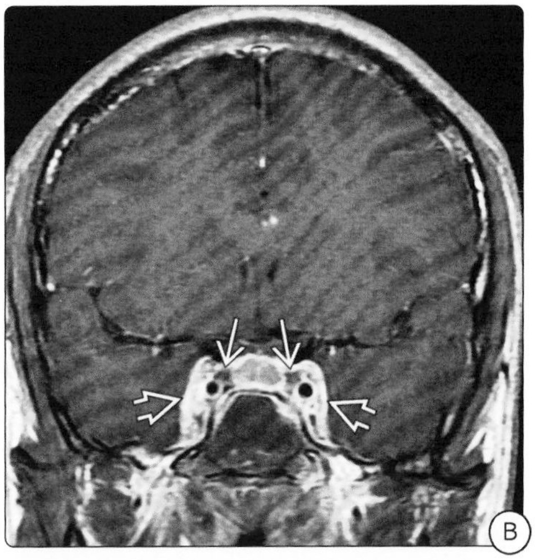

***(9-38B)** Coronal T1 C+ FS in the same case shows bulging CS walls and a nonenhancing thrombus.*

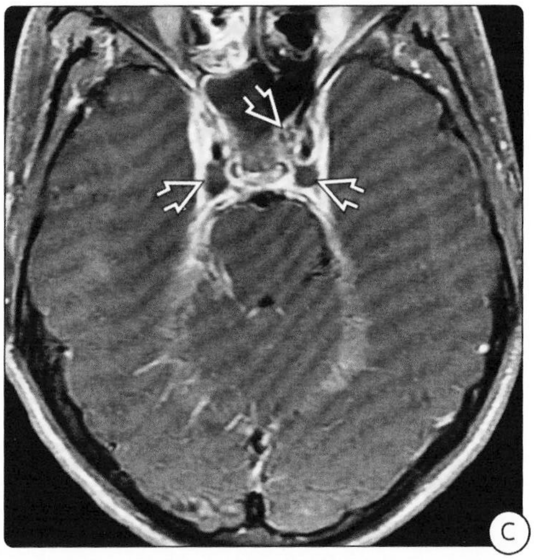

***(9-38C)** Axial T1 C+ FS shows intensely enhancing CS dura surrounding multiple foci of nonenhancing thrombus.*

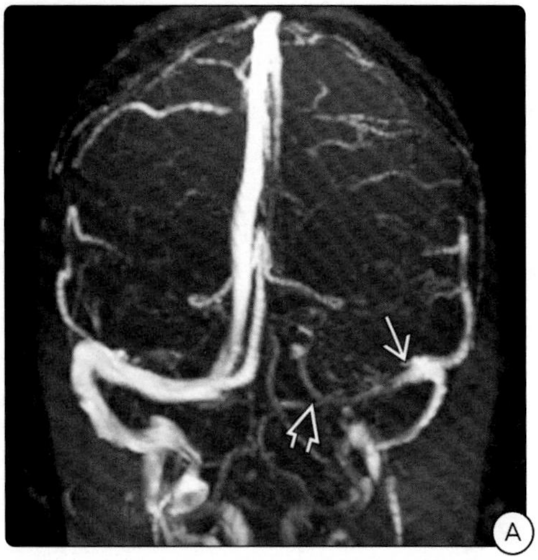

(9-39A) MR venogram in a 22y woman shows a dominant right TS. The left TS shows a "missing" segment, possible filling defect.

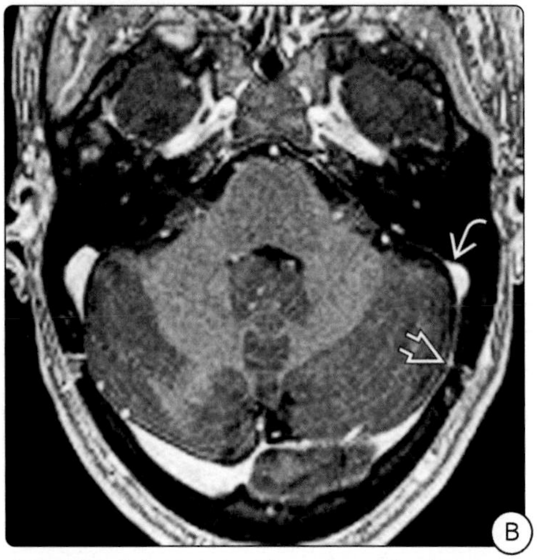

(9-39B) Axial MP-RAGE shows hypoplastic but patent left TS and a small sigmoid sinus.

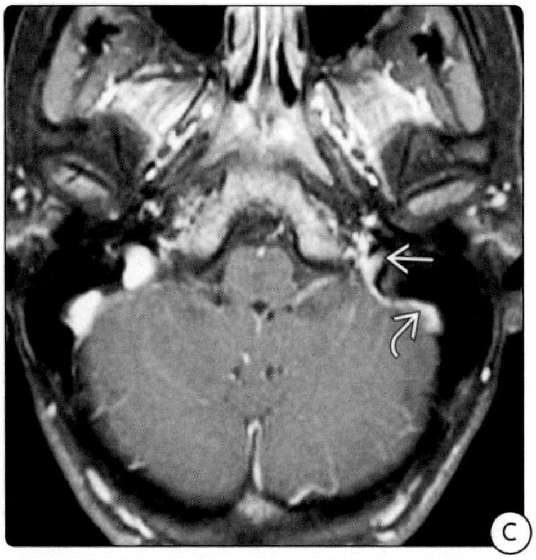

(9-39C) T1 C+ FS shows that the left sigmoid sinus and jugular bulb are hypoplastic. "Missing" left TS is a normal variant (hypoplasia).

Arachnoid Granulations and Septations

Another key differential diagnosis of DST is **giant arachnoid granulation** (AG). Giant AGs are round or ovoid short-segment filling defects that exhibit CSF-like attenuation on NECT and do not enhance on CECT scans **(9-40A)**.

MR appearance of AGs is more problematic than its CT findings. Giant AGs often do not follow CSF signal intensity (SI) on all sequences **(9-40B)**. CSF-incongruent SI is seen on at least one sequence (usually FLAIR) in 80% of MRs. Even large AGs do not fill the entire sinus **(9-40C)**, as most thrombi do, and, unlike clots, may show central linear enhancement. Brain tissue may *herniate* into the dural venous sinuses, often part of a complex giant AG.

Septations or **trabeculations** are fibrotic bands looking like linear filling defects in sinuses. One to five septa are in 30% of TSs, most often right TS.

Other Venous Occlusion Mimics

Less common entities can mimic dural sinus or cerebral vein occlusion: elevated hematocrit, unmyelinated brain, diffuse cerebral edema, and SDH.

High Hematocrit

The most common cause of a false-positive diagnosis of DST on NECT scan is an elevated hematocrit (i.e., patients with polycythemia vera or longstanding right-to-left cardiac shunts) **(9-41)**. This causes the appearance of a hyperdense sinus relative to the brain parenchyma. However, the intracranial arteries in patients with high hematocrits are also similarly hyperdense.

Unmyelinated Brain

Infants and young children often have *higher* hematocrits than adults, with relatively *lower* density of their unmyelinated brains. High-attenuation blood vessels *and* low-attenuation brain make all vascular structures (including dural sinuses and cortical veins) seem relatively hyperdense to dural sinus.

Diffuse Cerebral Edema

Diffuse cerebral edema with decreased attenuation of the cerebral hemispheres makes the dura and all the intracranial vessels—both veins *and* arteries—appear relatively hyperdense compared with the low-density brain.

Subdural Hematoma

Acute SDH that layers along the straight sinus and medial tentorium can cause hyperdensity that may mimic DST on NECTs. Dense thrombus surrounds the less dense flowing blood in the SSS and sinus confluence, mimicking an "empty delta" sign, seen *only* on contrast-enhanced scans!

CEREBRAL VENOUS OCCLUSION MIMICS

Common

- *Anatomic variant*: hypoplastic sinus segment (TS most common); segmented, multichanneled sinus (sinus confluence)
- *Flow artifacts*, *arachnoid granulations*, septations

Less Common

- *High-density blood* (elevated hematocrit): physiologic (infants, high altitude); polycythemia vera; longstanding right-to-left cardiac shunts
- *Low-density brain*: physiologic (unmyelinated); pathologic (diffuse cerebral edema)
- *Subdural hematoma*: layers along dura, sinuses; "empty delta" sign (NECT, not CECT)

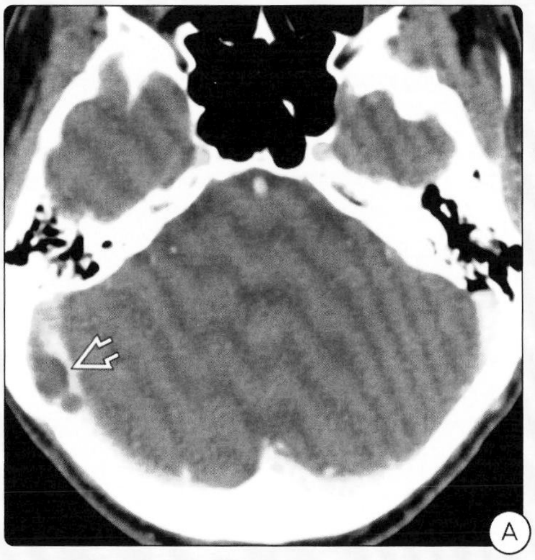

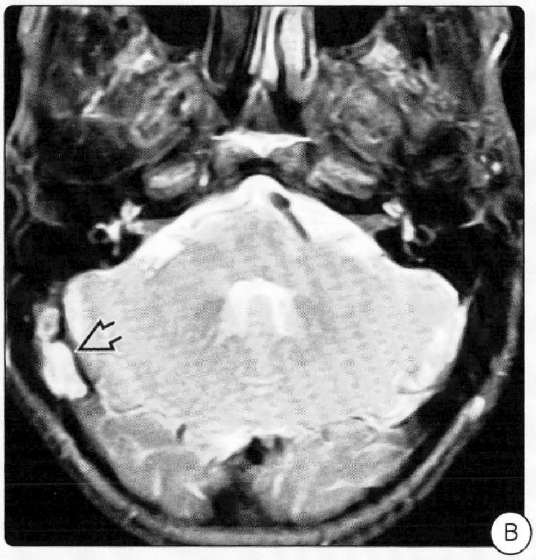

(9-40A) *Axial CTV shows a large CSF-density multiloculated filling defect* ➡ *in the right transverse-sigmoid sinus junction.* ***(9-40B)*** *T2WI in the same case shows that the mass is heterogeneously hyperintense* ⇨, *approximating the signal intensity of CSF.*

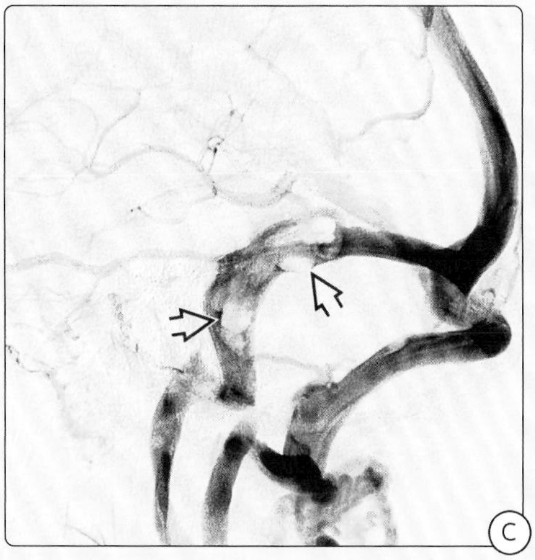

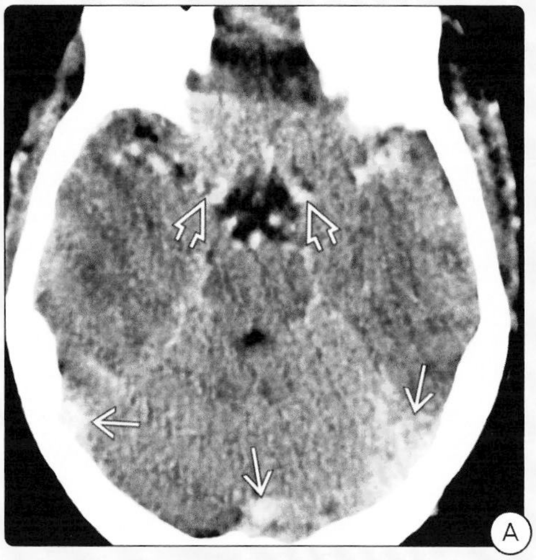

(9-40C) *Venous-phase internal carotid DSA shows large filling defects in the right TS-SS* ⇨. *There are giant arachnoid granulations.* ***(9-41A)*** *Axial NECT in a patient with high hematocrit shows symmetric hyperdensity in the dural sinuses* ➡ *and cranial arteries* ➡.

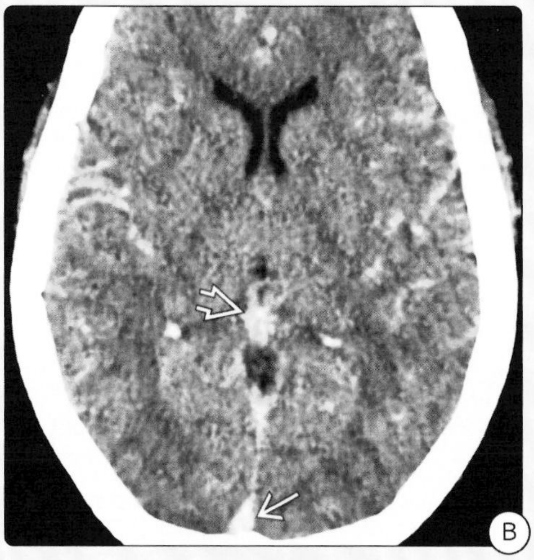

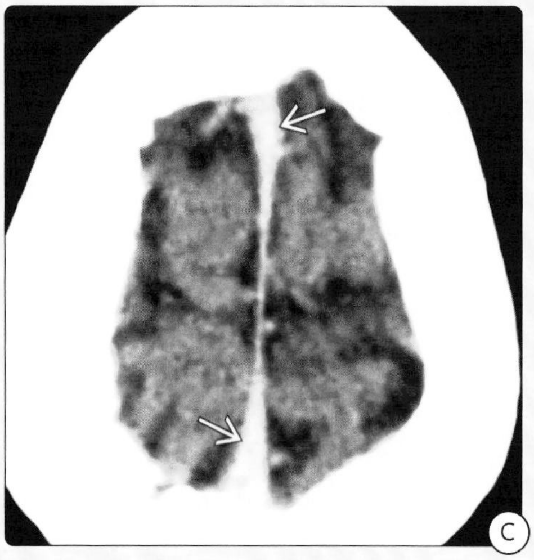

(9-41B) *More cephalad scan shows dense ICVs VofG* ➡, *and SS* ➡. *The middle carotid arteries in both sylvian fissures look as though this were a CECT scan.* ***(9-41C)*** *NECT scan shows the exceptionally hyperdense SSS* ➡. *Polycythemia makes all cerebral vessels look abnormally dense.*

Selected References

Normal Venous Anatomy and Drainage Patterns

Cheng Y et al: Normal anatomy and variations in the confluence of sinuses using digital subtraction angiography. Neurol Res. 39(6):509-515, 2017

Durst CR et al: Prevalence of dural venous sinus stenosis and hypoplasia in a generalized population. J Neurointerv Surg. 8(11):1173-1177, 2016

Kuijf HJ et al: Quantification of deep medullary veins at 7 T brain MRI. Eur Radiol. 26(10):3412-8, 2016

Lublinsky S et al: Automated cross-sectional measurement method of intracranial dural venous sinuses. AJNR Am J Neuroradiol. 37(3):468-74, 2016

Sahin H et al: Bilateral thalamic developmental venous variations (DVVs) draining into same internal cerebral vein: a case report and review with emphasis on DVVs with outflow restriction. Surg Radiol Anat. 38(6):711-6, 2016

Tortora D et al: Variability of cerebral deep venous system in preterm and term neonates evaluated on MR SWI venography. AJNR Am J Neuroradiol. ePub, 2016

Barboza MA et al: Intracranial venous collaterals in cerebral venous thrombosis: clinical and imaging impact. J Neurol Neurosurg Psychiatry. 86(12):1314-8, 2015

Liu MC et al: Time-resolved magnetic resonance angiography in the evaluation of intracranial vascular lesions and tumors: a pictorial essay of our experience. Can Assoc Radiol J. 66(4):385-92, 2015

Schuchardt F et al: In vivo analysis of physiological 3D blood flow of cerebral veins. Eur Radiol. 25(8):2371-80, 2015

Kopelman M et al: Intracranial nonjugular venous pathways: a possible compensatory drainage mechanism. AJNR Am J Neuroradiol. 34(7):1348-52, 2013

Cerebral Venous Thrombosis

Dural Sinus Thrombosis

Konakondla S et al: New developments in the pathophysiology, workup, and diagnosis of dural venous sinus thrombosis (DVST) and a systematic review of endovascular treatments. Aging Dis. 8(2):136-148, 2017

Schuchardt F et al: Acute cerebral venous thrombosis: three-dimensional visualization and quantification of hemodynamic alterations using 4-dimensional flow magnetic resonance imaging. Stroke. 48(3):671-677, 2017

Sheth SA et al: Venous collateral drainage patterns predict clinical worsening in dural venous sinus thrombosis. J Neurointerv Surg. ePub, 2017

Slasky SE et al: Venous sinus thrombosis in blunt trauma: incidence and risk factors. J Comput Assist Tomogr. ePub, 2017

Sadigh G et al: Diagnostic performance of MRI sequences for evaluation of dural venous sinus thrombosis. AJR Am J Roentgenol. 206(6):1298-306, 2016

Sari S et al: MRI diagnosis of dural sinus-cortical venous thrombosis: immediate post-contrast 3D GRE T1-weighted imaging versus unenhanced MR venography and conventional MR sequences. Clin Neurol Neurosurg. 134:44-54, 2015

Bonneville F: Imaging of cerebral venous thrombosis. Diagn Interv Imaging. 95(12):1145-50, 2014

Superficial Cerebral Vein Thrombosis

Boukobza M et al: Radiological findings in cerebral venous thrombosis presenting as subarachnoid hemorrhage: a series of 22 cases. Neuroradiology. 58(1):11-6, 2016

Kim J et al: Isolated cortical venous thrombosis as a mimic for cortical subarachnoid hemorrhage. World Neurosurg. 89:727.e5-7, 2016

Ritchey Z et al: Pediatric cortical vein thrombosis: frequency and association with venous infarction. Stroke. 47(3):866-8, 2016

Ban SP et al: Isolated cortical vein thrombosis with long cord sign. J Korean Neurosurg Soc. 58(5):476-8, 2015

Shastri M et al: Cortical venous thrombosis presenting with subarachnoid haemorrhage. Australas Med J. 8(5):148-53, 2015

Singh R et al: Isolated cortical vein thrombosis: case series. J Neurosurg. 1-7, 2015

Deep Cerebral Venous Thrombosis

Benifla M et al: Unilateral postoperative deep cerebral venous thrombosis with complete recovery: a report of 2 cases. Pediatr Neurosurg. 52(3):205-210, 2017

Taoka T et al: Structure of the medullary veins of the cerebral hemisphere and related disorders. Radiographics. 37(1):281-297, 2017

Cavernous Sinus Thrombosis/Thrombophlebitis

Pannu AK et al: Danger triangle of face and septic cavernous sinus thrombosis. J Emerg Med. ePub, 2017

Wang YH et al: A review of eight cases of cavernous sinus thrombosis secondary to sphenoid sinusitis, including a 12-year-old girl at the present department. Infect Dis (Lond). 49(9):641-646, 2017

Pandey S et al: Bulging and pulsating conjunctiva. JAMA Neurol. 73(4):472-3, 2016

Weerasinghe D et al: Septic cavernous sinus thrombosis: case report and review of the literature. Neuroophthalmology. 40(6):263-276, 2016

Venous Occlusion Mimics

Sinus Variants

Battal B et al: Brain herniations into the dural venous sinus or calvarium: MRI findings, possible causes and clinical significance. Eur Radiol. 26(6):1723-31, 2016

Han K et al: Diagnosis of transverse sinus hypoplasia in magnetic resonance venography: new insights based on magnetic resonance imaging in combined dataset of venous outflow impairment case-control studies: post hoc case-control study. Medicine (Baltimore). 95(10):e2862, 2016

Arachnoid Granulations and Septations

Rodrigues JR et al: Brain herniation into giant arachnoid granulation: an unusual case. Case Rep Radiol. 2017:8532074, 2017

Battal B et al: Brain herniations into the dural venous sinuses or calvarium: MRI of a recently recognized entity. Neuroradiol J. 27(1):55-62, 2014

De Keyzer B et al: Giant arachnoid granulations mimicking pathology. A report of three cases. Neuroradiol J. 27(3):316-21, 2014

Vasculopathy

The generic term "vasculopathy" literally means blood vessel pathology—of any kind, in any vessel (artery, capillary, or vein).

Because diseases such as atherosclerosis are so prevalent, evaluating the craniocervical vessels for vasculopathy is one of the major indications for neuroimaging. Large vessel atherosclerotic vascular disease (ASVD) is the single most prevalent vasculopathy in the head and neck, whereas carotid stenosis or embolization from ASVD plaques are the most common causes of ischemic strokes.

With the advent and widespread availability of multidetector CT angiography, high-resolution noninvasive imaging of the cervical and intracranial vasculature has become common. Digital subtraction angiography (DSA) is now rarely used for diagnostic purposes and is generally performed only as part of a planned endovascular intervention.

In this chapter, we discuss diseases of the craniocervical arteries, first laying a foundation with normal gross and imaging anatomy of the aortic arch and great vessels. We then address the topic of atherosclerosis, starting with a general discussion of atherogenesis. Extracranial ASVD and carotid stenosis are followed by a brief overview of intracranial large and medium artery ASVD.

So-called microvascular ASVD is probably even more common than large vessel disease and its clinical burden vastly underestimated. The section on atherosclerosis concludes with a consideration of arteriolosclerosis.

The broad spectrum of nonatheromatous vasculopathy is then addressed. Finally, we devote the last section of this chapter to non-ASVD diseases of the cerebral macro- and microvasculature. While arteriolosclerosis is by far the most common cause of small vessel vascular disease, nonatherogenic microvasculopathies such as amyloid angiopathy can have devastating clinical consequences.

Normal Anatomy of the Extracranial Arteries

Aortic Arch and Great Vessels

The aorta has four major segments: the ascending aorta, transverse aorta (mostly consisting of the aortic arch), aortic isthmus, and descending aorta.

Aortic Arch

The aortic arch (AA) lies in the superior mediastinum, beginning at the level of the second right sternocostal articulation. It then curves backward and to

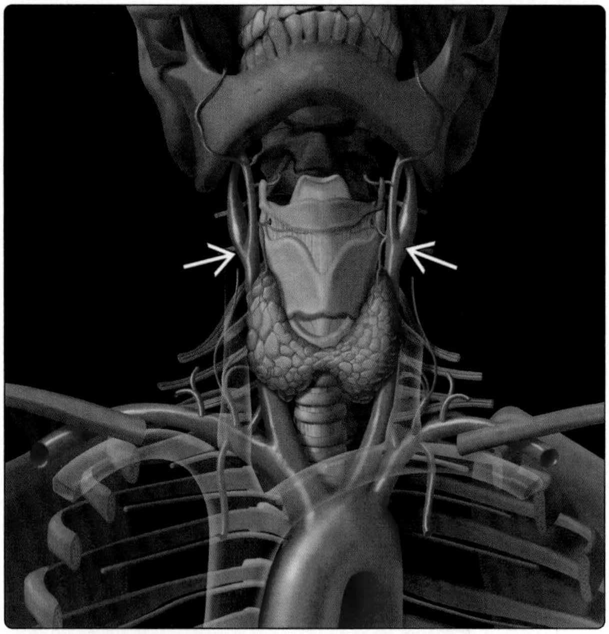

(10-1) AP graphic shows normal aortic arch, its relationship to adjacent structures. Right CCA arises from brachiocephalic trunk, whereas left CCA originates from arch. CCA bifurcations ➡ are around C3-4 level with ICAs initially lateral to ECAs.

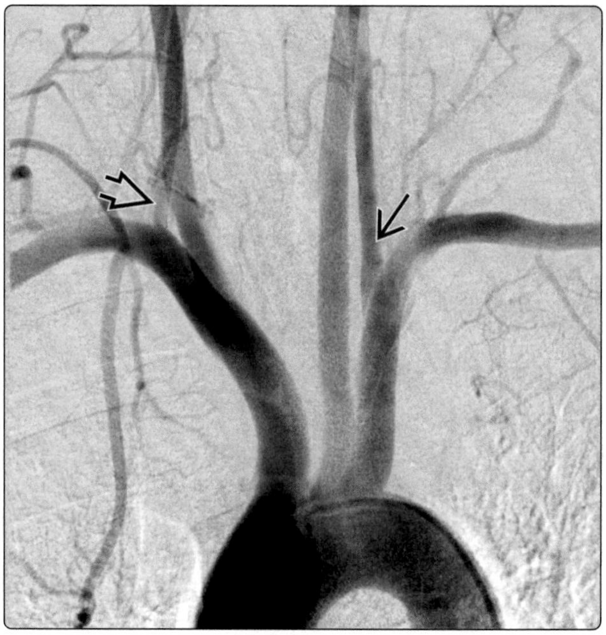

(10-2) DSA shows normal aortic arch, branches. The left vertebral artery (VA) ➡ arises from the proximal left subclavian artery (SCA) and is usually dominant. The right VA ➡ arises from the SCA distal to its origin from the brachiocephalic trunk.

the left over the pulmonary hilum. The AA thus has two curvatures, one that is convex upward and another that is convex forward and curving to the left.

The AA is anatomically related to a number of important structures **(10-1)**. Cervical sympathetic branches and the left CN X (vagus nerve) lie in front of the AA. The trachea, left recurrent laryngeal nerve, esophagus, thoracic duct, and vertebral column lie behind the arch. The great vessels lie above the AA, as does the left brachiocephalic vein. The pulmonary bifurcation, ligamentum arteriosum, and left recurrent laryngeal nerve all lie below the arch.

Great Vessels

Three major vessels arise from the AA. From right to left, these are the brachiocephalic trunk, the left common carotid artery (CCA), and the left subclavian artery (SCA) **(10-2)**. Collectively, these are known as the "great vessels."

Brachiocephalic Trunk. The brachiocephalic trunk (BCT), also called the innominate artery, is the first and largest branch of the AA. It ascends anterior to the trachea. Near the sternoclavicular joint, the BCT bifurcates into the **right SCA** and **right CCA**.

Major branches of the right SCA are the **right internal thoracic (mammary) artery**, **right vertebral artery** (right VA), **right thyrocervical trunk**, and **right costocervical trunk**. The right CCA bifurcates into its two terminal branches, the **right internal carotid artery** (ICA) and **right external carotid artery** (ECA).

Left Common Carotid Artery. The left CCA arises from the apex of the AA just distal to the BCT origin. The left CCA ascends to the left of the trachea, then bifurcates into the left ECA and left ICA near the upper border of the thyroid cartilage. The left CCA lies anteromedial to the internal jugular vein.

Left Subclavian Artery. The left SCA arises from the AA a few millimeters distal to the left CCA origin. The left SCA ascends into the neck, passing lateral to the medial border of the anterior scalene.

Major branches of the left SCA are the **left internal thoracic (mammary) artery**, **left VA**, **left thyrocervical trunk**, and **left costocervical trunk**.

Vascular Territory

The AA and great vessels supply the neck, skull, scalp, and the entire brain.

Normal Variants

The "classic" AA with three "great vessels" originating separately from the arch is seen in 80% of cases **(10-2)**. In 10-25% of cases, the left CCA shares a common V-shaped origin with the BCT (commonly referred to as a "bovine arch," a misnomer, as this configuration bears no resemblance to the AA branching pattern seen in ruminants). The left CCA arises from the proximal BCT in another 5-7% of cases. The left CCA and left SCA share a common origin (a left brachiocephalic trunk) in 1-2%. The left VA originates directly from the AA—not the left SCA—in 0.5-1.0% of cases **(10-3)**.

Three thoracic aorta "lumps and bumps" are normal anatomic variants that should not be mistaken for pathology. The **aortic isthmus** is a narrowed segment just distal to the left SCA and proximal to the site of the fetal ductus arteriosis. An **aortic spindle** is a circumferential bulge in the aorta just beyond the

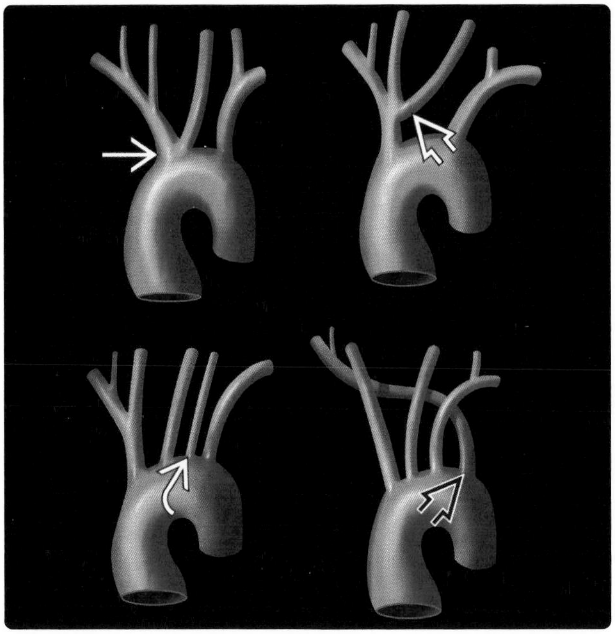

(10-3) Four arch variants are depicted: brachiocephalic trunk (BCT) and R ICA arising from V-shaped common origin, L ICA arising from BCT, L VA arising directly from arch, aberrant R SCA arising from arch as fourth "great vessel".

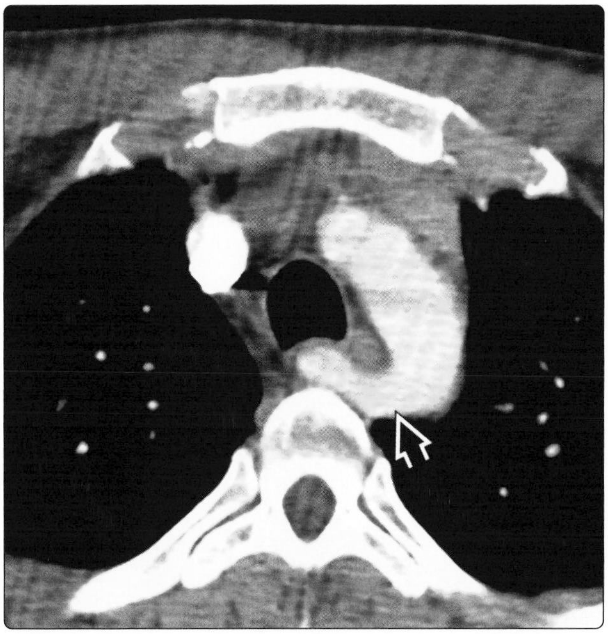

(10-4) Axial source image from a thoracic CTA shows aberrant right SCA arising as the last vessel from the aortic arch and passing behind the trachea.

ductus. Both the aortic isthmus and spindle typically disappear after two postnatal months but can persist into adulthood. A **ductus diverticulum** is a focal bulge along the anteromedial aspect of the aortic isthmus and is seen in 10% of adults.

Anomalies

Only the four most common AA anomalies are briefly discussed here. The most common congenital arch anomaly—seen in 0.5-1.0% of cases—is a **left AA with an aberrant right SCA**. Here the right SCA is the last—not the first—branch to arise from the AA **(10-4)**. Occasionally the aberrant right SCA arises from a dilated, diverticulum-like structure (Kommerell diverticulum). An aberrant right SCA is not associated with congenital heart disease.

Other important anomalies include a **right AA with mirror image branching**, which is strongly associated with cyanotic congenital heart disease (98% prevalence). Two anomalies that are rarely associated with congenital heart disease include a **right AA with aberrant left SCA** and a **double aortic arch** (DAA). In a DAA, each arch gives rise to a ventral carotid artery and a dorsal SCA (symmetric "four-artery" sign).

Cervical Carotid Arteries

The CCAs and their branches provide the major blood supply to much of the neck, all of the face, and the entire brain.

The right CCA arises at the sternoclavicular level and courses superiorly and anteromedially to the internal jugular veins. From its origin at the aortic arch, the left CCA ascends in front of, then lateral to, the trachea. It branches into the left ICA and ECA at the level of the upper thyroid cartilage. The CCA bifurcations are often about C3-C4 or C4-C5 level **(10-1)**.

Internal Carotid Artery

The cervical ICA is entirely extracranial and is designated as the C1 segment. In 90% of cases, the cervical ICA arises from the CCA posterolateral to the ECA.

The C1 ICA has two parts, the carotid bulb and the ascending segment. The **carotid bulb** is the most proximal aspect of the cervical ICA and is seen as a prominent focal dilatation with a cross-sectional area nearly twice as large as that of the distal ICA.

Slipstreams from the CCA strike the CCA bifurcation and divide, with approximately 30% of the flow passing into the ECA. The majority of the flow enters the anterior part of the proximal ICA and continues cephalad. A smaller slipstream actually reverses direction in the bulb, temporarily slowing and stagnating before reestablishing normal antegrade laminar flow with the central slipstream.

The **ascending ICA segment** courses cephalad in the carotid space, a fascially defined tubular sheath that contains all three layers of the deep cervical fascia. The cervical ICA has no normal branches in the neck.

External Carotid Artery

Each ECA has eight major branches **(10-5)**.

The first ECA branch is usually the **superior thyroid artery**, which may also arise from the CCA bifurcation. The superior thyroid artery arises anteriorly from the ECA and courses inferiorly to supply the superior thyroid and larynx. The **ascending pharyngeal artery** arises posteriorly from the ECA (or CCA bifurcation) and courses superiorly between the ECA

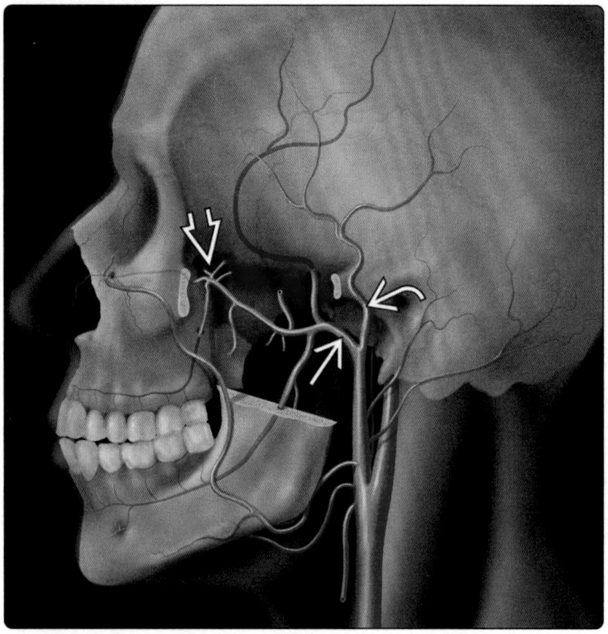

(10-5) Graphic shows that the two terminal ECA branches are the superficial temporal ➡ and maxillary ➡ arteries. The maxillary artery divides into its distal branches within the pterygopalatine fossa ➡.

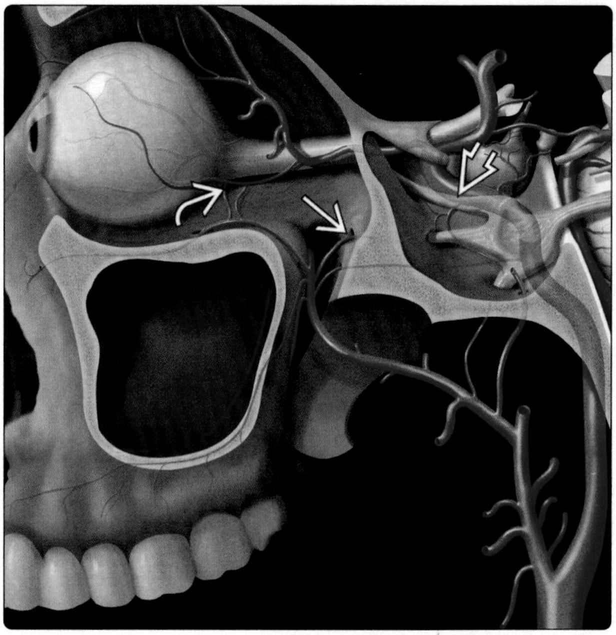

(10-6) Graphic shows numerous anastomoses between the ECA and cavernous ICA, including via the artery of the foramen rotundum ➡, lateral mainstem artery ➡, and ophthalmic artery ➡.

and ICA to supply the naso- and oropharynx, middle ear, dura, and CN IX-CN XI.

The **lingual artery** is the third ECA branch. It loops anteroinferiorly, then courses superiorly to supply the tongue, oral cavity, and submandibular gland. The **facial artery** arises just above the lingual artery, curving around the mandible before it passes anterosuperiorly to supply the face, palate, lips, and cheek.

The next two branches arise from the posterior surface of the ECA. The **occipital artery** courses posterosuperiorly between the skull base and C1 to supply the scalp, upper cervical musculature, and posterior fossa meninges. The **posterior auricular artery** is a smaller branch that also arises from the posterior ECA above the occipital artery. It courses superiorly to supply the ear and scalp.

The superficial temporal artery and maxillary artery are the two terminal branches of the ECA. The **superficial temporal artery** runs superiorly behind the mandibular condyle and loops over the zygoma to supply the scalp.

The **maxillary artery** is the larger of the two terminal ECA branches. Its first major branch is the *middle meningeal artery*, which runs superiorly and enters the calvaria through the foramen spinosum to supply the cranial meninges.

After giving off the middle meningeal artery, the maxillary artery courses anteromedially in the masticator space and then loops into the pterygopalatine fossa, where it terminates by dividing into branches that supply the deep face, paranasal sinuses, and nose.

Numerous anastomotic channels exist between all extracranial branches of the ECAs (except the superior thyroid and lingual arteries) and intracranial branches of the ICAs or musculospinal branches of the VAs **(10-6)**. These anastomoses (summarized in the box below) both provide an important pathway for collateral blood flow and pose a potential risk for intracranial embolization during neurointerventional procedures.

ECA-ICA-VA ANASTOMOSES

Ascending Pharyngeal Artery
- Tympanic branch → petrous ICA
- Several rami → cavernous ICA
- Odontoid arch/musculospinal branches → VA

Facial Artery
- Ophthalmic artery (OA) → intracranial ICA

Occipital Artery
- Transosseous perforators to VA
- To muscular branches of VAs

Posterior Auricular Artery
- Stylomastoid branch to petrous ICA

Superficial Temporal Artery
- Transosseous perforators → anterior falx artery → OA

Maxillary Artery
- Vidian artery → petrous ICA
- Middle meningeal artery → inferolateral trunk → cavernous ICA
- Artery of foramen rotundum → inferolateral trunk → cavernous ICA
- Middle/recurrent meningeal arteries → OA → intracranial ICA
- Deep temporal → OA → intracranial ICA

Atherosclerosis

Atherosclerotic vascular disease (ASVD) is by far the most common cause of mortality and severe long-term disability in industrialized countries, so it is difficult to overemphasize its importance. It affects all arteries, of all sizes, in all parts of the body.

The principal cause of cerebral infarction is atherosclerosis and its sequelae. Over 90% of large cerebral infarcts are caused by thromboemboli secondary to ASVD.

We begin our discussion with an overview of the etiology, biology, and pathology of atherogenesis. We then focus on extracranial ASVD before concluding with a brief discussion of the clinical and imaging manifestations of intracranial ASVD, including its microvascular manifestations.

Atherogenesis and Atherosclerosis

Terminology

The term "atherosclerosis" was originally coined to describe progressive "hardening" or "sclerosis" of blood vessels. The term "atheroma" (Greek for porridge) designates the material deposited on or within vessel walls. "Plaque" is used to describe a focal atheroma together with its epiphenomena, such as ulceration, platelet aggregation, and hemorrhage.

Atherogenesis is the degenerative process that results in atherosclerosis. **Atherosclerosis** is the most common pathologic process affecting large elastic arteries (e.g., the aorta) and medium-sized muscular arteries (e.g., the carotid and vertebral arteries). **Arteriolosclerosis** describes the effects of atherogenesis on smaller arteries (and is treated

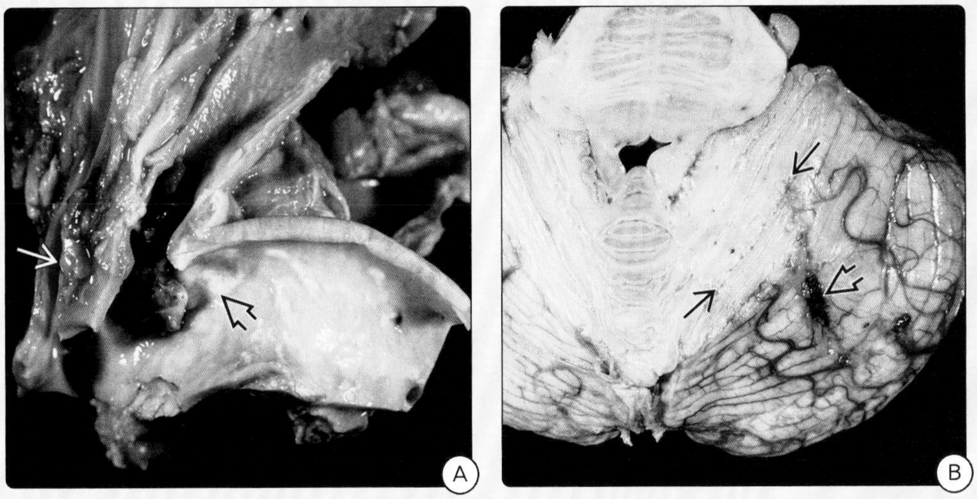

***(10-7A)** Autopsy specimen demonstrates extensive calcification and atherosclerotic vascular disease (ASVD) of the aortic arch ⇨ and proximal great vessels ➡.* ***(10-7B)** Section through the cerebellum, pons in the same case shows old hemorrhagic ⇨ and subacute embolic infarcts ⇨ in the left cerebellar hemisphere.*

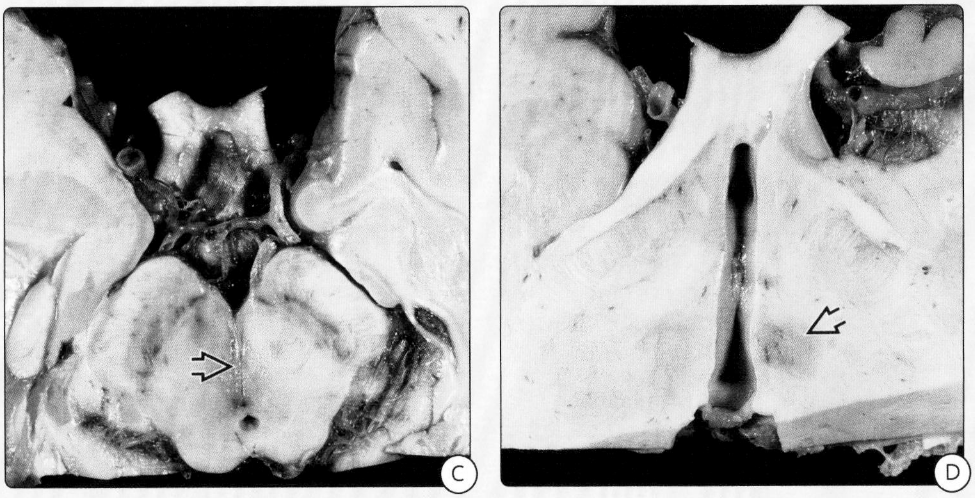

***(10-7C)** Section through the midbrain in the same case shows an old midline penetrating artery infarction ⇨, possibly secondary to an artery of Percheron occlusion.* ***(10-7D)** More cephalad section through the inferior third ventricle shows a subacute inferomedial thalamic infarct ⇨, consistent with artery of Percheron occlusion. (Courtesy R. Hewlett, MD.)*

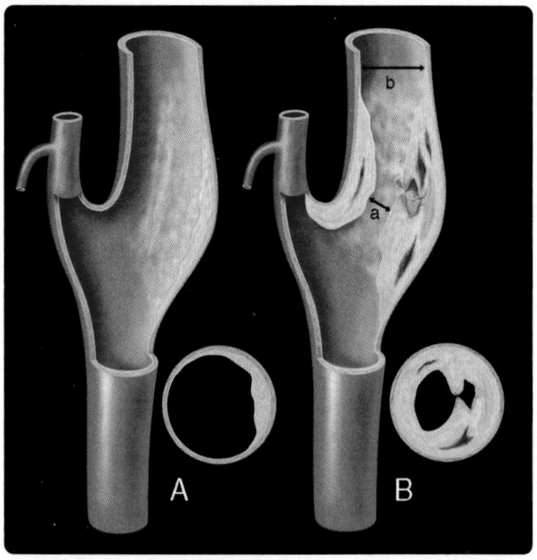

(10-8) (A) Mild ASVD with "fatty streaks." (B) Severe ASVD; % stenosis = (b - a)/b x 100; b = normal lumen, a = residual lumen diameter.

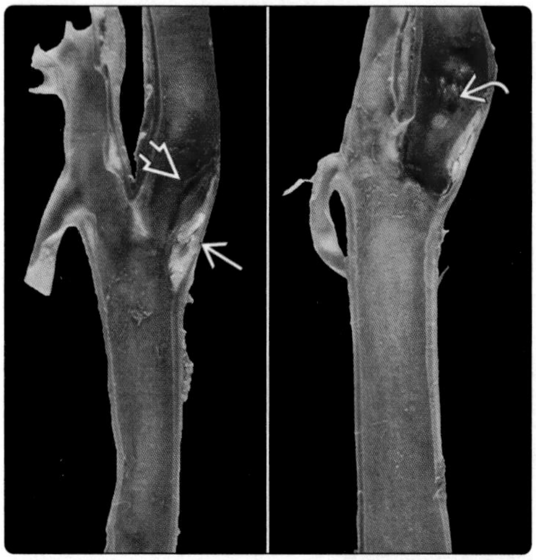

(10-9) (L) Stable ASVD shows fatty plaque, intact intima. (R) Initially "at-risk" plaque now shows ulceration, disrupted intima.

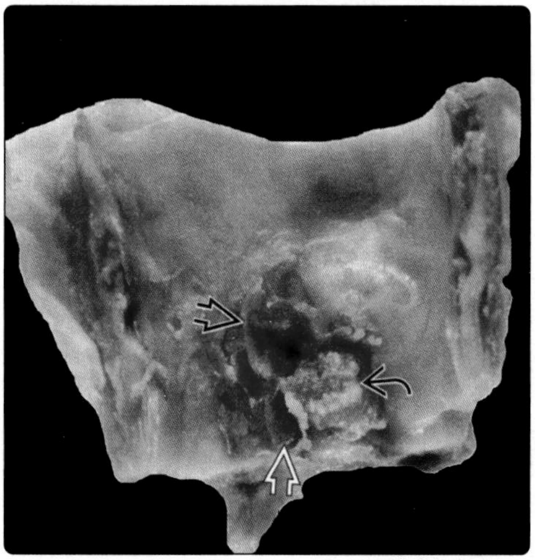

(10-10) Carotid endarterectomy shows ulcerated intima, calcification, intraplaque hemorrhage. (Courtesy J. Townsend, MD.)

separately at the end of this section). **ASVD** is the generic term describing atherosclerosis in any artery, of any size, in any area of the body.

Etiology

General Concepts. Atherosclerosis is a complex, slowly developing process that begins in the early teenage years and progresses over decades. Its causes are multifactorial but appear to be a combination of lipid retention, oxidation, and modification, which in turn incites chronic inflammation. Plasma lipids, connective tissue fibers, and inflammatory cells accumulate at susceptible sites in arterial walls, forming focal atherosclerotic plaques.

Active inflammatory, innate immune, and adaptive immune mechanisms all play a key role in ASVD development. Chronic exposure to low-density lipoproteins (LDLs) modified by oxidation activates endothelial cells, inducing expression of adhesion molecules, matrix metalloproteinases, and inflammatory genes. Monocyte accumulation and macrophage differentiation are also induced as part of the inflammatory process.

Neoangiogenesis is closely associated with plaque progression and is likely the primary source of intraplaque hemorrhage. Angiogenic factors cause vasa vasorum proliferation, formation of immature vessels, and loss of capillary basement membranes. Red blood cells leak into the plaque, inducing further inflammation and increasing the risk of plaque ulceration and rupture.

Genetics. The process of ASVD plaque development is the same regardless of race/ethnicity, sex, or geographic location. However, the *rate* at which plaques develop is faster in patients with genetic predisposition and acquired risk factors, such as hypertension, smoking, type 2 diabetes, and obesity.

No single predisposing mutation for ASVD has yet been identified. To date, most investigators conclude that ASVD probably reflects the interaction of multiple intrinsic (genetic) and extrinsic (environmental) factors. A genome-wide association approach has identified multiple foci that influence the risk of systemic ASVD, especially in the setting of incidental coronary heart disease.

Pathology

Location. The entire vasculature is exposed to similar environmental and genetic influences. In theory, ASVD lesions should occur randomly, with every artery—from large elastic arteries to arterioles—equally at risk of developing ASVD. Instead, ASVD occurs preferentially at highly predictable locations. In the extracranial vasculature, the most common sites are the proximal internal carotid arteries (ICAs) and common carotid artery (CCA) bifurcations, followed by the aortic arch and great vessel origins **(10-7)**.

The proximal ICA exhibits an anatomic feature unlike that found in any other vessel, i.e., the **carotid bulb**. This focal postbifurcation enlargement—together with the CCA branching angle—promotes both flow separation and recirculation/stasis in the bulb. The unusual flow patterns generated by this unique geometry result in increased particle residence time and low, oscillating wall shear stresses in the outer wall of the carotid bulb. This may account for the unusually high prevalence of atheromas at this particular location.

Size and Number. ASVD plaques vary in size from small, almost microscopic lipid deposits to large, raised, fungating, ulcerating lesions that can extend over several centimeters and dramatically narrow the parent vessel lumen. Most plaques are 0.3-1.5 cm in diameter. With ASVD, multiple lesions in multiple locations are the rule.

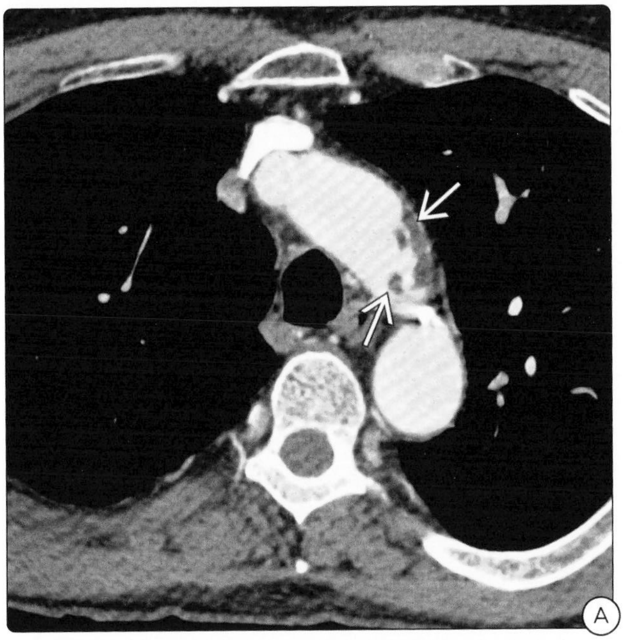

(10-11A) Axial CTA source image shows irregular, ulcerated atherosclerotic plaque ➡ along the aortic arch, proximal descending thoracic aorta.

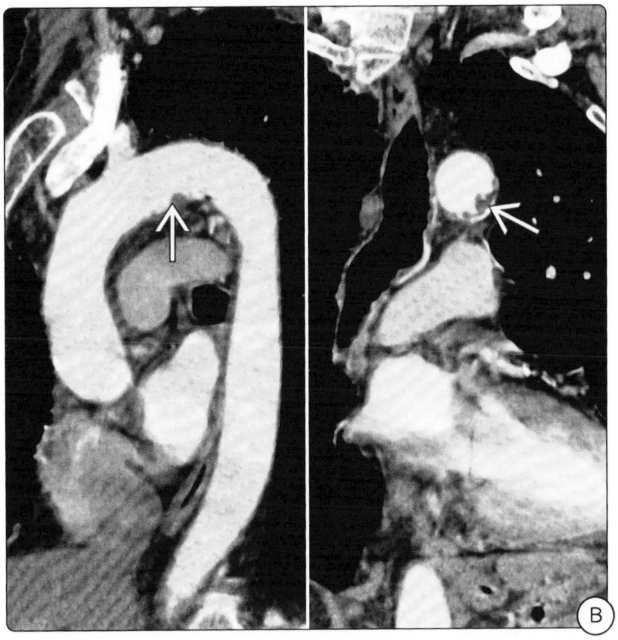

(10-11B) (L) "Candy cane" and (R) coronal views in the same case show the plaque ➡ along the lesser curvature of the aortic arch. (Courtesy G. Oliveira, MD.)

Gross Pathology. ASVD plaques develop in stages (**10-8**). The first detectable lesion is lipid deposition in the intima, seen as yellowish "fatty streaks." Other than "fatty streaks" and slightly eccentric but smooth intimal thickening, visible changes at this early stage are minimal.

Microscopic Features. ASVD plaques are classified histopathologically as "stable," "vulnerable," or "ulcerated."

Stable plaques. Uncomplicated **stable plaques**—the basic lesions of atherosclerosis—consist of cellular material (smooth muscle cells, monocytes, and macrophages), lipid (both intracellular and extracellular deposits), and an overlying fibrous cap (composed of collagen, elastic fibers, and proteoglycans). The intima covering a stable plaque is thickened, but its exterior surface remains intact, without disruption or ulceration. No intraplaque hemorrhage is present (**10-9**).

Vulnerable plaques. As a necrotic core of lipid-laden foam cells, cellular debris, and cholesterol gradually accumulates under the elevated fibrous cap, the cap thins and becomes prone to rupture (**"vulnerable" plaque**) (**10-9**).

Proliferating small blood vessels also develop around the periphery of the necrotic core. **Neovascularization** can lead to **subintimal hemorrhage** with rapid expansion, which increases pressure inside the plaque, promotes increasing lipid deposition, and enlarges the necrotic core, further weakening the overlying fibrous cap.

Ulcerated plaques. Plaque **ulceration** occurs when the fibrous cap weakens and ruptures through the intima, releasing necrotic debris (**10-10**). Slowly swirling blood within the ulcerated denuded endothelium first allows platelets and fibrin to aggregate. An intermittent Bernoulli effect then pulls the aggregates into the rapidly flowing main artery slipstream, causing arterioarterial embolization to distal intracranial vessels.

Clinical Issues

Epidemiology and Demographics. Although atherogenesis actually begins in the mid-teens, most patients with symptomatic lesions are middle-aged or elderly. However, atherosclerosis is increasingly common in younger patients, contributing to the rising prevalence of strokes in patients younger than 45 years.

There is a moderate male predominance. Although all ethnicities are affected, African Americans are at highest risk for ASVD.

Presentation. The clinical presentation of craniocervical ASVD is highly variable. As ASVD is generally a slowly progressive disorder, many lesions remain asymptomatic until they cause hemodynamically significant stenosis or thromboembolic disease. A carotid bruit may be the first clinically detectable sign of ICA stenosis. Transient ischemic attacks (TIAs) and "silent strokes" are common precursors of large territorial infarcts.

Natural History. The natural history of ASVD is also highly variable. ICA occlusion poses an especially high risk for eventual stroke, with over 70% of these patients eventually experiencing ischemic cerebral infarction.

Treatment Options. Treatment options include prevention, medical therapy (lipid-lowering regimens), and surgery or endovascular therapy (see below).

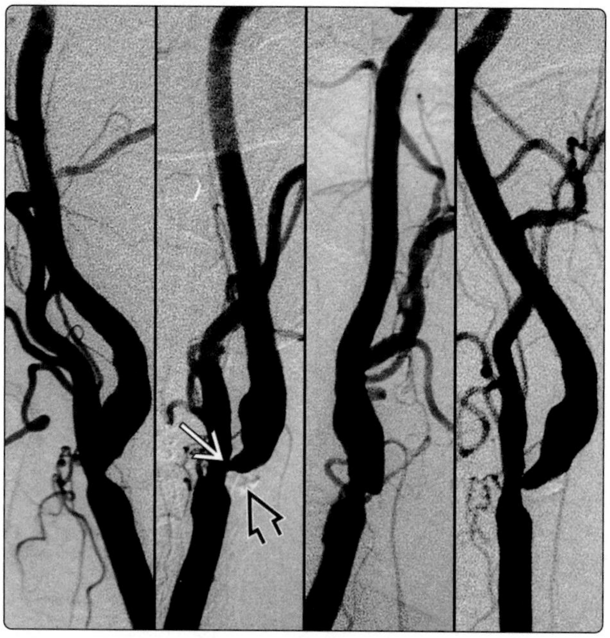

***(10-12)** Four-view DSA shows the importance of multiple projections to profile maximum proximal ICA stenosis ➡ and calcified plaque ⇨.*

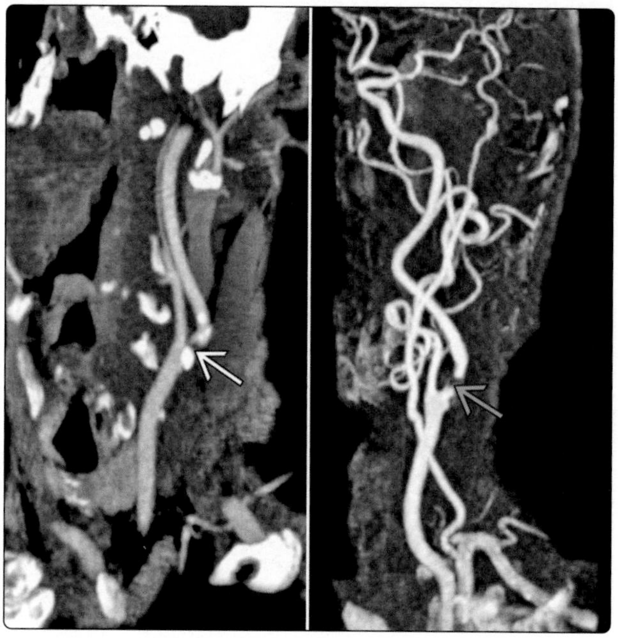

***(10-13)** (L) DSA shows critical ICA stenosis ➡. (R) MRA in the same case shows a "flow gap" ⇨ characteristic of a high-grade flow-limiting lesion.*

Extracranial Atherosclerosis

Extracranial ASVD is the single largest risk factor for stroke. That risk starts with the aortic arch.

Because DSA carries a small but definite risk, noninvasive imaging modalities are preferable screening procedures to evaluate patients for extracranial atherosclerosis and its complications. The major noninvasive options are CTA, high-resolution MRA, and ultrasound (US). Each technique has its advocates, advantages, disadvantages, cost considerations, and special "use case" scenarios. Many investigators recommend duplex US as the initial screening test in patients with recent TIAs or minor ischemic stroke, followed by CTA for those with positive results.

In-depth analysis and comparison of the many available vascular imaging modalities are beyond the scope of this book. We focus instead on ASVD in major anatomic sites, using examples of each technique as appropriate to demonstrate the relevant pathology.

Aortic Arch and Great Vessels

The aortic arch is an underrecognized source of intracranial ischemic strokes. Complete imaging evaluation of patients with thromboembolic infarcts in the brain should include investigation of the aortic arch.

Etiology. Aortic ASVD is more common in the descending thoracic aorta than in the ascending aorta or arch **(10-11)**. However, late diastolic retrograde flow from complex plaques in the proximal descending aorta distal to the left subclavian artery (SCA) origin can reach all supraaortic arteries. Retrograde flow extends to the left SCA orifice in nearly 60% of cases, the left CCA in 25%, and the brachiocephalic trunk in 10-15%.

Aortic emboli involve the left brain in 80% of cases and show a distinct predilection for the vertebrobasilar circulation. This striking geographic distribution is consistent with thromboemboli arising from ulcerated plaques in the descending aorta that are then swept by retrograde flow into left-sided arch vessels.

Epidemiology. Arch atherosclerosis is a documented independent risk factor for stroke, found on imaging studies in 10-20% of patients with acute ischemic infarcts and 25% of fatal strokes at autopsy. Ulcerated aortic plaques are present at autopsy in 60% of patients who died from cerebral infarction of unknown etiology. Aortic ASVD constitutes the only probable source of retinal emboli or cerebral infarction in nearly 25% of patients with "cryptogenic stroke," i.e., no likely cardiac or carotid source can be identified.

Imaging. The aortic arch and proximal descending aorta should be visualized together with the extracranial and intracranial vasculature. Some investigators now advocate a comprehensive "triple rule-out" CTA for acute ischemic stroke that also includes the heart and coronary arteries. Intravenous contrast is necessary to define the presence of mural thrombus, determine plaque extent, and evaluate the aortic wall for complications such as ulceration, aneurysm, and dissection.

The most common general imaging finding in aortic ASVD is irregular mural thickening with calcifications. Imaging features of aortic ASVD that are strongly correlated with stroke include atheromas located proximal to the left subclavian ostium,

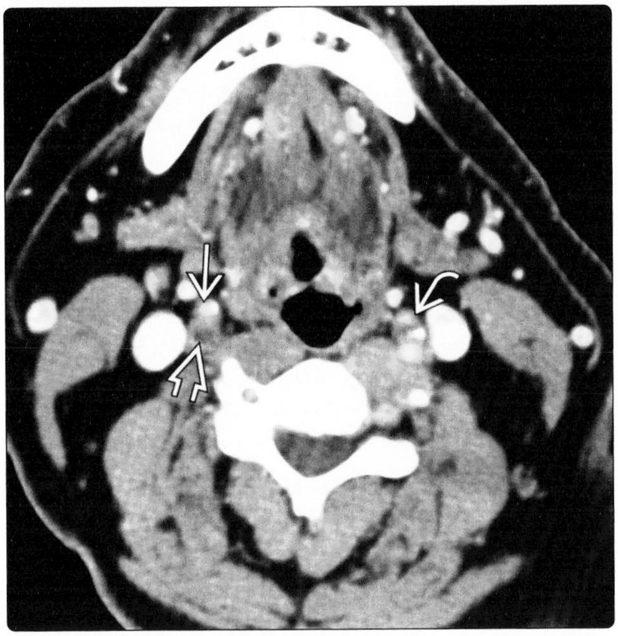

(10-14) CECT in a 60y man with stroke shows a very faint dot of enhancement ➡ in the right proximal ICA. High-grade stenosis is caused by a "soft" ASVD plaque with hypodense lipid ➡. The left ICA ➡ is irregular, stenotic.

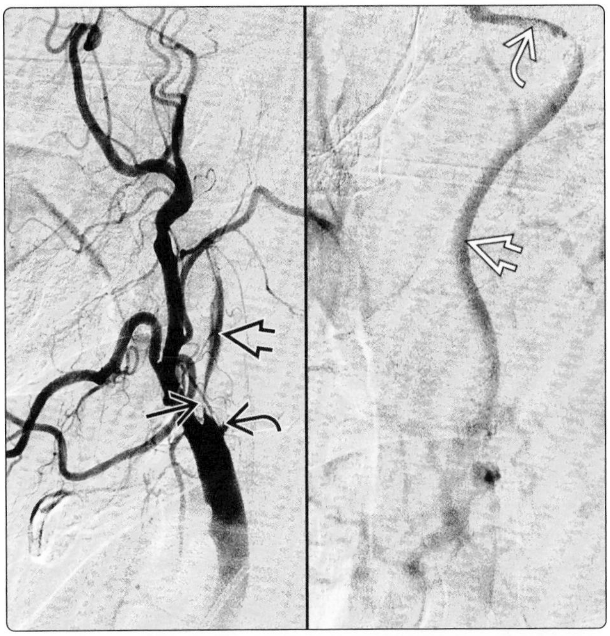

(10-15) (L) DSA shows ulcerated plaque ➡ causing high-grade, near-total stenosis ➡ with a "string" sign ➡. (R) Late phase shows the distal cervical ICA ➡. Filling defects ➡ are caused by thrombus.

plaques at least 4 mm in diameter that protrude into the aortic lumen, and the presence of mobile/oscillating thrombi.

Carotid Bifurcation/Internal Carotid Arteries

Between 20-30% of all ischemic infarcts are caused by carotid artery stenosis **(10-12)**. Therefore, determining the degree of carotid stenosis on imaging studies is now both routine and required.

Three studies have shown the benefits of endarterectomy in patients with definable carotid stenosis: the North American Symptomatic Carotid Endarterectomy Trial (NASCET), the European Carotid Surgery Trial (ECST), and the Asymptomatic Carotid Atherosclerosis Group (ACAS).

Although these studies used DSA as the gold standard for determining percentage of stenosis, recent studies have demonstrated a linear relationship between direct millimeter carotid stenosis measures on CTA and derived percentage of stenosis as defined by NASCET. These studies have demonstrated the efficacy of carotid endarterectomy, angioplasty, or stenting in symptomatic patients with ICA stenosis of 70% or greater.

Carotid stenosis is classified as moderate (50-69%), severe (70-93%), and "preocclusive" or critical (94-99%) **(10-13)** **(10-15)**. Patients with critical stenosis are at high risk for embolic stroke as long as the ICA lumen is patent.

In addition to stenosis degree, several recent studies have demonstrated the importance of also assessing the morphologic features of ASVD plaques. Rupture of an "at-risk" plaque with a large necrotic core under a thin fibrous cap is responsible for the majority of acute thrombi. As distal embolization from proximal ASVD-related clots is a common cause of cerebral ischemia/infarction, *identifying rupture-prone "vulnerable" plaques is at least as important as determining stenosis!*

CT Findings. The most common imaging findings in extracranial ASVD are mural calcifications, luminal irregularities, varying degrees of vessel stenosis, occlusion, and thrombosis. Elongation, ectasia, and vessel tortuosity can occur with or without other changes of ASVD.

NECT scans easily show vessel wall calcifications. Smooth plaques and extensive coalescent calcifications are associated with *decreased* risk of plaque rupture. Large atherosclerotic plaques may demonstrate one or more subintimal low-density foci. These represent the lipid-rich core of a "soft" plaque **(10-14)**. High-density subintimal foci indicate intraplaque hemorrhage. Both findings carry increased risk of plaque rupture and concomitant distal embolization.

CECT and CTA source images display the carotid lumen in cross section. Nonstenotic smooth luminal narrowing is the most common finding in ASVD. Ulcerations—seen as irregularly shaped contrast-filled outpouchings from the lumen—are detected with 95% sensitivity and 99% specificity. Occlusion and intraluminal thrombi are also readily demonstrated.

CTA is as accurate as DSA in determining ICA stenosis. Although some carotid stenoses are irregularly shaped and noncircular, measurement of the narrowest stenosis is a reasonably reliable predictor of cross-sectional area. Differentiating total from near occlusion is essential, as patients with occlusion are usually treated medically, whereas

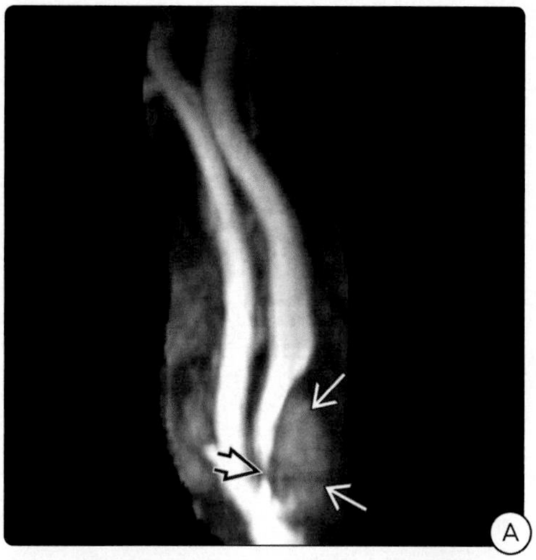

(10-16A) Oblique 3.0-T MRA shows very high-grade stenosis of the right carotid artery with a "flow gap" ⇨ caused by a large ASVD plaque ➡.

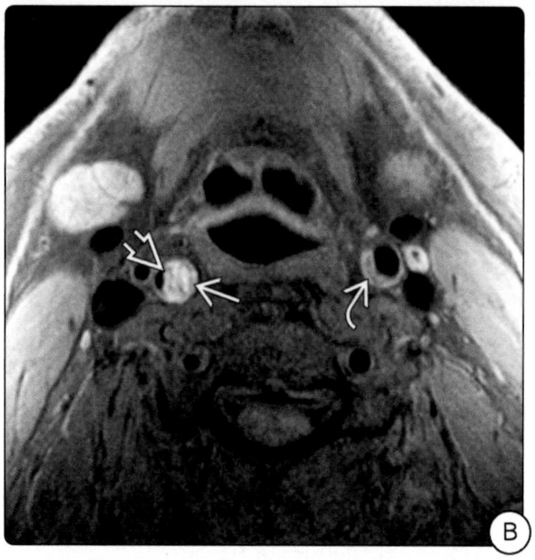

(10-16B) MP-RAGE shows intraplaque hemorrhage ➡ with tiny residual lumen ➡ in the R ICA, subintimal hemorrhage ➡ in the L ICA.

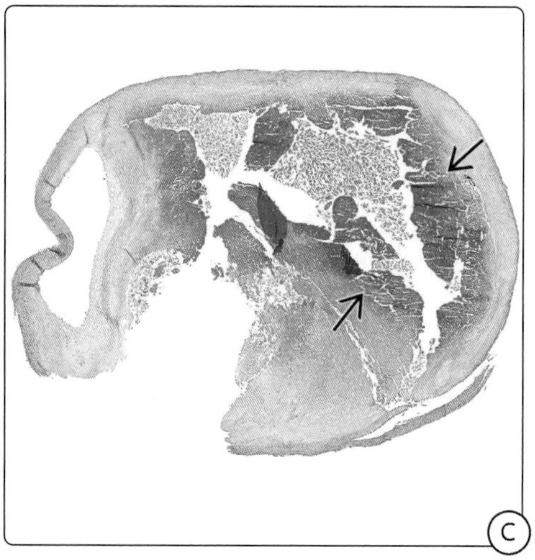

(10-16C) Right ICA endarterectomy shows that plaque hyperintensity is due to acute hemorrhage ⇨, not lipid. (Courtesy S. McNally, MD.)

patients with high-grade lesions are eligible for emergent surgery or endovascular treatment.

In addition to calculating percentage of stenosis **(10-8)**, plaque morphologic characteristics should be described in detail, as decision making is not based solely on stenosis degree. By itself, stenosis does not define complete stroke risk in symptomatic patients with < 70% stenosis or across all levels of stenoses in asymptomatic patients.

MR Findings. High-resolution MR imaging can be used to characterize carotid plaques, allowing identification of individual plaque components, including lipids, hemorrhage, fibrous tissue, and calcification. Intraplaque hemorrhage has been identified as an independent risk factor for ischemic stroke at *all* degrees of stenosis, including symptomatic patients with low-grade lesions (< 50%). Therefore accurate characterization of plaque morphology is important for patient management.

High signal intensity on T1-weighted fat-suppressed scans, MRA source images, or MP-RAGE sequences represents hemorrhage into complicated "vulnerable" atherosclerotic plaques, not lipid accumulation **(10-16)**. Unlike intraparenchymal brain bleeds, plaque hemorrhages may remain hyperintense up to 18 months. Vulnerable plaques are usually hyperintense on T2WI, whereas stable plaques are isointense on both T1- and T2WI.

T1 C+ FS scans may show enhancement around plaque margins, consistent with neovascularity in a vulnerable "at-risk" plaque.

Contrast-enhanced or unenhanced 2D TOF MRA is 80-85% sensitive and 95% specific for the detection of ICA > 70% ICA stenosis. Signal loss with a "flow gap" occurs if the stenosis is > 95%. Compared with CTA and DSA, MRA tends to overestimate the degree of stenosis.

DSA. Although DSA is generally considered the gold standard of vascular imaging—especially for documenting carotid stenosis/occlusion prior to surgical or endovascular intervention—it is no longer generally used as an initial screening procedure. DSA is occasionally utilized for the detailed assessment of collateral circulation patterns.

Plaque ulceration is seen on DSA as surface irregularity in the opacified vessel lumen **(10-15)**. The reported sensitivity of detecting plaque ulceration on DSA varies between 50-85%. Surface irregularity on DSA is associated with increased stroke risk at all degrees of stenosis.

Carotid stenosis can be identified and calculated on DSA. At least two or more views are required to profile the maximal stenosis **(10-12)**. The NASCET calculation for percentage of stenosis is the normal lumen diameter minus the minimal residual lumen diameter divided by the normal lumen diameter multiplied by 100 **(10-8)**. A 2-mm residual lumen with a 10-mm diameter represents an 80% stenosis.

"Tandem lesions" are stenoses distal to a more proximal lesion and are seen in approximately 2% of patients with hemodynamically significant cervical ICA stenosis. The most common site for a "tandem lesion" is the cavernous ICA.

Carotid thrombosis is seen as an intraluminal filling defect in the contrast column **(10-15)**. Carotid occlusion is seen as contrast ending blindly in a blunted, rounded, or pointed pouch in the proximal ICA.

High-grade stenosis causes very slow antegrade flow with delayed contrast washout. A **"string" sign** is present when only a "trickle" ("string") of antegrade flow is detected at DSA or color Doppler. The string sign—also called carotid pseudocollusion or preocclusion—represents > 95% stenosis **(10-15)**. Such patients are at especially high short-term risk for stroke.

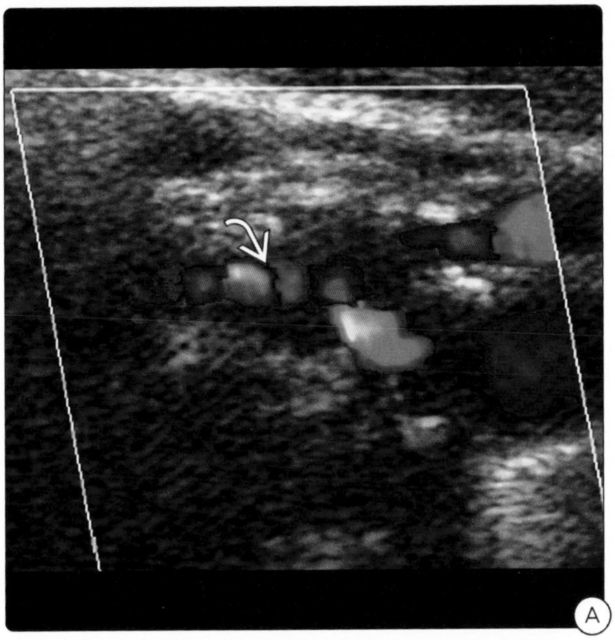

(10-17A) Longitudinal color Doppler ultrasound shows high-grade ICA stenosis. The arterial lumen is significantly narrowed with "aliasing" flow artifact ➡ because of increased flow velocity.

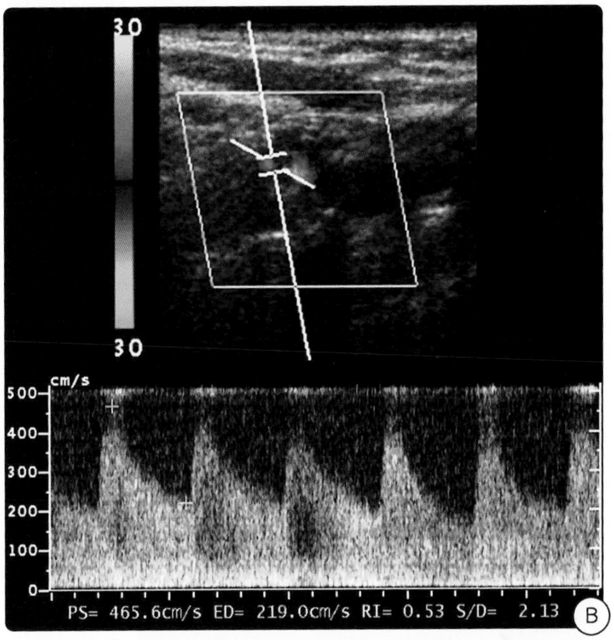

(10-17B) Spectral Doppler analysis in the same case shows findings of stenosis. Both peak systolic velocity and end-diastolic velocity are markedly increased, consistent with stenosis > 70%. (Courtesy S. S. M. Ho, MBBs.)

Examining the late venous phase of the DSA is critical to document subtle arterial patency, as this will determine whether emergent endarterectomy or stenting is a treatment option.

Ultrasound. US imaging includes grayscale US, color Doppler with color velocity imaging, power Doppler, and spectral Doppler analysis **(10-17)**.

Grayscale ultrasound. Grayscale US shows a fatty or "soft" plaque as hypoechoic, whereas a fibrous plaque is mildly echogenic. Calcified plaque is highly echogenic with distal shadowing. An ulcerated plaque appears as a focal crypt with sharp or overhanging edges. Occluded vessels show absent flow with echogenic material filling the vessel lumen.

Color Doppler. Stenosis < 50% shows relatively uniform intraluminal color hues at and distal to the stenosis. Stenosis greater than 50% shows mildly disturbed intraluminal color hues at and distal to the stenosis.

Stenosis > 70% shows color scale shift or "aliasing" caused by elevated velocity at the stenosis together with significant poststenotic turbulence. Occluded vessels show absent color flow, whereas high-grade near-occlusions may show a thin "trickle" of color.

Power Doppler. Power Doppler is useful in detecting low-velocity flow at and distal to preocclusive stenoses. Power Doppler is especially helpful in differentiating patent, preocclusive (high-grade) stenosis from occlusion.

Spectral Doppler. Spectral Doppler is useful for estimating the degree of stenosis from velocity parameters. Peak systolic velocity (PSV) is the most common, recommended measurement. Other useful measurements include the systolic velocity ratio (SVR), which is ICA stenosis/normal CCA, and end-diastolic velocity (EDV). PSV and EDV rise with increasing stenosis.

High-grade, near-occlusive stenoses demonstrate variable velocity. High flow resistance may actually decrease the PSV, so diagnosis is based on color Doppler appearance and damped waveforms distal to the stenosis.

VELOCITY PARAMETERS

In < 50% Stenosis
- PSV < 125 cm/s; EDV < 40 cm/s; SVR < 2.0

In 50-69% Stenosis
- PSV = 125-229 cm/s; EDV = 40-99 cm/s; SVR = 2.0-3.9

In ≥ 70% Stenosis
- PSV > 230 cm/s; EDV > 100 cm/s; SVR ≥ 4.0

Vertebral Arteries

ASVD in the extracranial vertebral arteries accounts for up to 20% of all posterior circulation ischemic strokes. Because the risk of selective vertebral artery (VA) catheterization in the presence of vasculopathy is 0.5-4.0%, noninvasive imaging with CTA or MRA is preferable. However, the tortuous course of the VA, great variability in normal caliber, thick bony covering, and presence of adjacent veins all create special challenges for the radiologist. The right VA is adequately visualized from its origin to the basilar confluence in only 75% of patients, and the left VA is well seen in approximately 70%.

Although mid- and distal cervical segment lesions occur, extracranial ASVD is most common at or near the VA origin

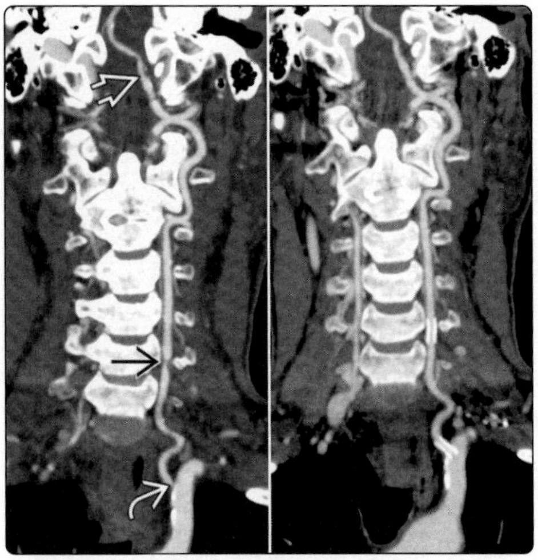

(10-18) (L) Severe VA origin ➨, moderate midcervical stenosis ➞. Intracranial ASVD ➨. (R) Post-stent CTA. (Courtesy C. Baccin, MD.)

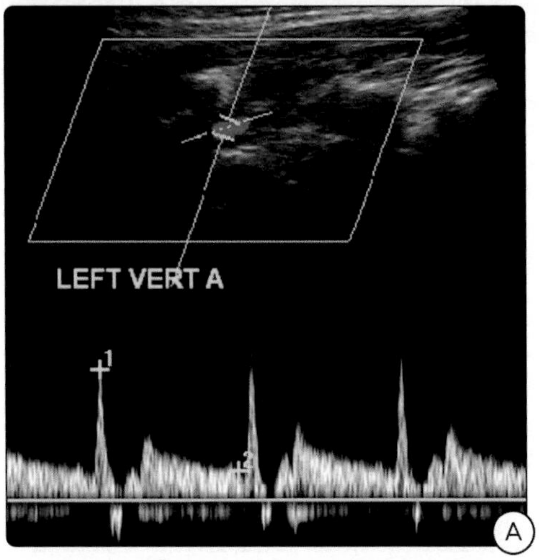

(10-19A) Longitudinal color Doppler ultrasound shows mild subclavian steal when the patient rests the arm.

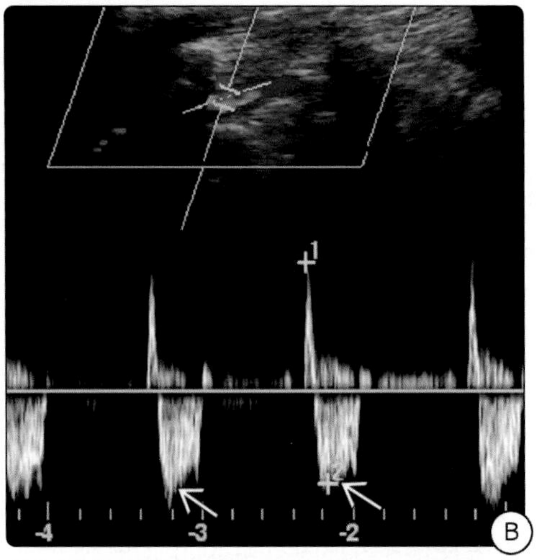

(10-19B) Steal is aggravated after arm exercise. Doppler waveform alternates with increasing retrograde flow ➨. (Courtesy S. S. M. Ho, MBBs.)

(10-18). Calcification and stenosis are the most common findings. CTA, MRA, color Doppler sonography, and DSA can all provide diagnostic images.

A special type of VA pathology is called **subclavian steal**. Here the SCA or brachiocephalic trunk is severely stenotic or occluded *proximal* to the vertebral artery origin. Flow reversal in the affected VA occurs as blood is recruited (i.e., "stolen") from the opposite VA, crosses the basilar artery (BA) junction, and flows in retrograde fashion down the VA into the SCA to supply the shoulder and arm distal to the stenosis/occlusion **(10-20)**.

Subclavian steal can be complete or partial, symptomatic or occult, and is often an incidental finding. Symptomatic patients present with posterior circulation symptoms secondary to vertebrobasilar insufficiency and brainstem ischemia. Episodic dizziness, diplopia, dysarthria, nausea, and visual disturbances are typical and are aggravated by exercise of the affected arm and shoulder. Significant blood pressure differential (> 20 mm Hg) between arms is usually associated with symptomatic subclavian steal.

Noninvasive imaging of subclavian steal can be problematic. Because superior saturation bands are applied in 2D TOF MRA, reversed flow direction in a VA can mimic occlusion. Standard TOF MRA alone may not be adequate to differentiate *reversed* flow from *absent* flow, so confirmation and quantification with additional imaging—either bolus-timed or direction-encoded phase-contrast MRA, color Doppler US, or DSA—are required **(10-19)**.

DSA shows a severely stenotic or occluded VA with collateral filling from the contralateral VA through the BA junction and/or multiple enlarged, unnamed muscular branches.

On the basis of hemodynamic changes in the VA, three degrees of subclavian steal are recognized on US. In occult steal, symptoms are absent, hemodynamic changes are minimal, and the only finding may be systolic deceleration. In moderate or partial steal, power Doppler spectrum shows alternating or partially reversed flow. In complete steal, VA flow is completely reversed. Dynamic tests with exercise are recommended for confirmation and treatment considerations.

Differential Diagnosis

The major differential diagnoses of extracranial ASVD include dissection, dissecting aneurysm, vasospasm, and fibromuscular dysplasia (FMD). All usually spare the carotid bulb.

Dissection (either traumatic or spontaneous) is more common in young/middle-aged patients and occurs in the *middle* of extracranial vessels. Extracranial dissections typically terminate at the exocranial opening of the carotid canal. Most are smooth or display minimal irregularities, whereas calcifications and ulcerations—common in carotid plaques—are absent.

Midsegment vessel narrowing with a focal mass-like outpouching of the lumen is typical of **dissecting aneurysm**. **Vasospasm** is more common in the intracranial vessels. When it involves the cervical carotid or vertebral arteries, it also typically spares the proximal segments.

FMD spares the carotid bulb and usually affects the middle or distal aspects of the extracranial carotid and vertebral arteries. A "string of beads" appearance is typical. Long-segment tubular narrowing is less common and may reflect coexisting dissection.

Less common mimics of extracranial ASVD include congenital hypoplasia and small vessel size secondary to reduced distal run off. Congenital **internal carotid artery hypoplasia**, featuring a small ipsilateral bony carotid canal, is rare. A congenital **hypoplastic vertebral artery** is common and considered a normal variant. Here the VA often terminates in the posterior inferior cerebellar artery, and the contralateral VA is typically large. If both posterior cerebellar arteries (PCAs) have a so-called fetal origin from the ICAs and the P1 PCA segments are absent, the entire vertebrobasilar system may appear relatively hypoplastic.

Diminished distal flow—"run off"—occurs when intracranial pressure becomes markedly elevated or if there is severe vasospasm of the intracranial vessels. The lumen of the affected cervical vessel diminishes in proportion to the reduced run off.

EXTRACRANIAL ATHEROSCLEROSIS

Etiology
- Multifactorial, progressive disease
- Plasma lipids accumulate in susceptible sites
- Lipids incite inflammatory response

Pathology
- Predictable locations
  - Carotid bifurcation, proximal ICA (carotid "bulb")
  - Aortic arch, great vessel origins
- First sign = fatty streaks, intimal thickening
- Stable plaque
  - Subintimal smooth muscle cells, macrophages accumulate
  - Fibrous cap formed under intact intima
- "Vulnerable" plaque
  - Necrotic core of cellular debris, cholesterol ± calcifications
  - Plaque thins, becomes prone to rupture
  - Neovascularization, subintimal hemorrhage
- Ulcerated plaque
  - Fibrous cap ruptures through intima
  - Denuded intima → platelet, fibrin aggregates
  - May embolize to intracranial circulation

Clinical Issues
- Identifiable risk factors in patients with ischemic stroke
  - Older age (> 60 years)
  - Diabetes mellitus
  - Elevated LDL
  - Hypertension
  - ± History of heart disease

Intracranial Atherosclerosis

One of the most serious and disabling manifestations of ASVD is stroke. Most acute ischemic strokes are thromboembolic, most often secondary to cardiac sources or plaques in the cervical ICA.

Many clinicians focus on extracranial carotid artery disease, considering intracranial ASVD (IASVD) a relatively infrequent cause of stroke. However, recent studies have demonstrated that IASVD accounts for 5-10% of all ischemic strokes. Nearly half of all patients with fatal cerebral infarction have at least one intracranial plaque-associated luminal stenosis at autopsy **(10-21)**.

With an expanding variety of treatment options now available, accurate delineation of IASVD is imperative for individualized patient care. In this section, we briefly review the manifestations of IASVD ranging from asymptomatic vascular ectasias to fusiform aneurysms and life-threatening but potentially treatable stenoocclusive disease.

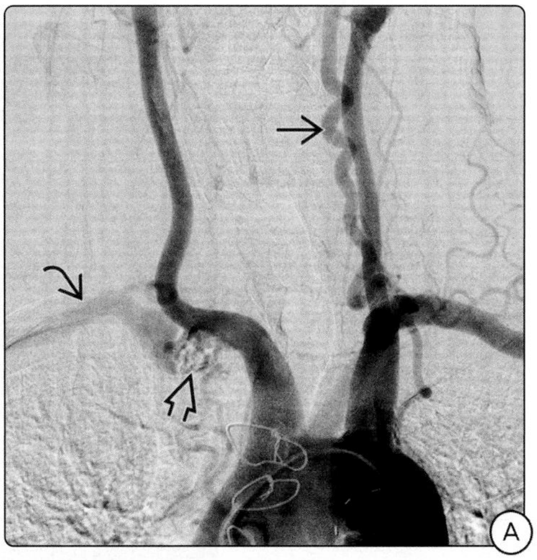

(10-20A) *DSA shows Ca++ ⇒, faint contrast in distal SCA ⇗. The right VA is unopacified. The left VA is enlarged and tortuous →.*

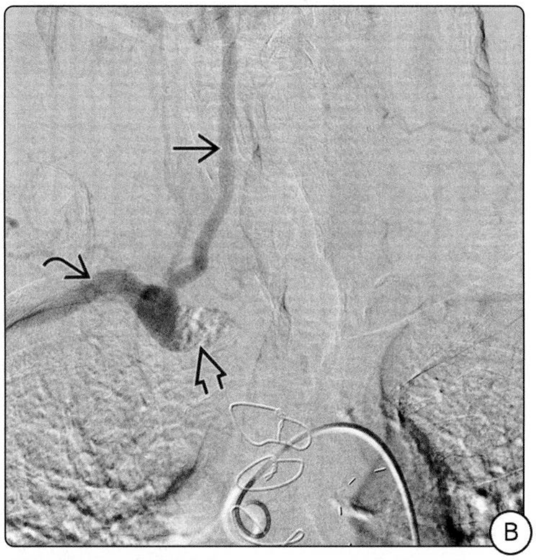

(10-20B) *Retrograde filling of right VA → and SCA ⇗ distal to calcification ⇒ and high-grade stenosis shows classic subclavian steal.*

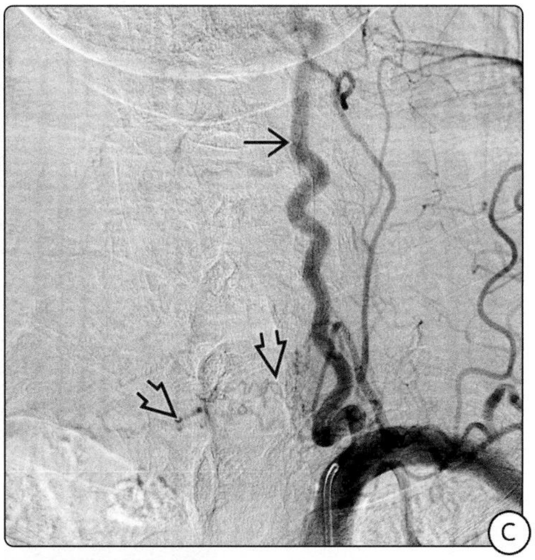

(10-20C) *Left SCA angiogram shows prominent VA →, muscular branches ⇒ collateralizing to the right SCA vascular distribution.*

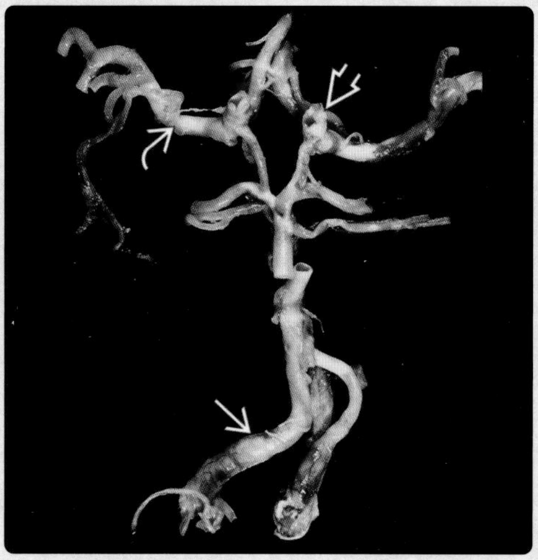

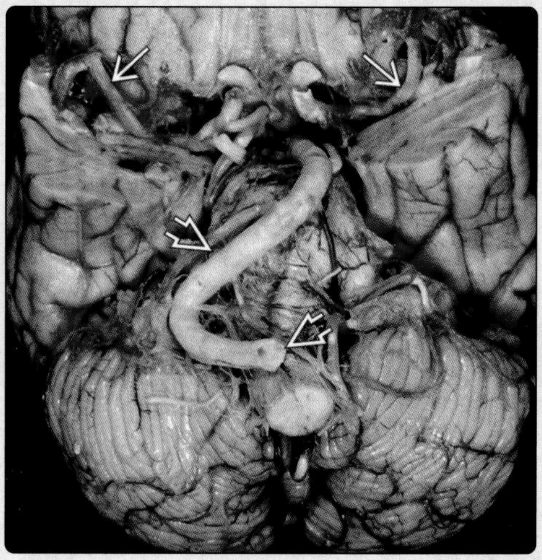

***(10-21)** Autopsy case shows the distribution of intracranial ASVD. Most severe disease is in the vertebrobasilar system, ICAs, and proximal MCAs. (Courtesy R. Hewlett, MD.)* ***(10-22)** Autopsy case of vertebrobasilar dolichoectasia (VBD) shows yellow atheromatous plaques in an extremely tortuous basilar artery. Note the mild ectasia of both middle cerebral arteries. (Courtesy R. Hewlett, MD.)*

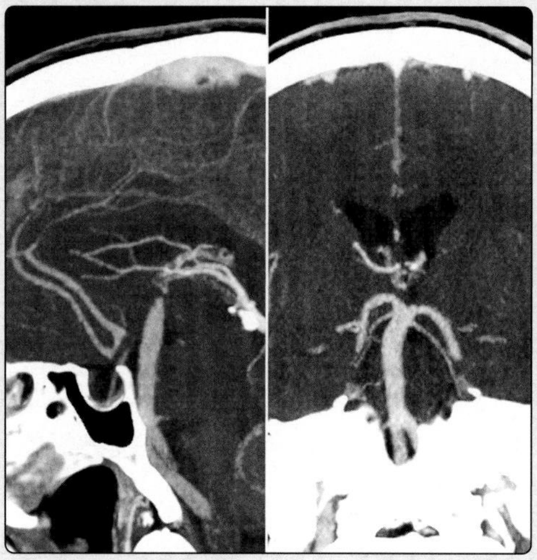

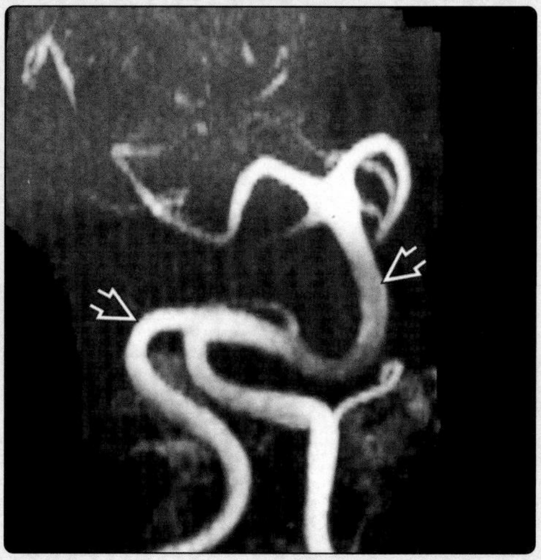

***(10-23)** Lateral (L) and AP (R) CTAs in a 49y man with VBD show an enlarged, elongated vertebrobasilar artery.* ***(10-24)** Coronal TOF MRA in a 54y woman with trigeminal neuralgia shows extreme tortuosity of the vertebrobasilar system. Note the smooth appearance of the lumen. Other than the VBD, the patient's entire MR was normal.*

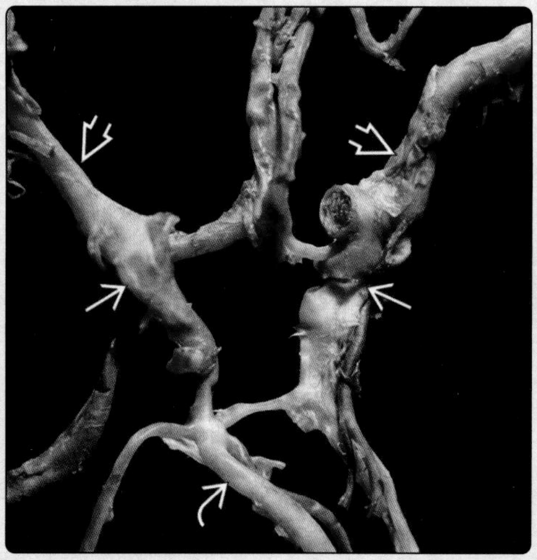

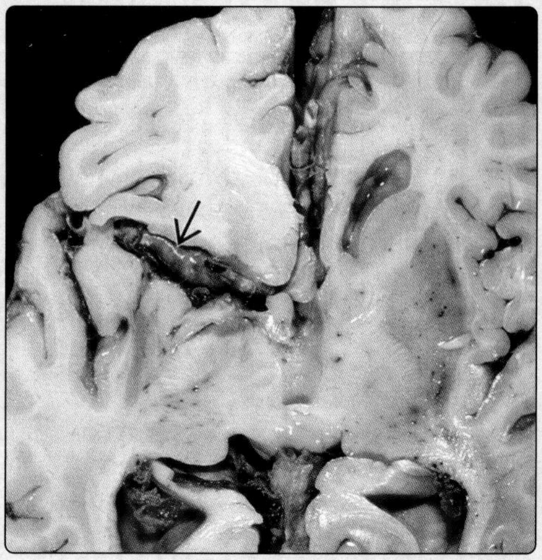

***(10-25)** Autopsy case demonstrates ASVD fusiform ectasias of the ICAs and MCAs. The posterior (vertebrobasilar) circulation is relatively spared. (Courtesy R. Hewlett, MD.)* ***(10-26)** Autopsy case shows extreme ectasia of the horizontal MCA segment. (Courtesy R. Hewlett, MD.)*

Ectasia

Generalized nonfocal vessel elongation is called "ectasia," "dolichoectasia," "arteriectasis," or "dilative arteriopathy." Elongated, tortuous vessels are common manifestations of advanced atherosclerosis throughout the body and also occur in both the cervical and intracranial arteries. When ectasia occurs in the posterior circulation, it is termed "vertebrobasilar dolichoectasia" **(10-22)**.

Many—if not most—ectatic intracranial vessels are asymptomatic and discovered incidentally at autopsy or on imaging studies **(10-23)**. These vascular enlargements are most common in middle-aged and elderly patients.

Ectasias can involve any part of the intracranial circulation but are most common in the vertebrobasilar arteries **(10-24)** and supraclinoid ICA **(10-25)**. Multifocal disease is common. Ectasias may extend from the BA and ICA into the proximal M1 or P1 segments **(10-26)**. Imaging findings of uncomplicated ectasias are one or more elongated arteries that do not demonstrate focal aneurysmal dilatation.

Atherosclerotic Fusiform Aneurysm

Atherosclerotic fusiform aneurysms (FAs) are focal arterial enlargements that are usually superimposed on an ectatic artery. ASVD FAs are most common in the vertebrobasilar circulation. When they occur in the anterior circulation, they can produce a rare but dramatic manifestation called a giant "serpentine" aneurysm. ASVD FAs are discussed in detail in Chapter 6.

Intracranial Stenoocclusive Disease

The advent of effective endovascular techniques to treat intracranial stenoocclusive disease has made detection and accurate delineation of IASVD as important as identifying and characterizing extracranial ASVD.

Epidemiology. Atherosclerosis that causes large artery intracranial occlusive disease (LAICOD) is now a well-defined yet relatively neglected and poorly understood stroke subtype. Recent studies have shown that the overall prevalence of IASVD in patients with concurrent extracranial disease varies between 20% and 50%, and 12% of patients have diffuse (multifocal) IASVD.

Between 8-10% of all strokes in North America are related to LAICOD. The prevalence of IASVD is especially high in African Americans, Hispanics, and Asians, in whom some studies have demonstrated a preponderance of intracranial stenosis relative to extracranial carotid stenosis. Insulin resistance and metabolic syndrome are significant risk factors for intracranial vs. extracranial ASVD.

Clinical Issues. Overall, symptomatic patients with moderate to severe stenosis (i.e., 70-99%) in the intracranial circulation have a 25% 2-year risk for recurrent stroke.

Clinical course varies significantly with stenosis sublocation. The vessel-specific mean overall annual mortality is 6.8% for middle cerebral artery stenosis, 11.6% for vertebrobasilar stenosis, and 12.4% for intracranial ICA stenosis.

Symptomatic IASVD generally has a poor prognosis, as conservative (i.e., medical) management frequently fails. Stroke recurrence rates in patients with IASVD treated with either warfarin or aspirin are unacceptably high. Among patients with symptomatic IASVD who fail antithrombotic therapy, the subsequent rates of stroke or vascular death are even higher, up to 45% per year.

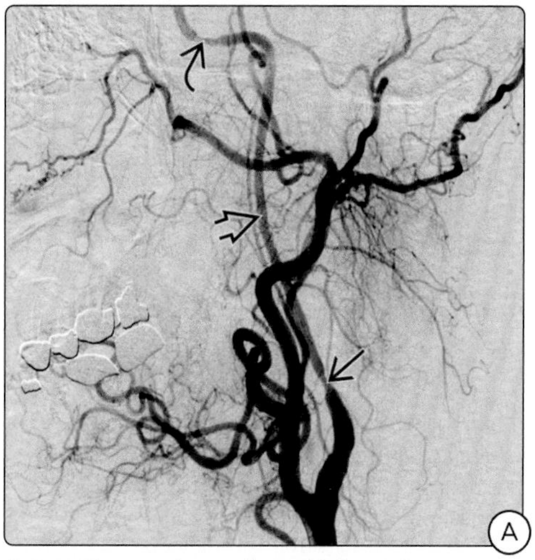

***(10-27A)** Lateral DSA shows high-grade narrowing of the cervical ICA, small distal ICA (from reduced flow), "tandem" stenosis.*

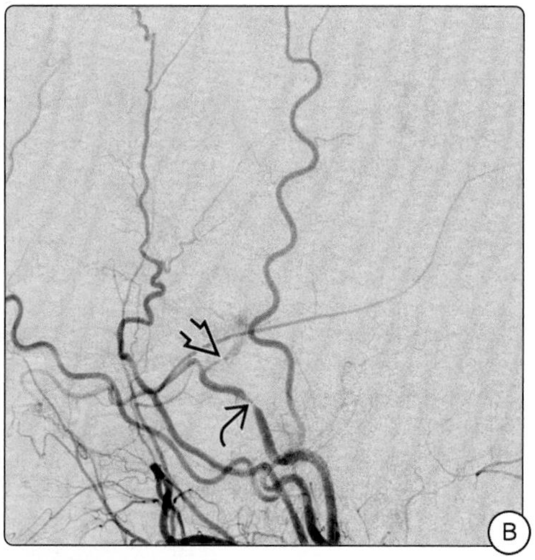

***(10-27B)** Intracranial view shows the high-grade cavernous ICA stenosis together with near-complete occlusion of the supraclinoid ICA.*

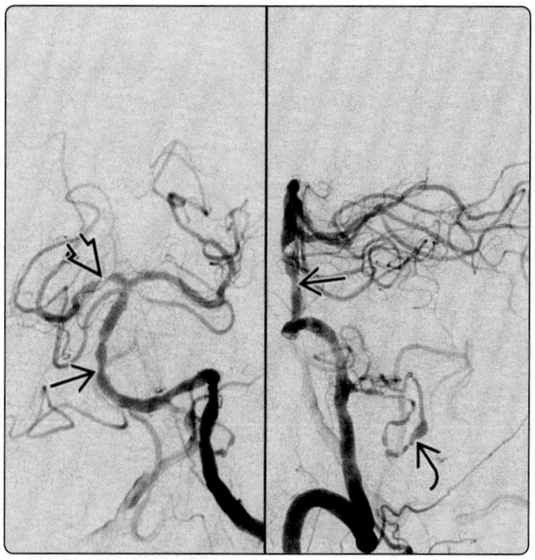

***(10-28)** (L) AP, (R) lateral DSA show extensive changes of ASVD in the vertebrobasilar artery, proximal right PCA, and PICA.*

The availability of endovascular techniques such as intracranial angioplasty has opened new treatment avenues for LAICOD. A variety of balloon-expandable, drug-eluting, and self-expanding stents are also now available as options.

Imaging. Mural calcifications are common on NECT with patterns varying from scattered stippled foci to thick continuous linear ("railroad track") deposits.

Angiography has been the traditional tool for diagnosing IASVD **(10-27)** **(10-28)**. Solitary or multifocal stenoses alternating with areas of poststenotic dilatation are typical findings. When atherosclerosis affects distal branches of the major intracranial vessels, the appearance can mimic that of vasculitis (see below).

Imaging the *intracranial* circulation in patients with a hemodynamically significant *extracranial* stenosis is imperative. A "tandem" stenosis—defined as any lesion with an *intracranial* stenosis greater than 50% in the same vascular distribution distal to a primary *extracranial* stenosis—is present in 20% of patients **(10-27)** **(10-31)**.

High-resolution "black blood" 3D vessel wall MR directly depicts IASVD and is a reliable tool for identifying IASVD and measuring plaque burden. Intramural hemorrhage and irregular, noncircumferential short-segment enhancing foci are common findings **(10-29)**. At least one IASVD lesion as been found in one-third of patients in a recent population-based study.

Differential Diagnosis. The major differential diagnoses of IASVD are vasculitis, vasospasm, and dissection.

Vasculitis occurs at all ages but is more common in middle-aged patients. Vasculitis and ASVD appear virtually identical on angiography (MRA, CTA, or DSA). Remember: the most common cause of a vasculitis-like pattern in an older patient isn't vasculitis; it's ASVD!

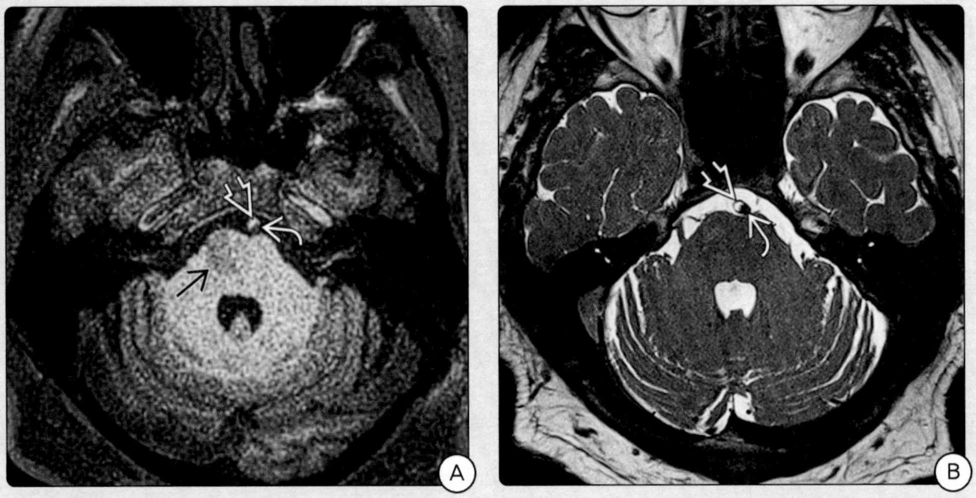

***(10-29A)** Axial T1 FS in a patient with a subacute right pontine infarct ➔ shows a crescent of T1 shortening ➡ in the basilar artery wall causing narrowing of the lumen ➡. **(10-29B)** Thin-section T2 space in the same case shows that the subacute mural hematoma is hyperintense ➡. Note narrowed residual lumen of the basilar artery ➡.*

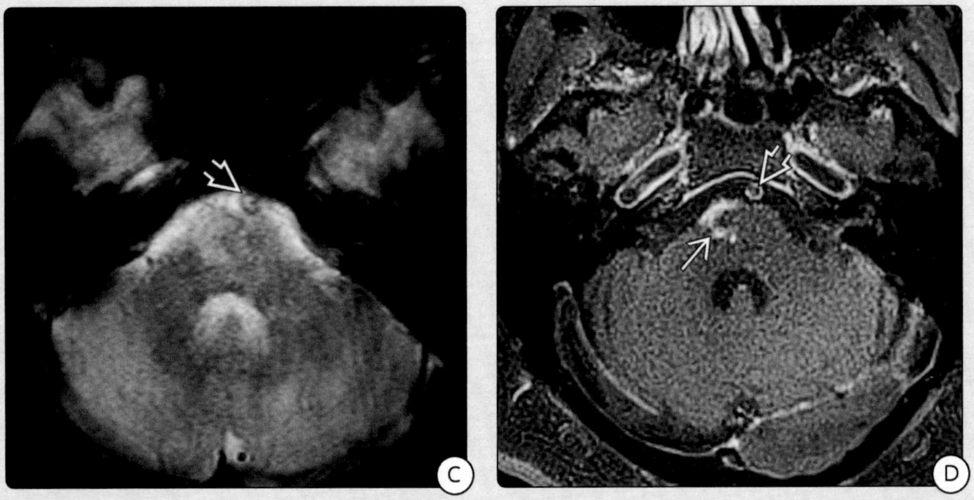

***(10-29C)** T2* GRE shows "blooming" ➡ of the mural hematoma. **(10-29D)** T1 C+ FS vessel wall imaging shows incomplete crescentic enhancement ➡ of the basilar artery wall. The subacute pontine infarct also enhances ➡. This is ASVD with wall inflammatory response.*

INTRACRANIAL ATHEROSCLEROSIS (ICASVD)

Epidemiology
- Found in one-third of patients in population-based imaging studies
  - Causes 8-10% of strokes in USA, Europe
  - > 50% in Asia

Clinical Issues
- Moderate/severe stenosis → 25% 2-year stroke risk

Imaging
- Mural Ca++
- Irregular narrowing ± ulcerations
- Deep watershed ischemia, lacunae
- High-resolution vessel wall imaging
  - Wall hemorrhage
  - Enhancement irregular, short segment, noncircumferential

Vasospasm spares the cavernous ICA and is usually more diffuse than ASVD. A history of trauma, subarachnoid hemorrhage, or drug abuse (typically with sympathomimetics) is common. **Intracranial dissection**—especially in the anterior circulation—is rare and usually occurs in young patients.

Arteriolosclerosis

Terminology

Arteriolosclerosis is also known as **small vessel disease** or—less specifically—cerebral microvascular disease. Arteriolosclerosis is a microangiopathy that typically affects small arteries (i.e., arterioles), especially in the subcortical and deep cerebral white matter (WM).

The term **leukoaraiosis** is sometimes used by neurologists to designate the confluent WM lesions associated with arteriolosclerosis, i.e., small vessel vascular disease. This is one

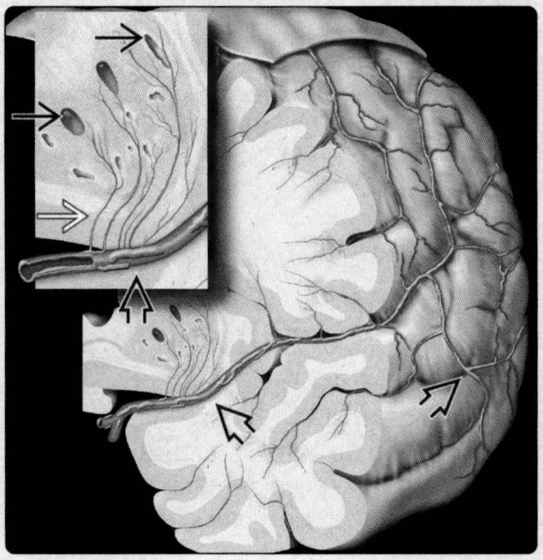

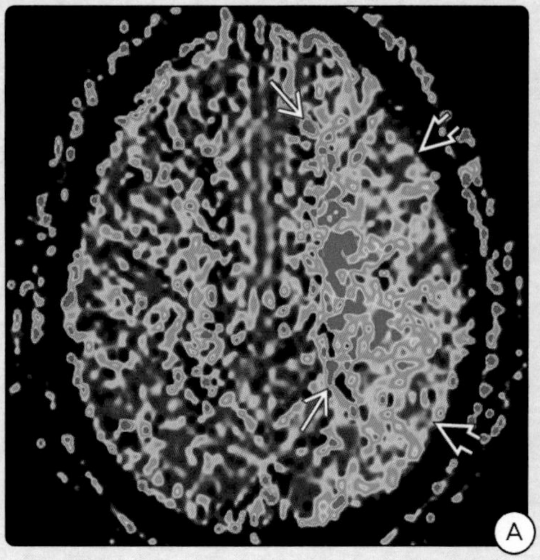

(10-30) Coronal graphic shows atherosclerotic plaques involving the major intracranial arteries and their branches. Inset shows penetrating (lenticulostriate) arteries and lacunar infarcts . (10-31A) CT perfusion in a 68y man in the ER with "stroke" shows significantly prolonged MTT in the deep white matter of the left hemisphere with relative sparing of the overlying cortex .

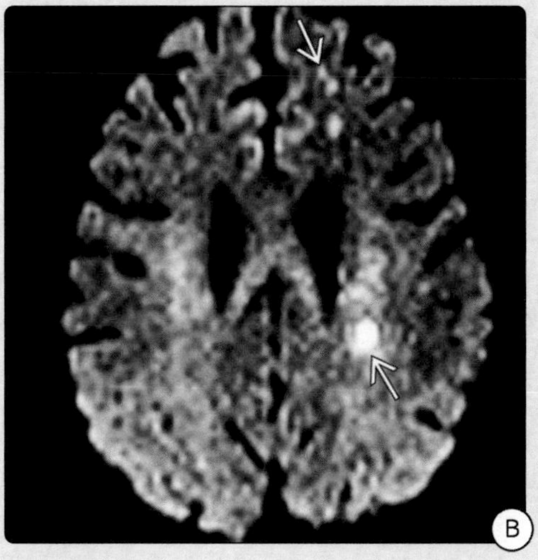

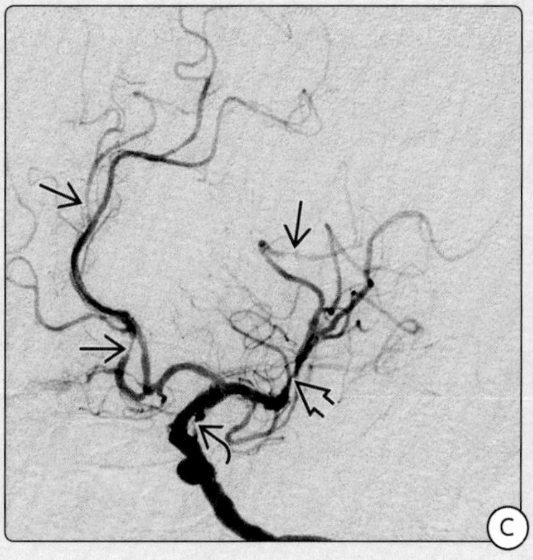

(10-31B) DWI in the same case shows multiple foci of restricted diffusion in the left hemisphere white matter. (10-31C) Oblique left carotid DSA shows severe ASVD in the distal ICA as well as the ACA and MCA . High-grade stenosis of the M2 MCA is present . This is intracranial ASVD with acute multiple lacunar infarcts in the deep watershed.

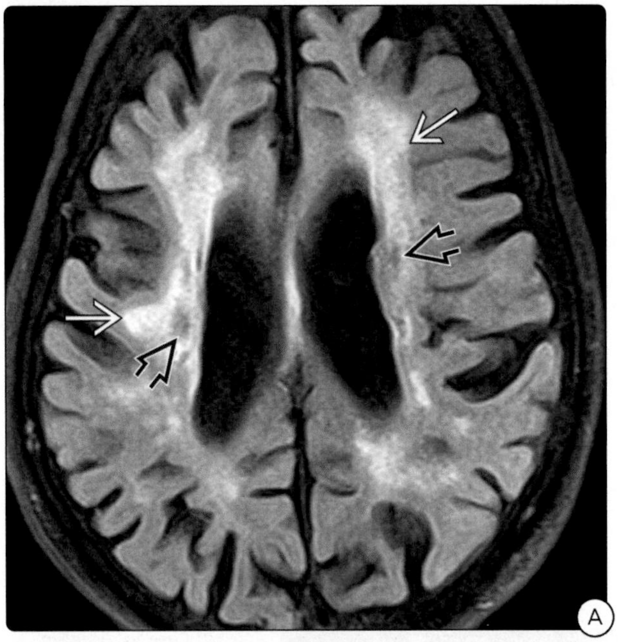

***(10-32A)** Axial FLAIR scan in an elderly demented patient with chronic hypertension and small vessel vascular disease shows volume loss, confluent periventricular white matter (WM) hyperintensities ➡, and multiple lacunar infarcts ⇨.*

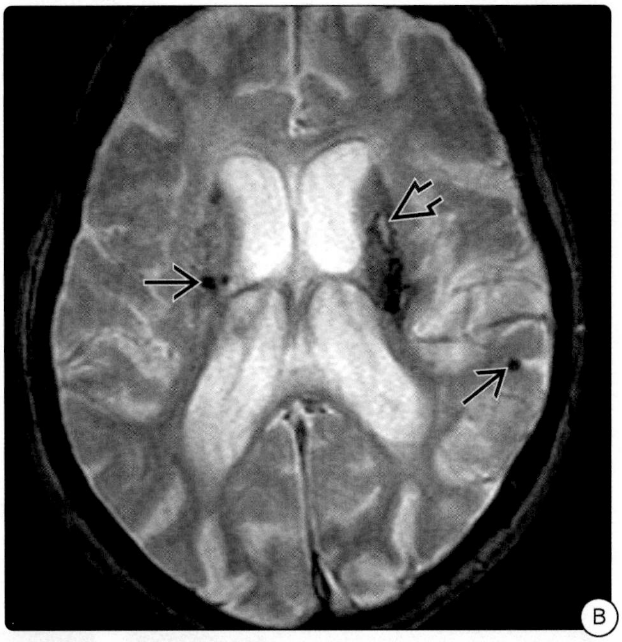

***(10-32B)** T2* GRE scan in the same patient demonstrates multifocal hypointensities, which are characteristic of cerebral microbleeds ⇨, and old hypertensive basal ganglia hemorrhage ⇨.*

of the most grossly visible markers that aging and vascular risk factors inflict on the brain.

Etiology and Pathology

Aging, chronic hypertension, hypercholesterolemia, and diabetes mellitus are the most common factors that predispose to cerebral microvascular disease. Genetic risk factors include the *APOE*E4* genotype.

Gross pathologic features of cerebral arteriolosclerosis include generalized volume loss, multiple lacunar infarcts, and deep WM spongiosis. Stenosis or occlusion of small vessels by arteriolosclerosis and lipohyalinosis probably results in WM microinfarctions **(10-30)**.

The microscopic correlates of the deep periventricular WM lesions identified on imaging studies have a spectrum of findings. Degenerated myelin (myelin "pallor"), axonal loss with increased extracellular fluid, lipofibrohyalinosis with small vessel occlusion, gliosis, spongiosis, and enlarged perivascular spaces can all be present in varying degrees.

Clinical Issues

The clinical manifestations of cerebral small vessel vascular disease vary widely and range from normal or minimal cognitive impairment to severe dementia. Although there is a relatively poor correlation between the degree of WM changes on imaging studies and cognitive performance, the severity of small vessel disease at autopsy correlates significantly with the degree of cognitive impairment.

Imaging

Imaging studies typically reflect WM rarefaction and spongiosis associated with varying degrees of generalized volume loss.

CT. Patchy and/or confluent WM hypodensities that spare the cortex are typical findings on NECT. Periventricular lesions have a broad or confluent base with the ventricular surface and are especially prominent around the atria of the lateral ventricles. Lesions are almost always nonenhancing on CECT.

MR. Patchy or confluent periventricular and subcortical WM hypointensities are seen on T1WI. The lesions are hyperintense on T2WI and are especially prominent on FLAIR **(10-32A)**. T2* (GRE, SWI) sequences often demonstrate multifocal "blooming" hypointensities, especially in the presence of chronic hypertension **(10-32B)**.

Differential Diagnosis

The most important differential diagnosis is **normal age-related hyperintensities**. Scattered periventricular WM lesions are almost universal after age 65.

Other significant differential considerations include **enlarged perivascular (Virchow-Robin) spaces** (PVSs). Prominent PVSs can be seen in patients of all ages and in virtually all locations, although they do increase with age. **Demyelinating disease** typically causes ovoid or triangular periventricular lesions that commonly involve the callososeptal interfaces, which are rarely involved by arteriolosclerosis.

Nonatheromatous Vascular Diseases

Although atherosclerotic vascular disease (ASVD) is by far the most common disease to affect the craniocervical vasculature, a number of other nonatheromatous disorders can affect the brain, causing stroke or stroke-like symptoms. In this section, we briefly discuss some of the most important entities, including nonatherosclerotic aging phenotypes, fibromuscular dysplasia (FMD), vasculitis, and non-ASVD noninflammatory vasculopathies such as cerebral amyloid disease.

Nonatherosclerotic Aging Phenotypes

Although ASVD increases with age, atherosclerosis is not the only arterial phenotype described in aging brain arteries. The main physiologic stimulus for brain arterial aging is probably chronic physiologic wall shear stresses.

Nonatherosclerotic age-associated degenerative phenotypes generally consist of elastin loss and internal elastic lamina (IEL) fragmentation. Although some of these changes may also overlap with atherosclerosis, the typical finding is that of intimal thickening without evidence of lipid deposition **(10-33)**.

Non-ASVD-associated imaging findings include progressive luminal dilation and vessel enlargement with elongation/ectasia and concentric intimal thickening **(10-34)**.

Fibromuscular Dysplasia

Terminology

FMD is an uncommon segmental nonatherosclerotic, noninflammatory disease of unknown etiology. FMD is a

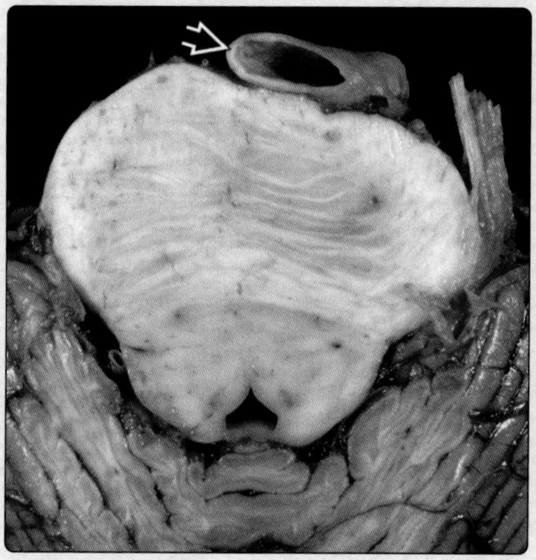

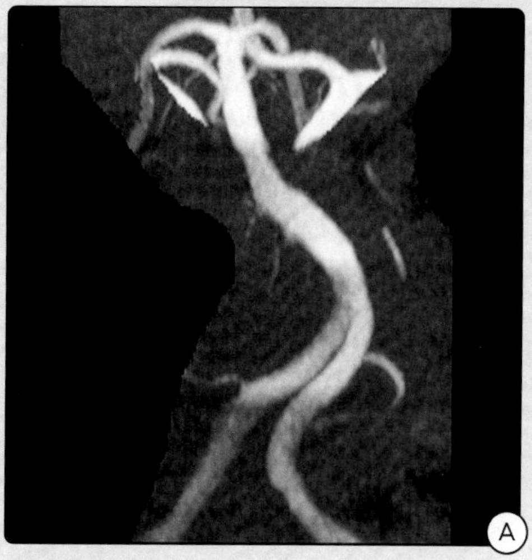

***(10-33)** Autopsy case shows basilar ectasia with elongation, enlargement with no visible changes of ASVD in the thickened but smooth arterial wall. **(10-34A)** Coronal 2D TOF MRA in a patient with a subacute pontine perforating artery infarct shows VBD with only minimal irregularities of the visualized lumen.*

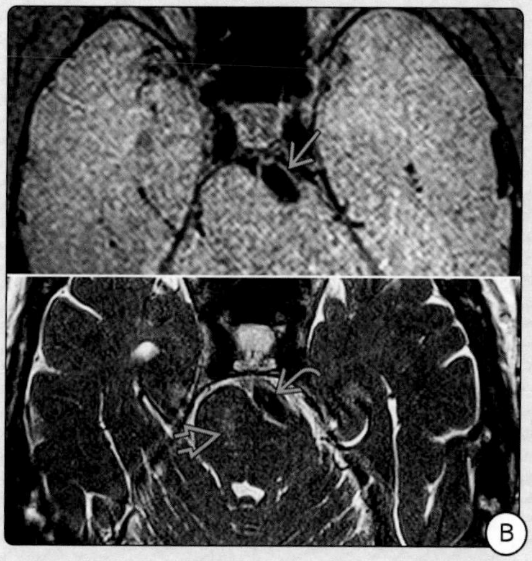

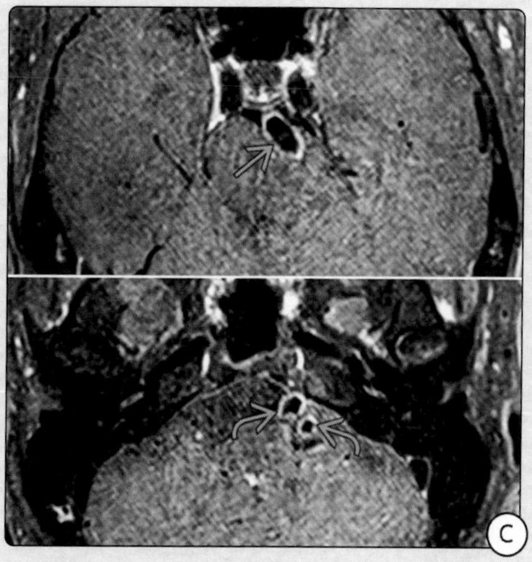

***(10-34B)** Precontrast T1 FS (top), T2 space (bottom) in the same case show that the basilar wall is isointense on T1 and moderately hyperintense on T2. Pontine infarct is faintly visible. **(10-34C)** High-resolution T1 C+ "black blood" vessel wall imaging shows circumferential enhancement of the basilar (top) and vertebral arteries (bottom); presumed nonatherosclerotic aging phenotype with inflammatory changes.*

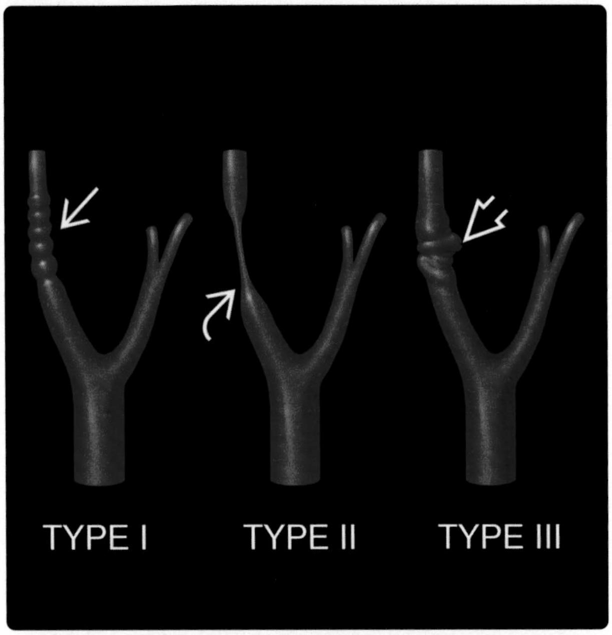

(10-35) Carotid bifurcation shows the principal subtypes of fibromuscular dysplasia (FMD). Type 1 appears as alternating areas of constriction and dilatation ➡, type 2 as tubular stenosis ➡, and type 3 as focal corrugations ± diverticulum ➡.

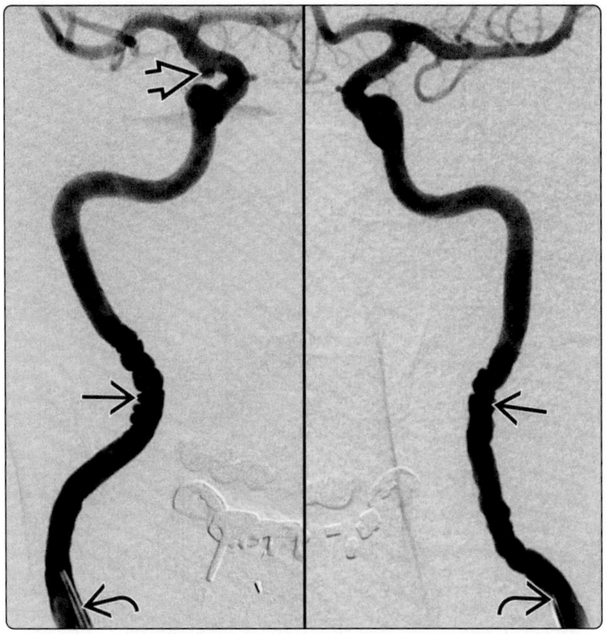

(10-36) AP DSA demonstrates type 1 FMD in both ICAs with sparing of the bulbs ➡, "string of beads" appearance in midcervical segments ➡, small unruptured saccular aneurysm ➡ of the right supraclinoid ICA.

polyvascular disease that affects medium and large arteries in many areas of the body.

Etiology

The exact pathoetiology of FMD remains unknown. A variant in the phosphatase/actin 1 regulator gene *PHACTR1* has recently been identified as a susceptibility locus for FMD. FMD has a complex inheritance pattern and is more common in first-degree relatives of patients with the disease, but most patients have no family history of FMD.

Pathology

Location. Although virtually any artery in any location can be affected, FMD affects some arteries far more than others. The renal arteries are affected in 75% of cases; about 35% of these are bilateral. Patients with known renal artery FMD often have cerebrovascular disease (and vice versa).

The cervicocephalic vessels are involved in up to 75% of cases. The internal carotid artery (ICA) is the most common site; vertebral artery (VA) FMD is seen in 20% of cases. Approximately half of all cervicocephalic FMD cases involve more than one artery (usually either both ICAs or one ICA and a VA). Intracranial FMD is very rare.

FMD carries an increased risk of developing intracranial saccular aneurysms. Intracranial saccular aneurysms are present in approximately 7-10% of patients with cervical FMD.

Size and Number. Size varies from small focal lesions with minimal beading to extensive disease involving most of the vessel 1-2 cm distal to its origin. Multiple arterial systems are involved in 25-30% of cases. When multisystem disease is present, the renal arteries are almost always involved.

Staging, Grading, and Classification. FMD is classified histologically into three categories according to which arterial wall layer is affected (media, intima, or adventitia) **(10-35)**. Several forms can also coexist in the same patient.

By far the most common type (type 1) is **medial fibroplasia**, accounting for approximately 60-85% of all FMD cases, and is mainly discovered in women between 30-50 years of age. The media has alternating thin and very thick areas formed by concentric rings of extensive fibrous proliferations and smooth muscle hyperplasia. The intima, IEL, and adventitia are normal. Inflammatory cells are absent.

Intimal fibroplasia (type 2) accounts for less than 10% of FMD cases and is mainly found in children. Focal band-like and smooth long-segment narrowings both occur. Histologically, the intima is markedly thickened by circumferential or eccentric collagen deposition. The IEL is preserved, and the media and adventitia are normal. Lipid and inflammatory components are absent.

Adventitial (periarterial) fibroplasia (type 3) is the least common type of FMD, accounting for less than 5% of cases. Dense collagen replaces the delicate fibrous tissue of the adventitia and may infiltrate the adjacent periarterial tissues.

Because as much as 5% of angiographically diagnosed FMD cases have histologic confirmation, the American Heart Association has recommended classifying FMD based on imaging appearance alone as simply either focal or multifocal.

Clinical Issues

Epidemiology. Once thought to be a relatively rare vasculopathy, overall prevalence of FMD is estimated between 4-6% in the renal arteries and 0.3-3.0% in the cervicocephalic arteries. FMD is identified in 0.5% of all patients screened with CTA for ischemic neurologic symptoms.

FMD primarily affects individuals between the ages of 20 and 60 years. Mean age in the U.S. Registry is 52 years.

Sex disparity in FMD is striking with a 9:1 female predominance. Although FMD is less common in men, it is associated with a higher incidence of dissections and aneurysms.

Presentation. Sudden onset of high blood pressure in a young woman is a classic presentation of renal FMD. FMD is found in about 1% of hypertensive patients and is the second leading cause of renovascular hypertension (after ASVD).

Carotid or vertebral FMD typically presents at an older age, generally around 50 years. Cervical FMD can present with headache, pulsatile tinnitus/bruit, dizziness, neck pain, transient ischemia attack, stroke, or dissection (often with Horner syndrome, i.e., ptosis, pupil constriction, and facial anhidrosis). Between 5-6% of patients are asymptomatic at the time of diagnosis.

Natural History and Treatment. The natural history of FMD is unclear, as many cases are now discovered incidentally on imaging studies. Overall, 1 of 5 patients with FMD will have dissections and 1 of 5 patients will have aneurysms.

To date, no prospective randomized trials have compared the efficacy of different treatment options. "Watch and wait" for patients with renal FMD without hypertension and with normal renal function is common, as is antiplatelet therapy for asymptomatic individuals with cervical FMD. Percutaneous balloon angioplasty is recommended for patients with recent-onset or resistant hypertension, transient ischemic attacks (TIAs), or stroke. Surgery is generally used only to treat aneurysms.

Imaging

Technical Considerations. In the past, DSA was considered the gold standard for the diagnosis of FMD. However, CTA accurately depicts FMD in the cervicocephalic arteries and also allows visualization of the intracranial vessels to detect the presence of associated aneurysms. TOF MRA can be problematic, as artifacts caused by patient motion or in-plane flow and susceptibility gradients can mimic the appearance of FMD.

Because multisystem disease is common, patients with newly diagnosed carotid and/or vertebral FMD should also have their renal arteries examined. The prevalence of renal FMD is 40-45% in patients with cephalocervical disease.

Imaging Findings. Imaging findings vary with FMD subtype. Between 80-90% of patients demonstrate findings typical for type 1 FMD (medial fibroplasia). An irregular "corrugated" or "string of beads" appearance with alternating areas of constriction and dilatation that are wider than the normal lumen is the typical appearance **(10-36)** **(10-37)** **(10-38)**. In type 2 (intimal fibroplasia), a smooth, long-segment tubular narrowing is present. In type 3 (adventitial) FMD, asymmetric diverticulum-like outpouchings from one side of the artery are present **(10-39)**.

All three cervical FMD subtypes spare the carotid bifurcations and great vessel origins, involve the middle segments, and are most common at the C1-C2 level. Complications of cervicocephalic FMD include dissection, intracranial aneurysm with or without subarachnoid hemorrhage (SAH) **(10-39)**, and arteriovenous fistulas. Other less common manifestations of FMD include vascular loops and fusiform vascular ectasias.

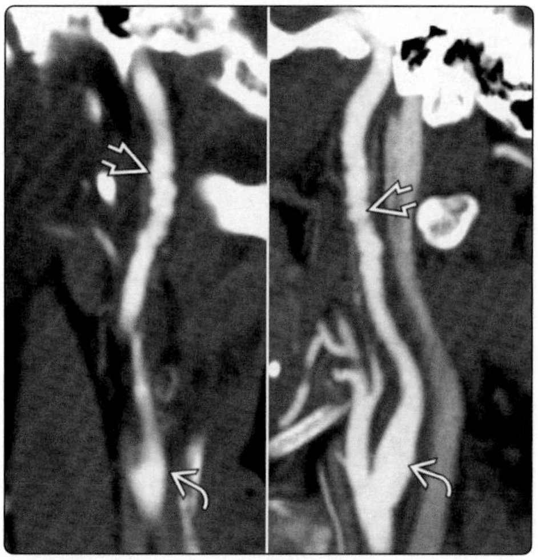

***(10-37)** AP (L), lateral (R) CTAs show typical changes of type 1 FMD in both carotid arteries. Note sparing of bulbs.*

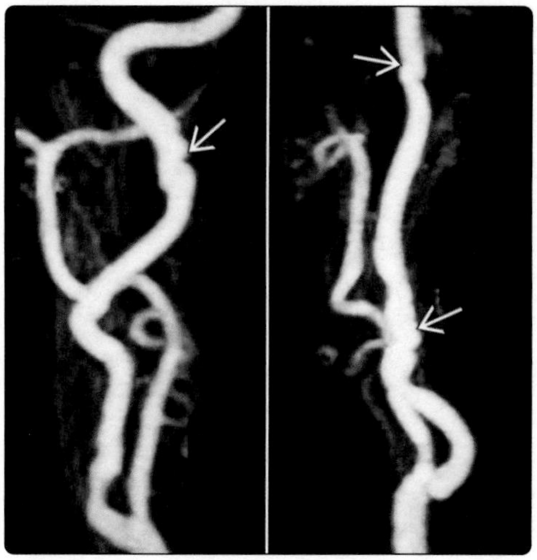

***(10-38)** TOF MRA shows another case of FMD with "string of beads" appearance in both cervical carotid arteries.*

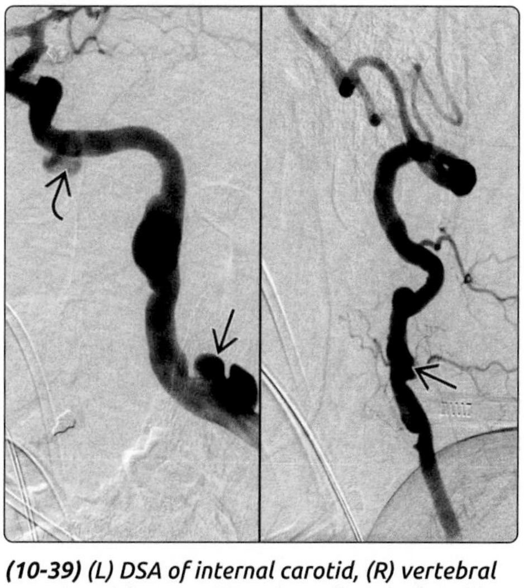

***(10-39)** (L) DSA of internal carotid, (R) vertebral arteries with type 3 FMD show diverticulum-like outpouchings, saccular aneurysm.*

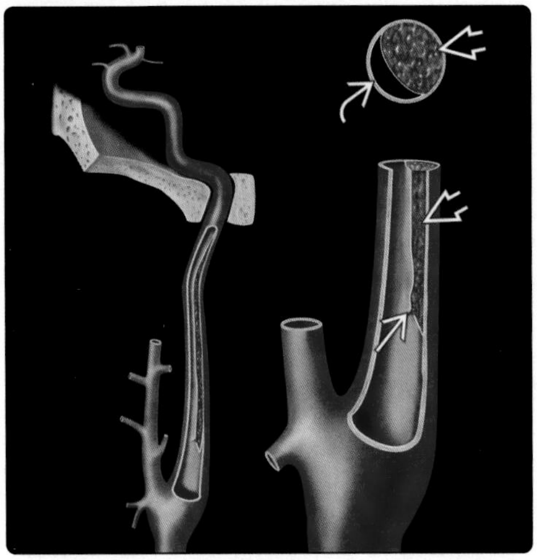

(10-40) Extracranial ICA dissection shows intimal tear ➡, subintimal thrombus ➡ compressing residual lumen ➡. Bulb is spared.

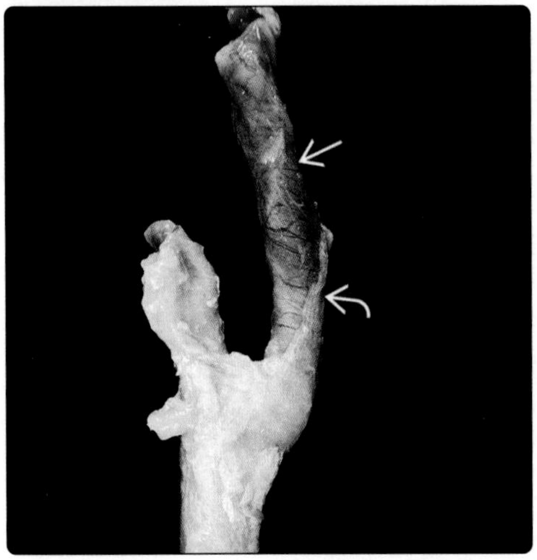

(10-41) Extracranial ICA dissection shows extensive mural thrombus ➡. Dissection begins ➡ distal to the bulb. (Courtesy R. Hewlett, MD.)

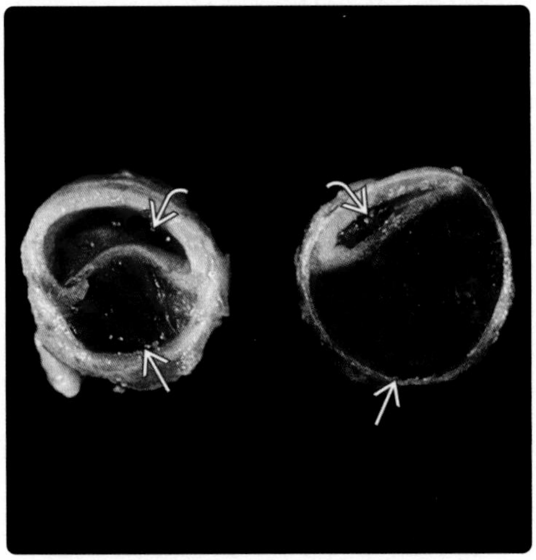

(10-42) Axial sections show carotid dissection with subintimal hematoma ➡, compressed residual lumen ➡. (Courtesy R. Hewlett, MD.)

FIBROMUSCULAR DYSPLASIA

Pathology
- Nonatherosclerotic, noninflammatory arteriopathy
- *PHACTR1* mutations recently identified
  - 10% familial
  - Complex pattern of inheritance
- Commonly affects medium-sized/large arteries
  - Renal 75%
  - Cervical arteries 75%
  - ICA 50%, VA 20-25%
  - Multiple vessels 50%
  - Intracranial very rare
- Classified by affected arterial wall layer
  - Type 1: medial fibroplasia
  - Type 2: intimal fibroplasia
  - Type 3: adventitial (periarterial) fibroplasia

Clinical Issues
- Any age, but 20-60 years most common
- F:M = 9:1
- Presentation
  - Can be asymptomatic, incidental (0.5% of cervical CTAs)
  - Most common = renovascular hypertension
  - Headache, pulsatile tinnitus
  - Neck pain, Horner syndrome
  - Stroke
- Natural history
  - 1 in 5 will have dissection
  - 1 in 5 will develop saccular aneurysm

Imaging
- Midsegments of cervical ICA, VA affected
- Spares carotid bulbs, usually terminates before entering skull base
- Appearance
  - "String of beads" (type 1) = 60-85%
  - Smooth, long-segment narrowing (type 2) = 10%
  - Adventitial (periarterial narrowing) ≤ 5%

Differential Diagnosis
- Atherosclerosis (involves bulb > midsegment)
- Arterial "standing waves" (type of vasospasm)
- Dissection (can occur with FMD)

Differential Diagnosis

The major differential diagnosis of FMD is **atherosclerosis**. FMD is most common in young women, a group that is generally at low risk for ASVD. FMD involves the middle to distal portions of the affected arteries, not the origins.

Arterial standing waves are a form of transient vasospasm that can be misinterpreted as type 1 FMD on catheter angiograms. The regular "corrugated" appearance contrasts with the irregular "string of beads" of FMD **(10-44A)**. Standing waves resolve spontaneously on repeat angiography (including CTA or MRA) or after the administration of vasodilators.

The smooth, tapered "tubular" narrowing of type 2 (intimal FMD) can be difficult to distinguish from **spontaneous dissection**, which also occurs as a complication of FMD. Other **nonatherosclerotic vasculopathies**, such as Takayasu arteritis and giant cell arteritis, can mimic tubular (i.e., intimal) FMD.

Dissection

Craniocervical arterial dissection (CAD) is the most common cause of ischemic stroke in young and middle-aged adults. Timely therapy can reduce the immediate stroke risk and mitigate long-term sequelae of craniocervical dissections, so imaging diagnosis is crucial to patient management.

Terminology

A **dissection** is a tear in at least one layer of the vessel wall that permits blood to penetrate into and delaminate (split apart or "dissect") wall layers **(10-40)**. CAD is characterized by an intramural hematoma that may narrow or occlude the vessel lumen **(10-41)** **(10-42)**. CAD is strongly associated with ischemic events, primarily artery-to-artery embolism, so early diagnosis and appropriate treatment are essential.

A **dissecting aneurysm** is a dissection characterized by an outpouching that extends beyond the vessel wall. Most occur with subadventitial dissections and are more accurately designated as **pseudoaneurysms** (i.e., they lack all normal vessel wall components).

Etiology

CAD can be extracranial or intracranial.

Almost 60% of *extracranial* dissections are "spontaneous," i.e., nontraumatic. Blunt or penetrating injury is common, but sports activities or cervical manipulations have also been implicated. Unusual etiologies with putative mechanical stress have given rise to unique terms such as "beauty parlor stroke" and "bottoms-up stroke."

Most nontraumatic dissections occur secondary to an underlying vasculopathy, such as FMD, Marfan syndrome, or other connective tissue disorder (e.g., Ehlers-Danlos type 4). Less common predisposing conditions include hypertension, migraine headaches, vigorous physical activity, hyperhomocysteinemia, and recent pharyngeal infection.

Intracranial dissections can be either traumatic or spontaneous. Iatrogenic dissections (typically secondary to endovascular procedures) are becoming increasingly common.

Pathology

Location. Dissections typically occur in the most mobile segment of a vessel, often starting or ending where the vessel transitions from a relatively free position to a position fixed by an encasing bony canal. The extracranial ICA is the most common overall site in the head and neck. Extracranial ICA dissections spare the carotid bulb and often extend up to—but only occasionally into—the skull base **(10-44A)**. Vertebral dissections are most common between the skull base and C1 and between C1 and C2.

Once thought to be rare—accounting for just 1-2% of all cervicocephalic dissections—recent statistics indicate intracranial dissections may be at least as common as their extracranial counterparts. The most frequently involved site is the VA. Dissections in the anterior circulation are even less common. They almost always involve the supraclinoid ICA, with or without extension into the proximal middle cerebral artery (MCA).

Size and Number. Dissections can be limited to a focal intimal tear and small subintimal hematoma. Most are solitary, long-segment lesions that extend for several centimeters. Approximately 20% involve two or more vessels. Multiple dissections are more common if an underlying vasculopathy such as Marfan, Ehlers-Danlos type 4, or FMD is present.

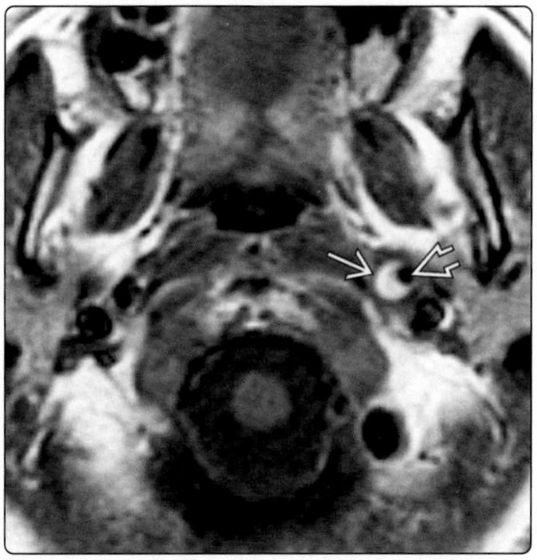

***(10-43)** Axial T1WI shows subacute subintimal hematoma, crescent-like hyperintensity around narrow "flow void" of midcervical ICA.*

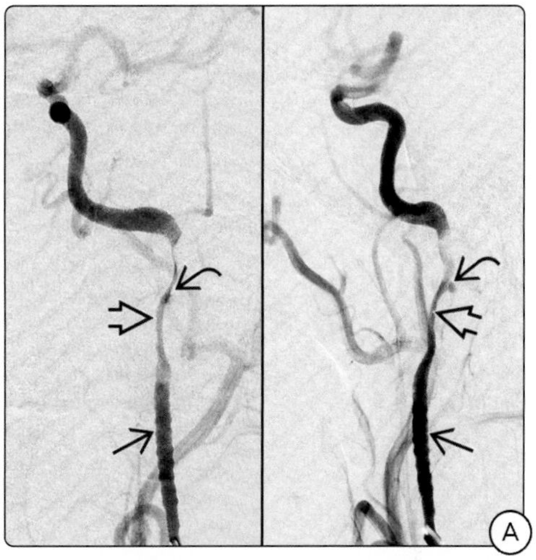

***(10-44A)** (L) AP, (R) lateral DSA show cervical ICA dissection to skull base, pseudoaneurysm, arterial "standing waves".*

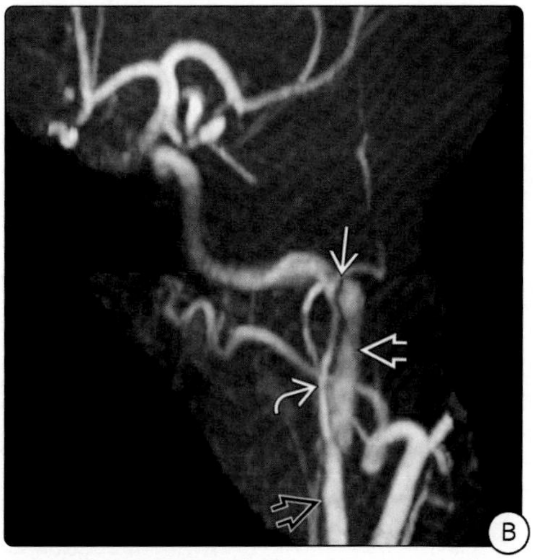

***(10-44B)** 2D TOF MRA in the same case clearly depicts dissection flap, lumen, subintimal hematoma. Proximal ICA is normal.*

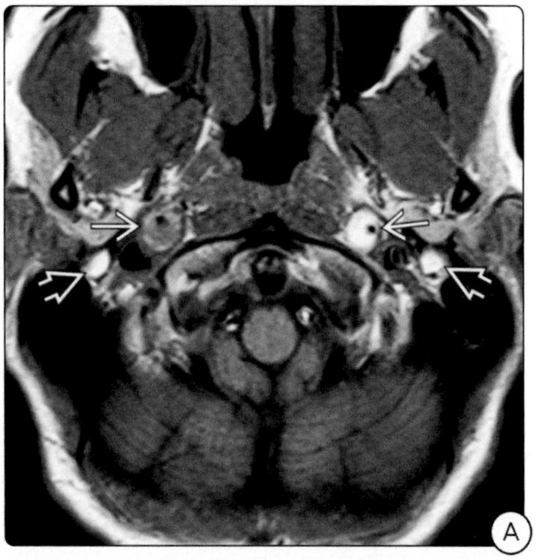

(10-45A) T1WI in Marfan shows dissection of both cervical ICAs ➡, both VAs ➡ with mural thrombus around tiny residual "flow voids."

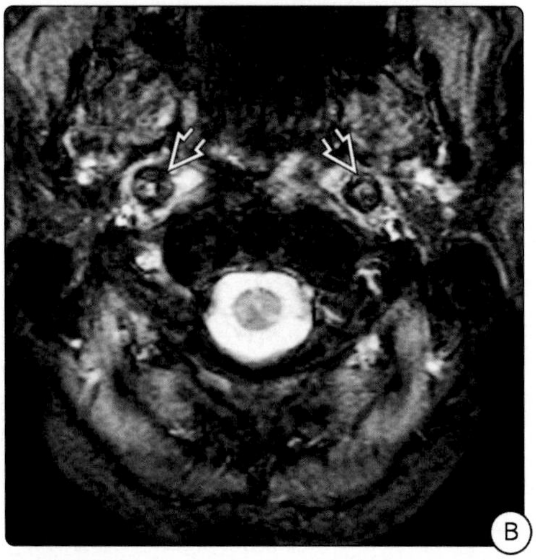

(10-45B) T2 GRE in the same patient demonstrates that the mural thrombus around the distal cervical ICAs "blooms" ➡.*

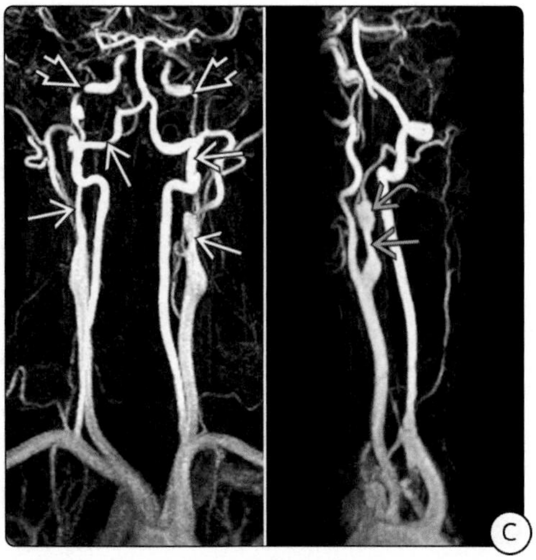

(10-45C) (L) MRA shows dissections in cervicocephalic vessels ➡, petrous ICAs ➡. (R) Left ICA dissection ⇨, pseudoaneurysm ⇨.

Gross Pathology. An intimal tear permits dissection of blood into the vessel wall, resulting in a medial or subendothelial hematoma. The hematoma narrows and may occlude the parent vessel lumen **(10-42)**. Occasionally dissections—especially in the VA—extend through the adventitia and present with SAH.

Clinical Issues

Epidemiology and Demographics. The annual incidence of ICA dissection is 2.5-3.0 cases per 100,000. The incidence of VA dissection is approximately half that of the ICA.

Although dissections occur at all ages, most are found in young and middle-aged adults. Peak age is 40 years. Carotid dissections are more common in men, whereas vertebral dissections are more common in women.

CAD accounts for approximately 2% of all ischemic strokes. In young and middle-aged patients with no or minimal ASVD risk factors, dissections may account for 10-25% of all ischemic strokes.

Presentation. Neck pain and headache are the most common symptoms. One or more lower cranial nerve palsies including postganglionic Horner syndrome may occur. Pulsatile tinnitus is a less frequent presentation.

Natural History. The natural history of most extracranial CADs is benign. Approximately 90% of stenoses resolve, and 60% of all occlusions recanalize. The risk of recurrent dissection is low; 2% in the first month, then 1% per year thereafter (usually in another vessel).

Persistent headache, pulsatile tinnitus, postganglionic Horner syndrome, and ischemic stroke are uncommon but well-recognized complications of CAD.

Intracranial CAD is much more problematic. Stroke is more common, and spontaneous recanalization is less frequent.

Treatment Options. Anticoagulation is the recommended treatment for extracranial arterial dissection. Six months of antiplatelet therapy in asymptomatic patients with stable imaging findings is common. Intravenous heparin with oral warfarin is an option, as is endovascular stenting. The treatment of intracranial CAD is controversial.

Imaging

Both lumen-opacifying procedures (e.g., CTA, conventional DSA, MRA) and cross-sectional techniques that visualize the vessel wall itself (e.g., CT, MR) should be used to delineate the full extent of disease.

General Features. Dissections can present as stenosis, occlusion, or aneurysmal dilatation.

CT Findings. NECT may show crescent-shaped thickening caused by the wall hematoma. Approximately 20% of VA dissections cause posterior fossa SAH.

CECT may show narrowing of the dissected vessel with or without aneurysmal dilatation.

MR Findings. T1WI with fat saturation is the best sequence for demonstrating CAD. A hyperintense crescent of subacute blood adjacent to a narrowed "flow void" in the patent lumen is typical **(10-43)**. T2WI may show laminated layers of thrombus that "blooms" on T2* **(10-45)**.

At least half of all patients with cervicocephalic dissections have cerebral or cerebellar infarcts, best depicted on DWI. Multiple ipsilateral foci of diffusion restriction are typical findings.

Angiography. Extracranial ICA dissections typically spare the carotid bulb, beginning 2-3 cm distal to the bifurcation and terminating at the exocranial opening of the carotid canal **(10-44A)**. Vertebral dissections are most common around the skull base and upper cervical spine.

CTA and MRA demonstrate an eccentrically narrowed lumen surrounded by a crescent-shaped mural thickening. A dissection flap can sometimes be identified **(10-44B)**. Pseudoaneurysms are common. An opacified double lumen ("true" plus "false" lumen) occurs in less than 10% of cases.

The most common finding on DSA is a smooth or slightly irregular, tapered midcervical narrowing **(10-44A)**. CAD with occlusion shows a flame-shaped "rat-tail" termination. Occasionally a subtle intimal tear or flap, a double lumen, narrowed or occluded true lumen, or pseudoaneurysm can be identified. If the dissection is subadventitial and does not narrow the vessel lumen, DSA can appear entirely normal; the paravascular hematoma must be detected on cross-sectional imaging.

Intracranial dissections are more difficult to diagnose than their extracranial counterparts **(10-46B)**. They are significantly smaller, and findings are often subtle **(10-47)**.

DISSECTION

Terminology
- Vessel wall tear → blood penetrates into, splits layers apart
  - Intramural hematoma formed
  - With or without pseudoaneurysm

Pathoetiology
- "Spontaneous" (nontraumatic) 60%, traumatic 40%
  - Underlying vasculopathy (FMD, Marfan, etc.) 40%
- Location
  - Extracranial ICA (spares bulb, usually terminates at skull base)
  - Vertebral artery (skull base-C1, C1-C2 most common)
  - Intracranial = extracranial (vertebral > > carotid)
  - Multiple arteries 20% (look for underlying vasculopathy)
- Gross pathology
  - Medial or subendothelial > subadventitial hematoma

Clinical Issues
- Most common cause of stroke in young, middle-aged adults
  - 2% of all ischemic strokes
- Peak age = 40 years
- Neck pain, headache
- 90% of stenoses, 60% of occlusions resolve
- Recurrent dissection rare (usually different vessel)

Imaging Findings
- Eccentric, crescent-shaped mural hematoma
  - Hyperintense on T1 FS
  - "Blooms" on T2*
  - Look for infarcts on DWI
- Long segment, smooth narrowing of vessel lumen typical
- ± Pseudoaneurysm

Differential Diagnosis
- Type 2 (intimal) FMD
- Atherosclerosis (involves bulb)
- Thrombosis without dissection
- Vasospasm

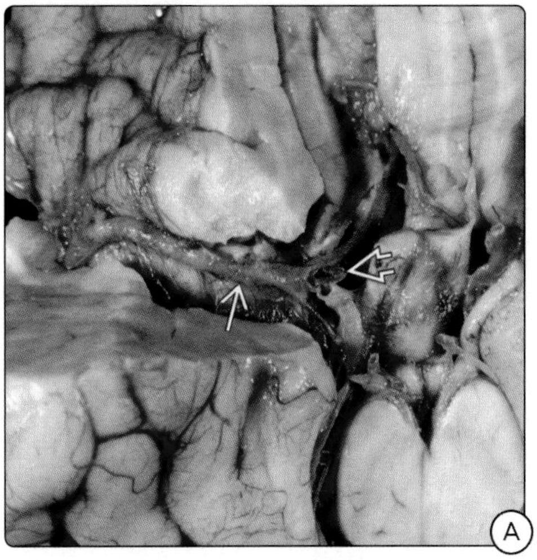

***(10-46A)** Autopsy case shows intracranial dissection extending from the supraclinoid ICA ➡ into the horizontal (M1) MCA segment ➡.*

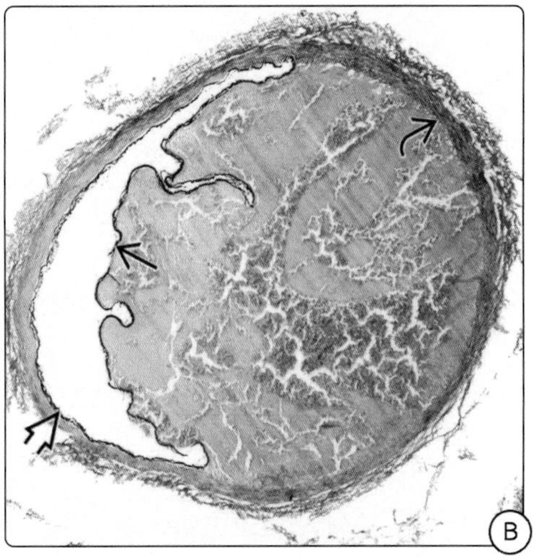

***(10-46B)** MCA shows organizing hematoma between intima, IEL ➡, and muscularis ➡; lumen ➡ is narrowed. (Courtesy R. Hewlett, MD.)*

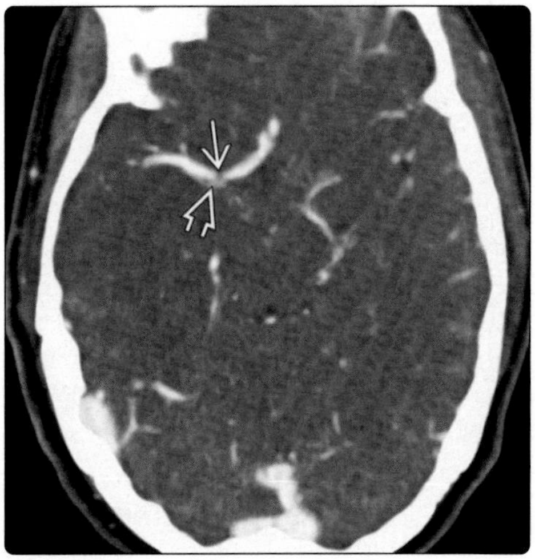

***(10-47)** CTA in a patient with supraclinoid ICA dissection shows hyperdense clot ➡ surrounding a very narrow distal ICA ➡.*

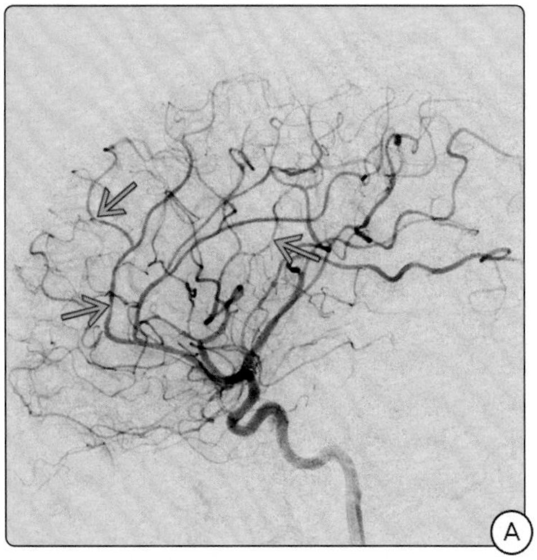

***(10-48A)** DSA in a 35y woman with thunderclap headache shows only multifocal "beaded" arterial segments ➱.*

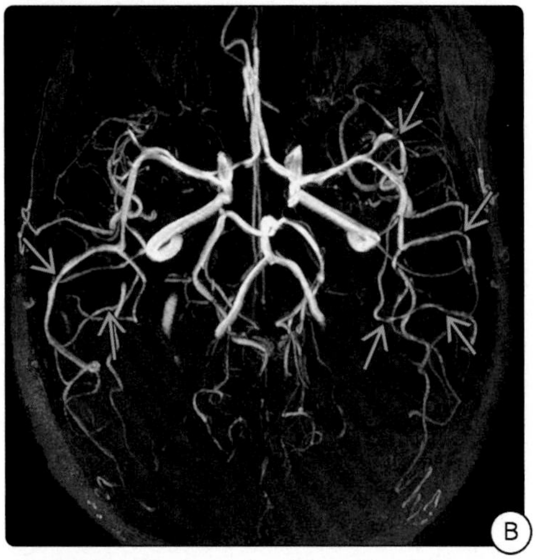

***(10-48B)** DSA 3 days later shows dramatic worsening with multiple bilateral "beaded" 2nd- and 3rd-order MCA branches ➱.*

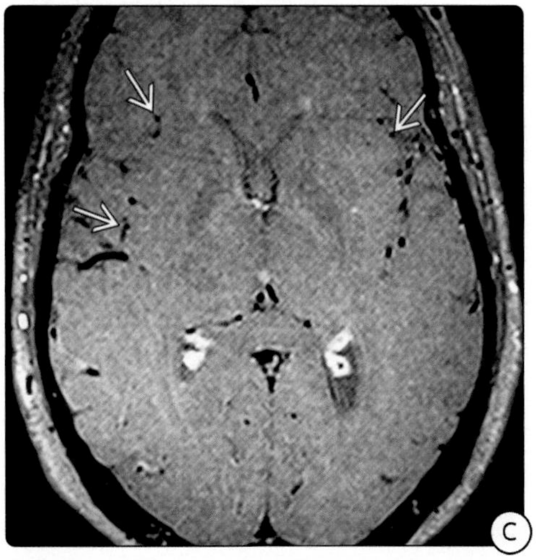

***(10-48C)** High-resolution "black blood" contrast-enhanced vessel wall imaging shows constricted vessels with no wall enhancement ➡; RCVS.*

Differential Diagnosis

The major differential diagnosis of *extracranial* arterial dissection is type 2 (intimal) **FMD**. A common complication of FMD is dissection, so the two conditions are interrelated and may be indistinguishable on imaging studies alone. Although multiple dissections do occur, they are much less common than multifocal FMD; careful evaluation of the other cervicocephalic vessels for typical changes of FMD may be helpful.

Atherosclerosis is more common than dissection in older patients. ASVD typically involves the great vessel origins and carotid bulb, sites that are almost always spared by dissection. As ASVD is a systemic disorder, multiple vessels in multiple vascular distributions are usually affected. Dissection, on the other hand, is solitary unless an underlying vasculopathy such as Marfan or Ehlers-Danlos syndrome is present **(10-45B)**.

Arterial **thrombosis** without an underlying dissection can cause tapered "rat-tail" narrowing or occlusion. Imaging findings of isolated thrombosis are difficult to distinguish from those of dissection complicated by a secondary superimposed thrombosis.

Vasospasm or reduced distal flow can cause diffuse narrowing of the extracranial vessels. Catheter-induced vasospasm during angiography typically resolves quickly.

Vasospasm and atherosclerosis are the major differential diagnostic considerations for *intracranial* dissections. Both affect multiple vessels in several vascular distributions, whereas intracranial CAD almost always is limited to the supraclinoid ICA and proximal MCA.

Vasoconstriction Syndromes

Vasospasm with multifocal foci of arterial constriction and dilation is a common, well-recognized complication of aneurysmal SAH (aSAH) and is the most common cause of severe cerebral vasoconstriction (see Chapter 6). Vasospasm and vasospasm-like arterial constrictions can also occur in the absence of aSAH, trauma, or infection.

Terminology

Reversible cerebral vasoconstriction syndrome (RCVS) now encompasses what was once considered a group of distinct clinical entities including Call-Fleming syndrome, postpartum angiopathy, drug-induced angiopathy, migrainous vasospasm, and thunderclap headache with reversible vasospasm.

The International Headache Society diagnostic criteria for RCVS include severe acute headache, a uniphasic disease course, no evidence for *aneurysmal* SAH (*convexal* SAH is common), normal/near normal CSF, and imaging demonstration of segmental cerebral artery vasoconstrictions that resolve within 3 months.

Etiology

The exact etiology of RCVS is unknown. Some authors posit that, rather than representing a single specific disease entity, the broad heterogeneity of clinical and imaging manifestations associated with RCVS suggests that it may represent a common end point of numerous diverse disease processes.

RCVS may result from deregulation in vascular tone induced by sympathetic overactivity (including sympathomimetic medications and recreational drugs), endothelial dysfunction, and oxidative stress.

Brain biopsies have demonstrated no histopathologic evidence for vasculitis or inflammatory infiltrates within the constricted, diffusely thickened vessel walls often associated with RCVS.

REVERSIBLE CEREBRAL VASOCONSTRICTION SYNDROME (RCVS)

Terminology
- Vasospasm with multifocal arterial constrictions
- RCVS now encompasses several entities
  - Call-Fleming syndrome
  - Postpartum angiopathy
  - Drug-induced angiopathies
  - Migrainous vasospasm, etc.

Pathoetiology
- Unknown
  - May represent end point of several disease processes
- Dysregulated vascular tone
- No histopathologic evidence for vasculitis, inflammation

Clinical Issues
- International Headache Society criteria for RCVS
  - Severe acute headache ("thunderclap" characteristic, nonspecific)
  - Uniphasic course
  - No evidence for aSAH
  - Normal/near normal CSF
  - Imaging shows segmental vasoconstrictions, resolve in 3 months
- Demographics
  - 20-50 years most common
  - F:M = 2.5:1.0
- Other: vasoactive medications, pregnancy, etc. 25-60%

Imaging Findings
- Multifocal arterial constrictions
  - Multiple vascular territories involved
- "Beaded" appearance
  - Characteristic but nonspecific
- High-resolution vessel wall imaging
  - No/minimal enhancement
  - ± Thickened wall, reduced lumen
- Other
  - cSAH
  - Strokes

Differential Diagnosis
- Posterior reversible encephalopathy syndrome (PRES)
  - Overlaps, often coexists with RCVS
- aSAH-related vasospasm
- Vasculitis
  - Concentric, long-segment wall enhancement

Clinical Issues

RCVS most commonly affects patients between the ages of 20-50 years although cases have also been reported in children and older adults. There is a slight female predominance (2.5:1.0).

Although "thunderclap" headache is characteristic, it is not specific for RCVS. A waxing and waning course with repeated episodes during 1-3 weeks is common.

A history of migraine headaches is elicited in 20-40% of cases. An exogenous "trigger" such as vasoactive medications and postpartum state is reported in 25-60% of cases.

Imaging

The diagnosis of RCVS requires demonstration of multifocal segmental arterial constrictions in multiple vascular territories on CTA, MRA, or DSA **(10-48)**. A "beaded" appearance with multifocal areas of narrowing interspersed with normal segments is typical. Initial imaging may be unremarkable during the first week after symptom onset, so repeat examination may be necessary.

High-resolution vessel wall imaging typically shows no or minimal enhancement **(10-48)**.

Convexal (cortical) SAH (cSAH) is identified in about one-third of cases, whereas strokes are seen in 6-39% and concomitant PRES in 9-38%.

Differential Diagnosis

RCVS and posterior reversible encephalopathy syndrome (**PRES**) overlap in both their clinical and imaging features and may occur concurrently. PRES-like reversible cerebral edema is seen in up to one-third of RCVS cases, and RCVS-like vasoconstrictions can be identified in the majority of PRES patients.

The other major differential diagnoses of RCVS are **aSAH-related vasospasm** and CNS vasculitis. RCVS-associated thunderclap headaches are often relapsing-remitting. aSAH typically occurs in the basal cisterns; isolated cSAH is rare. In aSAH, the vasospasm is typically long-segment narrowing of arteries in/around the circle of Willis. In RCVS, the segmental vasoconstrictions preferentially involve the more distal (second- and third-order) branches.

Vessel wall imaging can help distinguish RCVS from **vasculitis**. Concentric or tram-track wall enhancement is common in vasculitis; it is mild or absent in RCVS.

Vasculitis and Vasculitides

Terminology

The generic terms "vasculitis" and "angiitis" denote inflammation of blood vessels affecting arteries, veins, or both. The plural "vasculitides" is a more generic term that is often used interchangeably. "Arteritis" is more specific and refers solely to inflammatory processes that involve arteries.

Classification

Classifying vasculitis is difficult and controversial. The two most widely used classifications are the 1990 American College of Rheumatology (ACR) criteria and the 2007 Chapel Hill Consensus Conference (CHCC) criteria.

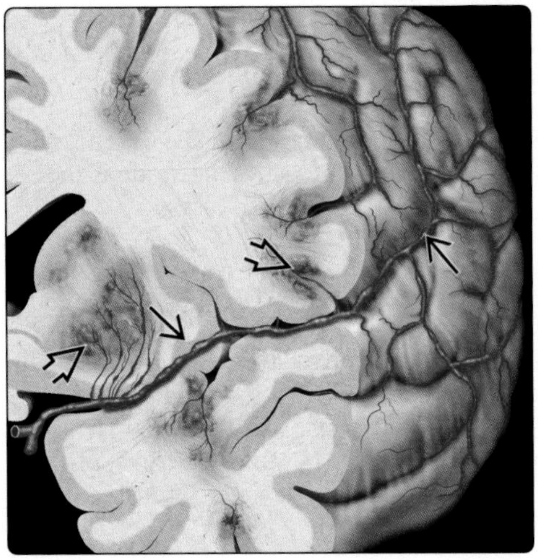

(10-49) Graphic shows vasculitis ➡ with multifocal infarcts, scattered hemorrhages ⇨ in the basal ganglia and at the GM-WM junction.

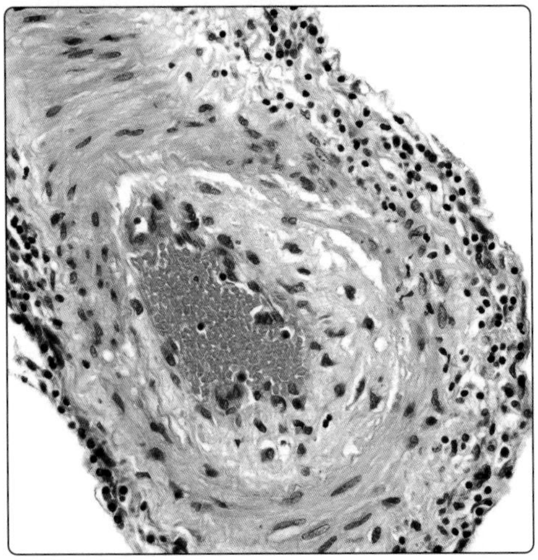

(10-50) Photomicrograph shows thick vessel wall with inflammation and necrosis, the cardinal features of vasculitis. (Courtesy R. Hewlett, MD.)

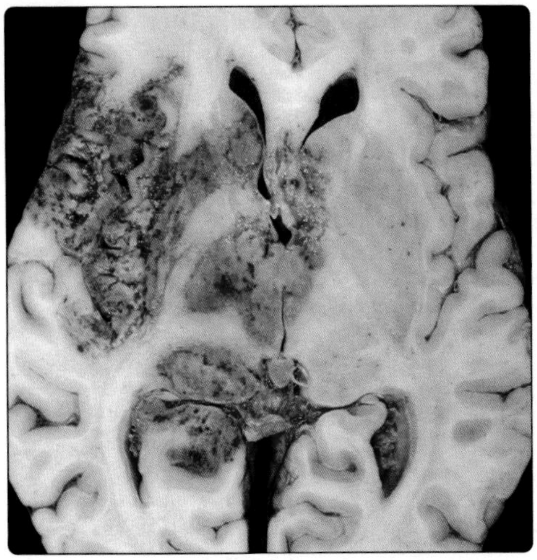

(10-51) Autopsy specimen shows vasculitis with multifocal cortical, basal ganglia lesions characterized by necrosis, petechial hemorrhages.

The ACR identified seven widely accepted types of vasculitis: giant cell arteritis, Takayasu arteritis, Wegener granulomatosis, Churg-Strauss syndrome, polyarteritis nodosa, Henoch-Schönlein purpura, and hypersensitivity vasculitis. This system was developed prior to the recognition of antineutrophil cytoplasmic autoantibodies (ANCAs), which now play a key role in the differential diagnosis of patients with small vessel vasculitis.

The CHCC further differentiated immune-complex-mediated vasculitides and cryoglobulinemic vasculitis, recognized ANCA-associated vasculitis, and distinguished microscopic polyangiitis from polyarteritis nodosa.

Etiology

Vasculitis can be caused by infection, collagen-vascular disease, immune complex deposition, drug abuse, and even neoplasms (e.g., lymphomatoid granulomatosis). The general pathologic features of many vasculitides are quite similar **(10-49)**. As a result, the definitive diagnosis depends primarily on hematologic and immunohistochemical characteristics. Other "surrogate" clinical markers such as glomerulonephritis and granulomatous inflammation of the airways have recently been added to help distinguish among the various vasculitides.

Isolated CNS vasculitis in which thorough clinical and laboratory examination does not identify another disorder causing the vascular inflammation is called **primary arteritis of the CNS (PACNS)**. This contrasts with the many *secondary* causes of CNS vasculitis.

Pathology

Although the vasculitides are a heterogeneous group of CNS disorders, they are characterized histopathologically by two cardinal features: inflammation and necrosis in blood vessel walls **(10-50)**. Infarcts in multiple vascular distributions are common **(10-51)**.

PACNS is definitively diagnosed by histopathologic examination of CNS blood vessels although its sensitivity may be less than 50%. Granulomatous vasculitis—the most common histopathologic subtype of PACNS—is characterized by mononuclear infiltrates with granulomas and multinucleated cells.

Imaging

As imaging in most vasculitides is similar regardless of etiology, this discussion will focus on the general features of vasculitis as it affects the brain.

CT Findings. NECT scans are relatively insensitive and are often normal. In a few cases, the first imaging manifestation of vasculitis is SAH (especially cSAH).

Multifocal hypodensities in the basal ganglia and subcortical white matter that demonstrate patchy enhancement on CECT are common.

MR Findings. Involvement of the cortex/subcortical white matter together with the basal ganglia is strongly suggestive of vasculitis. T1 scans can be normal or show multifocal cortical/subcortical and basal ganglia hypointensities. T2/FLAIR scans demonstrate hyperintensities in the same areas **(10-52A)**. T2* (GRE, SWI) may show parenchymal microhemorrhages **(10-52B)** and/or SAH in some cases.

Patchy enhancement with punctate and linear lesions is common on T1 C+ scans **(10-52C)**. Dural and leptomeningeal thickening/enhancement occur in some cases of granulomatosis with polyangiitis. Acute lesions with cerebral ischemia show multiple foci of diffusion restriction in the cortex, subcortical white matter, and basal ganglia.

High-resolution "black blood" vessel wall imaging shows thickening and multifocal homogeneous smooth, intense, concentric enhancement of the vessel wall.

Angiography. DSA is more sensitive than either CTA or MRA but not as sensitive as high-resolution vessel wall imaging.

Findings include multifocal irregularities, stenoses, and vascular occlusions **(10-53)**. In the past, luminal irregularity has been the imaging standard for characterization and diagnosis of CNS vasculitis. However, it is neither sensitive nor specific for vasculitis and should not be used to diagnose or exclude the disease.

Pseudoaneurysm formation and branch occlusions occur but are less common than luminal irregularities. Although the circle of Willis and horizontal segments of the anterior, middle, and posterior cerebral arteries can be affected, the distal branches of these vessels are most frequently involved.

Differential Diagnosis

The major differential diagnosis of vasculitis is ASVD.

ASVD typically occurs in older patients and involves larger, more proximal intracranial arteries (e.g., the carotid siphon and vertebral and basilar arteries). ASVD sometimes affects second- and third-order branches. Vessel wall imaging usually shows mild noncircumferential or no wall enhancement.

Vasospasm can also mimic vasculitis. However, vasospasm most commonly affects the major cerebral vessels. A history of trauma or SAH is common but not invariably present. **RCVS** and **postpartum angiopathy** can be indistinguishable from vasculitis.

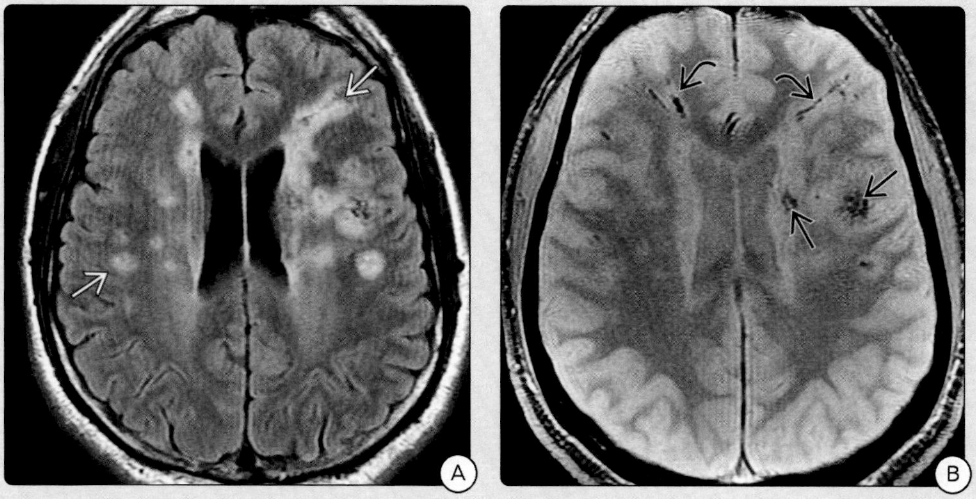

***(10-52A)** Axial FLAIR in a 29y man with headaches and transient neurological symptoms shows multiple bilateral hyperintensities in the caudate nuclei and subcortical and deep white matter. **(10-52B)** T2* GRE shows bilateral "blooming" hypointensities. The linear configuration of some of the lesions suggests vascular etiology.*

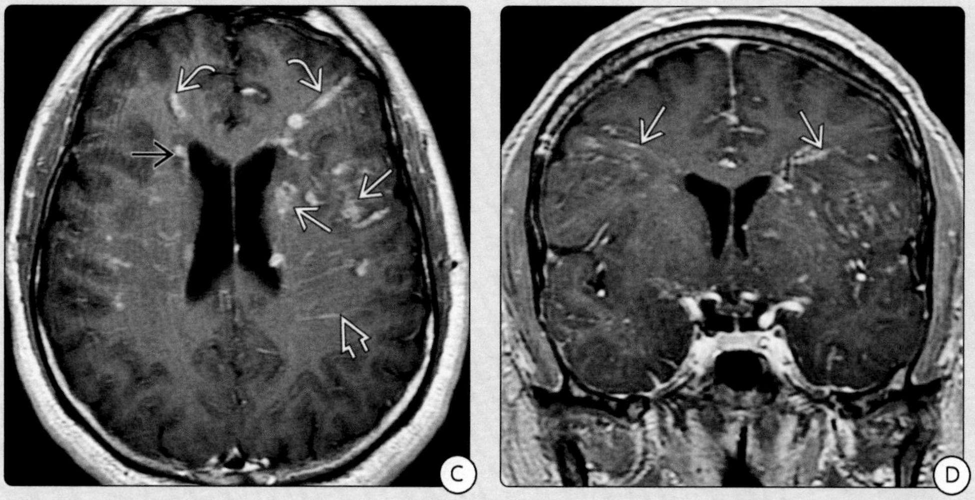

***(10-52C)** Axial T1 C+ MR shows numerous punctate, patchy, and linear enhancing foci. Note linear enhancement of small penetrating vessels. **(10-52D)** Coronal T1 C+ shows the prominent linear pattern of enhancement, suggesting a diffuse vascular process. This is biopsy-proven PACNS.*

Other Macro- and Microvasculopathies

A broad spectrum of both inherited and acquired noninflammatory, nonatherosclerotic diseases can involve the intracranial vasculature. In this section, we briefly review a few of the more important miscellaneous vasculopathies that affect both large and small cerebral vessels.

Sickle Cell Disease

Sickle cell disease (SCD) is one of the best characterized human monogenic disorders and the most common worldwide cause of childhood stroke. African American and African Brazilian children are among the most affected children outside of continental Africa.

Etiology and Pathology. Red blood cell abnormalities underlie the complex pathophysiology of SCD. SCD is an inherited, autosomal-recessive chronic hemolytic anemia caused by a point mutation in the β-globin gene cluster.

Ion balance dysregulation with cellular dehydration concentrates and polymerizes sickle hemoglobin. The rigid RBCs hemolyze, and their vasculotoxic products contribute to dysregulated vasomotor function, inflammation, and endothelial adhesiveness.

Damage to the endothelium of small vessels with progressive fibrosis, narrowing, and eventually occlusion are the end result of SCD vasculopathy. The brain microvasculature also assumes an inflammatory, procoagulant state that probably contributes to the high incidence of ischemic stroke in patients with SCD.

Clinical Issues. The most common CNS complication of SCD is stroke. Other neurologic manifestations of SCD include decreased cognitive function ("silent stroke") and headache.

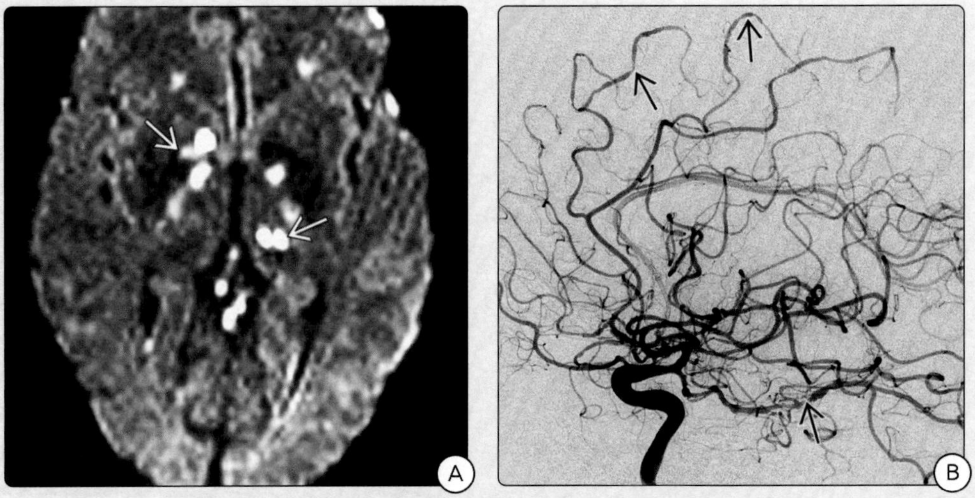

***(10-53A)** DWI in a patient with streptococcal meningitis shows multiple foci of restricted diffusion ➡ in the basal ganglia. Other images (not shown) demonstrated multiple peripheral lesions in the cortex and subcortical white matter. **(10-53B)** Right internal carotid artery angiogram, lateral view, arterial phase, shows multifocal segmental "beaded" areas of arterial narrowing and dilatation ⇨, classic findings of vasculitis.*

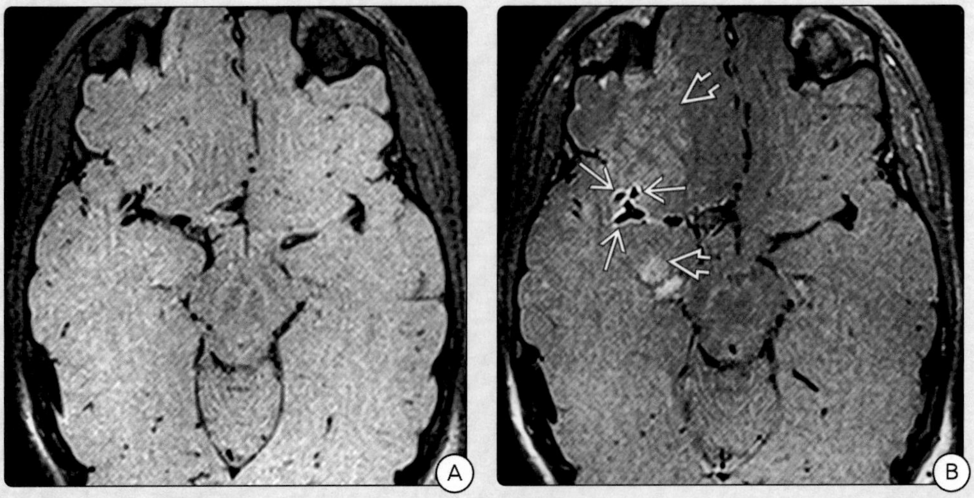

***(10-54A)** Precontrast high-resolution vessel wall imaging in a 14y girl with a "wake-up" stroke 3 days prior to the study shows no abnormality. **(10-54B)** Axial T1 C+ "black blood" shows intense circumferential and linear enhancement in the right MCA vessel walls ➡. Note enhancement in the subacute infarct ➡. This is proven antineutrophil cytoplasmic autoantibody vasculitis causing the MCA stroke.*

Most patients experience repeated ischemic events with worsening motor and intellectual deficits.

Approximately 75% of SCD-related strokes are ischemic, and 25% are hemorrhagic. Stroke risk is highest between the ages of 2 and 5 years.

Chronic transfusion, chelation for iron overload, and treatment with hydroxyurea for stroke prophylaxis are promising new treatments for SCD.

Imaging. A diffusely thickened calvaria with expanded diploic space secondary to increased hematopoiesis is a frequent finding, as is reconversion of "yellow" to "red" (hematopoietic) marrow **(10-55A)**.

Generalized volume loss with sulcal and ventricular enlargement together with multiple hypodensities in the cortex and cerebral white matter is common on NECT scans. CECT scans may show punctate enhancing foci in the basal ganglia and deep white matter from enlarged "moyamoya" type collaterals.

MR scans often demonstrate subcortical and white matter hyperintensities along the deep watershed zone on T2/FLAIR **(10-55B)**. A moyamoya-like pattern with supraclinoid ICA stenosis may develop with especially severe SCD **(10-55C)**. In such cases, an "ivy" sign with serpentine hyperintensities in the cerebral sulci from leptomeningeal collaterals can be seen on FLAIR.

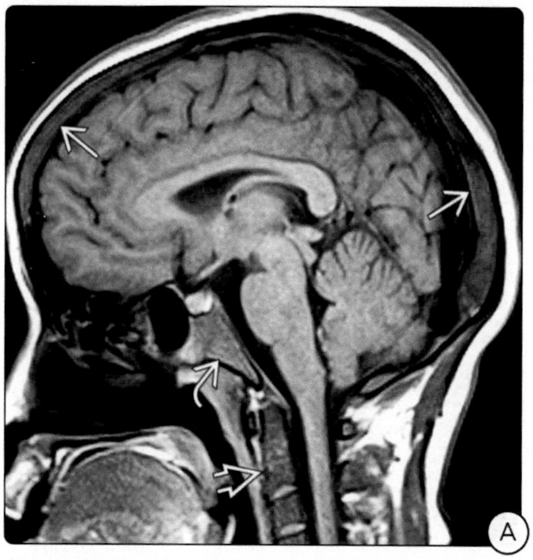

***(10-55A)** T1WI in 29y woman with SCD shows thick calvaria with hypointense marrow ➡. Clivus ➡, vertebral bodies ➡ are hypointense.*

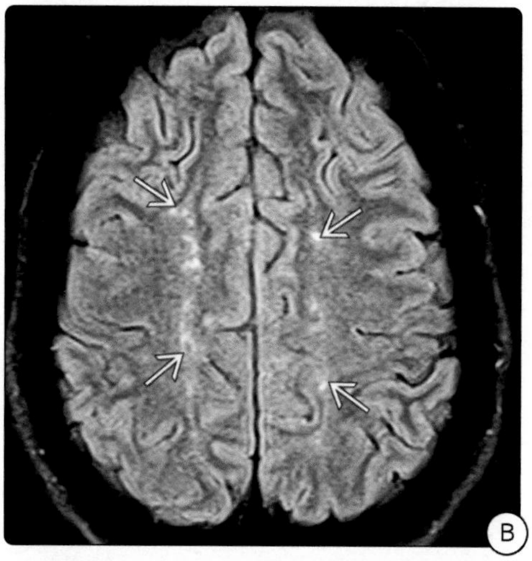

***(10-55B)** FLAIR scan in the same patient shows punctate hyperintensities in both watershed zones ➡, a common finding in SCD.*

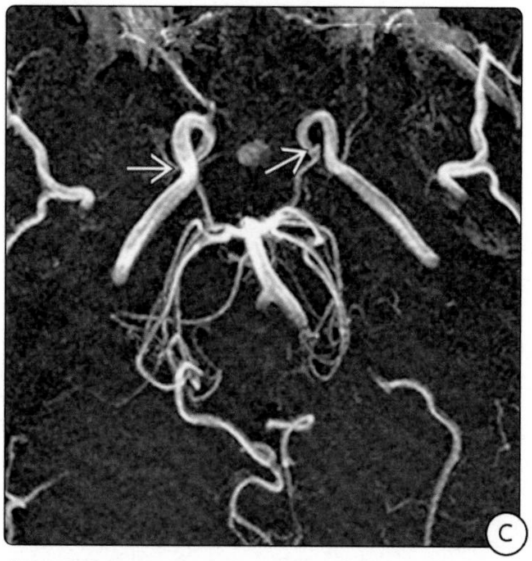

***(10-55C)** Submentovertex MIP of the MRA in the same patient shows occlusion of both supraclinoid ICAs ➡.*

SICKLE CELL DISEASE

Pathoetiology

- Ion balance dysregulation, cellular dehydration concentrate/polymerize sickle hemoglobin
- "Sickled" RBCs hemolyze, release vasculotoxic products
  - Platelet activation
  - Inflammation, ↑ adhesiveness, damage endothelium
  - Fibrosis, vasoconstriction, occlusion result

Clinical Issues

- Most common worldwide cause of childhood stroke
- Acute and chronic anemia
- Neurocognitive impairment common

Imaging

- Stroke
  - 75% ischemic, 25% hemorrhagic
  - Watershed zone WM hyperintensities
- In severe cases
  - ICAs occluded
  - "Moyamoya"-type basal collaterals develop

Moyamoya Disease

Terminology. Moyamoya disease (MMD) is an idiopathic progressive arteriopathy characterized by stenosis of the distal (supraclinoid) ICAs and formation of an abnormal vascular network at the base of the brain **(10-56)**. Multiple enlarged "telangiectatic" lenticulostriate, thalamo-perforating, leptomeningeal, dural, and pial arteries develop as compensatory circulation. These "moyamoya collaterals" can become so extensive that they resemble the "puff of smoke" from a cigarette, the Japanese term for which the disease is named **(10-57)**.

Etiology. The pathophysiology of MMD has been extensively investigated. Approximately 5-10% of Asian MMD cases are familial. Recent genome-wide and locus-specific association studies have identified a variant of the ring finger 213 gene (*RNF213*) as an important susceptibility gene in East Asians

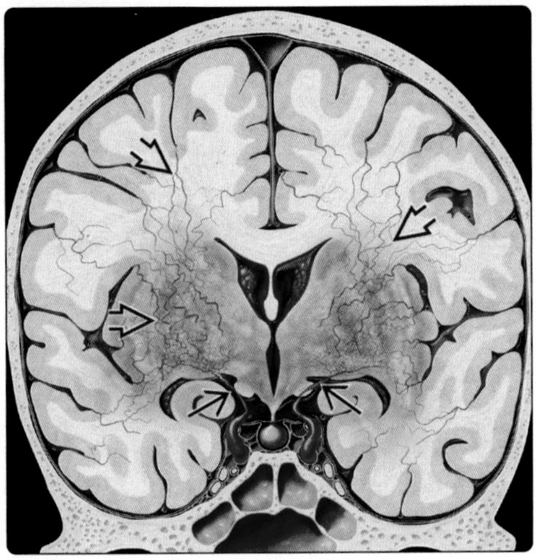

(10-56) MMD shows severely narrowed supraclinoid ICAs ⇒, striking "puff of smoke" from extensive basal ganglia, WM collaterals ⇒.

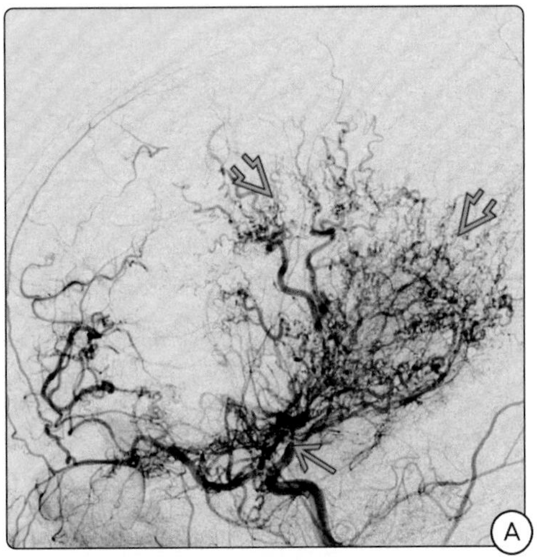

(10-57A) MMD in a 3y child shows near-total supraclinoid ICA stenosis ⇒ with innumerable tortuous enlarged moyamoya-like collaterals ⇒.

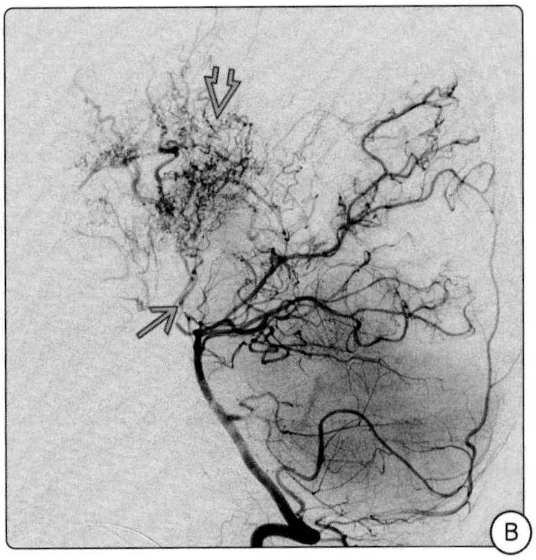

(10-57B) Vertebral angiogram in the same patient shows moyamoya-like collaterals ⇒ from enlarged thalamoperforating arteries ⇒.

with MMD. *RNF213* encodes a protein that is involved in proper vascular development.

MMD is also associated with several genetically transmitted disorders, including neurofibromatosis type 1, trisomy 21 (Down syndrome), and a spectrum of hemoglobinopathies such as sickle cell anemia. Collagen vascular diseases including Marfan and Ehlers-Danlos syndromes have also been associated with MMD.

Moyamoya-*like* collateral vessels can develop with any slowly progressive arteriopathy that affects the major intracranial arteries. When this pattern occurs with a known disease association, it is sometimes termed "pseudo-moyamoya" to distinguish it from "true" (i.e., idiopathic) MMD.

Pathology. The pathologic changes of MMD are very different from those of ASVD and vasculitis. The terminal ICAs show severe stenosis with concentric and eccentric fibrocellular intimal thickening without significant inflammatory cell infiltration. Subintimal lipid deposition, hemorrhage, and necrosis are absent. The internal elastic lamina is typically tortuous and stratified.

Clinical Issues. MMD is most prevalent in Japan and Korea, where its estimated incidence is 0.35-0.54 per 100,000 people. MMD is increasingly diagnosed worldwide, but its incidence in Europeans is estimated at one-tenth that of the Japanese population.

Moyamoya has two peak ages of presentation. Two-thirds of cases occur in children, and at least half of these occur under the age of 10 years. Between one-quarter and one-third present in adults with peak presentation in the fifth decade.

The clinical features of MMD in children differ from those in adults. When MMD presents in childhood, the initial symptoms are usually ischemic. In adults, approximately half of all patients develop intracranial hemorrhage from rupture of the fragile moyamoya collateral vessels. The other 50% present with TIAs or cerebral infarcts.

MMD is relentlessly progressive, and long-term outcome is generally poor. Even relatively "asymptomatic" patients commonly have cognitive disturbances and silent ischemic infarcts. Cerebral revascularization surgery, primarily encephalo-duro-arterio-synangiosis in children and superficial temporal artery-MCA bypass in adults, has been performed with some success.

Imaging. Multiple enhancing punctate "dots" (CECT) or "flow voids" (MR) in the basal ganglia are the most striking findings in MMD. T1 and T2 scans show markedly narrowed supraclinoid ICAs with multiple tortuous, serpentine "flow voids" **(10-58A)** **(10-58B)**. The appearance of multiple tiny collateral vessels in enlarged CSF spaces has been likened to "swimming worms in a bare cistern."

An "ivy" sign with sulcal hyperintensity from slow flow in leptomeningeal collaterals is sometimes seen on FLAIR and correlates with decreased vascular reserve in the affected hemisphere.

Multiple microbleeds can be detected on T2* GRE scans in 15-40% of patients and are associated with increased risk of overt cerebral hemorrhage. Susceptibility-weighted imaging (SWI) shows increased conspicuity of deep medullary veins, an appearance dubbed the "brush" sign.

T1 C+ scans often show contrast stagnating in slow-flowing collateral vessels both in the brain parenchyma and over its surface **(10-58C)**.

Diffusion tensor imaging (DTI) demonstrates loss of microstructural integrity in normal-appearing white matter, seen as lowered FA and elevated ADC.

pMR may demonstrate chronic cerebral hypoperfusion in the ICA territories, seen as increased relative cerebral blood volume secondary to compensatory vasodilatation and delayed TTP due to proximal vessel stenosis.

DSA, CTA, and MRA show predominantly anterior circulation disease with marked narrowing of both supraclinoid ICAs ("bottle neck" sign). The PCAs are less commonly involved. Prominent deep-seated lenticulostriate and thalamoperforator collaterals are present, forming the "puff of smoke" appearance characteristic of moyamoya. Numerous transosseous and transdural collaterals from the extracranial to intracranial circulation may develop.

MOYAMOYA DISEASE

Terminology
- Moyamoya = "puff of smoke"

Etiology and Epidemiology
- Ring finger 213 (*RNF213*) mutation in East Asians
- Progressive arteriopathy → stenosis supraclinoid ICAs

Pathology
- Fibrocellular intimal thickening
- No inflammation, hemorrhage, lipid deposition

Clinical Issues
- Worldwide distribution, most common in Japan
- Children (70%, usually < 10 years)
  - TIAs, stroke
- Adults (30%)
  - Hemorrhage > stroke
- Relentless course
- Revascularization (encephalo-duro-arterial-synangiosis, extracranial-intracranial bypass)

Imaging
- Stenosis/occlusion of supraclinoid ICAs
- Innumerable basal collaterals
- Atrophy
- Strokes (chronic, acute)
- Hemorrhage
  - Parenchymal
  - Subarachnoid

Moyamoya-Like Vascular Collaterals
- Moyamoya disease
- Radiation therapy
- NF1
- Trisomy 21
- Sickle cell disease
- Slowly progressive ASVD

Differential Diagnosis. The differential diagnosis of idiopathic ("true") moyamoya disease includes other slowly developing occlusive vasculopathies. **Radiation therapy**, **neurofibromatosis type 1**, **trisomy 21**, **sickle cell disease**, and even **atherosclerosis** may develop multiple small moyamoya-like collateral vessels.

Classic moyamoya typically affects *both* supraclinoid ICAs while sparing the posterior circulation. A unilateral **"aplastic"** or **twig-like M1 MCA** is a rare nonprogressive congenital anomaly that should be differentiated from MMD. Degenerative stenoocclusive disease with **"segmental" high-grade stenosis** or occlusion of the M1 MCA with a network of small vessels

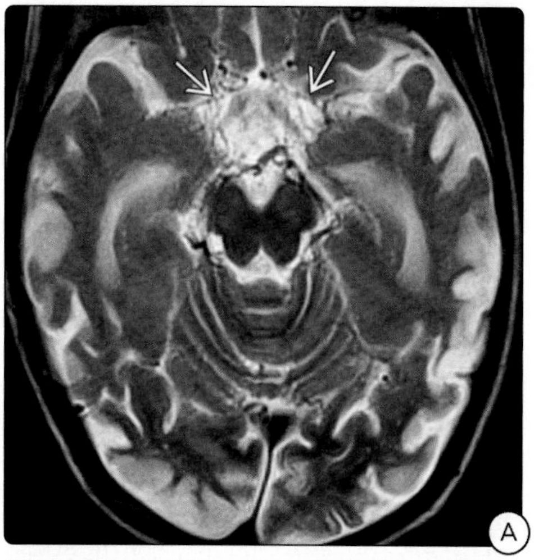

***(10-58A)** T2WI shows attenuated, almost thread-like supraclinoid ICAs, MCAs ➡ with marked cortical atrophy, enlarged temporal horns.*

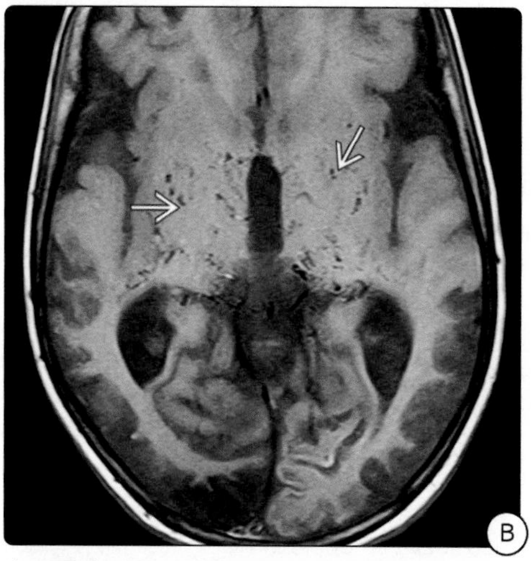

***(10-58B)** T1WI in the same patient shows multiple "flow voids" from enlarged moyamoya collaterals in the basal ganglia, thalami ➡.*

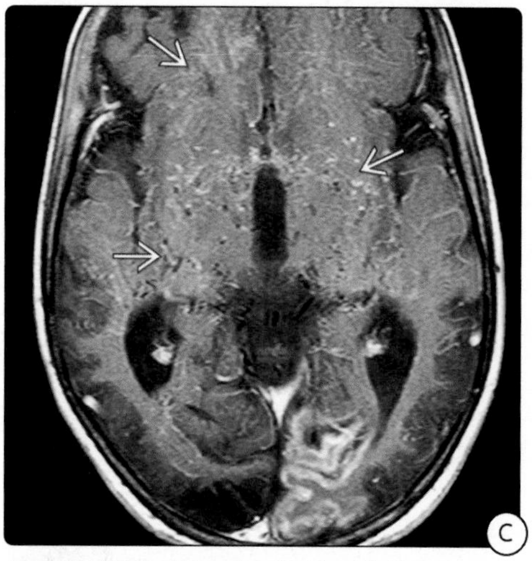

***(10-58C)** T1 C+ shows "puff of smoke" (punctate/serpentine enhancing vessels in BG, thalami, deep WM ➡). (Courtesy H. Els, MD.)*

bridging the gap between the horizontal and distal segments should also be differentiated from MMD.

CADASIL

CADASIL is the acronym for **c**erebral **a**utosomal **d**ominant **a**rteriopathy with **s**ubcortical **i**nfarcts and **l**eukoencephalopathy. CADASIL is an autosomal-dominant disease of the cerebral microvasculature that primarily affects smooth muscle cells in penetrating cerebral and leptomeningeal arteries.

Etiology and Pathology. CADASIL is caused by highly stereotyped missense point mutations in the *NOTCH3* gene. Fourteen distinct familial forms of CADASIL have been identified with mutations in different *NOTCH3* exons. These mutations all cause an odd number of cysteine residues within an epidermal growth factor repeat in the extracellular domain of *NOTCH3*.

The pathologic hallmark of CADASIL is accumulation of granular osmiophilic material in the basement membranes of small arteries and arterioles that causes severe fibrotic thickening and stenosis. Long penetrating cerebral arteries and their branches are especially affected. At autopsy, mild to moderate diffuse cerebral atrophy with multiple lacunar infarcts in the periventricular white matter, basal ganglia, thalamus, midbrain, and pons is present.

Clinical Issues. Although symptoms are restricted to the CNS, arterial changes of CADASIL are systemic. While its exact prevalence is unknown, CADASIL has been identified as the most common monogenic heritable cause of lacunar stroke and vascular dementia in adults. At initial presentation, only 35% of patients have a first-degree relative with known CADASIL.

The classic clinical presentation involves a young to middle-aged adult without identifiable vascular risk factors ("cryptogenic stroke"). The main clinical manifestations are recurrent ischemic strokes (60-85%), migraine headache with aura (which occurs in 25-75% of cases and is often the earliest manifestation of the disease), psychiatric disturbances (20-40%), and progressive cognitive impairment (20-40%). Although symptom onset is generally in the third decade, CADASIL can present in children.

Between 5-10% of CADASIL patients develop epileptic seizures, typically late in the disease course. A small number of patients present with an acute reversible encephalopathy syndrome with fever, confusion, coma, and seizure lasting several days.

CADASIL generally follows a progressive course, causing disability and dementia in 75% of cases. CADASIL patients who have a high lesion burden on baseline MR studies are at high risk for more rapid disease progression.

Imaging. Imaging is important in raising the possible diagnosis of CADASIL, as characteristic patterns may precede overt symptoms by more than a decade. The typical findings are multiple lacunar infarcts in the basal ganglia and high signal intensity lesions in the subcortical and periventricular white matter (WM).

NECT scans can be normal early in the disease course or show hypodense foci in the affected regions.

Bilateral, multifocal T2 and FLAIR hyperintensities in the periventricular and deep WM begin to appear by age 20. Although these findings are nonspecific, involvement of the **anterior temporal lobe** and **external capsule** has high sensitivity and specificity in differentiating CADASIL from the much more common sporadic cerebral small vessel disease (primarily arteriolosclerosis and lipohyalinosis) **(10-59A)**. DTI can demonstrate ultrastructural tissue damage with reduced FA even in "normal-appearing" WM.

Lacunar infarcts in the subcortical WM, basal ganglia, thalamus, internal capsule, and brainstem are found in 75% of patients between 30-40 years of age and increase in both number and prominence with age. Mild to moderate generalized cerebral atrophy is a relatively late finding and is independently associated with the extent of cognitive decline.

Cerebral microbleeds (CMBs) are found on T2* scans in 25% of patients between 40 and 50 years old and are seen in nearly 50% of patients over 50. Cortical superficial siderosis is absent.

Differential Diagnosis. The clinical diagnosis of CADASIL is often elusive, with at least one-third of all patients initially misdiagnosed with MS, dementia, or CNS vasculitis. Using electron microscopy to detect granular osmiophilic deposits in skin biopsy specimens is highly reliable, and immunostaining for NOTCH3 increases both sensitivity and specificity to over 90%.

The imaging differential diagnosis of CADASIL includes sporadic subcortical arteriosclerotic encephalopathy, mitochondrial encephalomyopathy with lactic acidosis and stroke-like episodes (MELAS), vasculitis, and antiphospholipid syndromes. **Subcortical arteriosclerotic encephalopathy** is a hypertension-associated disorder that causes WM disease and lacunar infarcts. Unlike CADASIL, the lesions generally do not involve the anterior temporal WM.

MELAS typically shows cortical and subcortical lesions and may present acutely as hyperintense gyral swelling on T2/FLAIR that resolves with clinical recovery. **Antiphospholipid syndromes** and **protein S deficiency** can both present in young and middle-aged adults. Cortical and lacunar infarcts, vasculitis-like findings on DSA, dural sinus thromboses, and WM hyperintensities on T2/FLAIR are common.

Other hereditary small vessel diseases of the cerebral vasculature can mimic CADASIL. A second known single-gene disorder that directly affects cerebral small vessels is termed **CARASIL** (**c**erebral **a**utosomal-**r**ecessive **a**rteriopathy with **s**ubcortical **i**nfarcts and **l**eukoencephalopathy). Most CARASIL cases have been reported in Japanese patients.

CADASIL

Pathoetiology
- Autosomal dominant
- *NOTCH3* missense mutation
- Osmophilic granule deposition in small arteries/arterioles
  - Thickening, stenosis
  - Occlusion, WM rarefaction

Clinical Issues
- Most common monogenic heritable cause of stroke/vascular dementia
- Recurrent ischemic strokes in young/middle-aged adults
  - Identifiable vascular risk factors absent ("cryptogenic stroke")
  - Only 35% have first-degree relative with known CADASIL

Imaging
- Imaging abnormalities at least 10 years before overt symptoms develop
- Multiple lacunae
  - Basal ganglia, subcortical WM, thalami, brainstem
- T2/FLAIR
  - Universal "leukoaraiosis"
  - Patchy, confluent hyperintensities
  - Anterior temporal, external capsule high sensitivity, specificity

Behçet Disease

Behçet disease (BD) is a chronic, idiopathic, relapsing-remitting, multisystem, inflammatory vascular disease that is characterized mainly by skin lesions. The CNS is involved in 20-25% of patients. When BD occurs in the CNS, it is termed neuro-Behçet disease (NBD).

Etiology and Pathology. CNS involvement in NBD is divided into parenchymal and nonparenchymal lesions. Parenchymal NBD is mainly a meningoencephalitis, with lesions in the brainstem, hemispheres, spinal cord, or meningoencephalitic lesions.

Nonparenchymal manifestations of NBD include dural sinus thrombosis, arterial occlusion, and/or aneurysms. Dural sinus and cortical vein thrombosis with intracranial hypertension is found in 10-35% of patients. Occlusion and pseudoaneurysm formation involving the intra- and extracranial arteries has been reported in NBD but is rare compared with venous disease.

Typical histologic findings of NBD are perivascular necrosis with mild inflammatory infiltrates and oligodendroglial degeneration.

Clinical Issues. While BD is most common in the Mediterranean region, the Middle East, and East Asia (especially Japan), it has a worldwide distribution. NBD typically affects young adults and has a moderate male predominance.

The major clinical features of BD are mucocutaneous recurrent oral and genital ulcers, aphthous stomatitis, ophthalmologic lesions such as uveitis and iridocyclitis, and multiple arthralgias **(10-60)**. Parenchymal NBD typically presents with pyramidal symptoms, whereas nonparenchymal disease usually causes elevated intracranial pressure secondary to dural sinus occlusion.

The clinical course of BD is typically chronic and may span up to a decade, although fulminant disease with rapid clinical deterioration has been reported. Neurologic involvement usually occurs months to years following systemic disease but is the initial presentation in 5% of patients. Overall mortality of NBD is low (5%).

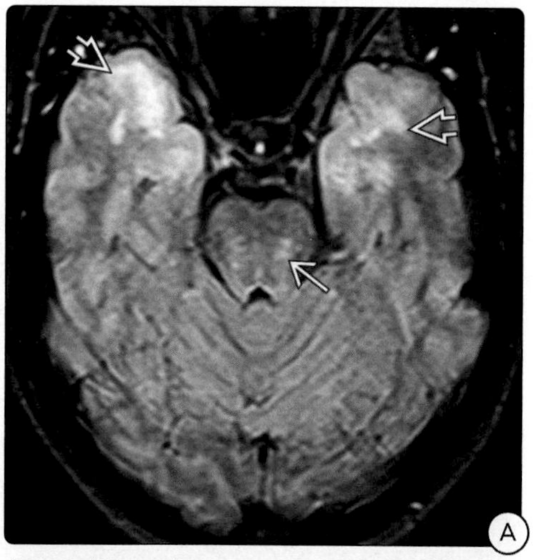

(10-59A) *FLAIR in a 32y woman w/ repeat strokes shows patchy/confluent WM hyperintensities in anterior temporal lobes ➡ and pons ➡.*

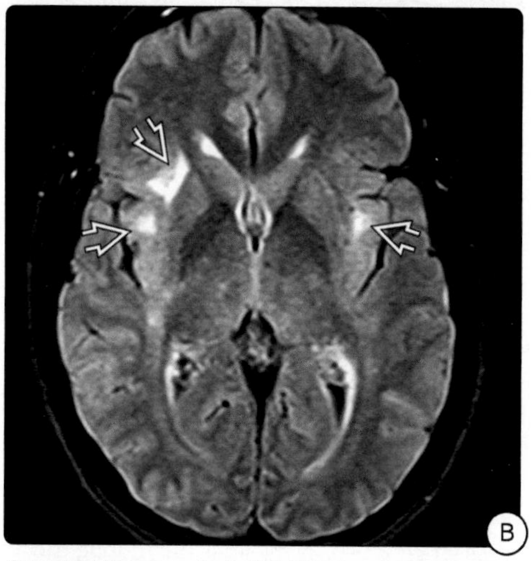

(10-59B) *More cephalad FLAIR scan in the same case demonstrates lesions in both external capsules ➡.*

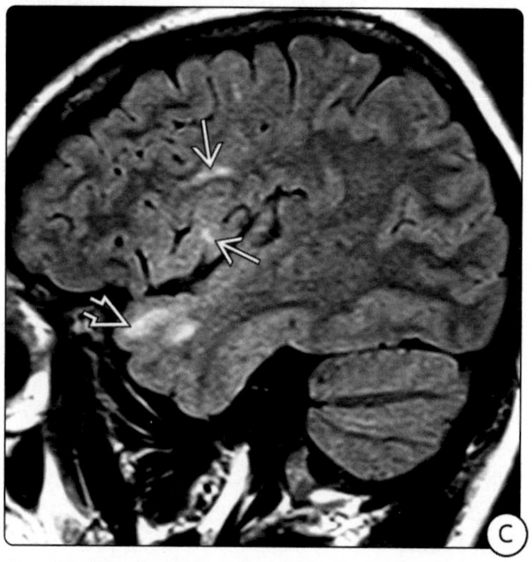

(10-59C) *Sagittal FLAIR shows anterior temporal subcortical WM ➡, external capsule lesions ➡; proven CADASIL with NOTCH3 mutation.*

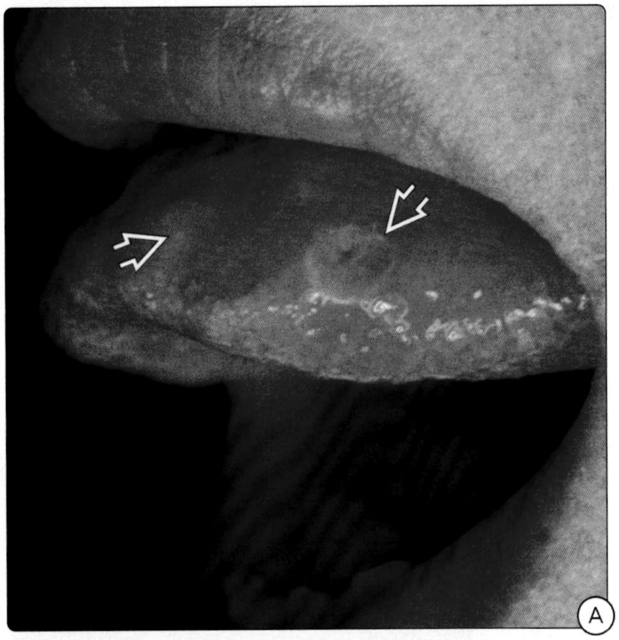

(10-60A) Clinical photograph of a patient with Behçet disease (BD) shows the classic oral ulcers ➡ involving the tongue and oral mucosa.

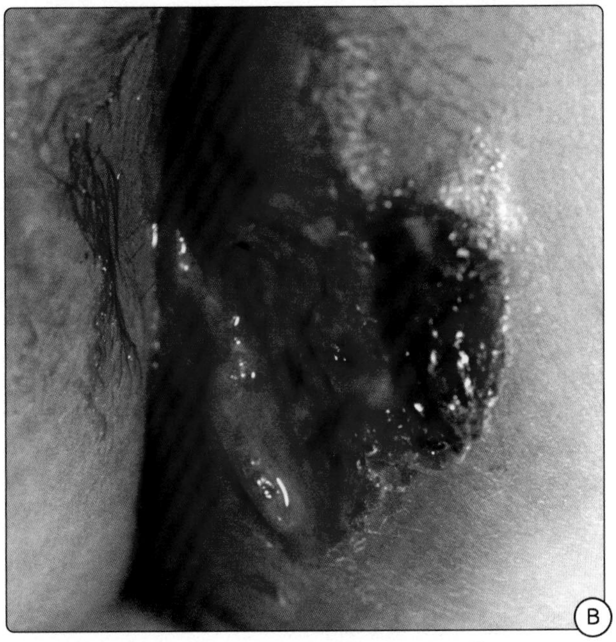

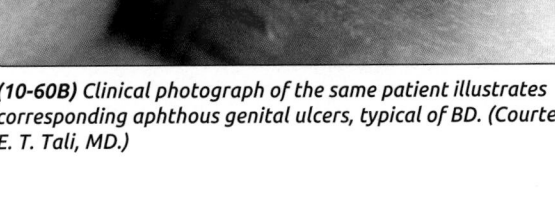

(10-60B) Clinical photograph of the same patient illustrates corresponding aphthous genital ulcers, typical of BD. (Courtesy E. T. Tali, MD.)

Imaging. Although any part of the CNS can be affected, brainstem involvement—especially of the cerebral peduncles—is typical and occurs in 50% of cases **(10-60)**. The thalamus and basal ganglia are the second most common sites of involvement, followed by the cerebral hemispheric white matter. Between 10-50% of NBD cases demonstrate focal lesions in the spinal cord.

Typical MR findings are small circular, linear, crescent-shaped, or irregular foci of T2/FLAIR hyperintensity in the midbrain. Mass effect is usually minimal, but, during the acute phase, large brainstem and/or basal ganglia lesions can exhibit significant mass effect, extending into the diencephalon and mimicking neoplasm.

Mild to moderate patchy enhancement following contrast administration is common; strong, uniform enhancement is rare.

Differential Diagnosis. The major differential diagnosis of BD includes **multiple sclerosis, sarcoidosis, neoplasm**, and **systemic inflammatory disease**. Oligoclonal bands are absent in the CSF, and the myelin basic protein is typically normal, helping distinguish BD from MS. Skin lesions are generally absent in sarcoid, whereas serum angiotensin-converting enzyme levels are usually (but not invariably) elevated.

Widespread brainstem involvement extending into the cerebral peduncles, thalami, basal ganglia, and periventricular WM has been reported and can mimic gliomatosis cerebri or lymphoma. Biopsy may be required to distinguish BD from neoplasm.

Systemic inflammatory diseases such as **systemic lupus erythematosus, antiphospholipid syndrome**, and **Sjögren disease** can resemble BD when they involve the CNS. Skin lesions are common in these disorders, but the oral and genital aphthous ulcers seen in BD are absent.

Sweet syndrome, also known as acute febrile neutrophilic dermatosis, is a multisystem inflammatory disorder that often manifests as a vasculitis presenting with painful erythematous skin plaques, fever, and leukocytosis. Neuro-Sweet and NBD can appear identical on MRI, with T2/FLAIR hyperintensities in the brainstem and basal ganglia. The CNS involvement in neuro-Sweet is usually transient, mimicking a relapsing and remitting encephalitis, whereas NBD usually follows a much more chronic, slowly progressive course.

Systemic Lupus Erythematosus

Terminology. Systemic lupus erythematosus (SLE or "lupus") is a multisystem complex autoimmune disorder that affects the respiratory, cardiovascular, gastrointestinal, genitourinary, and musculoskeletal systems, as well as the CNS. Most diagnoses of lupus are established on the basis of systemic findings and laboratory abnormalities with imaging playing an important but ancillary role in diagnosis and management.

When overt CNS symptoms are present, the disorder is termed CNS lupus (CNS SLE) or neuropsychiatric systemic lupus erythematosus (NPSLE).

Etiology. SLE is an autoimmune disorder characterized by immune complex deposition, vasculitis, and vasculopathy. Multiple components of the immune system are affected, including the complement system, T suppressor cells, and cytokine products. Circulating autoantibodies may be produced for many years before overt clinical SLE symptoms emerge.

Activation of the complement system, together with formation and deposition of immune complexes in tissues, recruits B lymphocytes, resulting in formation of autoantibodies. Normal immune suppression fails, resulting in an unchecked autoimmune response. Immune system dysfunction also results in frequent infections and increased prevalence of lymphoreticular malignancy.

CNS lupus is generally considered an angiopathic disease, although neural autoimmune damage, demyelination, and thromboembolism may be contributing factors. Lupus-related cerebral ischemia/infarction can result from coagulopathy (secondary to antiphospholipid syndrome), accelerated atherosclerosis (often associated with corticosteroid treatment), thromboembolism (secondary to Libman-Sacks endocarditis), or a true primary lupus vasculitis.

Pathology. The most frequent gross findings in patients with NPSLE are generalized volume loss with cortical atrophy and enlarged ventricles. Focal atrophy, cerebral infarcts, and hemorrhage are also common.

Lupus angiitis/vasculitis is characterized histopathologically by marked endothelial hyperplasia and obliterative intimal fibrosis in small arteries and arterioles. Occlusive fibrin thrombi without histologic evidence of vasculitis can also occur.

Clinical Issues. SLE affects one out of every 700 white female patients and one out of every 245 black female patients. CNS SLE occurs at all ages, with peak onset between the second and fourth decades. In adults, over 90% of patients are female. In children, the F:M ratio is 2-3:1.

Lupus onset can be insidious, and early clinical diagnosis can be elusive. Diagnostic criteria for SLE have been established by the American College of Rheumatology and include malar or discoid rash, oral and/or nasal ulcers, arthritis, serositis, renal disease, and vasculitis.

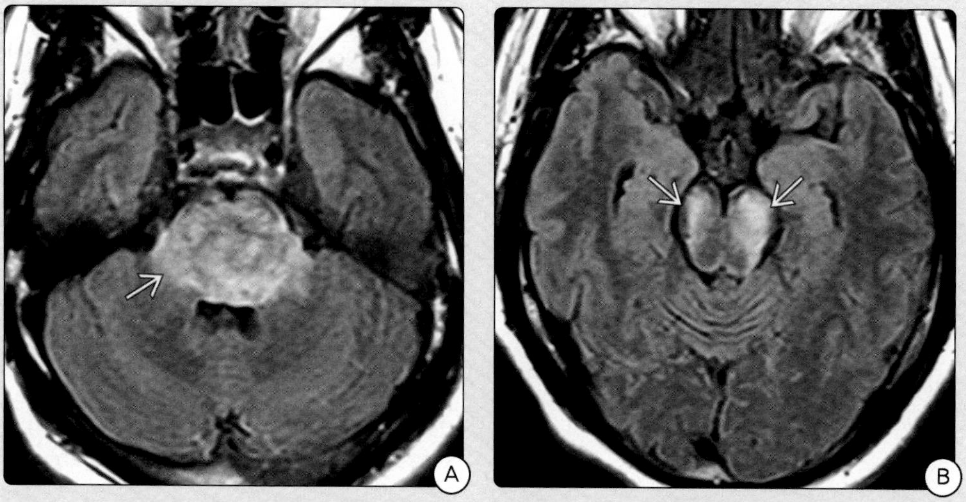

***(10-61A)** Axial FLAIR scan in a 30y man with fever, oral ulcers, and bilateral upper extremity weakness shows a heterogeneously hyperintense mass in the pons ➡. **(10-61B)** The lesions extend cephalad into both cerebral peduncles ➡, which also appear enlarged. Additional lesions were present in the basal ganglia (not shown).*

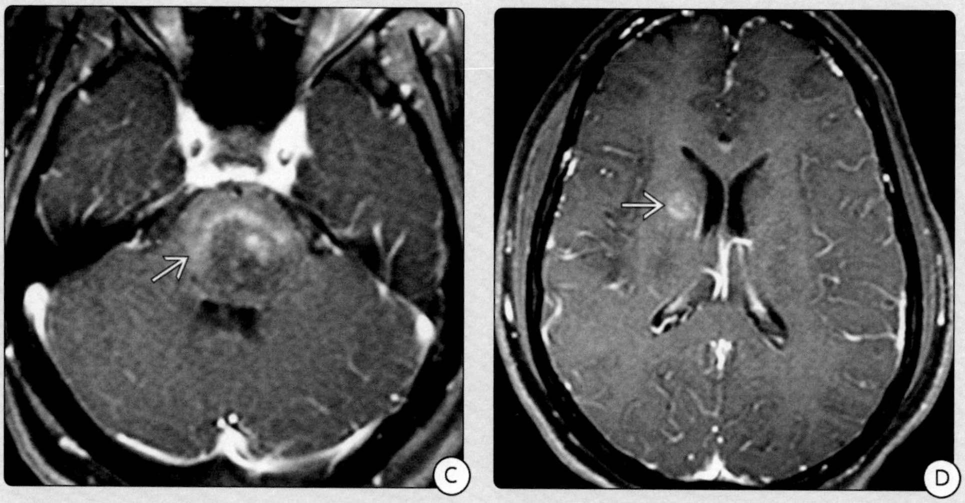

***(10-61C)** Axial T1 C+ FS scan in the same patient shows that the pontine mass ➡ enhances moderately but heterogeneously. **(10-61D)** T1 C+ FS scan shows a ring-enhancing lesion in the right caudate nucleus and anterior limb of the internal capsule ➡. This is biopsy-proven Behçet disease.*

CNS lupus occurs in 30-40% of cases and can be a serious, potentially life-threatening manifestation of SLE. Indeed, CNS lupus accounts for 15-20% of lupus-related deaths.

Imaging. Imaging abnormalities occur in 25-75% of NPSLE patients and are associated with disease severity/activity, increasing age, and documented neurologic events.

Initial NECT scans are often normal or show scattered patchy cortical/subcortical hypodensities. Large territorial infarcts and dural sinus occlusions occur but are less common. Spontaneous intracranial hemorrhages can occur in SLE patients with uremia, thrombocytopenia, and hypertension.

MR findings vary from normal to striking. The most common finding, seen in 25-50% of newly diagnosed NPSLE patients, is that of multiple small subcortical and deep WM hyperintensities on T2/FLAIR **(10-62)**. Large confluent lesions that resemble acute disseminated encephalomyelitis (ADEM) occur but are generally seen only in patients with CNS symptoms **(10-63)**. Diffuse cortical, basal ganglia, and brainstem lesions—suggestive of vasculopathy or vasculitis—are also common.

Acute lesions demonstrate transient enhancement on T1 C+ studies and restricted diffusion. pMR in patients with NPSLE shows elevated cerebral blood volume and cerebral blood flow.

Dural venous sinus and cortical/deep venous thrombosis occur in 20-30% of NPSLE cases. Systemic hypertension is common in SLE patients. Posterior reversible encephalopathy syndrome (PRES) is a rare but treatable manifestation of CNS lupus.

Differential Diagnosis. The imaging differential diagnosis of NPSLE is broad and includes **arteriolosclerosis** ("small vessel disease"), **multiple sclerosis, Susac syndrome**, non-lupus **antiphospholipid syndromes, Lyme disease**, and **other vasculitides** such as primary angiitis of the CNS.

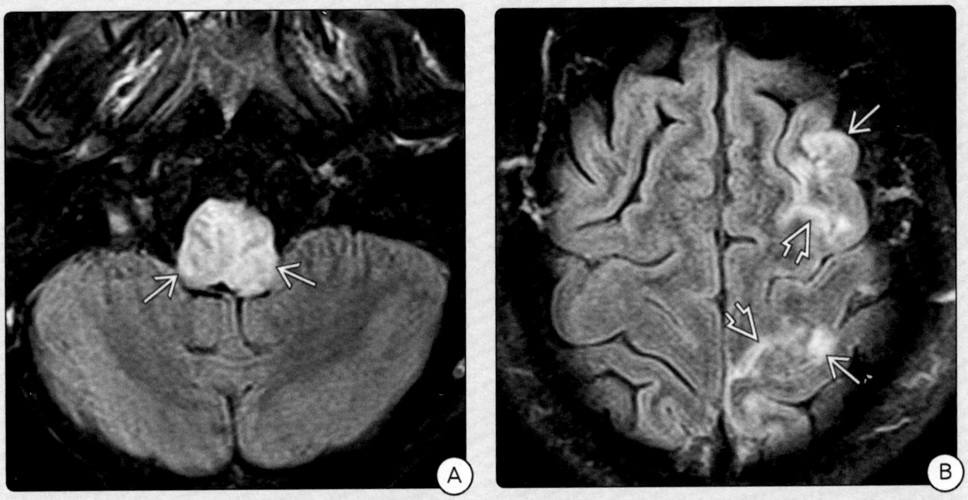

***(10-62A)** Axial FLAIR scan in a 33y woman with acute exacerbation of her CNS lupus shows confluent hyperintensity expanding the medulla ➡. **(10-62B)** FLAIR scan through the vertex in the same patient shows patchy cortical and subcortical hyperintensities in the left frontal and parietal lobes ➡. Mild mass effect with sulcal effacement ➡ is present. The right hemisphere appears normal.*

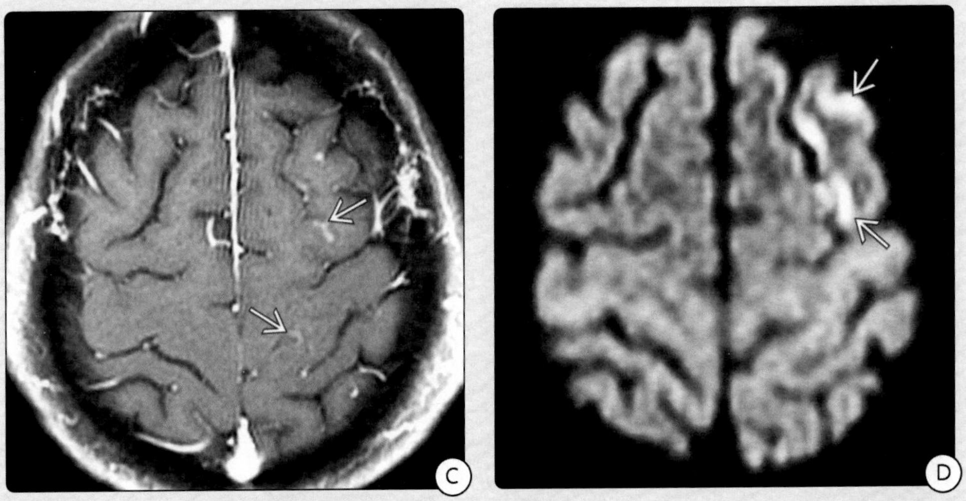

***(10-62C)** T1 C+ FS scan in the same patient shows mild patchy enhancement in the cortex and subcortical white matter of the left hemisphere ➡. **(10-62D)** DWI shows foci of restricted diffusion in the right frontal cortex ➡.*

There is a significant overlap of lupus with antiphospholipid syndrome (APS); between 25-40% of SLE patients have APS (see below). While there are no universally accepted diagnostic imaging criteria for NPSLE, the presence of multifocal infarcts and "migratory" edematous areas is suggestive of the disease.

Antiphospholipid Syndrome

Terminology and Etiology. APS is a multisystem disorder characterized by arterial or venous thrombosis, early strokes, cognitive dysfunction, and pregnancy loss. APS with widespread livedo reticularis and ischemic cerebrovascular episodes is called **Sneddon syndrome**.

Clinical Issues. The spectrum of antiphospholipid-mediated syndromes reflects end-organ injury due to microangiopathic disease and endothelial dysfunction. Variable clinical manifestations include skin disease (livedo reticularis rash, splinter hemorrhages); cardiac, pulmonary, and renal involvement; hematologic disorders; and neuropsychiatric symptoms.

The diagnosis of APS requires the presence of at least one clinical criterion (e.g., vascular thrombosis or pregnancy morbidity) and one laboratory finding, i.e., persistently positive lupus anticoagulant, antiphospholipid antibodies (e.g., anticardiolipin antibodies), or anti-β2 glycoprotein 1 antibody.

Mean age of onset is 50 years. There is a 2:1 female predominance (women with APS are often initially diagnosed because of pregnancy loss). A rare complication of APS is HELLP syndrome (**h**emolysis, **e**levated **l**iver enzymes, **l**ow **p**latelets).

CNS involvement in APS is common. Manifestations of CNS APS include cerebrovascular disease with arterial thrombotic events (early-onset TIA, stroke) or venous occlusions, MS-like syndromes, seizure, headache, and cognitive dysfunction. A rare "catastrophic" APS is characterized by multiorgan

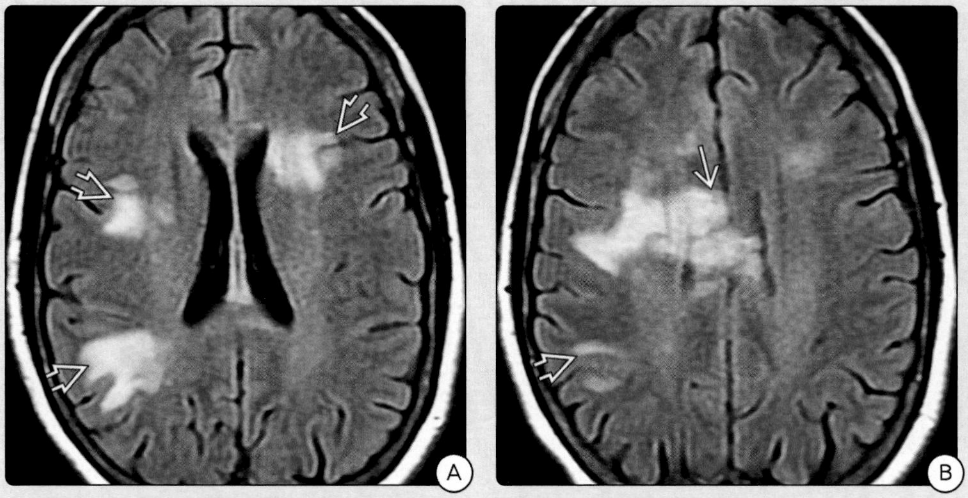

***(10-63A)** Axial FLAIR scan in a 55y woman with unusual neuropsychiatric symptoms shows patchy and confluent hyperintensities in the subcortical and deep periventricular white matter ➡. **(10-63B)** Axial FLAIR scan in the same patient shows subcortical white matter lesions ➡ in addition to "fluffy" confluent lesions that cross the corpus callosum ➡ and resemble acute disseminated encephalomyelitis.*

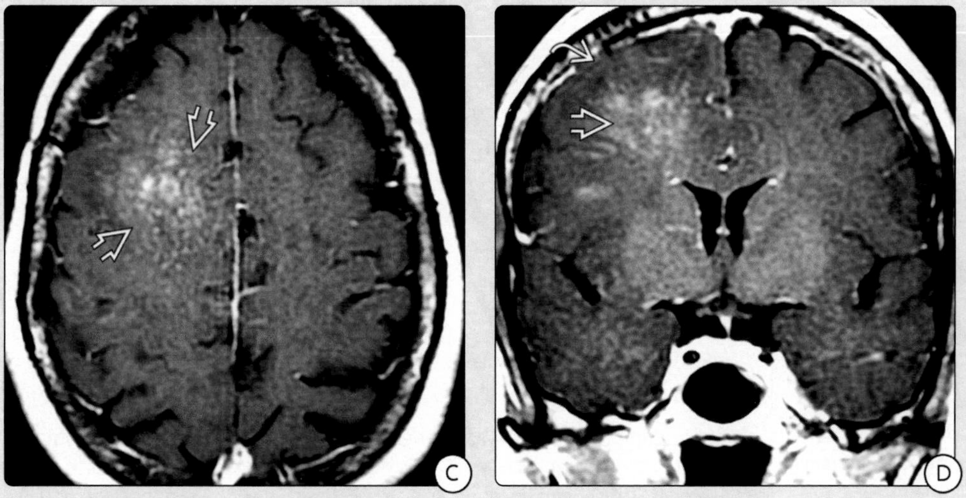

***(10-63C)** Coronal T1 C+ scan in the same patient shows mild punctate and linear foci of enhancement in the subcortical and deep cerebral white matter ➡. **(10-63D)** Coronal T1 C+ shows patchy and linear enhancing foci in the subcortical white matter ➡. Note the burr hole ➡ from biopsy. Histopathologic examination disclosed CNS lupus vasculitis.*

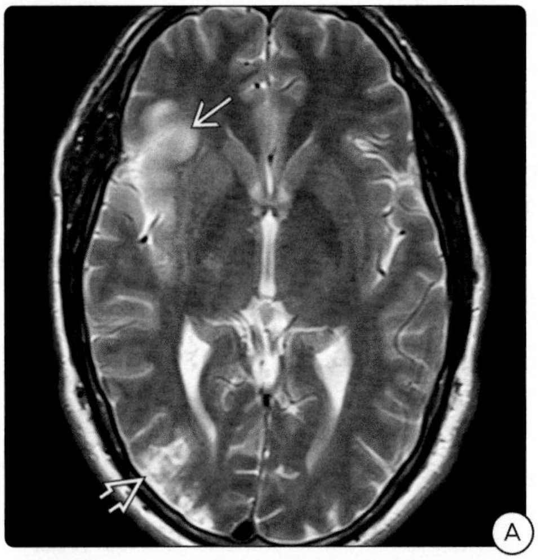

***(10-64A)** Axial T2WI in a 36y man w/ documented APS and multiple strokes shows acute gyral edema, parietal encephalomalacia.*

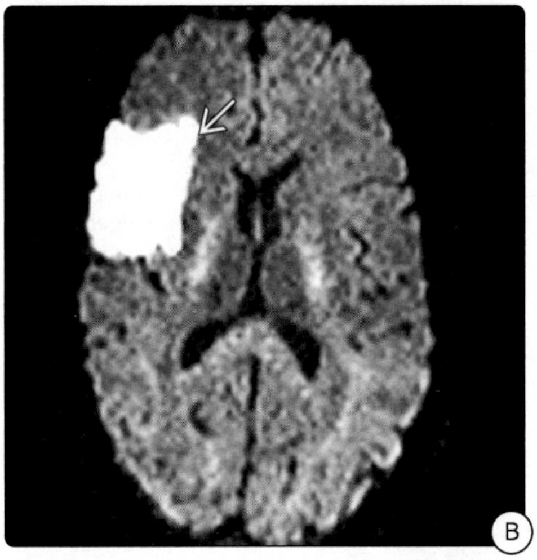

***(10-64B)** DTI trace image in the same patient shows acute restriction in the anterior division of the right middle cerebral artery.*

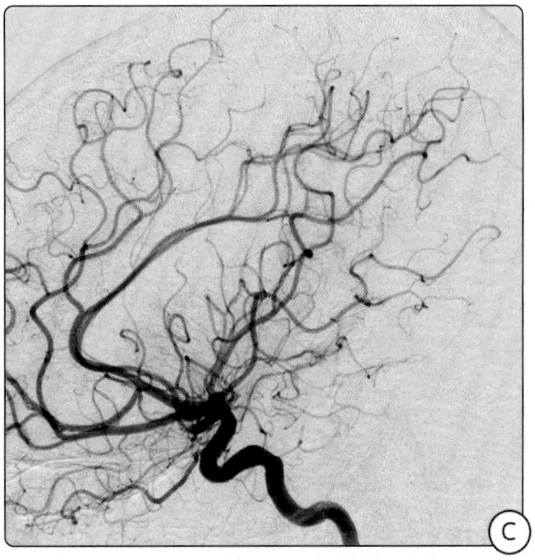

***(10-64C)** Lateral DSA in the same patient clearly demonstrates no evidence of vasculitis.*

accelerated and widespread vessel occlusions and has a mortality rate approaching 50%. Catastrophic acute CNS APS can cause acute encephalopathy as well as arterial and venous infarcts.

Imaging. Mixed-age multifocal cortical/subcortical infarcts, parietal-dominant atrophy with relative sparing of the frontal and temporal lobes, and "too many for age" deep WM hyperintensities on T2/FLAIR scans are typical findings in APS **(10-64)**. Both arterial and venous thromboses are common.

Differential Diagnosis. APS in the CNS can be difficult to distinguish from **multiple sclerosis**. The absence of callososeptal lesions is a helpful differential feature. **Multi-infarct ("vascular") dementia** usually lacks the parietal-dominant atrophy of APS. **SLE** commonly occurs with APS and may present with similar clinical and imaging findings.

Cerebral Amyloid Disease

Terminology. Cerebral amyloid disease encompasses a heterogeneous group of biochemically and genetically diverse CNS disorders. Cerebral amyloid disease occurs in several forms. By far, the most common is an age-related microvasculopathy termed **cerebral amyloid angiopathy** (CAA), also known as congophilic angiopathy. Amyloid deposition in neuritic plaques is also a prominent feature of **Alzheimer disease** (AD).

Uncommon manifestations of CNS amyloid disease include a focal, tumefactive mass-like lesion called an **amyloidoma.** Rarely, cerebral amyloid disease presents as an **amyloid β-related angiitis** (ABRA) with diffuse inflammatory changes that primarily affect the white matter. ABRA is also known as CAA-related inflammation.

Etiology. CAA is caused by the accumulation of aggregated Aβ in small cerebral vessels. Aβ is derived from proteolytic cleavage of amyloid precursor protein. Two amino acid species, a 42-aa length (Aβ42) and a shorter 40-aa (Aβ40) length, are associated with amyloid-related brain disease. Aβ42 is principally found in AD-associated neuritic plaques, whereas the shorter, relatively more soluble Aβ40 is the major form found in CAA.

Imbalance between Aβ production and clearance is considered a key element in the formation of CNS amyloid deposits. These deposits accumulate in the abluminal portion of the muscular layer and adventitia of cerebral arterioles and capillaries, causing progressive disruption of the neurovascular unit. The geographic distribution of Aβ deposits corresponds anatomically to the perivascular drainage pathways by which interstitial fluid and solutes are eliminated from the brain.

Aβ transport between the neuropil and cerebral circulation is blocked in CAA. Failure to clear Aβ from the brain has two major consequences: (1) intracranial hemorrhages associated with rupture of Aβ-laden vessels in CAA and (2) altered neuronal function caused by pathologic accumulation of Aβ and other soluble metabolites in AD. The most frequent vascular abnormality seen in AD is CAA.

Genetics. Amyloid precursor protein is encoded by the *APP* gene on chromosome 21.

CAA can be primary or secondary, sporadic or familial. Sporadic CAA is much more common than familial CAA and is strongly associated with presence of the *APOE*E4* allele.

Hereditary forms of CAA are generally familial and occur as an autosomal-dominant disorder with several recognized subtypes, including Dutch, Italian, Flemish/British, and Icelandic subtypes. Hereditary CAA is generally more severe and earlier in onset compared with the sporadic disease form.

Secondary CAA has been associated with hemodialysis, medullary thyroid carcinoma, and type 2 diabetes.

Pathology. CAA is characterized by progressive deposition of Aβ fibrils in the walls of small to medium-sized arteries and penetrating arterioles, with preferential involvement of the supratentorial cortex and leptomeninges. The cerebellum, brainstem, and basal ganglia are relatively spared.

Gross pathologic findings include major lobar hemorrhages (most commonly frontal or frontoparietal), cortical petechial hemorrhages, small cerebral infarcts, and white matter ischemic lesions **(10-65)**.

Microscopic features include a "smudgy" eosinophilic thickening of leptomeningeal and cortical vessels **(10-66)**. Severe cases can demonstrate vessel "splitting" (a "lumen within a lumen" appearance), fibrinoid necrosis, pseudoaneurysm formation, and thrombosis. Aβ-related angiitis demonstrates mural and perivascular inflammatory changes with necrosis, variable numbers of multinucleated giant cells, epithelioid histiocytes, eosinophils, and lymphocytes.

On Congo red stains, CAA vessels have a salmon-colored "congophilic" appearance. A characteristic yellow-green color ("birefringence") appears when the affected vessels are viewed using polarized light **(10-67)**. Immunohistochemistry using antibodies against Aβ is positive. Amyloid-laden blood vessels are also immunoreactive for matrix metalloproteinase-19.

Clinical Issues. CAA causes 5-20% of all nontraumatic cerebral hemorrhages and is now recognized as a major cause of spontaneous intracranial hemorrhage and cognitive impairment in the elderly.

Advancing age is the strongest known risk factor for developing CAA. Sporadic CAA usually occurs in patients older than 55 years, whereas the hereditary forms present one or two decades earlier. Patients with Aβ-related angiitis also tend to be younger than those with sporadic, noninflammatory CAA.

Autopsy studies show a CAA prevalence of 20-40% in nondemented and 50-60% in demented elderly populations. CAA is present in over 90% of AD patients at postmortem examination.

The most common clinical manifestations of CAA are focal neurologic deficits (with recurrent lobar hemorrhages) and cognitive impairment (with multiple chronic microbleeds).

The clinical presentation of patients with CAA-related inflammation (e.g., ABRA) differs, usually resembling an autoimmune-mediated vasculitis or a subacute meningoencephalitis. Headache and cognitive decline are common. Occasionally ABRA patients have a more fulminant course characterized by rapidly progressive dementia, seizure, and focal neurologic deficits. Three-quarters of patients with biopsy-proven ABRA respond to corticosteroid therapy, so establishing the correct histopathologic diagnosis is crucial for patient management.

Imaging. Imaging findings vary with the type of cerebral amyloid disease. CAA is by far the most common form; amyloidomas and ABRA are rare.

CT. NECT scans in patients with acute manifestations of CAA typically show a hyperdense lobar hematoma with varying peripheral edema. Multiple irregular confluent white matter hypointensities together with generalized volume loss are common. Enhancement on CECT is rare in cerebral amyloid disease and occurs only if a focal mass ("amyloidoma") or ABRA is present.

Occasionally, patients with CAA can present with so-called convexal subarachnoid hemorrhage (cSAH) **(10-68)**. In cSAH, the basal cisterns appear

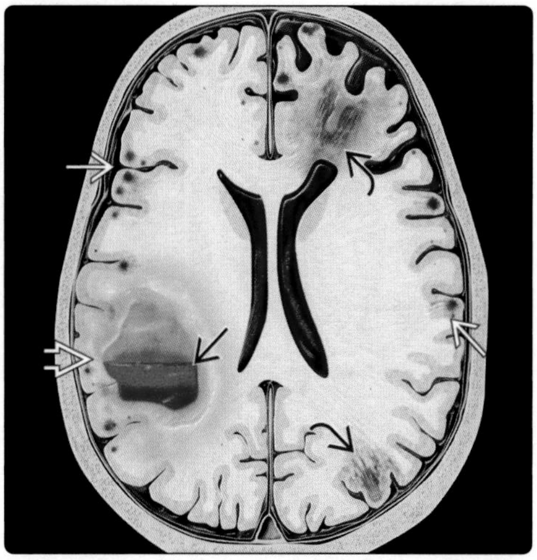

***(10-65)** Acute hematoma ➡ with fluid level ⇒; microbleeds ➡, old lobar hemorrhages ⇨ are typical findings in cerebral amyloid disease.*

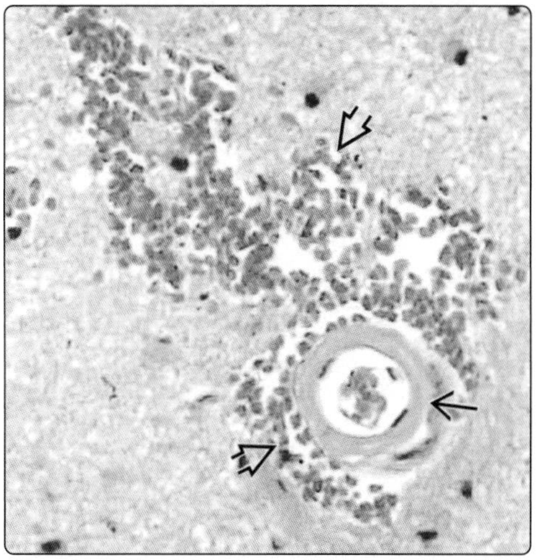

***(10-66)** High-power H&E shows thickened arteriole ⇒ w/ perivascular hemorrhages ⇨, normal for cerebral amyloid angiopathy (CAA).*

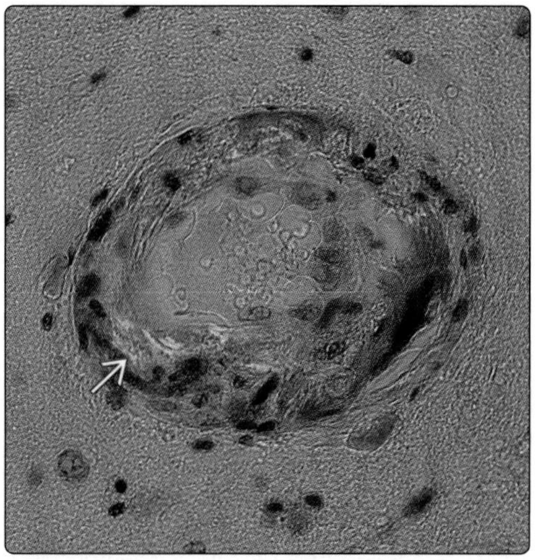

***(10-67)** Congo red stain in polarized light shows thickened arteriole w/ apple-green birefringence ➡. CAA. (Courtesy B. K. DeMasters, MD.)*

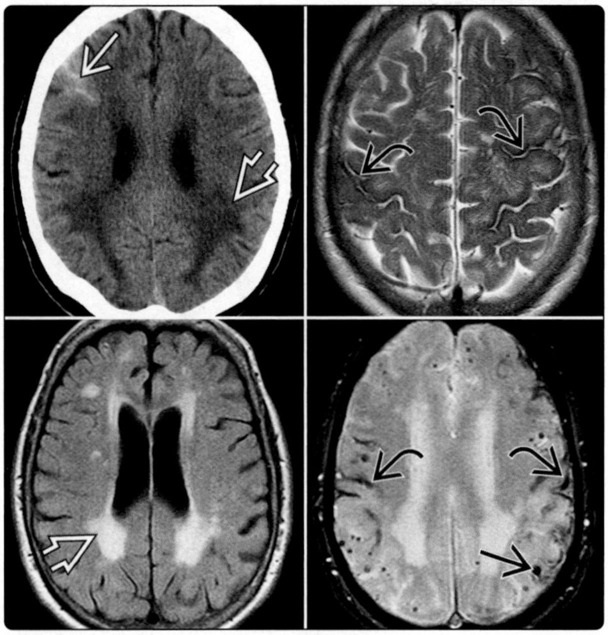

(10-68) Scans in a patient with headache and CAA show cSAH ➡, confluent WM lesions ➡, superficial siderosis ➡, and microbleeds ➡. (Courtesy M. Castillo, MD.)

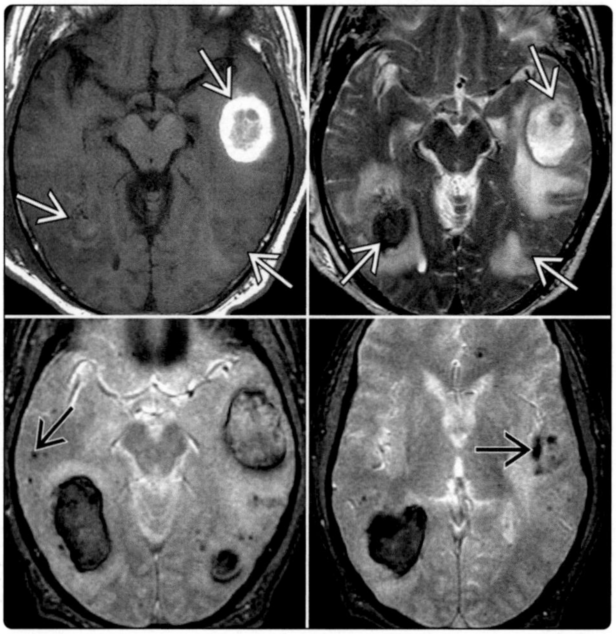

(10-69) MR scans demonstrate multiple lobar hemorrhages of different ages ➡, multifocal peripheral "blooming black dots" ➡ that are classic for CAA.

normal, but one or more adjacent convexity sulci demonstrate curvilinear hyperdensity consistent with blood.

MR. Signal intensity of a CAA-associated lobar hematoma varies with clot age **(10-69)**. Acute hematomas are isointense on T1WI and iso- to hypointense on T2WI.

The vast majority of patients with CAA have focal or patchy confluent WM hyperintensity on T2/FLAIR. Lobar lacunae are present in 25% of cases. Larger, asymmetric areas of confluent WM hyperintensity on T2/FLAIR with or without microhemorrhages are characteristic of ABRA. Mass effect is typically absent unless ABRA or a focal amyloid mass ("amyloidoma") is present.

In addition to residua from lobar hemorrhages **(10-69)**, T2* (GRE, SWI) sequences demonstrate multifocal punctate "blooming black dots" in the leptomeninges, cortex, and subcortical WM **(10-70E)**. The basal ganglia and cerebellum are relatively spared.

Both ABRA and amyloidoma may show such striking enhancement on T1 C+ that they mimic meningitis, encephalitis, or neoplasm **(10-70) (10-71)**.

Nuclear medicine. Patients with CAA have significantly decreased cerebral perfusion on 99m Tc-ECD SPECT studies. In vivo evaluation of CAA with PET amyloid imaging agents, such as carbon 11-labeled Pittsburgh Compound B (11C PiB), has good overall agreement between 11C PiB and either very low or high $A\beta$ loads.

Coregistered PET and T2* MR also demonstrate significantly increased 11C PiB retention at microbleed sites, indicating that microbleeds occur preferentially in regions of concentrated amyloid deposition.

CEREBRAL AMYLOID DISEASE

Pathology

- $A\beta40$ deposited in meningeal, cortical arterioles
  - "Congophilic" angiopathy
  - Mural, perivascular inflammation common
- Vessel walls thicker but weaker
- Lobar bleeds
- Perivascular microhemorrhages

Clinical Issues

- Causes 5-20% of spontaneous intracranial hemorrhages in elderly patients
  - ↑ Age = strongest risk factor
  - Most patients > 55 years old
- Normotensive, demented older adult typical

Imaging

- Classic NECT findings
  - Lobar hemorrhages of different ages
  - Convexal subarachnoid hemorrhage
- MR shows multifocal microbleeds
  - "Blooming" hypointensities on T2*
  - Typically cortical, meningeal (pial)
  - Cerebellum, brainstem, basal ganglia generally spared
  - Cortical superficial siderosis common
- Less common = $A\beta$-related inflammatory angiitis
  - T2/FLAIR parenchymal hyperintensity
  - Edema, mass effect
  - ± T2* "blooming" microbleeds
  - ± Sulcal-cisternal enhancement
- Rare = intracerebral amyloidoma (focal mass)

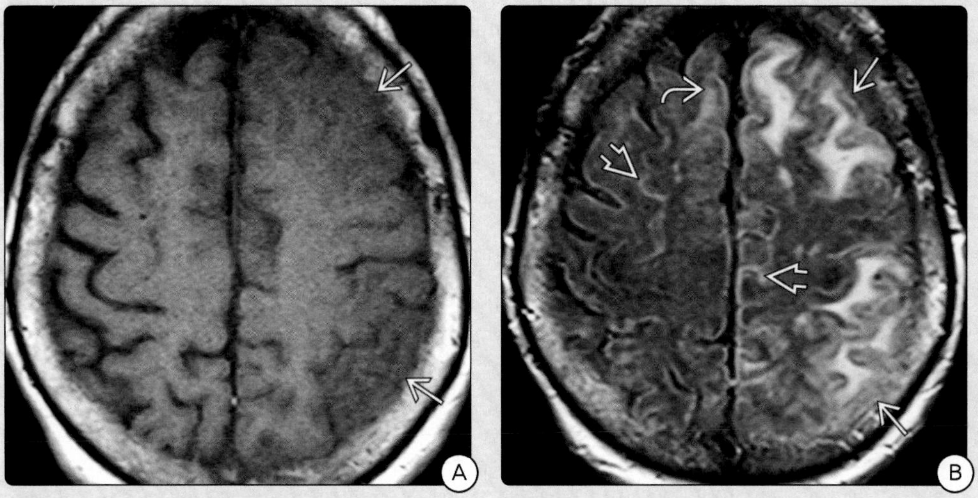

(10-70A) *T1WI in an 83y normotensive man with rapidly progressive dementia and right-sided weakness shows hypointense swollen gyri in the left hemisphere together with effacement of the adjacent sulci.* ***(10-70B)*** *FLAIR shows striking confluent WM hyperintensity in the left frontal, parietal lobes with patchy cortical and subcortical hyperintensities in the right hemisphere. The sulci in both hemispheres are also hyperintense.*

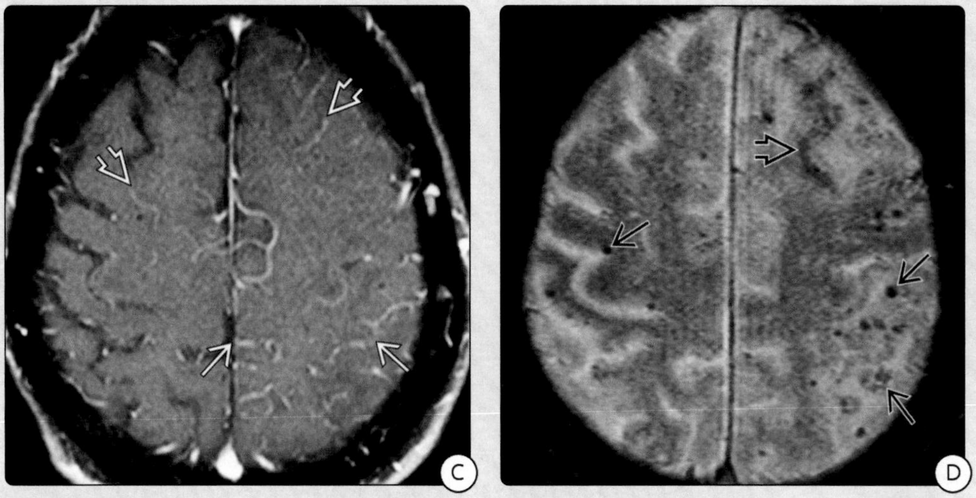

(10-70C) *T1 C+ FS shows extensive sulcal enhancement, especially over the left hemisphere.* ***(10-70D)*** *T2* GRE scan shows multiple "blooming" cortical/subcortical hypointensities and linear hypointensity along the left hemisphere sulci, suggestive of superficial (cortical) siderosis.*

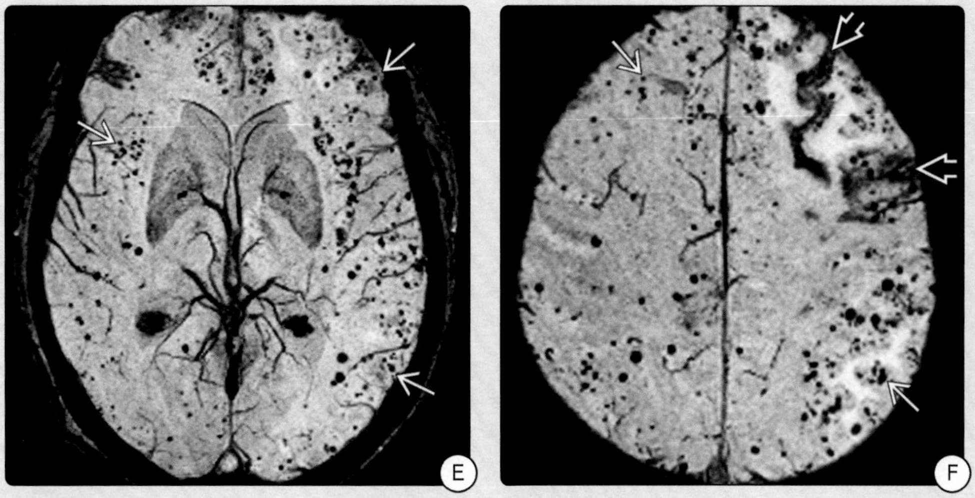

(10-70E) *T2* SWI scan shows innumerable peripheral "blooming black dots" in both hemispheres with sparing of the basal ganglia and thalami.* ***(10-70F)*** *T2* SWI through the corona radiata shows additional areas of siderosis and numerous microhemorrhages. Because of cerebral edema, mass effect, and sulcal enhancement, this case represents CAA-related inflammation (amyloid β-related angiitis, ABRA).*

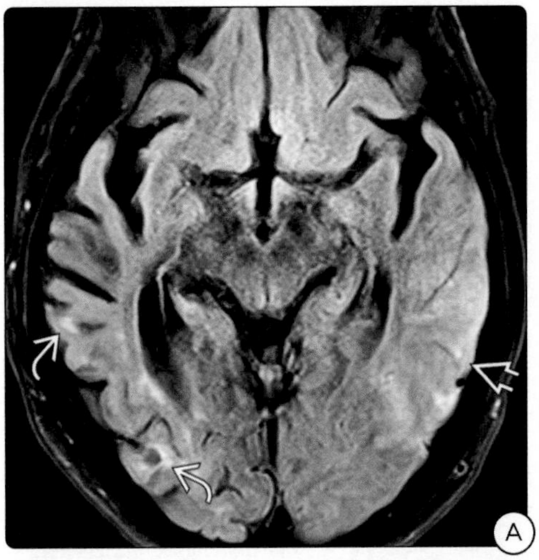

(10-71A) ***FLAIR in an 82y man shows atrophy, a few cortical/subcortical hyperintensities . Left temporal lobe is swollen and hyperintense .***

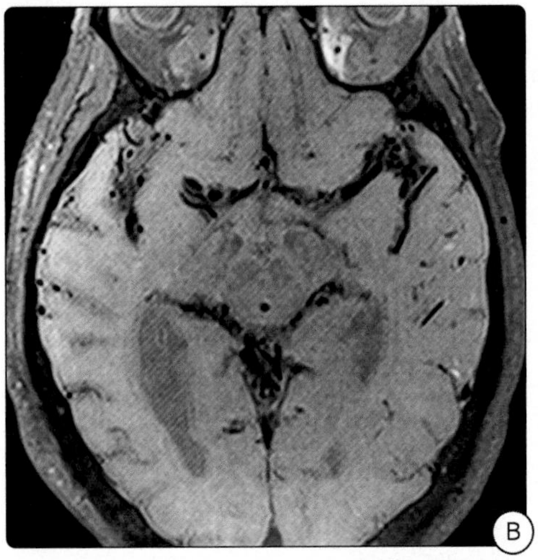

(10-71B) ***Precontrast axial high-resolution vessel wall imaging using "black blood" T1WI was performed on this patient.***

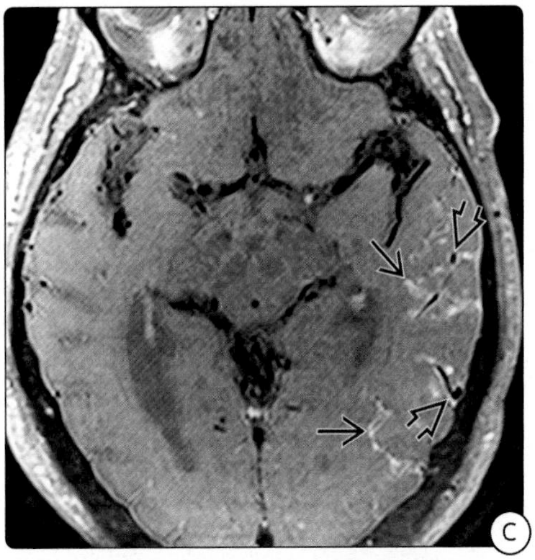

(10-71C) ***"Black blood" T1 C+ shows that MCA walls enhance , sulcal-cisternal enhancement . This is inflammatory amyloid angiopathy.***

Differential Diagnosis. The major differential diagnosis of CAA is **chronic hypertensive encephalopathy** (CHtnE). The microbleeds associated with CHtnE often involve the basal ganglia and cerebellum. Peripheral microbleeds occur but are less common than CAA-related microhemorrhages, which typically affect the cortex and leptomeninges.

Hemorrhagic lacunar infarcts can demonstrate "blooming" hemosiderin deposits. The basal ganglia and deep cerebral WM are the most common sites, helping distinguish these infarcts from the peripheral microbleeds of CAA.

Multiple cavernous angiomas (Zabramski type 4) typically involve the subcortical WM, basal ganglia, and cerebellum. The cortex is a less common site. "Locules" of blood with fluid-fluid levels and hemorrhages at different stages of evolution are often present in addition to multifocal "blooming black dots" on T2*.

Hemorrhagic metastases at the GM-WM junction can resemble CAA. The multifocal microbleeds typical of CAA lack mass effect, peripheral edema, and enhancement.

Because of their mass effect, edema, and enhancement patterns, ABRA and amyloidoma are difficult to distinguish from **infection** or **neoplasm** without biopsy.

Thrombotic Microangiopathies

Terminology. Thrombotic microangiopathy (TMA) represents a final common pathway of a diverse group of disorders characterized by microvascular occlusive thrombosis and vasculopathy. The TMAs are manifested as microangiopathic hemolytic anemia and thrombocytopenia.

There are four types of lesions described in TMA: (1) von Willebrand factor-platelet thrombi without microangiopathy, seen in **thrombotic thrombocytopenic purpura (TTP)**; (2) fibrin-platelet thrombi, seen in **disseminated intravascular coagulation (DIC)**; (3) microangiopathy with variable fibrin thrombi, seen in **hemolytic uremic syndrome (HUS);** and (4) intravascular clusters of cancer cells.

There are two HUS subtypes, classic and atypical. Classic HUS is associated with Shiga toxin, and **atypical HUS (aHUS)** occurs secondary to complement pathway dysregulation.

Because TTP and aHUS have overlapping clinical features, the term HUS-TTP has been used in the past. However, aHUS and TTP are histologically distinct entities and have different molecular pathophysiology.

Etiology. In TTP, an acquired inherited deficiency of the von Willebrand factor-cleaving protease ADAMTS-13 results in aggregations of platelets and ultralarge von Willebrand multimers to form platelet-rich thrombi throughout the microvasculature. Assessment of ADAMTS-13 activity is now routinely performed in patients with acute TMA and is helpful in differentiating TTP from other causes of TMA.

In aHUS, dysregulation of the alternative complement pathway leads to complement-mediated endothelial cell damage. TMA and acute renal injury without ADAMTS-13 deficiency or inhibitors are characteristic.

Multiple triggers such as infection with septicemia and segmental microvascular necrosis, drugs, toxins, cancer, chemotherapy, bone marrow transplantation, and pregnancy have all been associated with TMAs. A classic toxin-induced TMA is HUS following enterohemorrhagic *Escherichia coli* O104:H4 infection. Here extremely powerful toxins known as verotoxins or

Shiga toxins cause widespread vascular endothelial injury that in turn leads to multiorgan infarcts and hemorrhages.

Pathology. Biopsy is rarely performed in TMA. TMAs are characterized hematologically by platelet aggregation, profound thrombocytopenia, microcirculatory occlusions with ischemia or infarctions, microangiopathic hemolytic anemia, and microhemorrhages in multiple organs.

Gross pathology demonstrates multiple widespread foci of necrosis and hemorrhage. Arteriolar and capillary wall thickening, endothelial swelling and fragmentation, subendothelial accumulation of protein and cellular debris, and multiple platelet-fibrin occlusive thrombi are characteristic histopathologic findings **(10-72)**.

Clinical Issues. TMAs are rare. The overall incidence is estimated at less than 1:1,000,000 per year. Although the TMAs share a common pathophysiology, the clinical findings vary depending on the underlying disease.

DIC is the most common TMA, causing 80% of all cases. DIC is associated with a spectrum of comorbid pathologies including infection, tumor, vascular abnormalities, obstetrical and neonatal complications, massive tissue necrosis, and drug reactions. DIC is characterized clinically by thrombosis and/or hemorrhage at multiple sites.

TTP is the least common TMA. TTP is primarily a disease of children but can also affect young adults. Approximately half of all patients develop CNS symptoms, usually seizures and/or fluctuating neurologic deficits. Fever, renal insufficiency, and a purpuric rash over the trunk and limbs are common. The classic laboratory triad consists of thrombocytopenia, elevated lactate dehydrogenase, and schistocytosis. The majority of TTP patients have ADAMTS13 deficiency.

Although their symptoms often overlap, CNS disease is more common in TTP, whereas renal involvement predominates in HUS. aHUS is defined by the triad of mechanical hemolytic anemia, thrombocytopenia, and renal impairment. Complement dysregulation—not ADAMTS13 deficiency—is characteristic of aHUS.

Imaging. Multifocal cortical and subcortical ischemic and hemorrhagic infarcts are typical. NECT scans can be normal early in the disease course. Positive findings include peripheral poorly defined irregular hypoattenuating foci or hemorrhage with relatively well-delineated hyperdensities surrounded by variable edema **(10-73A)**. Mixed patterns with both hypo- and hyperdense lesions are also common.

Signal intensity on MR varies with clot age. Multifocal cortical/subcortical hyperintensities on T2/FLAIR are common in acute TMA **(10-75A)**. The most sensitive sequence is T2* (GRE, SWI) **(10-75B)**. Punctate "blooming" hypointensities are typical **(10-73B)** **(10-75B)**. DWI shows multiple foci of diffusion restriction.

aHUS, TTP, and pregnancy- or drug-associated TMA can all cause a PRES-like imaging pattern with posterior cortical/subcortical or brainstem hyperintensities. DWI in these cases is typically but not invariably normal.

Differential Diagnosis. The major differential diagnosis of TMAs, especially aHUS and TTP, is **acute hypertensive encephalopathy** (e.g., PRES). Both aHUS and TTP can cause a PRES-like syndrome with identical imaging findings. Clinical history and laboratory findings should distinguish between these two entities.

Multiple cerebral infarcts,especially septic emboli, can mimic the peripheral cortical lesions of TMA. Hemorrhagic septic emboli are typically not as diffuse as TMA-associated lesions. However, **septicemia with segmental**

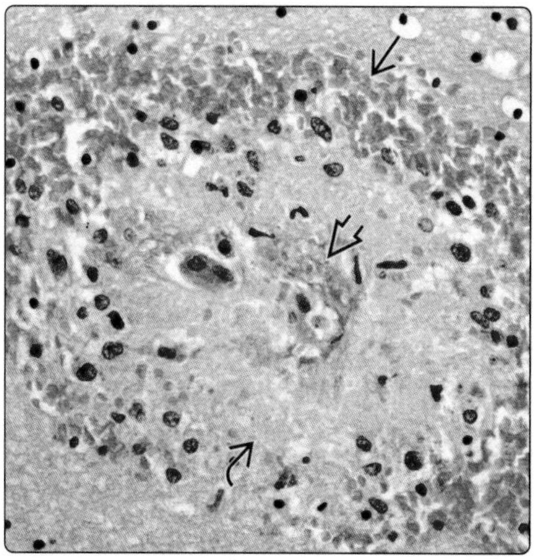

(10-72) H&E of DIC shows thickened, thrombosed arteriole ➲ with perivascular necrosis ➲, surrounding hemorrhage ➲.

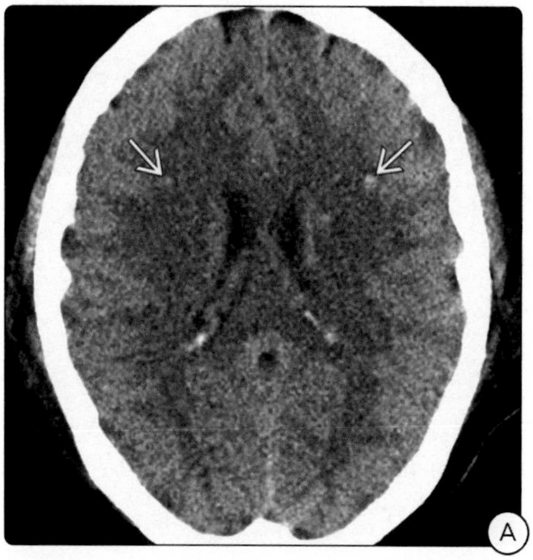

(10-73A) NECT in meningococcemia sepsis shows a few scattered punctate hyperdensities in the deep white matter ➲.

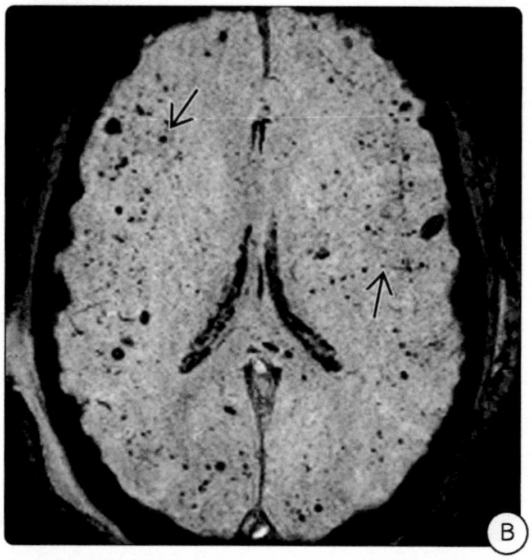

(10-73B) T2 SWI in the same case shows innumerable microbleeds ➲ in both the cortex, WM. This is DIC.*

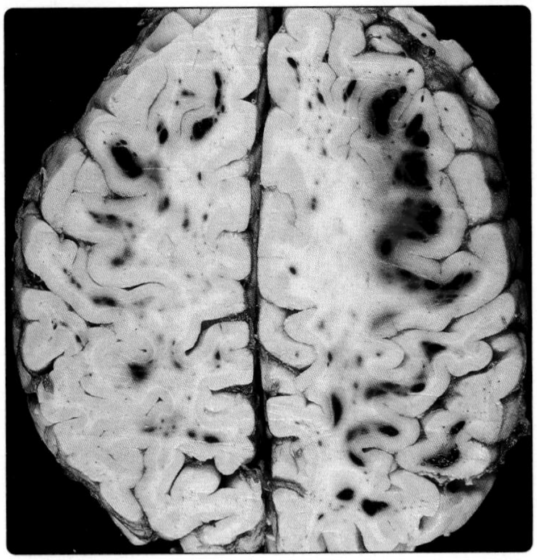

(10-74) *Autopsy of septicemia DIC shows multiple subcortical hemorrhages. (Courtesy R. Hewlett, MD.)*

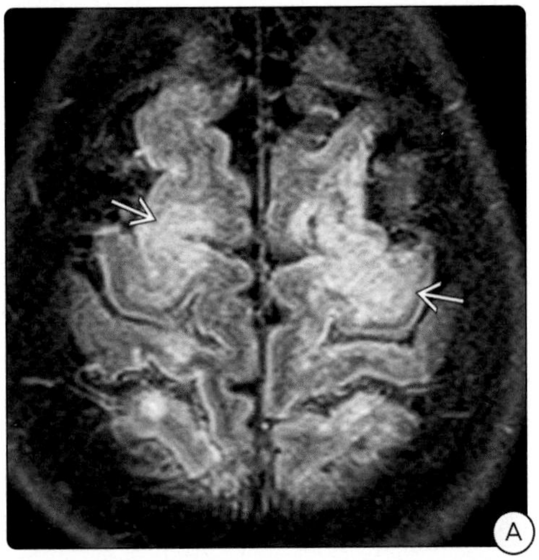

(10-75A) *FLAIR in strep pneumonia and sepsis, DIC shows bilateral cortical/subcortical hyperintensities ➔.*

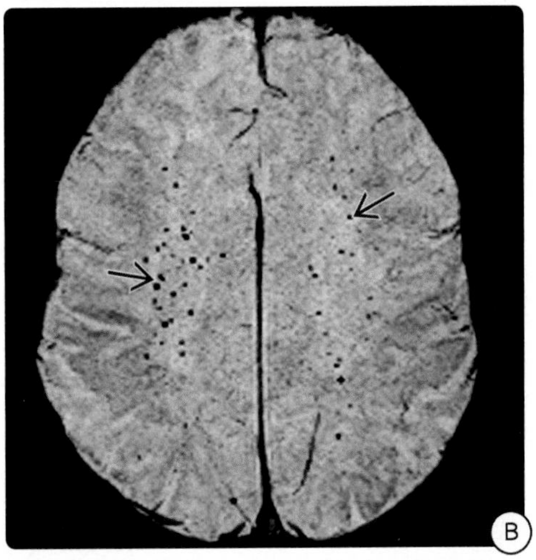

(10-75B) *SWI in 54y woman with chronic renal failure shows more "blooming" foci in the corona radiata ➔; microhemorrhages in HUS/TTP.*

microvascular necrosis can cause a diffuse hemorrhagic encephalopathy that may be exacerbated by DIC.

Antiphospholipid antibody syndrome complicated by HELLP syndrome can mimic TMA.

Cortical venous thrombosis with or without dural sinus occlusion can cause multiple peripheral hemorrhages. The hemorrhages and infarcts in TMA are typically more diffuse, and evidence for dural sinus thrombosis is absent.

THROMBOTIC MICROANGIOPATHIES

Terminology
- Microvascular occlusive disorders with
  - Thrombocytopenia
  - Intravascular hemolysis
  - Ischemic organ damage
- Major types
  - Disseminated intravascular coagulopathy
  - HUS (both Shiga-associated and complement-associated aHUS)
  - TTP

Etiology
- Endothelial cell injury
- Multiple triggers
  - Infection (e.g., septicemia, enterohemorrhagic *E. coli*)
  - Drugs
  - Cancer or chemotherapy
  - Pregnancy

Imaging
- Cortical/subcortical ischemic infarcts
- Multifocal microhemorrhages

Differential Diagnosis
- PRES
- Septic emboli
- Antiphospholipid antibody syndrome

Selected References

Normal Anatomy of the Extracranial Arteries

Aortic Arch and Great Vessels

Arazińska A et al: Right aortic arch analysis - anatomical variant or serious vascular defect? BMC Cardiovasc Disord. 17(1):102, 2017

Boufi M et al: Morphological analysis of healthy aortic arch. Eur J Vasc Endovasc Surg. 53(5):663-670, 2017

Girsowicz E et al: Anatomical study of healthy aortic arches. Ann Vasc Surg. ePub, 2017

Natsis K et al: The aberrant right subclavian artery: cadaveric study and literature review. Surg Radiol Anat. 39(5):559-565, 2017

Atherosclerosis

Atherogenesis and Atherosclerosis

Brown RA et al: Current understanding of atherogenesis. Am J Med. 130(3):268-282, 2017

McNally JS et al: Magnetic resonance imaging detection of intraplaque hemorrhage. Magn Reson Insights. 10:1-8, 2017

Extracranial Atherosclerosis

Cole JW: Large artery atherosclerotic occlusive disease. Continuum (Minneap Minn). 23(1, Cerebrovascular Disease):133-157, 2017

Xu Y et al: Co-existing intracranial and extracranial carotid artery atherosclerotic plaques and recurrent stroke risk: a three-dimensional multicontrast cardiovascular magnetic resonance study. J Cardiovasc Magn Reson. 18(1):90, 2016

Intracranial Atherosclerosis

Banerjee C et al: Stroke caused by atherosclerosis of the major intracranial arteries. Circ Res. 120(3):502-513, 2017

Baradaran H et al: Quantifying intracranial internal carotid artery stenosis on MR angiography. AJNR Am J Neuroradiol. 38(5):986-990, 2017

Harteveld AA et al: High-resolution intracranial vessel wall MRI in an elderly asymptomatic population: comparison of 3T and 7T. Eur Radiol. 27(4):1585-1595, 2017

Nonatheromatous Vascular Diseases

Fibromuscular Dysplasia

De Groote M et al: Fibromuscular dysplasia - results of a multicentre study in Flanders. Vasa. 46(3):211-218, 2017

Green R et al: Differences between the pediatric and adult presentation of fibromuscular dysplasia: results from the US Registry. Pediatr Nephrol. 31(4):641-50, 2016

Kiando SR et al: PHACTR1 is a genetic susceptibility locus for fibromuscular dysplasia supporting its complex genetic pattern of inheritance. PLoS Genet. 12(10):e1006367, 2016

Varennes L et al: Fibromuscular dysplasia: what the radiologist should know: a pictorial review. Insights Imaging. 6(3):295-307, 2015

Dissection

Larsson SC et al: Prognosis of carotid dissecting aneurysms: results from CADISS and a systematic review. Neurology. 88(7):646-652, 2017

Zhang FL et al: Dissection extending from extra- to intracranial arteries: a case report of progressive ischemic stroke. Medicine (Baltimore). 96(21):e6980, 2017

Kobayashi H et al: Extracranial and intracranial vertebral artery dissections: a comparison of clinical findings. J Neurol Sci. 362:244-50, 2016

Vasoconstriction Syndromes

Cappelen-Smith C et al: Reversible cerebral vasoconstriction syndrome: recognition and treatment. Curr Treat Options Neurol. 19(6):21, 2017

Coffino SW et al: Reversible cerebral vasoconstriction syndrome in pediatrics: a case series and review. J Child Neurol. 32(7):614-623, 2017

Lee MJ et al: Blood-brain barrier breakdown in reversible cerebral vasoconstriction syndrome: Implications for pathophysiology and diagnosis. Ann Neurol. 81(3):454-466, 2017

Miller TR et al: Reversible cerebral vasoconstriction syndrome, part 1: epidemiology, pathogenesis, and clinical course. AJNR Am J Neuroradiol. 36(8):1392-9, 2015

Miller TR et al: Reversible cerebral vasoconstriction syndrome, part 2: diagnostic work-up, imaging evaluation, and differential diagnosis. AJNR Am J Neuroradiol. 36(9):1580-8, 2015

Vasculitis and Vasculitides

Bond KM et al: Intracranial and extracranial neurovascular manifestations of Takayasu arteritis. AJNR Am J Neuroradiol. 38(4):766-772, 2017

Brinjikji W et al: Intracranial vessel wall imaging for evaluation of steno-occlusive diseases and intracranial aneurysms. J Neuroradiol. 44(2):123-134, 2017

Mossa-Basha M et al: Vessel wall imaging for intracranial vascular disease evaluation. J Neurointerv Surg. 8(11):1154-1159, 2016

Other Macro- and Microvasculopathies

de Amorim LC et al: Stroke in systemic lupus erythematosus and antiphospholipid syndrome: risk factors, clinical manifestations, neuroimaging, and treatment. Lupus. 26(5):529-536, 2017

Matsuda Y et al: RNF213 p.R4810K Variant and intracranial arterial stenosis or occlusion in relatives of patients with moyamoya disease. J Stroke Cerebrovasc Dis. S1052-3057(17)30177-5, 2017

Pasi M et al: Distribution of lacunes in cerebral amyloid angiopathy and hypertensive small vessel disease. Neurology. 88(23):2162-2168, 2017

Wollenweber FA et al: Cortical superficial siderosis in different types of cerebral small vessel disease. Stroke. 48(5):1404-1407, 2017

Bendapudi PK et al: An algorithmic approach to the diagnosis and management of the thrombotic microangiopathies. Am J Clin Pathol. 145(2):152-4, 2016

DeBaun MR et al: Central nervous system complications and management in sickle cell disease. Blood. 127(7):829-38, 2016

Phillips EH et al: The role of ADAMTS-13 activity and complement mutational analysis in differentiating acute thrombotic microangiopathies. J Thromb Haemost. 14(1):175-85, 2016

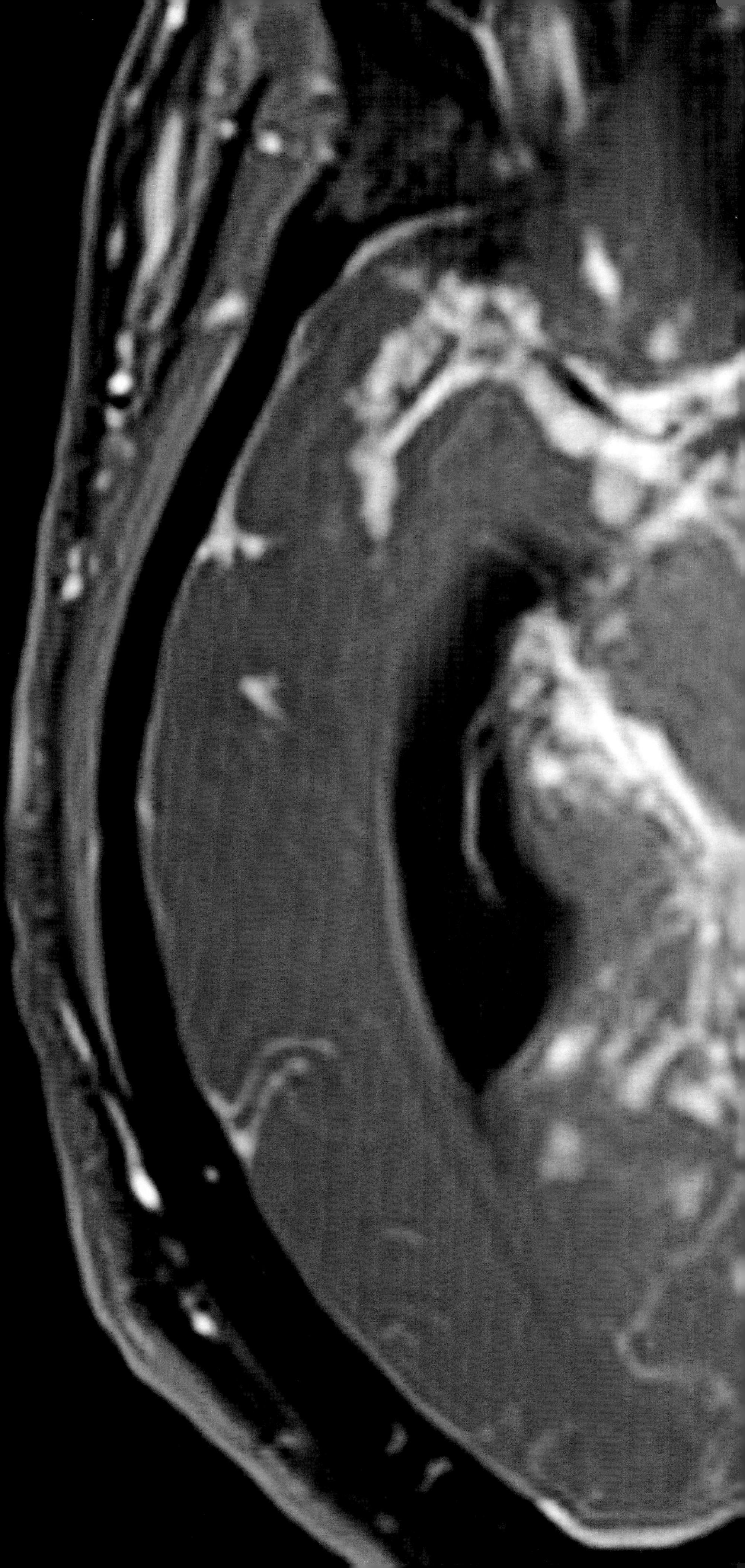

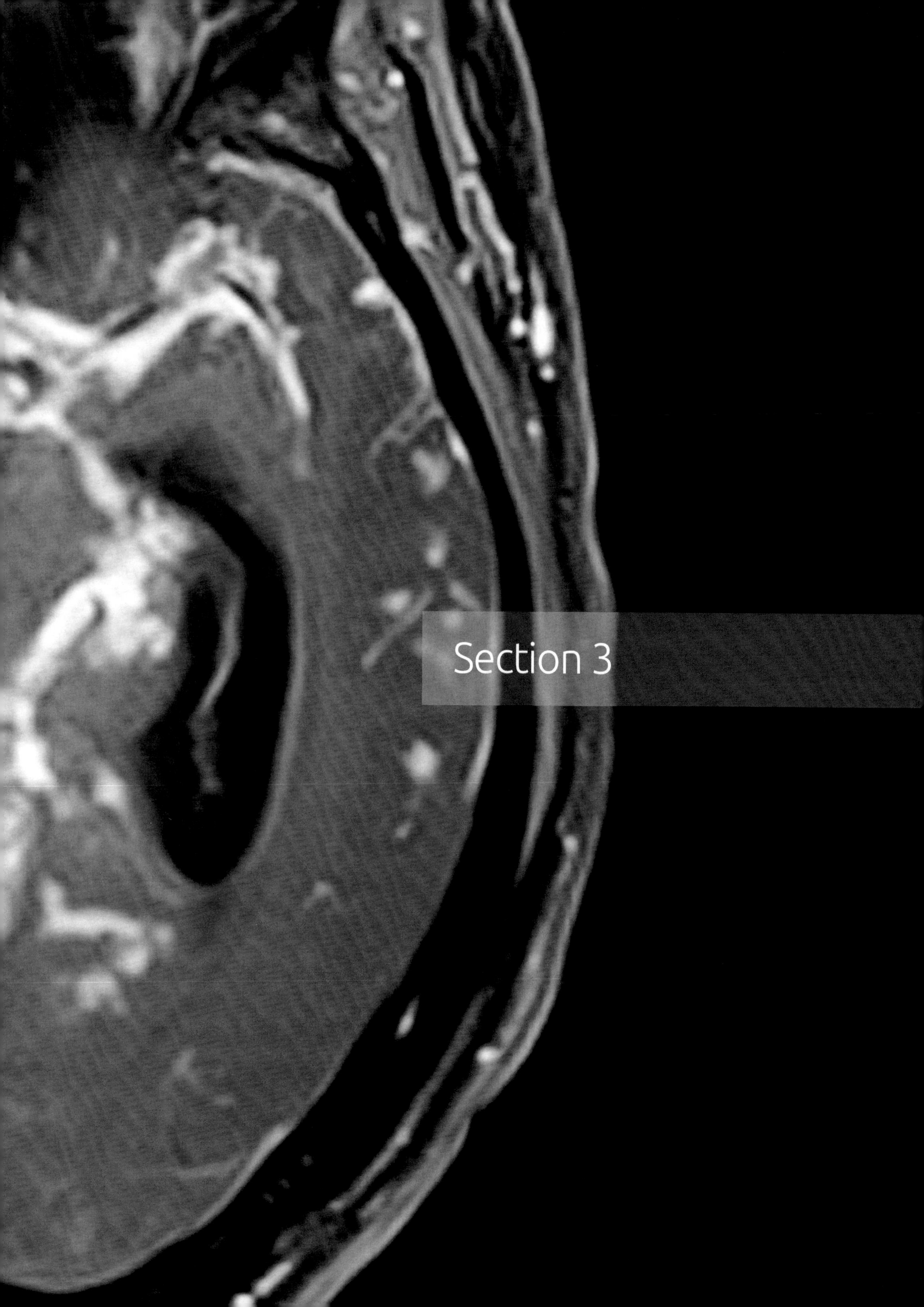

Section 3

Section 3

Infection, Inflammation, and Demyelinating Diseases

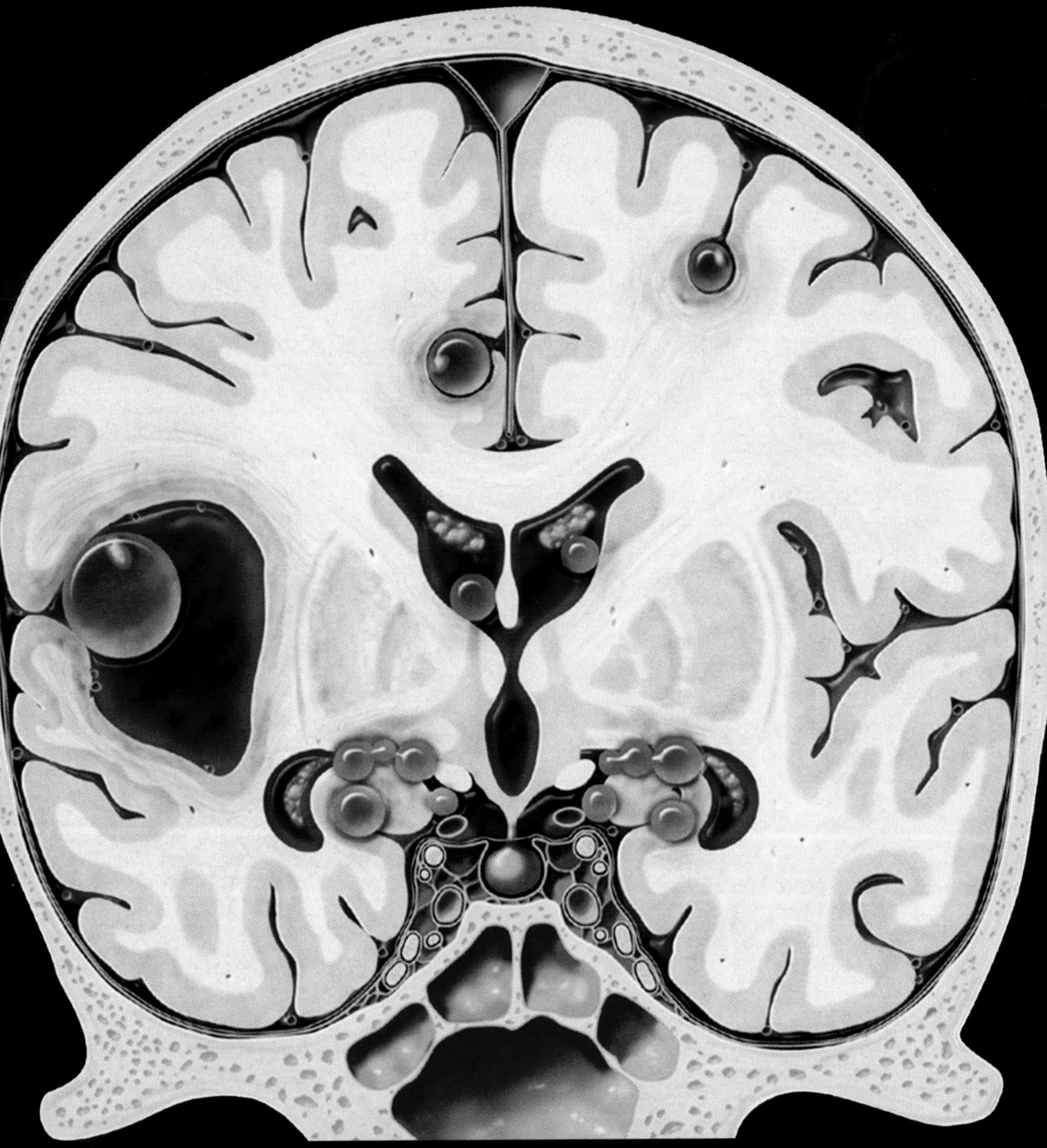

Approach to Infection, Inflammation, and Demyelination

The plague (both literal and figurative) of infectious diseases has been a threat to humankind for millennia. Parasitic infestations have been identified in Egyptian mummies from the Old Kingdom and still affect people today. Our ancient enemies—tuberculosis and malaria—once seemed to be under relative control. But are they? Absolutely not. One in three people in the world has been infected with M. tuberculosis.

In the antibiotic era, once-dreaded infections may seem a distant memory. But are they truly relegated to the medical history scrap heap? Hardly.

I once heard Dr. Joshua Lederberg, who shared the 1958 Nobel Prize in Physiology or Medicine for his discoveries concerning recombination and organization of bacterial genes, make a very telling comment. He remarked, "We are in an 'evolutionary foot race' with our closest competitors, viruses and bacteria." Guess who's winning? One doesn't need to be a genius to guess just *who* is winning ... and it isn't us humans!

Widespread use of antibiotics had its inevitable result. Adaptive evolution has rendered some organisms resistant even to the "antibiotics of last resort." Outbreaks of diverse multidrug-resistant organisms, once rare, are reported with increasing frequency. Methicillin-resistant *Staphylococcus aureus* (MRSA) and vancomycin-resistant *Enterococcus* (VRE) have achieved significant rates of colonization and infection in most intensive care units. To date, interventions aimed at reducing transmission of resistant bacteria in such high-risk settings have been relatively ineffective.

Misuse or mismanagement of first-line drugs has also resulted in the development of multidrug-resistant TB (MDR TB). MDR TB and the recent emergence of extensively drug-resistant TB (XDR TB) jeopardize the major gains achieved by several decades of TB control. The significant progress made in reducing TB-related deaths in immunocompromised patients is also threatened by these developments.

Although any part of the human body can become inflamed or infected, the brain has long been considered an "immunologically protected" site because of the blood-brain barrier. Although CNS infections are considerably less common than their systemic counterparts, the brain is by no means invulnerable to onslaught from pathogenic organisms.

The role of medical imaging in the emergent evaluation of intracranial infection ideally should be supportive, not primary. But in many health care facilities worldwide, triage of acute CNS disease frequently uses brain imaging as an initial noninvasive "screening procedure." Therefore, the

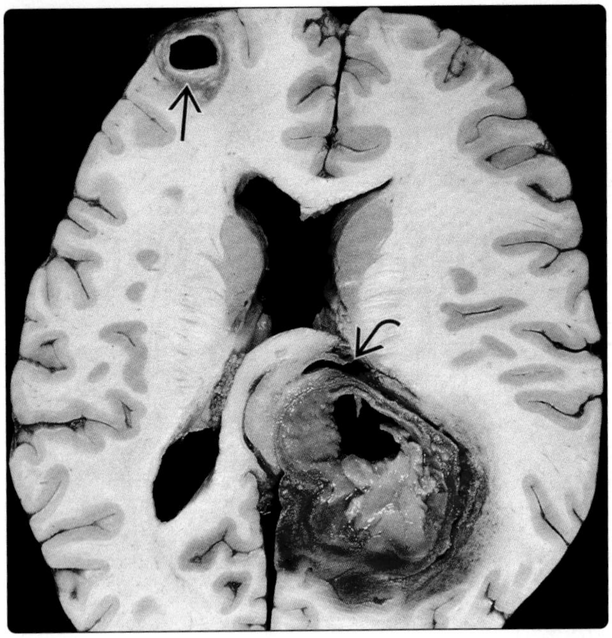

***(11-1)** Note small, well-encapsulated frontal lobe abscess ⇒ with a larger, less well-defined lesion in the contralateral hemisphere. The large abscess ruptured into the ventricle ⇒, causing pyocephalus and death. (Courtesy R. Hewlett, MD.)*

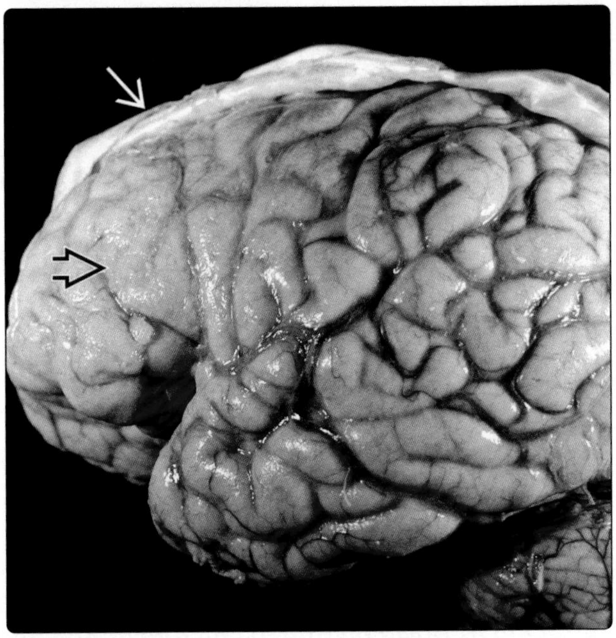

***(11-2)** Autopsy specimen shows the dura ⇒ reflected up to reveal a purulent-appearing collection in the underlying subdural space ⇒. Findings are typical for a pyogenic subdural empyema. (Courtesy R. Hewlett, MD.)*

radiologist may be the first—not the last—to recognize the presence of possible CNS infection.

In this part, we devote chapters 12 and 13 to CNS infections. HIV/AIDS is covered in Chapter 14. The last chapter, Chapter 15, considers the surprisingly broad spectrum of noninfectious idiopathic inflammatory and demyelinating disorders that affect the CNS.

INFECTION, INFLAMMATION, AND DEMYELINATING DISORDERS

CNS Infections
- Overview and classification
- Congenital, pyogenic, viral infections
- TB, fungal, parasitic, emerging infections

HIV/AIDS
- HIV infection
- Opportunistic infections
- AIDS-defining neoplasms

Demyelinating and Inflammatory Diseases
- MS, variants and mimics
- Postinfectious demyelination
- Inflammatory-like disorders

CNS Infections

The concept that the brain was an "immune privileged" organ in which the blood-brain barrier (BBB) was a relative fortress that restricted pathogen entry and limited inflammation has recently undergone significant revision. Lymphocytes circulate through the normal healthy brain, immune responses can occur without lasting consequence, and cross-talk between the brain and extra-CNS organs is both extensive and robust.

Evidence has also recently emerged that there is extensive CSF and interstitial fluid (ISF) exchange throughout the brain, a process now termed "glymphatics."

A pathway of waste removal from the CNS does exist and is facilitated by CSF entering the brain parenchyma and spinal cord via aquaporin 4 water channels on astrocytes that surround the brain vasculature. This wave of CSF entry drives ISF toward the perivenous space, where it collects and drains through lymphatic channels in the dural sinuses through foramina at the skull base to the deep cervical lymph nodes. The process flushes extracellular debris (including β-amyloid) from the parenchyma.

The presence of these drainage systems within the CNS is evidence that there is a constant flow and exchange of proteins within the brain and the blood. CD4+ central and effector memory T cells are found in healthy CSF. The brain is therefore not a "privileged organ" that is immunologically isolated from the rest of the body but rather is actively monitored by—and accessible to—blood-borne lymphocytes and their mediators.

A surprising large number of pathogens, including many neurotropic viruses, can infect the CNS. Well over 200 different organisms have been described as causing CNS infections of one type or another. Routes of entry include transsynaptic spread (e.g., herpes viruses), "hiding" within blood-borne lymphocytes that access the brain (e.g., HIV and JC viruses), and using the choroid plexus as a gateway into the CNS.

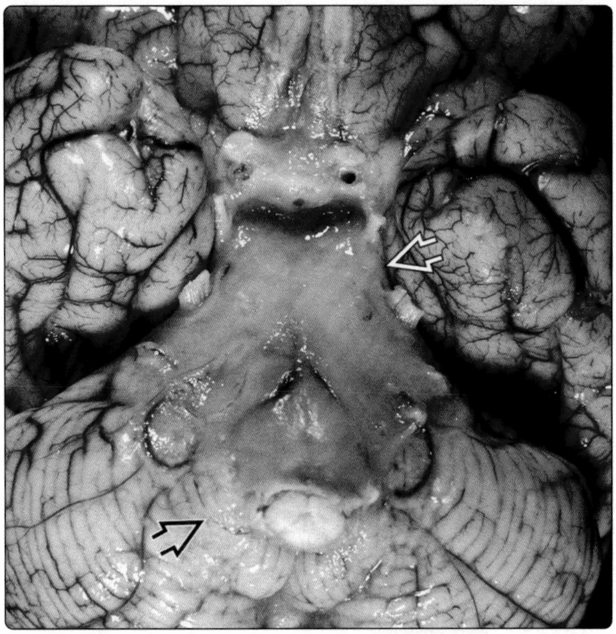

***(11-3)** Autopsy case of tuberculous meningitis shows thick exudate filling the basal cisterns ➡ and covering the pial surfaces of the frontal/temporal lobes and cerebellum ⇨. (Courtesy R. Hewlett, MD.)*

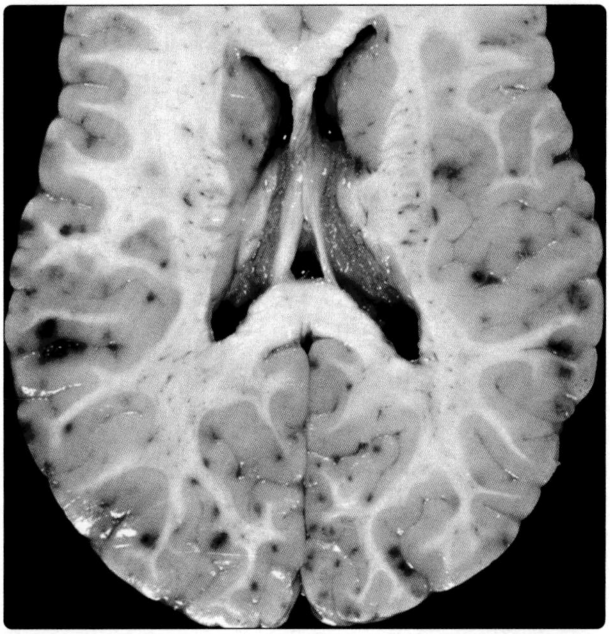

***(11-4)** Axial cut section of autopsied brain in a patient with septicemia shows multifocal petechial hemorrhages, primarily in the cortex and gray-white matter interfaces. (Courtesy R. Hewlett, MD.)*

Imaging plays an increasingly key role in the evaluation of potential CNS infections. However, imaging findings are often nonspecific, so a careful history and appropriate clinical-laboratory investigations are necessary for accurate diagnosis and appropriate treatment.

CNS infections can be classified in several ways. The most common method is to divide them into congenital/neonatal and acquired infections. Categorizing infections purely according to disease category, i.e., pyogenic, viral, granulomatous, parasitic, etc., is also very common. As imaging findings overlap considerably, this system is of little help to the radiologist.

In this text, we follow a combination of classifications. We first subdivide infections into congenital and acquired disorders. Congenital infections are discussed in Chapter 12. Because this is a relatively short discussion, we combine these with acquired pyogenic and viral infections.

Our discussion of pyogenic infections begins with the meninges (meningitis). We follow with a consideration of focal brain infections (cerebritis, abscess), the often lethal complication of ventriculitis (pyocephalus) **(11-1)**, and pus collections in the extraaxial spaces (subdural/epidural empyemas) **(11-2)**. We then focus on the CNS manifestations of acquired viral infections.

In Chapter 13, we consider the pathogenesis and imaging of tuberculosis, fungal infections, and parasitic and protozoal infestations. We conclude this second chapter on infections with a brief discussion of spirochetes and emerging CNS infections (e.g., the rare hemorrhagic viral fevers).

HIV/AIDS

In the more than three decades since AIDS was first identified, the disease has become a worldwide epidemic. With the development of effective combination antiretroviral therapies, HIV/AIDS has evolved from a virtual death sentence to a chronic but manageable disease—if the treatment is (1) available and (2) affordable. As treated patients with HIV/AIDS now often survive for a decade or longer, the imaging spectrum of HIV/AIDS has also evolved.

Treated HIV/AIDS as a chronic disease looks very different from HIV/AIDS in so-called high-burden regions of the world. In such places, HIV in socioeconomically disadvantaged patients often behaves as an acute, fulminant infection. Comorbid diseases such as TB, malaria, or overwhelming bacterial sepsis are common complications and may dominate the imaging presentation.

Complications of HAART treatment have created their own set of recognized disorders, such as immune reconstitution inflammatory syndrome (IRIS). In Chapter 14, we consider the effect of HIV itself on the CNS (HIV encephalitis), as well as opportunistic infections, IRIS, miscellaneous manifestations of HIV/AIDS, and HIV-associated neoplasms.

Demyelinating and Inflammatory Diseases

The final chapter in this part is devoted to demyelinating and noninfectious inflammatory diseases of the CNS.

First, let us be clear on terminology. *Infection* is caused by microorganisms. *Inflammation* is not synonymous with infection. Inflammation (from the Latin meaning "to ignite" or "set alight") is the response of tissues to a variety of pathogens (which may or may not be infectious microorganisms). The inflammatory "cascade" is complex and multifactorial. It involves the vascular system, immune system, and cellular responses, such as microglial activation, the primary component of the brain's innate immune response.

The CNS functions as a unique microenvironment that responds differently than the body's other systems to infiltrating immune cells. The brain white matter is especially susceptible to inflammatory disease. Inflammation can be acute or chronic, manageable or life-threatening. Therefore, imaging plays a central role in the identification and follow-up of neuroinflammatory disorders.

The bulk of Chapter 15 is devoted to multiple sclerosis **(11-5)**. Also included is a discussion of MS variants **(11-6)** and the surprisingly broad spectrum of idiopathic (noninfectious) inflammatory demyelinating diseases (IIDDs), such as neuromyelitis optica. Susac syndrome is a retinocochleocerebral vasculopathy that is often mistaken for MS on imaging studies, so it too is discussed in the context of IIDDs.

Postinfection, postvaccination, autoimmune-mediated demyelinating disorders are considered next. Acute disseminated encephalomyelitis (ADEM) and its most fulminant variant, acute hemorrhagic leukoencephalitis (AHLE), are delineated in detail.

We close the chapter with a discussion of neurosarcoid and inflammatory pseudotumors, including the rapidly expanding category of IgG4-related disorders.

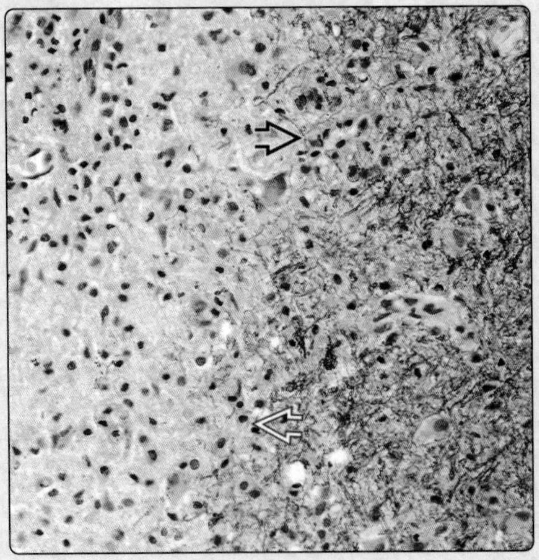

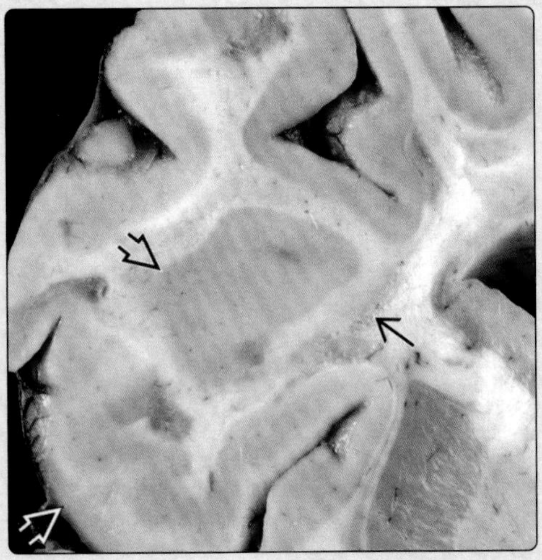

***(11-5)** H&E/Luxol fast blue stain emphasizes the sharp interface between lesion (pale-staining tissue ➔) and normal parenchyma (blue-staining tissue ➔) typical of most demyelinating plaques. (Courtesy B. K. DeMasters, MD.) **(11-6)** Gross autopsy with close-up view of "tumefactive" demyelinating disease ➔ shows peripheral necrosis ➔ with mass effect on the adjacent gyrus ➔. (Courtesy B. K. DeMasters, MD.)*

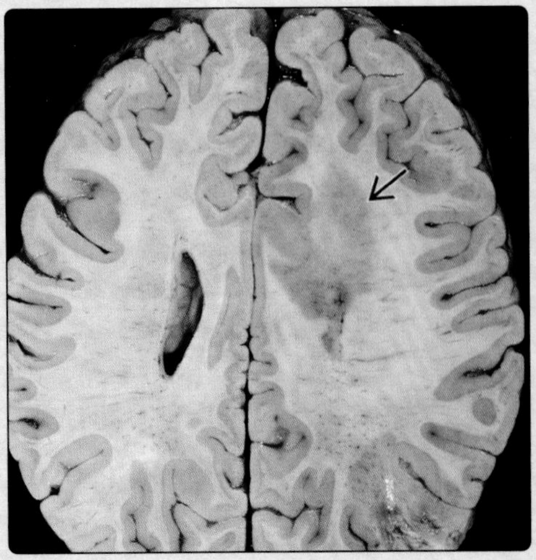

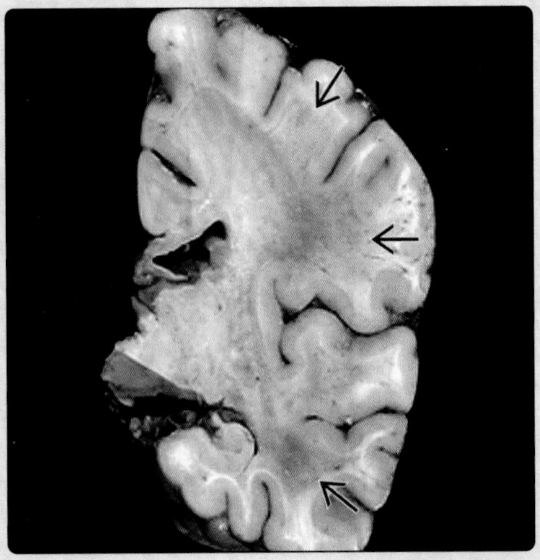

***(11-7)** Axial autopsied brain shows a solitary "horse-show" postinfectious tumefactive demyelinating lesion ➔. **(11-8)** Coronal gross pathology in a case of severe multiple sclerosis shows confluent demyelination in the subcortical white matter ➔. Note sparing of the subcortical U-fibers.*

Congenital, Acquired Pyogenic, and Acquired Viral Infections

Infectious diseases can be conveniently divided into congenital/neonatal and acquired infections. There are unique infectious agents that affect the developing brain. The stage of fetal development at the time of infection is often more important than the causative organism. The clinical manifestations of fetal and neonatal infection and long-term neurologic consequences compared with infections that affect the more mature or fully developed brain will be emphasized below.

We then delineate the first major category of acquired infections, i.e., pyogenic infections. We start with meningitis, the most common of the pyogenic infections. Abscess, together with its earliest manifestations (cerebritis), is discussed next, followed by considerations of ventriculitis (a rare but potentially fatal complication of deep-seated brain abscesses) and intracranial empyemas.

We close the chapter with a discussion of the pathologic and imaging manifestations of acquired viral infections.

Congenital Infections

Parenchymal calcifications are the hallmark of most congenital infections and have been reported with cytomegalovirus (CMV) **(12-2A)**, toxoplasmosis **(12-6A)**, congenital herpes simplex virus (HSV) infection **(12-8A)**, rubella **(12-15)**, congenital varicella-zoster virus **(12-17)**, Zika virus **(12-12B)**, and lymphocytic choriomeningitis virus (LCMV) **(12-16)**.

Infections of the fetal brain result in a spectrum of injury and malformation that depends more on the timing of infection than the infectious agent itself. Infections early in fetal development (e.g., during the first trimester) usually result in miscarriage, severe brain destruction, and/or profound malformations such as anencephaly, agyria, and lissencephaly.

When infections occur later in pregnancy, encephaloclastic manifestations and myelination disturbance (e.g., demyelination, dysmyelination, and hypomyelination) predominate. Microcephaly with frank brain destruction and widespread encephalomalacia are common **(12-11A)**.

With few exceptions (toxoplasmosis and syphilis), most congenital/perinatal infections are viral and are usually secondary to transplacental passage of the infectious agent. Zika virus is a relative newcomer to the list of viruses recognized as a cause of congenital CNS infection and is capable of causing profound brain destruction and resultant microcephaly. Zika virus infection

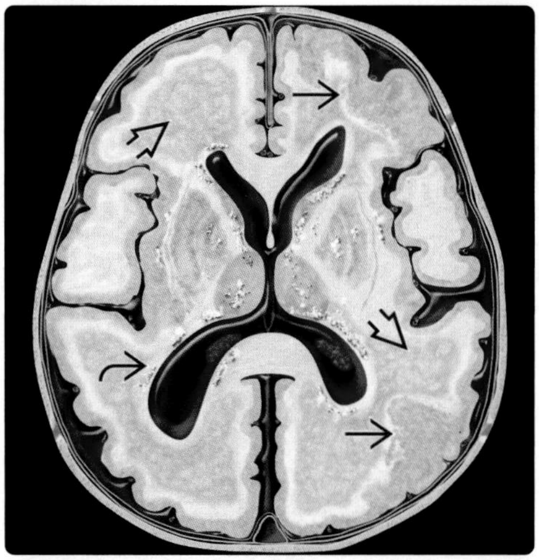

***(12-1)** Congenital CMV is shown with periventricular parenchymal calcifications, damaged white matter, dysplastic cortex.*

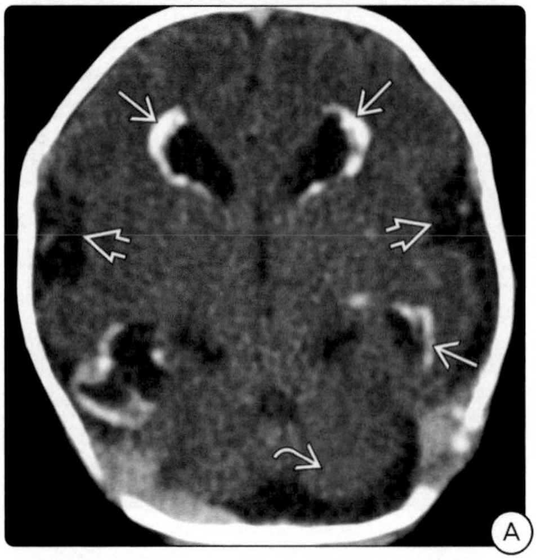

***(12-2A)** NECT in a newborn with CMV shows broad sylvian fissures, periventricular Ca++, and cerebellar hypoplasia.*

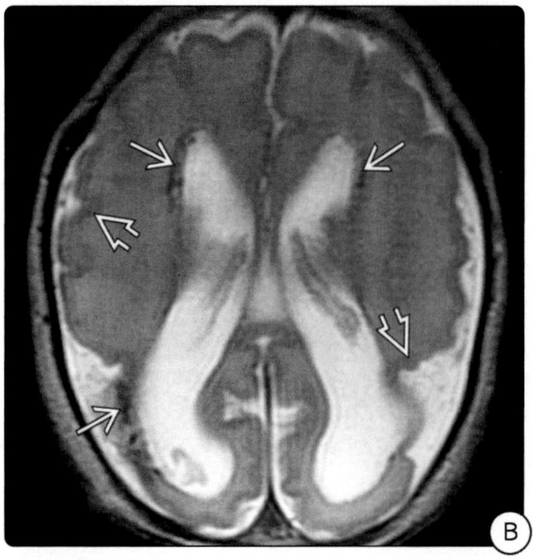

***(12-2B)** T2WI in the same patient shows ventriculomegaly, periventricular Ca++, and simplified gyral pattern (polymicrogyria).*

represents the first reported congenital CNS infection to be mostly transmitted by mosquitoes.

Six members of the herpesvirus family cause neurologic disease in children: HSV-1, HSV-2, varicella-zoster virus (VZV), Epstein-Barr virus (EBV), CMV, and human herpesvirus 6 (HHV-6).

Aside from CMV, HSV-2, Zika virus, and congenital HIV (vertically transmitted), congenital CNS infections have become less common due to immunization programs, prenatal screening, and global infection surveillance.

Here, an overview of the TORCH infections and important non-TORCH congenital/perinatal CNS infections is presented, beginning with the most globally common of the congenital infections, congenital CMV infection.

TORCH Infections

Terminology

Congenital infections are often grouped together and simply called **TORCH** infections—the acronym for **to**xoplasmosis, **r**ubella, **c**ytomegalovirus, and **h**erpes. If congenital **s**yphilis is included, the grouping is called TORCH(S) or (S)TORCH.

Etiology

In addition to the recognized "classic" TORCH(S) infections, a host of new organisms have been identified as causing congenital and perinatal infections. These include Zika virus, LCMV, human Parvovirus B19, human parechovirus, hepatitis B, VZV, tuberculosis, HIV, and the parasitic infection toxocariasis.

Imaging

CMV, toxoplasmosis, rubella, Zika virus, VZV, lymphocytic choriomeningitis virus, and HIV may all cause parenchymal calcifications. The location and distribution of the calcifications may strongly suggest the specific infectious agent. CMV causes periventricular calcifications, cysts, cortical clefts, polymicrogyria (PMG), schizencephaly, and white matter injury. Early CNS infection with Zika virus leads to severe microcephaly and calcifications at the gray matter-white matter junction. Rubella and HSV cause lobar destruction, cystic encephalomalacia, and nonpatterned calcifications. Congenital syphilis is relatively rare, causing basilar meningitis, arterial strokes, and scattered dystrophic calcifications. Congenital HIV is associated with basal ganglia calcification, atrophy, and aneurysmal arteriopathy.

TORCH(S), Zika virus, and LCMV infections should be considered in newborns and infants with microcephaly, parenchymal calcifications, chorioretinitis, and intrauterine growth restriction **(12-1)**.

Congenital Cytomegalovirus

CMV is the leading cause of nonhereditary deafness in children and is the most common cause of congenital brain infection in developed countries.

Terminology and Etiology

Congenital CMV infection is also called CMV encephalitis. CMV is a ubiquitous DNA virus that belongs to the human herpesvirus family.

Pathology

The timing of the gestational infection determines the magnitude of brain insult. Early gestational CMV infection causes germinal zone necrosis with subependymal cysts and dystrophic calcifications. White matter volume loss occurs at all gestational ages and can be diffuse or multifocal. Malformations of cortical development are very common, with PMG having the greatest prevalence **(12-2B)**.

Microscopic examination shows cytomegaly with viral inclusions in the nuclei and cytoplasm. Patchy and focal cellular necrosis, particularly of germinal matrix cells, is typical of first-trimester infection. Vascular inflammation and thrombosis are also common.

Clinical Issues

Epidemiology. CMV is the most common of all congenital infections. Between 0.25-1.00% of newborn infants shed CMV in their urine or saliva at birth. This translates to nearly 35,000 viral-shedding newborns annually. Of these, 10% develop CNS or systemic symptoms and signs. Up to 4,000 newborns in the USA are annually confirmed to have symptomatic CMV infection (e.g., congenital CMV disease). This later category has significant long-term neurodevelopmental sequelae.

Presentation and Natural History. With advances in fetal imaging, particularly fetal MR, many of the CNS imaging manifestations of congenital CMV infection that have have been chronicled in the newborn and infant are elegantly depicted antenatally (e.g., PMG, germinolytic cysts, and cerebellar dysgenesis).

Symptomatic newborns and infants may exhibit microcephaly, jaundice, hepatosplenomegaly, chorioretinitis, and rash. Asymptomatic newborns with congenital CMV infection may show microcephaly and otherwise initially appear developmentally normal. Sensorineural hearing loss, seizures, and developmental delay are the major long-term risks.

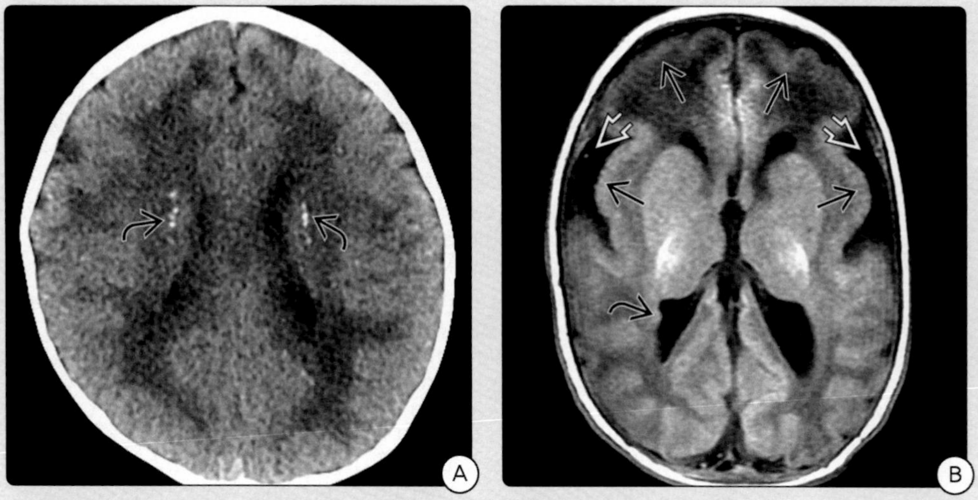

***(12-3A)** NECT in a microcephalic infant with confirmed congenital CMV infection and hearing loss (SNHL) shows caudostriatal → Ca++. **(12-3B)** T1WI in an infant with congenital CMV, shows broad sylvian fissures →, diffuse polymicrogyria (PMG) →, and gray matter (GM) heterotopia →. Note T1 prolongation within frontal white matter.*

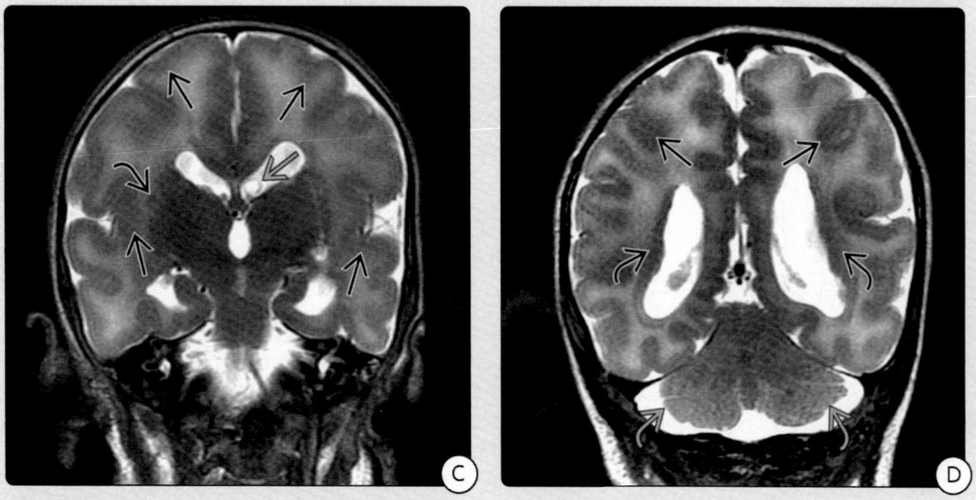

***(12-3C)** T2WI in the same patient demonstrates diffuse PMG →, GM heterotopia →, and vertical hippocampi. Note the left tela choroidea germinolytic cyst →. **(12-3D)** T2WI in the same microcephalic infant shows GM heterotopia →, PMG →, and cerebellar hypoplasia →. Note ventriculomegaly.*

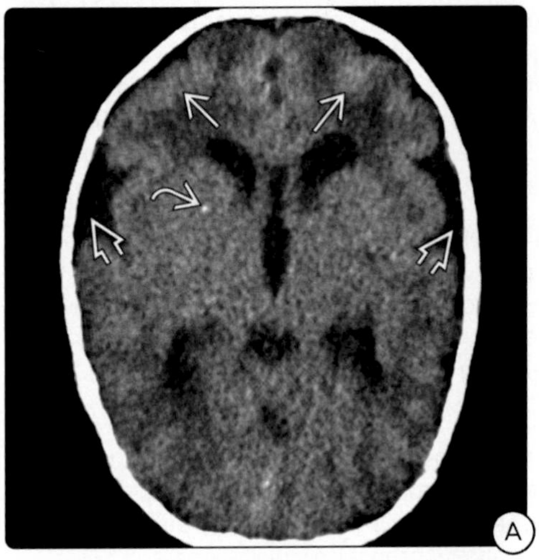

(12-4A) NECT shows a solitary calcification, broad sylvian fissures, and simplified gyri (PMG) in an infant with CMV.

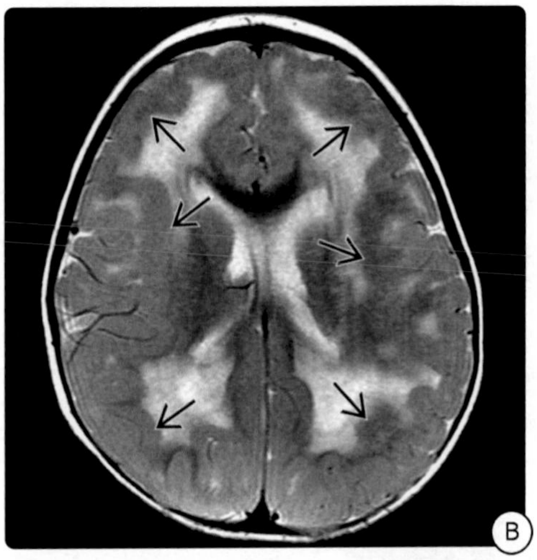

(12-4B) T2WI showing diffuse, asymmetric white matter (WM) T2 prolongation. Bilateral diffuse polymicrogyria is present.

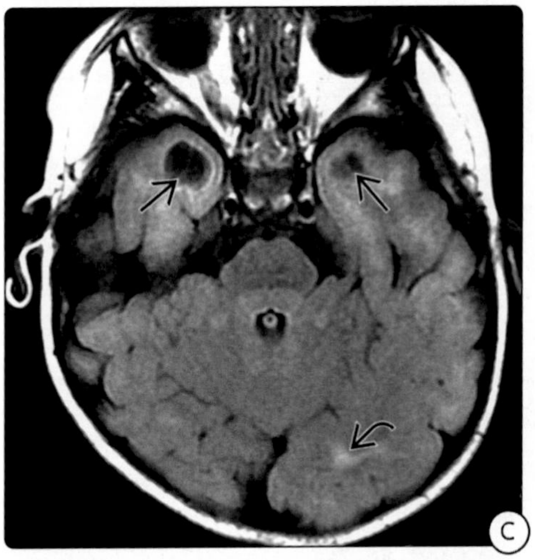

(12-4C) AXIAL T2 FLAIR image demonstrates bilateral temporal lobe cysts and scattered WM hyperintensities.

Newborns with systemic manifestations (e.g., hepatosplenomegaly, petechiae, and jaundice) have a slightly worse overall prognosis. Greater than half of all neonates with systemic signs and symptoms also have CNS involvement. The vast majority of these newborns that demonstrate microcephaly, ventriculomegaly, cortical malformations (e.g., PMG), white matter abnormalities, and parenchymal calcifications have major neurodevelopmental sequelae (e.g., cerebral palsy, epilepsy, and mental retardation).

Treatment Options. Early (before gestational week 17) maternal hyperimmunoglobulin therapy improves the outcome of fetuses from women with primary CMV infection. The use of antiviral agents is also being explored for the treatment of symptomatic congenital CMV beyond the neonatal period. Antiviral agents that specifically target CMV are ganciclovir, valganciclovir (VGVC), foscarnet, and cidofovir. VGVC is well tolerated and may improve or help preserve auditory function in infected infants.

Imaging

General Features. Imaging features of congenital CMV are protean, including microcephaly, ventriculomegaly, germinolytic cysts, cortical malformations (e.g., PMG), Ca++, cerebellar and hippocampal dysgenesis, and white matter abnormalities. As a general rule, the earlier the fetal infection, the more severe the findings **(12-1) (12-4)**.

CT Findings. NECT scans show intracranial calcifications and ventriculomegaly in the majority of symptomatic infants. Calcifications are predominantly periventricular, with a predilection for the germinal matrix zones, particularly the caudostriatal regions **(12-2A)**. Calcifications vary from numerous bilateral thick calcifications to faint punctate unilateral foci **(12-2A) (12-3A) (12-4A)**. Calcification may be entirely absent (e.g., some NECT series of proven congenital CMV CNS disease report the prevalence of intracranial Ca++ at 66%). Therefore, the absence of intracranial Ca++ does not exclude diagnosis of congenital CMV. NECT may also demonstrate cortical clefting and other features reflecting underlying cortical malformation (e.g., PMG).

MR Findings. MR remains the most sensitive imaging tool and examination of choice to depict the magnitude of congenital CNS CMV findings. MR shows the broad range of CMV-induced CNS abnormalities. This includes microcephaly with ventriculomegaly, cortical migrational and organizational abnormalities (the most common of which is PMG), cysts (germinal zone and pretemporal), parenchymal calcifications, white matter abnormalities (dysplastic and demyelinating), hippocampal dysgenesis, and cerebellar dysgenesis. It bears reemphasizing that cortical migrational and organizational abnormalities are present in approximately 10-50% of congenital CMV cases and range from minor dysgenesis with focal cortical clefting, simplified gyral pattern and "open" lateral cerebral/sylvian fissures (e.g. PMG), to more severe manifestations including agyria, lissencephaly, and schizencephaly.

PMG in most congenital CMV infection imaging reviews remains the most common imaging abnormality that will be detected, more common than calcification.

T1WI shows microcephaly and enlarged ventricles and cysts with a predilection for the periventricular germinal zones and pretemporal white matter. Cortical abnormalities such as cerebellar and hippocampal dysgenesis are well depicted **(12-3C) (12-3D)**. Also, subependymal hyperintense foci of T1 shortening caused by the periventricular calcifications may be seen. White matter hypointensities correspond to regions of demyelination and dysplasia. Sagittal midline T1WI shows a diminished cranial-to-facial ratio, indicating microcephaly. 3D T1WI techniques (e.g., 3D-SPGR) with isotropic axial and coronal reformations aide in detecting cortical, hippocampal, and cerebellar abnormalities (e.g., PMG) **(12-3)** **(12-4)**.

T2WI and FLAIR images show myelin delay, white matter destruction, demyelination, and white matter volume loss with focal, patchy, or confluent hyperintensities at sites of white matter abnormality. Periventricular (e.g., germinal zone and anterior temporal lobe) cysts are common **(12-4)** **(12-5)**. The pretemporal white matter cysts often begin as regions of T1 and T2 prolongation **(12-4C)** **(12-5C)**. T2WI also demonstrates the indistinct gray matter/white matter interface characteristic of PMG and characterizes other patterns of cortical organizational and migrational disturbance **(12-3C)**. Coronal T2WI and FLAIR demonstrate the patterns of vertically dysmorphic hippocampi and cerebellar dysgenesis **(12-3)**. Calcifications appear as foci of T2 shortening (e.g., hypointensity) **(12-1)**.

SWIs, including SWI-filtered phase maps, are able to distinguish paramagnetic substances (blood products as hypointense) from diamagnetic substances (calcification as hyperintense). Thus, SWI represents a valuable MR sequence in the imaging evaluation of suspected congenital CNS infections.

Fetal MR is more sensitive than US in the early detection of CMV-associated CNS abnormalities.

Ultrasound. Cranial sonography is useful for evaluation of the neonatal and infant brain (up to 6-8 months of age). In the setting of congenital CMV infection, cranial sonography may be technically challenging, as microcephaly (due to poor brain growth and brain destruction) is associated with overlapping sutures and diminished size of the anterior and posterior fontanelles, which represent the probe contact points for sonography. When an acoustic window is present, enlarged ventricles, periventricular hyperechogenic foci that correspond to the subependymal calcifications seen on NECT and MR (SWI), may be seen.

Other findings include germinal zone cysts (germinolytic), which may be present along the caudostriatal grooves in the periventricular zones and in the anterior temporal white matter. Lenticulostriate mineralizing vasculopathy appearing as linear and branching hyperechogenicities within the thalami and basal ganglia although not pathognomonic for CMV occurs in 25-30% of congenital CMV infections.

CONGENITAL CMV INFECTION SPECTRUM OF IMAGING ABNORMALITIES

- Calcifications (caudostriatal and periventricular)
- Cerebellar hypoplasia
- Cerebral cortical abnormalities
  - Polymicrogyria
  - Cortical cleft dysplasia
  - Schizencephaly
  - Lissencephaly
  - Pachygyria
  - Hippocampal dysplasia
- Cysts (germinolytic and anterior temporal)
- White matter abnormality

Differential Diagnosis

The differential diagnosis of congenital CMV includes other TORCH and non-TORCH infections, including toxoplasmosis, Zika virus, and LCMV. **Toxoplasmosis** is much less common than CMV and typically causes scattered parenchymal calcifications, not the dominant subependymal

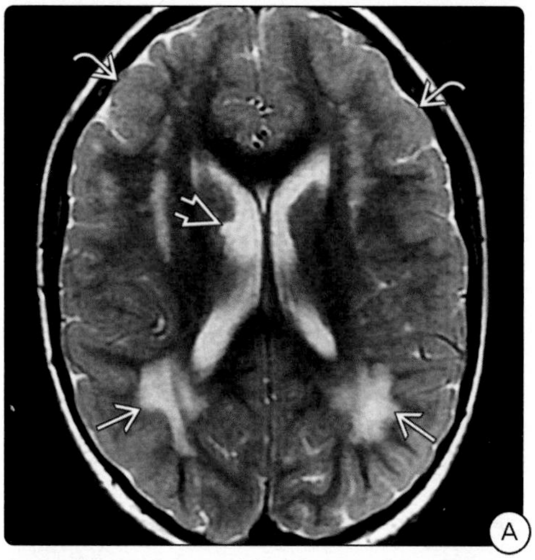

(12-5A) T2WI in a 3y girl with CMV shows WM hyperintensities ➡, germinolytic cyst ➡, and malformations of cortical development ➡.

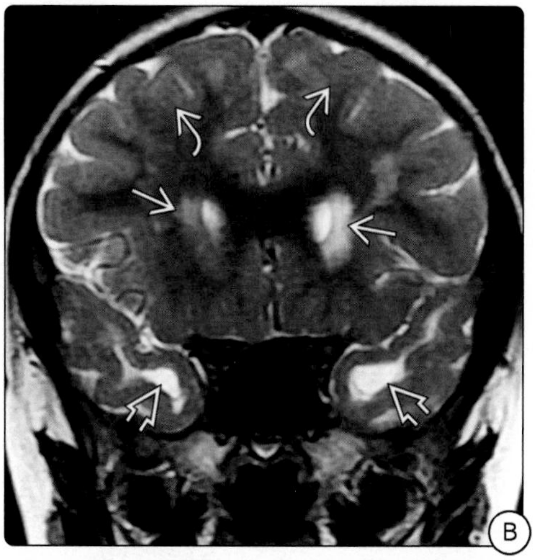

(12-5B) Coronal T2WI in the same patient shows periventricular WM hyperintensities ➡, anterior temporal lobe cysts ➡, and bilateral PMG ➡.

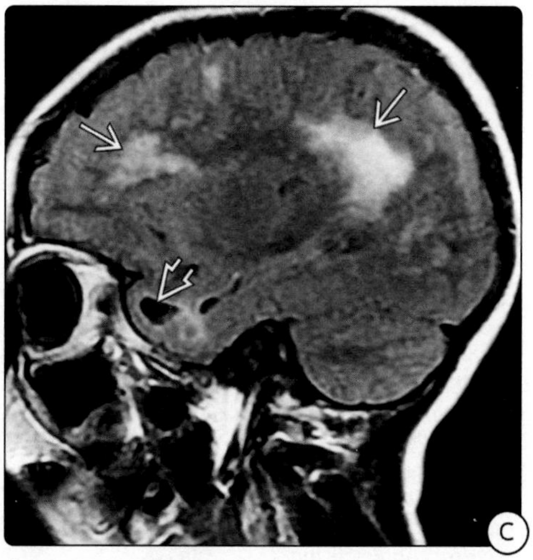

(12-5C) Sagittal T2 FLAIR shows multifocal WM hyperintensities ➡ and anterior temporal lobe cysts ➡.

pattern observed in CMV. Microcephaly and cortical dysplasia are also significantly less common in congenital toxoplasmosis. Up to 50% of toxoplasmosis patients have hydrocephalus. **Zika** and **LCMV** may display an array of imaging abnormalities that are precise mimics of congenital CMV disease.

Zika Virus Infection. Ca++ is universal, occurring at the at the GM/WM junctions. Additionally, ventriculomegaly, malformations of cortical development (e.g., PMG), occipital pseudocysts, callosal dysgenesis, myelination disturbance, and brainstem and cerebellar hypoplasia are frequently reported.

LCMV. CT and MR findings may mimic CMV. LCM may cause necrotizing ependymitis and aqueductal obstruction with resultant hydrocephalus and macrocephaly, like 50% of congenital toxoplasmosis cases **(12-16)**.

Pseudo-TORCH Syndromes. Some genetic disorders mimic the imaging abnormalities of congenital infections. Adams-Oliver, Baraitser-Reardon, Aicardi-Goutières syndrome, RNAse T2-deficient leukoencephalopathy, Coats plus syndrome, leukoencephalopathy, cerebral calcification, and cysts are rare, mostly autosomal-recessive demyelinating and degenerative disorders. Basal ganglia and brainstem calcifications are more common than the subependymal pattern characteristic of CMV, Zika, or LCMV.

Pseudo-TORCH syndromes, unlike congenital infections, show *progressive decline* in neurological status and *advancing imaging abnormalities.* **Pseudo-TORCH syndromes** typically lack malformations of the cortex (e.g. PMG) that are so common in many of the congenital infections.

Congenital Toxoplasmosis

Etiology and Pathology

Congenital toxoplasmosis is caused by intrauterine infection with *Toxoplasma gondii*, one of the world's most common

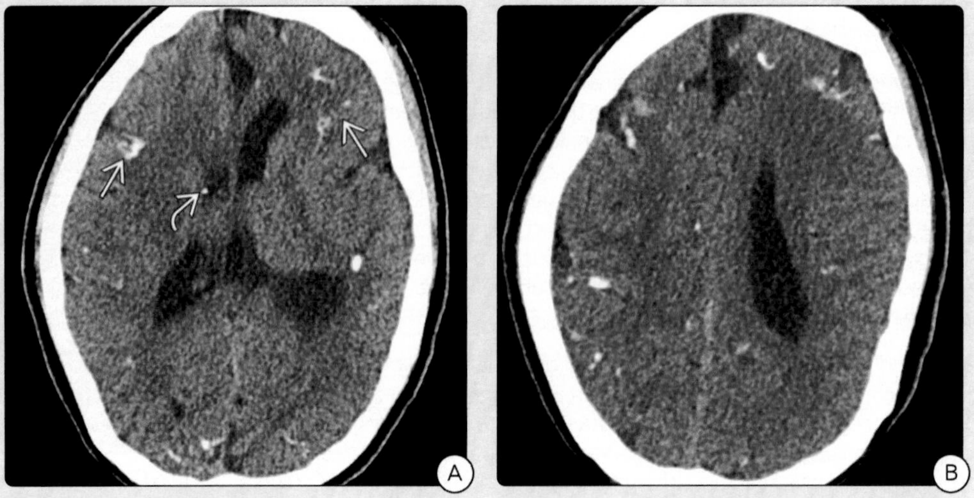

***(12-6A)** Axial NECT image from a 12y developmentally delayed girl with known congenital toxoplasmosis shows that punctate and linear calcifications primarily involve the cerebral cortex and subcortical white matter ➡. A single periventricular calcification is present ➥, contrasting this case with CMV. **(12-6B)** Axial NECT from the same girl shows scattered calcifications. Cortical anomalies are uncommon in congenital toxoplasmosis.*

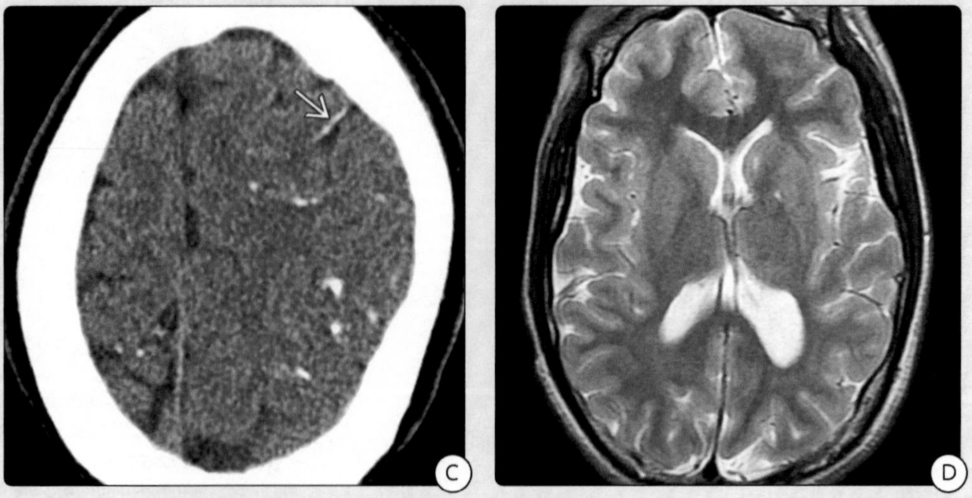

***(12-6C)** Axial NECT through cerebral convexities shows peripheral nature of the calcifications in this child with congenital toxoplasmosis. The linear "tram-track" calcification pattern described in some cases is nicely demonstrated here ➡. **(12-6D)** Axial T2WI in same girl shows normal hemispheric cortex without evidence of malformation, typically seen with CMV. Hydrocephalus is more common in toxoplasmosis.*

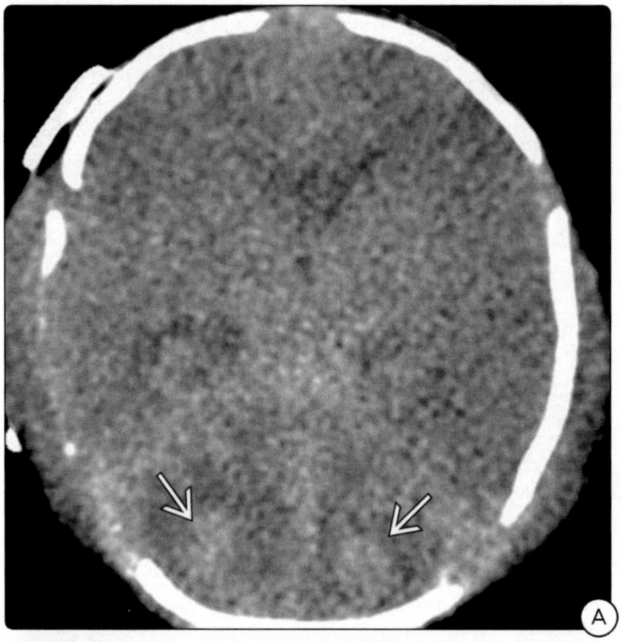

(12-7A) NECT shows 13d neonate with fever, lethargy, respiratory distress, hypoglycemia, and hepatomegaly, showing diffuse cerebral edema. Note the focal hyperattenuation (hemorrhage) within the cerebellar hemispheres .

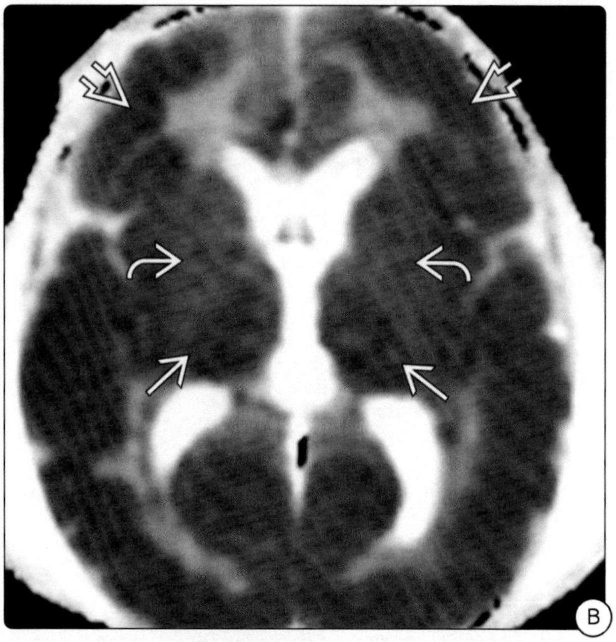

(12-7B) ADC map in the same neonate shows widespread symmetric diffusion restriction in the cortex , basal ganglia , and thalami . CSF PCR was positive for herpes simplex virus (HSV). This is disseminated congenital HSV infection.

obligate intracellular parasites. Infected domestic cats (e.g., the parasite's ultimate host) represent a major source of human infection, endemic in some developed countries (e.g., France). The infection in humans is usually acquired from the ingestion of contaminated water or undercooked food products (usually fresh fruit, vegetables, and meat) or by direct contact with the feces of an infected cat (e.g., gardening, litter box, or the child's sandbox).

Ependymitis leading to aqueductal obstruction and hydrocephalus with resultant macrocephaly is seen in approximately 50% of congenital toxoplasmosis. A diffuse inflammation of the meninges is present with large and small granulomatous lesions. Unlike CMV, malformations of cortical development are rare.

Clinical Issues

Toxoplasmosis is the second most common congenital infection. Approximately 5 in 1,000 pregnant women are infected with it. Estimates of the risk of fetal transmission vary from 10-100%.

Congenital toxoplasmosis causes severe chorioretinitis, jaundice, hepatosplenomegaly, growth retardation, and brain damage. Chorioretinitis is often severe. Infants with subclinical infection at birth are at risk for seizures, as well as delayed cognitive, motor, and visual defects.

Imaging and Differential Diagnosis

With some exceptions, imaging features of congenital toxoplasmosis resemble those of CMV, Zika, and LCMV. NECT scans show extensive parenchymal calcifications that often appear "scattered" throughout the brain parenchyma **(12-6)** unlike the germinal zone calcifications of CMV or subcortical calcifications of Zika virus infection. MR scans may show multiple subcortical cysts, porencephaly, and ventriculomegaly (hydrocephalus) often due to inflammatory debris and aqueductal obstruction. There is a notable lack of cortical malformations in those affected with congenital toxoplasmosis **(12-6D)** in contradistinction to those afflicted with congenital CMV disease **(12-2B)**.

Malformations of cortical development that are so common in Zika virus, congenital CMV, and LCMV infections are rare in toxoplasmosis.

Herpes Simplex Virus: Congenital and Neonatal Infections

Terminology

CNS involvement in HSV infection is called **congenital** or **neonatal HSV** when it involves neonates. In contradistinction, herpes simplex encephalitis (HSE) (HSE is also sometimes called herpes simplex virus encephalitis) describes encephalitis in individuals beyond the first postnatal month. In this section, we discuss neonatal HSV. HSE is discussed subsequently with other acquired viral infections.

Etiology

Herpes simplex viruses (HSV-1 and HSV-2) are double-stranded DNA viruses and members of the family *Herpesviridae* that infect humans. Approximately 2,000 infants in the USA annually are diagnosed with neonatal infections with either HSV-1 or HSV-2. The morbidity and mortality in

(12-8A) *A 4-week-old infant born to an HSV-2-positive mother had several days of fever and lethargy. T1WI shows multiple bilateral cortical ➡ and basal ganglia ➡ foci of T1 shortening, suggestive of subacute hemorrhage.* **(12-8B)** *More cephalad scan in the same patient shows additional areas of cortical T1 shortening ➡. Susceptibility-weighted MR with filtered phase maps aids in differentiating hemorrhage from calcification.*

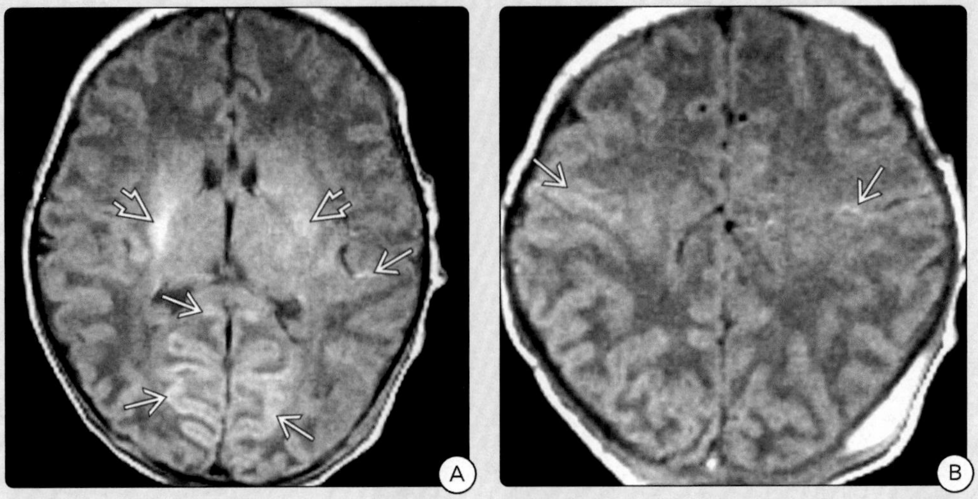

(12-8C) *T2WI in the same infant, 1 month later shows extensive multicystic encephalomalacia with blood-fluid levels ➡. Note ribbon-like T2 shortening within the cortex ➡ reflecting hemorrhage and or Ca++.* **(12-8D)** *T2WI through the convexity in the same patient illustrates holohemispheric cystic encephalomalacia ⇨ underlying regions of gyral T2 shortening ➡. This case illustrates early and late changes of congenital HSV.*

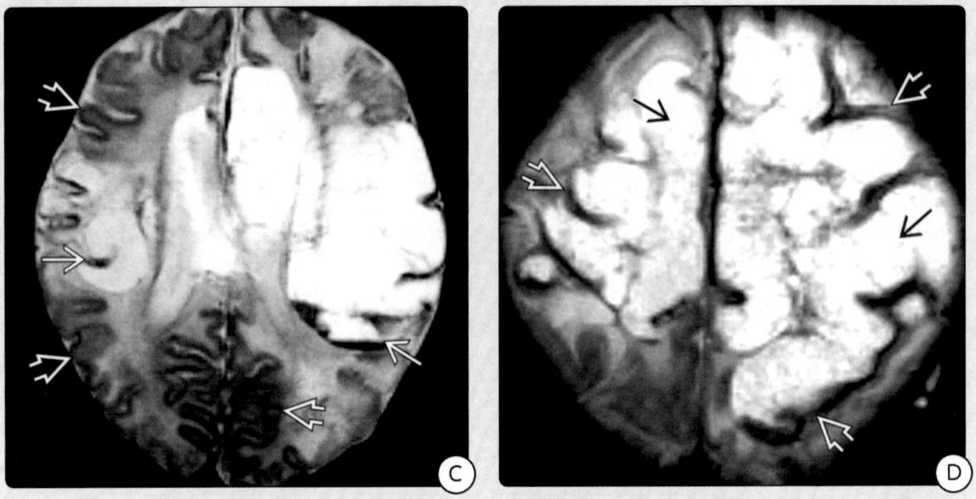

(12-9) *Autopsied brain from an infant with end-stage HSV shows markedly enlarged ventricles and extensive holohemispheric cystic encephalomalacia ⇨.* **(12-10)** *Coronal FLAIR in a microcephalic infant with a history of peripartum HSV-2 shows extensive cerebral hemispheric cystic encephalomalacia ➡ and gliosis ➡. Note the passive ventricular enlargement.*

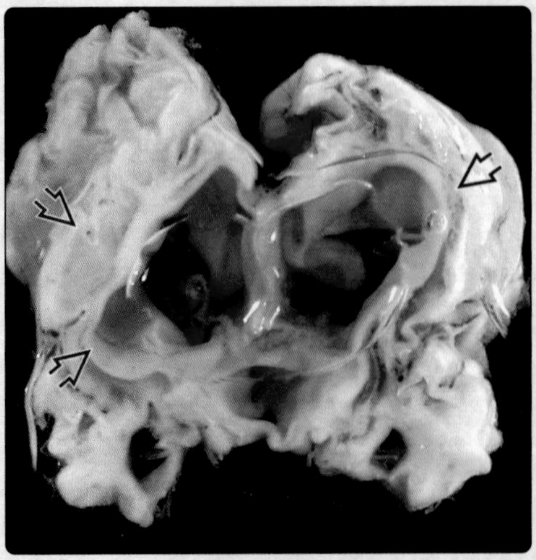

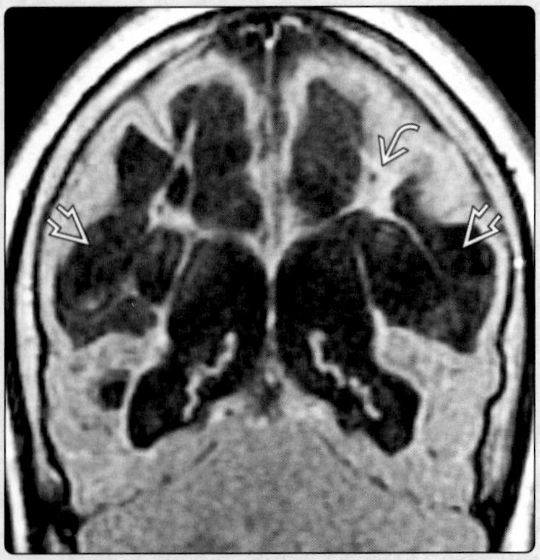

neonatal HSV-2 encephalitis is significantly worse compared with HSV-1 encephalitis. These are lifelong viral infections.

Pathology

Neonatal HSV encephalitis is a diffuse disease, without the predilection for the temporal lobes and limbic system seen in older children and adults.

Early changes include meningoencephalitis with necrosis, hemorrhage, and microglial proliferation. Atrophy with gross cystic encephalomalacia and parenchymal calcifications is typical of late-stage HSV. Near-total loss of brain substance with hydranencephaly is seen in severe cases.

Clinical Issues

Epidemiology. HSV-2 is one of the most prevalent sexually transmitted infections worldwide. Approximately 2% of women acquire HSV-2 annually. The majority are asymptomatic, and most are completely unaware of the disease. Neonatal HSV infections are vertically transmitted, occurring in approximately 1 in 3,200 deliveries in the United States. Prevalence is higher in African Americans, low-income mothers, and mothers with multiple sexual partners.

The vast majority (85%) of neonatal HSV is acquired at parturition, and 10% is contracted postnatally. Only 5% of cases are due to **in utero** transmission. Those who have contracted their infection in utero may manifest the congenital infection syndrome, namely microcephaly, skin rash or scarring, and cataracts. The risk is increased with primary maternal infection during the third trimester and can be decreased by cesarean delivery.

Presentation. Neonatal HSV infection causes three clinicopathological disease patterns: (1) skin, eye, and mouth disease; (2) encephalitis; and (3) disseminated disease with or without CNS disease. Approximately 50% of all infants with neonatal HSV will have CNS involvement, either isolated or as part of disseminated disease.

Clinicians must have a high index of suspicion for neonatal HSV infection. Only two-thirds of the infected neonates with HSV encephalitis show a herpetic skin rash. This disseminated infection presents with lethargy, poor feeding, jaundice, hepatomegaly, seizures, and respiratory distress. The fontanelle may bulge. Onset of symptoms in perinatal HSV infection is 2-4 weeks following delivery (peak = 16 days). The definitive diagnosis is based on detecting HSV DNA in the serum or CSF (e.g., PCR). Note that **as many as 25%** of neonates with HSV encephalitis have **negative PCR studies**.

Natural History. Death by 1 year of age occurs in approximately 50% of untreated neonates with overt CNS disease and 85% with disseminated infection. Half of surviving infants have permanent deafness, vision loss, cerebral palsy, and/or epilepsy.

Treatment Options. Prompt administration of antiviral therapy with high-dose acyclovir significantly reduces morbidity, especially in infants with disseminated disease, and should be initiated whenever perinatal HSV encephalitis is suspected even when the initial PCR is "negative." In such a case, empiric therapy with acyclovir should be initiated, lumbar puncture repeated, and PCR performed.

Imaging

Unlike childhood or adult HSE, neonatal HSV CNS infection is much more diffuse. Both gray and white matter are affected. HSV is known to damage many brain regions with necrosis, cellular debris, hemorrhage, macrophage and mononuclear inflammatory cellular infiltration, calcification, and hypertrophied astrocytes. Interestingly, the pial-glial membrane remains intact, and the ependyma and choroid plexuses are spared, in contrast to CMV **(12-7)**.

ALERT: The radiologist should strongly consider neonatal HSV encephalitis when cranial imaging at 2-3 weeks of neonatal life shows unexplained diffuse cerebral edema, with leptomeningeal enhancement, without or with cerebral parenchymal hemorrhage. Early MR with diffusion is advised **(12-7)**.

CT Findings. NECT may be normal early in the disease or show diffuse hypoattenuation involving both cortex and subcortical white matter reflecting cerebral edema **(12-7A)**. Hemorrhages may present as multifocal punctate, patchy, and curvilinear regions of hyperattenuation in the basal ganglia, white matter, and cortex **(12-7A)**.

MR Findings. MR without and with intravenous MR contrast (with a critical eye to DWI abnormalities) is the imaging procedure of choice in suspected cases of neonatal HSV, with recognition that the normal unmyelinated neonatal white matter presents a challenge in the early detection of HSV encephalitis.

HSV encephalitis is nonpatterned. In the acute and subacute stages of this disease, multifocal lesions (67%), deep gray matter involvement (58%), hemorrhage (66%), "watershed" pattern of injury (40%), and the occasional involvement of the brainstem and cerebellum have been reported.

DWI and ADC maps detect early cellular necrosis and are key, not only for the initial diagnosis of neonatal HSV encephalitis, but also to detect rare CNS relapses. In half of all patients, DWI demonstrates bilateral or significantly more extensive disease than seen on conventional MR **(12-7B)**. Areas of restricted diffusion may be the only positive imaging findings in early cases. Late-stage disease shows severe volume loss with enlarged ventricles and multicystic encephalomalacia **(12-9)** **(12-10)**.

In the early stages, diffuse cerebral edema may predominate. T1WI may be normal or show hypointensity (T1 prolongation) in affected areas. Proton density and FSE T2 sequences show hyperintensity in the cortex, white matter, and basal ganglia.

Warning: FLAIR sequences at less than 8 months of age underestimate parenchymal pathology, particularly within the hemispheric white matter. Hemorrhagic foci are common (66%) within 1 week of clinical diagnosis and best detected with T2* sequences (e.g., GRE, SWI), SWI being six times more sensitive to detect parenchymal Ca++.

Neurological Manifestations of Herpes Virus Infections Beyond 4 Weeks

Virus	Immunocompetent Hosts	Immunosuppressed Hosts
CMV	Meningoencephalitis	Retinitis, microglial nodular encephalitis
EBV	Meningoencephalitis, cerebellitis, optic neuritis, brainstem encephalitis	EBV, primary CNS lymphomas
HHV-6	Febrile seizures (< 2 years), hippocampi and amygdala, extratemporal involvement	Meningoencephalitis, leukoencephalitis, acute necrotizing encephalitis
HSV-1	Limbic structures involved, asymmetric bilateral, vascular territory involvement	Encephalitis
HSV-2	Aseptic meningitis	May have myelitis
VZV	Cerebellitis, vasculitis (stroke) (basal ganglia), multifocal leukoencephalopathy	Multifocal leukoencephalopathy

(Table 12-1) *CMV = cytomegalovirus; EBV = Epstein-Barr virus; HHV = human herpesvirus; HSV = herpes simplex virus; VZV, varicella zoster virus.*

Foci of patchy enhancement, typically a meningeal pattern of enhancement, are common on T1 C+ scans. In later stages, T1 shortening and T2 hypointensity with "blooming" on T2* GRE/SWI secondary to hemorrhagic foci may develop **(12-8)**.

MRS early in HSV encephalitis shows elevated lactate, lipids, choline, and excitatory neurotransmitters. NAA is reduced.

Ultrasound. Acutely, ultrasound demonstrates diffuse edema ("salt and pepper" pattern). Less common are linear echoes in the basal ganglia, similar to CMV.

Differential Diagnosis

The major differential diagnoses for neonatal HSV are **other TORCH and non-TORCH infections**. Neonates with HSV are usually normal for the first few days after delivery. Brain scans are normal or minimally abnormal early in the disease course. Calcifications and migrational anomalies are absent.

Because the initial imaging features of acute and subacute HSV encephalitis are often so nonspecific and may manifest with generalized cerebral edema, metabolic, toxic, and hypoxic ischemic insults must also be considered in the differential diagnosis.

In some cases, HSV causes watershed distribution ischemic injury in areas remote from the primary herpetic lesions and may be difficult to distinguish from partial protracted or mild to moderate **hypoxic-ischemic injury** (HII). However, term infants with HII typically follow a different clinical course, becoming symptomatic in the immediate postnatal period. Profound HII preferentially affects the perirolandic cortex and sulcal depths, white matter, hippocampi, and deep gray nuclei, including the ventrolateral thalami. Hemorrhage with "blooming" on T2* GRE is uncommon in neonatal HII.

Zika Virus Infection

Etiology

Zika virus is a single-stranded RNA *Flavivirus*, closely related to Dengue fever, yellow fever, West Nile virus, and Chikungunya. The virus is mostly transmitted by infected female mosquito vector bites, particularly *Aedes aegypti* mosquitos. It can also be transmitted through blood contamination perinatally and sexually. Zika virus has been directly linked to severe fetal microcephaly in infants born to infected mothers.

Pathology

Like CMV, Zika virus crosses the fetal-placental barrier and has been isolated from the brain and CSF of microcephalic newborns and the placental tissue and amniotic fluid. The virus leads to neurotoxicity and in experimental models impaired human neurosphere growth. Fetal germinal matrix tissue is a target for Zika virus. As with other congenital CNS infections, the timing of infection dictates the scope and magnitude of brain injury and malformation.

Clinical Issues

The diagnosis of Zika virus infection in the adult is complicated by the fact that up to 80% of infected individuals are asymptomatic. The symptoms when present are nonspecific and mild. Headache, rash, and fever may be reported. Conjunctivitis and Guillain-Barré syndrome are uncommon clinical manifestations of the infection.

Compared with congenital CMV disease, brain involvement with Zika virus infection tends to routinely cause severe brain damage, indicating a poor prognosis for neurologic outcome. The affected newborn shows microcephaly, a nonspecific term that refers to a smaller than expected head for normal gestational age. In Zika virus infection and other congenital infections, insults to the developing brain lead to microencephaly (small brain), which results in a small head (microcephaly). Also, associated overlapping sutures, closed fontanelles, and redundant scalp skin folds may be clinically observed. Seizures, poor feeding, hypotonia, and lethargy are nonspecific common clinical features among severely affected newborns.

Imaging

Cerebral parenchymal calcifications are universally present. The cerebral hemispheric GM-WM junction is the most

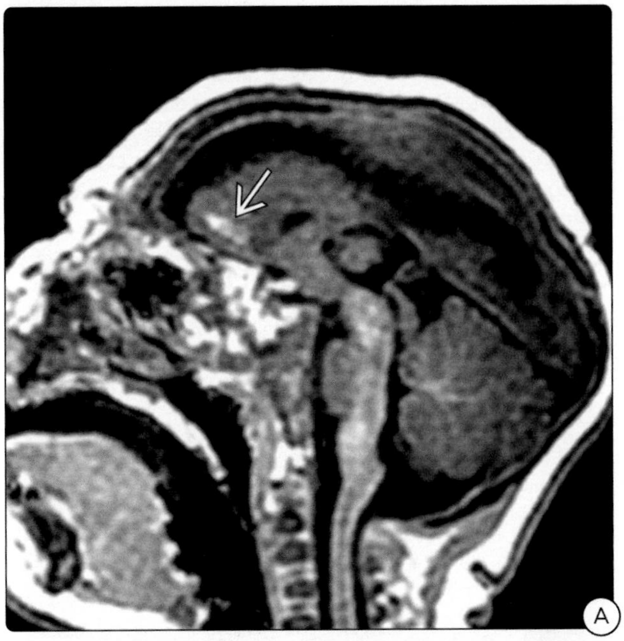

(12-11A) Sagittal T1WI shows diminished cranio-to-facial ratio secondary to microencephaly in congenital Zika viral infection. T1 shortening at GM-WM junction ➡ reflects Ca++. (Courtesy L. Brandao, MD.)

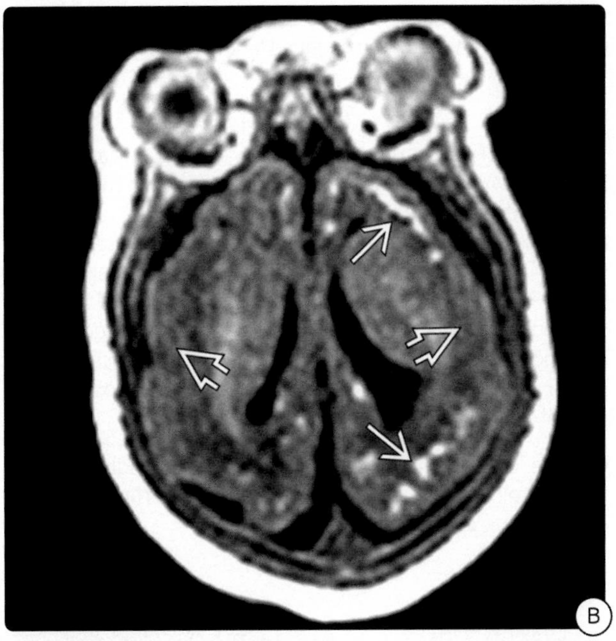

(12-11B) T1WI shows T1 shortening at the GM-WM junctions ➡ reflecting Ca++. Note the smooth brain surface, shallow sulci, and hazy GM-WM transitions consistent with PMG ⇨. (Courtesy L. Brandao, MD.)

common location **(12-12)**. Other sites include the basal ganglia/thalami, brainstem, and cerebellum. Cerebral, cerebellar, and brain stem volume loss, ventriculomegaly, and resultant microencephaly are seen. Disorders of the corpus callosum and cortex are common. Polymicrogyria (PMG), lissencephaly, and pachygyria are also seen. PMG is reported in up to 65% of affected newborns. Other reported abnormalities include occipital periventricular cysts, demyelination, microphthalmia, and cataracts.

MR is the most comprehensive tool to depict parenchymal calcifications (e.g., SWI with filtered phase maps), cortical migration, organizational abnormalities, ventriculomegaly, white mater myelination, developmental anomalies of the corpus callosum, and orbital abnormalities **(12-11)**. The US acoustical window is often limited by the small or closed fontanelles and sutural overlap seen in severe microcephaly. NECT, although sensitive for the detection of calcification, will underestimate presence and extent of cortical malformations and exposes the neonate to ionizing radiation.

Differential Diagnosis

Congenital CMV presents with microcephaly, PMG, and Ca++ at caudostriatal groove. **Toxoplasmosis** presents with macrocephaly, hydrocephalus, scattered Ca++, and lack of cortical malformations. **LCMV** presents with microcephaly and macrocephaly, scattered Ca++, PMG, and "negative" TORCH tests. **Pseudo-TORCH** presents with microcephaly, scattered Ca++ including brainstem and basal ganglia, which progresses, atrophy, and lack of cortical malformations.

Lymphocytic Choriomeningitis Virus

Etiology

Congenital lymphocytic choriomeningitis virus (LCMV) is an arenavirus and member of the *Arenaviridae* family of viruses. Rodents are the principal reservoir for this viral infection. The geographic range is broad with many cases reported from rural environments. The overall incidence of congenital LCMV is unknown.

Pathology

LCMV has a strong tropism for neuroblasts. Additionally, LCM causes necrotizing ependymitis similar to that seen in cases of congenital toxoplasmosis. The range of injury and malformation includes microencephaly (e.g., CMV-like), periventricular calcification, hydrocephalus, cortical dysplasia, and focal cerebral destruction. High rates of chorioretinitis and hydrocephalus are observed, thus often mimicking the imaging features of toxoplasmosis.

Clinical Issues

Unlike many other congenital CNS infections, hepatosplenomegaly, jaundice, and skin rash (e.g., petechial/purpuric) are absent in congenital LCMV. High rates of congenital hydrocephalus (likely secondary to the exudative ependymitis and aqueductal obstruction) and chorioretinitis are observed in LCMV.

Diagnosing LCMV requires the detection of LCMV-specific serologic responses (IgG and IgM). Detecting LCM viral-specific-IgG strongly suggests congenital infection. Such testing is not routine in the TORCH(S) laboratory inquiry. Thus, confirming LCMV requires nuanced laboratory assessment.

Imaging

The imaging findings of congenital LCMV infection can mimic those of CMV or toxoplasmosis **(12-16)**. Timing of the infection dictates the pattern of CNS injury. Unlike toxoplasmosis, malformations of cortical development do occur with LCMV. Hydrocephalus and calcifications can be shown with US, NECT, and MR. Malformations in cortical development are best displayed with MR. MR represents the imaging gold standard for the comprehensive characterization of injury and malformation for LCMV and all other congenital CNS infections.

Consider congenital LCMV infection when the imaging findings mimic CMV, Zika, or toxoplasmosis and the clinical and serologic evaluation is "normal."

Differential Diagnosis

Toxoplasmosis lacks cortical malformations, **congenital CMV** typically shows caudostriatal groove or periventricular Ca++ and PMG, **Zika virus** Ca++ is most common at the GM/WM junction, and **psuedo-TORCH** Ca++ involves the brainstem, basal ganglia, WM, and cortex and lacks cortical malformations.

Congenital (Perinatal) HIV

The imaging presentation of congenital HIV infection is quite different from the findings in acquired HIV/AIDS. Congenital HIV resembles the other congenital viral infections and is therefore discussed here. Acquired HIV/AIDS is considered separately (see Chapter 14).

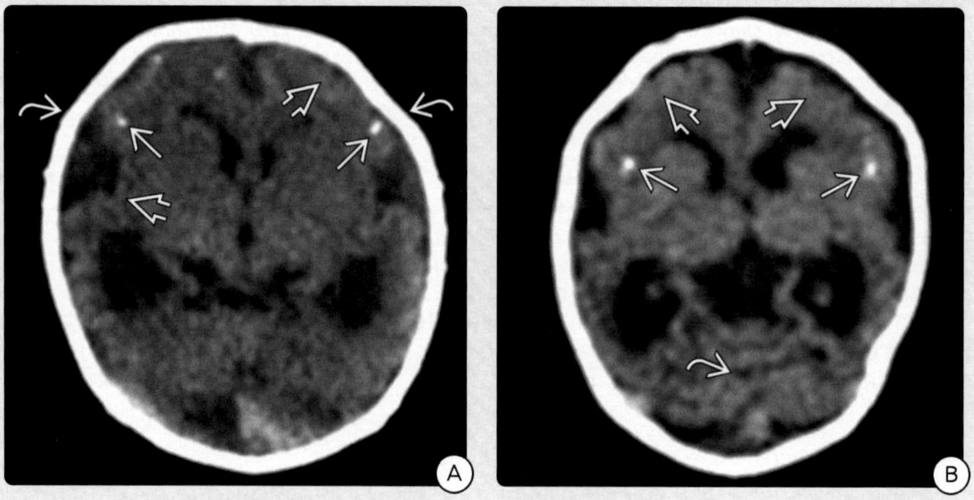

***(12-12A)** Axial NECT shows Zika-infected neonate. Peripheral Ca++ involves cortex and GM-WM junctions. Broad sylvian fissures, simplified gyral pattern (PMG), and ventriculomegaly are seen. Note the coronal sutural overlap due to microencephaly. **(12-12B)** NECT shows another microencephalic newborn showing Ca++ at GM-WM junctions. Diffuse PMG, ventriculomegaly, and rhombencephalosynapsis are seen.*

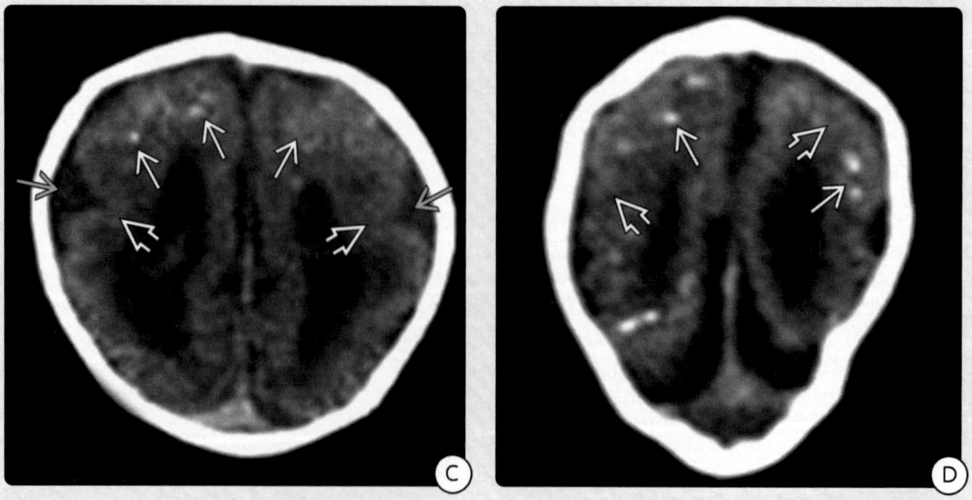

***(12-12C)** NECT shows numerous GM-WM junction calcifications, diffuse polymicrogyria (PMG) causing simplified gyral pattern, enlarged primitive-appearing sylvian fissures, and ventriculomegaly. **(12-12D)** Coronal NECT shows characteristic peripheral Ca++, ventriculomegaly, and holohemispheric polymicrogyria. (Courtesy A. Pessoa, MD.)*

SELECTED CONGENITAL AND PERINATAL INFECTIONS: NEUROIMAGING FINDINGS AND COMMON CAUSES

Cytomegalovirus
- Microcephaly, Ca++ at caudostriatal groove, polymicrogyria (PMG), cysts, WM abnormalities, cerebellar hypoplasia, vertical hippocampi

Toxoplasmosis
- Macrocephaly, hydrocephalus, scattered Ca++, lack of cortical malformations

Herpes Simplex Virus
- Early-diffuse cerebral edema, multifocal lesions, DWI abnormalities, hemorrhage, watershed infarctions, leptomeningeal enhancement, late cystic encephalomalacia

LCMV
- May precisely mimic features of CMV, negative routine TORCH testing

Zika Virus
- Microcephaly, ventriculomegaly, Ca++ at GM-WM junctions, cortical malformations

Rubella
- Microcephaly, Ca++ (basal ganglia, periventricular, and cortex) may cause lobar destruction

Varicella Zoster
- Necrosis of WM, deep GM nuclei, cerebellum ventriculomegaly, cerebellar aplasia, PMG

Syphilis
- Basilar meningitis, stroke, scattered Ca++

HIV
- Atrophy, basal ganglia Ca++, fusiform arteriopathy

Human Parechovirus
- Confluent periventricular WM abnormality mimic of perinatal periventricular leukomalacia

Human Parvovirus B19
- WM, cortical, and BG injury in setting of severe fetal anemia

Etiology

The causative agent is the retrovirus human immunodeficiency virus type 1 (HIV). At least 90% of congenital HIV cases are vertically transmitted (mother-to-child transmission). A minority (approximately 10%) might be due to blood transfusions, other blood products given therapeutically, or organ/tissue transplantation. Most infants become infected at birth or during the third trimester. Occasionally older infants are infected during breast feeding.

Pathology

The most characteristic gross finding is generalized brain volume loss with symmetric enlargement of the ventricles and subarachnoid spaces. Multiple foci of microglia, macrophages, infiltration of microglial nodules, and multinucleated giant cells containing viral particles are typical. Patchy myelin pallor and vacuolization are common. Mineralizing microangiopathy with basal ganglia calcifications and endothelial hypertrophy with gross cerebral vasculopathy are seen in some cases.

Clinical Issues

Epidemiology. Congenital HIV infection is diminishing as highly active antiretroviral therapy (HAART) becomes more widely available. Children account for just 2% of all HIV/AIDS patients in the USA and Europe but still represent 5-25% of cases worldwide. Congenital and acquired CMV infections are strong independent correlates of mother-to-child HIV transmission.

Presentation and Natural History. Symptoms generally begin around 3 months of life. Developmental delay, progressive motor dysfunction, and failure to thrive are the most common CNS symptoms. Hepatosplenomegaly, lymphadenopathy, and parotid lymphoepithelial cysts are common manifestations of congenital HIV.

Without antiretroviral therapy, infants and children with HIV encephalopathy show acquired microcephaly, progressive motor dysfunction, cognitive and developmental delay, apathy, dementia, hyperreflexia, ataxia, weakness, myoclonus, and/or seizures. Approximately 20% of infected infants die. Opportunistic infections are less common in HIV-infected children compared with adults; however, stroke is more common. Secondary CNS complications of congenital HIV include primary CNS lymphoma, stroke, opportunistic infection, and aneurysmal arteriopathy.

Imaging

The most striking and consistent finding is atrophy, particularly in the frontal lobes. Bilaterally symmetric basal ganglia calcifications are common **(12-13)**. Calcifications can be identified in the hemispheric white matter and cerebellum.

Ectasia and fusiform enlargement of intracranial arteries are found in 3-5% of cases **(12-14)**. Secondary VZV infectious vasculopathy has been implicated in the development of aneurysmal arteriopathy in HIV. Strokes with foci of restricted diffusion and subarachnoid hemorrhage may occur as complications of the underlying vasculopathy.

Differential Diagnosis

The differential diagnosis of congenital HIV is other TORCH infections. **CMV** is characterized by periventricular calcifications, microcephaly, and cortical dysplasia. Other than volume loss, the brain in congenital HIV appears normal. **Toxoplasmosis** is much less common than CMV and causes scattered parenchymal calcifications, not symmetric basal ganglia lesions. **Pseudo-TORCH** Ca++ involves cortex and WM, basal ganglia, brainstem, and cerebellum.

Other Congenital Infections

Rubella (German Measles)

Humans are the only reservoir for the rubella virus. Transmission is via virus-contaminated respiratory secretions.

Prior to widespread implementation of measles-mumps-rubella vaccine, epidemics of rubella occurred globally in 6- to 9-year intervals. With the advent of effective vaccination programs, the worldwide prevalence of congenital rubella syndrome (CRS) has declined dramatically. Approximately 100,000 infants are born with CRS, mostly in countries with low national vaccination rates.

Early in utero infection (e.g., particularly in the first trimester) results in miscarriage, fetal death, or congenital malformations in surviving infants. Late infection causes generalized brain volume loss, dystrophic calcifications, and regions of demyelination and/or gliosis.

The triad CRS includes ophthalmic (e.g., retinopathy, cataracts, microphthalmia), auditory (e.g., sensorineural deafness), and cardiac (e.g., patent ductus arteriosis, pulmonary artery stenosis) findings. Other clinical findings in CRS include craniofacial defects, microcephaly, and thrombocytopenic purpura.

Imaging findings are nonspecific, and, like other congenital infections, the timing of infection dictates the magnitude of destructive changes. Reported findings include microcephaly, parenchymal calcifications including cortical calcifications **(12-15)**, delayed myelination, periventricular and basal ganglia cysts, frontal-dominant white matter lesions (NECT hypoattenuating and MR T2 hyperintense), and atrophy, and, in severe cases, total brain destruction has been described.

Congenital Syphilis

Congenital syphilis (CS) is caused by transplacental passage of the *Treponema pallidum* spirochete from untreated mothers with syphilis. Infection occurs typically in the second and third trimesters.

Up to 60% of infants infected with CS are asymptomatic at birth. Symptoms typically develop later in infancy with early signs and symptoms including jaundice, hepatosplenomegaly, and rash. Later craniofacial signs and symptoms include saddle

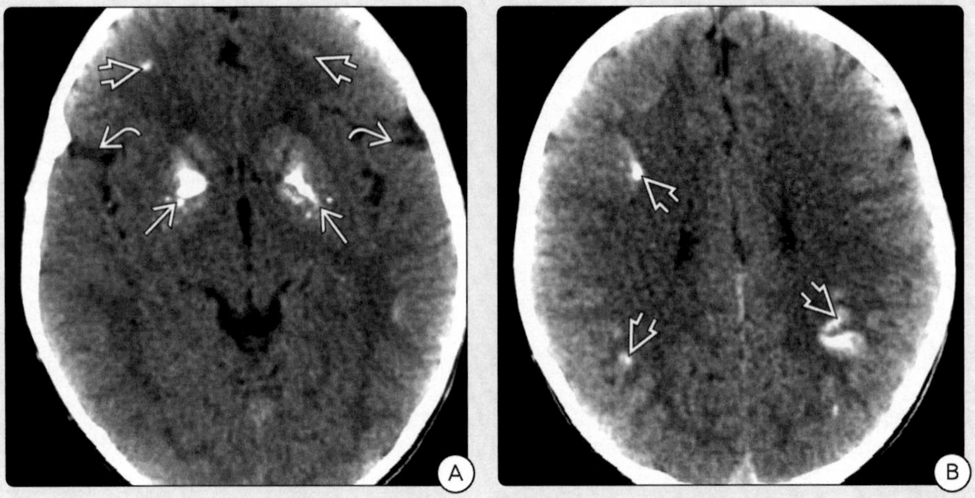

***(12-13A)** Axial NECT scan in a 5y child with congenital HIV shows bilateral symmetric calcifications in the basal ganglia ➔ and the subcortical white matter ➔. Prominent lateral cerebral fissures ➔ reflect atrophy. **(12-13B)** Axial NECT scan in the same patient shows fairly symmetric punctate and curvilinear calcifications at the gray-white matter junctions ➔ caused by mineralizing microangiopathy. (Courtesy V. Mathews, MD.)*

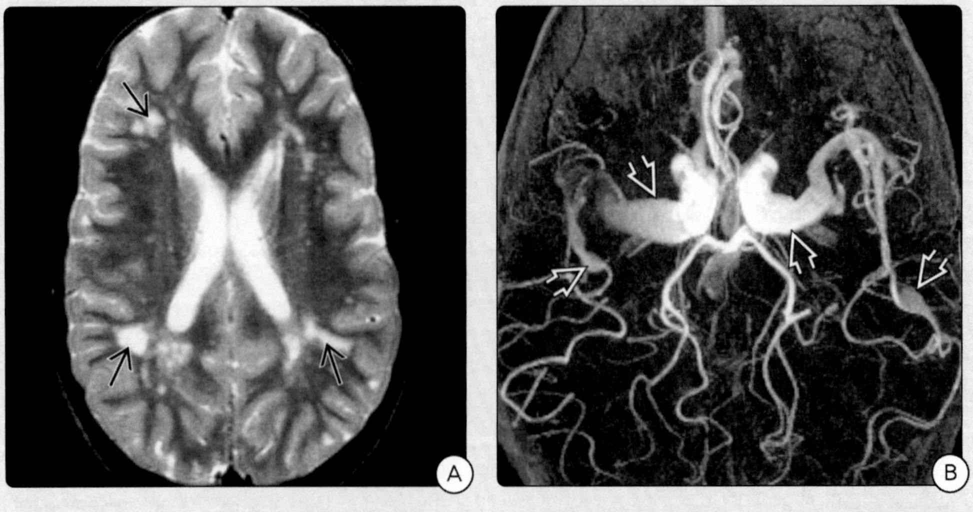

***(12-14A)** Axial T2WI MR in an 11y child demonstrates late manifestations of congenital HIV. Note prominent ventricles and sulci as well as multifocal white matter hyperintensities ➔. **(12-14B)** Submentovertex view of an MRA obtained in the same patient shows striking multicentric fusiform arteriopathy in both middle cerebral arteries ➔.*

nose deformity, frontal bossing, rhagades (scars around the mouth and nose), Hutchinson teeth, seizures, stroke, and signs of increased intracranial pressure. The most common imaging findings in CS are hydrocephalus and meningitis with leptomeningeal enhancement.

Imaging findings in CS include leptomeningeal enhancement, hydrocephalus, and cerebral infarction. Cisternal exudative meningitis can as a result of gumma formation lead to hypothalamic and pituitary dysfunction.

Congenital Varicella Zoster Virus Infection

In unimmunized populations, the rate of varicella infection (chickenpox) acquired through contact with respiratory secretions of infected children ranges between 1-3 per 1,000 pregnancies. Less than 2% of these pregnancies result in congenital varicella zoster syndrome. Neonates and infants with this congenital infection, like infants with congenital HSV and LCMV infections, generally lack the signs and symptoms of congenital infection, such as jaundice, hepatosplenomegaly, and skin rash (e.g., petechial/purpuric). Congenital varicella infection prior to 20 postconceptional weeks may lead to spontaneous abortion or embryopathic insults, including microcephaly secondary to cerebral destruction, chorioretinitis, limb and digit hypoplasia, and a distinctive pattern of skin scarring known as cicatrix.

Imaging findings in congenital varicella zoster infection include microcephaly, parenchymal calcifications, ventriculomegaly, polymicrogyria, and nonpatterned necrosis of white matter, lobar cortical and subcortical tissues, and deep gray nuclei. Similar necrotic lesions have been described in the cerebellum, leading to cerebellar atrophy **(12-17)**. MR is the most sensitive imaging tool to fully appraise injury.

Congenital/Perinatal Human Parechovirus Infection

Parechovirus is a picornavirus that can cause encephalitis and permanent injury to the developing CNS. It shows tropism for the periventricular white matter (e.g., leukotropic). The neonate may present with a sepsis-like illness, rash, fever, irritability, and seizures. CSF pleocytosis is uncommon, unlike most cases of meningoencephalitis. At present, no specific antiviral therapy is available.

Imaging findings in perinatal parechovirus infection include detection of bilateral confluent white matter abnormalities. NECT shows low-attenuation regions, and MR acutely demonstrates restricted diffusion as well as T1 and T2 prolongation. These leukotropic changes have been mistaken for perinatal white matter hypoxic ischemic injury in the preterm newborn.

Congenital Human Parvovirus B19

Human Parvovirus B19 is one well-documented cause of severe fetal anemia and a known cause of fetal death. The virus is also known to affect patients with immunologic disorders such as sickle cell anemia. Human Parvovirus B19 is the only known Parvovirus that is pathogenic to humans. The risk of maternal to fetal transmission is greatest in the first and second trimesters.

Imaging findings as a result of severe fetal anemia and intracranial resistive indices (transcranial Doppler US) drop. Resultant cerebral injury (e.g., ischemia, infarction, or severe diffuse destruction) may occur.

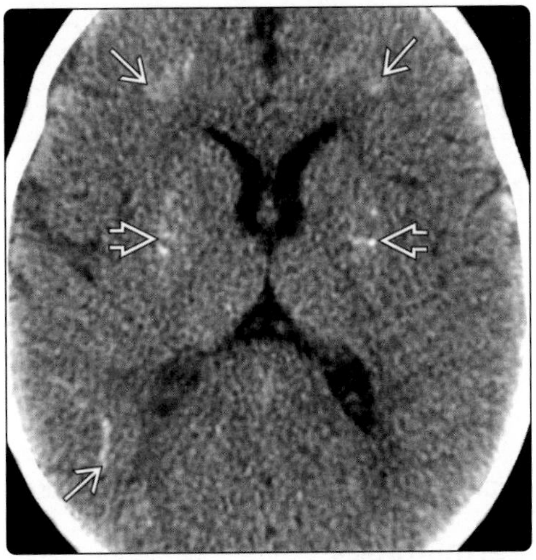

***(12-15)** NECT scan in an 18m boy with congenital rubella shows subtle subcortical ➡ and basal ganglia calcifications ⇨.*

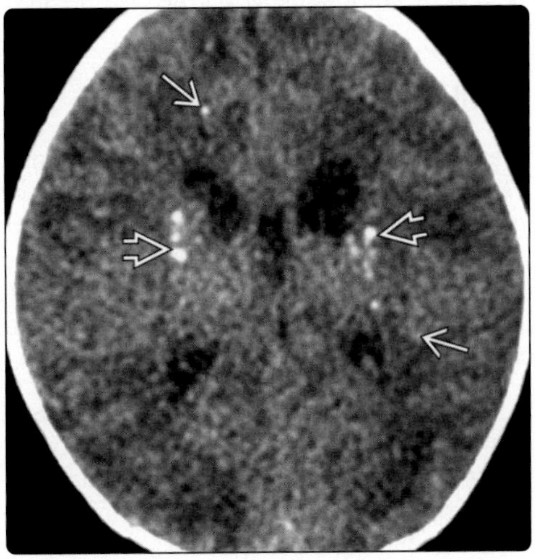

***(12-16)** NECT in an infant with congenital lymphocytic choriomeningitis shows focal parenchymal ➡ and periventricular Ca++ ⇨.*

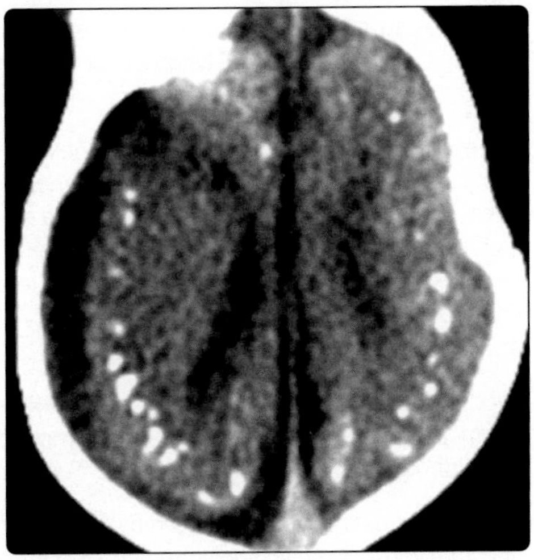

***(12-17)** NECT shows extreme microcephaly, extensive subcortical calcifications, and undersulcated brain in congenital VZV infection.*

Acquired Pyogenic Infections

Meningitis

Meningitis is a worldwide disease that leaves up to half of all survivors with permanent neurologic sequelae. Despite advances in antimicrobial therapy and vaccine development, bacterial meningitis represents a significant cause of morbidity and mortality. Infants, children, and the elderly or immunocompromised patients are at special risk. In this section, we focus on the etiology, pathology, and imaging findings of this potentially devastating disease.

Terminology

Meningitis is an acute or chronic inflammatory infiltrate of meninges and CSF. **Pachymeningitis** involves the dura-arachnoid; **leptomeningitis** affects the pia and subarachnoid spaces.

Etiology

Meningitis can be acquired in several different ways. *Hematogeneous spread* from remote systemic infection is the most common route. Direct *geographic extension* from sinusitis, otitis, or mastoiditis is the second most common method of spread. *Penetrating injuries* and *skull fractures* (especially of the skull base) are rare but important causes of meningitis.

Regardless of origin, all bacteria have to breach the blood-brain barrier (BBB) and blood-CSF barrier to invade the CNS. Bacterial binding to brain endothelial cells is a prerequisite for successful penetration into the CSF. Once accomplished, this results in meningeal inflammation, increased BBB permeability, CSF pleocytosis, and infiltration of the nervous tissue itself.

Many different infectious agents can cause meningitis. Most cases are caused by acute pyogenic (bacterial) infection. Meningitis can also be acute lymphocytic (viral) or chronic (tubercular or granulomatous).

The most common responsible agent varies with age, geography, and immune status. Group Bβ-hemolytic streptococcal meningitis is the leading cause of newborn meningitis in developed countries, whereas enteric, gram-negative organisms (typically *Escherichia coli*, less commonly *Enterobacter* or *Citrobacter*) cause the majority of cases in developing countries.

Vaccination has significantly decreased the incidence of *Haemophilus influenzae* meningitis, so the most common cause of childhood bacterial meningitis is now *Neisseria meningitidis*.

Adult meningitis is typically caused by *Streptococcus pneumoniae* or *N. meningitidis* (meningococci). The tetravalent meningococcal vaccine used to vaccinate adolescents in the USA does not contain serotype B, the causative organism of one-third of all cases of meningococcal disease in industrialized countries.

Listeria monocytogenes, *S. pneumoniae*, gram-negative bacilli, and *N. meningitidis* affect adults over the age of 55 as well as individuals with chronic illnesses.

Tuberculous meningitis is common in developing countries and in immunocompromised patients (e.g., HIV/AIDS patients and solid organ transplant recipients).

NEONATAL BACTERIAL MENINGITIS: COMMON CAUSES AND IMAGING

Group B Streptococcus
- Leptomeningeal enhancement, ischemic/infarctive injuries, white matter lesions (scattered or confluent)

Citrobacter species
- Rapidly cavitating lesions of the cerebral white matter, "squared" rim-enhancing abscesses

Enterobacter species
- Like *Citrobacter* shows tropism for cerebral white matter, large rim-enhancing cavitary lesions

Escherichia coli
- Basal meningitis, ventriculitis, cerebral abscess, and hydrocephalus

Listeria Monocytogenes
- Granulomatous involvement of meninges, choroid plexus, and subependymal regions

BACTERIAL MENINGITIS IN INFANTS: COMMON CAUSES

Infants
- Gram positive
  - Group B streptococcus (*Streptococcus agalactiae*)
  - *Staphylococcus aureus*
  - *Staphylococcus epidermidis*
- Gram negative
  - *Escherichia coli*
  - *Citrobacter species*
  - *Listeria monocytogenes*
  - *Pseudomonas aeruginosis*

BACTERIAL MENINGITIS IN CHILDREN: COMMON CAUSES

Older Children and Adolescents
- *Haemophilus influenzae type B*
- *Non-type B or nontypable Haemophilus influenzae*
- *Mycobacterium tuberculosis*
- *Neisseria meningitides*
- *Streptococcus pneumoniae*

Pathology

Location. The basal cisterns and subarachnoid spaces are the CSF spaces most commonly involved by meningitis, followed by the cerebral convexity sulci **(12-18)** **(12-19)** **(12-20)** **(12-22)**.

Gross Pathology. Cloudy CSF initially fills the subarachnoid spaces, followed by development of a variably dense purulent exudate that covers the pial surfaces. Vessels within the exudate may show inflammatory changes and necrosis.

Microscopic Features. The meningeal exudate contains the inciting organisms, inflammatory cells, fibrin, and cellular debris. The underlying brain parenchyma is often edematous, with subpial astrocytic and microglial proliferation.

Meningoencephalitis shows inflammatory changes in the pia, and the perivascular spaces may act as a conduit for extension from the pia into the underlying brain parenchyma.

Clinical Issues

Epidemiology and Demographics. Bacterial infections of the CNS are neurologic emergencies. These include meningitis, brain abscess, empyemas, and suppurative dual sinus thrombophlebitis (see Chapter 9).

Pyogenic meningitis is the most common cause of acute febrile encephalopathy. The overall prevalence of meningitis is estimated at 3:100,000 in industrialized countries. In the United States, meningitis is diagnosed in 62:100,000 emergency department visits.

Presentation. Presentation depends on patient age. In adults, fever (≥ 38.5°C) and either headache, nuchal rigidity, or altered mental status are the most common symptoms. Although less than half of all patients present with the classic triad of fever, neck stiffness, and altered mental status, nearly 100% will have at least one of these symptoms. Vomiting is another common but underrecognized manifestation of CNS infection.

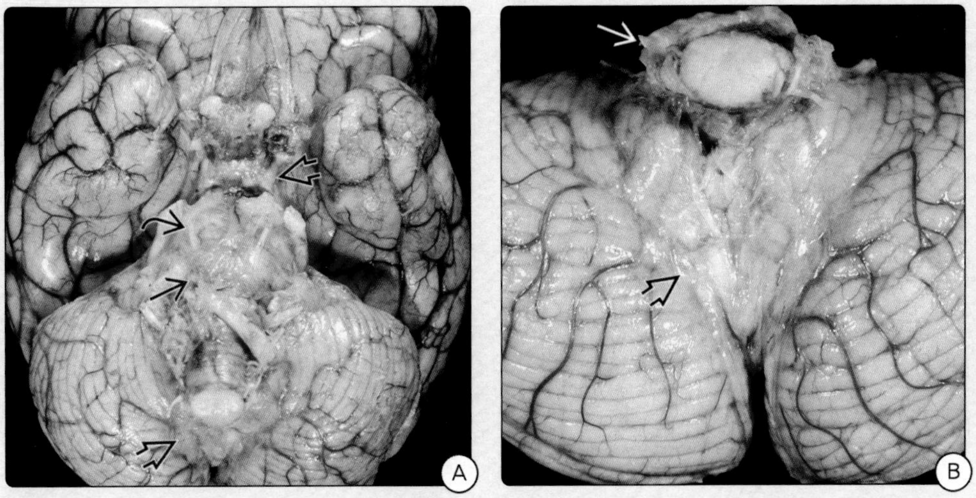

***(12-18A)** Autopsied brain shows typical changes of severe meningitis with dense purulent exudate covering the pons ⇨, coating the cranial nerves ⇨, and filling the basal cisterns ⇨. **(12-18B)** As seen in this autopsy photo, the exudate coats the medulla ➡ and completely fills the cisterna magna ⇨. (Courtesy R. Hewlett, MD.)*

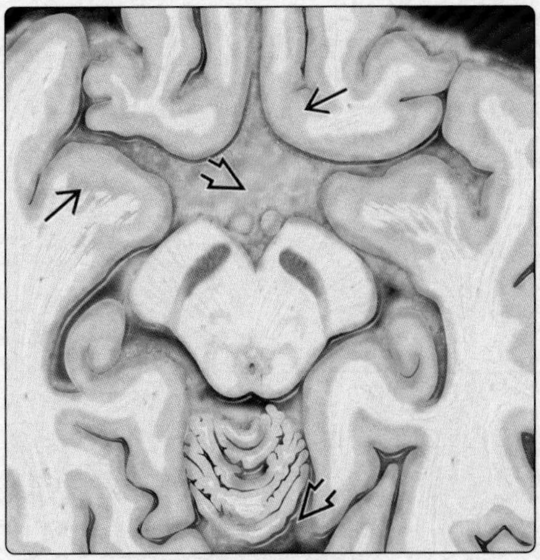

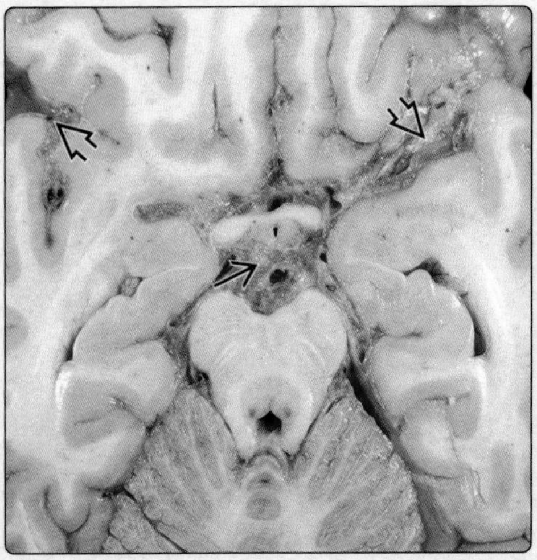

***(12-19)** Graphic of meningitis shows purulent exudate involving the leptomeninges and filling the basal cisterns and sulci ⇨. The underlying brain is mildly hyperemic ⇨. Venous and arterial spasm/occlusion may result in parenchymal infarction. **(12-20)** Axial autopsy section shows meningitis with exudate completely filling the suprasellar cistern ⇨ and sylvian fissures ⇨. (Courtesy R. Hewlett, MD.)*

Fever, lethargy, poor feeding, and irritability are common among infected infants. Children with *N. meningitidis* infection may develop a purpuric rash. Diffuse intravascular coagulopathy (DIC) may develop with meningococcal or *H. Influenzae* meningitis. Seizures occur in 30% of patients.

CSF shows leukocytosis (mainly polymorphonuclear cells), elevated protein, and decreased glucose. A normal C-reactive protein has a high negative predictive value in the diagnosis of bacterial meningitis.

Natural History. Despite rapid recognition and effective therapy, meningitis still has significant morbidity and mortality rates. Death rates from 15-25% have been reported in disadvantaged children with poor living conditions.

Complications are both common and numerous. **Extraventricular obstructive hydrocephalus** is one of the earliest and most common complications. The choroid plexus can become infected, causing choroid plexitis and then **ventriculitis**. Infection can also extend from the pia along the perivascular spaces into the brain parenchyma itself, causing **cerebritis** and then **abscess**.

Sub- and epidural **empyemas** or sterile **effusions** may develop. **Cerebrovascular complications** of meningitis include vasculitis, thrombosis, and occlusion of both arteries and veins.

Treatment Options. Specific antibiotic therapy should be based on culture and sensitivity.

Imaging

General Features. The "gold standard" for the diagnosis of bacterial meningitis is CSF analysis. Remember: **Imaging is neither sensitive nor specific for the detection of meningitis!** Therefore, imaging should be used in conjunction with—and not as a substitute for—appropriate clinical and laboratory evaluation.

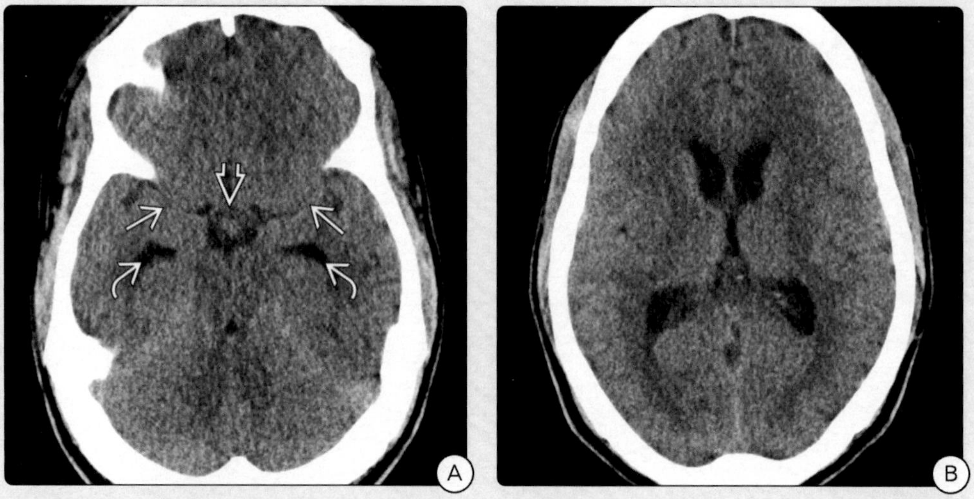

***(12-21A)** NECT in a 25y man with headache and fever shows mild enlargement of both temporal horns. CSF in the suprasellar cistern appears mildly hyperdense ("dirty"), and the sylvian fissures appear effaced. **(12-21B)** More cephalad NECT shows that the lateral and third ventricles are slightly enlarged. Note poor visualization of the superficial sulci, leading to a somewhat "featureless" appearance. Scan was initially read as normal.*

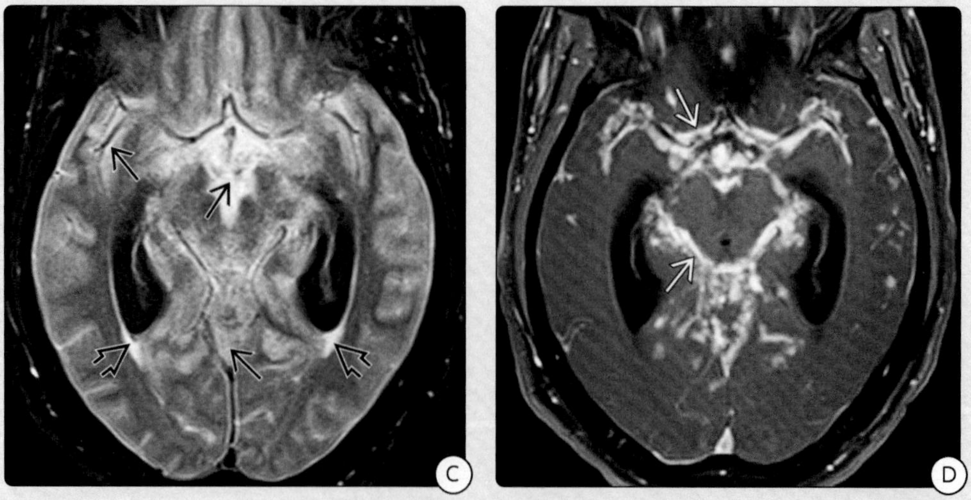

***(12-21C)** The patient returned 3 weeks later with increasing headaches and altered mental status. FLAIR shows the basal cisterns, and sulci are all hyperintense. Progressive hydrocephalus is noted, and transependymal interstitial edema is seen. **(12-21D)** T1 C+ FS in the same case shows diffuse linear and nodular sulcal-cisternal enhancement. This is pyogenic meningitis and has led to associated hydrocephalus.*

Imaging studies are best used to confirm the diagnosis and assess possible complications. Whereas CT is commonly employed as a screening examination in cases of headache and suspected meningitis, both the primary and acute manifestations of meningitis as well as secondary complications are best depicted on MR.

CT Findings. Initial NECT scans may be normal or show only mild ventricular enlargement **(12-21B)** **(12-25A)**. "Blurred" ventricular margins indicate acute obstructive hydrocephalus with accumulation of extracellular fluid in the deep white matter. Bone CT should be carefully evaluated for sinusitis and otomastoiditis.

As the cellular inflammatory exudate develops, it replaces the normally clear CSF. Subtle effacement of surface landmarks may occur as sulcal-cisternal CSF becomes almost isodense with brain **(12-21A)**. In rare cases, subtle hyperattenuation may be present in the basal subarachnoid spaces.

CECT may show intense enhancement of the inflammatory exudate as it covers the brain surfaces, extending into and filling the sulci.

MR Findings. The purulent exudates of acute meningitis are isointense with underlying brain on T1WI, giving the appearance of "dirty" CSF. The exudates are isointense with CSF on T2WI and do not suppress on FLAIR. Hyperintensity in the subarachnoid cisterns and superficial sulci on FLAIR is a typical but nonspecific finding of meningitis **(12-21C)**.

DWI is especially helpful in meningitis, as the purulent subarachnoid space exudates usually show restriction **(12-23B)**. pMR may demonstrate multiple regions of increased cerebral blood flow.

Pia-subarachnoid space enhancement occurs in 50% of patients **(12-21D)**. A curvilinear pattern that follows the gyri and sulci (the "pial-cisternal" pattern) is typical **(12-23A)** and is more common than dura-arachnoid enhancement.

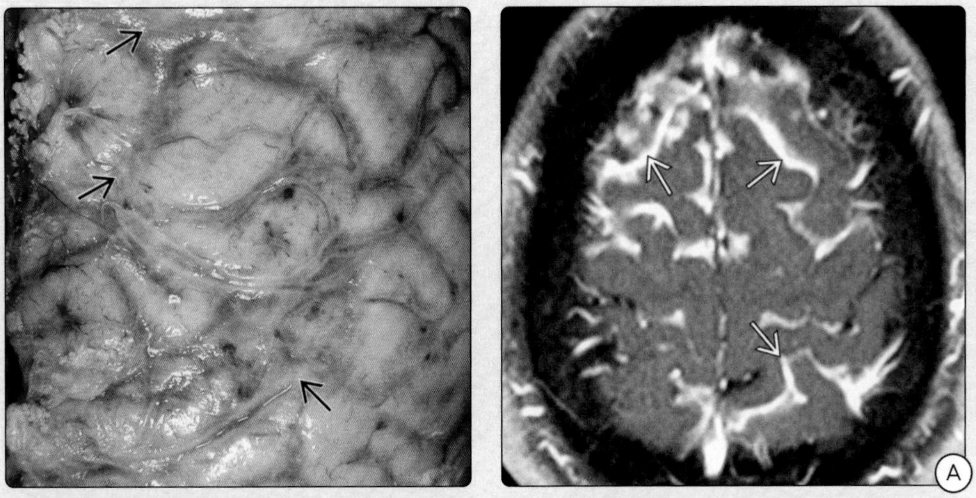

***(12-22)** Autopsy case with close-up view shows typical changes of pyogenic meningitis. The convexity sulci are filled with purulent exudate ⇒. (Courtesy R. Hewlett, MD.) **(12-23A)** T1 C+ FS scan in a case of acute pyogenic meningitis shows that diffuse, intensely enhancing exudate fills the convexity sulci ➡. FLAIR imaging is also sensitive in detecting SAS pathology.*

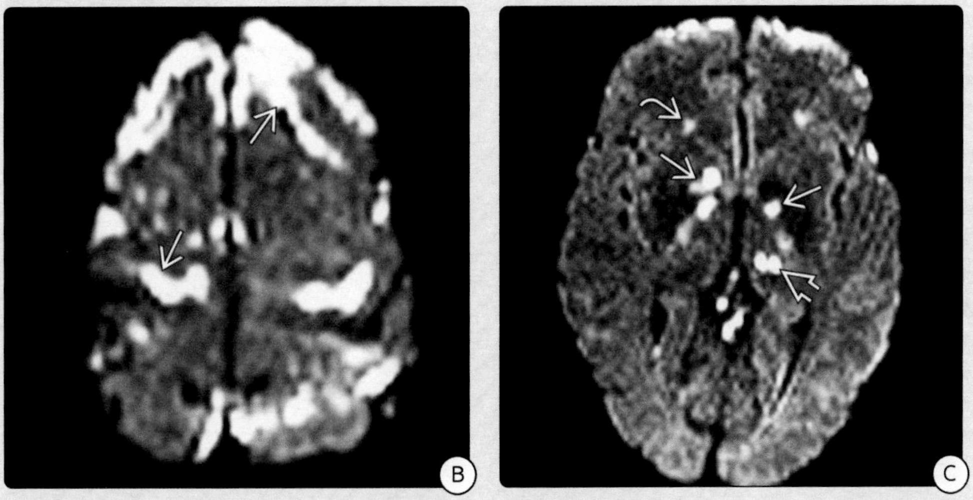

***(12-23B)** DWI in the same patient shows that the viscous pus filling the convexity sulci restricts strongly ➡. This is streptococcal meningitis with secondary vasculitis. **(12-23C)** DWI in the same case shows multifocal acute basal ganglia ➡, thalamic ➡, and deep parenchymal infarcts ➡.*

(12-24A) DWI in neonate with confirmed E. coli meningitis shows posterior fossa hyperintense subdural collections (empyemas) →. (12-24B) DWI in the same patient shows viscous dependent ventricular debris (ventriculitis) →. Note the vasogenic edema (increased diffusivity) within the occipital lobe ↪.

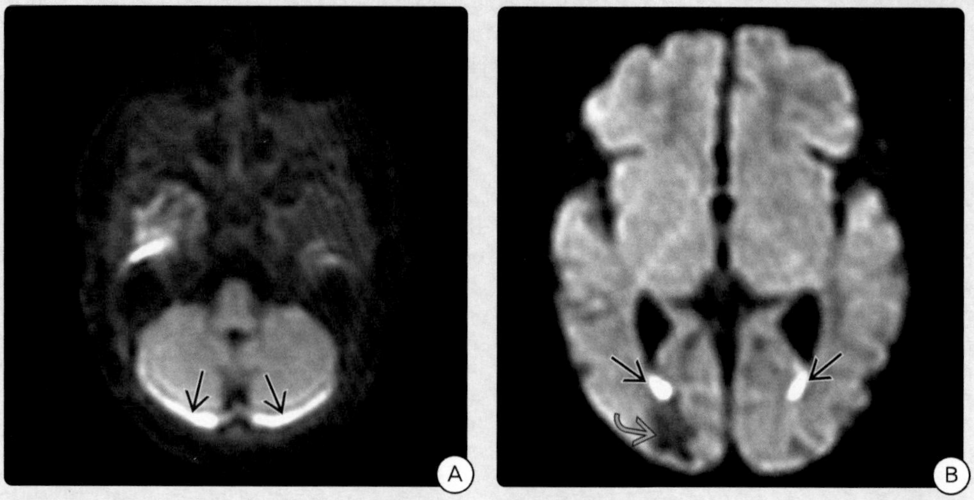

(12-24C) DWI in the same patient shows a focal hyperintensity within the right occipital lobe consistent with abscess ⇒. Note the lateral ventricular dilation (hydrocephalus). (12-24D) FLAIR in the same patient shows right occipital sulcal and cortical FLAIR hyperintensity → and expansion of the SASs with complex CSF signal ↪. Note early ventricular enlargement.

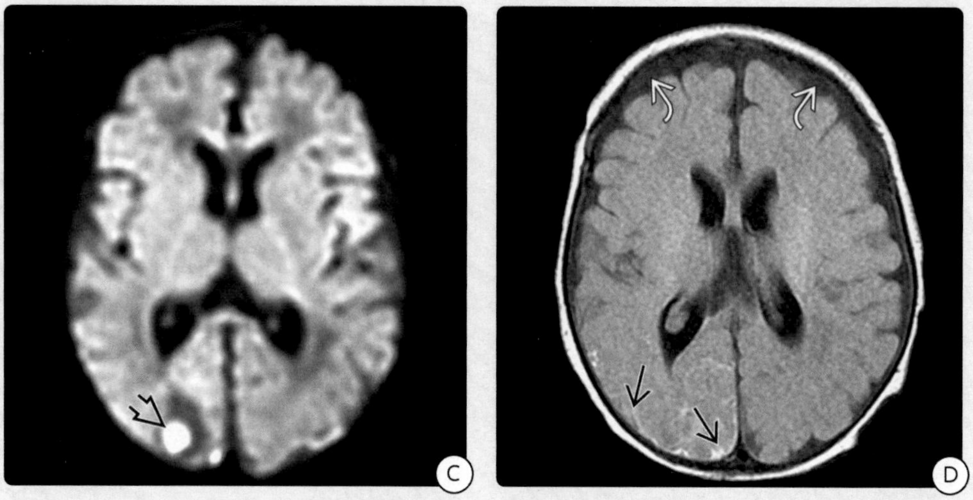

(12-24E) Enhanced T1WI in the same patient with E. coli meningitis shows retrocerebellar subdural empyemas →. Note the thick enhancing meningeal → and endosteal dura ↪. (12-24F) Enhanced T1WI in the same patient shows a rim-enhancing occipital lobe abscess ⇒ and leptomeningeal enhancement →. Early hydrocephalus is also noted.

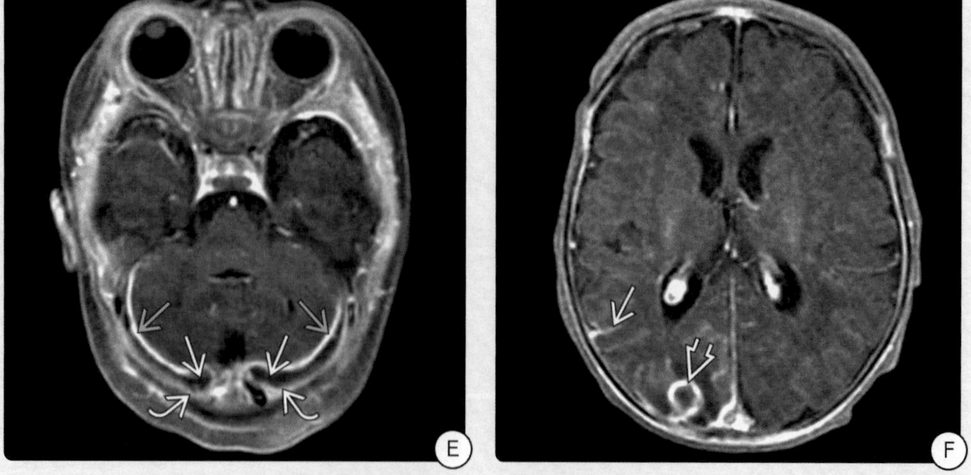

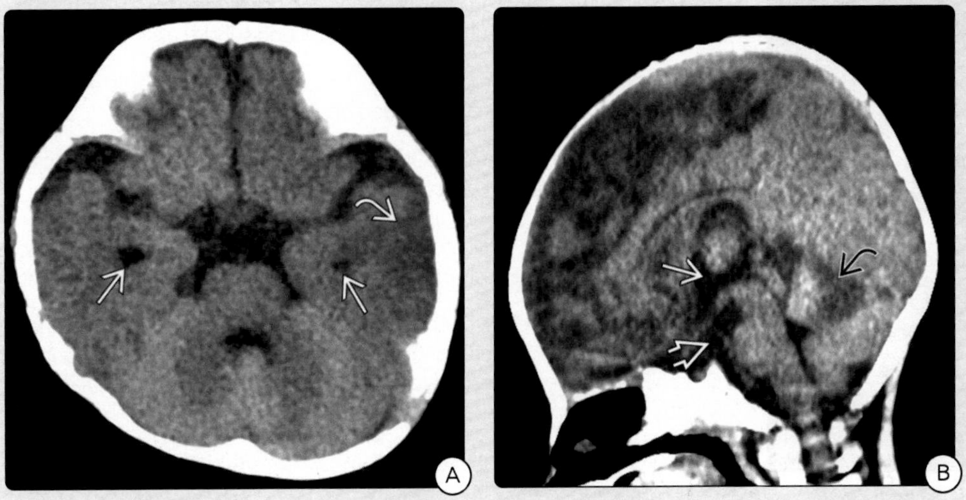

***(12-25A)** NECT shows a 3m infant with fever and focal seizure. Temporal horn dilation and left temporal lobe hypoattenuation are seen. **(12-25B)** NECT sagittal reformation shows superior vermian hypoattenuation (infarction). Note the prominence of the third ventricle and basal cisterns.*

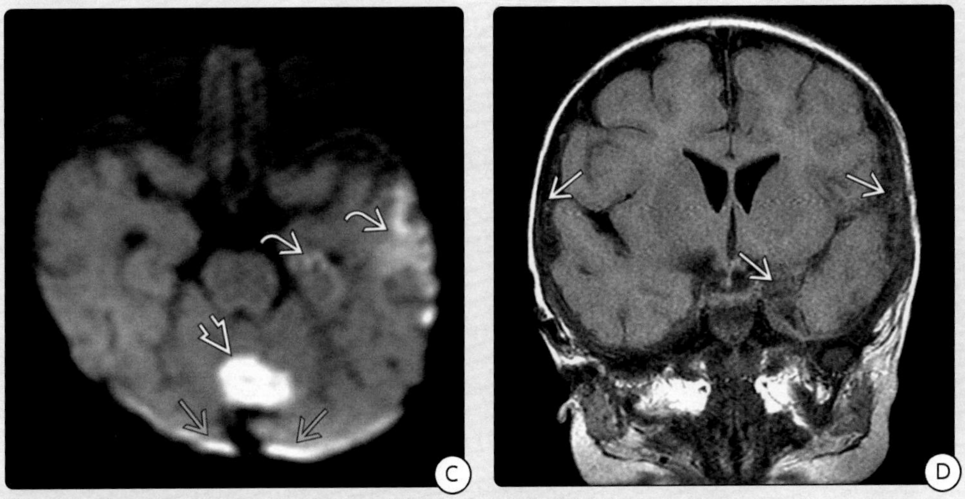

***(12-25C)** DWI in the same patient shows vermian and left temporal lobe hyperintensities confirmed on ADC maps as regions of ischemia/infarction. Note retrocerebellar subdural collections (empyemas). DWI is useful in cases of suspected meningitis. **(12-25D)** FLAIR in the same patient shows expanded "dirty" CSF signal throughout the subarachnoid spaces. Note the enlarged frontal horns with normal FLAIR CSF signal.*

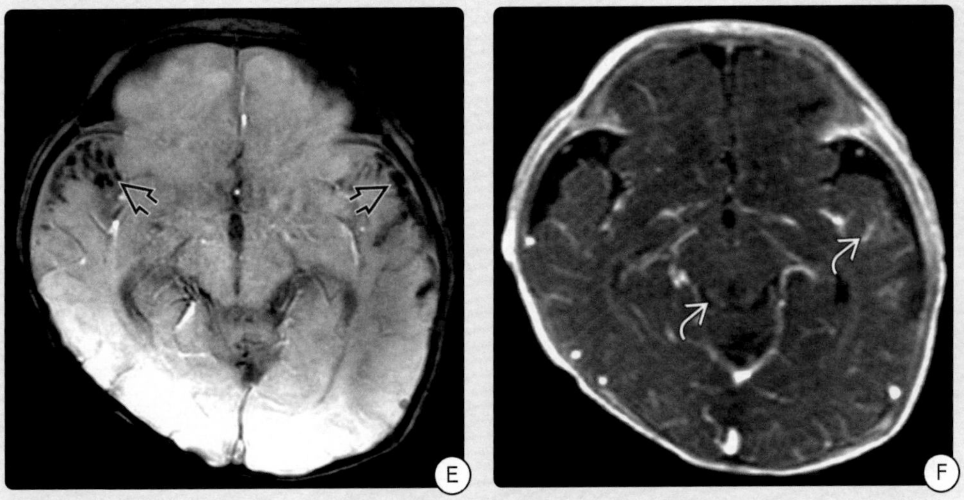

***(12-25E)** SWI in the same patient shows numerous tubular hypointensities within the lateral cerebral fissures and adjacent to the temporal lobes consistent with slow venous flow or thrombosis. **(12-25F)** Enhanced T1WI in the same patient, with confirmed Group B Strep meningitis, shows regions of leptomeningeal enhancement.*

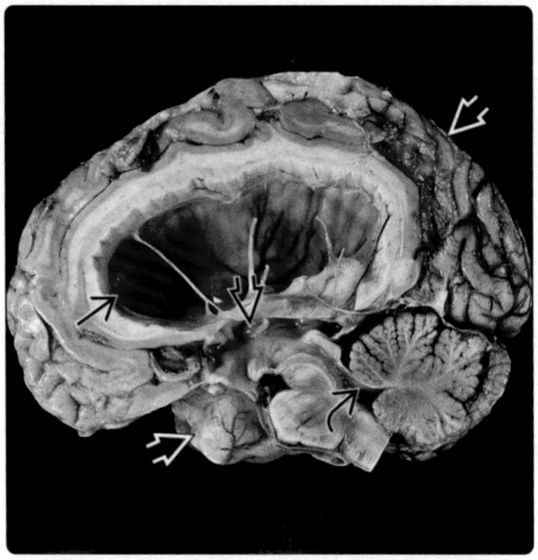

(12-26) Autopsy of meningitis with EVOH shows lateral, 3rd, 4th ventricular, aqueductal dilation. (Ellison, Neuropath, 3e.)

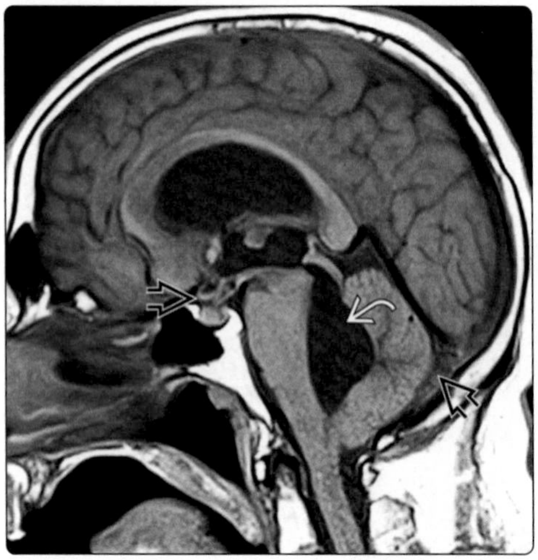

(12-27) Sagittal T1WI shows basilar meningitis. Lateral, 3rd ventricles are enlarged; 4th ventricle appears "ballooned" or obstructed.

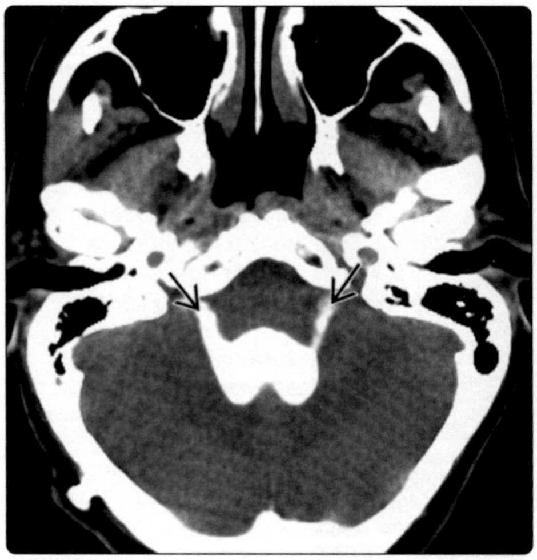

(12-28) CT ventriculogram shows dilated 4th ventricle, obstructed outflow at foramina of Luschka. EVOH is secondary to meningitis.

Postcontrast T2-weighted FLAIR and delayed postcontrast T1-weighted sequences may be helpful additions in detecting subtle cases.

Angiography. Irregular foci of constriction and dilatation characteristic of vasculitis can sometimes be identified on CTA or DSA.

Complications of Meningitis. Other than hydrocephalus, complications from meningitis are relatively uncommon. Postmeningitis reactive **effusions**—sterile CSF-like fluid pockets—develop in 5-10% of children treated for acute bacterial meningitis. Effusions are generally benign lesions that regress spontaneously over a few days and do not require treatment.

Effusions can occur either in the subdural (most common) or subarachnoid spaces. The frontal, parietal, and temporal convexities are the most common sites. NECT shows bilateral crescentic extraaxial collections that are iso- to slightly hyperdense compared with normal CSF.

Effusions are iso- to slightly hyperintense to CSF on T1WI and isointense on T2WI. They are often slightly hyperintense relative to CSF on FLAIR. Effusions usually do not enhance on T1 C+ but occasionally demonstrate enhancement along the medial (cerebral) surfaces of the lesions. Effusions do not restrict on DWI, differentiating them from subdural empyemas **(12-24)**.

Less common complications include pyocephalus (ventriculitis), empyema **(12-46)**, cerebritis and/or abscess **(12-24)**, venous occlusion, and ischemia **(12-23C)**. All are discussed separately below.

Differential Diagnosis

The major differential diagnosis of infectious meningitis is noninfectious meningitis. Other causes of meningitis include **noninfectious inflammatory disorders** (e.g., rheumatoid or systemic lupus erythematosus-associated meningitis, IgG4-related disease, drug-related aseptic meningitis, and multiple sclerosis) and neoplastic or **carcinomatous meningitis**. All can appear identical on imaging, so correlation with clinical information and laboratory findings is essential. **Remember**: *Sulcal/cisternal FLAIR hyperintensity is a nonspecific finding and can be seen with a number of different entities (see box below).*

CAUSES OF HYPERINTENSE CSF ON FLAIR

Common
- Blood
  - Subarachnoid hemorrhage
- Infection
  - Meningitis
- Artifact
  - Susceptibility; flow
- Tumor
  - CSF metastases

Less Common
- High inspired oxygen
  - 4-5x signal with 100% O_2
- Prominent vessels
  - Stroke (pial collaterals); "ivy" sign (moyamoya); pial angioma (Sturge-Weber)

Rare But Important
- Fat (ruptured dermoid)
- Gadolinium in CSF
  - Renal failure; blood-brain barrier leakage

Abscess

Terminology

A cerebral abscess is a localized infection of the brain parenchyma.

Etiology

Most abscesses are caused by hematogeneous spread from an extracranial location (e.g., lung or urinary tract infection and endocarditis). Abscesses may also result from penetrating injury or direct geographic extension from sinonasal and otomastoid infection. These typically begin as extraaxial infections such as empyema (see below) or meningitis (see above) and then spread into the brain itself.

Abscesses are most often bacterial, but they can also be fungal, parasitic, or (rarely) granulomatous. Although myriad organisms can cause abscess formation, the most common agents in immunocompetent adults are *Streptococcus* species,*Staphylococcus aureus*, and pneumococci. *Enterobacter* species like *Citrobacter* are a common cause of cerebral abscess in neonates. *Streptococcus intermedius* is emerging as an important cause of cerebral abscess in immunocompetent children and adolescents. In 20-30% of abscesses, cultures are sterile, and no specific organism is identified.

Proinflammatory molecules such as tumor necrosis factor-α and interleukin-1β induce various cell adhesion molecules that facilitate extravasation of peripheral immune cells and promote abscess development.

Bacterial abscesses are relatively uncommon in immunocompromised patients. *Klebsiella* is common in diabetics, and fungal infections by *Aspergillus* and *Nocardia* are common in transplant recipients. In patients with HIV/AIDS, toxoplasmosis and tuberculosis are the most common opportunistic infections.

In children, predisposing factors for cerebral abscess formation include meningitis, uncorrected cyanotic heart disease, sepsis, suppurative pulmonary infection, paranasal sinus or otomastoid trauma or suppurative infections, endocarditis, and immunodeficiency or immunosuppression states.

Pathology

Four general stages are recognized in the evolution of a cerebral abscess: (1) focal suppurative encephalitis/early cerebritis, (2) focal suppurative encephalitis/late cerebritis, (3) early encapsulation, and (4) late encapsulation. Each has its own distinctive pathologic appearance, which in turn determines the imaging findings.

Focal Suppurative Encephalitis. Sometimes also called the **"early cerebritis"** stage of abscess formation, in this earliest stage, suppurative infection is focal but not yet localized **(12-29)**. An unencapsulated, edematous, hyperemic mass of leukocytes and bacteria is present for 1-3 days after the initial infection **(12-30)**.

Focal Suppurative Encephalitis With Confluent Central Necrosis. The next stage of abscess formation is also called **"late cerebritis"** and begins 2-3 days after the initial infection **(12-31)**. This stage typically lasts between a week and 10 days.

Patchy necrotic foci within the suppurative mass form, enlarge, and then coalesce into a confluent necrotic mass. By days 5-7, a necrotic core is surrounded by a poorly organized, irregular rim of granulation tissue consisting of inflammatory cells, macrophages, and fibroblasts. The surrounding brain is edematous and contains swollen reactive astrocytes.

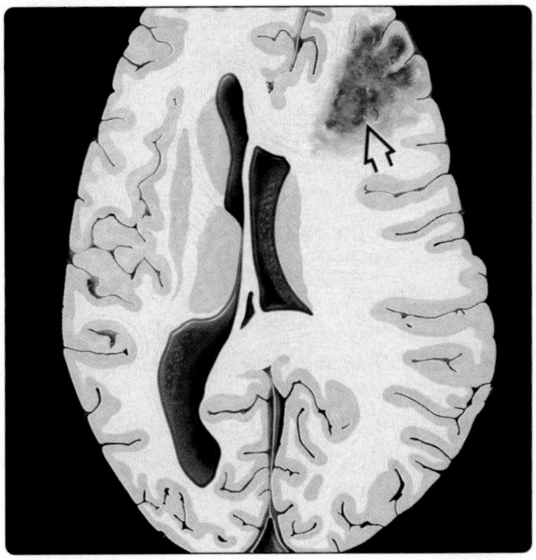

***(12-29)** Graphic of early cerebritis shows focal unencapsulated mass of petechial hemorrhage, inflammatory cells, and edema ⇒.*

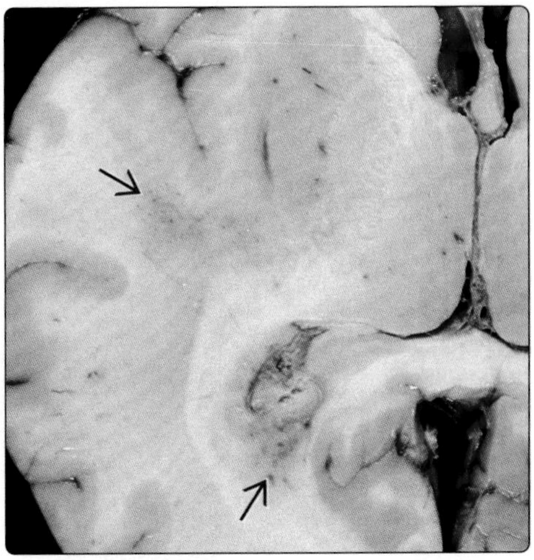

***(12-30)** Autopsy specimen shows foci of early cerebritis, unencapsulated edema, and petechial hemorrhages ⇒. (Courtesy R. Hewlett, MD.)*

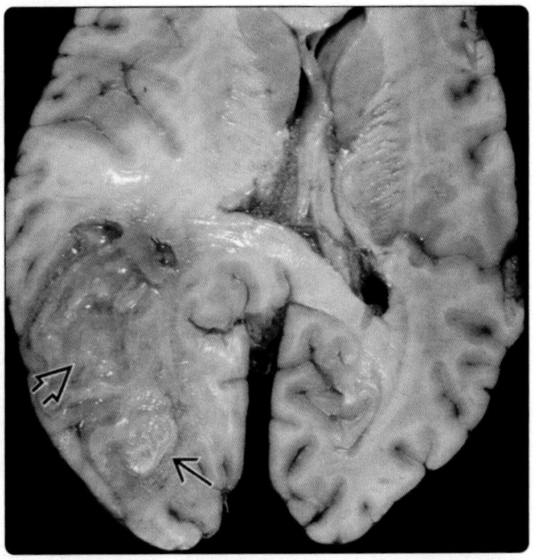

***(12-31)** Autopsied late cerebritis demonstrates coalescing lesion with some central necrosis ⇒, the beginnings of an ill-defined abscess rim ⇒.*

BRAIN ABSCESS: PATHOLOGY AND EVOLUTION

Stages
- Focal suppurative encephalitis (days 1-2)
  - Edematous, suppurative mass
  - No visible necrosis or capsule
- Focal suppurative encephalitis with confluent central necrosis (days 2-7)
  - Necrotic foci form, begin to coalesce
  - Poorly organized irregular rim
- Early encapsulation (days 5-14)
  - Coalescent core
  - Well-defined wall of fibroblasts, collagen
- Late encapsulation (> 2 weeks)
  - Wall thickens, then shrinks
  - Inflammation; edema decreases/disappears

Early Encapsulation. The **"early capsule"** stage starts around 1 week. Proliferating fibroblasts deposit reticulin around the outer rim of the abscess cavity. The abscess wall is now composed of an inner rim of granulation tissue at the edge of the necrotic center **(12-34)** and an outer rim of multiple concentric layers of fibroblasts and collagen **(12-35)**. The necrotic core liquefies completely by 7-10 days, and newly formed capillaries around the mass become prominent.

Late Capsulation. The **"late capsule"** stage begins several weeks following infection and may last for several months.

With treatment, the central cavity gradually involutes and shrinks. Collagen deposition further thickens the wall, and the surrounding vasogenic edema disappears. The wall eventually contains densely packed reticulin and is lined by sparse macrophages. Eventually only a small gliotic nodule of collagen and fibroblasts remains.

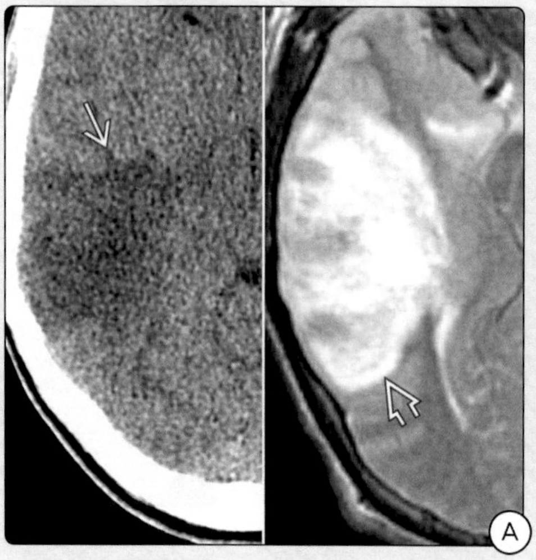

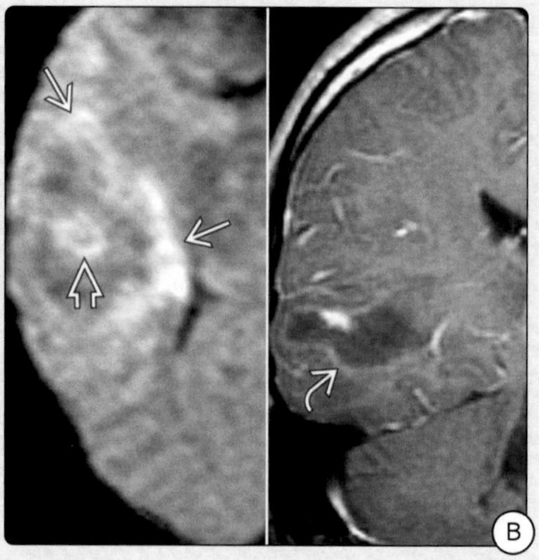

***(12-32A)** (L) NECT shows ill-defined hypoattenuation ➡ and mass effect within the right temporal lobe. Arterial infarction was suspected. (R) T2WI shows a hyperintense right temporal lobe mass ⇨. **(12-32B)** (L) DWI shows restricted diffusion at the periphery ➡, center ⇨ of the lesion. (R) Coronal T1 C+ shows a faint rim of peripheral enhancement ↗. Early cerebritis stage of abscess formation.*

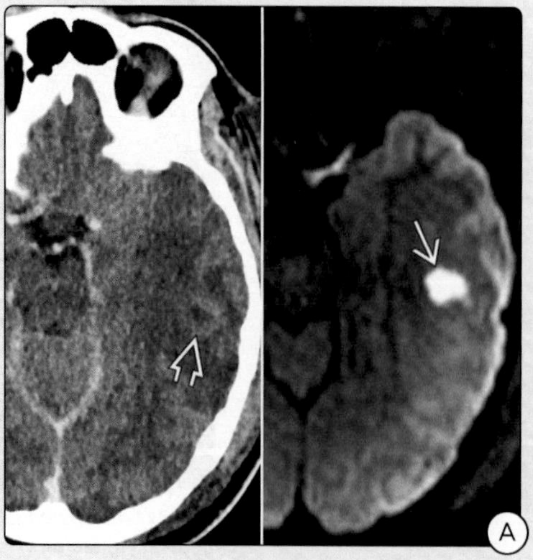

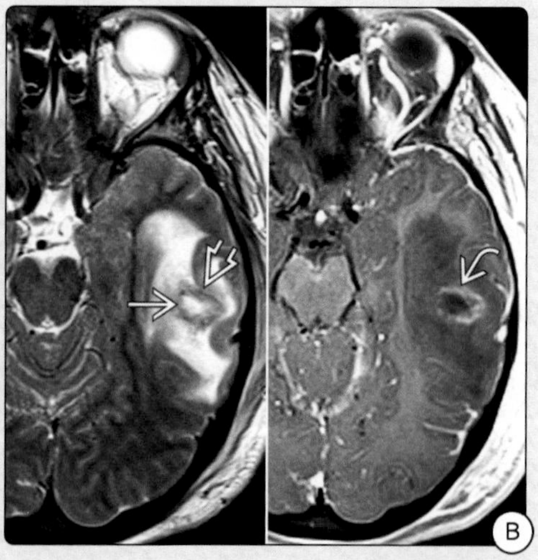

***(12-33A)** (L) CECT shows faint, ill-defined left temporal lobe ring enhancing lesion with peripheral edema ⇨. (R) DWI MR shows strong diffusion restriction ➡ in the center of the mass. **(12-33B)** (L) The mass exhibits a hyperintense center ➡, hypointense periphery ⇨ on T2WI. (R) Irregular, poorly defined enhancing rim ↗ is seen on T1 C+ FS. This is the late cerebritis stage of abscess formation.*

Clinical Issues

Demographics. Brain abscesses are rare. Only 2,500 cases are reported annually in the USA. Brain abscesses occur at all ages but are most common in patients between the third and fourth decades. Almost 25% occur in children under the age of 15 years. The M:F ratio is 2:1 in adults and 3:1 in children.

Presentation and Prognosis. Headache, seizure, and focal neurologic deficits are the typical presenting symptoms. Fever is common but not universal. CSF cultures may be normal early in the infection.

Brain abscesses are potentially fatal but treatable lesions. Rapid diagnosis, stereotactic surgery, and appropriate medical treatment have reduced mortality to 2-4%.

Imaging

General Features. Imaging findings evolve with time and are related to the stage of abscess development. MR is more sensitive than CT and is the procedure of choice.

Early Cerebritis. Very early cerebritis may be invisible on CT. A poorly marginated cortical/subcortical hypodense mass is the most common finding **(12-32A)**. Early cerebritis often shows little or no enhancement on CECT.

Early cerebritis is hypo- to isointense on T1WI and hyperintense on T2/FLAIR. T2* GRE may show punctate "blooming" hemorrhagic foci. Patchy enhancement may or may not be present. DWI shows diffusion restriction **(12-32B)**.

Late Cerebritis. A better-delineated central hypodense mass with surrounding edema is seen on NECT. CECT typically shows irregular rim enhancement **(12-33A)**.

Late cerebritis has a hypointense center and an iso- to mildly hyperintense rim on T1WI. The central core of the cerebritis is hyperintense on T2WI, whereas the rim is relatively hypointense. Intense but somewhat irregular rim enhancement is present on T1 C+ images **(12-33B)**.

Late cerebritis restricts strongly on DWI **(12-33A)**. MRS shows cytosolic amino acids (0.9 ppm), lactate (1.3 ppm), and acetate (1.9 ppm) in the necrotic core **(12-38)**. The abscess wall demonstrates low rCBV on pMR.

BRAIN ABSCESS IMAGING: CEREBRITIS STAGES

Early Cerebritis
- CT
  - Ill-defined hypodense mass on NECT
  - Usually no enhancement
- MR
  - T2/FLAIR heterogeneously hyperintense
  - T2* ± petechial hemorrhage; DWI + (often mild)
  - T1 C+ may show patchy enhancement

Late Cerebritis
- CT
  - Round/ovoid hypodense mass on NECT
  - ± Thin, irregular ring on CECT
- MR
  - T2/FLAIR hyperintense center, hypointense irregular rim
  - T2* GRE hypointense rim; DWI ++
  - Moderate/strong but irregular enhancing rim

Early Capsule. Abscesses are now well-delineated round or ovoid masses with liquefied, hyperintense *cores* on T2/FLAIR. The *rims* of abscesses are usually thin, complete, smooth, and

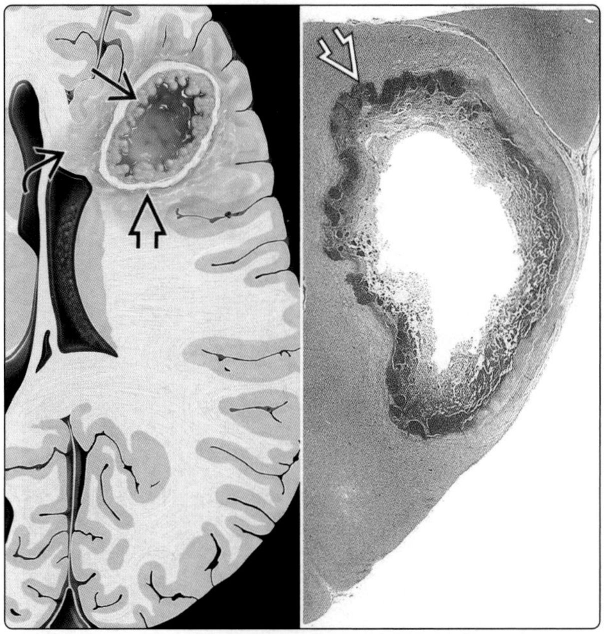

(12-34) (L) Graphic shows edema surrounding early capsule abscess. Well-defined double-layered wall surrounds a central core of necrosis, inflammatory debris . (R) Micrograph shows double-layered abscess wall . (Ellison, Neuropath, 3e.)

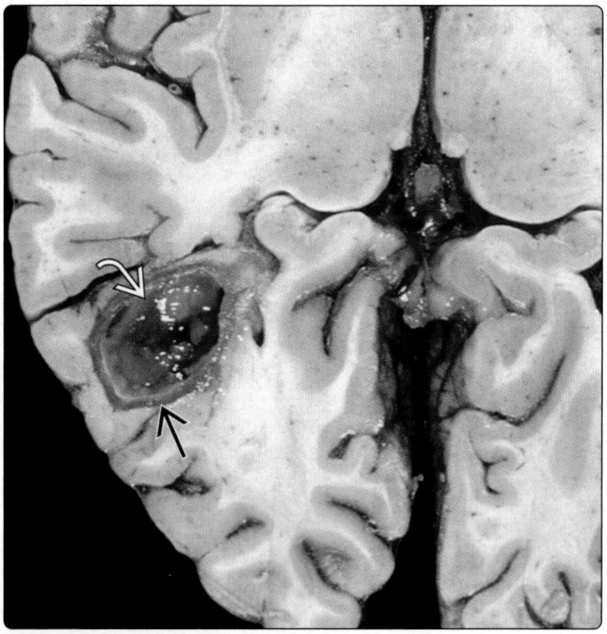

(12-35) Abscess at early capsule stage is shown. Necrotic core is surrounded by a double-layered, well-developed capsule . (Courtesy R. Hewlett, MD.)

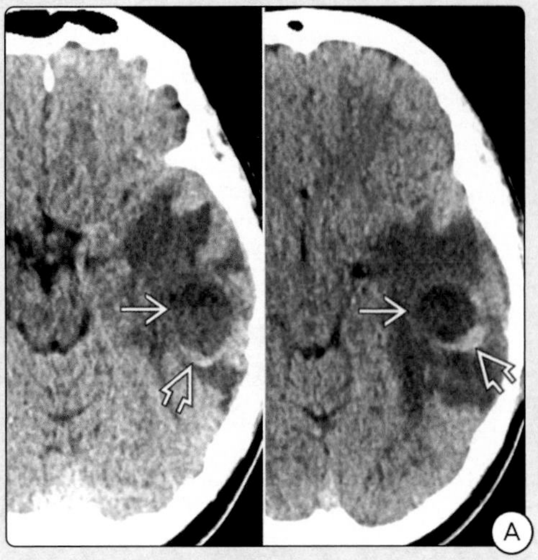

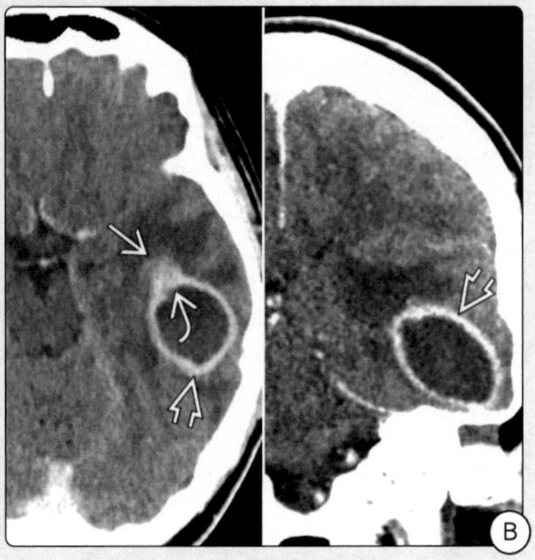

(12-36A) *(L and R) NECT scans show large, well-defined lesion with hyperdense rim and a hypodense center.* ***(12-36B)*** *Axial (L), coronal (R) CECT scans show complete, well-delineated rim enhancement. The abscess has progressed from late cerebritis to the early capsule stage. Note wall defect with adjacent area of new cerebritis.*

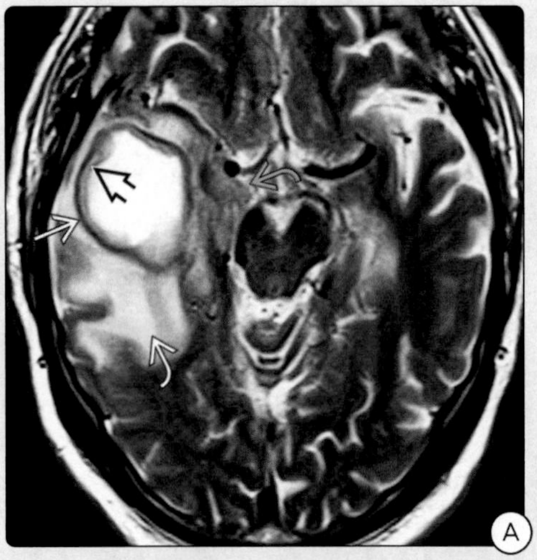

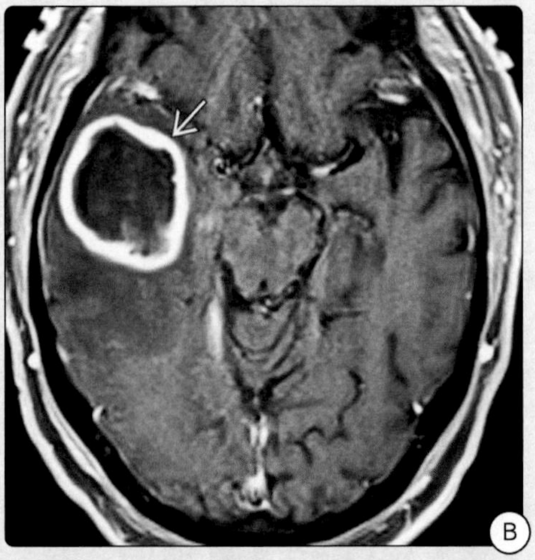

(12-37A) *T2WI in early capsule stage of abscess development shows classic "double rim" sign with hypointense outer rim and mildly hyperintense inner rim surrounding very hyperintense necrotic core. Note peripheral edema and mass effect (uncal herniation).* ***(12-37B)*** *T1 C+ FS in the same case shows intense enhancement of the well-developed abscess capsule.*

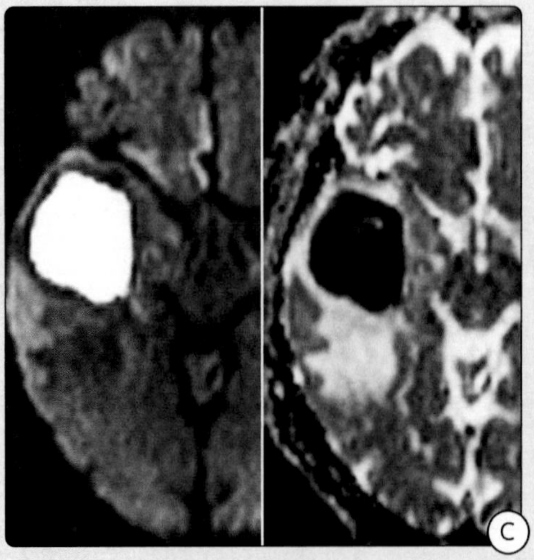

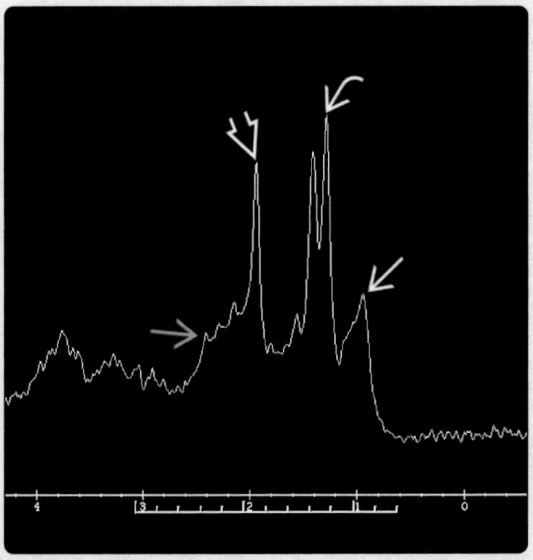

(12-37C) *DWI (L) and ADC map (R) in the same case show that necrotic contents of the abscess cavity restrict strongly, whereas the wall of the capsule itself does not.* ***(12-38)*** *MRS in another late cerebritis/early capsule abscess with TR 2,000 TE 35 shows amino acids (valine, leucine, isoleucine) at 0.9 ppm, acetate at 1.9 ppm, lactate at 1.3 ppm, and succinate at 2.4 ppm.*

hypointense on T2WI. A "double rim" sign demonstrating two concentric rims, the outer hypointense and the inner hyperintense relative to cavity contents, is seen in 75% of cases **(12-37A)**.

The necrotic core of encapsulated abscesses restricts strongly on DWI. T1 C+ sequences show a strongly enhancing rim **(12-24)** **(12-37B)** that is thinnest on its deepest (ventricular) side and "blooms" on T2*.

Late Capsule. With treatment, the abscess cavity gradually collapses while the capsule thickens even as the overall mass diminishes in size. The shrinking abscess often assumes a "crenulated" appearance, much like a deflated balloon **(12-39A)**.

Contrast enhancement in the resolving abscess may persist for months, long after clinical symptoms have resolved **(12-39)**.

BRAIN ABSCESS IMAGING: CAPSULE STAGES

Early Capsule
- Well-defined mass + strongly-enhancing rim
- Core: T2/FLAIR hyperintense, DWI +++
- Wall: "Double rim" sign (hyperintense inner, hypointense outer)

Late Capsule
- Wall thickens, cavity and edema reduce
- Enhancing focus may persist for months

Differential Diagnosis

The differential diagnosis of abscess varies with its stage of development. Early cerebritis is so poorly defined that it can be difficult to characterize and can mimic many lesions, including **cerebral ischemia** or neoplasm.

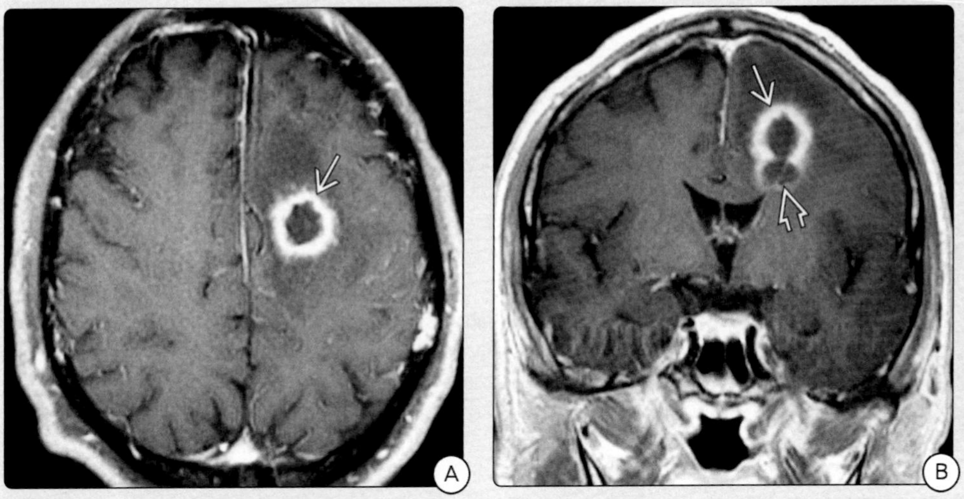

***(12-39A)** Axial T1 C+ FS scan in a 65y man with a history of dental abscess, headaches for 2-3 weeks shows a left posterior frontal thick-walled ring-enhancing mass ➡. Findings are consistent with late capsule stage of abscess development. **(12-39B)** Coronal T1 C+ FS scan in the same case shows the abscess wall ➡ is thinnest on its deepest side ➡, next to the lateral ventricle. Note edema and mass effect on the ventricle.*

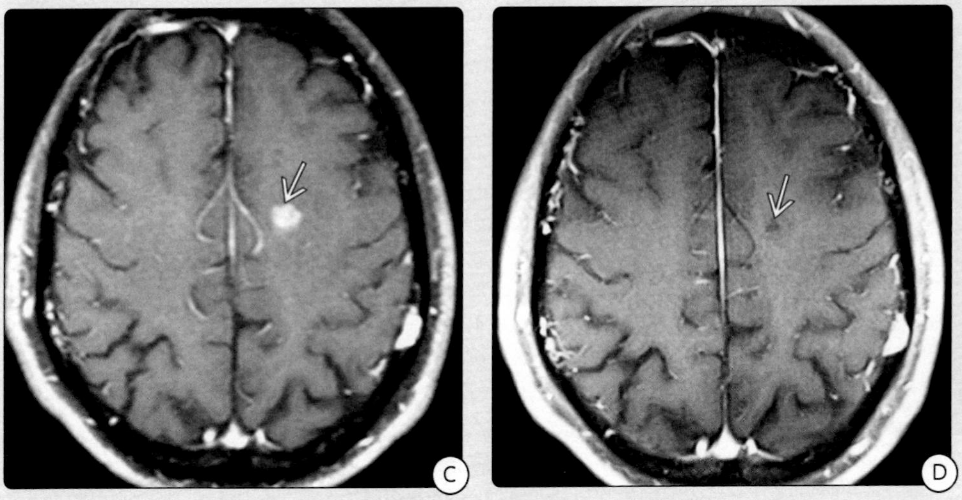

***(12-39C)** The patient was treated with intravenous antibiotics for 6 weeks. Follow-up scan at the end of treatment shows a small residual enhancing nodule ➡ with almost complete resolution of the surrounding edema. **(12-39D)** Follow-up T1 C+ FS scan 1 year later shows that only a small hypointense nonenhancing focus remains ➡.*

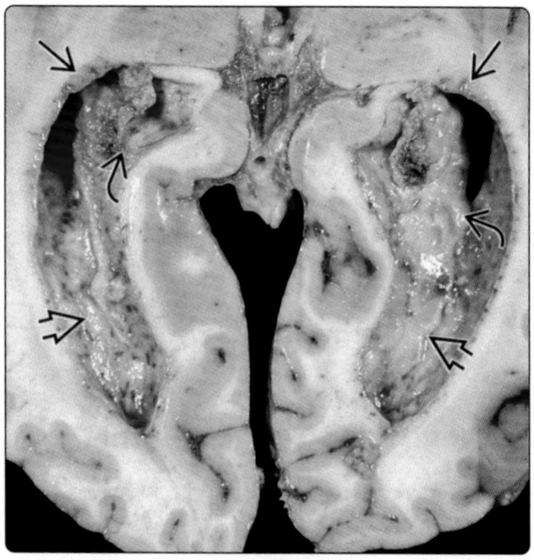

***(12-40)** Autopsy of IVRBA shows ependymal infection, choroid plexitis, pus adhering to ventricular walls. (Courtesy R. Hewlett, MD.)*

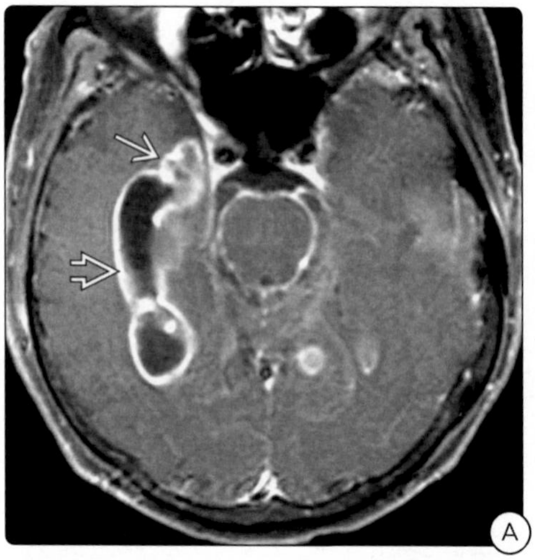

***(12-41A)** Axial T1 C+ FS scan shows meningitis and an abscess with intraventricular rupture (ventriculitis).*

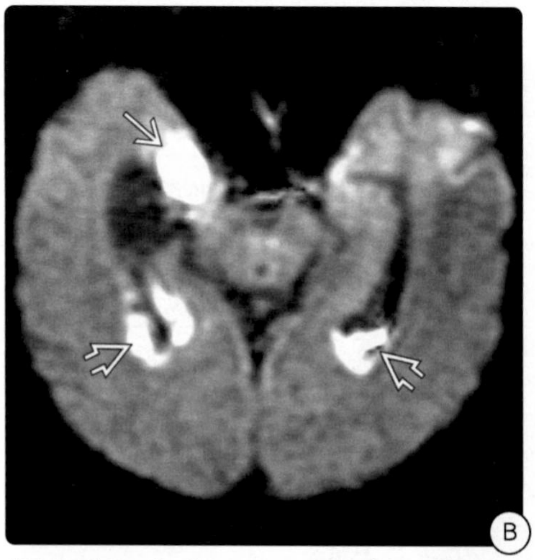

***(12-41B)** DWI in the same patient shows that the abscess viscous contents and ventricular purulent debris restrict.*

Once a ring develops around the necrotic center, the differential diagnosis is basically that of a generic ring-enhancing mass. Although there are many ring-enhancing lesions in the CNS, the most common differential diagnosis is infection vs. **neoplasm (glioblastoma or metastasis)**.

Tumors have increased rCBV in their "rind," usually do not restrict (or if they do, not as strongly as an abscess), and do not demonstrate cytosolic amino acids on MRS.

Less common entities that can appear as a ring-enhancing mass include **demyelinating disease**, in which the ring is usually incomplete and "open" toward the cortex. Resolving hematomas can exhibit a vascular, ring-enhancing pattern.

BRAIN ABSCESS: DIFFERENTIAL DIAGNOSIS

Early Cerebritis
- Encephalitis (may be indistinguishable)
- Stroke
  - Vascular distribution
  - Usually involves both cortex, WM
- Neoplasm (e.g., diffusely infiltrating low-grade astrocytoma)
  - Usually doesn't enhance or restrict

Late Cerebritis/Early Capsule
- Neoplasm
  - Primary (glioblastoma)
  - Metastasis
- Demyelinating disease
  - Incomplete ("horseshoe") enhancement

Ventriculitis

Primary intraventricular abscess is rare. A collection of purulent material in the ventricle is more likely due to intraventricular *rupture* of a brain abscess (IVRBA), a catastrophic complication. Ventriculitis also occurs as a complication of meningitis and neurosurgical procedures such as external ventricular drainage. Recognition and prompt intervention are necessary to treat this highly lethal condition.

Terminology

Ventriculitis is also called **ependymitis, pyocephalus**, and (less commonly) ventricular empyema.

Etiology

Infection of the ventricular ependyma most often occurs when a pyogenic abscess ruptures through its thin, medial capsule into the adjacent ventricle. Risk of IVRBA increases if an abscess is deep-seated, multiloculated, and/or close to the ventricular wall. A reduction of 1 mm between the ventricle and brain abscess increases the rupture rate by 10%.

Ventriculitis can also occur as a complication of meningitis, usually via spread of infection through the choroid plexus (choroid plexitis) into the CSF. In the pediatric population, ventriculitis is common in newborns with *E. coli* and group B *streptococcus* meningitis, and infants and young children with typable and non-typable *Haemophilus* species.

Nosocomial meningitis/ventriculitis is a rare but potentially devastating complication following neurosurgical interventions. Patients who require external ventricular drainage (EVD) are at special risk for development of device-related meningitis and ventriculitis. The infection rate of EVDs is high, even with antibiotic-impregnated devices. Reported incidences range from 5-20%.

The most common pathogens causing ventriculitis are *Staphylococcus*, *Streptococcus*, and *Enterobacter*. Infections are often multidrug resistant and difficult to treat.

Pathology

Autopsy examination shows that the ependyma, subependymal region, and choroid plexus are congested and covered with pus **(12-40)**. Hemorrhagic ependymitis may be present. Hydrocephalus with pus obstructing the aqueduct is common.

Clinical Issues

Epidemiology and Demographics. The incidence of IVRBA varies. Recent studies estimate that intraventricular rupture occurs in up to 35% of brain abscesses. Male patients are more commonly affected than female patients.

Presentation. Clinical features of IVRBA can be indistinguishable from those of brain abscesses without intraventricular rupture. In general, headaches are more severe and are accompanied by signs of meningeal irritation. Rapid deterioration of clinical status is typical.

Natural History and Treatment Options. Image-guided stereotactic aspiration is the simplest, safest method to obtain pus for culture and to decompress the abscess cavity. The combination of third-generation cephalosporins and metronidazole is the mainstay of initial empirical antimicrobial treatment. The choice of definitive antibiotics depends on culture results.

Despite aggressive medical and surgical management, many patients do poorly and succumb to the disease. Overall mortality is 25-85%. Only 40% of patients survive with good functional outcome.

Imaging

Ventriculomegaly with a debris level in the dependent part of the occipital horns together with periventricular hypodensity is the classic finding on NECT scans. The ventricular walls may enhance on CECT.

MR should be the first-line imaging modality in cases of suspected ventriculitis. Irregular ventricular debris that appears hyperintense to CSF on T1WI and hypointense on T2WI with layering in the dependent occipital horns is typical.

The most sensitive sequences are FLAIR and DWI. A "halo" of periventricular hyperintensity is usually present on both T2WI and FLAIR scans. DWI shows striking diffusion restriction of the layered debris **(12-41B)**.

Ependymal enhancement is seen in only 60% of cases and varies from minimal to moderate **(12-41A)**. When present, ependymal enhancement tends to be relatively smooth, thin and linear rather than thick and nodular.

Differential Diagnosis

The differential diagnosis of IVRBA is limited. Sudden deterioration of a patient with a known cerebral abscess together with intraventricular debris and pus on MR is almost certainly IVRBA.

Ependymal enhancement *without* intraventricular debris and pus is a nonspecific finding on imaging studies. Mild, thin, linear enhancement of the periventricular and ependymal veins is normal, especially around the frontal horns, septi pellucidi, and atria of the lateral ventricles.

Primary malignant CNS neoplasms such as **glioblastoma multiforme** and **primary CNS lymphoma** can spread along the ventricular ependyma, giving it a thick or nodular "lumpy-bumpy" appearance. **Germinoma** and **metastasis** from an extracranial primary neoplasm can both cause irregular ependymal thickening and enhancement.

Empyemas

Extraaxial infections of the CNS are rare but potentially life-threatening conditions. Early diagnosis and prompt treatment are essential to maximize neurologic recovery.

Terminology

Empyemas are pus collections that can occur in either the subdural or epidural space.

Etiology

The pathophysiologic basis of empyemas varies with patient age. Empyemas in infants and young children are most commonly secondary to bacterial meningitis.

In older children and adults, over two-thirds of empyemas occur as extension of infection from paranasal sinus disease. Infection can erode directly through the thin posterior wall of the frontal sinus, which is half the thickness of the anterior wall **(12-42)**. Infection may also spread indirectly in retrograde fashion through valveless bridging emissary veins.

Approximately 20% of empyemas in older children and adults are secondary to otomastoiditis. Rare causes of empyemas include penetrating head trauma, neurosurgical procedures, or hematogenous spread of pathogens from a distant extracranial site.

The most common organisms are staphylococci and streptococci.

Pathology

Location. Subdural empyemas (SDEs) are much more common than epidural empyemas (EDEs). The most common locations are the frontal and frontoparietal convexities. Peritentorial collections are rare but important locations for SDEs. In unusual cases, SDEs may be complicated by cerebritis or abscess in the adjacent brain.

Size and Number. Empyemas vary in size and extent. They range from small, focal epidural collections **(12-42)** to

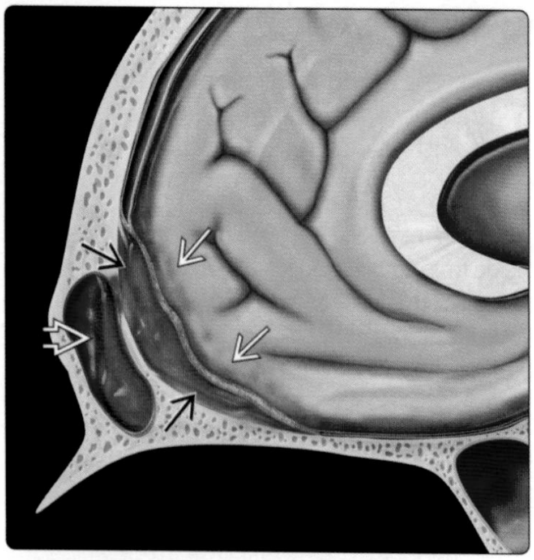

***(12-42)* Purulent frontal sinusitis ➡ with extension into epidural space causes epidural empyema ➡ and frontal lobe cerebritis ➡.**

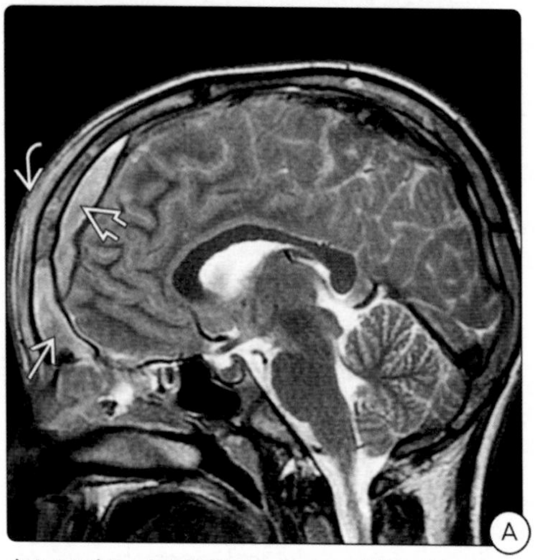

***(12-43A)* Sagittal T2WI is from a child with frontal sinusitis ➡ causing scalp cellulitis ➡ and epidural empyema ➡.**

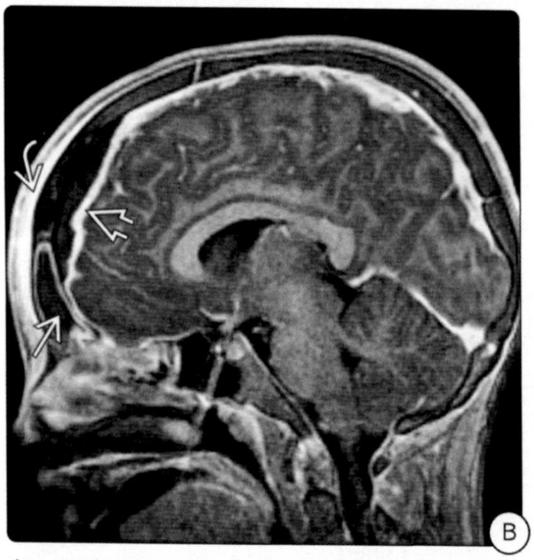

***(12-43B)* T1 C+ scan shows the frontal sinusitis ➡, cellulitis ➡, and enhancing endosteal dura ➡ displaced by the epidural empyema.**

extensive subdural infections that spread over most of the cerebral hemisphere and extend into the interhemispheric fissure.

Multiple lesions including mixed intra- and extradural collections are seen in 15-20% of cases. Loculated and/or multiple unilateral collections are more common than separate bilateral empyemas.

Gross and Microscopic Features. The most common gross appearance of an empyema is an encapsulated, thick, yellowish, purulent collection lying between the dura and the arachnoid. Early empyemas may be unencapsulated collections of cloudy, more fluid-like material.

Microscopic features are those of nonspecific inflammatory infiltrate with varying amounts of granulation tissue.

Clinical Issues

Epidemiology. SDEs and EDEs are rare in the developed world due to the early and judicious use of antibiotics. The incidence of extraaxial CNS infections is higher in patients with limited access to medical care.

Demographics. Extraaxial CNS infections can occur at any age but tend to occur at a significantly earlier age than brain abscesses. Male patients are more often affected than female patients. An adolescent boy with significant headache and fever should elicit a high index of suspicion for sinusitis complications and prompt immediate imaging evaluation.

Presentation. The most common clinical presentation is headache, followed by fever and altered sensorium. Preceding symptoms of sinusitis or otomastoiditis are common. Meningismus, seizures, and focal motor signs are also frequent.

"Pott puffy tumor"—a fluctuant ("doughy"), tender erythematous swelling of the frontal scalp—is considered a specific sign for frontal bone osteomyelitis with a subperiosteal abscess. Most occur in the setting of untreated frontal sinusitis. If the posterior table of the sinus is breached, an EDE may form. "Pott puffy tumor" is seen in up to one-third of patients with frontal EDE. Orbital cellulitis is a less common but significant sign of empyema.

Natural History and Treatment Options. The interval between initial infection (usually sinusitis) and onset of the empyema is typically 1-3 weeks. EDEs have a better prognosis than SDEs. Once established, untreated empyemas can spread quite rapidly, extending from the extraaxial spaces into the subjacent brain. Besides cerebritis and abscess formation, the other major complication of empyema is cortical vein thrombosis with venous ischemia.

Surgical drainage and rapid initiation of empiric intravenous antibiotic therapy (initially vancomycin and a third-generation cephalosporin) has been shown to reduce mortality. Mortality of treated empyemas is still significant, ranging from 10-15%.

Imaging

Imaging is essential to the early diagnosis of empyema. NECT scans may be normal or show a hypodense extraaxial collection **(12-45A)** that demonstrates peripheral enhancement on CECT **(12-44A)**. Bone CT should be evaluated for signs of sinusitis and otomastoiditis **(12-47A)**.

MR is the procedure of choice for evaluating potential empyemas. T1 scans show an extraaxial collection that is mildly hyperintense relative to CSF. SDEs are typically crescentic and lie over the cerebral hemisphere. The extracerebral space is widened, and the underlying sulci are compressed by the collection. SDEs often extend into the interhemispheric fissure but do not cross the midline.

EDEs are biconvex and usually more focal than SDEs. The inwardly displaced dura can sometimes be identified as a thin hypointense line between the epidural collection and the underlying brain **(12-43)**. In contrast to SDEs, frontal EDEs may cross the midline, confirming their epidural location **(12-47B)**.

Empyemas are iso- to hyperintense compared with CSF on T2WI and are hyperintense on FLAIR **(12-45B)**. Hyperintensity in the underlying brain parenchyma may be caused by cerebritis or ischemia (either venous or arterial).

SDEs typically demonstrate striking diffusion restriction on DWI **(12-45D)**. EDEs are variable but usually have at least some restricting component **(12-44C)**.

Empyemas show variable enhancement depending on the amount of granulomatous tissue and inflammation present **(12-24)**. The encapsulating membranes, especially on the outer margin, enhance moderately strongly **(12-43B)** **(12-44B)** **(12-45C)**.

Differential Diagnosis

The major differential diagnosis of extraaxial empyema is a nonpurulent extraaxial collection such as subdural effusion, subdural hygroma, and chronic subdural hematoma.

A **subdural effusion** is usually postmeningitic, is typically bilateral, and does not restrict on DWI. Because of its increased proteinaceous contents, effusions are typically hyperintense to CSF on FLAIR.

A **subdural hygroma** is a sterile, nonenhancing, nonrestricting CSF collection that occurs with a tear in the arachnoid, allowing escape of CSF into the subdural space. Hygromas are usually posttraumatic or postsurgical and behave exactly like CSF on imaging studies.

A **chronic subdural hematoma** (cSDH) is hypodense on NECT. Signal intensity varies with chronicity. Early cSDHs are hyperintense compared with CSF on both T1WI and T2/FLAIR. They may show some residual blood that "blooms" on T2* (GRE, SWI). The encapsulating membranes enhance and may show diffusion restriction. In contrast to SDEs, the cSDH contents themselves typically do not restrict on DWI. Very longstanding cSDHs look similar to CSF and may show little or no residual evidence of prior hemorrhage.

EMPYEMAS

Pathology
- Subdural empyemas (SDEs) > > epidural empyemas (EDEs)
- EDE focal (usually next to sinus, mastoid)
- SDE spreads diffusely along hemispheres, tentorium/falx

Imaging
- Bone CT: look for sinus, ear infection
- EDE is focal, biconvex, can cross midline
- SDE is crescentic, covers hemisphere, may extend into interhemispheric fissure
- SDEs restrict strongly on DWI; EDEs variable

Differential Diagnosis
- Chronic SDH, subdural hygroma, effusion

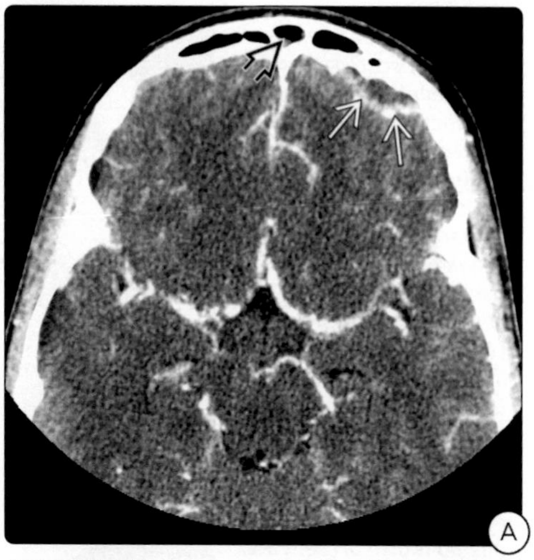

***(12-44A)** CECT shows frontal sinusitis (small fluid level) and biconvex lentiform epidural fluid collection with enhancing rim.*

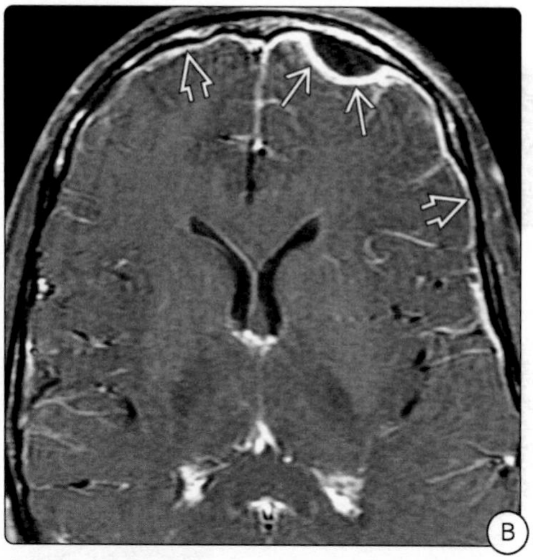

***(12-44B)** Axial T1 C+ FS in the same patient shows displaced thickened endosteal dura. Note reactive dural thickening.*

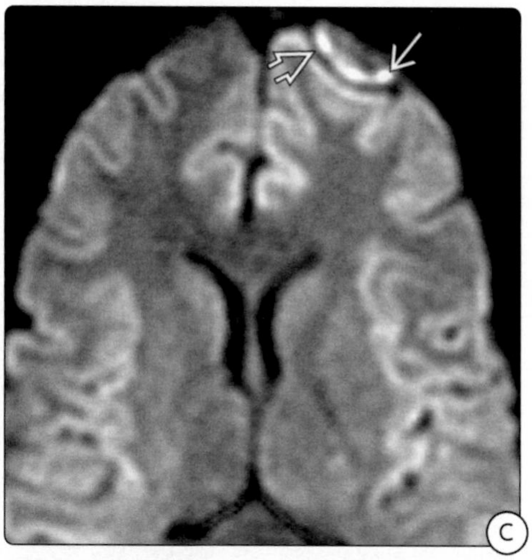

***(12-44C)** DWI shows a small hyperintense crescent of epidural pus that lies immediately outside the thick displaced dura.*

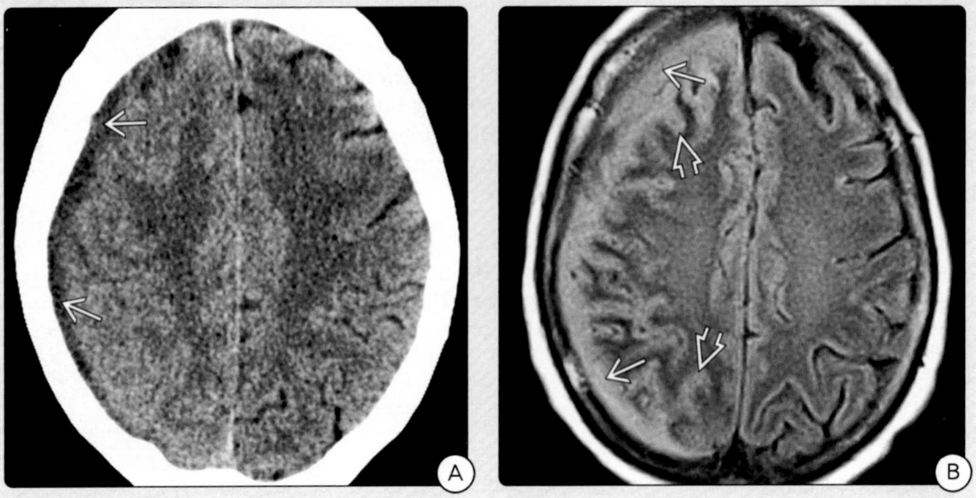

***(12-45A)** NECT in a 51y man with acute sinusitis who developed severe headache and altered mental status shows a hypoattenuating subdural collection → that compresses underlying brain. Fluid is slightly hyperattenuating compared with sulcal CSF.* ***(12-45B)** FLAIR in the same patient shows that the fluid collection → does not suppress. The underlying sulci are hyperintense, suggesting meningitis. Cortical edema is also present →.*

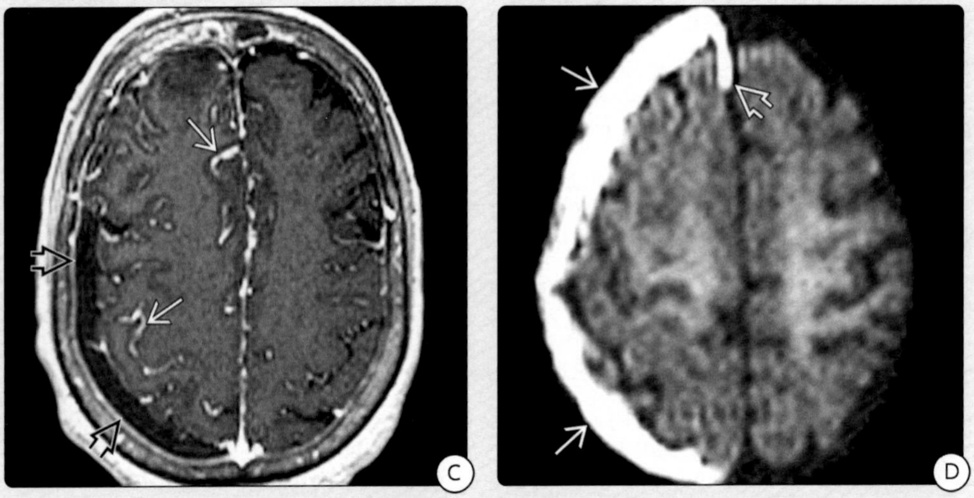

***(12-45C)** Axial T1 C+ SPGR for stereotactic aspiration shows outer endosteal dural enhancement →. Leptomeningeal enhancement → is consistent with meningitis.* ***(12-45D)** Axial DWI shows that the subdural empyema → restricts strongly and uniformly. Interhemispheric extension → does not cross midline. Subdural empyema was drained at craniotomy, and S. pneumoniae was cultured.*

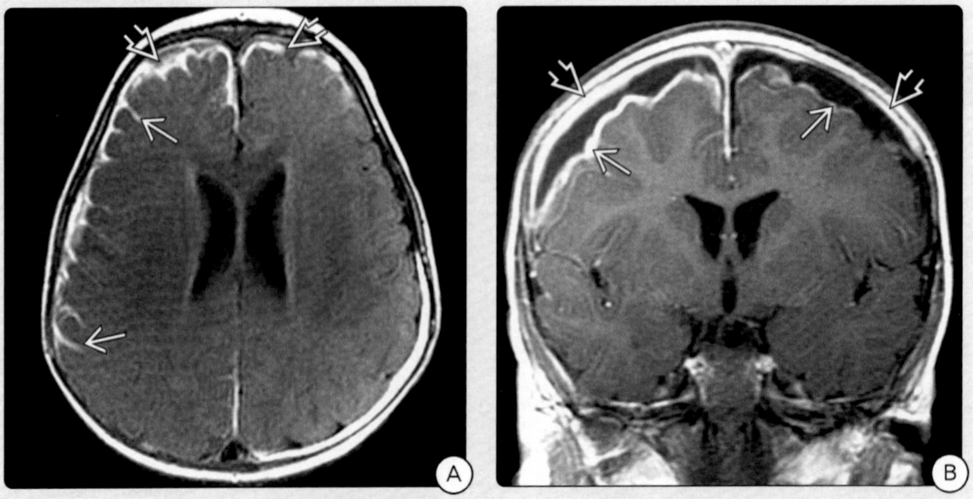

***(12-46A)** Axial T1 C+ scan in a child with pyogenic meningitis shows pia-subarachnoid space enhancement that follows the surfaces of the brain, extending into the sulci →. A small bifrontal fluid subdural collection (empyema) → is present.* ***(12-46B)** Coronal T1 C+ image shows that the meningitis extends over the convexal surfaces of the brain →. The subdural collections are encased by a thickened dura →. Subdural empyemas restrict on DWI; effusions do not.*

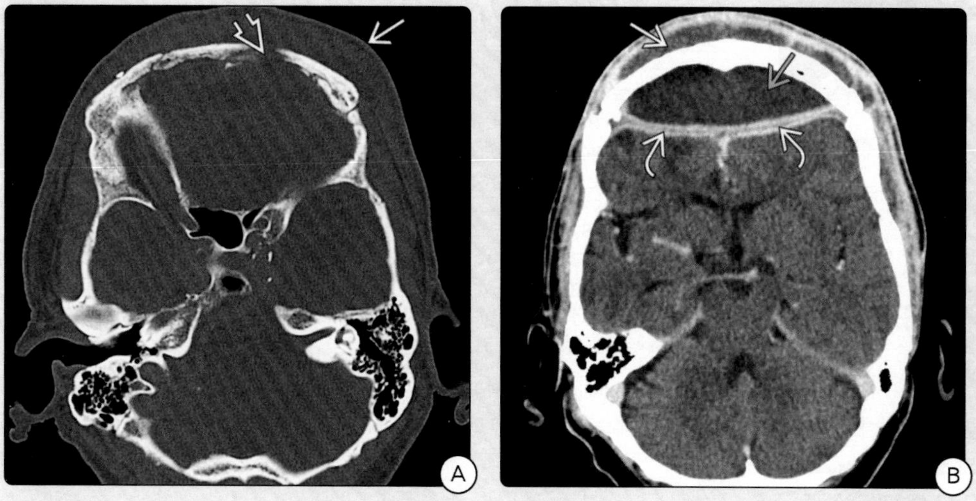

*(**12-47A**) A 66y man developed headaches and frontal scalp swelling several weeks after resection of an anterior fossa meningioma. Bone CT shows soft tissue scalp mass ➡ and bone destruction ➡ suspicious for osteomyelitis. (**12-47B**) CECT shows a subperiosteal abscess ➡ and large bifrontal epidural empyema ➡. Note thin film of intradural fluid ➡ between layers of periosteal and meningeal dura. It's frontal sinusitis with Pott puffy tumor.*

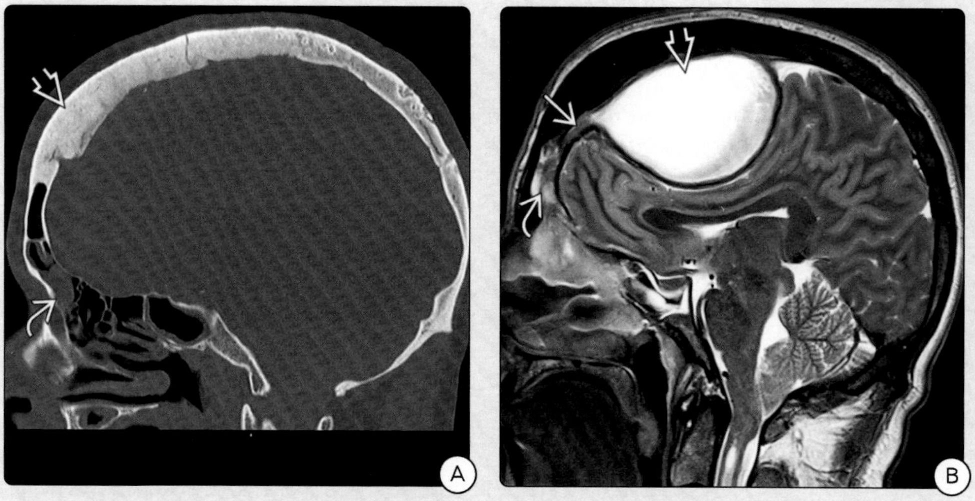

*(**12-48A**) Sagittal bone CT in a patient with frontal sinusitis ➡ and chronic headaches shows diffuse thickening and sclerosis ➡ of the frontal and anterior parietal bones. Findings suggest chronic osteomyelitis. (**12-48B**) Sagittal T2WI in the same patient shows a huge epidural fluid collection ➡ connecting directly ➡ to the infected frontal sinus ➡. DWI helps characterize pyogenic nature of sinus fluid.*

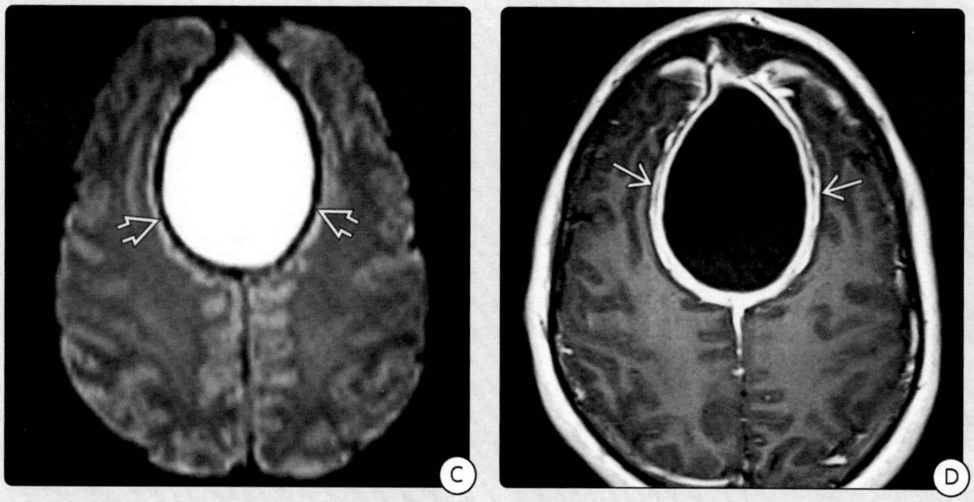

*(**12-48C**) Axial DWI in the same case shows that the interhemispheric fluid collection restricts (confirmed on ADC map) and splays apart thickened dura ➡. (**12-48D**) T1 C+ MR in the same patient shows that the thickened, intensely enhancing dura ➡ surrounds the nonenhancing epidural abscess.*

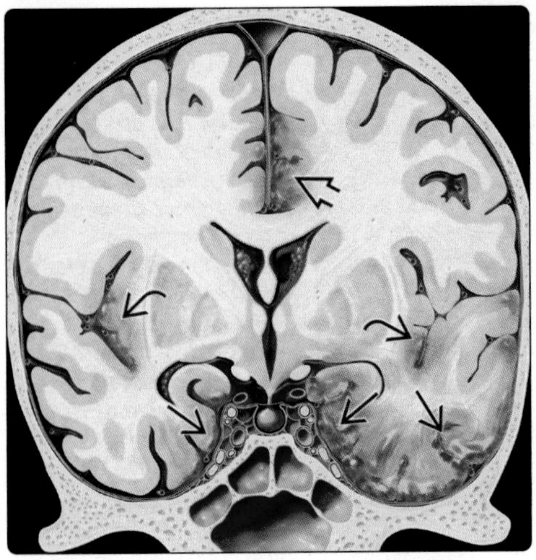

(12-49) Graphic shows herpes encephalitis with bilateral, asymmetric involvement of temporal lobes ➡, cingulate gyri ➡, and insula ➡.

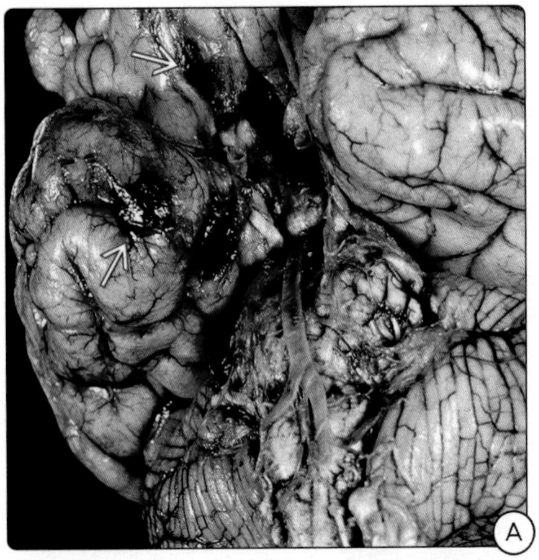

(12-50A) Autopsy of HSE shows hemorrhagic lesions in the basal medial temporal lobes and subfrontal regions ➡. (Courtesy R. Hewlett, MD.)

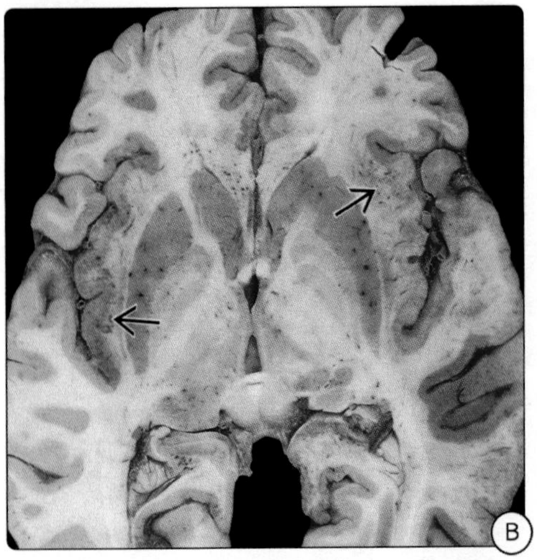

(12-50B) Axial section in the same case shows petechial hemorrhages in insular cortex of both temporal lobes ➡. (Courtesy R. Hewlett, MD.)

Acquired Viral Infections

A number of both familiar and and less well-known but emerging viruses can cause CNS infections. In this section, we focus on neurotropic herpes virus infections, which can promote acute fulminant CNS disease and become latent with the potential of reactivation that may last for decades.

Eight members of the herpes virus family are known to cause disease in humans. These are herpes simplex virus 1 (HSV-1) and HSV-2, varicella-zoster virus (VZV), Epstein-Barr virus (EBV), cytomegalovirus (CMV), and human herpes virus (HHV)-6, HHV-7, and HHV-8. Each has its own disease spectrum, clinical setting, and imaging findings.

HSV-1 typically involves the skin and facial mucosa, whereas HSV-2 is primarily associated with genital infection. HHV-6 and HHV-7 are increasingly recognized as major causes of morbidity and mortality in transplant recipients, whereas EBV and HHV-8 (also known as Kaposi sarcoma-associated herpesvirus) have proven oncogenic potential.

Congenital HSV-2 and CMV were both considered earlier, as their manifestations in newborn infants differ from those of acquired herpesvirus infections. HSV-1 and HHV-6 are discussed in this section. VZV and EBV are discussed later in the chapter under Miscellaneous Acute Viral Encephalitides.

In children, more than 100 viral species have either directly or indirectly been associated with CNS infection. In addition to viruses mentioned above, many other viruses have been implicated as important agents associated with pediatric encephalitis, including *Influenzae* A and B, adenovirus, respiratory syncytial virus (RSV), H1N1, parainfluenzae, and human metapneumovirus (HMPV)—a group collectively called the *respiratory viruses*. Most viruses reach the pediatric CNS hematogenously and enter the CNS via the choroid plexus or directly through the vascular endothelium.

Herpes Simplex Encephalitis

Terminology

CNS involvement in HSV infection is called congenital or neonatal HSV when it involves neonates but is designated herpes simplex encephalitis (HSE) in all individuals beyond the first postnatal month. HSE is also sometimes called HSV encephalitis.

Etiology

After the neonatal period, over 95% of HSE is caused by reactivation of HSV-1, an obligate intracellular pathogen. The virus initially gains entry into cells in the nasopharyngeal mucosa, invades sensory lingual branches of the trigeminal nerve, then passes in retrograde fashion into the trigeminal ganglion. It establishes a lifelong latent infection within sensory neurons of the trigeminal ganglion, where it can remain dormant indefinitely.

Genetic errors in Toll-like receptor 3 (*TLR3*) have been linked to HSE infection susceptibility. "Relapsing HSE" is often an NMDA receptor encephalitis triggered by antecedent HSV infection.

Pathology

Location. HSE has a striking affinity for the limbic system **(12-49)**. The anterior and medial temporal lobes, insular cortex, subfrontal area, and cingulate gyri are most frequently affected **(12-50A)**. Bilateral but asymmetric disease is typical **(12-50B)**. Extratemporal, extralimbic involvement occurs but is more common in children compared with adults. When it occurs, extralimbic HSE most often involves the parietal cortex. Brainstem-predominant infection is uncommon. The basal ganglia are usually spared.

Gross Pathology. HSE is a fulminant, hemorrhagic, necrotizing encephalitis. Massive tissue necrosis accompanied by numerous petechial hemorrhages and severe edema is typical. Inflammation and tissue destruction are predominantly cortical but may extend into the subcortical white matter. Advanced cases demonstrate gross temporal lobe rarefaction and cavitation.

Microscopic Features. Perivascular lymphocytic cuffing with diffuse neutrophil infiltration into the necrotic parenchyma is typical. Large "owl's-eye" viral inclusions in neurons, astrocytes, and oligodendrocytes are seen in the acute and subacute phases. Tissue destruction with neuronophagia and apoptosis is striking.

Clinical Issues

Epidemiology. HSV-1 is the most common worldwide cause of sporadic (i.e., nonepidemic) viral encephalitis. Overall prevalence is 1-3:1,000,000.

Demographics. HSE may occur at any age. It follows a bimodal age distribution, with one-third of all cases occurring between the ages of 6 months and 3 years and one-half seen in patients older than 50. There is no sex predilection.

Presentation. A viral prodrome followed by fever, headache, seizures, behavioral changes, and altered mental status is typical.

Natural History. HSE is a devastating infection with mortality rates ranging from 50-70%. Rapid clinical deterioration with coma and death is typical. Nearly two-thirds of survivors have significant neurologic deficits despite antiviral therapy.

Treatment Options. Antiviral therapy with intravenous acyclovir should be started immediately if HSE is suspected. Definitive diagnosis requires PCR confirmation. CSF PCR is 96-98% sensitive.

HERPES SIMPLEX ENCEPHALITIS (HSE)

Etiology
- > 95% caused by HSV-1

Pathology
- Necrotizing, hemorrhagic encephalitis
- Limbic system
    - Anteromedial temporal lobes, insular cortex
    - Subfrontal region, cingulate gyri

Imaging
- Bilateral > unilateral; asymmetric > symmetric
- FLAIR most sensitive
- DWI shows restriction

Imaging

CT Findings. NECT is often normal early in the disease course. Hypodensity with mild mass effect in one or both temporal lobes and the insula may be present **(12-51A)**. CECT is usually negative, although patchy or gyriform enhancement may develop after 24-48 hours **(12-51C)**.

MR Findings. MR is the imaging procedure of choice. T1 scans show gyral swelling with indistinct gray-white interfaces **(12-52A)**. T2 scans

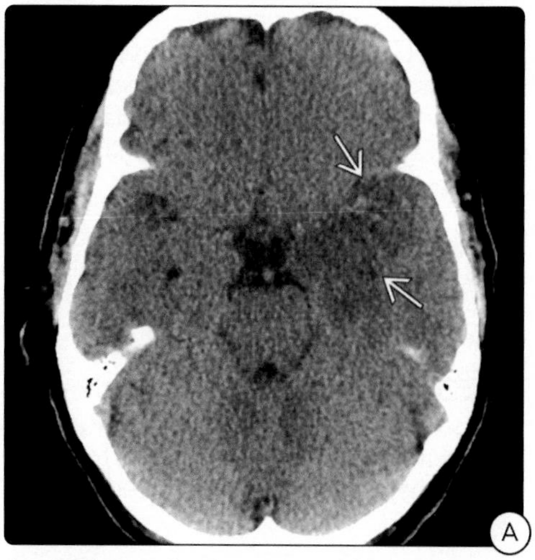

***(12-51A)** NECT in 60y woman with altered mental status shows an ill-defined low attenuation temporal lobe mass ➡, but was called normal.*

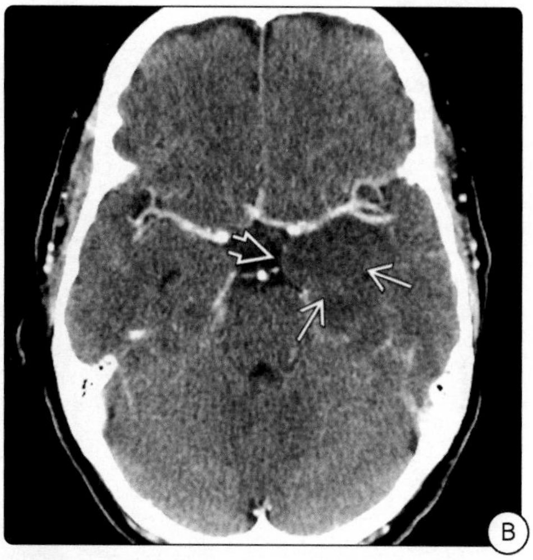

***(12-51B)** CECT in the same case obtained 48 hours later shows a hypoattenuating temporal lobe mass ➡. Note uncal herniation ➡.*

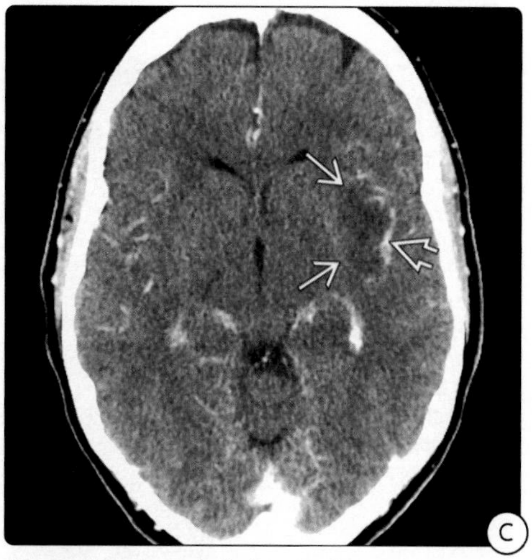

***(12-51C)** More cephalad CECT shows a hypoattenuating insular mass ➡ with superficial gyriform enhancement ➡.*

demonstrate cortical/subcortical hyperintensity with relative sparing of the underlying white matter. FLAIR is the most sensitive sequence and may be positive before signal changes are apparent on either T1- or T2WI. Bilateral but asymmetric involvement of the temporal lobes and insula is characteristic of HSE but is not always present.

T2* (GRE, SWI) may demonstrate petechial hemorrhages after 24-48 hours **(12-53)**. Gyriform T1 shortening, volume loss, and confluent curvilinear "blooming" foci on T2* are seen in the subacute and chronic phases of HSE.

HSE shows restricted diffusion early in the disease course **(12-52B)**, sometimes preceding visible FLAIR abnormalities. Enhancement varies from none (early) to intense gyriform enhancement several days later **(12-52D)**.

Differential Diagnosis

The major differential diagnoses for HSE are neoplasm, acute cerebral ischemia, status epilepticus, other encephalitides (especially HHV-6), and paraneoplastic limbic encephalitis. Primary neoplasms such as **diffusely infiltrating astrocytoma** usually involve white matter or white matter plus cortex.

Acute cerebral ischemia-infarction occurs in a typical vascular distribution, involving both the cortex and white matter. Onset is typically sudden compared with HSE, and a history of fever or a viral prodrome with flu-like illness is lacking. Especially in immunocompromised patients, late acute/subacute HSE itself can have a "pseudo-ischemic" appearance caused by widespread dead or dying neurons.

Status epilepticus is usually unilateral and typically involves just the cortex. Postictal edema is transient but generally more widespread, often involving most or all of the hemispheric cortex.

(12-52A) MR in the same patient as on the prior page shows left temporal lobe hypointensity on T1WI (L), hyperintensity on FLAIR (R). (12-52B) DWI in the same case shows restricted diffusion in the anterior temporal lobe cortex (L) and insular cortex (R).

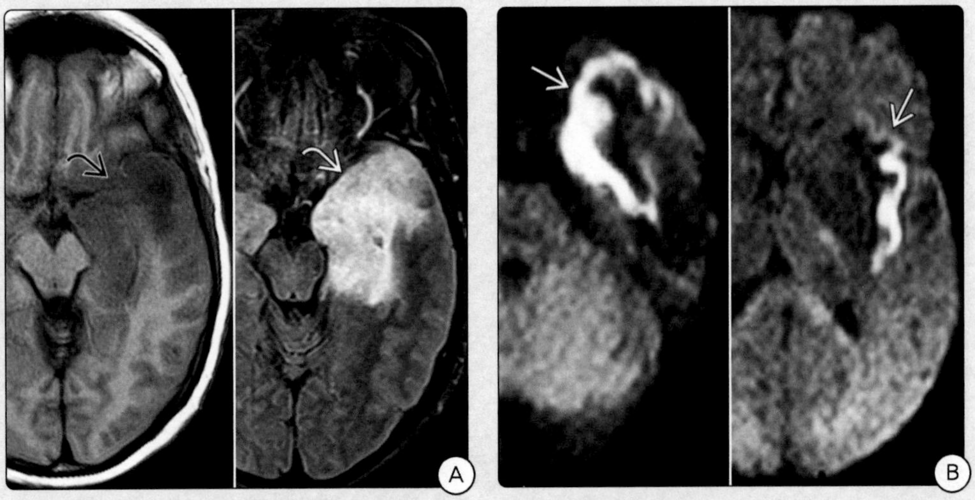

(12-52C) T1 C+ FS shows gyriform enhancement in the left insula and low-attenuation edema. (12-52D) Coronal T1 C+ shows gyriform cortical enhancement but also pial (leptomeningeal) enhancement. This is PCR-proven HSE meningoencephalitis. Note the ipsilateral ventricular compression and displacement.

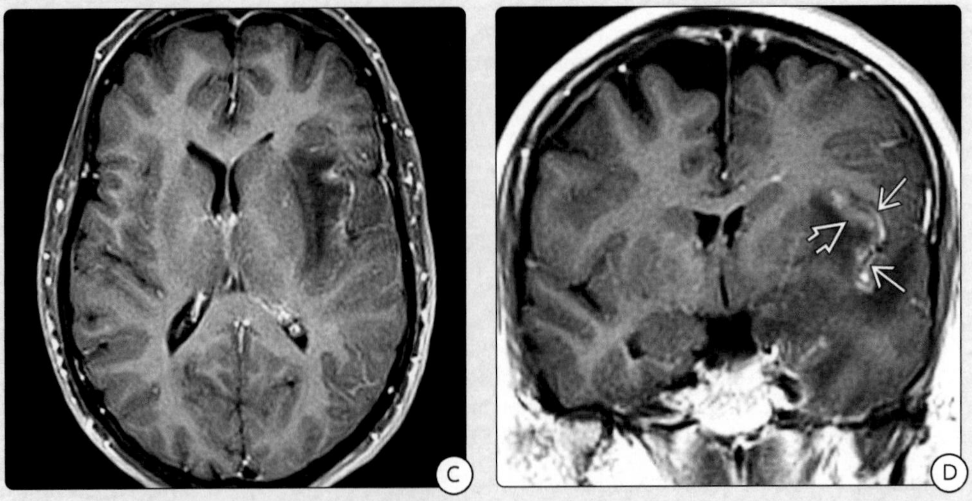

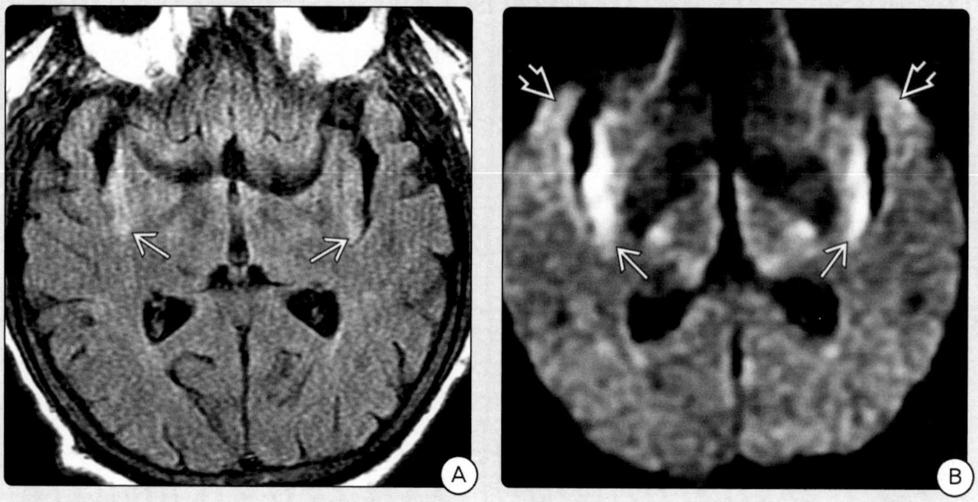

(12-53A) *A 68y man presented to the ED with viral prodrome and confusion. Initial NECT scan (not shown) was negative. FLAIR shows hyperintensity in both insular cortices ➡.* ***(12-53B)*** *DWI shows marked diffusion restriction in both insular cortices ➡. Somewhat less striking hyperintensity is seen in both anterior temporal lobes ➡.*

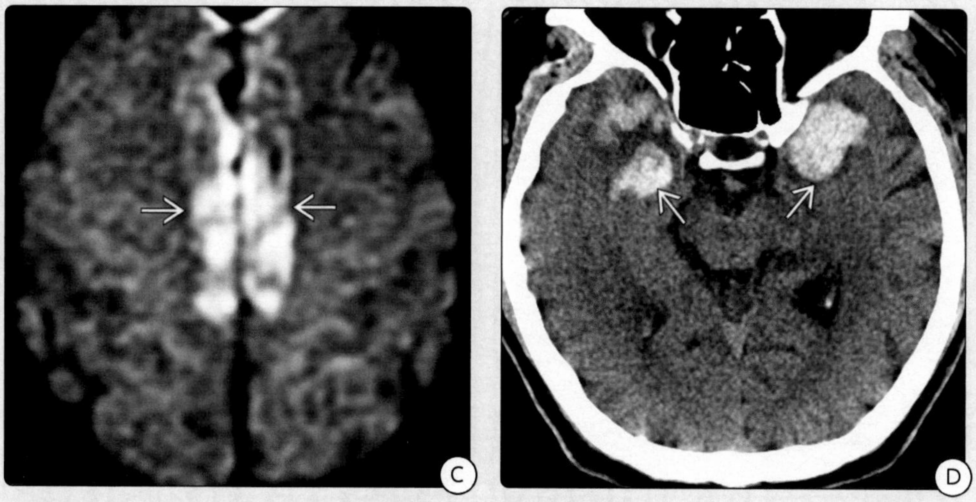

(12-53C) *More cephalad DWI in the same patient shows symmetric restricted diffusion in both cingulate gyri ➡. Because of the strong suspicion for HSE, the patient was placed on antiviral agents. PCR was positive for HSV-1.* ***(12-53D)*** *Despite treatment, the patient did poorly. Repeat NECT scan 2 weeks later shows confluent hemorrhages in both anteromedial temporal lobes ➡.*

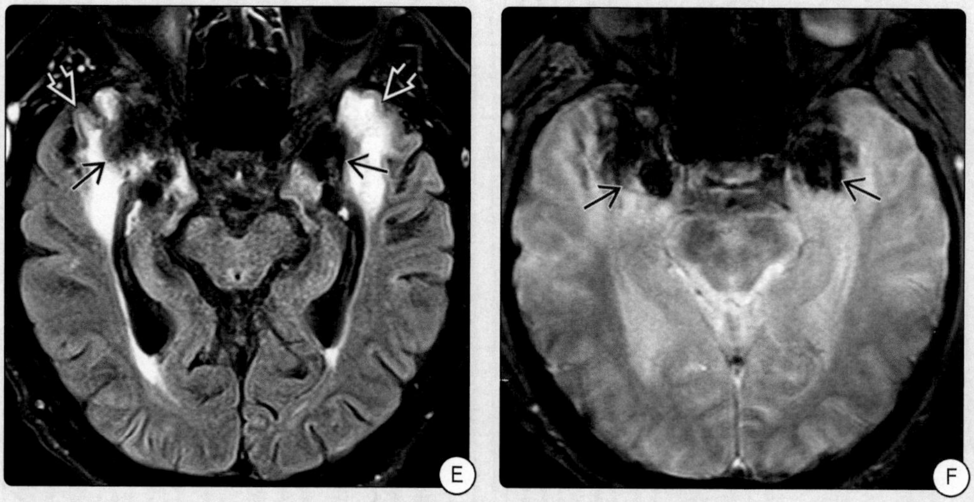

(12-53E) *FLAIR performed 5 months later shows severe atrophy. Temporal lobe confluent hyperintensities ➡ with patchy foci of marked hypointensity ➡ are consistent with encephalomalacia and chronic hemorrhage.* ***(12-53F)*** *T2* GRE shows marked confluent "blooming" in both anterior temporal lobes ➡ from the old hemorrhages. Similar findings were present in the insular cortex and cingulate gyri (not shown).*

HHV-6 encephalitis usually involves just the medial temporal lobes, but, if extrahippocampal lesions are present, it may be difficult to distinguish from HSE solely on the basis of imaging findings.

Antibody-mediated CNS disorders such as **limbic encephalitis** and **autoimmune encephalitis** often have a more protracted, subacute onset and frequently present with altered mental status of unclear etiology. In some cases, imaging findings may be virtually indistinguishable from those of HSE.

HHV-6 Encephalopathy

Etiology

More than 90% of the general population is seropositive for HHV-6 by 2 years of age. Most primary infections are asymptomatic, after which the virus remains latent.

Clinical Issues

HHV-6 can become pathogenic in immunocompromised patients, especially those with hematopoietic stem cell or solid organ transplantation. The median interval between transplantation and onset of neurologic symptoms is 3 weeks. Patients typically present with altered mental status, short-term memory loss, and seizures.

Imaging

NECT scans are typically normal. MR shows predominant or exclusive involvement of one or both medial temporal lobes (hippocampus and amygdala) **(12-54)**. Extrahippocampal disease is less common than with HSE. Transient hyperintensity of the mesial temporal lobes on T2WI and FLAIR with restriction on DWI is typical. T2* (GRE, SWI) scans show no evidence of hemorrhage.

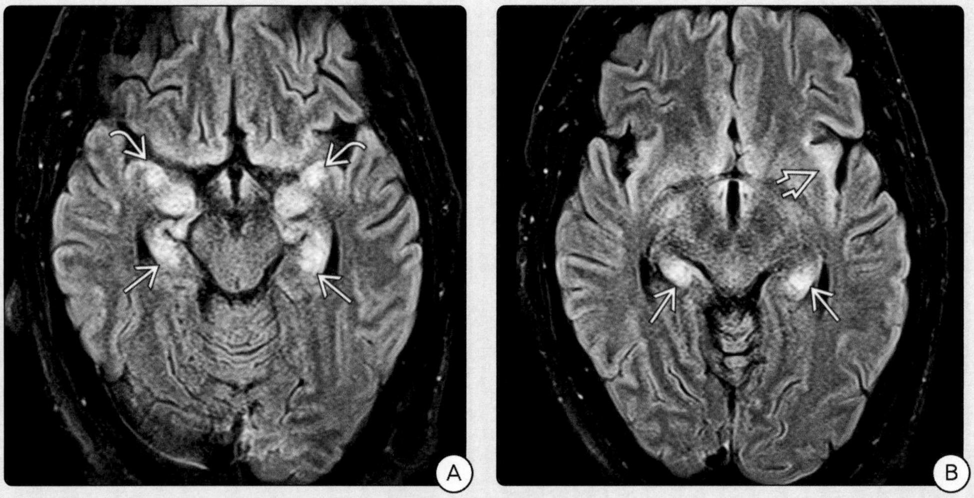

***(12-54A)** Axial FLAIR in a 43y man with proven HHV-6 encephalitis shows bilaterally symmetrical hyperintensity in the hippocampi and anteromedial temporal lobes, including the amygdalae. **(12-54B)** More cephalad FLAIR shows involvement of the hippocampal tails and left insular cortex.*

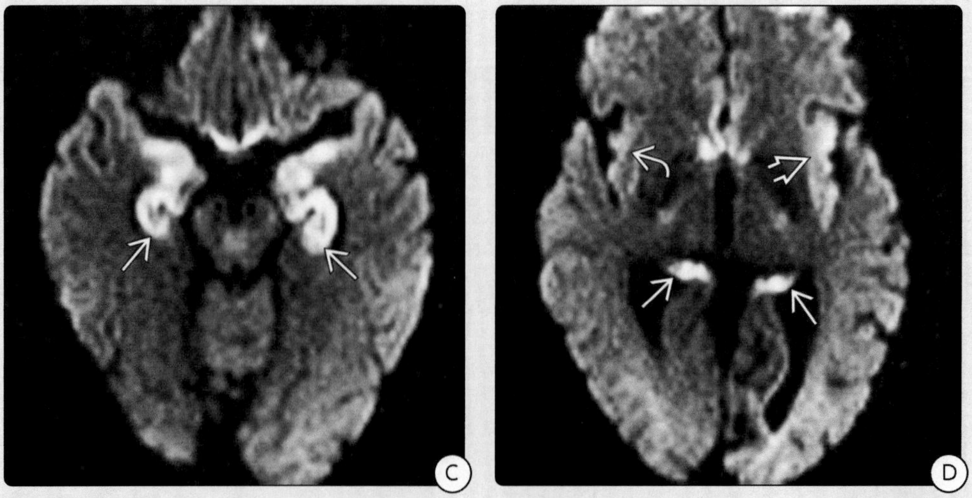

***(12-54C)** DWI shows strong, symmetric diffusion restriction in the hippocampi, medial temporal lobes, and amygdalae. **(12-54D)** DWI shows restricted diffusion in the hippocampal tails and left insular cortex. There is also mild involvement of the right insular cortex. This is variant HHV-6 encephalitis with extrahippocampal involvement.*

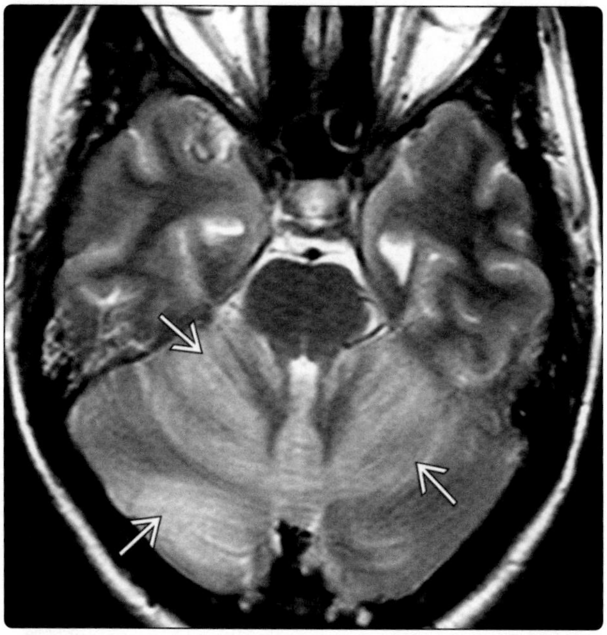

(12-55) T2WI in a 9y girl with a 2-week history of ear infection, headaches, confusion, and ataxia shows acute cerebellitis. Note edema and mass effect, seen as hyperintensity in both cerebellar hemispheres ➡. PCR was positive for VZV.

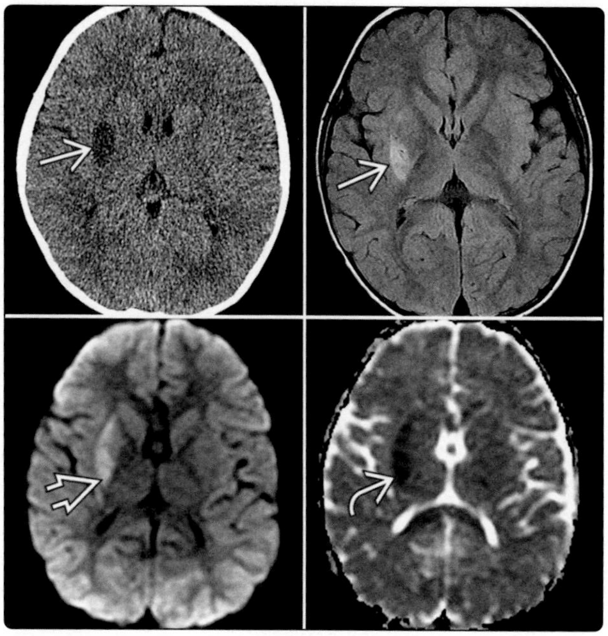

(12-56) VZV vasculitis with basal ganglia infarct in a 4y girl is shown. NECT and FLAIR scans show putaminal infarct ➡ that restricts, as shown on DWI ➡ and ADC ➡.

Differential Diagnosis

The major differential diagnosis is **HSE**. The disease course of HSE is more fulminant. Extratemporal involvement and hemorrhagic necrosis are common in HSE but rare in HHV-6 encephalopathy. In contrast to HSE, in HHV-6, MR abnormalities tend to resolve with time. **Postictal hippocampal hyperemia** is transient, and extrahippocampal involvement is absent.

HHV-6 ENCEPHALITIS

Clinical Issues
- Patients often immunocompromised
  - Hematopoietic stem cell, solid organ transplants

Imaging Findings
- Bilateral medial temporal lobes
  - Symmetric > asymmetric involvement
  - Extratemporal lesions less common than in HSE
- T2/FLAIR hyperintense
- Restricts on DWI

Differential Diagnosis
- HSE, limbic encephalitis
- Postictal hyperemia

Miscellaneous Acute Viral Encephalitides

Viral encephalitis is a medical emergency. Prognosis depends on both the specific pathogen and host immunologic status. Timely, accurate diagnosis and prompt therapy can improve survival and reduce the likelihood of brain injury.

Many viruses can cause encephalitis. Over 100 different viruses in more than a dozen families have been implicated in CNS infection. HSV-1, EBV, mumps, measles, and enteroviruses are responsible for most cases of encephalitis in immunocompetent patients.

Viral infection of the CNS is almost always part of generalized systemic disease. Most viruses infect the brain via hematogeneous spread. Others—such as some of the herpesviruses and rabies virus—are neurotropic and spread directly from infected mucosa or conjunctiva along nerve roots into the CNS.

CSF or serum analysis with pathogen identification by PCR amplification establishes the definitive diagnosis. Nevertheless, imaging is essential to early diagnosis and treatment.

The most common nonepidemic viral encephalitis, herpes encephalitis, was discussed earlier. In this section, we consider additional examples of viral CNS infections. We begin with two other members of the herpesvirus family—VCV and EBV. We then turn our attention to selected sporadic and epidemic encephalitides.

Varicella-Zoster Encephalitis

The incidence of VZV infection has decreased significantly since the introduction of a live attenuated VZV vaccine in 1995. Yet despite widespread vaccination rates, VZV continues to cause CNS disease. VZV, which causes chickenpox (varicella) and shingles (zoster), also causes Bell palsy, Ramsay-Hunt syndrome, meningitis, encephalitis, myelitis, Reye syndrome, and postherpetic neuralgia.

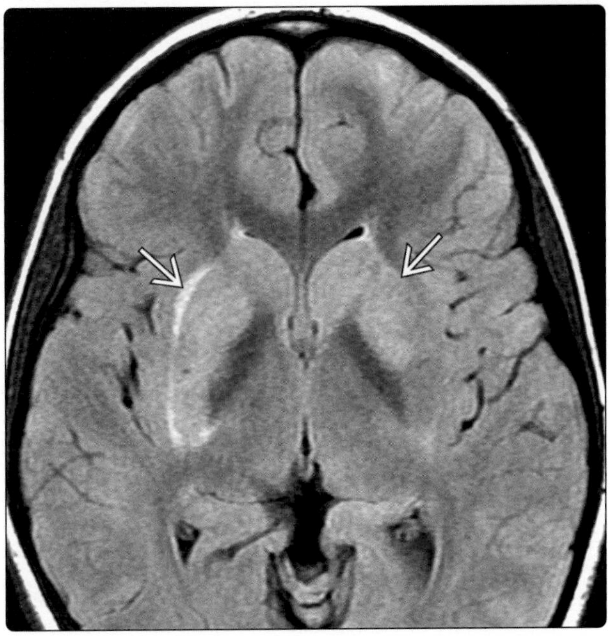

***(12-57)** FLAIR image in a 13y girl with fever and headache shows bilateral hyperintensities in the basal ganglia ➡. PCR was positive for EBV. EBV may affect the optic nerves and chiasm as well.*

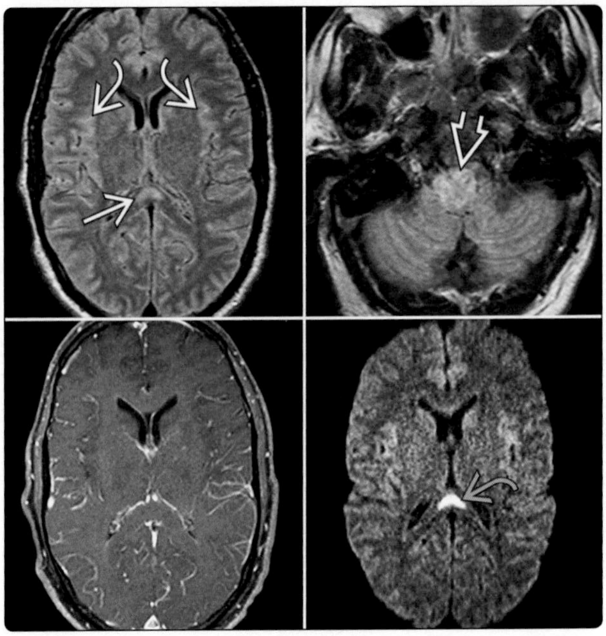

***(12-58)** FLAIR image of EBV encephalitis in a 29y man with headache, fever, diplopia, and somnolence shows sulcal hyperintensities ➡, focal lesion in CC splenium ➡, medulla ➡. WM lesions don't enhance; splenium lesion restricts on DWI ➡.*

VZV may cause a vasculopathy of both intra- and extracerebral arteries. Ischemic or hemorrhagic strokes, aneurysms, subarachnoid and parenchymal hemorrhages, arterial ectasias, and dissections have all been described.

VZV encephalitis has a wide age range with a median age at diagnosis of 46 years. Between 25-30% of patients are under 18 years of age.

Symptoms generally begin 10 days after chickenpox rash or varicella vaccination. Note, however, that many patients with CNS VZV disease present without the characteristic accompanying zoster rash.

Meningitis is the most frequent overall manifestation (50% of cases) and the most common clinical presentation in immunocompetent patients (90%). Encephalitis is the second most common CNS presentation (42%) but the most common manifestation in immunodeficient patients (67%). The most common presentation in children is acute cerebellar ataxia. Acute disseminated encephalomyelitis (ADEM) is rare (8%).

Cerebellitis with diffuse cerebellar swelling and hyperintensity on T2/FLAIR scan is common **(12-55)**. Children may develop multifocal leukoencephalopathy with patchy foci of T2/FLAIR hyperintensity. VZV vasculopathy with stroke causes multifocal cortical, basal ganglia, and deep white matter hyperintensities **(12-56)**. Enhancement on T1 C+ FS scans is variable in VZV encephalitis, and, when it occurs, it is typically patchy and mild. Restriction on DWI is common.

Epstein-Barr Encephalitis

EBV causes infectious mononucleosis. Uncontrolled proliferation of EBV-infected B cells results in posttransplant lymphoproliferative disease (PTLD). EBV is found in more than 90% of PTLD cases occurring within the first posttransplant year.

Mononucleosis is usually a benign, self-limiting disease. Neurologic complications occur in less than 7% of cases, but occasionally CNS disease can be the sole manifestation of EBV infection. Seizures, polyradiculomyelitis, transverse myelitis, encephalitis, cerebellitis, meningitis, and cranial nerve palsies have all been described as complications of EBV.

EBV has a predilection for deep gray nuclei. Bilateral diffuse T2/FLAIR hyperintensities in the basal ganglia and thalami are common **(12-57)**. Patchy white matter hyperintensities are seen in some cases. EBV can also cause a transient, reversible lesion of the corpus callosum splenium that demonstrates restriction on DWI **(12-58)**.

The differential diagnosis of EBV includes ADEM and other viral infections, especially West Nile virus.

West Nile Virus Encephalitis

West Nile virus (WNV) is a mosquito-borne Flavivirus that causes periodic epidemics of febrile illness and sporadic encephalitis in Africa, the Mediterranean basin, Europe, and southwest Asia. The first outbreak in the Western hemisphere occurred in New York in 1999. Since then, WNV has spread across North America and into parts of Central and South America. WNV is now the most common cause of epidemic meningoencephalitis in North America.

WNV cycles between mosquito vectors and bird hosts; humans are incidental hosts. Transmission increases in warmer months; in the Northern hemispheres, peak activity is from July through October. Nearly 80% of human WNV infections are clinically silent. Mild, self-limited fever is seen in 20%. Less

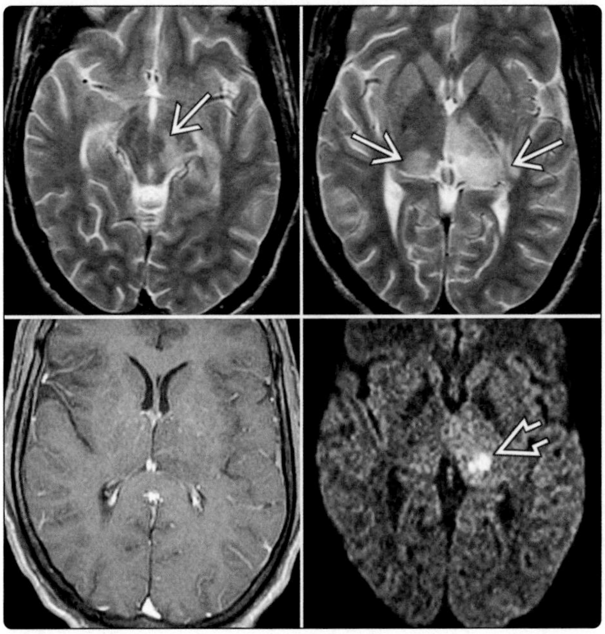

(12-59) Typical findings of West Nile virus (WNV) encephalitis include bilateral but asymmetric nonenhancing lesions in the basal ganglia and midbrain . DWI may demonstrate restriction . WNV is also tropic for spinal cord GM.

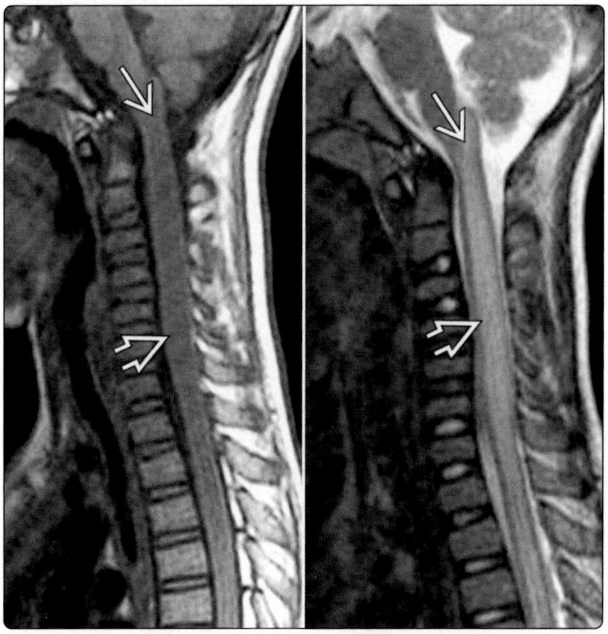

(12-60) Sagittal T1 (L) and T2 (R) scans show findings of rabies encephalomyelitis. Note involvement of the medulla and cervicothoracic spinal cord . (Courtesy R. Ramakantan, MD.)

than 1% of patients develop neuro-invasive disease. Immunosuppressed patients and the elderly are at higher risk.

WNV CNS infection can result in meningitis, encephalitis, and acute flaccid paralysis/poliomyelitis. The definitive diagnosis is made by PCR.

Bilateral hyperintensities on T2/FLAIR in the basal ganglia, thalami, and brainstem are typical **(12-59)**. WNV may cause a transient corpus callosum splenium lesion. Lesions restrict on DWI but rarely enhance.

Rabies Encephalitis

Rabies encephalitis is caused by a neurotropic RNA virus of the Rhabdoviridae family and is a significant public health problem in developing countries.

Nearly 55,000 deaths due to rabies encephalitis occur annually, 99% of them in Asia and Africa. The dog is the major vector and viral reservoir, although other mammals (e.g., bats, wolves, raccoons, skunks, and mongooses) may act as major hosts. The virus is abundant in the saliva of the infected animal and is deposited in bite wounds.

The virus replicates in muscle tissues at the wound, then infects motor neurons, and accesses the CNS by retrograde axoplasmic flow.

Human rabies encephalitis is a rapidly fulminant disease that is invariably fatal once clinical symptoms become evident. The history and clinical presentation are highly suggestive, but the definitive diagnosis requires laboratory confirmation of rabies antigen or rabies antibodies or isolation of the virus from biologic samples.

Rabies virus has a predilection for the brainstem, thalami, and hippocampi. MR shows poorly delineated hyperintensities in the dorsal medulla and upper spinal cord **(12-60)**, pontine tegmentum, periaqueductal gray matter, midbrain, medial thalami/hypothalami, and hippocampi. Hemorrhage and enhancement are generally absent, helping differentiate rabies from Japanese encephalitis and other viral encephalitides.

Influenza-Associated Encephalopathy

Influenza-associated encephalitis or encephalopathy (IAE) is characterized by high fever, convulsions, severe brain edema, and high mortality. It usually affects children younger than 5 years. Onset of neurologic deterioration occurs a few days to a week after the first signs of influenza infection. Many viruses have been reported as causing IAE, most recently H3N2 and influenza A (H1N1, also known as swine flu). The morbidity and mortality are particularly impressive among patients with trisomy 21 **(12-68)**.

Imaging studies are abnormal in the majority of cases. Symmetric bilateral thalamic lesions **(12-61)**, hemispheric edema, and reversible lesions in the corpus callosum splenium and WM are common. Findings resembling posterior reversible encephalopathy syndrome (PRES) have also been reported.

Acute Necrotizing Encephalopathy

Acute necrotizing encephalopathy (ANE) is a more severe, life-threatening form of IAE characterized by high fever, seizures, and rapid clinical deterioration within 2 or 3 days after symptom onset. The disease is often fatal. Most cases occur in children or young adults.

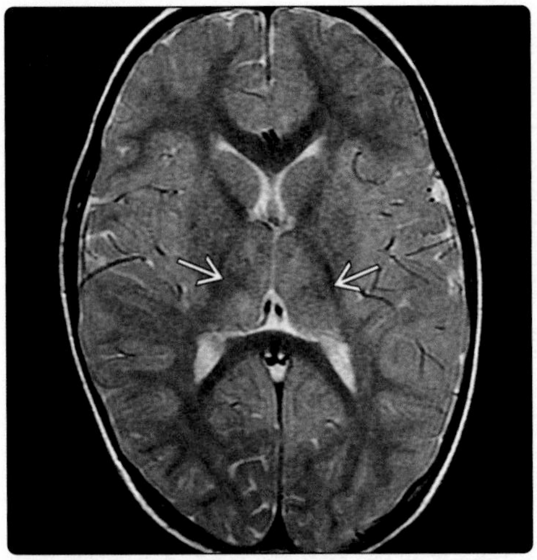

(12-61) T2WI in a 2y girl with influenza-associated encephalopathy (IAE) shows bithalamic fluffy hyperintensities ➡.

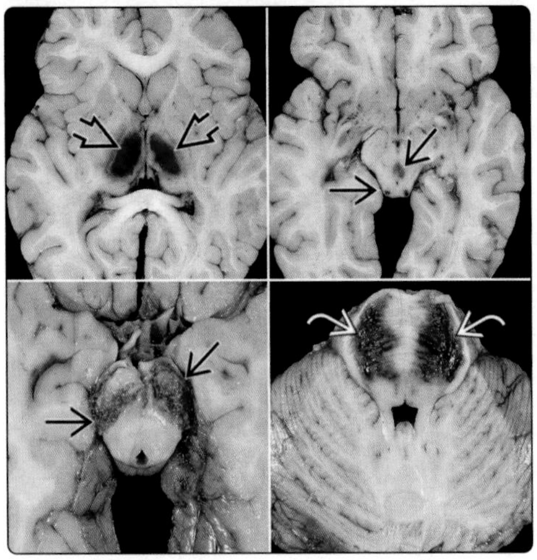

(12-62) Autopsied case of ANE shows symmetric hemorrhagic necrosis in thalami ➡, midbrain ➡, and pons ➡. (Courtesy R. Hewlett, MD.)

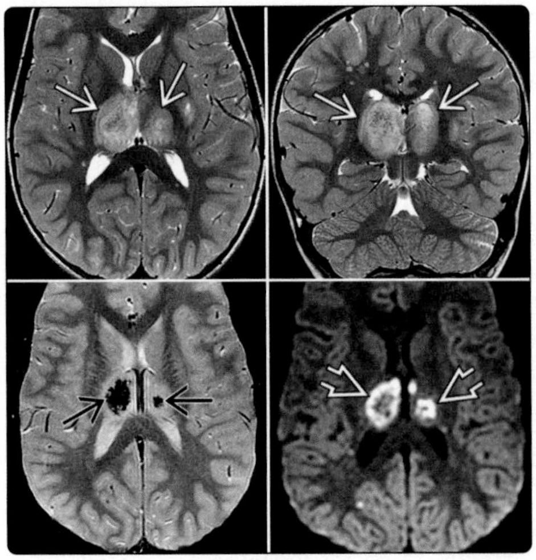

(12-63) ANE in obtunded 4y girl w/ influenza A shows bithalamic T2WI hyperintense lesions ➡, hemorrhage on T2 ➡, diffusion restriction ➡.*

ANE causes symmetric, often hemorrhagic, brain necrosis. The thalami, midbrain tegmentum, and pons are most severely affected **(12-62)**. Periventricular white matter, cerebellar, and spinal cord involvement has been reported in some cases.

CT may be normal early in the disease course. Bilaterally symmetric hyperintensity in the thalami is seen on T2/FLAIR **(12-63)**. The midbrain, pons, cerebellum, and deep cerebral white matter are frequently involved. T2* (GRE, SWI) shows "blooming" foci of petechial hemorrhage, most often in the thalami. Restriction on DWI has been described in some cases.

Miscellaneous Infectious Viral Encephalitides

A host of other viral encephalitides have been identified. Whereas some (such as rotavirus encephalitis) are widespread, others (e.g., Japanese encephalitis, LaCrosse encephalitis, Nipah virus encephalitis) currently have a more restricted geographic distribution.

Encephalitis caused by a member of the pediatric *respiratory virus group* **(Table 12-2)** often demonstrates basal ganglia and thalamic T2 prolongation and variable diffusivity changes on MR.

Arthropod-borne (ticks and mosquitoes) viruses represent an underappreciated cause of encephalitis in older pediatric patients and adults. Most of these viruses are from the *Flaviviridae* family. MR demonstrates T2 hyperintense lesions of the thalami, substantial nigra, basal ganglia, brainstem, cerebellum, and cerebral cortical and hemispheric WM.

Chronic Encephalitides

Some viruses cause acute, fulminating CNS infection. Others have a more insidious onset, producing a "slow" chronic infection. Some—such as the measles virus—can cause both. In this section, we briefly consider two chronic encephalitides: the measles reactivation syndrome called subacute sclerosing panencephalitis and Rasmussen encephalitis.

Subacute Sclerosing Panencephalitis

Subacute sclerosing panencephalitis (SSPE) is a rare progressive encephalitis that occurs years after measles virus infection. A few cases in immunocompromised patients occur following immunization. The measles virus infects neurons and remains latent for years. Why and how reactivation occurs are not fully understood.

Measles virus disproportionately affects children in regions with low measles vaccination rates. Almost all patients are children or adolescents; adult-onset SSPE occurs but is rare. There is a 2:1 male predominance. SSPE is rare in developed countries where vaccination rates are high.

On average, clinical manifestations appear 6 years after measles virus infection. Symptom onset is often insidious, with behavioral and cognitive deterioration, myoclonic seizures, and progressive motor impairment. Elevated measles antibody titers in CSF establish the diagnosis.

SSPE shows relentless progression **(12-64)**. More than 95% of patients die within 5 years, most within 1-6 months after symptom onset. To date, there is no effective treatment.

Imaging may be normal in the early stages of the disease, so normal MR does not exclude SSPE. Inflammatory infiltrates in cortical gray matter are the major pathologic findings in early SSPE; gray matter reduction in the frontotemporal cortex may occur before other lesions become apparent **(12-65)**. Other abnormal findings eventually develop, with bilateral but asymmetric cortical and subcortical white matter and periventricular and

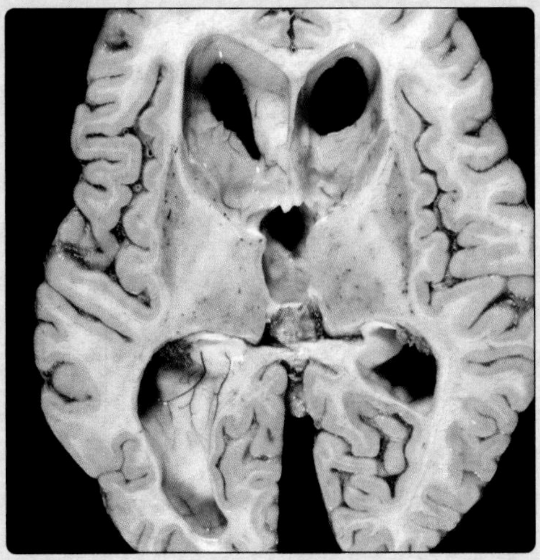

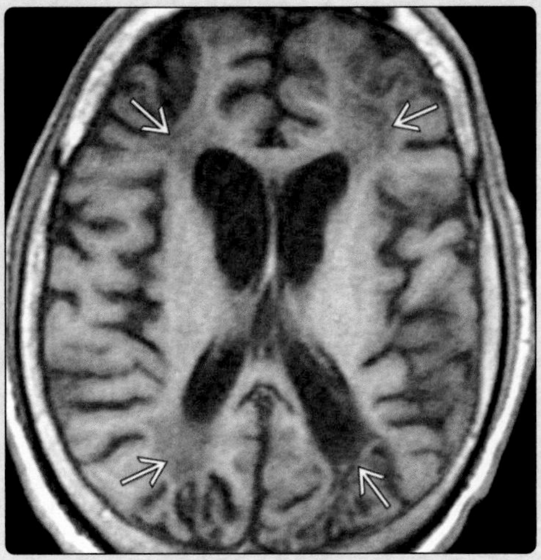

(12-64) *Autopsy of SSPE shows grossly enlarged ventricles and sulci with striking volume loss in basal ganglia and cerebral WM. In the occipital poles, the WM is so thin the ventricles almost contact the cortical GM.* ***(12-65)*** *T1WI in a 16y boy with deteriorating school performance and behavioral change shows diffuse atrophy with bifrontal and bioccipital hypointensities →. CSF was positive for measles antibodies.*

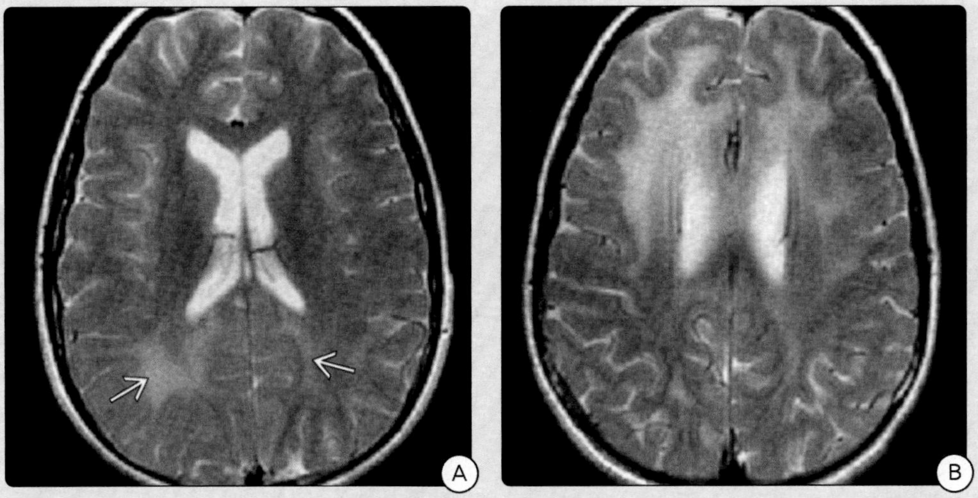

(12-66A) *Axial T2WI in a 13y child with unexplained cognitive decline and progressive motor impairment shows bilateral asymmetric WM hyperintensities in both occipital lobes →. The frontal WM appears normal. The ventricles are mildly enlarged for the patient's age.* ***(12-66B)*** *T2WI in the same child 6 months later shows WM hyperintensities having spread to involve both the frontal and parietal lobes. CSF was positive for measles antibodies.*

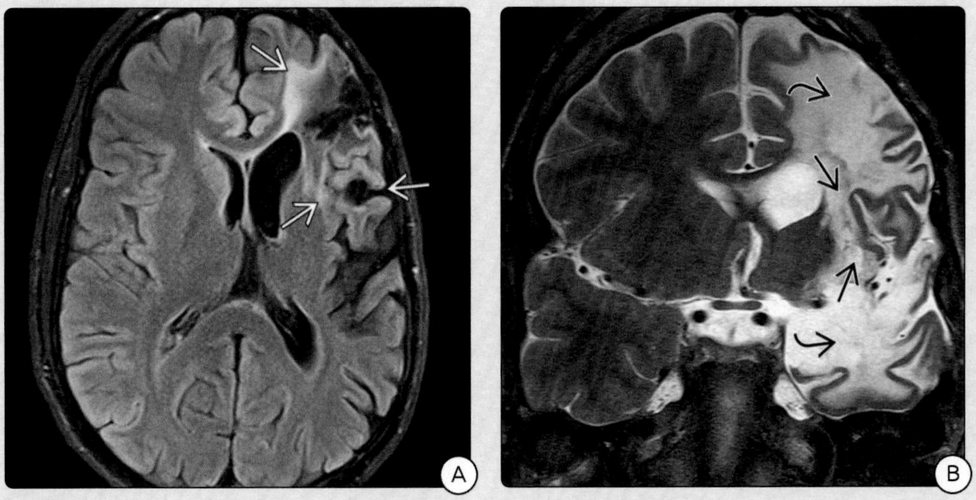

(12-67A) *Axial FLAIR in a 23y patient with medically refractory epilepsy secondary to RE shows left frontotemporal lobe volume loss with left lateral ventricle, sulcal enlargement. Note hyperintensity in WM, BG, insular cortex →.* ***(12-67B)*** *Coronal T2WI in the same patient shows fronto-temporal and insular atrophy → well. This is Rasmussen encephalitis. Note extensive WM hyperintensity, reflecting combination of edema and gliosis →.*

Imaging Features of Selected Causes of Acute Pediatric Encephalitis

Disorder	Imaging Findings
Bartonella henselae (cat scratch disease)	May cause vasculitis and stroke, T2 hyperintense lesions in thalami, basal ganglia, and WM
Epstein-Barr virus encephalitis	Shows tropism for deep gray matter structures, nonspecific involvement of cortex and hemispheric WM, cause of optic neuritis
Arthropod-borne encephalitis	Bilateral thalamic, symmetric or asymmetric T2 hyperintensities, without or with putamen and caudate involvement
HSV encephalitis, children and adolescence	Limbic system involvement, asymmetric–bilateral hemorrhage, deep gray matter spared
Japanese encephalitis	T2 prolongation of lesions involving thalami and hypothalami, minimal enhancement, reduced diffusion of lesions
Lyme disease	Subcortical WM T2 hyperintense lesions, periventricular WM lesions that mimic MS, nerve root and meningeal enhancement
Measles encephalomyelitis	Predominant involvement of thalami, corpus striatum, and cerebral cortex with T2 hyperintense lesions
Mycoplasma pneumoniae encephalitis	Leptomeningeal infiltration, may resemble primary angiitis enhancement of nerve roots, subcortical WM T2 hyperintense lesions
Nonpolio enteroviruses	Diverse, rhombencephalitis, leptomeningeal enhancement, cerebellar T2 hyperintense lesions
West Nile virus encephalitis	Bilateral basal ganglia and thalamic T2 hyperintense lesions

(Table 12-2) *WM = white matter.*

basal ganglia hyperintensity on T2/FLAIR sequences **(12-66)**. Diffuse atrophy with ventricular and sulcal enlargement ensues as the disease progresses. MRS shows decreased NAA and choline with elevated myoinositol and glutamine/glutamate.

Rasmussen Encephalitis

Rasmussen encephalitis (RE) is also called chronic focal (localized) encephalitis. RE is a rare progressive chronic encephalitis characterized by drug-resistant epilepsy, progressive hemiparesis, and mental impairment.

The exact etiology of RE is unknown. Viral infection or autoimmune disease such as **NMDA receptor encephalitis** following HSV infection have been suggested as possible etiologies. Biopsy findings are nonspecific, with leptomeningeal and perivascular lymphocytic infiltrates, microglial nodules, neuronal loss, and gliosis. Patients are clinically normal until seizures begin, usually between the ages of 14 months and 14 years. Peak onset is between 3 and 6 years. Neurologic deficits are progressive, and the seizures often become medically refractory. Treatment options have included immunomodulatory therapy, focal cortical resection, and functional hemispherectomy.

Initial imaging studies are usually normal. With time, hyperintensity on T2/FLAIR develops in the cortex and subcortical white matter of the affected hemisphere **(12-67)**. The disease is characterized by unilateral progressive cortical atrophy. Basal ganglia atrophy is seen in the majority of cases. MRS findings are nonspecific with decreased NAA and increased Cho. Myoinositol may be mildly elevated.

CHRONIC ENCEPHALITIDES

Subacute Sclerosing Panencephalitis (SSPE)
- Measles virus reactivation
- Occurs years after initial infection
- Almost always fatal
- WM hyperintensity
- Progressive atrophy

Rasmussen Encephalitis
- Etiology unknown (viral, autoimmune)
- Medically refractory epilepsy
- Unilateral
- WM hyperintensity, volume loss

MISCELLANEOUS NEUROTROPIC VIRUS INFECTIONS

Varicella-Zoster Encephalitis
- After chickenpox or vaccination
- Cortex, GM-WM junction, deep gray nuclei
- Cerebellitis, leukoencephalopathy, vasculopathy

Epstein-Barr Virus Encephalitis
- Rare mononucleosis complication
- Bilateral BG, midbrain, WM/splenium
- Cranial nerves, myelitis, polyneuropathies

West Nile Virus Encephalitis
- Most common epidemic meningoencephalitis in North America
- Bilateral BG, thalami, brainstem
- Cranial nerves, spinal cord/cauda equina

Rabies Encephalitis
- Developing > > developed countries
- Gray matter predominates
- Brainstem, thalami, spinal cord; limbic system

Influenza-Associated Encephalopathy (IAE)
- H1N1 (influenza A or "swine flu")
- Bilateral thalami, corpus callosum splenium
- Acute necrotizing encephalopathy
  - More fulminant form of IAE (often fatal)

Nipah Virus
- Multifocal T2/FLAIR hyperintensities
- ± DWI restriction, enhancement

Rotavirus Encephalitis
- Common GI pathogen in children
- Cerebellitis, corpus callosum splenium

Japanese Encephalitis
- Most common human endemic encephalitis
  - Korea, Japan, India, Southeast Asia
- Bilateral thalami, BG, substantia nigra, hippocampi
- High morbidity, mortality

LaCrosse Encephalitis
- School-aged children (Midwest USA)
- Mimics herpes simplex encephalitis but more benign

Chikungunya Encephalitis
- CHIKV-associated CNS disease
- Flavivirus related to dengue, West Nile, Japanese encephalitis
- Usually < 1 year and > 65 years
- 15-20% fatality
- Multifocal T2/FLAIR WM hyperintensities, DWI restriction

Zika Virus
- *A. aegypti* mosquito
- A flavivirus similar to dengue, West Nile virus, etc.
- Transmitted congenitally, sexually, blood products
- Microcephaly in newborn
- May cause Guillain-Barré syndrome, possibly other neurologic disorders

Dengue Virus
- Can cause dengue hemorrhagic fever, dengue shock syndrome
- BG, thalami, temporal lobes, pons, cord

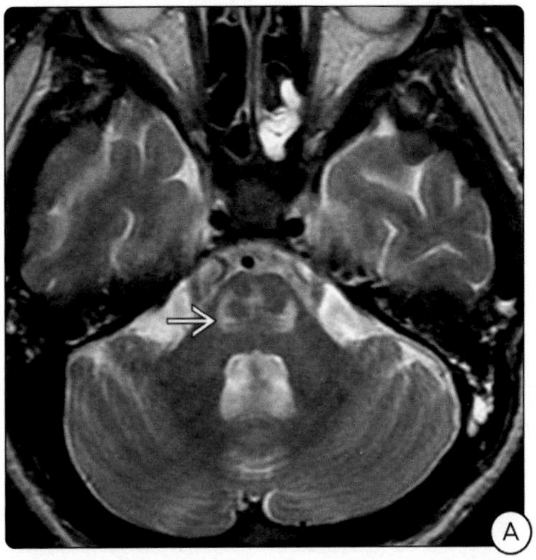

***(12-68A)** Axial T2WI in a 15y comatose boy with trisomy 21 and flu-like symptoms shows pontine hyperintensity ➡ resembling CPM.*

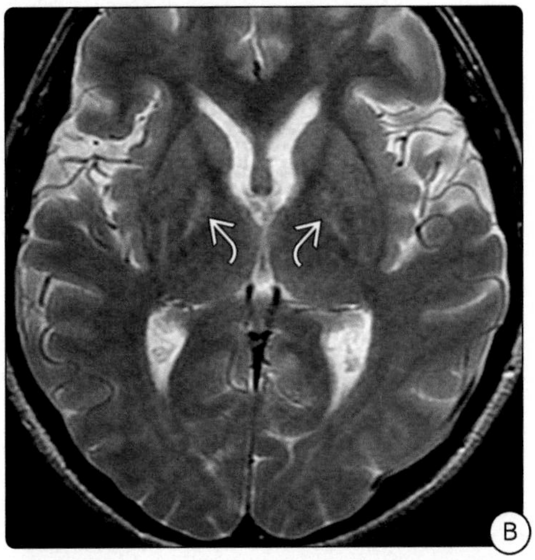

***(12-68B)** More cephalad T2WI shows bilateral hyperintensities in the globi pallidi ➡ but otherwise appears normal.*

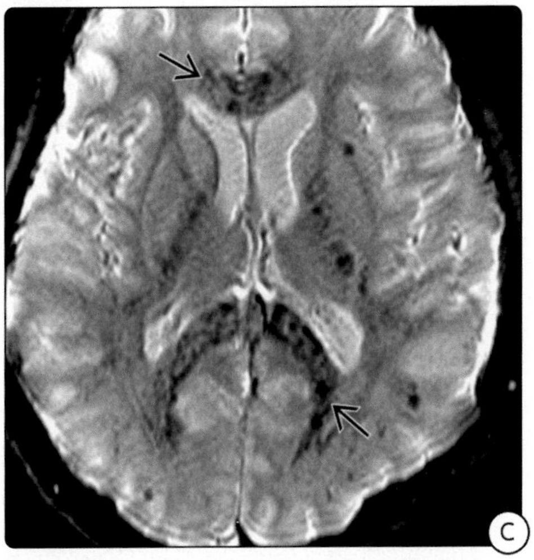

***(12-68C)** T2*GRE shows extensive cerebral microbleeds ➡, predominately in the white matter. This is PCR+ for H1N1 virus.*

Selected References

Congenital Infections

Lee J: Malformations of cortical development: genetic mechanisms and diagnostic approach. Korean J Pediatr. 60(1):1-9, 2017

Kahle KT et al: Hydrocephalus in children. Lancet. 387(10020):788-99, 2016

Arbelaez A et al: Congenital brain infections. Top Magn Reson Imaging. 23(3):165-72, 2014

Parmar H et al: Pediatric intracranial infections. Neuroimaging Clin N Am. 22(4):707-25, 2012

Congenital Cytomegalovirus

Kawasaki H et al: Pathogenesis of developmental anomalies of the central nervous system induced by congenital cytomegalovirus infection. Pathol Int. 67(2):72-82, 2017

Herpes Simplex Virus: Congenital and Neonatal Infections

Harris JB et al: Neonatal herpes simplex viral infections and acyclovir: an update. J Pediatr Pharmacol Ther. 22(2):88-93, 2017

Zika Virus Infection

Yun SI et al: Zika virus: an emerging flavivirus. J Microbiol. 55(3):204-219, 2017

Coyne CB et al: Zika virus - reigniting the TORCH. Nat Rev Microbiol. 14(11):707-715, 2016

Congenital (Perinatal) HIV

Muller WJ: Treatment of perinatal viral infections to improve neurologic outcomes. Pediatr Res. 81(1-2):162-169, 2017

Other Congenital Infections

Yazigi A et al: Fetal and neonatal abnormalities due to congenital rubella syndrome: a review of literature. J Matern Fetal Neonatal Med. 30(3):274-278, 2017

Acquired Pyogenic Infections

Meningitis

Dorsett M et al: Diagnosis and treatment of central nervous system infections in the emergency department. Emerg Med Clin North Am. 34(4):917-942, 2016

Wong AM et al: Arterial spin-labeling perfusion imaging of childhood meningitis: a case series. Childs Nerv Syst. 32(3):563-7, 2016

Shih RY et al: Bacterial, fungal, and parasitic infections of the central nervous system: radiologic-pathologic correlation and historical perspectives. Radiographics. 35(4):1141-69, 2015

Mohan S et al: Imaging of meningitis and ventriculitis. Neuroimaging Clin N Am. 22(4):557-83, 2012

Abscess

Brook I: Microbiology and treatment of brain abscess. J Clin Neurosci. 38:8-12, 2017

Sonneville R et al: An update on bacterial brain abscess in immunocompetent patients. Clin Microbiol Infect. ePub, 2017

Ventriculitis

Hazany S et al: Magnetic resonance imaging of infectious meningitis and ventriculitis in adults. Top Magn Reson Imaging. 23(5):315-25, 2014

Empyemas

Mattogno PP et al: Intracranial subdural empyema: diagnosis and treatment update. J Neurosurg Sci. ePub, 2017

Patel NA et al: Systematic review and case report: intracranial complications of pediatric sinusitis. Int J Pediatr Otorhinolaryngol. 86:200-12, 2016

Acquired Viral Infections

Boucher A et al: Epidemiology of infectious encephalitis causes in 2016. Med Mal Infect. 47(3):221-235, 2017

Koeller KK et al: Viral and prion infections of the central nervous system: radiologic-pathologic correlation: from the radiologic pathology archives. Radiographics. 37(1):199-233, 2017

Shives KD et al: Molecular mechanisms of neuroinflammation and injury during acute viral encephalitis. J Neuroimmunol. 308:102-111, 2017

Herpes Simplex Encephalitis

Gnann JW Jr et al: Herpes simplex encephalitis: an update. Curr Infect Dis Rep. 19(3):13, 2017

Nosadini M et al: Herpes simplex virus-induced anti-N-methyl-D-aspartate receptor encephalitis: a systematic literature review with analysis of 43 cases. Dev Med Child Neurol. ePub, 2017

Kaewpoowat Q et al: Herpes simplex and varicella zoster CNS infections: clinical presentations, treatments and outcomes. Infection. 44(3):337-45, 2016

Soares BP et al: Imaging of herpesvirus infections of the CNS. AJR Am J Roentgenol. 206(1):39-48, 2016

Miscellaneous Acute Viral Encephalitides

Koeller KK et al: Viral and prion infections of the central nervous system: radiologic-pathologic correlation: from the radiologic pathology archives. Radiographics. 37(1):199-233, 2017

Lin D et al: Reversible splenial lesions presenting in conjunction with febrile illness: a case series and literature review. Emerg Radiol. ePub, 2017

Saxena V et al: West Nile virus. Clin Lab Med. 37(2):243-252, 2017

Shives KD et al: Molecular mechanisms of neuroinflammation and injury during acute viral encephalitis. J Neuroimmunol. 308:102-111, 2017

Yun SI et al: Zika virus: an emerging flavivirus. J Microbiol. 55(3):204-219, 2017

Al-Qahtani AA et al: Zika virus: a new pandemic threat. J Infect Dev Ctries. 10(3):201-7, 2016

Billioux BJ et al: Neurological complications of Ebola virus infection. Neurotherapeutics. 13(3):461-70, 2016

Yoganathan S et al: Acute necrotising encephalopathy in a child with H1N1 influenza infection: a clinicoradiological diagnosis and follow-up. BMJ Case Rep. 2016:bcr2015213429, 2016

Tuberculosis and Fungal, Parasitic, and Other Infections

Overview

Infectious diseases are increasingly worldwide phenomena, with what once seemed exclusively local indigenous diseases rapidly spreading around the globe. New pathogens have emerged, as viruses such as HIV—almost unheard of 30 years ago—have become global health concerns. The rise in food and waterborne pathogens is unmistakable. Immigration and widespread travel have resulted in formerly exotic "tropical diseases" such as neurocysticercosis and other parasitic infections becoming commonplace.

In this chapter, we continue the delineation of acquired infections that we began in Chapter 12 with pyogenic and viral CNS infections. We first turn our attention to mycobacterial infections, focusing primarily on tuberculosis. We follow with an in-depth discussion of fungal and parasitic infections. We close the chapter with a brief consideration of miscellaneous and emerging CNS infections to remind us that the "hot zone" is right outside our windows, no matter where we live!

Mycobacterial Infections

Mycobacteria are small, rod-shaped, acid-fast bacilli with more than 125 recognized species. They are divided into three main groups, each with a different signature disease: (1) *Mycobacterium tuberculosis* (tuberculosis), (2) nontuberculous mycobacteria ("atypical" mycobacterial spectrum infections), and (3) *M. leprae* (leprosy). Each group has different pathologic features, clinical manifestations, and imaging findings.

Of the three groups, the so-called *M. tuberculosis* complex is responsible for the vast majority of human mycobacterial infections. It causes more than 98% of CNS tuberculosis (TB) and is therefore the major focus of our discussion. We follow with a brief review of nontuberculous mycobacterial infection and its rare manifestations in the head and neck. Leprosy causes peripheral neuropathy but virtually never affects the CNS and is not considered further.

Tuberculosis

Etiology

Most TB is caused by *M. tuberculosis*. Less common species that are also considered part of the *M. tuberculosis* complex include *M. africanum, M. microti, M. canetti,* and *M. bovis*. Human-to-human transmission is typical. Animal-to-human transmission via *M. bovis*, a common pathogen in the past, is now rarely encountered. Neurotuberculosis is secondary to hematogeneous spread from extracranial infection, most frequently in the lungs.

CNS TB begins with the development of small TB ("Rich") foci in the subpial or subependymal surfaces of the brain and spinal cord. Rupture of a Rich focus into the subarachnoid space causes meningitis, vasculitis, and occasionally encephalitis.

Pathology

CNS TB has several distinct pathologic manifestations. Acute/subacute TB **meningitis** (TBM) constitutes 70-80% of cases. An inflammatory reaction ("exudate") with a variable admixture of exudative, proliferative, and necrotizing components in the subarachnoid cisterns is the typical finding **(13-1)**. Rarely, TBM presents as an isolated pachymeningitis with focal or diffuse dura-arachnoid thickening.

The second most common manifestation of neurotuberculosis is a focal parenchymal infection with central caseating necrosis (TB granuloma or **tuberculoma**).

The least common manifestation of CNS TB is "abscess," which contains macrophages and liquefied necrotic debris. (As it usually does not contain pus with neutrophils, most TB "abscesses" are more correctly called pseudoabscesses.) TB **pseudoabscesses** are rare in immunocompetent patients but are found in 20% of patients coinfected with TB and HIV.

Location. TBM has a striking predilection for the basal cisterns although exudates in the superficial convexity sulci do occur.

Tuberculomas are space-occupying masses of granulomatous tissue. The majority occur in the cerebral hemispheres, especially the frontal and parietal lobes and basal ganglia. Occasionally, CNS TB presents as a focal dural **(13-11)**, intraventricular (choroid plexus), or isolated calvarial lesion.

TB abscesses can be found anywhere in the brain, from the hemispheres to the midbrain to the cerebellum.

Size and Number. Tuberculomas vary in size. The majority are small (less than 2.5 cm), and the "miliary" nodules are often just a few millimeters in diameter. "Giant" tuberculomas can reach 4-6 cm.

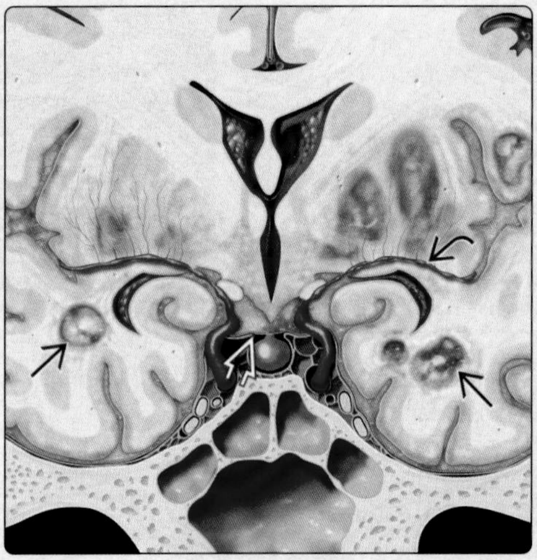
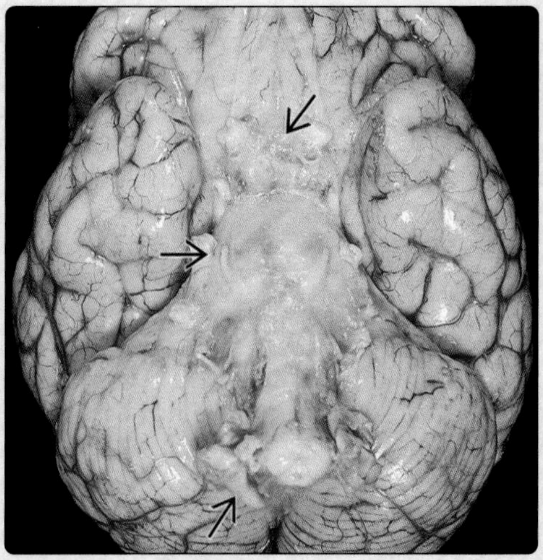

***(13-1)** Coronal graphic shows basilar TB meningitis (TBM) and tuberculomas, which often coexist. Note the vessel irregularity and early basal ganglia ischemia related to arteritis. **(13-2)** Autopsy case shows typical findings of TBM with dense exudates extending throughout the basal cisterns. Gross appearance is indistinguishable from that of pyogenic meningitis. (Courtesy R. Hewlett, MD.)*

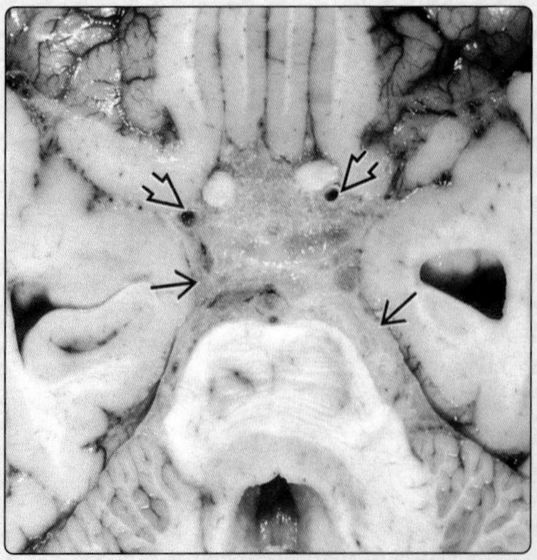
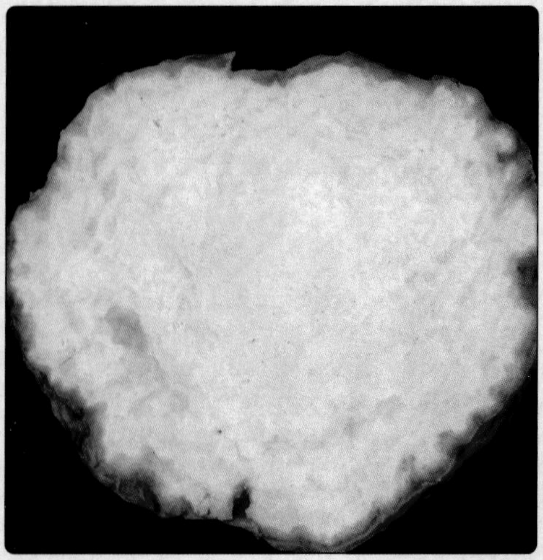

***(13-3)** Axial section through the suprasellar cistern in another autopsied case of TBM shows thick exudate filling the suprasellar cistern and coating the pons. Note the extremely small diameter of the supraclinoid internal carotid arteries due to TB vasculitis. (Courtesy R. Hewlett, MD.) **(13-4)** Surgically resected TB gumma shows the solid "cheesy" appearance of a caseating granuloma. (Courtesy R. Hewlett, MD.)*

Tuberculomas also vary in number, ranging from a solitary lesion to innumerable small "miliary" lesions.

Gross Pathology. TBM is seen as a dense, diffuse, glutinous exudate that accumulates in the basal cisterns, coating the brain surfaces and cranial nerves **(13-2)**. The suprasellar/chiasmatic region, ambient cisterns, and interpeduncular fossa are most commonly involved **(13-3)**.

Tuberculomas have a creamy, cheese-like, necrotic center surrounded by a grayish granulomatous rim **(13-4)**.

Microscopic Features. Edema, perivascular infiltrates, and microglial reaction are common in brain tissue immediately under the tuberculous exudate.

The inflammatory exudate encases major vessels and their perforating branches, invading vessel walls and causing a true panarteritis (sometimes called "endarteritis obliterans"). Vessel occlusions with secondary infarcts are identified in 40% of autopsied cases of TBM, most commonly in the basal ganglia and internal capsule. Large territorial infarcts are less common.

Mature tuberculomas demonstrate central caseating necrosis with a surrounding capsule that contains fibroblasts, multinucleated giant cells (generally Langerhans type), epithelioid histiocytes, plasma cells, and lymphocytes. Acid-fast bacilli may be difficult to identify.

TB abscesses consist of vascular granulation tissue with acid-fast bacilli, liquefied necrotic debris, and macrophages.

Clinical Issues

Epidemiology. TB is endemic in many developing countries and is reemerging in developed countries because of widespread immigration and HIV/AIDS. Worldwide, 8-10 million new cases are reported each year. The highest prevalence is in Southeast Asia, which accounts for one-third of all cases.

CNS infections account for only 10% of all TB infections but are among the most devastating of its many manifestations. One of the most common "brain tumors" in endemic countries is tuberculoma, which accounts for 10-30% of all brain parenchymal masses.

CNS TB occurs in both immunocompetent and immunocompromised patients. Among people with latent TB infection, HIV is the strongest known risk factor for progression to active TB. In TB and HIV/AIDS coinfection, each disease also greatly amplifies the lethality of the other.

Demographics. CNS TB occurs at all ages, but 60-70% of cases occur during the first two decades. There is no sex predilection.

Presentation. The most common manifestation of active CNS TB is meningitis (TBM). Presentation varies from fever and headache with mild meningismus to confusion, lethargy, seizures, and coma. Symptoms of increased intracranial pressure are common.

Cranial neuropathies, especially involving CNs II, III, IV, VI, and VII, are common.

Diagnosis. CSF shows low glucose, elevated protein, and lymphocytic pleocytosis. Acid-fast bacilli can sometimes be identified visually in CSF smears. Positive ELISA (sensitive) or Western blot (specific) immunoconfirmation as well as PCR or growth and identification of *M. tuberculosis* in cultures are the most common methods for establishing a definitive diagnosis of TBM.

Natural History and Treatment. Prognosis is variable and depends on the patient's immune status as well as treatment. Untreated TB can be fatal in 4-8 weeks. Even with treatment, one-third of patients deteriorate within 6 weeks. Overall mortality is 25-30% and is even higher in drug-resistant TB.

Multidrug-resistant TB (MDR TB) is resistant to at least two of the first-line anti-TB drugs, isoniazid and rifampin. **Extensively drug-resistant TB (XDR TB)** is defined as TB that is resistant to isoniazid and rifampin, any fluoroquinolone, and at least one of three injectable second-line drugs (i.e., amikacin, kanamycin, or capreomycin).

Common complications of CNS TB include hydrocephalus (70%) and stroke (up to 40%). The majority of survivors have long-term morbidity with seizures, mental retardation, neurologic deficits, and even paralysis.

CNS TB: ETIOLOGY, PATHOLOGY, AND CLINICAL ISSUES

Etiology
- *Mycobacterium tuberculosis* complex
  - Vast majority caused by *M. tuberculosis*
  - Other mycobacteria (e.g., *M. bovis*) rare
- Human-to-human transmission
- Hematogeneous spread from extracranial site
  - Lung > GI, GU
  - Other: bone, lymph nodes

Pathology
- TB meningitis (70-80%)
  - Exudative, proliferative, necrotizing inflammatory reaction
  - Basal cisterns > convexity sulci
- Tuberculoma (TB granuloma) (20-30%)
  - Caseating necrosis
  - Cerebral hemispheres, basal ganglia
- Pseudoabscess (rare)

Epidemiology and Demographics
- 8-10 million new cases annually
- All ages, but 60-70% in children < 20 years
- CNS TB in 2-5% of cases
- 10-30% of brain parenchymal masses in endemic areas

Presentation and Diagnosis
- Fever, headache, meningismus, signs of ↑ intracranial pressure
- PCR best, most rapid definitive diagnosis

Prognosis
- Overall mortality (25-30%)
- Worse with MDR or XDR TB

Imaging

General Features. Early diagnosis and treatment are necessary to reduce the significant morbidity and mortality associated with CNS TB. As CT scans may be normal in the earliest stages of TBM, contrast-enhanced MR is the imaging procedure of choice.

CT Findings

TB meningitis. Nonspecific hydrocephalus is the most frequent finding on NECT. "Blurred" ventricular margins indicate extracellular fluid accumulation in the subependymal white matter. As the disease progresses, iso- to mildly hyperdense basilar and sulcal exudates replace and efface the normal hypodense CSF **(13-5A)**. CECT usually shows intense enhancement of the basilar meninges and subarachnoid spaces **(13-5B)**.

Patients who deteriorate during treatment often develop new hydrocephalus, infarcts, exudates, or tuberculomas.

Tuberculoma. NECT scans show one or more iso- to slightly hyperdense round, lobulated, or crenated masses with variable perilesional edema. Calcification can be seen in healed granulomas **(13-6)**. CECT scans demonstrate punctate, solid, or ring-like enhancement **(13-7)**.

Abscess. TB abscesses are hypodense on NECT with significant mass effect and surrounding edema. Ring enhancement is seen on CECT.

MR Findings

TB meningitis. Basilar exudates are isointense with brain on T1WI, giving the appearance of "dirty" CSF. FLAIR scans show increased signal intensity in the sulci and cisterns. Marked linear or nodular meningeal enhancement is seen on T1 C+ FS sequences **(13-8)**. Focal or diffuse dura-arachnoid

***(13-5A)** NECT in a 6m child with tuberculous meningitis shows acute obstructive hydrocephalus with dilated temporal horns ➡ and effacement of the sylvian fissures with slightly hyperdense exudate ➡. **(13-5B)** CECT in the same case shows thick enhancing exudates throughout the basilar cisterns but most striking in the sylvian fissures ➡.*

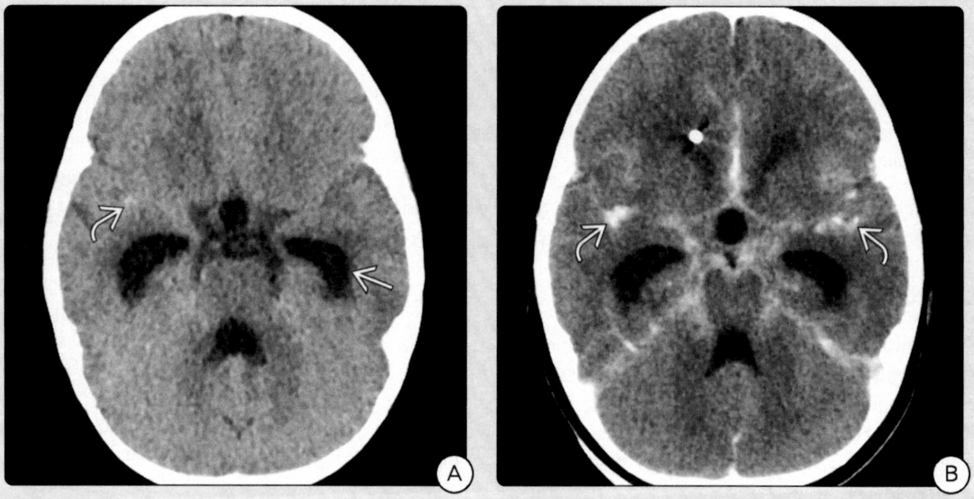

***(13-6)** Two different axial images from an NECT scan in a patient with CNS TB shows two calcified healed granulomas ➡. There was no evidence of active TBM. (Courtesy R. Ramakantan, MD.) **(13-7)** CECT scan in a 6y immunocompetent boy shows multiple small punctate-enhancing tuberculomas ➡.*

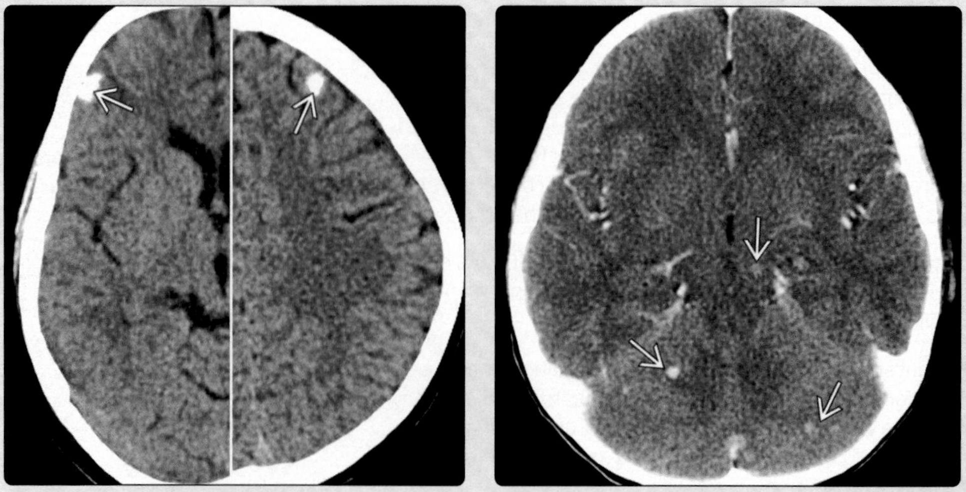

enhancement (pachymeningitis) with or without involvement of the underlying subarachnoid spaces may occur but is uncommon.

Tuberculous exudates often extend into the brain parenchyma along the perivascular spaces, causing a meningoencephalitis.

Vascular complications occur in 20-50% of cases. The "flow voids" of major arteries may appear irregular or reduced. Parenchyma adjacent to meningeal inflammation may demonstrate necrosis. Penetrating artery infarcts with enhancement and restricted diffusion are common.

Cranial nerve involvement is seen in 17-40% of cases. The optic nerve and CNs III, IV, and VII are most commonly affected. The affected cranial nerves appear thickened and enhance intensely on postcontrast images.

Tuberculoma. The most common parenchymal lesion in CNS TB is tuberculoma. Most TB granulomas are solid caseating, necrotizing lesions that appear hypo- or isointense with brain on T1WI and hypointense on T2WI **(13-9A)**. Liquefied areas may be T2 hyperintense with a hypointense rim and resemble abscess **(13-10A)**.

Enhancement is variable, ranging from small punctate foci to multiple rim-enhancing lesions. Mild to moderate round or lobulated ring-like enhancement around a nonenhancing center is the most typical pattern **(13-9B)** **(13-10B)**. pMR shows elevated relative cerebral blood volume in the cellular, hypervascular, enhancing rim. Solid caseating tuberculomas do not restrict on DWI although liquefied foci may restrict.

MRS can be very helpful in characterizing tuberculomas and distinguishing them from neoplasm or pyogenic abscess. A prominent decrease in NAA:Cr with a modest decrease in NAA:Cho is typical. A large lipid peak with absence of other metabolites such as amino acids and succinate is seen in 85-90% of cases **(13-10C)**.

Cerebritis and Abscess. Focal TB cerebritis is very rare. TB abscesses are also uncommon and can be solitary or multiple. They are often multiloculated, are typically larger than granulomas (> 3 cm), and can resemble neoplasm. TB abscesses are hypodense with peripheral edema and mass effect on NECT and show moderate ring enhancement on CECT.

Unlike tuberculomas, TB abscesses are usually hyperintense to brain on T2/FLAIR and restrict on DWI. A ring-enhancing multiloculated lesion or multiple separate lesions is the typical finding on T1 C+ images. MRS shows lipid and lactate peaks without evidence of cytosolic amino acids.

Differential Diagnosis

The major differential diagnosis of *TBM* is **pyogenic or carcinomatous meningitis**, as their imaging findings can be indistinguishable. **Carcinomatous meningitis** is usually seen in older patients with a known systemic or primary CNS neoplasm.

Neurosarcoidosis can also mimic TBM. Infiltration of the pituitary gland, infundibulum, and hypothalamus is common.

The major differential diagnosis of multiple parenchymal *tuberculomas* is **neurocysticercosis** (NCC). NCC usually shows multiple lesions in different stages of evolution. Tuberculomas can also resemble pyogenic **abscesses** or **neoplasms** **(13-11)** **(13-12)** **(13-13)**. Abscesses restrict on DWI. Tuberculomas have a large lipid peak on MRS and lack the elevated Cho typical of neoplasm.

TB *abscesses* appear identical to pyogenic abscesses on standard imaging studies. Both show restricted diffusion. MRS of TB abscesses shows no evidence of cytosolic amino acids, the spectral hallmark of pyogenic lesions.

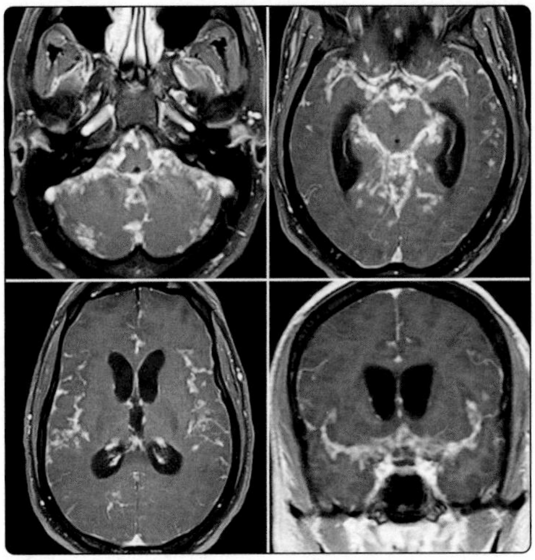

***(13-8)** T1 C+ FS scans show TBM with hydrocephalus, enhancing exudate throughout the basal cisterns and subarachnoid spaces.*

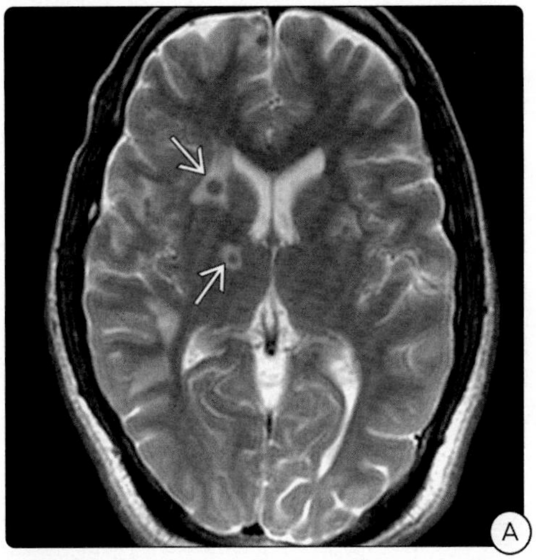

***(13-9A)** T2WI demonstrates multifocal tuberculomas as hypointense foci surrounded by edema ➡.*

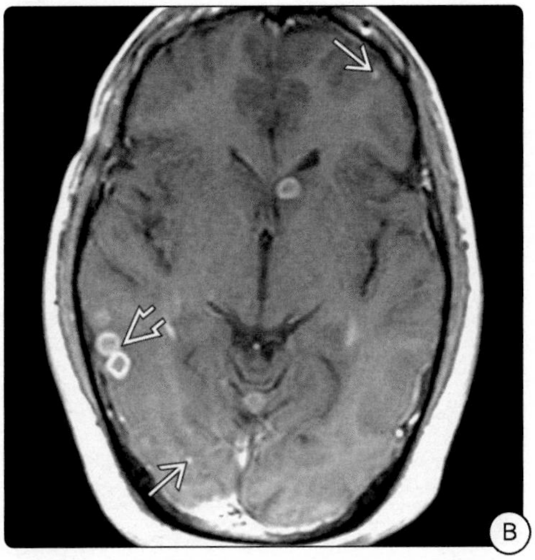

***(13-9B)** T1 C+ scan in the same case illustrates additional lesions with punctate ➡, ring enhancement ➡. (Courtesy R. Ramakantan, MD.)*

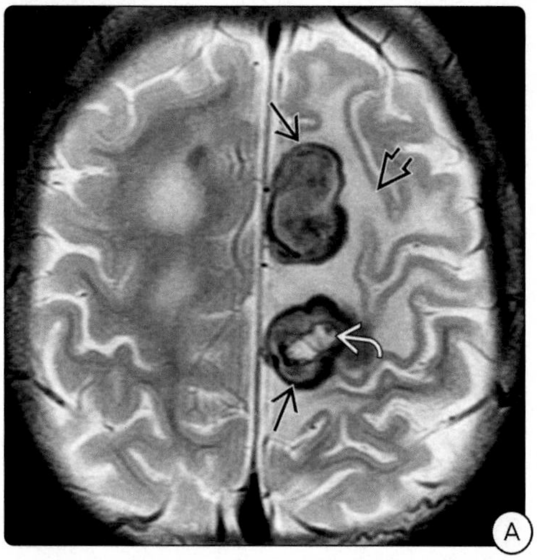

(13-10A) *Axial T2WI shows hypointense caseating tuberculomas → and edema →. Central liquefaction is hyperintense →.*

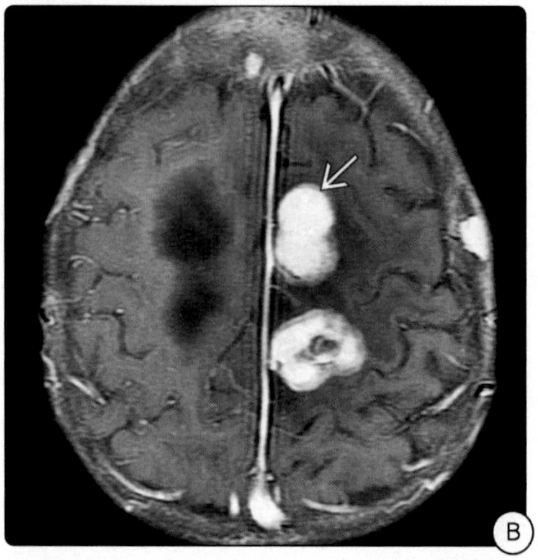

(13-10B) *T1 C+ FS scan demonstrates both solid → and thick rim enhancement.*

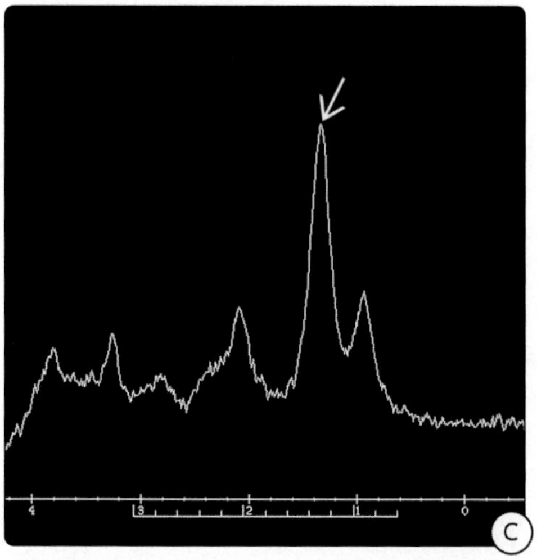

(13-10C) *MRS, with TE = 35 ms, demonstrates decreased NAA and prominent lipid lactate peak →.*

CNS TUBERCULOSIS: IMAGING AND DIFFERENTIAL DIAGNOSIS

General Features

- Best procedure = contrast-enhanced MR
- Findings vary with pathology
  - TB meningitis (TMB)
  - Tuberculoma
  - Abscess
- Combination of findings (usually TBM, tuberculoma)

CT Findings

- TBM
  - Can be normal in early stages!
  - Nonspecific hydrocephalus common
  - "Blurred" ventricular margins
  - Effaced basilar cisterns, sulci
  - Iso-/mildly hyperdense exudates
  - Thick, intense pia-subarachnoid space enhancement
  - Can cause pachymeningopathy with diffuse dura-arachnoid enhancement
  - Look for secondary parenchymal infarcts
- Tuberculoma
  - Iso-/hyperdense parenchymal mass(es)
  - Round, lobulated > irregular margins
  - Variable edema
  - Punctate, solid, or ring enhancement
  - May cause focal enhancing dural mass
  - Chronic; healed may calcify
- Abscess
  - Hypodense mass
  - Perilesional edema usually marked
  - Ring enhancement

MR Findings

- TBM
  - Can be normal
  - "Dirty" CSF on T1WI
  - Hyperintense on FLAIR
  - Linear, nodular pia-subarachnoid space enhancement
  - May extend via perivascular spaces into brain
  - Vasculitis, secondary infarcts common
  - Penetrating arteries > large territorial infarcts
- Tuberculoma
  - Hypo-/isointense with brain on T1WI
  - Most are hypointense on T2WI
  - Rim enhancement
  - Rare = dural-based enhancing mass
  - Large lipid peak on MRS
- Abscess
  - T2/FLAIR hyperintense
  - Striking perilesional edema
  - Rim, multiloculated enhancement

Differential Diagnosis

- TBM
  - Pyogenic, carcinomatous meningitis
  - Neurosarcoid
- Tuberculoma
  - Neurocysticercosis
  - Primary or metastatic neoplasm
  - Pyogenic abscess
  - Dural-based mass can mimic meningioma

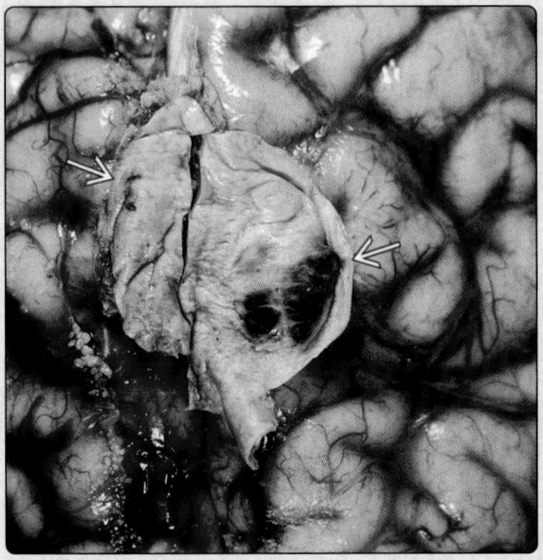

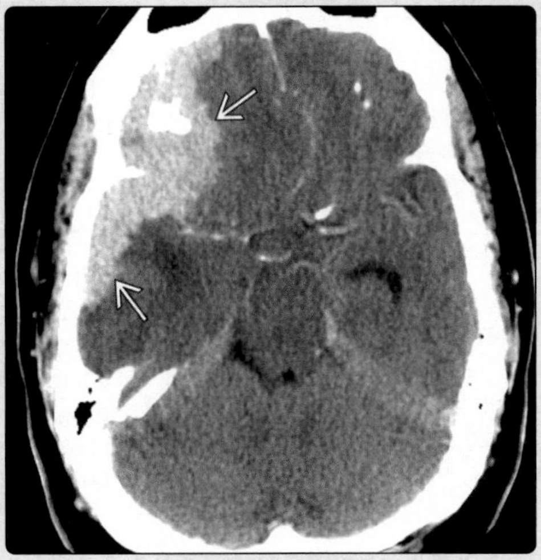

(13-11) Gross autopsy case shows TB as a focal dural mass ➡. Appearance is indistinguishable from that of meningioma. (13-12) CECT scan in a case of proven dura-based TB inflammatory pseudotumor shows extensive en plaque enhancing right frontotemporal mass ➡. (Courtesy A. Sillag, MD.)

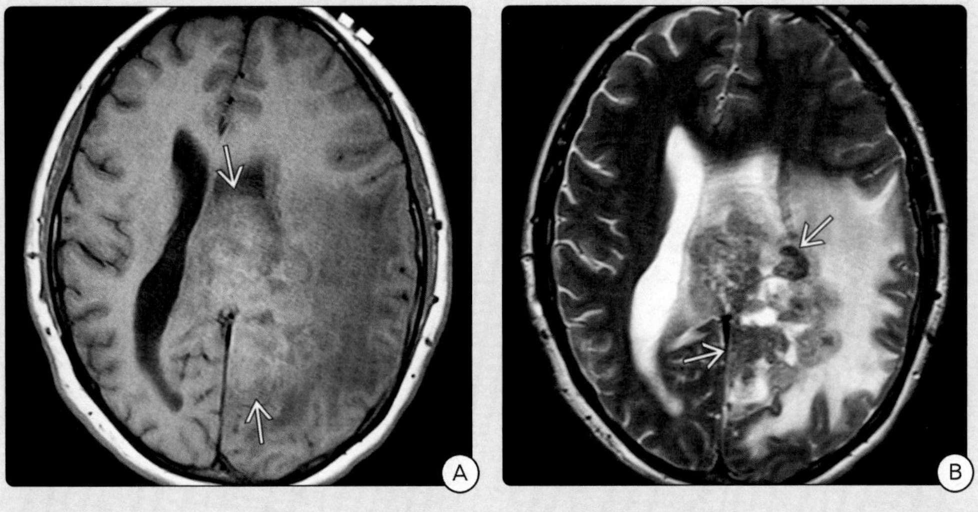

(13-13A) Axial T1WI in a 21y postpartum woman with seizures shows a mixed hypo-, iso-, and hyperintense mass ➡ in the corpus callosum and left parietooccipital lobe. (13-13B) Axial T2WI in the same case shows that the mixed signal intensity mass has several areas that appear strikingly hypointense ➡.

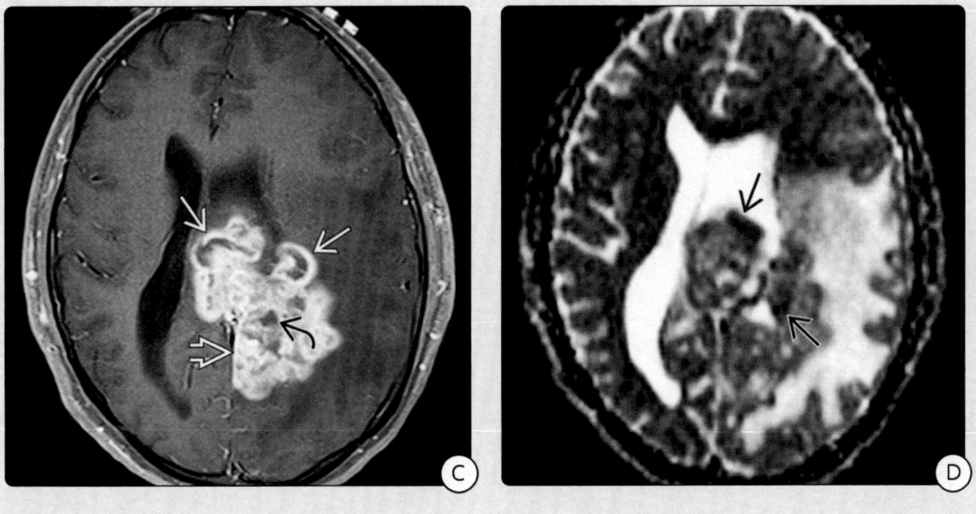

(13-13C) T1 C+ FS MR shows that the mass has multiple conglomerate foci of ring ➡ and solid ⇨ enhancement surrounding nonenhancing areas ↷. (13-13D) ADC map shows some foci of restricted diffusion ➡. Pathology disclosed granulomas with large, multifocal areas of coalescing necrosis. Although the causative organism was never identified, the most likely diagnosis was considered to be TB granuloma.

Nontuberculous Mycobacterial Infections

Nontuberculous mycobacteria (NTM) are ubiquitous organisms that are widely distributed in water and soil. The most prevalent NTM capable of causing disease in humans is *Mycobacterium avium* complex. Human disease is usually caused by environmental exposure, not human-to-human spread.

Compared with *M. tuberculosis*, NTM infections are uncommon. Most are caused by two closely related "atypical" mycobacteria, *M. avium* and *M. intracellulare*, which are collectively called *M. avium-intracellulare complex* (MAIC). Less common NTM include *M. abscessus*, *M. fortuitum*, and *M. kansasii*.

The most common manifestation of MAIC infection is pulmonary disease, which usually occurs in adults with intact systemic immunity. Disseminated systemic infections are primarily seen in immunocompromised patients.

Three disease patterns are seen in the head and neck: (1) chronic cervical lymphadenitis, (2) immune reconstitution inflammatory syndrome (IRIS), and (3) CNS disease **(13-14)**.

Nontuberculous Cervical Lymphadenitis

Clinical Issues. Subacute or chronic neck infection is by far the most common manifestation of MAIC in the head and neck. Children younger than 5 years and immunocompromised adults are typically affected. Most patients are afebrile and present with a painless, slowly enlarging submandibular or preauricular mass. Chest radiographs show no evidence of pulmonary TB.

Imaging. NECT scans demonstrate one or more enlarged, isodense, solid, or cystic-appearing level I and II lymph node(s). Unilateral disease is more common than bilateral disease.

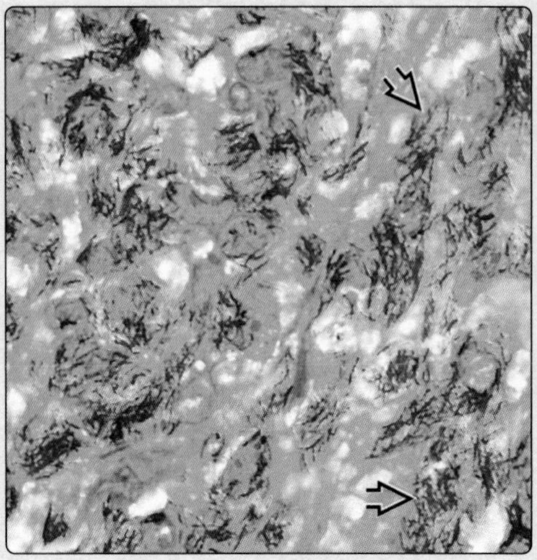

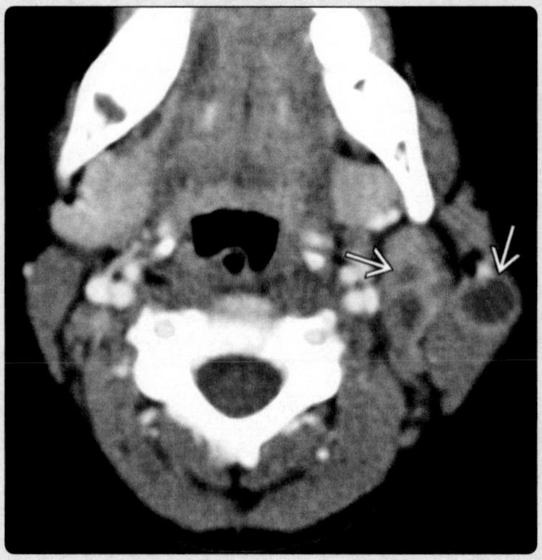

***(13-14)** Biopsy specimen of a CNS mycobacterial spindle cell pseudotumor from a patient with AIDS shows large numbers of acid-fast bacilli that fill epithelioid histiocytes. Granulomas, multinucleated giant cells are absent. (Courtesy B. K. DeMasters, MD.)* ***(13-15)** Axial CECT in a 2y girl with a painless left neck mass shows multiple ring-enhancing lymph nodes with low-attenuation centers; non-TB mycobacterial adenitis.*

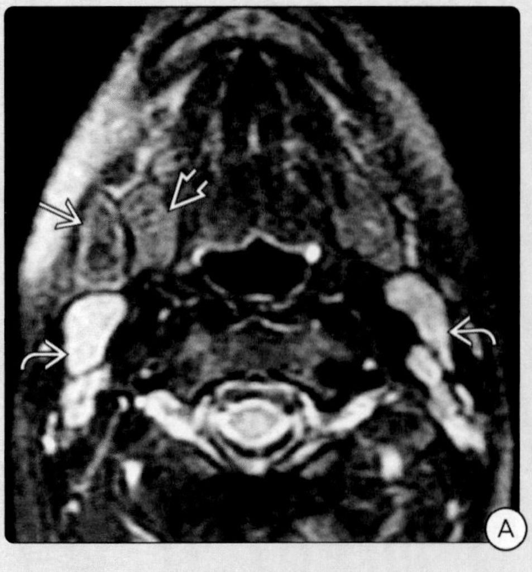

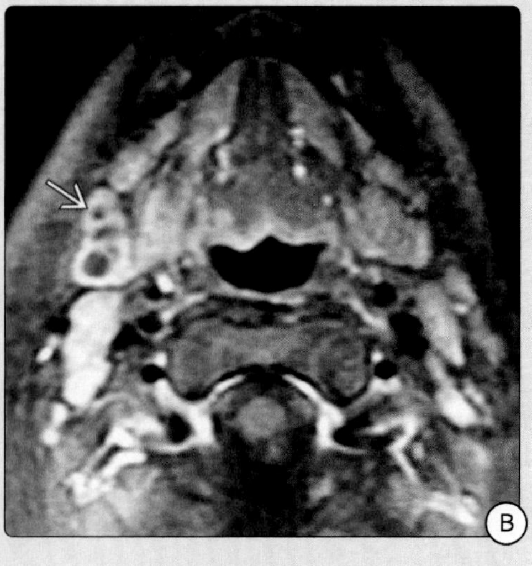

***(13-16A)** T2WI FS scan in a 2y boy with a 5-month history of cervical adenopathy shows enlarged level II lymph nodes and an enlarged, heterogeneous, less hyperintense lymph node lateral to the right submandibular gland.* ***(13-16B)** T1 C+ FS scan demonstrates peripheral enhancement and central necrosis in the nodal mass. The enlarged level II nodes enhance homogeneously. This is non-TB mycobacterial adenitis.*

Inflammatory changes in the surrounding tissues are minimal or absent.

Rim enhancement is common on CECT **(13-15)**. Occasionally, fistulization to the skin occurs.

MR shows hyperintense, cystic-appearing lymph node(s) with minimal surrounding inflammation on fat-saturated T2WI **(13-16A)**. T1 C+ FS illustrates marked peripheral enhancement around the nonenhancing necrotic centers **(13-16B)**.

Differential Diagnosis. The major differential diagnosis of nontuberculous cervical lymphadenitis is **suppurative lymphadenopathy**. Patients present with fever and painful mass(es). Cellulitis with stranding of fat and adjacent structures is common.

Tuberculosis causes 95% of cervical lymphadenitis cases in adults but only 8% in children. Half of all cases occur in immunocompromised patients. Imaging studies demonstrate multiple enlarged posterior triangle and internal jugular nodes. Bilateral lesions are typical. Coexisting pulmonary disease is common.

Less common mimics are cat scratch disease and second branchial cleft cysts. **Cat scratch disease** presents 1-2 weeks following the incident and is seen as reactive adenopathy in regional nodes draining the lesion. **Second branchial cleft cyst** can mimic a cystic lymph node but is located between the submandibular gland and sternocleidomastoid muscle.

MAIC-Associated IRIS

Atypical microbacterial IRIS outside the CNS is common, usually occurring as pulmonary disease and/or lymphadenitis, but MAIC-associated CNS IRIS is very rare. Reported findings are perivascular granulomatous inflammation with multiple enhancing parenchymal lesions on T1 C+ scans.

CNS Disease

MAIC is an important AIDS-defining opportunistic infection that commonly occurs in patients with CD4 lymphocyte counts < 50 cells/μL.

MAIC causes a localized mass-like inflammatory lesion called a mycobacterial spindle cell pseudotumor. The most common sites are the lymph nodes, lungs, and skin. Most reported cases in the head and neck are found in the nose and orbit.

At biopsy, mycobacterial pseudotumors contain sheets of epithelioid histiocytes with mixed inflammatory cell infiltrate and little necrosis. Innumerable acid-fast intracellular organisms can be demonstrated, but granulomas and multinucleated giant cells are absent **(13-14)**.

Intracranial lesions are uncommon. Imaging studies usually show an enhancing, dural-based mass that mimics meningioma or neurosarcoidosis. Cases of MAIC meningitis and brain abscess have been reported but are exceptionally rare.

NONTUBERCULOUS MYCOBACTERIAL INFECTION

Etiology and Clinical Issues
- Non-TB mycobacteria (NTM)
  - "Atypical" mycobacteria
  - Most common = *M. avium, M. intracellulare*
  - Collectively termed *M. avium-intracellulare complex* (MAIC)
- Pulmonary disease (immunocompetent)
- Disseminated systemic disease (immunocompromised)
- Head and neck disease less common; CNS rare

Nontuberculous Cervical Lymphadenitis
- Subacute/chronic lymphadenopathy
- Immunocompetent children < 5 years
- Typical presentation: Painless submandibular, preauricular mass
- Imaging shows enlarged, ring-enhanced node(s)

Immune Reconstitution Inflammatory Syndrome
- HIV(+) patient with disseminated MAIC placed on HAART
- Usually involves lungs, lymph nodes
- CNS disease very rare
  - Disseminated enhancing parenchymal lesions

CNS Disease Due to NTM
- Clinical issues
  - CNS MAIC < < < CNS TB
  - Immunocompromised adults
- Pathology
  - Mass-like (mycobacterial spindle cell pseudotumor)
  - Histiocytes, inflammatory cells, intracytoplasmic acid-fast bacilli
  - Lymph nodes, lungs, skin > > nose and orbit > CNS
- Imaging
  - Focal dural-based mass
  - Can mimic meningioma, neurosarcoid

Fungal Infections

Fungi are ubiquitous organisms with worldwide distribution. Most CNS fungal infections are opportunistic, resulting from inhalation of fungal spores and pulmonary infection followed by hematogeneous dissemination. Once uncommon, their prevalence is rising as the number of immunocompromised patients increases worldwide.

Terminology

CNS fungal infections are also called cerebral mycosis. A focal "fungus ball" is also called a mycetoma or fungal granuloma.

Etiology

Fungal Pathogens. A number of fungal pathogens can cause CNS infections. The most common are *Coccidioides immitis, Aspergillus fumigatus, Cryptococcus neoformans, Histoplasma capsulatum, Candida albicans*, and *Blastomyces dermatitidis.*

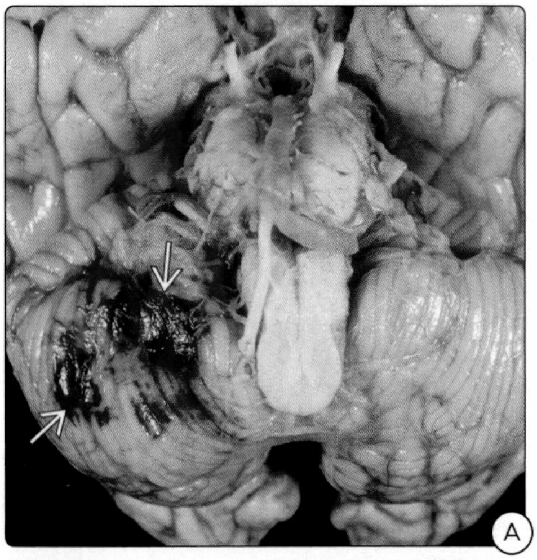

(13-17A) Autopsy case demonstrates multiple hemorrhagic infarcts ➡ typical of fungal infection.

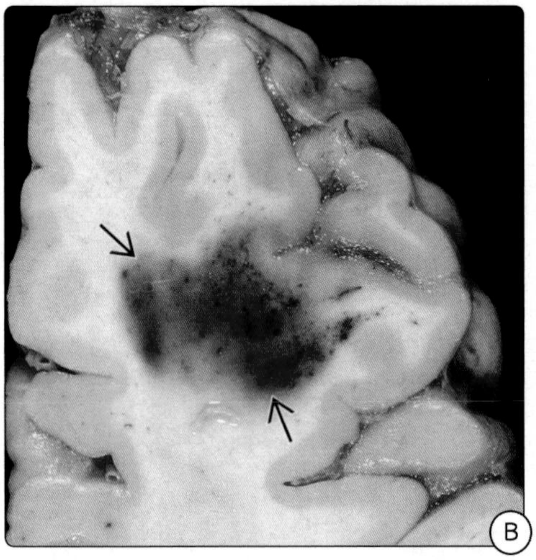

(13-17B) Axial section of cerebral hemisphere in the same case shows a hemorrhagic subcortical infarct ➡. (Courtesy R. Hewlett, MD.)

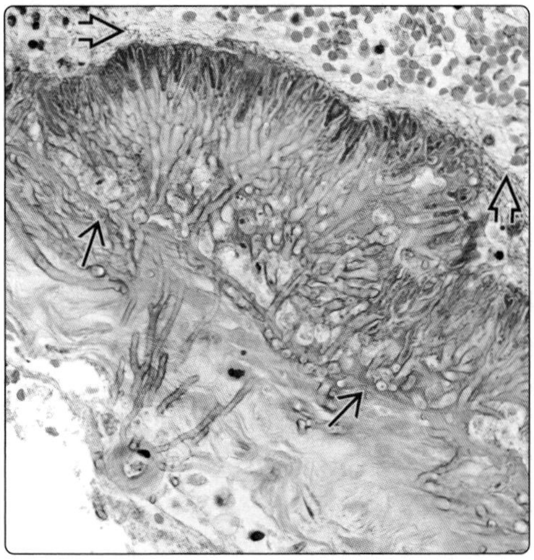

(13-18) Corona-like arrays of Aspergillus ➡ penetrate the wall of a leptomeningeal blood vessel ➡. (Courtesy B. K. DeMasters, MD.)

Members of the Zygomycetes class (especially the *Mucor* genus) can also become pathogenic.

The specific agents vary with immune status. Candidiasis, mucormycosis, and cryptococcal infections are usually opportunistic infections. They occur in patients with predisposing factors such as diabetes, hematologic malignancies, and immunosuppression. Coccidioidomycosis and aspergillosis affect both immunocompetent (often elderly) and immunocompromised patients.

Environmental Exposure. Aside from *C. albicans* (a normal constituent of human gut flora), most fungal infections are initially acquired by inhaling fungal spores in contaminated dust and soil.

Coccidioidomycosis occurs in areas with low rainfall and high summer temperatures (e.g., Mexico, southwestern United States, some parts of South America), whereas histoplasmosis and blastomycosis occur in watershed areas with moist air and damp, rotting wood (e.g., Africa, around major lakes and river valleys in North America).

Systemic and CNS Infections. Sufficiently large numbers of inhaled spores can produce pulmonary infection. In immunocompetent patients, fungi such as *Blastomycosis* and *Histoplasma* are usually confined to the lungs, where they cause focal granulomatous disease.

Hematogeneous spread from the lungs to the CNS is the most common route of infection, and cryptococcal meningitis is the most common fungal disease of the CNS.

Fungal sinonasal infections may invade the skull base and cavernous sinus directly. Sinonasal disease with intracranial extension (rhinocerebral disease) is the most common pattern of *Aspergillus* and *Mucor* CNS infection.

Disseminated fungal disease usually occurs only in immunocompromised patients.

Pathology

CNS mycoses have four basic pathologic manifestations: diffuse meningeal disease (most common), solitary or multiple focal parenchymal lesions (common), disseminated nonfocal parenchymal disease (rare), and focal dura-based masses (rarest).

Location. The meninges are the most common site, followed by the brain parenchyma and spinal cord.

Size and Number. Parenchymal mycetomas vary in size from tiny (a few millimeters) to 1 or 2 cm. Large lesions are rare although multiple lesions are common.

Gross Pathology. The most common gross finding is basilar meningitis with congested meninges. Parenchymal fungal infections can be either focal or disseminated. Fungal abscesses are encapsulated lesions with a soft tan or thick mucoid-appearing center, an irregular reddish margin, and surrounding edema. Disseminated disease is less common and causes a fungal cerebritis with diffusely swollen brain.

Hemorrhagic infarcts, typically in the basal ganglia or at the gray-white matter junction, are common with angioinvasive fungi **(13-17)**. On rare occasions, fungal infections can produce dura-based masses that closely resemble meningioma.

Microscopic Features. Microscopic features of CNS fungal infections vary with the specific agent **(13-18)**. *Blastomyces, Histoplasma, Cryptococcus,* and *Candida* are yeasts. *Aspergillus* has branching septated hyphae, whereas

Mucor has broad nonseptated hyphae. *Candida* has pseudohyphae. *Coccidioides* has sporangia that contain endospores.

Fungal abscesses exhibit central coagulative necrosis with moderate amounts of acute (polymorphonuclear leukocytic) or chronic (lymphohistiocytic) inflammation mixed with variable numbers of fungal organisms. Abscesses are surrounded by a rim of granulation tissue, perivascular hemorrhage, and thrombosed vessels. Fungal granulomas are less common and are characterized by the presence of multinucleated giant cells. Extraaxial fungal infections are characterized predominantly by spindle cell proliferations.

Clinical Issues

Epidemiology. Epidemiology varies with the specific fungus. Many infections are both common and asymptomatic (e.g., approximately 25% of the entire population in the USA and Canada are infected with *Histoplasma*).

Candidiasis is the most common nosocomial fungal infection worldwide. *Aspergillosis* accounts for 20-30% of fungal brain abscesses and is the most common cerebral complication following bone marrow transplantation. *Mucor* is ubiquitous but generally infects only immunocompromised patients.

Demographics and Presentation. Immunocompetent patients have a bimodal age distribution with fungal infections disproportionately represented in children and older individuals. There is a slight male predominance. Immunocompromised patients of all ages and both sexes are at risk.

Nonspecific symptoms such as weight loss, fever, malaise, and fatigue are common. Many patients initially have symptoms of pulmonary infection. CNS involvement is presaged by headache, meningismus, mental status changes, and/or seizure.

CLINICAL FEATURES, COMMON AGENTS, TYPICAL PATHOLOGY OF FUNGAL INFECTIONS

Normal/Immunocompetent
- *Blastomyces* (meningitis, abscess)
- *Histoplasma* (meningitis, abscess)
- *Coccidioides* (meningitis, meningoencephalitis)

HIV/AIDS, TNF Treatment
- *Cryptococcus* (meningoencephalitis, gelatinous pseudocysts)
- *Histoplasma* (meningitis)

Neutropenia
- *Candida* (meningitis, abscess)
- *Aspergillus* (abscess, hemorrhagic infarcts)

Hematopoietic Stem Cell Transplant/Steroids
- *Aspergillus* (abscess, hemorrhagic infarcts)
- *Mucor* (sinus infection, abscess, infarcts ± hemorrhage)
- *Nocardia* (abscess, meningitis)

Solid Organ Transplant
- *Candida* (meningitis, abscess)
- *Aspergillus* (abscess, hemorrhagic infarcts)
- *Cryptococcus* (meningoencephalitis)
- *Nocardia* (abscess, meningitis)

Neurosurgery
- *Candida* (abscess)

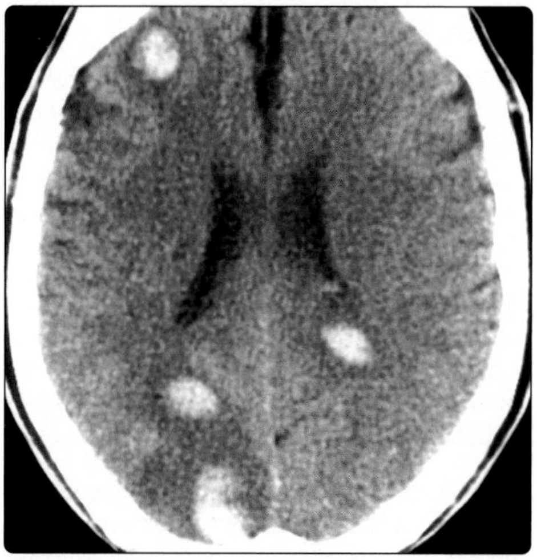

***(13-19)** NECT scan shows multifocal hemorrhages. Angioinvasive aspergillosis was documented at surgery.*

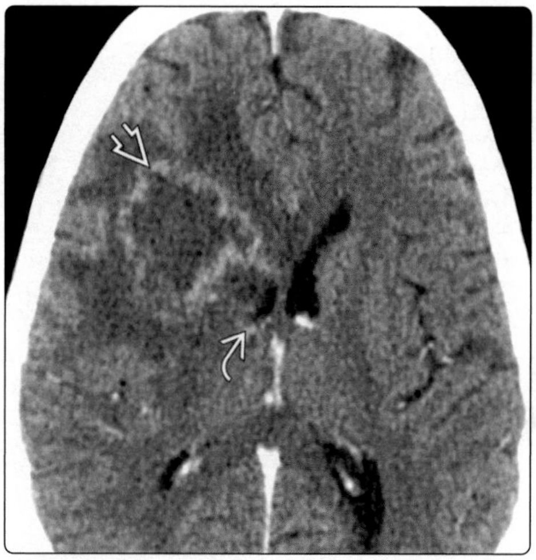

***(13-20)** CECT scan shows an irregular, crenulated enhancing lesion ➡ with edema, ventriculitis ↗. This is a solitary aspergilloma.*

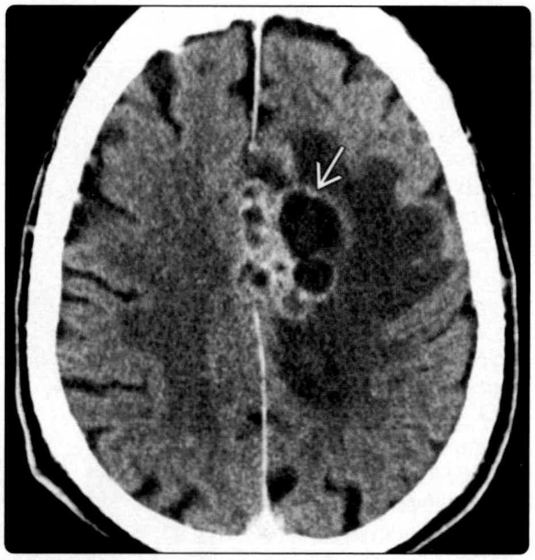

***(13-21)** CECT shows multiloculated ring-enhancing mass lesion ➡ with edema. Nocardia abscess was found at surgery.*

Imaging

General Features. Findings vary with the patient's immune status. Well-formed fungal abscesses are seen in immunocompetent patients. Imaging early in the course of a rapidly progressive infection in an immunocompromised patient may show diffuse cerebral edema more characteristic of encephalitis than fungal abscess.

CT Findings. Findings on NECT include hypodense parenchymal lesions caused by focal granulomas or ischemia. Hydrocephalus is common in patients with fungal meningitis. Patients with coccidioidal meningitis may demonstrate thickened, mildly hyperdense basal meninges.

Disseminated parenchymal infection causes diffuse cerebral edema. Multifocal parenchymal hemorrhages are common in patients with angioinvasive fungal species **(13-19)** **(13-27)**.

Diffuse meningeal disease demonstrates pia-subarachnoid space enhancement on CECT. Multiple punctate or ring-enhancing parenchymal lesions are typical findings of parenchymal mycetomas **(13-20)** **(13-21)**.

Mycetoma in the paranasal sinuses is usually seen as a single opacified hyperdense sinus that contains fine round to linear calcifications. Fungal sinusitis occasionally becomes invasive, crossing the mucosa to involve blood vessels, bone, orbit, cavernous sinuses, and intracranial cavities. Focal or widespread bone erosion with adjacent soft tissue infiltration can mimic neoplasm. Bone CT with reconstructions in all three standard planes is helpful to assess skull base involvement, and T1 C+ FS MR is the best modality to delineate disease spread beyond the nose and sinuses **(13-28)**.

MR Findings. Fungal meningitis appears as "dirty" CSF on T1WI. Parenchymal lesions are typically hypointense on T1WI but demonstrate T1 shortening if subacute hemorrhage is

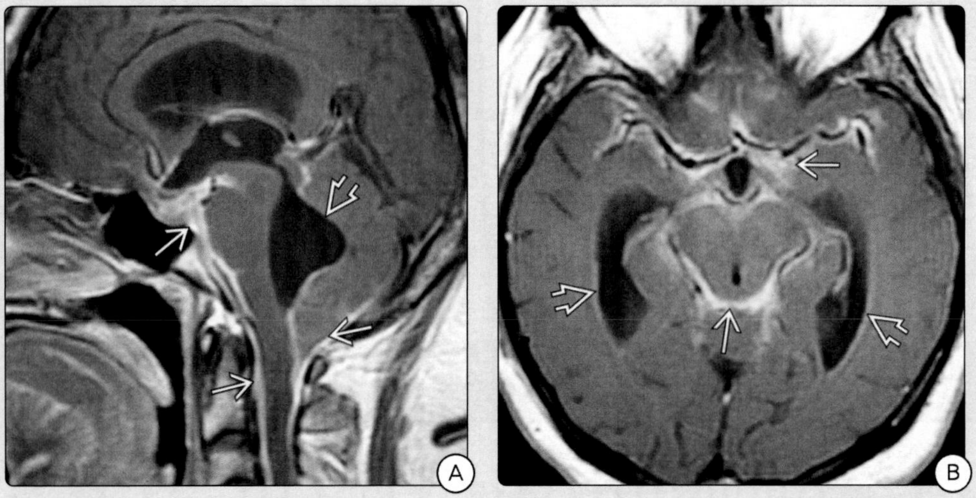

***(13-22A)** Sagittal T1 C+ scan in a 30y man with cocci meningitis/ventriculitis shows obstructive hydrocephalus with marked enlargement of 4th ventricle ➡. Thick enhancing exudate ➡ entirely fills suprasellar and prepontine cisterns and cisterna magna and extends inferiorly around the cervical spinal cord. **(13-22B)** Axial T1 C+ scan in the same patient shows extensive enhancement in the basal and ambient cisterns ➡. Note ependymitis ➡.*

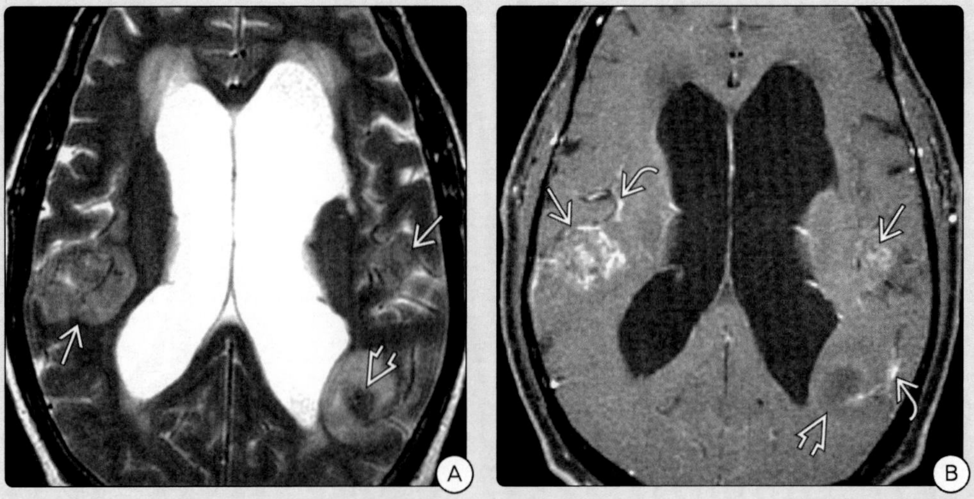

***(13-23A)** Axial T2WI in a patient with cocci meningitis shows hydrocephalus, multiple areas of cortical/subcortical hyperintensity ➡. Note focal hypointense central area ➡ in one of the lesions. **(13-23B)** T1 C+ FS in the same case shows patchy areas of enhancement ➡. The hemorrhagic lesion seen on the T2WI shows a faint, incomplete rim of enhancement ➡. This is cocci meningitis ➡ with early cerebritis.*

present. Irregular walls with nonenhancing projections into the cavity are typical.

T2/FLAIR scans in patients with fungal cerebritis show bilateral but asymmetric cortical/subcortical white matter and basal ganglia hyperintensity **(13-23A)**. Focal lesions (mycetomas) show high signal foci that typically have a peripheral hypointense rim, surrounded by vasogenic edema. T2* scans may show "blooming" foci caused by hemorrhages or calcification **(13-26)**. Focal paranasal sinus and parenchymal mycetomas usually restrict on DWI **(13-28D)**.

T1 C+ FS scans usually show diffuse, thick, enhancing basilar leptomeninges **(13-22)**. Angioinvasive fungi may erode the skull base, cause plaque-like dural thickening, and occlude one or both carotid arteries **(13-29)** **(13-30)**. Parenchymal lesions show punctate, ring-like, or irregular enhancement **(13-23B)** **(13-25)** **(13-26)**.

MRS shows mildly elevated Cho and decreased NAA. A lactate peak is seen in 90% of cases, whereas lipid and amino acids are identified in approximately 50%. Multiple peaks resonating between 3.6 and 3.8 ppm are common and probably represent trehalose.

Differential Diagnosis

The major differential is **pyogenic abscess(es)** and **tuberculoma**. **TB** can appear similar to fungal abscesses on standard imaging studies. Gross hemorrhage is more common with fungal than either pyogenic or tubercular abscesses. Fungal abscesses have more irregularly shaped walls and internal nonenhancing projections. Resonance between 3.6 and 3.8 ppm on MRS is typical.

Other mimics of fungal abscesses are primary **neoplasm** (e.g., glioblastoma with central necrosis) or metastases.

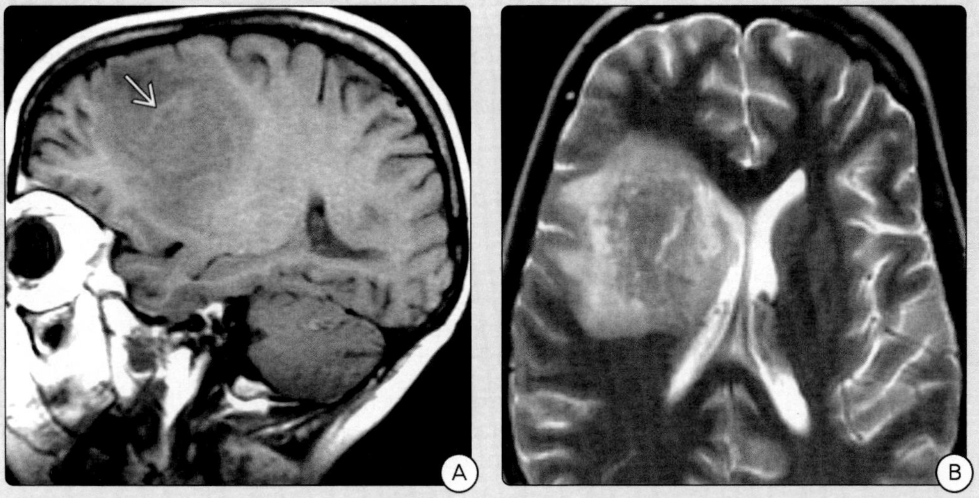

***(13-24A)** Sagittal T1WI in the same case as Figure 13-20 shows hypointense edema surrounding a mildly hyperintense rim. **(13-24B)** Axial T2WI shows that the lesion is mostly hypointense relative to cortex.*

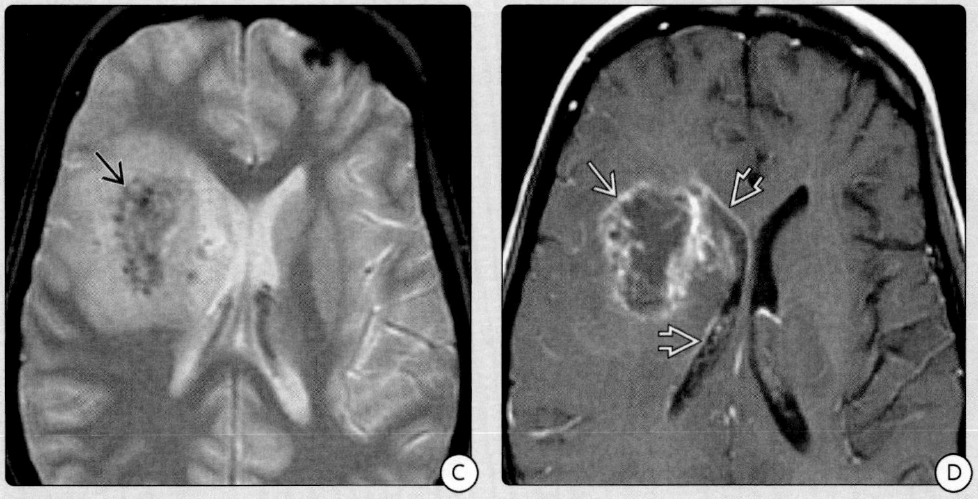

***(13-24C)** T2* GRE shows multiple punctate "blooming" foci within the mass, consistent with petechial hemorrhages. **(13-24D)** Axial T1 C+ shows the irregular, crenulated enhancing rim that surrounds the central nonenhancing lesion core. Note extension into the lateral ventricle with diffuse ependymal enhancement. Aspergilloma was found at surgery and confirmed by histopathology.*

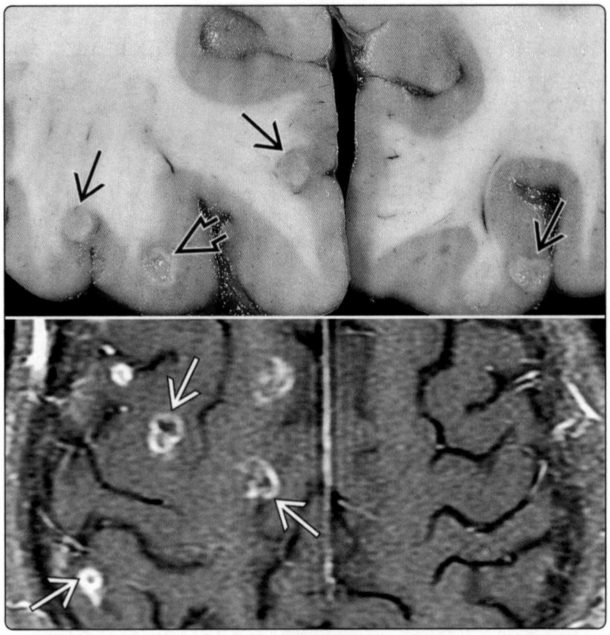

(13-25) (Top) Autopsy case demonstrates multiple solid, necrotic Nocardia abscesses in the cortex, gray-white matter junctions. (Bottom) T1 C+ FS shows multiple ring-enhancing fungal abscesses.

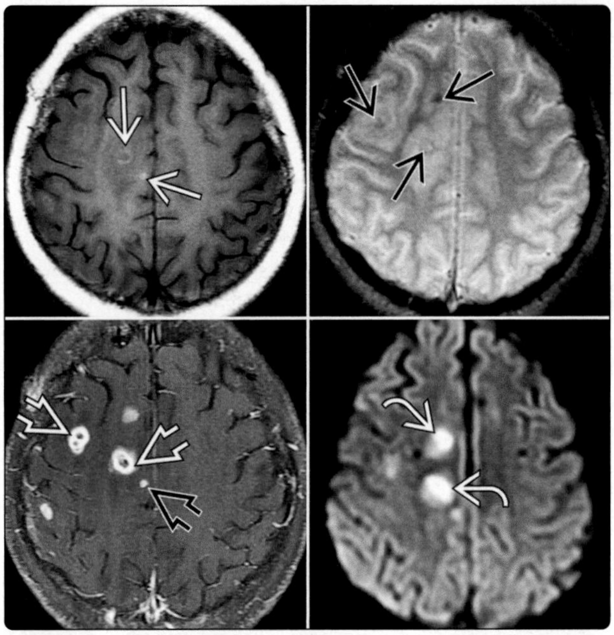

(13-26) Aspergillus abscesses are in an immunosuppressed patient. Axial T1WI shows punctate and ring-like hyperintense foci with "blooming" on T2. Punctate and rim enhancement is seen on T1 C+ FS. Lesions restrict on DWI.*

FUNGAL INFECTIONS: IMAGING AND DIFFERENTIAL DIAGNOSIS

CT

- Meningitis
  - Iso-/hyperdense meninges
- Abscess
  - Hypodense center
  - Hyperdense rim
  - Variable hemorrhage (angioinvasive infections)
- Sinonasal disease
  - Hyperdense (mycetoma)
  - May demonstrate Ca++
  - ± Bone destruction
  - ± Intracranial extension

MR

- Meningitis
  - "Dirty" CSF
  - Isointense with brain on T1WI
  - Hyperintense on T2/FLAIR
- Abscess
  - Hypointense center, hyperintense rim on T1WI
  - Hyperintense center, hypointense rim on T2WI
  - Hemorrhagic "blooming" foci on T2* common
  - Restriction on DWI
  - Strong enhancement on T1 C+
  - MRS lactate in 90%, lipids and amino acids in 50%; multiple peaks at 3.6-3.8 ppm

Differential Diagnosis

- Pyogenic, granulomatous meningitis
- Pyogenic abscess
- Neoplasm (primary, metastatic)

Parasitic Infections

Once considered endemic only in countries with poor sanitation and adverse economic conditions, parasitic diseases have become a global health concern, exacerbated by widespread travel and immigration.

With the exception of neurocysticercosis, CNS parasitic disease is rare. When they infest the brain, parasites can cause very bizarre-looking masses that can mimic neoplasm.

Neurocysticercosis

Cysticercosis is the most common parasitic infection in the world, and CNS lesions eventually develop in 60-90% of patients with cysticercosis.

Terminology

When cysticercosis infects the CNS, it is termed neurocysticercosis (NCC). A "cysticercus" cyst in the brain is actually the secondary larval form of the parasite. The "scolex" is the head-like part of a tapeworm, bearing hooks and suckers. In the larval form, the scolex is invaginated into one end of the cyst, which is called the "bladder."

Etiology

Most NCC cases are caused by encysted larvae of the pork tapeworm *Taenia solium* and are acquired through fecal-oral contamination. Humans become infected by ingesting *T. solium* eggs. The eggs hatch and release their larvae that then disseminate via the bloodstream to virtually any organ in the body.

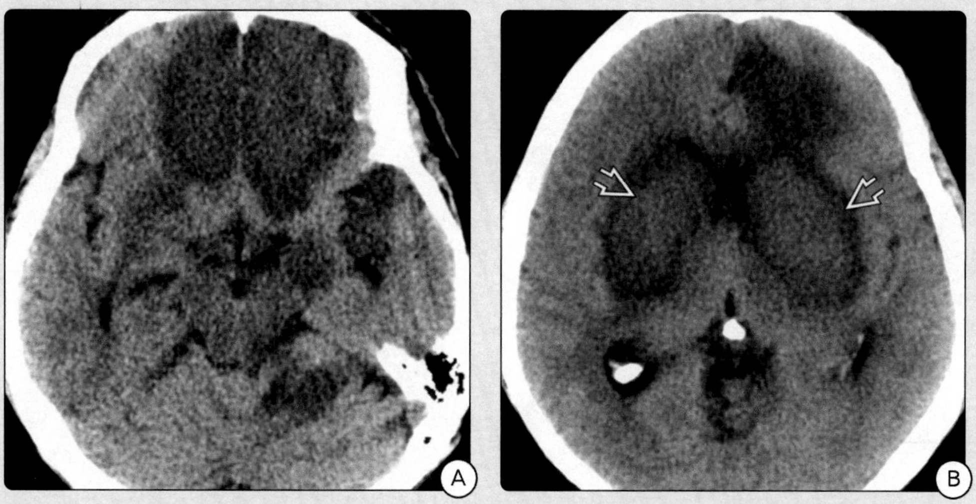

***(13-27A)** NECT scan of angioinvasive aspergillosis shows hypodense infarcts in the cerebellum, midbrain, and frontal and temporal lobes. **(13-27B)** Axial NECT scan in the same patient shows that the basal ganglia infarcts exhibit some hemorrhagic transformation ➡.*

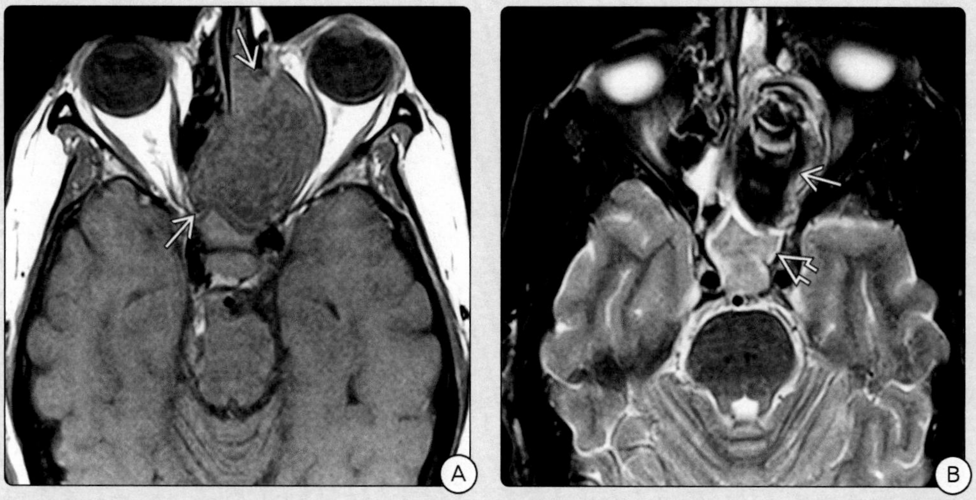

***(13-28A)** Series of images demonstrates a focal sinonasal mycetoma. Axial T1WI shows an expansile, destructive isointense mass ➡ in the nose and ethmoid sinus. The lesion invades the left orbit and extends posteriorly, obstructing the sphenoid sinus. **(13-28B)** The lesion is somewhat mixed signal intensity on T2WI FS but mostly appears profoundly hypointense ➡. Note obstructive changes in the sphenoid sinus ➡.*

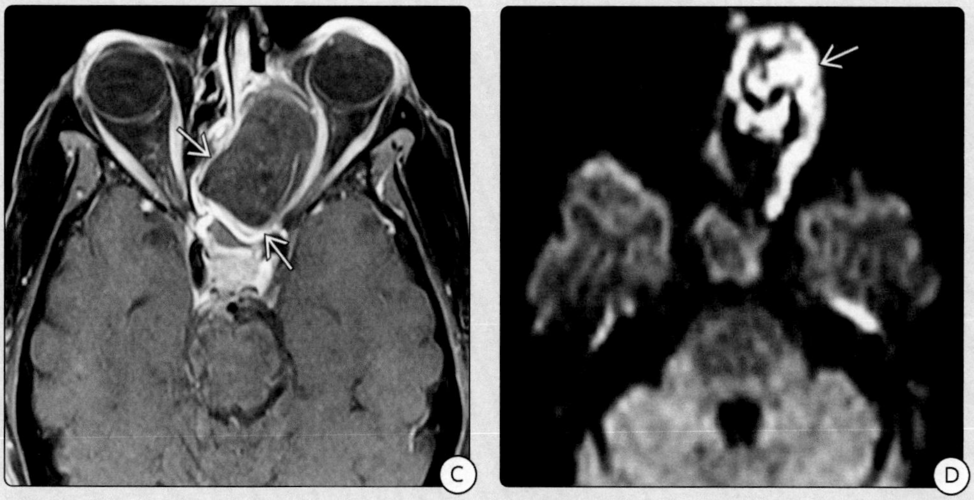

***(13-28C)** T1 C+ FS scan shows peripheral enhancement around the margins of the mass ➡. **(13-28D)** The mass shows diffusion restriction ➡.*

***(13-29)** Close-up view shows autopsied cavernous sinus with invasive fungal sinusitis occluding the left cavernous internal carotid artery ➡. (Courtesy R. Hewlett, MD.)* ***(13-30A)** Bone CT is of a patient with poorly controlled diabetes and invasive mucormycosis. Note bone invasion, destruction at orbital apex and sphenoid sinus ➡.*

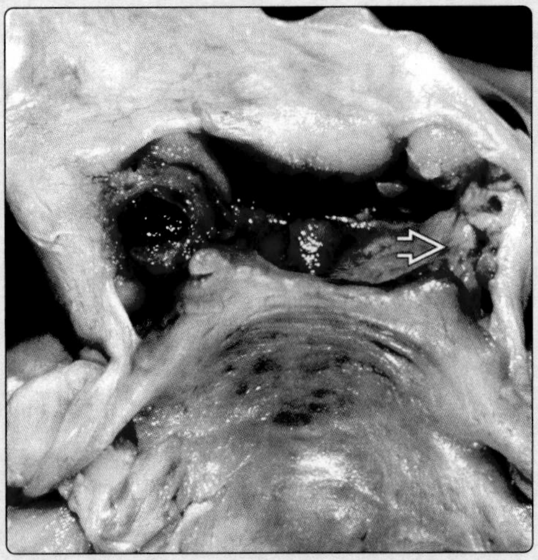

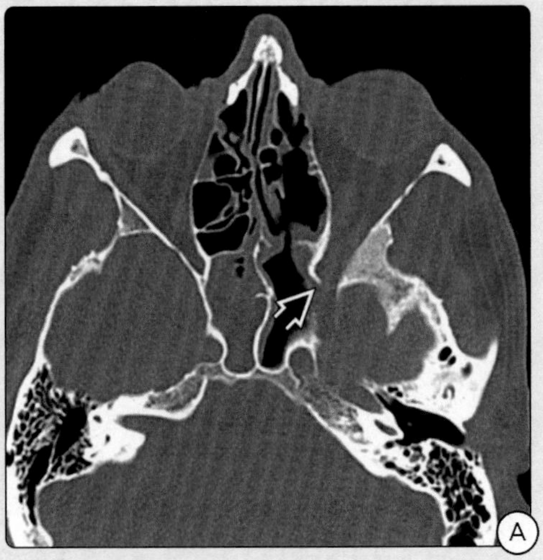

***(13-30B)** Axial T2WI FS shows normal right cavernous internal carotid artery "flow void" ➡ with left cavernous sinus mass and occluded internal carotid artery ➡.* ***(13-30C)** T1 C+ FS scan in the same patient shows the left cavernous sinus invasion ➡ and occluded carotid artery ➡.*

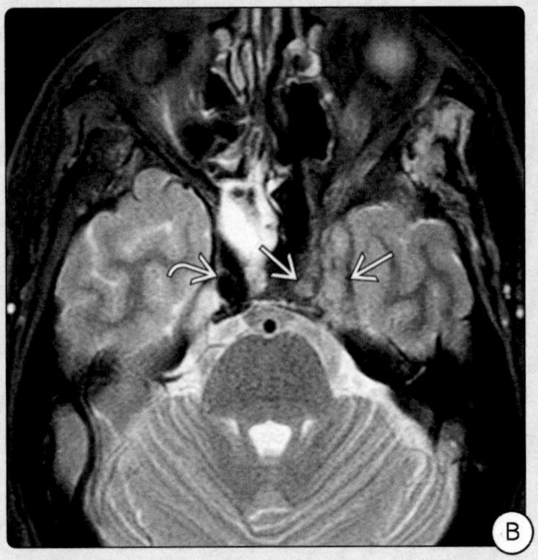

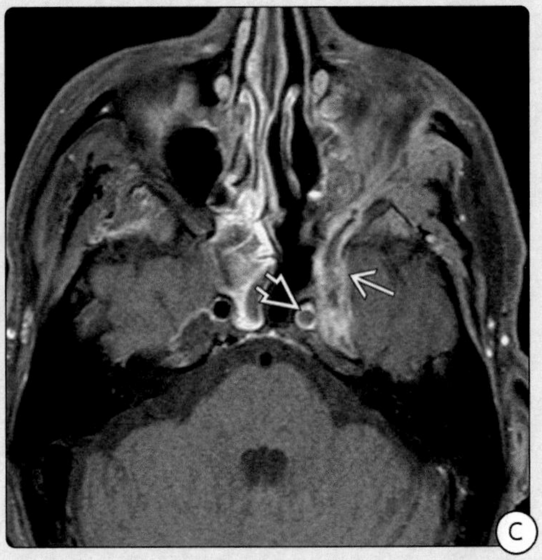

***(13-30D)** T1 C+ FS scan through the top of the cavernous sinus shows the invaded enhancing left side ➡ with absent flow void ➡ (compare to the normal right side ➡).* ***(13-30E)** Coronal T1 C+ FS shows the normal right cavernous ICA ➡, the occluded left ICA ➡, and the cavernous sinus infiltration ➡. Invasive sinonasal mucormycosis in a diabetic patient is a potentially lethal lesion. This patient died from a massive left middle cerebral artery stroke shortly after the scan.*

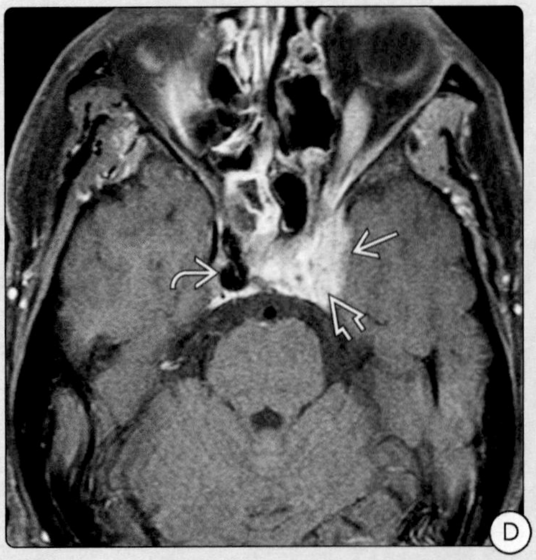

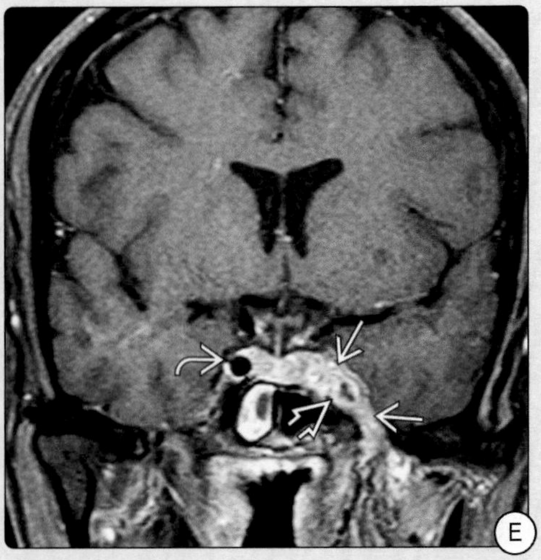

Pathology

Location. *T. solium* larvae are most common in the CNS, eyes, muscles, and subcutaneous tissue. The intracranial subarachnoid spaces are the most common CNS site, followed by the brain parenchyma and ventricles (fourth > third > lateral ventricles) **(13-31)**. NCC cysts in the depths of sulci may incite an intense inflammatory response, effectively "sealing" the sulcus over the cysts and making them appear intraaxial.

Size and Number. Most parenchymal NCC cysts are small (a few millimeters to 1 cm). Occasionally, multiple large NCC cysts up to several centimeters can form in the subarachnoid space (the "racemose" form of NCC that resembles a bunch of grapes). Either solitary (20-50% of cases) or multiple small cysts may occur.

Gross Pathology. Four stages of NCC development and regression are recognized. Patients may have multiple lesions at different stages of evolution.

In the **vesicular stage**, viable larvae (the cysticerci) appear as translucent, thin-walled, fluid-filled cysts with an eccentrically located, whitish, invaginated scolex **(13-32)** **(13-33)**.

In the **colloidal vesicular stage**, the larvae begin to degenerate. The cyst fluid becomes thick and turbid. A striking inflammatory response is incited and characterized by a collection of multinucleated giant cells, macrophages, and neutrophils. A fibrous capsule develops, and perilesional edema becomes prominent.

The **granular nodular stage** represents progressive involution with collapse and retraction of the cyst into a granulomatous nodule that will eventually calcify. Edema persists, but pericystic gliosis is the most common pathologic finding at this stage.

In the **nodular calcified stage**, the entire lesion becomes a fibrocalcified nodule **(13-34)**. No host immune response is present.

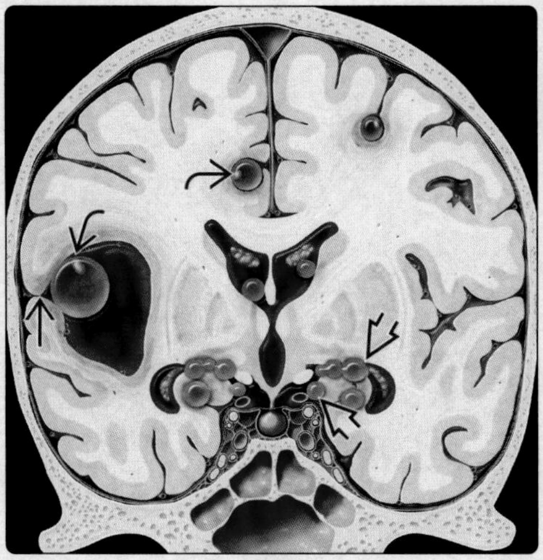

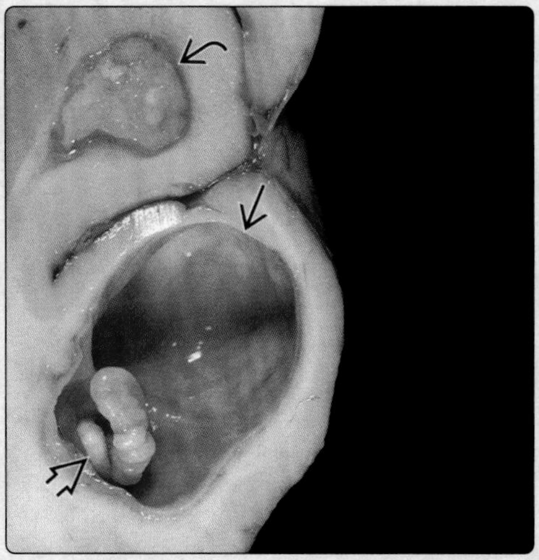

***(13-31)** This is NCC. Convexity cysts have scolex and surrounding inflammation, which, around the largest cyst, "seals" the sulcus, makes it appear parenchymal. "Racemose" cysts without scolices are seen in basal cisterns. **(13-32)** NCC in vesicular stage has a clear fluid-filled cyst and white eccentrically positioned scolex. Note the 2nd granular nodular lesion. (Courtesy R. Hewlett, MD.)*

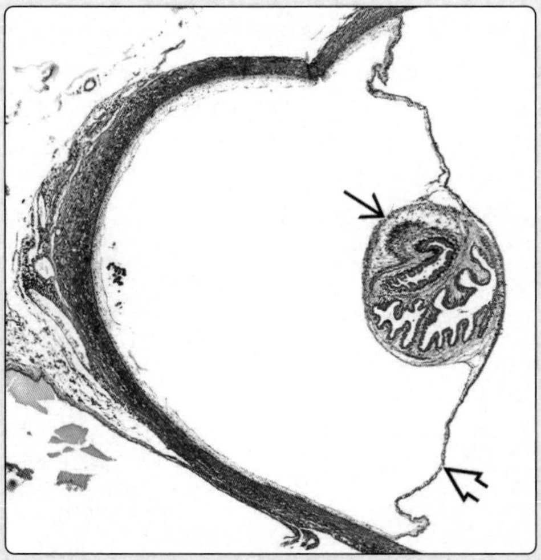

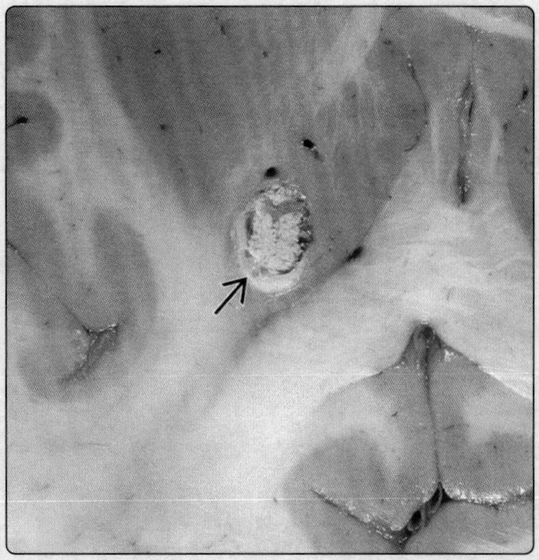

***(13-33)** Low-power photomicrograph of cysticercus shows the invaginated scolex lying within the thin-walled cyst, also known as the bladder. (Courtesy B. K. DeMasters, MD.) **(13-34)** Close-up view shows a nodular calcified NCC cyst. Note the lack of inflammation and lack of mass effect. (Courtesy R. Hewlett, MD.)*

NEUROCYSTICERCOSIS: GROSS PATHOLOGY

Location, Size, Number
- Subarachnoid > parenchyma > ventricles
- Usually < 1 cm
  - Subarachnoid ("racemose") cysts can be giant
- Multiple > solitary
  - Can have multiple innumerable tiny ("miliary") cysts

Development Stages
- Vesicular (quiescent, viable larva) = cyst + scolex
- Colloidal vesicular (dying larva)
  - Intense inflammation, edema
- Granular nodular (healing) = cyst involutes, edema ↓
- Nodular calcified (healed)
  - Quiescent, fibrocalcified nodule
  - No edema

Clinical Issues

Epidemiology. In countries where cysticercosis is endemic, calcified NCC granulomas are found in 10-20% of the entire population. Of these, approximately 5% (400,000 out of 75 million) will become symptomatic.

Demographics. NCC occurs at all ages, but peak symptomatic presentation is between 15 and 40 years. There is no sex or race predilection.

Presentation. NCC has a range of clinical manifestations. Signs and symptoms depend on number and location of larvae, developmental stage, infection duration, and presence or absence of host immune response.

Seizures/epilepsy are the most common symptoms (80%) and are a result of inflammation around degeneration cysts. Headache (35-40%) and focal neurologic deficit (15%) are also

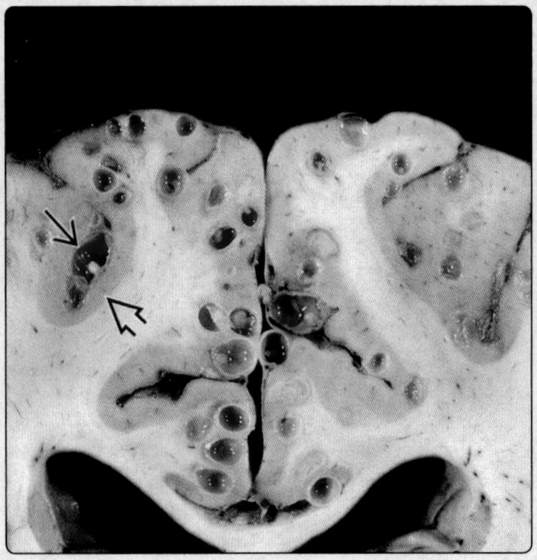
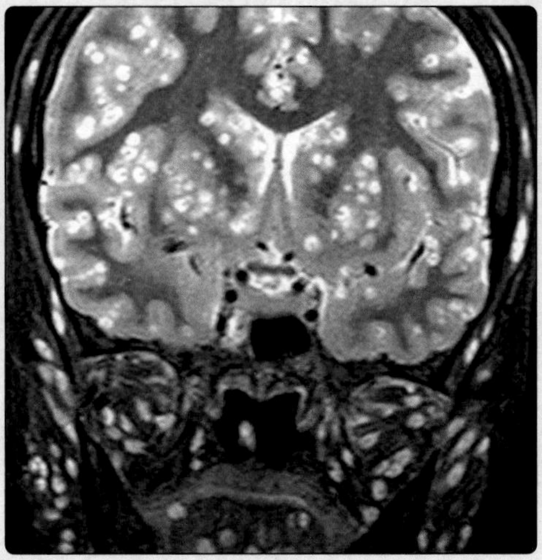

***(13-35)** Disseminated NCC with many cysts, mostly in the subarachnoid space, shows cyst with scolex in the depth of frontal sulcus ➡ surrounded by cortex ➡, making a subarachnoid cyst appear intraparenchymal. **(13-36)** T2WI shows disseminated vesicular NCC with "salt and pepper." Innumerable tiny hyperintense cysticerci with scolices (seen as small black dots inside cysts) are present; perilesional edema is absent.*

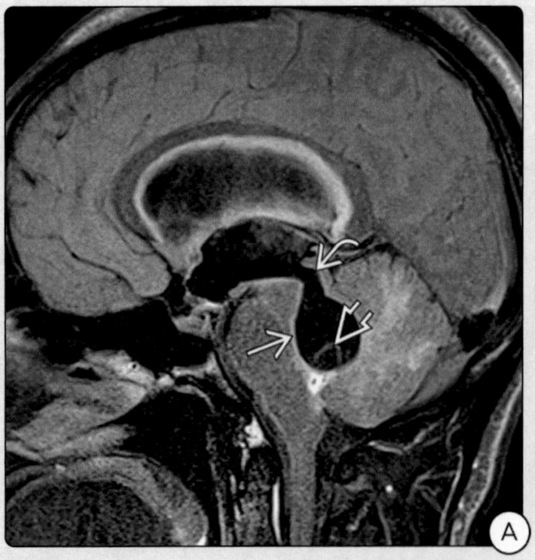

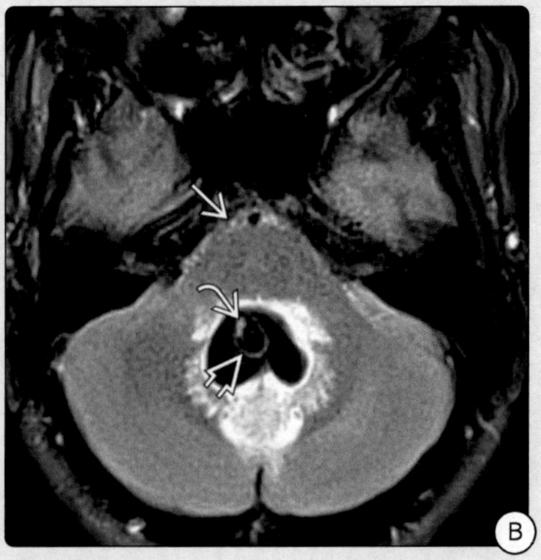

***(13-37A)** Sagittal FLAIR in a 26y woman with headaches shows obstructive hydrocephalus with enlargement of the lateral, third, and fourth ventricles ➡ as well as the aqueduct ➡. A solitary NCC cyst ➡ is visible in the bottom of the 4th ventricle. **(13-37B)** Axial FLAIR shows cyst wall ➡, scolex ➡, and interstitial fluid around the obstructed 4th ventricle. FLAIR hyperintensity ➡ in the basal cisterns indicates meningitis.*

common. Between 10-12% of patients exhibit signs of elevated intracranial pressure.

NCC—particularly the subarachnoid forms—can also cause cerebral vascular diseases. These include cerebral infarction, TIAs, and cerebral hemorrhage.

Natural History. During the early stages of the disease, patients are frequently asymptomatic. Many patients remain asymptomatic for years. The average time from initial infestation until symptoms develop is 2-5 years. The time to progress through all four stages varies from 1-9 years with a mean of 5 years.

Treatment Options. Oral albendazole with or without steroids, excision/drainage of parenchymal lesions, and endoscopic resection of intraventricular lesions are treatment options.

Imaging

General Features. Imaging findings depend on several factors: (1) life cycle stage of *T. solium* at presentation, (2) host inflammatory response, (3) number and location of parasites, and (4) associated complications such as hydrocephalus and vascular disease.

Vesicular (quiescent) stage. NECT shows a smooth thin-walled cyst that is isodense to CSF. There is no surrounding edema and no enhancement on CECT.

MR shows that the cyst is isointense with CSF on T1 and T2/FLAIR. The scolex is discrete, nodular, and hyperintense ("target" or "dot in a hole" appearance) and may restrict on DWI. Enhancement is typically absent. Disseminated or "miliary" NCC has a striking "salt and pepper brain" appearance **(13-35)** **(13-36)** with notable lack of perilesional edema.

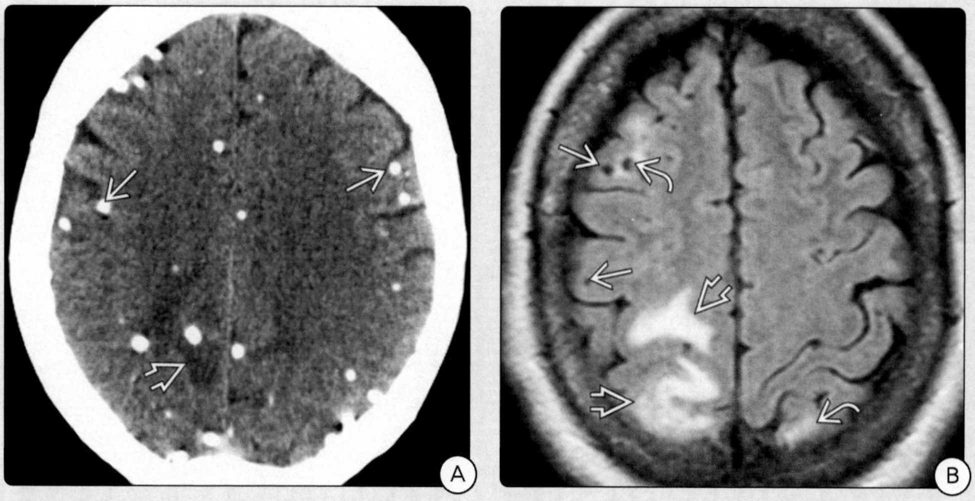

(13-38A) *NECT scan in a patient with NCC shows multiple nodular calcified lesions ➡. A few demonstrate adjacent edema ➡.* ***(13-38B)*** *FLAIR scan shows a few hypointense foci ➡ caused by quiescent NCC in the nodular calcified stage. Several foci of perilesional edema are apparent around lesions in the colloidal vesicular stage ➡, whereas minimal residual edema surrounds lesions in the granular nodular stage ➡.*

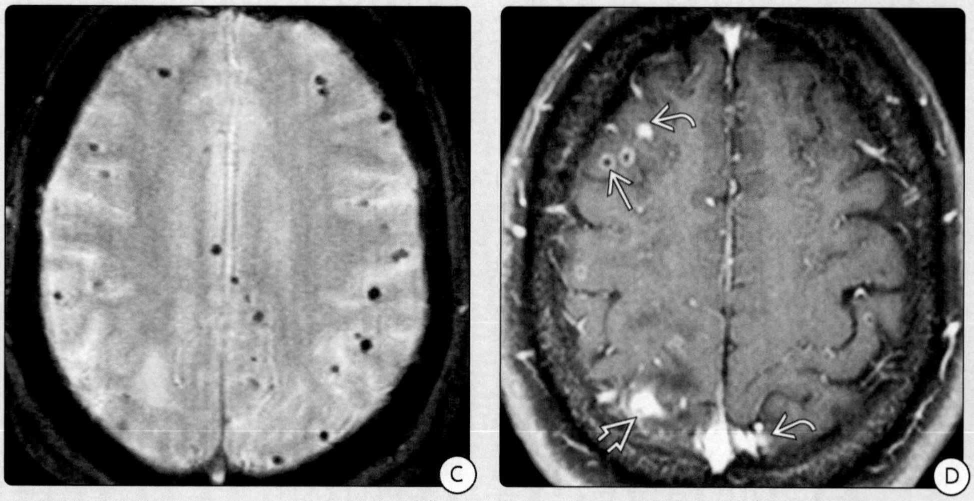

(13-38C) *T2* GRE scan shows multiple "blooming black dots" characteristic of nodular calcified NCC.* ***(13-38D)*** *T1 C+ FS scan shows faint ring-like ➡ and nodular ➡ enhancement of healing granular nodular NCC cysts. "Shaggy" enhancement with adjacent edema ➡ is characteristic of degenerating larvae in the colloidal vesicular stage. Multiple lesions in different stages of evolution are characteristic of NCC.*

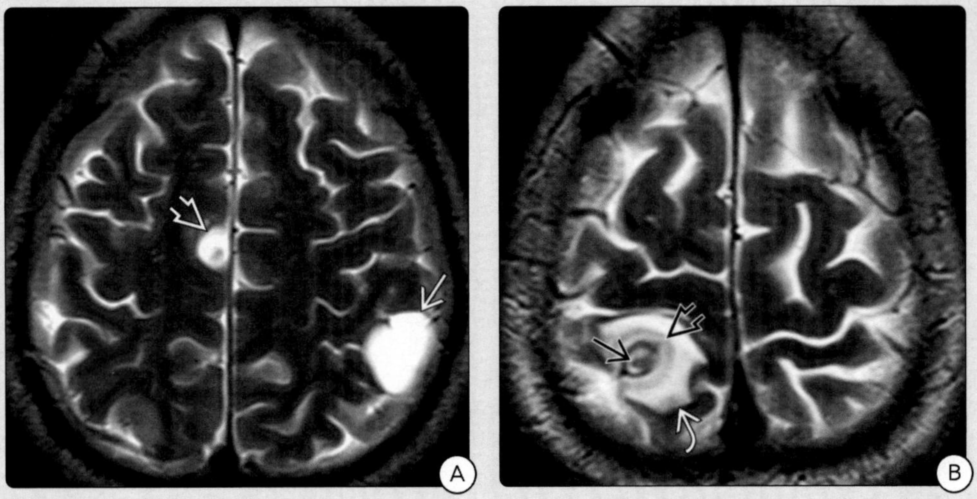

***(13-39A)** Series of images in a 41y Hispanic man with seizures show NCC cysts in different stages. This axial T2WI demonstrates a vesicular (cyst + scolex, no edema) and a cyst in the granular nodular stage. **(13-39B)** More cephalad scan shows an intrasulcal NCC cyst in colloidal vesicular stage with a nodule (scolex) and thick, mixed hypo- and hyperintense intense cyst wall. The surrounding edema is striking.*

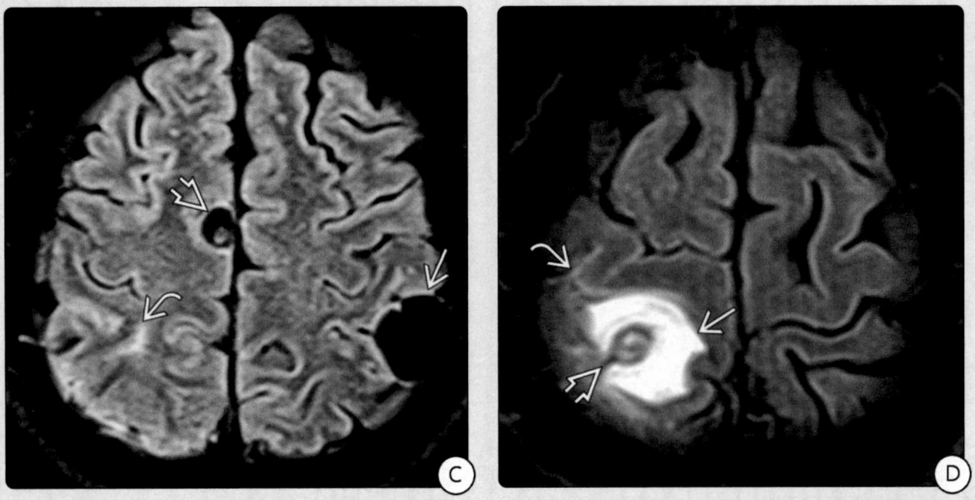

***(13-39C)** Axial FLAIR scan shows the vesicular NCC cyst with its scolex. The granular nodular cyst has minimal residual edema. Group of FLAIR hyperintense sulci represents leptomeningeal inflammation from the colloidal vesicular cyst above. **(13-39D)** More cephalad FLAIR MR shows that the colloidal vesicular cyst + nodule has striking edema and adjacent hyperintense sulci.*

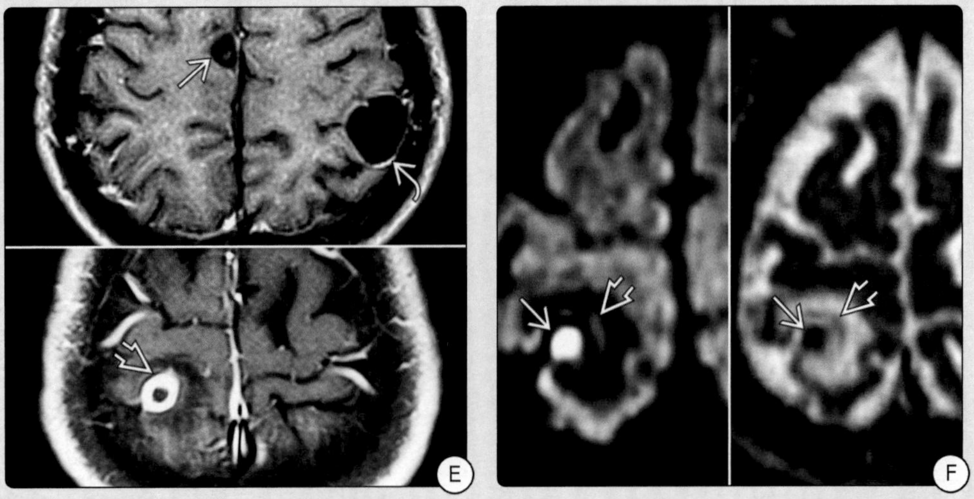

***(13-39E)** (Top) Axial T1 C+ FS shows no enhancement of vesicular NCC cyst, faint rim enhancement of granular nodular cyst wall. (Bottom) More cephalad scan shows the granular nodular cyst has thick, intense rim enhancement. **(13-39F)** Axial DWI (L) and ADC map (R) through the colloidal vesicular cyst show that the central viscous cavity of the cyst restricts strongly. Mild restriction in the enhancing capsule is present.*

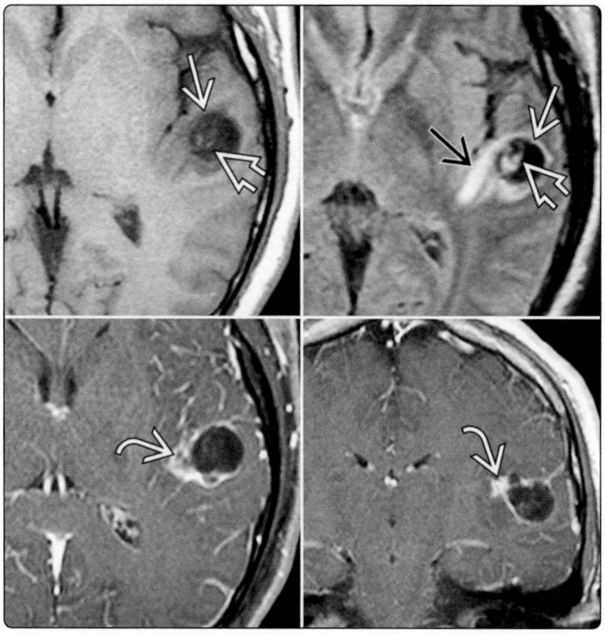

(13-40) Solitary degenerating colloidal vesicular NCC cyst with scolex demonstrates perilesional edema, "shaggy" enhancement.

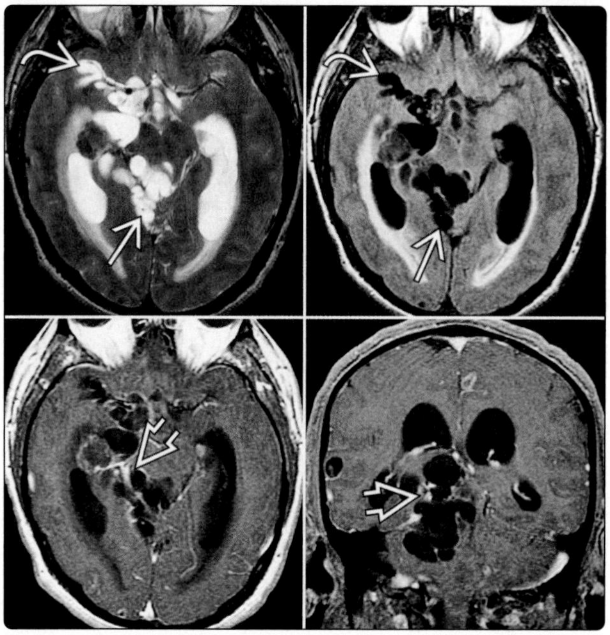

(13-41) "Racemose" NCC shows numerous variable-sized cysts fill the ambient cistern, sylvian fissure. Note hydrocephalus, meningeal reaction with mild/moderate rim enhancement around the "bunch of grapes" cysts.

Colloidal vesicular stage (dying scolex). Cyst fluid is hyperdense relative to CSF on NECT and demonstrates a ring-enhancing capsule on CECT. Moderate to marked edema surrounds the degenerating dying larvae.

MR shows that the cyst fluid is mildly hyperintense to CSF on T1WI and that the scolex appears hyperintense on FLAIR **(13-37)**. Moderate to marked surrounding edema is present **(13-38B)** and may even progress to a diffuse encephalitis.

Enhancement of the cyst wall is typically intense, ring-like, and often slightly "shaggy" **(13-38D)** **(13-40)**. Restricted diffusion in the scolex and viscous degenerating cyst can be present **(13-39)**.

Granular nodular (healing) stage. NECT shows mild residual edema. CECT demonstrates a progressively involuting, mildly to moderately enhancing nodule.

The cyst wall appears thickened and retracted, and the perilesional edema diminishes substantially, eventually disappearing. Nodular or faint ring-like enhancement is typical at this stage **(13-38D)**.

Nodular calcified (inactive) stage. A small calcified nodule without surrounding edema or enhancement is seen on CT **(13-38A)**. Shrunken, calcified lesions are seen as hypointensities on T1WI and T2WI. Perilesional edema is absent.

"Blooming" on T2* GRE is seen and may show multifocal "blooming black dots" if multiple calcified nodules are present **(13-38C)**. Quiescent lesions do not enhance on T1 C+.

Special Features. "Racemose" NCC shows multilobulated, variably sized, grape-like lesions in the basal cisterns. Most cysts lack an identifiable scolex. Arachnoiditis with fibrosis and scarring demonstrates rim enhancement around the cysts and along the brain surfaces. Obstructive hydrocephalus is common **(13-41)**.

NCC-associated vasculitis with stroke is a rare but important complication of "racemose" NCC that can mimic tuberculosis. Most infarcts involve small perforating vessels although large territorial infarcts have been reported.

Intraventricular NCC is associated with poor prognosis. Intraventricular cysts may be difficult to detect on CT. FLAIR and CISS are the most sensitive sequences for detecting the cysts on MR. The fourth ventricle is the most common site (50-55%) **(13-37)** followed by the third ventricle (25-30%), lateral ventricle (10-12%), and aqueduct (8-10%).

Differential Diagnosis

The differential diagnosis of NCC depends on lesion type and location. Subarachnoid/cisternal NCC can resemble **TB meningitis**. In contrast to NCC, the thick purulent basilar exudates typical of TB are solid and lack the cystic features of "racemose" NCC. **Carcinomatous meningitis** and **neurosarcoid** are also rarely cystic.

Abscess and **multifocal septic emboli** can resemble parenchymal NCC cysts but demonstrate a hypointense rim on T2WI and restrict strongly on DWI. A succinate peak on MRS helps distinguish a degenerating NCC cyst from abscess.

A giant parenchymal colloidal-vesicular NCC cyst with ring enhancement can mimic **neoplasm, tuberculoma**, or **toxoplasmosis**.

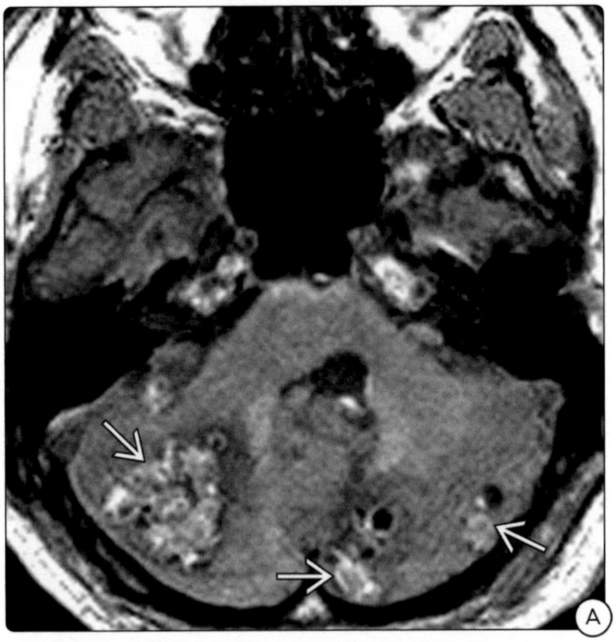

(13-42A) T1 C+ scan in a 20y man with alveolar echinococcosis demonstrates cauliflower-like clusters of multiple small, irregular, ring-enhancing cysts .

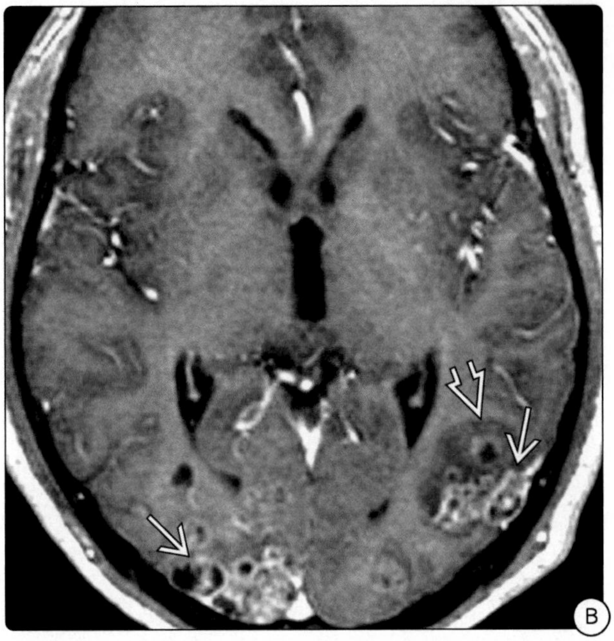

(13-42B) More cephalad T1 C+ scan shows additional collections of enhancing cysts , edema . FLAIR scans (not shown) demonstrated edema around all of the clusters. (Courtesy M. Thurnher, MD.)

The differential diagnosis of intraventricular NCC cyst includes **colloid cyst** (solid), **ependymal cyst** (cystic but lacks a scolex), and **choroid plexus cyst.**

> **NEUROCYSTICERCOSIS: IMAGING AND DIFFERENTIAL DIAGNOSIS**
>
> **Imaging**
> - Varies with stage
>   - Vesicular: Cyst with "dot" (scolex), no edema, no enhancement
>   - Colloidal vesicular: Ring enhancement, edema striking
>   - Granular nodular: Faint rim enhancement, edema decreased
>   - Nodular calcified: CT Ca++, MR "black dots"
> - Common to have lesions in different stages
>
> **Differential Diagnosis**
> - Parenchymal (colloidal vesicular) cyst = neoplasm, toxoplasmosis, TB
> - "Racemose" (subarachnoid) NCC = pyogenic/TB meningitis
> - Intraventricular cyst = ependymal, choroid plexus cysts

Echinococcosis

Terminology and Etiology

Infection by *Echinococcus* is called echinococcosis.

Two species of *Echinococcus* tapeworms, *E. granulosis* (EG) and *E. multilocularis/alveolaris* (EM/EA), are responsible for most human CNS infections. EG infestation is also called **hydatid disease** or hydatid cyst (HC). Infection with EM/EA is also known as **alveolar echinococcosis**.

Epidemiology

After NCC, echinococcosis is the second most common parasitic infection that involves the CNS. Humans—most often children—become accidental intermediate hosts by ingesting eggs in soil contaminated by excrement from a definitive host. Approximately 1-2% of patients with EG and 3-5% of patients with EM/EA develop CNS disease.

EG usually affects children, whereas EM/EA is more common in adults.

Pathology

The gross appearances of EG and EM/EA differ. EG typically produces a well-delineated cyst **(13-43)**. EM/EA has numerous irregular small cysts and appears as an infiltrative, invasive, neoplasm-like lesion in both liver and brain.

Hydatid cysts can be uni- or multilocular with "daughter cysts." The wall of a hydatid cyst has three layers: an outer dense fibrous pericyst, a middle laminated membranous ectocyst, and an inner germinal layer (the endocyst). It is the germinal layer that can produce "daughter cysts."

Imaging

The most common imaging appearance of HC is that of a large, unilocular, thin-walled cyst without calcification, edema, or enhancement on CT. Occasionally, a single large cyst will contain multiple "daughter cysts" **(13-45)**.

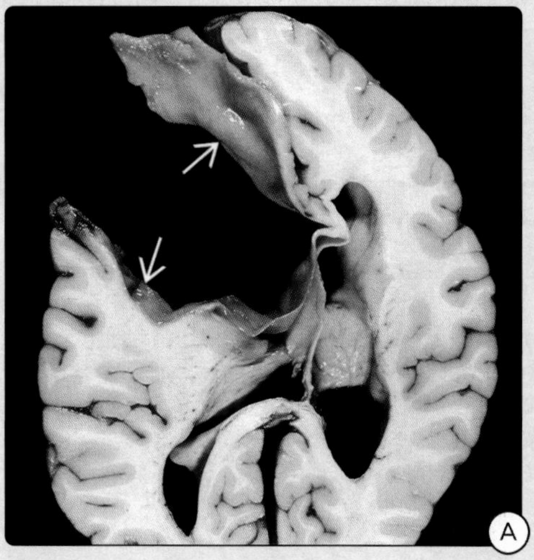

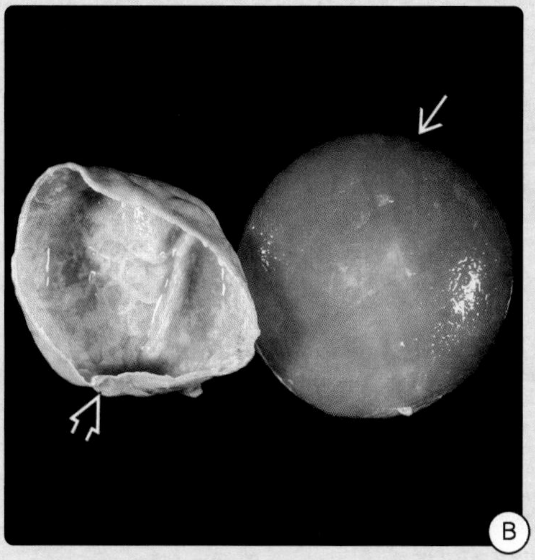

(13-43A) *Autopsy case shows brain after the removal of a huge unilocular hydatid cyst. Note the well-demarcated border between the cyst cavity and the brain. There is no surrounding edema, and the mass effect relative to the size of the cyst is minimal.* ***(13-43B)*** *Photograph of the external cyst wall with cut view of the cyst shows the typical thin wall of a classic hydatid cyst. (Courtesy R. Hewlett, MD.)*

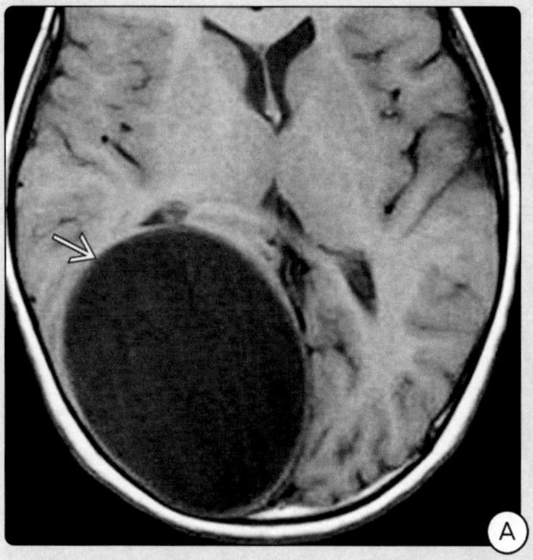

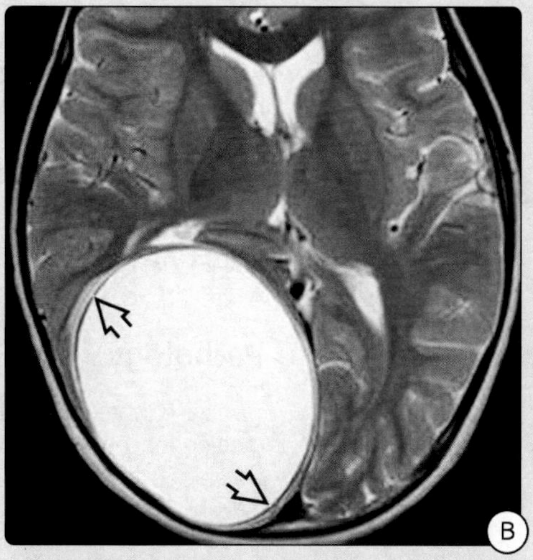

(13-44A) *Axial T1WI shows a unilocular hydatid cyst. Mass effect relative to the overall cyst size is only moderate.* ***(13-44B)*** *T2WI in the same patient nicely demonstrates the typical three-layered cyst wall. (Courtesy R. Hewlett, MD.)*

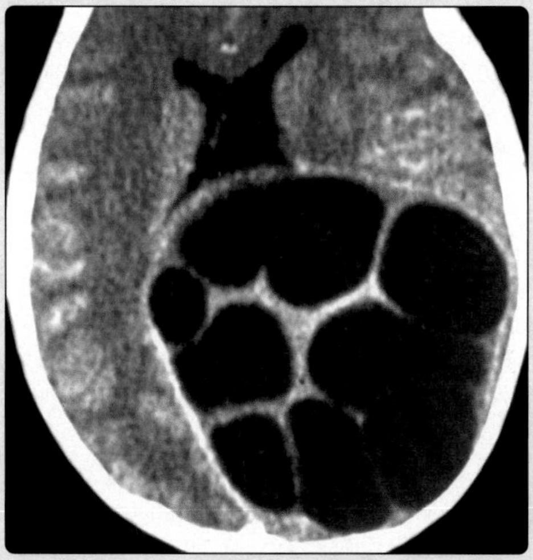

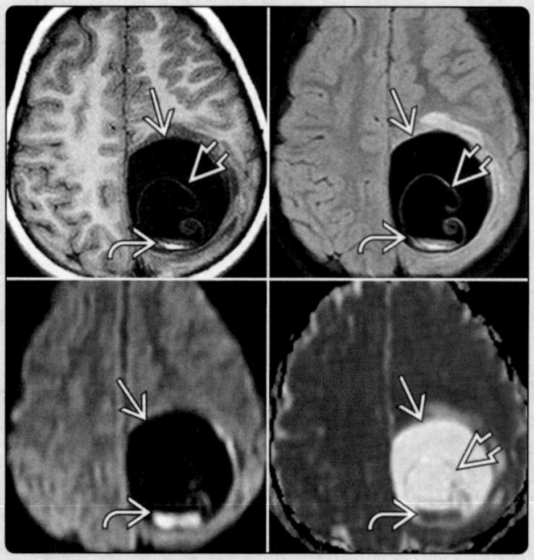

(13-45) *CECT scan shows a multiloculated hydatid cyst that contains multiple "daughter cysts." (Courtesy S. Nagi, MD.)* ***(13-46)*** *Series of axial MR scans with T1WI, FLAIR, DWI, and ADC (clockwise from top left corner) shows a hydatid cyst with detached germinal membrane and hydatid "sand" in the dependent part of the cyst. Surrounding edema and mass effect are minimal.*

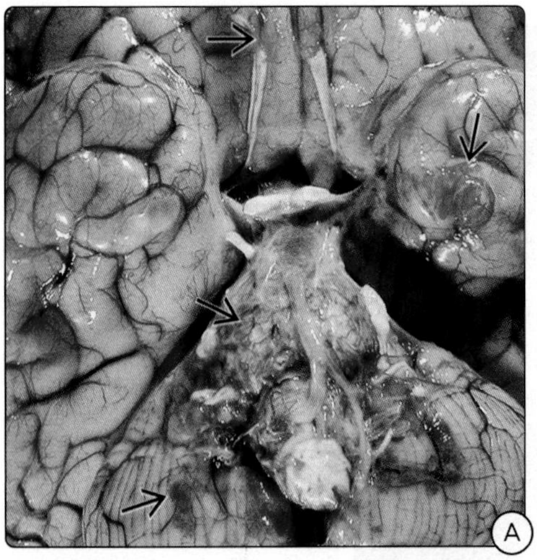

(13-47A) Gross pathology from a patient with amebic meningoencephalitis shows multiple basilar hemorrhagic exudates →.

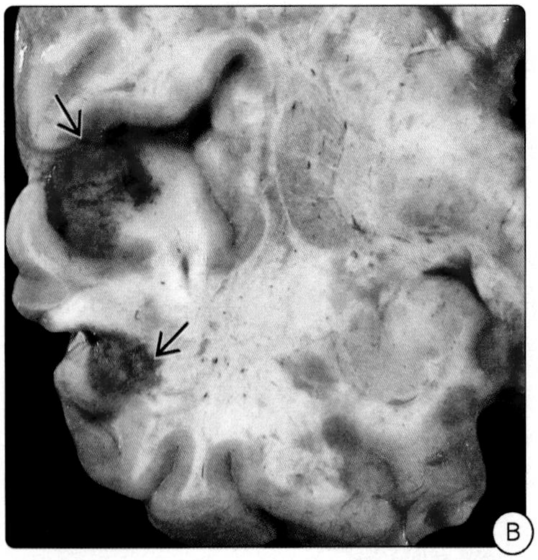

(13-47B) Coronal cut section in the same case demonstrates numerous focal parenchymal hemorrhages →.

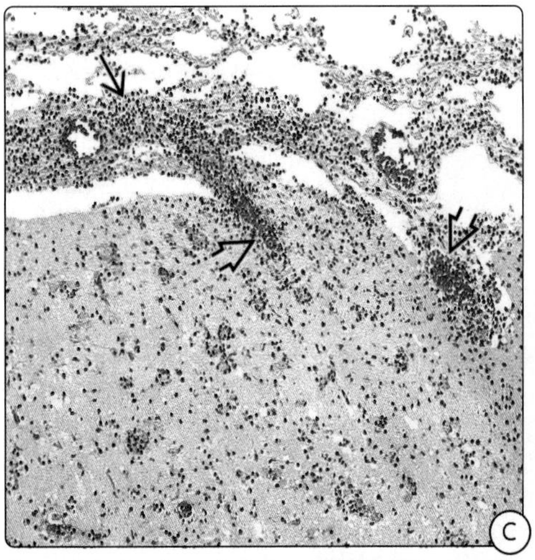

(13-47C) Histology shows meningitis →, hemorrhage/inflammatory cells in Virchow-Robin spaces →. (Courtesy B. K. DeMasters, MD.)

MR shows that cyst fluid is isointense with CSF on T1WI and T2WI **(13-44)**. Sometimes a detached germinal membrane and hydatid "sand" can be seen in the dependent portion of the cyst **(13-46)**.

EA consists of numerous irregular cysts that—unlike HC—are not sharply demarcated from surrounding brain and usually enhance following contrast administration. Irregular peripheral or ring-like, heterogeneous, nodular, and cauliflower-like patterns have been reported **(13-42)**.

Differential Diagnosis

The differential diagnosis of a supratentorial intraaxial cystic mass is extensive and includes cystic neoplasms, abscess, parasitic cysts, and neuroglial cysts. Of these, the most difficult to distinguish from HCs are neuroglial cysts and porencephalic cysts. **Neuroglial cysts** are rarely as large as HCs. **Porencephalic cysts** are literally "holes in the brain" adjacent to—and usually connected with—an enlarged ventricle.

Amebiasis

Terminology and Etiology

Amebae are free-living organisms that are distributed worldwide. Species of the *Acanthamoeba* (Ac) genus are found in soil and dust, fresh or brackish water, and a variety of other locations ranging from hot tubs and hydrotherapy pools to air conditioning units, contact lens solutions, and dental irrigation units. *Balamuthia mandrillaris* is a soil-dwelling organism. *Naegleria fowleri* is found in both soil and fresh water. *Entamoeba histolytica* (EH) occurs in food or water contaminated with feces.

Up to 10% of the population worldwide is infected with EH, but CNS disease is rare.

Pathology

Two basic types of CNS amebic infection occur: primary amebic meningoencephalitis (PAM) and granulomatous amebic encephalitis (GAE). Amebic abscess occurs but is relatively uncommon in Western and industrialized countries.

Gross autopsies of PAM show a necrotizing, hemorrhagic meningitis and angiitis with focal lesions in the orbitofrontal **(13-48)** and temporal lobes, brainstem, and upper spinal cord **(13-47)**. Numerous trophozoites are present, but no cysts are seen because of disease acuity.

GAE demonstrates granulomatous inflammation with multinucleated giant cells, trophozoites, and cysts. An amebic abscess has pus with trophozoites at the edge of the lesion.

Clinical Issues

PAM is an acute, rapidly progressive, necrotizing hemorrhagic meningoencephalitis caused by *N. fowleri*. Healthy children and immunocompetent young adults swimming in warm fresh water during the summer are the typical patients, presenting with fever, headache, and altered mental status. *N. fowleri* invades the olfactory mucosa and enters the brain along the olfactory nerves. PAM is almost always fatal. Death within 48-72 hours is typical.

GAE is a subacute to chronic condition usually caused by one of six *Acanthamoeba* species or *B. mandrillaris*. GAE shows no seasonal predilection. GAE is generally associated with immunodeficiency (e.g., HIV/AIDS, organ transplantation) and chronic debilitating conditions such as malnutrition and diabetes. Presentation ranges from headache and chronic low-grade fever to

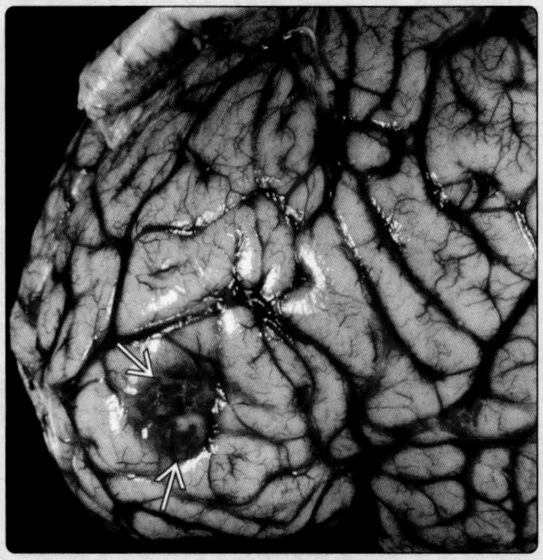

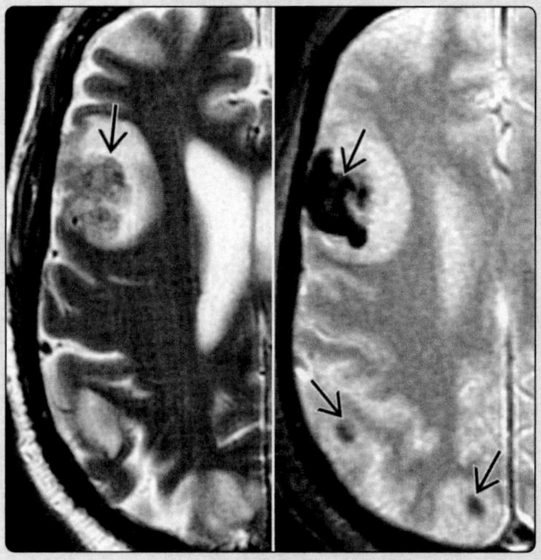

***(13-48)** Lateral view of an autopsied brain from a patient with amebic encephalitis shows focal parenchymal hemorrhage →. **(13-49)** (L) T2WI and (R) T2* GRE in another patient show multiple parenchymal hemorrhages → with "blooming." Biopsy disclosed amebic granuloma.*

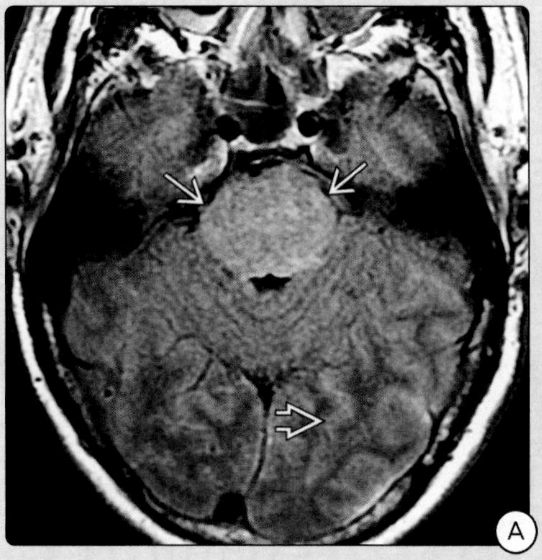

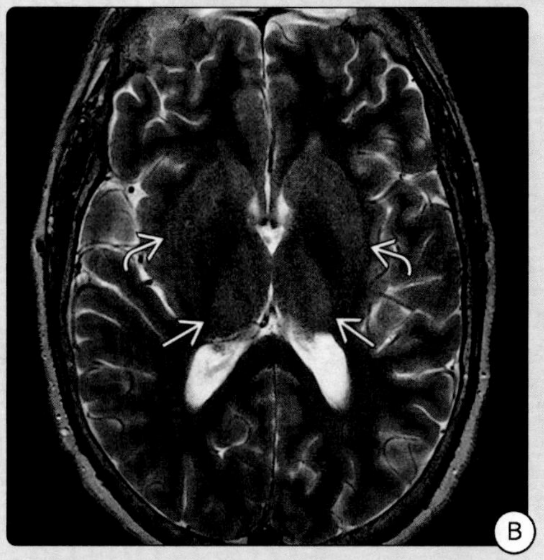

***(13-50A)** A 60y man with URI and fever spiking to 103° developed altered mental status. He rapidly declined and became comatose with GCS 3. Axial FLAIR shows strikingly swollen, hyperintense pons → and diffuse sulcal hyperintensity →. **(13-50B)** T2WI in the same case shows swollen, hyperintense basal ganglia → and thalami →.*

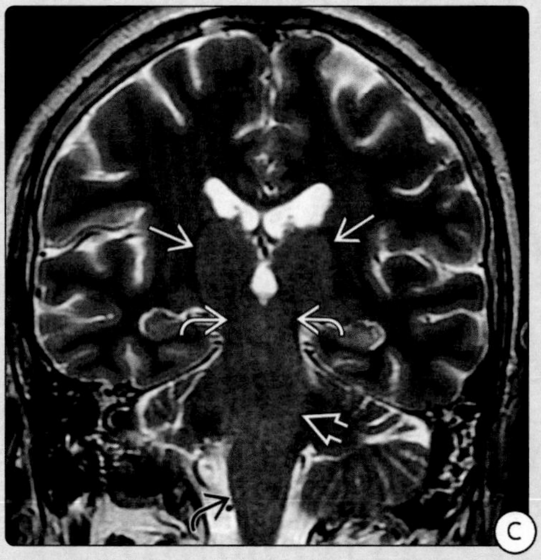

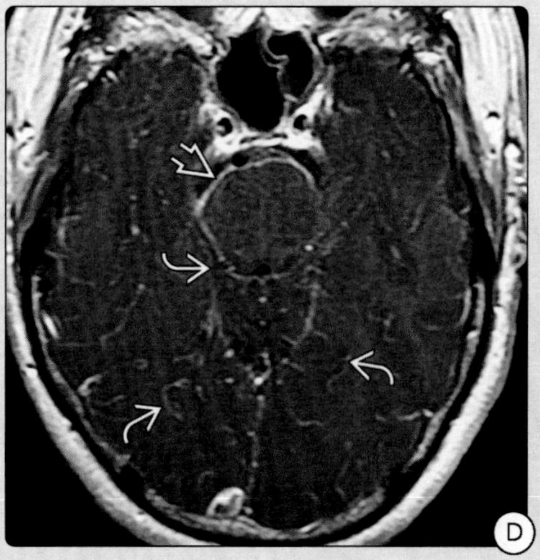

***(13-50C)** Coronal T2WI shows hyperintensity in both thalami →, midbrain →, pons →, and medulla →. **(13-50D)** T1 C+ shows diffuse enhancement along the surface of the pons → and throughout the cerebral sulci →. Imaging diagnosis was meningoencephalitis of unknown etiology. The patient expired 5 days after admission. Autopsy disclosed primary amebic encephalitis.*

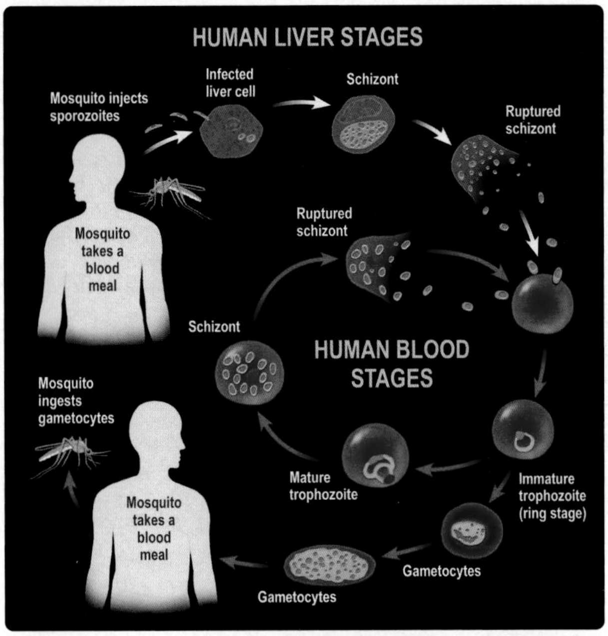

(13-51) Sporozoites inoculated into blood infect the liver cells. When mature, they rupture the cells, releasing merozoites that infect RBCs. Merozoites develop into trophozoites or gametocytes, which are then ingested by uninfected mosquitoes.

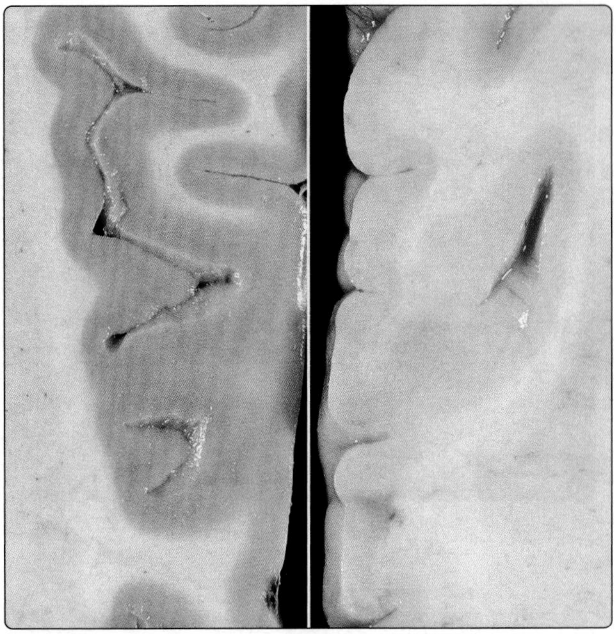

(13-52) Classic "slate gray" edematous cortex of cerebral malaria (L) compared with normal brain (R). (Courtesy R. Hewlett, MD.)

fulminant infection (with *B. mandrillaris*). Focal symptoms are present for an average of 2 or 3 months.

Amebic abscess in the CNS is rare even in endemic areas and is usually caused by *E. histolytica*. Most patients have intestinal or liver infection. In contrast to GAE, amebic abscess is not related to immunodeficiency, and most infected patients are immunocompetent.

Symptoms are nonspecific and include headache, altered mental status, and meningeal symptoms.

Imaging

A broad spectrum of imaging findings in amebic meningoencephalitis has been described, including meningeal exudates, multifocal hemorrhagic parenchymal lesions **(13-49)**, and pseudotumoral lesions with necrosis.

PAM demonstrates findings of leptomeningitis with sulcal obliteration and enhancement, especially along the perimesencephalic cisterns **(13-50D)**. Multifocal parenchymal lesions with involvement of posterior fossa structures, diencephalon, and thalamus are typical **(13-50)**. Necrotizing angiitis with hemorrhages and frank infarction is seen in some cases.

GAE demonstrates a multifocal pattern with discrete lesions at the corticomedullary junction and/or a pseudotumoral pattern with a solitary mass-like lesion.

Amebic abscesses are usually located in the basal ganglia or at the gray-white matter junction. Solitary or multiple irregularly shaped ring-enhancing hemorrhagic lesions are the typical imaging finding.

Differential Diagnosis

The imaging features of amebiasis are nonspecific. Amebic abscesses and meningoencephalitis can mimic disease caused by other pyogenic, parasitic, and granulomatous infections. Multifocal parenchymal and pseudotumoral lesions can mimic neoplasm.

Malaria

Terminology and Etiology

Cerebral malaria (CM) is caused by infection with the protozoan parasite *Plasmodium* and is transmitted by infected *Anopheles* mosquitoes. Four species cause human disease: *P. falciparum*, *P. vivax*, *P. ovale*, and *P. malariae*. Of these, *P. falciparum* has the most severe morbidity and mortality and causes 95% of all CM cases.

The life cycle of a malaria parasite involves the female *Anopheles* mosquito and a human host. Sporozoites are inoculated into humans during the mosquitoes' "blood meal." The sporozoites invade and replicate asexually in liver cells, maturing into schizonts that rupture and release merozoites. The merozoites infect red blood cells (RBCs). Merozoites can develop into trophozoites, which undergo asexual reproduction in the blood, or into gametocytes, which reproduce sexually in deep tissue capillaries. Gametocytes are ingested by mosquitoes, and the cycle is repeated over and over again **(13-51)**.

Pathology

Grossly the brain appears swollen, and its external surface is often a characteristic dusky dark red. Deposition of malaria pigment can give the cortex a slate gray color **(13-52)**. Petechial hemorrhages are often seen in the subcortical white matter, corpus callosum, cerebellum, and brainstem **(13-55)**.

The major microscopic feature is sequestration of parasitized RBCs in the cerebral microvasculature **(13-53)**. Perivascular ring and punctate microhemorrhages are common. Diagnostic black malarial pigment ("hemozoin bodies") within sequestered, hemoglobin-depleted "ghost" RBCs is common. Malaria parasites remain intravascular, so encephalitic inflammatory changes are absent.

Clinical Issues

Epidemiology and Demographics. Falciparum malaria is a leading cause of poor health, neurodisability, and death in tropical countries. Approximately 40% of the world's population is at risk. Between 250 and 500 million new cases of malaria develop every year, and more than half a million people die from the disease. The majority of cases occur in sub-Saharan Africa, where children under 5 years of age are most affected. Peak prevalence is between 1 and 3 years.

Severe malaria develops in 1% of symptomatic malaria infections. Of these, CM is the most severe manifestation. The incidence of CM is 1,120 per 100,000 per year in endemic areas. Malaria causes approximately one million deaths each year.

Malaria is generally restricted to tropical and subtropical areas with altitudes under 1,500 meters and to travelers or immigrants coming from endemic areas. A few isolated cases of "airport malaria" have been reported. For such cases, falciparum malaria occurred in individuals who never traveled outside the country but became infected by imported anopheline mosquitoes at or around an international airport.

Presentation and Natural History. The incubation period from infection to symptom development is 1-3 weeks. Shaking chills followed by cyclical high fever and profuse

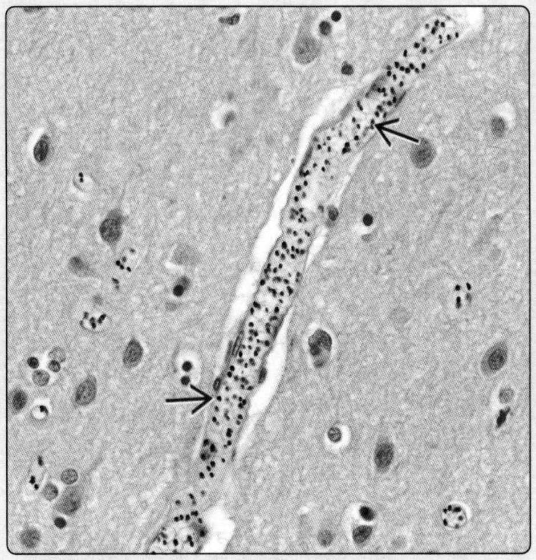

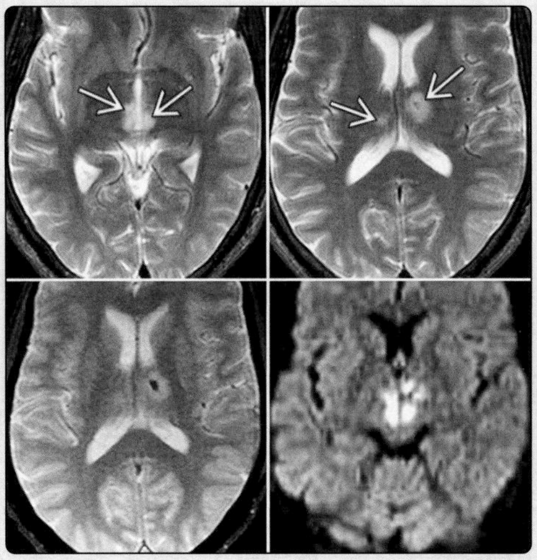

***(13-53)** In cerebral malaria, parasites convert metabolized hemoglobin to hemozoin ("malarial pigment"), seen here as tiny black "dots" in sequestered red blood cells →. (Courtesy B. K. DeMasters, MD.) **(13-54)** Scans in a patient with malaria show T2 basal ganglia hyperintensities → that "bloom" on T2* GRE and restrict on DWI. (Courtesy R. Ramakantan, MD.)*

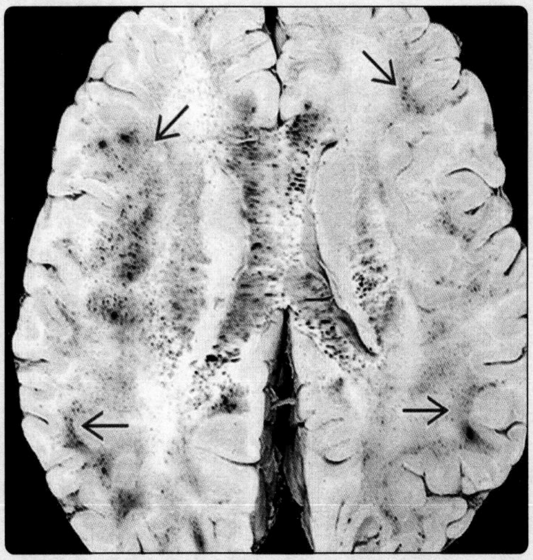

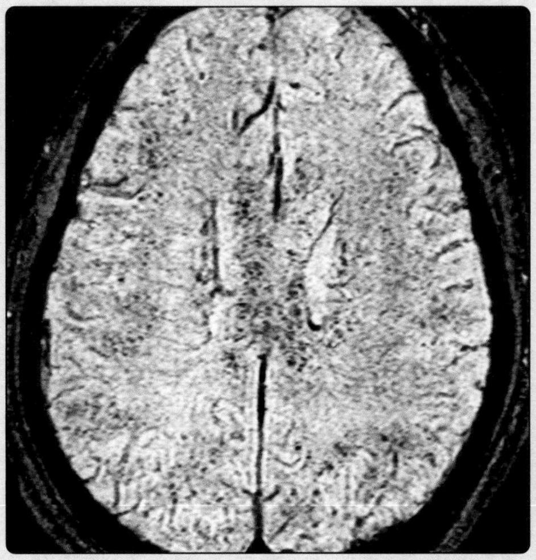

***(13-55)** Cerebral malaria shows innumerable petechial white matter hemorrhages → in the subcortical, deep white matter. (Courtesy L. Chimelli: A morphological approach to the diagnosis of protozoal infections of the CNS. Patholog Res Int. 2011.) **(13-56)** T2* SWI in a patient with cerebral malaria shows innumerable punctate "blooming" microhemorrhages throughout the white matter. (Courtesy K. Tong, MD.)*

sweating are typical and correspond temporally to RBC lysis after schizonts mature. *P. falciparum*, *P. ovale*, and *P. vivax* are characterized by fever every 48 hours, whereas *P. malariae* cycles every 72 hours.

Prognosis is variable. Individuals with sickle cell trait generally have milder disease. In other cases, headache, altered sensorium, and seizures develop and can be followed within 1-2 days by impaired consciousness, coma, and death. Mortality in CM is 15-20% even with appropriate therapy. Although many surviving patients recover completely, between 10-25% of affected children have long-term neurologic deficits.

P. falciparum relapse is rare. *P. vivax* and *P. ovale* can relapse, as dormant liver stages allow the parasite to survive during colder periods. Active forms can arise months to years later.

Imaging

Imaging findings on NECT vary from normal to striking. The most typical finding is focal infarcts in the cortex, basal ganglia, and thalami. Gross hemorrhage can occur but is rare. Diffuse cerebral edema is seen in severe CM and is especially prevalent in children.

MR shows focal hyperintensities in the basal ganglia, thalami, and white matter on T2/FLAIR **(13-54)**. Confluent hyperintensities can occur in severe cases although large territorial infarcts are rare.

T2* scans demonstrate multifocal "blooming" petechial hemorrhages in the basal ganglia and cerebral white matter. These linear and punctate hypointensities are especially striking on susceptibility-weighted imaging (SWI) **(13-55) (13-56)**. Malarial lesions generally do not enhance on T1 C+.

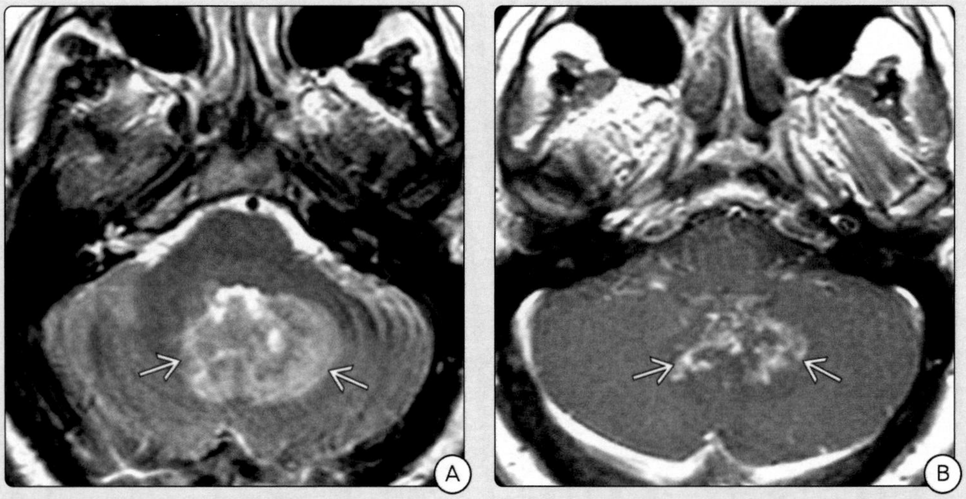

(13-57A) *Axial T2WI in a 34y man with schistosomiasis shows a mixed hypo- and hyperintense lesion involving the vermis and both cerebellar hemispheres.* ***(13-57B)*** *Axial T1 C+ scan shows a patchy "arborization" pattern of enhancement.*

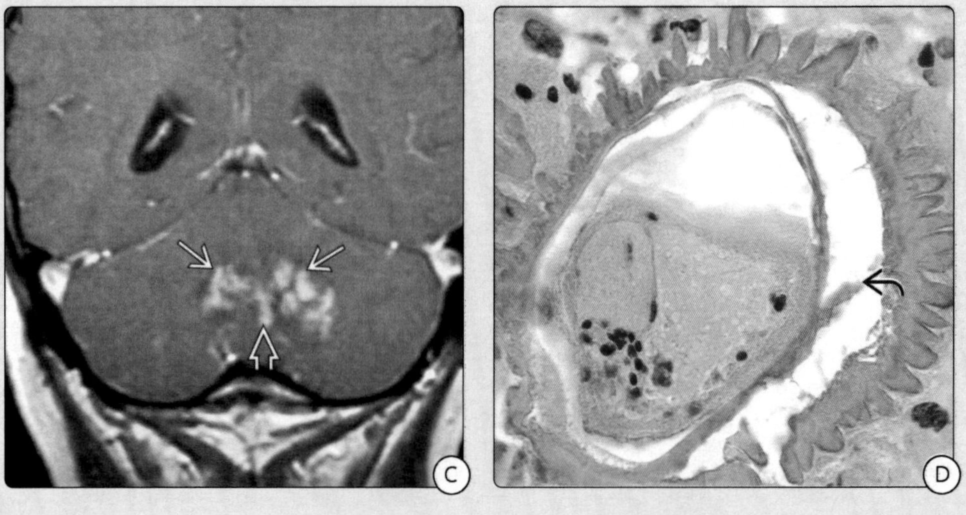

(13-57C) *Coronal T1 C+ shows patchy enhancement around a central linear focus, suggesting an "arborization" pattern.* ***(13-57D)*** *Microscopic view from the biopsied lesion shows the encysted S. mansoni with the classic lateral spine. (Courtesy D. Kremens, MD, S. Galetta, MD.)*

Differential Diagnosis

CM is a clinical diagnosis and should be considered in any patient with a febrile illness and impaired consciousness who lives in—or has recently traveled to—endemic malaria areas!

Differential diagnosis varies with patient age. The major imaging differential diagnosis of CM in adults is **multiple cerebral emboli/infarction**, which more commonly involves the gray-white matter junction or cortex. Multifocal white matter petechial hemorrhages on T2* are nonspecific and can be seen in **fat emboli** syndrome, **acute hemorrhagic leukoencephalitis**, **diffuse vascular injury**, and **thrombotic microangiopathies** such as disseminated intravascular coagulopathy.

The major differential diagnosis of CM in children is **acute necrotizing encephalopathy** and **infantile bilateral striatal necrosis**. These are generally influenza-associated diseases and follow flu-like respiratory infection or rotavirus gastroenteritis.

Other Parasitic Infections

Several parasites that affect humans invade the CNS, particularly if humans serve as intermediate or nonpermissive hosts. Schistosomiasis, paragonimiasis, sparganosis, trichinosis, and trypanosomiasis can occasionally involve the CNS. Although these parasitic infestations can occur at any age, they most commonly affect children and young adults.

Brain involvement is relatively uncommon. Common clinical features of CNS parasitoses include headache, epilepsy, and impaired consciousness. When CNS infestations occur, these parasites are associated with significant mortality and morbidity. Because imaging often resembles neoplasm, a history of travel to—or residence in—an endemic area is key to the diagnosis.

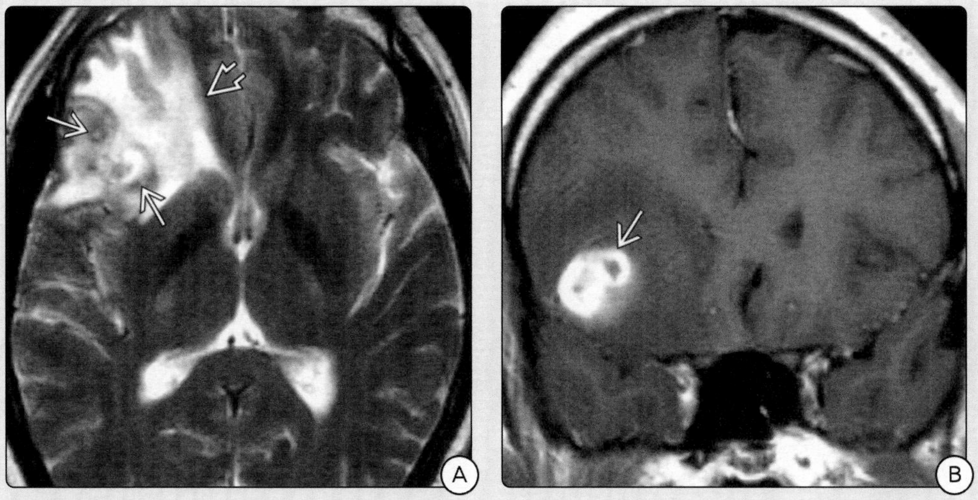

***(13-58A)** Axial T2WI in a young man from southeast Asia shows a heterogeneous right frontal lobe mass with intralesional hypointensities, suggesting hemorrhage. Moderate perilesional edema is present. **(13-58B)** Coronal T1 C+ shows conglomerate ring-enhancing lesions. Paragonimiasis granuloma was found at surgery.*

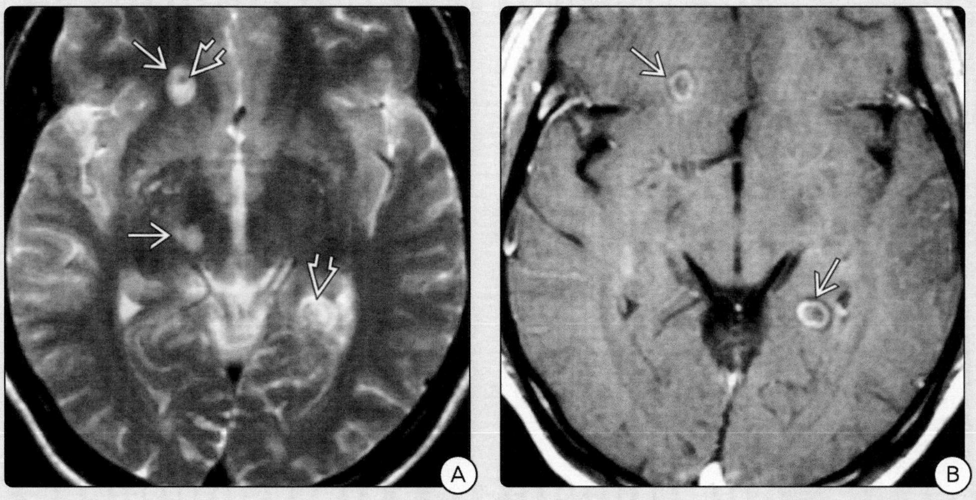

***(13-59A)** Axial T2WI in a patient with known sparganosis shows multiple ring-like hyperintensities with central hypointense foci. **(13-59B)** Axial T1 C+ scan in the same patient shows nonspecific ring enhancement. No "tunnel" sign was present. (Courtesy M. Castillo, MD.)*

Schistosomiasis

Schistosomiasis, also known as bilharziasis, is a trematode (fluke) infection that affects more than 200 million people worldwide.

Several *Schistosoma* species cause human disease. *Schistosoma haematobium* is endemic in Africa, especially the Nile River basin. *S. mansoni* is also endemic in Africa (the midcontinent and lake region), South America, and the Caribbean **(13-57D)**. *S. japonicum* is endemic in China, and *S. mekongi* is endemic in Southeast Asia.

Schistosoma species have a complex life cycle. Ova in human urine and feces hatch in fresh water and enter snails as their intermediate host. Snails release motile larvae (cercariae) that infect humans wading or swimming in infested water. The larvae penetrate skin and migrate to the liver or lungs, where they mature. Adult worms migrate to venous plexuses in the intestines (*S. mansoni, S. japonicum*) or bladder (*S. hematobium*).

The mature worms release eggs, which can be shed in urine or feces. Eggs can also disseminate to ectopic sites, including the brain. Focal meningeal and firm parenchymal masses are the typical gross pathologic findings. On microscopic examination, schistosome eggs show no spine (*S. japonicum*) or a terminal (*S. haematobium*) or lateral (*S. mansoni*) spine.

Typical imaging findings of neuroschistosomiasis are single or multiple conglomerated heterogeneous lesion(s) with edema and mass effect. A central linear enhancement surrounded by multiple punctate nodules (an "arborized" appearance) on T1 C+ MR **(13-57C)** has been described as characteristic.

Paragonimiasis

Paragonimiasis is another snail-borne trematode infection. Humans become infected by eating undercooked fresh water

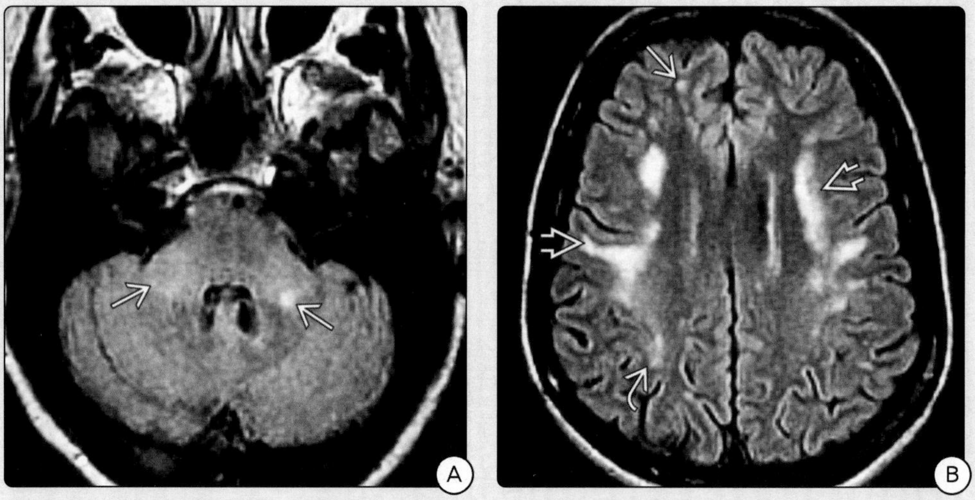

***(13-60A)** Series of axial FLAIR images demonstrates the multifocal T2/FLAIR white matter hyperintensities persisting 1 year after complete clinical response to treatment. Lesions are present in both middle cerebellar peduncles ➡. **(13-60B)** More cephalad scan in the same case shows multifocal punctate ➡ and patchy ➡ and confluent ➡ lesions in the subcortical and deep periventricular white matter.*

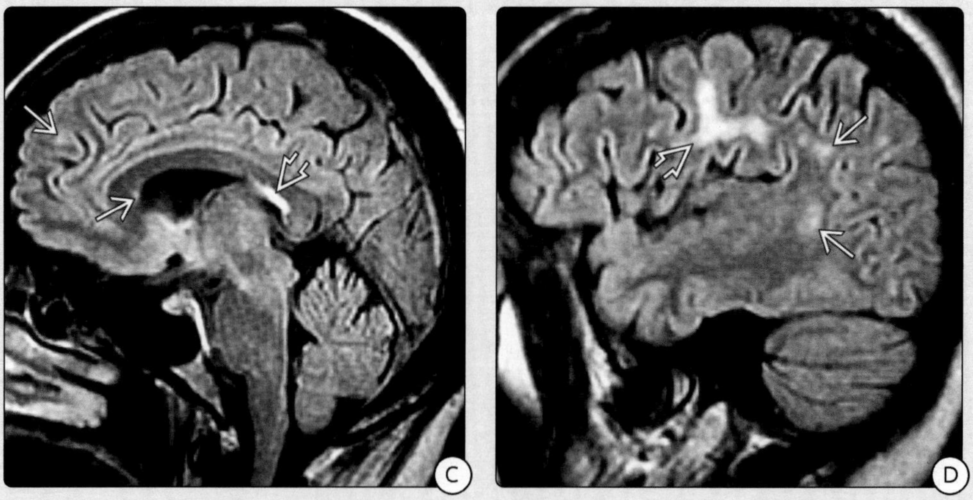

***(13-60C)** Midline sagittal FLAIR in the same case shows punctate lesions in the subcortical white matter and corpus callosum ➡. A larger confluent lesion in the corpus callosum ➡ is present just anterior to the splenium. **(13-60D)** More lateral FLAIR in the same case shows multiple punctate ➡ and confluent ➡ lesions in the subcortical white matter. Note sparing of the subcortical U fibers. This is documented Lyme disease.*

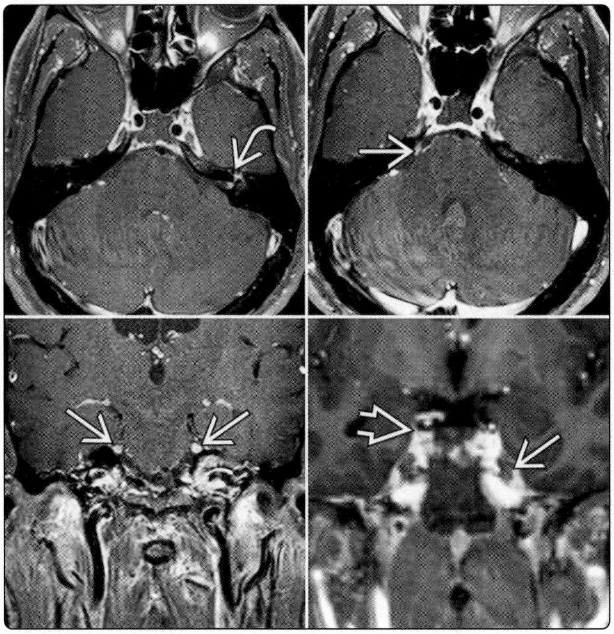

(13-61) Axial (top), coronal (bottom) T1 C+ FS scans in a patient with Lyme disease demonstrate left CN VII, bilateral CN V, and left CN III enhancement. (Courtesy P. Hildenbrand, MD.)

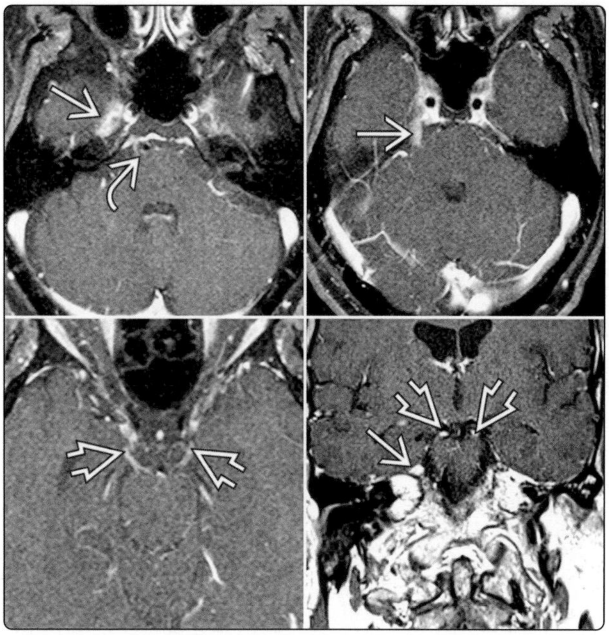

(13-62) T1 C+ FS scans in a patient with Lyme disease and multiple cranial nerve palsies show enhancement of the right fifth and sixth CNs as well as both oculomotor nerves. (Courtesy P. Hildenbrand, MD.)

crabs or crayfish contaminated by *Paragonimus westermani*, a lung fluke endemic in Asia and Central and South America. Worms penetrate the skull base foramina and meninges, then directly invade the brain, where they elicit a granulomatous inflammatory reaction. Adolescent boys are most commonly affected.

Imaging shows a heterogeneous mass with multiple conglomerated ring-enhancing lesions surrounded by edema **(13-58)**. Intralesional hemorrhage is common.

Sparganosis

Sparganosis is a rare parasitic infection caused by the larval cestode of *Spirometra mansoni*. Nearly half of all reported cases are due to ingestion of raw or undercooked frogs or snakes. Sparganosis is endemic in Southeast Asia, China, Japan, and Korea.

Imaging studies show an irregularly shaped mass, usually in the cerebral white matter, surrounded by edema. The most common imaging finding is the "tunnel" sign, a hollow tube ("tunnel") several centimeters long created by the burrowing worm. The "tunnel" is surrounded by an enhancing rim of reactive inflammatory granulomatous tissue. The second most common feature of cerebral sparganosis is a conglomerate mass of ring- or bead-like enhancing lesions **(13-59)**.

Sparganosis is typically characterized by the simultaneous presence of new and old lesions. Lesions in different stages of evolution from acute infection to cortical atrophy with white matter volume loss and calcifications around degenerated/dead worms are typical of this particular parasitic infestation.

Differential Diagnosis

Most parasitic infections share several common features. They usually present as mass-like lesions with edema and multiple "conglomerate" ring-enhancing foci. **Metastasis** and **glioblastoma multiforme** are two common neoplasms that can appear very similar to parasitic masses. **Inflammatory granulomas** (e.g., TB granulomas) can also mimic parasitic granulomas and are often endemic in the same geographic areas.

Miscellaneous and Emerging CNS Infections

Spirochete Infections of the CNS

Two spirochete species can cause significant CNS disease: *Borrelia* (e.g., Lyme disease, relapsing fever borreliosis) and *Treponema* (neurosyphilis).

Lyme Disease

Terminology. Lyme disease (LD) is also known as Lyme borreliosis. LD with neurologic disease is called Lyme neuroborreliosis (LNB) or neuro-Lyme disease. **Relapsing fever borreliosis** is a multisystem disease that infects a variety of tissues including the CNS (rare).

Lyme disease is a multisystem inflammatory disease caused by *B. burgdorferi* in the United States and *B. garinii* or *B. afzelii* in Europe. LD is a zoonosis maintained in animals such as field mice and white-tailed deer.

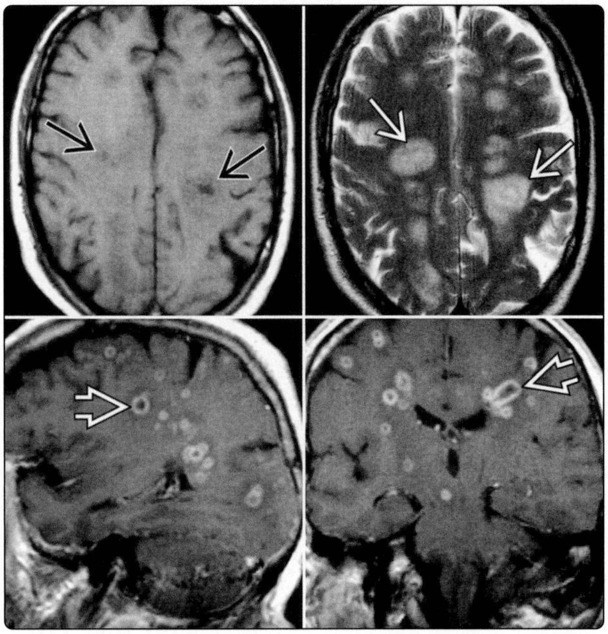

(13-63) (Upper L) T1 shows bilateral iso-/hypodense WM lesions ➙. (Upper R) T2 shows bilateral "fluffy" hyperintense lesions ➙ in the corona radiata. Sagittal (lower L) and coronal (lower R) show multifocal ring enhancement ➙; rickettsial encephalitis.

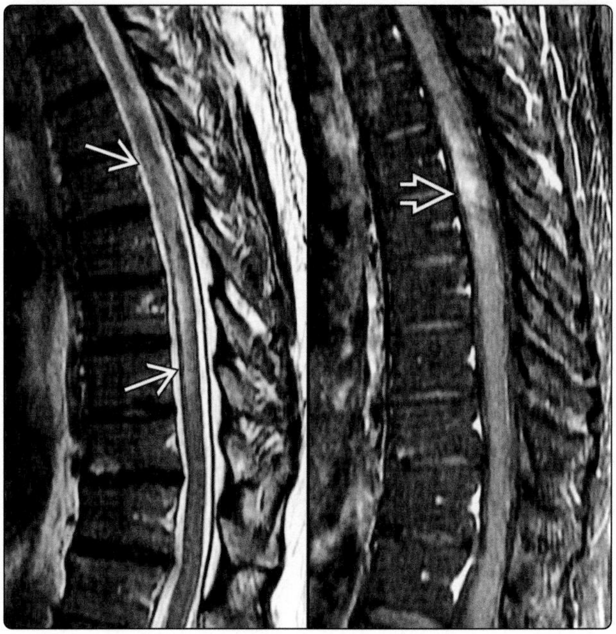

(13-64) Sagittal T2WI (L) and T1 C+ FS scan (R) of the thoracic cord show hyperintense cord lesions ➙ with patchy enhancement ➙. This is documented Lyme disease. (Courtesy P Hildenbrand, MD.)

LD is transmitted to humans by bite of *Ixodes* ticks and requires at least 36 hours of tick attachment as the spirochete moves from the tick midgut to the salivary glands to be transmitted. Most cases result from the bite of an infected nymph (about the size of a poppy seed) and may easily go unnoticed.

Relapsing fever (RF) borreliosis is caused by arthropod-borne spirochetes of the genus *Borrelia*. The major agents vary worldwide. In North America, RF is generally caused by *B. hermsii* and *B. turicatae* and is transmitted by tick bites. Small mammals (principally rodents) and birds are the reservoir organisms.

Etiology. The precise mechanism of CNS involvement is unclear. Direct brain infection/invasion, antigen-driven autoimmune-mediated mechanisms, and vasculitis-like processes have been postulated.

Clinical Issues

Epidemiology and demographics. LD is now the most common tick-borne disease in the United States and Europe with 20,000 new cases reported each year.

Prevalence varies significantly with geography. Between 90-95% of cases in the United States occur in the Mid-Atlantic states, the Northeast, and the upper Midwest (primarily Minnesota and Wisconsin). Occurrence peaks during the early summer, especially May and June.

LD occurs at all ages, but peak presentation is between 16 and 60 years. Thirty percent of cases occur in children.

Presentation. North American LD occurs in stages. Stage 1 occurs between 2 and 30 days after the initial tick bite and is characterized by erythema migrans—a characteristic round, outwardly expanding, target-like ("bull's-eye") rash—and "summer flu" symptoms such as fever, headache, and malaise. Migrating myalgias and pain in large joints may develop ("Lyme arthritis").

Stage 2 occurs 1-4 months after infection and presents with neurologic and cardiac symptoms. Neurologic symptoms develop in approximately 10-15% of cases, whereas cardiac involvement occurs in 8%. Stage 3 can occur several years following the initial infection and manifests as arthritic and chronic neurologic symptoms.

The classic triad of North American LNB consists of aseptic meningitis, cranial neuritis, and radiculoneuritis. Uni- or bilateral facial palsy is common and helps differentiate LNB from other disorders. Erythema migrans, "Lyme arthritis," and carditis are also common.

The most common symptom in children is headache, followed by facial nerve palsy and meningismus.

The most common presentation of European LNB is the triad of Bannwarth syndrome: lymphocytic meningitis, cranial neuropathy, and painful radiculitis. Erythema migrans, "Lyme arthritis," and carditis are all uncommon manifestations of European LD.

Natural history. The diagnosis and treatment of chronic LD are controversial. To date, there is no systematic evidence that *B. burgdorferi* can be identified in patients with chronic symptoms following treated LD (posttreatment Lyme disease syndrome, or PTLDS). Multiple randomized prospective trials have demonstrated no durable or significant benefit in treating PTLDS patients with prolonged courses of antibiotics.

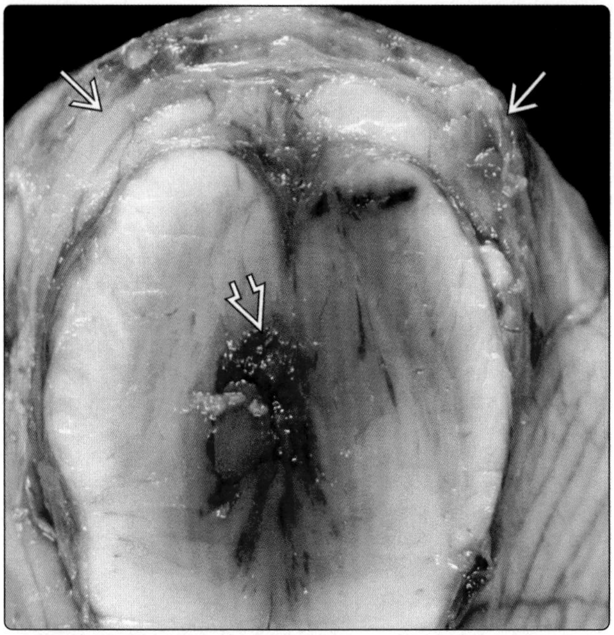

(13-65) Close-up view of autopsied brain demonstrates the typical findings of meningovascular syphilis. Exudate covers the pons →. A syphilitic gumma ⇨ is also present. (Courtesy R. Hewlett, MD.)

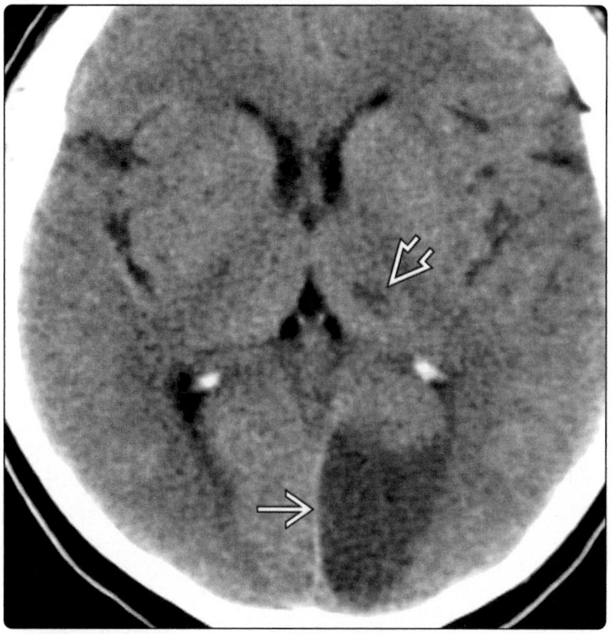

(13-66) NECT scan in a patient with meningovascular syphilis shows left occipital → and thalamic infarcts ⇨. DSA (not shown) disclosed vasculitis-like findings. (Courtesy P. Hildenbrand, MD.)

Diagnosis. Both the American Academy of Neurology (AAN) and the European Federation of Neurological Societies have recommended criteria for the diagnosis of LMB. In addition to all of the criteria included in the AAN, the European Federation requires CSF pleocytosis, evidence for intrathecal *B. burgdorferi* antibody, and no other "obvious reasons" for the neurologic symptoms other than Lyme for the definite diagnosis of LD.

DIAGNOSIS OF LYME NEUROBORRELIOSIS

American Academy of Neurology Recommendations

- Possible exposure to *Ixodes* ticks in Lyme-endemic area
- One or more of the following:
  - Erythema migrans
  - Immunologic evidence of exposure to *Borrelia burgdorferi*
  - Histopathologic, microbiologic, or PCR proof of *B. burgdorferi* infection
- Occurrence of a clinical disorder within the realm of those associated with Lyme disease (no other apparent cause)

European Federation of Neurological Societies

- Definite neuroborreliosis = all of below:
  - Neurologic symptoms suggestive of Lyme neuroborreliosis without other obvious reasons
  - CSF pleocytosis
  - Intrathecal *B. burgdorferi* antibody production
- Possible neuroborreliosis = 2 of the above

Pathology. Findings of meningitis and radiculitis predominate. Microscopic features include nonspecific perivascular T-lymphocytic cuffing and plasma cell infiltrates with axonal degeneration. Lymphocytes and plasma cells accumulate in autonomic ganglia of the peripheral nervous system. Spirochetes can be identified in the leptomeninges, nerve roots, and dorsal root ganglia, but not in the CNS parenchyma.

Imaging. Approximately 12-15% of patients with untreated *B. burgdorferi* infection develop CNS involvement. NECT and CECT scans in these patients are usually normal. MR findings vary with clinical syndrome.

Cranial Neuropathy. The most common clinical presentation of early LNB in the USA is facial palsy and is commonly misdiagnosed as Bell palsy.

Cranial nerve involvement is especially common in North American LNB. CN VII is the most frequently involved **(13-61)**, followed by CNs V and III. Involvement of other cranial nerves is less common.

Unilateral disease is more common than bilateral disease although multiple nerves can be affected **(13-62)**. Uniform enhancement on T1 C+ FS is the typical finding.

Encephalopathy. The most common MR finding is multiple small (2-8 mm) subcortical and periventricular white matter hyperintensities on T2/FLAIR **(13-60)**. These are identified in approximately half of all patients with LNB. Large "tumefactive" lesions are uncommon.

Enhancement of LNB white matter lesions varies from none to moderate **(13-63)**. Occasionally "horseshoe" or incomplete ring enhancement occurs and can mimic demyelinating disease.

Myelitis and Radiculitis. Spinal cord involvement by *B. burgdorferi* is very rare but is more common in European LD.

Diffuse or multifocal hyperintense lesions on T2WI with patchy cord and linear nerve root enhancement are typical **(13-64)**.

In European LNB, enhancement of cauda equina and lower spinal cord nerve roots is more common than cranial nerve enhancement.

Rare Manifestations. Rare reported manifestations of LNB include cerebral vasculitis with stroke, intracranial hypertension, chronic progressive encephalitis, and Borrelial lymphocytoma (predominately seen in Europe).

Differential Diagnosis. The major differential diagnosis of LNB is demyelinating disease. **Multiple sclerosis** (MS) frequently involves the periventricular white matter. Callososeptal involvement is more common in MS compared with LNB. Cranial nerve enhancement—especially CN VII—is less common than with LNB.

Susac syndrome typically involves the middle layers of the corpus callosum and is often accompanied by sensorineural hearing loss (rare in LNB) and visual symptoms.

Vasculitis involves the basal ganglia more than LNB does and rarely affects the cranial nerves.

Neurosyphilis

Terminology and Etiology. Syphilis is a chronic systemic infectious disease caused by the spirochete *Treponema pallidum*. Syphilis is usually transmitted via sexual contact although some cases of vertical transmission from mother to fetus have been reported. Neurosyphilis (NS) is also called neurolues. A focal syphilitic granuloma is called a gumma.

Epidemiology and Demographics. Once expected to be eradicated with the use of penicillin, syphilis has become dramatically more prevalent since 2000, primarily because of HIV/AIDS. Syphilis and HIV have emerged as important

(13-67A) *Axial T2WI in a 47y HIV-positive man with trigeminal neuralgia shows a mixed iso-/hyperintense mass involving the pons, cerebellum, and trigeminal nerve.* ***(13-67B)*** *Axial T1 C+ FS demonstrates pial enhancement surrounding the medulla and extending into the left internal auditory canal.*

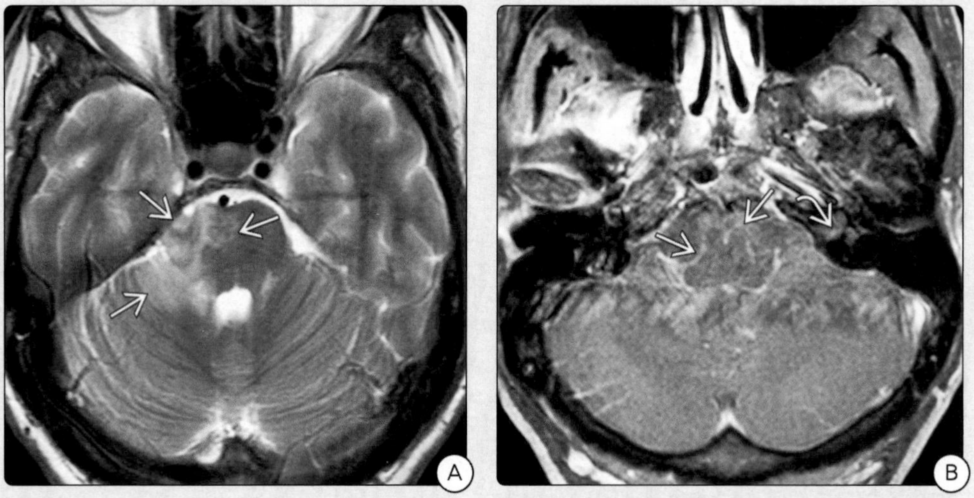

(13-67C) *More cephalad T1 C+ FS scan in the same patient shows intense enhancement in the pons and cerebellum with extension into Meckel cave and thickening of the adjacent dura.* ***(13-67D)*** *Coronal T1 C+ scan demonstrates the syphilitic gumma, adjacent dural thickening, and enhancement in both internal auditory canals. The patient's CD4 count at the time of imaging was 200. This is biopsy-proven meningovascular syphilis.*

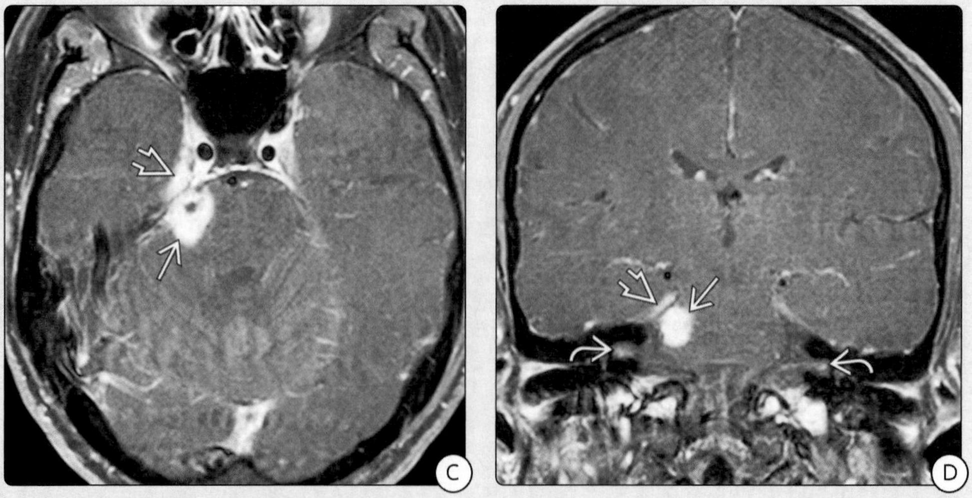

copathogens with reciprocal augmentation in both transmission and disease progression. HIV-positive patients tend to experience more aggressive symptomatology and are at greater risk of developing neurologic disease.

The M:F ratio is 2:1. Most patients are between 18 and 64 years with a mean age of slightly over 50 years. Congenital syphilitic gummatous lesions are exceptionally rare.

Clinical Issues. Between 5-10% of patients with untreated syphilis develop NS. *T. pallidum* disseminates to the CNS within days after exposure, although symptomatic NS can occur up to 25 years after the initial chancre. Peak occurrence is 15 years after primary infection.

NS has been divided into five major but overlapping clinicopathologic categories, i.e., asymptomatic, meningeal, meningovascular, parenchymatous, and gummatous. Neuropsychiatric disturbances are the most common presentation. Clinical manifestations can occur during any stage of the infection.

Early NS generally presents as meningovascular disease. Late NS is associated with chronic syphilis in the brain and spinal cord but rarely presents with classic tabes dorsalis or general paresis. Neuropsychiatric disturbances, primarily cognitive impairment and personality change, are common.

CSF Venereal Disease Research Laboratory (VDRL) tests are specific but not especially sensitive tests for NS. CSF VDRL is positive in just over 60% of cases. *T. pallidum* hemagglutination assay is positive in 80-85%.

Pathology. Brain syphilitic gumma is a completely curable disease, so appropriate diagnosis is essential for patient treatment.

Syphilitic gummata consist of a dense inflammatory infiltrate with large numbers of lymphocytes and plasma cells surrounding a central caseous necrotic core. Vascular proliferation, endarteritis with intimal thickening, and perivascular inflammation are characteristic findings. The definitive histologic diagnosis is obtained using fluorescent isothiocyanate-labeled monoclonal antibodies or PCR.

Gummata probably arise from excessive response of the cell-mediated immune system. Nearly two-thirds are located along brain surfaces, especially over the cerebral convexities. Direct extension from syphilitic meningovascular pial inflammation into the adjacent brain along the penetrating perivascular spaces is the probable mechanism. Dural thickening and inflammation adjacent to cerebral gummata are common.

Imaging. Two neuroimaging patterns should alert the neuroradiologist to the possible diagnosis of cerebral gummas: dural-based lesions that can mimic meningiomas and medial temporal lobe abnormalities that can mimic herpes encephalitis.

Syphilitic gummata are hypodensity or mixed-density lesions on NECT that enhance intensely on CECT. A ring-like or diffuse enhancement pattern is typical.

MR shows the gummata are hypointense on T1 and heterogeneously hyperintense on T2WI. Marked enhancement on T1 C+ is seen, and a dural "tail" is present in one-third of cases **(13-67)**.

Meningovascular syphilis may also cause a vasculopathy with lacunar or territorial infarcts that are indistinguishable from thromboembolic strokes **(13-66)**.

Differential Diagnosis. Because of their relative rarity, syphilitic gummata are most commonly misdiagnosed as **primary** or **metastatic neoplasms**. HIV/AIDS patients who have positive blood/CSF syphilis titers and a cerebral mass lesion with characteristic imaging findings might warrant an empiric trial of intravenous penicillin G with follow-up imaging.

SPIROCHETE CNS INFECTIONS

Lyme Disease (Neuroborreliosis)
- 12-15% develop CNS infection
- Cranial neuropathy
  - CN VII > V, III; others less common
  - Can affect multiple nerves
  - Smooth, linear enhancement on T1 C+
- Encephalopathy
  - T2/FLAIR punctate/confluent subcortical/deep white matter hyperintensities in 50%
  - Less common = tumefactive lesions ("fluffy" lesions, ring or incomplete ring enhancement)
- Myelitis/radiculopathy
  - Most common manifestation in European Lyme disease
  - Patchy cord enhancement
  - Multiple nerve roots may enhance

Neurosyphilis
- Increasing prevalence with AIDS epidemic
  - 75% men having sex with men
  - 50% coinfected with HIV
  - Can develop even with treated uncomplicated syphilis
- Dural-based gummas (mimics meningioma)
- Medial temporal lobe lesions (mimics herpes encephalitis)

Emerging CNS Infections

Emerging infections are diseases that are literally emerging to infect humans. Some of these are zoonoses (i.e., diseases transmitted from animals to humans), whereas others are insect borne. Most rarely affect the CNS, but, when they do, the results can be disastrous. Examples of the latter include the hemorrhagic viral fevers such as Korean hemorrhagic fever, Rift Valley fever, hantavirus, dengue, and Ebola.

Listeriosis

Listeriosis is an emerging food-borne zoonotic infection caused by *Listeria monocytogenes*, a gram-positive facultative intracellular bacterium that dwells in soil, vegetation, or animal reservoirs. There are six species of Listeria, only one of which—*L. monocytogenes*—is pathogenic in humans.

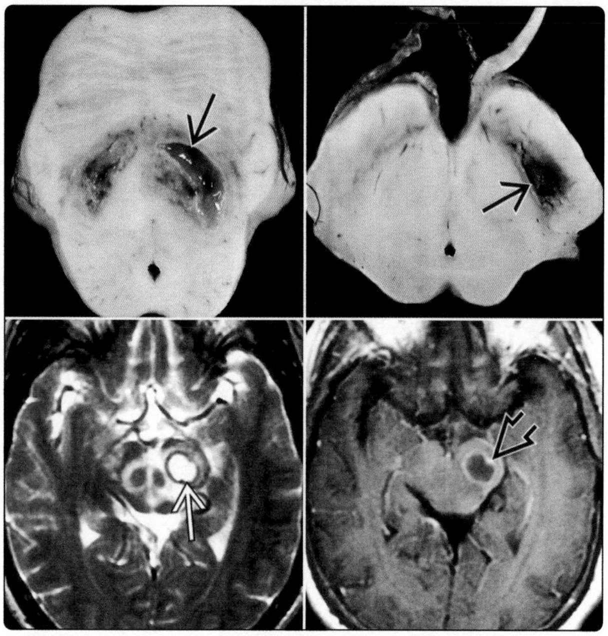

(13-68) Listeriosis shows classic findings of midbrain abscess ➙. T2WI (L), T1 C+ (R) a few days before death show focal hyperintense mass in left cerebral peduncle with hypointense rim ➙, perilesional edema, ring enhancement ➙.

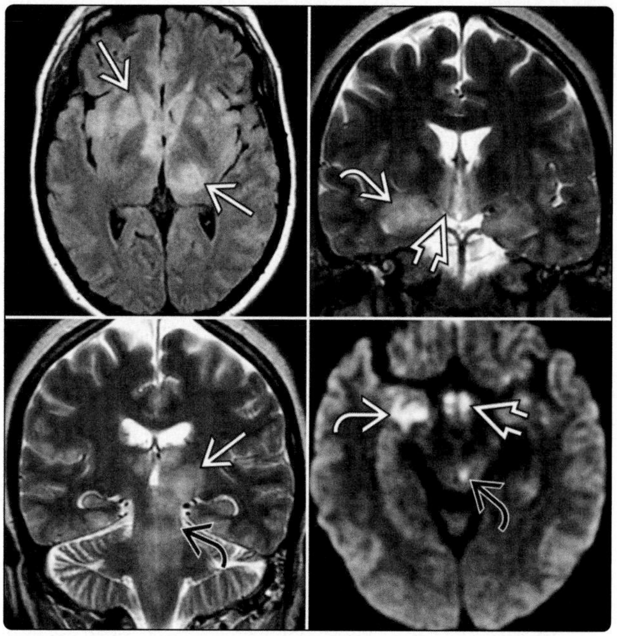

(13-69) FLAIR, T2WI, and DWI illustrate imaging findings of Dengue fever with bilateral, multifocal lesions in the basal ganglia and thalami ➙, medial temporal lobes ➙, midbrain and pons ➙, and hypothalamus ➙. (Courtesy D. Bertholdo, MD.)

Listeria causes gastroenteritis, mother-to-fetus infection, septicemia, and CNS infection in immunocompromised individuals, pregnant women, and newborns.

CNS listeriosis shows a specific tropism for the meninges and brainstem. Symptoms include fever, headache, cranial nerve palsies, vertigo, and somnolence. Once symptoms of CNS disease develop, the mortality rate is 25-30%.

Imaging findings are generally nonspecific. CNS listeriosis can occur as meningitis, encephalitis, cerebritis, or abscess. In the appropriate clinical setting, a solitary focal midbrain, pons, or medulla T2/FLAIR hyperintense, ring-enhancing mass with significant perilesional edema should suggest the possibility of *L. monocytogenes* abscess **(13-68)**.

Multiple abscesses occur in approximately 20-25% of cases. They tend to be located in the same hemisphere and appear distributed along the white matter fiber tracts of the brain. This distinct pattern may allow for earlier diagnosis and possibly improve patient outcome.

Hemorrhagic Viral Fevers

The Centers for Disease Control and Prevention (CDC) has identified six biologic agents as "category A" (easily disseminated or transmitted from person to person, resulting in high mortality rate and potential for major public health risk): anthrax, smallpox, botulism, tularemia, viral hemorrhagic fever, and plague. Of these, the **viral hemorrhagic fevers** are the most likely to affect the CNS **(13-70)**.

Filoviruses such as **Ebola** and **Marburg** are single-stranded RNA viruses that cause acute hemorrhagic fever with high mortality rates. Currently, there are no licensed vaccines or therapeutics to counter human Filovirus infections.

During the 2015 Ebola epidemic in West Africa, it became apparent that many patients likely died from acute fulminant meningoencephalitis, which was not initially recognized because of multiorgan involvement. Most are never imaged. The full range of neurologic sequelae in survivors is still being characterized in ongoing studies.

Hemorrhagic fevers with known CNS complications include dengue hemorrhagic fever/dengue shock syndrome and hantavirus with renal syndrome.

The flaviviruses—primarily **dengue** and **Zika virus**—are some of the most important emerging viral infections with high global disease incidence and the potential for rapid spread beyond nonendemic regions.

Dengue is increasingly common. Transmitted by *Aedes* mosquitoes, approximately 40% of the world's population is at risk of infection.

The clinical spectrum of dengue ranges from asymptomatic infection to life-threatening dengue hemorrhagic fever and dengue shock syndrome. Approximately 10% of patients with serologically confirmed dengue infection develop neurologic complications. In endemic areas, dengue has become the most frequent cause of encephalitis, surpassing even Herpes simplex virus.

Imaging studies may show multiple ischemic or hemorrhagic strokes **(13-69)**. Meningitis, encephalitis, ADEM, Guillain-Barré syndrome, and pituitary apoplexy have been reported in some cases.

Zika virus (ZIKV) is related to dengue, Chikungunya, West Nile, yellow fever, and Japanese encephalitis viruses. Brazil is the epicenter of the current ZIKV epidemic, which is rapidly spreading across the Americas. ZIKV is primarily a vector-borne disease carried by the *Aedes* mosquito. ZIKV can be transmitted congenitally, sexually, and through contaminated blood.

ZIKV causes severe microcephaly in infants born to infected mothers (congenital Zika syndrome). It has been reported to cause meningoencephalitis, myelitis, and Guillain-Barré syndrome in adults. To date, reported imaging findings are nonspecific.

Many patients with **hantavirus** or **Korean hemorrhagic fever** renal syndromes develop CNS symptoms such as acute psychiatric disorders, epilepsy, and meningismus. Autopsy studies demonstrate pituitary hemorrhage in 37%, pituitary necrosis in 5%, and brainstem hemorrhage in nearly 70%. In the few reported cases, MR showed pituitary hemorrhage and reversible splenium lesion in the corpus callosum.

MISCELLANEOUS/EMERGING CNS INFECTIONS

Listeriosis
- Predilection for meninges, midbrain/brainstem

Hemorrhagic Viral, Tick-Borne Disorders
- Filovirus infections
  - Ebola, Marburg, Rift Valley
- Flavivirus infections
  - Dengue, Zika virus (ZIKV), Japanese encephalitis, West Nile fever
  - Dengue = multiple hemorrhagic foci, strokes, meningoencephalitis, pituitary apoplexy
  - ZIKV = microcephaly (infants); meningoencephalitis, myelitis, Guillain-Barré (adults)
- Togavirus
  - Chikungunya = axonal spread from skin/nose to limbic system, subventricle zone

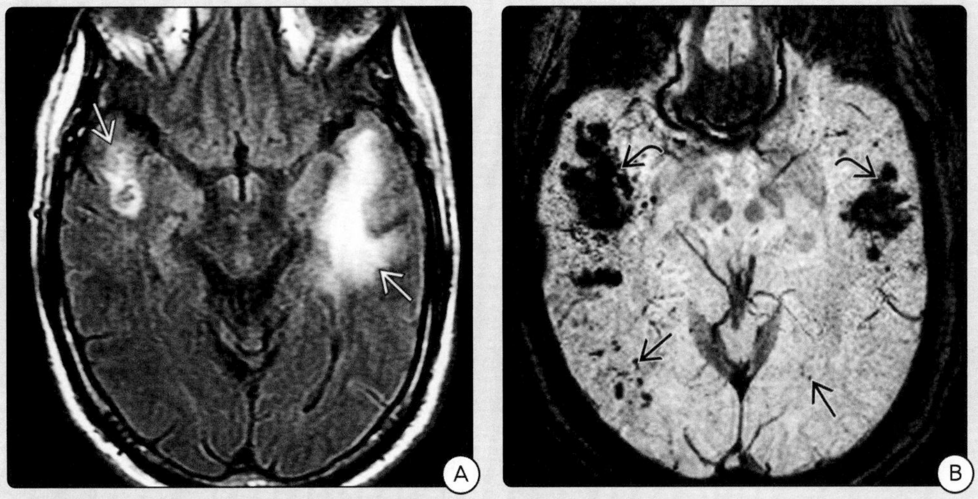

***(13-70A)** Axial FLAIR in a 38y man with altered mental status, progressive decline, and a seizure shows bilateral hyperintense lesions ➡ in the white matter of both temporal lobes. **(13-70B)** SWI MIP obtained several days after the patient lapsed into a coma shows bilateral lobar hematomas ➡ and numerous scattered petechial microhemorrhages ➡.*

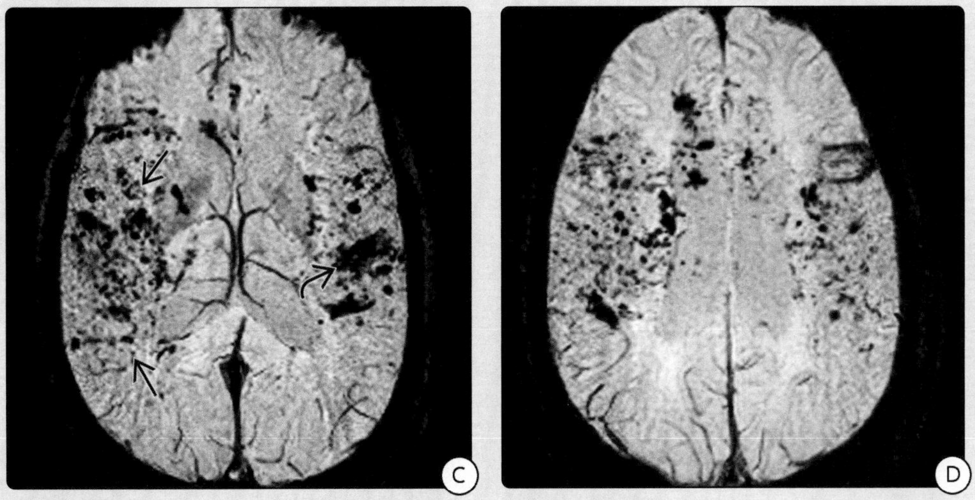

***(13-70C)** More cephalad T2*SWI MIP shows additional confluent hemorrhages ➡ and scattered microbleeds ➡. The basal ganglia are largely spared. **(13-70D)** More cephalad SWI shows numerous microhemorrhages. Fulminant hemorrhagic encephalitis is most likely viral. Inciting organism was not identified despite extensive laboratory investigation.*

Selected References

Mycobacterial Infections

Tuberculosis

Chandra SR et al: Factors determining the clinical spectrum, course and response to treatment, and complications in seronegative patients with central nervous system tuberculosis. J Neurosci Rural Pract. 8(2):241-248, 2017

Chaudhary V et al: Central nervous system tuberculosis: an imaging perspective. Can Assoc Radiol J. 68(2):161-170, 2017

Erdem H et al: The burden and epidemiology of community-acquired central nervous system infections: a multinational study. Eur J Clin Microbiol Infect Dis. ePub, 2017

Li D et al: Magnetic resonance imaging characteristics and treatment aspects of ventricular tuberculosis in adult patients. Acta Radiol. 58(1):91-97, 2017

Synmon B et al: Clinical and radiological spectrum of intracranial tuberculosis: a hospital based study in Northeast India. Indian J Tuberc. 64(2):109-118, 2017

Xiao Y et al: A scoring system to effectively evaluate central nervous system tuberculosis in patients with military tuberculosis. PLoS One. 12(5):e0176651, 2017

Patil S et al: Immunoconfirmation of central nervous system tuberculosis by blotting: a study of 300 cases. Int J Mycobacteriol. 4(2):124-30, 2015

Sanei Taheri M et al: Central nervous system tuberculosis: an imaging-focused review of a reemerging disease. Radiol Res Pract. 2015:202806, 2015

Psimaras D et al: Solitary tuberculous brain lesions: 24 new cases and a review of the literature. Rev Neurol (Paris). 170(6-7):454-63, 2014

Nontuberculous Mycobacterial Infections

Sood G et al: Outbreaks of nontuberculous mycobacteria. Curr Opin Infect Dis. ePub, 2017

Vu A et al: Toll-like receptors in mycobacterial infection. Eur J Pharmacol. 808:1-7, 2017

Heraud D et al: Nontuberculous mycobacterial adenitis outside of the head and neck region in children: a case report and systematic review of the literature. Int J Mycobacteriol. 5(3):351-353, 2016

Wu UI et al: A genetic perspective on granulomatous diseases with an emphasis on mycobacterial infections. Semin Immunopathol. 38(2):199-212, 2016

Chowdhary M et al: Intracranial abscess due to Mycobacterium avium complex in an immunocompetent host: a case report. BMC Infect Dis. 15:281, 2015

Lee YC et al: Mycobacterium avium complex infection-related immune reconstitution inflammatory syndrome of the central nervous system in an HIV-infected patient: case report and review. J Microbiol Immunol Infect. 46(1):68-72, 2013

Fungal Infections

Aljuboori Z et al: Fungal brain abscess caused by "black mold" (Cladophialophora bantiana) - a case report of successful treatment with an emphasis on how fungal brain abscess may be different from bacterial brain abscess. Surg Neurol Int. 8:46, 2017

Baeesa SS et al: Invasive orbital apex aspergillosis with mycotic aneurysm formation and subarachnoid hemorrhage in immunocompetent patients. World Neurosurg. 102:42-48, 2017

Swinburne NC et al: Neuroimaging in central nervous system infections. Curr Neurol Neurosci Rep. 17(6):49, 2017

Ulett KB et al: Cerebral cryptococcoma mimicking glioblastoma. BMJ Case Rep. 2017, 2017

Bakhshaee M et al: Acute invasive fungal rhinosinusitis: our experience with 18 cases. Eur Arch Otorhinolaryngol. 273(12):4281-4287, 2016

Cadena J et al: Invasive aspergillosis: current strategies for diagnosis and management. Infect Dis Clin North Am. 30(1):125-42, 2016

Farmakiotis D et al: Mucormycoses. Infect Dis Clin North Am. 30(1):143-63, 2016

Marzolf G et al: Magnetic resonance imaging of cerebral aspergillosis: imaging and pathological correlations. PLoS One. 11(4):e0152475, 2016

Shi M et al: Fungal infection in the brain: what we learned from intravital imaging. Front Immunol. 7:292, 2016

Vallabhaneni S et al: The global burden of fungal diseases. Infect Dis Clin North Am. 30(1):1-11, 2016

Panackal AA et al: Fungal infections of the central nervous dystem. Continuum (Minneap Minn). 21(6 Neuroinfectious Disease):1662-78, 2015

Shih RY et al: Bacterial, fungal, and parasitic infections of the central nervous system: radiologic-pathologic correlation and historical perspectives. Radiographics. 35(4):1141-69, 2015

Parasitic Infections

Carrizosa Moog J et al: Epilepsy in the tropics: emerging etiologies. Seizure. 44:108-112, 2017

Finsterer J et al: Parasitoses of the human central nervous system. J Helminthol. 87(3):257-70, 2013

Neurocysticercosis

Meng Q et al: Disseminated cysticercosis. N Engl J Med. 375(26):e52, 2016

Ripp K et al: The masquerading cyst: extraparenchymal neurocysticercosis presenting as acute meningitis. Am J Med. 129(3):e1-3, 2016

Venkat B et al: A comprehensive review of imaging findings in human cysticercosis. Jpn J Radiol. 34(4):241-57, 2016

Mahale RR et al: Extraparenchymal (racemose) neurocysticercosis and its multitude manifestations: a comprehensive review. J Clin Neurol. 11(3):203-11, 2015

Santos GT et al: Reduced diffusion in neurocysticercosis: circumstances of appearance and possible natural history implications. AJNR Am J Neuroradiol. 34(2):310-6, 2013

Echinococcosis

Bali B et al: Preoperative diagnosis of cerebral hydatid cyst and its therapeutic implications. J Neurosurg Sci. 60(1):137-9, 2016

Taslakian B et al: Intracranial hydatid cyst: imaging findings of a rare disease. BMJ Case Rep. 2016:bcr2016216570, 2016

Stojkovic M et al: Cystic and alveolar echinococcosis. Handb Clin Neurol. 114:327-34, 2013

Amebiasis

Visvesvara GS: Infections with free-living amebae. Handb Clin Neurol. 114:153-68, 2013

Malaria

Carrizosa Moog J et al: Epilepsy in the tropics: emerging etiologies. Seizure. 44:108-112, 2017

Strangward P et al: A quantitative brain map of experimental cerebral malaria pathology. PLoS Pathog. 13(3):e1006267, 2017

Wassmer SC et al: Severe malaria: what's new on the pathogenesis front? Int J Parasitol. 47(2-3):145-152, 2017

Yusuf FH et al: Cerebral malaria: insight into pathogenesis, complications and molecular biomarkers. Infect Drug Resist. 10:57-59, 2017

Hora R et al: Cerebral malaria - clinical manifestations and pathogenesis. Metab Brain Dis. 31(2):225-37, 2016

O'Brien MD et al: Lesson of the month 1: post-malaria neurological syndromes. Clin Med (Lond). 16(3):292-3, 2016

Other Parasitic Infections

Liao H et al: Imaging characteristics of cerebral sparganosis with live worms. J Neuroradiol. 43(6):378-383, 2016

Xia Y et al: Characteristic CT and MR imaging findings of cerebral paragonimiasis. J Neuroradiol. 43(3):200-6, 2016

Yu Y et al: Cerebral sparganosis in children: epidemiologic and radiologic characteristics and treatment outcomes: a report of 9 cases. World Neurosurg. 89:153-8, 2016

Lescano AG et al: Other cestodes: sparganosis, coenurosis and Taenia crassiceps cysticercosis. Handb Clin Neurol. 114:335-45, 2013

Pittella JE: Pathology of CNS parasitic infections. Handb Clin Neurol. 114:65-88, 2013

Miscellaneous and Emerging CNS Infections

Spirochete Infections of the CNS

Garkowski A et al: Cerebrovascular manifestations of Lyme neuroborreliosis-a systematic review of published cases. Front Neurol. 8:146, 2017

Ho EL et al: Neurosyphilis increases HIV-associated central nervous system inflammation but does not explain cognitive impairment in HIV-infected individuals with syphilis. Clin Infect Dis. ePub, 2017

Koedel U et al: Lyme neuroborreliosis. Curr Opin Infect Dis. 30(1):101-107, 2017

Zhong X et al: Neuropsychiatric features of neurosyphilis: frequency, relationship with the severity of cognitive impairment and comparison with Alzheimer disease. Dement Geriatr Cogn Disord. 43(5-6):308-319, 2017

Drago F et al: Neurosyphilis: from infection to autoinflammation? Int J STD AIDS. 27(4):327-8, 2016

Firlag-Burkacka E et al: High frequency of neurosyphilis in HIV-positive patients diagnosed with early syphilis. HIV Med. 17(5):323-6, 2016

Ramgopal S et al: Lyme disease-related intracranial hypertension in children: clinical and imaging findings. J Neurol. 263(3):500-7, 2016

Sarbu N et al: White matter diseases with radiologic-pathologic correlation. Radiographics. 36(5):1426-47, 2016

Koedel U et al: Lyme neuroborreliosis-epidemiology, diagnosis and management. Nat Rev Neurol. 11(8):446-56, 2015

Marques AR: Lyme neuroborreliosis. Continuum (Minneap Minn). 21(6 Neuroinfectious Disease):1729-44, 2015

Marra CM: Neurosyphilis. Continuum (Minneap Minn). 21(6 Neuroinfectious Disease):1714-28, 2015

Hildenbrand P et al: Lyme neuroborreliosis: manifestations of a rapidly emerging zoonosis. AJNR Am J Neuroradiol. 30(6):1079-87, 2009

Emerging CNS Infections

Billioux BJ: Neurological complications and sequelae of Ebola virus disease. Curr Infect Dis Rep. 19(5):19, 2017

Décard BF et al: Listeria rhombencephalitis mimicking a demyelinating event in an immunocompetent young patient. Mult Scler. 23(1):123-125, 2017

El-Abassi R et al: Whipple's disease. J Neurol Sci. 377:197-206, 2017

Singh MV et al: Preventive and therapeutic challenges in combating Zika virus infection: are we getting any closer? J Neurovirol. 23(3):347-357, 2017

Brasil P et al: Guillain-Barré syndrome associated with Zika virus infection. Lancet. 387(10026):1482, 2016

Pal S et al: Clinico-radiological profile and outcome of dengue patients with central nervous system manifestations: a case series in an Eastern India tertiary care hospital. J Neurosci Rural Pract. 7(1):114-24, 2016

Williamson PR et al: CNS infections in 2015: emerging catastrophic infections and new insights into neuroimmunological host damage. Lancet Neurol. 15(1):17-9, 2016

Arslan F et al: The clinical features, diagnosis, treatment, and prognosis of neuroinvasive listeriosis: a multinational study. Eur J Clin Microbiol Infect Dis. 34(6):1213-21, 2015

Bojanowski MW et al: Spreading of multiple Listeria monocytogenes abscesses via central nervous system fiber tracts: case report. J Neurosurg. 123(6):1593-9, 2015

Peregrin J et al: Primary Whipple disease of the brain: case report with long-term clinical and MRI follow-up. Neuropsychiatr Dis Treat. 11:2461-9, 2015

Compain C et al: Central nervous system involvement in Whipple disease: clinical study of 18 patients and long-term follow-up. Medicine (Baltimore). 92(6):324-30, 2013

Denizot M et al: Encephalitis due to emerging viruses: CNS innate immunity and potential therapeutic targets. J Infect. 65(1):1-16, 2012

HIV/AIDS

In this chapter, we explore the "many faces" of HIV/AIDS as it affects the central nervous system (CNS). We start by placing the disease in its epidemiologic and demographic context, then turn our attention to the pathology and imaging spectrum of CNS HIV/AIDS.

We next discuss the manifestation of HIV itself in the brain, i.e., HIV encephalitis. We follow with a consideration of unusual but important associated findings, such as HIV vasculopathy, HIV-associated bone marrow changes, and benign salivary gland lymphoepithelial lesions.

We then consider the broad spectrum of opportunistic infections that complicate HIV/AIDS and what happens when an HIV-positive patient is also coinfected with TB, another sexually transmitted disease, or malaria.

Long-term survivors with treated AIDS and the phenomenon of immune reconstitution inflammatory syndrome (IRIS) are then presented. We conclude the chapter by discussing neoplasms that occur in the setting of HIV/AIDS (the so-called AIDS-defining malignancies).

Overview

Introduction

It has been more than 30 years since a new syndrome associated with profound suppression of cell-mediated immunity was first identified. The causative agent, a retrovirus, was given the appropriate name of human immunodeficiency virus (HIV), and the syndrome it caused was named acquired immunodeficiency syndrome (AIDS).

It required nearly a decade to develop highly active multidrug, multiclass treatment regimens for HIV/AIDS. Highly active antiretroviral therapy (HAART), also called combination antiretroviral therapy (cART), has resulted in a dramatic decline in mortality for treated patients. Overall AIDS-related deaths have dropped by nearly 20% in the last 10 years.

In wealthy, industrialized countries where widespread access to HAART is readily available, HIV/AIDS has evolved from a virtual death sentence to a chronic but manageable disease. Survival in these countries has increased from a mean of 10.5 years to 22.5 years in a single decade. That's the good news. The bad news? Progress is fragile and unevenly distributed. In many less-developed "high-burden" parts of the world, HIV incidence is still rising in epidemic numbers. The personal and socioeconomic consequences of the HIV/AIDS epidemic have been devastating.

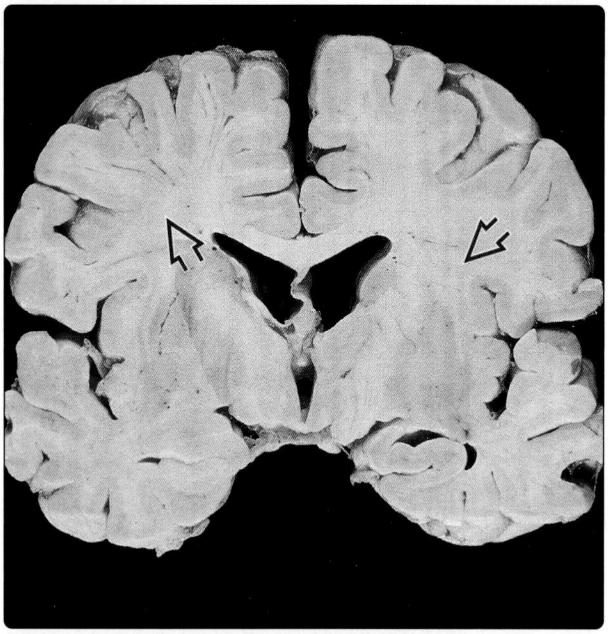

(14-1) Coronal autopsy of HIVE shows generalized volume loss with enlargement of the lateral ventricles, sylvian fissures. "Hazy," poorly defined abnormalities are present in WM ⇨ but spare the subcortical U-fibers. (Courtesy B. K. DeMasters, MD.)

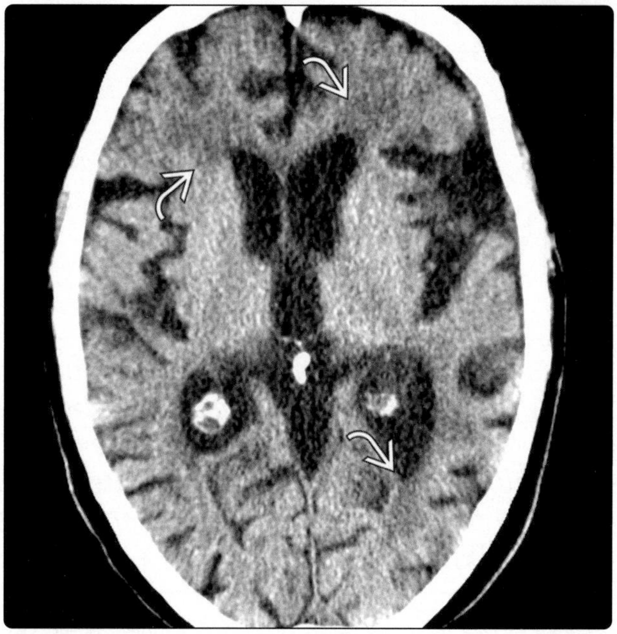

(14-2) Axial NECT scan in a 38y man with longstanding HIV/AIDS shows gross cerebral atrophy and multifocal hypodensities ➡ in the subcortical white matter.

Epidemiology

Summaries of the global AIDS epidemic indicate that, in 2015 (the most recent year for which complete data are available), the number of people living with HIV totaled over 35 million.

The enormous investments in the HIV response over the past 15 years are paying huge dividends. In 2014, new HIV infections were estimated at 2 million, 40% lower than the peak in 1997. Approximately 1.2 million infected individuals die each year from HIV/AIDS and its complications, a decrease of 42% from the peak in 2004.

Despite the notable success of the global HIV program, over 22 million infected individuals are still not accessing antiretroviral therapy. Of these, nearly 70% are in sub-Saharan Africa, and 3.4 million are children under the age of 15 years. Women now account for almost 52% of adult cases globally, and adolescent girls and young women in sub-Saharan Africa are being infected at twice the rate as that of boys and men of the same age.

These disparities mean that socioeconomic determinants of health affect both the prevalence and manifestations of HIV/AIDS. The same disease can have vastly different consequences—and therefore imaging appearances—in different parts of the world.

Although AIDS deaths are declining with the expanding access to antiretroviral therapy, these gains are being challenged by increasing morbidity and mortality associated with coinfection and comorbidity from other diseases. Tuberculosis is still the leading cause of hospitalization of adults and children living with HIV and remains the leading cause of HIV-related deaths.

Demographics

HIV is transmitted through unprotected sexual intercourse (anal or vaginal), transfusion of contaminated blood, and sharing of contaminated needles, as well as between mother and infant during pregnancy, childbirth, and breastfeeding.

HIV prevalence varies widely with geography, race/ethnicity, and sex. Sub-Saharan Africa accounts for nearly 70% of the global prevalence of HIV, disproportionately affecting women and young people. As a result of improved therapeutics and monitoring, HIV infections are also a growing concern in the elderly.

The most recently available data indicate that homosexual and bisexual men remain the population most heavily affected by HIV in the United States. New infection rates have been relatively stable since 2006 but are disproportionately higher in African American men compared with African American women, as well as higher in white men compared with white women.

Individuals with sexually transmitted diseases (including chlamydia, gonorrhea, syphilis, herpes, and human papillomavirus) are more likely than uninfected persons to acquire HIV infection. Approximately 10% of patients with hepatitis C are coinfected with HIV.

HIV Infection

HIV is a neurovirulent infection that has both direct and indirect effects on the CNS. Neurologic complications can arise from the HIV infection itself, from opportunistic infections or neoplasms, and from treatment-related metabolic derangements.

In this section, we consider the effects of the HIV virus itself on the brain. Extracranial manifestations of HIV/AIDS may also be identified on brain imaging studies, so we discuss these as well.

HIV Encephalitis

Between 75-90% of HIV/AIDS patients have demonstrable HIV-induced brain injury at autopsy **(14-1)**. Although many patients remain asymptomatic for variable periods, brain infection is the initial presenting symptomatology in 5-10% of cases. Approximately 25% of treated HIV/AIDS patients develop moderate cognitive impairment despite good virologic response to therapy.

Terminology

HIV encephalitis (HIVE) and HIV leukoencephalopathy (HIVL) are the direct result of HIV infection of the brain. Opportunistic infections are absent early although coinfections or multiple infections are common later in the disease course.

HIV-associated neurocognitive disorders (HANDs) are the most frequent neurologic manifestations of HIVE and HIVL. The term "acquired immunodeficiency dementia complex" refers specifically to HIV-associated dementia.

Etiology

HIV is a pathogenic neurotropic human RNA retrovirus. **HIV-1** is responsible for most cases of HIV/AIDS. **HIV-2** infection is predominantly a disease of heterosexuals and is found primarily in West Africa. Unless otherwise noted in this discussion, "HIV" or "HIV infection" refers to HIV-1 infection.

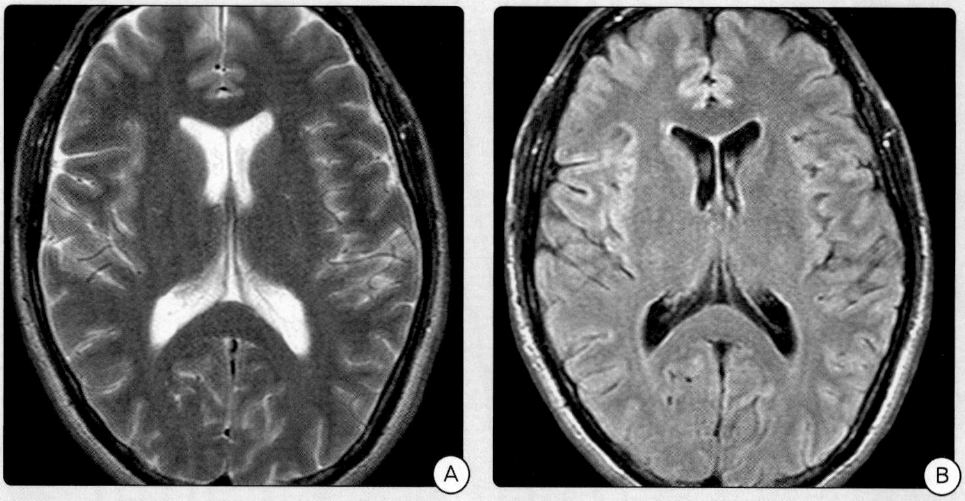

***(14-3A)** Axial T2WI in a 45y man with early dementia shows minimal enlargement of the lateral ventricles and sulci. **(14-3B)** Axial FLAIR shows no evidence of white matter hyperintensities.*

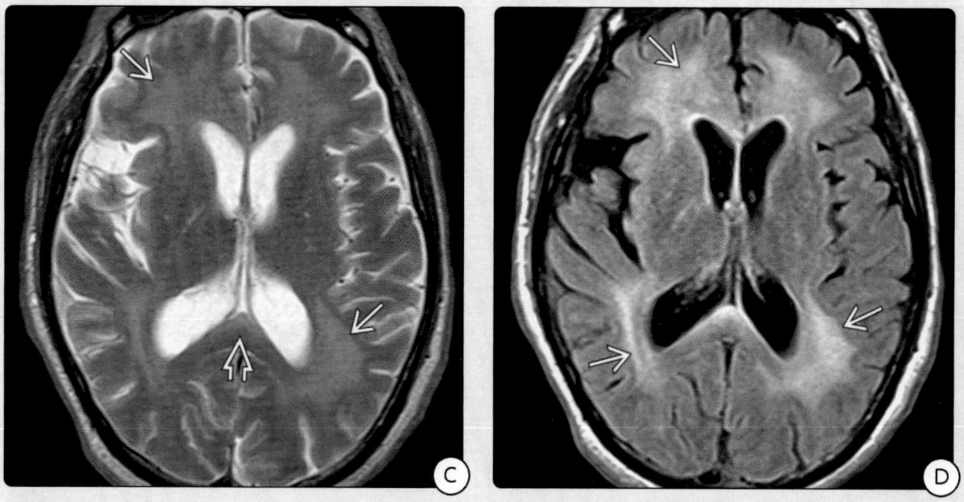

***(14-3C)** Four years later, the same patient has developed severe HIV-associated dementia. Axial T2WI shows significantly increased volume loss, reflected by the enlarged lateral ventricles and sulci. Symmetric confluent hyperintensities have developed in the cerebral white matter ⇒ and corpus callosum splenium ⇒. **(14-3D)** FLAIR shows the dramatic interval WM changes of severe HIV encephalitis ⇒. U-fibers are spared.*

HIV initially infects Langerhans (dendritic) cells in the skin and mucous membranes. Its envelope protein gp120 binds to CD4 receptors in these dendritic cells, which then migrate to lymphoid tissues and infect CD4-positive T cells. The virus proliferates in and then destroys the infected T cells. A burst of viremia develops within days and leads to widespread tissue dissemination.

The two major targets of viral infection are lymphoid tissue—especially T cells—and the CNS. HIV crosses the blood-brain barrier (BBB) both as cell-free virus and infected monocytes and T cells, which migrate across the intact BBB, penetrating the brain within 24-48 hours after initial exposure.

HIV infects astrocytes but does not directly infect neurons. However, once inside the brain, the HIV-infected monocytes and T cells produce proinflammatory cytokines such as TNF and IL-1β, which in turn further activate resident microglia and astrocytes.

The CNS-resident astroglia and microglia become activated, proliferate, and change to have an inflammatory expression signature. These activated cells, along with monocyte-derived perivascular macrophages, are the main contributors to neuroinflammation in HIV infection.

Neurons can be injured indirectly by viral proteins and neurotoxins. The activated cells also release neurotoxic factors such as excitatory amino acids and inflammatory mediators, resulting in neuronal dysfunction and cell death. However, neurons can be injured indirectly by viral proteins and neurotoxins. Some non-CNS peripheral reservoirs of virus also persist and may play an active role in ongoing brain injury, even with adequate treatment.

Pathology

Gross Pathology. Brain pathology in HIV/AIDS varies with patient age and disease acuity. In early stages, the brain appears grossly normal. Advanced HIVE results in generalized

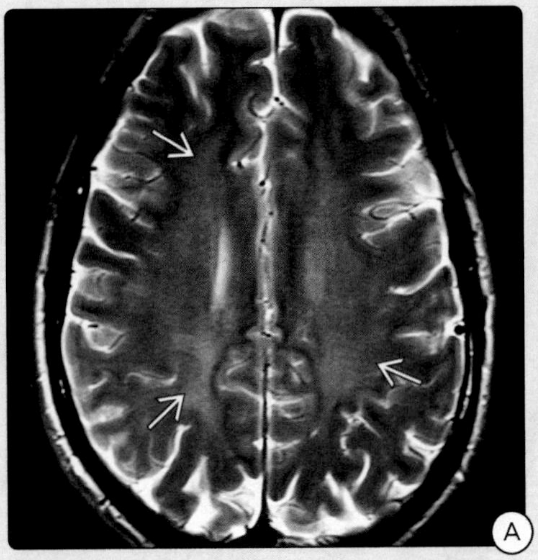

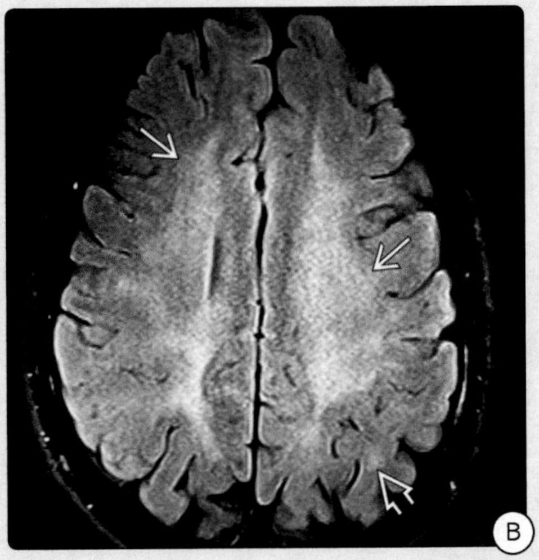

***(14-4A)** T2WI in a 43y man with HIV/AIDS and mild early cognitive impairment shows diffuse, confluent, bilaterally symmetric hyperintensity in the cerebral white matter ➡. Note sparing of the subcortical U-fibers. **(14-4B)** FLAIR scan in the same patient shows the "hazy" confluent white matter hyperintensity ➡ characteristic of HIVE. No atrophy is present, and—with the exception of a single focal left parietal lesion ➡—the subcortical WM is spared.*

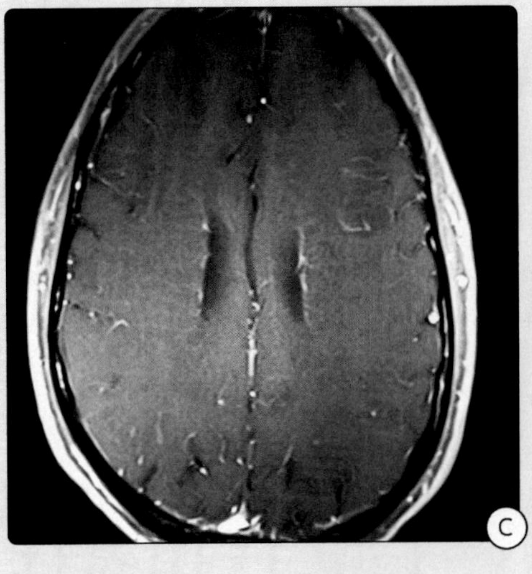

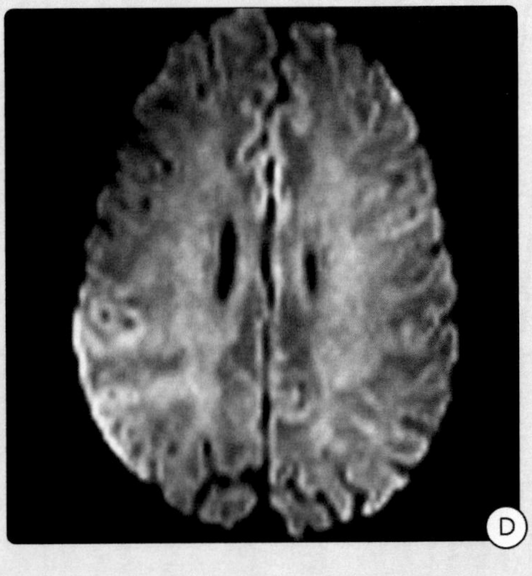

***(14-4C)** Axial T1 C+ FS in the same patient shows no parenchymal or meningeal enhancement. **(14-4D)** Axial DWI shows no evidence of restricted diffusion. The slight hyperintensity in the hemispheric white matter is not true diffusion restriction; rather, it is secondary to T2 "shine-through."*

brain volume loss ("atrophy") with enlarged ventricles and subarachnoid spaces **(14-1)**.

Microscopic Features. HIVE is characterized by gliosis, microglial clusters, perivascular macrophage accumulation, and multinucleated giant cells. The multinucleated giant cells contain viral antigens and are immunoreactive for the envelope protein gp120.

Immune activation (encephalitis) is often disproportionate to the amount of HIV virus present in the brain. Disseminated patchy foci of white and gray matter damage with myelin pallor and diffuse myelin loss are prominent features.

HIVL is characterized by ill-defined, diffuse myelin pallor with poorly demarcated areas of myelin loss. Lesions are most prominent in the deep periventricular white matter and corona radiata.

Clinical Issues

Epidemiology. Almost 60% of all AIDS patients eventually develop overt neurologic manifestations. Although combination antiretroviral therapy (cART) has significantly improved survival, approximately 15-25% of treated patients develop moderate cognitive impairment or full-blown AIDS dementia complex. In countries with widespread access to cART, AIDS dementia complex has become the most common neurologic complication of HIV infection.

Demographics. Both adult and pediatric HIV-positive patients can develop HIVE. From one-third to two-thirds of adult AIDS patients and 30-50% of pediatric cases are affected. The sex distribution of HIVE reflects that of HIV and varies with geographic region.

Age is consistently identified as a risk factor for HIV-related cognitive impairment. There is growing evidence that abnormal brain proteins accumulate in HIV-positive brains.

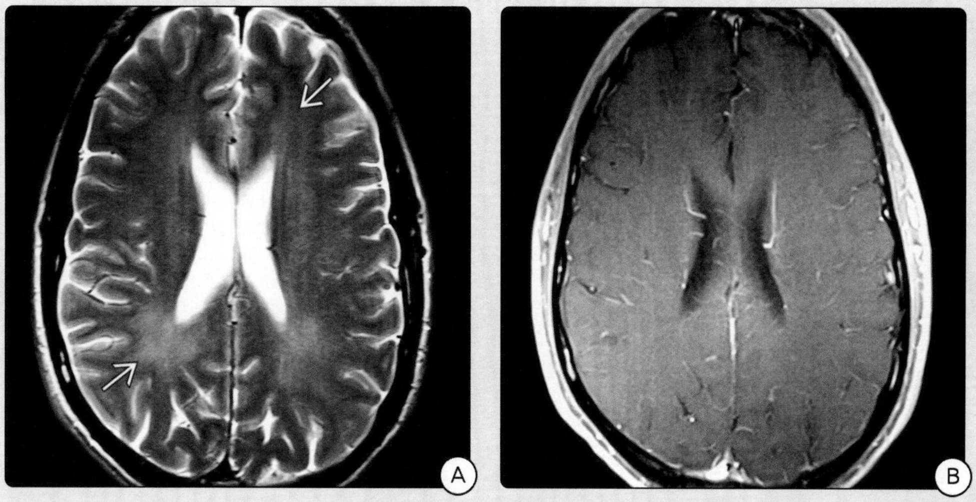

***(14-5A)** Axial T2WI in an HIV/AIDS patient on HAART shows diffuse hazy deep and periventricular WM hyperintensity ➡. The subcortical U-fibers are spared. **(14-5B)** T1 C+ in the same case shows no abnormal enhancement. This is typical HIV encephalitis.*

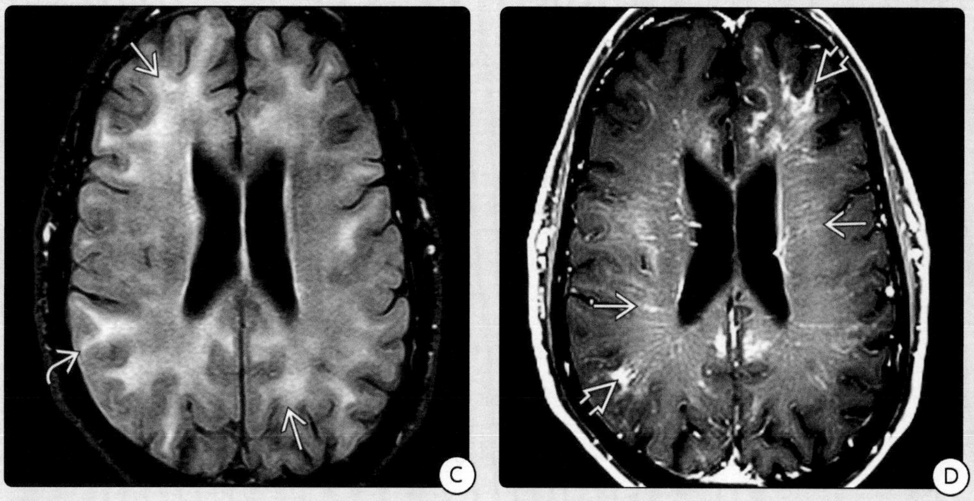

***(14-5C)** After 9 years on HAART, the patient discontinued his therapy and became acutely encephalopathic. FLAIR shows confluent WM hyperintensity extending throughout both hemispheres ➡ with involvement of U-fibers ➡. **(14-5D)** T1 C+ FS shows linear enhancement along medullary veins ➡ with patchy subcortical enhancing foci ➡. PCR was negative for JCV, and biopsy disclosed fulminant acute on chronic HIV encephalitis.*

Excess hyperphosphorylated tau, amyloid, and α-synuclein have all been identified and may contribute to the development of accelerated neurodegenerative syndromes and AIDS dementia complex.

Presentation. Some patients develop symptoms of an acute retroviral syndrome (ARVS) during the initial viremia. ARVS develops 2-4 weeks after infection and consists of sore throat, fever, lymphadenopathy, nausea, rashes, and variable neurologic changes.

HANDs develop as intermediate and long-term complications. Early brain infection with HIV is often asymptomatic, and cognitive and functional performances are both initially normal. Full-blown HIV-associated dementia causes advanced cognitive impairment and marked impact on daily function.

Natural History. Slowly progressive impairment of fine motor control, verbal fluency, and short-term memory is characteristic. Severe deterioration and subcortical dementia may develop in the final stages.

The latency period for HIV-2 infection is generally longer, and the viral loads are lower than with HIV-1. Immunodeficiency therefore evolves more slowly.

HIV ENCEPHALITIS: TERMS, ETIOLOGY, AND CLINICAL ISSUES

Terminology
- HIV encephalitis (HIVE)
  - Direct results of HIV brain infection
  - HIV-associated neurocognitive disorders (HANDs)
  - Most serious is AIDS dementia complex

Etiology
- HIV is neurotropic retrovirus
  - Most human infections caused by HIV-1
  - HIV-2 primarily in West Africa
- Cell-free virus, HIV-infected monocytes, T cells cross blood-brain barrier in 24-48 hours
- HIV infects astrocytes and microglia, but not neurons
  - Activated astrocytes, microglia + perivascular macrophages → neuroinflammation
  - Neurons indirectly injured by viral proteins, cytokines, neurotoxins

Clinical Issues
- Epidemiology
  - 60% of AIDS patients develop neurologic disease
  - 15-25% of highly active antiretroviral therapy (HAART)-treated patients develop AIDS dementia complex
- Presentation
  - Acute retroviral syndrome rare
  - More common = slow progressive impairment

Treatment Options. cART has decreased HIV/AIDS morbidity and mortality. It does not prevent development of HIVE but does decrease its overall severity.

A further advance is the potentially game-changing potential of preexposure prophylaxis (using antiretroviral drugs to prevent HIV infection). Experts believe a strategic approach using a combination of antiretroviral therapy with preexposure prophylaxis could almost eliminate HIV transmission to HIV-negative sexual and drug-using partners.

Imaging

General Features. HIVE does not cause mass effect. Even in the post-HAART era, the most common finding remains generalized progressive volume loss that is disproportionate to the patient's age. Cortical thinning and bilateral white matter lesions are the most common parenchymal abnormalities.

CT Findings. NECT scans may be normal in the early stages. Mild to moderate atrophy with patchy or confluent white matter hypodensity develops as the disease progresses **(14-2)**. HIVE does not enhance on CECT.

MR Findings. Generalized volume loss with enlarged ventricles and sulci is best appreciated on T1WI or thin-section inversion recovery sequences. Reduced gray matter volume in the medial and superior frontal gyri has been identified as a possible early imaging marker for HIVE. White matter signal intensity is generally normal or near normal on T1WI.

T2/FLAIR initially shows bilateral, patchy, relatively symmetric white matter hyperintensities. With time, confluent "hazy," ill-defined hyperintensity in the subcortical and deep cerebral white matter develops, and volume loss ensues **(14-3)**. HIVE usually does not enhance on T1 C+ and usually shows no restriction on DWI **(14-4)**. In fulminant cases, perivenular enhancement may indicate acute demyelination **(14-5)**.

Advanced imaging modalities may show early changes of HIVE not readily apparent on standard MR. MRS demonstrates neuronal damage as decreased NAA. mI, a marker of glial activation, is often elevated. Other reported early changes in HIVE include increased choline-to-creatine (Cho:Cr) ratios bilaterally in the frontal gray and white matter, in the left parietal white matter, and in total Cho:Cr ratio.

DTI shows that patients with AIDS-related dementia exhibit significantly elevated mean and radial diffusivity in the parietal white matter compared with nondemented patients with HIVE. Radial diffusivity is affected to a much greater extent than axial diffusivity, suggesting that demyelination is the prominent disease process in white matter.

Differential Diagnosis

The major differential diagnosis of HIVE is **progressive multifocal leukoencephalopathy** (PML). PML has patchy white matter lesions that can be unilateral or bilateral and appear as strikingly asymmetric hyperintensities on T2/FLAIR. Both the hemispheric and posterior fossa white matter are commonly affected. PML often involves the subcortical U-fibers, which are usually spared in HIVE.

Coinfections with other infectious agents are common in HIVE and may complicate the imaging appearance. **Cytomegalovirus** (CMV) can also cause a diffuse white matter encephalitis and ependymitis. **Toxoplasmosis** causes multifocal punctate and "target" or ring-enhancing lesions

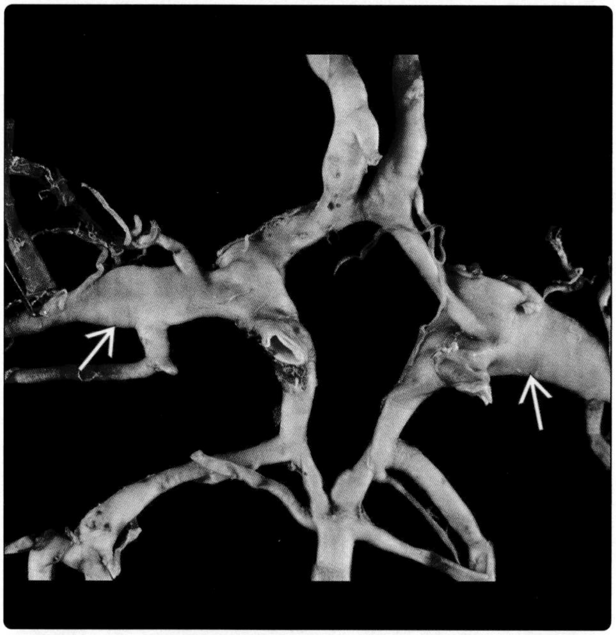

(14-6) ***Autopsy case in a hemophiliac child with AIDS and HIV vasculopathy shows striking fusiform dilatation of both middle cerebral arteries ➡, as well as all components of the circle of Willis. (Courtesy L. Rourke, MD.)***

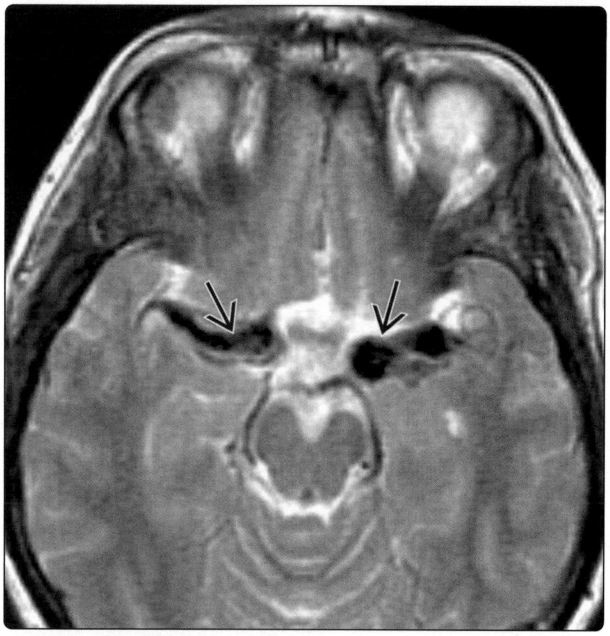

(14-7) ***Axial T2WI in a 13y boy with congenital HIV/AIDS who presented acutely with bilateral upper and lower extremity weakness and a facial droop shows markedly enlarged "flow voids" of both middle cerebral arteries ➡.***

that are more prominent in the basal ganglia. **Herpes encephalitis** and **human herpesvirus-6 (HHV-6) encephalitis** both involve the temporal lobes, especially the cortex.

HIV ENCEPHALITIS: IMAGING AND DDx

NECT
- Normal or atrophy ± white matter (WM) hypodensity

MR
- Volume loss with ↑ sulci, ventricles
- T2/FLAIR "hazy" WM symmetric hyperintensity
  - Spares subcortical U-fibers
- No mass effect
- Usually no enhancement
  - Possible exception = acute fulminant HIVE

Differential Diagnosis
- Progressive multifocal leukoencephalopathy (PML)
  - Coinfection with HIVE common
  - Usually asymmetric
  - Often involves U-fibers
- Opportunistic infections
  - Coinfection with HIVE common
  - CMV causes encephalitis, ependymitis
  - Toxoplasmosis: Multiple enhancing rings
  - Herpes, HHV-6 usually involve temporal lobes

Other Manifestations of HIV/AIDS

Vasculopathy

Cardiovascular disease has long been recognized as a consequence of HIV infection. While the etiology and pathogenesis of the cardiovascular disease are unknown, HIV affects every aspect of the cardiac axis, causing a spectrum of disease ranging from cardiomyopathy and myocarditis to peripheral vascular disease. HIV-associated vasculopathy is an increasingly recognized clinical entity, causing high morbidity and increasing mortality.

Stroke is an uncommon but growing cause of mortality and morbidity in HIV/AIDS patients. Autopsy series have found a 4-29% prevalence of cerebral infarction in patients with documented HIV/AIDS. Many of these strokes are due to non-HIV CNS coinfection, lymphoma, cardioembolic sources, or primary vasculitis. Approximately 5-6% are true HIV-associated vasculopathy with small vessel intimal thickening, mineralization, and perivascular inflammatory infiltrates.

HIV vasculopathy (HIV-V) and varicella-zoster virus (VZV) vasculitis are uncommon but increasingly important causes of stroke in the HIV/AIDS population.

HIV Vasculopathy. Striking nonatherosclerotic fusiform ectasias of the major intracranial arteries occur, usually in children with congenital HIV/AIDS **(14-6)** **(14-7)**. HIV-V is generally associated with large hemispheric strokes.

VZV Vasculopathy. CNS VZV vasculopathy (VZV-V) affects both large and small cerebral vessels. Large vessel disease is most common in immunocompetent individuals, whereas small vessel disease usually develops in immunocompromised patients. Overt neurologic disease often occurs months after zoster and sometimes presents without any history of zoster rash. The diagnosis can be confirmed by finding anti-VZV antibody in CSF.

HIV/AIDS patients with VZV-V are generally younger than those with HIV-V. In contrast to those associated with HIV-V, most strokes associated with VZV-V are small, deep-seated, subcortical infarcts. Large cortical hemispheric strokes are relatively rare.

HIV/AIDS Bone Marrow Changes

The calvaria and skull base, as well as part of the facial bones and upper cervical spine, are visible on sagittal T1-weighted brain MRs **(14-8)**. The cranium and mandible alone account for approximately 13% of active (red) marrow in adult humans. Add the cervical spine plus facial bones, and these structures together represent 15-20% of all bone marrow activity; therefore, carefully examining all the bones visible on brain MRs may provide important information regarding hematopoietic status.

Bone marrow abnormalities are common in HIV/AIDS patients and have been implicated in the brain injury underlying cognitive deterioration and dementia. Anemia before AIDS onset is strongly predictive of HIV-associated dementia (HAD). Escalation in monocyte trafficking from bone marrow into the brain in late-stage infection may represent a critical determinant of HAD neuropathogenesis.

Pathology. Pathologic processes alter the composition of bone marrow, causing a relative increase in cellular hematopoietic tissue and a corresponding replacement of adipose tissue. Extracellular hemosiderin, hypercellularity, and increased numbers of monocytes and macrophages all contribute significantly to marrow hypercellularity.

The most common skeletal abnormalities in HIV/AIDS patients are myelodysplasia (69% of biopsy specimens), evidence of reticuloendothelial iron blockade (65%), hypercellularity (53%), megaloblastic hematopoiesis (38%), lymphocytic aggregates (36%), plasmacytosis (25%), fibrosis (20%), and granulomas (13%). Most of the marrow abnormalities associated with HIV infection are related directly to the infection itself or its complications, not to therapeutic intervention.

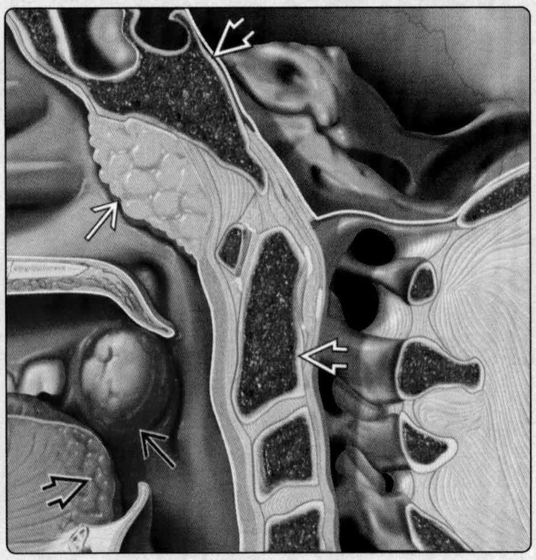

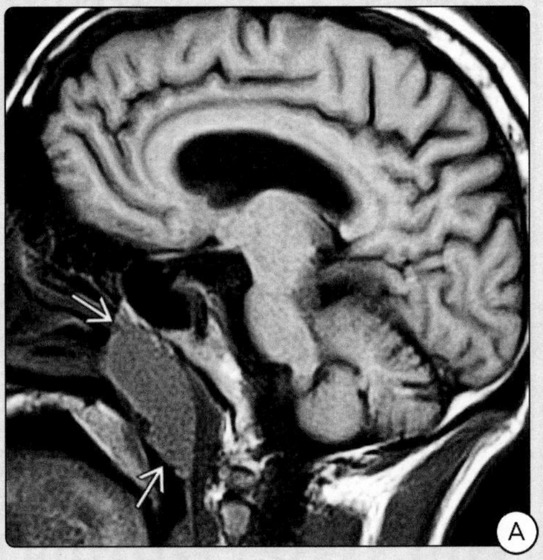

***(14-8)** Other H&N manifestations of HIV/AIDS include prominent lymphoid tissue (adenoids ➡, tonsils ⇨, Waldeyer ring ⇨) and reconversion of yellow to red (hematopoietic) marrow in the cervical spine and skull ➡. **(14-9A)** Sagittal T1WI in a 43y man with longstanding HIV/AIDS shows unusually prominent adenoids ➡.*

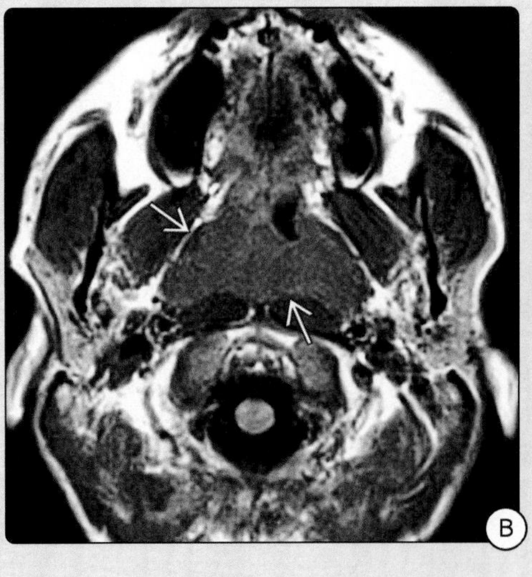

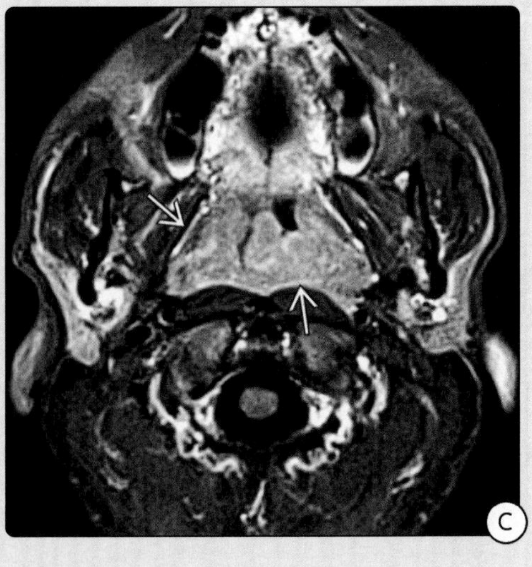

***(14-9B)** Axial T1WI in the same case shows that the upper nasopharynx is almost completely filled with enlarged adenoidal tissue ➡. **(14-9C)** Axial T1 C+ FS shows that the enlarged tonsils ➡ enhance strongly and uniformly.*

Imaging. Subtle changes in bone marrow may be difficult to detect on conventional MR images. Imaging findings that suggest marrow abnormalities are nonspecific. The prolonged T1 relaxation times alter signal intensity of hematopoietic bone marrow. Fatty T1 hyperintense "yellow" marrow is replaced with T1 hypointense tissue. The calvaria and clivus appear mottled or "gray." The affected vertebral bodies appear hypointense relative to the intervertebral discs (the "bright disc" sign).

Hypercellular bone marrow in HIV/AIDS patients may demonstrate reduced mean diffusivity on quantitative imaging before any grossly visible changes become apparent.

Benign Lymphoepithelial Lesions

Salivary gland disease is an important manifestation of HIV infection. Most lesions represent either benign nonneoplastic lymphoepithelial cysts or reactive lymphoid hyperplasia.

Benign lymphoepithelial lesions of the salivary glands include a spectrum of disorders ranging from the lymphoepithelial sialadenitis (LESA) of Sjögren syndrome to lymphoepithelial cysts (LEC) to both HIV-related and -unrelated cystic lymphoid hyperplasia (CLH).

LESA, LEC, and CLH share a common microscopic appearance characterized by epimyoepithelial islands and/or epithelium-lined cysts in a lymphoid stroma. However, they differ greatly regarding their etiology, clinical presentation, and management.

Benign lymphoepithelial lesions of HIV (BLL-HIV) are nonneoplastic cystic masses that enlarge salivary glands. Bilateral lesions are common. The parotid glands are most frequently affected **(14-10)**.

NECT scans show multiple bilateral well-circumscribed cysts within enlarged parotid glands. A thin enhancing rim is present on CECT scans **(14-11)**. The cysts are homogeneously

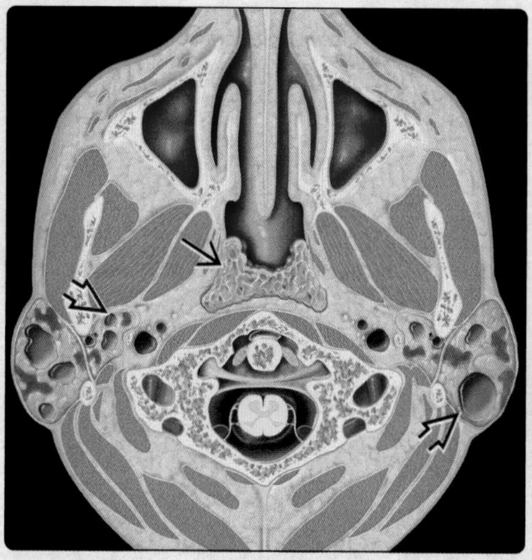

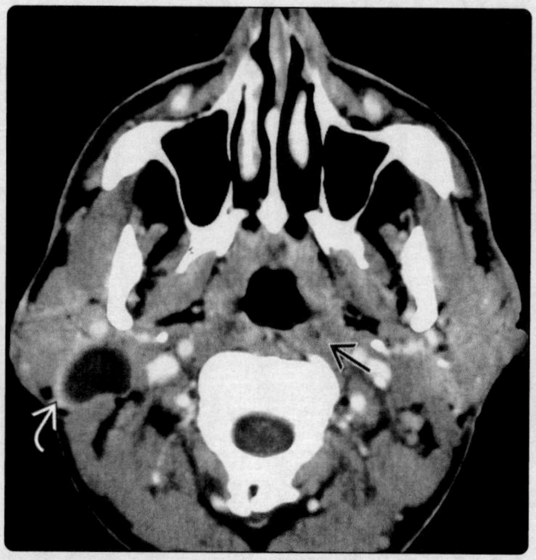

***(14-10)** Axial graphic shows typical lymphoid and lymphoepithelial lesions of HIV/AIDS. Note the hyperplastic tonsils ⇨ and multiple cysts in the superficial and deep lobes of both parotid glands ⇨. **(14-11)** Axial CECT scan in a 33y man with HIV/AIDS shows a large right parotid cyst with enhancing rim ➡ and an enlarged Waldeyer ring ⇨.*

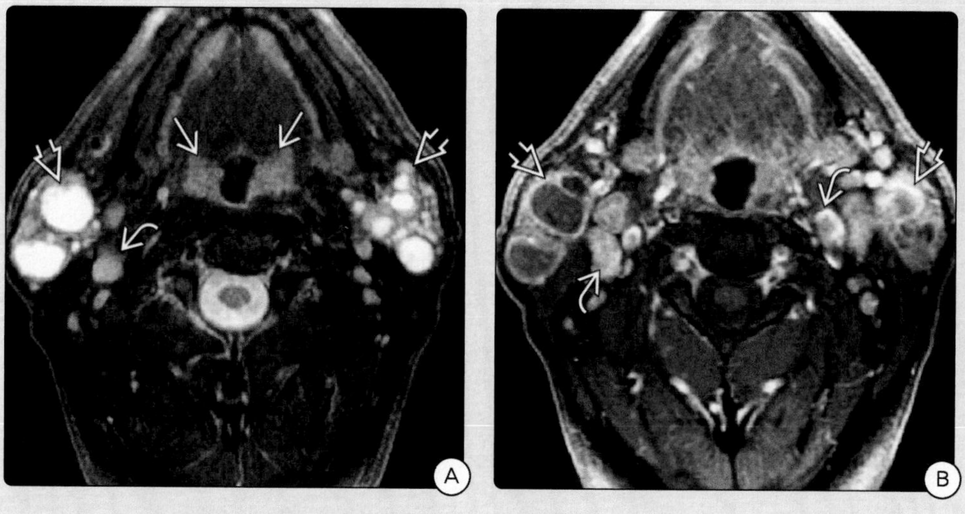

***(14-12A)** Axial T2WI in a 31y HIV-positive man shows hyperplastic Waldeyer ring ➡, prominent deep cervical lymph nodes ➡, and multiple variably sized cysts ➡ in both parotid glands. **(14-12B)** Axial T1 C+ FS scan in the same patient shows rim-enhancing cysts in both parotid glands ➡ and enlarged deep cervical lymph nodes ➡.*

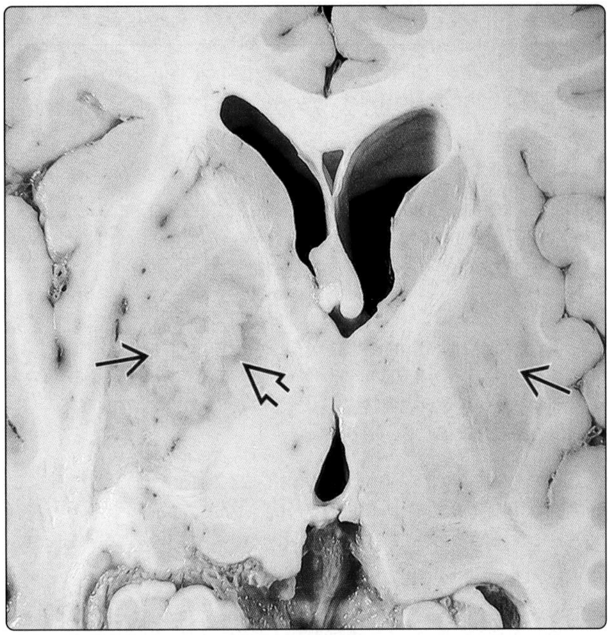

(14-13) Axial gross pathology from an HIV-positive patient shows ill-defined toxoplasmosis abscesses in both basal ganglia ➡. Note hemorrhage ➡ surrounding central necrosis in the right lesion. (Courtesy R. Hewlett, MD.)

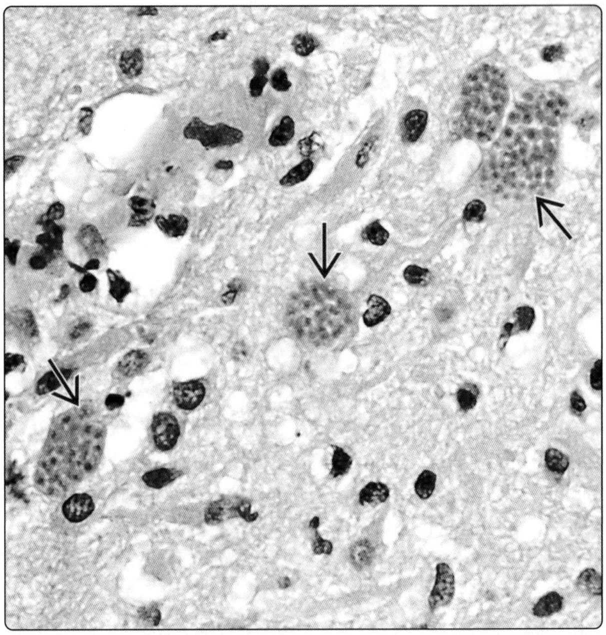

(14-14) Hematoxylin and eosin photomicrograph of toxoplasmosis reveals multiple encysted organisms ➡. (Courtesy B. K. DeMasters, MD.)

hyperintense on T2WI and demonstrate rim enhancement on T1 C+ **(14-12A)**.

Lymphoid Hyperplasia

Lymphoid hyperplasia is common in patients with HIV/AIDS. Immunohistochemistry, fluorescent in situ hybridization, and transmission electron microscopy have all identified HIV in lymph nodes, tonsils, and adenoidal tissue. Histologic evaluation of adenoids and tonsils excised from HIV/AIDS patients demonstrates a spectrum of changes including florid follicular hyperplasia, follicle lysis, attenuated mantle zone, and the presence of multinucleated giant cells.

Affected patients can be asymptomatic or present with a nasopharyngeal mass, nasal stuffiness or bleeding, hearing loss, or cervical lymphadenopathy.

Lymphoid hyperplasia of Waldeyer ring is the most common finding observed on brain MR. Unusually prominent tonsils and adenoids in a patient over 25-30 years of age should raise suspicion of HIV infection **(14-9)**.

The differential diagnosis of benign reactive lymphoid hyperplasia in HIV/AIDS patients is lymphoma.

Opportunistic Infections

With the advent of highly active antiretroviral therapy (HAART), the prevalence of CNS opportunistic infections has decreased five- to tenfold. Nevertheless, these infections and HIV coinfections such as tuberculosis continue to create substantial morbidity.

Toxoplasmosis

Toxoplasmosis (toxo) is the most common opportunistic infection and overall cause of a mass lesion in patients with HIV/AIDS.

Terminology and Etiology

Toxo is caused by the ubiquitous intracellular parasite *Toxoplasma gondii*. Between 20-70% of the population is seropositive for *T. gondii*, so infection in HIV/AIDS patients generally represents reactivation of latent infection.

T. gondii is an obligate intracellular parasite. Although any mammal can be a carrier and act as an intermediate host, cats are the definitive host. Humans become infected when the organism is accidentally ingested. The parasites rapidly multiply as tachyzoites. When the tachyzoites invade the CNS, they become bradyzoites and form parenchymal cysts.

Pathology

Location, Size, and Number. CNS toxo most commonly involves the basal ganglia, thalami, corticomedullary junctions, and cerebellum **(14-13)**.

Multifocal lesions are more common than solitary ones. In contrast to lymphoma, only 15-20% of toxo lesions present as solitary masses. Although large lesions do occur, most lesions are small and average between 2-3 cm in diameter.

Gross and Microscopic Features. The macroscopic appearance of CNS toxo in patients with HIV/AIDS is that of poorly circumscribed necrotizing abscesses with a hyperemic border and soft yellowish contents **(14-13)**.

Microscopic features include coagulative necrosis, encysted toxo organisms, numerous free tachyzoites, and minimal host inflammatory response **(14-14)**.

Clinical Issues

Demographics. Toxo prevalence varies widely. In countries in which HAART is widely available, its prevalence has diminished fourfold over the past decade, decreasing from 25% to 3-10%.

The overall prevalence of toxo in resource-poor regions is much higher. In Africa, 35-50% of all HIV/AIDS patients develop CNS toxoplasmosis. Immunocompromised patients are most likely to develop toxo when their CD4 counts fall below 200.

Presentation. Most HIV/AIDS patients with toxo present with focal neurologic findings superimposed on symptoms of global encephalopathy such as headache, confusion, and lethargy. Mild hemiparesis is the most common focal abnormality. Chorea is relatively rare.

Natural History and Prognosis. CNS toxo is fatal if left untreated, yet early institution of therapy can be curative. Treated patients usually improve significantly within 2-4 weeks. In resource-poor socioeconomic environments, median survival is only 28 months.

Imaging

CT Findings. The most common finding on NECT scan is multiple ill-defined hypodense lesions in the basal ganglia or thalamus with moderate to marked peripheral edema **(14-15A)**.

Enhancement on CECT is closely correlated to CD4 count. In patients with counts under 50, enhancement is absent or faint. Enhancement becomes more pronounced as the CD4

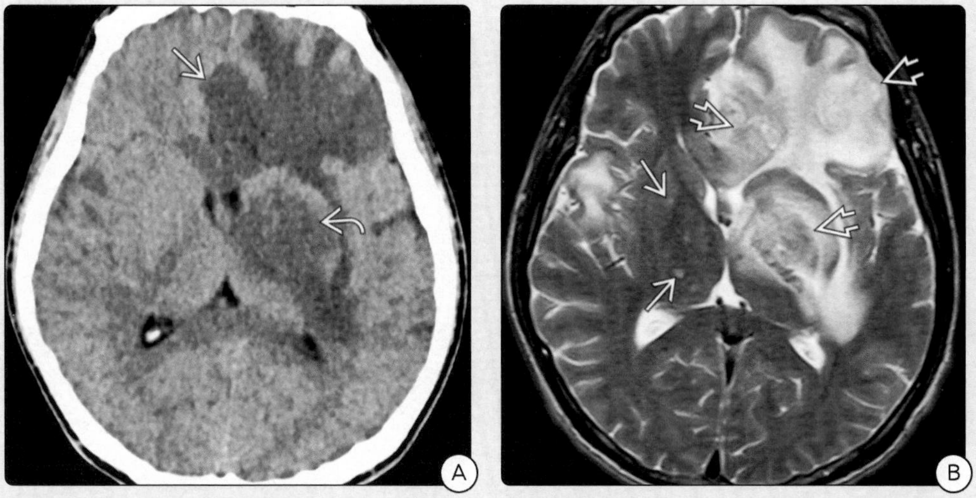

***(14-15A)** NECT in a 33y HIV-positive man in the ER with altered mental status shows hypodense masses in the left basal ganglia ➔ and frontal lobe ➔ with marked peripheral edema. **(14-15B)** T2WI in the same case shows three separate masses ➔ that are surrounded by marked edema and appear very heterogeneous in signal intensity. Several small hyperintensities are also present in the right basal ganglia and thalamus ➔.*

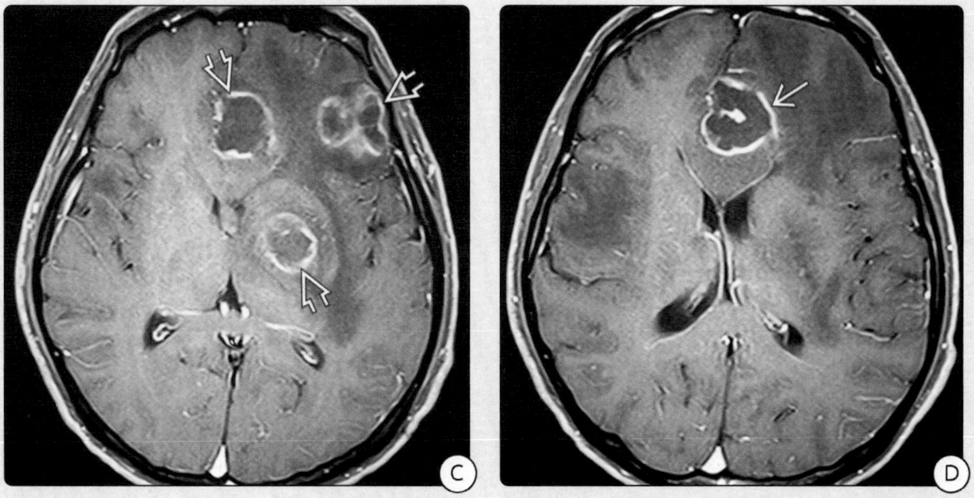

***(14-15C)** T1 C+ FS scan in the same case demonstrates irregular ring-enhancing lesions ➔. **(14-15D)** More cephalad T1 C+ demonstrates a classic "target" sign lesion with a peripheral rim of enhancement ➔ surrounding a central enhancing nodule. This is toxoplasmosis.*

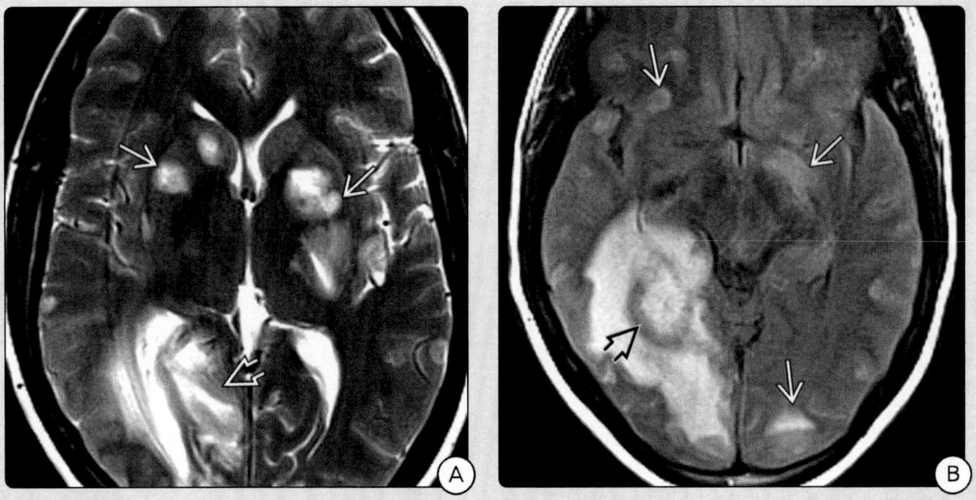

(14-16A) *T2WI in an HIV-positive patient with toxoplasmosis shows multiple hyperintense lesions in both basal ganglia, as well as a larger confluent lesion around the occipital horn of the right lateral ventricle.* ***(14-16B)*** *FLAIR scan in the same patient shows multiple small, mostly hyperintense WM lesions. A large "tumefactive" lesion with a hypointense rim, hyperintense center, and striking peripheral edema is present.*

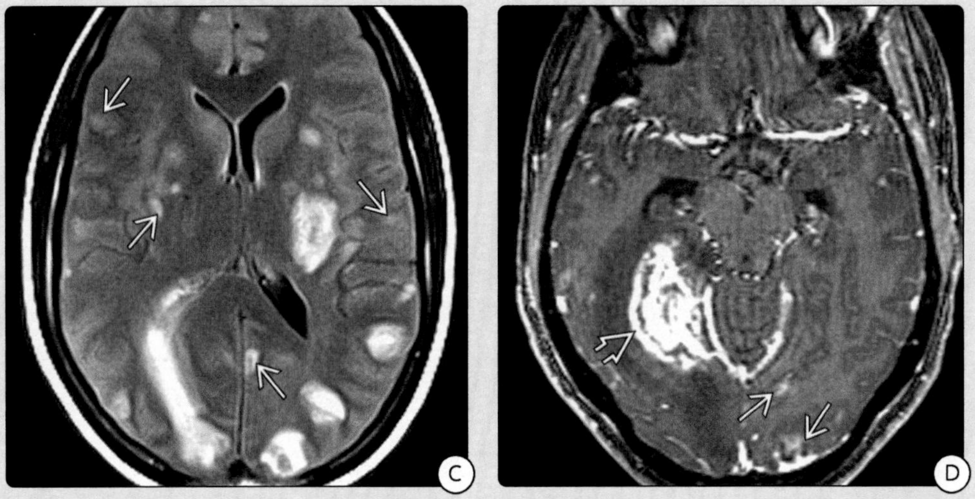

(14-16C) *More cephalad FLAIR scan in the same patient shows large, heterogeneously hyperintense lesions but numerous smaller foci scattered throughout the brain in the cortex and subcortical white matter.* ***(14-16D)*** *T1 C+ FS scan shows that the "tumefactive" lesion enhances strongly but heterogeneously. Several other enhancing lesions are present.*

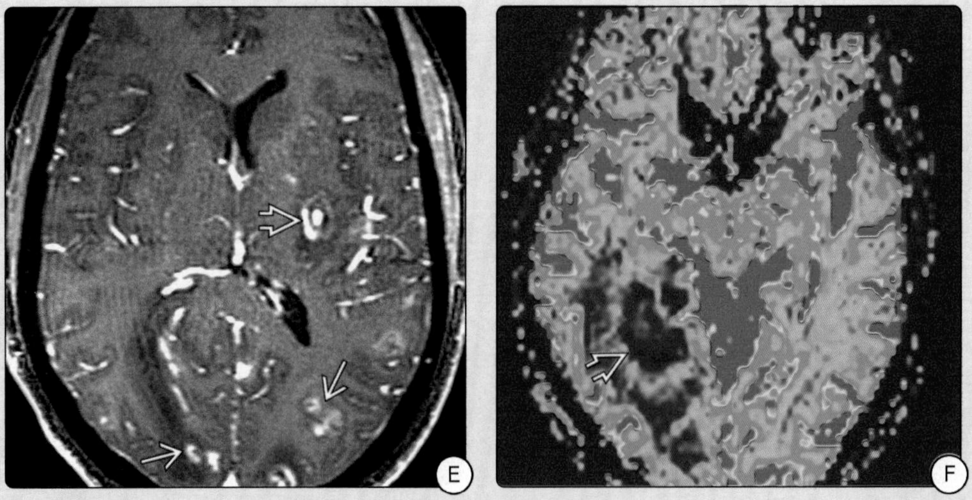

(14-16E) *More cephalad T1 C+ FS scan in the same patient demonstrates additional enhancing lesions, including a "target" lesion in the left basal ganglia.* ***(14-16F)*** *pMR scan in the same patient shows that the "tumefactive" lesion has markedly reduced relative cerebral blood volume, consistent with toxoplasmosis rather than lymphoma.*

count rises. Multiple punctate and ring-enhancing masses are the most common finding.

MR Findings. T1WI shows a hypointense mass that occasionally demonstrates mild peripheral hyperintensity caused by coagulative necrosis or hemorrhage.

Alternating concentric zones of hyper- and hypointensity with marked perilesional edema are seen on T2WI **(14-15B)**. The central T2 hyperintensity corresponds histologically to necrotizing abscess. As a toxo abscess organizes, intensity diminishes, and eventually the lesion becomes isointense relative to white matter. Perilesional hyperintensity represents edema with demyelination.

One or more nodular and ring-enhancing masses are typical on T1 C+ **(14-15C)**. A ring-shaped zone of peripheral enhancement with a small eccentric mural nodule represents the "eccentric target" sign **(14-15D)**. The enhancing nodule is a collection of concentrically thickened vessels, whereas the rim enhancement is caused by an inflamed vascular zone that borders the necrotic abscess cavity.

Disseminated toxoplasmosis encephalitis, also called microglial nodule encephalitis, produces multifocal T2 hyperintensities in the basal ganglia and subcortical white matter. Enhancement may be absent or minimal despite fulminant disease.

MRS findings are nonspecific and often show a lipid-lactate peak. Toxo shows reduced relative cerebral blood volume (rCBV) on SPECT and pMR scans **(14-16)**.

Differential Diagnosis

The major differential diagnosis is **primary CNS lymphoma** (PCNSL). CNS toxo typically presents with multifocal lesions. AIDS-related CNS toxo also has positive findings on serology in 80% of cases, and CSF PCR is definitive. Solitary toxo lesions

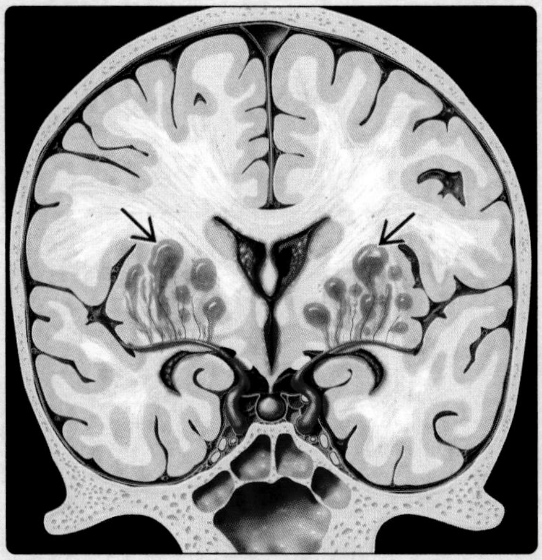

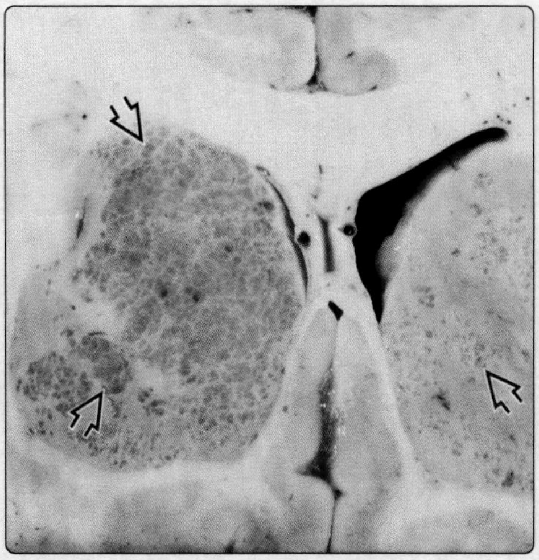

***(14-17)** Coronal graphic shows multiple dilated perivascular spaces ➡ filled with gelatinous mucoid-appearing material characteristic of cryptococcal infection in HIV/AIDS patients. **(14-18)** Coronal autopsied brain in HIV/AIDS shows innumerable tiny cryptococcal gelatinous pseudocysts in the basal ganglia ➡. (Courtesy A. T. Yachnis, Neuropathology, 2014.)*

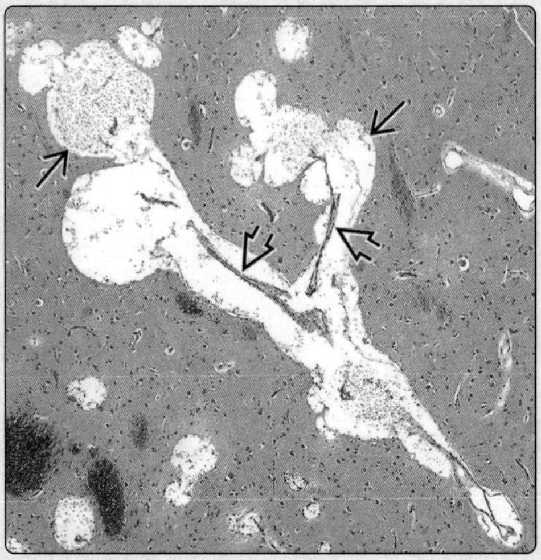

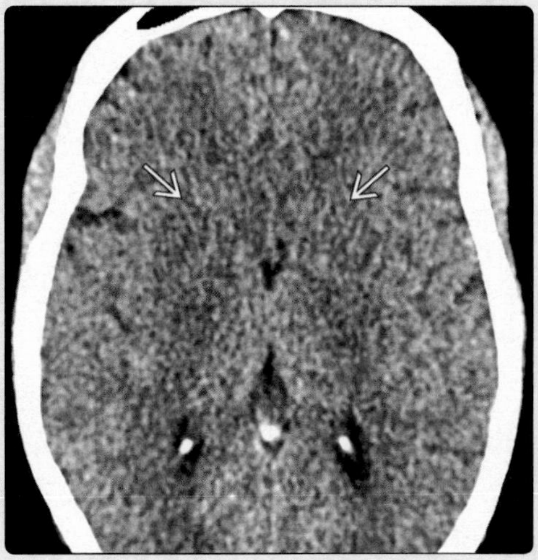

***(14-19)** Photomicrograph shows a branching vessel cut in longitudinal section ➡ surrounded by enlarged perivascular spaces stuffed full of cryptococcal gelatinous pseudocysts ➡. (Courtesy B. K. DeMasters, MD.) **(14-20)** Axial NECT scan in an HIV-positive patient shows hypodense basal ganglia ➡. (Courtesy N. Omar, MD.)*

are uncommon. Approximately 70% of isolated CNS masses in HIV/AIDS patients are PCNSL.

Cryptococcosis

Fungal infections can be life-threatening in immunocompromised patients, especially those with HIV/AIDS. Although many different fungi can cause CNS infection, the most common fungi to affect patients with HIV/AIDS are *Candida albicans*, *Aspergillus* species, and *Cryptococcus neoformans* (crypto). Cryptococcosis in immunocompetent patients was briefly discussed in Chapter 13. Here we focus on its appearance in immunocompromised patients.

Etiology and Epidemiology

Crypto is excreted in mammal and bird feces and is found in soil and dust. It is a ubiquitous fungus with worldwide distribution. The lungs are usually the primary infection site. CNS infection occurs when organisms circulating in the blood are deposited in the subarachnoid cisterns and perivascular spaces.

Crypto is the third most common CNS infectious agent in HIV/AIDS patients, after HIV and *T. gondii*. Prior to HAART, crypto CNS infections occurred in 10% of HIV patients, but it is now relatively rare in developed countries. Crypto usually occurs when CD4 counts drop below 50-100 cells/μL.

Pathology

CNS cryptococcal infection takes three main forms: meningitis, gelatinous pseudocysts **(14-17)**, and focal mass lesions called cryptococcomas. Cryptococcomas and meningitis are the most common forms in immunocompetent patients, whereas meningitis and gelatinous pseudocysts are the most common forms in HIV/AIDS patients **(14-18)**.

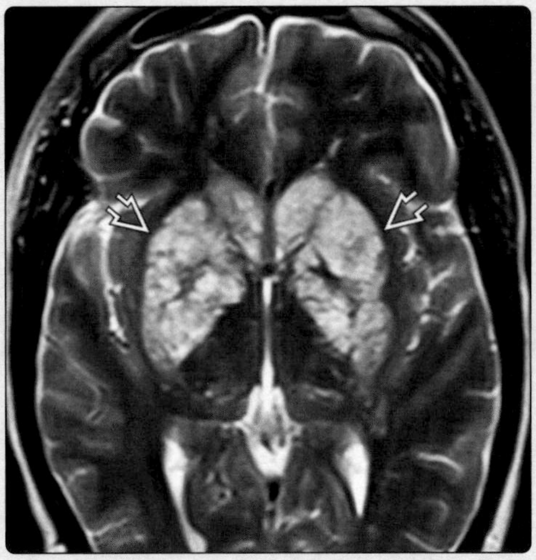

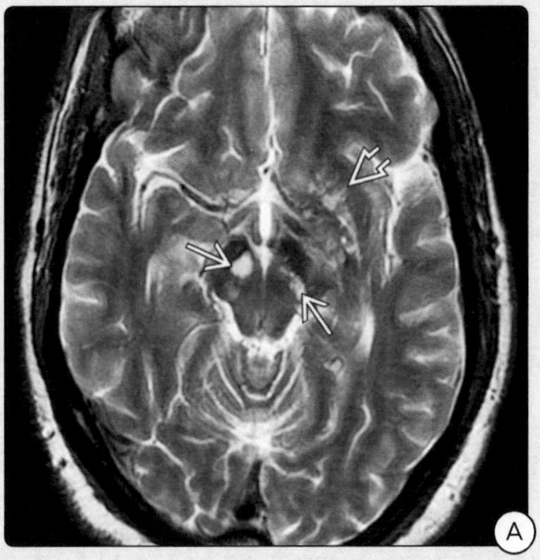

***(14-21)** T2WI in the same patient as Figure 14-20 shows that the lentiform nuclei and the heads of both caudate nuclei are grossly expanded by innumerable hyperintense cysts ➡ characteristic of cryptococcal gelatinous pseudocysts. (Courtesy N. Omar, MD.) **(14-22A)** Axial T2WI in a 55y man with HIV/AIDS shows enlarged perivascular spaces in both cerebral peduncles ➡ and in the left anterior perforated substance ➡.*

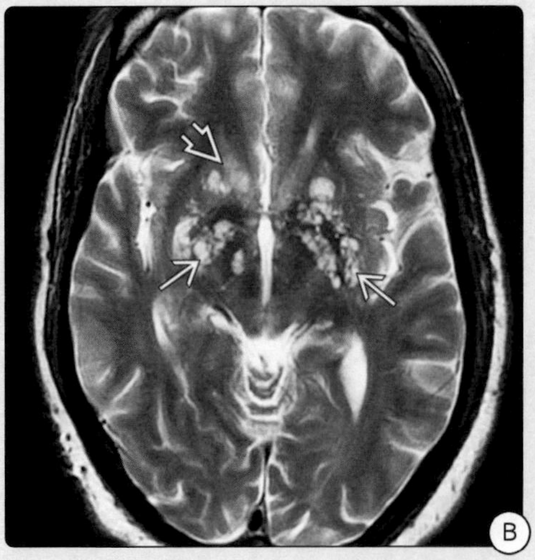

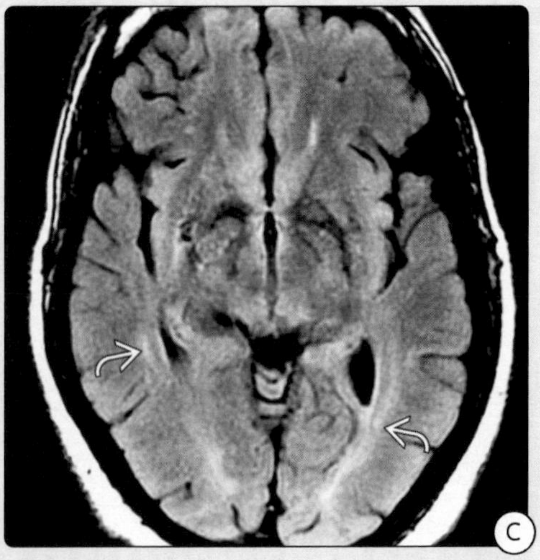

***(14-22B)** Axial T2WI in the same patient shows multiple gelatinous pseudocysts in both lenticular nuclei ➡, as well as the head of the right caudate nucleus ➡. **(14-22C)** FLAIR scan in the same patient shows that the pseudocysts suppress. Note "hazy" hyperintensity in the cerebral white matter ➡ consistent with HIVE. (Courtesy T. Markel, MD.)*

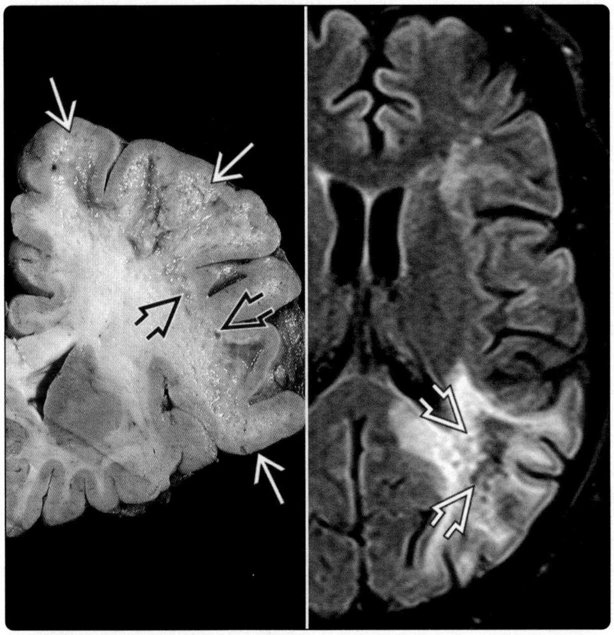

(14-23) (L) Autopsy of advanced PML shows coalescent subcortical demyelinated foci ➡ with multiple tiny cavities ⇨. (R) FLAIR of PML shows "spongy-appearing" hyperintense subcortical WM with multiple small hypointense cysts ➡.

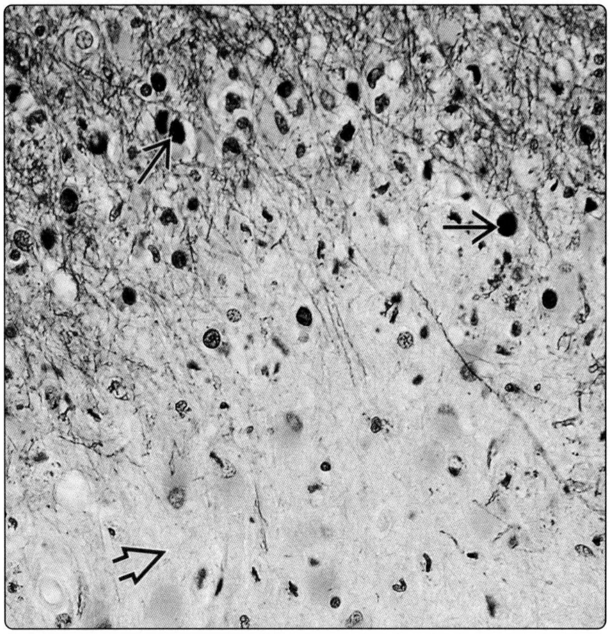

(14-24) Dark infected oligodendrocytes ⇨ are concentrated at the edge of the pink-appearing demyelinated foci ⇨ in this classic microscopic image of PML. (Both cases courtesy B. K. DeMasters, MD.)

In crypto meningitis or meningoencephalitis, the meninges become thickened and cloudy. Gelatinous mucoid-like cryptococcal capsular polysaccharides and budding yeast accumulate within dilated perivascular spaces (PVSs) **(14-19)**. Multiple gelatinous pseudocysts occur in the basal ganglia, midbrain, dentate nuclei, and subcortical white matter.

Clinical Issues

Crypto in patients with HIV/AIDS typically presents as meningitis or meningoencephalitis. Common symptoms are headache, seizure, and blurred vision. Focal neurologic deficits are uncommon.

Imaging

NECT scans often show hypodensity in the basal ganglia **(14-20)**. Enhancement varies with immune status. CECT scans in immunocompromised patients typically show no enhancement.

Cryptococcal gelatinous pseudocysts are hypointense to brain on T1WI and very hyperintense on T2WI **(14-21)**. The lesions generally follow CSF signal intensity and suppress on FLAIR **(14-22)**. Perilesional edema is generally absent. Lack of enhancement on T1 C+ is typical although mild pial enhancement is sometimes observed.

Differential Diagnosis

Enlarged PVSs are a common normal finding in virtually all patients and are seen at all ages. They can occur in clusters and typically follow CSF signal intensity. Enlarged PVSs do not enhance. In HIV/AIDS patients with CD4 counts under 20, symmetrically enlarged PVSs should be considered cryptococcal infection and treated as such.

Toxo usually has multifocal ring- or "target"-like enhancing lesions with significant surrounding edema. **Tuberculosis** usually demonstrates strong enhancement in the basal meninges. Tuberculomas are generally hypointense on T2WI. **Primary CNS lymphoma** in HIV/AIDS patients often shows hemorrhage, necrosis, and ring enhancement. Solitary lesions are more common than multifocal involvement.

Progressive Multifocal Leukoencephalopathy

Terminology

Progressive multifocal leukoencephalopathy (PML) is an opportunistic infection caused by the JC virus (JCV), a member of the Papovaviridae family. The virus was named "JC" after it was first isolated from autopsied brain tissue from a patient named John Cunningham.

Over the past two decades, the spectrum of JCV CNS infection has expanded beyond "classic" PML. Some investigators have suggested distinguishing between classic PML (cPML) and inflammatory PML (iPML). Other neurotropic forms of JCV infection include JCV encephalopathy (JCE), JC meningitis (JCM), and JCV infection of the cerebellar granular layer (JCV granule cell neuronopathy).

Etiology

JCV is a ubiquitous virus that circulates widely in the environment, primarily in sewage. More than 85% of the adult population worldwide has antibodies against JCV.

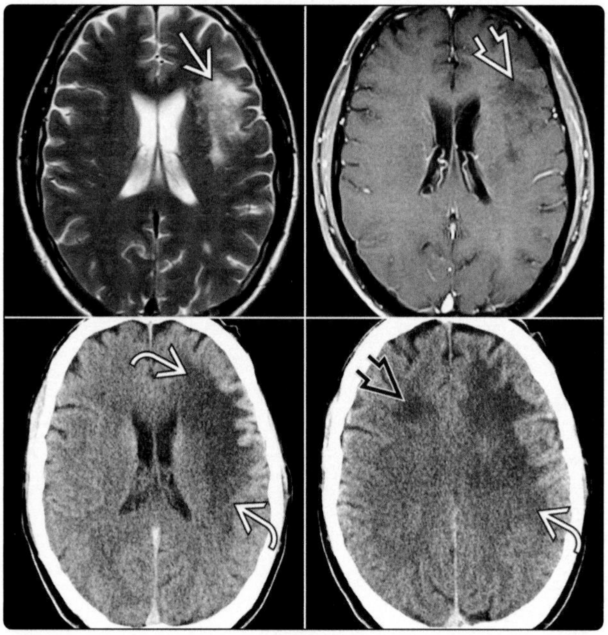

(14-25) cPML in a 32y HIV-positive man is shown. Confluent left frontal T2 hyperintensity spares cortex, does not enhance. NECT 6 weeks later shows the left frontal lesion has increased in size, and a new right frontal hypodensity is present.

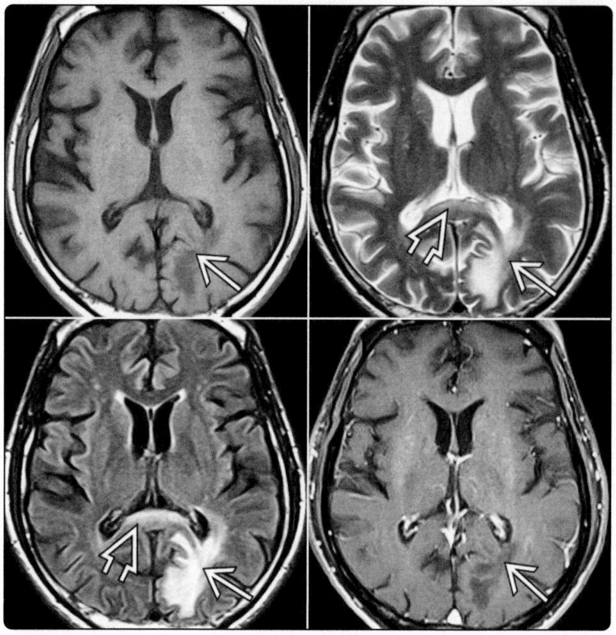

(14-26) MR in a clinically deteriorating 46y HIV-positive patient with a CD4 count < 10 cells/µL shows a confluent nonenhancing left occipital lesion that crosses the corpus callosum. CSF was PCR-positive for JC virus.

Asymptomatic infection is probably acquired in childhood or adolescence and remains latent until the virus is reactivated.

In some immunocompromised patients, the reactivated JCV becomes neurotropic and infects oligodendrocytes, causing a progressive demyelinating encephalopathy, i.e., PML.

Three phases in the development of PML have been identified. The first phase is the primary but clinically inapparent infection. In the second phase, the virus persists as a latent peripheral infection, primarily in the kidneys, bone marrow, and lymphoid tissue. The third phase is that of reactivation and dissemination with hematogeneous spread to the CNS.

HIV-induced immunodeficiency is now the most common predisposing factor for symptomatic JCV infection and is responsible for 80% of all cases. PML also occurs in the setting of collagen vascular disease, immunosuppression for solid organ or bone marrow transplantation, chemotherapy with rituximab for hematologic malignancies, and treatment with the immunosuppressive agent natalizumab for multiple sclerosis or Crohn's disease.

The expanding spectrum of PML now also includes patients *without* severe depletion of cellular immunity. This generally occurs in conditions with less overt immunodeficiency such as idiopathic CD4 lymphocytopenia, systemic lupus erythematosus, cirrhosis, psoriasis, and even pregnancy. Cases of PML in the absence of *any* documented immunodeficiency have also been reported.

Pathology

Location. Activated JCV almost exclusively affects oligodendrocytes, causing multifocal asymmetric demyelination with a predilection for the frontal and parietooccipital white matter.

Size and Number. Initial PML lesions are small, generally measuring a few millimeters in diameter. As the disease progresses, small foci coalesce into confluent lesions that can occupy large volumes of white matter.

Gross Pathology. Early lesions appear as small yellow-tan round to ovoid foci at the gray-white matter junction. The cortex remains normal. With lesion coalescence, large spongy-appearing depressions in the cerebral and cerebellar white matter appear **(14-23)**. Unlike ischemic infarcts, PML lesions are rarely completely cavitated.

Microscopic Features. Demyelination ranges from myelin pallor to severe loss. Pale-staining demyelinating foci are bordered by large infected oligodendrocytes with violaceous nuclear inclusions **(14-24)**. With the exception of cerebellar granular neurons, neuronal infection is rare.

Clinical Issues

Epidemiology. In the pre-HAART era, PML affected between 3-7% of HIV-positive patients and caused 18% of all CNS-related AIDS deaths. The increasingly widespread use of HAART has significantly reduced the prevalence of PML in patients with HIV/AIDS. The incidence has dropped from 0.7 to 0.07 per 100 person-years in the decade since the institution of HAART.

The incidence of natalizumab-associated PML is estimated at 1:1,000. Risk increases with duration of exposure.

Presentation and Natural History. Until recently, PML was the only known manifestation of CNS JCV infection. Newly

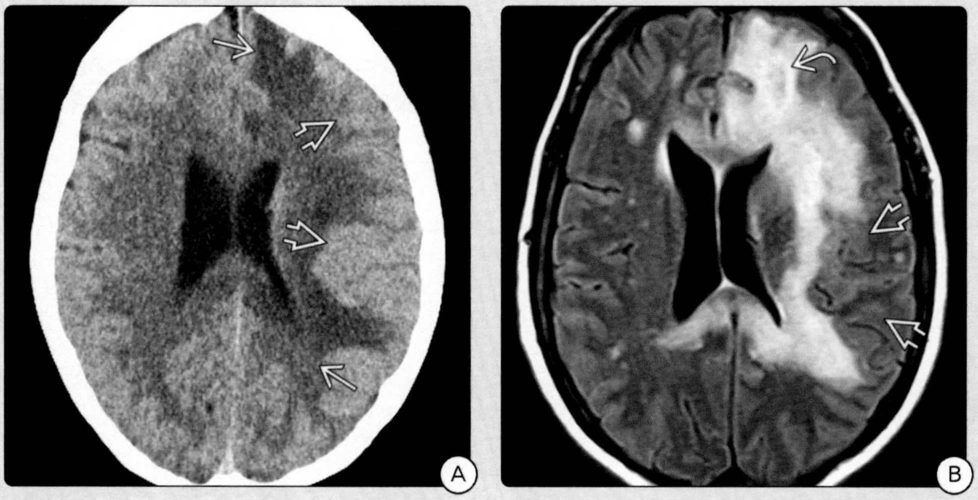

***(14-27A)** 54y woman on chemotherapy for acute myeloid leukemia developed headaches and visual problems. Axial NECT shows extensive hypodense lesion occupying most of the left hemisphere WM ➡. Note cortical swelling ➡, mass effect on left lateral ventricle. **(14-27B)** FLAIR shows confluent WM hyperintensity crossing corpus callosum, sulcal obliteration, cortical hyperintensity ➡. Note focal ring-like lesion ➡ in the left frontal lobe.*

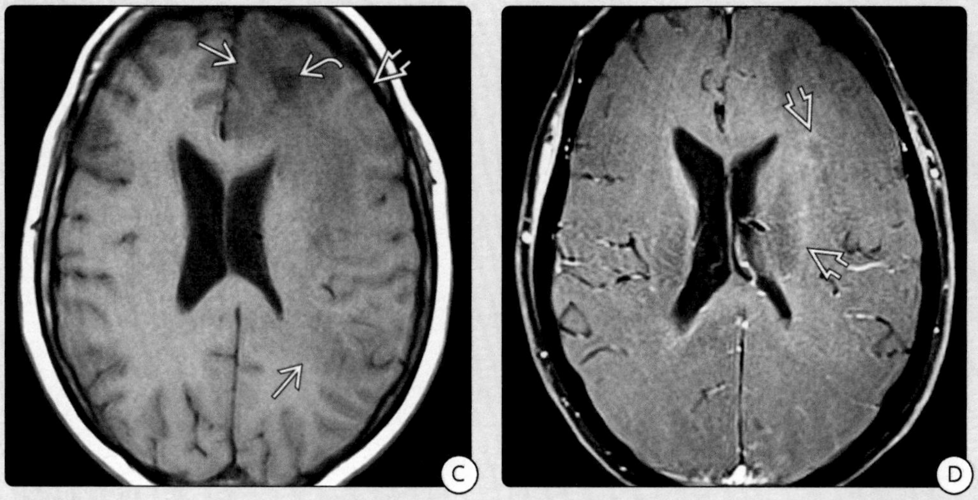

***(14-27C)** Axial T1WI shows ill-defined white matter hypointensity ➡ with effacement of the left superficial sulci ➡ and a focal hypointense left frontal mass ➡. **(14-27D)** T1 C+ FS shows faint but definite enhancement around the advancing margins of several lesions ➡.*

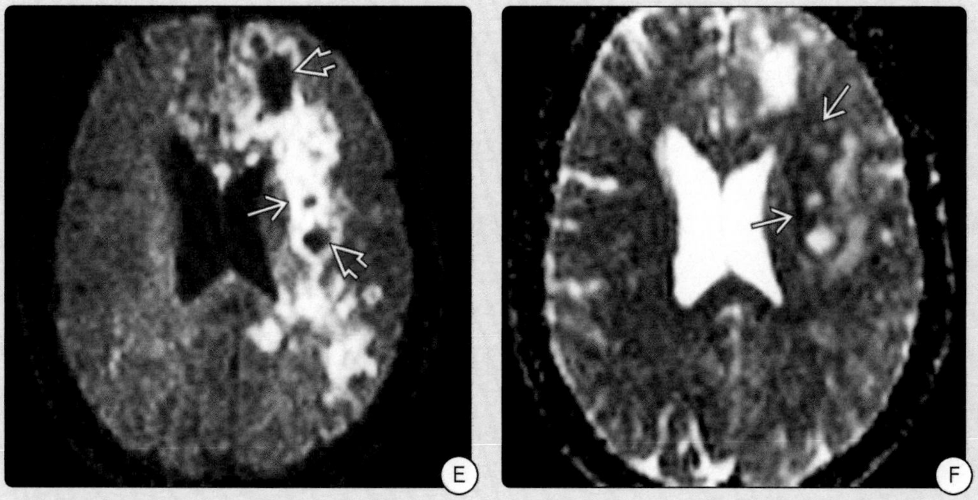

***(14-27E)** DWI shows restricted diffusion in many new white matter lesions ➡, whereas the centers of several older lesions ➡—including the ring-like area in the left frontal lobe—do not restrict. **(14-27F)** ADC shows restriction in the active margins of inflammation ➡. The patient's CSF PCR was positive for JC virus. With the mass effect and subtle enhancement, this was thought to represent the inflammatory PML variant.*

recognized presentations include PML-associated immune reconstitution inflammatory syndrome (IRIS, see below). Rare presentations include JCE, JCM, and an oligodendrocyte-sparing cerebellar syndrome associated with isolated infection of cerebellar granule cell neurons ("JCV granule cell neuronopathy").

The most common symptoms of PML are altered mental status, headache, lethargy, motor deficits, aphasia, and gait difficulties. In approximately 25% of patients, PML is the initial manifestation of AIDS and can appear early in the disease course while CD4 counts are above 200 cells/μL.

PML in untreated HIV/AIDS patients is often fatal with death in 6-8 months. HAART may stabilize the disease and improve overall survival, but PML is still the second most common cause of all AIDS-related deaths, second only to lymphoma.

PML in natalizumab-treated MS carries a high morbidity and mortality rate. Drug withdrawal and plasma exchange therapy have been used with some success to increase survival in these patients.

PML: ETIOLOGY AND PATHOLOGY

Etiology
- Caused by JC virus (JCV)
  - Ubiquitous; > 85% of adults have JCV antibodies
  - Acquired in childhood, latent until reactivated
- Most common predisposing condition = HIV (80%)
- Less common = collagen vascular disease, immunosuppression, MS treated with natalizumab (20%)
- Rare = systemic lupus erythematosus, pregnancy

Pathology
- Almost exclusively affects oligodendrocytes
- Multifocal demyelination

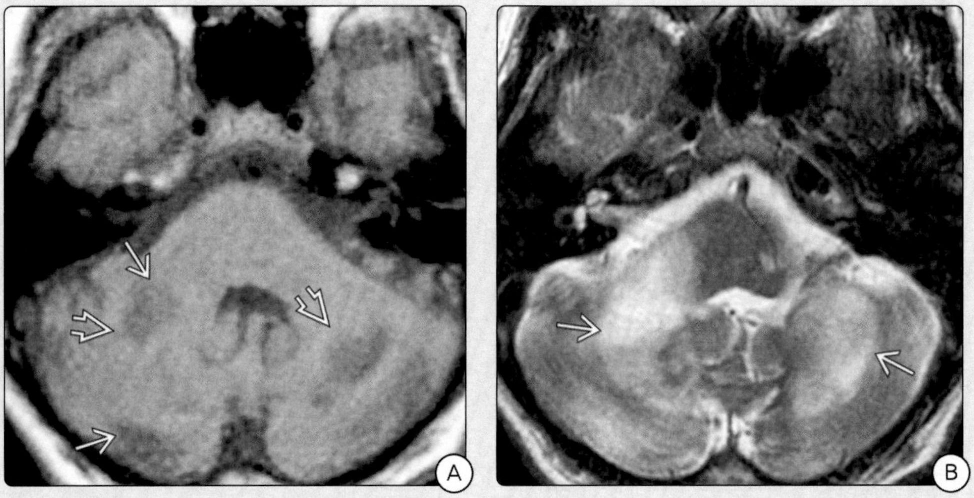

***(14-28A)** Axial T1WI MR in a 42y HIV-positive woman with cerebellar classic PML and gait difficulties shows several hypointense lesions in the cerebellum ➡. Note faint hyperintensity along the margins of the more anterior cerebellar lesions ➡. **(14-28B)** Axial T2WI in the same patient shows the characteristic involvement of both middle cerebellar peduncles ➡.*

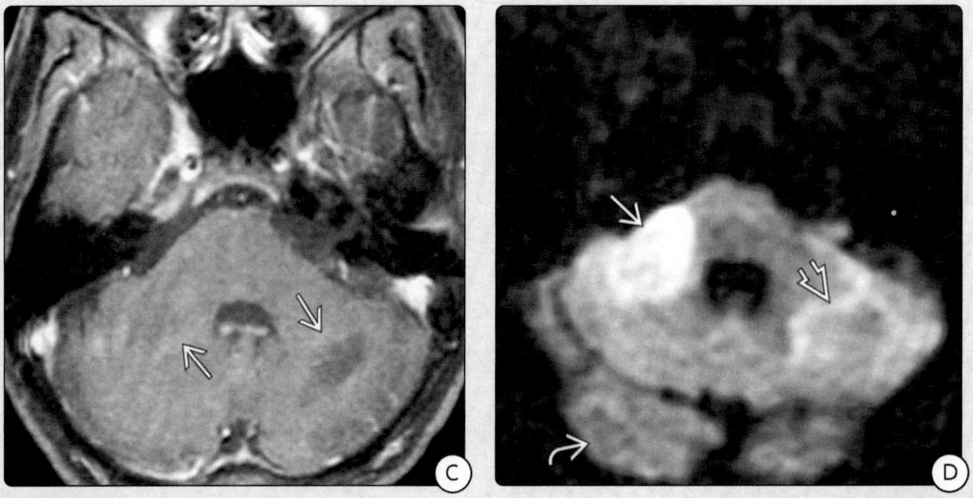

***(14-28C)** Axial T1 C+ FS scan shows very faint rim enhancement around the lesions ➡. **(14-28D)** DWI in the same patient shows lesions in three different stages. The right posterior cerebellar lesion ➡ shows no restriction, the right middle cerebellar peduncle lesion ➡ restricts strongly and uniformly, and the left cerebellar lesion shows restriction around the lesion's rim ➡.*

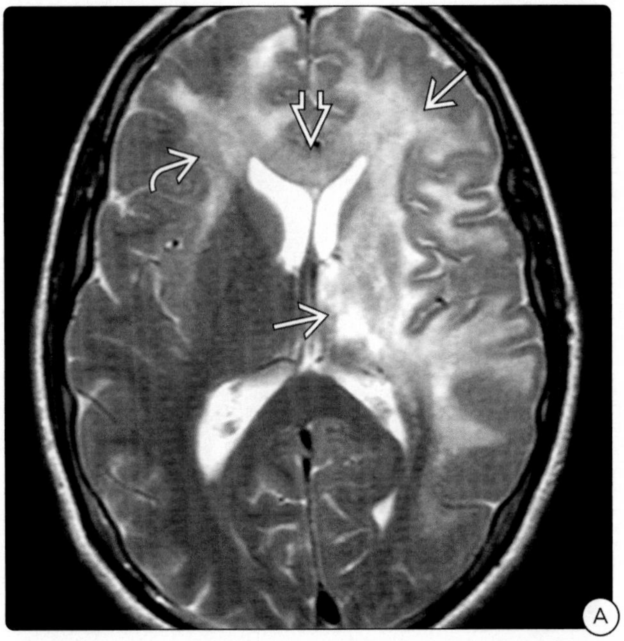

(14-29A) 27y HIV-positive man developed acute confusion, right-sided weakness. Axial T2WI shows confluent heterogeneous hyperintensity in left cerebral WM, basal ganglia that crosses the corpus callosum to involve the right frontal lobe.

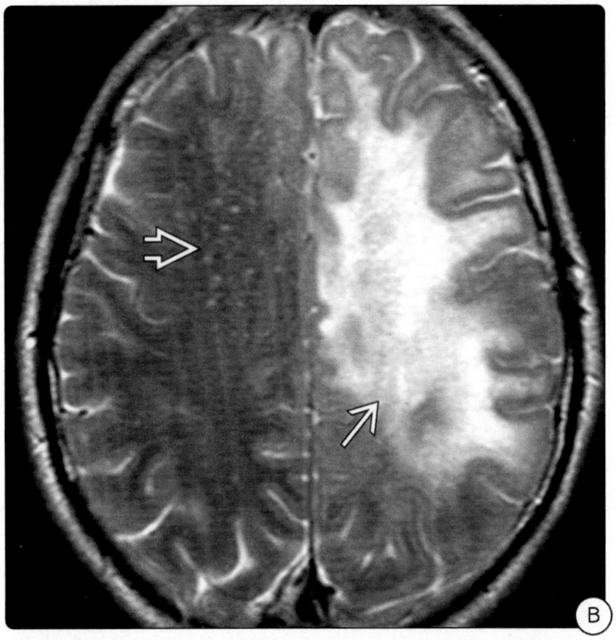

(14-29B) More superior image shows the inhomogeneously hyperintense nature of the lesion. Tiny hyperintense microcysts are present in the right frontal white matter. This is acute inflammatory PML.

Imaging

General Features. Imaging plays a key role in the diagnosis and follow-up of JCV infections. cPML can appear as solitary or multifocal widespread lesions. Any area of the brain can be affected, although the supratentorial lobar white matter is the most commonly affected site. The posterior fossa white matter—especially the middle cerebellar peduncles—is the second most common location. In occasional cases, a solitary lesion in the subcortical U-fibers is present.

Extent varies from small scattered subcortical foci to large bilateral but asymmetric confluent white matter lesions. In the early acute stage of infection, some mass effect with focal gyral expansion can be present. At later stages, encephaloclastic changes with atrophy and volume loss predominate.

CT Findings. More than 90% of cPML cases show hypodense areas in the subcortical and deep periventricular white matter on NECT **(14-25)**; 70% are multifocal. PML lesions generally do not enhance on CECT.

MR Findings

Classic PML. Multifocal, bilateral but asymmetric, irregularly shaped hypointensities on T1WI are typical. The lesions are heterogeneously hyperintense on T2WI **(14-26)** and typically extend into the subcortical U-fibers all the way to the undersurface of the cortex, which remains intact even in advanced disease **(14-27)**. Smaller, almost microcyst-like, very hyperintense foci within and around the slightly less hyperintense confluent lesions represent the characteristic spongy lesions seen in more advanced PML **(14-29)**.

PML generally does not enhance on T1 C+ scans, although faint peripheral rim-like enhancement occurs in 5% of all cases **(14-28)**. The exception is hyperacute PML in the setting of IRIS (see below) and in MS patients on natalizumab. In these cases, striking foci with irregular rim enhancement are frequently—but not invariably—present. Corticosteroids significantly decrease the prevalence and intensity of enhancement.

Appearance on DWI varies according to disease stage. In newly active lesions, DWI restricts strongly. Slightly older lesions show a central core with low signal intensity and high mean diffusivity (MD) surrounded by a rim of higher signal intensity and lower MD. Chronic "burned out" lesions show increased diffusion due to disorganized cellular architecture **(14-28)**.

DTI shows reduced fractional anisotropy consistent with disorganized white matter structure. As cPML lesions are comparatively avascular, pMR demonstrates reduced rCBV compared with unaffected white matter.

Findings on MRS are nonspecific, with decreased NAA reflecting neuronal loss. Increased choline, consistent with myelin destruction, and a lipid-lactate peak from necrosis are often present. Myoinositol is variable but may be elevated, consistent with inflammatory change.

Inflammatory PML. Imaging findings in iPML are identical to those of cPML except that the lesions demonstrate peripheral enhancement and/or mass effect **(14-27)** **(14-29)**. Acute iPML may have relatively increased vascularity and rCBV caused by the inflammatory angiogenic effect. In some patients, lesions may demonstrate features of iPML early and then evolve to cPML later in the disease course.

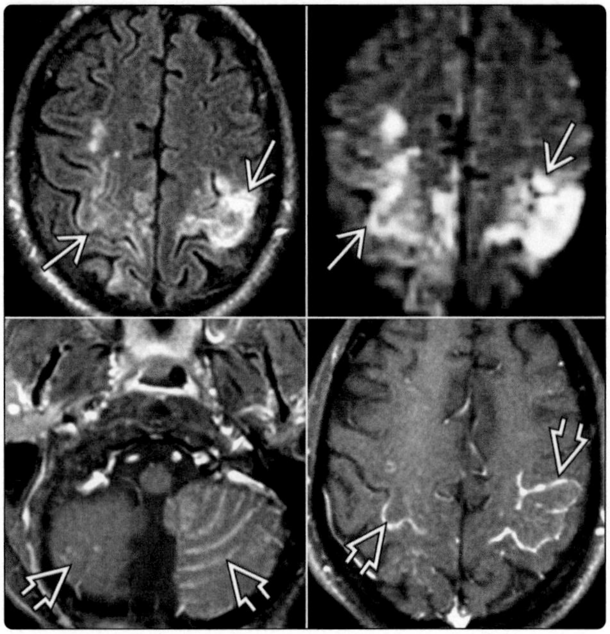

(14-30) CMV meningoencephalitis is shown in a 32y HIV-positive man. FLAIR shows hyperintensity in both parietal lobes, corresponding restriction on DWI ➔. T1 C+ scans show enhancement in the posterior fossa, convexity sulci ➔.

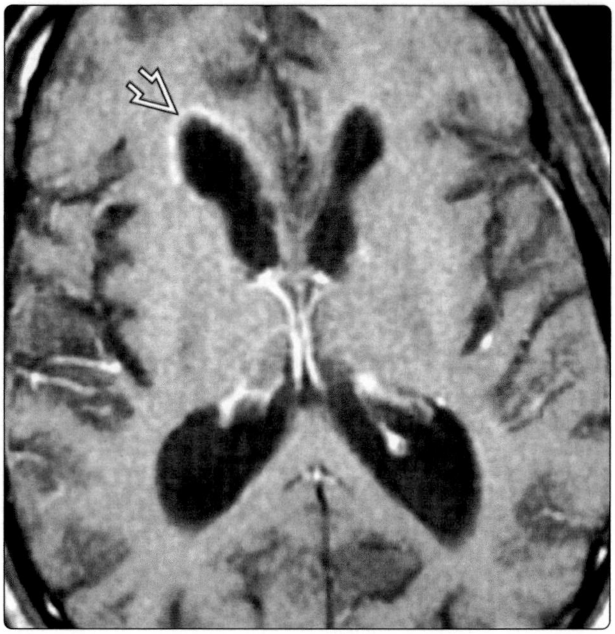

(14-31) T1 C+ scan in a patient with HIV encephalitis shows generalized volume loss. Note striking ependymal enhancement ➔, atypical for HIV encephalitis. This is CMV ventriculitis.

Miscellaneous JCV infections. JCV meningitis has no distinguishing features from other meningitides, demonstrating nonspecific sulcal-cisternal hyperintensity on FLAIR and enhancement on T1 C+ FS scans.

JCE initially affects the hemispheric gray matter, then extends into the subcortical white matter. JCV infection of the cerebellar granular layer is seen as cerebellar atrophy with T2 hyperintensity in the affected folia.

PML: CLINICAL FEATURES, IMAGING, AND DDx

Clinical Features

- PML pre-HAART = 3-7% of HIV(+); now sharply reduced
- Major CNS JCV syndrome = classic PML
- Others = iPML, JC encephalitis/meningitis

Imaging

- Multifocal WM lesions
  - Bilateral but asymmetric
  - Involve subcortical U-fibers
  - Spare cortex
- Usually no mass, no enhancement (unless iPML)

Differential Diagnosis

- HIV encephalitis (doesn't involve U-fibers)
- IRIS (PML-IRIS most common)
- Other opportunistic infections (e.g., cytomegalovirus)

Differential Diagnosis

The major differential diagnosis of cPML is **HIV encephalitis (HIVE)**. HIVE demonstrates more symmetric WM disease while sparing the subcortical U-fibers. **IRIS** is usually more acute and demonstrates strong but irregular ring-like enhancement.

Other Opportunistic Infections

A number of other infectious/inflammatory processes can cause or exacerbate preexisting CNS disease in patients with HIV/AIDS. These include cytomegalovirus (CMV), sexually transmitted diseases (especially neurosyphilis), tuberculosis, fungal infections, malaria, and bacterial abscesses. In this section, we focus on acquired CMV infection (congenital CMV was discussed in Chapter 12), the "deadly intersection" between HIV/AIDS and TB coinfection, and the "triple collision" when HIV, TB, and malaria all overlap.

Cytomegalovirus

CMV is a member of the herpesvirus family. While it is a ubiquitous virus, CMV typically remains latent until reactivated. Several risk factors predispose patients to the development of overt CMV CNS disease: T-cell depletion syndromes, anti-thymocyte globulin, allogenic stem cell transplants, and HIV/AIDS. All cause severe, protracted T-cell immunodeficiency.

CNS CMV is a late-onset disease in immunocompromised patients. With increasing use of HAART, less than 2% of HIV/AIDS patients develop overt symptoms of CMV infection. Patients with CD4 counts under 50 cells/μL are most at risk.

Mortality in CNS CMV is high despite therapy with a combination of antiviral drugs. Ganciclovir-resistant CMV has developed, making prophylactic therapy difficult in high-risk patients.

In contrast to congenital CMV in which the virus causes parenchymal calcifications, acquired CMV most commonly manifests as meningoencephalitis and ventriculitis/ependymitis. Although the imaging findings of meningoencephalitis resemble those of other infections **(14-30)**, enhancement along the ventricular ependyma in an immunocompromised patient is highly suggestive of CMV **(14-31)**.

Retinitis and myelitis with radiculitis are the two most frequent extracranial presentations.

Tuberculosis

TB is one of the most devastating coinfections in immunocompromised patients and is the main cause of morbidity and mortality in HIV-infected patients worldwide. The emergence of multidrug-resistant and extensively drug-resistant TB (MDR TB and XDR TB) has occurred almost entirely in patients coinfected with HIV.

More than one-third of all HIV/AIDS patients worldwide are coinfected with TB, and this deadly combination is disproportionately prevalent in highly endemic, resource-limited regions such as sub-Saharan Africa.

HIV is the most powerful known risk factor for reactivation of latent TB to active disease. HIV patients who are coinfected with TB have a 100 times greater risk of developing active TB compared with non-HIV patients. Conversely, the host immune response to TB enhances HIV replication and accelerates disease progression.

In turn, TB coinfection exacerbates the severity and accelerates the progress of HIV. In such patients, AIDS can behave as an acute fulminating illness with meningitis, bacterial abscesses, sepsis, coma, and death **(14-32)**. Mortality approaches 100%, and median survival is measured in days to a few weeks.

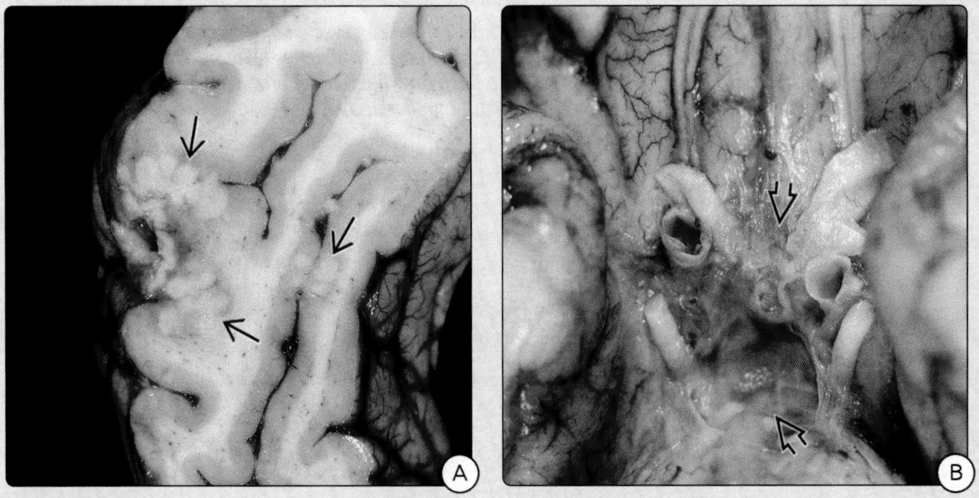

(14-32A) *Series of autopsy images, all from the same patient, shows the "cascade" of catastrophes caused by HIV-TB coinfection. Several of many multiple old healed granulomas ⇨ from prior CNS TB are shown in this axial section obtained through the temporal lobe.* ***(14-32B)*** *The patient became HIV positive, which reactivated his latent TB, causing severe tuberculous meningitis ⇨, as seen on this view of the basilar cisterns.*

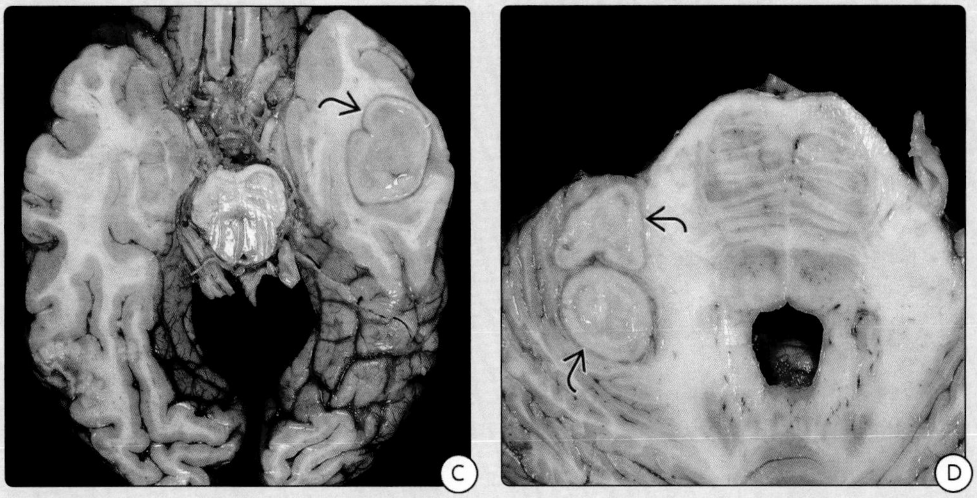

(14-32C) *With his immune system severely weakened, the patient became septic and developed several acute pyogenic abscesses. Note that the abscess in the temporal lobe ⇨ is relatively poorly encapsulated.* ***(14-32D)*** *Two other abscesses are shown in the cerebellum ⇨. The ultimate cause of death was acute overwhelming sepsis. (Courtesy R. Hewlett, MD.)*

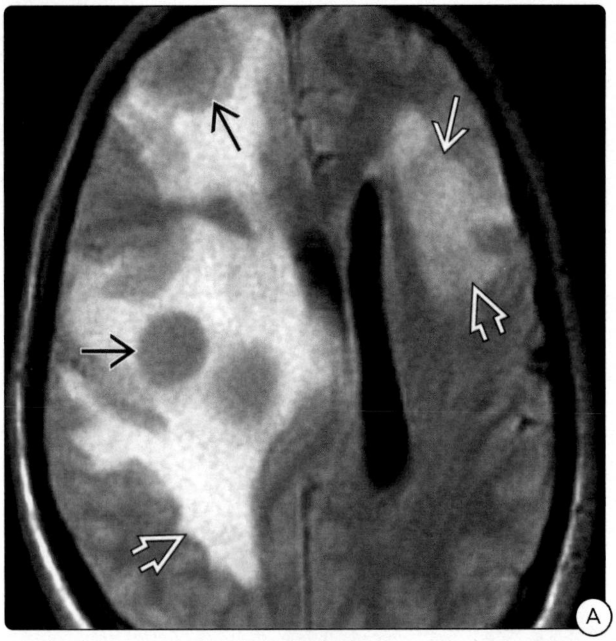

***(14-33A)** An HIV-positive patient with CD4 count < 50 cells/µL had rapidly progressive left-sided weakness, decreased mental status. FLAIR shows several hypointense and 1 hyperintense lesion with marked mass effect, significant edema.*

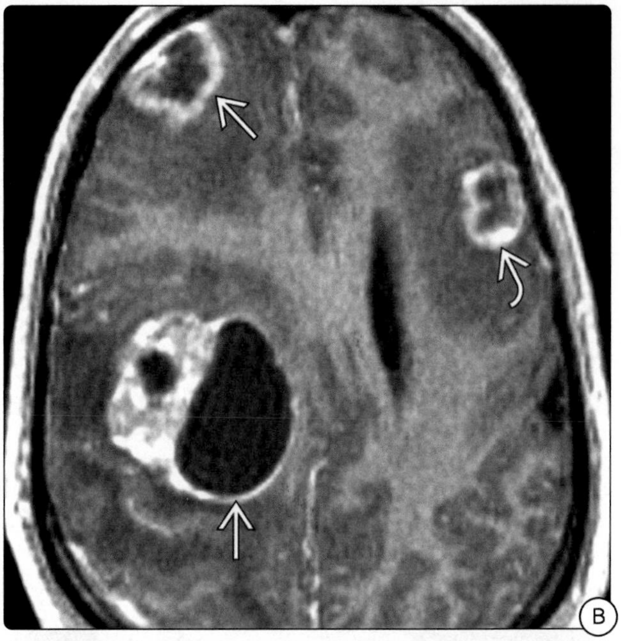

***(14-33B)** Axial T1 C+ scan in the same patient shows multiple rim-enhancing masses. This severely immunocompromised patient had both granulomas and a pseudoabscess in the setting of fulminant reactivated TB. (Courtesy S. Candy, MD.)*

TB is treated *first* in HIV-related infection both to preserve the effectiveness of HAART and to prevent the development of TB-IRIS (see below).

The typical imaging findings in HIV-associated CNS TB may differ slightly from those in immunocompetent patients, looking like TB "gone wild" with multiple parenchymal granulomas and pseudoabscesses **(14-33)**.

Immunocompromised patients with CD4 counts under 200 cells/µL mount a significantly attenuated immunologic response. Although meningitis is the most common manifestation of HIV-associated CNS TB, enhancement of meningeal inflammation, tuberculomas, and pseudoabscesses are often mild or absent even though greater numbers of acid-fast bacilli are present.

Malaria

The global burden of malaria remains high, and coinfection with multiple pathogenic organisms is common in endemic areas. HIV/AIDS and malaria have a bidirectional, synergistic interaction with each magnifying the deleterious effects of the other.

Seroprevalence of HIV-1 is high in patients with severe malaria. HIV-coinfected patients generally have a higher parasite burden, more complications, and a significantly higher case mortality rate.

In-hospital parasitemia, renal impairment, and clinical deterioration are common in these coinfected patients, so early identification of both infections is important for management.

HIV, TB, and malaria are three pandemics that overlap in resource-poor tropical countries. The least deadly condition is HIV infection without the other two comorbid disorders. The most deadly combinations are HIV-TB and HIV-TB-malaria.

MISCELLANEOUS OPPORTUNISTIC INFECTIONS

Cytomegalovirus (CMV)
- Herpesvirus family
- Develops in 2% of HIV/AIDS patients
- CD4 count usually < 50 cells/µL
- Imaging
  - Meningitis
  - Ventriculitis/ependymitis

Tuberculosis
- 1/3 of HIV/AIDS patients coinfected
- HIV most powerful known risk factor for reactivating latent TB
  - 100x risk than for non-AIDS patients
- TB enhances HIV replication, accelerates disease
  - May present as acute, fulminant, fatal infection
  - TB "gone wild"

Malaria
- HIV coinfection worsens outcome
- "Triple combination" of HIV-TB-malaria more deadly than HIV-malaria

Immune Reconstitution Inflammatory Syndrome

Terminology

CNS immune reconstitution inflammatory syndrome (IRIS) is a T-cell-mediated encephalitis that occurs in the setting of treated HIV or autoimmune disease (e.g., multiple sclerosis). CNS IRIS is also called neuro-IRIS.

Etiology

Most investigators consider neuro-IRIS a dysregulated immune response and pathogen-driven disease whose clinical expression depends on host susceptibility, the intensity and quality of the immune response, and the specific characteristics of the "provoking pathogen" itself.

IRIS occurs when forced immune reconstitution causes an exaggerated response to infectious (or sometimes noninfectious antigens) with massive destruction of virus-infected cells. IRIS develops in two distinct scenarios, "unmasking" IRIS and "paradoxical" IRIS. Both differ in clinical expression, disease management, and prognosis although their imaging manifestations are similar.

"Unmasking" IRIS occurs when antiretroviral therapy reveals a subclinical, previously undiagnosed opportunistic infection. Immune restoration leads to an immune response against a living pathogen. Here brain parenchyma is damaged by both the replicating pathogen and the incited immune response.

"Paradoxical" IRIS occurs when a patient who has been successfully treated for a recent opportunistic infection unexpectedly deteriorates after initiation of antiretroviral therapy. Here there is no newly acquired or reactivated

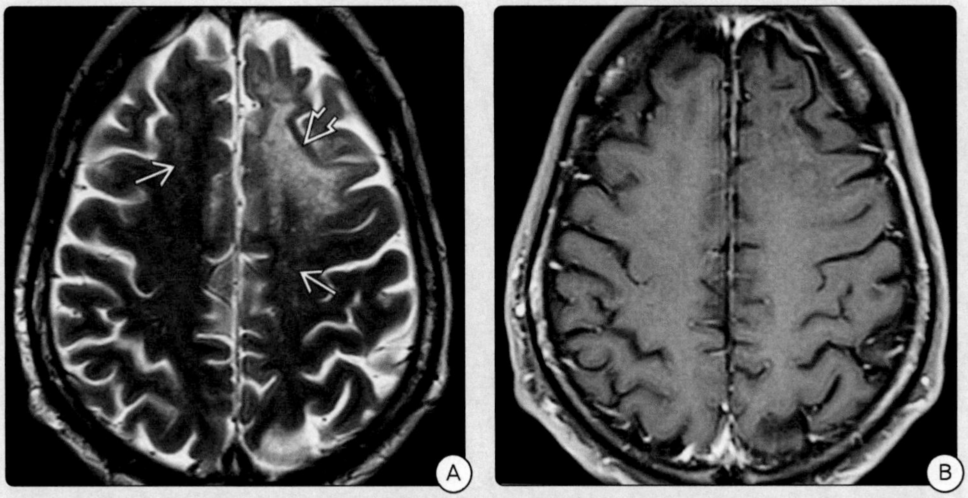

***(14-34A)** Baseline T2WI in a 40y man with untreated HIV/AIDS for 8 years shows diffuse volume loss and bifrontal hyperintense subcortical white matter lesions with both confluent ⇨ and round ➡, "punctate" lesions. **(14-34B)** Axial T1 C+ shows that none of the lesions enhance. The patient was placed on combination antiretroviral treatment (cART).*

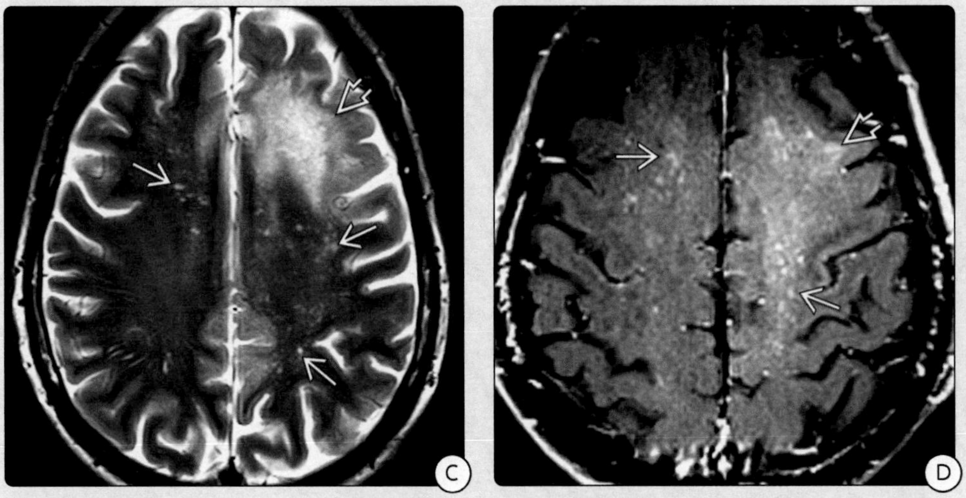

***(14-34C)** The patient deteriorated 5 weeks after beginning cART. Repeat T2WI shows enlargement of the confluent left frontal lesion ⇨ with interval appearance of innumerable punctate hyperintensities ➡ scattered throughout the subcortical and deep white matter of both hemispheres. **(14-34D)** T1 C+ FS shows that the confluent ⇨ and punctate lesions ➡ enhance. CSF was positive for JC virus. This is PML-IRIS.*

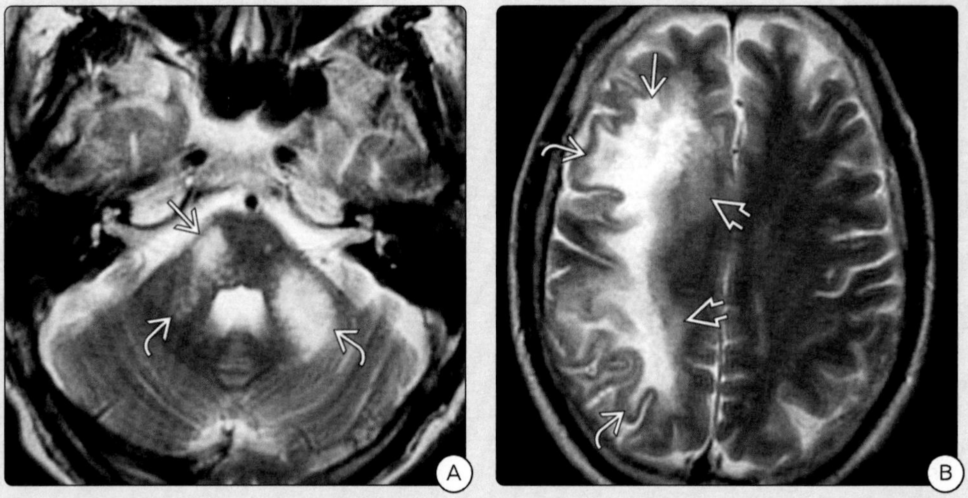

***(14-35A)** Axial T2WI in a 56y man with HIV/AIDS who deteriorated 8 weeks after HAART shows patchy hyperintense lesions in the pons ➡ and major cerebellar peduncles ↷. **(14-35B)** More cephalad T2WI through the corona radiata shows a confluent hyperintense lesion ➡ surrounded by hazy, less hyperintensity ⇗ in the right cerebral hemisphere. Note involvement of the subcortical U-fibers ↷.*

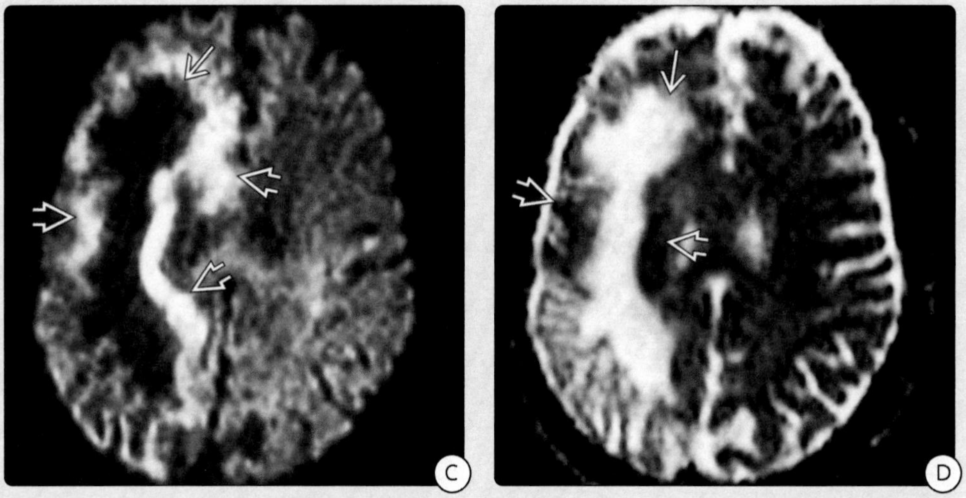

***(14-35C)** DWI in the same case shows a central area of T2 "black out" ➡ surrounded by an irregular area of restricted diffusion ⇗ along the periphery of the lesion. **(14-35D)** ADC shows T2 "shine-through" ➡ in the center of the lesion with surrounding hypointensity ⇗, indicating true restricted diffusion.*

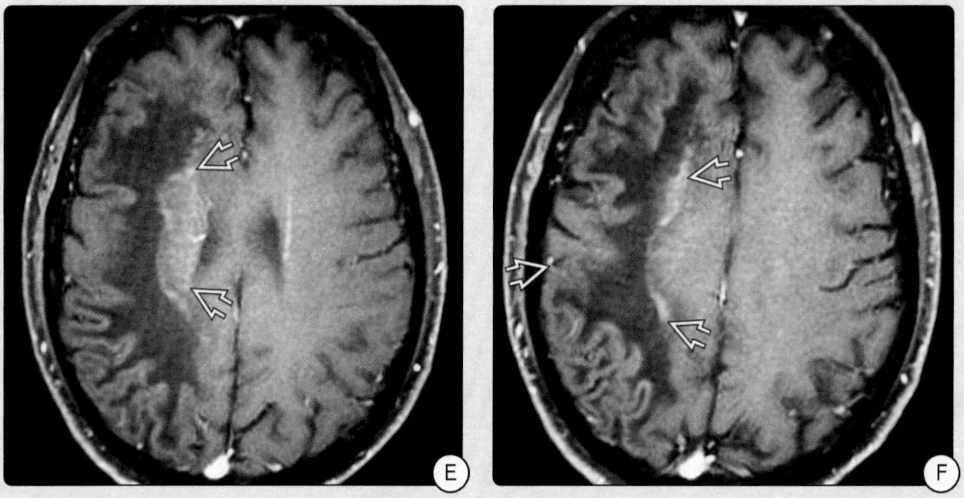

***(14-35E)** T1 C+ FS shows enhancement ⇗ along the medial side of the lesion. **(14-35F)** More cephalad T1 C+ FS shows additional areas of strong contrast enhancement ⇗. CSF PCR was positive for JC virus, so the imaging diagnosis of PML-IRIS was confirmed.*

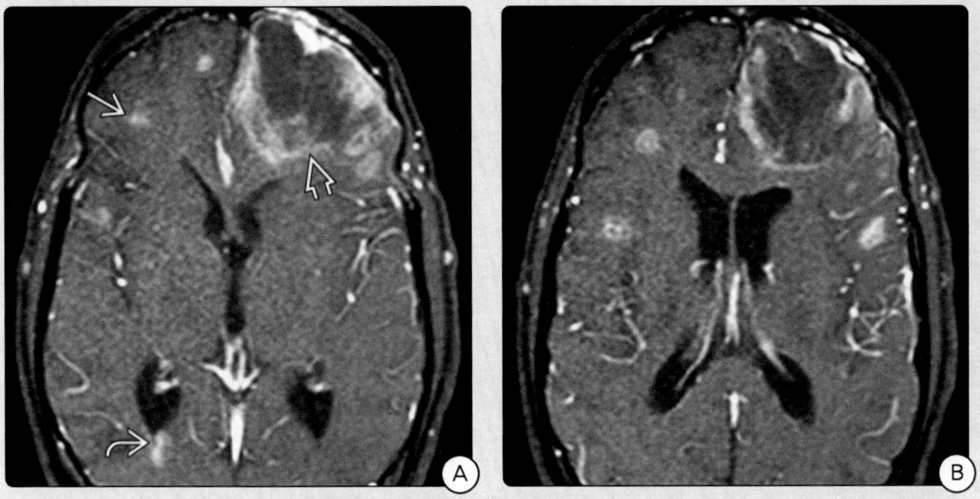

(14-36A) *A 38y HIV-positive man with a remote history of cardiac Chagas disease experienced acute worsening 2 weeks following initiation of HAART. T1 C+ FS scan shows multiple ring-like and nodular enhancing lesions and ventriculitis.* ***(14-36B)*** *More cephalad scan shows additional lesions.*

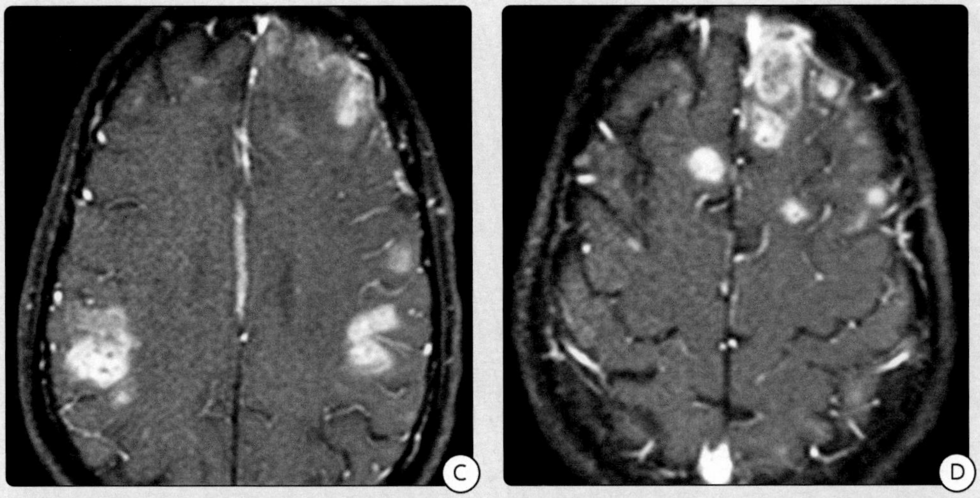

(14-36C) *Multiple heterogeneously enhancing lesions are seen at the gray-white matter interfaces of both hemispheres.* ***(14-36D)*** *Axial T1 C+ FS scan through the vertex shows many more lesions.*

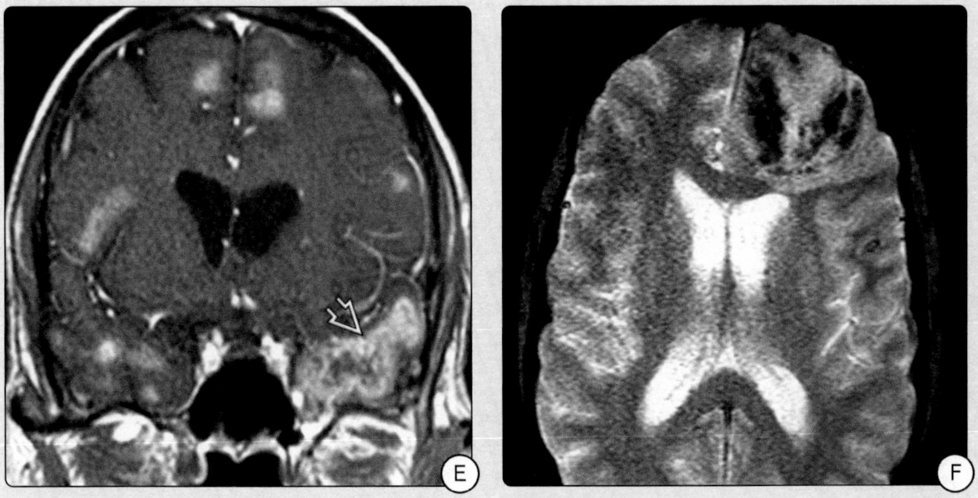

(14-36E) *Coronal T1 C+ scan shows multiple enhancing foci at the gray-white matter interfaces, as well as a large necrotic-looking left temporal lobe mass.* ***(14-36F)*** *T2* GRE scan shows multiple large and small hemorrhages. This is parasite-IRIS from reactivation of latent Chagas disease.*

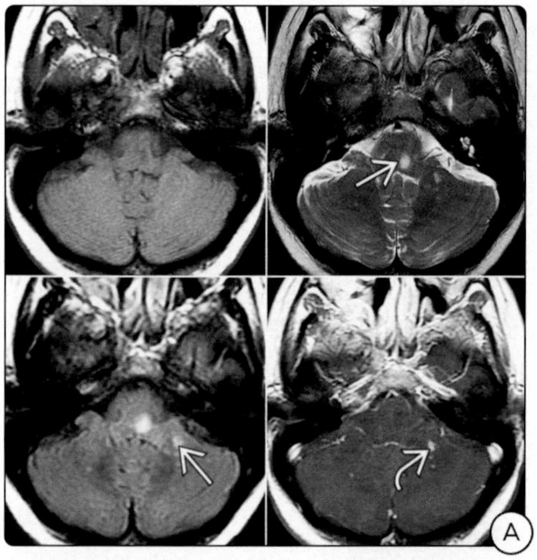

(14-37A) Baseline of natalizumab-associated PML-IRIS in MS shows posterior fossa lesions ➡ with solitary focus of punctate enhancement ➡.

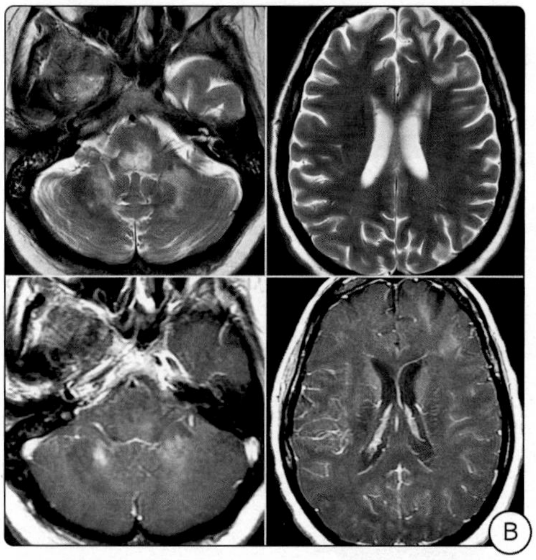

(14-37B) Three months later, symptoms had progressed. Existing lesions have enlarged, and new lesions have appeared.

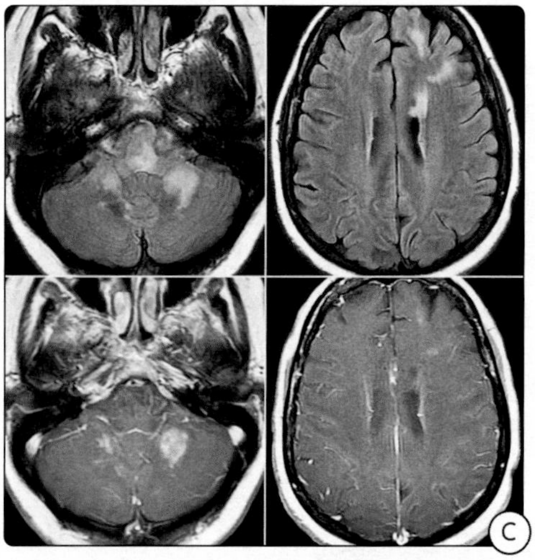

(14-37C) Following plasmapheresis and immunoadsorption treatment, the disease stabilized.

infection. The recovering immune response targets persistent pathogen-derived antigens or self-antigens and causes tissue damage.

Several different underlying pathogens have been identified with IRIS. The most common are JC virus (PML-IRIS), tuberculosis (TB-IRIS), and fungal infections, especially *Cryptococcus* (crypto-IRIS). Some parasitic infections—such as toxoplasmosis—are relatively common in HIV/AIDS patients but rarely associated with IRIS.

Not all neurotropic viruses cause IRIS. HIV itself rarely causes neuro-IRIS. Herpes viruses (e.g., herpes simplex virus, varicella-zoster virus, cytomegalovirus) are all rarely reported causes of neuro-IRIS.

An unusual type of IRIS occurs in MS patients treated with natalizumab who subsequently develop PML. Natalizumab-related PML is managed by discontinuation of the drug and instituting plasmapheresis/immunoadsorption (PLEX/IA) **(14-37)**. Neurologic deficits and imaging studies in some patients worsen during subsequent immune reconstitution, causing **natalizumab-associated PML-IRIS**. Two types are recognized: patients with early PML-IRIS (IRIS develops *before* institution of PLEX/IA) and patients with late PML-IRIS (IRIS develops *after* treatment with PLEX/IA). Neurologic outcome is generally worse in early PML-IRIS with a mortality rate approaching 25%.

Pathology

There are no specific histologic features or biomarkers for neuro-IRIS; rather, the diagnosis is established on the basis of clinical manifestations, exclusion of other disorders, and imaging or histopathologic evidence of inflammatory reaction.

Clinical Issues

Epidemiology. Between 15-35% of AIDS patients beginning HAART develop IRIS. Of these, approximately 1% develop neuro-IRIS. The two most important risk factors are a low CD4 count and a short time interval between treatment of the underlying infection and the commencement of antiretroviral therapy. The highest risk is in patients with a count less than 50 cells/μL.

Epidemiology varies according to the specific "provoking pathogen." The most common cause of neuro-IRIS is JC virus. Latent virus is reactivated when patients become immunodeficient. The reactivated virus infects oligodendrocytes, causing the lytic demyelination characteristic of PML. Nearly one-third of patients with preexisting PML worsen after beginning HAART and are considered to have "unmasking" **PML-IRIS.**

TB-IRIS occurs in 15% of patients who are coinfected with TB if antiretroviral therapy is initiated before the TB is adequately treated. Inflammasome activation underlies the immunopathogenesis of TB-IRIS. Almost 20% of TB-IRIS patients develop neurologic involvement characterized by meningitis, tuberculomas, and radiculomyelopathies. TB-IRIS is associated with a mortality rate of up to 30%.

"Paradoxical" **crypto-IRIS** affects 20% of HIV-infected patients in whom antiretroviral therapy was initiated after treatment of neuromeningeal cryptococcosis. The major manifestation of crypto neuro-IRIS is aseptic recurrent meningitis. Parenchymal cryptococcomas are rare.

Despite the high prevalence of parasitic infestations in resource-poor countries, only a few cases of parasite-associated neuro-IRIS have been reported. All have been caused by *T. gondii*.

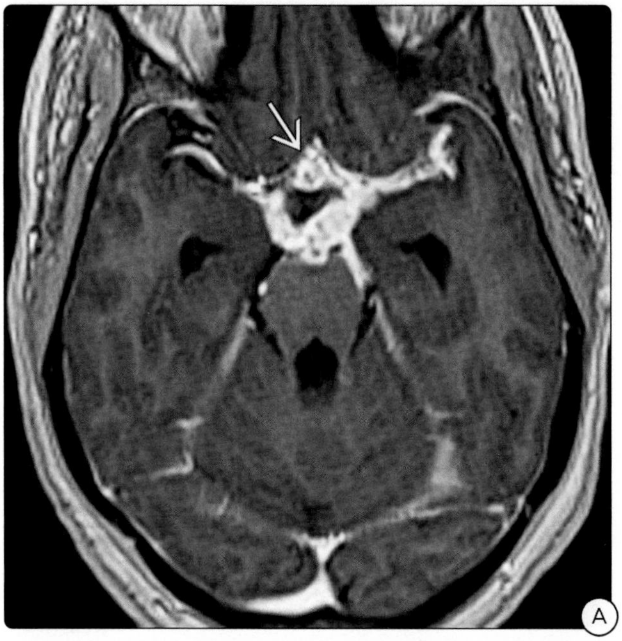

(14-38A) A 36y woman with TB meningitis, newly diagnosed HIV was placed on anti-TB medications. Two months later cART was initiated. She acutely deteriorated in 4 weeks. Axial T1 C+ SPGR scan shows diffuse thick basilar cistern enhancement ➡.

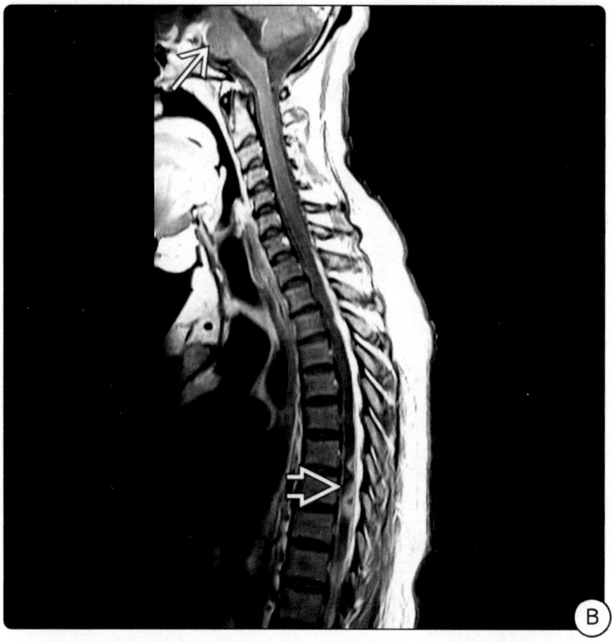

(14-38B) Sagittal T1 C+ MR of the spine shows that the TB meningitis ➡ also involves the spinal cord ➡. This is an example of TB-IRIS. (Courtesy S. Candy, MD.)

Natalizumab-associated IRIS is rare. To date, approximately 50 cases have been reported. Most are PML-IRIS.

Presentation. Neuro-IRIS is a polymorphic condition with heterogeneous clinical manifestations. The most common presentation is clinical deterioration of a newly treated HIV-positive patient despite rising CD4 counts and diminishing viral loads.

Natural History and Treatment Options. Given that a low CD4 T-cell count is a major risk factor for developing IRIS, starting HAART at a count of > 350/μL will prevent most cases.

Systemic IRIS is usually mild and self-limited. Prognosis in neuro-IRIS is variable. Corticosteroids and cytokine neutralization therapy have been used for treatment of neuro-IRIS with mixed results and are controversial.

Patients with neuro-IRIS may die within days to weeks. Mortality from PML-IRIS exceeds 40%, whereas that of crypto-IRIS is about 20%. TB-IRIS mortality is slightly lower (13%).

Imaging

A widespread pattern of confluent and linear or "punctate" perivascular hyperintensities on T2/FLAIR is virtually pathognomonic of PML-IRIS. A "punctate" pattern of enhancement is typical in the acute stage **(14-34)**.

Bizarre-looking parenchymal masses and progressively enlarging, enhancing lesions are also common in PML-IRIS and are seen in slightly less than half of all cases **(14-35)**.

IMMUNE RECONSTITUTION INFLAMMATORY SYNDROME (IRIS)

Terminology and Etiology

- Neuro-IRIS
  - "Unmasking" IRIS (HAART "unmasks" existing subclinical opportunistic infection)
  - "Paradoxical" IRIS (treated infection worsens after HAART)
- Pathogens associated with neuro-IRIS
  - JC virus (PML-IRIS) most common
  - Tuberculosis (TB-IRIS) next most common
  - Fungi (crypto-IRIS)
  - Drugs (natalizumab-associated PML-IRIS)
  - Parasites (rare, except for toxo-IRIS)
  - Neurotropic viruses (e.g., HIV, herpesviruses) rarely cause IRIS

Epidemiology

- 15-35% of AIDS patients starting HAART develop IRIS
- Of these, 1% develop neuro-IRIS
- CD4 count < 50 cells/μL = sharply increased risk of IRIS

Imaging

- "Punctate" pattern of T2/FLAIR hyperintensities
  - "Punctate" pattern of enhancement on T1 C+
- Confluent disease extending into subcortical U-fibers
  - Variable mass-like enhancement, often bizarre and "wild"

Differential Diagnosis

- Non-IRIS-associated opportunistic infections
- AIDS-defining malignancies
  - Especially lymphoma

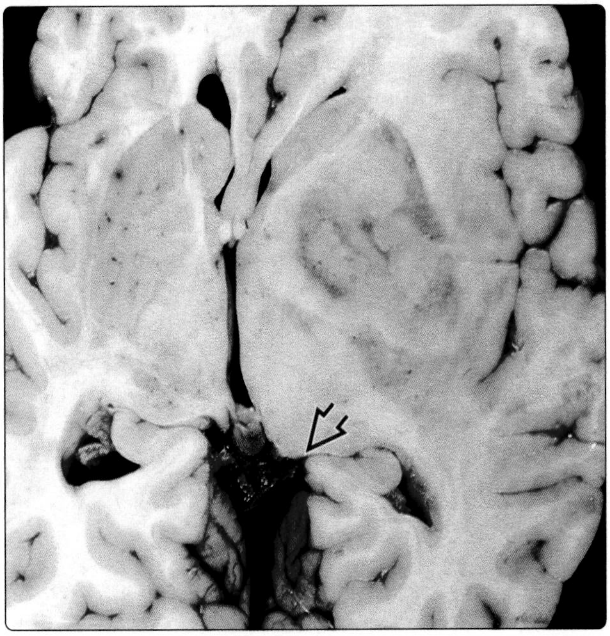

(14-39) Autopsy case of AIDS-related PCNSL shows a solitary mass in the basal ganglia with central necrosis and peripheral hemorrhage ⇒. (Courtesy R. Hewlett, MD.)

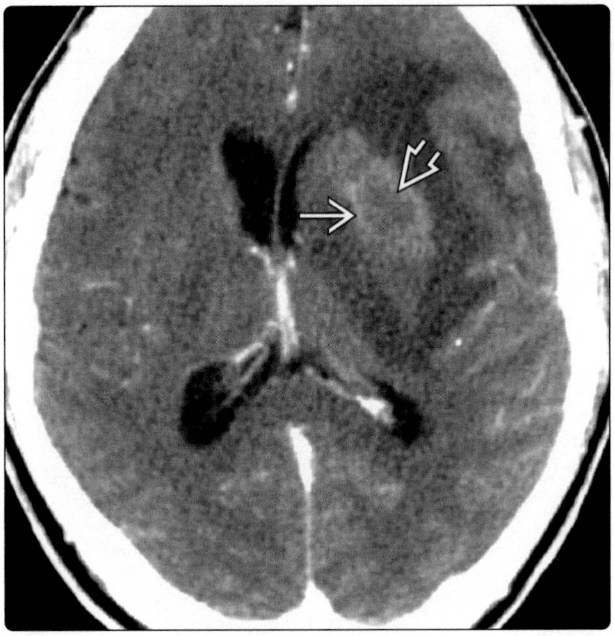

(14-40) Axial CECT scan in a different HIV-positive patient shows a solitary mass in the left basal ganglia with central necrosis ⇒ and mild rim enhancement ➡. Perilesional edema is marked. Biopsy disclosed PCNSL.

TB-IRIS patients can develop florid TB pseudoabscesses (TB "gone wild") and/or rapidly increasing enhancement in the basilar meninges **(14-38)**. Less common types of IRIS include fungal-IRIS and parasite-IRIS **(14-36)**.

Differential Diagnosis

The major imaging differential diagnosis of neuro-IRIS is **non-IRIS-associated opportunistic infection**. Contrast enhancement in combination with mass effect is more typical of IRIS but may be absent early in the disease course.

Neoplasms in HIV/AIDS

In HIV-positive patients, both Epstein-Barr virus (EBV) and human herpesvirus-8 (HHV-8; also known as Kaposi sarcoma-associated herpesvirus or KSHV) have been implicated in the development of a wide range of tumors.

EBV is associated with several malignancies including Hodgkin and non-Hodgkin lymphomas. EBV plays an especially prominent role in the development of lymphoma in patients with HIV or transplant-related immunosuppression.

KSHV-associated diseases include Kaposi sarcoma (KS), primary effusion lymphoma, and multicentric Castleman disease.

AIDS-defining malignancies (ADMs) include non-Hodgkin lymphomas, KS, and cervical cancer. The introduction of combination antiretroviral therapy (cART) has dramatically modified the natural history of HIV infection, causing a marked decline in the incidence of ADMs. In the United States and Europe, ADMs peaked in the mid-1990s and have since declined substantially. Recent statistics from South Africa show that, if cART is started before advanced immunodeficiency develops, the cancer burden in HIV-positive patients (especially children) can be substantially reduced.

In this text, we briefly discuss the two AIDS-defining malignancies that can affect the scalp, skull, and brain: primary central nervous system lymphomas (PCNSLs) and KS.

HIV-Associated Lymphomas

Compared with other cancers, cART has had a substantial but relatively smaller impact on the prevalence of lymphoma, which remains the most common ADM in the cART era.

HIV-associated PCNSLs are typically the diffuse large B-cell non-Hodgkin type. Malignancy risk is linked to the patient's immune status and increases with CD4 counts less than 50-100 cells/μL.

PCNSLs are the second most common cerebral mass lesion in AIDS (exceeded only by toxoplasmosis) and develop in 2-6% of patients. PCNSLs cause approximately 70% of all *solitary* brain parenchymal lesions in HIV/AIDS patients.

PCNSLs present as single or (less commonly) multiple masses. More than 90% are supratentorial, with preferential location in the basal ganglia and deep white matter abutting the lateral ventricle. PCNSLs often cross the corpus callosum. Central necrosis and hemorrhage are common in AIDS-related lymphomas **(14-39)**, which is reflected in the imaging findings **(14-40) (14-41D)**.

The major differential diagnosis is **toxoplasmosis**. Toxoplasmosis is more commonly multiple, and lesions often exhibit the "eccentric target" sign, i.e., an eccentrically located nodule within a ring-enhancing mass. DSC-pMR is helpful in distinguishing PCNSL from toxoplasmosis; lymphoma typically has increased relative cerebral blood volume (rCBV), whereas toxoplasmosis does not. PET and SPECT are also helpful imaging adjuncts, as lymphoma is "hot" but toxo is "not."

Kaposi Sarcoma

KS is the most common sarcoma in immunosuppressed patients. The next most frequent non-KS sarcoma is leiomyosarcoma, followed by angiosarcoma and fibrohistiocytic tumors.

KS develops from a combination of factors: HHV-8 infection (also known as KS-associated herpesvirus), altered immunity, and an inflammatory or angiogenic milieu. EBV infection is common in patients with HIV-associated leiomyosarcomas.

There has been a marked decline in the incidence of AIDS-related KS since the advent of antiretroviral therapy. Transplant-related KS often resolves after reduction of immunosuppression, highlighting the role of cellular immune response in the control of HHV-8 infection.

KS is the most common neoplasm in untreated AIDS patients. Overall, the most common site is the skin **(14-42)**, followed by mucous membranes, lymph nodes, and viscera. Classic KS is an indolent tumor with purplish or dark brown plaques and nodules, usually on the extremities. AIDS-associated KS is much more aggressive. Lesions most commonly occur on the face, genitals, and mucous membranes **(14-43)**.

Cranial KS is unusual and much less common than CNS lymphoma. When it occurs, cranial KS is typically seen as a localized scalp thickening **(14-44)** or an infiltrating soft tissue mass in the skin of the face and neck. Calvarial invasion is unusual. KS is isointense with muscle on T1WI, hyperintense on T2WI, and enhances strongly on CECT or T1 C+ MR.

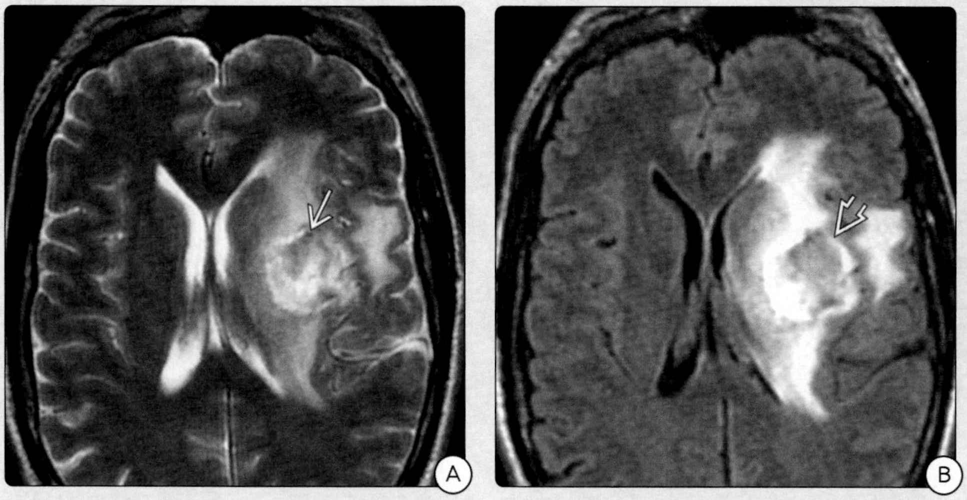

***(14-41A)** Axial T2WI in an HIV/AIDS patient who developed right-sided weakness shows a solitary heterogeneous mass → at the junction of the left basal ganglia and deep white matter. **(14-41B)** The center of the lesion is isointense → with brain on FLAIR.*

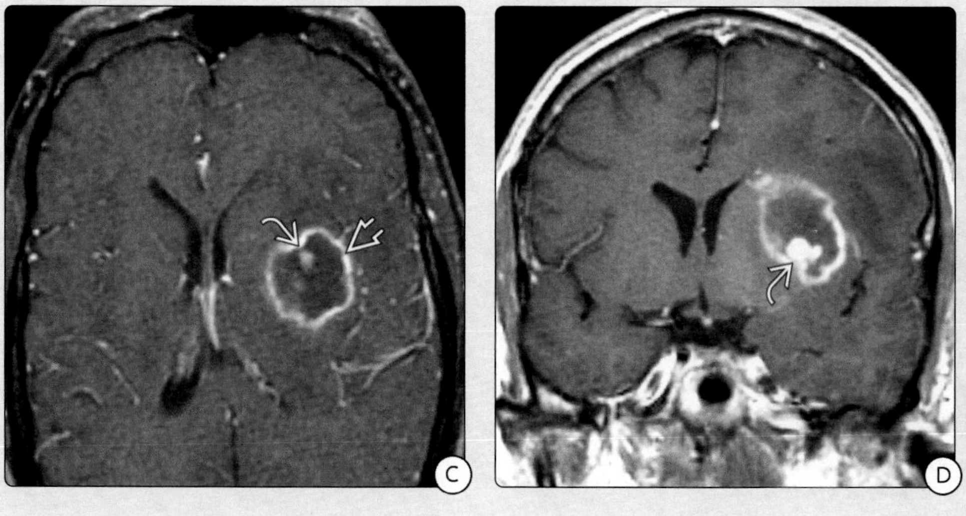

***(14-41C)** Axial T1 C+ FS scan shows an irregular rim of enhancement → around the central necrotic area and an eccentric enhancing nodule → within the necrotic mass. **(14-41D)** Because the coronal T1 C+ showed an "eccentric target" appearance → of the lesion, imaging diagnosis was toxoplasmosis (even though a solitary lesion is statistically more likely to be PCNSL). Anti-toxo therapy was ineffective. Biopsy showed diffuse large B-cell lymphoma.*

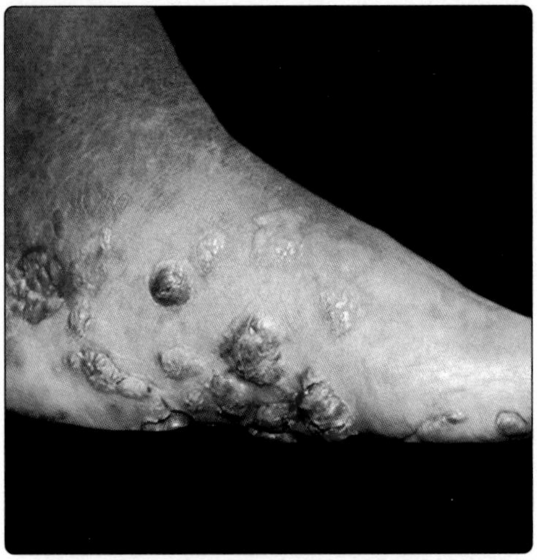

(14-42) *Clinical photograph shows classic Kaposi sarcoma (KS) presenting with multiple nodular skin lesions. (Courtesy T. Mentzel, MD.)*

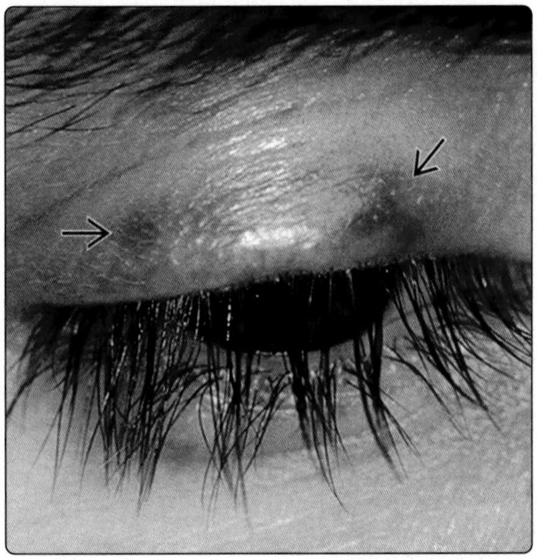

(14-43) *AIDS-related KS can present in unusual anatomic sites, like this small reddish lesion ⇒ on the upper eyelid. (Courtesy T. Mentzel, MD.)*

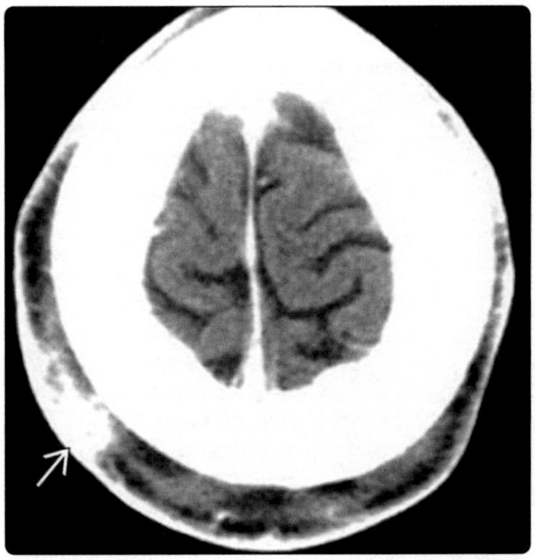

(14-44) *CECT scan demonstrates KS of the scalp in this AIDS patient. Note infiltration of the skin and subcutaneous tissues ➡.*

AIDS-DEFINING MALIGNANCIES

HIV-Associated Lymphoma

- Etiology and pathology
  - Often associated with EBV
  - Most are diffuse large B-cell non-Hodgkin lymphoma type
- Clinical issues
  - Second most common mass lesion in AIDS
  - Occurs in 2-6% of HIV/AIDS patients
  - 70% of solitary CNS masses in HIV(+) patients
- Imaging
  - Hemorrhage, necrosis common
  - Supratentorial (90%)
  - Basal ganglia, deep WM (often crosses corpus callosum)
  - Often ring-enhancing
  - Increased rCBV

Kaposi Sarcoma

- Etiology and pathology
  - Associated with HHV-8
  - Most common sarcoma in immunosuppressed
- Clinical issues
  - Antiretrovirals seriously reduce prevalence
  - Skin, mucous membranes, lymph nodes, scalp
- Imaging
  - Localized scalp thickening
  - Infiltrating soft tissue mass in skin of face or neck

Selected References

HIV Infection

Hileman CO et al: Inflammation, immune activation, and antiretroviral therapy in HIV. Curr HIV/AIDS Rep. 14(3):93-100, 2017

Henderson D et al: Neurosurgery and human immunodeficiency virus in the era of combination antiretroviral therapy: a review. J Neurosurg. 1-11, 2016

Lee AM et al: Safety and diagnostic value of brain biopsy in HIV patients: a case series and meta-analysis of 1209 patients. J Neurol Neurosurg Psychiatry. 87(7):722-33, 2016

HIV Encephalitis

Boban J et al: Proton chemical shift imaging study of the combined antiretroviral therapy impact on neurometabolic parameters in chronic HIV infection. AJNR Am J Neuroradiol. 38(6):1122-1129, 2017

Boban J et al: HIV-associated neurodegeneration and neuroimmunity: multivoxel MR spectroscopy study in drug-naïve and treated patients. Eur Radiol. ePub, 2017

Caruana G et al: The burden of HIV-associated neurocognitive disorder (HAND) in post-HAART era: a multidisciplinary review of the literature. Eur Rev Med Pharmacol Sci. 21(9):2290-2301, 2017

Cysique LA et al: White matter measures are near normal in controlled HIV infection except in those with cognitive impairment and longer HIV duration. J Neurovirol. ePub, 2017

Eggers C et al: HIV-1-associated neurocognitive disorder: epidemiology, pathogenesis, diagnosis, and treatment. J Neurol. ePub, 2017

Tang Z et al: Identifying the white matter impairments among ART-naïve HIV patients: a multivariate pattern analysis of DTI data. Eur Radiol. ePub, 2017

Vera JH et al: PET brain imaging in HIV-associated neurocognitive disorders (HAND) in the era of combination antiretroviral therapy. Eur J Nucl Med Mol Imaging. 44(5):895-902, 2017

Other Manifestations of HIV/AIDS

Diaconu IA et al: Diagnosing HIV-associated cerebral diseases - the importance of Neuropathology in understanding HIV. Rom J Morphol Embryol. 57(2 Suppl):745-750, 2016

Opportunistic Infections

Low A et al: Incidence of opportunistic infections and the impact of antiretroviral therapy among HIV-infected adults in low- and middle-income countries: a systematic review and meta-analysis. Clin Infect Dis. 62(12):1595-603, 2016

Maziarz EK et al: Cryptococcosis. Infect Dis Clin North Am. 30(1):179-206, 2016

Offiah CE et al: Spectrum of imaging appearances of intracranial cryptococcal infection in HIV/AIDS patients in the anti-retroviral therapy era. Clin Radiol. 71(1):9-17, 2016

Progressive Multifocal Leukoencephalopathy

Hodel J et al: Punctate pattern: a promising imaging marker for the diagnosis of natalizumab-associated PML. Neurology. 86(16):1516-23, 2016

Other Opportunistic Infections

Bell LC et al: In vivo molecular dissection of the effects of HIV-1 in active tuberculosis. PLoS Pathog. 12(3):e1005469, 2016

Fehintola FA et al: Malaria and HIV/AIDS interaction in Ugandan children. Clin Infect Dis. 63(3):423-4, 2016

Immune Reconstitution Inflammatory Syndrome

Marais S et al: Inflammasome activation underlying central nervous system deterioration in HIV-associated tuberculosis. J Infect Dis. 215(5):677-686, 2017

Sainz-de-la-Maza S et al: Incidence and prognosis of immune reconstitution inflammatory syndrome in HIV-associated progressive multifocal leucoencephalopathy. Eur J Neurol. 23(5):919-25, 2016

Bauer J et al: Progressive multifocal leukoencephalopathy and immune reconstitution inflammatory syndrome (IRIS). Acta Neuropathol. 130(6):751-64, 2015

Tanaka T et al: Central nervous system manifestations of tuberculosis-associated immune reconstitution inflammatory syndrome during adalimumab therapy: a case report and review of the literature. Intern Med. 54(7):847-51, 2015

Neoplasms in HIV/AIDS

McKenna C et al: TB or not to be? Kikuchi-Fujimoto disease: a rare but important differential for TB. BMJ Case Rep. 2017, 2017

Omer A et al: An integrated approach of network-based systems biology, molecular docking, and molecular dynamics approach to unravel the role of existing antiviral molecules against AIDS-associated cancer. J Biomol Struct Dyn. 35(7):1547-1558, 2017

Bohlius J et al: Incidence of AIDS-defining and other cancers in HIV-positive children in South Africa: Record Linkage Study. Pediatr Infect Dis J. 35(6):e164-70, 2016

Sugita Y et al: Primary central nervous system lymphomas and related diseases: pathological characteristics and discussion of the differential diagnosis. Neuropathology. 36(4):313-24, 2016

Brickman C et al: Cancer in the HIV-infected host: epidemiology and pathogenesis in the antiretroviral era. Curr HIV/AIDS Rep. 12(4):388-96, 2015

Pinzone MR et al: Epstein-barr virus- and Kaposi sarcoma-associated herpesvirus-related malignancies in the setting of human immunodeficiency virus infection. Semin Oncol. 42(2):258-71, 2015

HIV-Associated Lymphomas

Karia SJ et al: AIDS-related primary CNS lymphoma. Lancet. 389(10085):2238, 2017

Lin TK et al: Primary CNS lymphomas of the brain: a retrospective analysis in a single institute. World Neurosurg. ePub, 2017

Kaposi Sarcoma

Auten M et al: Human herpesvirus 8-related diseases: histopathologic diagnosis and disease mechanisms. Semin Diagn Pathol. 34(4):371-376, 2017

Demyelinating and Inflammatory Diseases

In the previous chapters, we discussed congenital and acquired infections. Here, we focus on the surprisingly broad spectrum of noninfectious inflammatory, autoimmune/autoantibody-mediated, and demyelinating disorders that can affect the CNS.

CNS inflammatory syndromes have been classified in numerous ways: by presentation (clinically isolated vs. polysymptomatic disease), pattern (monofocal or multifocal), geography (brain vs. spinal cord vs. peripheral nervous system), disease severity (from asymptomatic to severe), and disease course (monophasic, multiphasic, relapsing-remitting, progressive, etc.).

In this chapter, we follow a simplified approach, dividing our discussion into multiple sclerosis (MS) and its variants, postinfection/postvaccination inflammatory disorders, autoimmune/autoantibody-mediated disorders, and inflammatory-like disorders such as neurosarcoidosis and pseudotumors.

We begin with MS, delineating its etiology and pathology, epidemiology and clinical phenotypes, imaging appearance, and differential diagnosis. Following our detailed discussion of MS itself, we delineate several special variants such as Marburg and Schilder disease and Balo concentric sclerosis.

We then turn our attention to postinfection and postvaccination inflammatory syndromes. We focus on two particularly important entities: Acute disseminated encephalomyelitis (ADEM) and the fulminant, highly lethal acute hemorrhagic encephalomyelitis (AHEM).

The recent recognition of autoimmune encephalitis and autoantibody-mediated diseases as important disorders with overlapping neurological and imaging features is then addressed. Here we discuss neuromyelitis optica (also known as Devic disease or aquaporin-4 antibody disease) and nonparaneoplastic autoantibody-mediated CNS disorders such as anti-GAD limbic encephalitis. Susac syndrome—an immune-mediated microvascular endotheliopathy that can closely resemble MS—is also included here.

The chapter concludes by discussing three important inflammatory-like disorders of unknown or uncertain etiology: neurosarcoidosis, idiopathic inflammatory pseudotumors, and chronic inflammatory demyelinating polyneuropathy.

Multiple Sclerosis and Variants

The growing recognition that multiple sclerosis (MS) is not a single entity but a clinical spectrum comprising different subtypes has led to shifting paradigms in understanding its pathogenesis and implementing personalized, patient-centered treatment strategies.

Multiple Sclerosis

Terminology

MS is a progressive neurodegenerative disorder characterized histopathologically by multiple inflammatory demyelinating foci called "plaques."

Etiology

General Concepts. MS is a multifactorial disease whose precise pathogenesis remains unknown. It is influenced by a complex interplay of genetic susceptibility and epigenetic and postgenomic events. Environmental factors with diverse, population-specific levels of prevalence-latitude gradient also play a prominent role.

Autoimmune-Mediated Demyelination. Immune dysregulation in MS involves "cross-talk" between the innate and adaptive immune systems. Dendritic cells (DCs) function as antigen-presenting cells. Antigen binding to their surface activates the DCs, which then migrate across the BBB and communicate with naive CD4+ T cells. Proinflammatory cytokines and T-cell-mediated macrophage and resident microglia activation play a critical role in inflammatory demyelination, both in the initial and sustained immune responses to myelin antigens.

Environmental Factors. Epstein-Barr virus (EBV) exposure, chemicals, smoking, diet, and geographic variability all contribute to MS risk.

The risk of MS also varies across race and geographic regions. MS occurs less often in nonwhites compared with whites. MS frequency also increases with increasing latitude and is most common in temperate climates.

Genetics. MS is a partially heritable autoimmune disease. The strongest identified genetic risk factor is the human leukocyte antigen (*HLA-A*) gene with different HLA alleles in different

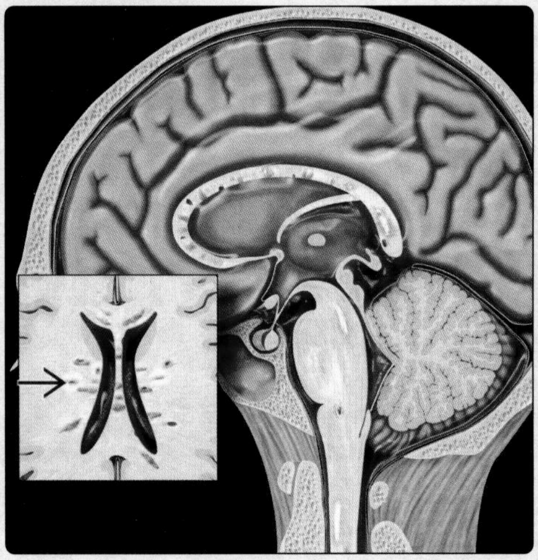

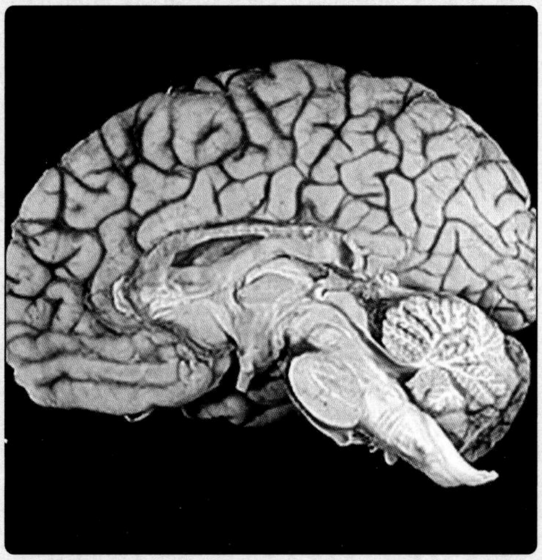

(15-1) Sagittal graphic illustrates multiple sclerosis plaques involving the corpus callosum, pons, and spinal cord. Note the characteristic perpendicular orientation of the lesions → at the callososeptal interface along penetrating venules. (15-2) Sagittal autopsied brain in a case with chronic multiple sclerosis (MS) shows a thinned corpus callosum with multiple lesions at the callososeptal interface.

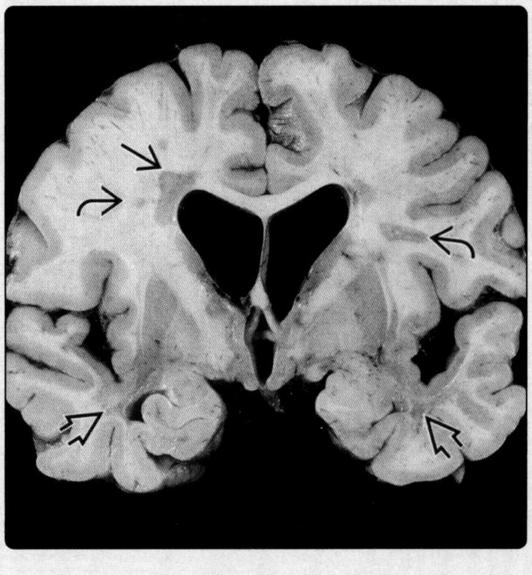

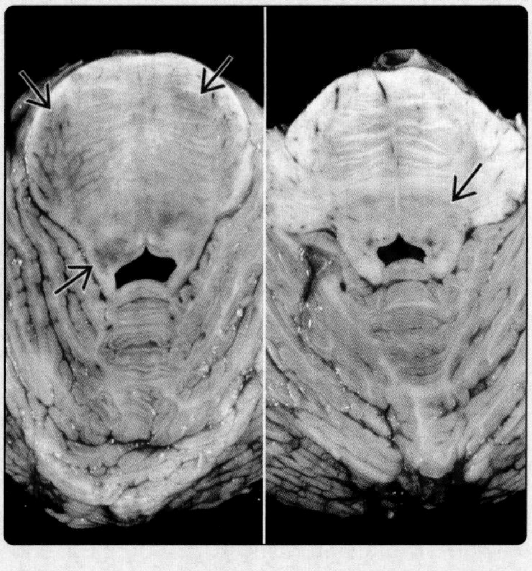

(15-3) Coronal autopsied brain shows periventricular patchy → and confluent → demyelinating plaques. Ovoid plaques → demonstrate the characteristic perpendicular orientation along medullary veins. Note atrophy with moderate ventricular and sulcal enlargement. (R. Hewlett, MD.) (15-4) Extensive confluent demyelinating plaques in the pons → are present in this autopsied MS case. (Courtesy R. Hewlett, MD.)

subpopulations and ethnicities. Genome-wide association studies have pinpointed nearly 200 single nucleotide polymorphisms that contribute to MS pathogenesis. However, all the identified risk loci together account for only 50% of the inherited MS risk.

Epigenetic modifications represent the bridge between genetic and environmental factors, but their precise role in MS initiation, progression, and response to treatment remains to be elucidated.

Pathology

Location. Most MS plaques are supratentorial. Less than 10% occur in the posterior fossa although infratentorial lesions are relatively more common in children.

MS plaques in the deep cerebral white matter are linear, round, or ovoid lesions that are oriented perpendicular to the lateral ventricles **(15-1)** **(15-5)**. Between 50-90% of all supratentorial lesions occur at or near the callososeptal interface and adjacent to the lateral ventricles **(15-2)** **(15-3)**. Centripetal perivenular extension is common, causing the appearance of "Dawson fingers" radiating outward from the lateral ventricles.

Other commonly affected areas include the subcortical U-fibers, brachium pontis, brainstem **(15-4)**, and spinal cord. Gray matter (cortex and basal ganglia) lesions are seen in 10% of cases.

Gross Pathology. Acute MS plaques are a tan-yellow color and have ill-defined margins with a granular texture. Chronic inactive plaques have more distinctly defined borders and are grayish in color with scarred and excavated, depressed centers **(15-6)**.

MULTIPLE SCLEROSIS

Location
- Supratentorial (90%), infratentorial (10%) (higher in children)
- Deep cerebral/periventricular white matter
- Predilection for callososeptal interface
- Perivenular extension (Dawson fingers)

Size and Number
- Multiple > solitary
- Mostly small (5-10 mm)
- Giant "tumefactive" plaques can be several centimeters
  - 30% of "tumefactive" MS lesions solitary

Microscopic Features. Histopathologically, MS plaques typically demonstrate (1) relatively sharp borders, (2) macrophage infiltrates (both interstitial and perivascular), and (3) perivascular chronic inflammation **(15-7)** **(15-8)**. Photomicrographs with Luxol fast blue stains contrast the "robin's-egg blue" of normally myelinated white matter **(15-9)** and the pale-staining, almost pinkish areas of myelin loss **(15-10)**.

Acute lesions are often hypercellular, with foamy macrophages and prominent perivascular T-cell lymphocytic cuffing. Normal-appearing white matter also frequently demonstrates changes, including microglial activation, T-cell infiltration, and perivascular lymphocytic cuffing.

Chronic plaques range from chronic active to chronic silent lesions. Chronic active lesions have continuing inflammation around their outer borders. Chronic silent ("burned out")

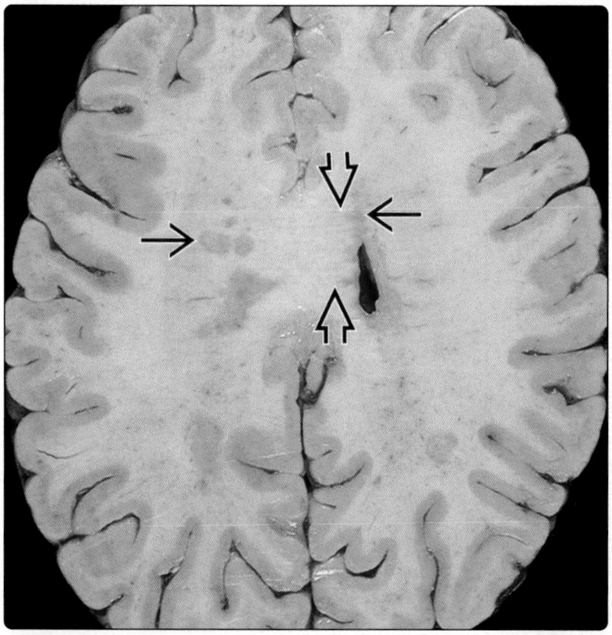

***(15-5)** Axial autopsy section shows typical ovoid, grayish MS plaques oriented perpendicularly and adjacent to the lateral ventricles →, along medullary (deep white matter) veins ⇒. (Courtesy R. Hewlett, MD.)*

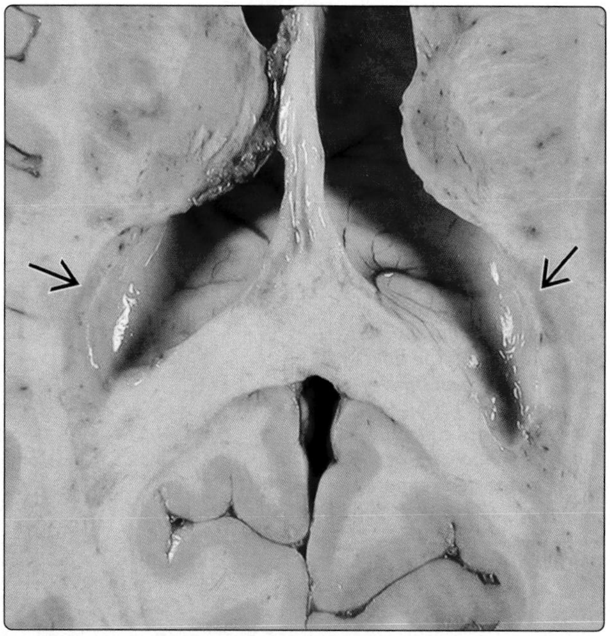

***(15-6)** Close-up axial view of autopsied brain shows confluent periventricular demyelinating plaques →. (Courtesy R. Hewlett, MD.)*

lesions are characterized by hypocellular regions, myelin loss, absence of active inflammation, and glial scarring.

MULTIPLE SCLEROSIS: PATHOLOGY

Gross Pathology

- Active: yellow-tan, ill-defined margins ± edema
- Chronic: grayish, flat
  - Longstanding lesions are depressed, excavated

Microscopic Features

- Plaques characterized by
  - Relatively sharp borders
  - Macrophages
  - Perivascular chronic inflammation
  - Reactive astrocytes
- Chronic: inflammation around borders
  - Longstanding plaques characterized by glial scarring, no active inflammation

Clinical Issues

Epidemiology. MS is the most frequent primary demyelinating pathology in the CNS, affecting approximately 350,000 people in the USA and 2.5 million worldwide. It is the most common chronic nontraumatic neurologic disease among young and middle-aged people in the developed world. The risk of MS is increased 15-35 times in first-order relatives of patients with clinically definite MS compared with the general population.

Demographics. Onset typically occurs in young to middle-aged adults from 20-40 years of age. Although median age at initial diagnosis is approximately 30 years, up to 10% of all patients with MS become symptomatic in childhood. Between 10-25% of children initially diagnosed as having acute disseminated encephalomyelitis (ADEM) are ultimately diagnosed with MS.

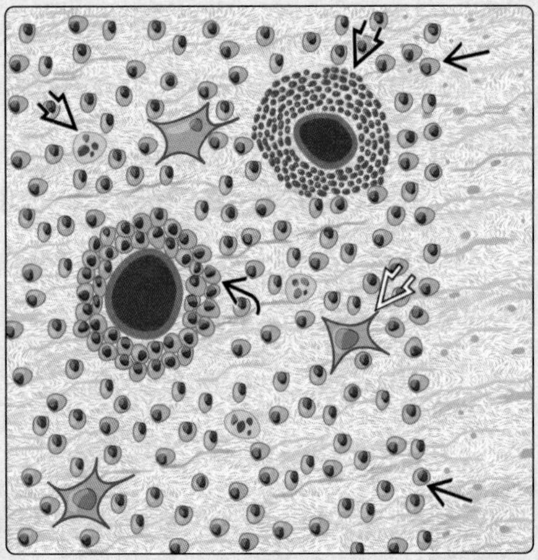

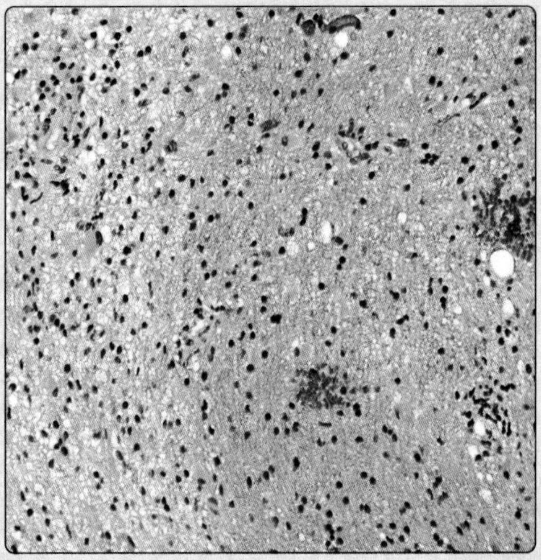

(15-7) Graphic of demyelinating plaque shows sharp border with normal brain ➡ and interstitial and perivascular macrophages ⇨. Perivascular chronic inflammation ↗ and scattered stellate reactive astrocytes ➡ are present. (15-8) H&E section of MS plaque shows relatively sharp border between plaque on left and normal white matter on the right.

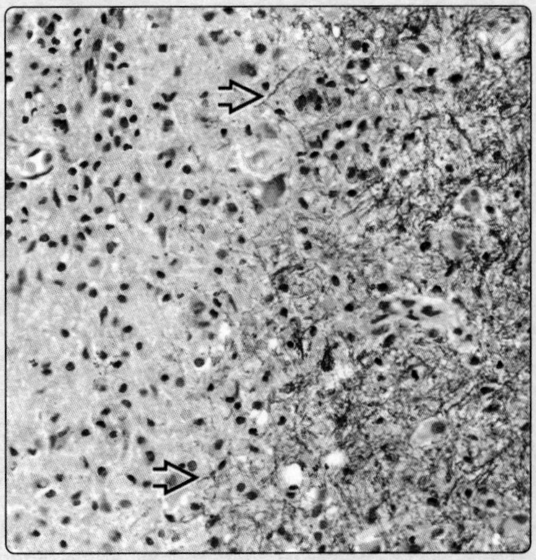

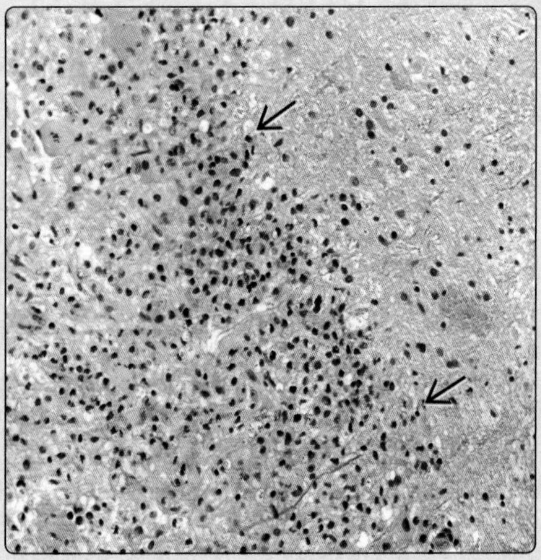

(15-9) H&E/Luxol fast blue stain of a demyelinating plaque emphasizes sharp interface ⇨ between lesion on the left (pale staining) and normal parenchyma on the right. (15-10) A chronic active ("smoldering") MS lesion shows a dense collection of macrophages ➡ at the edge of the demyelinated plaque. (All three cases courtesy B. K. DeMasters, MD.)

The overall F:M ratio is 1.77:1.00, but it is higher (3-5:1) in children. Caucasians of Northern European descent living in temperate zones are the most commonly affected ethnic group. MS is significantly less common in Asians and Africans. For example, African American men have a 40% lower MS risk than white men.

Presentation. Clinical presentation varies with heterogeneous neurologic manifestations, evolution, and disability. The interplay between inflammatory and neurodegenerative processes typically results in intermittent neurologic disturbances followed by progressive accumulation of disabilities.

The first attack of MS (most commonly optic neuritis, transverse myelitis, or a brainstem syndrome) is known as a clinically isolated syndrome. Half of patients with optic neuritis eventually develop MS.

Clinical MS Subtypes. Several major MS subtypes are recognized. From least to most severe they are as follows: radiologically isolated syndrome (**RIS**), clinically isolated syndrome (**CIS**), relapsing-remitting MS (**RR-MS**), relapsing progressive MS (**RP-MS**), secondary-progressive MS (**SP-MS**), and primary-progressive MS (**PP-MS**).

Some investigators also consider postvaccination (allergic) demyelination (ADEM) and neuromyelitis optica as part of the MS disease spectrum, but they are considered separately (see below).

Radiologically Isolated Syndrome. MS is now recognized as having a variable presymptomatic period of (at least) years and possibly even decades. The widespread use of MR in a broad spectrum of clinical settings (e.g., headache assessment) has led to increased recognition of individuals with incidental brain lesions consistent with MS.

RIS is a new subtype described at the very left (i.e., mildest) of the demyelinating disease spectrum. RIS refers to MR findings of spatial dissemination of T2/FLAIR lesions suggestive of MS in persons with no history of neurologic symptoms and with a normal neurologic examination.

Assessment of MR findings should be performed in the appropriate clinical context. Half of the patients with RIS are initially imaged because of headache, and the white matter lesions are considered "incidental" findings.

Some patients have demonstrable but asymptomatic cognitive impairment or axonal loss, suggesting the earliest subclinical stage of MS. Progression rate from RIS to clinically definite MS varies. About two-thirds of patients with RIS develop new lesions on follow-up imaging, and a third develop neurologic symptoms within 5 years.

Presence of oligoclonal bands in the CSF, younger age (≤ 37 years old), male sex, and abnormal visual evoked potentials are reported predictors of developing clinical disease.

By definition, patients with RIS have dissemination in space. When a clinical attack occurs in these patients, a diagnosis of MS can be made. Until that occurs, most experts agree that MS should not be diagnosed solely on the basis of MR findings.

Clinically Isolated Syndrome. CIS refers to a first episode of neurologic symptoms that (1) lasts at least 24 hours and (2) is caused by inflammation or demyelination in the CNS.

CIS can be monofocal or multifocal. In monofocal CIS, a single neurologic sign or symptom (e.g., optic neuritis) is caused by a single lesion. Multifocal CIS is characterized by more than one sign or symptom (e.g., an attack of optic neuritis accompanied by extremity paresthesias) caused by lesions in more than one location.

Disease progression to MS varies. Patients with MR-negative CIS have a 20% chance of developing MS.

If patients with CIS have MR evidence for typical brain lesions, the chance of developing clinically definite MS is 60-80%. If imaging demonstrates old lesions in a different location, dissemination in time is established, and the criteria for establishing MS are fulfilled (see below).

Relapsing-Remitting MS. The vast majority—about 85%—of all MS patients experience relapses alternating with remission phases and are classified as having RR-MS. Attacks ("relapses" or "exacerbations") are followed by periods of partial or complete recovery. New MR lesions often occur as part of a relapse but may also occur without symptoms.

Relapsing-Progressive MS. RP-MS is also known as secondary-progressive MS. In RP-MS, there is progressive worsening of neurologic function (accumulation of disability) over time.

Almost half of RR-MS patients enter an RP-MS stage within 10 years. By 25 years following initial diagnosis, 90% of RR-MS cases become the RP-MS subtype.

Primary-Progressive MS. PP-MS is characterized by worsening neurologic function from the outset and lacks periods of remission. Approximately 5-10% of patients have PP-MS.

Patients with PP-MS tend to have fewer brain lesions but more lesions in the spinal cord. In PP-MS, men and women are equally affected.

Natural History. Natural history varies. The majority of MS patients follow a protracted course with gradual deterioration and increasing disability. Approximately one-third have an initial episode followed by normal or near-normal function. Acute rapid neurologic deterioration without remission is uncommon.

Approximately two-thirds of patients with RIS show evidence of imaging progression; one-third develop neurologic symptoms within 5 years. Cortical and cervical cord lesions are important predictors of conversion to clinically definite MS. Pregnancy seems to shorten the time to conversion from RIS in some patients.

MULTIPLE SCLEROSIS: CLINICAL ISSUES

Demographics
- Peak = 20-40 years (10% in childhood)
- F:M ≈ 2:1
- Wide ethnic, geographic variation

Presentation
- Sensory, motor disturbances
- Optic neuritis (50% eventually develop MS)

Clinical Subtypes
- Radiologically isolated syndrome
- Clinically isolated syndrome
- Relapsing-remitting MS
- Relapsing-progressive MS (a.k.a. secondary-progressive)
- Primary-progressive MS

Imaging

General Features. MS plaques vary in size. Although most are small—between 5 and 10 mm—large lesions can reach several centimeters in diameter. MS plaques are usually multiple although 30% of giant "tumefactive" plaques initially occur as solitary lesions. These "tumefactive" MS plaques are relatively more common in children and young adults compared with middle-aged and older patients.

Tissue loss with generalized brain atrophy is common. Atrophy begins early in the disease and progresses throughout its course. Enlarged ventricles and sulci with white matter volume loss and a thinned corpus callosum are typical findings.

CT Findings. NECT is often normal early in the disease course, especially with mild cases. Solitary or multiple ill-defined white matter hypodensities may be present. Acute or subacute lesions may show mild to moderate punctate, patchy, or ring

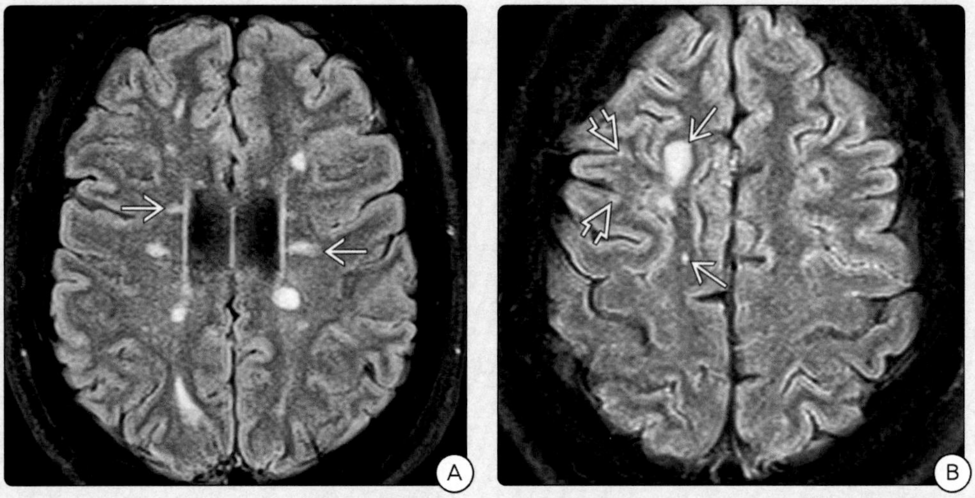

***(15-11A)** Axial FLAIR MR in a 30y woman with intermittent vague symptoms of numbness and tingling in her face and hands shows multiple ovoid subcortical and deep periventricular hyperintensities with several demonstrating a distinct perpendicular orientation to the lateral ventricles ➔ (Dawson fingers). **(15-11B)** More cephalad FLAIR in the same case shows additional lesions in the corona radiata ➔ and subtle lesions in the cortical gram ➔.*

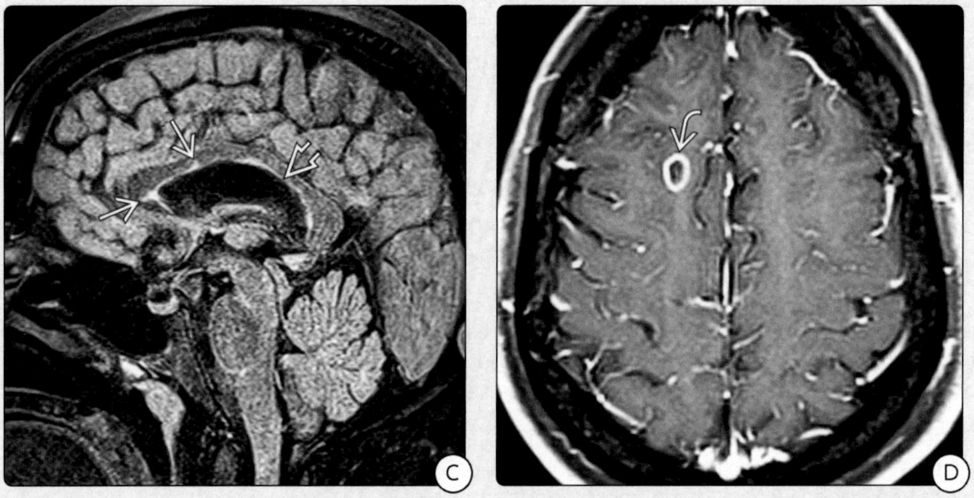

***(15-11C)** Sagittal FLAIR demonstrates several triangle-shaped hyperintensities ➔ at the callososeptal interface and a "dot-dash" appearance ➔ along the ventricle. **(15-11D)** T1 C+ FS in the same case showed a solitary ring-enhancing lesion ➔. The imaging appearance satisfies the revised 2010 McDonald and 2016 MAGNIMS modified criteria for the diagnosis of MS.*

enhancement on CECT. Enhancement increases with delayed or double-dose scans.

MR Findings. Over 95% of patients with clinically definite MS have positive findings on MR scans. Therefore, MR is the procedure of choice for both initial evaluation and treatment follow-up. The most recent revised McDonald criteria for MS diagnosis rely on MR to demonstrate dissemination in both space and time (see below).

T1WI. Most MS plaques are hypo- or isointense on T1WI **(15-12)**. The hypointensity ("black holes") correlates with axonal destruction. T1 hyperintensity is an independent predictor of atrophy, disability, and advancing disease. A faint, poorly delineated peripheral rim of mild hyperintensity secondary to lipid peroxidation and macrophage infiltration often surrounds sharply delineated hypointense "black holes." This gives many subacute and chronic lesions a characteristic "beveled" or "lesion-within-a-lesion" appearance **(15-13)**.

Chronic and severe cases typically show moderate volume loss and generalized atrophy. The corpus callosum becomes progressively thinner and is best delineated on sagittal T1WI.

T2/FLAIR. T2WI shows multiple hyperintense linear, round, or ovoid lesions surrounding the medullary veins that radiate centripetally away from the lateral ventricles **(15-11)**. Larger lesions often demonstrate a very hyperintense center surrounded by a slightly less hyperintense peripheral area **(15-15B)** and variable amounts of perilesional edema.

MS plaques often assume a distinct triangular shape with the base adjacent to the ventricle on sagittal FLAIR or T2WI images. One of the earliest findings is alternating areas of linear hyperintensity along the ependyma on sagittal FLAIR, known as the "ependymal 'dot-dash'" sign **(15-11)**.

Cortical demyelinating lesions are common and present in early MS and may even precede the appearance of classic white matter plaques in some patients!

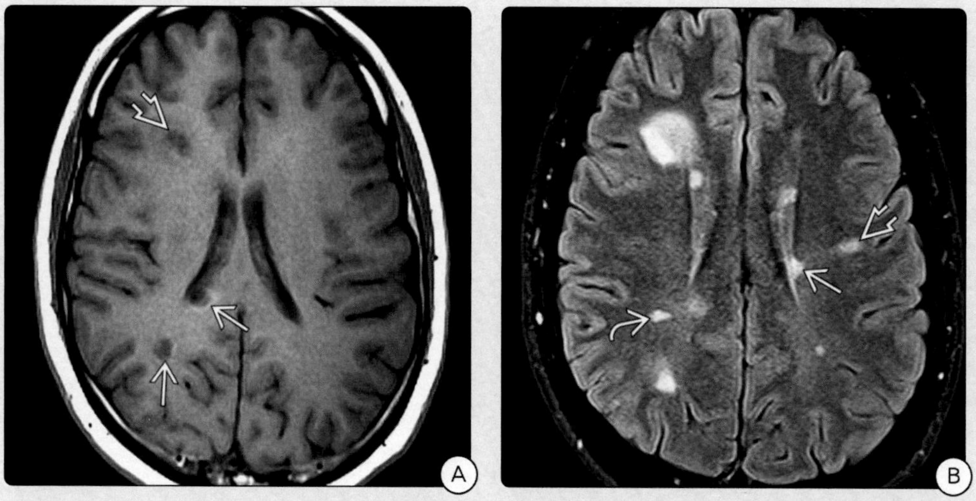

***(15-12A)** Axial T1WI in a 32y man with severe headaches following a viral prodrome shows multiple hypointense lesions in the deep white matter ➡. Note faint rim of T1 shortening ➡ around two of the lesions. **(15-12B)** FLAIR MR in the same case shows multiple round and ovoid hyperintensities ➡. Note triangle shape ➡ and perpendicular orientation ➡ of lesions following the course of deep medullary veins.*

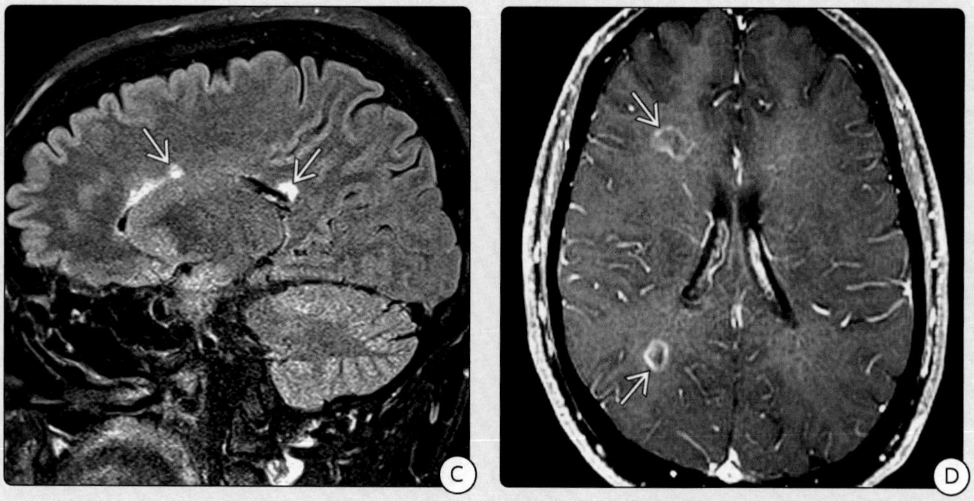

***(15-12C)** Sagittal FLAIR in the same case demonstrates the triangle shape of the periventricular lesions ➡. **(15-12D)** T1 C+ FS showed irregular rim enhancement ➡ of some—but not all—of the lesions. Patient was subsequently proven to have definite MS.*

Basal ganglia hypointensity is seen in 10-20% of chronic moderate to severe MS cases and is probably secondary to degenerative changes with heavy metal ion deposition.

T1 C+. MS plaques demonstrate transient enhancement during active demyelination. Punctate, nodular, linear, and rim patterns are seen **(15-12)** **(15-14)** **(15-15)**. A prominent incomplete rim ("horseshoe") of enhancement with the "open" nonenhancing segment facing the cortex can be present, especially in large "tumefactive" lesions **(15-16)** **(15-17)** **(15-18)**. Leptomeningeal enhancement occurs in some cases and may be a surrogate marker for cortical demyelination.

Enhancement disappears within 6 months in more than 90% of lesions. Steroid administration significantly reduces lesion enhancement and conspicuity and may render some lesions virtually invisible.

DWI. The overwhelming majority of acute plaques show normal or *increased* diffusivity. Although occasionally acute MS plaques can demonstrate restriction on DWI **(15-14F)**, such an appearance is atypical and should not be considered a reliable biomarker of plaque activity.

MRS. MRS may allow early distinction between relapsing-remitting and secondary-progressive MS. Secondary-progressive MS shows decreased NAA in normal-appearing gray matter consistent with axonal/neuronal loss or dysfunction.

Myoinositol levels are elevated in acute lesions and are also increased in normal-appearing white matter. "Tumefactive" MS shows nonspecific findings (elevated choline, decreased NAA, and high lactate).

Advanced Imaging Techniques. Some studies using DTI have reported reduced longitudinal diffusivity in areas of axonal injury. Others have used magnetization transfer imaging (MTI)

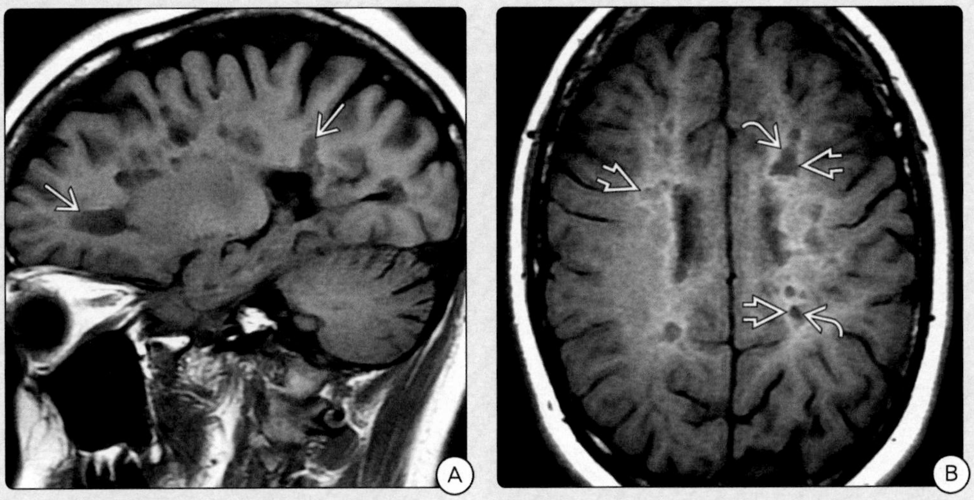

***(15-13A)** Sagittal T1WI in a 19y woman with longstanding MS shows findings of chronic "burned out" disease. Volume loss with multiple hypointense ovoid and triangular lesions in the deep periventricular white matter is present. **(15-13B)** Axial T1WI shows the ill-defined hyperintense rims surrounding the plaques, giving the distinct "lesion-within-a-lesion" appearance.*

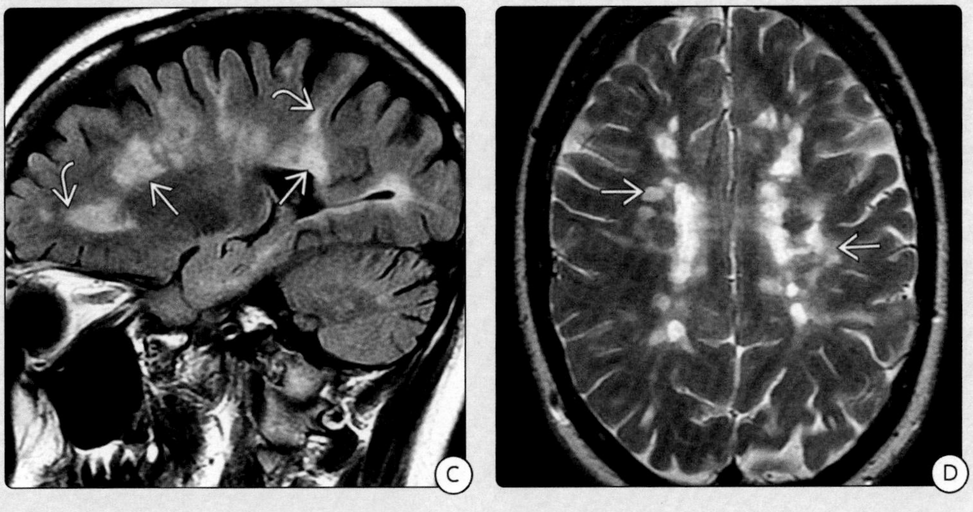

***(15-13C)** FLAIR shows the characteristic triangle configuration of typical deep white matter MS plaques seen in the sagittal plane. The broad bases of the triangles are oriented toward the ventricular surface with the apices pointing toward the cortex. **(15-13D)** T2WI shows the ovoid perivenular plaques that are oriented perpendicular to the lateral ventricles, as seen in the axial plane.*

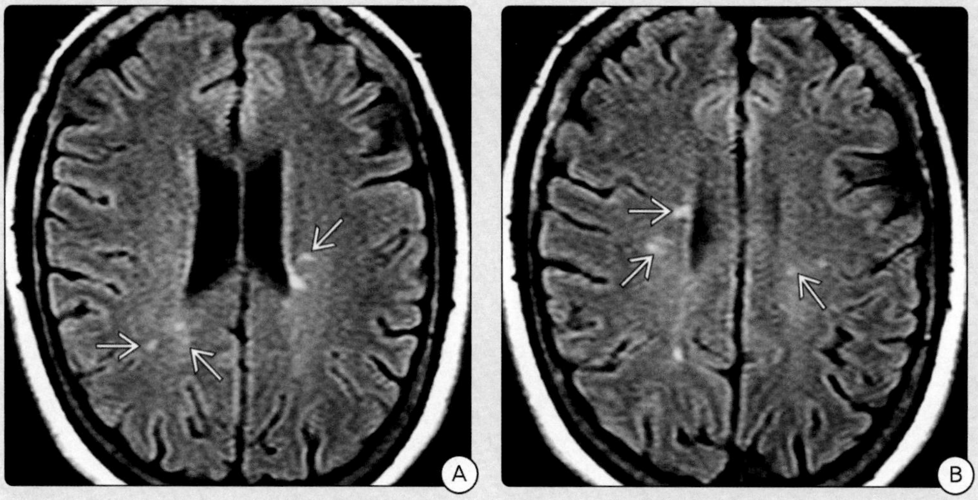

(15-14A) *Axial FLAIR scan in a middle-aged patient with a multiyear history of vague numbness and tingling shows a few scattered periventricular white matter hyperintensities* ➡. ***(15-14B)*** *Axial FLAIR in the same patient shows additional lesions* ➡. *Their ovoid shape, perivenular extension, and perpendicular orientation are highly suggestive of MS.*

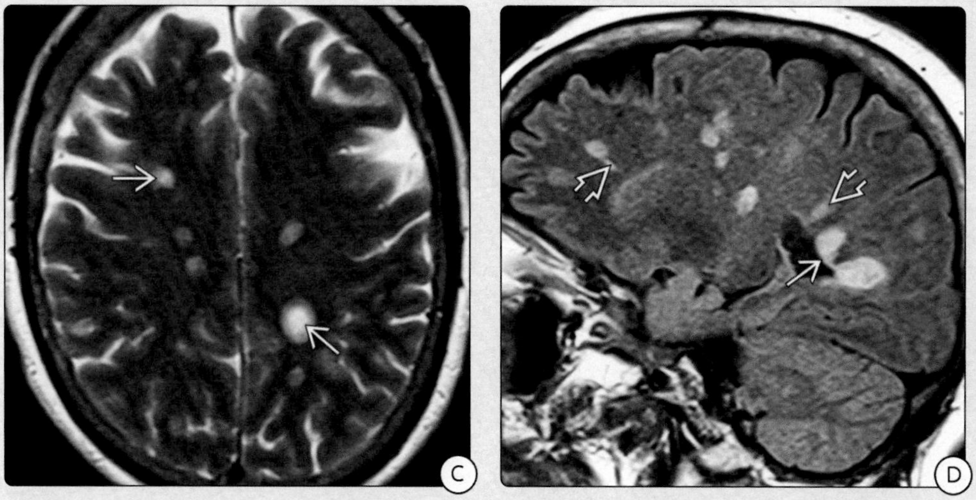

(15-14C) *Patient presented 2 years later with acute exacerbation of symptoms accompanied by confusion and disorientation. Note additional WM lesions with very hyperintense centers* ➡ *surrounded by slightly less hyperintense rims.* ***(15-14D)*** *Sagittal FLAIR shows multiple deep WM lesions. Note triangle-shaped occipital lesions with broad bases at the ventricular surface* ➡. *Ovoid-shaped lesions* ➡ *surrounding medullary veins are present.*

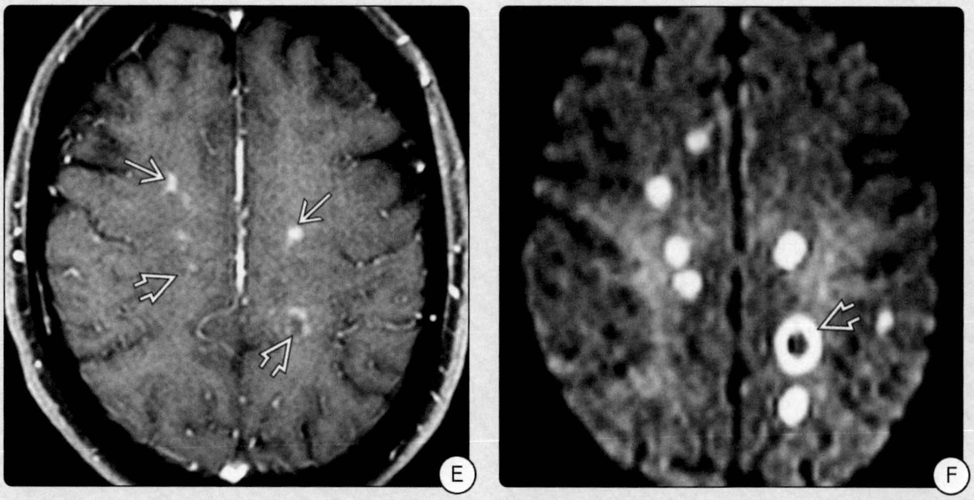

(15-14E) *T1 C+ FS scan shows punctate* ➡ *and incomplete rim enhancement* ➡ *in some of the lesions.* ***(15-14F)*** *DWI shows multiple foci of diffusion restriction. The left parietal lesion with incomplete ("horseshoe") rim enhancement shows diffusion restriction in the periphery* ➡ *surrounding a nonrestricting hypointense core. This is biopsy-proven MS.*

(15-15A) *Axial FLAIR in a 28y man with 3 weeks of visual symptoms shows several hypointense white matter lesions ➡. The left hemisphere lesions demonstrate a more hypointense center surrounded by a less hypointense rim.* ***(15-15B)*** *T2WI shows additional lesions ➡. The large left frontal lesion has a very hyperintense center surrounded by a thin hypointense rim ➡ and peripheral edema.*

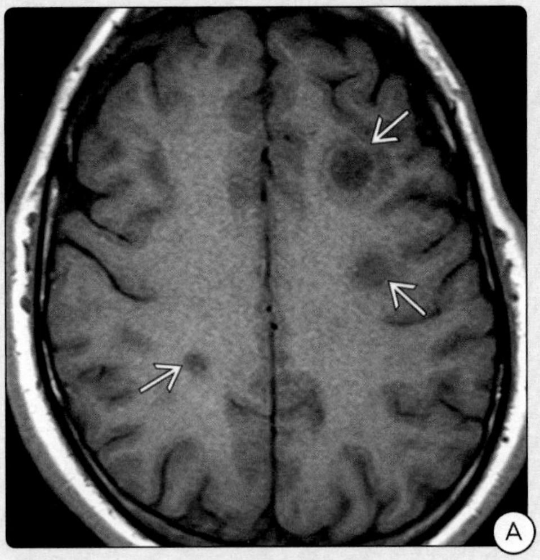

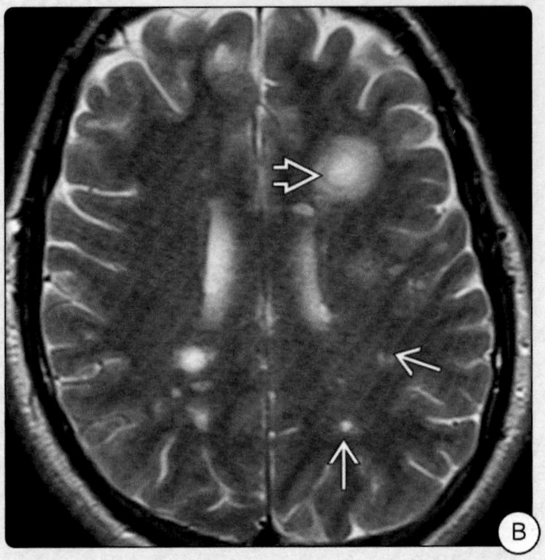

(15-15C) *Sagittal FLAIR shows small triangle-shaped hyperintensities at callososeptal interface ➡. Note alternating areas of hyper- and isointensity along undersurface of the corpus callosum ➡, the "dot-dash" sign of early MS.* ***(15-15D)*** *Axial T1 C+ FS shows multiple enhancing lesions in posterior fossa ➡, incomplete rim-enhancing lesion ➡ and an infiltrating lesion at the root entry zone of left trigeminal nerve ➡.*

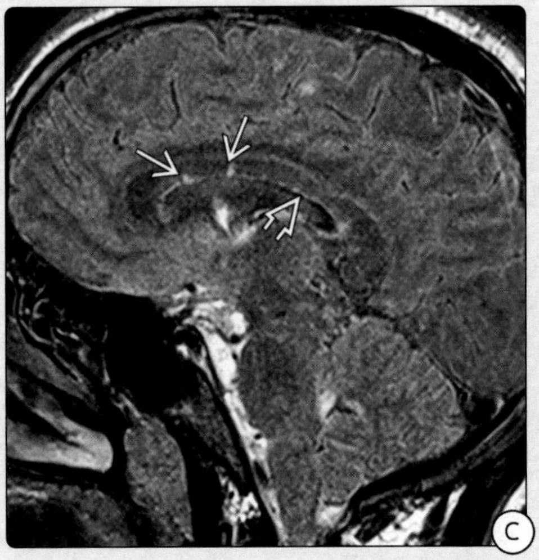

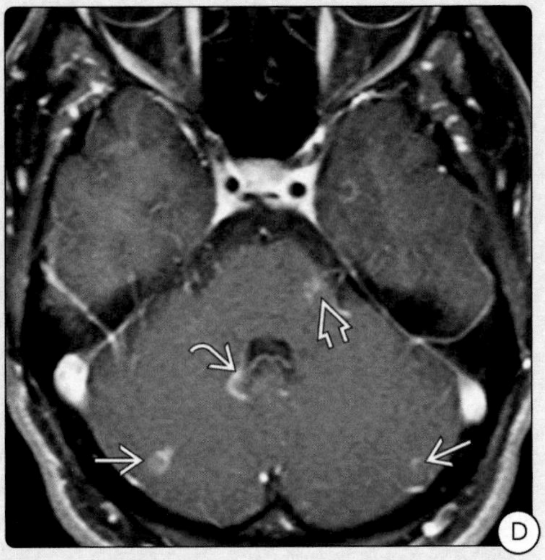

(15-15E) *Axial T1 C+ FS shows multiple foci of punctate and ring enhancement in the cerebral white matter. Note "target" appearance of the left frontal lesion ➡. CSF findings were consistent with a diagnosis of MS. The patient was placed on high-dose steroids.* ***(15-15F)*** *Repeat T1 C+ FS scan obtained 5 days later shows almost complete fading of the contrast-enhancing lesions. Steroids can dramatically reduce enhancement of MS lesions.*

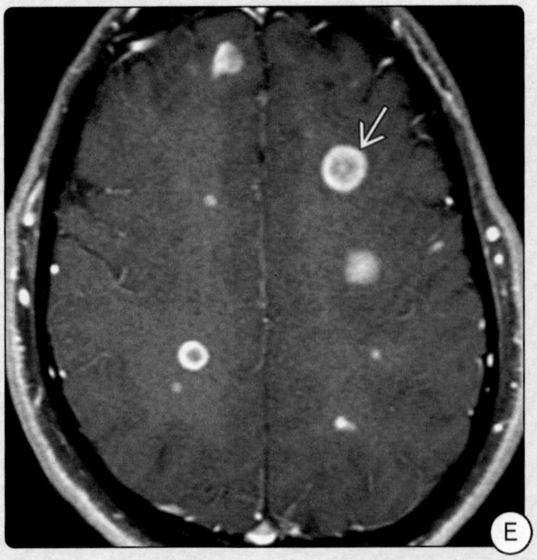

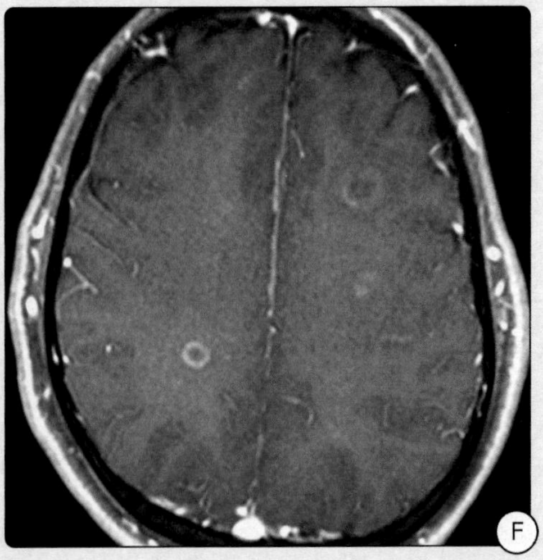

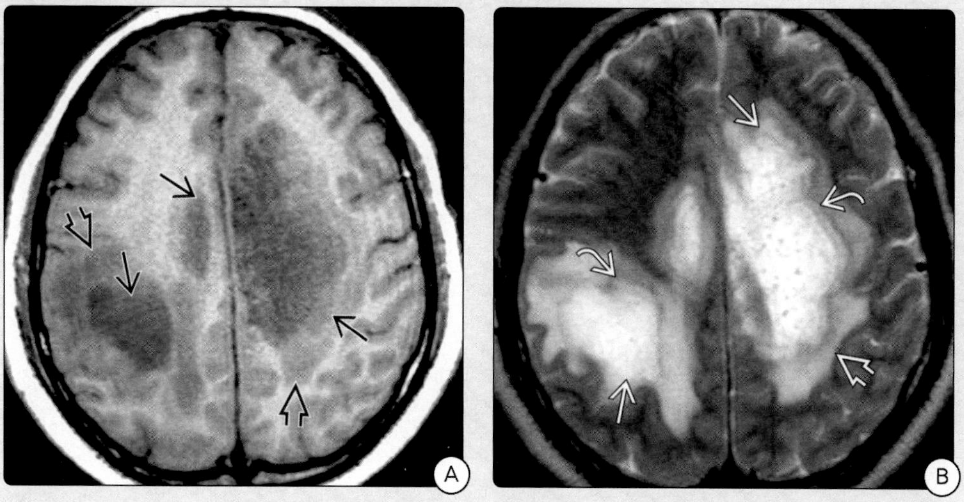

(15-16A) *Series of images demonstrates "tumefactive" MS. Axial T1WI shows large heterogeneously hypointense lesions in both cerebral hemispheres with significant perilesional edema.* ***(15-16B)*** *T2WI shows that the lesions are very hyperintense and surrounded by a thin hypointense rim and perilesional edema.*

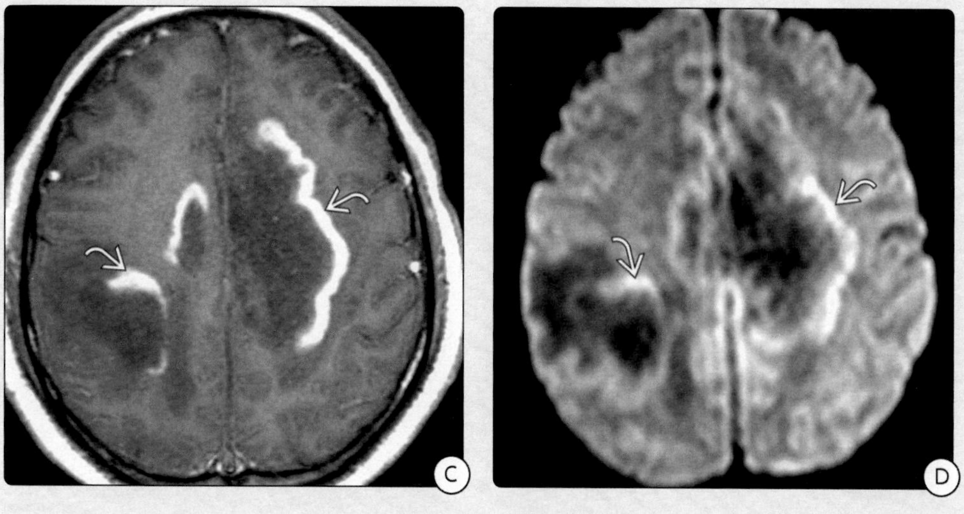

(15-16C) *The hypointense rims of the lesion show striking but incomplete ring enhancement.* ***(15-16D)*** *DWI shows that the enhancing rims restrict moderately.*

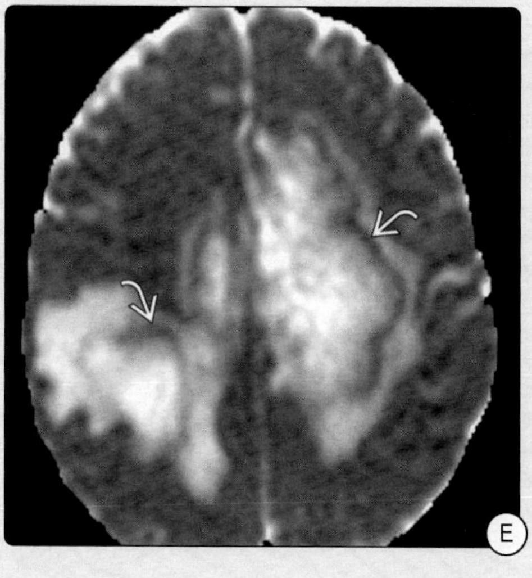

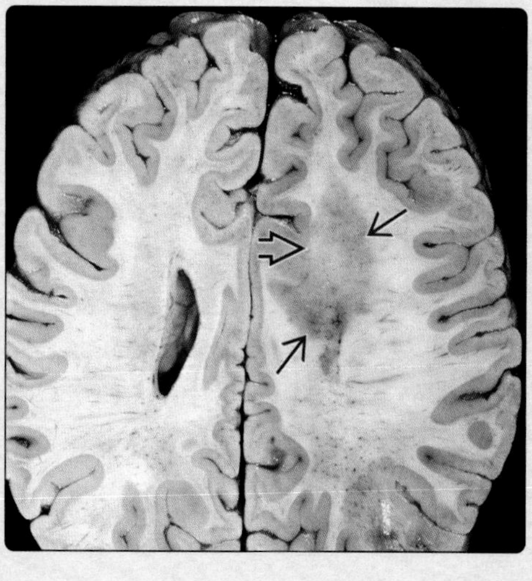

(15-16E) *The rims demonstrate low ADC values in this patient with biopsy-proven "tumefactive" MS. (Courtesy P. Rodriguez, MD.)* ***(15-17)*** *Autopsy specimen in another case demonstrates typical findings of "tumefactive" demyelination with a horseshoe-shaped demyelinating mass, the "open" end toward the cortex. (Courtesy R. Hewlett, MD.)*

to detect subtle myelin loss in nonlesional tissue (i.e., normal-appearing white matter).

MULTIPLE SCLEROSIS: IMAGING

CT
- Patchy/confluent hypodensities
- Mild/moderate, patchy, ring enhancement

MR
- Hypointense on T1WI ± faint hyperintense rim
- Very hyperintense center on T2WI, slightly less hyperintense rim
  - Callososeptal interface
  - Triangular on sagittal
  - Ovoid, perivenular on axial
  - Subpial, intracortical lesions common
- Active plaques enhance ("tumefactive" partial rim)
- Steroids suppress enhancement

2010 McDONALD CRITERIA FOR MS DIAGNOSIS

Dissemination in Space
- ≥ 1 T2 hyperintense lesion(s)
- In at least 2 of the following 4 areas
  - Periventricular
  - Juxtacortical
  - Infratentorial
  - Spinal cord

Dissemination in Time
- *Either* new T2 or Gd-enhancing lesion(s) on follow-up MR
- *Or* simultaneous presence of
  - Asymptomatic Gd-enhancing *and*
  - Nonenhancing lesions at any time

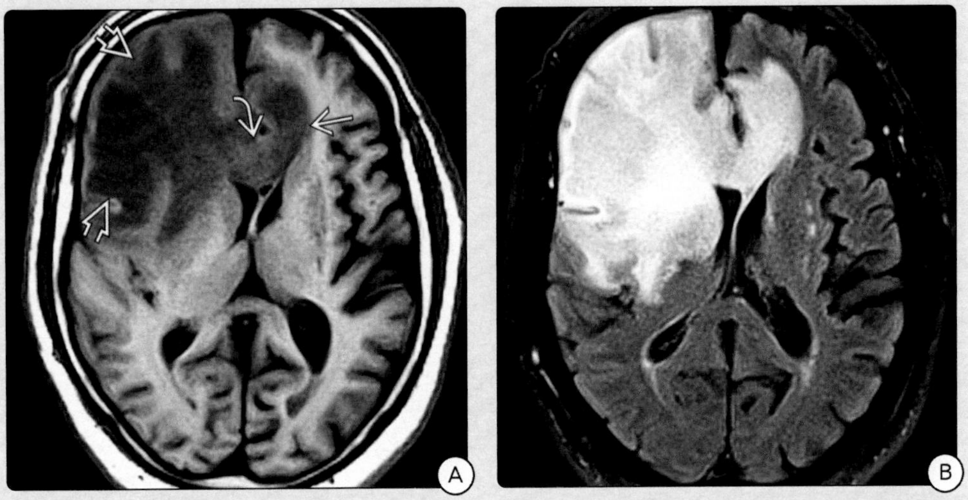

***(15-18A)** Axial T1WI in a 77y man with 2 days of progressive confusion shows a large hypointense right frontal lobe mass ➡ that thickens and crosses the corpus callosum ➡ and extends into the white matter of the left frontal lobe ➡. **(15-18B)** FLAIR in the same case shows that the huge mass is heterogeneously hyperintense. Note that, compared with the size of the lesion, the mass effect is relatively minor.*

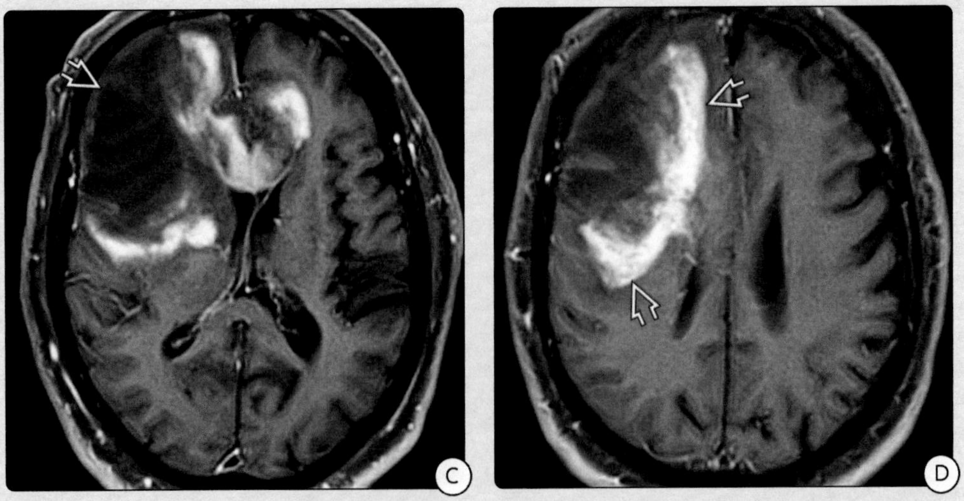

***(15-18C)** T1 C+ FS shows that the mass enhances strongly but very heterogeneously, with significant nonenhancing areas ➡ near the cortex of the right frontal lobe. **(15-18D)** More cephalad T1 C+ shows a thick, incomplete rim of enhancement ➡. Imaging diagnosis was tumefactive demyelination. Because of the patient's age and location of the mass, biopsy was performed. Pathologic diagnosis was tumefactive demyelination.*

2016 MAGNIMS RECOMMENDED MODIFICATIONS TO 2010 McDONALD CRITERIA FOR MS DIAGNOSIS

Dissemination in Space
- ≥ 3 or more periventricular lesions
- Add additional cardinal location (optic nerve) to CNS areas
- Expand juxtacortical location to cortical/juxtacortical
  - Use advanced imaging techniques to visualize cortical lesions
- Recommend whole spinal cord imaging
- No distinction between symptomatic vs. asymptomatic MR lesions
- Use same criteria for PP-MS and relapse-onset MS

Dissemination in Time
- No changes needed
- Nonenhancing black holes not useful for dissemination in time in adults
  - May help distinguish children with MS from ADEM

MR Criteria for the Diagnosis of MS. MR is now an integral part of the diagnostic evaluation of patients with suspected MS. The diagnosis relies on proof of disease dissemination in space and time and exclusion of disorders that can mimic MS. The 2010 revised McDonald criteria and the revised 2016 modifications suggested by the European collaborative research network that studies MR in MS (MAGNIMS) are summarized in the blue boxes on the facing page.

Differential Diagnosis

Multifocal T2/FLAIR "white spots" are nonspecific imaging findings and have a broad differential diagnosis. Hyperintensities in the correct location (callososeptal interface, periventricular) or of the correct shape (triangular) may represent "radiologically isolated" early MS. It is helpful to suggest whether such lesions do or do not meet McDonald criteria.

Multifocal enhancing white matter lesions can be caused by acute disseminated encephalomyelitis (ADEM), autoimmune-mediated vasculitis, and Lyme disease. **ADEM** usually has a history of viral prodrome or recent vaccination. **Vasculitis** often preferentially involves the basal ganglia and spares the callososeptal interface. **Lyme disease** (LD) can appear identical to MS. Cranial nerve enhancement is more common in LD than in MS.

Susac syndrome (see below) is often mistaken for MS on imaging studies, as both have multifocal T2/FLAIR white matter hyperintensities and both commonly affect young adult women. Lesions in Susac syndrome preferentially involve the middle of the corpus callosum, not the callososeptal interface.

"Tumefactive" MS can mimic **abscess** or **neoplasm** (**glioblastoma multiforme** or **metastasis**). *"Tumefactive" demyelination often has an incomplete or "horseshoe" pattern of enhancement.* **Progressive multifocal leukoencephalopathy** (PML) and **immune reconstitution inflammatory syndrome** (PML-IRIS) occur in a few MS patients treated with natalizumab. Irregular, "wild" enhancement in such cases may be difficult to distinguish from acute "tumefactive" MS.

MS: DIFFERENTIAL DIAGNOSIS

Multifocal T2/FLAIR Hyperintensities
- ADEM
- Lyme disease
- Vasculitis
- Susac syndrome

Mass-Like ("Tumefactive") Lesion(s)
- Neoplasm
  - Glioblastoma multiforme
  - Metastases
- PML/PML-IRIS
  - HIV/AIDS
  - Natalizumab-treated MS
- Medication-related
  - Enbrel

Multiple Sclerosis Variants

Major MS variants are (1) Marburg disease (acute, severe, fulminant MS) (**MD**), (2) Schilder disease (**SD**), and Balo concentric sclerosis (**BCS**).

Marburg Disease

Terminology, Clinical Issues, Pathology. MD is an acute fulminant MS variant characterized by rapid, relentless progression and an exceptionally severe clinical course that usually leads to death within 1 year. Patients are typically young adults.

Marked lymphocytic infiltrates **(15-19)** with inflammatory changes in the perivenular spaces **(15-20)** lead to acute, sometimes fulminant demyelination **(15-21)**.

MARBURG DISEASE

Clinical Issues
- Rare acute fulminate MS variant
  - Rapid neurologic deterioration
  - Monophasic, relentless progression
  - Death usually within 1 year
- Usually young adults

Pathology and Imaging
- Multifocal > solitary disease
  - Characterized by coalescent white matter plaques
  - Brain (including posterior fossa), spinal cord lesions
- Lesions characterized by massive inflammation, necrosis
- Imaging shows diffusely disseminated disease
  - Large cavitating lesions
  - Incomplete ("open") enhancing rim
  - Multiple other patchy enhancing foci

Imaging. Imaging shows multifocal diffusely disseminated disease with focal and confluent white matter hyperintensities on T2/FLAIR. Strong patchy enhancement on T1 C+ is typical, and large, cavitating, incomplete, ring-enhancing, "tumefactive" lesions are common **(15-22)**.

Schilder Disease

Terminology and Clinical Issues. SD—also known as myelinoclastic diffuse sclerosis—is a rare subacute or chronic demyelinating disorder characterized by one or more inflammatory demyelinating white matter plaques. SD is typically a disease of childhood and young adults. Median age at presentation is 18 years, with a slight female predominance.

Although SD is considered to be a variant of MS, clinical features are atypical for MS, and the disease is usually monophasic with a low rate of recurrence. Signs of increased intracranial pressure, aphasia, and behavioral symptoms are typical. CSF is usually normal, and there is no history to suggest acute disseminated encephalomyelitis (ADEM) (i.e., no fever, infection, or preceding vaccination). Approximately 15% of cases progress to MS.

Pathology. Solitary unilateral masses are present in two-thirds of cases. Most are large lesions, measuring several centimeters in diameter.

The histopathologic features of SD consist of white matter demyelination, lymphocytic perivascular infiltrates, and microglial proliferation.

Imaging. Imaging shows a subcortical hypodense lesion on NECT scans. MR shows a hypointense lesion on T1WI that is hyperintense on T2/FLAIR. Rim enhancement—often the incomplete or "open ring" pattern—is seen during the acute inflammatory stage.

The lesion rim usually restricts on DWI during the acute phase. MRS is nonspecific, showing a decreased but present NAA peak with increased Cho:Cr ratio. Lactate and lipid-lactate complexes are common.

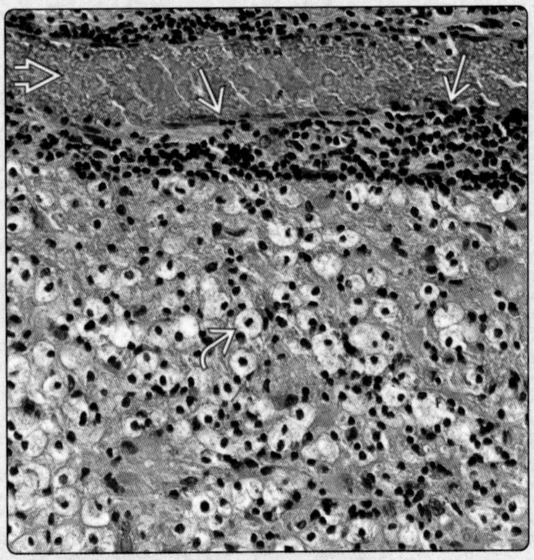

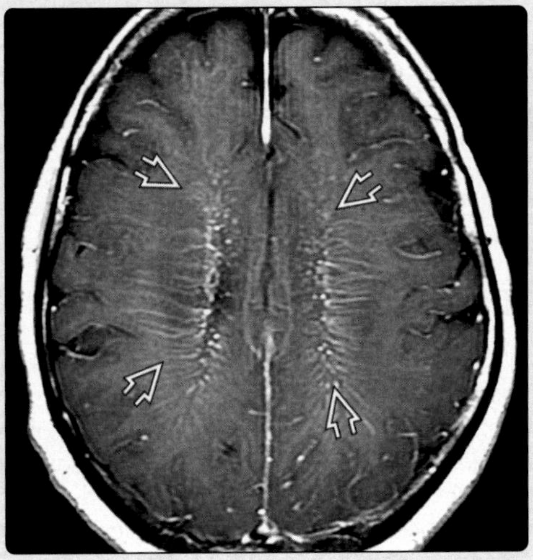

***(15-19)** H&E shows venule ➡ with marked perivascular lymphocytic cuffing ➡, striking macrophage infiltrates ➡ in acute, fulminant demyelination. Findings can raise concern for vasculitis, intravascular lymphoma. **(15-20)** T1 C+ FS in hyperacute demyelination (from fulminant MS or ADEM, PML-IRIS, etc.) can show striking enhancement, enlargement of deep medullary veins ➡. Findings can mimic vasculitis and intravascular lymphoma.*

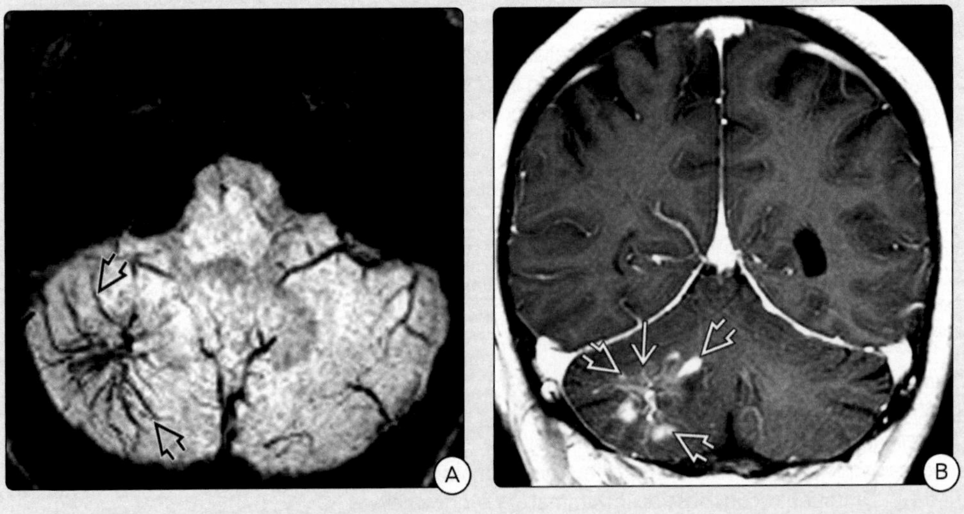

***(15-21A)** Axial T2* SWI in a 56y woman with cerebellar symptoms shows the typical "Medusa head" of a developmental venous anomaly (DVA) in the right cerebellar hemisphere ➡. **(15-21B)** Coronal T1 C+ shows multiple "fluffy" enhancing lesions ➡ surrounding the DVA ➡. Biopsy proved acute demyelinating disease with extensive perivenular plaques. Demyelination typically occurs along perivenular spaces.*

Differential Diagnosis. The differential diagnosis of SD can be difficult. "**Tumefactive" MS** can appear identical to SD on imaging studies. SD often mimics intracranial neoplasm or abscess both in clinical presentation and on imaging studies. **Pyogenic abscess** generally shows strong diffusion restriction in the lesion core. Perfusion MR may be helpful in distinguishing SD from **metastasis** and **glioblastoma multiforme**.

Balo Concentric Sclerosis

Terminology. BCS is generally considered an atypical or variant form of MS and occurs as a discrete, concentrically layered white matter lesion. It is often described as having an "onion ring" or "whorled" appearance.

Clinical Features. BCS is usually characterized by acute onset and rapid clinical deterioration. Peak presentation is between 20 and 50 years. The F:M ratio is approximately 2:1 and is most common in patients of east Asian origin.

Although patients can present with classic focal symptoms of MS, nonspecific findings such as headache and seizures are the most commonly reported presenting symptoms.

BCS prognosis varies. Once considered a rapidly progressive, invariably fatal disease, BCS may also follow a relatively benign course with substantial or complete recovery.

Pathology. The pathologic hallmark of BCS is its peculiar pattern of lamellar or concentric rings. Large plaques with alternating rims of demyelination and myelin preservation give the lesion its characteristic appearance **(15-23)**. BCS can occur as a solitary mass or, less commonly, as multiple lesions.

Imaging. Imaging studies reflect the distinctive gross pathology of BCS and vary with disease stage. Acute lesions have significant surrounding edema. Two or more alternating bands of differing signal intensities are seen on T2WI and resemble a "whirlpool" of concentric rings. The actively

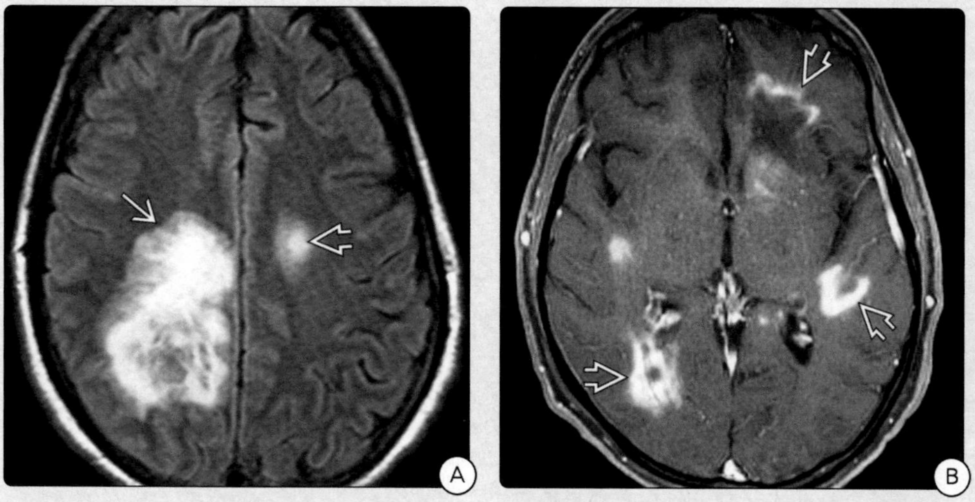

(15-22A) A 26y man presented with a short history of visual disturbances and left upper extremity weakness followed by rapid onset of numbness and quadriplegia. Axial FLAIR shows a large heterogeneously hyperintense lesion in the right parietal WM ➡ with a smaller lesion on the left ➡. (15-22B) Axial T1 C+ FS in the same case shows multiple bilateral incomplete ring-enhancing lesions ➡ in the deep and periventricular WM.

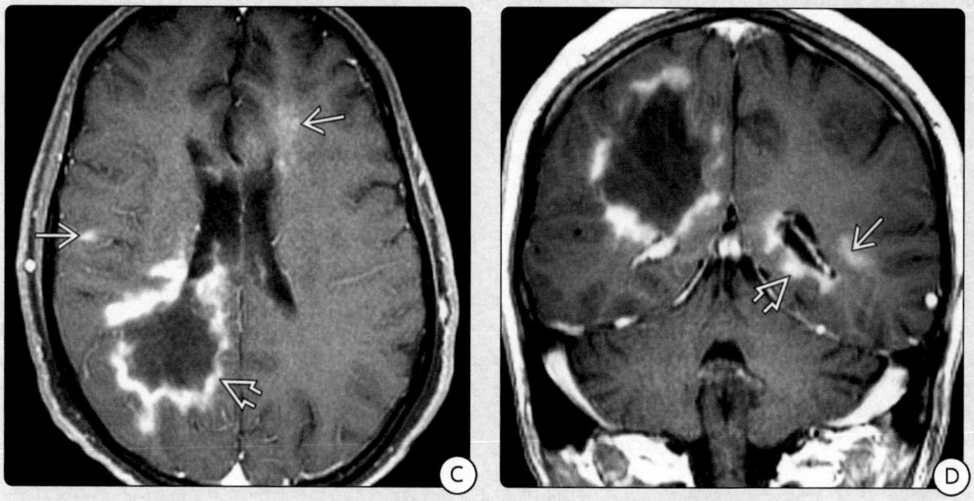

(15-22C) T1 C+ FS through the ventricles shows the necrotic, cavitating, acutely enhancing right parietal "tumefactive" mass ➡. Other enhancing foci are present ➡. (15-22D) Coronal T1 C+ scan shows extension around the left ventricle ➡ in addition to other enhancing foci ➡. This is the Marburg variant of MS.

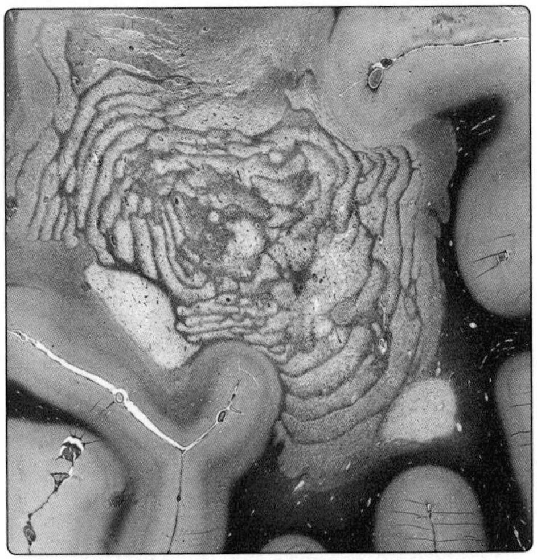

(15-23) Balo concentric sclerosis with rings of demyelinated areas alternate with blue layers of preserved myelin. (Courtesy B. K. DeMasters.)

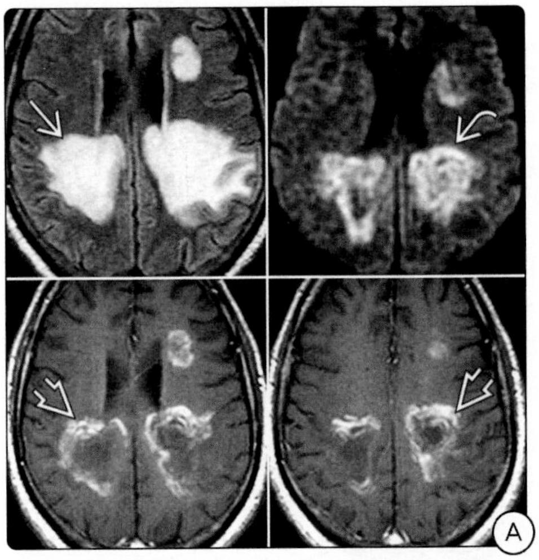

(15-24A) Acute Balo concentric sclerosis lesions are hyperintense on FLAIR ➡, restrict on DWI ➡, show concentric "onion bulb" enhancement ➡.

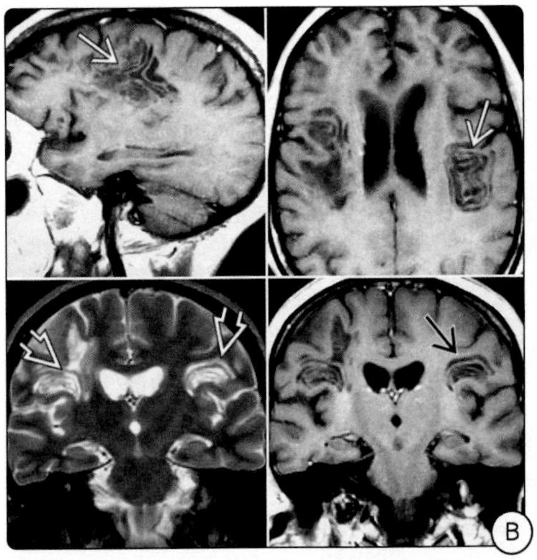

(15-24B) Follow-up scans show alternating rings of iso- and hyperintensity on T1 ➡ and T2WI ➡, no enhancement ➡. (Courtesy P. Rodriguez, MD.)

demyelinating layers enhance on T1 C+ sequences **(15-24A)**. Other more typical MS-like plaques can also be present.

Subacute or chronic BCS shows two or more alternating bands of iso- and hypointensity on T1WI. The concentric layers appear iso- and hyperintense on T2WI **(15-24B)**. Chronic BCS does not enhance on T1 C+.

OTHER MS VARIANTS

Schilder Disease
- Myelinoclastic diffuse sclerosis
  - Rare acute/subacute demyelinating disorder
  - Lesions may resolve; 15% progress to MS
- Young adults
  - Mean age at onset = 18 years
- Clinical features atypical for MS, ADEM
  - CSF normal
  - No history of fever, flu, vaccination
- Solitary > multifocal lesions
- Lesions look like "tumefactive" MS
- Differential diagnosis: neoplasm, abscess

Balo Concentric Sclerosis
- Concentric rings of demyelination/myelin preservation
  - Resemble tree trunk or onion bulb
  - Solitary > multifocal
- "Whirlpool" hyperintense concentric rings on T2WI
  - Minimal mass effect, edema
- Actively demyelinating layers enhance

Postinfection and Postimmunization Demyelination

Postinfectious demyelinating disorders, **acute disseminated encephalomyelitis (ADEM)** and **acute hemorrhagic leukoencephalopathy (AHLE)**, are considered part of the inflammatory demyelinating disease spectrum. A serious, potentially life-threatening type of acute encephalopathy in children, **acute necrotizing encephalopathy (ANE)**, is also included in this discussion.

Acute Disseminated Encephalomyelitis

Terminology

ADEM is a postinfection, postimmunization disorder that is also called parainfectious encephalomyelitis. Once considered a purely monophasic illness, recurrent and **multiphasic forms (MDEM)** of ADEM are now recognized.

Etiology

The immunohistopathologic features of ADEM mimic those of experimental allergic encephalitis, an induced autoimmune disease precipitated by myelin antibodies. Therefore, most investigators consider ADEM an immune-mediated CNS demyelinating disorder.

Pathology

Location. As the name implies, ADEM can involve both the brain and spinal cord. White matter lesions usually predominate, but basal ganglia involvement is seen in nearly half of all cases. Spinal cord lesions are found in 10-30%.

A rare ADEM variant, acute infantile bilateral striatal necrosis, occurs 1-2 weeks following a respiratory illness. Viral and streptococcal infections have been implicated and cause enlarged hyperintense basal ganglia, caudate nuclei, and internal/external capsules.

Size and Number. Lesion size varies from a few millimeters to several centimeters ("tumefactive" ADEM), and lesions have a punctate to flocculent configuration. Multiple lesions are more common than solitary lesions.

Gross Pathology. Small lesions are often inapparent on gross examination. Large "tumefactive" lesions cause a gray-pink white matter discoloration and often extend all the way to the cortex-white matter junction **(15-25)**. Mass effect is minimal compared with lesion size. Gross intralesional hemorrhage is rare and is more characteristic of AHLE than ADEM.

Microscopic Features. "Sleeves" of pronounced perivenular demyelination with macrophage-predominant inflammatory infiltrates are typical. The outer margins of ADEM lesions are indistinct compared with the relatively well-delineated edges of multiple sclerosis (MS) plaques. Viral inclusion bodies are generally absent, unlike viral encephalitis.

Clinical Issues

Epidemiology and Demographics. ADEM is second only to MS as the most common acquired idiopathic inflammatory demyelinating disease. Unlike MS, there is no female predominance. ADEM occurs most commonly in spring and autumn.

ADEM can occur at any age but—perhaps because of the frequency of immunizations and antigen exposure—is more common in childhood, with peak occurrence between 5 and 8 years of age. The overall estimated incidence is 0.8 per 100,000 persons annually. The incidence of childhood ADEM is estimated at 2-10 cases per million children per year. Between 10-25% of children with ADEM are eventually diagnosed with MS.

Presentation. Symptoms typically occur a few days to a few weeks following antigenic challenge (e.g., infection or vaccination). The majority of children with ADEM have a nonspecific febrile illness preceding onset. Viral exanthema is usually absent. Unlike MS, optic neuritis is rare.

Natural History. Disease course and outcome vary. **Monophasic ADEM** is the most common type. However, the disease sometimes follows an atypical course, waxing and waning over a period of several months.

Approximately 25% of patients initially diagnosed with ADEM experience a relapse. **Recurrent ADEM** is characterized by a second episode occurring within 2 years after the initial illness and involving the *same* anatomic area(s) as the original illness.

Multiphasic ADEM (MDEM) is characterized by one or more subsequent events that involve a *different* anatomic area as demonstrated by a new lesion on MR or a new focal neurologic deficit. MDEM is more common in children and is frequently associated with myelin oligodendrocyte glycoprotein (MOG) seropositivity.

More than half of all patients recover completely within 1 or 2 months after onset, whereas approximately 20% experience some residual functional impairment. Overall mortality in recent series is low.

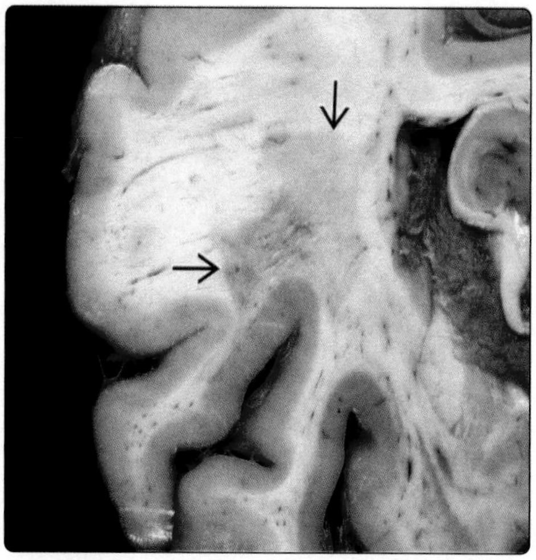

***(15-25)** Autopsy shows necrotizing demyelination ➡ typical of post-infection, post-vaccination disorders. (Courtesy R. Hewlett, MD.)*

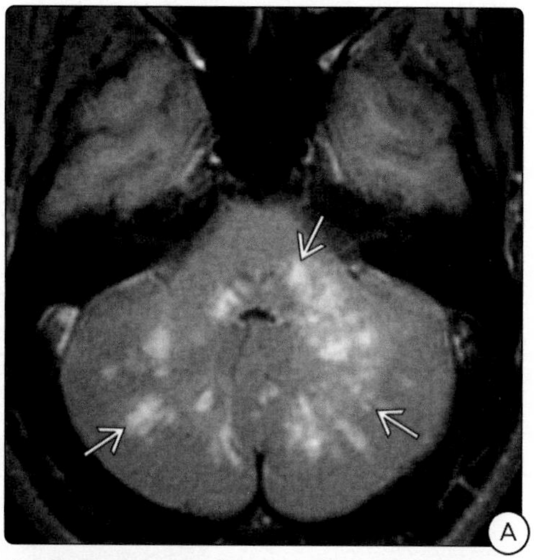

***(15-26A)** T1 C+ FS of 37y woman with headache, unsteady gait 2 weeks after URI shows multifocal patchy enhancing foci in pons, cerebellum ➡.*

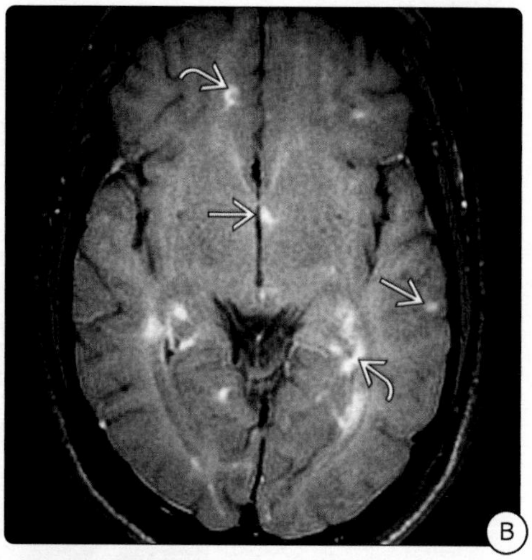

***(15-26B)** Axial T1 C+ FS scan shows several punctate ➡ and incomplete ring-enhancing lesions ➡ in both hemispheres. This is ADEM.*

ACUTE DISSEMINATED ENCEPHALOMYELITIS (ADEM)

Etiology and Pathology
- Postinfection, postimmunization
- Immune-mediated perivenular demyelination

Clinical Issues
- Second only to MS as acquired demyelinating disease
- No female predominance
- Occurs at all ages, but children 5-8 years old most affected
- Course, outcome vary
  - Monophasic ADEM: most common (> 70%)
  - Recurrent ADEM: second episode, same site (10%)
  - Multiphasic ADEM: multiple episodes, different sites (10%)
- Recover completely (> 50%)
- Mortality (1-2%)

Imaging

CT Findings. NECT is usually normal. CECT may show multifocal punctate or partial ring-enhancing lesions.

MR Findings. Multifocal hyperintensities on T2/FLAIR are the most common findings and vary from small round/ovoid foci to flocculent "cotton ball" lesions with very hyperintense centers surrounded by slightly less hyperintense areas with "fuzzy" margins **(15-27)**. Bilateral but asymmetric involvement is typical. Basal ganglia and posterior fossa lesions are common.

Enhancement varies from minimal to striking. Punctate, linear, ring, and incomplete ring patterns all occur **(15-26)** **(15-29)**. Large "tumefactive" lesions with horseshoe-shaped enhancement resemble "tumefactive" MS **(15-28)**. Cranial nerve enhancement is relatively common. Acute lesions may show restriction on DWI. MRS is nonspecific with low NAA and elevated lactate.

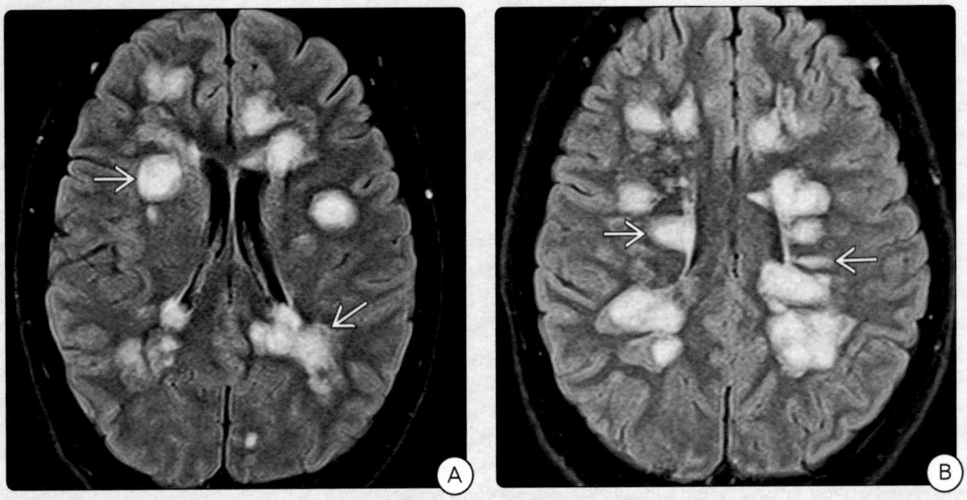

(15-27A) FLAIR in a 21y acutely encephalopathic man with confusion following viral infection shows bilateral white matter lesions with a "fluffy" appearance and "fuzzy" margins ➡. (15-27B) More cephalad FLAIR shows additional "fluffy" lesions oriented perpendicularly to the lateral ventricles ➡.

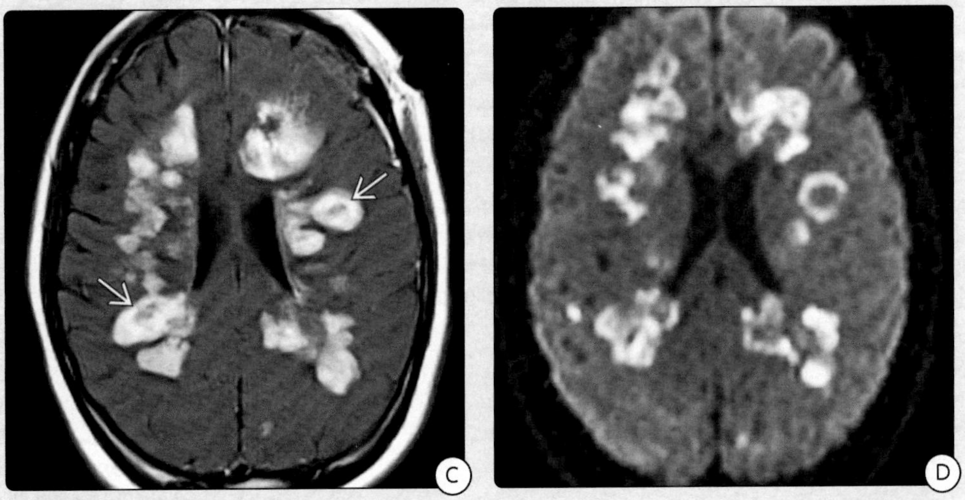

(15-27C) T1 C+ shows that the lesions enhance intensely but heterogeneously. Some have a ring-like appearance ➡. (15-27D) DWI shows acute diffusion restriction in the lesions. Biopsy disclosed demyelinating disease, most likely ADEM.

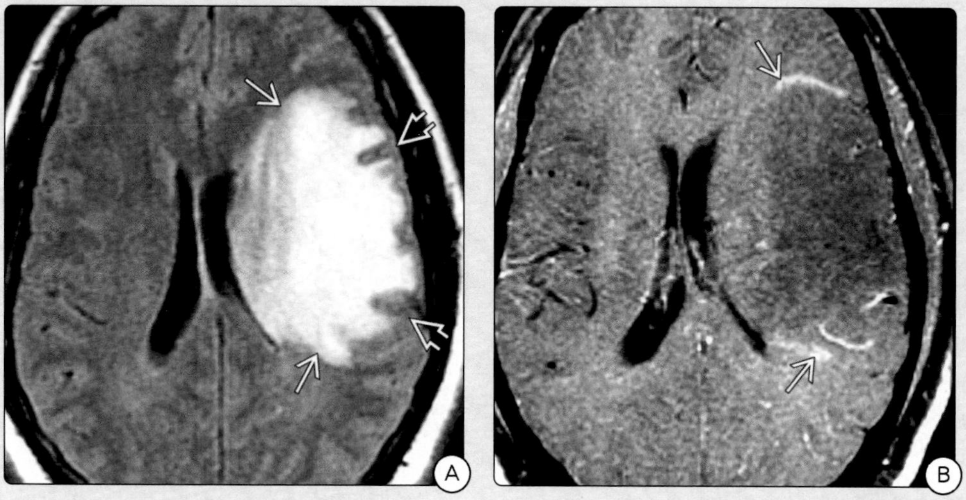

(15-28A) *FLAIR scan in a patient of acute "tumefactive" MS shows a large confluent hyperintense mass that exclusively involves the white matter ➡, sparing the cortex ➡. No other lesions were present.* ***(15-28B)*** *T1 C+ FS in the same patient shows partial rim enhancement around the mostly nonenhancing mass ➡. Biopsy disclosed acute demyelinating disease without evidence of neoplasm or infection.*

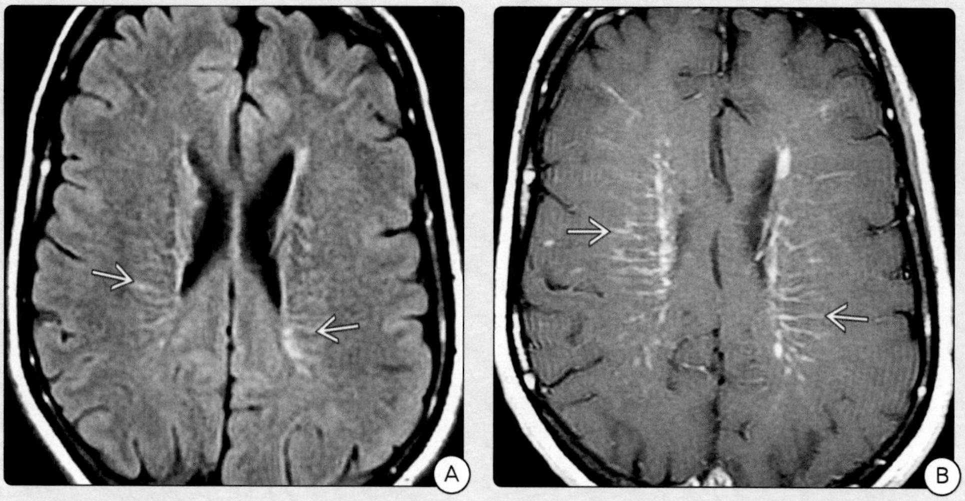

(15-29A) *Multiphasic ADEM is illustrated in this case of a 52y woman who presented with left-sided headache, retroorbital pain, and visual loss. Axial FLAIR scan shows enlarged hyperintense perivenular spaces ➡ in the deep cerebral white matter.* ***(15-29B)*** *Axial T1 C+ scan in the same patient shows striking linear enhancement ➡ along the deep medullary veins and perivascular spaces.*

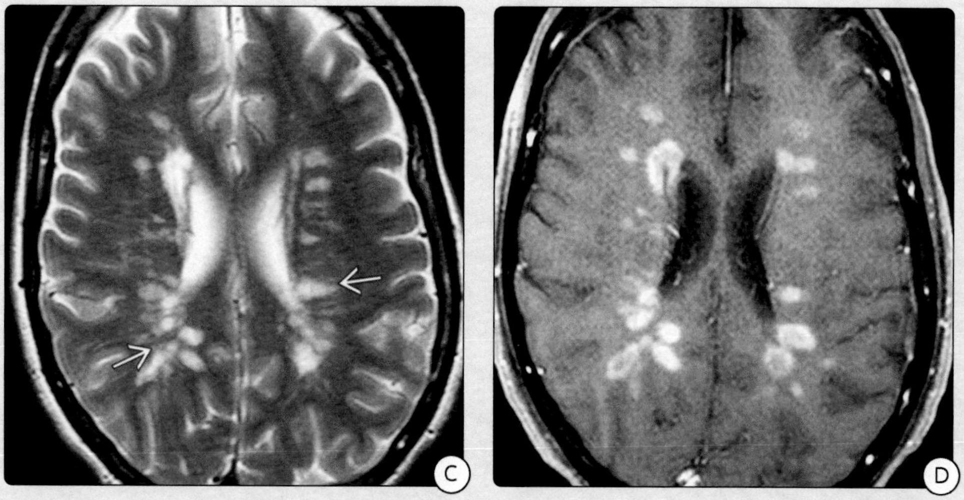

(15-29C) *Repeat scan was done 4 months later due to worsening symptoms. Axial T2WI shows multiple ovoid and triangular hyperintensities ➡ oriented perpendicular to lateral ventricles, considered characteristic for perivenular demyelination.* ***(15-29D)*** *Axial T1 C+ FS shows ovoid hyperintensities with ring, punctate, and linear enhancement. Biopsy found demyelinating disease most consistent with ADEM.*

Differential Diagnosis

The major differential diagnosis of ADEM is **MS**. "Tumefactive" lesions—including those with incomplete ring enhancement—occur in both disorders. ADEM is more common in children and often has a history of viral infection or immunization. MS more commonly involves the callososeptal interface and typically has a relapsing-remitting course, whereas most (but not all!) cases of ADEM are monophasic.

Neuromyelitis optica spectrum disorder (NMOSD) may be difficult to distinguish from recurrent ADEM. **MOG antibody-associated demyelination** may overlap with some forms of NMOSD.

Although very rare, **treatment-associated demyelinating diseases** with TNF-α inhibitors such as etanercept can mimic ADEM and NMOSD on imaging studies **(15-30)**. Demyelination associated with anti-TNF agents typically develops from 1 week to 12 months after treatment initiation.

ADEM: IMAGING

Brain
- Multifocal T2/FLAIR hyperintensities
  - Bilateral but asymmetric white matter lesions
  - Most lesions small, round/ovoid
  - Hazy flocculent "cotton balls" (> 2 cm, usually in children)
  - ± Basal ganglia, posterior fossa, cranial nerves
- Enhancement varies from none to striking
  - Multifocal punctate, linear, partial ring
  - Can be perivenular
  - Large lesions ("tumefactive") less common

Spinal Cord
- Patchy/longitudinally extensive T2 hyperintensity
- Strong but patchy enhancement

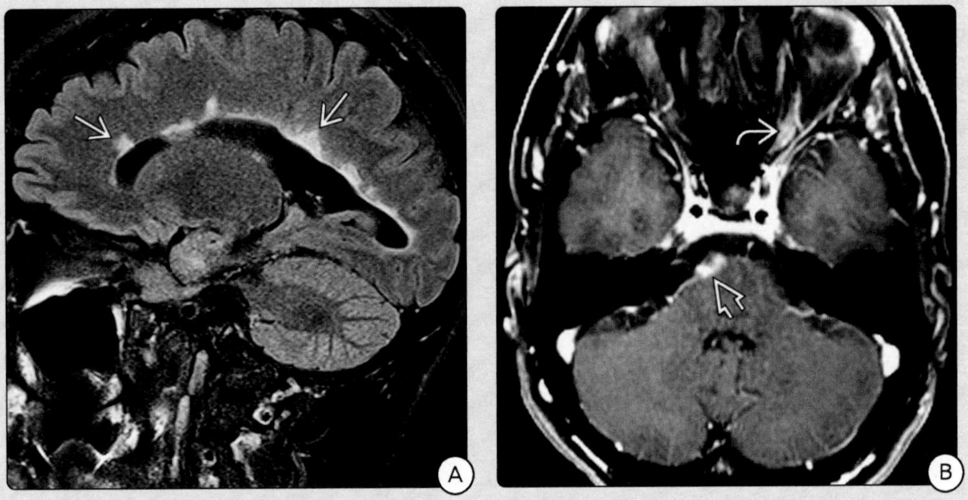

***(15-30A)** A 44y woman on etanercept for her rheumatoid arthritis complained of vision problems and numbness/tingling in her upper extremities. Sagittal FLAIR shows classic triangle-shaped demyelinating lesions along the callososeptal interface and ventricular ependyma. **(15-30B)** T1 C+ FS in the same case shows enhancement in the left optic nerve and pons.*

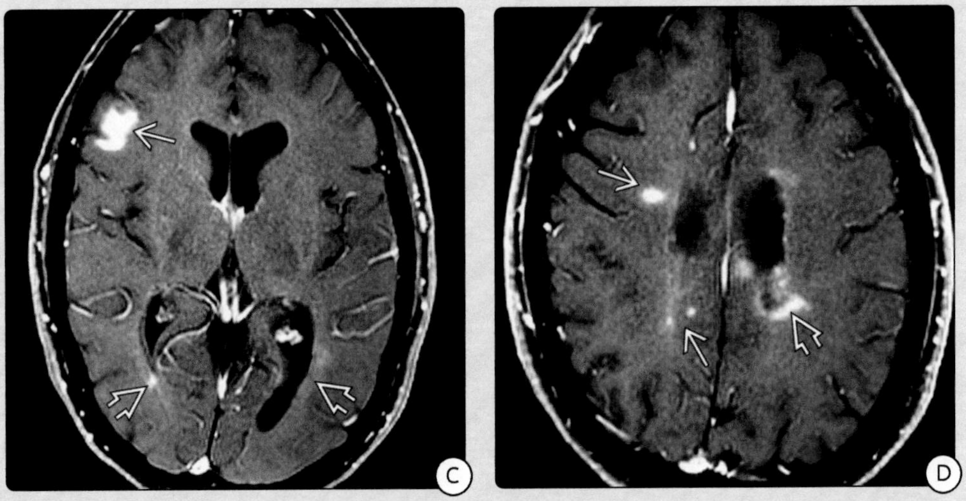

***(15-30C)** More cephalad scan in the same case shows a large enhancing lesion in the left frontal subcortical white matter. Additional enhancing foci are present along the ventricular ependyma. **(15-30D)** More cephalad T1 C+ FS scan shows additional lesions, including a partial ring-enhancing mass adjacent to the left lateral ventricle. This is anti-TNF treatment-associated demyelination.*

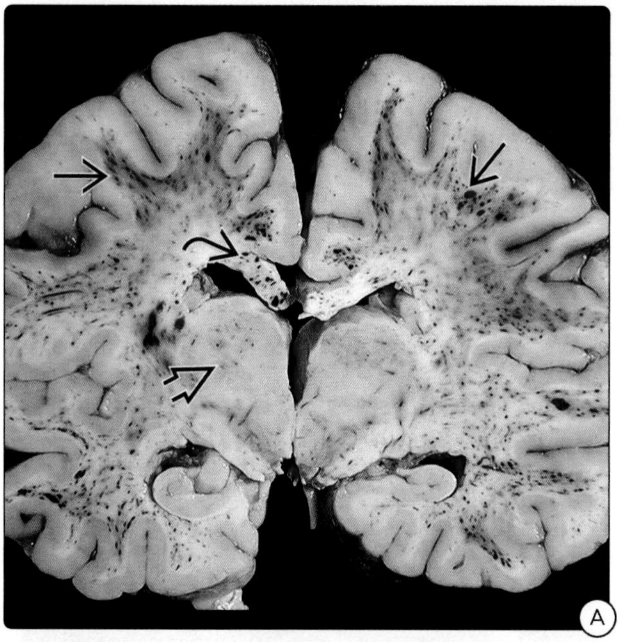

***(15-31A)** Coronal autopsy of AHLE shows innumerable bilaterally symmetric petechial WM hemorrhages → extending into subcortical U-fibers. Note lesions in corpus callosum ↷. The cortex is completely spared but not the deep gray nuclei ⇨.*

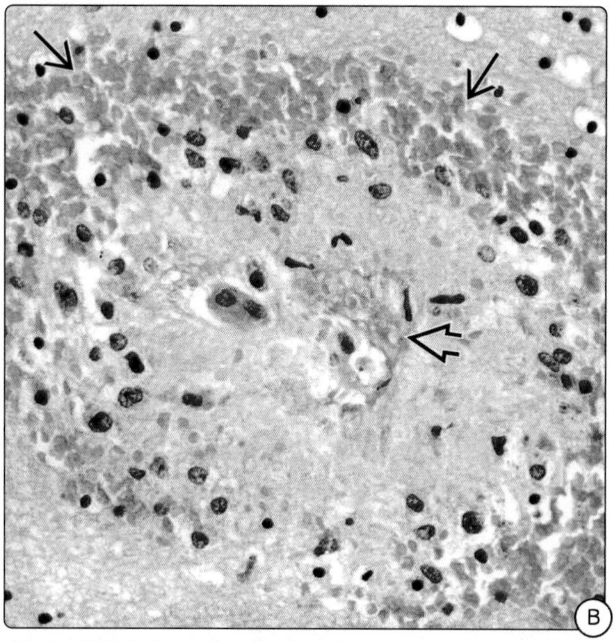

***(15-31B)** H&E photomicrograph in the same case shows a ring of perivascular hemorrhage → surrounding a thrombosed vessel ⇨. (Courtesy R. Hewlett, MD.)*

Acute Hemorrhagic Leukoencephalitis

Terminology

AHLE is also known as acute hemorrhagic leukoencephalopathy, acute hemorrhagic encephalomyelitis (AHEM), and Weston Hurst disease.

Some investigators include AHLE as part of the ADEM spectrum—as a hyperacute, exceptionally severe, extremely fulminant manifestation of ADEM. Because the histologic and imaging features of AHLE differ significantly from ADEM, in this text we consider AHLE separately from ADEM.

Etiology

AHLE is a fulminant demyelinating disease of unknown etiology. History of a viral prodrome or flu-like illness is common but not invariably present. Cross reactivity between myelin basic protein moieties and various infectious agent antigens probably causes an acute autoimmune-mediated demyelination.

Pathology

Location. AHLE predominantly affects the white matter but may involve both the brain and spinal cord. Both the cerebral hemispheres and posterior fossa structures are affected. Despite its name, AHLE may affect the gray matter. Basal ganglia involvement is common, but the cortical gray matter is generally (but not invariably) spared.

Size and Number. AHLE has two distinct manifestations: focal macroscopic parenchymal hemorrhages and innumerable petechial microbleeds. A few cases combine features of both.

Gross Pathology. The typical gross appearance is that of marked brain swelling with diffuse confluent and/or petechial hemorrhages **(15-31A)**. Hemorrhages are typically present in the leptomeninges, cerebral hemispheres (predominately the white matter), and cerebellum. The large arteries are normal without evidence for aneurysm or subarachnoid bleeding.

Microscopic Features. Findings vary with disease acuity. Fibrinoid necrosis of vessel walls with perivascular hemorrhages and mononuclear inflammatory cell cuffing are the pathologic hallmarks of fulminant AHLE **(15-31B)**. Diffuse, mostly neutrophilic infiltrates are typical, in contrast to the macrophage-predominant infiltrates typical of ADEM. Perivascular demyelination may occur in cases with a longer duration.

Clinical Issues

Epidemiology and Demographics. AHLE is considerably less common than ADEM. Approximately 2% of all ADEM cases are of the hyperacute hemorrhagic type that could be considered consistent with AHLE. Although AHLE occurs at all ages, most patients are children and young adults.

Presentation and Natural History. Most AHLE cases begin with a viral illness or vaccination followed by rapid neurologic deterioration. Fever and lethargy with increasing somnolence, decreased mental status, impaired consciousness, and long-tract signs are the most common clinical symptoms.

Untreated AHLE has a very poor prognosis. Rapid clinical deterioration and death usually occur within days to a week after symptom onset. Mortality is 60-80%. The disease course is fulminant and almost always fatal if untreated.

Treatment Options. Aggressive treatment with intravenous high-dose corticosteroids, immunoglobulin, cyclophosphamide, and plasmapheresis has been used with some success in a few cases.

Imaging

Imaging evaluation plays a key role in patients with a clinical history that suggests possible AHLE.

CT Findings. NECT may be normal unless macroscopic confluent hemorrhages are present. Petechial microhemorrhages are generally invisible, but white matter edema with diffuse, relatively asymmetric hypodensity in one or both hemispheres may be present.

MR Findings. T1 scans are often normal unless lobar hemorrhage is present. T2/FLAIR findings vary from subtle to striking. Multifocal scattered or confluent hyperintensities as well as bilateral confluent hyperintensity of the cerebral white matter are typical but nonspecific findings **(15-32)**.

Although large lobar confluent hemorrhages are easily identified on most standard sequences **(15-33)** **(15-34)**, T2* scans are the key to diagnosis. SWI sequences are more sensitive than GRE, especially when only microbleeds are present **(15-32D)**.

Multifocal punctate and linear "blooming" hypointensities in the corpus callosum that extend through the full thickness of the hemispheric white matter to the subcortical U-fibers are typical findings on T2*. Striking sparing of the overlying cortex is common. Additional lesions are frequently present in the basal ganglia, midbrain, pons, and cerebellum.

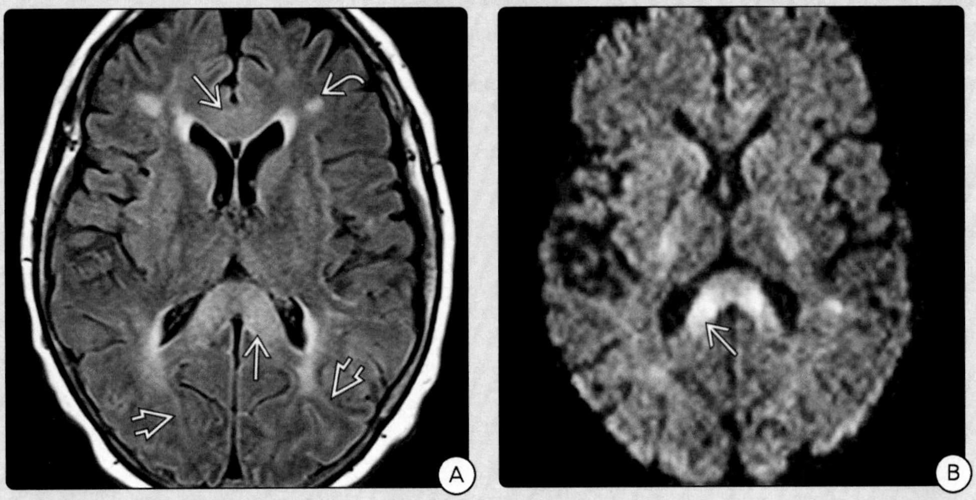

***(15-32A)** A 69y woman had a viral exanthem followed several days later by lethargy and progressive decline in mental status. Axial FLAIR shows confluent hyperintensity in splenium and genu of the corpus callosum ➡, together with bifrontal focal hemispheric white matter lesions ➡ and subtle confluent hyperintensity in the occipital subcortical white matter ➡. **(15-32B)** DWI shows restricted diffusion in the corpus callosum splenium ➡.*

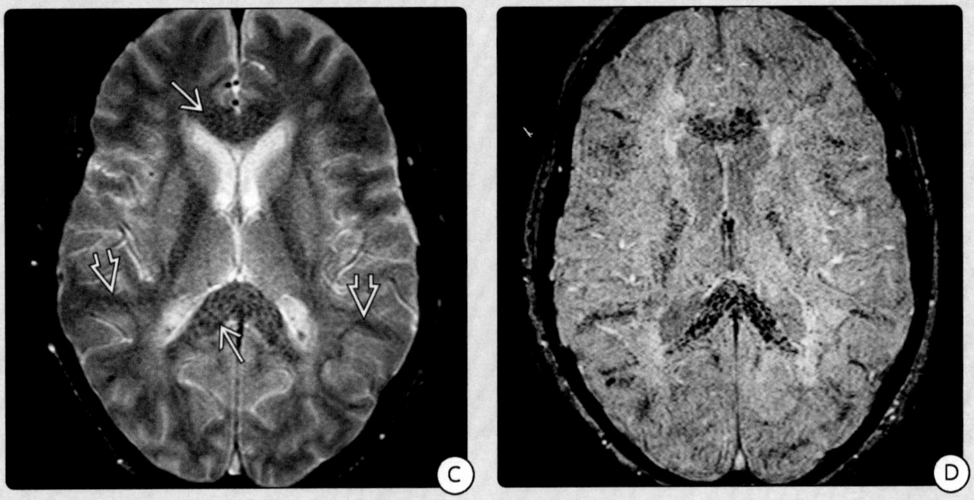

***(15-32C)** T2* GRE shows punctate hypointensities in the corpus callosum ➡ with subtle "blooming" in the subcortical WM ➡. **(15-32D)** The patient continued to deteriorate, so repeat MR with SWI was obtained. Innumerable bilaterally symmetric punctate and linear "blooming" hypointensities are seen throughout the WM with striking sparing of cortical gray matter. AHLE was diagnosed on imaging and confirmed with biopsy.*

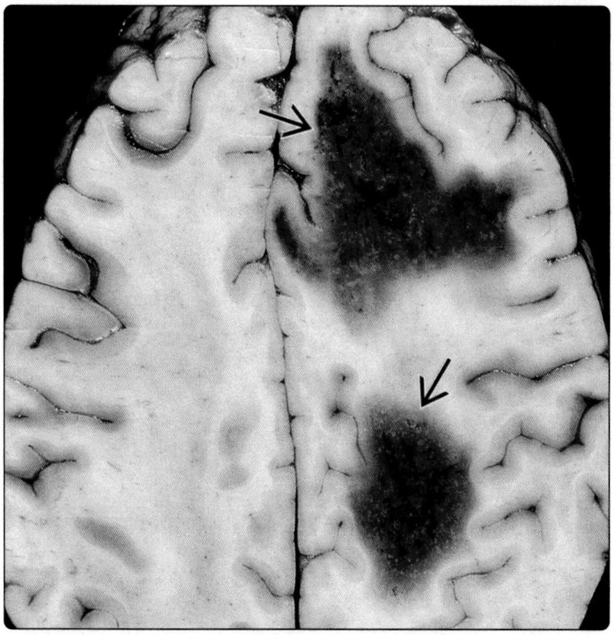

(15-33) Autopsy case shows two areas of gross hemorrhagic necrosis →. Findings, clinical history of prior flu-like illness with rapidly progressive clinical course are characteristic of AHLE. (Courtesy R. Hewlett, MD.)

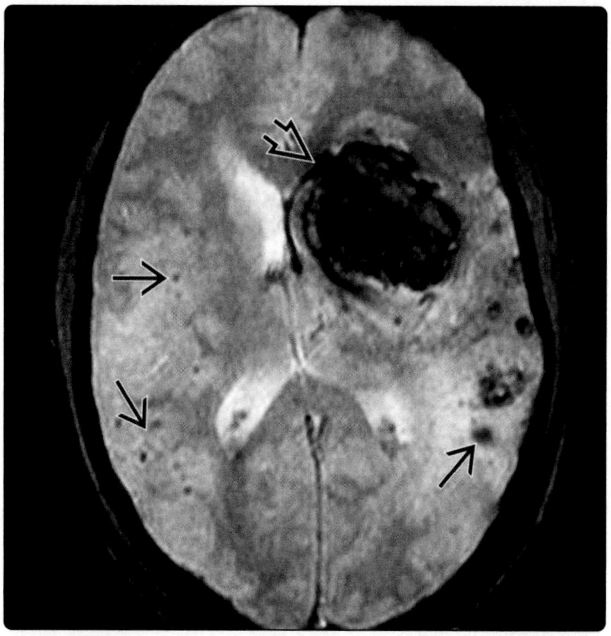

(15-34) T2* GRE scan in a patient with rapid decline after a flu-like illness shows a large left frontal hemorrhage ⇨ with numerous "blooming" foci → in multiple WM lesions. This is AHLE. (Courtesy R. Ramakantan, MD.)

Enhancement on T1 C+ occurs in 50% of cases and ranges from linear perivascular space enhancement to larger patchy or confluent foci.

Differential Diagnosis

The major differential diagnosis of AHLE is **ADEM**. Both share a number of similar features. However, ADEM usually follows a much less fulminant course and does not demonstrate the characteristic lobar or perivascular hemorrhages of AHLE.

Other entities that should be considered in the differential diagnosis include **fulminant MS, acute necrotizing encephalopathy (ANE)**, and **macrophage activation syndrome**.

Acute fulminant **MS** (Marburg type) is not characterized by high fever or marked leukocytosis. The prominent hemorrhagic foci on MR seen with AHLE are absent.

ANE is most common in young children, is often associated with influenza, and results from a para- or postinfectious "cytokine storm." Strikingly symmetric thalamic necrosis with bilateral T2/FLAIR hyperintensities and bithalamic hemorrhages is common. Basal ganglionic and cortical hemorrhages are rare in AHLE.

Petechial microhemorrhages similar to those seen in AHLE can be found in a number of other disorders, including diffuse vascular injury, disseminated intravascular coagulopathy, fat emboli, thrombotic thrombocytopenic purpura, sepsis, vasculitis, hemorrhagic viral fevers, malaria, and rickettsial diseases.

ACUTE HEMORRHAGIC LEUKOENCEPHALITIS (AHLE)

Terminology
- Also called acute hemorrhagic encephalomyelitis (AHEM), Weston Hurst disease

Etiology and Pathology
- Similar to ADEM (viral/postviral autoimmune-mediated condition)
- May represent fulminant form of ADEM

Clinical Issues
- Rare; 2% of ADEM cases
- All ages affected, especially children/young adults
- Fever, lethargy, impaired consciousness
- Rapidly progressive, often lethal course

Imaging
- General features
  - White matter edema
  - Focal macroscopic hemorrhages or multifocal microbleeds
- MR procedure of choice
  - Multifocal scattered or confluent lesions on T2/FLAIR
  - Corpus callosum, cerebral white matter, pons, cerebellum ± basal ganglia
  - Cortical gray matter generally spared
  - T2* (GRE, SWI) depicts microbleeds
  - 50% show variable enhancement

Differential Diagnosis
- ADEM
- Fulminant MS (Marburg type)

Autoimmune Encephalitis

The autoimmune encephalitides are an important, newly recognized disease "family" with a spectrum of related disorders that share overlapping clinical features and imaging findings. Most—but not all—are characterized by limbic dysfunction and varying involvement of the temporal lobes and neocortex.

The autoimmune encephalitides are differentiated by specific antibody subtypes and can be paraneoplastic or nonparaneoplastic. Paraneoplastic-associated disorders such as anti-Hu and anti-Ma encephalitis are discussed in Chapter 27. Nonneoplastic autoimmune encephalitis is discussed here. Because of its unique imaging findings, aquaporin-4 (AQP4) and neuromyelitis optica spectrum disorder (NMOSD) are discussed separately in this section.

Autoimmune Encephalitis

In addition to paraneoplastic and non-tumor-associated disorders, the autoimmune encephalitides are further subdivided according to the cellular location of their neuronal antigens.

Group I antibodies target intracellular antigens, whereas Group II antibodies target cell surface antigens. Group I antibodies are more closely associated with underlying malignancy although **anti-glutamic acid decarboxylase (GAD)** disease targets intracellular antigens but is most commonly associated with nonneoplastic conditions such as type 1 diabetes mellitus.

Terminology

The autoimmune encephalitides are differentiated by—and named according to—specific antibody subtypes that cause immune-mediated attacks on the CNS.

(15-35A) Axial FLAIR in a 71y woman with progressively decreased mental status shows hyperintensity in both anteromedial temporal lobes ➡ and the right hippocampus ⮫. (15-35B) More cephalad FLAIR in the same case shows hyperintensity in the right insular cortex ➡ and external capsule ⮫.

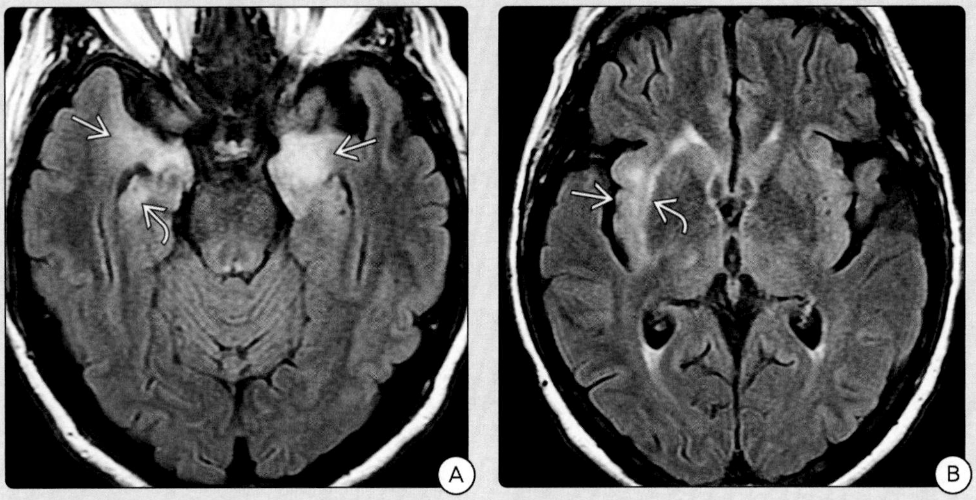

(15-35C) DWI shows no evidence for restricted diffusion. (15-35D) Follow-up FLAIR 6 months later shows bilateral but asymmetric mesial temporal sclerosis ➡ with gliotic brain surrounding enlarged temporal horns ⇨. This is limbic encephalitis. An unidentified neuronal-specific antibody was found on CSF autoantibody studies.

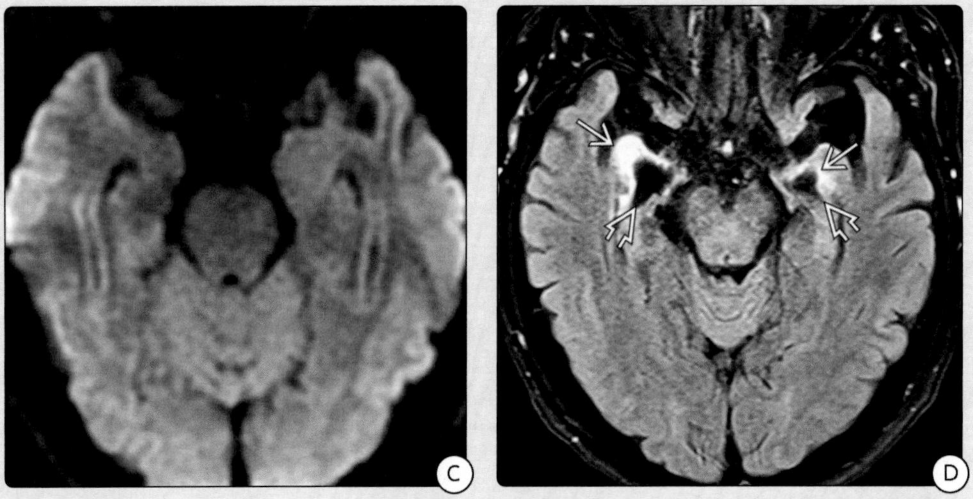

Etiology

The major antigens responsible for inciting autoimmune encephalitis are an ever-expanding group of antibodies that is shown in the box below.

Antibodies against cell-surface antigens such as **AQP4** and **voltage-gated potassium channels (VGKC-complex)** including the **leucine-rich glioma inactivated 1 (LGI1)** are among the commonest autoantibodies in patients with nonneoplastic autoimmune-mediated CNS disease.

Another common group of autoimmune disorders are those with ion channel antigens. These include **N-methyl, D-aspartate receptor (NMDAR or NMDAr)** and **γ-aminobutyric acid receptor (GABAr)** encephalitis, which has a higher association with cancer (e.g., small-cell lung cancer) than other group II autoantibodies.

Less common subtypes include **anti-glutamate receptor 3 (GluR3)** autoantibodies (associated with Rasmussen encephalitis) and **voltage-gated calcium channel (VGCC)** encephalitis.

NONNEOPLASTIC AUTOIMMUNE ENCEPHALITIS

Group I

- Intracellular antigens
- Often associated with underlying malignancy
- Examples
  - Anti-Hu, anti-Ma
  - Anti-Ri (breast, small cell lung), anti-Yo (ovarian, breast)
  - Anti-GAD (usually *NOT* associated with malignancy)

Group II

- Cell-surface antigens
- Malignancy less common
- Examples
  - NMDAr, GABAr
  - VGKC (including LGI1), VGCC
  - GluR3 (Rasmussen)

Pathology

Regardless of the etiology and antibody profile, the autoimmune encephalitides have a distinct predilection for the limbic system.

Clinical Issues

Antigenic specificities appear to determine the associated clinical syndromes. The most common presentation is subacute cognitive dysfunction and altered mental status. Seizures and medically intractable epilepsy are also common, especially in VGKC-complex encephalitis.

NMDAr encephalitis is typically characterized by an initial viral-like prodrome followed by psychiatric symptoms, amnesia, and seizures. Nonneoplastic NMDAr is more common and often occurs in young women. Between 25-50% of older women have an ovarian teratoma or carcinoma.

Less common presentations include stiff leg or stiff person syndromes and cerebellar ataxia.

Imaging

Imaging findings are variable. The most common pattern is that of limbic encephalitis. T2/FLAIR hyperintensity in one or both medial temporal lobes is typical **(15-35)**. Extralimbic involvement with structures such as the cortex, striatum, and diencephalon varies. For example, cortical involvement is

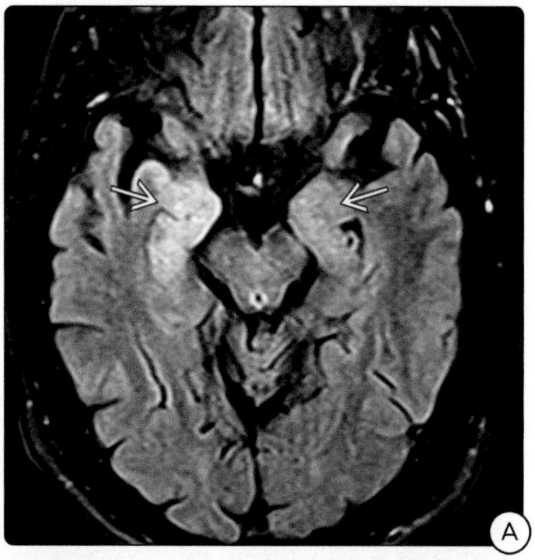

***(15-36A)** FLAIR in a 68y man with seizures, LGI1-encephalitis shows bilateral but asymmetric medial temporal lobe hyperintensities ➡.*

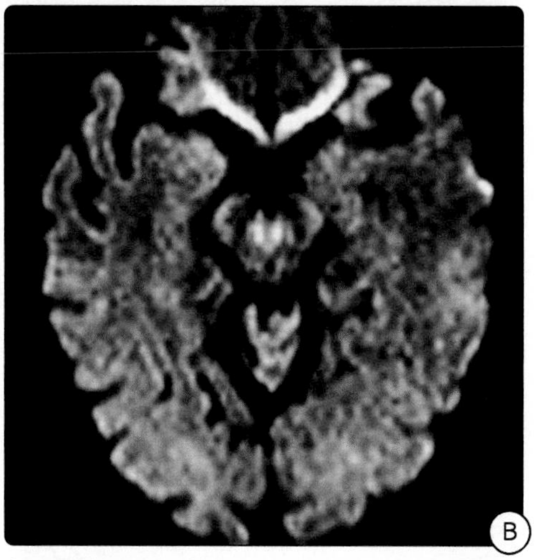

***(15-36B)** DWI in the same case shows no evidence for restricted diffusion.*

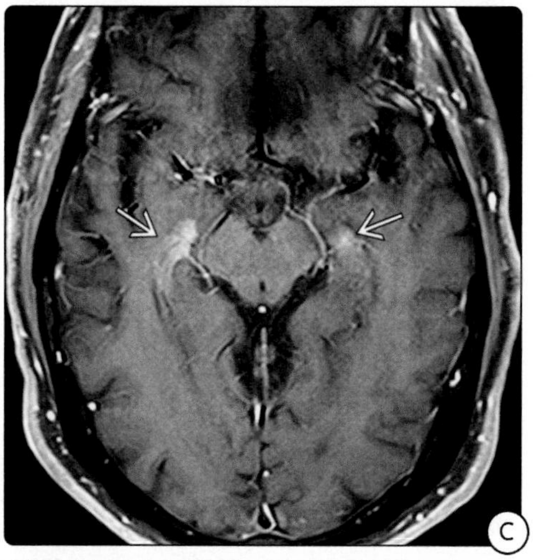

***(15-36C)** T1 C+ FS in the same case shows asymmetric enhancement ➡ in both medial temporal lobes.*

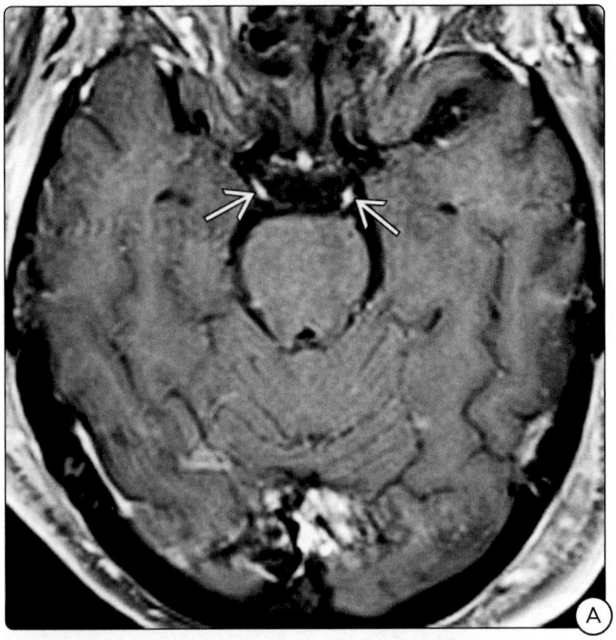

(15-37A) T1 C+ in a patient with ataxia, limb weakness, and ophthalmoplegia demonstrates that both oculomotor nerves enhance ➡. Other CNs including the right CN V and both CN VIIs enhanced (not shown).

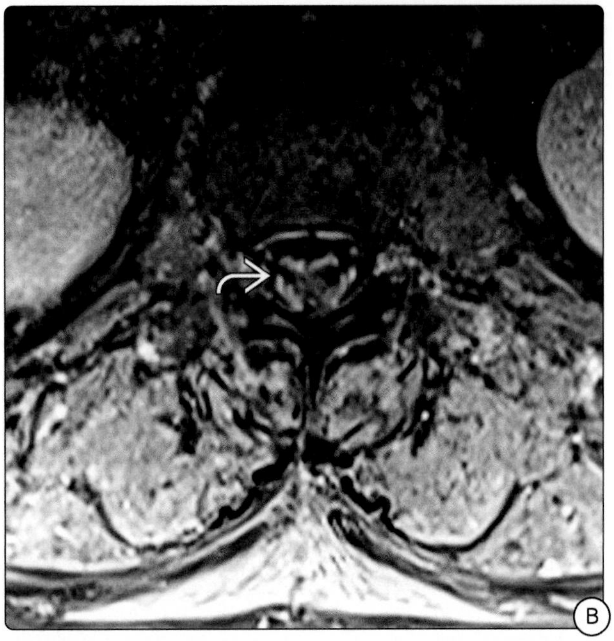

(15-37B) T1 C+ FS of the conus medullaris in the same case demonstrates striking enhancement of both the anterior and posterior spinal nerve roots ➡. This is Miller-Fisher variant of Guillain-Barré spectrum.

common in VGCC encephalitis, whereas it is very rare in VGKC encephalitis.

Diffusion restriction is variable but often absent. Enhancement on T1 C+ occurs in approximately 25% of cases **(15-36)** and is frequently associated with subsequent development of mesial temporal sclerosis.

A subset of patients will have no neuroimaging findings despite severe neuropsychiatric dysfunction. In these patients, serum/CSF antibody testing may be definitive

Differential Diagnosis

The differential diagnosis of autoimmune encephalitis includes **herpes simplex encephalitis, HHV-6 encephalitis**, and systemic autoimmune disorders such as SLE, antiphospholipid antibody syndrome, and thyroid encephalopathy.

Guillain-Barré Spectrum Disorders

Miller Fisher syndrome (MFS) (acute ophthalmoplegia and ataxia) and **Bickerstaff brainstem encephalitis (BBE)** are rare inflammatory disorders that are now considered subtypes of **Guillain-Barré syndrome (GBS)** (acute onset of limb weakness). All three variants are now considered autoimmune-mediated encephalitides associated with **anti-GQ1b antibody syndrome**. Approximately 10% of patients are GQ1b-seronegative, and many are positive for antibodies against glutamic acid decarboxylase (**anti-GAD**).

Guillain-Barré spectrum disorders (GBSDs) are typically preceded by a prodromal illness. Clinical features vary with subtype, but progressive limb weakness and diplopia are common. The disease course is usually monophasic with recurrences reported in 4-7% of GBS, 12% of MFS, and 25% of patients with BBE.

Brain MR findings are nonspecific. Enhancement of one or more cranial nerves may occur in the acute stage of MFS inflammatory demyelinating neuropathy **(15-37)**. Patchy or confluent moderately extensive T2/FLAIR hyperintensity in the midbrain and pons may be present in BBE.

The differential diagnosis of GBSD includes NMOSD and Listeria brainstem rhombencephalitis.

Neuromyelitis Optica Spectrum Disorder

Terminology

Neuromyelitis optica spectrum disorder (NMO)—formerly known as **Devic syndrome**—is a severe form of acute demyelinating disease that preferentially involves the spinal cord and optic nerves with relative sparing of the cerebral white matter.

In 2015, an international consensus panel revised the diagnostic criteria for NMO and broadened the disease name to **NMO spectrum disorder** (NMOSD). In the past, the criteria for a diagnosis of NMO required both optic neuritis and transverse myelitis. The revised criteria (see below) allow other symptoms such as postrema syndrome (intractable hiccups or nausea and vomiting) and brainstem syndromes (double vision or ataxia) to be included.

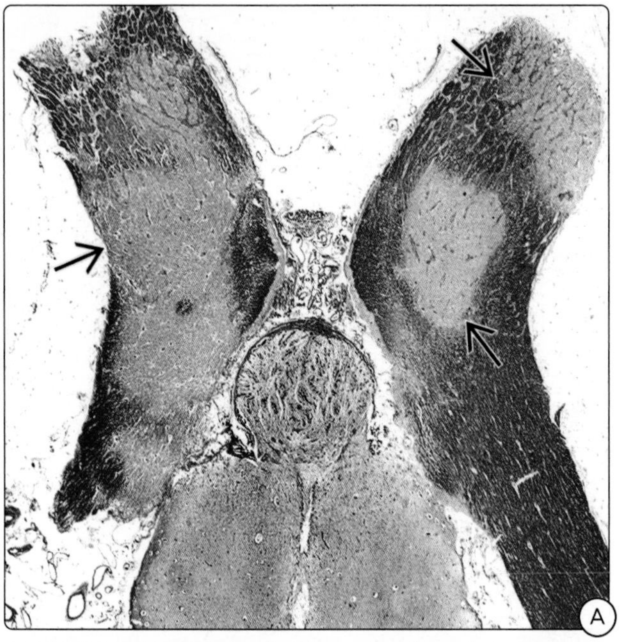

A

(15-38A) Luxol fast blue stain of a section through the optic chiasm shows classic demyelinating foci characteristic of neuromyelitis optica ➡.

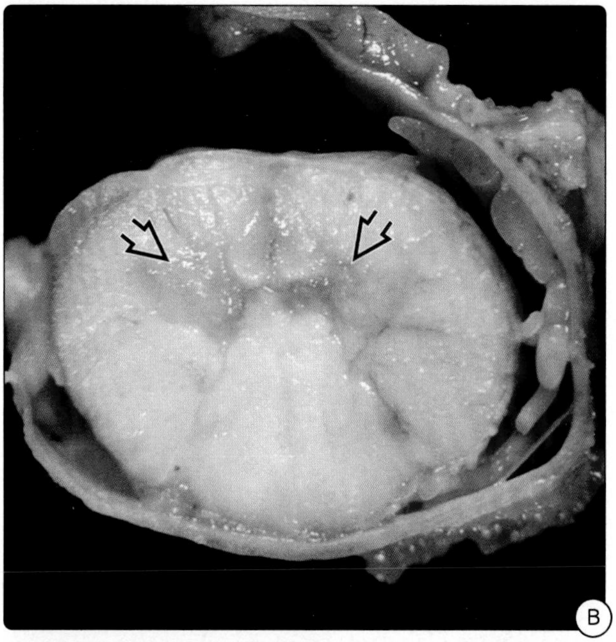

B

(15-38B) Axially sectioned spinal cord in the same case demonstrates cavitating central cord lesions ➡. (Courtesy R. Hewlett, MD.)

Etiology

The most common form of NMOSD is a primary autoantibody-mediated astrocytopathy characterized by the presence of antibodies to aquaporin-4 (AQP4). AQP4 is the most abundant water channel in the CNS and is located in the foot processes of astrocytes surrounding the blood-brain barrier.

A specific biomarker of the disease, NMO-IgG, is 90% specific and 70-75% sensitive for NMOSD. NMO-IgG is almost always negative in MS and other autoimmune disorders, such as Sjögren syndrome and systemic lupus erythematosus.

AQP4-IgG-negative NMOSD is less common. Some of these patients have antibodies to myelin oligodendrocyte glycoprotein (MOG). **MOG antibody-associated disease** targets oligodendrocytes, not astrocytes, and may be a separate biologic entity.

Pathology

Location. In classic NMOSD, one or both optic nerves are involved together with the spinal cord **(15-38)**. The cervical cord is most commonly affected, and lesions typically extend over three or more consecutive segments. Brain lesions are not uncommon and tend to cluster around the third and fourth ventricles and the dorsal midbrain/aqueduct of Sylvius.

Microscopic Features. Selective AQP4 immunoreactivity loss and vasculocentric complement and immunoglobulin deposition are characteristic. Antibody-independent AQP4 loss also occurs in other demyelinating conditions, namely Balo disease and some cases of MS.

It is the *immunohistochemical* staining pattern of NMO-IgG that is diagnostic. NMO-IgG binds to the abluminal face of microvessels at sites of immune complex deposition in NMOSD lesions. Actively demyelinating NMO lesions demonstrate vessel hyalinization, a finding not present in MS or ADEM. In addition, eosinophils are commonly found in NMOSD biopsies but are rare in MS.

Clinical Issues

Epidemiology and Demographics. In contrast to the striking geographical distribution of MS, NMOSD is a worldwide disease. It is common in Asia, and, in UK and USA studies, 10-50% of patients with NMOSD are non-Caucasian.

Another distinguishing feature from MS is age at symptom onset. Patients with NMOSD are on average 10 years older than patients with MS. Mean age at initial diagnosis is around 40 years.

Between 15-20% of patients with NMOSD are over age 60 at onset. The F:M ratio for AQP4-positive NMOSD is 8-9:1.

Between 10-25% of NMOSD patients are seronegative for AQP4 **(15-41)**. Seronegative NMO is equally distributed among the sexes.

Presentation and Natural History. NMOSD is classically characterized by severe uni- or bilateral optic neuritis and transverse myelitis occurring simultaneously at disease onset. Involvement of other CNS regions is now recognized as part of the NMOSD spectrum.

NMOSD follows an unpredictable course, but prognosis is generally worse than for MS. The vast majority of cases (85-90%) are relapsing, but NMOSD occasionally occurs as a monophasic illness. Relapsing NMOSD generally results in severe residual injury that accumulates with each subsequent attack.

Almost 30% of NMOSD patients are initially misdiagnosed with MS. NMO-IgG seropositivity is detected in 3-5% of patients who have a clinically isolated syndrome at the time of initial presentation.

Treatment Options. Accurate diagnosis is essential because some drugs used for MS can worsen NMOSD. Recent studies suggest that the therapeutic options in NMO should be immunosuppressive rather than immunomodulatory drugs. Plasma exchange can be used in severe cases.

2015 REVISED NMOSD DIAGNOSTIC CRITERIA: AQP4-IgG POSITIVITY

AQP4-IgG positivity plus 1 core clinical characteristic

- Optic neuritis
- Acute myelitis
- Area postrema syndrome
    - Unexplained hiccups, or nausea and vomiting
- Acute brainstem syndrome
- Symptomatic narcolepsy or diencephalic clinical syndrome
    - With NMOSD-typical diencephalic MR lesions
- Symptomatic cerebral syndrome
    - With NMOSD-typical brain lesions

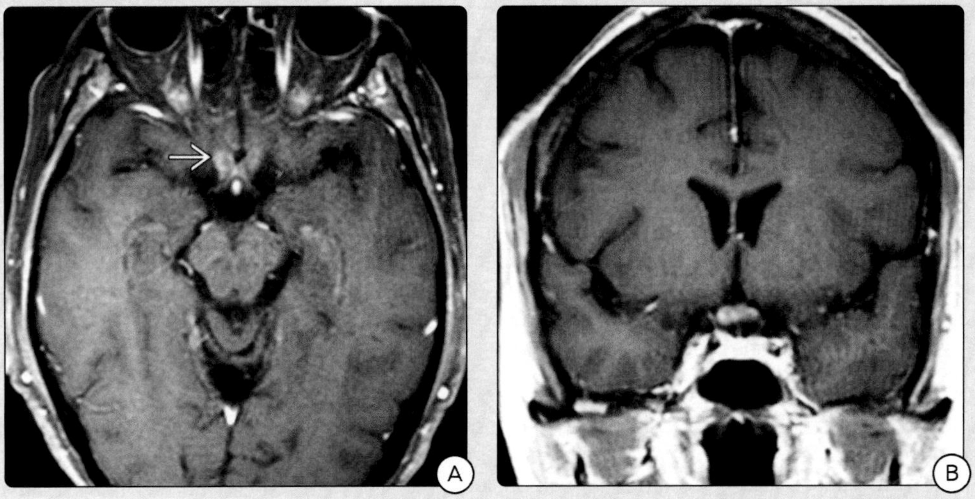

***(15-39A)** Axial T1 C+ FS in a patient with serologically proven neuromyelitis optica (NMO) shows optic chiasm enhancement ➡. **(15-39B)** Coronal T1 C+ scan in the same patient confirms the optic chiasm enhancement. T2/FLAIR scans (not shown) showed no evidence of other lesions.*

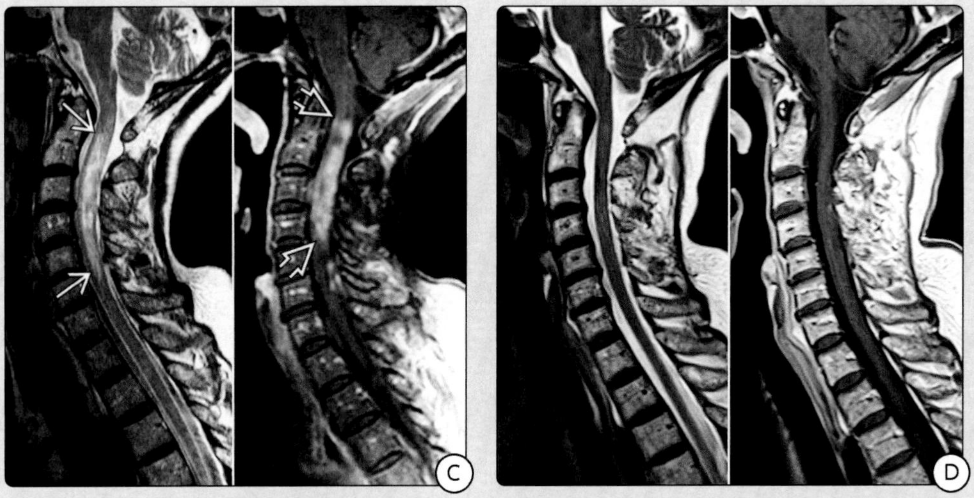

***(15-39C)** (L) Sagittal T2WI in the same case shows a swollen cord with confluent hyperintense lesion extending from C1-C5 ➡. (R) T1 C+ shows patchy enhancement ➡. **(15-39D)** Repeat study after 3 months of immunosuppressive therapy shows that the lesions have completely resolved.*

2015 NMOSD CRITERIA: AQP4-IgG NEGATIVITY

If AQP4-IgG negative

- At least 2 core clinical characteristics; 1 must be
  - Optic neuritis, longitudinally extensive transverse myelitis, or area postrema syndrome
- *If acute optic neuritis*, MR with
  - Normal brain or nonspecific WM lesions or
  - T2 hyperintense or T1 C+ enhancing optic nerve lesion involving optic chiasm or > 50% of optic nerve
- *If acute myelitis*, MR with
  - Intramedullary lesion over 3 contiguous segments
  - Or focal atrophy of at least 3 contiguous segments
- *If area postrema* syndrome, MR with
  - Dorsal medulla/area postrema lesion(s)
- *If acute brainstem* syndrome, MR with
  - Periependymal brainstem lesions

Imaging

The most common MR findings are (1) a hyperintense, enhancing cord lesion that extends over three or more contiguous vertebral segments and (2) optic nerve hyperintensity and/or enhancement, consistent with acute optic neuritis **(15-39)**.

Dorsal medulla and periependymal posterior fossa lesions are characteristic findings in NMOSD with area postrema syndrome and acute brainstem syndrome, respectively. Between 30-60% of NMO patients also have nonspecific T2/FLAIR hyperintensities in the cerebral white matter, so this finding does *not* exclude the diagnosis.

The major differential diagnosis of NMOSD is MS. The brain is more involved in **MS**, whereas multisegmental contiguous spinal cord disease is typical of NMOSD.

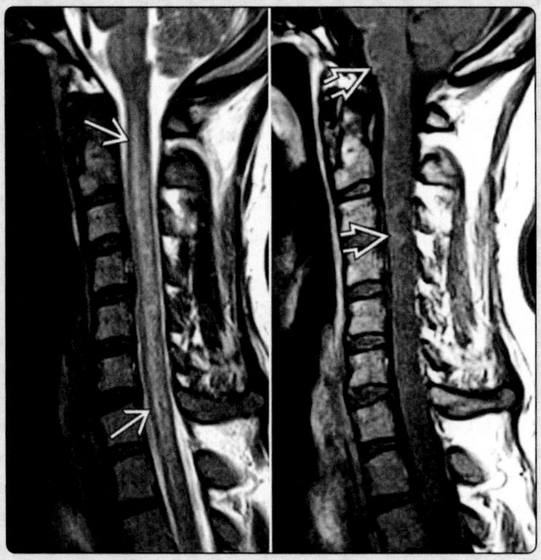

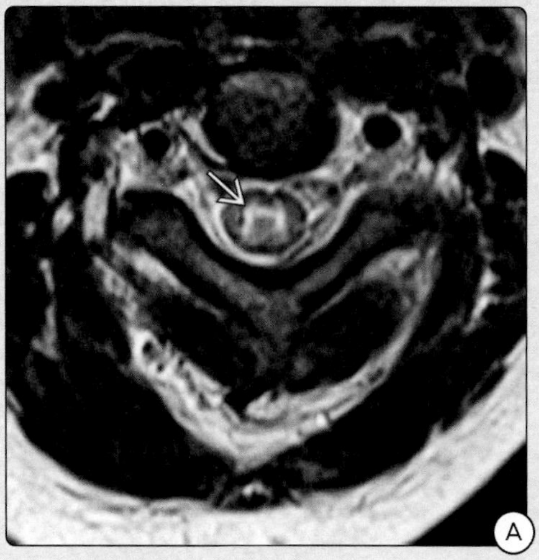

*(15-40) (L) Sagittal T2WI in a 30y woman with "transverse myelitis" shows confluent hyperintensity ➔ involving the entire central cervical spinal cord. (R) Sagittal T1 C+ FS shows faint patchy enhancement in the cord, anterior medulla ➔. The cord appears slightly swollen on both sequences. **(15-41A)** Axial T2WI in the same case shows an H-shaped hyperintensity ➔ involving the central gray matter.*

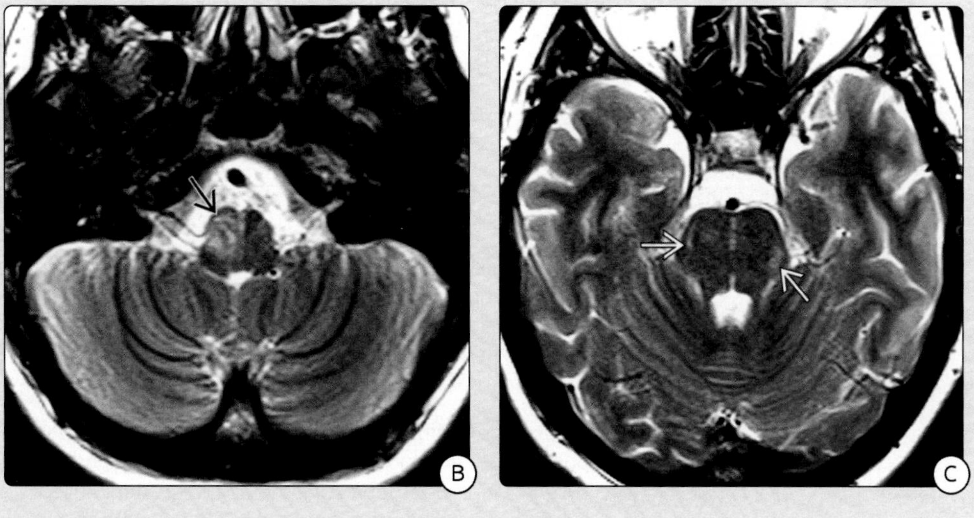

*(15-41B) T2WI in the same case shows hyperintensity ➔ in the right medulla. **(15-41C)** More cephalad T2WI shows multifocal patchy hyperintensities in the pons ➔. After a second attack, evaluation established the diagnosis of antigen-negative NMO spectrum disorder (NMOSD).*

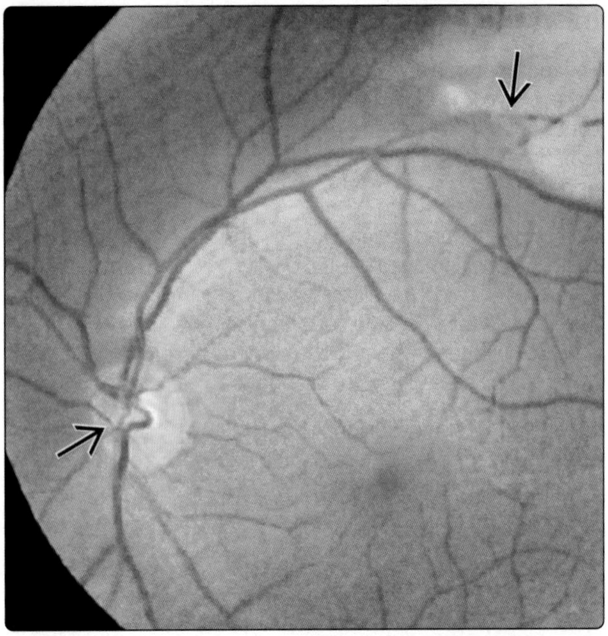

(15-42) Funduscopic examination demonstrates multiple retinal artery branch occlusions and irregularities ➡. (Courtesy K. Digre, MD.)

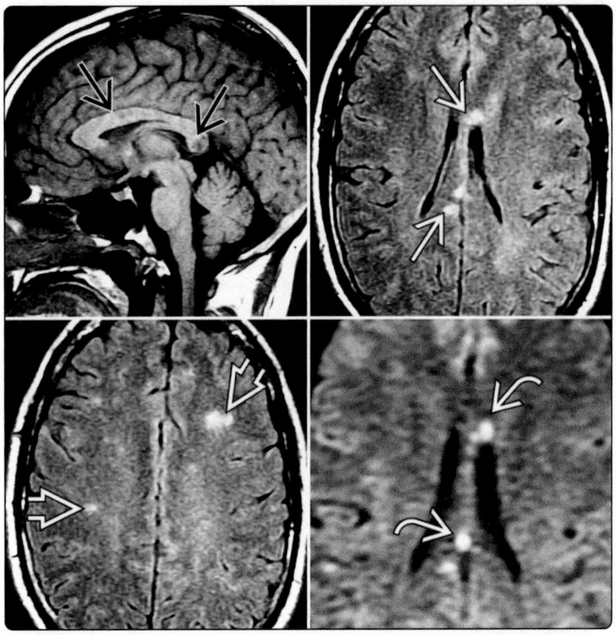

(15-43) Classic findings of Susac syndrome with middle callosal "holes" on sagittal T1WI ➡, multifocal ovoid callosal ➡ and WM hyperintensities ➡ on FLAIR, and diffusion restriction on DWI ➡. (Courtesy P. Rodriguez, MD.)

Susac Syndrome

Susac syndrome (SS) is often mistaken for MS on imaging studies. While most investigators have concluded that SS is a multisystem autoimmune endotheliopathy with microvascular occlusions and not a true primary demyelinating disorder, it is included in this chapter both because it is considered an autoimmune disorder and some of its imaging findings resemble MS.

Terminology

SS is also known as retinocochleocerebral vasculopathy, RED-M (for **r**etinopathy, **e**ncephalopathy, and **d**eafness-associated **m**icroangiopathy), and SICRET (**s**mall **i**nfarcts of **c**ochlear, **r**etinal, and **e**ncephalic **t**issue).

Pathology

The findings are those of a microangiopathy with microinfarcts. The infarcts can be acute or subacute and involve either the cortex or white matter or both. The microvasculature is abnormal. Intraluminal hyaline thrombi, perivascular inflammatory changes with aggregates of macrophages, and prominent swollen, activated endothelial cells are typical histologic features of SS.

Clinical Issues

Epidemiology. SS is a rare disorder. Its true prevalence is unknown, but the incidence is probably more common than previously thought given that many SS cases have been misdiagnosed as MS.

Demographics. SS predominantly affects young adult women between 20-40 years of age. Mean age at presentation is 35 years. The F:M ratio is 3-5:1.

Presentation. Presentation is variable. The classic clinical triad in SS consists of acute or subacute encephalopathy, sensorineural hearing loss, and branch retinal artery occlusions **(15-42)** although many patients do not initially present with the full triad.

In 50% of cases, migraine-like headache is a heralding symptom. Waxing and waning changes in mental status with memory impairment, confusion, and behavioral and psychiatric disturbances are common, often dominant features.

Hearing loss is typically low to medium frequency and can be uni- or bilateral, symmetric or asymmetric. Associated vertigo, ataxia, and nystagmus are common.

Inflamed retinal arterioles with branch retinal artery occlusions are typically present at fluorescein angiography.

Muscle and skin lesions ("livedo racemosa") have also been reported in patients with SS.

Natural History. The clinical course of SS is unpredictable. It is often but not invariably self-limited, resolving within 2-4 years. Some patients have a relapsing-remitting course, whereas others experience permanent neurologic deficits (most commonly deafness and impaired vision).

Treatment Options. The management goal is to prevent permanent neurologic damage. Early, aggressive, and sustained immunosuppressive therapy is recommended. Intravenous glucocorticoids with the addition of immune globulin or cyclophosphamide in refractory cases have produced a good response in many patients.

Imaging

CT Findings. NECT and CECT scans are usually normal. Temporal bone CT is helpful to exclude other causes of sensorineural hearing loss.

MR Findings. Sagittal T1WI in patients with chronic SS may show typical "punched-out" hypointense lesions in the middle layers of the corpus callosum **(15-43)**. T2/FLAIR shows multiple periventricular and deep white matter hyperintensities in over 90% of cases **(15-44)**. Almost 80% show corpus callosal involvement with lesions that typically involve the middle of the corpus callosum and spare the undersurface **(15-45)**. Basal ganglia lesions occur in 70% of cases and brainstem lesions in nearly one-third **(15-44)**.

Acute SS lesions show punctate enhancement on T1 C+. Leptomeningeal enhancement occurs in 30% of patients. DTI shows widespread white matter disruption with focal damage to the corpus callosum genu.

Differential Diagnosis

The major imaging differential diagnoses of SS are MS, ADEM, and Lyme disease. **MS** preferentially involves the undersurface of the corpus callosum, which is usually spared in SS. Auditory involvement with hearing loss is unusual in MS.

ADEM and **Lyme disease** rarely involve the middle layers of the corpus callosum. ADEM is generally monophasic, preceded by a viral prodrome or history of vaccination.

Vasculitis and **thromboembolic infarcts** are other differential considerations. Both rarely affect the corpus callosum.

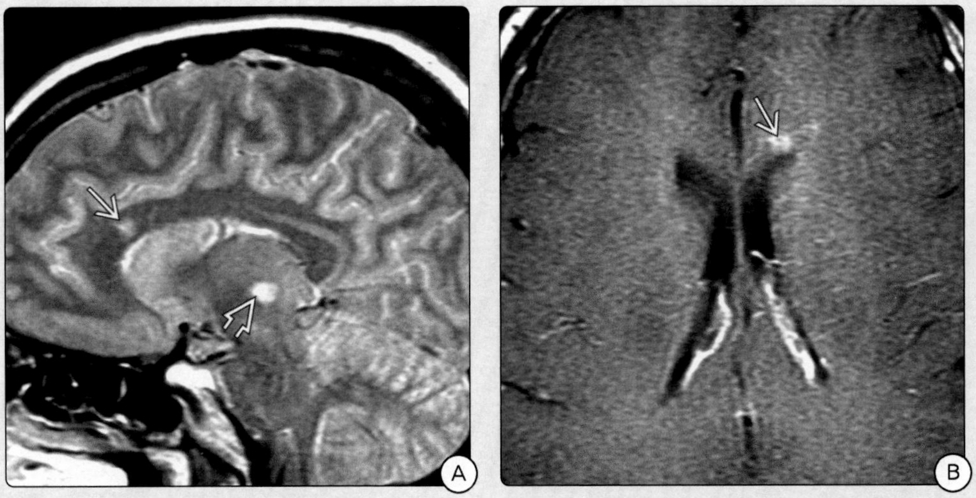

***(15-44A)** A 27y woman presented with headaches, blurred vision, dizziness, and buzzing and ringing in both ears. Sagittal T2WI shows hyperintense foci, one in the middle of the corpus callosum genu ➡ and a second lesion in the thalamus ➡. **(15-44B)** Axial T1 C+ shows that the corpus callosum genu lesion ➡ enhances.*

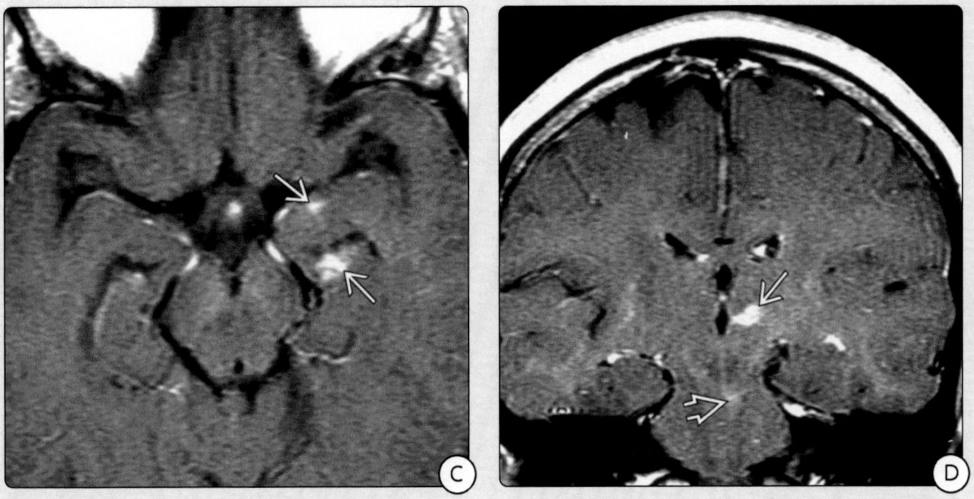

***(15-44C)** Close-up view of axial T1 C+ through the suprasellar cistern shows two additional enhancing lesions ➡ in the left temporal lobe. **(15-44D)** Coronal T1 C+ shows that the left thalamic lesion ➡ enhances. Another small enhancing lesion is present in the midpons ➡. Imaging findings plus clinical history are virtually diagnostic of Susac syndrome.*

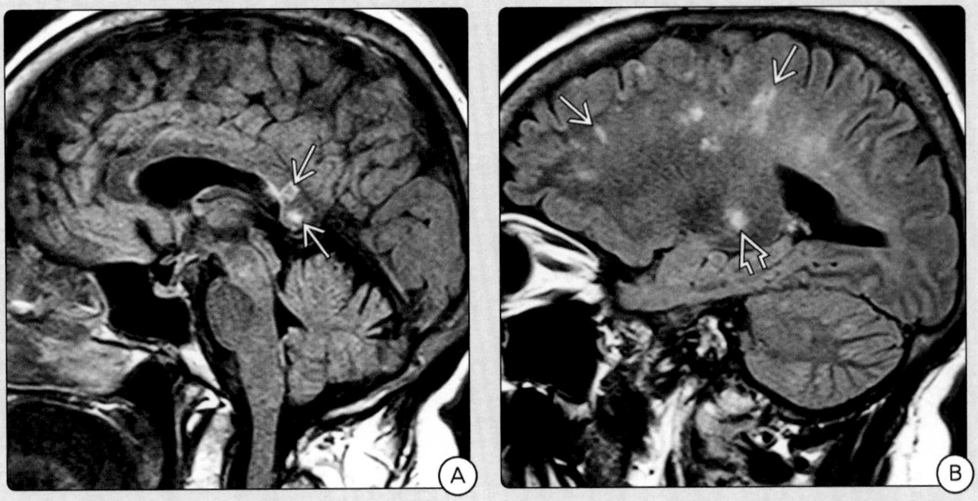

(15-45A) *Series of FLAIR scans demonstrates progressive disease in a patient with Susac syndrome. Initial sagittal FLAIR scan shows two hyperintense lesions in the middle of the corpus callosum splenium ➡.* ***(15-45B)*** *More lateral scan demonstrates multiple punctate and ovoid hyperintensities in the subcortical and deep white matter ➡. A lesion is also present in the thalamus ➡.*

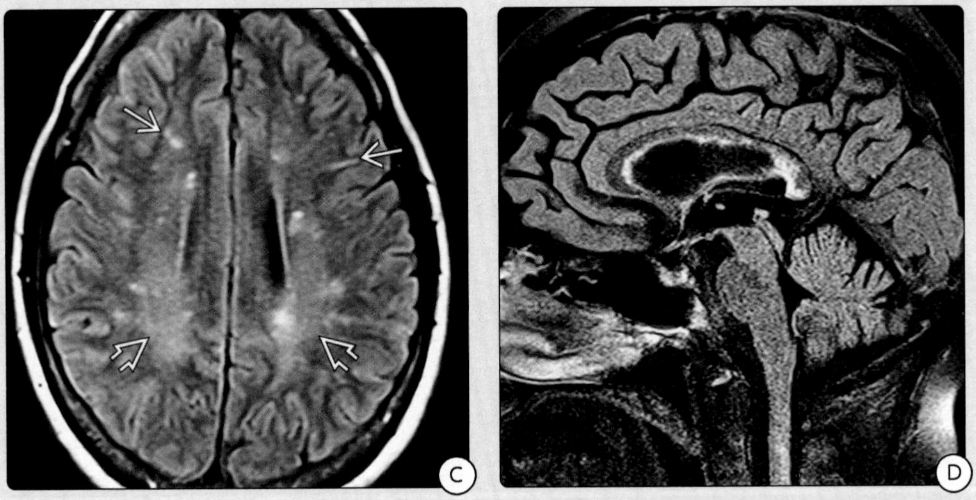

(15-45C) *Axial FLAIR shows multiple punctate, ovoid hyperintensities ➡. There are also confluent deep white matter lesions of lesser hyperintensity in both parietal lobes ➡.* ***(15-45D)*** *The patient's symptoms continued to worsen. Nearly 18 months later, she was almost completely blind and deaf. Repeat sagittal FLAIR scan shows marked interval volume loss with thin corpus callosum and widened sulci.*

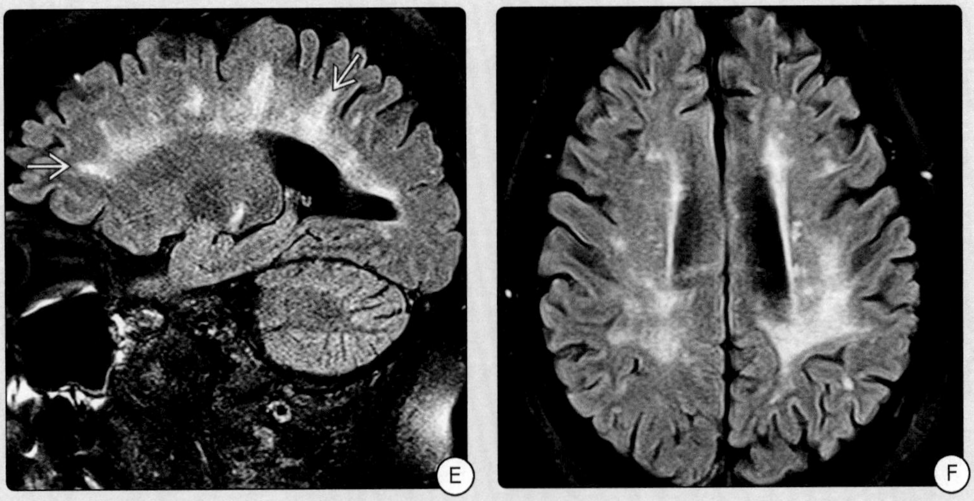

(15-45E) *Sagittal FLAIR now shows confluent deep periventricular WM lesions ➡ that involve most of the corona radiata but spare the subcortical association fibers. Lateral ventricle is rather enlarged compared to the comparable scan from 18 months prior.* ***(15-45F)*** *Axial FLAIR now shows sulcal widening, enlargement of lateral ventricles, confluent WM disease. Severe progression in Susac syndrome is rare but clinically devastating.*

SUSAC SYNDROME

Etiology and Pathology
- Immune-mediated occlusive microendotheliopathy

Clinical Issues
- F > > M
- Clinical triad
  - Headache, encephalopathy
  - Sensorineural hearing loss
  - Vision abnormalities

Imaging and DDx
- T2/FLAIR WM hyperintensities (> 90%)
  - Involvement of corpus callosum (CC) (80%)
  - Middle of CC > > callososeptal interface
- Basal ganglia lesions (70%)
- Variable enhancement (usually punctate)
- DDx = MS, ADEM, Lyme disease, vasculitis

CLIPPERS

CLIPPERS is the acronym for **c**hronic **l**ymphocytic **i**nflammation with **p**ontine **p**erivascular **e**nhancement **r**esponsive to **s**teroids. CLIPPERS is a rare disorder first described in 2010 as a distinct form of brainstem encephalitis with predominant T-cell pathology.

The hallmark of CLIPPERS is the presence of widespread foci of perivascular inflammation dominated by CD4+ T cells in the brainstem and cerebellum. Histopathologic evidence for lymphoma or demyelinating disease is absent.

Patients typically present with subacute brainstem symptoms such as gait ataxia, diplopia, facial paresthesias, and nystagmus. Mean age at onset is is 40-50 years. There is a minor male predominance in reported case series.

Multifocal T2/FLAIR hyperintensities with punctate or curvilinear enhancement on T1 C+ "peppering" the pons and

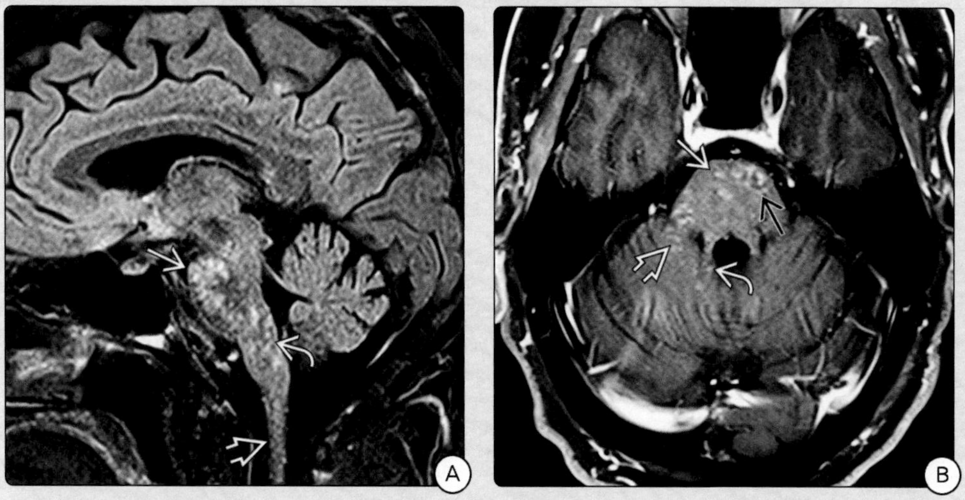

(15-46A) Sagittal FLAIR in a 52y man with diplopia, dysarthria, and facial numbness shows multiple punctate hyperintensities "peppering" the pons ➔, medulla ➔, and extending into the upper cervical spinal cord ➔. (15-46B) T1 C+ FS shows punctate ➔ and curvilinear ➔ foci of contrast enhancement. Note extension into the cerebellum ➔ and superior cerebellar peduncle ➔.

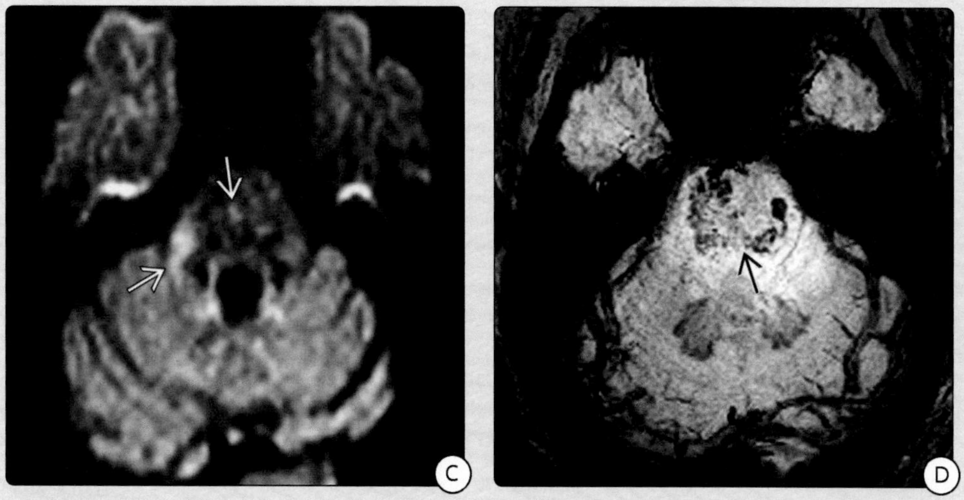

(15-46C) DWI shows scattered foci of restricted diffusion ➔. (15-46D) Axial T2* SWI MIP shows multiple hemorrhagic foci ➔ in the pons. The patient responded dramatically to steroids, but cessation of GCS treatment resulted in disease recurrence. CLIPPERS was diagnosed on the basis of imaging findings and GCS responsiveness.

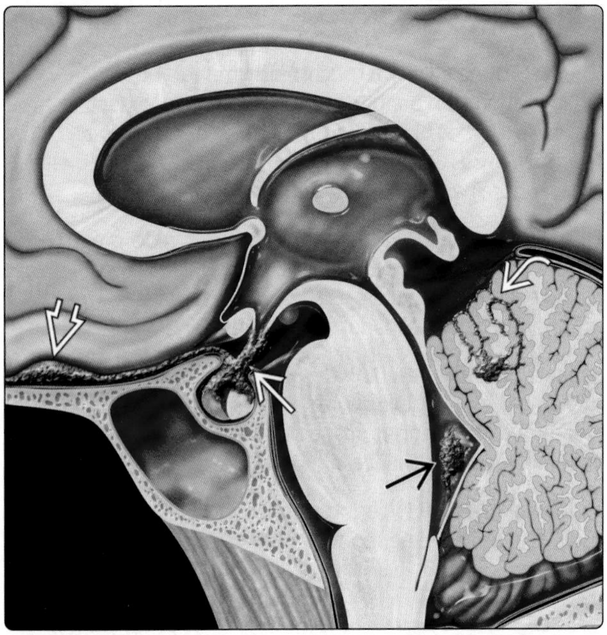

(15-47) Graphic illustrates common neurosarcoid locations: (1) infundibulum, extending into the pituitary ➡, (2) plaque-like dura-arachnoid thickening ➡, and (3) synchronous lesions of the superior vermis ➡ and fourth ventricle choroid plexus ➡.

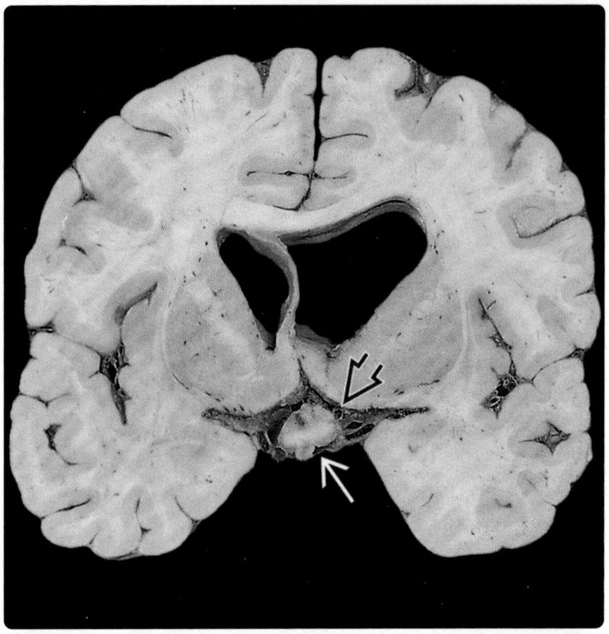

(15-48) Autopsy of neurosarcoidosis demonstrates gelatinous infiltration of the leptomeninges ➡ around the thickened hypothalamus and optic chiasm ➡. (Courtesy Ellison, Neuropathology, 3e.)

cerebellum are typical **(15-46)**. Occasionally lesions are also found in the midbrain, basal ganglia and thalami, cerebral hemispheres, cranial nerves, and spinal cord. There is a clear geographic gradient of lesser inflammation with increasing distance from the brainstem and cerebellum.

Foci of restricted diffusion may occur in the acute phase. Punctate microbleeds in the affected areas are sometimes identified on T2* SWI sequences.

The clinical and imaging differential diagnosis of CLIPPERS is broad. It includes **autoimmune encephalitis** and **Bickerstaff brainstem encephalitis, vasculitis, intravascular lymphoma, lymphomatoid granulomatosis, neuro-Behçet, neurosarcoidosis, CNS histiocytosis, multiple sclerosis**, and **NMOSD**.

Dramatic response to glucocorticosteroids (GCSs) supports the diagnosis of CLIPPERS although relapses are common after cessation of immunosuppression. GCS therapy failure is a strong indication for an alternative diagnosis.

Inflammatory-Like Disorders

Neurosarcoidosis

Terminology

Sarcoidosis ("sarcoid") is a multisystem inflammatory disorder characterized by discrete noncaseating epithelioid granulomas. It can involve virtually any organ but has a propensity for the lungs, lymph nodes, and skin. When sarcoidosis affects the CNS it is termed "neurosarcoid" (NS).

Etiology

The etiology of sarcoidosis remains unknown. Although the initiating event in its pathogenesis remains elusive, the prevailing view is that genetically susceptible individuals develop sarcoidosis following exposure to presently unidentified antigens. A reactive inflammatory cascade ensues that appears to be driven primarily through CD4-positive T cells.

Pathology

Location. The CNS is involved in approximately 5% of cases, usually in combination with disease elsewhere. Only 5-10% of NS cases are confined to the CNS and occur without evidence of systemic sarcoidosis.

Sarcoid can involve any part of the nervous system or its coverings. The most common location is the leptomeninges, especially around the base of the brain. Diffuse leptomeningeal thickening with or without more focal nodular lesions is seen in about 40% of cases **(15-47)**.

The hypothalamus and infundibulum are also favored intracranial sites **(15-48)**. NS can involve cranial nerves, eye and periorbita, bone, the ventricles and choroid plexus, and the brain parenchyma itself. Both supra- and infratentorial compartments are affected. Sarcoid can also involve the spinal leptomeninges, cord, and nerve roots.

Size and Number. NS lesions vary in size from tiny granulomas that infiltrate along the pia and perivascular spaces to large dura-based masses that closely resemble meningiomas. Multiple lesions are more common than solitary lesions.

Gross Pathology. The gross appearance varies widely and depends on location. Somewhat nodular diffuse basilar leptomeningeal thickening is common **(15-48)**. Extension of the granulomas into the brain perivascular spaces is a frequent finding **(15-51)**, as are infiltration and enlargement of the hypothalamus and infundibulum. Single or multifocal discrete, firm, yellow-tan granulomas are typical findings.

Fibrocollagenous tissue becomes progressively more prominent with longstanding disease and may result in dense meningeal fibrosis, seen as a pachymeningopathy with or without focal dural masses.

Microscopic Features. Sarcoid granulomas are noncaseating collections with central aggregates of epithelioid histiocytes and multinucleated giant cells together with variable numbers of benign-appearing lymphocytes and plasma cells. There is no histologic or immunohistochemical evidence of infection or neoplasm.

Clinical Issues

Epidemiology and Demographics. NS has a bimodal age distribution. The largest peak occurs during the third and fourth decades with a second smaller peak in patients—especially women—over the age of 50 years. There is a moderate female predominance.

Sarcoidosis is distributed worldwide although prevalence varies significantly with geography and ethnicity. African Americans and Northern European Caucasians have the highest disease incidence. In the USA, the lifetime risk in African Americans is nearly threefold higher than in Caucasians.

Presentation. Symptoms vary with location. The most common presentation of NS is isolated or multiple cranial

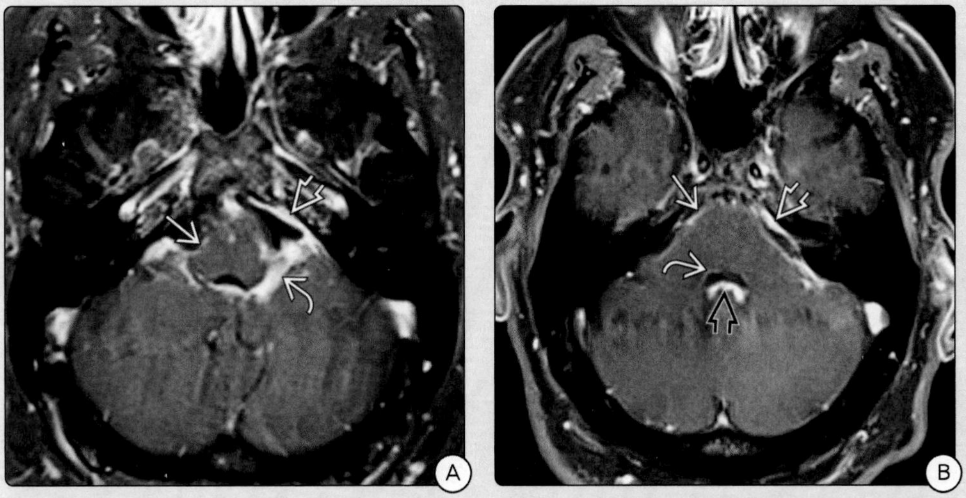

***(15-49A)** Axial T1 C+ FS in a 56y woman with proven neurosarcoid shows thickening and enhancement along the choroid plexus, dura, and pial surface of the medulla. **(15-49B)** More cephalad T1 C+ FS shows thickened, enhancing dural plaque. Lesions are also present along the pial surface of the pons, the choroid plexus of the fourth ventricle, and the ventricular ependyma.*

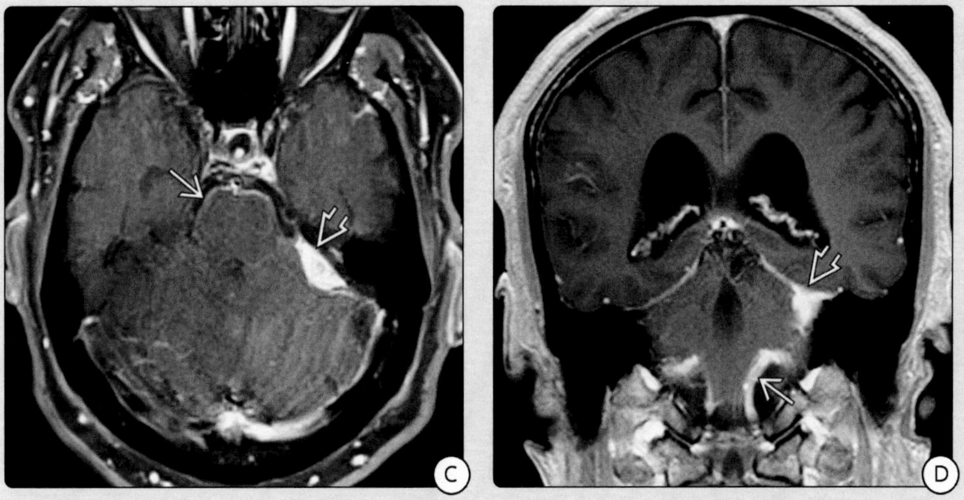

***(15-49C)** More cephalad axial T1 C+ FS scan shows the pial involvement. A mass-like enhancing dural plaque at the left cerebellopontine angle (CPA) cistern resembles a meningioma. **(15-49D)** Coronal T1 C+ scan in the same case shows the extensive leptomeningeal enhancement and the CPA dural plaque.*

nerve deficits, seen in 50-75% of patients. Involvement of virtually every cranial nerve has been reported. The facial and optic nerves are the most frequently affected.

Nonspecific symptoms of NS include headache, fatigue, seizures, encephalopathy, cognitive deficits, and psychiatric disturbances. Symptoms of pituitary/hypothalamic dysfunction such as diabetes insipidus or panhypopituitarism are seen in 10-15% of cases.

Diagnosing NS may be difficult because the clinical features can be nonspecific and elevated serum angiotensin-converting enzyme (ACE) levels are seen in less than half of all cases. The diagnosis of definite NS requires histologic confirmation, so most diagnoses of NS are "possible" or "probable."

Natural History. Nearly two-thirds of patients experience a self-limited monophasic illness. One-third follow a chronic remitting-relapsing course with the development of additional granulomas.

Treatment Options. Most patients with NS respond to corticosteroids. Second-line treatment with immunosuppressive agents and third-line treatment with monoclonal antibodies against TNF-α have been tried with variable success.

Imaging

General Features. Systemic sarcoidosis has protean manifestations and is one of the great mimickers of many other diseases. NS is no different, and findings vary widely. Specific imaging features are described below and summarized according to frequency in the accompanying box.

CT Findings. Depending on the amount of fibrosis present, NS can appear slightly hyperdense relative to normal brain parenchyma on NECT scan. Leptomeningeal disease may enhance on CECT, resembling tuberculosis or pyogenic meningitis. Dura-based masses are typically modestly hyperdense and enhance strongly and uniformly on CECT.

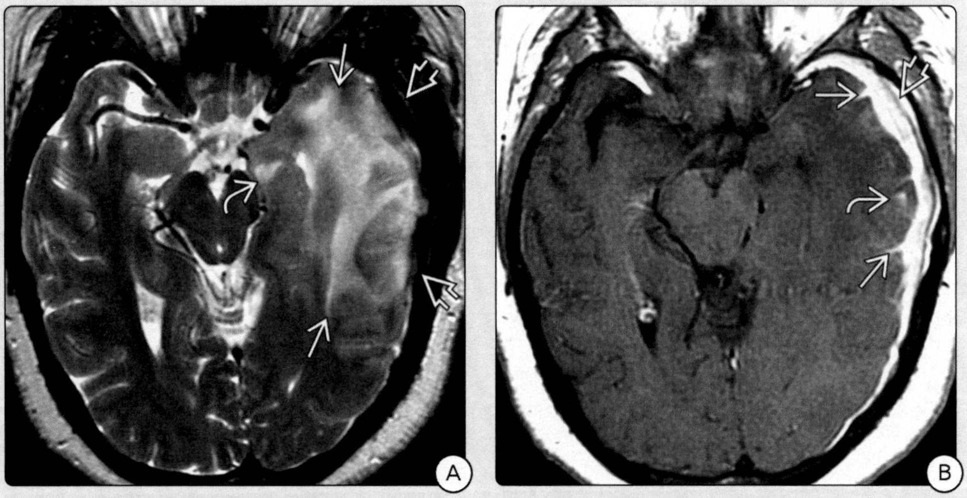

(15-50A) Axial T2WI in a 44y woman with worsening headaches, diplopia shows extensive edema in enlarged left temporal lobe with early uncal, hippocampal herniation. Very hypointense dural thickening is along entire surface of middle cranial fossa. (15-50B) Axial T1 C+ shows intense dura-arachnoid thickening and enhancement. Note involvement of underlying sulci with some parenchymal enhancement.

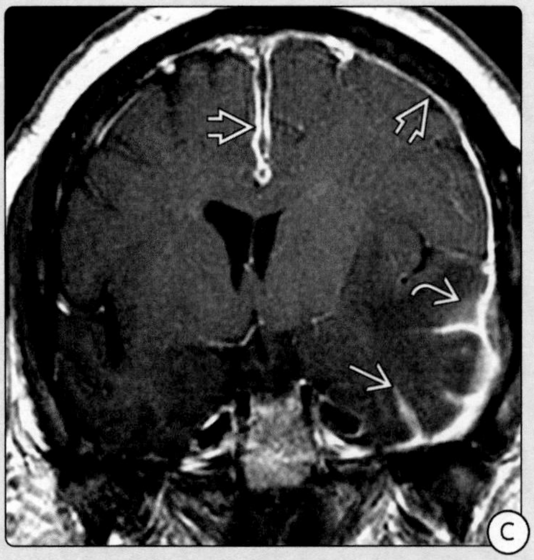

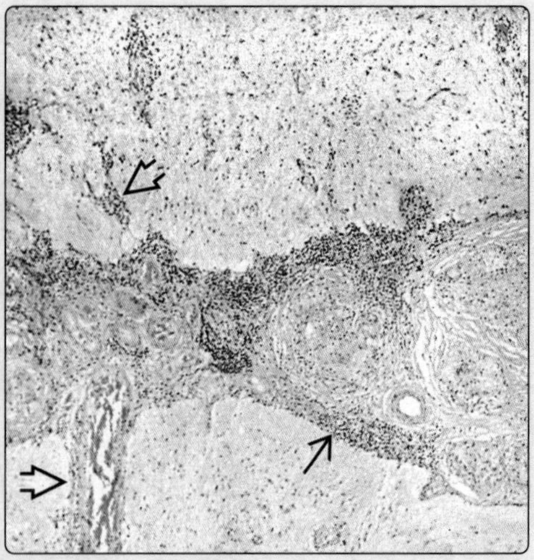

(15-50C) Coronal T1 C+ shows enhanced thickened pia. Extensive dura-arachnoid thickening and enhancement in underlying parenchyma are apparent. Biopsy proved neurosarcoid with brain invasion. (15-51) Photomicrograph of another case has extensive pial infiltration by noncaseating sarcoid granulomas. Note extension along penetrating perivascular spaces into brain parenchyma. (Courtesy S. Aydin, MD.)

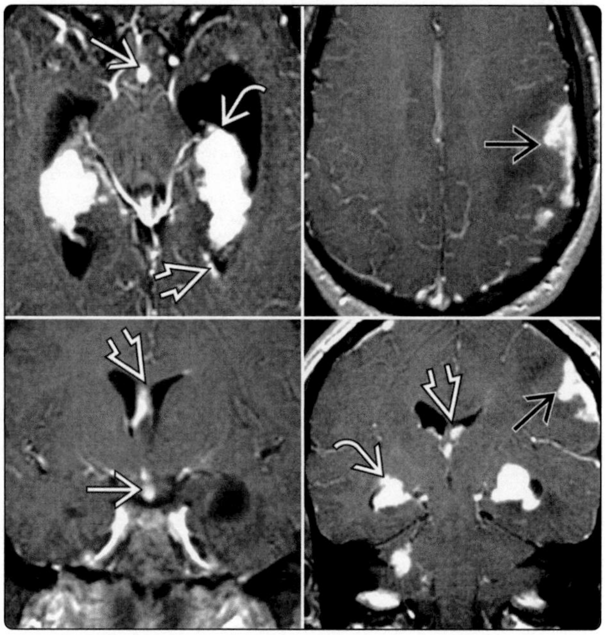

(15-52) Collage of T1 C+ scans shows neurosarcoidosis with involvement of the infundibulum, choroid plexus, ependyma, and meninges.

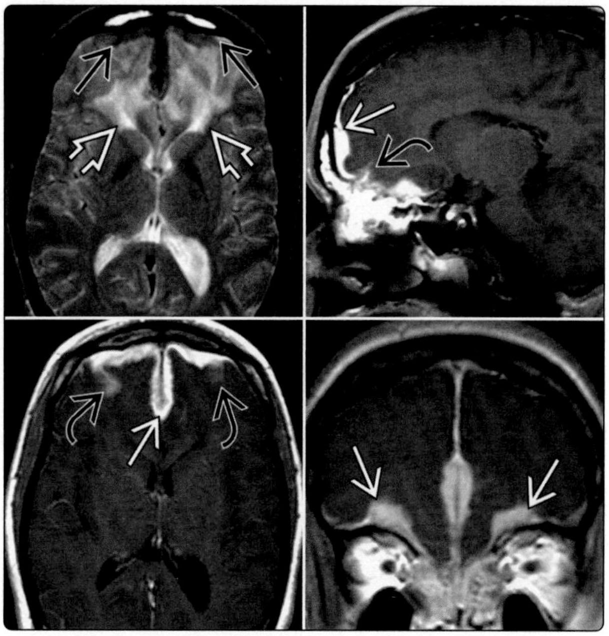

(15-53) Neurosarcoidosis with dura-arachnoid thickening is hypointense on T2WI and enhances strongly and uniformly. Parenchymal extension along perivascular spaces causes edema and enhancement.

Sarcoidosis involving the calvaria or skull base is uncommon. Well-circumscribed "punched-out" lesions with nonsclerotic margins can be seen on bone CT.

MR Findings. NS is isointense with brain on T1WI and hyperintense relative to CSF. Sulci filled with leptomeningeal infiltrates appear effaced. Dura-based masses resemble meningiomas, so large lesions sometimes create a distinct CSF-vascular "cleft" between the lesion and the brain. More often, the subarachnoid space is filled, and the border between the sarcoid and brain is indistinct.

Signal intensity on T2 depends on the amount of fibrocollagenous material present. Longstanding dural lesions are relatively hypointense. Parenchymal infiltration along the perivascular spaces causes a vasculitis-like reaction with edema, mass effect, and hyperintensity on T2/FLAIR.

The most common finding on T1 C+ scans is nodular or diffuse pial thickening, found in approximately one-third to one-half of all cases **(15-49)**.

Half of NS patients eventually develop parenchymal disease. Hypothalamic and infundibular thickening with intense enhancement is seen in 5-10% of cases. Multifocal nodular enhancing masses or more diffuse perivascular infiltrates may develop **(15-50)**. Solitary parenchymal or dura-based masses are less common **(15-53)**. In rare cases, coalescing granulomas form a focal expansile mass ("tumefactive" NS).

NS may cause solitary or multifocal thickened enhancing cranial nerves as well as enhancing masses in the ventricles and choroid plexus **(15-52)**.

NEUROSARCOID: IMAGING

Most Common

- Linear/nodular leptomeningeal enhancement
  - Predilection for basilar cisterns
- Parenchymal enhancing lesions
  - Thick enhancing hypothalamus/pituitary stalk, gland
  - Perivascular infiltrating or mass-like lesions
- Cranial nerve enhancement (CN VII, CN II most common)

Less Common

- Solitary or multiple dura-based masses
  - Diffuse/plaque-like or focal mass
- Diffuse/focal nonenhancing T2/FLAIR hyperintensities

Rare But Important

- "Tumefactive" parenchymal masses
- Choroid plexus mass(es)

Differential Diagnosis

The differential diagnosis of NS depends on lesion location. **Meningitis**—especially TB meningitis—can look very similar to NS of the basilar leptomeninges. **Carcinomatous meningitis** can also resemble leptomeningeal NS.

The differential diagnosis of dura-based NS includes **meningioma**, **lymphoma**, and **intracranial inflammatory pseudotumor (IIP)**, whereas hypothalamic/infundibular/pituitary NS may look like **histiocytosis** or lymphocytic **hypophysitis**.

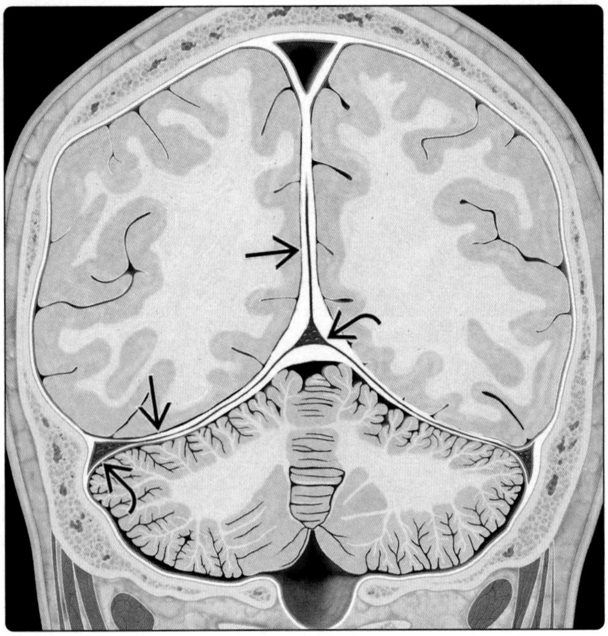

(15-54) Coronal graphic depicts fibrocollagenous falcotentorial thickening around chronically thrombosed dural venous sinuses, the etiology of the so-called "Eiffel by night" sign.

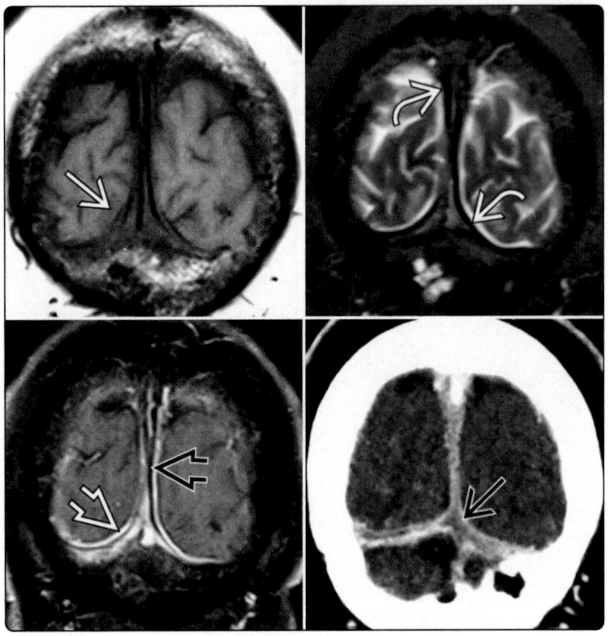

(15-55) Chronic DST with "Eiffel by night sign." Top L: T1WI shows thick falcotentorial dura, which is very hypointense on STIR (R). Bottom L: T1 C+ FS shows enhancing thickened dura around nonenhancing sinus. R: CTV shows chronic DST.

Coalescent parenchymal NS looks like **primary CNS lymphoma** or **metastases**, whereas multifocal enhancing lesions can resemble **multiple sclerosis**, **metastases**, and **intravascular lymphoma**. The differential diagnosis of solitary or multiple cranial NS is broad and includes infection, demyelinating disease, and neoplasm.

Intracranial Inflammatory Pseudotumors

"Intracranial inflammatory pseudotumor" (IIPT) is an umbrella term that encompasses a spectrum of infectious, reactive, and reparative processes. IIPTs have variously been known as idiopathic hypertrophic pachymeningopathy, plasma cell granulomas, and inflammatory myofibroblastic tumors.

If their etiology is unknown, IIPTs are designated as "idiopathic" although a growing number of these lesions now have known causes such as **chronic dural sinus thrombosis, inflammatory myofibroblastic tumor**, and **IgG4-related disease (see below).**

Grossly, IIPTs can exhibit focal or diffuse dura-arachnoid thickening. IIPTs are firm, yellowish, and typically exhibit a somewhat lobulated or nodular surface.

Histopathologically, IIPTs are benign nonneoplastic mass-like cellular aggregates that consist of a dense fibroinflammatory infiltrate with a prominent fibrocollagenous stroma and polyclonal (not monoclonal) mononuclear infiltrates. There is no evidence for granuloma, vasculitis, or neoplasm. Inflammatory myofibroblastic tumors (IMTs) consist of dense fibrosis with spindle cell proliferations and a variable lymphoplasmacytic infiltrate.

IIPs can affect any part of the CNS but are typically meninges-based lesions that can be isolated or locally invasive. A common imaging finding is thickened dura along the posterior falx and tentorium **(15-54)** that is T2 hypointense and exhibits strong enhancement around a central nonenhancing area, an appearance that has been dubbed the "Eiffel by night" sign. Chronic dural sinus occlusion is present in nearly half of all cases and can be identified on CTV or MRV.

Focal mass-like dura-arachnoid thickening is the typical imaging finding with IMTs. IMTs are typically isointense on T1WI, hypointense on T2WI, and enhance strongly and homogeneously on T1 C+ FS sequences **(15-57)**. Approximately 10% of intracranial IMTs invade the adjacent brain.

The differential diagnosis of noninvasive IIP with a dural-based mass includes en plaque **meningioma, neurosarcoid**, and **dural metastases**. Rare entities in the differential diagnosis include **tuberculosis**.

The imaging finding of dura-arachnoid thickening is nonspecific. The differential diagnosis includes **intracranial hypotension**, **prior surgery**, **dural sinus thrombosis**, **chronic subdural hematoma**, and residua of **chronic meningitis** (among the many entities that can cause this appearance on imaging studies).

Invasive IIPs behave aggressively and may simulate **malignant neoplasm** or **fungal infection**. Bone CT shows lytic, permeative destruction adjacent to a dural-based soft tissue mass. The definitive diagnosis requires biopsy, as there are no pathognomonic imaging characteristics. IIPs are discussed in detail and extensively illustrated in Chapter 26.

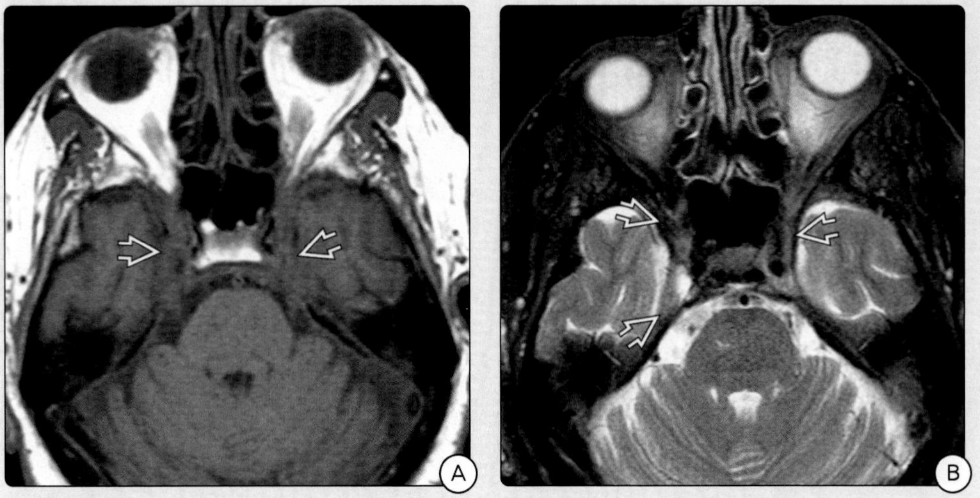

***(15-56A)** Axial T1WI in an 81y man with decreasing vision in his left eye shows isointense mass diffusely infiltrating both cavernous sinuses. **(15-56B)** T2 FS in the same case shows that the infiltrating tissue is slightly hypointense compared with the brain.*

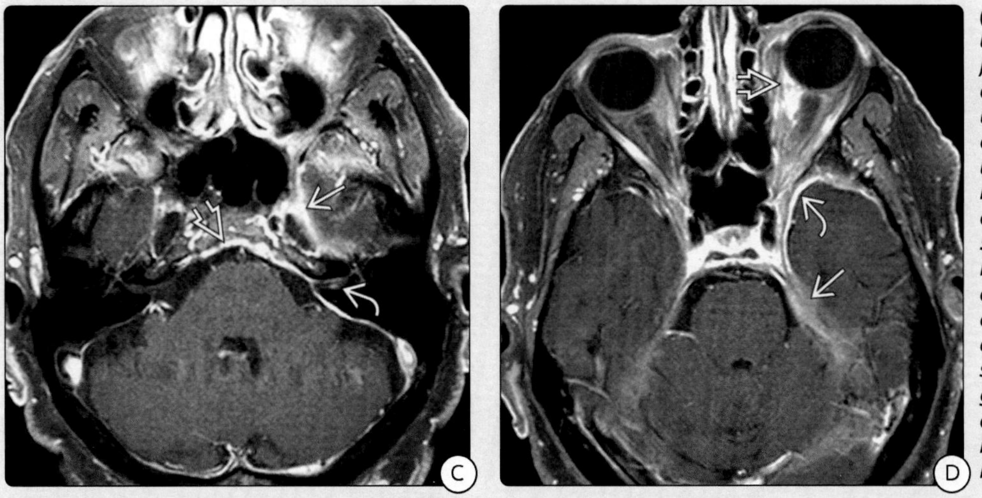

***(15-56C)** T1 C+ FS scan through the posterior fossa shows sheet-like dural thickening along the left cavernous sinus, clivus, and petrous temporal bone, extending into the left internal auditory canal. **(15-56D)** More cephalad T1 C+ FS shows the plaque-like dura-arachnoid thickening along the tentorium and cavernous sinus/left sphenoid wing. The left globe is mildly proptotic, and there is an infiltrating intraconal retrobulbar mass.*

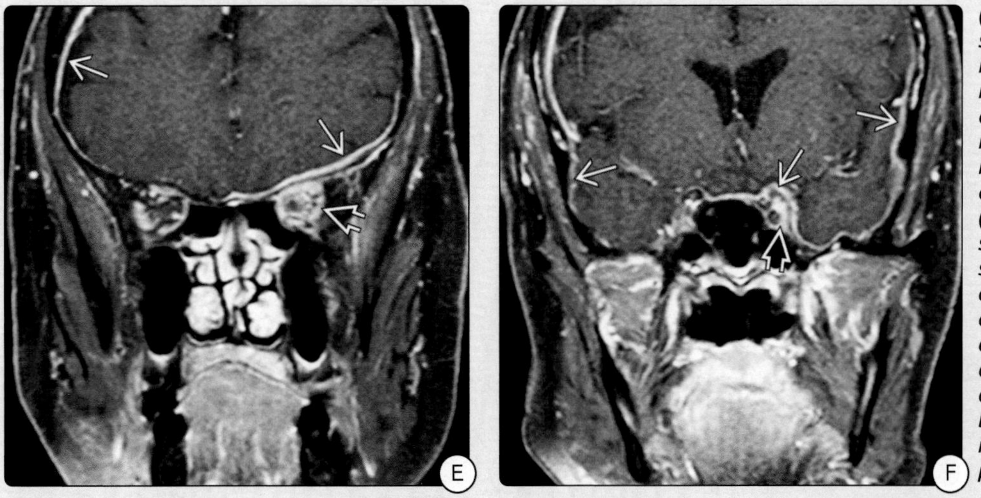

***(15-56E)** Coronal T1 C+ FS shows the enhancing, infiltrating intraconal mass surrounding and encasing the left optic nerve sheath. Note diffuse intracranial dura-arachnoid thickening. **(15-56F)** More posterior scan in the same case shows diffuse dura-arachnoid thickening and infiltrating mass extending through the left orbital apex into the cavernous sinus. This is biopsy-proven inflammatory pseudotumor.*

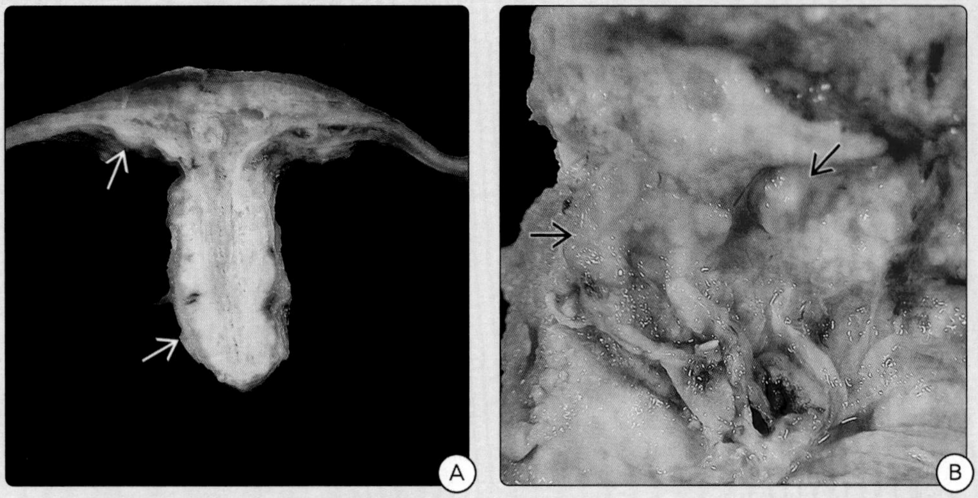

(15-57A) *Gross autopsy of inflammatory myofibroblastic tumor shows nodular thickening along the falx and adjacent dura →.* ***(15-57B)*** *Close-up view of the dissected dura shows the firm, nodular thickening → along its surface.*

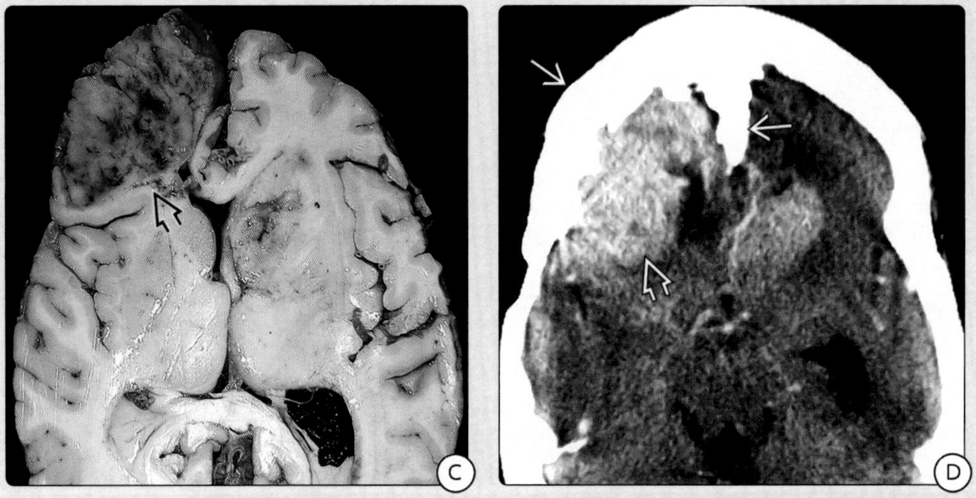

(15-57C) *Autopsy section shows dural-based mass ⇒.* ***(15-57D)*** *CECT scan shows thickened, irregular skull → with an underlying enhancing dural-based mass → that appears to be invading the adjacent brain.*

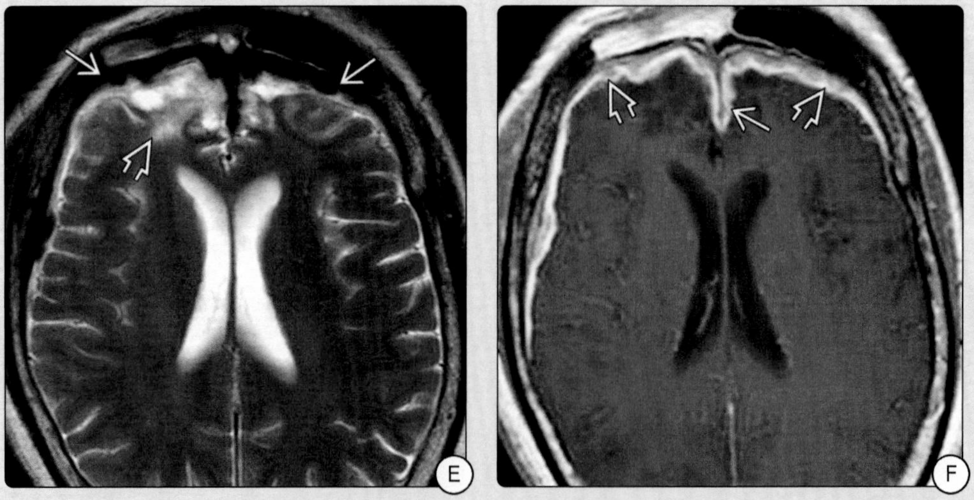

(15-57E) *T2WI shows a nodular, very hypointense mass along the dura →. Note hyperintensity in the underlying frontal lobes →, suggesting parenchymal invasion by the dural-based mass.* ***(15-57F)*** *T1 C+ MR shows the nodular, thickened dura extending around the anterior falx → and around both frontal lobes →. Invasive inflammatory myofibroblastic tumor was diagnosed at autopsy. Compare to gross findings.*

IgG4-Related Disease

IgG4-related disease (IgG4-RD) is a multisystem, multifocal fibrosclerotic inflammatory disorder that is primarily tumefactive or "mass-like," less often diffusely infiltrative.

IgG4-RD most commonly involves the lung and retroperitoneal spaces. The most common head and neck sites are the orbit and salivary glands. Sinonasal IgG4-RD can present as a permeative destructive, locally invasive mass that mimics sinonasal lymphoma. Some cases exhibit bone destruction with invasion of the orbit or intracranial compartment.

Isolated intracranial IgG4-RD has been described in pituitary gland and stalk, cranial nerves, cavernous sinus, and dura **(15-58)** **(15-60)**.

The major differential diagnosis of orbit IgG4-RD is **orbital lymphoproliferative disorders**. These include IIP, benign lymphoepithelial lesion, mucosa-associated lymphoid tissue (MALT), and diffuse large B-cell lymphoma.

Chronic Inflammatory Demyelinating Polyneuropathy

A rare type of localized autoimmune demyelinating disease, **chronic inflammatory demyelinating polyneuropathy (CIDP)**, is characterized by repeated episodes of demyelination and remyelination with "onion bulb" hypertrophy of the affected nerves. CIDP usually affects spinal and peripheral nerve roots but occasionally involves cranial nerves.

CIDP is characterized by chronic progressive or relapsing symmetric sensorimotor involvement. Clinically, CIDP is often initially diagnosed as Guillain-Barré syndrome, Bickerstaff encephalitis, or multiple sclerosis.

Diffuse thickening with striking hyperintensity on T2/STIR and mild to moderate enhancement of one or more cranial nerves are the typical imaging manifestations of intracranial CIDP **(15-59)**. Parenchymal demyelinating foci consistent with multiple sclerosis are commonly—but not invariably—present.

The imaging differential diagnosis of intracranial CIDP includes the hereditary neuropathies such as **Charcot-Marie-Tooth** disease. Other disorders that can mimic CIDP include **neurosarcoidosis** and cranial nerve infiltration secondary to **lymphoma** or **metastases**. **Multiple sclerosis, Lyme disease**, and **acute disseminated encephalomyelitis** (ADEM) can all cause cranial nerve enhancement but typically do not cause the striking symmetric enlargement that characterizes CIDP.

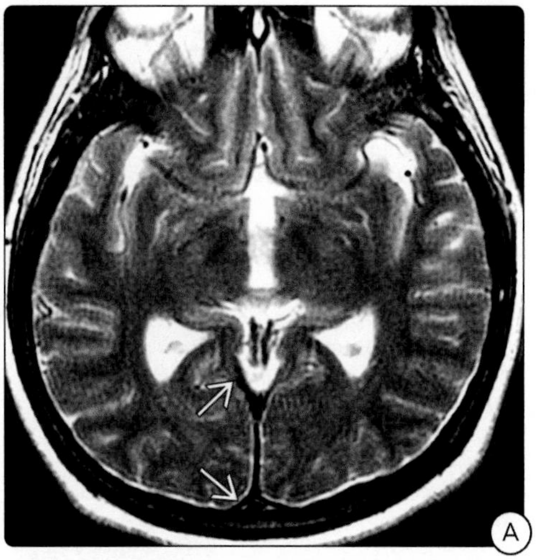

***(15-58A)** T2WI in a 51y woman with tinnitus shows hypointense falcotentorial dural thickening ➡.*

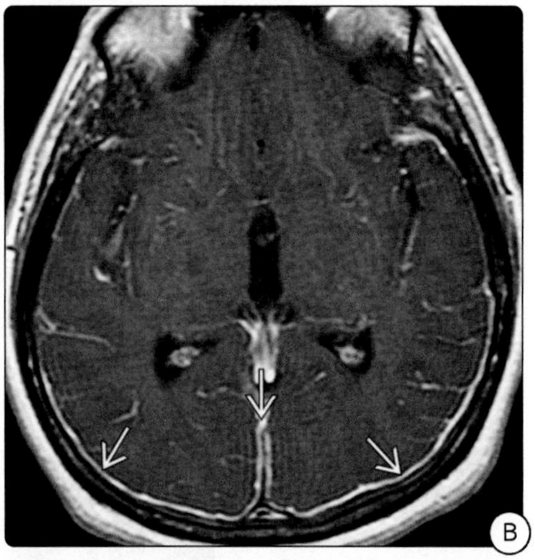

***(15-58B)** T1 C+ MR shows linear falcotentorial dura-arachnoid thickening ➡.*

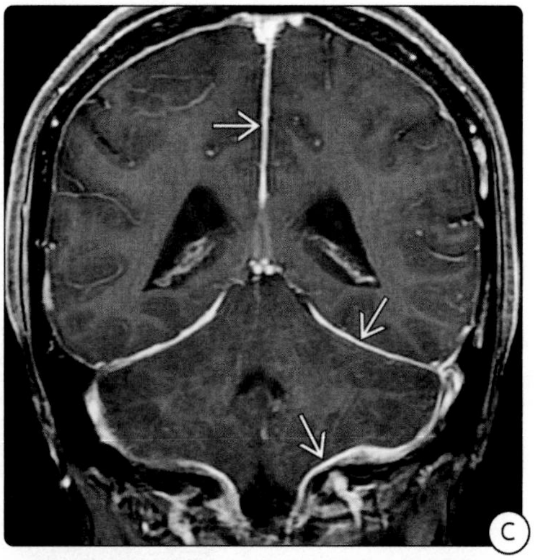

***(15-58C)** Coronal shows dural thickening ➡. Biopsy showed fibroinflammatory change. Restaining 10 years later showed IgG4-RD.*

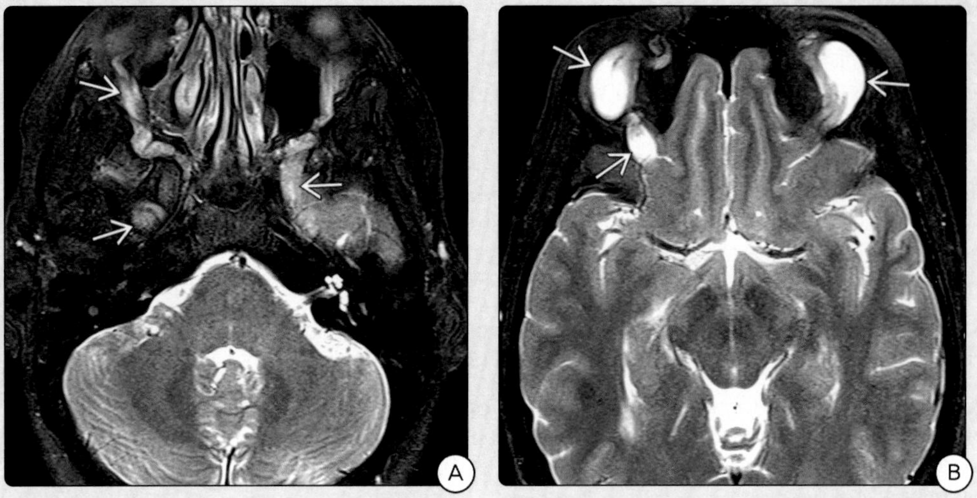

(15-59A) *Chronic inflammatory demyelinating polyneuropathy (CIDP) in a 23y woman with bilateral trigeminal nerve deficits shows striking hyperintensity and fusiform enlargement of both CN Vs ➡ on this T2-weighted fat-suppressed scan.* ***(15-59B)*** *Image through the midbrain and upper orbits in the same patient shows hugely enlarged, markedly hyperintense ophthalmic nerves ➡.*

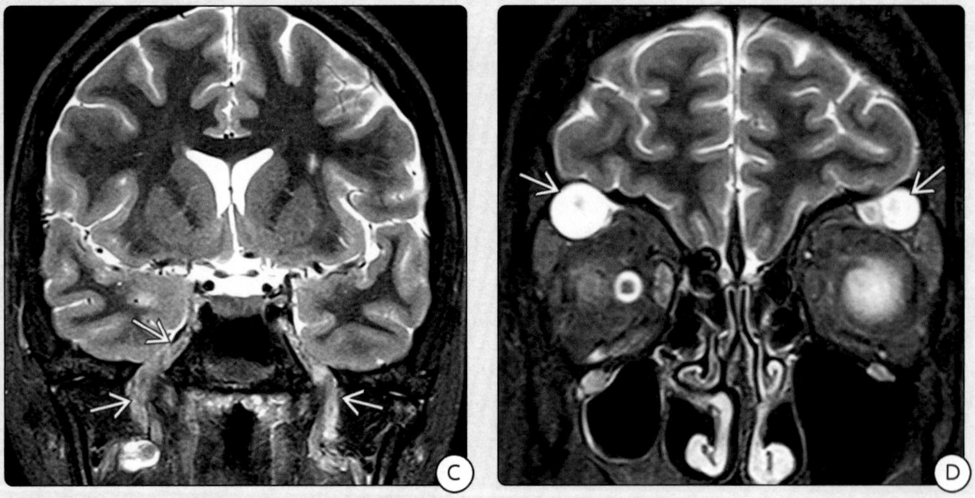

(15-59C) *Coronal STIR scan in the same patient shows fusiform rope-like enlargement and moderate hyperintensity of both mandibular nerves, extending from the Meckel cave into the deep face ➡.* ***(15-59D)*** *Coronal STIR scan through the orbits shows the massively but symmetrically enlarged hyperintense ophthalmic nerves ➡.*

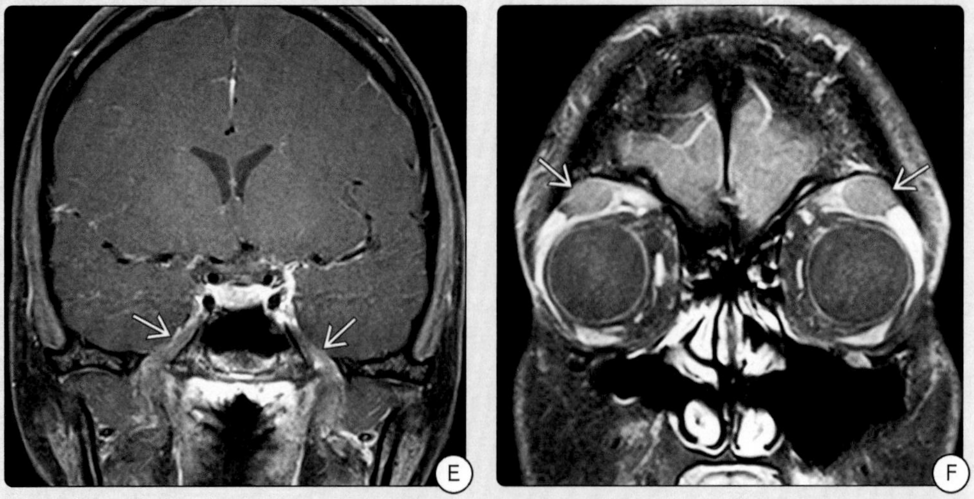

(15-59E) *Coronal T1 C+ FS shows that the enlarged trigeminal nerves enhance moderately ➡ but somewhat heterogeneously.* ***(15-59F)*** *Coronal T1 C+ FS shows mild to moderate enhancement of both ophthalmic divisions of CNV ➡. The patient had been diagnosed with MS, but no brain lesions were identified. CNS CIDP was confirmed at biopsy.*

Selected References

Multiple Sclerosis and Variants

Filippi M et al: MRI criteria for the diagnosis of multiple sclerosis: MAGNIMS consensus guidelines. Lancet Neurol. 15(3):292-303, 2016

Frederick MC et al: Tumefactive demyelinating lesions in multiple sclerosis and associated disorders. Curr Neurol Neurosci Rep. 16(3):26, 2016

Golan D et al: Shifting paradigms in multiple sclerosis: from disease-specific, through population-specific toward patient-specific. Curr Opin Neurol. 29(3):354-61, 2016

Ozgen H et al: Oligodendroglial membrane dynamics in relation to myelin biogenesis. Cell Mol Life Sci. 73(17):3291-310, 2016

Grigoriadis N et al: A basic overview of multiple sclerosis immunopathology. Eur J Neurol. 22 Suppl 2:3-13, 2015

Karussis D: The diagnosis of multiple sclerosis and the various related demyelinating syndromes: a critical review. J Autoimmun. 48-49:134-42, 2014

Multiple Sclerosis

Brownlee WJ et al: Diagnosis of multiple sclerosis: progress and challenges. Lancet. 389(10076):1336-1346, 2017

Dekker I et al: Brain and spinal cord MR imaging features in multiple sclerosis and variants. Neuroimaging Clin N Am. 27(2):205-227, 2017

Parnell GP et al: The multiple sclerosis (MS) genetic risk factors indicate both acquired and innate immune cell subsets contribute to MS pathogenesis and identify novel therapeutic opportunities. Front Immunol. 8:425, 2017

Sadovnick AD et al: Genetic modifiers of multiple sclerosis progression, severity and onset. Clin Immunol. 180:100-105, 2017

Tenembaum SN: Pediatric multiple sclerosis: distinguishing clinical and MR imaging features. Neuroimaging Clin N Am. 27(2):229-250, 2017

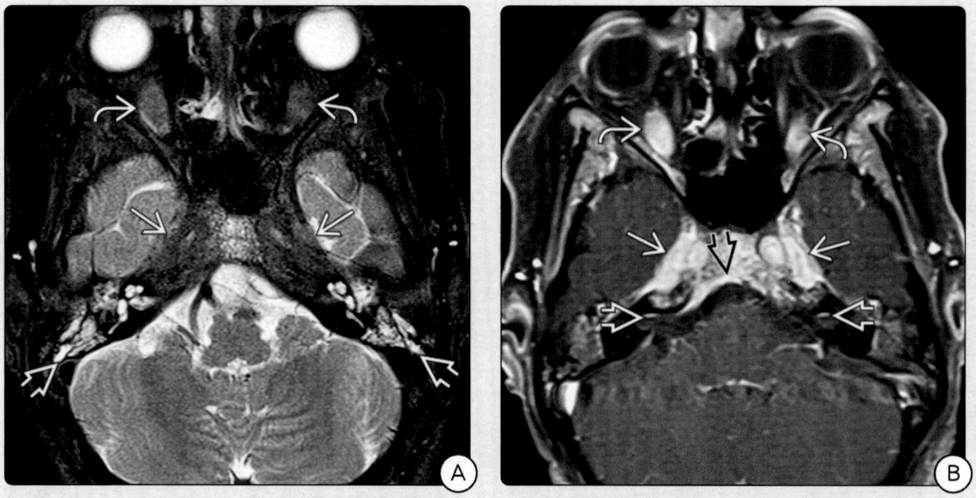

***(15-60A)** Axial T2 FS MR in a 26y woman with headache, proptosis, and right CN VI palsy shows hypointense diffusely infiltrating mass in both cavernous sinuses and orbital apices. Bilateral serous otitis media is present. **(15-60B)** T1 C+ FS in the same case shows that the cavernous sinus and orbital apex masses enhance strongly. Also note clival dura-arachnoid thickening with linear enhancement in both internal auditory canals.*

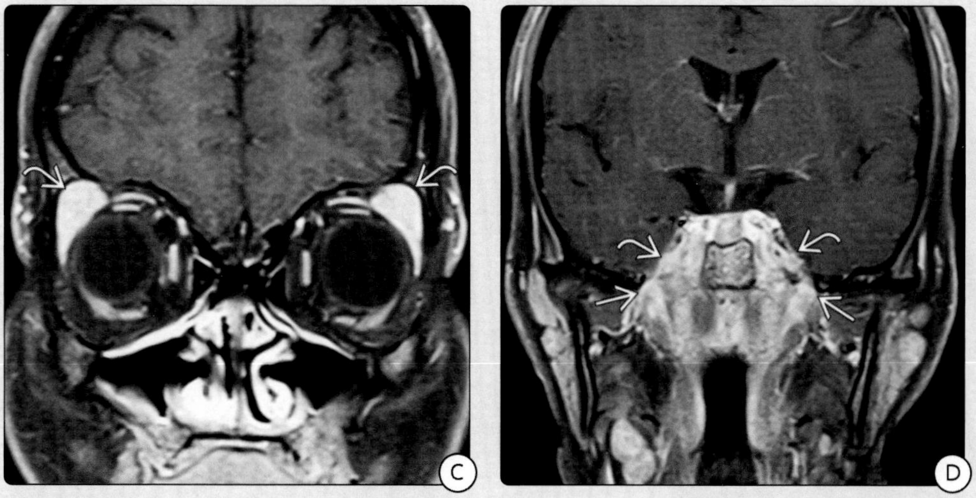

***(15-60C)** Coronal T1 C+ FS shows markedly enlarged, intensely enhancing lacrimal glands. **(15-60D)** More posterior T1 C+ FS scan shows that the cavernous sinus infiltrating mass involves both Meckel caves and extends through the foramen ovale into the nasopharynx, obstructing the eustachian tubes. This is biopsy-proven IgG4-related disease (IgG4-RD).*

Sarbu N et al: White matter diseases with radiologic-pathologic correlation. Radiographics. 36(5):1426-47, 2016

Multiple Sclerosis Variants

Dekker I et al: Brain and spinal cord MR imaging features in multiple sclerosis and variants. Neuroimaging Clin N Am. 27(2):205-227, 2017

Maraş Genç H et al: Long-term clinical and radiologic follow-up of Schilder's disease. Mult Scler Relat Disord. 13:47-51, 2017

Frederick MC et al: Tumefactive demyelinating lesions in multiple sclerosis and associated disorders. Curr Neurol Neurosci Rep. 16(3):26, 2016

Hardy TA et al: Atypical inflammatory demyelinating syndromes of the CNS. Lancet Neurol. 15(9):967-981, 2016

Sarbu N et al: White matter diseases with radiologic-pathologic correlation. Radiographics. 36(5):1426-47, 2016

Nunes JC et al: The most fulminant course of the Marburg variant of multiple sclerosis-autopsy findings. Mult Scler. 21(4):485-7, 2015

Hardy TA et al: Baló's concentric sclerosis. Lancet Neurol. 13(7):740-6, 2014

Rahmlow MR et al: Fulminant demyelinating diseases. Neurohospitalist. 3(2):81-91, 2013

Postinfection and Postimmunization Demyelination

Acute Disseminated Encephalomyelitis

Abu Libdeh A et al: Acute disseminated encephalomyelitis: a gray distinction. Pediatr Neurol. 68:64-67, 2017

Kaunzner UW et al: An acute disseminated encephalomyelitis-like illness in the elderly: Neuroimaging and neuropathology findings. J Neuroimaging. 27(3):306-311, 2017

Wong YY et al: Evolution of MRI abnormalities in paediatric acute disseminated encephalomyelitis. Eur J Paediatr Neurol. 21(2):300-304, 2017

Berzero G et al: Diagnosis and therapy of acute disseminated encephalomyelitis and its variants. Expert Rev Neurother. 16(1):83-101, 2016

Koelman DL et al: Acute disseminated encephalomyelitis in 228 patients: a retrospective, multicenter US study. Neurology. 86(22):2085-93, 2016

Zhu TH et al: Demyelinating disorders secondary to TNF-inhibitor therapy for the treatment of psoriasis: A review. J Dermatolog Treat. 1-8, 2016

Bevan CJ et al: Fulminant demyelinating diseases of the central nervous system. Semin Neurol. 35(6):656-66, 2015

Rahmlow MR et al: Fulminant demyelinating diseases. Neurohospitalist. 3(2):81-91, 2013

Acute Hemorrhagic Leukoencephalitis

Berzero G et al: Diagnosis and therapy of acute disseminated encephalomyelitis and its variants. Expert Rev Neurother. 16(1):83-101, 2016

Koelman DL et al: Acute disseminated encephalomyelitis in 228 patients: a retrospective, multicenter US study. Neurology. 86(22):2085-93, 2016

Nabi S et al: Weston-Hurst syndrome: a rare fulminant form of acute disseminated encephalomyelitis (ADEM). BMJ Case Rep. 2016, 2016

Ramanathan S et al: Anti-MOG antibody: the history, clinical phenotype, and pathogenicity of a serum biomarker for demyelination. Autoimmun Rev. 15(4):307-24, 2016

Bevan CJ et al: Fulminant demyelinating diseases of the central nervous system. Semin Neurol. 35(6):656-66, 2015

Robinson CA et al: Early and widespread injury of astrocytes in the absence of demyelination in acute haemorrhagic leukoencephalitis. Acta Neuropathol Commun. 2:52, 2014

Autoimmune Encephalitis

Autoimmune Encephalitis

Celicanin M et al: Autoimmune encephalitis associated with voltage-gated potassium channels-complex and leucine-rich glioma-inactivated 1 antibodies - a national cohort study. Eur J Neurol. ePub, 2017

Kalman B: Autoimmune encephalitides: a broadening field of treatable conditions. Neurologist. 22(1):1-13, 2017

Kelley BP et al: Autoimmune encephalitis: pathophysiology and imaging review of an overlooked diagnosis. AJNR Am J Neuroradiol. 38(6):1070-1078, 2017

Varley J et al: Autoantibody-mediated diseases of the CNS: structure, dysfunction and therapy. Neuropharmacology. ePub, 2017

Brenton JN et al: Antibody-mediated autoimmune encephalitis in childhood. Pediatr Neurol. 60:13-23, 2016

Graus F et al: A clinical approach to diagnosis of autoimmune encephalitis. Lancet Neurol. 15(4):391-404, 2016

Lancaster E: The diagnosis and treatment of autoimmune encephalitis. J Clin Neurol. 12(1):1-13, 2016

Guillain-Barré Spectrum Disorders

Ishii J et al: Recurrent Guillain-Barré syndrome, Miller Fisher syndrome and Bickerstaff brainstem encephalitis. J Neurol Sci. 364:59-64, 2016

Renaud M et al: Chronic Bickerstaff's encephalitis with cognitive impairment, a reality? BMC Neurol. 14:99, 2014

Neuromyelitis Optica Spectrum Disorder

Akaishi T et al: Neuromyelitis optica spectrum disorders. Neuroimaging Clin N Am. 27(2):251-265, 2017

Anadure R et al: Recurrent longitudinally extensive myelitis and aquaporin-4 seronegativity - the expanding spectrum of neuromyelitis optica. J Clin Diagn Res. 11(4):OD05-OD07, 2017

Peschl P et al: Myelin oligodendrocyte glycoprotein: deciphering a target in inflammatory demyelinating diseases. Front Immunol. 8:529, 2017

Ran Y et al: Anti-NMDAR encephalitis followed by seropositive neuromyelitis optica spectrum disorder: a case report and literature review. Clin Neurol Neurosurg. 155:75-82, 2017

Weinshenker BG et al: Neuromyelitis spectrum disorders. Mayo Clin Proc. 92(4):663-679, 2017

Hinson SR et al: Autoimmune AQP4 channelopathies and neuromyelitis optica spectrum disorders. Handb Clin Neurol. 133:377-403, 2016

Hyun JW et al: Evaluation of the 2015 diagnostic criteria for neuromyelitis optica spectrum disorder. Neurology. 86(19):1772-9, 2016

Kleiter I et al: Neuromyelitis optica: evaluation of 871 attacks and 1,153 treatment courses. Ann Neurol. 79(2):206-16, 2016

Sepúlveda M et al: Neuromyelitis optica spectrum disorders: comparison according to the phenotype and serostatus. Neurol Neuroimmunol Neuroinflamm. 3(3):e225, 2016

Wingerchuk DM et al: International consensus diagnostic criteria for neuromyelitis optica spectrum disorders. Neurology. 85(2):177-89, 2015

Susac Syndrome

Kleffner I et al: Diagnostic criteria for Susac syndrome. J Neurol Neurosurg Psychiatry. 87(12):1287-1295, 2016

Kothari N et al: Branched retinal artery occlusions and Susac syndrome. JAMA Neurol. 73(7):884-5, 2016

Vishnevskia-Dai V et al: Susac syndrome: clinical characteristics, clinical classification, and long-term prognosis. Medicine (Baltimore). 95(43):e5223, 2016

Vodopivec I et al: Clinical features, diagnostic findings, and treatment of Susac syndrome: a case series. J Neurol Sci. 357(1-2):50-7, 2015

CLIPPERS

Blaabjerg M et al: Widespread inflammation in CLIPPERS syndrome indicated by autopsy and ultra-high-field 7T MRI. Neurol Neuroimmunol Neuroinflamm. 3(3):e226, 2016

Taieb G et al: Punctate and curvilinear gadolinium enhancing lesions in the brain: a practical approach. Neuroradiology. 58(3):221-35, 2016

Dudesek A et al: CLIPPERS: chronic lymphocytic inflammation with pontine perivascular enhancement responsive to steroids. Review of an increasingly recognized entity within the spectrum of inflammatory central nervous system disorders. Clin Exp Immunol. 175(3):385-96, 2014

Simon NG et al: Expanding the clinical, radiological and neuropathological phenotype of chronic lymphocytic inflammation with pontine perivascular enhancement responsive to steroids (CLIPPERS). J Neurol Neurosurg Psychiatry. 83(1):15-22, 2012

Inflammatory-Like Disorders

Neurosarcoidosis

Ait-Oufella H et al: Leptomeningeal infiltration, the hallmark of neurosarcoidosis. Am J Med. ePub, 2017

Balevic SJ et al: Islands of inflammation: neurosarcoidosis. Am J Med. 130(2):157-160, 2017

Ibitoye RT et al: Neurosarcoidosis: a clinical approach to diagnosis and management. J Neurol. 264(5):1023-1028, 2017

Fritz D et al: Clinical features, treatment and outcome in neurosarcoidosis: systematic review and meta-analysis. BMC Neurol. 16(1):220, 2016

Leonhard SE et al: Neurosarcoidosis in a tertiary referral center: a cross-sectional cohort study. Medicine (Baltimore). 95(14):e3277, 2016

Rao R et al: Neurosarcoidosis in pediatric patients: a case report and review of isolated and systemic neurosarcoidosis. Pediatr Neurol. 63:45-52, 2016

Shimizu K et al: Isolated neurosarcoidosis presenting with multiple cranial nerve palsies. Surg Neurol Int. 7:44, 2016

Bagnato F et al: Neurosarcoidosis: diagnosis, therapy and biomarkers. Expert Rev Neurother. 15(5):533-48, 2015

Intracranial Inflammatory Pseudotumors

Li J et al: Role of IgG4 serology in identifying common orbital lymphoproliferative disorders. Int J Ophthalmol. 9(2):275-7, 2016

Dash GK et al: Clinico-radiological spectrum and outcome in idiopathic hypertrophic pachymeningitis. J Neurol Sci. 350(1-2):51-60, 2015

Desai SV et al: Sinonasal and ventral skull base inflammatory pseudotumor: a systematic review. Laryngoscope. 125(4):813-21, 2015

Okano A et al: Intracranial inflammatory pseudotumors associated with immunoglobulin G4-related disease mimicking multiple meningiomas: a case report and review of the literature. World Neurosurg. 83(6):1181.e1-4, 2015

Thomas B et al: 'Eiffel-by-Night': a new MR sign demonstrating reactivation in idiopathic hypertrophic pachymeningitis. Neuroradiol J. 20(2):194-5, 2007

IgG4-Related Disease

Thompson A et al: Imaging of IgG4-related disease of the head and neck. Clin Radiol. ePub, 2017

Rice CM et al: Intracranial spread of IgG4-related disease via skull base foramina. Pract Neurol. 16(3):240-2, 2016

Wick CC et al: IgG4-related disease causing facial nerve and optic nerve palsies: case report and literature review. Am J Otolaryngol. 37(6):567-571, 2016

Joshi D et al: Cerebral involvement in IgG4-related disease. Clin Med. 15(2):130-4, 2015

Toyoda K et al: MR imaging of IgG4-related disease in the head and neck and brain. AJNR Am J Neuroradiol. 33(11):2136-9, 2012

Chronic Inflammatory Demyelinating Polyneuropathy

Grimm A et al: Giant nerves in chronic inflammatory polyradiculoneuropathy. Muscle Nerve. 55(2):285-289, 2017

Rajabally YA et al: Hereditary and inflammatory neuropathies: a review of reported associations, mimics and misdiagnoses. J Neurol Neurosurg Psychiatry. 87(10):1051-60, 2016

Abe Y et al: Characteristic MRI features of chronic inflammatory demyelinating polyradiculoneuropathy. Brain Dev. 37(9):894-6, 2015

Al-Bustani N et al: Recurrent isolated sixth nerve palsy in relapsing-remitting chronic inflammatory demyelinating polyneuropathy. J Clin Neuromuscul Dis. 17(1):18-21, 2015

Okuzumi A et al: Ophthalmic nerve hypertrophy in chronic inflammatory demyelinating polyradiculoneuropathy. Neurology. 82(17):1566-7, 2014

Kale HA et al: Magnetic resonance imaging findings in chronic inflammatory demyelinating polyneuropathy with intracranial findings and enhancing, thickened cranial and spinal nerves. Australas Radiol. 51 Spec No, 2007

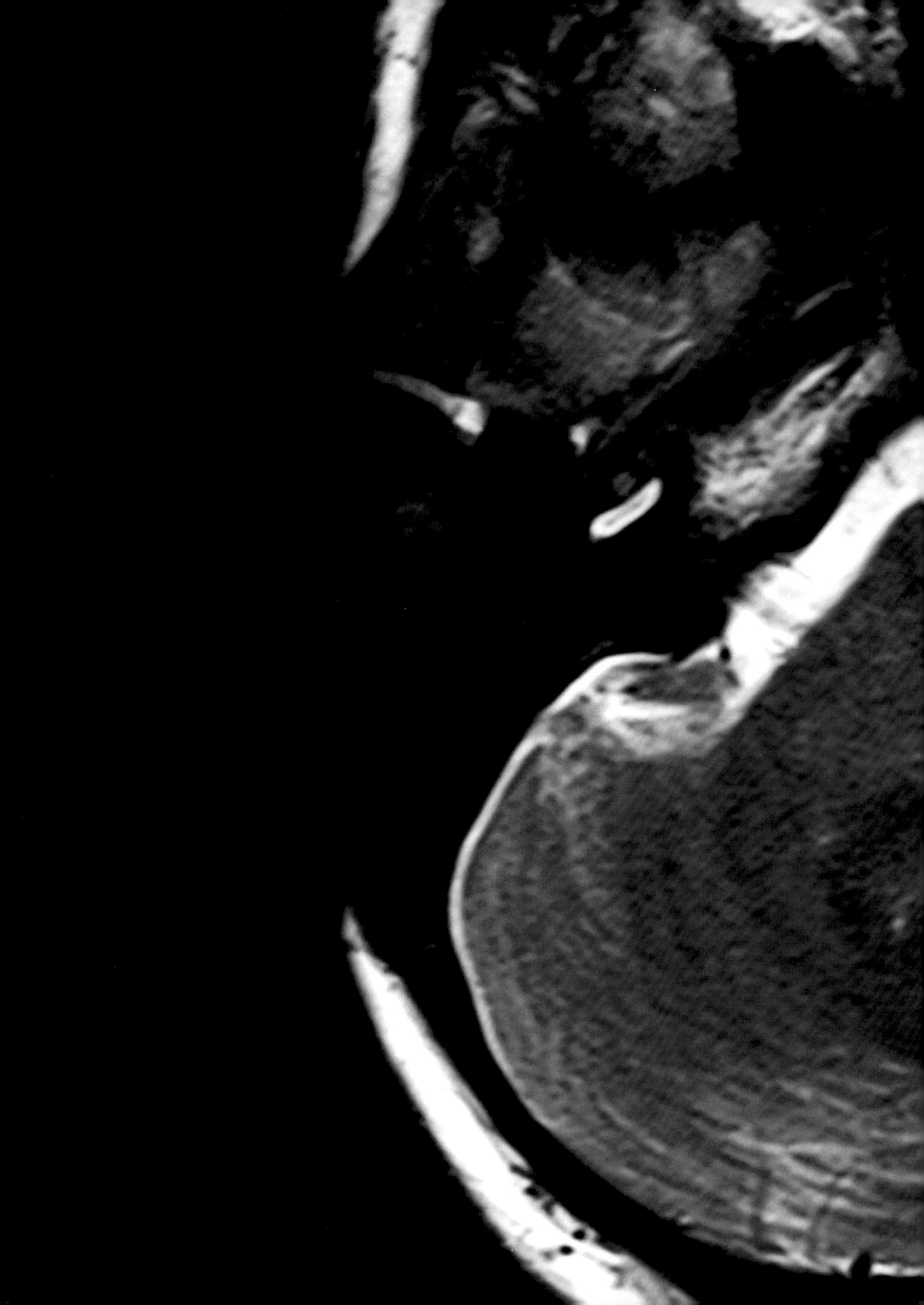

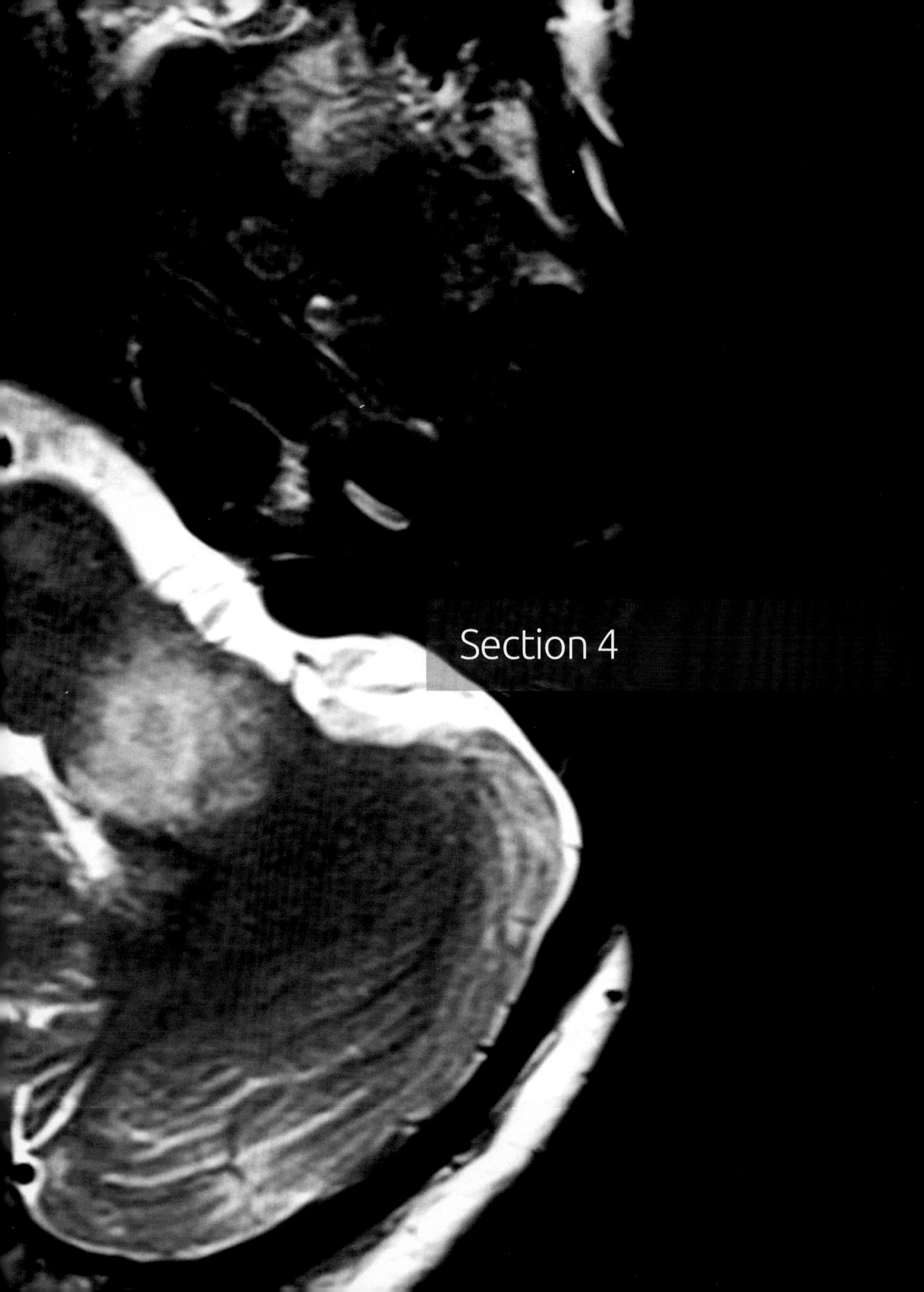

Section 4

Section 4

Neoplasms, Cysts, and Tumor-Like Lesions

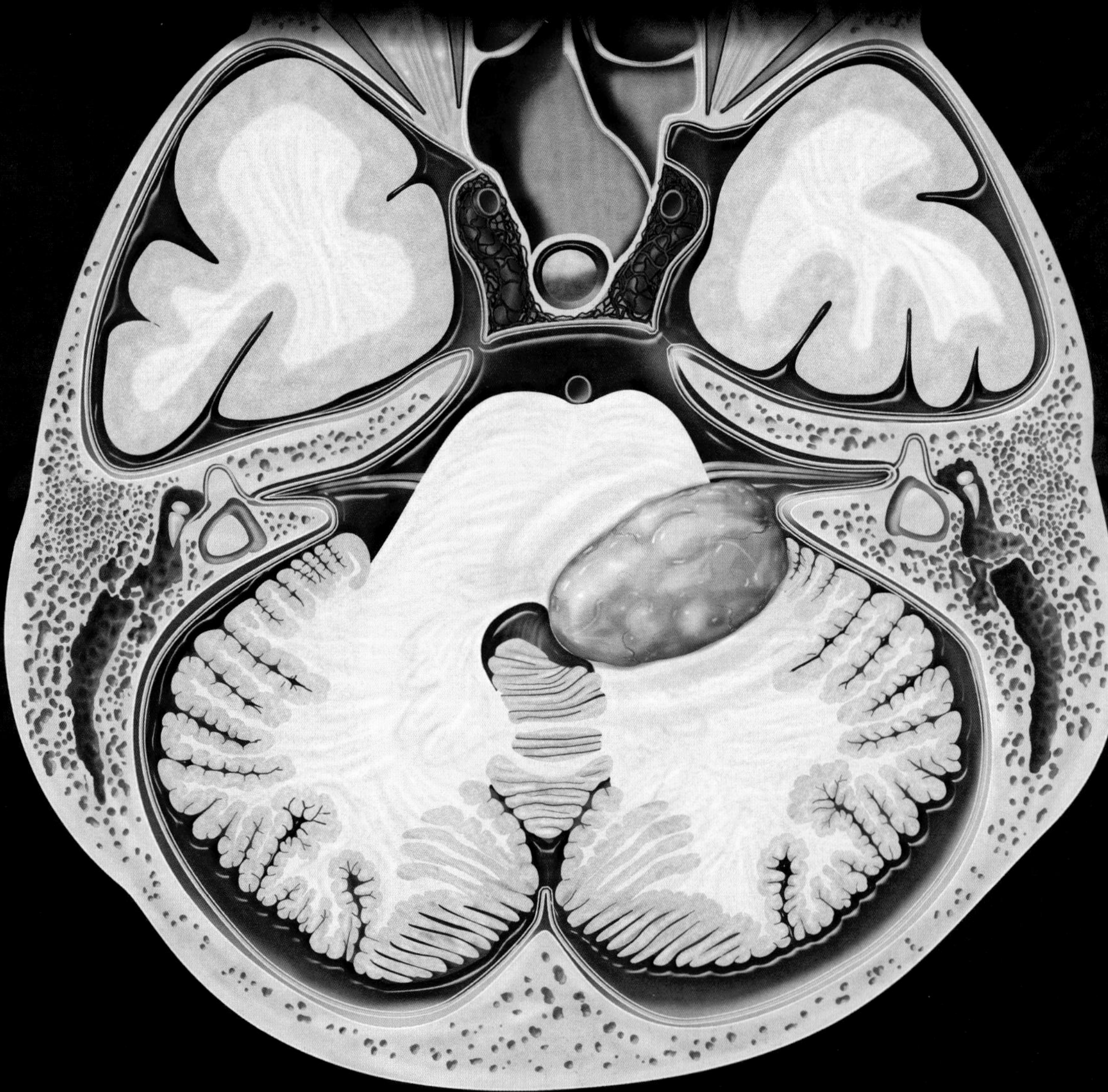

Introduction to Neoplasms, Cysts, and Tumor-Like Lesions

The most widely accepted classification of brain neoplasms is sponsored by the World Health Organization (WHO). Since 1986, a working group of world-renowned neuropathologists has convened approximately every 7 years for an editorial and consensus update conference on brain tumor classification and grading. The results are then published by the International Agency for Research on Cancer (IARC) as the WHO Classification of Tumours of the Central Nervous System.

The fourth edition was published in 2007 and added eight new tumor entities plus four new variants to the existing classification schema. The 2016 CNS WHO update—the version followed in this text—represents a dramatic paradigm shift in the way brain tumors are classified.

All prior systems were based on the concept that tumors could be classified according to their phenotypic similarities with different putative cells of origin. These were largely microscopic features and immunohistochemical (IHC) expression of lineage-associated proteins. They were then graded on a scale of I-IV according to their observed level of differentiation. Hence the lineage of astrocytomas was presumed to be from astrocytes, oligodendrogliomas from oligodendrocytes, etc **(16-1)**.

Rapid progress in elucidating tumor genetics (e.g., data from The Cancer Genome Atlas, genome-wide association studies, and next-generation sequencing panels) has fundamentally altered the classification of CNS neoplasms. Most primary CNS neoplasms are now thought to arise from genetically altered stem cells **(16-2)**. The 2016 WHO integrates both genotypic and phenotypic (i.e., histologic) parameters, incorporating both into the newly updated classification schema.

The increasing availability of immunohistochemical surrogates for identifying molecular genetic alterations in CNS neoplasms makes applying the new 2016 WHO criteria an integral part of modern neuropathology. Familiarity with these new criteria is essential for radiologists and clinical neuroscientists alike.

Classification and Grading of CNS Neoplasms

Historically, brain tumors have been both classified and graded. **Classification** traditionally assigned CNS neoplasms to discrete categories

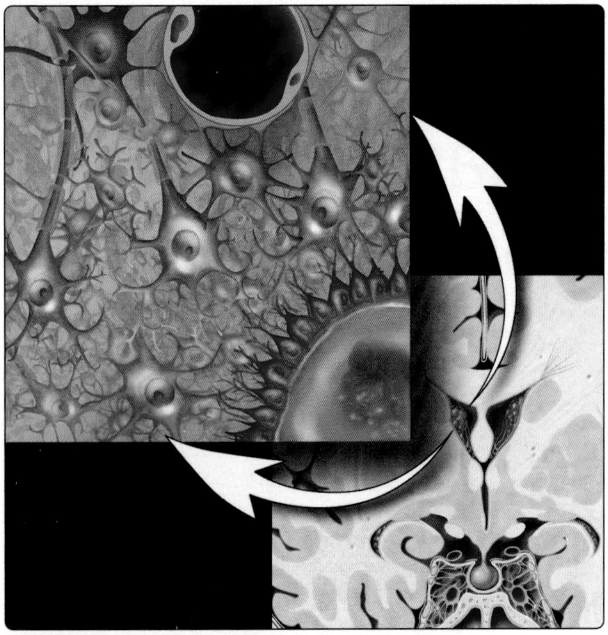

(16-1) The neuropil consists of astrocytes, oligodendrocytes, neurons, microglia, choroid plexus, and ependymal cells. Mature cells of each type were once thought to undergo malignant transformation, producing corresponding neoplasms.

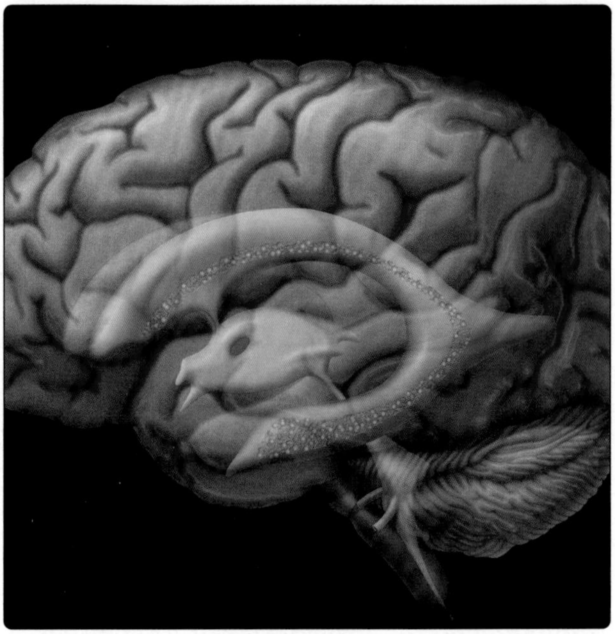

(16-2) Graphic depicts neural stem cells in yellow, shown arising from the subventricular zone just under the ependyma of the lateral ventricles. Primary CNS neoplasms are now thought to arise from these indigenous stem cells and microglia.

based on the histologic similarity of tumor cells to normal or embryonic constituents of the nervous system.

Brain tumor classification is now based on a combination of histology and molecular diagnostics. There are two major ways to identify the genetic signatures of brain tumors: by (1) direct interrogation of the mutated DNA itself or (2) immunohistochemistry, which assesses the *effects* of the mutated genes on proteins.

Direct interrogation by DNA (Sanger) sequencing, PCR amplification, or pyrosequencing is relatively expensive and unavailable at many medical centers, meaning tissue samples must be sent out to reference laboratories.

Immunohistochemistry (IHC) is a convenient, relatively inexpensive way to detect the protein products of specific oncogenic mutations. It is robust, reproducible, and much more widely available as a surrogate for molecular genetic alterations. A number of mutant-specific antibodies are now available and are in routine use in most major medical centers.

Histologic **grading** is used as a means of predicting the biologic behavior of tumors and—together with molecular features—remains an important guide to therapeutic decisions. The 2016 World Health Organization (WHO) tumor grade determinations are still made largely on the basis of histologic criteria. This introduces some inconsistencies, e.g., an IDH-wild-type diffuse astrocytoma is a grade II neoplasm, but its biologic behavior is more like an anaplastic astrocytoma (grade III) or glioblastoma (IV) **(Table 16-1)**.

Most recognized tumor entities have been assigned WHO grades and International Classification of Diseases for Oncology (ICD-O) codes, but a number of other tumors remain ungraded or have been given only provisional codes.

Demographics of CNS Neoplasms

The incidence of CNS tumors peaks among young children (those aged younger than 5 years) **(16-3)** and then again in the fifth to seventh decades of life. They are only the seventh most common neoplasm in adults (20+ years), yet malignant brain tumors contribute disproportionately to mortality and morbidity in cancer patients. CNS tumors are now the second leading cause of cancer-related mortality in men aged 20-39 years and the fifth leading cause in women.

The incidence rates of childhood cancers have risen steadily, driven largely by increases in leukemia and CNS tumors. According to the most recent Central Brain Tumor Registry of the United States (CBTRUS), primary CNS tumors are now the most common of all solid neoplasms in children and adolescents (0-19 years) and the second leading cause of cancer mortality in individuals aged younger than 20 years.

Prevalence of specific tumor types varies with location. The most common anatomic location of all intracranial tumors is the meninges, followed by the cerebral hemispheres, sellar region, cranial nerves, brainstem, and cerebellum **(16-5)**. Meningiomas are the most common histologic subtype of primary CNS neoplasm, followed by gliomas and pituitary adenomas **(16-6)**.

Tumor prevalence also varies significantly with age. Approximately half of all adult brain tumors are primary neoplasms, while half represent metastatic spread from extra-CNS tumors **(16-7)**. Overall, the most common primary brain tumor in adults is meningioma, followed by astrocytomas and pituitary neoplasms **(16-6)**. However, the most common *malignant* CNS neoplasm is glioblastoma **(16-8)**, which

Selected CNS Glial Neoplasms and WHO Grades

Neoplasm	Grade
DIFFUSE ASTROCYTIC AND OLIGODENDROGLIAL TUMORS	
Diffuse astrocytoma, IDH-mutant	II
Diffuse astrocytoma, IDH-wild-type	II*
Anaplastic astrocytoma, IDH-mutant	III
Anaplastic astrocytoma, IDH-wild-type	III*
Glioblastoma, IDH-wild-type	IV
Glioblastoma, IDH-mutant	IV
Diffuse midline glioma, *H3 K27M*-mutant	IV
Oligodendroglioma, IDH-mutant and Ip/19q-codeleted	II
Anaplastic oligodendroglioma, IDH-mutant and Ip/19q-codeleted	III
OTHER ASTROCYTIC TUMORS	
Pilocytic astrocytoma	I
Pilomyxoid astrocytoma	N/A
Subependymal giant cell astrocytoma	I
Pleomorphic xanthoastrocytoma	II
Anaplastic pleomorphic xanthoastrocytoma	III
EPENDYMAL TUMORS	
Subependymoma	I
Myxopapillary ependymoma	I
Ependymoma	II
Ependymoma, *RELA* fusion-positive	II/III
Anaplastic ependymoma	III

Neoplasm	Grade
OTHER GLIOMAS	
Choroid glioma of the third ventricle	II
Angiocentric glioma	I
Astroblastoma	N/A
CHOROID PLEXUS TUMORS	
Choroid plexus papilloma	I
Atypical choroid plexus papilloma	II
Choroid plexus carcinoma	III
NEURONAL AND MIXED NEURONAL-GLIAL TUMORS	
Dysembryoplastic neuroepithelial tumor	I
Gangliocytoma	I
Multinodular and vacuolated tumor (pattern)	I
Ganglioglioma	I
Anaplastic ganglioma	III
Dysplastic cerebellar gangliocytoma (Lhermite-Duclos disease)	I
Desmoplastic infantile astrocytoma and ganglioma	I
Rosette-forming glioneuronal tumor	I
Diffuse leptomeningeal glioneuronal tumor	N/A
Central neurocytoma	II

(Table 16-1) *N/A = tumor not assigned a grade by the World Health Organization. *Behaves more like IDH wild-type GBM. Modified from Louis DN: WHO classification and grading of tumors of the central nervous system. In: Louis DN et al: WHO Classification of Tumors of the Central Nervous System. Lyon, France: IARC, 2016, pp. 12-13.*

represents about half of all malignant brain tumors and more than 55% of all CNS gliomas **(16-9)**.

In children age 0-4 years old, the most frequently reported tumor type is embryonal neoplasm. The most common overall childhood cancers (ages 0-19 years) are pilocytic astrocytoma and embryonal tumors (two-thirds of which are medulloblastoma) **(16-10)**.

PRIMARY CNS NEOPLASMS BY LOCATION

- Meninges, 36%
- Cerebral hemispheres, 31%
- Sellar region, 17%
- Cranial nerves, 7%
- Brainstem, cerebellum, 4%
- Spinal cord/cauda equina, 3%
- Ventricles, 1%
- Miscellaneous, 1%

The incidences of primary CNS neoplasms by location, histologic group, and age are illustrated in the pie charts and shaded boxes. Statistics are from the CBTRUS statistical report and, because of rounding, may not add up to 100%.

PRIMARY CNS NEOPLASMS BY HISTOLOGIC GROUP

- Meningioma, 36%
- Astrocytoma, 21%
- Pituitary, 16%
- Nerve sheath, 8%
- Oligodendroglioma, 3%
- Ependymal, 2%
- Embryonal, 1%
- All others, 11%

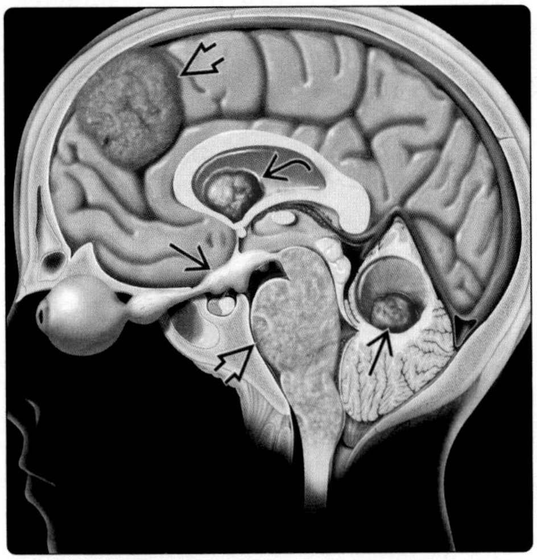

(16-3) Childhood astrocytomas are mostly pilocytic ➞. Diffuse astrocytomas ➞ are less common. SEGA in TS is shown ➞.

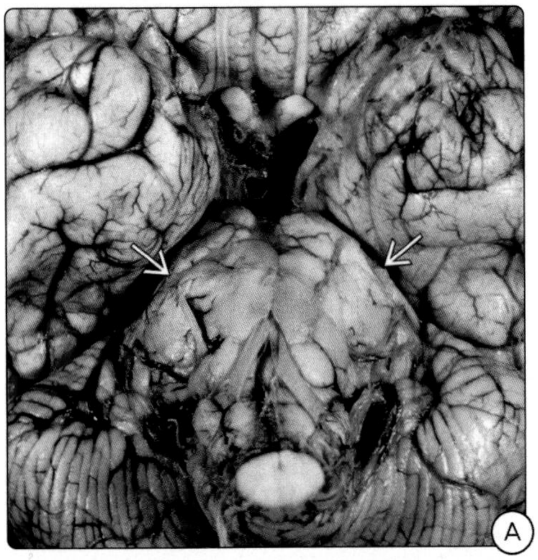

(16-4A) Autopsy shows pediatric diffuse intrinsic pontine glioma with "fat" pons ➞. Most are IDH wild-type histone-mutant tumors.

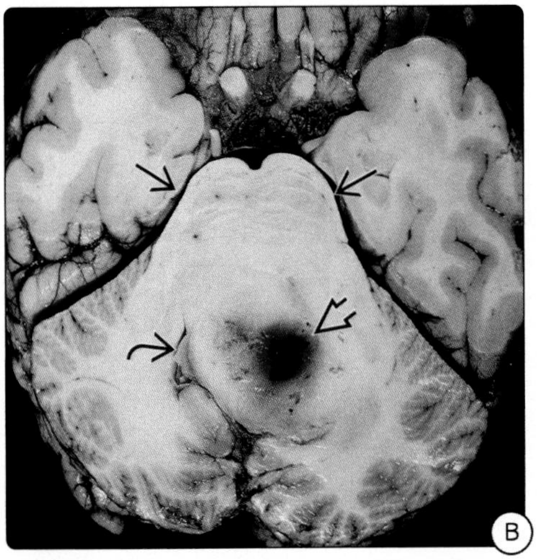

(16-4B) DIPG shows enlarged pons ➞, tumor compressing the 4th ventricle ➞. Hemorrhagic focus ➞ was GBM. (Courtesy R. Hewlett, MD.)

BRAIN TUMOR INCIDENCE BY AGE GROUP

Children (0-14 years old)

- Pilocytic astrocytoma, 18%
- Embryonal neoplasms, 15%
  - Two-thirds = medulloblastoma
- Malignant glioma, NOS, 15%
- Diffuse astrocytoma, 11%
- Neuronal/mixed glioneuronal, 6%
- Ependymal, 6%
- Nerve sheath, 5%
- Pituitary, 4%
- Craniopharyngioma, 4%
- Germ cell, 4%
- Glioblastoma, 3%
- Meningioma, 2%
- Oligodendroglioma, 1%
- All others, 5%

Adolescents (15-19 years old)

- Pituitary, 27%
- Pilocytic astrocytoma, 10%
- Other astrocytoma, 8%
- Neuronal, mixed glioneuronal, 8%
- Nerve sheath, 6%
- Meningioma, 5%
- Germ cell, 4%
- Ependymal, 4%
- Embryonal tumors, 4%
- Glioblastoma, 3%
- Craniopharyngioma, 2%
- Oligodendroglioma, 2%
- Lymphoma, 1%

Adults (20+ years old)

- Metastatic, 50%
- Primary, 50%
  - Meningioma, 18%
  - Glioblastoma, 7%
  - Pituitary, 7%
  - Nerve sheath tumor, 4%
  - Other astrocytoma, 3%
  - Lymphoma, 2%
  - Oligodendroglioma, 2%
  - All other, 7%

Gliomas

Primary CNS neoplasms are divided into several general groups. Gliomas—second only to meningiomas in incidence—are one of the most heterogeneous group of neoplasms.

Glial neoplasms constitute one of the most heterogeneous groups of brain tumors and are the most common overall malignant brain tumor. Tumors of putative glial cell origin were originally called "gliomas" (because of their supposed derivation from glue-like glial cells).

The neuropil contains several subtypes of glial cells: astrocytes, oligodendrocytes, ependymal cells, and modified ependymal cells that form the choroid plexus. In the past, each subtype was thought to give rise to a specific type of "glioma." In this rather simplistic view, abnormal astrocytes were considered the source of astrocytomas, oligodendrocytes the source of oligodendrogliomas, etc. **(16-1)**.

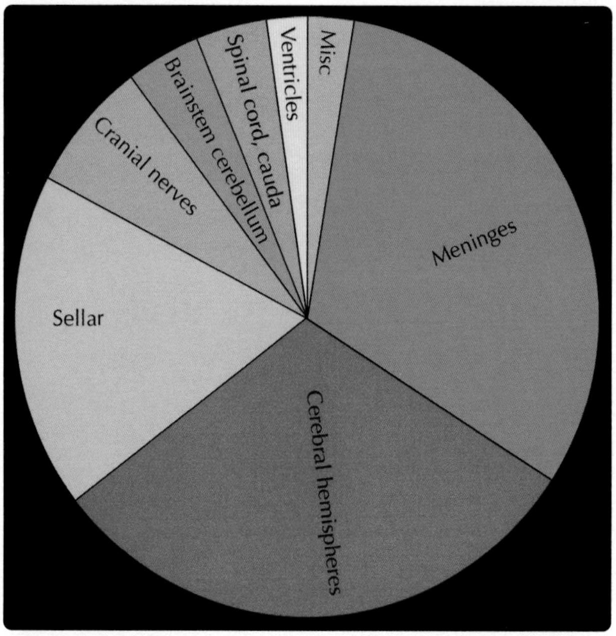

(16-5) Graph indicates percentage of primary brain tumors by location. The most common overall site is the cranial meninges followed by the cerebral hemispheres and sellar region. All other locations account for less than 25% of primary CNS neoplasms.

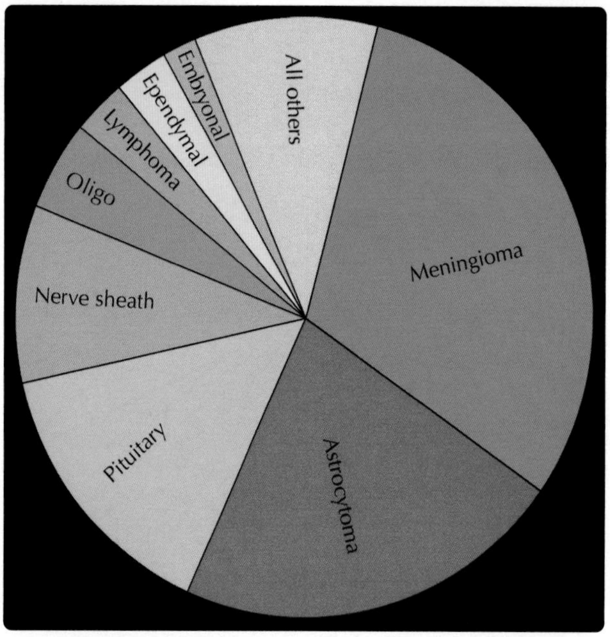

(16-6) Graph represents primary CNS neoplasms by histologic subtypes. Meningiomas are the most common group followed by astrocytomas and pituitary tumors. All other histologic groups comprise about one-third of the total.

A paradigm shift in our understanding of cancer origins has occurred over the last few years. Many—if not most—primary neoplasms of the brain parenchyma are now thought to arise from **pluripotential neural stem cells** (NSCs). These NSCs persist in two areas of the postnatal brain: the subventricular zone—the region located under the ependyma of the brain ventricles—and the dentate gyrus of the hippocampus **(16-2)**.

Normal neurogenesis and gliogenesis continue throughout life. Brain NSCs have a high rate of proliferation and are thus prone to genetic errors. When these brainstem cells mutate, they become tumor progenitor cells (tumor stem cells) that can generate phenotypically diverse neoplasms.

Data from The Cancer Genome Atlas identified a mutation in isocitrate dehydrogenase (IDH) as an early "driver mutation" in gliomagenesis. Mutated IDH converts a normal metabolite, α-ketoglutarate, to D-2-hydroxyglutarate (2-HG). 2-HG is an "oncometabolite" that alters cellular epigenetic profiles and induces "broad metabolic reprogramming." In the 2016 WHO, IDH status—which can be reliably determined using IHC—is the major characteristic identifying diffusely infiltrating astrocytic and oligodendroglial tumors.

In the 2016 WHO, astrocytomas that have a more circumscribed growth pattern (e.g., pilocytic astrocytoma, pleomorphic xanthoastrocytoma, and subependymal giant cell astrocytomas) are now separated from the diffusely infiltrating gliomas (e.g., astrocytomas and oligodendrogliomas). The latter are nosologically more similar than are diffuse astrocytoma and pilocytic astrocytoma. The "family trees" in the "new WHO" have been redrawn to reflect this new understanding.

Entity-defining glioma mutations may also differ in children versus adults. In prior WHO classifications, pediatric diffuse gliomas were grouped together with their adult counterparts despite long-recognized differences in biologic behavior. Although they look the same under the microscope, they have distinct and very different underlying genetic abnormalities.

The 2016 WHO has therefore designated a narrowly defined group of diffusely infiltrating tumors that are characterized by a specific mutation in histone H3 genes as a new, separate entity (H3 K27M-mutant diffuse midline glioma). In time, other pediatric gliomas that appear similar to adult neoplasms may be given separate diagnostic categories (e.g., pediatric oligodendrogliomas, which often lack the entity-defining 1p19q codeletion of adult oligodendrogliomas).

Astrocytomas

There are many histologic types and subtypes of astrocytomas. Astrocytomas can be relatively localized (and generally behave more benignly) or diffusely infiltrating with an inherent tendency to malignant degeneration **(16-4)**.

The most common astrocytomas are diffusely infiltrating neoplasms in which no distinct border between tumor and normal brain is present (even though the tumor may look discrete on imaging studies). Diffuse astrocytomas are now divided into IDH-mutant and IDH-wild-type tumors. Diffuse astrocytomas are designated as WHO grade II neoplasms with the caveat that an IDH wild-type grade II astrocytoma behaves more like a III (anaplastic) or IV astrocytoma (i.e., glioblastoma).

Anaplastic astrocytomas are also subdivided into IDH-mutant or wild-type and designated as WHO grade III, whereas glioblastomas are grade IV neoplasms.

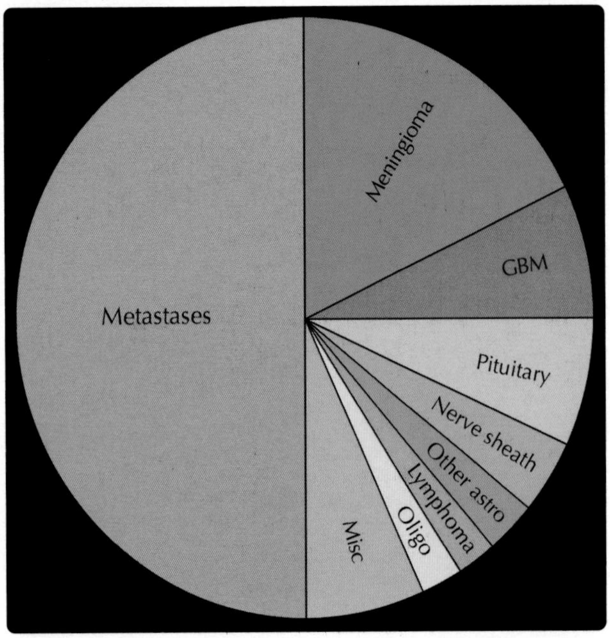

(16-7) Graph depicts the relative prevalence of all intracranial tumors in adults. Roughly half are metastases from systemic cancers; the other half are primary neoplasms.

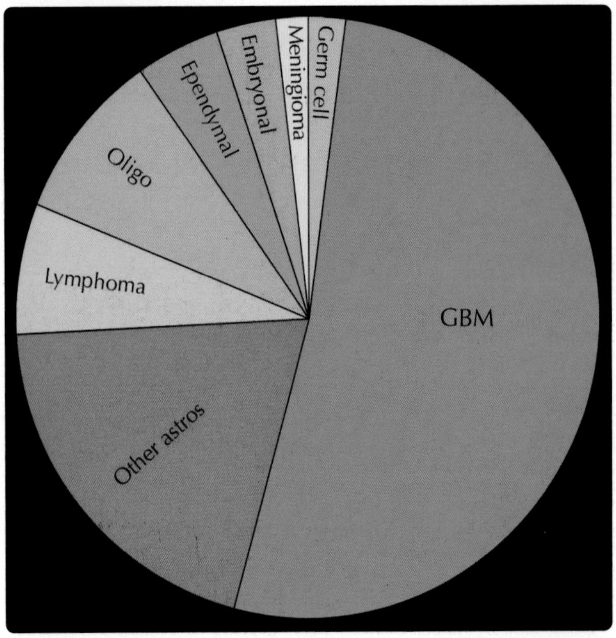

(16-8) When all malignant primary CNS neoplasms are grouped together regardless of age, glioblastoma and other malignant astrocytomas (diffuse fibrillary, anaplastic astrocytomas) far outweigh all other types combined.

All diffusely infiltrating astrocytomas have an inherent tendency to malignant progression, but, grade for grade, IDH-mutant neoplasms behave better than IDH-wild-type tumors. *Note that there is no such thing as a grade I diffusely infiltrating astrocytoma.*

The more localized astrocytic tumors are less common than the diffusely infiltrating astrocytomas. Two of the localized tumors, pilocytic astrocytoma (PA) and subependymal giant cell astrocytoma (SEGA), are designated WHO grade I neoplasms. Neither displays a tendency to malignant progression although a variant of PA, pilomyxoid astrocytoma, may behave more aggressively.

Patient age has a significant effect on neoplasm type and location. This is especially true for astrocytomas. Astrocytomas in adults tend to be malignant (e.g., anaplastic astrocytomas, glioblastomas) and to affect the cerebral hemispheres. In contrast, PAs are tumors of children and young adults. They are common in the cerebellum and around the third ventricle but rarely occur in the hemispheres **(16-3)**.

Nonastrocytic Glial Neoplasms

Oligodendrogliomas, ependymomas, and choroid plexus tumors are all considered nonastrocytic glial neoplasms.

Oligodendroglial Tumors. Oligodendroglial tumors are IDH-mutant and have a category-defining mutation, 1p19q codeletion. Two grades are recognized: a well-differentiated WHO grade II neoplasm (oligodendroglioma) and a WHO grade III neoplasm (anaplastic oligodendrogliomas).

Ependymal Tumors. Ependymal tumors vary from WHO grade I to III. Subependymoma, a benign-behaving neoplasm of middle-aged and older adults that occurs in the frontal horns and fourth ventricle, is a WHO grade I tumor. So is myxopapillary ependymoma, a tumor of young and middle-aged adults that is almost exclusively found at the conus, cauda equina, and filum terminale of the spinal cord.

Ependymoma, generally a slow-growing tumor of children and young adults, is a WHO grade II neoplasm that may arise anywhere along the ventricular system and in the central canal of the spinal cord. Anaplastic ependymomas are biologically more aggressive, have poorer prognosis, and are designated WHO grade III neoplasms.

Infratentorial ependymomas, typically arising within the fourth ventricle, occur predominantly in children. Supratentorial ependymomas are more common in the cerebral hemispheres than the lateral ventricle and are usually tumors of young children.

Each ependymoma subtype is developmentally and molecularly distinct, has a predilection for a specific anatomic location, and has specific identifiable genetic mutations. Ependymomas and a newly described tumor, *RELA* fusion-positive ependymoma, are discussed in detail in Chapter 18.

Choroid Plexus Tumors. Choroid plexus tumors are papillary intraventricular neoplasms derived from choroid plexus epithelial cells. Almost 80% of choroid plexus tumors are found in children and are one of the most common brain tumors in children under the age of 3 years.

Choroid plexus tumors are divided into choroid plexus papillomas (CPPs), which are WHO grade I tumors, atypical choroid plexus papilloma (WHO grade II), and choroid plexus carcinomas (CPCas), designated WHO grade III. CPPs are five to ten times more common than CPCas. Both CPPs and CPCas

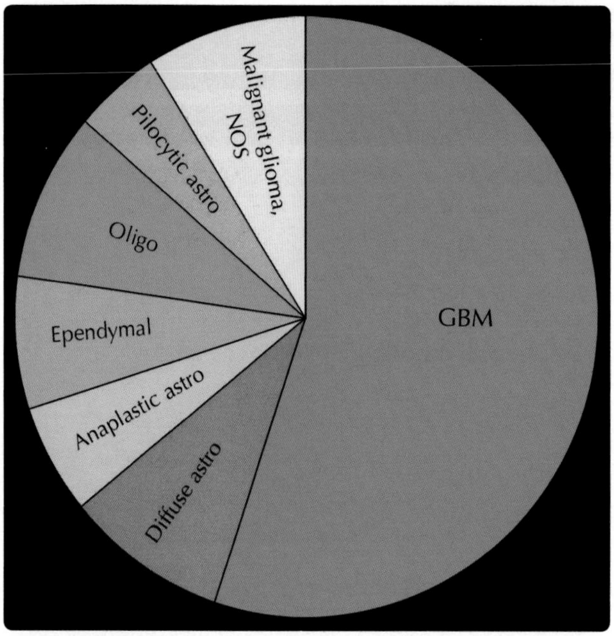

(16-9) More than half of all CNS glial neoplasms are glioblastomas. Of the nonastrocytic gliomas, oligodendrogliomas are the most common subtype.

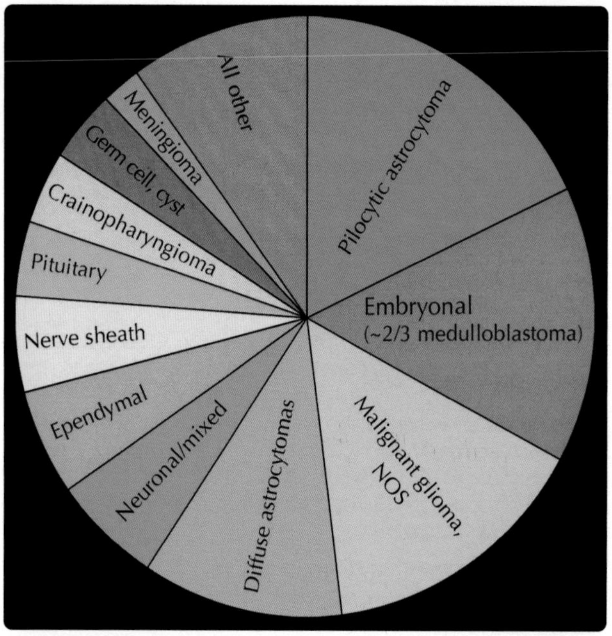

(16-10) Graph depicts brain tumors in children from newborn to age 14. Pilocytic astrocytoma and embryonal neoplasms are the most common types. Compared with adults, malignant gliomas are rare, and metastases are insignificant.

can spread diffusely through the CSF, so the entire neuraxis should be imaged before surgical intervention.

Other Gliomas. Other gliomas include chordoid glioma of the third ventricle, angiocentric glioma, and astroblastoma.

CNS GLIOMAS

- Glioblastoma, 55%
- Diffuse astrocytoma, 9%
- Anaplastic astrocytoma, 6%
- Oligodendroglial tumors, 9%
- Ependymal tumors, 7%
- Pilocytic astrocytoma, 5%
- Malignant glioma, NOS, 9%

Neuronal and Mixed Neuronal-Glial Tumors

Neuroepithelial tumors with ganglion-like cells, differentiated neurocytes, or poorly differentiated neuroblastic cells are characteristic of this heterogeneous group.

This group includes dysembryoplastic neuroepithelial tumor (DNET), and ganglion cell neoplasms include gangliocytoma, ganglioglioma, and dysplastic cerebellar gangliocytoma (Lhermitte-Duclos disease). Other tumors in this category are desmoplastic infantile astrocytoma and ganglioglioma, neurocytoma, papillary glioneuronal tumor, rosette-forming glioneuronal tumor, and cerebellar liponeurocytoma.

One new tumor entity—diffuse leptomeningeal glioneuronal tumor—and one pattern, multinodular and vacuolating neuronal tumor of the cerebrum (considered a distinct pattern of gangliocytoma), have been added to the 2016 WHO classification.

Tumors of the Pineal Region

Pineal region neoplasms account for less than 1% of all intracranial neoplasms and can be germ cell tumors or pineal parenchymal tumors. Pineal parenchymal tumors are less common than germ cell tumors. Germ cell neoplasms do occur in other intracranial sites but are discussed together with pineal parenchymal neoplasms.

Pineocytoma is a very slowly growing, well-delineated pineal parenchymal tumor that is usually found in adults. Pineocytomas are WHO grade I. Pineal parenchymal tumor of intermediate differentiation (PPTID) is intermediate in malignancy. PPTIDs can be either WHO grade II or III neoplasms **(Table 16-2)**.

Pineoblastoma is a highly malignant primitive embryonal tumor mostly found in children. Highly aggressive and associated with early CSF dissemination, pineoblastomas are WHO grade IV neoplasms.

Papillary tumor of the pineal region (PTPR) is a rare neuroepithelial tumor of adults. PTPRs are designated as WHO grade II or III neoplasms.

Embryonal Tumors

The embryonal tumor group includes medulloblastoma, embryonal tumors, and atypical teratoid/rhabdoid tumors (AT/RTs). All are highly malignant invasive tumors. All are WHO grade IV and are mostly tumors of young children.

Pineal, Embryonal, and Selected Mesenchymal CNS Neoplasms

Neoplasm	Grade
PINEAL PARENCHYMAL TUMORS	
Pineocytoma	I
Pineal parenchymal tumor of intermediate differentiation	II/III
Pineoblastoma	IV
EMBRYONAL NEOPLASMS	
Medulloblastomas, genetically defined	--
Medulloblastoma, WNT-activated	IV
Medulloblastoma, SHH-activated	IV
Medulloblastoma, group 3	IV
Medulloblastoma, group 4	IV
Embryonal tumors with multilayered rosettes, *C19MC*-altered	IV
Medulloepithelioma	IV
CNS embryonal tumor, NOS	IV
Atypical teratoid/rhabdoid tumor	IV
TUMORS OF CRANIAL/PARASPINAL NERVES	
Schwannoma	I
Neurofibroma	I
Perineurioma	I
Malignant peripheral nerve sheath tumor (MPNST)	II/III/IV

Neoplasm	Grade
MENINGIOMAS	
Meningioma	I
Atypical meningioma	II
Anaplastic (malignant) meningioma	III
MESENCHYMAL, NONMENINGOTHELIAL TUMORS	
Solitary fibrous tumor/hemangiopericytomas	--
Grade 1	I
Grade 2	II
Grade 3	III
Hemangioblastoma	I
Hemangioma	I
Inflammatory myofibroblastic tumor	N/A
Benign/malignant fibrous histiocytoma	N/A
Lipoma	I
Sarcomas (many types)	III/IV
Chondroma	N/A
Chondrosarcoma	N/A

(Table 16-2) *N/A = tumor not assigned a grade by the World Health Organization.*
Modified from Louis DN: WHO classification and grading of tumors of the central nervous system. In: Louis DN et al: WHO Classification of Tumors of the Central Nervous System. Lyon, France: IARC, 2016, pp. 12-13.

Embryonal tumors have undergone major restructuring in the 2016 WHO. Two alternative ways of looking at medulloblastoma—as genetically defined or histologically defined—are included. Some of the genetically defined and recognized histologic variants are associated with dramatically different prognoses and therapeutic implications.

The term "primitive neuroectodermal tumor" has been eliminated, and a new tumor, embryonal tumor with multilayered rosetted, C19MC-altered, has been recognized.

Meningeal Tumors

Meningeal tumors are the second largest category of primary CNS neoplasms. They are divided into meningiomas and mesenchymal, nonmeningothelial tumors (i.e., tumors that are *not* meningiomas).

Meningiomas

Meningiomas arise from meningothelial (arachnoidal) cells. Most are attached to the dura but can occur in other locations (e.g., choroid plexus of the lateral ventricles).

Although meningiomas have many histologic subtypes (e.g., meningothelial, fibrous, psammomatous), each with a different ICD-O code, the current WHO schema classifies them rather simply. Most meningioma subtypes are benign, have a low risk of recurrence and/or aggressive growth, and are grouped together as WHO grade I neoplasms.

Atypical meningiomas, as well as the chordoid and clear cell variants, are WHO grade II tumors. Anaplastic (malignant) meningiomas, including the papillary and rhabdoid subtypes, correspond to WHO grade III.

Both WHO grade II and III meningiomas have a greater likelihood of recurrence and/or aggressive behavior. The WHO classification also notes that meningiomas of any subtype or grade with a high proliferation index and/or brain invasion have a greater likelihood of aggressive behavior.

Mesenchymal Nonmeningothelial Tumors

Both benign and malignant nonmeningothelial mesenchymal tumors can originate in the CNS. Most correspond to tumors of soft tissue or bone. Generally, both a benign and malignant (sarcomatous) type occur. Lipomas and liposarcomas,

Miscellaneous Selected CNS Primary Neoplasms and WHO Grades

Neoplasm	Grade
LYMPHOMAS	
Diffuse large B-cell lymphoma of CNS	N/A
Immunodeficiency-associated CNS lymphomas *AIDS-related (large B cell)* *EBV-positive (large B cell)* *Lymphomatoid granulomatosis*	
Intravascular large B-cell lymphoma	N/A
MALT lymphoma of the dura	N/A
HISTIOCYTIC TUMORS	
Langerhans cell histiocytosis	
Erdheim-Chester disease	
Rosai-Dorfman disease	N/A
Juvenile xanthogranuloma	N/A

Neoplasm	Grade
GERM CELL TUMORS	
Germinoma	N/A
Embryonal carcinoma	
Teratoma *Mature* *Immature* *Malignant*	
Mixed germ cell tumor	
SELLAR REGION TUMORS	
Craniopharyngioma *Adamantinomatous craniopharyngioma* *Papillary craniopharyngioma*	I
Granular cell tumor	I
Pituicytoma	I
Spindle cell oncocytoma	I

(Table 16-3) *N/A = tumor not assigned a grade by the World Health Organization.*
Modified from Louis DN: WHO classification and grading of tumors of the central nervous system. In: Louis DN et al: WHO Classification of Tumors of the Central Nervous System. Lyon, France: IARC, 2016, pp. 12-13.

chondromas and chondrosarcomas, osteomas and osteosarcomas are examples.

A major change in 2016 is consolidating solitary fibrous tumor (SFT) and hemangiopericytoma (HPC) into a single entity (SFT/HPC) with three grades. Grade I corresponds to the low cellularity, spindle cell lesion traditionally diagnosed as SFT. Grade II corresponds to the tumor previously diagnosed in the CNS as hemangiopericytoma, and grade III is used to designate SFT/HPCs with malignant features.

Primary melanocytic neoplasms of the CNS are rare. They arise from leptomeningeal melanocytes and can be diffuse or circumscribed, benign or malignant.

Tumors of Cranial (and Spinal) Nerves

Schwannoma

Schwannomas are benign encapsulated nerve sheath tumors that consist of well-differentiated Schwann cells. They can be solitary or multiple. Multiple schwannomas are associated with neurofibromatosis type 2 (NF2) and schwannomatosis, a syndrome characterized by multiple schwannomas but lacking other features of NF2.

Intracranial schwannomas are almost always associated with cranial nerves (CN VIII is by far the most common) but occasionally occur as parenchymal lesions. Schwannomas do not undergo malignant degeneration and thus are designated WHO grade I neoplasms **(Table 16-3)**.

Neurofibroma

Neurofibromas (NFs) are diffusely infiltrating extraneural tumors that consist of Schwann cells and fibroblasts. Solitary scalp neurofibromas occur, and multiple NFs or plexiform NFs occur as part of neurofibromatosis type 1. NFs correspond histologically to WHO grade I. Plexiform NFs may degenerate into malignant peripheral nerve sheath tumors (MPNSTs). MPNSTs are graded from WHO II to IV, the same three-tiered system used for soft tissue sarcomas.

WHO Changes

Changes to the 2007 WHO include recognizing melanotic schwannoma as a distinct entity rather than a schwannoma variant, recognition of hybrid nerve sheath tumors, and designation of two histologic subtypes of MPNST.

Lymphomas and Histiocytic Tumors

With the onset of the HIV/AIDS era and increasing drug-induced immunocompromised states, some neuropathologists predicted that lymphoma would soon become the most common malignant intracranial neoplasm, surpassing glioblastoma. Although their incidence has increased slightly over the past two decades, lymphomas are still significantly less common than glioblastoma and other malignant astrocytomas.

The 2016 CNS WHO has expanded the classification of systemic lymphomas and histiocytic neoplasms to parallel those in the corresponding hematopoietic/lymphoid WHO classification **(Table 16-3)**.

MALIGNANT PRIMARY CNS NEOPLASMS

- Glioblastoma, 46%
- All other astrocytomas, 17%
- Lymphoma, 6%
- Oligodendroglioma, 7%
- Ependymal neoplasms, 4%
- Embryonal neoplasm, 3%
- Meningioma, 1%
- Germ cell neoplasm, 1%

Germ Cell Tumors

Intracranial germ cell tumors (GCTs) are morphologic and immunophenotypic homologs of germinal neoplasms that arise in the gonads and extragonadal sites. From 80-90% occur in adolescents. Most occur in the midline (pineal region, around the third ventricle).

Germinomas are the most common intracranial GCT. Teratomas differentiate along ectodermal, endodermal, and mesodermal lines. They can be mature, immature, or occur as teratomas with malignant transformation. Other miscellaneous GCTs include the highly aggressive yolk sac tumor, embryonal carcinoma, and choriocarcinoma.

Germ cell tumors are discussed in detail with tumors of the pineal region.

Sellar Region Tumors

The sellar region is one of the most anatomically complex areas in the brain. However, the official WHO classification of sellar region tumors includes only craniopharyngioma and rare tumors such as granular cell tumor of the neurohypophysis, pituicytoma, and spindle cell oncocytoma of the adenohypophysis.

The sellar region contains many structures besides the craniopharyngeal duct and infundibular stalk that give rise to masses seen on imaging studies. The most common of these masses—pituitary adenoma—is not part of the WHO classification but is included here, as are variants (such as pituitary hyperplasia) and nonneoplastic tumor-like masses (e.g., hypophysitis and hypothalamic hamartoma) that can mimic neoplasms.

Pituitary Adenoma

Pituitary adenomas account for the majority of sellar/suprasellar masses in adults and the third most common overall intracranial neoplasm in this age group. Pituitary adenomas are classified by size as microadenomas (≤ 10 mm) and macroadenomas (≥ 11 mm).

Craniopharyngioma

Craniopharyngioma is a benign (WHO grade I), often partially cystic neoplasm that is the most common nonneuroepithelial intracranial neoplasm in children. It shows a distinct bimodal age distribution with the cystic adamantinomatous type seen mostly in children and a smaller peak in middle-aged adults. The less common papillary type is usually solid and found almost exclusively in adults.

Miscellaneous Sellar Region Tumors

Granular cell tumor of the neurohypophysis, also called choristoma, is a rare tumor of adults that usually arises from the infundibulum. Pituicytomas are glial neoplasms of adults that also usually arise within the infundibulum. Spindle cell oncocytoma of the adenohypophysis is an oncocytic nonendocrine neoplasm. All of these rare tumors are WHO grade I. The diagnosis is usually histologic, as differentiating these tumors from each other and from other adult tumors such as macroadenoma can be problematic.

Metastatic Tumors

Metastatic neoplasms represent nearly half of all CNS tumors. In Chapter 27, we consider the "many faces" of CNS metastatic disease as well as the intriguing topic of paraneoplastic syndromes.

Paraneoplastic neurologic syndromes (PNSs) are rare nervous system dysfunctions in cancer patients that are not due to metastases or local effects of a tumor. Classic PNSs with "onconeural" antibodies and several recently described nonparaneoplastic encephalitides are likewise included in Chapter 27.

Intracranial Cysts

Cysts are common findings on neuroimaging studies and, for purposes of discussion, included in this part of the text. Although our focus is primarily neoplasms, nonneoplastic CNS cysts can sometimes be confused with "real" brain tumors and are often considered in the differential diagnosis of mass lesions in specific anatomic locations.

We therefore take an anatomic- and imaging-based approach to intracranial cysts. Here the key consideration is not cyst wall histopathology (as in brain neoplasms) but anatomic location **(16-11)**.

There are four key anatomy-based questions to pose when considering the imaging diagnosis of an intracranial cyst. (1) Is the cyst extra- or intraaxial? (2) Is it supra- or infratentorial? (3) Is it midline or off-midline? (4) If the cyst is intraaxial, is it in the brain parenchyma or inside the ventricles?

Although many cysts can be found in multiple locations, each type has its own "preferred" (i.e., most common) site. The three major anatomic sublocations are the extraaxial spaces (including the scalp and skull), the brain parenchyma, and the cerebral ventricles.

Extraaxial Cysts

This is the second largest group of nonneoplastic cysts. The chapter on nonneoplastic cysts considers these first, beginning from the scalp and skull and proceeding inward to

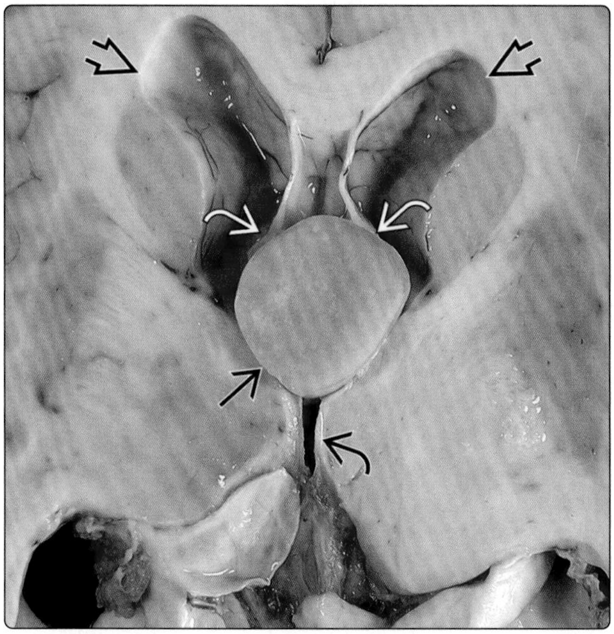

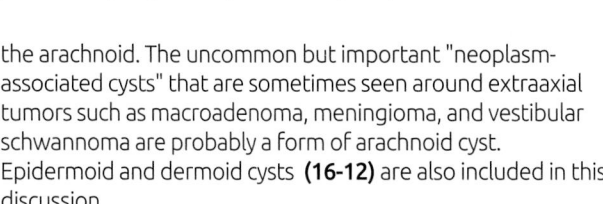

***(16-11)** A gelatinous cyst ➩ at the foramen of Monro splays the fornices ➡ and enlarges the lateral ventricles ➩, whereas the third ventricle ➩ is normal. Location is virtually pathognomonic for colloid cyst. (Courtesy R. Hewlett, MD.)*

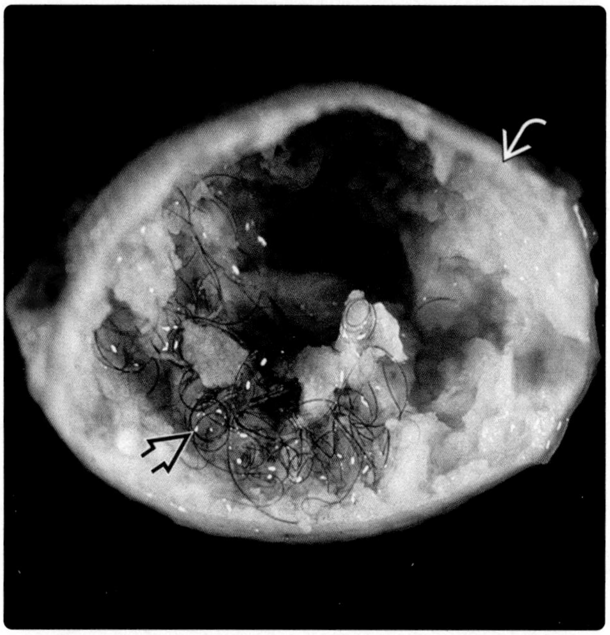

***(16-12)** Gross pathology of a resected dermoid cyst shows thick, greasy sebaceous and keratin debris ➡. Note tangles of hair ➩ within the well-delineated cyst.*

the arachnoid. The uncommon but important "neoplasm-associated cysts" that are sometimes seen around extraaxial tumors such as macroadenoma, meningioma, and vestibular schwannoma are probably a form of arachnoid cyst. Epidermoid and dermoid cysts **(16-12)** are also included in this discussion.

Intraaxial (Parenchymal) Cysts

The most common parenchymal cysts are enlarged perivascular spaces and hippocampal sulcus remnants, followed by porencephalic (encephaloclastic) cysts. Neuroglial cysts—parenchymal cysts lined by nonneoplastic gliotic brain—are relatively uncommon.

Intraventricular Cysts

Intraventricular cysts are less common than cysts in the brain parenchyma. The most common intraventricular cysts are choroid plexus cysts, which are almost always incidental findings on imaging studies. Colloid cysts are the second most common cyst but the most important to diagnose because they can suddenly and unexpectedly obstruct the foramen of Monro **(16-11)**. Acute obstructive hydrocephalus and even death can result.

INTRACRANIAL CYSTS

Extraaxial Cysts
- Arachnoid cyst
  - Choroid fissure cyst
- Epidermoid cyst
- Dermoid cyst
- Neurenteric cyst
- Pineal cyst
- Nonneoplastic tumor-associated cyst

Intraaxial (Parenchymal) Cysts
- Enlarged perivascular spaces
- Hippocampal sulcus remnants
- Neuroglial cyst
- Porencephalic cyst

Intraventricular Cysts
- Choroid plexus cyst
- Colloid cyst
- Ependymal cyst

Selected References

Classification and Grading of CNS Neoplasms

Sahm F et al: WHO 2016 Classification: changes and advancements in the diagnosis of miscellaneous primary CNS tumours. Neuropathol Appl Neurobiol. ePub, 2017

Bielle F: Building diagnoses with four layers: WHO 2016 classification of CNS tumors. Rev Neurol (Paris). 172(4-5):253-5, 2016

Chhabda S et al: The 2016 World Health Organization Classification of Tumours of the Central Nervous System: what the paediatric neuroradiologist needs to know. Quant Imaging Med Surg. 6(5):486-489, 2016

Louis DN et al (eds), WHO Classification of Tumours of the Central Nervous System. Lyon, France: International Agency for Research on Cancer, 2016

Louis DN et al: The 2016 World Health Organization Classification of Tumors of the Central Nervous System: a summary. Acta Neuropathol. 131(6):803-20, 2016

Demographics of CNS Neoplasms

Gittleman HR et al: Trends in central nervous system tumor incidence relative to other common cancers in adults, adolescents, and children in the United States, 2000 to 2010. Cancer. 121(1):102-12, 2015

Ostrom QT et al: CBTRUS Statistical Report: primary brain and central nervous system tumors diagnosed in the United States in 2008-2012. Neuro Oncol. 17 Suppl 4:iv1-iv62, 2015

Gliomas

Condello S et al: The hunt for elusive cancer stem cells. Oncotarget. 8(24):38076-38077, 2017

Perry A et al: Histologic classification of gliomas. Handb Clin Neurol. 134:71-95, 2016

Shoemaker LD et al: Neural stem cells (NSCs) and proteomics. Mol Cell Proteomics. 15(2):344-54, 2016

Zacher A et al: Molecular diagnostics of gliomas using next generation sequencing of a glioma-tailored gene panel. Brain Pathol. 27(2):146-159, 2017

Tanboon J et al: The diagnostic use of immunohistochemical surrogates for signature molecular genetic alterations in gliomas. J Neuropathol Exp Neurol. 75(1):4-18, 2016

Tumors of the Pineal Region

Plant AS et al: Pediatric malignant germ cell tumors: a comparison of the neuro-oncology and solid tumor experience. Pediatr Blood Cancer. 63(12):2086-2095, 2016

Raleigh DR et al: Histopathologic review of pineal parenchymal tumors identifies novel morphologic subtypes and prognostic factors for outcome. Neuro Oncol. 19(1):78-88, 2016

Embryonal Tumors

Chiang JC et al: Molecular pathology of paediatric central nervous system tumours. J Pathol. 241(2):159-172, 2017

Chhabda S et al: The 2016 World Health Organization Classification of Tumours of the Central Nervous System: what the paediatric neuroradiologist needs to know. Quant Imaging Med Surg. 6(5):486-489, 2016

Lymphomas and Histiocytic Tumors

Sugita Y et al: Primary central nervous system lymphomas and related diseases: pathological characteristics and discussion of the differential diagnosis. Neuropathology. 36(4):313-24, 2015

Sellar Region Tumors

Saeger W et al: Emerging histopathological and genetic parameters of pituitary adenomas: clinical impact and recommendation for future WHO classification. Endocr Pathol. 27(2):115-22, 2016

Intracranial Cysts

Taillibert S et al: Intracranial cystic lesions: a review. Curr Neurol Neurosci Rep. 14(9):481, 2014

Adeeb N et al: The intracranial arachnoid mater : a comprehensive review of its history, anatomy, imaging, and pathology. Childs Nerv Syst. 29(1):17-33, 2013

Osborn AG, Preece MT: Intracranial cysts: radiologic-pathologic correlation and imaging approach. Radiology 239(3):650-64, 2006.

Astrocytomas

Gliomas account for slightly less than one-third of all intracranial neoplasms and over 80% of the primary malignant ones. Almost three-quarters of gliomas are astrocytomas. Astrocytomas are the single largest group of neoplasms that arise within the brain itself.

Astrocytomas form a surprisingly diverse group of neoplasms with many different histologic types and subtypes. These fascinating tumors differ widely in preferential location, peak age, clinical manifestations, morphologic features, biologic behavior, and prognosis.

General Features of Astrocytomas

Introduction

We introduce astrocytomas with a brief discussion of their putative origin, classification (by both histologic phenotype and genotype), grading, and importance of age and location in determining astrocytoma tumor subtypes.

For purposes of our discussion, astrocytomas are organized into two general categories: a relatively "localized," comparatively more benign-behaving group and a "diffusely infiltrating," more biologically aggressive group. This distinction is somewhat arbitrary and imperfect, as some "circumscribed" astrocytomas occasionally become more aggressive and infiltrate adjacent structures despite their low-grade histology.

Origin of Astrocytomas

Astrocytomas were originally named for their putative origin from the stellate-shaped cells—"astrocytes"—that are the dominant component of the neuropil (vastly outnumbering neurons). It was once assumed that astrocytes could undergo both hyperplasia (nonneoplastic "reactive astrocytosis") and neoplastic transformation.

There is now considerable evidence that diffuse astrocytomas do *not* arise from neoplastic transformation of normal mature astrocytes. Instead, they probably develop from distinct populations of precursor "glioma-initiating" cells that possess stem cell properties.

Characteristics of cancer stem cells include (1) capacity for self-renewal, (2) differentiation potential, (3) high tumorigenicity, (4) drug resistance, and (5) radioresistance.

Glioma stem-like cells (GSCs or glioma-initiating cells) maintain these general properties of cancer stem cells, express genes characteristic of neural stem

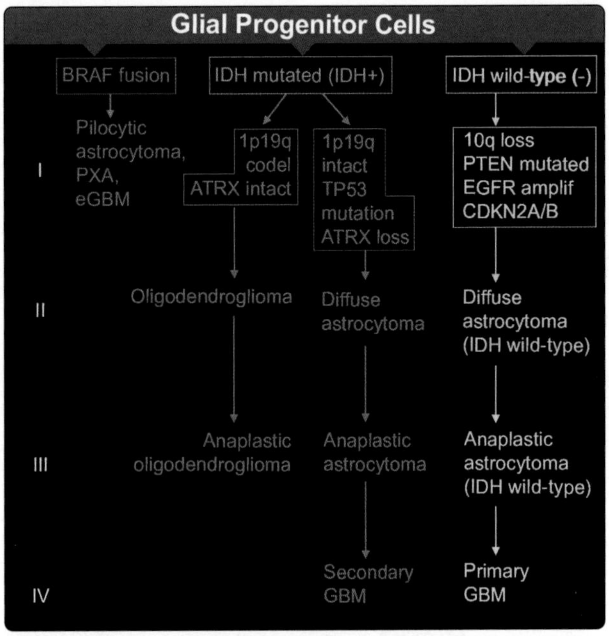

(17-1) Glioma cell lines are shown with "driver" mutation IDH+. Subsequent mutations lead either to astrocytomas (blue) or oligodendrogliomas (green). IDH-wild-type astrocytoma grades II/III lead to primary glioblastoma (GBM).

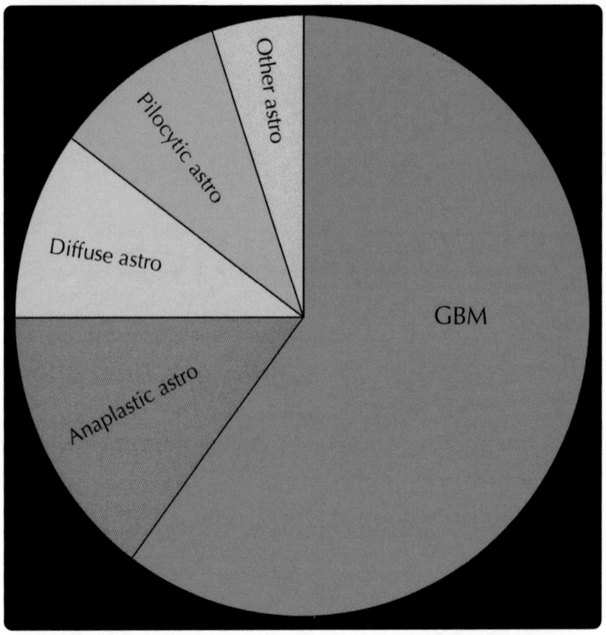

(17-2) Graphic shows % of astrocytomas. Glioblastoma (green) represents over half of all astrocytomas. AA is the next most common astrocytoma. "Other astrocytomas" such as pleomorphic xanthoastrocytoma and SEGA are relatively rare.

cells, and then differentiate into phenotypically diverse populations including neuronal, astrocytic, and oligodendroglial lineages.

Investigators have identified populations of GSCs within glioblastomas that are treatment-resistant and retain tumorigenetic abilities. These GSCs share critical signaling pathways with normal human neural stem cells but with distinct alterations characteristic for their tumor subgroups. At least three types of putative GSCs have been proposed, each of which gives rise to a specific set of glial neoplasms as discussed below.

Classification and Grading of Astrocytomas

Although tumor staging is commonly used for neoplasms elsewhere in the body, CNS neoplasms are first classified (into specific tumor types) and then graded (a measure of malignancy).

Classification

In the past, classification was based almost exclusively on histologic phenotype. Now, once the initial diagnosis of a diffuse glioma is established by long-established histologic criteria, gliomas (whether astrocytic or not) are grouped into subtypes according to the presence or absence of specific genetic parameters.

The initial entity-defining genetic marker in gliomas is **isocitrate dehydrogenase (IDH)** mutation status **(17-1)**. IDH1 and IDH2 are homodimers that are a key part of the citric acid cycle. IDH metabolizes isocitrate to α-ketoglutarate (α-KG). *Mutated* IDH converts α-KG to D-2-hydroxyglutarate (2-HG), which is an oncometabolite.

The vast majority of IDH-mutant diffuse astrocytomas, as well as the World Health Organization (WHO) grade III and IV tumors that evolve from them, also have class-defining loss-of-function mutations in *TP53* and *ATRX*. *ATRX* (alpha-**t**halassemia-**m**ental retardation **x**-linked gene) loss is associated with epigenomic dysregulation and telomere dysfunction. *TP53* (**t**umor **p**rotein **p53**) is a tumor suppressor gene and is the most frequently mutated gene in human cancers, found in more than 50% of cases.

In the 2016 WHO "family tree," IDH-mutant gliomas are separated by other, mutually exclusive genetic mutations into **astrocytomas (IDH-mutated, 1p19q intact, ATRX loss)** and **oligodendrogliomas (IDH-mutated, 1p19q codeletion, ATRX intact).** We discuss astrocytomas in this chapter; oligodendrogliomas are grouped with other nonastrocytic glial neoplasms and discussed in Chapter 18.

Localized Astrocytomas. Astrocytomas with a more circumscribed or localized growth pattern (e.g., pilocytic astrocytoma, pleomorphic xanthoastrocytoma, and subependymal giant cell astrocytoma) lack IDH mutations and often exhibit *BRAF* fusion. This group represents between 10 and 15% of astrocytomas **(17-2)**.

IDH-Mutant Astrocytomas. The vast majority of astrocytomas grow more rapidly, diffusely infiltrate adjacent tissues, and display an inherent propensity to undergo malignant degeneration. Approximately 85% of diffusely infiltrating astrocytomas are the IDH-mutant.

IDH-Wild-Type Astrocytomas. The less common IDH wild-type astrocytomas lack IDH mutation and are characterized by

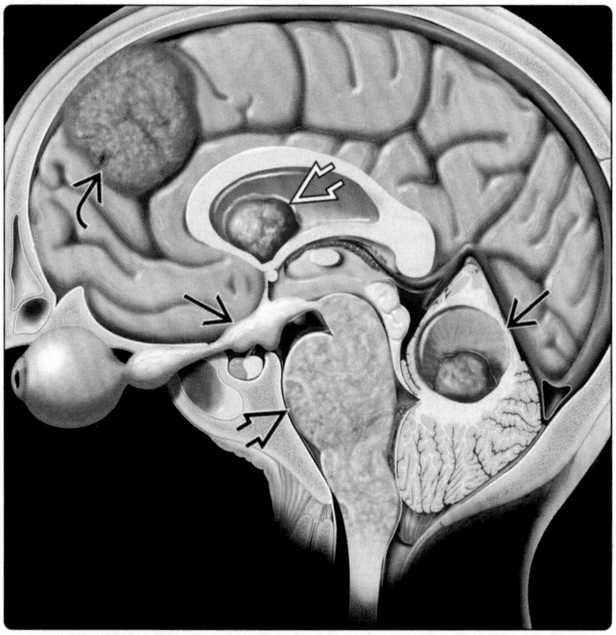

(17-3) Childhood pilocytic astrocytomas occur in the cerebellum and hypothalamus/optic nerves. H3 K27M mutant glioma is the most common pontine tumor. Hemispheric astrocytomas and SEGAs are relatively uncommon.

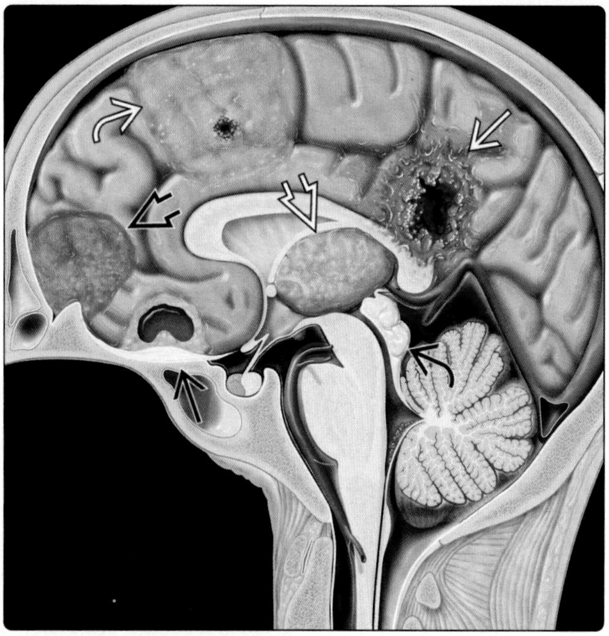

(17-4) Adult GBM and AA are common in cerebral hemispheres, corpus callosum; DA predominates in frontal lobe, brainstem/tectum. PXA with cyst, meningeal reaction, thalamic H3 K27M-mutant midline glioma are shown.

a different group of genetic abnormalities (e.g., *PTEN* mutation, *EGFR* amplification, etc).

Histone H3-Mutant Gliomas. A fourth "family" of gliomas lacks IDH mutation and is characterized by mutations in histone H3 genes, a diffuse growth pattern, and midline location.

Grading

The WHO grading system assigns astrocytomas from grades I to grade IV. Grade I lesions have low proliferative potential and generally long progression-free survival. Only two relatively circumscribed histologic subtypes of astrocytomas—pilocytic and subependymal giant cell astrocytomas—are designated as **WHO grade I** neoplasms.

All diffusely infiltrating astrocytomas are *at least* WHO grade II neoplasms, and the vast majority are grades III-IV. Tumors with cytologic atypia alone (i.e., diffuse astrocytomas) are considered **WHO grade II**. If anaplasia and mitotic activity are also present, they are considered **WHO grade III** (i.e., anaplastic astrocytoma). Tumors that additionally demonstrate microvascular proliferation (defined either as endothelium multilayering—not simple hypervascularity—or "glomeruloid" vasculature) and/or necrosis are **WHO grade IV** neoplasms (i.e., glioblastoma).

Distinguishing a grade II from a grade III astrocytoma on the basis of histologic features alone can be difficult. Neuropathologists add a measure of cellular proliferation called the Ki-67 proliferation index as a surrogate estimate for subsequent biologic behavior of the tumor.

Age and Location in Astrocytomas

Diffuse astrocytomas in childhood look microscopically like their adult counterparts yet exhibit distinctly different biologic behaviors. One of the most striking is the effect of age on both astrocytoma subtype and preferred location. Some astrocytomas (such as pilocytic astrocytoma) occur almost exclusively in children, whereas others (e.g., glioblastoma) are far more common in adults. In addition, it is becoming increasingly apparent that there are also site-specific genetic differences even among histologically similar tumor subtypes.

There is also a very strong anatomic preference with some tumors in certain age groups occurring frequently in some locations and very rarely in others. Approximately 75% of all primary brain tumors in children occur in the posterior fossa, whereas the reverse is the case in adults.

Astrocytomas in children are typically localized tumors that occur most commonly in the posterior fossa or optic pathway. The highly lethal H3 K27M-mutant diffuse midline glioma occurs in the pons or thalamus. Hemispheric diffuse astrocytomas are relatively less uncommon **(17-3)**.

The vast majority of adult astrocytomas are diffusely infiltrating (grades II-IV), almost exclusively supratentorial, and located in the cerebral hemispheres **(17-4)**.

Childhood Astrocytomas

Brain and CNS tumors are the most common cancer among those aged 0-19 years. Astrocytomas account for nearly half of all intracranial neoplasms in this age group.

Newborns and Infants. Astrocytomas of any type are very rare in newborns and infants. When they occur in this age group, they tend to be supratentorial, rather than the preferential infratentorial location seen in older children. Congenital astrocytomas are large, bulky, highly malignant hemispheric neoplasms **(17-45)**. **Glioblastoma** is the most common congenital astrocytoma.

A rare variant of pilocytic astrocytoma called **pilomyxoid astrocytoma** also presents primarily in infants under 1 year of age, usually occurring as a large H-shaped hypothalamic mass that extends laterally into one or both temporal lobes.

Children. The vast majority of childhood astrocytomas are low-grade gliomas (LGGs). Over 90% are **pilocytic astrocytomas** (PA, WHO grade I), whereas less than 10% are **diffuse astrocytomas** (DA, WHO grade II). Malignant astrocytomas (WHO grades III-IV) are rare in children.

In contrast to their adult counterparts, pediatric LGGs generally lack IDH and *ATRX* or *TP53* mutations. They rarely undergo pathologic progression to a diffuse astrocytic tumor of higher grade (e.g., anaplastic astrocytoma or glioblastoma).

Besides PA, the only other grade I astrocytoma that commonly occurs in children is **subependymal giant cell astrocytoma** (SEGA). SEGAs virtually always occur in the setting of tuberous sclerosis. SEGAs are almost exclusively found in the lateral ventricle near the foramen of Monro, attached to the septi pellucidi.

In addition to specific tumor types, childhood astrocytomas have a particularly strong predilection for certain anatomic locations **(17-3)**. After the age of 1-2 years, more than half are infratentorial; the cerebellum and the brainstem are the most common sites. Cerebellar and tectal plate astrocytomas are usually PAs, whereas most brainstem "gliomas" are the H3 K27M-mutant diffuse midline gliomas **(17-63)**.

The second most common overall astrocytoma site in children clusters around the third ventricle, hypothalamus, and optic chiasm. Most astrocytomas in this location are pilocytic, including the rare pilomyxoid variant.

The cerebral hemispheres are the least common site of astrocytomas in children. The astrocytoma most frequently seen here is the diffuse astrocytoma (WHO grade II), which is usually a tumor of older children and young adults. Hemispheric PAs occur but are quite rare.

Astrocytomas in Young Adults

The most common of all primary CNS neoplasms in patients between the ages of 18 and 30 years is **IDH-mutant diffuse astrocytoma** (WHO grade II). Most occur in the hemispheric white matter, most commonly in the frontal or temporal lobes. **Pilocytic astrocytoma** still occurs in the late teens to early 20s, but its incidence declines sharply with increasing age.

Pleomorphic xanthoastrocytoma (PXA) is a WHO grade II-III neoplasm. PXAs are usually cortically based hemispheric tumors that present with epilepsy. PXAs are more common in young adults than in children.

Adult Astrocytomas

In contrast to astrocytomas in children, astrocytomas in patients over the age of 30 years are mostly supratentorial and occur primarily in the cerebral hemispheres **(17-4)**.

PAs are rare in adults. Most adult astrocytomas are IDH-mutant astrocytomas. In general, the older the patient, the higher the tumor grade. **IDH-mutant diffuse astrocytoma** (WHO grade II) predominates in young adults, whereas **anaplastic astrocytoma** (WHO grade III) and **glioblastoma** (WHO grade IV) are much more common in middle-aged and older adults.

AGE AND ASTROCYTOMAS

Newborn/Infant
- Rare
- Supratentorial > > infratentorial
- Large, bulky hemispheric mass
- Most common = glioblastoma
- Less common = pilomyxoid astrocytoma
- Rare = pilocytic astrocytoma

Children/Young Adults
- Common
- Infratentorial > supratentorial
- Pilocytic > diffusely infiltrating astrocytoma > subependymal giant cell astrocytoma (SEGA)
- Pilocytic astrocytoma
  - Cerebellum, fourth ventricle > pons, medulla
  - Optic chiasm/hypothalamus > tectum
  - Hemispheric pilocytic astrocytoma, rare
- Diffuse astrocytoma
  - Mostly IDH-mutant
  - Cerebral hemispheres > brainstem > cerebellum
- SEGA
  - Most at/around foramen of Monro
  - Look for signs of tuberous sclerosis
- H3 K27M-mutant midline glioma
  - 75% of diffuse intrinsic pontine gliomas
  - Most IDH-wild-type
  - Worst survival of all pediatric brain tumors

Middle-Aged/Older Adults
- The older the patient, the more malignant the astrocytoma
- Glioblastoma > anaplastic > > diffuse astrocytoma
- Usually involve hemispheric white matter
- Posterior fossa very rare

Localized Astrocytomas

In this section, we consider the relatively "localized" or circumscribed astrocytomas. Localized astrocytomas are significantly less common than diffusely infiltrating astrocytomas.

Recall that only two localized astrocytomas, **pilocytic astrocytoma** (PA) and **subependymal giant cell astrocytoma**, are designated as WHO grade I neoplasms. WHO grade I tumors have low proliferative potential, can often be cured with surgical resection alone, and do not display an inherent tendency to malignant progression. Remote metastases are very rare, and, in the uncommon instances when they occur, the metastases generally maintain their bland (i.e., grade I) histologic features.

Pilomyxoid astrocytoma (PMA) is a rare but more aggressive PA variant that often grows more rapidly and has a less favorable prognosis. Because it has unique gene expression as well as histopathologic and clinical features that differ from those of PA, PMA is discussed separately.

Pilocytic Astrocytoma

Terminology

PA, sometimes termed "juvenile pilocytic astrocytoma" or "cystic cerebellar astrocytoma," is a well-circumscribed, typically slow-growing glioma of young patients.

Etiology

Genetics of PA. There is increasing evidence that PAs from different locations in the brain may arise from region-specific neural stem/progenitor cells and that different genes are expressed in different "site-specific" locations.

PAs can be sporadic or syndromic. PAs that develop in patients with neurofibromatosis type 1 (NF1) have different mutations from non-NF1-associated PAs. The genetic changes for both occur in genes whose protein products function to regulate cell growth through the RAS downstream signaling pathway.

RAS transmits its growth-promoting signals through downstream effectors, primarily the BRAF/MEK/MAPK and AKT pathways. Although these two different downstream effectors can function independently, both converge on the mammalian target of rapamycin (mTOR) complex to result in increased mTOR hyperactivation and cell proliferation.

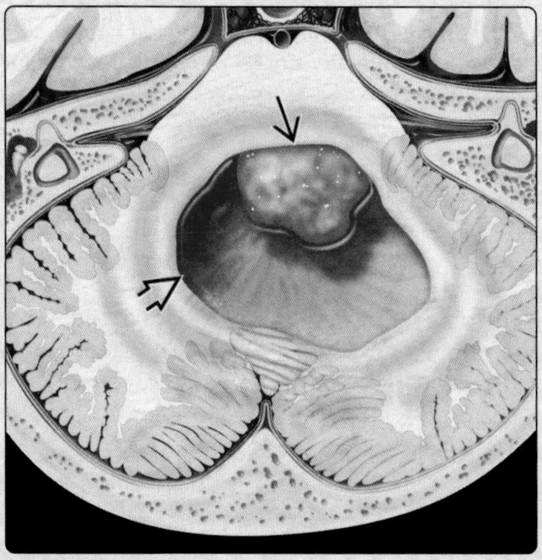

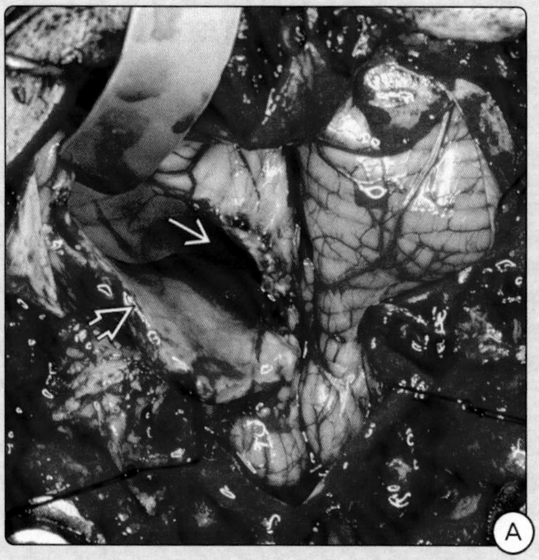

***(17-5)** Graphic shows typical cerebellar pilocytic astrocytoma with vascular-appearing tumor nodule →, large nonneoplastic cyst ⇒. Cyst wall consists of compressed but otherwise histologically normal brain parenchyma. **(17-6A)** Intraoperative photo shows cerebellar hemisphere cyst ⇒ held open by a retractor. Cyst wall consists of compressed brain parenchyma. A reddish nodule → is visible.*

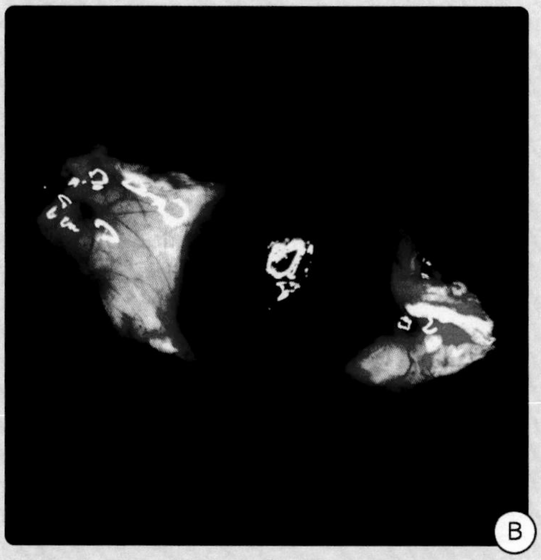

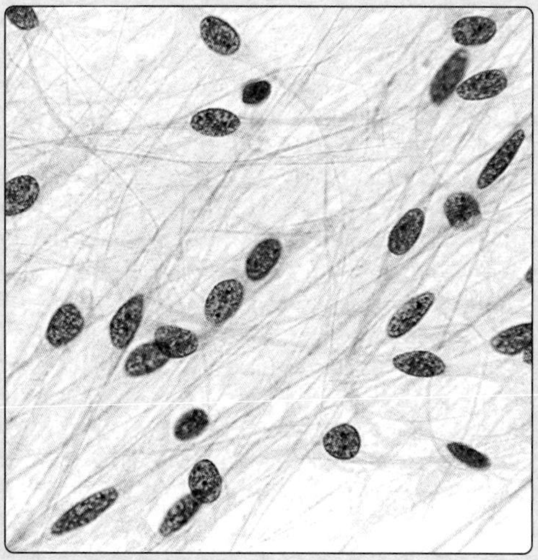

***(17-6B)** Gross pathology of the cyst wall nodule in the same case shows a very vascular-appearing, well-delineated mass attached to the wall. (Courtesy R. Hewlett, MD.) **(17-7)** PAs are characterized by bipolar fibrillar or hair-like (pilocytic) cells with long, narrow processes. (Courtesy P. Burger, MD.)*

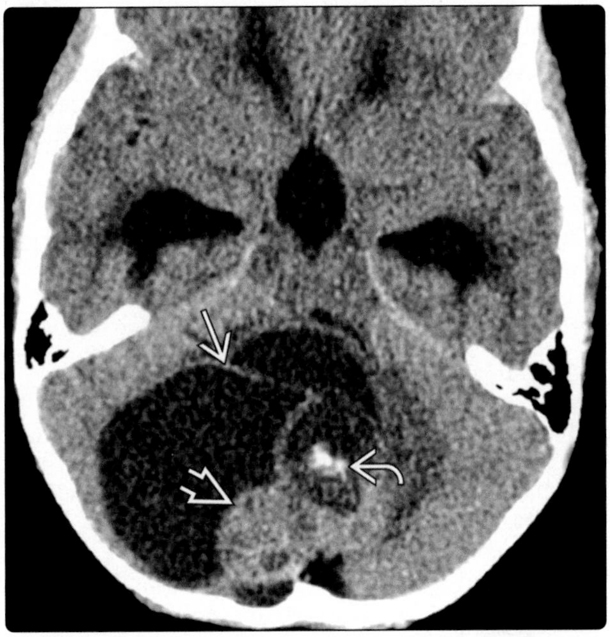

(17-8) NECT scan shows a posterior fossa PA with cysts, solid tumor nodule, Ca++, and associated obstructive hydrocephalus.

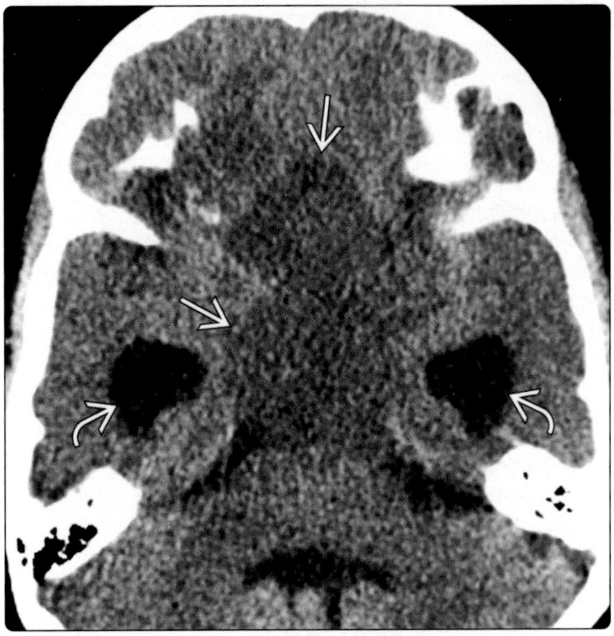

(17-9) Axial NECT of a hypothalamic-optic chiasmatic PA shows well-delineated lobulated hypodensity filling the suprasellar cistern. The mass causes obstructive hydrocephalus, seen as symmetrically enlarged temporal horns.

NF1-Associated Pilocytic Astrocytomas. Approximately 15% of NF1 patients develop PAs, most commonly in the optic nerves/tracts ("optic pathway gliomas"). The *NF1* gene, located on the long arm of chromosome 17, encodes neurofibromin. Neurofibromin functions to inactivate RAS. When biallelic mutational inactivation of this tumor suppressor gene occurs, the result is overactivity of the RAS and MAPK pathways.

Sporadic Pilocytic Astrocytomas. NF1 mutations are rare in sporadic PAs. Nearly all cerebellar PAs have a *BRAF* gene fusion, which leads to activation of the downstream MEK signaling cascade, which in turn increases progression through the cell cycle and leads to increased cell growth.

Pathology

Location. PAs may arise anywhere in the neuraxis but have a distinct predilection for certain sites. The cerebellum is the most common location, accounting for nearly 60% of all PAs **(17-5)**.

The second most common site is in and around the optic nerve/chiasm and hypothalamus/third ventricle, which together account for between one-quarter and one-third of all PAs. The third most common location is the pons and medulla. PAs also occur in the tectum, where they may cause aqueductal stenosis.

The cerebral hemispheres are a reported but uncommon location of PA. When they occur outside the posterior fossa, optic pathway, or suprasellar region, PAs tend to be cortically based cysts with a tumor nodule.

Gross Pathology. PAs are typically well-circumscribed grayish tumors with both firm and softer mucoid areas. Focal calcification may be present.

Sometimes PAs form a mural nodule in association with a cyst **(17-5)**. The walls of most PA-associated cysts usually consist of compressed but otherwise normal brain parenchyma with the neoplastic element confined to the mural tumor nodule **(17-6)**. Cyst contents are typically a protein-rich xanthochromic fluid.

Cystic PAs are preferentially located in the cerebellum and (less commonly) the cerebral hemispheres. A solid, more infiltrative appearance is common in the optic pathways and hypothalamus. Frank invasion of surrounding brain is typically absent or limited to a narrow border immediately adjacent to the neoplasm.

Microscopic Features. The classic finding of PA is a "biphasic" pattern of two distinct astrocyte populations. The dominant type is composed of compact, hair-like ("pilocytic") bipolar cells with Rosenthal fibers [electron-dense glial fibrillary acidic protein (GFAP)-positive cytoplasmic inclusions] **(17-7)**. Intermixed are loosely textured, hypocellular, GFAP-negative areas that contain multipolar cells with microcysts. Telangiectatic or glomeruloid vascular proliferation is common.

Ki-67/MIB-1 is typically less than 5%, indicating low proliferative potential.

Rare anaplastic PA variants do occur in children but are more common in adults. In palisading necrosis, increased cellularity, cytologic atypia, more than five mitoses per high-powered field, and a high Ki-67 or MIB-1 proliferative index are features that suggest anaplastic PA.

Staging, Grading, and Classification. PA is a WHO grade I tumor. Tumor dissemination occasionally occurs but is rare. Criteria for anaplasia or assigning a WHO grade higher than I are not well established.

Clinical Issues

Epidemiology. PA accounts for 5-10% of all gliomas and is the most common primary brain tumor in children. PAs represent nearly 25% of all CNS neoplasms and 85% of posterior fossa astrocytomas in this age group. PAs in the cerebral hemisphere are rare and tend to affect an older group of patients than the cerebellar or optic pathway PAs.

Demographics. More than 80% of PAs occur in patients under 20. The peak incidence is in "middle-aged" children between the ages of 5 and 15 years. There is no sex predilection.

Presentation. Symptoms vary with location. Cerebellar PAs often present with headache, morning nausea, and vomiting, as intraventricular obstructive hydrocephalus is common. Ataxia, visual loss, and cranial nerve palsies also occur.

Optic pathway PAs typically present with visual loss. An uncommon presentation of a PA involving the hypothalamus is diencephalic syndrome, a rare but potentially lethal cause of failure to thrive despite adequate caloric intake.

Pontine and medullary PAs are uncommon but typically present with multiple cranial nerve palsies.

Natural History. PAs generally grow slowly. Ten-year survival exceeds 90%, even with partially resected tumors. Almost half of residual tumors show spontaneous regression or arrested long-term growth.

Rare cases of disseminated grade I PA have been reported. However, some cases that were initially diagnosed as "aggressive" or "atypical" PA may be pilomyxoid astrocytoma

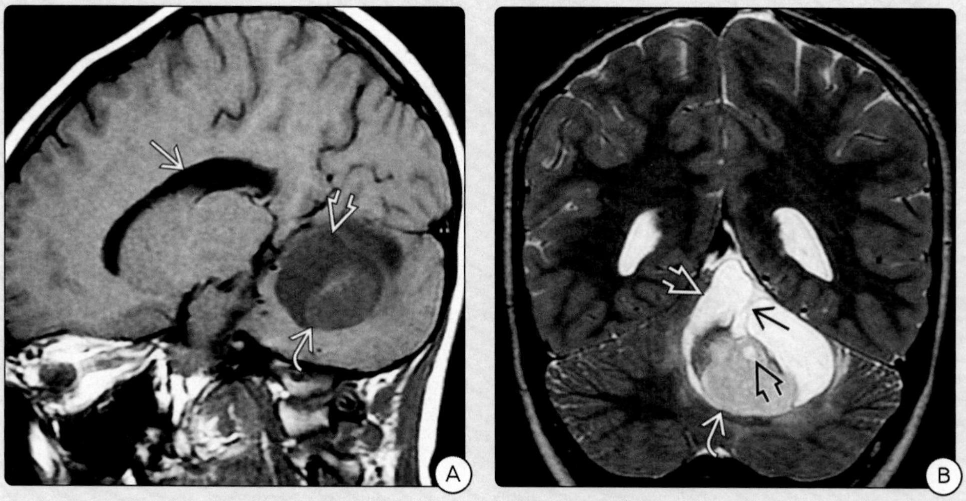

(17-10A) Sagittal T1WI in a child with headaches shows a cystic mass in the cerebellar hemisphere. The cyst fluid ➡ is hyperintense relative to CSF in the lateral ventricle ➡, which does not appear enlarged. A nodule ➡ is present within the cyst. (17-10B) Coronal T2WI shows that the cyst ➡ appears to be partially septated ➡ with a solid mixed signal intensity nodule ➡ that contains a small cystic component ➡.

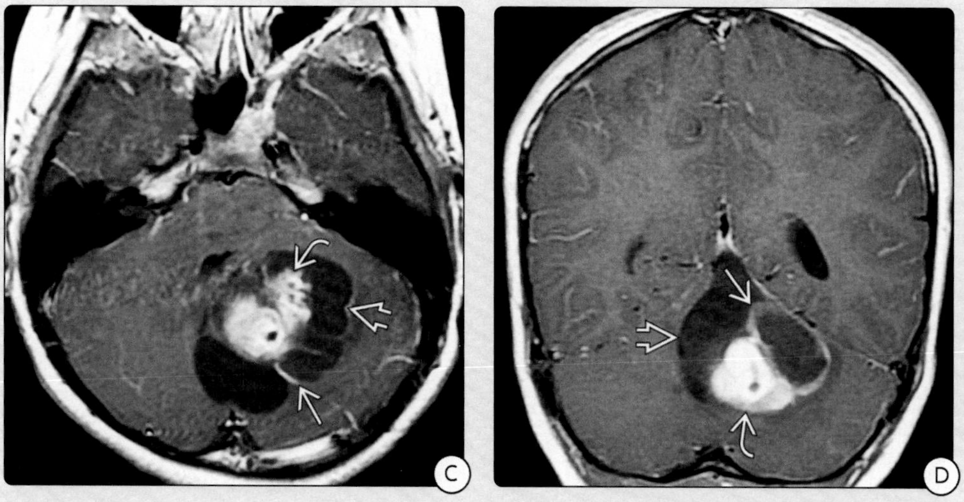

(17-10C) Axial T1 C+ shows that the cyst nodule ➡ enhances strongly but heterogeneously. Some enhancement of the cyst wall ➡ and internal septations ➡ is present. (17-10D) Coronal T1 C+ shows that the cyst wall is mostly nonenhancing ➡, while the cyst nodule ➡ and some internal septations ➡ enhance strongly. Pathology disclosed pilocytic astrocytoma, BRAF V600E mutation.

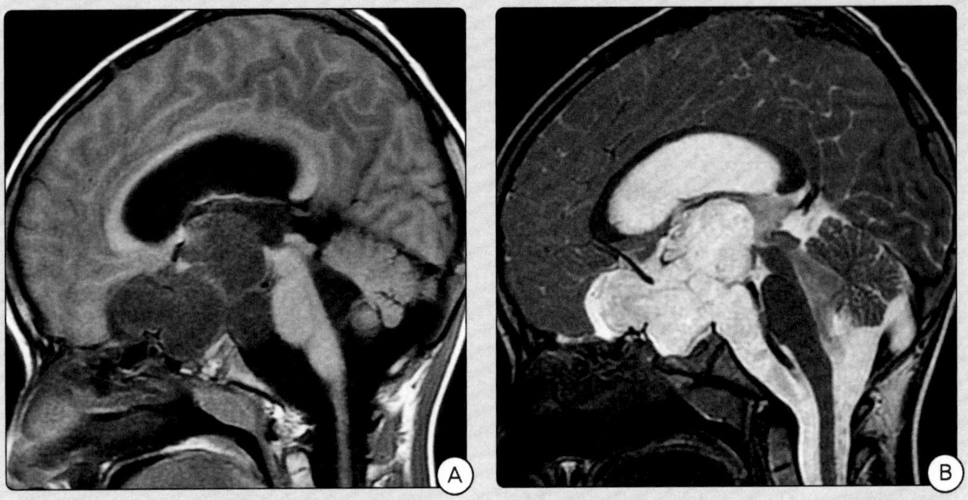

(17-11A) *A 7y boy had 2 months of morning vomiting, headache, visual difficulties. NECT showed a large lobulated suprasellar mass. Sagittal T1WI shows a hypointense hypothalamic mass that widens and largely fills the sella, extends dorsally in front of the pons. Moderate obstructive hydrocephalus is present.* ***(17-11B)*** *Sagittal T2WI in the same case shows that the mass is extremely hyperintense.*

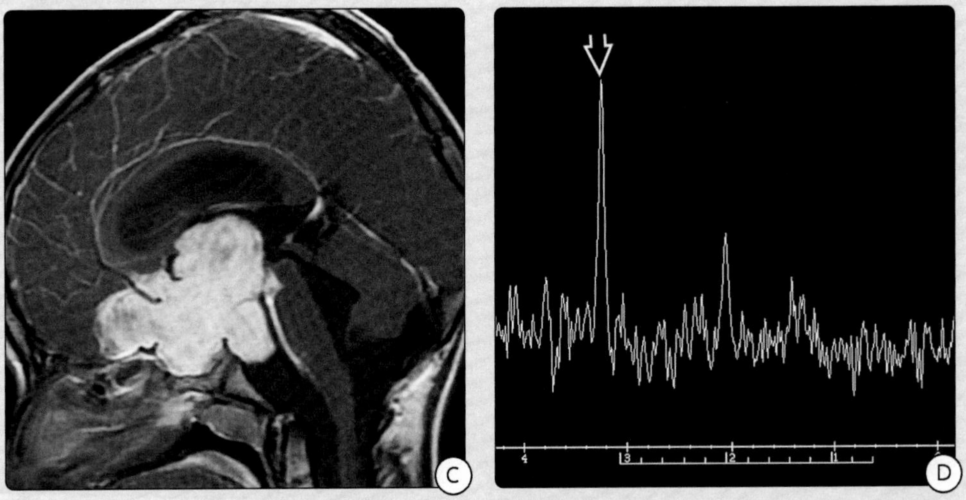

(17-11C) *Sagittal T1 C+ MR shows that the mass enhances intensely, slightly heterogeneously.* ***(17-11D)*** *MRS in the same case with TR 1500 TE 288 shows a "pseudomalignant" spectrum with a markedly elevated choline peak ➡, a common finding in PA. Imaging diagnosis was chiasmatic-hypothalamic PA. Biopsy confirmed a pilocytic astrocytoma, WHO grade I.*

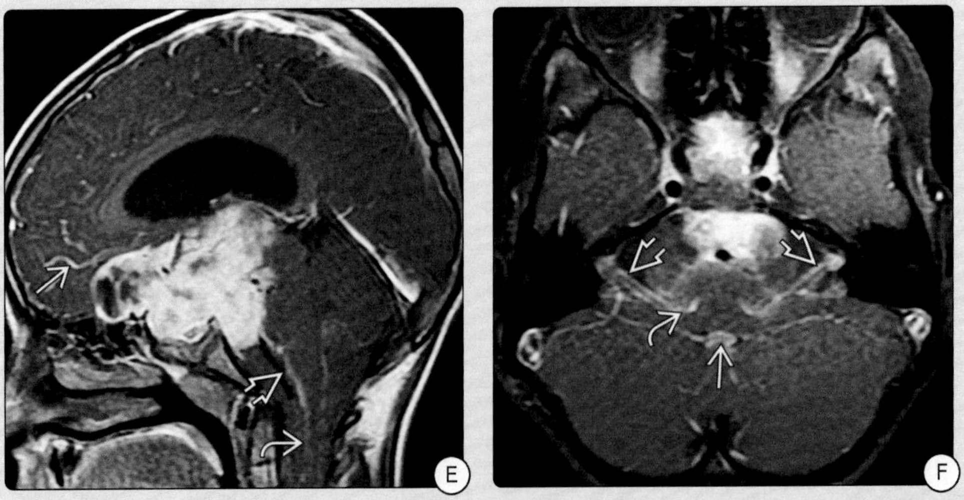

(17-11E) *Sagittal T1 C+ MR obtained 2 months later shows diffuse pial enhancement with tumor along the interhemispheric fissure ➡, coating the brainstem ➡ and cervical cord ➡.* ***(17-11F)*** *Axial T1 C+ FS shows metastatic tumor in the fourth ventricle ➡, coating the medulla ➡ as well as the 7th and 8th cranial nerves ➡. Despite CSF dissemination, the patient is alive 4 years later.*

(PMA). PMAs generally have an earlier age of onset, more aggressive clinical course, and poorer prognosis than PA.

Imaging

Similar to clinical presentation, imaging findings vary with PA location. The most common appearance of a posterior fossa PA is a well-delineated cerebellar cyst with a mural nodule.

PAs in and around the optic nerve, chiasm, third ventricle, and tectum tend to be solid, infiltrating, and less well marginated **(17-14)**. When they occur in these locations, PAs tend to expand the affected structures, which maintain their underlying anatomic configuration.

PAs in the tectum expand the collicular plate and may cause aqueductal obstruction **(17-61)**. The rare hemispheric PA typically presents as a cortically based lesion, usually a cyst with a mural nodule **(17-15)**.

CT Findings. NECT scans show a mixed cystic/solid **(17-8)** or solid mass **(17-9)** with focal mass effect and little, if any, adjacent edema. Calcification occurs in 10-20% of cases. Hemorrhage is uncommon; if present, the tumor may be a PMA rather than PA.

Most PAs enhance on both CT and MR scans. The most common pattern, seen in approximately half of all cases, is a nonenhancing cyst with a strongly enhancing mural nodule. A solid enhancing mass with central necrosis is seen in 40%, and 10% show solid homogeneous enhancement. If delayed scans are obtained, a contrast-fluid level may accumulate within the cyst.

MR Findings. Cystic PAs are usually well-delineated and appear slightly hyperintense to CSF on both T1- and T2WI. They do not suppress completely on FLAIR. The mural nodule is iso-/hypointense on T1WI and iso-/hyperintense on T2WI. Solid PAs appear iso- or hypointense to parenchyma on T1WI and hyperintense on T2/FLAIR. Posterior extension along the

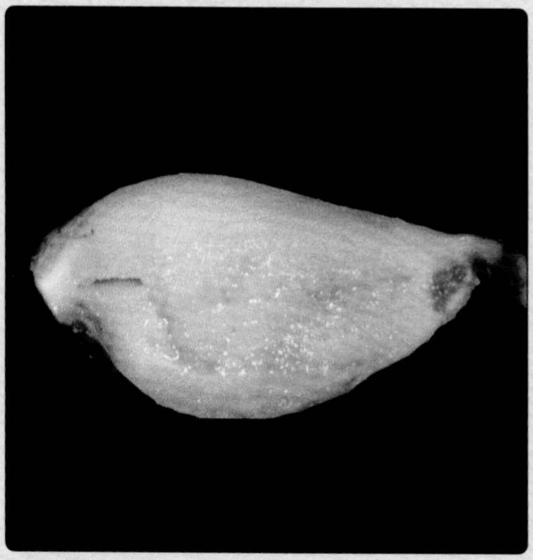

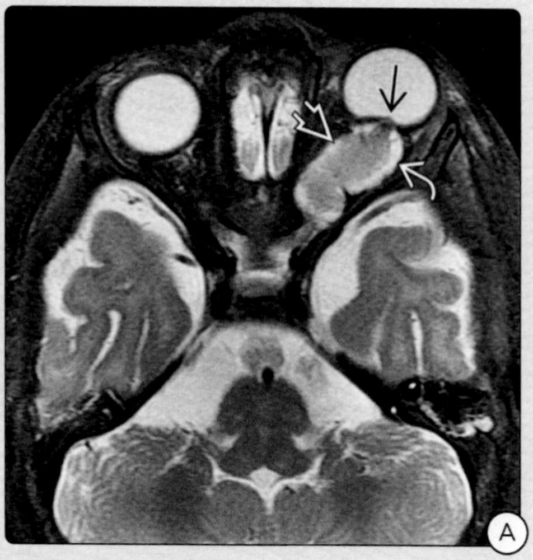

(17-12) Gross pathology of an optic nerve "glioma" shows fusiform enlargement of the optic nerve. Most optic nerve gliomas are pilocytic astrocytomas. Less commonly, they are WHO grade II diffusely infiltrating astrocytomas. (Courtesy R. Hewlett, MD.) (17-13A) T2WI in a 6m infant with NF1 shows a thickened, tortuous left optic nerve ➡ and dilated sheath ➡ with intraocular protrusion of the optic nerve head ⇨.

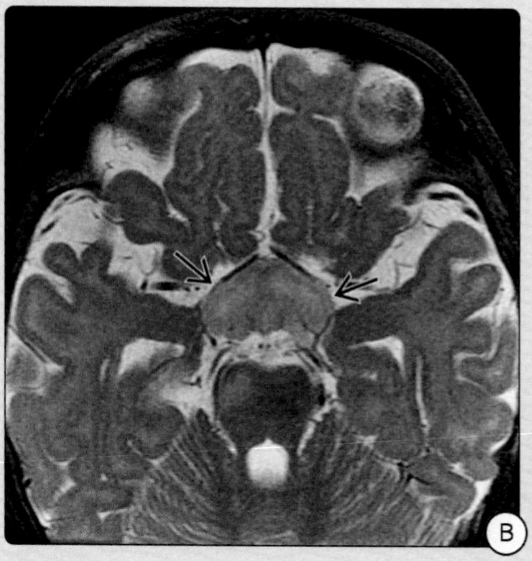

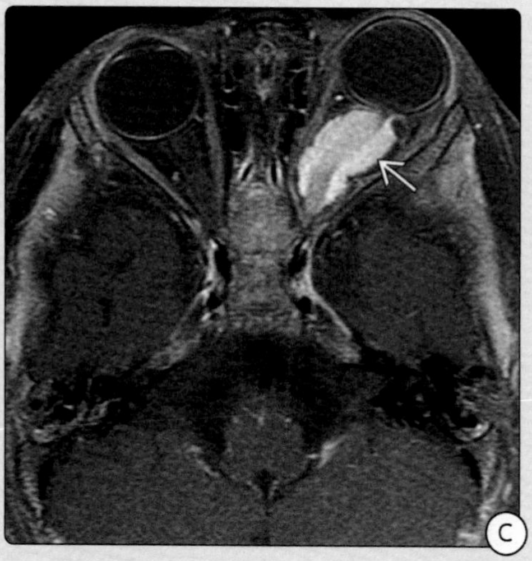

(17-13B) More cephalad T2WI shows that the optic chiasm is enlarged, infiltrated by tumor ⇨. (17-13C) T1 C+ FS shows that the left optic nerve is enlarged, infiltrated with enhancing tumor ➡. This is NF1-associated pilocytic astrocytoma.

optic radiations is not uncommon with a suprasellar PA and does not denote malignancy.

PAs contain numerous capillaries with fenestrations and open endothelial tight junctions that permit the escape of large macromolecules across the blood-brain barrier. They may therefore show striking enhancement following contrast administration. Intense but heterogeneous enhancement of the nodule in a cystic PA is typical **(17-10)**. Enhancement of the cyst wall itself varies from none to moderate. A variant pattern is a solid mass with central necrosis and a thick peripherally enhancing "rind" of tumor.

PAs in the optic nerve **(17-12)**, optic chiasm, and hypothalamus/third ventricle show quite variable enhancement (from none to striking) **(17-13)**, whereas hemispheric PAs generally present with a cyst plus an enhancing mural nodule.

MRS in PAs often shows elevated Cho, low NAA, and a lactate peak—paradoxical findings that are more characteristic of malignant neoplasms than this clinically benign-behaving tumor **(17-11)**. pMR shows low to moderate rCBV.

Angiography. Solid PAs are usually avascular, whereas cystic PAs may show moderately intense, prolonged vascular staining of the mural nodule. Arteriovenous shunting with "early draining" veins is uncommon.

Differential Diagnosis

The differential diagnosis of PA depends on location. Posterior fossa PAs can resemble **medulloblastoma**, especially when they are mostly solid midline tumors. Medulloblastomas typically restrict on DWI, whereas PAs do not.

Ependymoma is a plastic-appearing tumor that extrudes out the foramen of Magendie and lateral recesses. The imaging

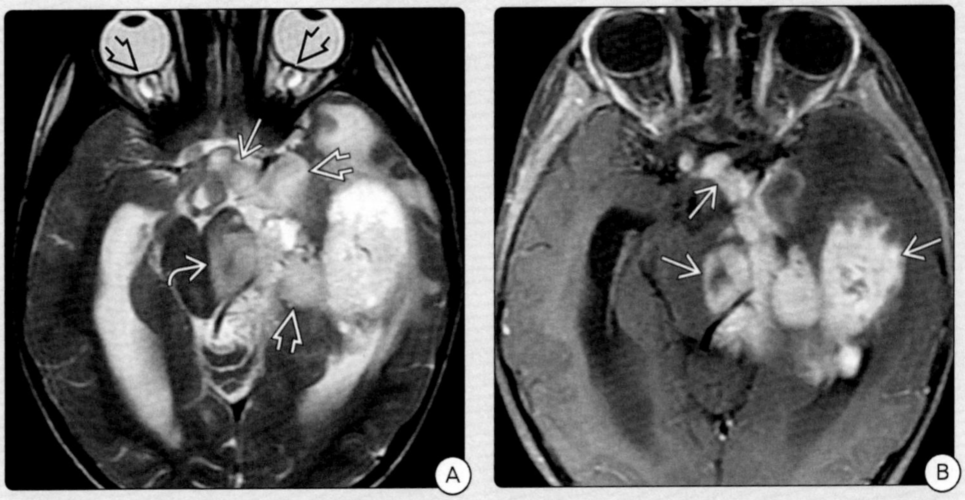

***(17-14A)** T2WI in a 4y girl shows a heterogeneously hyperintense mass infiltrating the optic chiasm, left midbrain, and medial temporal lobe, causing obstructive hydrocephalus and dilated optic nerve sheaths with flattened globes. **(17-14B)** T1 C+ FS shows the intensely but heterogeneously enhancing mass. Histopathology disclosed pilocytic astrocytoma with BRAF V600F mutation.*

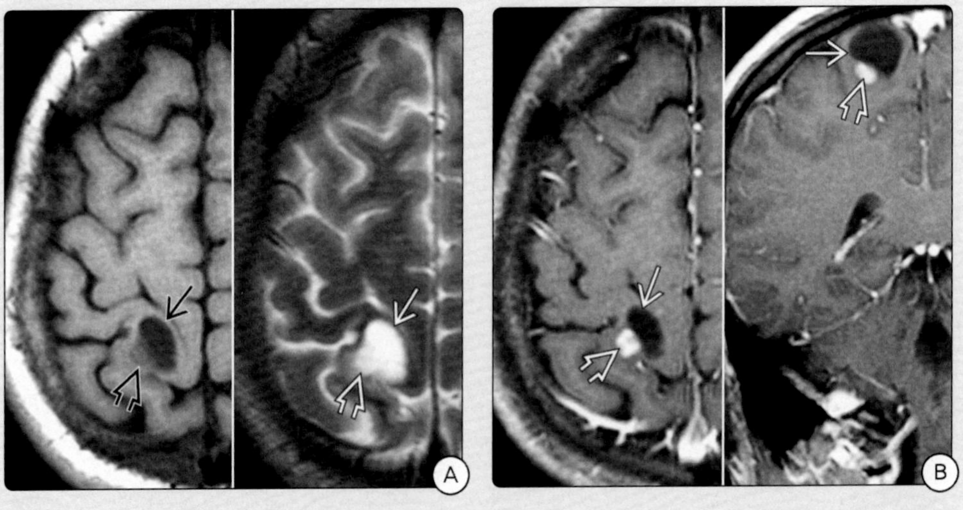

***(17-15A)** (L) T1WI in a 19y man with NF1 shows a cystic lesion in the right parietal lobe with a small less hypointense solid component. (R) T2WI shows that the cyst and nodule are both hyperintense. **(17-15B)** Sagittal (L), coronal (R) T1 C+ scans show the solid nodule enhances intensely, cyst wall does not. Surgery disclosed pilocytic astrocytoma, WHO grade I. Most common site for PA, especially in NF1, is the optic chiasm/nerves.*

appearance of **hemangioblastoma** (HGBL) can resemble PA, but HGBLs are tumors of middle-aged adults rather than children. HGBLs have significant peritumoral edema and markedly elevated rCBV.

The major differential diagnosis of hypothalamic PAs is **PMA**. PMAs tend to occur in younger children and infants. Hemorrhage is rare in PA but relatively common in PMA. **Demyelinating disease** and postviral inflammation can mimic visual pathway PAs. Optic neuritis can cause enlargement and enhancement of the optic nerves and chiasm.

The differential diagnosis of a hemispheric PA with a "nodule plus cyst" appearance is **ganglioglioma**. Gangliogliomas are generally cortically based and often calcify. **Pleomorphic xanthoastrocytomas** (PXA) can present with a solid "nodule plus cyst" but are tumors of young adults, not children. PXAs often incite meningeal reaction ("dural tail" sign).

Pilomyxoid Astrocytoma

Pilomyxoid astrocytoma (PMA) is a rare, recently described neoplasm that is considered a variant of pilocytic astrocytoma (PA). PMA has a unique histologic appearance and differs from PA in its presentation, imaging appearance, and clinical course.

Genetically, PMA and PA also differ. PMAs are usually negative for *BRAF* and overexpress the developmental genes *H19*, IGH2BP3/*IMP3*, and *DACT2*.

Pathology

Location. Although PMAs may occur anywhere along the neuraxis, they have a strong geographic predilection for the suprasellar region. Almost 60% center in the hypothalamus/optic chiasm, often extending into both temporal lobes **(17-16)**.

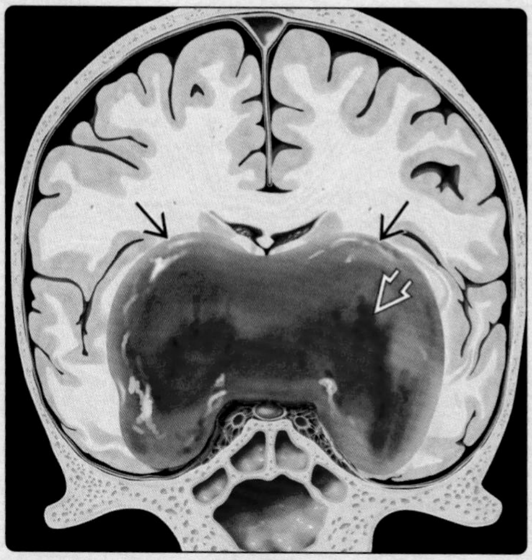

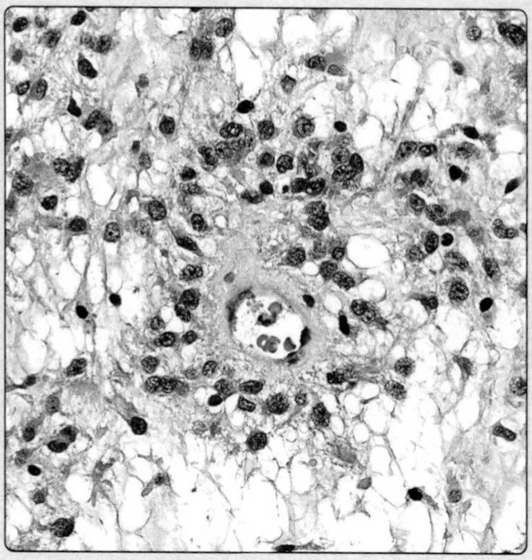

***(17-16)** PMA has bulky H-shaped hypothalamic/chiasmatic region mass extending to temporal lobes. Shiny myxoid matrix ⇨ and hemorrhage ➡ are seen. **(17-17)** Loose perivascular formations in a basophilic myxoid matrix are classic histologic features of PMA. (Courtesy P. Burger, MD.)*

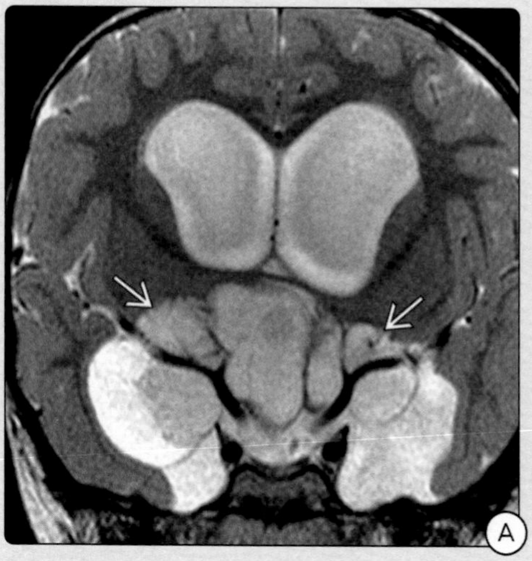

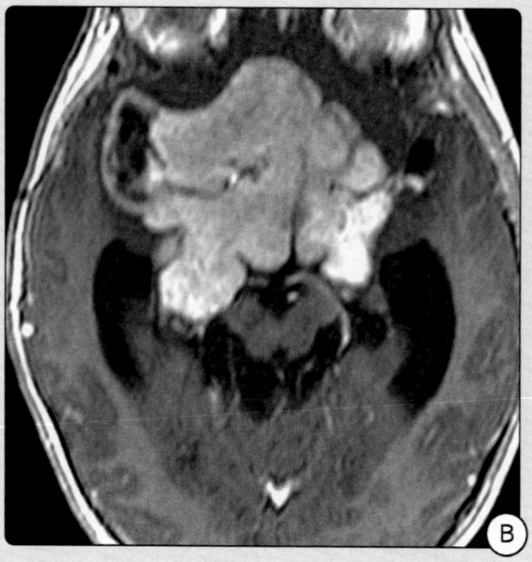

***(17-18A)** Coronal T2WI shows a large lobulated PMA ➡ that involves the hypothalamus and both medial temporal lobes. **(17-18B)** Axial contrast-enhanced SPGR in the same case shows the intensely enhancing H-shaped configuration of a hypothalamic PMA. (Courtesy M. Thurnher, MD.)*

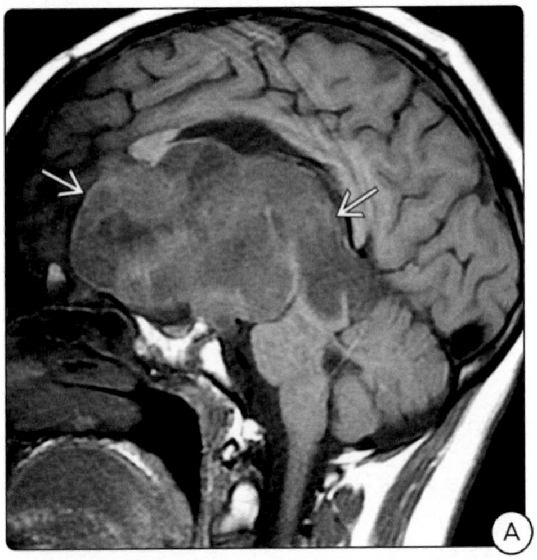

(17-19A) T1WI in a 10y girl diagnosed at age 2y with a hypothalamic/optic chiasm PA shows a huge mixed signal intensity suprasellar mass ➡.

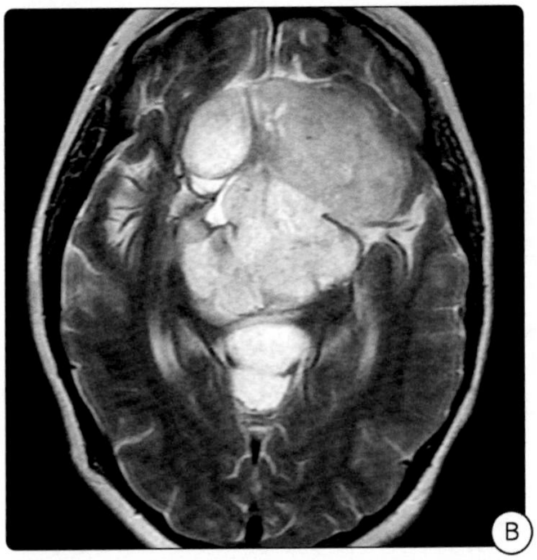

(17-19B) Axial T2WI in the same case shows that the mass is heterogeneously hyperintense.

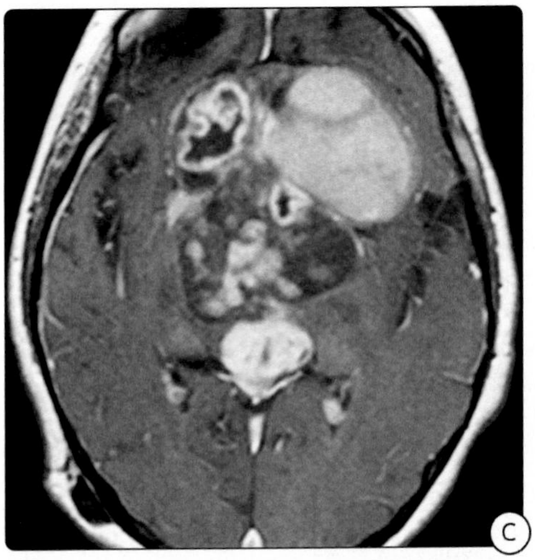

(17-19C) T1 C+ MR shows that the mass has mixed solid, cystic, ring-enhancing portions. Rebiopsy disclosed PMA.

About 40% of PMAs occur in atypical locations, mostly the cerebral hemispheres. In contrast to PA, PMAs in the cerebellum or fourth ventricle are rare.

Gross Pathology. PMAs are generally large, bulky, but relatively well-circumscribed masses. A glistening appearance caused by the myxoid component is common. Hemorrhage and necrosis are more common than with PA.

Microscopic Features. Rosenthal fibers and the characteristic biphasic pattern of PA are absent. Instead, PMAs consist of monomorphic piloid tumor cells embedded in a striking, mucopolysaccharide-rich myxoid matrix. There is little, if any, compact fibrillar tissue.

The neoplastic cells often display an angiocentric pattern that some investigators consider almost pathognomonic of PMA **(17-17)**. PMAs are GFAP and vimentin positive. MIB-1 is usually in the 1-2% range.

Staging, Grading, and Classification. Because of its more aggressive behavior and more frequent CSF dissemination, many neuropathologists consider PMA a grade II neoplasm although the most recent WHO has not made a definite grade assignment.

FEATURES THAT DISTINGUISH PMA FROM PA

Genetics
- High expression of *H19*, IGF2BP3 (*IMP3*)
- Low expression of *BRAF* fusion

Pathology
- Piloid cells + myxoid background
- Angiocentric growth
- May be WHO grade II

Clinical Issues
- More common in infants, children < 2 years
- Often more aggressive behavior
    - Occasionally may demonstrate progressive maturation to PA
    - Some may dedifferentiate to glioblastoma
- CSF dissemination more common

Imaging
- May occur anywhere along neuraxis
    - Nearly 75% in hypothalamus/optic chiasm
    - Atypical locations more common in older patients
- Large, bulky, H-shaped tumor
    - May extend laterally toward/into temporal lobes
- Heterogeneously hyperintense on T1/FLAIR
- Hemorrhage on T2* more common
- Enhancement intense, more homogeneous

Differential Diagnosis
- The major DDx for PA and PMA is diffuse astrocytoma (DA)
    - DA more common in older children, young adults (20-45 years)
    - DA in cerebral hemispheres > hypothalamus, cerebellum

Clinical Issues

Epidemiology. The exact incidence of PMA is unknown but is estimated at 0.5-1.0% of all astrocytomas, considerably less common than PA. Between 5-10% of cases diagnosed histologically as "aggressive" PAs may actually be PMAs.

Demographics. Although PMA has a relatively wide age range, it typically occurs at an earlier mean age than PA. Suprasellar PMAs are typically tumors

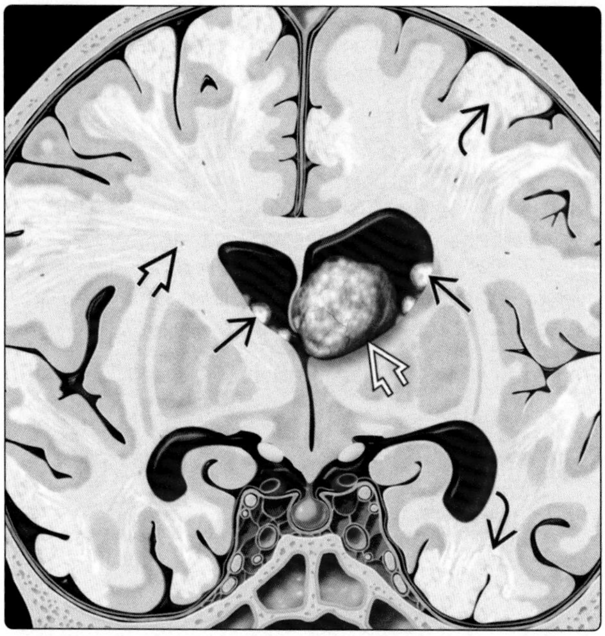

(17-20) Coronal graphic shows a SEGA ➡ in a patient with tuberous sclerosis. Note subependymal nodules ➡ and cortical tubers ➡ with "blurring" of the gray-white interface. Prominent radial glial bands ➡ are also present in the medullary WM.

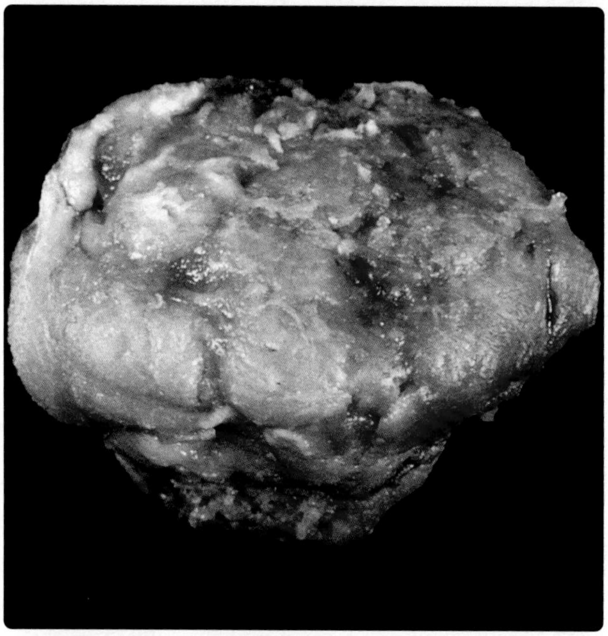

(17-21) Gross specimen of SEGA shows that they are resectable, discrete masses that lend themselves to complete or near-complete resection. (From DP2: Neuropathology.)

of infants and children younger than 4 years. Median age at presentation is 2 years. PMAs in atypical locations are more common in adolescents and young adults.

Presentation. Clinical presentation is often insidious. Infants may present with signs of increased intracranial pressure, failure to thrive, and diencephalic syndrome. Hypothalamic dysfunction and visual disturbances are common.

Natural History. Patients with PMAs generally have a worse prognosis that those with PA. Posttreatment recurrence rate is higher, progression-free interval is smaller, and overall survival is shorter.

Imaging

Compared with PAs, PMAs are more often solid and are primarily hypodense on NECT. Intratumoral hemorrhage is seen in nearly half of all cases; calcification is rare.

PMAs are iso- to hypointense on T1WI and hyperintense on T2/FLAIR **(17-18A)**, reflecting the high proportion of myxoid matrix in these tumors. Peritumoral edema is minimal or absent. Approximately 20% of PMAs demonstrate evidence of intratumoral hemorrhage on T2* (GRE, SWI), which is very rare in PAs.

Diffusion restriction is absent, and ADC values are relatively high, reflecting the low cellularity histology characteristic of both PAs and PMAs.

PMAs demonstrate strong, generally homogeneous enhancement after contrast administration **(17-18B)**. Occasionally large lesions may exhibit heterogeneous enhancement **(17-19)**. CSF dissemination is common with PMA, so the entire neuraxis should be imaged prior to surgical intervention.

Subependymal Giant Cell Astrocytoma

Subependymal giant cell astrocytoma (SEGA) is a localized, circumscribed, WHO grade I astrocytic tumor that mostly occurs in patients with tuberous sclerosis complex (TSC) **(17-20)**.

Terminology

SEGA is a neuroglial tumor composed of spine to large cells that occurs near the foramen of Monro.

Etiology

The origin of SEGAs and their relationship to the subependymal hamartomas that are a near-constant feature of TSC are controversial. Although there are histologic similarities between the two lesions, mitotic figures are found only in SEGAs.

Genetics

TSC-Associated SEGAs. The majority of SEGAs in patients with TSC have biallelic inactivation of the *TSC1* or *TSC2* genes. The *TSC1* and *TSC2* genes encode the tumor suppressor proteins hamartin and tuberin, respectively. Mutations prevent the hamartin/tuberin heterodimer from deactivating Rheb, leading to mammalian target of rapamycin genes (mTOR) upregulation. mTOR upregulation leads to uncontrolled cell growth and protein synthesis. Phosphorylation-driven inactivation of the tuberous sclerosis complex-2 protein (*TSC2*, tuberin) promotes cell growth in a TOR-dependent manner.

Nonsyndromic SEGAs. Between 10 and 20% of patients with SEGA do not have other features of TSC. SEGAs with low levels of *TSC1* somatic mosaicisms may occur without other presentations of the disease. Isolated nonsyndromic SEGAs have also been reported in patients *without* demonstrable germline or tumor mutations in *TSC1* or *TSC2* on sequencing.

Pathology

Location. Nearly all SEGAs are located in the lateral ventricles, adjacent to the foramen of Monro **(17-23)**.

Size and Number. SEGAs vary in size from tiny to lesions measuring several centimeters in diameter. The average tumor size is 10-15 mm. Most SEGAs are solitary lesions. So-called double SEGAs occur in up to 20% of cases.

Gross Pathology. SEGAs are well-circumscribed, multilobulated solid intraventricular masses that rarely hemorrhage or undergo necrosis **(17-21)**. Calcification is common.

Microscopic Features. SEGA tumor cells display a wide spectrum of astroglial phenotypes that may be indistinguishable from subependymal nodules (SENs). Large pyramidal cells that resemble astrocytes or ganglion cells are typical. Nuclei are large, round, and usually eccentric with open chromatin and prominent nucleoli. Mitoses are variable but generally few in number, so MIB-1 is low.

Staging, Grading, and Classification. SEGAs are WHO grade I neoplasms.

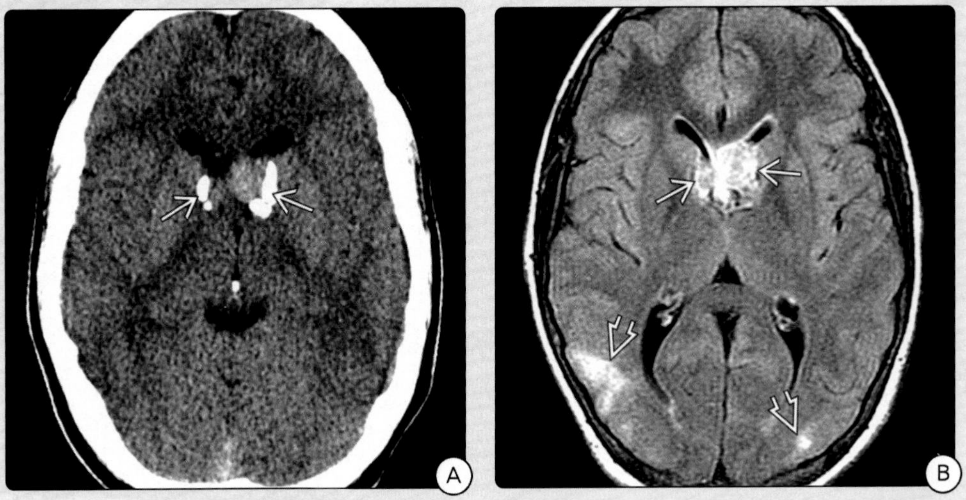

(17-22A) NECT scan in a child with tuberous sclerosis complex shows slightly hyperdense calcified masses in the frontal horns of both lateral ventricles ➡. (17-22B) FLAIR scan in the same patient shows that the masses ➡ are heterogeneously hyperintense. Again note the cortical tubers ➡.

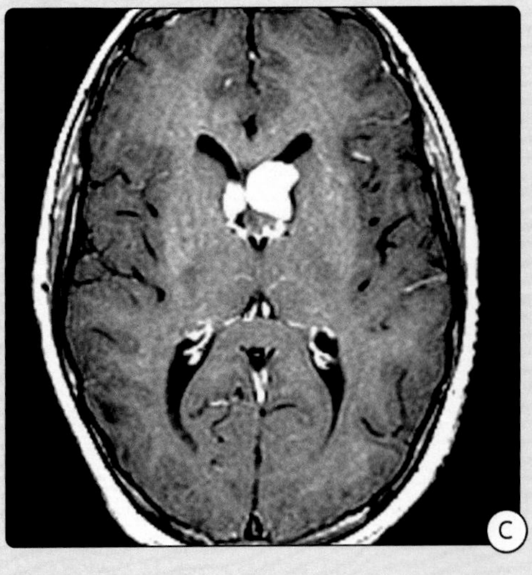

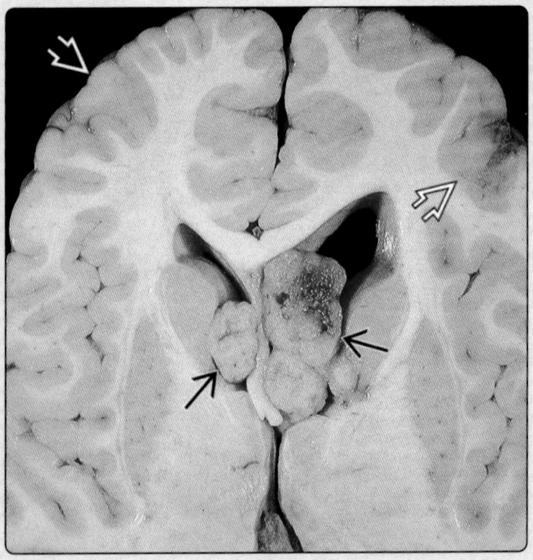

(17-22C) T1 C+ shows the intense enhancement of the masses. Subependymal giant cell astrocytomas are here shown in a tuberous sclerosis complex patient. (17-23) Axial autopsy in a patient with tuberous sclerosis shows cortical tubers ➡, bilateral SEGAs ➡. Note that left frontal horn is enlarged, but the tumor remains circumscribed and noninvasive. (Courtesy R. Hewlett, MD.)

Clinical Issues

Epidemiology. SEGAs arise in a relatively small proportion (10-20%) of patients with TSC but cause up to 25% of the morbidity associated with this condition.

Demographics. SEGAs generally occur in the setting of TSC and typically develop during the first two decades of life. Mean age at diagnosis is 11 years. Sporadic SEGAs without obvious tuberous sclerosis stigmata occur but are extremely rare.

Presentation. Epilepsy in tuberous sclerosis patients is related to cortical tubers, not SEGA. SEGAs are generally asymptomatic until they cause obstructive hydrocephalus. Headache, vomiting, and loss of consciousness are typical symptoms.

Natural History. Prognosis is generally good, as SEGAs are benign lesions that grow slowly and rarely infiltrate adjacent brain. Many patients with SEGAs have small lesions that may remain relatively stable. Median growth rate generally ranges from 2.5-5.6 mm per year.

The clinical course of SEGA, however, is not invariably so benign. The main concern is obstructive hydrocephalus, which may develop suddenly and result in rapidly rising intracranial pressure.

Treatment Options. When imaging findings are indeterminate and a lesion near the foramen of Monro cannot be clearly identified as an SEN or SEGA, close interval follow-up imaging (initially every 6 months, then annually if there is no evidence of growth) is recommended. A lesion in this location should be treated as soon as it shows evidence of enlargement.

Surgical resection has been the treatment of choice, as regrowth rates after complete tumor removal are very low. However, not all SEGAs can be resected completely. Biologically targeted pharmacotherapy with mTOR inhibitors such as sirolimus and everolimus has provided a safe and efficacious treatment option. SEGAs can recur a few months after drug discontinuation, so continued therapy may be necessary to avoid recurrence.

Imaging

The most important ancillary imaging findings to identify are those of TSC (see Chapter 39). In the absence of a known family history, mental retardation, epilepsy, or cutaneous stigmata, imaging may provide the first clues to the diagnosis of TSC.

CT Findings. SEGAs are hypo- to isodense, variably calcified lesions near the foramen of Monro **(17-22A)**. Calcified SENs may be seen along the lateral ventricle margins, especially the caudothalamic grooves. Hydrocephalus is present in 15% of cases. "Blurred" lateral ventricle margins indicate severe obstructive hydrocephalus with transependymal CSF migration.

SEGAs demonstrate strong but heterogeneous enhancement. An enhancing lesion at the foramen of Monro on CECT scan should be considered SEGA until proven otherwise.

MR Findings. SEGAs are hypo- to isointense compared with cortex on T1WI and heterogeneously iso- to hyperintense on T2WI. Larger SEGAs may have prominent "flow voids." Strong but heterogeneous enhancement is typical.

FLAIR is especially useful for detecting subtle CNS features of TSC such as SENs, cortical tubers, and white matter radial migration lines. Streaky linear hyperintensities extending through the white matter to the subjacent ventricle or wedge-shaped hyperintensities underlying expanded ("clubbed") gyri are typical **(17-22B)**.

SEN enhancement is much more visible on MR than on CT. Between 30-80% of SENs enhance following contrast administration **(17-22C)**, so enhancement alone is insufficient to distinguish an SEN from a SEGA. Although a mass at the foramen of Monro larger than 10-12 mm in diameter is usually a SEGA **(17-24)**, only progressive enlargement is sufficient to differentiate a SEGA from an SEN.

SUBEPENDYMAL GIANT CELL ASTROCYTOMA

Etiology, Genetics
- 5-15% of patients with TSC develop SEGA
- 80-90% of SEGAs are associated with TSC
  - Biallelic inactivation of *TSC1* or *TSC2* genes
  - Loss of hamartin or tuberin immunoexpression
  - Activation of mTOR pathway
- Sporadic SEGAs without TSC = 10-20%

Pathology
- Circumscribed, multinodular mass at foramen of Monro
- Does not infiltrate brain
- WHO grade I

Clinical Issues
- Mean age = 11 years
- Seizures, ↑ intracranial pressure

Imaging Findings
- Ca++ on NECT, enhance on CECT
- T1 iso-/hypointense, T2/FLAIR hyperintense
- May have prominent vascular "flow voids"
- Strong, heterogeneous enhancement
- Look for signs of TSC

Differential Diagnosis

The major differential diagnosis of SEGA in a patient with TSC is a benign nonneoplastic **SEN**. SENs remain stable and do not need to be treated, whereas SEGAs gradually enlarge and eventually require surgical treatment. SEGAs arise only near the foramen of Monro, whereas SENs can be located anywhere around the ventricular wall, especially along the caudothalamic groove. Although SENs are much more common than SEGAs, a partially calcified enhancing lesion at the foramen of Monro larger than 5 mm is more likely to be a SEGA than an SEN.

*(**17-24A**) Sagittal T2WI in a 7y girl with headaches, morning nausea, and vomiting shows a heterogeneous, lobulated mass → in the lateral ventricle. Severe obstructive hydrocephalus with upward bowing of the corpus callosum → is present. (**17-24B**) Axial T2WI in the same case shows the heterogeneous mass has prominent internal "flow voids →," obstructs the foramen of Monro, and causes periventricular fluid accumulation in the left frontal lobe.*

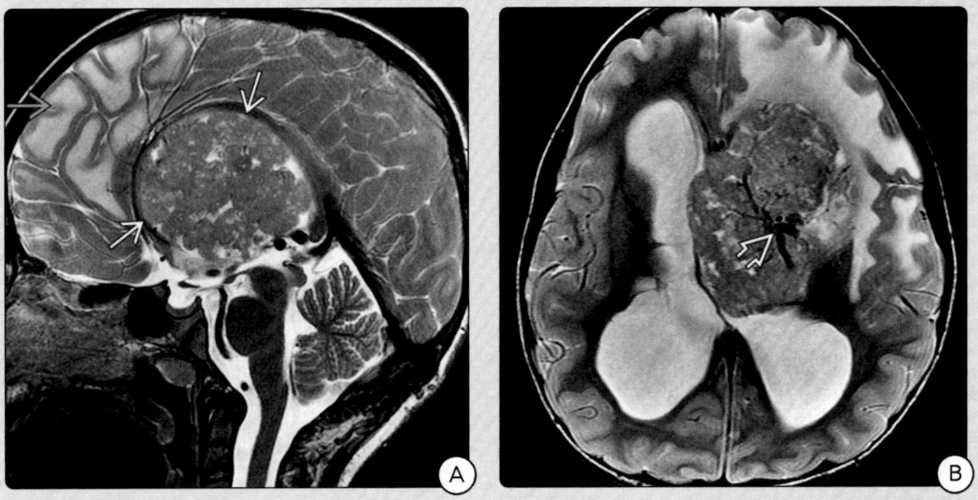

*(**17-24C**) T1 C+ FS MR shows that the mass enhances intensely but very heterogeneously. (**17-24D**) Axial pMR in the same case shows that the mass exhibits markedly elevated rCBV →.*

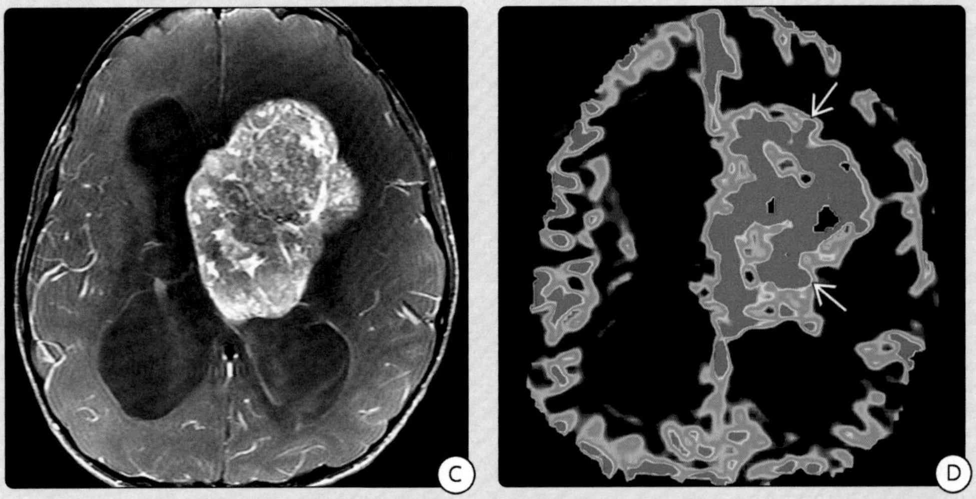

*(**17-24E**) Coronal T2WI shows the prominent vascular "flow voids" → intrinsic to the mass. The margin between the lateral ventricle and brain → is indistinct, and there is significant associated edema →. (**17-24F**) AP view of left internal carotid angiogram shows a very hypervascular mass with irregular, enlarged arteries → and early draining veins →. A large SEGA without brain invasion was removed at surgery.*

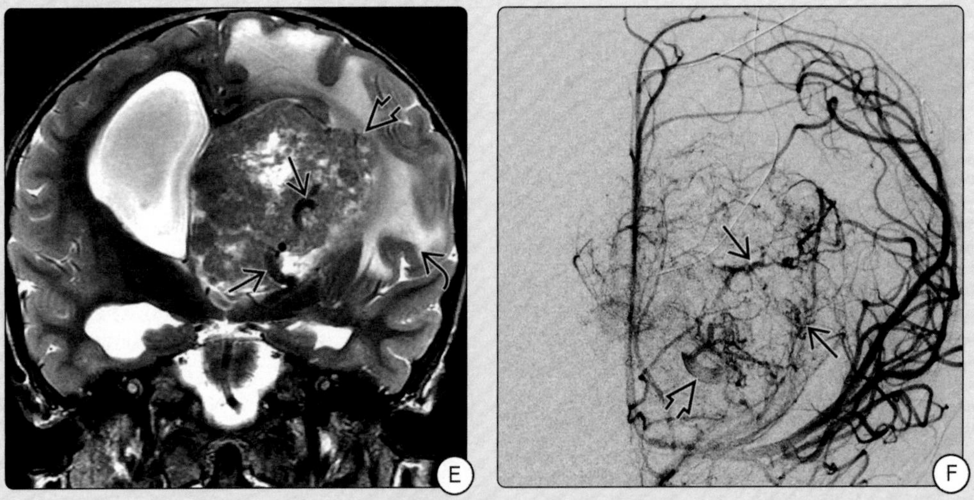

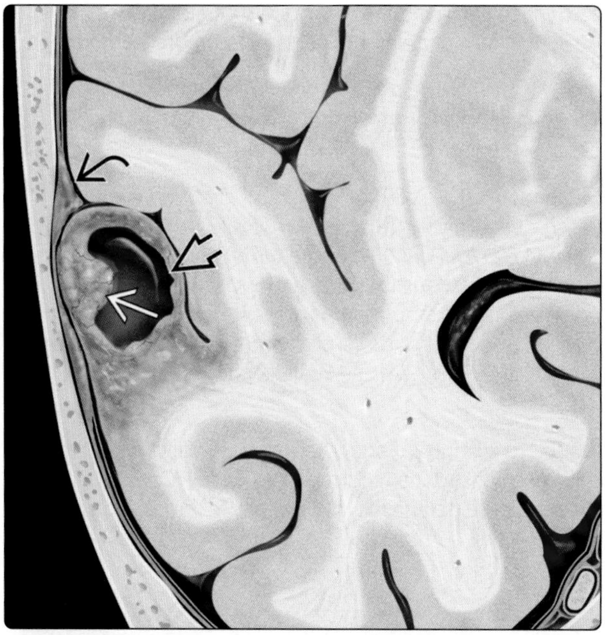

(17-25) Coronal graphic depicts pleomorphic xanthoastrocytoma with cyst, nodule abutting pial surface, and reactive thickening of the adjacent dura-arachnoid.

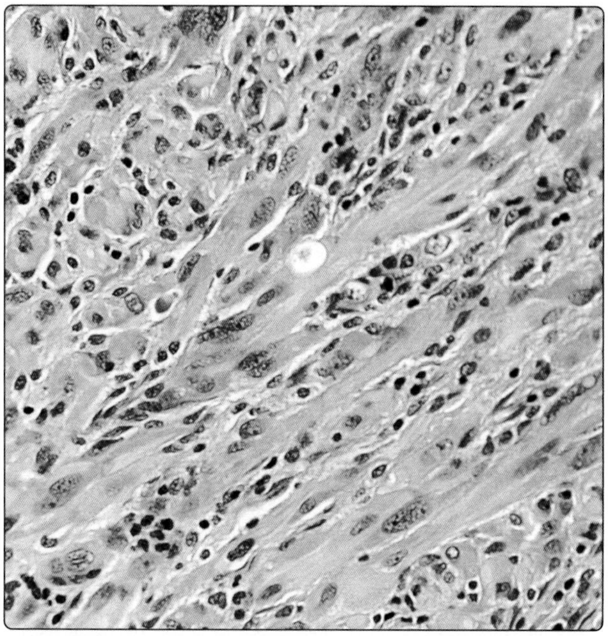

(17-26) Classic histologic features of PXA include somewhat fascicular architecture and cells that appear pleomorphic but not "monstrous." The bulk of the lesion is compact, noninfiltrating. (Courtesy P. Burger, MD.)

Other lateral ventricle masses that should be included in the differential diagnosis are **subependymoma** (a tumor of middle-aged and elderly patients) and **central neurocytoma** (a "bubbly" tumor that arises in the lateral ventricle body). Low-grade **diffusely infiltrating astrocytoma** can arise in the septi pellucidi or fornices, but these tumors typically neither calcify nor enhance.

Pleomorphic Xanthoastrocytoma

Terminology

Pleomorphic xanthoastrocytoma (PXA) is a rare astrocytic glioma with large pleomorphic, frequently multinucleated cells and xanthomatous change.

Etiology

PXAs are sometimes associated with cortical dysplasia and typically express neuronal markers. Possible origin from multipotent neuroectodermal precursor cells or from a preexisting hamartomatous lesion has been postulated.

PXAs lack IDH and H3 histone mutations. More than half have *BRAF* point mutations, a feature they share with pilocytic astrocytoma and ganglioglioma.

Pathology

Location. Over 95% of PXAs are supratentorial hemispheric masses. Most are superficial cortically based, seizure-associated neoplasms. The temporal lobe is the most common site (40-50%), and involvement of the adjacent leptomeninges is common. Other frequent locations include the frontal (33%) and parietal (20%) lobes. Cerebellar and spinal cord PXAs have been reported but are very rare.

Size and Number. PXAs are usually solitary lesions although a few multicentric lesions have been reported. Most are small; lesions greater than 3 cm are uncommon.

Gross Pathology. The most common gross appearance is that of a relatively discrete partially cystic mass with a mural nodule that abuts or is attached to the leptomeninges **(17-25)**. Dural invasion is rare. The deep tumor margins may be indistinct with focal parenchymal infiltration into the adjacent subcortical white matter.

Microscopic Features. The most striking features of PXA are its pleomorphism, dense reticulin network, compact architecture, and lipidization of tumor cells. Fibrillary and giant, multinucleated, neoplastic astrocytes are intermixed with large, lipid-containing, GFAP-positive cells **(17-26)**. Necrosis is rare.

Almost all PXAs are GFAP positive and show S100 immunoreactivity. Neuronal markers such as synaptophysin and neurofilament protein are often present. Mitotic figures are rare or absent.

Staging, Grading, and Classification. PXAs are WHO grade II tumors. PXAs that display anaplastic features including higher cellularity and increased mitoses are designated WHO grade III tumors (see below).

Clinical Issues

Epidemiology. PXA is a rare tumor, accounting for slightly less than 1% of all astrocytomas.

Demographics. PXAs are generally tumors of children and young adults; mean age at diagnosis is 22 years.

Presentation. Because of its characteristic superficial cortically based location, the most common presentation is longstanding epilepsy.

Natural History. Recurrence following gross total resection is uncommon. Mitotic activity and extent of resection are the only predictors of subsequent biologic behavior. Overall 5-year survival is approximately 80%, and the 10-year survival rate is 70%.

Imaging

CT Findings. NECT scans show a well-delineated, peripheral, cortically based mass that contacts the leptomeninges. Two imaging patterns are common. A "cyst + nodule" configuration is present in 70% of cases, and a predominantly solid mass with intratumoral cysts is seen in 30%. The overlying skull may be thinned and remodeled on bone CT. Calcifications are present in 40% of cases, but gross intratumoral hemorrhage is rare.

The mural nodule of a PXA shows moderate to intense enhancement on CECT.

MR Findings. The solid component of a PXA is heterogeneously hypo- or isointense relative to cortex on T1WI **(17-27A)**. Over 90% of the tumor nodules demonstrate heterogeneous hyperintensity on T2WI and FLAIR. If calcifications or hemorrhage is present, "blooming" on T2* can be seen. The cystic portions of PXA are usually hyperintense relative to CSF on T2WI and FLAIR sequences **(17-27B)** **(17-27C)**.

Moderate enhancement of the tumor nodule is typical following contrast administration **(17-27D)**. Over 90% of PXAs abut the pia and may incite reactive thickening of the

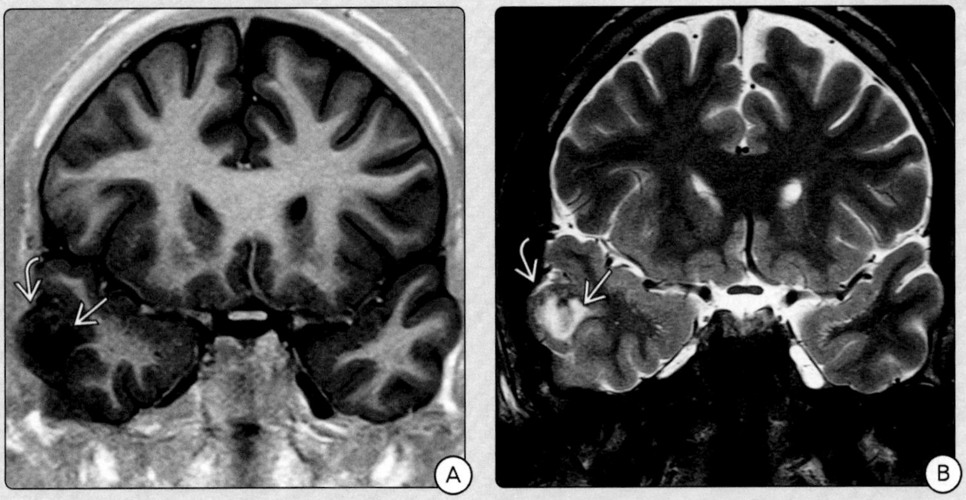

***(17-27A)** Coronal inversion recovery scan in a 19y man with longstanding temporal lobe epilepsy shows a partially cystic right temporal lobe mass ➡ that remodels the adjacent calvaria ➡. **(17-27B)** Coronal T2WI shows that the lesion ➡ is predominantly hyperintense. The smooth remodeling of the adjacent calvaria ➡ can be especially well appreciated on this image.*

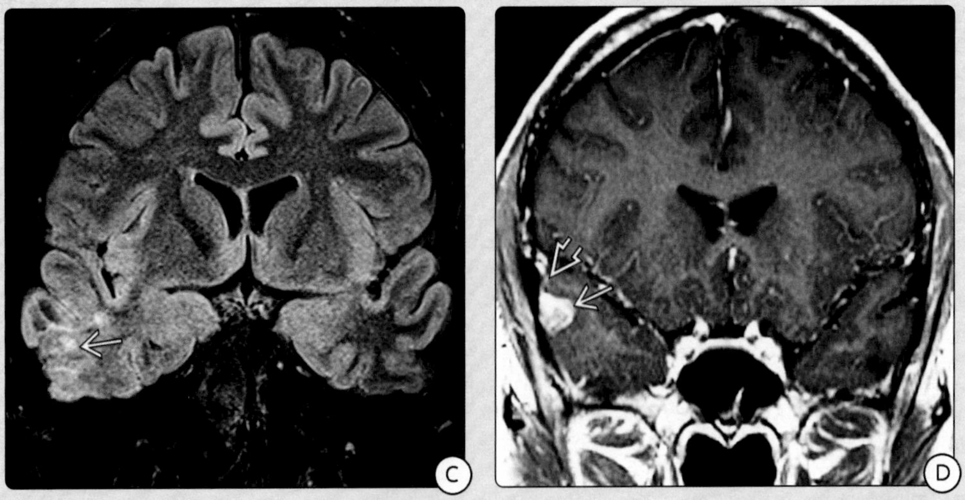

***(17-27C)** Coronal FLAIR scan shows that the lesion is heterogeneously hyperintense ➡. **(17-27D)** Coronal T1 C+ scan demonstrates an enhancing nodule ➡ that abuts the dura, causing minimal thickening and enhancement ➡. WHO grade II pleomorphic xanthoastrocytoma was removed at surgery.*

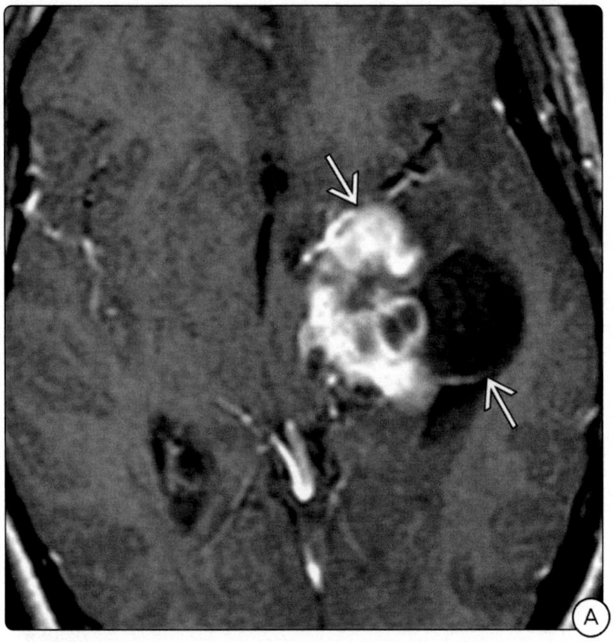

(17-28A) T1 C+ FS in a 27y woman with seizures shows a mixed solid, cystic mass in the left medial temporal lobe ➡. Histopathology disclosed PXA with anaplastic features.

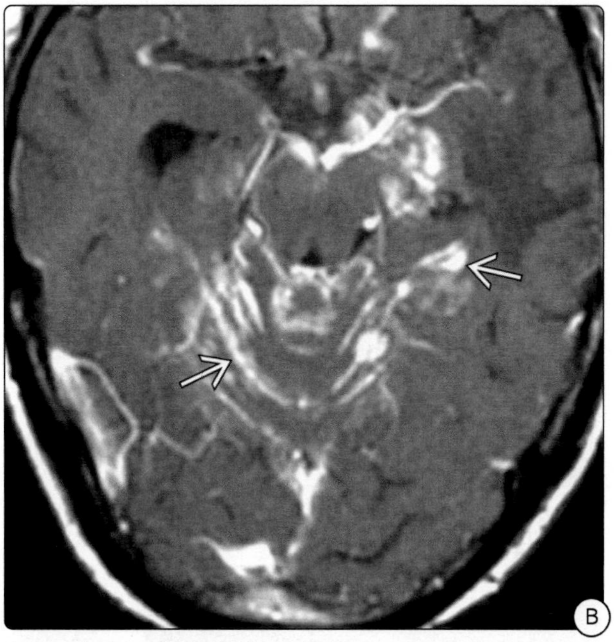

(17-28B) The patient was lost to follow-up but returned 18 months later with severe headaches, multiple cranial nerve palsies. T1 C+ shows diffuse CSF metastases ➡. She expired 2 years after initial diagnosis. This was PXA, WHO grade III.

adjacent dura. A "dural tail" sign was seen in 15-50% of cases in reported series.

Differential Diagnosis

The major differential diagnosis of PXA is **ganglioglioma**, another cortically based tumor that often causes epilepsy. Other less common tumors with a "cyst + nodule" appearance can mimic PXA, including hemispheric **pilocytic astrocytoma. Dysembryoplastic neuroepithelial tumor (DNET)** has a similar presentation and age range but typically has a multicystic "bubbly" appearance.

Diffuse (low-grade) fibrillary astrocytoma usually involves the white matter and does not involve the meninges. **Oligodendroglioma** can present as a slow-growing cortical-white matter junction lesion that remodels the adjacent calvaria, but the "cyst + nodule" pattern is usually absent.

CORTICALLY BASED TUMORS WITH "CYST + NODULE"

Common
- Ganglioglioma
- Metastasis

Less Common
- Pilocytic astrocytoma
- Pleomorphic xanthoastrocytoma
- Glioblastoma multiforme

Rare
- Hemangioblastoma
- Desmoplastic infantile astrocytoma/ganglioglioma
- Papillary glioneuronal tumor
- Schwannoma

Anaplastic Pleomorphic Xanthoastrocytoma

A PXA that has anaplastic features with more than five mitoses per ten high-power fields is now recognized as an anaplastic pleomorphic xanthoastrocytoma (aPXA), WHO grade III.

aPXAs sometimes have epithelioid features and share common histologic, immunohistochemical, molecular, and clinical characteristics found in a rare glioblastoma variant, epithelioid glioblastoma. aPXAs typically do not show *IDH1* gene mutation or *EGFR* amplification and often harbor *BRAF* mutations.

Few aPXAs with imaging findings have been reported. Large, more heterogeneous-appearing masses are typical. As leptomeningeal spread is common with these more aggressive tumors, complete craniospinal imaging should be obtained either at the time of diagnosis or on short interval follow-up **(17-28)**.

Diffuse Astrocytomas

WHO grade II diffuse astrocytomas, WHO grade III anaplastic astrocytomas, and WHO grade IV glioblastomas are each divided into two subtypes depending on the presence or absence of IDH mutation. If IDH mutation status is unknown, these tumors are designated as diffuse astrocytoma, not otherwise specified (NOS).

We begin this discussion with **IDH-mutant** astrocytomas. IDH-mutant tumors account for approximately 90% of WHO grade

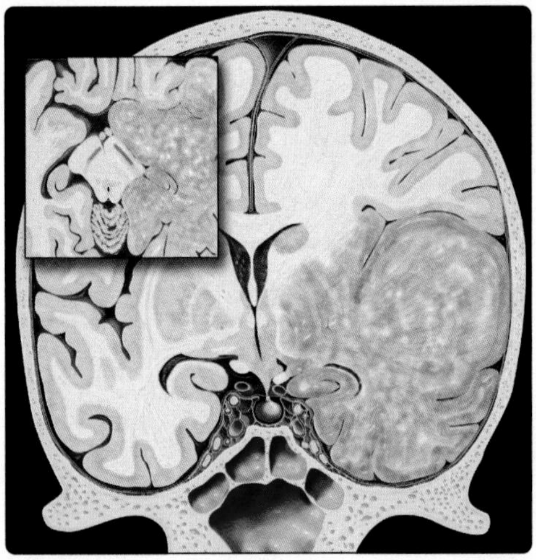

(17-29) Diffusely infiltrating astrocytoma (WHO grade II) is shown expanding the temporal lobe, infiltrating cortex/subcortical WM.

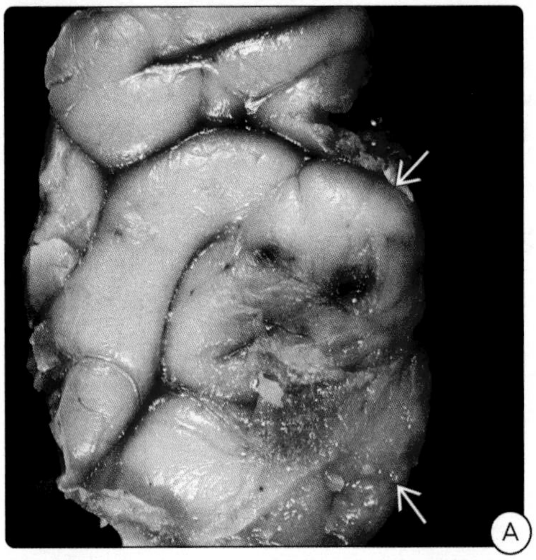

(17-30A) Surgical specimen from resected infiltrating DA shows expansion of cortex ➡, mass effect on underlying gyri.

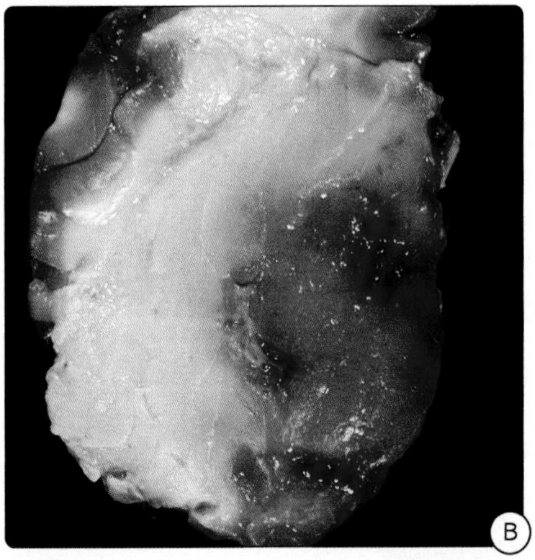

(17-30B) Cut section shows tumor infiltrates cortex, subcortical WM; no clear border between normal, abnormal brain. (R. Hewlett, MD.)

II and III astrocytomas and are discussed first. We then follow with their **IDH-wild-type** counterparts and a discussion of **glioblastoma** (most of which are also IDH-wild-type) and **gliosarcoma**.

We then conclude this chapter with a discussion of pediatric brainstem tumors and the newly recognized, highly malignant **diffuse midline glioma, H3 K27M-mutant.**

Diffuse Astrocytoma, IDH-Mutant

Terminology

Diffuse astrocytoma, IDH-mutant (IDH-mutant DA) is a diffusely infiltrating astrocytoma with a mutation in either the *IDH1* or *IDH2* gene that corresponds histologically to WHO grade II. IDH-mutant DAs tend to grow slowly but have an intrinsic tendency for malignant progression to IDH-mutant anaplastic astrocytoma (AA) and (eventually) IDH-mutant glioblastoma (GBM).

The terms "low-grade astrocytoma" and "fibrillary astrocytoma" are no longer used.

Etiology

IDH-mutant DAs develop from a distinct population of precursor cells in the frontal subventricular zones. In addition to *IDH1* mutation, these tumors also typically harbor class-defining loss-of-function mutations in *ATRX* and *TP53.*

Pathology

Location. Although IDH-mutant DAs can arise anywhere, the cerebral hemispheres are the most common overall site **(17-29)** with a preferential location in the frontal lobes. Almost 20% involve the deep gray nuclei.

Size and Number. Frontal lobe IDH-mutant DAs may become rather large before producing symptoms. Temporal lobe lesions are often smaller at initial presentation because of their propensity to cause partial complex seizures.

Gross Pathology. All diffuse astrocytomas are infiltrating lesions with ill-defined borders. Enlargement and distortion of invaded structures are typical. Gray-white matter interfaces are blurred **(17-30)**. Occasional cysts and calcification may be present. Hemorrhage is rare.

Microscopic Features. Well-differentiated fibrillary astrocytes in a loosely structured, often microcystic tumor matrix is the classic appearance. Mitotic activity is rare or absent, and the MIB-1 index is low.

Immunohistochemistry is essential in establishing the diagnosis of IDH-mutant DA. By definition, IDH-1 positivity is present in all cases. *TP53* mutation and *ATRX* loss are characteristic but not required for the diagnosis. 1p/19q codeletion (characteristic for oligodendrogliomas) is absent.

Staging, Grading, and Classification. IDH-mutant DAs are WHO grade II neoplasms.

Clinical Issues

Clinical features (i.e., age at presentation and survival) are essentially similar for both IDH-mutant DA and AA.

Epidemiology. DAs (the vast majority of which are IDH-mutant) account for between 10 and 15% of astrocytomas in adults.

Demographics. The mean age at presentation is mid-30s (range 20-50 years).

Presentation. Symptoms are location dependent. Seizure is the most common presentation of hemispheric lesions.

Natural History. Recurrence following surgical resection is common. Large series have shown that the mean survival of IDH-mutant DAs is nearly 11 years, almost identical with IDH-mutant AAs.

IDH-MUTANT DIFFUSE ASTROCYTOMAS

Terminology
- Formerly known as low-grade astrocytoma or diffuse astrocytoma

Etiology
- Glioma cancer stem cell
- Molecular genetics
  - *IDH1/2* mutated
  - *ATRX* loss, *TP53* mutated
  - 1p/19q intact (not codeleted)

Pathology
- Supratentorial (frontal lobe most common)
- Infiltrating, ill-defined borders
- WHO grade II
- Inherent tendency to undergo malignant degeneration

Clinical Issues
- 10-15% of astrocytomas
- Age = 20-45 years (mean = 38 years)
- Overall survival = 11 years
  - Not significantly different from IDH+ anaplastic astrocytoma

Imaging

CT Findings. NECT shows an ill-defined homogeneous mass that is hypodense relative to white matter. Calcification is seen in 20% of cases. Gross cystic change and hemorrhage are rare. CECT shows no enhancement.

MR Findings. Most IDH-mutant DAs are frontal lobe predominant and tend to infiltrate the white matter with relative sparing of the overlying cortex. Moderate mass effect with adjacent gyral expansion is common.

DAs are typically hypointense on T1WI **(17-31A)** and hyperintense on T2/FLAIR **(17-31B)**. Note that, although diffusely infiltrating astrocytomas may appear somewhat circumscribed on MR, neoplastic cells generally infiltrate adjacent normal-appearing brain.

T2* scans may show "blooming" foci if calcification is present. IDH-mutant DAs do not enhance following contrast administration **(17-31C)** and do not restrict on DWI.

MRS shows elevated choline, low NAA, and a high mI:Cr ratio. 3T MRS may exhibit an elevated 2-hydroxyglutarate peak (2-HG) resonating at 2.25 ppm.

Dynamic contrast-enhanced (DCE) MR perfusion shows relatively low rCBV. Foci of increased rCBV may represent areas of early malignant degeneration.

Differential Diagnosis

The definitive diagnosis of IDH-mutant DA requires histologic confirmation and molecular profiling. The major *imaging* differential diagnoses are other astrocytomas and oligodendroglioma.

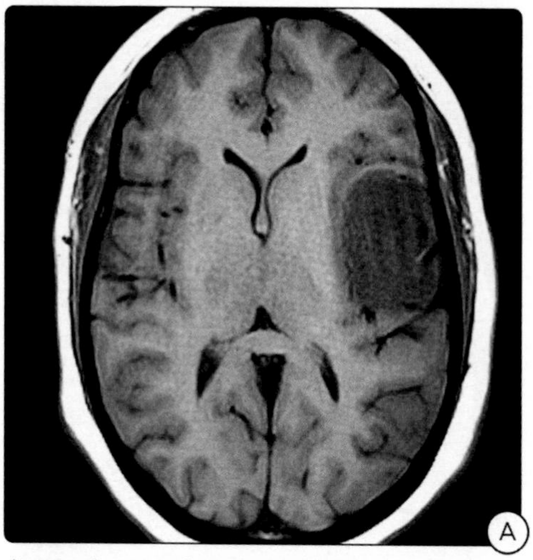

***(17-31A)** T1WI of a 28y man shows hypointense left temporal lobe mass compressing the external capsule and basal ganglia. MR ruled out stroke.*

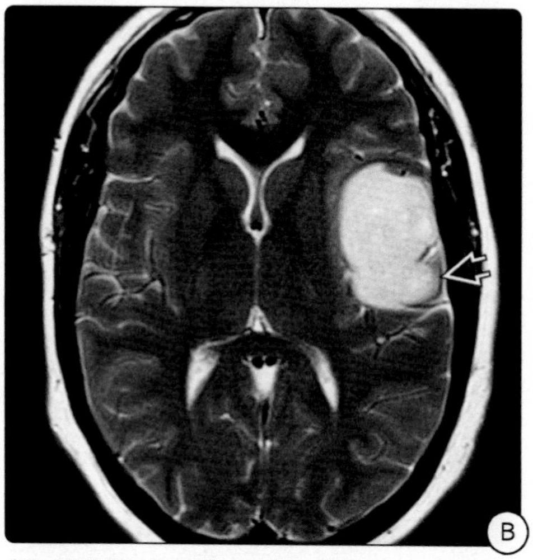

***(17-31B)** T2WI configuration of the mass is more round than wedge-shaped, and a thin, compressed layer of cortex ➡ overlies the mass.*

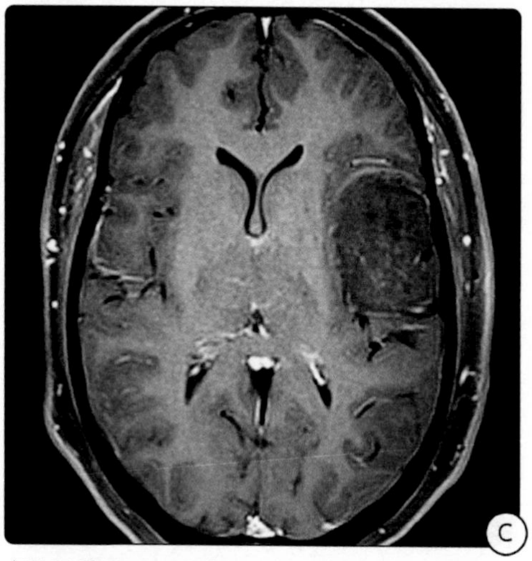

***(17-31C)** T1 C+ FS shows no enhancement. This is WHO grade II astrocytoma, IDH-mutated, both p53 and PTEN positive.*

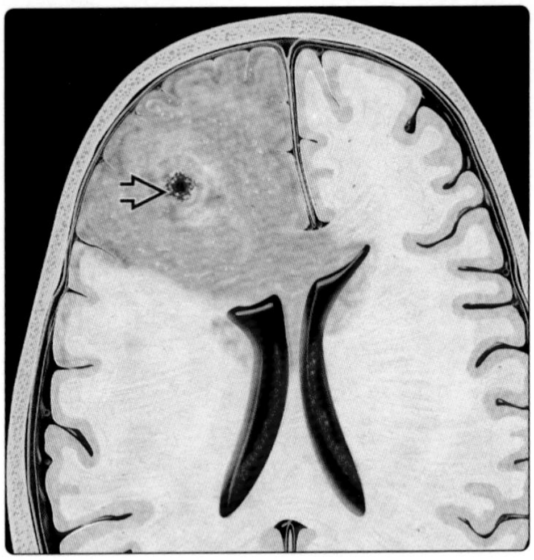

(17-32) Anaplastic astrocytoma (WHO grade III) diffusely infiltrates the right frontal lobe. Focal area of degeneration into GBM is depicted ➡.

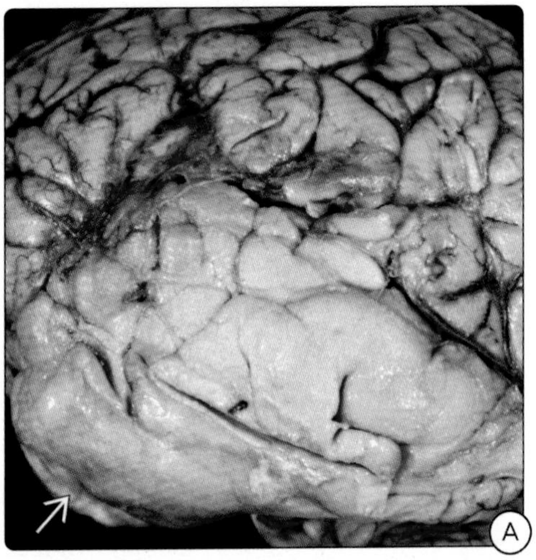

(17-33A) Autopsy case of anaplastic astrocytoma shows massive expansion of the entire temporal lobe ➡. (Courtesy R. Hewlett, MD.)

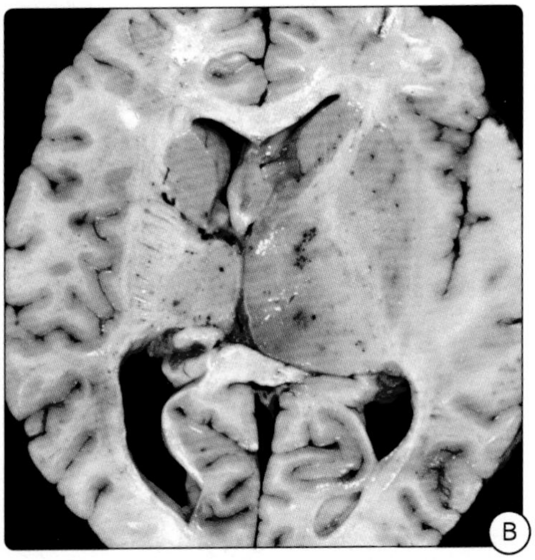

(17-33B) Axial section shows that the mass is poorly marginated and infiltrates both gray and white matter. (Courtesy R. Hewlett, MD.)

IDH-mutant anaplastic astrocytoma, a WHO grade III neoplasm, is indistinguishable from grade II DA on the basis of imaging findings.

Pilocytic astrocytoma is generally more circumscribed and much better demarcated than a DA. Pilocytic astrocytomas often has a "cyst + nodule" configuration rather than an infiltrating appearance and demonstrates moderate to strong enhancement following contrast administration.

Oligodendroglioma is generally cortically based, more often calcifies, and frequently has enhancing foci.

Nonneoplastic masses that can mimic IDH-mutant DA include acute stroke and encephalitis. **Acute cerebral ischemia-infarction** typically involves both cortex and subcortical white matter and occurs in specific vascular distribution. **Encephalitis** with T2/FLAIR hyperintensity shows enhancement on T1 C+. Both acute strokes and encephalitis exhibit restricted diffusion on DWI sequences.

IMAGING OF IDH-MUTANT DIFFUSE ASTROCYTOMAS

Imaging Features

- Hypodense on NECT
- No enhancement on CECT
- Hypointense on T1, hyperintense on T2/FLAIR
- No enhancement, hemorrhage
- MRS shows 2-HG peak at 2.25 ppm
- Low rCBV
  - Foci of ↑ rCBV suspicious for malignant degeneration

Differential Diagnosis

- IDH-mutant anaplastic astrocytoma
- Pilocytic astrocytoma
- Oligodendroglioma
- Nonneoplastic
  - Acute cerebral ischemia-infarction
  - Encephalitis

Anaplastic Astrocytoma, IDH-Mutant

Terminology

Anaplastic astrocytoma, IDH-mutant (IDH-mutant AA) is a diffusely infiltrating astrocytoma with anaplasia, significant proliferative activity, and a mutation in either the *IDH1* or *IDH2* gene. IDH-mutant AAs have an inherent tendency for malignant progression to IDH-mutant glioblastoma **(17-32) (17-36)**.

Pathology

The basic molecular features are similar to those of IDH-mutant DAs. By definition, mutations in *IDH1* or *IDH2* are present in all tumors. *TP53* and *ATRX* loss are present in the majority of tumors. 1p/19q are not codeleted.

The principal histopathologic features of IDH-mutant AA are those of a diffusely infiltrating astrocytoma that has increased mitotic activity. The Ki-67 proliferation index is usually in the 5-10% range.

Location. The most common site of IDH-mutant AA is the cerebral hemispheres, especially the frontal and temporal lobes **(17-33A)**. Involvement of the deep gray nuclei is common in larger lesions **(17-33B)**.

Gross Pathology. IDH-mutant AAs vary greatly in size and are usually solitary but widely infiltrating lesions. Multifocal AAs occur but are rare.

Gross expansion of the affected brain without frank tissue destruction is typical. The adjacent gyri are enlarged, and tumor often extends into the basal ganglia. Consistency varies from rubbery to fleshy, highly cellular tumors with poorly delineated margins. Cysts and intratumoral hemorrhage are rare.

Microscopic Features. IDH-mutant AAs are characterized by moderate to markedly increased cellularity, increased mitotic activity compared with the WHO grade II equivalent, and distinct nuclear atypia. Microvascular proliferation and necrosis are absent. Ki-67 (MIB-1) is elevated, generally in the 5-15% range, but can overlap with values for low-grade diffuse astrocytoma and glioblastoma.

Staging, Grading, and Classification. IDH-mutant AA corresponds histologically to WHO grade III.

Clinical Issues

Prior to the IDH era, the median survival for all AAs was 3-5 years. Recent studies show that the symptoms, mean age at diagnosis, and length of progression-free survival are similar to those of IDH-mutant diffuse astrocytomas.

IDH-MUTANT ANAPLASTIC ASTROCYTOMA

Etiology
- Begins as IDH-mutant diffuse (grade II) astrocytoma
  - Undergoes malignant degeneration to anaplastic astrocytoma
  - Maintains IDH-mutant status throughout life

Pathology
- WHO grade III
  - IDH-mutant, *ATRX* loss
- Hypercellular
- Anaplasia
- Increased mitoses
  - Ki-67 5-10%
- Lacks necrosis, microvascular proliferation

Clinical Issues
- Overall survival not statistically different from IDH-mutant diffuse astrocytoma (DA)

Imaging
- Similar to IDH-mutant DA
- Enhancing focus, any areas of ↑ rCBV likely represent malignant degeneration

Imaging

Imaging features and differential diagnosis of IDH-mutant AAs are similar to—and generally indistinguishable from—those of IDH-mutant diffuse astrocytomas.

CT Findings. IDH-mutant AAs are ill-defined low-density lesions on NECT. The majority do not enhance on CECT. When present, enhancement is usually focal, patchy, poorly delineated, and heterogeneous.

MR Findings. Most IDH-mutant AAs are hypointense on T1WI **(17-34A)** and hyperintense on T2/FLAIR **(17-34B)**. The margins may appear grossly discrete, but tumor cells invariably infiltrate adjacent brain. Hemorrhage and calcification are uncommon, so T2* "blooming" is typically absent.

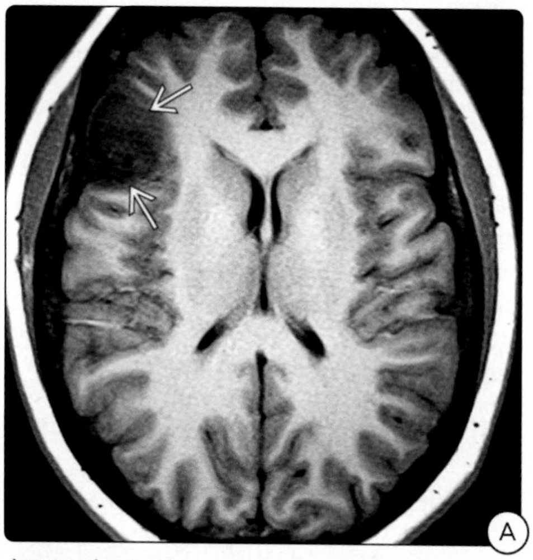

***(17-34A)** T1WI in a 45y woman with seizure shows well-delineated hypointense mass in right frontal lobe cortex, subcortical white matter.*

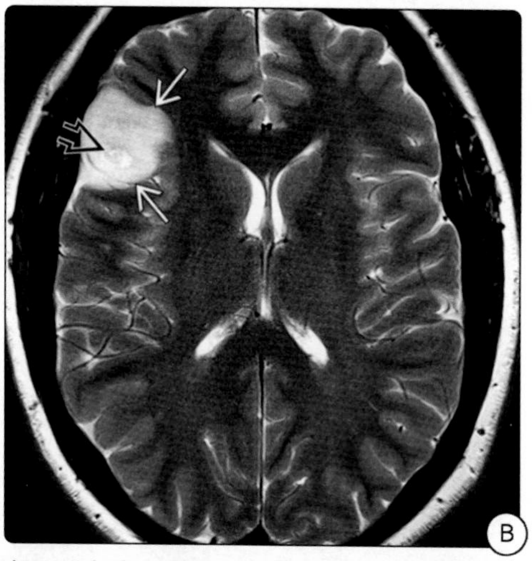

***(17-34B)** The mass appears hyperintense, relatively well circumscribed. Note small central focus of heterogeneous signal intensity.*

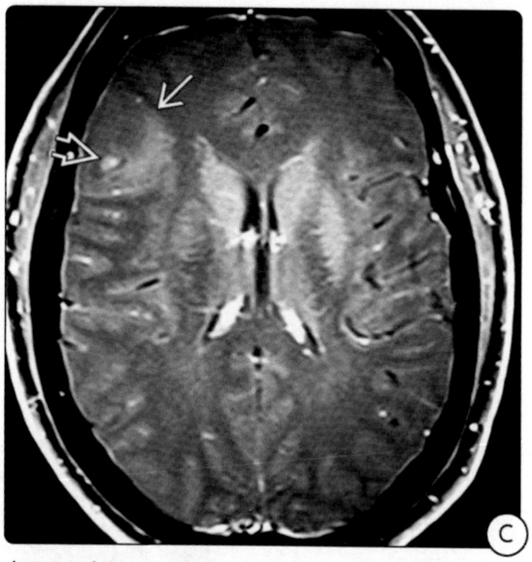

***(17-34C)** T1 C+ FS shows enhancement in center of mass. WHO grade III IDH-mutated AA was resected. Patient is alive 3 years later.*

Contrast enhancement varies from none to moderate. Between 50-70% show some degree of enhancement. Focal **(17-34C)**, nodular, homogeneous, patchy, or even ring-enhancing patterns may be seen.

IDH-mutant AAs generally do not restrict on DWI. MRS shows elevated choline, decreased NAA, and a 2-HG peak at 2.25 ppm. DTI can be helpful in delineating early WM tract invasion. Perfusion MR shows increased rCBV in the most malignant parts of the tumor. Color choline maps are helpful in guiding stereotactic biopsy, improving diagnostic accuracy with decreased sampling error.

Diffuse Astrocytoma, IDH-Wild-Type

Terminology

IDH-wild-type diffuse astrocytomas (DAs) are, by definition, diffusely infiltrating astrocytomas without *IDH* gene mutations.

Etiology

IDH-wild-type DAs, AAs, and GBM all probably arise from a line of glioma progenitor cells that is genetically distinct from the IDH-mutant line.

More than 75% of adult IDH-wild-type astrocytomas carry mutations similar to those of IDH-wild-type GBMs. *EGFR*, *H3F3A* (histone), and *TERT* mutations are associated with poor outcome, whereas *MYB* amplification is more favorable.

Pathology

IDH-wild-type DAs are WHO grade II neoplasms but come with the caveat that, in this instance, WHO grade does not correlate well with biologic behavior.

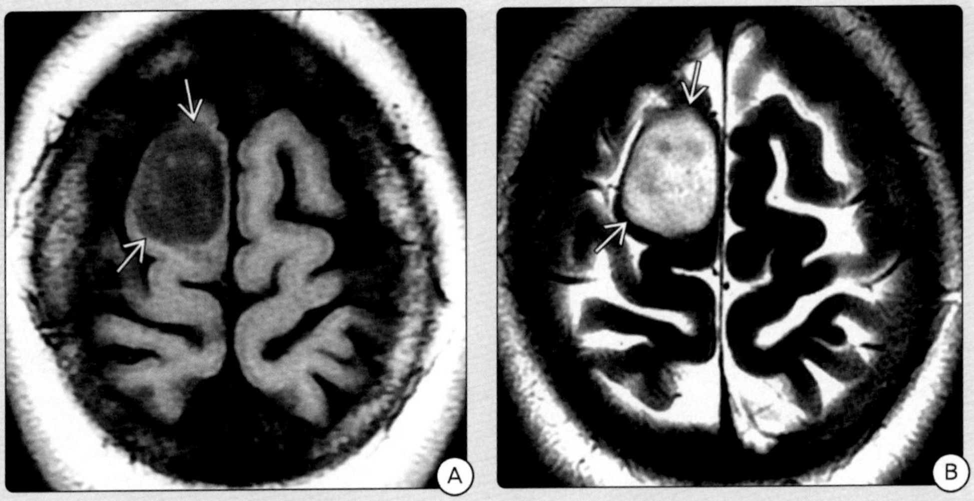

***(17-35A)** Axial T1WI in a 24y woman with seizures shows a hypodense mass in the right frontal lobe ➡. **(17-35B)** T2WI in the same case shows that the mass is heterogeneously hyperintense, with sharply delineated borders ➡.*

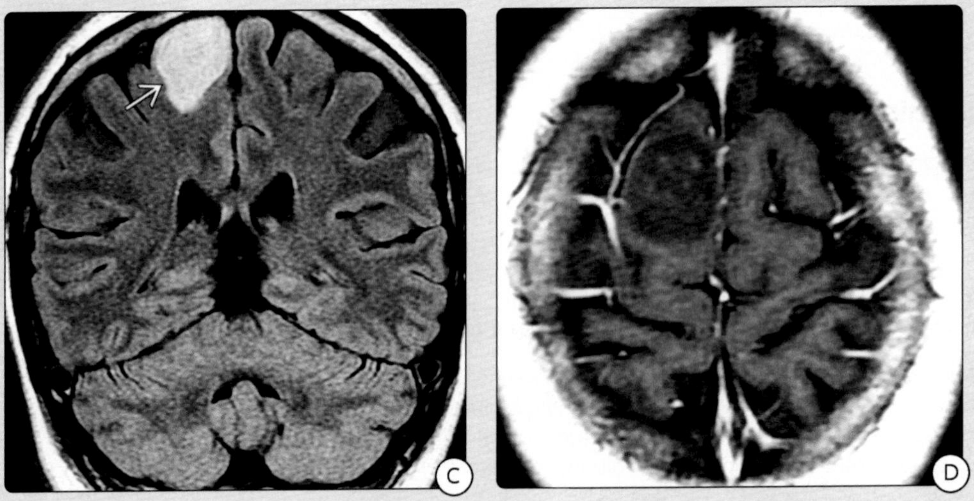

***(17-35C)** Coronal FLAIR shows that the hyperintense mass ➡ is relatively discrete. **(17-35D)** Axial T1 C+ MR shows no evidence for enhancement. The mass was completely resected. Pathology showed IDH-wild-type WHO grade II diffuse astrocytoma. p53 was positive, but MIB-1 was 20%. The patient is alive and disease-free 3 years later.*

Clinical Issues

Grade for grade, IDH-wild-type astrocytomas behave worse than their IDH-mutated counterparts. Thus, a grade II IDH-wild-type DA or AA will behave more like GBM (a WHO grade IV neoplasm).

Imaging

Standard imaging findings and differential diagnosis are similar to those of IDH-mutant DA. An infiltrating expansile mass that predominantly involves the hemispheric white matter is typical **(17-35)**. MRS shows absence of a 2-HG peak.

Anaplastic Astrocytoma, IDH-Wild-Type

IDH-wild-type anaplastic astrocytoma (IDH-wild-type AA) is uncommon, accounting for only 20% of all AAs. Most have an identical gross/microscopic and imaging appearance to IDH-mutant tumors while sharing the molecular and clinical features of IDH-wild-type glioblastoma or H3 K27M-mutant midline glioma (see below) **(17-36)**.

In the past, diffuse gliomas with a unique pattern of widespread brain invasion were designated as **gliomatosis cerebri** (GC). By definition, three or more lobes with frequent bihemispheric, basal ganglionic, and/or infratentorial extension were involved **(17-37)**.

Although IDH-mutant tumors occasionally exhibit this widespread infiltrative pattern, the majority of adult tumors that would once have been designated as GCs are IDH-wild-type AAs **(17-38)**. GC does not represent a distinct molecular entity and is no longer considered a separate diagnosis.

GCs in children are distinct from those in adults **(17-39)** but share genetic, epigenetic, and imaging **(17-40)** characteristics with other pediatric infiltrative high-grade gliomas.

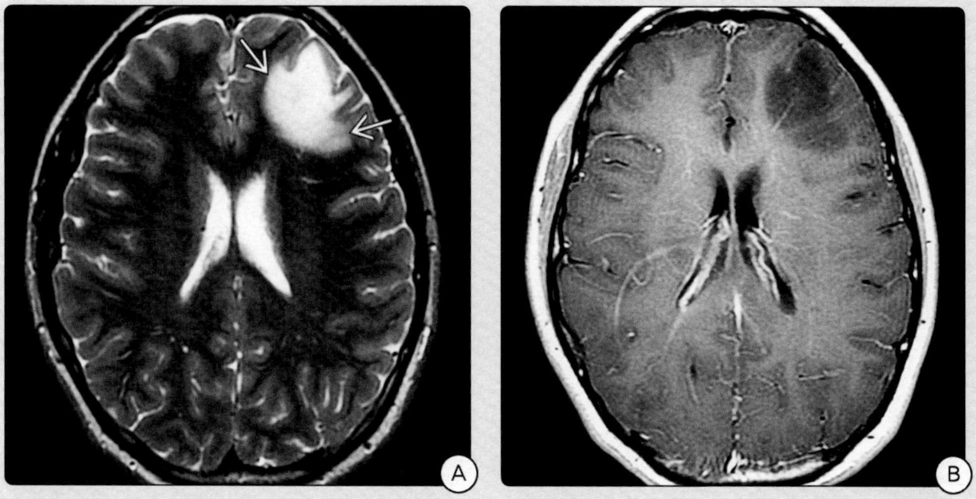

***(17-36A)** A 15y girl with minor head trauma had an NECT scan (not shown) that demonstrated a hypodense left frontal mass. T2WI shows a hyperintense mass ➔ predominately involving the subcortical and deep WM. **(17-36B)** T1 C+ FS shows no enhancement. Surgery disclosed IDH-wild-type anaplastic astrocytoma, WHO grade III.*

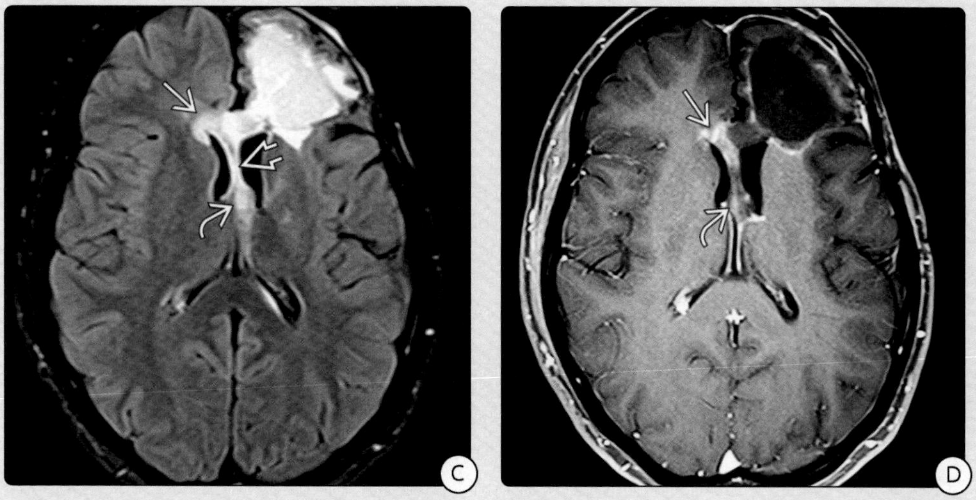

***(17-36C)** The patient was disease-free for 3 years, but the tumor recurred. Axial FLAIR shows hyperintense tumor crossing the corpus callosum ➔, infiltrating the septum pellucidum ➔ and fornix ➔. **(17-36D)** T1 C+ FS shows nodular enhancement around the resection cavity and enhancement in the corpus callosum ➔ and fornix ➔. Reoperation disclosed IDH-wild-type GBM.*

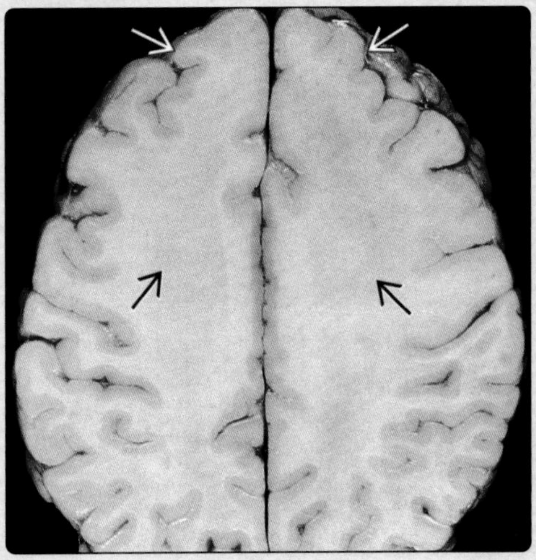

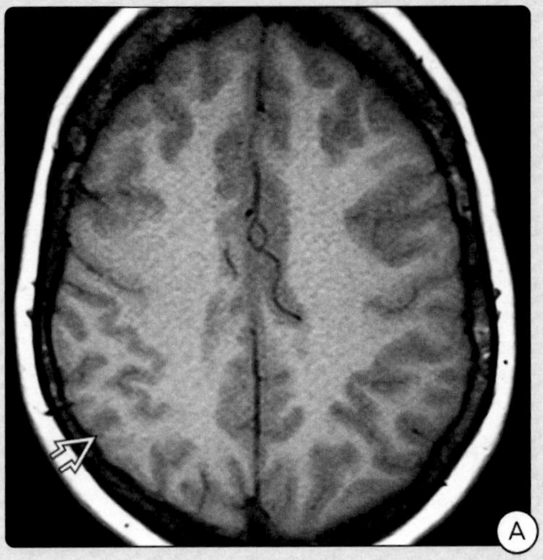

(17-37) Autopsy case shows gliomatosis cerebri infiltrating the WM →, cortex of both frontal lobes. Compare the effaced GM-WM interfaces ➡ with the more normal-appearing parietal cortex. (Courtesy R. Hewlett, MD.) (17-38A) Axial T1WI in a patient with gliomatosis cerebri shows asymmetry between the normal-appearing right parietal cortex ➡ and the thickened cortex in the rest of the hemispheres.

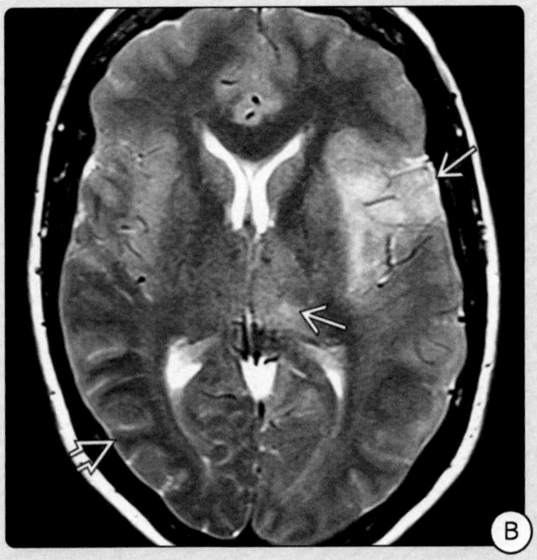

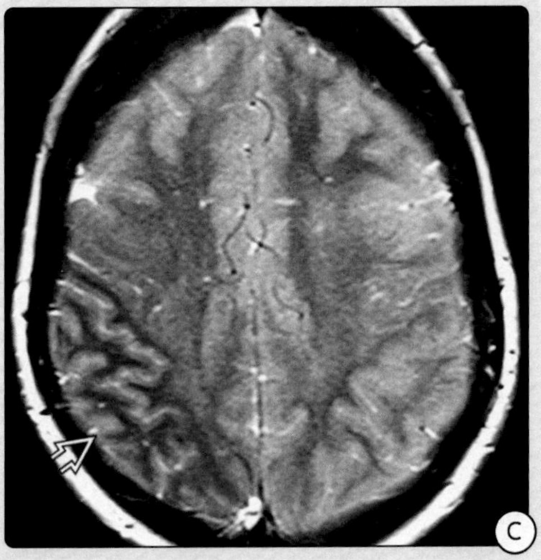

(17-38B) T2WI in the same patient shows hyperintensity in both temporal lobes, thalami, and cortex of both hemispheres →. Only the right parietal cortex ➡ appears spared. (17-38C) Scan through the upper corona radiata shows expanded hyperintense cortex, "hazy" hyperintensity in the underlying WM. Again, only the right parietal lobe ➡ appears relatively spared. Although abnormal, the basic underlying cerebral architecture is preserved.

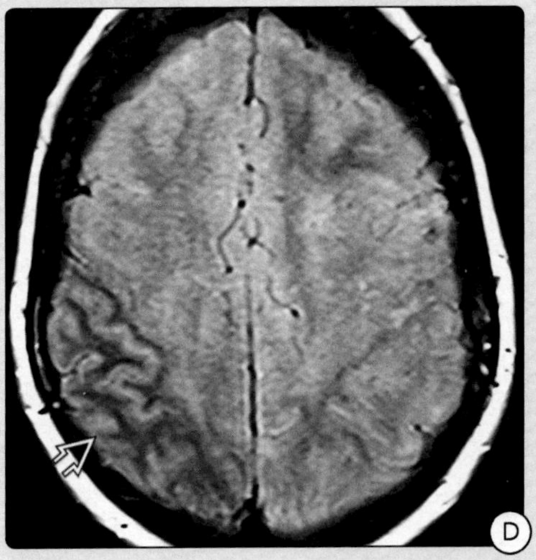

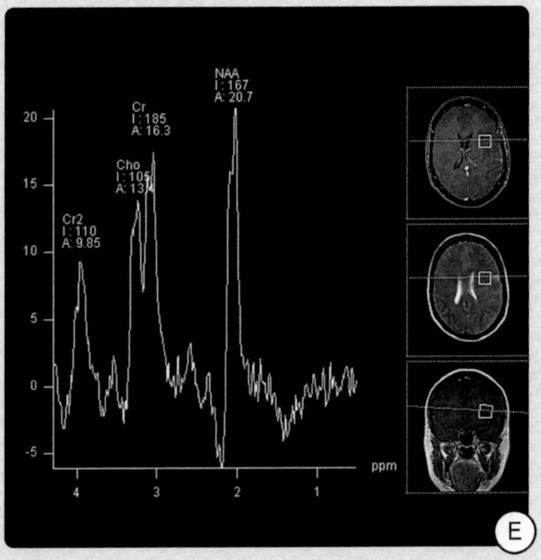

(17-38D) FLAIR scan demonstrates that the diffusely infiltrating mass extends throughout the cortex and corona radiata of both hemispheres. Only the right parietal lobe appears relatively uninvolved ➡. (17-38E) MRS shows almost normal appearance. Because gliomatosis cerebri infiltrates between and around normal tissue, spectra are often unrevealing. WHO grade II gliomatosis cerebri was found at biopsy.

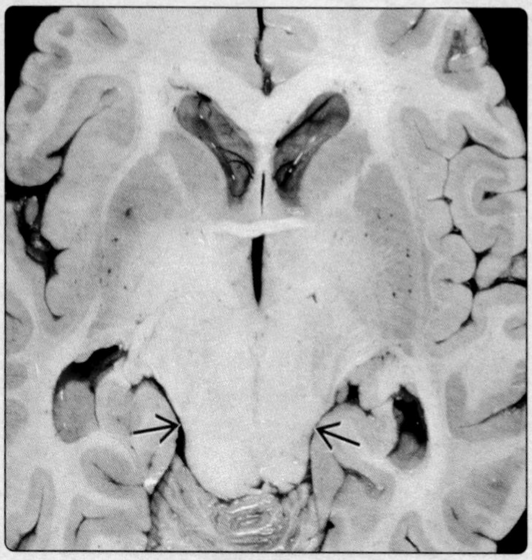

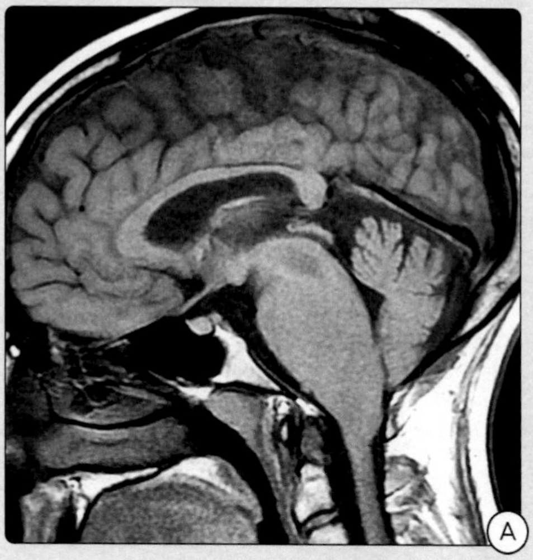

***(17-39)** Gliomatosis cerebri can sometimes begin in the posterior fossa and then extend upward through the midbrain into the thalami. In this autopsy specimen, the midbrain is expanded ⇨, and both thalami are infiltrated by tumor. (Courtesy R. Hewlett, MD.)* ***(17-40A)** Sagittal T1WI shows a 26y neurologically normal woman with headaches. An extensive mass diffusely expands the midbrain, pons, medulla, and upper cervical spinal cord.*

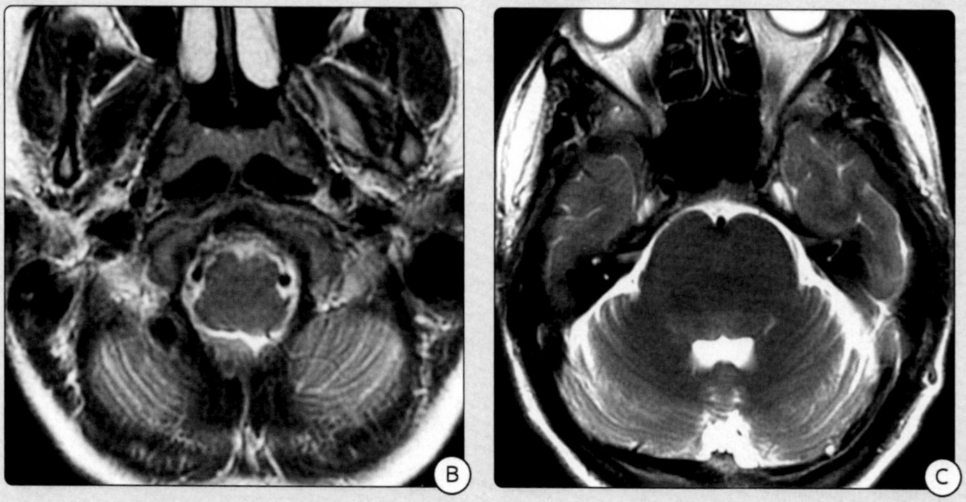

***(17-40B)** Axial T2WI shows that the medulla is grossly enlarged but that its overall signal intensity is only slightly increased.* ***(17-40C)** T2WI through the middle of the pons shows striking enlargement without definite signal abnormality.*

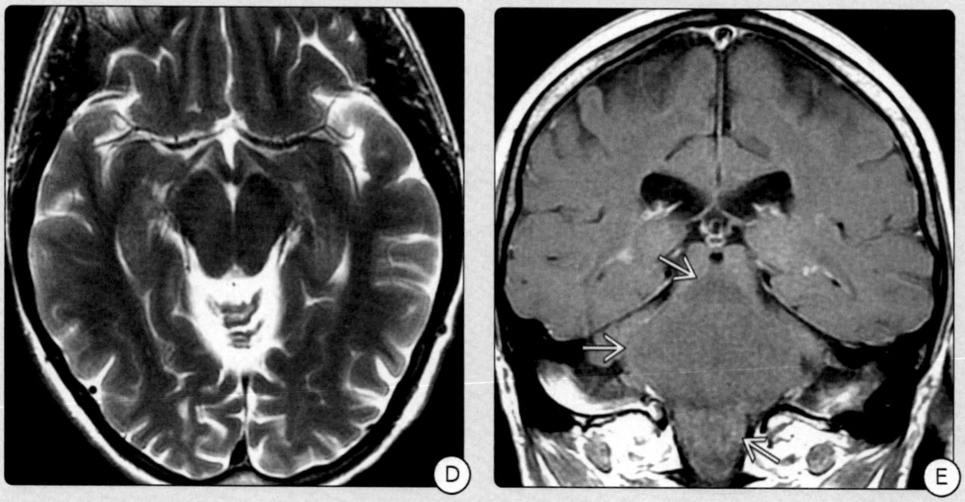

***(17-40D)** More cephalad T2WI shows midbrain is almost twice its normal size; aqueduct remains patent, no sign of obstructive hydrocephalus.* ***(17-40E)** Coronal T1 C+ shows no sign of enhancement, but slight hypointensity is seen in expanded medulla, pons, midbrain ➔. Because tumor involved midbrain, hindbrain, spinal cord, this was diagnosed as probable low-grade (WHO II) gliomatosis cerebri. No biopsy was performed.*

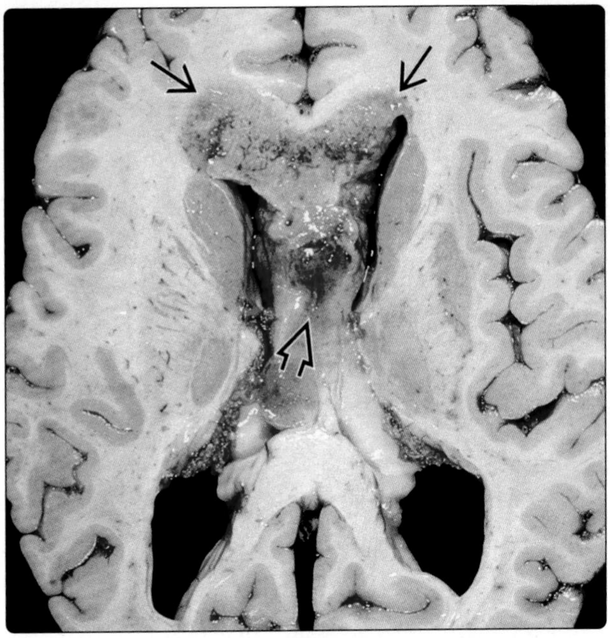

(17-41) Autopsy specimen shows "butterfly" glioblastoma multiforme ➡ crossing corpus callosum genu, extending into and enlarging fornix ⮕. (Courtesy R. Hewlett, MD.)

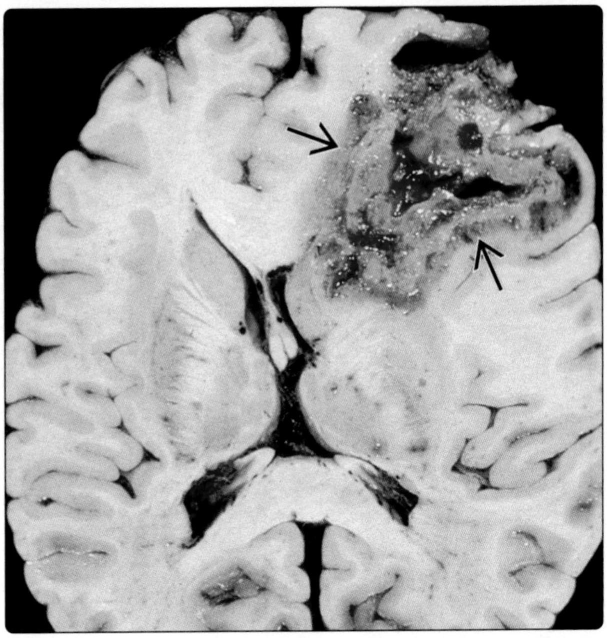

(17-42) Autopsy specimen shows classic primary glioblastoma multiforme with hemorrhage, viable "rind" of tumor ➡ surrounding a necrotic core. (Courtesy R. Hewlett, MD.)

ANAPLASTIC ASTROCYTOMA, IDH-WILD-TYPE

Etiology, Pathology
- Same glial progenitor line as IDH-DA, GBM
- Can exhibit widespread infiltrative pattern
  - Most cases of "gliomatosis cerebri" are IDH-AAs
  - No longer separate diagnosis
- Degeneration into IDH-wild-type GBM, often in < 2y

Imaging
- Widespread, infiltrative T2/FLAIR hyperintense
- Often exhibits foci of contrast enhancement

Glioblastoma, IDH-Wild-Type

IDH-wild-type glioblastoma (GBM) is the most common and most malignant of all astrocytomas, accounting for over 95% of GBMs.

Terminology

IDH-wild-type GBM is sometimes called **"IDH-wild-type primary glioblastoma"** to distinguish it from IDH-mutant GBMs, which arise from lower-grade IDH-mutant astrocytomas.

Etiology

IDH-wild-type GBMs are putative de novo lesions, with no recognizable lower-grade precursor tumor. However, many of the genetic alterations that characterize IDH-wild-type GBMs (e.g., *TERT* promoter mutations, *EGFR* and *PTEN* mutations, loss of chromosomes 10p and 10q, etc.) are also present in the majority of grade II and III wild-type astrocytomas, suggesting that they may constitute a continuum of the same disease.

Three inherited cancer syndromes—namely **neurofibromatosis type 1** (NF1), **Li-Fraumeni**, and **Turcot syndrome**—demonstrate an enhanced propensity to develop IDH-wild-type GBMs.

Pathology

Location. In contrast to IDH-mutant GBMs (see below), IDH-wild-type GBMs are distributed throughout the cerebral hemispheres. They preferentially involve the subcortical and deep periventricular white matter, easily spreading across compact tracts such as the corpus callosum and corticospinal tracts. Symmetric involvement of the corpus callosum is common, the so-called "butterfly glioma" pattern **(17-41)**.

Size and Number. IDH-wild-type GBMs vary widely in size. Because they spread quickly and extensively along compact white matter tracts, up to 20% appear as multifocal lesions at the time of initial diagnosis. Between 2-5% of multifocal GBMs are true synchronous, independently developing tumors.

Gross Pathology. The most frequent appearance is a reddish-gray tumor "rind" surrounding a central necrotic core **(17-42)**. Mass effect and peritumoral edema are marked. Increased vascularity and intratumoral hemorrhage are common.

Microscopic Features. Necrosis and microvascular proliferation are the histologic hallmarks of GBMs, distinguishing them from anaplastic astrocytomas.

Varied tumor cells comprise GBMs. Pleomorphic fibrillary astrocytes, gemistocytes, bipolar bland-appearing but

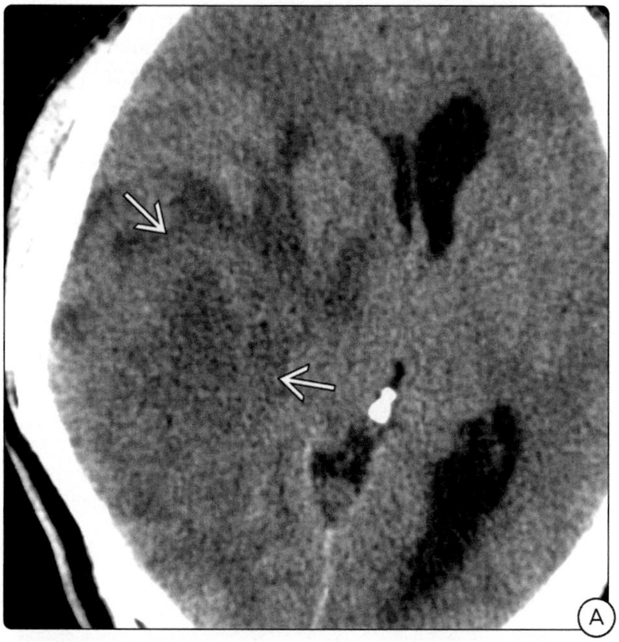

(17-43A) *NECT scan shows typical findings of GBM with a large, mixed iso-/hypodense mass ➡ that compresses and displaces lateral ventricles.*

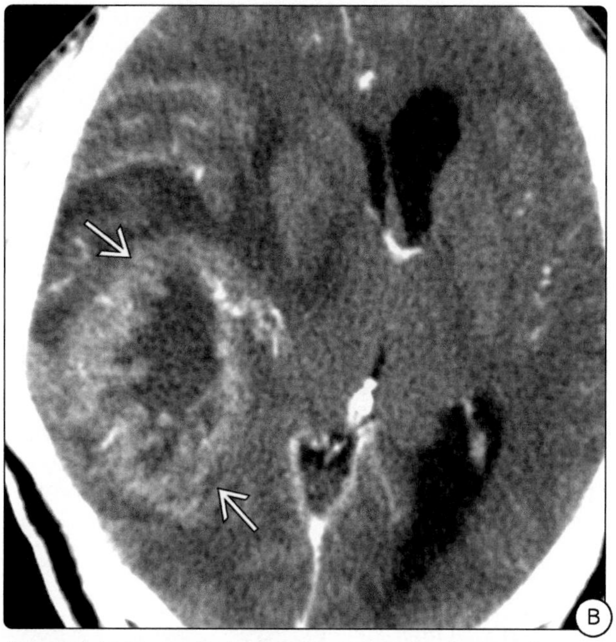

(17-43B) *CECT scan in the same patient shows the irregular enhancing "rind" of tissue ➡ surrounding the nonenhancing necrotic core of the tumor.*

mitotically active small cells (including "microglia"), and large bizarre multinucleated giant cells are all common features.

GBMs generally have a high proliferation index (MIB-1), almost always > 10%.

Staging, Grading, and Classification. GBMs are WHO grade IV neoplasms.

Clinical Issues

Demographics. GBM is the most common malignant brain tumor in adults, representing between 12 and 15% of all intracranial neoplasms and 60-75% of astrocytomas.

GBMs can occur at any age (including in neonates and infants), but peak age is 55-85 years. IDH-wild-type GBMs tend to occur in older adults (peaking between 60 and 75 years), whereas IDH-mutant GBMs occur a decade or two earlier. The M:F ratio is essentially equal.

Presentation. Presentation varies with location. Seizure, focal neurologic deficits, and mental status changes are the most common symptoms. Headache from elevated intracranial pressure is also common.

Approximately 2% of GBMs present with sudden stroke-like onset caused by acute intratumoral hemorrhage. Underlying GBM should always be a diagnostic consideration in an older normotensive patient with a spontaneous, unexplained intracranial hemorrhage.

Natural History. GBM is a relentless, progressive disease. Mean survival in patients with IDH-wild-type GBM is under 1 year. *MGMT* promoter methylation is a strong predictor for response to alkylating agents and correlates with somewhat better survival.

Imaging

General Features. The vast majority of IDH-wild-type GBMs demonstrate a thick, irregular, enhancing "rind" of tumor surrounding a necrotic core.

In rare cases, no dominant mass is present. Instead, tumor extends diffusely throughout the cerebral white matter. Confluent and patchy white matter hyperintensities on T2/FLAIR scans mimic small vessel vascular disease. An even rarer variant is "primary diffuse leptomeningeal gliomatosis." Here tumor extends diffusely around the brain surfaces, mostly between the pia and the glia limitans of the cortex.

CT Findings. Most IDH-wild-type GBMs demonstrate a hypodense central mass surrounded by an iso- to moderately hyperdense rim on NECT **(17-43A)**. Hemorrhage is common, but calcification is rare. Marked mass effect and significant hypodense peritumoral edema are typical ancillary findings.

CECT shows strong but heterogeneous irregular rim enhancement **(17-43B)**. Prominent vessels in highly vascular GBMs are seen as linear enhancing foci adjacent to the mass.

MR Findings. T1WI shows a poorly marginated mass with mixed signal intensity. Subacute hemorrhage is common. T2/FLAIR shows heterogeneous hyperintensity with indistinct tumor margins and extensive vasogenic edema. Necrosis, cysts, hemorrhage at various stages of evolution, fluid/debris levels, and "flow voids" from extensive neovascularity may be seen. T2* imaging often shows foci of susceptibility artifact **(17-45)**.

T1 C+ shows strong but irregular ring enhancement surrounding a central nonenhancing core of necrotic tumor **(17-44)**. Nodular, punctate, or patchy enhancing foci outside the main mass represent macroscopic tumor extension into adjacent structures. Microscopic foci of viable tumor cells are invariably present far beyond any demonstrable areas of enhancement or edema on standard imaging sequences.

Most GBMs do not restrict on DWI. DTI may show reduced fractional anisotropy and disrupted white matter tracts from tumor invasion. MRS usually shows elevated choline, decreased NAA and mI, and a lipid/lactate peak resonating at 1.33 ppm. pMR shows elevated rCBV in the tumor "rind" and increased vascular permeability.

Angiography. Angiography shows a prominent capillary phase tumor "blush," enlarged/irregular-appearing vessels, and "pooling" of contrast. Arteriovenous shunting is common, seen as "early draining" veins.

Patterns of GBM Spread. GBM is the most common primary CNS neoplasm that causes "brain-to-brain" metastases **(17-46)**. Although some primary tumors such as medulloblastoma, ependymoma, and germinoma tend to disseminate almost exclusively through CSF pathways, GBMs are notorious for their ability to spread via multiple routes. Because GBM spreads so rapidly and viable tumor cells are present throughout much of the normal-appearing brain, many neuropathologists and oncologists consider GBM a "whole-brain" disease.

White Matter Spread. The most common route of GBM spread is through the white matter **(17-51)**. Dissemination along compact white matter tracts such as the corpus callosum, fornices, anterior commissure, and corticospinal tract can result in tumor implantation in geographically remote areas such as the pons, cerebellum, medulla, and spinal cord **(17-47)**. Viable tumor cells are dispersed into (and beyond) the visible peritumoral edema.

(17-44A) Axial T1WI in a 71y woman with confusion, decreasing mental status shows a large hypointense right frontal lobe mass. Note presence of some prominent "flow voids" within the mass. (17-44B) T2WI in the same case shows the mass is mixed iso- and hyperintense. Note prominent "flow voids" in and adjacent to the mass.

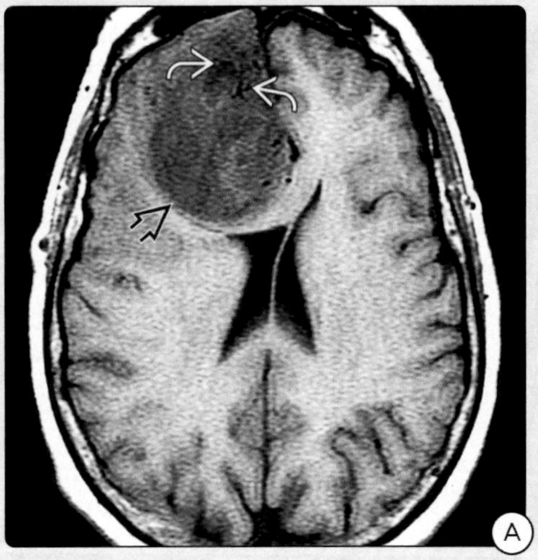

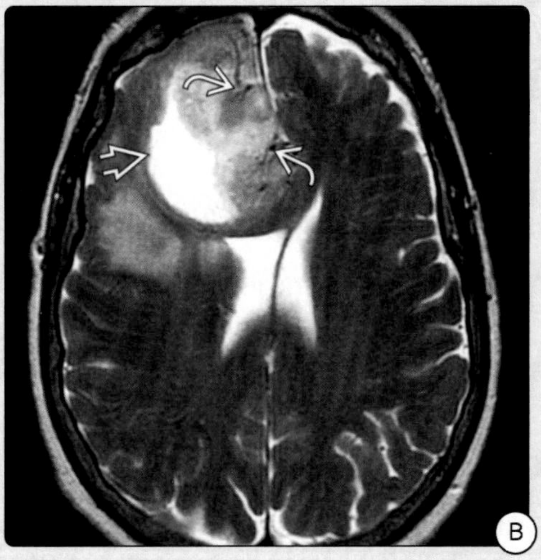

(17-44C) Axial T1 C+ shows a thick "rind" of enhancing tumor surrounding a nonenhancing central necrotic cavity. The mass directly abuts and invades the dura. Note enhancing "dural tails" extending away from the mass. (17-44D) Coronal T1 C+ FS shows dural invasion. Imaging diagnosis was gliosarcoma. WHO grade IV IDH-wild-type GBM with MIB-1 > 70% was found at histopathology without evidence for a sarcomatous component.

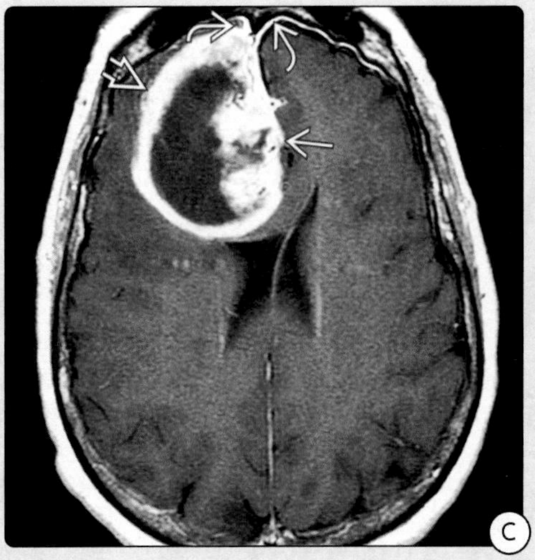

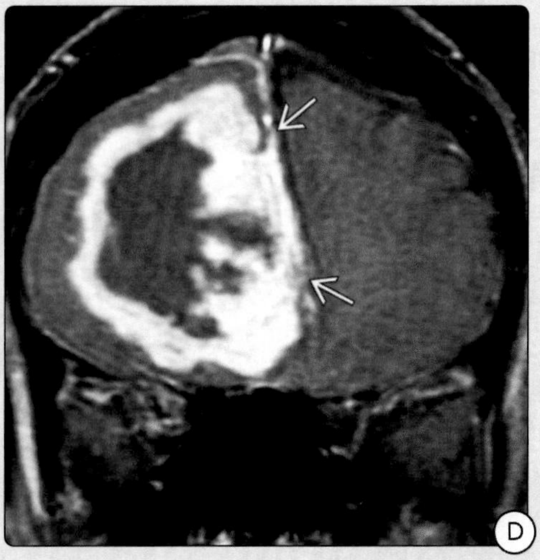

CSF Dissemination. GBM often seeds the CSF, filling the sulci and cisterns **(17-52)**. Diffuse coating of cranial nerves and the pial surface of the brain is also common. This appearance of "carcinomatous meningitis" may be indistinguishable on imaging studies from pyogenic meningitis **(17-48)**.

"Drop metastases" can extend inferiorly into the spinal canal, covering the spinal cord, thickening nerves, and causing focal mass-like deposits within the thecal sac.

Ependymal and Subependymal Spread. GBM spread along the ventricular ependyma also occurs but is less common than diffuse CSF dissemination. The interior of the ventricles—most often the lateral ventricles—is coated with enhancing tumor and resembles pyogenic ventriculitis on contrast-enhanced imaging.

Subependymal tumor spread also occurs, producing a thick neoplastic "rind" as tumor "creeps" and crawls around the ventricular margins **(17-49)**.

Skull-Dura Metastases. Direct invasion of GBM through the pia and into the dura-arachnoid is rare. In exceptional cases, tumor erodes into and sometimes even through the calvaria, extending into the subgaleal soft tissues.

Extra-CNS Metastases. Hematogeneous spread of GBM to systemic sites occurs but is rare. Bone marrow (especially the vertebral bodies), liver, lung, and even lymph node metastases can occur **(17-50)**.

Differential Diagnosis

The major neoplasm that should be distinguished from GBM is **metastasis**. Metastases are often multiple and tend to occur peripherally at the gray-white matter junction. Even large metastases are round or ovoid, not infiltrating like GBM.

Other GBM mimics include anaplastic astrocytoma, anaplastic oligodendroglioma, and primary CNS lymphoma. **Anaplastic astrocytomas** generally do not enhance although some do

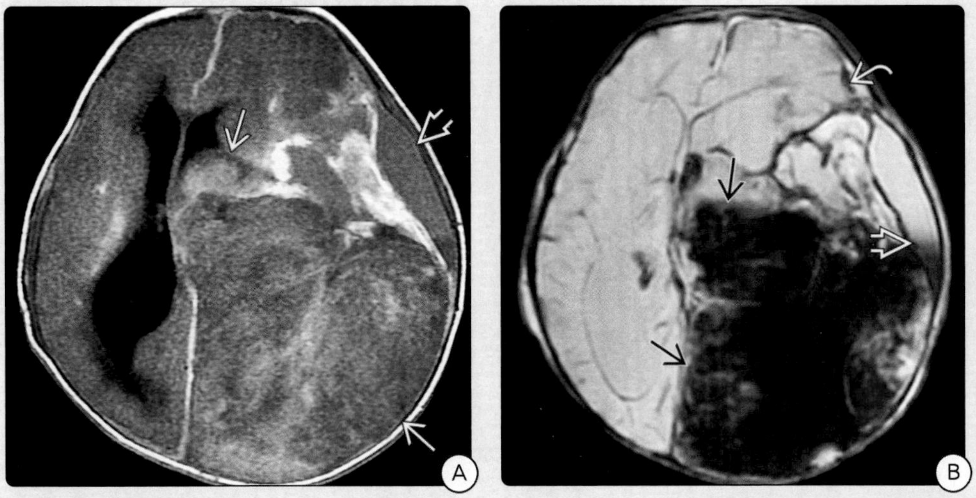

***(17-45A)** Axial T1 FLAIR scan in a newborn infant with macrocephaly shows a very heterogeneous-appearing holohemispheric mass. An extraaxial fluid collection is present overlying the left hemisphere. **(17-45B)** T2* scan in the same case shows significant "blooming" throughout most of the mass. Note superficial siderosis and blood-fluid level in the extraaxial collection.*

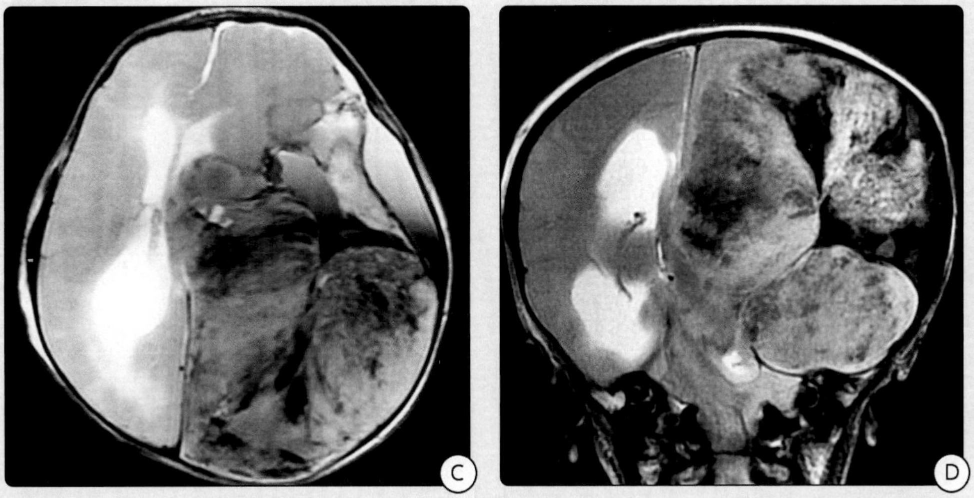

***(17-45C)** T2WI shows the mass is extremely heterogeneous. The only remaining normal brain in the left hemisphere is the frontal lobe. **(17-45D)** Coronal T2WI confirms the heterogeneous signal intensity in the bizarre-appearing mass. Preoperative diagnosis was embryonal neoplasm. GBM was found at surgery. Congenital GBMs are often very bulky heterogeneous-appearing tumors.*

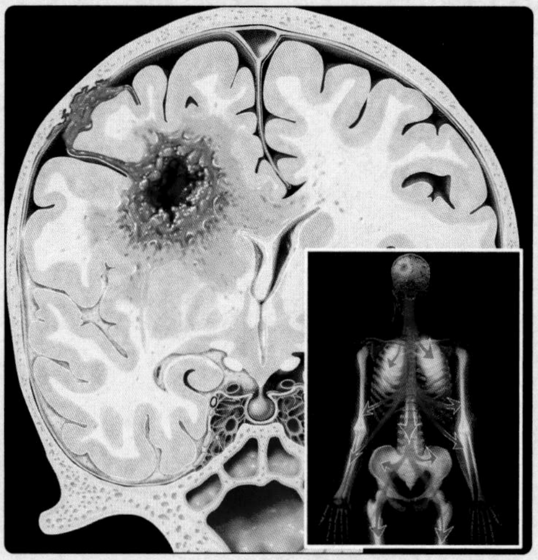

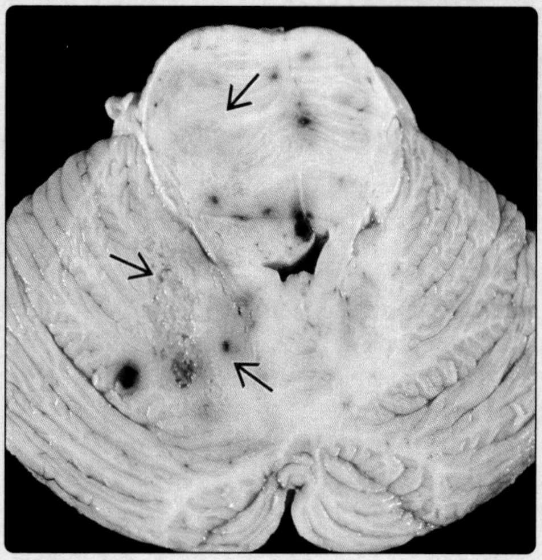

(17-46) *Graphic shows potential GBM routes of spread. Preferential tumor spread is along compact WM tracts but can be ependymal, subpial, diffuse CSF ("carcinomatous meningitis"). Dural, skull invasion, extracranial metastases rarely occur.* ***(17-47)*** *Autopsy shows patterns of GBM dissemination. Axial section through pons and cerebellum shows multiple discrete foci of parenchymal tumor ➔. (Courtesy E. T. Hedley-Whyte, MD.)*

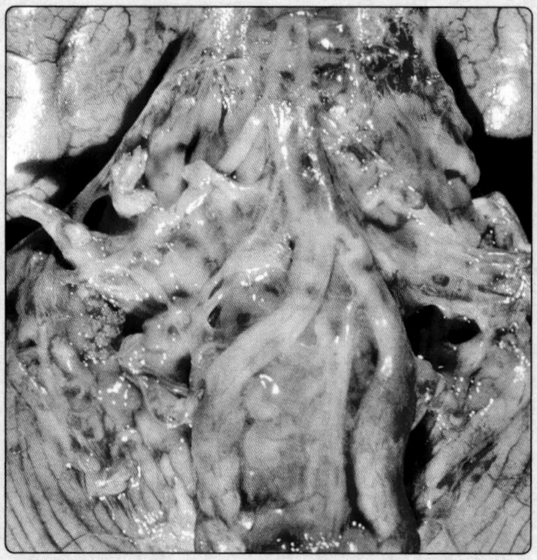

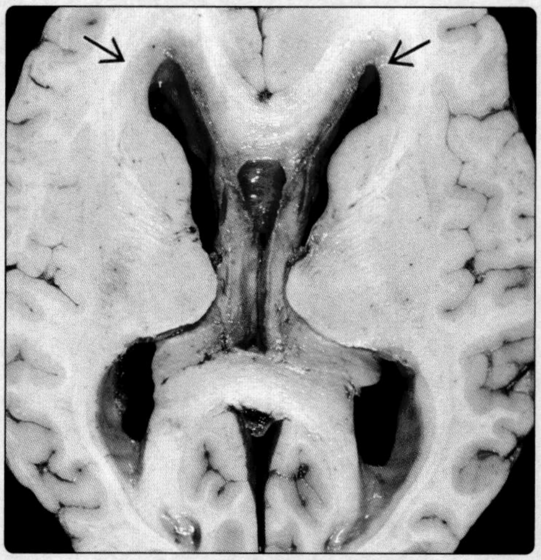

(17-48) *"Carcinomatous meningitis" from GBM coats the surface of the brainstem and cerebellum, basilar artery, and cranial nerves. Gross appearance is virtually indistinguishable from that of pyogenic meningitis. (Courtesy R. Hewlett, MD.)* ***(17-49)*** *Glioblastoma has spread around both lateral ventricles in a thick band of subependymal tumor ➔. (Courtesy R. Hewlett, MD.)*

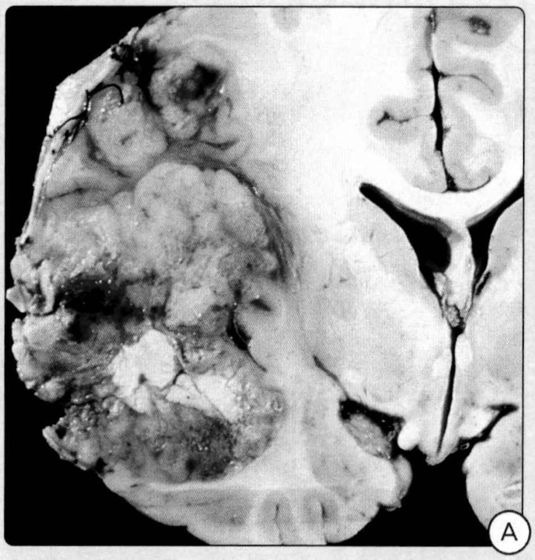

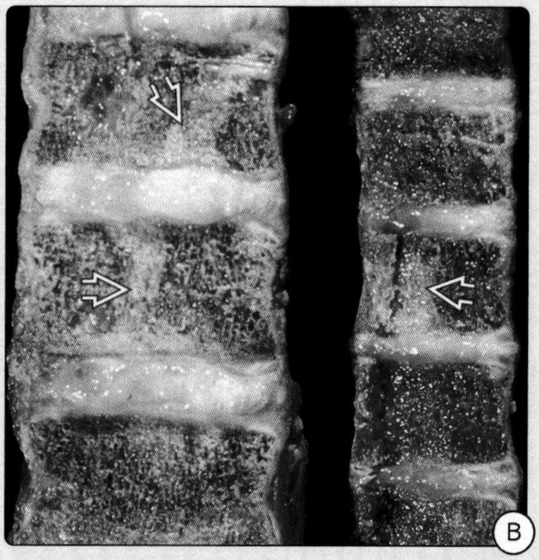

(17-50A) *Coronal autopsied brain shows a necrotic, hemorrhagic temporal lobe GBM.* ***(17-50B)*** *Lumbar (L) and thoracic (R) spine in the same case show multiple metastases in the vertebral bodies ➔. Extracranial spread of GBM is rare although documented in this case. (Courtesy E. T. Hedley-Whyte, MD.)*

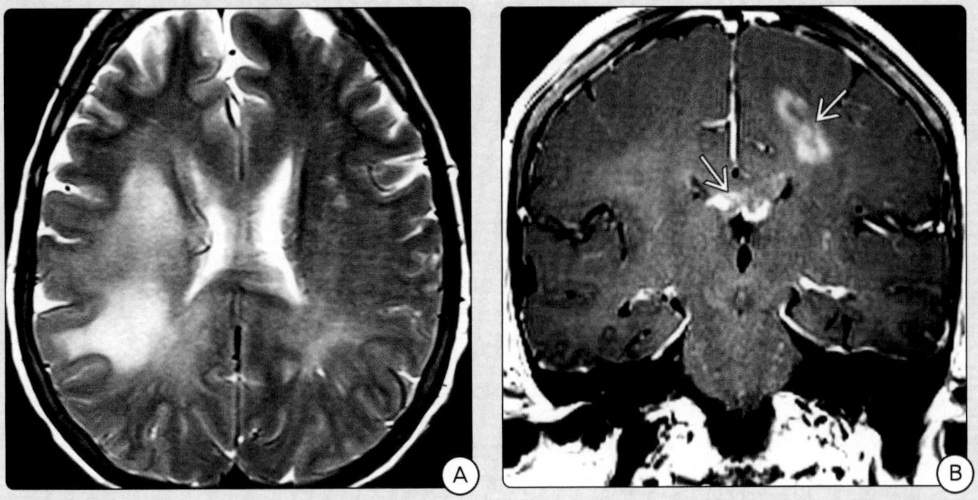

(17-51A) T2WI shows diffuse confluent and patchy WM hyperintensity in this elderly patient with increasing confusion, left-sided weakness. (17-51B) Coronal T1 C+ in the same patient shows enhancement in the left hemispheric WM and corpus callosum ➡. Biopsy disclosed diffusely infiltrating GBM.

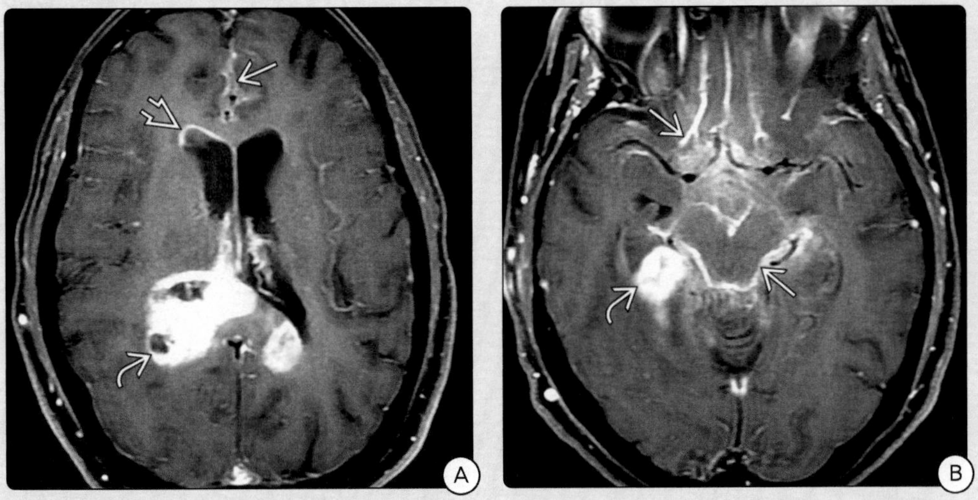

(17-52A) Series of T1 C+ FS scans demonstrates GBM ➡ with widespread CSF dissemination. Note ependymal ➡, sulcal-cisternal ➡ enhancement. (17-52B) Lower T1 C+ FS scan shows the primary tumor ➡ together with a diffuse coating of midbrain, enhancement throughout the suprasellar cistern extending into both sylvian fissures and olfactory sulci ➡.

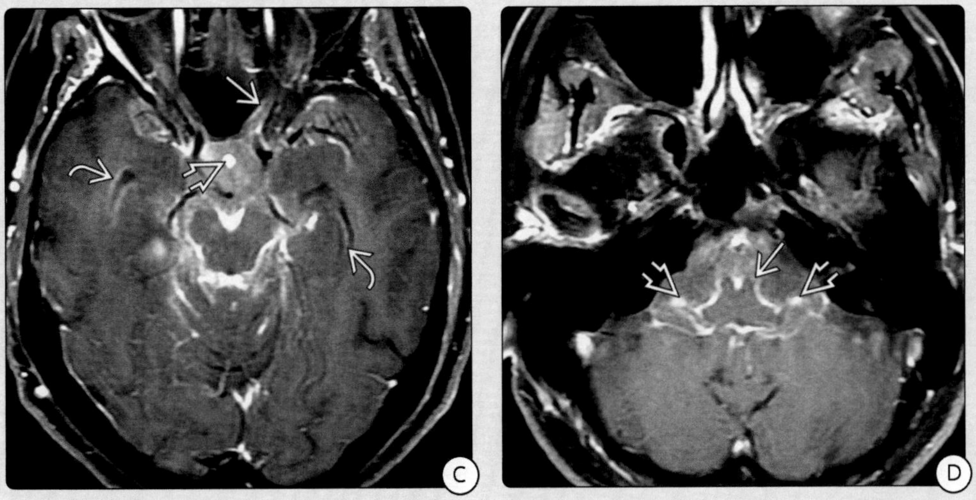

(17-52C) Enhancing tumor thickens, coats infundibular stalk ➡, extends along optic nerve sheath into orbit ➡, fills interpeduncular cistern. Note ependymal spread around both temporal horns ➡. (17-52D) Medulla is diffusely coated with tumor ➡; enhancing tumor is seen along CNs IX-XI ➡. GBM can spread throughout CSF space ("carcinomatous meningitis"). Numerous "drop metastases" to the lumbosacral sac were also present.

and may be difficult to distinguish from GBM on imaging alone.

Anaplastic oligodendroglioma may infiltrate white matter in a manner similar to GBM and may be difficult to diagnose without biopsy. **Primary CNS lymphoma** often involves the corpus callosum but is rarely necrotic in the absence of HIV/AIDS.

The major nonneoplastic differential diagnosis of GBM is **abscess**. Abscesses typically have thinner, more regular rims and restrict on DWI. MRS often shows succinate and cytosolic amino acids, which are rare in GBM.

"Tumefactive" demyelination in the subcortical white matter may demonstrate peripheral rim enhancement. A "horseshoe" pattern, often draped around a sulcus, is common. An incomplete rim with the open segment pointing toward the sulcus and cortex is typical for "tumefactive" demyelination.

Glioblastoma, IDH-Mutant

IDH-mutant glioblastoma (IDH-mutant GBM) is much less common than IDH-wild-type GBM, accounting for approximately 5-10% of cases.

Terminology

IDH-mutant GBMs are also called "secondary GBMs," as they almost invariably develop from lower-grade IDH-mutant astrocytic tumors.

Etiology

IDH mutation is an early event in gliomagenesis, and it persists throughout the progression from IDH-mutant diffuse and anaplastic astrocytomas to GBM. *TP53* mutations and *ATRX* loss are common, but *EGFR* amplification is absent.

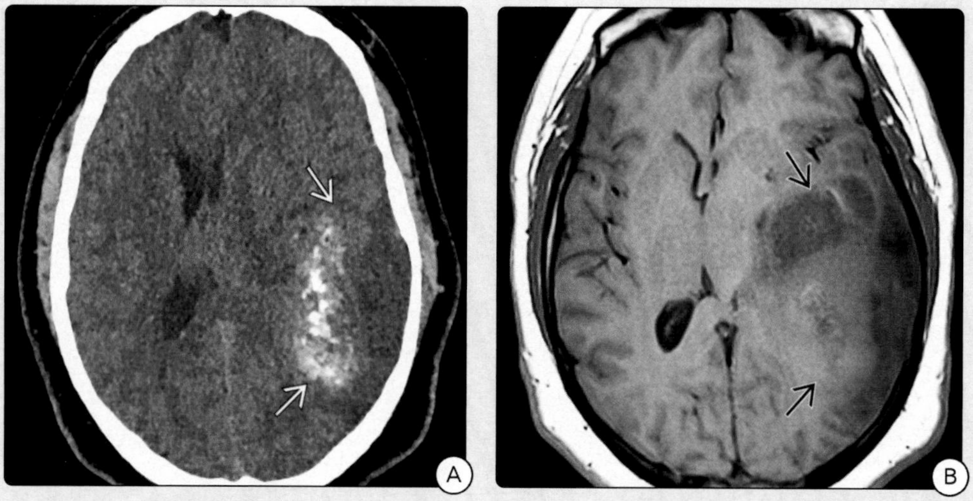

***(17-53A)** Axial NECT scan in a 26y man with right superior quadrantanopsia shows a partially calcified mixed density mass ➡ in the left temporoparietal region. **(17-53B)** T1WI in the same case shows a mixed signal intensity mass ⇨ that involves both the gray and white matter.*

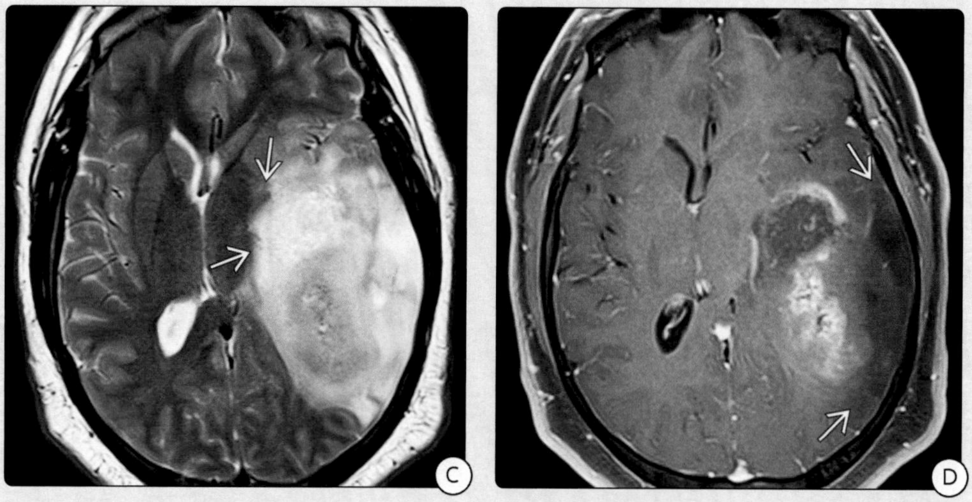

***(17-53C)** T2WI and FLAIR showed mass involves virtually all of the temporal and parietal lobes, extending medially into the basal ganglia and thalamus ➡. **(17-53D)** T1 C+ FS shows the mass has patchy areas of enhancement, but the majority of the mass does not enhance ➡. The presence of calcification and large nonenhancing areas are typical for secondary GBMs. Tumor was an IDH-mutated GBM that arose in a lower-grade astrocytoma.*

If standard R132H immunohistochemistry is *IDH1* negative, next-generation sequencing is recommended to detect a noncanonical *IDH1* or any *IDH2* mutation.

GLIOBLASTOMA: IDH-WILD-TYPE VS. IDH-MUTANT

IDH-Wild-Type GBM
- Also called "primary" GBM
  - Arises de novo
  - *IDH1* negative, *PTEN* mutated, *EGFR* amplified
- > 95% of all GBMs
- Peak age = 55-85 years
  - Survival < 1 year
- Pathology
  - Necrosis, microvascular proliferation
  - WHO grade IV
- Imaging
  - Anywhere in hemispheres
  - Thick irregular enhancing tumor "rind" around central necrotic core
  - Hemorrhage common

IDH-Mutant GBM
- Also called "secondary" GBM
  - Arises from malignant degeneration of lower-grade tumor
  - *IDH1* mutated, *TP53* mutated, *ATRX* loss
- ≈ 5% of GBMs
- Peak age = 45 years
  - Survival 2-3 years
- Pathology
  - Similar to IDH-wild-type but less palisading necrosis
  - WHO grade IV
- Imaging
  - Predilection for frontal lobe
  - Less prominent necrosis
  - Significant nonenhancing areas
  - MRS shows 2-HG at 2.25 ppm

Pathology

In contrast to the similar appearance of IDH-mutant and wild-type diffuse and anaplastic astrocytomas, IDH-mutant GBMs generally look different from IDH-wild-type tumors.

Location. In contrast to IDH-wild-type GBMs, IDH-mutant GBMs have a strong predilection for the frontal lobe, similar to the preferential localization of WHO grade II diffuse astrocytomas.

Gross Pathology. IDH-mutant GBMs diffusely infiltrate the brain but hemorrhage, and the large regions of central necrosis so characteristic of IDH-wild-type GBMs are usually absent.

Microscopic Features. With some exception, histologic features of IDH-mutant GBMs resemble those of IDH-wild-type tumors. Palisading necrosis is less frequent; focal areas of oligodendroglioma-like components are more common.

Staging, Grading, and Classification. IDH-mutant GBMs correspond histologically to WHO grade IV.

Clinical Issues

IDH-mutant GBMs arise at a significantly younger age (mean = 45 years) and have a better prognosis compared with their IDH-wild-type counterparts. Mean overall survival is 2-3 years.

Imaging

IDH-mutant GBMs show a distinct (but not exclusive) predilection for the frontal lobes. Significant nonenhancing areas are typically present, and the classic thick tumor rind surrounding a large central necrotic core that characterizes IDH-wild-type GBMs is generally absent **(17-53)**. Exceptions are common, so molecular profiling is still necessary to establish the definitive diagnosis.

MRS may disclose a 2-HG peak resonating at 2.25 ppm.

Gliosarcoma

Terminology

Gliosarcoma (GS) is a GBM variant characterized by a biphasic tissue pattern with areas of glial (gliomatous) and mesenchymal (sarcomatous) differentiation.

Etiology

GS was once thought to be a "collision tumor" with the astrocytic and sarcomatous portions arising separately and independently but in close geographic proximity. More recent evidence shows that similar cytogenetic alterations are present in both components and therefore are monoclonal in origin. The sarcomatous areas are most likely a result of phenotypic change in the GBM cells rather than the coincidental development of two genetically distinct, separate neoplasms.

GS can be primary or secondary. Most GSs are primary tumors and arise de novo. Secondary GSs occur in patients with previously resected and irradiated GBMs or as radiation-induced tumors in patients without any prior history of GBM.

The genetic profile of GS is generally similar to that of a primary GBM with *PTEN* mutations/deletion, *TP53* mutations, and *CDK4* and *MDM2* amplification. *EGFR* amplification is uncommon. *MGMT* methylation and *IDH1* mutation are rare.

Pathology

GS is characterized by a biphasic tissue pattern. Areas that exhibit both neoplastic glial and metaplastic mesenchymal elements are present within the same tumor. The gliomatous element may be geographically separated from—or intermingled with—the mesenchymal component **(17-54)**.

Gross Pathology. The temporal lobe is the most common site (nearly half of all cases) followed by the frontal (20%) and parietal lobes (15%).

Two gross phenotypic subtypes have been recently described. One is meningioma-like with a superficial location and relatively well-circumscribed solid (predominately sarcomatous) tumor mass. The other subtype is a deeply

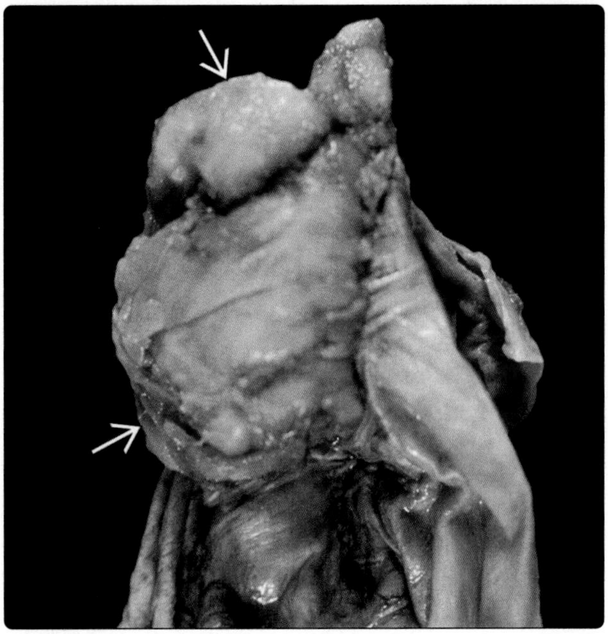

(17-54) Autopsy case of gliosarcoma demonstrates a dura-based tumor nodule ➡ that appears very similar to meningioma. (Courtesy Rubinstein Collection, AFIP Archives.)

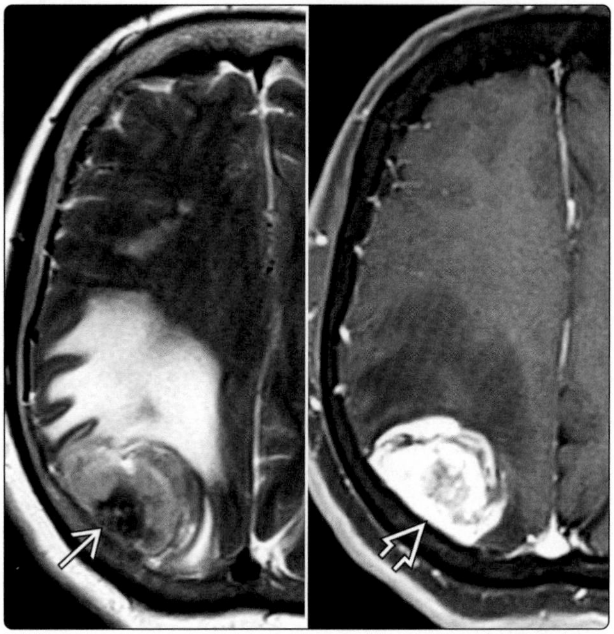

(17-55) T2WI (L), T1 C+ FS (R) in a 74y woman show a mixed hypo-/hyperintense right parietal mass ➡ that abuts the dura, enhances intensely but heterogeneously ⇨. Preop diagnosis was atypical meningioma; GS WHO grade IV, IDH-wild-type.

located neoplasm that resembles a GBM with a necrotic center and hypervascular tumor rind.

Microscopic Features. Histologically, the glial component meets the usual criteria for GBM (see above). The mesenchymal component may display a wide variety of morphologic features with fibroblastic, cartilaginous, osseous, muscle, or adipose cell lineage.

Staging, Grading, and Classification. GSs are WHO grade IV neoplasms.

Clinical Issues

GSs are rare, accounting for approximately 2-4% of all GBMs. Peak age is the fifth to seventh decades (mean age = 60 years). There is a 2.5:1 M:F predominance.

Prognosis is grim with an overall survival of 13 months. Median survival for the meningioma-like phenotype is slightly longer.

Local recurrence following surgical resection is typical, occurring in almost 90% of cases. In contrast to GBM, extracranial metastases are relatively common, occurring in 10-15% of cases.

GLIOSARCOMA

Terminology
- GS = GBM with glial (gliomatous), mesenchymal (sarcomatous) differentiation

Etiology
- *Not* a "collision tumor"
- Same cytogenetic profiles in both components
  - Similar to GBMs (most GSs are *IDH1* wild-type)

Pathology
- Biphasic tissue pattern
  - Neoplastic glial, metaplastic mesenchymal elements
- Two gross phenotypes
  - Meningioma-like with superficial location, relatively circumscribed
  - GBM-like with deep location, necrotic center + hypervascular tumor rind

Clinical Issues
- Rare (2-4% of GBMs)
- Mean age = 60 years
- Overall survival = 13 months

Imaging
- Can look like aggressive meningioma or GBM ± dural invasion

Imaging

The most common appearance is a peripherally located heterogeneously enhancing solid mass with moderate to

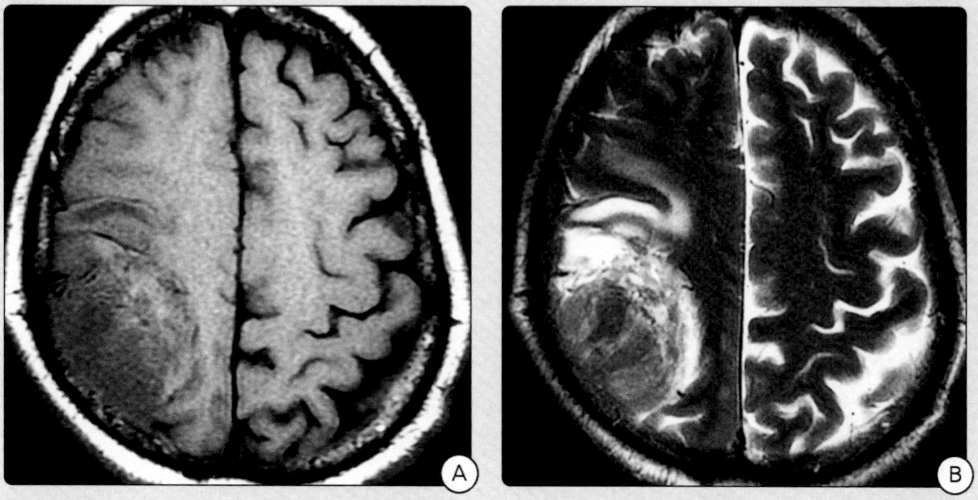

(17-56A) *Axial T1WI in a 72y man with headache and left-sided weakness shows a mixed iso-/hypo-/hyperintense right parietal mass with a broad base that abuts the dura and locally invades the calvarium.* ***(17-56B)*** *T2WI in the same case shows the central part of the mass is mixed iso-/hypointense, while the periphery is hyperintense.*

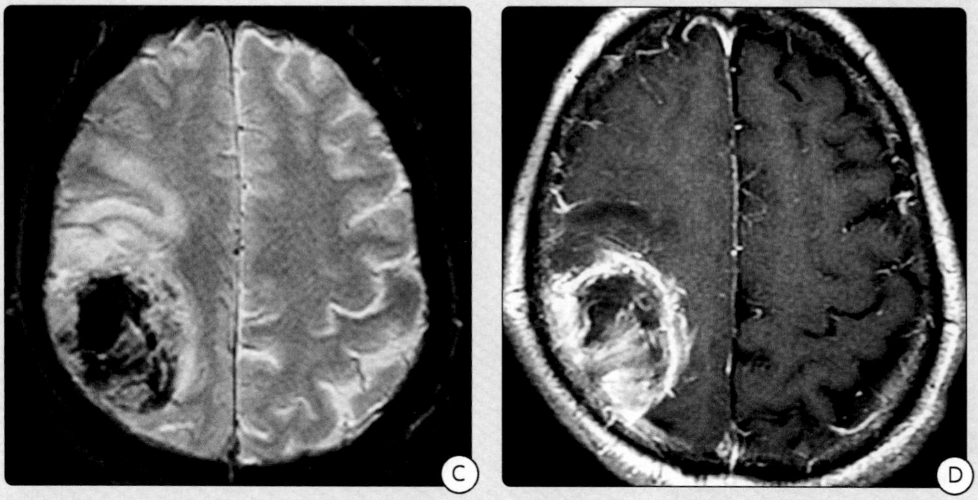

(17-56C) *T2* GRE shows that the center of the mass exhibits significant "blooming," suggesting hemorrhage.* ***(17-56D)*** *T1 C+ MR in the same case shows a thick enhancing rind of tumor that surrounds a necrotic, hemorrhagic core. Note invasion of the adjacent skull, suggestion of dural tail. This is gliosarcoma, IDH1-wild-type.*

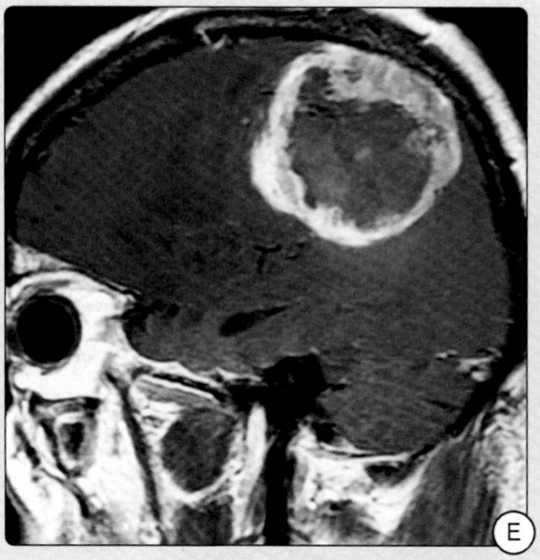

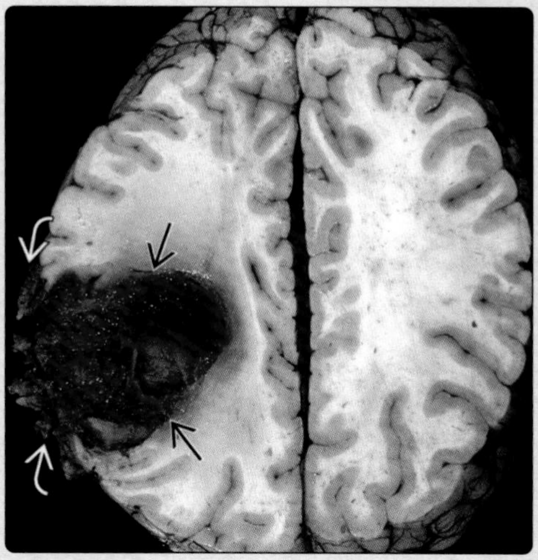

(17-56E) *Sagittal T1 C+ MR in the same patient shows similar findings.* ***(17-57)*** *Axial autopsied brain shows necrotic, hemorrhagic GBM ⇨ with dural invasion ➲. Gross pathology and imaging findings can be indistinguishable from gliosarcoma.*

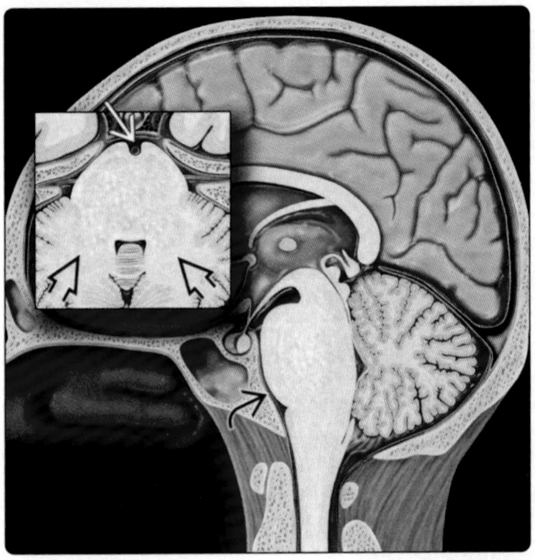

(17-58) DIPG expands pons ⇨ and medulla, wrapping around basilar artery ➡ and extending into both middle cerebellar peduncles ⇨.

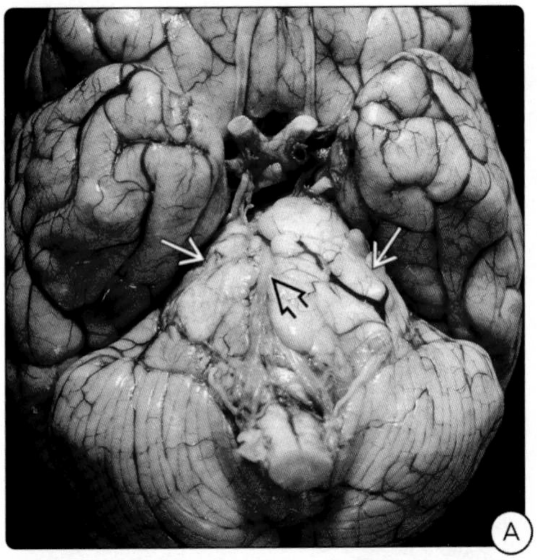

(17-59A) Autopsy specimen shows a diffuse pontine glioma expanding the pons ➡, almost completely encasing the basilar artery ⇨.

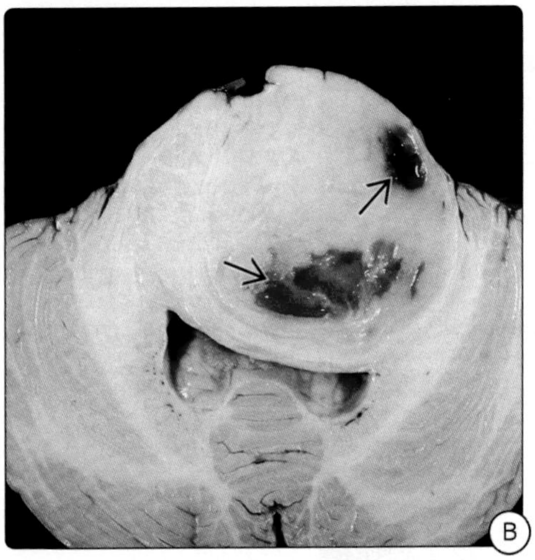

(17-59B) Cut section shows infiltrating tumor. This was AA (WHO III) with necrotic, hemorrhagic foci of GBM ⇨. (Courtesy R. Hewlett, MD.)

marked surrounding edema **(17-55)**. GSs often abut the meninges **(17-56)** but may not demonstrate dural attachment or obvious invasion.

Many cases arise deep within the cerebral hemispheres remote from the dura-arachnoid. These tumors exhibit a central necrotic core surrounded by a thick, irregular rind of enhancement and may be indistinguishable from GBM.

Differential Diagnosis

The major differential diagnoses of GS are **anaplastic meningioma** and **glioblastoma with dural invasion (17-57)**. **Other sarcomas, dural metastases, lymphoma, plasmocytoma**, and **neurosarcoid** can all present as dura-based lesions with variable brain invasion.

GSs that arise deep within the brain parenchyma and do not abut the meninges are usually indistinguishable from **GBM**.

Pediatric Diffuse Gliomas

In the past, diffusely infiltrating gliomas in children were lumped together with their adult counterparts. Although microscopically similar, their biologic behaviors are often very different.

Advances in molecular genetics have disclosed that similar-appearing neoplasms also have their own set of distinct genetic alterations. For example, when oligodendrogliomas occur in children, they frequently lack the 1p19q codeletions that characterize adult tumors. Most pediatric high-grade gliomas lack *IDH1* mutation.

Unlike adult high-grade astrocytomas, pediatric high-grade astrocytomas frequently arise in the midline (pons, thalamus, and spinal cord). A newly defined entity that is characterized by midline location and mutations in the histone H3 gene includes tumors that were previously referred to as diffuse intrinsic pontine glioma (DIPG) and is now officially recognized as **diffuse midline glioma, H3 K27M-mutant**.

Pediatric brainstem gliomas (BSGs) account for 10% of pediatric brain tumors and can involve the midbrain, pons, or medulla. Most are astrocytic neoplasms, but their histologic subtypes, genetic profiles, and prognosis vary substantially. Therefore, pediatric diffuse gliomas may differ from their adult counterparts, and also *not all pediatric BSGs are the same—geography, molecular profile, tumor grade, and patient outcome are remarkably variable!*

Pathology

Pediatric BSGs are divided into two groups by location. The most common location is the pons (two-thirds of cases). These pontine gliomas are called **DIPGs (17-58)**. Approximately 80% are high-grade tumors **(17-59)**. Intrapontine histologic variation is common. Different areas of WHO grade II, III, and IV astrocytoma can all occur within the densely tumor-packed pons. Most of these DIPGs exhibit histone mutations (see below) and are IDH-wild-type.

Midline non-brainstem diffuse high-grade gliomas are less common. They involve the midbrain (15%) or the medulla/pontomedullary junction (20%). These tumors share many clinical and biologic features with DIPGs and have a similarly dismal prognosis.

Disease-defining somatic mutations in *H3F3A*, *HIST1H3B*, and *ACVR1* are present in virtually 100% of DIPGs and are conserved across all midline locations (e.g., pons, midbrain, tectum, and lower brainstem). Similar mutations are present in 50% of pediatric thalamic GBMs.

The second group of midline gliomas consists of focal, much less aggressive tumors that are confined predominately to the tectal plate/periaqueductal region and often remain stable over long periods of time.

Tectal gliomas are frequently found in older children and young adults, typically presenting with symptoms of obstructive hydrocephalus rather than cranial neuropathy. Most tectal gliomas are pilocytic astrocytomas (WHO grade I neoplasms) or IDH-mutant diffuse WHO grade II astrocytomas (10-20%).

BRAINSTEM GLIOMAS

Pathology
- Children (10% of childhood brain tumors)
  - 2/3 in pons (diffusely infiltrating pontine glioma, DIPG)
  - Most are H3 (histone) mutant, IDH-wild-type
- Adults (uncommon)
  - 60% medulla, 30% pons, 10% midbrain/tectum
  - Low grade > high grade

Prognosis
- Children
  - Among most lethal of childhood cancers
  - H3 mutant DIPG = poor prognosis; < 10% survive 2 years
  - WHO grade varies (poor correlation with survival)
- Adults: generally better prognosis

Imaging
- "Fat" pons, tectum, or medulla
  - T2/FLAIR hyperintensity
  - Enhancement often absent/minimal in pediatric brainstem gliomas (BSGs)
  - Enhancement common in adult BSGs

Differential Diagnosis
- Brainstem encephalitis
- Demyelinating disease
- Metabolic disease (e.g., osmotic demyelination)
- Intracranial hypotension
  - Brainstem "sagging" → "fat" pons

Clinical Issues

DIPGs are among the most lethal of all childhood cancers. Aggressive local and distant metastatic spread is common. Overall, median survival is less than 1 year despite multimodal therapies.

Outcome correlates more accurately with histone 3 mutation status than with WHO grade. Survival in children with WHO grade II tumors with H3.3 mutation is comparable to patients with WHO grade IV GBMs **(17-62)**, whereas the outcome in patients with WHO grade IV tumors but wild-type H3.3 is similar to low-grade IDH wild-type astrocytomas.

Adult DIPGs are rare, accounting for approximately 2% of all intracranial neoplasms. Most are IDH-wild-type anaplastic astrocytomas or GBMs. Survival is similar to supratentorial IDH-wild-type tumors of similar grade and histology.

Imaging

DIPGs expand and diffusely infiltrate the pons. They have indistinct margins and are hypointense on T1WI and hyperintense on T2/FLAIR. DIPGs often expand anteriorly, enfolding and sometimes almost completely engulfing the basilar artery **(17-60)**. Foci of necrosis and even intratumoral

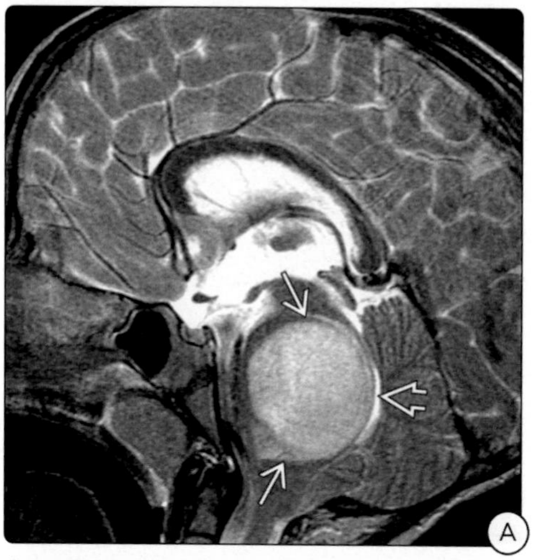

***(17-60A)** T2WI in a child with diffuse pontine glioma shows a hyperintense mass ➡ expanding pons, displacing fourth ventricle ➡ posteriorly.*

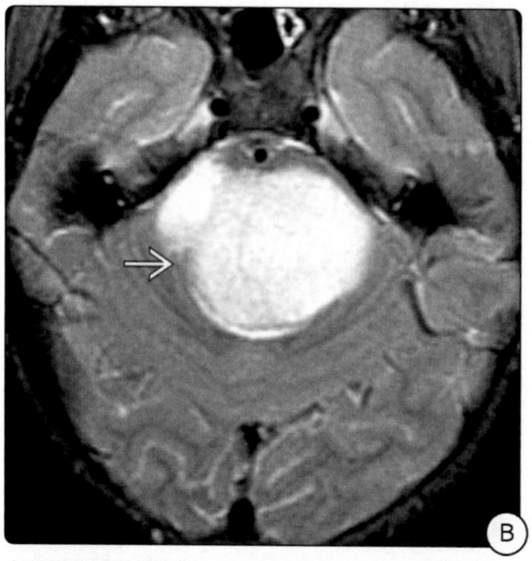

***(17-60B)** T2 FS shows mass is hyperintense with poorly defined margins ➡. This is WHO grade II diffusely infiltrating astrocytoma.*

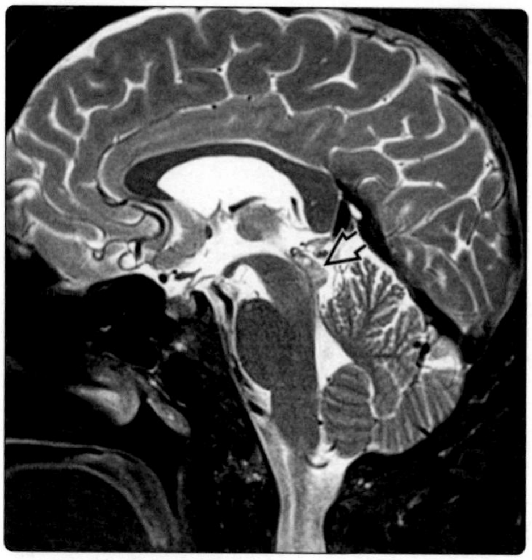

***(17-61)** Sagittal T2WI shows incidental finding of presumed tectal glioma ➡ in a 50y woman. The lesion has remained unchanged over 5 years.*

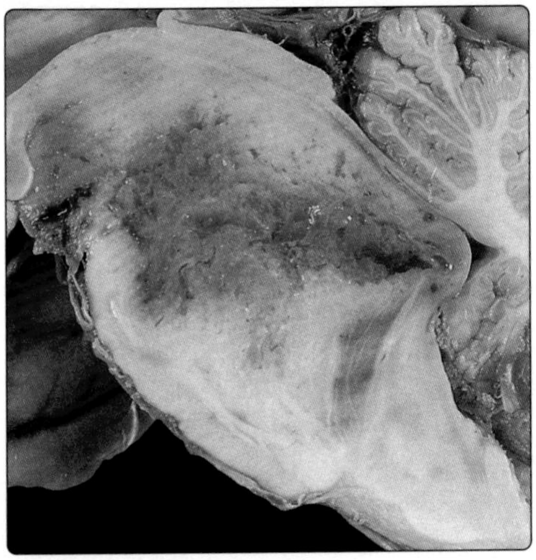

(17-62) Autopsied case of pediatric DIPG shows diffusely expanded pons, CSF metastases. (From Ellison, Neuropathology, 2013.)

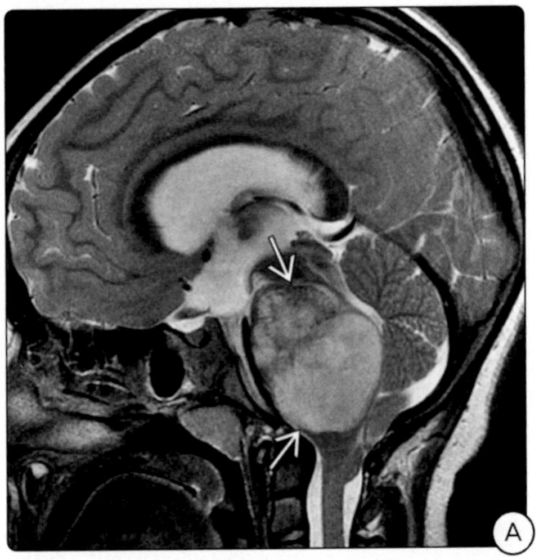

(17-63A) Sagittal T2WI in a 5y girl with multiple cranial nerve palsies shows heterogeneous hyperintense tumor ➡ expanding entire pons.

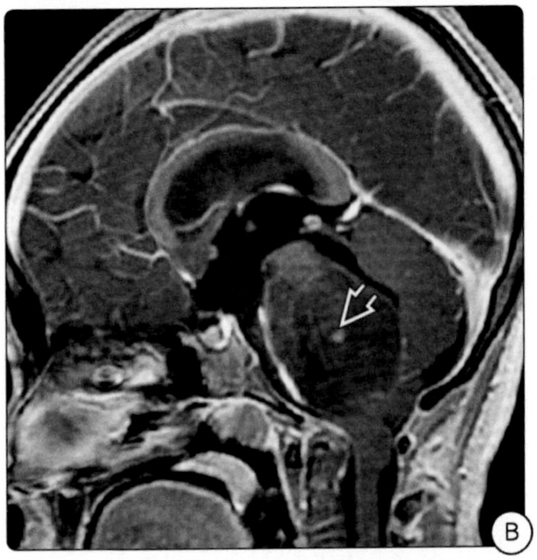

(17-63B) Sagittal T1 C+ FS shows single focus of mild enhancement in the tumor ➡. This is proven diffuse midline glioma, H3 K27M-mutant.

hemorrhage may be present. Most DIPGs show either no or relatively little patchy enhancement **(17-63)**.

Tectal gliomas are discrete, well-marginated lesions that focally enlarge the colliculi or midbrain tegmentum and often obstruct the cerebral aqueduct. They are iso- to hypointense on T1WI and hyperintense on T2/FLAIR **(17-61)**. Contrast enhancement is minimal or absent. Tectal gliomas are indolent lesions that typically remain stable in size over many years.

Differential Diagnosis

The general differential diagnosis of pediatric BSG is **brainstem encephalitis, demyelinating disease** (MS, ADEM), **neurofibromatosis type 1** (NF1), and **osmotic demyelination**.

A "fat" pons can be mimicked by **intracranial hypotension**. Brain "sagging" can make the midbrain and pons look abnormally large on axial images. Signal intensity is normal on T2/FLAIR. Look for ancillary signs of intracranial hypotension, such as dural-venous engorgement, effacement of the suprasellar cistern, subdural hematoma(s), and acquired tonsillar herniation.

Diffuse Midline Glioma, H3 K27M-Mutant

Terminology

An H3 K27M-mutant diffuse glioma is an infiltrative, high-grade glioma with predominantly astrocytic differentiation and a K27M mutation. Midline or paramedian locations are typical. The brainstem, thalamus, and spinal cord are the most common sites. H3 K27M-mutant diffuse midline glioma is mostly a tumor of children but can also occur in adults.

Etiology

The majority of DIPGs and thalamic GBMs are histone H3 variant tumors. This molecularly defined set of neoplasms is characterized by K27M mutations in the histone H3 gene *H3F3A*. p53 overexpression and *ATRX* loss (except in pontine gliomas) are commonly associated findings.

The K27M mutation appears to be mutually exclusive with *IDH1* mutation and *EGFR* amplification. *BRAF* mutation is rare.

Pathology

Gross Pathology. Symmetric or asymmetric fusiform enlargement of the pons is typical for DIPGs **(17-62)**. The thalami are the second most common intracranial site. Other reported locations include the spinal cord, third ventricle, hypothalamus, pineal region, and cerebellum.

Pontine tumors may extend superiorly into the thalami or inferiorly into the upper cervical cord. Occasionally, H3-mutant tumors exhibit diffuse spread with a gliomatosis cerebri pattern. Leptomeningeal dissemination occurs in approximately 40% of cases.

Microscopic Features. The vast majority of H3 midline gliomas exhibit astrocytic morphology, but a wide spectrum of morphologic variations has been reported. Focal areas of necrosis, hemorrhage, and microvascular proliferation may be present. Mitotic figures are high.

H3 K27M-mutant diffuse gliomas are WHO grade IV neoplasms.

Clinical Issues

H3 K27M-mutant gliomas can occur at any age but are location dependent. Median age at diagnosis with pontine tumors is 7 years, whereas non-brainstem (primarily thalamic and spinal) histone-mutant gliomas average two decades older.

For diffuse midline gliomas in general, H3 K27M mutation generally confers a worse prognosis than that of IDH-wild-type astrocytomas. Less than 10% of patients with DIPGs survive longer than 2 years. In thalamic diffuse midline gliomas, high-grade histology is associated with short overall survival regardless of histone gene status.

Imaging

Imaging features of H3 K27M-mutant brainstem gliomas are those described above for DIPGs **(17-63)**.

Thalamic diffuse H3-mutant gliomas show an enlarged thalamus with T2/FLAIR hyperintensity. Enhancement is variable but typically minimal or patchy and usually involves <25% of the tumor **(17-64)**. Leptomeningeal dissemination and "brain-to-brain" metastases are common in all H3 K27M-mutant midline gliomas, so the entire neuraxis should be visualized on initial evaluation.

Differential Diagnosis

The differential diagnosis for pontine diffuse midline gliomas, H3 K27M-mutant, is the same as delineated above for DIPGs.

The differential diagnosis for unilateral thalamic H3 K27M-mutant glioma is the same for other IDH-wild-type WHO grade II and III astrocytomas (see above). Bithalamic tumors can resemble nonneoplastic disorders, such as internal cerebral vein thrombosis, artery of Percheron infarct, and Wernicke encephalopathy.

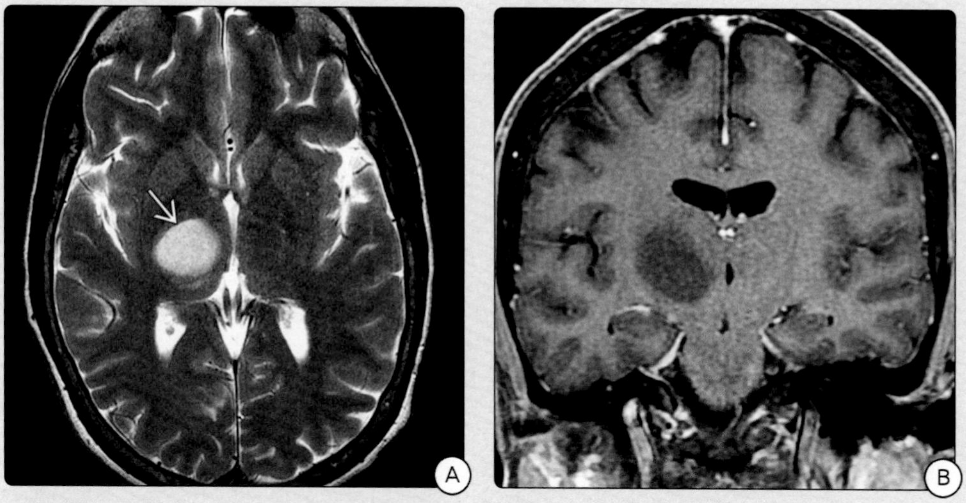

***(17-64A)** T2WI shows a hyperintense right thalamic mass ➡. **(17-64B)** Coronal T1 C+ FS in the same case shows no enhancement. Stereotaxic biopsy disclosed anaplastic astrocytoma, IDH-wild-type.*

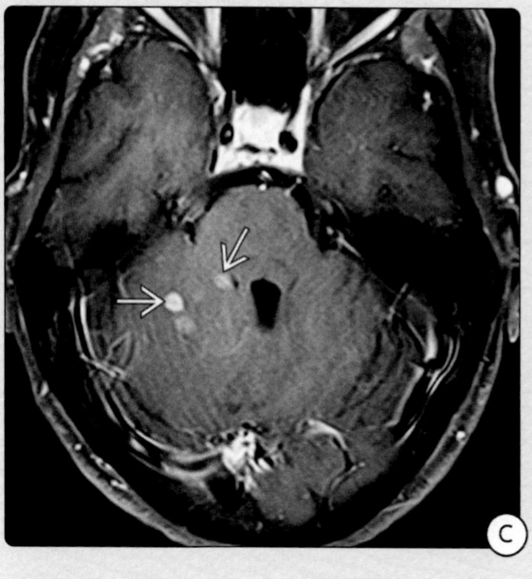

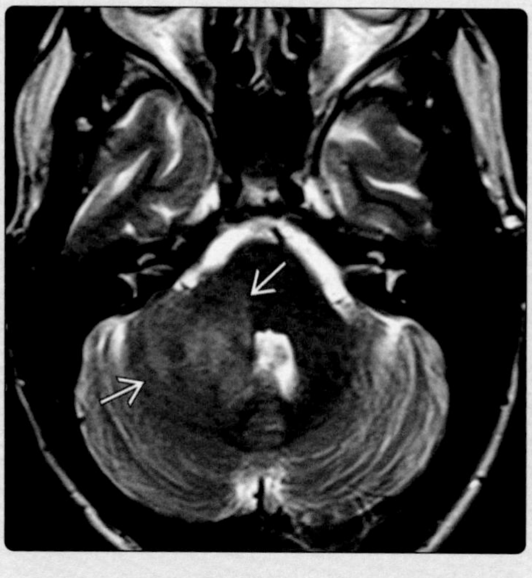

***(17-64C)** T1 C+ FS shows multiple metastases ➡. Case was subsequently identified as an H3 K27M-mutant high grade glioma. This mutation is present in two-thirds of unilateral high-grade thalamic astrocytomas. **(17-65)** Eighteen months later the patient developed cerebellar symptoms. Antemortem T2WI shows a mildly hyperintense mass in the right brachium pontis and cerebellar hemisphere ➡.*

Selected References

General Features of Astrocytomas

Origin of Astrocytomas

Bischof J et al: Cancer stem cells: the potential role of autophagy, proteolysis, and cathepsins in glioblastoma stem cells. Tumour Biol. 39(3):1010428317692227, 2017

Capdevila C et al: Glioblastoma multiforme and adult neurogenesis in the ventricular-subventricular zone: a review. J Cell Physiol. 232(7):1596-1601, 2017

Ludwig K et al: Molecular markers in glioma. J Neurooncol. ePub, 2017

Classification and Grading of Astrocytomas

Capdevila C et al: Glioblastoma multiforme and adult neurogenesis in the ventricular-subventricular zone: a review. J Cell Physiol. 232(7):1596-1601, 2017

Karsy M et al: New molecular considerations for glioma: IDH, ATRX, BRAF, TERT, H3 K27M. Curr Neurol Neurosci Rep. 17(2):19, 2017

Hattori N et al: World Health Organization grade II-III astrocytomas consist of genetically distinct tumor lineages. Cancer Sci. 107(8):1159-64, 2016

Louis DN et al: The 2016 World Health Organization Classification of Tumors of the Central Nervous System: a summary. Acta Neuropathol. 131(6):803-20, 2016

Localized Astrocytomas

Pilocytic Astrocytoma

Sexton-Oates A et al: Methylation profiling of paediatric pilocytic astrocytoma reveals variants specifically associated with tumour location and predictive of recurrence. Mol Oncol. ePub, 2017

Tomić TT et al: A new GTF2I-BRAF fusion mediating MAPK pathway activation in pilocytic astrocytoma. PLoS One. 12(4):e0175638, 2017

Bonfield CM et al: Pediatric cerebellar astrocytoma: a review. Childs Nerv Syst. 31(10):1677-85, 2015

Spennato P et al: Posterior fossa tumors in infants and neonates. Childs Nerv Syst. 31(10):1751-72, 2015

Pilomyxoid Astrocytoma

Rosenfeld A et al: A case series characterizing pilomyxoid astrocytomas in childhood. J Pediatr Hematol Oncol. 38(2):e63-6, 2016

Alkonyi B et al: Differential imaging characteristics and dissemination potential of pilomyxoid astrocytomas versus pilocytic astrocytomas. Neuroradiology. 57(6):625-38, 2015

Kleinschmidt-DeMasters BK et al: Pilomyxoid astrocytoma (PMA) shows significant differences in gene expression vs. pilocytic astrocytoma (PA) and variable tendency toward maturation to PA. Brain Pathol. 25(4):429-40, 2015

Subependymal Giant Cell Astrocytoma

Arroyo MS et al: Acute management of symptomatic subependymal giant cell astrocytoma with everolimus. Pediatr Neurol. 72:81-85, 2017

Appalla D et al: Mammalian target of rapamycin inhibitor induced complete remission of a recurrent subependymal giant cell astrocytoma in a patient without features of tuberous sclerosis complex. Pediatr Blood Cancer. 63(7):1276-8, 2016

Krishnan A et al: Cross-sectional imaging review of tuberous sclerosis. Radiol Clin North Am. 54(3):423-40, 2016

Pachow D et al: The mTOR signaling pathway as a treatment target for intracranial neoplasms. Neuro Oncol. 17(2):189-99, 2015

Ouyang T et al: Subependymal giant cell astrocytoma: current concepts, management, and future directions. Childs Nerv Syst. 30(4):561-70, 2014

Pleomorphic Xanthoastrocytoma

Jiménez-Heffernan JA et al: Cytologic features of pleomorphic xanthoastrocytoma, WHO grade II. A comparative study with glioblastoma. Diagn Cytopathol. 45(4):339-344, 2017

Lohkamp LN et al: MGMT promoter methylation and BRAF V600E mutations are helpful markers to discriminate pleomorphic xanthoastrocytoma from giant cell glioblastoma. PLoS One. 11(6):e0156422, 2016

Ida CM et al: Pleomorphic xanthoastrocytoma: natural history and long-term follow-up. Brain Pathol. 25(5):575-86, 2015

Anaplastic Pleomorphic Xanthoastrocytoma

Vaubel RA et al: Recurrent copy number alterations in low-grade and anaplastic pleomorphic xanthoastrocytoma with and without BRAF V600E mutation. Brain Pathol. ePub, 2017

Alexandrescu S et al: Epithelioid glioblastomas and anaplastic epithelioid pleomorphic xanthoastrocytomas-same entity or first cousins? Brain Pathol. 26(2):215-23, 2016

Diffuse Astrocytomas

Maus A et al: Glutamate and α-ketoglutarate: key players in glioma metabolism. Amino Acids. 49(1):21-32, 2017

Paul Y et al: DNA methylation signatures for 2016 WHO classification subtypes of diffuse gliomas. Clin Epigenetics. 9:32, 2017

Ceccarelli M et al: Molecular profiling reveals biologically discrete subsets and pathways of progression in diffuse glioma. Cell. 164(3):550-63, 2016

de la Fuente MI et al: Integration of 2-hydroxyglutarate-proton magnetic resonance spectroscopy into clinical practice for disease monitoring in isocitrate dehydrogenase-mutant glioma. Neuro Oncol. 18(2):283-90, 2016

Reuss DE et al: IDH mutant diffuse and anaplastic astrocytomas have similar age at presentation and little difference in survival: a grading problem for WHO. Acta Neuropathol. 129(6):867-73, 2015

Diffuse Astrocytoma, IDH-Mutant

Capdevila C et al: Glioblastoma multiforme and adult neurogenesis in the ventricular-subventricular zone: a review. J Cell Physiol. 232(7):1596-1601, 2017

Richardson TE et al: Rapid progression to glioblastoma in a subset of IDH-mutated astrocytomas: a genome-wide analysis. J Neurooncol. ePub, 2017

Venteicher AS et al: Decoupling genetics, lineages, and microenvironment in IDH-mutant gliomas by single-cell RNA-seq. Science. 355(6332), 2017

Lima GL et al: Incidental diffuse low-grade gliomas: from early detection to preventive neuro-oncological surgery. Neurosurg Rev. 39(3):377-84, 2016 von Deimling A et al: Diffuse astrocytoma, IDH-mutant. In: Louis DN et al (eds), WHO Classification of Tumours of the Central Nervous System. Lyon, France: International Agency for Research on Cancer, 2016, pp 18-23

Anaplastic Astrocytoma, IDH-Mutant

Ballester LY et al: Molecular classification of adult diffuse gliomas: conflicting IDH1/IDH2, ATRX and 1p/19q results. Hum Pathol. ePub, 2017

Leu K et al: Perfusion and diffusion MRI signatures in histologic and genetic subtypes of WHO grade II-III diffuse gliomas. J Neurooncol. ePub, 2017

Pekmezci M et al: Adult infiltrating gliomas with WHO 2016 integrated diagnosis: additional prognostic roles of ATRX and TERT. Acta Neuropathol. 133(6):1001-1016, 2017

Robinson C et al: IDH1-mutation in diffuse gliomas in persons age 55 years and over. J Neuropathol Exp Neurol. 76(2):151-154, 2017

de la Fuente MI et al: Integration of 2-hydroxyglutarate-proton magnetic resonance spectroscopy into clinical practice for disease monitoring in isocitrate dehydrogenase-mutant glioma. Neuro Oncol. 18(2):283-90, 2016

Diffuse Astrocytoma, IDH-Wild-Type

Abudumijiti A et al: Adult IDH wild-type lower-grade gliomas should be further stratified. Neuro Oncol. ePub, 2017

Broniscer A et al: Gliomatosis cerebri in children shares molecular characteristics with other pediatric gliomas. Acta Neuropathol. 131(2):299-307, 2016

Herrlinger U et al: Gliomatosis cerebri: no evidence for a separate brain tumor entity. Acta Neuropathol. 131(2):309-19, 2016

von Deimling A et al: Anaplastic astrocytoma, IDH-mutant. In: Louis DN et al (eds), WHO Classification of Tumours of the Central Nervous System. Lyon, France: International Agency for Research on Cancer, 2016, pp 24-27

Anaplastic Astrocytoma, IDH-Wild-Type

Leu K et al: Perfusion and diffusion MRI signatures in histologic and genetic subtypes of WHO grade II-III diffuse gliomas. J Neurooncol. ePub, 2017

Glioblastoma, IDH-Wild-Type

Filbin MG et al: Gliomas genomics and epigenomics: arriving at the start and knowing it for the first time. Annu Rev Pathol. 11:497-521, 2016

Kalkan R: The importance of mutational drivers in GBM. Crit Rev Eukaryot Gene Expr. 26(1):19-26, 2016

Louis DN et al: Glioblastoma, IDH-wildtype. In: Louis DN et al (eds), WHO Classification of Tumours of the Central Nervous System. Lyon, France: International Agency for Research on Cancer, 2016, pp 28-51

Mandel JJ et al: Impact of IDH1 mutation status on outcome in clinical trials for recurrent glioblastoma. J Neurooncol. 129(1):147-54, 2016

Glioblastoma, IDH-Mutant

Richardson TE et al: Rapid progression to glioblastoma in a subset of IDH-mutated astrocytomas: a genome-wide analysis. J Neurooncol. ePub, 2017

Gliosarcoma

Meyer RM et al: Glioblastoma recurrence, progression, and dissemination as a purely subdural gliosarcoma. J Neurooncol. 132(3):521-522, 2017

Castelli J et al: Prognostic and therapeutic factors of gliosarcoma from a multi-institutional series. J Neurooncol. 129(1):85-92, 2016

Pediatric Diffuse Gliomas

Clerk-Lamalice O et al: MRI evaluation of non-necrotic T2-hyperintense foci in pediatric diffuse intrinsic pontine glioma. AJNR Am J Neuroradiol. ePub, 2016

Hoffman LM et al: Spatial genomic heterogeneity in diffuse intrinsic pontine and midline high-grade glioma: implications for diagnostic biopsy and targeted therapeutics. Acta Neuropathol Commun. 4:1, 2016

Klimo P Jr et al: Malignant brainstem tumors in children, excluding diffuse intrinsic pontine gliomas. J Neurosurg Pediatr. 17(1):57-65, 2016

Nikbakht H et al: Spatial and temporal homogeneity of driver mutations in diffuse intrinsic pontine glioma. Nat Commun. 7:11185, 2016

Tisnado J et al: Conventional and advanced imaging of diffuse intrinsic pontine glioma. J Child Neurol. 31(12):1386-93, 2016

Panditharatna E et al: Clinicopathology of diffuse intrinsic pontine glioma and its redefined genomic and epigenomic landscape. Cancer Genet. 208(7-8):367-73, 2015

Theeler BJ et al: Adult brainstem gliomas: correlation of clinical and molecular features. J Neurol Sci. 353(1-2):92-7, 2015

Diffuse Midline Glioma, H3 K27M-Mutant

Aboian MS et al: Imaging characteristics of pediatric diffuse midline gliomas with histone H3 K27M mutation. AJNR Am J Neuroradiol. 38(4):795-800, 2017

Meyronet D et al: Characteristics of H3 K27M-mutant gliomas in adults. Neuro Oncol. ePub, 2017

Nakata S et al: Histone H3 K27M mutations in adult cerebellar high-grade gliomas. Brain Tumor Pathol. ePub, 2017

Yoshimoto K et al: Prevalence and clinicopathological features of H3.3 G34-mutant high-grade gliomas: a retrospective study of 411 consecutive glioma cases in a single institution. Brain Tumor Pathol. ePub, 2017

Broniscer A et al: Bithalamic gliomas may be molecularly distinct from their unilateral high-grade counterparts. Brain Pathol. ePub, 2016

Solomon DA et al: Diffuse midline gliomas with histone H3-K27M mutation: a series of 47 cases assessing the spectrum of morphologic variation and associated genetic alterations. Brain Pathol. 26(5):569-80, 2016

Nonastrocytic Glial Neoplasms

Nonastrocytic gliomas (NAGs) represent a broad spectrum of neoplasms derived from neural stem cells or glial progenitor cells that maintain glial characteristics. This group of neoplasms is significantly smaller than the astrocytomas but nevertheless comprises an important class of tumors that range from relatively well-circumscribed and biologically indolent neoplasms (e.g., choroid plexus papilloma) to highly malignant tumors such as anaplastic oligodendrogliomas and ependymomas.

As a group, NAGs occur in patients of all ages. Some—such as choroid plexus papilloma—are usually tumors of young children, often under the age of five. In contrast, oligodendrogliomas tend to be tumors of adults.

Different ependymoma subtypes affect different age groups and arise in location-specific sites. Cellular ependymoma is usually a childhood tumor, whereas subependymoma is typically a tumor of older adults.

The paramount importance of correct, specific glioma diagnosis relates to treatment decisions and prognosis.

We first discuss oligodendroglial tumors and their entity-defining molecular markers. We follow with a discussion of ependymomas and their location-specific subtypes, including the newly recognized *RELA* fusion-positive ependymoma.

Tumors of the choroid plexus, which itself is derived from modified ependymal cells, constitute the third group of neoplasms included in this chapter. Lastly, we briefly consider a miscellaneous group of uncommon nonastrocytic glial tumors called "other gliomas" in the current WHO classification. To date, this group includes astroblastoma, chordoid glioma (of the third ventricle), and angiocentric glioma.

Oligodendrogliomas

Oligodendrocytes are found predominantly in the white matter. Their primary function is the production and maintenance of myelin.

Tumors morphologically resembling oligodendrocytes—oligodendrogliomas, OGs—are the third most common type of glial neoplasm (after anaplastic astrocytoma and glioblastoma).

Histologically, oligodendroglial tumors constitute a spectrum ranging from well-differentiated, relatively indolent tumors to frankly malignant neoplasms with rapid growth. OGs are currently classified into two types: a

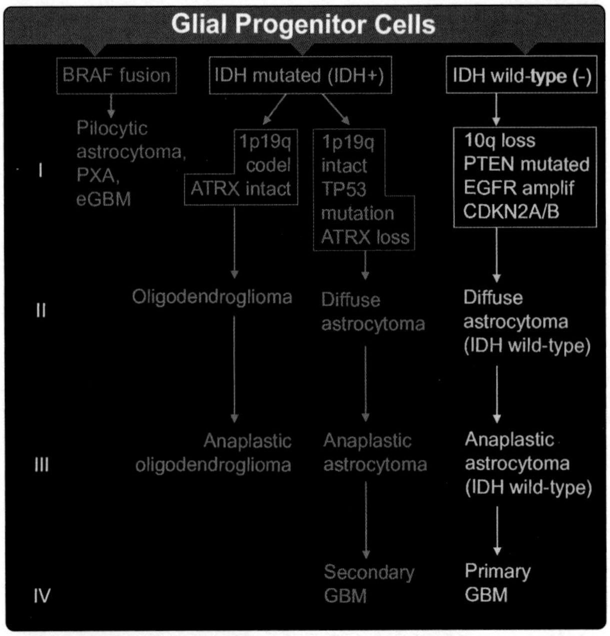

***(18-1)** Graphic shows glial progenitor cells and gliomagenesis. After the "driver" IDH mutation, oligodendrocyte progenitor cells undergo sequential mutations to give rise to oligodendrogliomas (shown in green).*

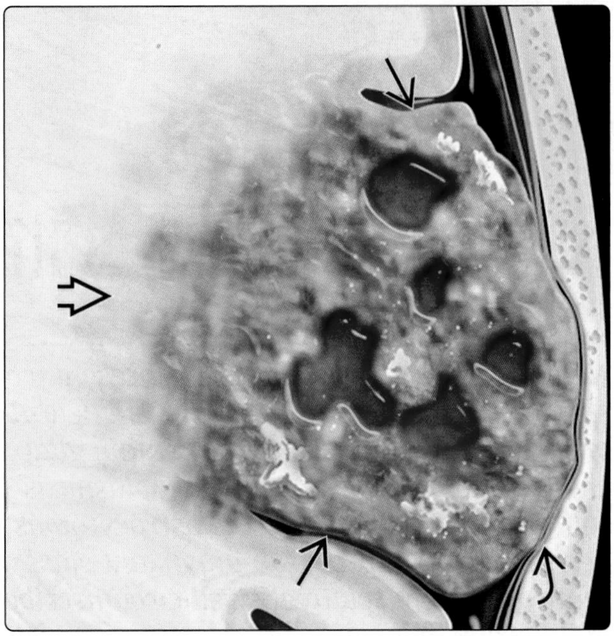

***(18-2)** Oligodendrogliomas (OGs) are poorly demarcated, cortically based "fleshy" masses ➡ that infiltrate cortex and subcortical white matter ⇨. Remodeling of adjacent bone ↪ is common.*

well-differentiated tumor (OG) and a malignant variant (anaplastic OG).

Oligodendroglioma, IDH-Mutant and 1p/19q Codeleted

Terminology

Like other neoplasms, OGs develop as a result of genetic and molecular alterations that accumulate with tumor progression. OGs are diffusely infiltrating, slow-growing gliomas with specific entity-defining molecular markers, i.e., *IDH1* or *IDH2* mutation plus deletion of chromosomal arms 1p and 19q (termed 1p/19q codeletion).

Etiology

Genetics. OGs and diffuse astrocytomas share the same early "driver" IDH mutation. OGs then diverge, undergoing subsequent genetic alterations (1p and 19q losses) that distinguish them from astrocytomas as well as from other gliomas **(18-1)**. Virtually all 1p/19q-codeleted tumors also carry *TERT* mutations. OGs typically retain *ATRX* nuclear expression and lack *TP53* mutation. *EGFR* amplifications are mutually exclusive with 1p/19q codeletion and IDH mutations, so they are also absent in OGs.

Childhood tumors that histologically resemble OG often are IDH-wild-type and do not exhibit 1p/19q codeletion. They are incompletely characterized but often have *FGFR1*, *MYB*, or *MYBL1* alterations (see below).

Only a tiny fraction of oligodendroglial tumors occur in the setting of single-gene hereditary syndromes. OGs develop in approximately 10% of patients with biallelic **Lynch syndrome**, a multitumor colorectal cancer syndrome caused by germline mutations in one of the mismatch repair genes. Lynch syndrome confers a fourfold increased risk of brain tumors, most commonly glioblastomas.

Pathology

Location. Most OGs arise at the gray-white matter junction **(18-2)**. The vast majority (85-90%) are supratentorial. The most common site is the frontal lobe (50-65%) followed by the parietal, temporal, and occipital lobes. Posterior fossa and spinal cord OGs are uncommon.

OGs in children often involve unusual sites such as the posterior fossa and spinal cord.

Primary leptomeningeal OGs have been reported but are now considered a newly recognized and codified entity, diffuse leptomeningeal glioneuronal tumor (discussed in the following chapter).

Gross Pathology. OGs are typically solid, soft, "fleshy," cortically based tan-to-pink masses. They are poorly circumscribed and blend gradually into adjacent structures, blurring the gray-white matter boundary and expanding one or more gyri **(18-3)**. Extension through the glia limitans to the pial surface is common.

Calcification is frequent, and zones of cystic degeneration are common. However, frank necrosis is rare. Intratumoral hemorrhage is common, especially with larger or more aggressive OGs.

Microscopic Features. OGs vary in cellularity. Most are highly cellular lesions with closely packed, "back-to-back" sheets of small cells, whereas others are relatively paucicellular. Uniform

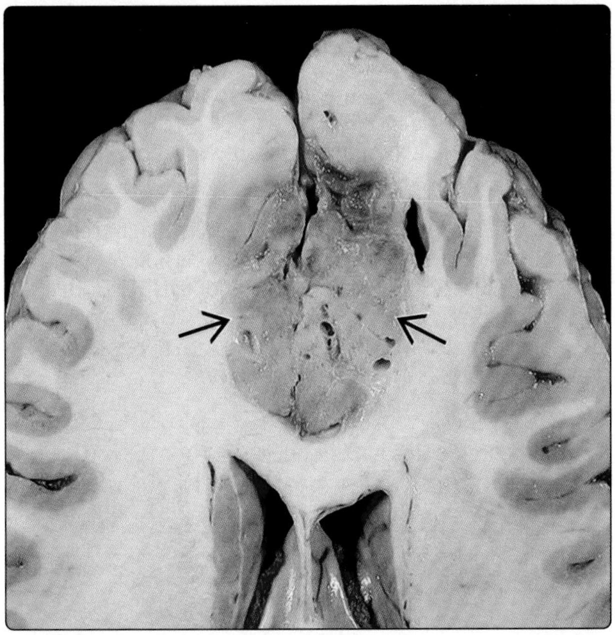

(18-3) Autopsy specimen of oligodendroglioma shows typical cortical/subcortical "fleshy" mass →. (Courtesy R. Hewlett, MD.)

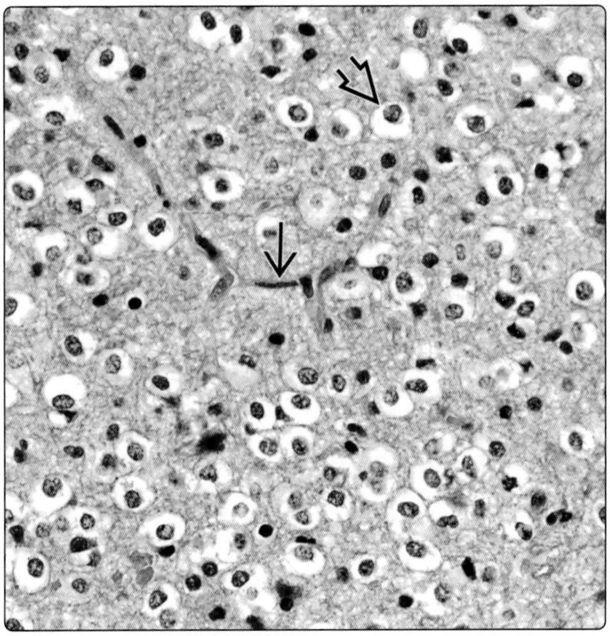

(18-4) Classic microscopic features of OG include a closely packed population of uniform tumor cells with "fried egg" appearance → and the "chicken-wire" pattern → of the microvasculature. (From DP2: Neuropathology.)

round or slightly oval hyperchromatic nuclei surrounded by a prominent perinuclear "halo" of clear watery cytoplasm give OGs a classic "fried egg" appearance **(18-4)**. A branching network of delicate angulated capillaries ("chicken-wire" pattern) is often present, but florid microvascular proliferation is absent.

Staging, Grading, and Classification. So-called "canonical oligodendrogliomas" (IDH-mutated, 1p/19q codeleted) without necrosis, florid microvascular proliferation, or marked mitotic activity (Ki-67 index < 5%) are designated as WHO grade II neoplasms.

Clinical Issues

Epidemiology. OGs account for 2-5% of all primary CNS neoplasms and 5-20% of gliomas. Approximately half of oligodendroglial tumors are WHO grade II neoplasms, and half are grade III (anaplastic OG, discussed below).

OGs are primarily tumors of adults, with only 1-5% occurring in children. Most OGs arise between the ages of 35 and 55 with a peak incidence between 40 and 45 years. There is a moderate male predominance.

Presentation. Because OGs commonly involve the cortical gray matter, seizures are the most common presenting symptom. Headache is the second most common presentation.

Natural History. OGs are slow-growing but locally aggressive neoplasms. The 5-year survival rate is nearly 80%, and median survival time is 10-12 years. OGs are relatively indolent tumors but eventually fatal in most cases.

Local recurrence following resection is very common. Diffuse CSF dissemination is rare. Malignant degeneration to anaplastic OG or glioblastoma occurs in some patients.

Treatment Options. Gross total resection is the primary treatment and improves outcome no matter the histologic grade or genetic status. IDH-mutant, 1p/19q codeleted OGs are chemosensitive; combined radio- and chemotherapy is standard treatment.

Imaging

General Features. OGs are seen as round or oval, relatively sharply delineated masses that involve the cortex and subcortical white matter.

CT Findings. OGs are most often peripheral and cortically based. Focal gyral expansion with thinning and remodeling of the overlying calvaria is common. Almost two-thirds are hypodense on NECT scan **(18-5A)**, while one-third exhibit mixed density patterns.

Coarse nodular or clumped calcification is seen in 70-90% of cases. Gyriform Ca++ is very suggestive. Cystic degeneration occurs in 20%. Gross hemorrhage and peritumoral edema are less common and do not indicate malignant degeneration.

Enhancement varies from none to moderate; approximately 50% of OGs demonstrate some degree of enhancement. A patchy multifocal pattern is typical.

MR Findings. OGs often appear relatively well delineated and are usually hypointense relative to gray matter on T1WI. They are typically heterogeneously hyperintense on T2/FLAIR **(18-5B) (18-5C)**. Vasogenic edema is uncommon. Calcification is seen as "blooming" foci on T2* sequences.

Many OGs do not enhance on T1 C+ **(18-5D)**. Moderate heterogeneous enhancement is seen in approximately half of all cases. OGs do not restrict on DWI.

MRS shows moderately elevated Cho and decreased NAA with an elevated 2-HG peak resonating at 2.25 ppm.

Perfusion MR is often used to predict the type and WHO grade of brain neoplasms. Low-grade OGs are more highly vascular and metabolically active than astrocytomas of comparable grade. OGs may display high relative cerebral blood volume (rCBV) foci that reflect the prominent "chicken wire" vascularity characteristic of IDH-mutated,1p/19q-codeleted OGs. Therefore, *an elevated rCBV in an OG does not necessarily indicate high-grade histopathology!*

Differential Diagnosis

The major differential diagnosis of OG is **diffuse astrocytoma**. Although the two may be indistinguishable, diffusely infiltrating astrocytomas more commonly involve the white matter—less often the cortex—and do not enhance.

Differentiation of a WHO grade II OG from **anaplastic oligodendroglioma** (AO) may be difficult on the basis of imaging alone. Hemorrhage and necrosis are more common in AO than OG but are not definitive.

Other cortically based, slow-growing tumors that typically present with seizures include **ganglioglioma** and **dysembryoplastic neuroepithelial tumor (DNET)**. Both are more common in children and young adults. Gangliogliomas are more common in the temporal lobe with a "cyst + nodule" appearance. DNETs are typically "bubbly" and may have associated cortical dysplasia.

Central neurocytoma is indistinguishable from OG on light microscopy and requires immunohistochemical stains (e.g.,

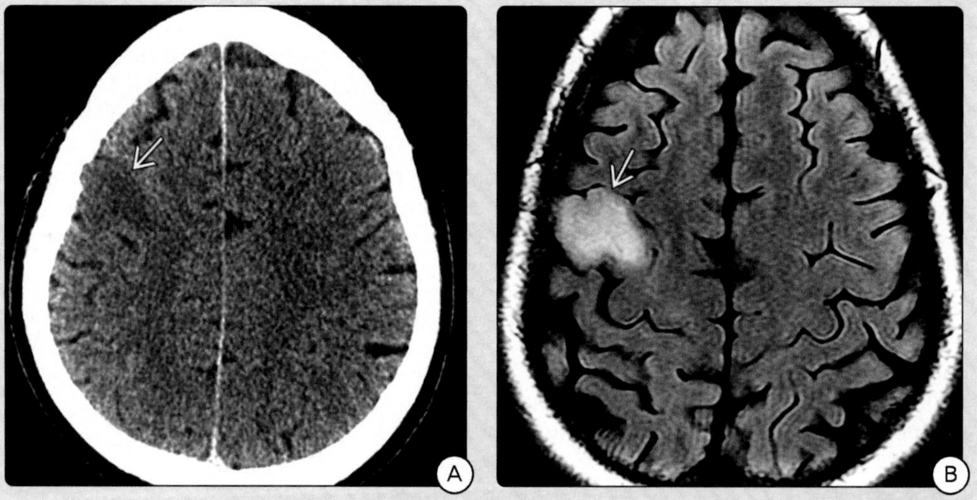

***(18-5A)** NECT in a 31y woman with a first-time seizure shows a wedge-shaped hypodensity ➡ in the right posterior frontal lobe. **(18-5B)** Axial FLAIR in the same case shows that the mass is hyperintense ➡ and involves the cortex, infiltrating the underlying white matter and expanding the overlying gyrus.*

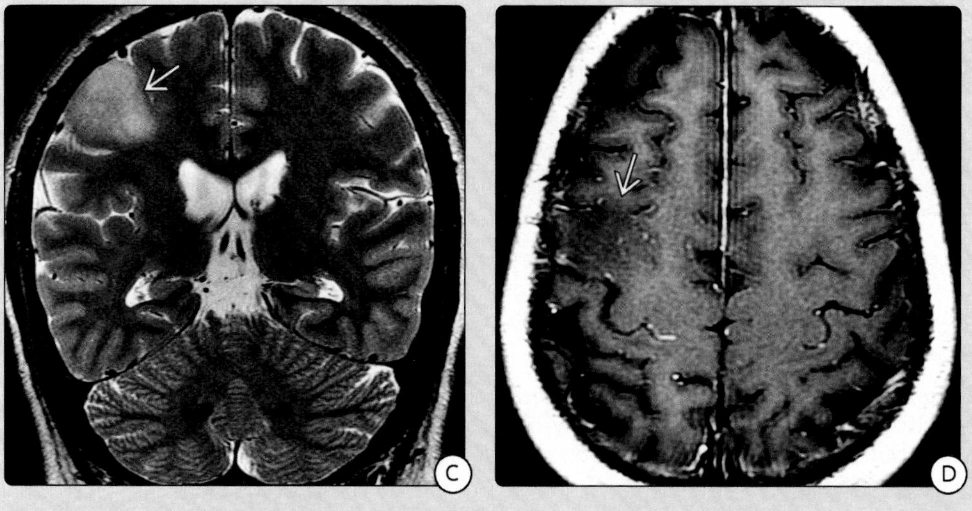

***(18-5C)** Coronal T2WI shows that the heterogeneously hyperintense mass ➡ extends to the cortical surface and deep into the subcortical white matter. **(18-5D)** T1 C+ MR shows that the mass ➡ is hypointense and does not enhance. WHO grade II oligodendroglioma, IDH-mutant 1p/19q codeleted was found at histopathology.*

synaptophysin) for diagnosis. Most central neurocytomas are intraventricular, whereas OGs are lobar, typically cortically based masses.

Extraventricular neurocytoma is a very rare, cortically based variant that does not necessarily exhibit the "bubbly" pattern so typical of its intraventricular counterpart; it may be indistinguishable from an OG on imaging.

OLIGODENDROGLIOMA

Pathology
- Molecular genetics
  - "Canonical" OGs IDH-mutated, 1p/19q codeletion
- General features
  - 85-90% in cerebral hemispheres (most common = frontal lobes)
  - Arise at gray-white matter junction
  - Diffusely infiltrate cortex
  - Poorly circumscribed
- Microscopic features
  - "Fried egg" cells with "chicken-wire" vascularity
  - WHO grade II

Clinical Issues
- Epidemiology
  - Third most common primary brain tumor (2-5%)
  - Mostly middle-aged adults (rare in children)
- Common presentation = seizures, headache
- Grow slowly; survival 10-12 years

Imaging
- Relatively well delineated
- Ca++ 70%; hemorrhage, edema uncommon
- 50% enhance

Anaplastic Oligodendroglioma, IDH-Mutant and 1p/19q Codeleted

Terminology

An IDH-mutant and 1p/19q codeleted OG with focal or diffuse histologic features of anaplasia is designated as anaplastic oligodendroglioma (AO).

Etiology

AOs can develop either de novo or arise from progression of a preexisting WHO grade II OG. Mean time to progression from a WHO II OG to WHO grade III AO is approximately 6-7 years.

AOs have the same basic immunoprofile as WHO grade II OGs. In addition to the IDH mutations, 1p/19q codeletion, and *TERT* promoter mutations, AOs usually have additional subsequent genetic alterations. 9p LOH and polysomies are common, whereas *EGFR* amplification is absent.

Pathology

Location. AOs demonstrate the same preference for the frontal lobe as do OGs. The temporal lobe is the second most common site.

Gross Pathology. Other than the presence of necrotic foci, the macroscopic features of AO are similar to those of grade II OGs **(18-7)**.

Microscopic Features. Focal or diffuse features of malignancy are present. AOs have higher cell density with more nuclear pleomorphism and

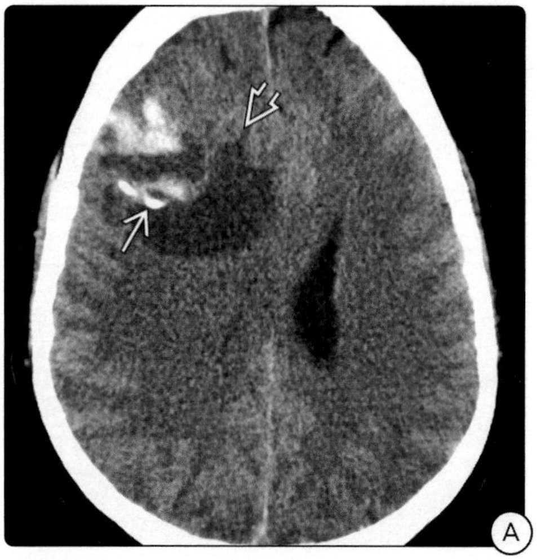

***(18-6A)** NECT in a 39y man with headache shows a mixed-density right frontal mass ➡ with prominent calcifications ➡.*

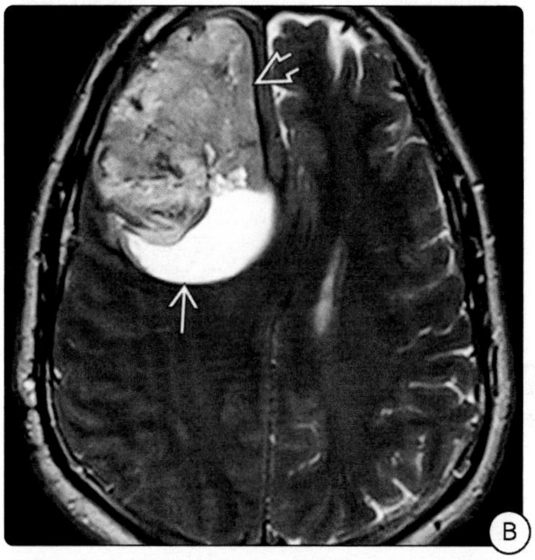

***(18-6B)** T2WI shows bright fluid in cystic portion ➡, heterogeneous SI in solid part of mass ➡. Mass extends to cortical surface of frontal lobe.*

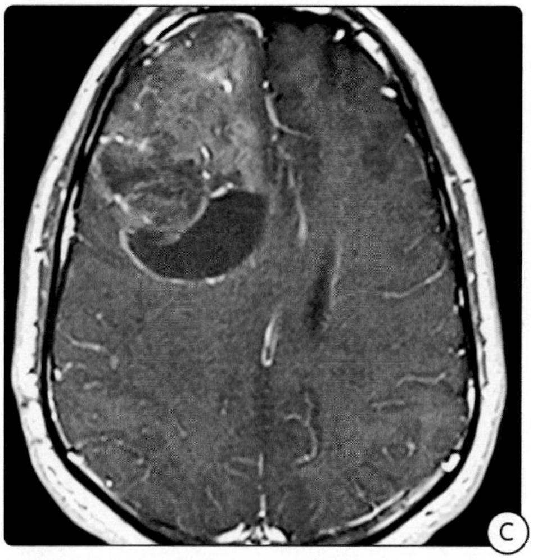

***(18-6C)** T1 C+ enhances in solid tumor, with rim enhancement around cyst; this is anaplastic OG, WHO grade III, IDH-mutant 1p/19q codeleted.*

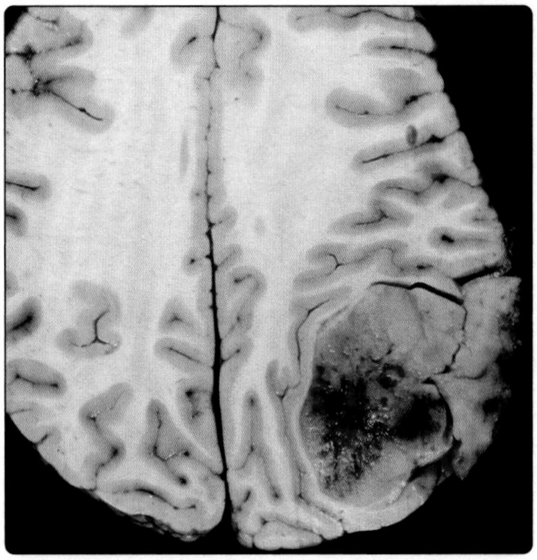

(18-7) Gross pathology of AO involves cortex and subcortical WM. Areas of hemorrhagic necrosis are present. (Courtesy R. Hewlett, MD.)

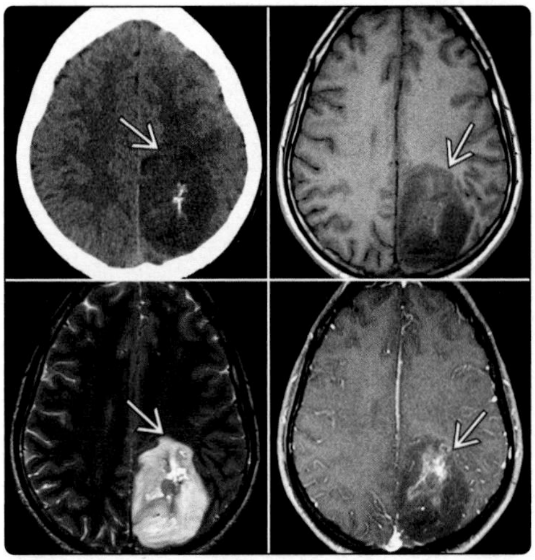

(18-8) Imaging in a 37y man shows relatively well-demarcated left parietal mass ➡. This is WHO grade II oligodendroglioma.

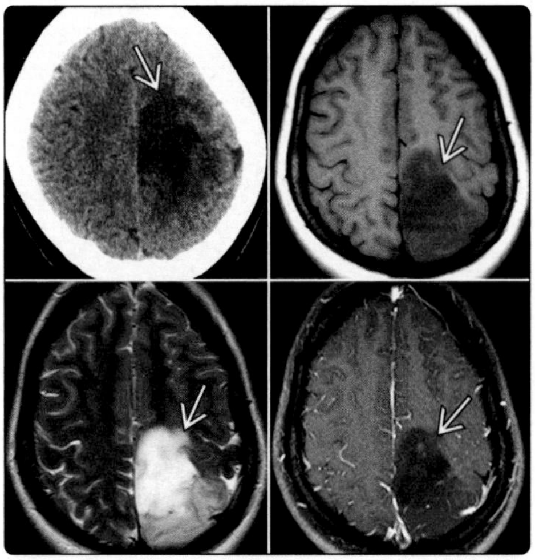

(18-9) Imaging in a 24y woman shows a mass ➡ that looks like the oligodendroglioma in Figure 18-8. This is AO, WHO grade III.

hyperchromatism than OGs. Cystic degeneration and necrosis with or without pseudopalisading are common. Microvascular proliferation is common and sometimes florid.

Proliferative activity is higher than with OGs, usually > 5%. Although there is no accepted cut-off value for distinguishing AO from OG, labeling indices in the 7-10% or higher range are typical.

Staging, Grading, and Classification. AOs are WHO grade III tumors.

Clinical Issues

Epidemiology. Between 25-35% of all oligodendroglial tumors are anaplastic. AOs account for 1-2% of all primary brain tumors.

Presentation. Patients with AOs are approximately 6 years older than patients with OGs and are very rare in children. Mean age at presentation is 50 years. Clinical symptoms are indistinguishable from those of OG, with seizure and headache the most common presentations.

Natural History. Survival time varies from a few months to as much as a decade. Mean survival is 4 years with an overall 5-year and 10-year survival rate of 52% and 40%, respectively. Surgical resection followed by upfront combined radiotherapy and chemotherapy has improved overall survival.

Imaging

The general imaging features of AO are very similar to those of OG and do not reliably predict tumor grade **(18-8)** **(18-9)**. Peritumoral edema, hemorrhage, and foci of cystic degeneration are more common. Enhancement is variable, ranging from none to striking **(18-6)**.

As OGs are often quite vascular, rCBV may be misleading. MRS is more helpful, with a Cho:Cr ratio greater than 2.33 suggestive of AO.

Differential Diagnosis

The major differential diagnosis of AO is **oligodendroglioma**. Tumor contrast enhancement is not helpful in distinguishing AO from low-grade OG. **Anaplastic astrocytoma** or even **glioblastoma** may also be difficult to differentiate from AO on the basis of imaging findings alone.

ANAPLASTIC OLIGODENDROGLIOMA

Genetics, Pathology
- IDH-mutated and 10/19q codeleted
- Necrosis, microvascular proliferation
- Increased mitoses (Ki-67 greater than 5%)
- WHO grade III

Imaging
- Can be indistinguishable from OG
- Generally more heterogeneous, enhancement

Oligodendroglioma Lacking IDH Mutation and 1p/19q Codeletion

A small subset of histologically classic OGs and AOs lack IDH mutation and 1p/19q codeletion on molecular testing, suggesting that they represent a different disease. These include the majority of "oligodendroglial-like" neoplasms in children and adolescents, which are biologically as well as genetically distinct from their adult counterparts.

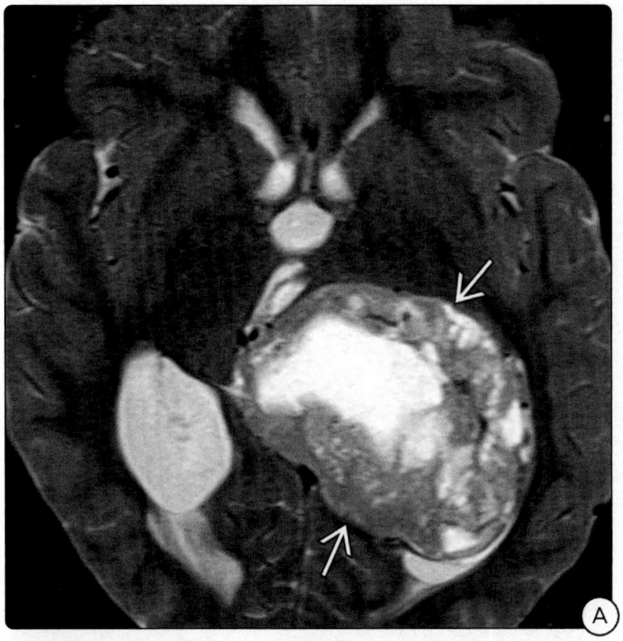

(18-10A) ***Axial T2 FS MR in an 8y boy shows a large, heterogeneously hyperintense mass ➡ in the left thalamus that is causing obstructive hydrocephalus. The mass appears relatively well demarcated, with little surrounding edema.***

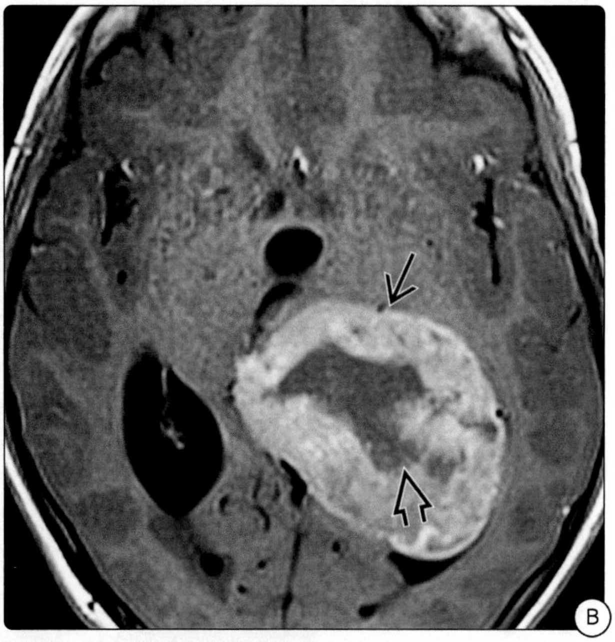

(18-10B) ***T1 C+ MR shows a thick rind of enhancing tumor ➡, central necrotic core ➡. This is AO, WHO III, 1p19q nondeleted. Nuclear Olig-2 and ATRX were positive, but IDH, H3.3, and p53 negative; MIB-1 was 10%. (Courtesy M. Warmuth-Metz, MD.)***

Some pediatric OGs carry the oncogenic *BRAF* fusion genes, similar to many pilocytic astrocytomas and other low-grade gliomas, including the disseminated OG-like leptomeningeal neoplasms. Degeneration of OGs into AO is less common than in adults.

OGs that lack IDH mutation and 1p/19q codeletion appear similar to canonical OGs on histopathology. IDH-1-negative AOs with nondeleted 1p/19q have a poor prognosis and may resemble GBM on imaging studies **(18-10)**.

Oligoastrocytoma

Oligoastrocytoma (OA) is a tumor with two morphologically distinct admixed neoplastic cell types. The mixed or ambiguous cellular differentiation in such tumors precludes designation as either diffuse astrocytoma or OG.

In the 2016 WHO, the diagnosis of OA is discouraged. Most neoplasms with histologic features suggesting both an astrocytic and an oligodendroglial component can be definitively classified as either astrocytoma **or** OG using molecular testing.

Tumors with combined IDH mutation and 1p/19q codeletion are classified as IDH-mutant and 1p/19q OG, irrespective of a mixed or ambiguous histology. Tumors with IDH mutation that lack 1p/19q codeletion are classified as IDH-mutant diffuse astrocytoma, also irrespective of mixed or ambiguous histology. Loss of *ATRX* nuclear expression also supports the diagnosis of IDH-mutant astrocytoma. *TP53* mutation is mutually exclusive with 1p/19q codeletion and also helps support the diagnosis.

Ependymal Tumors

Ependymal tumors are a heterogeneous group of neoplasms that can arise anywhere in the neuraxis. The genetics of ependymal tumors is still being delineated, and the molecular alterations that lead to ependymoma oncogenesis have not been completely elucidated. Recent evidence suggests that ependymomas have localization as well as grade-specific expression signatures, possibly related to different stem cell radial glia in all three craniospinal compartments.

Despite histopathologic similarities among ependymomas at different anatomical sites, its molecular biology is heterogeneous. *Supratentorial and posterior fossa ependymomas are distinct diseases*, with distinct genetic, transcriptional, and epigenetic alterations.

Using DNA methylome profiling, some neuropathologists have devised a molecular classification that results in nine ependymoma subgroups, three in each anatomical compartment of the CNS (spine, posterior fossa, and supratentorial). Stem cells isolated from ependymomas also have distinct populations that are unique to specific anatomic sites, which explains the predominant locations of different tumor types in different age groups **(18-11)**.

To date, a prognostic and reproducible classification of ependymomas has not been established. In this text, we use the 2016 WHO classification, which is still primarily organized by histopathology but also recognizes one new genetically defined ependymoma subtype, *RELA* fusion-positive ependymoma.

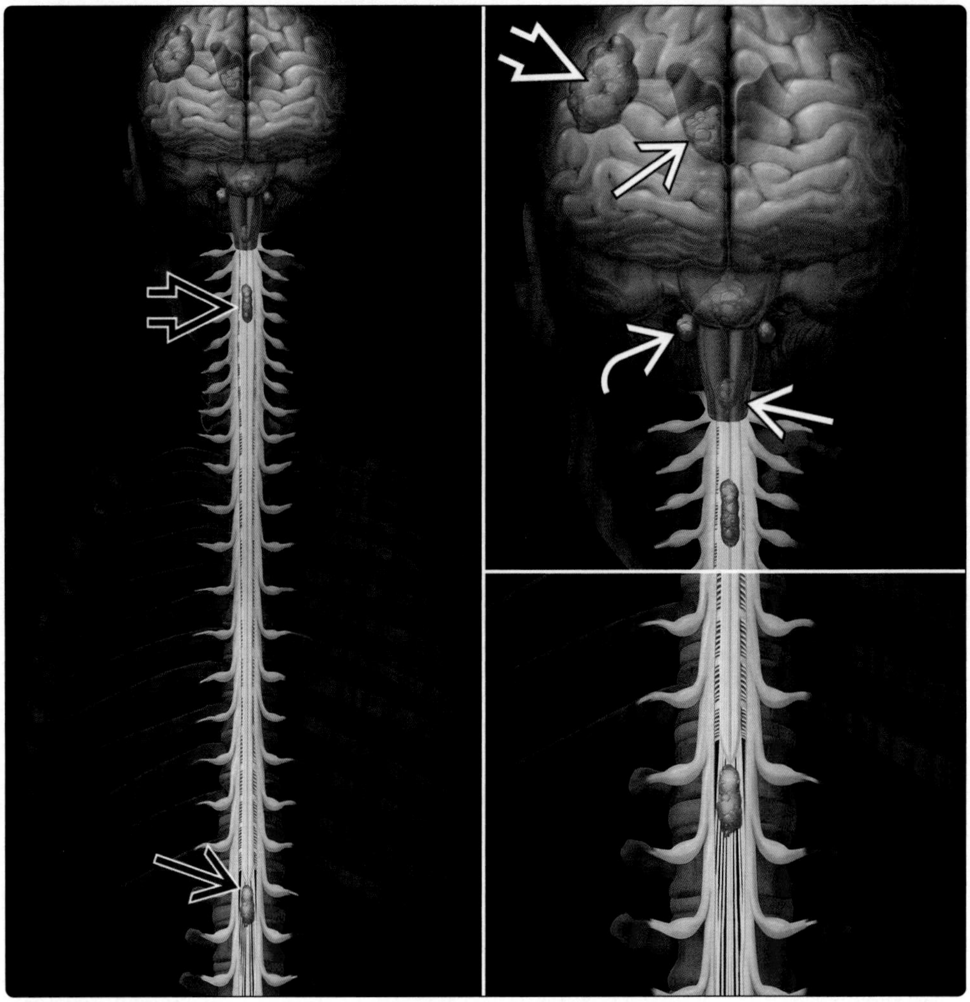

(18-11) Graphic shows ependymoma subtype and correlation with geographic localization. Subependymomas are found in the frontal horn of the lateral ventricle (ST-SE) and obex (PF-SE) ➡. Supratentorial EPNs ➡ are most often RELA- or YAP-fusion tumors. Posterior fossa ependymomas ➡ are PF-EPN-A or B. Spinal ependymomas can be myxopapillary ➡ (SP-MPE), which occur almost exclusively in the conus/filum terminale, or cellular/anaplastic ependymomas ➡ (SP-EPN), which occur in the central canal of the spinal cord and are intramedullary neoplasms.

The WHO classifies tumors that exhibit ependymal differentiation into five distinct tumor types: subependymoma (SE), myxopapillary ependymoma, ependymoma, *RELA* fusion-positive ependymoma, and anaplastic ependymoma.

We discuss all these tumors in this section, starting with the most common subtype, **ependymoma**. We follow with a consideration of **anaplastic ependymoma** and **RELA fusion-positive ependymoma**. The fourth histopathologic subtype that occurs in the brain is **SE**. Finally, although it is almost exclusively an intraspinal tumor, we also briefly consider **myxopapillary ependymoma**.

Ependymoma

Posterior fossa (PF) ependymomas can be either SEs (see below) or "classic" ependymomas. Two PF ependymoma groups can be distinguished and are designated **PF-EPN-A** and **PF-EPN-B**. Although they appear similar at gross pathology and on imaging studies, they differ in both age and biologic behavior.

Pathology

Location. Approximately 60% of ependymomas are *infratentorial*. Of these, 95% are found in the fourth ventricle. The remainder occur as cerebellopontine angle (CPA) lesions.

Between 30-40% of ependymomas are *supratentorial*. In 60% of cases, they arise from the lateral or third ventricles. In 40% of cases, they arise in the cerebral hemispheres without a visible connection to the ventricular system.

Approximately 10% of ependymomas occur in the *spine*. Spinal ependymomas differ genetically from their intracranial counterparts and have a more favorable prognosis.

Size and Number. Ependymomas are solitary neoplasms. Size varies, but most supratentorial ependymomas are large bulky neoplasms that exceed 4 cm in diameter at presentation.

Gross Pathology. Posterior fossa ependymomas are reddish-tan or gray in color and form relatively well-demarcated, lobulated masses. PF-EPNs have a "plastic" appearance, extruding through the foramina of Luschka and Magendie to fill the cisterns and encase cranial nerves and blood vessels **(18-12) (18-13) (18-14)**.

Calcification, cyst formation, and hemorrhage are common.

Microscopic Features. The most characteristic microarchitectural feature of ependymoma is the presence of perivascular pseudorosettes, in which tumor cells are arranged radially around blood vessels.

Neuropathologists recognize three ependymoma variants (papillary, clear cell, and tancytic), but these lack clinicopathologic significance.

Typical ependymoma vasculature is relatively mature and shows little angiogenic activity compared with malignant gliomas or the anaplastic variant of ependymoma.

Staging, Grading, and Classification. Ependymomas are designated as WHO grade II neoplasms. However, the utility of histologic grading of ependymoma for treatment stratification is controversial, as there is no consistent association of tumor grade with patient outcome.

Clinical Issues

Epidemiology. Ependymomas represent 3-9% of all gliomas. Ependymoma accounts for approximately 10% of CNS neoplasms in children and 30% of all brain tumors in children under the age of 3 years. Ependymoma is the third most common posterior fossa tumor of childhood (after medulloblastoma and astrocytoma).

Demographics. PF-EPN-A ependymomas are almost exclusively found in young children (median age = 3 years), and male patients predominate, nearly 2:1. Patients in the PF-EPN-B subgroup are mostly adolescents and young adults (median age = 30 years) with a slight female predominance.

Presentation. Symptoms are location dependent. Fourth ventricle ependymomas commonly cause intraventricular obstructive hydrocephalus and present with headache, vomiting, and papilledema. Ataxia is common. Supratentorial

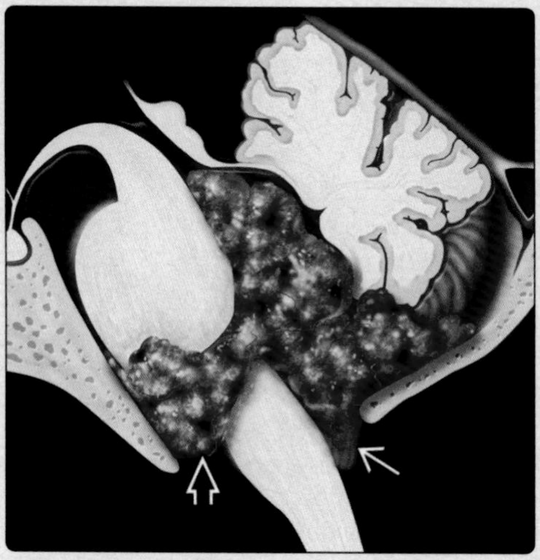

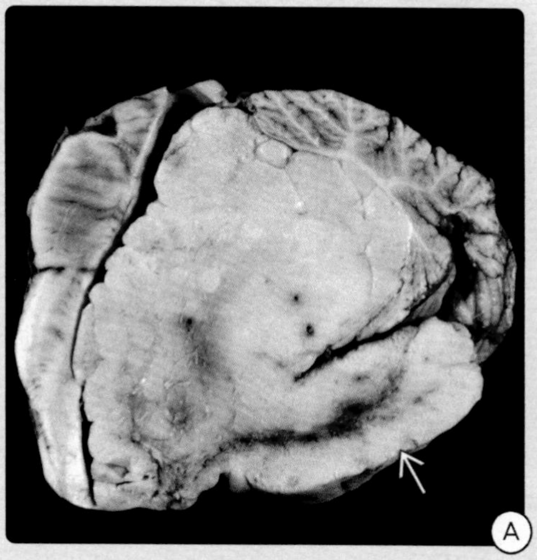

(18-12) Graphic depicts "classic" cellular ependymoma of the fourth ventricle extending through the foramen of Magendie into the cisterna magna ➡, around the pons under the brachium pontis, and through the lateral recesses into the cerebellopontine angle cisterns ➡. (18-13A) Sagittal autopsy case shows ependymoma filling the fourth ventricle, elevating the vermis, extending posteroinferiorly to fill the cisterna magna ➡.

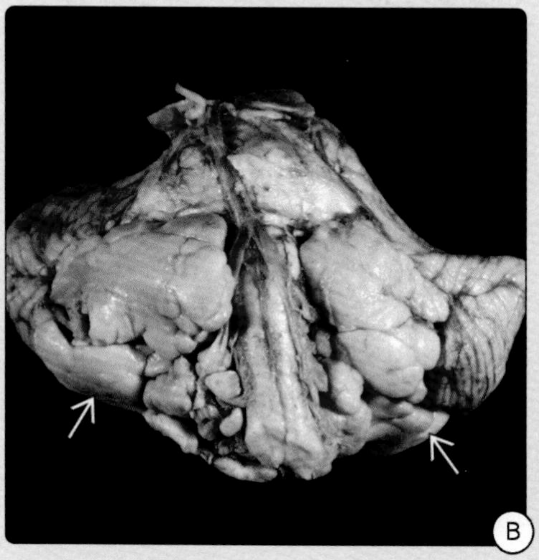

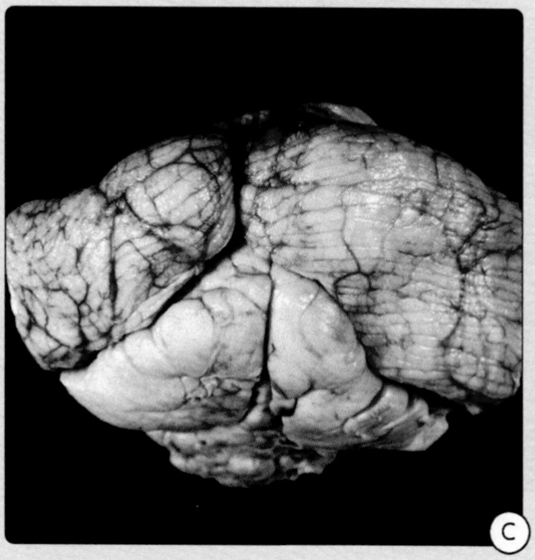

(18-13B) Coronal view in the same case shows massive tumor extension through both foramina of Luschka into the cerebellopontine angle cisterns ➡. (18-13C) Posterior view shows tumor bulging through the foramen of Magendie, completely filling the cisterna magna. Posterior fossa ependymomas squeeze out the foramina of the fourth ventricle, oozing like toothpaste into the surrounding CSF spaces. (Courtesy E. Ross, MD.)

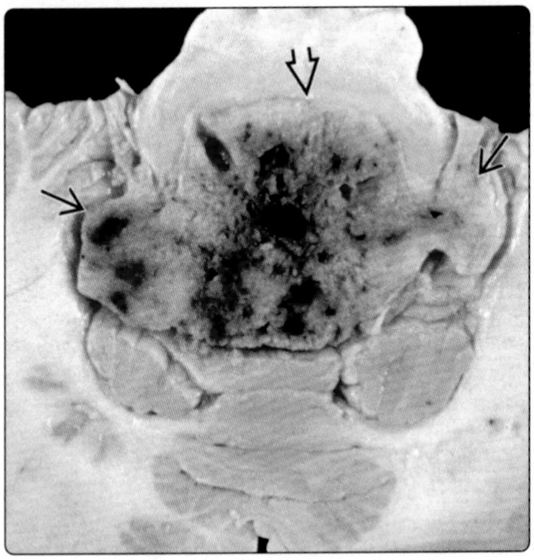

(18-14) Ependymoma fills 4th ventricle, extends through lateral recesses to foramina of Luschka. (Courtesy E. Ross, MD.)

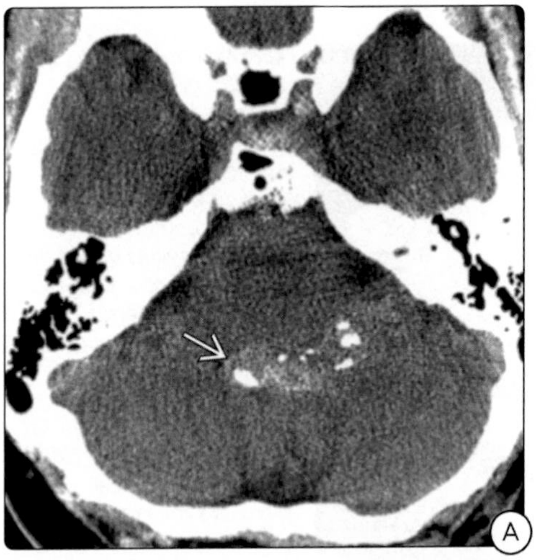

(18-15A) Axial NECT scan shows partially calcified mass in inferior 4th ventricle.

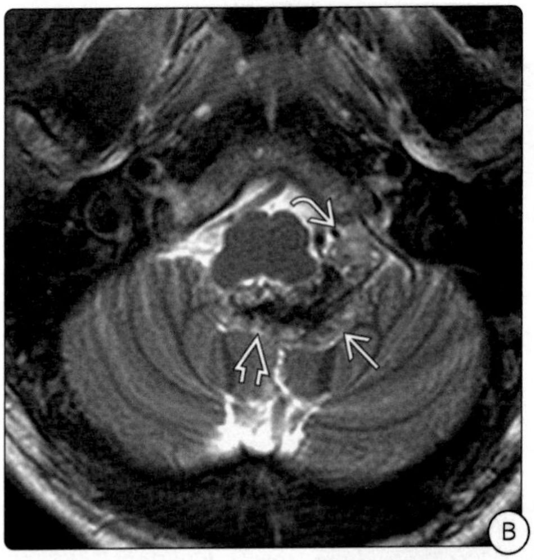

(18-15B) T2WI shows "plastic" nature of the mass extruding through the lateral recess into the adjacent CPA. This is ependymoma.

parenchymal ependymomas present with seizures and focal neurologic deficits.

Natural History. Patients with ependymoma exhibit a wide range of clinical outcomes. Overall 5-year survival for the PF-EPN-A subgroup is approximately 50%, whereas it is 85-90% for the PF-EPN-B group.

Correlation between tumor grade and outcome is controversial, but the overall survival rate of patients with WHO grade II ependymoma is slightly better than that of patients with anaplastic ependymoma.

Treatment Options. Maximum cytoreduction surgery followed by conformal radiotherapy—not cranial spinal irradiation—is the standard treatment. Adjuvant therapy is generally reserved for recurrent tumor.

EPENDYMOMA

Location
- 60-70% posterior fossa
- 30-40% supratentorial

Pathology
- From fourth ventricle → cisterna magna, CPA
- WHO grade II

Clinical Issues
- 10% of childhood brain tumors
- PF-EPN-A
  - Median age = 3 years, M:F = 2:1
  - Ataxia, hydrocephalus
  - 5-year survival 50%
- PF-EPN-B
  - Older children, adults (median age = 30 years)
  - 5-year survival 85-90%

Imaging

General Features. *Infratentorial* ependymomas are relatively well-delineated "plastic" tumors that typically arise from the floor of the fourth ventricle and extrude through the outlet foramina. They extend laterally through the foramina of Luschka toward the CPA cistern **(18-15)** and posteroinferiorly through the foramen of Magendie into the cisterna magna.

Sagittal images disclose a mass that fills most of the fourth ventricle and extrudes inferiorly into the cisterna magna **(18-16A)**. Axial and coronal images show lateral extension toward or into the CPA cisterns **(18-16B)** **(18-16C)**.

Obstructive hydrocephalus is a frequent accompanying feature of infratentorial ependymoma. Extracellular fluid often accumulates around the ventricles, giving the appearance of "blurred" margins.

CSF dissemination is a key factor in staging, prognosis, and treatment of ependymoma. The only statistically significant preoperative imaging predictor of patient outcome is evidence of tumor spread. Therefore, *preoperative imaging of the entire cranial-spinal axis should be performed in any child with a posterior fossa neoplasm*, especially if medulloblastoma or ependymoma is suspected.

Supratentorial ependymomas are generally large, bulky, aggressive-looking hemispheric tumors. Gross cyst formation, calcification, and hemorrhage are more common compared with their infratentorial counterparts.

CT Findings. Ependymomas are generally mixed density on NECT scans with hypodense intratumoral cysts intermixed with iso- and hyperdense soft tissue portions. Coarse calcification occurs in approximately half of all ependymomas. Macroscopic hemorrhage can be identified in approximately 10% of cases.

Most ependymomas show mild to moderate heterogeneous enhancement.

MR Findings. Ependymomas are generally heterogeneously hypointense relative to brain parenchyma on T1WI and hyperintense on T2/FLAIR **(18-17)**. Following contrast administration, most ependymomas enhance. Areas of strong, relatively homogeneous enhancement are intermixed with foci of minimal or no enhancement.

T2* imaging (GRE, SWI) commonly demonstrates "blooming" foci that can be caused by calcification and/or old hemorrhage. An ependymoma may bleed, causing nonaneurysmal subarachnoid hemorrhage and siderosis around the tumor and along the pial surfaces of the cerebellum.

Most ependymomas do not restrict on DWI although foci of restricted diffusion can be identified in some cases.

General MRS metabolite ratios are nonspecific. Elevated choline and reduced NAA are common in ependymoma, as in many other brain tumors. Perfusion MR generally demonstrates markedly elevated cerebral blood volume with poor return to baseline.

EPENDYMOMA: IMAGING

Infratentorial Ependymoma
- Fills fourth ventricle
- Extends into CPA, cisterna magna
- Obstructive hydrocephalus
- Cysts, Ca++ (50%), hemorrhage (10%) on NECT
- Mixed signal intensity, strong enhancement on MR
- "Blooming" foci on T2* common
- Usually does not restrict on DWI

Supratentorial Ependymoma
- Most are *RELA* fusion-positive ependymoma
- Usually large, bulky, aggressive-looking
    - Gross cysts, Ca++, hemorrhage common
- Poor prognosis

Differential Diagnosis

Differential diagnosis of ependymoma is location dependent.

The major differential diagnosis of *infratentorial* ependymoma is **medulloblastoma.** Medulloblastomas are more common and typically arise from the roof of the fourth ventricle (not from the floor, as is typical of ependymoma). Medulloblastomas are hyperdense on NECT, often demonstrate diffusion restriction, and more frequently show evidence of CSF dissemination at the time of initial diagnosis. Cysts, hemorrhage, and calcification are less common in medulloblastoma compared with ependymoma.

Pilocytic astrocytoma is a common posterior fossa tumor in children and young adults but is more often found in the cerebellar hemispheres.

The major differential diagnosis of *supratentorial* ependymoma is **anaplastic astrocytoma** or **glioblastoma**. **Astroblastoma** is typically a tumor of older children and young adults that has a mixed solid-cystic "bubbly" appearance. In very young children, **primitive neuroectodermal tumor** and **atypical teratoid/rhabdoid tumor** can cause hemispheric masses that closely resemble parenchymal ependymoma.

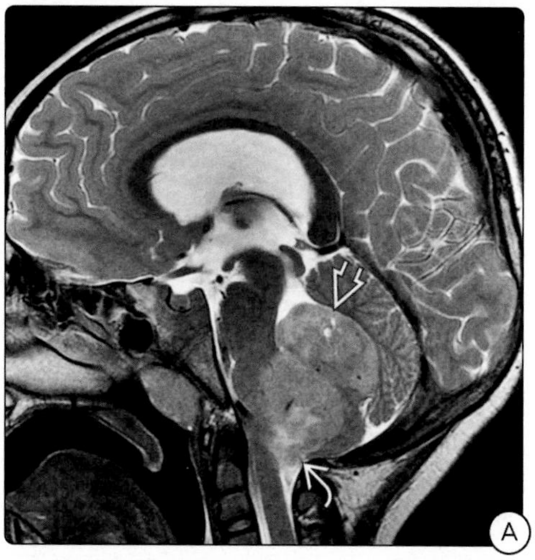

***(18-16A)** T2WI in a 3y girl with headache, vomiting shows a hyperintense 4th ventricle mass ⇨ extending through foramen of Magendie ➩.*

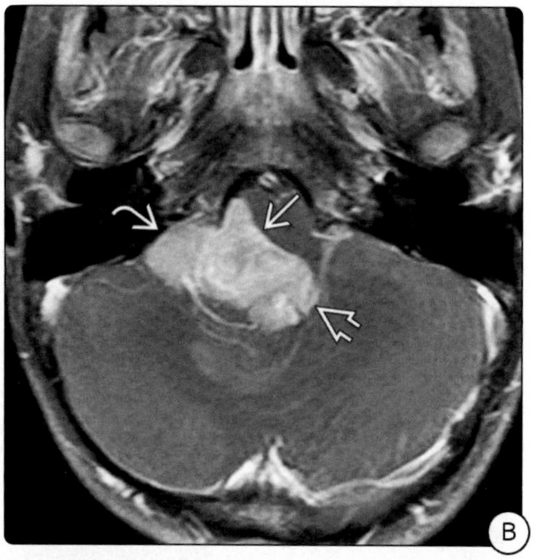

***(18-16B)** Axial T1 C+ FS shows that the intensely enhancing 4th ventricle mass ⇨ extends through the foramen of Luschka ⇨ into the CPA ➩.*

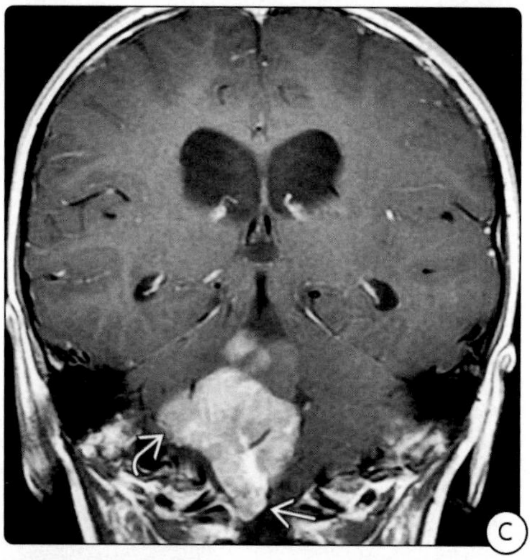

***(18-16C)** Coronal T1 C+ shows the extension into the CPA cistern ➩, cisterna magna ⇨. This is ependymoma (PF-EPN-A).*

Anaplastic Ependymoma

Anaplastic ependymoma is characterized by more rapid growth, vascular proliferation, increased cellularity, higher mitotic activity, and less favorable outcome compared with the typical cellular ependymoma. Anaplastic ependymomas are designated WHO grade III neoplasms. Although no association between grade and biologic behavior has been established, miRNA expression may predict overall and event-free survival.

Anaplastic ependymoma is a neuropathologic diagnosis, as imaging findings are indistinguishable from those of cellular ependymoma **(18-17)**.

Ependymoma, *RELA- and YAP1-* Fusion-Positive

Ependymoma, *RELA* fusion-positive is a new, genetically defined ependymoma subtype that has been recognized by the 2016 WHO. The tumor is a large, heterogeneous-appearing mass that occurs almost exclusively in the cerebral hemispheres **(18-18)** and accounts for nearly 70% of childhood supratentorial ependymomas (ST-EPN-RELA). A smaller subgroup with *YAP1* fusion **(18-19)** has been described but not yet officially recognized.

ST-EPN-RELA tumors have been assigned WHO grade II or III, depending on the degree of anaplasia.

ST-EPN-RELA median age at presentation is 8 years, but this tumor can also occur in adults. ST-EPN-YAP1 median age is 14 years. The 5-year survival for ST-EPN-RELA ependymoma is

(18-17A) FLAIR scan in a 3y boy shows a mixed signal intensity mass ➡ in the inferior fourth ventricle that extends anterolaterally through both foramina of Luschka into the cerebellopontine angle cisterns ➡. (18-17B) Sagittal T1 C+ scan in the same patient shows the heterogeneously enhancing fourth ventricle mass ➡ extruding posteroinferiorly through the foramen of Magendie into the cisterna magna ➡.

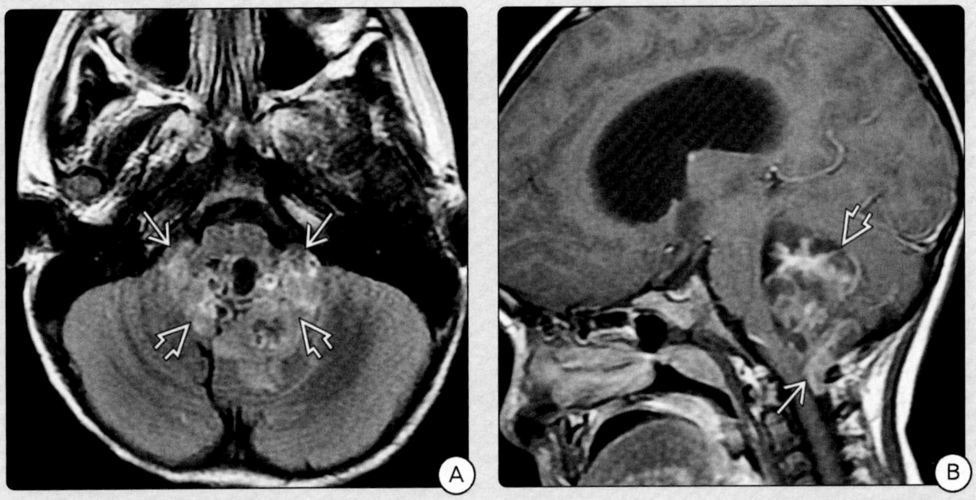

(18-17C) Axial T1 C+ FS scan in the same patient shows mixed cystic, solid enhancing tumor ➡ that expands, fills the fourth ventricle ➡. (18-17D) Coronal T1 C+ scan shows tumor extending inferiorly from the fourth ventricle into the cisterna magna ➡, laterally through the foramina of Luschka ➡. Note obstructive hydrocephalus ➡. Histopathology showed anaplastic ependymoma (WHO grade III), PF-EPN-A. The child survived 2 years.

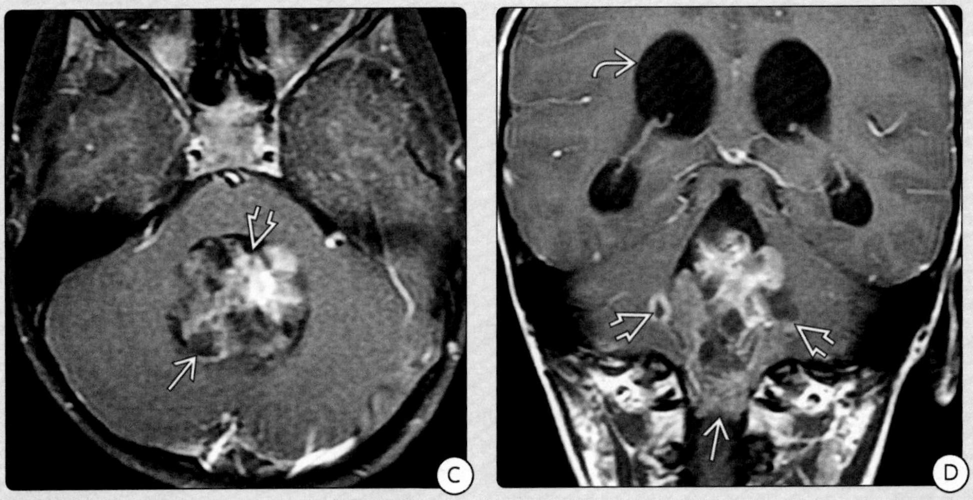

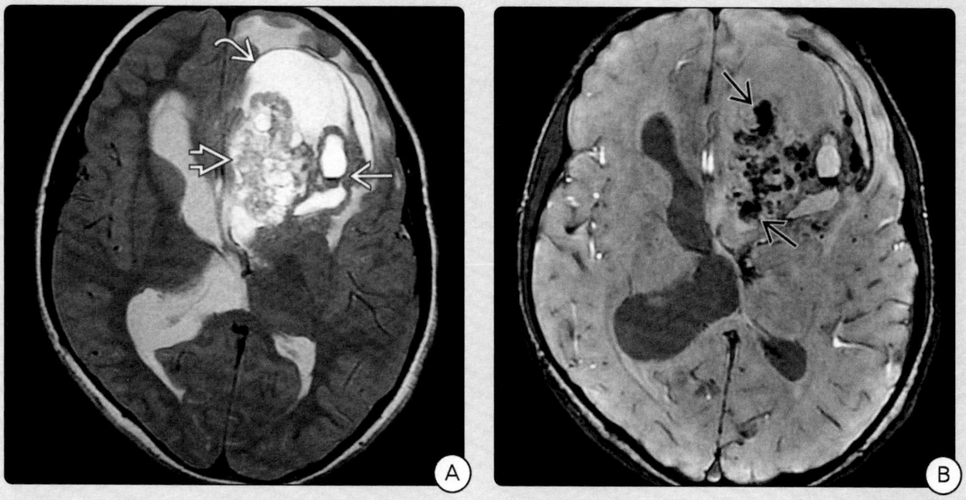

***(18-18A)** Axial T2WI in an 11y girl with 6 weeks of nausea and vomiting shows a large mixed cystic ➡ and solid ➡ mass occupying almost the entire left frontal lobe. Note hemorrhage with blood-fluid levels ➡ in several of the cysts. **(18-18B)** T2* SWI shows multiple hemorrhagic foci ➡ in the mass.*

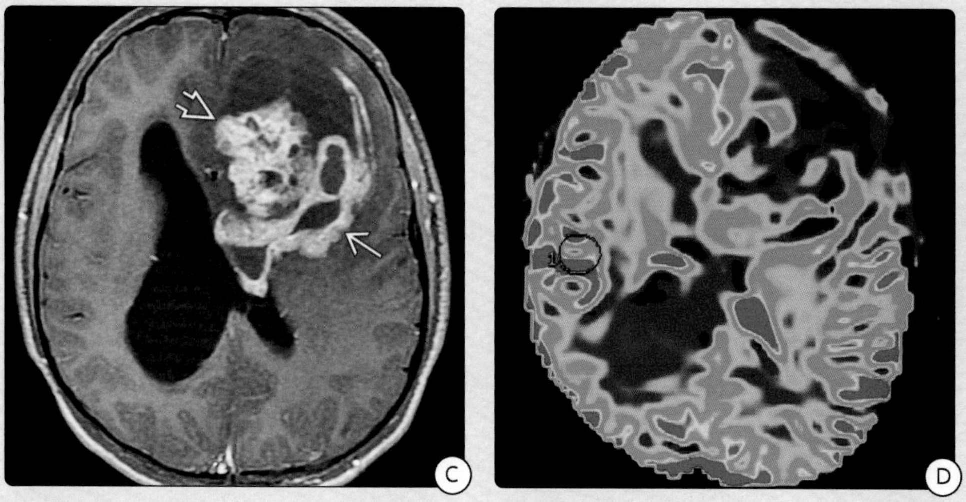

***(18-18C)** T1 C+ FS in the same case shows thick, irregular rinds of enhancing tumor ➡ around the cystic portions of the mass. The solid portion ➡ enhances heterogeneously. **(18-18D)** DSC dynamic perfusion MR shows low relative cerebral blood volume in the mass. Ependymoma, RELA fusion-positive was found at pathology.*

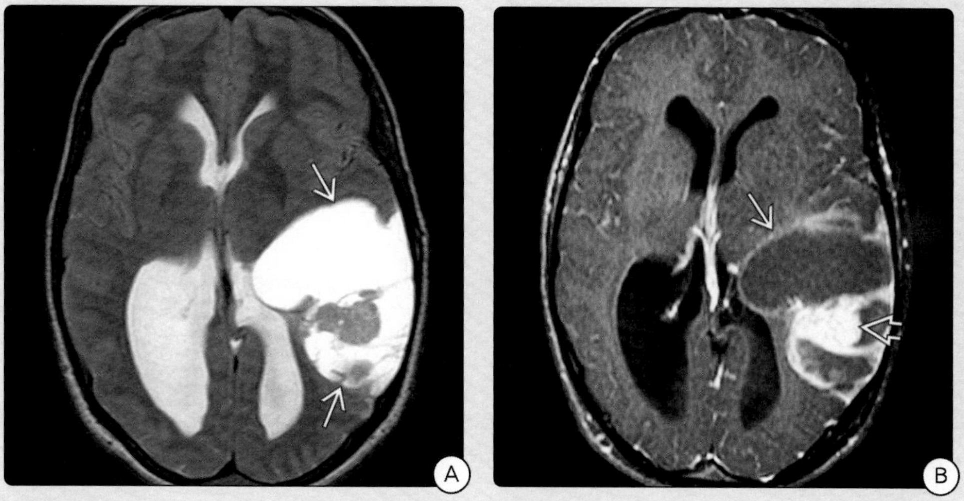

***(18-19A)** T2WI from MR initially obtained in 2004 in a 28y woman with a supratentorial ependymoma shows a large mass in the left hemisphere ➡. **(18-19B)** T1 C+ FS shows mixed solid ➡, cystic ➡ enhancement. Some supratentorial ependymomas have an excellent prognosis. Most are associated with YAP1 fusions.*

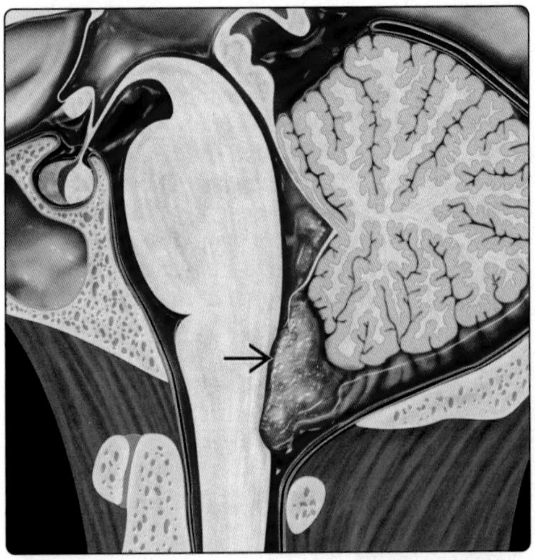

(18-20) Graphic depicts subependymoma of the inferior fourth ventricle ⇒ at the level of the obex.

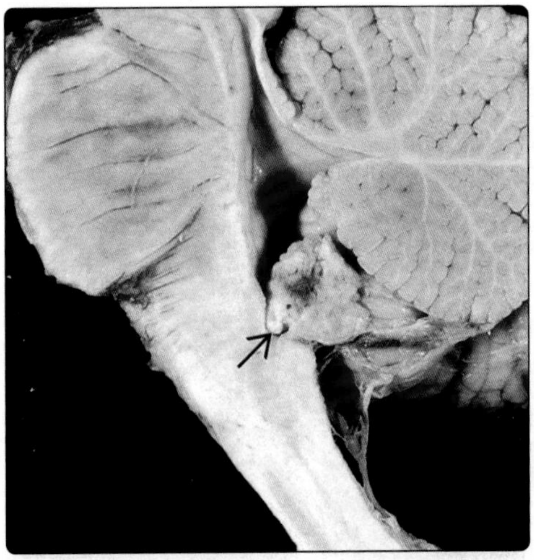

(18-21) Sagittal autopsy section shows incidental finding of a small fourth ventricle subependymoma ⇒. (Courtesy P. Burger, MD.)

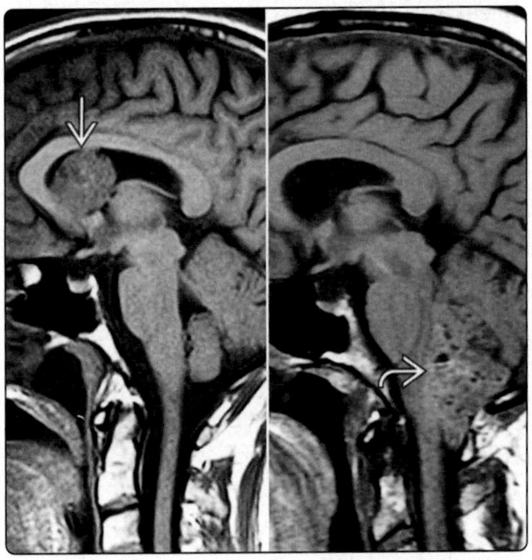

(18-22) Sagittal T1WIs show locations of subependymoma in the frontal horn of the lateral ventricle ➡ (L), obex of 4th ventricle ➡ (R).

50%. In a small reported group of ST-EPN-YAP1 ependymomas, all patients survived, and only one recurred.

Subependymoma

Terminology

Subependymomas (SEs) are rare, benign, slow-growing, noninvasive tumors that are often found incidentally at imaging or autopsy.

Etiology

The origin of SEs is unclear. They may arise from pluripotential ependymal-glial precursor cells, astrocytes in the subependymal plate, or a preexisting hamartomatous lesion. A specific mutation on the *TRPS1* gene may play a role in at least some cases.

Pathology

Location. SEs are usually located within or adjacent to an ependyma-lined space. Nearly half of all cases occur in the frontal horn of the lateral ventricle, near the foramen of Monro, where they are often attached to the septi pellucidi **(18-26)**. The fourth ventricle is the second most common site **(18-20) (18-21)** followed by the occipital horn of the lateral ventricle **(18-24)**. Parenchymal and intramedullary intraspinal SEs occur but are uncommon.

Size and Number. SEs are solitary tumors. Most are less than 2 cm, although some tumors may reach several centimeters in diameter. A few cases of very large biventricular SEs that fill both lateral ventricles have been reported. Because the posterior fossa is more anatomically constrained, infratentorial tumors are generally smaller than their supratentorial counterparts.

Gross Pathology. SEs are solid, round to somewhat lobulated, well-delineated, gray-tan masses. Calcification, cysts, and hemorrhage are common in larger lesions.

Microscopic Features. Bland nuclei in a dense fibrillary stroma with variable microcystic degeneration is typical. MIB-1 labeling is less than 1%.

Staging, Grading, and Classification. SEs are designated as WHO grade I neoplasms.

Clinical Issues

Epidemiology. SEs are found in 0.5-1.0% of autopsies and account for 8.0% of all ependymomas.

Demographics. SEs are tumors of middle-aged and older adults. They are very rare in children. As with other ependymomas, there is a moderate male predominance.

Presentation. The majority of SEs are asymptomatic and discovered incidentally. Approximately 40% cause symptoms, mostly related to CSF obstruction or mass effect.

Natural History. SEs exhibit an indolent growth pattern, expanding slowly into a ventricular space. Larger tumors may cause obstructive hydrocephalus, but they rarely invade adjacent brain. Recurrence is rare after gross total resection.

Treatment Options. "Watchful waiting" with serial imaging is appropriate in asymptomatic patients. Complete surgical resection of symptomatic SEs is the procedure of choice.

Imaging

General Features. SEs are well-demarcated nodular masses that may expand the ventricle but usually cause little mass effect. Large lesions may cause obstructive hydrocephalus.

CT Findings. SEs are iso- to slightly hypodense compared with brain on NECT scans. Calcification and intratumoral cysts may be present, especially in larger lesions. Hemorrhage is rare. Little or no enhancement is seen on CECT.

MR Findings. SEs are hypo- to isointense compared with brain on T1WI **(18-22)**. Intratumoral cysts are common in larger lesions. SEs are heterogeneously hyperintense on T2/FLAIR **(18-23)**. Peritumoral edema is usually absent. T2* (GRE, SWI) may show "blooming" foci, probably secondary to calcification. Hemorrhage is seen in 10-12%. Enhancement varies from none or mild to moderate **(18-27)**.

SEs do not restrict on DWI. MRS shows normal choline with mildly decreased NAA.

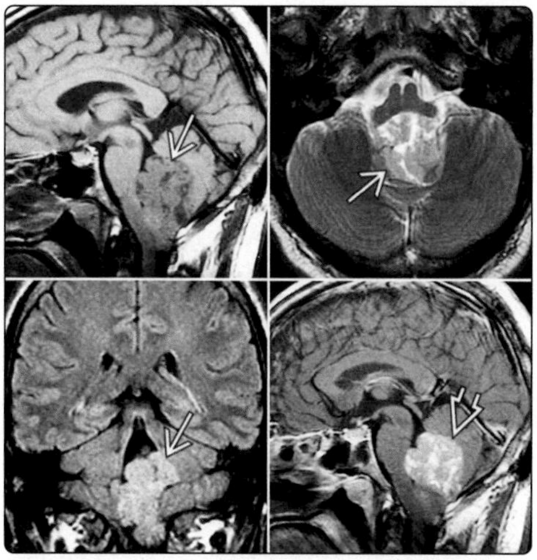

***(18-23)** Subependymoma MR has 4th ventricle mass ➡ w/ T1 iso-/hypointensity, T2/FLAIR hyperintensity, strong enhancement ➡.*

Differential Diagnosis

The differential diagnosis of SE varies with age and SE location. In older patients, the major differential is intraventricular **metastasis**. Most intraventricular metastases arise in the choroid plexus. In young to middle-aged adults, **central neurocytoma** should be considered. Central neurocytoma is typically found in the body of the lateral ventricle, not the frontal horn or inferior fourth ventricle, and has a characteristic "bubbly" appearance. **Choroid plexus papilloma** usually occupies the body, not the inferior fourth ventricle.

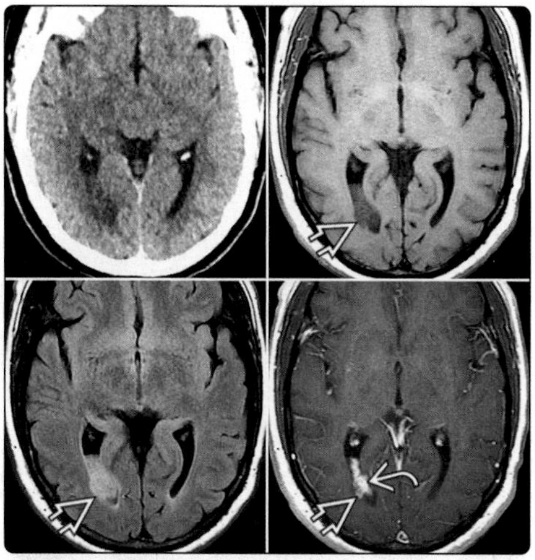

***(18-24)** Occipital horn subependymoma is shown. NECT, T1, FLAIR, and T1 C+ FS show enhancement ➡ and parenchymal invasion ➡.*

SUBEPENDYMOMA

Pathology
- Can be found in all three anatomic compartments
  - Posterior fossa (fourth ventricle) > supratentorial (frontal horn) > spine
  - WHO grade I

Clinical Issues
- Middle-aged, older adults
- Often asymptomatic, discovered incidentally

Imaging Features
- Often Ca++; hemorrhage rare
- Iso-/hypointense on T1WI, hyperintense on T2WI
- Variable enhancement

In children, **ependymoma** and (in patients with tuberous sclerosis) **subependymal giant cell astrocytoma** are considerations. **Choroid plexus papillomas** in children are usually in the atrium of the lateral ventricle. Choroid plexus papilloma also has a frond-like appearance and typically shows intense uniform enhancement.

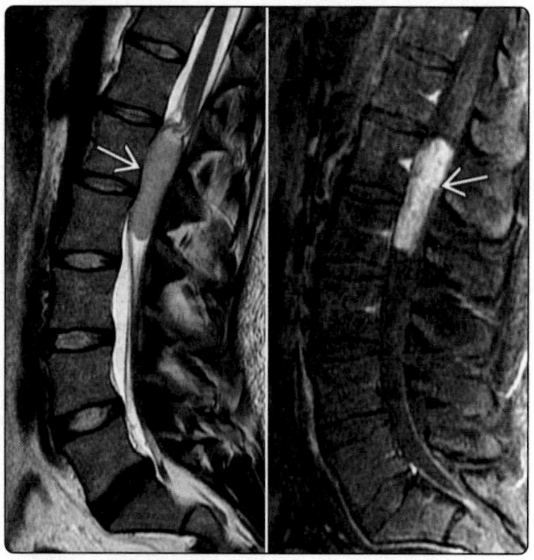

***(18-25)** Sagittal T2WI (L), T1 C+ FS (R) show classic myxopapillary ependymoma of the cauda equina ➡.*

Myxopapillary Ependymoma

Myxopapillary ependymoma (MPE) is a very slow-growing type of ependymoma that occurs mostly in young adults. It is almost exclusively a tumor of the conus medullaris, cauda equina, and filum terminale of the spinal cord **(18-25)**.

Myxopapillary ependymomas correspond to WHO grade I. In the typical myxopapillary ependymoma, elongated GFAP-positive cells are in a papillary arrangement around a fibrovascular core that contains both hyalinized blood vessels and myxoid degeneration. MIB-1 labeling index is low, generally less than 1%. No anaplastic variant of myxopapillary ependymoma is recognized.

Despite its benign histopathologic profile, 50% of MPEs in children have leptomeningeal disease at the time of initial diagnosis, so complete neuraxis imaging should be performed prior to surgery. Although disseminated tumor and/or recurrent or progressive disease after surgery are common, overall survival is excellent.

Primary intracranial myxopapillary ependymomas are exceptionally rare but have been reported in the ventricles and brain parenchyma. Imaging findings are nonspecific but generally those of a cyst with enhancing nodule.

Choroid Plexus Tumors

Choroid plexus epithelium shares a common embryologic origin with ependymal cells. Hence choroid plexus tumors are considered tumors of neuroepithelial tissue and comprise an important subgroup of the nonastrocytic gliomas.

Three histologic subtypes of choroid plexus neoplasms are recognized: choroid plexus papilloma (CPP), atypical choroid plexus papilloma (aCPP), and choroid plexus carcinoma (CPCa).

In addition to histopathology in the diagnosis of choroid plexus tumors, recent methylation profiling studies have revealed three clinically distinct molecular subgroups of choroid plexus tumors: pediatric low-risk choroid plexus tumors (cluster 1), adult low-risk choroid plexus tumors (cluster 2), and pediatric high-risk choroid plexus tumors (cluster 3). Cluster 1 (young age, mainly supratentorial

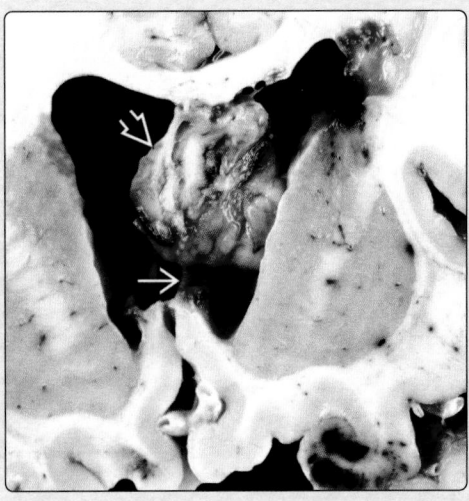

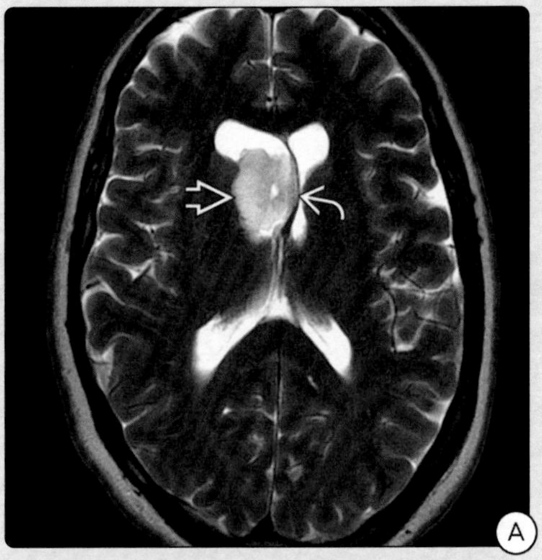

(18-26) Coronal gross pathology shows well-delineated frontal horn mass ➔ attached to the septum pellucidum ➔. This is subependymoma (ST-SE). (18-27A) Axial T2WI shows a well-demarcated hyperintense frontal horn mass ➔ that seems to be attached to the septum pellucidum ➔.

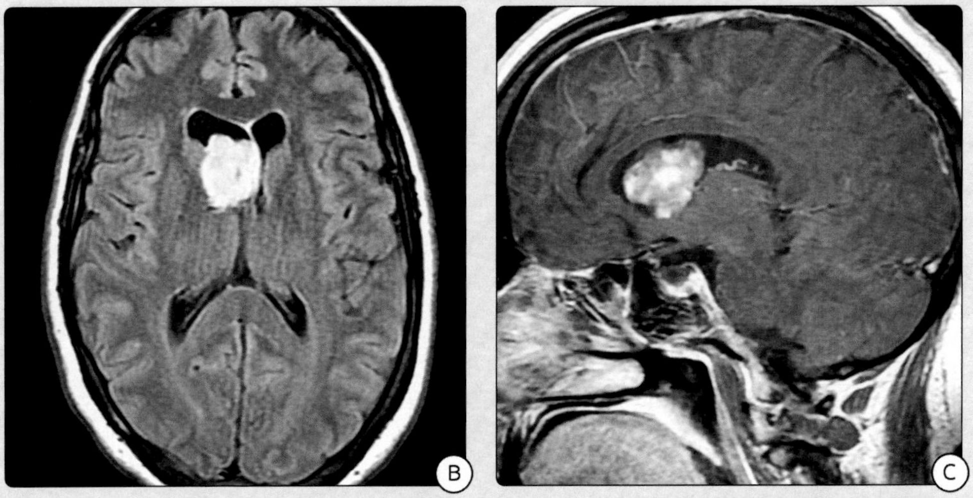

(18-27B) FLAIR shows that the mass is very hyperintense. There is no evidence for periventricular fluid accumulation. (18-27C) Parasagittal T1 C+ shows that the lobulated mass enhances heterogeneously, appears confined to the frontal horn of the ventricle. This is subependymoma (ST-SE), WHO grade I.

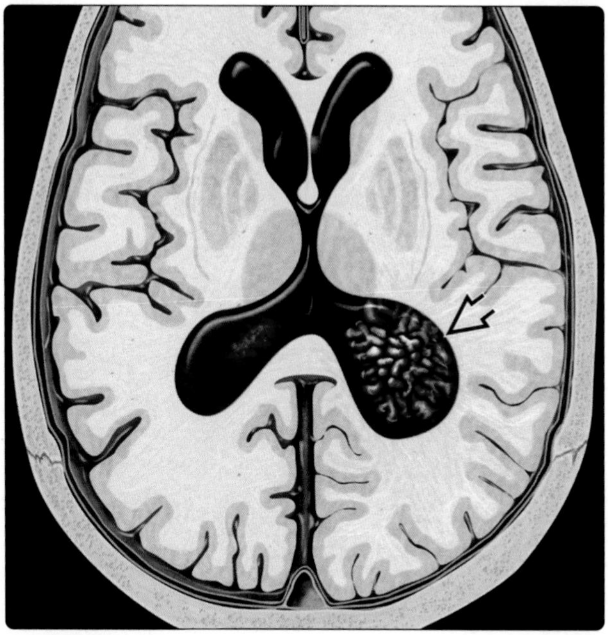

(18-28) Axial graphic depicts a frond-like mass ➲ in the atrium of the left lateral ventricle. The ventricles are moderately enlarged from overproduction of CSF. This is a choroid plexus papilloma.

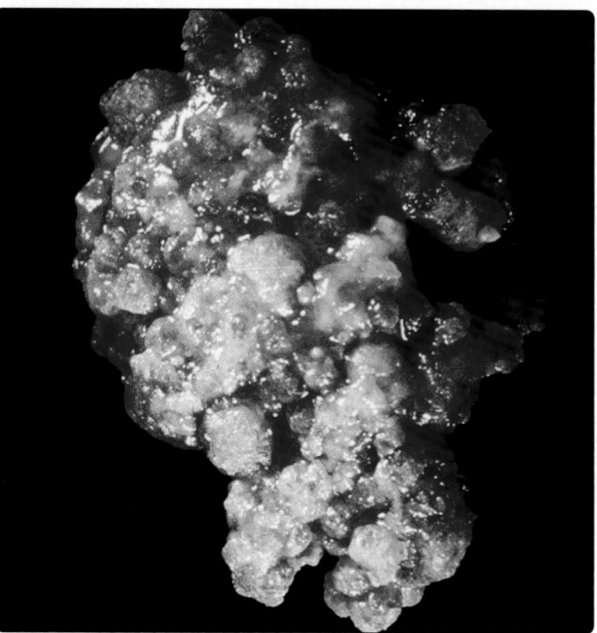

(18-29) Resected choroid plexus papilloma exhibits classic "cauliflower-like" gross appearance. Multiple vascular papillary excrescences are typical. (From Fuller et al., Practical Surgical Neuropathology: A Diagnostic Approach, 6th ed.)

location) and cluster 2 (adult age, mainly infratentorial location) are characterized by low risk of tumor progression. Cluster 3 (young age, supratentorial location) is characterized by choroid plexus tumors with a higher risk of progression and includes many aCPPs and basically all CPCas.

In this section, we discuss each of these types with the major focus on choroid plexus papilloma—the most common primary choroid plexus tumor.

Choroid Plexus Papilloma

Terminology

Choroid plexus papilloma (CPP) is the most benign of the choroid plexus neoplasms.

Etiology

General Concepts. Congenital CPPs are common and may develop when the differentiating fetal choroid plexus is transiently ciliated.

Genetics. Genomic analysis of CPPs suggests a role of genes involved in the development and biology of plexus epithelium (i.e., *OTX2* and *TRPM3*).

Choroid plexus tumors—especially carcinomas—occur in patients with **Li-Fraumeni syndrome**, a cancer predisposition syndrome caused by *TP53* germline mutation. *SMARCB1* mutations with INI1 protein alterations and CPPs have been described in the **rhabdoid predisposition syndrome**. Both mutations are very rarely identified in sporadic CPPs.

CPPs also occur as part of **Aicardi syndrome**, an X-linked dominant syndrome that occurs almost exclusively in female patients. Aicardi syndrome is defined by the triad of infantile spasms, corpus callosum agenesis, and pathognomonic chorioretinal abnormalities (lacunae). Since it was first described in 1965, new features such as cortical malformations, gray matter heterotopias, CPPs, and choroid plexus cysts have been identified and added to the Aicardi spectrum. The prevalence of CPPs in Aicardi syndrome is estimated at 3-5%. Bilateral and triventricular CPPs occur in 1% of cases.

Pathology

Location. CPPs arise wherever choroid plexus is normally found, occurring in proportion to the amount of choroid plexus normally present in each location. Therefore, the vast majority arise in the lateral (50%) and fourth (40%) ventricles. The trigone is the most common overall site **(18-28)**. A few large CPPs involve multiple locations. Triventricular CPP is seen in 5% of cases and originates in the third ventricle, extending cephalad through the foramen of Monro into both lateral ventricles.

Only 5-10% of all CPPs occur in locations other than the lateral and fourth ventricles. Just 5% are found in the third ventricle. CPPs are occasionally found as primary cerebellopontine angle (CPA) tumors, in which tufts of choroid plexus extrude through the foramina of Luschka into the adjacent CPA cisterns. Extraventricular CPPs are extremely rare. They have been reported in the brainstem, cerebellum, pituitary fossa, and septi pellucidi.

There is a strong effect of age on CPP location. More than 80% of all CPPs in infants arise in the atrium of the lateral ventricle. The fourth ventricle and CPA cisterns are more

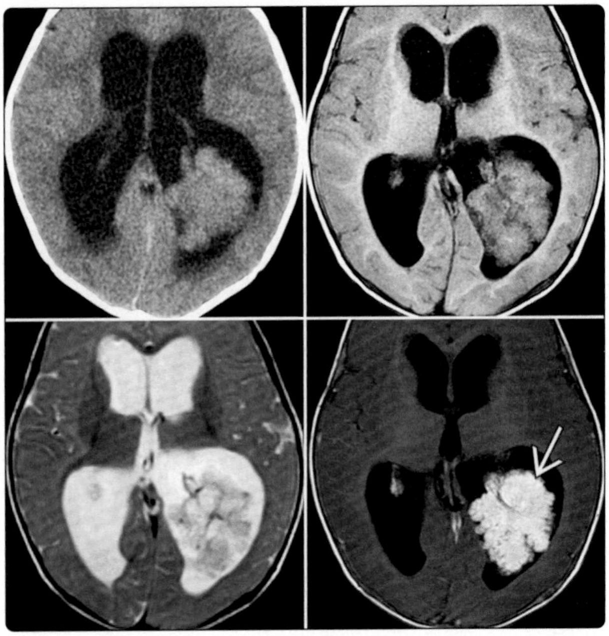

***(18-30)** NECT scan and a series of MRs demonstrate the typical appearance of choroid plexus papilloma. The lobulated intraventricular mass enhances strongly →. Note hydrocephalus caused by overproduction of CSF.*

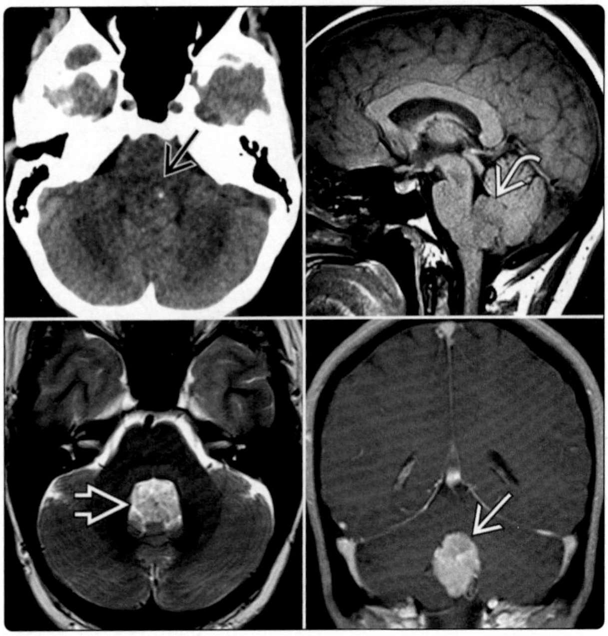

***(18-31)** A 39y woman had a calcified 4th ventricle mass → discovered incidentally on a head CT for trauma. The mass is well demarcated on T1WI →, hyperintense on T2WI →, and enhances intensely →; choroid plexus papilloma (WHO grade I).*

typical locations in adults. The lateral ventricles are an exceptionally rare site of CPP in older patients.

Size and Number. CPPs are usually solitary tumors, varying in size from small to huge masses. Occasionally, multiple noncontiguous lesions are seen, but most represent CSF dissemination from the primary tumor site. Multiple CPPs arise independently, as synchronous tumors are rarely seen.

Gross Pathology. CPPs are well-circumscribed papillary or cauliflower-like masses that may adhere to—but usually do not invade through—the ventricular wall. Cysts and hemorrhage are common.

Microscopic Features. Histologically, the architecture of CPPs closely resembles that of normal nonneoplastic choroid plexus. A core of fibrovascular connective tissue covered by a single layer of uniform benign-appearing epithelial cells is typical. Cytokeratins, vimentin, and podoplanin are expressed by virtually all CPPs.

Mitotic activity is very low, with MIB-1 less than 1%. CPPs are generally confined to the ventricle of origin and rarely exhibit an infiltrative growth pattern.

Staging, Grading, and Classification. CPPs are WHO grade I neoplasms.

Clinical Issues

Epidemiology. CPPs are rare lesions, accounting for less than 1% of all primary intracranial neoplasms. However, CPPs represent 10-20% of brain tumors occurring in the first year of life.

Demographics. Median age at presentation is 1.5 years for lateral and third ventricular CPPs, 22.5 years for fourth ventricle CPPs, and 35.5 years for CPA CPPs. There is a very slight male predominance.

Presentation. CPPs tend to obstruct normal CSF pathways. Infants present with increased head size and raised intracranial pressure. Children and adults may experience headache, nausea, and vomiting.

CPP can also present as a fetal brain tumor and is the fifth most common congenital brain neoplasm (after teratoma, astrocytoma, craniopharyngioma, and primitive neuroectodermal tumor). Macrocephaly with a large intracranial mass and hydrocephalus is the most common presentation.

Natural History. Surgical resection is often curative. The recurrence rate following gross total resection is low, only about 5-6%. Malignant progression of CPP to choroid plexus carcinoma has been reported but is rare.

Imaging

General Features. A well-delineated, lobulated intraventricular mass with frond-like papillary excrescences is typical. *Diffuse leptomeningeal dissemination is uncommon but does occur with histologically benign CPPs, so preoperative imaging of the entire neuraxis is recommended!*

CHOROID PLEXUS PAPILLOMA

Pathology
- Lateral ventricle (50%, usually children)
- Fourth ventricle, CPA cistern (40%, usually adults)
- Third ventricle (10%, children)
- Lobulated, frond-like configuration
- WHO grade I

Clinical Issues
- 13% of brain tumors in first year of life
- Mean age = 1.5 years for CPPs in lateral, third ventricle
- Symptoms of obstructive hydrocephalus common
- Occurs with Aicardi, Li-Fraumeni, rhabdoid predisposition syndromes

Imaging Findings
- CT
  - Iso-/hyperdense lobulated mass
  - Hydrocephalus common
  - Ca++ (25%)
  - CECT shows intense enhancement
- MR
  - Iso-/hypointense on T1
  - Iso-/hyperintense on T2/FLAIR
  - "Flow voids" common
  - May show "blooming" foci on T2*
  - Intense enhancement, no restriction
  - Occasionally demonstrates CSF dissemination (image entire neuraxis preoperatively!)

CT Findings. The majority of CPPs are iso- to hyperdense compared with brain on NECT scans **(18-30)**. Calcification is seen in 25% of cases. Hydrocephalus—either obstructive or caused by CSF overproduction—is common. CECT scans show intense homogeneous enhancement.

MR Findings. A sharply marginated lobular mass that is iso- to slightly hypointense relative to brain is seen on T1WI. CPPs are iso- to hyperintense on T2WI and FLAIR. Linear and branching internal "flow voids" reflect the increased vascularity common in CPPs. T2* (GRE, SWI) may show hypointense foci secondary to calcification or intratumoral hemorrhage.

Intense homogeneous enhancement is seen following contrast administration **(18-31)**. CPPs generally do not restrict on DWI. MRS may show elevated myoinositol (mI).

Rare CPP variants include purely cystic CPP and cystic extraaxial metastases from an intraventricular CPP. In purely cystic CPP, a large, often mobile cyst with intensely enhancing mural nodules is attached to the choroid plexus. It can cause sudden obstructive hydrocephalus. Purely cystic extraaxial metastases from CPP are seen as nonenhancing cisternal CSF-like cysts that resemble multiple parasitic cysts, most commonly neurocysticercosis.

Ultrasound. CPPs appear as well-defined, lobular, hyperechoic intraventricular masses on transcranial US.

Differential Diagnosis

The major differential diagnoses of CPP are **atypical choroid plexus papilloma** and **choroid plexus carcinoma** (CPCa). Both share similar imaging features on standard MR sequences. CPCa has a higher cerebral blood flow than CPP on pMR. CPCa is also far more likely to invade brain parenchyma than CPP. CSF dissemination occurs with all three histologic types of choroid

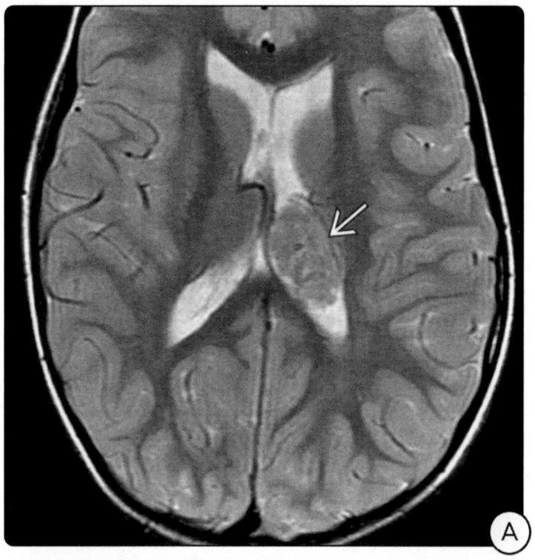

***(18-32A)** T2WI of the same patient shows that the mass ➡ is isointense with gray matter.*

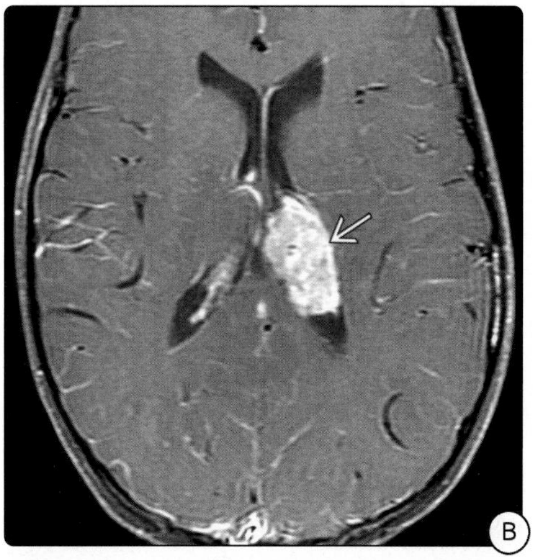

***(18-32B)** The mass ➡ enhances intensely on T1 C+ FS. Atypical choroid plexus papilloma (WHO grade II) was histopathologically identified.*

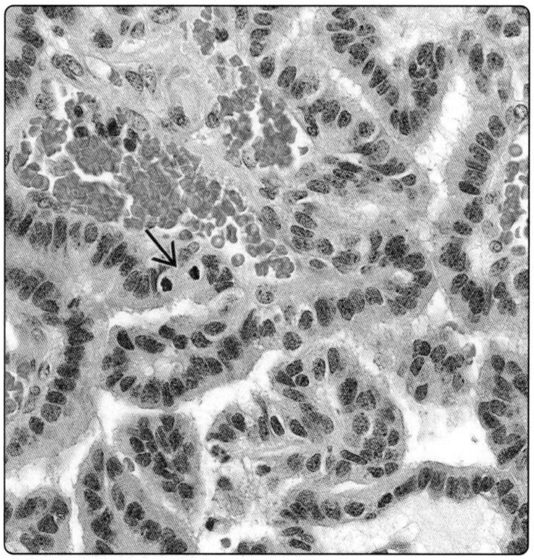

***(18-33)** CPPs are atypical based on ↑ mitotic activity ➡ (> WHO grade I CPPs). 2+ mitoses/10 HPF is threshold, met here. (P. Burger, MD.)*

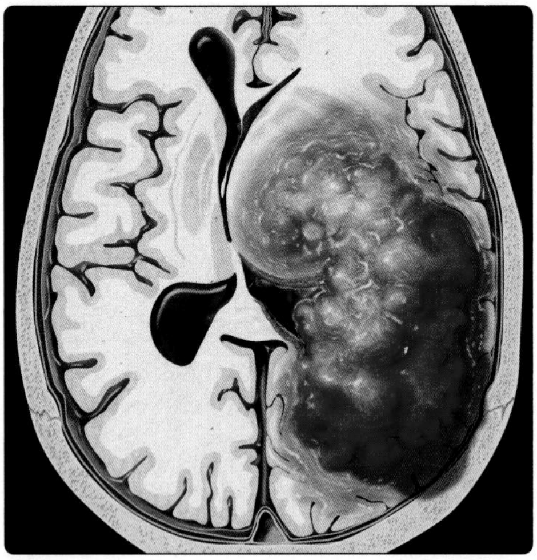

(18-34) ***Graphic has choroid plexus carcinoma; hemorrhagic, highly vascular mass fills atrium of lateral ventricle, invades parenchyma.***

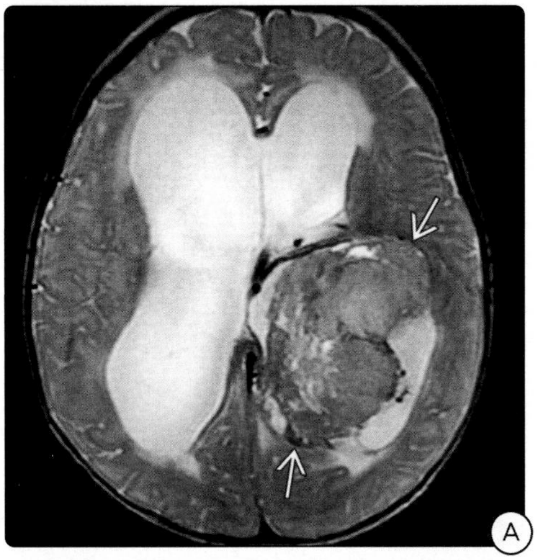

(18-35A) ***T2WI in an 8m girl with macrocrania, vomiting shows severe hydrocephalus, large mass in the atrium of the left lateral ventricle.***

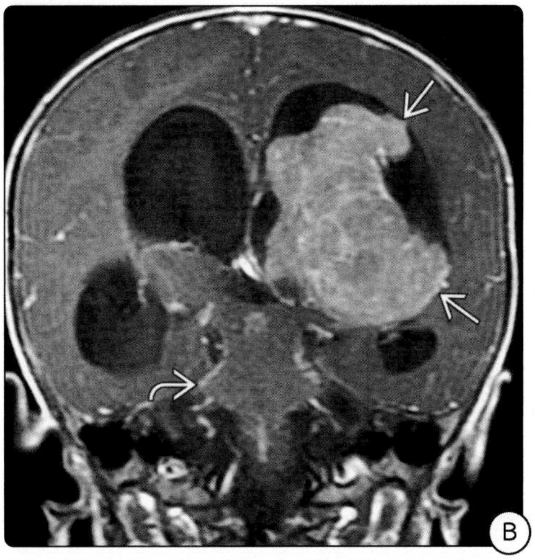

(18-35B) ***T1 C+ shows intense but heterogeneous enhancement in the mass. Note diffuse CSF spread. This is choroid plexus carcinoma.***

plexus tumors and is therefore neither a distinguishing feature nor a reliable predictor of malignancy.

Choroid plexus hyperplasia, also called **villous hypertrophy of the choroid plexus**, is a very rare cause of CSF overproduction and shunt-resistant hydrocephalus. Diffuse villous hyperplasia may result in CSF production exceeding three liters per day. Unlike CPP, most cases of choroid plexus hyperplasia are bilateral and diffusely enlarge the entire length of the choroid plexus.

Choroid plexus xanthogranulomas are benign incidental lesions that occur commonly in the lateral ventricular choroid plexus. They consist of desquamated epithelial cells with accumulated lipid together with macrophages and multinucleated foreign body giant cells. In contrast to most CPPs, they are found primarily in middle-aged and older patients. On imaging they appear as bilateral multiloculated cysts within the enhancing choroid plexus glomus.

Choroid plexus metastasis occurs in middle-aged and older adults and is not in the differential diagnosis of a pediatric CPP.

CHOROID PLEXUS PAPILLOMA: DIFFERENTIAL DIAGNOSIS

Children
- Atypical choroid plexus papilloma
- Choroid plexus carcinoma
- Villous hyperplasia

Adults
- Choroid plexus xanthogranulomas
- Metastases

Atypical Choroid Plexus Papilloma

Atypical choroid plexus papilloma (aCPP) is a recently recognized neoplasm that is intermediate in malignancy between CPP (WHO grade I neoplasm) and choroid plexus carcinoma (WHO grade III neoplasm). aCPPs represent approximately 15% of all choroid plexus tumors.

The main distinguishing histopathologic feature of aCPP is increased mitotic activity with elevated MIB-1 labeling **(18-33)**. Increased cellularity and nuclear pleomorphism are common.

aCPPs in methylation clusters 1 and 2 typically demonstrate no tumor progression, whereas those in cluster 3 have a less favorable outcome.

Only a few imaging cases of aCPP have been reported. All have the lobulated papillary appearance with strong uniform enhancement that also characterizes CPP **(18-32)**. Imaging findings to date do not discriminate between aCPP and CPP, so the definitive diagnosis depends on histopathology.

Choroid Plexus Carcinoma

Terminology

Choroid plexus carcinoma (CPCa) is a rare malignant tumor that occurs almost exclusively in young children.

Etiology

Genetics. Nearly half of all CPCas harbor *TP53* mutations. The *TP53*-mutated tumor genome is associated with significant risk of progression and poor outcome.

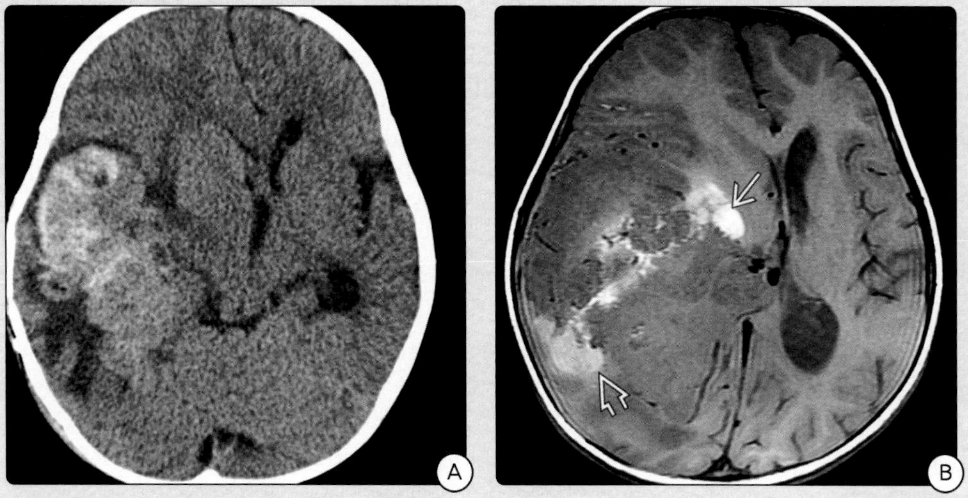

(18-36A) *NECT scan in a 2y girl with a large head and papilledema shows a predominantly hyperdense lobulated mass in the right lateral ventricle invading adjacent brain.* ***(18-36B)*** *T1WI shows that the mass is mostly iso- and hypointense, but areas of variable hyperintensity suggest hemorrhage ➡ and proteinaceous fluid in cysts ➡.*

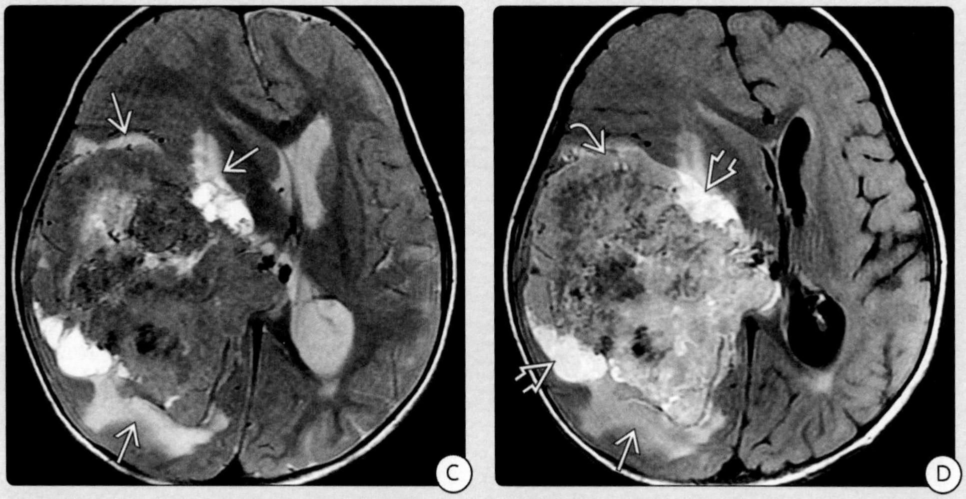

(18-36C) *T2WI shows the extremely heterogeneous nature of the mass. Gross tumor invasion of the brain parenchyma with surrounding edema ➡ is present.* ***(18-36D)*** *FLAIR scan depicts the mass ➡, surrounding edema ➡, hemorrhage, and/or cyst formation ➡.*

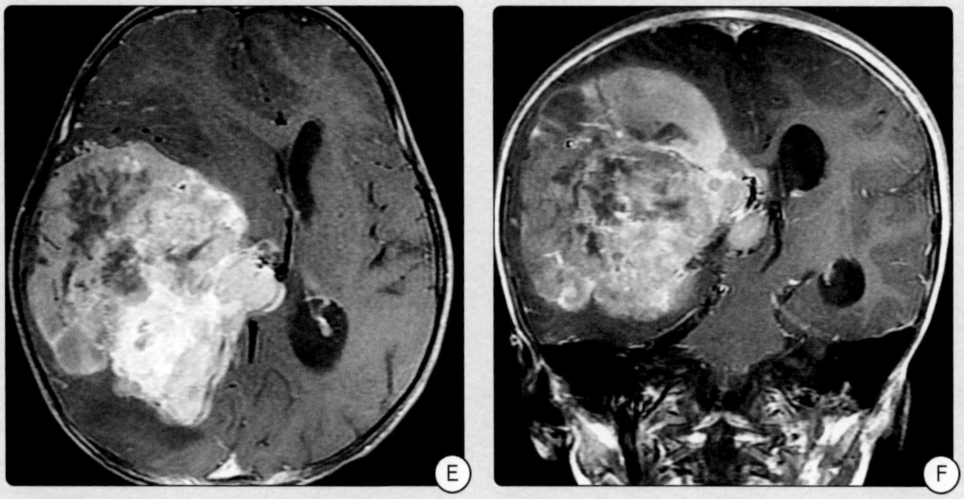

(18-36E) *T1 C+ FS scan shows that the mass enhances intensely but heterogeneously.* ***(18-36F)*** *Coronal T1 C+ scan shows the extent of tumor invasion into the adjacent parenchyma. This is choroid plexus carcinoma.*

All CPCas fall into methylation cluster 3 and are associated with a mean progression-free survival of 55 months.

Pathology

Gross Pathology. CPCa almost always arises in the lateral ventricle. This heterogeneous, bulky intraventricular tumor often displays gross hemorrhage and necrotic foci. Invasion into adjacent brain parenchyma is common **(18-34)**.

Microscopic Features. Frank cytologic features of malignancy are seen, including frequent mitoses (generally at least 5-10 per high-power field), increased cellular density, nuclear pleomorphism, loss of papillary architecture, and necrosis. MIB-1 is elevated, ranging from 15% to 20%.

Immunohistochemical and genetic features show some overlap between CPCa and atypical teratoid/rhabdoid tumor.

Staging, Grading, and Classification. CPCa is a WHO grade III neoplasm.

Clinical Issues

Epidemiology. Although CPCa is uncommon, representing less than 1% of all pediatric brain tumors, it accounts for 5% of supratentorial neoplasms. CPCa represents 20-40% of all primary choroid plexus neoplasms.

Demographics. Between 70-80% of CPCas arise in children younger than 3 years. Median age at diagnosis is 18 months.

Presentation. The most common symptoms—nausea, vomiting, headache, and obtundation—are caused by obstructive hydrocephalus.

Natural History. Prognosis in patients with these aggressive tumors is generally dismal, especially those with incomplete resection of a *TP53*-mutated genotype.

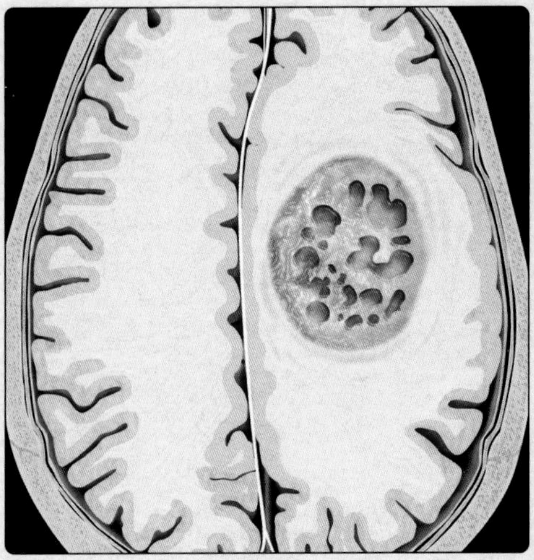

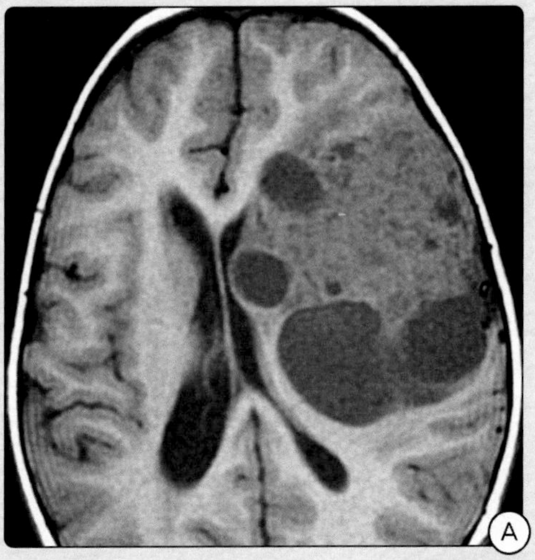

***(18-37)** Graphic depicts astroblastoma as a relatively well-circumscribed hemispheric mass with multiple intratumoral cysts. **(18-38A)** Axial T1WI shows typical findings of astroblastoma with innumerable tiny and multiple large cysts.*

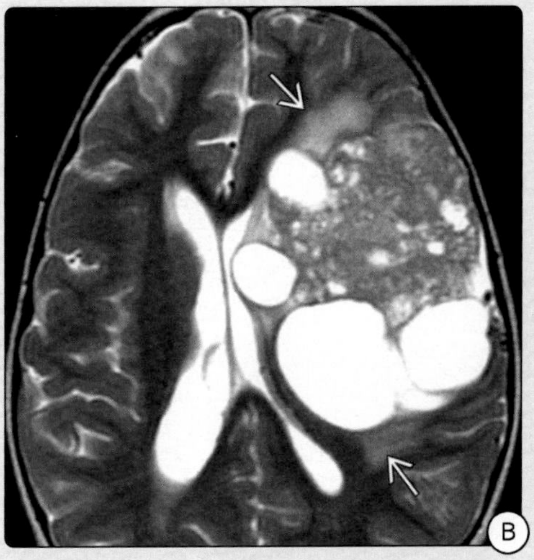

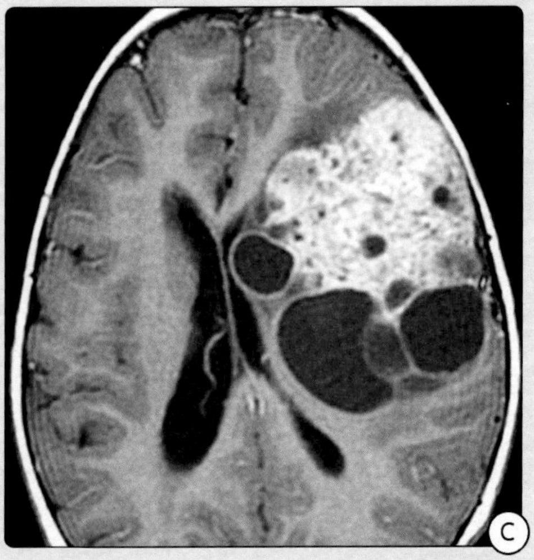

***(18-38B)** T2WI shows that, relative to the size of the mass, there is little peritumoral edema ➡. **(18-38C)** T1 C+ shows that the solid portions of the mass enhance, whereas the cysts do not.*

Imaging

CPCa often invades through the ventricular ependyma into adjacent brain. Edema, necrosis, intratumoral cysts, and hemorrhage are common **(18-36)**. Enhancement is typically strong but heterogeneous. CSF dissemination is common **(18-35)**.

Differential Diagnosis

The major differential diagnoses are **choroid plexus papilloma (CPP)** and **atypical choroid plexus papilloma (aCPP)**. Imaging features of all three primary choroid plexus tumors overlap. CSF spread occurs with both benign and malignant varieties. CPP rarely invades the brain, so the presence of frank parenchymal invasion and accompanying edema suggests CPCa.

OTHER CHOROID PLEXUS NEOPLASMS

Atypical Choroid Plexus Papilloma
- WHO grade II
- Imaging findings similar to those of choroid plexus papilloma

Choroid Plexus Carcinoma
- Rare
- Children less than 3 years (70-80%)
- WHO grade III
- Imaging
  - Invades through ependyma
  - Edema, necrosis, cysts, hemorrhage common
  - Strong heterogeneous enhancement
  - CSF dissemination common

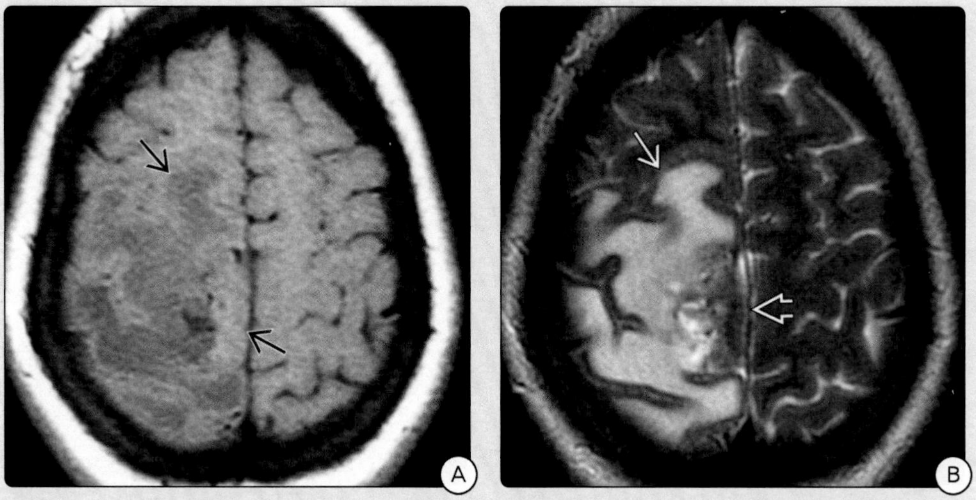

(18-39A) *Axial T1WI in a 22y woman with headaches and left-sided weakness shows a mixed iso-/hypointense mass in the right cerebral hemisphere →.* ***(18-39B)*** *T2WI in the same case shows a mixed iso-/hyperintense mass → with striking edema ⇨.*

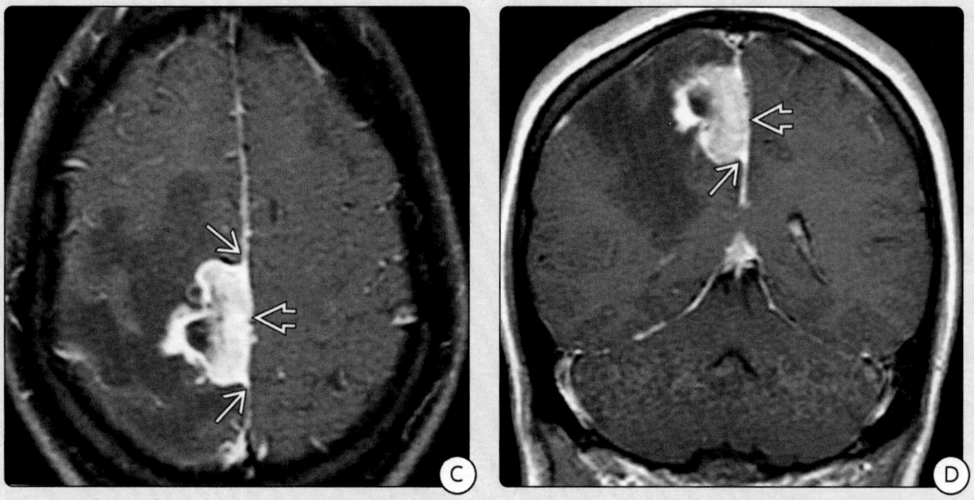

(18-39C) *T1 C+ FS shows that the intensely enhancing mass ⇨ abuts the dura with small dural "tails" →.* ***(18-39D)*** *Coronal T1 C+ MR shows the dural-based intensely enhancing mass ⇨ and dural "tail" →. Preoperative diagnosis was meningioma. Astroblastoma was found at pathology.*

Other Neuroepithelial Tumors

"Other neuroepithelial tumors" is an eclectic group of uncommon neoplasms that currently includes astroblastoma, chordoid glioma of the third ventricle, and angiocentric glioma.

Astroblastoma

Terminology

Astroblastoma (AB) is a rare glial neoplasm that mainly affects children, adolescents, and young adults. Although its precise etiology and exact histogenesis are controversial, AB is recognized as a distinct entity.

Pathology

Grossly, ABs are firm, often cystic hemispheric parenchymal masses **(18-37)**. Even though the name "astroblastoma" implies astrocytic lineage, it has overlapping features with astrocytomas, ependymomas, and sometimes other glial neoplasms.

Unlike ependymomas and angiocentric gliomas, ABs demonstrate distinctive astroblastic pseudorosettes and are usually Olig2 immunopositive. IDH is also negative, and ABs only occasionally exhibit MGMT promoter methylation. *BRAF* V600E mutations are common, suggesting that ABs may be ontologically related to other cortically based low-grade tumors of children and young adults.

Although some investigators recognize subsets of low-grade and high-grade ABs, no WHO grade has been assigned to date. Recent studies suggest that so-called "higher grade" ABs have significantly poorer survival.

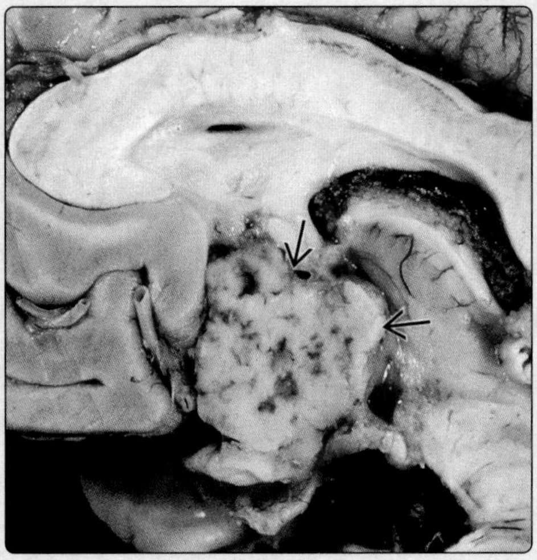

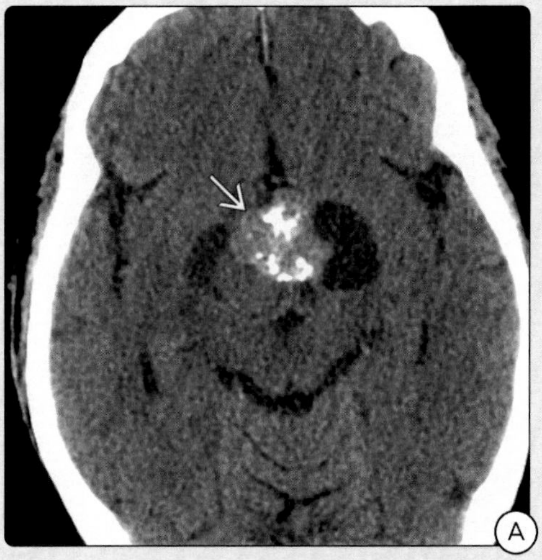

(18-40) Midline sagittal autopsy specimen shows chordoid glioma as a lobulated mass ⇨ that fills the third ventricle. (Courtesy P. Burger, MD.) (18-41A) NECT scan shows a lobulated, hyperdense, partially calcified midline mass ➡ in the inferior third ventricle.

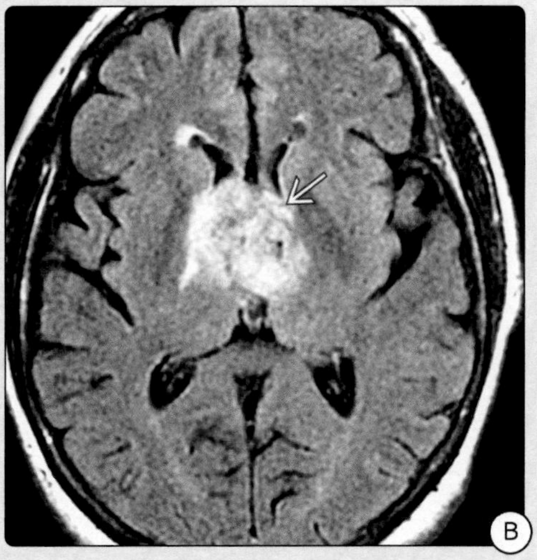

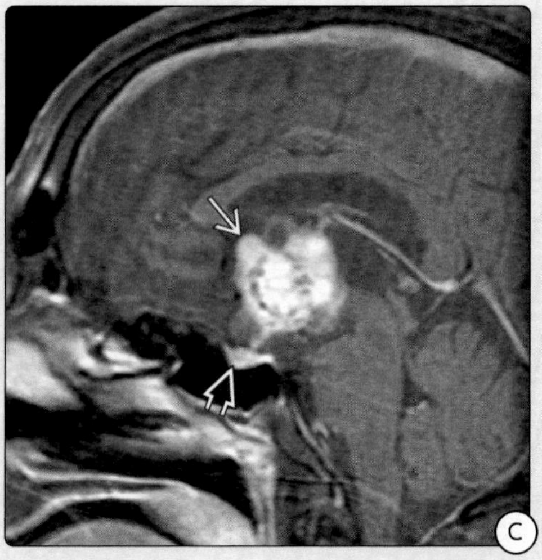

(18-41B) FLAIR scan in the same patient shows that the mass ➡ is heterogeneously hyperintense. (18-41C) Sagittal T1 C+ scan shows that the mass ➡ is well marginated and enhances intensely but somewhat heterogeneously. The infundibular stalk and pituitary gland ➡ appear entirely normal. Chordoid glioma of the third ventricle was the histopathologic diagnosis.

Clinical Issues

Astroblastomas account for less than 1% of all primary brain tumors and 0.5-3.0% of gliomas. Although they can occur at any age, most ABs are found in children and young adults. Median age at diagnosis is 14 years. The M:F ratio is 1:2.

Despite its ominous-sounding name, the biologic behavior of AB is quite variable. Patients with low-grade tumors and gross total resection often have good long-term overall survival rates.

Imaging

General Features. Astroblastoma is almost exclusively a supratentorial, often superficially located hemispheric tumor that is typically well demarcated. Surrounding edema is minimal or absent. Most astroblastomas exhibit both solid and cystic components, frequently giving them a characteristic "bubbly" appearance.

CT Findings. Astroblastomas are hyperdense on NECT (85%), and almost three-quarters exhibit punctate/psammomatous or dense globular calcifications.

MR Findings. Astroblastoma is hypo- to isointense compared with white matter on T1WI and heterogeneously hyperintense on T2/FLAIR **(18-38)**. A mixed "bubbly" appearance, caused by intratumoral cysts, is common. Hemorrhage, including blood-fluid levels in the cystic components, can be present. Restricted diffusion has been described. MR spectroscopy is nonspecific.

Heterogeneous enhancement following contrast administration is typical. The combination of peripheral rim and solid nodular enhancement gives some lesions a "signet ring" appearance. Some peripherally located astroblastomas incite dural reaction, causing a "dural tail" sign **(18-39)**.

Differential Diagnosis

While the overall imaging findings of astroblastoma are somewhat nonspecific, the combination of age (10-30 years), anatomic location (cerebral hemisphere), and a "bubbly" appearance may suggest the diagnosis.

Other entities that resemble astroblastoma vary with age. In young children, **astrocytoma, hemispheric ependymoma**, and **atypical teratoid/rhabdoid tumor** should be considered. In older children and young adults, **oligodendroglioma** and **pleomorphic xanthoastrocytoma** are in the differential diagnosis. Astroblastomas that abut the dura and have a "dural tail" can resemble atypical **meningioma**.

Chordoid Glioma of the Third Ventricle

Chordoid glioma (CG) is a rare adult tumor that is distinguished by its location (third ventricular region), stereotypical histology (both glial and chordoid elements), and characteristic imaging features.

Etiology

Although the precise etiology of CGs is unclear, ultrastructural studies are most consistent with an ependymal histogenesis. Recent studies suggest that CGs may arise from the organum vasculosum of the lamina terminalis.

There are no known risk factors or syndromic associations.

Pathology

Location. CGs arise in the anterior aspect of the third ventricle adjacent to the lamina terminalis. The smallest reported CG was 1.5 cm, and the largest measured 7.0 cm in maximum diameter.

Gross Pathology. CGs are solid, round or slightly lobulated, semitranslucent masses that are tan-gray and moderately vascular **(18-40)**. Many CGs are grossly encapsulated.

Microscopic Features. The general appearance is that of a chordoid architecture with myxoid background. Cords and clusters of round or fusiform epithelioid neoplastic cells with abundant eosinophilic cytoplasm are suspended in a variably mucinous, often vacuolated, lymphoplasmacytic-rich matrix.

CGs resemble chordomas or chordoid meningiomas microscopically. However, unlike these similar-appearing tumors, CGs show strong diffuse immunoreactivity for the glial marker GFAP. Most are positive for an epithelial membrane antigen and CD34 but are usually negative for neurofilament protein. IDH-1 immunostaining is negative.

Mitoses are rare, and MIB-1 labeling index is low.

Staging, Grading, and Classification. CGs are WHO grade II neoplasms.

Clinical Issues

Epidemiology. CG is rare, representing less than 1% of all gliomas.

Demographics. CG is a tumor of middle-aged adults (35-60 years old). There is a 2:1 F:M ratio.

Presentation. Clinical presentation of CG varies from asymptomatic to aggressive. Headache, nausea, and memory impairment are common. On neurologic examination, visual field deficit is the most common abnormality. Endocrine disturbances are seen in 10-15% of patients. Most cases show slow, mild progression.

Natural History and Treatment. CGs are slow-growing tumors. Because they are frequently attached to the hypothalamus and floor of the third ventricle, resection is often subtotal. The most common postoperative complication is hypothalamic dysfunction with diabetes insipidus and obesity.

Imaging

General Features. Radiologic features of reported CGs are remarkably consistent. Most CGs are well-demarcated ovoid masses that are confined to the anterior third ventricle and are clearly separate from the pituitary gland and infundibulum. Most tumors abut the lamina terminalis, which may be its anatomic site of origin. CGs are often continuous with the hypothalamus inferiorly, but gross brain invasion is rare. Enhancement is typically strong and relatively uniform.

CT Findings. CGs are moderately hyperdense compared with brain on NECT. Strong, homogeneous enhancement is typical. Occasional cases with calcification have been reported. Hydrocephalus is present in 10-15% of cases.

MR Findings. Sagittal MR demonstrates that the tumor is clearly separated from the pituitary gland and infundibular stalk, which it often displaces posteriorly. CGs are typically isointense with brain on T1WI and slightly hyperintense on T2WI. Strong uniform enhancement is typical **(18-41)**. Intratumoral cysts are seen in 25% of cases, but hemorrhage is rare.

Differential Diagnosis

Primary third ventricular tumors in adults are all uncommon, as are **metastases** in this location. As CGs are clearly separate from the pituitary gland, macroadenoma is usually not in the differential diagnosis although a few purely third ventricular **pituitary macroadenomas** and **craniopharyngiomas** have been reported. **Chordoid meningioma** can look just like a CG, but the third ventricle is a rarely reported site for a rare meningioma variant.

Tuber cinereum (TC) hamartomas are most common in preadolescent male patients with precocious puberty. Although TC hamartomas are isointense with brain on T1- and T2WI, they do not enhance. As CGs are tumors of adults, childhood hypothalamic tumors such as adamantinomatous **craniopharyngioma** and **pilocytic astrocytoma** are not diagnostic considerations.

(18-42A) Axial T2WI in a patient with seizures shows a wedge-shaped hyperintense cortical, subcortical mass in the right parietal lobe ➡. (18-42B) FLAIR scan shows the mass ➡ as well as thickening of the adjacent gyri ➡.

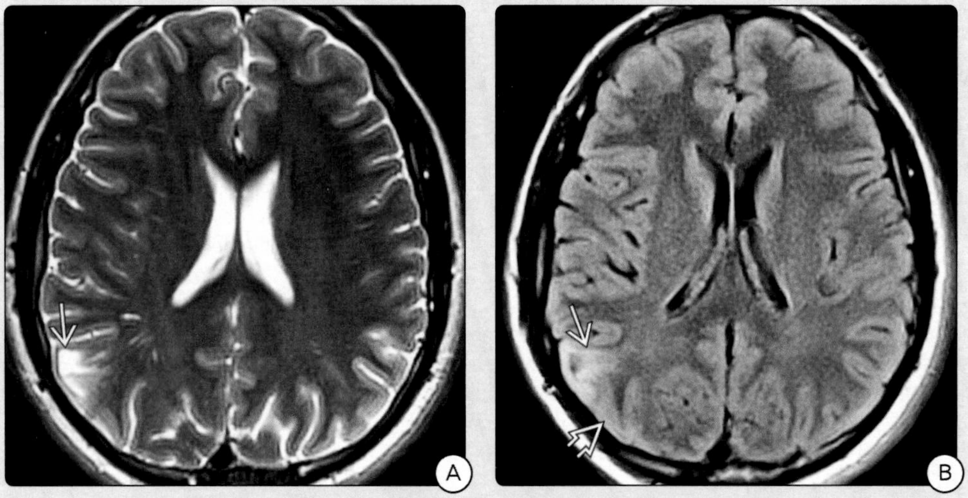

(18-42C) T1 C+ shows that the mass ➡ does not enhance. (18-42D) ADC map shows that the mass does not demonstrate diffusion restriction. Angiocentric glioma was the histologic diagnosis. The adjacent gyral thickening noted on the FLAIR scan probably represents associated focal cortical dysplasia, a finding commonly associated with angiocentric glioma. (All four images courtesy M. Castillo, MD.)

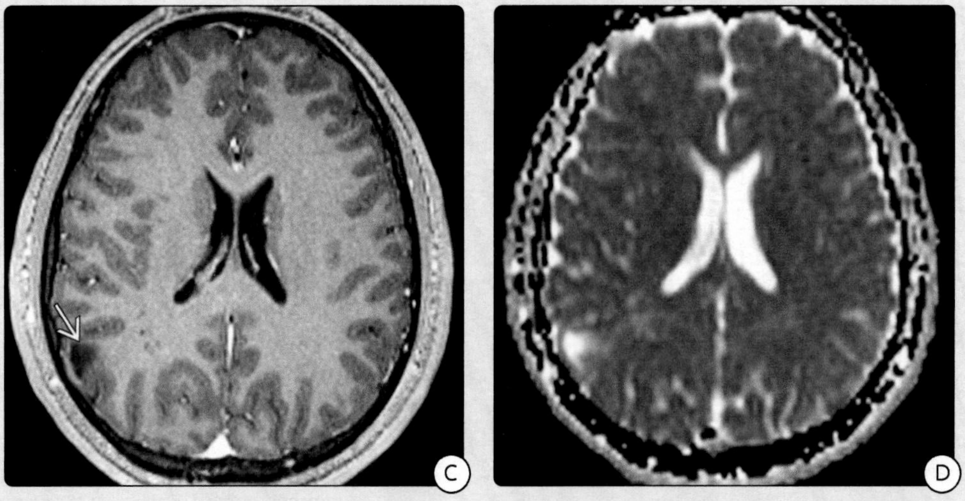

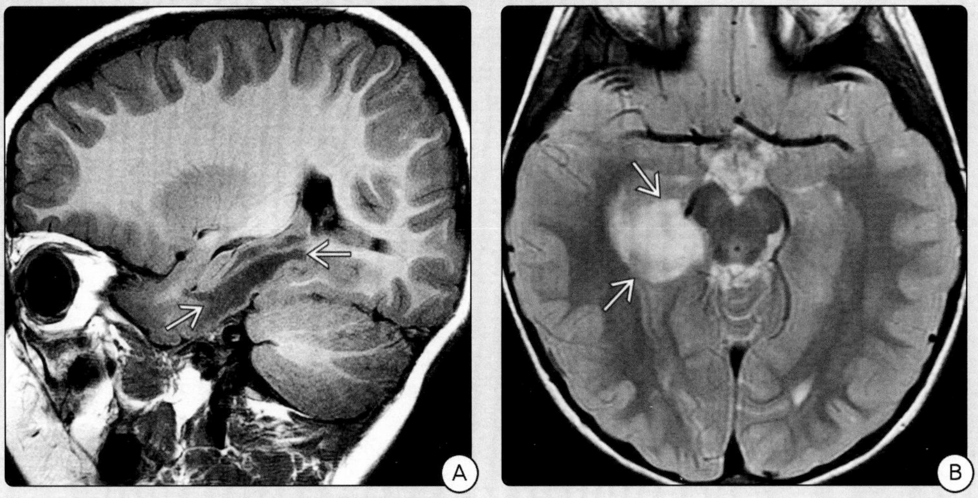

(18-43A) *Sagittal T1WI in a 5y boy with temporal lobe epilepsy shows a hypointense mass ➡ in the left temporal lobe.* **(18-43B)** *Axial T2WI in the same case shows a rather ill-defined hyperintense mass ➡ in the right temporal lobe.*

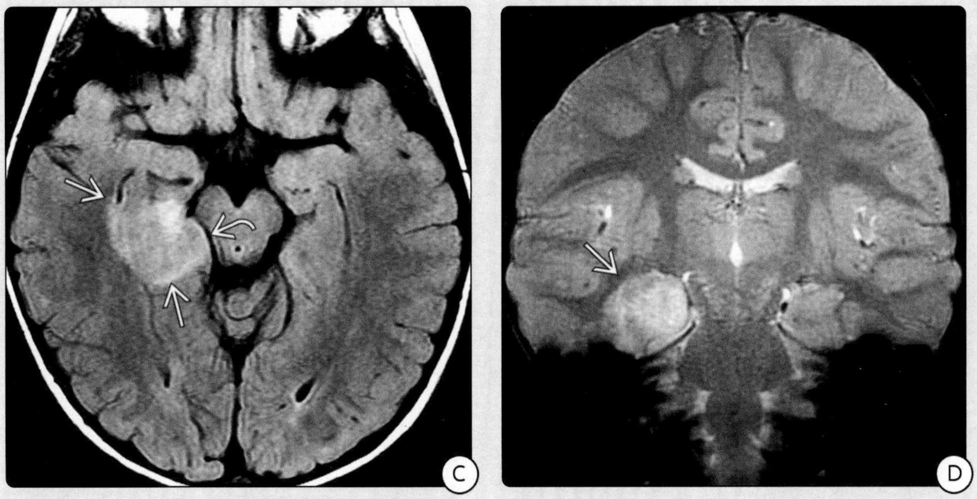

(18-43C) *The lesion ➡ is hyperintense on FLAIR and appears slightly expansile, with some mass effect of the hippocampus on the midbrain ➦.* **(18-43D)** *Coronal T2* shows no evidence for blooming hypointensity to suggest hemorrhage or calcification in the mass ➡.*

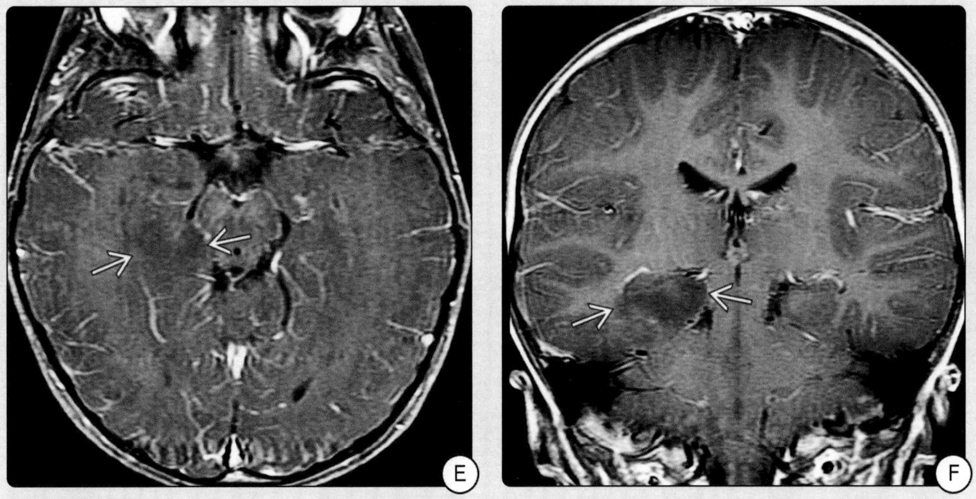

(18-43E) *Axial T1 C+ FS shows the ill-defined hypointense mass ➡ and shows no evidence for enhancement.* **(18-43F)** *Coronal T1 C+ in the same case shows no evidence of enhancement in the slightly expansile hypointense mass ➡. The mass was resected, and angiocentric glioma was found at pathologic examination.*

Angiocentric Glioma

Angiocentric glioma (AG) is an epilepsy-associated low-grade glioma. Because of its uncertain histogenesis, the WHO groups AG together with astroblastoma and chordoid glioma in the category "other gliomas."

Terminology

Angiocentric glioma has also been called "angiocentric neuroepithelial tumor."

Etiology

Recent studies have identified *MYB-QKI* fusions as a specific and single candidate driver event in angiocentric gliomas. Tumorigenesis is promoted through three mechanisms: *MYB* activation by truncation, enhancer translocation driving aberrant *MYB-QKI* expression, and hemizygous loss of the tumor suppressor *QKI*.

Clinical Issues

AGs are typically tumors of children and young adults. More than 95% of patients present with intractable focal epilepsy. Surgical excision is generally curative.

Pathology

AGs are superficial, cortically based tumors. The most common locations are the frontal and temporal lobes. AGs are characterized by elongated bipolar spindle cells with a striking angiocentric orientation. Adjacent focal cortical dysplasia is common. MIB-1 is generally less than 1%. AGs are WHO grade I neoplasms.

Imaging

NECT shows a solid, cortically based tumor with variable attenuation. Calcification may be present, but necrosis, hemorrhage, and intratumoral cysts are absent.

MR demonstrates a diffusely infiltrating expansile cortical mass without sharply demarcated borders **(18-42)**. Most AGs are hyperintense on T2/FLAIR. A subtle rim of T1 shortening and stalk-like extension toward the ventricle have been described in some cases. Enhancement is generally absent **(18-43)**. Focal cortical dysplasia can often be identified adjacent to the tumor.

Differential Diagnosis

AG is similar in appearance to other low-grade cortically based neoplasms in children/young adults who present with longstanding epilepsy. The major differential diagnoses include **dysembryoplastic neuroepithelial tumor (DNET)** as well as **ganglioglioma** and **oligodendroglioma**. All are more common than AG.

OTHER NEUROEPITHELIAL TUMORS

Astroblastoma
- Pathology
  - Features overlap with ependymoma, astrocytoma
  - Olig2 is positive, but IDH, MGMT are negative
  - *BRAF* V600E mutation common
  - No WHO grades assigned
  - More aggressive "higher grade" tumors have reduced survival
- Clinical Features
  - Usually children, young adults 10-30 years old
  - M:F = 1:2
  - Gross total resection often has good long-term survival
- Imaging Findings
  - Superficial location common
  - Well-demarcated, mixed "bubbly" appearance common
  - Variable enhancement but usually heterogeneous
- Differential Diagnosis
  - Diffuse astrocytoma; pleomorphic xanthoastrocytoma; supratentorial ependymoma

Chordoid Glioma of the Third Ventricle
- Pathology
  - Lobulated solid mass
  - Moderately vascular
  - Neoplastic epithelioid cells in mucinous background
  - GFAP+ but IDH-
  - WHO grade II
- Clinical Features
  - Middle-aged adults
  - M:F = 1:2
  - Presentation usually hypothalamic dysfunction
- Imaging Findings
  - Ovoid T2/FLAIR mildly hyperintense 3rd ventricle mass
  - Clearly separate from pituitary, infundibulum
  - Strong, uniform enhancement typical
- Differential Diagnosis
  - 3rd ventricle macroadenoma, craniopharyngioma; chordoid meningioma

Angiocentric Glioma
- Pathology
  - *MYB-QK1* fusion
  - Cortically based
  - Usually frontal, temporal lobes
- Clinical Features
  - Children, young adults
  - > 95% present with intractable epilepsy
- Imaging Findings
  - Expansile cortical mass without sharp borders
  - T2/FLAIR hyperintense
  - Subtle rim of T1 shortening common
  - May have "stalk-like" extension toward ventricle
  - Usually doesn't enhance

Selected References

Oligodendrogliomas

Halani SH et al: Defining neoplastic diseases differently: an emerging paradigm from The Cancer Genome Atlas lower-grade gliomas project. Mol Cell Oncol. 3(2):e1074333, 2016

Reifenberger G et al: Oligodendroglioma, IDH-mutant and 1p/19q codeleted. In: Louis DN et al (eds), WHO Classification of Tumours of the Central Nervous System. Lyon, France: International Agency for Research on Cancer, 2016, pp 60-77

Roth RM et al: Discordant mismatch repair protein immunoreactivity in Lynch syndrome-associated neoplasms: a recommendation for screening synchronous/metachronous neoplasms. Am J Clin Pathol. 146(1):50-6, 2016

Tanboon J et al: The diagnostic use of immunohistochemical surrogates for signature molecular genetic alterations in gliomas. J Neuropathol Exp Neurol. 75(1):4-18, 2016

Ellenbogen JR et al: Genetics and imaging of oligodendroglial tumors. CNS Oncol. 4(5):307-15, 2015

Oligodendroglioma, IDH-Mutant and 1p/19q Codeleted

Komori T: Pathology of oligodendroglia: an overview. Neuropathology. ePub, 2017

Yoon HJ et al: Differential diagnosis of oligodendroglial and astrocytic tumors using imaging results: the added value of perfusion MR imaging. Neuroradiology. ePub, 2017

Smits M: Imaging of oligodendroglioma. Br J Radiol. 89(1060):20150857, 2016

Oligodendroglioma Lacking IDH Mutation and 1p/19q Codeletion

Wu CT et al: Oligodendrogliomas in children: clinical experiences with 20 patients. J Pediatr Hematol Oncol. 38(7):555-8, 2016

Kumar A et al: Oncogenic KIAA1549-BRAF fusion with activation of the MAPK/ERK pathway in pediatric oligodendrogliomas. Cancer Genet. 208(3):91-5, 2015

Ependymal Tumors

Bi Z et al: Clinical, radiological, and pathological features in 43 cases of intracranial subependymoma. J Neurosurg. 122(1):49-60, 2015

Pajtler KW et al: Molecular classification of ependymal tumors across all CNS compartments, histopathological grades, and age groups. Cancer Cell. 27(5):728-43, 2015

Ependymoma

Pajtler KW et al: The current consensus on the clinical management of intracranial ependymoma and its distinct molecular variants. Acta Neuropathol. 133(1):5-12, 2017

Tsangaris GT et al: Pediatric ependymoma: a proteomics perspective. Cancer Genomics Proteomics. 14(2):127-136, 2017

Ellison DW et al: Ependymoma. In: Louis DN et al (eds), WHO Classification of Tumours of the Central Nervous System. Lyon, France: International Agency for Research on Cancer, 2016, pp 106-112

Lee CH et al: The similarities and differences between intracranial and spinal ependymomas : a review from a genetic research perspective. J Korean Neurosurg Soc. 59(2):83-90, 2016

Thompson YY et al: Posterior fossa ependymoma: current insights. Childs Nerv Syst. 31(10):1699-706, 2015

Anaplastic Ependymoma

Zakrzewska M et al: Altered microRNA expression is associated with tumor grade, molecular background and outcome in childhood infratentorial ependymoma. PLoS One. 11(7):e0158464, 2016

Ependymoma, RELA- and YAP1-Fusion-Positive

Louis DN et al: The 2016 World Health Organization Classification of Tumors of the Central Nervous System: a summary. Acta Neuropathol. 131(6):803-20, 2016

Cachia D et al: C11orf95-RELA fusion present in a primary supratentorial ependymoma and recurrent sarcoma. Brain Tumor Pathol. 32(2):105-11, 2015

Subependymoma

Fischer SB et al: TRPS1 gene alterations in human subependymoma. J Neurooncol. ePub, 2017

Nguyen HS et al: Intracranial subependymoma: a SEER analysis 2004-2013. World Neurosurg. 101:599-605, 2017

Zhou S et al: Neuroradiological features of cervical and cervicothoracic intraspinal subependymomas: a study of five cases. Clin Radiol. 71(5):499.e9-15, 2016

Jain A et al: Subependymoma: clinical features and surgical outcomes. Neurol Res. 34(7):677-84, 2012

Myxopapillary Ependymoma

Khan NR et al: Primary seeding of myxopapillary ependymoma: different disease in adult population? Case report and review of literature. World Neurosurg. 99:812.e21-812.e26, 2017

Bandopadhayay P et al: Myxopapillary ependymomas in children: imaging, treatment and outcomes. J Neurooncol. 126(1):165-74, 2016

Celano E et al: Spinal cord ependymoma: a review of the literature and case series of ten patients. J Neurooncol. 128(3):377-86, 2016

Chen X et al: Spinal myxopapillary ependymomas: a retrospective clinical and immunohistochemical study. Acta Neurochir (Wien). 158(1):101-7, 2016

Choroid Plexus Tumors

Choroid Plexus Papilloma

Bahar M et al: Choroid plexus tumors in adult and pediatric populations: the Cleveland Clinic and University Hospitals experience. J Neurooncol. 132(3):427-432, 2017

Shi YZ et al: Atypical choroid plexus papilloma: clinicopathological and neuroradiological features. Acta Radiol. 284185116676651, 2017

Abdulkader MM et al: Disseminated choroid plexus papillomas in adults: a case series and review of the literature. J Clin Neurosci. 32:148-54, 2016

Paulus W et al: Choroid plexus papilloma. In: Louis DN et al (eds), WHO Classification of Tumours of the Central Nervous System. Lyon, France: International Agency for Research on Cancer, 2016, pp 124-127

Safaee M et al: Choroid plexus papillomas: advances in molecular biology and understanding of tumorigenesis. Neuro Oncol. 15(3):255-67, 2013

Atypical Choroid Plexus Papilloma

Thomas C et al: Methylation profiling of choroid plexus tumors reveals 3 clinically distinct subgroups. Neuro Oncol. 18(6):790-6, 2016

Choroid Plexus Carcinoma

Thomas C et al: Methylation profiling of choroid plexus tumors reveals 3 clinically distinct subgroups. Neuro Oncol. 18(6):790-6, 2016

Dangouloff-Ros V et al: Choroid plexus neoplasms: toward a distinction between carcinoma and papilloma using arterial spin-labeling. AJNR Am J Neuroradiol. 36(9):1786-90, 2015

Other Neuroepithelial Tumors

Astroblastoma

Lehman NL et al: Morphological and molecular features of astroblastoma, including BRAFV600E mutations, suggest an ontological relationship to other cortical-based gliomas of children and young adults. Neuro Oncol. 19(1):31-42, 2017

Mallick S et al: Patterns of care and survival outcomes in patients with astroblastoma: an individual patient data analysis of 152 cases. Childs Nerv Syst. ePub, 2017

Aldape KD et al: Astroblastoma. In: Louis DN et al (eds), WHO Classification of Tumours of the Central Nervous System. Lyon, France: International Agency for Research on Cancer, 2016, pp 121-122.

Cunningham DA et al: Neuroradiologic characteristics of astroblastoma and systematic review of the literature: 2 new cases and 125 cases reported in 59 publications. Pediatr Radiol. 46(9):1301-8, 2016

Chordoid Glioma of the Third Ventricle

Erwood AA et al: Chordoid glioma of the third ventricle: report of a rapidly progressive case. J Neurooncol. 132(3):487-495, 2017

Brat DJ, Fuller GN: Chordoid glioma of the third ventricle. In: Louis DN et al (eds), WHO Classification of Tumours of the Central Nervous System. Lyon, France: International Agency for Research on Cancer, 2016, pp 116-118

Bongetta D et al: Chordoid glioma: a rare radiologically, histologically, and clinically mystifying lesion. World J Surg Oncol. 13:188, 2015

Morais BA et al: Chordoid glioma: case report and review of the literature. Int J Surg Case Rep. 7C:168-71, 2015

Angiocentric Glioma

Ampie L et al: Clinical attributes and surgical outcomes of angiocentric gliomas. J Clin Neurosci. 28:117-22, 2016

Bandopadhayay P et al: MYB-QKI rearrangements in angiocentric glioma drive tumorigenicity through a tripartite mechanism. Nat Genet. 48(3):273-82, 2016

Neuronal and Glioneuronal Tumors

As previously discussed, neuroepithelial tumors are the largest group of CNS neoplasms. By definition, the term "neuroepithelial tumor" encompasses all neoplasms that are derived from glial or neuronal precursor stem cells.

Pure glial neoplasms—astrocytomas and the heterogeneous group of nonastrocytic gliomas—were considered in the preceding two chapters. We now turn our attention to the next major group of primary CNS neoplasms, i.e., neuroepithelial tumors with ganglion-like cells and/or differentiated neurocytes.

Pineal parenchymal tumors and embryonal tumors with poorly differentiated proliferating neuroblasts, the last two subgroups of neuroepithelial tumors, are discussed in Chapters 20 and 21, respectively.

Glioneuronal Tumors

The recognition of new low-grade gliomas that contain distinct neurocytic elements has broadened the spectrum of glioneuronal tumors. Neuronal and mixed glioneuronal tumors have varying morphologic patterns and biologic behavior. Glioneuronal tumors are less common than pure glial neoplasms (e.g., astrocytomas and oligodendrogliomas), accounting for 0.5-2.0% of all primary brain tumors. As a group, glioneuronal neoplasms are often associated with seizures, less biologically aggressive than most other glial tumors, and generally have a more favorable prognosis.

Most tumors in the neuronal and mixed glioneuronal category are designated as WHO grade I. More aggressive glioneuronal tumors that morphologically resemble malignant gliomas but show immunohistochemical evidence of some neuronal differentiation are uncommon. These anaplastic gangliogliomas are the only tumor in this category that are assigned WHO grade III. There are no glioneuronal tumors that are designated as WHO grade IV neoplasms.

We begin this section by discussing the most common histologically mixed glioneuronal neoplasm, **ganglioglioma**. We then briefly consider **desmoplastic infantile tumors** that have astrocytic and/or ganglion cell elements.

We then consider **dysembryoplastic neuroepithelial tumor (DNET)**, now recognized as one of the more common causes of temporal lobe epilepsy. We conclude the section by discussing two rare glioneuronal tumors (**rosette-forming glioneuronal tumor** and **papillary glioneuronal tumor**) and the newly recognized **diffuse leptomeningeal glioneuronal tumor**.

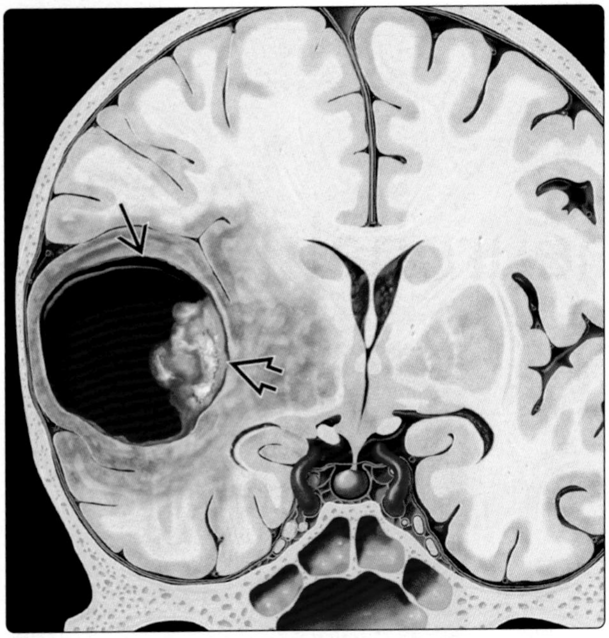

(19-1) Coronal graphic depicts typical ganglioglioma of the temporal lobe with cyst → and a partially calcified mural nodule →.

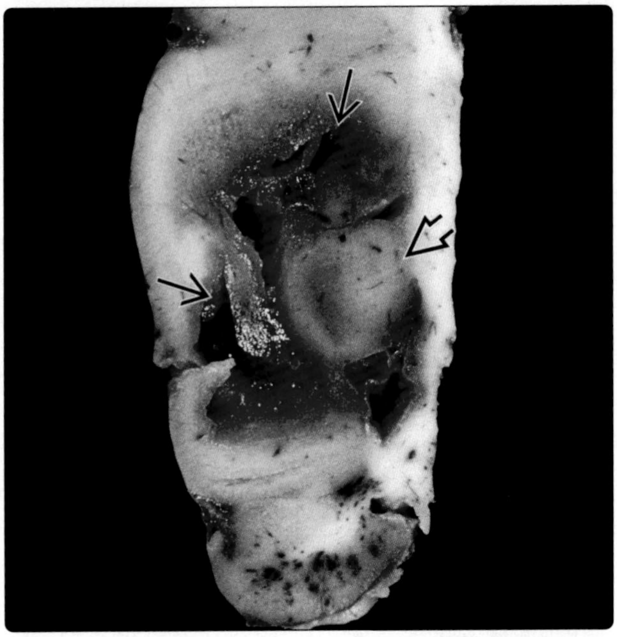

(19-2) Partial temporal lobectomy specimen with ganglioglioma shows tumor nodule →, partially collapsed cysts →. Hemorrhage is primarily surgical. (Courtesy R. Hewlett, MD.)

Overview of Ganglion Cell Tumors

Ganglion cell tumors are benign, well-differentiated neoplasms characterized by the presence of dysplastic ganglion cells. Two types of ganglion cell tumors are recognized, gangliocytomas and gangliogliomas. Gangliocytomas—ganglion cell tumors that demonstrate *exclusive* ganglion cell composition—are relatively rare and are discussed in the following section together with neuronal neoplasms and tumor-like lesions.

The vast majority of ganglion cell tumors are histologically mixed lesions that contain *both* neoplastic ganglion cell and glial elements. These neoplasms are called **gangliogliomas** and designated as WHO grade I. More aggressive tumors (i.e., those with substantial mitotic activity, microvascular proliferation, and occasional necrosis), called **anaplastic gangliomas**, are assigned WHO grade III.

Ganglioglioma

Terminology

Ganglioglioma (GG) is a well-differentiated, slow-growing tumor composed of dysplastic ganglion cells and neoplastic glial cells.

Etiology

Etiology and Molecular Genetics. Molecular genetics suggest that the neuronal and glial components in GGs both derive from a common precursor cell. The most frequent genetic alterations are *BRAF* V600E mutation (40-60%). *H3F3A* mutations occur in midline pediatric grade 1 GGs but have a better outcome than the diffuse pontine gliomas.

GG has been reported in Turcot syndrome as well as neurofibromatosis type 1 and neurofibromatosis type 2.

Pathology

Location. GGs occur throughout the CNS. Most are located superficially, and more than 75% arise in the temporal lobe **(19-1)**. The next most common site is the frontal lobe, the location for 10% of GGs. A few GGs have been reported in the ventricles.

Approximately 15% of GGs are found in the posterior fossa, usually either in the brainstem or cerebellum. GGs also occur as cerebellopontine angle cistern and intramedullary cord lesions.

Size and Number. GGs are solitary lesions that virtually never metastasize unless they undergo malignant transformation. They vary in size from 1-6 cm.

Gross Pathology. GGs are superficially located, firm, grayish-tan neoplasms that often expand the cortex **(19-2)**. The most common appearance is that of a cyst with mural nodule or a solid tumor. Calcification is common, but gross hemorrhage and frank necrosis are rare.

Microscopic Features. The histologic hallmark of GG is its combination of neuronal and glial elements, which can be intermixed or geographically separated. Varying numbers of dysplastic neurons are interspersed with the glial component, which constitutes the proliferative and neoplastic element of the tumor. Astrocytic cells with pilocytic or fibrillary-like features are the most common glial element.

Mitotic figures are rare. MIB-1 reflects the proliferating glial component and varies from 1-3%.

Immunohistochemistry staining demonstrates both neuronal features (i.e., synaptophysin expression) and glial features [glial fibrillary acidic protein (GFAP)-positive cells). Approximately 75% of GGs exhibit immunoreactivity for the stem cell epitope CD34. GGs are IDH-negative.

Malignant features in GGs are uncommon but—when present—almost invariably involve the glial component. Sarcomatous change occurs but is rare.

Staging, Grading, and Classification. GGs are benign and designated as WHO grade I neoplasms. GGs with anaplastic features correspond histologically to WHO grade III. Criteria for an intermediate grade of GG (WHO grade II) have been discussed but not established. Malignant transformation of grade I GG occurs but is rare (see below).

Clinical Issues

Epidemiology. GG is the most common mixed glioneuronal tumor but accounts for just 1.0-1.5% of all primary brain tumors. GGs are more common in children and represent between 5-10% of pediatric CNS neoplasms.

Demographics. GG is predominantly a tumor of children and young adults; 80% of patients are younger than 30 years. Peak presentation is 15-20 years. There is no sex predilection.

Presentation. Chronic, pharmacologically resistant temporal lobe epilepsy is present in the majority of cases. Seizures are generally the complex partial type.

Natural History. GGs are typically very slow-growing neoplasms. Recent studies have shown that GGs with nonseizure presentation and atypical imaging findings are less amenable to gross total resection and are associated with worse outcomes despite WHO grade I status.

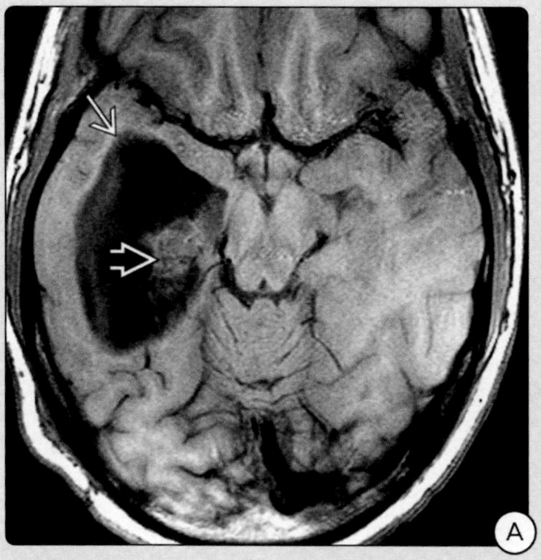

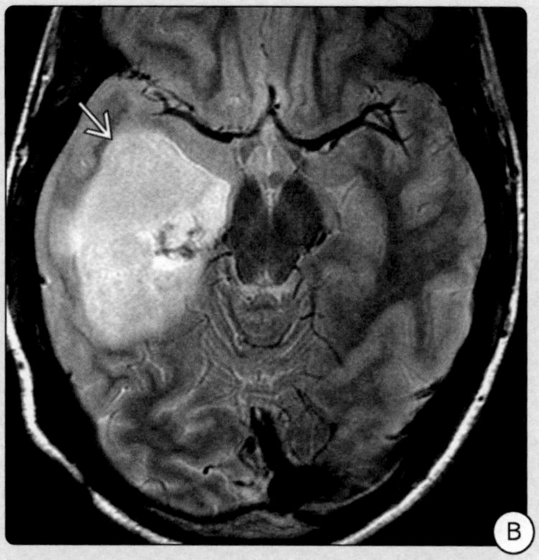

***(19-3A)** Axial T1WI in a 15y boy with right temporal lobe epilepsy shows a large mass with cystic and heterogeneous-appearing solid components. **(19-3B)** Axial PD in the same case shows that the cyst is hyperintense compared with the adjacent brain.*

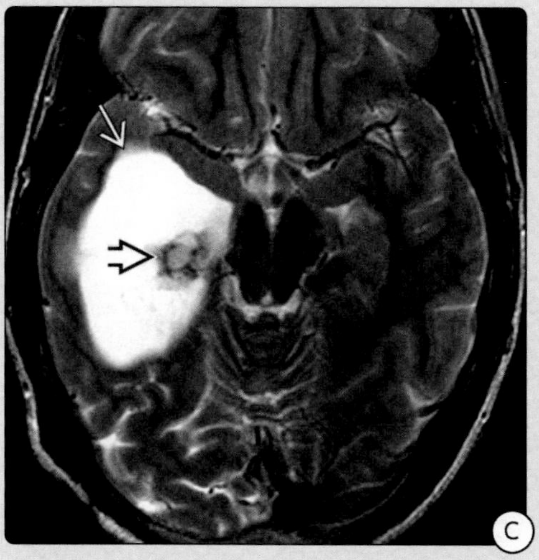

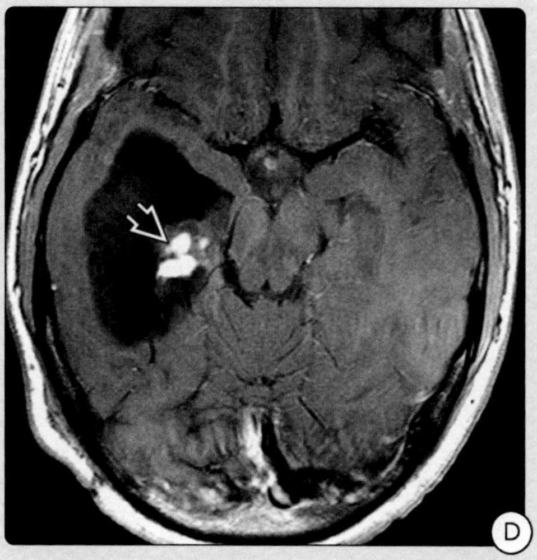

***(19-3C)** T2WI in the same case shows the hyperintense cyst. The nodule is mixed hypo- and hyperintense compared with the brain. **(19-3D)** T1 C+ MR shows that parts of the nodule enhance, whereas the cyst wall does not. Pathologic diagnosis was ganglioglioma, WHO grade I.*

Malignant degeneration is uncommon, occurring in 1-5% of cases.

Treatment Options. Complete surgical resection is generally curative, with 80% of patients becoming seizure-free after tumor removal. The vast majority of patients experience a 5-year recurrence-free survival.

Imaging

General Features. GGs are cortically based superficial parenchymal lesions that have two general imaging patterns: (1) a well-defined solid or partially cystic mass with mural nodule **(19-3)** and (2) a diffusely infiltrating, less well-delineated mass with ill-defined borders and patchy enhancement uncommonly occurring.

CT Findings. GGs display varying attenuation on NECT. A cystic component is seen in nearly 60% of cases. Approximately 30% have a well-circumscribed hypodense cyst with isodense mural nodule, whereas 40% are primarily hypodense. Between 30-50% of GGs calcify. Hemorrhage is rare.

Only 50% of GGs enhance following contrast administration. Patterns vary from solid, rim, or nodular to cystic with an enhancing nodule.

MR Findings. Compared with cortex, GGs are hypo- to isointense on T1WI and hyperintense on T2/FLAIR. Surrounding edema is generally absent. Focal cortical dysplasia adjacent to the tumor occurs in some cases.

Enhancement varies from none or minimal to moderate but heterogeneous. The classic pattern is a cystic mass with an enhancing mural nodule. Homogeneous solid enhancement also occurs. Ill-defined, patchy enhancement is atypical and associated with a worse clinical outcome **(19-4)**.

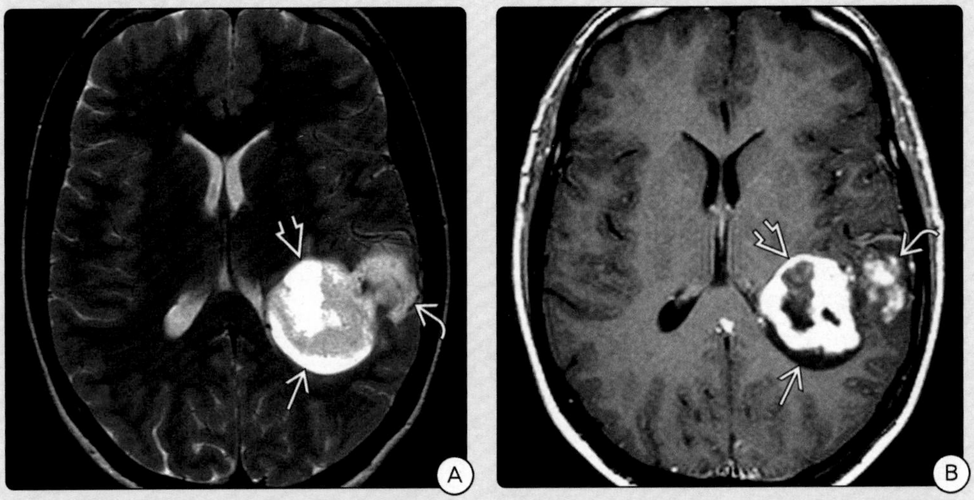

***(19-4A)** Axial T2WI in a 30y woman with seizures shows an ill-defined heterogeneously hyperintense left parietal mass ➡ and cyst ➡ extending superficially toward the cortex ➡. **(19-4B)** T1 C+ shows a large mixed cystic-solid enhancing mass ➡ with an adjacent nonenhancing cyst ➡. Ill-defined patchy enhancement extends from the mass to the cortex ➡.*

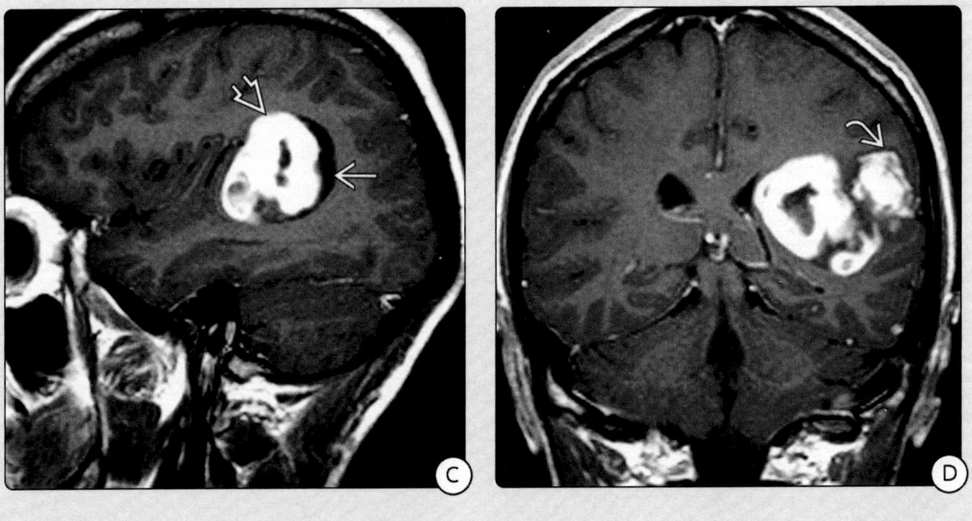

***(19-4C)** Sagittal T1 C+ shows the solid ➡, cystic ➡ nature of the mass. **(19-4D)** Coronal T1 C+ shows that the patchy, ill-defined enhancement extends toward the cortex ➡. This is a ganglioglioma, WHO grade I, but MIB-1 = 5%. Biopsy of tumor recurrence 3 years later showed anaplastic features that were not present on the original histopathology.*

Differential Diagnosis

The major differential consideration is **diffuse astrocytoma**. Note that diffuse infiltrating astrocytoma typically does not enhance. A supratentorial hemispheric **pilocytic astrocytoma** can present as a cyst with an enhancing nodule. Calcification in pilocytic astrocytoma is rare compared with GG.

Pleomorphic xanthoastrocytoma (PXA) often has a "cyst + mural nodule" and resembles GG. PXA often has a dural "tail," helping to distinguish it from other epilepsy-inducing cortical neoplasms.

Dysembryoplastic neuroepithelial tumor (DNET) is a superficial cortical neoplasm that typically has a multicystic "bubbly" appearance. A hyperintense rim surrounding the mass on FLAIR scan is common. In contrast to GG, enhancement is rare.

Oligodendroglioma is typically more diffuse and less well delineated than GG. Oligodendrogliomas with a "cyst + mural nodule" configuration are uncommon. When they do occur, they are difficult to distinguish from GG on imaging studies alone.

CAUSES OF TEMPORAL LOBE EPILEPSY

Most common = mesial temporal sclerosis

Tumor-associated temporal lobe epilepsy
- Ganglioglioma (40%)
- DNET (20%)
- Diffuse low-grade astrocytoma (20%)
- Other (20%)
  - Pilocytic astrocytoma
  - Pleomorphic xanthoastrocytoma
  - Oligodendroglioma

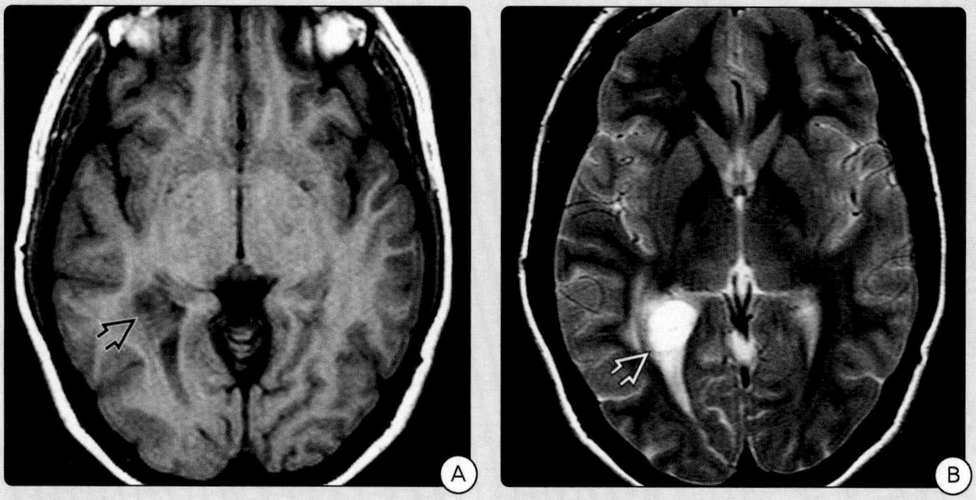

*(**19-5A**) T1WI in a 28y woman with headaches shows a mixed iso-/hypointense mass ➡ in or adjacent to the atrium of the right lateral ventricle. (**19-5B**) T2WI in the same case shows that the mass ➡ is very hyperintense.*

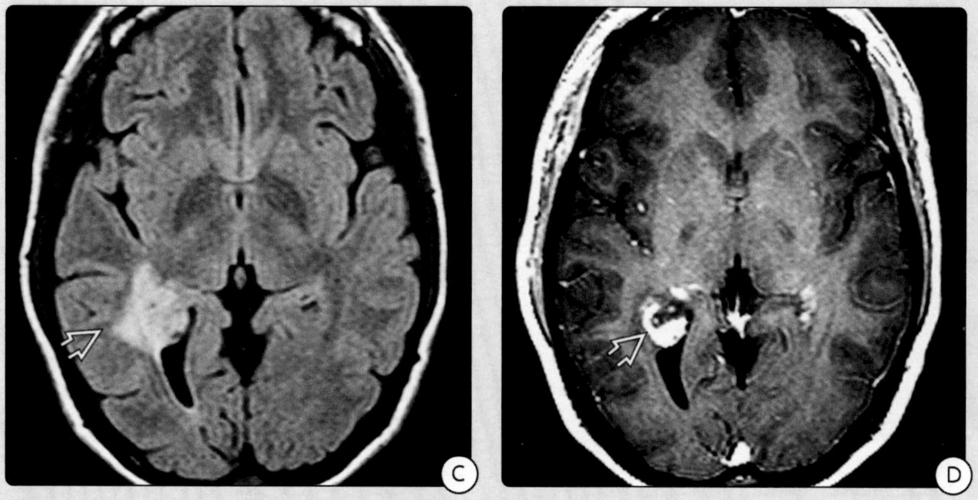

*(**19-5C**) FLAIR shows that the mass is very hyperintense and appears to extend into the deep periventricular white matter ➡. (**19-5D**) T1 C+ shows that the mass ➡ enhances intensely but heterogeneously. Pathology disclosed anaplastic ganglioglioma, WHO grade III.*

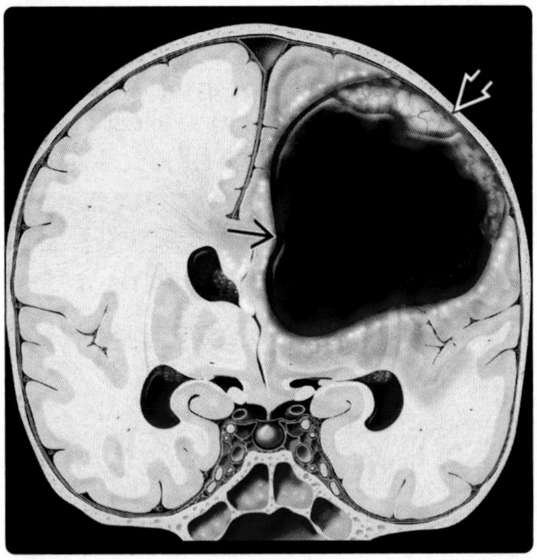

(19-6) Graphic depicts desmoplastic infantile astrocytoma/ganglioma with large mixed cystic, solid component abutting the dura.

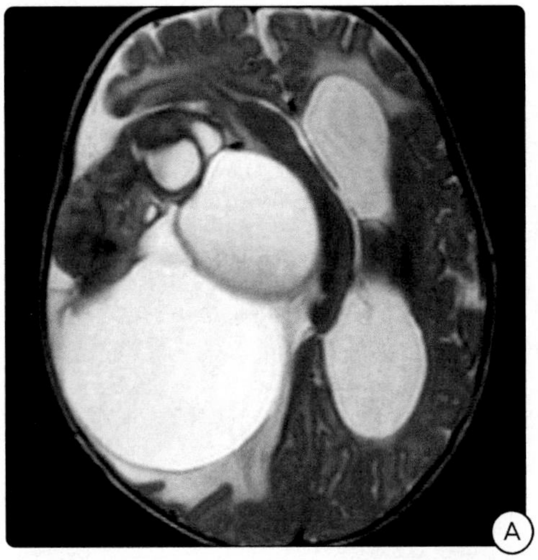

(19-7A) T2WI in a 10m infant shows obstructive hydrocephalus, huge mixed cystic, solid mass in the right cerebral hemisphere.

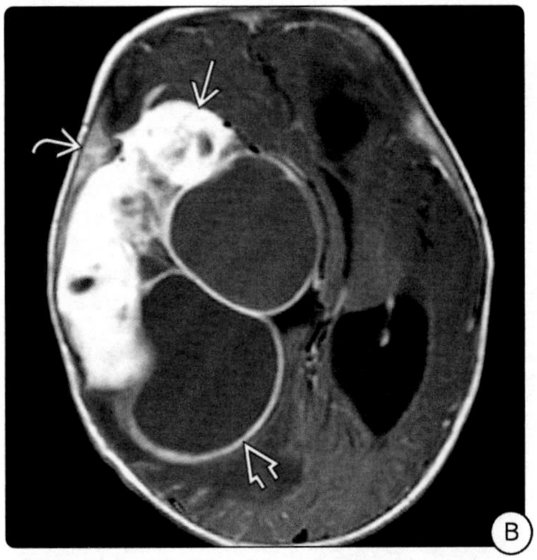

(19-7B) T1 C+ shows the solid mass abuts, thickens the dura-arachnoid and enhances intensely, as do the cyst walls; DIA.

Anaplastic Ganglioglioma

Anaplastic ganglioglioma (AGG) is a rare, aggressive glioneuronal tumor that represents approximately 6% of all GGs. Markers to predict anaplastic transformation of GGs are poorly defined although H3 histone mutation (K27M in *H3F3A*) has been reported in one case of GG with spontaneous malignant transformation.

AGGs are composed of dysplastic ganglion cells and an anaplastic (usually glial) component. Malignant changes almost invariably involve the glial component and include increased cellularity, cellular pleomorphism, and frequent mitoses with occasional necrotic foci. AGGs are WHO grade III neoplasms.

AGGs most commonly affect children and young adults. Most reported cases are supratentorial, highly epileptogenic tumors. The temporal lobe is the most common site, but cases have been reported within the spinal cord and ventricles **(19-5)**. Radiologic findings are nonspecific and overlap those of GG and diffuse astrocytomas. Recurrence following surgery is common, often resulting in diffuse craniospinal metastases.

GANGLIOGLIOMAS

Ganglioglioma
- Terminology
  - Well-differentiated, slow-growing tumor
  - Biphasic tumor with variable combination of neuronal, glial elements
- Etiology and Genetics
  - Both components share common progenitor stem cell
  - *BRAF* V600E mutation
  - IDH1(-), 1p/19q not codeleted
- Pathology
  - Dysplastic ganglion cells + neoplastic glial cells
  - Superficial, corticocentric
  - Solid or mixed cystic/solid
  - Temporal, frontal lobes > parietal > brainstem, ventricles
  - Usually noninfiltrative
  - Few/no mitoses (MIB-1 = 1-3%)
  - WHO grade I
- Clinical Issues
  - Most common mixed glial-neuronal neoplasm
  - 1% of all primary brain tumors but 10% in children
  - Common presentation = seizures
  - Children, young adults
- Imaging Findings
  - Well-delineated (often temporal lobe) mass
  - Cyst + enhancing nodule most common

Anaplastic Ganglioglioma
- Etiology
  - Most are malignant transformation of previously diagnosed benign GG
  - 8-10% of GGs
- Pathology
  - Dysplastic ganglion cells + anaplastic glial component
  - Increased cellularity, mitoses
  - Vascular proliferation, necrosis
  - WHO grade III
- Imaging Findings
  - Atypical location common (i.e., deep rather than cortical)
  - Often larger, more infiltrative/poorly demarcated

Desmoplastic Infantile Astrocytoma/Ganglioglioma

Terminology

Intracranial desmoplastic infantile tumors are rare, usually benign, mostly cystic lesions of young children that often have a radiologically aggressive appearance. Two histologic forms of desmoplastic infantile tumors have been described: desmoplastic infantile astrocytoma (DIA) and desmoplastic infantile ganglioglioma (DIG). Because elements of both types are often present in a single lesion, the WHO considers DIA/DIG a single tumor entity.

Pathology

DIA/DIGs are large, bulky, supratentorial hemispheric masses with a median diameter approaching 8 cm. They are sharply demarcated, mixed cystic-solid tumors that involve the superficial cortex and the adjacent leptomeninges, often appearing attached to the dura **(19-6)**. The frontal and parietal lobes are the most common sites.

Microscopically, DIA/DIGs have three distinct components: spindle cells in a "desmoplastic" stroma, plump astrocytes with glassy cytoplasm, and a variable neuronal component, usually clusters of undifferentiated neuronal or ganglion cells. Tumors without a ganglion cell component are termed DIA.

Mitotic activity is rare. DIA/DIG is designated as a WHO grade I tumor.

Clinical Issues

DIA/DIGs primarily occur in children under the age of 5 years, with a large majority presenting within the first year of life. Between 20-25% occur in children older than 24 months.

Increasing head circumference with tense bulging fontanelles in a lethargic infant with "sunset eyes" is the typical presentation.

Most intracranial neoplasms that present in infants and neonates are associated with poor outcome. In contrast, DIA/DIG has a benign prognosis and very rarely metastasizes. Gross total resection generally results in long-term survival. Some DIA/DIGs even regress spontaneously after partial debulking.

Approximately 15% of children with DIA/DIG develop leptomeningeal spread and die.

Imaging

Imaging discloses a massive, heterogeneous, peripherally located mixed cystic-solid supratentorial mass. The cystic portion is usually located relatively deep inside the hemispheric white matter, whereas the solid portion is typically peripheral, often directly abutting the dura.

CT shows a cystic hypoattenuating portion with a mixed-density solid component. Calcification has been reported in a few cases but is uncommon. Hemorrhage, necrosis, and peritumoral edema are rare.

MR shows a large, often multilobulated or septated cystic mass with a solid plaque-like dura-based component. The solid mass is often iso-/hypointense on T2WI and enhances strongly but often heterogeneously **(19-7)**. Adjacent dural thickening ("dural tail" sign) is common. Approximately 25% of cases show at least some cyst wall enhancement.

Even though they are benign neoplasms, DIA/DIGs may exhibit restricted diffusion.

MRS is nonspecific. Most cases demonstrate reduced NAA and elevated Cho. Few cases with pMR have been reported, but increased relative cerebral blood volume/flow has been reported compared with the peritumoral region and contralateral normal white matter.

Differential Diagnosis

The most common overall cause of a large, bulky, heterogeneous hemispheric mass in an infant is **teratoma**. Teratoma is much more heterogeneous appearing than DIA/DIG and often extends extracranially. **Primitive neuroectodermal tumor** (PNET) is another common congenital brain neoplasm. Teratomatous and PNET-related cysts are rarely as large as those of DIA/DIG, and their solid portions generally do not abut the dura.

RELA-fusion ependymoma often calcifies, hemorrhages, and typically occurs in older children and adults.

DESMOPLASTIC INFANTILE ASTROCYTOMA/GANGLIOGLIOMA

Terminology
- Two forms of desmoplastic infantile tumors
  - Desmoplastic infantile astrocytoma (DIA)
  - Desmoplastic infantile ganglioglioma (DIG)

Pathology
- Rare benign glioneuronal tumor
- Prominent desmoplastic leptomeningeal stromal reaction
  - Fibroblasts, collagen-rich matrix
  - Low-grade spindle cells
- Neuroepithelial cells (can appear relatively poorly differentiated)
  - Neoplastic astrocytes (DIA)
  - Variably mature neuronal component (DIG)
- Ki-67 usually < 2%
- WHO grade I

Clinical Issues
- Most present in first year of life

Imaging Findings
- Typically large, bulky supratentorial mass
- Multiple cysts, solid components

Differential Diagnosis
- Teratoma
- *RELA*-fusion ependymoma

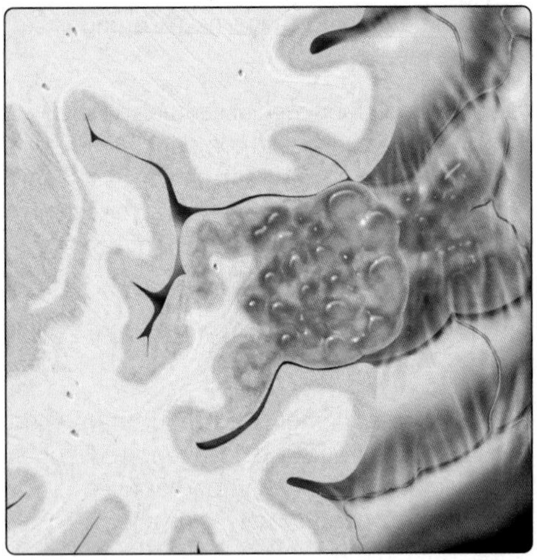

(19-8) Graphic depicts DNET with multicystic and multinodular components.

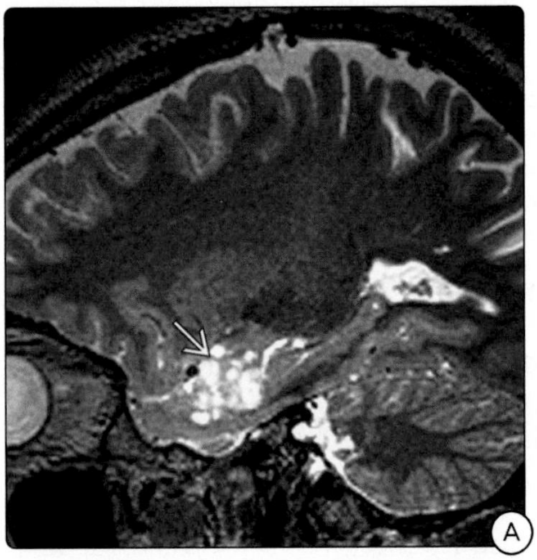

(19-9A) Sagittal T2WI shows a "bubbly" temporal lobe mass ➡.

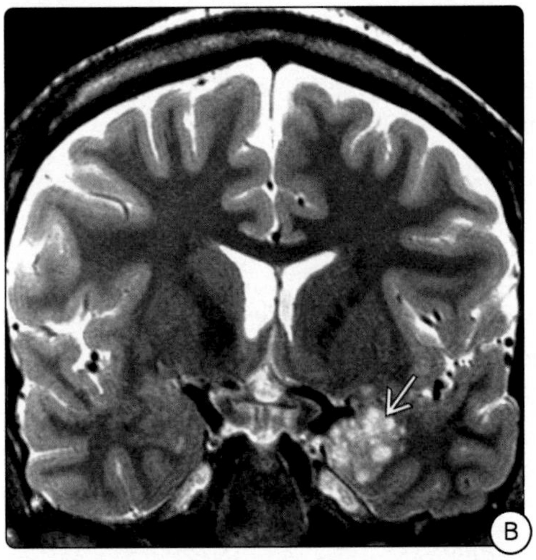

(19-9B) Coronal T2WI in the same patient shows a cortically based, "bubbly" mass with the typical appearance of a DNET ➡.

DNET

Ganglioglioma and dysembryoplastic neuroepithelial tumor (DNET) are the two most common long-term epilepsy-associated tumors. DNET was originally identified in the surgical specimens from young patients with medically refractory epilepsy. The 2016 WHO classification includes DNET in the category of "neuronal and mixed neuronal-glial tumors."

Terminology

DNET is a benign, usually cortically based lesion characterized by a multinodular architecture **(19-8)**. Because DNET is often associated with cortical dysplasia, some neuropathologists believe it may be a congenital malformation rather than a true neoplastic lesion.

Etiology

Most investigators believe DNETs have a dysontogenetic/malformative origin. Although the exact histogenesis remains unknown, whole-exome sequencing has shown that *FGFR1* alterations and MAP kinase pathway activation are key events in the pathogenesis of DNET. *BRAF* V600E mutations occur in 30-60% of cases. *TP53* and IDH mutations are absent. Whole-arm 1p/19q codeletion is also absent.

Pathology

Location. DNETs can be located in any part of the supratentorial cortex. Between 45-50% are located in the temporal lobes, whereas one-third occur in the frontal lobes. Rare cases have been reported in other sites such as the lateral ventricle, and an unusual "diffuse" form of DNET has been described.

Size and Number. DNETs are generally solitary lesions and vary in size from millimeters to several centimeters. A few tumors that involve a large portion of the affected lobe have been reported. Multifocal DNETs affecting different sites in the CNS have been reported.

Gross Pathology. DNETs are intracortical tumors that thicken and expand the gyri. The glioneuronal component often has a viscous consistency together with single or multiple firmer nodules **(19-10)**.

Microscopic Features. The histologic hallmark of DNET is its "specific glioneuronal element" (SGNE). "Simple" DNETs consist of the SGNE and nodular areas. A multinodular architecture with columns or nodules of bundled axons oriented perpendicularly to the cortex and lined by oligodendrocyte-like cells is characteristic. Neurons appear to float in a pale, mucinous-appearing matrix adjacent to these columns. Cytologic atypia, necrosis, and mitoses are rare. The Ki-67-labeling index is usually less than 1-2%.

"Complex" DNETs have additional features, including cortical dysplasia. The adjacent cortex is dysplastic in nearly 80% of DNETs.

Staging, Grading, and Classification. DNETs are WHO grade I neoplasms. Malignant transformation is rare although anaplasia has been reported after radiation and/or chemotherapy.

Clinical Issues

DNET is a tumor of children and young adults. Both familial and sporadic forms occur. DNETs occasionally occur in patients with neurofibromatosis type 1 or XYY syndrome.

DNET: ETIOLOGY AND PATHOLOGY

Etiology
- *FGFR1*, *BRAF* mutations

Pathology
- Benign (WHO grade I)
- Rare (< 1% of all neuroepithelial tumors)
- Location
  - Supratentorial, superficial
  - Intracortical
  - Temporal lobe most common site
- Multinodular architecture, heterogeneous cellular composition
  - Specific glioneuronal element
  - Oligodendrocyte-like cells in mucoid matrix with interspersed "floating" neurons
- Frequently associated with cortical dysplasia
  - Classified as ILAE FCD type IIIb

The vast majority of patients present before age 20 years, typically with pharmacologically resistant partial complex seizures. Although DNETs account for only 1% of all neuroepithelial tumors, they are second only to ganglioglioma as a cause of temporal lobe epilepsy.

DNETs show little or no growth over time. Even simple lesionectomy is generally successful. Because cortical dysplasia is frequently associated with DNET, however, a more aggressive resection is advocated by many epilepsy surgeons. Removing epileptogenically active areas around the tumor increases seizure-free outcome.

Long-term clinical follow-up usually demonstrates no tumor recurrence, even in patients with subtotal resection.

Imaging

General Features. DNET has a distinct appearance on neuroimaging studies. A well-demarcated, triangular,

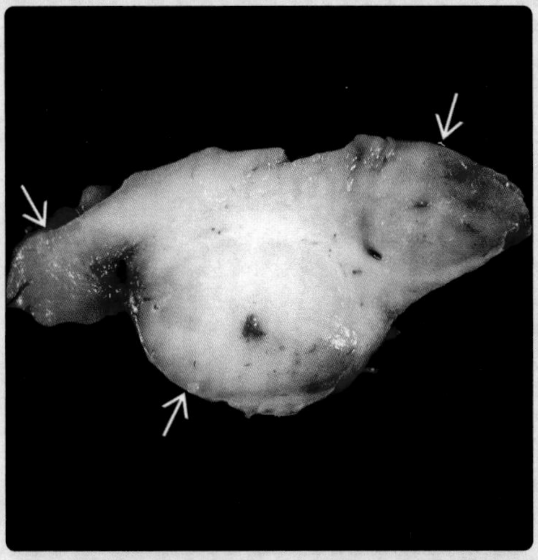

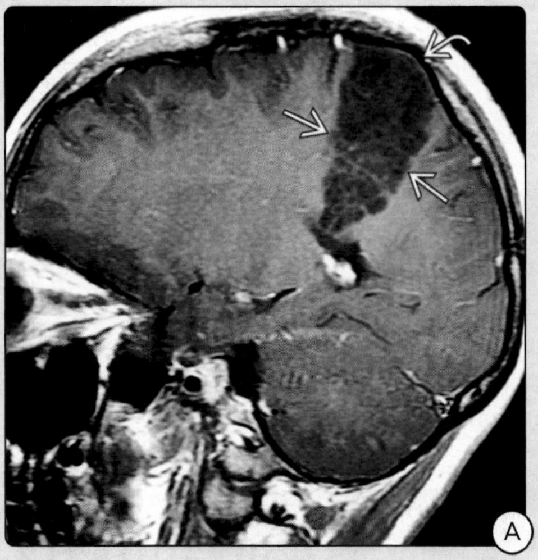

A

***(19-10)** Resected surgical specimen shows the typical nodular, somewhat "mucinous-appearing" cysts ➔ of a DNET. (Courtesy R. Hewlett, MD.) **(19-11A)** Sagittal T1 C+ in a 14y boy with longstanding right body complex partial seizures shows a wedge-shaped, superficially located "bubbly" mass ➔. The mass is hypointense and shows no enhancement. Note adjacent calvarial remodeling ➔.*

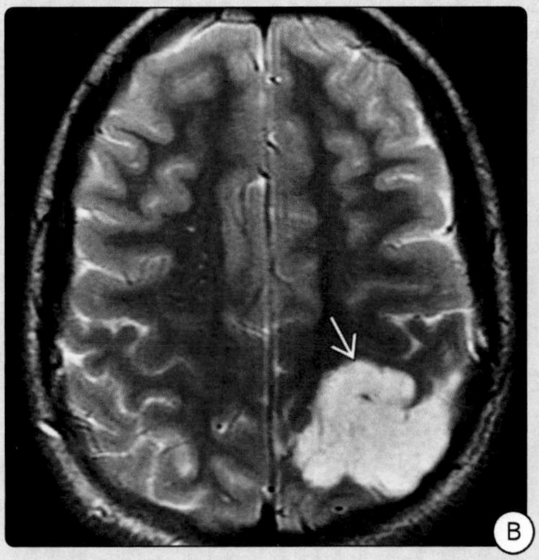

B

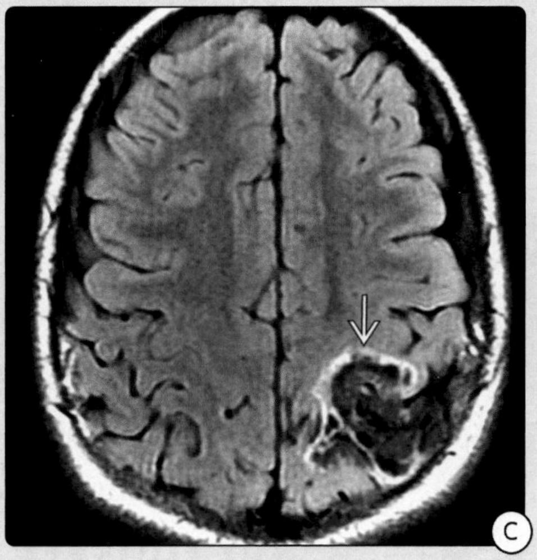

C

***(19-11B)** T2WI in the same case shows that the "bubbly-appearing" mass ➔ is very hyperintense and sharply demarcated. There is no surrounding edema. **(19-11C)** FLAIR in the same case shows that the mass is heterogeneously hypointense with a hyperintense rim ➔. Classic DNET was found at surgery.*

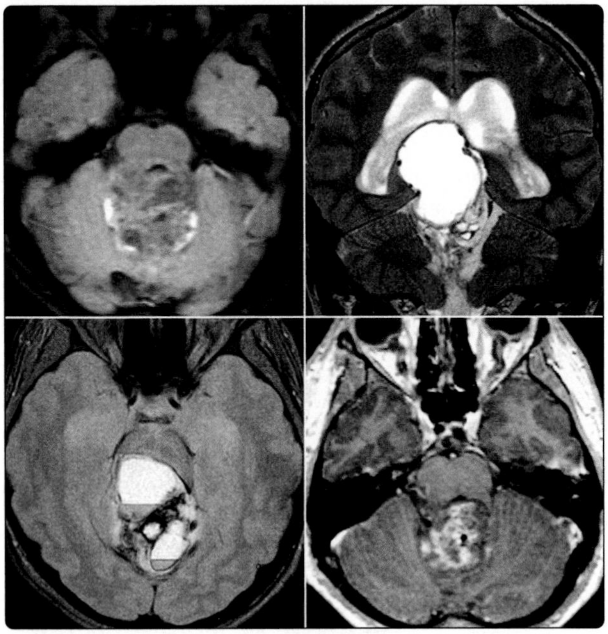

(19-12) RGNT is a very heterogeneous tumor with cysts, hemorrhage, fluid-fluid levels, and patchy enhancement. (Courtesy M. Thurnher, MD.)

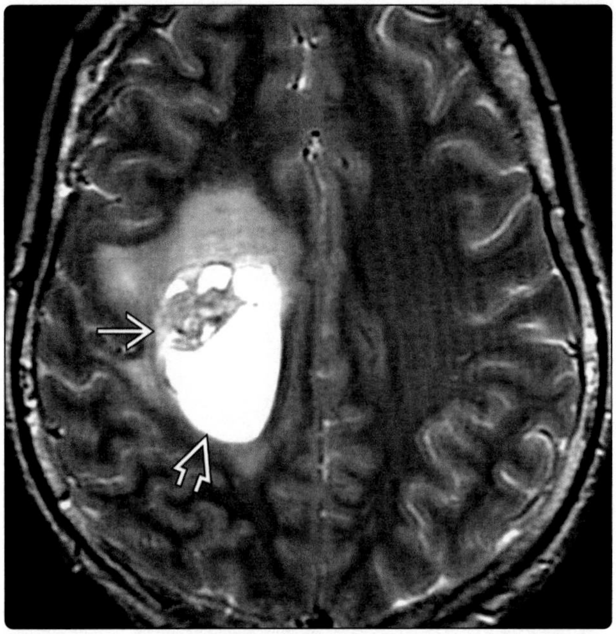

(19-13) T2WI of PGNT shows a well-circumscribed cystic ➡ mass with mural nodule ➡ in the right hemisphere. (Courtesy F. J. Rodriguez, MD.)

"pseudocystic" or "bubbly" cortical/subcortical mass in a young patient with longstanding complex partial epilepsy is highly suggestive of the diagnosis **(19-9)**.

CT Findings. NECT scans disclose a hypodense cortical/subcortical mass. Calcification is seen in 20% of cases. Gross intratumoral hemorrhage is rare. Focal bony scalloping or calvarial remodeling is common with tumors adjacent to the inner table of the skull.

DNET: CLINICAL ISSUES AND IMAGING

Clinical Issues
- Most patients < 20 years
  - Intractable, drug-resistant epilepsy
  - Second most common tumor-associated temporal lobe epilepsy
- Grows slowly, surgery usually curative
- Recurrence, malignant transformation very rare

Imaging
- Wedge-shaped cortical/subcortical mass
- "Points" toward ventricle
- Multicystic/septated "bubbly" appearance
  - Hyperintense on T2WI
  - Rim of hyperintensity on FLAIR
  - Edema absent
  - Usually doesn't enhance

MR Findings. A multilobulated, hypointense, "bubbly" cortical mass that may involve the subcortical white matter is seen on T1WI. DNETs are strikingly hyperintense on T2WI with a multicystic or septated appearance.

DNETs are hyperintense compared with normal cortex on FLAIR scans. A characteristic, even more hyperintense rim along the tumor periphery is present in 75% of cases **(19-11)**. Peritumoral edema is absent.

"Blooming" on T2* (GRE, SWI) occurs in a few cases, more likely related to calcification than to hemorrhage.

DNETs generally show little or no enhancement on T1WI C+. When present, enhancement is generally limited to a mild nodular or punctate pattern.

MRS shows decreased NAA without elevated Cho or Cho:Cr ratio.

Differential Diagnosis

The main imaging differential diagnoses are **focal cortical dysplasia, ganglioglioma,** and **multinodular and vacuolating neuronal tumor of the cerebrum (MVNT)**. The "bubbly" appearance of DNET and FLAIR hyperintense rims are helpful distinguishing features. MVNTs are typically multifocal and occur in the deep layers of the cortex and adjacent white matter.

The rare **angiocentric glioma** closely resembles DNET on imaging, but a hyperintense rim is seen on T1WI, not FLAIR.

Rosette-Forming Glioneuronal Tumor

Terminology

Rosette-forming glioneuronal tumor (RGNT) is a rare, slow-growing glioneuronal tumor that was originally described as occurring only in the fourth ventricle but is now recognized in other anatomic locations as well.

Pathology

RGNTs are generally infratentorial midline lesions. The most common—but by no means the only—location is the fourth ventricle and/or cerebellar vermis. The pineal region is the second most common site. Size varies from 1 or 2 cm to large bulky tumors that occasionally exceed 4 cm in diameter.

The pathologic hallmark of RGNT is its biphasic histology. Two distinct components are present. One consists of uniform neurocytes that form rosettes and/or perivascular pseudorosettes. The other is astrocytic and resembles pilocytic astrocytoma (PA). Despite their histologic similarity with PA, *BRAF* mutations have not been described in intracranial RGNTs. *IDH1/2* is negative, and 1p/19q is not codeleted.

MIB-1 labeling index is low. Local invasion and CSF dissemination are rare. RGNTs are WHO grade I neoplasms.

Clinical Issues

RGNT is a tumor of young and middle-aged adults. Mean age at diagnosis is 33 years. Typical presenting symptoms are headache and ataxia.

Imaging

The imaging appearance of a classic RGNT is more ominous than its benign pathology and biologic behavior would indicate. A heterogeneous-appearing mass centered within the fourth ventricle or vermis is the typical finding **(19-12)**. A multicystic appearance with hemorrhage on T2* (GRE or SWI), blood-fluid levels, and calcification is common.

A moderate peripheral/heterogeneous pattern of enhancement following contrast administration is typical. CSF dissemination with multiple satellite lesions may occur, so imaging the complete neuraxis is appropriate whenever an RGNT is suspected.

Differential Diagnosis

Because of its location and typical age at onset, the differential diagnosis of RGNT is limited. **Metastasis** is always a consideration but rare in young adults. Primary infratentorial midline neoplasms in this age group are uncommon.

Ependymoma with cysts and hemorrhage may resemble RGNT. **Pilocytic astrocytoma** is generally found in younger patients and rarely hemorrhages. **Choroid plexus papilloma** does occur in the fourth ventricle in adults, but its intense contrast enhancement and distinctive frond-like papillary architecture help distinguish it from RGNT.

Papillary Glioneuronal Tumor

Initially considered a ganglioglioma variant, papillary glioneuronal tumor (PGNT) is now recognized as a distinct entity. It is a rare, relatively well-circumscribed, clinically indolent tumor of the cerebral hemispheres that primarily affects young adults.

Similar to RGNTs, PGNTs are biphasic tumors with both astrocytic and neuronal elements. The distinguishing feature of PGNT is the presence of glial fibrillary acidic protein (GFAP)-positive neoplastic glial cells lining hyalinized vascular pseudopapillae. Synaptophysin-positive interpapillary collections of neurocytes, large neurons, and intermediate-sized "ganglioid" cells are present.

PGNT is designated as a WHO grade I neoplasm. A few reported cases have shown atypical histologic features or late biologic progression.

Imaging findings in PGNT are nonspecific. Most tumors are located in the deep periventricular white matter **(19-13)**. A well-circumscribed cyst with enhancing nodule is the most common reported appearance although mixed cystic and solid as well as completely solid masses have been reported. The major differential diagnosis is ganglioglioma, which has a virtually identical imaging appearance to PGNT.

Diffuse Leptomeningeal Glioneuronal Tumor

Terminology

Diffuse leptomeningeal glioneuronal tumor (DLGNT) is a rare primary glioneuronal neoplasm that is characterized by widespread, plaque-like leptomeningeal growth. Because these tumors often exhibit an oligodendroglial-like cytology, they have also been termed diffuse oligodendroglial-like leptomeningeal neoplasm or leptomeningeal oligodendrogliomatosis. Some investigators have termed the process diffuse leptomeningeal neuroepithelial tumor.

Etiology

The etiology of DLGNTs is unknown. The most frequently identified genetic alteration is *BRAF* fusion. *IDH1/2* mutations are absent. 1p/19q codeletion and isolated 1p deletion have been reported in some cases.

Pathology

Widespread diffuse leptomeningeal tumor spread with multifocal extension along the perivascular (Virchow-Robin) spaces is typical, as is infiltration of the cranial nerves. Tumor often coats the spinal cord and nerve roots.

DLGNTs are diffusely positive for both GFAP and synaptophysin. Scattered cells may be positive for oligodendrocyte transcription factor (OLIG2) and Neu-N.

No WHO grade has been assigned to DLGNTs. The vast majority of these rare tumors are low-grade lesions with MIB-1 < 1%. A subset shows anaplastic features with increased mitoses and glomeruloid microvascular proliferation.

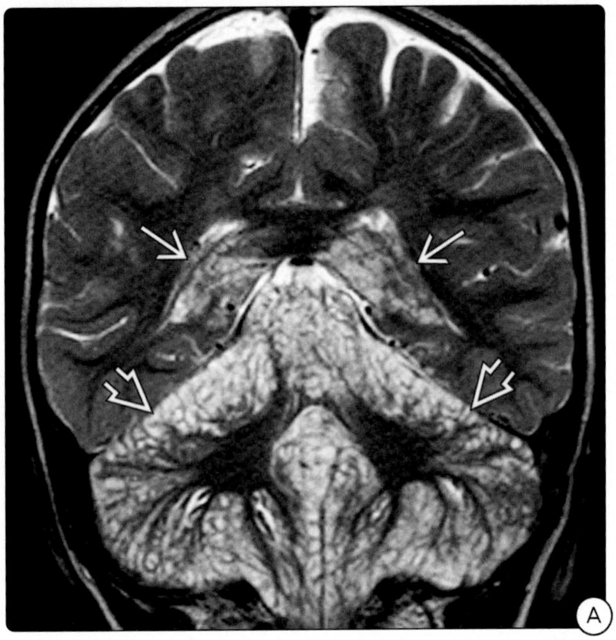

(19-14A) Coronal T2WI in a 5y boy with DLGT shows innumerable tiny hyperintense cysts studding the cerebellar folia and ventricular ependyma.

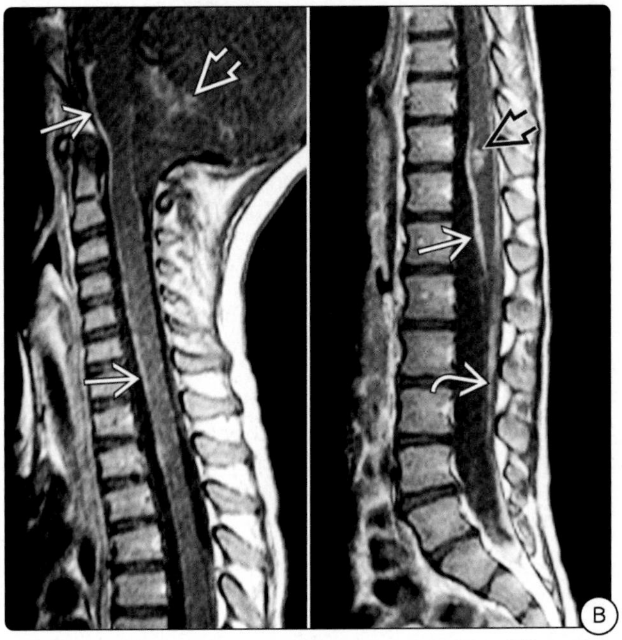

(19-14B) Sagittal T1 C+ scans in the same case show diffuse pial enhancement, enhancement of the cerebellar lesions, and cauda equina. Note enhancing mass in conus; diffuse leptomeningeal glioneuronal tumor. (Courtesy S. Blaser, MD.)

Clinical Issues

Age at presentation varies from 2-7 years with a mean of 4 years. A few cases in adults have been reported. Signs and symptoms of slowly developing communicating hydrocephalus (i.e., headache, nausea, vomiting, and papilledema) are typical. CSF examination typically shows elevated protein but no malignant cells.

Prognosis is variable. Lesions tend to be indolent or slowly progressive although anaplastic transformation has been reported in a few cases.

Imaging

Moderate to severe obstructive hydrocephalus is common. Innumerable small cystic T2/FLAIR hyperintense nodules coating the pial surface of the spinal cord and brain—especially in/around the cerebellar folia—are typical **(19-14A)**. Widespread, extensive thickening and enhancement of the intracranial and spinal leptomeninges is present on T1 C+ sequences **(19-14B)**. Intraventricular and occasionally intraparenchymal lesions (especially in the spinal cord) have been reported.

Differential Diagnosis

The differential diagnosis of DLGNT is limited. Severe **pyogenic or tubercular meningitis** may cause extensive leptomeningeal thickening and enhancement but rarely presents as multifocal leptomeningeal T2/FLAIR hyperintense cysts.

Neurocysticercosis is rarely as diffusely disseminated as DLGNT. Occasionally, cystic **metastases** from intracranial primary neoplasms (e.g., choroid plexus tumors) can mimic DLGNT.

Neuronal Tumors

As a group, tumors that exhibit exclusive ganglion cell or neurocytic differentiation account for just 0.5-1.0% of all primary brain tumors. Two general categories of neuronal tumors are recognized: gangliocytoma and neurocytoma.

We begin our discussion of ganglion cell tumors with the pure ganglion cell neoplasm, **gangliocytoma**, and a unique, newly described pattern of ganglion cell tumor called **multinodular and vacuolating neuronal tumor of the cerebrum**.

We close the chapter with a discussion of cerebellar gangliocytomas. Also called "dysplastic cerebellar gangliocytoma," they are better known as **Lhermitte-Duclos disease** (LDD).

Gangliocytoma

Terminology

Gangliocytoma (GCyt) is a benign, well-circumscribed neoplasm that contains only differentiated ganglion cells. No glial component is present. Transitional forms between GCyt and ganglioglioma exist without clear distinction between the two entities.

Dysplastic GCyts of the cerebellum—also known as Lhermitte-Duclos disease (LDD)—are a major CNS manifestation of Cowden syndrome (an autosomal-dominant familial tumor syndrome that causes a spectrum of hamartomas and neoplasms). These are discussed separately below.

Etiology

The etiology of GCyt is unknown although it is considered a developmental tumor.

Pathology

Location. Although they can occur anywhere, nearly three-quarters of supratentorial GCyts occur in the temporal lobe. Other reported sites include the brainstem, sellar region, and spinal cord.

Gross and Microscopic Features. GCyts can be solid or mixed solid and cystic lesions. Microscopically, GCyts consist of bizarre-appearing mature ganglion cells. Mitoses are few or absent. Immunoreactivity to CD34, a stem cell marker, is positive in the majority of GCyts. GCyts are WHO grade I neoplasms.

Clinical Issues

GCyt occurs most frequently in children and young adults under the age of 30 years. Most patients present with pharmacoresistant epilepsy.

GCyts grow slowly, if at all. Surgical resection is generally curative and results in long-term progression-free survival.

Imaging

GCyts are mixed density on NECT, often containing both cystic and solid components **(19-15A)**. Calcification is common, occurring in about one-third of cases. Hemorrhage and necrosis are absent.

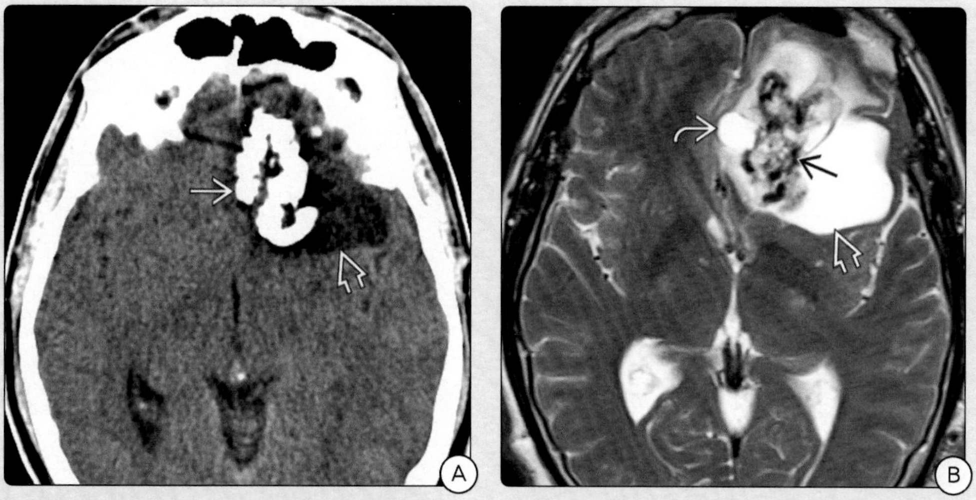

***(19-15A)** NECT scan in a 29y man with seizures shows a partially calcified ➡, partially cystic ➡ left frontal lobe mass. **(19-15B)** T2WI in the same patient shows that the partially calcified solid portion of the mass ⇨ has very heterogeneous signal intensity. A large cyst ➡ and a smaller one ➡ are associated with the mass. Edema is minimal considering the large size of the tumor.*

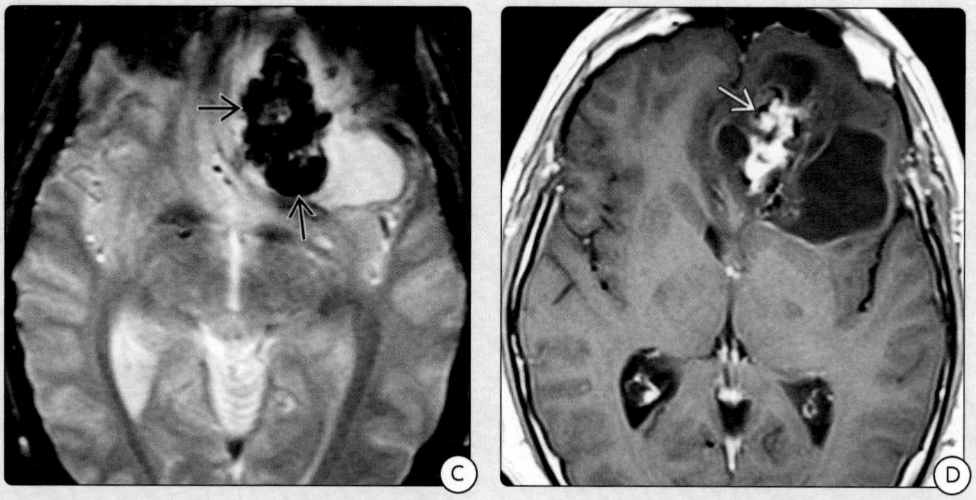

***(19-15C)** T2* GRE shows that the densely calcified solid portion "blooms" ⇨. **(19-15D)** The tumor nodule shows mild patchy enhancement ➡. Preoperative diagnosis was ganglioglioma. This was pathologically proven gangliocytoma. (Courtesy N. Agarwal, MD.)*

GCyts are hypo- to isointense relative to cortex on T1WI and hyperintense on T2/FLAIR **(19-15)**. Enhancement varies from none to striking homogeneous enhancement in the solid portions of the tumor.

Differential Diagnosis

The major differential diagnosis of GCyt is **ganglioglioma**. Gangliogliomas are often cortical, epilepsy-inducing tumors with both a cystic and enhancing solid component.

Ganglioglioma may be indistinguishable from GCyt on imaging studies.

Cortical dysplasia, another common cause of refractory epilepsy in young patients, follows gray matter on all sequences and does not enhance.

Multinodular and Vacuolating Tumor of the Cerebrum

Terminology

Multinodular and vacuolating neuronal tumor of the cerebrum (MVNT) is a recently described clinicopathologic lesion with uncertain class assignment. The 2016 WHO includes MVNT as a "pattern" of gangliocytoma.

Etiology

The etiology of MVNTs is unknown, and it is unclear whether it represents a true neoplasm or is a hamartomatous/malformative process ("quasi-tumor").

Recent studies have demonstrated that MVNTs express widespread nuclear immunolabeling for HuC/HuD neuronal antigens, OLIG2, and internexin-a (INA). These markers are all

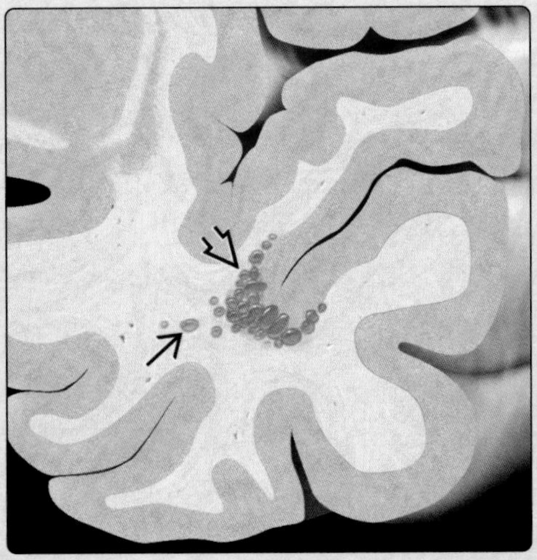

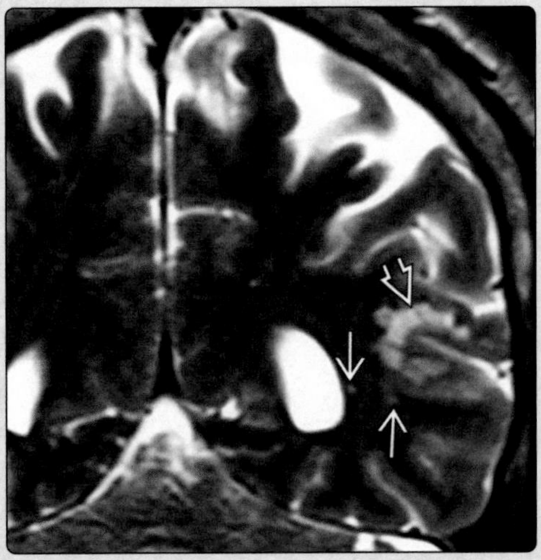

(19-16) Graphic depicts MVNT pattern of gangliocytoma, seen as clustered and scattered variably sized cystic-appearing nodules on the inner cortex, superficial white matter. (19-17) Coronal T2WI shows a cluster of variably sized cysts in the superficial white matter that hugs the inner cortex in a distinct U-shaped configuration. Note similar-appearing scattered nodules in the deep white matter, typical pattern of MVNT.

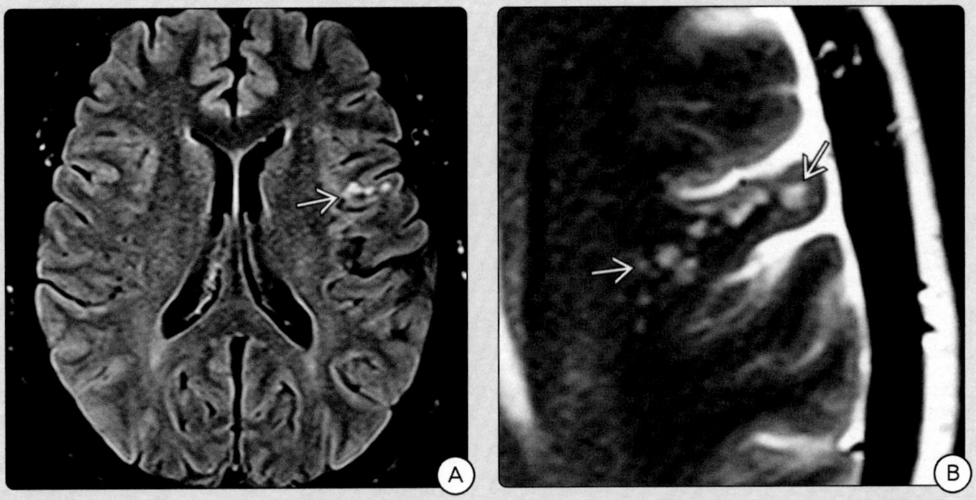

(19-18A) Axial FLAIR in a patient with headache and a nonfocal neurologic examination shows several discrete subcortical nodules that do not suppress and do not cause mass effect. (19-18B) Close-up view of the T2WI in the same case shows that the scattered hyperintense nodules are variably sized, located along the deep margin of the cortical ribbon and subcortical white matter. This was presumed MVNT.

associated with neurogenesis at earlier stages of neuronal development. Mature neuronal markers including synaptophysin and neurofilament are often absent or only weakly positive.

Pathology

Grossly, MVNTs consist of multiple discrete and coalescent nodules exhibiting varying degrees of matrix vacuolization. They are located primarily within the deep cortical ribbon and superficial subcortical white matter, although separate nodules sometimes occur in the deep and periventricular WM **(19-16)**.

Histopathologically, MVNTs are characterized by ambiguous to recognizably neuronal cells and/or dysplastic ganglion cells with cytoplasmic vacuoles.

MVNTs are glial fibrillary acidic protein (GFAP) negative. Molecular genetics have failed to demonstrate alterations in IDH, *BRAF*, and 1p19q.

Clinical Issues

Many cases of MVNT are discovered incidentally on imaging studies. Seizures and headache are the principal clinical manifestations.

Imaging

MVNTs are benign, nonaggressive-appearing lesions that remain stable over serial imaging. CT scans are usually normal without evidence for calcification or mass effect.

MR scans show a unique pattern of multiple, variably sized (usually small) discrete and coalescent nodules along the inner cortical ribbon and subcortical white matter **(19-17)** **(19-18)**.

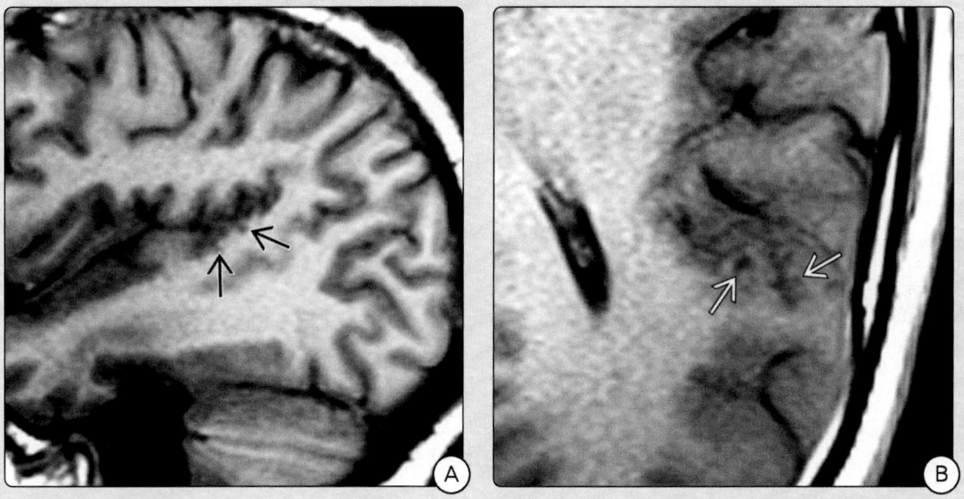

***(19-19A)** Sagittal T1WI in a 48y man with headaches and a remote history of resected cavernous malformation in the contralateral hemisphere shows several discrete nodules → along the undersurface of the cortex of the temporal lobe. The nodules are isointense with cortex. **(19-19B)** Close-up view of an axial T1WI in the same case shows multiple tiny discrete isointense/mildly hypointense nodules → in the deep cortex.*

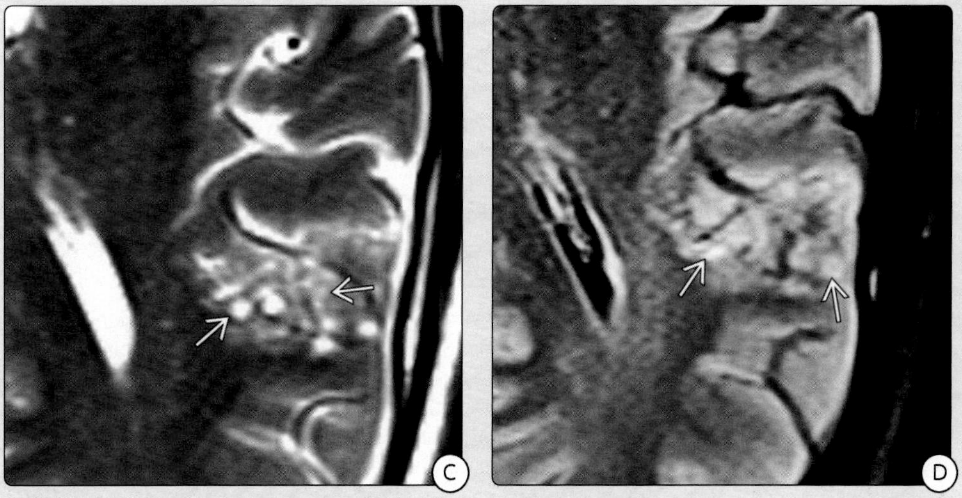

***(19-19C)** T2WI shows that the variably-sized nodules → are hyperintense relative to the overlying cortex. **(19-19D)** Close-up view of FLAIR sequence in the same case shows that the deep intra- and subcortical nodules → do not suppress. This almost tiger-striped appearance is also typical of MVNT. An incidental finding was presumed MVNT pattern of gangliocytoma. Findings have been stable for 5 years.*

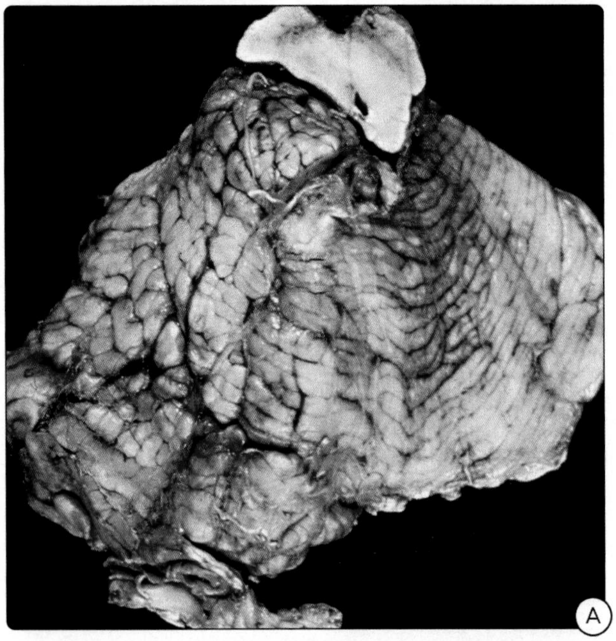

(19-20A) *Autopsy specimen shows dysplastic cerebellar gangliocytoma expanding the cerebellar hemisphere. (Courtesy AFIP Archives.)*

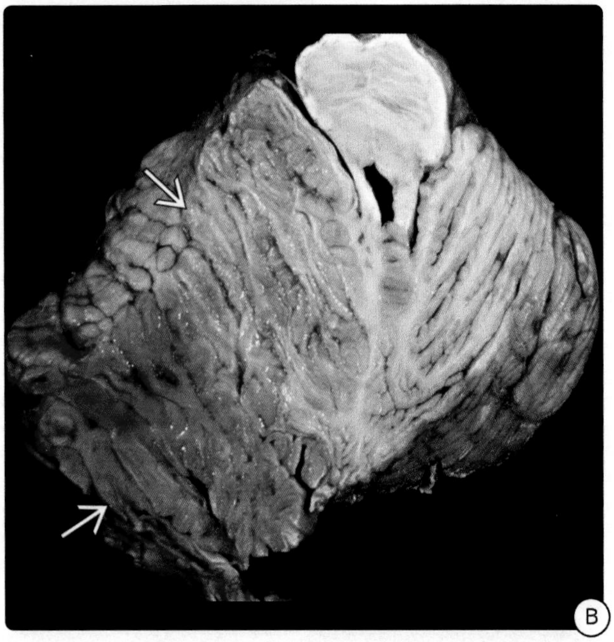

(19-20B) *Cut section through the mass shows grossly thickened cerebellar folia ➡. (Courtesy AFIP Archives.)*

The nodules are isointense with gray matter on T1WI and hyperintense on T2/FLAIR **(19-19)**.

MULTINODULAR AND VACUOLATING TUMOR OF THE CEREBRUM (MVNT)

Terminology
- 2016 WHO considers MVNT a "pattern" of gangliocytoma
- True neoplasm vs. "quasi-tumor" (malformation, hamartoma)

Pathology
- Discrete, coalescent vacuolated nodules
- Deep cortical ribbon/subcortical white matter
- Small neurons and/or dysplastic ganglion cells
- Benign, nonaggressive (WHO grade I)

Clinical Issues
- Often found incidentally on imaging
- Most common = headache, seizure

Imaging Features
- Multiple discrete small T2/FLAIR hyperintense nodules
  - Tiny "bubbles"
- Along undersurface of cortex
  - Form "cup" around cortex
  - Ribbon of U-shaped hyperintensity
- Can be imbedded in FLAIR hyperintense white matter
- Normal MRS, DWI

Differential Diagnosis
- DNET (larger, surface of cortex)
- Cortical dysplasia/hamartoma

MVNTs do not suppress on FLAIR and may be embedded in FLAIR hyperintense white matter. A characteristic appearance is that of a ribbon-like or nodular pattern that "cups" the undersurface of the cortex in a U-shaped configuration **(19-17)**. Occasionally, more diffuse confluent gyriform or "tiger stripe" T2/FLAIR hyperintensity infiltrates the cortex.

Mass effect and edema are absent. Enhancement is minimal or absent. MRS and pMR are usually normal.

Differential Diagnosis

The major differential diagnoses of MVNT include dysembryoplastic neuroepithelial tumor (DNET) and focal cortical dysplasia. **DNET** typically involves the whole cortical ribbon and extends to the surface. The nodules of MVNT are typically smaller, with multiple scattered discrete nodules rather than the solid coalescent mass of DNET.

Most foci of **cortical dysplasia** are isointense with gray matter on all sequences. MVNTs may represent hamartomas or malformative lesions.

Dysplastic Cerebellar Gangliocytoma

Terminology

Dysplastic cerebellar gangliocytoma is a rare benign cerebellar mass composed of dysplastic ganglion cells. Dysplastic cerebellar gangliocytoma is also known as **Lhermitte-Duclos disease** (LDD). Other terms for LDD include granular cell hypertrophy, granulomolecular hypertrophy of the cerebellum, cerebellar hamartoma, diffuse ganglioneuroma, or gangliomatosis of the cerebellum.

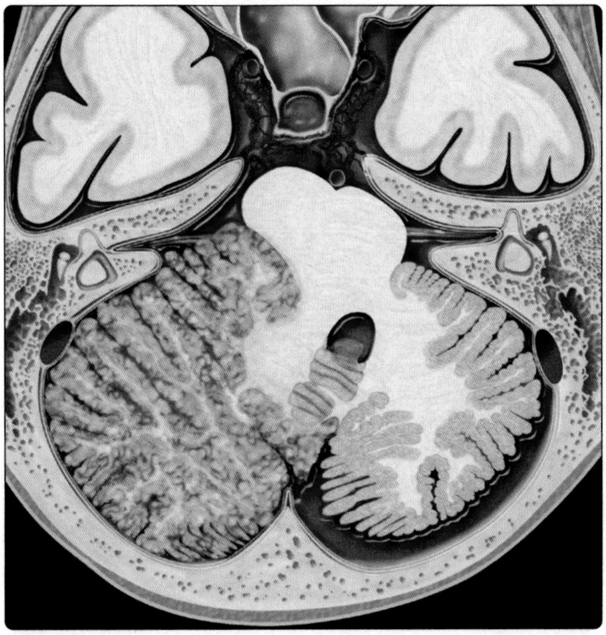

(19-21) Graphic depicts dysplastic cerebellar gangliocytoma (Lhermitte-Duclos disease).

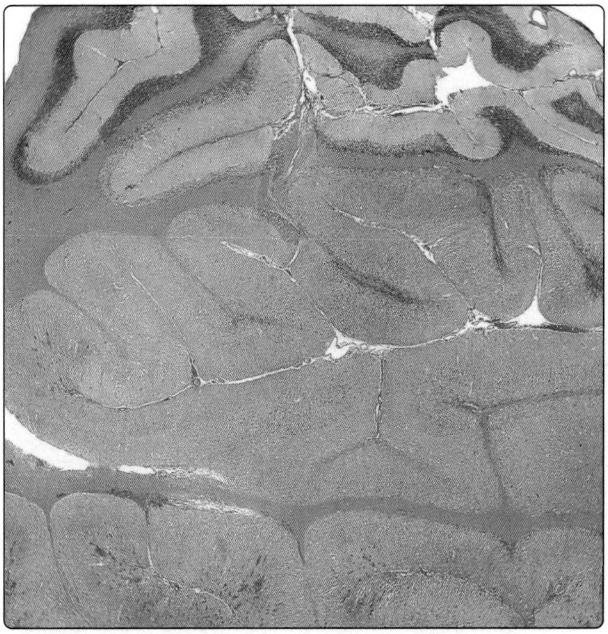

(19-22) Folia expansion in LDD is best appreciated at low magnification, a view in which the thickness of the affected cerebellar cortex, loss of dark-staining internal granule cells are readily apparent. (Courtesy F. J. Rodriguez, MD.)

LDD may occur as part of the multiple hamartoma syndrome called **Cowden syndrome** (CS). When LDD and CS occur together, they are sometimes called Cowden-Lhermitte-Duclos or **COLD syndrome**. CS is also known as **multiple hamartoma-neoplasia syndrome** or **PTEN hamartoma tumor syndrome**.

CS is an autosomal-dominant phacomatosis. The vast majority of patients have hamartomatous neoplasms of the skin combined with neoplasms and hamartomas of multiple other organs. Breast, thyroid, endometrium, and gastrointestinal cancers are the most prevalent other neoplasms in CS.

Etiology

General Concepts. Whether LDD constitutes a neoplastic, malformative, or hamartomatous lesion is debated. The majority of LDD cases are sporadic, but the association of LDD with CS favors a hamartomatous origin.

Approximately 40% of dysplastic cerebellar gangliocytomas occur as part of CS.

Genetics. CS is caused by a *PTEN* germline mutation that results in cellular proliferation of ectodermal, mesodermal, and endodermal tissues. CS is characterized by multiple hamartomas and malignant neoplasms.

Pathology

Location. LDD is always infratentorial, usually involving the cerebellar hemisphere or the vermis. Large lesions involve both. The brainstem is a rare site for LDD.

Size and Number. Dysplastic cerebellar gangliocytomas often become very large, displacing the fourth ventricle and causing obstructive hydrocephalus. The vast majority are unilateral although a few cases of LDD with bilateral lesions of the cerebellar hemispheres have been reported.

Gross Pathology. The gross appearance of LDD is a tumor-like mass that expands and replaces the normal cerebellar architecture **(19-20)**. On cut section, the cerebellar folia are markedly widened and have a grossly "gyriform" appearance **(19-21)**.

Microscopic Features. LDD is characterized by marked disruption of the normal cerebellar cortical layers. Diffuse hypertrophy of the granular cell layer with absence of the Purkinje layer of the cerebellum is typical **(19-22)**. Progressive hypertrophy of the granular cell neurons with increased myelination of their axons in an expanded molecular layer is also characteristic. Mitoses and necrosis are absent.

Staging, Grading, and Classification. It is unclear whether dysplastic cerebellar gangliocytoma (LDD) is neoplastic or hamartomatous. If neoplastic, LDD corresponds to WHO grade I.

Clinical Issues

Epidemiology. The prevalence of LDD is unknown. The incidence of CS with *PTEN* mutation is estimated at 1 in 250,000.

Demographics. LDD occurs in all age groups, but most cases occur in adults between 20-40 years. The average age at diagnosis is 34 years. There is no sex predilection.

Presentation. Patients may be asymptomatic or present with symptoms of increased intracranial pressure such as

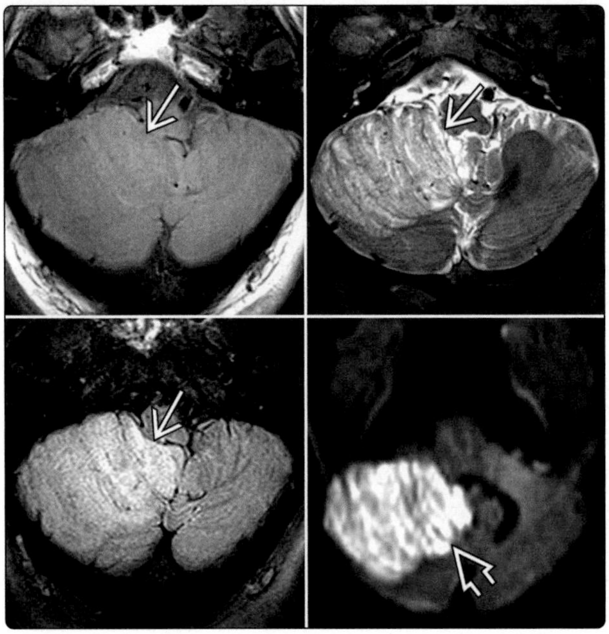

(19-23) Series of MRs in a patient with LDD shows typical findings of thickened cerebellar folia and mass effect ➡. LDD is cellular and may show restricted diffusion ➡.

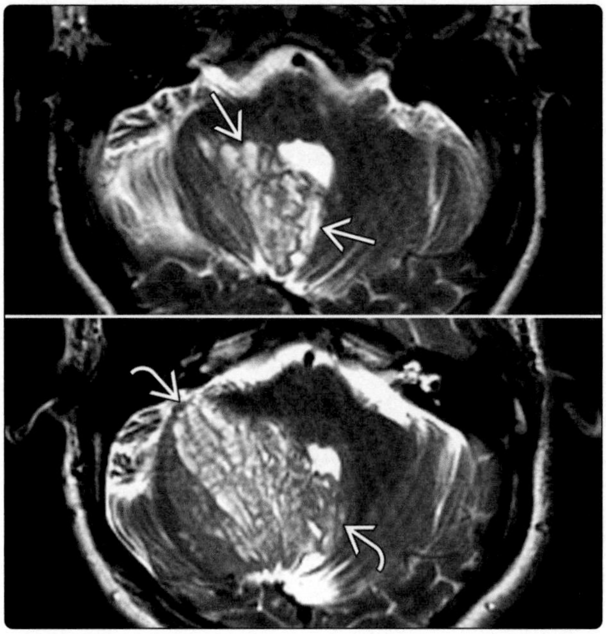

(19-24) (Top) Initial T2WI in a 16y girl shows typical "tiger stripe" pattern ➡ of LDD. (Bottom) T2WI obtained 16 years later when patient exhibited increasing ataxia shows lesion ➡ has increased in the interval. Surgical resection confirmed LDD.

headache, nausea, and vomiting. Cranial nerve palsies, gait disturbance, and visual abnormalities are also common.

Natural History. LDD enlarges very slowly over many years **(19-24)**. No cases of metastatic spread or CSF dissemination have been reported.

Treatment Options. Shunting or surgical debulking are options for symptomatic patients with hydrocephalus. Because LDD is not encapsulated and blends gradually into normal cerebellar tissues, complete resection is difficult and the complication rate is high. Cerebellar mutism has been reported after LDD resection.

Imaging

General Features. A nonenhancing unilateral cerebellar mass in a middle-aged patient that demonstrates a prominent "tiger stripe" pattern on MR is typical of LDD.

CT Findings. Most cases of LDD are hypodense on NECT. Mass effect with compression of the fourth ventricle, effacement of the cerebellopontine angle cisterns, and obstructive hydrocephalus is common. Calcification is rare. Necrosis and hemorrhage are absent. CECT generally shows no appreciable enhancement.

LDD is moderately hypermetabolic on FDG PET/CT scans.

MR Findings. An expansile cerebellar mass with linear hypointense bands on T1WI is typical. T2WI shows the nearly pathognomonic "tiger stripe" pattern of alternating inner hyperintense and outer hypointense layers in enlarged cerebellar folia **(19-23)**.

T2* (GRE, SWI) demonstrates prominent venous channels surrounding the grossly thickened folia. T1 C+ shows striking linear enhancement of these abnormal veins in between the folia.

DWI may show restricted diffusion, probably reflecting the hypercellularity and increased axonal density characteristic of LDD. PWI shows increased relative cerebral blood volume, reflecting the prominent enlarged interfolial veins, not malignancy. MRS shows normal or slightly reduced NAA and normal Cho:Cr ratios. A lactate doublet may be present. LDD can appear hypermetabolic on F-18 FDG PET imaging.

High-definition fiber tractography has been reported as a powerful surgical planning tool in LDD, allowing maximal lesion resection without damage to the unaffected tracts.

Differential Diagnosis

Imaging findings of LDD are so characteristic that the diagnosis can usually be established without biopsy confirmation. While the suggested differential diagnosis has included medulloblastoma and subacute cerebellar infarction, generally these should not be confused with LDD.

Medulloblastoma, especially the Shh desmoplastic variant, may present as a lateral cerebellar mass but usually occurs in younger patients and rarely displays the "tiger stripes" so characteristic of LDD. **Cerebellar infarction** is confined to a specific vascular territory, and symptom onset is acute or subacute rather than chronic. Occasionally, **ganglioglioma** occurs in the posterior fossa and may mimic LDD. Gangliogliomas typically enhance and, although sometimes bizarre-appearing, rarely demonstrate prominent "tiger stripes."

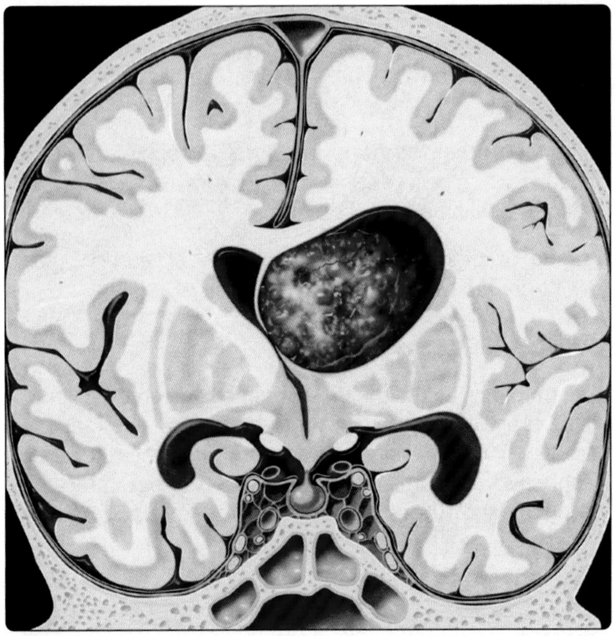

(19-25) Coronal graphic depicts central neurocytoma as a multicystic, relatively vascular, occasionally hemorrhagic mass in the body of the lateral ventricle.

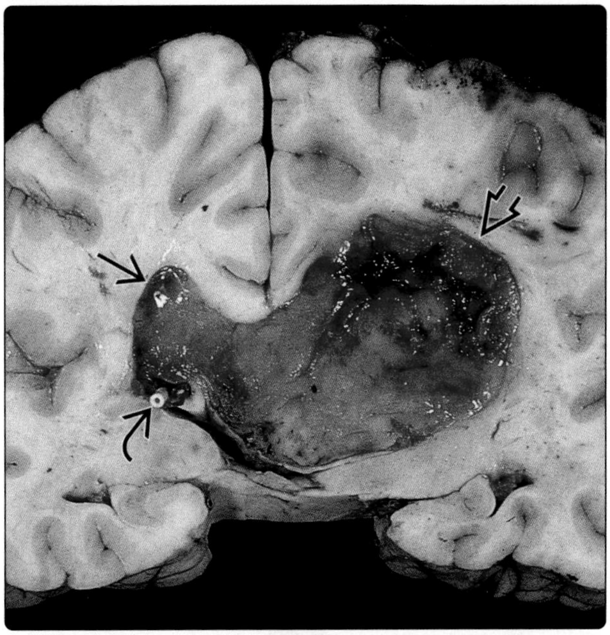

(19-26) Coronal autopsy shows a vascular, flesh-appearing central neurocytoma expanding the left lateral ventricle, crossing through the foramen of Monro to fill right lateral ventricle. Note ventricular shunt. (Neuropathology, 2013.)

CEREBRAL GANGLIOCYTOMAS

Gangliocytoma
- Pathology
  - Rare tumor composed of differentiated ganglion cells
  - Temporal lobe (75%)
  - WHO grade I
- Clinical Issues
  - Most patients < 30 years
  - Epilepsy
- Imaging Findings
  - "Cyst + nodule" or solid
  - No hemorrhage, necrosis
  - Ca++ frequent, enhancement variable

Multinodular and Vacuolating Tumor of the Cerebrum
- Unique pattern of gangliocytoma (see box above)
- T2/FLAIR hyperintense "bubbles" along inner surface of cortex

Dysplastic Cerebellar Gangliocytoma
- Terminology
  - Lhermitte-Duclos disease (LDD)
  - LDD + multiple hamartomas = Cowden-Lhermitte-Duclos (COLD)
- Pathology
  - Enlarged, thick "gyriform" cerebellar folia
  - Hypertrophied granular layer, absent Purkinje
  - WHO grade I
- Imaging Findings
  - Mass with laminated, "tiger stripe" appearance
  - Linear enhancement of veins around thickened folia

A few rare **cerebellar cortical dysplasias** can mimic LDD. However, these malformations do not demonstrate progressive enlargement and rarely cause mass effect with hydrocephalus.

A few cases of posterior fossa **tuberous sclerosis complex** (TSC) that mimic LDD have been reported. However, these patients are generally younger and have other stigmata of TSC.

Central Neurocytoma

An unusual benign-acting intraventricular neoplasm of young adults, originally thought to be an oligodendroglioma subtype, is now recognized as a tumor of neuronal lineage and has been given the name **central neurocytoma (CNC)**. Similar-appearing neoplasms in the brain parenchyma are less common and are termed **extraventricular neurocytoma**. In this section, we consider both these benign neurocytic neoplasms.

Terminology

CNC is a well-differentiated neuroepithelial tumor with mature neurocytic elements.

Etiology

The precise origin of CNCs is unknown. Bipotential precursor cells of the periventricular germinal matrix are capable of both neuronal and glial differentiation and may be the etiology of these unusual neoplasms. The 1p,19q codeletions characteristic of oligodendroglioma are absent.

Pathology

Location. CNCs are tumors of the lateral ventricle body, usually attached to the septi pellucidi and arising near the foramen of Monro **(19-25)**.

Size and Number. CNCs vary in size from small to huge and extending through the foramen of Monro to involve the contralateral ventricle.

Gross Pathology. The gross appearance of CNC is similar to that of oligodendroglioma. A well-defined, lobulated, moderately vascular intraventricular mass is characteristic **(19-27)**.

Microscopic Features. The histologic hallmark of CNC is its remarkable nuclear uniformity with round uniform cells arranged in sheets or lobules. Prominent zones of fine delicate neuropil may be present in between the tumor lobules.

MIB-1 is generally less than 2%. A labeling index of more than 2% or increased mitoses with microvascular proliferation and necrosis have been associated with increased risk of tumor recurrence.

Immunohistochemistry is positive for synaptophysin. OLIG2 is negative, which helps distinguish CNC from oligodendroglioma.

Staging, Grading, and Classification. Central neurocytoma is a WHO grade II neoplasm.

Clinical Issues

Epidemiology. CNC is the most common primary intraventricular neoplasm of young and middle-aged adults, accounting for nearly half of all cases. Overall, they are rare neoplasms that represent between 0.25-0.50% of intracranial neoplasms and 10% of all intraventricular tumors.

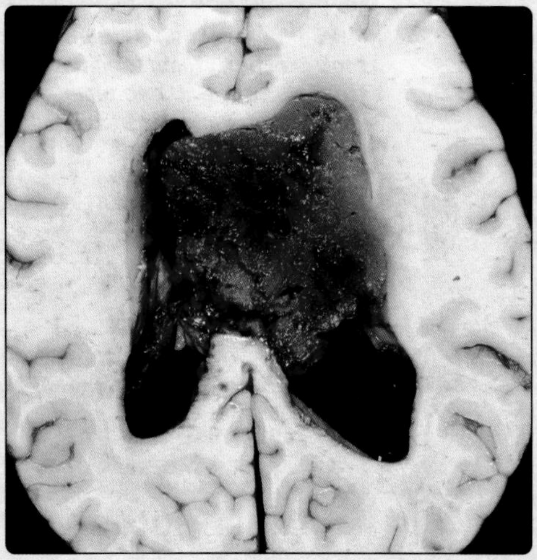

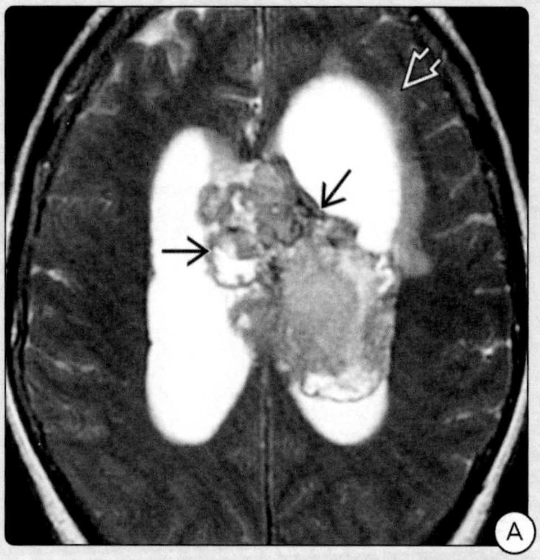

(19-27) Autopsy case shows a large hemorrhagic neoplasm confined to the lateral ventricles. This is a central neurocytoma. (Courtesy R. Hewlett, MD.) (19-28A) Axial T2WI shows a biventricular mass of mixed signal intensity ➙ causing moderate obstructive hydrocephalus. Note subependymal fluid accumulation in the left frontal lobe ➙. There is no periventricular "halo" around the remainder of the lateral ventricles.

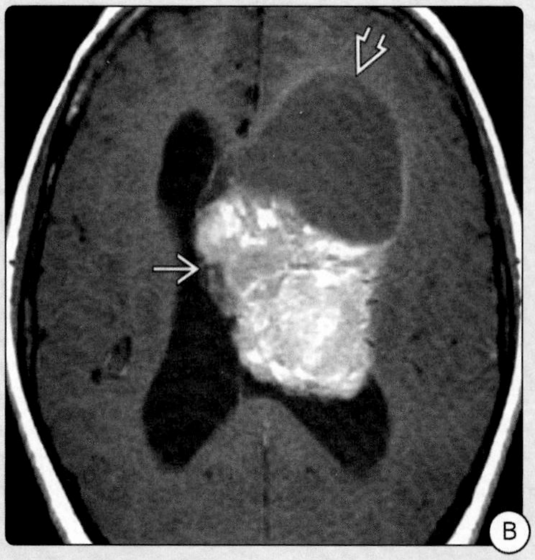

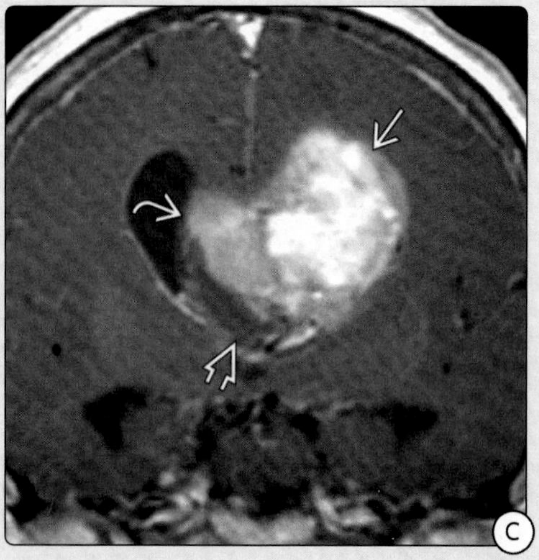

(19-28B) T1 C+ scan shows that the mass ➙ enhances strongly but heterogeneously. The large "cyst" seen on the T2WI is an entrapped frontal horn of the left lateral ventricle that contains proteinaceous fluid ➙. (19-28C) Coronal T1 C+ scan shows that the mass crosses from the body of the left lateral ventricle ➙, passes through the foramen of Monro ➙, and balloons into the right lateral ventricle ➙. This is a central neurocytoma.

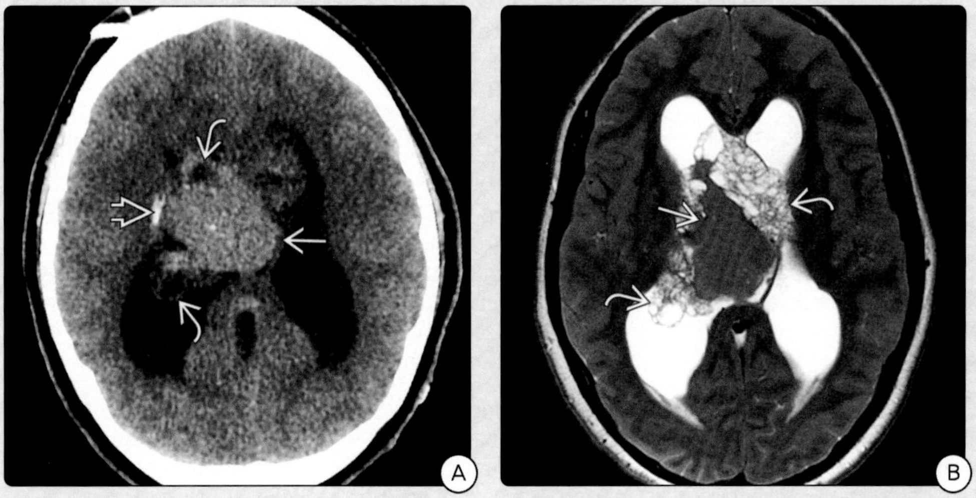

***(19-29A)** NECT in an 18y woman in the emergency room with 1 month of increasingly severe headaches shows a biventricular mass with hyperdense and hypodense components with focal calcifications. **(19-29B)** T2WI in the same case shows obstructive hydrocephalus. The mass has a large solid component and contains multiple variably sized hyperintense cysts with a "soap bubble" appearance.*

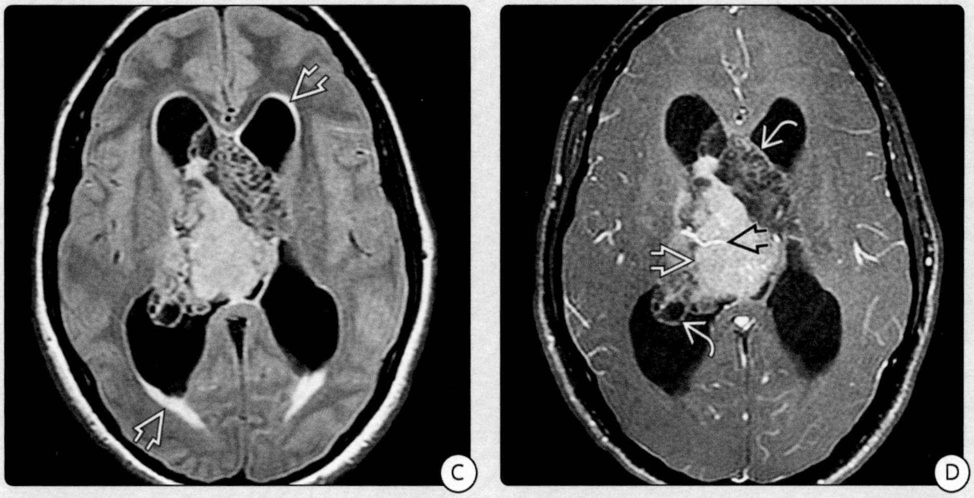

***(19-29C)** FLAIR shows periventricular fluid accumulation and multiple cysts with fluid that suppresses incompletely. **(19-29D)** T1 C+ FS shows that the solid portion of the mass enhances intensely, as do the walls of the variably sized cysts. Note the prominent vessel supplying the solid portion of the mass.*

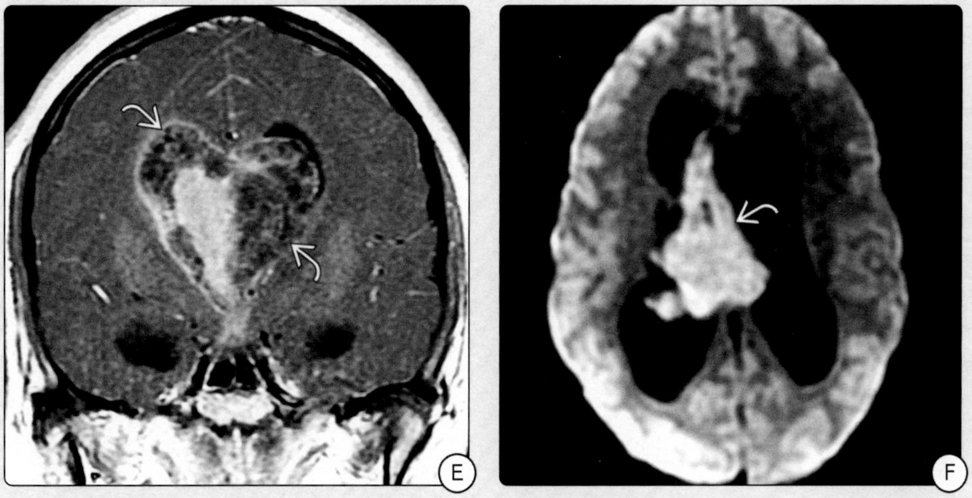

***(19-29E)** Coronal T1 C+ shows the typical "soap bubble" appearance of central neurocytoma. **(19-29F)** DWI shows restricted diffusion in some of the solid portions of the tumor. Pathologic diagnosis was central neurocytoma, WHO grade I.*

Demographics. CNCs are generally tumors of young adults and are rarely diagnosed in children or the elderly. Nearly three-quarters of all patients present between the ages of 20 and 40 years. Mean age at presentation is 30 years. There is no sex predilection.

Presentation. Symptoms are usually those of increased intracranial pressure. Headache, mental status changes, and visual disturbances are common. Focal neurologic deficits are rare. Some CNCs are found incidentally at imaging.

Natural History. CNCs are slow-growing tumors that rarely invade adjacent brain parenchyma. Sudden ventricular obstruction or acute intratumoral hemorrhage may cause abrupt clinical deterioration and even death. CSF dissemination has been reported but is very rare.

Treatment Options. Complete surgical resection is the treatment of choice. The extent of resection is the most important prognostic factor. Recurrence is rare. Five-year survival rate is 90%.

Imaging

General Features. A "bubbly" mass in the body or frontal horn of the lateral ventricle is classic for CNC.

CT Findings. NECT shows a mixed-density solid and cystic intraventricular neoplasm that is attached to the septi pellucidi. Obstructive hydrocephalus is common. Calcification is present in 50-70% of cases. Frank intratumoral hemorrhage occurs but is rare. CNCs show moderately strong but heterogeneous enhancement on CECT.

MR Findings. CNCs are heterogeneous masses that are mostly isodense with gray matter on T1WI. Intratumoral cysts and prominent vascular "flow voids" are common. A "bubbly" appearance on T2WI is typical **(19-28)**. CNCs are heterogeneously hyperintense on FLAIR and demonstrate

(19-30A) Sagittal T2WI in a 7y boy with seizures shows multiple hyperintense cysts in the inferior temporal gyrus ➡. (19-30B) Coronal T2WI in the same patient shows a relatively discrete cystic mass in the right medial temporal lobe ➡. Preoperative diagnosis was DNET. This was extraventricular neurocytoma found by histopathology. (Courtesy A. Rossi, MD.)

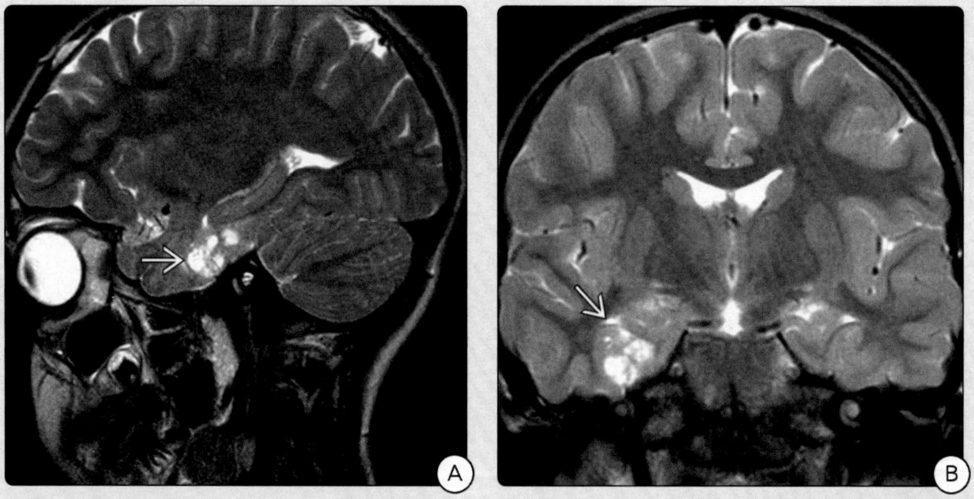

(19-31A) FLAIR scan in a 61y woman with headaches and right-sided weakness shows a hyperintense mass ➡ adjacent to the left lateral ventricle. Proteinaceous fluid in the necrotic center ⮫ does not suppress. (19-31B) T1 C+ scan shows thick, nodular, rim enhancement. Histopathology showed frequent mitoses, endothelial proliferation. This was synaptophysin-positive anaplastic extraventricular neurocytoma. (Courtesy J. Boxerman, MD.)

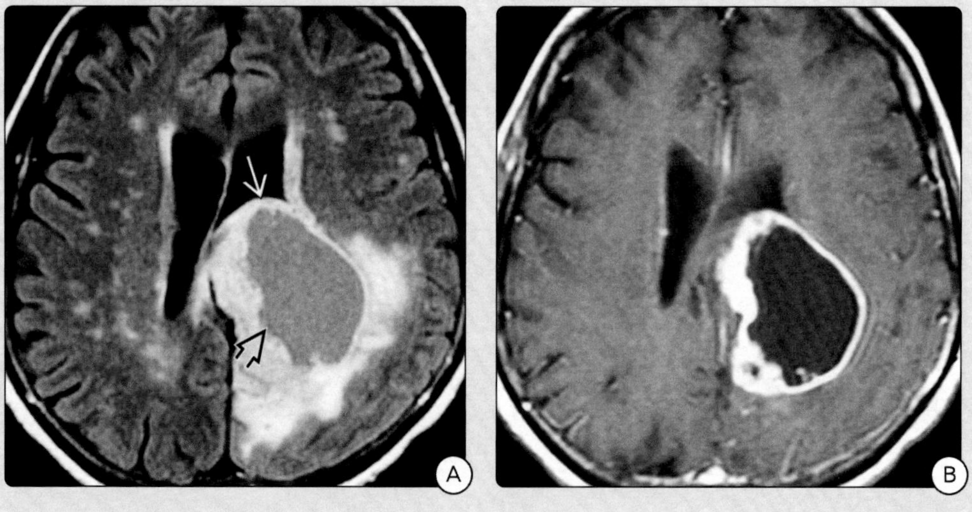

moderate to strong but heterogeneous enhancement following contrast administration **(19-29)**.

Decreased NAA and modestly elevated Cho are present on MRS. The presence of some NAA and glycine along with an inverted alanine peak at 1.5 ppm with a TE of 135 ms is highly suggestive of neurocytoma.

Differential Diagnosis

The major differential diagnosis of CNC is **subependymoma**. Subependymoma is more common in the inferior fourth ventricle, but supratentorial subependymomas are typically located adjacent to the foramen of Monro and may appear very similar. CNCs are tumors of younger adults, whereas subependymoma is more common in older adults.

Supratentorial cellular **ependymoma** occurs in children and is mostly a parenchymal, not intraventricular, lesion.

Subependymal giant cell astrocytoma also occurs in a similar location, adjacent to the foramen of Monro. Clinical and other imaging stigmata of tuberous sclerosis (i.e., subependymal nodules and cortical tubers) are usually present.

An intraventricular **metastasis** usually occurs in older patients. Choroid plexus is a more common site than the lateral ventricle body. **Meningioma** is also more common in the ventricular trigone (choroid plexus glomus) than the frontal horn or body.

True intraventricular **oligodendroglioma** is rare. As the imaging appearance is indistinguishable from CNC, the diagnosis of intraventricular oligodendroglioma is established on the basis of immunohistochemistry and genetic studies. Oligodendrogliomas are synaptophysin-negative and often show mutations of *OLIG2* and 1p,19q.

Extraventricular Neurocytoma

Terminology

Neoplasms that resemble central neurocytomas (CNCs) have been reported outside the ventricular system. In 2007, the WHO categorized these uncommon tumors as extraventricular neurocytoma (EVNCT).

Pathology

EVNCTs are histologically identical to CNCs. As the only definable distinguishing feature from CNC is location, both tumors are given the same pathologic code (WHO grade II).

Some authors have reported a wider variability in morphologic features, cellularity, proliferation rate, and outcome compared with CNCs. When atypical histologic features with necrosis, vascular proliferation, and mitoses (> 3 per 10 high-powered fields) are present, these variants are often called "atypical" EVNCT. A WHO grade for these more aggressive variants has not been established.

Clinical Issues

EVNCTs are generally tumors of young adults. The most common presenting symptom is epilepsy. Some studies have suggested that EVNCTs behave more aggressively than CNCs with poorer long-term outcome.

Imaging

EVNCTs vary widely in imaging appearance. They are usually located in the cerebral hemispheres or the parasellar region, where they resemble pituitary macroadenoma. Some tumors resemble CNCs or dysembryoplastic neuroepithelial tumors (DNETs) with a T2 hyperintense "bubbly" appearance **(19-30)**. Others have a "cyst + nodule" configuration similar to ganglioglioma.

A few extraventricular neurocytomas appear as large, heterogeneous, enhancing parenchymal neoplasms that are difficult to distinguish from high-grade astrocytoma, primitive neuroectodermal tumor (PNET), or supratentorial ependymoma and probably represent "atypical" EVNCTs **(19-31)**.

Differential Diagnosis

The atypical location makes the diagnosis challenging, as EVNCTs can mimic virtually any parenchymal neoplasm. The "soap bubble" appearance of a classic **central neurocytoma** is often inconspicuous or absent, and, when it is present, it can mimic **DNET**. Thick, irregular rim enhancement can be indistinguishable from **anaplastic astrocytoma** or **glioblastoma**.

Sellar or parasellar EVNCTs can be difficult to distinguish on imaging studies from pituitary **macroadenoma**. Less common primary pituitary tumors such as pituicytoma, granular cell tumor of the sellar region, or spindle cell oncocytoma are also similar in imaging appearance to sellar EVNCTs.

Selected References

Glioneuronal Tumors

Tomita T et al: Glioneuronal tumors of cerebral hemisphere in children: correlation of surgical resection with seizure outcomes and tumor recurrences. Childs Nerv Syst. 32(10):1839-48, 2016

Ganglioglioma

Breton Q et al: BRAF-V600E immunohistochemistry in a large series of glial and glial-neuronal tumors. Brain Behav. 7(3):e00641, 2017

Becker AJ et L: Ganglioglioma. In: Louis DN et al (eds), WHO Classification of Tumours of the Central Nervous System. Lyon, France: International Agency for Research on Cancer, 2016, pp 138-41

Pagès M et al: Co-occurrence of histone H3 K27M and BRAF V600E mutations in paediatric midline grade I ganglioglioma. Brain Pathol. ePub, 2016

Varshneya K et al: A national perspective of adult gangliogliomas. J Clin Neurosci. 30:65-70, 2016

Anaplastic Ganglioglioma

Lüdemann W et al: Pediatric intracranial primary anaplastic ganglioglioma. Childs Nerv Syst. 33(2):227-231, 2017

Terrier LM et al: Natural course and prognosis of anaplastic gangliogliomas: a multicenter retrospective study of 43 cases from the French Brain Tumor Database. Neuro Oncol. 19(5):678-688, 2017

Zanello M et al: Clinical, imaging, histopathological and molecular characterization of anaplastic ganglioglioma. J Neuropathol Exp Neurol. 75(10):971-980, 2016

Desmoplastic Infantile Astrocytoma/Ganglioglioma

Samkari A et al: Desmoplastic infantile astrocytoma and ganglioglioma: case report and review of the literature. Clin Neuropathol. 36 (2017)(1):31-40, 2017

Bianchi F et al: Supratentorial tumors typical of the infantile age: desmoplastic infantile ganglioglioma (DIG) and astrocytoma (DIA). A review. Childs Nerv Syst. 32(10):1833-8, 2016

DNET

Kasper BS et al: New classification of epilepsy-related neoplasms: the clinical perspective. Epilepsy Behav. 67:91-97, 2017

Sontowska I et al: Dysembryoplastic neuroepithelial tumour: insight into the pathology and pathogenesis. Folia Neuropathol. 55(1):1-13, 2017

Pietsch T et al: Dysembryoplastic neuroepithelial tumour. In: Louis DN et al (eds), WHO Classification of Tumours of the Central Nervous System. Lyon, France: International Agency for Research on Cancer, 2016, pp 132-5

Rivera B et al: Germline and somatic FGFR1 abnormalities in dysembryoplastic neuroepithelial tumors. Acta Neuropathol. 131(6):847-63, 2016

Rosette-Forming Glioneuronal Tumor

Beuriat PA et al: Rosette-forming glioneuronal tumor outside the fourth ventricle: a case-based update. Childs Nerv Syst. 32(1):65-8, 2016

Hainfellner JA et al: Rosette-forming glioneuronal tumour. In: Louis DN et al (eds), WHO Classification of Tumours of the Central Nervous System. Lyon, France: International Agency for Research on Cancer, 2016, pp 150-1

Kitamura Y et al: Comprehensive genetic characterization of rosette-forming glioneuronal tumors: independent component analysis by tissue microdissection. Brain Pathol. ePub, 2016

Medhi G et al: Imaging features of rosette-forming glioneuronal tumours (RGNTs): a series of seven cases. Eur Radiol. 26(1):262-70, 2016

Papillary Glioneuronal Tumor

Zhao RJ et al: Clinicopathologic and neuroradiologic studies of papillary glioneuronal tumors. Acta Neurochir (Wien). 158(4):695-702, 2016

Diffuse Leptomeningeal Glioneuronal Tumor

Dodgshun AJ et al: Disseminated glioneuronal tumors occurring in childhood: treatment outcomes and BRAF alterations including V600E mutation. J Neurooncol. 128(2):293-302, 2016

Reifenberger G et al: Diffuse leptomeningeal glioneuronal tumor. In: Louis DN et al (eds), WHO Classification of Tumours of the Central Nervous System. Lyon, France: International Agency for Research on Cancer, 2016, pp 152-5

Neuronal Tumors

Gangliocytoma

Capper D et al: Gangliocytoma. In: Louis DN et al (eds), WHO Classification of Tumours of the Central Nervous System. Lyon, France: International Agency for Research on Cancer, 2016, pp 136-7

Multinodular and Vacuolating Tumor of the Cerebrum

Cathcart SJ et al: Multinodular and vacuolating neuronal tumor: a rare seizure-associated entity. Am J Surg Pathol. ePub, 2017

Fukushima S et al: Multinodular and vacuolating neuronal tumor of the cerebrum. Brain Tumor Pathol. 32(2):131-6, 2015

Dysplastic Cerebellar Gangliocytoma

Eberhart CG et al: Dysplastic cerebellar gangliocytoma (Lhermitte-Duclos disease). In: Louis DN et al (eds), WHO Classification of Tumours of the Central Nervous System. Lyon, France: International Agency for Research on Cancer, 2016, pp. 142-3

Fernandes-Cabral DT et al: High-definition fiber tractography in the evaluation and surgical planning of Lhermitte-Duclos disease: a case report. World Neurosurg. 587:e9-587.e13, 2016

Central Neurocytoma

Lee SJ et al: Central neurocytoma: a review of clinical management and histopathologic features. Brain Tumor Res Treat. 4(2):49-57, 2016

Zacharoulis S et al: Central versus extraventricular neurocytoma in children: a clinicopathologic comparison and review of the literature. J Pediatr Hematol Oncol. 38(6):479-85, 2016

Choudhri O et al: Atypical and rare variants of central neurocytomas. Neurosurg Clin N Am. 26(1):91-8, 2015

Donoho D et al: Imaging of central neurocytomas. Neurosurg Clin N Am. 26(1):11-9, 2015

Pineal and Germ Cell Tumors

The pineal region is located in the middle of the brain. Because there are so many critical structures that surround this small gland, operating on pineal region lesions poses a challenge to neurosurgeons, and accurate preoperative assessment is essential. The posterior third ventricle, midbrain, thalamus, vein of Galen, internal cerebral vein, quadrigeminal plate, and tentorial apex are all critical structures in the adjacent "neighborhood."

The pineal gland consists of pineal parenchymal cells, astrocytes, and sympathetic neurons. A number of other cells can also be found adjacent to the pineal gland. These include ependymal cells (lining the third ventricle), choroid plexus cells, arachnoid cells that form the velum interpositum, and astrocytes in the brainstem, thalamus, and corpus callosum splenium.

Lesions of the pineal region include a broad spectrum of both neoplasms and nonneoplastic entities. This histologic diversity reflects the broad range of normal cell types that reside within the gland and its adjacent structures.

The pineal region may also be the site of neoplasms that are more commonly found elsewhere. Metastases, neuronal tumors, endothelial tumors, and lymphomas are all occasionally seen. Congenital lesions such as epidermoid and dermoid cysts as well as lipomas can also occur.

Overall, pineal region tumors are rare, accounting for 1-3% of all intracranial neoplasms. Despite their histologic complexity, neoplasms in this region can be grouped into three simple overarching categories. The two most important groups arise from cells within the pineal gland itself: (1) tumors of pineal parenchymal cells and (2) germ cell tumors (GCTs).

The third group of pineal region lesions is composed of tumors of "other cell" origin. These include metastases and rare tumors that arise from pineal astrocytes or ependyma-like cells. Tumors and nonneoplastic masses may also arise from adjacent structures in close proximity. They include entities such as tentorial apex meningioma, aneurysmal dilatation of the vein of Galen, and nonneoplastic cysts (including cysts of the pineal gland itself).

We begin our discussion with a brief review of normal gross and imaging anatomy of the pineal region. Understanding normal pineal region anatomy is critical for correct imaging diagnosis. The differential diagnoses are very different for a mass *inside* the pineal gland versus a mass that lies in the same general region but is *outside* the gland.

We then turn our attention to the two major groups of neoplasms, pineal parenchymal tumors and GCTs. GCTs occupy a separate category in the WHO classification. However, because the pineal gland is by far the most common site for GCTs and because the differential diagnosis of an intrinsic pineal

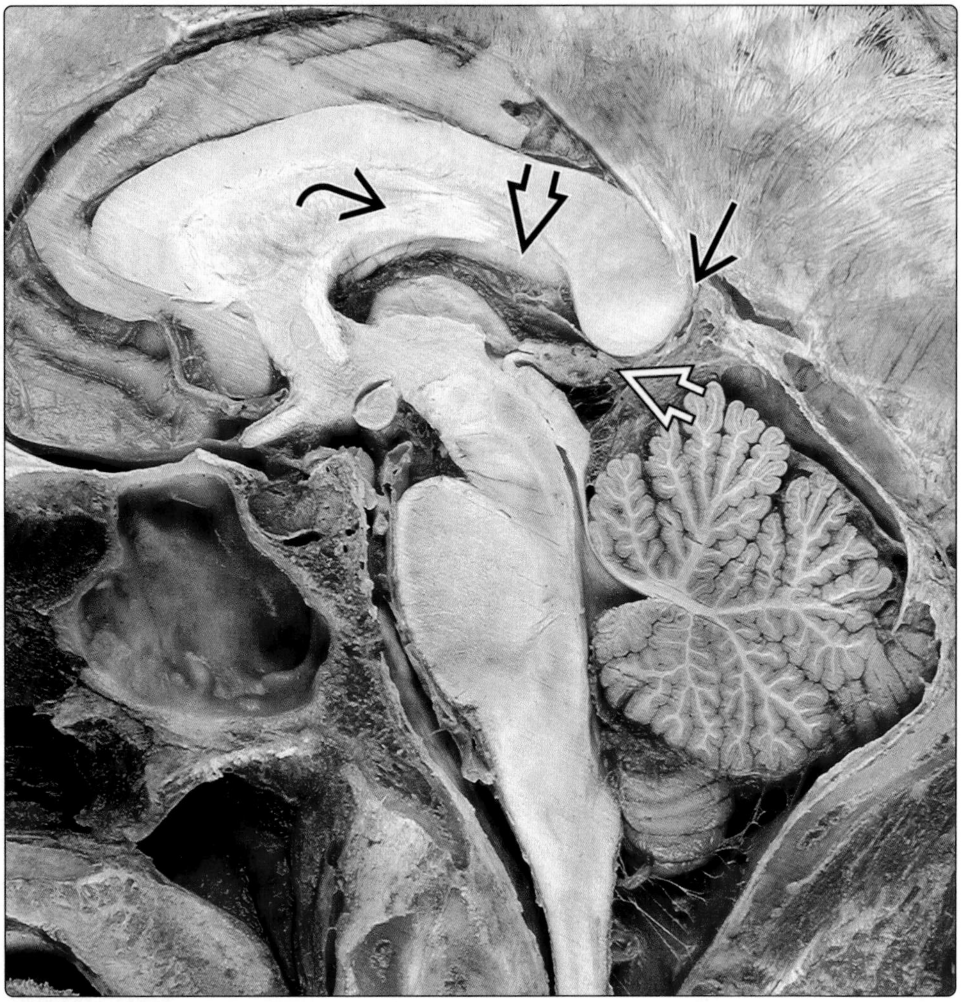

***(20-1)** Sagittal midline section demonstrates the anatomic complexity of the pineal region. The pineal gland ➡ is adjacent to the tentorial apex and vein of Galen ➡, lying behind the third ventricle below the velum interpositum (VI) ➡. The VI lies below the fornix ➡, contains the internal cerebral veins, and helps form the roof of the third ventricle. (Courtesy M. Nielsen, MS.)*

gland tumor includes both pineal parenchymal tumors and pineal GCTs, we consider them together in this chapter.

We close our discussion with a brief discussion of "other cell" tumors in the pineal gland and a differential diagnosis of pineal region masses.

Pineal Region Anatomy and Histology

The pineal region is located under the falx cerebri, near its confluence with the tentorium cerebelli. This anatomically complex region encompasses the pineal gland itself, adjacent CSF spaces (the third ventricle and subarachnoid cisterns), brain parenchyma (corpus callosum splenium, quadrigeminal plate, upper vermis), arteries (medial and lateral posterior choroidal), veins (internal cerebral veins, vein of Galen), dural sinuses (inferior sagittal sinus, straight sinus), and meninges (dura and arachnoid) **(20-1)**.

Gross Anatomy

We begin our discussion of the pineal region with the pineal gland itself, then consider its relationship to the normal structures that surround it.

Pineal Gland

The pineal gland, also called the hypophysis cerebri, is a small round or triangular endocrine organ that nestles between the superior colliculi. It is attached to the diencephalon and posterior wall of the third ventricle by the pineal stalk. It has other connections to the habenular and posterior commissures. The pineal gland also connects with other important structures, including the hypothalamus, hippocampi, amygdala, and brainstem.

The main vascular supply to the pineal gland is derived from branches of the medial posterior choroidal artery. The gland lacks a capillary blood-brain barrier.

Microscopically, 95% of the pineal gland consists of specialized neurons called **pinealocytes** that are arranged in cords or lobules separated by a fibrovascular stroma. Pinealocytes have both photosensory and neuroendocrine functions. The pinealocytes are interspersed with astrocytes and numerous

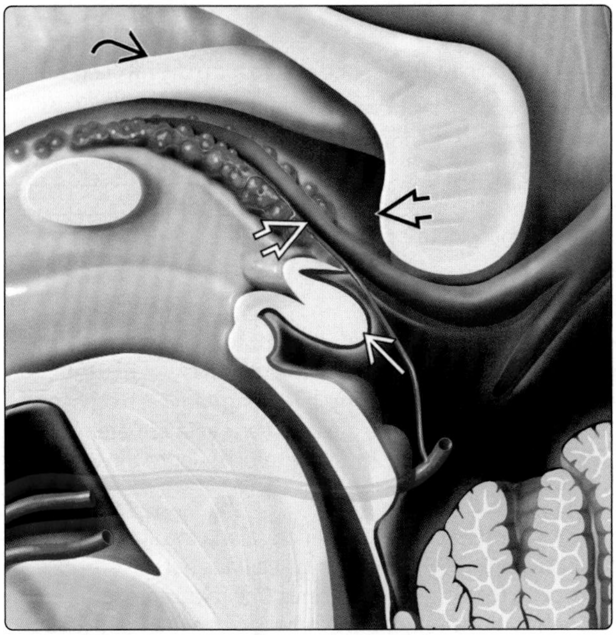

(20-2) Sagittal graphic depicts the normal anatomy of the pineal region. The pineal gland ➡ abuts the posterior third ventricle and lies below the fornix ➡, velum interpositum ➡, and internal cerebral vein ➡.

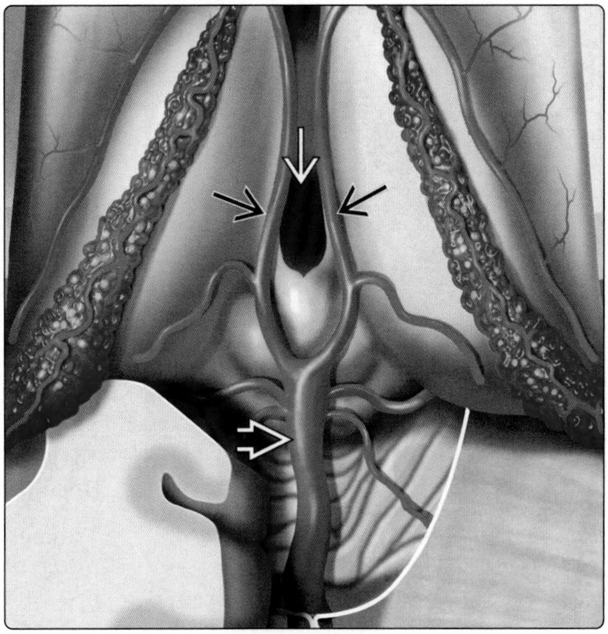

(20-3) Axial graphic shows the velum interpositum ➡ opened into the roof of the third ventricle, paired internal cerebral veins ➡, and vein of Galen ➡.

blood vessels. Fine sand-like calcifications are commonly deposited within the pineal parenchyma.

The major hormone produced by the pineal gland is melatonin. **Melatonin** plays an important role in the synchronization of seasonal reproductive rhythms and entrainment of circadian cycles. Influenced by the dark/light cycle, the protein-coupled metabotropic melatonin receptors MT1 and MT2 are the primary mediators of its physiologic actions.

Third Ventricle and Commissures

The pineal gland abuts the posterior third ventricle. The third ventricle has two small posterior CSF outpouchings that abut the pineal gland. The more prominent **supra-pineal recess** lies above the pineal gland and below the corpus callosum splenium. The smaller **pineal recess** points posteriorly, directly into the gland.

Two commissural fiber tracts relate to the pineal gland. The **habenular commissure** lies just above the pineal gland, immediately below the suprapineal recess. The **posterior commissure** lies below the gland.

Fornix

The fornices are part of the limbic system. The two fornices, together with the fimbria, are the smallest and innermost of three nested C-shaped arches that surround the diencephalon and basal ganglia. The fornices provide the primary efferent outputs from the hippocampus.

Each **fornix** has four parts. The **crura** arch under the corpus callosum splenium forms part of the medial wall of the lateral ventricles. The **commissure** connects the two crura, which then converge to form the body. The **body** is attached to the inferior surface of the corpus callosum. The bodies of the fornices curve inferiorly, forming the **columns** or "pillars" of the fornices. The fornices terminate in the mammillary bodies.

The commissure and bodies of the fornices lie above the velum interpositum (VI), internal cerebral veins, and pineal gland **(20-2)**.

Velum Interpositum

The **tela choroidea** is a thin translucent bilaminar membrane that forms the **VI** **(20-1)**. The VI stretches (and thus is "interposed") between the bodies of the two fornices. The VI forms the roof of the third ventricle and is closed anteriorly at the foramen of Monro. If it is open posteriorly, it forms a CSF-filled space that communicates directly with the quadrigeminal cistern. This normal variant is called a **cavum of the velum interpositum** or **cistern of the velum interpositum.**

The VI extends laterally over the thalami, where it becomes "tacked down" at the choroid fissures and continuous with the choroid plexus of the lateral ventricles. The VI covers the pineal gland and habenular commissure but is not directly attached to these structures.

Quadrigeminal Cistern

The **quadrigeminal cistern** is a rhomboid-shaped CSF space that lies dorsal to the tectal (quadrigeminal) plate and pineal gland. It is continuous inferiorly with the superior vermian cistern and laterally with the two ambient cisterns. Anteriorly it connects directly with the **cistern of the VI.**

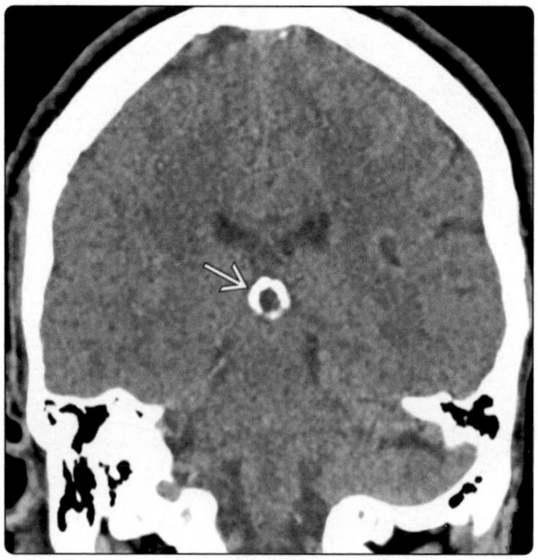

(20-4) Coronal NECT in a patient with minor head injury shows a 14-mm Ca++ cystic pineal gland ➡. This is a normal variant.

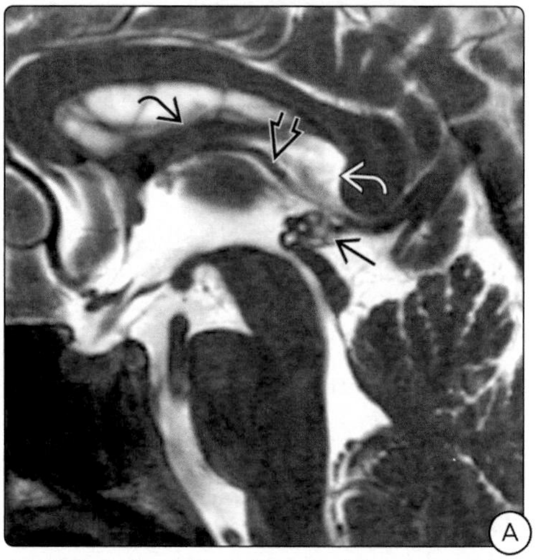

(20-5A) Sagittal T2WI shows multicystic pineal gland ➡ behind third ventricle, below ICV ➡, velum interpositum ➡, and fornix ➡.

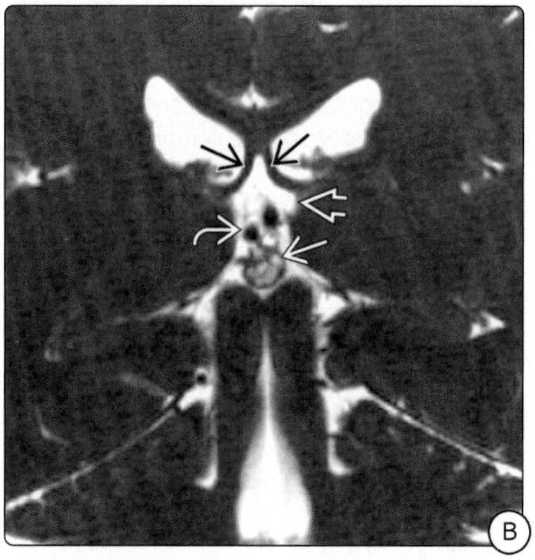

(20-5B) Coronal T2WI shows pineal gland ➡ below internal cerebral veins ➡, velum interpositum ➡, and fornices ➡.

Meninges

Infoldings of the inner (meningeal) layer of the dura form the **falx cerebri** and **tentorium cerebelli**. These two dural leaves unite just behind the corpus callosum splenium to form the **falcotentorial junction**.

A loosely adherent, thin, almost transparent layer of **arachnoid** closely follows the dura and forms the outer border of the subarachnoid spaces. The arachnoid does not invaginate into the sulci or CSF cisterns.

Veins and Venous Sinuses

The **internal cerebral veins** (ICVs) are paired, paramedian veins that course posteriorly between the dorsal and ventral membranous layers of the VI. The ICVs terminate in the quadrigeminal cisterns by uniting with each other and the basal veins of Rosenthal to form the great cerebral **vein of Galen** **(20-3)**. The ICVs lie above the pineal gland, which lies anteroinferior to the vein of Galen **(20-2)**.

The **inferior sagittal sinus** (ISS) courses posteriorly along the inferior (free) margin of the falx cerebri. The ISS and vein of Galen unite at the falcotentorial junction to form the **straight sinus**. The falcotentorial junction, together with the leaves of the tentorium cerebelli, forms the "roof" of the quadrigeminal cistern.

Arteries

The **medial posterior choroidal arteries** arise from the P2 segments of the posterior cerebral arteries. They curve laterally around the brainstem, enter the tela choroidea, and run anteromedially along the roof of the third ventricle. Branches of the medial posterior choroidal arteries provide the main arterial supply to the pineal gland.

Parenchyma

The **corpus callosum splenium** lies above and behind the pineal gland. The **tectal (quadrigeminal) plate** lies below it. The **thalami** lie inferolateral to the pineal gland.

Normal Imaging

Pineal Calcification on NECT

Physiologic pineal gland calcification ("concretions") is common **(20-4)**. Primary mineralization occurs in an organic matrix formed by pinealocytes. Pineal calcification increases with age. Reported prevalence is 1% in children under age 6 years, 8% in patients under age 10, and 40% in patients under 30. More than half of all adults have calcified pineal glands.

The diameter of normal pineal glands is usually ≤ 10 mm, but glands measuring 14-15 mm are not uncommon.

MR of the Pineal Region

Thin-section, small field-of-view sagittal T2WI is the ideal sequence for imaging the pineal gland and adjacent structures. The contrast between CSF in the posterior third ventricle in front, the velum interpositum above, and the quadrigeminal cistern posteriorly allows maximum delineation of the gland **(20-5)**.

An easy way to recall the relationship of the pineal gland to its adjacent structures can be identified using sagittal T2WI. From top down, the mnemonic "**f**amous **V.I.P.**" identifies the **f**ornix, **v**elum interpositum, **i**nternal cerebral veins, and **p**ineal gland. Lesions in the fornix, VI, and ICVs will all displace the pineal gland inferiorly.

Lesions that arise from the tectal plate displace the pineal gland anterosuperiorly, whereas third ventricle masses displace it posteriorly. Knowing the normal gross anatomy helps make it simple!

Histology

The pineal gland has a unique morphology that differs considerably from the rest of the CNS. The gland is encased in a pial capsule and exhibits a loosely lobulated arrangement with a prominent intralobular fibrovascular and glia stroma.

The normal pineal gland is densely cellular and is composed mainly of pinocytes surrounded by connective tissue septa. Pinocytes are a specialized type of neuroepithelial cell, closely related to neurons, that have photosensory and neuroendocrine functions. Pinocytes stain avidly with neuronal immunohistochemical markers (e.g., synaptophysin and neurofilament protein).

At least four other cell types have been identified in the pineal gland, including interstitial cells and small numbers of fibrillary astrocytes.

Germ cells are *not* normal pineal gland constituents, and primitive germ cell elements are not found in fetal pineal glands. The theory that germ cell neoplasms arise from primordial germ cells that failed to migrate properly during the first few weeks of embryonic development is probably incorrect. More recent hypotheses implicate native stem cells of pluripotent or neural type as the source of neoplastically transformed germ cell elements.

Pineal Parenchymal Tumors

In North America and Europe, pineal *region* tumors represent less than 1% of all primary intracranial neoplasms but 3-8% of pediatric tumors. In Asia, they account for 3-3.5% of brain tumors. Despite their rarity, a broad spectrum of neoplasms can arise from the pineal gland itself or structures that are in its vicinity.

Most tumors of the pineal *gland* are germ cell neoplasms, which account for approximately 40% of all pineal tumors and are discussed separately. Pineal parenchymal tumors (PPTs) are intrinsic primary neuronal tumors that arise from pinealocytes or their precursors. PPTs account for less than 0.2% of all brain tumors but cause approximately 15-30% of pineal gland tumors.

PPT grading is based on the presence or absence of mitoses and neurofilament staining. Three grades are recognized: (1) **pineocytoma**, (2) **pineal parenchymal tumor of intermediate differentiation (PPTID)**, and (3) **pineoblastoma**, the most malignant parenchymal cell tumors.

In the most recent epidemiologic studies, pineocytomas account for 13-15% of pineal parenchymal neoplasms (probably an underrepresentation, as many presumed cases are not resected or biopsied). PPTIDs represent nearly two-thirds of cases, and pineoblastomas account for approximately 20%.

The very rare **papillary tumor of the pineal region** (PTPR), with which we conclude our discussion of PPTs, resembles pineocytoma but actually arises from the subcommissural organ.

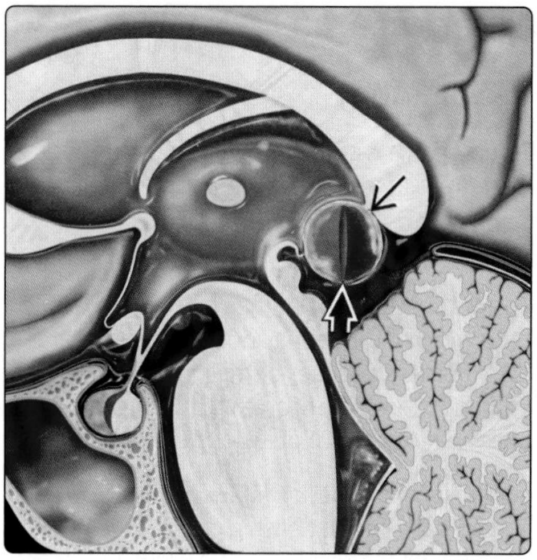

***(20-6)** Graphic depicts pineocytoma. The cystic center is lined by a rim of solid, partially calcified tumor ⇒. Hemorrhage ➡ is not uncommon.*

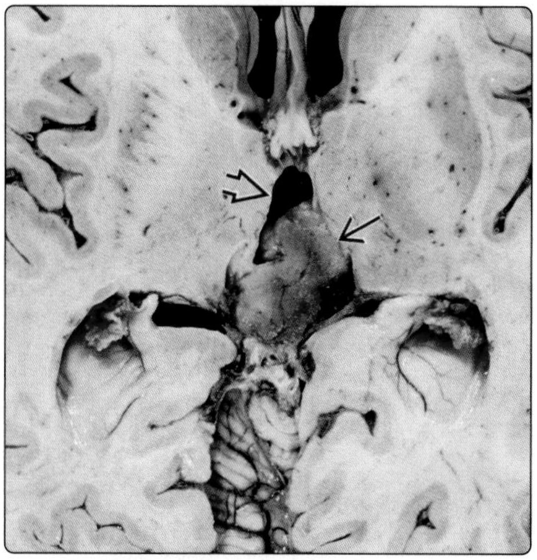

***(20-7)** Autopsy case shows pineocytoma as a well-demarcated lobulated mass ⇒ behind the third ventricle ⇒. (Courtesy B. Horten, MD.)*

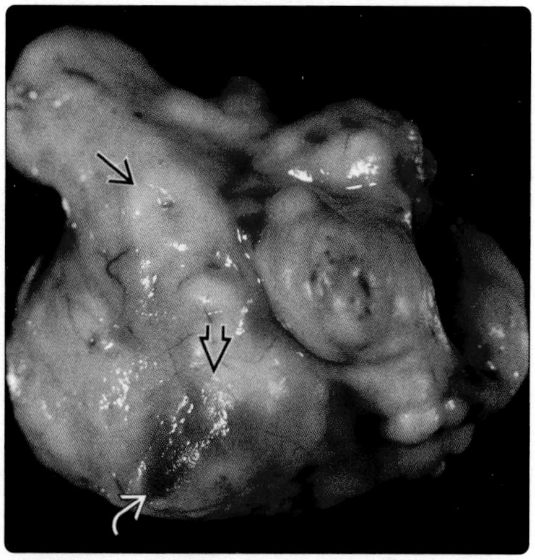

***(20-8)** Resected pineocytoma shows multiple cysts ⇒, solid nodules ⇒, and intratumoral hemorrhage ➡. (Courtesy R. Hewlett, MD.)*

Pineocytoma

Terminology

Pineocytoma is a slow-growing and well-differentiated PPT composed of mature cells that resemble normal pinealocytes.

Etiology

The ontogeny of the human pineal gland recapitulates the phylogeny of the retina and the pineal organ. PPTs mimic the developmental stages of the pineal gland, with immunoexpression profiles that indicate that they are biologically linked to pinealocytes.

No consistent genetic mutations have been described to date, and no definite relationship of pineocytoma with the *RB1* gene has been established. No syndromic associations have been demonstrated.

Pathology

Location and Size. Pineocytomas are located behind the third ventricle and rarely invade it or adjacent structures **(20-6)** **(20-7)**. Pineocytomas vary in size. Although "giant" tumors have been reported, most are smaller than 3 cm in diameter.

Gross Pathology. Pineocytomas are well-circumscribed, round or lobular, gray-tan masses that may display intratumoral cysts or hemorrhagic foci **(20-8)**.

Microscopic Features. Pineocytomas are composed of small uniform cells that closely resemble pinealocytes. Large "pineocytomatous rosettes" are the most characteristic feature.

Immunopositivity for neuronal markers such as synaptophysin, neuron-specific enolase, and neurofilament protein (NFP) is typical.

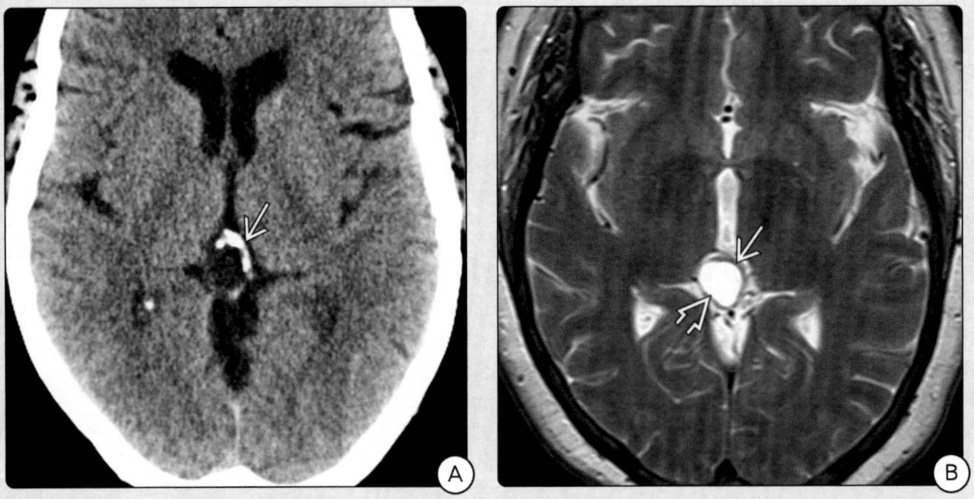

(20-9A) NECT scan shows the typical findings of pineocytoma. The cystic-appearing pineal mass "explodes" calcifications toward the periphery of the lesion →. (20-9B) T2WI in the same patient shows a cyst → surrounded by a thin rim of solid tissue →.

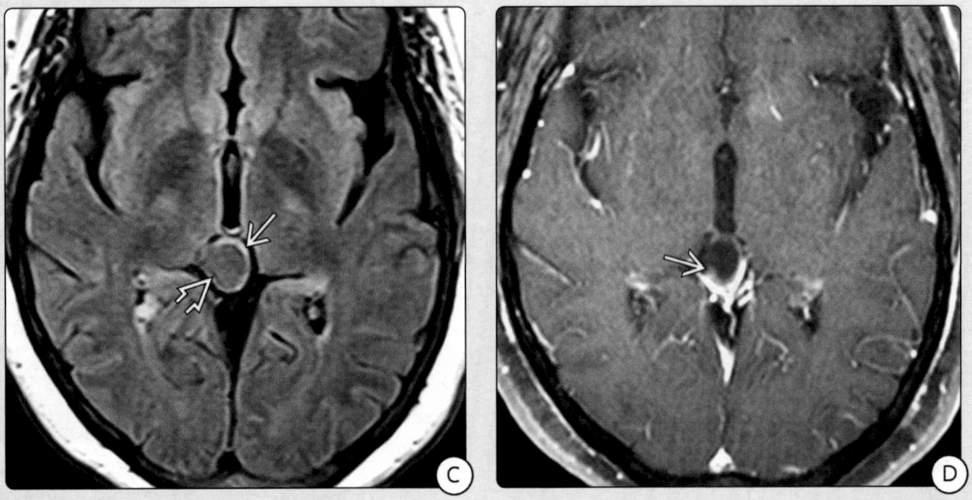

(20-9C) FLAIR scan shows that the cyst wall → is mildly hyperintense and that the cyst fluid → does not suppress. (20-9D) T1 C+ FS demonstrates that the cyst wall enhances →. This is pathologically proven pineocytoma, WHO grade I.

Pineocytoma and the normal pineal gland may appear very similar, and histologic differentiation between the two may be difficult, especially in small tissue samples.

Staging, Grading, and Classification. Pineocytoma is positive for both synaptophysin and neurofilament and shows no mitoses. Pineocytomas are WHO grade I neoplasms.

Clinical Issues

Epidemiology. Pineocytoma is the most common PPT, accounting for 15-60% of all primary PPTs.

Demographics. Pineocytomas occur at all ages but are mostly tumors of adults. Mean age at diagnosis is 43 years. There is a slight female predominance (M:F = 0.6:1).

Presentation. Many small pineocytomas are discovered incidentally on imaging studies. Larger lesions may compress adjacent structures or cause hydrocephalus. Headache and Parinaud syndrome (paralysis of upward gaze) are common in symptomatic patients.

Natural History. Pineocytomas grow very slowly and often remain stable in size over many years. Gross total resection is the major prognostic factor with reported 5-year survival rates between 90 and 100%.

Treatment Options. "Watchful waiting" is common with small lesions. Imaging is usually obtained only if the patient's symptoms change. Complete surgical resection is generally curative, without recurrence or metastatic tumor spread.

Imaging

CT Findings. Pineocytomas are globular, well-delineated masses that are mixed iso- to hypodense on NECT scans. Calcifications typically appear "exploded" toward the periphery of the pineal gland **(20-9A)**.

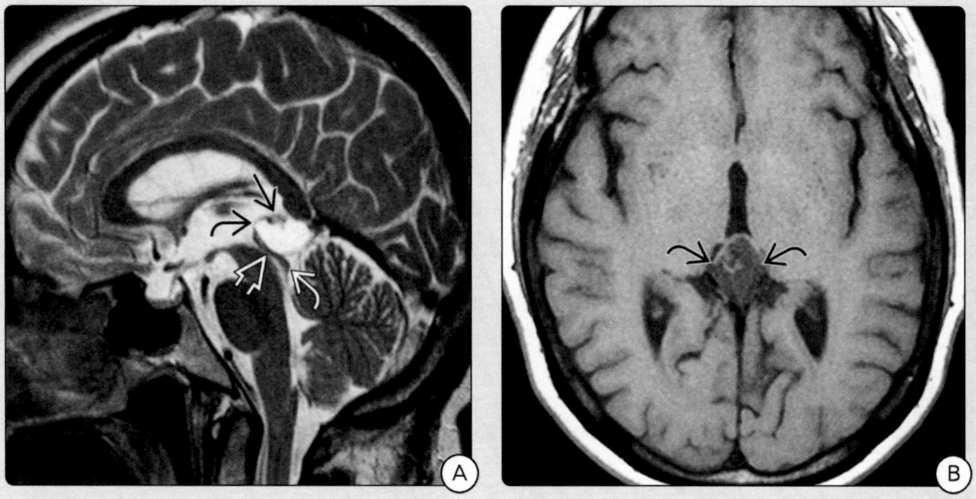

***(20-10A)** Sagittal T2WI in a 58y woman with headaches and a normal neurologic examination shows a mixed cystic and solid pineal mass that compresses the tectal plate. The cerebral aqueduct is patent. **(20-10B)** Axial T1WI in the same case shows that the cystic portion of the mass is hyperintense compared with CSF in the adjacent third ventricle.*

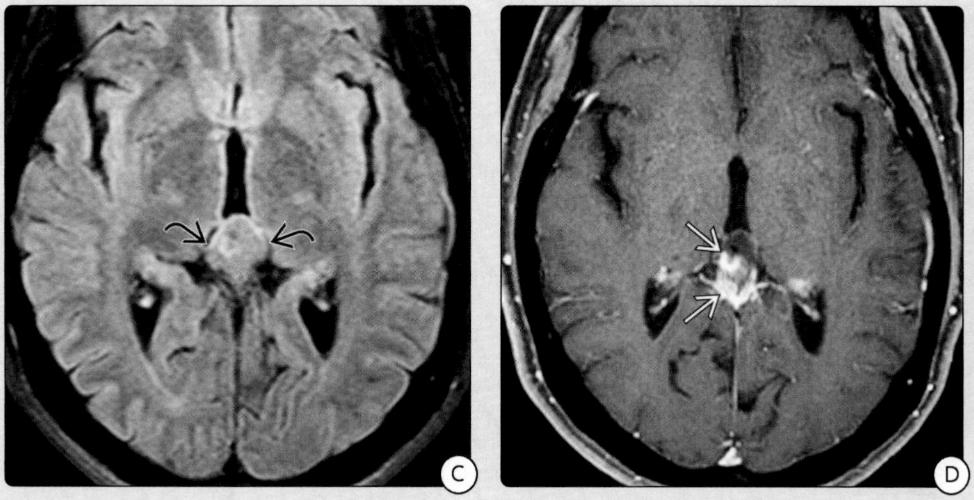

***(20-10C)** Axial FLAIR MR in the same case shows that fluid in the cyst does not suppress. There is no evidence for obstructive hydrocephalus. **(20-10D)** Axial T1 C+ FS MR shows strong but heterogeneous enhancement in the solid portions of the mass. The lesion has remained stable for several years. This is presumed (not proven) pineocytoma.*

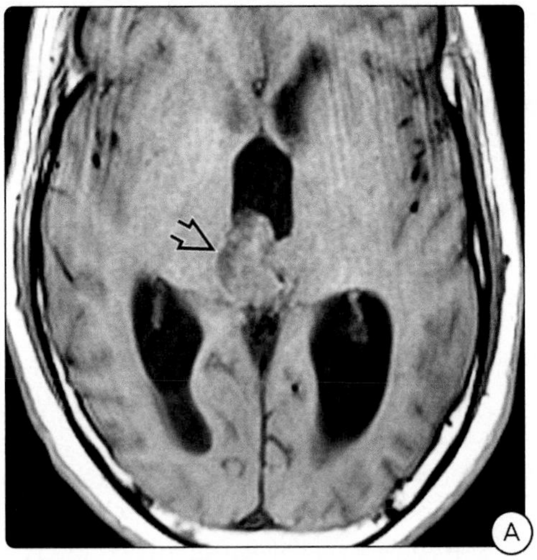

(20-11A) Axial T1WI in a 57y man with headaches shows a lobulated mixed iso-/hypointense pineal mass ⇨ causing obstructive hydrocephalus.

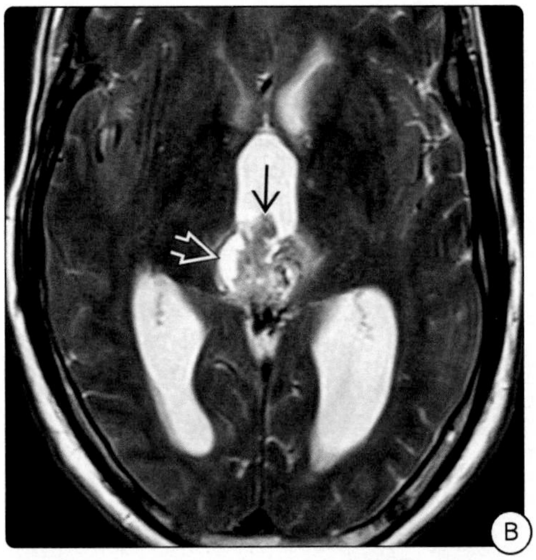

(20-11B) An axial T2WI scan in the same case shows both solid ⇨ and cystic ➡ portions of the mass.

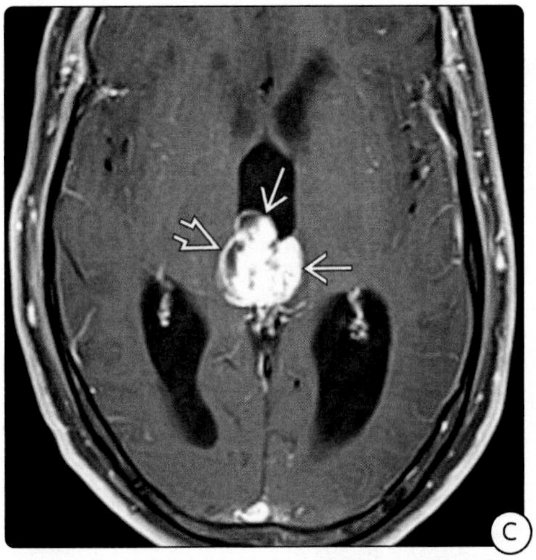

(20-11C) Axial T1 C+ FS scan shows the solid portions of the mass ➡ and cyst ➡ enhance strongly. This is PPTID, WHO grade II.

MR Findings. Pineocytomas are well-demarcated round or lobular masses that are iso- to hypointense on T1WI and hyperintense on T2WI and FLAIR **(20-9B)** **(20-9C)**. T2* GRE may show "blooming" foci secondary to calcification or hemorrhage. Pineocytomas typically enhance avidly with solid, rim, or even nodular patterns **(20-9D)** **(20-10)**.

Differential Diagnosis

The major differential diagnosis of pineocytoma is a benign, nonneoplastic **pineal cyst**. Pineal cysts may be indistinguishable from pineocytomas on imaging studies. **Germinoma** typically "engulfs" rather than "explodes" the pineal calcifications, is most common in male adolescents, and enhances intensely and uniformly. **Pineal parenchymal tumor of intermediate differentiation** (PPTID) is a tumor of middle-aged and older patients. The imaging appearance of PPTIDs is more "aggressive" than that of pineocytoma (see below).

PINEOCYTOMA

Pathology
- Most 1-3 cm
- Well-demarcated, round/lobulated
- WHO grade I

Clinical Issues
- Adults (mean = 40 years)
- Grows very slowly, often stable for years

Imaging
- CT
  - Mixed iso-/hypodense
  - Pineal Ca++ "exploded"
- MR
  - Iso-/hypointense on T1, hyperintense on T2
  - Cysts common, may hemorrhage
  - Variable enhancement (solid, rim, nodular)

Differential Diagnosis
- Benign pineal cyst (may be indistinguishable)
- Germinoma ("engulfs" Ca++, male adolescents)
- PPTID (more "aggressive looking")

Pineal Parenchymal Tumor of Intermediate Differentiation

Some pineal lesions both look worse and behave more aggressively than pineocytomas but are still less malignant than pineoblastomas. In 2007, the WHO formally recognized a new tumor, pineal parenchymal tumor of intermediate differentiation (PPTID), which is intermediate in malignancy between pineocytoma and pineoblastoma.

Terminology

PPTID supersedes the terms "atypical" or "aggressive" pineocytoma.

Pathology

Grossly, PPTID is a large, heterogeneous mass with peripheral calcification and variable cystic changes. Microscopically, PPTIDs are moderate to highly cellular tumors that exhibit dense lobular architecture. Two morphologic subtypes, small cell and large cell, have been recently described.

PPTIDs can be either WHO grade II or III although definite histologic grading criteria remain to be defined.

Clinical Issues

Epidemiology and Demographics. PPTIDs are the most common pineal parenchymal tumor, representing between half and two-thirds of all cases. PPTIDs can occur at any age but are typically tumors of middle-aged adults.

Natural History. Diplopia, Parinaud syndrome, and headache are the most common presenting symptoms. Biologic behavior is variable, and long-term survival—even with subtotal resection—is common. Tumors tend to enlarge slowly over many years and recur locally although CSF dissemination may occur.

Treatment Options. Treatment of PPTID is controversial. Stereotactic biopsy followed by surgical resection is the most common treatment. The role of adjuvant chemotherapy or radiotherapy is undetermined.

Imaging

General Features. PPTIDs have a more "aggressive" imaging appearance than pineocytoma **(20-11)**. Extension into adjacent structures (e.g., the ventricles and thalami) is common. Size varies from less than 1 cm to large masses that are 4-6 cm in diameter. CSF dissemination is uncommon but does occur, so imaging evaluation of the entire neuraxis should be performed prior to surgical intervention.

CT Findings. NECT scans show a hyperdense mass that "engulfs" pineal gland calcifications. PPTIDs generally enhance strongly and uniformly.

MR Findings. PPTIDs are mixed iso- and hypointense on T1WI, isointense with gray matter on T2WI, and hyperintense on FLAIR. T2* (GRE, SWI) scans may show hypointense "blooming" foci. Enhancement is generally strong but heterogeneous on T1 C+ **(20-12)**. MRS shows elevated Cho and decreased NAA. A lactate peak may be present.

Differential Diagnosis

The major differential diagnosis of PPTID is **pineocytoma**. A more aggressive-appearing pineal mass in a middle-aged or older adult is most consistent with PPTID. **Pineoblastoma** is typically a tumor of younger patients. **Germinoma** is more common in male adolescents. **Papillary tumor of the pineal region** can appear identical on imaging studies but is very rare.

PINEAL PARENCHYMAL TUMOR OF INTERMEDIATE DIFFERENTIATION

Pathology
- 50-68% of pineal parenchymal tumors
- WHO grade II or III

Clinical Issues
- Middle-aged adults

Imaging
- Appears more "aggressive" than pineocytoma
- Usually larger, more heterogeneous
- May disseminate via CSF

Differential Diagnosis
- Pineocytoma > > pineoblastoma
- Germinoma

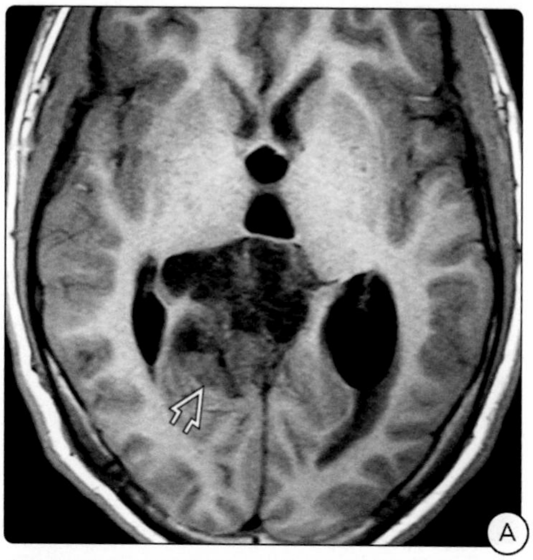

***(20-12A)** Axial T1WI in a 21y man with Parinaud syndrome shows a large heterogeneous mass causing moderate obstructive hydrocephalus.*

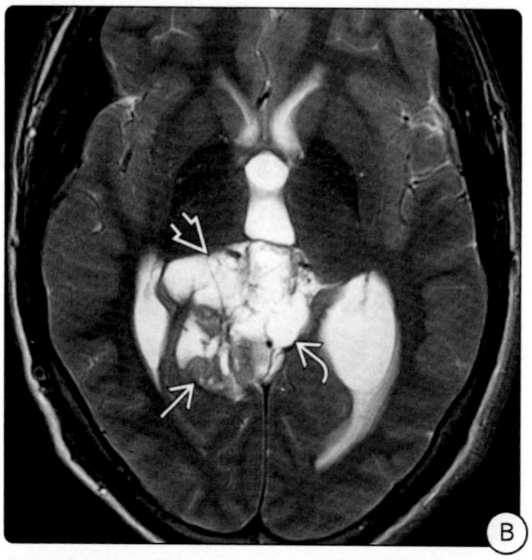

***(20-12B)** T2WI shows numerous hyperintense cysts and solid isointense nodules comprising the mass.*

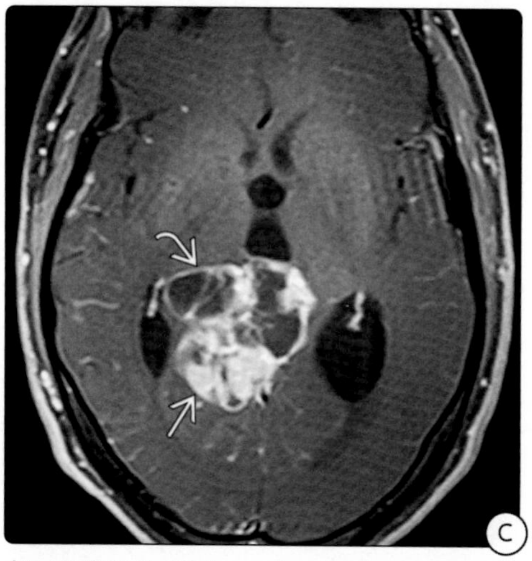

***(20-12C)** T1 C+ FS shows strong enhancement of the solid portions of the mass and cyst walls. Pathology was PPTID, WHO grade III.*

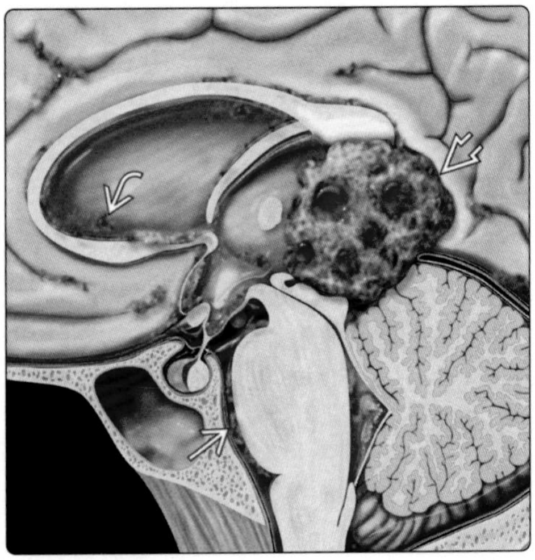

(20-13) Sagittal graphic depicts pineoblastoma ➡ with CSF dissemination into ventricles ➡, subarachnoid spaces ➡.

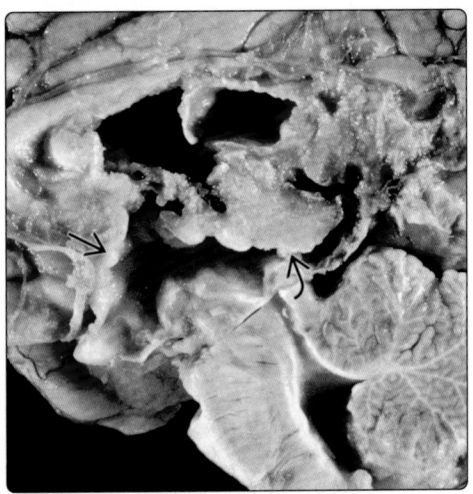

(20-14) Autopsied pineoblastoma ➡ shows dissemination with metastases coating lateral, third ventricles ➡. (Courtesy B. Horten, MD.)

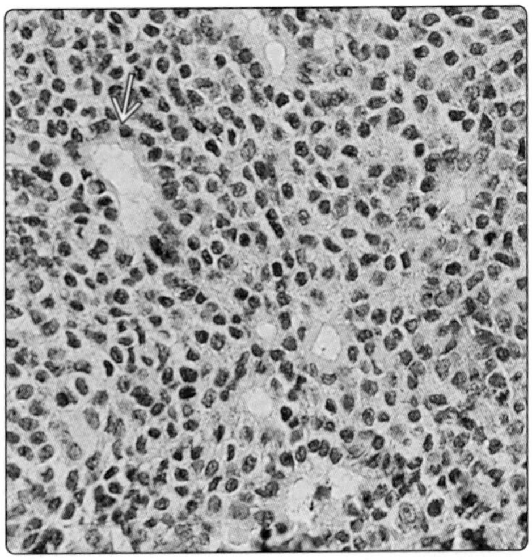

(20-15) Pineoblastoma is composed of sheets of small blue undifferentiated cells with occasional rosettes ➡. (Courtesy B. K. DeMasters, MD.)

Pineoblastoma

Terminology

Pineoblastoma (PB) is a poorly differentiated, highly embryonal neoplasm of the pineal gland.

Etiology

Along with the less malignant pineal parenchymal tumors, PBs share morphologic and immunohistochemical features with embryonic cells of the developing human pineal gland and retina.

PBs are known to occur in patients with *RB1* gene abnormalities. PBs also occur in patients with familial (bilateral) retinoblastoma (the so-called "trilateral retinoblastoma syndrome"), and cases have been reported in familial adenomatous polyposis. Patients with **DICER1 syndrome** are at increased risk for developing PBs.

Pathology

Gross Pathology. A soft, friable, diffusely infiltrating tumor that invades adjacent brain and obstructs the cerebral aqueduct is typical **(20-13)**. Necrosis and intratumoral hemorrhage are common, as is CSF dissemination with sheet-like coating of the brain and spinal cord **(20-14)**.

Microscopic Features. PBs are highly cellular neoplasms that resemble other embryonic neoplasms. Undifferentiated small round blue cells with hyperchromatic nuclei and a high nuclear-to-cytoplasmic ratio are the dominant histologic feature of PB. Occasional Homer-Wright rosettes (neuroblastic differentiation) or Flexner-Wintersteiner rosettes (retinoblastic differentiation) can be identified **(20-15)**. Mitotic activity varies but is generally high.

Staging, Grading, and Classification. PB are WHO grade IV neoplasms.

Clinical Issues

Epidemiology. PBs comprise 0.5-1.0% of primary brain tumors, 15% of pineal region neoplasms, and 20-35% of pineal parenchymal tumors.

Demographics. Although they can occur at any age, PBs are decidedly more prevalent in children. Most present in the first two decades.

Presentation. Symptoms of elevated intracranial pressure such as headache, nausea, and vomiting are typical. Parinaud syndrome is common.

Natural History. PBs are the most primitive and biologically aggressive of all the pineal parenchymal tumors. Prognosis is poor with a median survival of 16-25 months. CSF dissemination is frequent at the time of initial diagnosis and the most common cause of death.

Treatment Options. Surgical debulking with adjuvant chemotherapy and craniospinal radiation comprise the typical regimen.

Imaging

General Features. PBs are large, bulky, aggressive-looking pineal region masses that invade adjacent brain and usually cause obstructive hydrocephalus. CSF dissemination is common, so the entire neuraxis should be imaged prior to surgical intervention.

CT Findings. A large, hyperdense, inhomogeneously enhancing mass with obstructive hydrocephalus is typical. If pineal calcifications are present, they appear "exploded" toward the periphery of the tumor **(20-16A)**.

MR Findings. PBs are heterogeneous tumors that frequently demonstrate necrosis and intratumoral hemorrhage. They are usually mixed iso- to hypointense compared with brain on T1WI and mixed iso- to hyperintense on T2WI **(20-17)**. They enhance strongly but heterogeneously. Because they are densely cellular tumors, restriction on DWI is common **(20-16B)**.

Differential Diagnosis

The major differential diagnosis of PB is **PPTID**. PBs tend to occur in children. CSF dissemination at diagnosis is more common. **Germinoma** may mimic PB on imaging studies, as it also frequently demonstrates CSF spread. Germinomas are more common in adolescent and young adult male patients. They tend to "engulf" rather than "explode" pineal calcifications.

Nongerminomatous malignant germ cell tumors are a heterogeneous group of tumors that may be indistinguishable on imaging studies from PBs. Elevated tumor markers such as α-fetoprotein and β-human chorionic gonadotropin—all usually negative in germinoma and PB—are helpful in establishing the diagnosis.

Pineal anlage tumors are a peculiar, very rare malignant pineal tumor of infants and young children. Pineal anlage tumors exhibit both PB-like neuroectodermal and ectomesenchymal elements (striated muscle, fibrous and adipose tissue, and cartilaginous islands). No endodermal components are present, distinguishing these unusual tumors from teratomas.

Imaging shows a mixed solid and cystic pineal region mass that typically causes obstructive hydrocephalus. Imaging findings are indistinguishable from other pineal parenchymal tumors such as pineocytoma and PPTID. Age is the only characteristic suggesting this rare neoplasm.

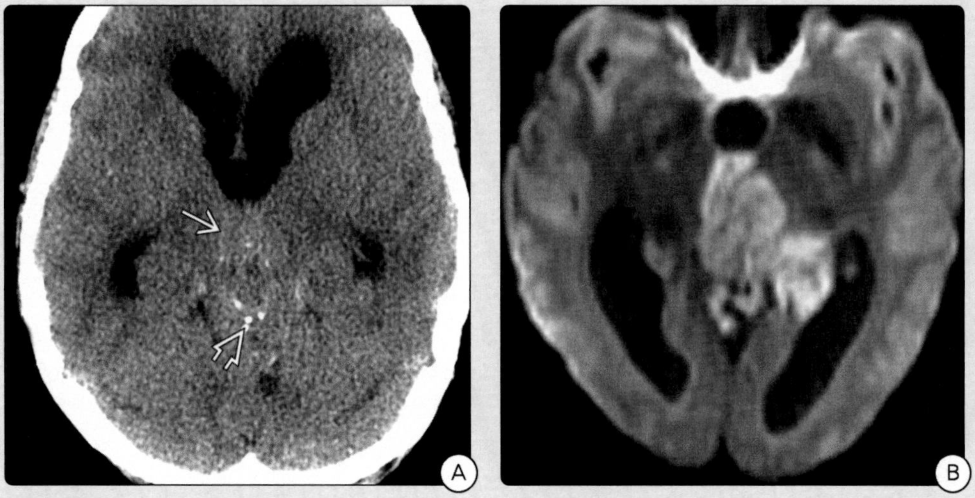

***(20-16A)** NECT of pineoblastoma shows an ill-defined, slightly hyperdense pineal region mass ➡ causing obstructive hydrocephalus. Some calcifications ➡ are seen toward the periphery of the mass. **(20-16B)** DWI in the same patient shows moderate diffusion restriction, consistent with high cellularity.*

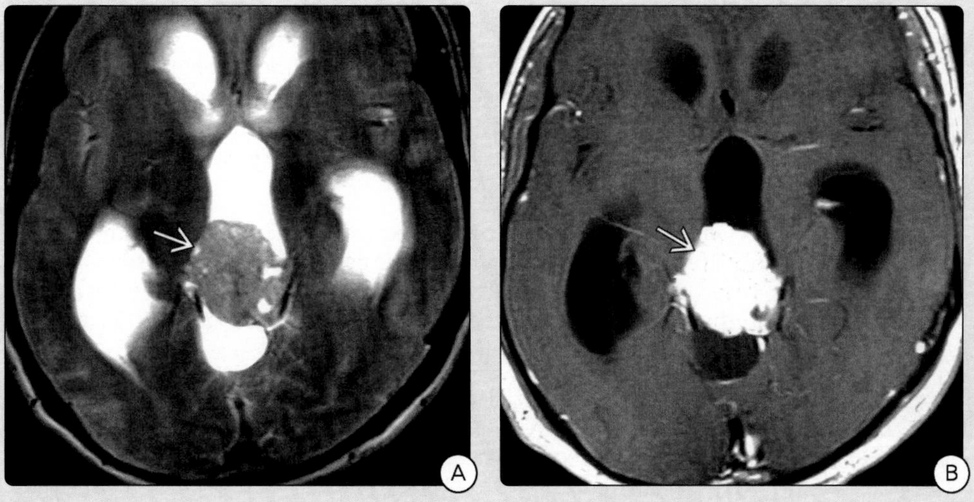

***(20-17A)** T2WI in another patient with pineoblastoma shows a large pineal mass ➡ that causes severe obstructive hydrocephalus. **(20-17B)** T1 C+ scan in the same patient shows that the lesion ➡ enhances intensely, uniformly. (Courtesy R. Hewlett, MD.)*

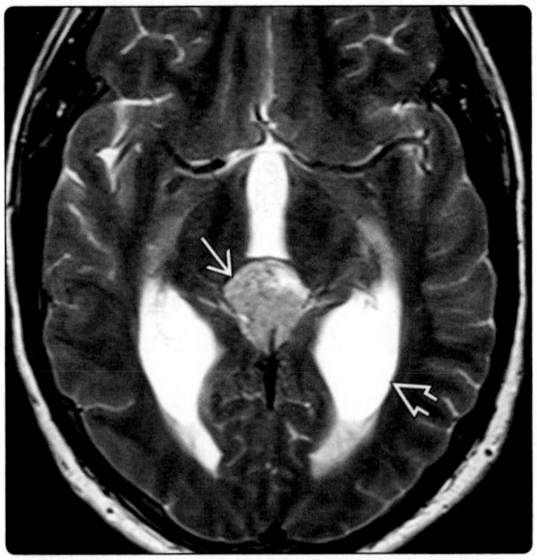

(20-18) T2WI in 43y man w/ headache, nausea, vomiting for 11 days shows hyperintense pineal mass ➡, acute obstructive hydrocephalus ➡.

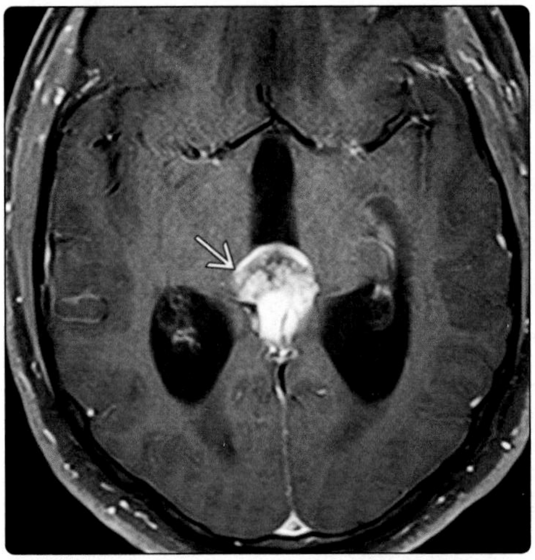

(20-19) T1 C+ FS shows mass ➡ enhances intensely, heterogeneously, no evidence for CSF spread. This is pineoblastoma, WHO grade IV.

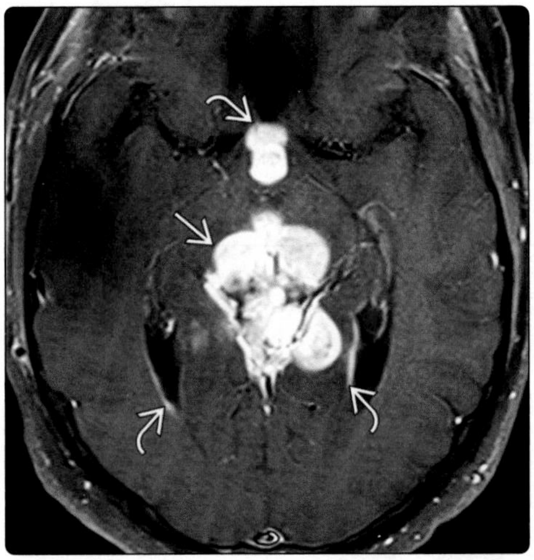

(20-20) The patient deteriorated 5 weeks later. Repeat T1 C+ FS shows mass ➡ has increased significantly, and there is CSF dissemination ➡.

PINEOBLASTOMA

Etiology
- Cells of embryonic pineal gland/retina
- Genetic susceptibility
  - *RB1* mutation
  - Familial adenomatous polyposis
  - *DICER1* germline mutation

Pathology
- Most primitive, malignant of all PPTs
- Diffusely infiltrates adjacent structures
- Early, widespread CSF dissemination common
- WHO grade IV

Clinical Issues
- 15% of pineal region tumors
- 20-35% of PPTs
- All ages but primarily children (< 20 years old)
- Prognosis generally poor

Imaging
- CT
  - Inhomogeneously hyperdense
  - Ca++ "exploded"
- MR
  - Large, bulky, aggressive-looking
  - Necrosis, intratumoral hemorrhage common
  - Enhances strongly, heterogeneously
  - Restricts on DWI (densely cellular)
  - Look for CSF spread (image entire neuraxis)

Papillary Tumor of the Pineal Region

Papillary tumor of the pineal region (PTPR) is a rare neuroepithelial tumor that arises from the subcommissural organ in the posteroinferior wall of the third ventricle **(20-21)**. PTPRs are adult tumors; mean age at diagnosis is 32 years.

Typical chromosomal alterations as well as specific DNA methylation and mRNA expression profiles have been recently delineated that allow differentiation of PTPR from close histopathologic mimics such as ependymoma and PPTID. Chromosome 10 losses are the most common genetic alteration. Several subcommissural organ-related genes such as transcription factor SPDEF are overexpressed in PTPRs.

Macroscopically, PTPRs are indistinguishable from pineocytoma although they are easily differentiated microscopically. PTPRs show distinct papillary architecture with pseudostratified columnar epithelium. Grading of PTPRs has yet to be defined, but, in the 2016 WHO, PTPRs correspond to grade II or III neoplasms.

Outcome is complicated by local recurrence. Two subgroups with differential methylation profiles have been identified. Progression-free survival in patients with a low frequency of hypermethylated genes is nearly three times longer than those with higher methylation levels (125 months vs. 43 months, respectively).

Only a few PTPRs with imaging findings have been reported. PTPRs tend to be large, relatively well circumscribed, and often partially cystic. Strong but heterogeneous enhancement is typical **(20-22)**. No features that would distinguish these tumors from pineal parenchymal tumors of intermediate

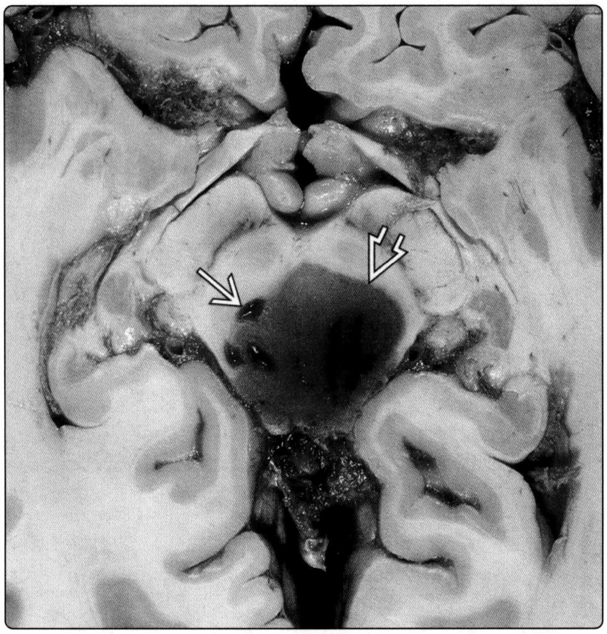

***(20-21)** Autopsy of a posterior third ventricular mass that invades midbrain tegmentum shows cysts ➡, hemorrhage ➡. Microscopy showed ependymal differentiation. Tumor would now likely be classified as PTPR. (Courtesy R. Hewlett, MD.)*

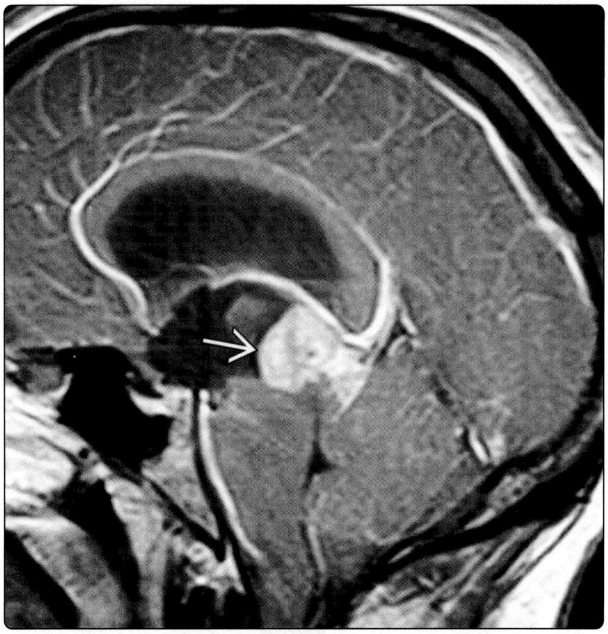

***(20-22)** Sagittal T1 C+ scan of a PTPR shows an enhancing pineal mass ➡ causing obstructive hydrocephalus. These imaging findings are nonspecific. (Courtesy P. Burger, MD.)*

differentiation, the major imaging differential diagnosis, have been described.

PAPILLARY TUMOR OF THE PINEAL REGION

Etiology and Pathology
- Probably arises from subcommissural organ
  - In posteroinferior wall of third ventricle
  - Ependymal differentiation
  - Chromosome 10 loss
  - Transcription factor SPDEF overexpressed
- WHO grade II or III
  - Histologic grading criteria not yet defined

Clinical Features
- Adults
  - Mean age at diagnosis = 32 years
- Local recurrence common; CSF dissemination rare
  - Two subgroups defined by methylation profiling
  - Hypermethylated tumors have shorter progression-free survival

Imaging
- Nonspecific
- Large, lobulated, heterogeneously enhancing mass

Differential Diagnosis
- Pineal parenchymal tumor of intermediate differentiation
- Germinoma

Germ Cell Tumors

Overview of Germ Cell Tumors

Intracranial germ cell tumors (GCTs) are rare neoplasms that vary in histologic differentiation, prognosis, and clinical behavior.

GCTs are divided into two basic groups, germinomas and nongerminomatous germ cell tumors. Germinomas comprise the larger group and represent approximately two-thirds of all GCTs. The smaller group consists of *non*germinomatous GCTs (NGGCTs), which includes both teratomas and a heterogeneous group of "other" nongerminomatous malignant germ cell neoplasms.

We begin with an overview of intracranial GCTs, then discuss germinomas, teratomas, and the "other" germ cell tumors in greater detail.

Terminology

Intracranial GCTs are morphologic and immunophenotypic homologs of similar neoplasms that arise in the gonads and extragonadal sites. They are given the same names as their extracranial counterparts, i.e., germinoma, embryonal carcinoma, yolk sac tumor, choriocarcinoma, teratoma, and mixed GCT.

Etiology

As the normal mature pineal gland does not contain germ cells, GCTs were once thought to arise from "aberrant migration" of cells from at least one of the three primordial germ layers (ectoderm, mesoderm, and endoderm). Recent genome-wide studies show that primary intracranial GCTs have a methylation profile strongly resembling that of primordial germ cells at the migration phase.

Pure germ cell tumors and NGGCTs as well as CNS and testicular GCTs show similar mutational profiles, suggesting that all GCTs share a common molecular pathogenesis. The dominant genetic drivers of GCTs regardless of site of origin are activation of the mitogen-activated protein kinase (MAPK) and/or phosphoinositide 3-kinase (PI3K) pathways, indicating that they develop from a common ancestral cell.

Pathology

Although GCTs can arise in many intracranial locations, they have a distinct affinity for the midline (i.e., the pineal region, around the third ventricle, and the pituitary infundibulum) or very near the midline (i.e., basal ganglia).

GCTs are classified according to histologic features and immunohistochemical profiles. They vary in malignancy from mature teratomas to poorly differentiated, highly aggressive neoplasms such as embryonal carcinoma, choriocarcinoma, and endodermal sinus (yolk sac) tumors. Histologically mixed lesions are common.

Clinical Issues

GCTs account for 0.5-3.5% of all brain tumors but 3-8% of primary CNS neoplasms in children. Prevalence is location dependent. In Asia, GCTs cause 8-15% of pediatric brain tumors.

GCTs are generally tumors of children and young adults; 80-90% of patients are younger than 20 years of age. Many GCTs secrete oncoproteins such as α-fetoprotein or β-hCG, so laboratory evaluation and imaging are both key to diagnosis. Prognosis and treatment vary with tumor type.

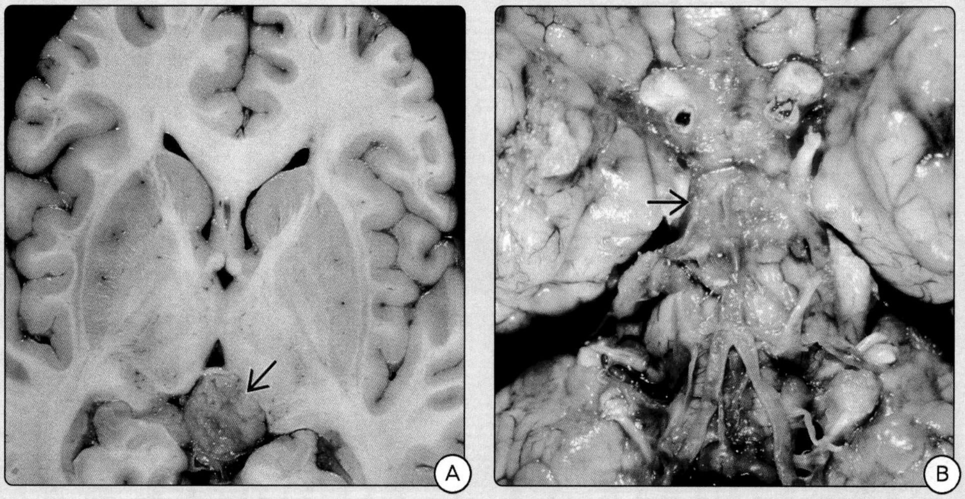

(20-23A) Autopsy specimen shows a pineal germinoma ➔.(Courtesy R. Hewlett, MD.) (20-23B) Submentovertex view of the basal cisterns in the same case shows diffuse CSF tumor ("carcinomatous meningitis") filling the suprasellar cistern ➔ and coating the brain. (Courtesy R. Hewlett, MD.)

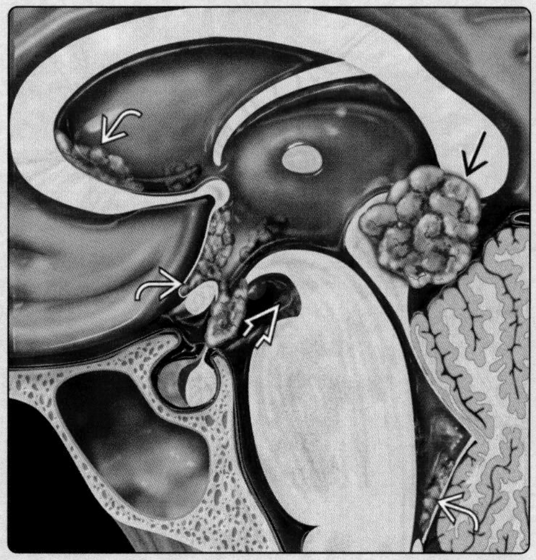

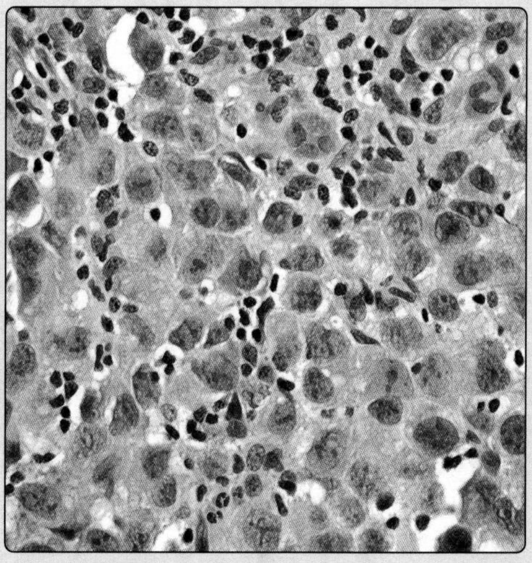

(20-24) Sagittal graphic depicts typical pineal germinoma ➔. CSF dissemination to the third, lateral, and fourth ventricles ➔ is common, as is subarachnoid tumor spread ➔. (20-25) Classic germinoma consists of large round cells with prominent nucleoli, admixed with small lymphocytes. (Courtesy T. Tihan, MD.)

INTRACRANIAL GERM CELL TUMORS

Pathology
- Homologs of gonadal neoplasms
  - Germinoma, teratoma, choriocarcinoma, etc.
- Neoplastic correlates of primitive ectoderm, mesoderm, endoderm
- Propensity to arise in/near midline

Clinical Issues
- 3-8% of primary CNS tumors in children
  - More common in Asia (9-15% of pediatric brain tumors)
- Generally affect children, young adults
  - 80-90% < 20 years old
- Many secrete oncoproteins (α-fetoprotein, β-hCG)
- Treatment, prognosis vary with tumor type

Germinoma

Terminology

Although germinomas are also called dysgerminoma or extragonadal seminoma, "germinoma" is the preferred term. The old name, "atypical teratoma," is confusing and no longer used.

Pathology

Location. Intracranial germinomas have a distinct predilection for midline structures **(20-23)**. Between 80-90% "hug" the midline, extending along the midline axis from the pineal gland to the suprasellar region. One-half to two-thirds are found in the pineal region with the suprasellar region the second most frequent location, accounting for one-quarter to one-third of germinomas.

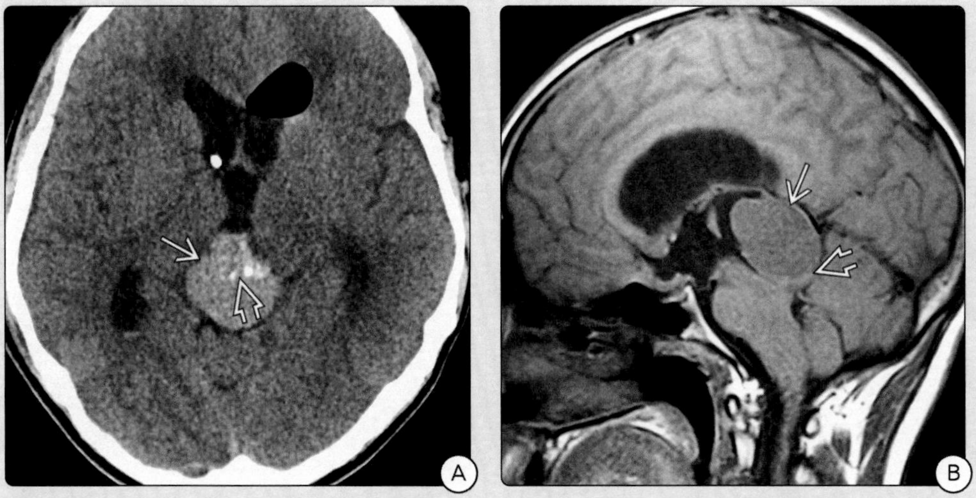

***(20-26A)** Post-ventriculostomy NECT scan in a 19y man shows hyperdense pineal mass ➡ "engulfing" pineal gland calcifications ⇨. **(20-26B)** Sagittal T1WI in the same patient shows a well-defined pineal mass ➡ compressing the tectal plate inferiorly ⇨, causing severe obstructive hydrocephalus.*

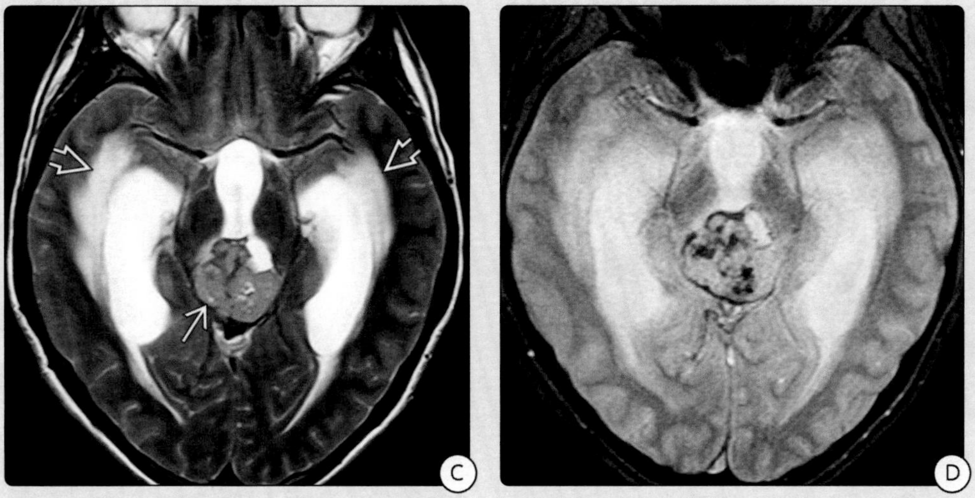

***(20-26C)** T2WI in the same patient shows mixed signal intensity in the mass ➡. Note severe obstructive hydrocephalus with "halo" of fluid around both temporal horns ⇨. **(20-26D)** T2* shows "blooming" hypointensities around and within the mass, probably a combination of hemorrhage and calcification.*

Nongerminomatous subtypes predominate at other sites. Off-midline germinomas occur in only 5-10% of cases. The basal ganglia and thalami are the most common off-midline sites.

Size and Number. Size at diagnosis varies with location. Some infundibular stalk germinomas become symptomatic (usually causing central diabetes insipidus) before they can be detected on high-resolution contrast-enhanced MRs. Pineal germinomas that do not invade the tectum or cause hydrocephalus can be as large as several centimeters at the time of initial diagnosis.

Approximately 20% of intracranial germinomas are multiple. The most frequent combination is a pineal plus a suprasellar ("bifocal" or "double midline") germinoma **(20-24)**. Whether these are metastatic or synchronous lesions is debated.

Gross Pathology. Germinomas are generally solid, friable, tan-white masses that often infiltrate adjacent structures. Intratumoral cysts, small hemorrhagic foci, and CSF dissemination are common **(20-23)**.

Microscopic Features. Germinomas are histologically similar to ovarian dysgerminoma and testicular seminoma. A pure germinoma consists of large, relatively undifferentiated cells with prominent nucleoli arranged in monomorphous sheets or lobules separated by fine fibrovascular septa.

Nearly all germinomas have a biphasic pattern of abundant reactive lymphocytes—usually dominated by T cells—intermixed with large round germinoma cells with prominent nucleoli **(20-25)**. Some tumors exhibit such a florid lymphoplasmacellular reaction that it can obscure the neoplastic elements. Occasionally germinomas provoke an intense granulomatous response that mimics sarcoidosis or tuberculosis.

Mitotic activity is common and may even be conspicuous, but frank necrosis is rare.

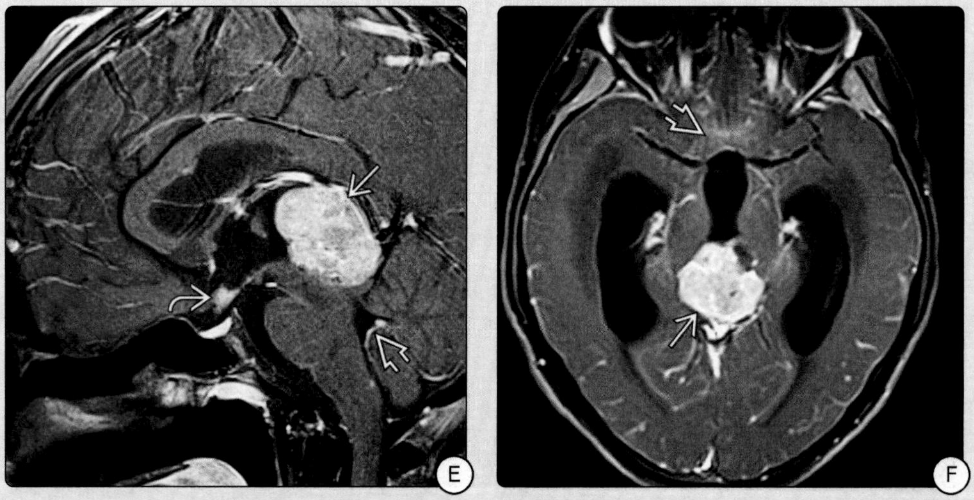

(20-26E) Sagittal T1 C+ FS scan in the same patient shows that the mass ➡ enhances intensely. Note tumor in the anterior recesses of the third ventricle ➡ and along the floor of the fourth ventricle ➡. (20-26F) Axial T1 C+ FS shows the enhancing mass ➡ and sulcal-cisternal enhancement ➡ suggesting CSF dissemination.

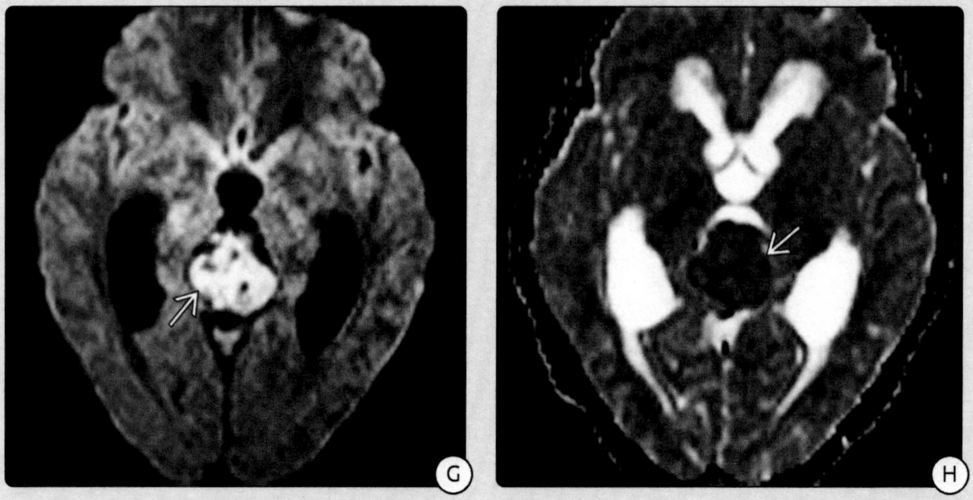

(20-26G) DWI shows diffusion restriction ➡. (20-26H) ADC map shows moderate restriction ➡ consistent with a highly cellular mass. This was confirmed as germinoma.

Clinical Issues

Epidemiology. Germinoma is the most common intracranial GCT and accounts for 1-2% of all primary brain tumors.

Demographics. More than 90% of patients are younger than 20 years of age at initial diagnosis. Peak presentation is 10-14 years. The M:F ratio for pineal germinoma is 10:1. Suprasellar germinomas have no sex predilection.

Presentation. Presentation varies with location. Pineal germinomas typically present with headache and Parinaud syndrome. The most common presentation for suprasellar germinoma is central diabetes insipidus. Visual loss and precocious puberty are other presentations.

CSF cytology is rarely positive for tumor cells. Elevated serum or CSF markers (α-fetoprotein, β-HCG) are rare in pure germinomas but common with mixed GCTs.

Natural History. CSF dissemination and invasion are common, but pure germinomas have a very favorable response to radiation therapy. The five-year survival for treated patients with pure germinoma is greater than 90%.

Germinomas that contain syncytiotrophoblastic giant cells have a higher recurrence rate and reduced long-term survival.

Treatment Options. Histologic documentation followed by radiation therapy is the standard first-line treatment. Adjuvant chemotherapy is reserved for disseminated tumors although the KIT/RAS and AKT1/mTOR pathways are potential therapeutic targets.

"Relapsed" patients are often salvaged with either standard-dose chemotherapy and reirradiation or high-dose chemotherapy plus autologous stem cell rescue, with or without reirradiation. Patients with relapsed germinoma have better overall survival than relapsed NGGCTs.

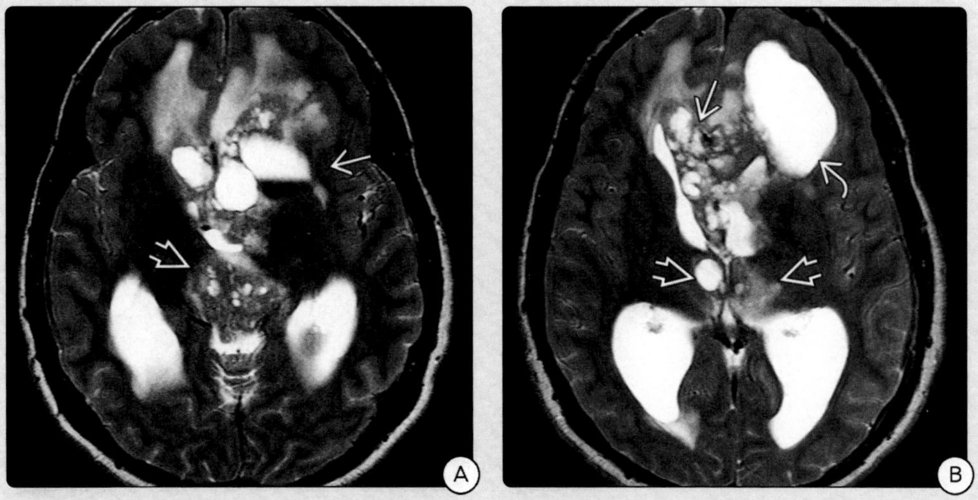

***(20-27A)** Axial T2WI in a 24y man with severe headaches shows two bizarre-appearing masses: one in the pineal gland has multiple cysts ➡. The other tumor—in the basal ganglia and corpus callosum—has multiple cysts, some of which contain hemorrhage ➡. **(20-27B)** The basal ganglionic-corpus callosum mass contains multiple small cysts ➡ and a large cyst in the left frontal lobe ➡. The pineal mass extends anteriorly into the medial thalami ➡.*

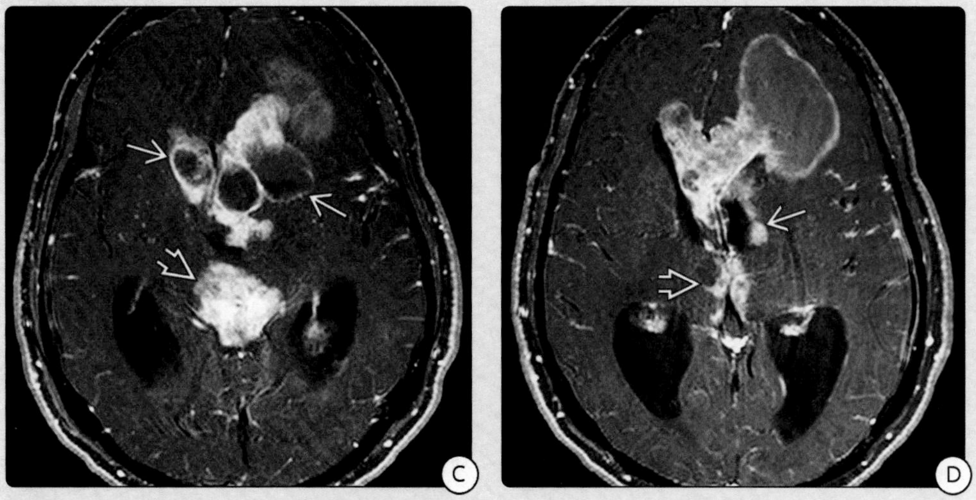

***(20-27C)** T1 C+ FS in the same case shows that the pineal/thalamic mass enhances intensely ➡. The cyst walls of the basal ganglionic-callosal-frontal lobe mass also enhance ➡. **(20-27D)** More cephalad T1 C+ shows enhancing tumor along the ependymal surfaces of the left frontal horn ➡ and third ventricle/thalami ➡. This is a germinoma.*

(20-28A) Sagittal FLAIR in a 16y boy with headaches, Parinaud syndrome shows a pineal mass with surrounding hyperintensity extending into the tectal plate and corpus callosum splenium. *(20-28B)* Axial FLAIR in the same case shows the pineal mass, surrounding hyperintensity extending into both thalami. Obstructive hydrocephalus with periventricular fluid accumulation is present.

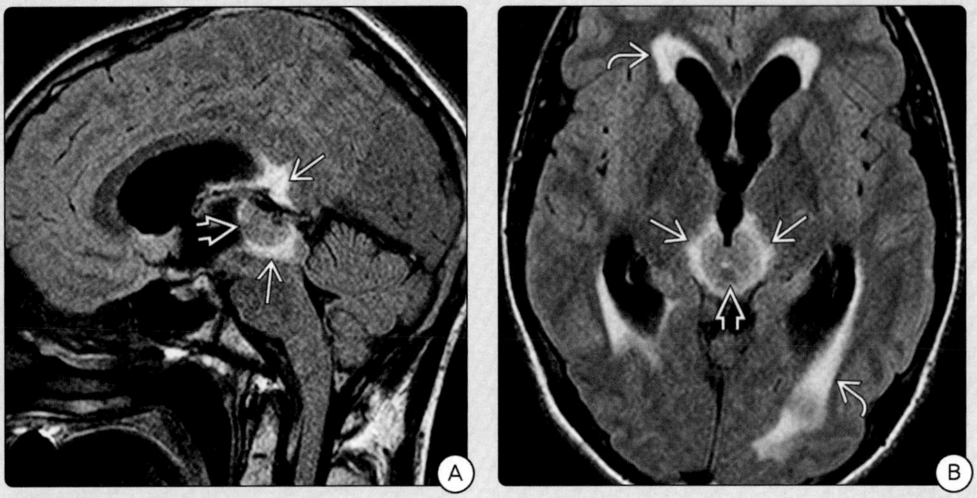

(20-28C) Axial T2WI in the same case shows that the pineal mass contains multiple small cysts and is surrounded by hyperintensity extending into both thalami. *(20-28D)* Coronal T2WI demonstrates the striking perilesional hyperintensity that surrounds the pineal mass.

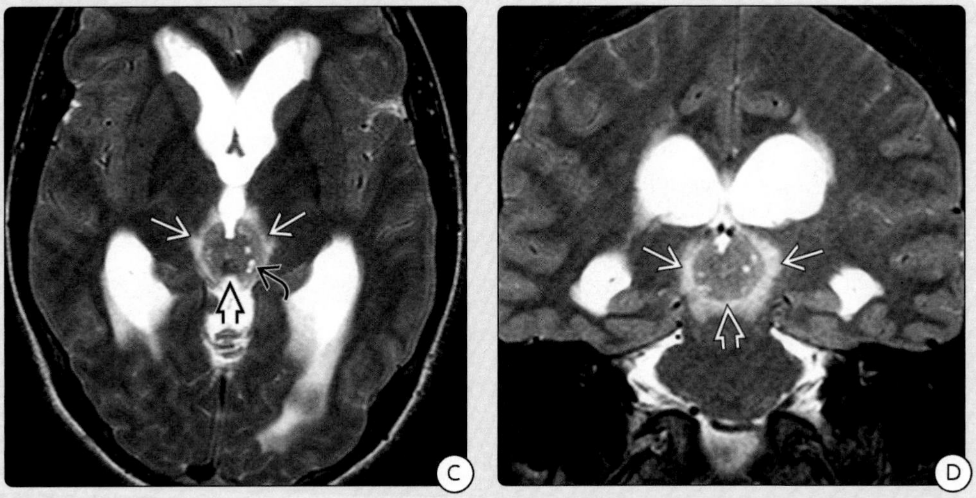

(20-28E) Axial T1 C+ FS shows that the pineal mass enhances strongly and appears well delineated. *(20-28F)* Coronal T1 C+ FS shows that the mass enhances, while the perilesional hypointensity does not. Initial stereotaxic biopsy disclosed only granulomatous inflammation. Repeat biopsy confirmed germinoma.

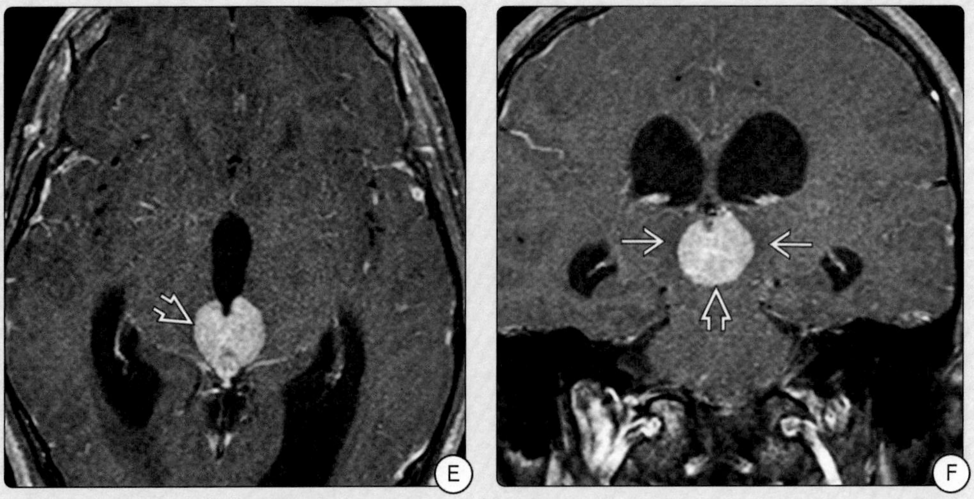

GERMINOMA: PATHOLOGY AND CLINICAL ISSUES

Pathology
- Involve midline structures (80-90%)
- Pineal > > suprasellar > basal ganglia
- Can be multiple (20%)
  - Most common = pineal + suprasellar
- Biphasic microscopic pattern
  - Prominent population of reactive lymphocytes
  - Large primordial germ cells with prominent nucleoli
- "Inflammatory" germinoma
  - Intense granulomatous response
  - Can cause confusion with TB, sarcoid

Clinical Issues
- 1-2% of all neoplasms (more common in Asia)
- Most common intracranial GCT
- > 90% of patients < 20y
- Pineal germinoma, M:F = 3-10:1; suprasellar, M = F
- May cause diabetes insipidus before infundibular lesion seen at imaging!

Imaging

General Features. CSF dissemination is common, so the entire neuraxis should be imaged in patients with suspected germinoma. MR is the procedure of choice for complete delineation of germinoma extent. Caution: some suprasellar germinomas may present with diabetes insipidus long before lesions are visible on MR. In such cases, serial imaging should be performed.

CT Findings. Because nearly all germinomas contain numerous lymphocytes, they are typically hyperdense compared with brain on NECT. They appear to be "draped" around the posterior third ventricle. Obstructive hydrocephalus is variable. Pineal calcifications are "engulfed" and surrounded by tumor **(20-26A)**.

Strong uniform enhancement on CECT is typical. Nearly 20% of germinomas are multiple, so look carefully for a second lesion in the suprasellar region (anterior 3rd ventricle recesses, infundibular stalk) **(20-26E)**!

MR Findings. Germinomas are iso- to slightly hyperintense to cortex on T1- and T2WI **(20-26)**. Variably sized intratumoral cysts are common, especially in larger and "ectopic" lesions. Hemorrhage is generally uncommon except in basal ganglionic germinomas **(20-27)**. T2* (GRE, SWI) may show "blooming" due to intratumoral calcification. Enhancement is strong and usually homogeneous. Because of their high cellularity, germinomas may show restricted diffusion **(20-26)**.

"Inflammatory" germinomas may show extensive, nonenhancing peritumoral T2/FLAIR hyperintensity that extends into adjacent structures, such as the midbrain and thalami **(20-28)**. In such cases, biopsies—especially small stereotaxic samples—may disclose only granulomatous reaction and be mistaken for TB or neurosarcoid.

Differential Diagnosis

The major differential diagnosis of pineal germinoma is **mixed germ cell tumor** as well as **nongerminomatous germ cell tumors**. NGGCTs tend to be larger than germinomas at diagnosis, contain T1 hyperintense foci, enhance more strongly, and have higher mean ADC values. Bifocal lesions are almost always germinomas.

Some **pineoblastomas** may appear similar to germinoma but "explode" rather than "engulf" pineal calcifications. **Pineal parenchymal tumor of intermediate differentiation** usually occurs in middle-aged and older adults.

The major differential diagnosis of suprasellar germinoma is **Langerhans cell histiocytosis** (LCH). Both are common in children, often cause diabetes insipidus, and may be indistinguishable on imaging studies alone. However, LCH does not produce oncoproteins. **Neurosarcoidosis** in an adult can cause a suprasellar mass that resembles germinoma.

GERMINOMA: IMAGING AND DDx

CT
- NECT: Hyperdense, "engulfs" pineal Ca++
- CECT: Enhances strongly, uniformly

MR
- T1 iso-/hypointense, T2 iso-/hyperintense
- Inflammatory germinomas may have extensive peritumoral T2/FLAIR hyperintensity
- GRE shows Ca++, hemorrhage
- Often restricts on DWI
- Enhances intensely, heterogeneously
- CSF spread common (look for other lesions)
  - Anteroinferior 3rd ventricle, infundibular stalk
- Image entire neuraxis before surgery!

Differential Diagnosis
- Nongerminomatous GCT
- PPTs (pineoblastoma, PPTID)
- Histiocytosis (stalk lesion in child)
- Neurosarcoidosis (stalk lesion in adult)

Teratoma

Teratomas are tridermic masses that originate from "misenfolded" or displaced embryonic stem cells. Teratomas recapitulate somatic development and differentiate along ectodermal, mesodermal, and endodermal cell types.

Although they may originate anywhere in the body, teratomas are most commonly found in sacrococcygeal, gonadal, mediastinal, retroperitoneal, cervicofacial, and intracranial locations. Teratomas preferentially involve the midline; intracranial lesions most often arise in the pineal or suprasellar region.

Teratomas account for 2-4% of primary brain tumors in children and almost half of all congenital (perinatal) brain tumors. They account for more than 60% of prenatally detected parenchymal brain tumors.

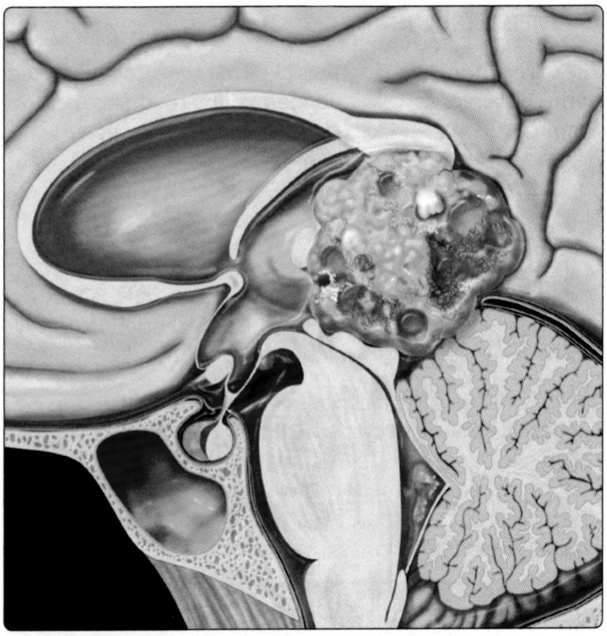

(20-29) Graphic showcases a pineal teratoma with the typical heterogeneous tissue components (cysts, solid tumor, calcifications, fat, etc.).

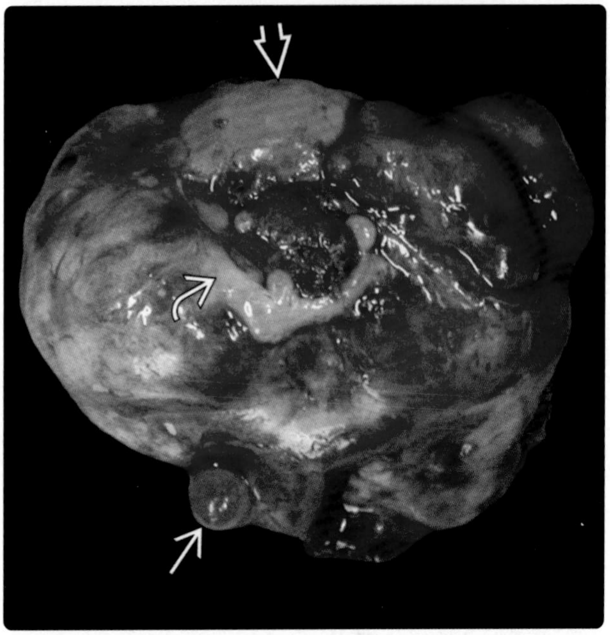

(20-30) Gross pathology of pineal teratoma shows a well delineated heterogeneous mass with a lobulated surface containing cysts ➡, fat ➡, and connective tissue ➡. (From Ellison, Neuropathology, 3e.)

Teratomas are more common in Asians and male patients. They have two peaks in age distribution. Ten percent occur before 5 years of age; nearly half occur from 5-15 years of age. Age at diagnosis is an important prognostic feature, independent of tumor location. Peri- or antenatal presentation is associated with higher risk of adverse outcome. Clinical behavior also varies significantly with tumor size.

There are three recognized types of teratoma. These range from a benign well-differentiated "mature" teratoma to an immature teratoma to a teratoma with malignant differentiation. All three share some imaging features, such as complex masses with striking heterogeneity in density and/or signal intensity. Cysts and hemorrhage are common.

Mature Teratoma

Mature teratomas are well-demarcated lobulated tumors that are composed entirely of fully differentiated adult-type elements from two or three embryonic germ layers. Ectodermal elements such as skin, hair, and dermal appendages (e.g., sebaceous glands) as well as CNS tissue are common **(20-29)**. Mesodermal elements such as cartilage, bony spicules, teeth, adipose tissue, and muscle may be prominent features. Mucinous-appearing intratumoral cysts are common and are often lined with respiratory or gastrointestinal epithelium **(20-30)**.

Mitotic activity is low or absent. A mature teratoma is a WHO grade I lesion.

The size of a mature teratoma varies from relatively small pineal lesions to huge holocranial lesions with massive extracranial extension into the orbit, face, ears, and oral cavity. The intracranial component of these craniofacial teratomas may become so large that there is virtually complete loss of normal intracranial architecture. In such cases, normal brain structures are basically unrecognizable.

Imaging shows a complex-appearing multiloculated lesion with fat, calcification, numerous cysts, and other tissues **(20-31)**. Hemorrhage is common. Enhancement is variable.

Immature Teratoma

Immature teratomas contain a complex admixture of at least some fetal-type tissues from all three germ cell layers in combination with more mature tissue elements **(20-32)** **(20-33)**. It is common to have cartilage, bone, intestinal mucous, and smooth muscle intermixed with primitive neural ectodermal tissue. Hemorrhage and necrosis are common.

Giant immature teratomas are congenital lesions usually seen in a fetus or newborn. Most are associated with stillbirth, perinatal death, or significant morbidity after attempted surgical resection.

The fetal ultrasound diagnosis of intracranial teratoma can generally be established relatively early in pregnancy (15-16 weeks). Macrocephaly, progressive hydrocephalus, and polyhydramnios are common. A rapidly growing heterogeneous mass with mixed hyper- and hypoechogenic features is typical.

CT or MR demonstrate almost complete replacement of brain tissue by a complex mixed-density or signal intensity mass **(20-34)** **(20-35)**.

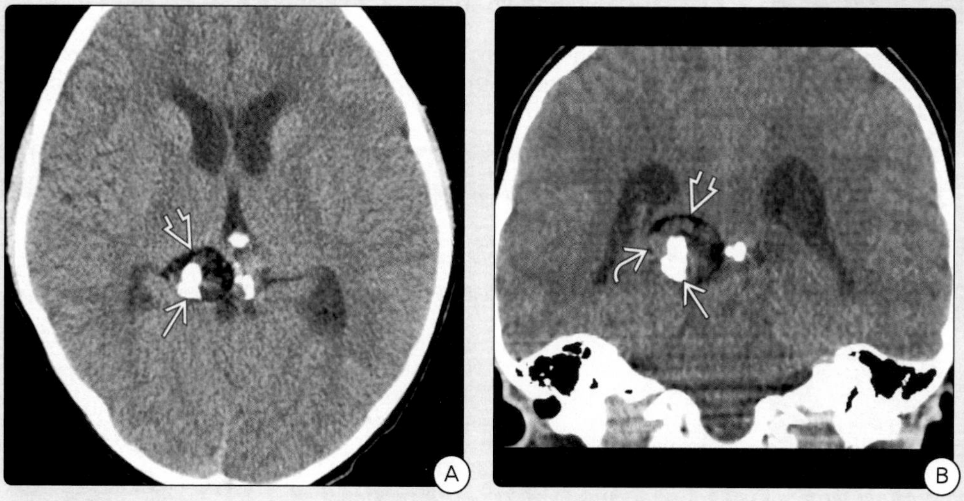

***(20-31A)** Axial NECT in an 8y boy with headaches, nausea, and vomiting shows a very heterogeneous mass in the pineal region. Hypodense fat-attenuation tissue ➾ surrounds a densely calcified component ➾ that grossly resembles a tooth. **(20-31B)** Coronal reformatted NECT shows that the pineal region mass contains very hypodense fat-like tissue ➾, isodense solid components ➾, and the tooth-like calcified hyperdensity ➾.*

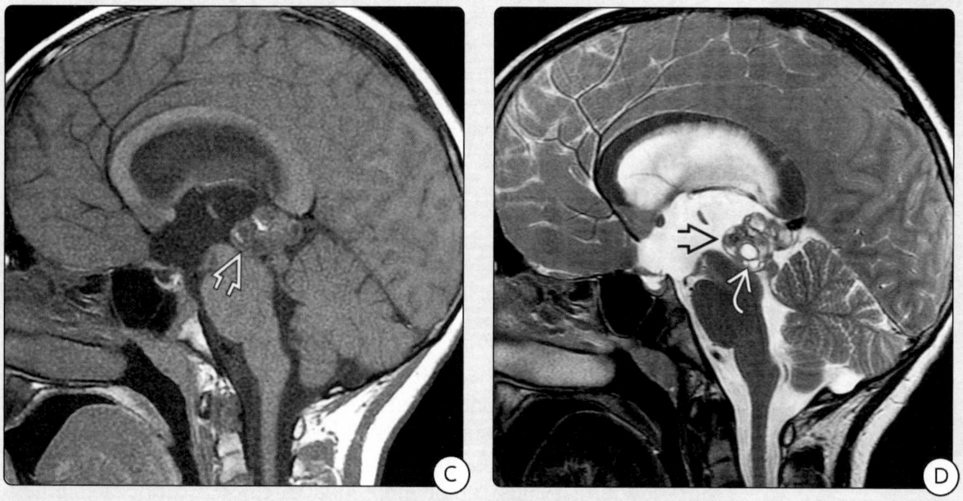

***(20-31C)** Sagittal T1WI in the same case shows a well-delineated, lobulated pineal mass ➾ containing very heterogeneous signal intensities. The mass is causing moderate obstructive hydrocephalus. **(20-31D)** Sagittal T2WI shows that the heterogeneous-appearing mass ➾ also contains numerous cysts ➾.*

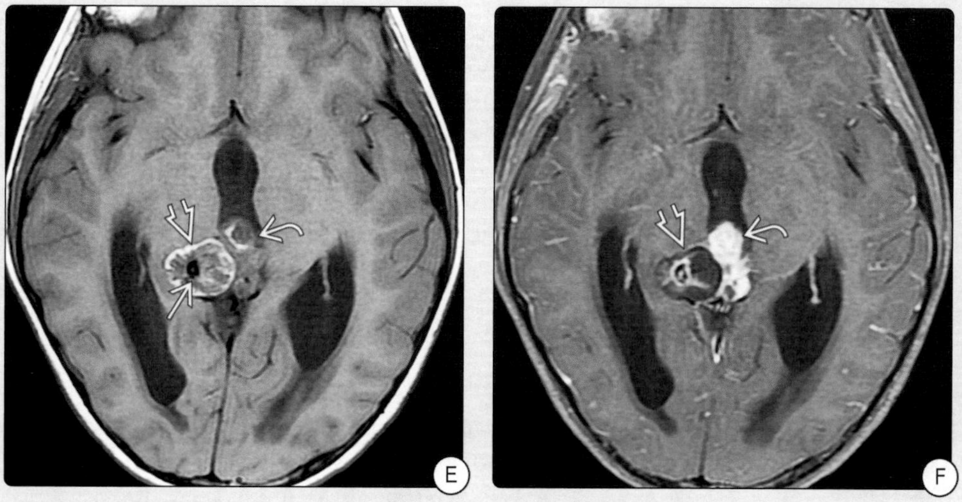

***(20-31E)** Axial T1WI shows T1 shortening around the periphery of the mass ➾ consistent with fat. The internal signal void ➾ is caused by the densely calcified component. A lobulated mixed signal intensity component is present in the posterior 3rd ventricle ➾. **(20-31F)** T1 C+ FS shows that the fat suppresses ➾ and the lobulated component enhances strongly ➾. Mature teratoma was removed at surgery.*

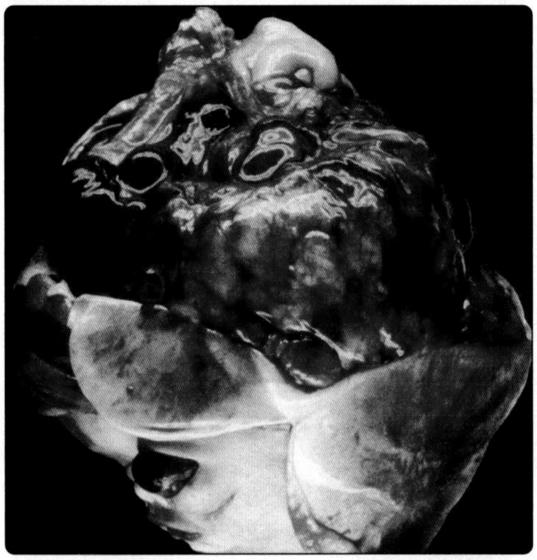

(20-32) Fetal autopsy case shows a large intra- and extracranial immature teratoma with multiple cysts and hemorrhage.

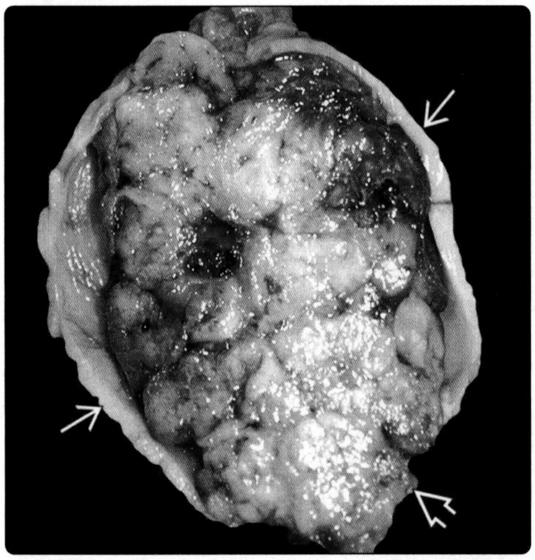

(20-33) Autopsy of congenital teratoma shows a heterogeneous mass ➔ occupying most of the brain ➔. (Courtesy T. Tihan, MD.)

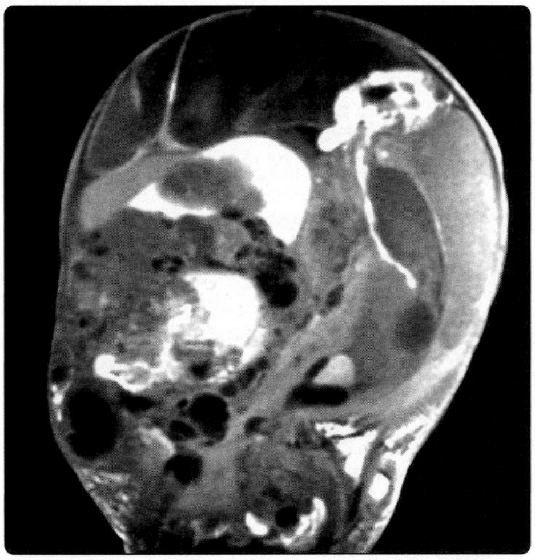

(20-34) Postmortem T1WI of a newborn shows a complex holocranial mass of mixed signal intensity. This is immature teratoma.

Teratoma With Malignant Transformation

Teratomas with malignant transformation generally arise from immature teratomas and contain somatic-type cancers such as rhabdomyosarcoma or undifferentiated sarcoma.

INTRACRANIAL TERATOMAS

Pathology
- Arise from totipotential germ cells
- Tridermic with cells derived from all 3 germ cell layers
- 3 types
  - Mature teratoma (most common; well differentiated)
  - Immature teratoma (some incompletely differentiated tissue)
  - Teratoma with malignant transformation

Clinical Issues
- Only 3-4% of all teratomas are in CNS
- 40-50% of all congenital brain tumors

Imaging
- Large holocranial/extracranial lesion in newborn?
  - Most likely teratoma
  - Distorts skull/brain, splits sutures
  - Intracranial structures may be unrecognizable
  - May extend through skull base into oral cavity
  - Mixed density/signal intensity
  - Cysts, hemorrhage common
- Pineal teratoma
  - Mixed density, signal intensity
  - Fat, Ca++, bone, cysts common
  - Often causes obstructive hydrocephalus

Other Germ Cell Neoplasms

Germinomas are by far the most common of the germ cell neoplasms. Nongerminomatous malignant germ cell tumors (NGMGCTs) are rare neoplasms that contain undifferentiated epithelial cells and are often mixed with other germ cell elements (most often germinoma). These include **yolk sac (endodermal sinus) tumor, embryonal carcinoma, choriocarcinoma**, and **mixed germ cell tumor**.

NGMGCTs generally occur in adolescents with a peak incidence at 10-15 years of age. Prognosis is usually poor with overall survival less than 2 years.

Differentiating intracranial germ cell neoplasms on the basis of imaging studies alone is problematic. All intracranial GCTs—whether benign or malignant—tend to "hug" the midline. Many express different oncoproteins, so immunohistochemical profiling is an essential part of diagnosis.

Yolk Sac Tumor

Yolk sac (endodermal sinus) tumors represent just 2% of all intracranial GCTs. Yolk sac tumors are composed of primitive epithelial cells in a loose, variably cellular myxoid matrix. Peak occurrence is in the second decade. Imaging features are nonspecific.

Embryonal Carcinoma

Embryonal carcinoma is another tumor that contains large, anaplastic epithelioid cells that are arranged in sheets, cords, and nests.

Imaging findings are nonspecific and may be indistinguishable from germinoma **(20-36)**.

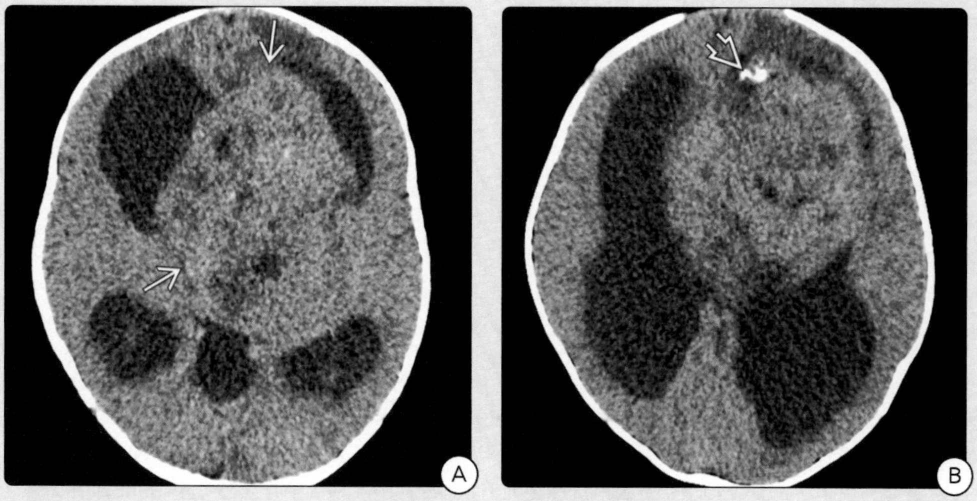

***(20-35A)** Axial NECT in a newborn with macrocephaly shows a mixed-density midline mass → expanding and obstructing the lateral and third ventricles. **(20-35B)** More cephalad NECT shows a focus of calcification → in the mass.*

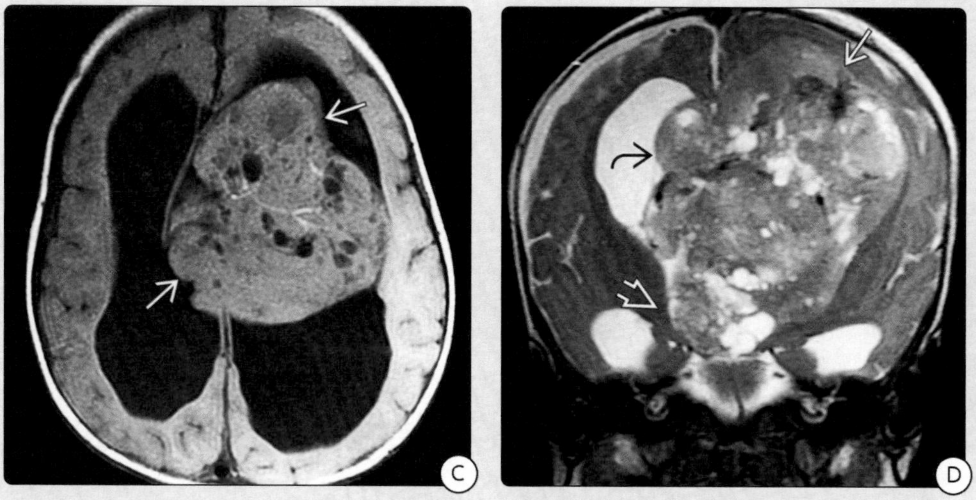

***(20-35C)** Axial T1WI shows that the lobulated mass → is relatively well demarcated and exhibits hypo-, iso-, and hyperintense foci. **(20-35D)** The mass is very heterogeneous-appearing on this coronal T2WI. Note that the mass fills most of the left lateral ventricle →, extends across the midline into the right lateral ventricle →, and inferiorly through the foramen of Monro into the third ventricle →.*

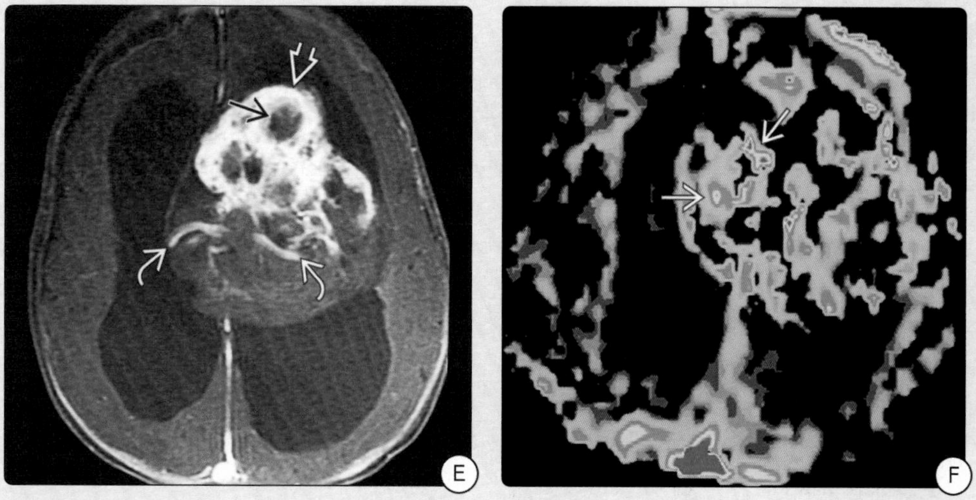

***(20-35E)** Axial T1 C+ FS shows that part of the mass enhances strongly but heterogeneously →. Note intratumoral cysts → and tubular enhancement from prominent neovascularity →. **(20-35F)** MR perfusion in the same case shows some intratumoral foci of elevated rCBV →. Immature teratoma was found at surgery.*

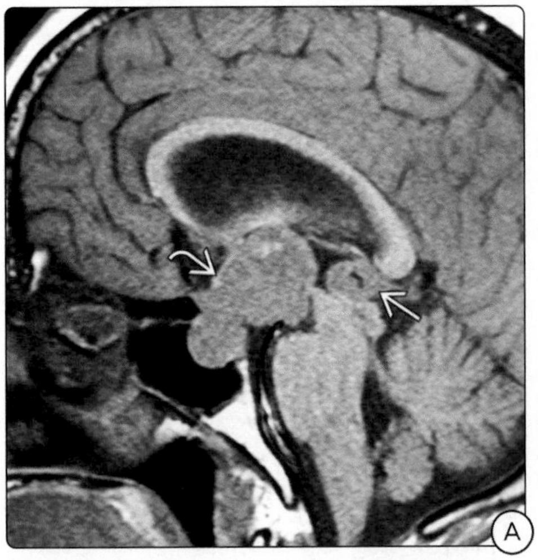

***(20-36A)** Sagittal T1WI in a 22y man with headaches, diabetes insipidus shows a sellar/suprasellar mass, pineal lesion.*

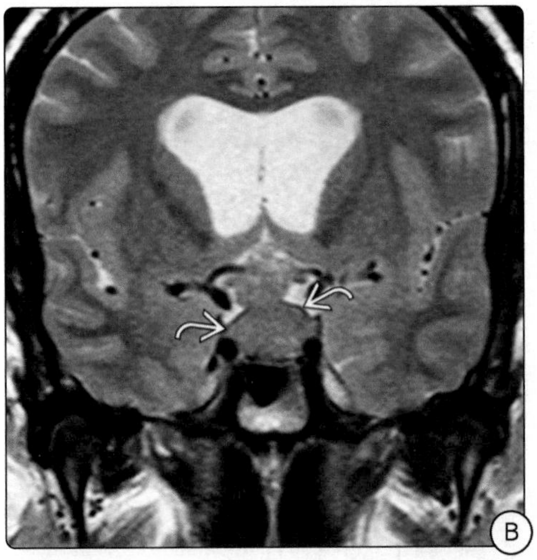

***(20-36B)** Coronal T2WI shows that the intra/suprasellar mass appears moderately hypointense.*

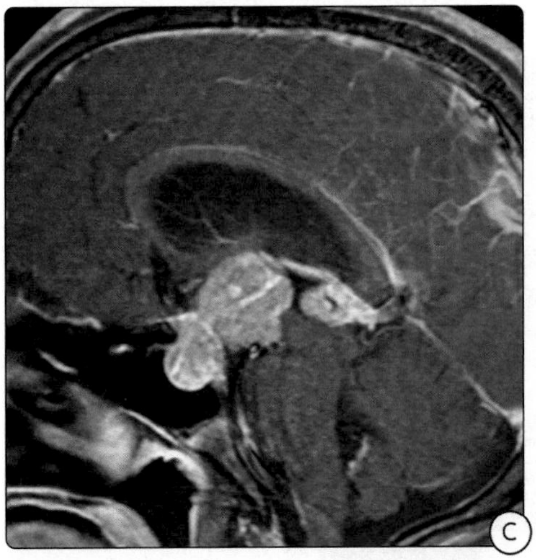

***(20-36C)** Both masses enhance strongly but heterogeneously on T1 C+ FS. This is embryonal carcinoma.*

Choriocarcinoma

Most choriocarcinomas develop within or outside the uterus following a gestational event ("gestational" choriocarcinoma). Nongestational choriocarcinomas can arise from germ cells in gonadal or extragonadal midline locations.

CNS choriocarcinoma can be primary or metastatic, arising from an extracranial site such as the retroperitoneum or mediastinum. Primary intracranial choriocarcinoma (PICCC) is the rarest, most malignant of all the intracranial GCTs.

PICCCs are dimorphic tumors characterized by extraembryonic differentiation along cytotrophoblastic and syncytiotrophoblastic lines. They are composed of mononucleated trophoblastic cells admixed with large multinucleated syncytiotrophoblastic cells. Hemorrhage, necrosis, fibrosis, and neovascularity are common.

PICCCs typically present in patients 3-20 years of age. There is a nearly 4:1 male predominance. Precocious puberty is the most common presentation in male patients. Markedly elevated serum hCG/β-hCG levels are strongly suggestive of PICCC.

The most common sites of PICCC are the pineal and suprasellar regions. MR is helpful for tumor localization, characterization, and preoperative evaluation, but the findings are nonspecific. Intratumoral hemorrhages with stripe-like or patchy hypointensities on T2WI are common. Heterogeneous rim and nodular enhancement is seen in most cases. Extraneural/CSF metastases are common.

Mixed Germ Cell Tumor

Mixed GCTs are composed of any of the above histologic subtypes, often together with germinomatous elements. Mixed GCTs are more common than any pure germ cell lesion except for germinoma. Imaging findings are nonspecific **(20-37)**.

"Other Cell" Pineal and Pineal Region Neoplasms

Miscellaneous Pineal Neoplasms

Rarely, tumors arising within the pineal gland are composed of neoplastic elements other than parenchymal or germ cells. Primary glial neoplasms such as astrocytoma (including glioblastoma) **(20-38)** and oligodendroglioma **(20-39)** can occur within the pineal gland itself as can melanoma arising from pineal melanocytes **(20-40)**. Metastases from extracranial sources also occasionally present as pineal masses **(20-41)**.

In general, imaging findings with intrinsic pineal gland masses are nonspecific and do not permit differentiation between the broad spectrum of histologic types, so biopsy is necessary to guide patient management.

Miscellaneous Pineal Region Masses

Neoplasms and nonneoplastic masses in the pineal region can also originate from nongland structures such as the tectal plate, third ventricle, meninges of the tentorial apex, and the CSF spaces **(20-42)** **(20-43)**. A general approach to evaluating pineal region masses is delineated in the box below.

APPROACH TO PINEAL REGION MASSES

Key Questions to Consider

- Is the mass in the pineal gland itself?
  - If not, can you determine its anatomic origin?
- What is the patient's age, sex?
- Is there serum or CSF evidence of oncoproteins?
- Is there imaging evidence for other lesions?
  - Pineal + suprasellar usually = germinoma
  - Pineal + CSF spread usually = GCT, metastasis

Pineal Gland Mass

- Common
  - Pineal cyst (nonneoplastic)
- Less common
  - Pineocytoma
  - Germinoma
- Rare but important
  - Pineal parenchymal tumor of intermediate differentiation
  - Pineoblastoma
  - "Trilateral retinoblastoma"
  - Teratoma (mature or immature)
  - Nongerminomatous malignant germ cell tumor
  - Papillary tumor of the pineal region
  - Glioma (astrocytoma, oligodendroglioma)
  - Metastasis
  - Melanoma

Pineal Region Mass

- Common
  - Intrinsic masses of the pineal *gland* itself (see above)
- Less common (masses *outside* pineal gland)
  - Arachnoid cyst
  - Dermoid cyst
  - Epidermoid cyst
  - Astrocytoma (tectal glioma)
  - Meningioma (tentorial apex)
  - Lipoma
  - Metastasis
- Rare but important
  - Vascular malformation (vein of Galen malformation, dural arteriovenous fistula)
  - Vertebrobasilar dolichoectasia
  - Basilar tip aneurysm
  - Schwannoma (CNs III, IV)

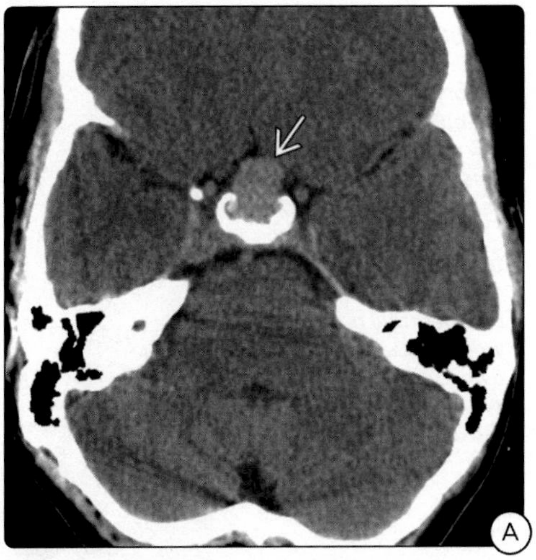

***(20-37A)** NECT in a 19y man with diabetes insipidus shows a partially calcified hyperdense suprasellar mass.*

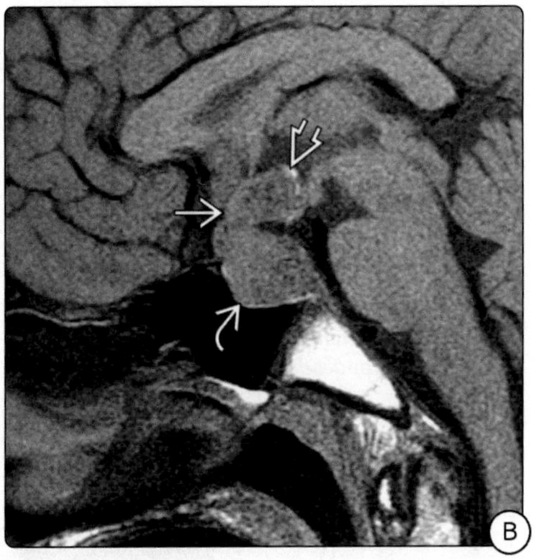

***(20-37B)** Sagittal T1WI shows mass infiltrates pituitary gland, infundibulum/third ventricle, contains scattered foci of T1 shortening.*

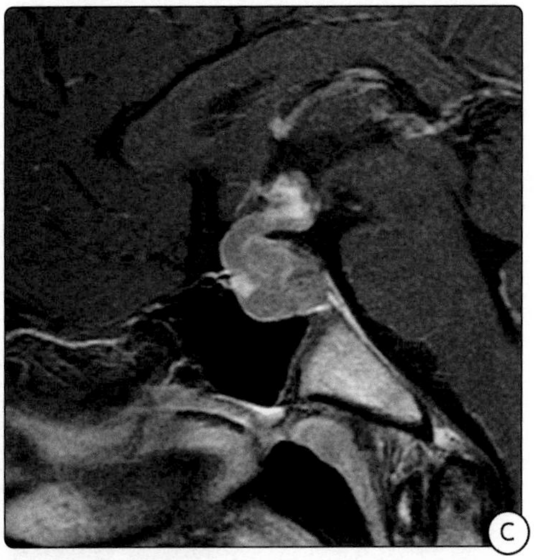

***(20-37C)** The mass enhances on T1 C+ FS. Mixed germ cell tumor with germinomatous and mature teratomatous elements was found at surgery.*

*(**20-38A**) Axial T2WI in a 56y man with 4-week history of headache, diplopia shows a mixed iso- and hyperintense mass in the posterior third ventricle/pineal region. (**20-38B**) T1 C+ FS in the same case shows that the mass enhances strongly. Preoperative diagnosis was PPTID. Anaplastic astrocytoma, IDH wild-type, was found at histopathology.*

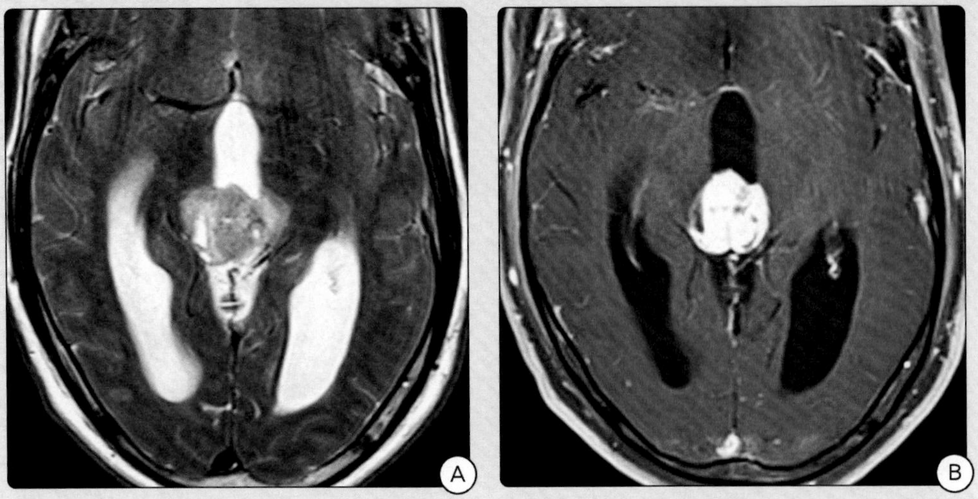

*(**20-39A**) Axial T2WI in a 37y man with Parinaud syndrome shows a mixed signal mass in the pineal region. (**20-39B**) T1 C+ in the same case shows mixed solid, cystic enhancing portions of the mass. Preoperative diagnosis was PPTID. Oligodendroglioma was found at histopathology.*

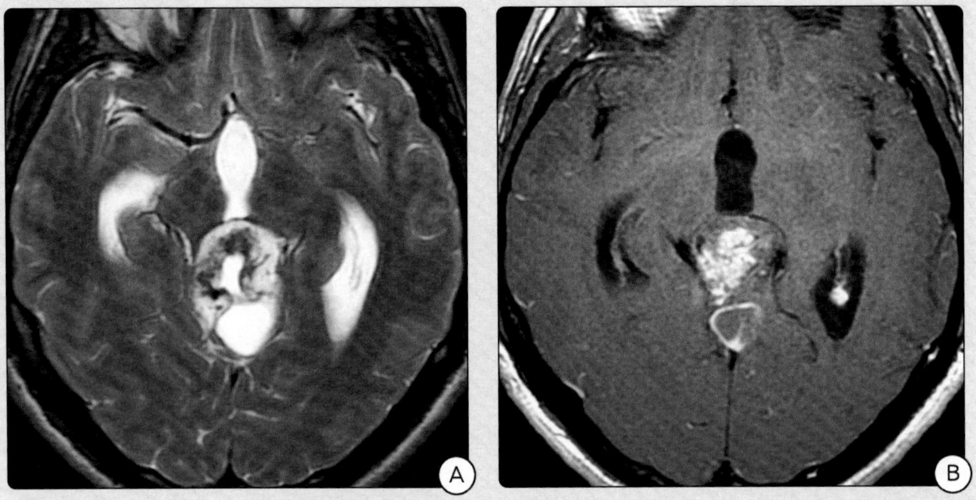

*(**20-40A**) Axial T2WI in a 68y man with headache and altered mental status shows acute obstructive hydrocephalus caused by a mixed signal mass in the pineal region. (**20-40B**) T1 C+ FS in the same case shows the mass enhances strongly. Stereotaxic biopsy revealed melanoma. No systemic source could be identified, so this is a presumed primary melanoma of the pineal gland.*

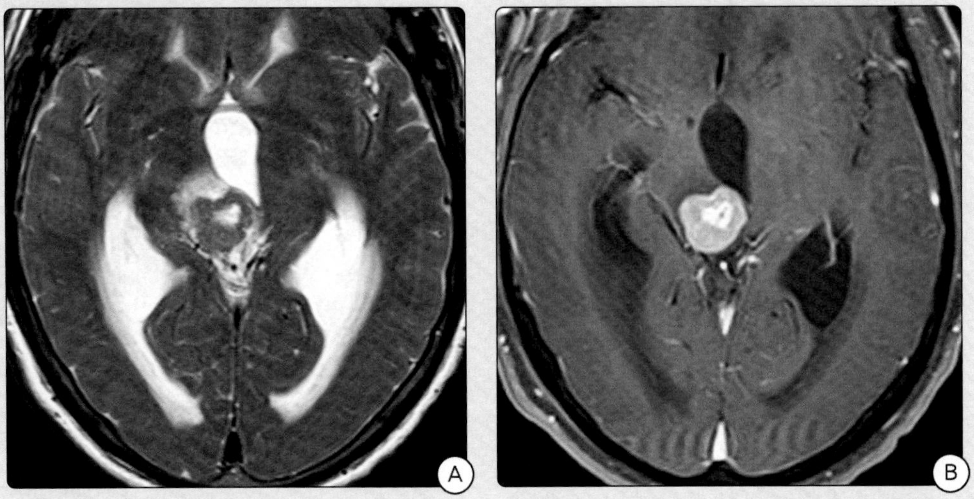

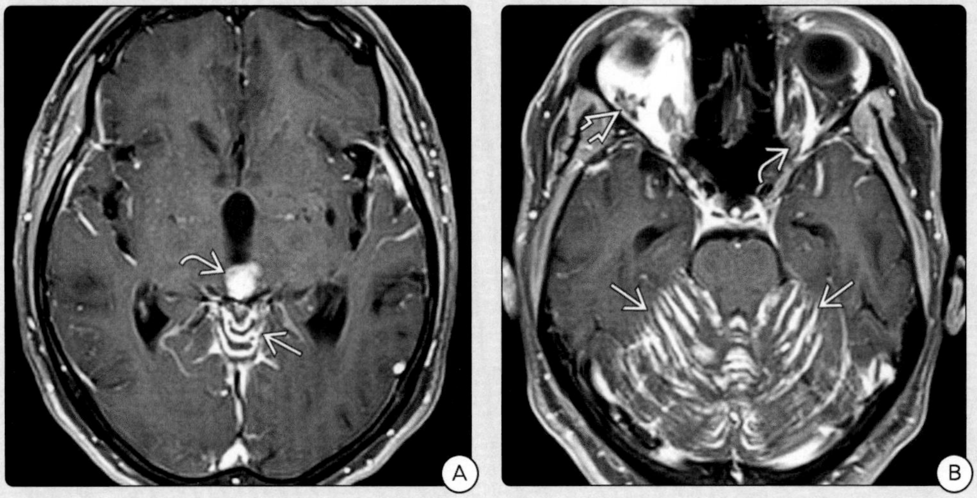

***(20-41A)** T1 C+ FS in a 63y woman with breast cancer, headaches, and Parinaud syndrome shows enhancing pineal mass and a pial tumor in the superior vermis. **(20-41B)** More inferior T1 C+ shows diffuse CSF spread outlining the cerebellar folia. Note metastasis to the right orbit and CSF spread along left optic nerve sheath.*

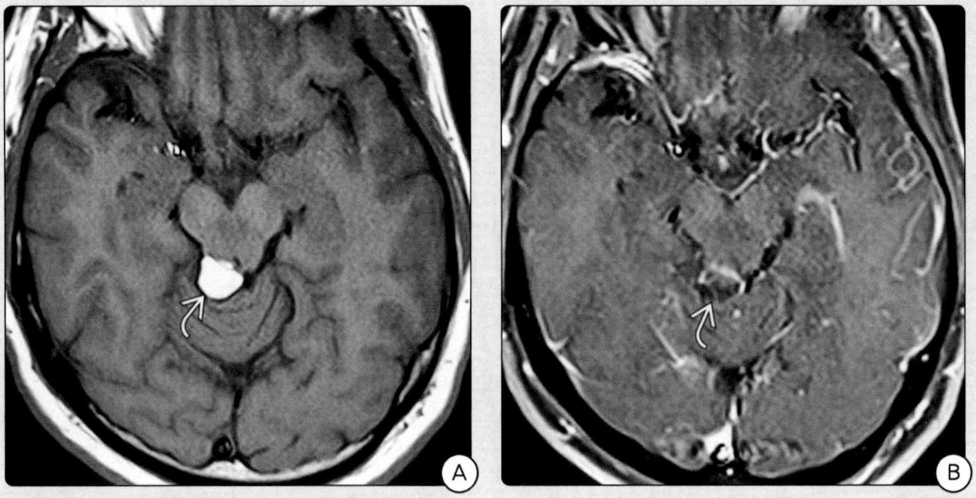

***(20-42A)** Axial T1WI in a patient scanned for stroke-like symptoms shows a well-delineated hyperintense mass that abuts the tectal plate. **(20-42B)** Axial T1 C+ FS in the same case shows that the tectal plate mass suppresses. This is quadrigeminal plate lipoma, incidental finding.*

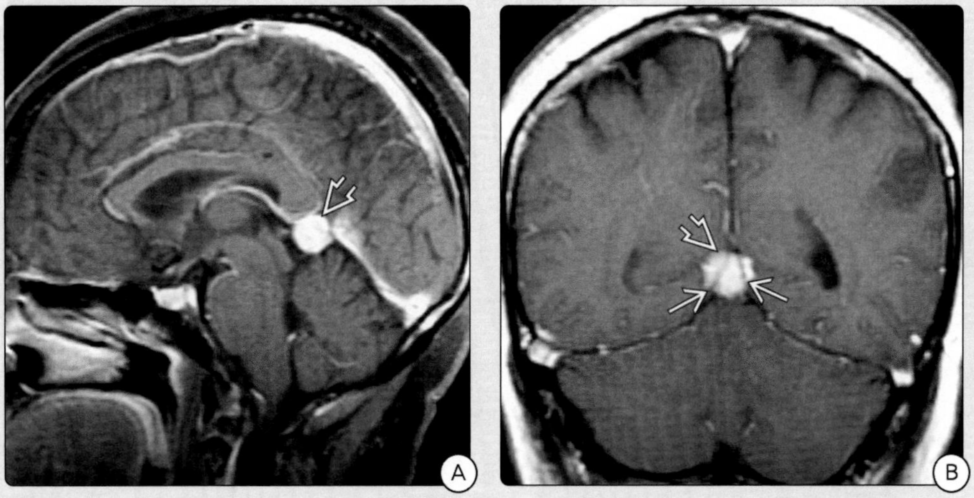

***(20-43A)** Sagittal T1 C+ FS in a 50y woman with headaches shows a well-demarcated, intensely enhancing mass in the pineal region (quadrigeminal cistern) near the tentorial apex. **(20-43B)** Coronal T1 C+ shows that the intensely enhancing mass straddles the leaves of the tentorium cerebelli. This is tentorial apex meningioma, incidental finding.*

Selected References

Pineal Region Anatomy and Histology

Shoja MM et al: History of the pineal gland. Childs Nerv Syst. 32(4):583-6, 2016

Jiménez-Heffernan JA et al: Cytologic features of the normal pineal gland of adults. Diagn Cytopathol. 43(8):642-5, 2015

Gross Anatomy

Matsuo S et al: Midline and off-midline infratentorial supracerebellar approaches to the pineal gland. J Neurosurg. 126(6):1984-1994, 2017

Meyer FB et al: Introduction to microsurgery of the third ventricle, pineal region, and tentorial incisura. Neurosurg Focus. 40 Video Suppl 1:1, 2016

Normal Imaging

Galluzzi P et al: MRI-based assessment of the pineal gland in a large population of children aged 0-5 years and comparison with pineoblastoma: part I, the solid gland. Neuroradiology. 58(7):705-12, 2016

Sirin S et al: MRI-based assessment of the pineal gland in a large population of children aged 0-5 years and comparison with pineoblastoma: part II, the cystic gland. Neuroradiology. 58(7):713-21, 2016

Whitehead MT et al: Physiologic pineal region, choroid plexus, and dural calcifications in the first decade of life. AJNR Am J Neuroradiol. 36(3):575-80, 2015

Pineal Parenchymal Tumors

Tamrazi B et al: Pineal region masses in pediatric patients. Neuroimaging Clin N Am. 27(1):85-97, 2017

Mottolese C et al: Incidence of pineal tumours. A review of the literature. Neurochirurgie. 61(2-3):65-9, 2015

Ostrom QT et al: CBTRUS Statistical Report: primary brain and central nervous system tumors diagnosed in the United States in 2008-2012. Neuro Oncol. 17 Suppl 4:iv1-iv62, 2015

Pineocytoma

Nakazato Y et al: Pineocytoma. In: Louis DN et al (eds), WHO Classification of Tumours of the Central Nervous System. Lyon, France: International Agency for Research on Cancer, 2016, pp. 170-172

Pineal Parenchymal Tumor of Intermediate Differentiation

Raleigh DR et al: Histopathologic review of pineal parenchymal tumors identifies novel morphologic subtypes and prognostic factors for outcome. Neuro Oncol. 19(1):78-88, 2017

Amato-Watkins AC et al: Pineal parenchymal tumours of intermediate differentiation - an evidence-based review of a new pathological entity. Br J Neurosurg. 30(1):11-5, 2016

Kang YJ et al: Integrated genomic characterization of a pineal parenchymal tumor of intermediate differentiation. World Neurosurg. 85:96-105, 2016

Pineoblastoma

Bueno MT et al: Pediatric imaging in DICER1 syndrome. Pediatr Radiol. ePub, 2017

Parikh KA et al: Pineoblastoma-the experience at St. Jude Children's Research Hospital. Neurosurgery. ePub, 2017

Gener MA et al: Clinical, pathological, and surgical outcomes for adult pineoblastomas. World Neurosurg. 84(6):1816-24, 2015

Papillary Tumor of the Pineal Region

Heim S et al: Papillary tumor of the pineal region: a distinct molecular entity. Brain Pathol. 26(2):199-205, 2016

Germ Cell Tumors

Overview of Germ Cell Tumors

Fukushima S et al: Genome-wide methylation profiles in primary intracranial germ cell tumors indicate a primordial germ cell origin for germinomas. Acta Neuropathol. 133(3):445-462, 2017

Wu CC et al: MRI features of pediatric intracranial germ cell tumor subtypes. J Neurooncol. ePub, 2017

Germinoma

Pérez-Ramírez M et al: Pediatric pineal germinomas: epigenetic and genomic approach. Clin Neurol Neurosurg. 152:45-51, 2017

Ichimura K et al: Recurrent neomorphic mutations of MTOR in central nervous system and testicular germ cell tumors may be targeted for therapy. Acta Neuropathol. 131(6):889-901, 2016

Rosenblum MK et al: Germ cell tumors. In: Louis DN et al (eds), WHO Classification of Tumours of the Central Nervous System. Lyon, France: International Agency for Research on Cancer, 2016, pp. 286-291

Teratoma

Algahtani H et al: Teratoma of the nervous system: a case series. Neurocirugia (Astur). ePub, 2017

Nariai H et al: Prenatally diagnosed aggressive intracranial immature teratoma-clinicopathological correlation. Fetal Pediatr Pathol. 35(4):260-4, 2016

Robles Fradejas M et al: Fetal intracranial immature teratoma: presentation of a case and a systematic review of the literature. J Matern Fetal Neonatal Med. 1-8, 2016

DasGupta S et al: Central nervous system teratomas in infants: a report of two cases. Indian J Pathol Microbiol. 58(1):89-92, 2015

Other Germ Cell Neoplasms

Murray MJ et al: A pipeline to quantify serum and cerebrospinal fluid microRNAs for diagnosis and detection of relapse in paediatric malignant germ-cell tumours. Br J Cancer. 114(2):151-62, 2016

Zhang S et al: Clinical and radiologic features of pediatric basal ganglia germ cell tumors. World Neurosurg. 95:516-524.e1, 2016

Jinguji S et al: Long-term outcomes in patients with pineal nongerminomatous malignant germ cell tumors treated by radical resection during initial treatment combined with adjuvant therapy. Acta Neurochir (Wien). 157(12):2175-83, 2015

"Other Cell" Pineal and Pineal Region Neoplasms

Lensing FD et al: Pineal region masses--imaging findings and surgical approaches. Curr Probl Diagn Radiol. 44(1):76-87, 2015

Smith AB et al: From the archives of the AFIP: lesions of the pineal region: radiologic-pathologic correlation. Radiographics. 30(7):2001-20, 2010

Embryonal Neoplasms

Malignant brain tumors are the second leading cause of death in pediatric cancer patients. The most common of these tumors are the embryonal neoplasms, a heterogeneous group of primitive neoplasms with protean histopathologic manifestations.

The rapidly evolving molecular classification of brain tumors has fundamentally changed the understanding of embryonal neoplasms. In the 2016 World Health Organization schema, the classification of the largest group of embryonal neoplasms—medulloblastoma—was revised to reflect both recognized histopathologic variants and clinically relevant molecular subgroups.

Embryonal neoplasms other than medulloblastomas have also undergone substantial changes. The term primitive neuroectodermal tumor (PNET) has been removed from the diagnostic lexicon, and the tumors formerly included in this category have been redefined using molecular data.

The 2016 WHO classification now recognizes three general categories of embryonal tumors: (1) medulloblastoma, (2) other (non-medulloblastoma) embryonal tumors, and (3) atypical teratoid/rhabdoid tumor. All three are discussed in this chapter.

Medulloblastoma

Medulloblastoma Overview

Medulloblastoma (MB) is the most common malignant CNS neoplasm of childhood and the second most common overall pediatric brain tumor (after astrocytoma). As a group, MBs accounts for approximately 20% of childhood CNS neoplasms.

It is now recognized that the pathologically defined entity historically known as MB is not a single tumor entity but a heterogeneous clustering of multiple distinct, clinically relevant molecular subgroups based on transcriptome or methylome profiling. International consensus now recognizes four molecular subgroups. Three of the four subgroups have at least one further level of hierarchy. Each distinct MB molecular subgroup differs in its demographics, recommended treatments, and clinical outcomes (see below).

In addition to genetically defined MBs, the 2016 WHO retained a histopathologic MB classification because of its clinical utility when molecular (i.e., genetic) analysis is either limited or unavailable. We discuss both systems below.

Histologically Defined Classification of Medulloblastoma

MB is defined as an embryonal neuroepithelial tumor that arises in the cerebellum or dorsal brain stem and consists of densely packed small round undifferentiated ("blue") cells. Moderate nuclear pleomorphism and a high mitotic index (MIB-1 or Ki-67) are characteristic.

The 2016 WHO classification recognizes **classic medulloblastoma** and three medulloblastoma histopathologic variants: (1) **desmoplastic/nodular medulloblastoma**, (2) **medulloblastoma with extensive nodularity**, and (3) **large cell/anaplastic medulloblastoma**.

All MBs are designated as WHO grade IV neoplasms irrespective of their histologic or genetic subtype.

Classic Medulloblastoma. Classic MBs account for approximately 70% of all MBs. They exhibit highly cellular sheets and lobules of uniform small round "blue cells" with neuroblastic (Homer-Wright) rosettes and perivascular pseudorosettes. Mitotic figures are variable **(21-1)**.

Desmoplastic/Nodular Medulloblastoma and Medulloblastoma With Extensive Nodularity. The term "desmoplastic" refers to the growth of fibrous or connective tissue. The **desmoplastic/nodular MB** variant accounts for 15-20% of MBs. This variant is characterized by abundant islands of reticulin fibers interspersed in a background of less differentiated small round blue cells **(21-2)**. In instances in which the nodules predominate, the variant is known as **medulloblastoma with extensive nodularity (MBEN)**.

Large Cell/Anaplastic Medulloblastoma. The **large cell/anaplastic MB** variant accounts for approximately 10% of MBs. Large anaplastic-appearing cells with nuclear pleomorphism, high mitotic activity, and abundant apoptosis are characteristic **(21-3)**.

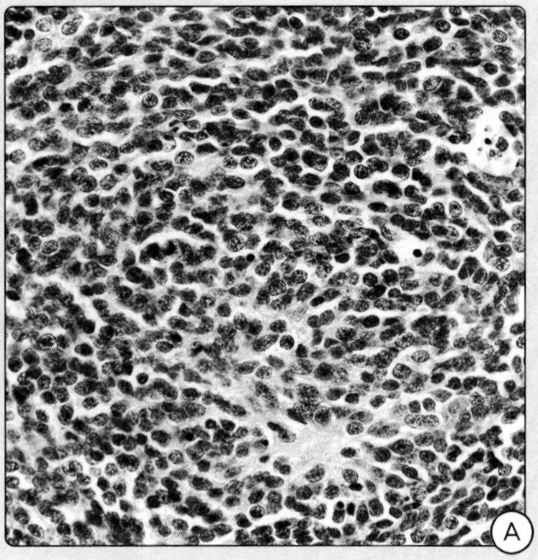

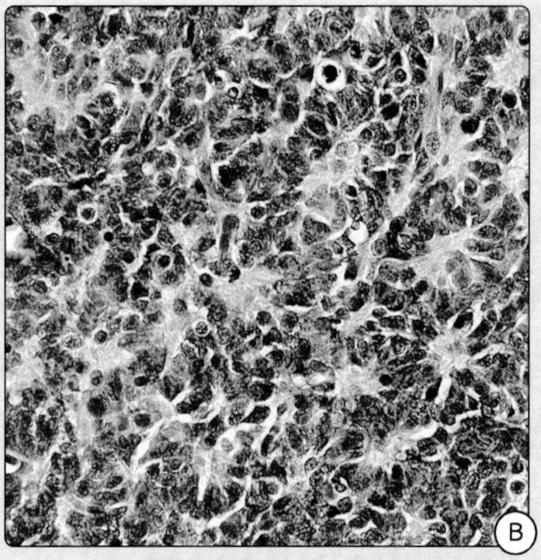

***(21-1A)** Classic medulloblastomas (MBs) are formed of sheets of small, uniform "round blue cells" with little nuclear pleomorphism. Mitoses are relatively few although this is a WHO grade IV neoplasm. (From DP: Neuropathology, 2e.)* ***(21-1B)** Homer-Wright (neuroblastic) rosettes with fibrillar cores are characteristic of classic MBs. (From DP: Neuropathology, 2e.)*

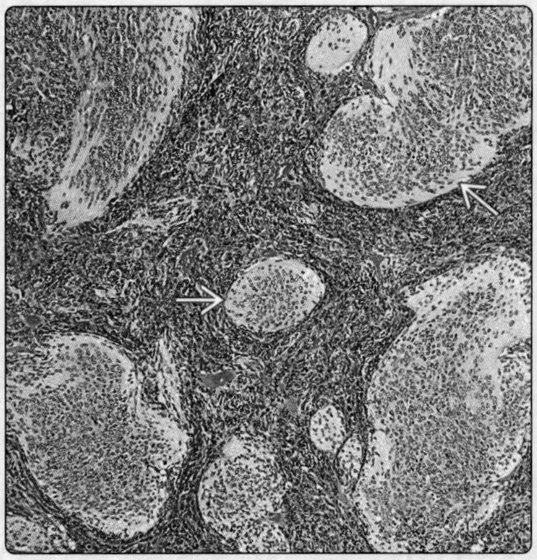

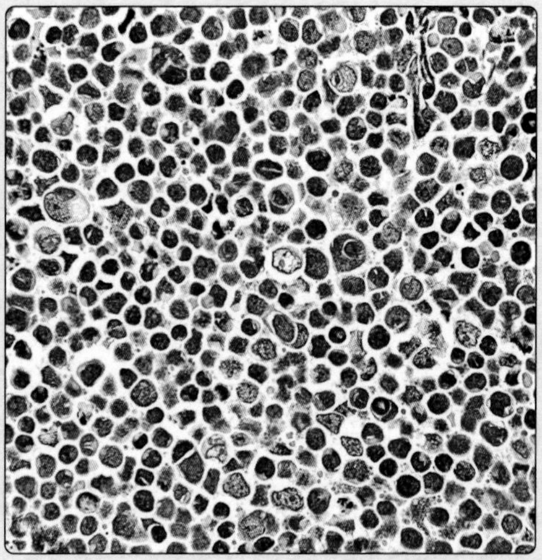

***(21-2)** The desmoplastic/nodular MB variant contains pale-staining reticular-laden islands ➡ surrounded by the darker blue, less differentiated background of extranodular tissue. (From DP: Neuropathology, 2e.)* ***(21-3)** Large cell/anaplastic MBs contain large anaplastic-appearing cells with prominent nucleoli. (From DP: Neuropathology, 2e.)*

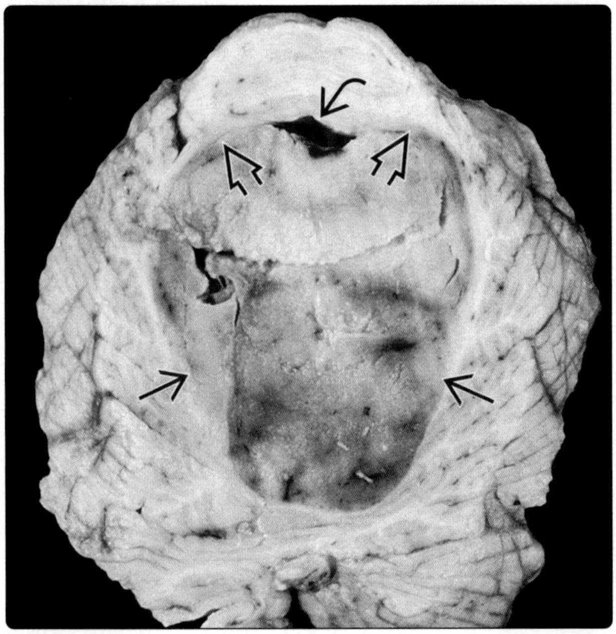

(21-4) Autopsy specimen demonstrates a large medulloblastoma ⇒ nearly filling the fourth ventricle with some sparing of the uppermost aspect of the ventricle ⇒. Pons is compressed anteriorly ⇒. (Courtesy R. Hewlett, MD.)

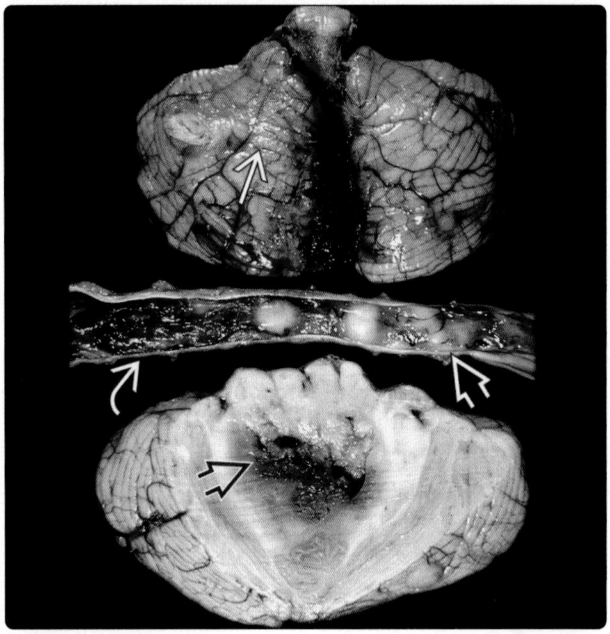

(21-5) CSF spread is from MB. Cut section shows in situ tumor expanding, filling 4th ventricle ⇒. Glistening, translucent "sugar icing" metastases coat cerebellum ⇒; "drop" metastases along spinal cord ⇒, cauda equina ⇒. (Courtesy R. Hewlett, MD.)

Genetically Defined Classification of Medulloblastomas

Molecular classification is redefining the risk stratification of patients with MB. MB is a genetically heterogeneous disease with four main molecular subgroups. All four MB subtypes have different origins, preferred anatomic locations, and demographics, as well as dramatically different prognosis and therapeutic implications.

The two named pathways are the WNT-activated and SHH-activated pathways. Two non-WNT, non-Shh groups are designated as simply "group 3" and "group 4."

WNT-Activated Medulloblastomas. WNT-activated medulloblastoma (WNT-MB) is the smallest molecular subgroup (10%) and appears strikingly different from the other MBs. WNT MBs are lateralized tumors that arise from the lower rhombic lip in the dorsolateral primitive brainstem around the foramen of Luschka **(21-12)**.

Loss of chromosome 6 and activating mutations in the WNT signaling pathway are typical. Almost 90% of WNT-MBs have somatic mutations in the *CTNNB1* gene. Germline mutations in the WNT pathway inhibitor, *APC*, predispose individuals to develop MB in the setting of **Turcot syndrome**.

WNT MBs are very rare in infants but more common in children (7-14 years of age) and young adults. They almost always exhibit classic histology. Childhood patients with WNT MBs consistently show a favorable prognosis (5-year survival > 90%), and reduced intensity risk-adapted therapies are currently being studied.

SHH-Activated MBs. The SHH subgroup accounts for 25-30% of MBs. **SHH-activated MBs** arise from granule neuron precursor cells (GNPCs), which are found in the external granular layer of the cerebellum until early in the second postnatal year. GNPC proliferation is dependent on SHH signaling pathway activation. Because of their rhombic lip origin, SHH MBs are often located laterally within the cerebellar hemispheres **(21-6)**. The vermis is the second most common site.

SHH-MBs have significantly enriched desmoplastic or nodular pathology compared with all other subgroups. *TP53* mutations, *MYCN* amplifications, and large cell anaplastic histology are significantly more frequent in childhood SHH MBs compared with SHH MBs in infants in whom desmoplastic/nodular and classical histologies predominate.

For risk stratification purposes in patients younger than 16, SHH-activated MB is now split into two age-dependent subgroups: infants (< 4.3 years) and children (> 4.3 years).

SHH-MBs associated with *MYCN* and *GLI1* amplifications or *TP53* mutation have a poor prognosis even when treated with high-dose craniospinal radiation and adjuvant chemotherapy.

Individuals with germline mutations in the SHH receptor *PTCH1* have **basal cell nevus (Gorlin) syndrome** and are predisposed to develop SHH-activated MBs.

Non-WNT/Non-SHH Medulloblastoma. Non-WNT/non-SHH MBs are classic or large cell/anaplastic tumors that cluster into two groups ("group 3" and "group 4") defined by transcriptome, methylome, and microRNA profiles. There is significant clinicobiological overlap between the two groups.

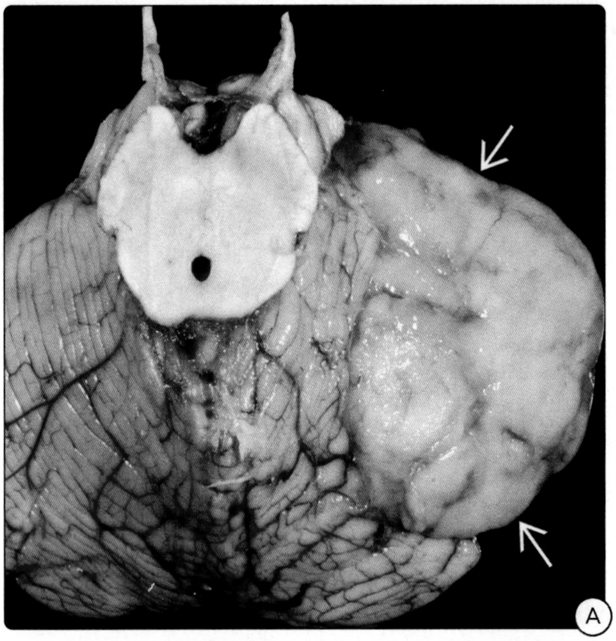

(21-6A) Autopsy specimen from an adult shows desmoplastic medulloblastoma as a firm, fibrous-appearing, somewhat lobular and laterally located mass ➡ in the cerebellar hemisphere. (Courtesy R. Hewlett, MD.)

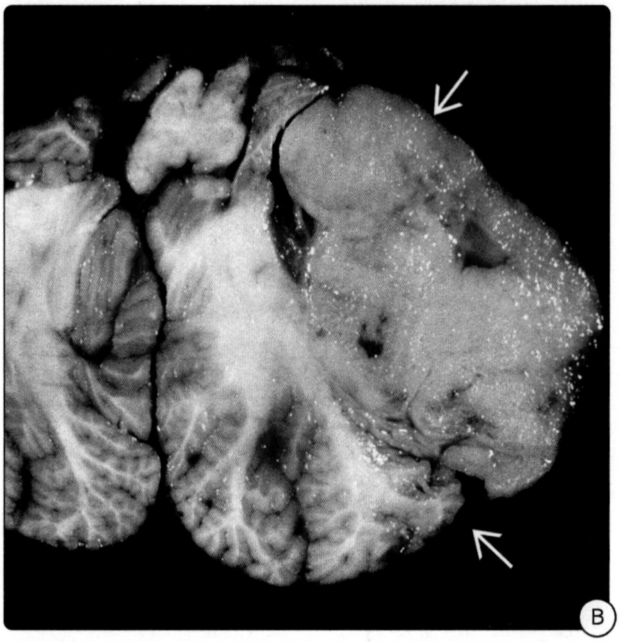

(21-6B) Cut section shows the classic desmoplastic medulloblastoma located in the lateral cerebellar hemisphere ➡. Most tumors in this location are SHH-activated. (Courtesy R. Hewlett, MD.)

MEDULLOBLASTOMA CLASSIFICATION

Histologically Defined Medulloblastomas

- Classic medulloblastoma
- Medulloblastoma variants
  - Desmoplastic/nodular medulloblastoma
  - Medulloblastoma with extensive nodularity
  - Large cell/anaplastic medulloblastoma

Genetically Defined Medulloblastomas

- WNT-activated medulloblastoma
- SHH-activated medulloblastomas
  - *TP53* mutant
  - *TP53* wild-type
- Non-WNT/non-SHH medulloblastomas
  - Group 3 medulloblastoma
  - Group 4 medulloblastoma

Group 3 is the third largest MB subgroup (20-25%). Group 3 tumors are common in infants but exceedingly rare in adults. There is a 2:1 M:F predominance. Most exhibit classical histopathology. *MYC* amplification is common, and approximately 50% of patients present with metastases **(21-10)**.

Group 3 MBs have the worst outcome of all four molecular subtypes. *MYC* amplification is the only risk factor significantly associated with progression-free survival in this group.

Group 4 is the largest (about 35%) of the four molecular MB subgroups. Most Group 4 MBs exhibit classic histology. Large cell/anaplastic variants do occur but are uncommon, whereas desmoplastic histology is rare. Group 4 MBs affect all ages but are most common in children. The M:F ratio is 2:1. A minority of Group 4 MBs present with metastasis. Prognosis is intermediate.

Classic Medulloblastoma

Pathology

Location. More than 85% of classic MBs (CMBs) arise in the midline **(21-4)**. They are located within the fourth ventricle and focally infiltrate the dorsal brainstem and vermis. Occasionally, CMB occurs as a diffusely infiltrating lesion without a focal dominant mass **(21-7)**.

Posteroinferior extension into the cisterna magna is common. Unlike ependymoma, lateral extension into the cerebellopontine angle is rare.

Size and Number. CMBs vary in size. Most tumors are between 2 and 4 cm at the time of initial diagnosis.

Gross Pathology. CMBs are relatively well-defined pink or grayish masses that typically fill the fourth ventricle, displacing and compressing the pons anteriorly **(21-4)**. Small scattered foci of necrosis and hemorrhage may be present.

Microscopic Features. CMBs are highly cellular tumors. Dense sheets of uniform cells with round or oval hyperchromatic pleomorphic nuclei surrounded by scanty cytoplasm are the typical appearance ("small round blue cell tumor") **(21-1A)**. Neuroblastic (Homer-Wright) rosettes—radial arrangements of tumor cells around fibrillary processes—are found in 40% of cases **(21-1B)**.

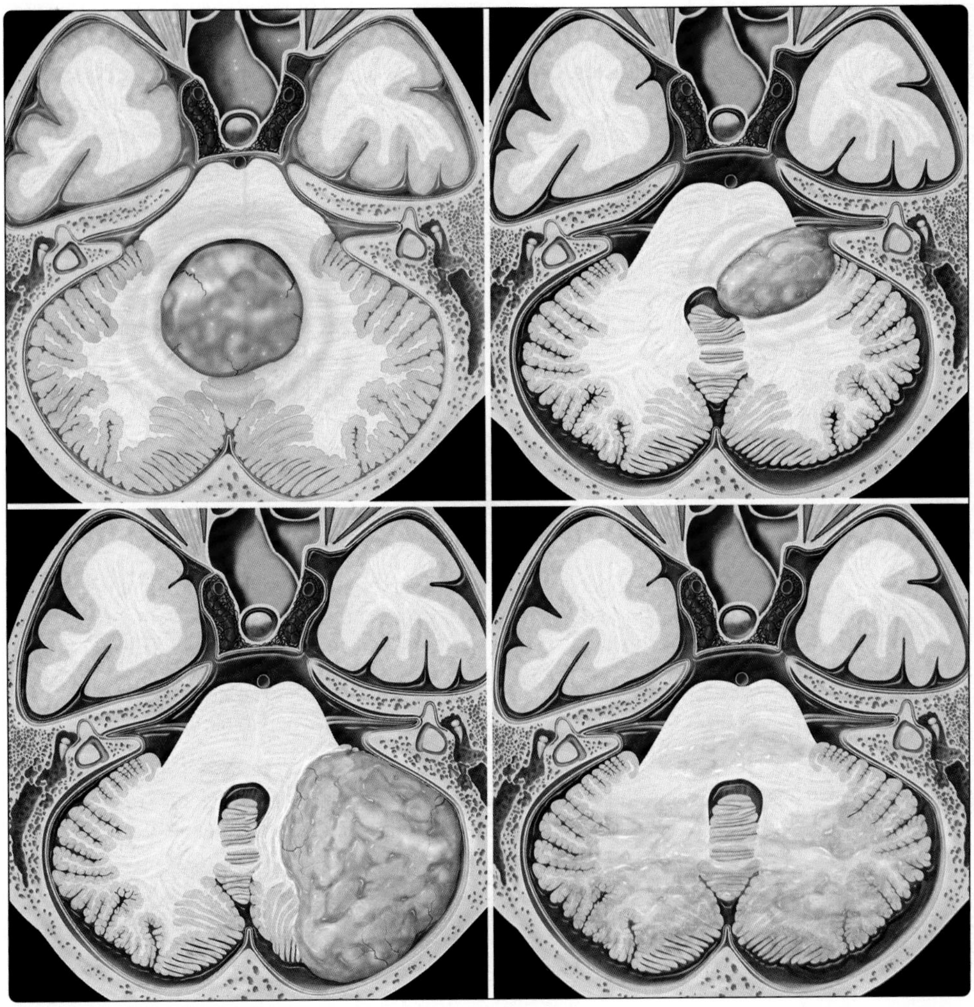

(21-7) (Upper left) Graphic depicts classic medulloblastoma in the midline fourth ventricle with CSF spread. All molecular subgroups and all histologies can be located here, but the most common subtypes are groups 3 and 4 (compare to Figure 21-9). (Upper right) Graphic depicts a medulloblastoma in the cerebellar peduncle/CPA cistern. This location is classic for WNT medulloblastoma (compare to Figures 21-10 and 21-12). (Lower left) Graphic depicts a medulloblastoma in the lateral cerebellar hemisphere. This is the classic location for desmoplastic medulloblastoma, SHH molecular subtype (compare to Figure 21-11). (Lower right). Graphic depicts a nonfocal, diffusely infiltrating medulloblastoma (compare to Figure 21-13). Groups 3 and 4 can be diffusely infiltrating with no dominant mass. Group 4 MBs are sometimes characterized by exhibiting minimal or no enhancement on T1 C+ FS (compare to Figure 21-9).

CLASSIC MEDULLOBLASTOMA

Terminology
- Classic medulloblastoma (CMB)

Etiology
- All four molecular subtypes represented
  - Almost all WNT-activated MBs are CMBs
- CMBs from dorsal midbrain → fourth ventricle

Pathology
- Midline (> 85%, fourth ventricle)
- "Small round blue cell tumor"
- Neuroblastic (Homer-Wright) rosettes
- WHO grade IV

Clinical Features
- MB = 20% of all pediatric brain tumors
- CMBs = 70% of all MBs
- Most common malignant posterior fossa childhood neoplasm
- Most CMBs in patients < 10 years
  - Second peak in patients 20-40 years
- Low risk if WNT activated

Clinical Issues

Epidemiology and Demographics. MBs cause 10% of all pediatric brain tumors and are the most common malignant posterior fossa childhood neoplasm. CMBs account for 70% of MBs. Most occur before age 10 years. There is a second, smaller peak in adults aged 20-40 years.

Presentation. The most common clinical manifestations of MB are vomiting (90%) and headache (80%). Psychomotor regression, ataxia, strabismus, and spasticity are common. The median interval between symptom onset and diagnosis is 2 months.

Because of their location, MBs tend to compress the fourth ventricle and cause obstructive hydrocephalus. In one-third of children younger than 3 years, the diagnosis is made only after life-threatening signs of intracranial hypertension appear.

Natural History. CMBs occur in all four principal molecular subgroups. Risk varies with subgroup. Almost all WNT-activated MBs exhibit classic histology and are considered low-risk neoplasms. Overall survival is excellent with surgical resection and adjuvant chemotherapy. SHH-activated *TP53*-mutant MBs with classic histology are considered standard risk.

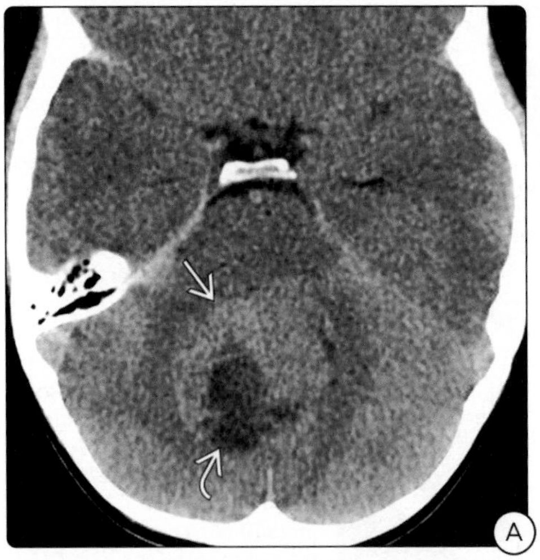

(21-8A) NECT shows a mostly hyperdense midline posterior fossa mass ➡ with intratumoral cysts ↪.

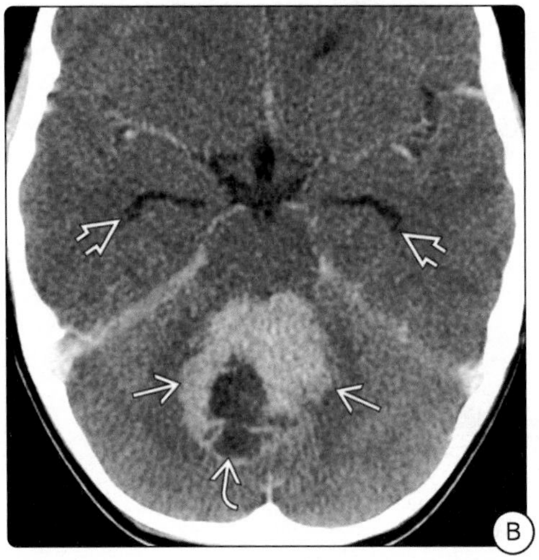

(21-8B) The solid portion ➡ enhances strongly on CECT, whereas the cyst ↪ does not. Note the mild enlargement of the temporal horns ⇨.

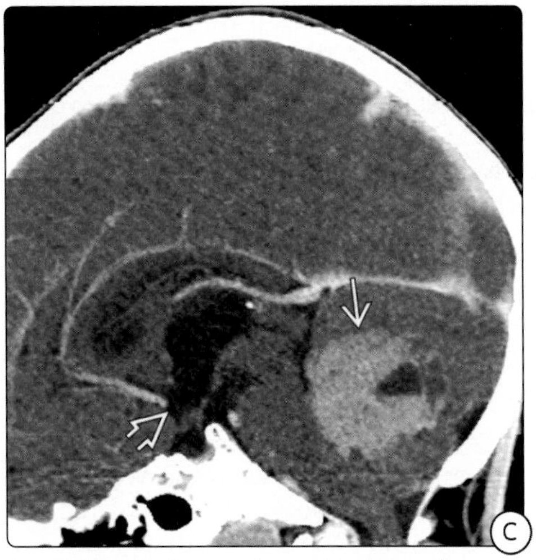

(21-8C) Sagittal CECT shows the obstructing midline mass ➡ causes moderate hydrocephalus ⇨. This is classic MB, WHO IV, standard risk.

Imaging

General Features. CMBs have relatively defined margins on imaging studies. Despite this appearance, 40-50% have CSF dissemination at the time of initial diagnosis **(21-5)**. Preoperative contrast-enhanced MR of the entire neuraxis is recommended.

CT Findings. NECT scans show a moderately hyperdense, relatively well-defined mass in the midline posterior fossa **(21-8A)** or around the foramen of Luschka (WNT-subgroup MB). Cyst formation (40%) and calcification (20-25%) are common **(21-9A)**. Gross hemorrhage is rare. Strong but heterogeneous enhancement is seen on CECT **(21-8B)**.

If dense tentorial or falcine calcifications are present, the patient should be evaluated for basal cell nevus (Gorlin) syndrome.

MR Findings. Almost all CMBs are hypointense relative to gray matter on T1WI and hyperintense on T2WI **(21-9B)**. Peritumoral edema is present in one-third of cases. Obstructive hydrocephalus with periventricular accumulation of CSF is common and best delineated on FLAIR.

Enhancement patterns show striking variation, ranging from minimal to patchy to marked. Two-thirds of CMBs show marked enhancement, whereas one-third show only subtle, marginal, or linear enhancement **(21-9D)**.

Occasionally, CMBs present as diffusely infiltrating cerebellar masses with multifocal scattered T2/FLAIR hyperintensities and minimal or no enhancement **(21-13)**.

Because of their dense cellularity, CMBs often show moderate restriction on DWI **(21-9C)**. pMR shows low rCBV and increased permeability on K2 maps.

CLASSIC MEDULLOBLASTOMA: IMAGING AND DIFFERENTIAL DIAGNOSIS

CT
- Hyperdense on NECT
- Cysts (40%)
- Ca++ (20-25%)
- Hemorrhage rare
- Enhances strongly, heterogeneously

MR
- Hypo- on T1, hyperintense on T2
- Often restricts on DWI
- Enhancement: none to strong

Differential Diagnosis
- Medulloblastoma variant
- Atypical teratoid/rhabdoid tumor
- Lhermitte-Duclos disease (adults)

Differential Diagnosis

The major differential diagnosis of CMB in children is a **medulloblastoma variant**. A posterior fossa **atypical teratoid/rhabdoid tumor (AT/RT)** may be indistinguishable from CMB on imaging studies alone.

Choroid plexus papilloma (CPP) of the fourth ventricle is rare in children but can be hyperdense on NECT and enhance strongly on CECT. The front-like papillary configuration is often apparent on MR, and looking for a myoinositol peak on MRS can provide helpful distinguishing features.

Lhermitte-Duclos disease (LDD) can be seen in children but is more common in young adults. LDD and desmoplastic MB may resemble one another although the striated pattern of LDD is quite characteristic.

The differential diagnosis of MB in adults differs. The most common parenchymal posterior fossa mass in adults is **metastasis**.

Medulloblastoma With Extensive Nodularity

MBs with extensive nodularity (MBENs) occur almost exclusively in infants, and most all are Shh pathway MBs. The expanded lobular ("nodular") architecture of MBENs is the major histologic feature that differentiates them from CMB and desmoplastic MB.

Imaging studies demonstrate striking nodularity. Off-midline or paramidline location is more common. T1 C+ MR scans show multifocal grape-like tumor masses that enhance strongly and uniformly.

Desmoplastic/Nodular Medulloblastoma

Desmoplastic MB (DMB) is an MB variant characterized by nodules of neuronal maturation in a dense intercellular reticulin fiber network. There is a strong association between desmoplastic histology and Shh subtype; almost all adult and 90% of infant DMBs belong to the Shh subgroup.

DMBs account for 15-20% of MBs, but prevalence varies significantly with patient age. DMBs cause about 40% of MBs in infants but only 10% of adult MBs.

The vermis is the customary location in children. Adult DMBs are often located laterally within the cerebellar hemispheres **(21-11)**. DMBs have a somewhat better prognosis than classic, anaplastic, or large cell MBs.

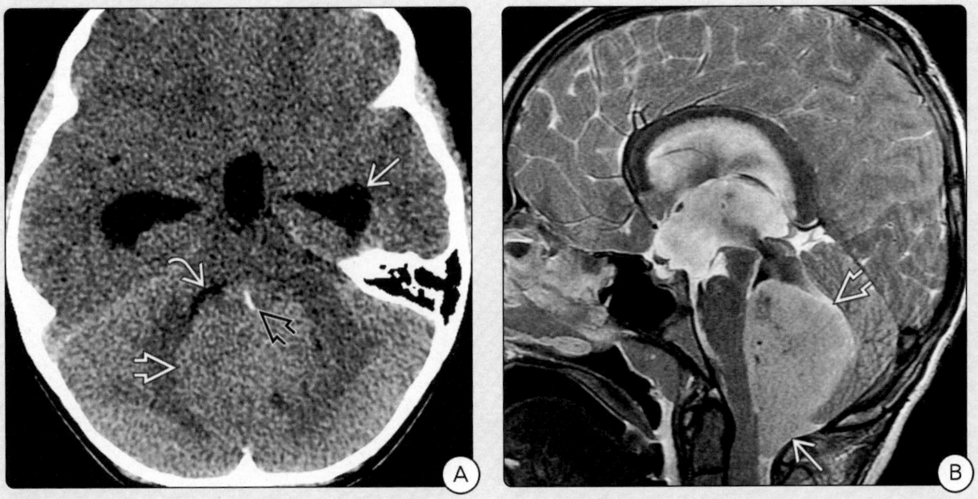

***(21-9A)** NECT in an 8y boy with confusion, headache, and 3 weeks of vomiting shows a mildly hyperdense mass ➡ in the midline posterior fossa that fills the fourth ventricle ➡. Obstructive hydrocephalus ➡ and a small focus of calcification ➡ in the mass are present. **(21-9B)** Sagittal T2WI shows that the mass ➡ fills the fourth ventricle and extends posteroinferiorly through the foramen of Magendie into the cisterna magna ➡.*

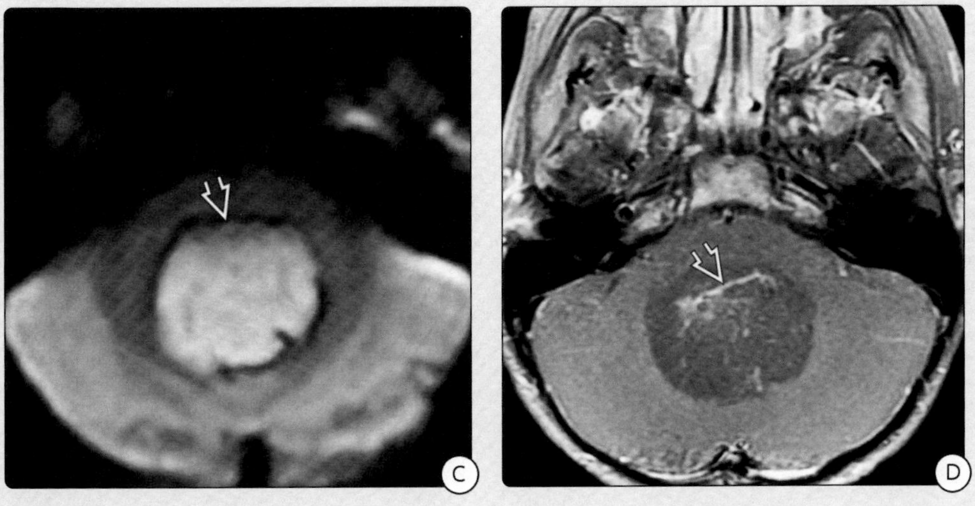

***(21-9C)** Axial DWI in the same case shows that the mass ➡ exhibits uniformly restricted diffusion. **(21-9D)** Axial T1 C+ FS shows mild irregular enhancement ➡ in the center of the mass. This is group 4, classic histology, WHO grade IV, standard risk.*

Imaging findings that suggest DMB include off-midline location (adults), multiple peripheral small cysts, and focal areas of T2/FLAIR iso- or hypointensity that enhance on T1 C+.

Large Cell/Anaplastic Medulloblastoma

Large cell MB (LCMB) is the rarest histologic variant, accounting for just 2-4% of cases. LCMBs have considerable cytologic overlap with anaplastic MBs and are often grouped together as "large cell/anaplastic medulloblastoma" (LC/A MB). LC/A MBs are generally Shh, group 3, or group 4 molecular subtypes. Both LCMBs and anaplastic MBs have a dismal prognosis.

Marked but inhomogeneous enhancement is typical. There are no reported imaging features that distinguish LCMB from anaplastic MB.

MEDULLOBLASTOMA VARIANTS

Desmoplastic Medulloblastoma
- SHH-activated
- Young children, second peak in young adults
- Off-midline location in adults, vermis in children

Medulloblastoma With Extensive Nodularity (MBEN)
- Infants
- Off-midline or paramidline > midline
- Multifocal grape-like tumor masses

Large Cell/Anaplastic Medulloblastoma (LC/A)
- All molecular subtypes represented except WNT-activated (very rare)
    - Most group 3, SHH/*TP53*-mutant MBs
    - Generally high-risk tumors (early CSF spread)
- No distinctive imaging features

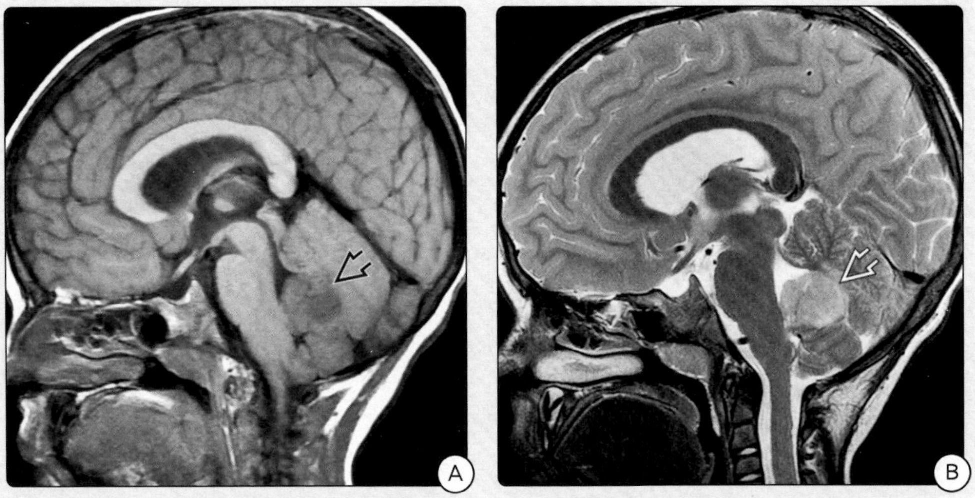

***(21-10A)** Sagittal T1WI in a 4y boy with vomiting and bulging fontanelle shows a mixed iso- and hypointense mass in the midline posterior fossa. **(21-10B)** Sagittal T2WI in the same case shows that the mass bulges into the 4th ventricle and is iso- to mildly hyperintense compared with gray matter.*

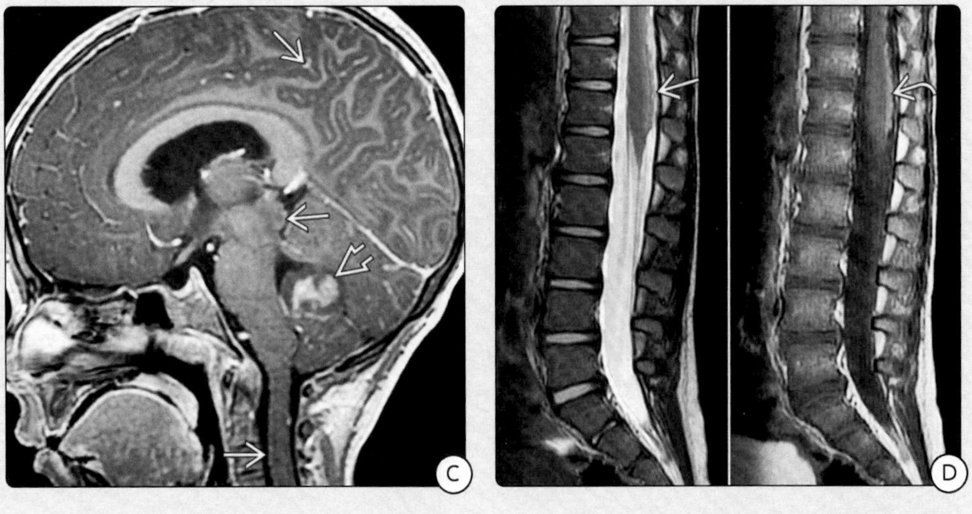

***(21-10C)** Sagittal T1 C+ shows strong but patchy enhancement in the mass. Note subtle pial enhancement along the tectum, in the hemispheric sulci, and coating the spinal cord. **(21-10D)** Sagittal T2WI (L) shows thickened nodular "lumpy-bumpy" hyperintensity along the distal spinal cord. Sagittal T1 C+ (R) shows that these are enhancing pial metastases. This is group 3 MB with CSF dissemination at initial presentation.*

Other CNS Embryonal Tumors

CNS embryonal neoplasms other than medulloblastoma (MB) are a heterogeneous group of tumors composed of poorly differentiated cells that may express neuronal and/or glial markers. These non-MB embryonal tumors have undergone substantial alterations in classification, with deletion of the term primitive neuroectodermal tumor (PNET) and the recognition that many embryonal neoplasms display amplification of the C19MC region on chromosome 19.

In addition to many pediatric CNS embryonal tumors that were formerly designated as PNETs, the new group of **C19MC-amplified embryonal tumors** (ETMRs) includes entities variously called ETANTR (**e**mbryonal **t**umor with **a**bundant **n**europil and **t**rue **r**osettes), ependymoblastoma, and medulloepithelioma.

Embryonal Tumor With Multilayered Rosettes, C19MC-Altered

Terminology

ETMRs are aggressive CNS embryonal tumors that are characterized histologically by multilayered rosettes and genetically by amplification or fusion in the C19MC locus at 19q13.42.

Pathology

Approximately 70% of ETMRs are supratentorial masses that appear relatively well demarcated with little surrounding edema. Tumors are often more than 5 cm in diameter, and some are massive lesions that occupy much of the cerebral

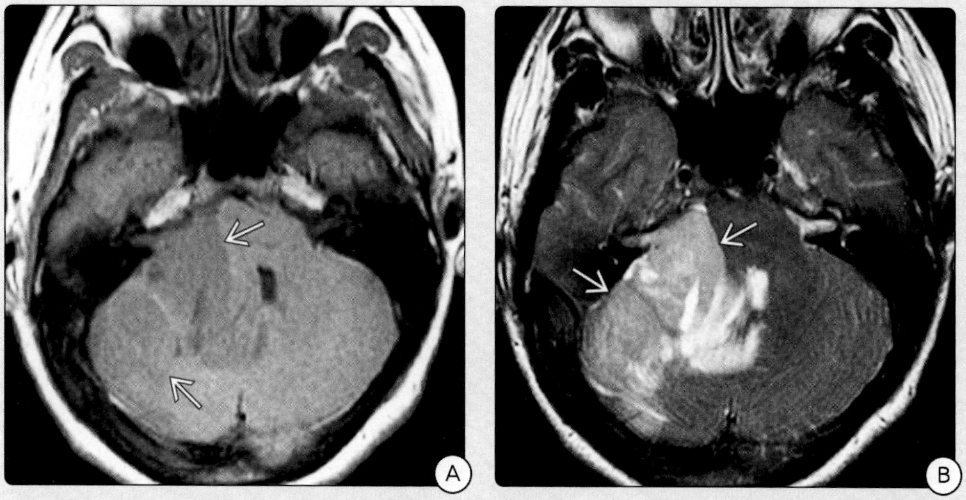

***(21-11A)** Axial T1WI in a 24y woman with headaches and dizziness shows a mildly hypointense mass ➔ in the right cerebellar hemisphere. **(21-11B)** T2WI in the same case shows that the mass ➔ is hyperintense compared with cortex.*

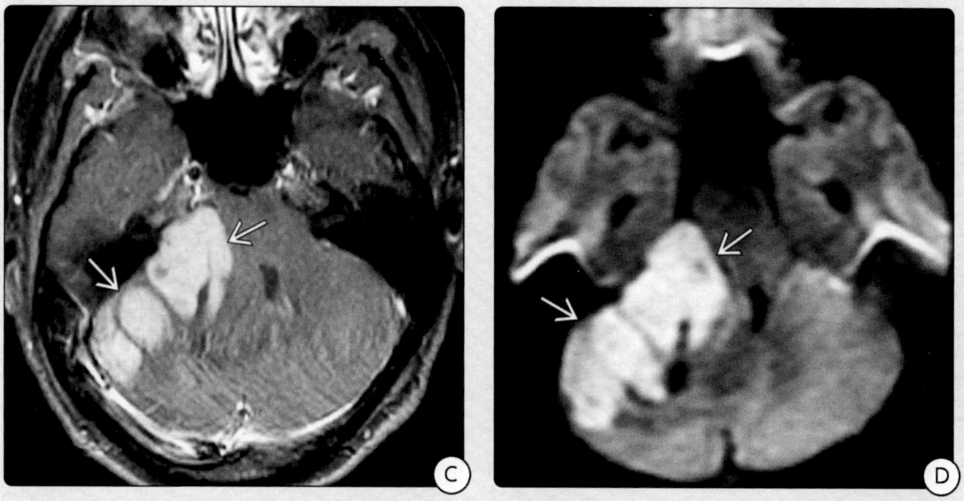

***(21-11C)** T1 C+ FS in the same case shows strong, uniform enhancement in the solid, lobulated-appearing mass ➔. **(21-11D)** DWI shows that the mass restricts strongly and uniformly ➔. Desmoplastic medulloblastoma was found at surgery. Most desmoplastic medulloblastomas in the lateral cerebellum are SHH-activated, low-risk tumors of children and adults.*

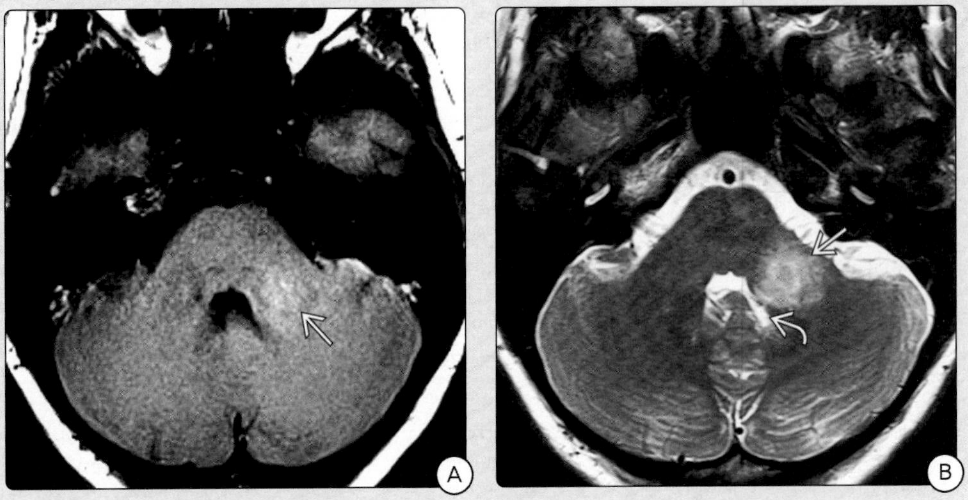

***(21-12A)** Axial T1WI in a 22y woman with headaches shows an ill-defined hyperintense mass ➡ in the left brachium pontis. **(21-12B)** T2WI in the same case shows that the mass ➡ is heterogeneously hyperintense and compresses and displaces the lateral recess of the fourth ventricle ↪ but does not invade it.*

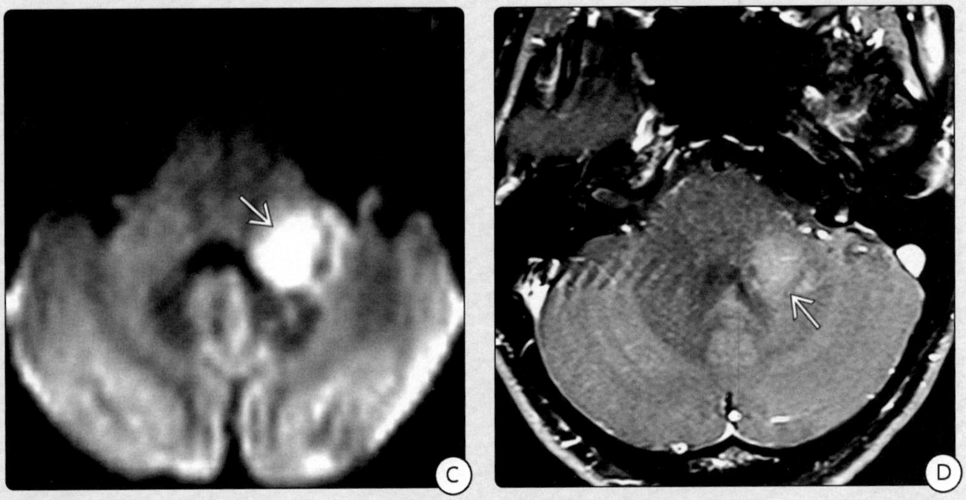

***(21-12C)** Axial DWI in the same case shows that the mass ➡ restricts strongly. Surgery disclosed classic histology, WNT-activated. This is considered a low-risk tumor. The patient is alive and well 5 years later. **(21-12D)** Axial T1 C+ FS shows mild enhancement in the brachium pontis mass ➡.*

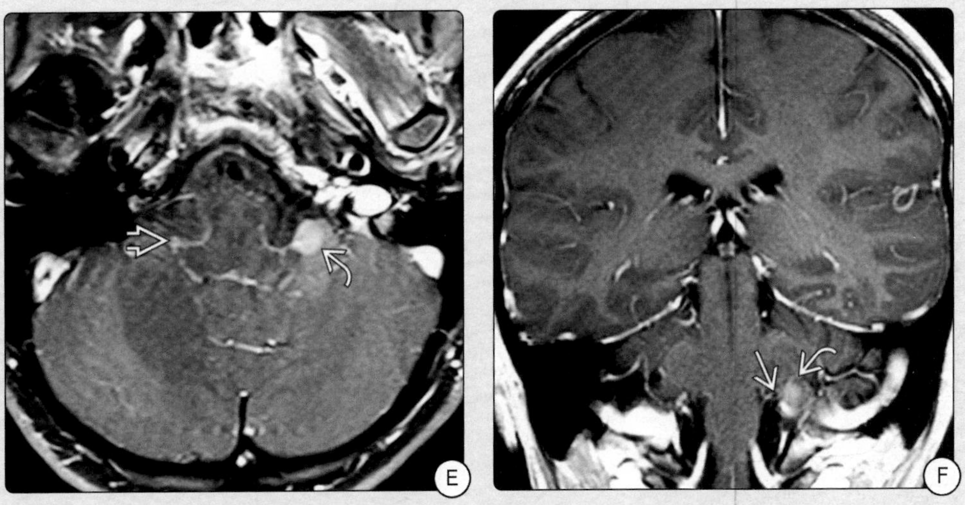

***(21-12E)** More inferior axial T1 C+ FS shows an enhancing mass ↪ near the left foramen of Luschka. Note pial enhancement ⇨, suggesting CSF metastases. **(21-12F)** Coronal T1 C+ shows that the enhancing mass ↪ is immediately adjacent to the foramen of Luschka ➡. This is WNT medulloblastoma, classic histology. The patient is alive 3 years after initial diagnosis.*

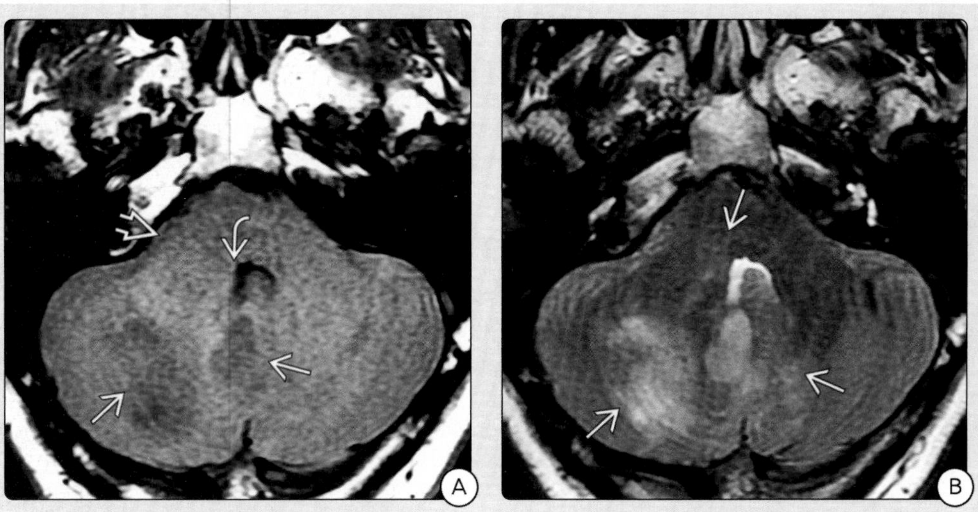

(21-13A) *Axial T1WI in a 32y man with ataxia shows expansion and deformity of the right pons and brachium pontis ➡. Note mass effect on the 4th ventricle ➡ and ill-defined hypointensities in the right cerebellar hemisphere and vermis ➡.* ***(21-13B)*** *Axial T2WI in the same case shows multifocal patchy hyperintensities in both cerebellar hemispheres, the vermis, and the pons ➡.*

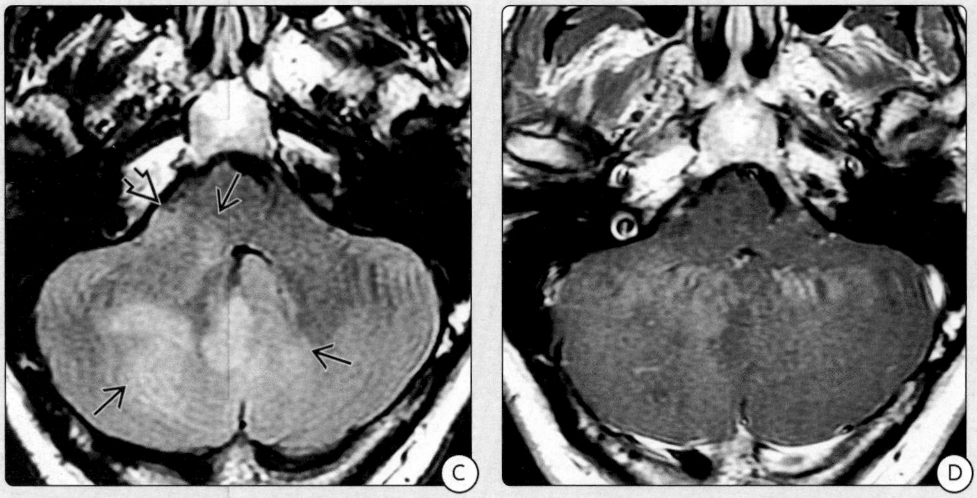

(21-13C) *FLAIR in the same case shows the extensive patchy hyperintensities ➡, misshapen right pons, and brachium pontis ➡.* ***(21-13D)*** *T1 C+ FS shows no enhancement.*

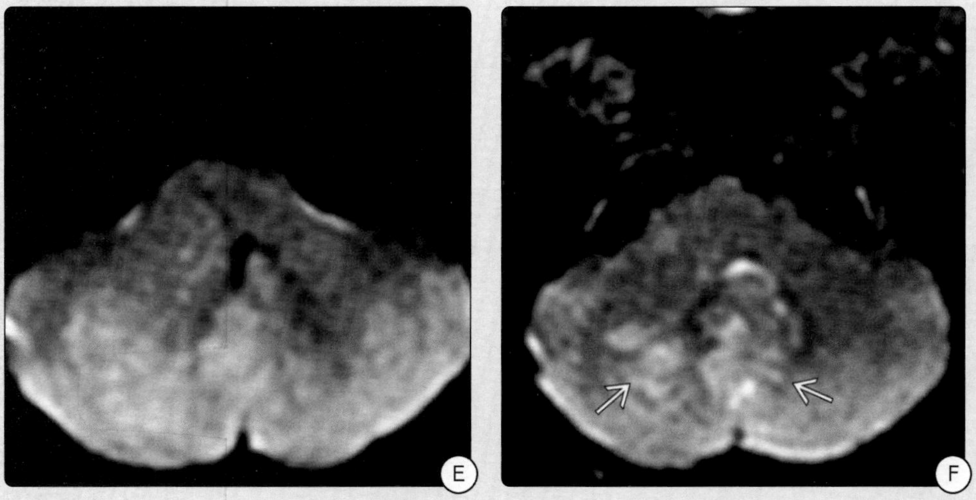

(21-13E) *DWI shows no evidence for restricted diffusion.* ***(21-13F)*** *Axial ADC shows patchy foci of T2 "shine through" ➡ without evidence for restricted diffusion. This is biopsy-proven classic histology medulloblastoma, WHO IV. Molecular profile was not obtained. Occasionally a diffusely infiltrating medulloblastoma presents without a dominant enhancing mass.*

hemispheres. The cerebellum and brainstem are the primary site in 30% of cases.

On cut section, ETMRs are soft grayish pink to purplish masses that frequently contain areas of necrosis **(21-14)**. Intratumoral cysts and hemorrhage are common.

Microscopically, ETMRs contain abundant neuropil and true rosettes with a pseudostratified neuroepithelium surrounding a central round or slit-like lumen. Mitoses are frequent, and CSF dissemination is common. Most ETMRs exhibit high LIN28A protein expression, considered a potent diagnostic immunohistochemical marker for this neoplasm.

C19MC-altered ETMR corresponds histologically to WHO grade IV.

Clinical Issues

Almost all ETMRs occur under the age of 4 years, with the majority occurring in the first 2 years of life. Increasing head circumference and signs of elevated intracranial pressure are common. Headache, nausea, vomiting, and visual disturbances are typical presenting symptoms.

Imaging

General Features. ETMRs grow rapidly and are often very large, heterogeneous-appearing masses that cause gross distortion and effacement of the underlying brain architecture **(21-15)**.

CT Findings. A complex, heterogeneously iso- to hyperdense mass with mixed cystic and solid components is typical on NECT. Necrosis and intratumoral hemorrhages are common, as are dystrophic calcifications. CECT scans show moderate but heterogeneous enhancement.

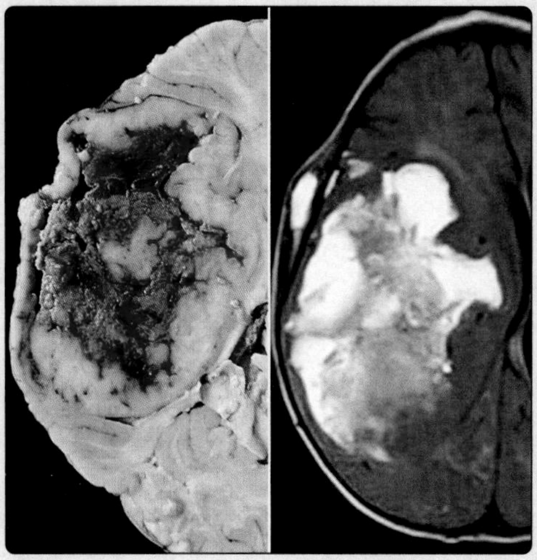

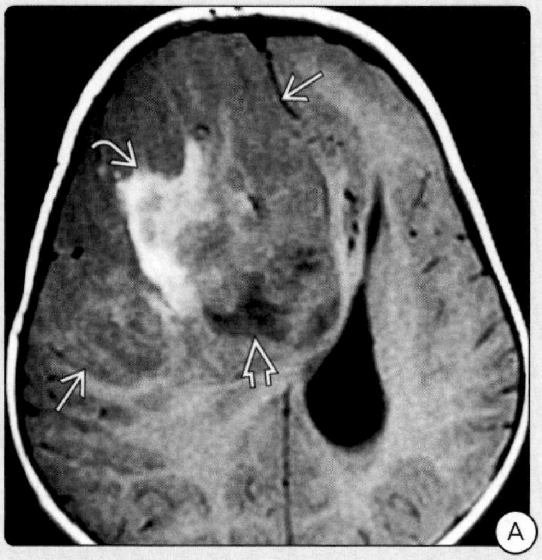

***(21-14)** Autopsy (L) and antemortem FLAIR scan (R) in an 8m infant with a supratentorial embryonal neoplasm show a large, aggressive-looking hemispheric mass with confluent areas of necrosis and hemorrhage. There is relatively little peritumoral edema. (Courtesy R. Hewlett, MD.) **(21-15A)** Axial T1WI in an infant with macrocephaly shows a very large right frontal mass ➔ with areas of necrosis ⇨ and hemorrhage ⤻.*

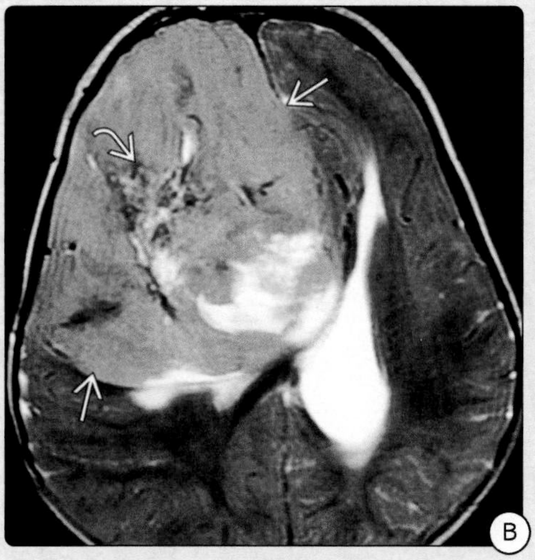

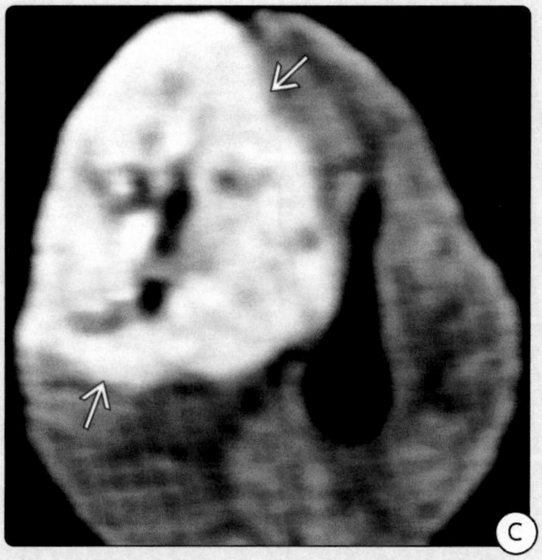

***(21-15B)** T2WI in the same patient shows that the mass is relatively well demarcated ➔ and mostly hyperintense with heterogeneously hypointense foci of hemorrhage ⤻. **(21-15C)** The lesion restricts on DWI ➔. This is a supratentorial embryonal neoplasm (formerly designated as PNET). (Courtesy G. Hedlund, DO.)*

MR Findings. All sequences exhibit heterogeneous signal intensity with T1 shortening **(21-15A)** and T2* blooming secondary to intratumoral hemorrhage. T2/FLAIR hyperintensity in cystic or necrotic segments and isointensity in the solid portions of the mass are typical. Peritumoral edema is typically minimal or absent **(21-16)**.

Because of their relatively dense cellularity, C19MC-altered ETMRs may show foci of moderately restricted diffusion **(21-15C)** **(21-16D)**. pMR shows areas of elevated rCBV and vascular permeability.

Heterogeneous enhancement with solid and rim enhancement is typical **(21-17)** **(21-18)**.

Differential Diagnosis

The differential diagnosis of C19MC-altered ETMR in infants and children includes other bulky hemispheric masses, including **AT/RT, RELA fusion-positive ependymoma, astroblastoma, glioblastoma**, and the rare **CNS neuroblastoma** or **ganglioneuroblastoma**.

Other CNS Embryonal Tumors

To date, medulloblastoma, C19MC-altered ETMRs, and atypical teratoid/rhabdoid tumor (AT/RT) are the only genetically defined CNS embryonal neoplasms in the 2016 WHO.

Several rare CNS embryonal tumors *without* current molecular classification in the 2016 WHO include **medulloepithelioma, CNS neuroblastoma (NB),** and **CNS ganglioneuroblastoma**. Embryonal tumors that lack the specific histopathologic features or molecular alterations that define other CNS neoplasms are designated as **CNS embryonal tumor, NOS.**

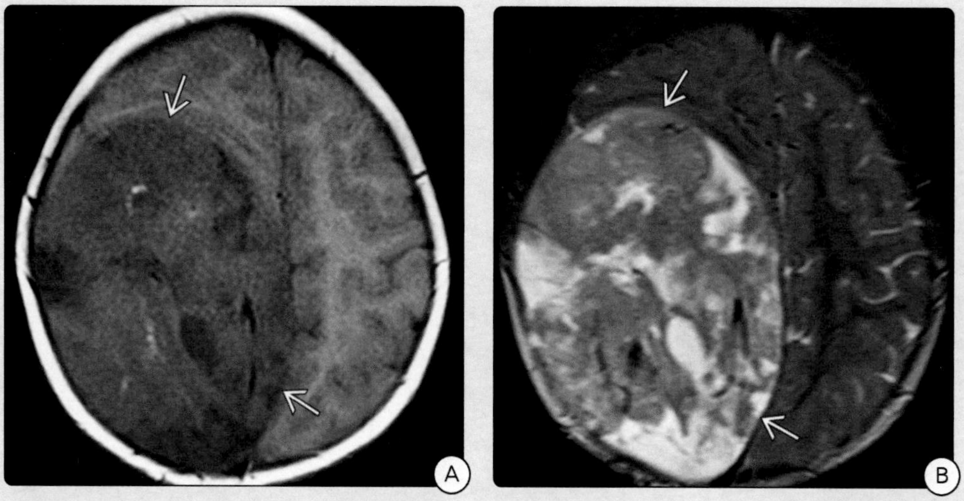

***(21-16A)** Axial T1WI in a 2y girl shows a large mass of mixed signal intensity ➡ that occupies most of the right cerebral hemisphere. **(21-16B)** Axial T2 FS MR in the same case shows that the mass is very heterogeneously hyperintense ➡ and relatively well demarcated. There is no discernible surrounding edema.*

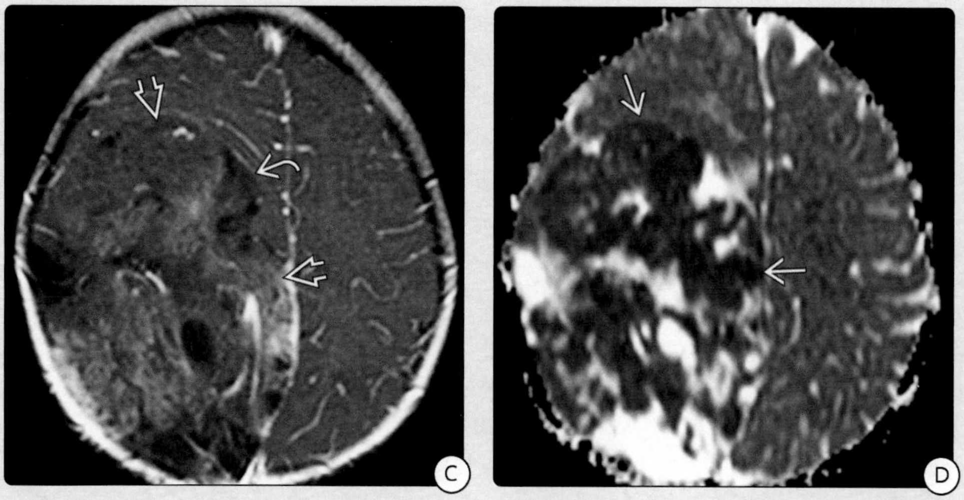

***(21-16C)** Axial T1 C+ MR shows mild to moderate patchy enhancement ➡ in some portions of the mass, whereas others show little or no enhancement ➡. **(21-16D)** ADC map shows that solid portions of the tumor ➡ exhibit restricted diffusion. Embryonal tumor with multilayered rosettes, C19MC-altered, was documented. (Courtesy M. Warmuth-Metz, MD.)*

Medulloepithelioma

Medulloepithelioma (ME) is an embryonal tumor characterized by papillary tubular arrangements of neoplastic neuroepithelium that mimic the embryonic neural tube. C19MC alterations are rare or absent. Mitotic figures are common with MIB-1 often exceeding 50%.

Almost all patients are younger than 5 years at the time of diagnosis. Half are under the age of two. Symptoms of elevated intracranial pressure are the typical presentation.

MEs are often massive tumors that replace much of the affected hemisphere and appear very heterogeneous on both CT and MR. Cysts, calcification, and sometimes hemorrhagic foci are common. There are no imaging features that distinguish MEs from C19MC-altered ETMRs.

CNS Neuroblastoma

Craniocerebral NB can be either secondary or primary. Secondary disease is far more common than primary CNS NB and so is discussed first. NB is notorious for its diverse manifestations (one of the "great mimickers") and can masquerade as primary neurologic disease in a child with an unexplained neurologic disorder.

Secondary (Metastatic) Neuroblastoma. NB is a neuroendocrine tumor that arises from neural crest elements, usually within the adrenal gland or sympathetic nervous system. It is the most common extracranial solid cancer in childhood and the most common overall cancer of infants. NB accounts for 10-15% of all childhood malignancies, following leukemia and primary brain tumors in prevalence.

Clinical Issues. Metastases are present in almost 70% of NB patients at the time of initial diagnosis. Skeletal metastases are the most common manifestation. Approximately 25%

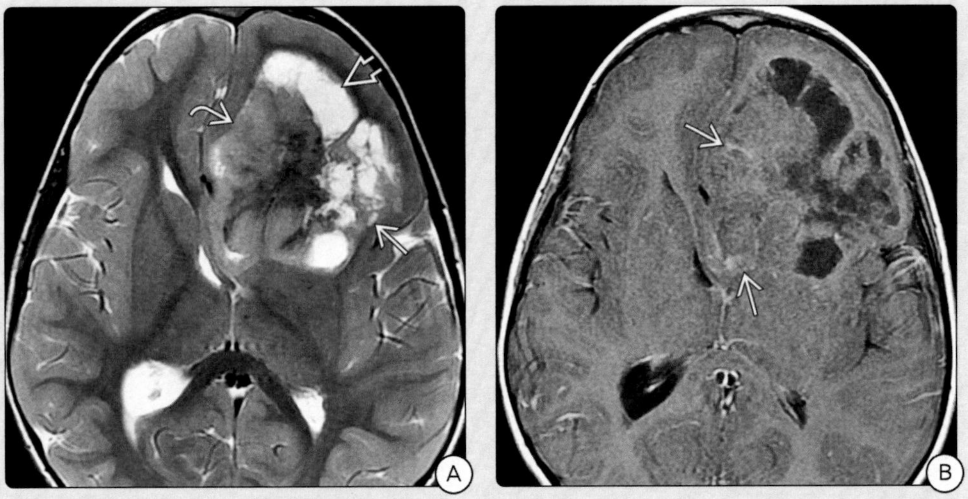

***(21-17A)** Axial T2WI in 3y child shows large, very heterogeneous left frontal lobe mass with both solid ➭, mixed cystic/solid ➡, and cystic-appearing portions ➡. **(21-17B)** T1 C+ FS shows minimal enhancement in solid ➡ portions of mass. Histologic diagnosis was ETANTR. In new 2016 WHO, this would either be C19MC-amplified embryonal tumor or designated as CNS embryonal tumor, NOS. (Courtesy T. Poussaint, MD.)*

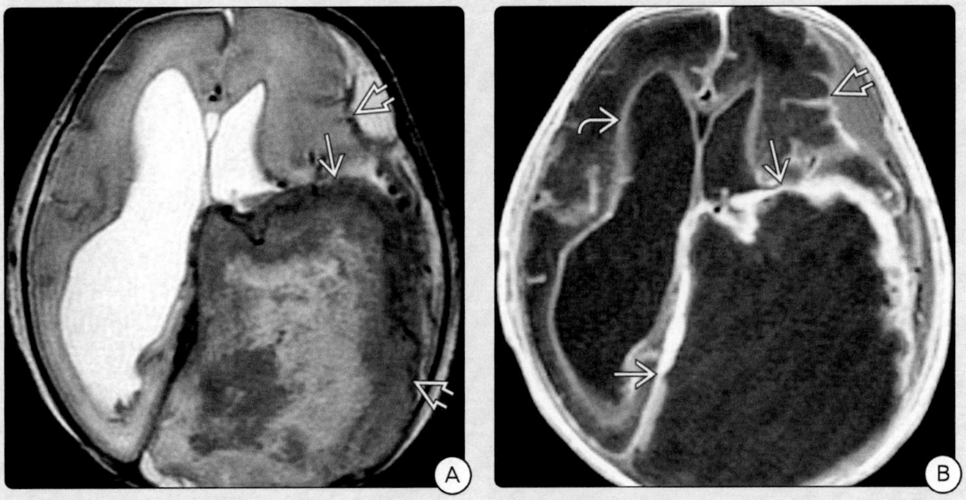

***(21-18A)** T2WI in newborn with macrocrania, nystagmus, periodic breathing, and bulging fontanelle shows predominantly necrotic, partially hemorrhagic hemisphere mass ➡ with hemosiderin staining ➡ around mass and over the cerebrum. **(21-18B)** This T1WI C+ shows the rim of the tumor enhances ➡. Note enhancement over the pia ➡ and around the ventricular ependyma ➭. This is CNS embryonal neoplasm, NOS. (Courtesy G. Hedlund, DO.)*

occur in the orbit, calvaria, and skull base. The classic clinical manifestation of orbital metastatic NB is a child with proptosis and "raccoon eyes."

CNS involvement by metastatic NB is uncommon and generally occurs as a late complication of stage IV disease (3-year risk = 8%). CNS NB metastases are usually detected at the time of disease recurrence rather than initial diagnosis.

Imaging. NECT shows one or more hyperdense soft-tissue masses with orbit, skull, scalp, and/or extradural components. Bone CT shows fine "hair on end" spicules of the periosteal bone that project from the skull or greater sphenoid wings **(21-19)**. Multiple bilateral lesions involving both the inner and outer tables of the skull are typical. Lytic defects and widened indistinct sutures are other common findings.

MR shows an extraaxial mass that is heterogeneously hypointense to brain on both T1- and T2WI. Strong enhancement following contrast administration is typical. Linear hypointensities that represent the "hair on end" bony spicules can sometimes be identified within the strongly enhancing masses **(21-20)**.

CNS lesions are uncommon, appearing as a parenchymal **(21-21)**, an intraventricular, or even a spinal cord mass. Disseminated leptomeningeal disease is rare.

Nuclear medicine studies are helpful in the early evaluation of NB. Metaiodobenzylguanidine (MIBG) imaging is the most sensitive and specific imaging modality to determine primary and metastatic disease. F18 FDG PET is helpful in depicting stage I and II NB.

The major imaging differential diagnosis of NB metastatic to the calvaria is **leukemia**. Both often have dura- or calvaria-based masses, but parenchymal lesions are much more common with leukemia than with NB.

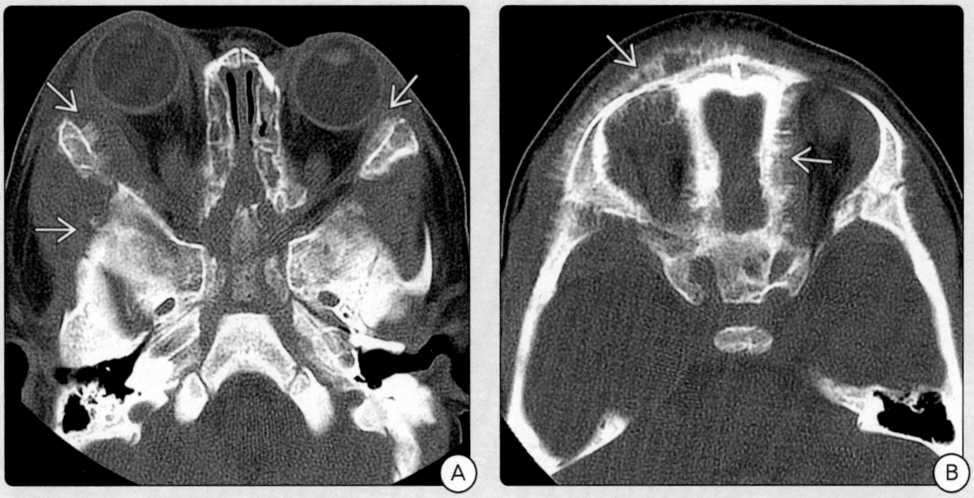

***(21-19A)** Axial bone CT is of a 9m boy with proptosis, stage IV suprarenal neuroblastoma identified on abdominal CT (not shown). Note the striking orbital spiculated periostitis with adjacent soft tissue masses ➡. (Courtesy S. Blaser, MD.) **(21-19B)** More cephalad scan in the same patient shows the classic "hair on end" appearance ➡ of metastatic neuroblastoma. (Courtesy S. Blaser, MD.)*

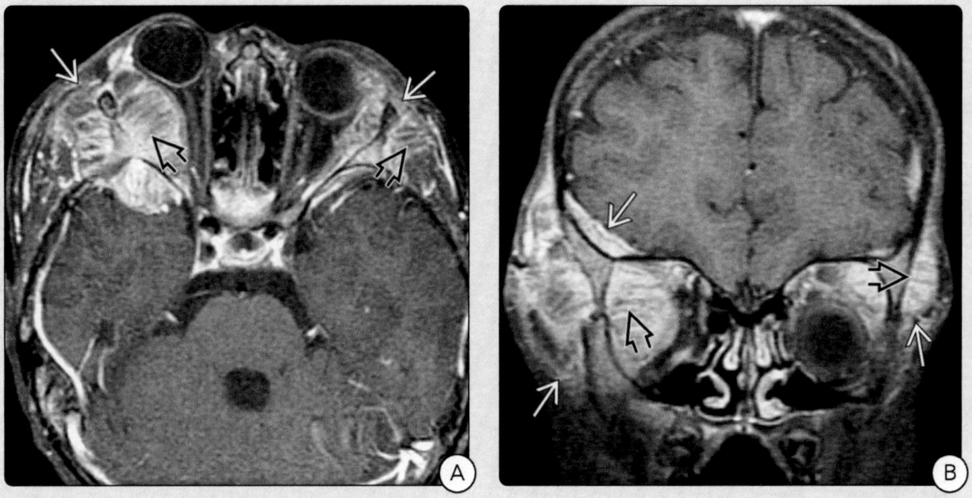

***(21-20A)** T1 C+ FS in metastatic neuroblastoma shows bilateral enhancing soft tissue masses ➡ and "hair on end" neoplastic periostitis ⇨. **(21-20B)** Coronal T1 C+ FS shows metastases ➡ with striking "hair on end" neoplastic periosteitis ⇨. (Courtesy C. Y. Ho, MD.)*

Other lesions that can present with lytic bone lesions include **Langerhans cell histiocytosis** (LCH). Both can present with dura-based masses, but the spiculated periosteal reaction of metastatic NB is absent in LCH.

Primary CNS Neuroblastoma. Primary CNS NB is much less common than secondary disease. If a supratentorial embryonal neoplasm displays *only* neuronal differentiation, then by definition it is a cerebral NB. Imaging findings are indistinguishable from those of other PNETs, i.e., a large hemispheric mass with necrosis, hemorrhage, and strong but heterogeneous enhancement following contrast administration.

Esthesioneuroblastoma

Terminology. Esthesioneuroblastoma (ENB)—also known as **olfactory neuroblastoma**—is a rare malignant neuroectodermal tumor that arises in the superior nasal cavity **(21-22)**. ENBs are a type of "small round blue cell tumor" that may be difficult to differentiate from other tumors such as lymphoma and Ewing sarcoma.

Etiology. ENBs are tumors of neural crest origin that probably arise from basal cells of the olfactory epithelium. There are no known risk factors.

ENBs and other sinonasal neuroendocrine tumors (sinonasal neuroendocrine carcinoma, sinonasal undifferentiated carcinoma) overexpress *ASCL1*. The neurotrophin receptors TrkA and TrkB are also strongly expressed in almost all ENBs. TrkB overexpression participates in tumorigenesis through ERK and Akt pathway activation.

Pathology. As they are primarily extracranial neoplasms, ENBs are not graded according to WHO criteria. ENBs appear grossly as submucosal lobulated, moderately vascular masses.

The modified Kadish classification is used for staging and recognizes four stages: stage A, tumors that are localized to

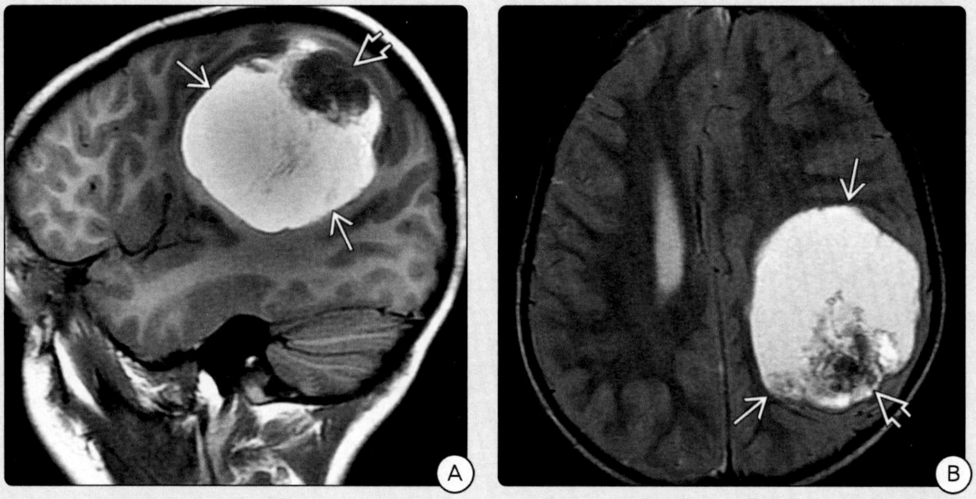

***(21-21A)** Sagittal T1WI in a 3y girl with seizures and systemic metastases from an extensive retroperitoneal neuroblastoma shows a hyperintense cystic-appearing parietal mass ➡ with a solid hypointense mural nodule ➡. **(21-21B)** Axial T2WI in the same case shows that the cyst contents are hyperintense ➡, whereas the irregularly shaped nodule ➡ is hypointense compared with adjacent cortex.*

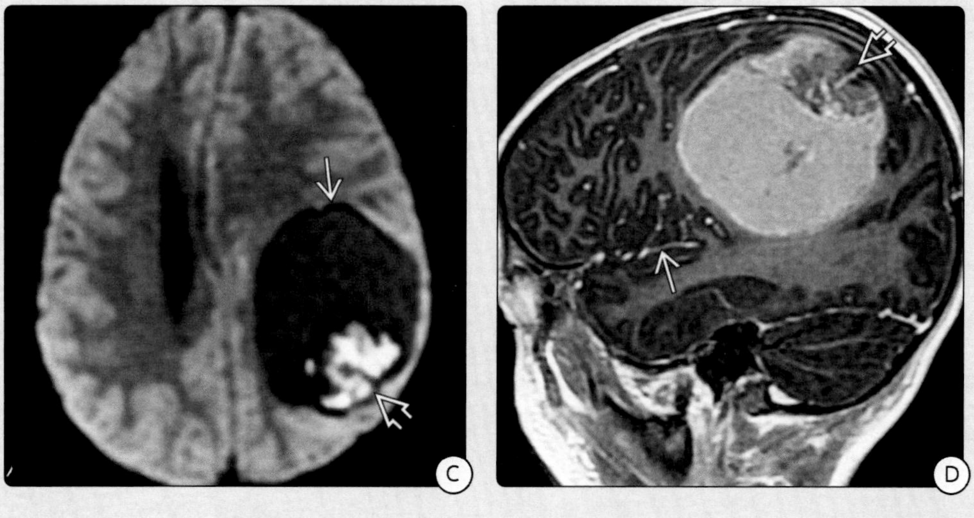

***(21-21C)** DWI in the same case shows facilitated diffusion in the cyst ➡ and restricted diffusion in the hypercellular tumor nodule ➡. **(21-21D)** Sagittal T1 C+ SPGR shows that the tumor nodule demonstrates mild enhancement ➡. Note diffuse sulcal enhancement from CSF metastases ➡. Parenchymal metastases from extracranial neuroblastoma are rare.*

the nasal cavity; stage B, nasal cavity and paranasal sinuses; stage C, orbital and intracranial extension; stage D, cervical and distant metastases.

Histologic grading uses the Hyams system with grades I-IV based on nuclear pleomorphism, mitoses, and necrosis. ENBs are divided into low-grade (Hyams I-III) and high-grade (Hyams IV) tumors.

Low-grade ENBs feature a lobular architecture with neurofibrillary intercellular matrix and pseudorosette formation. Mild nuclear pleomorphism with infrequent mitoses is typical. Electron microscopy demonstrates neurosecretory granules. To date, no studies clearly prove molecular differences between low- and high-grade ENBs.

Clinical Issues. ENBs account for approximately 2-3% of all nasal cavity tumors.

ENBs have a wide age range with a bimodal peak in the second and sixth decades of life. ENB is usually not a diagnostic consideration in children.

The most common symptoms are nasal obstruction and epistaxis. ENBs with intracranial extension may present with headache, proptosis, and cranial neuropathies.

Overall 5-year survival rate is approximately 75% but varies with Kadish stage. Five-year survival ranges from over 90% (Kadish A) to under 35% (Katish D). Local recurrence is common (30%). Nodal and/or distant metastases to lung, bone, and liver develop in 10-30% of patients.

Imaging. The typical finding in ENB is a superior nasal cavity mass at the cribriform plate. A "dumbbell" shape—the upper portion in the anterior cranial fossa and the lower portion in the nose with the narrowest aspect at the cribriform plate—is seen with large masses **(21-22)**.

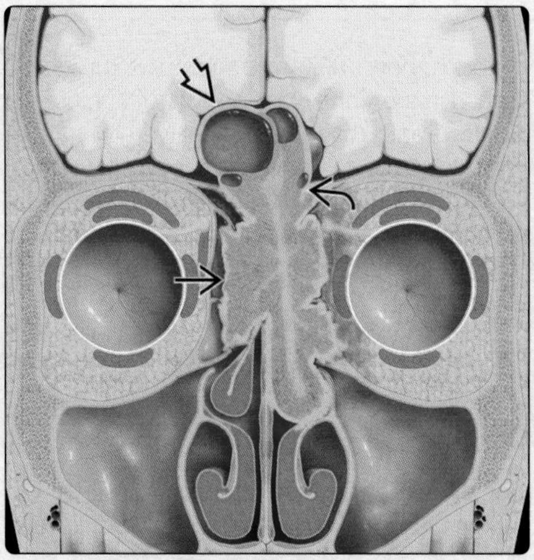

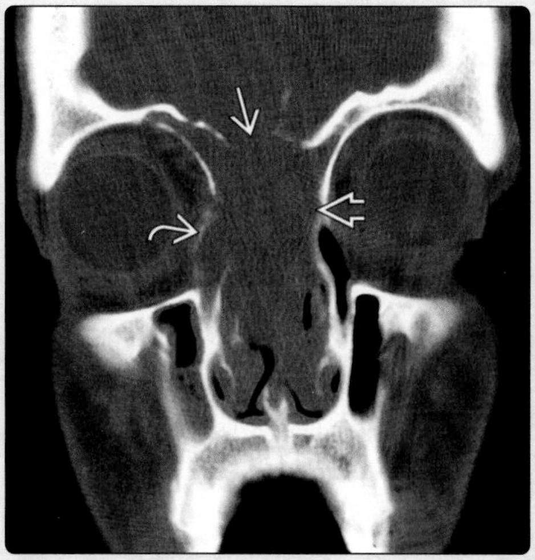

***(21-22)** Coronal graphic depicts esthesioneuroblastoma (ENB) as a large nasal mass → with cephalad intracranial extension → through the cribriform plate →. **(21-23)** Coronal bone CT shows an ENB filling the upper nasal cavity and ethmoid sinuses →. The lesion extends through the anterior skull base →. The right lamina papyracea is thinned and laterally displaced →. (From DI: Head and Neck, 3e.)*

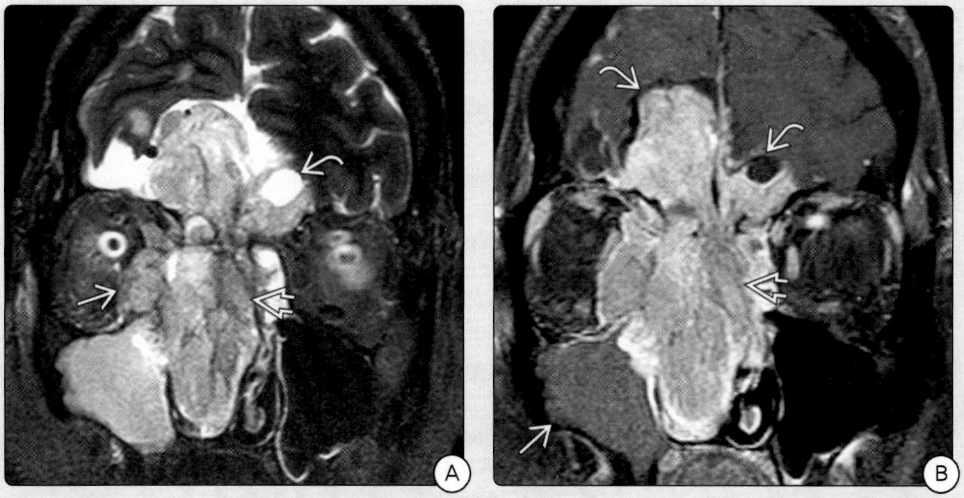

***(21-24A)** Coronal T2 FS in a 47y woman shows a classic ENB → filling the nasal cavity and ethmoid sinuses. The lesion extends superiorly into the anterior cranial fossa and laterally into the right orbit →. Note cysts at the tumor-brain interface →, a common finding with ENBs. **(21-24B)** Coronal T1 C+ FS in the same case shows the ENB → enhances strongly, moderately uniformly. Note tumor-associated cysts →, obstructed right maxillary sinus →.*

CT Findings. Bone CT shows expansile bone remodeling mixed with bone destruction, especially of the cribriform plate **(21-23)**. Speckled intratumoral calcification is unusual. A homogeneously enhancing mass on CECT is typical.

MR Findings. ENB is hypo- to isointense compared with brain on T1WI and iso- to hyperintense on T2WI. Areas of cystic degeneration and intratumoral hemorrhage are common. Some large ENBs that extend intracranially have benign nonneoplastic tumor-associated cysts around their superior and lateral margins at the tumor-brain interface. ENBs generally enhance strongly and relatively uniformly **(21-24)**.

ENB spread to cervical lymph nodes is common, typically spreading first to level II nodes, with frequent involvement of level I, level III, and retropharyngeal nodal groups at later stages. Nodes harboring metastatic disease are predominantly solid and demonstrate avid contrast enhancement.

PET/CT. 18F FDG PET/CT is a useful adjunct to conventional imaging in the initial staging or subsequent restaging of ENB. Nodal and distant metastatic disease, as well as local recurrence obscured by treatment changes on standard imaging, can be depicted. PET/CT changes previously assigned disease stage and alters patient management in nearly 40% of cases with more than one-third of tumors upstaged.

Differential Diagnosis. The major differential diagnoses of ENB with intracranial extension are **sinonasal squamous cell carcinoma** (SCCa) and **sinonasal neuroendocrine carcinoma** (SNEC). Sinonasal SCCa is more common in the maxillary antrum than in the nose and does not enhance as intensely as ENB. SNECs develop in the superior or posterior nasal cavity, often extending into the maxillary or ethmoid sinuses. Patients with **sinonasal adenocarcinoma** often have a history of occupational or wood dust exposure.

Sinonasal undifferentiated carcinoma (SNUC) may be difficult to distinguish from ENB on imaging alone. **Sinonasal non-Hodgkin lymphoma** is typically hyperdense on NECT, restricts on DWI, and rarely extends directly superiorly into the skull base and anterior fossa. **Sinonasal melanoma** favors the lower nasal cavity as its site of origin (septum, turbinates). T1 hyperintensity and T2 hypointensity are classic MR findings.

Anterior skull base (cribriform plate) **meningioma** typically causes hyperostosis and exhibits a "sunburst" pattern of vascularity with the central tumor supplied by dural branches of the carotid arteries. Peritumoral cysts are not a distinguishing feature, as they occur with both meningiomas and ENBs.

New Molecularly Defined Embryonal Neoplasms

A significant proportion of tumors originally diagnosed as CNS-PNETs demonstrate ambiguous small-cell morphology, making it difficult to classify on the basis of histology alone and highlighting the diagnostic necessity of utilizing molecular markers.

In addition to the well-recognized molecularly defined CNS embryonal neoplasms, recent studies have identified four new tumor entities with specific genetic alterations and distinct histopathologic and clinical features. These new molecularly defined entities have been designated as **CNS neuroblastoma with FOXR2 activation** (CNS NB-*FOXR2*), **CNS Ewing sarcoma family tumor with CIC alteration** (CNS EFT-*CIC*), **CNS high-grade neuroepithelial tumor with MN1 alteration** (CNS HGNET-*MN1*), and **CNS high-grade neuroepithelial tumor with BCOR alteration** (CNS HGNET-*BCOR*).

All these tumors are rare, WHO grade IV malignant neoplasms that tend to affect infants and young children although they may also occur in adolescents and adults. They typically present as large, bulky supratentorial hemispheric masses that are characterized by imaging findings that are indistinguishable from other CNS embryonal neoplasms.

Malignant Rhabdoid Tumors

Malignant rhabdoid tumors (MRTs) are aggressive tumors that were first described in the kidneys and soft tissues of infants and young children. Cranial rhabdoid tumors were subsequently recognized as a distinct pathologic entity and termed atypical teratoid/rhabdoid tumor (AT/RT). AT/RTs are separated from other CNS embryonal neoplasms and non-CNS MRTs by distinct immunohistochemical, histopathologic, and molecular features.

Atypical Teratoid/Rhabdoid Tumor

Terminology

AT/RT is a malignant CNS embryonal tumor composed of poorly differentiated elements and malignant rhabdoid cells.

Etiology

AT/RT is now a genetically-defined tumor characterized by deletions and biallelic inactivating mutations of the *SMARCB1/*SNF5 gene. Loss of the SMARCB1 protein in AT/RT results in unopposed expression of *LIN28B* (a key gene in embryonic development and for the maintenance of pluripotency in stem cells) and related oncogenes such as CCND1.

AT/RT is not a homogeneous disease even though these tumors are all characterized by the prototypic loss of expression of *SMARCB1* (or *SMARCA4* in the rare *SMARCB1* wild-type cases). Molecular profiling has identified three epigenetically and clinically distinct AT/RT subgroups, currently designated as ATRT-TYR, ATRT-SHH, and ATRT-MYC.

ATRT-TYRs have broad *SMARCB1* deletions exhibiting overexpression of melanosomal genes. ATRT-SHH tumors have focal *SMARCB1* aberrations with overexpression of SHH pathway. ATRT-MYCs also have focal *SMARCB1* deletions but overexpress the *MYC* and HOX clusters.

Pathology

Location. AT/RTs occur in both the supra- and infratentorial compartments. Location is correlated with epigenetic subgroup.

Slightly more than half of AT/RTs are supratentorial, usually occurring in the cerebral hemispheres **(21-25)** although cases in other sites (including the suprasellar cistern, ventricles **(21-26)**, and pineal gland **(21-27)**) have been reported. Most supratentorial AT/RTs are ATRT-MYC or ATRT-SHH subtypes.

Posterior fossa AT/RTs preferentially occur in the cerebellar hemispheres **(21-28)** although they can occur in the fourth ventricle, where they mimic medulloblastoma **(21-29)**. Other less frequent sites include the cerebellopontine angle and brainstem. All three molecular subgroups can occur in the infratentorial compartment although the posterior fossa is the site of almost 75% of ATRT-TYR neoplasms.

AT/RT: ETIOLOGY AND PATHOLOGY

Etiology

- Loss of expression of *SMARCB1* protein (INI1) required for diagnosis
    - *SMARCB1* wild-type has *SMARCA4* mutations
- Loss of part or all of chromosome 22
- 3 epigenetically distinct AT/RT subgroups
    - ATRT-TYR, ATRT-SHH, ATRT-MYC

Pathology

- Supratentorial ~ 50%
    - Most are ATRT-MYC or ATRT-SHH
- Infratentorial ~ 50%
    - All 3 subgroups (75% of ATRT-TYR)
- Poorly differentiated neuroepithelial elements + rhabdoid cells
- WHO grade IV

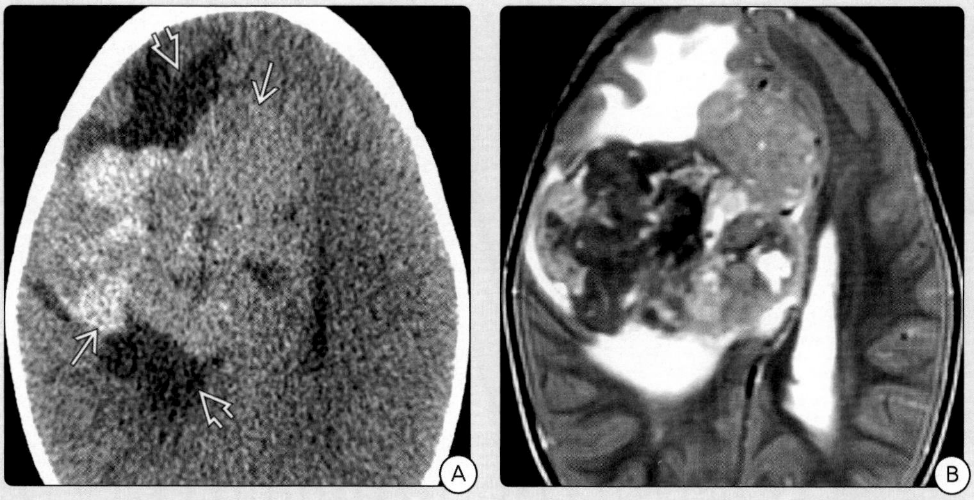

***(21-25A)** NECT in an 18m girl with vomiting for 1-2 weeks shows a mixed, mostly hyperdense right frontal mass ➡ with marked vasogenic edema ⇨. **(21-25B)** T2WI shows that the mass has mixed, mostly hypo- and isointense signal intensity.*

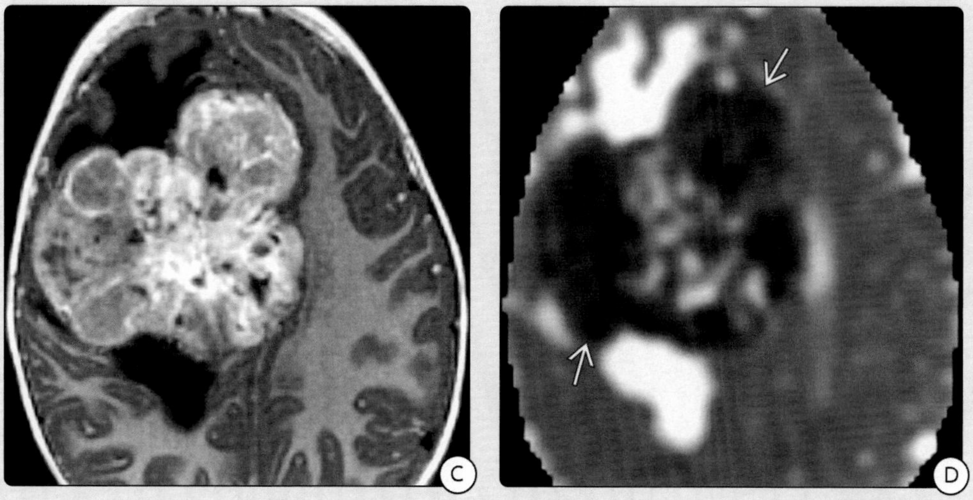

***(21-25C)** T1 C+ shows diffuse but very heterogeneous enhancement. **(21-25D)** ADC map shows marked diffuse restriction ➡ due to the high cellularity of the tumor. MRS (not shown) demonstrated elevated Cho and lactate. Histologic diagnosis was atypical teratoid/rhabdoid tumor (AT/RT). (Courtesy B. Jones, MD.)*

Gross Pathology. The gross appearance—a large, soft, fleshy, hemorrhagic, necrotic mass—is similar to that of other CNS embryonal neoplasms.

Microscopic Features. AT/RTs are composed of poorly differentiated neural, epithelial, and mesenchymal elements together with prominent rhabdoid cells. Loss of nuclear staining for INI1 is diagnostic of AT/RT.

Clinical Issues

Epidemiology. AT/RT accounts for 1-2% of all pediatric brain tumors. Most occur in children under 5 years of age. Peak incidence is between birth and 2 years, and some investigators suggest that AT/RT accounts for at least 10% of all CNS neoplasms in infants. AT/RT does occur in adults but is rare. There is a moderate male predominance.

AT/RT can occur sporadically or in **rhabdoid tumor predisposition syndrome** (RTPS). RTPS is a familial cancer syndrome characterized by a markedly increased risk of developing MRTs—including AT/RT—caused by loss or inactivation of the *SMARCB1* gene (less commonly, the mutation involves the *SMARCA4* gene). Pedigree analysis supports an autosomal-dominant inheritance pattern with incomplete penetrance.

Patients with RTPS may develop an AT/RT with a synchronous renal or extrarenal MRT. Children with RTPS and AT/RT are even younger, have more extensive disease, and experience more rapid progression. Other CNS tumors associated with RTPS include choroid plexus carcinoma and rhabdoid meningioma.

Natural History. AT/RT is a highly malignant tumor with generally poor prognosis. Median survival is around 17 months. Most children die within 6 to 8 months despite aggressive therapy. Survival in adults is somewhat better, averaging 2 years.

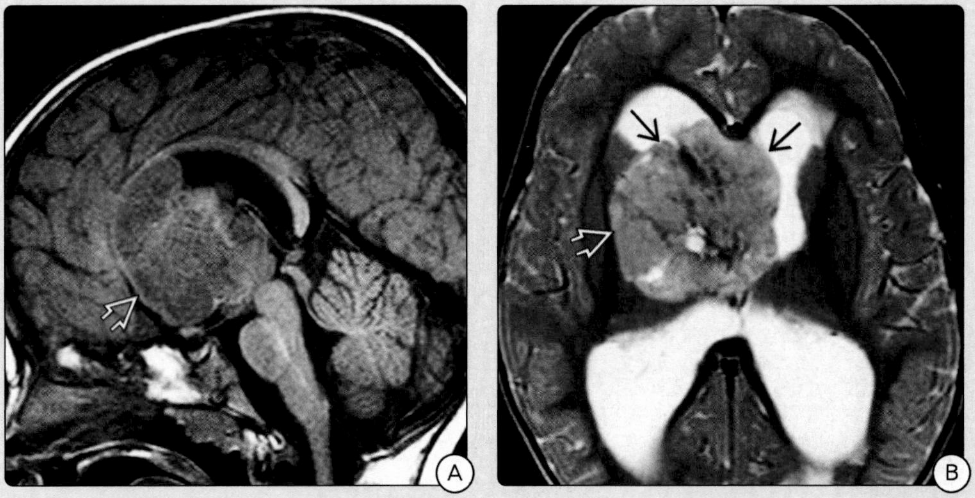

***(21-26A)** Sagittal T1WI in an 18m girl with vomiting and lethargy shows a large lobulated, mixed-signal-intensity mass in the third ventricle. **(21-26B)** Axial T2WI in the same case shows that the mass is heterogeneously hyperintense and extends into the frontal horns of both lateral ventricles, causing severe obstructive hydrocephalus.*

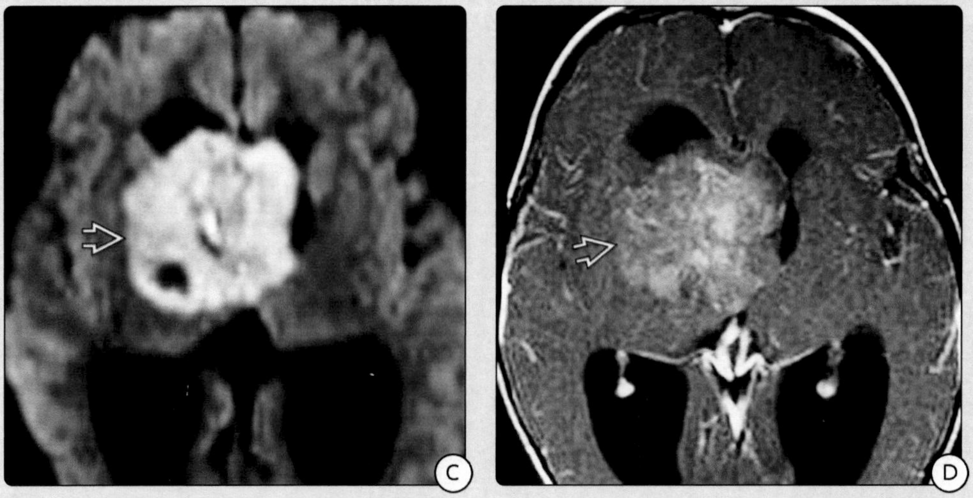

***(21-26C)** Axial DWI in the same case shows that the mass exhibits strong diffusion restriction. **(21-26D)** Axial T1 C+ FS in the same case shows that the mass enhances moderately but quite heterogeneously. AT/RT was found at surgery. The patient survived 11 months.*

AT/RT: CLINICAL ISSUES

Epidemiology
- 1-2% of pediatric brain tumors
    - Children < 5 years, most < 2 years
    - 10% of CNS neoplasms in infants
    - Occasionally occur in adults (rare)

Rhabdoid Tumor Predisposition Syndrome
- Malignant rhabdoid tumors
- Choroid plexus carcinoma

Imaging

General Features. AT/RT shares many imaging features with other embryonal tumors, i.e., they are densely cellular neoplasms that frequently contain hemorrhage, necrosis, cysts, and calcifications. A moderately large, bulky tumor with mixed solid and cystic components and heterogeneous density/signal intensity is typical.

CSF dissemination is common, so the entire neuraxis should be imaged prior to surgical intervention.

CT Findings. NECT scan shows a mildly to moderately hyperdense mass with cysts and hemorrhagic foci **(21-25A)** **(21-27)**. Calcification and obstructive hydrocephalus—especially with posterior fossa AT/RT—are common **(21-29A)**. Enhancement is typically strong but heterogeneous.

MR Findings. AT/RTs are heterogeneously hypo- to isointense to brain on T1WI and iso- to hyperintense on T2WI **(21-25)**. "Blooming" foci on T2* (GRE, SWI) are common. Mild to moderate diffusion restriction is present **(21-25D)**. MRS shows elevated Cho and decreased or absent NAA.

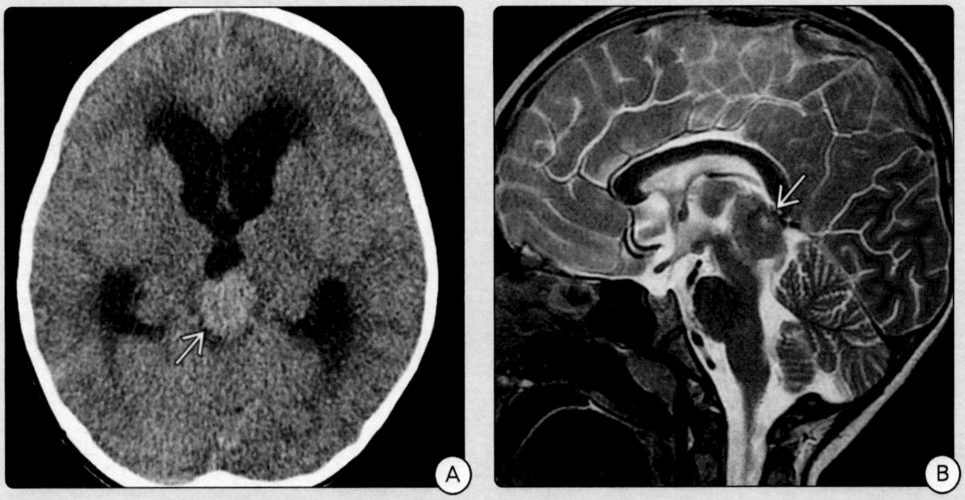

(21-27A) Axial NECT in a 4y girl with a 1-month history of headache and vomiting shows a hyperdense mass ➡ in the pineal region, causing severe obstructive hydrocephalus. (21-27B) Sagittal T2WI in the same case shows a pineal gland mass ➡ that appears isointense with the adjacent brain.

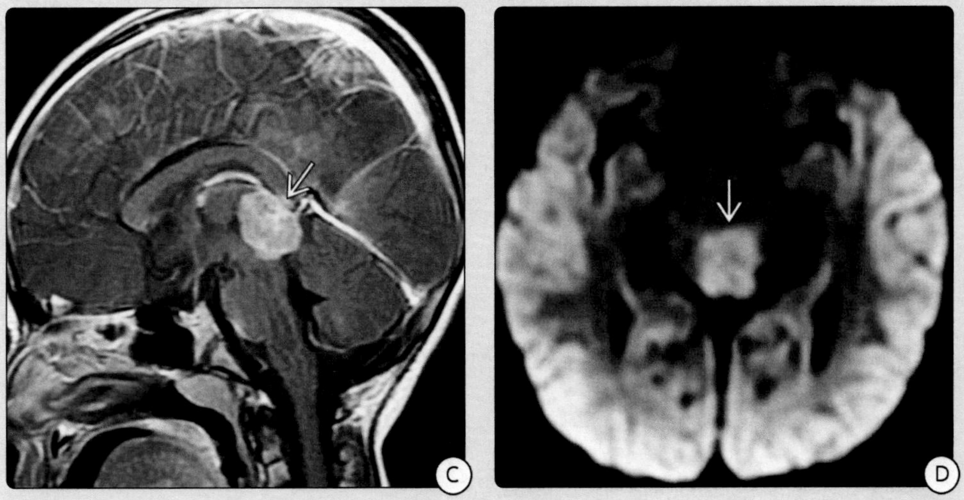

(21-27C) Sagittal T1 C+ in the same case shows that the mass ➡ enhances strongly but slightly heterogeneously. (21-27D) Axial DWI shows the mass ➡ exhibits restricted diffusion. Preoperative diagnosis was pineoblastoma. AT/RT was found at surgery. The patient is alive 11 months after surgery with adjuvant chemotherapy.

Enhancement on T1 C+ is strong but heterogeneous **(21-26)**. Leptomeningeal spread is present in 15-20% of cases at the time of initial imaging.

Differential Diagnosis

The major differential diagnosis for supratentorial AT/RT includes **C19MC-altered embryonal neoplasm, RELA-fusion ependymoma, teratoma,** and **malignant astrocytoma**. As all of these may be bulky—even massive—tumors with very heterogeneous imaging appearance, definitive diagnosis requires biopsy and *SMARCB1* (INI1) staining.

The major differential diagnosis for posterior fossa AT/RT is **medulloblastoma**. These tumors can look virtually identical on imaging studies **(21-29) (21-30)**.

AT/RT: IMAGING AND DIFFERENTIAL DIAGNOSIS

Imaging

- Heterogeneous, hyperdense on NECT
- Heterogeneous on both T1, T2
- Enhances strongly but heterogeneously
- CSF spread in 15-20% at diagnosis
- Restricts on DWI

Differential Diagnosis

- DDx of *supratentorial* AT/RT
  - CNS embryonal tumor, C19MC-altered
  - *RELA*-fusion ependymoma, teratoma, malignant astrocytoma
- DDx of *posterior fossa* AT/RT
  - Medulloblastoma (midline AT/RT may be indistinguishable)

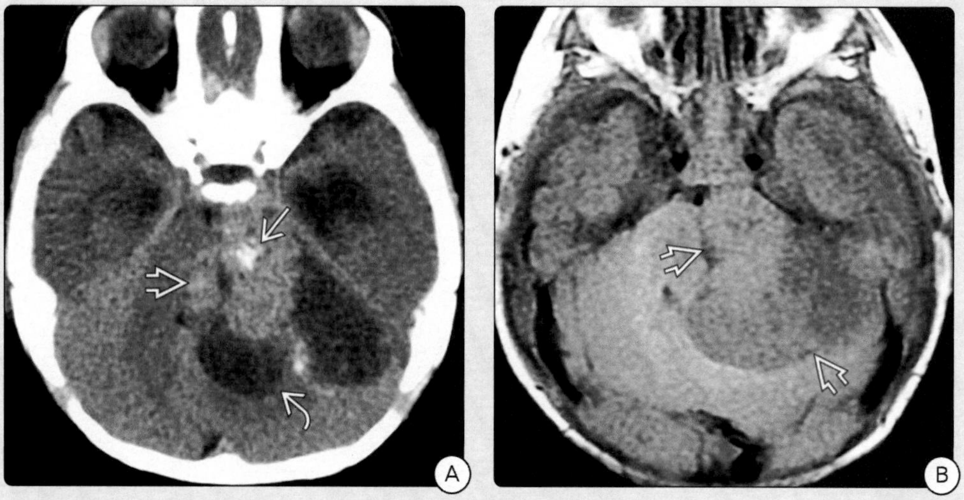

***(21-28A)** NECT in a 4m boy with vomiting, head tilt, and bulging fontanelle shows a partially solid ➡, partially cystic-appearing ➡ posterior fossa mass that exhibits focal calcifications ➡. **(21-28B)** Axial T1WI in the same case shows that the mass ➡ is mixed iso-/hypointense compared with gray matter.*

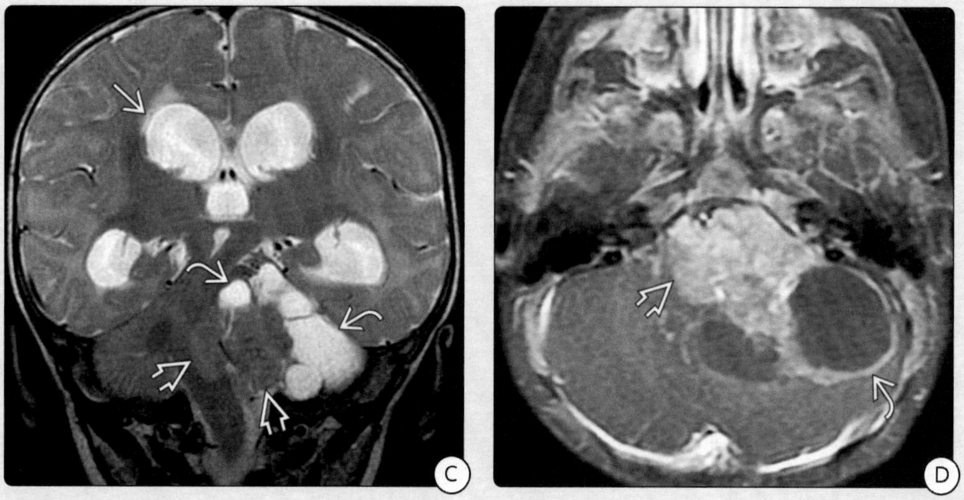

***(21-28C)** Coronal T2WI in the same case shows that the mixed solid ➡, cystic ➡ mass is causing severe obstructive hydrocephalus ➡. **(21-28D)** Axial T1 C+ FS shows the solid components ➡ of the mass enhancing strongly but heterogeneously. The cysts exhibit rim enhancement ➡. This is AT/RT, WHO grade IV.*

Other CNS Neoplasms With Rhabdoid Features

CNS embryonal tumor with rhabdoid features is a highly malignant neoplasm composed of poorly differentiated elements and rhabdoid cells with *SMARCB1* or *SMARCA4* expression. These extremely rare tumors correspond histologically to WHO grade IV.

Rhabdoid meningioma is an uncommon WHO grade III meningioma subtype that contains sheets of rhabdoid cells. Most have high proliferative indices and exhibit other cytologic features of malignancy. Rhabdoid meningiomas are very rare in infants and retain INI1 staining, which differentiates them histopathologically from AT/RT.

CNS NEOPLASMS WITH RHABDOID FEATURES

Rhabdoid Glioblastoma
- GBM + rhabdoid cells (*SMARCB1* loss)
- Younger than typical GBM
- Extracranial metastases common

Embryonal Neoplasm With Rhabdoid Features
- WHO IV tumor with differentiated rhabdoid cells
- *SMARCB1/4* mutation

Rhabdoid Meningioma
- Rhabdoid features without *SMARCB1* mutation

Rhabdoid Predisposition Syndrome
- *SMARCB1* germline mutation/deletion
- AT/RT, choroid plexus carcinoma, medulloblastoma

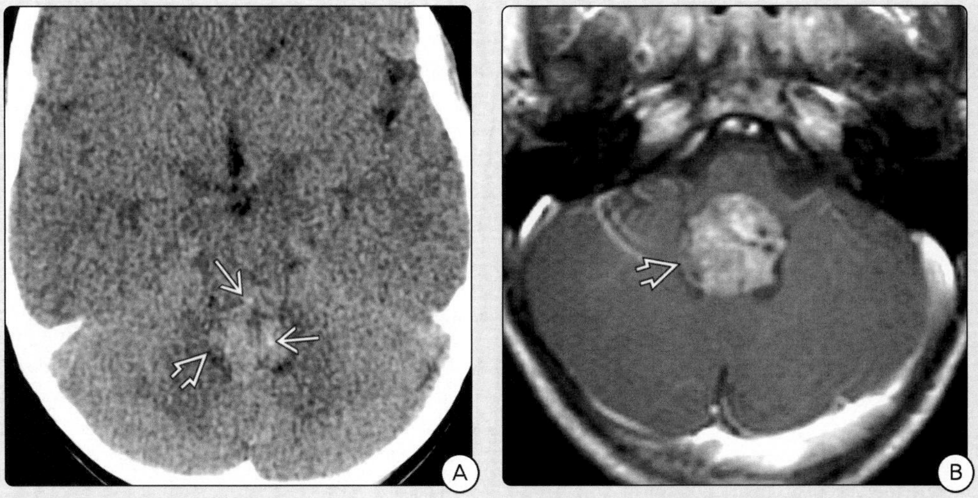

***(21-29A)** NECT in a 3y boy with morning emesis for 4-6 weeks shows a hyperdense mass ➡ in the fourth ventricle. Note intratumoral calcifications ➡. There is no evidence for obstructive hydrocephalus. **(21-29B)** T1 C+ shows that the mass ➡ enhances heterogeneously. Preoperative diagnosis was medulloblastoma. Histologic examination revealed AT/RT, WHO grade IV.*

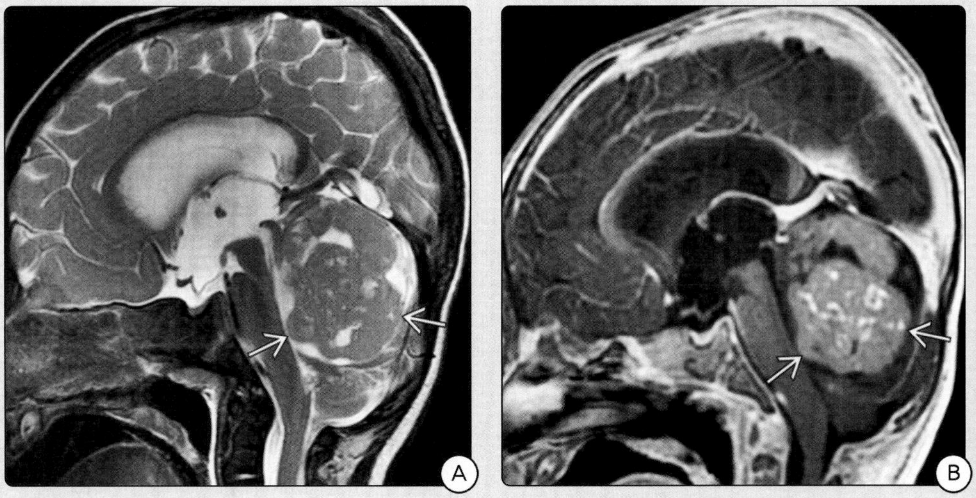

***(21-30A)** Sagittal T2WI in a 6m girl with lethargy and vomiting shows a heterogeneous-appearing mass ➡ in the fourth ventricle causing severe obstructive hydrocephalus. **(21-30B)** Sagittal T1 C+ in the same case shows that the mass ➡ enhances very heterogeneously. Preoperative diagnosis was medulloblastoma. AT/RT was found at surgery. Imaging findings of posterior fossa AT/RTs can be indistinguishable from MB.*

Selected References

Medulloblastoma

Borowska A et al: Medulloblastoma: molecular pathways and histopathological classification. Arch Med Sci. 12(3):659-66, 2016

Medulloblastoma Overview

Juhnke BO et al: Refining medulloblastoma subgroups. Lancet Oncol. ePub, 2017

Schwalbe EC et al: Novel molecular subgroups for clinical classification and outcome prediction in childhood medulloblastoma: a cohort study. Lancet Oncol. ePub, 2017

Classic Medulloblastoma

Brandão LA et al: Posterior fossa tumors. Neuroimaging Clin N Am. 27(1):1-37, 2017

Ellison DW et al: Medulloblastoma. In: Louis DN et al (eds), WHO Classification of Tumours of the Central Nervous System. Lyon, France: International Agency for Research on Cancer, 2016, pp. 184-188

Ellison DW et al: Medulloblastoma, classic. In: Louis DN et al (eds), WHO Classification of Tumours of the Central Nervous System. Lyon, France: International Agency for Research on Cancer, 2016, p. 194

Kijima N et al: Molecular classification of medulloblastoma. Neurol Med Chir (Tokyo). 56(11):687-697, 2016

Medulloblastoma With Extensive Nodularity

Giangaspero F et al: Medulloblastoma with extensive nodularity. In: Louis DN et al (eds), WHO Classification of Tumours of the Central Nervous System. Lyon, France: International Agency for Research on Cancer, 2016, pp. 198-199

Gessi M et al: Medulloblastoma with extensive nodularity: a tumor exclusively of infancy? Neuropathol Appl Neurobiol. 43(3):267-270, 2016

Desmoplastic/Nodular Medulloblastoma

Pietsch T et al: Desmoplastic/nodular medulloblastoma. In: Louis DN et al (eds), WHO Classification of Tumours of the Central Nervous System. Lyon, France: International Agency for Research on Cancer, 2016, pp. 195-197

Large Cell/Anaplastic Medulloblastoma

Huang PI et al: Large cell/anaplastic medulloblastoma is associated with poor prognosis-a retrospective analysis at a single institute. Childs Nerv Syst. ePub, 2017

Ellison DW et al: Large cell/anaplastic medulloblastoma. In: Louis DN et al (eds), WHO Classification of Tumours of the Central Nervous System. Lyon, France: International Agency for Research on Cancer, 2016, p. 200

Other CNS Embryonal Tumors

McLendon R et al: Other CNS embryonal tumors. In: Louis DN et al (eds), WHO Classification of Tumours of the Central Nervous System. Lyon, France: International Agency for Research on Cancer, 2016, pp. 206-208

Embryonal Tumor With Multilayered Rosettes, C19MC-Altered

Horwitz M et al: Embryonal tumors with multilayered rosettes in children: the SFCE experience. Childs Nerv Syst. 32(2):299-305, 2016

Korshunov A et al: Embryonal tumour with multilayered rosettes, C19MC-altered. In: Louis DN et al (eds), WHO Classification of Tumours of the Central Nervous System. Lyon, France: International Agency for Research on Cancer, 2016, pp. 201-205

Other CNS Embryonal Tumors

Czapiewski P et al: Genetic and molecular alterations in olfactory neuroblastoma - implications for pathogenesis, prognosis and treatment. Oncotarget. 7(32):52584-52596, 2016

Dublin AB et al: Imaging characteristics of olfactory neuroblastoma (esthesioneuroblastoma). J Neurol Surg B Skull Base. 77(1):1-5, 2016

Nalavenkata SB et al: Olfactory neuroblastoma: fate of the neck–a long-term multicenter retrospective study. Otolaryngol Head Neck Surg. 154(2):383-9, 2016

Malignant Rhabdoid Tumors

Atypical Teratoid/Rhabdoid Tumor

Ud Din N et al: Atypical teratoid/rhabdoid tumor of brain: a clinicopathologic study of eleven patients and review of literature Asian Pac J Cancer Prev. 18(4):949-954, 2017

Choi SA et al: LIN28B is highly expressed in atypical teratoid/rhabdoid tumor (AT/RT) and suppressed through the restoration of SMARCB1. Cancer Cell Int. 16:32, 2016

Judkins AR et al: Atypical teratoid/rhabdoid tumour. In: Louis DN et al (eds), WHO Classification of Tumours of the Central Nervous System. Lyon, France: International Agency for Research on Cancer, 2016, pp. 209-212

Torchia J et al: Integrated (epi)-genomic analyses identify subgroup-specific therapeutic targets in CNS rhabdoid tumors. Cancer Cell. 30(6):891-908, 2016

Other CNS Neoplasms With Rhabdoid Features

Gelal MF et al: Magnetic resonance imaging features of rhabdoid glioblastomas. Clin Neuroradiol. 26(3):329-40, 2016

Miyahara M et al: Glioblastoma with rhabdoid features: report of two young adult cases and review of the literature. World Neurosurg. 86:515.e1-9, 2016

Tumors of the Meninges

The cranial meninges give rise to a broad spectrum of neoplasms that usually occur as extraaxial masses (i.e., outside the brain parenchyma but inside the skull). Tumors of the cranial meninges are divided into three basic pathologic groups: (1) meningiomas and meningioma variants, (2) mesenchymal nonmeningothelial tumors, and (3) melanocytic tumors.

Meningioma is the most common of all intracranial neoplasms. Meningiomas (benign, atypical, and anaplastic) are by far the largest group of meningothelial neoplasms. Although meningiomas are physically attached to the dura, they actually arise from arachnoid "cap" cells rather than from the dura itself.

Both benign and malignant mesenchymal nonmeningothelial tumors can originate within the CNS. These uncommon tumors correspond histologically to tumors of soft tissue or bone found elsewhere in the body. **Solitary fibrous tumor/hemangiopericytoma, hemangioblastoma,** and **hemangioma** are also now included in this subgroup.

The third group features the rare **primary melanocytic lesions** of the cranial meninges, including focal melanocytoma and diffuse leptomeningeal melanocytosis.

Anatomy of the Cranial Meninges

The cranial meninges consist of the dura mater, the arachnoid, and the pia.

Dura

The dura mater—also called the pachymeninx—is a continuous fibrous sheet that lines the calvaria and spine. As its name implies (Latin for "tough mother"), the dura is a comparatively tough covering that provides significant protection against injury and infection. It is also the most important site for CSF turnover.

Neurosurgeons traditionally view the cranial dura as a simple bilaminar structure with an **outer ("periosteal") layer** and an **inner ("meningeal") layer**. The periosteal layer is firmly attached to the cranial vault, especially at sutures. The inner (meningeal) layer folds inward to form the falx cerebri, tentorium cerebelli, and diaphragma sellae. The two layers separate to contain the dural venous sinuses (see Chapter 9).

Anatomists have identified *three* different layers of dura at light microscopy. The **outer dural border layer**, which is just 2 μm thick, is the thinnest layer

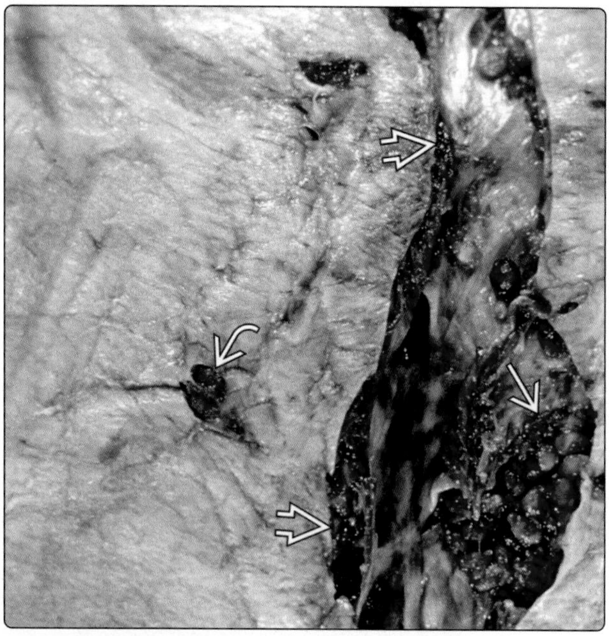

(22-1) Close-up view of dura ➡, opened to show the superior sagittal sinus with numerous arachnoid granulations protruding into the sinus ➡. Note the small parasagittal venous lake with arachnoid granulation ➡. (Courtesy E. Ross, MD.)

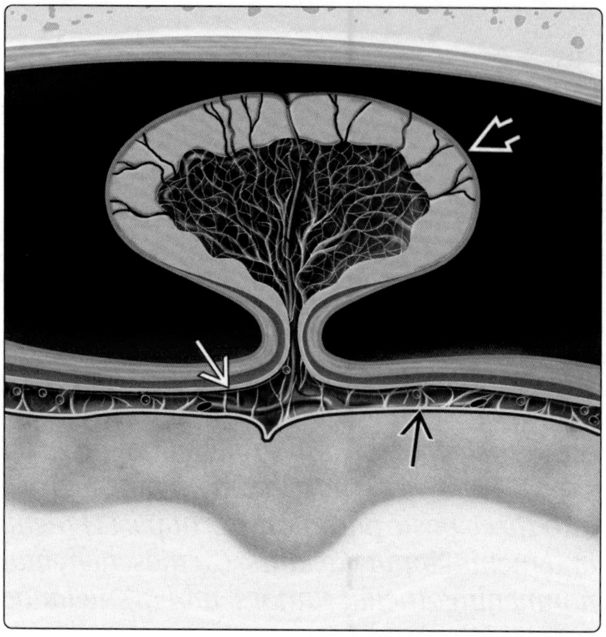

(22-2) Graphic demonstrates pia ➡, arachnoid ➡, and arachnoid granulation projecting into venous sinus ➡. CSF from subarachnoid space is covered by a "cap" of arachnoid cells.

and consists of fibroblasts, collagen, and elastic fibers. The middle layer, called the **fibrous dura**, is well vascularized. Its thickness varies according to location and patient age (more prominent in infants than in adults). The innermost layer is called the **dural border cell layer**. This inner layer is 8 µm thick and is composed of only cells that adhere to the arachnoid trabeculae.

Scanning electron microscopy reveals that the dura actually consists of *five* layers, each with different constituents and patterns of organization. The outermost (**bone surface layer**) abuts the inner table of the skull. The next three components (an **external median layer**, a **vascular layer**, and an **internal median layer**) comprise the middle layer recognized by anatomists as the fibrous dura. Highly ordered collagen fibers in the median layer are arranged in three directions to form the three different layers.

The innermost layer, which is called the **arachnoid layer**, faces the arachnoid membrane itself. The arachnoid layer consists of tortuous collagen bundles that are not oriented in any common direction.

Arachnoid and Arachnoid Granulations

The **arachnoid** is a thin translucent membrane that is loosely attached to the innermost dural layer and follows its contours all the way around the inside of the skull. The outermost layer of arachnoid cells intermingles with cells of the inner dura but can be easily detached from the dura, forming a space (subdural or interdural space) between these two layers of the meninges.

Specialized villous outpouchings of the arachnoid protrude into dural venous sinuses **(22-1)**. These arachnoid granulations (AGs) are covered with a layer of specialized, metabolically active arachnoid cells called arachnoid "cap" cells **(22-2)**. AGs and contiguous diploic veins are distributed throughout the cranium and permit resorption of CSF into the venous system.

The largest AGs lie along the superior sagittal sinus but are present in other venous sinuses as well. AGs are also common in the temporal bone. Approximately 10-15% completely penetrate the dura to make direct contact with the inner cortical surface.

Pia Mater

The **pia** is the innermost layer of the cranial meninges. The pia covers the surface of the brain and adheres to the cortex relatively tightly, following gyral convolutions. The pia invaginates along penetrating vessels to form the perivascular (Virchow-Robin) spaces (PVSs).

Recent studies have shown that the PVSs form a complicated intraparenchymal network distributed over the whole brain, connecting the cerebral convexities, basal cisterns, and ventricular system. PVSs may play a significant role both in providing drainage routes for cerebral metabolites and in maintaining normal intracranial pressure.

Meningomas

Meningiomas are the most common of all brain tumors, accounting for over a third of all primary intracranial neoplasms. The WHO subdivides meningiomas into

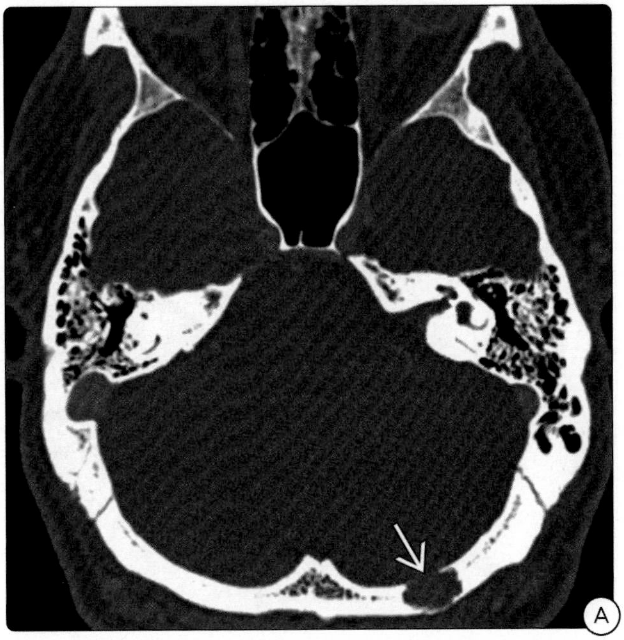

(22-3A) A 34y man had a CT angiogram for trauma. A well-delineated scalloped lesion ➡ in the left occipital squama is likely an intraosseous arachnoid granulation.

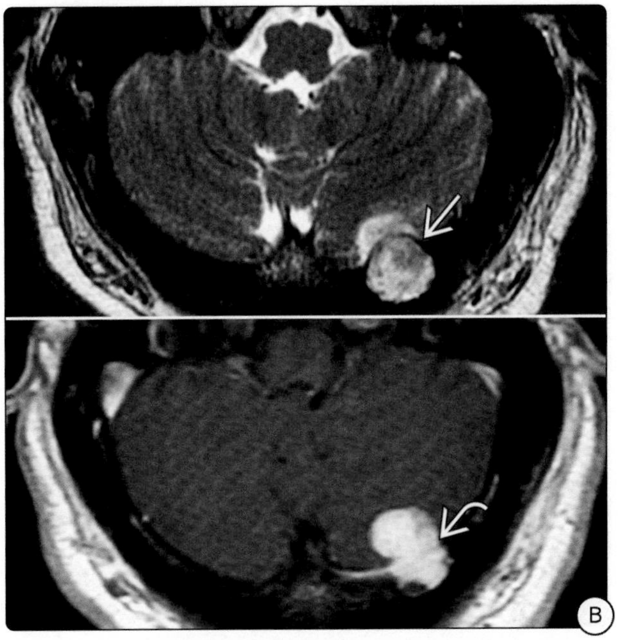

(22-3B) 14 years later the patient was reimaged. Note occipital expansile T2 hyperintense dumbbell-shaped mass ➡ (top) that enhances intensely ➡ (bottom); this is meningioma originating from an intraosseous arachnoid granulation.

meningioma and meningioma variants. Meningioma is a benign lesion with nonaggressive growth and a low recurrence risk and corresponds histologically to WHO grade I. These histologically and biologically benign meningiomas are by far the most common type.

Meningioma variants include benign histologic subtypes such as meningothelial, fibrous, transitional, psammomatous, microcystic, secretory, and angiomatous meningiomas. All of these variants are classified as WHO grade I neoplasms.

In contrast, other meningioma variants are associated with more aggressive clinical behavior and less favorable outcomes. **Atypical meningioma** corresponds to WHO grade II. Other WHO grade II variants include chordoid and clear cell meningiomas.

The most aggressive form of meningioma, corresponding to WHO grade III, is **anaplastic ("malignant") meningioma**. Other WHO grade III variants include papillary and rhabdoid meningiomas.

We consider all three grades of meningioma in this section.

Meningioma

Terminology

Benign meningiomas are also called common or typical meningiomas (TM).

Etiology

Meningiomas arise from progenitor cells that give rise to arachnoid meningothelial ("cap") cells positioned outside the thin arachnoid layer that covers the brain and spinal cord **(22-3)**.

Ionizing radiation is the only established environmental risk factor for meningioma. People who were exposed in childhood are at higher risk. The dose-related time interval to tumor development varies from 20 to 40 years. Many of these tumors have chromosome 7 monosomy.

Meningiomas are cytogenetically heterogeneous tumors. Next-generation genomic analyses have identified driver mutations in five genes, which classify meningiomas into mutually exclusive groups with distinctive clinical correlations.

NF2 Mutant Meningiomas. The most common cytogenetic alteration in meningioma is monosomy of chromosome 22, an early event in meningioma tumorigenesis. *NF2* mutations are detected in most meningiomas associated with type 2 neurofibromatosis (NF2) and are found in up to 60% of sporadic meningiomas. *NF2* mutations occur in approximately equal frequency among all three WHO grades.

NF2 mutant meningiomas have biallelic inactivation of the *NF2* tumor suppressor gene and subsequent loss of its protein product Merlin. Merlin is capable of modulating a wide range of signaling pathways, including the Ras/Raf/MEK, Rac/PAK/JNK, and Wnt/β-catenin pathways.

NF2 mutant meningiomas usually exhibit fibrous or transitional histology and originate along the posterior or superior cerebral hemispheres, the posterior and lateral skull base, and the spinal cord.

Non-NF2 Meningiomas. Non-NF2 meningiomas have mutations in other "driver genes." To date, four mutations (*TRAF7*, *KLF4*, *AKT1*, and *SMO*, which activates Hedgehog

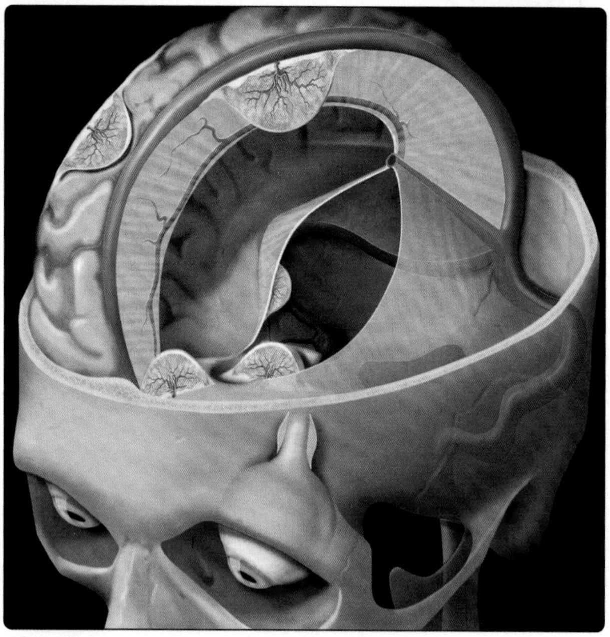

***(22-4)** The most common meningioma sites are convexity, parafalcine, followed by sphenoid ridge, olfactory groove, sella/parasellar region. 8-10% are infratentorial. Extracranial sites include optic nerve sheath, nose, and paranasal sinuses.*

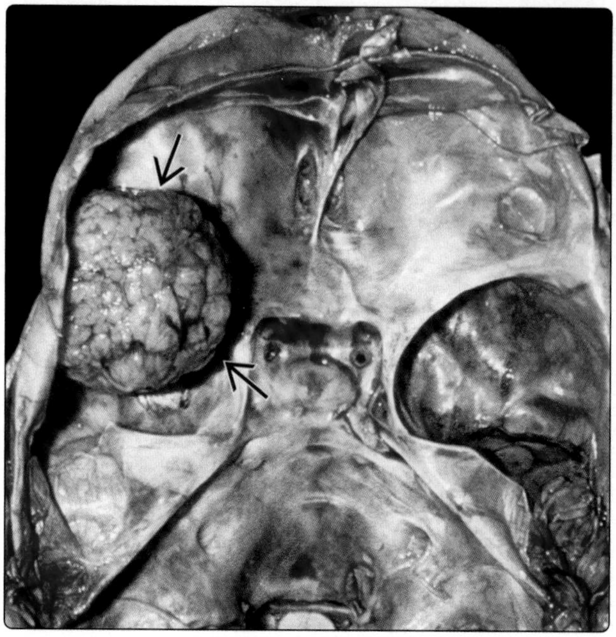

***(22-5)** Autopsy specimen demonstrates classic globose meningioma ⇒ as a round, "bosselated" mass with a flat surface toward the dura. (Courtesy R. Hewlett, MD.)*

signaling) have been identified. These non-NF2 meningiomas are usually benign and originate from the medial skull base and anterior cerebral hemispheres. Meningothelial, secretory, and microcystic histologies are common.

Pathology

Location. Meningiomas can occur at virtually any site within the CNS **(22-4)**. Over 90% of intracranial meningiomas are supratentorial. The most common location is parasagittal/convexity, accounting for almost half of all meningiomas.

Between 15-20% are located along the sphenoid ridge **(22-5)**. Other common locations near the skull base include the olfactory groove and sellar/parasellar region (including the cavernous sinus). Less common supratentorial sites include the ventricles (usually in the choroid plexus glomus) and pineal region (tentorial apex).

Approximately 8-10% of intracranial meningiomas occur in the posterior fossa. The cerebellopontine angle is by far the most common infratentorial site followed by the jugular foramen and foramen magnum, usually from the clivus or craniocervical junction. Meningiomas rarely arise from the squamous portion of the occipital bone.

Between 1-2% of meningiomas are extracranial. Sites include the orbit (optic nerve sheath), paranasal sinuses, and nose. A few TMs arise within the skull ("intradiploic" or "intraosseous" meningioma) and are most common where arachnoid granulations occur.

MENINGIOMA: LOCATION

General

- Supratentorial (90%), infratentorial (8-10%)
- Multiple (10%; neurofibromatosis type 2, meningiomatosis)

Sites

- Most common (60-70%)
  - Parasagittal (25%)
  - Convexity (20%)
  - Sphenoid ridge (15-20%)
- Less common (20-25%)
  - Posterior fossa (8-10%)
  - Olfactory groove (5-10%)
  - Parasellar (5-10%)
- Rare (2%)
  - Intraventricular
  - Pineal region/tentorial apex
  - Extracranial (optic nerve sheath, sinuses, nose)
  - Intraosseous (diploic space, often associated with arachnoid granulations)

Size and Number. Meningiomas vary widely in size. Most are small (less than 1 cm) and found incidentally. Some—especially those arising in the anterior fossa from the olfactory groove—may attain large size before causing symptoms.

Meningiomas can be solitary (90%) or multiple. Multiple meningiomas occur in **NF2** as well as in **multiple meningiomatosis syndrome**.

Gross Pathology. Meningiomas have two general configurations: a round ("globose") **(22-5)** **(22-6)** **(22-7)** and a

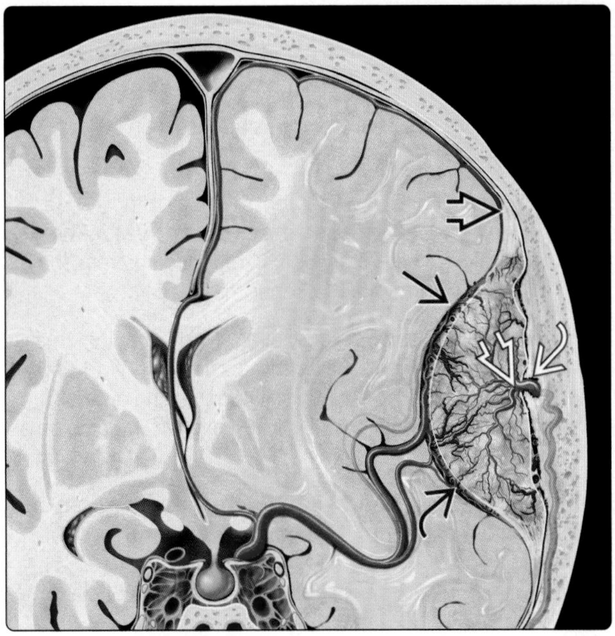

(22-6) Classic meningioma has a broad base toward dura, reactive dural thickening (dural "tail") ➲, enostotic "spur" ➲, CSF-vascular "cleft" ➲. MMA supplies tumor core in "sunburst" pattern ➲; pial vessels supply periphery ➲.

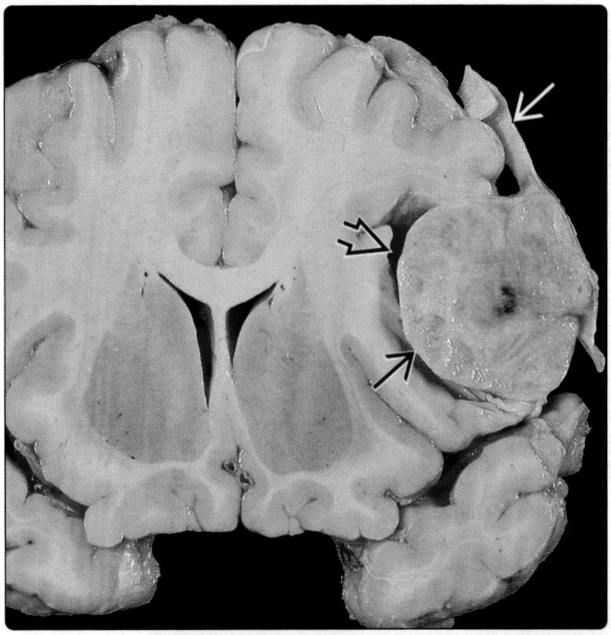

(22-7) Autopsy specimen shows classic globose meningioma ➲. Note prominent CSF-vascular cleft ➲ and reactive dural thickening ➲ ("dural tail" sign).

flat, sheet-like or carpet-like ("en plaque") appearance **(22-15)**. Most TMs are well-demarcated firm, rubbery, or gritty masses that have a broad base of dural attachment. As they grow, TMs typically invaginate toward adjacent brain. A CSF-vascular "cleft" is usually present between the tumor and underlying cortex **(22-6)** **(22-7)**. Although histologically benign meningiomas very occasionally invade the brain, this is uncommon.

Meningiomas often cause reactive nonneoplastic thickening of the adjacent dura ("dural tail" sign on imaging) **(22-9)** **(22-10)**. They commonly invade dural venous sinuses and may extend through the dura to involve the skull, inducing calvarial hyperostosis.

Although small "microcysts" are not uncommon in TMs, gross cystic change is rare. Frank hemorrhage is uncommon, occurring in only 1-2% of cases.

Rarely, metastasis from an extracranial primary to a meningioma occurs. Such **"collision tumors"** are typically lung or breast metastases to a histologically typical meningioma.

Microscopic Features. Meningiomas exhibit a wide spectrum of histologic appearances. The 2016 WHO classification lists many subtypes of typical meningioma. The most common are the **meningothelial, fibrous**, and mixed or **transitional** variants.

All TMs are benign WHO grade I tumors and by definition carry a low risk of recurrence and aggressive growth. Their mitotic index is low, with MIB-1 usually less than 1%.

Histologically benign-appearing TMs that show gross or microscopic brain invasion are designated as grade II neoplasms (see below).

Clinical Issues

Epidemiology. Recent epidemiologic data suggest that meningioma is the most frequently diagnosed primary brain tumor, accounting for over one-third of all reported CNS tumors. Typical meningiomas account for 90-95% of these tumors.

Many TMs are small and discovered incidentally, often at imaging. The lifetime risk of developing meningioma is approximately 1%, and meningiomas are found in 1-3% of autopsies.

Multiple meningiomas are common in patients with NF2 and non-NF2 hereditary multiple meningioma syndromes. Sporadic multiple (i.e., not syndromic) meningiomas occur in about 10% of cases.

Demographics. Meningiomas are classically tumors of middle-aged and older adults. Peak occurrence is in the sixth and seventh decades (mean = 65 years). Although meningioma accounts for slightly less than 3% of primary brain tumors in children, meningioma still represents the most common dura-based neoplasm in this age group. Many (but by no means all) are related to NF2. NF2-related meningiomas occur at a significantly younger age compared with nonsyndromic meningiomas.

Meningioma is one of the few brain tumors that exhibits a female predominance. Women are almost twice as likely men to develop WHO grade I meningiomas. The F:M ratio varies with age, peaking at 3.5-4:1 in premenopausal women in the 35- to 44-year age group.

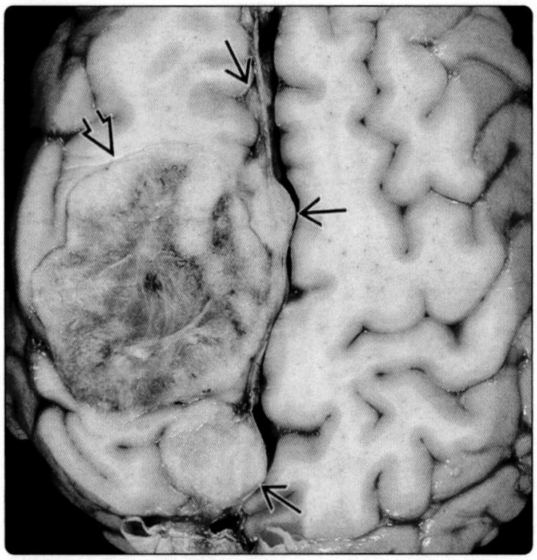

(22-8) Autopsied meningiomatosis shows meningioma invaginating into brain, multiple falcine meningiomas. (R. Hewlett, MD.)

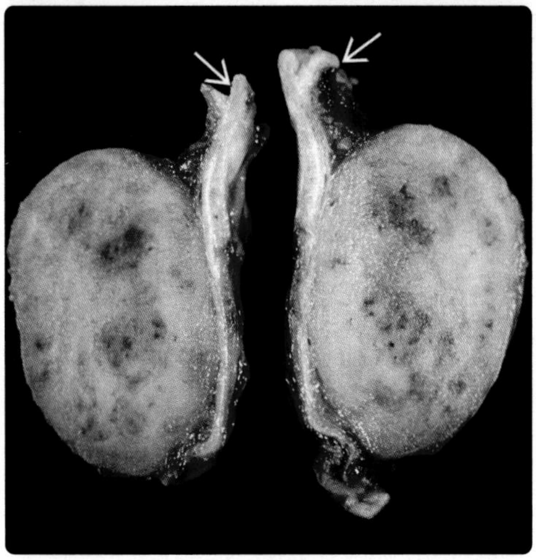

(22-9) Meningioma in cut section shows attachment to dura, reactive dural thickening ("dural tail" sign). (Courtesy R. Hewlett, MD.)

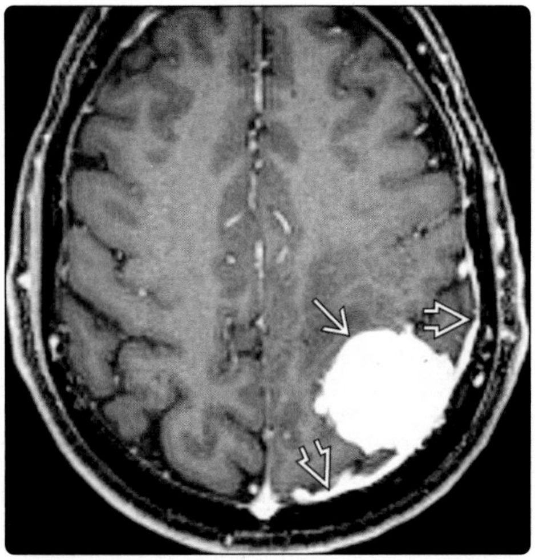

(22-10) Axial T1 C+ shows strongly enhancing typical meningioma. Adjacent dural thickening ("dural tail" sign) is common.

Most WHO grade I meningiomas have progesterone receptors, and progesterone receptor expression is inversely associated with meningioma grade.

Presentation. Symptoms relate to size and tumor site. Less than 10% of meningiomas become symptomatic.

Natural History. Longitudinal studies have demonstrated that most meningiomas under 2.5 cm grow very slowly—if at all—over 5 years. The majority of small, asymptomatic, incidentally discovered meningiomas show minimal growth and are usually followed with serial imaging.

Malignant degeneration of a TM into an atypical or anaplastic meningioma is rare. Extracranial metastases are exceptionally rare, occurring in 1 in 1,000 cases. When they do occur, metastases are generally to the lung or axial skeleton. Metastases from both benign and atypical/malignant meningiomas have been reported.

Treatment Options. A neurosurgeon once stated, "Like the impressions on a finger tip, each meningioma is different." Stratified treatment risk-benefit ratios vary, not just with tumor type and grade, but also with size and location, vascular supply, and presence or absence of a brain/tumor cleavage plane.

Image-guided surgery with resection of symptomatic lesions is generally curative. The major factor associated with meningioma recurrence is subtotal resection.

Recent microexpression data have identified a differentially expressed gene, *DCC* (deleted in colorectal cancer), that may constitute a biomarker associated with benign meningiomas that are at risk for progression.

Stereotactic radiosurgery or chemotherapy with progesterone antagonists may be options in patients with TMs in critical locations such as the cavernous sinus.

MENINGIOMA: CLINICAL ISSUES

Epidemiology
- Most common intracranial primary neoplasm
  - 36% of all primary CNS neoplasms
- Most are asymptomatic
  - Found incidentally at imaging/autopsy (1-3%)
- Solitary (> 90%)
  - Multiple in NF2, meningiomatosis

Demographics
- F:M = 2:1
  - Sex difference greatest prior to menopause
- Median age at diagnosis = 65 years
- Rare in children unless NF2

Natural History
- Grows slowly
- Rarely metastasizes

Imaging

General Features. The general appearance of a TM is a round or lobulated, sharply demarcated, extraaxial dura-based mass that buckles the cortex inward. A discernible CSF-vascular "cleft" is usually present, especially on MR. Parenchymal invasion is uncommon. When present, it indicates atypical meningioma, WHO grade II. Rarely, a meningioma is pedunculated and invaginates into the brain, which may make it difficult to distinguish from an intraaxial primary tumor.

Meningioma-associated cysts are found in 4-7% of cases. These can be intra- or extratumoral. Occasionally pools of CSF are trapped between the tumor and adjacent brain.

CT Findings

NECT. Almost three-quarters of meningiomas are mildly to moderately hyperdense compared with cortex **(22-13)**. About one-quarter are isodense **(22-14A)**. Hypodense meningiomas occur but are uncommon **(22-19A)**. Frank necrosis or hemorrhage is rare.

Peritumoral vasogenic edema, seen as confluent hypodensity in the adjacent brain, is present in about 60% of all cases.

Approximately 25% of TMs demonstrate calcification **(22-11)** **(22-12)**. Focal globular or more diffuse sand-like ("psammomatous") calcifications occur.

Bone CT may show hyperostosis that varies from minimal to striking. Hyperostosis is often but not invariably associated with tumor invasion. Striking enlargement of an adjacent paranasal sinus may occur with skull base meningiomas **(22-17)**. Bone lysis or frank destruction can also occur. Bone involvement by meningioma occurs with both benign and malignant meningiomas and is not predictive of tumor grade.

CECT. The vast majority of meningiomas enhance strongly and uniformly **(22-13)**.

MR Findings

General Features. The majority of meningiomas are isointense with cortex on all sequences. Between 10-25% of cases demonstrate changes suggestive of cyst formation or necrosis although frank hemorrhage is uncommon.

T1WI. Meningiomas are typically iso- to slightly hypointense compared with cortex. Predominant hypointensity on T1WI and hyperintensity on T2WI suggest the microcystic variant of TM **(22-19)**.

T2WI. Most TMs are iso- to moderately hyperintense compared with cortex **(22-21A)**. These are associated with a "soft" consistency at surgery, whereas T2/FLAIR hypointense tumors tend to be "hard" and somewhat gritty. Densely fibrotic and calcified meningiomas (appearing as "brain rocks" on NECT) can be very hypointense.

The CSF-vascular "cleft" **(22-6)** is especially well delineated on T2WI and is seen as a hyperintense rim interposed between the tumor and brain **(22-21A)**. A number of "flow voids" representing displaced vessels are often seen within the "cleft."

Sometimes a "sunburst" pattern that represents the dural vascular supply to the tumor can be identified radiating toward the periphery of the mass **(22-20)**.

FLAIR. Meningioma signal intensity varies from iso- to hyperintense relative to brain. FLAIR is very useful for depicting peritumoral edema, which is found with approximately half of all TMs. Peritumoral edema is related to the presence of pial blood supply and VEGF expression, not tumor size or grade. Some small meningiomas incite striking peritumoral edema, whereas some very large masses exhibit virtually none.

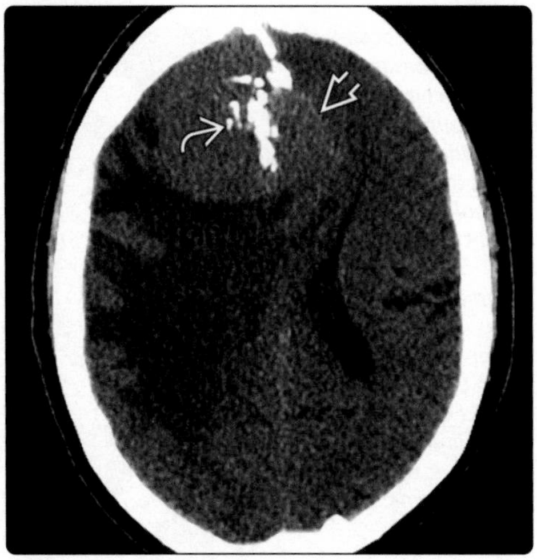

(22-11) Axial NECT in a 67y woman with headaches shows a slightly hyperdense, heavily calcified right frontal mass.

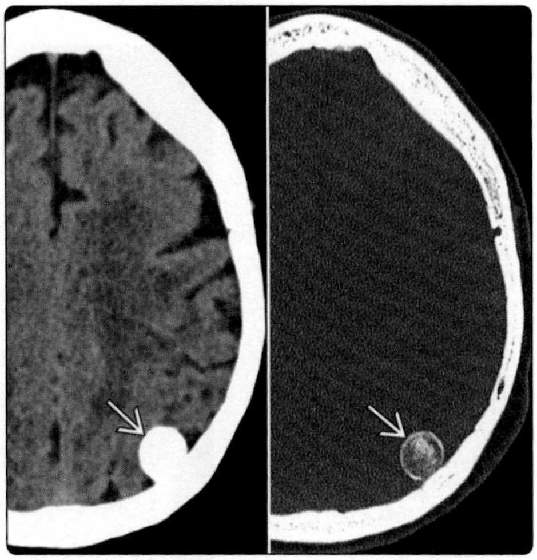

(22-12) NECT in 88y woman with soft tissue (L), bone algorithm (R) shows densely calcified meningioma. This is an incidental finding.

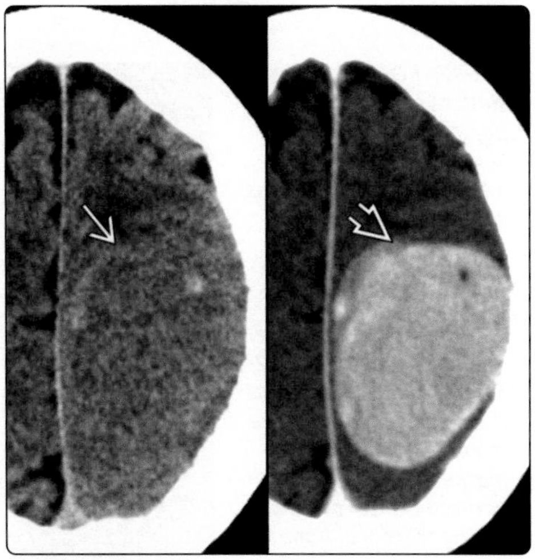

(22-13) NECT (L) and CECT (R) show isodense left convexity mass that enhances uniformly. This is classic meningioma, WHO grade I.

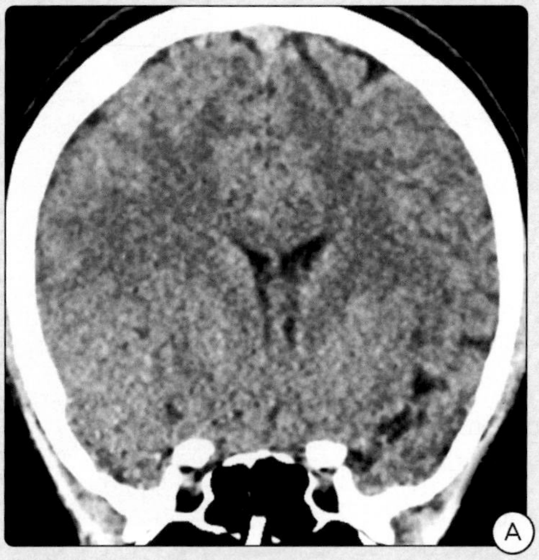
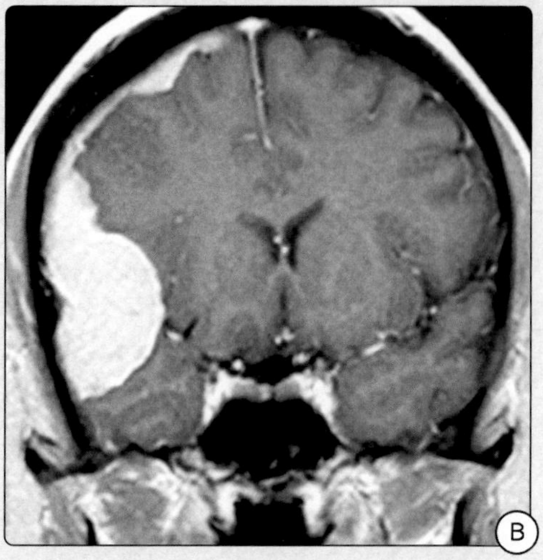

***(22-14A)** Coronal NECT in a 43y woman with headaches shows subtle effacement of the right sylvian fissure with slight left to right subfalcine herniation of the lateral ventricles. **(22-14B)** Coronal T1 C+ MR in the same case shows extensive "en plaque" meningioma. Because they are often isodense with cortex, noncalcified meningiomas can be difficult to detect on NECT scans.*

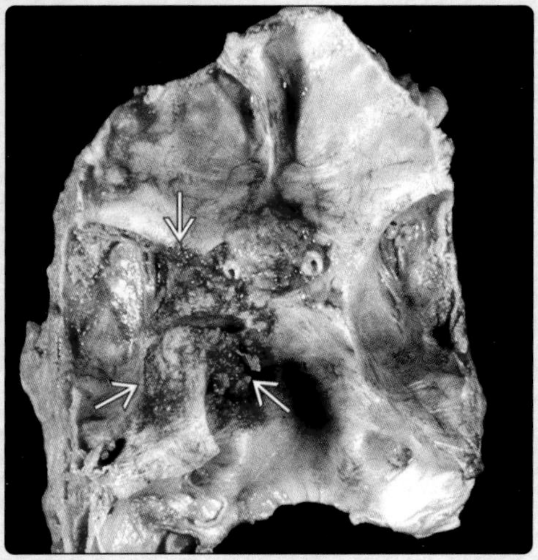
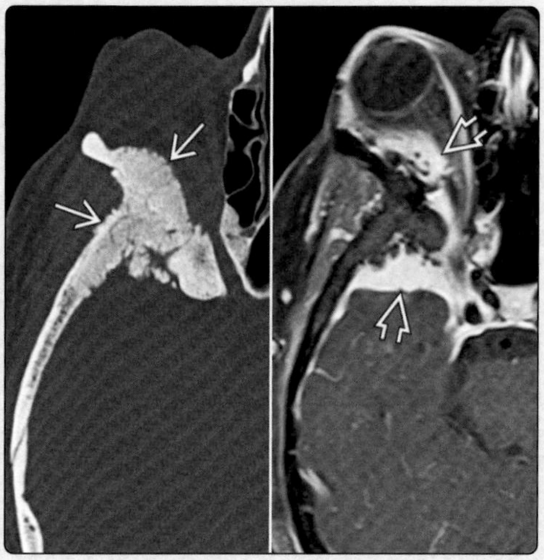

***(22-15)** Autopsy specimen shows an extensive skull base "en plaque" meningioma. Such tumors often affect more than one compartment and infiltrate and thicken bone. The sphenoid wing and orbit are favored sites. (Courtesy R. Hewlett, MD.) **(22-16)** (L) Bone CT shows striking hyperostosis of the sphenoid wing in a middle-aged woman with proptosis. (R) T1 C+ FS shows enhancing "en plaque" meningioma.*

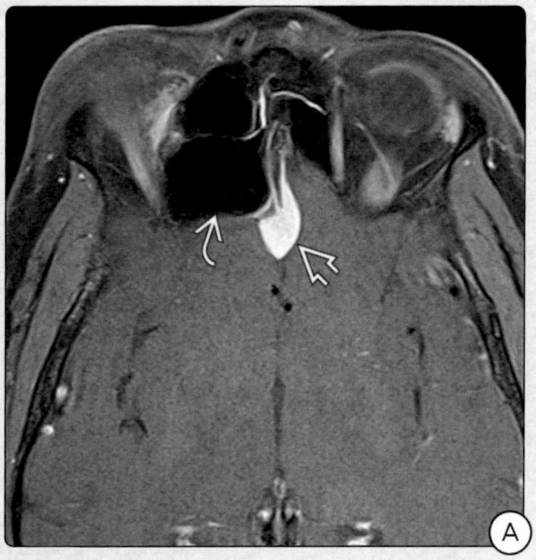
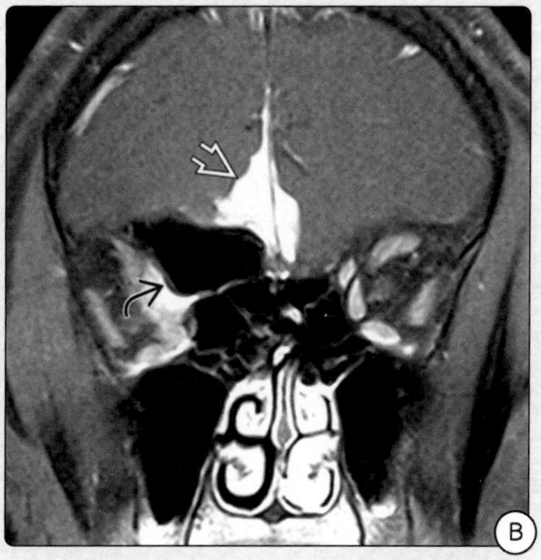

***(22-17A)** Occasionally skull base meningiomas adjacent to a paranasal sinus cause massive enlargement of the sinus, a condition known as pneumosinus dilatans. This relatively small meningioma caused massive enlargement of the frontal sinus. **(22-17B)** Coronal T1 C+ FS in the same case shows the meningioma and markedly enlarged aerated orbital plate of the right frontal bone.*

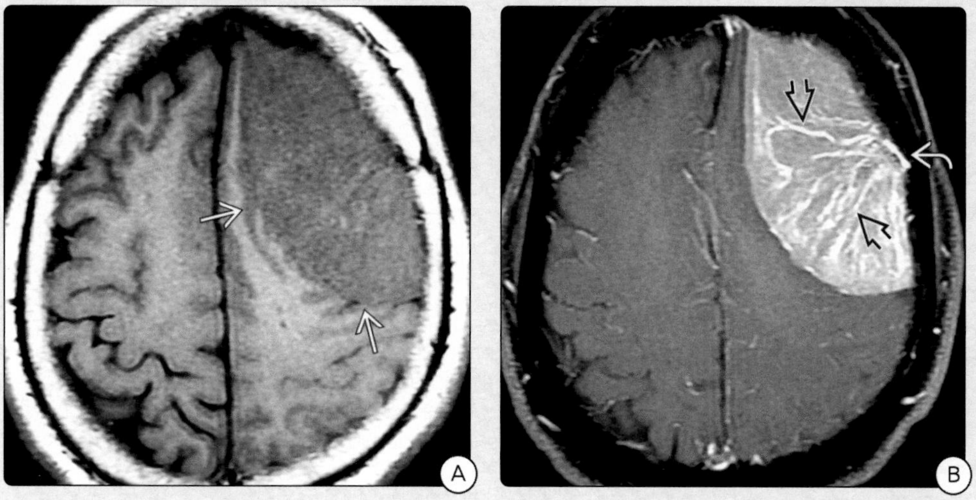

***(22-18A)** Large-convexity meningioma is shown with typical MR findings. The tumor has a flat base toward the dural surface and "buckles" the cortex and GM-WM interface inward ➡. Meningiomas are most commonly isointense with cortex on T1WI. **(22-18B)** T1 C+ FS scan shows that the tumor enhances intensely. Especially well seen is the even more hyperintense "sunburst" of vessels ⇨ that supplies the tumor, radiating outward from the enostotic "spur" ↩.*

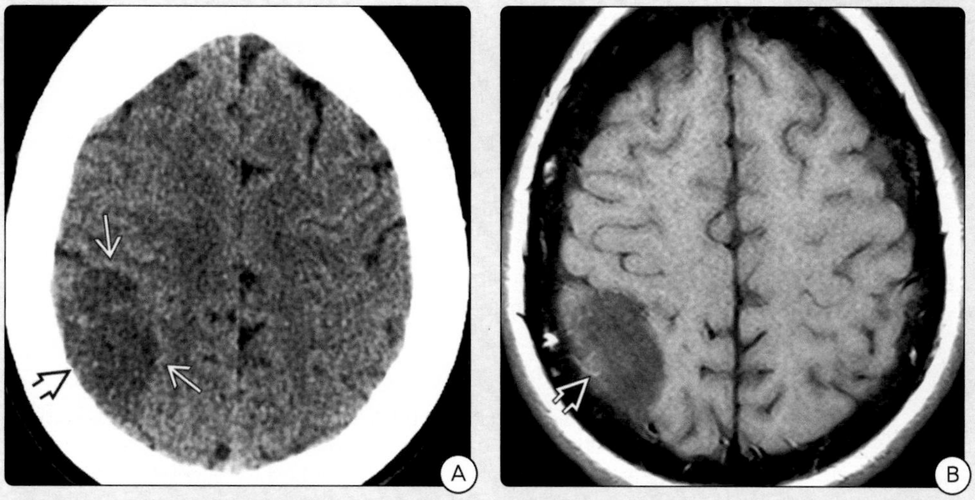

***(22-19A)** Axial NECT in a 48y woman with headaches shows a hypodense right parietal mass ⇨. Note inward displacement of the adjacent cortex ➡, suggesting that the mass is extraaxial. **(22-19B)** T1WI in the same case shows that the mass ⇨ is hypointense relative to the adjacent brain.*

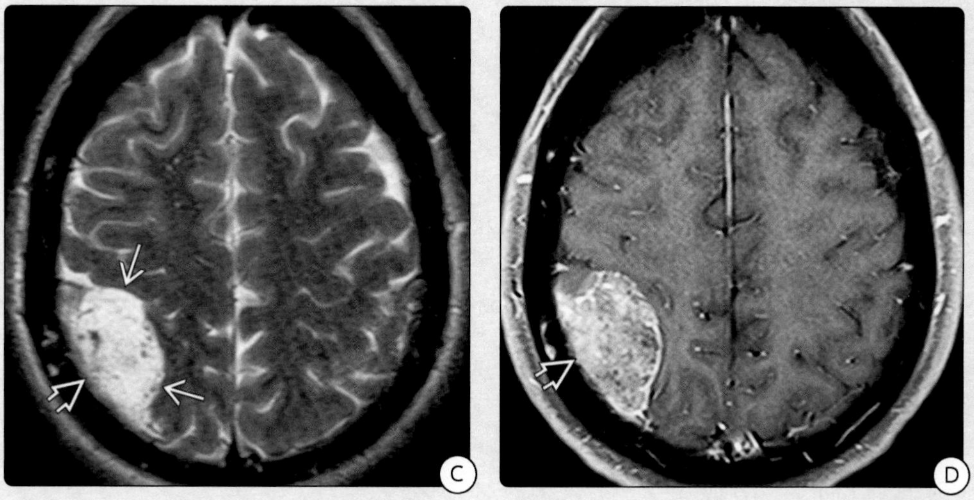

***(22-19C)** T2WI in the same case shows that the mass ⇨ has a broad base toward the dura and is very hyperintense compared with the adjacent brain. The smooth inward "buckling" of the cortex ➡ caused by the mass is striking. **(22-19D)** T1 C+ FS MR shows strong but heterogeneous "bubbly" enhancement of the mass ⇨. This is microcystic meningioma, WHO grade I.*

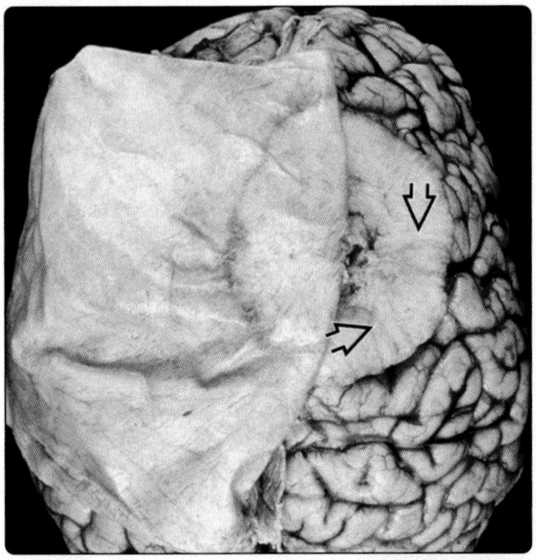

(22-20) Autopsy shows convexity meningioma with dural attachment, "sunburst" of vessels radiating outward . (Courtesy AFIP Archives.)

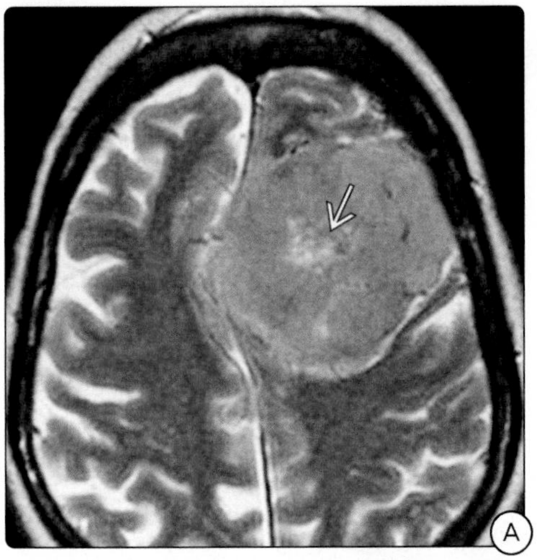

(22-21A) T2WI shows an isointense convexity meningioma. Central hyperintensity is where dural vessels enter the mass (see Figure 22-6).

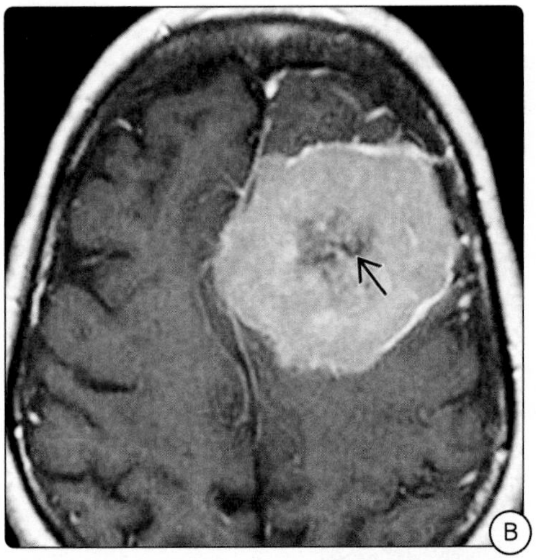

(22-21B) T1 C+ shows that the mass enhances intensely. Note the "flow voids" in the vascular center of the mass .

Pools of CSF trapped in the cleft between tumor and brain (nonneoplastic "peritumoral cysts") are usually proteinaceous and may not suppress completely on FLAIR.

T2* (GRE, SWI). T2* sequences are helpful to depict intratumoral calcification. "Blooming" secondary to intratumoral hemorrhage is rare.

T1 C+. Virtually all meningiomas, including densely calcified "brain rocks" and intraosseous tumors, demonstrate at least some enhancement following contrast administration. Over 95% enhance strongly and homogeneously **(22-14B)**.

A dural "tail" is seen in the majority of meningiomas and varies from a relatively focal area adjacent to the tumor **(22-10)** to dural thickening and enhancement that extends far beyond the site of tumor attachment. The dural "tail" often enhances more intensely and more uniformly than the tumor itself. A "dural tail" sign is not pathognomonic of meningioma.

Most of the enhancing dural "tail" represents benign, reactive dural thickening. Tumor extending 1 cm beyond the base of the tumor is rare.

Nonenhancing *intratumoral* cysts are seen in 5% of cases. Nonneoplastic *peritumoral* cysts do not enhance. Enhancement around the rim of a cyst suggests the presence of marginal tumor in the cyst wall, so complete cyst resection is recommended if technically feasible.

DWI. Most meningiomas do not restrict on DWI.

Perfusion MR. Perfusion MR may be helpful in distinguishing TM from atypical/malignant meningiomas. High rCBV in the lesion or in the surrounding edema suggests a more aggressive tumor grade.

MRS. Alanine (Ala, peak at 1.48 ppm) is often elevated in meningioma although glutamate-glutamine (Glx, peak at 2.1-2.6 ppm) and glutathione (GSH, peak at 2.95 ppm) may be more specific potential markers.

Angiography

CTA, MRA/MRV. CTA is very helpful in detecting dural venous sinus invasion or occlusion. Although it may be helpful in depicting the general status of the vascular supply to a meningioma, DSA is best for detailed delineation of tumor vascularity prior to embolization or surgery. Tumor invasion of major dural venous sinuses is especially well depicted on MRV.

DSA. The classic angiographic appearance of a meningioma is a radial "sunburst" of vessels extending from the base of the tumor toward its periphery. Dural vessels supply the core or center of the lesion, radiating outward from the vascular pedicle of the tumor **(22-22A)**. Pial vessels from internal carotid artery branches may become "parasitized" and supply the periphery of the mass **(22-22C)**.

A prolonged vascular "blush" that persists late into the venous phase is typical. In some cases, arteriovenous shunting with the appearance of "early draining" veins occurs **(22-22B)**. Careful examination of the venous phase should be conducted to detect dural sinus invasion or occlusion.

Preoperative embolization with tumor devascularization may substantially reduce operative time and blood loss. Careful delineation of tumor blood supply, including "dangerous" extra- to intracranial anastomoses, is essential to procedure success.

MENINGIOMA: IMAGING

General
- Round or flat ("en plaque"), dura-based
- Extraaxial mass with "cleft" between tumor, brain

CT
- Hyperdense (70-75%)
- Calcified (20-25%)
- Cysts (peri- or intratumoral) (10-15%)
- Hemorrhage rare
- > 90% enhance

MR
- Usually isointense with gray matter
- CSF-vascular "cleft"
- ± Vascular "flow voids"
- Strong, often heterogeneous enhancement (> 98%)
- Dural "tail" (60%)

Angiography
- "Sunburst" vascularity
- Dural arteries to outside, pial to inside
- Prolonged, dense vascular "blush"

Differential Diagnosis

The major differential diagnosis of typical meningioma is **atypical** or **malignant meningioma**. Although there are no pathognomonic imaging features that reliably distinguish TM from these more aggressive variants, TMs are statistically far more common. Malignant meningiomas typically invade the brain and may exhibit a "mushrooming" configuration (see below).

Dural metastasis, usually from a breast or lung primary, may be virtually indistinguishable from meningioma on imaging studies.

Other meningioma mimics include **granuloma** (TB, sarcoid) and focal **idiopathic hypertrophic pachymeningitis**. Solitary dural granulomas are rare. Idiopathic hypertrophic pachymeningitis is uncommon. Most cases are found in or around the skull base, particularly the orbit, cavernous sinus, and posterior fossa (clivus/cerebellopontine angle). Idiopathic hypertrophic pachymeningitis can invade bone and may be virtually indistinguishable from "en plaque" meningioma.

Rare entities that can closely resemble meningioma include hemangioma and solitary fibrous tumor/hemangiopericytoma. A **hemangioma of the dura** or **venous sinuses** is a true vasoformative neoplasm that can resemble meningioma. Most hemangiomas are very hyperintense on T2WI, whereas most meningiomas are iso- to mildly hyperintense. Delayed slow centripetal "filling in" of the mass on dynamic contrast-enhanced MR is suggestive of hemangioma.

Intracranial solitary fibrous tumor/hemangiopericytoma is relatively rare. Most are found adjacent to the dura, venous sinuses, or choroid plexus. Solitary fibrous tumor may be indistinguishable on imaging studies from typical meningioma.

Extramedullary hematopoiesis (EMH) can present as confluent or multifocal dura-based disease resembling "en plaque" solitary or multiple meningiomatosis. EMH occurs in the setting of chronic anemia or marrow depletion disorders.

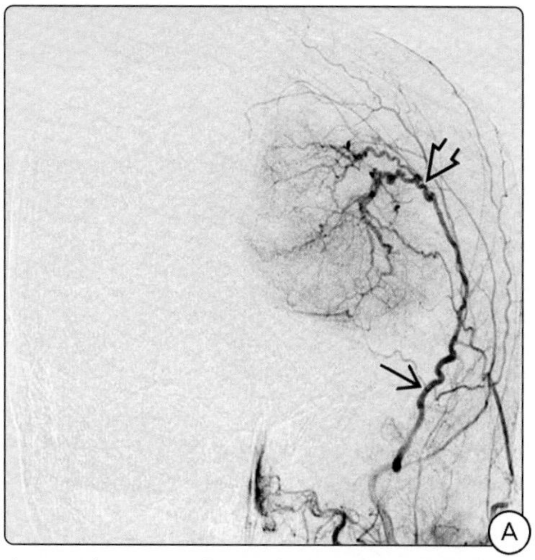

***(22-22A)** AP DSA of ECA shows enlarged middle meningeal artery with "sunburst" of vessels supplying meningioma.*

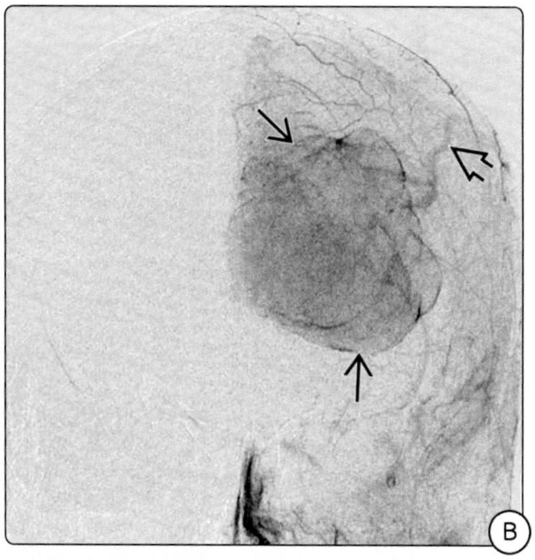

***(22-22B)** Later phase of ECA DSA shows prolonged vascular "blush" characteristic of meningioma. "Early draining" vein is seen.*

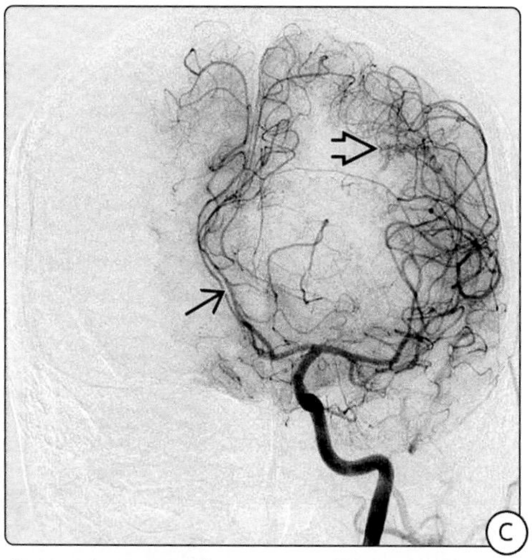

***(22-22C)** ICA DSA shows mass effect with the ACA shifted. Only minimal supply to periphery of tumor is coming from pial MCA branches.*

MENINGIOMA MIMICS

Common
- Metastasis
  - Most common = breast, lung, colon, prostate
- Lymphoma

Less Common
- Granuloma
  - TB, sarcoid most common
  - Other (less common) = plasma cell granuloma, Rosai-Dorfman disease

Rare But Important
- IgG4-related disease
- Dural/venous sinus hemangioma
- Solitary fibrous tumor/hemangiopericytoma
- Gliosarcoma, other sarcoma (e.g., Ewing)
- Extramedullary hematopoiesis

Atypical Meningioma

Terminology

Atypical meningioma (AM) is intermediate in grade between benign and malignant forms and is defined histopathologically (see below).

Etiology

There is a significant correlation between the number of inactivating *NF2* mutations and tumor grade. Almost 60% of AMs show gain of chromosome arm 1q.

Pathology

Location. Most atypical and malignant meningiomas arise from the calvaria. The skull base is a relatively uncommon location for these more aggressive lesions.

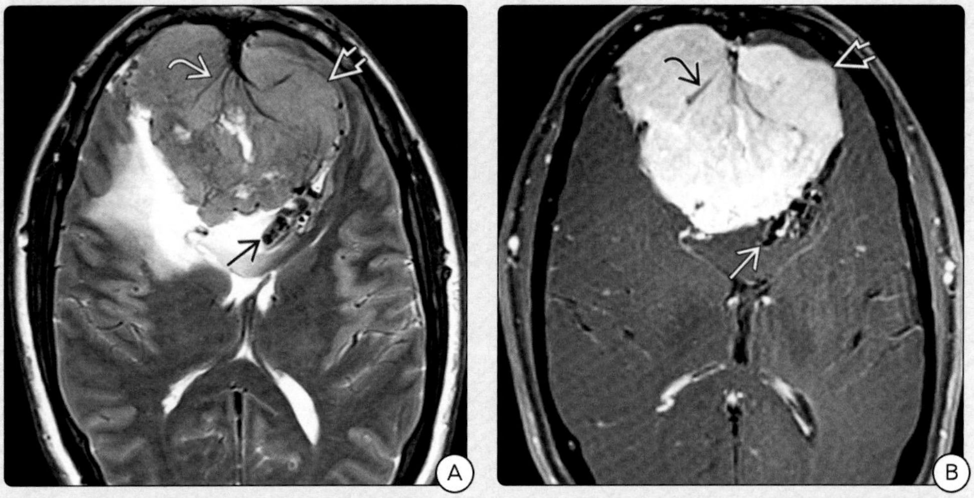

***(22-23A)** Axial T2WI in a 43y man shows a lobulated bifrontal mass that is mostly isointense with cortex. Note prominent "sunburst" vessels within the mass and in the CSF-vascular "cleft". **(22-23B)** T1 C+ FS in the same case shows that the well-delineated mass enhances intensely, mostly uniformly. Note prominent "flow voids" within the tumor as well as the in the CSF-vascular cleft.*

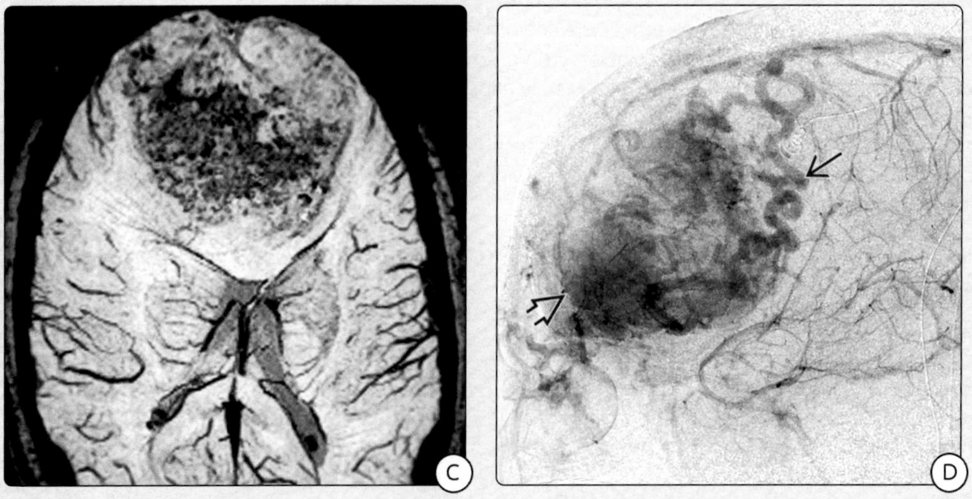

***(22-23C)** Axial MIP of T2* SWI MR shows that the tumor is remarkably vascular, filled with innumerable enlarged vessels with slow flow causing the susceptibility artifact. **(22-23D)** Venous phase of lateral DSA in the same case shows an intense, prolonged vascular tumor "stain". Note multiple enlarged, tortuous draining veins around the mass. Clear cell meningioma, WHO grade II, was found at surgery.*

Gross Pathology. Approximately half of all atypical meningiomas invade the adjacent brain. In such cases, there is no intervening layer of leptomeninges between the invading tumor and underlying parenchyma.

Microscopic Features. The 2016 WHO now recognizes brain invasion together with a mitotic count of four or more mitoses per high-power field as sufficient criteria for diagnosing atypical meningioma. Clusters or irregular finger-like protrusions of tumor cells infiltrating the underlying parenchyma are present. Brain invasion is also strongly correlated with the presence of other histopathologic criteria of atypia (see below).

Atypical meningioma can also be diagnosed on the presence of three or more of the following histologic features: foci of spontaneous necrosis, sheeting (loss of whorling or fascicular architecture with a patternless or sheet-like growth), prominent nucleoli, high cellularity, and small cells (tumor clusters with high nuclear:cytoplasmic ratio).

Some meningioma subtypes are classified as WHO grade II tumors simply because of their greater likelihood of recurrence and/or more aggressive behavior. These include the **chordoid** and **clear cell** meningioma subtypes.

All atypical meningiomas are WHO grade II neoplasms.

Clinical Issues

Epidemiology. AMs represent 10-15% of all meningiomas.

Demographics. AMs tend to occur in slightly younger patients compared with TMs. Pediatric meningiomas tend to be more aggressive. In contrast with TMs, AMs display a slight male predominance.

A new autosomal-dominant tumor predisposition syndrome with heterozygous loss-of-function germline mutations in the *SMARCE1* tumor suppressor gene causes spinal and intracranial clear cell meningiomas. Symptomatic male

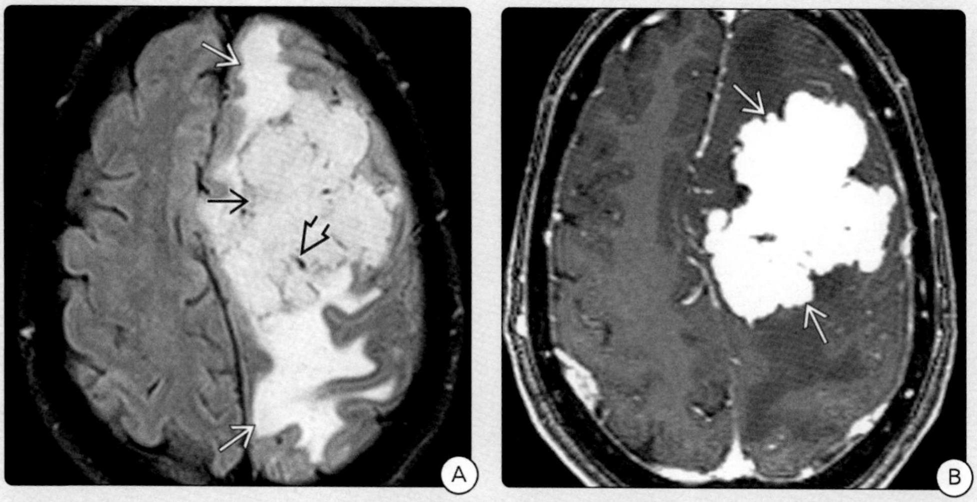

***(22-24A)** FLAIR scan in a 68y woman with right-sided weakness shows a hyperintense, lobulated convexity mass ➡ with numerous "flow voids" ➡, edema ➡. **(22-24B)** T1 C+ FS demonstrates that the mass ➡ enhances intensely and uniformly. Coronal T1 C+ (not shown) demonstrated that the mass was attached to the dura and exhibited a "dural tail" sign.*

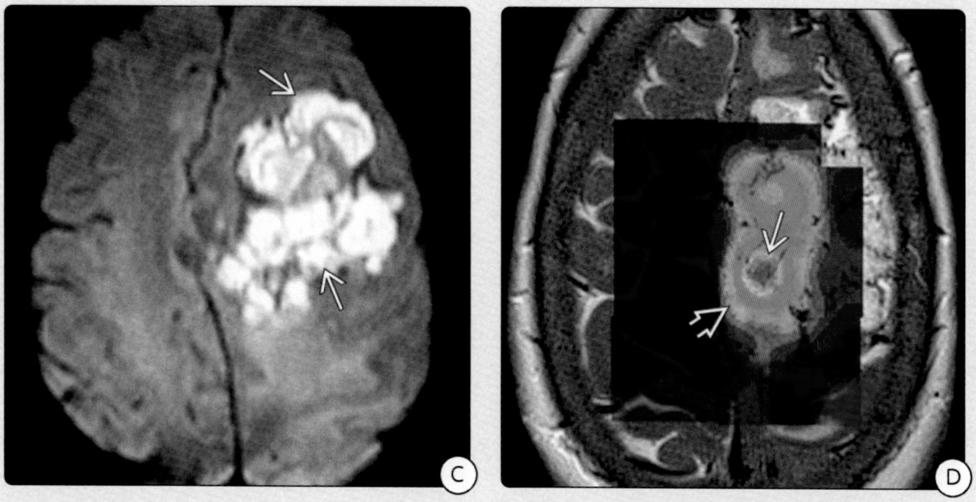

***(22-24C)** The mass ➡ shows restricted diffusion, consistent with high cellularity. **(22-24D)** MRS shows markedly elevated Cho, decreased NAA. Choline map shows the elevated Cho ➡ with the highest levels in the center of the lesion ➡. This is atypical meningioma, clear cell type, WHO grade II. (Courtesy M. Thurnher, MD.)*

patients develop tumors in childhood, whereas carrier female patients develop tumors in adolescence or early adulthood.

Natural History. AMs are generally associated with a higher recurrence rate (25-30%) and shorter recurrence-free survival compared with TMs. The Simpson and modified Shinsu grading systems are the best predictors of recurrence after resection. Grade I represents macroscopically complete tumor removal including excision of its dural attachment and any abnormal bone. Grades II-IV represent progressively less complete resection, and grade V is simple decompression, with or without biopsy.

Imaging

General Features. A good general rule is that it is difficult—if not impossible—to predict meningioma grade on the basis of imaging findings **(22-29)**. However, because brain invasion is a frequent (but not always visible) feature of AMs, the CSF-vascular "cleft" typically seen in TMs is often compromised or absent.

CT Findings. AMs are usually hyperdense with irregular margins. Minimal or no calcification is seen, and frank bone invasion with osteolysis is common. Tumor may invade through the skull into the scalp.

MR Findings. Tumor margins are usually indistinct with no border between the tumor and the underlying cortex. A CSF-vascular "cleft" is often absent or partially effaced. Peritumoral edema and cyst formation are common but nonspecific findings **(22-23)**. Contrast enhancement is strong but often quite heterogeneous.

ADC is significantly lower in atypical and malignant meningiomas compared with TMs. Perfusion MR may show elevated rCBV, especially in the peritumoral edema **(22-24)**. MRS often shows elevated alanine.

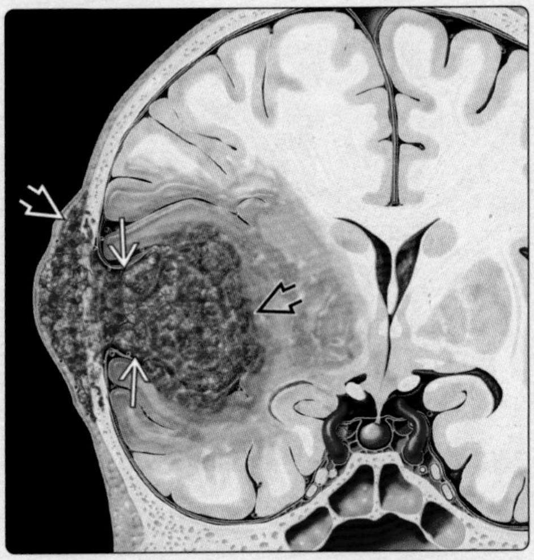
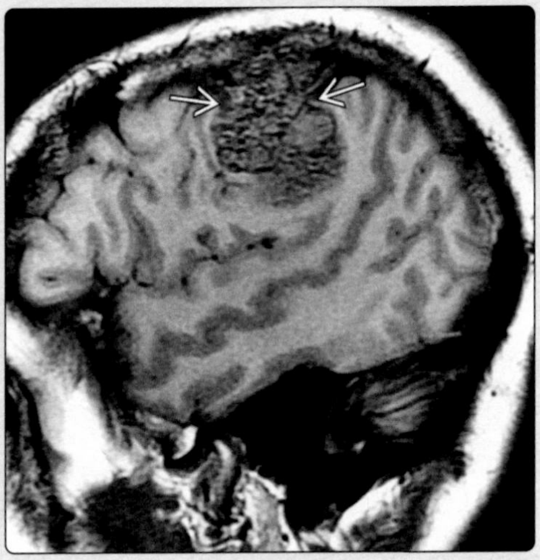

(22-25) Graphic shows malignant meningioma invading brain ➾ without CSF-vascular "cleft." The tumor also penetrates dura, invades calvarium, has a significant extracranial component ➾. Note "mushroom" configuration ➡, which may suggest more aggressive meningioma. (22-26) Sagittal T1WI in a 50y man with left-sided weakness shows mixed iso-/hypointense extraaxial mass "mushrooming" ➡ into brain.

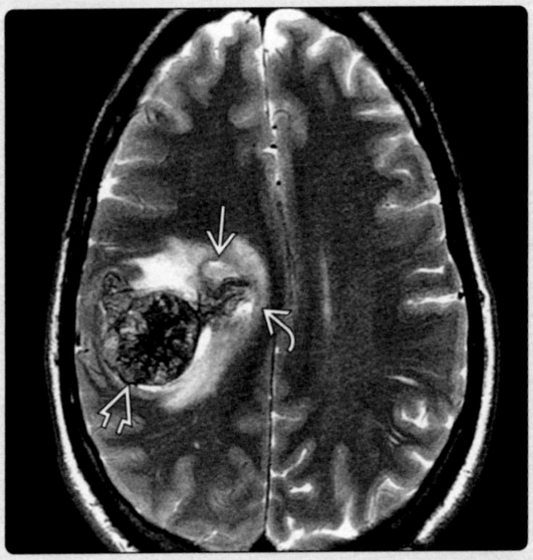
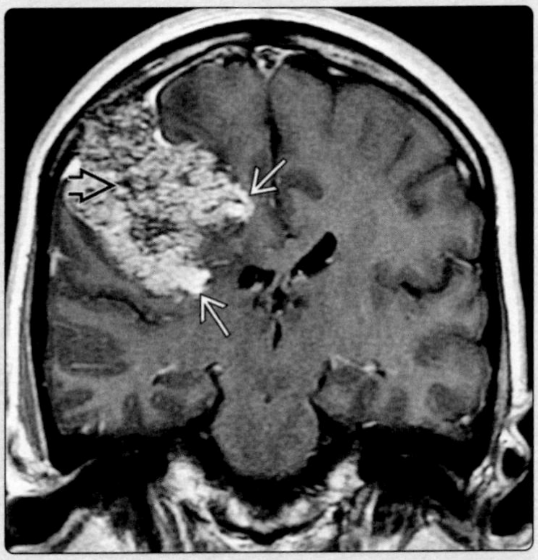

(22-27) Axial T2WI shows the very heterogeneous signal of the lesion ➾, "mushroom" of focal brain invasion ➡ with adjacent edema ➾. (22-28) Coronal T1 C+ MR shows that an intensely enhancing lesion contains numerous "flow voids" ➾ and invades adjacent brain ➡. This is papillary meningioma, WHO grade III.

Differential Diagnosis

Because it is difficult to determine meningioma tumor grade on the basis of imaging findings alone, the major differential diagnosis of AM is **typical meningioma. Dural metastasis** and **malignant meningioma** can also be indistinguishable from AM. **Sarcomas**, such as gliosarcoma in older patients and Ewing and osteogenic sarcoma in young patients, may also be difficult to distinguish from biologically aggressive meningiomas.

Anaplastic Meningioma

Terminology

Anaplastic meningioma—also called malignant meningioma—exhibits overtly malignant cytology and/or markedly elevated mitotic activity.

Etiology

Chromosomal mutations are increased compared with AMs. Several genes have been associated with malignant progression in meningioma. Homozygous deletions or mutations of the tumor suppressor genes *CDKN2A* (ARF) and *CDKN2B* are found in most anaplastic meningiomas. A new meningioma-associated tumor suppressor gene *NDRG2* is downregulated in anaplastic meningioma and atypical meningiomas with aggressive clinical behavior.

Pathology

Most anaplastic meningiomas invade the brain and exhibit histologic features of frank malignancy **(22-25)**. These include increased cellular atypia with bizarre nuclei and markedly elevated mitotic index (more than 20 mitoses per 10 high-power fields). Malignant meningioma subtypes include

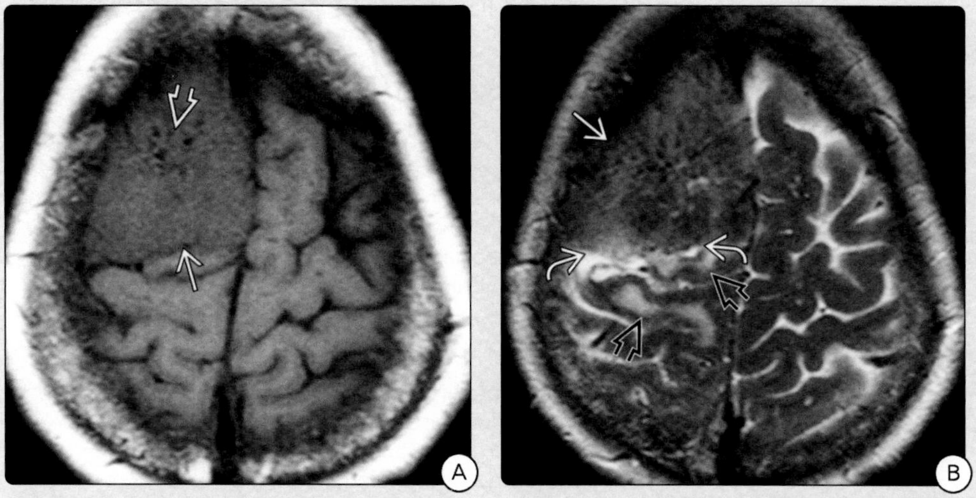

***(22-29A)** Axial T1WI in a 68y woman with headaches shows a right frontal mass that is isointense with cortex and exhibits a central cluster of "flow voids". **(22-29B)** Axial T2WI in the same case shows that the mass appears mildly hypointense and has a relatively well-demarcated CSF-vascular "cleft" between the mass and adjacent brain. Mild edema is present in the WM of the adjacent gyri.*

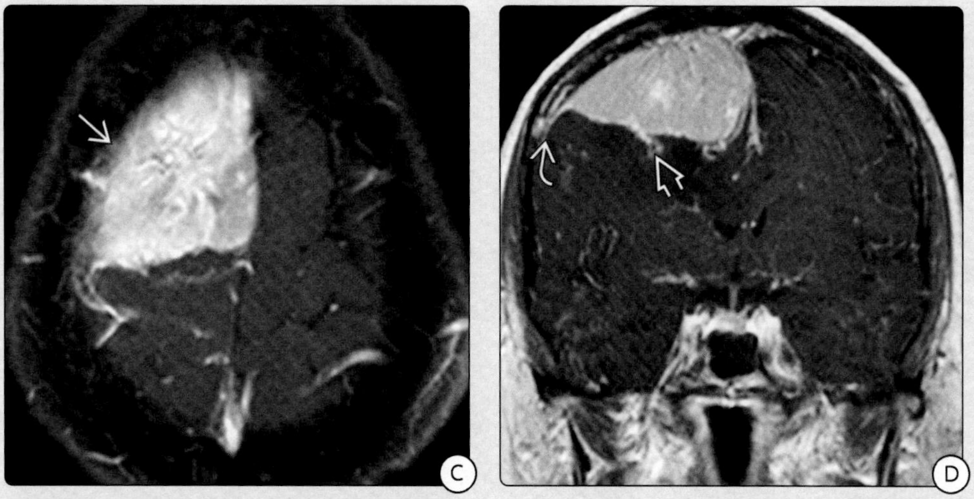

***(22-29C)** Axial T1 C+ FS shows that the mass enhances intensely, relatively uniformly. **(22-29D)** Coronal T1 C+ shows that the intensely enhancing mass has a relatively inconspicuous associated dural "tail". There is a small area of enhancement in the adjacent brain, suggesting focal parenchymal invasion. This is WHO grade III malignant meningioma.*

papillary and **rhabdoid** meningiomas as well as meningiomas of any histologic subtype with a high proliferation index.

Anaplastic meningioma corresponds histologically to WHO grade III.

Clinical Issues

Epidemiology. Frankly malignant meningiomas are rare, representing only 1-3% of all meningiomas. Malignant meningiomas have a striking male predominance.

Natural History. Prognosis is poor. Recurrence rates following tumor resection range from 50-95%. Survival times range from 2-5 years and vary depending on resection extent.

Imaging

General Features. The imaging triad of extracranial mass, osteolysis, and "mushrooming" intracranial tumor is present in most—but not all—cases of anaplastic meningioma. Calcification is rare, and contrast enhancement is typically heterogeneous.

Differential Diagnosis

The main differential diagnosis of anaplastic meningioma is **metastasis. Atypical meningioma** can be indistinguishable from malignant meningioma on imaging studies alone, as brain invasion occurs in both.

Solitary fibrous tumor/hemangiopericytoma, gliosarcoma, and **sarcomas** such as meningeal fibrosarcoma can all mimic anaplastic meningioma.

Nonmeningothelial Mesenchymal Tumors

CNS nonmeningothelial mesenchymal neoplasms correspond to soft tissue or bone tumors found elsewhere in the body. They can be tumors of adipose, fibrous, histiocytic, cartilaginous, or vascular tissues and can also arise from muscle or bone. Both benign and malignant varieties of each type occur, ranging from benign (WHO grade I) to highly malignant (WHO grade IV) sarcomatous neoplasms.

Nonmeningothelial mesenchymal tumors rarely involve the CNS. When they do, they are usually extraaxial lesions. We discuss these tumors in two groups, benign and malignant neoplasms.

Benign Mesenchymal Tumors

Terminology

Benign mesenchymal tumors (BMTs) correspond in name and histology to their extracranial counterparts. Osteocartilaginous tumors such as chondroma, osteochondroma, and osteoma are the most common BMTs that occur within the CNS. Pure fibrous tumors such as fibromatosis and solitary fibrous tumor are rare, as are mixed fibrohistiocytic tumors such as benign fibrous histiocytoma (also termed fibrous xanthoma).

Etiology

Intracranial BMTs usually originate from the meninges (typically the dura), choroid plexus, or skull base. The cranial meninges contain primitive pluripotential mesenchymal cells that can give rise to a broad spectrum of nonmeningothelial mesenchymal tumors. Most are supratentorial; the falx is the most common site.

The skull base and clivus develop by enchondral ossification. **Chondromas** and **enchondromas** usually arise from cartilaginous synchondroses in the skull base. Therefore, the central skull base, especially the sella/parasellar region, is the most common site. Less commonly, chondromas can arise from the dura or falx. **Osteochondromas** also typically arise in or near the skull base.

In contrast to the skull base, the calvarial vault develops by membranous ossification. **Osteomas** are benign tumors that arise from membranous bone. In the head, the paranasal sinuses and calvaria are the most common sites.

Pathology

The macro- and microscopic appearance of BMTs depends on their cell type and is similar to their extracranial soft tissue counterparts. For example, **chondromas** and **enchondromas** are sharply demarcated "bosselated" tumors that generally have a broad flat base and grossly resemble cartilage. **Osteochondromas** appear as a sessile or pedunculated cartilage-capped bony exostosis. **Osteomas** resemble dense lamellar bone.

Solitary fibrous tumors (SFTs) can arise anywhere but are generally dura based. SFTs and hemangiopericytoma are now considered to constitute a continuous pathologic spectrum and are discussed separately below.

BMTs are all WHO grade I neoplasms.

Clinical Issues

Epidemiology. With the exception of hemangiomas and lipomas, cranial mesenchymal nonmeningothelial tumors are all rare. Together, these BMTs account for less than 1% of all intracranial neoplasms. Overall, **chondroma/enchondroma** is the most common benign osteocartilaginous tumor of the skull base. **Osteoma** is the most common benign osseous tumor of the calvaria.

Most BMTs occur as solitary nonsyndromic lesions. Multiple BMTs generally occur as part of inherited tumor syndromes. Multiple osteomas occur as part of **Gardner syndrome** (together with skin tumors and colon polyps). Multiple enchondromas or "enchondromatosis" are part of **Ollier disease**. Enchondromas associated with soft tissue hemangiomas are found in **Maffucci syndrome**.

Demographics. BMTs can occur at any age. The peak age for chondroma is the second to fourth decades. Osteomas are more common in middle-aged patients. In general, there is no sex predilection.

Presentation. Most BMTs are asymptomatic and discovered incidentally. Others such as osteomas may present as a longstanding skull "bump." Occasionally large BMTs, especially those arising within or near the skull base, cause cranial nerve palsies.

Natural History. Most BMTs can be completely resected and have a favorable prognosis. Malignant degeneration is generally rare. Multiple osteochondromas ("osteochondromatosis") have a higher propensity to undergo malignant transformation. The risk increases as the number and size of the lesions increase.

Treatment Options. Unless cosmetically deforming, small BMTs such as osteomas are generally of no clinical significance and are left alone. The treatment for symptomatic BMTs is complete surgical resection.

Imaging

General Features. Imaging findings vary with tumor type. Most BMTs are benign-appearing nonaggressive masses of the scalp, skull, or dura that resemble their counterparts found elsewhere in the body.

CT Findings. Chondroma/enchondromas of the skull base are sessile, smoothly lobulated, expansile masses that contain curvilinear matrix calcifications and sometimes mature bone **(22-30)**. Slight enhancement on CECT may occur.

Osteochondromas are sessile or pedunculated bony masses that are contiguous with and project from their underlying bone of origin. Osteochondromas may exhibit a "cap" of matrix with speckled calcification that enhances mildly following contrast administration.

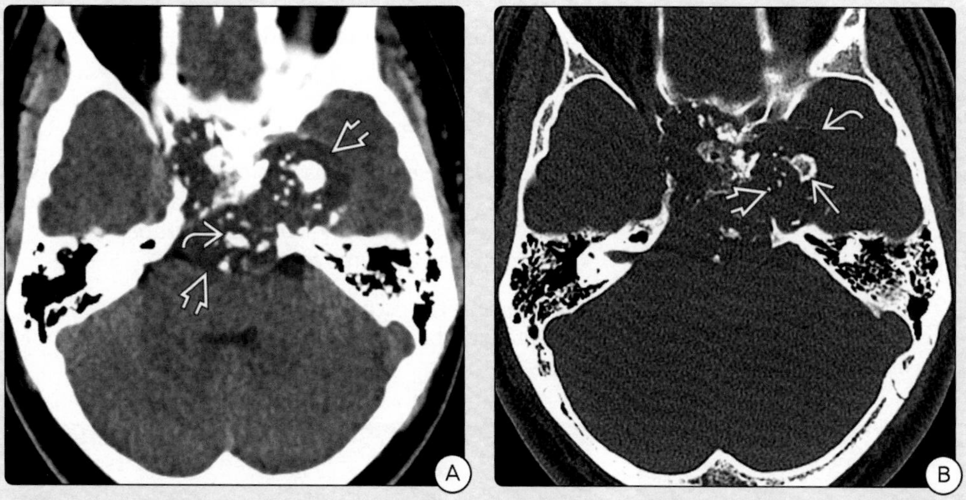

***(22-30A)** NECT in a 21y man with blurred vision shows a hypodense central skull base mass with numerous matrix calcifications. **(22-30B)** Bone CT in the same case shows erosion of the central skull base and anterior clinoid processes by the mass. Note matrix mineralization, calcified arcs, and dysplastic cortical bone within the mass.*

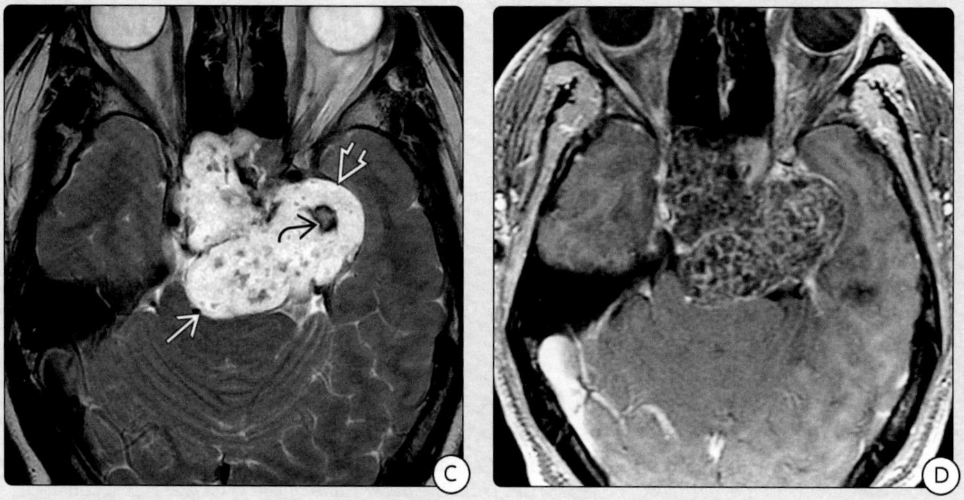

***(22-30C)** Axial T2FS MR in the same case shows that the lobulated mass is well delineated and extremely hyperintense and compresses/displaces the pons posteriorly. Dysplastic cortical bone within the mass is well seen. **(22-30D)** T1 C+ FS shows a "bubbly" enhancement pattern within the mass. Pathology showed enchondroma with foci of chondrosarcoma arising within the mass.*

Osteomas are seen as dense masses of well-demarcated mature lamellar bone. They occur in paranasal sinuses—the most common site—or the calvarium **(22-31)**.

MR Findings. All BMTs are typically well-delineated, noninvasive-appearing masses with variable signal intensity on both T1- and T2WI. A "ring and arc" pattern of contrast enhancement can be seen with chondromas. BMTs generally do not incite dural reaction, so a "dural tail" sign is absent.

Hemangioma

Terminology

Hemangiomas are benign nonmeningothelial mesenchymal tumors. They are common vascular neoplasms that closely resemble normal vessels and are found in all organs of the body **(22-32)**. Hemangiomas are completely different from—and should not be confused with—cavernous angiomas, which are vascular malformations rather than neoplasms.

Etiology

Hemangiomas probably arise by endothelial hyperplasia and hamartomatous-like proliferation.

Pathology

Location. Intracranial hemangiomas can be located in different cranial compartments but are almost always extraaxial. They are found in the calvarium **(22-33)**, dural venous sinuses, and dura.

Size and Number. Hemangiomas vary in size from microscopic to massive. Transspatial extension across different anatomic compartments (e.g., scalp and skull, soft tissues, orbit, and cavernous sinus) is common. Multicentric lesions are uncommon in the CNS.

Gross Pathology. Hemangiomas are nonencapsulated, vascular-appearing, reddish-brown lesions. When they involve the calvaria, radiating spicules of lamellar bone are interspersed with vascular channels of varying sizes **(22-33)**. Hemangiomas of the venous sinuses and dura do not contain bone but otherwise resemble calvarial hemangiomas, consisting of large vascular channels in a soft, compressible mass.

Microscopic Features. Hemangiomas are classified on the basis of their dominant vessels and can be capillary, cavernous, or mixed lesions. Most intracranial hemangiomas are cavernous and contain large, endothelium-lined spaces separated by fibrous septa. True intracranial capillary hemangiomas are very rare and consist of smaller vessels without fibrous septa.

Staging, Grading, and Classification. Hemangiomas are WHO grade I neoplasms.

Clinical Issues

Demographics. Hemangiomas represent only about 1% of all bone tumors. Most are found in the spine; the diploic space of the calvaria is the most common intracranial site. Dural and venous sinus hemangiomas are rare.

Hemangiomas can occur at any age although the peak presentation is between the fourth and fifth decades. The M:F ratio is 1:2-4.

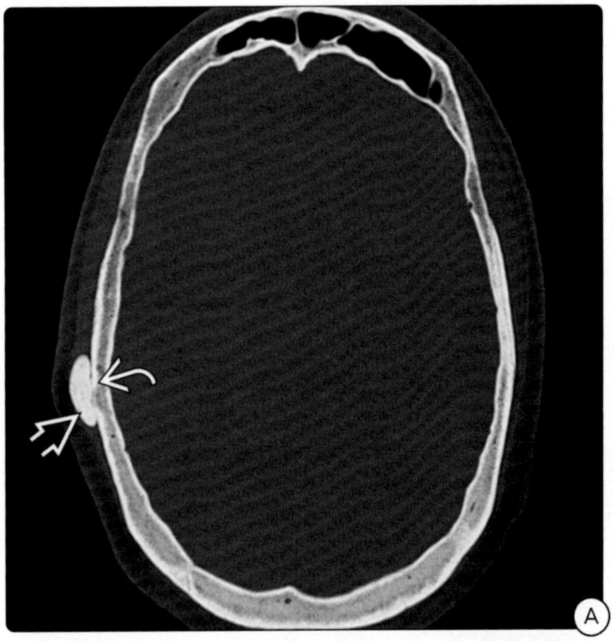

(22-31A) Axial bone CT of a 42y woman with a longstanding "lump" on her head shows a smooth, well-delineated hyperdense mass that can clearly be seen to arise directly from the cortex of the calvarium.

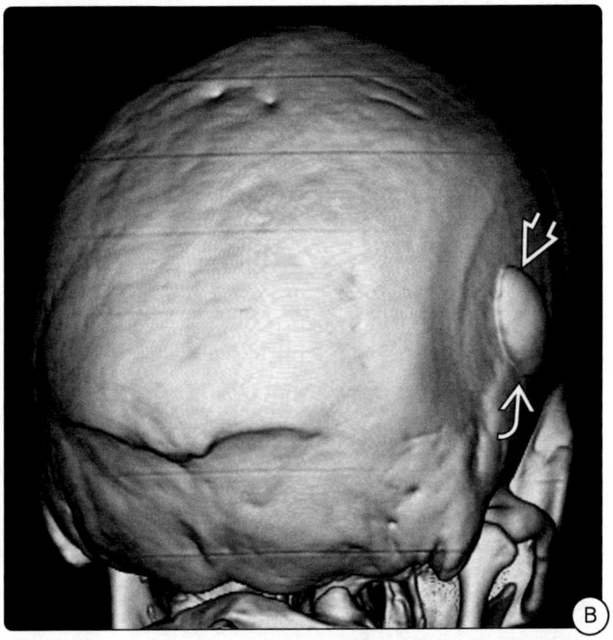

(22-31B) 3D shaded surface rendering shows that the bony mass arises from the outer table of the skull. This is calvarial osteoma.

Presentation. Most calvarial hemangiomas are asymptomatic, limited to the diploic space, and do not extend beyond the inner and outer tables **(22-34)**. Large lesions may present as painless firm masses. Scalp hemangiomas presenting with Kasabach-Merritt syndrome (consumptive coagulopathy due to sequestration and destruction of clotting factors within the lesion) have been reported.

Cavernous sinus hemangiomas can be asymptomatic but often present with headache, diplopia, or other cranial neuropathies such as anisocoria.

Intracranial hemangiomas occasionally occur as part of **POEMS** syndrome, a rare multisystem disease with typical features of **p**olyneuropathy, **o**rganomegaly, **e**ndocrinopathy, **m**onoclonal plasma-proliferative disorders, and **s**kin changes.

Natural History. Hemangiomas typically grow very slowly and do not undergo malignant degeneration. Pregnancy or hormone administration may trigger enlargement.

Capillary hemangiomas of infancy (usually in the skin, scalp, orbit, or oral mucosa and only rarely involving the brain) appear within a few months of birth, grow rapidly, plateau, and then involute.

Treatment Options. Calvarial hemangiomas are typically left alone unless tumor growth is demonstrated. The treatment of venous sinus hemangiomas is much more problematic. These highly vascular lesions bleed easily, and surgical mortality is high. Radiation (gamma knife surgery) has been used with some success in a few reported cases and may become the primary treatment choice for hemangiomas in critical locations such as the cavernous sinus.

Imaging

CT Findings. A calvarial hemangioma is seen as a sharply marginated, expansile diploic mass on NECT. Some lesions isolated to the scalp may have no underlying bony involvement.

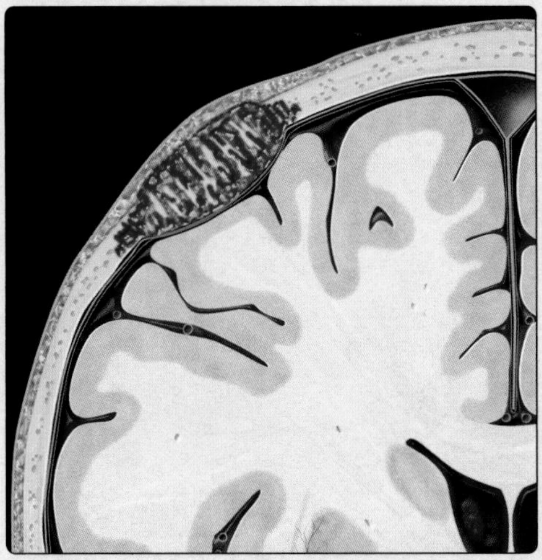

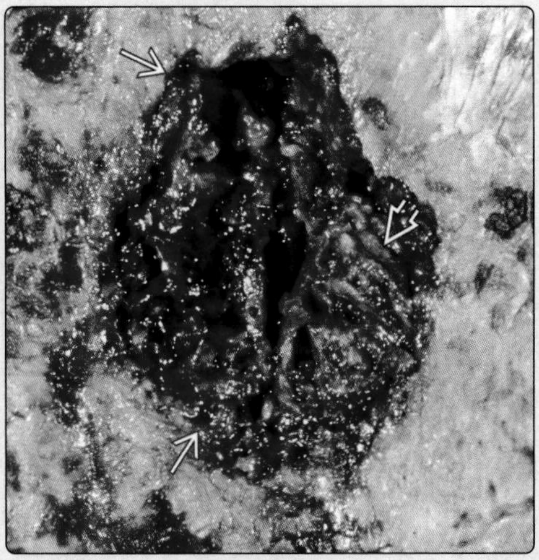

(22-32) *Coronal graphic depicts typical hemangioma of the calvaria as spicules of lamellar bone interspersed with vascular channels.* ***(22-33)*** *Photograph of resected calvarial hemangioma shows an unencapsulated, very vascular-appearing mass ➡ with radiating spicules of bone ➡.*

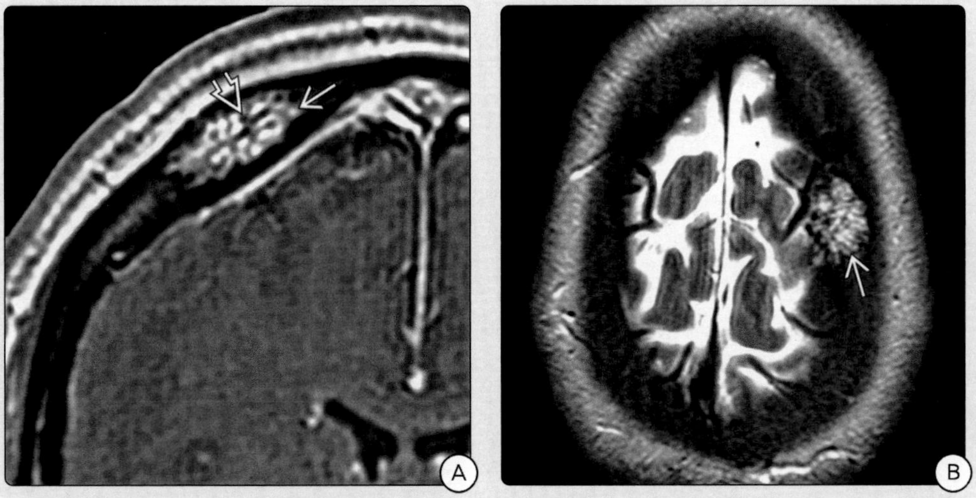

(22-34A) *Coronal T1 C+ FS scan shows a typical calvarial hemangioma ➡ that slightly expands the diploic space. The vascular channels enhance intensely, whereas the "dots" of bone spicules within the lesion ➡ do not.* ***(22-34B)*** *Axial T2WI of another calvarial hemangioma shows that the mass ➡ is mostly very hyperintense. The hypointense "dots" of radiating bone spicules give the lesion a striped appearance.*

Bone CT shows that the inner and outer tables are thinned but usually intact. A thin sclerotic margin may surround the lesion. "Spoke-wheel" or reticulated hyperdensities caused by fewer but thicker trabeculae are present within the hemangioma, giving it a "honeycomb" or "jail bars" appearance.

On CECT, foci of intense enhancement interspersed with focal hypodensities caused by the residual thickened trabeculae are typical.

MR Findings. Mixed hypo- to isointensity is the dominant pattern on T1WI. Scattered hyperintensities usually are caused by fat—not hemorrhage—within the lesion. Most hemangiomas are markedly hyperintense on T2WI **(22-35)**.

Contrast-enhanced scans show diffuse intense enhancement. Dynamic scans show slow centripetal "filling in" of the lesion **(22-36)**.

Angiography. Dural and venous sinus hemangiomas can closely resemble meningiomas, with slow, persistent contrast accumulation in the capillary and venous phases of the angiogram.

Differential Diagnosis

The differential diagnosis of calvarial hemangioma includes "holes in the skull" caused by venous lakes and arachnoid granulations, burr holes, dermoids, eosinophilic granuloma, and metastasis.

The major differential diagnosis for dural/venous sinus hemangioma is **meningioma**. Except for the microcystic variant, meningiomas do not display the marked hyperintensity on T2WI seen in most hemangiomas. Hemangiomas also exhibit the classic "filling in" from the periphery to the center of the lesion on rapid-sequence dynamic contrast-enhanced T1WIs.

***(22-35A)** Axial bone CT in a 32y woman with headaches shows an extensive "salt and pepper" lesion ➡ that causes slight expansion of the right parietal diploë. **(22-35B)** Axial T1WI in the same case shows that the extensive lesion ⇨ is slightly hyperintense compared with the normal diploic space. The cortex appears thinned in some areas ➡ but is largely intact.*

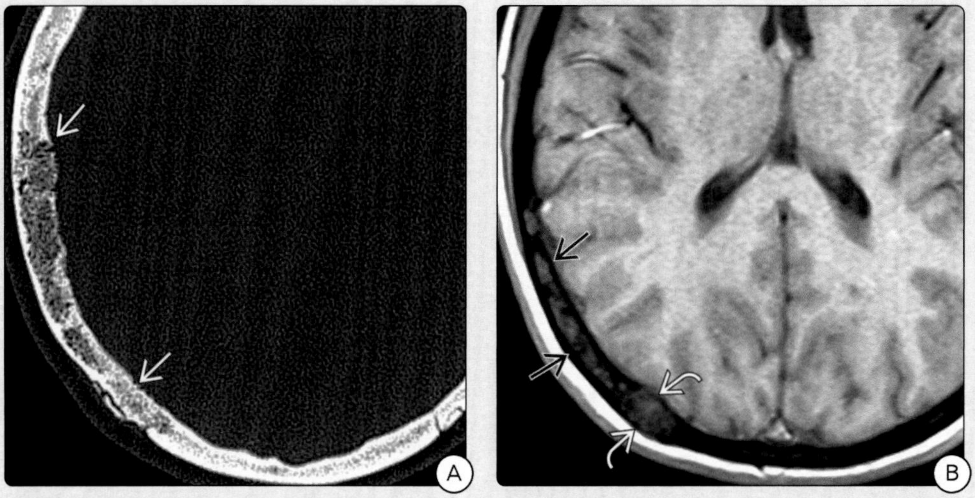

***(22-35C)** Axial T2WI in the same case shows that the extensive diploic space lesion ➡ has a very hyperintense but "speckled" appearance and has focally thinned and broken through cortex ➡. **(22-35D)** Axial T1 C+ FS MR shows that the lesion enhances intensely ➡ and has a striated or "speckled" appearance ➡. This is calvarial hemangioma.*

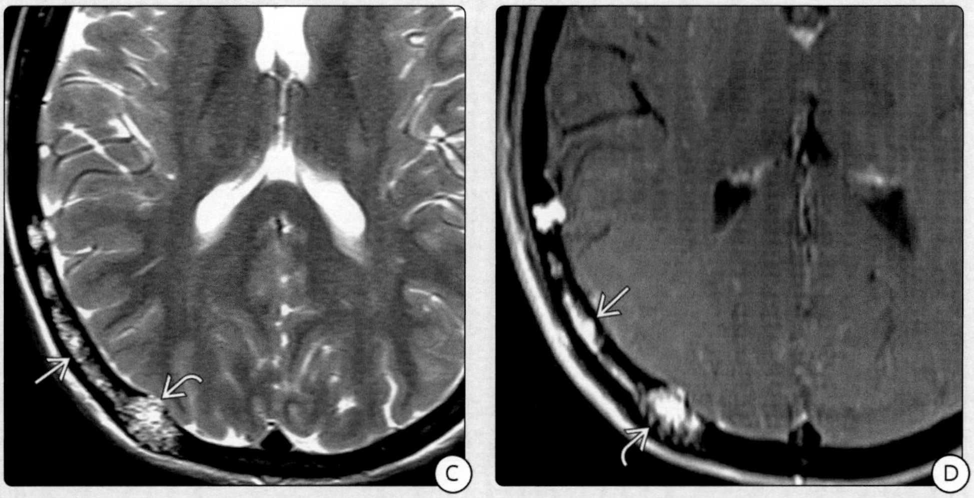

CALVARIAL AND DURAL HEMANGIOMAS

Pathology
- Benign vasoformative neoplasm with capillary-type growth pattern
- Calvarium (diploic space) more than dura, dural venous sinuses

Clinical Features
- Any age, mostly small/asymptomatic

Imaging Findings
- CT: Radiating "spoke-wheel" bone spicules
- MR: T2 "honeycomb" hyperintensities
  - Dynamic T1 C+ shows "filling in" of lesion

Differential Diagnosis
- Calvarial = venous channels, arachnoid granulations, etc.
- Dura/venous sinus = meningioma

Malignant Mesenchymal Tumors

Malignant mesenchymal nonmeningothelial tumors are the malignant version of the soft tissue and bone tumors described above. Most are WHO grade IV neoplasms.

Terminology

Malignant mesenchymal tumors (MMTs) include mostly **sarcomas** (of many histologic types) and other neoplasms such as **undifferentiated pleomorphic sarcoma/malignant fibrous histiocytoma** (MFH).

Etiology

Most investigators posit pluripotential meningeal mesenchymal cells as the origin of MMTs. These cells are capable of giving rise to the spectrum of histologic types seen in nonmeningothelial neoplasms.

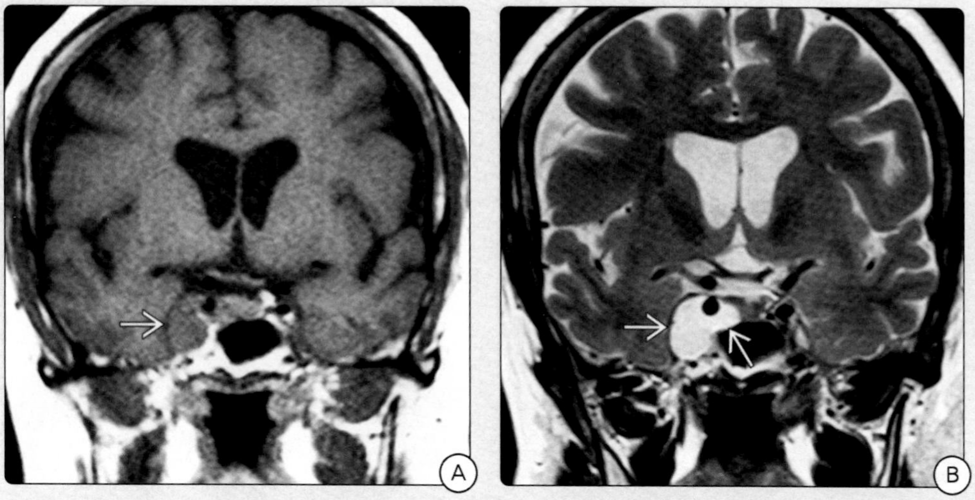

(22-36A) *Coronal T1WI in a 66y woman with diagnosis of meningioma on outside MR shows a mass in the right cavernous sinus ➡ that is isointense with gray matter.* ***(22-36B)*** *Coronal T2WI in the same case shows that the mass ➡ is extremely and uniformly hyperintense.*

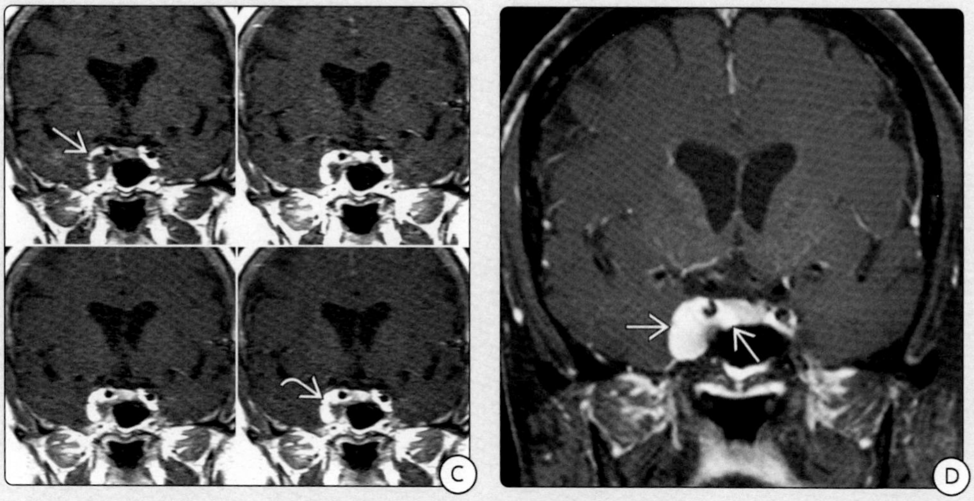

(22-36C) *Dynamic contrast-enhanced fat-saturated T1WIs show progressive "filling in" of mass by contrast with the periphery of the lesions filling first ➡, followed by centripetal (central) enhancement of the rest of the lesion with time ➡.* ***(22-36D)*** *T1 C+ FS scan 5 min after contrast injection for the dynamic sequence shows that the entire mass ➡ now enhances intensely, uniformly. This is cavernous sinus hemangioma. Surgery was cancelled.*

Prior radiation therapy is a known cause of MMTs, most commonly fibrosarcomas. The Epstein-Barr virus may play a role in developing smooth muscle tumors, which occasionally occur in immunocompromised patients.

Pathology

Location. Most intracranial MMTs arise in the dura or skull base **(22-37)**. Some arise in the scalp or calvaria. Chondrosarcomas classically arise from the petrooccipital fissure **(22-38)**.

Gross Pathology. Most intracranial sarcomas invade the brain. Necrosis and gross hemorrhage are common.

Microscopic Features. Most MMTs are composed of small, undifferentiated mesenchymal cells that may be difficult to distinguish from one another by light microscopy. Electron microscopy and immunohistochemistry may be helpful.

Clinical Issues

Epidemiology. MMTs are rare tumors. In the aggregate, they represent 0.5-2.0% of intracranial neoplasms.

Demographics. MMTs can occur at any age. Some (such as rhabdomyosarcoma and Ewing sarcoma) are much more common in children than adults. Chondrosarcomas are tumors of young adults with a mean age of 37 years at presentation. Fibrosarcomas are more common in middle-aged adults.

There is no sex predilection for most MMTs. Ewing sarcoma is more common in male patients.

Presentation. Clinical symptoms vary with tumor location.

Natural History. Prognosis depends on tumor type and grade. Most MMTs grow rapidly, and prognosis is generally poor. Many recur locally, sometimes years after initial treatment, and metastases outside the CNS are not uncommon.

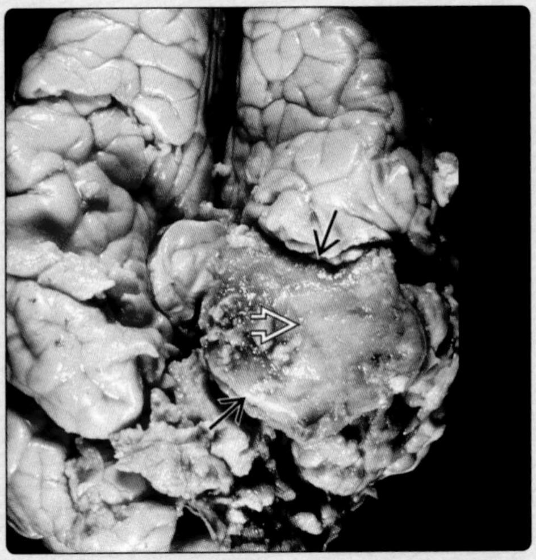

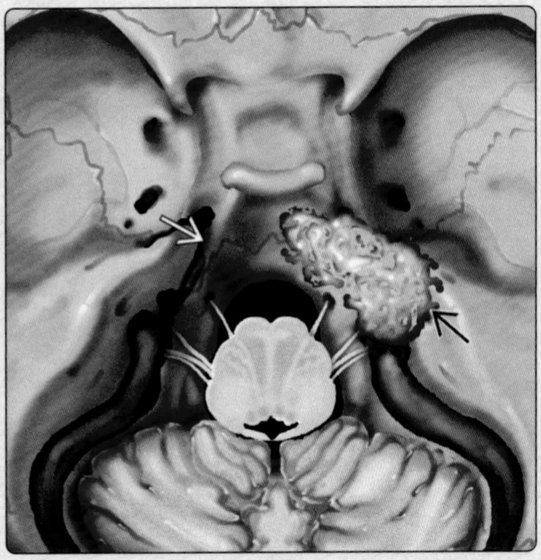

***(22-37)** Large skull base mass invades the brain. Note the cartilaginous-appearing components. This is chondrosarcoma. (Courtesy AFIP Archives.)* ***(22-38)** Graphic depicts skull base chondrosarcoma centered in the left petrooccipital fissure (compare to the normal right side).*

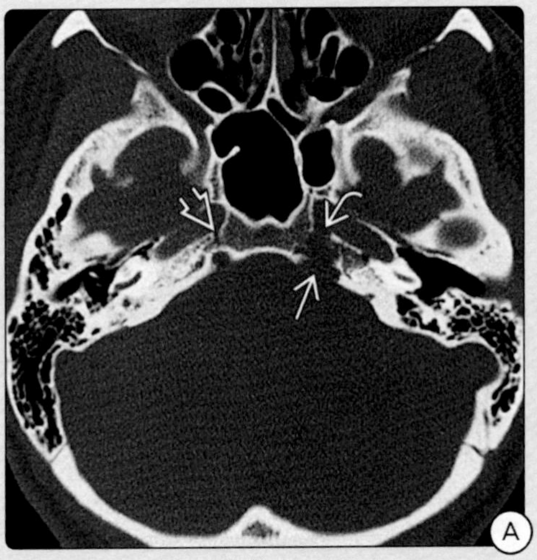

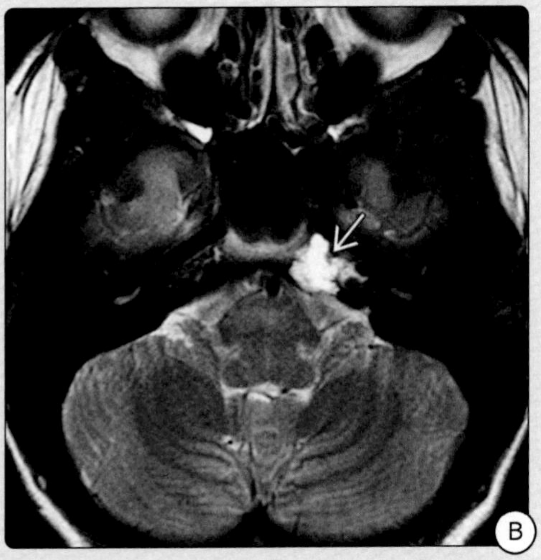

***(22-39A)** Axial bone CT in a 25y woman with sixth nerve palsy shows an erosive, destructive lesion of the left petro-occipital fissure. The wall of the petrous ICA segment is dehiscent. Compare to normal right petro-occipital fissure.* ***(22-39B)** Axial T2WI in the same case shows a lobulated, hyperintense mass at the left petrous apex centered over the petro-occipital fissure. This is chondrosarcoma.*

The exception to this general rule is skull base chondrosarcomas. Most are well to moderately differentiated low-grade lesions and are slow-growing, locally invasive tumors that rarely metastasize. High-grade chondrosarcomas are more aggressive tumors that frequently metastasize and have a much poorer prognosis.

Imaging

General Features. Imaging findings of MMTs are those of highly aggressive dural, skull base **(22-39)**, calvarial, or scalp lesions that invade adjacent structures **(22-40)**. Although intracranial sarcomas may appear grossly circumscribed, local parenchymal invasion is present at surgery.

CT Findings. NECT scans show a mixed-density soft tissue mass that causes lysis of adjacent bone **(22-41A)**. Chondrosarcoma may have stippled calcifications or classic "rings and arcs." Sometimes "sunburst" calcifications can be seen in osteosarcomas. Periosteal reaction is generally absent, with the exception of Ewing sarcoma.

Most MMTs enhance strongly but quite heterogeneously **(22-41)**.

MR Findings. Other than suggesting a highly aggressive mass, there are no MR findings specific for MMTs. Fibrous, chondroid, and osteoid tissue are often very hypointense on both T1- and T2WI. FLAIR is very helpful in demonstrating brain invasion.

Most MMTs enhance strongly but heterogeneously. Foci of necrosis are common.

Angiography. Some MMTs such as angiosarcomas are highly vascular. Others show little or no neovascularity and are seen primarily as a nonspecific avascular mass.

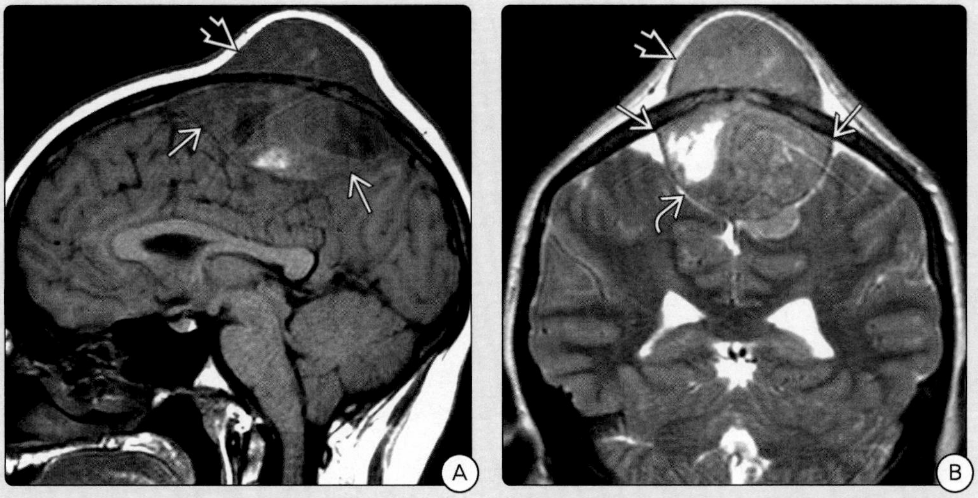

***(22-40A)** Sagittal T1WI of a child with a head "lump" shows a large subcutaneous soft tissue mass ➡ that invades the underlying calvarium and extends into the epidural space ➡. **(22-40B)** Coronal T2WI in the same case shows the invasive transdural, transcalvarial mass of mixed signal intensity ➡. The dura is displaced inward ➡, and a thin rim of CSF ➡ separates most of the mass from the underlying brain.*

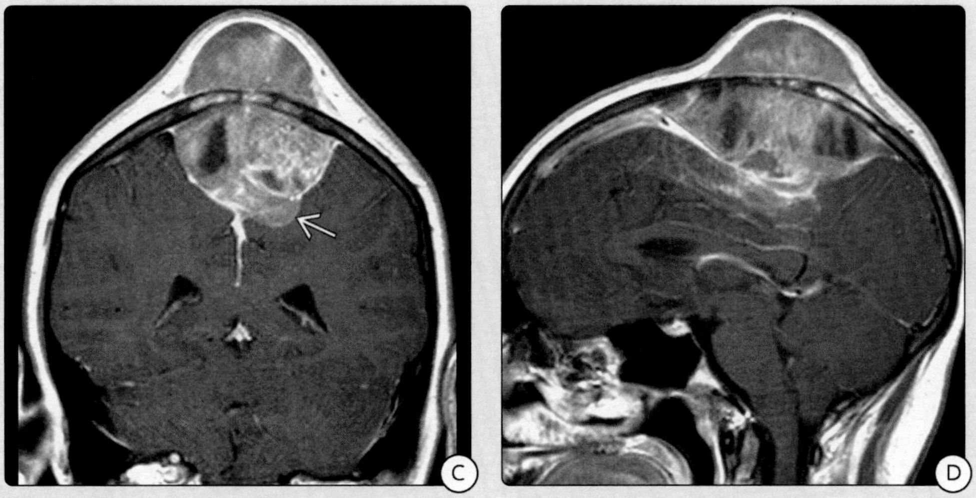

***(22-40C)** The mass enhances strongly but very heterogeneously on T1 C+. Note focal invasion through the dura into the underlying brain ➡. **(22-40D)** Sagittal T1 C+ scan shows the heterogeneous, aggressive appearance of the mass. This is Ewing sarcoma.*

*(**22-41A**) Axial bone CT in a 64y woman with a "lump" on her head shows a destructive soft tissue mass → centered on the right parietal bone. No reactive bone formation or intratumoral calcifications are present. (**22-41B**) Axial CECT in the same case shows that the mass → enhances strongly but heterogeneously, with central nonenhancing areas ⇨ suggestive of necrosis.*

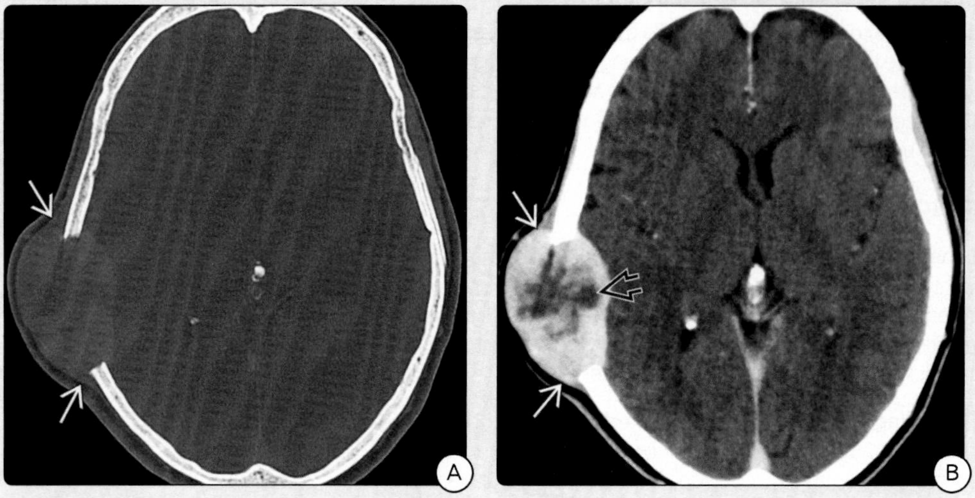

*(**22-41C**) T1WI in the same case shows that the mass → is isointense with cortex and buckles the dura → and underlying cortex medially. (**22-41D**) Axial T2WI in the same case shows that the mass is heterogeneously iso- and hypointense.*

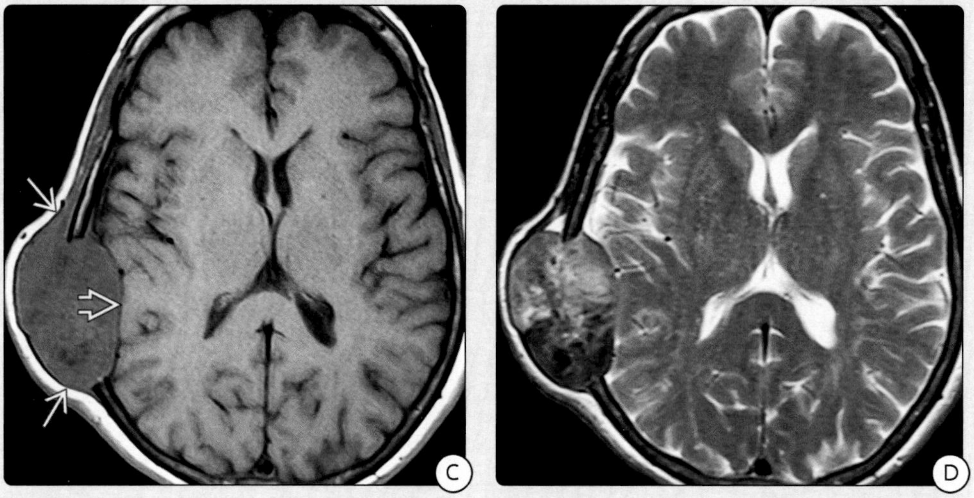

*(**22-41E**) T1 C+ FS shows that the mass → enhances intensely with a nonenhancing central necrotic core ⇨. Note subtle "tails" of reactive dural thickening, enhancement ↷. (**22-41F**) DWI shows no evidence for restricted diffusion. Fibrosarcoma with fascicles of malignant spindle cells was found at surgery.*

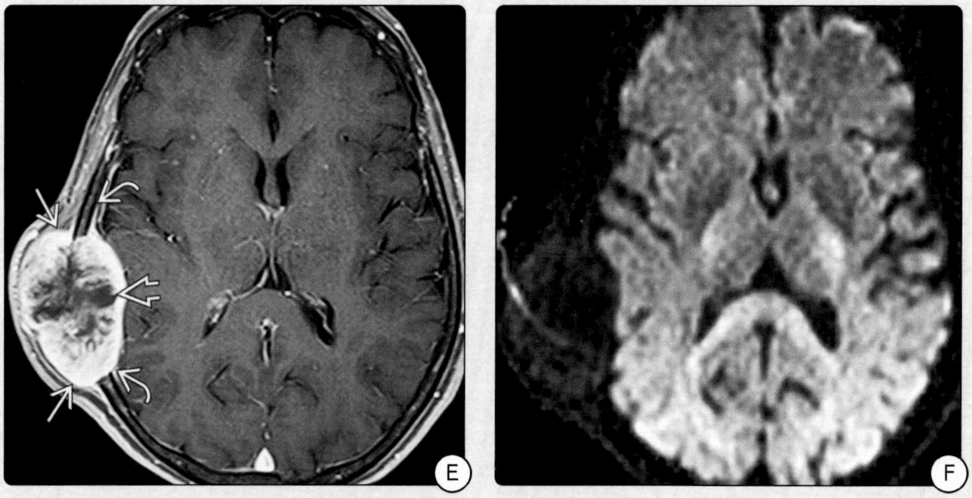

Differential Diagnosis

There are no characteristic radiologic findings that distinguish most MMTs from other aggressive neoplasms such as **malignant meningioma** or **metastases**. Sarcoma subtypes are difficult to identify on the basis of imaging findings alone. For example, a histologically definite liposarcoma may demonstrate virtually no imaging features that would suggest the presence of fat.

Solitary Fibrous Tumor/Hemangiopericytoma

Terminology

Solitary fibrous tumor (SFT) represents a continuum of mesenchymal tumors with increasing cellularity. Because SFTs and hemangiopericytomas (HPCs) share the same molecular genetic profile, the 2016 WHO has created the combined term **solitary fibrous tumor/hemangiopericytoma (SFT/HPC)** to describe such lesions. Three grades of increasing malignancy are assigned to these tumors (see below).

Although relatively rare, SFT/HPC is the most common primary intracranial nonmeningothelial mesenchymal neoplasm. These tumors are very cellular, highly vascular neoplasms known for their aggressive clinical behavior, high recurrence rates, and distant metastases even after gross total surgical resection.

Etiology

Most meningeal SFT/HPCs have a genomic inversion at 12q13, which leads to a fusion of the *NAB2* and *STAT6* genes.

Pathology

Location. Most SFT/HPCs are dura based, usually arising from the falx or tentorium. The most common site is the occipital

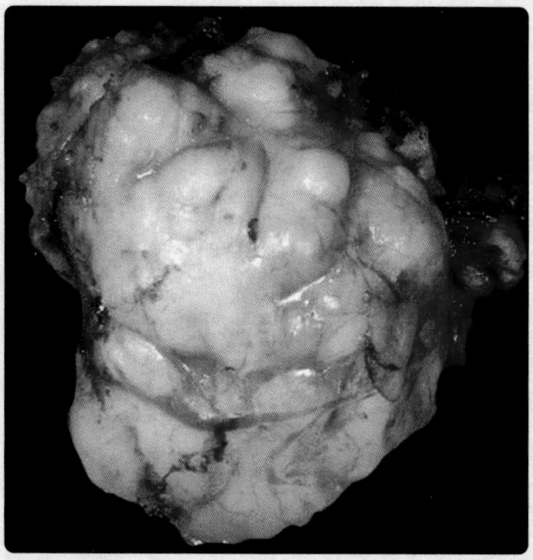

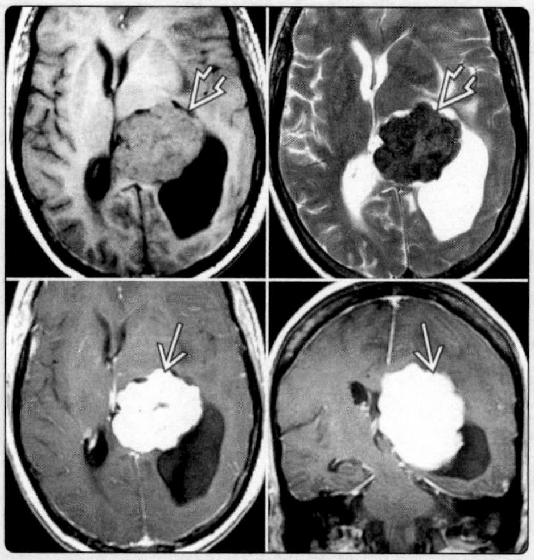

***(22-42)** Solitary fibrous tumors are firm, well-circumscribed masses that can appear identical to meningioma. (Courtesy E. Rushing, MD.) **(22-43)** A T1 iso-, T2 hypointense mass ➡ that enhances strongly and uniformly ➡ is seen in the atrium of the left lateral ventricle. Final diagnosis was solitary fibrous tumor and/or hemangiopericytoma, grade I.*

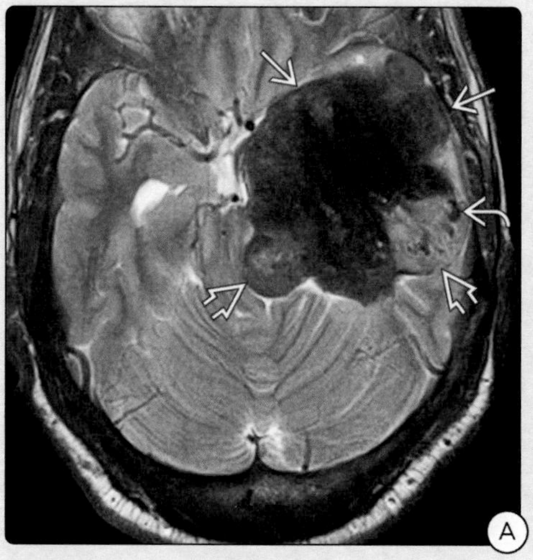

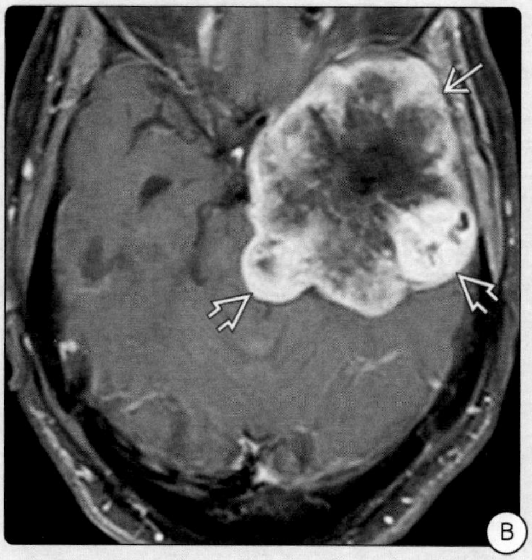

***(22-44A)** T2WI shows a large, well-delineated bosselated left middle cranial fossa mass. The mass ➡ is extremely hypointense except for two areas ➡ where it is nearly isointense with cortex. Note prominent "flow voids" in one of the nodules ➡. **(22-44B)** T1 C+ FS shows the periphery of the mass ➡ and nodules ➡ enhances intensely, while the central part of the mass does not. This is solitary fibrous tumor, WHO grade I. (Courtesy R. Hewlett, MD.)*

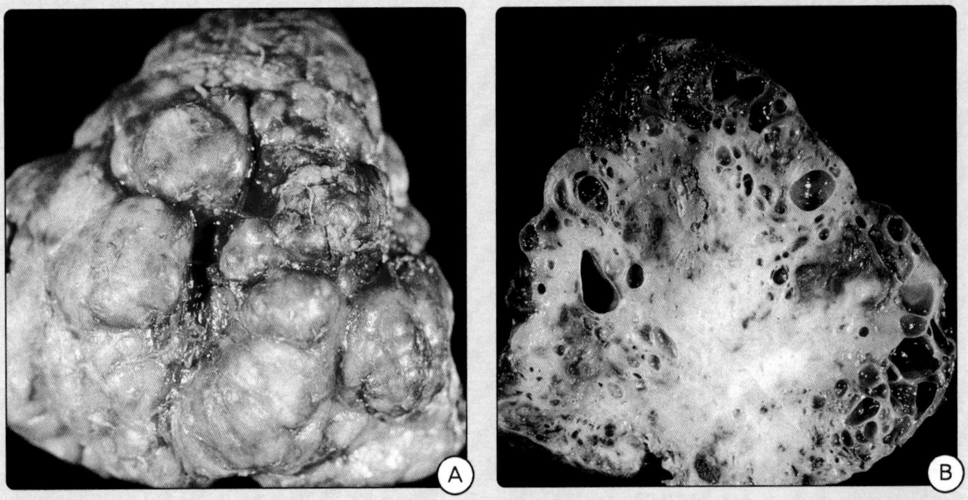

***(22-45A)** Resected specimen of hemangiopericytoma shows "bosselated" configuration. This tumor would now correspond to SFT/HPC, WHO grade II. **(22-45B)** Cut section through the specimen shows multiple cysts and enlarged vascular channels. (Courtesy R. Hewlett, MD.)*

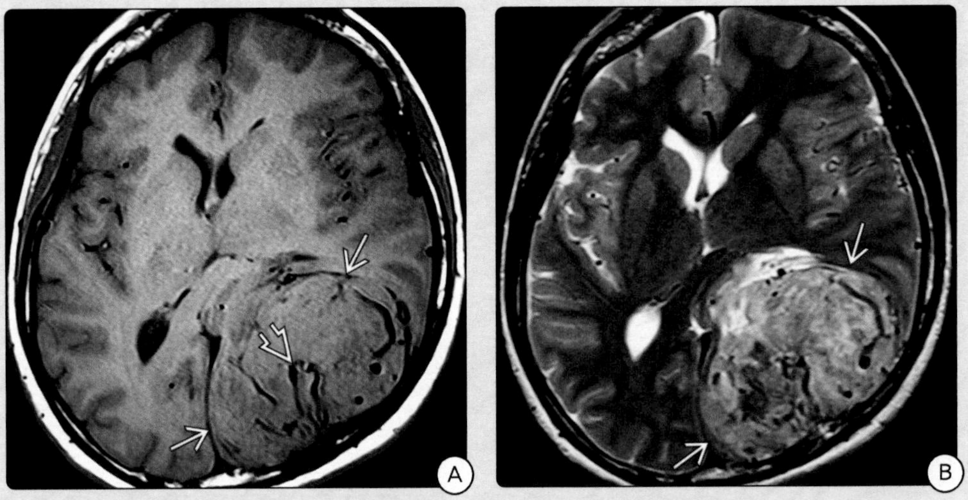

***(22-46A)** Axial T1WI in a 21y woman with vision problems shows a huge left parieto-occipital mass that is mostly isointense with the underlying brain. Note prominent "flow voids" within the mass. **(22-46B)** Axial T2WI in the same case shows that the large mass is displacing brain around it, suggesting that it is extraaxial in origin.*

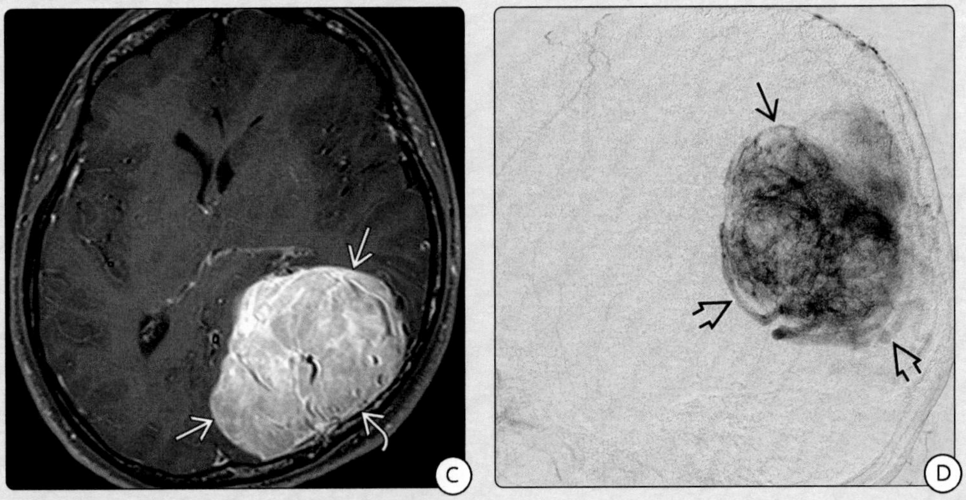

***(22-46C)** Axial T1 C+ FS shows that the intensely but heterogeneously enhancing mass has a broad base that abuts the dura. **(22-46D)** Late venous-phase DSA of the selective left external carotid angiogram shows an extremely vascular mass with prolonged tumor staining. Note prominent draining veins . This is SFT/hemangiopericytoma, WHO grade III (previously diagnosed as anaplastic hemangiopericytoma).*

region, where they often straddle the transverse sinus. Intraparenchymal SFT/HPCs occur in the cerebrum and spinal cord, often without a discernible dural attachment. The cerebral ventricles are another common site.

Size and Number. SFT/HPCs are almost always solitary lesions. They are relatively large tumors, reaching up to 10 cm in diameter. Lesions more than 4-5 cm are not uncommon.

Gross Pathology. SFTs are solid, lobulated, relatively well-demarcated neoplasms **(22-42)**. HPCs contain abundant vascular spaces **(22-45)**. Intratumoral hemorrhage is common.

Microscopic Features. *STAT6* nuclear expression can be detected by immunohistochemistry and confirms the diagnosis of SFT/HPC. Histologic features vary from a solitary fibrous tumor phenotype with patternless fascicular architecture and abundant collagen to the HPC phenotype characterized by high cellularity and prominent branching vessels.

Most tumors with the SFT phenotype are low-grade lesions. Mitoses are rare, with Ki-67 mostly in the 1-4% range. Anaplasia is uncommon.

Tumors with the HPC phenotype are highly cellular, containing dense masses of swirling cells, dilated slit-like "staghorn" blood vessels, and an abundant network of reticulin fibers. Necrosis is common. Nuclear atypia and mitotic activity vary.

Staging, Grading, and Classification. Three grades of SFT/HPC are recognized in the 2016 WHO. Grade I corresponds to the highly collagenous, low-cellularity spindle cell lesion previously diagnosed as **solitary fibrous tumor**. Grade II corresponds to the more cellular tumor with "staghorn" vasculature that was previously diagnosed as **hemangiopericytoma**.

Grade III SFT/HPC represents what was termed **anaplastic hemangiopericytoma**. More than five mitoses per ten high-power fields are present, and Ki-67 is usually 10% or more.

Clinical Issues

Epidemiology. HPCs are rare tumors, accounting for less than 1% of all primary intracranial neoplasms and 2-4% of all meningeal tumors.

Demographics. Meningeal HPCs generally occur at a slightly younger age than meningiomas. Mean age at diagnosis is 43 years. There is a slight male predominance.

Natural History. Even with complete resection, local recurrence is the rule. The majority of meningeal HPCs eventually metastasize extracranially to bone, lung, and liver. There is no significant difference in survival between grade II and grade III HPCs.

Treatment Options. Surgical resection with radiation therapy or radiosurgery is the treatment of choice.

Imaging

CT Findings. HPCs are hyperdense extraaxial masses that invade and destroy bone. Extracalvarial extension under the scalp is common. Calcification and reactive hyperostosis are absent.

Strong but heterogeneous enhancement is typical.

SOLITARY FIBROUS TUMOR/HEMANGIOPERICYTOMA

Terminology, Etiology
- Solitary fibrous tumor (SFT)/hemangiopericytoma (HPC)
  - Spectrum of tumors sharing common molecular features
  - *NAB2* and *STAT6* fusion → *STAT6* nuclear expression (can be detected by IHC)

Pathology
- SFT/HPC WHO grade I
  - Collagenous, low-cellularity spindle cell lesion
  - Previously diagnosed as solitary fibrous tumor
- SFT/HPC WHO grade II
  - More cellular, "staghorn" vasculature
  - Previously diagnosed in CNS as hemangiopericytoma
- SFT/HPC WHO grade III
  - 5 or more mitoses/HPF
  - Previously anaplastic hemangiopericytoma

Clinical Features
- Rare (< 1% of CNS primary neoplasms)
  - But are most common CNS nonmeningothelial mesenchymal tumor
  - SFT/HPC grades II, III recur, metastasize

Imaging Findings
- SFT/HPC grade I hypointense on T2WI
- SFT/HPC II resembles aggressive meningioma
  - Calcification absent
  - Iso- to mildly hyperintense on T1WI
  - Iso- to heterogeneously hyperintense on T2WI
  - Very vascular, prominent "flow voids"
  - Enhances strongly but heterogeneously
  - "Dural tail" sign usually absent

Differential Diagnosis
- SFT/HPC I = meningioma
- SFT/HPC II, III
  - Atypical/malignant meningioma
  - Dural metastases
  - Gliosarcoma
  - Malignant mesenchymal tumor

MR Findings. Low-grade intracranial SFTs are circumscribed masses that are usually dura-based and resemble meningioma. Lesions are isointense with gray matter on T1WI and have variable signal intensity on T2WI. A mixed hyper- and hypointense pattern is common. Collagen-rich areas can be very hypointense **(22-44)**. Avid enhancement following contrast administration is typical **(22-43)**.

Most HPCs demonstrate mixed signal intensity on all sequences. They tend to be predominantly isointense to gray matter on T1 scans and iso- to hyperintense on T2 scans **(22-46)**. Prominent "flow voids" are almost always present.

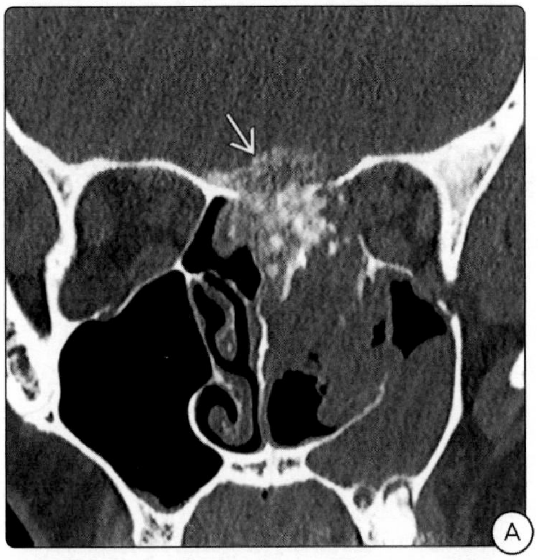

***(22-47A)** Coronal bone CT in a 36y woman shows a partially ossified destructive mass in the upper nasal vault, anterior cranial fossa ➡.*

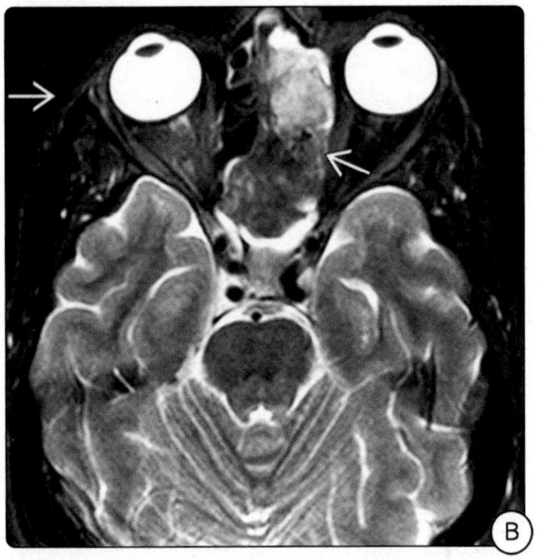

***(22-47B)** Axial T2 FS demonstrates that the lobulated mass ➡ is hypointense compared with the brain.*

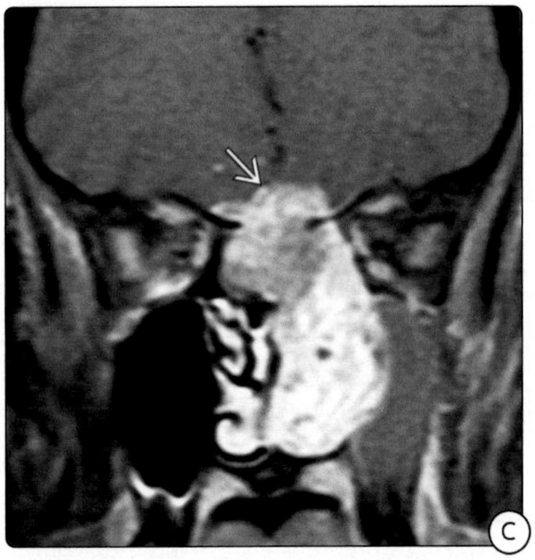

***(22-47C)** T1 C+ FS shows the strongly enhancing mass ➡. Malignant phosphaturic mesenchymal tumor was diagnosed on histopathology.*

Contrast enhancement is marked but heterogeneous. Nonenhancing necrotic foci are common. A "dural tail" sign is absent.

Angiography. HPCs may invade and occlude dural sinuses, so CTV or MRV are helpful noninvasive techniques for delineating patency.

DSA shows HPCs as hypervascular masses with prominent vascularity, "early draining" veins, and intense prolonged tumor "staining" **(22-46D)**. HPCs usually recruit blood supply from both dural and pial vessels.

Differential Diagnosis

The major differential diagnosis of low-grade SFT is typical (WHO grade I) meningioma. The major differential of HPC is a highly vascular aggressive meningioma, particularly an **atypical** or **malignant meningioma**. HPCs rarely calcify or cause hyperostosis, and a "dural tail" sign is typically absent.

Dural metastases with skull invasion can be indistinguishable from HPC. Rare neoplasms that can resemble HPC include **gliosarcoma** and **malignant mesenchymal tumors**.

Rarely, an intracranial SFT/HPC or malignant mesenchymal tumor can cause severe hypophosphatemia and metabolic bone disease not explained by any other metabolic or hereditary disease. These **osteomalacia-inducing tumors** (OITs) can be confused with aggressive meningioma **(22-47)**. OITs secrete fibroblast growth factor 23, resulting in a paraneoplastic syndrome of hypophosphatemic osteomalacia. The most common intracranial OITs are phosphaturic mesenchymal tumors and SFT/HPCs. Most are preferentially located within the anterior cranial fossa.

Primary Melanocytic Lesions

Primary melanocytic tumors of the CNS are very rare with an estimated incidence of 0.9 per 10 million. Focal melanotic masses span a morphologic spectrum from low-grade melanocytoma to malignant melanoma. By far the most frequent melanocytic CNS lesions are metastases from extracranial malignant melanomas.

Primary CNS melanomas are thought to originate from leptomeningeal melanocytes, which are preferentially located at the base of the brain, ventral medulla, and along the upper cervical spinal cord. They can present as focal nodular masses or diffuse leptomeningeal infiltrates. Diffuse leptomeningeal melanotic infiltrates also occur in meningeal melanocytosis/melanomatosis (neurocutaneous melanosis) **(22-48)**.

Melanocytoma and Melanoma

Melanocytomas account for less than 0.1% of all CNS neoplasms. Recent studies have shown that melanocytomas carry *GNAQ/GNA11* mutations and present with copy number variants in chromosomes 3 and 6.

Melanocytomas are solitary, darkly pigmented, low-grade tumors that do not invade adjacent brain. Preferred sites are the posterior fossa (skull base, cerebellopontine angle), temporal lobe, Meckel cave (with nevus of Ota), and spinal cord/nerve roots. Melanocytomas rarely undergo malignant transformation.

Melanomas frequently demonstrate *TERT* promoter mutations and frequently harbor additional oncogene mutations. Prognosis is variable for melanocytic tumors of intermediate differentiation and poor for melanoma.

Melanotic lesions are hyperdense on NECT and enhance strongly on CECT. The paramagnetic properties of melanin cause T1 shortening, so hyperintensity on T1WI and hypointensity **(22-49)** on T2WI are characteristic.

The major differential diagnosis for primary melanocytic lesions of the brain is **metastatic malignant melanoma**.

Diffuse Meningeal Melanocytosis/Melanomatosis

Diffuse leptomeningeal melanocytosis and melanomatosis are usually features of neurocutaneous melanosis (NCM), a rare neurocutaneous syndrome of childhood. Most patients present with numerous congenital melanotic nevi of the skin.

Diffuse melanocytic lesions appear as dense, thick, black confluent aggregates that fill the subarachnoid spaces and coat the pia.

Bilateral T1 hyperintense foci in the amygdala is an early sign of NCM **(22-49A)**. Diffuse leptomeningeal enhancement and extension into the brain parenchyma via the perivascular spaces can occur and usually indicate malignant transformation with poor prognosis **(22-49B)**.

Melanotic Neuroectodermal Tumor of Infancy

Also known as melanotic progonoma or retinal anlage tumor, melanotic neuroectodermal tumor of infancy (MNTI) is a rare tumor that usually arises from the maxilla, mandible, or cranial vault. Most patients present within the first year of life.

MNTIs are neural crest tumors that exhibit biphasic histology with melanin-containing and neuroblast-like cells. They are generally considered benign but can grow rapidly and be locally aggressive with intracranial extension, mimicking solitary fibrous tumor/hemangiopericytoma or sarcoma **(22-50)**. Malignant degeneration occurs but is uncommon.

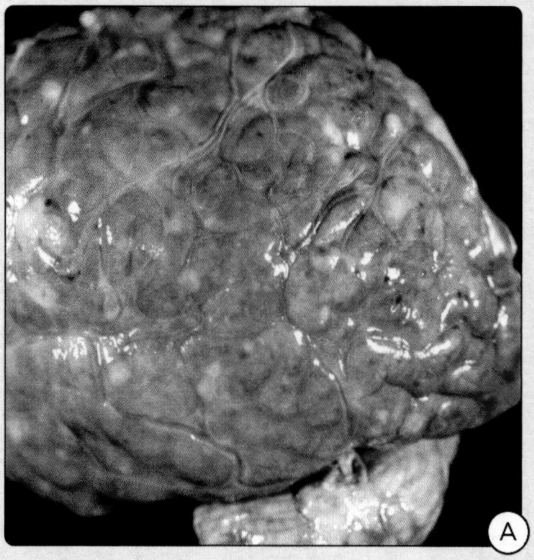

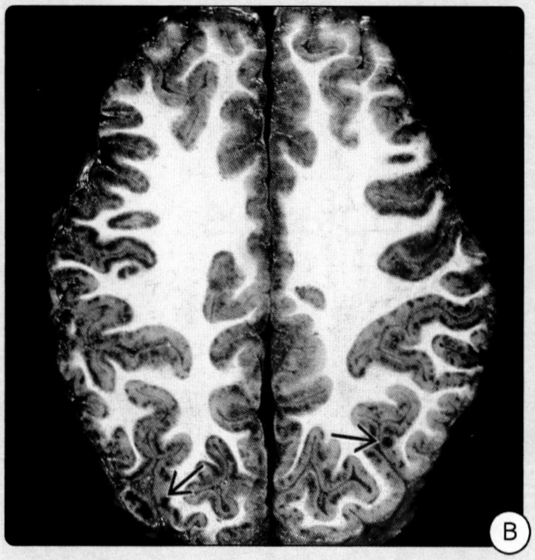

***(22-48A)** Autopsy specimen shows diffuse leptomeningeal melanosis with gray-black discoloration of the entire brain surface. (Courtesy R. Hewlett, MD.) **(22-48B)** Axial section from the same specimen shows that the gyri are enlarged, studded with innumerable tiny black nodules ⇒ representing tumor extension via perivascular spaces. This is diffuse primary leptomeningeal malignant melanocytosis. (Courtesy R. Hewlett, MD.)*

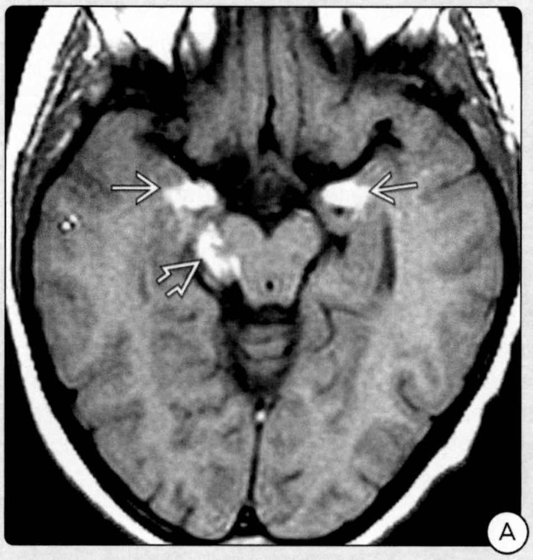

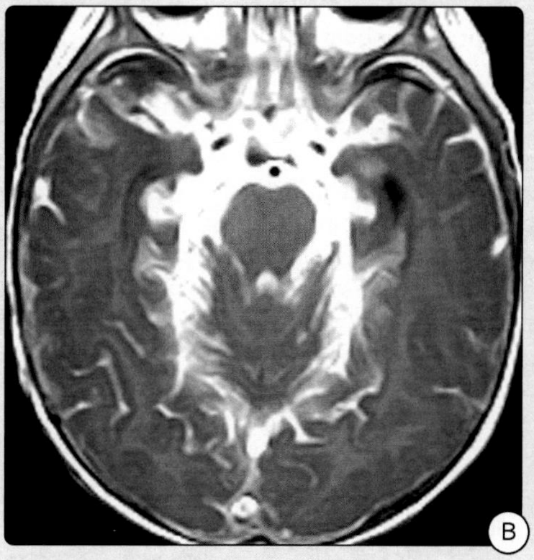

***(22-49A)** T1WI in a patient with neurocutaneous melanosis shows characteristic ovoid hyperintensities in the amygdala of both temporal lobes ➡. Another focus of melanotic deposition with T1 shortening ➡ is seen along the midbrain. (Courtesy S. Blaser, MD.) **(22-49B)** T1 C+ scan in the same patient shows diffuse, thick leptomeningeal enhancement. (Courtesy S. Blaser, MD.)*

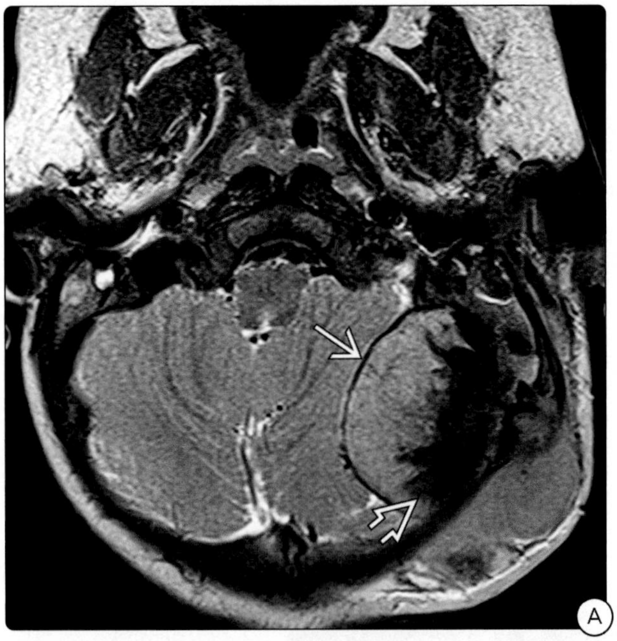

(22-50A) Axial T2WI in a 3m infant with a "bump" on the left side of the head shows an aggressive-appearing mass ➡ centered on the left occipital bone. Note intracranial extradural extension ➡.

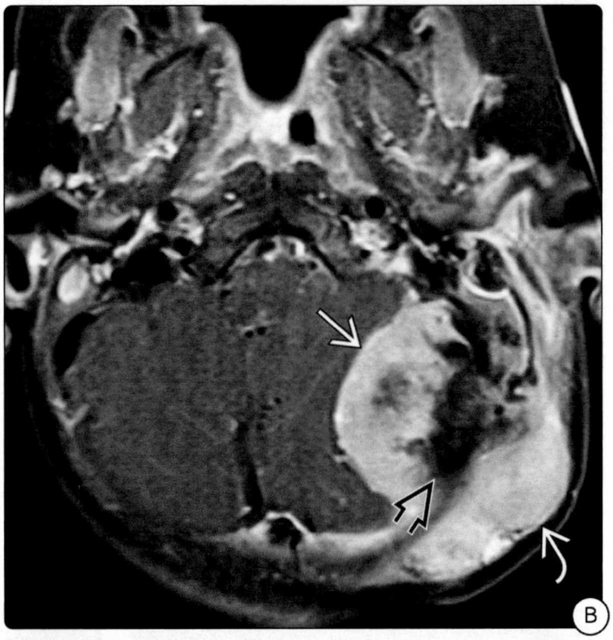

(22-50B) T1 C+ FS shows that the intra- ➡, extracranial ➡ components of the calvarial mass ➡ enhance intensely. This is melanotic progonoma (melanotic neuroectodermal tumor of infancy). (Courtesy T. Poussaint, MD.)

Other Related Neoplasms

Hemangioblastoma

Terminology

Hemangioblastoma (HGBL) is also known as capillary hemangioma. Although the term "blastoma" suggests malignant, highly aggressive lesions, HGBLs are benign, slow-growing, relatively indolent vascular neoplasms. HGBL occurs in both sporadic and multiple forms.

Multiple HGBLs are almost always associated with the autosomal-dominant inherited cancer syndrome **von Hippel-Lindau disease** (VHL). A rare non-VHL form of multiple disseminated HGBLs is termed **leptomeningeal hemangioblastomatosis**.

Etiology

The precise etiology of HGBLs remains unknown. *VHL* gene mutations (losses or inactivations) are present in 20-50% of sporadic HGBLs. Multiple key angiogenic pathways (including VEGF/VEGFR2 and Notch/Dll4) are massively activated in HGBL and contribute synergistically to the tumor's abundant vascularization.

Pathology

Location. HGBLs can occur in any part of the CNS, although the vast majority (90-95%) of intracranial HGBLs are located in the posterior fossa. The cerebellum is by far the most common site (80%) followed by the vermis (15%). Approximately 5% occur in the brainstem, usually the medulla.

The nodule of an HGBL is superficially located and typically abuts a pial surface **(22-51)**.

Supratentorial tumors are rare, accounting for 5-10% of all HGBLs. Most are clustered around the optic pathways and occur in the setting of VHL.

Size and Number. Hemangiomas vary in size from tiny to large, especially when associated with a cyst. Unless they are syndromic, HGBLs are solitary lesions. If more than one HGBL is present, the patient by definition has VHL. A positive family history or presence of other VHL markers (such as visceral cysts, retinal angioma, renal cell carcinoma) should prompt genetic screening.

Gross Pathology. The common appearance is that of a beefy red, vascular-appearing nodule that abuts a pial surface **(22-52)**. A variably sized cyst is present in 50-60% of cases. Cyst fluid is typically yellowish, and the cyst wall is usually smooth. Approximately 40% of HGBLs are solid tumors.

Microscopic Features. HGBLs contain two different cell types, stromal and vascular cells. Generally it is the stromal (not the vascular) cells that are the neoplastic element of an HGBL.

The cyst wall of most HGBLs is nonneoplastic, composed of compressed brain with fibrillary neuroglia devoid of tumor cells. The intratumoral cyst fluid shares a proteomic fingerprint with normal serum and has no proteins in common with HGBL tumor tissue. Cyst formation in HGBLs is therefore a result of vascular leakage from tumor vessels, not tumor liquefaction or active secretion.

Mitoses in HGBLs are few or absent, so proliferation rates are low, too (usually MIB-1 less than 1). HGBL is a WHO grade I neoplasm. There is no recognized atypical or anaplastic variant.

HEMANGIOBLASTOMA: PATHOLOGY AND CLINICAL ISSUES

Pathology
- Posterior fossa (90-95%)
  - Cerebellum most common site
- Cyst + nodule (60%), solid (40%)

Clinical Issues
- Epidemiology/demographics
  - Uncommon (1.0-2.5% of primary brain tumors)
  - 7% of all adult primary posterior fossa tumors
  - Peak age = 30-65 years (younger with VHL), rare < 15 years
- Presentation/natural history
  - May cause hydrocephalus
  - Dysmetria, ataxia
  - 5% have secondary polycythemia
  - Slow, "stuttering" growth
  - Metastasis rare

Clinical Issues

Epidemiology. HGBL accounts for 1.0-2.5% of primary CNS neoplasms and approximately 7% of all primary posterior fossa tumors in adults. It is the second most common infratentorial parenchymal mass in adults (after metastasis).

Between 25-40% of HGBLs are associated with VHL.

Demographics. HGBL is generally a tumor of adults between the ages of 30 and 65 years. Pediatric HGBLs are rare. VHL-associated HGBLs tend to present at a significantly younger age but are still relatively rare in children under the age of 15. There is a slight male predominance.

Presentation. Most symptoms in patients with the cystic form of HGBL are caused by the cyst, not the neoplastic nodule. Headache is the presenting symptom in 85% of cases. HGBLs produce erythropoietin, which causes secondary polycythemia in approximately 5% of patients.

Natural History and Treatment Options. Because HGBLs exhibit a "stuttering" growth pattern, they frequently are stable lesions that can remain asymptomatic for long intervals. Imaging progression alone is not an indication for treatment although tumor/cyst growth rates can be used to predict symptom formation and future need for treatment.

Although HGBLs show no intrinsic tendency to metastasize, there are sporadic reports of intraspinal dissemination. Complete en bloc resection is the procedure of choice. Total resection eliminates tumor recurrence although new HGBLs may develop in the setting of VHL.

Imaging

General Features. HGBLs have four basic imaging patterns: (1) solid HGBLs without associated cysts, (2) HGBLs with intratumoral cysts, (3) HGBLs with peritumoral cysts (nonneoplastic cyst with solid tumor nodule), and (4) HGBLs associated with both peri- and intratumoral cysts (nonneoplastic cyst with cysts in the tumor nodule). A nonneoplastic peritumoral cyst with solid nodule is the most common pattern, seen in 50-65% of cases. The second most common pattern is the solid form, seen in about 40% of cases.

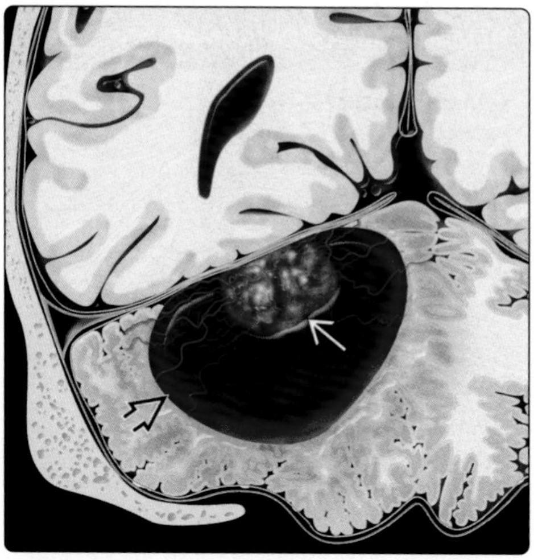

***(22-51)** Graphic depicts typical HGBL with cyst wall ⇨ composed of compressed cerebellum. Vascular tumor nodule ➡ abuts pial surface.*

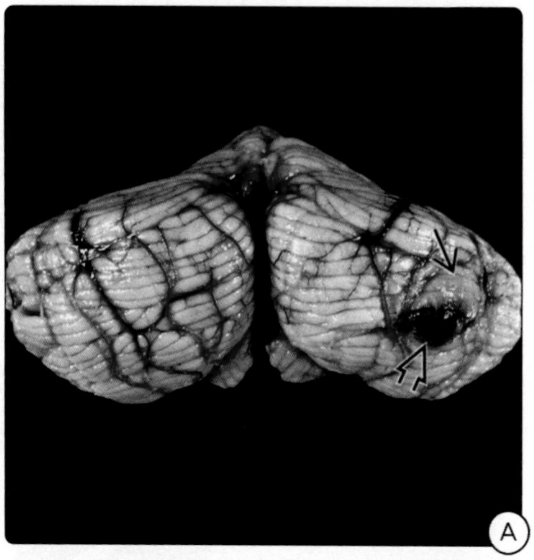

***(22-52A)** Autopsy specimen shows superficial nodule abutting the pia ⇨, hemorrhagic cyst ⇨ of a typical HGBL. (Courtesy E. Ross, MD.)*

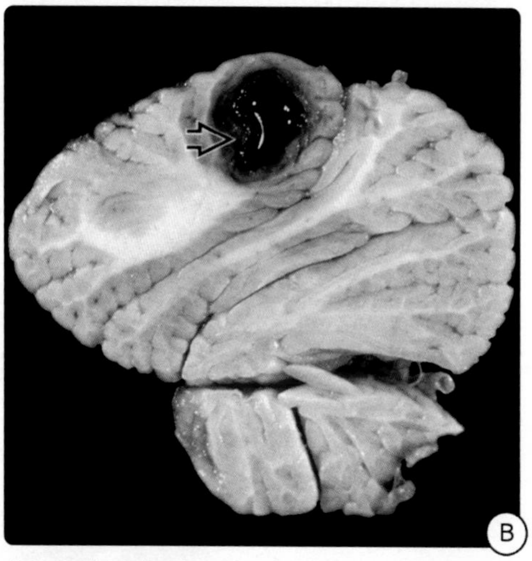

***(22-52B)** Sagittal section in the same case shows the hemorrhagic cyst ⇨. The tumor nodule is not visible. (Courtesy E. Ross, MD.)*

HEMANGIOBLASTOMA: IMAGING

General Features

- "Cyst + nodule" (60%)
  - Nodule abuts pial surface
- Solid (40%)

CT

- Low-density cyst
- Strongly enhancing nodule

MR

- Cyst
  - Fluid slightly hyperintense to CSF
  - Wall usually nonneoplastic
- Nodule
  - Isointense to brain
  - "Flow voids" common
  - Enhances intensely

CT Findings. The most common appearance is a well-delineated iso- to slightly hyperdense nodule associated with a hypodense cyst. Calcification and gross hemorrhage are absent. The nodule enhances strongly and uniformly following contrast administration.

MR Findings. An isointense nodule with prominent "flow voids" is seen on T1WI. If an associated peritumoral cyst is present, it is typically hypointense to parenchyma on T1WI but hyperintense compared with CSF **(22-53)**.

Compared with brain parenchyma, the tumor nodule of an HGBL is moderately hyperintense on T2WI and FLAIR. Intratumoral cysts and prominent "flow voids" are common. The cyst fluid is very hyperintense on both T2WI and FLAIR **(22-53)**.

Occasionally an HGBL hemorrhages. If present, blood products "bloom" on T2*.

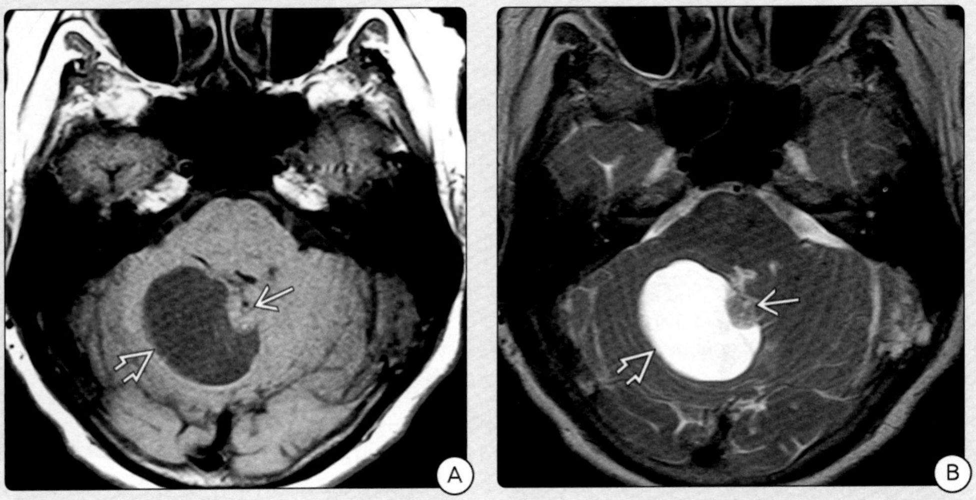

***(22-53A)** Axial T1WI in a 70y woman with ataxia shows a cystic cerebellar mass ➡ with a mural nodule ➡. **(22-53B)** Axial T2 FS MR in the same case shows that the cyst fluid ➡ is very hyperintense, while the nodule is mostly isointense ➡ with adjacent brain.*

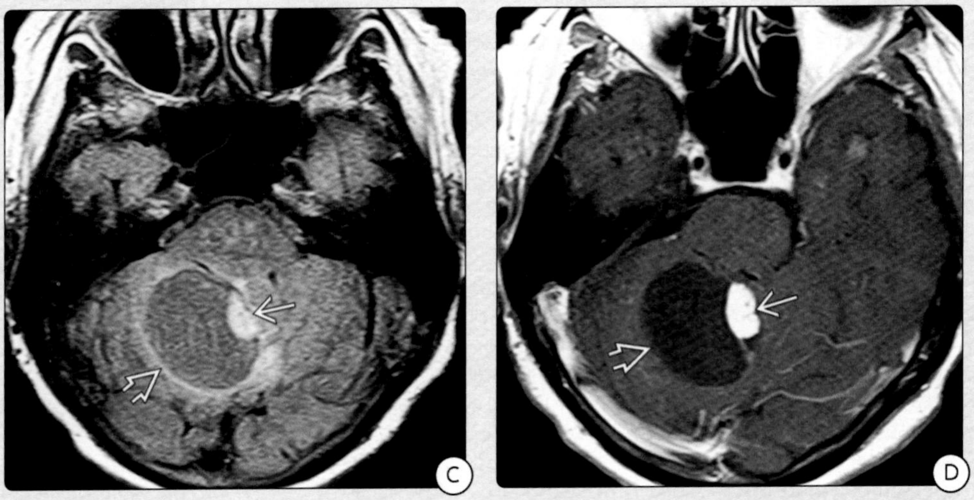

***(22-53C)** FLAIR shows that the fluid ➡ does not suppress, and the mural nodule ➡ is hyperintense to brain parenchyma. **(22-53D)** T1 C+ MR shows that the mural nodule enhances intensely ➡, while the cyst wall does not exhibit any contrast enhancement ➡. This is solitary hemangioblastoma, WHO grade I.*

Intense enhancement of the nodule—but not the cyst itself—is typical **(22-53D)**. Cyst wall enhancement should raise the possibility of tumor involvement, as compressed, nonneoplastic brain does not enhance.

Noncystic HGBLs enhance strongly but often heterogeneously **(22-54)**. Multiple HGBLs are seen in VHL and vary from tiny punctate to large solid tumors (see Chapter 40).

Supratentorial HGBLs are rare. Most occur around the optic nerves or chiasm. HGBL occasionally occurs as a hemispheric mass with a "cyst + nodule" appearance **(22-56)**.

Angiography. The most common appearance is that of an intensely vascular tumor nodule that shows a prolonged vascular "blush" **(22-55)**. "Early draining" veins are common. If a tumor-associated cyst is present, vessels appear displaced and "draped" around an avascular mass.

Differential Diagnosis

The differential diagnosis of HGBL varies with age. In a middle-aged or older adult, the statistically most common cause of an enhancing posterior fossa intraaxial (parenchymal) mass is **metastasis**, not HGBL! DWI and DSC-PWI are helpful in the characterization and differentiation of HGBL from brain metastases. HGBL has higher minimum ADC values and relative ADC ratios compared with metastases.

A cerebellar mass with "cyst + nodule" in a child or young adult is most likely a **pilocytic astrocytoma**, not HGBL or metastasis. Occasionally a **cavernous malformation** can mimic an HGBL with hemorrhage.

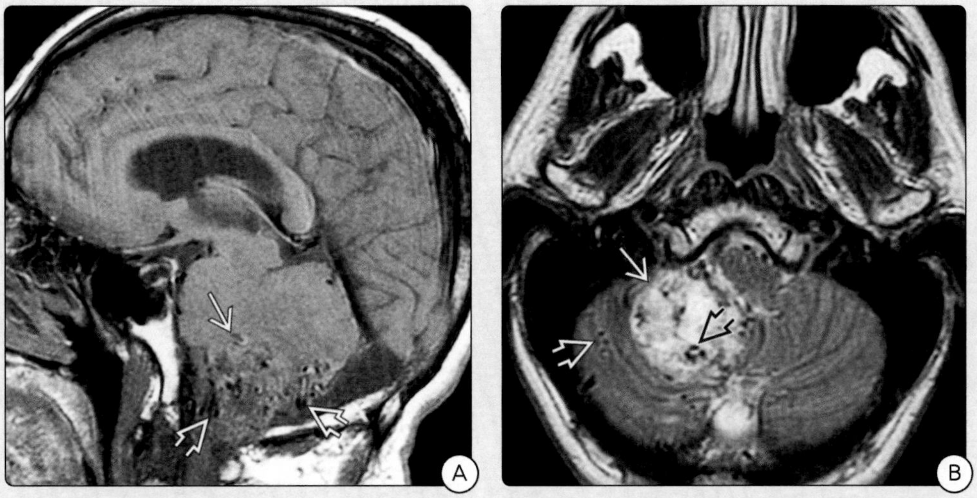

(22-54A) Sagittal T1WI in a 63y man with vertigo shows a posterior fossa mass with numerous prominent "flow voids". (22-54B) Axial T2WI in the same case shows that the mass is very hyperintense. Prominent "flow voids" are seen within the mass and adjacent cerebellum.

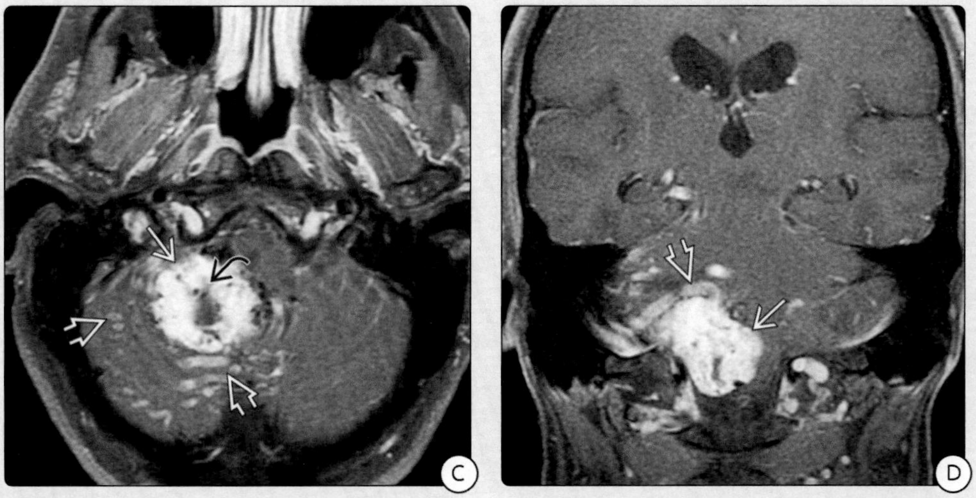

(22-54C) Axial T1 C+ FS in the same case shows that the mass enhances intensely, appears solid with an area of central necrosis. Note numerous prominent serpentine enhancing vessels in the adjacent cerebellum. (22-54D) Coronal T1 C+ FS shows the solid mass, prominent draining vein. This is hemangioblastoma, WHO grade I.

Selected References

Anatomy of the Cranial Meninges

Liebo GB et al: Brain herniation into arachnoid granulations: clinical and neuroimaging features. J Neuroimaging. 26(6):592-598, 2016

Bucchieri F et al: Lymphatic vessels of the dura mater: a new discovery? J Anat. 227(5):702-3, 2015

Mortazavi MM et al: Anatomical variations and neurosurgical significance of Liliequist's membrane. Childs Nerv Syst. 31(1):15-28, 2015

Tsutsumi S et al: Cranial arachnoid protrusions and contiguous diploic veins in CSF drainage. AJNR Am J Neuroradiol. 35(9):1735-9, 2014

Adeeb N et al: The intracranial arachnoid mater : a comprehensive review of its history, anatomy, imaging, and pathology. Childs Nerv Syst. 29(1):17-33, 2013

Adeeb N et al: The pia mater: a comprehensive review of literature. Childs Nerv Syst. 29(10):1803-10, 2013

Adeeb N et al: The cranial dura mater: a review of its history, embryology, and anatomy. Childs Nerv Syst. 28(6):827-37, 2012

Meningomas

Meningioma

Starr CJ et al: Meningioma mimics: five key imaging features to differentiate them from meningiomas. Clin Radiol. ePub, 2017

Zakhari N et al: Uncommon cranial meningioma: key Iimaging features on conventional and advanced imaging. Clin Neuroradiol. 27(2):135-144, 2017

Boukobza M et al: Cystic meningioma: radiological, histological, and surgical particularities in 43 patients. Acta Neurochir (Wien). 158(10):1955-64, 2016

Gerkes EH et al: A heritable form of SMARCE1-related meningiomas with important implications for follow-up and family screening. Neurogenetics. 17(2):83-9, 2016

Gunel M et al: 218Meningioma driver mutations determine their anatomical site of origin. Neurosurgery. 63 Suppl 1:185, 2016

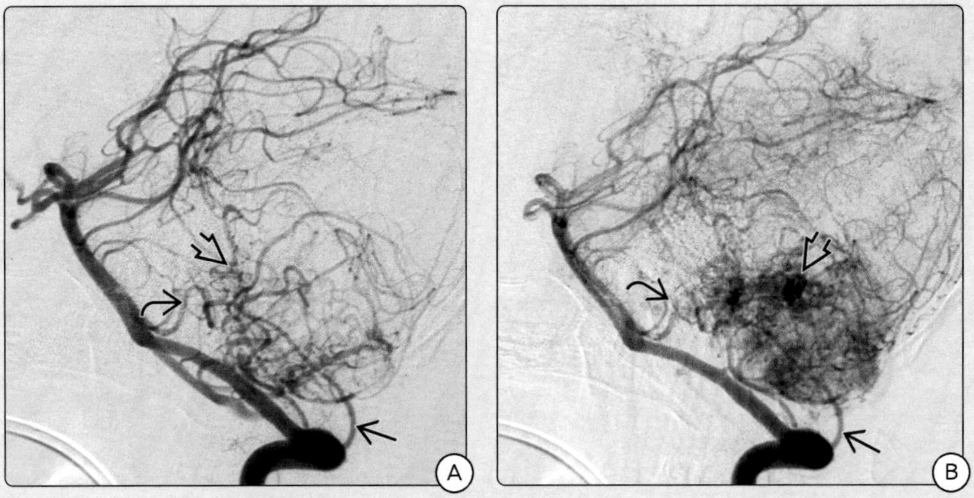

***(22-55A)** Early arterial phase, lateral view of a vertebrobasilar DSA shows a patient with cerebellar hemangioblastoma. Note vascular tumor mass → supplied primarily by enlarged branches of the anterior → and posterior inferior cerebellar arteries →. **(22-55B)** Late arterial phase in the same case shows the characteristic prolonged tumor "blush" → coming from branches of enlarged PICA → and AICA →.*

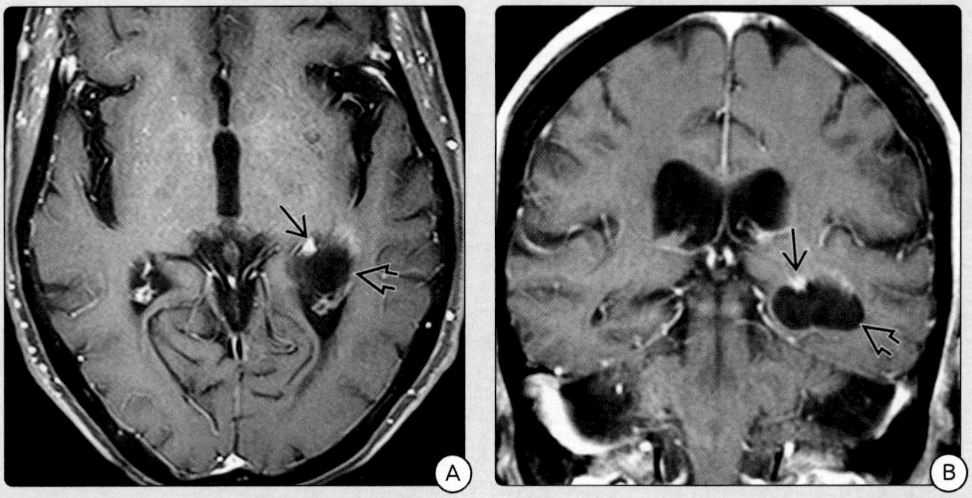

***(22-56A)** Axial T1 C+ FS in an 84y woman with a positive family history of VHL shows a cystic lesion → with an enhancing nodule → in the left posteromedial temporal lobe. **(22-56B)** Coronal T1 C+ MR in the same case shows that the cyst wall → does not enhance, but the nodule enhances strongly, uniformly →. Lesion has been stable for 5 years. This is presumed supratentorial hemangioblastoma in the setting of VHL.*

Louis DN et al: The 2016 World Health Organization Classification of Tumors of the Central Nervous System: a summary. Acta Neuropathol. 131(6):803-20, 2016

Pećina-Šlaus N et al: Molecular genetics of intracranial meningiomas with emphasis on canonical Wnt signalling. Cancers (Basel). 8(7), 2016

Perry A et al: Meningioma. In: Louis DN et al (eds), WHO Classification of Tumours of the Central Nervous System. Lyon, France: International Agency for Research on Cancer, 2016, pp 232-245

Yuzawa S et al: Genetic landscape of meningioma. Brain Tumor Pathol. 33(4):237-247, 2016

Di Vitantonio H et al: Cavernous hemangioma of the dura mater mimicking meningioma. Surg Neurol Int. 6(Suppl 13):S375-8, 2015

Domingues P et al: Genetic/molecular alterations of meningiomas and the signaling pathways targeted. Oncotarget. 6(13):10671-88, 2015

Atypical Meningioma

Garzon-Muvdi T et al: Atypical and anaplastic meningioma: outcomes in a population based study. J Neurooncol. ePub, 2017

Sahm F et al: DNA methylation-based classification and grading system for meningioma: a multicentre, retrospective analysis. Lancet Oncol. 18(5):682-694, 2017

Messerer M et al: Recent advances in the management of atypical meningiomas. Neurochirurgie. 62(4):213-22, 2016

Nanda A et al: Outcome of resection of WHO Grade II meningioma and correlation of pathological and radiological predictive factors for recurrence. J Clin Neurosci. 31:112-21, 2016

Anaplastic Meningioma

Kessler RA et al: Metastatic atypical and anaplastic meningioma: a case series and review of the literature. World Neurosurg. 101:47-56, 2017

Cimino PJ: Malignant progression to anaplastic meningioma: neuropathology, molecular pathology, and experimental models. Exp Mol Pathol. 99(2):354-9, 2015

Nonmeningothelial Mesenchymal Tumors

Antonescu CR et al: Mesenchymal, non-meningothelial tumors. In: Louis DN et al (eds), WHO Classification of Tumours of the Central Nervous System. Lyon, France: International Agency for Research on Cancer, 2016, pp 248-254

Benign Mesenchymal Tumors

Antonescu CR et al: Mesenchymal, non-meningothelial tumors. In: Louis DN et al (eds), WHO Classification of Tumours of the Central Nervous System. Lyon, France: International Agency for Research on Cancer, 2016, pp 248-254

Reinshagen C et al: Intracranial dural based chondroma. J Clin Neurosci. 25:161-3, 2016

Hemangioma

Kirmani AR et al: A unique case of calvarial hemangioma. Surg Neurol Int. 7(Suppl 14):S398-401, 2016

Wang X et al: Convexity dural cavernous haemangioma mimicking meningioma: a case report. Br J Neurosurg. 30(3):345-7, 2016

Malignant Mesenchymal Tumors

Fathalla H et al: Osteomalacia-inducing tumors of the brain: a case report, review and a hypothesis. World Neurosurg. 84(1):189.e1-5, 2015

Solitary Fibrous Tumor/Hemangiopericytoma

Ghose A et al: CNS hemangiopericytoma: a systematic review of 523 patients. Am J Clin Oncol. 40(3):223-227, 2017

Jiang N et al: Solitary fibrous tumor of central nervous system: clinical and prognostic study of 24 cases. World Neurosurg. 99:584-592, 2017

Choi J et al: Hemangiopericytomas in the central nervous system: a multicenter study of Korean cases with validation of the usage of STAT6 immunohistochemistry for diagnosis of disease. Ann Surg Oncol. 23(Suppl 5):954-961, 2016

Fritchie KJ et al: NAB2-STAT6 gene fusion in meningeal hemangiopericytoma and solitary fibrous tumor. J Neuropathol Exp Neurol. 75(3):263-71, 2016

Yalcin CE et al: Solitary fibrous tumor/hemangiopericytoma dichotomy revisited: a restless family of neoplasms in the CNS. Adv Anat Pathol. 23(2):104-11, 2016

Pang H et al: Morphologic patterns and imaging features of intracranial hemangiopericytomas: a retrospective analysis. Onco Targets Ther. 8:2169-78, 2015

Primary Melanocytic Lesions

Koelsche C et al: Melanotic tumors of the nervous system are characterized by distinct mutational, chromosomal and epigenomic profiles. Brain Pathol. 25(2):202-8, 2015

Jaiswal S et al: Primary melanocytic tumors of the central nervous system: a neuroradiological and clinicopathological study of five cases and brief review of literature. Neurol India. 59(3):413-9, 2011

Other Related Neoplasms

Hemangioblastoma

Franco A et al: CNS hemangioblastomatosis in a patient without von Hippel-Lindau disease. CNS Oncol. 6(2):101-105, 2017

Pierscianek D et al: Study of angiogenic signaling pathways in hemangioblastoma. Neuropathology. 37(1):3-11, 2017

Huntoon K et al: Biological and clinical impact of hemangioblastoma-associated peritumoral cysts in von Hippel-Lindau disease. J Neurosurg. 124(4):971-6, 2016

Plate KH et al: Hemangioblastoma. In: Louis DN et al (eds), WHO Classification of Tumours of the Central Nervous System. Lyon, France: International Agency for Research on Cancer, 2016, pp 254-257

She D et al: Differentiating hemangioblastomas from brain metastases using diffusion-weighted imaging and dynamic susceptibility contrast-enhanced perfusion-weighted MR imaging. AJNR Am J Neuroradiol. ePub, 2016

Cranial Nerves and Nerve Sheath Tumors

The 2016 WHO made relatively few changes in the way tumors of the cranial and paraspinal nerves are classified. The four basic categories of ***schwannoma, neurofibroma, perineurioma****, and* ***malignant peripheral nerve sheath tumor*** *were retained. A new category,* ***hybrid nerve sheath tumor****, was added, as such histologically combined tumors are increasingly recognized by neuropathologists. Because* ***melanotic schwannoma*** *is both clinically and genetically distinct from "conventional" schwannoma, it is also now classified as a distinct entity rather than a variant.*

With the exception of vestibular schwannoma, all intracranial nerve sheath tumors are rare. They occur ether sporadically or as part of tumor-associated familial tumor syndromes such as neurofibromatosis types 1 and 2.

The vast majority of nerve sheath neoplasms are benign. The two major tumor types that are found intracranially and at or near the skull base are schwannomas and neurofibromas. Both are discussed in detail here. The third type of benign tumor, perineurioma, is primarily a tumor of peripheral nerves and soft tissues, although rare cases involving cranial nerves have been reported. Perineurioma is briefly considered at the end of this chapter.

Malignant nerve sheath tumors—melanotic schwannoma and the rare intracranial malignant peripheral nerve sheath tumor (MPNST)—are also considered in this chapter.

More than 99% of intracranial nerve sheath tumors are associated with a cranial nerve. Because characteristic imaging findings of these tumors are location specific rather than generic, we begin this chapter with a review of normal cranial nerve anatomy.

Cranial Nerve Anatomy

In this section, we briefly cover cranial nerve (CN) anatomy, beginning our discussion with the upper cranial nerves (CNs I-VI). We then turn to the lower cranial nerves (CNs VII-XII). The function, anatomy, and key clinical/imaging points are delineated for the individual cranial nerves.

The intracranial anatomy of each nerve is discussed segment by segment, from its intraaxial location and exit from the brain, passage through the adjacent CSF cisterns, entrance into or exit from the skull base, and extracranial course. Remember: cranial nerves do *not* stop at the skull base! When imaging cranial neuropathies, it is critically important to image—and carefully evaluate—each segment, following the affected nerve all the way from its origin to its "functional endplate."

Upper Cranial Nerves

Olfactory Nerve (CN I)

Function. The olfactory nerve is a special visceral afferent involved with the sense of smell.

Anatomy. Unmyelinated fibers from bipolar receptor cells high in the nasal vault gather into fascicles, pierce the cribriform plate of the ethmoid bone, and then synapse in the olfactory bulb **(23-1)** **(23-5)**. The olfactory bulb passes posteriorly to the olfactory trigone **(23-4)**. Olfactory stria from the trigone pass into the brain with the largest tract, the lateral olfactory stria, terminating in the temporal lobe.

Olfactory nerves lack a layer of Schwann cells. Instead, special populations of glial cells called "olfactory ensheathing cells" (OECs) that are derived from precursor cells in the embryonic neural crest surround axons of the olfactory nerve. Similar to Schwann cells, Notch signaling pathway gene expression is important during OEC development. OECs resemble Schwann cells on light microscopy, but immunohistochemical staining distinguishes the two. OECs can both migrate and regenerate, enhancing axonal extension after injury.

Key Concepts. Coronal sinus CT that focuses on the nasal vault and cribriform plate is the best examination for isolated anosmia **(23-2)**. MR of the nose, anterior cranial fossae, and medial temporal lobes is the best examination for clinically complicated anosmia **(23-3)**.

Optic Nerve (CN II)

The optic nerve is technically a brain tract, not a true cranial nerve; it is ensheathed and myelinated by oligodendrocytes, not Schwann cells. Tumors of the optic nerve are

(23-1) This is cranial nerve (CN) I. Bipolar olfactory cells cross the cribriform plate and the synapse in the bulb. The olfactory tract divides into stria at the olfactory trigone. (23-2) Coronal bone CT shows the cribriform plate with fenestrations for olfactory bundles to cross from the nose to the synapse in olfactory bulbs.

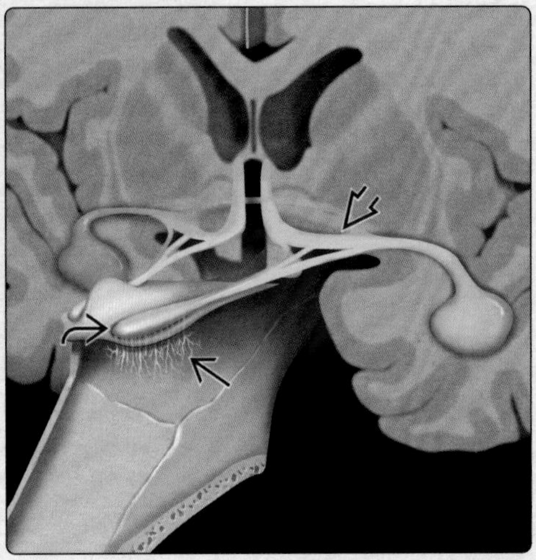

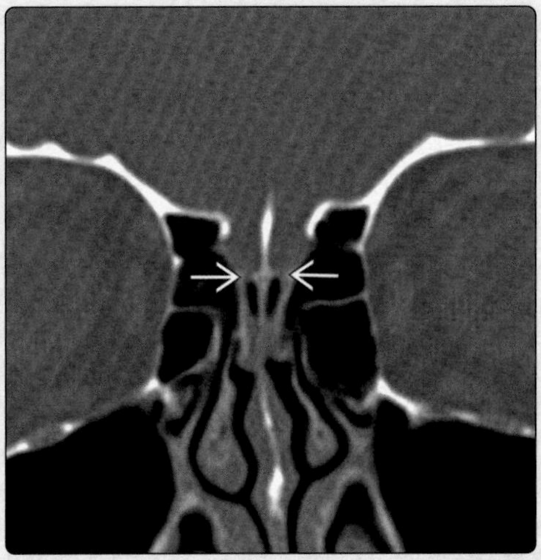

(23-3) Coronal T2FS shows normal olfactory bulbs and olfactory sulci. (23-4) This graphic shows olfactory tracts (CN I), optic chiasm, oculomotor (CN III), trochlear (CN IV), trigeminal, and abducens (CN VI) nerves.

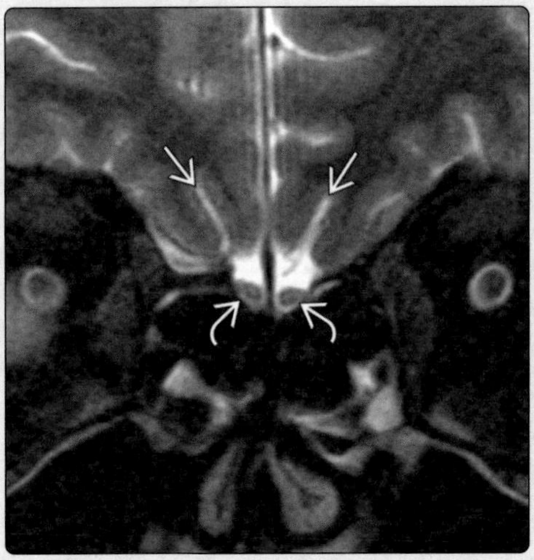

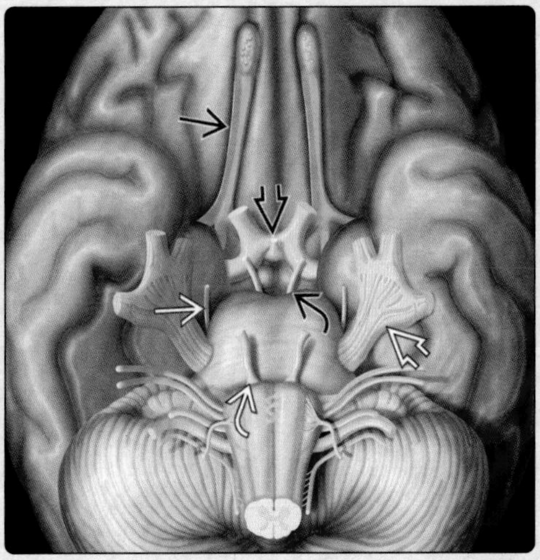

astrocytomas, not schwannomas, and were discussed in Chapter 17.

Function. The optic nerve is the nerve of vision.

Anatomy. The visual pathway consists of the globe/retina, optic nerve, optic chiasm, and retrochiasmal structures. The **intraocular segment** of CN II is surrounded by a sleeve of CSF that connects directly with the intracranial subarachnoid space (SAS). It is covered by the same three meningeal layers as the brain (dura, arachnoid, pia) **(23-9)**. The **intracanalicular segment** of the optic nerve passes through the optic canal **(23-5)** **(23-8)**. The **intracranial (cisternal) segment** extends from the optic canal to the optic chiasm.

The **optic chiasm** is an X-shaped structure that lies in the upper suprasellar cistern. Nerve fibers from the medial half of both retinas cross here, running posterolaterally to the opposite side **(23-11)** **(23-12)**.

The **optic tracts** are posterior extensions of the optic chiasm that curve around the cerebral peduncles. Their lateral bands synapse in the lateral geniculate body (LGB). Efferent axons from the LGB form the optic radiations (geniculocalcarine tracts). The **optic radiations** fan out as they pass posteriorly to terminate in the calcarine cortex (primary visual cortex) along the medial occipital lobes.

Key Concepts. Globe or optic nerve pathology results in **monocular visual loss**. Imaging focus should extend from the globe to the optic chiasm. Intrinsic or extrinsic lesions of the optic chiasm cause **bitemporal heteronymous hemianopsia**, i.e., loss of both temporal visual fields. Retrochiasmal pathology causes **homonymous hemianopsia**, i.e., vision loss that involves either the two right or the two left halves of both visual fields. A left-sided lesion causes *right* homonymous hemianopsia, whereas a right-sided lesion causes *left* homonymous hemianopsia.

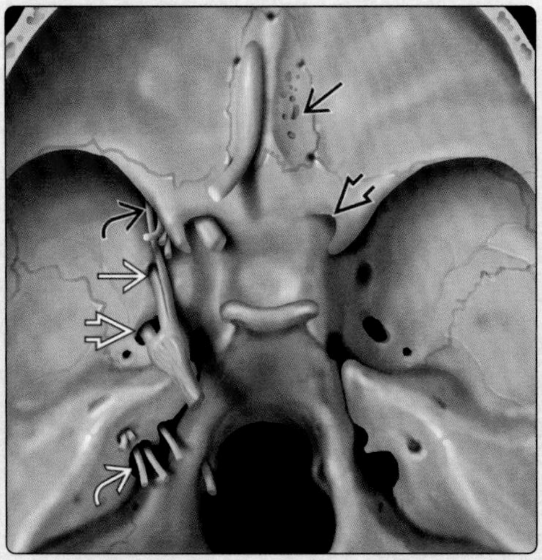

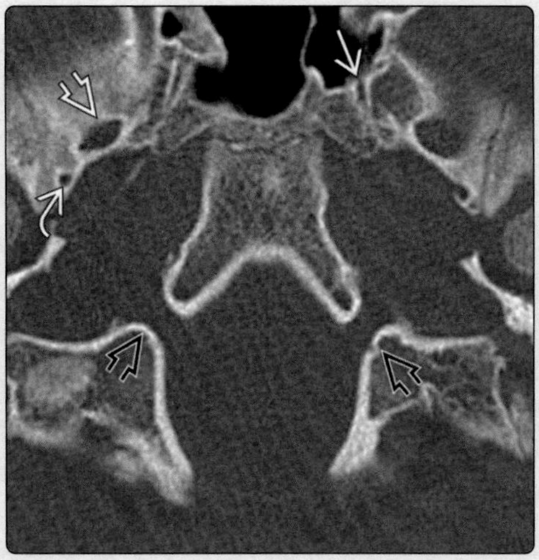

***(23-5)** Axial graphic depicts cranial nerves and the relationship to osseous foramina. Cribriform plate (CN I), optic canal (CN II), superior orbital fissure (SOF) (III, IV, V_1), rotundum (V_2), ovale (V_3), and jugular foramen (IX-XI) are shown. **(23-6)** Axial bone CT through the skull base shows foramen ovale (CN V_3), spinosum (middle meningeal artery), vidian canal, and hypoglossal canals.*

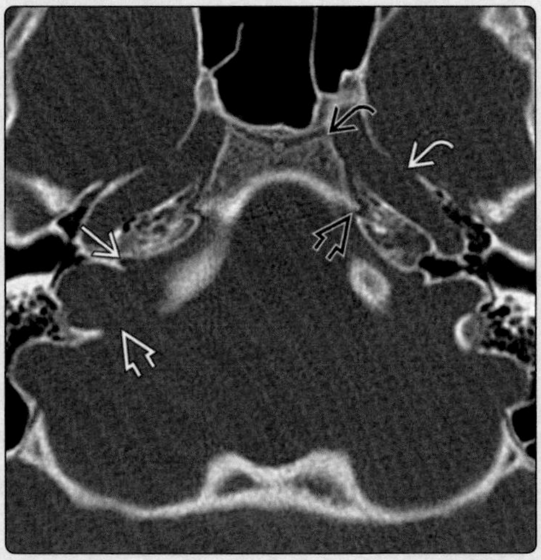

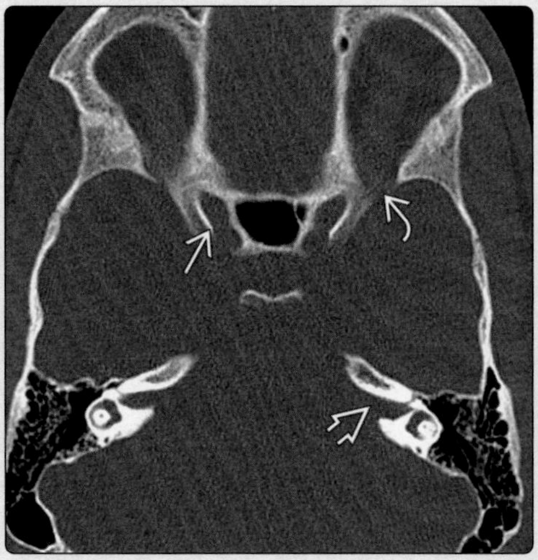

***(23-7)** Bone CT shows the jugular foramen with pars nervosa and pars vascularis. The petrous carotid canals and petro-occipital fissures are also visible. Note the presence of a sphenoccipital synchrondosis. **(23-8)** Bone CT shows the optic canals and internal auditory canals. The section is through the most cephalad aspect of the superior orbital fissures, which are barely visible.*

UPPER CRANIAL NERVES I AND II

Olfactory Nerve (CN I)
- Function = visceral afferent for smell
- Skull entrance = cribriform plate
- Key concept
  - Image the coronal plane from upper nose to temporal lobes

Optic Nerve (CN II)
- Function = vision
- Skull entrance = optic canal
- Key concepts
  - Myelinated brain tract
  - Not ensheathed by Schwann cells
  - Tumors are astrocytomas, not schwannomas

Papilledema is the ocular manifestation of increased intracranial pressure that is transmitted along the SAS of the optic nerve sheath complex. On imaging studies with moderate to severe papilledema, the posterior sclerae become flattened, and the optic nerve head may appear elevated. Accentuated tortuosity and elongation with dilatation of the perioptic SAS are common.

Oculomotor Nerve (CN III)

Function. The oculomotor nerve has both motor and parasympathetic functions. It innervates all the extraocular muscles except the lateral rectus and superior oblique muscles. Its parasympathetic fibers control pupillary sphincter function and accommodation.

Anatomy. The oculomotor nerve has four segments. Its **intraaxial segment** is in the midbrain. The oculomotor nucleus lies just in front of the periaqueductal gray matter. The fascicles of CN III course anteriorly through the red nucleus and substantia nigra, then exit the midbrain medial to the cerebral peduncles **(23-4)**.

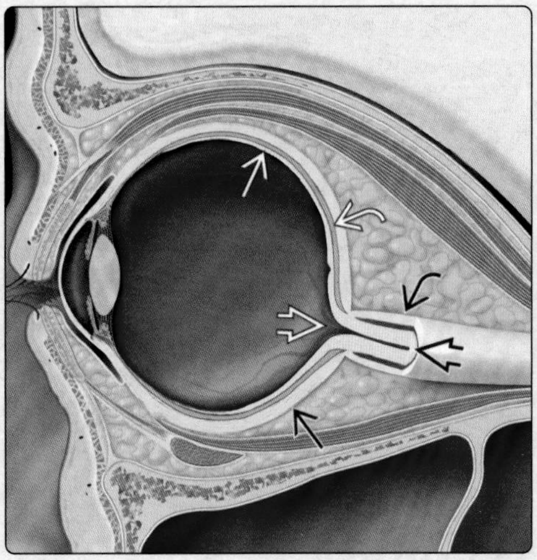

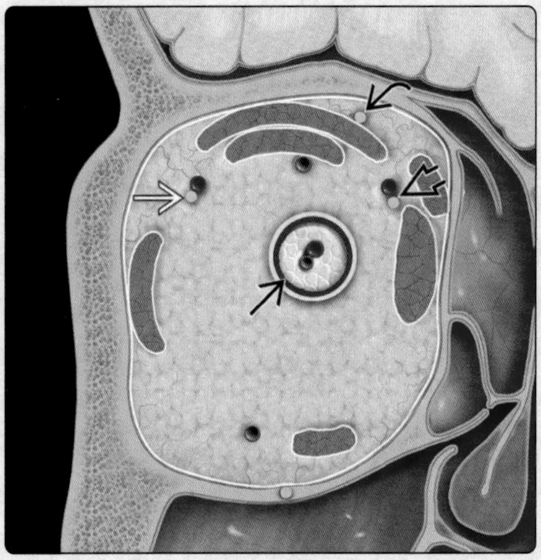

***(23-9)** Sagittal graphic depicts the globe with the optic nerve → inside its dura-arachnoid sheath →. The retina →, choroid →, sclera →, and central retinal artery/vein → are illustrated. The two extraocular muscles just under the orbital roof are the levator palpebrae and superior rectus. The inferior rectus is depicted below. **(23-10)** Coronal graphic shows optic nerve →, IV → frontal nerve (CN V_1) →, and the abducens nerve →.*

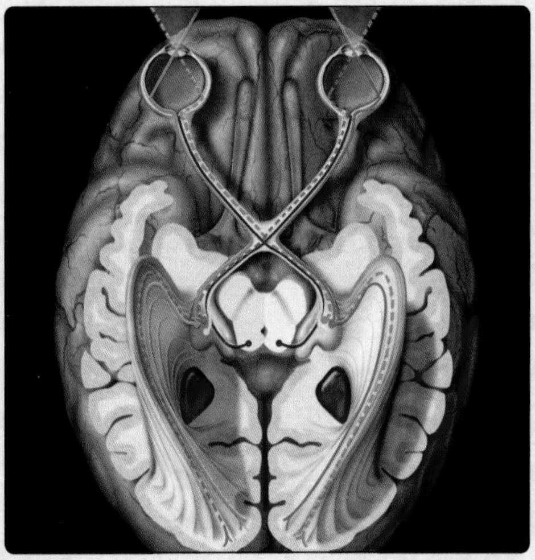

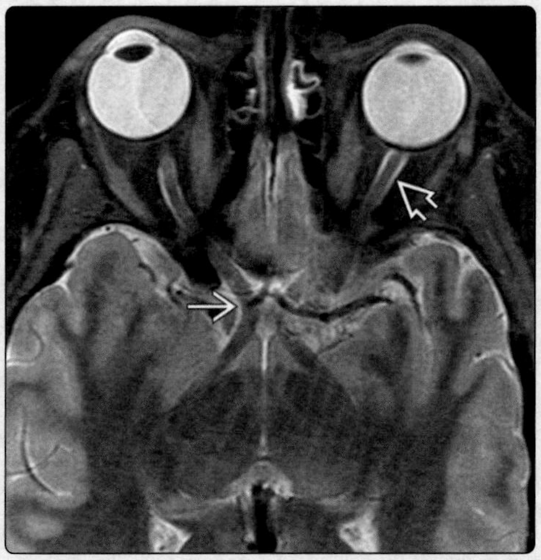

***(23-11)** Graphic depicts the visual system with the fields from the globes to the calcarine cortex. **(23-12)** Axial T2WI shows optic nerves surrounded by CSF in optic nerve sheath →. Optic chiasm → and tracts are also visible.*

The **cisternal segment** courses anteriorly toward the cavernous sinus, passing between the posterior cerebral and superior cerebellar arteries.

The **intracavernous segment** lies in the superolateral wall of the cavernous sinus and is surrounded by a thin sleeve of CSF (the **oculomotor cistern**) **(23-13)** **(23-15)** **(23-16)**. The oculomotor nerve exits the cavernous sinus through the superior orbital fissure **(23-5)**. Its **extracranial segment** passes through the tendinous annulus and then divides into superior and inferior branches. Preganglionic parasympathetic fibers follow the inferior branch to the ciliary ganglion.

Key Concepts. The pupilloconstrictor fibers of CN III are located in the periphery of the nerve, predominantly along its superolateral aspect. The cisternal segment of the oculomotor nerve lies in close proximity to the posterior communicating artery (PCoA). PCoA aneurysms often compress the third nerve, causing **a pupil-involving third nerve palsy. Pupil-sparing third nerve palsy** is commonly caused by microvascular infarction of the core of the nerve with relative sparing of its peripheral fibers.

Trochlear Nerve (CN IV)

Function. The trochlear nerve is a pure motor nerve that innervates the superior oblique muscle.

Anatomy. Like the oculomotor nerve, CN IV has four segments. Its **intraaxial segment** is also in the midbrain, anterior to the periaqueductal gray matter lying just below the oculomotor nerve nuclei. Its fascicles then course posteroinferiorly around the cerebral aqueduct and decussate within the superior medullary velum. The trochlear nerve exits the dorsal midbrain just below the inferior colliculi **(23-14)**.

The **cisternal segment** courses anteriorly in the ambient cistern, adjacent to the free edge of the tentorium. It then passes between the posterior cerebral and superior cerebellar arteries, just inferior to the oculomotor nerve, and enters the

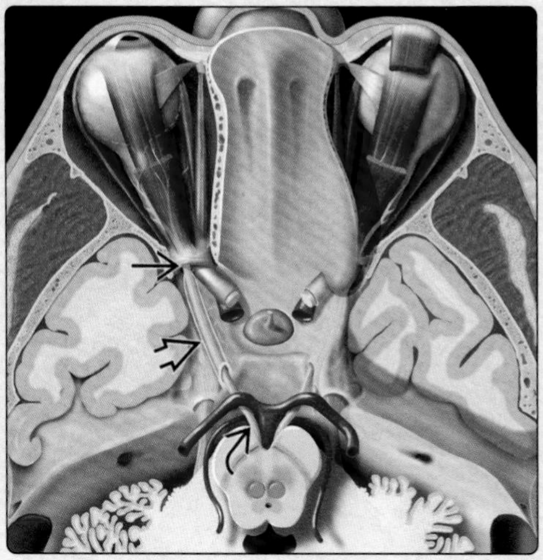

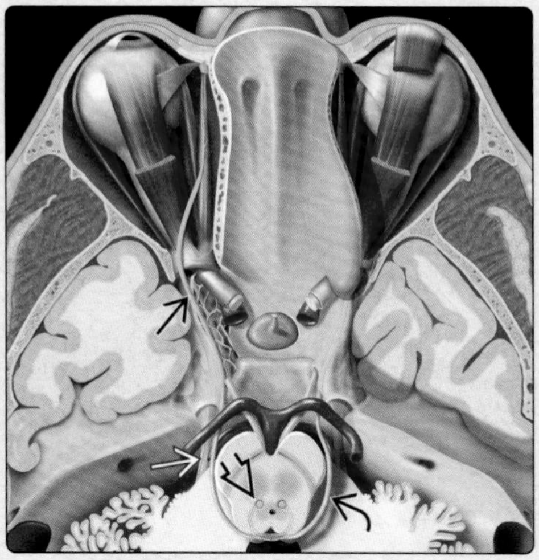

***(23-13)** Graphic shows oculomotor nuclei in midbrain (green) and nerve exiting between posterior and superior cerebellar arteries at interpeduncular fossa and coursing through CSF-filled oculomotor cistern in cavernous sinus to enter the orbit through the SOF. **(23-14)** Graphic shows trochlear nuclei, dorsally exiting and decussating trochlear nerves, trigeminal nerve (CN V), CN IV in cavernous sinus and orbit.*

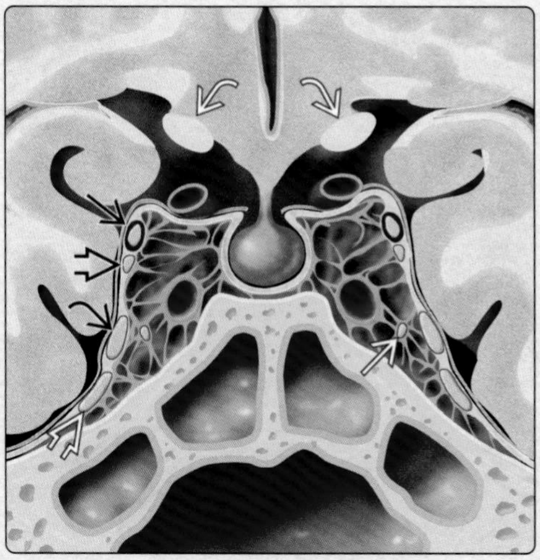

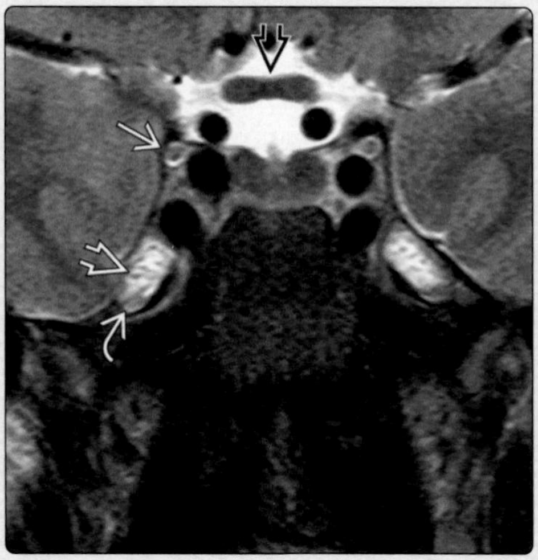

***(23-15)** Except CN VI, cavernous sinus CNs are in lateral dural wall. CNs III surrounded by CSF-filled oculomotor cistern, IV, V_1, and V_2 are shown. Optic tracts pass posteriorly from chiasm and curve around hypothalamus. **(23-16)** Coronal T2 shows CN III in the CSF-filled oculomotor cistern, fascicles of trigeminal nerve in Meckel cave, and gasserian ganglion. Optic chiasm is seen in suprasellar cistern.*

cavernous sinus (CS). The **cavernous segment** lies in the lateral dural wall, just below CN III **(23-15)**.

The trochlear nerve exits the CS through the superior orbital fissure together with CNs III and VI. The **extracranial segment** then passes above the tendinous annulus of Zinn (CNs III and VI pass through the ring) **(23-14)**.

Key Concepts. The long course of the cisternal segment and its proximity to the hard knife-like edge of the tentorium make the trochlear nerve especially vulnerable to injury during closed head trauma. Trochlear palsy causes superior oblique paralysis, resulting in outward rotation (extorsion) of the affected eye. The resulting diplopia and weakness of downward gaze causes most patients to compensate by tilting their heads away from the affected side. Look for trochlear neuropathy in patients with torticollis ("wry neck").

Trigeminal Nerve (CN V)

Function. The trigeminal nerve is a mixed sensory and motor nerve. It is the major sensory nerve of the head and face and innervates the muscles of mastication.

Anatomy. The trigeminal nerve has four segments: a ganglion (the semilunar ganglion) and three postganglionic divisions **(23-19)**.

The **intraaxial segment** has four nuclei (three sensory and one motor) that are located in the brainstem and upper cervical spinal cord (between C2 and C4).

CN V emerges from the lateral pons at the root entry zone. The **cisternal segment** courses anteriorly through the prepontine cistern. It then passes through a dural ring, the porus trigeminus, to enter Meckel cave **(23-17)** **(23-18)**.

The **interdural segment** lies entirely within **Meckel cave**, a CSF-filled, dura-arachnoid-lined outpouching from the

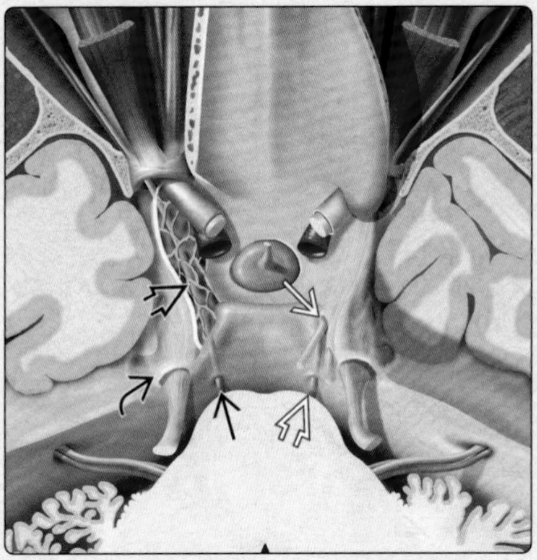

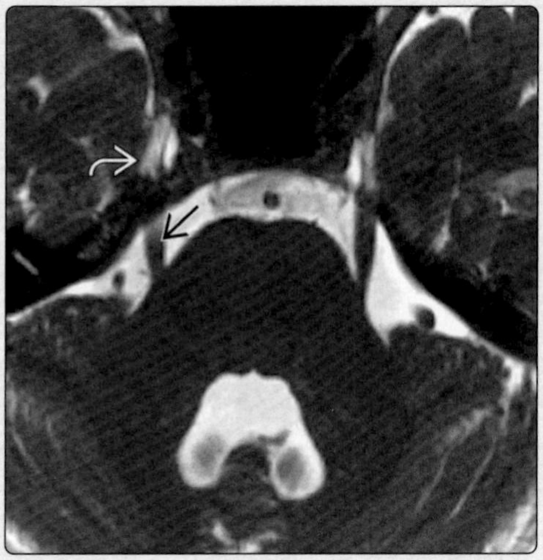

(23-17) *Axial graphic shows abducens nerve (CN VI) exiting at pontomesencephalic junction, coursing across the prepontine cistern to Dorello canal, ascending under the dura to cross the petrous apex, and course through the cavernous sinus to the SOF. CN V in Meckel cave, CN III, and CN IV are also shown.* ***(23-18)*** *Axial T2WI shows the cisternal and Meckel cave segments of the trigeminal nerve.*

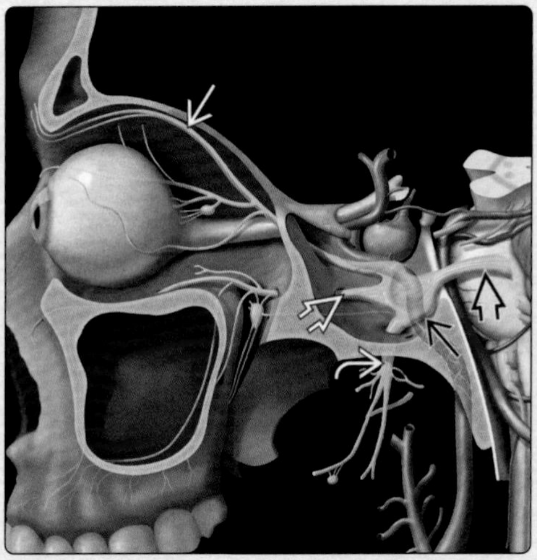

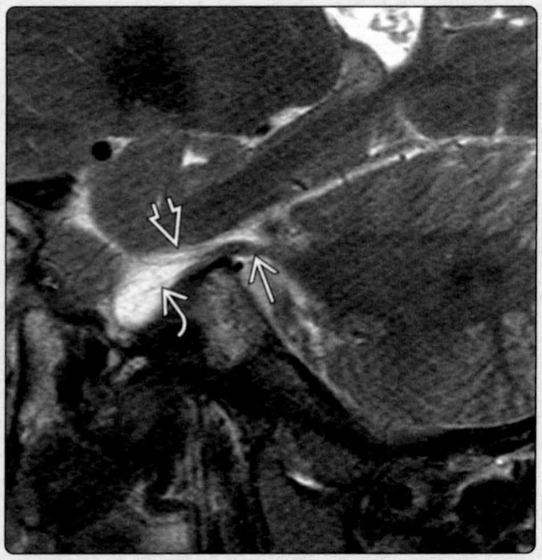

(23-19) *Graphic shows trigeminal nerve branches V_1, V_2, and V_3, cisternal segment, and the gasserian ganglion in Meckel cave.* ***(23-20)*** *Sagittal T2 FS MR shows the trigeminal nerve trunk as it crosses the cerebellopontine angle (CPA) cistern toward the pons. Meckel cave is CSF-filled and is continuous with the CPA cistern. Note individual nerve fascicles of CN V within Meckel cave.*

prepontine SAS. Once inside Meckel cave, CN V separates into several discrete fascicles **(23-16)** **(23-20)**. It then synapses in the **trigeminal (gasserian** or **semilunar) ganglion**, a small crescent of tissue that lies at the bottom of Meckel cave.

The **postganglionic segment** of CN V consists of three divisions: CN V_1 (ophthalmic nerve), CN V_2 (maxillary nerve), and CN V_3 (mandibular nerve).

The **ophthalmic nerve** lies in the lateral cavernous sinus wall just below CN IV. It passes anteriorly toward the orbital apex and exits the CS through the **superior orbital fissure**. The ophthalmic nerve is a pure sensory nerve, innervating the scalp, forehead, nose, and globe.

The **maxillary nerve** courses anteriorly in the lateral dural wall of the CS, just below CN V_1. It exits through the **foramen rotundum**, traversing the upper aspect of the pterygopalatine fossa. It enters the orbit and courses anteriorly in the infraorbital groove, exiting through the infraorbital foramen. The maxillary nerve supplies sensation to the cheek and upper teeth.

The **mandibular nerve** exits Meckel cave directly from the semilunar ganglion, passing inferiorly through the foramen ovale. Unlike the other two postganglionic divisions, CN V_3 does *not* pass through the CS. The mandibular nerve is both motor and sensory, supplying the muscles of mastication, the mylohyoid, and the anterior belly of the digastric. Its most important sensory innervations involve the teeth and tongue.

Key Concepts. Be alert for denervation atrophy (shrinkage, fatty infiltration) of the muscles of mastication. That may be the first imaging indication of CN V_3 neuropathy and should prompt further evaluation. (Meckel cave lesions are a common cause.)

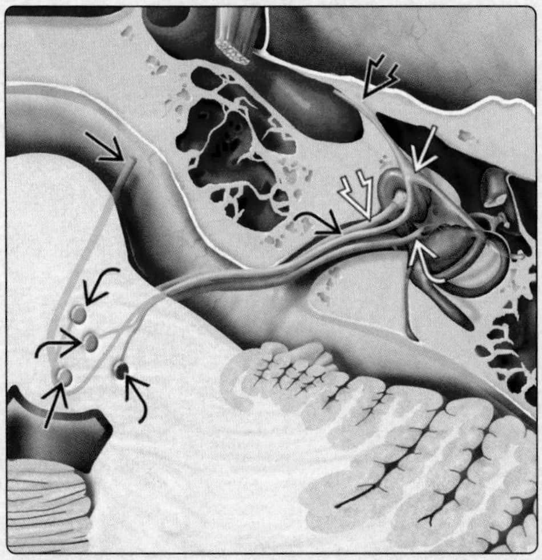

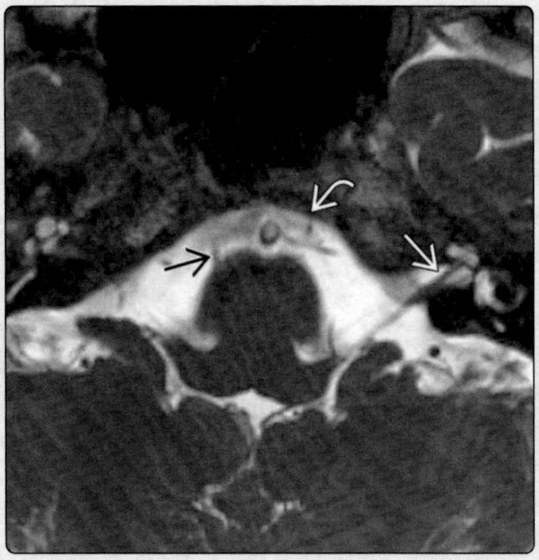

***(23-21)** CN VI nerve/nucleus is shown. CN VII nuclei/internal auditory canal (IAC) segment, geniculate ganglion, greater superficial petrosal nerve (GSPN), and CN VIII cochlear and vestibular nerves can all be seen. **(23-22)** Axial T2WI at the level of the pontomedullary junction shows the right VI nerve and the left CN VI as it heads into Dorello canal. The cochlear nerve is also well seen on this image.*

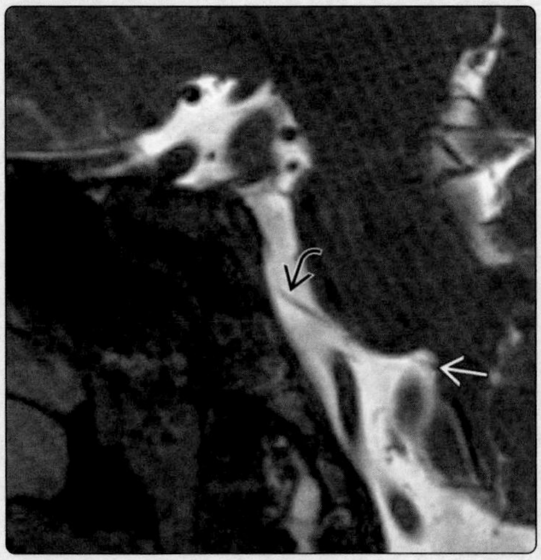

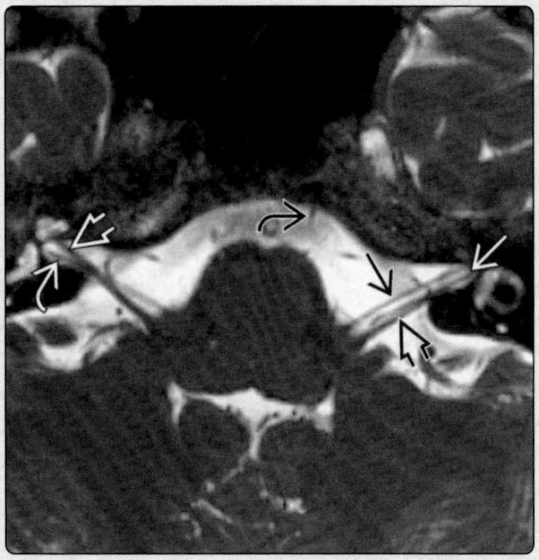

***(23-23)** Sagittal T2WI shows CN VI as it exits anteriorly from the pontomedullary junction and crosses the prepontine cistern toward Dorello canal. **(23-24)** T2WI shows left CN VI and VII, vestibulocochlear, and superior vestibular nerves, and right cochlear, inferior vestibular nerves.*

Abducens Nerve (CN VI)

Function. The abducens nerve is a pure motor nerve. It provides innervation to the lateral rectus muscle (abduction).

Anatomy. The abducens nerve has five segments. The **intraaxial segment** begins in the CN VI nuclei, which are located in the pons, just anterior to the fourth ventricle. Axons of CN VII loop around the abducens nuclei, creating the "bump" in the floor of the fourth ventricle called the facial colliculus **(23-21)**.

Fibers from the abducens nuclei course directly anteriorly, emerging from the brainstem just lateral to the midline at the pontomesencephalic junction.

The **cisternal segment** of CN VI ascends anterosuperiorly through the prepontine cistern, then penetrates the clival dura **(23-17)** **(23-23)**. The **interdural segment** of CN VI courses superiorly between the two layers of dura in a shallow channel known as **Dorello canal**. The abducens nerve then crosses over the top of the petrous apex just below the petrosphenoidal ligament to enter the CS.

The **cavernous segment** courses anteriorly within the CS itself, the only cranial nerve to do so (the others are embedded within the lateral dural wall). Inside the CS, the abducens nerve lies along the inferolateral aspect of the internal carotid artery **(23-15)**.

CN VI exits the CS through the superior orbital fissure. The **intraorbital segment** passes anteriorly through the tendinous ring that attaches the extraocular muscles.

Key Concepts. Simple (i.e., isolated) abducens palsy is the most common ocular motor nerve palsy. A "pseudo" sixth nerve palsy (inability to abduct the eye) is usually caused by an infiltrative lesion in the lateral rectus muscle itself.

(23-25) CN VII GSPN, chorda tympani, stapedius nerve, and stylomastoid foramen are all shown. Distal branches ramify within the parotid gland. (23-26) Solitary nucleus to chorda tympani (taste), superior salivatory nucleus to GSPN (lacrimation), and motor nucleus/nerve are all shown in this graphic.

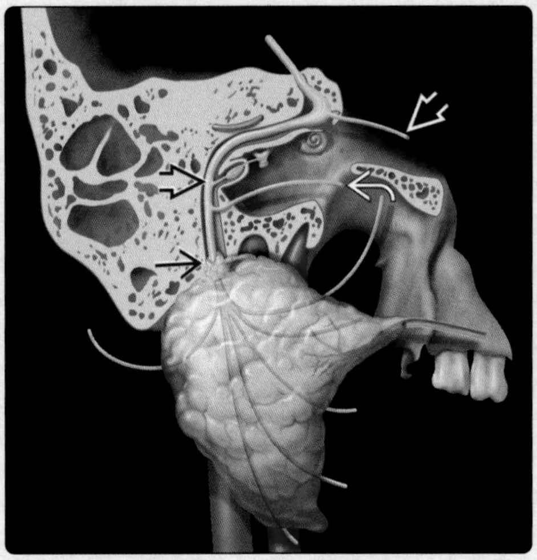

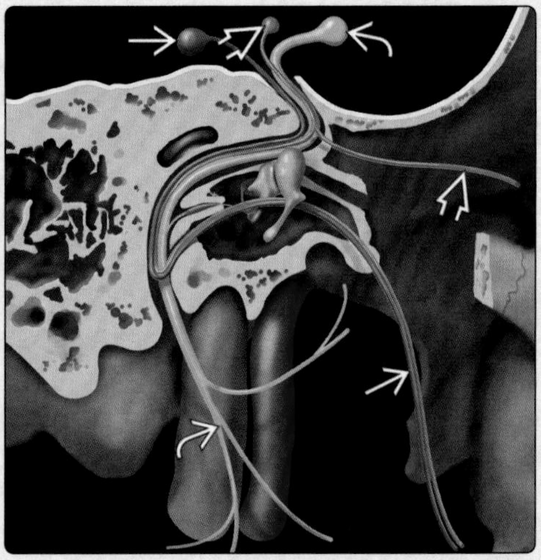

(23-27) Bone CT shows tympanic segment under lateral semicircular canal and the mastoid segment descending to the stylomastoid foramen. (23-28) Axial temporal bone CT shows the bony labyrinthine segment of CN VII and its anterior genu for the geniculate ganglion.

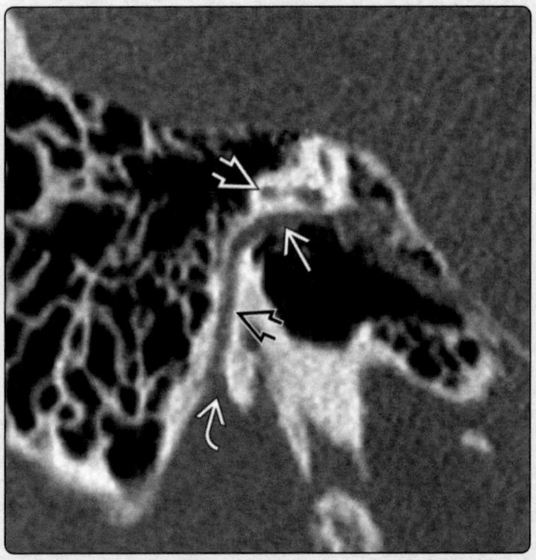

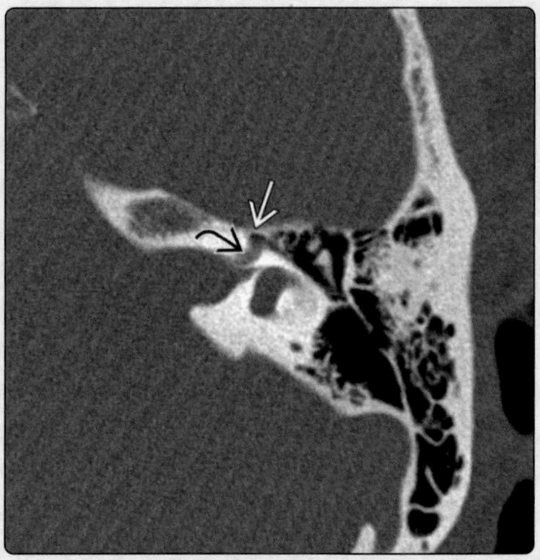

In its course over the petrous apex, the abducens nerve is vulnerable to increased intracranial pressure and inflammation in the adjacent temporal bone ("apical petrositis").

UPPER CRANIAL NERVES III-VI

Oculomotor Nerve (CN III)
- Function
  - Innervates all extraocular muscles, except lateral rectus, superior oblique
- Skull exit = superior orbital fissure (SOF)
- Key concept
  - Is neuropathy pupil-involving or pupil-sparing?

Trochlear Nerve (CN IV)
- Function = innervates superior oblique muscle
- Skull exit = SOF
- Key concept
  - Head tilt/torticollis can be caused by CN IV injury

Trigeminal Nerve (CN V)
- Function (mixed motor, sensory)
  - Innervates muscles of mastication
  - Sensory from head, face
- Skull exits
  - Ophthalmic (CN V_1) = SOF
  - Maxillary (CN V_2) = foramen rotundum
  - Mandibular (CN V_3) = foramen ovale
- Key concepts
  - Look at face!
  - Denervation atrophy of masticator muscles

Abducens Nerve (CN VI)
- Function = innervates lateral rectus
- Skull exit = SOF
- Key concepts
  - Intrinsic lateral rectus disease can mimic CN VI palsy
  - ↑ Intracranial pressure, apical petrositis can cause abducens palsy

Lower Cranial Nerves

Facial Nerve (CN VII)

Function. The facial nerve has multiple functions. It provides motor innervation to the muscles of facial expression. It provides parasympathetic innervation to the lacrimal, submandibular, and sublingual glands. It also provides a special sensory function, i.e., taste, to the anterior two-thirds of the tongue.

Anatomy. The facial nerve has four segments. The **intraaxial segment** consists of the facial nerve nuclei that lie in the ventrolateral pons. Efferent fibers from the motor nucleus loop dorsally around the abducens nucleus, then pass anterolaterally to exit the brainstem at the pontomedullary junction **(23-21)**.

The **cisternal segment** of CN VII courses laterally through the cerebellopontine angle (CPA) together with the vestibulocochlear nerve (CN VIII) to the internal auditory canal (IAC) **(23-24)**.

The **intratemporal facial nerve** follows a complex course, first coursing laterally as the *IAC segment* and the most anterosuperior of the four nerves within the IAC **(23-30) (23-34)**. It then exits the bony IAC, bending anteriorly and becoming the *labyrinthine segment*. At its most anterior bend (which is called the "anterior genu"), the facial nerve synapses in the geniculate ganglion and then courses posteriorly under the lateral semicircular canal as the *tympanic segment* **(23-25) (23-28)**. It curves inferiorly at the "posterior genu" and descends in the mastoid as the *mastoid segment* **(23-27)**.

The important intratemporal branches of the facial nerve from top to bottom are the **greater superficial petrosal nerve** (parasympathetic fibers that supply the lacrimal gland), the **stapedius nerve** (innervation of the stapedius muscle), and the **chorda tympani** (taste from the anterior two-thirds of the tongue) **(23-26)**.

The facial nerve exits the skull at the stylomastoid foramen, then enters the parotid gland. Once inside the gland, the **extracranial facial nerve** ramifies into its terminal motor branches, which innervate the muscles of facial expression **(23-25)**.

Key Concepts. Facial nerve enhancement within the CPA cistern or IAC is always abnormal. With the exception of the labyrinthine segment, a robust vascular plexus surrounds most of the intratemporal facial nerve. Therefore, the facial nerve is the only cranial nerve with segments that may exhibit some enhancement following contrast administration.

If the bony intratemporal CN VII canal is normal, mild enhancement of the geniculate ganglion and tympanic and mastoid segments is considered normal. The geniculate ganglion enhances in 75% of cases, and tympanic segment enhancement occurs in half of all cases. The mastoid segment nearly always enhances. Segmental facial nerve enhancement is more conspicuous at higher field strengths (3.0 T).

The first step in facial nerve imaging requires clinical input. When imaging is requested for "facial nerve palsy," detailed information is key. Typical Bell palsy (i.e., of short duration, uncomplicated by other CN neuropathy) does not need imaging.

It is essential to know whether a facial nerve deficit is central ("upper motor neuron") or peripheral ("lower motor neuron"). *Upper* (central or supranuclear) motor neuron injury, due to a parenchymal lesion above the brainstem, results in paralysis of the contralateral muscles of facial expression but spares the forehead. Stroke is a common cause of upper motor neuron facial palsy.

Lower motor neuron injury can involve CN VII at any point from its brainstem nucleus through its peripheral branches. Lower motor neuron facial palsy involves paralysis of all ipsilateral muscles of facial expression. In such cases, imaging should extend from the brainstem through the parotid gland.

If a lower motor neuron facial injury is present, further information regarding the so-called special functions of the facial nerve is essential. Are taste and lacrimation intact? Does

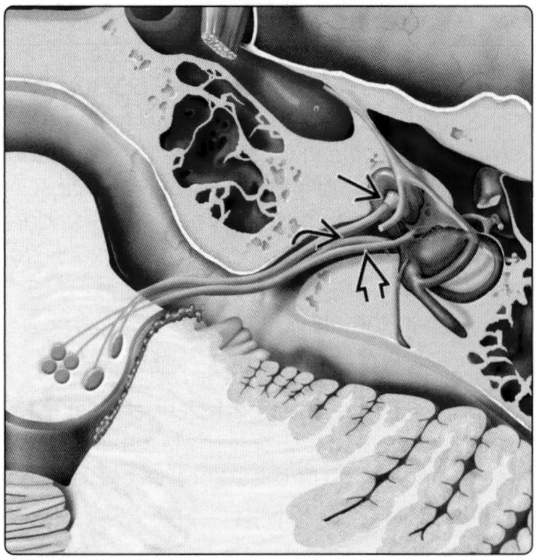

(23-29) CN VIII. Cochlear nerve/modiolus ➔, inferior ➔/superior ➔ vestibular nerves, nuclei in medulla, tracts in inferior cerebellar peduncle.

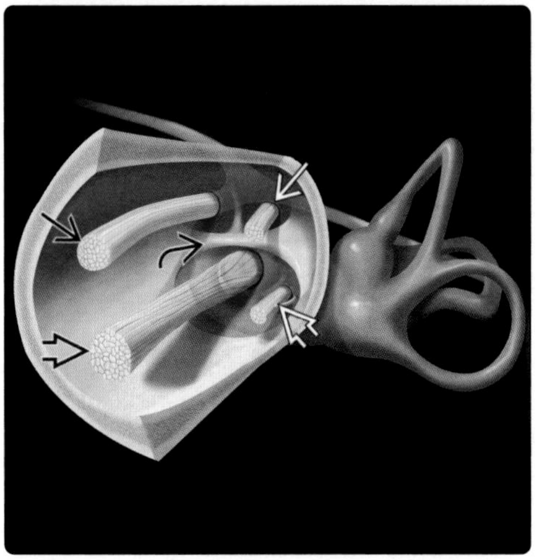

(23-30) Bony IAC with facial nerve (CN VII) ➔, cochlear nerve (CN VIII) ➔, superior ➔/inferior ➔ vestibular nerves, crista falciformis ➔.

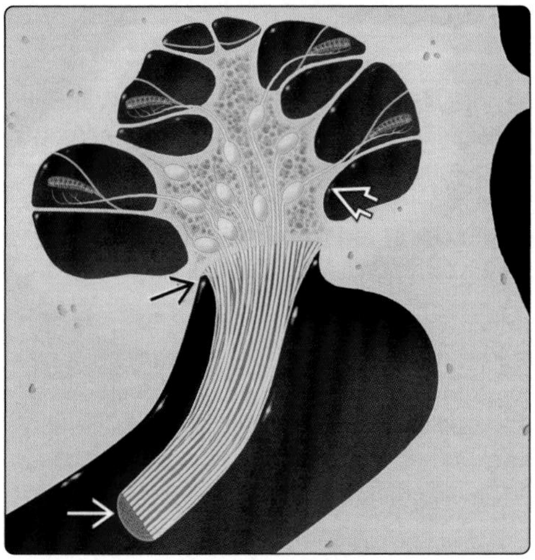

(23-31) Cochlea with modiolus ➔, cochlear nerve ➔, and aperture ➔. Spiral ganglion cells are shown in yellow within the modiolus.

the patient have hyperacusis? If these special functions are spared, the cause of a lower motor neuron facial palsy is extracranial.

If the special functions are affected, knowing exactly which ones are involved helps localize lesion extent. Malignant parotid tumors—especially adenoid cystic carcinoma—have a marked propensity to enter the stylomastoid foramen and invade up the intratemporal facial nerve.

The most distal of the intratemporal facial nerve branches is the chorda tympani, which is affected first. Loss of taste in the anterior tongue results. As tumor progresses more cephalad, the next affected branch is the stapedius nerve. Hyperacusis results. As tumor reaches the geniculate ganglion, the greater superficial petrosal nerve is compromised, resulting in problems with lacrimation.

A lesion proximal to the geniculate ganglion will cause facial paralysis and affect all three special functions.

If a complete lower neuron facial palsy is complicated by CN VI and/or CN VIII involvement, the lesion is most likely in the pons (CN VI) or CPA-IAC (CN VIII).

CRANIAL NERVES VII AND VIII

Facial Nerve (CN VII)

- Functions
  - Motor (muscles of facial expression)
  - Special sensory (taste, anterior 2/3 of tongue)
  - Parasympathetics (lacrimal, submandibular, sublingual glands)
- Skull exit
  - Exits through stylomastoid foramen into IAC along with CN VIII
- Key concepts
  - Typical Bell palsy does not require imaging
  - CN VII neuropathy? Ask if upper or lower motor neuron
  - Parotid malignancies "creep up" facial nerve
  - Special functions affected (taste, hyperacusis, lacrimation)?

Vestibulocochlear Nerve (CN VIII)

- Function = afferent sensory nerve
  - Hearing (cochlear nerve)
  - Balance (vestibular nerve)
- Skull entrance = internal auditory canal
  - Most anteroinferior = cochlear nerve
  - Posterior = superior, inferior vestibular nerves
- Key concepts
  - MR in vestibular nerve dysfunction usually negative
  - Unilateral sensorineural hearing loss with lesion on MR → 95% vestibulocochlear schwannomas

Vestibulocochlear Nerve (CN VIII)

Function. The vestibulocochlear nerve is purely sensory. It is the afferent sensory nerve responsible for hearing and the sense of balance.

Anatomy. CN VIII has two major components, the **cochlear nerve** and the **vestibular nerve (23-29) (23-30)**. Unlike the other cranial nerves, CN VIII is best described from outside to inside (peripheral to central).

The **cochlear nerve** arises from the spiral ganglion in the modiolus of the cochlea. Its fibers pass through the cochlear aperture into the IAC **(23-31)**. The cochlear nerve is the most anteroinferior of the four nerves in the IAC **(23-34)**. Near the opening of the IAC, the porus acusticus, the cochlear nerve joins the superior and inferior vestibular nerves to form the vestibulocochlear nerve.

The **vestibular nerve** arises from bipolar neurons in the vestibular ganglion at the IAC fundus. Its fibers coalesce to form the **superior** and **inferior vestibular nerves**, which are separated by a bony bar called the falciform (transverse) crest. The superior and inferior vestibular nerves course medially in the posterior aspect of the IAC **(23-32)** **(23-33)**. At the porus acusticus, they join with the cochlear nerve to form CN VIII.

CN VIII passes medially through the CPA cistern and enters the lateral brainstem at the pontomedullary junction to become the **intraaxial segment**. The cochlear nuclei are found in the restiform body at the lateral surface of the inferior cerebellar peduncle. The vestibular nuclei lie along the inferior floor of the fourth ventricle.

Key Concepts. At least 90-95% of all lesions that cause unilateral sensorineural hearing loss—and are detected on imaging—are vestibulocochlear schwannomas. Isolated vestibular nerve dysfunction (dizziness, vertigo, balance problems) usually does not have positive findings on MR. "Conductive" (intracochlear) hearing loss is best evaluated by high-resolution multiformatted temporal bone CT.

Glossopharyngeal Nerve (CN IX)

Function. The glossopharyngeal nerve is small but has complex functions. It is a special sensory nerve (responsible for taste in the posterior third of the tongue) as well as a regular sensory nerve (innervating middle ear, pharynx). It carries parasympathetic fibers to the parotid gland and is the motor supply to the stylopharyngeus muscle. Last but by no means least, it is viscerosensory to the carotid body and sinus.

Anatomy. Like most of the other cranial nerves, CN IX has four segments: intraaxial, cisternal, skull base, and extracranial.

CN IX has four nuclei. All are in the upper and middle medulla, anterolateral to the inferior fourth ventricle. The **intraaxial segment** consists of these nuclei plus their tracts. The tracts course anterolaterally from the nuclei to exit or enter the medulla in the postolivary sulcus.

The **cisternal segment** travels toward the jugular foramen, coursing just above the vagus nerve. The glossopharyngeal nerve exits the skull by passing into the anterior aspect (pars nervosa) of the jugular foramen **(23-7)** **(23-35)**. In its **skull base segment**, the glossopharyngeal nerve lies adjacent to the inferior petrosal sinus. Its **extracranial segment** courses inferiorly through the carotid space.

Key Concepts. In the coronal plane, the jugular tubercles and basiocciput form a construct that resembles the head, beak, and body of an eagle. CN IX (together with CNs X and XI) courses through the jugular foramen, which lies superolateral to the eagle's "head" and "beak." The hypoglossal canal lies under the eagle's "head," at the "neck" formed by the "beak" above and the "body" below **(23-36)** **(23-37)**.

Vagus Nerve (CN X)

Function. The vagus nerve is also a mixed nerve with sensory (ear, larynx, viscera), special (taste from epiglottis), motor (most of soft palate, superior and recurrent laryngeal nerves), and parasympathetic (regions of head/neck, thorax, abdominal viscera) functions.

Anatomy. The **intraaxial segment** of the vagus nerve lies in the inferior medulla. Its nuclei lie in front of the inferior fourth ventricle. Fibers to and from the nuclei exit the medulla in the postolivary sulcus. Its **cisternal segment** courses anterolaterally through the medullary cistern, lying between the glossopharyngeal nerve above and the bulbar portion of the spinal accessory nerve (CN XI) below.

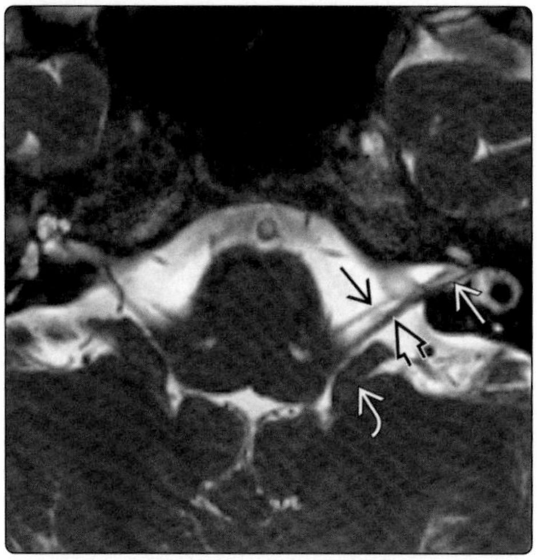

***(23-32)** Axial T2WI shows CN VII ⇒, vestibulocochlear nerve (CN VIII) ⇒, superior vestibular nerve ➡, flocculus of cerebellum ➡.*

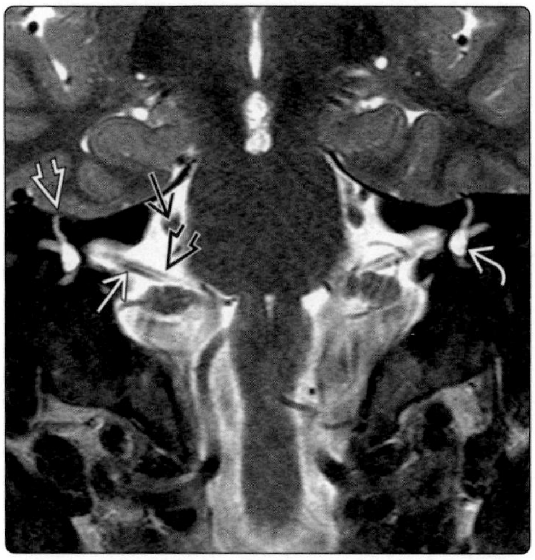

***(23-33)** Coronal T2WI shows CN V ⇒, CN VII ⇒, CN VIII ➡, vestibule ➡, and superior semicircular canal ➡.*

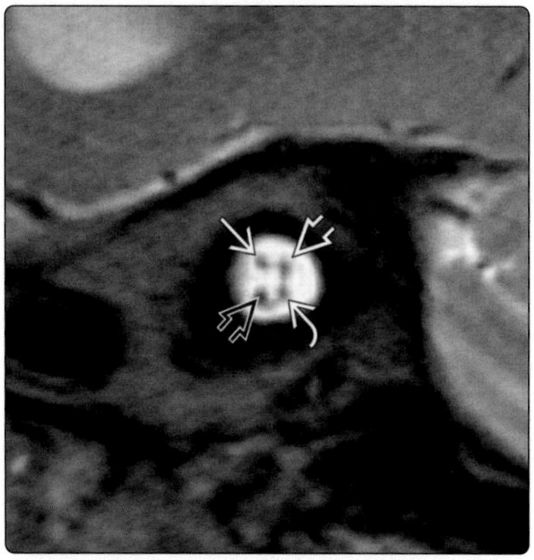

***(23-34)** Sagittal T2WI of mid IAC shows 4 nerves as "dots" in CSF: CN VII ➡, superior ➡ and inferior ➡ vestibular nerves, cochlear nerve ⇒.*

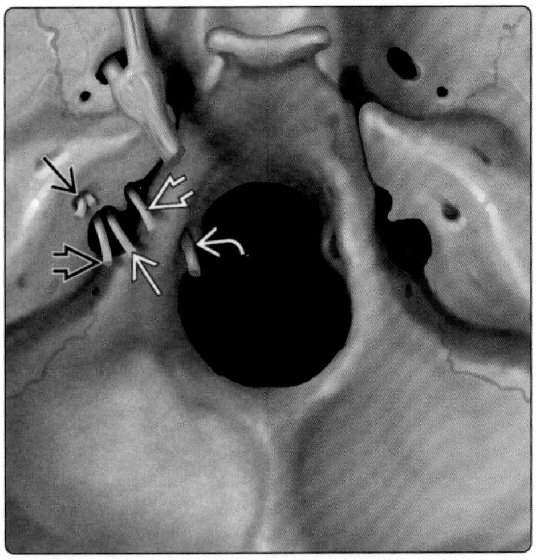

(23-35) Lower CNs, foramina are shown: CNs VII and VIII in IAC ⇒, CNs IX ⇒, X ⇒, XI ⇒ in jugular foramen, CN XII ⇒ in hypoglossal canal.

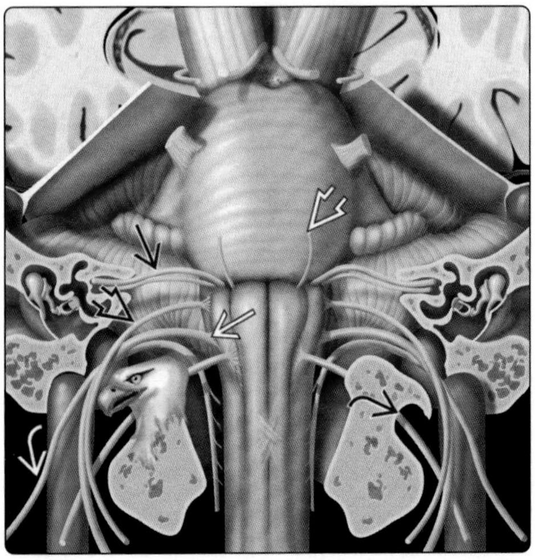

(23-36) CNs VI ⇒, VII, VIII ⇒, IX ⇒, X ⇒, XI ⇒, and XII ⇒ are shown. Jugular tubercle looks like the head of an eagle.

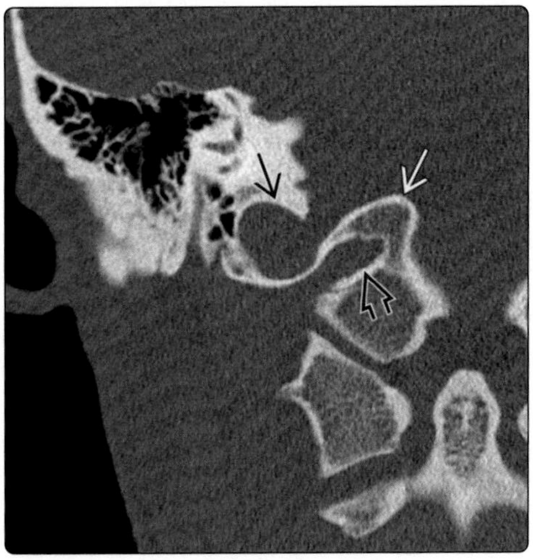

(23-37) CNs IX/X/XI exit jugular foramen ⇒ on top of jugular tubercle ⇒ (eagle's "head"). CN XII exits hypoglossal canal ⇒ under eagle's "beak."

Its **skull base segment** begins where CN X enters the posterior aspect (pars vascularis) of the jugular foramen. It lies anteromedial to the jugular bulb. CN X exits the jugular foramen into the carotid space. It descends, passing under the aortic arch on the left and the subclavian artery on the right. The recurrent laryngeal nerves on both sides then turn cephalad to course superiorly in the tracheoesophageal groove.

CRANIAL NERVES IX, X, AND XI

Glossopharyngeal Nerve (CN IX)

- Functions
  - Taste/sensation to posterior 1/3 of tongue
  - Sensory to middle ear/pharynx
  - Parasympathetic to parotid gland
  - Motor to stylopharyngeus
  - Viscerosensory to carotid body/sinus
- Skull exit
  - Jugular foramen (pars nervosa)
- Key concepts
  - Isolated CN IX neuropathy very rare
  - Usually occurs with CNs X, XI neuropathy
  - Look for medullary cistern, skull base lesion

Vagus Nerve (CN X)

- Functions
  - Sensory (ear, larynx, viscera)
  - Taste (epiglottis)
  - Motor (innervates soft palate, pharyngeal constrictors, larynx)
  - Parasympathetic (head/neck, thorax, abdomen)
- Skull exit
  - Jugular foramen (pars vascularis)
- Key concepts
  - Proximal neuropathy: image medulla to hyoid
  - Distal neuropathy: image through subclavian artery (right), aortopulmonary window (left)

Spinal Accessory Nerve (CN XI)

- Function
  - Motor to sternomastoid, trapezius
- Skull exit/entrance
  - Spinal component enters through foramen magnum
  - Unites with bulbar portion
  - Both exit through jugular foramen (pars vascularis)
- Key concepts
  - May be injured during radical neck dissection
  - Look for ipsilateral trapezius atrophy

Key Concepts. Proximal vagal neuropathy requires imaging from the medulla to the level of the hyoid. If multiple cranial nerves (CNs IX-XII) are affected, the culprit lesion is usually in the medullary cistern or skull base (jugular foramen), where all four nerves are in close proximity.

Distal vagal neuropathy is usually isolated and manifests as laryngeal dysfunction (look for a paramedian vocal cord). It requires imaging from the level of the hyoid all the way to the carina/aortopulmonary window on the left and the subclavian artery on the right.

Spinal Accessory Nerve (CN XI)

Function. The spinal accessory nerve is a pure motor nerve that innervates the sternomastoid and trapezius muscles.

Anatomy. CN XI has **two intraaxial segments** that arise from two different sets of nuclei, one in the medulla and the other in the proximal cervical cord. Bulbar fibers arise from the nucleus ambiguus in the medulla **(23-38)**. Spinal fibers originate from the spinal nucleus, a column of cells along the anterior horn extending from C1-C5 **(23-39)**.

The **two cisternal segments** of CN XI initially follow different courses. The bulbar fibers exit the medulla at the postolivary sulcus **(23-40)** and course anterolaterally through the basal cistern together with CNs IX and X. The spinal fibers emerge from the lateral aspect of the cervical spinal cord and course superiorly **(23-41)**. Both fiber bundles then unite in the basal cistern. The **skull base segment** of CN XI passes through the posterior part (pars vascularis) of the jugular foramen, together with the vagus nerve and jugular bulb **(23-44)**.

The **extracranial segment** begins as the glossopharyngeal nerve exits the jugular foramen into the carotid space.

Key Concepts. CN XI is often injured during radical neck dissection. Look for trapezius atrophy and compensatory hypertrophy of the ipsilateral levator scapulae.

Hypoglossal Nerve (CN XII)

Function. The hypoglossal nerve is a pure motor nerve that innervates both the intrinsic and most of the extrinsic (styloglossus, hyoglossus, genioglossus) tongue muscles. The only exception is the geniohyoid muscle, which is innervated by the C1 spinal nerve.

Anatomy. The hypoglossal nerve has four distinct segments. The intraaxial, cisternal, and skull base segments are relatively short. The extracranial segment is by far the longest and most complex portion of CN XII.

The **intraaxial segment** of CN XII begins at the hypoglossal nucleus. The hypoglossal nucleus lies just under the hypoglossal eminence of the inferior fourth ventricle. Fibers course anteriorly across the medulla and exit at the preolivary (ventrolateral) sulcus to enter the medullary (basal) cistern.

The **cisternal segment** extends from its exit at the medulla through the basal cistern to the entrance of the hypoglossal canal **(23-41)**. Accompanied by a prominent venous plexus, the **skull base segment** of CN XII passes through the **hypoglossal canal**, which is located in the occipital bone beneath the jugular tubercle and jugular foramen **(23-42)** **(23-43)**.

The **extracranial segment** of the hypoglossal nerve descends in the posterior aspect of the carotid space. It exits the carotid space between the carotid artery and the internal jugular vein, then runs anteroinferiorly toward the hyoid bone to provide motor innervation to the tongue muscles.

HYPOGLOSSAL NERVE (CN XII)

Function
- Motor to tongue muscles

Skull Exit = Hypoglossal Canal
- At base of occipital bone
- Below jugular tubercle, jugular foramen

Key Concepts
- Look for ipsilateral denervation tongue atrophy
- Shrunken, fatty infiltration

Key Clinical/Imaging Concepts. CN XII is most readily identified on axial images. The clival cortex takes an abrupt right-angle turn anterolaterally and

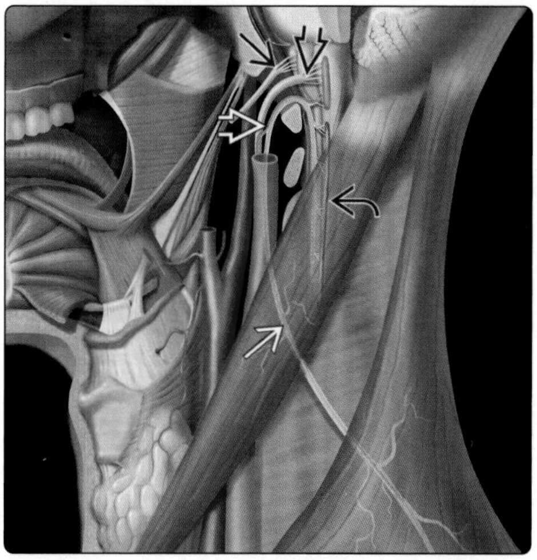

***(23-38)** CNs IX ➙, X ➙, XI ➙. Bulbar CN XI ➙ crosses to CN X and joins spinal root from spinal accessory nucleus of CN XI ➙ in jugular foramen.*

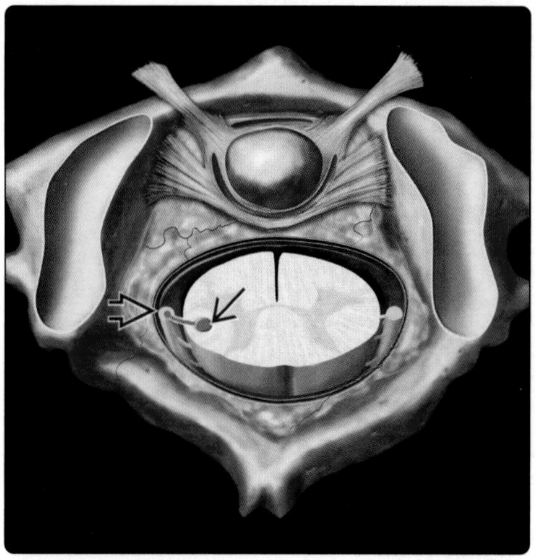

***(23-39)** The spinal nucleus of CN XI ➙ sends rootlets to form the spinal root of the accessory nerve ➙.*

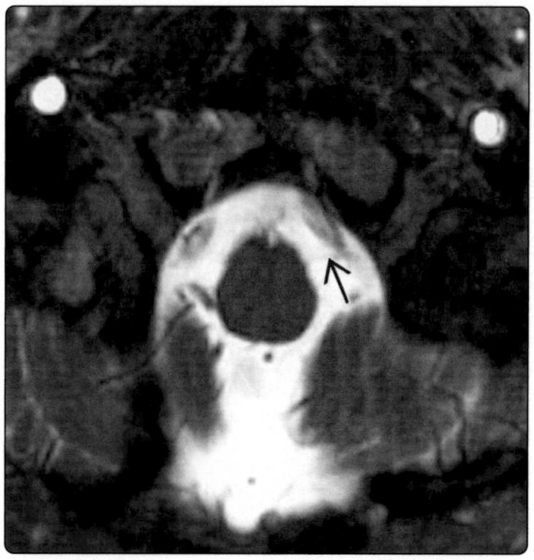

***(23-40)** Axial T2WI demonstrates the left bulbar CN XI segment ➙ exiting the postolivary sulcus.*

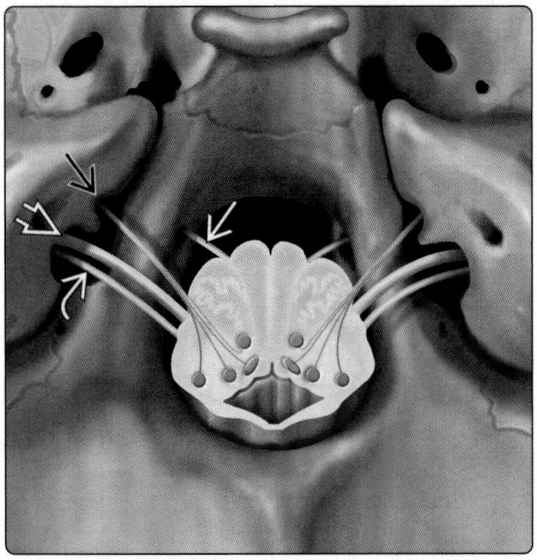

***(23-41)** CN XII exits medulla at preolivary sulcus. CN IX is in pars nervosa of jugular foramen . CNs X and XI are in the pars vascularis.*

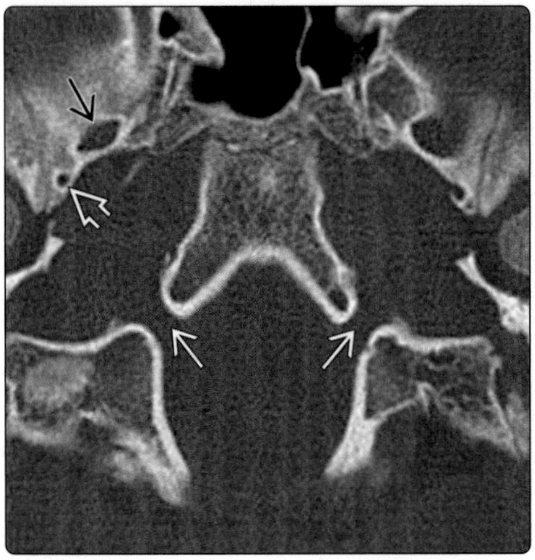

***(23-42)** Axial bone CT shows hypoglossal canals . Foramen ovale (CN V_3), foramen spinosum (middle meningeal artery) are also seen.*

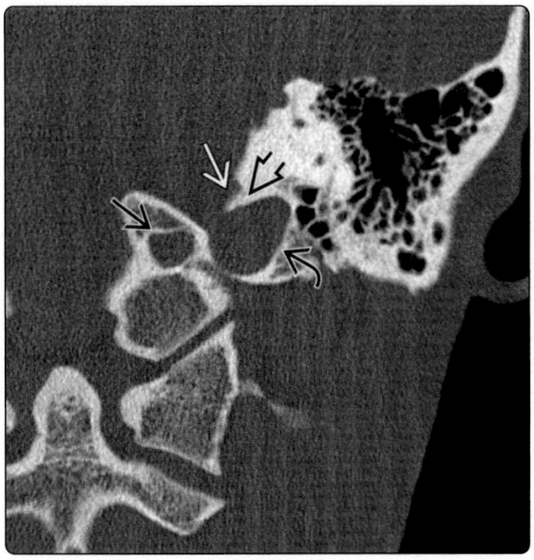

***(23-43)** Hypoglossal canal (CN XII exit), jugular foramen, jugular spine . CN IX exits pars nervosa , CNs X, XI exit pars vascularis .*

forms the medial wall of the short, obliquely oriented hypoglossal canal **(23-42)**.

In the coronal plane, the jugular tubercle and occipital condyle form a visual construct that resembles the head, beak, and body of an eagle. The hypoglossal canal and nerve are located between its "head" and "beak" **(23-37)** **(23-43)**.

A hypoglossal lesion causes atrophy of the ipsilateral tongue muscles. Look for fatty infiltration and volume loss.

Schwannomas

Neuropathologists now recognize four histologic subtypes of schwannoma: conventional, cellular, plexiform, and melanocytic. The vast majority of schwannomas that involve cranial nerves are the conventional type. With the exception of melanotic schwannoma, imaging findings do not distinguish between histologic subtypes. Rather, conventional intracranial schwannomas are distinguished—and discussed here—according to their cranial nerve of origin.

Because the pathology of intracranial schwannomas is similar, we discuss it and other shared features before delving into specific schwannomas.

Schwannoma Overview

Terminology

Schwannomas are benign slow-growing encapsulated tumors that are composed entirely of well-differentiated Schwann cells. Less common terms are neurinoma and neurilemmoma.

Etiology

General Concepts. Schwannomas originate from Schwann cells, which are derived from precursor cells in the embryonic neural crest. Schwannomas may arise along the course of any peripheral nerve or cranial nerves III-XII. Because the olfactory and optic nerves do not contain Schwann cells, schwannomas do not arise from CNs I and II. The rare reported cases of "olfactory groove schwannomas" are probably tumors that arise from olfactory ensheathing cells.

Schwann cells are also not a component of normal brain parenchyma. The exceptionally rare intraparenchymal schwannoma is thought to arise from neural crest remnants that later express aberrant Schwann cell differentiation. Intramedullary (spinal cord) schwannomas are more common than intraparenchymal brain schwannomas.

Genetics. The neurofibromatosis type 2 (NF2) tumor suppressor Merlin is a protein whose loss results in defective morphogenesis and tumorigenesis in multiple tissues. Genetic studies have linked both sporadic and NF2-associated schwannomas [especially vestibular schwannomas (VSs)] to the *NF2* tumor suppressor gene located on chromosome 22. Approximately half of NF2 cases represent new mutations, suggesting a high mutation rate in this gene.

Biallelic inactivation (the classic "two-hit mechanism") of the *NF2* gene is also detected in nearly all sporadic vestibular schwannomas and 50-70% of meningiomas.

Inherited Tumor Syndromes. The most common tumor predisposition syndrome that causes multiple schwannomas is **NF2**. The presence of bilateral VSs is pathognomonic of NF2. One VS and a first-degree relative

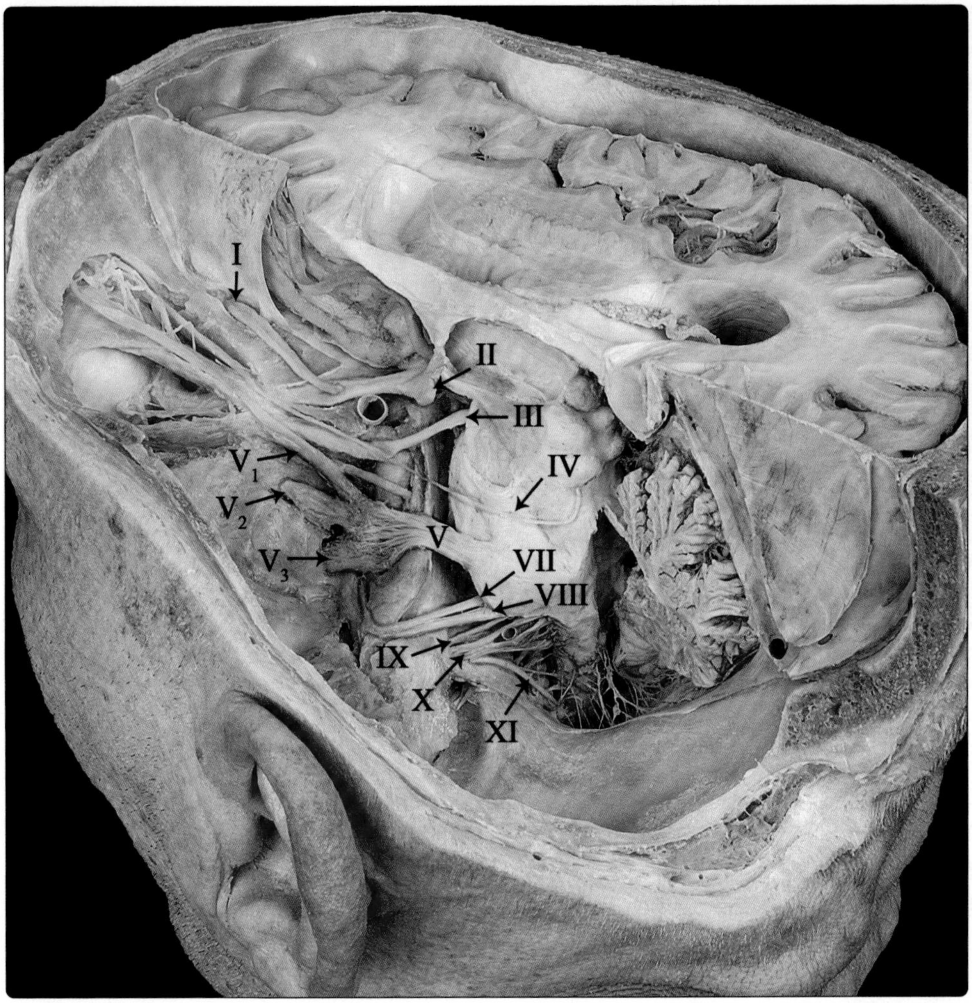

(23-44) Olfactory nerve (I), optic chiasm (II), oculomotor nerve (III), trochlear nerve (IV) coursing anteriorly in the ambient cistern, and the trigeminal nerve (V) with its ophthalmic (V_1), maxillary (V_2), and mandibular (V_3) branches are shown. Abducens (VI) and hypoglossal (XII) nerves are not visualized. CPA segments of the facial (VII) and vestibulocochlear (VIII) nerves are shown. Glossopharyngeal (IX), vagus (X), and spinal accessory (XI) nerves course toward the jugular foramen. (Courtesy M. Nielsen, MS.)

with NF2 or a VS in combination with another cranial nerve schwannoma, meningioma, or glioma is also indicative of NF2.

Schwannomatosis is a condition with multiple peripheral, often painful schwannomas without other features of NF2. These patients have no evidence of VS, no first-degree relative with NF2, and no known constitutional *NF2* mutation.

Schwannomatosis occurs in 2-4% of patients with schwannomas. Both sporadic and familial forms of schwannomatosis occur and can be associated with both nonvestibular intracranial and spinal schwannomas.

Patients with schwannomatosis tend to be younger than those who present with solitary schwannomas. The average age at onset is 28.5 years.

Plexiform schwannoma, also known as **multinodular schwannoma**, is a Schwann cell tumor in which multiple (2-50) circumscribed lesions occur along an affected nerve fascicle. Most are dermal-subcutaneous tumors of the extremities, trunk, head, and neck. Brain lesions have not been reported.

Approximately 90% of plexiform schwannomas are sporadic with 5% associated with NF2 and 5% with schwannomatosis. Unlike patients with NF1 and plexiform neurofibromas, there is no known predilection for malignant degeneration of plexiform schwannomas.

Carney complex (CNC) or Carney syndrome (MIM) is a rare autosomal-dominant syndrome characterized by pigmented lesions of the skin and mucosa, cardiac, cutaneous, and other myxomas, and multiple endocrine tumors. Melanotic schwannomas occur in up to 10% of patients with CNC.

Pathology

Location. Schwannomas arise at the glial-Schwann cell junction of CNs III-XII. The distance from the brain to the interface where the glial covering terminates and Schwann cell ensheathing begins varies with each cranial nerve. In some—such as the oculomotor nerve (CN III)—the junction is in close proximity to the brain. Here schwannomas arise close to the exit of the parent nerve from the brain. In others—such as the vestibulocochlear nerve (CN VIII)—the junction lies at some distance from the nerve exit or entrance into the brainstem.

Sensory nerves are much more commonly affected by schwannomas compared with pure motor cranial nerves. The vestibulocochlear nerve is by far the most common

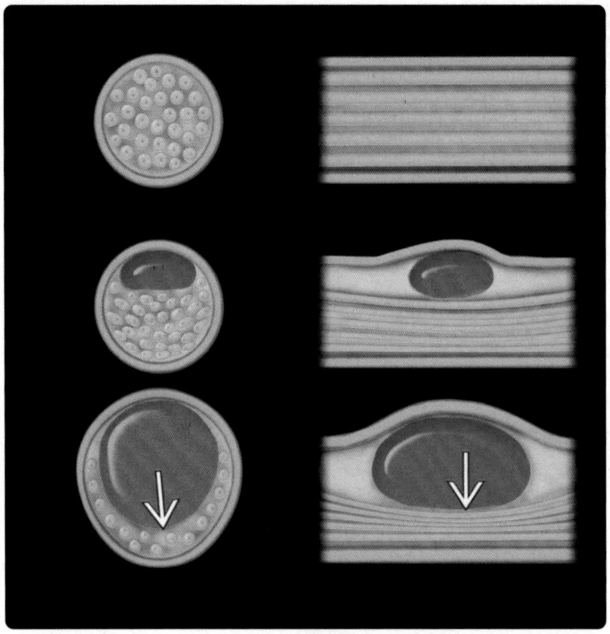

(23-45) Axial (L) and sagittal (R) graphics show a schwannoma arising within a unifascicular nerve. The tumor displaces other nerve fibers peripherally ➡.

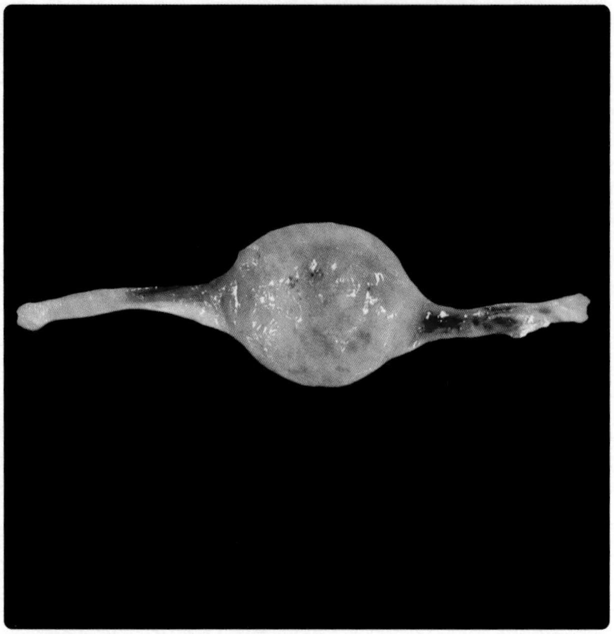

(23-46) Schwannomas are encapsulated by perineurium and epineural collagen and grow eccentrically to the nerve of origin. (From DP: Neuropathology, 2e.)

intracranial site (90%). The second most common site is the trigeminal nerve (CN V) (2-4%).

INTRACRANIAL SCHWANNOMAS

Synonyms
- Neurilemoma, neurinoma

Epidemiology
- Vestibular (CN VIII) most common (95%)
  - All other sites combined (1-5%)
- Trigeminal (CN V) second most common
- Jugular foramen (CNs IX, X, XI) third
- Hypoglossal (CN XII) fourth
- All others rare except in neurofibromatosis type 2
- Intraparenchymal schwannomas very rare

Pathology
- Arise at glial-Schwann cell junction
  - Distance from brain varies according to cranial nerve
- Benign encapsulated nerve sheath tumor
- Well-differentiated neoplastic Schwann cells
- Biphasic histology with 2 components
  - Compact, highly ordered cellularity ("Antoni A")
  - Less cellular, myxoid matrix ("Antoni B")

Schwannomas of cranial nerves other than CN VIII and CN V are very rare, accounting for just 1-2%. As a group, jugular foramen schwannomas (i.e., schwannomas arising from the glossopharyngeal, vagal, and spinal accessory nerves) are the third most common, followed by facial (CN VII) and hypoglossal (CN XII) schwannomas. In the absence of NF2, schwannomas of CNs III, IV, and VI are all very rare.

Intraparenchymal and intraventricular schwannomas occur but are extremely uncommon.

Size and Number. Most intracranial schwannomas are small, especially those that arise from motor nerves. Some, especially trigeminal schwannomas, can attain huge size and involve both intra- and extracranial compartments.

Most schwannomas occur singly in otherwise healthy individuals and are termed "sporadic" or "solitary" schwannomas. The presence of multiple schwannomas in the same individual suggests an underlying tumor predisposition syndrome.

Gross Pathology. Schwannomas arise eccentrically from their parent nerves and are smooth or nodular well-encapsulated lesions **(23-45)** **(23-46)**. Cystic change is common, as is yellow discoloration due to lipidization. Microhemorrhages occur, but gross macroscopic bleeds are rare.

Microscopic Features. A biphasic pattern is typical of **conventional schwannoma**. The "Antoni A" pattern consists of compact fascicles of elongated spindle cells that demonstrate occasional nuclear palisading (Verocay bodies). A less cellular, loosely textured, more haphazard arrangement with clusters of lipid-laden cells is called the "Antoni B" pattern **(23-48)**. Mitotic figures are rare. Immunohistochemistry is characterized by strong diffuse positivity for S100 protein.

Cellular schwannoma consists mostly of "Antoni A" tissue but lacks Verocay bodies. Such tumors may demonstrate hypercellularity and minor nuclear atypia. Frequent mitotic figures and increased proliferative indices can be seen in young children. Cellular schwannomas do not undergo malignant transformation.

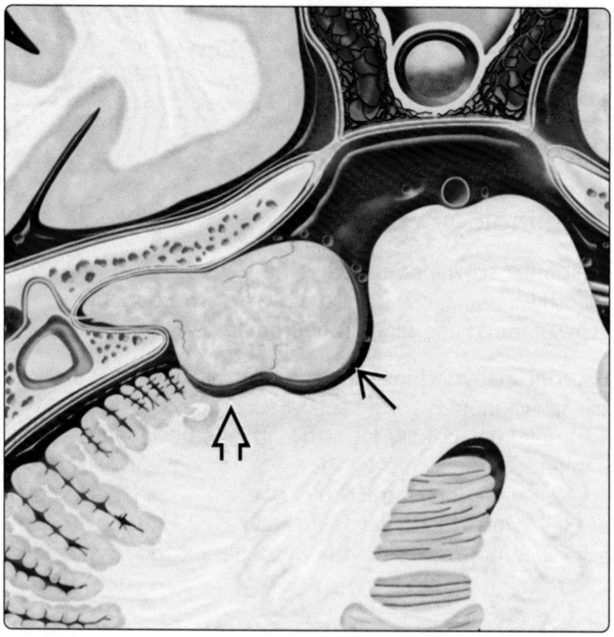

(23-47) Graphic of a large vestibular schwannoma shows the typical "ice cream on cone" morphology. Note the prominent CSF-vascular "cleft" between the middle cerebellar peduncle ➡ and the cerebellar hemisphere ⇨.

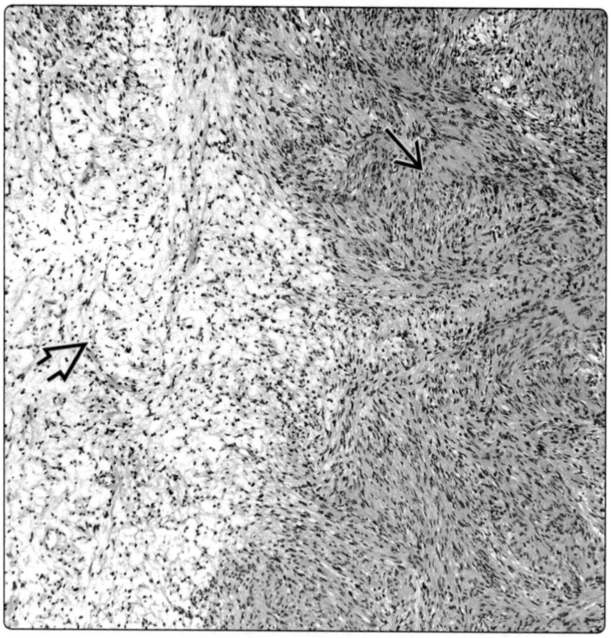

(23-48) The juxtaposition of the cellular "Antoni A" ➡ and loose "Antoni B" ⇨ patterns is classic for conventional schwannoma. (From DP: Neuropathology, 2e.)

Plexiform schwannoma can be either conventional or cellular type.

Staging, Grading, and Classification. Conventional schwannomas correspond to WHO grade I.

Clinical Issues

Epidemiology. The vast majority of schwannomas occur outside the CNS, most often in the skin and subcutaneous tissues. Intracranial schwannomas are relatively uncommon, constituting about 7% of all primary neoplasms.

Demographics. All ages are affected, but the peak incidence is in the fourth to sixth decades. Schwannomas do occur in children but are uncommon unless associated with NF2. There is no sex predilection.

Presentation. Many schwannomas are asymptomatic, and any symptoms are location specific. As schwannomas favor sensory nerves, motor symptoms are rare. Vestibular schwannoma, the most common intracranial schwannoma **(23-47)**, presents with sensorineural hearing loss (see below).

Natural History. Schwannomas are benign tumors that tend to grow very slowly. The exception is VSs in young patients with NF2. These tumors have higher MIB-1 indices.

Recurrence after complete surgical removal of a conventional schwannoma is uncommon. Roughly 30-40% of cellular schwannomas recur after subtotal resection but do not undergo malignant transformation.

Schwannomas rarely—if ever—undergo malignant degeneration. Most "malignant intracerebral schwannomas" are probably malignant peripheral nerve sheath tumors (see below).

Approximately 10% of melanotic schwannomas are malignant. In approximately half of these cases, the patients have **Carney complex**, an autosomal-dominant disorder characterized by lentiginous facial pigmentation, cardiac myxoma, and endocrine overactivity (e.g., precocious puberty, pituitary adenoma with acromegaly, and Cushing syndrome with multinodular adrenal hyperplasia).

Treatment Options. Depending on size, location, and symptoms, treatment options range from watchful waiting to surgery and stereotactic radiosurgery.

Imaging

General Features. Neuroimaging findings reflect their slow growth and benign biologic behavior. A well-circumscribed extraaxial mass that originates within or near a cranial nerve and displaces but does not invade adjacent structures is typical.

CT Findings. Most schwannomas exhibit low to intermediate attenuation on NECT scans and show smooth expansion/remodeling of osseous foramina on bone CT. Cystic change is common. Gross intratumoral hemorrhage is uncommon, and calcification is rare. Strong moderately heterogeneous enhancement after contrast administration is typical.

MR Findings. Schwannomas are generally isointense with cortex on T1WI and heterogeneously hyperintense on T2WI and FLAIR **(23-50A)**. Although macroscopic intratumoral hemorrhage is rare, T2* (GRE, SWI) scans often reveal "blooming" foci of microbleeds **(23-56)**.

Secondary changes of muscle edema or denervation with atrophy and fatty infiltration can occur with motor nerve schwannomas. Vagal nerve schwannomas may cause vocal cord paralysis.

Virtually all schwannomas enhance intensely. Approximately 15% have nonenhancing intratumoral cysts. Nonneoplastic peritumoral cysts occur in 5-10% of cases, especially with larger lesions **(23-55)**.

Differential Diagnosis

The differential diagnosis of a **solitary enlarged enhancing cranial nerve** includes schwannoma, multiple sclerosis, viral and postviral neuritis, Lyme disease, sarcoid, ischemia, and malignant neoplasms (metastases, lymphoma, and leukemia).

The most common cause of **multiple enhancing cranial nerves** is metastasis. NF2, neuritis (especially Lyme disease), lymphoma, and leukemia are significantly less common than metastasis. Rare but important causes include multiple sclerosis and chronic inflammatory demyelinating polyneuropathy, a disorder that usually affects spinal nerves but may occasionally involve cranial nerves.

Vestibular Schwannoma

Terminology

Vestibular schwannoma (VS) is the preferred term for a CN VIII schwannoma. VSs are also known as **acoustic schwannomas** and **acoustic neuromas**.

Focal **intralabyrinthine schwannomas**, also known as **inner ear schwannomas**, form a special subgroup of CN VIII schwannomas **(23-51)**. Intralabyrinthine schwannomas are named according to sublocation. Schwannomas within the cochlea are termed **intracochlear**. Lesions within the vestibule are called **intravestibular** schwannomas **(23-53)**. If a schwannoma involves *both* the vestibule and the cochlea, it is

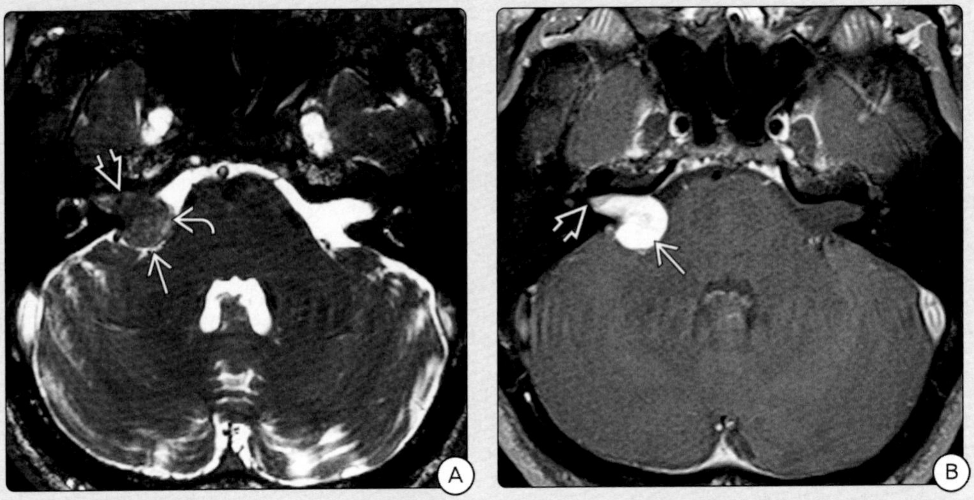

***(23-49A)** Thin-section CISS demonstrates a classic vestibular schwannoma (VS) with "ice cream on cone" appearance and thin CSF-vascular "cleft" where the tumor slightly indents the adjacent pons and middle cerebellar peduncle. **(23-49B)** Strong, relatively uniform enhancement is seen on T1 C+ FS scan. The tumor extends to the IAC fundus.*

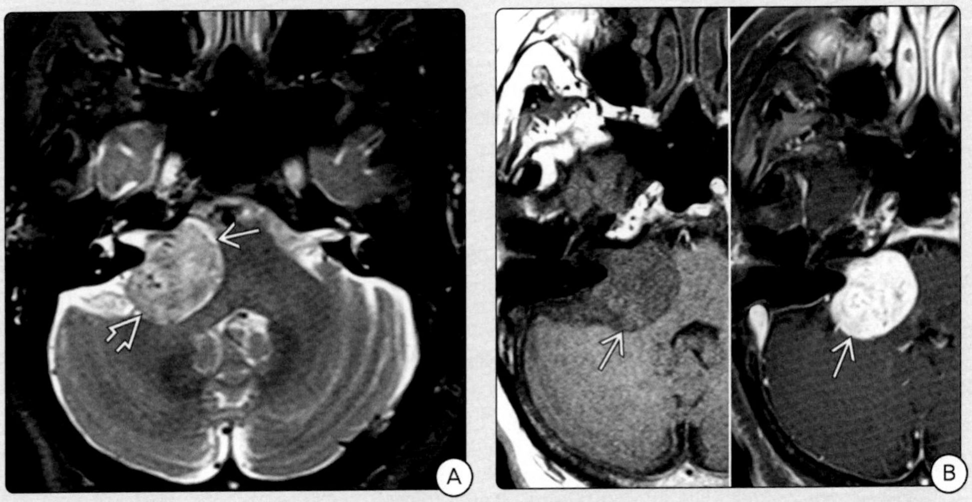

***(23-50A)** Axial T2 FS shows heterogeneously hyperintense signal of typical large VS. The tumor indents the pons and cerebellar peduncle, deforming the fourth ventricle. Note CSF "cleft" between the tumor and brainstem. **(23-50B)** Precontrast T1WI (L) and postcontrast T1 C+ FS (R) in the same case show that the tumor enhances intensely but somewhat heterogeneously. This is a VS with conventional histology.*

termed **vestibulocochlear**. A schwannoma that crosses the modiolus from the cochlea into the internal auditory canal (IAC) fundus is a **transmodiolar** schwannoma. If a lesion crosses from the vestibule into the IAC fundus, it is termed **transmacular**. Finally, an extensive schwannoma that crosses the entire inner ear from the IAC fundus to the middle ear is called **transotic (23-54)**.

Etiology

General Concepts. VSs arise from the vestibular portion of CN VIII at the glial-Schwann cell junction, inside the IAC near the porus acusticus. Schwannomas rarely arise from the cochlear portion of CN VIII.

Genetics. The pathogenesis underlying both familial and most sporadic VSs has been linked to mutation in a single gene, the neurofibromin 2 *(NF2)* gene located on chromosome 22. Nearly 60% of sporadic VSs have inactivating mutations of *NF2*.

Pathology

Location. VSs may occur at any location along the course of the nerve. Small VSs are often completely intracanalicular. Larger lesions frequently protrude medially through the porus acusticus into the cerebellopontine angle (CPA) cistern.

Size and Number. Small VSs are round or ovoid lesions that generally measure 2-10 mm in length. VSs that extend into the CPA cistern can become very large, up to 5 cm in diameter. Bilateral VSs are pathognomonic of NF2.

Clinical Issues

Epidemiology. VS is by far the most common intracranial schwannoma. VS is also the most common cerebellopontine cistern mass, accounting for 85-90% of lesions in this location.

Demographics. Peak presentation is 40-60 years of age. There is no sex predilection.

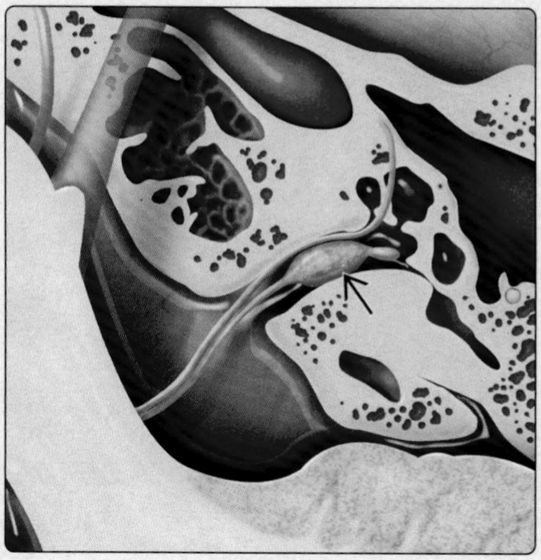

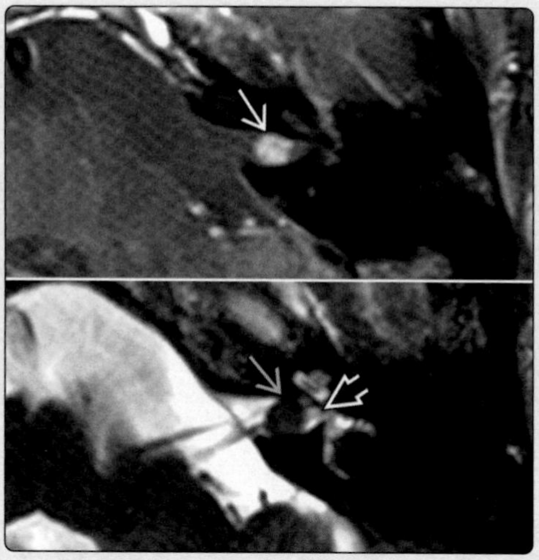

***(23-51)** Graphic depicts an intracanalicular VS as round or fusiform enlargement of the nerve ➡. **(23-52)** Small intracanalicular VS ➡ (top) is shown on axial T1 C+ scan. High-resolution axial T2WI (bottom) in the same patient nicely shows the VS as a round isointense mass in the IAC ➡. Note the fundal "cap" of CSF ➡.*

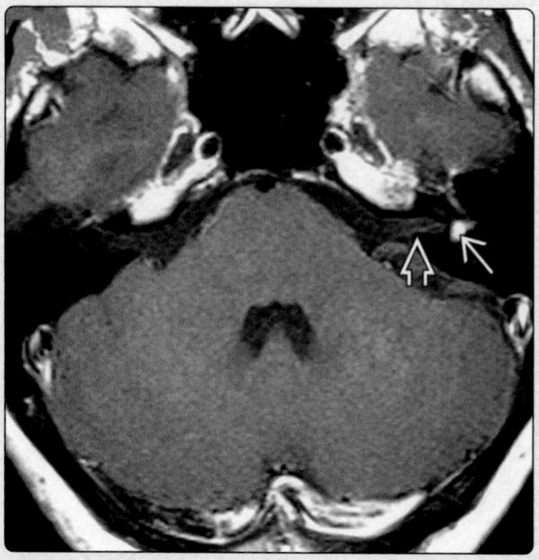

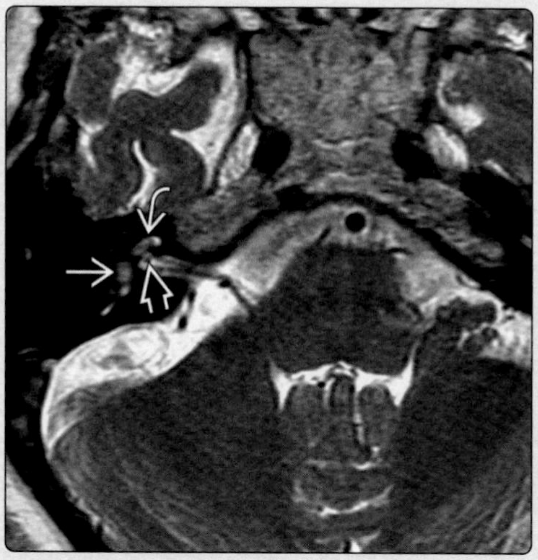

***(23-53)** Axial T1 C+ shows a tiny enhancing intralabyrinthine schwannoma ➡. Because the tumor involves only the vestibule, it is called an intravestibular schwannoma. The IAC ➡ is normal. **(23-54)** Axial T2WI shows a schwannoma that involves both the vestibule ➡ and the cochlea ➡. A tiny nodule of tumor ➡ can be seen at the IAC fundus, so this is a transotic schwannoma.*

Presentation. The most common presentation is in an adult with slowly progressive unilateral sensorineural hearing loss (SNHL). Small VSs may present initially with tinnitus. Large lesions often present with trigeminal and/or facial neuropathy.

Natural History. The growth rate of VSs varies. On average, they tend to enlarge between 1 or 2 mm per year. Approximately 60% grow very slowly (under 1 mm per year), whereas 10% of patients experience rapid enlargement of their lesions (more than 3 mm per year). Size and position at presentation also affect VS growth rate; intracanalicular VSs grow more slowly than extracanalicular lesions.

The growth rate of NF2-associated VSs is generally considered more aggressive compared with that of sporadic VSs.

Treatment Options. Treatment options vary. Watchful observation of small lesions with interval follow-up imaging is common, especially in older patients. Surgical removal or stereotactic radiotherapy are other possibilities. The surgical approach of choice varies with tumor size and location, as well as whether hearing preservation is possible.

Imaging

General Features. The classic imaging appearance of VS is an avidly enhancing mass that looks like "ice cream on a cone" **(23-49)**. Many VSs extend medially from their origin within the IAC. The intracanalicular part of the tumor represents the "cone." If a VS passes through the porus acusticus, it typically expands when it enters the CPA, forming the "ice cream" on the cone.

Precisely defining the size and extent of a VS is one of the most important goals of imaging. Some VSs remain as small slow-growing lesions that are entirely intracanalicular **(23-51)** **(23-53)**. Many intracanalicular VSs have a distinctive fundal "cap" of CSF interposed between the lesion and the modiolus **(23-52)**. Others grow laterally, extending deep into the IAC

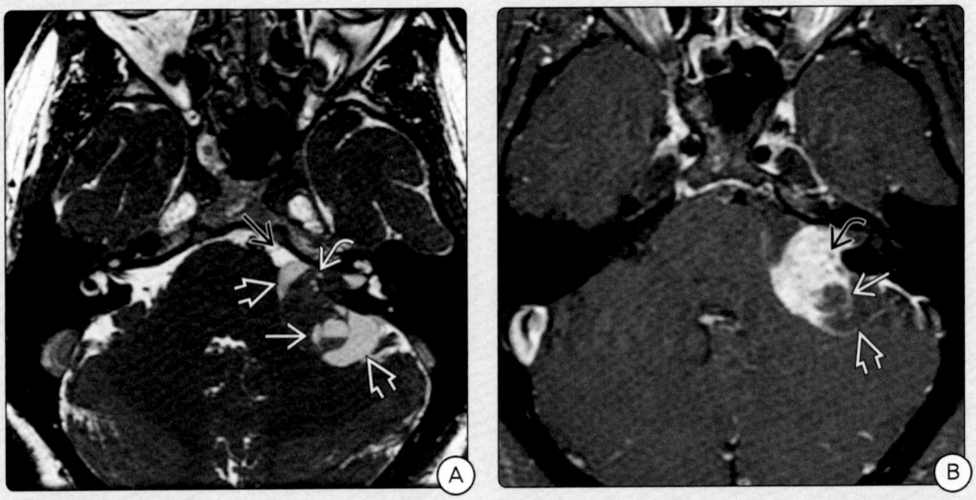

***(23-55A)** Axial FIESTA in a 31y man with headaches, left facial numbness shows large VS with intratumoral and marginal cysts with fluid-fluid level suggesting hemorrhage. Peritumoral cysts are present, exhibit different signal from normal CSF in CPA cistern. **(23-55B)** T1 C+ FS shows nonenhancing intratumoral cysts, rim enhancement along marginal and peritumoral cysts. This is cystic VS with intracystic hemorrhage.*

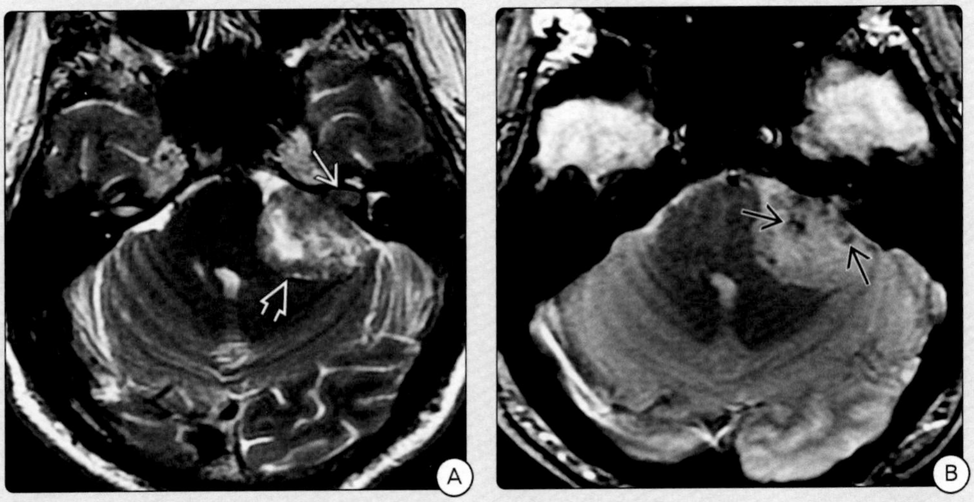

***(23-56A)** Axial T2WI in a 67y man with left-sided sensorineural hearing loss (SNHL) shows a very heterogeneous-appearing mass with a large CPA component, smaller intracanalicular component (classic "ice cream on cone"). **(23-56B)** T2* GRE shows multiple blooming foci of intratumoral hemorrhage. The lesion enhanced very heterogeneously on T1 C+ (not shown). This is hemorrhagic VS.*

fundus, and may eventually pass through the cochlear aperture into the modiolus **(23-54)**.

CT Findings. CT is generally negative unless lesions are large enough to expand the IAC or protrude into the CPA cistern. VSs are generally noncalcified, appear mildly hyperdense on NECT, and enhance strongly and relatively uniformly on CECT. Bone CT may show IAC enlargement on the symptomatic side.

MR Findings. Full-brain FLAIR with axial and coronal fat-saturated T1 C+ imaging of the CPA and ICA is the standard. A "screening" study for adults with uncomplicated unilateral SNHL is a common option and is generally limited to high-resolution T2WI, CISS, or FIESTA sequences. Detailed evaluation of the CPA/ICA can be performed with these sequences, reserving contrast-enhanced studies for patients with equivocal screening studies.

VSs are generally iso/hypointense with brain on T1WI **(23-50B)**. An intracanalicular VS appears as a hypointense filling defect within the bright CSF on CISS **(23-49A)**. Larger VSs are iso- to heterogeneously hyperintense on T2WI. Microhemorrhage on T2* is common although macroscopic hemorrhage is rare (0.4% of all newly diagnosed VSs but 5-6% of anticoagulated patients).

Virtually all VSs enhance strongly following contrast administration **(23-49B)**. A schwannoma-associated "dural tail" sign occurs but is rare compared with CPA meningiomas.

Special imaging sequences may be helpful in the preoperative planning for VS surgery. MR tractography with three-dimensional tumor modeling can depict the precise location of the CNs that surround large VSs.

Differential Diagnosis

The major differential diagnosis of VS is **CPA meningioma**. Most meningiomas "cap" the IAC and do not extend deep to the porus. However, a reactive dural "tail" in the IAC may make

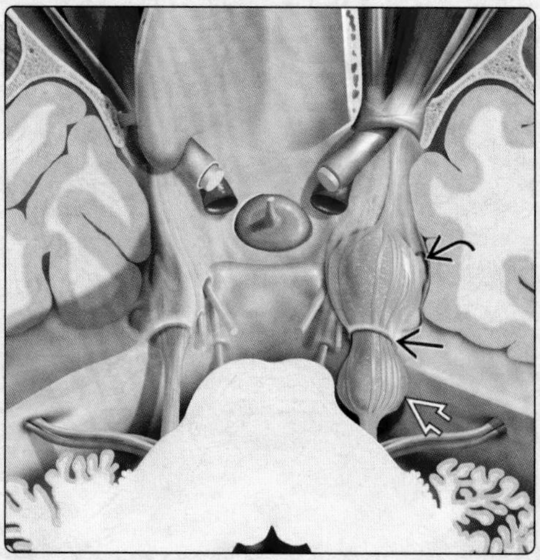

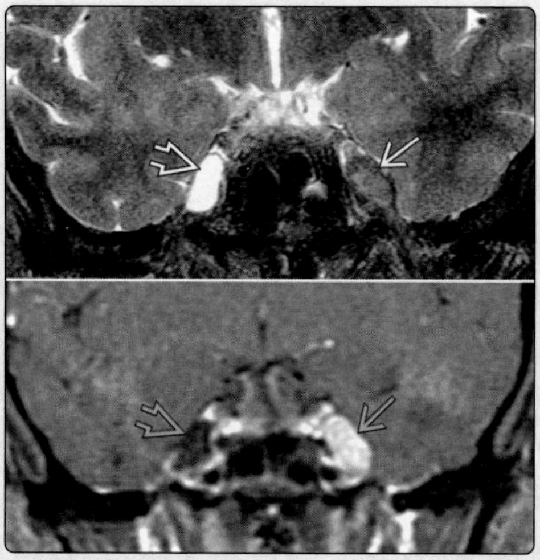

(23-57) *"Dumbbell" trigeminal schwannoma shows that cisternal tumor segment ➡ is constricted as it passes through porus trigeminus ⇨. Schwannoma then expands again ⇨ when it enters Meckel cave.* ***(23-58)*** *Coronal T2WI of left CN V schwannoma (top) shows "winking Meckel cave" sign. CSF-filled right side ➡ contrasts with tumor-filled left Meckel cave ➡. Schwannoma enhances ⇨, while right side ⇨ is normal (bottom).*

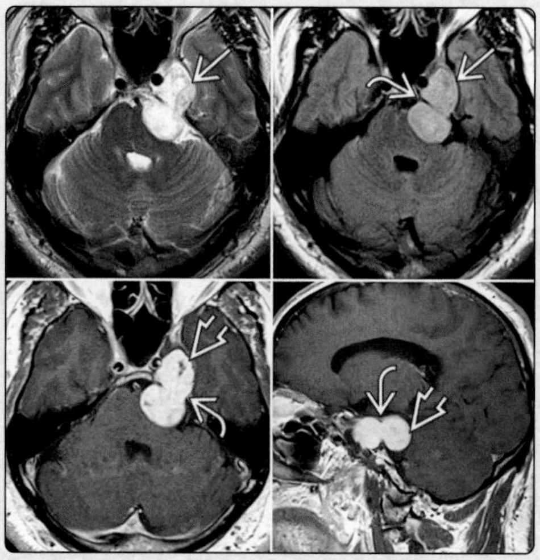

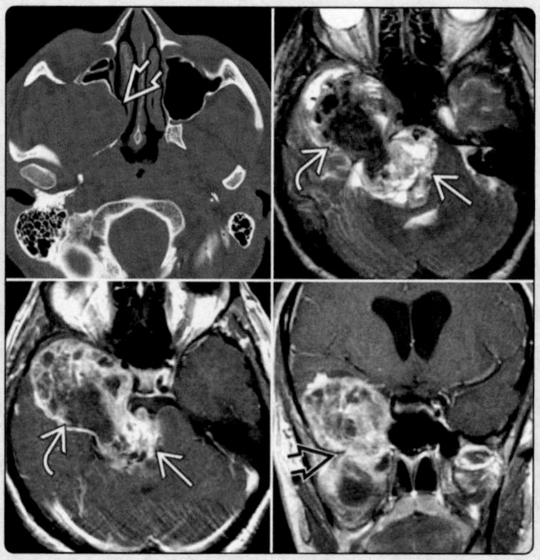

(23-59) *This is a large "dumbbell" trigeminal schwannoma. Tumor is hyperintense on T2WI, and FLAIR ➡ enhances strongly on T1 C+ ➡. Note prominent constriction by dural ring of the porus trigeminus ➡.* ***(23-60)*** *Giant "tricompartmental" schwannoma of CNs V_2 and V_3 with cystic and hemorrhagic changes enlarges pterygopalatine fossa ➡, extends from posterior fossa ➡ into middle fossa ➡, through foramen ovale into masticator space ⇨.*

distinction between VS and meningioma difficult unless other dural "tails" along the petrous ridge are also present.

A **facial nerve schwannoma** confined to the IAC may be difficult to distinguish from a VS. Facial nerve schwannomas are much less common and usually have a labyrinthine segment "tail." Beware: extension along the labyrinthine segment of the facial nerve means the schwannoma arises from CN VII and is not a VS.

Metastases can coat the facial and vestibulocochlear nerves within the IAC. Metastases are usually bilateral with other lesions present.

Other CPA masses such as **epidermoid cysts, arachnoid cysts,** and **aneurysms** can usually be distinguished easily from VS. VSs occasionally have prominent intramural cysts, but a completely cystic schwannoma without an enhancing tumor rim is very rare.

Trigeminal Schwannoma

Although trigeminal schwannomas are the second most common intracranial schwannoma, they are rare tumors. They may involve any part of the CN V complex, including extracranial peripheral divisions of the nerve. Nearly two-thirds of all Meckel cave tumors are schwannomas.

The principal presenting symptoms involve sensory impairment in one or more of the three divisions. Trigeminal neuralgia can occur but is uncommon.

Imaging

Trigeminal schwannomas arise from the junction of the gasserian ganglion and the trigeminal nerve root **(23-57)**. Small lesions may be confined to Meckel cave. They have a very characteristic appearance on coronal T2WI, the "winking Meckel cave" sign. Because at least 90% of each Meckel cave is normally filled with CSF, any lesion that fills the cave with soft

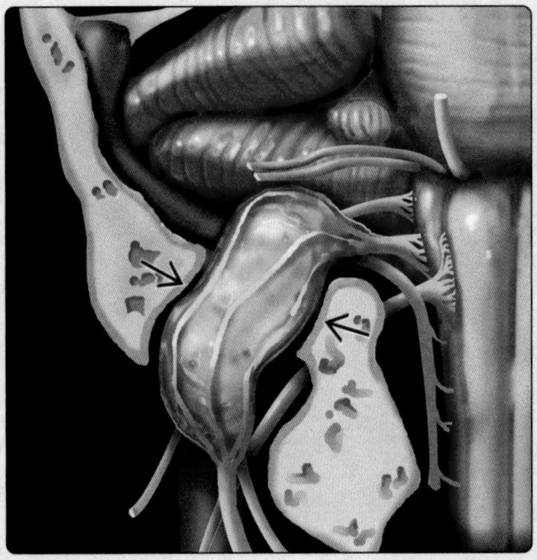

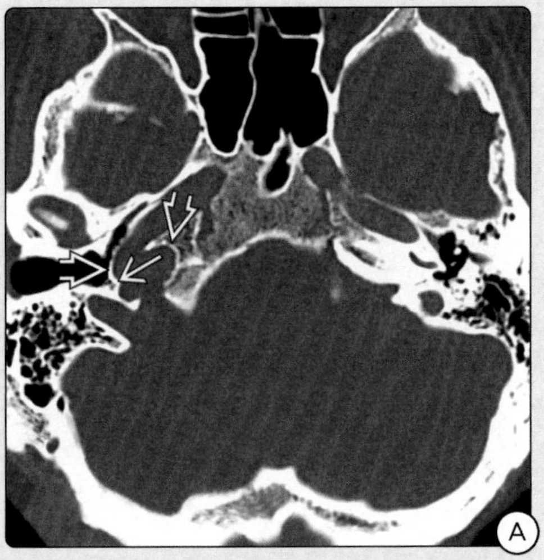

***(23-61)** Coronal graphic of a vagal schwannoma shows the tumor enlarging and remodeling the bony margins of the jugular foramen →. The "beak" of the "eagle" is eroded. **(23-62A)** NECT scan shows osseous remodeling of the right jugular foramen. The jugular spine → is eroded, but the surrounding cortex → appears intact (compare with Figure 23-6).*

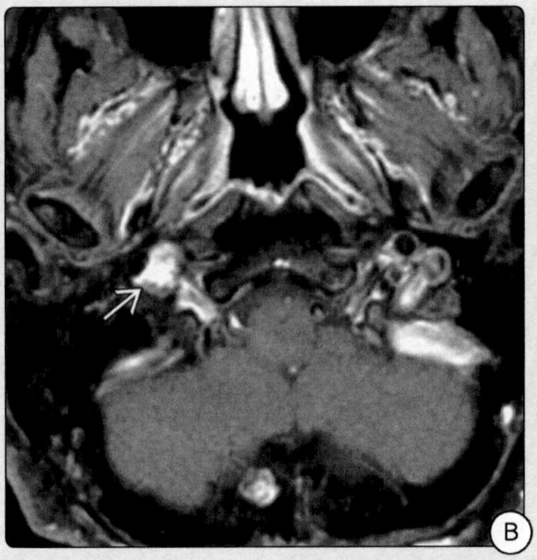

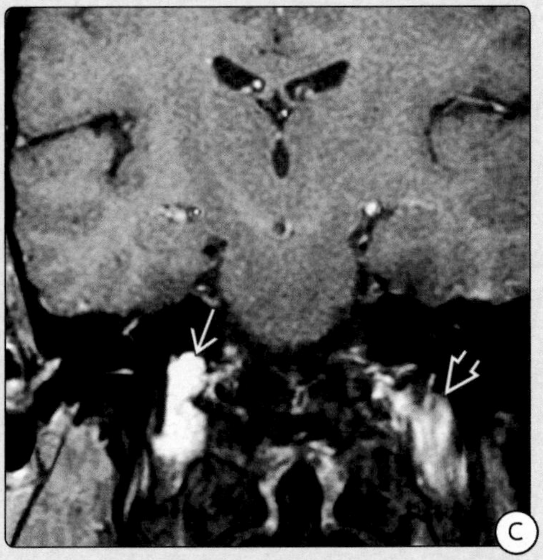

***(23-62B)** Axial T1 C+ FS scan shows an enhancing mass in the jugular foramen →. **(23-62C)** Coronal T1 C+ FS shows the intensely enhancing mass →. Contrast this with the normally enhancing left jugular bulb and vein →. At surgery, this jugular foramen schwannoma proved to be arising from the vagal nerve (CN X).*

tissue contrasts sharply with the bright signal on the opposite normal side **(23-58)**.

Bicompartmental tumors are common. Schwannomas that originate in Meckel cave can extend into the posterior fossa (through the porus trigeminus). These tumors have a characteristic "dumbbell" configuration **(23-59)**.

Less commonly, bicompartmental tumors extend from the middle fossa anteroinferiorly through the foramen ovale into the masticator space. Tumors that involve all three locations are uncommon and are termed "three-compartment" trigeminal schwannomas **(23-60)**.

Schwannomas that involve the mandibular division (CN V_3) may cause denervation atrophy of the muscles of mastication.

Differential Diagnosis

The appearance of a bi- or tricompartmental CN V schwannoma is distinctive. The major differential diagnoses of a Meckel cave schwannoma are **meningioma** and **metastasis**.

Jugular Foramen Schwannoma

Although schwannomas account for approximately 40% of all jugular foramen (JF) neoplasms, JF schwannomas constitute only 2-4% of all intracranial schwannomas.

Glossopharyngeal schwannomas are the most common JF schwannoma but are still rare, with just 42 cases reported between 1908 and 2008. The vast majority (85%) presented with vestibulocochlear symptoms secondary to compression and displacement, not CN IX symptoms. Glossopharyngeal schwannomas can occur anywhere along the course of CN IX, but the majority of symptomatic cases are intracranial/intraosseous.

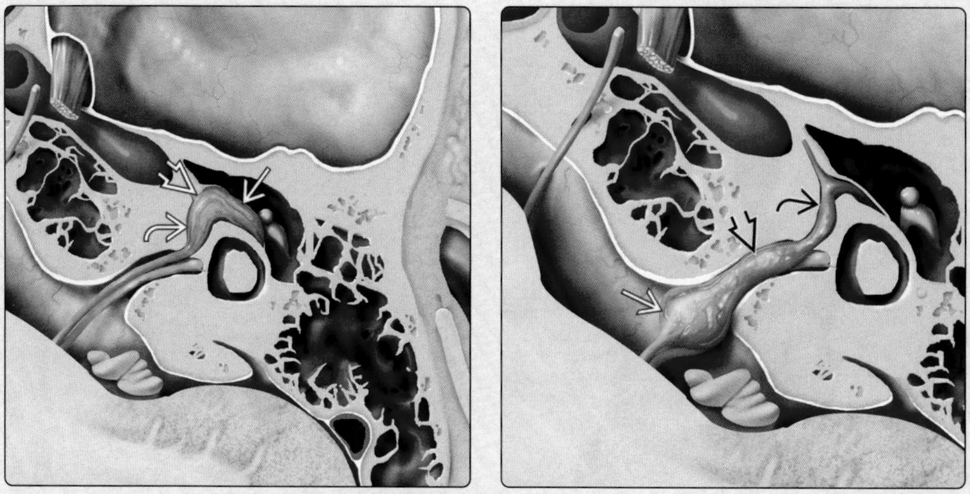

***(23-63)** Axial graphic depicts a small tubular facial nerve schwannoma involving the labyrinthine segment ➜, geniculate ganglion ➜, and anterior tympanic segment ➜ on CN VII. **(23-64)** Graphic depicts a larger facial nerve schwannoma with CPA ➜ and IAC ➜ segments. This can mimic a vestibular schwannoma ("ice cream on cone" appearance) except for the "tail" of tumor ➜ extending into the labyrinthine segment.*

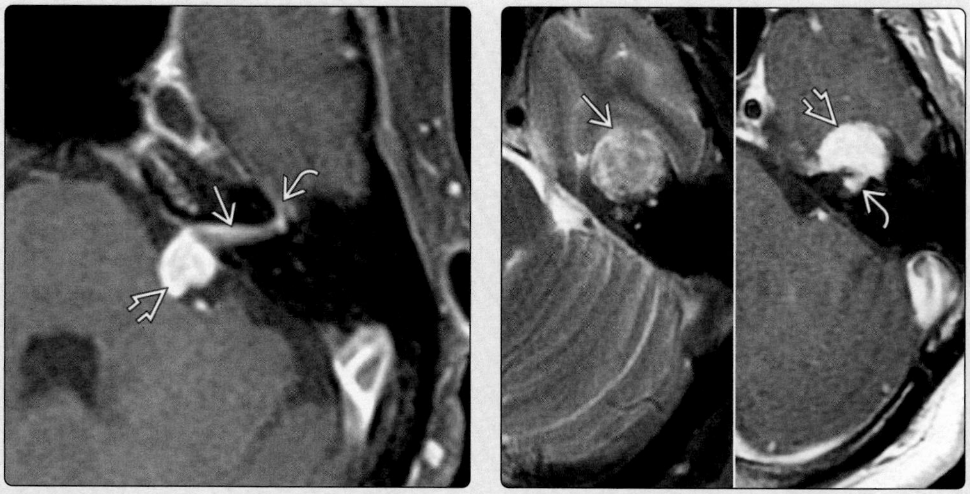

***(23-65)** Close-up view of T1 C+ FS scan shows a facial nerve schwannoma in the CPA ➜, extending into the IAC ➜ and geniculate ganglion ➜. **(23-66)** Geniculate fossa VII schwannoma is shown. T2WI (L) shows globular heterogeneously hyperintense mass ➜ tracking along the GSPN and extending extradurally into the middle cranial fossa. The labyrinthine ➜, geniculate ganglion ➜ segments (R) enhance intensely. (Courtesy P. Hildenbrand, MD.)*

*(**23-67A**) Sagittal T1 C+ FS shows intensely enhancing, subfrontal, "dumbbell" mass → extended through eroded cribriform plate into nasal cavity →. (**23-67B**) Axial T1 C+ in same patient shows well-circumscribed, intensely enhancing mass centered on cribriform plate. Diagnosis was olfactory nerve schwannoma. Most similar-appearing cases are likely olfactory ensheathing cell tumors, not schwannomas. (Courtesy G. Parker, MD.)*

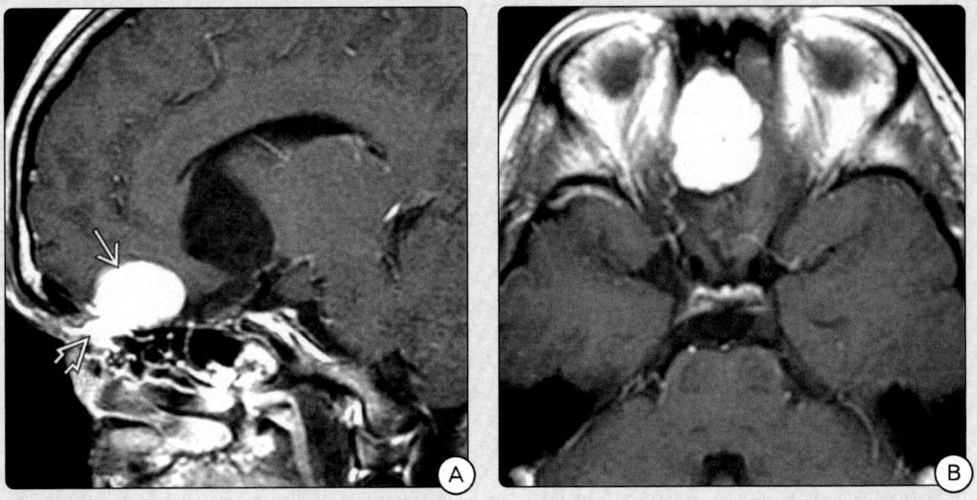

*(**23-68**) Coronal autopsy case shows incidental left oculomotor schwannoma → seen between posterior cerebral artery above → and superior cerebellar artery below →. Contrast with the normal right CN III →. (Courtesy E. T. Hedley-Whyte, MD.) (**23-69A**) Coronal T1WI C+ demonstrates the enlarged, enhancing right oculomotor nerve →.*

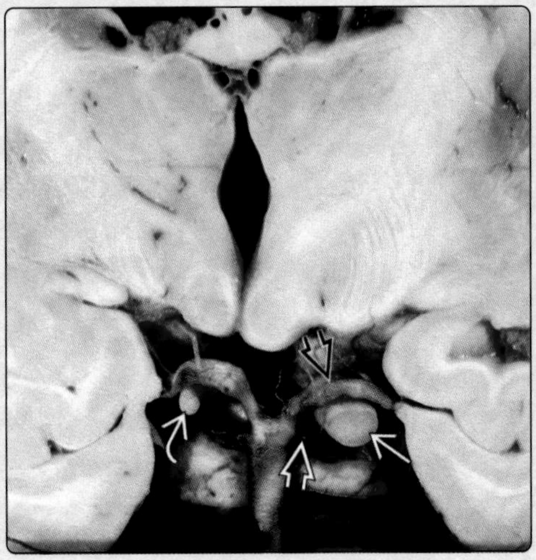

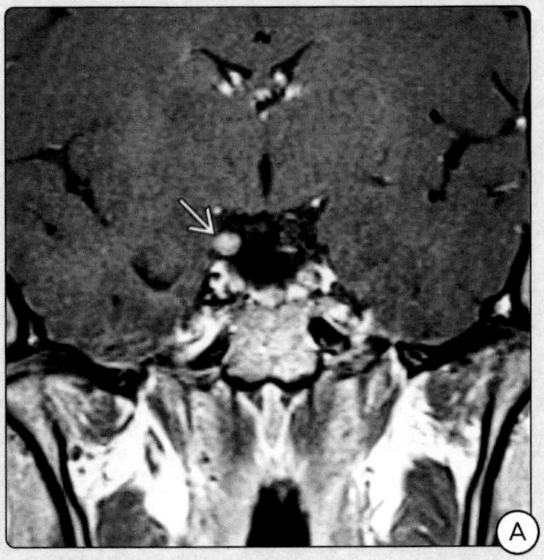

*(**23-69B**) Sagittal T1 C+ scan in the same patient shows tubular enlargement of the oculomotor nerve → extending from its midbrain exit to the cavernous sinus. (**23-69C**) Axial T1 C+ scan in the same patient shows the enlarged, intensely enhancing right oculomotor nerve →. The lesion was unchanged after 3 years. This was presumed schwannoma.*

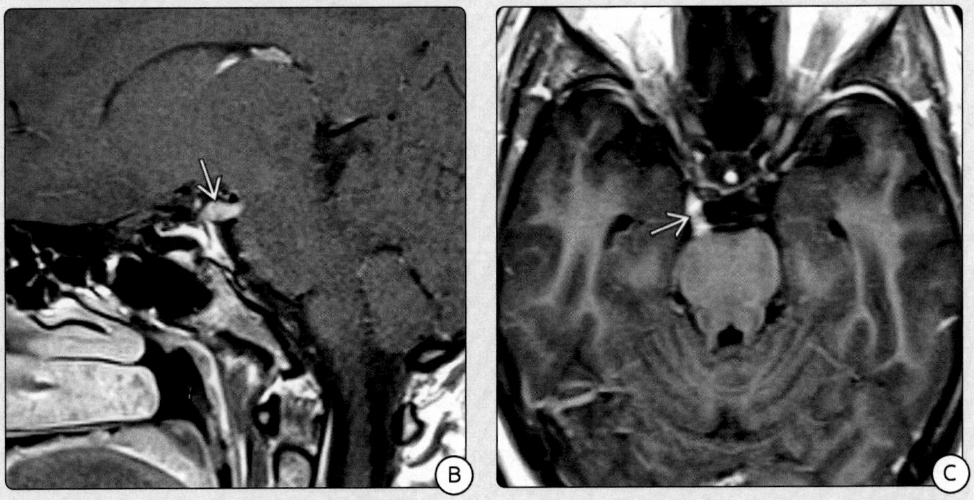

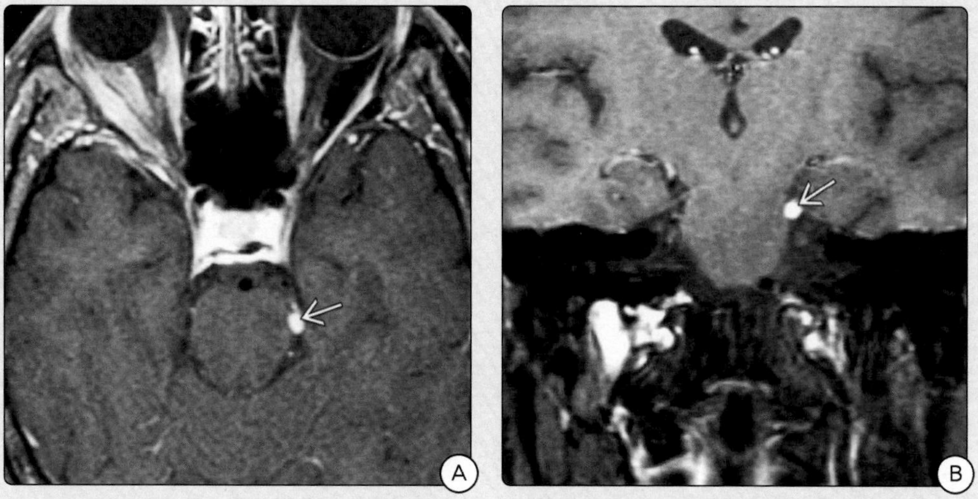

(23-70A) *Axial T1 C+ FS scan shows a small enhancing tumor in the left ambient cistern →.* **(23-70B)** *Coronal T1 C+ FS scan in the same patient shows that the tumor → lies along the expected course of CN IV. This was probable trochlear schwannoma.*

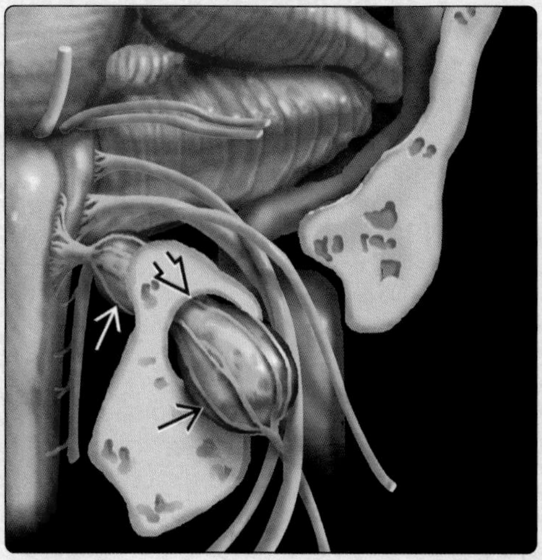

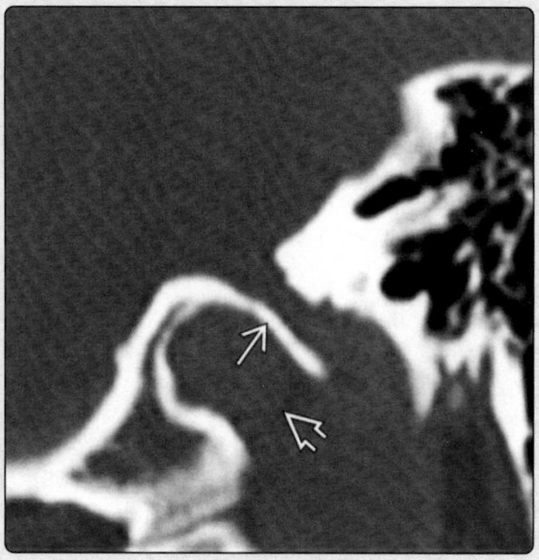

(23-71) *Graphic depicts hypoglossal schwannoma. CN XII schwannomas have a "dumbbell" shape with a cisternal segment →, relative constriction in the bony hypoglossal canal →, and a larger extracranial component →.* **(23-72)** *Coronal bone CT with hypoglossal schwannoma shows enlarged hypoglossal canal → with thinning, remodeling of the jugular tubercle → ("head" and "beak" of the "eagle," as seen in Figure 23-37).*

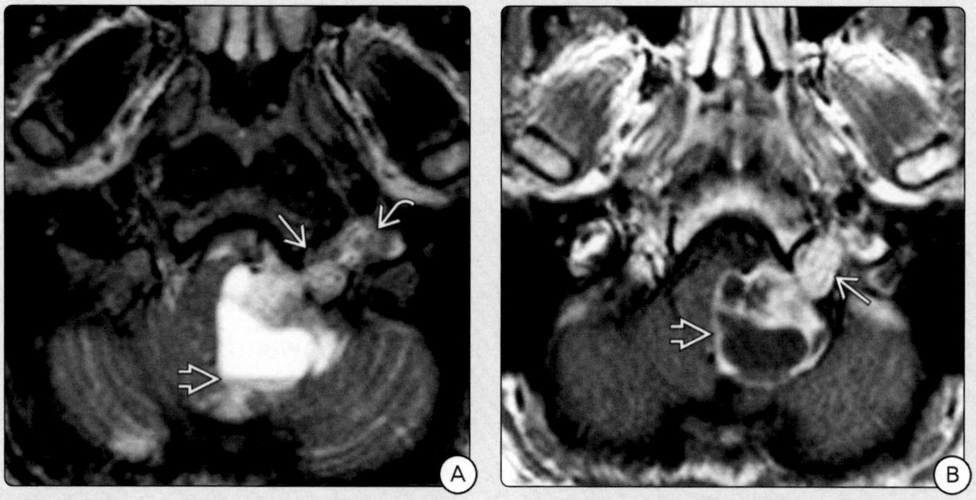

(23-73A) *Axial T2FS in a patient with excruciating left arm pain shows a heterogeneously hyperintense posterior fossa mass with a large partially cystic intracranial component that exhibits a blood-fluid level →. Note extension through an enlarged hypoglossal canal → into the high deep carotid space →.* **(23-73B)** *T1 C+ shows the partially cystic →, partially solid → enhancing mass. This is "dumbbell" hypoglossal schwannoma.*

Compared with their extracranial counterpart, intracranial **vagal schwannomas** are rare. Purely intracisternal ones are even more unusual. Most vagal schwannomas are "dumbbell" lesions that extend from the basal cistern through the jugular foramen into the high deep carotid space **(23-61)** **(23-62)**. When large, they may compress the ventrolateral medulla and cause refractory neurogenic hypertension.

Spinal accessory nerve schwannomas not associated with neurofibromatosis are very rare. They can be either intrajugular or intracisternal.

The major differential diagnoses of JF schwannoma include **meningioma, glomus jugulare tumor,** and **metastasis**. Only a JF schwannoma smoothly enlarges and remodels the jugular fossa.

Facial Nerve Schwannoma

Facial nerve schwannomas (FNSs) are rare lesions that can arise anywhere along the course of the facial nerve, from its origin in the CPA to its extracranial ramifications in the parotid space **(23-63)** **(23-64)**. Depending on their location along CN VII, FNSs display several imaging patterns. The most common presentation is facial neuropathy.

CPA-IAC FNSs are radiologically indistinguishable from vestibular schwannomas if they do not demonstrate extension into the labyrinthine segment of the facial nerve canal. Lesions that traverse the labyrinthine segment often have a "dumbbell" appearance.

Almost 90% of FNSs involve more than one facial nerve segment **(23-65)**. The **geniculate fossa** is the most common site, involved in more than 80% of all FNSs. The **labyrinthine** and **tympanic segments** are each involved in slightly over half of FNSs.

Geniculate fossa FNSs typically appear as a round or tubular enhancing mass in a smoothly enlarged facial nerve canal.

FNSs that track along the **greater superficial petrosal nerve** are seen as a round middle cranial fossa extraaxial mass **(23-66)**.

Tympanic segment FNSs often pedunculate into the middle ear cavity, losing their tubular configuration.

When the **mastoid segment** is involved, tumor may break into adjacent mastoid air cells and assume a more aggressive appearance, mimicking a malignant invasive tumor.

Schwannomas of Other Intracranial Nerves

Motor nerve schwannomas are much less common than those arising from sensory or mixed sensory-motor nerves. Less than 1% of intracranial schwannomas arise from CNs III, IV, VI, and XII.

"Other" cranial schwannomas resemble their more common counterparts on imaging studies. Most motor nerve schwannomas are small, round or ovoid, well-delineated, strongly enhancing lesions.

Olfactory (CN I) "Schwannoma"

The cells that ensheathe the intracranial olfactory nerve are actually modified glial cells, not Schwann cells (see above). Primary tumors of the CN I nerve sheath are very rare. Once termed "olfactory groove schwannoma" or "subfrontal schwannoma," many of these neoplasms are more accurately called "olfactory ensheathing cell (OEC) tumors." True schwannomas of the olfactory groove may arise from meningeal branches of the trigeminal nerve or anterior ethmoidal nerves, not CN I.

Tumors of CN I typically present with anosmia. Many reach large size, causing frontal lobe signs such as emotional lability and complex partial seizures **(23-67)**.

Esthesioneuroblastoma, also known as olfactory neuroblastoma, is a rare malignant tumor that arises in the superior nasal cavity from olfactory mucosa. Esthesioneuroblastoma is discussed with embryonal and neuroblastic tumors (see Chapter 21).

Optic Nerve (CN II) "Schwannoma"

Neoplasms of the optic nerve (a brain tract) are astrocytomas, not schwannomas. Intraorbital schwannomas arise from peripheral branches of CNs IV, V_1, or VI or from sympathetic or parasympathetic fibers (not the optic nerve).

Oculomotor (CN III) Schwannoma

Oculomotor schwannomas are rare but are the most common of all the pure motor nerve schwannomas **(23-68)**. They can be asymptomatic or present with diplopia.

The most frequent location of a CN III schwannoma is in the interpeduncular cistern near the nerve exit from the midbrain **(23-69)**. The second most common site is the cavernous sinus. Most intracranial oculomotor schwannomas are small, generally measuring less than 0.5 cm in diameter. Combined orbitocavernous sinus schwannomas are somewhat larger, extending from the orbit through the superior orbital fissure into the cavernous sinus.

Intraorbital schwannomas are rare. As a group, they account for just 1% of all orbital tumors. They typically present with slowly progressive proptosis and seldom develop diplopia.

Trochlear (CN IV) Schwannoma

Trochlear nerve schwannomas are uncommon **(23-70)**. They cause diplopia (isolated unilateral superior oblique palsy) and compensatory head tilt that may be misdiagnosed clinically as "wry neck." Most CN IV schwannomas are small and are either simply watched or treated with prism spectacles.

Abducens (CN VI) Schwannoma

Schwannomas of the abducens nerve are extremely rare. Most patients present with a history of diplopia.

Schwannomas can occur anywhere along the entire length of the nerve, including its intracavernous and orbital segments. Most are found in the cerebellopontine angle cistern, adjacent to the pontomesencephalic junction. They typically displace the facial/vestibulocochlear nerve complex posterosuperiorly and may be difficult to distinguish on imaging studies from schwannomas that arise from the cisternal segments of these nerves.

Hypoglossal (CN XII) Schwannoma

Hypoglossal tumors are the rarest of the "other" schwannomas, accounting for only 5% of all nonvestibular intracranial schwannomas **(23-71)**. Over 90% present with denervation hemiatrophy of the tongue.

Most CN XII schwannomas originate intracranially but can also extend extracranially as a "dumbbell" tumor that expands and remodels the hypoglossal canal **(23-72)**. Most are solid enhancing masses although cystic and even hemorrhagic CN XII schwannomas have been reported **(23-73)**.

Parenchymal Schwannomas

Because the brain parenchyma does not normally contain Schwann cells, so-called "ectopic" schwannomas not associated with cranial nerves are very rare (<1% of cases). Parenchymal schwannomas may arise from ectopic neural crest stem cells that become displaced during embryogenesis. Other possible etiologies include origin in the sympathetic nerve plexus that surrounds cerebral blood vessels.

Most intraparenchymal schwannomas are solitary and nonsyndromic. Approximately 15% are associated with NF2. The most common reported sites are the frontal and temporal lobes. Parenchymal schwannomas have also been described in the cerebellar hemispheres, vermis, brainstem, and cerebral ventricles **(23-75)**.

Pathologically, two-thirds of cases are either cystic or contain areas of cystic degeneration. The histology of parenchymal

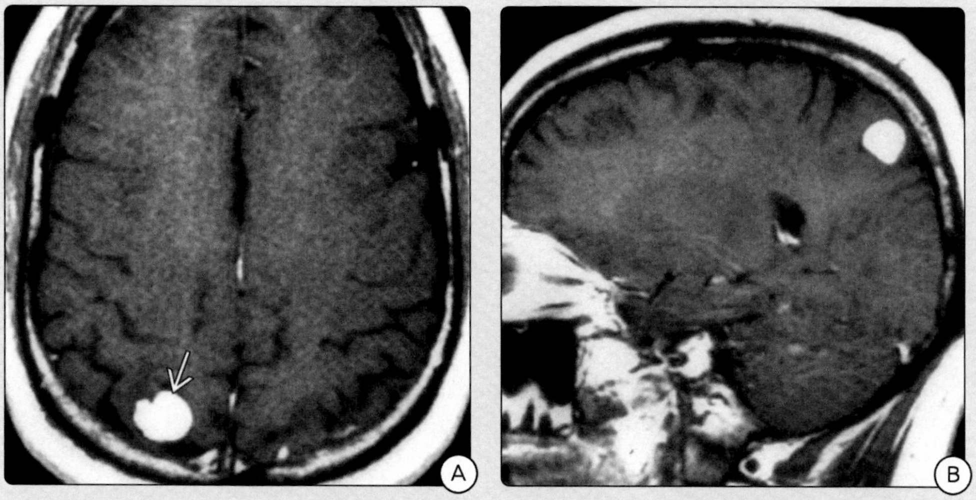

(23-74A) Axial T1 C+ scan shows a well-demarcated, enhancing parenchymal mass without edema. (23-74B) Sagittal T1 C+ scan in the same patient shows that the lesion is clearly intraaxial. Parenchymal schwannoma was diagnosed at histopathology.

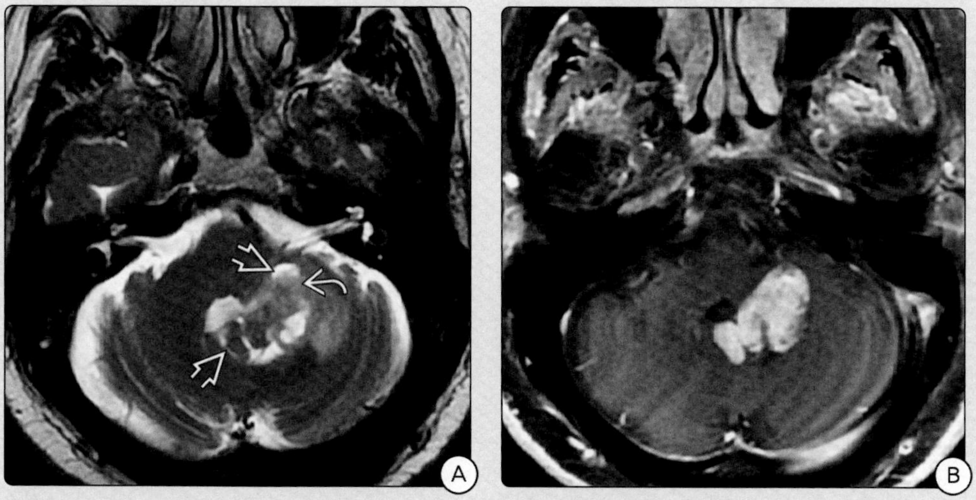

(23-75A) Axial T2WI in an 84y man with headaches shows a mass in the fourth ventricle extending anterolaterally through an enlarged lateral recess. (23-75B) T1 C+ FS in the same case shows that the mass enhances strongly but heterogeneously. Preoperative diagnosis was subependymoma. Conventional schwannoma was found at histopathology.

schwannoma is indistinguishable from that of other schwannomas.

On imaging studies, most intracranial parenchymal schwannomas appear well demarcated. The most common imaging pattern is that of a cyst with a mural nodule and peripheral enhancement. One-third are solid tumors with strong homogeneous or heterogeneous enhancement **(23-74)**. Peritumoral edema varies from none to moderate.

Melanotic Schwannoma

Melanotic schwannoma (MS) is a rare tumor composed of melanin-producing cells that have ultrastructural features resembling Schwann cells **(23-76)**. Cytological atypia with hyperchromasia and macronucleoli is common. Two histologic MS subtypes, psammomatous and nonpsammomatous, are recognized.

Paraspinal and extraneural locations (e.g., skin, soft tissues, bone, and viscera) are the most common sites. Craniofacial and intracranial MSs are very rare.

Peak age at diagnosis is about a decade younger compared with conventional schwannoma. MSs can be sporadic or syndromic. Approximately half of all patients with psammomatous MS have **Carney complex**, an autosomal-dominant disorder characterized by facial pigmentation, cardiac myxoma, and endocrine hyperactivity (including Cushing syndrome). Loss-of-function germline mutations of the *PRKAR1A* gene on chromosome 17q are characteristic. Malignant degeneration occurs in approximately 10% of PMSs associated with Carney complex.

Because melanin causes T1 shortening, most MSs are hyperintense on T1WI **(23-77)** and hypointense on T2WI **(23-78)**. Enhancement varies from minimal to striking.

(23-76) Gross pathology of melanotic schwannoma shows a well circumscribed mass with abundant bluish-black pigment ➡. (23-77A) Sagittal T1WI in a patient with left sensorineural hearing loss shows a hyperintense extraaxial mass ➡ in the prepontine/IAC cistern.

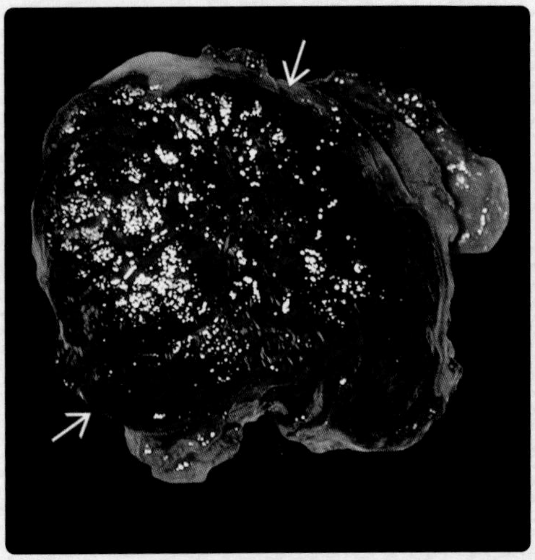

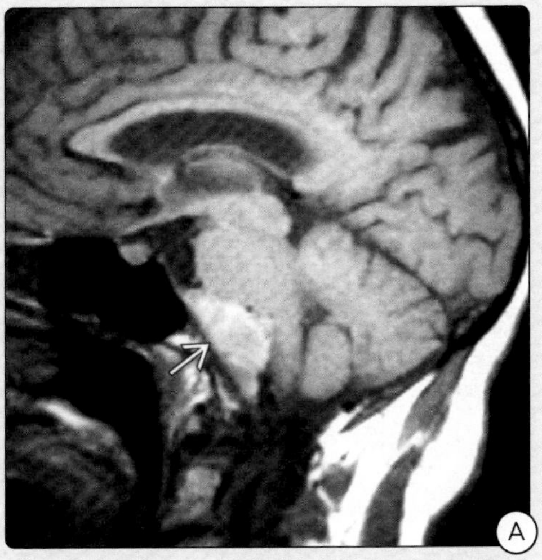

(23-77B) Axial T1WI (top) in the same case shows a heterogeneously hyperintense "ice cream on a cone" lesion in the left CPA/IAC. The lesion is hypointense on T2WI (bottom). Malignant melanotic schwannoma was removed. (23-77C) Axial T1 C+ obtained 3 months after the original surgery shows extensive enhancing recurrent tumor ➡. The patient died of disseminated metastases 6 months later.

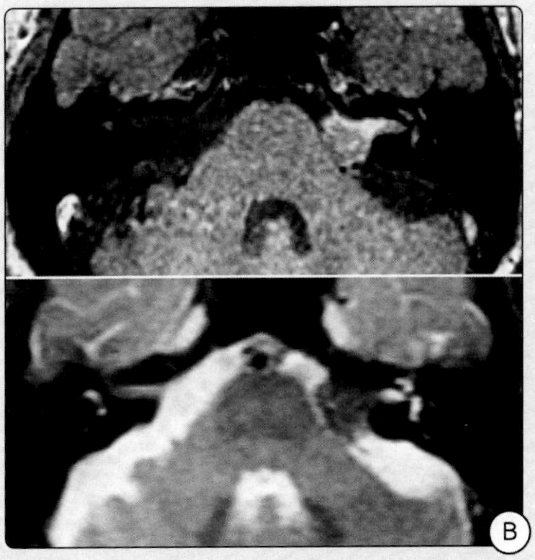

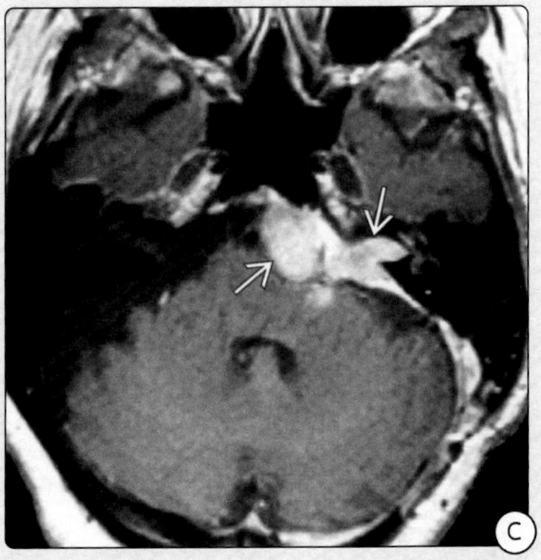

The main imaging differential diagnosis in melanotic schwannoma is **metastatic melanoma** and **hemorrhagic conventional schwannoma**.

Schwannomatosis

Nonsyndromic schwannomas are almost always solitary lesions. Multiple schwannomas occur in the setting of two familial tumor syndromes, **neurofibromatosis type 2** (NF2) and **schwannomatosis**. Bilateral vestibular schwannomas are pathognomonic of NF2. Multiple, mostly nonvestibular schwannomas in the absence of other NF2 features are characteristic of schwannomatosis. Both of these syndromes are discussed in Chapter 39.

Neurofibromas

Intracranial neurofibromas (NFs) are much less common than schwannomas. NFs can affect the scalp, skull, some cranial nerves (especially CN V_1), or—rarely—the brain. They are found at all ages. Both sexes are affected equally.

NFs can be solitary or multiple. Multiple NFs and plexiform NFs occur only in connection with neurofibromatosis type 1 (NF1).

The gross appearance of NFs is different from that of schwannomas. Schwannomas are well-delineated encapsulated lesions that arise eccentrically from their parent nerve. Schwannomas typically displace elements of the normal parent nerve to one side. In contrast, neurofibromas generally present as more diffuse nerve expansions. They display single or multiple fascicles that enter and leave the affected nerve. Axons of the parent nerve pass through

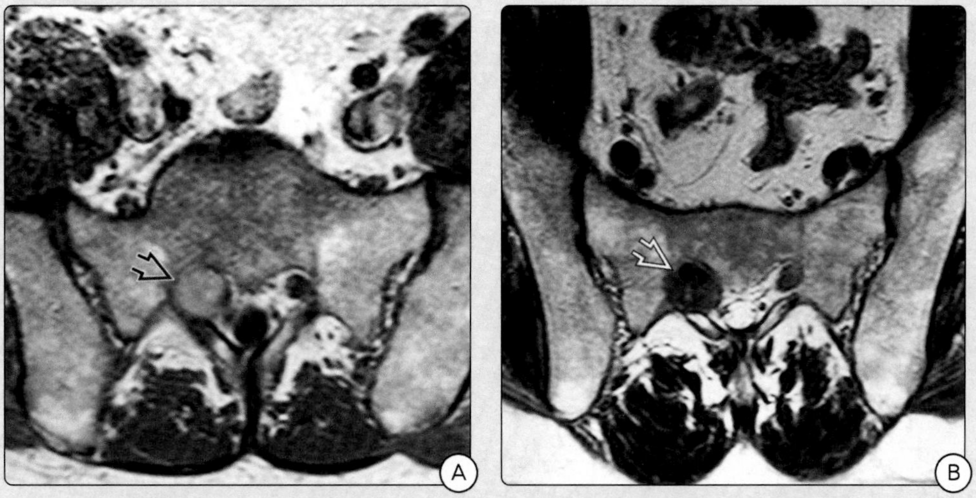

***(23-78A)** Axial T1WI in a 40y man with right sciatica shows a well-demarcated hyperintense mass in the right S1 nerve root. **(23-78B)** Axial T2WI in the same case shows that the mass is slightly lobulated and markedly hypointense.*

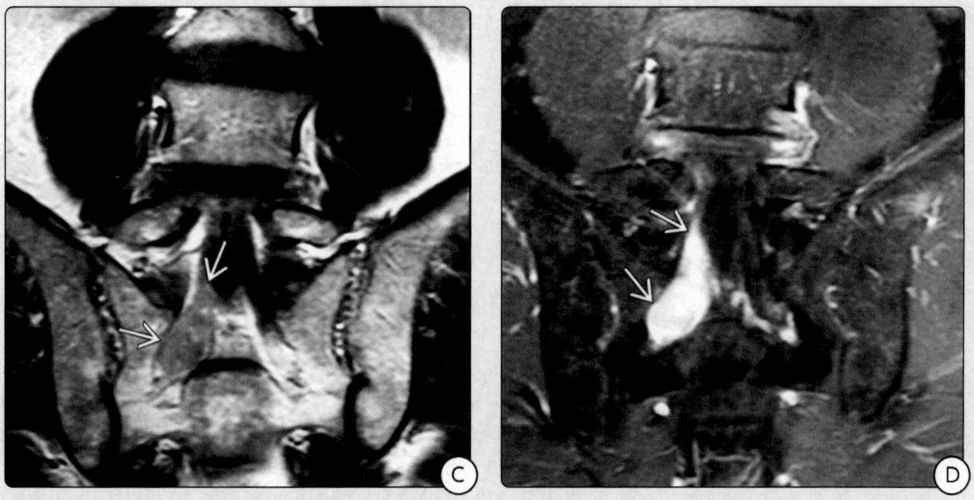

***(23-78C)** Coronal T1WI in the same case shows the hyperintense, fusiform expansile lesion of the right S1 nerve root. **(23-78D)** Coronal T1 C+ FS shows that the lesion enhances intensely. Benign melanotic schwannoma, nonpsammomatous type, was found at histopathology.*

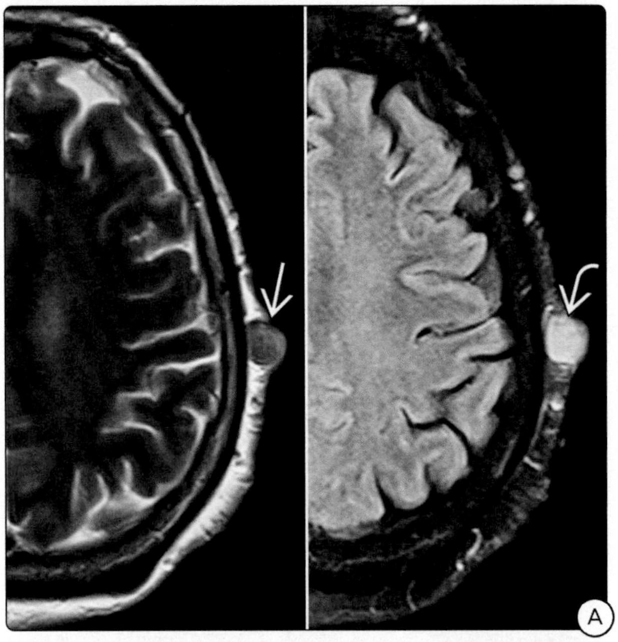

***(23-79A)** Axial T2WI (L) in a 62y woman with a solitary scalp neurofibroma shows that the well-demarcated mass extends from the calvarium to the skin surface. The neurofibroma is hyperintense on FLAIR (R).*

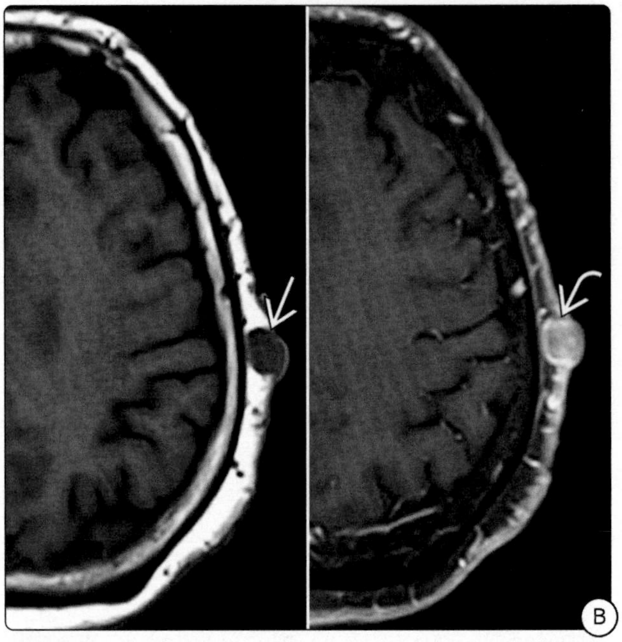

***(23-79B)** Axial precontrast T1WI (L) compared to the postcontrast fat-saturated scan (R) shows that the lesion enhances strongly in a somewhat "target" fashion.*

neurofibromas and are intermixed with tumor cells, distinguishing them from schwannoma.

The microscopic appearance of NFs also differs from that of schwannomas. Schwannomas are pure Schwann cell tumors. Neurofibromas consist of both Schwann cells and fibroblasts. NFs also contain other cell types, including perineural cells, mast cells, pericytes, endothelial cells, and smooth muscle cells. NFs also typically have a large amount of extracellular matrix with collagen.

In this section, we discuss both solitary and plexiform neurofibromas. Both neurofibromatosis types 1 and 2 are discussed in Chapter 39.

Solitary Neurofibroma

A solitary neurofibroma in the head and neck rarely—if ever—involves cranial nerves. Solitary neurofibromas affect patients of all ages and are usually sporadic (nonsyndromic). Most occur in the absence of NF1 and present as a painless scalp or skin mass.

Solitary neurofibromas are round or ovoid unencapsulated masses composed of Schwann cells and fibroblasts in a myxoid or collagenous matrix. Solitary neurofibromas are WHO grade I neoplasms.

Scalp solitary neurofibromas are seen on imaging studies as well-delineated, focal, enhancing masses that abut but do not invade the calvaria **(23-79)**.

Plexiform Neurofibroma

Terminology and Etiology

Plexiform neurofibromas (PNFs) are infiltrative intra- and extraneural neoplasms that occur almost exclusively in patients with NF1 **(23-80)**. Plexiform neurofibromas and neurofibromas of major nerves are considered potential precursors of malignant peripheral nerve sheath tumors (see below).

Pathology

Location. Approximately one-third of PNFs are found in the head and neck. Cranial PNFs usually involve CNs V, IX, or X. The most typical locations are the scalp, orbit, pterygopalatine fossa, and parotid gland. Scalp and orbital PNFs most commonly involve the ophthalmic branches of the trigeminal nerve. Parotid PNFs involve peripheral branches of the facial nerve.

Extracranial PNFs are often multicompartmental and do not respect fascial boundaries. Orbital PNFs may enlarge the superior orbital fissure and extend into the cavernous sinus as far as Meckel cave **(23-81)**.

Size and Number. PNFs are typically extensive, diffusely infiltrating lesions. Multiple variably sized lesions are typical.

Gross and Microscopic Features. Grossly, PNFs have a distinctive "bag of worms" appearance **(23-82)**. PNFs demonstrate a predominant intrafascicular growth pattern, with redundant loops of expanded nerve fascicles intermixed with collagen fibers and mucoid material **(23-83)**.

Staging, Grading, and Classification. PNFs are WHO grade I neoplasms.

Clinical Issues

PNFs are a major cause of morbidity in patients with NF1. Approximately 5% of PNFs eventually degenerate into malignant peripheral nerve sheath tumors.

Imaging

General Features. PNFs are poorly delineated worm-like soft tissue masses that diffusely infiltrate the scalp, orbit, or parotid gland.

CT Findings. PNFs infiltrate and enlarge soft tissues, typically the scalp and periorbita. They are generally isodense with muscle. Calcification and hemorrhage are rare.

CECT shows heterogeneous enhancement. Bone CT may show expansion of the superior orbital fissure and pterygopalatine fossa.

MR Findings. PNFs are isointense on T1WI and hyperintense on T2WI. Strong, sometimes heterogeneous enhancement is common **(23-84)**.

A "target" sign of hypointensity within an enhancing tumor fascicle is seen in some PNFs but is not pathognomonic.

Differential Diagnosis

The major differential diagnosis of PNF is **malignant peripheral nerve sheath tumor (MPNST)**. As many MPNSTs arise from PNFs, early differentiation may be difficult.

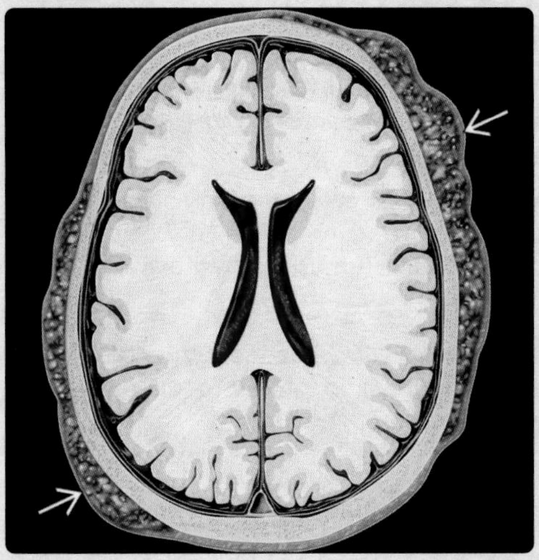

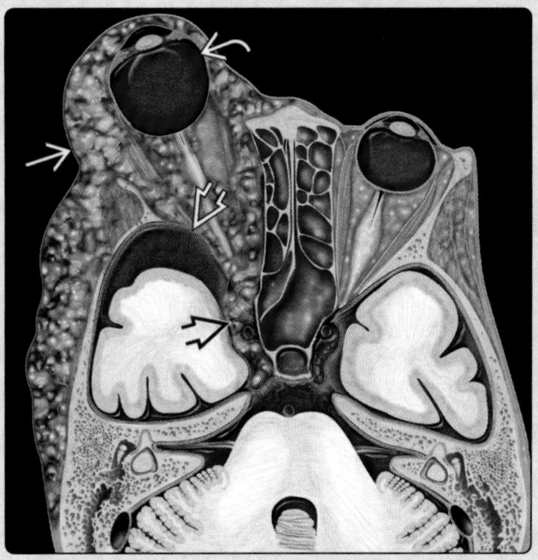

***(23-80)** Graphic depicts plexiform neurofibromas (PNFs) diffusely infiltrating and deforming the scalp ➡. **(23-81)** Axial graphic depicts extensive PNF ➡ of the right face and orbit, infiltrating the cavernous sinus ⇨ in a patient with neurofibromatosis type 1 (NF1). Buphthalmos ("cow eye") ➡ and sphenoid wing hypoplasia ➡ are other features of NF1 that are illustrated here.*

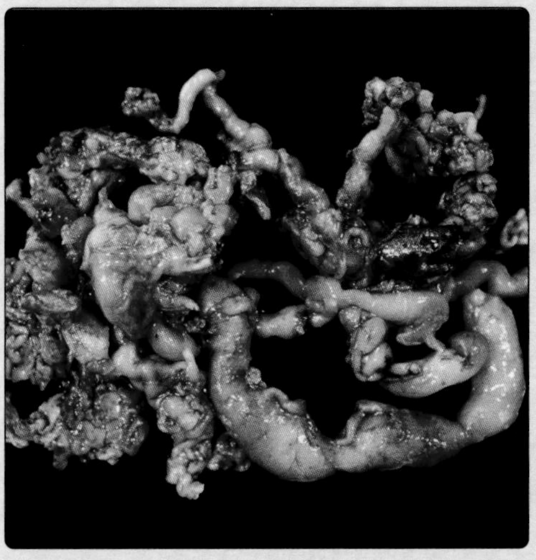

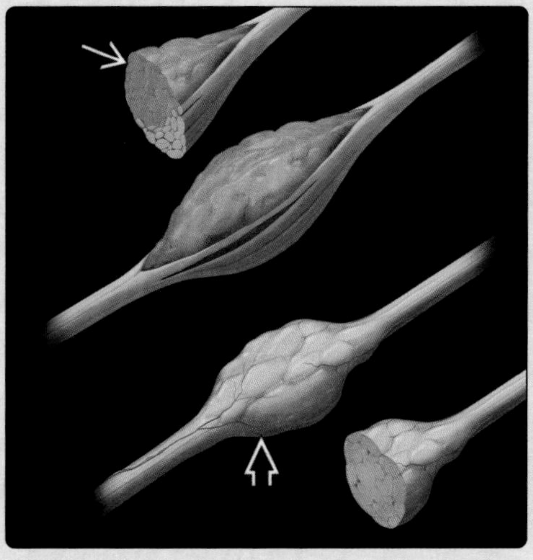

***(23-82)** Gross pathology shows plexiform neurofibroma with multiple enlarged, worm-like tumor fascicles. (Courtesy R. Hewlett, MD.) **(23-83)** Graphic depicts the difference between schwannoma (above) and neurofibroma (below). Schwannomas ➡ displace nerve fascicles, whereas neurofibromas ➡ infiltrate between fascicles.*

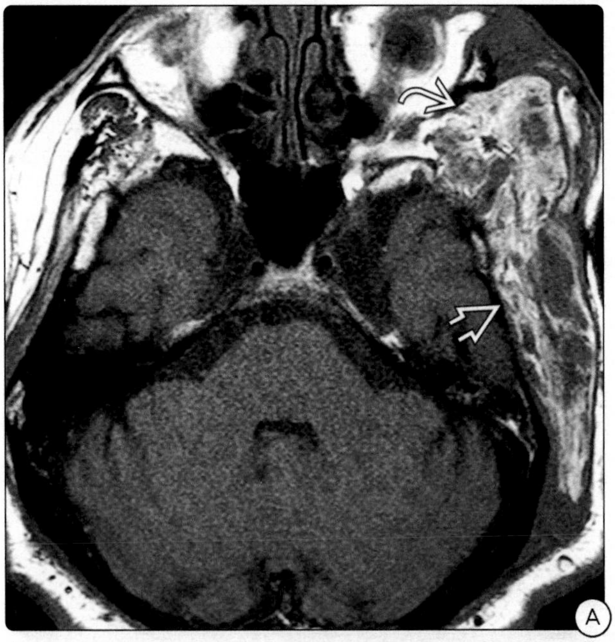

(23-84A) Axial T1WI in a patient with NF1 demonstrates a very large infiltrating mass in the left scalp ➡ that extends into the high deep masticator space ➡.

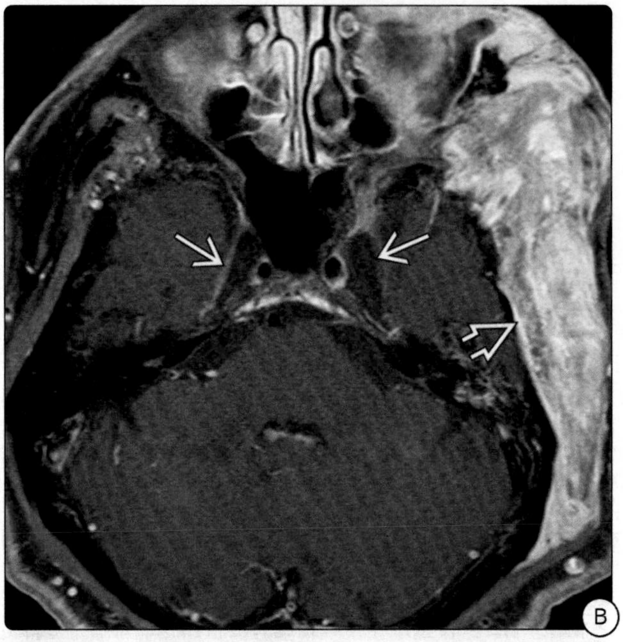

(23-84B) T1 C+ FS in the same case shows that the extensively infiltrating plexiform neurofibroma of the scalp ➡ enhances intensely but heterogeneously. Note patulous Meckel caves ➡, a finding of dural ectasia in some patients with NF1.

NEUROFIBROMA

Solitary Neurofibroma
- Most are sporadic (nonsyndromic)
- All ages (children to adults)
- Nodular to polypoid
- Scalp, skin
- Rarely (if ever) involves cranial nerves

Plexiform Neurofibroma
- Pathology
  - Composed of Schwann cells + fibroblasts, mucoid material
  - Fusiform, infiltrates nerve
  - Often multicompartmental
  - Does not respect fascial boundaries
- Clinical Issues
  - Usually diagnostic of NF1
  - "Sporadic" PNFs can occur without other signs of NF1, but most have *NF1* gene alterations
  - Risk of malignant degeneration in PNF = 5%
  - Rapid/painful enlargement, invasion? Suspect malignant peripheral nerve sheath tumor (MPNST)!
- Imaging
  - Multifocal scalp, orbit lesions most common
  - "Bag of worms" appearance
  - May enlarge superior orbital fissure, extend into CS
  - Intracranial involvement rare unless malignant degeneration
- Differential Diagnosis
  - MPNST (invasive)
  - Schwannoma (usually solitary; skin/scalp lesions, plexiform schwannoma rare)
  - Metastases

If a previously quiescent PNF enlarges rapidly or becomes painful, malignant degeneration into MPNST should be suspected. Most MPNSTs are invasive as well as infiltrating lesions.

Schwannomas are well-circumscribed solitary lesions that involve CNs, especially CN VIII. In contrast to PNF, scalp and orbital schwannomas are uncommon.

Basal cell carcinoma and infiltrating skin/scalp **metastases** without concomitant involvement of the underlying skull are rare.

Scalp **sarcomas** and **lymphomas** are also rare. When present, they are more diffusely infiltrating, homogeneous lesions without normal-appearing tissue interspersed within the mass.

Malignant Nerve Sheath Neoplasms

Malignant Peripheral Nerve Sheath Tumor

Terminology

A malignant peripheral nerve sheath tumor (MPNST) is any malignant tumor that arises from a peripheral nerve or shows nerve sheath differentiation. This term replaces designations such as malignant schwannoma, malignant neurofibroma, neurosarcoma, and neurofibrosarcoma.

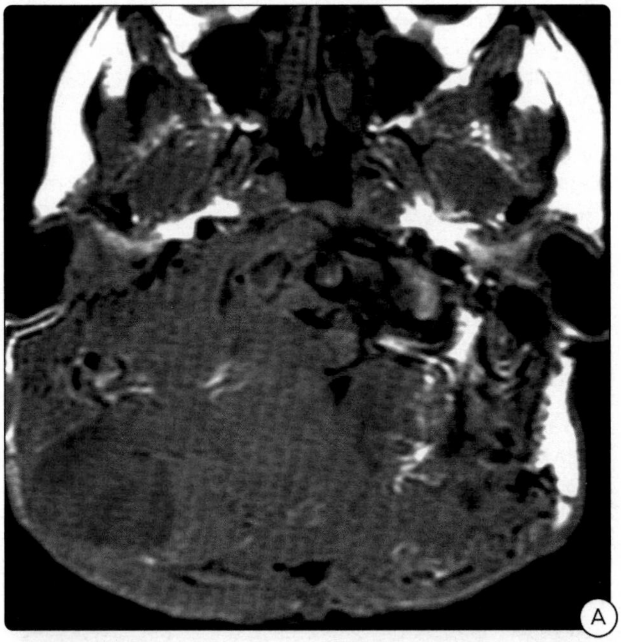

(23-85A) An NF1 patient with a longstanding PNF experienced rapid enlargement of the mass, which became painful. T1WI shows a massive soft tissue mass invading the skull base and upper cervical spine.

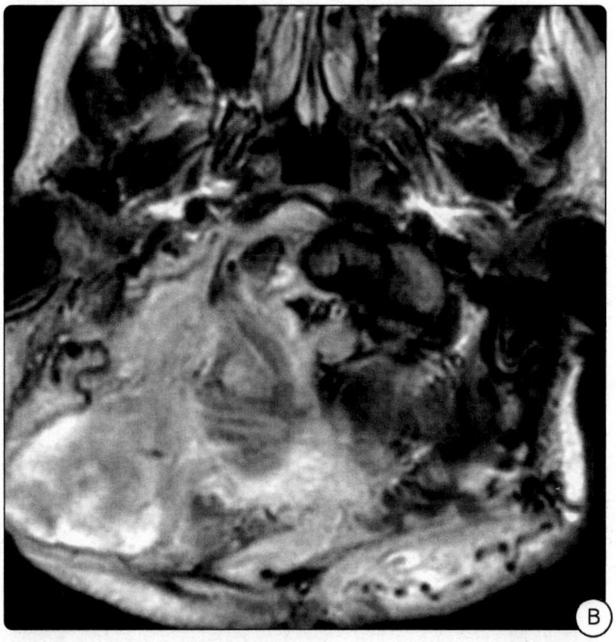

(23-85B) T1 C+ shows that the mass enhances intensely but very heterogeneously. The size, extent, and invasive nature of the mass were significantly different from prior baseline studies. Malignant peripheral nerve sheath tumor was found at biopsy.

When it occurs intracranially, an MPNST is sometimes called a malignant intracerebral nerve sheath tumor or a primary malignant intracranial nerve sheath tumor.

Etiology

Approximately half of all cranial MPNSTs occur sporadically, most likely from pluripotent neural crest cells. The other half arise from a preexisting benign nerve sheath tumor. Identifiable precursor lesions reported with MPNSTs include both plexiform and solitary intraneural neurofibroma. Malignant transformation of conventional or cellular schwannomas is exceptionally rare.

Approximately two-thirds of *peripheral* MPNSTs are associated with malignant degeneration of tumors associated with NF1. Diffuse loss of neurofibromin occurs in 90% of NF1-associated and 43% of sporadic MPNSTs. Genetic data suggest that combined inactivation of *NF1*, *CDKN2A*, and *PRCD* with aberrant activation of downstream RAS signaling is critical for MPNST pathogenesis.

The overall lifetime risk of developing an MPNST at any location in patients with NF1 is estimated at 8-13%. In a recent series of *intracranial* MPNSTs, 5 of 17 patients had NF1. Four had postirradiation MPNSTs.

Pathology

Location. MPNST is much more common in the peripheral or spinal nerves than in the cranial nerves. The most commonly affected cranial nerves are the vestibular, facial, and trigeminal nerves. Intracranial MPNSTs not associated with cranial nerves are extremely rare.

Size and Number. The majority of MPNSTs are over 5 cm, although intracranial lesions may be smaller at initial diagnosis.

Microscopic Features. MPNSTs vary greatly in appearance. The majority are widely infiltrating, hypercellular lesions that show proliferating malignant spindle cells with numerous mitoses. The 2016 WHO now recognizes two subtypes of MPNST: **epithelioid MPNST** and **MPNST with perineurial differentiation**. Other variants such as Triton tumor (an MPNST with rhabdomyoblastic differentiation) are considered histologic patterns, not subtypes.

Immunohistochemistry differentiates malignant tumors of nerve sheath derivation from soft tissue sarcomas. The majority of MPNSTs show diffuse, strong immunoreactivity for p53 protein along with S100 and collagen IV-laminin staining.

Staging, Grading, and Classification. There is no clinically validated and reproducible grading system for MPNSTs. Low-grade MPNSTs (15% of cases) are relatively well-differentiated tumors often arising in transition from neurofibroma. All the other MPNSTs are considered high-grade.

Clinical Issues

Epidemiology. MPNSTs are rare, accounting for only 0.001% of malignant neoplasms. MPNSTs that arise from cranial nerves are even rarer. Intracranial MPNSTs *not* associated with cranial nerves are exceptionally rare.

Demographics. Although they can occur at almost any age, sporadic MPNSTs are primarily tumors of middle-aged and older adults. Peak occurrence is in the fifth and sixth decades. NF1-associated MPNSTs occur earlier, with mean age 20-35 years. MPNSTs show a slight female predominance.

Natural History. Intracranial MPNSTs are fast-growing, aggressive, highly invasive tumors that generally have the same poor prognosis as those of spinal and peripheral nerves. MPNSTs are fatal in two-thirds of all patients. Most die as a result of disseminated metastases despite surgery, radiation, and chemotherapy.

Treatment Options. Total tumor resection with adjuvant radiotherapy is the treatment mainstay. Even with tumor-free margins, recurrence is common (40-70%). Survival of patients with subtotal tumor removal is generally less than 1 year.

Imaging

There are no obvious characteristics that would differentiate MPNST from benign nerve sheath tumor on a single baseline imaging study **(23-86)**. Gross necrosis or hemorrhage is rare. A few tumors may initially show frank brain or skull invasion, poor margination, and edema. MRS findings are nonspecific. Elevated choline is common.

It is the behavior on *serial* imaging studies that helps distinguish MPNST from benign nerve sheath tumors. Aggressive growth with brain and bone invasion is typical **(23-85)**.

CSF dissemination often rapidly ensues after the initial diagnosis is established. Distant extracranial metastases, most often to the lung, are common.

Differential Diagnosis

Small MPNSTs may be indistinguishable from benign nerve sheath tumors. The major differential diagnosis of a scalp or skull base MPNST is **plexiform neurofibromas**.

Both are diffusely infiltrating, poorly marginated lesions. When plexiform neurofibromas extend intracranially, they expand natural foramina and fissures but do not directly invade bone or brain. Rapid enlargement and bone destruction are more consistent with MPNST.

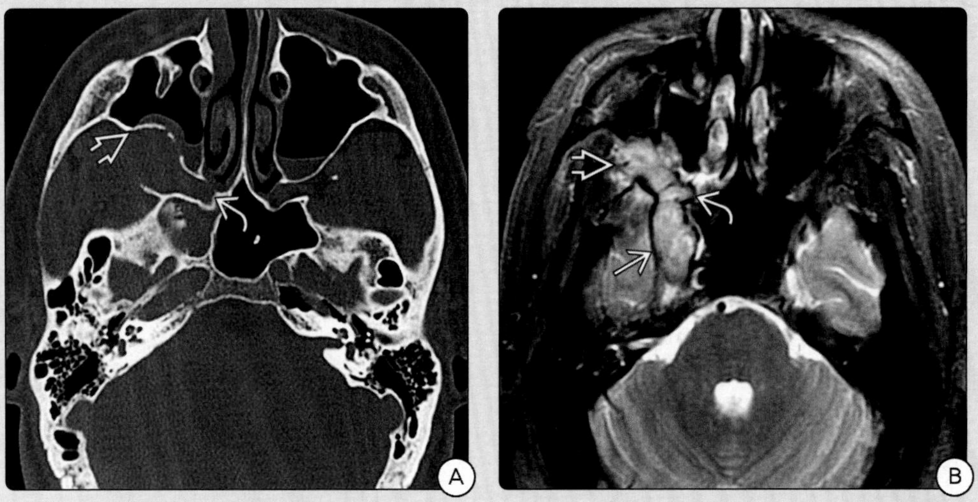

***(23-86A)** Axial bone CT in a 42y man with progressive numbness of his right cheek and jaw shows a mass in the high deep masticator space remodeling and partially eroding the posterior maxillary sinus wall ➡ and expanding the pterygopalatine fossa ➡. **(23-86B)** T2 FS shows a hyperintense fusiform mass in the masticator space ➡ extending posteriorly through the enlarged pterygopalatine fossa ➡ into the cavernous sinus ➡.*

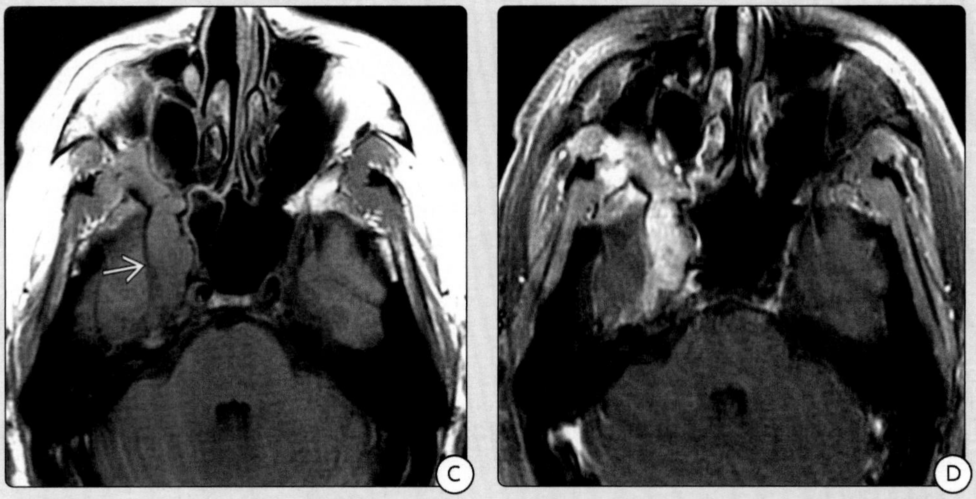

***(23-86C)** Axial T1WI shows that the fusiform mass ➡ expands the cavernous sinus and appears isointense with brain. **(23-86D)** T1 C+ FS in the same case shows that the mass enhances strongly, somewhat heterogeneously. Preoperative diagnosis was trigeminal schwannoma. Malignant peripheral nerve sheath tumor was found at histopathology.*

MALIGNANT PERIPHERAL NERVE SHEATH TUMOR

Terminology
- MPNST is the accepted term (replaces malignant schwannoma, neurofibrosarcoma)

Pathology
- Location
  - Peripheral/spinal > > cranial nerves
  - Vestibular, facial, trigeminal most common intracranial locations
- Features
  - Widely infiltrating
  - Malignant spindle cells, numerous mitoses
  - Immunohistochemistry distinguishes MPNST from other sarcomas
  - Low-grade (15%) MPNSTs more differentiated, often from neurofibroma
  - High-grade (85%) MPNSTs include spindle cell, pleomorphic, sarcomatous differentiation

Clinical Issues
- Rare; usually middle-aged, older adults
- Younger if neurofibromatosis type 1 associated
- Many arise de novo or from malignant degeneration of neurofibroma
- 8-13% risk of MPNST in plexiform neurofibroma

Imaging
- No distinctive imaging features
- Behavior on serial imaging best indicator
- Rapid aggressive growth
- Invasion, CSF dissemination

The rare brain parenchymal MPNST that is not associated with a cranial nerve is indistinguishable from other highly aggressive, invasive malignant neoplasms. The major differential diagnoses include **glioblastoma, gliosarcoma, fibrosarcoma,**and **malignant fibrous histiocytoma.**

Other Nerve Sheath Tumors

A number of other neoplasms and tumor-like conditions occasionally involve cranial nerves although most are much more common in peripheral nerves and soft tissues. Examples include perineurioma, solitary fibrous tumor, and neurofibrosarcoma.

Intraneural **perineuriomas** account for just 1% of nerve sheath tumors. Perineuriomas involving cranial nerves are very rare, usually involving extracranial branches of CNs V or VII. **Solitary fibrous tumors** that arise from intracranial cranial nerves are indistinguishable from schwannomas on imaging studies, so the definitive diagnosis is histopathologic. **Neurofibrosarcomas** are more properly considered malignant nerve sheath tumors (whether peripheral or intracranial).

Chronic interstitial demyelinating polyneuropathy (CIDP) and **Charcot-Marie-Tooth disease** are benign conditions that rarely affect cranial nerves. When they do, diffuse enlargement and enhancement of one or more cranial nerves can be seen **(23-87)** **(23-88)**.

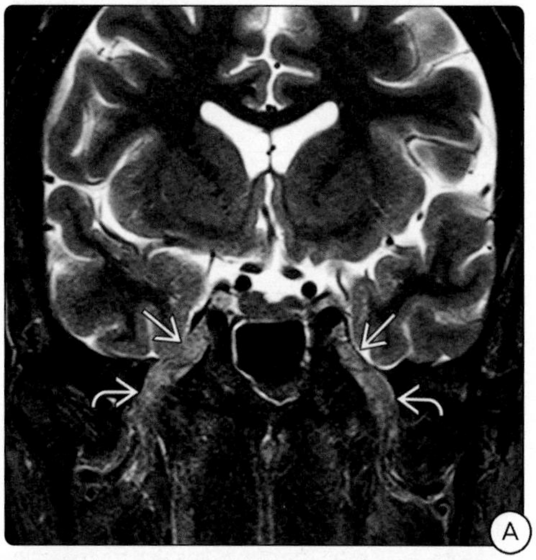

***(23-87A)** Coronal STIR shows symmetric, fusiform enlargement of both intra- and extracranial trigeminal nerve segments.*

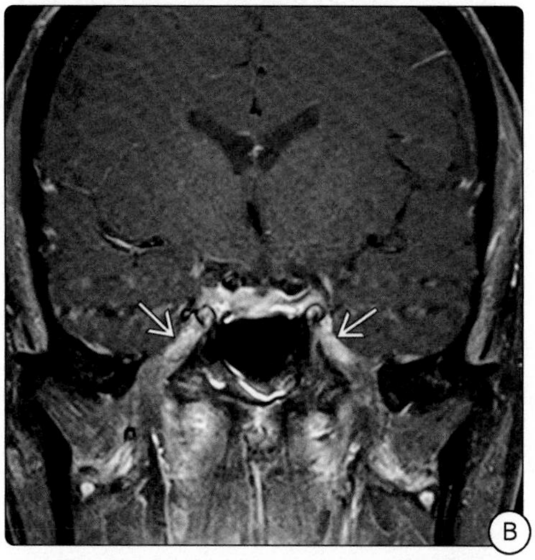

***(23-87B)** Coronal T1 C+ FS shows the enlarged, enhancing trigeminal nerves. This is chronic interstitial demyelinating polyneuropathy (CIDP).*

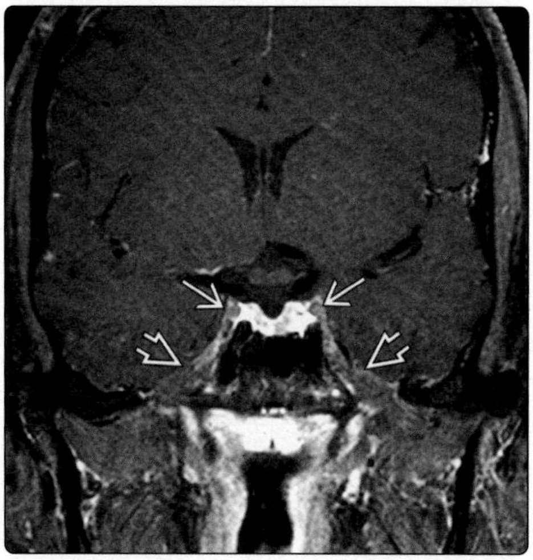

***(23-88)** Coronal T1 C+ FS in Charcot-Marie-Tooth disease shows symmetrically enlarged, enhancing oculomotor, trigeminal nerves.*

Selected References

Cranial Nerve Anatomy

Upper Cranial Nerves

Schwob JE et al: The stem and progenitor cells of the mammalian olfactory epithelium: Taking poietic license. J Comp Neurol. 525(4):1034-1054, 2017

Tsutsumi S et al: Visualization of the olfactory nerve using constructive interference in steady state magnetic resonance imaging. Surg Radiol Anat. 39(3):315-321, 2017

Elder C et al: Isolated abducens nerve palsy: update on evaluation and diagnosis. Curr Neurol Neurosci Rep. 16(8):69, 2016

Miller SR et al: Evidence for a Notch1-mediated transition during olfactory ensheathing cell development. J Anat. 229(3):369-83, 2016

Seeburg DP et al: The role of imaging for trigeminal neuralgia: a segmental approach to high-resolution MRI. Neurosurg Clin N Am. 27(3):315-26, 2016

Tantiwongkosi B et al: Imaging of ocular motor pathway. Neuroimaging Clin N Am. 25(3):425-38, 2015

Yu F et al: Advanced MR imaging of the visual pathway. Neuroimaging Clin N Am. 25(3):383-93, 2015

Lower Cranial Nerves

Haller S et al: Imaging of neurovascular compression syndromes: trigeminal neuralgia, hemifacial spasm, vestibular paroxysmia, and glossopharyngeal neuralgia. AJNR Am J Neuroradiol. 37(8):1384-92, 2016

Ong CK et al: The glossopharyngeal, vagus and spinal accessory nerves. Eur J Radiol. 74(2):359-67, 2010

Schwannomas

Schwannoma Overview

Ando T et al: Comparison between MR imaging findings of intracranial and extracranial schwannomas. Clin Imaging. 42:218-223, 2017

Antonescu CR et al: Schwannoma. In: Louis DN et al (eds), WHO Classification of Tumours of the Central Nervous System. Lyon, France: International Agency for Research on Cancer, 2016, pp 214-218

Skolnik AD et al: Cranial nerve schwannomas: diagnostic imaging approach. Radiographics. 36(5):1463-77, 2016

Vestibular Schwannoma

Caltabiano R et al: A mosaic pattern of INI1/SMARCB1 protein expression distinguishes schwannomatosis and NF2-associated peripheral schwannomas from solitary peripheral schwannomas and NF2-associated vestibular schwannomas. Childs Nerv Syst. 33(6):933-940, 2017

Coffey N et al: Imaging findings in sensorineural hearing loss: a pictorial essay. Can Assoc Radiol J. 68(2):106-115, 2017

Håvik AL et al: Genetic landscape of sporadic vestibular schwannoma. J Neurosurg. 1-12, 2017

Schulze M et al: Improvement in imaging common temporal bone pathologies at 3 T MRI: small structures benefit from a small field of view. Clin Radiol. 72(3):267.e1-267.e12, 2017

Daultrey CR et al: Size as a risk factor for growth in conservatively managed vestibular schwannomas: the Birmingham experience. Otolaryngol Clin North Am. 49(5):1291-5, 2016

Trigeminal Schwannoma

Agrawal A et al: Extracranial trigeminal schwannomas: a retrospective analysis. J Maxillofac Oral Surg. 16(2):164-169, 2017

Agarwal A: Intracranial trigeminal schwannoma. Neuroradiol J. 28(1):36-41, 2015

Facial Nerve Schwannoma

McRackan TR et al: Primary tumors of the facial nerve. Otolaryngol Clin North Am. 48(3):491-500, 2015

Schwannomas of Other Intracranial Nerves

Zhang Q et al: Intra- and extramedullary dumbbell-shaped schwannoma of the medulla oblongata: a case report and review of the literature. World Neurosurg. 98:873.e1-873.e7, 2017

Shin RK et al: Transient ocular motor nerve palsies associated with presumed cranial nerve schwannomas. J Neuroophthalmol. 35(2):139-43, 2015

Suthar PP et al: Isolated hypoglossal nerve schwannoma: an uncommon presentation of schwannoma. J Clin Diagn Res. 9(10):TJ01-2, 2015

Parenchymal Schwannomas

Luo W et al: Intracranial intraparenchymal and intraventricular schwannomas: report of 18 cases. Clin Neurol Neurosurg. 115(7):1052-7, 2013

Melanotic Schwannoma

Agarwalla PK et al: Pigmented lesions of the nervous system and the neural crest: lessons from embryology. Neurosurgery. 78(1):142-55, 2016

Spina A et al: Intracranial melanotic schwannomas. J Neurol Surg A Cent Eur Neurosurg. 76(5):399-406, 2015

Schwannomatosis

Kehrer-Sawatzki H et al: The molecular pathogenesis of schwannomatosis, a paradigm for the co-involvement of multiple tumour suppressor genes in tumorigenesis. Hum Genet. 136(2):129-148, 2017

Faucett EA et al: A diagnostic dilemma: multiple primary intracranial tumors without vestibular schwannomas. Ann Otol Rhinol Laryngol. 125(11):938-942, 2016

Neurofibromas

Perry A et al: Neurofibroma. In: Louis DN et al (eds), WHO Classification of Tumours of the Central Nervous System. Lyon, France: International Agency for Research on Cancer, 2016, pp 219-221

Röhrich M et al: Methylation-based classification of benign and malignant peripheral nerve sheath tumors. Acta Neuropathol. 131(6):877-87, 2016

Lymphomas and Hematopoietic and Histiocytic Tumors

The spectrum of hematopoietic neoplasms and tumor-like disorders that affect the CNS ranges from frankly malignant neoplasms like diffuse large B-cell lymphoma to nonneoplastic lesions such as extramedullary hematopoiesis.

For purposes of discussion, this chapter is divided into three major sections: (1) lymphomas and related disorders, (2) histiocytic tumors, and (3) hematopoietic tumors and tumor-like lesions (leukemias, plasma cell neoplasms, and extramedullary hematopoiesis). We begin our discussion with the largest group, **lymphomas and related disorders.**

Histiocytic tumors occasionally involve the CNS. These neoplasms and nonneoplastic tumor-like masses are composed of histiocytes that are microscopically identical to their extracranial counterparts. Both **Langerhans cell histiocytosis** and **non-Langerhans histiocytoses** such as Erdheim-Chester disease, Rosai-Dorfman disease, juvenile xanthogranuloma, and histiocytic sarcoma are considered in the second section.

Lastly, we then turn our attention to hematopoietic tumors and tumor-like lesions. Although the most recent WHO classification includes only malignant lymphomas and histiocytic tumors in the group of hematopoietic neoplasms, we include **leukemia** in this chapter even though CNS involvement is almost always secondary to systemic disease.

Plasma cell myeloma and **solitary plasmacytoma** affecting the skull and brain are also usually secondary to extracranial disease, but they are a form of mature B-cell neoplasms and hence are included here rather than in Chapter 27 on metastases. We conclude the chapter with a brief discussion of **extramedullary hematopoiesis**—benign, nonneoplastic proliferations of blood-forming elements—which can appear virtually identical to malignant hematopoietic neoplasms.

Lymphomas and Related Disorders

Lymphoid CNS lesions may occur either as primary tumors or metastatic deposits from extracranial disease. Together, lymphoid neoplasms comprise the sixth most common group of CNS malignancies. More than 95% are **diffuse large B-cell lymphomas** (DLBCLs).

The remaining 4-5% of primary CNS lymphoma (PCNSL) subtypes are T- and NK-/T-cell lymphomas and low-grade B-cell lymphomas such as mucosa-associated (MALT) lymphomas of the dura and marginal zone B-cell lymphomas that correspond to their systemic counterparts. MALT lymphoma of the dura and Hodgkin-type lymphomas (HLs) are uncommon in

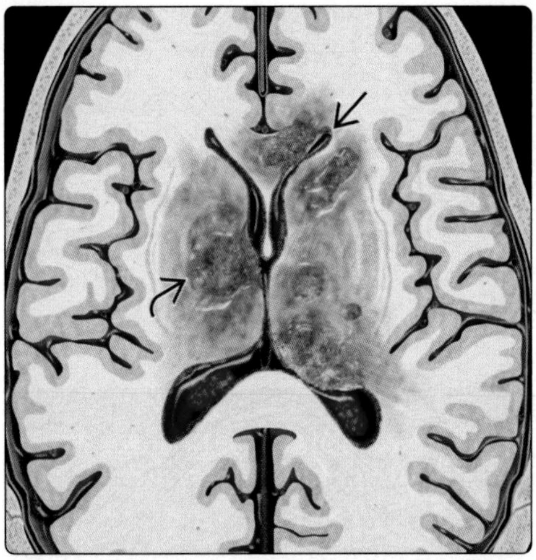

(24-1) This is PCNSL. Periventricular lesions ➡ are in BG, thalamus, corpus callosum with extensive subependymal spread of disease ➡.

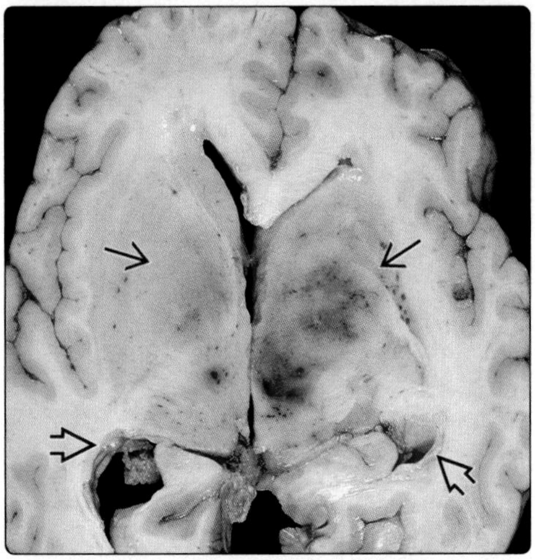

(24-2) Autopsy shows PCNSL with bilateral deep basal ganglionic, thalamic masses ➡, ependymal spread ➡. (Courtesy R. Hewlett, MD.)

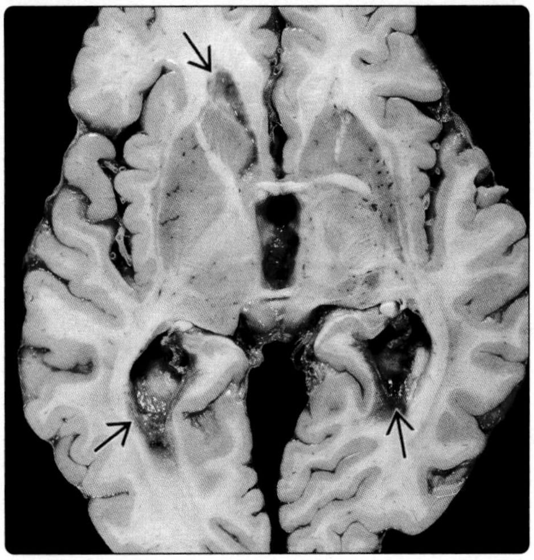

(24-3) Autopsy shows extensive ependymal spread of PCNSL around the lateral ventricles ➡.(Courtesy R. Hewlett, MD.)

the CNS. Most are seen as metastatic lesions in the setting of advanced systemic disease although rare primary CNS lesions have been described.

We begin this chapter by focusing on DLBCL. We then consider the fascinating spectrum of **immunodeficiency-associated CNS lymphomas** (including lymphomatoid granulomatosis and posttransplant lymphoproliferative disorder).

We follow the detailed discussion of DLBCL with a discussion of **intravascular large B-cell lymphoma**, an uncommon but increasingly well-recognized cause of unexplained cognitive decline in elderly patients. Uncommon primary CNS lymphomas such as low-grade B-cell lymphomas, T-cell and NK-/T-cell lymphomas, anaplastic large cell lymphoma, and MALT lymphoma of the dura are then briefly discussed.

We close this section with a brief review of CNS metastatic lymphoma. (Metastatic lymphoma is included here instead of in Chapter 27 with other metastatic disease, as its imaging appearance differs from that of other systemic cancers that spread to the brain.)

Diffuse Large B-Cell Lymphoma of the CNS

Terminology

A diffuse large B-cell lymphoma of the CNS (DLBCL) is an extranodal B-cell lymphoma that arises exclusively inside the CNS. By definition, disease outside the nervous system is absent at the time of initial diagnosis. The vast majority of primary CNS lymphomas (PCNSLs) are DLBCLs. For purposes of discussion, in this text, the terms PCNSL and DLBCL are used interchangeably.

2016 WHO CLASSIFICATION OF PRIMARY CNS LYMPHOMAS

Diffuse Large B-Cell Lymphoma of the CNS

Immunodeficiency-Associated CNS Lymphomas
- AIDS-related diffuse large B-cell lymphoma
- Epstein-Barr virus-positive diffuse large B-cell lymphoma, NOS
- Lymphomatoid granulomatosis
- Posttransplant lymphoproliferative disorder

Intravascular Large B-Cell Lymphoma

Miscellaneous Rare CNS Lymphomas
- Low-grade B-cell lymphomas
- T-cell and NK-/T-cell lymphoma
- Anaplastic large cell lymphoma

MALT Lymphoma of the Dura

Etiology

General Concepts. Whether PCNSL arises inside or as transformed B cells originating outside the brain is unclear. Although functional lymphatic vessels are present in the dural venous sinuses, the brain parenchyma itself lacks classic lymphatics and normally contains very few lymphocytes. So how and why lymphomas arise as primary CNS neoplasms in immunocompetent individuals is unknown.

What is clearly evident is that lymphoma cells—regardless of whether they originate within or outside the brain—exhibit a distinct, highly selective neurotropism for the CNS microenvironment and its vasculature. Intra- and perivascular tumor spread is common.

Most PCNSLs are mature B-cell lymphomas that have a late or postgerminal center of origin with blocked terminal B-cell differentiation. Persistent surface expression of both B-cell lymphoma 6 (BCL6) protein and interferon regulatory factor 4 (IRF4) along with immunoglobulin gene rearrangement indicates that most PCNSLs have an activated B-cell phenotype.

Genetics. No genetic predispositions to PCNSL have been identified. Next-generation sequencing has identified a number of mutated genes involved in B-cell proliferation and differentiation, but to date no true lymphomagenesis "driver mutations" similar to those of gliomagenesis have been pinpointed.

Over 80% of protein-changing mutations in CNS DLBCL are located in eight specific genes (including *PTEN, CTNNB1, ATM*, and *TP53*), pointing to the potential role of these genes in lymphomagenesis. Notably, CNS DLBCL shares certain gene mutations (e.g., *TP53* and *SMO*) with other solid brain tumors.

Epigenetic changes may also contribute to DLBCL pathogenesis, including aberrant hypermethylation of *DAPK1*.

Pathology

Location. DLBCL can affect any part of the neuraxis. Up to 75% all PCNSLs contact a CSF surface, either the ventricular ependyma or pia **(24-1)**. The cerebral hemispheres are the preferred site (85%). Lesions are often deep-seated with a predilection for the periventricular white matter, especially the corpus callosum. The basal ganglia and thalami are the next most common locations **(24-2)**. Tumor spread along the ventricular ependyma and into the choroid plexus is seen in some cases **(24-2) (24-3)**.

The hypothalamus, infundibulum, and pituitary gland are less common sites. Posterior fossa lesions and lesions of the spinal cord are relatively rare (15% of cases).

Primary DLBCL may also develop in the leptomeninges, calvarial vault, and central skull base although these areas are more commonly involved by metastatic spread from extracranial primary tumors (see below). Primary dura-based DLBCLs are very rare. Most are low-grade B-cell or MALT types.

Ocular lymphomas are almost always high-grade B-cell lymphomas. In contrast, lymphomas of the orbital adnexa are most often MALT-type tumors (see below).

Size and Number. DLBCL lesions vary in size from microscopic implants to large bulky masses.

Up to two-thirds of all PCNSLs are solitary lesions. Of the PCNSLs with multiple lesions, approximately half are bilateral.

Gross Pathology. Single or multiple hemispheric masses with a "fish flesh" consistency are typical. In contrast to astrocytomas, lymphomas tend to be relatively well demarcated rather than diffusely infiltrating lesions. Most are solid, pale lesions with occasional necroses and small hemorrhagic foci. Large confluent areas of frank necrosis and gross intratumoral hemorrhage are more common in AIDS-related PCNSLs (see below) **(24-10)**.

Occasionally, PCNSLs diffusely infiltrate large areas of the hemispheres without forming a focal cohesive mass. Widespread infiltration of lymphoma cells in both gray and white matter is characteristic. This condition—also known as **lymphomatosis cerebri**—is uncommon, occurring in less than 5% of cases, and is a pattern, not a distinct disease entity.

Microscopic Features. PCNSLs are highly cellular tumors. Microscopically, large atypical cells with large round to irregular nuclei with prominent nucleoli are typical. MIB-1 is high, often exceeding 50% (significantly higher than with glioblastoma). The WHO does not assign a grade to PCNSL.

Most PCNSLs exhibit a distinct predilection for blood vessels, with layering of tumor cells in and around vessels that extend from these perivascular cuffs into the adjacent parenchyma. This **"angiocentric" clustering** is often accompanied by prominent rings of reticulin in and around vessel walls.

The overwhelming majority of DLBCLs are positive on CD20 and CD45 immunostaining.

Reactive inflammatory infiltrates consisting of mature T and B cells are common. Occasionally, steroid-responsive **multifocal demyelinating "sentinel" lesions** that are indistinguishable from those seen in tumefactive multiple sclerosis or acute disseminated encephalomyelitis (ADEM) can be seen months or even several years before PCNSL is diagnosed.

Even small doses of corticosteroids can induce striking apoptosis in PCNSLs. **Steroid treatment preceding biopsy can obscure the diagnosis of PCNSL in up to 50% of cases!**

PCNSL: ETIOLOGY AND PATHOLOGY

Etiology
- CNS lacks lymphatics, normally contains few lymphocytes
- Precise origin in immunocompetent individuals unknown

Pathology
- 3-6% of all primary CNS neoplasms
- Vast majority (90-95%) are DLBCLs
  - Large atypical cells
  - CD20+, CD45+
  - MIB-1 > 50%
- Predilection for deep brain
  - Periventricular WM, basal ganglia
  - Perivascular lymphoid clusters also common
- Solitary (2/3), multiple (1/3)
  - Multiple compartments may be involved
- Focal > > diffusely infiltrating lesions (lymphomatosis cerebri)
- Hemorrhage, necrosis rare in immunocompetent patients
- "Sentinel" demyelinating lesion indistinguishable from MS or ADEM can precede PCNSL!
- Corticosteroids → ↑ apoptosis, can obscure diagnosis of PCNSL!

Clinical Issues

Epidemiology. Although PCNSLs account for only 3% of all malignant CNS neoplasms, worldwide prevalence is increasing as a result of the HIV/AIDS epidemic and the use of immunosuppressive therapies (see below).

Demographics. Although PCNSLs can occur at all ages, they are generally tumors of middle-aged and older adults. Peak age (in immunocompetent patients) is 60 years. There is an overall slight male predominance.

Presentation. Most patients with PCNSL present with focal neurologic deficits, altered mental status, and neuropsychiatric disturbances. Seizures are less common than in patients with other primary brain tumors.

Occasionally, PCNSL is preceded by demyelinating and inflammatory lesions similar to multiple sclerosis. Cases of so-called "sentinel lesions" occurring up to 2 years after initial presentation with demyelinating lesions have been reported.

Patients with nonfocal, diffusely infiltrating PCNSLs (lymphomatosis cerebri) typically present with generalized cognitive decline and rapidly progressive dementia. Memory deficits, ataxia, personality changes, and abnormal behaviors are common. Most patients are middle aged or elderly.

Natural History. CNS DLBCL has a significantly worse outcome than its systemic counterparts. CNS DLBCL is an aggressive tumor with a median survival of only a few months in untreated patients. In general, immunocompetent patients younger than 60 years fare slightly better than older patients and patients with acquired immunodeficiency syndromes.

Patients with lymphomatosis cerebri generally have a dire prognosis, with survival under 2 years uncommon.

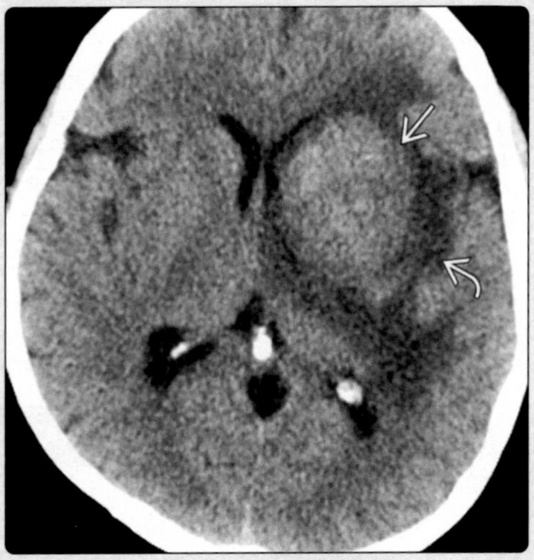

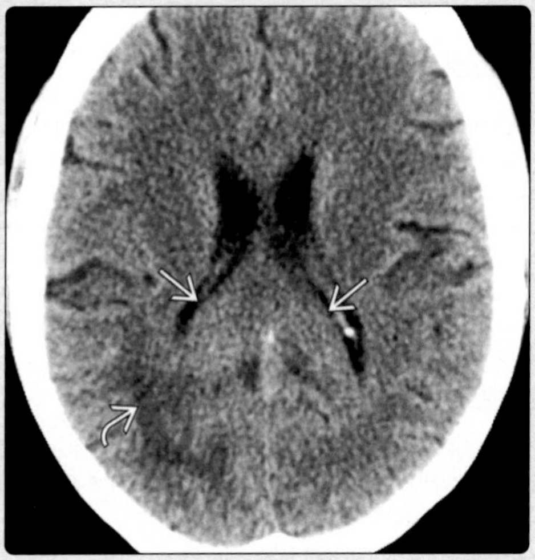

***(24-4)** NECT in a 63y woman with right-sided weakness shows a solitary hyperdense mass ➡ in the left BG with moderate edema ↪. **(24-5)** Axial NECT in a 63y woman with "stroke-like" presentation shows a grossly thickened corpus callosum splenium ➡ and right occipital confluent hypodensity ↪. Note that the "butterfly" mass is isodense with cortex and basal ganglia, not normal white matter. DLBCL was found at surgery.*

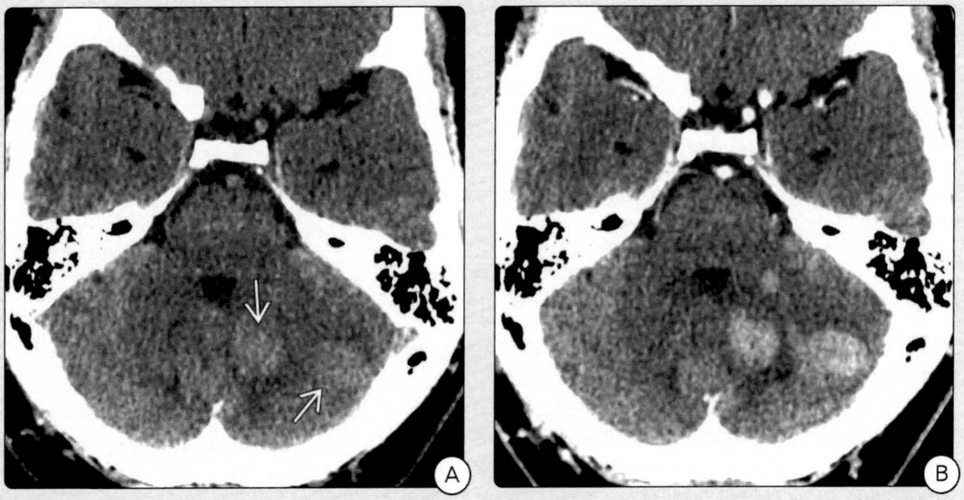

***(24-6A)** NECT scan in a patient with PCNSL shows hyperdense masses in the left cerebellum ➡. (Courtesy P. Hilenbrand, MD.) **(24-6B)** CECT shows multiple moderately enhancing masses in the cerebellum. (Courtesy P. Hildenbrand, MD.)*

Treatment Options. Early diagnosis is crucial for proper management of PCNSLs. As gross surgical resection does not improve prognosis, stereotactic biopsy for diagnostic confirmation and histologic tumor typing is recommended.

As with systemic non-Hodgkin lymphomas, treatment options for DLBCL include corticosteroids, high-dose methotrexate-based polychemotherapy, and radiation. Approximately 70% of patients initially respond to treatment, but relapse is very common. Progression-free survival is approximately 1 year, and overall survival is approximately 3 years. Only 20-40% of patients experience prolonged progression-free survival.

Antineoplastic agents designed specifically to treat B-cell malignancies and B-cell-driven diseases such as rheumatoid arthritis have been used with some success in selected cases. Rituximab is a chimeric murine/human monoclonal immunoglobulin G1 antibody that targets CD20, a cell-surface marker specifically found on B lymphocytes.

Imaging

General Features. Contrast-enhanced cranial MR is the modality of choice in evaluating patients with suspected PCNSL. As isolated spinal cord involvement is rare (3-4% of cases), spinal imaging is indicated only in patients with myelopathy or suspected diffuse meningeal dissemination.

Contrast-enhanced CT of the chest, abdomen, and pelvis or PET-CT is generally recommended in patients with suspected PCNSL to look for an extracranial source of disease.

CT Findings. All PCNSLs are highly cellular tumors. White matter or basal ganglia lesions in contact with a CSF surface are typical. Most lesions appear hyperdense compared with normal brain on NECT scans **(24-4)** **(24-5)**. Marked peritumoral edema is common, but gross necrosis, hemorrhage, and calcification are rare (2-5%) unless the patient is immunocompromised **(24-11A)**.

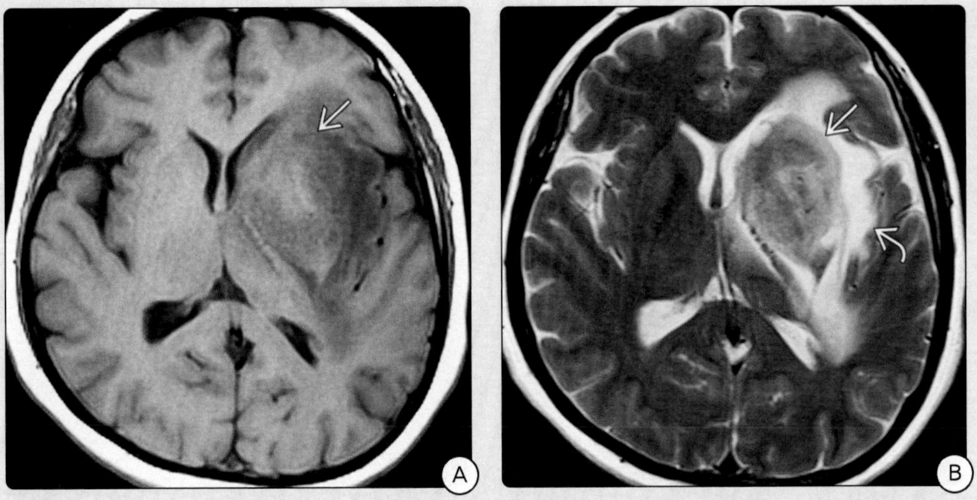

***(24-7A)** Axial T1WI shows a mass ➔ in the left basal ganglia that is mostly isointense with cortex. **(24-7B)** T2WI in the same case shows that the mass ➔ is mixed iso- to hypointense relative to cortex. A moderate amount of hyperintense peripheral edema ↪ is present.*

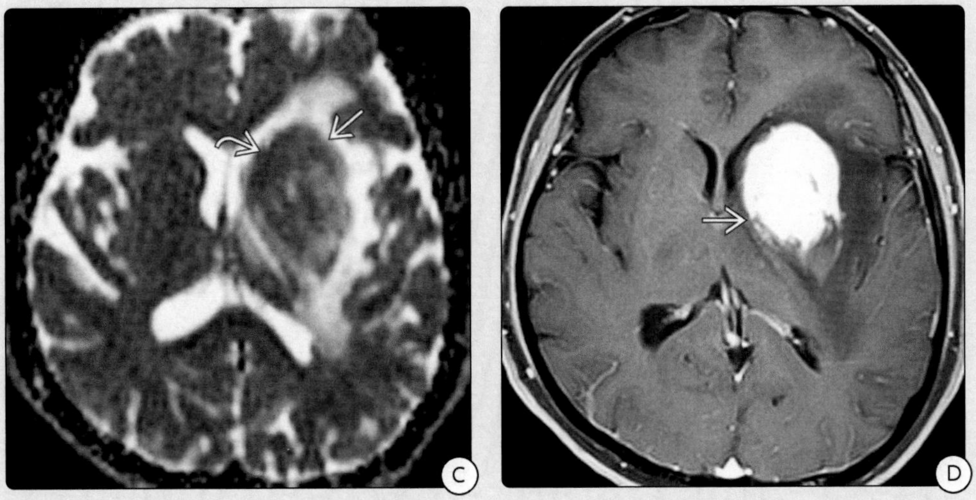

***(24-7C)** ADC map shows that the mass ➔ exhibits mild to moderate restricted diffusion ↪. **(24-7D)** T1 C+ FS shows that the mass ➔ enhances intensely and uniformly. DLBCL was found at surgery (same case as Figure 24-4).*

(24-8A) Axial T1WI in a 61y woman with DLBCL and no evidence for systemic disease on PET shows lesions in the basal ganglia and thalami ⇨ that appear isointense with gray matter. (24-8B) T2WI in the same case shows that the lesions ➡ appear isointense with gray matter, associated with some hyperintense peripheral edema ➡.

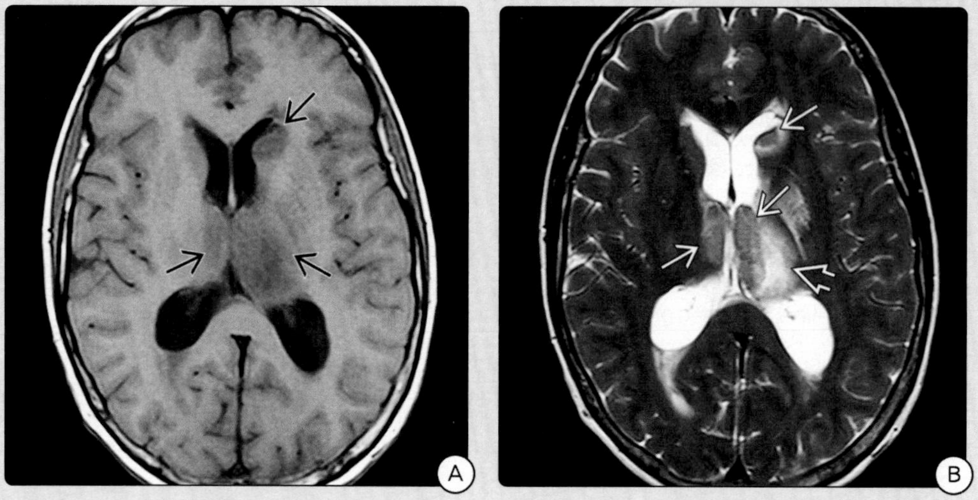

(24-8C) T1 C+ FS shows that the lesions ➡ enhance strongly and uniformly. (24-8D) The lesions ➡ show restricted diffusion with low ADC. Peritumoral edema ➡ is hyperintense because of "T2 shine-through."

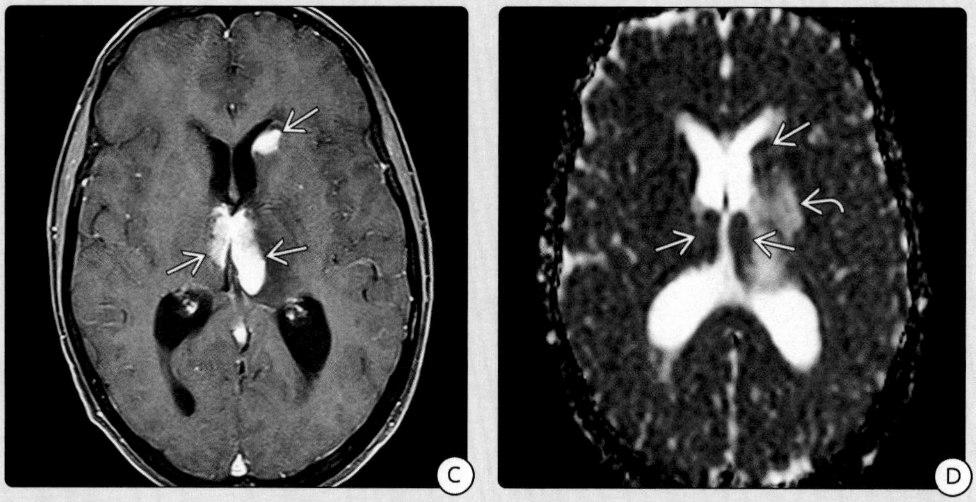

(24-8E) pMR shows no evidence for elevated rCBV in the lesions ➡. (24-8F) pMR with Ktrans shows elevated capillary permeability in the lesions ➡.

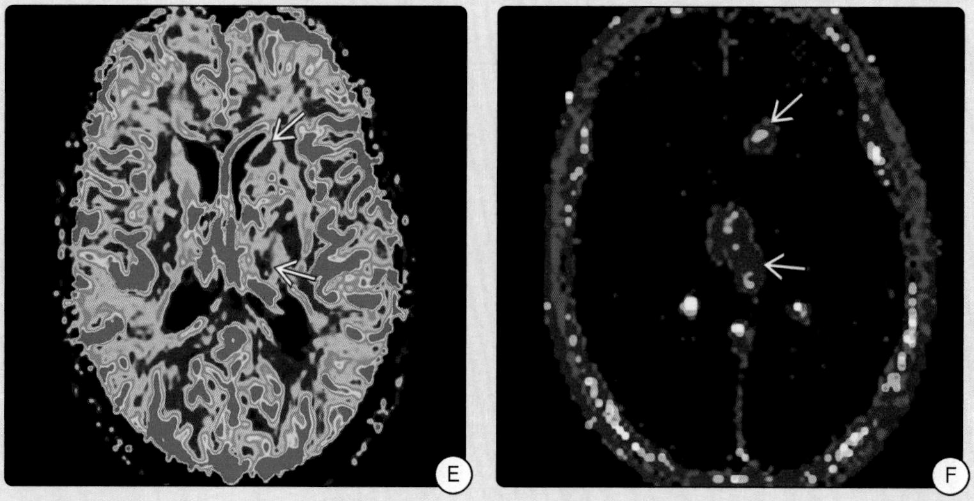

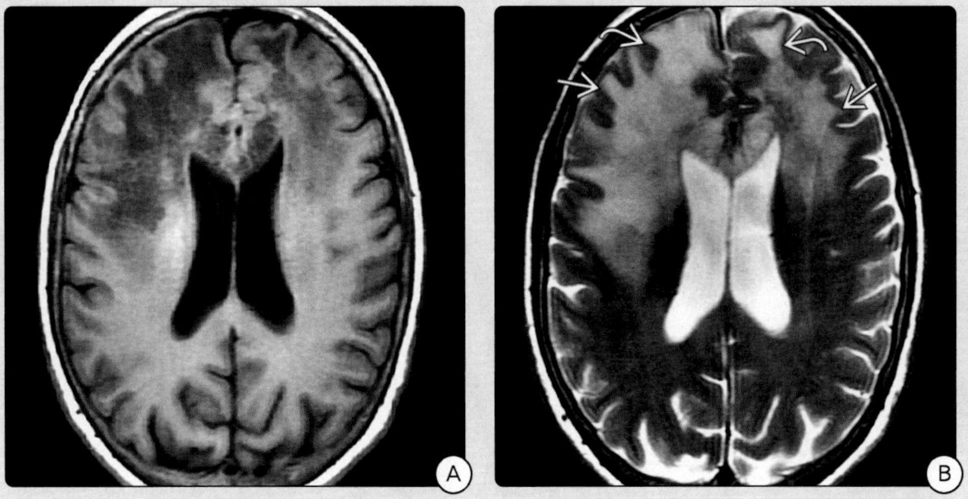

(24-9A) *Axial T1WI in a 64y woman with altered mental status and increasing confusion shows enlargement and diffuse confluent hypointensity in both frontal lobes and the corpus callosum genu.* ***(24-9B)*** *Axial T2WI in the same case shows confluent hyperintensity ➡ and gyral expansion of both frontal lobes ➡ with maintenance of the underlying architecture of the brain.*

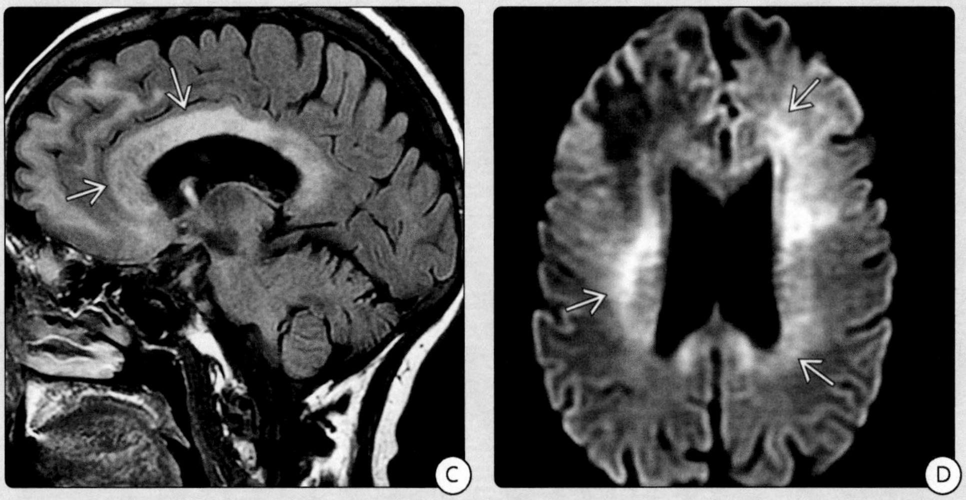

(24-9C) *Sagittal FLAIR in the same case shows infiltration and expansion of the corpus callosum ➡.* ***(24-9D)*** *DWI in the same case shows restricted diffusion throughout the periventricular WM ➡.*

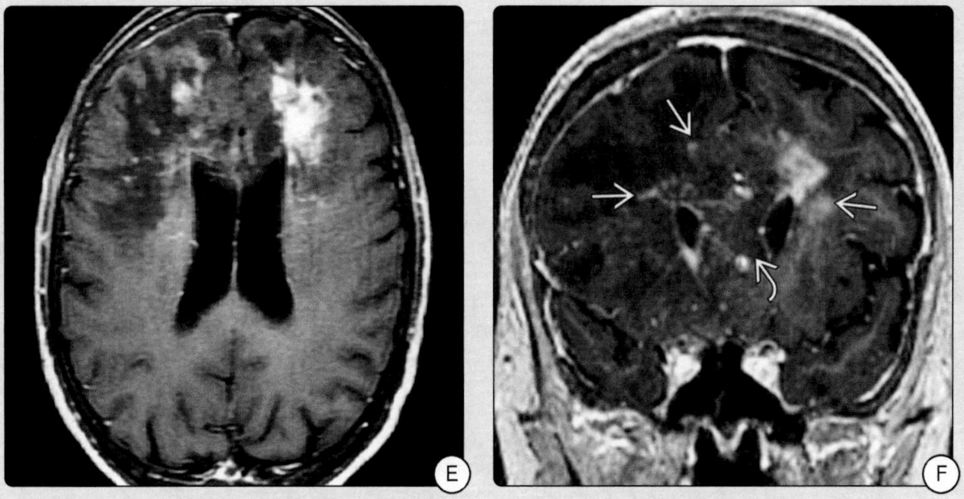

(24-9E) *T1 C+ FS shows patchy enhancement in both frontal lobes.* ***(24-9F)*** *Coronal T1 C+ SPGR shows that the thickened corpus callosum ➡ is largely nonenhancing, while there is patchy punctate and linear enhancement in the periventricular and deep WM ➡. Biopsy showed diffusely infiltrating DLBCL and lymphomatosis cerebri pattern.*

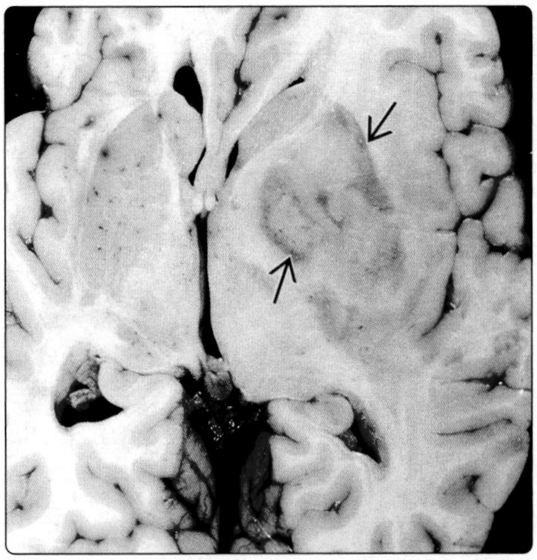

(24-10) Autopsy of PCNSL in HIV/AIDS shows hemorrhagic, necrotic left basal ganglia mass. (Courtesy R. Hewlett, MD.)

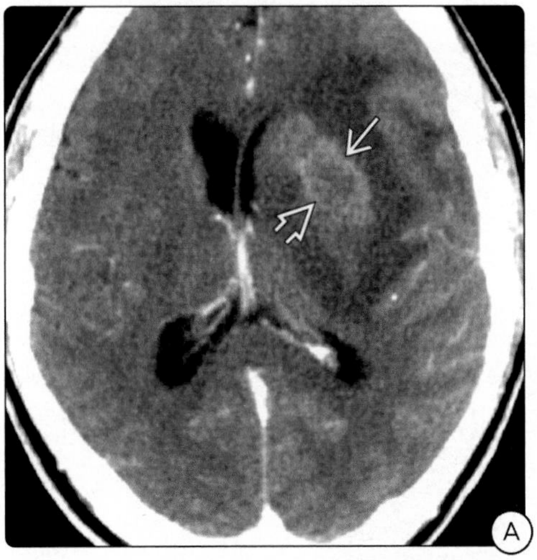

(24-11A) CECT scan shows necrosis and only faint rim enhancement in this HIV-positive patient with PCNSL.

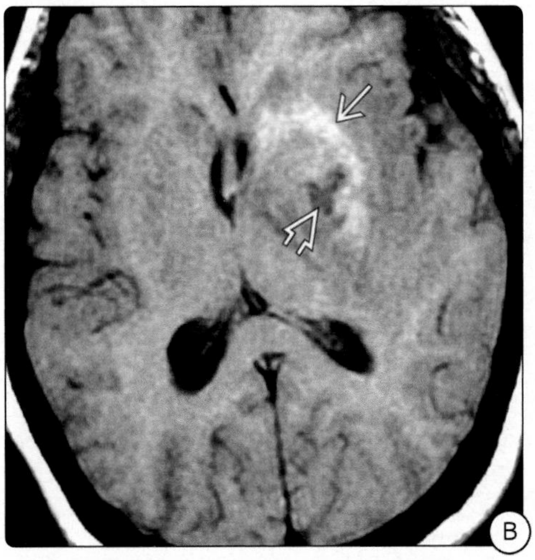

(24-11B) T1WI shows T1 shortening due to subacute hemorrhage with more acute hemorrhage in the necrotic core of the lesion.

DLBCLs in immunocompetent patients show mild to moderate, relatively homogeneous enhancement on CECT **(24-6)**. Irregular ring enhancement is rare unless the patient is immunocompromised.

MR Findings. Over three-quarters of DLBCLs in **immunocompetent** patients are iso- or slightly hypointense compared with gray matter on T1WI and isointense on T2WI **(24-7)**.

FLAIR signal is variable but usually iso- or hyperintense. Microhemorrhages with intratumoral "blooming" on T2* are present in 5-8% of cases, but gross hemorrhage is uncommon unless the patient is immunocompromised (see below).

Nearly all PCNSLs in immunocompetent patients enhance **(24-7D)**. Solid homogeneous or mildly heterogeneous enhancement is common; ring enhancement is rare. MRS typically demonstrates elevated choline and high lipids.

Because of their high cellularity, over 95% of PCNSLs show mild to moderate diffusion restriction with low ADC values **(24-7C)**. MRS is nonspecific, with elevated choline, reduced NAA and myoinositol, and prominent lipids. Tumor neovascularization is absent in PCNSLs; therefore, rCBV is relatively low, and permeability is not increased on DCE pMR even though the tumor is highly malignant **(24-8)**.

Diffusely infiltrating PCNSLs, also known as **lymphomatosis cerebri**, are uncommon. Patchy or confluent bihemispheric T2/FLAIR hyperintensities in the deep cerebral white matter and basal ganglia are typical **(24-9)**. Enhancement may be minimal or even absent on initial imaging in lymphomatosis cerebri, but patchy or nodular enhancing lesions are common on follow-up studies. Restricted diffusion is seen in two-thirds of cases.

Steroid administration significantly alters the imaging findings of PCNSLs. Significant cell lysis with tumor regression and normalization of the blood-brain barrier occurs in 40-85% of patients with **corticosteroid-treated PCNSLs**. Tumors typically diminish in size. Contrast enhancement also decreases or even disappears completely ("ghost tumor") although some T2 and FLAIR signal abnormalities may persist.

FDG PET Findings. Increased metabolism on FDG-PET is uncommon. However, occult systemic lymphomas are found in 5-8% of patients with putative PCNSL. In such cases, FDG PET and PET/CT fusion imaging are helpful in looking for extracranial lymphoma.

Differential Diagnosis

The major differential diagnosis of PCNSL is **glioblastoma** (GBM). Although both tumors often cross the corpus callosum, hemorrhage and necrosis are rare in PCNSL. Enhancement in immunocompetent patients with PCNSL is strong and relatively homogeneous, whereas a peripheral ring pattern is more typical of GBM. Advanced MR techniques such as DWI, MRS, and DCE pMR are helpful in distinguishing PCNSLs from other highly aggressive primary brain tumors.

The second most common differential diagnosis of PCNSL is **metastasis**. Dura-based PCNSLs may resemble **meningioma** or—due to their hyperdensity—even look like an acute epi- or subdural hematoma.

In patients with lymphomatosis cerebri who lack a dominant cohesive tumor mass, the differential diagnosis is much broader. Lymphomatosis cerebri can mimic **infectious or autoimmune inflammatory encephalitis, microvascular disease, toxic-metabolic processes,** and

neurodegenerative disorders. Callosal involvement favors lymphomatosis cerebri.

In the setting of solid organ or hematopoietic stem cell transplants, **lymphomatoid granulomatosis** and **posttransplant lymphoproliferative disorder** (PTLD) may closely resemble PCNSL. Biopsy is necessary for confirmation and patient management.

PCNSL: IMAGING AND DDx IN IMMUNOCOMPETENT PATIENTS

General Features
- Periventricular WM, basal ganglia common sites
  - 95% contact a CSF surface
- Cautions
  - Findings vary with immune status
  - Steroids may mask/↓ imaging findings!

CT
- Hyperdense on NECT
- Hemorrhage, necrosis rare

MR
- Generally isointense with GM on T1-, T2WI
- Petechial hemorrhage in immunocompetent patients
- Gross hemorrhage, necrosis rare
- Strong, relatively uniform enhancement
- Often restricts on DWI
- Lymphomatosis cerebri
  - Mimics diffuse WM disease with T2/FLAIR confluent hyperintensity
  - Enhancement can be subtle or patchy, occasionally absent

Differential Diagnosis
- Glioblastoma, metastasis
- Lymphomatosis cerebri
  - Microvascular disease
  - Encephalitis (infectious, inflammatory, autoimmune)
  - Toxic-metabolic disorders
  - Diffusely infiltrating glioma

Immunodeficiency-Associated CNS Lymphomas

Lymphomas associated with either inherited or acquired immunodeficiency are grouped together as immunodeficiency-associated CNS lymphomas. The immunodeficiency-associated CNS lymphomas include **AIDS-related diffuse large B-cell lymphoma, Epstein-Barr virus (EBV)-positive DLBCL** in elderly patients with no known immunodeficiency, **lymphomatoid granulomatosis**, and monomorphic or polymorphic **posttransplant lymphoproliferative disorders**.

Some lymphomas are linked to viral infections. PCNSLs associated with **EBV** account for 10-15% of all cases.

Congenital immunodeficiency syndromes increase the risk of lymphoma, as does severe acquired immunosuppression. Congenital immunodeficiency syndromes include **Wiskott-Aldrich syndrome** and **severe combined immunodeficiency**.

Autoimmune diseases linked to PCNSL include rheumatoid arthritis, Sjögren syndrome, and systemic lupus erythematosus.

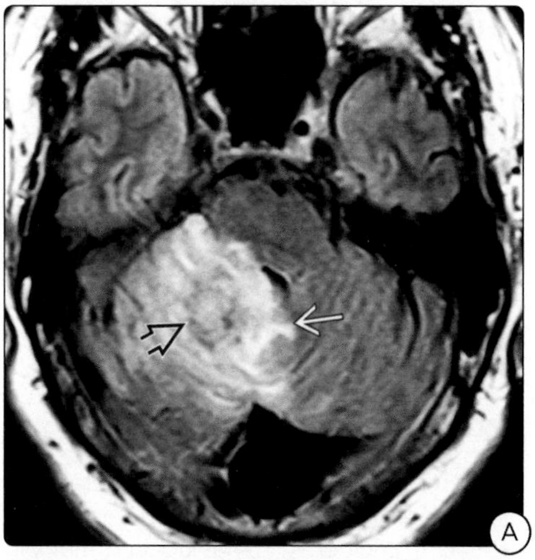

(24-12A) *FLAIR in a 43y HIV+ man with ataxia shows a solitary right cerebellar lesion ➾ with surrounding edema ➡, mass effect.*

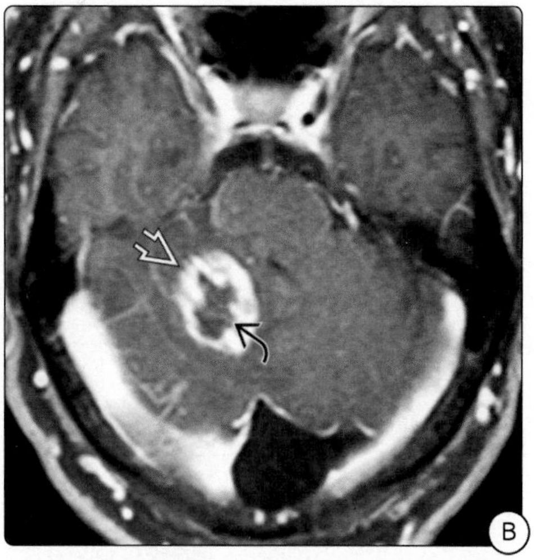

(24-12B) *T1 C+ FS in the same case shows a thick, irregular enhancing rim ➡ surrounding a core of necrotic nonenhancing tissue ➾.*

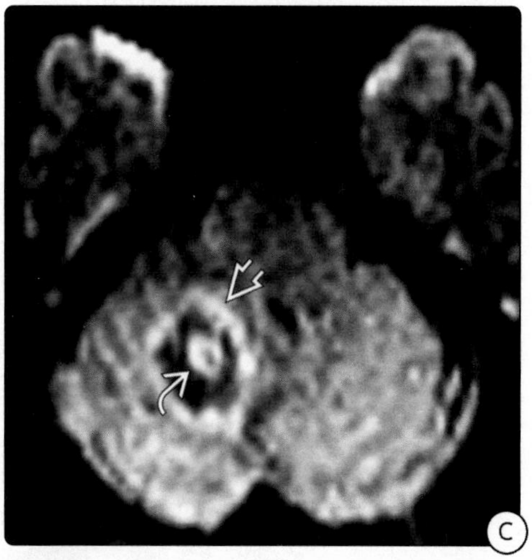

(24-12C) *DWI shows diffusion restriction in the rim ➡ and lesion core ➡. Immunodeficiency-related DLBCL was found at surgery.*

AIDS-Related Diffuse Large B-Cell Lymphoma

Although HIV-associated PCNSL has become rarer with the introduction of highly active antiretroviral therapy (HAART), between 2 and 12% of HIV/AIDS patients eventually develop CNS lymphoma, generally during the later stages of their disease. These patients can exhibit elevated levels of B-cell-stimulatory cytokines and other markers of immune activation several years prior to the diagnosis of systemic AIDS-associated non-Hodgkin B-cell lymphomas.

Pathology

With a few exceptions, AIDS-related CNS DLBCL shares the morphological features of PCNSL in immunocompetent patients. In addition to EBV association, multiple lesions are more common, as are larger, more confluent necrotic areas **(24-10)**.

Clinical Issues

Mean age at onset in patients with HIV/AIDS is 40 years, two decades younger than immunocompetent patients. Lymphomas in transplant recipients occur even earlier, generally between the ages of 35 and 40. Mean age of onset in children with inherited immunodeficiencies is 10 years.

Overall survival in HIV/AIDS and other immunocompromised patients with PCNSL is substantially diminished, no matter the age at presentation.

Imaging

Multiple lesions are common, as are more frequent and larger confluent areas of necrosis **(24-11A)**. Intratumor hemorrhage with T1 shortening and "blooming" on T2* scans is common **(24-11B)**. Enhancement is variable but often mild. Ring enhancement surrounding a nonenhancing core of necrotic tissue is typical **(24-12)**.

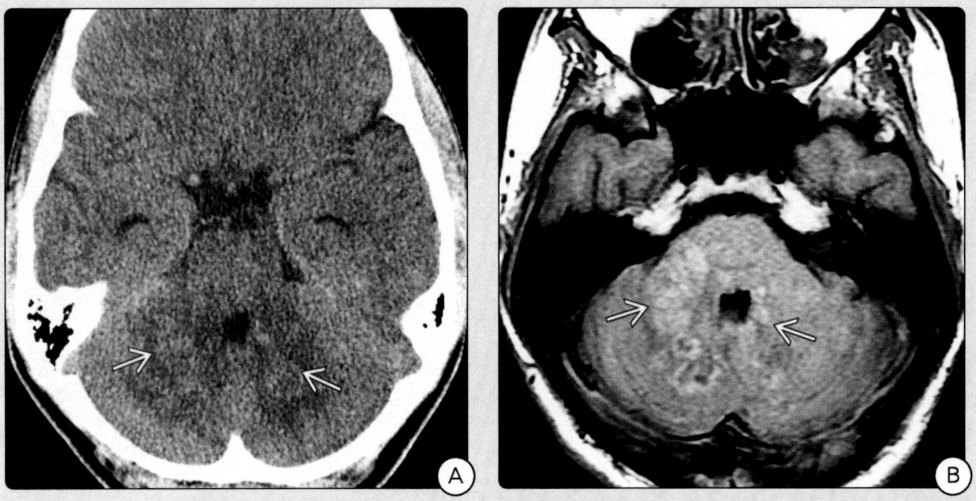

***(24-13A)** NECT scan in a 16y boy with fever, cough, and ataxia shows heterogeneous hypo-, isodense infiltrate ➡ in the white matter of both cerebellar hemispheres. **(24-13B)** Axial T1WI in the same patient shows that the multifocal cerebellar lesions are slightly hyperintense ➡.*

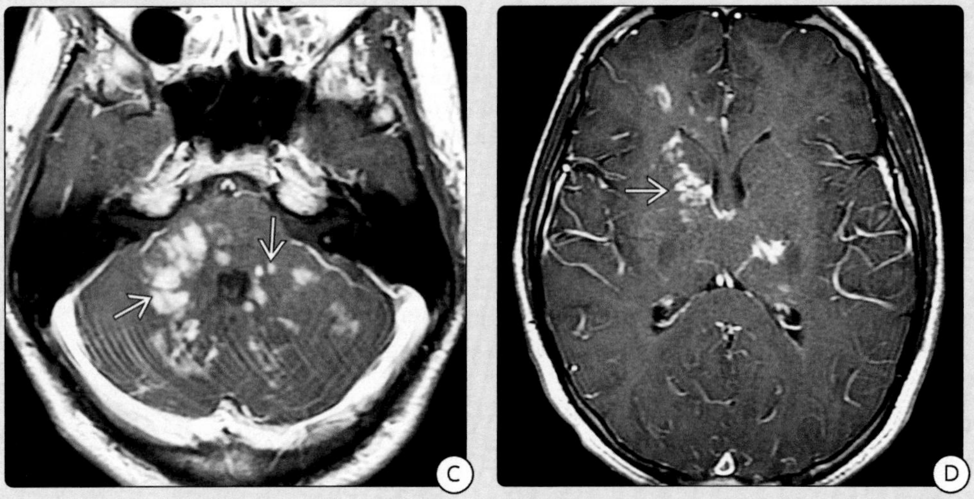

***(24-13C)** T1 C+ shows strong enhancement of the lesions ➡. **(24-13D)** More cephalad T1 C+ scan shows additional enhancing foci ➡ in the basal ganglia and hemispheric white matter. Imaging diagnosis was hemophagocytic lymphohistiocytosis. Biopsy disclosed lymphomatoid granulomatosis.*

Differential Diagnosis

In immunocompromised patients, the major differential diagnosis of PCNSL is **toxoplasmosis**. *A solitary ring-enhancing lesion in an HIV/AIDS patient is most often lymphoma,* whereas multiple lesions are more characteristic of toxoplasmosis. An "eccentric target" sign is suggestive of toxoplasmosis although necrotic lymphomas occasionally show an enhancing "ring with a nodule" pattern. Toxoplasmosis is hypometabolic on PET and pMR and often exhibits elevated ADC values with a ratio greater than 1:6.

Progressive multifocal leukoencephalopathy (PML) usually does not enhance. However, **acute PML** lesions and JC virus-associated **immune reconstitution inflammatory syndrome** (IRIS) may show ring enhancement. Enhancement often looks quite bizarre with multifocal poorly delineated partial rings of enhancement surrounding the demyelinating foci.

Lymphomatoid Granulomatosis

Terminology

Lymphomatoid granulomatosis (LYG) is a rare multisystem angiocentric and angioinvasive lymphoproliferative disorder characterized by atypical B-cell proliferations. LYG is now considered an immunodeficiency-related extranodal large B-cell lymphoma.

Etiology

EBV infection is a feature of most reported cases. LYG also occurs in the setting of HIV/AIDS and in patients on maintenance immunosuppression following solid organ transplantation. Inherited disorders such as Wiskott-Aldrich disease and congenital immunodeficiency syndrome are rare but reported causes of LYG.

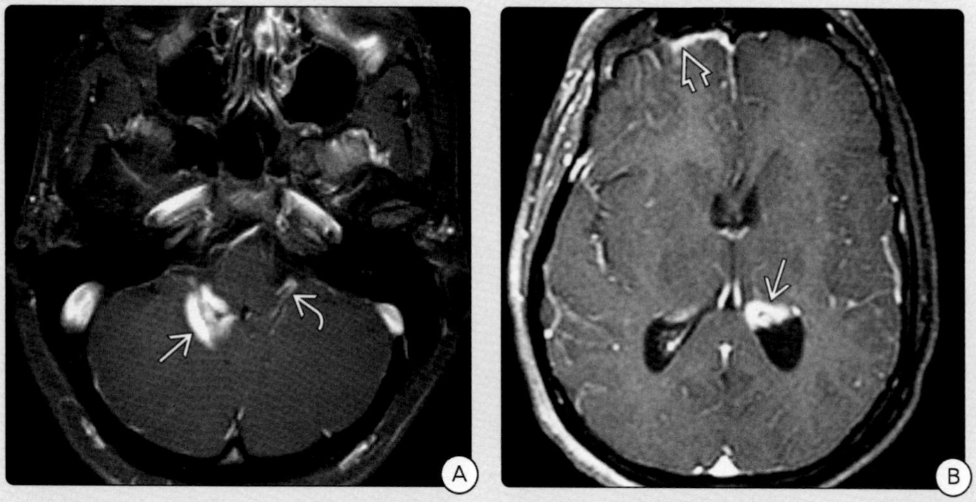

***(24-14A)** Axial T1 C+ FS in a 37y woman shows an enhancing mass in the right cerebellum and choroid plexus in 4th ventricle lateral recess ➡. A less conspicuous mass is present in the left foramen of Luschka ➡. **(24-14B)** More cephalad T1 C+ FS in the same case shows additional enhancing masses in the glomus of the left choroid plexus ➡ and right frontal dura-arachnoid ➡. This is biopsy-proven lymphomatoid granulomatosis.*

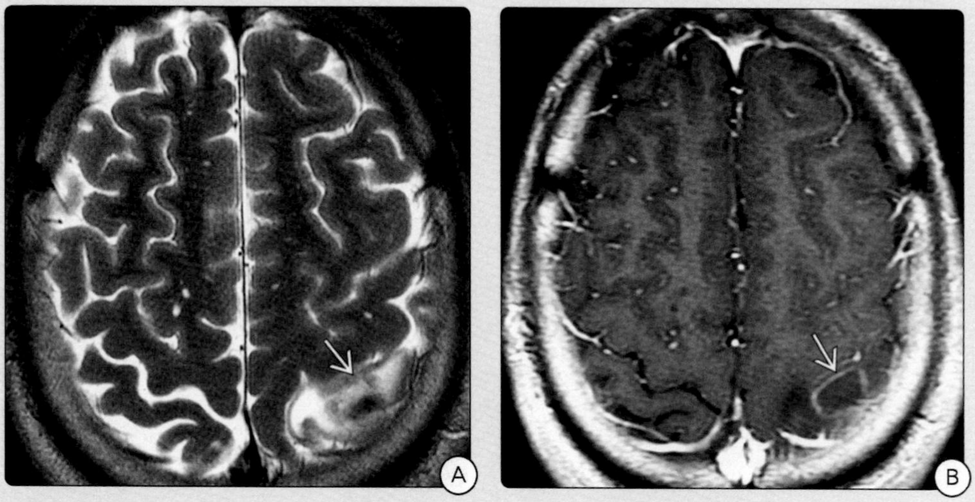

***(24-15A)** Axial T2WI in a 25y man with a grand mal seizure shows a mixed signal mass ➡ in the left parietal lobe. **(24-15B)** T1 C+ in the same case shows a ring-enhancing lesion ➡. DWI (not shown) did not demonstrate restricted diffusion. This is biopsy-proven Epstein-Barr virus (EBV)-related lymphomatoid granulomatosis.*

Pathology

The lung is the most commonly involved site, followed by the skin. The CNS is involved in about 25% of cases. Lesions range in size from a few millimeters up to 1 or 2 cm in diameter. Large focal masses are rare.

The classic histologic triad of LYG consists of nodular polymorphic lymphocytic infiltrate, angiitis, and granulomatosis with central necrosis.

LYG shares several histologic similarities with posttransplantation lymphoproliferative disorders (see below). Angiocentric and angiodestructive polymorphous infiltrates consisting predominantly of lymphocytes mixed with plasma cells, immunoblasts, and histiocytes are present.

LYG is graded on a scale of 1 to 3 based on the numbers of atypical EBV-positive B cells and necrosis compared with the background of reactive T lymphocytes.

Clinical Issues

Patients of all ages are affected, but peak occurrence is between the fourth and sixth decades. The typical patient is a middle-aged man with fever, dry cough, and weight loss. As clinical manifestations, laboratory data, and imaging are all nonspecific, biopsy is mandatory for definitive diagnosis.

Prognosis is generally poor in untreated patients with median survival of 14 months. Approximately half of patients with LYG respond to steroids and chemotherapeutic agents.

Imaging

Nearly half of patients with LYG have demonstrable brain lesions on MR. Imaging findings are nonspecific, and there is no direct correlation with LYG grade.

The most common abnormalities are multifocal T2/FLAIR nodular hyperintensities in the cerebral hemispheres, deep

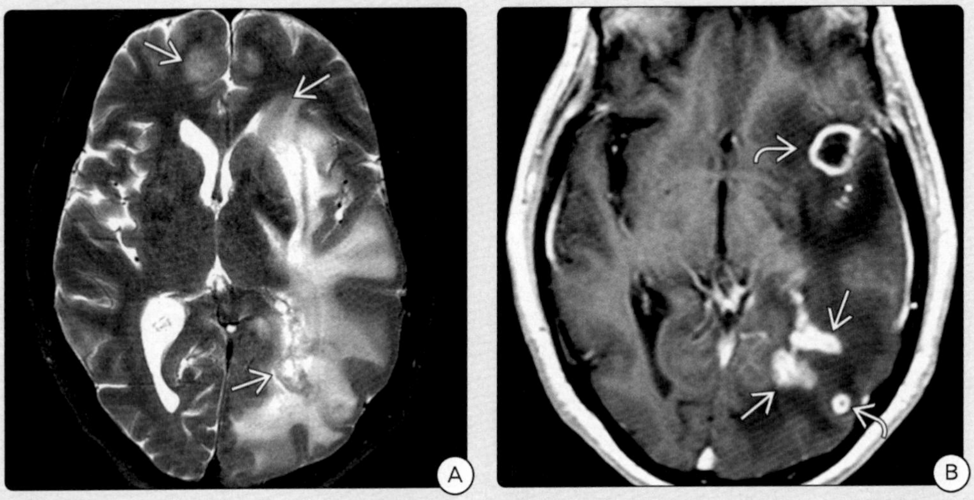

***(24-16A)** T2WI in a 66y woman with altered mental status 3 years after orthotopic liver transplant shows multiple heterogeneously hyperintense lesions ➡ and severe left hemisphere edema. (Courtesy P. Chapman, MD.) **(24-16B)** T1 C+ MR in the same case shows multiple solid ➡, ring-enhancing lesions ↪. (Courtesy P. Chapman, MD.)*

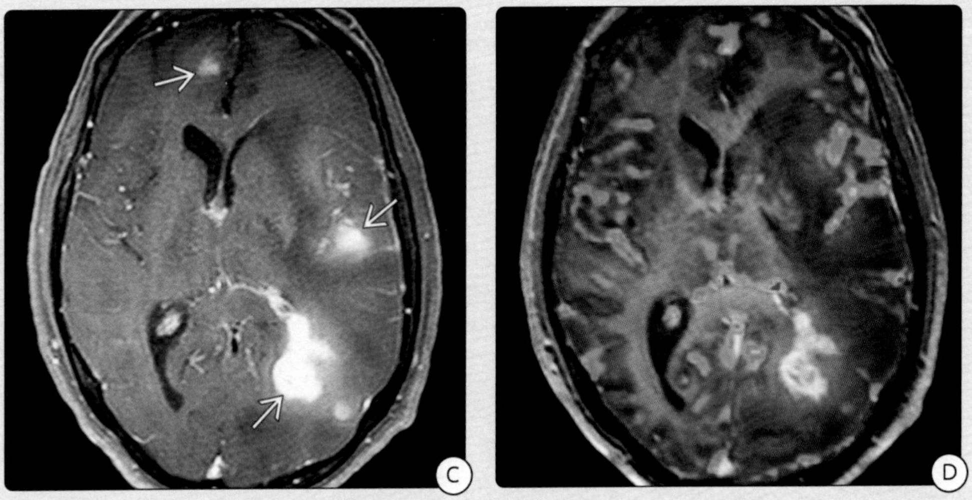

***(24-16C)** Delayed cephalad T1 C+ FS scan shows multiple enhancing lesions ➡. (Courtesy P. Chapman, MD.) **(24-16D)** Fused PET-contrast-enhanced MR image shows no evidence for increased metabolic activity in the lesions. Brain biopsy showed EBV+ PTLD. (Courtesy P. Chapman, MD.)*

gray nuclei, cerebellum, or spinal cord **(24-13)**. The second most common imaging finding in LYG is involvement of the leptomeninges and cranial nerves. Dura-based masses and choroid plexus lesions also occur **(24-14)**.

LYG typically enhances strongly. Both solid and ring-like patterns as well as multifocal punctate and nodular and linear enhancing foci have been described **(24-15)**.

Differential Diagnosis

The major differential diagnosis of LYG is **vasculitis**. Other considerations include diffusely infiltrating B-cell lymphoma **(lymphomatosis cerebri), intravascular lymphoma,** and nonneoplastic lymphoproliferative disorders such as **CLIPPERS** (**c**hronic **l**ymphocytic **i**nflammation with **p**ontine **p**erivascular **e**nhancement **r**esponsive to **s**teroids).

Posttransplant Lymphoproliferative Disorder

Posttransplant lymphoproliferative disorder (PTLD) is a potentially life-threatening complication of immunosuppressive therapy in patients with solid organ or hematopoietic cell transplantation.

The PTLD disease spectrum ranges from an infectious mononucleosis-like illness with reactive lymph node hyperplasia to malignant lymphoma. PTLDs are related to EBV.

Pathology

PTLDs can be polymorphic or monomorphic. **Polymorphic PTLD** consists of a heterogeneous cell population that may reflect the full range of B-cell maturation from prominent plasmacytic infiltrates to proliferating immunoblasts with

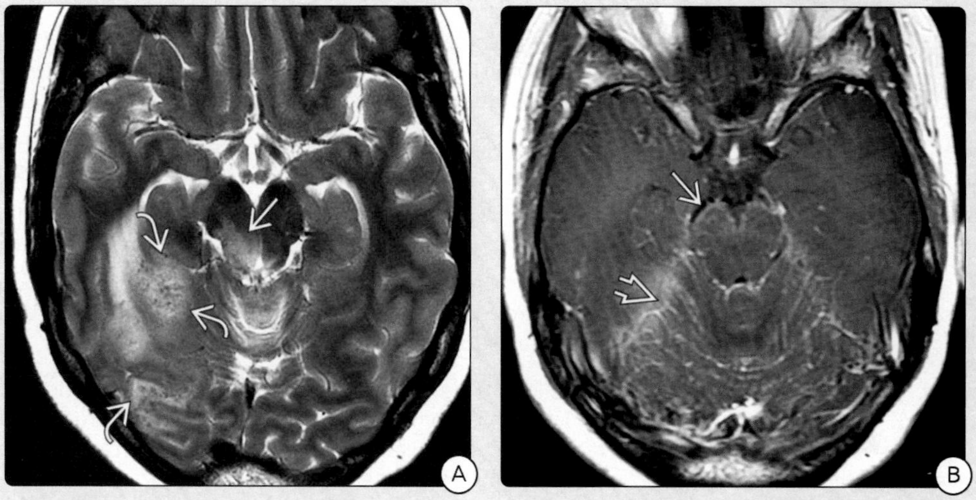

(24-17A) *Axial T2WI in a 28y woman who was immunosuppressed for rheumatoid arthritis shows multifocal confluent hyperintense lesions in the midbrain ➡ and right occipital lobe ⇨.* ***(24-17B)*** *T1 C+ in the same case shows diffuse linear and nodular enhancement along the midbrain ➡ and cerebellum ⇨.*

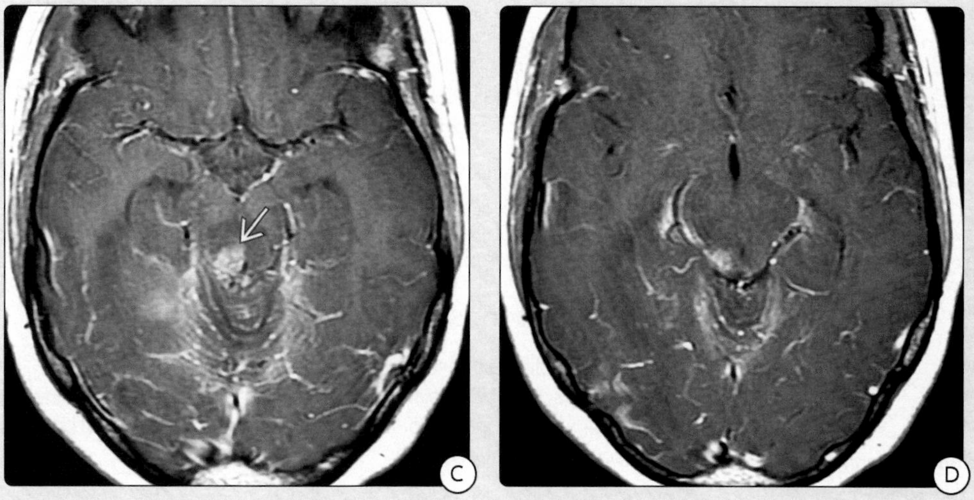

(24-17C) *More cephalad T1 C+ shows an enhancing mass in the midbrain ➡ as well as the linear and nodular cerebellar and occipital enhancement.* ***(24-17D)*** *More cephalad T1 C+ shows nodular, sulcal, mass-like enhancement along the midbrain, superior vermis, and right occipital lobe. This was biopsy-proven PTLD.*

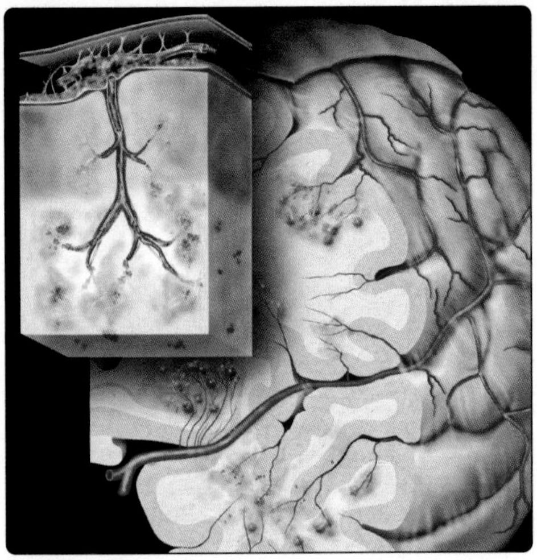

(24-18) Graphic depicts IVL. Malignant cells plug vessels, causing perivascular infiltrates and petechial hemorrhages.

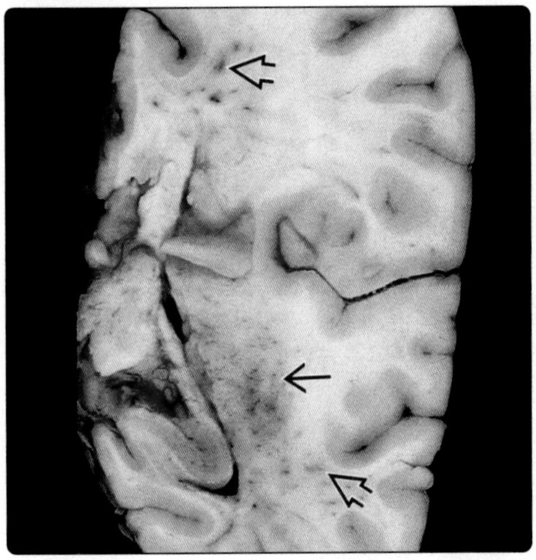

(24-19) Autopsied IVL shows punctate/linear grayish infiltrates, petechial and perivascular hemorrhages. (Courtesy R. Hewlett, MD.)

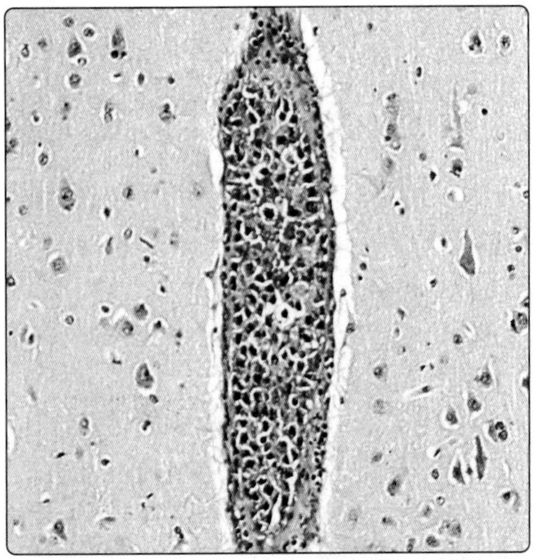

(24-20) Intravascular lymphoma completely fills brain arteriole with "small round blue cells." (Courtesy T. Tihan, MD.)

necrosis. Polymorphic PTLD does not fulfill the histologic criteria for lymphoma.

Monomorphic PTLD consists of large blastic cells with prominent nucleoli. Most monomorphic PTLDs are classified as diffuse large B-cell lymphomas.

Clinical Issues

Epidemiology. The overall prevalence of PTLD following solid organ transplantation is 0.5-2.5%. Up to 15-20% of patients who develop PTLD have CNS involvement. Isolated CNS PTLD is rare, occurring in less than 0.5% of transplant cases.

Demographics. Pediatric transplant recipients develop PTLD more frequently than adult patients because children are less likely to have EBV-specific immunity at transplantation. The frequency varies with the type of transplant, with the highest prevalence reported with multiorgan or intestinal (20%), lung or heart (8-20%), liver (4-15%), and kidney (1-8%) transplants. PTLD after hematopoietic cell transplantation accounts for less than 2% of cases.

Presentation. PTLD typically presents several years following transplantation. Symptoms very with tumor location.

Treatment Options. Because treatment regimens vary significantly, distinguishing polymorphic from monomorphic PTLD and malignant lymphoma is essential, often requiring biopsy for definitive diagnosis.

Reduction or cessation of immunosuppression is generally the first step in treating PTLD. Polymorphic PTLD usually responds well within 2 to 4 weeks. PTLD that fails to respond to reduced immunosuppression has a very high mortality rate (50-90%).

Most cases of monomorphic PTLD are unresponsive to immunosuppression withdrawal and require additional therapeutic modalities. Surgical resection, chemotherapy, and radiation therapy are possibilities.

Because CNS PTLD lesions are often resistant to the combination of drugs known as CHOP (cyclophosphamide, hydroxydaunomycin, Oncovin, and prednisone), radiotherapy is generally used in combination with agents such as high-dose methotrexate. High-dose rituximab, an anti-CD20 monoclonal antibody, may be effective in some patients.

Imaging

Imaging features of CNS PTLD resemble those of AIDS-related lymphoma. Most lesions are solitary masses that are hypointense to cortex on T1WI and heterogeneously hypo-/hyperintense on T2WI. Solid or ring-like enhancement is common following contrast administration **(24-16)** **(24-17)**. Lymphoma-related PTLDs usually show moderate restriction on DWI.

Extracranial head and neck PTLD results in a spectrum of findings. Bilateral cervical lymphadenopathy occurs in 75% of cases. Nodes often appear necrotic. Other manifestations include orbital involvement and sinonasal lesions that resemble polyposis or sinusitis.

Differential Diagnosis

The major differential diagnosis of PTLD is **primary CNS lymphoma**—especially AIDS-related lymphoma. The imaging differential diagnosis of CNS lesions in transplant recipients also includes **opportunistic infections** such as toxoplasmosis.

POSTTRANSPLANT LYMPHOPROLIFERATIVE DISORDER (PTLD)

Terminology and Etiology
- Complication of organ or stem cell transplants
  - Long-term maintenance immunosuppression
- Ranges from benign mono-like illness to malignant lymphoma

Pathology
- Monomorphic or polymorphic lymphoid proliferations
- Polymorphic PTLD has plasmacytic B-cell elements of varying maturity
- Monomorphic PTLD has blastic cells → large B-cell lymphoma

Clinical Issues
- 0.5-2.5% of patients with solid organ transplants
- 15-20% with PTLD have CNS involvement
- Presents several years after transplantation
- Children > adults

Imaging
- Brain findings resemble those of AIDS-related lymphoma
- Extracranial PTLD
  - Bilateral cervical adenopathy common
  - Orbital, sinonasal lesions

Intravascular (Angiocentric) Lymphoma

Intravascular lymphoma (IVL) is a rare subtype of DLBCL characterized by proliferating malignant cells within small and medium-sized vessels. Although it can involve any organ, IVL typically affects the skin and the CNS.

Terminology

IVL is also called angiocentric or angioendotheliotropic lymphoma, angiotropic large cell lymphoma, endovascular lymphoma, and malignant angioendotheliomatosis.

Etiology

IVL is an aggressive malignant lymphoma that usually arises from B cells. T cells or NK cells may occasionally be the cell of origin. A possible association of IVL (especially the NK type) with EBV has been reported.

Pathology

The gross macroscopic appearance varies from normal to small multifocal infarcts of varying ages scattered throughout the cortex and subcortical white matter **(24-18)**. Focal cerebral masses are rare. Petechial microhemorrhages may be present and are more common than confluent macroscopic bleeds **(24-19)**.

At histologic examination, markedly atypical cells with large round nuclei and prominent nuclei are found in small and medium-sized vessels **(24-20)**. Extension into the adjacent perivascular spaces is minimal or absent. CD20 staining is helpful in identifying tumor cells, especially when they are sparse and widely scattered.

Clinical Issues

Epidemiology. IVL is rare. CNS involvement occurs in 75-85% of patients.

Demographics. IVL is typically a tumor of middle-aged and elderly patients. Mean age at presentation is 60-65 years.

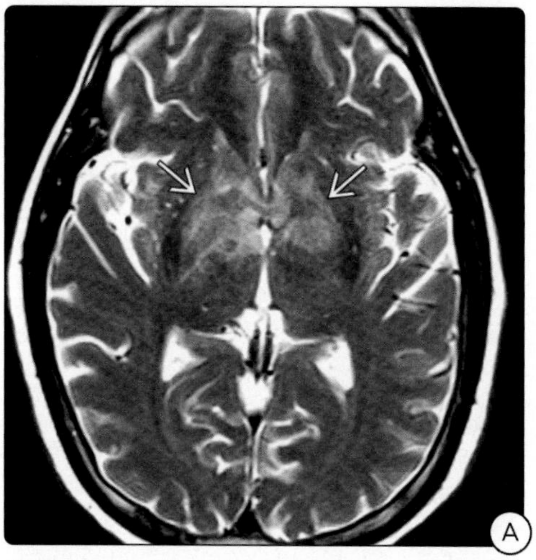

***(24-21A)** T2WI in a 61y man with progressive cognitive decline shows patchy hyperintensities in the basal ganglia and internal capsules.*

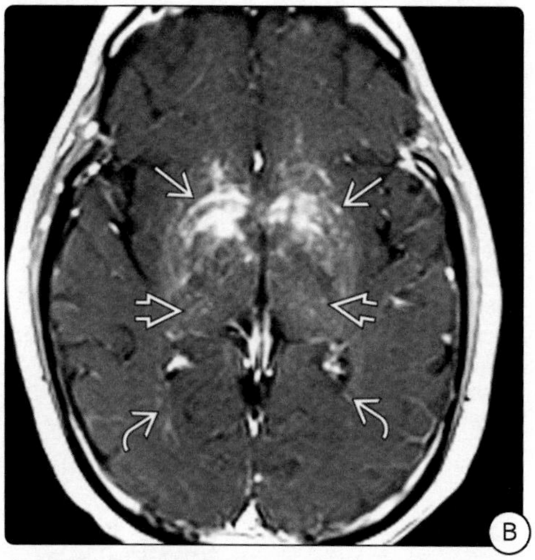

***(24-21B)** Axial T1 C+ shows punctate, linear, and patchy confluent foci of contrast enhancement in the basal ganglia, thalami, deep WM.*

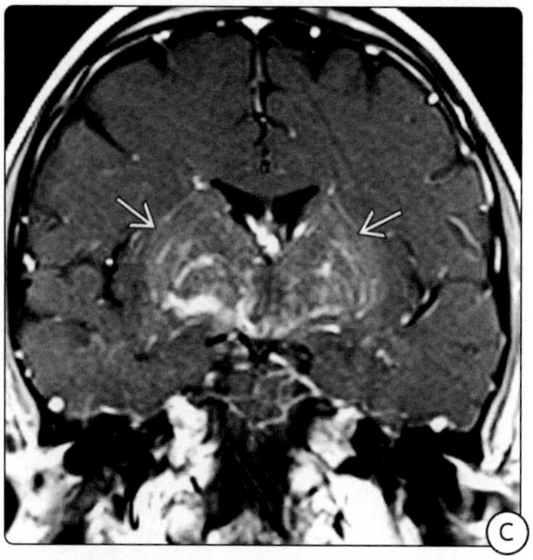

***(24-21C)** Coronal T1 C+ shows prominent curvilinear enhancement following penetrating arteries, intravascular DLBCL found at biopsy.*

Presentation. Sensory and motor deficits, neuropathies, and multiple stroke-like episodes are common symptoms. Some patients present with progressive neurological deterioration and cognitive decline characterized by confusion and memory loss. Skin changes with elevated plaques or nodules are present in half of all cases.

Natural History. Outcome is generally poor. By the time of initial presentation, most patients have advanced disseminated disease. IVL is a relentless, rapidly progressive disease with a high mortality rate. Mean survival is 7-12 months.

Treatment Options. Because IVL is a widely disseminated disease, systemic chemotherapy is the recommended treatment. High-dose chemotherapy with autologous stem cell transplantation is often used in younger patients.

Imaging

There are no pathognomonic neuroimaging findings for IVL. Ischemic foci with infarct-like lesions are the most common imaging finding. CT may be normal or nonspecific, demonstrating only scattered white matter hypodensities. MR shows multiple T2/FLAIR hyperintensities **(24-21A)**. Microhemorrhages are common, so "blooming" foci on T2* (GRE, SWI) are often present **(24-22)**. Linear/punctate enhancement oriented along perivascular spaces is suggestive of IVL **(24-21C)**. Multifocal areas of diffusion restriction may be present **(24-22D)**.

Differential Diagnosis

IVL is a "great imitator," both clinically and on imaging studies. Stereotactic biopsy is thus necessary to establish the definitive diagnosis. **Vasculitis** with punctate and linear enhancing foci

(24-22A) T2WI in a 60y man with a several-month history of increasing confusion and decreasing mental status shows multifocal ill-defined hyperintensities in the hemispheric WM ➡. (24-22B) FLAIR scan in the same patient shows several additional lesions. There was no evidence of cortical or basal ganglia hyperintensities.

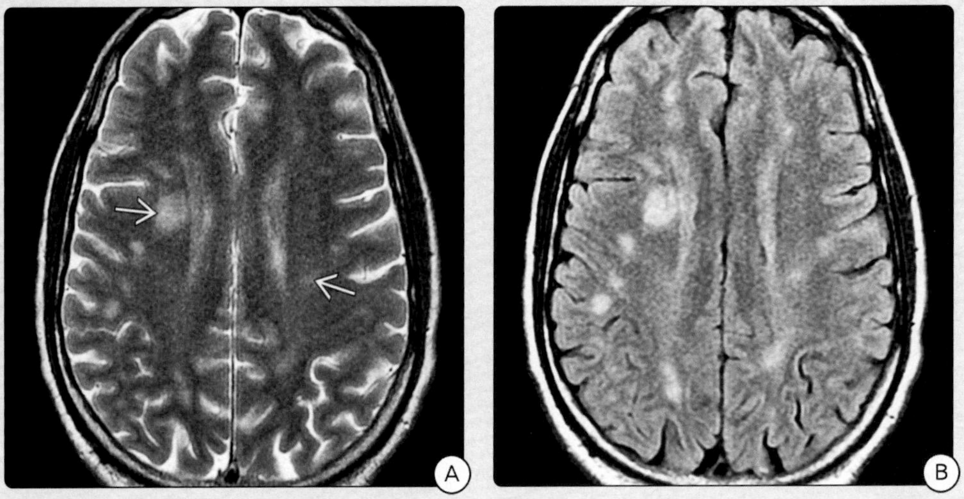

(24-22C) T2 GRE shows multiple tiny hemorrhagic foci ➡. (24-22D) DWI shows multiple foci of restricted diffusion in both hemispheres ➡. The patient died shortly after the scan was obtained. Autopsy demonstrated intravascular lymphoma.*

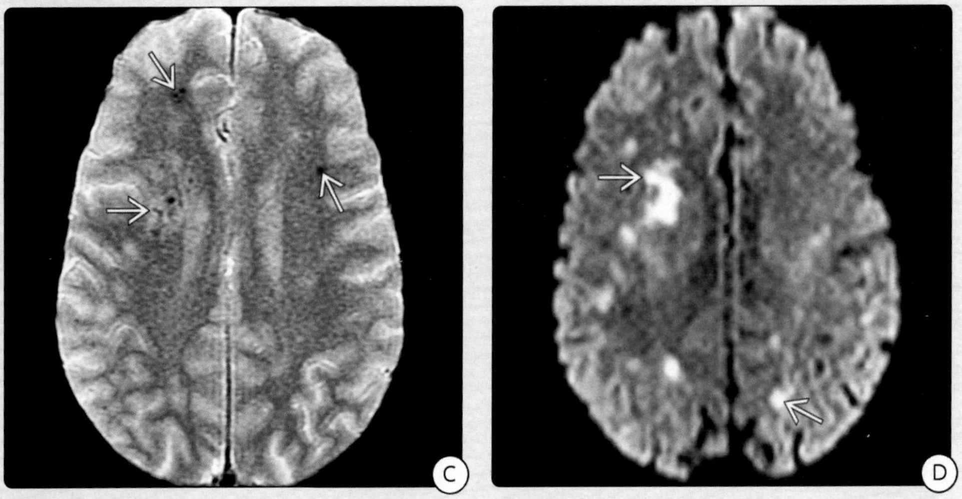

may be virtually indistinguishable from IVL on imaging studies alone.

PCNSL, especially in the setting of immunodeficiency syndromes, may mimic IVL. IVL is most often multifocal, whereas two-thirds of PCNSLs are solitary lesions. Diffuse multifocal PCNSL, especially when it occurs in the form of **lymphomatosis cerebri**, may be difficult to distinguish from IVL. Lymphomatosis cerebri often shows little or no enhancement.

Rapidly progressive leukoencephalopathy with confluent nonenhancing white matter lesions is a rare presentation of diffusely infiltrating CNS IVL and may mimic a cerebral **demyelinating disorder**.

Diffuse **subacute viral encephalitis** can likewise mimic IVL, especially on biopsy. Parenchymal **neurosarcoid** with perivascular nodular spread may also resemble IVL on imaging studies.

INTRAVASCULAR (ANGIOCENTRIC) LYMPHOMA

Pathology
- Small/medium-sized vessels filled with tumor
- Little/no parenchymal tumor
- Multifocal infarcts, microhemorrhages common

Clinical Issues
- Older patients with dementia, cognitive decline, TIAs
- Skin lesions (50%)

Imaging
- Multifocal T2/FLAIR hyperintensities
- Hemorrhages, foci of restricted diffusion
- Linear/punctate enhancement

Common Differential Diagnoses
- PCNSL
- Vasculitis

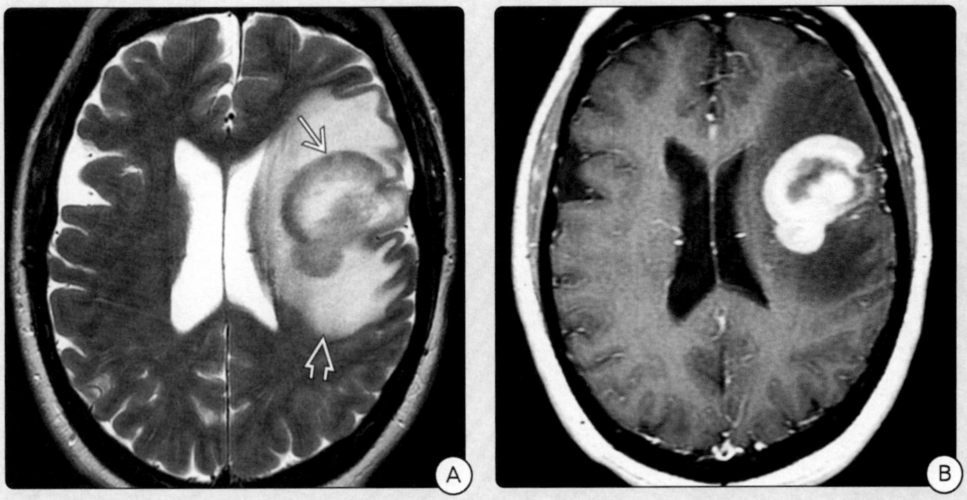

***(24-23A)** T2WI in a 52y woman with PCNSL, diffuse large T-cell type, shows hyper-, hypointense mass ➡ with striking peritumoral edema ⇨. **(24-23B)** The mass restricted on DWI (not shown). T1 C+ scan shows that the mass enhances strongly and relatively uniformly.*

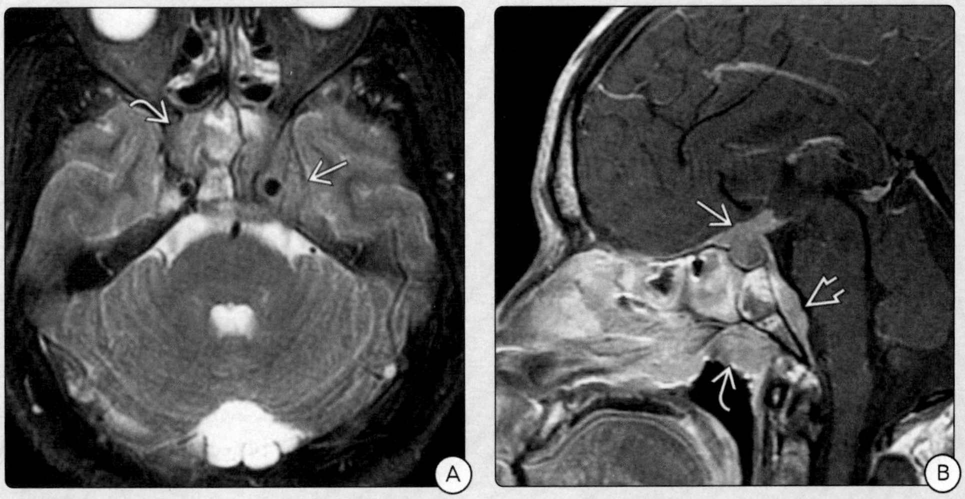

***(24-24A)** Axial T2 FS scan in a 26y man with EBV-positive extranodal NK-/T-cell lymphoma shows a hypointense mass ➡ invading the upper nasopharynx ⇨, skull base, and cavernous sinuses. **(24-24B)** Sagittal T1 C+ in the same case shows the enhancing nasopharyngeal mass ⇨ invading the skull base, extending intracranially to involve the pituitary gland and stalk ➡. Note dural mass along the clivus ⇨.*

Miscellaneous Rare CNS Lymphomas

Other than DLBCL, primary CNS lymphomas are rare. These include low-grade B- and T-cell lymphomas, high-grade T- and NK-/T-cell lymphomas (NKTCLs), and the exceptionally rare primary CNS Hodgkin and Burkitt lymphomas.

Low-grade lymphomas, most of which are of B-cell lineage, account for approximately 3% of all CNS lymphomas and almost exclusively affect immunocompetent adults. These tend to be indolent neoplasms with relatively longer survival compared with DLBCLs.

Primary CNS T-cell lymphomas and NKTCLs are very rare, accounting for approximately 2% of all PCNSLs. Most reported cases are associated with prior EBV infection. Imaging findings are generally indistinguishable from parenchymal DLBCL, with solitary, multifocal, or diffusely infiltrating masses **(24-23)**. Rare cases of primary NKTCLs presenting as diffuse leptomeningeal and cranial nerve enhancement have been reported. Approximately 7% of patients with peripheral T-cell lymphoma develop secondary CNS disease.

EBV-positive nasal-type extranodal NKTCL primarily affects young to middle-aged adult men. The upper aerodigestive tract (nasal cavity, nasopharynx, paranasal sinuses, and palate) is most commonly involved. Preferential sites of extranasal involvement include the skin, soft tissue, GI tract, and testis. Less than 3% of cases invade or metastasize to the CNS **(24-24)**. Prognosis is generally poor even with chemotherapy and radiation therapy.

MALT Lymphoma of the Dura

Extranodal marginal zone lymphomas of mucosa-associated lymphoid tissue (MALT lymphomas) in the head and neck are most often ocular adnexal tumors, occurring in the conjunctiva, lacrimal glands, orbit, and eyelids. The cranial meninges, especially the dura, are occasional intracranial sites

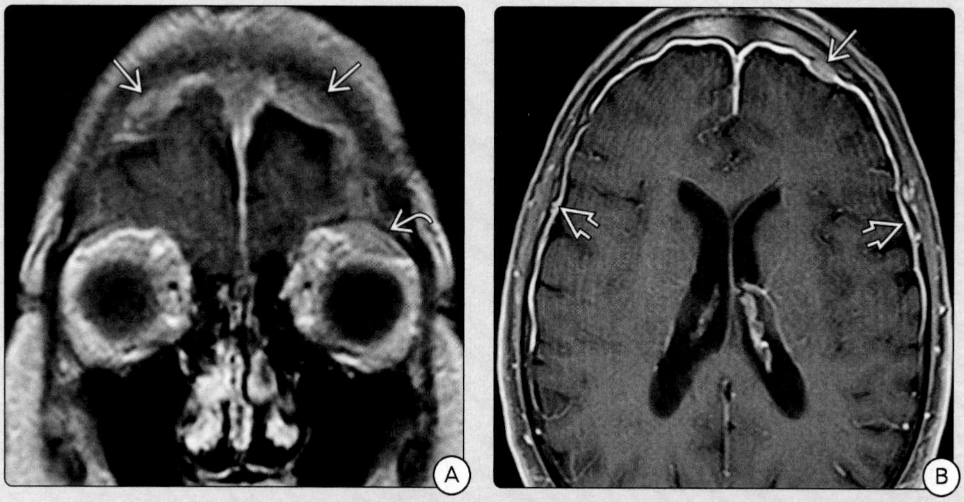

***(24-25A)** Coronal T1 C+ in a 73y woman with forehead swelling and blurry vision in her left eye shows orbital adnexal and dural-based masses . **(24-25B)** T1 C+ FS of the brain shows diffuse bilateral dura-arachnoid thickening and focal calvarial masses . Extranodal marginal zone lymphoma of mucosa-associated lymphoid tissue (MALT lymphoma) of the dura was found at surgery.*

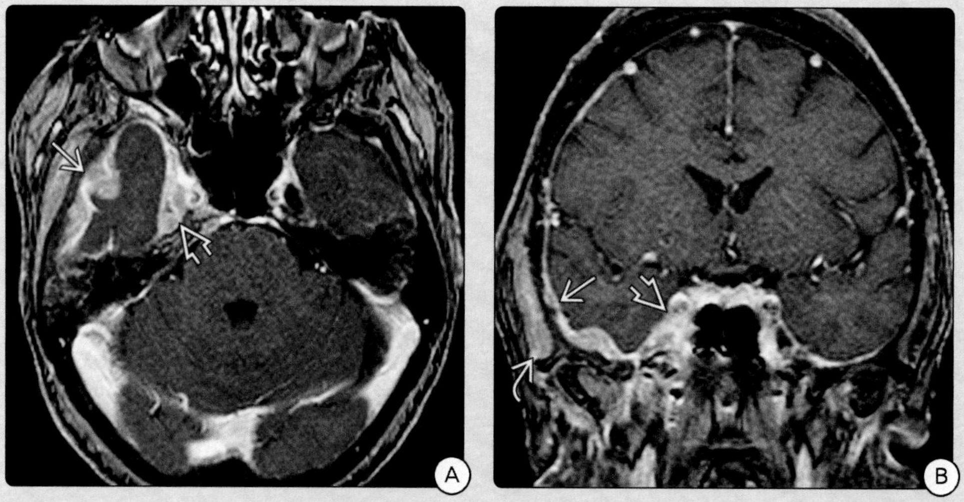

***(24-26A)** Axial T1 C+ FS in a 67y woman with blurry vision and right CN VI palsy shows a dural-based infiltrating mass in the right cranial fossa , cavernous sinus . **(24-26B)** Coronal T1 C+ FS in the same case shows the right cavernous sinus , middle fossa dura-arachnoid , and temporalis muscle thickening . This was MALT lymphoma of the dura.*

(24-25). Diffuse dura-arachnoid thickening with one or more meningioma-like masses is the most typical imaging finding **(24-26)**. Parenchymal lesions are rare. Prognosis is excellent, with a 5-year survival rate of 85%.

Metastatic Intracranial Lymphoma

Terminology

Metastatic intracranial lymphoma is also called secondary CNS lymphoma (SCNSL). Here the skull, meningeal, and brain lesions are all secondary to systemic lymphoma **(24-27) (24-28) (24-29) (24-30)**.

Clinical Issues

Aggressive high-grade tumors increase the risk of CNS spread. Between 3-5% of patients with diffuse large B-cell systemic lymphomas eventually develop CNS involvement. Approximately 80% of SCNSLs are caused by DLBCL.

Peak prevalence of metastatic CNS lymphoma is in the sixth and seventh decades. Prognosis is poor, especially in elderly patients. Systemic methotrexate has been recommended as the optimal treatment for isolated CNS relapse involving the brain parenchyma. Rituximab treatment may be effective in some cases.

Imaging

SCNSL is typically identified with neuroimaging. Metastatic lymphoma rarely presents as a parenchymal mass. In contrast with PCNSL, skull and dural involvement is much more frequent **(24-31) (24-32)**. Both calvarial vault and skull base metastases are common. Skull base metastases may extend inferiorly into the nose and paranasal sinuses or spread superolaterally into the cavernous sinus, Meckel cave, and pituitary gland/stalk.

Calvarial lesions often involve the adjacent scalp and epidural space. Dural "tails" are common. Involvement of the

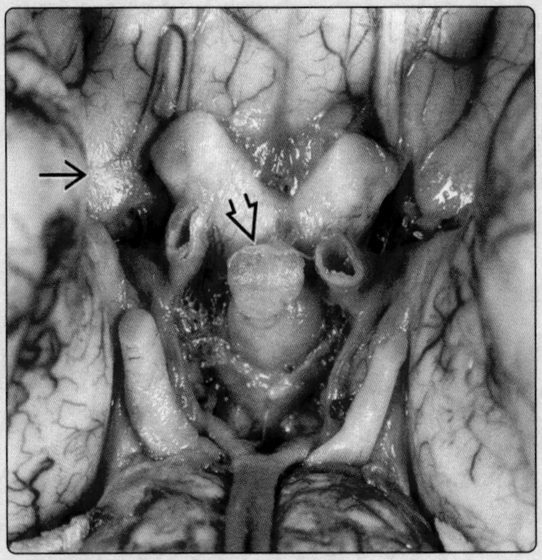

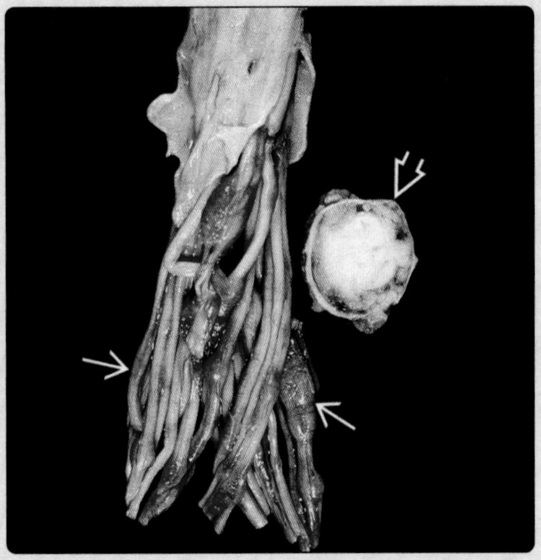

***(24-27)** Close-up view shows leptomeningeal metastases →. Metastatic lymphoma also thickens the infundibular stalk ⇨. The pituitary gland (not shown) was also involved by tumor. **(24-28)** Nodular, linear metastases from systemic lymphoma diffusely thicken the nerve roots of the cauda equina ➡. Axial section shows that the intradural, extramedullary space is filled with tumor ➡.*

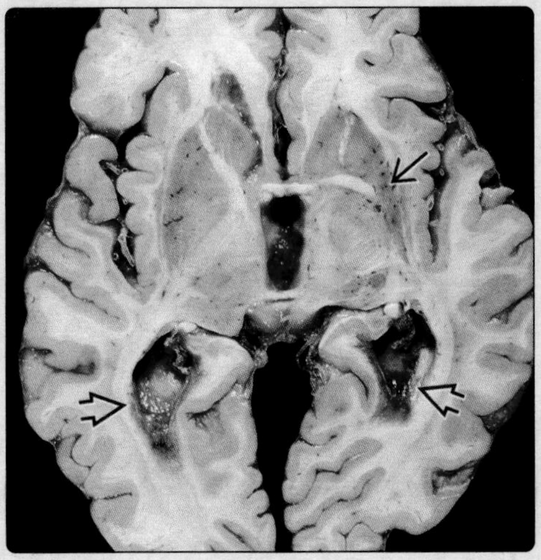

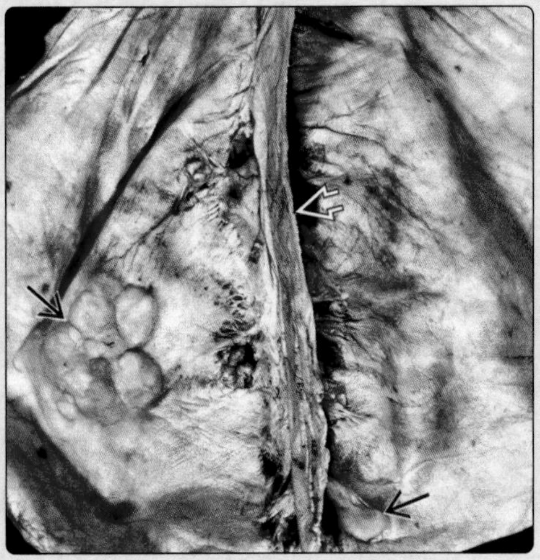

***(24-29)** Cut section through the ventricles shows that the ependymal surfaces of the lateral ventricles are coated with glistening tumor ⇨. The perivascular spaces in the basal ganglia are enlarged by cords of intravascular malignant lymphoma →. **(24-30)** Diffuse dural thickening ➡ with multiple focal deposits of lymphoma → resembles meningiomatosis. (Autopsy cases are courtesy R. Hewlett, MD.)*

leptomeninges and underlying brain parenchyma may occur as late complications. Parenchymal lesions in the absence of skull and dural disease are uncommon **(24-33)**.

SECONDARY (METASTATIC) INTRACRANIAL LYMPHOMA

- 80% from high-grade systemic B-cell lymphomas
- Skull, dural lesions > > brain parenchyma
  - Multicompartmental disease common
  - Calvaria + dural/epidural, scalp lesions
  - Skull base + nose, cavernous sinus/pituitary
- Leptomeningeal, CSF spread uncommon
  - Choroid plexus
  - Ventricular ependyma
- Spine "drop metastases" (3-5%)

Diffuse leptomeningeal tumor spread and disseminated CSF lesions are relatively uncommon. Tumor spread along the optic nerve sheath is rare. Cranial neuropathies with multifocal enhancing cranial nerves occur as a late complication. Intradural lesions in the spine ("drop metastases") occur in 3-5% of cases.

Histiocytic Tumors

Histiocytes belong to the group of mononuclear phagocytes and are defined as "tissue-resident" macrophages. Histiocytic CNS neoplasms are a heterogeneous group of tumors that are histologically and immunologically identical to their extracranial counterparts.

For decades, the histiocytoses were divided into Langerhans cell histiocytosis (LCH) and non-Langerhans cell histiocytoses. With the discovery of recurrent *BRAF* mutations in LCH—later also found in Erdheim-Chester disease—the histiocytoses are

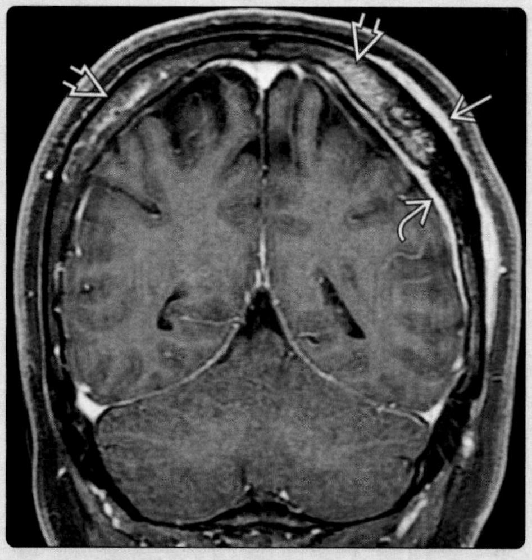

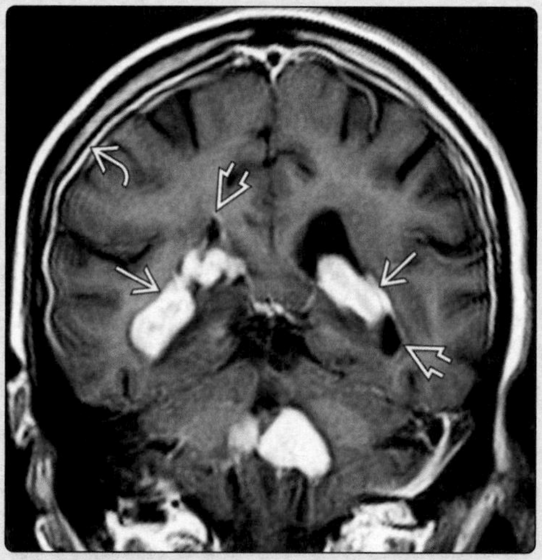

***(24-31)** Coronal T1 C+ FS in a patient with systemic DLBCL demonstrates enhancing metastatic lymphoma in the galea aponeurotica, calvarium, and dura-arachnoid. **(24-32)** Coronal T1 C+ in a 75y man with systemic DLBCL shows multiple choroid plexus and ependymal metastases. Diffuse dura-arachnoid metastases are also present.*

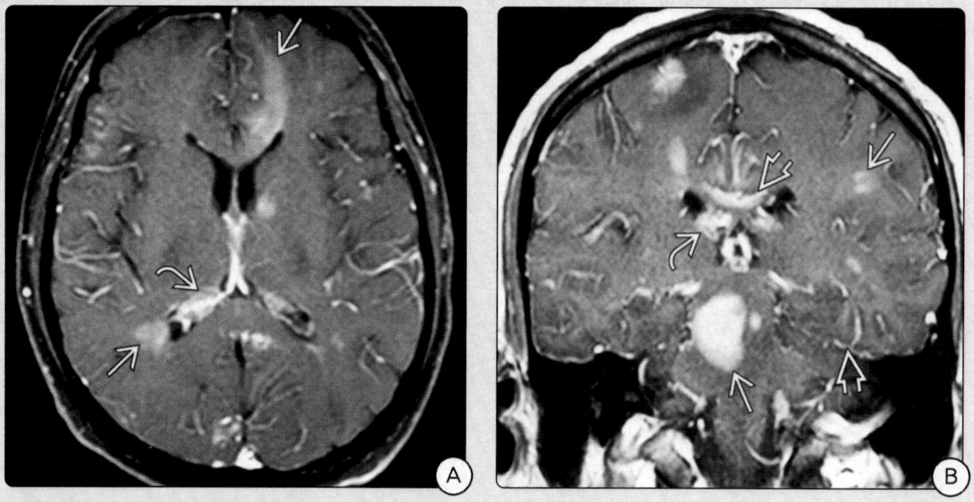

***(24-33A)** Axial T1 C+ FS in a patient with cutaneous T-cell lymphoma shows multifocal enhancing masses in the parenchyma and choroid plexus. **(24-33B)** Coronal T1 C+ in the same case shows multifocal parenchymal, choroid plexus, and pial metastases.*

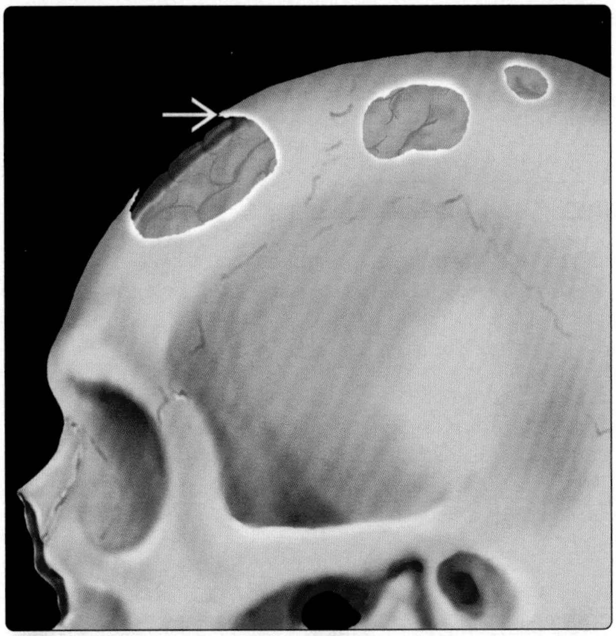

(24-34) Graphic depicts the well-defined lytic skull lesions that are characteristic of LCH. The lesions lack marginal sclerosis and show "beveled" edges ➡.

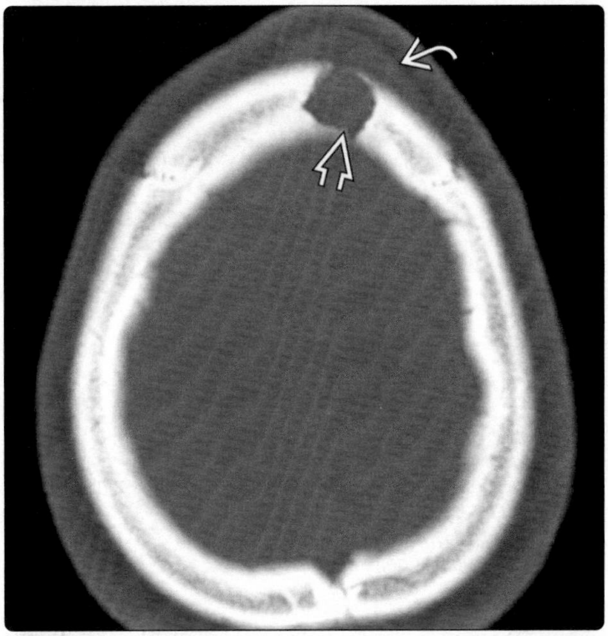

(24-35) Bone CT shows the classic appearance of LCH as a sharply marginated lytic calvarial lesion ➡. Note the associated soft tissue mass ➡.

now recognized as true neoplastic disorders with identifiable oncogenic drivers.

The histiocytoses are divided into five groups based on their histology, phenotype, and molecular alterations. The 2016 WHO classification recognizes five histiocytic tumors that affect the CNS: **Langerhans cell histiocytosis, Erdheim-Chester disease, Rosai-Dorfman disease, juvenile xanthogranuloma**, and **histiocytic sarcoma**. Because of its imaging similarities to these five recognized diseases, we also include a discussion of hemophagocytic lymphohistiocytosis in this section.

Langerhans Cell Histiocytosis

LCH can involve the CNS via direct invasion from the craniofacial bones, skull base, or meninges. Extraaxial masses of the hypothalamic-pituitary axis are also common, especially in the infundibular stalk. Parenchymal involvement is uncommon but portends high-risk disease.

LCH cells represent immature, partially activated dendritic Langerhans cells. Microglial cells are the intrinsic histiocytes of the brain and may participate in causing secondary neuronal damage, such as LCH-associated neurodegeneration.

Terminology

LCH is a clonal neoplastic proliferation of Langerhans cells. LCH was previously referred to as histiocytosis X.

Etiology

Between 50 and 60% of patients with LCH have *BRAF* V600E mutations, but the RAF-MEK-ERK pathway is activated in all patients. *MAP2K1*, which encodes MEK1, is mutated in 25% of cases.

Pathology

Location. Bone lesions are the most common manifestation of LCH (80-95% of cases) **(24-34)**. Fifty percent are monostotic.

The craniofacial bones and skull base are the most commonly affected sites (55%), followed by the hypothalamic-pituitary region (50%), cranial meninges (30%), and choroid plexus (5%). Approximately one-third of patients exhibit parenchymal lesions. A leukoencephalopathy-like pattern, often with degenerative changes in the dentate nuclei and/or basal ganglia, occurs in nearly one-third of all LCH cases.

Size and Number. Size ranges from small calvarial lesions to extensive infiltrating masses that involve most of the skull base. Multiple lesions are found in 50% of cases.

Gross Pathology. Lesions are yellowish-white and vary from discrete dura-based nodules to granular, poorly defined parenchymal infiltrates.

Microscopic Features. Two major subtypes of CNS lesions occur in LCH: tumorous lesions and degenerative lesions. **LCH-related tumefactions** contain a mixture of Langerhans cells and variable numbers of multinucleated histiocytes plus macrophages, lymphocytes, plasma cells, and occasionally eosinophils. Langerhans cells express S100 and vimentin as well as several histocyte markers.

LCH-related neurodegenerative lesions are most common in the brainstem and/or cerebellum. Langerhans cells are absent, while marked inflammatory changes with severe

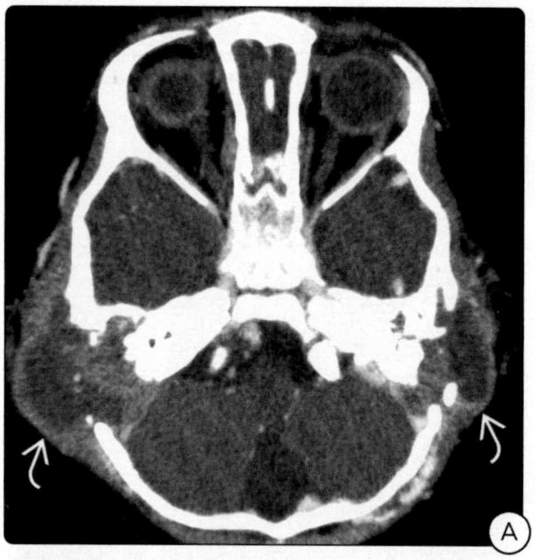

(24-36A) *CECT in 15m girl with mastoid region swelling, central DI, and ataxia shows bilateral destructive temporal bone masses ➡.*

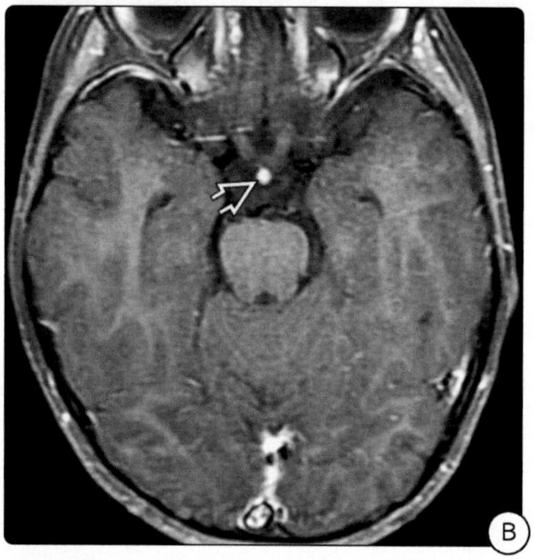

(24-36B) *Axial T1 C+ FS in the same case demonstrates a thickened, enhancing infundibular stalk ➡.*

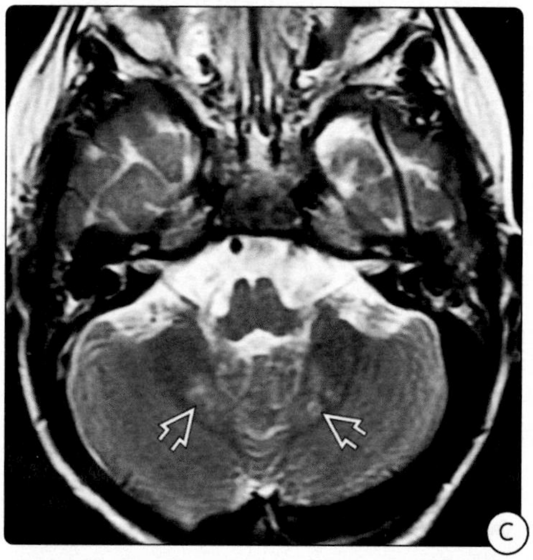

(24-36C) *T2WI shows patchy hyperintensities ➡ in the dentate nuclei representing autoimmune-mediated demyelination.*

neuronal and axonal loss are present. Lesions consist of lymphocytes, activated microglia, and gliosis.

Staging, Grading, and Classification. LCH is now classified on the basis of disease extent as unifocal, multifocal (usually polyostotic), and disseminated disease.

Clinical Issues

Epidemiology. LCH is rare. The prevalence in children is estimated at 0.5 per 100,000 per year. Most cases with isolated lesions present in young children under 2 years of age with a M:F predominance of 2:1. Multifocal disease onset is generally between 2 and 5 years of age.

Presentation. The clinical presentation of LCH ranges from a self-healing bone lesion to multisystem life-threatening disease. Skin and bone lesions are the most frequent overall manifestations of LCH. Neurological involvement occurs in 20-50% of cases. Although isolated LCH does occur, most cases of CNS LCH are diagnosed concurrently with multisystem disease.

The most common presenting symptom of CNS LCH is central diabetes insipidus (DI), occurring in approximately half of all patients with multisystem LCH. Between 8-10% of children with central DI have LCH. Other CNS-related findings include symptoms of increased intracranial pressure, cranial nerve palsies, seizures, visual disturbances, ataxia, and neurocognitive disturbances.

Natural History. Natural history and prognosis of **classic LCH** vary according to age at onset and whether the disease is isolated, multifocal, or disseminated. Solitary osseous lesions have the best prognosis, as spontaneous remission is relatively common. Overall survival rates are good although mortality in young children with multisystem disease approaches 15-20%.

Neurodegenerative LCH is generally a progressive disorder, with neurocognitive symptoms developing in about 25% of patients after 6 years. **Malignant LCH** exists but is very rare. Atypical organ involvement and an aggressive clinical course are characteristic.

LCH: ETIOLOGY, PATHOLOGY, AND CLINICAL FEATURES

Etiology
- Clonal neoplastic proliferation of Langerhans cells
- Most carry either *BRAF* V600E or *MAP2K1* mutations

Pathology
- Neoplastic Langerhans cells, variable histiocytes, and inflammatory cells
  - Craniofacial bones, 55%
  - Hypothalamic-pituitary stalk, 50%
  - Cranial meninges, 30%
  - Choroid plexus, 5%
- Nonneoplastic neurodegenerative changes
  - Cerebellum, basal ganglia, 35%

Clinical Features
- Solitary LCH children < 2 years old
- Multifocal LCH between 2 and 5 years
- Skin, bone lesions most common
- Central diabetes insipidus in 50%

Treatment Options. Therapeutic options depend on symptoms, location, and disease extent, ranging from simple surgical excision to radiation and chemotherapy.

Imaging

CT Findings. Craniofacial involvement is the most common presentation of CNS LCH. One or more sharply marginated lytic skull or facial bone defects are the most common manifestations on NECT **(24-35)**, present in 55% of cases. A "beveled" appearance with the inner table more affected than the outer is typical.

Geographic skull base destruction, often centered on the temporal bone, may be extensive **(24-36A)**. Associated soft tissue lesions may be small and relatively discrete, or they may be large, extensively infiltrating masses.

MR Findings. Soft tissue masses adjacent to calvarial vault or skull base lesions may show mild T1 shortening secondary to the presence of lipid-laden histiocytes.

Abnormalities of the hypothalamus and pituitary stalk are common. The posterior pituitary "bright spot" is often absent, and the infundibular stalk may appear thickened (> 3 mm) and nontapering **(24-36B)**. Lesions are slightly hyperintense on T2WI.

LCH enhances strongly and uniformly on T1 C+ scans. Look for a thickened enhancing infundibulum, dura-based masses, and choroid plexus involvement **(24-37)**. Punctate foci of parenchymal enhancement occur in approximately 15% of cases **(24-39)**, with the pons the most frequent site **(24-38)**.

Nontumorous neurodegenerative changes are common **(24-39A)**. Secondary cerebellar degeneration occurs in 25% of cases and is seen as bilaterally symmetrical confluent T2/FLAIR hyperintensities, typically in the dentate nuclei **(24-36C)**.

LCH: IMAGING

CT
- > 50% have lytic craniofacial lesion(s)
- "Beveled" lesion > geographic destruction

MR
- Soft tissue mass adjacent to bone lesion
- Hypothalamus/pituitary stalk
  - Absent posterior pituitary "bright spot"
  - Thickened (> 3 mm), nontapering stalk
- Enhancing lesions
  - Dura-based mass(es)
  - Choroid plexus
  - Punctate/linear parenchymal enhancing foci
- Nontumorous degenerative changes
  - Symmetric T2/FLAIR hyperintensity cerebellum/dentate nuclei, basal ganglia

Differential Diagnosis

The differential diagnosis varies with lesion site. Lytic calvarial lesions that may mimic LCH include **burr holes** and other **surgical defects, dermoid** and **epidermoids, leptomeningeal cysts,** and **infection**. With the exception of neuroblastoma, osseous **metastases** are relatively rare in children.

A thickened infundibular stalk can be seen with **germinoma**, the most important differential consideration in a child with central DI. Less common

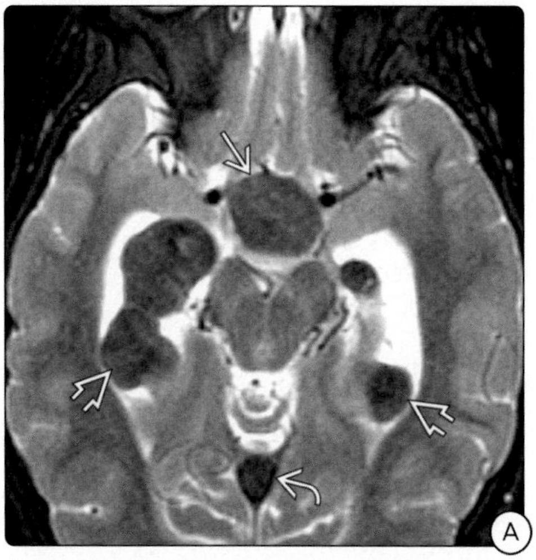

***(24-37A)** T2WI in a patient with LCH shows hypointense suprasellar ➡, choroid plexus ➡, and dural masses ➡.*

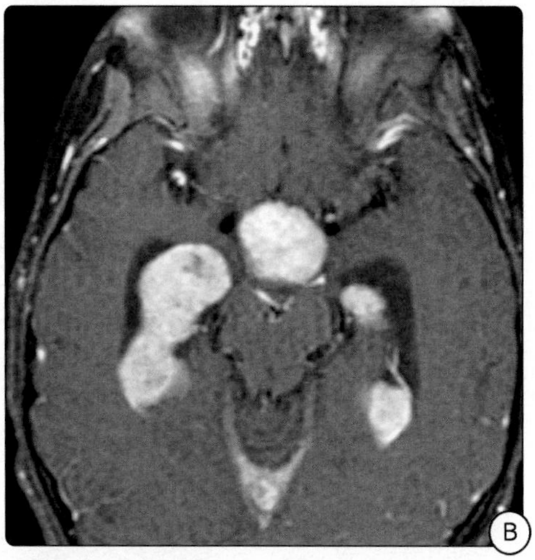

***(24-37B)** T1 C+ FS scan in the same patient shows that the lesions enhance intensely, slightly heterogeneously.*

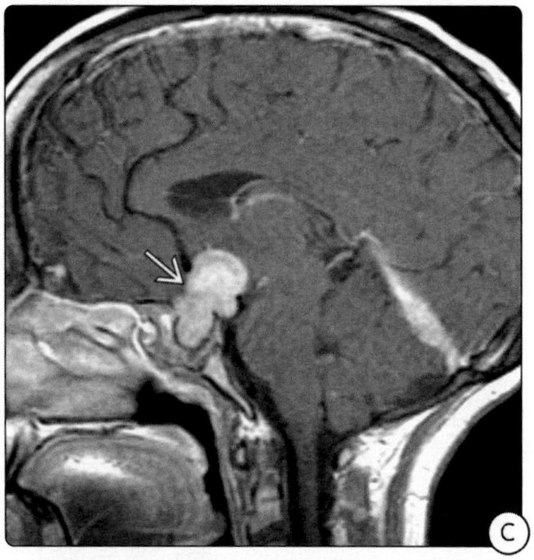

***(24-37C)** Sagittal T1 C+ shows the suprasellar mass involving the hypothalamus, infundibular stalk and infiltrating the pituitary gland ➡.*

lesions with a thick nontapering stalk include **neurosarcoid** (uncommon in children), **astrocytoma**, and **hypophysitis**.

Erdheim-Chester Disease

Terminology

Erdheim-Chester disease (ECD) is a rare non-LCH histiocytosis characterized by xanthomatous infiltrates of foamy histiocytes.

Etiology

As 50-60% of patients with ECD have *BRAF* V600E mutations and activating *MAP2K1* mutations are present in another 30%, the genetic parallels between ECD and LDH indicate a potential shared cell of origin for both conditions.

Pathology

Although it may affect multiple organs, ECD is most typically a disease of long bones. Extraskeletal manifestations occur in 50% of cases. Intracranial lesions are present in 10% of patients.

The brain, meninges, orbits, and sellar/juxtasellar region are all reported sites of ECD. Widespread infiltrative parenchymal lesions and dural thickening/meningioma-like mass(es) are the most common manifestations. Almost all patients with intracranial ECD also have facial and/or calvarial thickening.

Microscopically, ECD is characterized by infiltrates of lipid-laden neoplastic histiocytes, multinucleated giant cells, scant lymphocytes, and variable fibrosis or gliosis. The histiocytes are CD68 positive and negative for CD1a and S100 protein.

(24-38A) Axial T2WI in a 46y man with multiple cranial nerve palsies shows heterogeneously hyperintense mass infiltrating, expanding the pons and both middle cerebellar peduncles. (24-38B) More cephalad T2WI shows infiltration into the midbrain, the hypothalamus, and both medial temporal lobes.

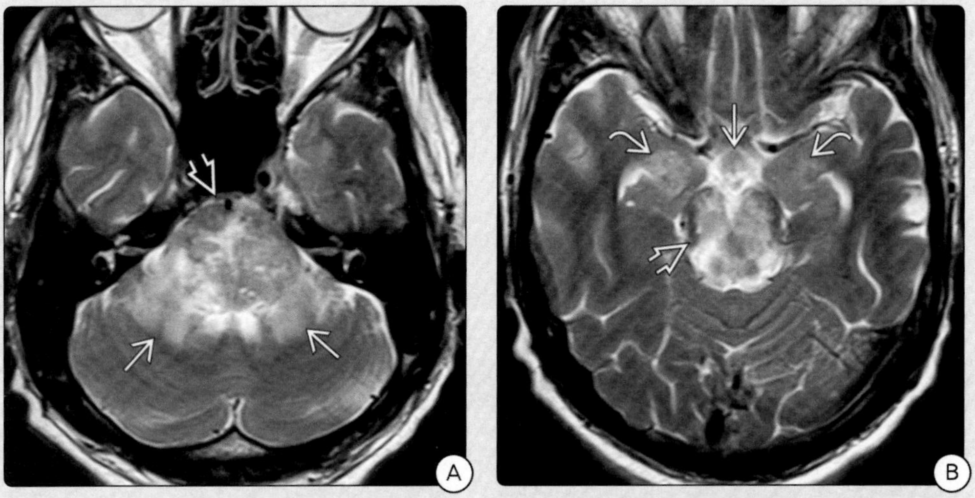

(24-38C) T1 C+ FS shows strong but patchy and solid nodular enhancement in the pons. (24-38D) More cephalad T1 C+ FS shows solid enhancement in the hypothalamus and patchy enhancement in the medial temporal lobes and midbrain. Biopsy disclosed LCH.

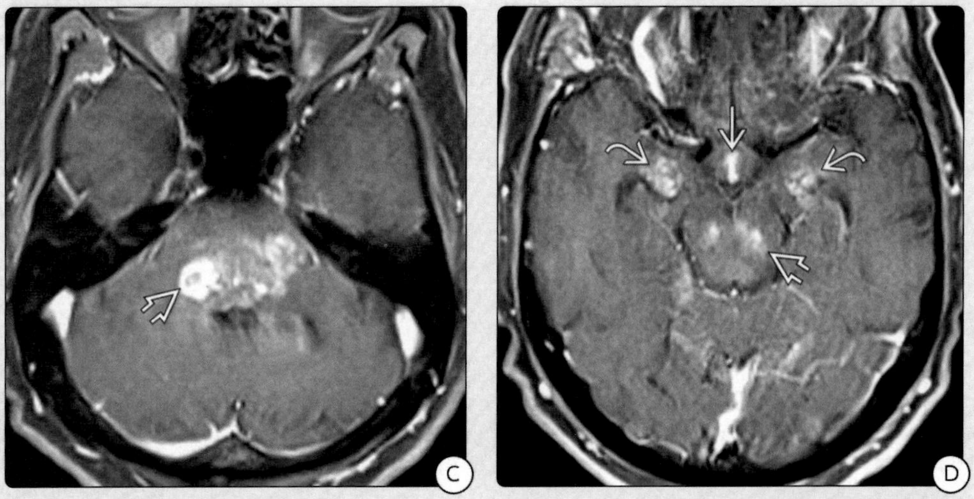

Clinical Issues

ECD usually occurs in adults over 55 years of age. Prognosis in ECD is generally poor although treatment with interferon-α has improved survival in some patients.

Imaging

The hypothalamic-pituitary axis is involved in 50-55% of intracranial ECD **(24-40)**. The pons and cerebellum—especially the dentate nuclei—are the second most common intraaxial location. Solitary or multiple dura-based masses with or without diffuse pachymeningeal thickening occur in almost 25% of cases **(24-40D)**. Osteosclerosis of the facial bones, calvaria, or vertebral column may be a specific feature suggesting the diagnosis.

Imaging in patients with hypothalamic-pituitary involvement shows absent posterior pituitary "bright spot" on T1WI. A focal suprasellar mass or nodular thickening of the infundibular stalk is common.

Meningioma-like dural masses are isointense on T1WI and iso- to hypointense on T2WI. Strong homogeneous enhancement is typical.

Between 15-20% of ECD cases demonstrate parenchymal lesions. Multifocal areas of T2/FLAIR hyperintensity that show mild nodular enhancement on T1 C+ are typical findings. Ependymal enhancement with deep linear extension into the lentiform nuclei has been described as a finding suggestive of ECD.

A unique finding with ECD is perivascular disease. Periaortic fibrosis and perivascular infiltration along the carotid arteries extending into the cavernous sinus may occur. These lesions are very hypointense on T2WI and enhance strongly and intensely.

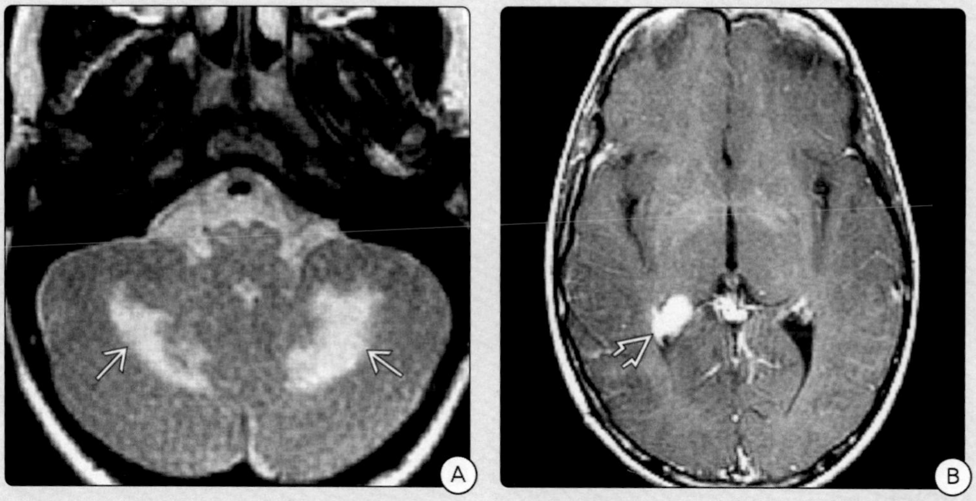

***(24-39A)** Axial T2WI in a child with systemic LCH shows bilateral symmetric hyperintensities in the cerebellum ➡. **(24-39B)** T1 C+ in the same case shows an enhancing mass ➡ in the right choroid plexus.*

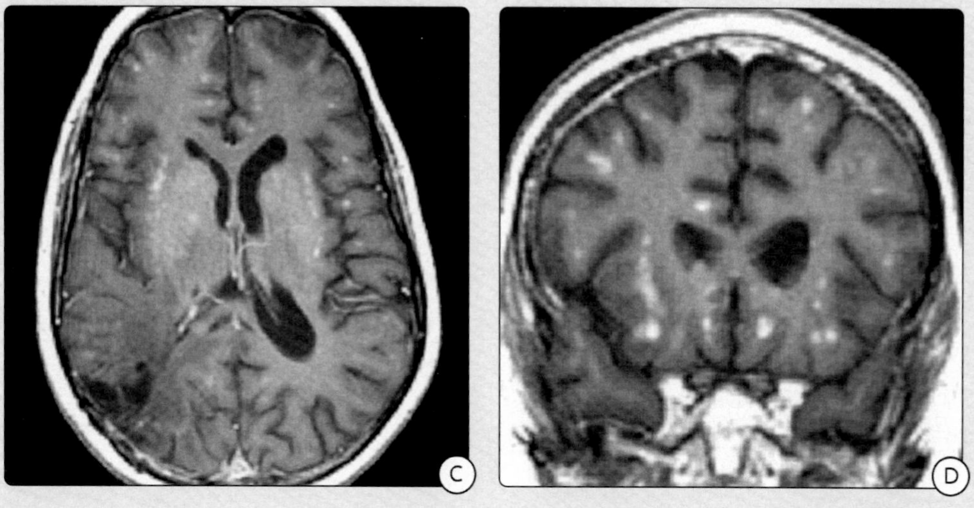

***(24-39C)** Axial T1 C+ shows multiple enhancing nodules in the subcortical and deep WM. Right parietal encephalomalacia is from biopsy of the brain and choroid plexus. **(24-39D)** Coronal T1 C+ in the same case shows the enhancing nodules. This is biopsy-proven parenchymal LCH with secondary degenerative changes in the cerebellum.*

Differential Diagnosis

The differential diagnosis of ECD includes **meningioma** and **LCH**. LCH is generally a disease of children, whereas ECD primarily affects middle-aged and older adults. Osteosclerosis of the facial bones and/or calvaria may be a unique feature of ECD although histologic analysis plays the definitive role in differentiating ECD from other histiocytoses. **Wegener granulomatosis** (WG) may mimic ECD with sinus, orbital, and meningeal lesions, but WG usually causes osteolysis, not osteosclerosis.

Rosai-Dorfman Disease

Terminology

Rosai-Dorfman disease (RDD), also called sinus histiocytosis with massive lymphadenopathy, is a rare benign histioproliferative disorder of unknown etiology. *BRAF* V600E mutations are absent.

Pathology

RDD is now defined by the accumulation of CD68-positive, S100-positive, and CDE1a-negative proliferating histiocytes with intact, mature hematolymphoid cells floating freely within their cytoplasm ("emperipolesis"). A prominent lymphoplasmatic infiltrate is also frequently present within the tumor mass. The most common immunotypic feature of RDD is uniform, strong expression of S-100 protein in the absence of CD1a expression.

Clinical Issues

RDD can occur at any age, but almost 80% of patients are younger than 20 years old at the time of initial diagnosis. Bilateral massive but painless cervical lymphadenopathy is the most common presentation. CNS involvement is rare and

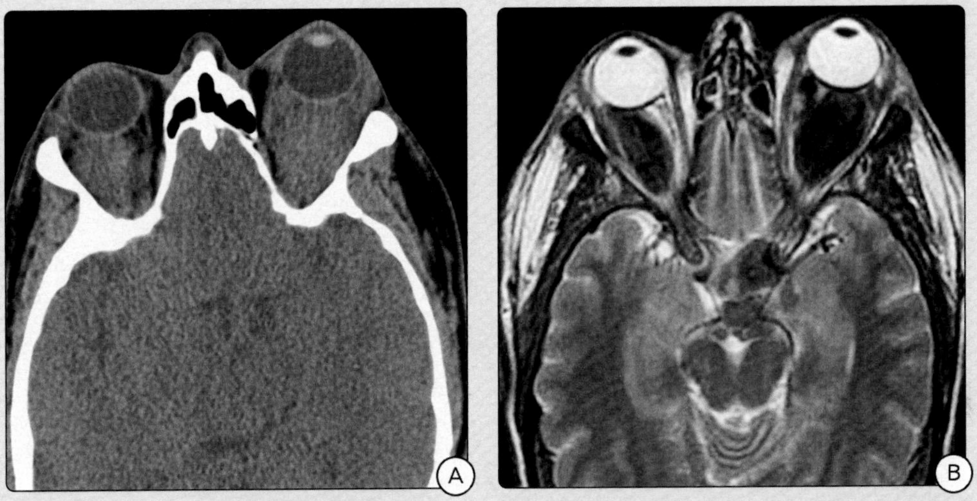

***(24-40A)** Axial NECT in a 39y man with proptosis shows bilateral intraconal retrobulbar soft tissue lesions. **(24-40B)** T2WI in the same case shows that the orbital lesions are very hypointense. Note well-delineated lobulated hypointense masses in the suprasellar cistern.*

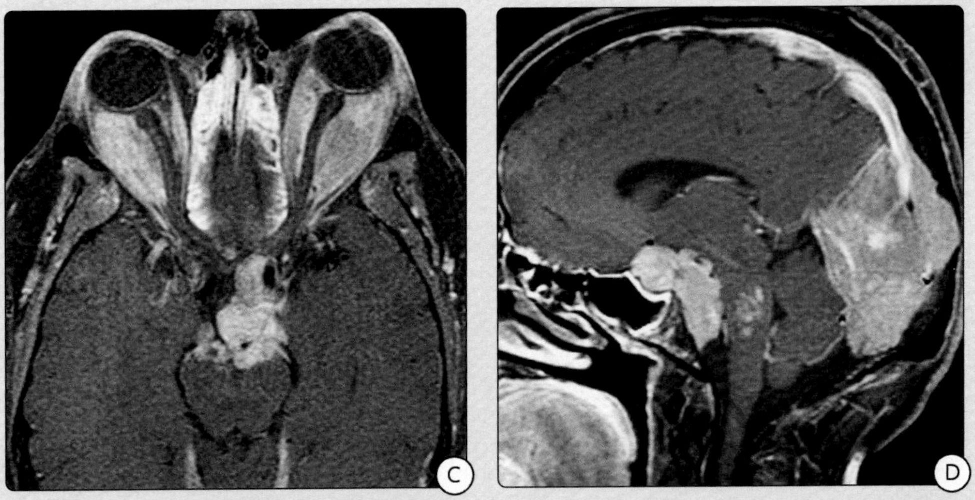

***(24-40C)** T1 C+ FS shows that the intraconal retrobulbar masses enhance intensely, as does the lobulated suprasellar mass. **(24-40D)** Sagittal T1 C+ FS in the same case shows extensive dural-based masses along falx, clivus, and diaphragma sellae and infiltrating the pituitary gland. Note enhancing lesions in the pons. This is biopsy-proven Erdheim-Chester disease.*

generally occurs *without* cervical adenopathy or other extranodal involvement.

Prognosis is generally favorable after surgical resection and/or corticosteroid treatment.

Imaging

RDD has a protean imaging appearance but most frequently presents as bilateral cervical lymphadenopathy. Extranodal involvement is seen in 50% of cases. The skin, nose, sinuses, and orbit (especially the eyelids and lacrimal glands) are often affected.

Intracranial RDD occurs in 5% of cases. Solitary or multiple dura-based masses that are moderately hyperdense on NECT and enhance strongly on CECT are typical findings. Sellar/suprasellar and intraspinal lesions are even less common. They can be isolated or occur in concert with more typical dura-based and/or orbital lesions.

RDD is typically isointense with gray matter on T1WI and iso- to slightly hypointense on T2WI. Lesions demonstrate high fractional anisotropy, low ADC, and mild "blooming" on SWI.

Intense homogeneous enhancement occurs following contrast administration **(24-41)**. Less commonly, multiple cranial and peripheral enhancing nerves can be identified.

pMR is decreased. FDG PET shows variable uptake. Nodal and lacrimal disease shows avid uptake, but other sites are often "cold" on FDG PET.

Differential Diagnosis

*Extra*cranial RDD closely resembles **non-Hodgkin lymphoma**. Reactive lymphadenopathy and TB adenopathy are common in children and may mimic RDD. Biopsy with histopathology is necessary for definitive diagnosis.

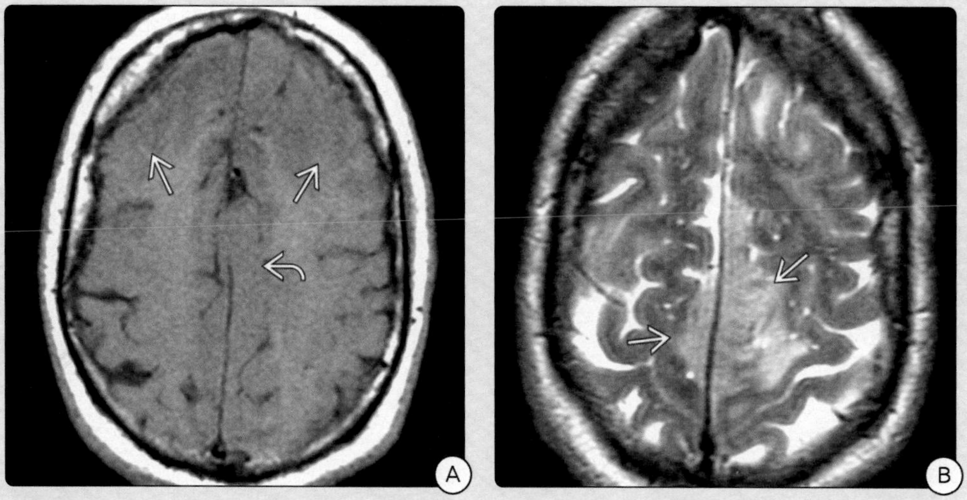

***(24-41A)** T1WI shows effaced sulci and GM-WM interfaces in both frontal lobes → and along the interhemispheric fissure ↪. **(24-41B)** T2WI shows lobulated parafalcine masses → that are iso- to slightly hyperintense relative to cortex.*

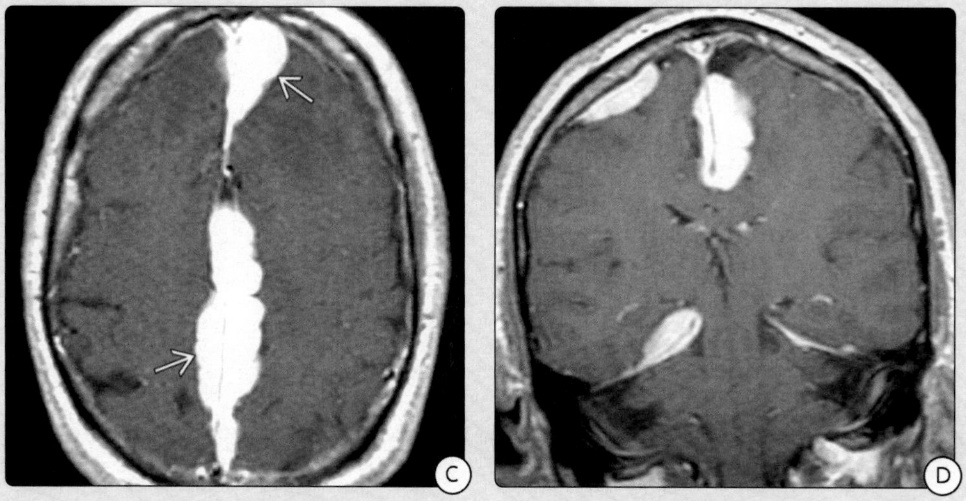

***(24-41C)** Axial T1 C+ shows extensive, lobulated, intensely enhancing frontal and parafalcine masses →. **(24-41D)** Coronal T1 C+ scan shows additional lesions over the convexity and along the leaves of the tentorium cerebelli. The patient had Rosai-Dorfman disease diagnosed by cervical lymph node biopsy.*

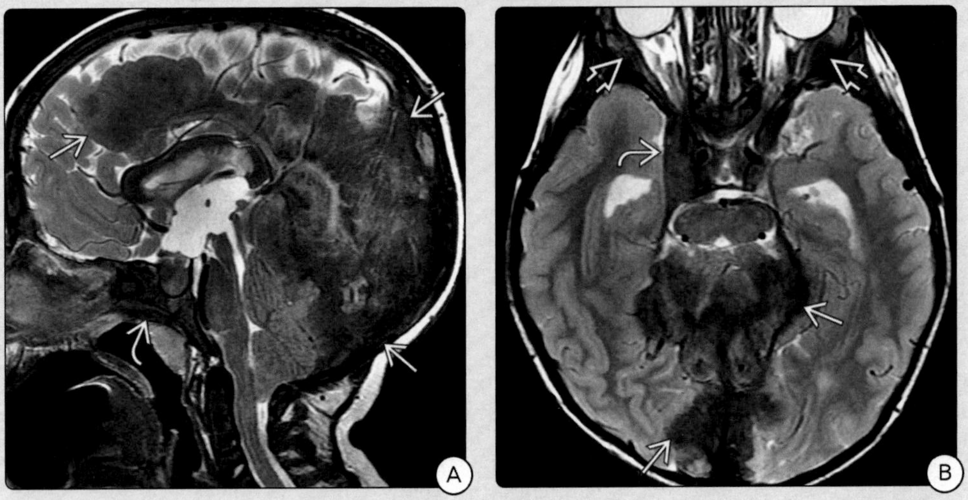

(24-42A) *Sagittal T2WI in a 7y boy with proven JXG shows multiple lobulated hypointense masses along the falx and tentorium. Note infiltration of skull base/cavernous sinus/pituitary gland.* ***(24-42B)*** *Axial T2WI in the same case shows lobulated, very hypointense masses along the falx and tentorium, as well as involvement of the cavernous sinus and orbits.*

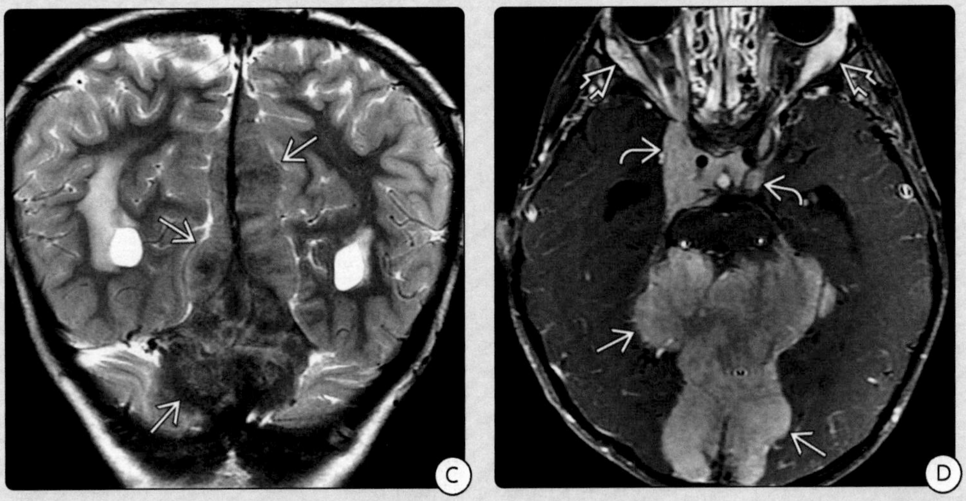

(24-42C) *Coronal T2WI shows the lobulated extraaxial masses along the falx cerebri and tentorium.* ***(24-42D)*** *Axial T1 C+ FS shows that the masses along the falx and tentorium as well as the lesions infiltrating the cavernous sinus and orbits all enhance intensely and uniformly.*

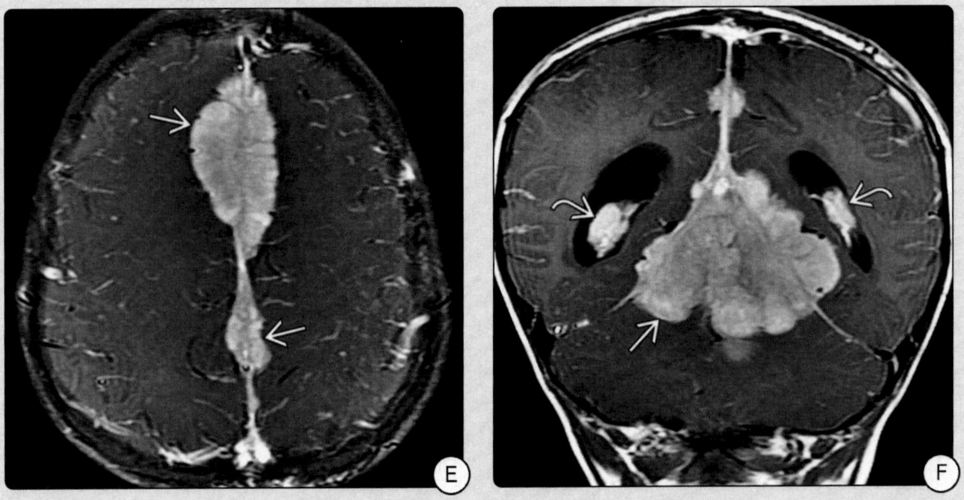

(24-42E) *More cephalad T1 C+ FS shows the lobulated enhancing masses along the falx. The imaging appearance is very similar to RDD, which occurs primarily in adults.* ***(24-42F)*** *Coronal T1 C+ shows the enhancing masses filling the tentorial incisura. Note additional lesions in the choroid plexi.*

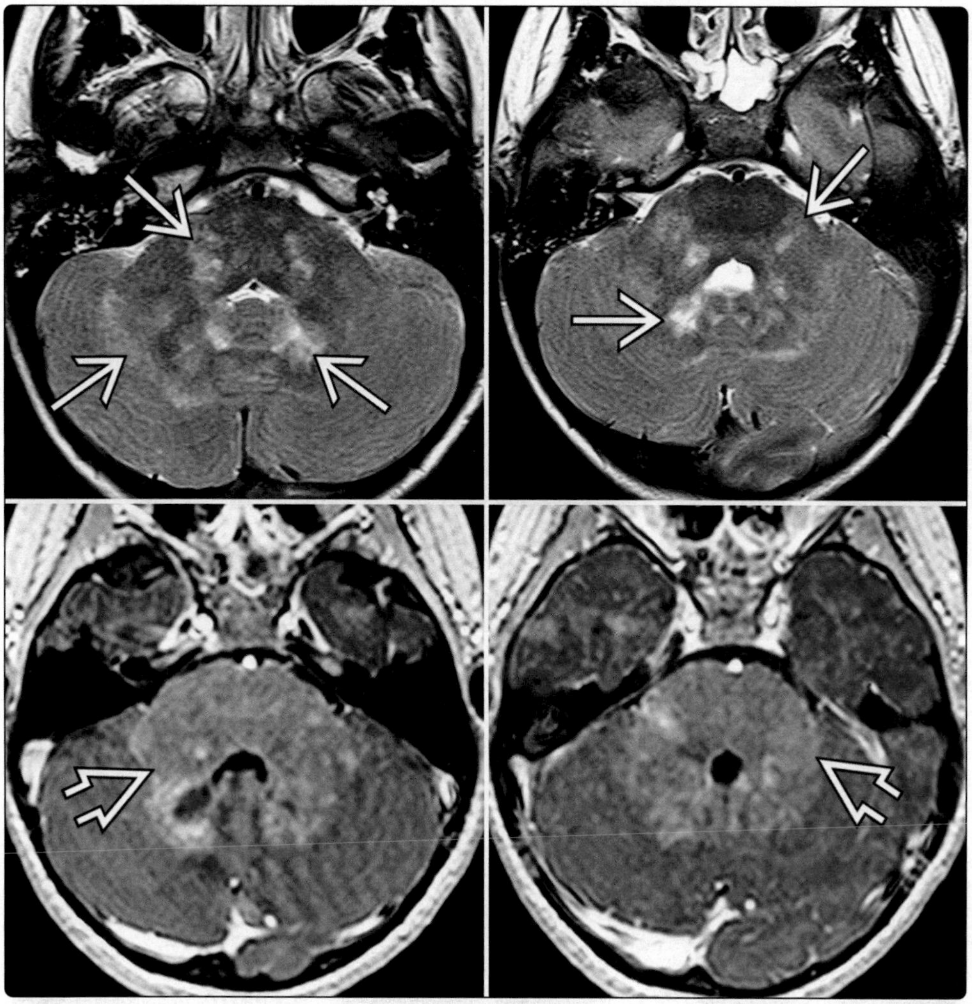

***(24-43)** (Top) T2 scans in a 2y child with high fever and seizures show multiple patchy hyperintensities ➡ expanding the pons and both middle cerebellar peduncles, extending into the dentate nuclei and cerebellar hemispheres. (Bottom) T1 C+ SPGR scans for stereotactic localization prior to biopsy show diffuse confluent and patchy enhancement ➡. Histopathologic diagnosis was hemophagocytic lymphohistiocytosis.*

The major imaging differential diagnosis of *intra*cranial RDD is **meningioma**. pMR is helpful in distinguishing RDD, which is generally hypometabolic. **Neurosarcoid** with dura-based and sellar/suprasellar involvement can mimic RDD, as can other dural-based masses such as **metastasis, plasma cell granuloma, infectious granuloma** (e.g., TB), and **IgG4-related disease**.

Juvenile Xanthogranuloma

Terminology

Juvenile xanthogranuloma (JXG) is now considered a family of lesions that spans a spectrum from papular xanthoma and xanthoma disseminatum to cephalic histiocytosis and spindle cell xanthogranuloma.

Pathology

JXG are soft, yellowish or tan lesions that are composed of round or spindled, variably vacuolated neoplastic histiocytes, scattered giant cells, lymphocytes, and occasional eosinophils. JXGs are CD68 positive, CD1a and S100 negative, and factor XIIIa positive.

Clinical Issues

JXG generally affects young children and is usually limited to the skin. JXG may arise in the brain or cranial meninges, either with or without cutaneous manifestations. Cerebral lesions have been associated with multifocal or systemic forms of the disease, with an occasionally fulminant or relentless progressive clinical course.

Imaging

Imaging findings with JXG vary. Disseminated white matter lesions resemble those of LCH. Lesions may also affect the sellar region, choroid plexus, orbits, and paranasal sinuses. A rare disseminated form of xanthoma, called xanthoma disseminatum, preferentially affects young adults. The pituitary-hypothalamic axis and dura are most commonly affected by this variant **(24-42)**.

Histiocytic Sarcoma

Histiocytic sarcoma is a rare, aggressive malignant neoplasm characterized by highly cellular noncohesive infiltrates of large, pleomorphic, mitotically active histiocytes. Reported cases of CNS histiocytic sarcoma have involved the brain parenchyma, meninges, and cavernous sinus. Isolated cases of

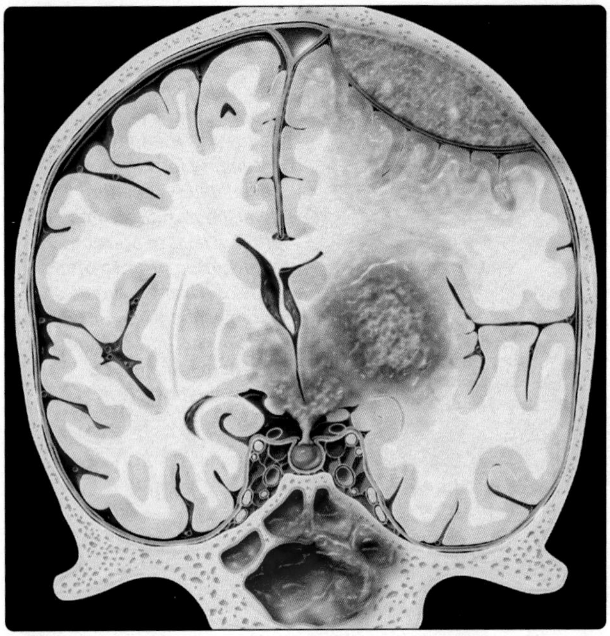

***(24-44)** Coronal graphic depicts the typical greenish discoloration of granulocytic sarcoma. Extradural and sinus disease is common. Parenchymal lesions in the basal ganglia, hypothalamus, and infundibular stalk are also illustrated.*

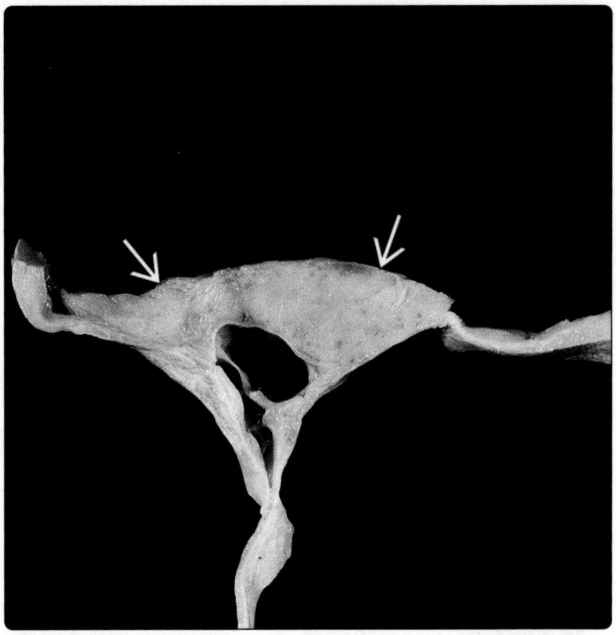

***(24-45)** Autopsy specimen shows dural thickening, infiltration, and focal masses ➡ in a patient who died from AML. (Courtesy R. Hewlett, MD.)*

radiation-associated histiocytic sarcoma involving the CNS have been reported.

Malignant fibrous histiocytoma is now considered a high-grade undifferentiated pleomorphic sarcoma and is no longer regarded as a true histiocytic lesion. Only isolated cases have been reported to involve the brain. Sarcomas and malignant mesenchymal tumors are discussed in detail in Chapter 22.

Hemophagocytic Lymphohistiocytosis

Hemophagocytic lymphohistiocytosis (HLH) is not a single disease but a clinical syndrome of life-threatening hyperinflammation. It can occur as a genetic defect (primary or familial HLH, which usually occurs in infancy as an autosomal-recessive disorder) or as a reactive infection-associated process caused by viruses such as EBV, H1N1, and Bunyavirus. CNS HLH occurs in 30-70% of cases.

Terminology

Secondary HLH is also known as macrophage activation syndrome.

Etiology

Unlike the other histiocytic disorders, there is no specific cell marker for HLH. Specific mutations linked to HLH include perforin (*FHL2*) and *UNC13D*-FHL3 gene mutations. The mutation for X-linked lymphoproliferative disorder involves the *SH2D1A* gene.

Although its pathogenesis is not fully understood, HLH may be mediated by excessive activation of CD8+ T lymphocytes and the release of cytokines such as TNF-α and interferon-γ.

Pathology

HLH is characterized by aggressive proliferation of activated macrophages and histiocytes that infiltrate the brain and meninges. Perivascular infiltration follows the initial leptomeningeal inflammation. Eventually, massive parenchymal infiltration, blood vessel destruction, and tissue necrosis ensue. Hemophagocytosis, the histologic hallmark of the disease, may be scant or even absent early in the disease course.

Clinical Issues

HLH is primarily a disease of infants and young children. Fever, hepatosplenomegaly, and cytopenias characterize the disease. The typical clinical presentation includes irritability, bulging fontanelle, seizures, cranial nerve palsies, ataxia, and hemiplegia. Primary HLH is lethal without allogenic stem cell transplantation. Secondary HLH is usually self-limited.

Imaging

CNS involvement is present in at least 75% of all HLH patients at the time of initial diagnosis. Imaging shows extensive confluent T2/FLAIR hyperintense infiltrates in the cerebellum and cerebral white matter **(24-43)**. Symmetric periventricular lesions without thalamic and brainstem involvement are common in primary HLH. Linear and nodular enhancement of parenchymal lesions and the pial surfaces of the brain is typical.

Hematopoietic Tumors and Tumor-Like Lesions

Leukemia

Leukemia is the most common form of childhood cancer, representing approximately one-third of all cases. Acute lymphoblastic leukemia (ALL) accounts for 80% and acute myeloid leukemia (AML) for most of the remaining 15-20%. Chronic myelocytic leukemia (CML) and lymphocytic leukemia are much more common in adults. Regardless of specific type, the general clinical features of leukemias are similar.

Once relatively uncommon, the prevalence of CNS involvement has risen with treatment advances that result in prolonged overall survival. Neurological symptoms in leukemia patients may be due to CNS involvement (direct or primary effects) or occur as treatment complications (secondary effects).

Treatment-related complications include white matter lesions, mineralizing microangiopathy, posterior reversible encephalopathy syndrome (PRES), secondary tumors, infections, and brain volume loss. These are considered separately in Chapter 30. Here we consider the direct effects of leukemia on the CNS.

Terminology

Leukemic masses containing primitive myeloblasts, promyelocytes, or myelocytes were initially called **chloromas** (for the greenish discoloration caused by high levels of myeloperoxidase in these immature cells). As 30% of the cells are other colors (white, gray, or brown), these tumors have been renamed **granulocytic (myeloid) sarcomas**.

Etiology

Granulocytic sarcoma is often diagnosed simultaneously with or immediately after the onset of acute leukemia. In patients without overt leukemia, granulocytic sarcoma usually presages the development of AML by several months. Other conditions that predispose to the development of granulocytic sarcoma are myelodysplastic syndromes and nonneoplastic myeloproliferative disorders, such as polycythemia vera, hypereosinophilia, and myeloid metaplasia.

Intracranial granulocytic sarcomas probably develop when neoplastic cells in the calvaria migrate via haversian canals through the periosteum and into the dura to form focal leukemic masses. If the pial-glial barrier is breached, tumor can spread directly or via the perivascular spaces into the underlying brain.

Extramedullary leukemia (EML) is common in children with leukemia. CNS involvement is rare and occurs either as leukemia cells within the CSF or as focal aggregates of immature myeloid cells that infiltrate bone and soft tissues.

Pathology

Location. EML can affect virtually any part of the body, including the skin, lymph nodes, stomach, and colon. Multiple lesions are common. Lesions of the vertebrae, orbits, and calvaria are more common than intracranial deposits, which are relatively rare.

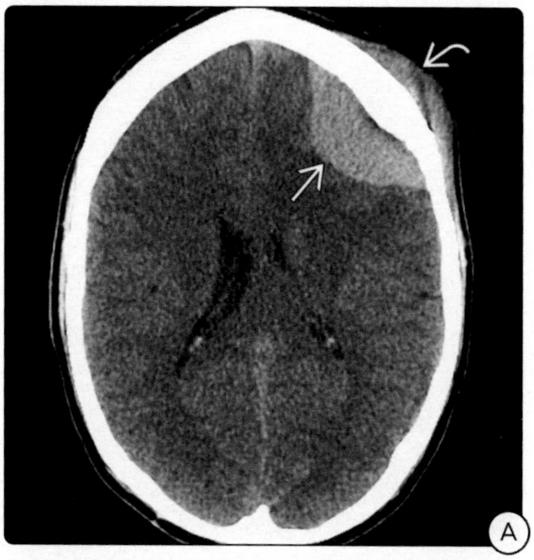

(24-46A) NECT in a 28y man with AML and a scalp "lump" shows left frontal subgaleal ➡ and hyperdense extraaxial mass ➡.

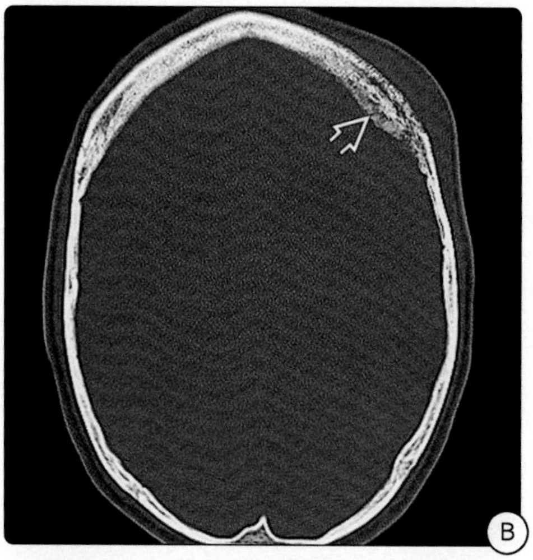

(24-46B) Bone CT with edge enhancement shows permeative, destructive changes in the adjacent calvarium ➡.

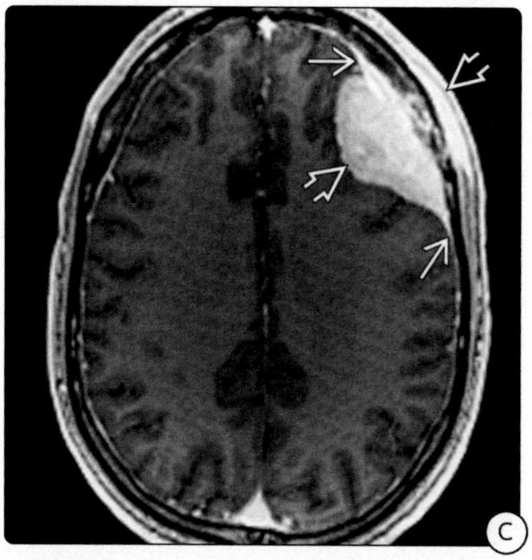

(24-46C) Prebiopsy T1 C+ SPGR shows the subgaleal/calvarial/epidural mass ➡ enhances intensely. Note small dural "tails" ➡; chloroma.

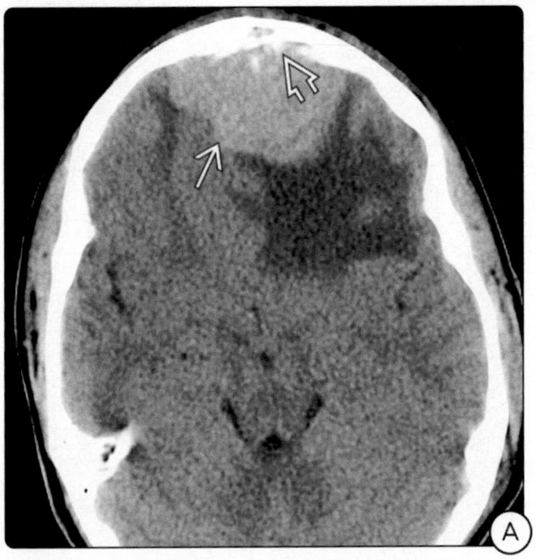

(24-47A) NECT scan in a child with AML shows a hyperdense midline frontal mass → with peritumoral edema and bone destruction →.

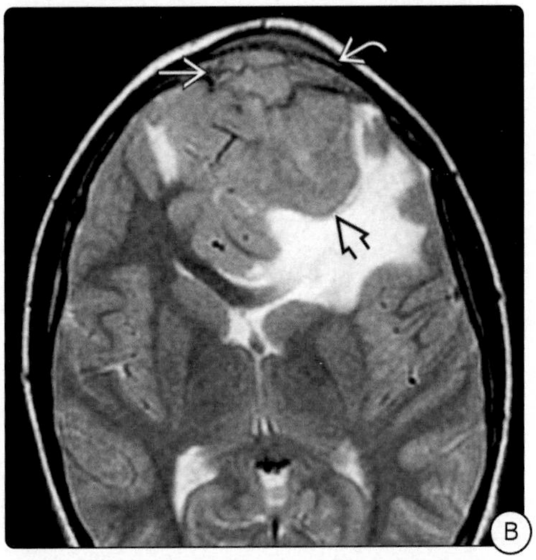

(24-47B) T2WI shows the mass →, permeative destructive bone lesion →, and parenchymal mass → that is isointense with cortex.

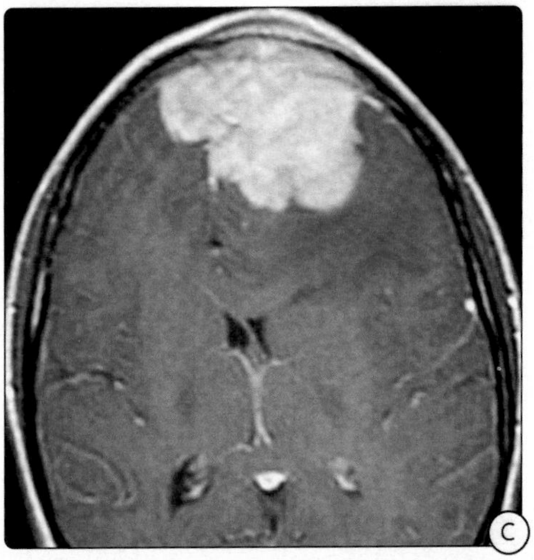

(24-47C) The lesion enhances strongly, mostly uniformly on T1 C+. This is granulocytic sarcoma ("chloroma").

Between 5-7% of patients with AML have asymptomatic CNS involvement as evidenced by positive CSF cytological analysis. Overt CNS leukemia presents in three forms: (1) meningeal disease ("carcinomatous meningitis"), (2) intravascular tumor aggregates with diffuse brain disease ("carcinomatous encephalitis"), and (3) focal tumor masses (granulocytic sarcoma).

Most intracranial lesions are located adjacent to malignant deposits in the orbits, paranasal sinuses, skull base, or calvaria. Intraaxial granulocytic sarcomas occur but are less common **(24-44)**.

Size and Number. Multifocal involvement is typical. Extraaxial lesions are generally large and seen as extensive bony infiltrates and dura-based masses **(24-45)**. Parenchymal lesions are usually smaller, ranging from a few millimeters to 1 or 2 cm.

Microscopic Features. Granulocytic sarcomas are highly cellular tumors that consist of leukemic myeloblasts and myeloid precursors embedded in a rich reticulin-fiber network. Monotonous tumor cells with large nuclei, prominent nucleoli, and scanty eosinophilic cytoplasm are typical. Nuclei are often pleomorphic. Multiple mitoses are typical, with MIB-1 labeling exceeding 50%.

Clinical Issues

Epidemiology and Demographics. Granulocytic sarcoma occurs in 3-10% of patients with AML and 1-2% of patients with CML. Intracranial and intraspinal lesions in the absence of systemic disease are very rare. Although granulocytic sarcoma can affect patients of virtually any age, 60% are younger than 15 years at the time of initial diagnosis.

Presentation. The typical clinical setting is that of a child with AML who develops headache or focal neurologic deficits. Meningeal disease may occur in adults with either acute or chronic myelogenous leukemia. Cranial nerve palsies are typical symptoms.

Natural History. Although the overall survival in treated AML is 40-50%, development of granulocytic sarcoma implies blastic transformation and poor prognosis. Transformation of chronic lymphocytic leukemia (CLL) into diffuse large non-Hodgkin lymphoma (Richter syndrome) is a rare but serious complication. Median survival in transformed CLL is 5 or 6 months despite multiagent therapy.

Treatment Options. Patients with AML presenting with granulocytic sarcoma may benefit from individually tailored regimens with risk-adapted chemotherapy, postinduction intensification of therapy, hematopoietic stem cell transplantation, and prolonged treatment maintenance.

Imaging

Imaging is key to the diagnosis of CNS involvement, as CSF studies may be negative.

CT Findings. Granulocytic sarcomas typically present as one or more iso- or hyperdense dura-based masses on NECT **(24-46A)**. Strong uniform enhancement is typical. Bone CT often shows infiltrating, permeative, destructive lucent lesions **(24-46B)**. An adjacent soft tissue mass may be present.

MR Findings. Nearly 75% of patients with leukemia and positive CSF cytology have abnormal findings on MR **(24-46C)** **(24-47)**. Pachymeningeal (30%), leptomeningeal (25%), cranial nerve (30%) **(24-50)**, and spinal meningeal (70%) types of enhancement are typical.

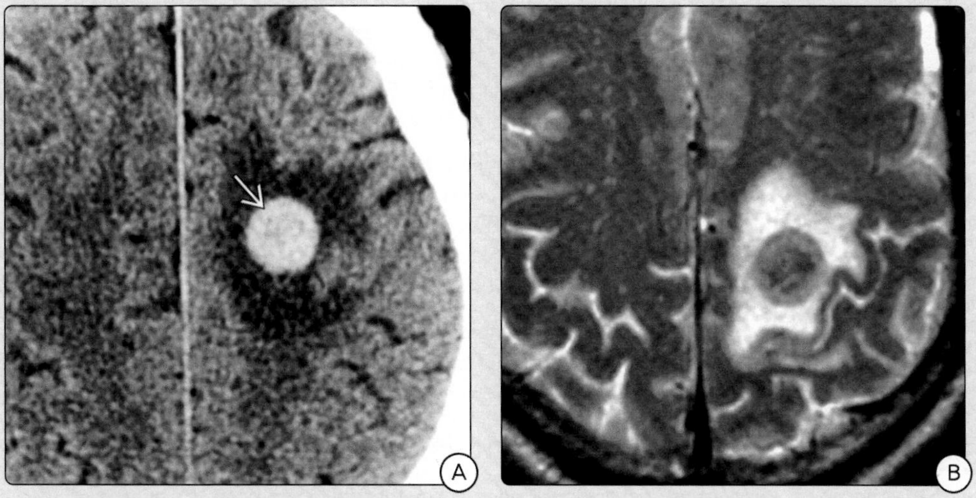

***(24-48A)** NECT scan in a child with AML shows a round, very hyperdense mass → in the left corona radiata. **(24-48B)** The lesion is hypointense on T2WI. "Chloroma" (granulocytic sarcoma) was found at biopsy.*

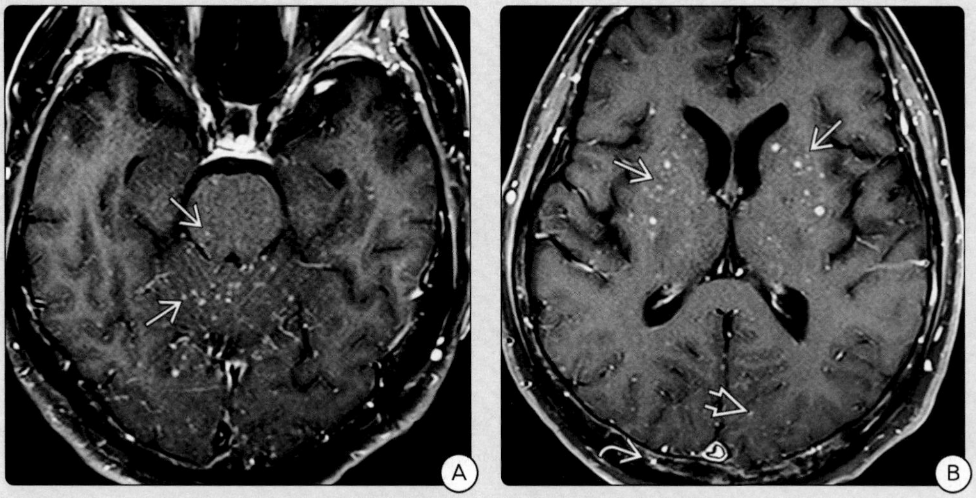

***(24-49A)** Axial T1 C+ FS in a 49y man with acute myelogenous leukemia and altered mental status shows innumerable punctate-enhancing lesions → in the pons and cerebellum. **(24-49B)** More cephalad T1 C+ FS in the same case shows additional enhancing lesions primarily clustered in the basal ganglia → with a few scattered lesions in the hemispheres ⇨. Multiple calvarial lesions are also present ↪.*

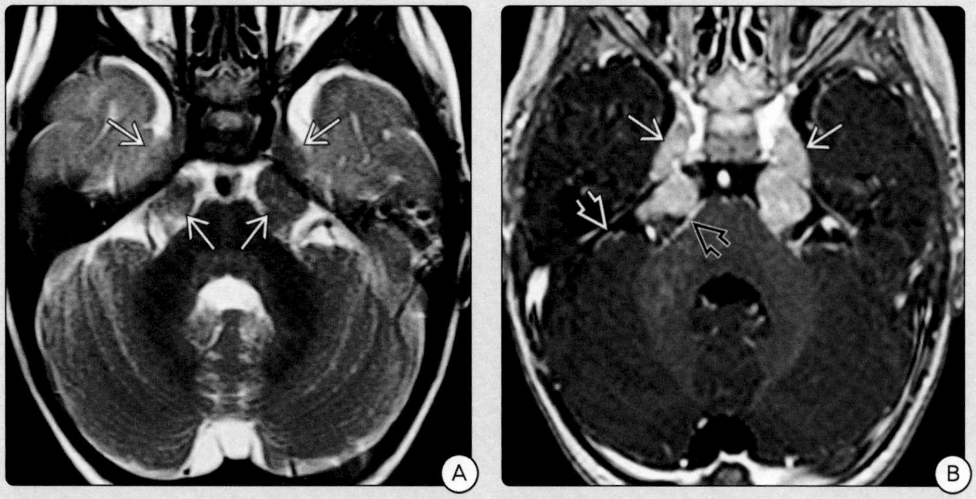

***(24-50A)** Axial T2WI in a 5y girl with leukemia and multiple cranial nerve palsies shows bilateral Meckel cave and cerebellopontine angle cistern lesions →. (Courtesy N. Agarwal, MD.) **(24-50B)** Axial T1 C+ SPGR image shows that the lesions enhance strongly, uniformly →. Note pial enhancement along the pons ⇨ and cerebellum ⇨. (Courtesy N. Agarwal, MD.)*

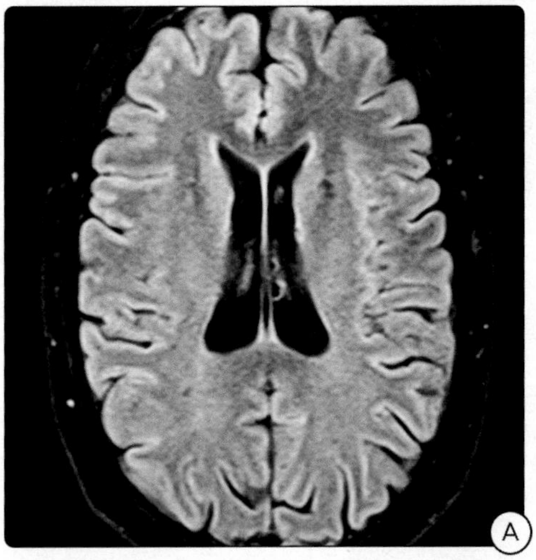

(24-51A) *FLAIR in a 26y man with ALL, HA, and altered mental status appears normal.*

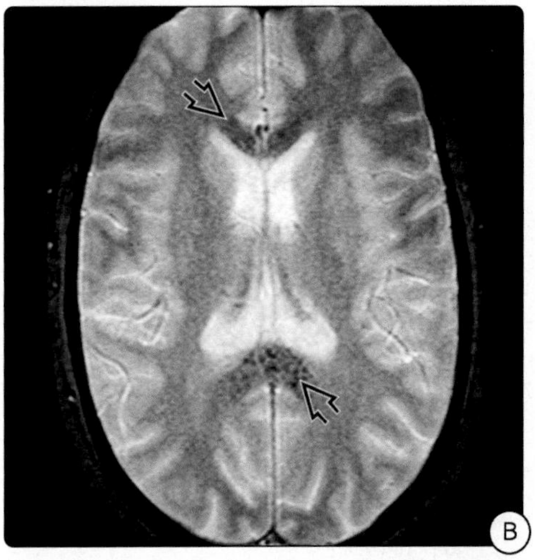

(24-51B) *T2* GRE in the same case shows punctate hypointensities in the corpus callosum ⇨.*

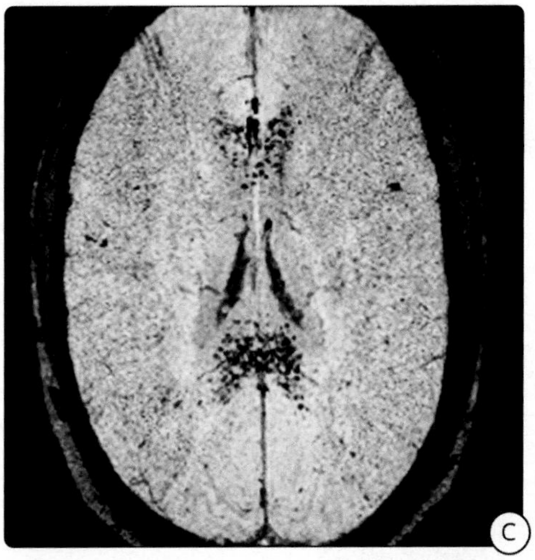

(24-51C) *T2* SWI shows innumerable blooming foci throughout the brain. These are leukemia-associated microbleeds.*

Parenchymal lesions ("chloroma") are much less common than meningeal disease. Chloromas are hypo- to isointense on T1WI and heterogeneously iso- to hypointense on T2/FLAIR **(24-48)** **(24-50)**. FLAIR is helpful in detecting pial, perivascular, and CSF spread. Hemorrhage is common and easily detected on T2* (GRE, SWI) imaging **(24-51)**.

Enhancement of parenchymal **(24-49)** and focal dural chloromas **(24-47C)** is typically strong and relatively homogeneous. Fat-saturated postcontrast T1 scans are especially helpful in detecting osseous involvement and delineating its extent. Because of its cellularity, granulocytic sarcoma often demonstrates diffusion restriction.

Nuclear Medicine Findings. Tc-99m MDP is commonly used to detect bone disease. Whole-body FDG PET or fused PET/CT shows avid uptake and is useful for initial staging as well as assessing treatment response.

Differential Diagnosis

Differential diagnosis depends on location. Dura-based granulocytic sarcomas may resemble **extraaxial hematoma, lymphoma,** or **meningioma**.

In younger children, **metastatic neuroblastoma** and **Langerhans cell histiocytosis** can mimic granulocytic sarcoma. **Extramedullary hematopoiesis** is a diagnostic consideration but is typically more hypointense than granulocytic sarcoma on T2WI.

Parenchymal granulocytic sarcomas or "chloromas" are much less common than dura-based lesions. The major differential diagnosis of granulocytic sarcoma is **lymphoma** or (in older patients) **metastasis**.

CNS LEUKEMIA

Terminology and Etiology

- Leukemia = most common childhood cancer
  - Acute lymphoblastic leukemia (ALL) (80%)
  - Acute myeloid leukemia (AML) (20%)
  - Chronic leukemias generally in adults
- CNS leukemias are extramedullary leukemias

Pathology and Clinical Issues

- CNS leukemia disease spectrum
  - Meningeal disease
  - Diffuse parenchymal disease (rare)
  - Granulocytic sarcoma (focal leukemic mass)
- Location
  - Extraaxial, dura-based > parenchymal
  - Typically by malignant deposits in skull, orbit, sinuses
  - Multiple lesions, multiple compartments typical
- Presentation varies; asymptomatic, positive CSF (5-7%)
  - CNS involvement in 3-10% of patients with AML

Imaging

- NECT
  - Permeative destructive bone lesions
  - Hyperdense dural masses (parenchymal disease rare)
- MR
  - Hypo-/isointense to brain on T1
  - Heterogeneously iso-/hyperintense on T2
  - ± Hemorrhage on T2* (GRE, SWI)
  - Enhances strongly
  - DWI often positive
- Whole-body FDG PET, PET/CT
  - Useful for staging, assessing treatment response

Plasma Cell Tumors

Plasma cell myeloma and related immunosecretory disorders are a group of B-cell clonal proliferations characterized by production of monoclonal immunoglobulin from immortalized plasma cells.

Three major forms of neoplastic plasma cell proliferations are recognized: (1) solitary bone plasmacytoma (SBP), (2) solitary extramedullary plasmacytoma (EMP), and (3) multiple myeloma (MM).

SBPs are sometimes simply called plasmacytoma or solitary plasmacytoma (SP). SPs are characterized by a mass of neoplastic monoclonal plasma cells in either bone or soft tissue without evidence of systemic disease. SPs are rare (5-10% of all plasma cell neoplasms) and are most commonly found in the vertebrae and skull.

EMP is usually seen in the head and neck, typically in the nasal cavity or nasopharynx.

Multifocal disease is **MM (24-52)**. **Plasmablastic lymphoma** is an uncommon, aggressive lymphoma that most frequently arises in the oral cavity of HIV-infected patients. Rarely, **atypical monoclonal plasma cell hyperplasia** occurs as an intracranial inflammatory pseudotumor (discussed in Chapter 28).

Etiology

Although the etiology of plasma cell tumors remains unknown, there is good evidence for a multistep transformation process that corresponds to clinically discernible disease stages.

Monoclonal gammopathy is a common asymptomatic precursor lesion that carries a 1% annual risk for progression to frank plasma cell neoplasms. Terminal stages in plasma cell neoplasms are characterized by increasing genetic complexity and independence from bone marrow stromal cells.

Pathology

Location. SBPs almost always occur in red marrow, most frequently in the spine. The skull is the next most common location in the head and neck.

EMPs in the presence of MM are uncommon (4-5% of cases) and rarely involve the CNS. Myelomatous involvement of the CNS is rare, with less than 1% of patients having identifiable CNS involvement (presence of atypical plasma cells in CSF and/or identification of meningeal or intraparenchymal disease on MR).

Gross and Microscopic Features. Gelatinous red-brown tissue replaces normal-appearing yellow marrow. Trabecular bone loss is usually apparent. Microscopic examination discloses monotonous sheets of uniform well-differentiated neoplastic plasma cells with eccentric nuclei and basophilic cytoplasm. At least 10% of the cells in a bone marrow biopsy specimen must be plasma cells for definitive diagnosis of MM.

Approximately 60% of MMs produce IgG, 20-25% produce IgA, and 15-20% produce free immunoglobulin light chains.

Staging, Grading, and Classification. The two most commonly used myeloma staging systems are the Durie-Salmon PLUS classification and the International Staging System (ISS). Durie-Salmon PLUS integrates clinical, laboratory, and histopathologic parameters with imaging features.

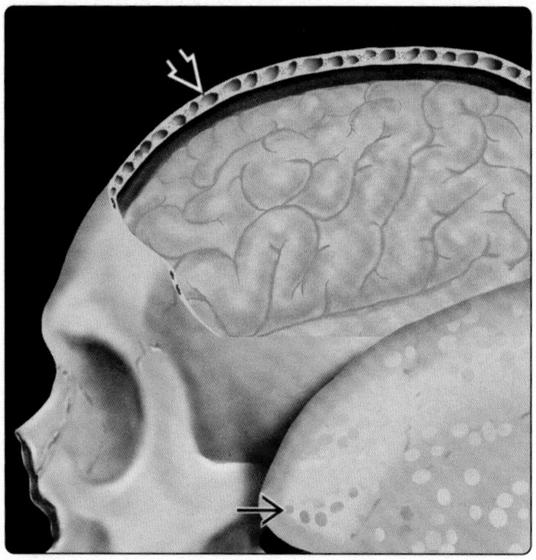

***(24-52)** Graphic shows multiple lytic foci characteristic of MM. Sagittal section shows the "punched-out" lesions in the diploic space.*

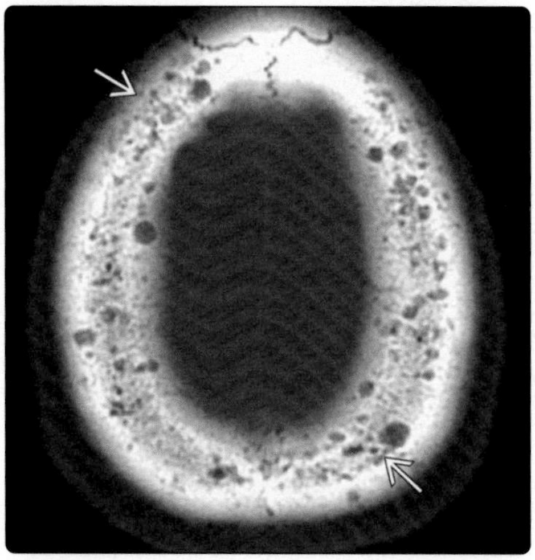

***(24-53)** Bone CT shows MM. Innumerable lytic "punched-out" lesions give the calvaria the characteristic "salt and pepper" appearance.*

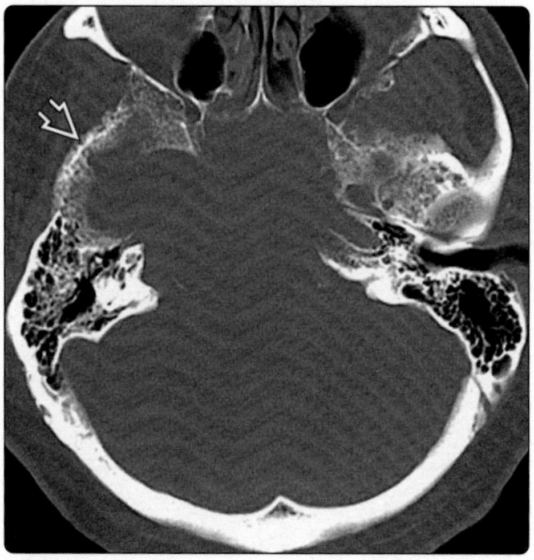

***(24-54)** NECT shows plasmacytoma with destruction of central BOS. Note "salt and pepper" look of the squamous temporal bone.*

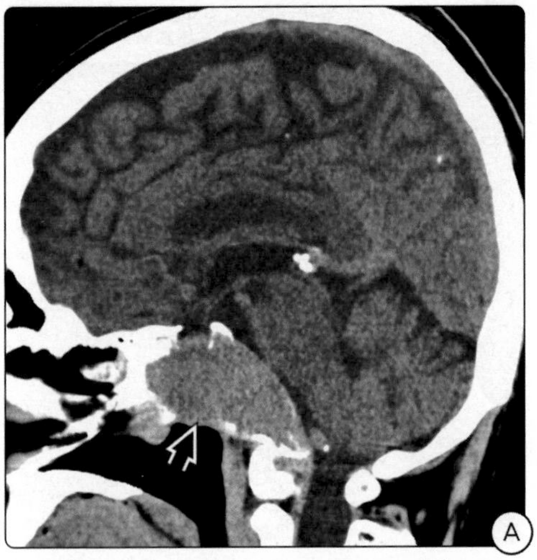

(24-55A) Sagittal NECT in a 67y man with multiple cranial neuropathies shows hyperdense, destructive central skull base mass ➔.

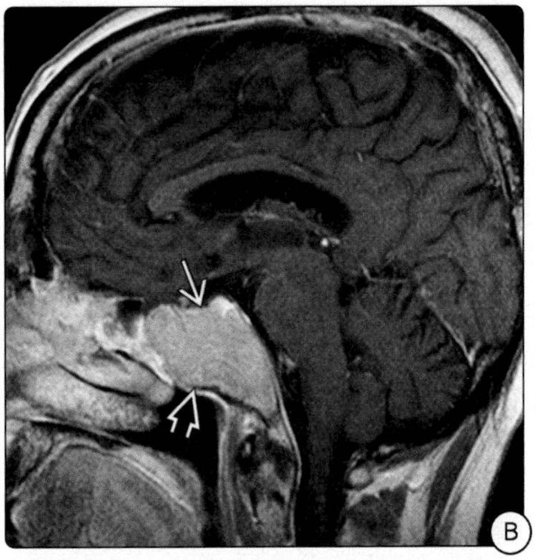

(24-55B) Sagittal T1 C+ MR shows the mass ➔ enhances intensely and uniformly. Note engulfment, infiltration of the pituitary gland ➔.

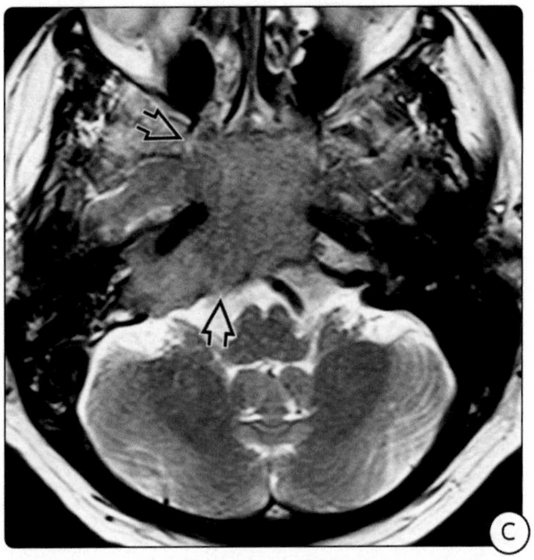

(24-55C) Axial T2WI shows the extent of the destructive mass ➔, which is mildly hypointense relative to GM. This is plasmacytoma.

Clinical Issues

Epidemiology. MM is the most common primary bone malignancy, accounting for approximately 10% of all hematologic malignancies. Almost half of all SBPs eventually progress to MM.

Intracranial MM is uncommon and is usually secondary, occurring mostly as extension into the dura and leptomeninges from osseous lesions in the calvaria, skull base, nose, or paranasal sinuses.

Primary CNS plasmacytoma is very rare. Waldenström macroglobulinemia (a.k.a. Bing-Neel syndrome) may form dural lesions that then invade the brain parenchyma.

Demographics. Prevalence varies with the type of plasma cell proliferation but generally rises with advancing age. Median age of patients with SBP or EMP is 55 years. The vast majority of patients with MM are older than 40 years with peak age at presentation in the seventh decade. There is a slight female predominance for SBP and a moderate male predominance in EMP and MM.

Presentation. The most common presentation is bone pain. Constitutional symptoms such as fever of unknown origin are common with MM. Cranial nerve involvement is rare but may develop secondary to skull base plasmacytoma.

Immunoelectrophoresis detects M protein in the serum and/or urine from 99% of patients.

Natural History. Many plasma cell tumors eventually transform into MM. The 5-year survival rate of MM is 20%. With newer treatment regimens, median survival has increased from 2 or 3 years to 4 years. Death is usually secondary to renal insufficiency, infection, and thromboembolic events.

Treatment Options. Treatment depends on disease stage. Evaluation of clinical, morphological, immunophenotypical, and cytogenetic features is necessary for individual risk assessment and appropriate therapy.

PLASMA CELL TUMORS: PATHOLOGY

Pathology
- Solitary bone plasmacytoma (SBP)
- Multifocal disease = multiple myeloma (MM)
- Red marrow sites (spine > skull)

Durie-Salmon PLUS Staging (MM)
- Monoclonal gammopathy
  - < 10% plasma cells in bone marrow
  - Normal marrow on MR, PET/CT
- Smoldering MM
  - ≥ 10% plasma cells in bone marrow
  - Limited marrow disease on MR, PET/CT
- MM
  - ≥ 10% plasma cells and/or plasmacytoma + end-organ damage
  - Focal or diffuse lesions on MR
  - ↑ FDG marrow uptake (multifocal or diffuse)

Imaging

Although radiography can only detect trabecular bone loss of more than 30-50%, skeletal surveys are still widely used for staging and surveillance of plasma cell tumors. CT is the best procedure for delineating lytic lesions in the skull base or calvaria.

MR is best used to evaluate the presence of diffuse marrow infiltration and define the extent of soft tissue disease. Whole-body MR is helpful in detecting systemic disease that would indicate the diagnosis of MM instead of solitary plasmacytoma.

CT Findings. SBPs are intramedullary soft tissue masses that produce lytic lesions centered in bone marrow. NECT shows a "punched-out" lesion without sclerotic margins or identifiable internal matrix. Cortical breakthrough with formation of a soft tissue mass adjacent to the lytic lesion may be present.

MM shows numerous lytic lesions **(24-53)**, usually centered in the spine, skull base, calvarial vault, or facial bones **(24-54)** **(24-55A)**. A variegated "salt and pepper" pattern is typical.

Diffuse osteopenia without focal lesions is seen in 10% of MM cases.

MR Findings. In staging MM, the extent of bone marrow involvement is assessed on T1WI. Whole-body MR has emerged as the most sensitive imaging modality for detecting diffuse and focal bony lesions.

Osseous lesions replace normal hyperintense fatty marrow and are typically hypointense on T1WI. T2 and fat-saturated sequences such as T2-weighted STIR imaging also highlight the extent of marrow infiltration **(24-55C)**. Focal and diffuse lesions appear hyperintense. Both SBPs and MM enhance strongly following contrast administration **(24-55B)**. Leptomeningeal and parenchymal disease occurs but is uncommon **(24-56)**.

Nuclear Medicine. Bone scintigraphy is not useful in evaluating MM, as lesions are often "cold" on Tc-99m scans. PET/CT is especially helpful for identifying and localizing extramedullary lesions. Sensitivity is 96% with a specificity of almost 80%.

Differential Diagnosis

Multiple "punched-out" destructive myeloma lesions can appear virtually identical to lytic **metastases**. Spine and skull base MM can resemble **leukemia** or non-Hodgkin **lymphoma. Invasive pituitary macroadenoma** may be difficult to distinguish from MM, as both are isointense with gray matter. An elevated prolactin is often present with macroadenoma, and the pituitary gland cannot be separated from the mass.

PLASMA CELL TUMORS: CLINICAL ISSUES, IMAGING, AND DDx

Clinical Issues
- Monoclonal gammopathy is common precursor lesion
- 1% annual risk of developing plasma cell neoplasm
- Generally older adults
- Approximately 50% of SBPs progress to MM
- MM 5-year survival = 20%

Imaging
- NECT
  - Solitary or multiple "punched-out" lytic lesion(s)
  - ± Soft tissue mass
- MR
  - Lesions replace normal fatty marrow
  - Hypointense on T1-, T2WI
  - Enhance on T1 C+ FS

Differential Diagnosis
- Lytic metastases (extracranial primary)
- Leukemia, lymphoma
- Invasive pituitary macroadenoma (central skull base)

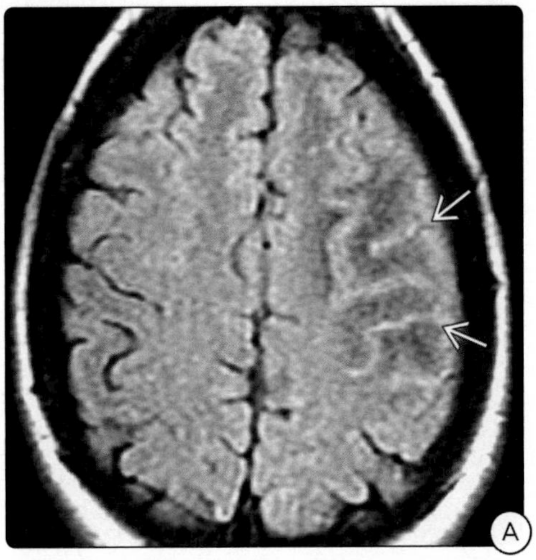

(24-56A) FLAIR in a patient with Waldenström macroglobulinemia shows hyperintense sulci, edema in the left hemisphere ➡.

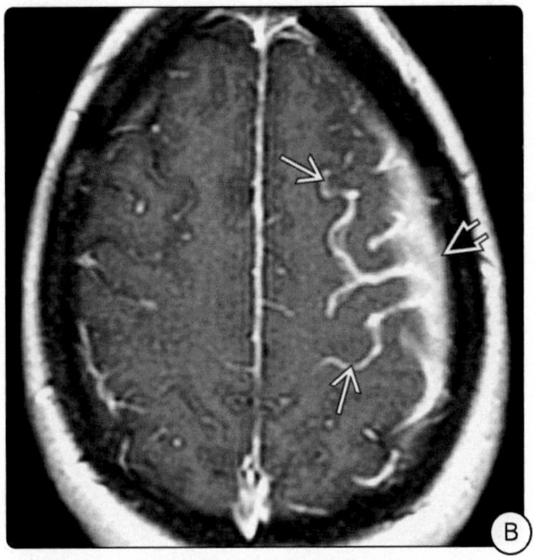

(24-56B) T1 C+ scan shows an enhancing dura-arachnoid mass ➡ with enhancement of the underlying sulci ➡.

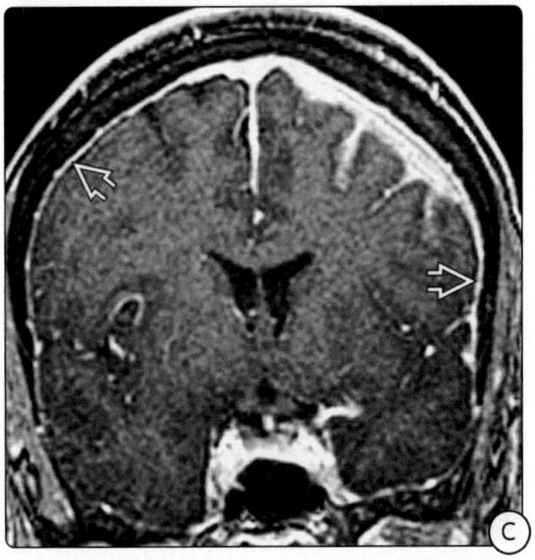

(24-56C) T1 C+ FS shows diffuse dura-arachnoid thickening ➡ and lymphoplasmacytic infiltrate in meninges. (Courtesy P. Hildenbrand, MD.)

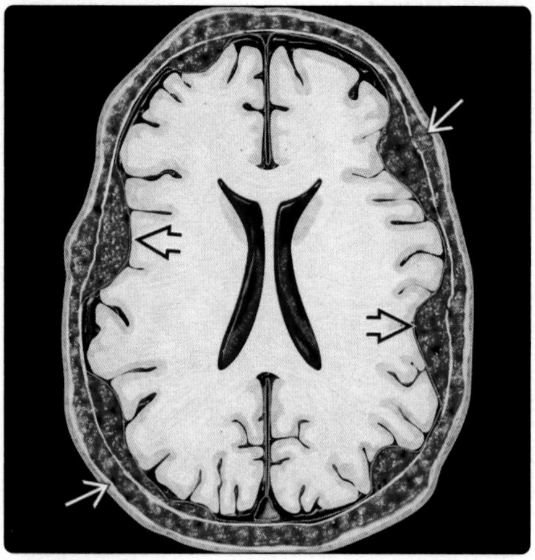

(24-57) Graphic shows extramedullary hematopoiesis, hematopoietic calvarial marrow ➡, and lobulated extraaxial masses ⇨.

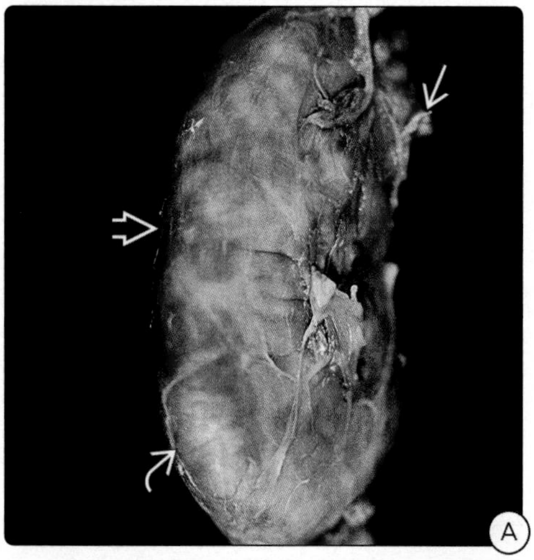

(24-58A) EMH shows smooth dura-based mass ⇨ with small dural "tails" ➡. Bluish discolorations ➡ are from blood-forming elements.

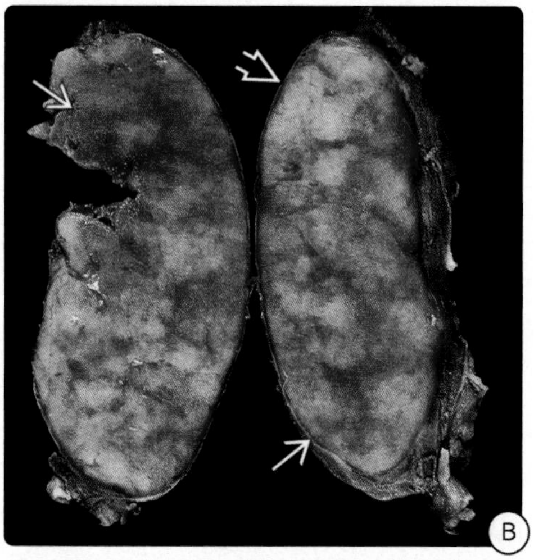

(24-58B) Sectioned nodule hematopoietic tissue is seen as red marrow ➡, scattered between fatty foci ➡. (Courtesy R. Hewlett, MD.)

Extramedullary Hematopoiesis

Extramedullary hematopoiesis (EMH) is the compensatory formation of blood elements due to decreased medullary hematopoiesis. Various anemias (thalassemia, sickle cell disease, hereditary spherocytosis, etc.) are the most common etiologies, accounting for 45% of cases. Myelofibrosis/myelodysplastic syndromes (35%) are the next most common underlying causes associated with EMH.

Multiple smooth, juxtaosseous, circumscribed, hypercellular masses are typical **(24-57)** **(24-58)**. The most common site is along the axial skeleton. The face and skull are the most common head and neck sites. The subdural space is the most common intracranial location.

EMH is hyperdense on NECT **(24-59A)**, enhances strongly and homogeneously on CECT, and may show findings of underlying disease on bone CT (e.g., "hair on end" pattern in thalassemia, dense bone obliterating the diploic space in osteopetrosis).

Round or lobulated subdural masses that are iso- to slightly hyperintense relative to gray matter on T1WI and hypointense on T2WI are typical **(24-59B)**. EMH enhances strongly and uniformly on postcontrast T1WI **(24-59C)**.

The major differential diagnoses of intracranial EMH are **dural metastases** and **meningioma**. **Neurosarcoid** and **lymphoma** are other considerations.

EXTRAMEDULLARY HEMATOPOIESIS

Etiology
- Decreased medullary hematopoiesis
- Compensatory formation of blood elements
- Anemias (45%), myelofibrosis/myelodysplasia (35%)

Pathology
- Multiple smooth juxtaosseous masses
- Spine, face, skull, dura

Imaging
- Hyperdense on NECT
- T1 iso-/hypo-, T2 hypointense
- Enhances strongly

Differential Diagnosis
- Dural metastases
- Meningioma
- Neurosarcoid
- Lymphoma

Selected References

Lymphomas and Related Disorders

Brandão LA et al: Lymphomas-Part 1. Neuroimaging Clin N Am. 26(4):511-536, 2016

Brandão LA et al: Lymphomas-Part 2. Neuroimaging Clin N Am. 26(4):537-565, 2016

Deckert M et al: Lymphomas. In: Louis DN et al (eds), WHO Classification of Tumours of the Central Nervous System. Lyon, France: International Agency for Research on Cancer, 2016, pp 272-277

Diffuse Large B-Cell Lymphoma of the CNS

Citterio G et al: Primary central nervous system lymphoma. Crit Rev Oncol Hematol. 113:97-110, 2017

Lin X et al: Diagnostic accuracy of T1-weighted dynamic contrast-enhanced-MRI and DWI-ADC for differentiation of glioblastoma and primary CNS lymphoma. AJNR Am J Neuroradiol. 38(3):485-491, 2017

Paydas S: Primary central nervous system lymphoma: essential points in diagnosis and management. Med Oncol. 34(4):61, 2017

Koeller KK et al: Extranodal lymphoma of the central nervous system and spine. Radiol Clin North Am. 54(4):649-71, 2016

Todorovic Balint M et al: Gene mutation profiles in primary diffuse large B cell lymphoma of central nervous system: next generation sequencing analyses. Int J Mol Sci. 17(5), 2016

AIDS-Related Diffuse Large B-Cell Lymphoma

Brunnberg U et al: HIV-associated malignant lymphoma. Oncol Res Treat. 40(3):82-87, 2017

Carbone A et al: Epstein-Barr virus associated lymphomas in people with HIV. Curr Opin HIV AIDS. 12(1):39-46, 2017

Karia SJ et al: AIDS-related primary CNS lymphoma. Lancet. 389(10085):2238, 2017

Brandão LA et al: Lymphomas-Part 2. Neuroimaging Clin N Am. 26(4):537-565, 2016

Lymphomatoid Granulomatosis

Koeller KK et al: Extranodal lymphoma of the central nervous system and spine. Radiol Clin North Am. 54(4):649-71, 2016

Low LK et al: B-cell lymphoproliferative disorders associated with primary and acquired immunodeficiency. Surg Pathol Clin. 9(1):55-77, 2016

Posttransplant Lymphoproliferative Disorder

Barrantes-Freer A et al: Diagnostic red flags: steroid-treated malignant CNS lymphoma mimicking autoimmune inflammatory demyelination. Brain Pathol. ePub, 2017

Morris J et al: A rare presentation of isolated CNS posttransplantation lymphoproliferative disorder. Case Rep Oncol Med. 2017:7269147, 2017

Degen D et al: Primary central nervous system posttransplant lymphoproliferative disease: an uncommon diagnostic dilemma. Nephrology (Carlton). 21(6):528, 2016

Intravascular (Angiocentric) Lymphoma

Sharma TL et al: Intravascular T-cell lymphoma: a rare, poorly characterized entity with cytotoxic phenotype. Neuropathology. ePub, 2017

Fonkem E et al: Neurological presentations of intravascular lymphoma (IVL): meta-analysis of 654 patients. BMC Neurol. 16:9, 2016

Miscellaneous Rare CNS Lymphomas

Termuhlen AM: Natural killer/T-cell lymphomas in pediatric and adolescent patients. Clin Adv Hematol Oncol. 15(3):200-209, 2017

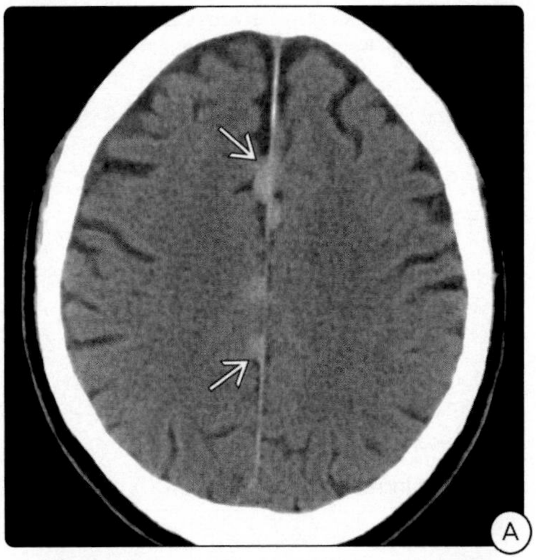

***(24-59A)** NECT of EMH shows several hyperdense nodules ➡ along the falx cerebri.*

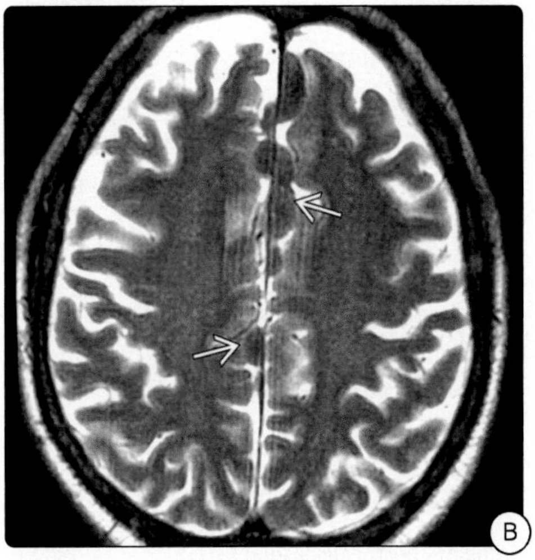

***(24-59B)** The lobulated lesions are very hypointense on T2WI ➡.*

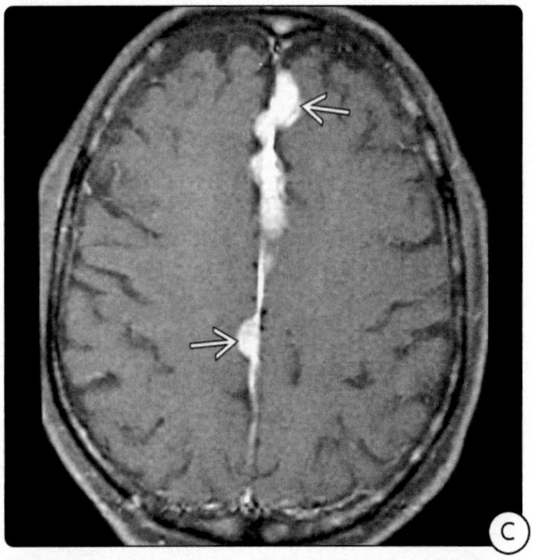

***(24-59C)** EMH enhances strongly, uniformly ➡ as shown on this T1 C+ FS scan in the same patient.*

Gurion R et al: Central nervous system involvement in T-cell lymphoma: A single center experience. Acta Oncol. 55(5):561-6, 2016

Menon MP et al: Primary CNS T-cell lymphomas: a clinical, morphologic, immunophenotypic, and molecular analysis. Am J Surg Pathol. 39(12):1719-29, 2015

MALT Lymphoma of the Dura

de la Fuente MI et al: Marginal zone dural lymphoma: the Memorial Sloan Kettering Cancer Center and University of Miami experiences. Leuk Lymphoma. 58(4):882-888, 2017

Douleh DG et al: Intracranial marginal zone B-cell lymphoma mimicking meningioma. World Neurosurg. 91:676.e9-676.e12, 2016

Metastatic Intracranial Lymphoma

Herr MM et al: Survival of secondary central nervous system lymphoma patients in the rituximab era. Clin Lymphoma Myeloma Leuk. 16(9):e123-e127, 2016

Korfel A et al: How to facilitate early diagnosis of CNS involvement in malignant lymphoma. Expert Rev Hematol. 1-11, 2016

Histiocytic Tumors

Haroche J et al: Histiocytoses: emerging neoplasia behind inflammation. Lancet Oncol. 18(2):e113-e125, 2017

Paulus W et al: Histiocytic tumors. In: Louis DN et al (eds), WHO Classification of Tumours of the Central Nervous System. Lyon, France: International Agency for Research on Cancer, 2016, pp 280-283

Ranganathan S: Histiocytic proliferations. Semin Diagn Pathol. 33(6):396-409, 2016

Langerhans Cell Histiocytosis

Porto L et al: Central nervous system imaging in childhood Langerhans cell histiocytosis - a reference center analysis. Radiol Oncol. 49(3):242-9, 2015

Erdheim-Chester Disease

Estrada-Veras JI et al: The clinical spectrum of Erdheim-Chester disease: an observational cohort study. Blood Adv. 1(6):357-366, 2017

Martineau P et al: The imaging findings of Erdheim-Chester disease: a multimodality approach to diagnosis and staging. World J Nucl Med. 16(1):71-74, 2017

Rosai-Dorfman Disease

Joshi SS et al: Cranio-spinal Rosai Dorfman disease: case series and literature review. Br J Neurosurg. 1-8, 2017

Luo Z et al: Characteristics of Rosai-Dorfman disease primarily involved in the central nervous system: 3 case reports and review of literature. World Neurosurg. 97:58-63, 2017

Juvenile Xanthogranuloma

Meshkini A et al: Systemic juvenile xanthogranuloma with multiple central nervous system lesions. J Cancer Res Ther. 8(2):311-3, 2012

Histiocytic Sarcoma

Jiang M et al: Lymphoma classification update: T-cell lymphomas, Hodgkin lymphomas, and histiocytic/dendritic cell neoplasms. Expert Rev Hematol. 10(3):239-249, 2017

Zanelli M et al: Primary histiocytic sarcoma presenting as diffuse leptomeningeal disease: case description and review of the literature. Neuropathology. ePub, 2017

Hemophagocytic Lymphohistiocytosis

Cai G et al: Central nervous system involvement in adults with haemophagocytic lymphohistiocytosis: a single-center study. Ann Hematol. 96(8):1279-1285, 2017

Hematopoietic Tumors and Tumor-Like Lesions

Keraliya AR et al: Imaging of nervous system involvement in hematologic malignancies: what radiologists need to know. AJR Am J Roentgenol. 205(3):604-17, 2015

Leukemia

Frishman-Levy L et al: Advances in understanding the pathogenesis of CNS acute lymphoblastic leukaemia and potential for therapy. Br J Haematol. 176(2):157-167, 2017

Murthy H et al: Diagnosis and management of leukemic and lymphomatous meningitis. Cancer Control. 24(1):33-41, 2017

Ranta S et al: Role of neuroimaging in children with acute lymphoblastic leukemia and central nervous system involvement at diagnosis. Pediatr Blood Cancer. 64(1):64-70, 2017

Arber DA et al: The 2016 revision to the World Health Organization (WHO) classification of myeloid neoplasms and acute leukemia. Blood. 127(20):2391-405, 2016

Guenette JP et al: MRI findings in patients with leukemia and positive CSF cytology: a single-institution 5-year experience. AJR Am J Roentgenol. 1-5, 2016

Plasma Cell Tumors

Paludo J et al: Myelomatous involvement of the central nervous system. Clin Lymphoma Myeloma Leuk. 16(11):644-654, 2016

Wilberger AC et al: Intracranial involvement by plasma cell neoplasms. Am J Clin Pathol. 146(2):156-62, 2016

Extramedullary Hematopoiesis

van der Bruggen W et al: PET in benign bone marrow disorders. Semin Nucl Med. 47(4):397-407, 2017

Roberts AS et al: Extramedullary haematopoiesis: radiological imaging features. Clin Radiol. 71(9):807-14, 2016

Sellar Neoplasms and Tumor-Like Lesions

The sellar region is one of the most anatomically complex areas in the brain. It encompasses the bony sella turcica and pituitary gland plus all the normal structures that surround it. Virtually any of these can give rise to pathology that ranges from incidental and innocuous to serious, potentially life-threatening disease.

At least 30 different lesions occur in or around the pituitary gland, arising from either the pituitary gland itself or the structures that surround it. These include the cavernous sinus and its contents, arteries (the circle of Willis), cranial nerves, meninges, CSF spaces (the suprasellar cistern and third ventricle), central skull base, and brain parenchyma (the hypothalamus).

Despite the overwhelming variety of lesions that can occur in this region, at least 75-80% of all sellar/juxtasellar masses are due to one of the "Big Five": macroadenoma, meningioma, aneurysm, craniopharyngioma, and astrocytoma. All other lesions combined account for less than one-quarter of sellar region masses. Entities such as germinoma, Rathke cleft cyst, and hypophysitis each cause 1-2% or less.

Some authors recommend using a mnemonic (such as SATCHMO for **s**arcoid, **a**neurysm or **a**denoma, **t**eratoma or **t**uberculosis, **c**raniopharyngioma or **c**yst, **h**ypophysitis or **h**amartoma or **h**istiocytosis, **m**eningioma or **m**etastasis, and **o**ptic glioma) to remember the spectrum of lesions that can occur in/around the sella. However, this list mixes rare with common lesions and is unhelpful in establishing a clinically tailored, radiologically appropriate differential diagnosis.

The previous chapters in this section focus on specific neoplasms as defined histopathologically. This chapter is different. Its focus is geography and location. The goal of this discussion is to present the anatomy of the sellar region and then discuss the various lesions that make their home in this anatomically varied "neighborhood."

We begin the chapter with a general overview that includes keys to diagnosis, clinical considerations, and helpful findings on imaging studies. We then consider the normal gross and imaging anatomy of the sellar region.

Next we discuss normal variants such as physiologic hypertrophy that can mimic pituitary pathology. Congenital lesions (such as tuber cinereum hamartoma) that can be mistaken for more ominous pathology are also delineated. Pituitary gland and infundibular stalk neoplasms are then discussed. A brief consideration of miscellaneous lesions such as lymphocytic hypophysitis, pituitary apoplexy, and the postoperative sella follows.

The goal of imaging is to determine precisely the location and characteristics of a sellar mass, delineate its relationship to—and involvement

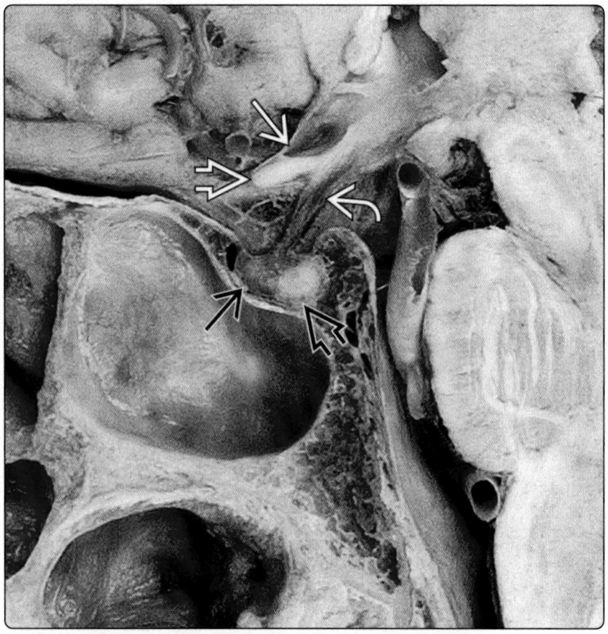

(25-1) Midline anatomic section depicts sella and surrounding structures. Adenohypophysis ➡, neurohypophysis ➡ are shown, along with the optic chiasm ➡ and optic ➡ and infundibular ➡ recesses of the third ventricle. (Courtesy M. Nielsen, MS.)

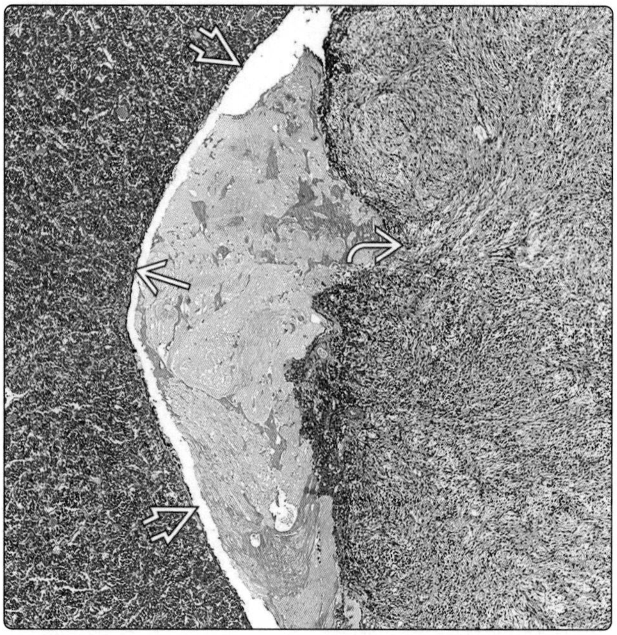

(25-2) Photomicrograph of a sectioned normal pituitary gland shows Rathke pouch remnant as a "cleft" ➡ between the anterior ➡ and posterior ➡ lobes of the pituitary gland. (Courtesy A. Ersen, MD, B. Scheithauer, MD.)

with—surrounding structures, and construct a reasonable, limited differential diagnosis to help direct patient management. We then conclude the chapter with a summary of—and approach to—a differential diagnosis of sellar masses.

When you finish this discussion, you should be able to look at an unknown sellar mass and offer a focused differential diagnosis, not simply a recital of all the possible lesions that can be found in this anatomically complex region!

Diagnostic Considerations

Anatomic sublocation is the single most important key to establishing an appropriate differential diagnosis of a sellar region mass. The first step is assigning a lesion to one of three anatomic compartments, identifying it as an (1) intrasellar, (2) suprasellar, or (3) infundibular stalk lesion.

The key to determining anatomic sublocation accurately is the question, "Can I find the pituitary gland separate from the mass?" If you can't, and the gland *is* the mass, the most likely diagnosis is macroadenoma.

If the mass is clearly *separate* from the pituitary gland, it is extrapituitary and therefore not a macroadenoma. Other pathologies such as meningioma in an adult or craniopharyngioma should be considered in such cases.

Clinical Considerations

The single most important clinical feature in establishing an appropriate differential diagnosis for a sellar region mass is **patient age**. Lesions that are common in adults (macroadenoma, meningioma, and aneurysm) are generally rare in children. A lesion in a prepubescent child—especially a boy—that looks like a macroadenoma is almost never a neoplasm. Nonneoplastic pituitary gland enlargement in children is much more common than tumors. Therefore, an enlarged pituitary gland in a child is almost always either normal physiologic hypertrophy or nonphysiologic nonneoplastic hyperplasia secondary to end-organ failure (most commonly hypothyroidism).

Some lesions that are common in children (e.g., opticochiasmatic/hypothalamic pilocytic astrocytoma and craniopharyngioma) are relatively uncommon in adults.

Sex is also important. Imaging studies of young menstruating female patients and postpartum women often demonstrate plump-appearing pituitary glands due to temporary physiologic hyperplasia.

Imaging Considerations

Imaging appearance is very helpful in evaluating a lesion of the sellar region. After establishing the anatomic sublocation of a lesion, look for imaging clues. Are other lesions present? Is the lesion calcified? Does it appear cystic? Does it contain blood products? Is it focal or infiltrating? Does it enhance? Does it enlarge or invade the sella turcica?

Sellar Region Anatomy

We briefly review the normal gross and imaging anatomy of the sellar region. Understanding normal anatomy forms the foundation for our subsequent consideration of sellar neoplasms and tumor-like lesions, the major topics of this chapter.

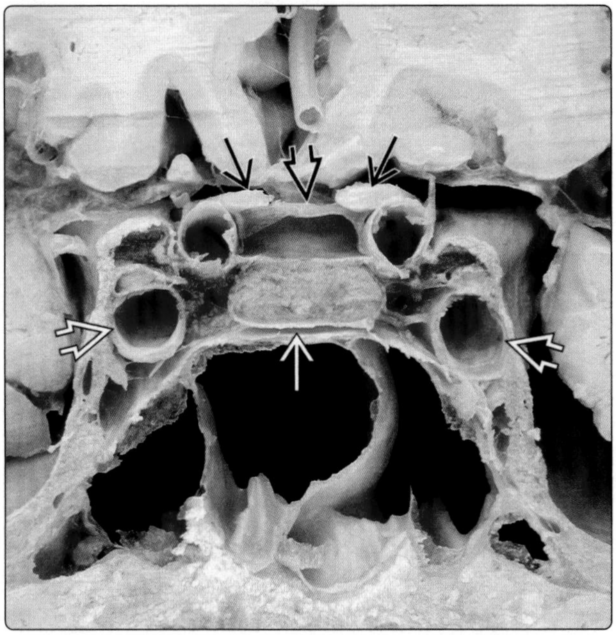

(25-3) Coronal gross section shows important structures adjacent to the pituitary gland. Cavernous, supraclinoid internal carotid arteries (ICAs) are shown, as are the diaphragma sellae and optic nerves. (Courtesy M. Nielsen, MS.)

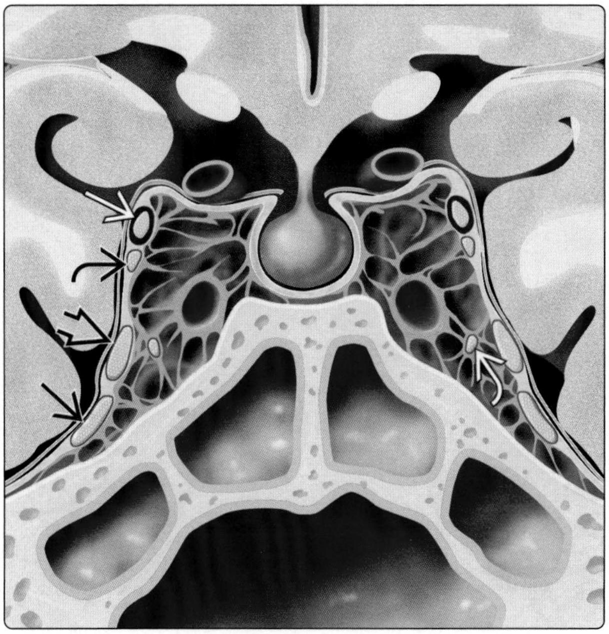

(25-4) Cranial nerves in the lateral dural wall of cavernous sinus include CNs III, IV, V_1, and V_2. Only CN VI is inside the cavernous sinus itself.

Gross Anatomy

Bony Anatomy

The **sella turcica** ("Turkish saddle") is a midline concavity in the basisphenoid of the central skull base that contains the pituitary gland. The sella is entirely embedded within the sphenoid bone. The anterior borders of the sella are formed by the tuberculum sellae and anterior clinoid processes of the lesser sphenoid wing, whereas the posterior border is formed by the dorsum sellae. The top of the dorsum sellae expands slightly posteriorly and laterally to form the posterior clinoid processes, which in turn form the upper margin of the clivus **(25-1)**.

The sellar floor is part of the sphenoid sinus roof, which is partially or completely aerated. The cavernous segments of the internal carotid arteries lie in shallow bony grooves (the **carotid sulci**) located inferolateral to the pituitary fossa **(25-3)**.

Meninges

The meninges in and around the sella form important anatomic landmarks. **Dura** covers the bony floor of the sella, separating it from the pituitary gland. A thin dural reflection borders the pituitary fossa laterally and forms the medial cavernous sinus wall.

A small circular dural shelf, the **diaphragma sellae** **(25-3)**, forms a roof over the sella that almost covers the pituitary gland. The diaphragma sellae has a variably sized central opening, the **diaphragmatic hiatus**, that transmits the pituitary stalk **(25-5)**. The mean diameter of the diaphragmatic hiatus is 7 mm.

A prominent basal **arachnoid** membrane, called the Liliequist membrane, forms trabeculae that cross the suprasellar cistern and cover the hypothalamus and diaphragma sellae. A sleeve of arachnoid reflects over the pituitary stalk, forming a thin hypophyseal cistern that can provide a surgical dissection plane in approaching suprasellar masses.

Pituitary Gland

The pituitary gland, also called the hypophysis, is a reddish-gray, bean-shaped gland with two distinct parts (sometimes called "lobes"): the anterior pituitary, also called the **adenohypophysis** (AH), and the posterior pituitary or **neurohypophysis** (NH) **(25-40)**.

The anterior and posterior pituitary lobes differ in embryologic origin, structure, and function but are joined together into a single gland, the hypophysis.

Anterior Pituitary Gland (Adenohypophysis). The AH, formerly called the anterior lobe, accounts for 75-80% of the total pituitary gland volume. The AH wraps anterolaterally around the NH in a U-shaped configuration. The AH is subdivided into three parts: the pars distalis (pars anterior), pars intermedia, and pars tuberalis.

The AH develops as an outgrowth—called **Rathke pouch**—of embryonic ectoderm that lines the roof of the buccal cavity **(25-2)**. This outgrowth subsequently detaches from the buccal cavity, and its anterior wall thickens to become the largest part of the AH called the **pars distalis**. The posterior wall differentiates into the **pars intermedia**, whereas the dorsolateral portions extend around the infundibulum as the **pars tuberalis**.

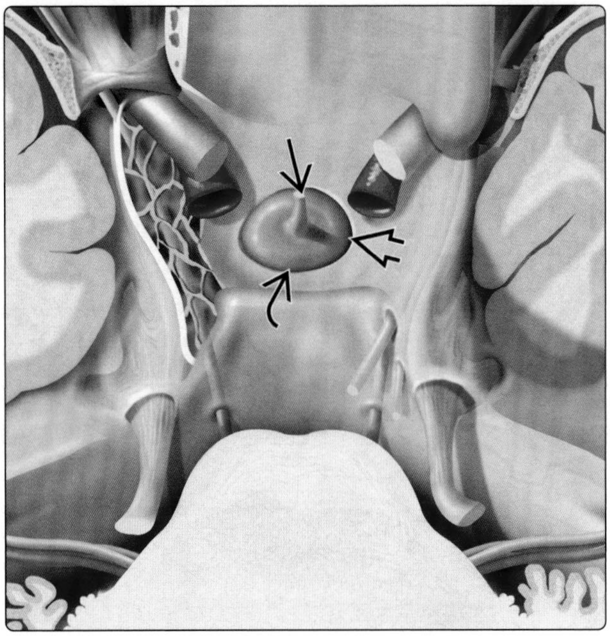

***(25-5)** Axial graphic depicts the pituitary gland ➡ and stalk ➡ from above seen through the opening of the diaphragma sellae ➡.*

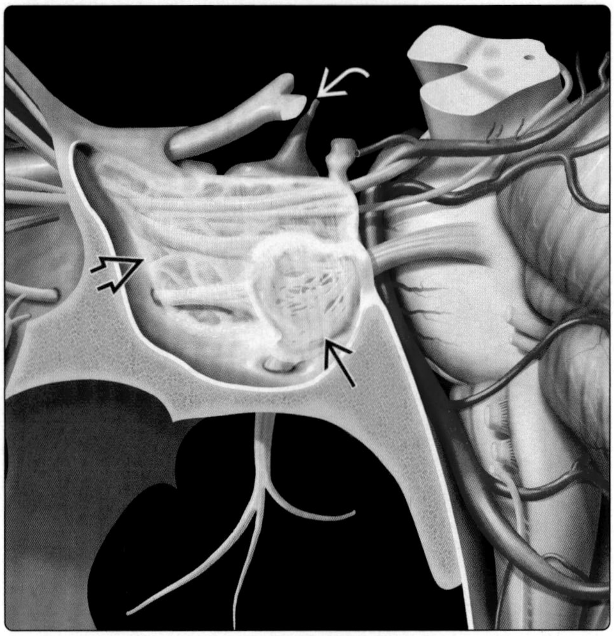

***(25-6)** Sagittal graphic depicts cranial nerves of the cavernous sinus ➡ lateral to the pituitary gland and stalk ➡. Meckel cave is filled with CSF and contains fascicles of CN V and the gasserian (semilunar) ganglion ➡.*

All three parts of the AH produce hormones. Most are tropins that regulate the function of other endocrine cells such as secretary cells in the gonads, thyroid, and adrenal cortex. All of the anterior pituitary hormones are regulated by hypothalamic-releasing hormones except prolactin (PRL), which is under the control of a dopaminergic circuit.

Cells in the pars distalis of the AH produce five different hormones: somatotropin (also known as growth hormone or GH), PRL, thyroid-stimulating hormone, follicle-stimulating hormone/luteinizing hormone (FSH/LH), and adrenocorticotrophic hormone (ACTH). In addition, the AH also has a substantial proportion of cells that do not express hormonal markers. These non-hormone-secreting cells are called chromophobes.

The pituitary gland of newborns already presents a full set of terminally differentiated hormone-producing cells. However, the postnatal gland undergoes extensive remodeling. Soon after birth, the AH enters a dramatic growth phase that significantly increases the size of the gland.

The adult pituitary gland can adapt its cellular composition in response to changing physiologic conditions.

Posterior Pituitary Gland (Neurohypophysis). The posterior pituitary or NH develops from the embryonic diencephalon (forebrain) as a downward extension of the hypothalamus. The posterior pituitary is subdivided into a large **pars nervosa** and smaller **infundibulum** (pituitary stalk).

The NH comprises 20-25% of the overall pituitary gland volume. The NH remains attached to the brain via the infundibulum, which inserts into the **median eminence of the hypothalamus**.

Most of the pars nervosa parenchyma consists of axonal terminations of neurons whose cell bodies are located in the hypothalamus. Neurons constitute approximately 75% of the posterior lobe. The remaining 25% of the posterior lobe consists of glial cells called **pituicytes**.

There are no intrinsic hormone-producing cells in the pars nervosa or pituitary stalk. Instead, the pars nervosa secretes two hormones that are formed in the hypothalamus: **antidiuretic hormone** (also called **vasopressin**) and **oxytocin**. Both hormones are synthesized as a larger precursor prohormone that also contains a carrier protein, **neurophysin**. The prohormone is transported down the axons of the hypothalamo-hypophyseal tract in the infundibulum, cleaved to its active form in the NH, and stored as secretory granules in the axon terminals.

Blood Supply

Arteries. Two sets of branches arise from the **internal carotid arteries** (ICAs) to supply the neurohypophysis. Single **inferior hypophyseal arteries** arise from the cavernous ICAs and supply most of the neurohypophysis. Several **superior hypophyseal arteries** arise from the supraclinoid ICAs with smaller contributions from the anterior and posterior cerebral arteries. The superior hypophyseal arteries mostly supply the median eminence of the hypothalamus and infundibular stalk.

There is no direct arterial supply to the AH.

Veins. The **hypophyseal portal system** consists of a primary capillary plexus in the median eminence of the pituitary hypothalamus and infundibulum and a secondary capillary plexus in the pars distalis of the AH. These are connected by long hypophyseal portal veins. Venous blood from both the anterior and posterior pituitary drains into the cavernous sinus.

The portal system forms an essential link between the hypothalamus and endocrine system; it is the route by which hypothalamic releasing and inhibitory hormones reach their target cells in the pars distalis of the AH to control pituitary function. The portal system also carries hypophyseal hormones from the gland to their endocrine targets and facilitates feedback control of secretion.

Hypothalamus and Third Ventricle

The **hypothalamus** lies directly above the pituitary gland, extending posteriorly from the lamina terminalis (anterior wall of the third ventricle) to the mammillary bodies. The **tuber cinereum** is part of the hypothalamus. It is the thin convex mass of gray matter that lies between the optic chiasm anteriorly and the mammillary bodies posteriorly. The infundibular stalk extends inferiorly from the tuber cinereum, gradually tapering as it descends to become continuous with the posterior pituitary lobe.

The **third ventricle** lies in the midline just above the hypothalamus. Two CSF-filled recesses of the third ventricle, the **optic** and **infundibular recesses**, project inferiorly toward the hypothalamus. The optic recess is more rounded and lies just in front of the **optic chiasm**. The infundibular recess is more conical and pointed, extending into the upper part of the pituitary stalk **(25-7A)**.

Cavernous Sinus, Cranial Nerves

Cavernous Sinus. The **cavernous sinuses** (CSs) are irregularly shaped, trabeculated venous compartments that lie along the lateral aspects of the sella turcica. The CSs are contained within a prominent lateral and a thin (often inapparent) medial dural wall. Important CS contents include the **cavernous ICA** segments and several cranial nerves.

Cranial Nerves. Here we briefly review the cranial nerves that course through the cavernous sinus. (Anatomy of all the cranial nerves is discussed in detail in Chapter 23.)

The **abducens cranial nerve** (CN VI) is the only cranial nerve that actually lies within the CS, inferolateral to the cavernous ICA. Cranial nerves III, IV, V_1, and V_2 all lie within the lateral dural wall **(25-4)**. The **oculomotor nerve** (CN III) is the most cephalad of the cavernous cranial nerves and is contained within a thin sleeve of CSF-filled arachnoid called the **oculomotor cistern**. The **trochlear nerve** (CN IV) lies just inferior to CN III.

Two divisions of the **trigeminal nerve** (CN V), the ophthalmic (V_1) and maxillary (V_2) divisions, lie inferior to the trochlear nerve. The mandibular nerve (CN V_3) does not enter the CS. The trigeminal ganglion lies within another arachnoid-lined CSF space, **Meckel cave**. CN V_3 exits inferiorly from the trigeminal (gasserian or semilunar) ganglion and passes through the foramen ovale into the masticator space **(25-6)**.

Imaging Technique and Anatomy

Technical Considerations

Appropriate imaging of the hypothalamic-pituitary axis is based on specific endocrine testing as suggested by clinical signs and symptoms. Thin-section (2-3 mm) multiplanar MR with a small field of view obtained before and after contrast administration, including dynamic as well as static sequences, is the best imaging procedure for hypothalamic-pituitary axis abnormalities **(25-7)**. CTA, MRA, DSA, and petrosal sinus sampling are supplemental techniques in selected cases.

Contrast-enhanced CT occasionally facilitates diagnosis of neuroendocrine abnormalities but is less sensitive than MR. Bone CT may be helpful in depicting the extent of bony involvement with invasive adenomas or differentiating lesions that arise in the basisphenoid.

Pituitary Size and Configuration

Overall height of the pituitary gland on coronal T1-weighted MR scans varies with both age and sex. In prepubescent children, 6 mm or less is normal. The upper limit of normal in men and postmenopausal women is 8 mm.

Physiologic hypertrophy during puberty and young menstruating female patients is common, with normal gland height reaching 10 mm. Pregnant and postpartum lactating female patients have even larger, superiorly convex pituitary glands that may measure up to 12-14 mm in height.

The infundibular stalk measures approximately 3-4 mm in diameter at the level of the optic chiasm and gradually tapers to about 2 mm as it descends to its insertion into the pituitary gland **(25-7F)**.

Signal Intensity of the Pituitary Gland

Pituitary gland signal intensity varies. With the exception of neonates (in whom the AH can be large and *very* hyperintense), the AH is typically isointense compared with cortex on both T1- and T2WI. The NH usually has T1 shortening (the so-called posterior pituitary "bright spot") caused by the presence of neurosecretory granules. The posterior pituitary "bright spot" does not contain lipid and does not suppress on fat-suppression techniques **(25-7E)**. Up to 20% of endocrinologically normal patients lack a posterior pituitary "bright spot."

The infundibular stalk is isointense with the pituitary except for a central hyperintensity on T2WI. The infundibular recess of the third ventricle extends inferiorly into the stalk for a variable distance.

Enhancement Patterns

The pituitary gland does not have a blood-brain barrier, so it enhances rapidly and intensely following contrast administration. Pituitary gland enhancement is slightly less intense than that of venous blood in the adjacent cavernous sinuses **(25-7D)**.

*(**25-7A**) 3.0-T sagittal T2WI shows pituitary and surrounding structures, optic chiasm, optic and infundibular recesses. (**25-7B**) Axial T1 C+ shows intensely enhancing venous blood and dura of cavernous sinus, slightly less intensely enhancing pituitary gland. Right CN III is a linear structure coursing anteriorly in the lateral dura. "Flow voids" of cavernous ICA normally lie in the carotid sulci lateral to the pituitary gland.*

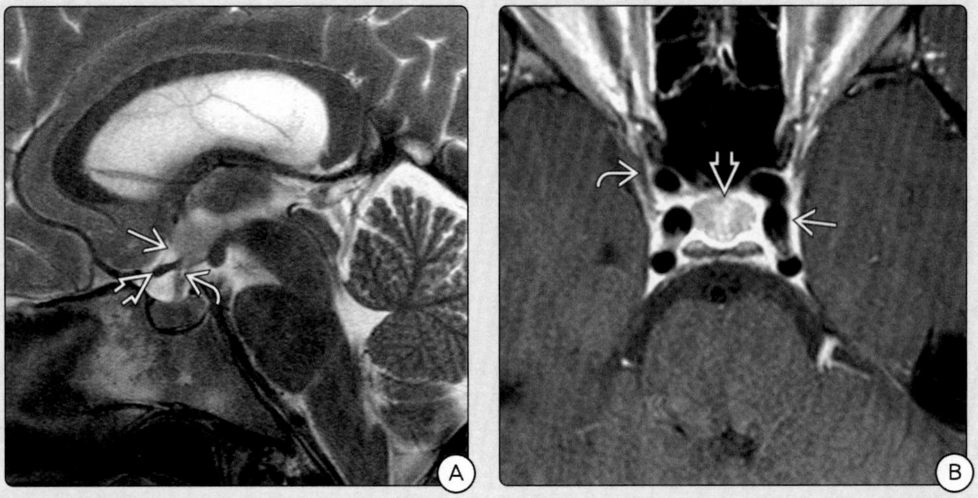

*(**25-7C**) Coronal T2WI shows hyperintensity of CSF in the oculomotor cisterns, Meckel caves. The "dots" inside Meckel caves are fascicles of the trigeminal nerve. Diaphragma sellae cover the sella. (**25-7D**) Coronal T1 C+ FS shows CN III as rounded filling defects at the upper outer corners of the cavernous sinus. The infundibular stalk and pituitary gland enhance less intensely than venous blood in the cavernous sinus.*

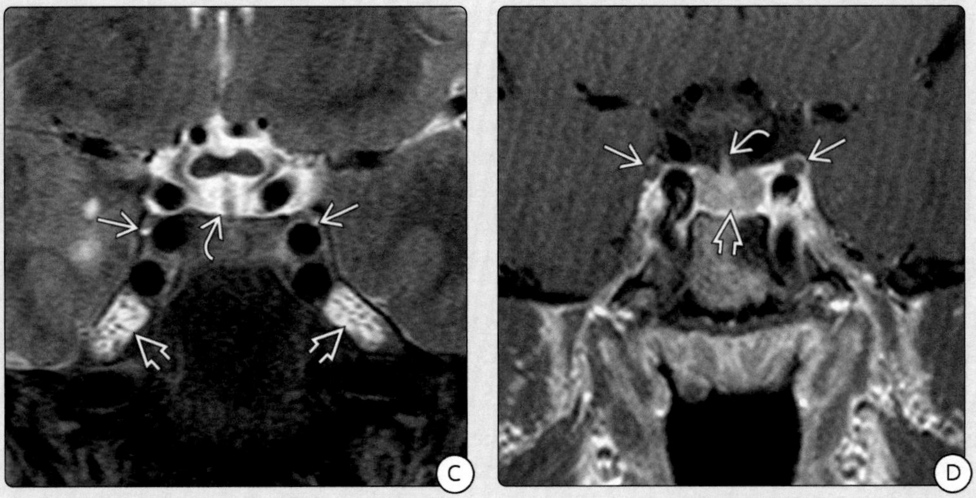

*(**25-7E**) Sagittal T1WI with fat saturation shows that the neurohypophysis remains bright, indicating that its hyperintensity is not fat but neurosecretory granules. (**25-7F**) Sagittal T1 C+ FS shows that the infundibular stalk and tuber cinereum of the hypothalamus lack a blood-brain barrier and enhance. Note normal tapering of the infundibulum as it courses inferiorly from the hypothalamus to the pituitary gland.*

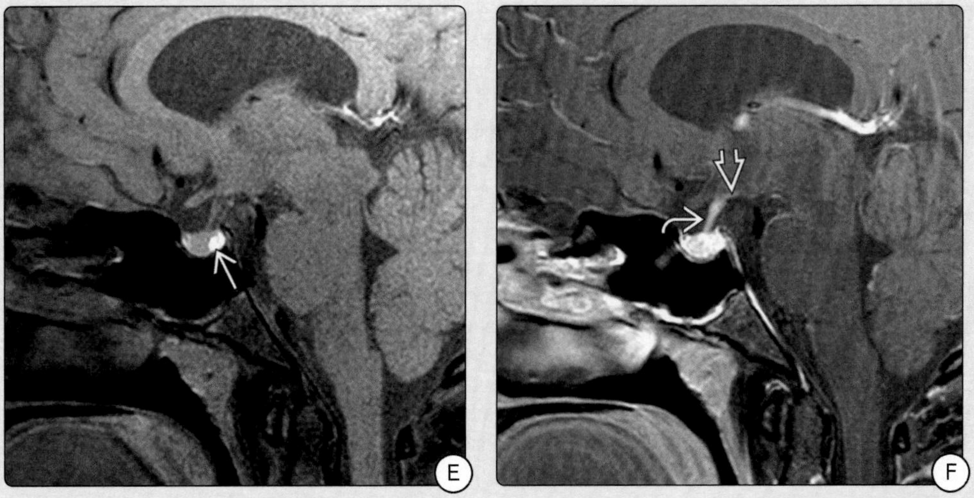

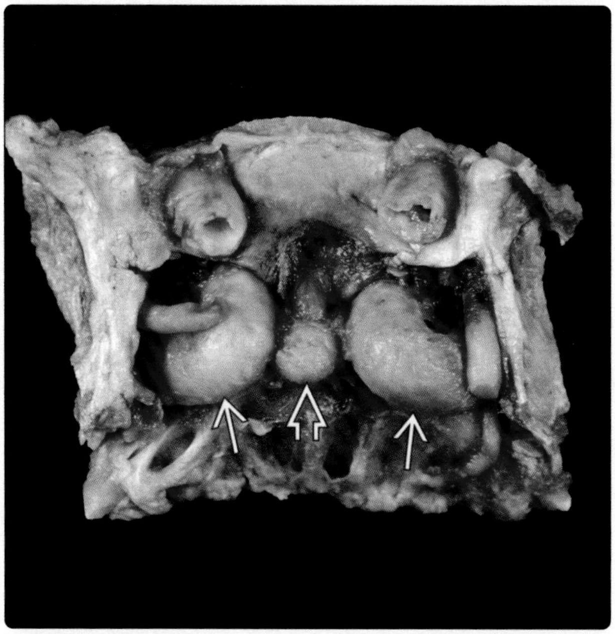

(25-8) Autopsy dissection of the central skull base shows medially positioned cavernous carotid arteries ➡ abutting and slightly compressing the pituitary gland ⇨. (Courtesy A. Ersen, MD, B. Scheithauer, MD.)

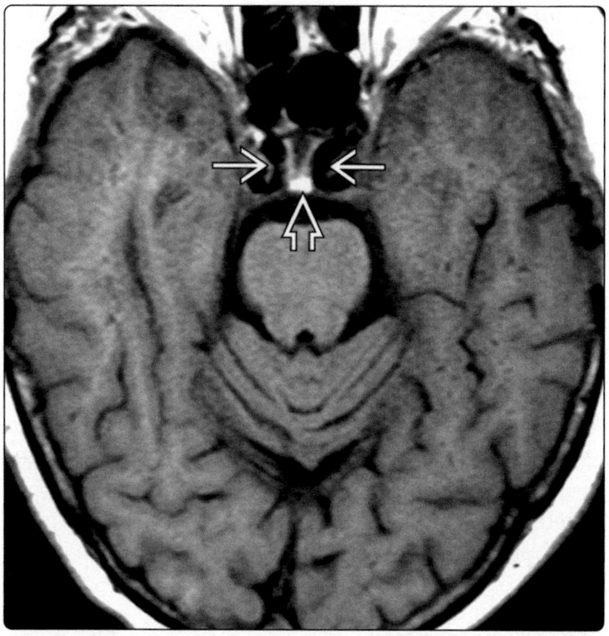

(25-9) Axial T1WI shows "kissing" carotids ➡ with compressed pituitary gland between them. The posterior pituitary "bright spot" ⇨ is seen squeezed upward between the carotid arteries.

The infundibular stalk and tuber cinereum of the hypothalamus also lack a blood-brain barrier and enhance on T1 C+ **(25-7F)**.

Pituitary "Incidentalomas"

Focal areas of hypointensity or nonenhancement are common on contrast-enhanced scans of the pituitary gland. They are seen in 15-20% of asymptomatic patients and have been dubbed pituitary "incidentalomas." Most are less than 1 cm in diameter ("microincidentalomas"). They can be caused by benign intrapituitary cysts as well as nonfunctioning microadenomas. Both are common at autopsy.

Although most pituitary "incidentalomas" are unsuspected imaging findings and generally of no clinical significance, recent endocrinologic guidelines recommend that patients with microincidentalomas undergo a thorough history, physical examination, and limited laboratory evaluation (i.e., PRL and IGF-1 levels). Patients with "macroincidentalomas" (more than 1 cm) should be evaluated for hypopituitarism and have formal visual field evaluation if the lesion abuts the optic nerves or chiasm.

If patients do not meet specified surgical criteria for removal, follow-up MR is recommended at 6 months for a "macroincidentaloma," 1 year for a "microincidentaloma," and progressively less frequently thereafter if the "incidentaloma" remains unchanged in size.

Normal Imaging Variants

A number of variants occur in the pituitary gland and around the sella turcica; these should not be mistaken for disease on imaging studies. Not all enlarged pituitary glands are abnormal! Pseudoenlargement of the pituitary gland can be caused by "kissing" carotids or an unusually shallow bony sella. Pituitary hyperplasia can be abnormal, but it can also be physiologic and normal. An empty sella is a common normal variant but can be a manifestation of idiopathic intracranial hypertension (pseudotumor cerebri).

"Kissing" Carotid Arteries

The cavernous internal carotid arteries (ICAs) normally lie lateral to the pituitary gland in the parasellar carotid sulci. Occasionally, the ICAs are positioned medially and actually course *inside* the bony sella **(25-8)**. These "kissing" carotid arteries may compress the pituitary gland, squeezing it upward and making it appear modestly enlarged. The presence of medially positioned ICAs is highly important in presurgical planning for transsphenoidal hypophysectomy, as normally positioned ICAs are not encountered in this approach **(25-9)**.

Pituitary Hyperplasia

Terminology

Pituitary hyperplasia is a nonneoplastic increase in adenohypophysial cell number. It can be normal (physiologic) or pathologic.

Etiology

Physiologic Hyperplasia. Physiologic increase in pituitary volume is common and normal in many circumstances. Physiologic hypertrophy of puberty and enlarged pituitary glands in young menstruating female patients is very common

(25-10) (25-11) (25-12) (25-13). Pituitary gland enlargement secondary to prolactin (PRL) cell hyperplasia also occurs during pregnancy and lactation or in response to exogenous estrogen treatment.

Pathologic Hyperplasia. Pathologic hyperplasia most commonly occurs in response to **end-organ failure**. Primary hypothyroidism is the most common cause of pathologic pituitary hyperplasia. Thyroid-stimulating hormone cell hyperplasia can be induced by longstanding primary hypothyroidism **(25-14)**. Adrenocorticotrophic hormone (ACTH) cell hyperplasia occurs with hypocortisolism in Addison disease. Gonadotroph hyperplasia occurs as a response to primary hypogonadism (Klinefelter or Turner syndromes).

Pathologic hyperplasia can also be induced by ectopic excess of releasing hormones. Growth hormone (GH) cell hyperplasia occurs with increased growth hormone-releasing hormone secreted by pancreatic islet cell tumor, pheochromocytoma, bronchial carcinoma, and thymic carcinoid tumor.

ACTH cell hyperplasia may be secondary to corticotropin-releasing hormone secretion from a hypothalamic hamartoma (see below), neuroendocrine tumor, or ACTH-dependent Cushing disease. Mammosomatotroph hyperplasia occurs in McCune-Albright syndrome and gigantism.

Pathology

Gross Pathology. The most common physiologic form of pituitary hyperplasia is diffuse PRL cell hyperplasia during pregnancy and lactation. The adenohypophysis is symmetrically enlarged, sometimes nearly twice or three times normal size, but otherwise appears grossly normal.

Clinical Issues

Epidemiology. With the exception of PRL cell hyperplasia in pregnancy, pituitary hyperplasia is rare.

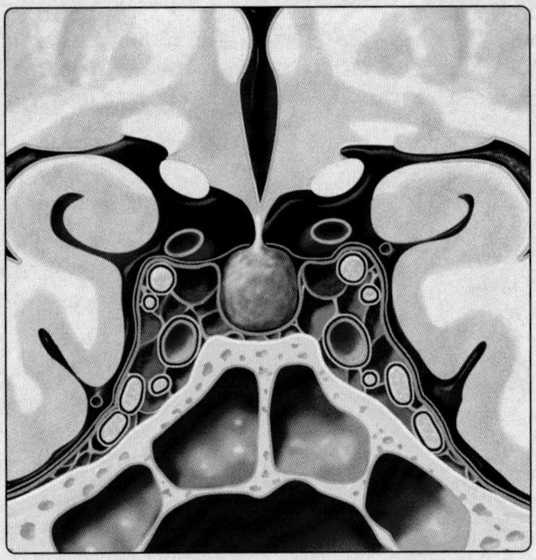

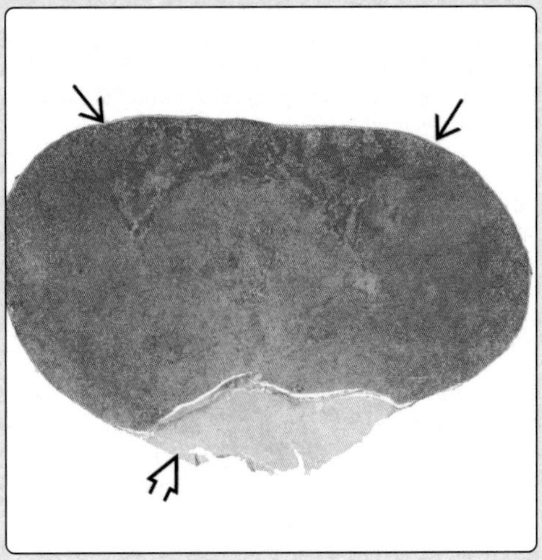

(25-10) Coronal graphic shows physiologic pituitary hyperplasia. The gland is uniformly enlarged and has a mildly convex superior margin. (25-11) Low-power photomicrograph shows an axial section of a pituitary gland with hyperplasia. The diffusely enlarged anterior lobe → dwarfs the neurohypophysis ⇨. (Courtesy A. Ersen, MD, B. Scheithauer, MD.)

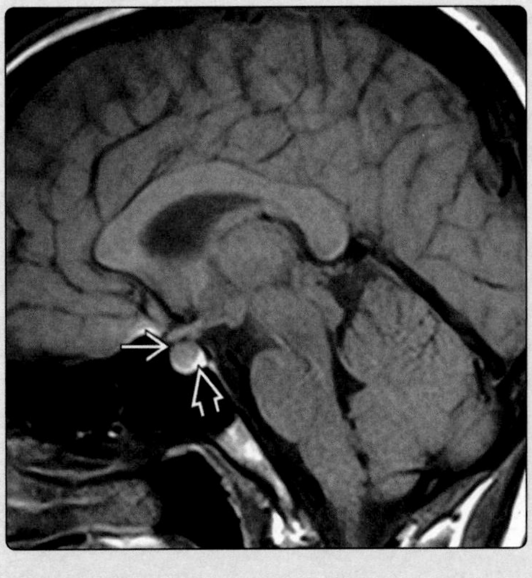

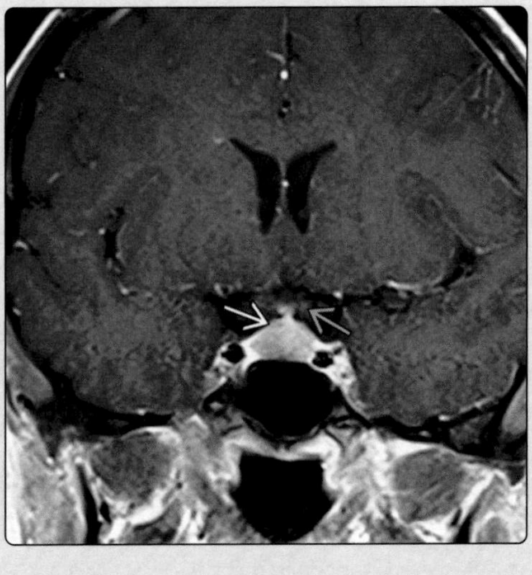

(25-12) Sagittal T1WI in a 16y girl shows normal upward bulging of the pituitary gland ➡. The sellar floor is intact. Note the normal hyperintensity of the neurohypophysis ⇨. (25-13) Coronal T1 C+ in the same patient shows the upwardly convex gland ➡ almost touching the optic chiasm →. The overall volume of the pituitary gland is almost twice the size of one in a postmenopausal woman.

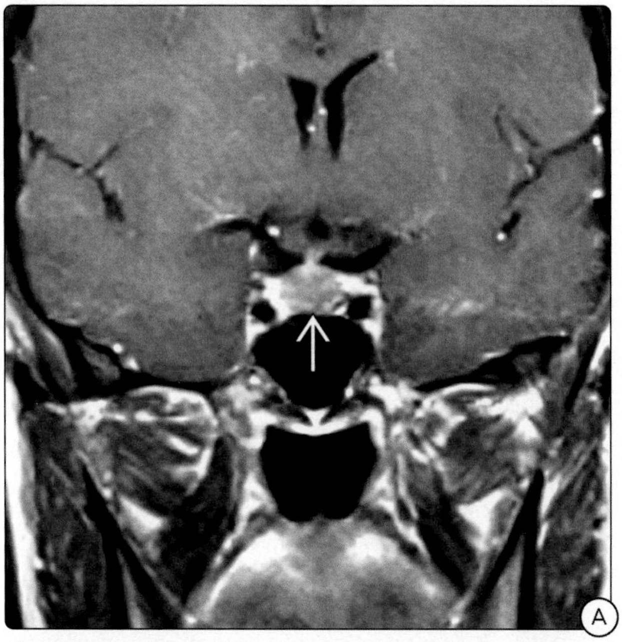

(25-14A) ***Coronal T1 C+ scan in a prepubescent male patient with hypothyroidism shows pituitary hyperplasia ➡ with an upwardly bulging gland that mimics macroadenoma.***

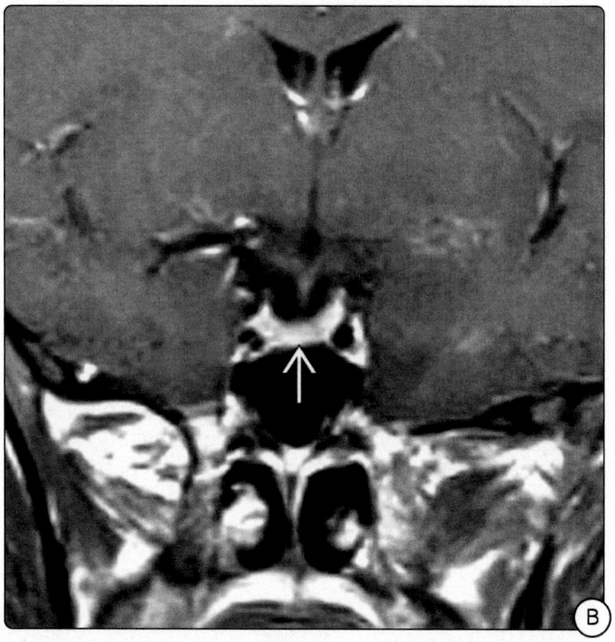

(25-14B) ***Repeat scan obtained a few weeks following initiation of thyroid hormone replacement shows that the pituitary gland returns to a normal size ➡.***

Demographics. Most patients are children or young adults. PRL cell hyperplasia is the most common etiology.

Presentation. Symptoms vary with the specific hormone. PRL cell hyperplasia causes hyperprolactinemia, whereas GH cell hyperplasia causes gigantism or acromegaly. ACTH cell hyperplasia causes Cushing disease.

Natural History. Normal physiologic hypertrophy does not require treatment. Pathologic hyperplasia is treated medically, and prognosis is excellent. There is no increase in prevalence of adenoma.

Imaging

Symmetric increase in pituitary gland size and overall volume without focal mass effect or bony erosion is the classic finding.

NECT scans show that the superior margin of the gland is convex upward, measuring 10-15 mm in height. There is no evidence of erosion of the bony sella turcica. Enhancement is strong and generally uniform on CECT.

MR demonstrates an enlarged gland that bulges upward and may even contact the optic chiasm. The enlarged pituitary is isointense with cortex on both T1- and T2WI. Dynamic contrast-enhanced MR scans with 2- to 3-mm slice thickness and small field of view show that the gland enhances homogeneously. Occasionally focal nodular enhancement is present, especially with ACTH cell hyperplasia.

Differential Diagnosis

Pituitary hyperplasia may be difficult to distinguish from **macroadenoma**. Age, sex, and endocrine status are helpful. Primary neoplasms of the pituitary gland are rare in children, whereas physiologic enlargement is common. **Remember**: *an enlarged pituitary gland in a prepubescent male patient is almost always hyperplasia, not adenoma!*

Lymphocytic hypophysitis can cause an enlarged pituitary gland. Lymphocytic hypophysitis is most common in pregnant and postpartum female patients and may be difficult to distinguish from physiologic PRL cell hyperplasia on imaging studies alone. If stalk enlargement is present, hypophysitis is more likely than hyperplasia.

Intracranial hypotension results in pituitary enlargement above the sella turcica in 50% of patients. These patients typically present with headaches related to decreased intracranial CSF pressure. The classic imaging appearance of intracranial hypotension includes diffuse dural thickening and enhancement, downward displacement of the brain through the incisura ("slumping midbrain"), and distension of the venous structures and dural sinuses.

Empty Sella

Terminology

An **empty sella** (ES) is an arachnoid-lined, CSF-filled protrusion that extends from the suprasellar cistern through the diaphragma sellae into the sella turcica **(25-15)**. An ES is rarely completely "empty"; a small remnant of flattened pituitary gland is almost always present at the bottom of the bony sella, even if it is inapparent on imaging studies. Therefore, the term "partially empty sella" is anatomically more accurate.

Etiology

An ES can be primary or secondary. A **primary empty sella** occurs when an unusually wide (sometimes called "incompetent") opening in the diaphragma sellae allows intrasellar herniation of arachnoid and CSF from the suprasellar cistern above into the sella turcica below **(25-16)**. Pulsatile CSF may gradually enlarge and deepen the sella, but the bony lamina dura separating the sella from the sphenoid sinus remains intact **(25-17)**.

A **secondary empty sella** occurs when pituitary volume is reduced with surgery, bromocriptine therapy, or radiation treatment. Less often, pituitary apoplexy (usually with pituitary macroadenoma) may leave the expanded bony sella largely empty with only a small remnant of infarcted hemorrhagic gland at the posteroinferior aspect of the sella.

Rarely, a child with perinatal insult resulting in diffuse neuronal necrosis in the hypothalamus may have a very thin hypophyseal stalk and a partially empty sella.

A rare but important cause of secondary ES is **Sheehan syndrome**. Sheehan syndrome is one of the most common causes of hypopituitarism in underdeveloped countries. It results from ischemic pituitary necrosis due to severe postpartum hemorrhage. The great majority of patients with Sheehan syndrome have an empty sella on CT or MR scan.

Clinical Issues

Epidemiology. The exact prevalence of ES is unknown. An ES is identified in 5-10% of cranial MR scans.

Demographics. Although ES can occur at any age, peak presentation is in the fifth decade. There is a 4:1 female predominance. The mean body mass index of patients with an

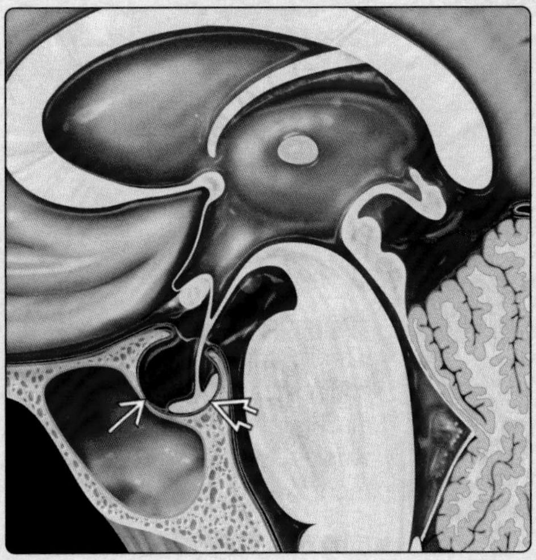

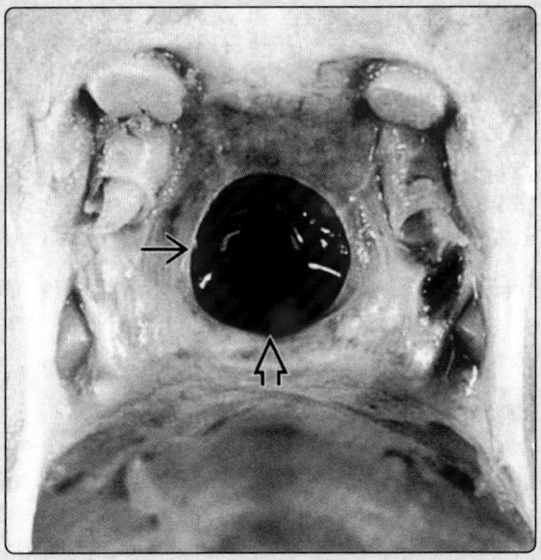

***(25-15)** Graphic depicts primary empty sella with CSF-filled arachnoid cistern protruding inferiorly into the enlarged sella turcica, flattening the pituitary gland posteroinferiorly against the sellar floor . **(25-16)** Autopsy specimen seen from above shows a wide opening of the diaphragma sellae with CSF-filled sella below . (Courtesy M. Sage, MD.)*

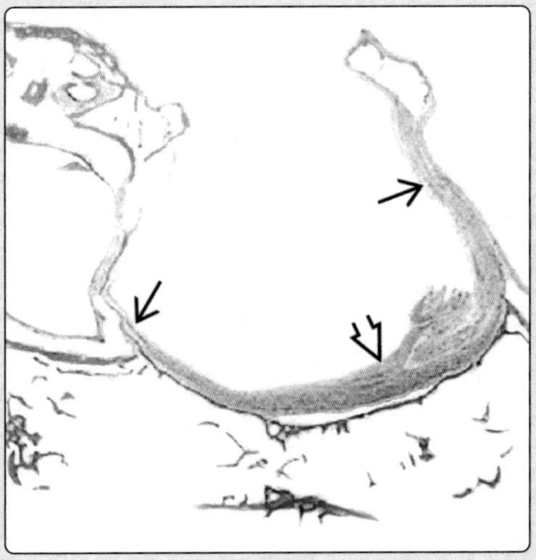

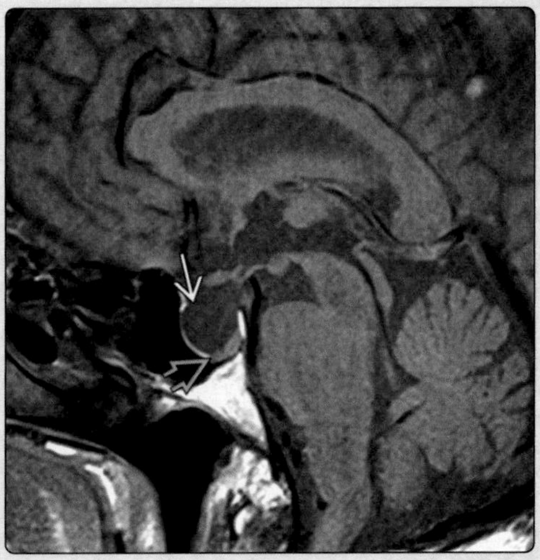

***(25-17)** Sagittal low-power photomicrograph shows a partially empty sella as an enlarged, mostly CSF-filled sella with the pituitary gland flattened against the sellar floor. (Courtesy W. Kucharczyk, MD.) **(25-18)** Sagittal T1 image shows a classic empty sella with an enlarged sella turcica in this 58y woman with Cushing syndrome. The pituitary gland is thinned and flattened against the sellar floor .*

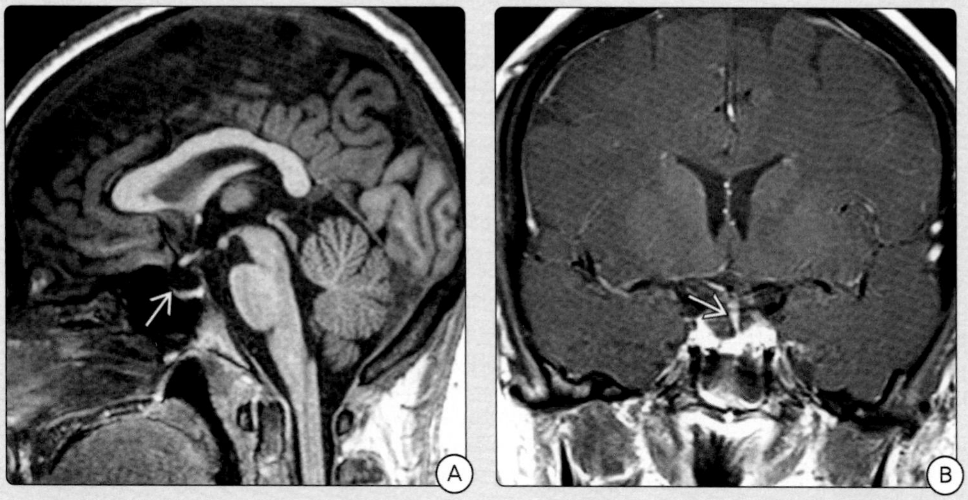

(25-19A) Sagittal T1WI in a 28y woman with complex partial seizures shows an incidental empty sella ➡. (25-19B) Coronal T1 C+ in the same patient shows that the stalk ➡ inserts off-midline, a normal variant. The patient's endocrine profile was normal.

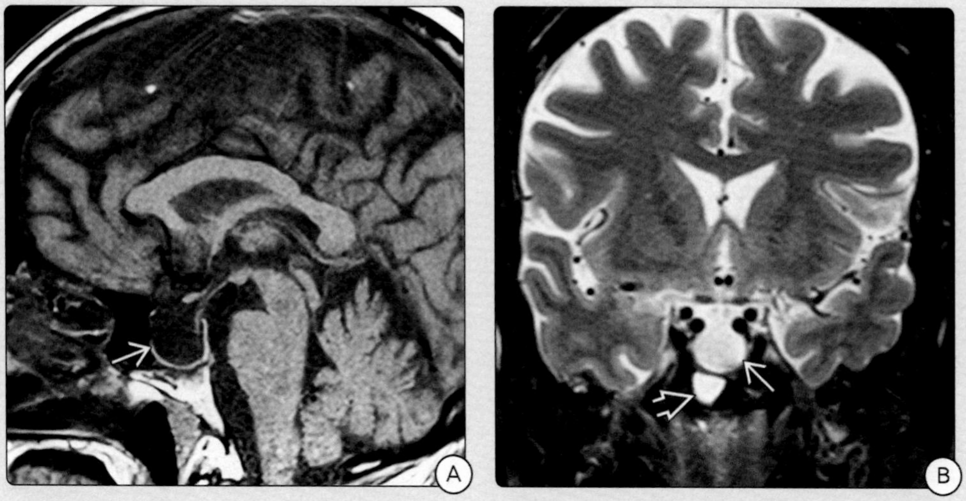

(25-20A) An empty sella is not always benign, as illustrated by this case of a 56y woman with a CSF leak. The enormous CSF-filled empty sella ➡ is much larger than the usual normal variant. (25-20B) Coronal T2WI in the same patient shows the CSF-filled sella turcica ➡ with a fluid collection ➡ below the thinned floor. Surgery confirmed a bony dehiscence, which was repaired.

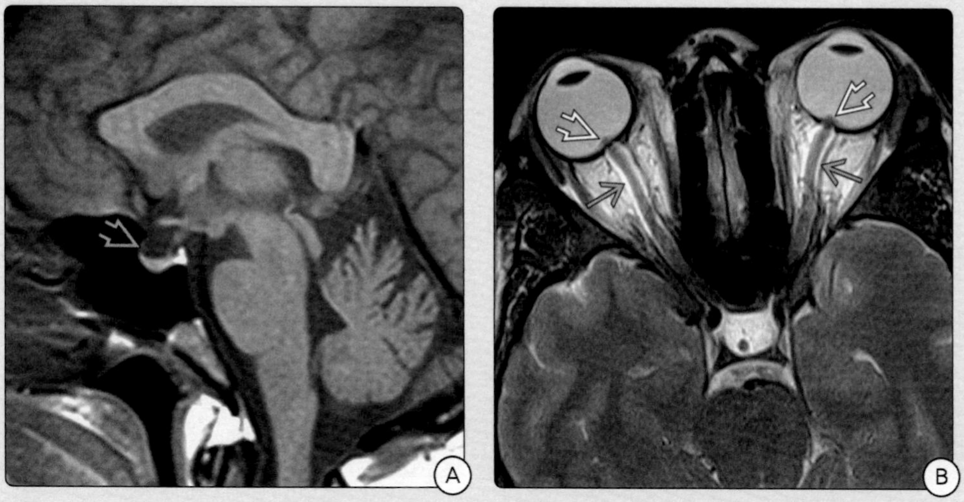

(25-21A) Sagittal T1WI shows a partially empty sella ➡ in this 24y woman with headaches. A normal pituitary gland in this young woman would have an upwardly convex margin. (25-21B) Axial T2WI of the orbits in the same patient shows dilated optic nerve sheaths ➡ around the nerves and protrusion of the optic nerve heads into posterior globes ➡ related to papilledema. These are classic findings of idiopathic intracranial hypertension.

empty or partially empty sella is significantly higher than of those without an ES.

Presentation. Most patients with ES are asymptomatic or have nonspecific symptoms such as headache **(25-19)**. However, primary ES may be associated with various clinical conditions ranging from mild endocrine disturbances to rhinorrhea or otorrhea. Between 18-20% of patients with primary ES have hyperprolactinemia, 5% have global anterior hypopituitarism, and 4% have isolated GH deficiency. Almost 80% of middle-aged obese women with spontaneous CSF otorrhea or rhinorrhea have an associated ES demonstrated on preoperative MR **(25-20)**. Patients with idiopathic intracranial hypertension commonly have an associated partially empty sella **(25-21)**.

Occasionally, patients present with visual disturbances caused by inferior displacement of the optic chiasm into the ES. Most such cases are secondary ES following transsphenoidal hypophysectomy for pituitary adenoma resection.

Treatment Options. Primary and secondary ES generally do not require definitive treatment. Hormone replacement may be needed in some cases. CSF rhinorrhea/otorrhea or optic chiasm displacement with severe visual compromise may necessitate surgical intervention.

Imaging

General Features. Imaging studies show intrasellar CSF with a thinned pituitary gland flattened against the sellar floor.

CT Findings. CSF-density fluid fills a sella that may be of normal size or moderately enlarged. The bony floor of the sella is intact in primary ES, but, in secondary ES, it often shows a surgical defect caused by transsphenoidal hypophysectomy. The infundibular stalk and pituitary remnant enhance normally on CECT scans. The stalk may be displaced off midline, appearing somewhat "tilted."

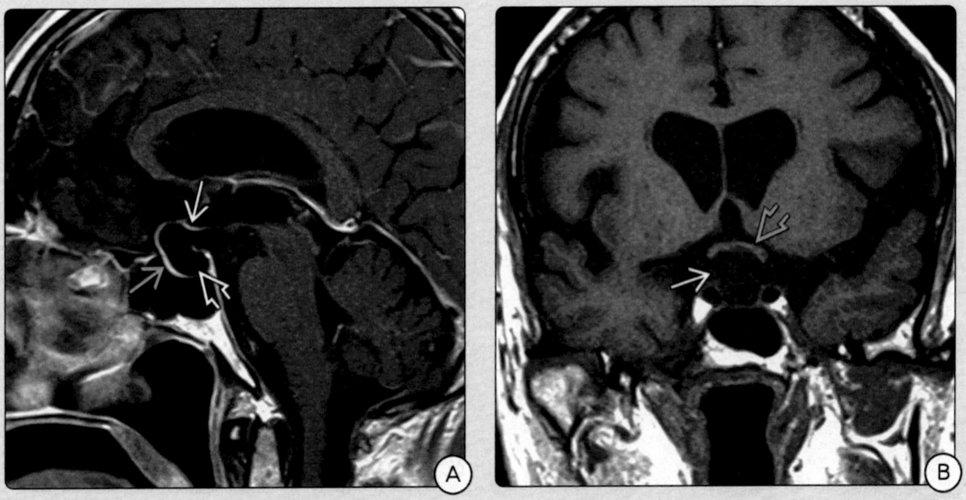

(25-22A) Sagittal T1 C+ MR image in a 73y man shows an arachnoid cyst filling the sella and suprasellar regions. Note the superior displacement of the infundibulum. The enhancing pituitary gland is flattened anteriorly within the sella turcica. (25-22B) Coronal T1WI in the same patient shows that the optic chiasm is displaced superiorly by the arachnoid cyst. The cyst follows CSF signal intensity on all MR sequences.

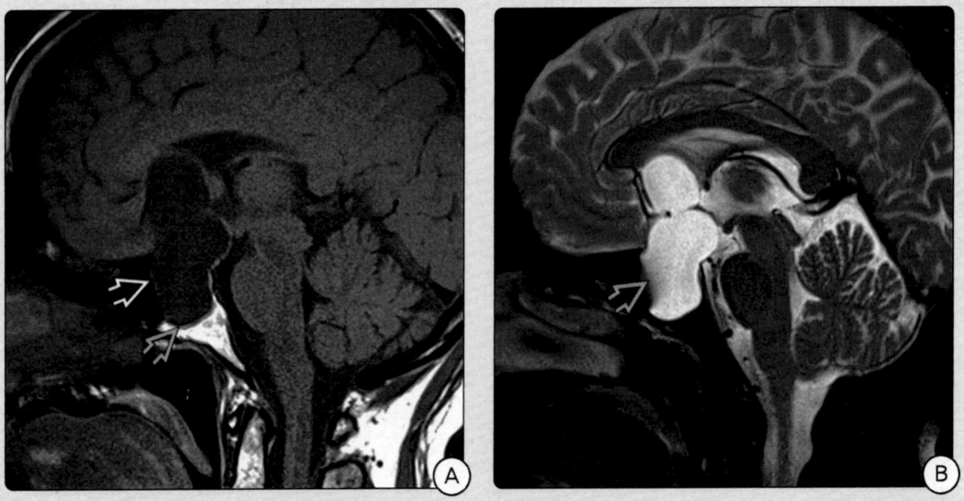

(25-23A) Sagittal T1WI shows a very large cystic mass filling the sella and suprasellar regions with mass effect on the adjacent brain. Note the enlarged, flattened sella turcica. (25-23B) Sagittal T2WI in the same patient shows that the arachnoid cyst follows CSF signal intensity. There was no enhancement of this cyst and no intracystic nodule to suggest a Rathke cleft cyst. Following cyst removal, the pituitary function returned to normal.

MR Findings. The intrasellar fluid behaves exactly like CSF on T1- and T2WI and suppresses completely on FLAIR. DWI shows no diffusion restriction. In severe cases, the optic chiasm and/or anterior third ventricle may appear herniated into—or retracted toward—the sella. If the ES is secondary to surgery, fat packing and scarring with adhesions may distort the imaging findings.

Differential Diagnosis

The major differential diagnosis of an ES is a suprasellar **arachnoid cyst** that may herniate into the sella turcica. The bony sella is often not simply enlarged but eroded and flattened. Although arachnoid cysts are often incidental, they are variably sized and usually become symptomatic when large, resulting in mass effect on the pituitary infundibulum and gland. Arachnoid cysts follow CSF signal intensity on all MR sequences and completely suppress on FLAIR images. Sagittal T2WI often shows an elevated, compressed third ventricle draped over the suprasellar arachnoid cyst **(25-22)** **(25-23)**.

The other major consideration of patients with an ES is **idiopathic intracranial hypertension** (IIH), also known as "pseudotumor cerebri." Both incidental ES and patients with IIH have an increased prevalence in obese female patients. Imaging findings also show some overlap, as both conditions often demonstrate an empty sella. In IIH, the optic nerve sheaths are often dilated, and the ventricles and CSF cisterns often appear smaller than normal. Patients with IIH will also typically have papilledema, which can be seen on MR as protrusion of the optic nerve papilla into the posterior globes **(25-21)**.

Increased intracranial pressure (↑ ICP) caused by obstructive hydrocephalus usually results in displacement of the enlarged anterior third ventricle recesses—not the suprasellar cistern—toward or into the bony sella. Transependymal CSF migration is common in ↑ ICP but absent in ES.

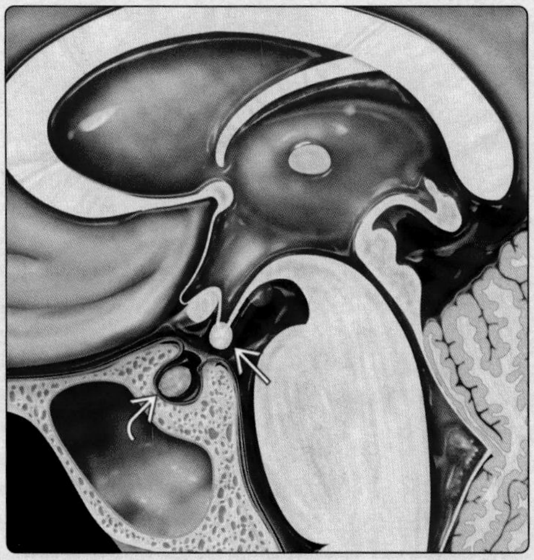

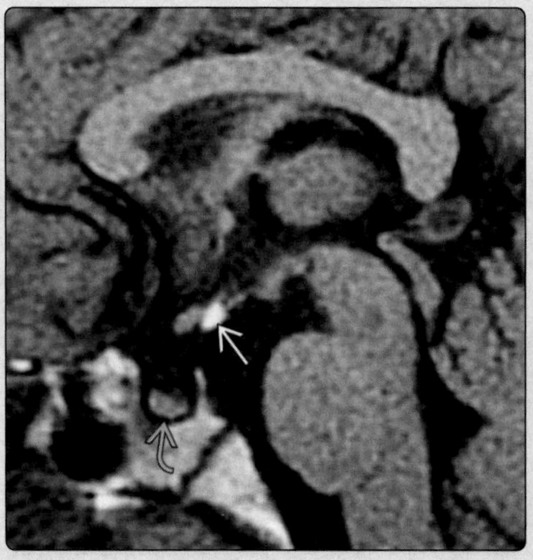

***(25-24)** Sagittal graphic demonstrates ectopia of the posterior pituitary gland ➡, located at the distal end of a truncated pituitary stalk. The sella turcica and adenohypophysis ⮫ are both small. **(25-25)** Sagittal T1WI shows an ectopic posterior pituitary gland at the hypothalamic median eminence ➡. The infundibulum is absent, and the anterior pituitary gland ⮫ is small. The normal posterior pituitary "bright spot" is not in its typical location.*

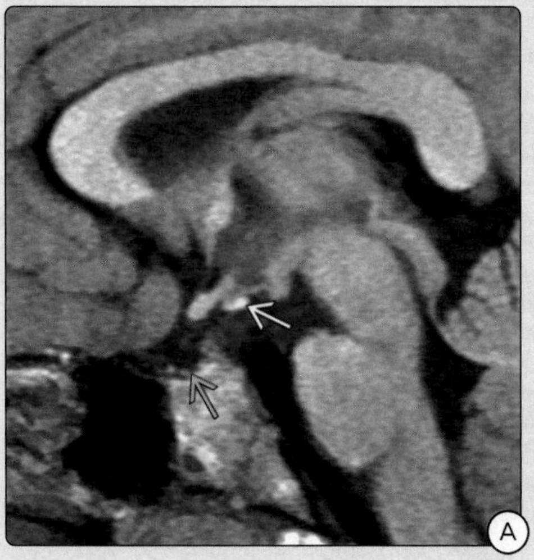

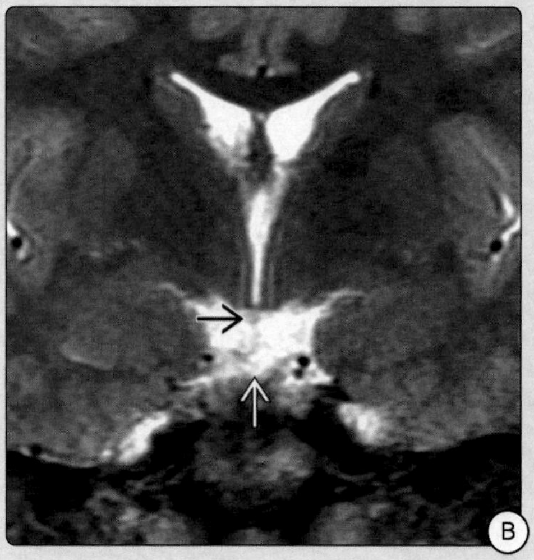

***(25-26A)** Sagittal T1WI in a 4y girl with panhypopituitarism shows more severe anomalies with almost no tissue in the sella ⇨, an absent stalk, and ectopic posterior pituitary in the hypothalamus ➡. **(25-26B)** Coronal T2WI in the same patient shows an almost inapparent pituitary gland ➡ and absent stalk with displaced neurohypophysis in the hypothalamus ⇨.*

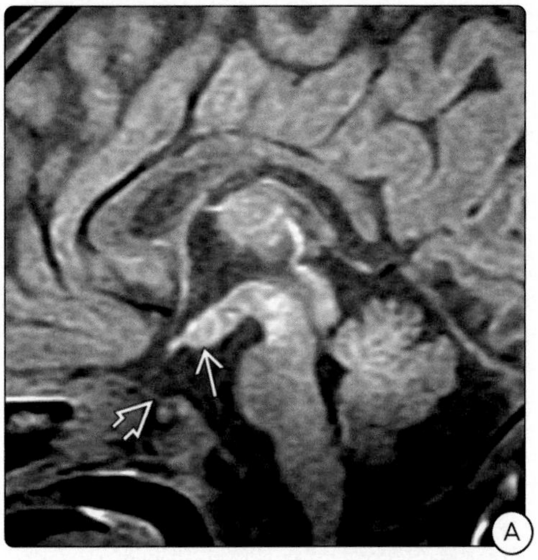

(25-27A) *Sagittal T1WI shows a thickened floor of the 3rd ventricle ➡ from fusion of the hypothalamus and an almost inapparent sella ➡.*

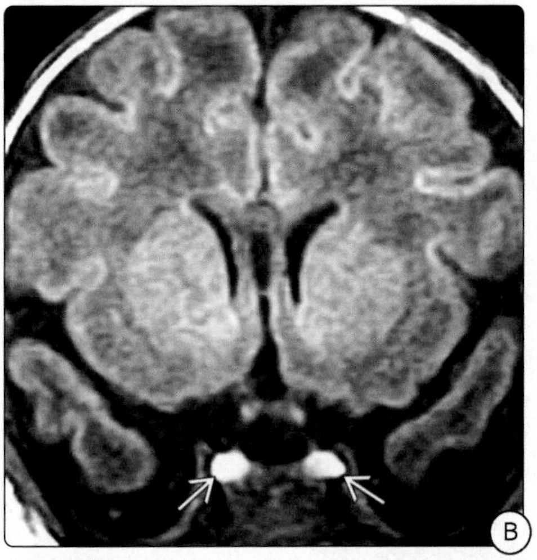

(25-27B) *Coronal T1WI in the same patient shows two laterally displaced hyperintense pituitary glands ➡.*

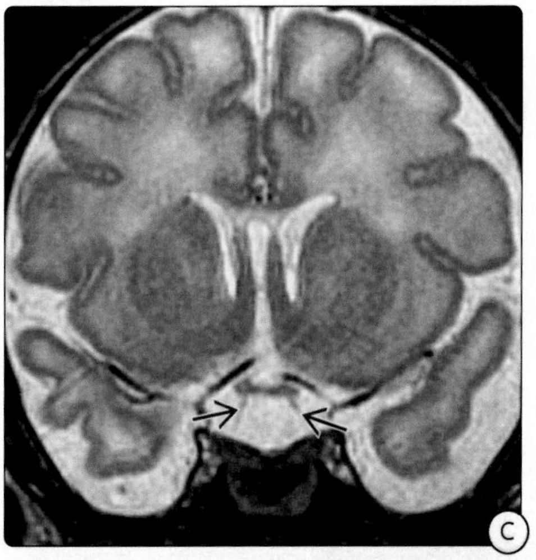

(25-27C) *Coronal T2WI in the same patient shows duplicated pituitary stalks ➡. A duplicated pituitary is a rare congenital anomaly.*

Congenital Lesions

Pituitary Anomalies

Complete absence of the pituitary gland and stalk is rare and nearly always fatal at or soon after birth. Pituitary hypoplasia is much more common **(25-24)**. Many affected children have growth hormone deficiency and short stature, i.e., they are "pituitary dwarfs." These patients can be treated with hormone replacement therapy, so accurate diagnosis and early recognition of this disorder are essential.

Pituitary Hypoplasia

A **hypoplastic pituitary gland** is the most frequent abnormality in children with *isolated* growth hormone deficiency, whereas **stalk abnormalities** are more common in children with *multiple* hormone deficiencies. Nearly 75% of children with hypopituitarism are male.

Imaging abnormalities include a small sella and anterior pituitary lobe, hypoplasia or absence of the stalk, and an "ectopic" posterior pituitary "bright spot" seen as displacement of the T1 hyperintense posterior lobe into the infundibulum or median eminence of the hypothalamus **(25-25)** **(25-26)**.

In general, the extent of MR abnormalities correlates with the severity of hormone deficiency. Patients with isolated GH deficiency are more likely to have a normal-sized adenohypophysis and infundibulum than those with multiple endocrine deficiencies.

Kallmann syndrome, also known as hypogonadotropic hypogonadism, is a neuronal migration disorder that results in hypoplastic or absent olfactory nerves and sulci. Various visual and septal anomalies as well as pituitary gland hypoplasia are common.

Pituitary Duplication

Pituitary duplication is a rare anomaly in which two pituitary stalks can be identified on the coronal view **(25-27B)** **(25-27C)**. The tuber cinereum of the hypothalamus and mammillary bodies are fused into a single thick mass that is best visualized on midline sagittal views **(25-27A)**. Associated craniofacial and craniocervical anomalies are common in these cases.

Unlike pituitary hypoplasia, pituitary duplication rarely causes hormone deficiencies. Instead, a spectrum of midline craniofacial and craniocervical segmentation and fusion anomalies are often seen. Female patients are more commonly affected.

Hypothalamic Hamartoma

Terminology

Hypothalamic hamartoma (HH), also known as diencephalic or **tuber cinereum hamartoma**, is a nonneoplastic congenital malformation associated with precocious puberty, behavioral disturbances, and gelastic seizures.

Etiology

HHs are an anomaly of neuronal migration that probably occurs between gestational days 33 and 41. A syndromic abnormality that occurs with HH, **Pallister-Hall syndrome** (PHS), is caused by *GLI3* frameshift mutations on chromosome 7p13.

Pathology

Location. The majority of HHs are located in the tuber cinereum, i.e., between the infundibular stalk in front and the mammillary bodies behind **(25-28)** **(25-29)**. They can be pedunculated **(25-30)** or sessile **(25-31)**. Pedunculated lesions extend inferiorly from the hypothalamus into the suprasellar cistern, whereas sessile HHs project from the floor of the third ventricle into its lumen.

Size and Number. HHs are solitary lesions that vary in size from a few millimeters **(25-32)** to huge mixed solid-cystic lesions measuring several centimeters in diameter **(25-33)** **(25-34)**.

Gross and Microscopic Features. HHs are well-defined round or ovoid soft tissue masses that resemble normal brain parenchyma. Histologically, HHs consist of well-differentiated small and large neurons interspersed with variable amounts of glial cells. Calcification, hemorrhage, and necrosis are rare although very large lesions often contain well-delineated cysts.

Staging, Grading, and Classification. The most common classification of HHs is morphologic. HHs can be pedunculated or sessile. **Pedunculated** HHs are attached to the tuber cinereum and project into the suprasellar cistern. **Sessile** HHs are attached to the floor of the third ventricle and often incorporate the mammillary bodies. Projection into the suprasellar cistern is variable.

Clinical Issues

Demographics. HHs are rare lesions although up to one-third of patients with central precocious puberty have an HH. There is a moderate male predominance.

Presentation. Most HHs present between 1 and 3 years of age. Three-quarters of patients with histologically verified HHs have precocious puberty, and 50% have seizures.

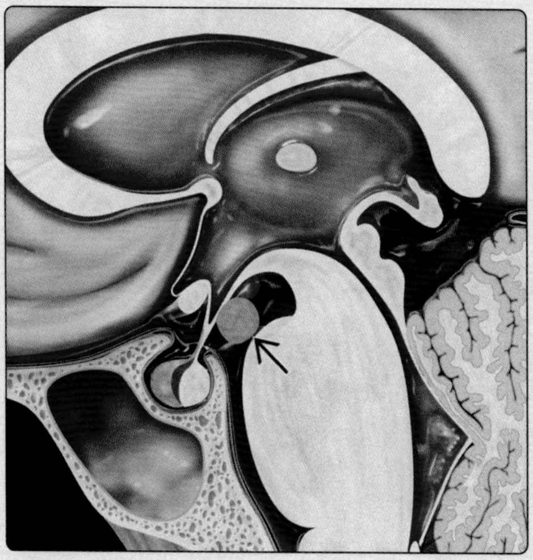

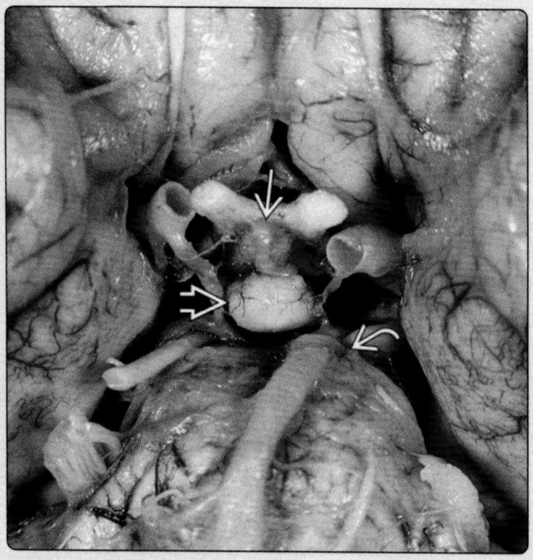

***(25-28)** Sagittal graphic shows a pedunculated hypothalamic hamartoma interposed between the infundibulum anteriorly and the mammillary bodies posteriorly. The mass resembles gray matter. **(25-29)** Submentovertex view shows a classic "collar button" pedunculated HH positioned between the infundibular stalk in front, mammillary bodies (not visible), and pons behind. (Courtesy R. Hewlett, MD.)*

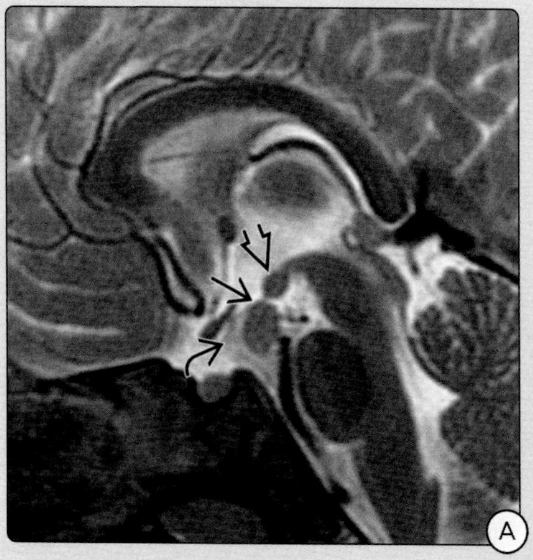

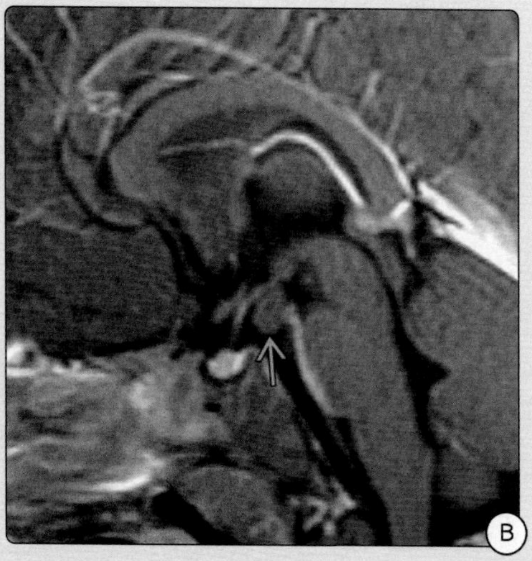

***(25-30A)** Sagittal T2WI in a 12m child with central precocious puberty shows a classic "collar button" hypothalamic hamartoma between the infundibular stalk and the mammillary bodies. The mass is isointense with gray matter. **(25-30B)** Sagittal T1 C+ in the same patient shows that the hypothalamic hamartoma does not enhance. If the mass enhanced, a glioma should be considered.*

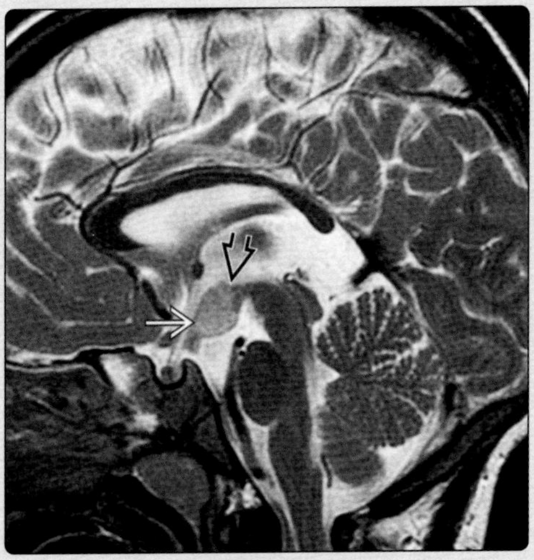

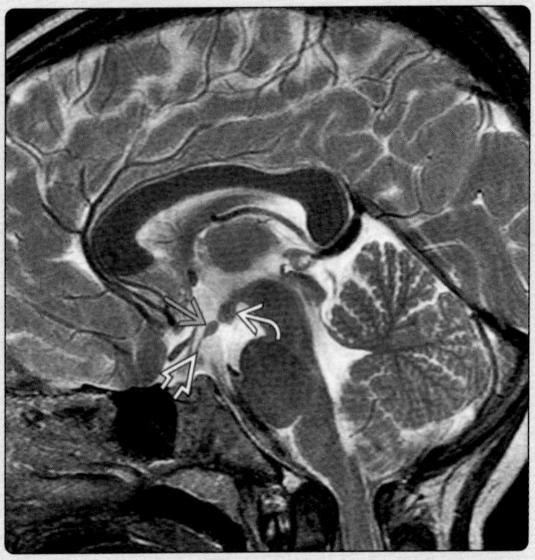

***(25-31)** Sagittal T2WI shows a classic sessile hypothalamic hamartoma bulging into the floor of the third ventricle. The mass is mildly hyperintense to gray matter, a normal feature of HH. Sessile lesions are more commonly associated with gelastic seizures.* ***(25-32)** Sagittal T2WI shows a tiny sessile hypothalamic hamartoma isointense to gray matter just behind the infundibulum and in front of the mammillary bodies.*

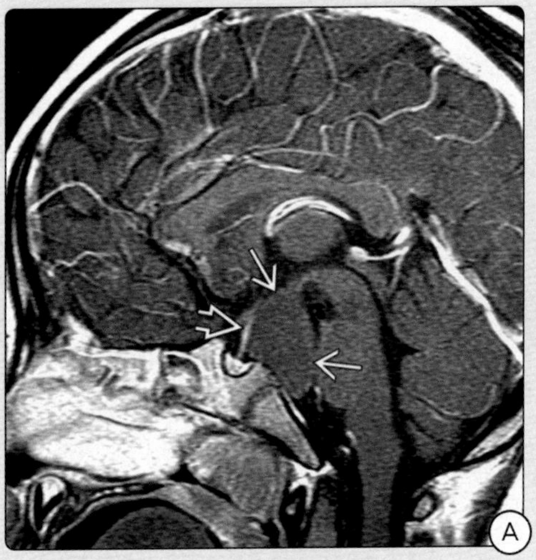

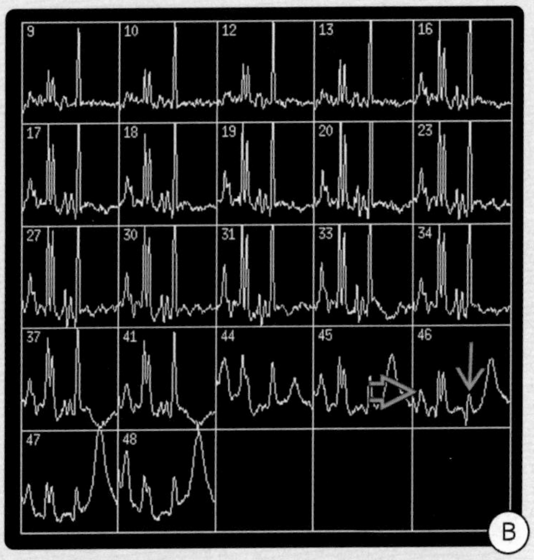

***(25-33A)** T1 C+ scan in a teenage male patient with hypogonadotropic hypogonadism shows a lobulated, nonenhancing mass in the suprasellar and prepontine cistern. The infundibular stalk is displaced anteriorly.* ***(25-33B)** Multivoxel MRS of the mass shows decreased NAA with elevated myoinositol in the voxel directly over the mass. Findings and history are consistent with a hypothalamic hamartoma.*

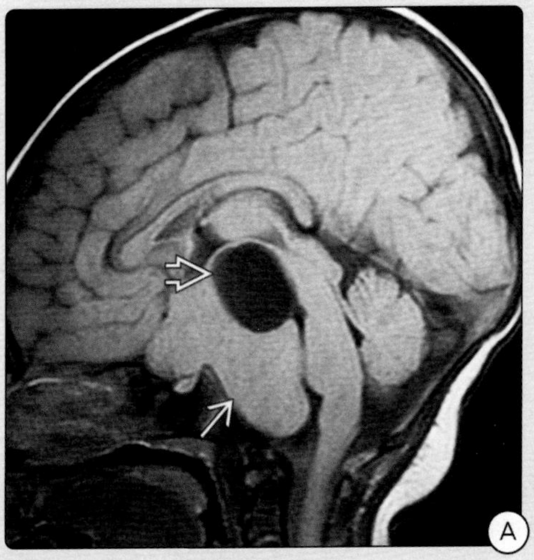

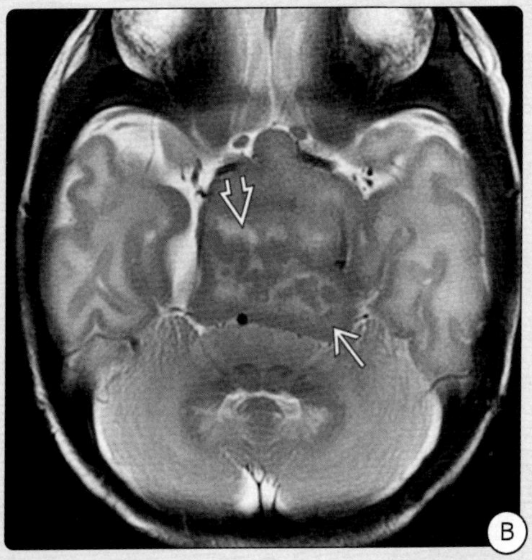

***(25-34A)** Sagittal T1WI shows an enormous hypothalamic hamartoma extending posteriorly behind the clivus. A CSF-like cyst is associated with the mass. (Courtesy R. Nguyen, MD.)* ***(25-34B)** T2WI in the same pediatric patient shows that the hamartoma is composed of dysplastic, disorganized gray matter with some unmyelinated white matter inside the lesion. (Courtesy R. Nguyen, MD.)*

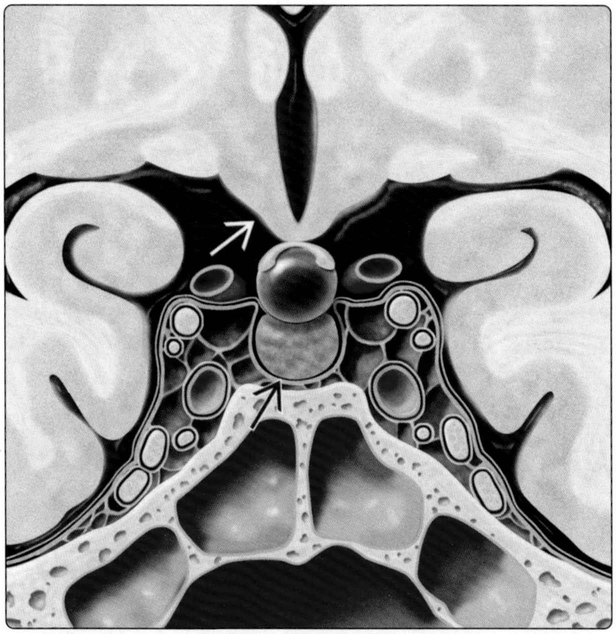

(25-35) Coronal graphic shows a typical suprasellar Rathke cleft cyst interposed between the pituitary gland ⇨ and the optic chiasm ➡.

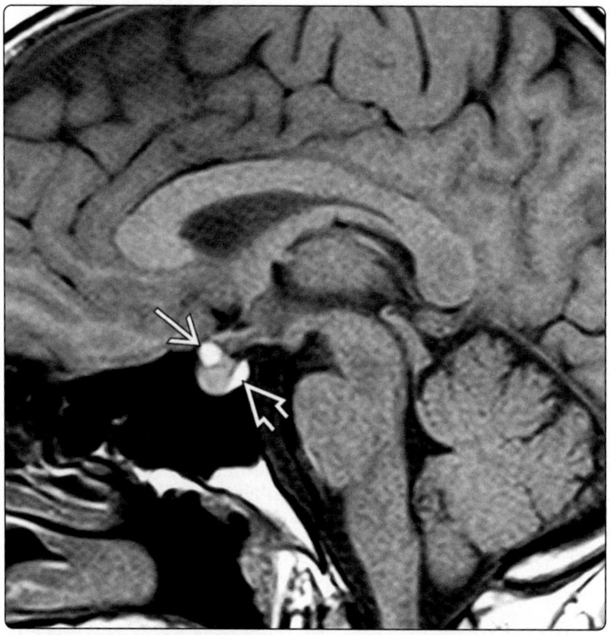

(25-36) Sagittal T1WI in an asymptomatic patient shows a tiny hyperintense suprasellar mass ➡ that appears separate from the pituitary gland "bright spot" of the neurohypophysis ➡. This is presumed Rathke cleft cyst.

HH-associated seizures are highly variable, age dependent, and often refractory to treatment. Gelastic seizures (ictal laughing fits) are the most common type and vary from facial grinning to intense contractions of the diaphragm accompanied by body shaking. These gelastic seizures are more common with sessile tumors, whereas precocious puberty is more often present in patients with small pedunculated lesions. Patients may present with both seizures and precocious puberty.

Anomalies associated with HH include holoprosencephaly. Patients with Pallister-Hall syndrome have digital malformations and other midline (epiglottis/larynx) and cardiac, renal, or anal anomalies in addition to the HH.

Natural History. HHs generally remain stable in size. Hormonal suppressive therapy, i.e., luteinizing hormone-releasing hormone agonists, is helpful in some cases. Failure of medical therapy or rapid lesion growth may necessitate surgery.

Imaging

General Features. A nonenhancing hypothalamic mass between the infundibular stalk and mammillary bodies is the classic imaging appearance of HH **(25-30)**.

CT Findings. NECT scan shows a homogeneous suprasellar mass that is isodense to slightly hypodense compared with brain. Intralesional cysts may be present in larger HHs. HHs do not enhance on CECT.

MR Findings. Pedunculated HHs are shaped like a collar button on sagittal T1WI, extending inferiorly into the suprasellar cistern. Signal intensity is usually isointense to normal gray matter on T1WI and iso- to slightly hyperintense on T2/FLAIR. The degree of T2 hyperintensity is directly related to the proportion of glial versus neuronal tissue in the lesion.

HHs do not enhance following contrast administration. If there is enhancement in the lesion, consider a glial tumor.

MRS shows mildly decreased NAA and slightly increased choline, consistent with reduced neuronal density and relative gliosis. Myoinositol is elevated, which is consistent with an increased glial component compared with normal brain.

Differential Diagnosis

The differential diagnoses of HH are craniopharyngioma and chiasmatic/hypothalamic astrocytoma. Clinical features are very helpful in distinguishing HH from these lesions.

Craniopharyngioma is the most common suprasellar mass in children. Over 90% of craniopharyngiomas are cystic, 90% calcify, and 90% show nodular and rim enhancement.

Optic pathway/hypothalamic pilocytic astrocytoma is the second most common pediatric suprasellar mass. Astrocytomas are hyperintense on T2/FLAIR and often enhance on T1 C+.

Rathke Cleft Cyst

Terminology

Rathke cleft cyst (RCC) is a benign endodermal cyst of the sellar region.

Etiology

RCCs are thought to arise from remnants of the fetal Rathke pouch. When the embryonic stomodeum (the primitive oral cavity) invaginates and extends dorsally, it forms the endoderm-lined craniopharyngeal duct. It meets an outgrowth from the third ventricle, giving rise to the hypophysis. The anterior wall of the pouch forms the anterior lobe and pars tuberalis, whereas the posterior wall forms the pars intermedia. The interposed lumen forms a narrow "cleft"—Rathke cleft—that normally regresses by the twelfth gestational week. If it persists and expands, it forms an RCC.

Pathology

Location. RCCs are limited to the sellar region. Approximately 40% are completely intrasellar, generally positioned between the anterior lobe and pars intermedia, whereas 60% are suprasellar **(25-35)** **(25-36)**.

Size and Number. Most symptomatic RCCs are 5-15 mm in diameter. Occasionally, an RCC becomes very large and can compress the optic chiasm and adjacent brain and erode into the skull base. An enlarged sella turcica may be seen with RCCs.

Gross Pathology. RCCs are smoothly lobulated, sharply marginated cysts. Cyst contents vary from clear and CSF-like to thick yellow inspissated mucoid material.

Microscopic Features. RCCs are endodermal (not ectodermal) cysts. They are lined by a single layer of ciliated cuboidal or columnar epithelium together with various amounts of goblet cells. On immunohistochemical studies, RCCs express cytokeratins 8 and 20.

Clinical Issues

Demographics. Although RCCs occur at all ages, mean age at presentation is 45 years.

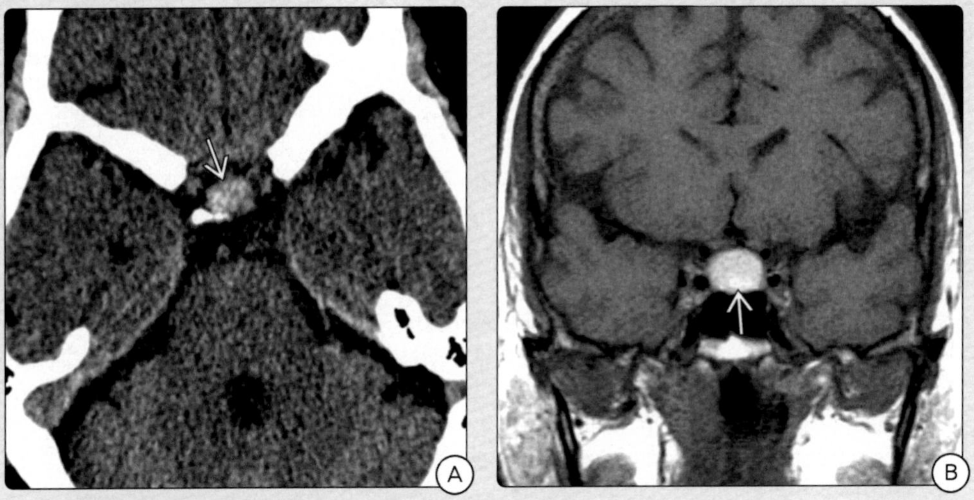

(25-37A) NECT scan shows a hyperdense mass projecting superiorly into the suprasellar cistern ➡. Only 5-10% of Rathke cleft cysts are hyperdense on CT. The lack of calcification helps differentiate a Rathke cleft cyst from a craniopharyngioma. (25-37B) Coronal T1WI scan in the same patient shows that the mass ➡ is homogeneously hyperintense.

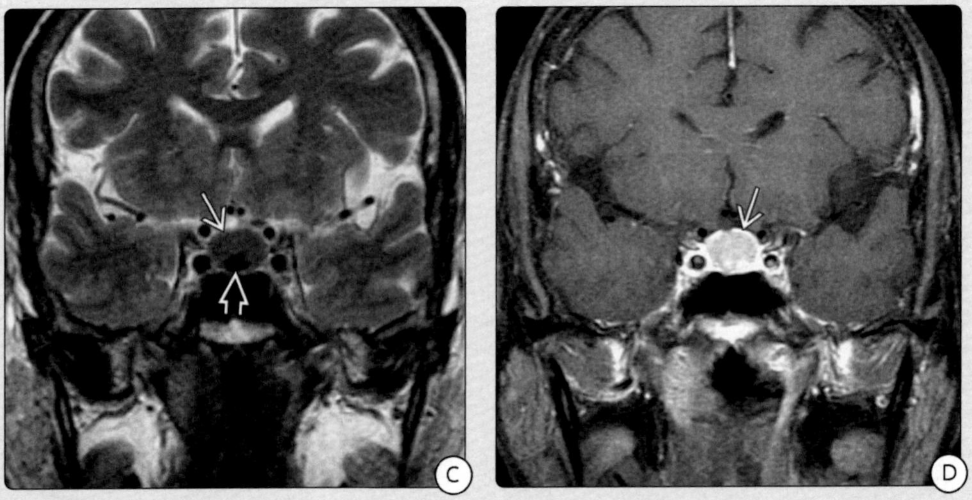

(25-37C) T2WI in the same patient shows that the cyst ➡ is hypointense and contains an even more hypointense intracystic nodule ➡. An intracystic nodule may be seen in up to 75% of patients with Rathke cleft cyst. (25-37D) A rim ("claw") of enhancing pituitary gland ➡ is seen around the cyst. Rathke cleft cyst with intracystic nodule was found at surgery. Lack of enhancement within the cyst and an intracystic nodule allow accurate preoperative diagnosis.

Presentation. Most RCCs are asymptomatic and discovered incidentally at imaging or autopsy. Symptomatic RCCs cause pituitary dysfunction (~70%), visual disturbances (~45-55%), and headache (~50%).

Occasionally RCCs present with "cyst apoplexy," usually—but not invariably—caused by sudden intracystic hemorrhage. Symptoms are generally indistinguishable from those of pituitary apoplexy.

Natural History. Most RCCs are stable and do not change in size or intensity characteristics. RCCs do not undergo malignant degeneration.

Imaging

CT Findings. NECT scans show a well-delineated round or ovoid mass within or just above the sella turcica. Three-quarters of RCCs are hypodense on NECT, whereas 20% are mixed hypo- and isodense. Between 5 and 10% are hyperdense **(25-37A)**. Calcification is uncommon compared with craniopharyngioma.

MR Findings. Signal intensity varies with cyst contents. Half of all RCCs are hypointense on T1WI, and half are hyperintense **(25-37B)**. The majority of RCCs are hyperintense on T2WI **(25-38A)**, whereas 25-30% are iso- to hypointense **(25-37C)**. Careful inspection reveals an intracystic nodule in 40-75% of cases **(25-37C)** **(25-38A)**.

RCCs are almost always hyperintense on FLAIR **(25-39A)**. An enhancing rim ("claw" sign) of compressed pituitary gland can often be seen surrounding the nonenhancing cyst **(25-37D)** **(25-38B)** **(25-39B)**.

Differential Diagnosis

The major differential diagnosis of RCC is **craniopharyngioma**. Floccular, rim, or nodular calcifications are common in craniopharyngioma, whereas RCCs rarely calcify. The rim or

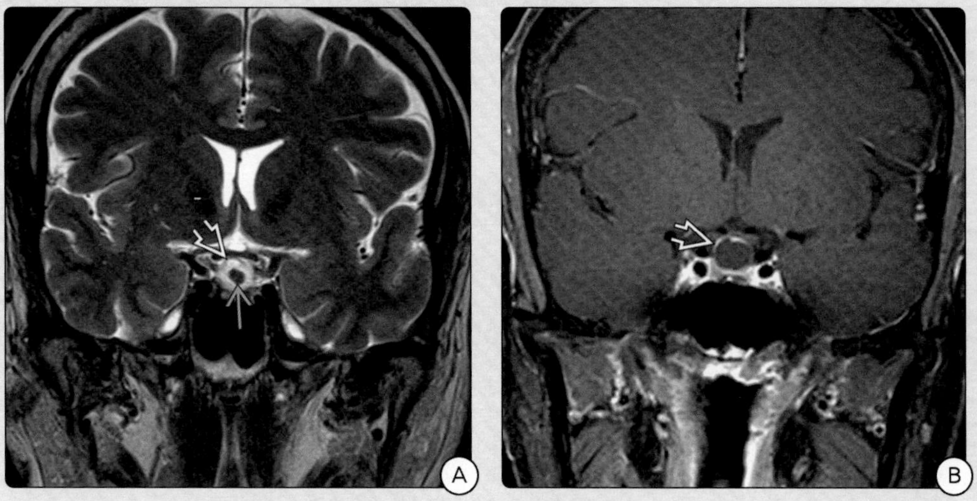

***(25-38A)** Coronal T2WI in a 62y woman with headaches shows a hyperintense intra- and suprasellar cyst ➡ with a hypointense intracystic nodule ⇨. **(25-38B)** Coronal T1 C+ MR in the same patient shows a cystic suprasellar mass with thin peripheral enhancement ➡ representing a "claw sign" related to compression of the adjacent normal pituitary gland by the Rathke cleft cyst.*

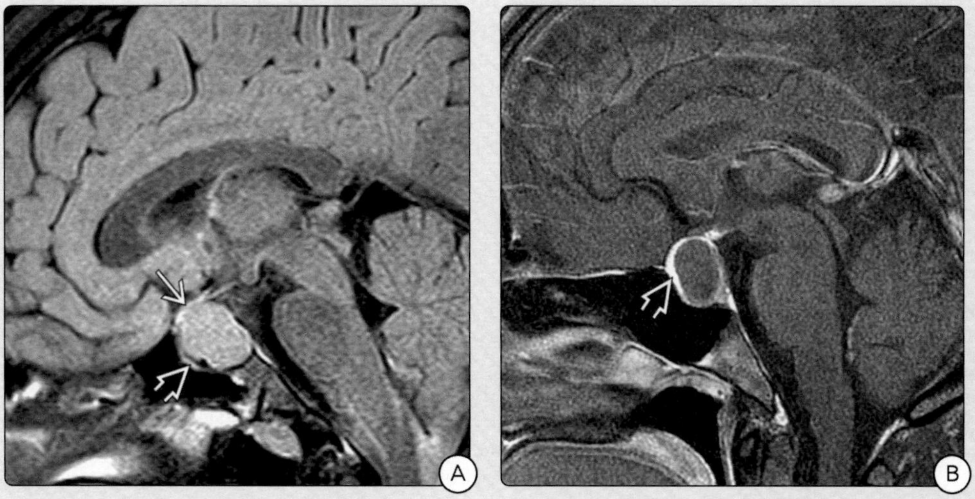

***(25-39A)** Sagittal FLAIR MR in a 19y woman with visual symptoms shows a hyperintense sellar and suprasellar mass ➡. Rathke cleft cysts are typically T2 and FLAIR hyperintense. Note the superior displacement of the optic chiasm ➡. **(25-39B)** Sagittal T1 C+ MR in a 42y patient with a Rathke cleft cyst shows the classic "claw sign" ➡ of compressed pituitary gland wrapping around the anterior aspect of the cyst.*

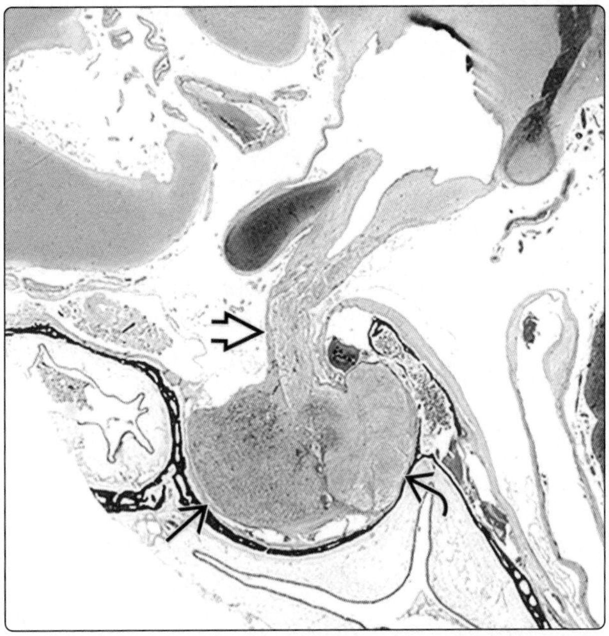

***(25-40)** Sagittal section through the pituitary gland shows the anterior ⇨ and posterior ⇨ pituitary lobes, as well as the infundibular stalk ⇨ connecting the hypothalamus to the neurohypophysis. (Courtesy A. Ersen, MD, B. Scheithauer, MD.)*

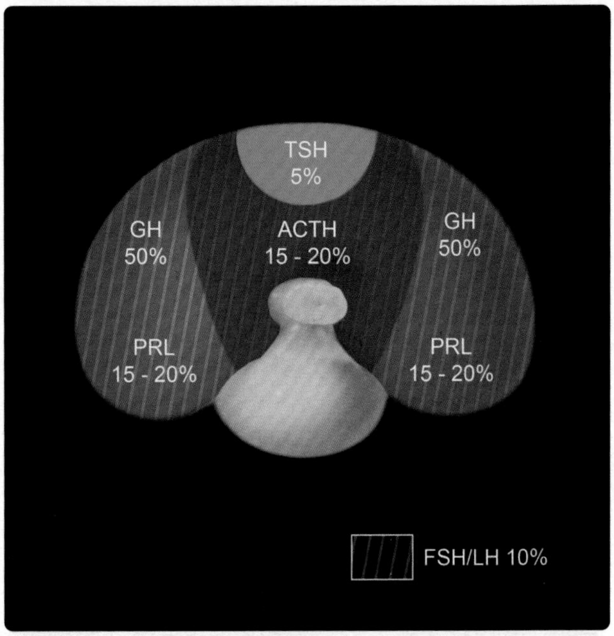

***(25-41)** Graphic depicts location of anterior pituitary lobe cells. Lateral wings contain mainly GH and PRL cells. Corticotrophs (ACTH) and thyrotrophs (TSH) are in the median mucoid wedge. FSH/LH cells are distributed diffusely.*

nodular enhancement in craniopharyngioma is generally thicker and more irregular than the "claw" of enhancing pituitary gland that surrounds the nonenhancing RCC.

A cystic pituitary adenoma—especially a **nonfunctioning cystic microadenoma**—can be difficult to distinguish from a small intrasellar RCC. Both rarely calcify; both are common etiologies for pituitary "incidentalomas" on MR scans. Neither requires treatment, so the distinction is largely academic.

Other nonneoplastic cysts that can occur in the sellar region are dermoid (fat, calcification common) and epidermoid cysts (rarely midline, usually CSF-like, DWI hyperintense), arachnoid cysts (larger, CSF-like, lacking an intracystic nodule), and inflammatory cysts (e.g., neurocysticercosis; multiple far more prevalent than solitary cysts).

RATHKE CLEFT CYST

Etiology and Pathology
- Remnant of embryonic Rathke cleft
- Intrasellar (40%), suprasellar (60%)
- Contents vary (CSF-like to thick mucoid)
- Endodermal lining + goblet cells

Imaging
- Hypointense (50%), hyperintense (50%) on T1WI
- Hyperintense on T2/FLAIR
- Look for
  - Intracystic nodule (40-75%)
  - "Claw" of enhancement representing stretched normal pituitary gland

Neoplasms

Pituitary Adenomas

Terminology

Pituitary adenomas are adenohypophysial tumors composed of secretory cells that produce pituitary hormones **(25-40)** **(25-41)**. **Microadenomas** are defined as tumors ≤ 10 mm in diameter, whereas larger adenomas are designated **macroadenomas** **(25-42)** **(25-43)** **(25-44)** **(25-45)**.

Etiology

General Concepts. Cells with multipotent progenitor/stem-cell-like properties have been identified in the adult pituitary gland and may play a key role in tumorigenesis. Alterations in the normal microenvironment of pituitary stem cells may trigger uncoordinated proliferation and subsequent formation of pituitary adenomas.

Genetics. Adenomagenesis is a multistep, multicausal process that includes both initiation and progression phases. A number of activated oncogenes and loss of tumor suppressor gene functions are involved. In addition, several endocrine factors at either the hypothalamic or systemic level may induce adenohypophysial cell proliferation.

Mutations in the aryl hydrocarbon receptor-interacting protein gene (*AIP*) have been identified in patients with familial isolated pituitary adenoma syndrome (see below) but are rare in patients with sporadic pituitary adenomas.

Familial Pituitary Tumor Syndromes. Most pituitary adenomas are sporadic tumors and occur in adults. Approximately 5% of all pituitary adenomas are familial.

Four recognized inherited familial tumor syndromes with specific identified genetic defects are associated with pituitary adenomas: multiple endocrine neoplasia type 1 (MEN1), Carney complex, McCune-Albright syndrome (MAS), and familial isolated pituitary adenoma (FIPA) syndrome.

MEN1 is an autosomal-dominant disease with highly penetrant germline mutations that predisposes patients to develop tumors in hormone-secreting cells. MEN1 is characterized by combinations of more than 20 different endocrine and nonendocrine tumors. Pituitary tumors occur in 15-40% of MEN1 patients. MEN1-associated adenomas are often plurihormonal (most commonly secreting prolactin and growth hormone, GH), larger, and more invasive neoplasms.

Carney complex is associated with spotty skin pigmentation, myxomas, endocrine tumors, and schwannomas. Adrenal involvement causing adrenocorticotrophic hormone (ACTH)-independent Cushing syndrome is seen in one-third to one-half of patients with Carney complex. GH-producing pituitary tumors are seen in 10%.

MAS is defined by the triad of gonadotropin-independent sexual precocity, café au lait skin lesions, and fibrous dysplasia. Tumors or nodular hyperplasia of a number of endocrine glands lead to hypersecretory syndromes such as acromegaly, hyperprolactinemia, and Cushing syndrome. MAS is caused by a postzygotic mutation in the *GNAS* gene.

FIPA is a recently described condition in which affected family members develop only pituitary tumors. It includes familial pituitary tumors that are *not* associated with MEN1 and Carney complex.

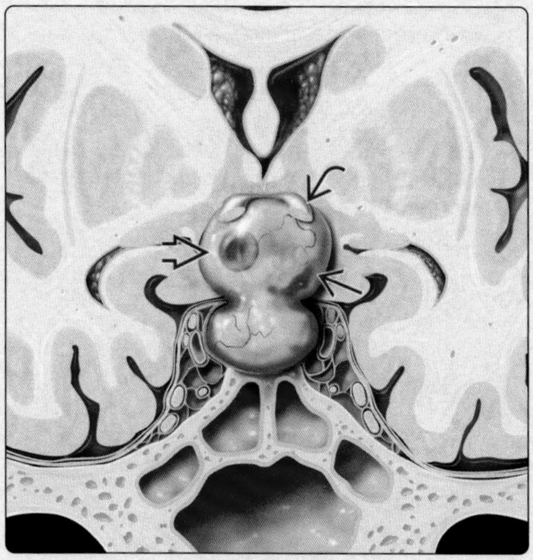

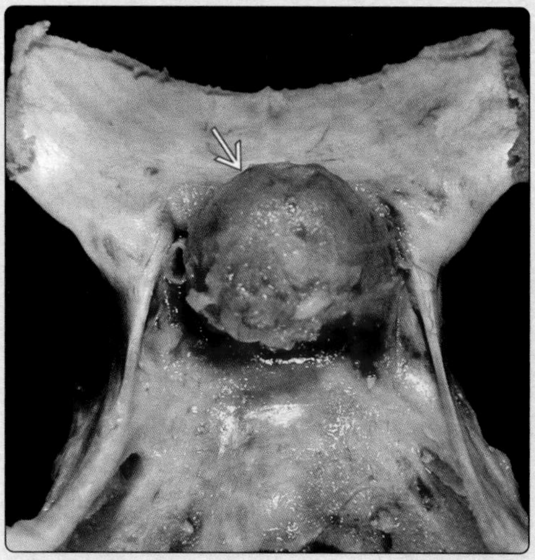

***(25-42)** Coronal graphic shows a snowman-shaped or "figure eight" sellar and suprasellar mass ⇨. Small foci of hemorrhage ⇨ and cystic change ⇨ are present within the lesion. The pituitary gland cannot be identified separately from the mass; indeed, the gland is the mass. **(25-43)** Autopsy specimen shows a macroadenoma ➡ protruding superiorly into the suprasellar cistern. (Courtesy R. Hewlett, MD.)*

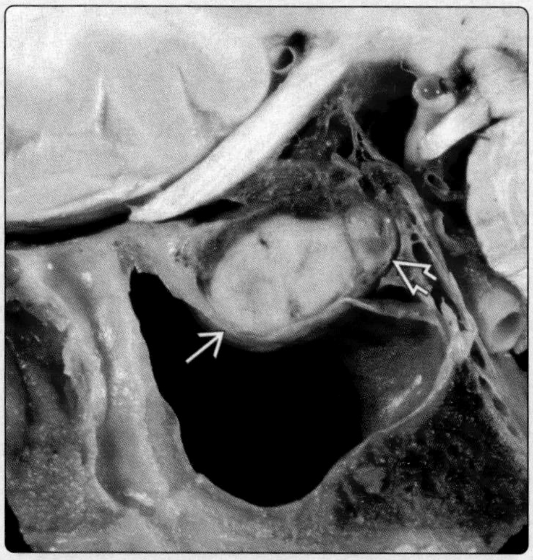

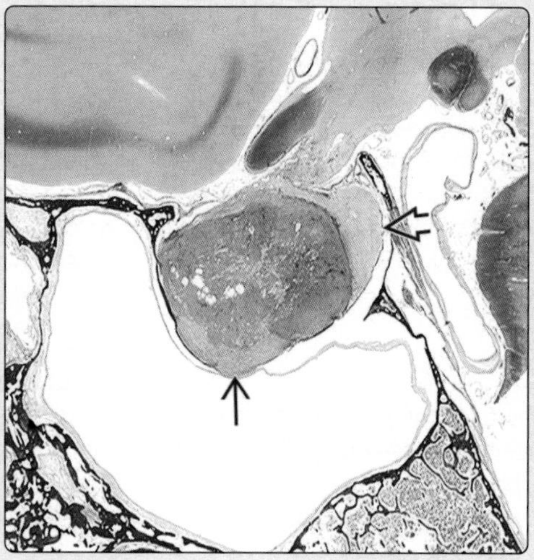

***(25-44)** Pituitary adenomas ➡ are well-circumscribed masses that compress and displace the normal pituitary gland ➡. (Courtesy A. Erson, MD, B. Scheithauer, MD.) **(25-45)** Sagittal low-power photomicrograph shows a prolactinoma eroding the sellar floor ⇨, compressing and displacing the normal pituitary gland posteriorly ⇨. (Courtesy A. Ersen, MD, B. Scheitauer, MD.)*

Functional Classification of Pituitary Adenomas

Adenoma Type	%	M:F	IHC Profile	Clinical Presentation
Sparsely granulated PRL cell adenoma	27.00	1.0:2.5	PRL	Female patients: amenorrhea-galactorrhea syndrome; male patients: sellar mass, hypogonadism
Densely granulated PRL cell adenoma	0.04	N/A	PRL	
Densely granulated GH cell adenoma	7.10	1.0:0.7	GH, α-subunit (PRL, TSH, LH, FSH)	Acromegaly (adult) or gigantism (child)
Sparsely granulated GH cell adenoma	6.20	1.0:1.1	GH (PRL, α-subunit)	Acromegaly (adult) or gigantism (child)
Mixed GH-PRL cell adenoma	3.50	1.0:1.1	GH, PRL (α-subunit, TSH)	Acromegaly + hyperprolactinemia
Mammosomatotroph adenoma	1.20	1.0:1.1	GH, PRL (α-subunit, TSH)	Acromegaly + hyperprolactinemia
Acidophil stem cell adenoma	1.60	1.0:1.5	PRL, GH	Hyperprolactinemia; acromegaly is uncommon
Densely granulated corticotroph adenoma	9.60	1.0:5.4	ACTH (LH, α-subunit)	Cushing disease, Nelson syndrome
Sparsely granulated corticotroph adenoma	Rare	N/A	ACTH	Cushing disease, Nelson syndrome
Thyrotroph adenoma	1.10	1.0:1.3	TSH (GH, PRL, α-subunit)	Hyperthyroidism
Gonadotroph adenoma	9.80	1.0:0.8	FSH, LH, α-subunit (ACTH)	Nonfunctioning sellar mass
Silent "corticotroph" adenoma subtype 1	1.50	1.0:1.7	ACTH	Nonfunctioning sellar mass, pituitary
Silent "corticotroph" adenoma subtype 2	2.00	1.0:0.2	β-endorphin, ACTH	Nonfunctioning sellar mass
Silent adenoma subtype 3	1.40	1.0:1.1	Any combination of anterior pituitary hormones	Female patients: mimics PRL-secreting adenoma; male patients: nonfunctioning sellar mass
Null cell adenoma	12.40	1.0:0.7	Immunoreactive (FSH, LH, TSH, α-subunit)	Nonfunctioning sellar mass
Oncocytoma	13.40	1.0:0.5	Immunonegative (FSH, LH, TSH, α-subunit)	Nonfunctioning sellar mass
Unclassified adenomas	1.80	N/A	N/A	Variable

(Table 25-1) *ACTH = adrenocorticotrophic hormone; FSH = follicle-stimulating hormone; GH = growth hormone; LH = luteinizing hormone; N/A = not available; PRL = prolactin; TSH = thyroid-stimulating hormone.*

Prolactinomas are found in 40% of all FIPA patients, somatotropinomas in 30%, and nonsecreting adenomas in 13%. In general, pituitary tumors in FIPA present earlier than sporadic pituitary adenomas, are significantly larger, and more often demonstrate cavernous sinus invasion.

Two FIPA subgroups have been identified based on genetic and phenotypic features. In 15-25% of cases, affected families have *AIP* gene mutations and autosomal-dominant inheritance. They typically develop growth hormone-secreting adenomas and prolactinomas, often in childhood. The second, much larger group has adult-onset disease and more varied types of adenoma. To date, no causative gene has been identified.

Pathology

Location. With rare exceptions, adenomas arise within the sella turcica. Reported ectopic sites include the sphenoid sinus (the most common site), nasopharynx, third ventricle, and suprasellar cistern. Such cases are designated **ectopic pituitary adenoma**.

Adenomas arise from the adenohypophysis. Specific sublocation follows the normal distribution of peptide-containing cells. Prolactinomas and growth-hormone secreting tumors—the two most common pituitary adenomas—tend to arise laterally within the adenohypophysis, whereas thyroid-stimulating hormone (TSH)- and ACTH-secreting tumors are more often midline.

Size and Number. Adenomas vary in size from microscopic lesions **(25-50A)** **(25-50B)** to giant tumors more than 5 cm that invade the skull base and extend into multiple cranial fossae. Pituitary adenomas are usually solitary lesions. Multiple synchronous pituitary adenomas are unusual. "Double" or even "triple" adenomas are found in 1% of autopsies but rarely diagnosed on preoperative MR scans.

Gross Pathology. Macroadenomas are red-brown, lobulated masses that often bulge upward through the opening of diaphragma sella **(25-43)** or, less commonly, extend laterally toward the cavernous sinus. Approximately half of macroadenomas contain cysts and/or hemorrhagic foci.

Microscopic Features. Histologic examination shows a uniform population of round, polygonal, or elongated cells

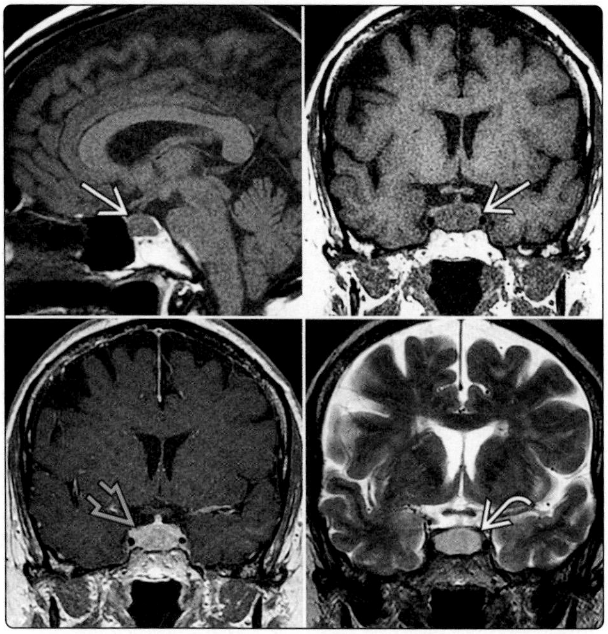

(25-46) Series of MRs shows a small macroadenoma that measured 12 mm in height. The mass is isointense with GM ➡ on T1- and T2WI ➡ and enhances strongly and uniformly ➡.

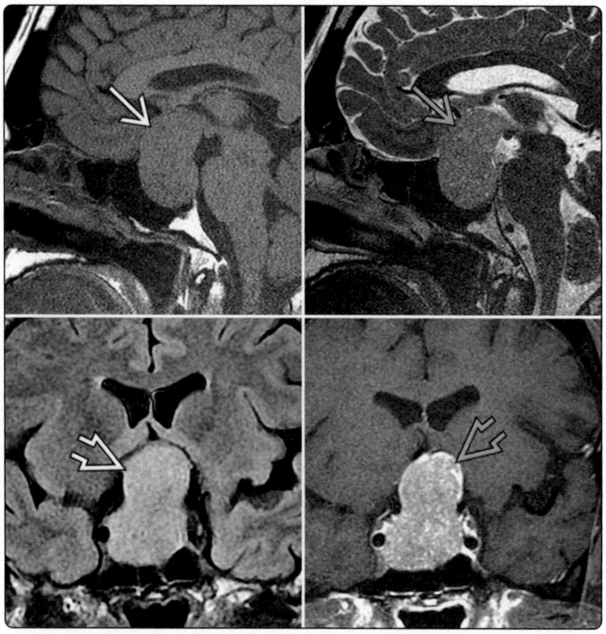

(25-47) Sagittal T1WI ➡, T2WI ➡, FLAIR ➡, and T1 C+ ➡ show a very large "snowman" or "figure eight" sellar and suprasellar mass. The pituitary gland cannot be identified as separate from the mass (macroadenoma).

with moderately abundant cytoplasm and inconspicuous nucleoli. Cellular atypia is uncommon, and mitoses are rare.

Staging, Grading, and Classification. Adenoma classification is now based on immunohistochemical profile and clinical presentation. The "tinctorial" characteristics of cells as seen on H&E preparations ("acidophilic," "basophilic," "chromophobic") are not precisely correlated with specific hormone production and are no longer used as diagnostic terms.

Pituitary adenomas are almost all WHO grade I tumors. MIB-1 and p53 immunoreactivity correlate with tumor invasion but do not indicate malignant transformation. Most adenomas are "typical" lesions with both MIB-1 and p53 under 3%. Adenomas with elevated MIB-1 greater than 3%, increased mitoses, and extensive p53 staining are considered atypical adenomas and correlate with early recurrence and more rapid regrowth **(25-54)**.

Clinical Issues

Epidemiology. Pituitary adenomas are among the most common of all CNS neoplasms, accounting for 10-15% of primary intracranial neoplasms. Approximately 60% of patients undergoing surgery have macroadenomas, and 40% have microadenomas. However, microadenomas are much more common than macroadenomas at autopsy. Clinically silent incidental microadenomas are identified in 15-25% of autopsies.

Demographics. Peak age of presentation is between the fourth and seventh decades. Only 2% of pituitary adenomas are found in children. Most of these occur in adolescent girls. PAs in prepubescent boys are very rare.

Presentation. Almost two-thirds of pituitary adenomas secrete a hormone (~ 40-50%% prolactin, 10% GH, 6% corticotropin, 1% thyrotropin) and cause typical hypersecretory syndromes. The remaining one-third do not produce a hormone and are referred to as nonfunctioning (or nonsecreting or null cell) adenomas **(Table 25-1)**.

Female patients with prolactinomas present with amenorrhea-galactorrhea syndrome, whereas male patients present with hypogonadism and impotence. GH-secreting tumors cause acromegaly in adults and gigantism in children. Patients with corticotroph tumors present with Cushing disease or Nelson syndrome (rapid enlargement of an adenoma following bilateral adrenalectomy). TSH-secreting adenomas cause hyperthyroidism.

Macroadenomas generally present with mass effect. Headache and visual disturbances are common. Diabetes insipidus is rarely associated with pituitary adenoma, so its presence should prompt consideration of an alternative diagnosis.

Natural History and Treatment. Although pituitary adenoma growth rates are quite variable, most enlarge slowly over a period of years. Malignant transformation is exceptionally rare.

Treatment options are numerous and include surgical resection, medical management, stereotactic radiosurgery, and conventional radiation therapy. Management strategy should be individualized for each patient.

Imaging

General Features. A sellar or combined intra- and suprasellar mass that cannot be identified separately from the pituitary

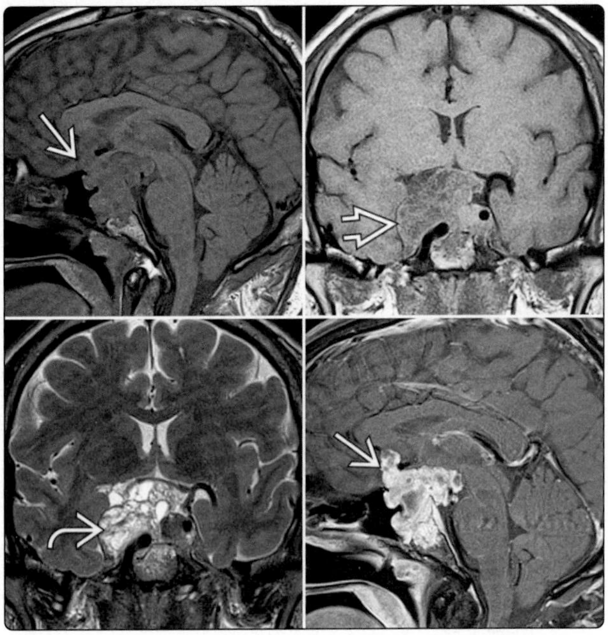

(25-48) Lobulated, invasive sellar/suprasellar mass ➡ has multiple medium/small-sized T2 hyperintense cysts ➡. Macroadenoma also invades the right cavernous sinus ➡.

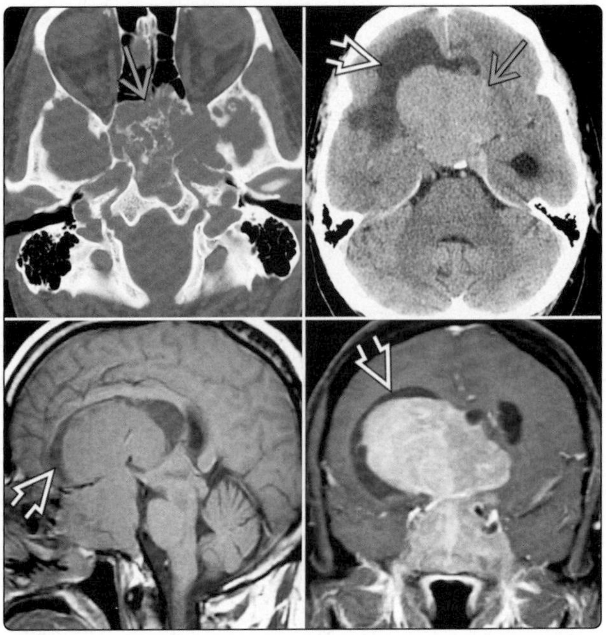

(25-49) Bone CT (top left), CECT (top right) show a huge invasive pituitary macroadenoma ➡. CECT, sagittal T1WI, coronal T1 C+ FS all show trapped pools of CSF ➡ adjacent to the tumor. These are nonneoplastic peritumoral cysts.

gland—the mass *is* the gland—is the most characteristic imaging finding.

CT Findings. Bone CT may show an enlarged, remodeled sella turcica. The lamina dura of the sellar floor is generally intact. Note, however, that "giant" pituitary adenomas may erode and extensively invade the skull base, mimicking metastasis or aggressive infection.

Pituitary adenomas demonstrate variable attenuation on NECT scans. Macroadenomas are usually isodense with gray matter, but cysts (15-20%) and hemorrhage (10%) are common. Calcification is rare (less than 2%). Moderate but heterogeneous enhancement of macroadenomas is typical on CECT, but small microadenomas may be invisible.

MR Findings

Macroadenomas. Macroadenomas are usually isointense with cortex **(25-46)** **(25-47)**. The posterior pituitary "bright spot" is absent (20%) or displaced into the supradiaphragmatic cistern (80%) on T1-weighted sagittal scans. Small cysts and hemorrhagic foci are common. Fluid-fluid levels can be present but are more common in patients with pituitary apoplexy.

Adenomas are generally isointense with gray matter on T2WI but can also demonstrate heterogeneous signal intensity **(25-48)**. Hyperintensity along the optic pathways on T2/FLAIR occurs in 15-20% of cases in which macroadenomas compress the optic chiasm. Hemorrhagic adenomas "bloom" on T2*.

Most macroadenomas enhance strongly but heterogeneously on T1 C+ **(25-49)**. Subtle dural thickening (a dural "tail") is present in 5-10% of cases.

Microadenomas. Unless they hemorrhage, small microadenomas may be inapparent on standard nonenhanced sequences. Many microadenomas appear slightly hypointense on T1 C+ **(25-51)** **(25-52)**. Others enhance more strongly and may become isointense with the enhancing pituitary gland, rendering them virtually invisible.

Microadenomas enhance more slowly than the normal pituitary tissue. This discrepancy in enhancement timing can be exploited by using thin-section coronal dynamic contrast-enhanced scans. Fast image acquisition during contrast administration can often discriminate between the slowly enhancing microadenoma and rapidly enhancing normal gland. Between 10-30% of microadenomas are seen only on dynamic T1 C+ imaging **(25-53)**.

Angiography. CTA in patients with suprasellar extension of macroadenoma may show the supraclinoid internal carotid and anterior choroidal arteries displaced laterally. DSA may demonstrate an enlarged meningohypophyseal trunk with prolonged vascular "stain" or "blush" in the tumor.

Cavernous/inferior petrosal venous sampling may be helpful in evaluating patients with ACTH-dependent Cushing syndrome.

Differential Diagnosis

The differential diagnosis of pituitary adenoma varies with size and patient demographics.

Pituitary Macroadenoma. The major differential diagnosis of pituitary macroadenoma is **pituitary hyperplasia**. Between 25 and 50% of endocrinologically normal women who are 18-35 years old have an upwardly convex pituitary gland on MR or CT examination. The height of the gland is usually at least 10 mm unless the patient is pregnant or lactating. Less commonly, end-organ failure (such as hypothyroidism) results in compensatory pituitary enlargement. *As adenomas are very rare in children, if a prepubescent female patient or young male patient has an "adenoma-looking" pituitary gland, endocrine work-up is mandatory!*

Tumors that can resemble pituitary adenoma include meningioma, metastasis, and craniopharyngioma. Meningioma and metastasis are very rare in children. **Meningioma** of the diaphragma sellae can usually be identified as clearly separate from the pituitary gland below. Additionally, a dural tail and diffuse avid enhancement may be seen. True isolated intrasellar meningiomas are very rare.

Metastasis to the stalk and/or pituitary gland from an extracranial primary neoplasm is uncommon. Lung and breast are the most common sources. Most pituitary metastases are secondary to spread from adjacent bone or the cavernous sinus, generally occurring as a late manifestation of known systemic tumor. Hematogeneous metastases to the pituitary gland do occur but are rare. CNS metastases elsewhere in the brain are common but not invariably present.

Craniopharyngioma is the most common suprasellar tumor of childhood, whereas pituitary adenomas in children are rare. Craniopharyngiomas in middle-aged adults are typically solid papillary tumors that do not calcify as the adamantinomatous ones do. Often in adults with craniopharyngioma, the pituitary gland can be identified as anatomically separate from the mass.

Pituitary carcinoma is exceedingly rare (see below). Because of this rarity, even the most aggressive-looking pituitary tumors are statistically far more likely to be adenomas than carcinomas.

Nonneoplastic entities that can mimic macroadenoma include aneurysm and hypophysitis. An **aneurysm** arises eccentrically from the circle of Willis and is usually not in the midline directly above the sella. Paramedian saccular aneurysms are hyperdense on NECT and may demonstrate rim calcification, whereas pituitary adenomas rarely calcify. A "flow void" with or without laminated clot along the aneurysm wall is common on MR.

Hypophysitis is much less common than macroadenoma but can appear virtually identical to an adenoma on imaging studies. Lymphocytic hypophysitis—the most common type—typically occurs in peripartum or postpartum female patients or as an autoimmune hypophysitis in patients treated with immunomodulating therapies (e.g., ipilimumab for metastatic malignant melanoma).

Pituitary Microadenoma. Pituitary microadenoma may be difficult to distinguish from incidental nonneoplastic intrapituitary cysts such as **Rathke cleft cyst** or **pars intermedia cyst**. Microadenomas enhance; cysts are seen as nonenhancing foci within the intensely enhancing pituitary gland. A small hemorrhagic microadenoma may appear identical to a Rathke cleft cyst that contains proteinaceous fluid, as both are hyperintense on T1WI.

PITUITARY ADENOMA: IMAGING AND DDx

CT

- Sella usually enlarged, remodeled, cortex intact
- Invasive adenomas erode, destroy bone
- Majority are isodense with brain
  - Cysts (15-20%)
  - Hemorrhage (10%)
  - Ca++ rare (1-2%)

MR

- Usually isointense with cortex
- Heterogeneous signal intensity common (cysts, hemorrhage)
- Strong, heterogeneous enhancement
- 10-30% of microadenomas seen only with dynamic T1 C+

Differential Diagnosis

- Pituitary hyperplasia (know patient age, sex!)
  - Physiologic (young/pregnant/lactating female patients)
  - Nonphysiologic (end-organ failure)
- Other tumors
  - Meningioma, craniopharyngioma, metastasis
  - Pituitary carcinoma *exceptionally* rare
  - Aggressive-looking adenoma is almost never malignant!
- Nonneoplastic lesions
  - Aneurysm
  - Hypophysitis

Pituitary Carcinoma

Pituitary carcinoma (PCa) is very rare, representing less than 0.2% of all operated adenohypophysial neoplasms. Its estimated prevalence is 4 per 1 million person-years. Most PCas arise as metastases from multiple recurring invasive adenomas; de novo malignancy is unusual. Survival is inversely proportionate with increasing age.

Conventional histologic criteria for malignancy (necrosis, nuclear atypia, pleomorphism, mitotic activity) are insufficient for diagnosis. A true PCa must exhibit either frank brain invasion or CSF/systemic metastases **(25-55)**.

PCa has no unique imaging features and may be indistinguishable from an invasive but histologically typical adenoma. Only documentation of craniospinal metastases or systemic tumor spread can confirm the diagnosis.

Pituitary Blastoma

Pituitary blastoma is a recently described pituitary tumor in neonates and infants characterized by large glandular structures that resemble Rathke epithelium and adenohypophysial cells. Arrested pituitary development and unchecked proliferation are the likely etiology of this unusual tumor.

Histology shows small undifferentiated blastema-like cells interspersed with large pituitary secretory cells. Mitotic activity is variable. Imaging findings are nonspecific and

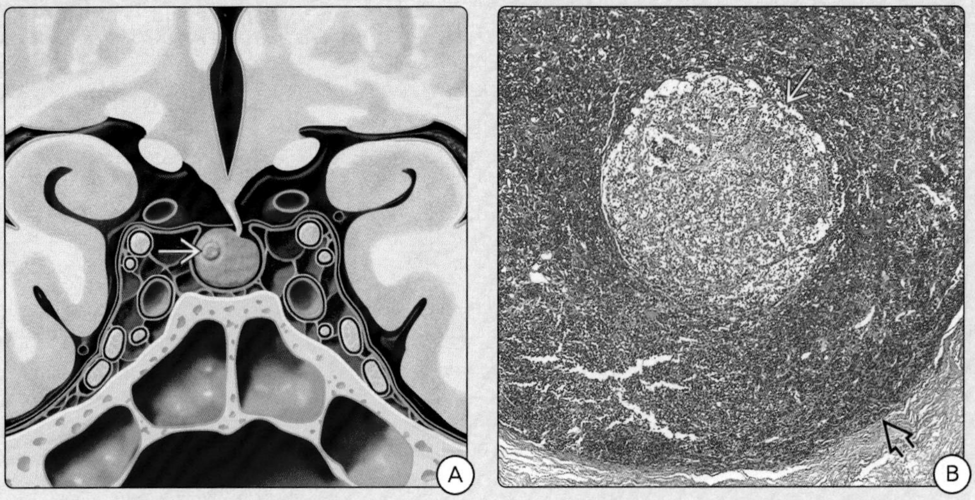

(25-50A) *Coronal graphic depicts a pituitary microadenoma ➡.* ***(25-50B)*** *Low-power photomicrograph of a pituitary gland at autopsy shows a small nonsecreting microadenoma ➡ surrounded by the normal adenohypophysis ⇨. Incidental asymptomatic microadenomas are common on imaging studies and at autopsy. (Courtesy J. Townsend, MD.)*

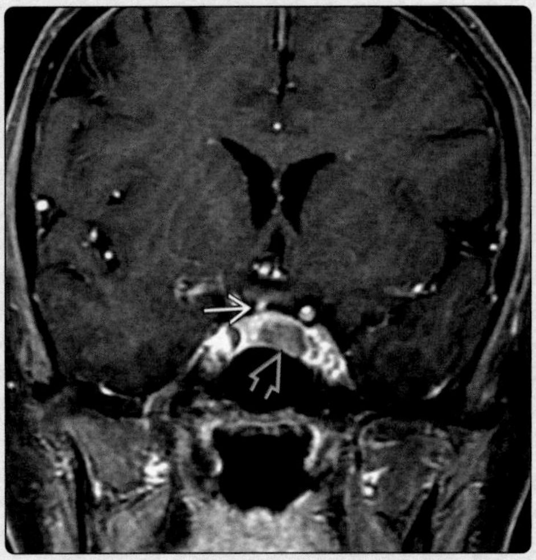

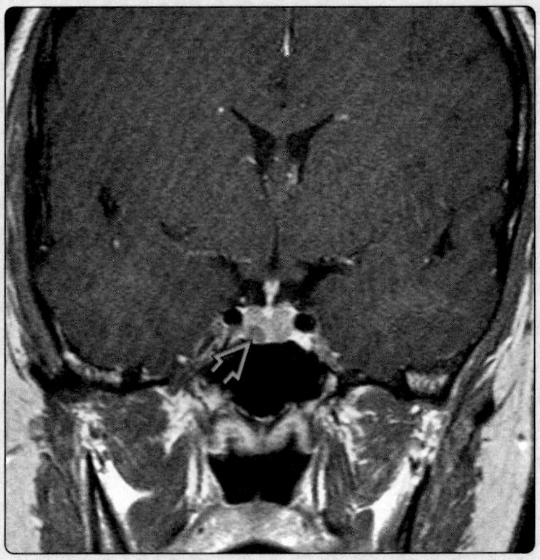

(25-51) *Coronal T1 C+ MR in a patient with amenorrhea and elevated prolactin shows a mass in the left pituitary gland ⇨ and displacement of the infundibulum ➡. The mass enhances more slowly than normal gland and appears relatively hypointense.* ***(25-52)*** *Coronal T1 C+ MR in a 36y woman with Cushing syndrome shows a right pituitary mass ⇨ related to her pituitary microadenoma. ACTH-secreting tumors are often centrally located within the gland.*

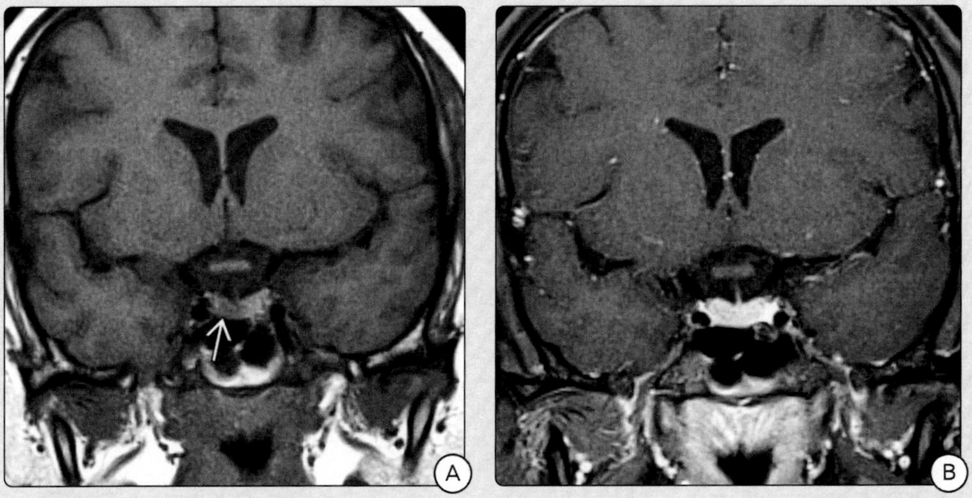

(25-53A) *Coronal T1WI in a patient with headache, amenorrhea, elevated prolactin demonstrates a hypointense mass ➡ in the right lateral pituitary gland.* ***(25-53B)*** *Standard T1 C+ FS in the same patient shows no abnormality. Dynamic enhanced MR technique may show an adenoma, as it enhances more slowly than the normal pituitary gland, which lacks a blood-brain barrier. Up to 30% of microadenomas may only be seen on dynamic T1 C+ MR.*

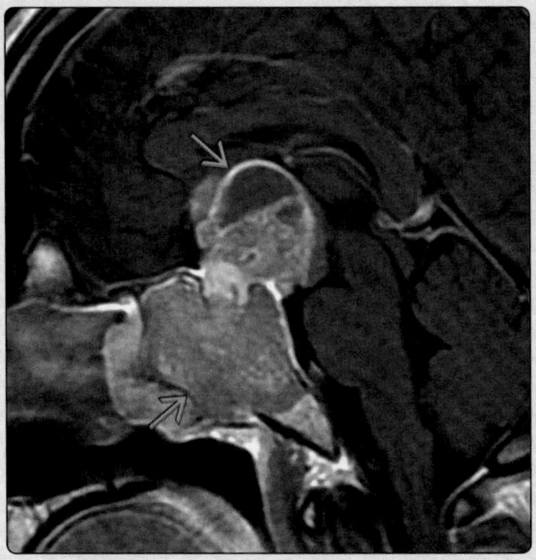
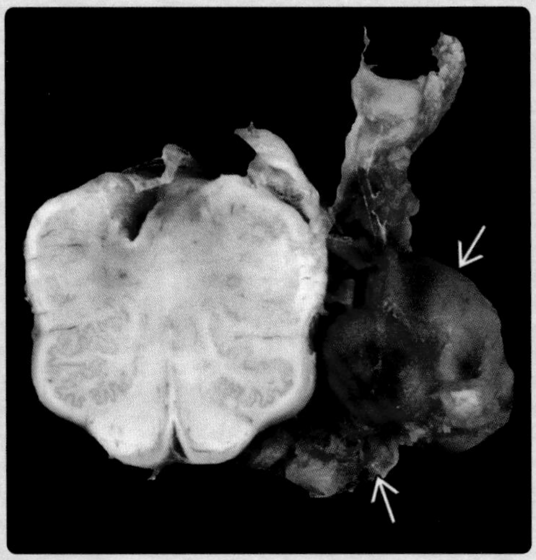

(25-54) *Sagittal T1 C+ image shows a large, heterogeneous invasive pituitary macroadenoma ⇨. Pathology showed a high MIB-1 index of 9% with necrosis and hemorrhage, diagnostic of an atypical adenoma.* ***(25-55)*** *Autopsy specimen shows a pituitary carcinoma with CSF "drop metastasis" ➡ along the medulla. CSF or systemic dissemination is required for diagnosis of a pituitary carcinoma. (Courtesy A. Ersen, MD, B. Scheithauer, MD.)*

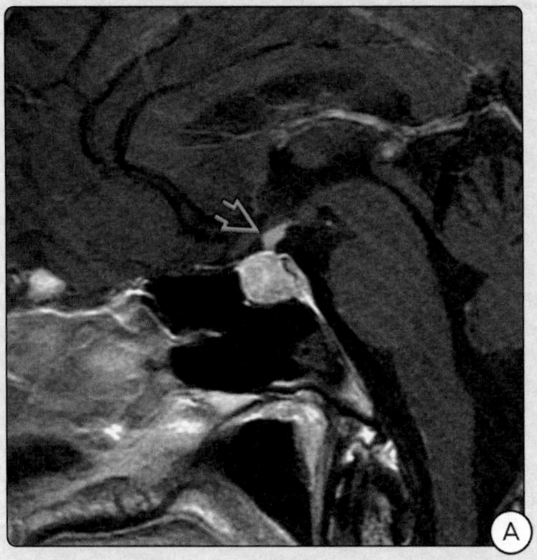

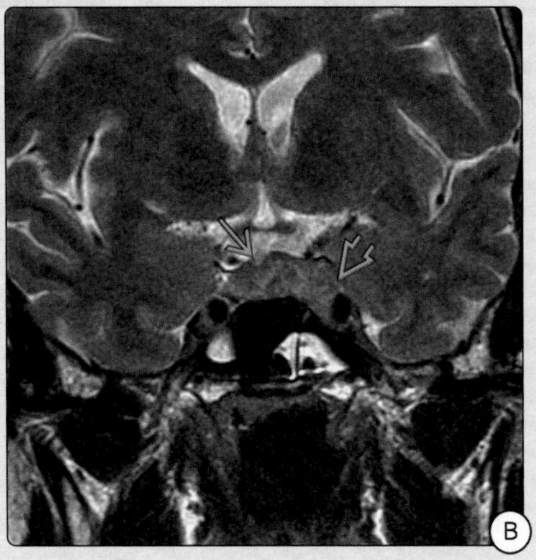

(25-56A) *Sagittal T1 C+ in a 58y man with diabetes insipidus shows diffuse pituitary gland enlargement and abnormal thickening and enhancement of the infundibulum ⇨.* ***(25-56B)*** *Coronal T2WI in the same patient shows a hypointense mass ⇨ with invasion into the cavernous sinus ⇨. The T2 low signal, stalk involvement, and infiltrative appearance help differentiate this lymphoma from the more common adenoma.*

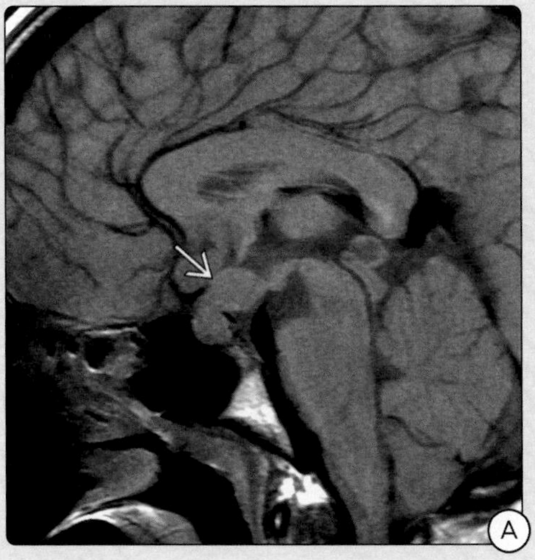

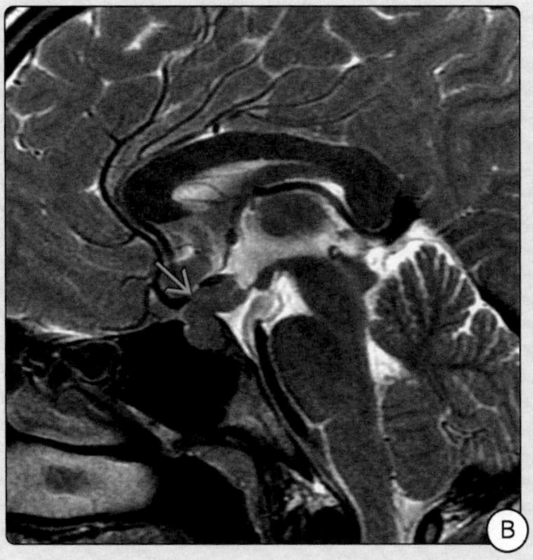

(25-57A) *Sagittal T1WI in a 14y girl with abnormal menses shows a diffusely abnormal pituitary infundibulum ➡ and absence of the posterior pituitary bright spot. There was diffuse enhancement after contrast (not shown).* ***(25-57B)*** *Sagittal T2WI in the same patient shows the hypointense infundibular mass ⇨. Considerations in this young patient include germinoma and Langerhans cell histiocytosis. Germinoma was found at biopsy.*

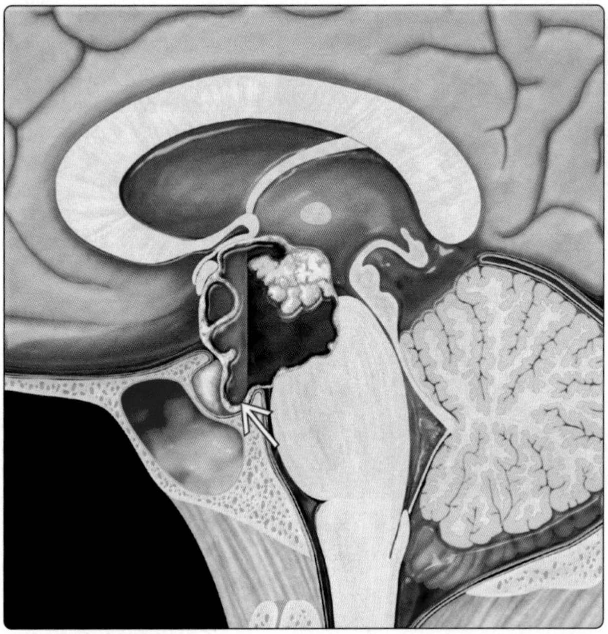

(25-58) Sagittal graphic shows a predominantly cystic, partially solid suprasellar mass with focal rim calcifications. Note the small intrasellar component and fluid-fluid level. The fluid, rich in cholesterol, is dark and viscous.

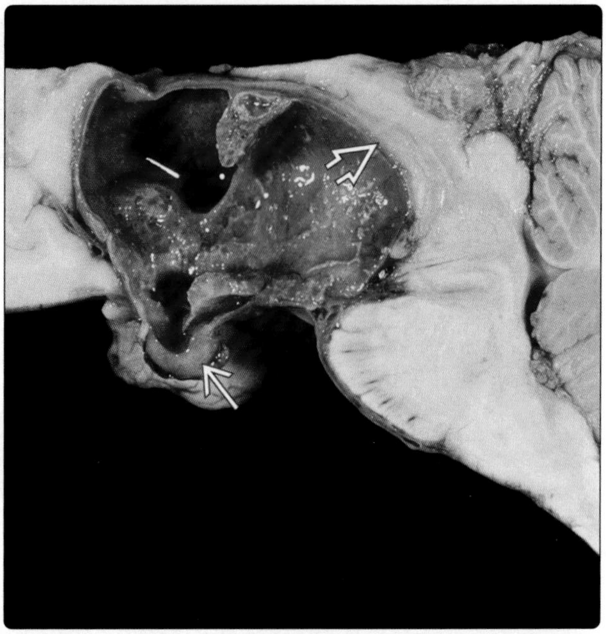

(25-59) Sagittal autopsy specimen of adamantinomatous craniopharyngioma shows a small solid intrasellar component and a large suprasellar cystic component that adheres to adjacent brain. (Courtesy R. Hewlett, MD.)

resemble those of macroadenoma. The few described cases show a heterogeneously enhancing sellar/suprasellar mass, often invading the cavernous sinus.

Lymphoma

Primary CNS lymphoma (PCNSL) is a rare variant of extranodal non-Hodgkin lymphoma restricted to the brain, spinal cord, eye, and meninges. The most common location for primary CNS lymphoma is along a CSF surface, typically in the periventricular white matter. The hypothalamus, infundibulum, and pituitary gland are less common sites for PCNSL. The vast majority of PCNSL is diffuse large B-cell lymphoma (90-95%). PCNSL is discussed in more detail in Chapter 24. This section will focus on the pituitary axis.

Imaging of PCNSL varies with immune status. In the immunocompetent patient, PCNSL is hyperdense on CT related to the high nuclear:cytoplasmic ratio. PCNSL is usually isointense or slightly hypointense on T1WI and isointense to gray matter on T2WI. PCNSL shows homogeneous enhancement on postcontrast MR and may appear more infiltrative than the more common pituitary adenoma **(25-56)**. DWI typically shows diffusion restriction related to the high cellularity. PCNSL involving the pituitary axis may affect the infundibulum, pituitary gland, or the hypothalamus. Patients often present with diabetes insipidus or panhypopituitarism.

Germinoma

A germinoma is the most common intracranial germ cell tumor, representing two-thirds of intracranial germ cell tumors and 1-2% of all primary brain tumors. Germinomas are located in the pineal region most commonly (50-65%) and the suprasellar region in approximately 25-35% of cases. Less common locations include the basal ganglia and thalami. Germinomas may present as synchronous pineal and suprasellar masses. Germinomas are tumors of young patients with the vast majority presenting in patients in the first two decades. The peak age at presentation is between 10-12 years old.

Germinomas are WHO grade II tumors that are typically treated with radiation therapy following a biopsy. Germinomas of the suprasellar region most commonly present with diabetes insipidus. Less common presenting signs include visual loss and hypothalamic-pituitary dysfunction with decreased growth and precocious puberty.

Germinomas of the suprasellar region are classically hyperdense on CT, similar to lymphoma. When involving the pituitary axis, a germinoma involves the infundibulum and/or neurohypophysis and often presents in a child with an absent posterior pituitary "bright spot" **(25-57)**. Diffuse enhancement of an enlarged infundibulum is the typical MR appearance. Diffusion restriction on DWI is typical.

Craniopharyngioma

Terminology and Etiology

Craniopharyngioma (CP) is a benign, often partly cystic sellar/suprasellar mass that probably arises from epithelial remnants of Rathke pouch. The molecular pathogenesis of CP is unknown. Reactivation of the Wnt signaling pathway may be one factor in the pathogenesis of adamantinomatous CPs.

Pathology

Location. Completely intrasellar CPs are rare. CPs are primarily suprasellar tumors (75%). A small intrasellar component is present in 20-25% of cases **(25-58)**. Occasionally, CPs (especially the papillary type) arise mostly or entirely within the third ventricle **(25-64)**.

Size and Number. CPs are solitary lesions that range in size from a few millimeters to several centimeters. Lesions larger than 5 cm are common. Giant CPs may extend into both anterior and middle cranial fossae **(25-63)**. Posteroinferior extension between the clivus and pons down to the foramen magnum can be seen in exceptionally large lesions.

Gross Pathology. Two types of craniopharyngiomas are recognized: adamantinomatous and papillary. About 90% of all CPs are adamantinomatous; 10% are papillary.

The typical gross appearance of an **adamantinomatous CP** is that of a multilobulated, partially solid but mostly cystic suprasellar mass **(25-59)** **(25-61)**. Multiple loculated cysts are common. The cysts often contain dark, viscous, "machinery oil" fluid rich in cholesterol crystals **(25-58)**. The surfaces of adamantinomatous CPs are often irregular and infiltrative, adhering to adjacent structures such as the hypothalamus.

Papillary CP is usually a discrete encapsulated mass with a smooth surface that does not adhere to adjacent brain. Papillary CPs are often solid, with a cauliflower-like configuration. When they contain cysts, the fluid is clear (unlike the "machinery oil" cholesterol-rich contents of adamantinomatous CPs).

Microscopic Features. Adamantinomatous CPs have a peripheral layer of palisading stratified squamous epithelium surrounding nodules of "wet" keratin. Cholesterol "clefts" and squamous debris are typical. Calcification is common.

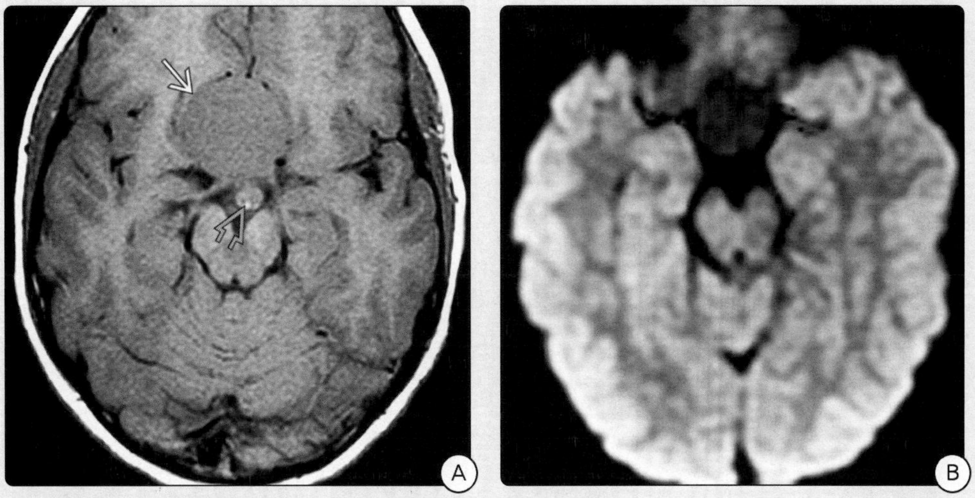

***(25-60A)** Axial T1WI in a 14y boy shows a large suprasellar mass ➡ that is mostly isointense with cortex except for a small nodular posterior excrescence that has a tiny hyperintense focus ➡. **(25-60B)** DWI image in the same patient shows no restriction.*

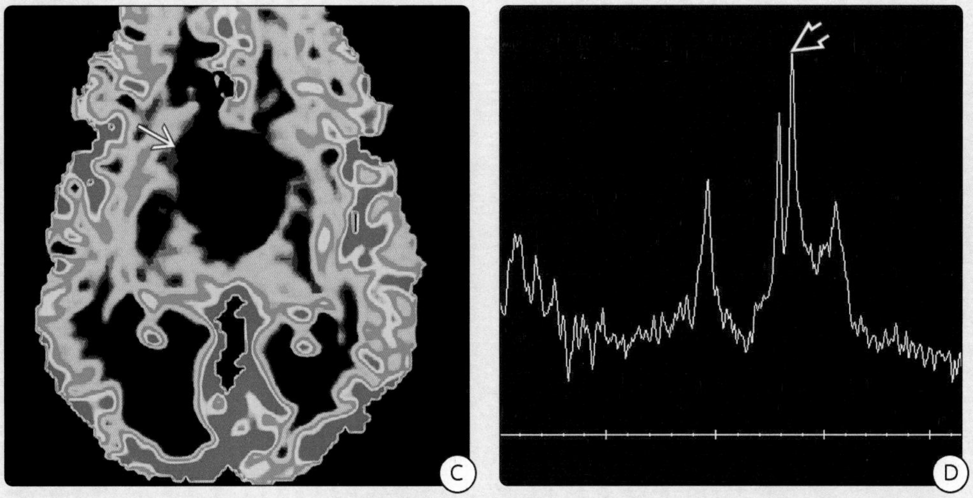

***(25-60C)** pMR in the same patient shows no evidence of elevated rCBV. The mass ➡ is essentially as avascular as the CSF-containing occipital horns of the lateral ventricles. **(25-60D)** MRS shows a very large lipid-lactate peak ➡ characteristic of the cholesterol and lipid contents of craniopharyngioma. Adamantinomatous craniopharyngioma was found at surgery.*

(25-61) *Axial autopsy specimen shows a mostly cystic craniopharyngioma ➡ in the suprasellar cistern. A small tumor nodule is present ➡. (Courtesy R. Hewlett, MD.)* ***(25-62A)*** *Axial NECT scan in a 7y boy with a 2-month history of visual problems presenting with acute near-total vision loss shows a typical cystic suprasellar mass with rim calcification ➡, suggesting craniopharyngioma.*

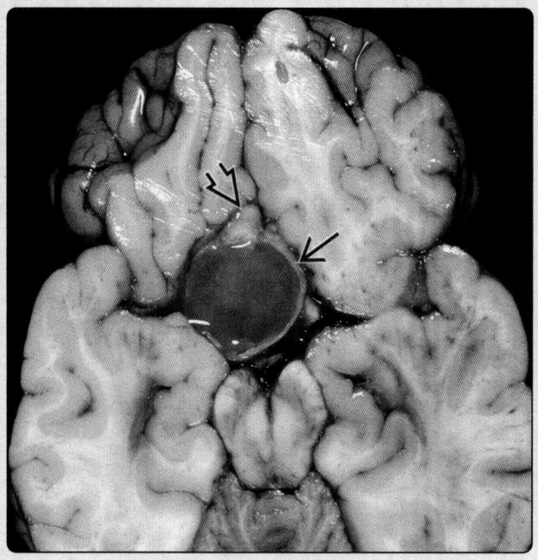

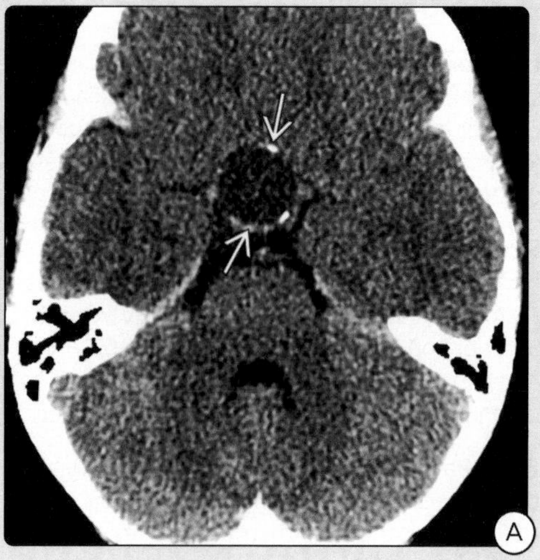

(25-62B) *Sagittal T1WI in the same patient shows a lobulated sellar and suprasellar mass ➡ that is nearly isointense with white matter in the corpus callosum.* ***(25-62C)*** *The mass ➡ is very hyperintense on sagittal T2WI. Some hypointense debris ➡ is present at the bottom of the mostly cystic mass. There is mild expansion of the sella turcica.*

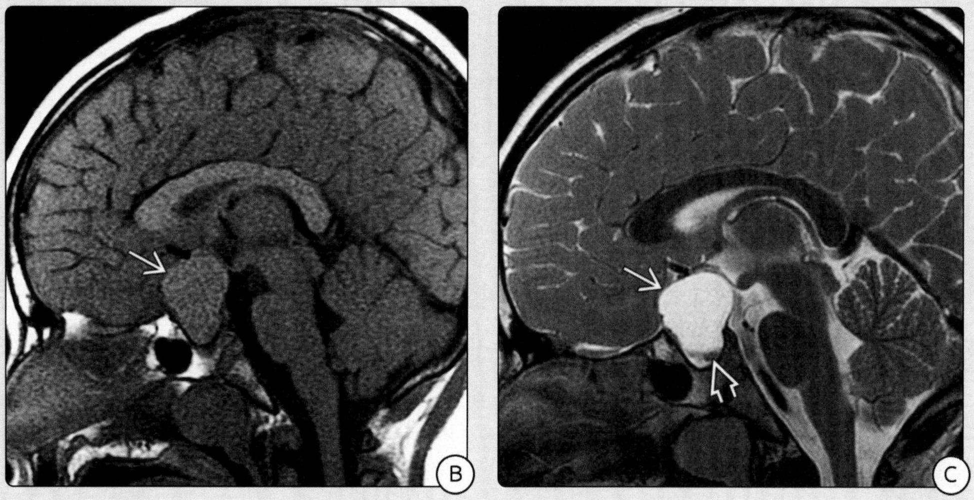

(25-62D) *Sagittal T1 C+ shows thin rim enhancement around the mass ➡.* ***(25-62E)*** *Coronal T1 C+ shows the thin enhancing tumor rim ➡ with a small tumor nodule ➡. Adamantinomatous craniopharyngioma was found at surgery. Craniopharyngioma is the most common nonglial tumor in children. The enhancing nodule helps differentiate this tumor from a Rathke cleft cyst.*

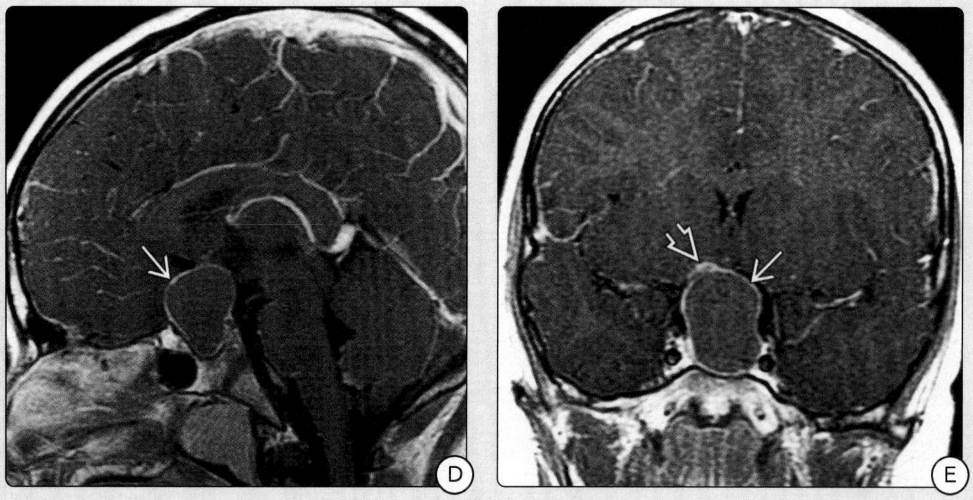

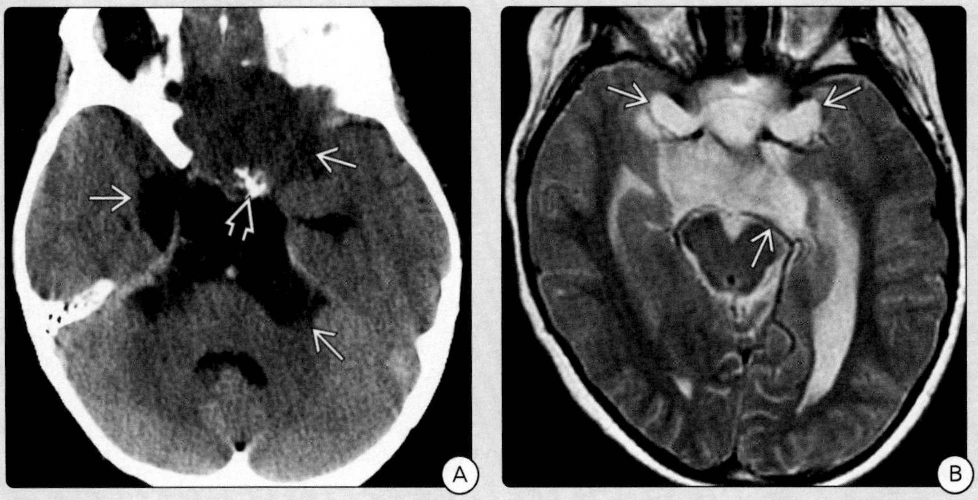

***(25-63A)** Axial NECT image in a 9y boy shows an extensive hypodense mass involving the anterior, middle, and posterior cranial fossae ➡. A small focus of calcification ⇨ is present inside the mass. **(25-63B)** Axial T2WI shows that the cysts are mostly hyperintense ➡ with mild local mass effect on the adjacent brain.*

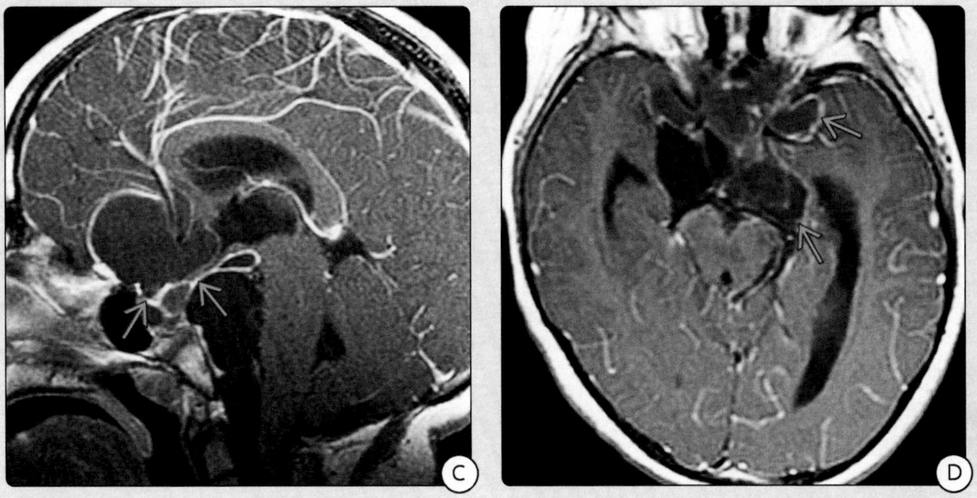

***(25-63C)** Sagittal T1 C+ in the same patient demonstrates some thin rim enhancement → around parts of the sellar and suprasellar mass. **(25-63D)** Axial T1 C+ confirms that thin rims of enhancement are present →. When a multicystic, bizarre-appearing mass in a child extends into several fossae, craniopharyngioma should be a consideration. Adamantinomatous craniopharyngioma was seen at resection.*

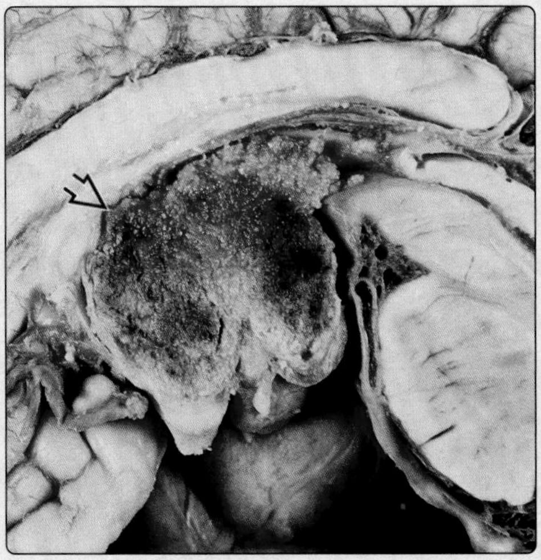

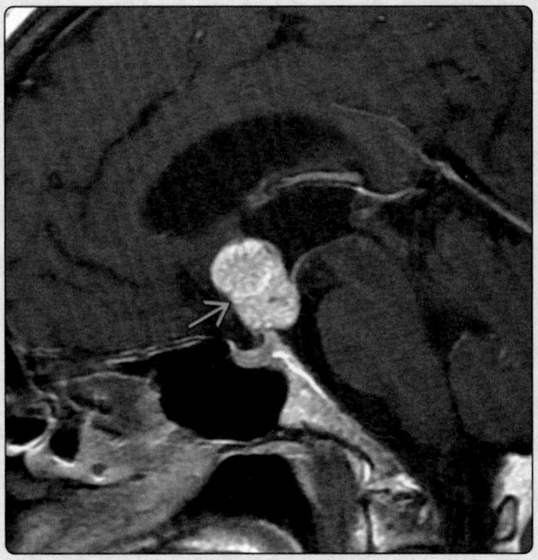

***(25-64)** Midline sagittal autopsy section shows a solid mass filling the third ventricle ⇨. This was papillary craniopharyngioma. (Courtesy B. Scheithauer, MD.) **(25-65)** Sagittal T1 C+ image in a 60y man shows a solidly enhancing mass in the anterior third ventricle →. Note that the pituitary gland is separate from the mass. Imaging is typical of a papillary craniopharyngioma.*

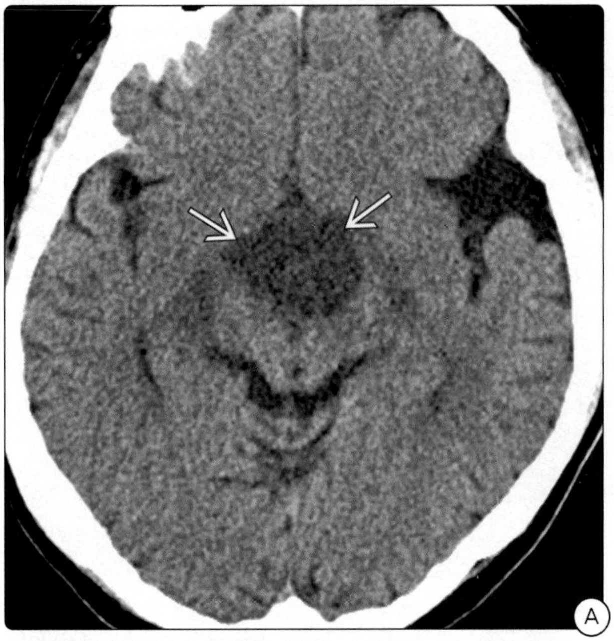

(25-66A) NECT in a 44y man with headaches and psychiatric symptoms shows a well-defined, hypodense, noncalcified mass ➡ in the suprasellar cistern.

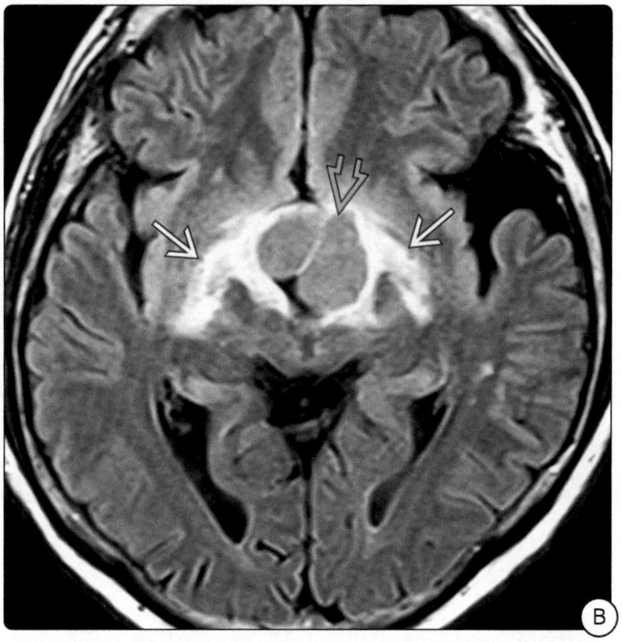

(25-66B) FLAIR scan shows that the mass ⇨ does not suppress. Note the hyperintensity in the hypothalamus and optic tracts ➡. Papillary craniopharyngioma was found at surgery. No parenchymal tumor invasion was present.

Papillary CPs have solid sheets of well-differentiated squamous epithelium. Crude epithelial pseudopapillae form around fibrovascular stromal cores. Occasional goblet cells are present.

Staging, Grading, and Classification. Both adamantinomatous and papillary craniopharyngiomas are WHO grade I neoplasms. MIB-1 is low.

CRANIOPHARYNGIOMA: ETIOLOGY AND PATHOLOGY

Etiology
- Epithelial remnants of Rathke pouch

Pathology
- 2 types
  - Adamantinomatous (90%)
  - Papillary (10%)
  - Both are WHO grade I
- Adamantinomatous
  - Multiple cysts
  - Squamous epithelium, "wet" keratin
  - Cholesterol-rich "machinery oil" fluid
- Papillary
  - Solid > > cystic (clear fluid)
  - Almost always adults (40-55 years old)

Clinical Issues

Epidemiology. CP is the most common nonglial neoplasm in children, accounting for 6-10% of all pediatric brain tumors and slightly more than half of suprasellar neoplasms.

Demographics. CPs occur nearly equally in children and adults. Adamantinomatous CPs have a bimodal age distribution with a large peak between 5 and 15 years and a second, smaller peak at 45-60 years. CPs are rare in newborns and infants; only 5% arise in patients between birth and 5 years of age.

Papillary CPs almost always occur in adults with a peak incidence between 40 and 55 years.

Presentation. Symptoms vary with tumor size and patient age. Patients most commonly present with visual disturbances, either with or without accompanying headache. Large tumors compress the infundibular stalk ("stalk effect") resulting in abnormal pituitary function (often with mild elevation of prolactin). Endocrine deficiencies including growth failure, delayed puberty, and diabetes insipidus are common.

Natural History. CPs are slow-growing neoplasms with a propensity to recur following surgery. More than 85% of patients survive at least 3 years following diagnosis. However, the recurrence rate at 10 years approaches 20-30% even in patients with gross total resection. Recurrence is significantly more common with larger and incompletely excised lesions.

Approximately half of long-term survivors experience reduced quality of life, mostly due to morbid hypothalamic obesity. Spontaneous malignant transformation to squamous cell carcinoma is rare. Most cases of CP malignant degeneration occur in patients with multiple recurrences and prior radiotherapy.

Treatment Options. Gross total resection is the best treatment option. Hypothalamic injury is the major risk, especially with large adamantinomatous CPs.

Imaging

General Features. A partially calcified, mixed solid and cystic extraaxial suprasellar mass in a child is the classic appearance. A compressed, displaced pituitary gland can sometimes be identified as separate from the mass.

CT Findings. Adamantinomatous CPs follow a "rule of ninety," i.e., 90% are mixed cystic/solid, 90% are calcified, and 90% enhance **(25-62)**.

Papillary CPs rarely calcify. They are often solid or mostly solid. When they contain intratumoral cysts, the cysts are usually smaller and less complex-appearing than those seen with adamantinomatous CPs.

MR Findings. Signal intensity varies with cyst contents **(25-60)**. Multiple cysts are common, and intracystic fluid within each cyst varies from hypo- to hyperintense compared with brain on T1WI **(25-62)**.

CP cysts are variably hyperintense on T2WI and FLAIR. The solid nodule is often calcified and moderately hypointense. Hyperintensity extending along the optic tracts is common and usually represents edema, not tumor invasion **(25-66)** **(25-67A)**.

The cyst walls and solid nodules typically enhance following contrast administration **(25-62)** **(25-67)**.

MRS shows a large lipid-lactate peak, characteristic of the cholesterol and lipid constituents of a CP. pMR shows low rCBV **(25-60)**.

CRANIOPHARYNGIOMA: CLINICAL ISSUES, IMAGING, AND DDx

Clinical Issues
- > 50% of pediatric suprasellar neoplasms
- Occurs equally in children, adults
  - Peak in children = 5-15 years; peak in adults = 40-55 years
  - Papillary type much more common in adults
- Slow growth
  - Recurrence common
  - Malignant transformation rare

Imaging
- CT
  - Can be giant (> 5 cm), involve multiple fossae
  - Adamantinomatous: 90% cystic, 90% calcify, 90% enhance
  - Papillary: solid > cystic
- MR
  - Variable signal on T1WI
  - Usually hyperintense on T2/FLAIR
  - Enhancement (nodular or rim) 90%
  - MRS: large lipid-lactate peak

Differential Diagnosis
- Rathke cleft cyst

Differential Diagnosis

The major differential diagnosis of CP is **Rathke cleft cyst** (RCC). RCCs do not calcify, appear to be much less heterogeneous, and do not show nodular enhancement. The ADC of RCC is significantly increased compared with that of cystic CPs. Immunohistochemistry is helpful, as RCCs express specific cytokeratins that CPs do not.

Hypothalamic/chiasmatic astrocytoma is usually a solid suprasellar mass that is clearly intraparenchymal. Calcifications and cysts are uncommon. These tumors are T2 hyperintense and have variable enhancement.

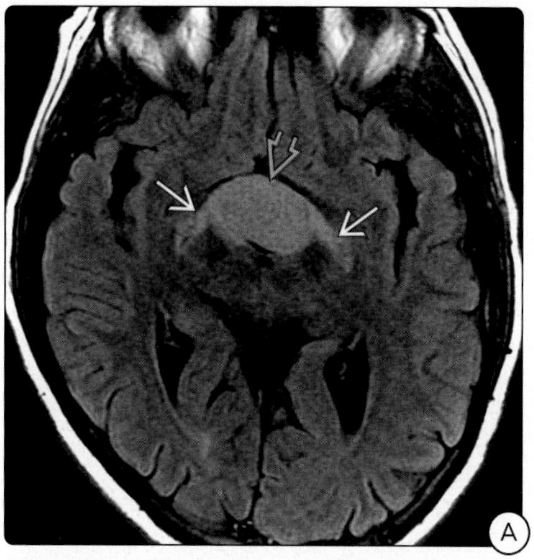

***(25-67A)** Axial FLAIR image in a 47y patient with headaches shows a suprasellar mass ⇨ with edema in the adjacent optic tracts ➡.*

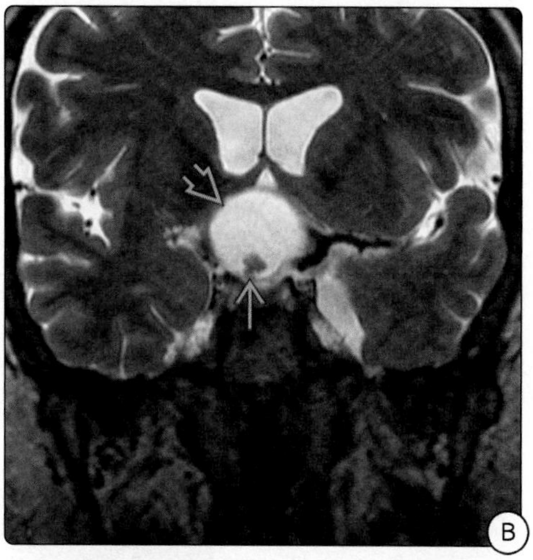

***(25-67B)** Coronal T2WI in the same patient shows the cystic mass ⇨ with a focal inferior nodule ⇨. No calcification was seen on CT (not shown).*

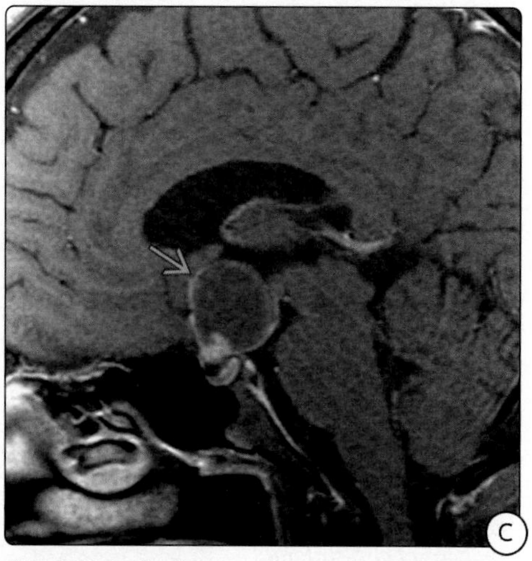

***(25-67C)** Sagittal T1 C+ shows enhancement of the suprasellar mass ⇨ and nodule at the anterior 3rd ventricle. This is craniopharyngioma.*

Pituitary adenoma is rare in prepubescent children (peak age period for CP). A **dermoid cyst** can be hyperintense on T1WI and may demonstrate calcification. An **epidermoid cyst** (EC) is usually off-midline with DWI restriction. Suprasellar ECs are uncommon. Neither dermoid nor epidermoid cysts enhance.

Nonadenomatous Pituitary Tumors

Primary nonadenomatous pituitary gland tumors are rare, poorly understood entities. The 2007 WHO Classification of Tumours of the Central Nervous System clarified matters, formally recognizing three histologically distinct pituitary region neoplasms: pituicytoma, spindle cell oncocytoma (SCO), and granular cell tumor. All are WHO grade I tumors. The 2016 WHO Classification of Tumours of the Central Nervous System further classified these three tumors, recognizing that all show nuclear expression of TTF1, suggesting that they all may constitute a spectrum of a single nosologic entity.

Pituicytoma

Previously also known as "choristoma" and "infundibuloma," pituicytoma arises from modified glial cells ("pituicytes") that reside in the infundibular stalk and neurohypophysis **(25-68)**.

Visual disturbance with or without headache is the most common presenting symptom. Patients with pituicytoma almost never present with diabetes insipidus, galactorrhea, or prolactinemia.

Pituicytoma can appear as either an intrasellar or a suprasellar mass. The majority of pituicytomas are isointense with brain on T1WI and hyperintense on T2WI. They usually arise along the infundibulum or neurohypophysis and enhance homogeneously following contrast enhancement **(25-69)**.

Pituicytoma is the only one of the nonadenomatous tumors that can present as a purely intrasellar mass. An intrasellar

(25-68) Sagittal graphic shows a pituicytoma involving the infundibular stalk and neurohypophysis. (25-69) Sagittal T1 C+ scan in a 22y woman with delayed growth and hypopituitarism shows an enhancing infundibular mass that is clearly separate from the pituitary gland. Imaging findings have remained stable over many years. This is presumed pituicytoma.

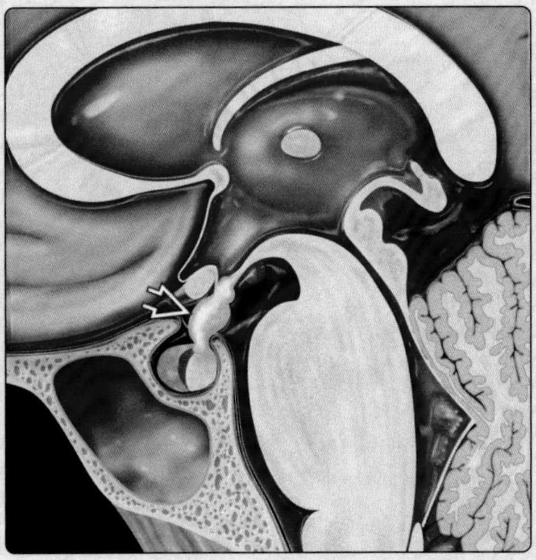

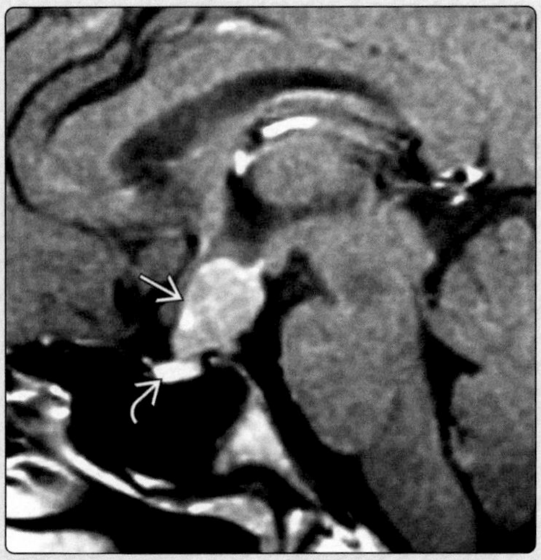

(25-70A) Sagittal T1WI in a 69y woman with headaches, visual symptoms shows a sellar-suprasellar mass that is well delineated and isointense with brain. The pituitary gland cannot be distinguished as separate from the mass. (25-70B) Coronal T1 C+ image shows that the lesion enhances strongly and uniformly. Preoperative diagnosis was pituitary macroadenoma. Spindle cell oncocytoma was diagnosed at histologic examination.

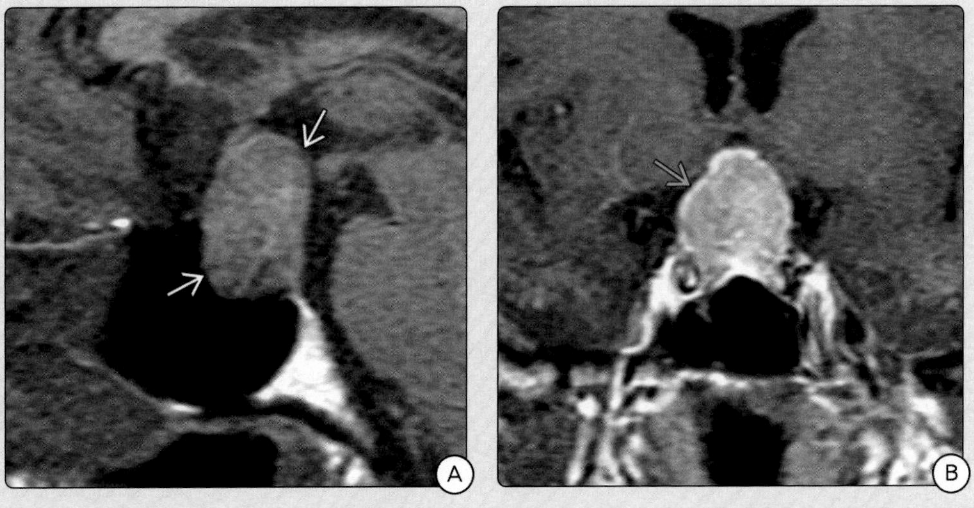

mass that is clearly separate from the anterior pituitary gland and enhances homogeneously is most likely a pituicytoma.

Spindle Cell Oncocytoma

SCO, also previously known as folliculostellate cell tumor, consists of "spindled" oncocytes containing granular, mitochondria-rich cytoplasm.

Visual disturbance, panhypopituitarism, and headache are the most common presenting symptoms. SCOs do not appear to cause diabetes insipidus.

To date, all pathologically proven cases have presented as mixed intrasellar and suprasellar infiltrating pituitary lesions. Imaging findings are similar to—and cannot be distinguished from—those of pituitary adenoma or lymphocytic hypophysis **(25-70)**.

Granular Cell Tumor

Like pituicytoma, granular cell tumor is a tumor of the neurohypophysis. Many granular cell tumors are asymptomatic and discovered incidentally at autopsy. Some enlarge with time, becoming symptomatic in middle-aged or older adults. Visual disturbance, headache, and amenorrhea are common. Similar to pituicytoma and SCO, granular cell tumors rarely present with diabetes insipidus, prolactinemia, or galactorrhea.

Granular cell tumors are typically suprasellar masses. They are hyperdense on NECT **(25-71A)** and isointense with brain on both T1- and T2WI. Granular cell tumors enhance strongly and homogeneously following contrast administration **(25-71)**.

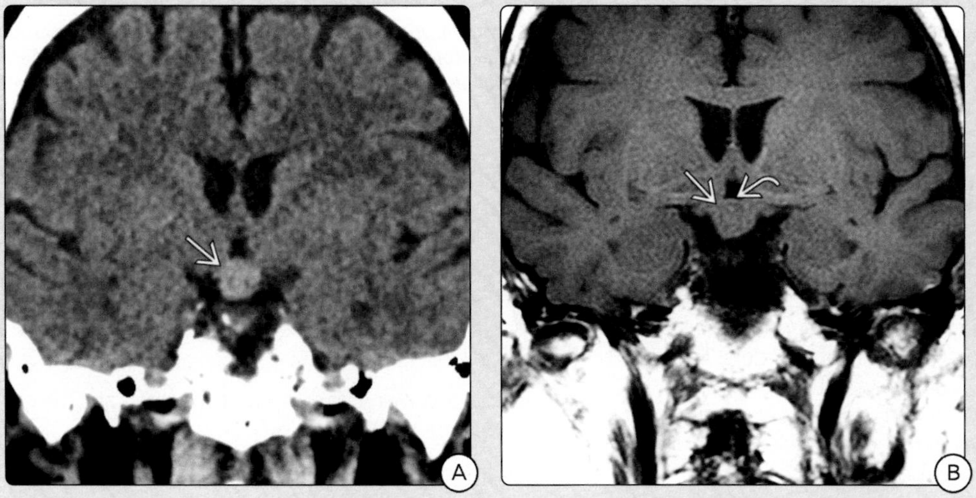

***(25-71A)** Coronal NECT in a 66y woman with headache and visual disturbances shows a well-delineated hyperdense suprasellar mass ➔. **(25-71B)** Coronal T1WI in the same case shows that the mass ➔ projects from the undersurface of the hypothalamus ➔, compresses the inferior third ventricle, and is homogeneously isointense with brain.*

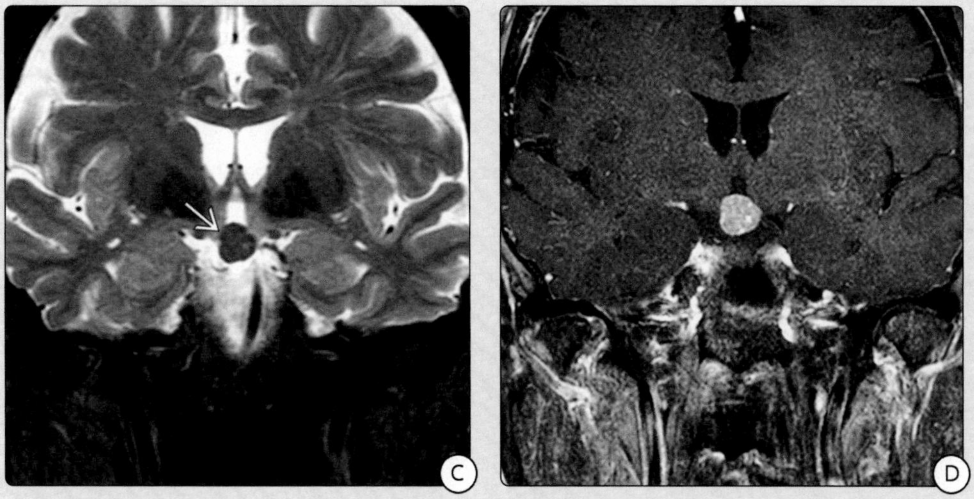

***(25-71C)** Coronal STIR in the same case shows that the well-delineated mass ➔ is slightly lobulated and mildly hypointense compared with white matter. **(25-71D)** Coronal T1 C+ FS shows that the mass enhances intensely and uniformly. Granular cell tumor of the neurohypophysis was diagnosed at histopathology.*

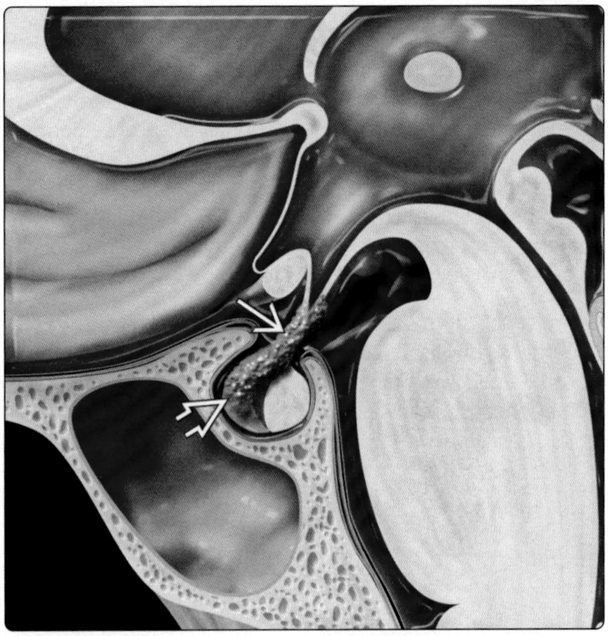

(25-72) Sagittal graphic shows lymphocytic hypophysitis. Note thickening of the infundibulum ➡ and infiltration into the anterior lobe of the pituitary gland ➡.

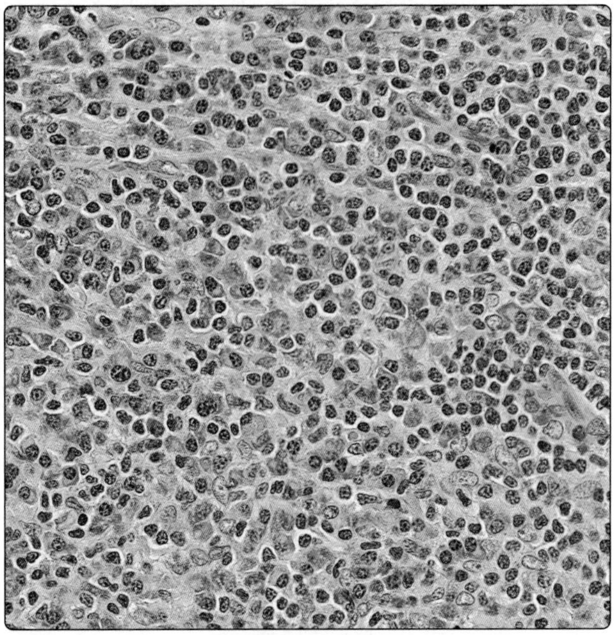

(25-73) Lymphocytic adenohypophysitis is typified by numerous infiltrating cytologically benign lymphocytes overrunning the gland. (Courtesy B. K. DeMasters, MD.)

Miscellaneous Lesions

Hypophysitis

Hypophysitis is an inflammation of the pituitary gland that comprises an increasingly complex group of disorders. There are two main histologic forms of hypophysitis: lymphocytic hypophysitis (LH) and nonlymphocytic hypophysitis. Recent reports of other variants broaden the hypophysitis spectrum even further. In this section, we focus on LH, the most common form. We then briefly discuss nonlymphocytic hypophysitis, including granulomatous hypophysitis and some of the newly described entities that are often characterized by plasma cell infiltrates.

Lymphocytic Hypophysitis

Terminology. LH is also called lymphocytic adenohypophysitis, primary hypophysitis, and stalkitis. A variant form of LH is called lymphocytic infundibuloneurohypophysitis (LINH).

Etiology. LH is an uncommon autoimmune inflammatory disorder of the pituitary gland that most often occurs in women of child-bearing age, usually late in pregnancy or shortly after childbirth. Immune competence is reestablished in the late pregnancy/peripartum period. Antipituitary antibodies co-react with both the pituitary gland and the placenta.

LH is also associated with other autoimmune disorders. Approximately 25% of patients have coexistent systemic inflammatory/autoimmune disease. Thyroiditis, polymyositis, type 1 diabetes, and psoriasis have all been associated with LH.

Pathology. The pituitary gland and stalk in LH appear diffusely enlarged and firm although inflammatory changes are predominantly or exclusively in the anterior lobe **(25-72)**. Microscopic features include a dense infiltrate mostly composed of T-cell lymphocytes **(25-73)**. Varying degrees of gland destruction and fibrosis may be present. Granulomas and giant cells are absent.

LINH typically involves *both* the neurohypophysis and the adenohypophysis **(25-76)**.

Clinical Issues. Between 80 and 90% of patients with LH are female; 30-60% of cases occur in the peripartum period. There is no adverse effect on the fetus.

The most common presenting symptoms are headache and multiple endocrine deficiencies with partial or total hypopituitarism. Diabetes insipidus is common. Adrenocorticotrophic hormone deficits often appear first. Hyperprolactinemia occurs in one-third of all patients, probably secondary to stalk compression.

Men, women past child-bearing age, and children are affected in 10-20% of cases. Middle-aged men typically present with diabetes insipidus.

Treatment is hormone replacement with or without corticosteroids.

Imaging. LH is typically both intrasellar and suprasellar. Adjacent dural or sphenoid sinus mucosal thickening is common.

Imaging shows a thickened, nontapering infundibular stalk. A rounded, symmetrically enlarged pituitary gland is common **(25-74)**. The sellar floor is intact, not expanded or eroded. The posterior pituitary "bright spot" is absent in 75% of cases. LH enhances intensely and uniformly.

HYPOPHYSITIS vs. NONSECRETING PITUITARY ADENOMA

Hypophysitis
- Clinical profile
  - Younger patients (mean: women = 35 years, men = 45 years)
  - Patient age < 40 years favors hypophysitis
  - Pregnant/peripartum patient
  - Diabetes insipidus common
- Smaller mass
- Symmetric pituitary expansion
- Loss of normal posterior pituitary "bright spot" (PPBS)
- Stalk enlarged, nontapering
- Homogeneous signal, strong enhancement

Pituitary Adenoma
- Clinical profile
  - Older patients (peak = 60 years)
  - Diabetes insipidus rare
- Larger mass
  - Volume > 6 cm^3 favors adenoma
- Asymmetric pituitary expansion
- PPBS generally preserved
- Stalk displaced but otherwise normal
- Heterogeneous signal, moderate enhancement

Differential Diagnosis. The major differential diagnosis for LH is nonsecreting **pituitary macroadenoma**. The distinction is important, as treatment differs significantly. LH is treated medically, whereas surgical resection is the primary treatment for pituitary macroadenoma. Macroadenomas can be giant, but LH only occasionally exceeds 3 cm in diameter. Clinical findings are also helpful, as LH commonly presents with diabetes insipidus **(25-76)**.

The stalk is usually normal in **pituitary hyperplasia**, although patient age and sex are similar. **Metastasis** usually occurs in older patients with known systemic primary tumor.

Granulomatous hypophysitis may occur secondary to infection, sarcoidosis, or Langerhans cell histiocytosis. Granulomatous hypophysitis is less common than LH, has a different epidemiologic profile, and tends to enhance more heterogeneously. **IgG4-** and **drug-related hypophysitis** is very rare.

Granulomatous Hypophysitis

Granulomatous hypophysitis has different epidemiologic characteristics than LH does. Granulomatous hypophysitis is equally common in both sexes, and there is no association with pregnancy.

Granulomatous hypophysitis can be primary (idiopathic) or secondary **(25-75)**. **Secondary granulomatous hypophysitis** is far more common than primary granulomatous hypophysitis and typically results from necrotizing granulomatous inflammation. Infectious/inflammatory secondary granulomatous hypophysitis can be caused by TB, sarcoid, fungal infection, syphilis, Langerhans cell histiocytosis, Wegener granulomatosis, Erdheim-Chester disease, granulomatous autoimmune hypophysitis, ruptured Rathke cleft cyst, or craniopharyngioma. Secondary granulomatous hypophysitis may also occur as a reaction to systemic inflammatory disorders, such as Crohn disease. Imaging findings are nonspecific, resembling those of LH or pituitary adenoma.

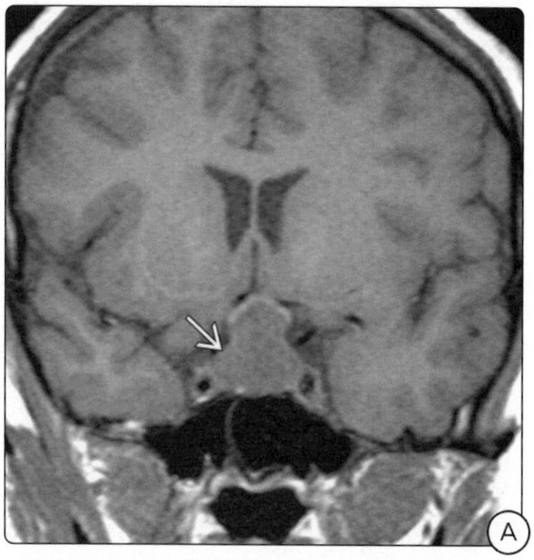

***(25-74A)** Coronal T1WI in a 19y pregnant woman with vision problems shows a "figure eight" or snowman-shaped intra- and suprasellar mass ➡.*

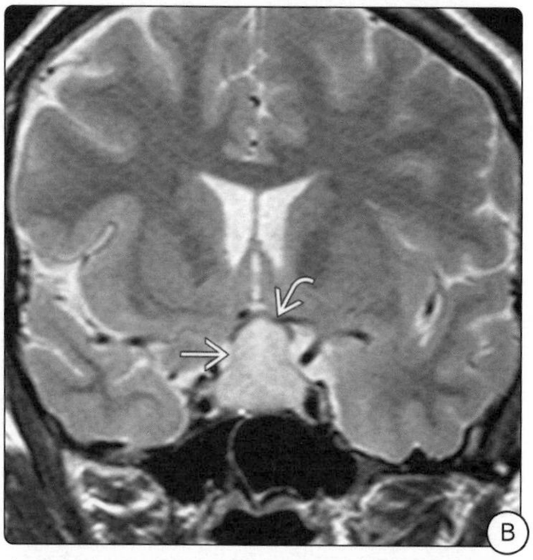

***(25-74B)** Coronal T2WI shows that the lesion ➡ is mildly hyperintense. Note elevation and draping of the optic chiasm ➡ over the mass.*

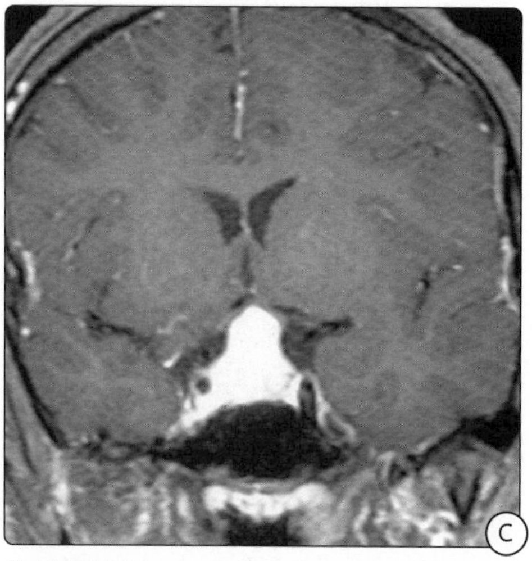

***(25-74C)** T1 C+ shows that the mass appears virtually identical to pituitary macroadenoma. This is lymphocytic hypophysitis.*

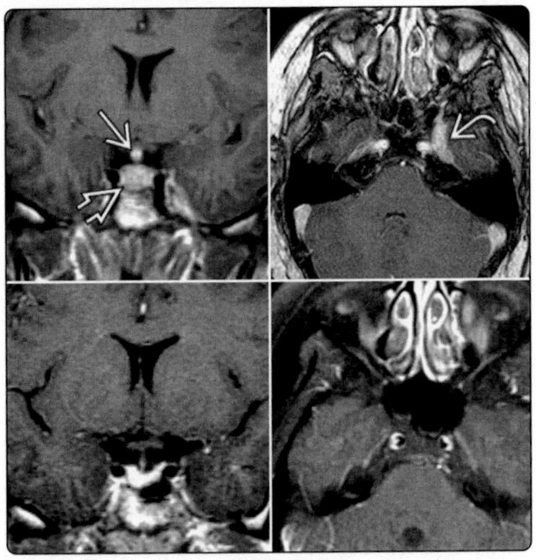

(25-75) This is granulomatous hypophysitis. (Top) Fat pituitary gland ➡, stalk ➡, and pseudotumor ➡. (Bottom) Steroids resolved it.

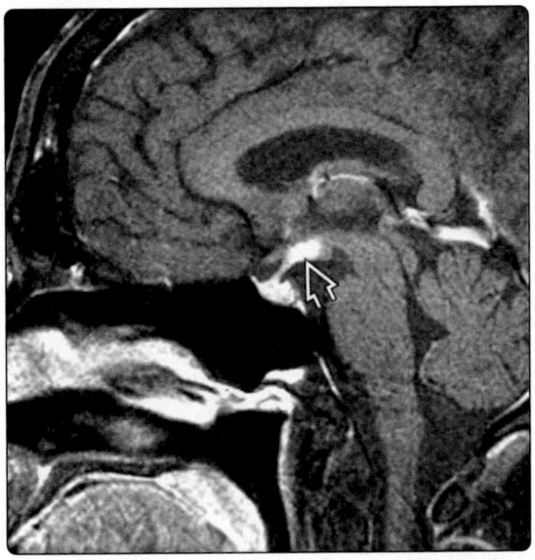

(25-76) LINH in a middle-aged man with diabetes insipidus is seen here as an enhancing mass ➡ in the hypothalamus.

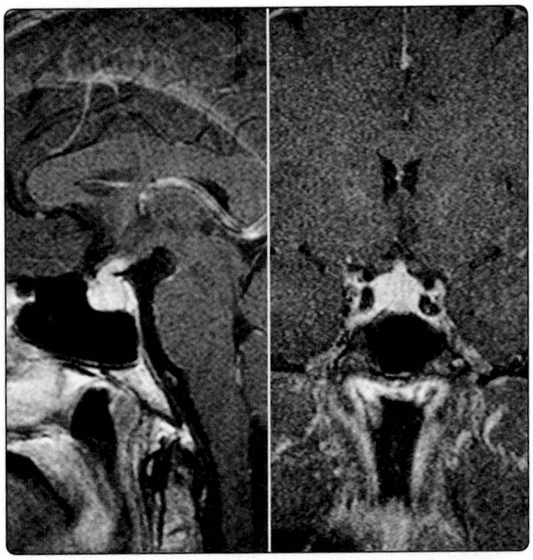

(25-77) Patient on ipilimumab for metastatic melanoma developed drug-induced hypophysitis with infiltration of the stalk and pituitary gland.

Primary granulomatous hypophysitis is a rare inflammatory disease without identifiable infectious organisms. The precise etiology of primary granulomatous hypophysitis is unknown. Nonnecrotizing granulomas with multinucleated giant cells, histiocytes, and various numbers of plasma cells and lymphocytes are typical. Primary granulomatous hypophysitis usually presents with diabetes insipidus. A symmetric sellar mass that enhances strongly but heterogeneously is seen on imaging studies.

Other Hypophysitis Variants

A number of new hypophysitis variants have been recently described. **IgG4-related hypophysitis** has a marked mononuclear infiltrate mainly characterized by increased numbers of IgG4-positive plasma cells. Imaging findings resemble those of lymphocytic infundibuloneurohypophysitis. The pituitary stalk and posterior pituitary lobe are enlarged and enhance intensely following contrast administration.

Drug-related hypophysitis has been reported in cases of cancer immunotherapy with antibodies that stimulate T-cell responses (e.g., ipilimumab) **(25-77)**. Clinicians and radiologists should be aware of autoimmune-induced hypophysitis as a complication of new treatments. Imaging of drug-related hypophysitis usually shows enlargement of the pituitary gland with or without infundibulum.

Langerhans Cell Histiocytosis

Terminology

Langerhans cell histiocytosis (LCH) is now considered a neoplastic disease with *BRAF* V600E mutations and LCH clonality. LCH is discussed in more detail in Chapter 24. This section focuses more specifically on the pituitary axis.

Clinical Issues

Presentation. Patients with pituitary axis LCH typically present with diabetes insipidus. There may be associated visual disturbances or hypothalamic dysfunction.

Demographics. LCH typically presents in patients less than 2 years of age. The peak age at onset is 1 year old for isolated LCH and between 2 and 5 years of age in multifocal disease. Female patients are more commonly affected 2:1.

Natural History. The overall survival rates of patients with LCH at 5, 15, and 20 years are 88%, 88%, and 77%, respectively. Late sequela are often present and include diabetes insipidus in 25% and growth failure in 20%. Therapeutic options depend on symptoms, location, and extent of disease. Patients with diabetes insipidus are treated with oral or nasal vasopressin. They may also be treated with chemotherapy and radiation therapy.

Imaging

The classic imaging of LCH of the pituitary axis is an absent posterior bright spot with a thickened, enhancing pituitary infundibulum **(25-78A)**. LCH may also present as a sellar and suprasellar mass **(25-78B)**.

Differential Diagnosis

The major differential diagnosis of LCH in a **child** is **germinoma**. Both LCH and germinoma may present with an absent posterior "bright spot" and a thickened, enhancing pituitary infundibulum. Germinomas typically present in young patients (peak of 10-12 years) with diabetes insipidus. There is significant imaging overlap of LCH and germinoma although the age of the patient can be a helpful distinguishing feature, as LCH is most common in the first 2 years of life.

In an **adult**, the major differential diagnosis of LCH affecting the pituitary axis is **neurosarcoid** or **hypophysitis**. **Neurosarcoid** patients often present with solitary or multifocal CNS masses as well as pulmonary hilar lymphadenopathy. Patients with neurosarcoid are usually between 20-30 years of age or over 50 years of age and have diabetes insipidus if the pituitary axis is affected. Although hypophysitis may present with loss of the normal pituitary "bright spot," **hypophysitis** usually affects the pituitary gland and the infundibulum, whereas LCH is usually centered in the infundibulum only. Additionally, patients with hypophysitis are typically young adults who may have another autoimmune disorder.

Neurosarcoid

Neurosarcoid is a multisystem inflammatory disease characterized by noncaseating epithelioid-cell granulomas. Neurosarcoid is discussed in more detail in Chapter 15. This section will focus on the pituitary axis.

Etiology

The etiology of neurosarcoid remains unknown. It may be related to stimulation of the immune system by one or more antigens and/or an abnormal immune response.

Pathology

Sarcoidosis may affect many body parts, especially the lymph nodes and lungs. The hilar lymph nodes are the most common site. The CNS is usually affected in combination with disease elsewhere. However, approximately 5-10% of neurosarcoid

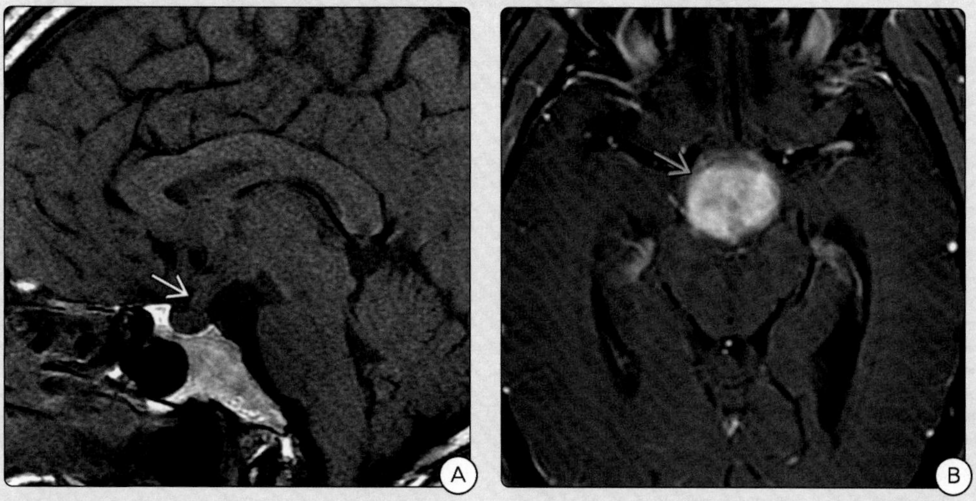

***(25-78A)** Sagittal T1WI in a young adult shows a thickened pituitary infundibulum ➡ with absence of a normal posterior pituitary bright spot, typical of Langerhans cell histiocytosis. **(25-78B)** Axial T1 C+ MR image in the same patient 9 months later shows an enhancing ⇨ suprasellar mass. Patient was lost to follow-up and returned with progressive pituitary dysfunction at the time of this MR. Langerhans cell histiocytosis was diagnosed at resection.*

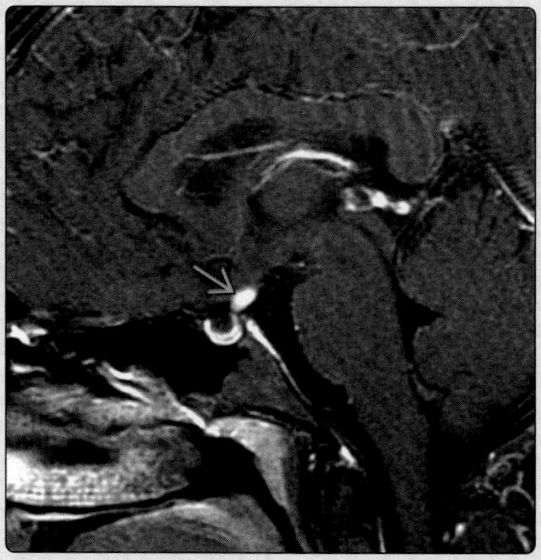

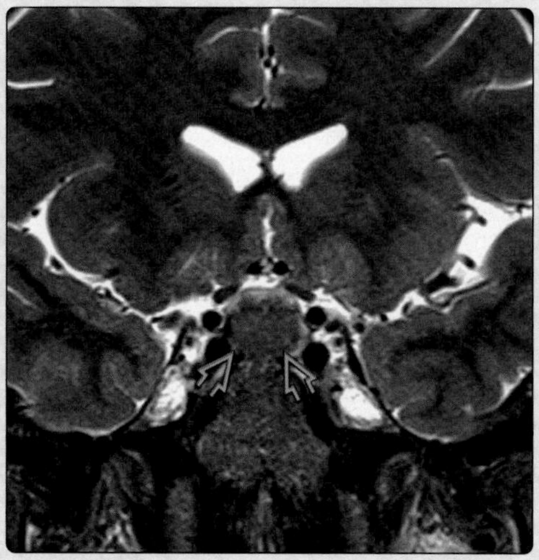

***(25-79)** Sagittal T1 C+ MR in a 50y woman with diabetes insipidus shows marked thickening of the infundibulum ⇨. Patient was diagnosed with neurosarcoid. Differential considerations include lymphocytic hypophysitis, lymphoma, and metastatic disease. **(25-80)** Coronal T2WI shows a hypointense sella/suprasellar mass ⇨ in this female patient with pituitary dysfunction. Neurosarcoid was diagnosed at resection.*

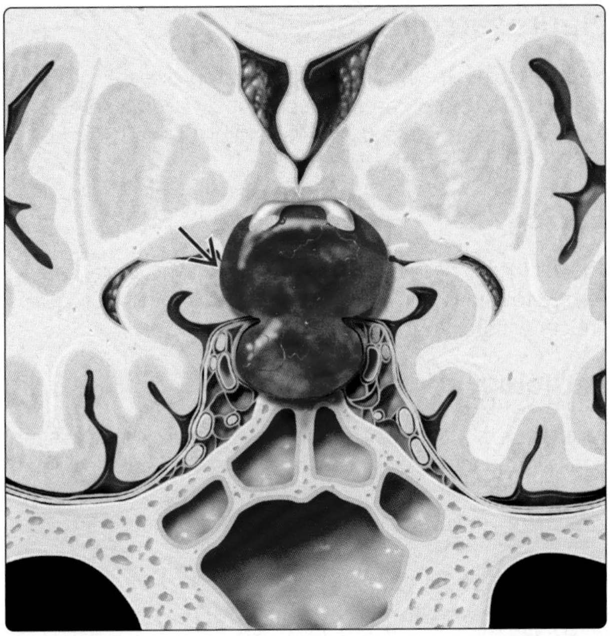

(25-81) Coronal graphic shows a macroadenoma with acute hemorrhage ➔, causing pituitary apoplexy.

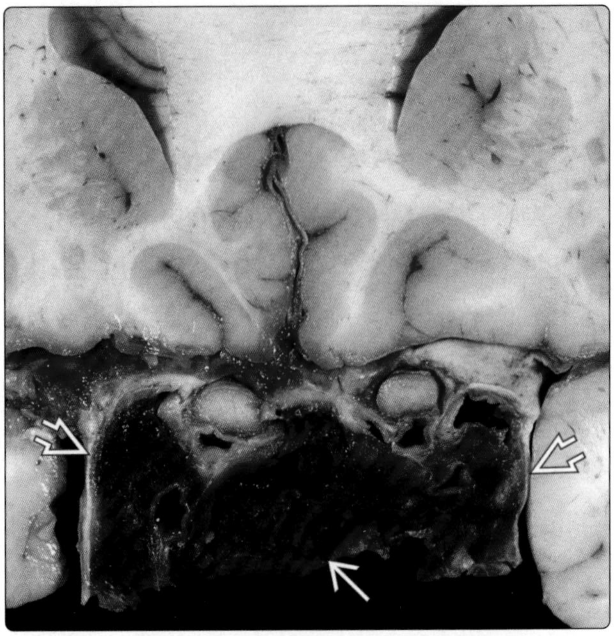

(25-82) Autopsy specimen of pituitary apoplexy shows hemorrhagic macroadenoma ➔ extending into both cavernous sinuses ➔. (Courtesy R. Hewlett, MD.)

cases are confined to the CNS and occur without systemic sarcoid.

Clinical Issues

Presentation. Sarcoid symptoms vary with lesion location. The CNS is involved in approximately 5-10% of sarcoid patients. Patients with lesions affecting the pituitary axis result in pituitary and hypothalamic dysfunction, including diabetes insipidus and panhypopituitarism.

Demographics. There is a bimodal age peak with the initial peak in the third and forth decades and a later peak age in women greater than 50 years old. In the United States, the lifetime risk of sarcoid in African Americans is nearly three times higher than in Caucasians. In Europe, Caucasians are most commonly affected. Sarcoidosis may occur in families.

Natural History. Neurosarcoid has a variable clinical course. It is often an indolent disease that is up to 50% asymptomatic. Approximately 65-70% of neurosarcoid patients have self-limited monophasic illness. The remainder of patients with neurosarcoid have a remitting-relapsing course. The majority of patients respond rapidly to steroids.

Imaging

Neurosarcoid may present as diffuse or focal dural (pachymeningeal) and/or leptomeningeal thickening and enhancement, pituitary infundibulum and/or hypothalamic thickening and enhancement, cranial nerve enhancement, brain parenchymal lesions, or less commonly choroid plexus lesions **(25-79)** **(25-80)**.

Differential Diagnosis

The main differential diagnoses for pituitary axis neurosarcoid are lymphocytic hypophysitis, lymphoma, and metastatic disease. Lymphocytic hypophysitis often presents with loss of the normal pituitary "bright spot" and shows abnormal enhancement in the pituitary gland and the infundibulum. Lymphoma often has an enhancing, infiltrative appearance and may affect the hypothalamus and pituitary gland as well as the infundibulum. Metastatic disease affecting the pituitary axis often has other sites of disease and a known primary cancer.

INFUNDIBULAR STALK MASSES

Adults

- Neurosarcoid (isolated stalk lesion rare)
- Hypophysitis ("stalkitis")
- Metastasis
- Lymphoma
- Pituicytoma

Children

- Germinoma (diabetes insipidus may occur before lesion is visible on MR!)
- Langerhans cell histiocytosis (look for other lesions)
- Ectopic neurohypophysis (displaced PPBS)
- Leukemia

Pituitary Apoplexy

Pituitary apoplexy (PAP) is a well-described acute clinical syndrome with headache, visual defects, and variable endocrine deficiencies. In some cases, profound pituitary insufficiency develops and may become life-threatening.

Etiology

PAP is caused by hemorrhage into—or ischemic necrosis of—the pituitary gland. A preexisting macroadenoma is present in 65-90% of cases, but PAP can also occur in microadenomas or histologically normal pituitary glands. What precipitates the hemorrhage or necrosis is unknown.

In rare cases, patients undergoing treatment with bromocriptine or cabergoline for pituitary adenoma have developed life-threatening PAP. More often, this medical therapy results in a subclinical hemorrhage into the adenoma.

Pathology

The most common gross appearance of PAP is that of a large intrasellar or combined intra- and suprasellar mass **(25-81)**. Between 85 and 90% of cases demonstrate gross hemorrhagic infarction **(25-82)**. Nonhemorrhagic ("bland") pituitary infarction causes an enlarged, edematous-appearing pituitary gland. Microscopic features are nonspecific and generally unremarkable.

Clinical Issues

Epidemiology and Demographics. PAP is rare, occurring in approximately 1% of all patients with pituitary macroadenomas. Peak age is 55-60 years. PAP is rare in patients under the age of 15 years. The M:F ratio is 2:1.

Presentation. Headache is almost universal in patients with PAP and is the most common presenting symptom, followed by nausea (80%) and visual field disturbance (70%). Hemorrhagic tumors that extend into the cavernous sinus may compress cranial nerves III, IV, V, and VI.

Almost 80% of patients with PAP have panhypopituitarism. Acute adrenal crisis with hypovolemia, shock, and disseminated intravascular coagulation may occur. Occasionally, diffuse subarachnoid hemorrhage may be seen.

Rarely, pituitary apoplexy with panhypopituitarism and diabetes insipidus develops in patients with **h**emolysis, **e**levated **l**iver enzymes, and **l**ow **p**latelet count (HELLP) syndrome.

Natural History. PAP varies from a clinically benign event to catastrophic presentation with permanent neurologic deficits. Coma or even death may ensue in severe cases.

Long-term survivors often have permanent pituitary insufficiency requiring hormone replacement (most commonly steroids or thyroid hormone). Almost half of all male patients with PAP require testosterone replacement.

Patients with pituitary adenomas and PAP may show recurrent pituitary tumor growth and therefore merit continued postoperative surveillance.

A rare variant of PAP is **Sheehan syndrome** (SS). Sheehan syndrome is acute postpartum ischemic necrosis of the anterior pituitary gland, typically caused by blood loss and hypovolemic shock during or after childbirth. SS may result in long-term loss of hormone function. Remote SS is a rare cause of partially empty sella on imaging studies.

Treatment Options. Surgical decompression is generally necessary in patients with compromised visual acuity. Supportive therapy with steroids and fluid/electrolyte/hormone replacement is often required.

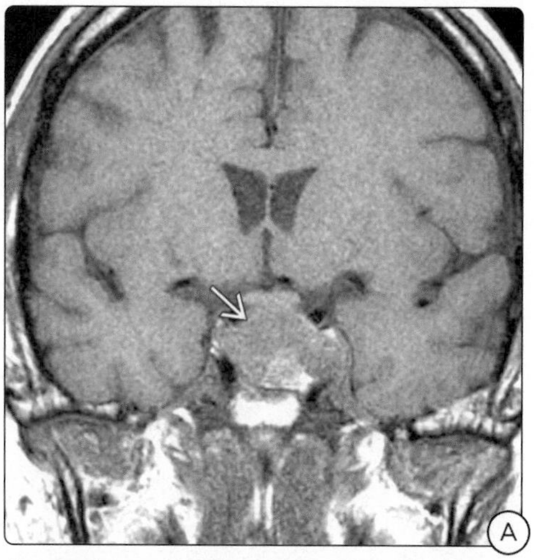

***(25-83A)** T1WI in a 68y man with "thunderclap" headache and visual changes shows mostly isointense intra- and suprasellar mass ➡.*

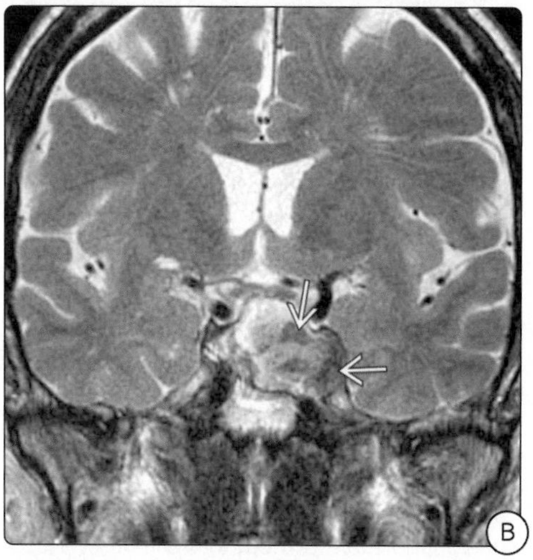

***(25-83B)** Coronal T2WI shows that the mass is very heterogeneous in signal intensity with multiple hemorrhagic foci ➡.*

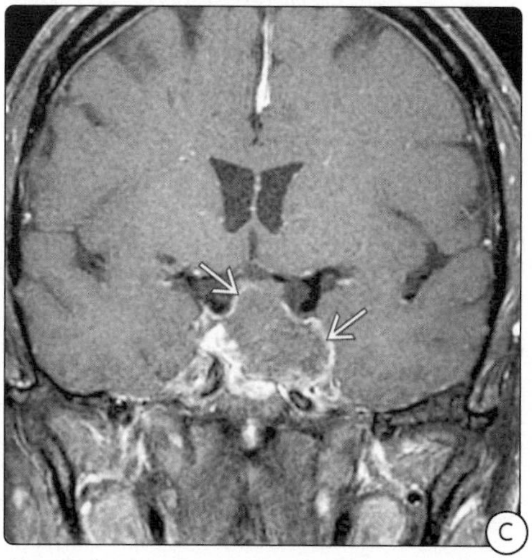

***(25-83C)** Coronal T1 C+ FS shows thin peripheral enhancement ➡, pituitary apoplexy with necrotic, hemorrhagic adenoma found at surgery.*

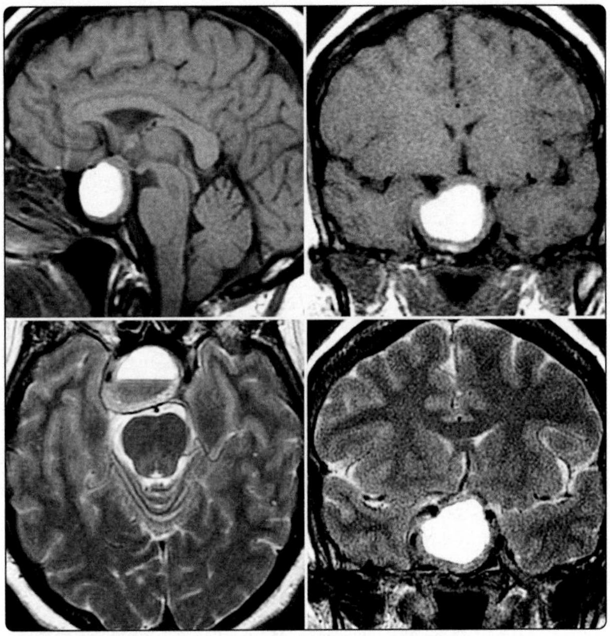

(25-84) Pituitary apoplexy in a 50y woman with 4 days of visual changes shows subacute hemorrhage in the pituitary gland with a blood-fluid level.

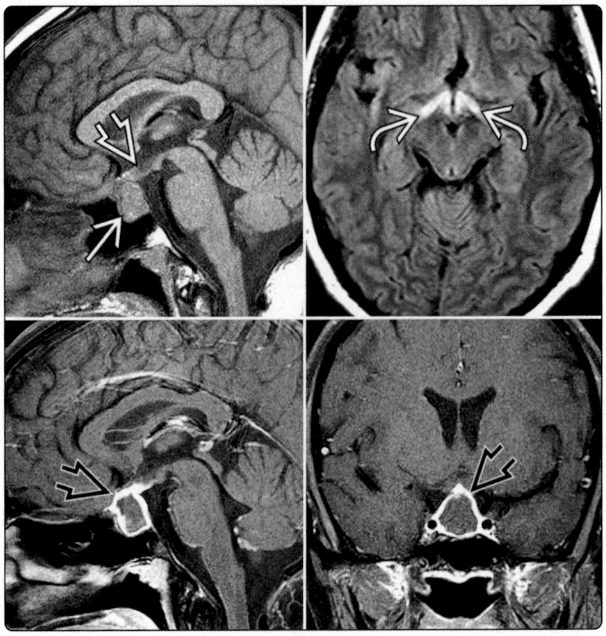

(25-85) (Top left) T1WI shows an enlarged pituitary gland ➡, thick hypothalamus ➡. (Top right) FLAIR hyperintensity is along both optic tracts ➡. (Bottom) Rim enhancement ➡ is shown. This is nonhemorrhagic pituitary apoplexy.

Imaging

General Features. An enlarged pituitary gland with peripheral rim enhancement is typical of pituitary apoplexy **(25-83)**. Gross intraglandular hemorrhage is common but not invariably present.

CT Findings. NECT scans are often normal. Hemorrhage into the pituitary gland with a hyperdense sellar/suprasellar mass can be identified in 20-25% of cases. Occasionally, subarachnoid hemorrhage into the basal cisterns can be identified.

MR Findings. MR is the procedure of choice to evaluate suspected PAP. Signal intensity depends on whether the PAP is hemorrhagic or nonhemorrhagic. Hemorrhage can be identified in 85-90% of cases **(25-84)**.

Signal intensity depends on clot age. Acute PAP is heterogeneously iso- to hypointense to brain on T1WI. Initially iso- to mildly hyperintense on T2WI, PAP rapidly becomes hypointense on T2WI. Acute compression of the hypothalamus and optic chiasm may cause visible edema along the optic tracts on T2/FLAIR scans.

"Blooming"/susceptibility artifact on T2* is common if blood products are present but may be obscured by artifact from the adjacent paranasal sinuses. T1 C+ shows rim enhancement **(25-85)**. Dural thickening and enhancement is seen in 50%, and mucosal thickening in the adjacent sphenoid sinus occurs in 80% of all patients. PAP usually restricts on DWI.

PITUITARY APOPLEXY

Etiology
- Hemorrhagic or nonhemorrhagic pituitary necrosis
- Preexisting macroadenoma (65-90%)

Clinical Issues
- Sudden onset
- Headache, visual defects
- Hypopituitarism (80%)
- Can be life-threatening
- Can result in permanent pituitary insufficiency
- Sheehan syndrome = postpartum pituitary necrosis

Imaging
- Enlarged pituitary
  - ± Hemorrhage (85-90%)
- Rim enhancement around nonenhancing gland
- May cause hypothalamic, optic tract edema

Differential Diagnosis
- Hemorrhagic macroadenoma without apoplexy
- Rathke cleft cyst apoplexy
- Pituitary abscess
- Acute thrombosed aneurysm

Differential Diagnosis

The major differential diagnosis of PAP is **hemorrhagic macroadenoma**. Focal hemorrhages in adenomas are common, but, in contrast to PAP, the clinical course is typically subacute or chronic. Most adenomas enhance strongly but heterogeneously, whereas PAP demonstrates rim enhancement around a predominantly nonenhancing, expanded pituitary gland.

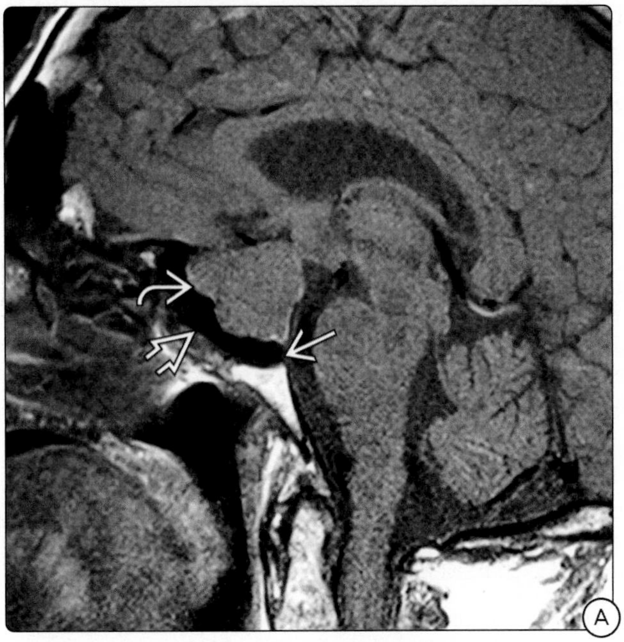

(25-86A) Sagittal T1WI in a patient with longstanding acromegaly shows well-aerated sphenoid sinus ➡ extending posteriorly to clivus ➡. Pneumatization is classified as postsellar. Note well-defined sellar bulge ➡ into sphenoid sinus.

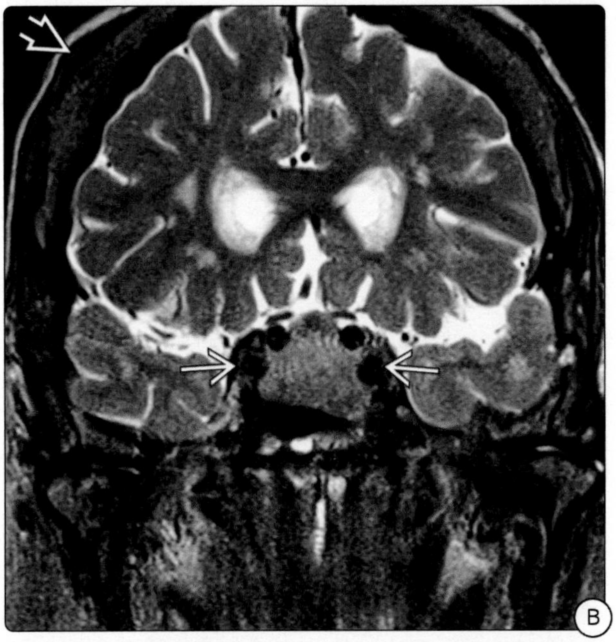

(25-86B) Coronal T2WI shows the exceptionally thick skull ➡ of this patient. The intercarotid distance ➡ measured 24 mm. Transsphenoidal surgery was successful because of the favorable anatomy.

Rathke cleft cyst (RCC) can contain thick proteinaceous fluid that appears hyperintense on T1WI and mimic intrapituitary hemorrhage. Most RCCs are asymptomatic and found incidentally. With some exceptions, RCCs that become symptomatic typically follow a subacute/chronic course. Apoplexy is a rare but distinct presentation caused by sudden hemorrhage into the cyst. RCC with apoplexy can mimic the symptoms of PAP, but the cyst can usually be identified as separate from the pituitary gland.

Pituitary abscess is a rare entity that may be difficult to distinguish from PAP with "bland" (ischemic) infarction. Clinical signs of infection may be minimal or absent. T1 shortening around the rim rather than the center of the mass is characteristic of abscess. Rim enhancement with restriction on DWI is typical for both pituitary abscess and PAP.

Acute thrombosis of a large intra- or parasellar **aneurysm** can present with panhypopituitarism and subarachnoid hemorrhage. "Mixed age" laminated clot is common, and a small residual "flow void" from the residual patent lumen can often be identified on MR.

Lymphocytic **hypophysitis** can cause a relatively sudden onset of symptoms and thus mimic PAP clinically. LH usually causes only modest gland enlargement. The pituitary enhances intensely and uniformly.

Pre- and Postoperative Sella

Two approaches are almost universally used in sellar surgery: traditional sublabial transsphenoidal surgery and minimally invasive completely endoscopic surgery. Image-guided surgery with robotics and stereotactic intraoperative MR is increasingly used with microsurgical and endoscopic techniques. Subfrontal craniotomy is now uncommon and is generally used only for lesions with very large supradiaphragmatic tumors.

Each of these techniques requires careful preoperative imaging evaluation. In this section, we focus on the preoperative evaluation for—and postoperative imaging of—transsphenoidal and endoscopic surgery. Both involve safely navigating the sphenoid sinus and avoiding the many critical structures in and around the sella.

Preoperative Evaluation

Most surgical approaches (transethmoid, transnasal, or transseptal) pass through the sphenoid sinus to reach the sella. Regardless of which operative technique—microscopic or endoscopic—is used, delineating sphenoid sinus anatomy and identifying anatomic variants that might impact surgery are important to successful patient outcome.

CT and MR each has a unique contribution to the full preoperative evaluation of sellar lesions. Multiplanar MR is the procedure of choice to characterize the lesion and define its extent. In concert with MR, preoperative CT helps define relevant bony anatomy.

Four key features of sphenoid sinus anatomy should be identified: the location and extent of pneumatization, the sellar configuration, any septation, and the intercarotid distance.

Pneumatization. Location and extent of sphenoid sinus pneumatization are the major concern. Pneumatization is classified as sellar (57%), postsellar (22%), presellar (21%), or conchal (2%). The specific type of pneumatization is generally determined from sagittal MRs **(25-86)**.

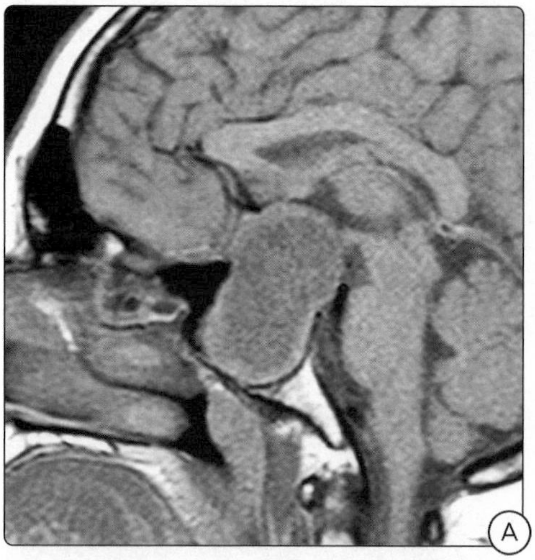

(25-87A) Preoperative sagittal T1WI shows a large sellar/suprasellar solid and cystic mass that expands, erodes, and deepens the sella turcica.

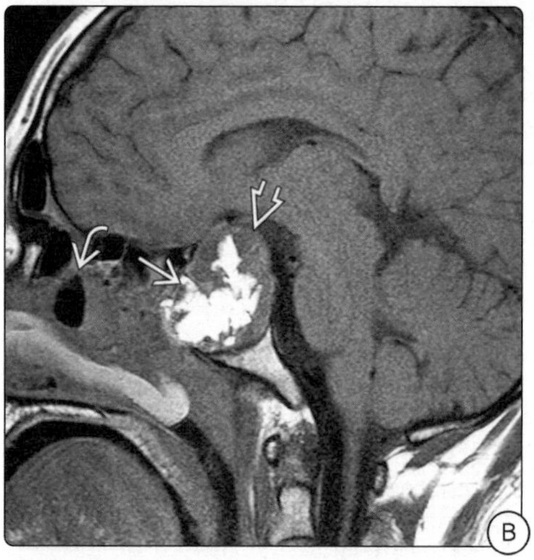

(25-87B) Postoperative T1 C+ scan after tumor debulking shows fat packing, residual tumor, and sphenoid air-fluid level.

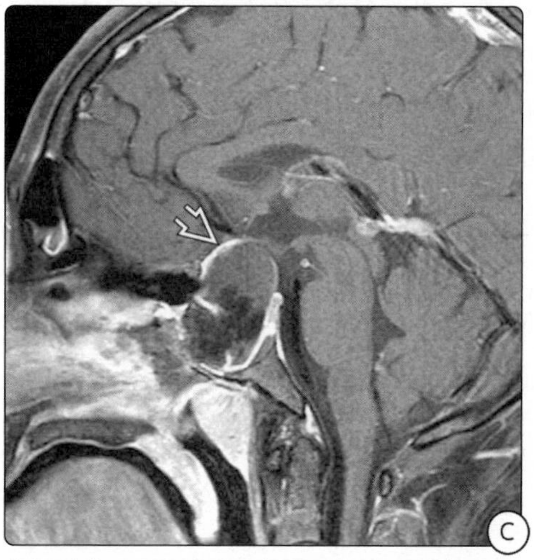

(25-87C) T1 C+ FS scan shows suppressed fat and a thin rim of enhancing tissue.

The rare conchal nonpneumatized sphenoid is important to recognize preoperatively, as it makes transsphenoidal surgery more difficult. At the opposite end of the spectrum, a highly pneumatized sphenoid sinus may make the surgery technically easier but also distorts the anatomic configuration, attenuating the bone and potentially uncovering the carotid arteries and optic nerves.

A pneumatized dorsum sellae can be penetrated during surgery, resulting in a CSF leak.

Sellar Configuration. The presence (well defined) or absence (ill defined) of sellar bulging in relation to the sellar floor and the degree of sphenoid pneumatization should be reported. Pneumatization of the planum sphenoidale and dorsum sellae should also be noted. These are determined from sagittal MR.

A prominent sellar bulge into a pneumatized sphenoid sinus is seen in 75% of patients **(25-86A)**. The other 25% have an absent or ill-defined sellar bulge. A well-pneumatized sphenoid sinus with a prominent sellar bulge facilitates surgery, which is further eased if the sellar floor is thinned or disrupted by tumor. Dorsum sellae pneumatization is present in the majority.

Septation. The presence or absence of an intersphenoid septum should be determined. If present, note whether there is a single intersinus septum or more than one septa. The position of the septal insertion (in the sellar floor, at the carotid canal, or at the optic canal) should be identified. This is best evaluated on both axial and coronal bone CT.

Axial scans show no septum in 10-11% of patients and a single intersphenoid septum in 70%. An accessory septum is seen in 10% of patients, and 7-9% have multiple septa.

The intersphenoid septum must be removed to expose the sellar floor, so determining its location is crucial. The septum is rarely located in the midline. It typically deviates to one side or the other, dividing the sphenoid sinus into two unequal cavities. This results in an asymmetric appearance of the sellar floor. In 30-40% of patients, the septum deviates quite laterally and terminates adjacent to the internal carotid artery.

Intercarotid Distance. The intercarotid distance is measured between the medial aspects of the two signal "voids" of the cavernous ICA segments as seen on midsellar coronal MR. Intercarotid distance varies widely, ranging from 10-12 mm to 30 mm (mean of 23 mm). Narrow distances (< 12 mm) increase the chance of vascular injury during transsphenoidal surgery.

Postoperative Evaluation

To evaluate the postoperative sella, thin-section, small FOV imaging in both the sagittal and coronal planes is mandatory. Precontrast T1- and T2WI images plus postcontrast fat-saturated sequences are standard.

The appearance on postoperative MR scans is complicated by hemorrhage, use of hemostatic agents, packing materials (muscle, fat, fascia lata), and residual tumor. Typical findings include a bony defect in the anterior sphenoid sinus wall, fluid and mucosal thickening in the sinus, fat packing within the sella turcica, hemorrhage, and varying amounts of residual mass effect **(25-87)**.

The first postoperative scan provides the baseline against with which subsequent imaging is compared. With time, hemorrhage evolves and resorbs, fat packing fibroses and retracts, and mass effect decreases. A partially empty sella with or without traction on the infundibular stalk and optic chiasm is typical in the months and years following the initial surgery.

Complications such as diabetes insipidus, stalk transection, and electrolyte disturbances are usually temporary. Long-term complications include CSF leaks and cranial neuropathy.

Differential Diagnosis of a Sellar Region Mass

In establishing a helpful differential diagnosis of a sellar mass, determining anatomic sublocation is the first, most important step. Is the lesion (1) intrasellar, (2) suprasellar, or (3) in the infundibular stalk? Or is it a combination of these locations?

Whether a sellar/suprasellar mass *is* the pituitary gland itself or is separate from the mass is the most important imaging task and the most helpful finding **(25-88)** **(25-89)** **(25-90)** **(25-91)**. Masses that can be clearly distinguished as separate from the pituitary gland are rarely—if ever—macroadenomas.

The most helpful clinical feature is patient age. Some lesions are common in adults but rarely occur in children. Sex and endocrine status are helpful ancillary clues. For example, pituitary macroadenomas rarely cause diabetes insipidus, but it is one of the most common presenting symptoms of hypophysitis.

Lastly, consider some specific imaging findings. Is the mass cystic? Is it calcified? What is the MR signal intensity? Does the lesion enhance?

Intrasellar Lesions

Intrasellar lesions can be mass-like or non-mass-like. Keep two concepts in mind: (1) not all "enlarged pituitary glands" are abnormal. Pituitary size and height vary with sex and age. A "fat" pituitary can also occur with intracranial hypotension. (2) Pituitary "incidentalomas" are common (identified in 15-20% of normal MR scans), often cystic microadenomas or Rathke cleft cysts.

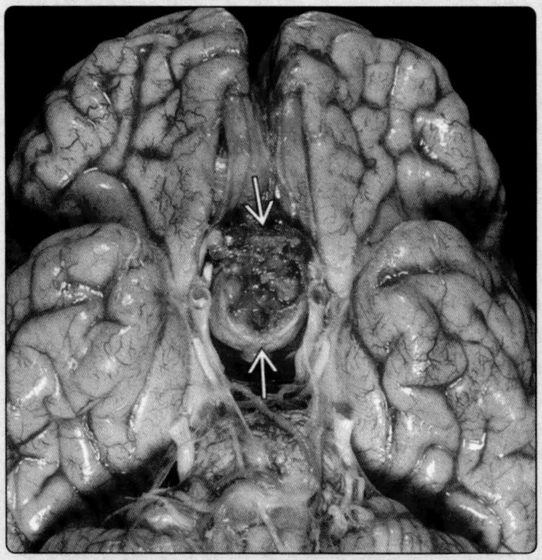
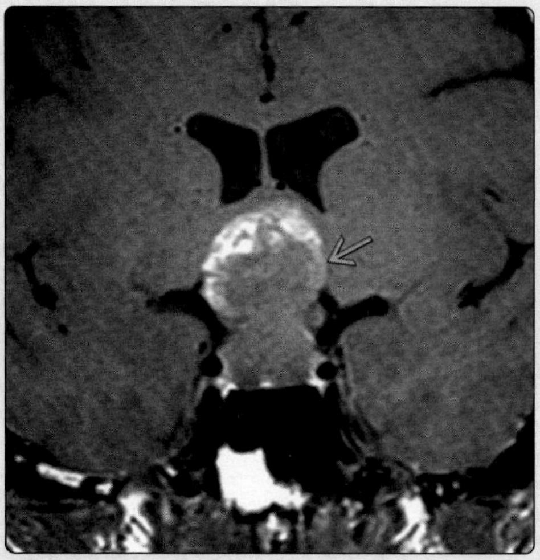

(25-88) *Submentovertex view of autopsied brain shows large intra- and suprasellar mass ➡. The pituitary gland cannot be separated from the mass and indeed is the mass. (Courtesy R. Hewlett, MD.)* ***(25-89)*** *Coronal T1WI shows the classic "snowman" or "figure eight" shape of a macroadenoma ⇨. The mass and gland are indistinguishable from each other.*

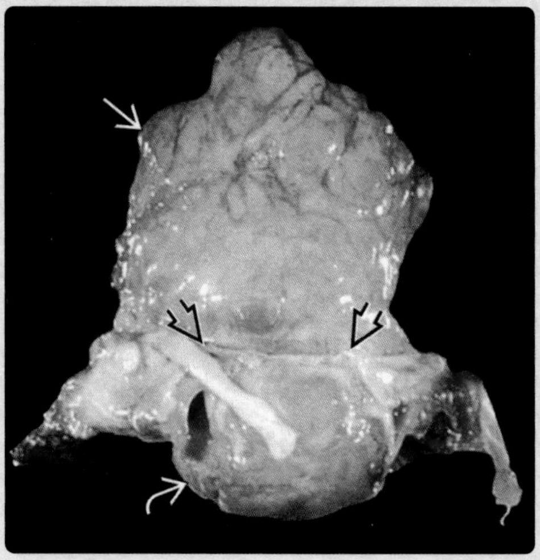
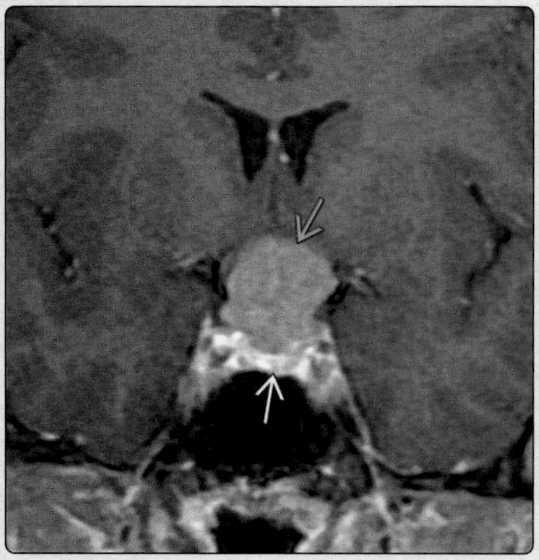

(25-90) *Coronal view shows autopsied suprasellar meningioma. The tumor ➡ is separated from the pituitary gland below ➡ by the diaphragma sellae ⇨, from which the meningioma arose. (Courtesy J. Paltan, MD.)* ***(25-91)*** *Coronal T1 C+ image of a suprasellar meningioma ⇨ shows that the tumor is separate from the more enhancing normal pituitary gland ➡.*

WHEN THE MASS *CANNOT* BE SEPARATED FROM THE PITUITARY GLAND
Common • Pituitary macroadenoma • Pituitary hyperplasia (physiologic, pathologic) **Less Common** • Neurosarcoid • Langerhans cell histiocytosis • Hypophysitis **Rare But Important** • Metastasis • Lymphoma • Germinoma

INTRASELLAR LESION
Common • Pituitary hyperplasia (physiologic, pathologic) • Pituitary microadenoma • Empty sella **Less Common** • Pituitary macroadenoma • Rathke cleft (or other) cyst • Craniopharyngioma • Neurosarcoid **Rare But Important** • Lymphocytic hypophysitis • Intracranial hypotension (venous congestion) • Vascular ("kissing" carotids, aneurysm) • Meningioma • Metastasis • Lymphoma

Common Suprasellar Masses

The five most common overall suprasellar masses, i.e., the "Big Five," are pituitary macroadenoma, meningioma, aneurysm, craniopharyngioma, and astrocytoma. Together they account for 75-80% of all sellar region masses. Three of the "Big Five" (the "Big Three")—adenoma, meningioma, aneurysm—are common in adults but rare in children **(25-92)** **(25-93)**.

COMMON SUPRASELLAR MASSES
Adults • Pituitary adenoma (mass = gland) • Meningioma (mass separate from gland) • Aneurysm ("flow void," pulsation artifact) **Children** • Craniopharyngioma (90% cystic, 90% calcify, 90% enhance) • Hypothalamic/optic chiasm astrocytoma (solid, no calcification)

Less Common Suprasellar Masses

The presence of some less common lesions can often be inferred from imaging studies.

LESS COMMON SUPRASELLAR MASSES
• Rathke cleft cyst (well delineated, separate from pituitary) • Arachnoid cyst (behaves just like CSF) • Dermoid cyst (looks like fat) • Neurocysticercosis (usually multiple)

Rare Suprasellar Masses

Keep these lesions in mind—they can mimic more common lesions, but the appropriate treatment differs sharply.

RARE BUT IMPORTANT SUPRASELLAR MASSES
• Hypophysitis (may look like adenoma) • Hypothalamic hamartoma ("collar button" between stalk, mammillary bodies) • Metastasis (systemic cancer; look for other lesions) • Lymphoma (often infiltrates adjacent structures)

Cystic Intra-/Suprasellar Mass

If an intra- or suprasellar mass is primarily or exclusively cystic, the differential diagnosis considerations change. The key issue is to distinguish a cystic mass that originates *within* the sella versus intrasellar extension *from* a suprasellar lesion **(25-94)**. Other than Rathke cleft cyst, completely intrasellar nonneoplastic cysts are rare, as is a totally intrasellar craniopharyngioma without suprasellar extension.

In a **child** with a suprasellar cystic mass, consider an enlarged third ventricle, craniopharyngioma, neurocysticercosis, and astrocytoma. In an **adult**, consider arachnoid cyst, neurocysticercosis, Rathke cleft cyst, adenoma, and aneurysm **(25-95)**.

CYSTIC *INTRA*SELLAR MASS
Common • Empty sella • Idiopathic intracranial hypertension **Less Common** • Cystic pituitary adenoma • Rathke cleft cyst • Neurocysticercosis cyst **Rare But Important** • Craniopharyngioma • Epidermoid cyst, arachnoid cyst • Pituitary apoplexy • Thrombosed aneurysm

CYSTIC *SUPRA*SELLAR MASS

Common

- Enlarged third ventricle
- Arachnoid cyst
- Craniopharyngioma
- Neurocysticercosis cyst

Less Common

- Rathke cleft cyst
- Dermoid cyst
- Epidermoid cyst

Rare But Important

- Pituitary macroadenoma, apoplexy
- Astrocytoma (usually solid)
- Ependymal cyst
- Aneurysm (patent or thrombosed)

CALCIFIED *SUPRA*SELLAR MASS

Common

- Atherosclerosis
- Craniopharyngioma
- Meningioma
- Aneurysm
    - Saccular
    - Fusiform, atherosclerotic

Less Common

- Neurocysticercosis
- Pilocytic astrocytoma
- Dermoid cyst

Rare But Important

- Macroadenoma
- Tuberculosis
- Chondroid tumor

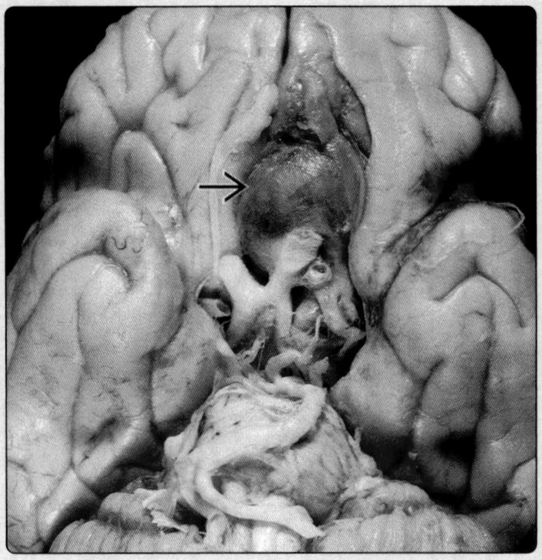

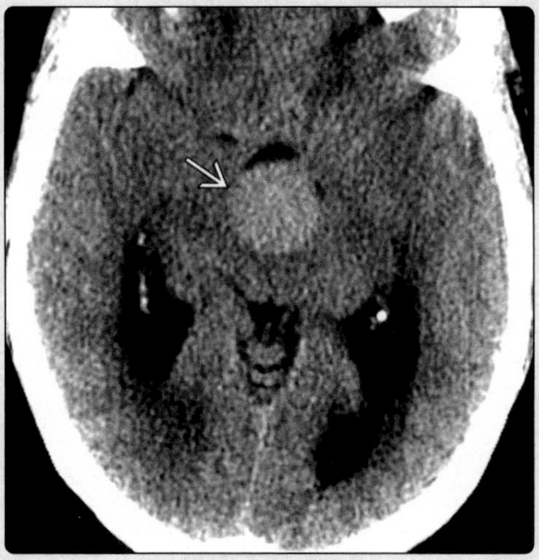

***(25-92)** Autopsy specimen demonstrates an unruptured suprasellar aneurysm ⇨. (Courtesy R. Hewlett, MD.) **(25-93)** NECT in a 55y man with headaches shows hyperdense noncalcified mass ➡ in the suprasellar cistern. Considerations in an adult include macroadenoma, meningioma, and aneurysm. This is large basilar tip aneurysm.*

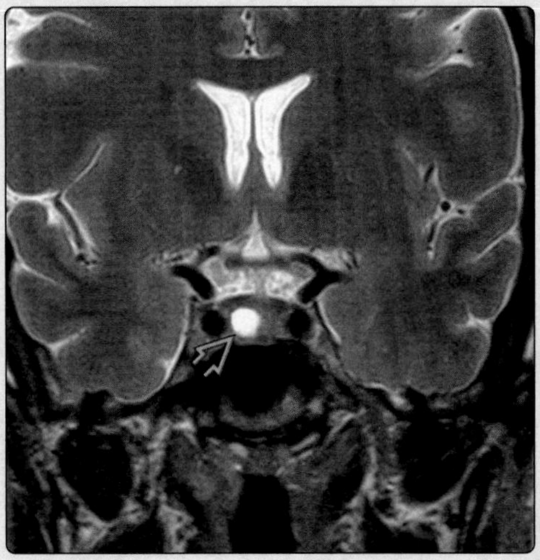

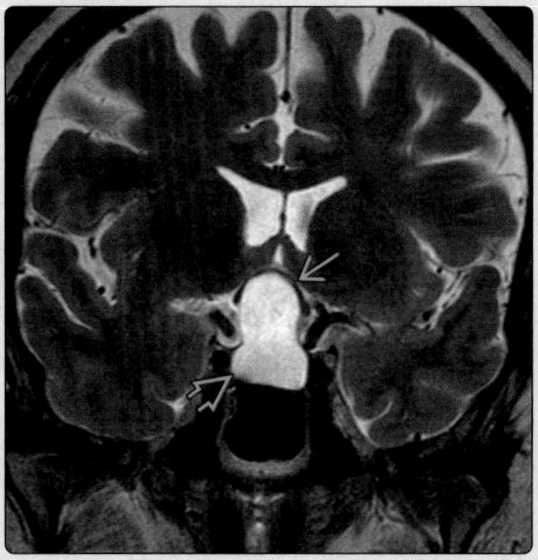

***(25-94)** Coronal T2WI shows a cystic intrasellar mass ⇨ in a young adult with elevated prolactin. Cystic microadenoma was found at resection. Imaging mimics a Rathke cleft cyst. **(25-95)** Coronal T2WI shows a cystic intra- and suprasellar mass ⇨. The optic chiasm ⇨ is elevated and draped over the cyst. Arachnoid cyst was found at surgery. ACs follow CSF signal intensity on all MR sequences.*

Selected References

Sellar Region Anatomy

Go JL et al: Imaging of the sella and parasellar region. Radiol Clin North Am. 55(1):83-101, 2017

Zamora C et al: Sellar and parasellar imaging. Neurosurgery. 80(1):17-38, 2017

Imaging Technique and Anatomy

Grajo JR et al: Multiple endocrine neoplasia syndromes: a comprehensive imaging review. Radiol Clin North Am. 54(3):441-51, 2016

Normal Imaging Variants

Pituitary Hyperplasia

Syro LV et al: Pathology of GH-producing pituitary adenomas and GH cell hyperplasia of the pituitary. Pituitary. 20(1):84-92, 2017

Kocova M et al: Diagnostic approach in children with unusual symptoms of acquired hypothyroidism. When to look for pituitary hyperplasia? J Pediatr Endocrinol Metab. 29(3):297-303, 2016

Empty Sella

Saindane AM et al: Factors determining the clinical significance of an "empty" sella turcica. AJR Am J Roentgenol. 200(5):1125-31, 2013

Congenital Lesions

Pituitary Anomalies

El Sanharawi I et al: High-resolution heavily T2-weighted magnetic resonance imaging for evaluation of the pituitary stalk in children with ectopic neurohypophysis. Pediatr Radiol. 47(5):599-605, 2017

Hypothalamic Hamartoma

Kameyama S et al: MRI-guided stereotactic radiofrequency thermocoagulation for 100 hypothalamic hamartomas. J Neurosurg. 124(5):1503-12, 2016

Rathke Cleft Cyst

Park M et al: Differentiation between cystic pituitary adenomas and Rathke cleft cysts: a diagnostic model using MRI. AJNR Am J Neuroradiol. 36(10):1866-73, 2015

Neoplasms

Pituitary Adenomas

Molitch ME: Diagnosis and treatment of pituitary adenomas: a review. JAMA. 317(5):516-524, 2017

Tamrazi B et al: Apparent diffusion coefficient and pituitary macroadenomas: pre-operative assessment of tumor atypia. Pituitary. 20(2):195-200, 2017

Lilja Y et al: Visual pathway impairment by pituitary adenomas: quantitative diagnostics by diffusion tensor imaging. J Neurosurg. 1-11, 2016

Sav A et al: Invasive, atypical and aggressive pituitary adenomas and carcinomas. Endocrinol Metab Clin North Am. 44(1):99-104, 2015

Pituitary Blastoma

Scheithauer BW et al: Pituitary blastoma: a unique embryonal tumor. Pituitary. 15(3):365-73, 2012

Lymphoma

Deckert et al: Lymphomas. In: Louis DN et al (eds), WHO Classification of Tumours of the Central Nervous System. Lyon, France: International Agency for Research on Cancer, 2016, pp 272-277

Tarabay A et al: Primary pituitary lymphoma: an update of the literature. J Neurooncol. 130(3):383-395, 2016

Germinoma

Rosenblum M et al: Germ cell tumours: germinoma. In: Louis DN et al (eds), WHO Classification of Tumours of the Central Nervous System. Lyon, France: International Agency for Research on Cancer, 2016, pp 286-291

Di Iorgi N et al: Pituitary stalk thickening on MRI: when is the best time to re-scan and how long should we continue re-scanning for? Clin Endocrinol (Oxf). 83(4):449-55, 2015

Craniopharyngioma

Wijnen M et al: Very long-term sequelae of craniopharyngioma. Eur J Endocrinol. 176(6):755-767, 2017

Buslei R et al: Tumours of the sellar region: craniopharyngioma. In: Louis DN et al (eds), WHO Classification of Tumours of the Central Nervous System. Lyon, France: International Agency for Research on Cancer, 2016, pp 324-328

Nonadenomatous Pituitary Tumors

Hagel C et al: Immunoprofiling of glial tumours of the neurohypophysis suggests a common pituicytic origin of neoplastic cells. Pituitary. 20(2):211-217, 2017

Brat D et al: Pituicytoma. In: Louis DN et al (eds), WHO Classification of Tumours of the Central Nervous System. Lyon, France: International Agency for Research on Cancer, 2016, pp 332-333

Fuller G et al: Granular cell tumour of the sellar region. In: Louis DN et al (eds), WHO Classification of Tumours of the Central Nervous System. Lyon, France: International Agency for Research on Cancer, 2016, pp 329-331

Lopes M et al: Spindle cell oncocytoma. In: Louis DN et al (eds), WHO Classification of Tumours of the Central Nervous System. Lyon, France: International Agency for Research on Cancer, 2016, pp 334-335

Miscellaneous Lesions

Hypophysitis

Kyriacou A et al: Lymphocytic hypophysitis: modern day management with limited role for surgery. Pituitary. 20(2):241-250, 2017

Langerhans Cell Histiocytosis

Paulus W et al: LCH. In: Louis DN et al (eds), WHO Classification of Tumours of the Central Nervous System. Lyon, France: International Agency for Research on Cancer, 2016, pp 280-281

Neurosarcoid

Anthony J et al: Hypothalamic-pituitary sarcoidosis with vision loss and hypopituitarism: case series and literature review. Pituitary. 19(1):19-29, 2016

Pituitary Apoplexy

Singh TD et al: Management and outcomes of pituitary apoplexy. J Neurosurg. 122(6):1450-7, 2015

Miscellaneous Tumors and Tumor-Like Conditions

Some important neoplasms that affect the calvaria, skull base, and cranial meninges are not included in the most recent standardized WHO classification of CNS tumors. This chapter covers several of these intriguing tumors as well as tumor-like lesions that do not easily fit into other sections of this text. Although infections, granulomatous disease, demyelinating disorders, and vascular diseases (among others) may sometimes mimic CNS neoplasms, they are treated separately in their own respective chapters.

We begin with *extra*cranial tumors and tumor-like conditions. These lesions mostly arise within the calvaria or skull base. We then turn our attention to an interesting group of *intra*cranial lesions that all mimic neoplasms, i.e., they are pseudotumors. These tumor-like lesions may arise within the meninges, CSF cisterns, or brain parenchyma. Some lesions may involve multiple compartments and can be intracranial, extracranial, or a combination of both.

Extracranial Tumors and Tumor-Like Conditions

Fibrous Dysplasia

Benign fibroosseous lesions of the craniofacial complex are represented by a variety of intraosseous disease processes. These include bone dysplasias, the most common of which is fibrous dysplasia (FD).

Terminology

FD is a benign dysplastic fibroosseous lesion that is also known as fibrocartilaginous dysplasia, osteitis fibrosa, and generalized fibrocystic disease of bone.

Etiology

General Concepts. FD is a developmental lesion with local arrest of normal structural/architectural development. Abnormal differentiation of osteoblasts results in replacement of normal marrow and cancellous bone by immature "woven" bone and fibrous stroma.

Genetics. Recent studies have demonstrated that FD is a neoplastic—not dysplastic—lesion. Activating mutations of the *GNAS1* gene result in

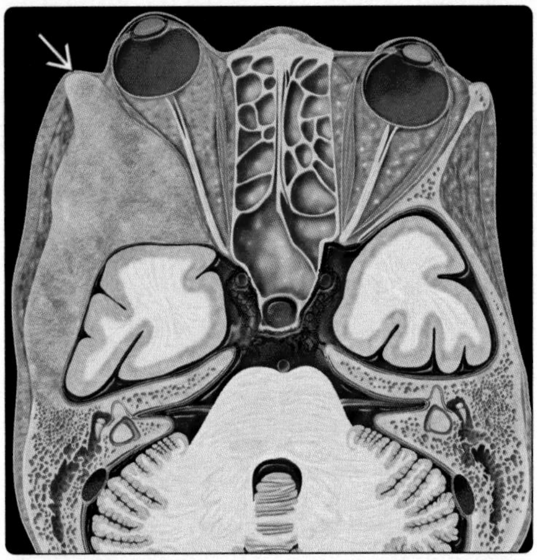

***(26-1)** FD is with expansion of lateral orbital rim ➡, sphenoid wing, temporal squamosa. Note exophthalmos, stretching of optic nerve.*

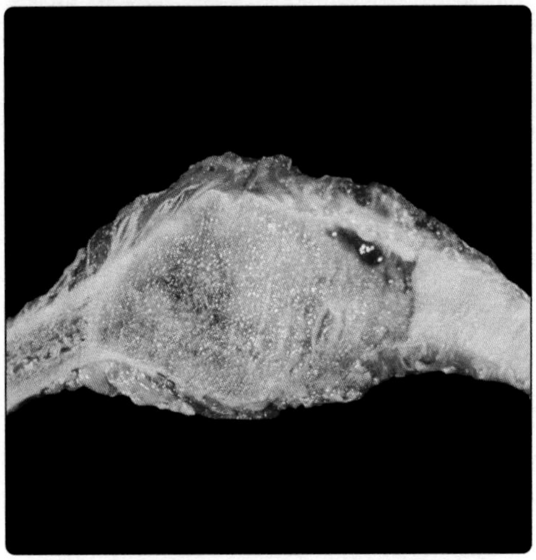

***(26-2)** FD in a rib is a solid tan tumor that expands bone, has "ground-glass" appearance. (Courtesy A. Rosenberg, MD, G. P. Nielsen, MD.)*

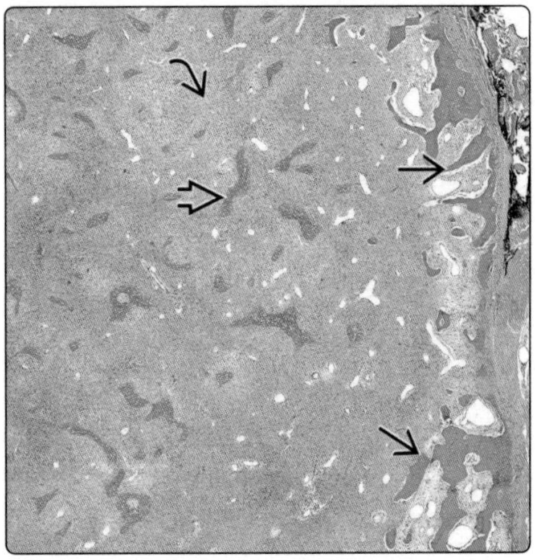

***(26-3)** FD shows "woven" bony trabeculae ⇨, fibrous stroma ⇨, reactive subperiosteal new bone ➡. (A. Rosenberg, MD, G. P. Nielsen, MD.)*

overexpression of the c-fos proto-oncogene, which contributes to the initiation and progression of FD.

Pathology

Location. Virtually any bone in the head and neck can be affected by FD. The skull and facial bones are the location of 10-25% of all monostotic FD lesions. The frontal bone is the most common calvarial site, followed by the temporal bone, sphenoid, and parietal bones. Involvement of the clivus is rare. The orbit, zygoma, maxilla, and mandible are the most frequent sites in the face **(26-1)**.

Size and Number. FD lesions range in size from relatively small—less than 1 cm—to massive lesions that involve virtually an entire bone. Altered osteogenesis may occur within a single bone ("monostotic FD") or multiple bones ("polyostotic FD"). **Monostotic FD** accounts for approximately 60-80% of all lesions; **polyostotic FD** occurs in 20-40% of cases.

Polyostotic FD with endocrinopathy is known as **McCune-Albright syndrome** (MAS) and occurs in 3-5% of cases. The classic MAS triad consists of multiple FD lesions, endocrine dysfunction (typically precocious puberty), and cutaneous hyperpigmentation ("café au lait spots").

Gross Pathology. FD is tan to whitish gray **(26-2)**. Depending on the relative amount of fibrous versus osseous content, texture varies from firm and rubbery to "gritty."

Microscopic Features. Fibrous and osseous tissues are admixed in varying proportions **(26-3)**. In the early stages, pronounced osteogenesis with thin osteoid anastomosing trabeculae rimmed with osteoblasts is seen. A stromal fibroblastic element with variable vascularity is interspersed between trabeculae of immature "woven" bone that resembles "Chinese letters."

Almost 60% of cases demonstrate different stromal patterns admixed with the usual fibroblastic elements. These include focal fatty metamorphosis (20-25%), myxoid stroma (15%), and calcifications (12%). Cystic degeneration occurs but is uncommon.

Clinical Issues

Epidemiology. FD is rare, representing approximately 1% of all biopsied primary bone tumors. It is the second most common pediatric primary skull lesion (after dermoid cysts).

Demographics. Although FD can present at virtually any age, most patients are younger than 30 years at the time of initial diagnosis. Polyostotic FD presents earlier; the mean age is 8 years. With the exception of FD as part of MAS, which affects female patients more than male patients, there is no sex predilection.

Presentation. Symptoms of craniofacial FD depend on lesion location. Painless osseous expansion with calvarial or facial asymmetry is common. Proptosis and optic neuropathy are common in patients with orbital disease. Conductive hearing loss and facial weakness are typical in patients with temporal bone FD. Mandibular FD typically presents with "cherubism."

Polyostotic FD may cause "leontiasis ossea" (lion-like physiognomy) or complex cranial neuropathies (secondary to severe narrowing of the neural foramina).

Natural History. Disease course varies. Monostotic lesions do not regress or disappear, but they generally stabilize at puberty. In contrast, polyostotic FD generally becomes less active after puberty although long bone deformities may progress, and microfractures may develop.

Malignant transformation is very rare,occurring in less than 1% of all FD cases and has been described in both the monostotic and polyostotic forms.

Treatment options for FD are limited. Recurrence is very high following curettage and bone grafting. Radiation therapy is generally avoided, as it may induce malignant transformation. Intravenous bisphosphonate therapy has been used to ameliorate the disease course with some reported success.

FIBROUS DYSPLASIA: PATHOLOGY AND CLINICAL ISSUES

Pathology

- Location, number
  - Any bone
  - Craniofacial (10-25%)
  - Solitary (60-80%) or polyostotic (20-40%)
- Gross pathology: "woven" bone
- Microscopic pathology
  - Variable admixture of fibrous, osseous components
  - Less common: fat, myxoid tissue, Ca++, cysts

Clinical Issues

- Rare (< 1% of biopsied bone tumors)
  - One of the most common fibroosseous lesions
- Monostotic patients < 30 years
- Polyostotic fibrous dysplasia
  - Younger (mean age = 8 years)
  - McCune-Albright (3-5%)
  - Craniofacial > calvarial involvement

Imaging

General Features. Most craniofacial lesions are monostotic. However, skeletal survey or whole-body MR is recommended to detect asymptomatic lesions in other bones that would indicate polyostotic disease or MAS.

Imaging findings depend on disease stage. In general, very early lesions are radiolucent and then undergo progressive calcification, resulting in a "ground-glass" appearance. Mixed patterns are common.

CT Findings. Nonaggressive osseous remodeling and thickening of the affected bone are typical. NECT shows a geographic expansile lesion centered in the medullary cavity. Abrupt transition between the lesion and adjacent normal bone is typical.

Bone CT appearance varies with the relative content of fibrous versus osseous tissue. FD can be sclerotic, cystic, or mixed (sometimes called "pagetoid"). A pattern with mixed areas of radiopacity and radiolucency is found in almost half of all cases **(26-4A)** **(26-5)**. The classic relatively homogeneous "ground-glass" appearance occurs in 25%. Densely sclerotic lesions are common in the skull base. Almost one-quarter of all FD cases have some cystic changes, seen as central lucent areas with thinned but sclerotic borders.

MR Findings. FD is usually homogeneously hypointense on T1WI. Signal intensity on T2WI is variable. Moderate hypointensity is characteristic of ossified and/or fibrous portions of the lesion **(26-4B)**. Active lesions may be heterogeneous and may have hyperintense areas on T2 or FLAIR **(26-5D)**. Cysts appear as rounded high signal foci.

Signal intensity following contrast administration varies depending on the lesion stage and ranges from no enhancement to diffuse, avid enhancement in active lesions **(26-4C)**.

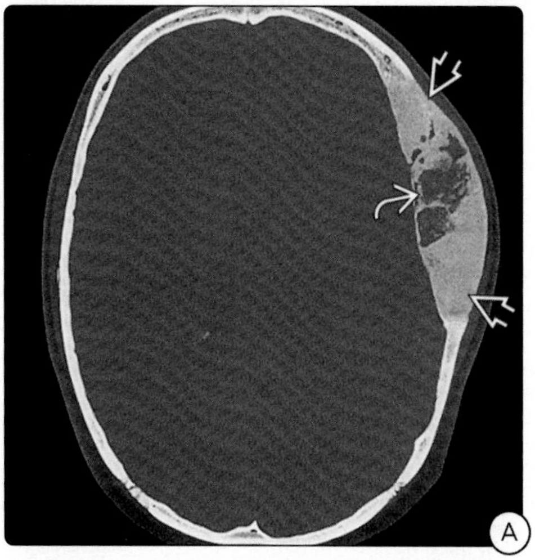

***(26-4A)** Bone CT in a 26y woman shows classic monostotic FD with "ground glass" appearance ➡, central noncalcified fibrous stroma ➡.*

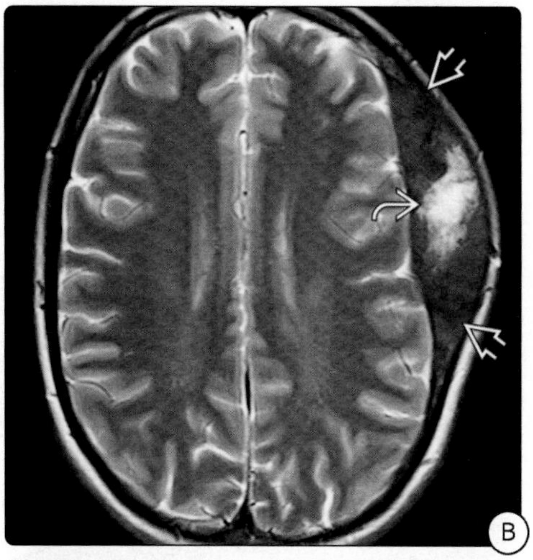

***(26-4B)** T2WI shows that dense, ossified bone is hypointense ➡, but a central area of active disease is hyperintense ➡.*

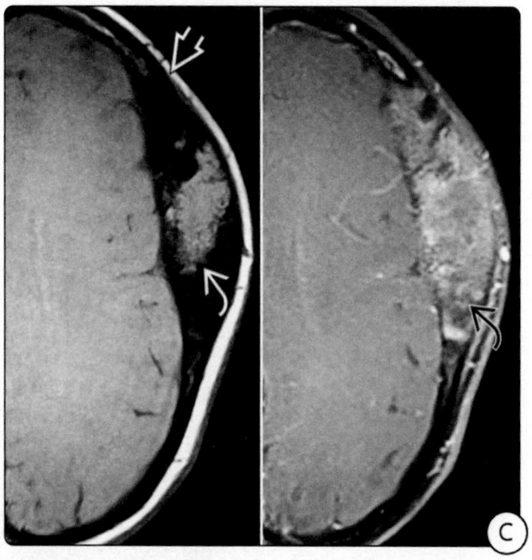

***(26-4C)** (L) T1WI in the same case shows hypointense periphery ➡, isointense center ➡. (R) T1 C+ FS shows most of mass ➡ enhances.*

Nuclear Medicine. FDG PET and 68Ga-PET/CT show increased metabolic activity in one or more sites and can mimic metastatic disease.

Differential Diagnosis

The major differential diagnoses for craniofacial FD are Paget disease and ossifying fibroma (OF).

Paget disease typically occurs in elderly patients and usually involves the calvaria and temporal bone. A "cotton wool" appearance is typical on digital skull radiographs and bone CT.

OF may mimic the cystic monostotic form of FD. OF has a thick, bony rim with a lower density center on bone CT and generally appears more mass-like and localized. Diffuse **sclerosing osteomyelitis** of the mandible may also resemble FD.

Intraosseous meningioma is another differential consideration. Intraosseous meningiomas are more common in the calvaria than in the skull base and facial bones. A strongly enhancing en plaque soft tissue mass is often associated with the bony lesion. A mixed sclerotic-destructive skull base **metastasis** may mimic FD. In most cases, an extracranial primary site is known.

The differential diagnosis of FD includes rare fibroosseous disorders that can affect the craniofacial bones. These include **osteitis deformans, florid osseous dysplasia, focal cementoosseous dysplasia,** and **periapical cemental dysplasia**.

Facial bone changes associated with hyperparathyroidism and **renal osteodystrophy** may present with a classic "ground-glass" appearance on both conventional radiography and CT. However, in contrast to FD, these changes are generalized and diffuse.

(26-5A) Bone CT in a 19y man with polyostotic FD and cranial nerve palsies shows multiple lesions in the facial bones and calvarium. (26-5B) More cephalad bone CT shows several lesions expanding the calvarium.

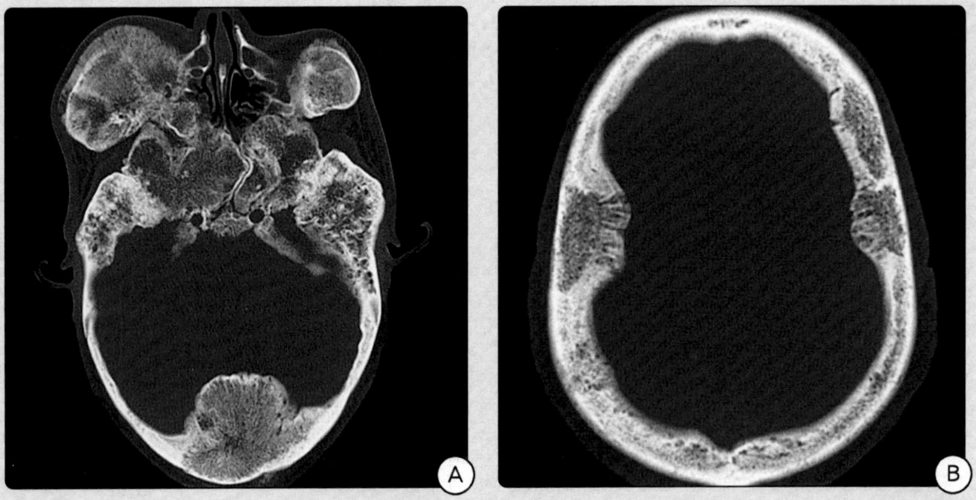

(26-5C) Sagittal reformatted bone CT shows the expansile, "ground glass" appearance of the skull base ➔ and calvarial lesions ➔. (26-5D) Sagittal T2WI shows that the expansile skull base ➔ and calvarial ➔ lesions are heterogeneously hyperintense. Note severe posterior fossa crowding with acquired tonsillar herniation ➔.

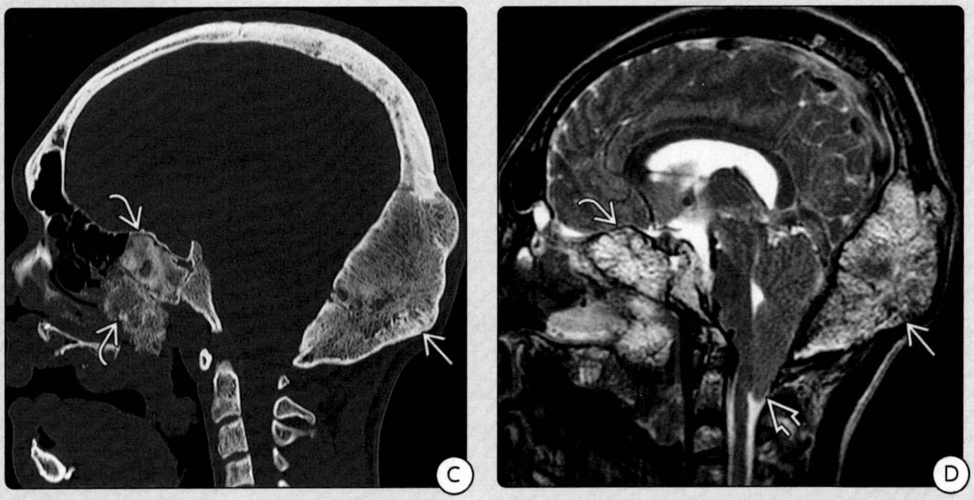

FIBROUS DYSPLASIA: IMAGING AND DDx

Imaging
- CT
  - Bone remodeled, expanded
  - "Ground-glass" appearance classic
  - Sclerotic, cystic, mixed ("pagetoid") changes
- MR
  - T1 hypointense, T2 variable (usually hypointense)
  - Enhancement varies from none to intense

Differential Diagnosis
- Paget disease (older patients)
- Ossifying fibroma, other benign fibroosseous lesions
- Intraosseous meningioma
- Renal osteodystrophy

Paget Disease

Terminology

Paget disease (PaD) of bone, also called osteitis deformans, is the most exaggerated example of abnormal osseous remodeling. PaD is characterized by rapid bone turnover within one or more discrete skeletal lesions.

Etiology

Genetic alterations occur in both classic Paget disease of the elderly and the uncommon familial Paget-like bone dysplasias that arise during childhood. All involve defective function of the molecular pathway that regulates osteoclastogenesis (the osteoprotegerin/TNFRSF11A or B/RANKL/RANK pathway).

Mutations in the gene encoding sequestosome 1 (*SQSTM1*) have been identified in one-third of patients with the familial form of FD and in a smaller proportion of patients with sporadic PaD. *SQSTM1* mutations affect functioning of the p62 phenotype, which increases the sensitivity of osteoclast precursors to osteoclastogenic cytokines, thus causing a predisposition to PaD. *SQSTM1* mutations are also strongly associated with PaD disease severity and complications.

Mutations in the valosin-containing protein gene (*VCP*) cause a unique disorder characterized by classic PaD, inclusion body myopathy, and frontotemporal dementia.

Pathology

Location, Size, and Number. The skull (both calvaria and skull base) is affected in 25-65% of patients **(26-6)**. In contrast to FD, PaD is more commonly polyostotic (65-90% of cases).

Gross Pathology. The pagetoid skull shows diffuse thickening **(26-7)**. Patches of fibrovascular tissue initially replace fatty marrow.

Microscopic Features. In the early lytic stage, active PaD is characterized by cellular fibroosseous lesions with minimally calcified osteoid trabeculae. Increased vascularity is common. Osteoblastic rimming is present together with osteoclastic resorptive lacunae. Osteoclasts are numerous and larger than normal; they also have increased numbers of nuclei.

In the inactive stage, bone turnover and excessive vascularity decrease and the trabeculae coarsen.

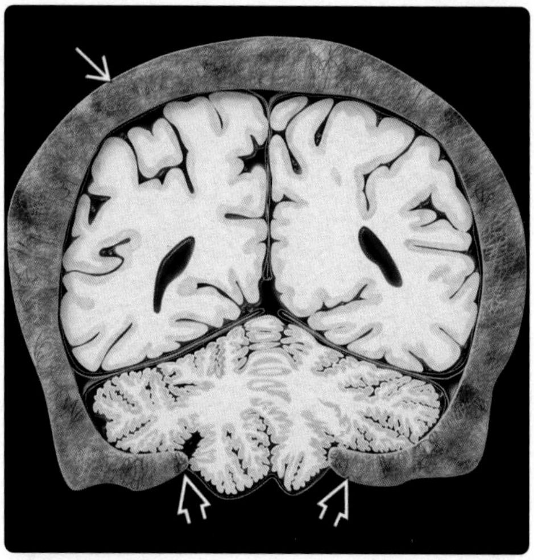

***(26-6)** Graphic shows diffuse Paget disease of the skull with severe diploic widening ➔ and basilar invagination ➔.*

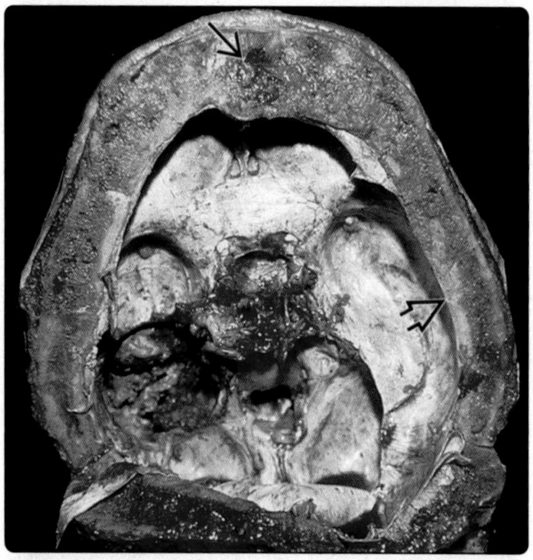

***(26-7)** Autopsied Paget disease shows calvarial thickening with sclerotic bone ➔, patches of fibrovascular tissue ➔. (From Dorfman, 2016.)*

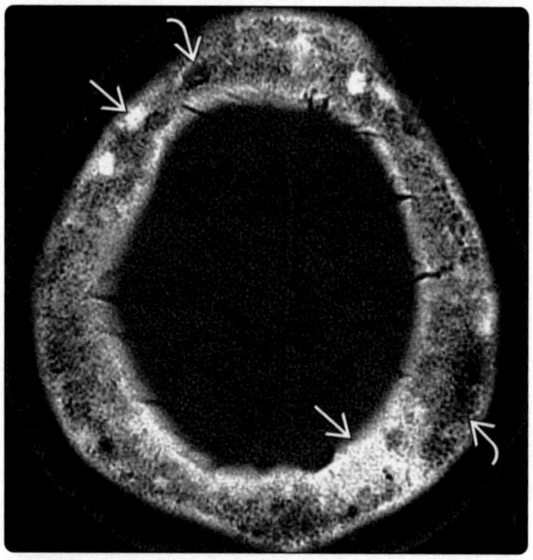

***(26-8)** Bone CT in a 63y woman with Paget disease shows thick calvarium with mixed sclerotic ➔ and lucent areas ➔.*

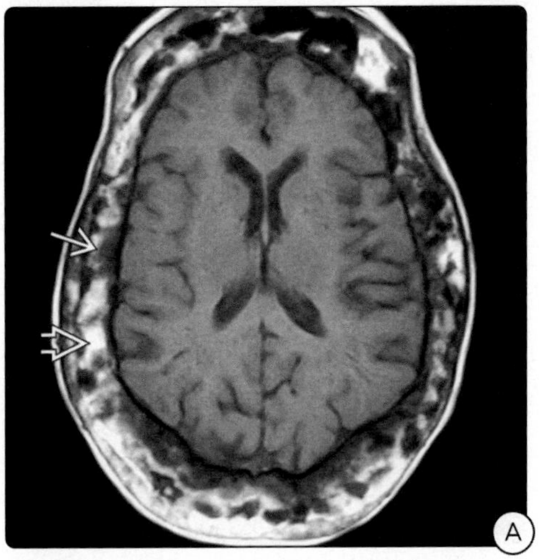

(26-9A) T1WI shows mixed hyper- ➡, hypointense ➡ diploic lesions in a calvarium massively expanded by Paget disease.

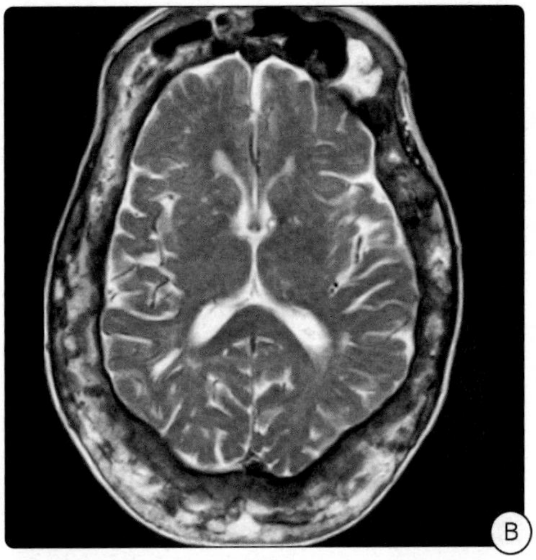

(26-9B) T2WI in the same case shows the extremely "mottled" heterogeneous appearance of calvarial Paget disease.

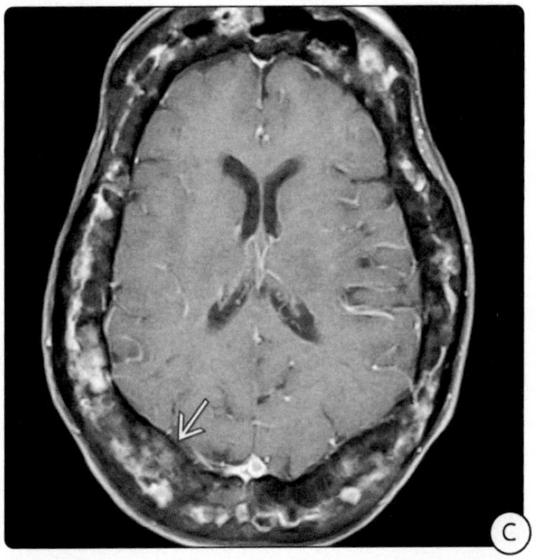

(26-9C) Patchy enhancement is seen on T1 C+ FS ➡, indicating that some active disease is present in this longstanding case.

Clinical Issues

Epidemiology. PaD is common, affecting up to 10% of individuals over the age of 80. It is especially prevalent in the United States, the British Isles, Canada, Australia, and some parts of Western Europe. PaD is rare in Asia and Africa.

Demographics. Classic PaD is a disease of the elderly. Most patients are 55-85 years of age with less than 5% of cases occurring in patients under the age of 40. There is a moderate male predominance.

Juvenile PaD, also known as idiopathic hyperphosphatasia, is an autosomal-recessive bone dysplasia. It begins in infancy or early childhood and is characterized by long bone widening, acetabular protrusion, pathologic fractures, and skull thickening.

Presentation. Presentation varies with location, and all bones of the craniofacial complex can be affected. Patients with calvarial PaD may experience increasing hat size. Cranial neuropathy is common with skull base lesions, most commonly affecting CN VIII. Patients may present with either conductive (ossicular involvement) or sensorineural hearing loss (cochlear involvement or bony compression).

Markedly elevated serum alkaline phosphatase is a constant feature, whereas calcium and phosphate levels remain within normal range.

Natural History. In the extracranial skeleton, osseous expansion with progressive skeletal deformity is typical. Osseous weakening leads to long bone deformities and fractures. In comparison, craniofacial PaD generally has a more benign course and may remain asymptomatic for many years.

Two neoplastic processes are associated with PaD: giant cell tumor (benign) and sarcoma (malignant). **Giant cell tumor** is an expansile intraosseous mass that usually occurs in the epiphyses and metaphyses of long bones in patients with longstanding polyostotic PaD. Giant cell tumors that arise secondarily in pagetoid bone are rare. Just 2% occur in the skull, where the most common site is the sphenoid bone. Involvement of the calvarial vault is rare.

Malignant transformation to **osteosarcoma** occurs in 0.5-1.0% of cases and is generally seen in patients with widespread disease. Most osteosarcomas are high grade and have already metastasized at the time of diagnosis. Only 15% of patients survive beyond 2 or 3 years.

Treatment Options. Bisphosphonates reduce bone turnover and have been effective in many cases of PaD.

Imaging

General Features. Imaging findings in PaD vary with disease stage. In the early active stage, radiolucent lesions develop in the calvaria, a condition termed **osteoporosis circumscripta**. Enlarged bone with mixed lytic and sclerotic foci and confluent nodular calcifications follows (the **"cotton wool"** appearance) in the mixed active stage. The final inactive or quiescent stage is seen as **dense bony sclerosis**.

CT Findings. In early PaD, bone CT shows well-defined lytic foci (osteoporosis circumscripta). Mixed areas of bony lysis and sclerosis then develop, producing the "cotton wool" appearance **(26-8)**. Varying degrees of dense bony sclerosis can develop.

In severe cases, the softened expanded skull base can produce basilar invagination.

MR Findings. Multifocal T1 hypointense lesions replace fatty marrow **(26-9A)**. Signal intensity on T2WI is often heterogeneous **(26-9B)**. Patchy enhancement on T1 C+ can occur in the advancing hypervascular zone of active PaD **(26-9C)**.

Nuclear Medicine. The active stage of PaD shows markedly increased uptake on Tc-99m bone scans. 18F-NaF PET/CT can also demonstrate high uptake in PD, mimicking metastatic disease.

Differential Diagnosis

FD may appear very similar to craniofacial PaD. However, PaD occurs mostly in the elderly and does not have the typical "ground-glass" appearance that often characterizes FD.

Sclerotic metastases may resemble PaD, but no trabecular coarsening or bony enlargement is present. The early lytic phase of PaD may resemble lytic metastases or multiple myeloma; neither enlarges the affected bone.

PAGET DISEASE

Pathology
- Monostotic (65-90%)
- Calvaria, skull base affected (25-60%)
- Fibroosseous tissue replaces fatty marrow

Clinical Issues
- Affects up to 10% of patients > 80 years
- Enlarging skull, CN VIII neuropathy common
- Malignant transformation (0.5-1.0%)
  - Sarcoma > giant cell tumor

Imaging
- Early: lytic ("osteoporosis circumscripta")
- Mid: mixed lytic, sclerotic ("cotton wool")
- Late: dense bony sclerosis

Differential Diagnosis
- Fibrous dysplasia (younger patients)
- Metastases, myeloma

Aneurysmal Bone Cyst

Terminology

Aneurysmal bone cysts (ABCs) are benign expansile multicystic lesions that typically develop in childhood or early adulthood. At least 70% of ABCs are primary lesions; the rest arise secondarily within a preexisting benign tumor such as giant cell tumor or osteoblastoma.

Pathology

The most common overall ABC location is the metaphysis of long bones (70-80% of cases) with the vertebrae (generally the posterior elements) the site of 15% of lesions.

The craniofacial bones are a relatively uncommon location. Lesions can occur in the jaws (maxilla, mandible), petrous temporal bone, basisphenoid, and paranasal sinuses. ABCs of the skull and orbit are rare, accounting for less than 1% of all cases.

ABCs consist of blood-filled cavernous spaces with intracystic hemorrhages of variable ages. Multiple variably sized cysts are separated by septa lined by

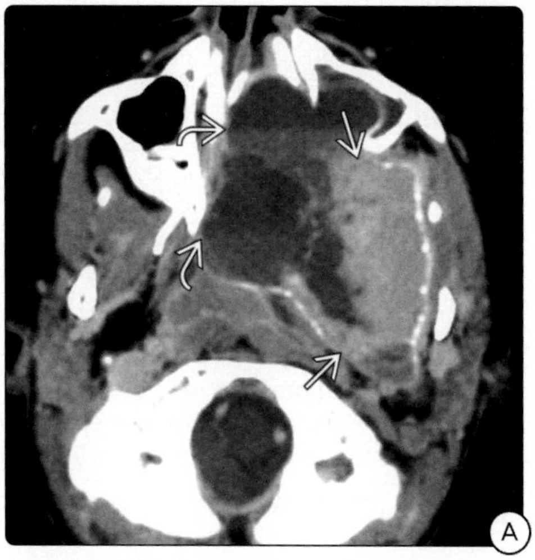

***(26-10A)** CECT shows an expansile mass with cysts and fluid-fluid levels ➡, solid portion exhibiting relatively uniform enhancement ➡.*

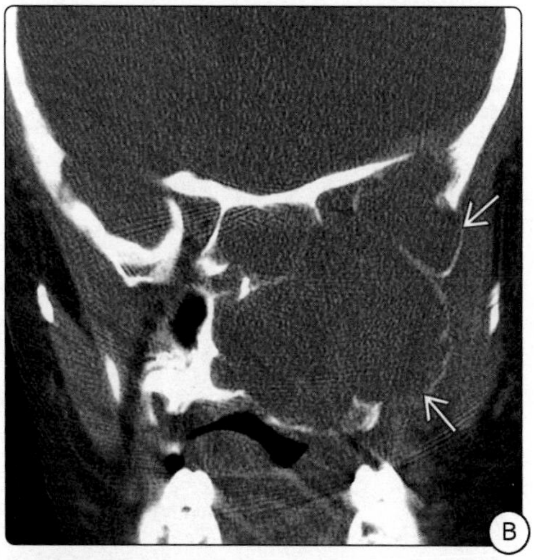

***(26-10B)** Coronal bone CT demonstrates a thin "eggshell" rim of expanded bone around the lesion ➡.*

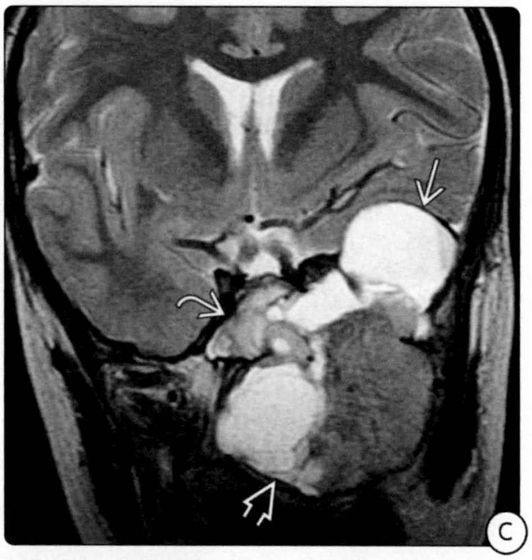

***(26-10C)** T2WI shows the lesion ➡ expands intracranially ➡, extends into sphenoid sinus ➡; aneurysmal bone cyst. (Courtesy A. Illner, MD.)*

endothelium, spindle-shaped fibroblasts, and scattered multinucleated giant cells.

Clinical Issues

ABCs represent 5% of all primary bone tumors and are the second most common pathologically proven bone tumor of childhood. About 70% occur in the first two decades, with a slight male predominance. Symptoms vary with location. Many lesions are asymptomatic or present with slowly progressive swelling.

Treatments for symptomatic ABC are curettage, cryosurgery, and bone graft. Recurrence rates are high, varying from 20-50%. Preoperative embolization may be helpful in selected cases.

Imaging

NECT scans show an eccentric lesion with expanded, remodeled, ballooned ("aneurysmally dilated") bone surrounded by a thin sclerotic rim **(26-10)**. Multiple cystic spaces with fluid-fluid levels are present **(26-11)**.

MR shows a multicystic lesion with a hypointense rim surrounding multiple fluid-filled spaces. Hemorrhages of varying ages with fluid-fluid levels are a prominent imaging feature, as are smaller cysts ("diverticula") that project from larger lesions. The surrounding rim and fibrous septa enhance following contrast administration **(26-11)**.

Differential Diagnosis

Some ABCs may have a phase of relatively rapid growth and can be mistaken clinically for a more aggressive lesion. The most important imaging differential diagnosis of ABC is **telangiectatic osteosarcoma** (OS), which may have fluid-fluid

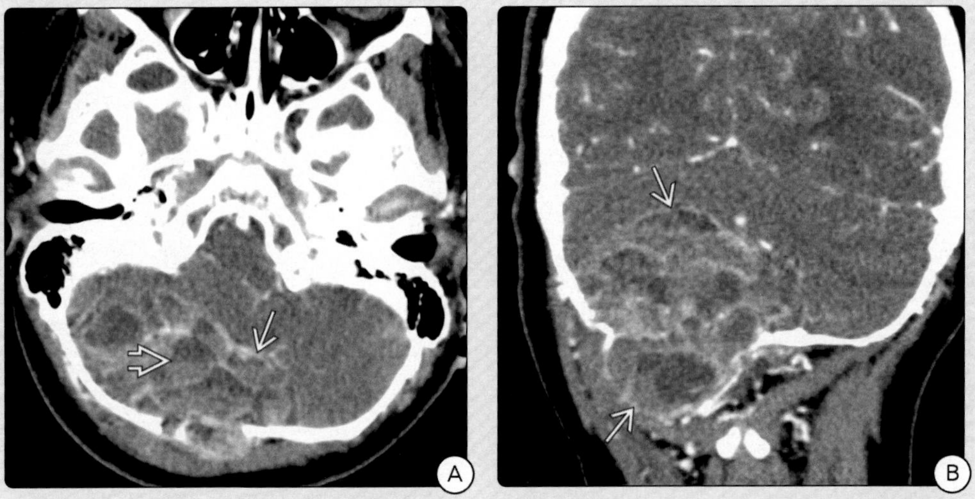

***(26-11A)** Axial CECT of an aneurysmal bone cyst demonstrates multiple cysts with fluid-fluid levels and enhancing rims. **(26-11B)** Coronal CECT shows that the mass is both intra- and extracranial. The dependent blood-fluid levels in the cysts are better appreciated on the axial scan.*

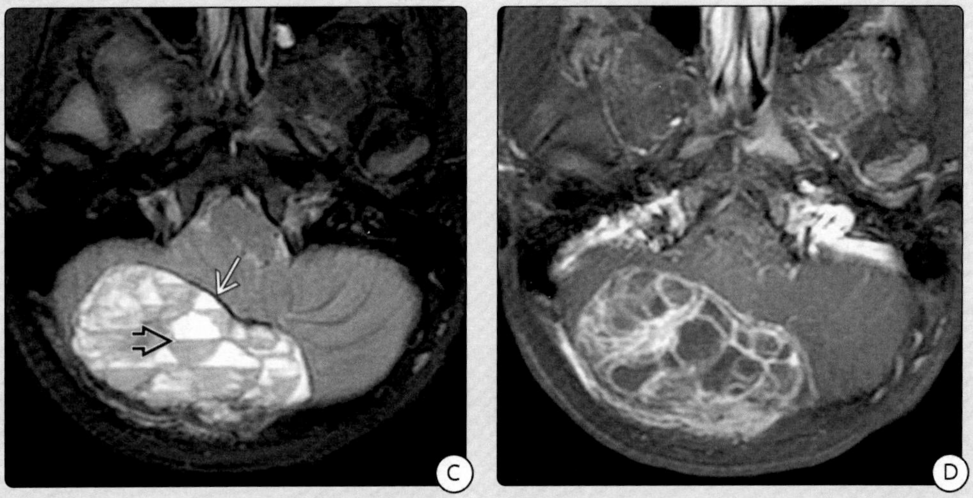

***(26-11C)** T2WI shows multiple cysts with blood-fluid levels. The thin black line draped over the mass is the displaced dura. **(26-11D)** T1 C+ FS shows the characteristic enhancement of the cyst walls and septations within the tumor.*

levels that resemble those of ABC. Incomplete margination, soft tissue mass, cortical destruction, and significant solid portions should suggest telangiectatic OS instead.

Giant cell tumor and **osteoblastoma** are associated with secondary ABC, and both show significant solid components.

Chordoma

Terminology

Chordomas are rare, locally aggressive primary malignant neoplasms with a phenotype that recapitulates the notochord.

Etiology

Skull base (clival) chordomas probably arise from the cranial end of primitive notochordal remnants. Subpopulations of cancer stem-like cells have been identified in some chordomas.

Signal transducer and activation of transcription (STAT) proteins regulate key cellular fates, including proliferation and apoptosis. *STAT3* is activated in chordoma.

Pathology

Chordomas are midline tumors that may arise anywhere along the primitive notochord. The sacrum is the most common site (50% of all chordomas) followed by the sphenooccipital (clival) region (35%) and spine (15%).

Most sphenooccipital chordomas are midline lesions **(26-12)**. Occasionally, a chordoma is predominantly extraosseous and arises off-midline, usually in the nasopharynx or cavernous sinus.

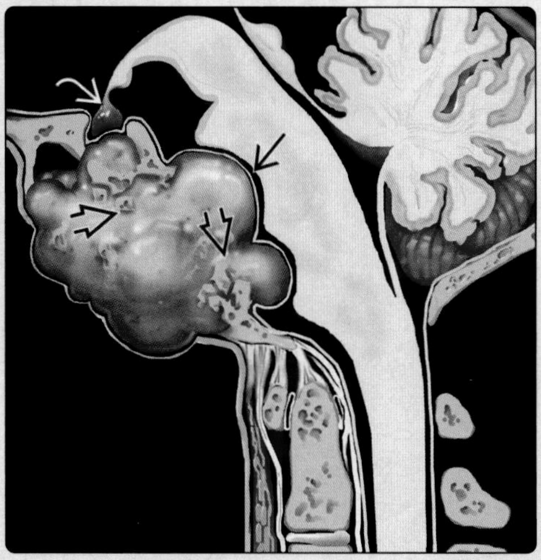

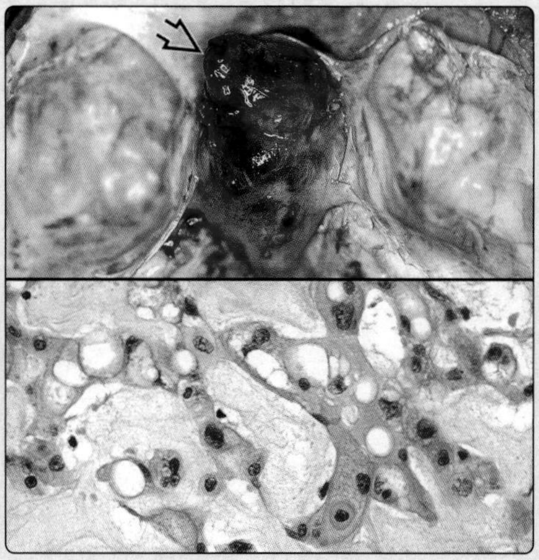

***(26-12)** Sagittal graphic shows an expansile, destructive, lobulated clival mass with a "thumb" of tumor indenting the pons. The pituitary gland is elevated by the tumor. Note the bone fragments "floating" in the chordoma. **(26-13)** (Top) Autopsy of clival chordoma shows lobulated mass invading sella. (Bottom) Microscopy shows physaliphorous cells with vacuolated cytoplasm. (From Ellison, Neuropathology, 2013).*

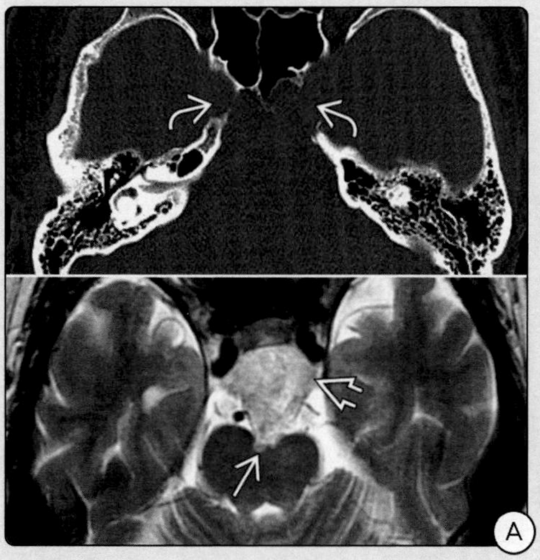

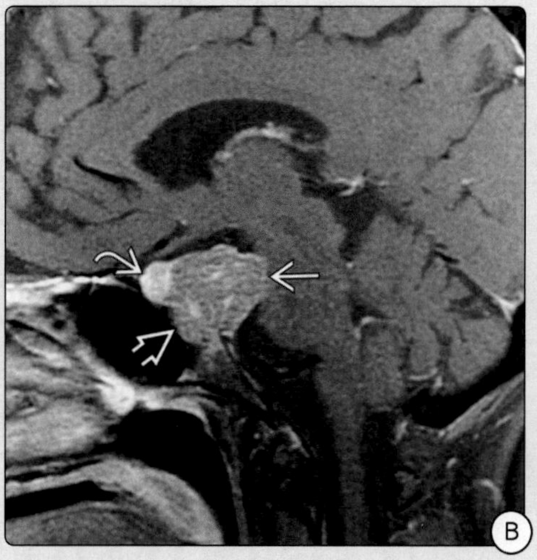

***(26-14A)** Axial bone CT (top) shows a destructive lesion in the central skull base. (Bottom) The lesion is heterogeneously hyperintense on T2WI. Note posterior extension indenting the pons. **(26-14B)** Sagittal T1 C+ FS in the same case shows that the destructive enhancing mass displaces the pituitary gland anteriorly and indents the pons posteriorly. This is chordoma.*

Three major histologic forms of chordoma are recognized: conventional ("classic"), chondroid, and dedifferentiated. Conventional chordoma is the most common type and consists of physaliphorous cells that contain mucin and glycogen vacuoles, giving a characteristic "bubbly" appearance to its cytoplasm **(26-13)**.

Chondroid chordomas have stromal elements that resemble hyaline cartilage with neoplastic cells nestled within lacunae. Dedifferentiated chordoma represents less than 5% of chordomas and typically occurs in the sacrococcygeal region, not the clivus.

Both conventional and chondroid chordomas are strongly immunopositive for the epithelial markers cytokeratin (especially CK8) and epithelial membrane antigen (EMA). Dedifferentiated chordomas exhibit *SMARCB1*/INI1 loss and are associated with dismal prognosis.

Clinical Issues

Chordomas account for 2-5% of all primary bone tumors but cause almost 40% of sacral tumors. Although chordomas may occur at any age, peak prevalence is between the fourth and sixth decades. There is a moderate male predominance.

Clival chordomas typically present with headaches and diplopia secondary to CN VI compression. Large chordomas may cause multiple cranial neuropathies, including visual loss and facial pain.

Although they grow slowly, chordomas are eventually lethal unless treated with aggressive resection and proton beam irradiation. The overall 5-year survival rate of patients following radical resection is 75%. Chondroid chordomas exhibit the most favorable outcomes, whereas dedifferentiated tumors are associated with the most rapid progression and poor overall survival.

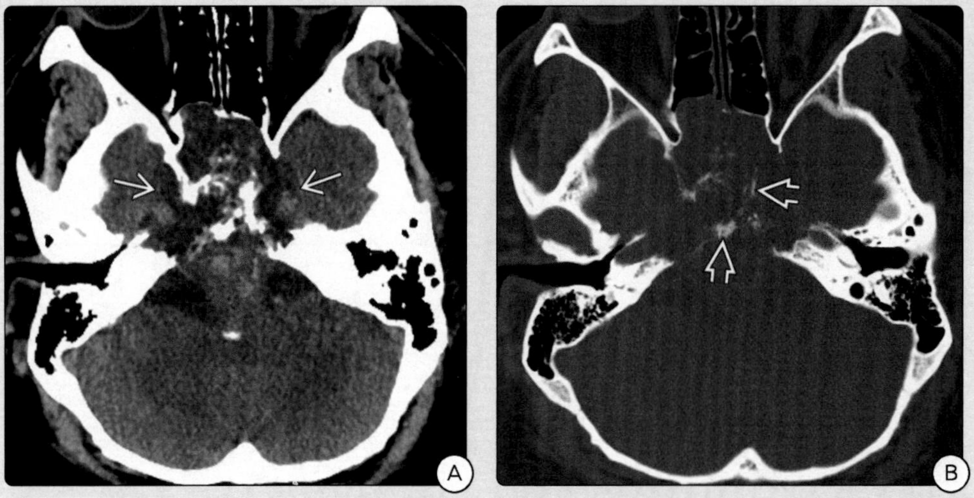

***(26-15A)** Axial NECT in a 39y man with multiple cranial nerve palsies shows destructive, heterogeneous-appearing central skull base mass ➡. **(26-15B)** Bone CT shows near-complete destruction of the sphenoid with eroded clivus and petrous apices. Some dysmorphic-appearing matrix mineralization ➡ is present within the mass.*

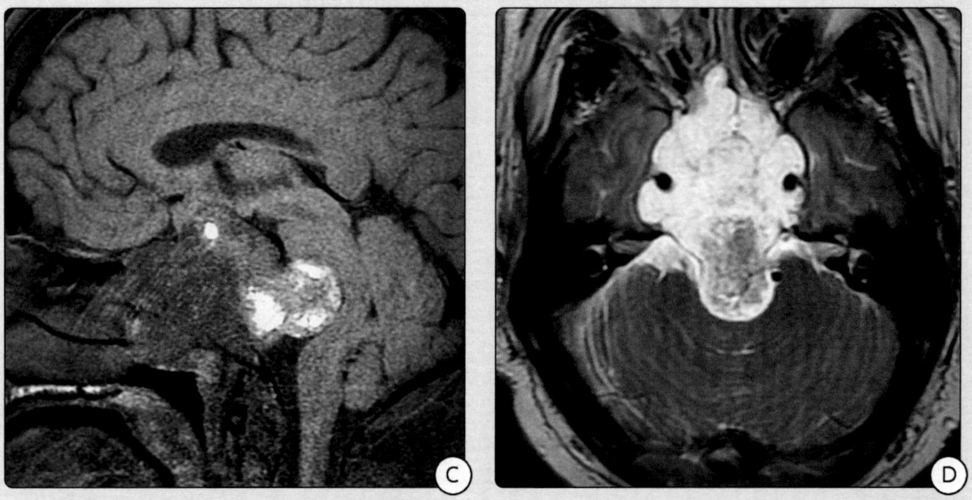

***(26-15C)** Sagittal T1WI shows that the mass has destroyed almost the entire sphenoid bone with "thumb" of tumor indenting the pons. **(26-15D)** Axial T2WI shows that the lobulated extradural mass is very hyperintense and displaces both carotid arteries laterally and the basilar artery posteriorly. Conventional chordoma was found at surgery.*

Imaging

NECT shows a relatively well-circumscribed, moderately hyperdense midline or paramedian clival mass with permeative lytic bony changes. Intratumoral calcifications generally represent sequestrations from destroyed bone.

Chordomas exhibit substantial heterogeneity on MR. Most conventional chordomas are typically intermediate to low signal intensity on T1WI. On sagittal images, a "thumb" of tumor tissue is often seen extending posteriorly through the cortex of the clivus and indenting the pons.

Conventional chordomas are very hyperintense on T2WI **(26-16B)**, reflecting high fluid content within the physaliphorous cells. Intratumoral calcifications and hemorrhage may cause foci of decreased signal within the overall hyperintense mass.

Moderate to marked but heterogeneous enhancement is typical after contrast administration. Increased tumor-to-pons postcontrast signal intensity is associated with more abundant blood supply and increased risk of tumor progression.

Recent studies have shown that MR grading of clival chordomas based on T2 hyperintensity and the degree of postcontrast enhancement relative to the adjacent pons may be useful in predicting more rapid tumor progression.

Differential Diagnosis

A large **invasive pituitary macroadenoma** can mimic CCh. CChs typically displace but do not invade the pituitary gland, whereas macroadenomas cannot be identified separate from the gland.

Signal intensity of a **skull base chondrosarcoma** is very similar to that of CCh. Chondrosarcomas typically arise off-midline, along the petrooccipital fissure. **Ecchordosis physaliphora** is a rare nonneoplastic notochordal remnant that may arise anywhere from the skull base to the sacrum. Most are small

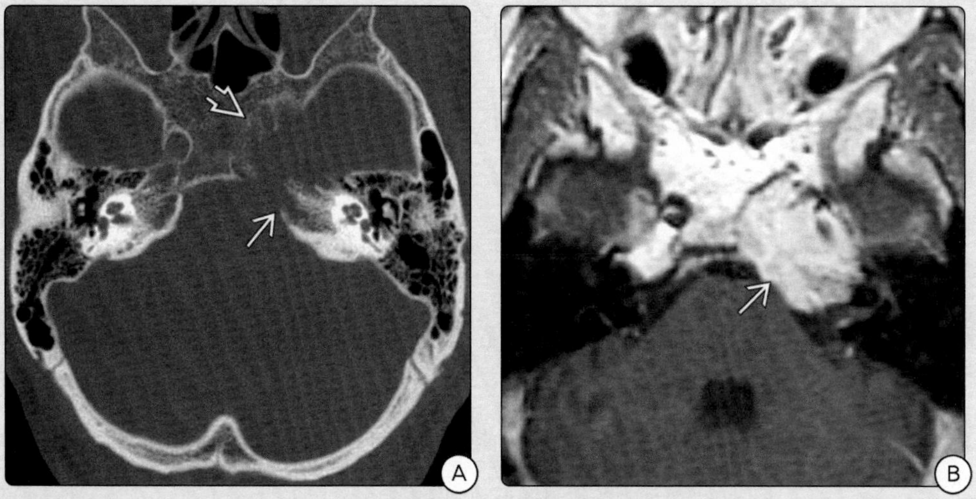

***(26-16A)** Bone CT shows lytic, destructive lesion along left basisphenoid ➡ and the petrous apex ➡. **(26-16B)** The mass ➡ enhances strongly on T1 C+. Lateral clival chordomas are less common than midline lesions. (Courtesy J. Curé, MD.)*

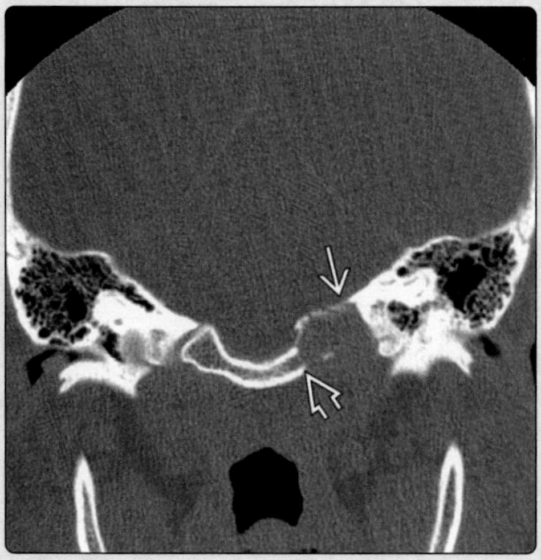

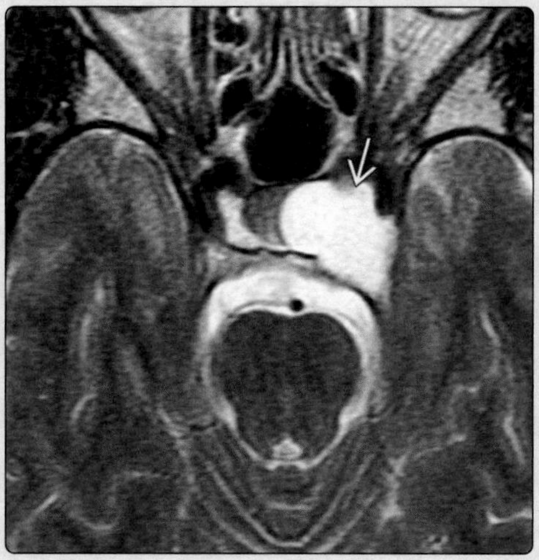

***(26-17)** Coronal bone CT clearly demonstrates the off-lateral location of the destructive mass eroding the clivus ➡ and the petrous apex ➡. **(26-18)** Axial T2WI demonstrates a hyperintense mass ➡ in the left cavernous sinus invading the sphenoid bone.*

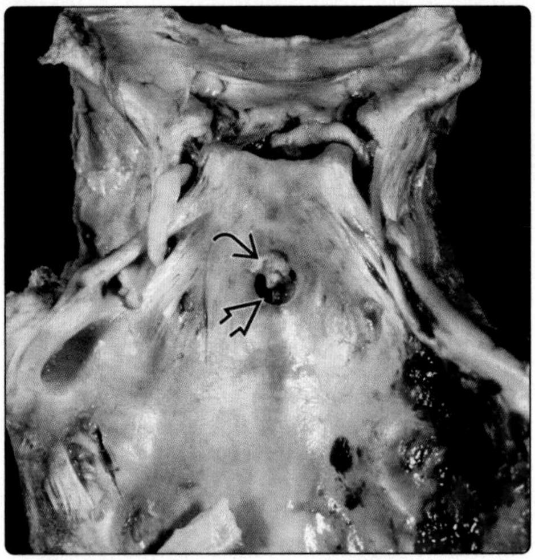

***(26-19)** Focal defect of bone and dura in mid-clivus ➡ is associated with a small ecchordosis physaliphora ➡. (Courtesy R. Hewlett, MD.)*

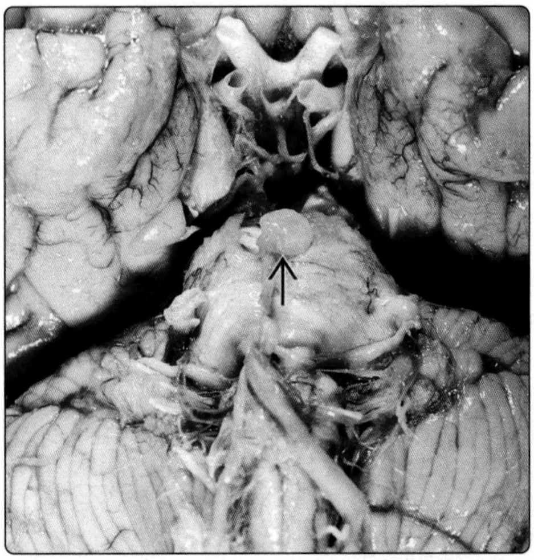

***(26-20)** Gelatinous-appearing nodule ➡ is in front of pons. Incidental finding is physaliphorous ecchordosis. (Courtesy R. Hewlett, MD.)*

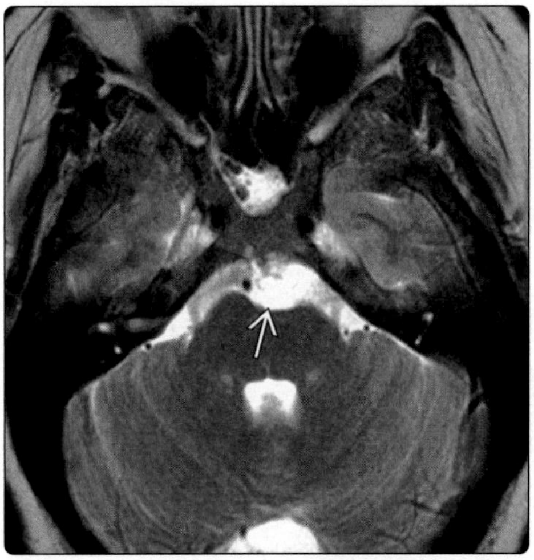

***(26-21)** T2WI shows lobulated, well-delineated, hyperintense midline mass ➡ indenting the pons. This is physaliphorous ecchordosis.*

and found incidentally at autopsy or imaging. They usually lie just in front of the pons and have a thin stalk-like connection to a smaller intraclival component (see below).

Skull base **metastases** and **plasmacytoma** are destructive lesions that are usually isointense with brain on all sequences. Predominantly intraosseous **meningioma** is rare in the skull base. It usually causes sclerosis and hyperostosis rather than a permeative destructive pattern.

CHORDOMA

Etiology
- Arises from cranial end of primitive notochordal remnants
- *STAT3* activation

Pathology
- Typically midline
  - 50% sacrum
  - 35% sphenooccipital (clivus)
  - 15% vertebral body
- Three types
  - Typical ("classic") with physaliphorous cells
  - Chondroid
  - Dedifferentiated (< 5%, usually sacral)

Clinical Features
- Any age but peak = 4th-6th decades
- Cranial neuropathies

Imaging Findings
- CT
  - Permeative destructive central BOS lesion
  - Often contains sequestered bony fragments
- MR
  - T1 hypointense, T2 hyperintense
  - "Thumb" of tumor extends posteriorly, indents pons
  - Variable, usually moderate enhancement

Differential Diagnosis
- Invasive pituitary macroadenoma
- Chondrosarcoma
- Ecchordosis physaliphora

Intracranial Pseudotumors

Ecchordosis Physaliphora

Ecchordosis physaliphora (EP) is a small (usually < 1 cm) gelatinous soft tissue mass that represents an ectopic notochordal remnant **(26-20)**. Ectopic notochordal rests can occur anywhere along the midline craniospinal axis from the dorsum sellae to the sacrococcygeal region. EPs are more common in the spine than the skull and are generally incidental findings at imaging or autopsy.

Histopathologically, EPs consist of physaliphorous cells imbedded in a myxoid matrix. The cells are characterized by large mucin-containing intracytoplasmic vacuoles. Necrosis and mitoses are absent.

Imaging features of EPs are quite characteristic. CT demonstrates a well-delineated hypodense, nonenhancing midline intraclival mass with scalloped sclerotic margins.

The key imaging feature of EP that distinguishes it from other similar-appearing lesions is the presence of a small pedicle or stalk that connects the clival lesion to an intradural component in the prepontine cistern. Best demonstrated on MR, EPs are hypointense to brain on T1WI and hyperintense relative to CSF on T2WI **(26-21)**. EPs do not enhance following contrast administration, and follow-up studies show no change in lesion size.

The major differential diagnosis of EP in the basisphenoid bone is **clival chordoma.** Chordomas are permeative destructive lesions. Other prepontine cistern lesions that can mimic EP include arachnoid, neurenteric, epidermoid, and dermoid cysts. **Arachnoid cysts** are much more common in the cerebellopontine angle cisterns and behave exactly like CSF on all sequences.

Neurenteric cysts are often slightly off-midline and somewhat lower, adjacent to the pontomedullary junction. **Epidermoid cysts** (ECs) are irregular, somewhat frond-like lesions that restrict on DWI. ECs are more common in the cerebellopontine angle cisterns. **Dermoid cysts** usually follow fat signal, not CSF.

Textiloma

Hemostatic elements that are introduced into the central nervous system occasionally induce an excessive inflammatory reaction that may be difficult to distinguish from recurrent or residual tumor on neuroimaging studies.

Terminology

Textiloma refers to a mass created by a retained surgical element (inadvertently or deliberately left behind) and its associated foreign body inflammatory reaction.

The terms "gossypiboma," "gauzoma," and "muslinoma" refer specifically to retained nonresorbable cotton or woven materials.

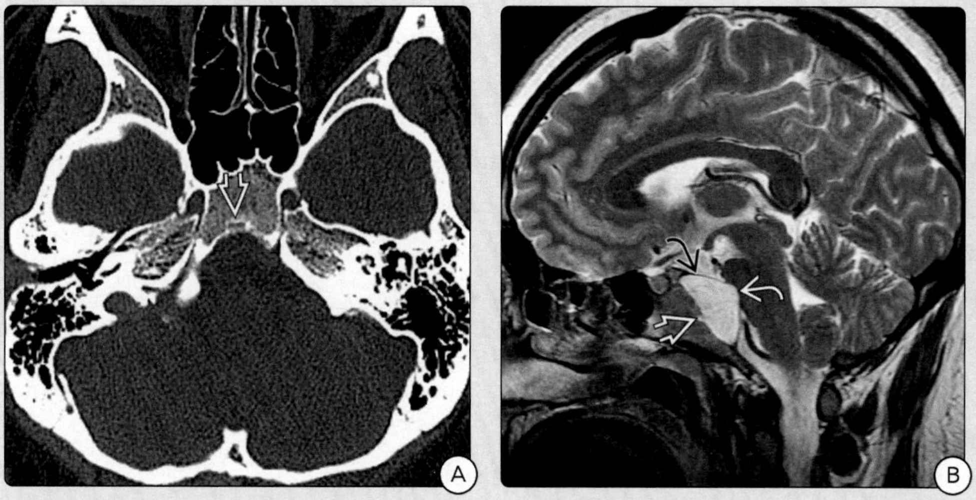

***(26-22A)** Bone CT in an 18y man with headaches and intermittent visual symptoms shows a small niche of bone with sclerotic margins ➔ in an otherwise intact clivus. **(26-22B)** Sagittal T2WI shows a large, very hyperintense mass ➔ elevating the clival dura ➔, displacing the pons posteriorly. Note small "stalk" ➔ extending into clivus.*

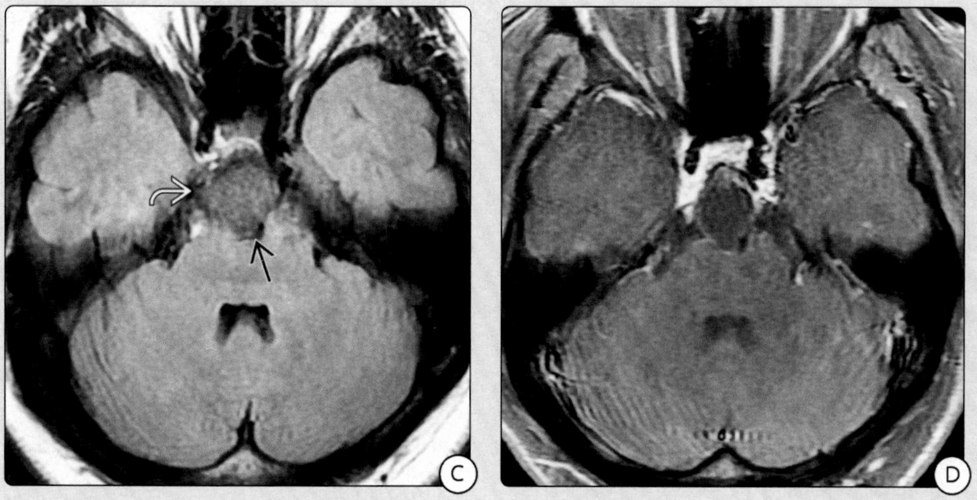

***(26-22C)** Axial FLAIR shows that the mass ➔ indents the pons ➔ and does not suppress. **(26-22D)** T1 C+ FS shows that the mass does not enhance. Physaliphora ecchordosis was proven at surgery.*

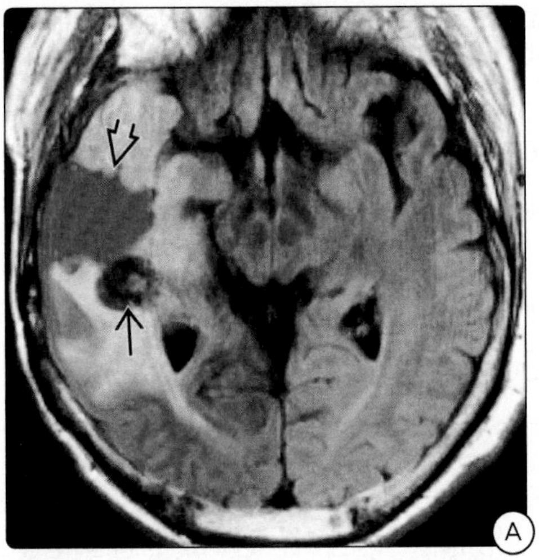

(26-23A) Axial FLAIR shows a hypointense mass ➡ adjacent to the tumor resection cavity ⇨.

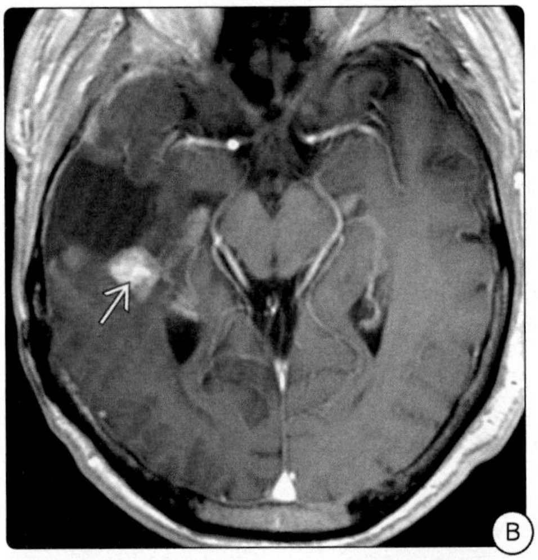

(26-23B) The lesion ➡ demonstrates solid but heterogeneous enhancement on T1 C+ FS.

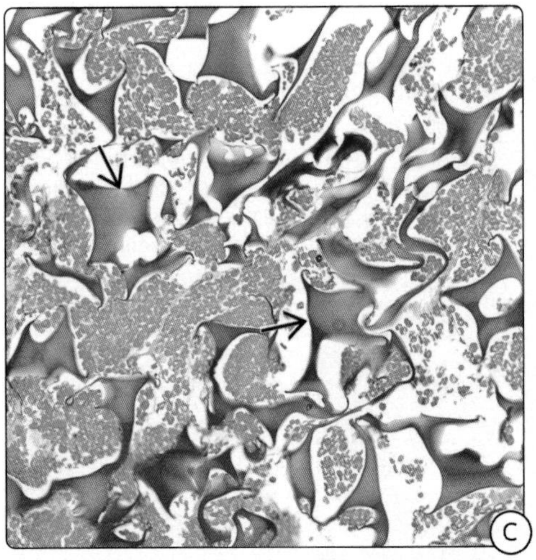

(26-23C) Histology (same case) shows amorphous spicules ➡ surrounded by blood. This is gelfoam textiloma. (Courtesy B. K. DeMasters, MD.)

Etiology

Hemostatic agents can be resorbable or nonresorbable. All classes of resorbable and nonresorbable agents may produce textilomas as an allergic response.

Resorbable agents include gelatin sponge, oxidized cellulose, and microfibrillar collagen. Nonresorbable agents include various forms of cotton pledgets, cloth (i.e., muslin), and synthetic rayon. Although bioabsorbable hemostats are often left in place, nonresorbable agents are typically removed prior to surgical closure. Any of these materials may induce an inflammatory reaction, creating a textiloma.

Pathology

Most textilomas occur within surgical resection sites or around muslin-reinforced aneurysms. Histologic examination typically shows a core of degenerating inert hemostatic agent surrounded by inflammatory reaction. Foreign body giant cells and histiocytes are often present. Each agent exhibits distinctive histologic features, often permitting specific identification **(26-23C)**.

Clinical Issues

Textilomas are uncommon. The highest reported prevalence is following abdominal and orthopedic surgery. Intracranial textilomas are rare with fewer than 75 reported cases.

Textilomas may be asymptomatic or cause symptoms that suggest tumor recurrence.

Imaging

Intracranial textilomas are almost always iso- or hypointense on T1WI. Approximately 45% are iso- and 40% are hypointense on T2/FLAIR **(26-23A)**. Some "blooming" on T2* may be present. All reported cases of textiloma enhance on postcontrast scans. Ring and heterogeneous solid enhancement patterns occur almost equally **(26-23B)**.

Differential Diagnosis

The major differential diagnosis is **recurrent neoplasm** or **radiation necrosis**. Residual or recurrent tumor can coexist with textiloma. If present, T2 hypointensity helps distinguish textiloma from neoplasm or **abscess**. Definitive diagnosis typically requires biopsy and histologic examination with both routine stains and polarized light.

Calcifying Pseudoneoplasm of the Neuraxis

Calcifying pseudoneoplasm of the neuraxis (CAPNON) is a rare but distinctive nonneoplastic lesion of the CNS. Calcifying pseudoneoplasms are also known as fibroosseous lesions, cerebral calculi, "brain stones," and "brain rocks."

CAPNONs are nonneoplastic, noninflammatory lesions. They are discrete intra- or extraaxial masses that contain various combinations of chondromyxoid and fibrovascular stroma, metaplastic calcification, and ossification.

CAPNONs have also been characterized as foreign body reactions with giant cells, tissue ossification, and the formation of lamellar bone or scattered psammoma bodies. The surrounding brain often exhibits inflammatory changes, with gliosis and edema leading to mass effect.

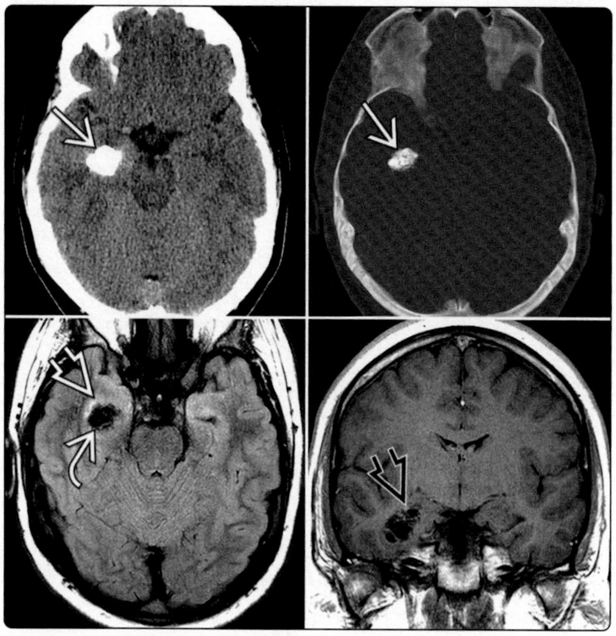

***(26-24)** NECT (upper L) and bone CT (upper R) show densely calcified mass ➡. FLAIR (lower L) shows that hypointense mass ➡ is surrounded by edema ➡, doesn't enhance ➡ (lower R). This is CAPNON. (Courtesy S. Blaser, MD.)*

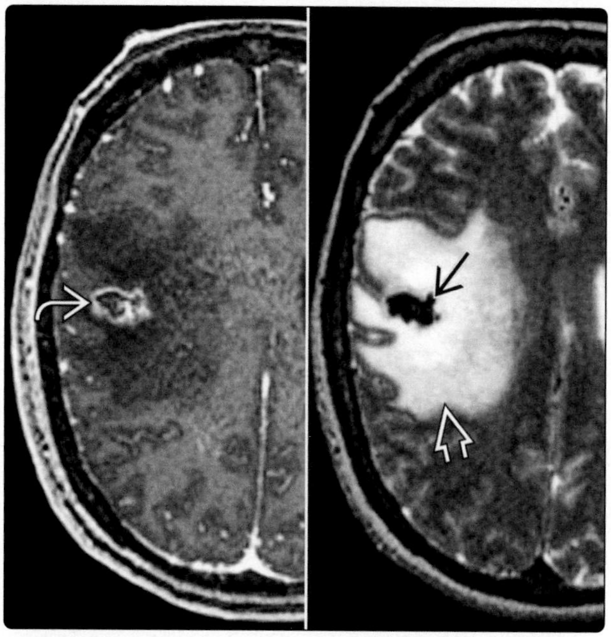

***(26-25)** Sometimes surgically proven CAPNONs are extremely hypointense on T2WI ➡, incite intense edema ➡, and exhibit rim enhancement ➡. (Courtesy B. K. Kleinschmidt-DeMasters, MD.)*

Positive immunoreactivity to vimentin and epithelial membrane antigen (EMA) are typical. GFAP and S-100 protein are typically negative, helping distinguish CAPNON from astrocytic neoplasms and meningioma.

Intracranial CAPNONs are usually asymptomatic and discovered incidentally on imaging studies although seizures and headache have been reported. A few cases have been reported in association with meningioangiomatosis and neurofibromatosis type 2.

Most CAPNONs are solitary lesions; multiple lesions have been described but are uncommon.

NECT scans demonstrate a densely calcified leptomeningeal, deep intrasulcal, or brain parenchymal "rock." The temporal lobe is the most common site.

On MR, CAPNONs demonstrate little mass effect, are isointense on T1WI, and are uniformly hypointense on T2WI and FLAIR. Mild "blooming" is seen on T2* GRE. Perilesional edema varies from none to extensive. Enhancement varies from none to moderate. Solid, linear, serpiginous, and peripheral rim-like enhancement patterns have all been reported.

The differential diagnosis of CAPNON includes an ossified vascular lesion—most often a **cavernous malformation**—and densely calcified neoplasm, such as **oligodendroglioma, meningioma,** and **choroid plexus papilloma** with osseous metaplasia. Although cavernous malformations can often be distinguished by their "popcorn" mixed hyperintensity on T2WI, biopsy is usually necessary for definitive diagnosis.

INTRACRANIAL PSEUDOTUMORS

Ecchordosis Physaliphora
- Ectopic notochord remnant
  - Dorsum sellae to sacrum
  - Physaliphorous cells, mucoid matrix
- Clival defect, sclerotic margins
- Stalk connects to hyperintense prepontine mass

Textiloma
- Foreign body reaction
  - Usually to hemostatic elements
  - Other = introduced embolic materials
- Iso-/hypointense on T2WI
- Ring, heterogeneous enhancement on T1 C+

Calcifying Pseudoneoplasm of the Neuraxis (CAPNON)
- Chondrocalcific or ossified mass
  - Usually in sulcus
- Very hypointense on T2/FLAIR
- Enhancement varies (none to rim-like)

Selected References

Extracranial Tumors and Tumor-Like Conditions

Fibrous Dysplasia

Couturier A et al: Craniofacial fibrous dysplasia: a 10-case series. Eur Ann Otorhinolaryngol Head Neck Dis. ePub, 2017

Kwee TC et al: Benign bone conditions that may be FDG-avid and mimic malignancy. Semin Nucl Med. 47(4):322-351, 2017

Yang L et al: Prevalence of different forms and involved bones of craniofacial fibrous dysplasia. J Craniofac Surg. 28(1):21-25, 2017

Zreik RT et al: Malignant transformation of polyostotic fibrous dysplasia with aberrant keratin expression. Hum Pathol. 62:170-174, 2017

Benhamou J et al: Prognostic factors from an epidemiologic evaluation of fibrous dysplasia of bone in a modern cohort: the FRANCEDYS Study. J Bone Miner Res. 31(12):2167-2172, 2016

Rossi DC et al: Extensive fibrous dysplasia of skull base: case report. Neurol Sci. 36(7):1287-9, 2015

Tehli O et al: Computer-based surgical planning and custom-made titanium implants for cranial fibrous dysplasia. Neurosurgery. 11 Suppl 2:213-9, 2015

Unal Erzurumlu Z et al: CT imaging of craniofacial fibrous dysplasia. Case Rep Dent. 2015:134123, 2015

Neelakantan A et al: Benign and malignant diseases of the clivus. Clin Radiol. 69(12):1295-303, 2014

Zhou SH et al: Gene expression profiling of craniofacial fibrous dysplasia reveals ADAMTS2 overexpression as a potential marker. Int J Clin Exp Pathol. 7(12):8532-41, 2014

Paget Disease

Cucchi F et al: 18F-sodium fluoride PET/CT in Paget disease. Clin Nucl Med. 42(7):553-554, 2017

Kwee TC et al: Benign bone conditions that may be FDG-avid and mimic malignancy. Semin Nucl Med. 47(4):322-351, 2017

Qi X et al: Familial early-onset Paget's disease of bone associated with a novel hnRNPA2B1 mutation. Calcif Tissue Int. ePub, 2017

Lalam RK et al: Paget disease of bone. Semin Musculoskelet Radiol. 20(3):287-299, 2016

Rai NP et al: Paget's disease with craniofacial and skeletal bone involvement. BMJ Case Rep. 2016:bcr2016216173, 2016

Aneurysmal Bone Cyst

Sodhi HB et al: Temporal aneurysmal bone cyst: cost-effective method to achieve gross total resection. Acta Neurochir (Wien). 158(8):1633-5, 2016

Motamedi MH et al: Assessment of 120 maxillofacial aneurysmal bone cysts: a nationwide quest to understand this enigma. J Oral Maxillofac Surg. 72(8):1523-30, 2014

Chordoma

Guler E et al: The added value of diffusion magnetic resonance imaging in the diagnosis and posttreatment evaluation of skull base chordomas. J Neurol Surg B Skull Base. 78(3):256-265, 2017

Kitamura Y et al: Genetic aberrations and molecular biology of skull base chordoma and chondrosarcoma. Brain Tumor Pathol. 34(2):78-90, 2017

Rassi MS et al: Pediatric clival shordoma: a curable disease that conforms to Collins' Law. Neurosurgery. ePub, 2017

Tian K et al: MR Imaging grading system for skull base chordoma. AJNR Am J Neuroradiol. 38(6):1206-1211, 2017

Zhai Y et al: Clinical features and prognostic factors of children and adolescent patients with clival chordomas. World Neurosurg. 98:323-32, 2017

Gulluoglu S et al: The molecular aspects of chordoma. Neurosurg Rev. 39(2):185-96; discussion 196, 2016

Hasselblatt M et al: Poorly differentiated chordoma with SMARCB1/INI1 loss: a distinct molecular entity with dismal prognosis. Acta Neuropathol. 132(1):149-51, 2016

Wang AC et al: STAT3 inhibition as a therapeutic strategy for chordoma. J Neurol Surg B Skull Base. 77(6):510-520, 2016

Intracranial Pseudotumors

Ecchordosis Physaliphora

Park HH et al: Ecchordosis physaliphora: typical and atypical radiologic features. Neurosurg Rev. 40(1):87-94, 2017

Ferguson C et al: A case study of symptomatic retroclival ecchordosis physaliphora: CT and MR imaging. Can J Neurol Sci. 43(1):210-2, 2016

Özgür A et al: Ecchordosis physaliphora: evaluation with precontrast and contrast-enhanced fast imaging employing steady-state acquisition MR imaging based on proposed new classification. Clin Neuroradiol. 26(3):347-53, 2016

Chihara C et al: Ecchordosis physaliphora and its variants: proposed new classification based on high-resolution fast MR imaging employing steady-state acquisition. Eur Radiol. 23(10):2854-60, 2013

Textiloma

Akpinar A et al: Textiloma (gossypiboma) mimicking recurrent intracranial abscess. BMC Res Notes. 8:390, 2015

Minks D et al: Suspected cerebral foreign body granuloma following endovascular treatment of intracranial aneurysm: imaging features. Neuroradiology. 57(1):71-3, 2015

Slater LA et al: Long-term MRI findings of muslin-induced foreign body granulomas after aneurysm wrapping. A report of two cases and literature review. Interv Neuroradiol. 20(1):67-73, 2014

Calcifying Pseudoneoplasm of the Neuraxis

Saha A et al: Calcifying pseudoneoplasm of the spine: imaging and pathological features. Neuroradiol J. ePub, 2017

Metastases and Paraneoplastic Syndromes

Brain metastases are rapidly increasing in incidence and are major complications of common cancers. Up to 40% of all patients with advanced cancers (particularly lung and breast) will eventually develop CNS involvement. Brain metastases are often ultimately responsible for patient mortality even in the face of controlled systemic disease.

CNS metastatic disease arises from numerous sources and has many different imaging "faces." We begin this chapter with an overview that includes the brain as a "sanctuary site" for CNS metastases. We focus on general features, including how and from where cranial metastases arise, the role of highly site-specific microRNAs in the metastatic "cascade," the effect of age on primary tumor type and CNS location, symptomatology, treatment options, and prognosis.

We follow with a discussion of cranial metastases by anatomic location, beginning with the brain parenchyma (the most common overall CNS location) and concluding with perineural tumor extension from head and neck cancers. We include an updated discussion of how metastatic neoplasms of unknown origin are characterized in the era of targeted therapies for tumors such as non-small cell lung cancer and melanoma.

We conclude with a consideration of the remote effects of cancer on the CNS and the increasingly important group of so-called paraneoplastic syndromes.

Metastatic Lesions

The incidence of CNS metastases is increasing worldwide. Brain metastases are, not only a leading cause of cancer mortality, but also as a group have become the most common CNS neoplasm in adults. Brain metastases are now 10 times more common than primary malignant CNS tumors with at least 170,000 new cases reported in the USA each year. Population aging, improved imaging techniques, and new treatment regimens that allow patients with primary systemic cancers to survive longer all contribute to this striking increase.

Overview

Terminology

Metastases are secondary tumors that arise from primary neoplasms at another site.

Etiology

Routes of Spread. CNS metastases can arise from both extra- and intracranial primary tumors. Metastases from **extracranial primary neoplasms** ("body-to-brain metastases") most commonly spread via **hematogeneous dissemination**.

Direct geographic extension from a lesion in an adjacent structure (such as squamous cell carcinoma in the nasopharynx) also occurs but is much less common than hematogeneous spread. Invasion usually proceeds along paths of least resistance, i.e., through natural foramina and fissures where bone is thin or absent. **Perineural** and **perivascular spread** are less common but important direct geographic routes by which head and neck tumors gain access to the CNS.

Primary intracranial neoplasms sometimes spread from one CNS site to another, causing brain-to-brain or brain-to-spine metastases. One typical example is spread of a malignant astrocytoma (e.g., glioblastoma) to other CNS sites. Spread occurs preferentially along compact white matter tracts such as the corpus callosum and internal capsule but can also involve the ventricular ependyma, pia, and perivascular spaces.

CSF dissemination with "carcinomatous meningitis" and "drop metastases" to the brain and spine occurs with both extra- and intracranial primary neoplasms.

Metastasis Formation. Although vascular dissemination of systemic tumor cells occurs readily, the development of brain metastases is far more complex than simply delivering a tumor embolism to an end organ. The brain is a biologically relatively protected ("sanctuary") site because of the blood-brain barrier. Most disseminated tumor cells do not immediately produce brain metastases.

The establishment, growth, and survival of metastases all depend on the interaction of tumor cells with multiple different host factors in the target organ microenvironment. Metastasis formation is a biologically complicated, genetically mediated process. A veritable cascade of events (the **metastatic "cascade"**) is required before brain metastases develop. There is also increasing evidence that specific microRNAs in the primary tumor are metastasis location-specific, including oncogenic microRNAs that seem to be specific for the CNS.

Specific receptors mediate attachment and subsequent infiltration of circulating tumor cells into the CNS. Once tumor cells enter the brain, they are surrounded and infiltrated by activated astrocytes. These astrocytes upregulate "survival genes" in tumor cells, rendering them highly resistant to chemotherapy.

If metastatic cells manage to colonize the inhospitable brain habitat, upregulated matrix proteins, cytokines, and various growth factors may create a microenvironment that actually promotes tumor growth. Inactivation of tumor suppressor genes with simultaneous activation of protooncogenes is typical. Upregulation and amplification of some genes such as *EGFR* is also common.

Origin of CNS Metastases. Both the source and the intracranial location of metastases vary significantly with patient age. Approximately 10% of all brain metastases originate from an unknown primary neoplasm at the time of initial diagnosis. In 10% of patients, the brain is the only site involved.

Children. The most common sources of cranial metastases in children are hematologic malignancies. In descending order of frequency, they are leukemia, lymphoma, and sarcoma (osteogenic sarcoma, rhabdomyosarcoma, and Ewing sarcoma).

The preferential locations are the skull and dura. Parenchymal metastases are much less common in children compared with adults.

Adults. Metastases from lung, breast, and melanoma account for at least two-thirds of all brain metastases in adults. The overall most common extracranial primary tumor that metastasizes to the brain parenchyma is lung cancer (especially adenocarcinoma and small cell carcinoma).

Breast cancer is the second most common primary tumor source, followed by melanoma, renal carcinoma, and colorectal cancer. In between one-quarter and one-third of cases, the primary tumor is unknown at the time of neurosurgical intervention.

Skull, dura, and spine metastases are typically caused by prostate, breast, or lung cancer, followed by hematologic malignancies and renal cancers.

CNS METASTASES: EPIDEMIOLOGY AND ETIOLOGY

Epidemiology
- Adults > > children
  - Metastases = most common CNS neoplasm in adults
  - 5x increase in past 50 years
  - Brain metastases occur in > 30-40% of cancer patients

Routes of Spread
- Most common = extracranial primary to CNS via
  - Hematogeneous dissemination
  - Direct geographic extension (nasopharynx, sinuses)
  - Perineural, perivascular spread
- Less common
  - Brain-to-brain from CNS primary
  - Brain-to-CSF from CNS primary
- Least common
  - Tumor-to-tumor metastasis
  - Sometimes called "collision tumor"
  - Most common "donor" tumor = breast, lung
  - Most common "recipient" tumor = meningioma

Origin
- 10% unknown primary at initial diagnosis
  - Children: leukemia, lymphoma, sarcoma
  - Adults: lung, breast cancer, melanoma, renal carcinoma, colorectal cancer

Pathology

Location. The brain parenchyma is the most common site (80%), followed by the skull and dura (15%). Diffuse leptomeningeal (pial) and subarachnoid space infiltration is relatively uncommon, accounting for just 5% of all cases.

The vast majority of parenchymal metastases are located in the cerebral hemispheres. Hematogeneous metastases have a special predilection for arterial border zones and the junction between the cortex and subcortical white matter **(27-1)** **(27-2)**. Between 3-5% are found in the basal ganglia. Rarely, tumor cells diffusely infiltrate the brain perivascular spaces, a process termed "carcinomatous encephalitis" **(27-4)**.

Only 15% of metastases are found in the cerebellum. The midbrain, pons, and medulla are uncommon sites (especially for solitary lesions) and account for less than 5% of metastases.

Other rare sites include the choroid plexus, ventricular ependyma, pituitary gland/stalk, and retinal choroid.

Size and Number. Although parenchymal metastases vary in size from microscopic implants to a few centimeters in diameter, most are between a few millimeters and 1.5 cm. Large hemispheric metastases are rare. In contrast, skull and dural metastases can become very large.

Approximately half of all metastases are solitary lesions, and half are multiple. About 20% of patients have two lesions, 30% have three or more, and only 5% have more than five lesions. Approximately 1% have such widespread dissemination that they have a "miliary" appearance.

Gross Pathology. The gross pathologic appearance of metastases varies according to tumor site.

Parenchymal Metastases. Parenchymal metastases are generally round, relatively circumscribed lesions that exhibit

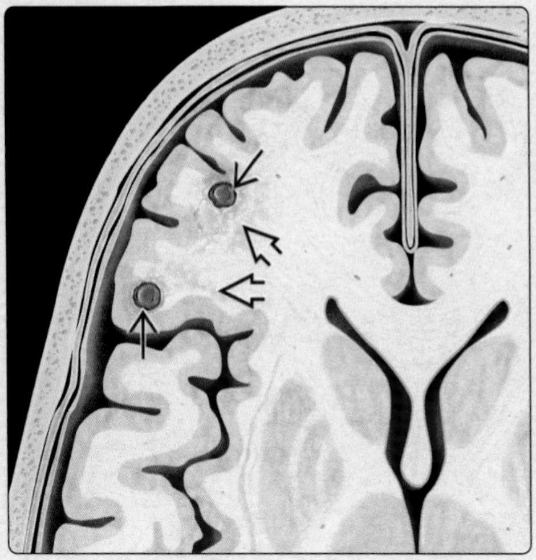

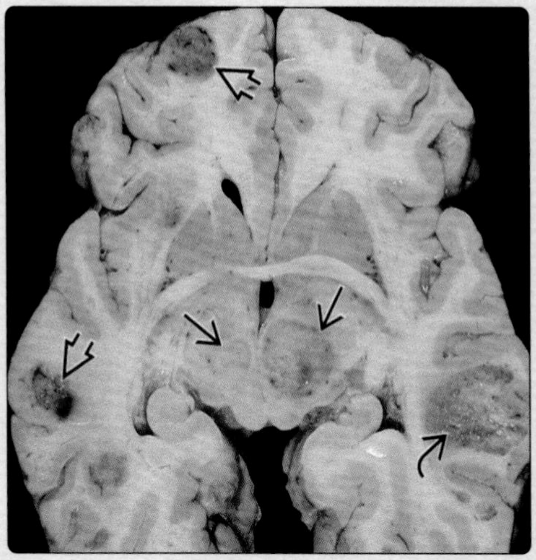

***(27-1)** Graphic shows parenchymal metastases ➔ with surrounding edema ⇨. The GM-WM junction is the most common location. Most metastases are round, not infiltrating. **(27-2)** Metastases from bronchogenic carcinoma show varied locations, appearances. GM-WM lesions show hemorrhage ⇨, midbrain lesions are gray-tan ➔, and another parenchymal metastasis shows necrosis ↗. (Courtesy R. Hewlett, MD.)*

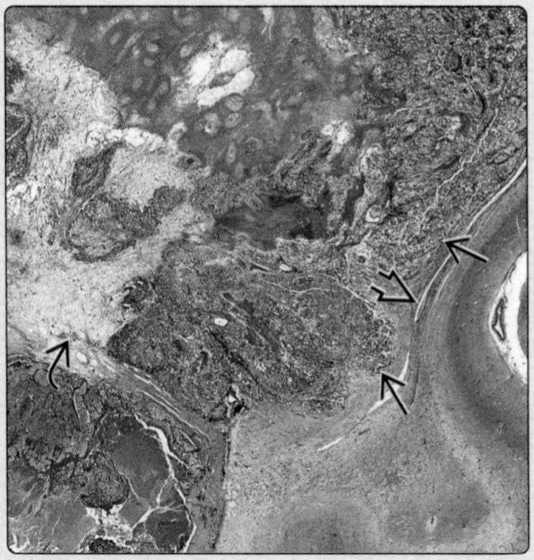

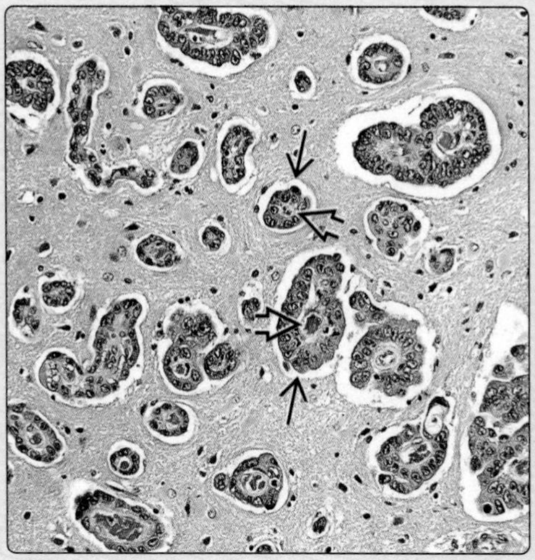

***(27-3)** Parenchymal metastases generally have sharp borders ➔ with adjacent brain ⇨. Necrosis ↗ is common and often extensive. (From DP: Brain, 3e.) **(27-4)** Perivascular spread of this metastatic adenocarcinoma is striking. Note cuffs of tumor cells ➔ surrounding innumerable small arteries and arterioles ⇨. (From DP: Brain, 3e.)*

sharp borders with the adjacent brain **(27-3)**. With the exception of melanotic melanoma, most are tan or grayish white. Some mucin-producing adenocarcinomas have a gelatinous appearance.

Inflammatory reactions to infiltrating tumor cells can alter the permeability and function of the brain neurovascular unit at the proliferating edge of the tumor. Peritumoral edema, necrosis, and mass effect range from none to striking.

The spatial distribution of parenchymal metastases is nonuniform, suggesting that vulnerability to metastases may differ among brain regions. For example, the parietooccipital lobes are the most common site for non-small cell lung cancers.

Hemorrhage varies with primary tumor type. Melanoma, renal cell carcinoma, and choriocarcinoma are especially prone to develop intratumoral hemorrhages. For example, compared with lung cancer, metastatic melanoma is five times more likely to hemorrhage.

Diffusely infiltrating parenchymal metastases are rare. When they occur, they may be grossly indistinguishable from anaplastic astrocytoma or glioblastoma. Small cell lung carcinoma is the most common tumor that causes such "pseudogliomatous" infiltration.

Skull/Dural Metastases. Calvarial and skull base metastases can be relatively well circumscribed or diffusely destructive, poorly marginated lesions **(27-5)** **(27-6)**. Head and neck tumors that extend intracranially by direct geographic invasion generally cause significant local bony destruction.

Dural metastases usually occur in combination with adjacent skull lesions, appearing as focal nodules or more diffuse, plaque-like sheets of tumor **(27-8)** **(27-9)** **(27-10)**. Dural metastasis without skull involvement is much less common.

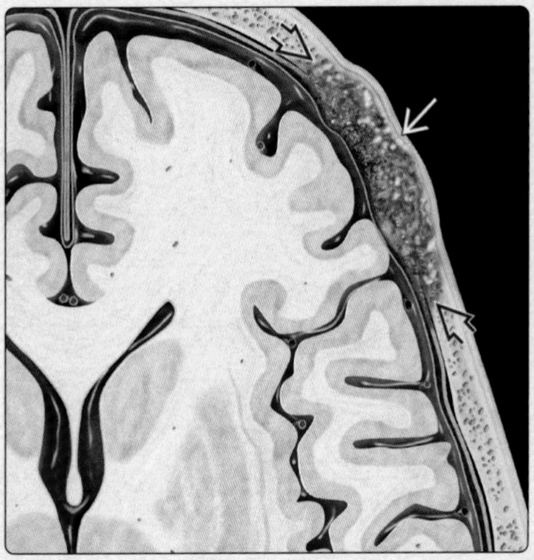

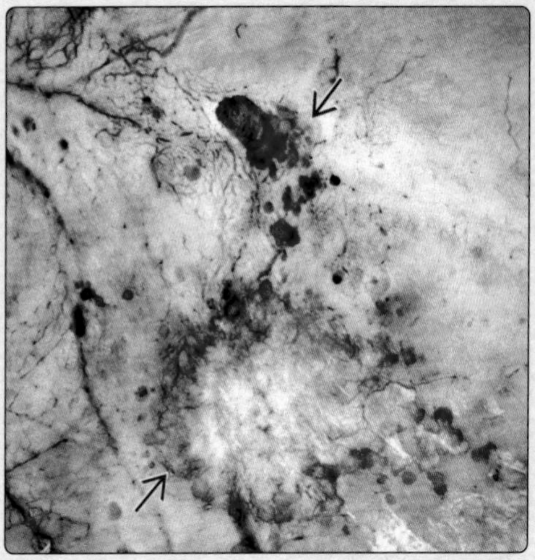

***(27-5)** Axial graphic illustrates a destructive skull metastasis expanding the diploic space and invading/thickening the underlying dura (light blue linear structure).* ***(27-6)** Skull metastases are seen here as permeative, lytic, and destructive lesions.*

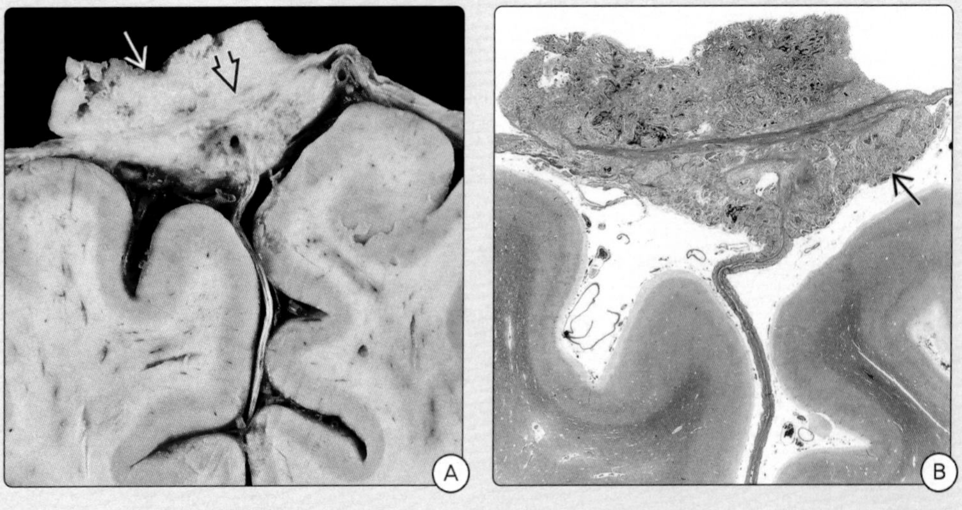

***(27-7A)** Metastatic tumor penetrates the dura and invades the superior sagittal sinus. The overlying skull (not shown) was involved. (Courtesy P. Burger, MD.)* ***(27-7B)** Low-power photomicrograph shows that the endocranial aspect of the tumor involves both the dura and underlying arachnoid. (Courtesy P. Burger, MD.)*

Most dural metastases also involve the subjacent arachnoid and are actually dura-arachnoid tumor deposits.

Leptomeningeal Metastases. The term "leptomeningeal metastases" actually describes metastases to the subarachnoid spaces and pia. Diffuse opacification of the leptomeninges with sugar-like coating of the pia is typical **(27-11)**. Multiple nodular deposits **(27-12)** and infiltration of the perivascular (Virchow-Robin) spaces with extension into the adjacent cortex may occur **(27-13)**. Rarely, metastatic tumor spreads under the pia (subpial spread).

Microscopic Features. Although metastases may display more marked mitoses and elevated labeling indices compared with their primary systemic source, they generally preserve the same cellular features.

Some metastases are more difficult than others to characterize on standard histopathologic studies. Apart from their morphologic features, ancillary immunohistochemical (IHC) analysis is the most effective tool for characterizing a metastatic neoplasm of unknown origin.

Recent advances have enabled delineation of actionable, clinically relevant genomic alterations within metastases that help identify the primary source. IHC characterization and new microRNA-based tests can identify the tumor origin in the majority of such cases. Molecular analysis is a further step that can be helpful.

In some instances, metastases harbor relevant genetic alterations that are not present in primary tumor biopsies. Genomic heterogeneity and molecular discordance between primary tumors and brain metastases are additional factors complicating potential targeted treatment regimens.

CNS METASTASES: PATHOLOGY

Location
- Adults
  - Brain (80%, cerebral hemispheres > > cerebellum)
  - Skull/dura (15%)
  - Pia ("leptomeningeal"), CSF (5%)
  - Other (1%)
- Children
  - Skull/dura > > brain parenchyma

Size
- Parenchymal metastases
  - Microscopic to a few centimeters (most 0.5-1.5 cm)
- Skull/dura metastases
  - Variable; can become very large

Number
- Solitary (50%)
- 2 lesions (20%)
- ≥ 3 lesions (30%)
  - Only 5% have > 5 lesions

Gross Pathology
- Round, well-circumscribed > > > infiltrating
- Variable edema, necrosis, hemorrhage

Microscopic Features
- Preserves general features of primary tumor
- May have more mitoses, elevated labeling indices

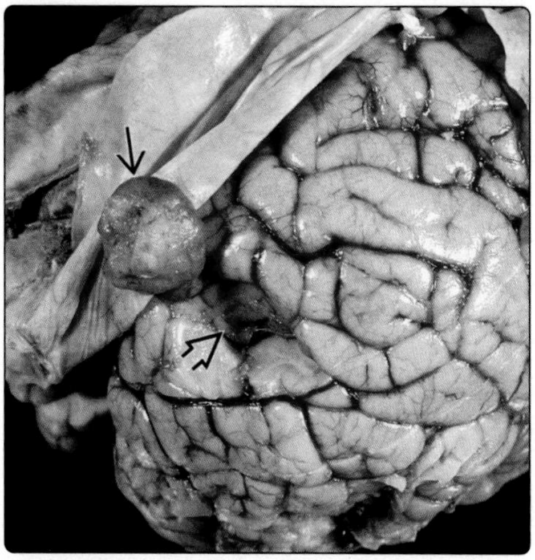

***(27-8)** Solitary dural metastasis indents the brain and appears identical to a meningioma. (Courtesy R. Hewlett, MD.)*

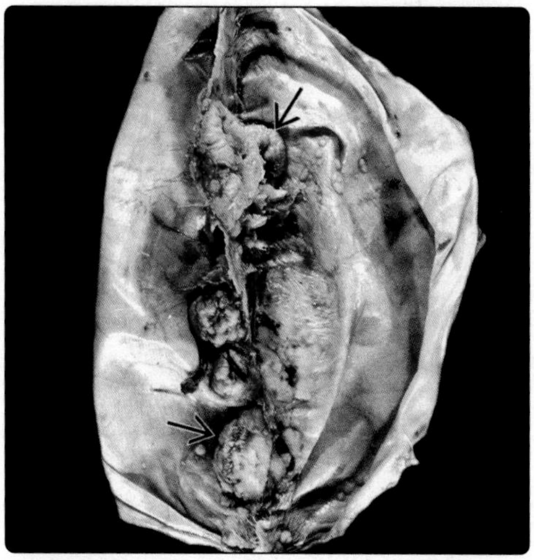

***(27-9)** Multiple dural metastases from breast carcinoma are shown. (Courtesy B. Horten, MD.)*

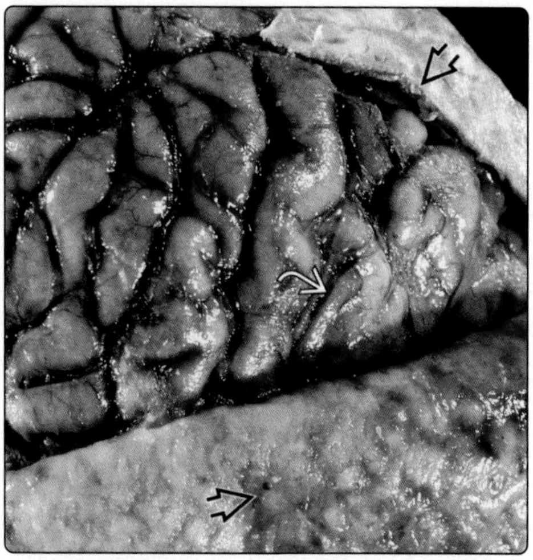

***(27-10)** Metastatic prostate cancer thickens the dura-arachnoid in a nodular pattern. The subarachnoid space and pia are also involved.*

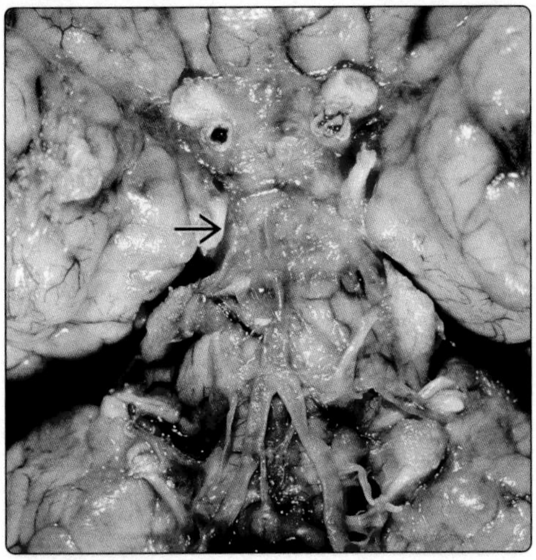

***(27-11)** Pia-subarachnoid ("leptomeningeal") metastases coat the brain, fill the subarachnoid cisterns ➡. (Courtesy R. Hewlett, MD.)*

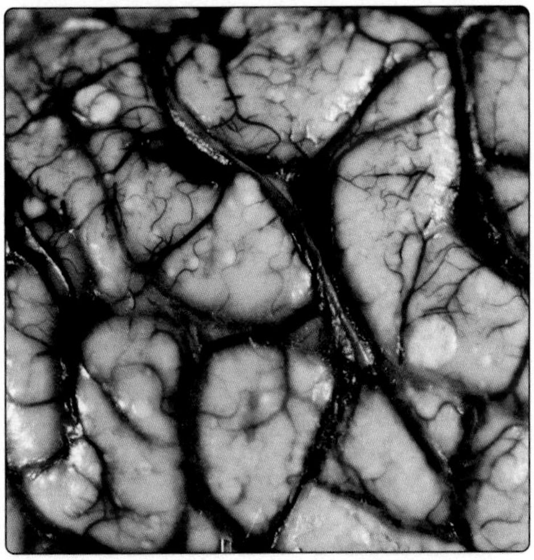

***(27-12)** Metastatic carcinoma shows many discrete tumor deposits on pia. (Courtesy P. Burger, MD, DP: Neuropathology, 2e.)*

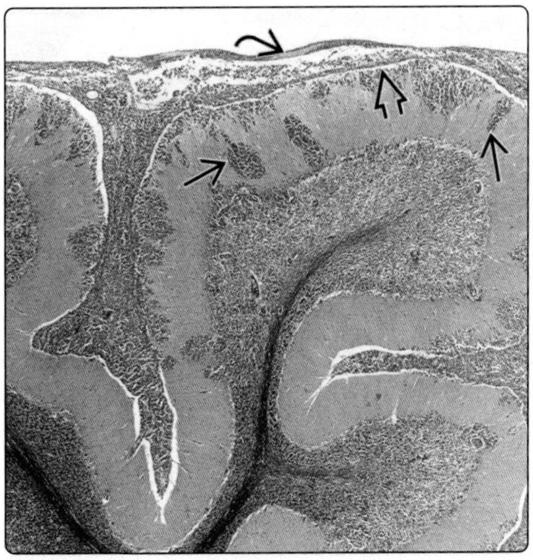

***(27-13)** Mets fill space between the arachnoid ↷ and pia ⇧ and extend along perivascular spaces into cortex ➡. (Courtesy P. Burger, MD.)*

Clinical Issues

Demographics. As treatments for primary systemic cancers improve, patients live longer, and the incidence of brain metastasis continues to increase.

Currently, up to 40% of patients with treated systemic cancers eventually develop brain metastases. The incidence is strongly age-related, ranging from less than 1:100,000 in patients younger than 25 years to more than 30:100,000 at age 60 years.

Peak prevalence is in patients over 65 years of age. Only 6-10% of children with extracranial malignancies develop brain metastases.

Skull/dura metastases have a bimodal distribution. There is a smaller peak in children and a much larger peak in middle-aged and older adults. Overall average age is 50 years, skewed by pediatric cases and young women with aggressive breast cancers.

Presentation. Symptoms vary with tumor site. Seizure and focal neurologic deficit are the most common presenting symptoms of parenchymal metastases. Half of all patients with skull/durae metastases present with headache. Seizure, sensory or motor deficit, cranial neuropathy, or a palpable mass under the scalp are other common symptoms.

Natural History. The natural history of parenchymal metastases is grim. Relentless progressive increase in both number and size of metastases is typical.

Median survival after diagnosis is short, generally averaging between 3 and 6 months. Median survival in patients with untreated metastases from lung cancer is around 1 month. Longer survival is associated with younger patient age, higher performance status, low systemic tumor activity, primary site, and presence of a solitary lesion.

Treatment Options. Treatment choice varies with the histologic type and number and location of metastases. General treatment aims are symptom prevention/palliation, improvement in quality of life, and—when possible—prolonged survival. Surgical resection, fractionated stereotactic radiosurgery, whole-brain radiation, and immuno- or chemotherapy are the most widely available options although many chemotherapeutic agents have limited blood-brain barrier penetration.

Recent advances in tumor immunology such as the discovery of monoclonal antibodies targeting immune checkpoints (immune checkpoint blockade, ICB) have opened promising new frontiers in the fight against cancer. Significant improvements in survival of patients with CNS metastases from metastatic melanoma, non-small cell lung cancer, and renal cell carcinoma have been reported using ICB in combination with radiation therapy.

Imaging

Imaging findings and differential diagnosis vary with metastasis location. Each anatomic site has special features; each is discussed separately below.

Determining tumor response to therapy and then differentiating response from recurrence or treatment-related changes on imaging studies can be challenging. Radiological guidelines such as RECIST and Macdonald criteria for response assessment in solid tumors are inadequate for the CNS. The updated Response Assessment in Neuro-Oncology (RANO) criteria are often used but remain controversial, particularly for assessing neuroinflammatory processes and the impact of vascular targeting agents.

Parenchymal Metastases

Terminology

Parenchymal metastases are secondary tumor implants that involve the brain parenchyma. Tumor in the perivascular (Virchow-Robin) spaces is included in our discussion of parenchymal metastases; intraventricular (ependymal and choroid plexus) metastases are discussed as miscellaneous metastases (see below).

Imaging

Conventional CT and MR are the most commonly used techniques for detecting brain metastases and monitoring treatment response.

CT Findings. Both soft tissue and bone algorithm reconstructions that should be performed as subtle calvarial lesions can easily be overlooked. Soft tissue reconstructions should be viewed with both narrow and intermediate ("subdural") window widths.

NECT. Most metastases are iso- to slightly hypodense relative to gray matter **(27-14A)**. Sometimes, edema is the most striking manifestation of metastases on NECT **(27-15)**. In the absence of edema or intratumoral hemorrhage, even moderately large metastases may be virtually invisible on NECT scans **(27-16)**. With the exception of treated metastases, calcification is rare.

Occasionally, the first manifestation of an intracranial metastasis is catastrophic brain bleeding. An underlying metastasis is a not uncommon cause of spontaneous intracranial hemorrhage in older adults **(27-17)**.

CECT. The vast majority of parenchymal metastases enhance strongly following contrast administration **(27-14B) (27-16B)**. Double-dose delayed scans may increase lesion conspicuity. Solid, punctate, nodular, or ring patterns can be seen.

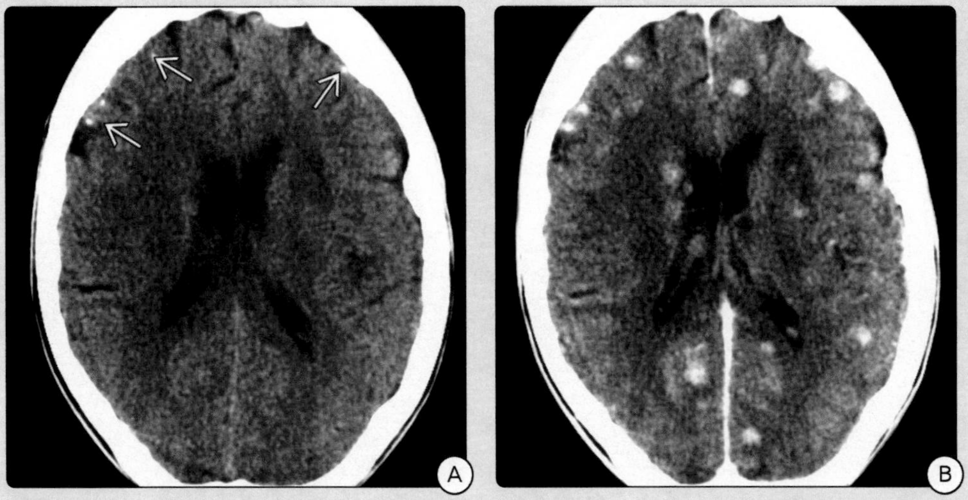

(27-14A) Axial NECT in a 63y woman with known breast carcinoma shows a few scattered bifrontal hyperdensities ➡. (27-14B) CECT scan shows "too numerous to count" enhancing metastases, most of which were isodense and completely invisible on the precontrast study.

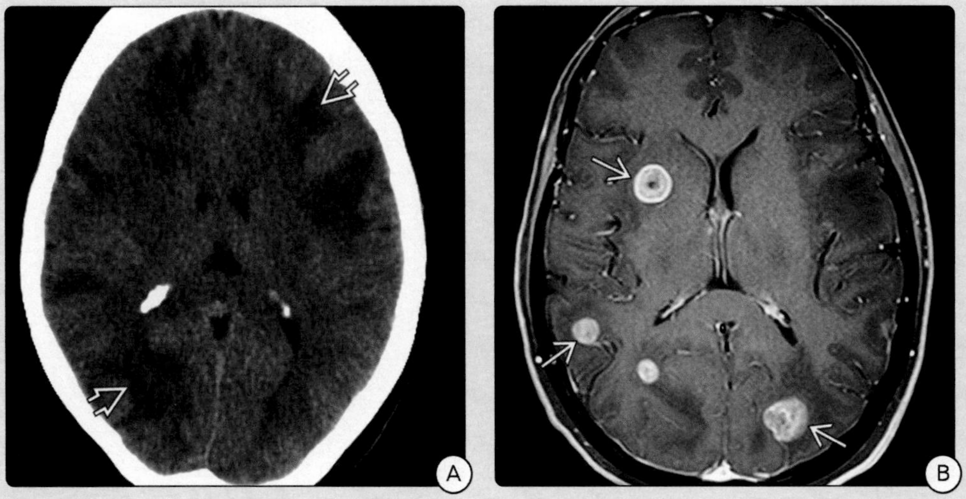

(27-15A) NECT in a 57y woman in the ER with seizure and altered mental status shows multiple patchy and confluent hypodensities ➡ in the subcortical and deep white matter of both hemispheres. (27-15B) A CECT was declined and emergency MR obtained to "look for stroke." T1 C+ FS shows multiple enhancing nodules ➡ as the cause for the edema. Chest, abdomen, and pelvis CT was normal. Biopsy disclosed adenocarcinoma.

MR Findings

T1WI. Most metastases are iso- to mildly hypointense on T1WI **(27-18A)**. The exception is melanoma metastasis, which has intrinsic T1 shortening and thus appears moderately hyperintense **(27-19)**. Subacute hemorrhagic metastases show disordered, heterogeneous signal intensity, often with bizarre-appearing intermixed foci of T1 hyper- and hypointensities **(27-20)**.

T2/FLAIR. Signal intensity on T2WI varies widely depending on tumor type, lesion cellularity, presence of hemorrhagic residua, and amount of peritumoral edema. Many metastases are very cellular neoplasms with high nuclear:cytoplasmic ratios and thus appear hypointense on T2WI and FLAIR **(27-18B)** **(27-18C)**. Exceptions are mucinous tumors, cystic metastases, and tumors with large amounts of central necrosis, all of which can appear moderately hyperintense. Some hyperintense metastases show little or no surrounding edema. Multiple small hyperintense metastases ("miliary metastases") can be mistaken for small vessel vascular disease unless contrast is administered.

T2*. Blood products and melanin contain metal ions including iron, copper, manganese, and zinc. Both subacute hemorrhage and melanin cause prominent signal intensity loss ("blooming") on T2* (GRE, SWI) images **(27-20)** **(27-23)**. Nearly 75% of melanoma metastases have either T1 hyperintensity or demonstrate susceptibility effect; 25% demonstrate both. Nonhemorrhagic nonmelanotic metastases do not become hypointense on T2* **(27-19)**.

T1 C+. Virtually all nonhemorrhagic metastases enhance following contrast administration **(27-15B)** **(27-18D)**. Patterns vary from solid, uniform enhancement to nodular, "cyst + nodule," and ring-like lesions **(27-21)** **(27-22)**. Multiple metastases in the same patient may exhibit different patterns **(27-20)**.

(27-16A) Axial NECT in a patient with headaches and nonfocal neurological symptoms appears almost normal except for anatomic distortion and asymmetry in the white matter of both temporal lobes caused by a nearly isodense parenchymal mass ➡. (27-16B) CECT in the same case shows that the mass enhances strongly ➡. Peritumoral edema is almost absent. Biopsy disclosed metastasis, primary unknown.

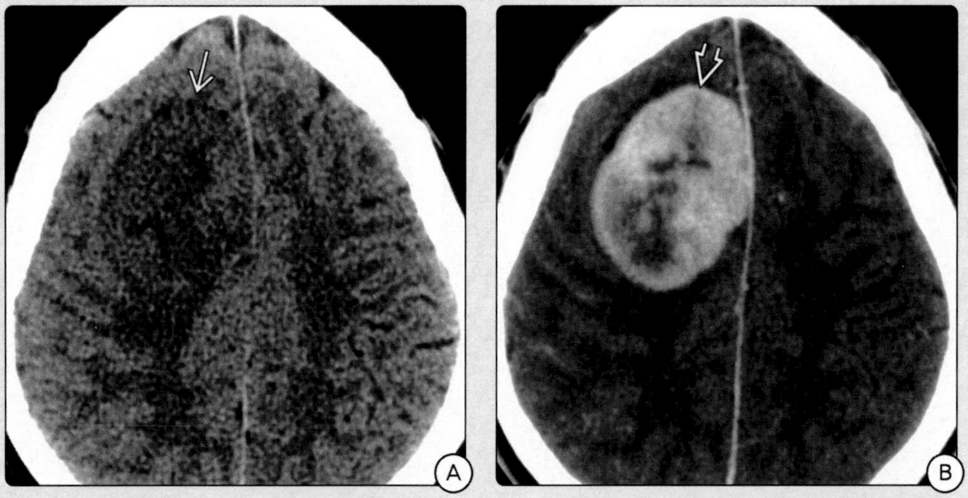

(27-17A) An 80y man was in the emergency department for "brain attack." NECT shows a large heterogeneously hyperdense left parietooccipital hematoma. (27-17B) CTA shows a "spot" sign of contrast accumulation ➡ within the expanding hematoma ➡. Actively bleeding metastatic adenocarcinoma, unknown primary, was found at surgery.

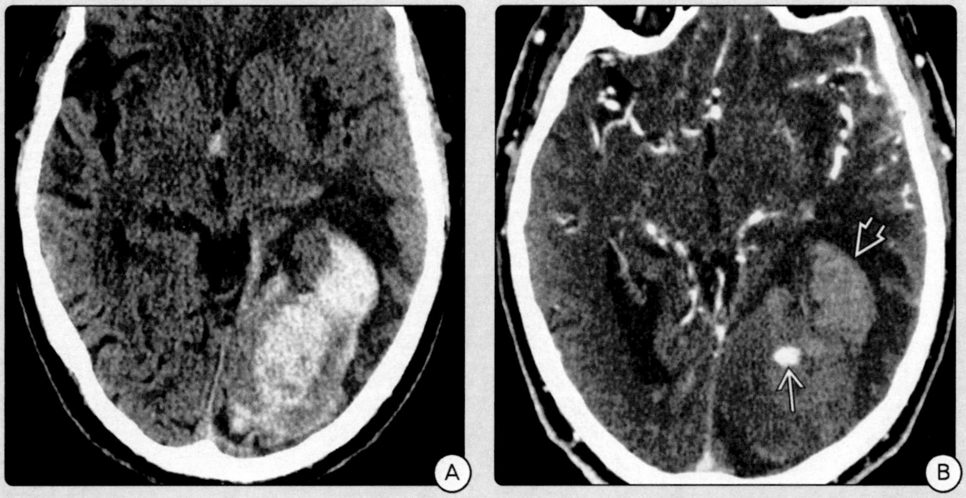

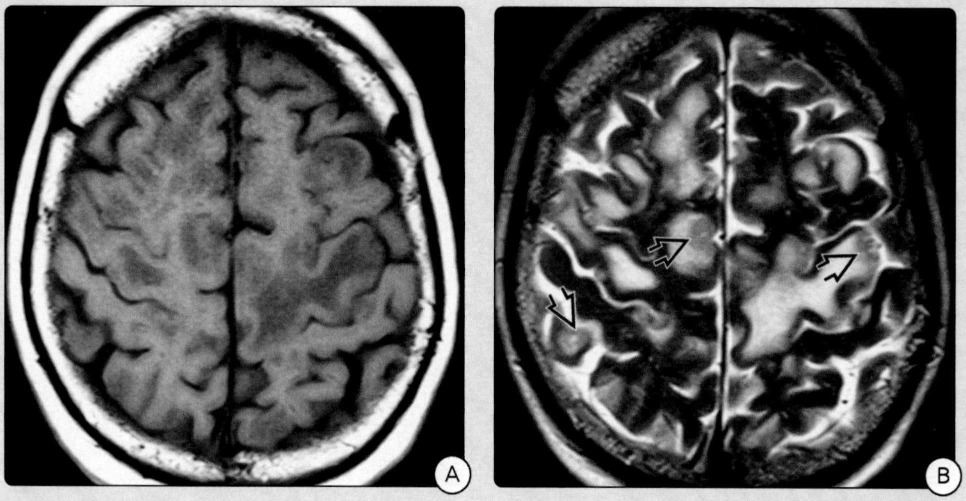

(27-18A) T1WI shows a 63y man with a urogenital primary carcinoma and a normal scan 6 months prior to presenting with seizure. Multiple hypointensities are visible in the subcortical WM of both hemispheres. (27-18B) Iso- to slightly hyperintense nodules at the GM-WM interfaces ➡ are surrounded by edema on this T2WI.

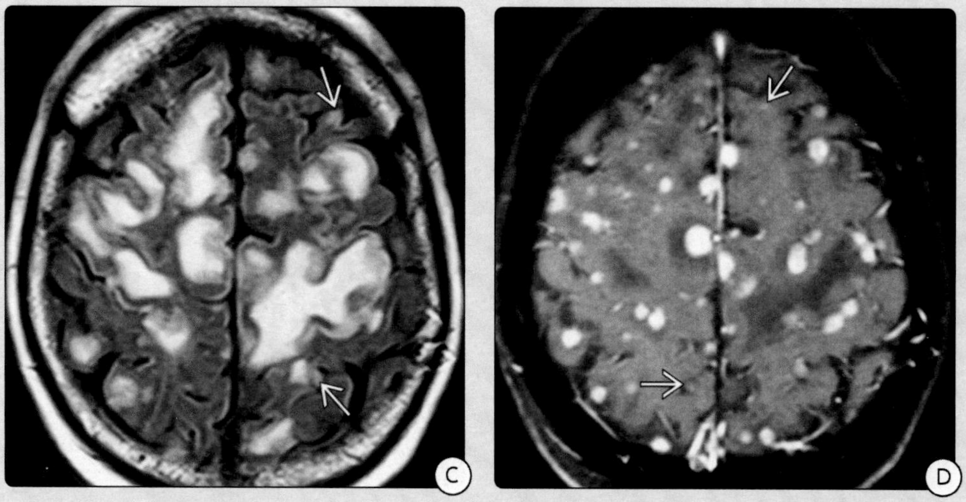

(27-18C) The nodules appear hyperintense on FLAIR. Additional small lesions in the cortex-subcortical white matter are seen ➡. (27-18D) The lesions enhance intensely on T1 C+ FS. A number of tiny enhancing foci ➡ that were not seen on T2 or FLAIR are identified.

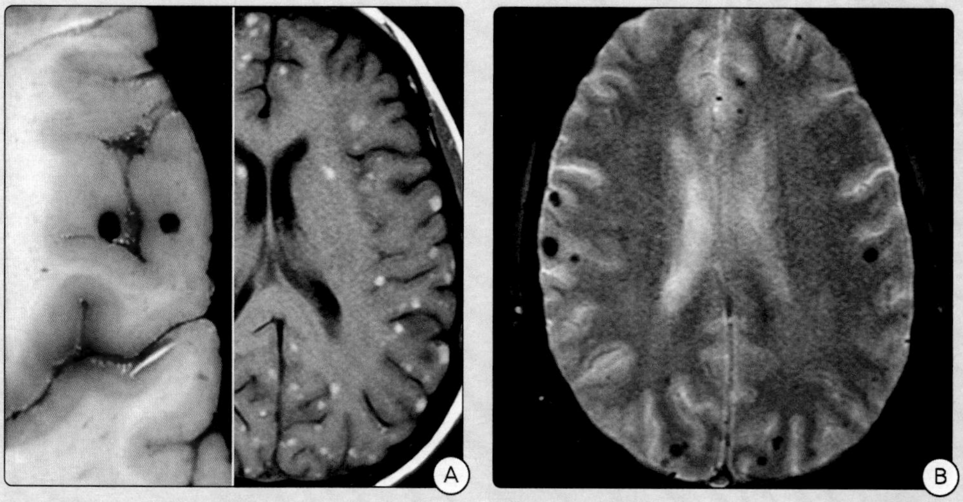

(27-19A) (L) Autopsy shows round black nodules in the cortex, GM-WM interface. This is melanoma metastasis. (Courtesy R. Hewlett, MD.) (R) T1WI in a patient with metastatic melanoma shows innumerable hyperintense metastases. (27-19B) T2 GRE in same patient shows that only a few of the metastases visible on the T1WI "bloom," indicating that most of the T1 shortening was secondary to melanin, not subacute hemorrhage.*

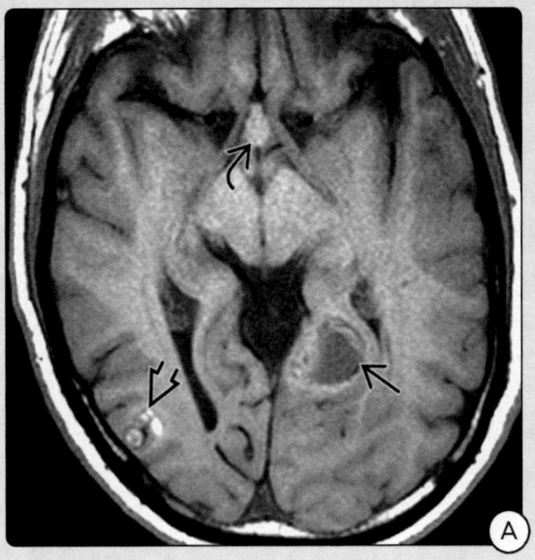

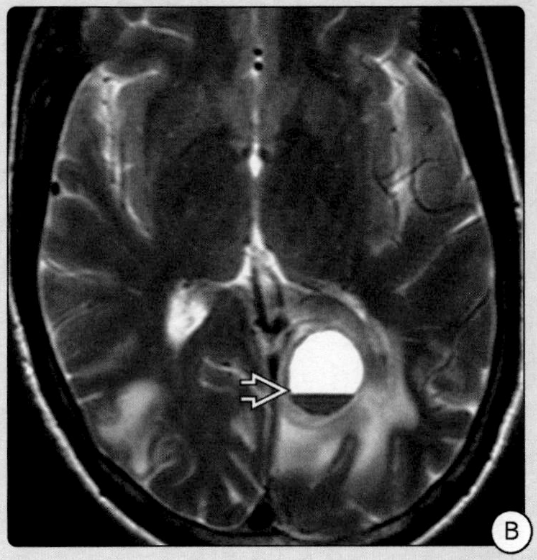

***(27-20A)** T1WI in another patient with metastatic melanoma shows three metastases, each with a different appearance. One has hemorrhages of different ages, resembles cavernous malformation. The second has central necrosis, and the infundibular metastasis is isointense with white matter. **(27-20B)** Slightly more cephalad T2WI in the same patient shows hemorrhage with fluid-fluid level in the necrotic metastasis.*

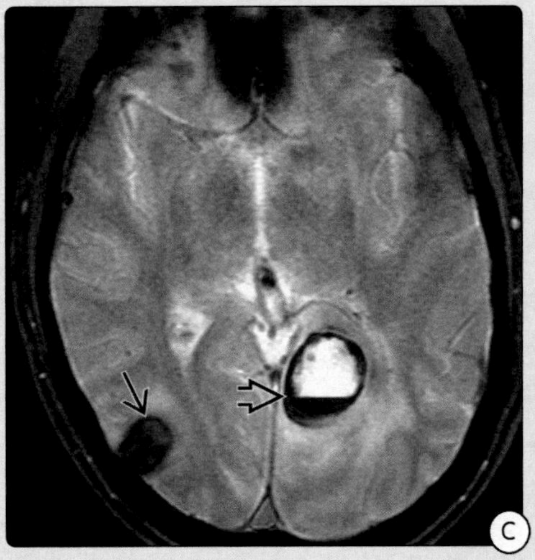

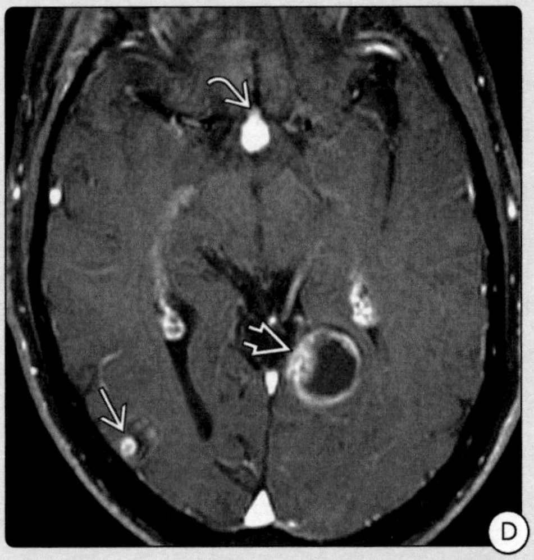

***(27-20C)** T2* GRE shows "blooming" around the rim of the necrotic metastasis, whereas the other hemorrhagic lesion shows nearly homogeneous signal loss. **(27-20D)** T1 C+ FS shows that the infundibular metastasis enhances strongly, uniformly. The necrotic metastasis shows a "cyst + nodule" configuration, whereas the smaller hemorrhagic metastasis shows a tiny ring of enhancement.*

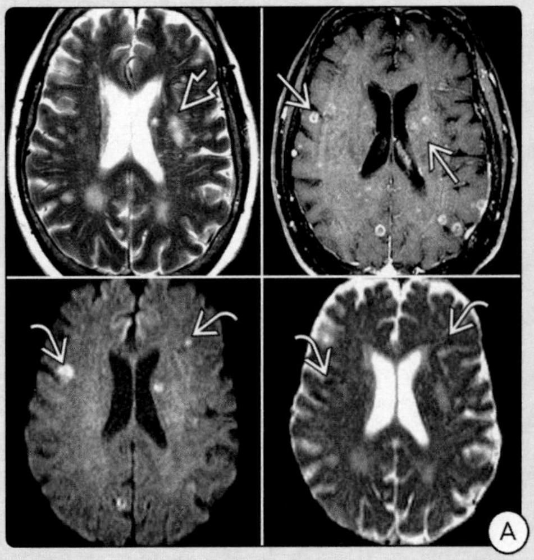

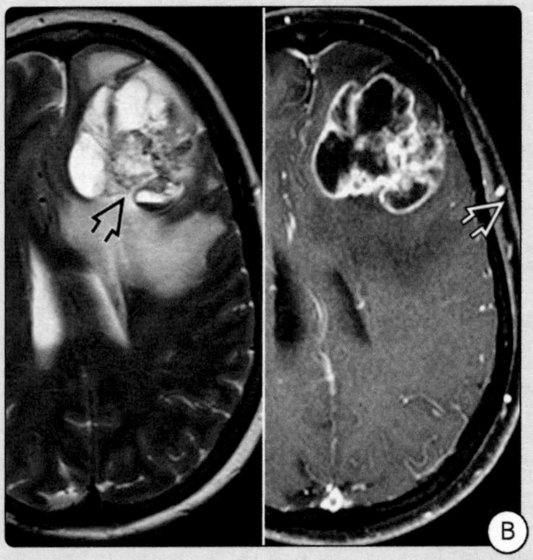

***(27-21A)** Two unusual cases show variations of mets. Mets from lung carcinoma in an elderly patient appear as nonspecific T2 hyperintensities but show punctate, ring enhancement on T1 C+ FS. Some show restriction on DWI. **(27-21B)** (L) T2WI shows infiltrating, cystic, hemorrhagic lesion. (R) T1 C+ FS shows bizarre multiloculated ring enhancement. Preop Dx was GBM; breast mets found at surgery.*

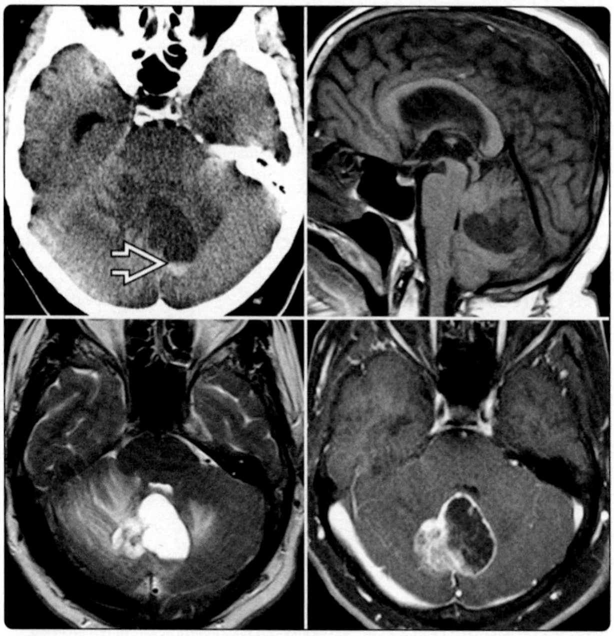

***(27-22)** A 63y man presented with severe headaches and papilledema. NECT scan shows a solitary posterior fossa mass with hemorrhage. MR scans show a "cyst + nodule" pattern. This was adenocarcinoma, unknown primary.*

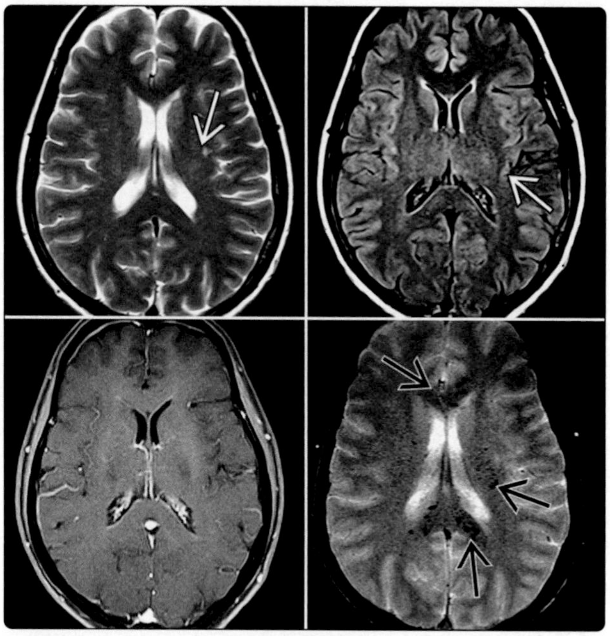

***(27-23)** Occasionally, metastases present with nonspecific encephalopathy. T2/FLAIR scans show a few scattered WM hyperintensities. No definite enhancement on T1 C+, multiple "blooming" foci on T2*. Metastases are from breast primary.*

Longitudinal studies have demonstrated that, in older patients, multifocal hyperintensities identified on T2-weighted or FLAIR scans that do not enhance following contrast administration virtually never turn out to be metastases.

The conspicuity of metastases can be increased on T1 C+ scans with fat suppression and magnetization transfer sequences. The use of double- and even triple-dose contrast-enhanced scans has been reported to increase sensitivity but is not in standard use. Contrast-enhanced T2 FLAIR is a new technique that improves sensitivity compared with contrast-enhanced inversion recovery (IR) and IR-prepared fast spoiled gradient echo (FSPGR) sequences.

DWI. With the exception of highly cellular neoplasms such as medulloblastoma and lymphoma, most *primary* brain tumors do not show restriction on DWI. Metastasis behavior on DWI is much more unpredictable. Well-differentiated adenocarcinoma metastases tend to be hypointense (nonrestricting), whereas more aggressive small and large cell neuroendocrine carcinomas are hyperintense on DWI **(27-21A)**. ADC values inversely reflect tumor cellularity, i.e., low ADC indicates high cellularity.

DTI with a combination of fractional anisotropy (FA) and ADC calculations may be helpful in distinguishing metastases from glioblastoma.

PWI. The differentiation of primary from solitary metastatic brain tumors using pMR is controversial. Some studies suggest that the diagnostic accuracy of MR—including rCBV measurement—is better at grading glial neoplasms than differentiating high-grade gliomas from solitary parenchymal metastases.

MRS. Prominent lipid signal is the dominating peak on MRS in the majority of brain metastases. However, lipid signal is also common in many cellular processes, including inflammation and necrosis. Choline is generally elevated, and Cr is depressed or absent in most metastases.

Molecular MR. Some MR contrast agents specifically target markers, such as endothelial vascular cell adhesion molecule-1 (VICAM-1), that are upregulated in vessels associated with brain metastases. Their use may permit early detection of micrometastases before lesions become apparent on standard gadolinium-enhanced sequences.

Nuclear Medicine Findings. Although it is effective for delineating systemic disease, standard PET/CT understages patients with brain metastases and fails to demonstrate a number of lesions easily detected on standard MR. Early results using new agents such as F18-DOPA show promise in detecting disease relapse after surgical treatment and/or radiotherapy.

Differential Diagnosis

The differential diagnosis of parenchymal metastases varies with imaging findings. The major differential diagnosis for punctate and ring-enhancing metastases is abscess. **Abscesses** and **septic emboli** typically restrict on DWI and show elevated amino acids and lactate on MRS.

Occasionally, **glioblastoma** (GBM) can mimic parenchymal metastases, especially a multifocal GBM with metachronous lesions or brain-to-brain tumor spread. Solitary GBM tends to be infiltrating, whereas metastases are almost always round and relatively well demarcated. GBMs are generally solitary and preferentially located in the deep cerebral white matter, whereas 50% of metastases are multiple, typically occurring at gray-white matter interfaces.

PARENCHYMAL METASTASES: IMAGING AND DDx

CT
- Variable density (most iso-, hypodense)
- Most enhance on CECT
- Perform bone CT for calvarial, skull base metastases

T1WI
- Most metastases: iso- to slightly hypointense
- Melanoma metastases: hyperintense
- Hemorrhagic metastases: heterogeneously hyperintense

T2/FLAIR
- Varies with tumor type, cellularity, hemorrhage
- Most common: iso- to mildly hyperintense
- Can resemble small vessel vascular disease

T2*
- Subacute blood, melanin "bloom"

T1 C+
- Almost all nonhemorrhagic metastases enhance strongly
- Solid, punctate, ring, "cyst + nodule"

DWI
- Variable; most common: no restriction
- Highly cellular metastases may restrict

MRS
- Most prominent feature: lipid peak
- Elevated Cho, depressed/absent Cr

Differential Diagnosis
- Most common: abscess, septic emboli
- Less common
    - Glioblastoma
    - Multiple embolic infarcts
    - Small vessel (microvascular) disease
    - Demyelinating disease
    - Multiple cavernous malformations

Primary infratentorial parenchymal brain tumors in adults are rare. No matter what the imaging findings are, *a solitary cerebellar mass in a middle-aged or older adult should be considered a metastasis until proven otherwise!* Even with a "cyst + nodule" appearance, which is classic for **hemangioblastoma**, metastasis should still be at the top of the differential diagnosis list.

Both metastases and **multiple embolic infarcts** share a predilection for arterial "border zones" and the gray-white matter interfaces. Most acute infarcts restrict strongly on DWI and rarely demonstrate a ring-enhancing pattern on T1 C+ scans. Chronic infarcts and age-related **small vessel microvascular disease** are hyperintense on T2WI and do not enhance following contrast administration.

Multiple sclerosis (MS) occurs in younger patients and is preferentially located in the deep periventricular white matter. An incomplete ring or "horseshoe" pattern of enhancement is more characteristic of MS and other demyelinating disorders than of metastasis.

Multiple **cavernous angiomas** can mimic hemorrhagic metastases. Hemorrhagic metastases generally show disordered evolution of blood products and an incomplete hemosiderin rim.

Skull and Dural Metastases

Terminology

The term "skull" refers both to the calvaria and to the skull base. As one cannot distinguish neoplastic involvement of the periosteal versus meningeal dural layers, we refer to these layers collectively as the "dura." In actuality, the arachnoid—the outermost layer of the leptomeninges—adheres to the dura, so it too is almost always involved any time tumor invades the dura.

Overview

The skull and dura are the second most common sites of CNS metastases from extracranial primary tumors. Calvarial and skull base metastases can occur either with or without dural involvement.

In contrast, dural metastases without coexisting calvarial lesions are less common. Between 8-10% of patients with advanced systemic cancer have dural metastases. Breast (35%) and prostate (15-20%) cancers are the most frequent sources. Single lesions are slightly more common than multiple dural metastases.

Imaging

General Features. Solitary or multiple focal lesions involve the skull, dura (and underlying arachnoid), or both. A less common pattern is diffuse neoplastic dura-arachnoid thickening, seen as a curvilinear layer of tumor that follows the inner table of the calvaria.

CT Findings. Complete evaluation requires *both* soft tissue and bone algorithm reconstructions of the imaging data **(27-24)**. Scans with soft tissue reconstruction obscure skull lesions, which may be invisible unless bone algorithms are utilized **(27-25)**. Soft tissue scans viewed with bone windows do not provide sufficient detail for adequate assessment.

NECT. Large dural metastases displace the brain inward, buckling the gray-white matter interface medially. Hypodensities in the underlying brain suggest parenchymal invasion or venous ischemia.

Bone CT usually demonstrates one or more relatively circumscribed intraosseous lesions. Permeative, diffusely destructive lesions are the second most common pattern. A few osseous metastases—mostly those from prostate and treated breast cancer—can be blastic and sclerotic.

CECT. The most common finding is a focal soft tissue mass centered on the diploic space. A biconvex shape with both subgaleal and dural extension is typical **(27-26)**. Most dural metastases enhance strongly.

MR Findings

T1WI. Hyperintense fat in the diploic space provides excellent, naturally occurring demarcation from skull metastases. Metastases replace hyperintense yellow marrow and appear as hypointense infiltrating foci **(27-27)**. Dural metastases thicken the dura-arachnoid and are typically iso- or hypointense to underlying cortex **(27-28)** **(27-29)**.

T2/FLAIR. Most skull metastases are hyperintense to marrow on T2WI, but the signal intensity of dural metastases varies. FLAIR hyperintensity in the underlying sulci suggests pia-subarachnoid tumor spread **(27-30)**. Hyperintensity in the underlying brain is present in half of all cases and suggests either tumor invasion along the perivascular spaces or compromise of venous drainage.

T1 C+. Nearly 70% of dural metastases are accompanied by metastases in the overlying skull **(27-31)**. Involvement of the adjacent scalp is also common. Contrast-enhanced T1WI should be performed with fat saturation (T1 C+ FS) for optimal delineation, as some calvarial lesions may enhance just enough to become isointense with fat.

Most dural metastases enhance strongly, appearing as biconvex masses centered along the adjacent diploic space. Dural "tails" are present in about half of all cases. Frank tumor invasion into the underlying brain is seen in one-third. Dural thickening can be smooth and diffuse or nodular and mass-like.

DWI. Hypercellular metastases with enlarged nuclei and reduced extracellular matrix may show diffusion restriction (hyperintense) and decreased ADC values (hypointense).

Nuclear Medicine Findings. Skull metastases are intensely positive on Tc-99m scan. Integrated FDG PET/CT scans have a very high positive predictive value for bone metastases, including calvarial lesions. Dural lesions are less well visualized.

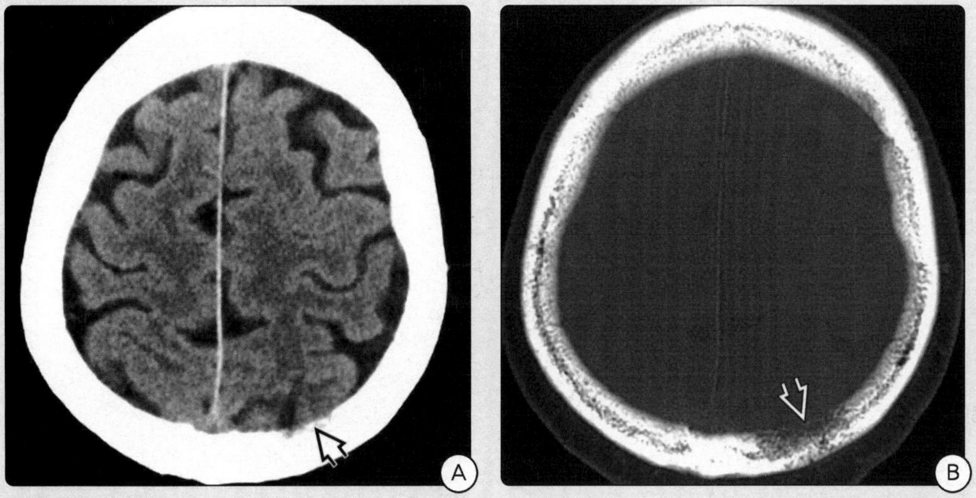

***(27-24A)** NECT scan in a 64y man with headache and no focal neurologic signs shows no abnormality of the brain parenchyma. A subtle irregularity of the left posterior parietal bone ➾ can be seen on soft tissue reconstruction (80 HU). **(27-24B)** Bone algorithm reconstruction shows a solitary permeative destructive lesion that extends through the inner, outer tables of the skull ➾. Metastasis is from lung carcinoma.*

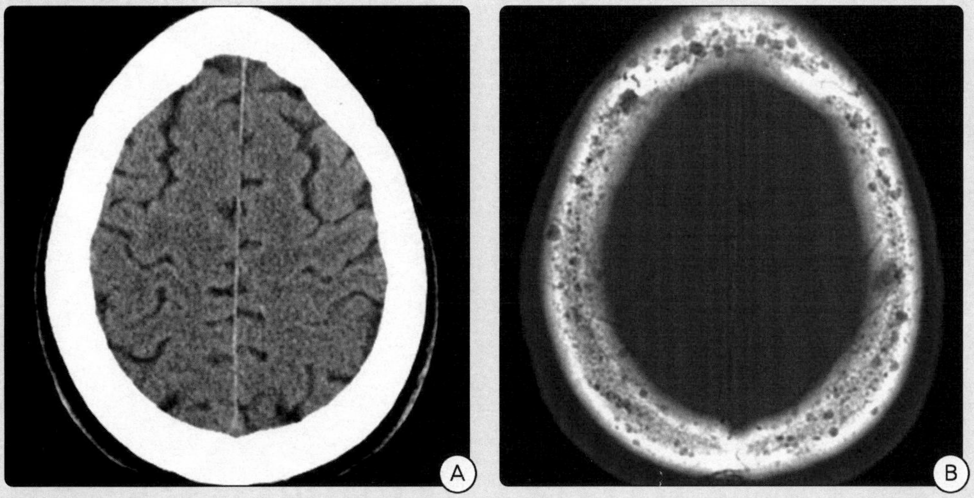

***(27-25A)** NECT scan with a soft tissue algorithm reconstruction, soft tissue windows (80 HU), shows no abnormalities in this 53y man with headaches. **(27-25B)** Bone algorithm reconstruction shows innumerable well-defined lytic lesions in the skull. This is multiple myeloma.*

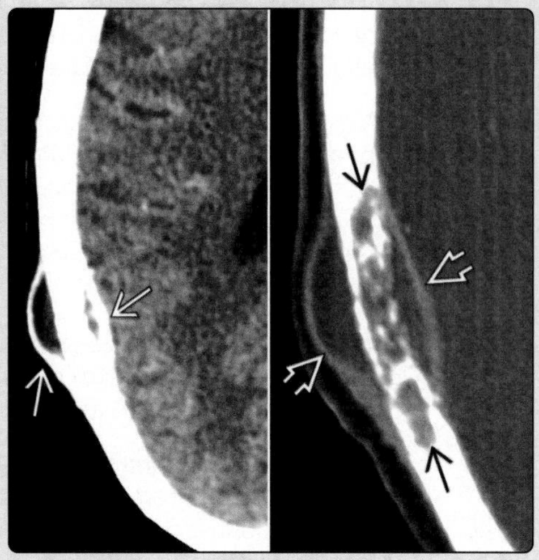

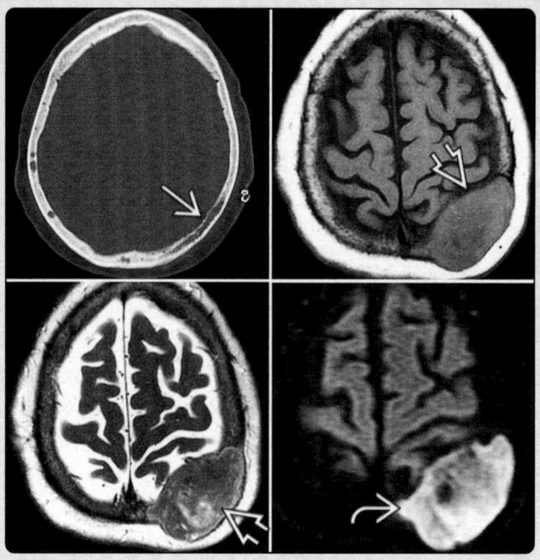

***(27-26)** (L) CECT with soft tissue windows shows a lesion ➡ centered on diploic space of calvaria. (R) Intermediate windows show extent of the lytic, destructive metastasis ⇨, better delineate the subgaleal and extradural components ➡. **(27-27)** Metastatic breast carcinoma to the skull, dura is seen as a permeative destructive lesion in the left parietal diploë ➡. Lesion is mostly isointense to brain on T1-, T2WI ➡ and restricts on DWI ➡.*

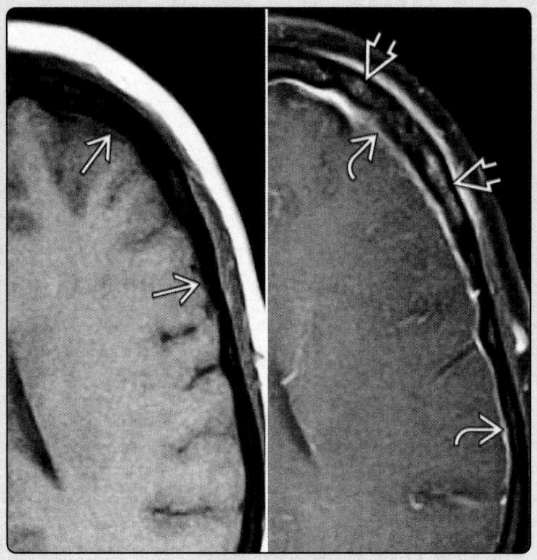

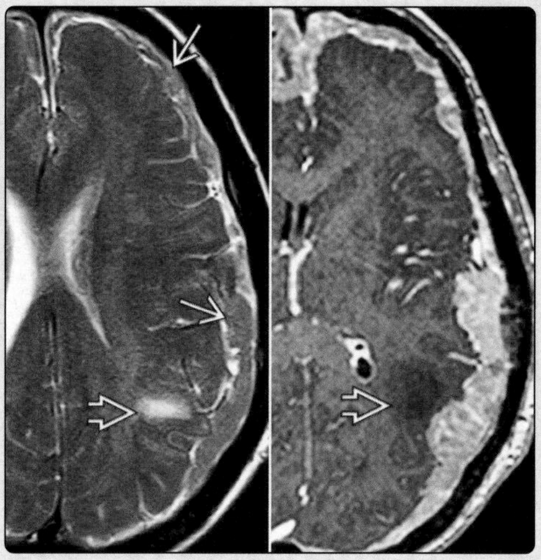

***(27-28)** (L) Subtle dura-arachnoid metastasis is seen here as mild thickening ➡. (R) Thickened dura ➡ enhances on T1 C+ FS. Enhancing lesions in the diploic space can now be identified ➡. **(27-29)** Metastases from prostate cancer thicken the dura, fill the subarachnoid space ➡. Edema ➡ indicates infiltration along the perivascular spaces into the brain parenchyma. (Courtesy N. Agarwal, MD.)*

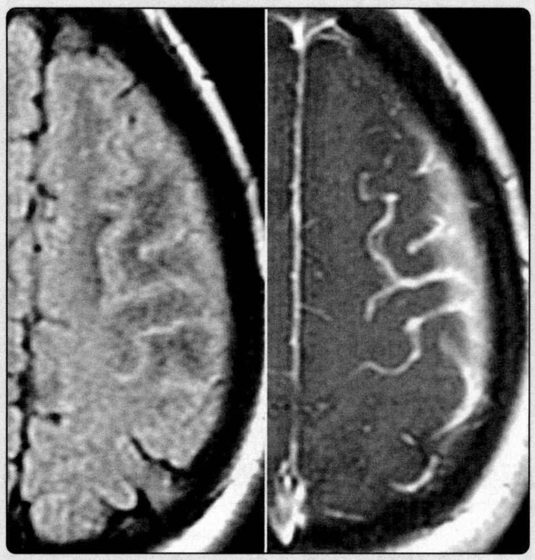

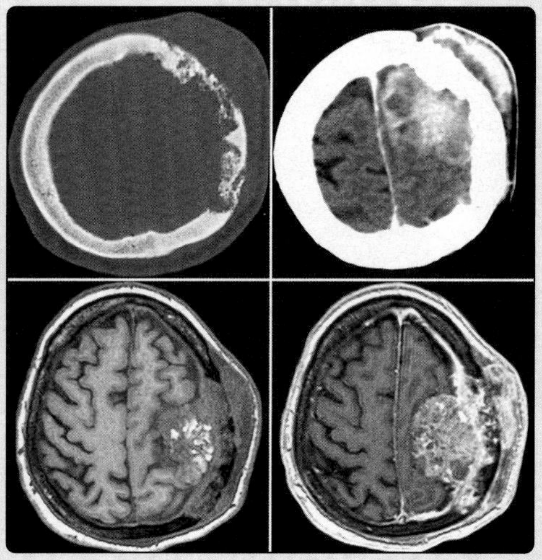

***(27-30)** Dura-arachnoid metastasis from Waldenström macroglobulinemia extends into the subarachnoid space and effaces the sulci. (Courtesy P. Hildenbrand, MD.) **(27-31)** Extensive calvarial, scalp, and dural metastasis from lung carcinoma is illustrated.*

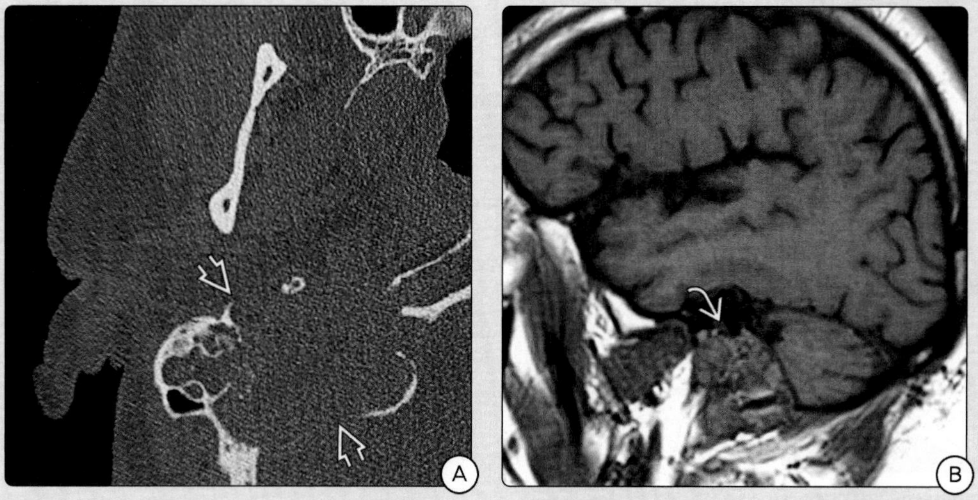

(27-32A) *Axial temporal bone CT in a patient with multiple right lower cranial nerve palsies shows a lytic, destructive mass ➡ that almost completely erodes the right temporal bone.* ***(27-32B)*** *Sagittal T1WI in the same case shows a heterogeneous, mostly isointense extradural mass ➡ with its epicenter in the right temporal bone.*

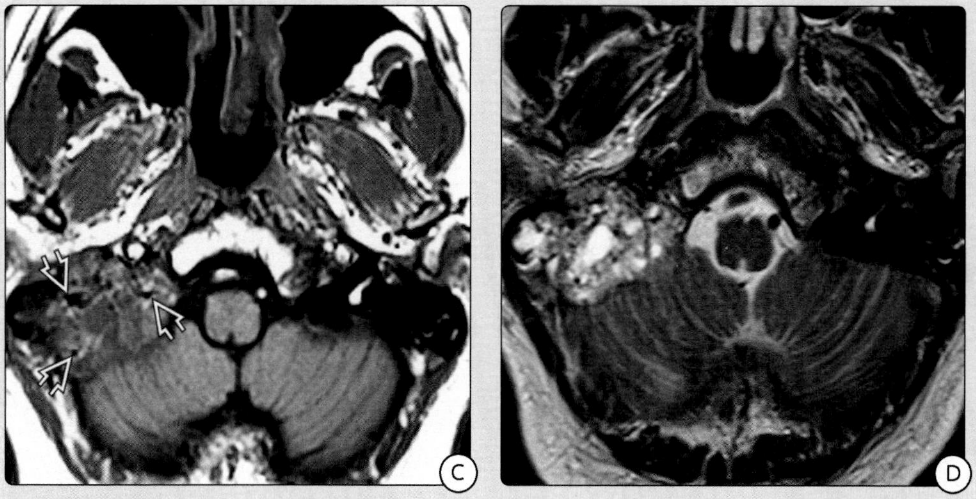

(27-32C) *Axial T1WI in the same case shows that the heterogeneous mass is mostly isointense with gray matter. A few "flow voids" ➡ are visible within the lesion.* ***(27-32D)*** *T2WI in the same case shows that the mass appears heterogeneously hyperintense, with some internal cysts and relatively few "flow voids."*

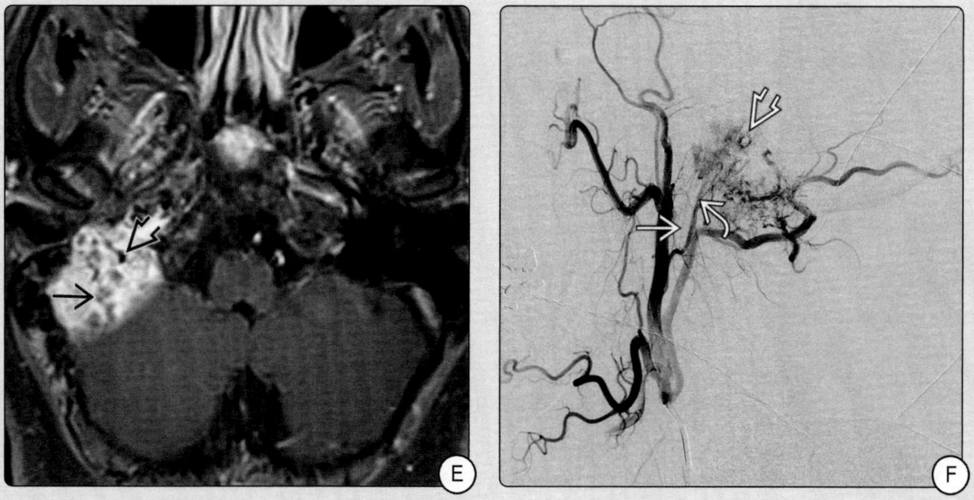

(27-32E) *T1 C+ FS shows that the mass enhances intensely, with a few internal nonenhancing areas ➡ and relatively few "flow voids" ➡.* ***(27-32F)*** *Lateral view of an external carotid angiogram, arterial phase, shows a vascular mass ➡ that is supplied by the posterior auricular ➡, penetrating branches of the occipital artery. The ascending pharyngeal artery ➡ appears normal. Metastatic renal cell carcinoma was found at surgery.*

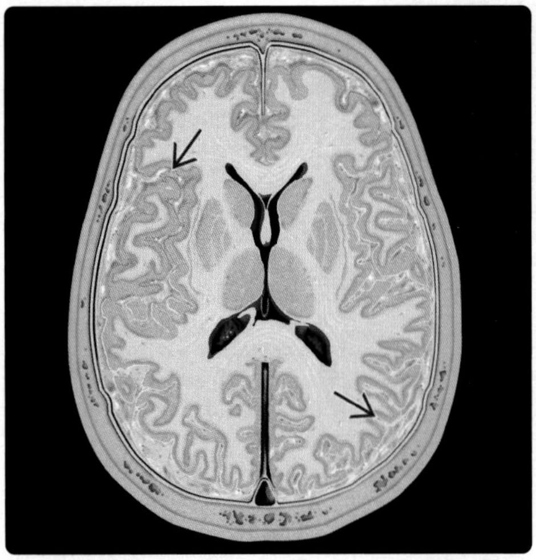

(27-33) Graphic depicts pia-subarachnoid space metastases in white, covering the brain surface and sulci and filling the subarachnoid spaces ➡.

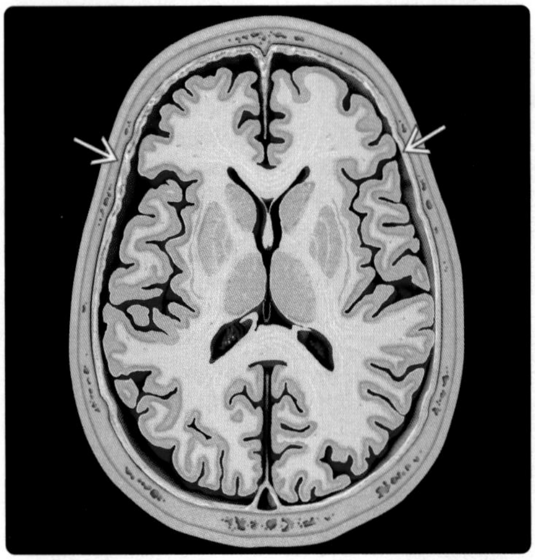

(27-34) This graphic depicts dura-arachnoid metastases as curvilinear thickening that follows the inner table of the skull ➡.

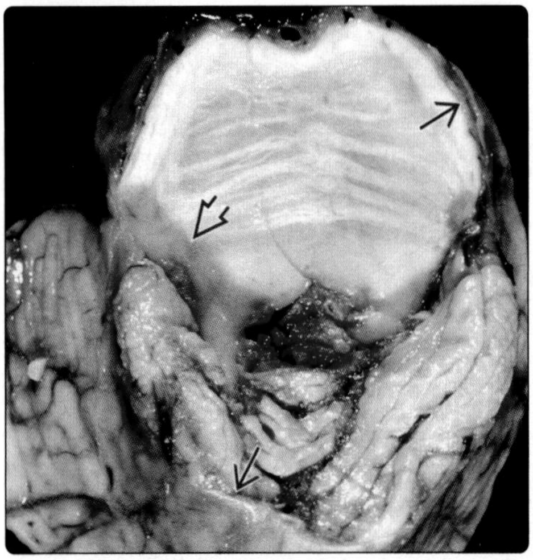

(27-35) Autopsy shows diffuse leptomeningeal metastases ("sugar icing") coating the brain surfaces ➡, filling the subarachnoid spaces ➡.

Angiography. DSA is rarely used unless a vascular lesion is suspected. Most metastases—especially those from renal cell carcinoma—are hypervascular **(27-32)**.

SKULL/DURA METASTASES

General Features
- Second most common site of CNS metastases
- Skull alone or skull + dura > > isolated dural metastases
- "Dural" metastases usually dura *plus* arachnoid!

CT
- Use both soft tissue, bone reconstructions
- Skull: permeative lytic lesion(s)
- Scalp, dura: biconvex mass centered on skull

MR
- T1WI: metastases replace hyperintense fat
- T2WI: most skull metastases hyperintense
- FLAIR: look for
  - Underlying sulcal hyperintensity (suggests pia-subarachnoid space tumor)
  - Parenchymal hyperintensity (suggests brain invasion along perivascular spaces)
- T1 C+
  - Use fat-saturation sequence
  - Skull/scalp/dural lesion(s) can be focal or diffuse, enhance strongly
  - "Dural tail" sign (50%)
  - Less common: diffuse dura-arachnoid thickening ("lumpy-bumpy" or smooth)
- DWI: hypercellular metastases may restrict

Differential Diagnosis
- Skull metastases
  - Surgical defect, venous lakes/arachnoid granulations
  - Myeloma
  - Osteomyelitis
- Dural metastases
  - Meningioma (solitary or multiple)

Differential Diagnosis

The differential diagnosis of skull and dura-arachnoid metastases depends on which compartment is involved and whether solitary or multiple lesions are present.

The major differential diagnoses for skull metastases are surgical defects and normal structures. A **surgical defect** such as a burr hole or craniotomy can be distinguished from a metastasis by clinical history and the presence of defects in the overlying scalp. **Venous lakes, vascular grooves, arachnoid granulations,** and sometimes even **sutures** can mimic calvarial metastases. Normal structures are typically well corticated, and the underlying dura is normal.

Myeloma can be indistinguishable from multiple lytic skull metastases. Skull base **osteomyelitis** is a rare but life-threatening infection that can resemble diffuse skull base metastases. ADC values are generally higher in infection than in malignant neoplasms.

The major differential diagnosis for solitary or multifocal dura-arachnoid metastases is **meningioma**. Metastases, especially from breast cancer, can be virtually indistinguishable from solitary or multiple meningiomas on the basis of imaging studies alone.

The differential diagnosis of diffuse dura-arachnoid thickening is much broader. Nonneoplastic pachymeningopathies such as meningitis, chronic subdural hematoma, and intracranial hypotension can all cause diffuse dura-arachnoid thickening. Metastatic dural thickening is generally—although not invariably—more "lumpy-bumpy" **(27-28)** **(27-29)**.

Leptomeningeal Metastases

Leptomeningeal cancer dissemination is a metastatic complication with growing impact in clinical oncology. Recent advances in therapeutic management have been achieved, so early diagnosis is critical for optimal treatment. In addition to CSF examination, contrast-enhanced MR of the entire neuraxis is recommended for complete pretreatment evaluation.

Terminology

The anatomic term "leptomeninges" refers to both the arachnoid *and* the pia. The widely used term "leptomeningeal metastases" (LM) is technically incorrect, as it is employed to designate the imaging pattern seen when tumor involves the subarachnoid spaces and pia **(27-33)**. Arachnoid metastases are almost always secondary to dura involvement and look quite different **(27-34)**.

For purposes of this discussion, pia-subarachnoid space metastases are referred to as LMs. Other synonyms include meningeal carcinomatosis, neoplastic meningitis, and carcinomatous meningitis.

Epidemiology and Etiology

LMs are uncommon, seen in only 5% of patients with **systemic cancers** **(27-11)**. The most common extracranial primary tumor causing LM is breast cancer **(27-36)**. The second most common source is small cell lung carcinoma. Although uncommon, leptomeningeal dissemination of melanoma carries an especially dire prognosis.

Intracranial primary tumors more commonly cause LM. In adults, the two most common are glioblastoma and lymphoma **(27-35)**. The most common intracranial sources of childhood LM are medulloblastoma and other embryonal tumors such as embryonal tumors with multilayered rosettes C19MC-altered, ependymoma, and germinoma.

Imaging

General Features. In contrast to dura-arachnoid metastases that "hug" the inner table of the calvaria, LM follow the brain surfaces, curving along gyri and dipping into the sulci. The general appearance on contrast-enhanced scans is as though the CSF "turns white" **(27-33)**.

CT Findings. NECT scans may be normal or show only mild hydrocephalus. Subtle sulcal-cisternal effacement with nearly isodense infiltrates can be seen replacing the hypodense CSF in some cases.

CECT scans may also be normal. Sulcal-cisternal enhancement, especially at the base of the brain, can be seen in some cases **(27-37A)**.

MR Findings. T1 scans may be normal or show only smudged "dirty" CSF **(27-38A)**. Most LMs are hyperintense on T2WI and may be indistinguishable from normal CSF.

FLAIR imaging shows loss of CSF suppression, resulting in nonspecific sulcal-cisternal hyperintensity **(27-38B)**. If tumor has extended from the pia into the perivascular spaces, underlying brain parenchyma may show hyperintense vasogenic edema.

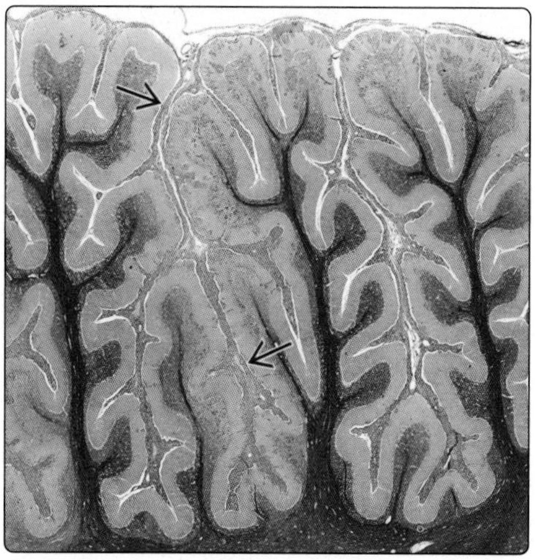

(27-36) Stain shows diffuse CSF breast carcinoma mets filling cerebellar sulci ⇒. (P. Burger, MD, DP: Neuropathology, 2e.)

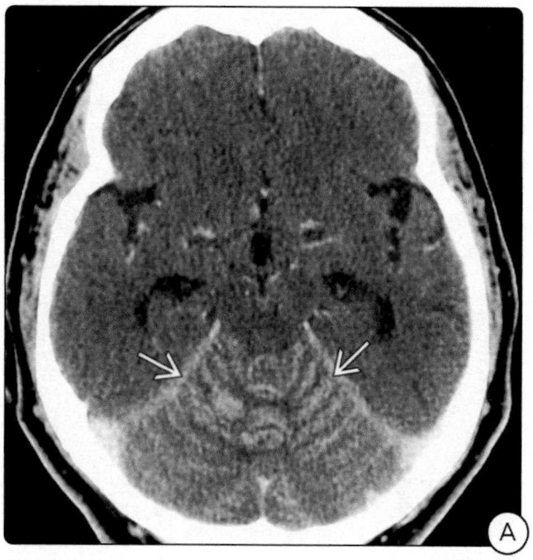

(27-37A) CECT in a 63y woman with headaches, breast cancer, shows enhancing metastases covering the pia over the cerebellum, vermis ⇒.

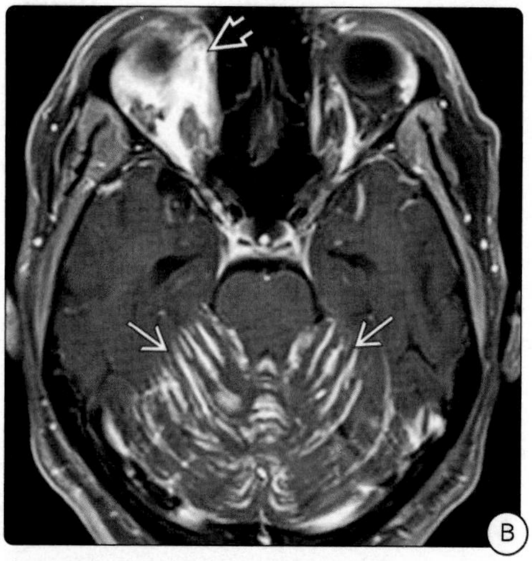

(27-37B) T1 C+ FS shows the enhancing leptomeningeal metastases ⇒ especially well. Also note metastasis to right orbit ⇒.

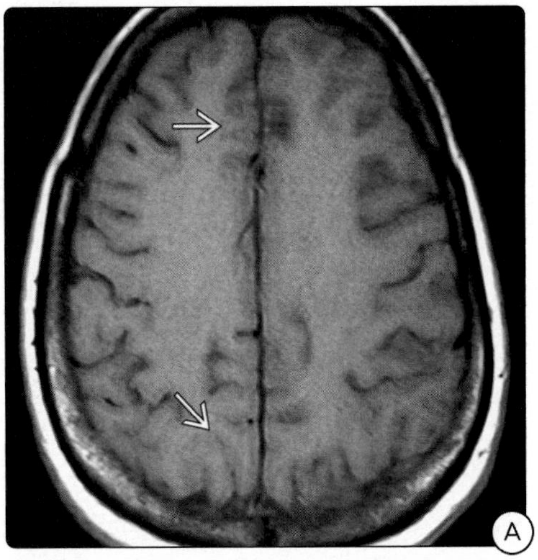

***(27-38A)** Axial T1WI in a 55y woman being staged for small cell lung carcinoma shows subtle effacement of CSF in the superficial sulci ➡.*

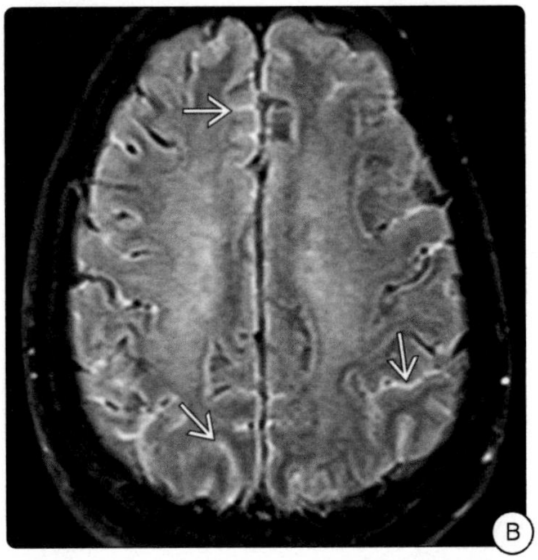

***(27-38B)** FLAIR MR scan demonstrates definite sulcal hyperintensity in multiple areas ➡.*

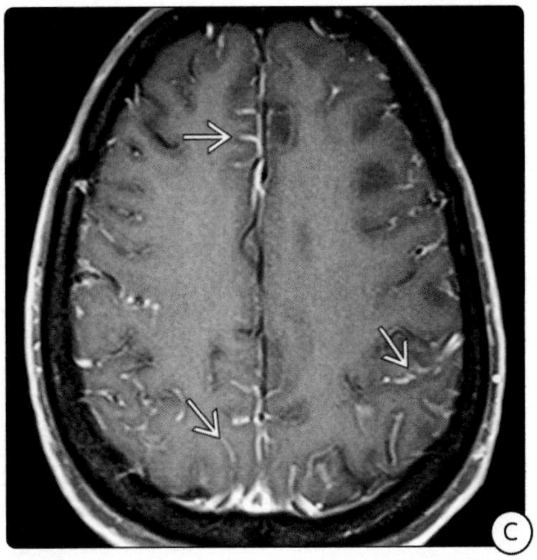

***(27-38C)** T1 C+ FS shows enhancement in the abnormal sulci ➡. CSF documented disseminated CSF metastases.*

Postcontrast T1 scans show meningitis-like findings. Smooth or nodular enhancement seems to coat the brain surface, filling the sulci **(27-38C)** and sometimes almost the entire subarachnoid space including the thecal sac **(27-39)**. Cranial nerve thickening with linear, nodular, or focal mass-like enhancement may occur with or without disseminated disease **(27-51)** **(27-52)**.

Tiny enhancing miliary nodules or linear enhancing foci in the cortex and subcortical white matter indicate extension along the penetrating perivascular spaces.

Differential Diagnosis

The major differential diagnosis of leptomeningeal metastases is **infectious meningitis**. It may be difficult or impossible to distinguish between carcinomatous and infectious meningitis on the basis of imaging findings alone. Other diagnostic considerations include **neurosarcoid**. Clinical history and laboratory features are essential elements in establishing the correct diagnosis.

LEPTOMENINGEAL METASTASES

General Features
- Pia + subarachnoid space metastases
- Uncommon
  - 5% of systemic cancers
  - More common with primary tumors (e.g., GBM, medulloblastoma, germinoma)

CT
- NECT: may be normal ± mild hydrocephalus
- CECT: sulcal-cisternal enhancement (looks like pyogenic meningitis)

MR
- T1WI: normal or "dirty" CSF
- T2WI: usually normal
- FLAIR: sulcal-cisternal hyperintensity (nonspecific)
- T1 C+: sulcal-cisternal enhancement (nonspecific)

Differential Diagnosis
- Meningitis
- Neurosarcoid

Miscellaneous Metastases

The three areas covered above (brain parenchyma, skull/dura-arachnoid, and pia-subarachnoid spaces) are—by far—the most common sites for CNS metastatic deposits. Nevertheless, there are several "secret" sites that may also harbor metastases. The CSF, ventricles and choroid plexus, pituitary gland/infundibular stalk, pineal gland, and eye are less obvious places where intracranial metastases occur and may escape detection. In this section, we briefly consider the location and imaging appearances of these metastases.

CSF Metastases

Circulating tumor cells in the CSF can be difficult to detect using routine cytological examination and are typically identified on imaging studies in the later stages of disease dissemination.

Both extra- and intracranial metastases can seed the CSF. Intracranial CSF metastases are usually seen as "dirty" CSF on T1WI and FLAIR, often occurring together with diffuse pial spread. "Drop metastases" into the spinal subarachnoid space are a manifestation of generalized CSF spread.

Ependymal spread around the ventricular walls occurs with primary CNS tumors much more often than with extracranial sources **(27-39)** **(27-40)**.

Ventricles/Choroid Plexus Metastases

Location. The lateral ventricle choroid plexus is the most common site for ventricular metastases, followed by the third ventricle. Only 0.5% of ventricular metastases occur in the fourth ventricle. Solitary choroid plexus metastases are more common than multiple lesions. Choroid plexus metastases usually occur in the presence of multiple metastases elsewhere in the brain. Occasionally, a metastatic deposit can lodge in the choroid plexus before parenchymal lesions become apparent.

Clinical Issues. Intraventricular metastases from extracranial malignancies are rare, accounting for just 1-5% of cerebral metastases and 6% of all intraventricular tumors. Most involve the choroid plexus; the ventricular ependyma is affected less frequently.

The most common primary sources in adults are renal cell carcinoma and lung cancer. Melanoma, stomach, and colon cancers and lymphoma are less common causes of choroid plexus metastases. Neuroblastoma, Wilms tumor, and retinoblastoma are the most common primary tumors in children. Prognosis is generally poor with most patients succumbing to systemic disease progression or to multifocal CNS disease.

Imaging. Choroid plexus metastases enlarge the choroid plexus and are iso- to hyperdense compared with normal choroid plexus on NECT scans. They enhance strongly but heterogeneously.

Choroid plexus metastases are often hypervascular, so hemorrhage is quite common. Most nonhemorrhagic choroid plexus metastases are hypointense to brain on T1WI and hyperintense on T2/FLAIR. Intense enhancement following contrast administration is typical. Choroid plexus metastases display a prolonged vascular "blush" on DSA.

Differential Diagnosis. In an older patient (especially one with known systemic cancer such as renal cell carcinoma), the differential diagnosis of a choroid plexus mass should always include metastasis. Other common choroid plexus lesions in older patients are **meningioma** and **choroid plexus xanthogranuloma**. Choroid plexus meningiomas enhance strongly and generally uniformly. Choroid plexus cysts (xanthogranulomas) are usually bilateral, multicystic-appearing lesions.

Although solitary metastasis to the third ventricle is rare, metastatic deposit to the choroid plexus in the foramen of Monro may mimic **colloid cyst**. Although the wall of a colloid cyst occasionally demonstrates rim enhancement, solid enhancement almost never occurs.

Pituitary Gland/Infundibular Stalk Metastases

Clinical Issues. Metastasis causes approximately 1% of all resected pituitary tumors and is found in 1-2% of autopsies. Breast and lung primaries account for two-thirds of cases, followed by GI tract adenocarcinomas. Most pituitary metastases involve the posterior lobe, probably because of its direct systemic arterial supply via the hypophyseal arteries (the anterior pituitary is mostly supplied by the hypophyseal portal venous system). Coexisting brain metastases are common, but solitary lesions do occur.

Signs and symptoms such as headache and visual disturbances can mimic those of pituitary macroadenoma although they often progress much more rapidly in patients with metastases. Clinical diabetes insipidus is common.

Imaging. A sellar mass with or without bone erosion, stalk thickening, loss of posterior pituitary "bright spot," and cavernous sinus invasion is typical but

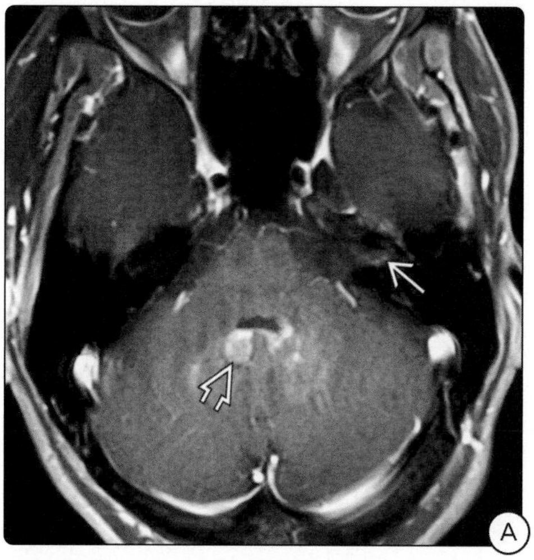

***(27-39A)** T1 C+ FS in a 23y man with glioblastoma shows CSF metastases in the fourth ventricle ⇨ and left IAC ➡.*

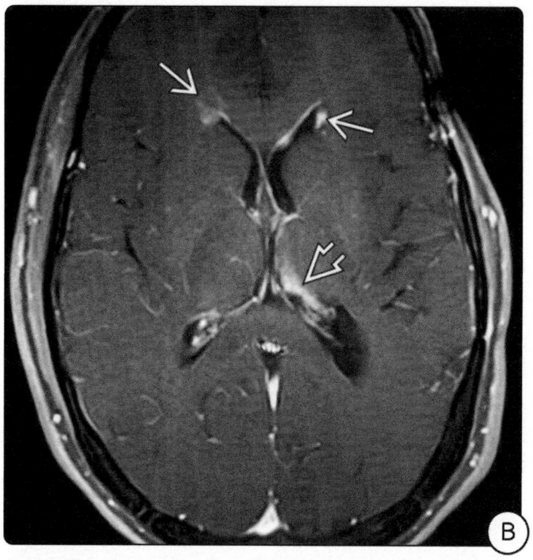

***(27-39B)** T1 C+ FS through the lateral ventricles shows diffuse ependymal ➡ and choroid plexus ⇨ metastases.*

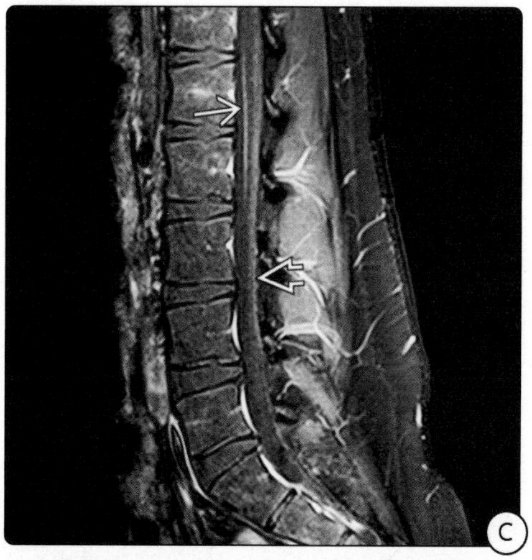

***(27-39C)** Sagittal T1 C+ FS shows diffuse CSF spread ("drop metastases") with tumor coating the conus ➡ and cauda equina ⇨.*

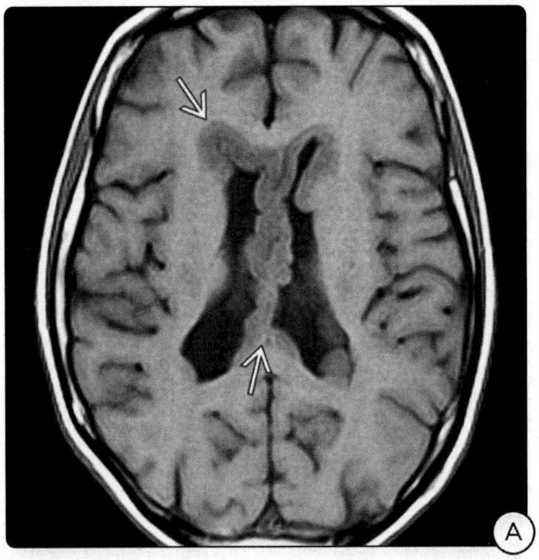

***(27-40A)** Axial T1WI in a 28y woman with a remote history of medulloblastoma shows diffuse nodular ependymal thickening ➡.*

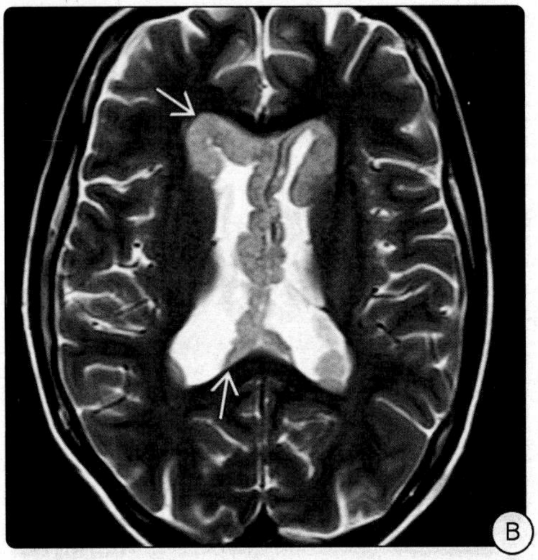

***(27-40B)** T2WI in the same case nicely demonstrates the subependymal nodules ➡, which appear isointense with gray matter.*

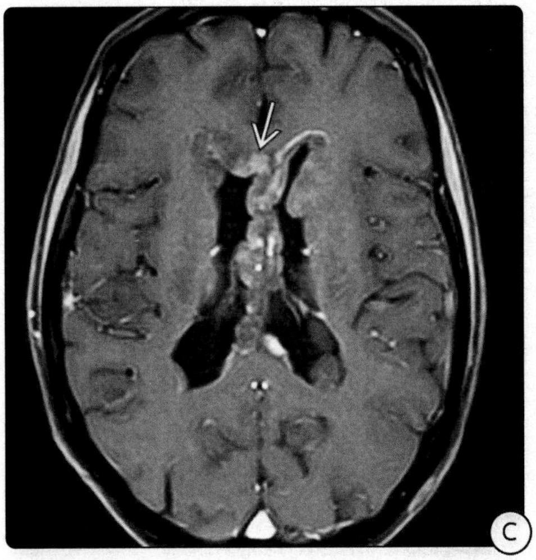

***(27-40C)** The nodules enhance heterogeneously on T1 C+ FS ➡. Metastatic medulloblastoma was documented by CSF.*

nonspecific. An infiltrating, enhancing pituitary and/or stalk mass is the most common finding **(27-41)**.

Differential Diagnosis. The major differential diagnosis of pituitary metastasis is **macroadenoma**. Macroadenomas rarely present with diabetes insipidus. In the setting of a known systemic cancer, rapid growth of a pituitary mass with onset of clinical diabetes insipidus is highly suggestive but certainly not diagnostic of metastasis. **Lymphocytic hypophysitis** can also resemble pituitary metastasis on imaging studies.

Pineal Gland Metastases

Although the pineal gland is a relatively common source of primary CNS tumors that seed the CSF, it is one of the rarest sites to harbor a metastasis. Only 0.3% of intracranial metastases involve the pineal gland. Lung, breast, skin (melanoma), and kidney are the most frequent sources **(27-42)**. When pineal metastases do occur, they are usually solitary lesions without evidence of metastatic deposits elsewhere and are indistinguishable on imaging studies from primary pineal neoplasms.

Ocular Metastases

Clinical Issues. Metastases to the eye are rare. The highly vascular uveal tract is the most common location if metastases are present. Within the uvea, the choroid is by far the most commonly affected site, accounting for nearly 90% of all ocular metastases. The iris (8-9%) and the ciliary body (2%) are other possible locations.

Breast cancer is the most common cause of ocular metastases, followed by lung cancer. The diagnosis of ocular metastases is based on clinical findings supplemented by imaging studies.

Imaging. CT and MR findings are nonspecific, demonstrating a posterior segment mass that often enhances strongly after contrast administration **(27-43)**. Whole-brain imaging is recommended, as 20-25% of patients with choroidal metastases have concurrent CNS lesions.

Differential Diagnosis. The differential diagnosis of choroidal metastasis includes other hyperdense posterior segment masses. Primary **choroidal melanoma** and **hemangioma** may appear similar on both CT and MR. Both metastasis and melanoma can penetrate the Bruch membrane. Ocular ultrasound may be helpful in diagnosing hemangioma. Melanoma and metastases may incite **hemorrhagic choroidal** or **retinal detachment**.

Direct Geographic Spread From Head and Neck Neoplasms

Cephalad spread from head and neck neoplasms such as **sinonasal squamous cell carcinoma, adenoid cystic carcinoma, non-Hodgkin lymphoma**, and **esthesioneuroblastoma** may extend intracranially. This direct extension is also called geographic or regional spread.

Sinonasal tumors gain access to the cranial cavity in three ways: (1) erosion superiorly through the relatively weak bone of the cribriform plate into the anterior cranial fossa, (2) direct extension into the pterygopalatine fossa (PTPF) with posterior spread into the cavernous sinus **(27-44)**, and (3) perineural tumor spread into the PTPF, cavernous sinus, and Meckel cave. We now briefly discuss sinonasal squamous cell carcinoma as the prototypical head and neck neoplasm with geographic intracranial spread. Perineural tumor spread is considered separately below.

Sinonasal Squamous Cell Carcinoma

Squamous cell carcinoma (SCCa) is an aggressive malignant epithelial tumor with squamous cell or epidermoid differentiation. SCCa is the most common sinonasal malignancy, accounting for 3% of all head and neck neoplasms. Almost all sinonasal SCCas occur in patients older than 40, with peak prevalence at 50-70 years. There is a moderate male predominance. Most patients present with symptoms of sinusitis refractory to medical therapy.

Risk factors for developing sinonasal SCCa include inhaled wood dust, metallic particles, and some chemicals. There is *no* direct link to smoking.

Pathology. Nearly three-quarters of sinonasal SCCas arise in the sinuses, whereas 25-30% arise primarily in the nose. The maxillary antrum is the most common site for sinonasal SCCa overall. Approximately 10% of sinus SCCas arise in the ethmoid sinuses.

Sinonasal SCCa that involves the brain is classified according to American Joint Committee on Cancer (AJCC) criteria rather than given a WHO grade. Nasal-ethmoidal SCCa that invades the cribriform plate is considered a T3 tumor. If the anterior cranial fossa is involved, the tumor is a T4a lesion. T4b tumors involve the dura, brain, middle cranial fossa, clivus, or cranial nerves other than the mandibular nerve (CN V_3).

Imaging. CT scans show a solid mass with irregular margins and bone destruction. Sinonasal SCCa is isointense with mucosa on T1WI and mildly to moderately hypointense on T2WI.

SCCa shows mild to moderate enhancement following contrast administration but enhances to a lesser extent than adenocarcinoma, esthesioneuroblastoma, and melanoma. Axial and sagittal T1 C+ fat-saturated images are recommended to detect perineural tumor spread (see below). Coronal T1 C+ FS images are recommended to delineate extension through the cribriform plate into the anterior cranial fossae **(27-45)**.

Differential Diagnosis. The differential diagnosis of sinonasal SCCa with intracranial extension includes **other malignancies** such as sinonasal adenocarcinoma, undifferentiated carcinoma, and non-Hodgkin lymphoma. Nonmalignant mimics of sinonasal SCCa that may extend intracranially include **invasive fungal sinusitis** and **Wegener granulomatosis**.

Perineural Metastases

Terminology

Perineural tumor (PNT) spread is defined as extension of malignant tumor along neural sheaths.

Etiology

Many head and neck cancers have a propensity to spread along nerve sheaths. Mucosal or cutaneous tumors such as SCCa and major/minor salivary gland malignancies such as adenoid cystic carcinoma all are prone to PNT spread. Other tumors such as melanoma and non-Hodgkin lymphoma also frequently spread along major nerve sheaths. Perineural invasion occurs in 2-6% of cutaneous head and neck basal carcinomas and SCCas.

PNT spread may be anterograde, retrograde, or both. "Skip" lesions and lesions that cross from one nerve to another are common.

Pathology

Location. The most common nerves to be affected by PNT are the maxillary division of the trigeminal nerve (CN V_2) **(27-46)** **(27-47)** and the facial nerve

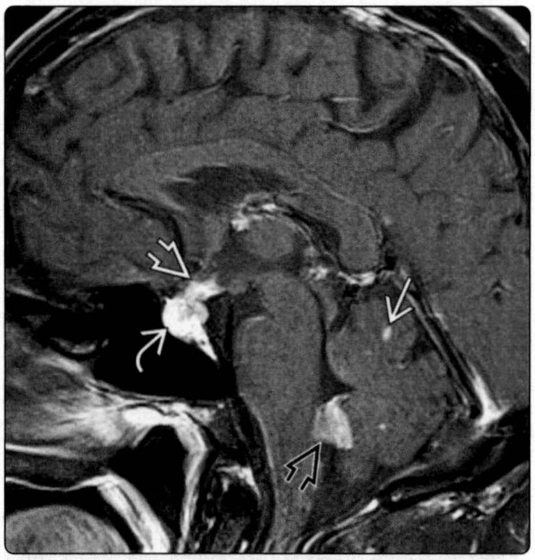

***(27-41)** T1 C+ FS shows metastases to pituitary gland/stalk, 3rd ventricle, 4th ventricle choroid plexus, and vermian folia.*

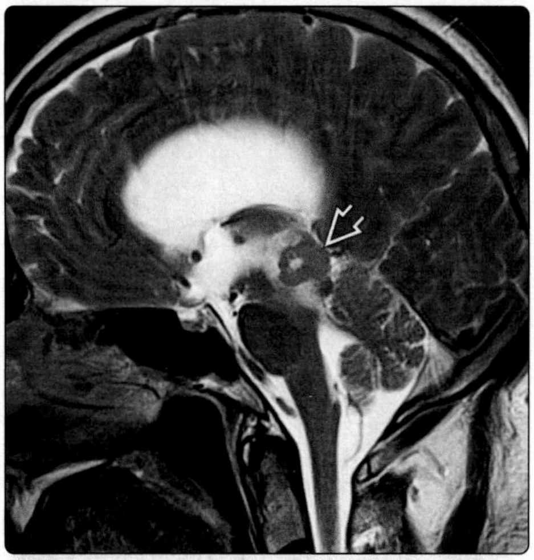

***(27-42)** Sagittal T2WI in a patient with melanoma shows metastasis to the pineal gland causing acute obstructive hydrocephalus.*

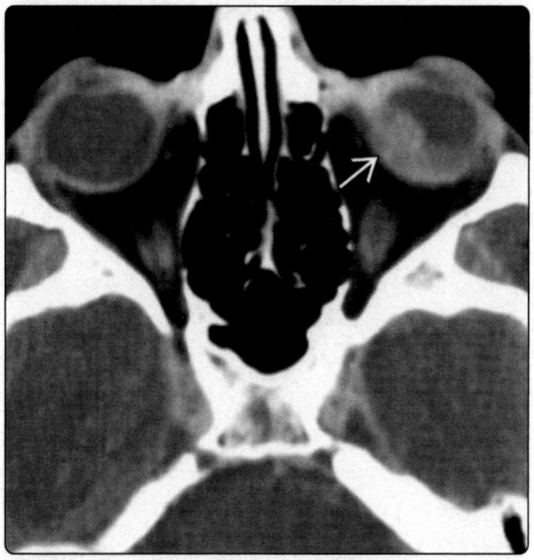

***(27-43)** CECT scan shows a lobulated enhancing mass in the posterior segment of the left globe. This was metastatic breast carcinoma.*

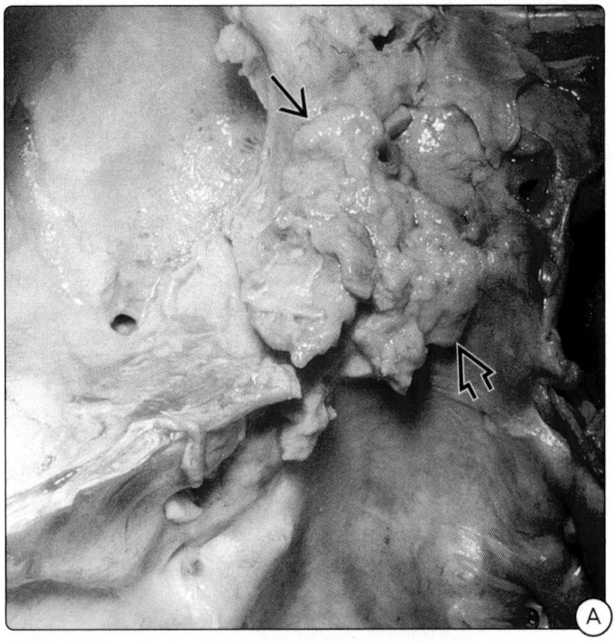

(27-44A) Autopsy specimen shows nasopharyngeal squamous cell carcinoma extending cephalad, eroding through the central skull base into the cavernous sinus ➡ and sellar floor ⇨.

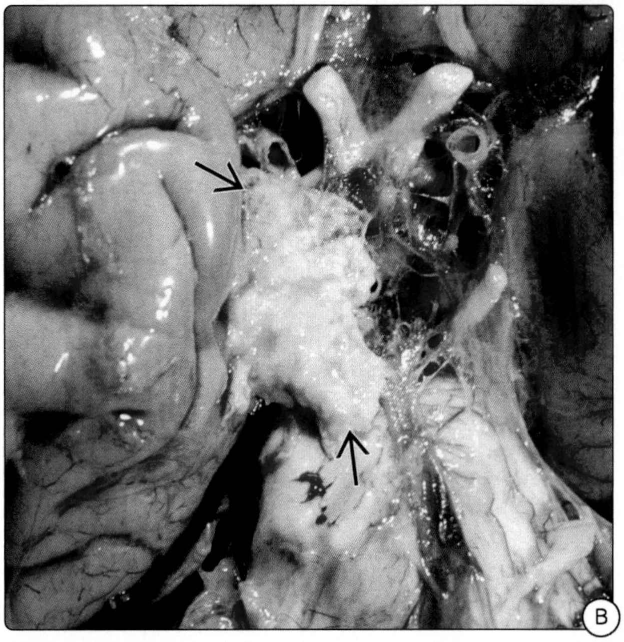

(27-44B) Tumor extends from the cavernous sinus along CN III into the suprasellar and prepontine cistern ➡. (Courtesy R. Hewlett, MD.)

(CN VII) **(27-48)**. SCCa or melanoma of the cheek can infiltrate the infraorbital division of CN V_2. Posterior spread into the PTPF allows access to the cavernous sinus and Meckel cave via the foramen rotundum.

The mandibular nerve (CN V_3) can be invaded by any masticator space malignancy. Retrograde spread up the nerve from an oral cavity mucosal SCCa is a classic example **(27-49)**.

Parotid gland malignancies such as adenoid cystic carcinoma can "creep" up the facial nerve all the way into the internal auditory canal.

Microscopic Features. Tumor extends along a nerve via the epineurium, expressing neural cell adhesion molecules and eventually invading the nerve itself.

Clinical Issues

Early PNT spread is often asymptomatic. Trigeminal pain and paresthesia, including denervation atrophy of the muscles of mastication, are common with CN V lesions. CN VII lesions present with facial weakness or paralysis. CN VII special functions are lost as tumor gradually spreads upward along the facial nerve canal.

Imaging

General Features. Tubular enlargement of the affected nerve together with widening of its bony canal or foramen is typical. If the nerve passes through a structure such as the PTPF that is normally filled with fat, the fat becomes "dirty" or effaced. *Look for denervation atrophy*—common with CN V_3 lesions—seen as small, shrunken muscles of mastication with fatty infiltration **(27-46)** **(27-50)**.

HEAD AND NECK TUMORS WITH CNS INVOLVEMENT

Direct Geographic Spread
- Etiology
  - Most common = sinonasal squamous cell carcinoma (SCCa)
  - Other = adenoid cystic carcinoma, undifferentiated carcinoma, non-Hodgkin lymphoma (NHL)
- Imaging
  - Soft tissue mass in nasopharynx/sinuses
  - Permeative destructive changes in skull base

Perineural Tumor Spread
- Etiology
  - Adenoid cystic carcinoma, SCCa, NHL most common
  - Can be antegrade, retrograde, or combination
- Location
  - CNs V_3, VIII most common
- Imaging
  - Look for denervation atrophy (e.g., pterygoid with V_3 involvement)
  - "Dirty fat" on T1WI (e.g., parapharyngeal space, pterygopalatine fossa)
  - "Fat nerve" ± involvement of Meckel cave
  - Enhancing tumor on T1 C+ FS

CT Findings. Bone CT shows smooth—not permeative destructive—enlargement of the affected foramen or canal. NECT may show abnormal soft tissue density replacing normal fat. CECT may show subtle soft tissue enhancement.

If tumor extends into the cavernous sinus, the walls may bulge outward, and Meckel cave may be filled with soft tissue instead of CSF **(27-46A)**.

MR Findings. The natural contrast provided by fat on T1WI is extremely helpful in detecting possible PNT. Obliterated fat—especially in the PTPF—is a key finding. PNT is often isointense with nerve and difficult to see on T2WI. Tumor spread into Meckel cave replaces the normal hyperintense CSF with isointense soft tissue.

Postcontrast T1 scans should be performed with fat saturation to increase conspicuity of the enlarged, strongly and uniformly enhancing nerve.

Differential Diagnosis

The major differential diagnosis of a solitary enlarged, enhancing cranial nerve in a middle-aged or older adult is perineural metastasis versus **schwannoma**. Schwannomas are tubular or fusiform enlargements that enhance strongly but heterogeneously. The vast majority of schwannomas are vestibulocochlear, whereas the trigeminal and facial nerves are the most common sites for perineural metastases. **Lymphoma** can involve a single cranial nerve but is more often multifocal.

Plexiform neurofibroma can infiltrate the orbital division of CN V but almost always occurs with neurofibromatosis type 1.

Neurosarcoid and **invasive fungal sinusitis** can infiltrate one or more cranial nerves. **Chronic inflammatory demyelinating polyneuropathy** (CIDP) usually involves spinal nerves but occasionally affects cranial nerves. Multiple enhancing CNs are more common than solitary involvement in CIDP. Other causes of multifocal cranial nerve enhancement include **multiple sclerosis, viral/postviral neuritis**, and **Lyme disease**.

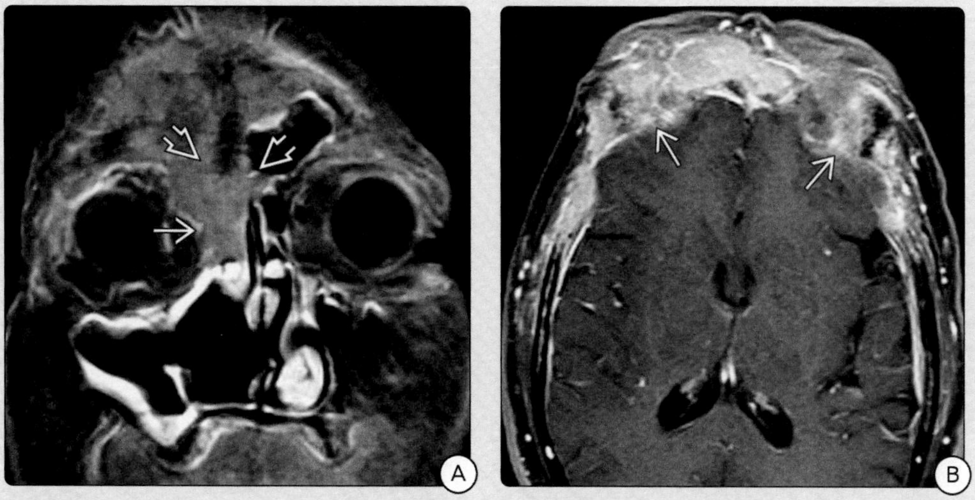

***(27-45A)** Recurrent nasopharyngeal squamous cell carcinoma shows cephalad extension into the right ethmoid sinus ➡ and both anterior cranial fossae ➡. **(27-45B)** Axial T1 C+ FS scan shows the massive extension of tumor into the frontal sinuses. The frontal bones are completely eroded. The dura is thickened and disrupted ➡ with tumor extending into and obliterating the underlying subarachnoid space.*

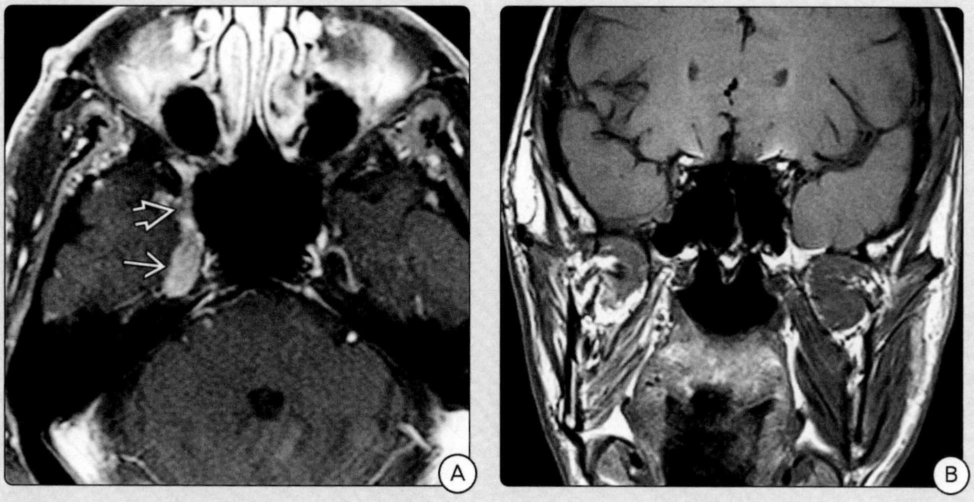

***(27-46A)** Enhancing lesion fills the right Meckel cave ➡, infiltrates and thickens CN V_2 ➡. CN V_3 (not shown) also demonstrated tumor involvement. **(27-46B)** Coronal T1 C+ shows that the ipsilateral muscles of mastication including the temporalis muscle are atrophic and fatty infiltrated compared with the normal-appearing left side. This was denervation atrophy.*

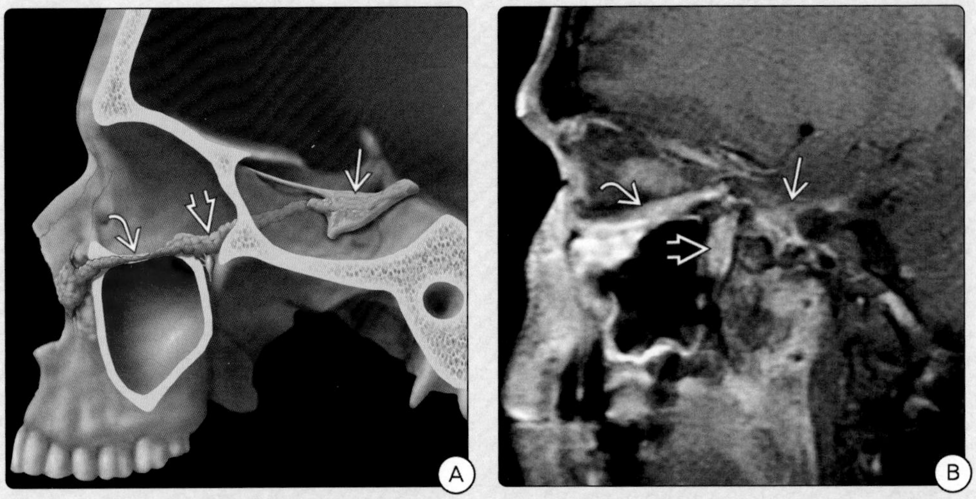

(27-47A) Sagittal graphic shows perineural tumor spread from a cheek malignancy "creeping" along the infraorbital nerve into the pterygopalatine fossa, through the foramen rotundum into the Meckel cave and gasserian ganglion. (27-47B) Sagittal T1 C+ FS shows tumor in the cheek spreading retrograde along the infraorbital nerve, filling the pterygopalatine fossa, extending into the foramen rotundum.

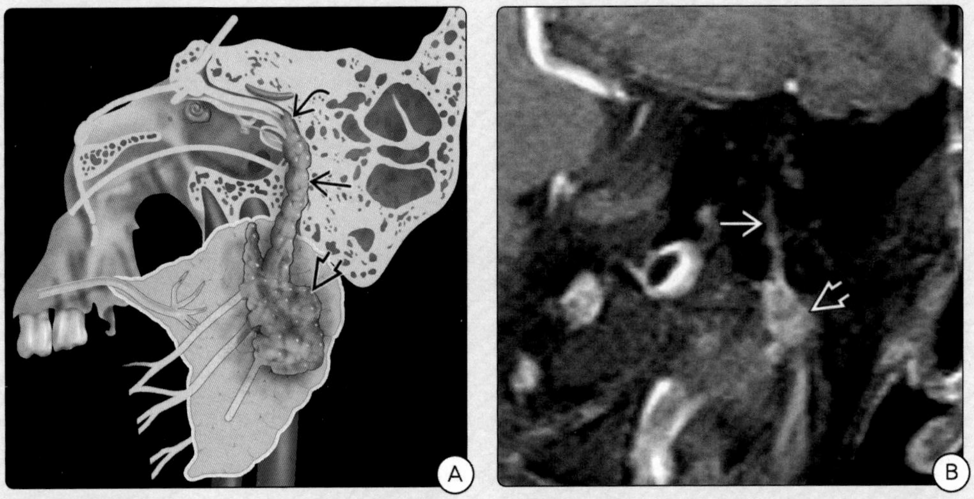

(27-48A) Oblique sagittal graphic depicts a parotid gland tumor spreading intracranially along the descending CN VII up to the posterior genu. (27-48B) Sagittal T1 C+ FS scan shows an enhancing parotid tumor extending along the descending portion of the facial nerve.

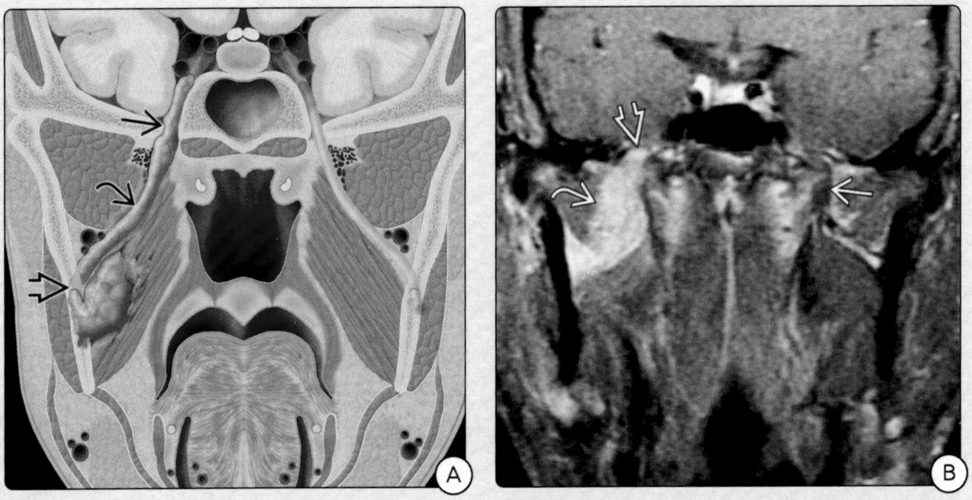

(27-49A) Coronal graphic shows a perineural tumor extending from masticator space into mandible along inferior alveolar nerve, then spreading along mandibular nerve (V_3) through foramen ovale into Meckel cave and gasserian ganglion. (27-49B) Coronal T1 C+ FS shows markedly thickened, enhancing mandibular nerve extending proximally into foramen ovale. Compare to normal, nonenhancing left CN V.

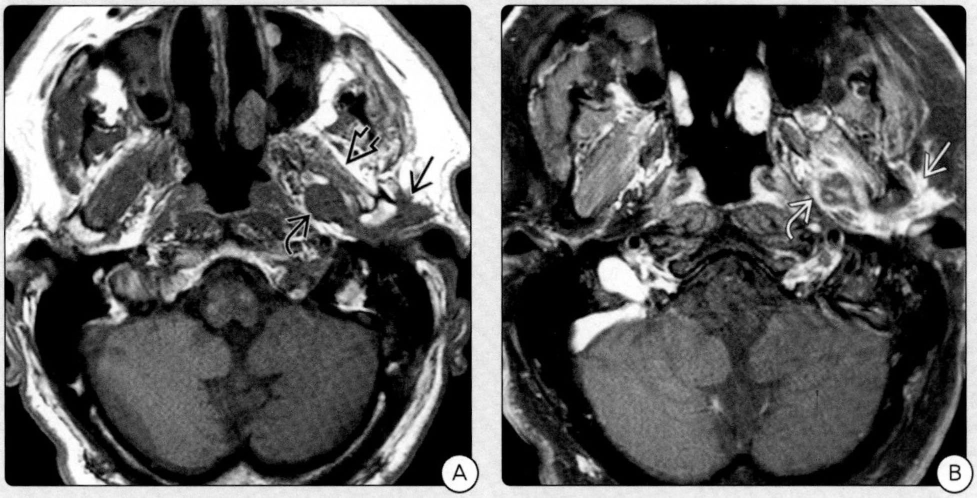

(27-50A) *Axial T1WI in a 77y man with history of facial paralysis 4 years prior followed by onset of facial numbness 1 year prior shows a mass from the left parotid* ➙ *infiltrating the parapharyngeal space* ➙*. Note atrophy of the left medial pterygoid muscle* ➙*.* ***(27-50B)*** *T1 C+ FS shows tumor infiltrating from the deep lobe of the parotid* ➙ *around the mandibular condyle into the left medial pterygoid muscle, parapharyngeal space* ➙*.*

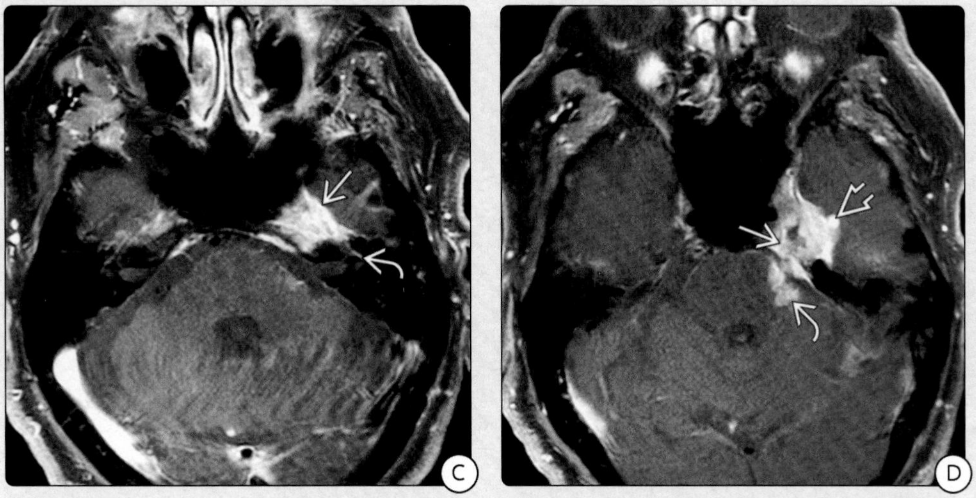

(27-50C) *More cephalad T1 C+ FS shows the tumor infiltrating the left Meckel cave and cavernous sinus* ➙*. Perineural tumor spread along greater superficial petrosal nerve extends into the labyrinthine segment of the facial nerve* ➙*.* ***(27-50D)*** *Enhancing tumor invades through cavernous sinus wall into the adjacent temporal lobe* ➙*. Tumor extends retrograde along the trigeminal nerve* ➙ *through the root entry zone into the pons* ➙*.*

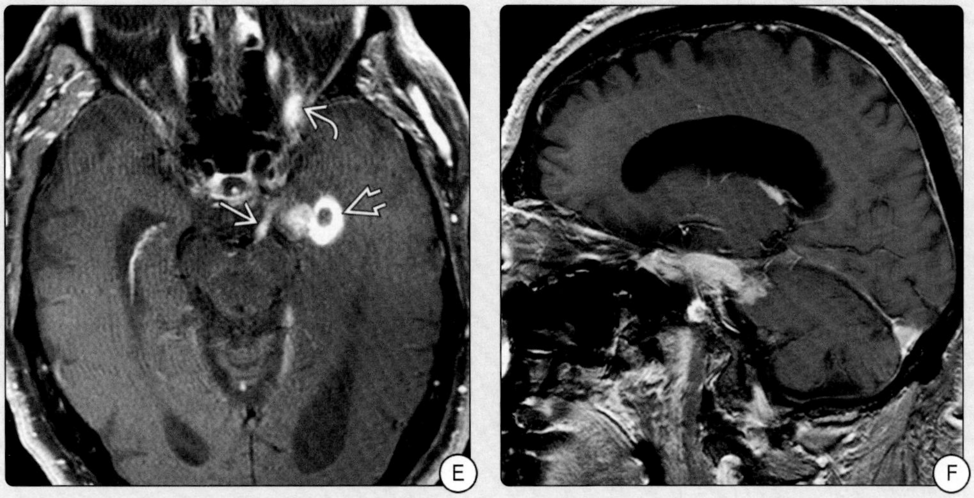

(27-50E) *More cephalad T1 C+ shows tumor invading into the orbit along* V_2 ➙ *and from the cavernous sinus retrograde along the trigeminal nerve* ➙*. Note tumor in the medial temporal lobe* ➙*.* ***(27-50F)*** *Sagittal T1 C+ FS shows the extent of tumor invasion from the orbital apex through the cavernous sinus and Meckel cave along the trigeminal nerve into the pontocerebellar angle.*

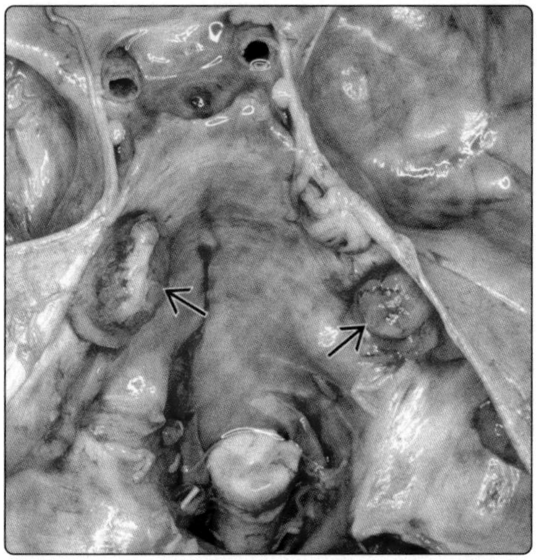

(27-51) Autopsy specimen shows bilateral IAC/CPA metastases to CNs VII and VIII ➲. This is colon carcinoma. (Courtesy R. Hewlett, MD.)

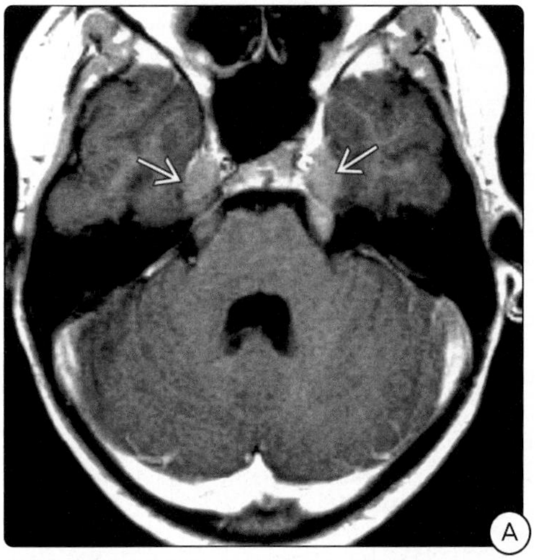

(27-52A) Axial T1 C+ scan shows that the cisternal, Meckel cave segments of both trigeminal nerves are thickened, enhance ➲.

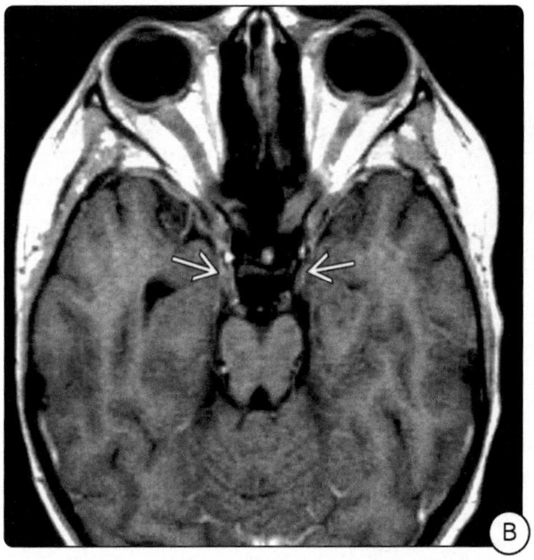

(27-52B) Axial T1 C+ in the same patient shows that both oculomotor nerves are also thickened ➲. This is acute lymphoblastic leukemia.

DIFFERENTIAL DIAGNOSIS OF ENLARGED/ENHANCING CRANIAL NERVES

Solitary Cranial Nerve

- Most common
  - Schwannoma
  - Metastasis (hematogenous, perineural)
- Less common
  - Neurofibromatosis type 1 (NF1) (plexiform neurofibroma)
  - Multiple sclerosis
  - Lymphoma
  - Viral/postviral neuritis (including acute disseminated encephalomyelitis)
  - Lyme disease
  - Neurosarcoid
- Rare but important
  - Ischemia, diabetes
  - Leukemia

Multiple Cranial Nerves

- Most common
  - NF2
  - Metastasis (hematogenous > perineural)
- Less common/rare
  - Lymphoma
  - Chronic interstitial demyelinating polyneuropathy
  - Langerhans cell histiocytosis (disseminated)

Paraneoplastic Syndromes

We close this chapter with a brief discussion of cancer-induced remote neurological effects, collectively called **paraneoplastic syndromes** or **paraneoplastic neurologic disorders** (PNDs). By definition, PNDs are not related to direct (local or metastatic) tumor invasion, adverse effects of chemotherapy, malnutrition, or infection. In a paraneoplastic syndrome, extra-CNS tumors exert their adverse influence on the brain not via metastasis but indirectly.

Most PNDs are mediated by antibodies against known neural antigens ("onconeuronal antibodies") although some cases appear to be mediated by nonhumoral mechanisms. The most commonly accepted theory of paraneoplastic immune-mediated neurologic injury is that primary tumors contain immune cells such as CD4+T cells, NK cells, macrophages, and dendritic cells. When tumor cells undergo apoptosis, the dendritic cells may phagocytose them and then travel to various lymphoid structures, where they present antigens to various T and even B cells. Activated T cells and autoimmune antibodies then cross the blood-brain barrier, where neurons can be targeted.

Paraneoplastic neurologic syndromes are rare, affecting less than 1% of all patients with systemic cancer. In most cases, a paraneoplastic syndrome is diagnosed only after other etiologies—primarily metastatic disease—have been excluded. However, in 70% of patients with PND, neurologic symptoms are the *first* manifestation of a tumor.

PNDs may involve any part of the CNS (brain, spinal cord) or peripheral nervous system although the temporal lobes seem to be the most favored site.

Several types of PND have been recognized. These include **paraneoplastic limbic encephalitis, paraneoplastic encephalomyelitis, paraneoplastic**

cerebellar degeneration, paraneoplastic opsoclonus-myoclonus, paraneoplastic sensorimotor neuropathy, retinopathy, stiff-person syndrome, and **Lambert-Eaton myasthenic syndrome**.

At least 60% of PND patients have various antineuronal antibodies that can be detected in the serum or CSF, but imaging may offer the first clues to the presence of a possible PND.

We first consider the most common paraneoplastic syndrome—paraneoplastic limbic encephalitis—and then discuss a few miscellaneous PNDs. We conclude with a brief mention of extralimbic paraneoplastic disorders and seronegative autoimmune syndromes that can mimic paraneoplastic limbic encephalitis.

Paraneoplastic Encephalitis/Encephalomyelitis

Paraneoplastic encephalitis/encephalomyelitis can involve the limbic system, brainstem (midbrain, pons, medulla), cerebellum, or spinal cord.

The most common form of paraneoplastic encephalomyelitis is paraneoplastic limbic encephalitis (PLE). Note that limbic encephalitis is a heterogeneous group of immune-mediated disorders that also includes *non*paraneoplastic autoimmune encephalitides such as anti-GAD and LGI1 encephalitis. The nonparaneoplastic autoimmune encephalitides were discussed in Chapter 15.

Four components are generally required for the diagnosis of PLE. These are (1) presence of neurologic symptoms, (2) diagnosis of cancer within 4 years from onset of the neurologic manifestations, (3) exclusion of other neurologic disorders, and (4) at least one of the following: CSF analysis showing inflammation with negative cytology, a temporal lobe lesion on brain MR, or epileptic activity in the temporal lobes on EEG.

Terminology

By definition, paraneoplastic limbic encephalitis is a limbic system disorder. The medial temporal lobes are preferentially involved, but the inferior frontal region, insular cortex, and cingulate gyrus can also be affected.

Etiology

The most frequent neoplasm associated with PLE is small cell lung cancer, identified in about half of all cases. Other associated tumors include testicular neoplasms (20%), breast carcinoma (8%), thymoma, and lymphoma.

Antineuronal antibodies are frequently but not invariably found in the CSF or serum of patients with PLE. The most common is the anti-Hu antibody, which is present in about half the patients with small cell lung cancer-associated PLE. Anti-Ma2 PLE is associated with testicular germ cell tumors.

Other neuronal autoantibodies include anti-Ri (breast, small cell lung cancer), anti-Yo (ovarian, breast), and anti-Ma2 (testicular germ cell cancer). These often affect the brainstem (midbrain, pons, medulla) either in isolation or as part of a more widespread autoantibody-mediated encephalitis.

Clinical Issues

Presentation. Neurological symptoms often precede identification of the inciting tumor by weeks or months. The nonspecific nature and diversity of symptoms add to the difficulty of diagnosing PLE. Symptoms gradually develop and evolve over a period of days to weeks. Confusion and short-term memory loss with relative preservation of other cognitive functions—with or without mood and behavioral changes—are typical. Complex partial seizures are common.

Pathology

The histologic features of PLE are similar to those of viral encephalitis and myelitis. A lymphoplasmacytic inflammatory infiltrate with variable degrees of neuronal loss is typical.

Imaging

MR is the procedure of choice in diagnosing PLE. T2/FLAIR shows hyperintensity in one or both medial temporal lobes **(27-53) (27-54)**.

PARANEOPLASTIC NEUROLOGICAL DISORDERS AND ANTINEURONAL ANTIBODIES

Paraneoplastic Limbic Encephalitis
- Primary autoantibody = anti-Hu (small cell lung)
- Other = anti-Ma2 (testicular germ cell)

Paraneoplastic Brainstem Encephalitis
- Anti-Hu, Anti-Ri (breast)
- Anti-NMDA (ovarian teratoma)

Paraneoplastic Cerebellar Degeneration
- Primary autoantibody = anti-Yo (ovarian, breast)
- Anti-Hu, anti-Ri, anti-Tr, or pmGLuR1 (Hodgkin lymphoma)
- Anti-VGCC (small cell lung)

Stiff-Person Syndrome
- Primary antineuronal antibody = anti-GAD65
- Other = anti-amphiphysin

Opsoclonus-Myoclonus Syndrome
- Primary antineuronal antibody = anti-Ri
- Other = anti-Yo, anti-Hu, anti-amphiphysin, anti-Nova 1/2

Differential Diagnosis

The major differential diagnosis of PLE is **herpes encephalitis**. Other causes of LE that can mimic PLE include **glutamic acid decarboxylase 65 (GAD65) autoantibody-associated LE**, **posttransplant acute limbic encephalitis** (PALE) syndrome, and **human herpesvirus 6 (HHV-6) encephalitis**.

Autoimmune nonparaneoplastic LE with positive GAD65 antibodies typically presents with seizures and/or status epilepticus. T2/FLAIR hyperintensity in both hippocampi and amygdalae is typical. Enhancement is generally absent.

HHV-6 encephalitis is associated with hematological malignancies such as Hodgkin and angioimmunoblastic T-cell lymphoma and leukemia.

Patients with neurologic manifestations that are unexplained by any other neurologic disorder should be tested for antineural antibodies. Paraneoplastic syndromes that affect the CNS and some of their major antineuronal antibodies are summarized in the box below. Although the sensitivity and specificity of these assays are not 100%, they can be helpful in establishing the diagnosis of a PND.

Miscellaneous Paraneoplastic Syndromes

Paraneoplastic Cerebellar Degeneration

Paraneoplastic cerebellar degeneration (PCD) is seen in less than 1% of cancers, typically with small cell lung carcinoma, Hodgkin lymphoma, breast cancer, and gynecologic malignancies.

PCD selectively affects the cerebellum and typically presents with ataxia and gait instability, vertigo, dizziness, and oscillopsia. Onset can be acute or subacute and occurs in the absence of brain metastases. Anti-Yo (the most common) or anti-Ri (antineuronal nuclear) antibodies may be detected in the serum and/or CSF of affected patients. Noncerebellar and psychiatric symptoms are more common with anti-Hu PCD.

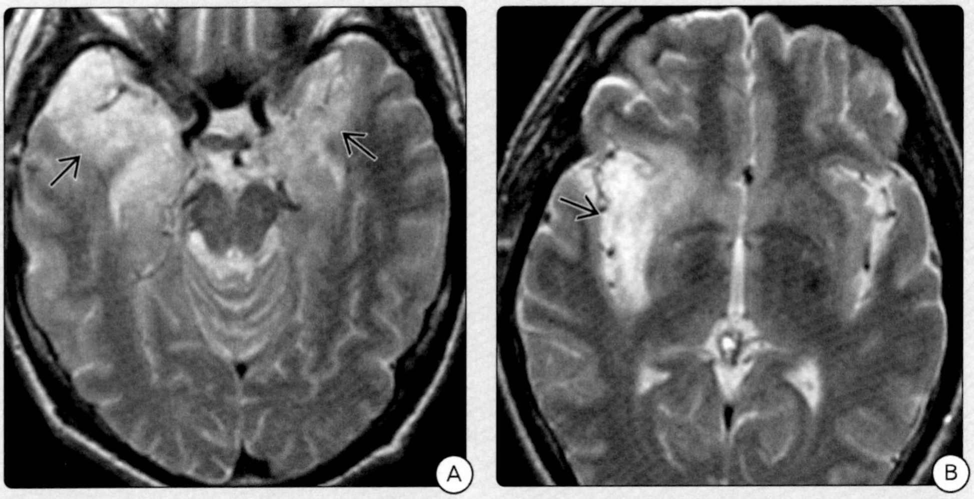

***(27-53A)** Axial T2WI in a 75y man with small cell lung cancer and paraneoplastic limbic encephalitis shows bilateral confluent hyperintensity in both anteromedial temporal lobes ⇒. **(27-53B)** More cephalad scan in the same patient shows that the right insular cortex and the extreme and external capsules are affected ⇒.*

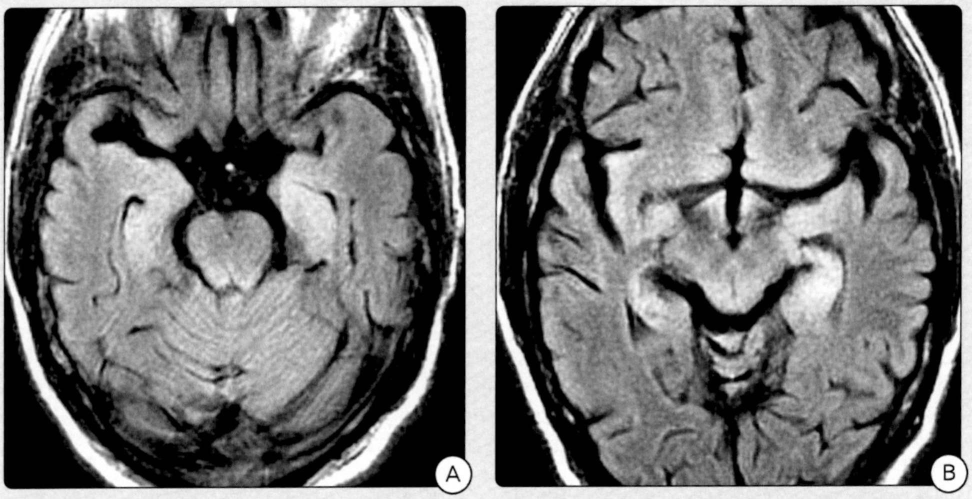

***(27-54A)** Axial FLAIR scan in a 67y man with documented voltage-gated potassium channel complex (VGKC) antibodies shows hyperintensity in both medial temporal lobes. **(27-54B)** More cephalad scan shows the extent of the hyperintensity, including involvement of the right insula.*

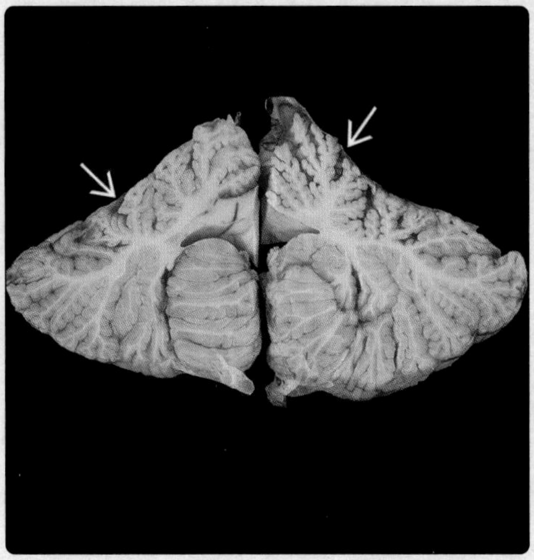

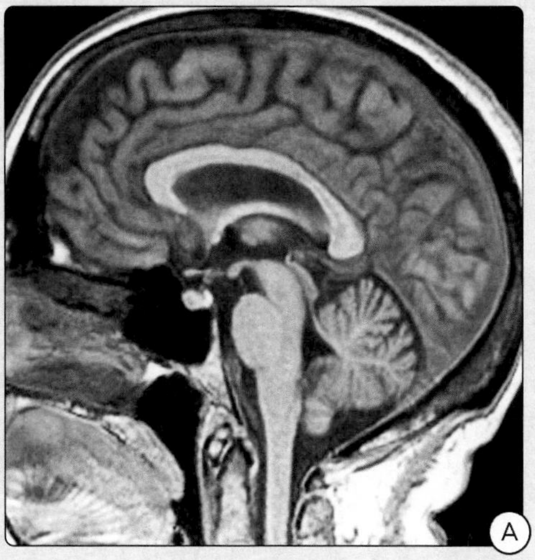

***(27-55)** Coronal autopsied case of paraneoplastic cerebellar degeneration in a patient with lung carcinoma shows cerebellar atrophy, seen here as shrunken folia and enlarged sulci ➔. (Courtesy R. Hewlett, MD.) **(27-56A)** Sagittal T1WI in a 53y woman with breast cancer and ataxia appears normal.*

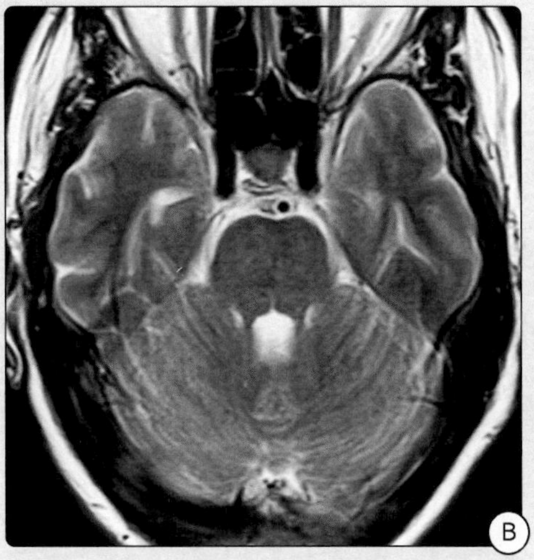

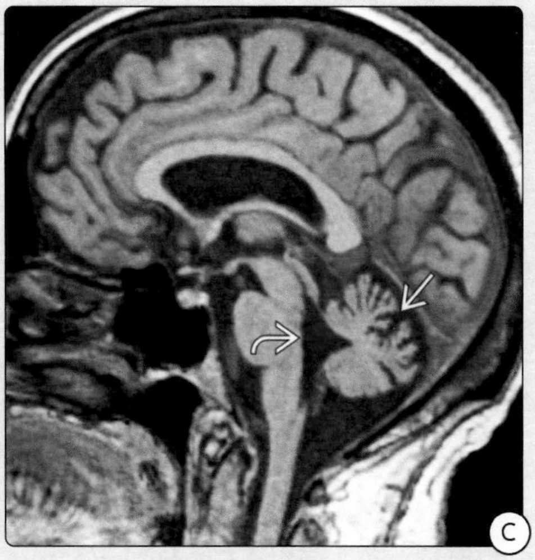

***(27-56B)** Axial T2WI in the same case appears normal. **(27-56C)** The patient's ataxia and cerebellar signs worsened. Sagittal MP-RAGE obtained 5 months later shows interval development of a markedly enlarged 4th ventricle ➔ and striking vermian atrophy ➔.*

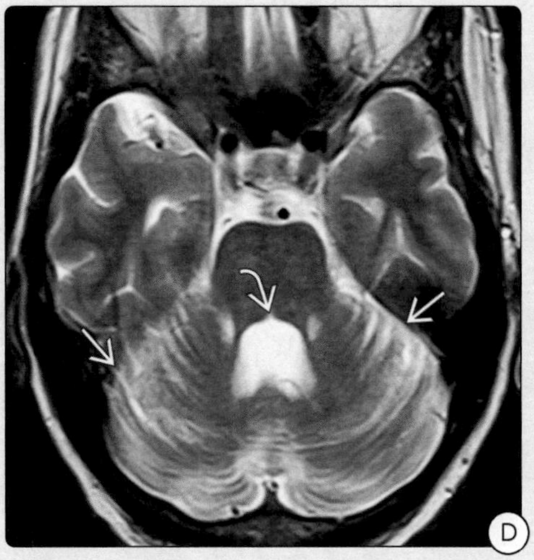

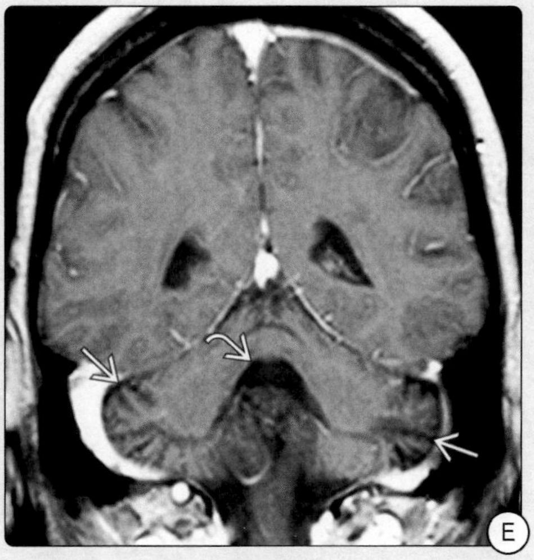

***(27-56D)** Axial T2WI shows the enlarged 4th ventricle ➔, shrunken cerebellar folia with enlarged sulci ➔. **(27-56E)** Coronal T1 C+ shows the enlarged 4th ventricle ➔ and shrunken cerebellar folia ➔. This is paraneoplastic cerebellar degeneration.*

Macroscopic abnormalities are generally minimal, most commonly enlargement of the cerebellar folia **(27-55)**. The microscopic hallmark of PCD is widespread severe loss of Purkinje cells with variable loss of granule cells. Inflammatory infiltrates are usually sparse or absent.

MR is normal ("remarkably unremarkable") in most patients. Some cases demonstrate transient cerebellar enlargement with focal or diffuse hyperintensity on FLAIR. Subacute or chronic PCD shows mild to moderate generalized cerebellar atrophy on MR **(27-56)** and hypometabolism on PET.

Stiff-Person Syndrome

Stiff-person syndrome (SPS), previously known as stiff-man syndrome, is a disorder characterized by fluctuating muscle rigidity and painful spasms. SPS is a reported paraneoplastic neurologic manifestation of breast cancer, especially invasive ductal carcinoma. About 90% of cases are associated with glutamic acid decarboxylase (anti-GAD) antibodies, an autoantibody that is also often seen in type 1 diabetes mellitus. Less commonly, paraneoplastic SPS is associated with anti-amphiphysin antibodies. The target antigen for anti-amphiphysin is a 128-kDa brain protein found at synapses.

Few imaging findings in SPS have been published. MR is usually normal although T2/FLAIR hyperintensity in the medial temporal lobe and F-FDG-PET uptake in the medial temporal lobes have been reported in patients with SPS and those with symptoms of paraneoplastic limbic encephalitis.

Paraneoplastic Opsoclonus-Myoclonus Syndrome

Paraneoplastic opsoclonus-myoclonus syndrome (OMS) is usually seen in children with neuroblastoma, less commonly in adults with breast or small-cell lung cancer. It is usually associated with anti-Ri antibodies that cross react with two antigens, Nova-1 and Nova-2, that are widely expressed in the CNS.

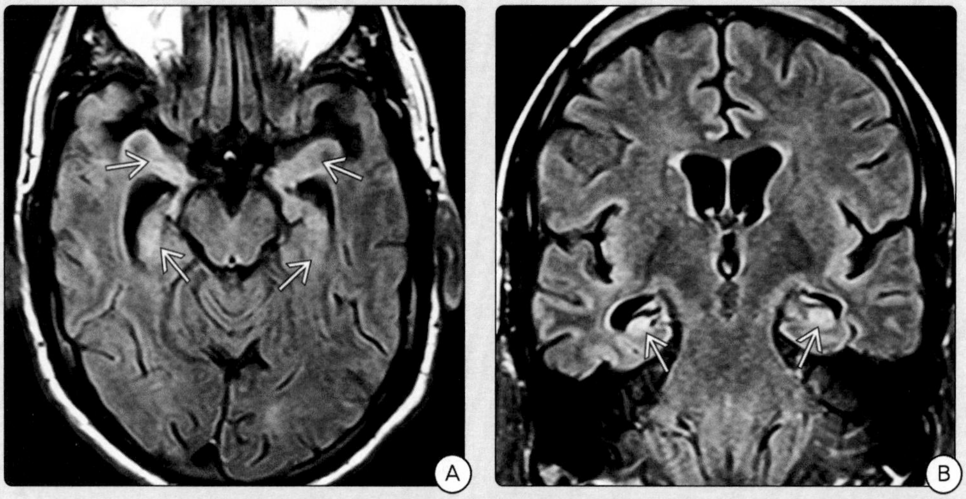

***(27-57A)** Axial FLAIR scan in a 32y man with a 6-month history of progressive dementia shows enlarged sylvian fissures, prominent temporal horns, and striking volume loss in both hippocampi. Bilaterally symmetric uncal-hippocampal hyperintensity is present ➡. **(27-57B)** Coronal FLAIR scan shows generalized supratentorial volume loss with symmetric hippocampal hyperintensity ➡.*

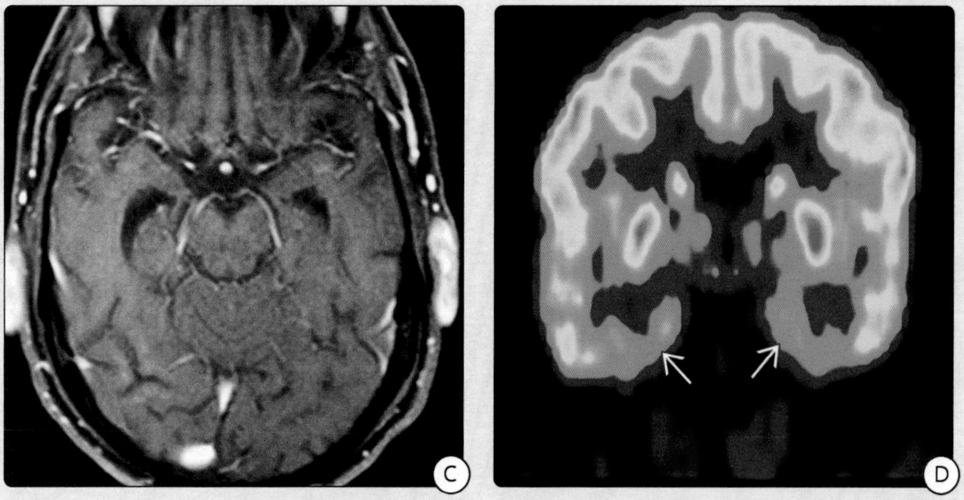

***(27-57C)** T1 C+ FS scan shows no evidence of enhancement. **(27-57D)** Coronal FDG PET scan shows strikingly reduced uptake in both medial temporal lobes ➡. Imaging diagnosis was paraneoplastic limbic encephalitis. Extensive evaluation for systemic neoplasm and infectious pathogens was negative. Final diagnosis was seronegative autoimmune limbic encephalitis (SNALE).*

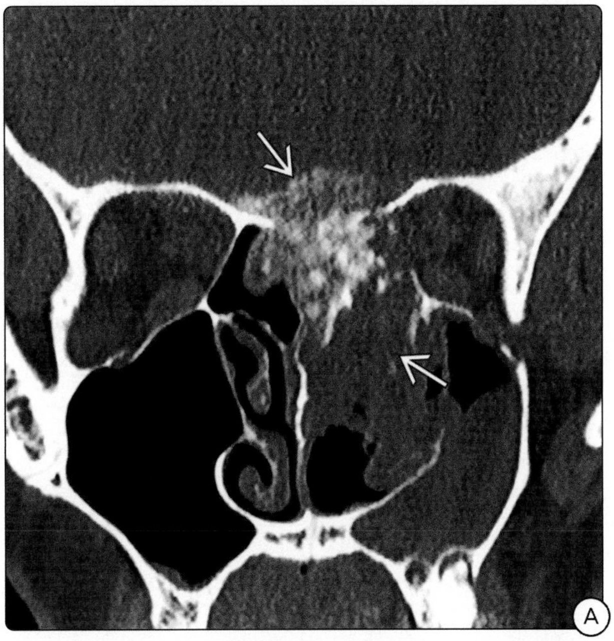

(27-58A) Coronal bone CT in a 36y woman with tumor-induced osteomalacia caused by a malignant phosphaturic mesenchymal tumor of the skull base shows the partially calcified destructive lesion of the sphenoethmoidal complex ➡.

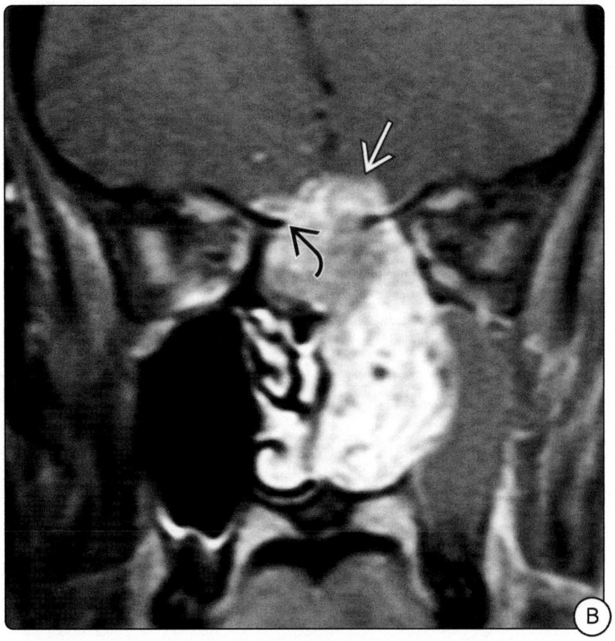

(27-58B) Coronal T1 C+ FS shows that the lesion erodes the planum sphenoidale ⇨ and extends intracranially ➡. Final histopathologic diagnosis was malignant solitary fibrous tumor causing TIO.

OMS is characterized by rapid involuntary conjugate eye movements (opsoclonus) and brief, involuntary muscle twitching (myoclonus) with or without ataxia, aphasia, strabismus, or mutism.

VGKC-Associated Encephalitis

Only 25-30% of patients with antibodies against VGKC-associated proteins such as LGI1 and Caspr2 have remote solid organ or hematologic malignancy, primarily small cell lung cancer and thymoma. Imaging findings are nonspecific and include T2/FLAIR hyperintensity in the limbic system and/or basal ganglia **(27-54)**. Reported cases of PET/CT show intense symmetrical uptake in the basal ganglia.

Lobar Extralimbic and Seronegative Autoimmune Paraneoplastic Encephalopathies

Lobar extralimbic paraneoplastic encephalopathies and seronegative autoimmune limbic encephalitis have received less attention than the more classic PLE and PCD syndromes. In these syndromes, exhaustive searches for infectious pathogens and autoantibodies are negative.

Imaging findings are similar to those of herpes encephalitis and paraneoplastic limbic encephalitis with uncal-hippocampal T2/FLAIR hyperintensity and hypometabolism on PET **(27-57)**. Some reported cases can resemble glioma with a focal mass-like enhancing lesion.

Oncogenic Osteomalacia

Oncogenic osteomalacia, also called tumor-induced osteomalacia (TIO), is an uncommon acquired paraneoplastic syndrome. It usually affects the limbs or axial skeleton but occasionally involves the skull base. Tumors that cause TIO are **phosphaturic mesenchymal tumors** with mixed connective tissue that secrete fibroblast growth factor 23 (FGF-23). **Hemangiopericytoma** (malignant solitary fibrous tumor) causes approximately 70-80% of TIO cases **(27-58)**.

IMAGING OF MAJOR PARANEOPLASTIC NEUROLOGICAL DISORDERS

Paraneoplastic Encephalomyelitis
- Limbic encephalitis most common form
- T2/FLAIR hyperintensity in one or both medial temporal lobes
- No enhancement on T1 C+

Paraneoplastic Cerebellar Degeneration
- Usually normal
- Subacute/chronic may show cerebellar atrophy

Stiff-Person Syndrome
- Usually normal
- SPS with limbic encephalitis may exhibit T2/FLAIR hyperintensity in medial temporal lobes
- F-FDG-PET may show hypermetabolism in medial temporal lobes

Voltage-Gated Potassium Channel-Complex Disorders
- Only 25% associated with systemic malignancy
- T2/FLAIR hyperintensity in medial temporal lobes, basal ganglia
- PET/CT intense uptake in basal ganglia

Selected References

Metastatic Lesions

Overview

Bekaert L et al: Histopathologic diagnosis of brain metastases: current trends in management and future considerations. Brain Tumor Pathol. 34(1):8-19, 2017

Dagogo-Jack I et al: Treatment of brain metastases in the modern genomic era. Pharmacol Ther. 170:64-72, 2017

Lowery FJ et al: Brain metastasis: unique challenges and open opportunities. Biochim Biophys Acta. 1867(1):49-57, 2017

Mostofa AG et al: The process and regulatory components of inflammation in brain oncogenesis. Biomolecules. 7(2), 2017

Schrijver WA et al: Unravelling site-specific breast cancer metastasis: a microRNA expression profiling study. Oncotarget. 8(2):3111-3123, 2017

Spreafico F et al: Proteomic analysis of cerebrospinal fluid from children with central nervous system tumors identifies candidate proteins relating to tumor metastatic spread. Oncotarget. ePub, 2017

D'Souza NM et al: Combining radiation therapy with immune checkpoint blockade for central nervous system malignancies. Front Oncol. 6:212, 2016

Wesseling P et al: Metastatic tumours of the CNS. In: Louis DN et al (eds), WHO Classification of Tumours of the Central Nervous System. Lyon, France: International Agency for Research on Cancer, 2016, pp 338-341, 2016

Lin NU et al: Response assessment criteria for brain metastases: proposal from the RANO group. Lancet Oncol. 16(6):e270-8, 2015

Parenchymal Metastases

Balendran S et al: Next-generation sequencing-based genomic profiling of brain metastases of primary ovarian cancer identifies high number of BRCA-mutations. J Neurooncol. ePub, 2017

Bekaert L et al: Histopathologic diagnosis of brain metastases: current trends in management and future considerations. Brain Tumor Pathol. 34(1):8-19, 2017

Sandler KA et al: Treatment trends for patients with brain metastases: does practice reflect the data? Cancer. 123(12):2274-2282, 2017

Leptomeningeal Metastases

Boire A et al: Complement component 3 adapts the cerebrospinal fluid for leptomeningeal metastasis. Cell. 168(6):1101-1113.e13, 2017

Le Rhun E et al: Neoplastic meningitis due to lung, breast, and melanoma metastases. Cancer Control. 24(1):22-32, 2017

Hyun JW et al: Leptomeningeal metastasis: clinical experience of 519 cases. Eur J Cancer. 56:107-14, 2016

Smalley KS et al: Managing leptomeningeal melanoma metastases in the era of immune and targeted therapy. Int J Cancer. 139(6):1195-201, 2016

Miscellaneous Metastases

Chen H et al: A rare case of small cell carcinoma of lung with intraventricular metastasis. Br J Neurosurg. 1-3, 2017

Konstantinidis L et al: Intraocular metastases--a review. Asia Pac J Ophthalmol (Phila). 6(2):208-214, 2017

Sánchez Orgaz M et al: Orbital and conjunctival metastasis from lobular breast carcinoma. Orbit. 1-4, 2017

Wendel C et al: Pituitary metastasis from renal cell carcinoma: description of a case report. Am J Case Rep. 18:7-11, 2017

Direct Geographic Spread From Head and Neck Neoplasms

Dundar Y et al: Skull base invasion patterns and survival outcomes of nonmelanoma skin cancers. J Neurol Surg B Skull Base. 78(2):164-172, 2017

Tashi S et al: The pterygopalatine fossa: imaging anatomy, communications, and pathology revisited. Insights Imaging. 7(4):589-99, 2016

Perineural Metastases

Badger D et al: Imaging of perineural spread in head and neck cancer. Radiol Clin North Am. 55(1):139-149, 2017

Barrera-Flores FJ et al: Perineural spread-susceptible structures: a non-pathological evaluation of the skull base. Eur Arch Otorhinolaryngol. 274(7):2899-2905, 2017

Moghimi M et al: Perineural pseudoinvasion: an unusual phenomenon in nonmalignancies. Adv Anat Pathol. 24(2):88-98, 2017

Panizza BJ: An overview of head and neck malignancy with perineural spread. J Neurol Surg B Skull Base. 77(2):81-5, 2016

Paraneoplastic Syndromes

Kelley BP et al: Autoimmune encephalitis: pathophysiology and imaging review of an overlooked diagnosis. AJNR Am J Neuroradiol. 38(6):1070-1078, 2017

Mauermann ML: Neurologic complications of lymphoma, leukemia, and paraproteinemias. Continuum (Minneap Minn). 23(3, Neurology of Systemic Disease):669-690, 2017

Sundermann B et al: Imaging workup of suspected classical paraneoplastic neurological syndromes: a systematic review and retrospective analysis of 18F-FDG-PET-CT. Acad Radiol. ePub, 2017

Fanous I et al: Paraneoplastic neurological complications of breast cancer. Exp Hematol Oncol. 5:29, 2016

Paraneoplastic Encephalitis/Encephalomyelitis

Fanous I et al: Paraneoplastic neurological complications of breast cancer. Exp Hematol Oncol. 5:29, 2016

Masangkay N et al: Brain 18F-FDG-PET characteristics in patients with paraneoplastic neurological syndrome and its correlation with clinical and MRI findings. Nucl Med Commun. 35(10):1038-46, 2014

Miscellaneous Paraneoplastic Syndromes

Martinez-Hernandez E et al: Clinical and immunologic investigations in patients with stiff-person spectrum disorder. JAMA Neurol. 73(6):714-20, 2016

van Sonderen A et al: From VGKC to LGI1 and Caspr2 encephalitis: the evolution of a disease entity over time. Autoimmun Rev. 15(10):970-4, 2016

Nonneoplastic Cysts

There are many types of intracranial cysts. Some are incidental and of no significance. Others may cause serious—even life-threatening—symptoms.

In this chapter, we consider a number of different intracranial cysts: cystic-appearing anatomic variants that can be mistaken for disease, congenital/developmental cysts, and a variety of miscellaneous cysts. We exclude parasitic cysts, cystic brain malformations, and cystic neoplasms, as they are discussed in their respective chapters.

The etiology, pathology, and clinical significance of nonneoplastic intracranial cysts are so varied that classifying them presents a significant challenge.

In a schema based on *etiology*, cysts are classified as normal anatomic variants (e.g., enlarged perivascular spaces), congenital lesions derived from embryonic ecto- or endoderm (colloid and neurenteric cysts), developmental inclusion cysts (e.g., dermoid and epidermoid cysts), and miscellaneous cysts that don't easily fit into any particular category (such as choroid plexus and tumor-associated cysts). Etiology is interesting but unhelpful in establishing an imaging-based diagnosis.

Categorizing cysts by the *histologic* characteristics of their walls—as is traditional in neuropathology texts—is again of little help when faced with the challenge of providing an appropriate differential diagnosis based on imaging findings alone.

An *imaging-based* approach to the classification of intracranial cysts is much more practical, as most intracranial cysts are discovered on CT or MR examination. This approach takes into account three easily defined features: (1) anatomic location, (2) imaging characteristics (i.e., density/signal intensity of the contents, presence/absence of calcification and/or enhancement), and (3) patient age. Of these three, anatomic location is the most helpful **(Table 28-1)**.

While many types of intracranial cysts occur in more than one anatomic location, some sites are "preferred" by certain cysts. In this chapter, we discuss cysts from the outside in, beginning with scalp and intracranial extraaxial cysts before turning our attention to parenchymal and intraventricular cysts.

There are four key anatomy-based questions to consider about a cystic-appearing intracranial lesion (see below). A summary chart based on these simple questions, together with the cysts discussed throughout the text, is included on the next page **(Table 28-1)**.

Intracranial Cystic-Appearing Lesions

	Supratentorial	Infratentorial
Extraaxial		
Midline	Pineal cyst Dermoid cyst Rathke cleft cyst Arachnoid cyst (suprasellar)	Neurenteric cyst Arachnoid cyst (retrocerebellar)
Off-midline	Arachnoid cyst (middle cranial fossa, convexity) Epidermoid cyst Tumor-associated cyst Trichilemmal ("sebaceous") cyst (scalp) Leptomeningeal cyst ("growing fracture")	Epidermoid cyst (CPA) Arachnoid cyst (CPA) Tumor-associated cyst
Intraaxial		
Parenchymal	Enlarged perivascular spaces Neuroglial cyst Porencephalic cyst Hippocampal sulcus remnants	Enlarged perivascular spaces (dentate nuclei)
Intraventricular	Choroid plexus cyst Colloid cyst Choroid fissure cyst Ependymal cyst	Epidermoid cyst (fourth ventricle, cisterna magna) Cystic ("trapped") fourth ventricle

(Table 28-1) *CPA = cerebellopontine angle. Leptomeningeal cyst, Rathke cleft cyst, and cystic/trapped fourth ventricle are discussed in chapters 2, 25, and 34, respectively. All the other entities listed in the table are considered here.*

FOUR KEY ANATOMY-BASED QUESTIONS

- Is the cyst extra- or intraaxial?
- Is the cyst supra- or infratentorial?
- If the cyst is extraaxial, is it midline or off-midline?
- If the cyst is intraaxial, is it in the brain parenchyma or inside the ventricles?

Scalp Cysts

Overview

A number of benign cutaneous cysts can present as scalp lesions. Most are not deliberately imaged, as the scalp is easily accessible to both visual and manual inspection. Nevertheless, scalp masses are not uncommonly identified on imaging studies intended to visualize intracranial structures. Imaging also becomes important when a scalp lesion is clinically felt to be potentially malignant, has a vascular component, or might be in anatomic continuity with intracranial contents.

Age is helpful in the differential diagnosis of nontraumatic scalp masses. In adults, the differential diagnosis includes skin carcinomas (basal and squamous cell), dermoid and epidermoid cysts, hemangiomas, and metastases. Trichilemmal ("sebaceous") cysts are common scalp masses in middle-aged and older patients.

The most common scalp mass in children is Langerhans cell histiocytosis, followed by epidermoid and dermoid cysts, scalp hemangiomas, and neurofibromas. Less common but important scalp lesions in children include cephalocele and sinus pericranii.

The three statistically most common scalp cysts are epidermoid cyst (50%), trichilemmal cysts (25-30%), and dermoid cysts (20-25%). Epidermoid and dermoid cysts are discussed later in the chapter. We discuss trichilemmal (pilar or "sebaceous") cysts of the scalp here.

Trichilemmal ("Sebaceous") Cyst

Terminology

Although the term "sebaceous cyst" is commonly used by radiologists, this type of cyst does not actually contain sebaceous material. Such cysts are more accurately called trichilemmal cysts (TCs). Rarely, TCs enlarge and proliferate. Proliferating TCs are known as pilar ("turban") tumors. Malignant TCs are referred to as "proliferating trichilemmal cystic carcinoma."

Etiology

TCs are derived from the outer root sheath of hair follicles, not sebaceous glands.

Pathology

As only 0.3% of sebaceous cysts sent for pathologic examination are malignant, routine pathologic evaluation of sebaceous cysts is now considered necessary only when clinical suspicion of malignancy exists. In such cases, the most common neoplasm is squamous cell carcinoma.

Location, Size, and Number. Most TCs are found within the dermis or subcutaneous tissue. They can be single or multiple and vary from a few millimeters to several centimeters.

Gross and Microscopic Features. TCs are characterized by a fibrous capsule lined by stratified squamous epithelium. The cyst contents consist primarily of waxy desquamated keratin. Lobules of squamous epithelium in the cyst wall suggest a proliferating TC.

Clinical Issues

Epidemiology and Demographics. TCs affect 5-10% of the population. Although they can occur at any age, most occur in elderly women.

Presentation and Natural History. TCs generally appear as hairless, mobile, slightly compressible, subcutaneous scalp masses.

TCs grow slowly and have often been present for years. Rarely, they become locally aggressive and may even invade bone. Malignant degeneration with distant metastasis is rare.

Treatment Options. Surgical excision is the major treatment. Incomplete excision may result in recurrence.

Imaging

General Features. These scalp masses are generally large, well-delineated, round or ovoid, but somewhat complex-appearing lesions.

CT Findings. TCs are sharply delineated solid, cystic, or mixed solid-cystic masses that are hyperdense compared with subcutaneous fat. Calcification is common and may be seen in punctate, curvilinear, or coarse forms **(28-1A)**. Sometimes calcifications layer in the dependent portion of larger cysts. Typical TCs do not enhance, nor do they remodel or invade the underlying calvaria.

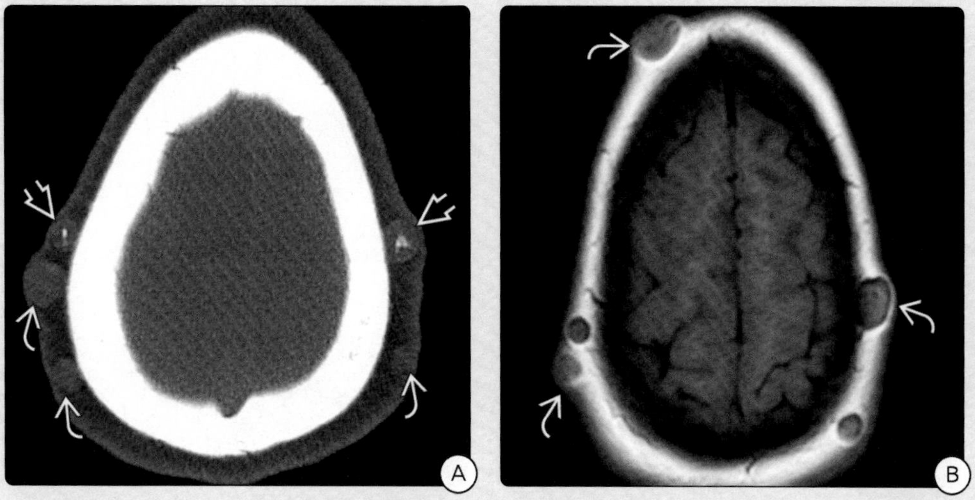

***(28-1A)** NECT with bone window in a patient being imaged for acute stroke shows incidental finding of five trichilemmal cysts. Two contain calcifications ➡, whereas the other three ➡ do not. The underlying skull is normal. **(28-1B)** Axial T1WI in the same case shows that the well-delineated scalp cysts ➡ are isointense with brain.*

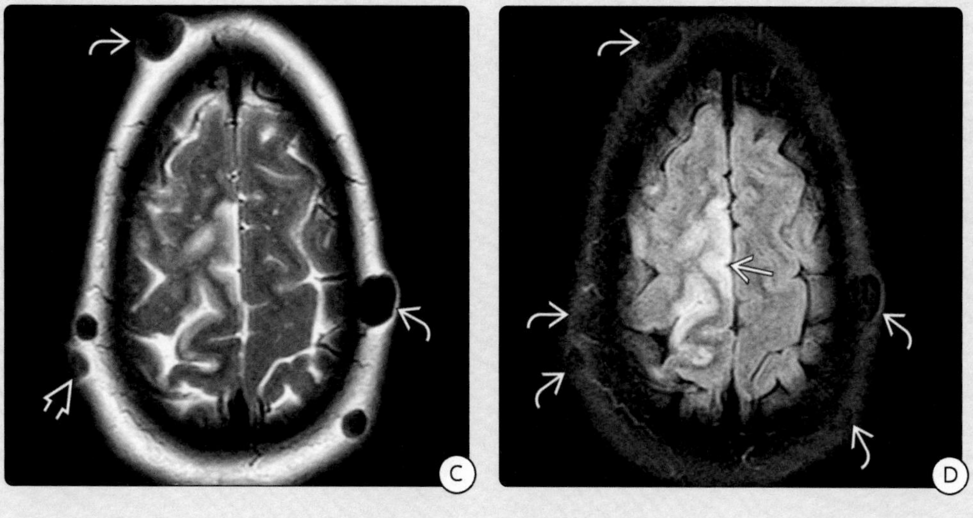

***(28-1C)** Most of the larger cysts appear quite hypointense ➡ on T2WI. One of the smaller cysts is heterogeneously hypointense ➡. **(28-1D)** The cysts are hypointense ➡ compared with brain on FLAIR. The patient's acute infarct is seen as cortical hyperintensity ➡.*

MR Findings. TCs are well-circumscribed scalp masses that appear incompletely surrounded by fat **(28-1B)**. They are generally isointense with brain and muscle on T1WI and inhomogeneously hypointense on T2WI **(28-1C)**.

TCs do not suppress on FLAIR **(28-1D)**. "Blooming" foci on T2* (GRE, SWI) are caused by calcifications, not hemorrhage.

Simple uncomplicated TCs do not enhance, although the proliferating variant may show significant enhancement with solid lobules interspersed with nonenhancing cystic foci.

Differential Diagnosis

In adults, the imaging differential diagnoses are benign and malignant scalp tumors. **Basal cell carcinomas** and **scalp metastases** are ill-defined, poorly delineated scalp masses that invade the subcutaneous soft tissues and may erode bone. Superficial ulceration is common. **Dermoid** and **epidermoid cysts** as well as **hemangiomas** are all much more common in the skull than in the scalp.

TCs are rare in children. In this age group, the most important lesions to differentiate from benign scalp cysts (usually dermoids/epidermoids, not TCs) are congenital brain malformations that protrude through skull defects and present as subcutaneous masses.

Cephaloceles contain variable combinations of brain/meninges/vessels. They vary in size from very large to small lesions ("atretic cephalocele").

Sinus pericranii is a compressible, bluish-tinged scalp mass that communicates with the intracranial venous system through a skull defect.

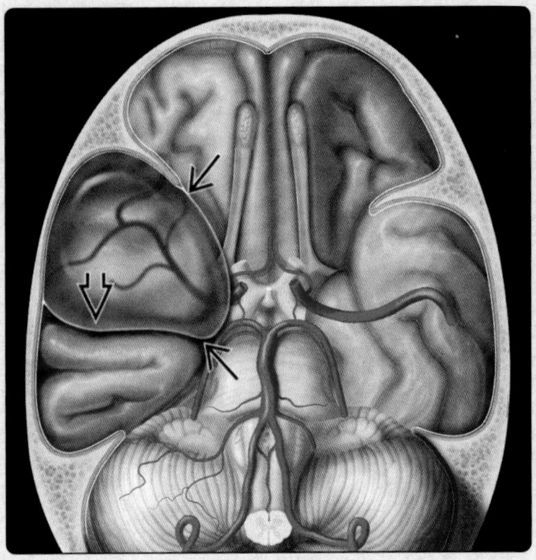

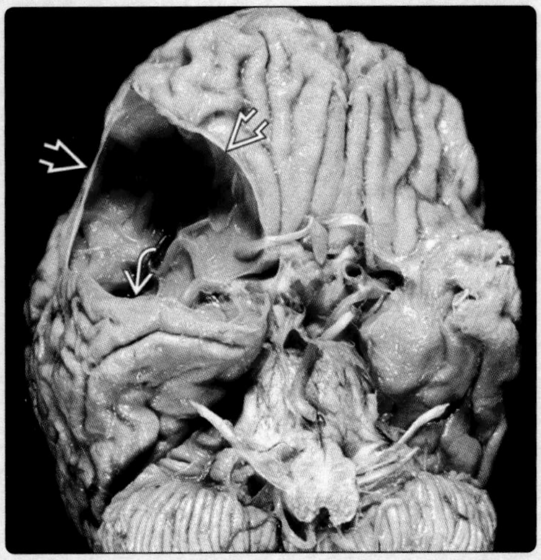

***(28-2)** Graphic depicts a middle cranial fossa arachnoid cyst. The arachnoid ⇒ splits and encloses CSF, the middle fossa is expanded, and the overlying bone is thinned. Note that the temporal lobe ⇒ is displaced posteriorly. **(28-3)** Autopsy specimen shows a classic middle fossa arachnoid cyst between layers of "duplicated" arachnoid ➡. The temporal lobe ➡ is displaced and hypoplastic. (Courtesy J. Townsend, MD.)*

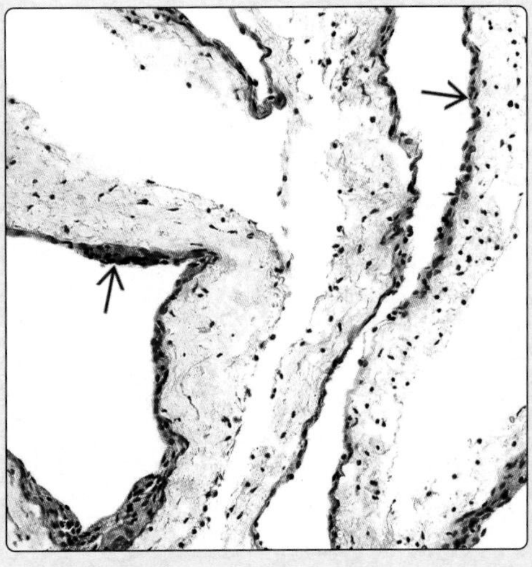

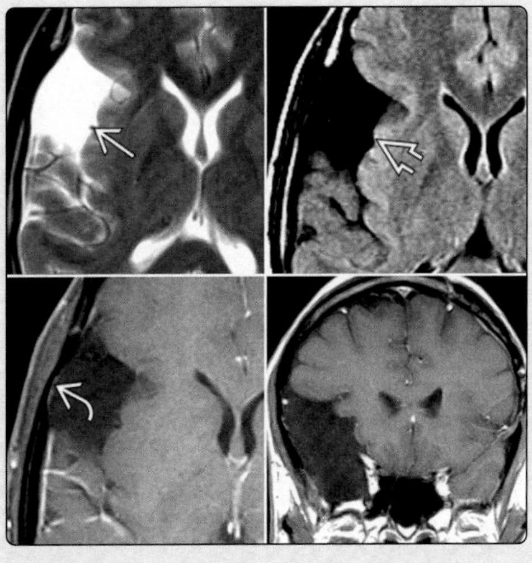

***(28-4)** An arachnoid cyst is lined by a single layer of mature arachnoid cells ⇒ under a delicate fibrous membrane. (Courtesy P. Burger, MD.) **(28-5)** Arachnoid cysts often have scalloped margins and are CSF-like on T2WI ➡. They suppress on FLAIR ➡, remodel the skull ➡, and do not enhance.*

Extraaxial Cysts

Extraaxial cysts are between the skull and brain. With few exceptions, most lie within the arachnoid membrane or in the subarachnoid space.

Determining sublocation of an extraaxial cyst (supra- vs. infratentorial, midline vs. off-midline) is helpful in establishing a meaningful differential diagnosis **(Table 28-1)**. For example, an arachnoid cyst is the only type that commonly occurs in the posterior fossa. Some extraaxial cysts are usually (although not invariably) off-midline. Others—pineal and Rathke cleft cysts—occur only in the midline.

We begin our discussion of extraaxial cysts with the most common type, arachnoid cyst.

Arachnoid Cyst

Although arachnoid cysts (ACs) occur throughout the neuraxis, the vast majority are intracranial.

Terminology

An AC, also known as a meningeal cyst, is a CSF-containing cyst lined by a layer of flattened arachnoid cells.

Etiology

General Concepts. The vast majority of ACs arise as anomalies of meningeal development. The embryonic endomeninges fail to merge and remain separated, forming a "duplicated" arachnoid. CSF is secreted by cells in the cyst wall and accumulates between the layers.

Less commonly, arachnoid loculations are acquired as a result of hemorrhage, infection, or surgery. Arachnoid-like cysts also

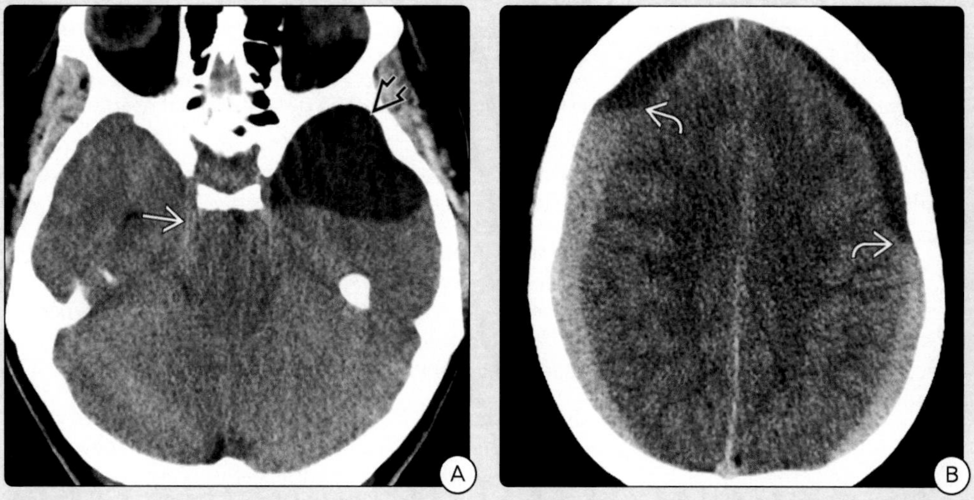

***(28-6A)** NECT in a 59y woman with severe headaches and confusion shows a CSF-density mass in the left middle cranial fossa ➲. Note "tight" appearance of brain, with basilar cistern effacement and midbrain compression ➲. **(28-6B)** More cephalad NECT in the same case shows mixed-density acute-on-chronic bilateral subdural hematomas (SDHs) ➲.*

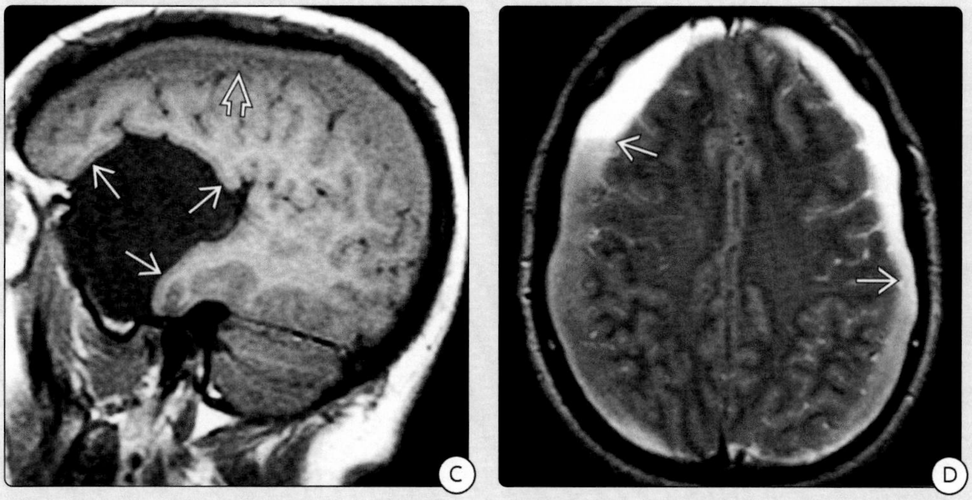

***(28-6C)** Sagittal T1WI in the same case shows the middle fossa arachnoid cyst displacing the temporal lobe cortex around it ➲. Note isointense SDH ➲. **(28-6D)** Axial T2WI shows the mixed-age SDHs with fluid-fluid levels ➲ between the chronic SDH above and the more acute component below. This is arachnoid cyst with associated bilateral SDHs.*

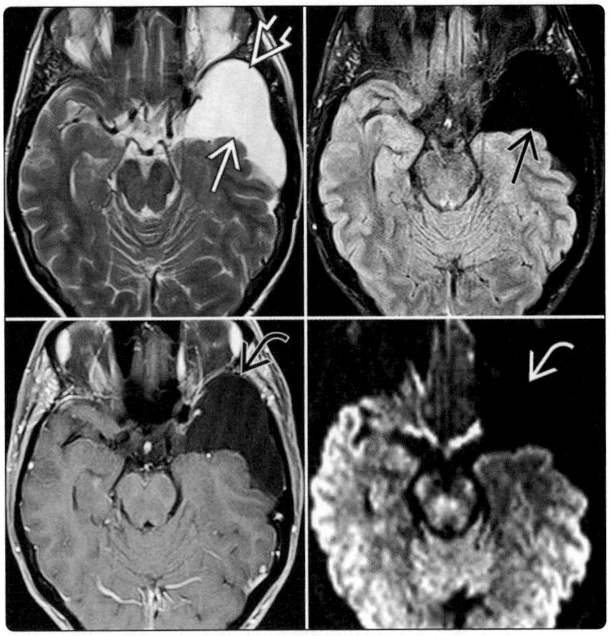

(28-7) T2WI (upper L) shows large AC ➡ that expands middle cranial fossa ➡, suppresses completely on FLAIR ➡ (upper R), does not enhance ➡ (lower L), and does not exhibit restricted diffusion ➡ (lower R). This is incidental finding in a 53y woman.

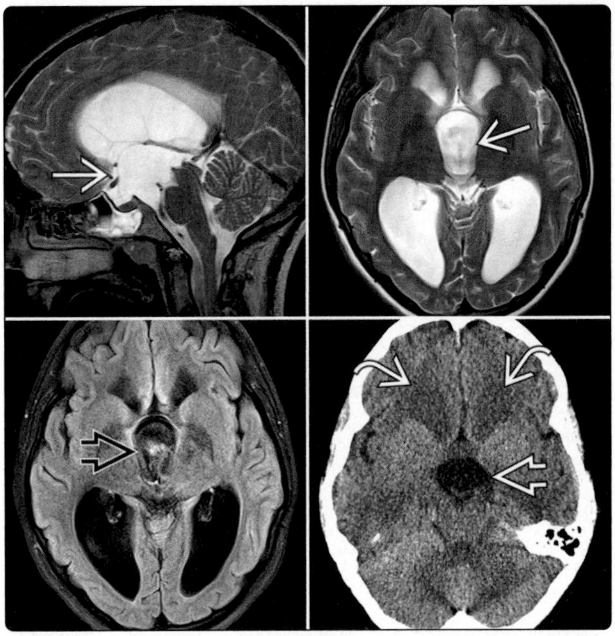

(28-8) Large CSF-filled suprasellar AC is shown on T2WI ➡. CSF pulsations in cyst do not suppress completely on FLAIR ➡. CT cisternogram shows dilute contrast in the lateral ventricles ➡, while the noncommunicating cyst ➡ does not opacify.

sometimes arise adjacent to extraaxial tumors such as meningiomas, schwannomas, and pituitary macroadenomas. These benign fluid-containing tumor-associated cysts are discussed separately.

There is a relationship between subdural hematomas (SDHs) and ACs although whether this is causative or coincidental is unclear. Traumatic SDHs can rupture into ACs. The converse—AC rupture causing a spontaneous SDH—occurs but is rare.

Genetics. Most ACs are sporadic and nonsyndromic. Syndromic ACs have been reported in association with acrocallosal, Aicardi, and Pallister-Hall syndromes.

Pathology

Location. Most ACs are supratentorial. They are usually off-midline and are the most common off-midline extraaxial supratentorial cyst **(28-2)**.

Nearly two-thirds are found in the middle cranial fossa, anteromedial to the temporal lobe **(28-3)**. Fifteen percent of ACs are found over the cerebral convexities, predominantly over the frontal lobes.

Midline ACs are relatively rare in the supratentorial compartment. The most frequent supratentorial midline location for ACs is the suprasellar cistern, followed by the quadrigeminal cistern and velum interpositum. Interhemispheric fissure ACs are typically associated with callosal anomalies.

Between 10-15% of ACs are found in the posterior fossa. The most common location is the cerebellopontine angle cistern, where ACs are the second most common cystic-appearing extraaxial mass (after epidermoid). The next most frequent site is retrocerebellar.

Size and Number. ACs vary in size, ranging from small incidental cysts to large space-occupying lesions. ACs are almost always solitary. Multiple meningeal cysts have been reported but are probably acquired, resulting from undetected meningitis.

Gross Pathology. ACs are well-marginated cysts filled with clear colorless fluid that resembles CSF. They are devoid of internal septations and are completely encased by a delicate translucent membrane.

Microscopic Features. ACs consist of a delicate fibrous membrane lined by a single layer of mature, histologically normal arachnoid cells **(28-4)**. Small inflammatory infiltrates occur but are rare.

ARACHNOID CYST: PATHOLOGY

Location
- Supratentorial (90%)
  - Middle fossa (67%)
  - Convexities (15%)
  - Other (5-10%): suprasellar, quadrigeminal cisterns
- Infratentorial (10-12%)
  - Mostly CPA cistern (second most common cystic CPA mass)
  - Less common = cisterna magna

Gross Pathology
- Thin translucent cyst wall bulging with clear fluid
- Lined by mature arachnoid cells

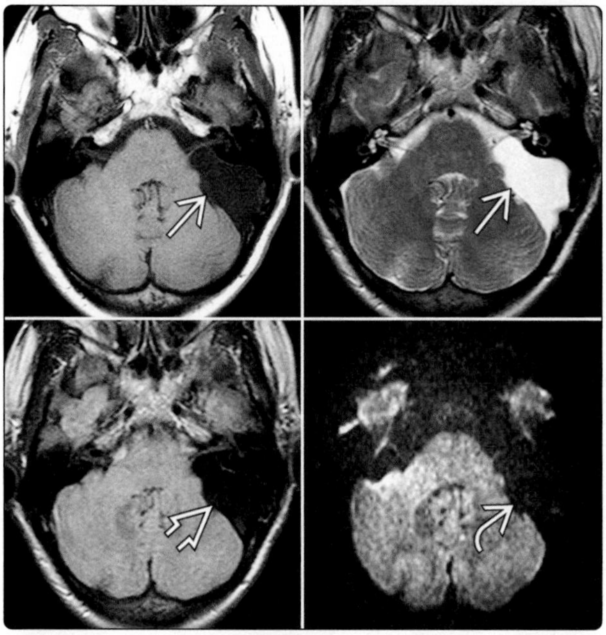

(28-9) *Left cerebellopontine angle arachnoid cyst is isointense with CSF on T1WI and T2WI ➡ and suppresses completely on FLAIR ➡. No diffusion restriction is seen on DWI ➡.*

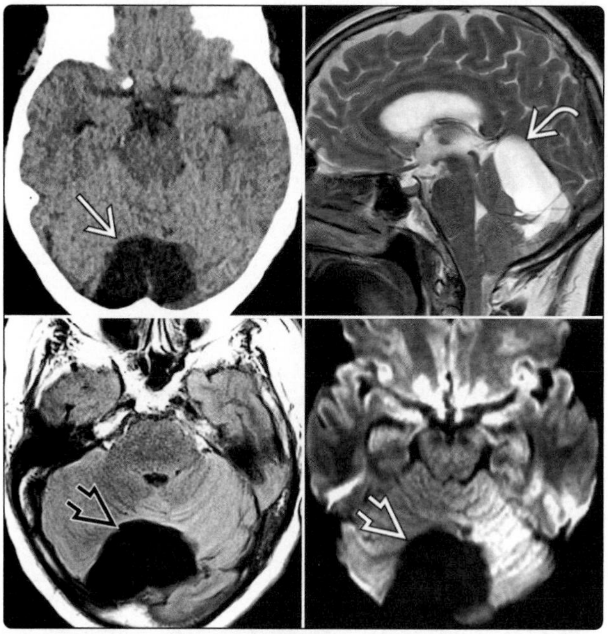

(28-10) *Large midline posterior fossa AC is isodense with CSF on NECT ➡. The unilocular AC ➡ compresses and displaces vermis and brainstem anteriorly. The cyst suppresses completely on FLAIR ➡ and does not restrict on DWI ➡.*

Clinical Issues

Epidemiology. ACs are the most common of all congenital intracranial cysts. They account for approximately 1% of all space-occupying intracranial lesions and are identified on imaging studies in 1-2% of patients.

Demographics. ACs can be seen at any age. Most (nearly 75%) are found in children and young adults. There is no sex difference.

Presentation. Most ACs are asymptomatic and found incidentally. Symptoms vary with size and location. Headaches are common in symptomatic ACs.

Some suprasellar ACs become very large and cause obstructive hydrocephalus.

Natural History. ACs are not associated with increased mortality. Most incidentally discovered ACs remain stable over many years. Enlargement—if any—is very gradual. Enlargement is strongly associated with younger age and rarely occurs in children older than 4 years at the time of initial diagnosis.

Hemorrhage—either traumatic or spontaneous—into an intracranial AC is rare but may cause sudden enlargement. The presence of an AC increases shear force on impact and may be a risk factor for intracystic bleeding. Recent studies have shown no significant role of location or shape of ACs on hemorrhage risk.

Treatment Options. Asymptomatic ACs are usually "leave me alone" lesions. Surgical options for symptomatic ACs include endoscopic resection or fenestration, open fenestration/marsupialization, or cystoperitoneal shunting with a programmable valve. Following shunting, 60% of ACs disappear completely; in half of these patients, it is possible to remove the shunt without shunt dependence.

Imaging

General Features. Uncomplicated ACs behave *exactly* like CSF on CT and MR **(28-5)**. FLAIR and DWI are the best sequences to distinguish cystic-appearing intracranial masses from one another.

CT Findings. Uncomplicated ACs are CSF density **(28-6A)**. If intracystic hemorrhage has occurred, the cyst fluid may be moderately hyperdense compared with CSF **(28-6B)**. Large middle cranial fossa ACs expand the fossa and cause temporal lobe hypoplasia or displacement **(28-6A)**.

With moderately large ACs, bone CT may show pressure remodeling of the adjacent calvaria. ACs do not cause frank bone invasion.

ACs do not enhance. Installation of intrathecal contrast ("CT cisternography") may be helpful in demonstrating communication with the subarachnoid space (SAS) **(28-8)**. Most symptomatic ACs do not demonstrate direct, free communication with the SAS and may require microsurgical decompression. Patients with completely communicating ACs may not need surgical intervention.

MR Findings. ACs are sharply marginated, somewhat scalloped-appearing lesions that parallel CSF signal intensity on all sequences. They are therefore isointense with CSF on T1- and T2-weighted images **(28-9)**. ACs cause moderate focal mass effect, displacing but not engulfing adjacent brain, vessels, and cranial nerves.

The internal appearance of an AC is intrinsically featureless, containing neither septations nor vessels.

ACs suppress completely with FLAIR **(28-10)**. Occasionally, CSF pulsations within large lesions may cause spin dephasing, producing heterogeneous signal intensity and significant propagation of phase artifact across the scan **(28-8)**.

ACs do not restrict on DWI and do not enhance. CSF flow imaging such as 2D cine PC may demonstrate communication between cyst and adjacent subarachnoid space.

Differential Diagnosis

The major differential diagnosis of AC is **epidermoid cyst** (EC). ECs are often almost—but not quite—exactly like CSF. They have a cauliflower-like, lobulated configuration instead of the sharply marginated borders of an AC. ECs engulf vessels and nerves, insinuating themselves along CSF cisterns. ECs do not suppress completely on FLAIR and typically show moderate to marked hyperintensity on DWI.

Enlarged subarachnoid spaces caused by brain volume loss are usually more diffuse CSF collections and do not cause mass effect on adjacent structures.

A **subdural hygroma** or **chronic subdural hematoma** (cSDH) is not precisely like CSF and is usually crescentic, not round or scalloped. cSDHs usually show evidence of prior hemorrhage, especially on T2* sequences, and may have enhancing encasing membranes.

A **porencephalic cyst** looks just like CSF, but it is intraaxial and lined by gliotic white matter that is often hyperintense on FLAIR. Rarely, **neurenteric cysts** can resemble ACs although they are usually hyperintense compared with CSF. Supratentorial neurenteric cysts are rare.

(28-11A) Axial T1WI in a 47y woman with right trigeminal neuralgia being evaluated for possible multiple sclerosis shows a well-delineated CSF-like mass ➡ medial to the left temporal horn. (28-11B) T2 FS in the same case shows that the cystic mass ➡ has the identical signal intensity as CSF in the adjacent cisterns.

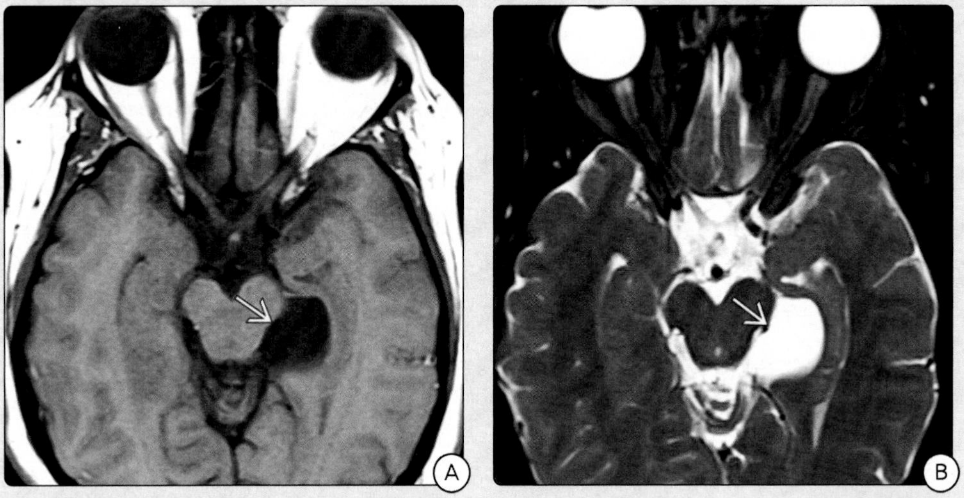

(28-11C) Axial FLAIR in the same case shows that the cyst ➡ suppresses completely. (28-11D) Sagittal FLAIR shows the typical "spindle-shaped" configuration of a choroid fissure cyst ➡. This was an incidental finding, unrelated to the patient's symptoms.

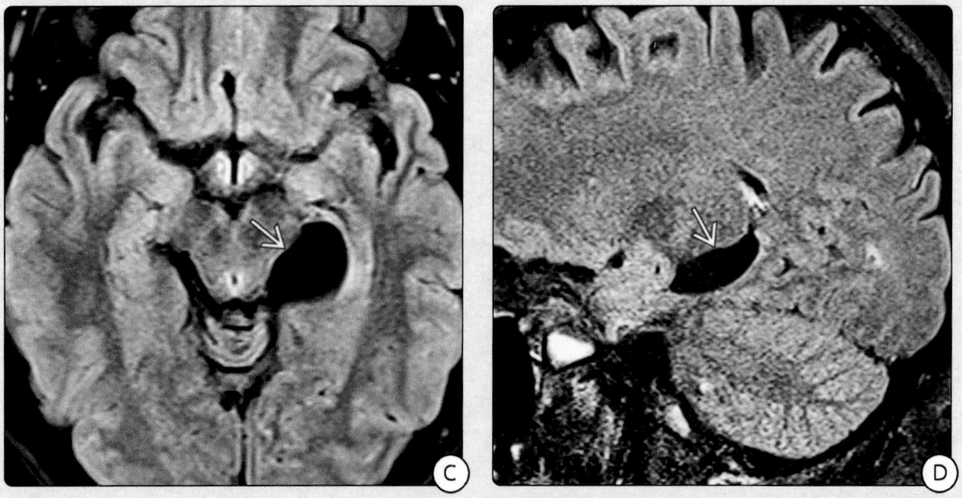

ARACHNOID CYST: CLINICAL ISSUES, IMAGING, AND DDx

Clinical Issues

- Most common nonneoplastic intracranial cyst
  - 1% of all intracranial masses
  - All ages; children + young adults (75%)
  - Prevalence = 2% on imaging studies
- Most do not communicate freely with subarachnoid space

Imaging

- Behaves *exactly* like CSF
- FLAIR/DWI best to distinguish from other cysts

Differential Diagnosis

- Most common = epidermoid cyst
- Less common
  - Enlarged subarachnoid spaces
  - Loculated subdural hygroma/hematoma
  - Porencephalic cyst
  - Neoplasm-associated cyst
- Rare = neurenteric cyst

Choroid Fissure Cyst

The choroid fissure is an infolding of CSF between the fornix and thalamus. It is normally a shallow, inconspicuous, C-shaped cleft that curves posterosuperiorly from the anterior temporal lobe all the way to the atrium of the lateral ventricle. The choroidal arteries and choroid plexus lie just medial to the choroid fissure.

A CSF-containing cyst can form anywhere along the choroid fissure. These "choroid fissure cysts" are probably caused by maldevelopment of the embryonic tela choroidea, a double layer of pia that invaginates through the choroid fissure to reach the lateral ventricles.

Choroid fissure cysts can therefore be regarded as a subtype of arachnoid cyst. We consider them separately because of their unique location and imaging appearance.

Imaging

Most choroid fissure cysts are discovered incidentally on imaging studies. They lie just medial to the temporal horn of the lateral ventricle between the hippocampus and diencephalon. Choroid fissure cysts follow CSF density/signal intensity on all sequences **(28-11)**. On axial and coronal images they are round to oval but on sagittal images have a distinctive, somewhat elongated "spindle" shape **(28-11D)**.

Epidermoid Cyst

Both congenital and acquired epidermoid cysts are found in the CNS. Although spinal epidermoid cysts (ECs) are often acquired lesions, intracranial ECs are always congenital in origin.

Terminology

An intracranial EC is an inclusion cyst that is derived from embryonic ectodermal elements. ECs cysts have incorrectly been called "tumors," but they are not neoplastic. The term "cholesteatoma" should be reserved for an acquired lesion arising as a complication of chronic otitis media.

Etiology

General Concepts. ECs arise during the third to fifth gestational weeks. Ectodermal cellular remnants caused by incomplete cleavage of neural from cutaneous ectoderm result in the inclusion of epiblasts in the neural tube. Congenital CPA epidermoids are derived from cells of the first branchial groove.

Pathology

Location. Extracranial ECs commonly involve the scalp, face, and neck. Over 90% of intracranial ECs are intradural and are almost always extraaxial **(28-12)**. ECs are more often off- or paramidline and have a predilection for the basal cisterns, where they insinuate themselves around cranial nerves and vessels.

The CPA cistern is the single most common site, accounting for nearly half of all intracranial ECs. The middle cranial fossa (sylvian fissure) and parasellar region together account for 10-15% of ECs. Less common locations are the cerebral ventricles, usually the fourth ventricle. Purely extradural intradiploic ECs account for 5-10% of cases. Parenchymal ECs do occur but are rare.

Gross Pathology. The outer surface of an EC is often shiny, resembling mother of pearl **(28-13)**. Multiple "cauliflower" excrescences are typical **(28-14)**. The cyst is filled with soft, waxy, creamy, or flaky material.

Microscopic Features. The cyst wall consists of an outer fibrous capsule lined by stratified squamous epithelium. The cyst contains concentric lamellae of keratinaceous debris and solid crystalline cholesterol. Dermal appendages (a characteristic of dermoid cysts) are absent.

Clinical Issues

Epidemiology. ECs represent 0.2-1.8% of primary intracranial tumors and tumor-like lesions. They are the most common intracranial developmental cyst and are four to nine times more common than dermoid cysts. Overall, EC is the third most common CPA mass (after vestibular schwannoma and meningioma) and the most common cystic mass in this location.

Demographics. Peak age of presentation is 20-60 years. Symptomatic ECs are rare in children. There is no sex predominance.

Presentation. ECs may remain clinically silent for many years. Symptoms are location dependent. Headache and cranial neuropathy (especially involving CNs V, VII, and VIII) are common features.

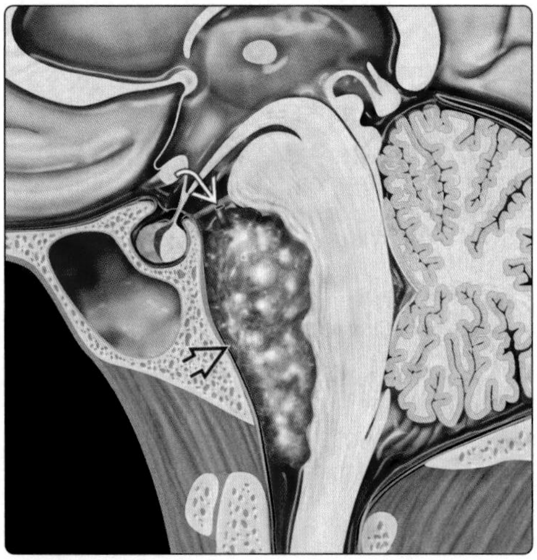

(28-12) Graphic shows a multilobulated epidermoid cyst within prepontine cistern encasing the basilar artery, displacing pons.

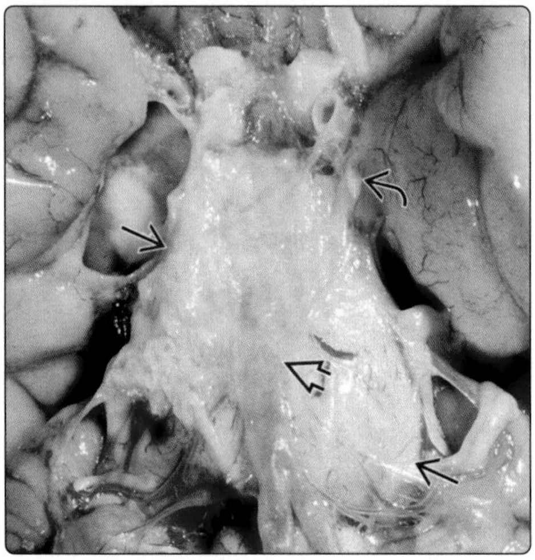

(28-13) Autopsy shows epidermoid cyst as a whitish, "pearly" tumor. Note the encased basilar artery, oculomotor nerves.

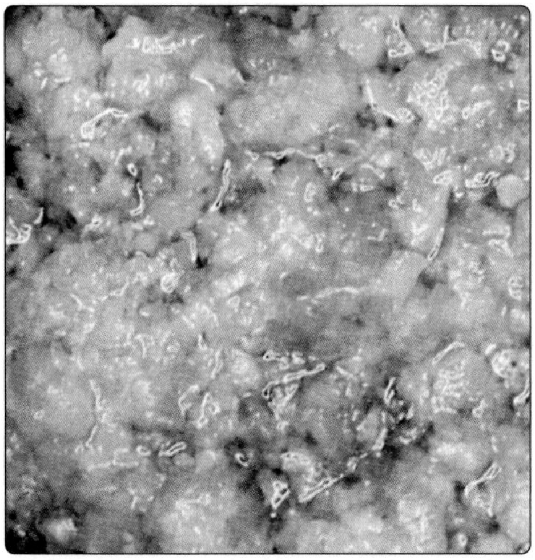

(28-14) Close-up view of a surgical specimen shows classic "cauliflower" appearance of the external surface of an epidermoid cyst.

Natural History. ECs grow very slowly via progressive accumulation of normally dividing epidermal cells and accretion of desquamated keratin. ECs often reach considerable size before becoming symptomatic. In contrast to dermoid cysts, rupture of an EC is rare. Malignant transformation occurs but is extremely rare.

Treatment Options. The insinuating characteristics of ECs make them difficult to resect. Although total resection minimizes the risk of postoperative aseptic meningitis, hydrocephalus, and tumor recurrence, aggressive surgery may be associated with cranial nerve or ischemic deficits.

EPIDERMOID CYST: ETIOLOGY, PATHOLOGY, AND EPIDEMIOLOGY

Etiology
- Congenital inclusion cyst
- Epithelial remnants in neural tube

Pathology
- Gross pathology
  - Insinuates in/around CSF cisterns
  - Encases vessels/cranial nerves
  - "Cauliflower-like" excrescences
  - "Pearly" whitish surface
  - Waxy, creamy, or flaky contents
- Microscopic pathology
  - Squamous epithelium + keratin debris, solid cholesterol
  - *NO* dermal appendages!

Epidemiology
- 0.2-1.8% of primary intracranial tumors
- Peak age 20-60 years
- Symptomatic ECs rare in children

Imaging

General Features. Epidermoid cysts resemble CSF on imaging. Irregular frond-like excrescences and an insinuating growth pattern in CSF cisterns are characteristic.

CT Findings. Over 95% of ECs are hypodense and appear almost identical to CSF on NECT scans. Calcification is present in 10-25%. Hemorrhage is very rare. Hyperdense "white" epidermoids are uncommon, representing 3% of reported lesions. Enhancement is rare.

MR Findings. ECs are iso- or slightly hyperintense compared with CSF on both T1- and T2-weighted sequences. Slight heterogeneity in signal intensity is often present **(28-15A)**.

"Atypical" epidermoids account for only 5-6% of cases. A "white" epidermoid is a rare type of EC that has a high protein content and may be hyperintense on T1WI and hypointense on T2WI. Enhancement is generally absent although mild peripheral enhancement can be seen in 25% of cases.

ECs either do not suppress at all or suppress incompletely on FLAIR **(28-15B)**. They restrict on DWI and are therefore moderately to strikingly hyperintense **(28-15C)**.

Differential Diagnosis

The major differential diagnosis is **arachnoid cyst (AC)**. ACs are smoothly marginated, behave *exactly* like CSF on all sequences, suppress completely on FLAIR, and do not restrict on DWI. The rare "white" epidermoid can mimic **neurenteric cyst**.

Parasitic cysts such as neurocysticercosis (NCC) are usually multiple and small and often contain a discernible scolex. Most NCC cysts are located within the depths of cerebral sulci or in the brain parenchyma. **Cystic neoplasms** are rarely mistaken for ECs, as the cyst wall and/or nodule enhances.

Dermoid cysts should not be confused with ECs. Dermoid cysts contain fat and dermal appendages and do not resemble CSF on imaging studies.

EPIDERMOID CYST: FEATURES, IMAGING, AND DDx

General Features
- Resembles CSF (vs. fat-like dermoid)
- Insinuates around/along CSF cisterns
- Encases, displaces vessels and cranial nerves

Location
- Intradural (90%), intradiploic (10%)
- CPA cistern most common site (~ 50%)

CT
- Hypodense (> 95%)

MR
- Slightly hyperintense to CSF on T1WI
- Does not suppress on FLAIR
- Restricts ("bright") on DWI

Differential Diagnosis
- Arachnoid cyst
  - Suppresses on FLAIR, restricts on DWI
- Other
  - Inflammatory cyst (e.g., neurocysticercosis)
  - Neurenteric cyst (not exactly like CSF)

Dermoid Cyst

Terminology

A dermoid cyst (DC) is a histologically benign cystic mass with mature squamous epithelium, keratinous material, and adnexal structures (hair follicles and sebaceous and sweat glands).

Etiology

General Concepts. Like epidermoid cysts, DCs are thought to arise from the inclusion of ectodermally committed cells at the time of neural tube closure (third to fifth week of embryogenesis). DCs grow slowly secondary to the production of hair and oils from the internal dermal elements.

Genetics. Most DCs are sporadic although there is a reported association with Goldenhar and Klippel-Feil syndromes.

Pathology

Location. DCs are usually extraaxial lesions that are most often found in the midline **(28-16)**. The suprasellar cistern is the most common site, followed by the posterior fossa and frontonasal region.

Gross Pathology. A dermoid cyst is a thick-walled unilocular cyst lined by stratified squamous epithelium. Sectioned DCs typically contain thick, greasy sebaceous material, keratin debris, and skin adnexa such as hair follicles **(28-17)**. Lipid and cholesterol elements floating on proteinaceous material may be present.

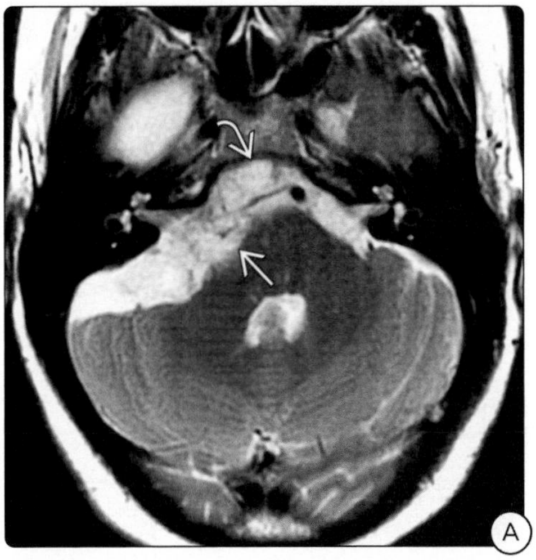

***(28-15A)** T2WI shows a lobulated, irregular hyperintense mass in the right CPA ➡ and basilar ⇨ cisterns. The CSF looks "dirty."*

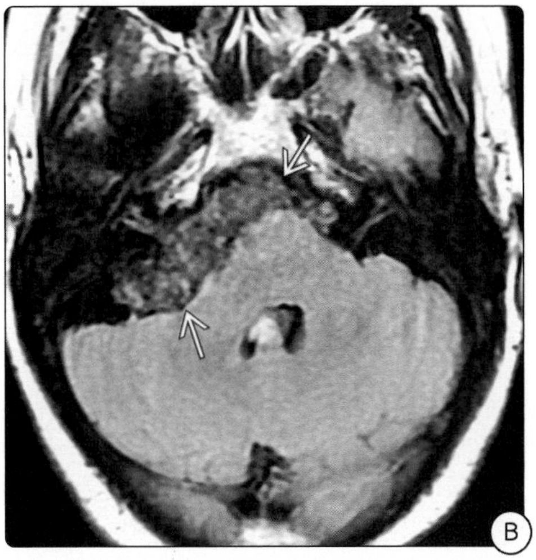

***(28-15B)** FLAIR demonstrates that the lobulated, cauliflower-like mass ➡ does not suppress.*

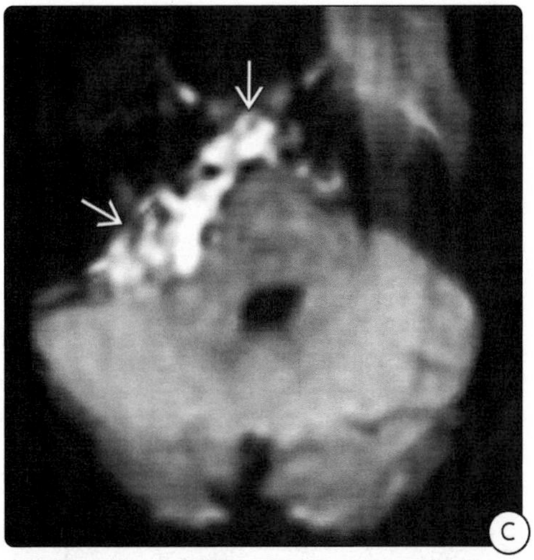

***(28-15C)** The mass ➡ restricts on DWI. This is a classic epidermoid cyst.*

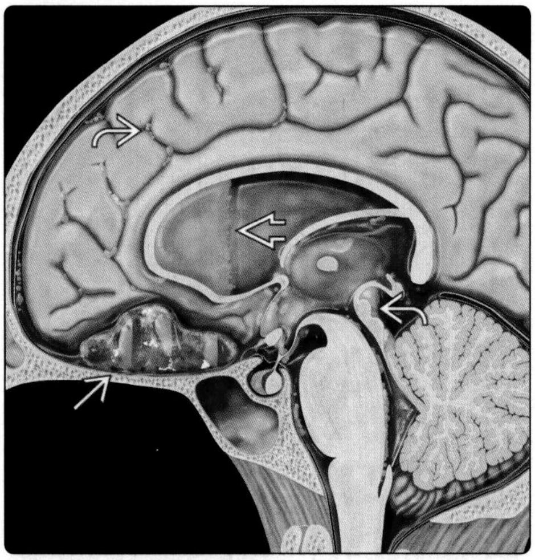

(28-16) Ruptured DC ➡ is heterogeneous fat-containing midline mass with ventricular fat-fluid level ➡ and fat droplets in SASs ➡.

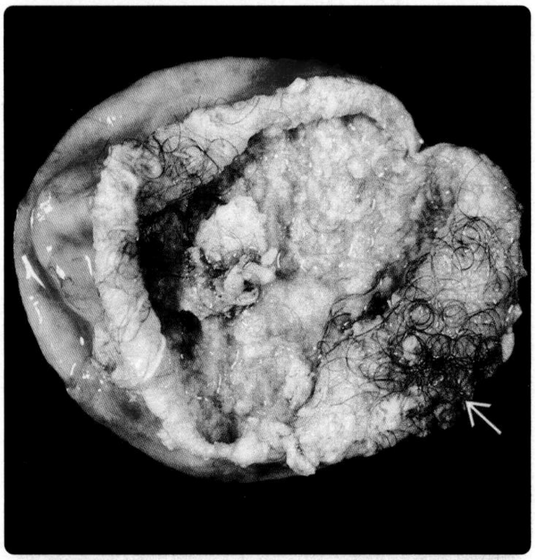

(28-17) Dermoid cyst contains thick, greasy sebaceous material, keratin debris, and hair ➡. (Courtesy R. Hewlett, MD.)

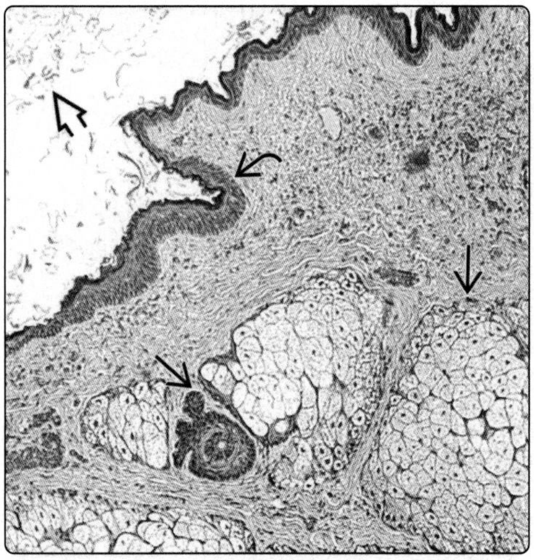

(28-18) Micrograph of dermoid cyst shows squamous epithelium ➡, dermal appendages ➡ in cyst wall, and keratin debris ➡ in cyst center.

Microscopic Features. The outer wall of a DC consists of squamous epithelium. The inner lining contains multiple sebaceous and apocrine glands, fat, and hair follicles **(28-18)**.

Clinical Issues

Epidemiology. DCs are much less common than epidermoid cysts, representing less than 0.5% of intracranial masses.

Demographics. Presentation occurs at significantly younger ages compared with epidermoids, peaking in the second to third decades.

Presentation. DCs often remain asymptomatic until they rupture. Although cyst rupture is usually not fatal, chemical meningitis with seizure, coma, vasospasm, infarction, and even death may ensue as a consequence.

Natural History. DCs typically grow very slowly although rapid enlargement with rupture has been reported. Cyst rupture is usually spontaneous but has also been associated with head trauma. Fat from a ruptured DC may persist for years. DCs occasionally degenerate into squamous cell carcinomas.

Treatment Options. Complete surgical resection is the goal, but residual tumor adherent to neurovascular structures is often left behind to minimize postoperative complications. Unlike epidermoid cysts, the recurrence rate after DC resection is very low.

Imaging

General Features. DCs resemble fat. A round, well-circumscribed lipid-containing mass is the usual appearance.

CT Findings. DCs are quite hypointense on NECT scans **(28-19A)**. Calcification of the capsule is seen in 20% of cases. With rupture, hypodense fatty "droplets" disseminate in the CSF cisterns and may cause discernible fat-fluid levels in the ventricles.

In infants with frontal DC, bone CT usually discloses a bifid crista galli with a large foramen cecum and sinus tract.

MR Findings. Signal intensity varies with fat content in the cyst. Most DCs are heterogeneously hyperintense on T1WI **(28-19B)**. T1WI is also the most sensitive sequence to detect disseminated fat "droplets" in the subarachnoid space, diagnostic of ruptured dermoid **(28-20)**. Fat suppression is helpful to confirm the presence of lipid elements.

Standard PD and T2 scans show increasingly more pronounced "chemical shift" artifact in the frequency-encoding direction as the time of repetition is lengthened. Fat is very hypointense on standard T2WI but is "bright" (hyperintense) on fast spin echo T2-weighted sequences. DCs demonstrate heterogeneous hyperintensity with linear or striated laminations if hair is present within the cyst.

Uncomplicated DCs are heterogeneously hyperintense on FLAIR. Ruptured DCs demonstrate subtle FLAIR sulcal hyperintensity **(28-20C)** and "bloom" on T2* GRE or SWI **(28-20D)**.

Most DCs do not enhance although ruptured DCs may cause significant chemical meningitis with extensive leptomeningeal reaction and enhancement.

Spectroscopy may show an elevated lipid peak at 0.9-1.3 ppm.

DERMOID CYST

Pathology
- Location
  - Usually extraaxial
  - Midline > off-midline
  - Suprasellar > posterior fossa > frontonasal
- Wall of squamous epithelium
  - Cyst contains fatty sebaceous material, keratin, skin adnexa

Clinical Findings
- Grow slowly
- Usually asymptomatic until rupture

Imaging
- NECT
  - Hypodense, Ca++ in 20%
  - "Fatty" droplets in cisterns if ruptured
- MR
  - Heterogeneously hyperintense on T1WI/FSE T2
  - Heterogeneously hyperintense on FLAIR
  - Ruptured DCs "bloom" on T2*GRE

Differential Diagnosis

The major differential diagnosis of DC is **epidermoid cyst**. Epidermoid cysts behave more like CSF on both CT and MR, whereas DCs resemble fat on imaging studies. Dermoids often rupture, spilling fatty droplets into the subarachnoid space. Epidermoid cyst rupture does occur but is much less common and may demonstrate high serum carbohydrate antigen CA 199.

Lipoma may resemble a DC but is generally much more homogeneous on MR and is often associated with other congenital malformations such as callosal dysgenesis.

Craniopharyngioma is often multicystic, extends into the sella, calcifies, and enhances. **Teratoma** may resemble a DC but most commonly occurs in the pineal gland and is much more heterogeneous on imaging than the typical DC.

DERMOID vs. EPIDERMOID CYST

Pathology
- *Both* dermoid, epidermoid contain squamous epithelium + keratin debris
- *Only* dermoid also contains fat, dermal appendages

Clinical Issues
- Dermoid cysts *less* common than epidermoids
- Dermoid cysts more common in children/young adults
- Dermoid cysts commonly rupture

Imaging
- DC behaves mostly like fat
  - Most often midline, supra- or juxtasellar
- Epidermoid cyst more like CSF
  - Most often midline
  - Most common site = posterior fossa (cerebellopontine angle cistern)

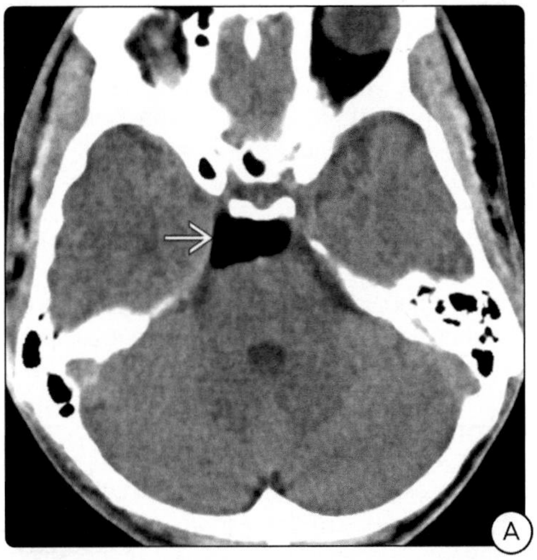

***(28-19A)** Axial NECT in a 20y man with severe headaches shows a very hypodense mass ➡ in the prepontine cistern.*

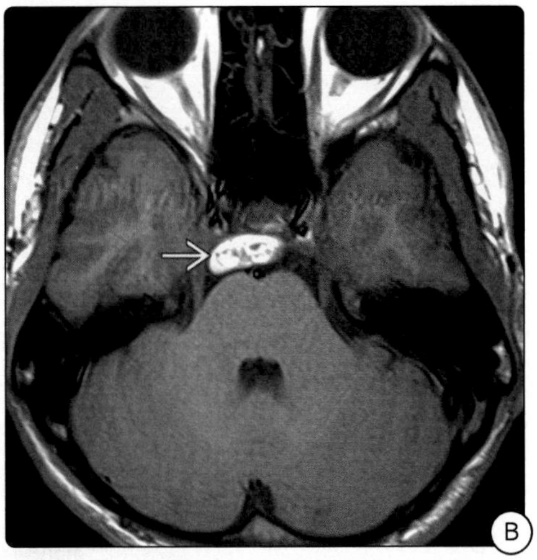

***(28-19B)** T1WI in the same case demonstrates that the mass ➡ is heterogeneously hyperintense.*

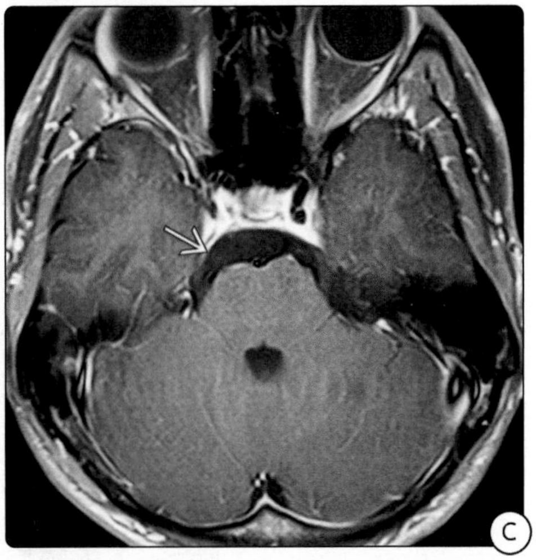

***(28-19C)** T1 C+ FS shows that the mass ➡ suppresses completely and does not enhance. This is dermoid cyst without evidence for rupture.*

Neurenteric Cyst

Neurenteric (NE) cysts are rare endodermal-derived developmental CNS lesions. They are significantly more common in the spine than in the brain.

Terminology

NE cyst is also called enterogenous cyst, enteric cyst, endodermal cyst, and neuroendodermal cyst. Other less common terms, primarily applied to intraspinal NE cysts, are gastrogenic and archenteric cysts.

Etiology

NE cysts, along with Rathke cleft and colloid cysts, are endodermally derived developmental lesions of the CNS. Immunohistochemical studies have demonstrated that NE cysts are most likely derived from embryonic multipotent endodermal cells. These cells freely migrate along the embryonic neuroectoderm, which lies just dorsal to the developing notochord. If the neuroectoderm fails to separate from the notochord, displaced nests of respiratory or alimentary tissue may ultimately form an NE cyst.

The most cephalad aspect of the notochord forms the clivus, which is why most intracranial NE cysts are found in the midline posterior fossa. The rare supratentorial NE cysts probably form when the traveling multipotent endodermal cells proceed over the notochord into the supratentorial area.

Pathology

Location. The most common CNS site is the spine. Intracranial NE cysts are rare, accounting for less than 25% of all cases. Almost 75% of these occur in the posterior fossa, and almost all are extraaxial. The typical location is midline or slightly off-midline, just anterior to the pontomedullary junction **(28-21)**. The lower CPA cistern is also a common site.

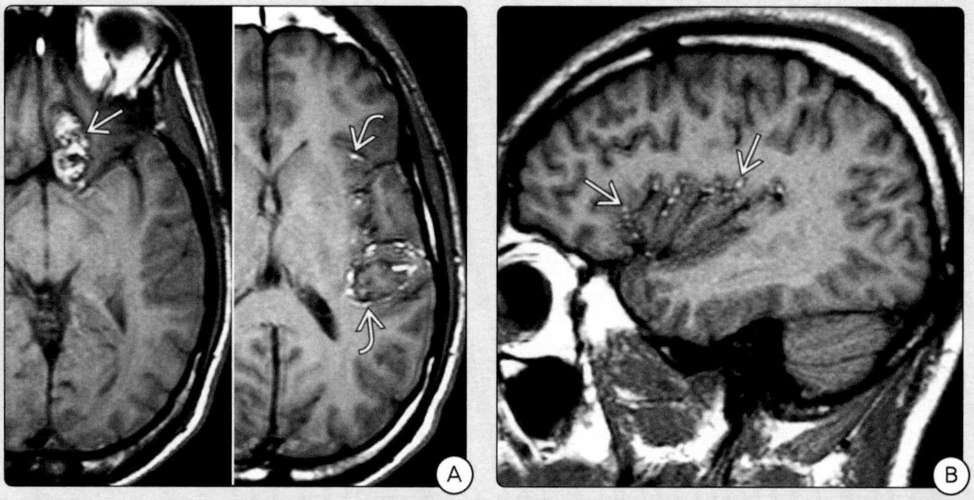

(28-20A) (L) Axial T1WI shows dermoid cyst as heterogeneously hyperintense paramedian mass ➡. (R) Cyst rupture has spilled T1 hyperintense fatty droplets into the sulci along the sylvian fissure ↪. (28-20B) Sagittal T1WI in the same case nicely shows hyperintense droplets from the ruptured dermoid along the sylvian fissure sulci ➡.

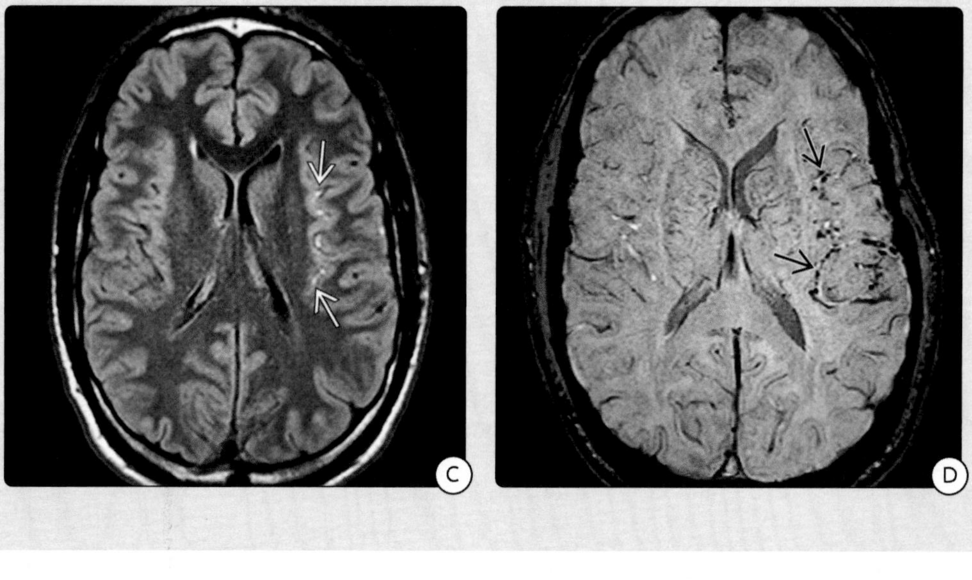

(28-20C) Droplets from the ruptured dermoid in the left sylvian fissure ➡ are hyperintense on FLAIR (compare to the normal-appearing right sylvian fissure). (28-20D) T2* SWI shows that the droplets exhibit "blooming" and appear as punctate hypointensities ➡ in the left sylvian fissure.

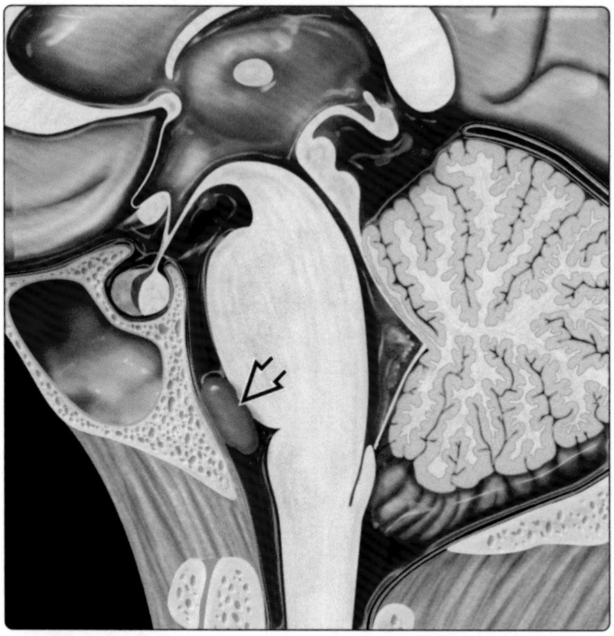

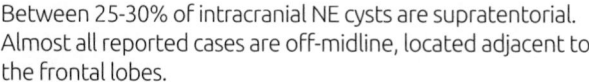

(28-21) Sagittal graphic shows a classic neurenteric cyst ➲. Intracranial neurenteric cysts are most often found near the midline, anterior to the brainstem.

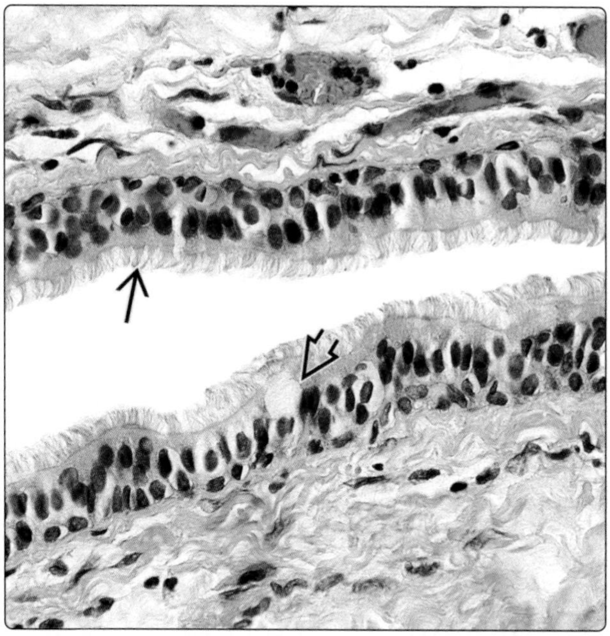

(28-22) Neurenteric (endodermal) cysts are mostly lined with pseudostratified ciliated epithelium ➲ and contain variable numbers of goblet cells ➲. (Courtesy P. Burger, MD.)

Between 25-30% of intracranial NE cysts are supratentorial. Almost all reported cases are off-midline, located adjacent to the frontal lobes.

Size and Number. NE cysts vary in size. Most are relatively small (1-3 cm in diameter). Occasionally, NE cysts can become very large (up to 9 cm), especially when they occur in the supratentorial compartment.

NE cysts are almost always solitary. "Seeding" or wide dissemination with multiple cysts spreading throughout the spinal canal is reported but rare.

Gross Pathology. NE cysts are typically well-delineated, smoothly marginated cysts. The wall is thin and translucent. Cyst contents range from clear colorless fluid that resembles CSF to thick viscous mucoid secretions.

Microscopic Features. NE cysts are lined by three cell types that resemble the respiratory tract (pseudostratified-ciliated), stomach (goblet-columnar), or respiratory bronchioles (simple cuboidal) **(28-22)**. A few cases of squamous metaplasia and even mucinous adenocarcinomas arising in an NE cyst have been reported.

Clinical Issues

Demographics. NE cysts occur in patients of all ages. Age distribution is bimodal, with a large peak in the third and fourth decades and a smaller peak in the first decade. Average age at presentation is 34 years. There is a slight male predominance.

Presentation. Posterior fossa NE cysts typically present with waxing and waning neck pain or occipital headaches. Headaches, behavior changes, and seizures have been reported with supratentorial lesions.

Natural History. NE cysts grow very slowly and are often stable for years.

Treatment Options. Small NE cysts are sometimes monitored with periodic imaging. Symptomatic cysts are excised. Total surgical removal is the treatment goal but may be difficult due to adhesion of the cyst membrane to critical neurovascular structures.

NEURENTERIC CYST: PATHOLOGY AND CLINICAL ISSUES

Location
- Posterior fossa (75%)
  - Extraaxial, midline/slightly off-midline
  - Anterior to pontomedullary junction
- Supratentorial (25%)
  - Extraaxial, adjacent to frontal lobes

Pathology
- Endodermal-derived congenital inclusion cyst
- Size varies from 1-9 cm
- Round/ovoid shape, smoothly marginated
- Wall contains mucin-secreting goblet cells

Clinical Issues
- Spinal NE cyst 3-4x more common than intracranial
- Asymptomatic or headache, neck pain

Imaging

General Features. NE cysts are all well delineated and round to ovoid. Density and signal intensity vary according to protein content of the cyst fluid. Most NE cysts are moderately proteinaceous and therefore often do not precisely parallel CSF.

CT Findings. Most NE cysts are iso- to slightly hyperdense compared with CSF. Hyperdense ("white") NE cysts are seen in about 25% of cases. Calcification and intracystic hemorrhage are absent. In contrast to spinal NE cysts, bony anomalies are rare. NE cysts do not enhance following contrast administration.

MR Findings. NE cysts are sharply demarcated lesions that displace but do not engulf adjacent neurovascular structures. The cyst wall itself is often inapparent. Signal intensity of cyst contents varies widely, depending on imaging sequence and protein content.

Cyst fluid is almost always iso- to hyperintense compared with CSF on T1WI **(28-23)**. Over 90% are hyperintense to CSF on PD and T2WI. Between 5-10%—typically NE cysts with inspissated, significantly dehydrated contents—are hypointense.

NE cysts do not suppress on FLAIR and are almost always hyperintense relative to CSF. As NE cysts almost never calcify or hemorrhage, T2* (GRE, SWI) sequences do not demonstrate "blooming."

Only a few reports of NE cysts have included DWI findings. In those cases, diffusion restriction was mild or absent.

Most NE cysts do not enhance following contrast administration. A few cases of mild posterior rim enhancement at the cyst-brain interface have been reported.

Differential Diagnosis

Other endodermal-derived cysts such as Rathke cleft (sella) and colloid cyst (foramen of Monro) are very location specific, and their anatomic sites do not overlap with those of NE.

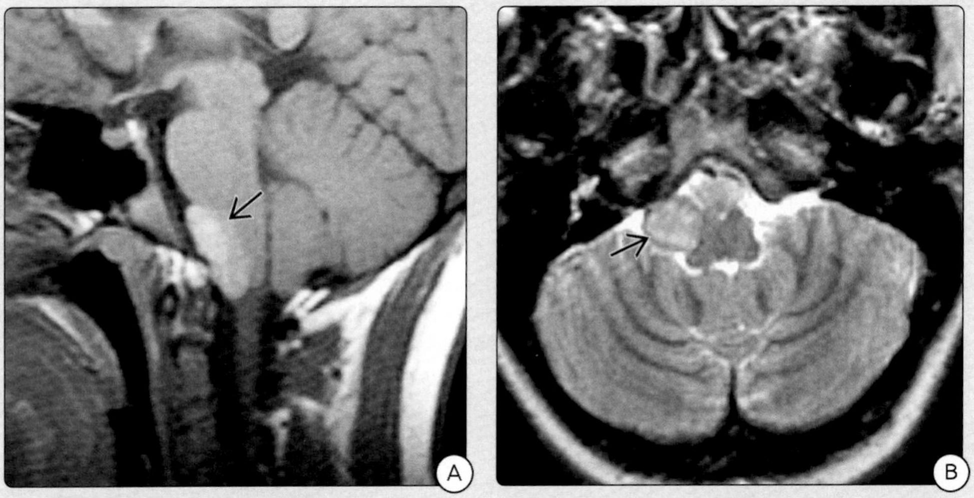

***(28-23A)** Sagittal T1WI of a neurenteric cyst shows a hyperintense ovoid midline mass ⇨ in front of the medulla. **(28-23B)** Axial T2WI shows that the mass ⇨ is well delineated. It is heterogeneously hypointense to CSF, suggesting inspissated contents. More typically NE cysts are hyperintense to CSF.*

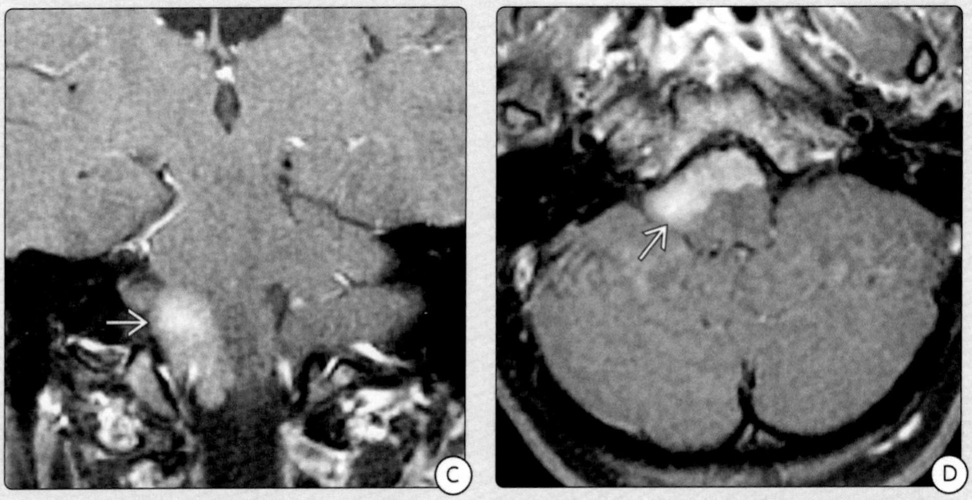

***(28-23C)** Coronal T1 C+ scan shows that the ovoid mass ➡ is well demarcated and hyperintense. **(28-23D)** Axial T1 C+ FS shows that the mass ➡ extends inferiorly to the lower medulla. The center of the mass is just slightly off-midline, a typical solution for a posterior fossa neurenteric cyst.*

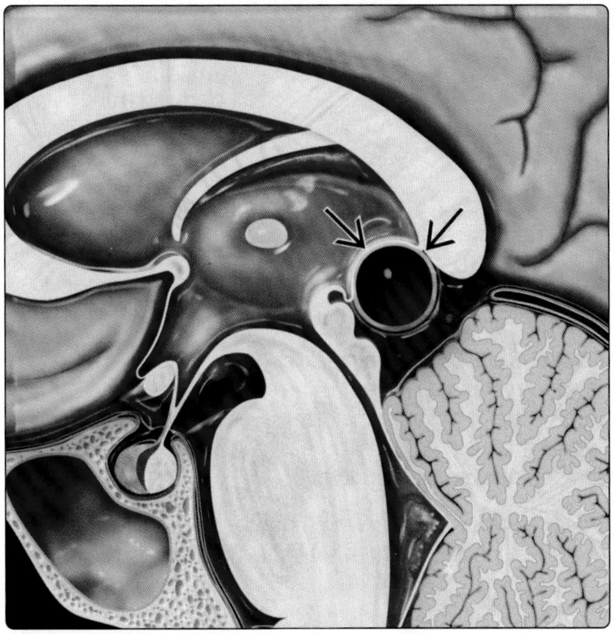

(28-24) Sagittal graphic shows a small cystic lesion within the pineal gland ⇒. Small benign pineal cysts are often found incidentally at autopsy or imaging.

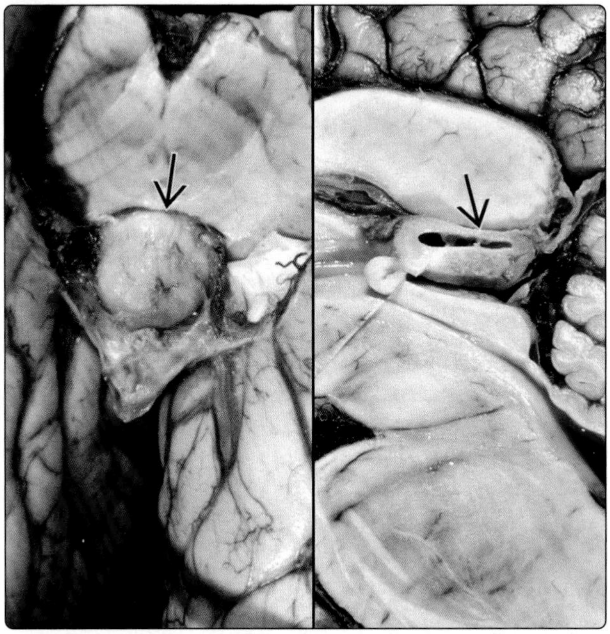

(28-25) Axial (L), sagittal (R) autopsy views of pineal cyst ⇒ show the typical location behind the tectal plate. (Courtesy E. T. Hedley-Whyte, MD.)

The major differential diagnosis of NE cyst is **epidermoid cyst (EC)**. ECs are insinuating lesions that have lobulated frond-like surfaces. Most restrict strongly on DWI. Posterior fossa ECs are usually more lateral than NE cysts, occurring more commonly in the CPA cistern than at the pontomedullary junction. Some reported cases of "white" epidermoids may actually have been NE cysts.

Arachnoid cyst follows CSF signal intensity on all sequences (e.g., suppresses completely on FLAIR) and does not restrict on DWI. **Schwannoma** is the most common extraaxial posterior fossa mass in adults. It typically enhances strongly and rarely occurs in the midline.

Ecchordosis physaliphora (EP) is a gelatinous-appearing notochordal remnant that typically occurs in the prepontine cistern and is attached to a visible defect in the dorsal clivus by a thin stalk-like pedicle (see Figures 26-19-22).

NEURENTERIC CYST: IMAGING AND DDx

CT
- NECT: Iso-/slightly hyperintense to CSF
- CECT: No enhancement

MR
- T1WI: Almost always iso-/slightly hyperintense to CSF
- PD, T2WI: Hyperintense to CSF (> 90%)
- FLAIR: Does not suppress
- DWI: Mild/no restriction

Differential Diagnosis
- Most common = epidermoid, arachnoid cysts
- Less common = schwannoma (cystic)
- Rare = ecchordosis physaliphora

Pineal Cyst

Modern imaging has resulted in a plethora of pineal "things" found on CT and especially MR. These lesions, often seen in patients with vague complaints and no symptoms referable to the pineal region, can be troublesome to both radiologists and referring clinicians.

Terminology

A pineal cyst (PC) is a benign glia-lined, fluid-containing cyst within the pineal gland parenchyma.

Etiology

The precise etiology of PCs is unknown. Theories include persistent coalescing embryonic pineal cavities and glial degeneration with cavitation.

Pathology

Location. An easy way to remember the normal midline anatomic structures in the pineal region—from top to bottom—is "**f**amous **V.I.P.**" for **f**ornix, **v**elum interpositum, **i**nternal cerebral veins, and **p**ineal gland (see Chapter 20). As expected, any pineal gland mass—including PCs—therefore lies below the fornix, velum interpositum, and internal cerebral veins, displacing them superiorly. Although PCs may compress the posterior third ventricle, most PCs exert little or no mass effect on the tectum and aqueduct, so hydrocephalus is rare except with very large cysts.

Size and Number. PCs are well-demarcated round or ovoid expansions within an otherwise normal-appearing pineal gland **(28-24)**. Most PCs are less than 10 mm in diameter. The largest reported PC is 4.5 cm. PCs are usually unilocular, but lesions containing multiple smaller cysts do occur.

Gross Pathology. The general appearance is that of a smooth, soft, tan-yellow pineal gland that contains a uni- or multilocular cyst **(28-25)**. Cyst fluid is clear to yellowish.

Microscopic Features. PCs are cavities of various sizes surrounded by an outer layer of attenuated pineal parenchyma. The inner layer is a sharply defined zone of finely fibrillar glial tissue with Rosenthal fibers. PCs have no ependymal or epithelial lining.

The inner surface of a pineal cyst cavity is often hemosiderin stained as the result of intralesional hemorrhage. There are no gross pathologic or histologic features that distinguish symptomatic from asymptomatic PCs.

Clinical Issues

Epidemiology. Cystic-appearing lesions in the pineal gland are common on MR scans, seen in one-half of children and over one-quarter of healthy adults. Between 25-40% of autopsied pineal glands contain cysts.

Demographics. PCs can occur at *any* age although they are more often discovered in middle-aged and older adults.

The overall F:M ratio is 2:1. The incidence among women ages 21-30 years is significantly higher than in any other group.

Presentation. Most PCs are clinically benign and asymptomatic, discovered incidentally at imaging or autopsy. Large PCs may obstruct the cerebral aqueduct, resulting in hydrocephalus and headache. Parinaud syndrome (tectal compression) is less common.

Pineal "apoplexy" occurs with sudden intracystic hemorrhage. Acute worsening of headaches combined with visual

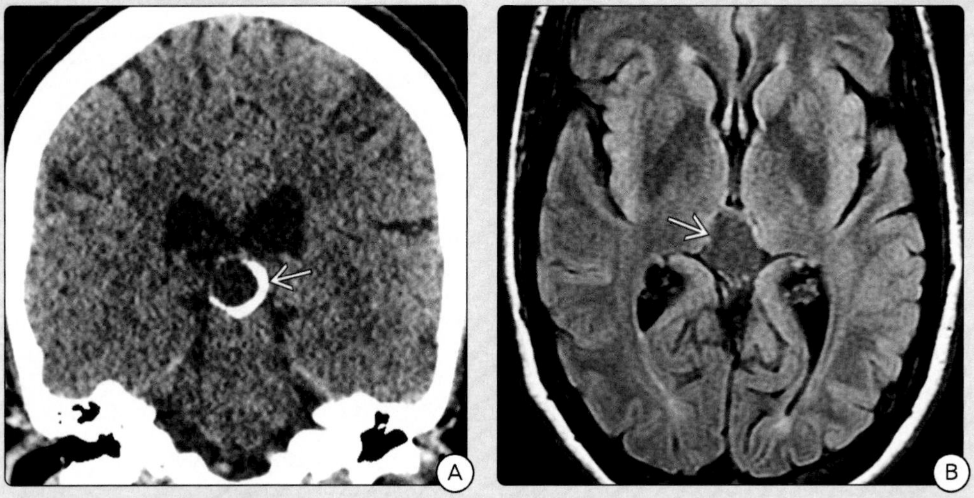

***(28-26A)** Coronal NECT in a 49y woman with chronic headaches shows a large cystic pineal gland with thick rim calcification ➡. **(28-26B)** Axial FLAIR in the same case shows that the fluid in the pineal cyst ➡ does not compress completely.*

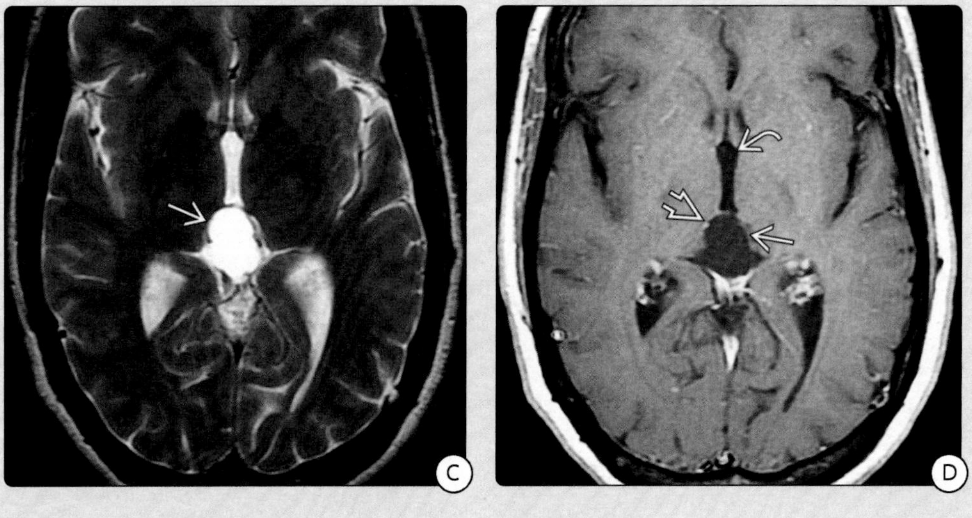

***(28-26C)** T2WI in the same case shows that the cyst fluid ➡ appears slightly hyperintense compared with CSF in the ventricles. **(28-26D)** T1 C+ shows that the cyst fluid ➡ is slightly hyperintense compared with CSF in the adjacent third ventricle ➡. Minimal enhancement of the cyst wall ➡ is present. This is nonneoplastic pineal cyst.*

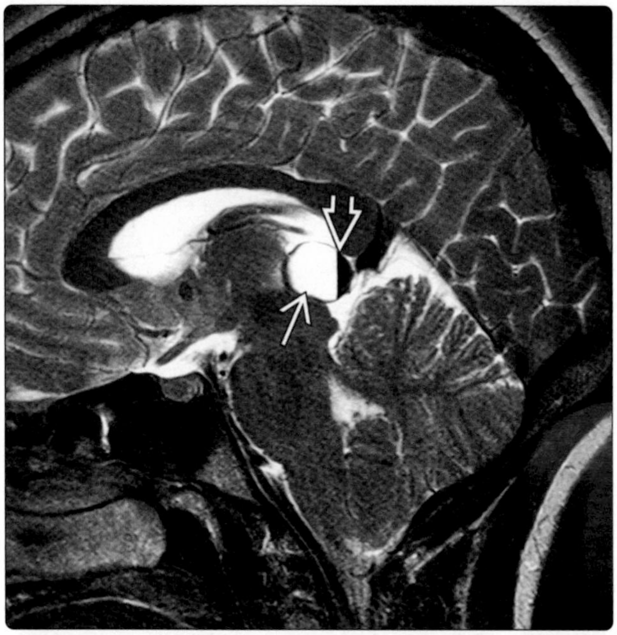

***(28-27)** Sagittal T2WI in a 17y girl with sudden onset of severe headache, visual difficulties shows a large pineal cyst ➡ with blood-fluid level ➡ indicating hemorrhage (cyst "apoplexy").*

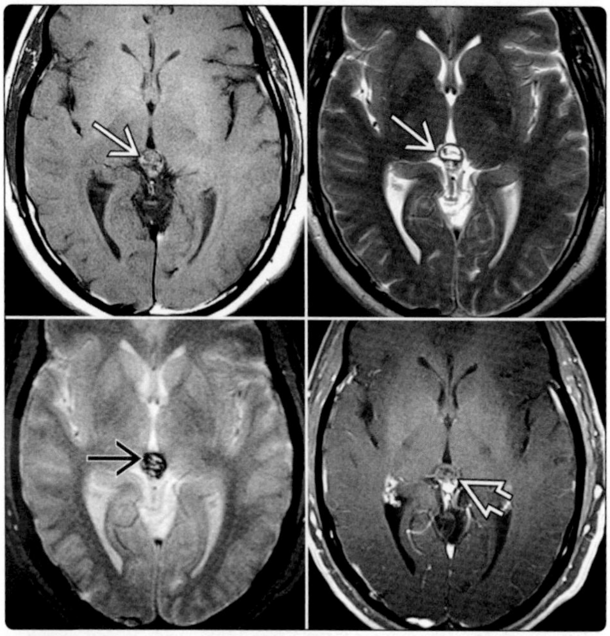

***(28-28)** Small pineal cyst is seen with hemorrhage ➡, "blooming" on T2* ⇨, with rim and nodular enhancement on T1 C+ FS ➡.*

symptoms can occur. A "thunderclap" headache may mimic symptoms of aneurysmal subarachnoid hemorrhage. Pineal "apoplexy" can result in acute intraventricular obstructive hydrocephalus. Rare cases result in sudden death.

Natural History. Serial follow-up of indeterminate cystic lesions of the pineal region shows, in most lesions, no significant change in size or character over time intervals from months to years. Most investigators recommend that incidentally identified PCs be followed clinically and do not require serial imaging. Patients with growing lesions, atypical contrast enhancement, or hemorrhage on MR are more likely to develop hydrocephalus and have malignant pathology, so follow-up serial MRs are recommended.

Treatment Options. Most PCs are "leave me alone" lesions. Symptomatic cysts may require stereotactic aspiration or biopsy/resection.

Imaging

CT Findings. At least 25% of PCs show calcification within the cyst wall **(28-26A)**. The cyst fluid is iso- to slightly hyperdense compared with CSF. A very hyperdense PC in a patient with severe headache should raise suspicion of hemorrhage with cyst "apoplexy."

The ventricles are usually normal. Large ventricles with "blurred" margins indicate acute obstructive hydrocephalus.

Enhancement is typical. Rim, crescentic, or nodular patterns have all been described with PCs.

MR Findings. Thin-section high-resolution sagittal and axial T2 scans are especially helpful for detecting and characterizing lesions in the anatomically complex pineal region.

As with other cysts, PC signal intensity varies with imaging sequence and cyst contents **(28-26)**.

Most PCs are small and cause minimal or no mass effect. Large cysts—or PCs with acute intracystic hemorrhage—may cause obstructive hydrocephalus. In such cases, PD and T2/FLAIR scans show "fingers" of hyperintensity extending into the periventricular white matter due to subependymal accumulation of brain interstitial fluid. These are especially well demonstrated on sagittal scans.

Between 50 and 60% of PCs are slightly hyperintense compared with CSF on T1WI. Approximately 40% are isointense with CSF. Approximately 1-2% are very hyperintense, which may indicate intracystic hemorrhage. A blood-fluid level may be present **(28-27)**.

The vast majority of PCs are hyperintense to CSF on intermediate (PD) sequences and iso- to slightly hyperintense on T2WI. Internal septations are visible in 20-25% of cases, and 10% are multicystic. If acute hemorrhage has occurred, intracystic blood may appear very hypointense.

PCs do not suppress completely on FLAIR and are moderately hyperintense relative to brain parenchyma. If intracystic hemorrhage has occurred, cyst fluid "blooms" on T2* (GRE, SWI) **(28-28)**. Rim calcifications may show mild "blooming."

Between one- and two-thirds of PCs enhance. The most common pattern is a thin circumferential rim of enhancement. Less common patterns include nodular, crescentic, or irregular enhancement.

PCs typically do not restrict on DWI. Neuronal markers are absent on MRS.

Differential Diagnosis

The most common differential diagnosis is **normal pineal gland**. Normal pineal glands often contain one or more small cysts and can have nodular, crescentic, or ring-like enhancement.

The most important pathologic entity to be differentiated from a PC is **pineocytoma**. Pineocytoma is a WHO grade I pineal parenchymal tumor that is usually solid or at least partially solid/cystic. Purely cystic pineocytomas are much less common and can be indistinguishable from PC on imaging. Pineocytomas can remain stable for many years without significant change on serial imaging.

Atypical imaging findings, focal invasion, or significant interval change in a presumed PC or pineocytoma should raise suspicion for the more aggressive **pineal parenchymal tumor of intermediate differentiation** (PPTID).

PINEAL CYST

Pathology
- Usually < 1 cm, unilocular > multicystic
- Wall contains attenuated pineal parenchyma
- Fluid clear to yellowish

Clinical Issues
- Common
  - 23% of normal MRs, 25-40% of autopsies
- Occur at any age; more common in adults
- Usually asymptomatic, found incidentally

Imaging
- Ca++ (25%)
- Fluid slightly hyperintense to CSF on MR
- Rim, nodular, or crescentic enhancement

Differential Diagnosis
- Normal pineal gland, pineocytoma

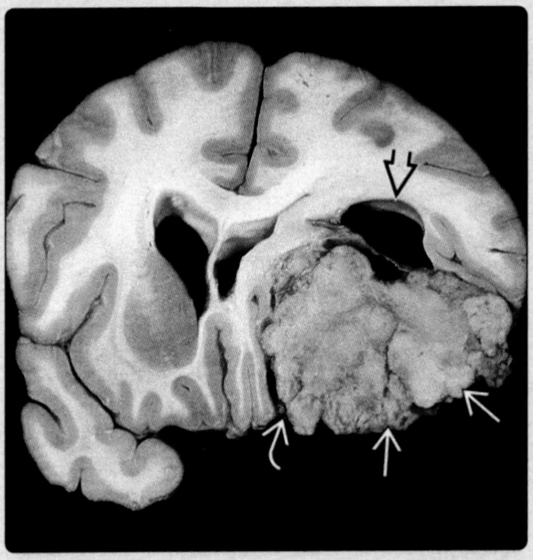

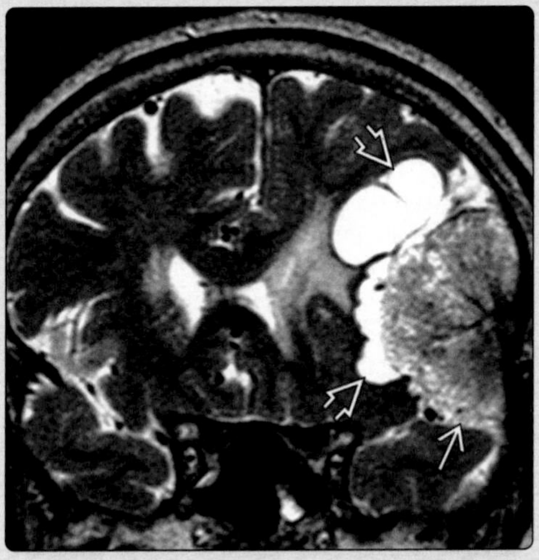

***(28-29)** Autopsy specimen shows a frontal meningioma → with CSF-vascular "cleft" → and a large tumor-associated cyst →. **(28-30)** Coronal T2WI shows a typical sphenoid wing meningioma → with hyperintense pools of trapped fluid → between the tumor and brain. (Courtesy M. Thurnher, MD.)*

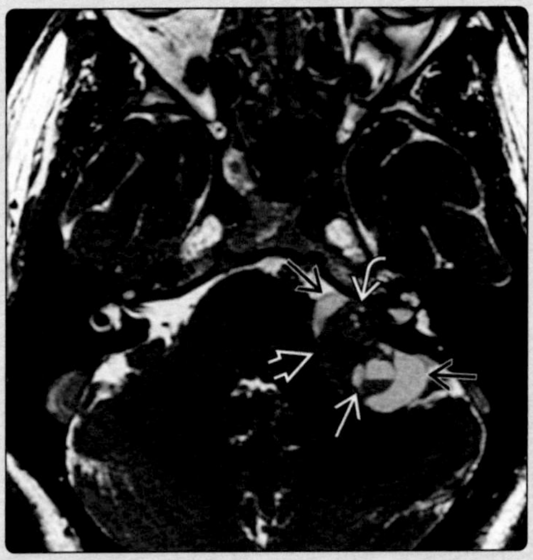

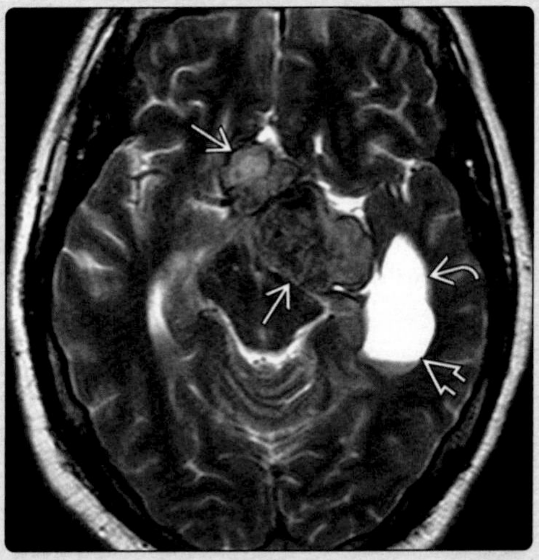

***(28-31)** FIESTA shows a large left vestibular schwannoma → with small intratumoral →, larger marginal cysts with blood-fluid levels →, and very prominent extratumoral cysts → in the cerebellopontine angle cistern that are different signal intensity from the adjacent normal CSF. **(28-32)** Axial T2WI shows a pituitary macroadenoma with suprasellar extension →, a prominent tumor-associated cyst → with a blood-fluid level →.*

Nonneoplastic Tumor-Associated Cysts

Terminology

Tumor-associated cysts (TACs) are benign cysts that are adjacent to, but not contained within, a neoplasm.

TACs are also referred to as peritumoral cysts. Surgeons sometimes call them "herald" cysts, as they are immediately adjacent to (and thus "herald" the presence of) a tumor mass.

Etiology

Whether TACs are true arachnoid cysts or fluid collections mostly lined by compressed gliotic brain is debatable. Cyst formation may also relate to blood-brain-barrier deficiency with peritumoral extravasation of water, electrolytes, and plasma proteins from altered microvessels.

TACs are usually associated with benign extraaxial tumors, such as meningioma, schwannoma, pituitary macroadenoma, and craniopharyngioma. TACs are found in both supra- and infratentorial compartments.

Pathology

Most TACs represent trapped, encysted "pools" of CSF adjacent to a large extraaxial neoplasm **(28-29)**. The contents of these peritumoral collections vary from clear CSF-like liquid to turbid proteinaceous fluid. The cyst wall generally consists of gliotic brain with reactive astrocytes and lymphocytes. No tumor cells are present.

Location. TACs are usually positioned at the tumor-brain interface between the mass and adjacent cortex.

Size and Number. TACs vary from small insignificant collections to very large cysts. Most are solitary, but occasionally multiple loculated fluid collections are trapped at the tumor-brain interface.

Clinical Issues

Unless a TAC becomes unusually large, symptoms are generally related to the neoplasm itself, not the TAC.

Imaging

General Features. The common appearance is one or more "pools" of trapped fluid surrounding an extraaxial tumor mass **(28-30)**.

CT Findings. TACs are hypodense to brain and usually iso- to slightly hyperdense compared with CSF. No calcification, hemorrhage, or enhancement is present.

MR Findings. Signal intensity varies with protein content. Most TACs are hypointense to brain on T1WI and very hyperintense on PD and T2WI **(28-32)**. Hemorrhage with blood-fluid levels may be present **(28-31)** **(28-32)**. Suppression on FLAIR is variable. Enhancement is minimal or absent and generally related to reactive inflammatory changes in the cyst wall, not tumor.

Differential Diagnosis

TACs must be distinguished from **cystic neoplasms, arachnoid cyst** (not tumor-associated), and **enlarged perivascular (Virchow-Robin) spaces** (see below). The latter two behave like CSF on imaging studies.

Parenchymal Cysts

Parenchymal (intraaxial) cysts are much more common than either their extraaxial or intraventricular counterparts. Once a cyst has been identified as lying within the brain itself, the differential diagnosis is limited. The most common parenchymal cysts—prominent perivascular spaces and hippocampal sulcus remnants—are anatomic variants. Neuroglial cysts and porencephalic cysts are relatively uncommon. All other nonneoplastic, noninfectious brain cysts are rare.

Enlarged Perivascular Spaces

By far the most common parenchymal brain "cysts" are enlarged perivascular spaces (PVSs). They vary from solitary, small, inconspicuous, and unremarkable to multiple, large, bizarre, alarming-looking collections of CSF-like fluid. They are often asymmetric, may cause mass effect, and have frequently been mistaken for multicystic brain tumors.

Terminology

PVSs are also known as Virchow-Robin spaces. PVSs are pia-lined spaces that accompany penetrating arteries and arterioles into the brain parenchyma. The PVSs do not communicate directly with the subarachnoid space.

Etiology

General Concepts. The brain PVSs form a complicated intraparenchymal network that is distributed throughout the cerebral hemispheres, midbrain, and cerebellum. They are filled with interstitial fluid (ISF), not CSF, and are thought to be a major pathway for ISF and cerebral metabolites to exit the brain. Recent evidence suggests the PVSs also perform an essential role in maintaining intracranial pressure homeostasis.

Precisely why some PVSs become enlarged is unknown. Most investigators believe ISF egress is blocked, causing cystic enlargement of the PVSs.

Genetics. Sporadic PVS enlargement has no known genetic predilection. Patients with Hurler, Hunter, or Sanfilippo disease accumulate undegraded mucopolysaccharides within enlarged PVSs. A few congenital muscular dystrophies have also been associated with cystic PVSs.

Pathology

Location. Although PVSs can be found virtually anywhere in the brain, they have a striking predilection for the inferior third of the basal ganglia, especially near the anterior commissure

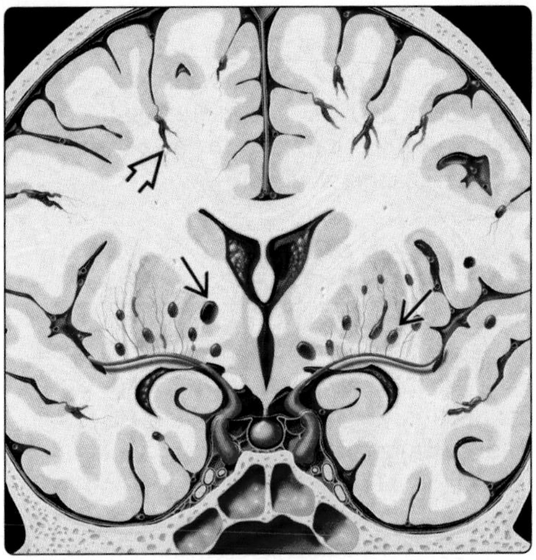

(28-33) Graphic shows normal PVSs along penetrating arteries in the basal ganglia ➡ and subcortical white matter ⇨.

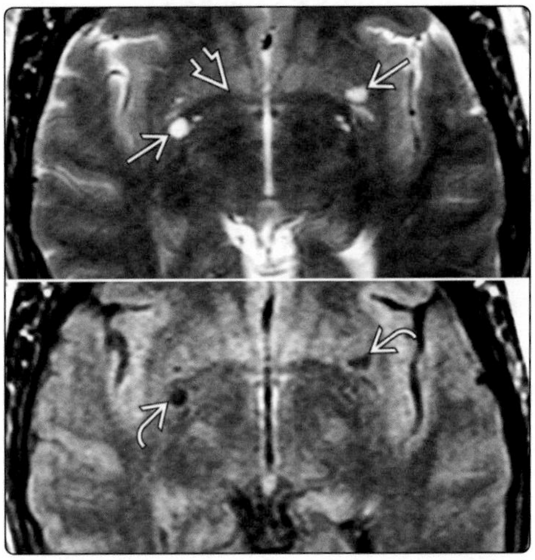

(28-34) (Top) T2WI shows perivascular spaces ➡ clustered around the anterior commissure ⇨. ISF-filled VRSs suppress on FLAIR ↪ (bottom).

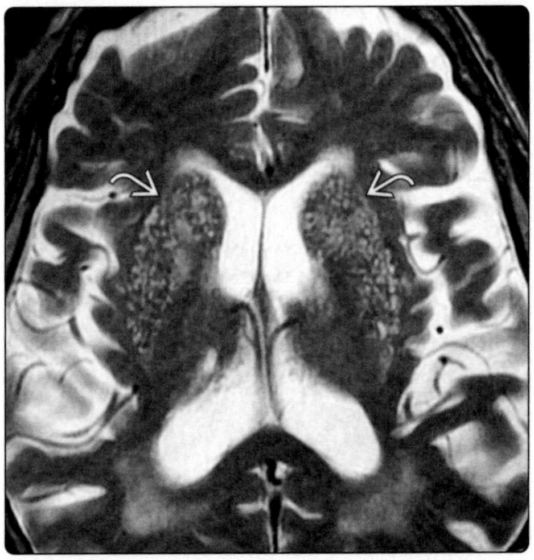

(28-35) Basal ganglia PVSs can become very prominent in older patients ↪, a condition termed "état criblé" or cribriform state.

(28-33). They are also common in the subcortical and deep white matter as well as the midbrain and dentate nuclei of the cerebellum.

Size and Number. Enlarged PVSs tend to occur in clusters. Collections of multiple variably sized PVSs are much more common than solitary unilocular lesions.

Most PVSs are smaller than 2 mm. PVSs increase in size and prevalence with age **(28-35)**. Giant so-called tumefactive PVSs measuring up to 9 cm in diameter have been reported.

Gross Pathology. Enlarged PVSs appear as collections of smoothly demarcated cysts filled with clear colorless fluid **(28-36)**.

Microscopic Features. PVSs are bounded by a single or double layer of invaginated pia. Cortical PVSs are lined by a single layer of pia, whereas two layers accompany lenticulostriate and midbrain arteries.

As a PVS penetrates into the subcortical white matter, it becomes fenestrated and discontinuous. The pial layer disappears completely at the capillary level.

The brain parenchyma surrounding enlarged PVSs is typically normal without gliosis, inflammation, hemorrhage, or discernible amyloid deposition.

Clinical Issues

Epidemiology. PVSs are the most common nonneoplastic parenchymal brain "cysts." With high-resolution 3.0-T MR, small PVSs are seen in nearly all patients **(28-34)**, in virtually every location, and at all ages. Between 25-30% of children have identifiable PVSs on high-resolution MR scans.

Demographics. Enlarged PVSs are more common in middle-aged and older patients and increase in both size and number with age **(28-35)**. Recent studies have linked enlarged PVSs with age, lacunar stroke subtype, and white matter lesions and consider them as an MR marker of cerebral small vessel disease.

Presentation. Most enlarged PVSs do not cause symptoms and are discovered incidentally on imaging studies or at autopsy. Neuropsychological evaluation is typically normal. Nonspecific symptoms such as headache, dizziness, memory impairment, and Parkinson-like symptoms have been reported in some cases, but their relationship to enlarged PVSs is unclear. Large PVSs in the midbrain may cause obstructive hydrocephalus and present with headache.

Natural History. Enlarged PVSs tend to be stable in size and remain unchanged over many years although a few cases of progressively enlarging PVSs have been reported.

Treatment Options. Enlarged PVSs are "leave me alone" lesions that should not be mistaken for serious disease. If midbrain PVSs cause obstructive hydrocephalus, the generally accepted treatment is to shunt the ventricles, not the cysts.

Imaging

General Features. The common pattern of enlarged PVSs is one or more clusters of variably sized CSF-like cysts. They commonly cause focal mass effect. For example, if they occur in the subcortical white matter, the overlying gyri are enlarged with concomitant compression of adjacent sulci **(28-38)**.

CT Findings. Enlarged PVSs are groups of round/ovoid/linear/punctate CSF-like lesions that do not demonstrate calcification or hemorrhage **(28-37)**. PVSs do not enhance following contrast administration.

MR Findings. Even though they are filled with ISF, PVSs closely parallel CSF signal intensity on all imaging sequences. Focal mass effect is common. Enlarged PVSs in the subcortical white matter expand overlying gyri **(28-38)** **(28-39)**. Enlarged PVSs in the midbrain may compress the aqueduct and third ventricle, resulting in intraventricular obstructive hydrocephalus **(28-36)**.

PVSs are isointense with CSF on T1-, PD, and T2WI. They suppress completely on FLAIR **(28-34)**. Edema in the adjacent brain is absent although 25% of "tumefactive" PVSs have minimal increased signal intensity around the cysts.

PVSs do not hemorrhage, enhance, or demonstrate restricted diffusion.

Differential Diagnosis

The major differential diagnosis is chronic **lacunar infarction**. Although they often affect the basal ganglia and suppress on FLAIR, lacunar infarcts do not cluster around the anterior commissure, are often irregular in shape, and frequently exhibit hyperintensity in the adjacent brain.

In some older patients, very prominent PVSs in the basal ganglia are present. This condition, called **"état criblé"** (cribriform state), should not be mistaken for multiple lacunar infarcts. PVSs are round/ovoid and regular in configuration, and the adjacent brain parenchymal is usually normal without gliosis or edema.

Infectious cysts (especially parenchymal neurocysticercosis cysts) are usually small. Although often multiple or multilocular, they typically do not occur in clusters of variably sized cysts as is typical for enlarged PVSs.

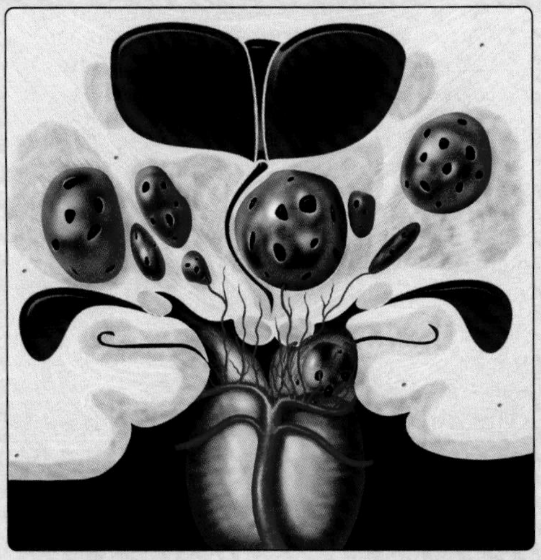

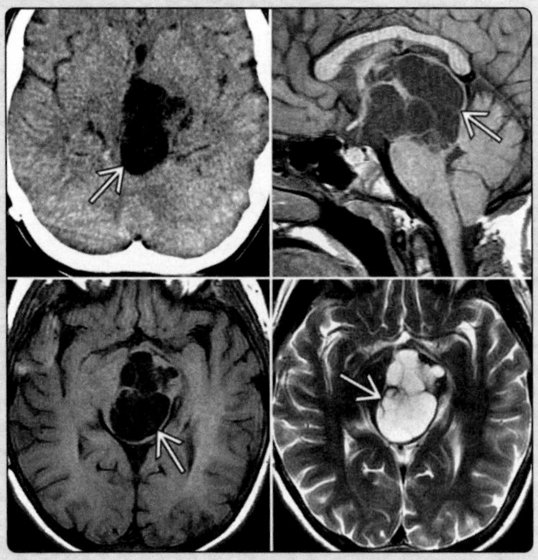

***(28-36)** Coronal graphic shows enlarged perivascular spaces in the midbrain and thalami that cause mass effect on the third ventricle and aqueduct with resulting hydrocephalus. **(28-37)** NECT and MR scans show a cluster of variably sized CSF-like cysts grossly expanding the midbrain. These are giant "tumefactive" perivascular spaces.*

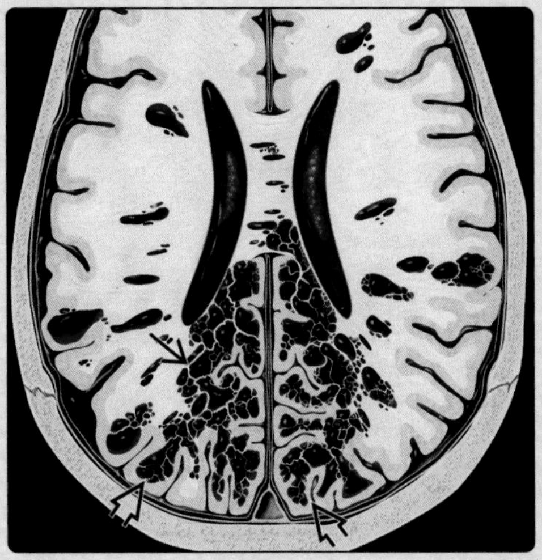

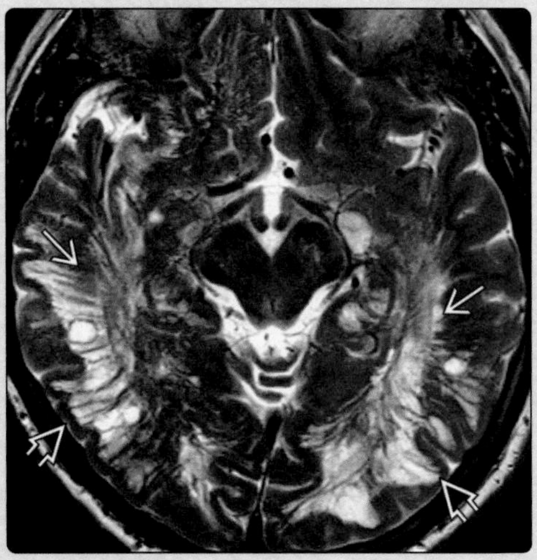

***(28-38)** Graphic depicts innumerable hemispheric enlarged PVSs in subcortical, deep white matter. Note that the overlying gyri are expanded but otherwise normal. **(28-39)** Axial T2WI in a 69y moderately demented man shows innumerable enlarged PVSs. Note sparing of overlying cortex, which appears expanded. (Courtesy M. Warmuth-Metz, MD.)*

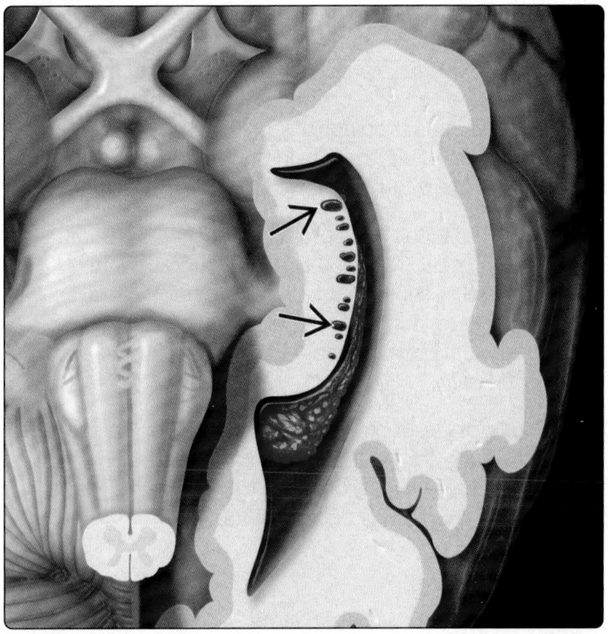

(28-40) Graphic of normal temporal lobe shows a string of cysts within the lateral hippocampus, along the residual cavity of the primitive hippocampal sulcus ⇒. Hippocampal sulcus remnant cysts are incidental, a normal finding.

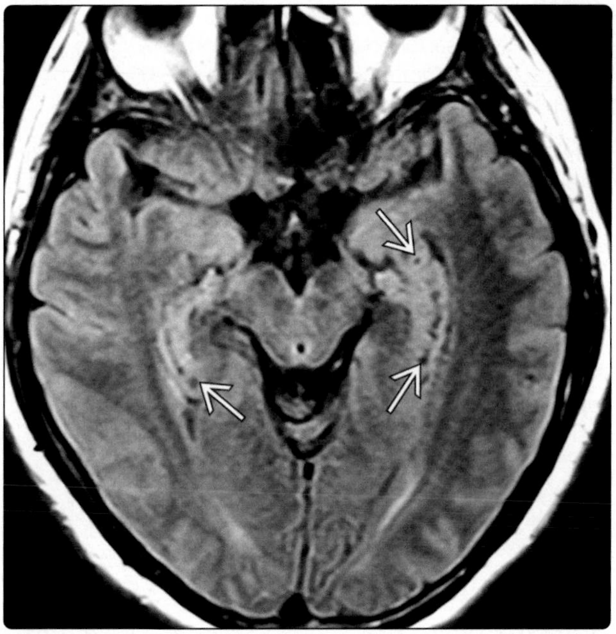

(28-41) Axial FLAIR scan shows hippocampal sulcus remnants as lines of tiny cysts ➡ medial to both temporal lobes. These contain CSF and therefore suppress completely on FLAIR.

ENLARGED PERIVASCULAR SPACES (PVSs)

Terminology
- Also known as Virchow-Robin spaces
- Found around penetrating blood vessels
- Lined by pia, filled with interstitial fluid
- Do not communicate directly with subarachnoid space

Pathology
- Normal PVSs common, < 2 cm
- Giant "tumefactive" PVSs up to 9 cm reported
- Basal ganglia, subcortical WM most common

Imaging
- Often bizarre-looking
- Occur in clusters
- Variably sized cysts
- Follow CSF

Hippocampal Sulcus Remnants

Terminology

Hippocampal sulcus remnants (HCSR) are also called hippocampal remnant cysts and hippocampal sulcal cavities.

Etiology

At 15 fetal weeks, the hippocampus normally unfolds and surrounds an "open" shallow fissure—the hippocampal sulcus—along the medial surface of the temporal lobe. The walls of the hippocampal sulcus gradually fuse, and the sulcus is eventually obliterated.

At times, some segments of the closing hippocampal sulcus fail to fuse. One or more residual cystic cavities remain and persist into adult life. These remnant cavities—hippocampal remnant cysts—are normal anatomic variants **(28-40)**.

Pathology

HCSRs are pia-lined cavities filled with CSF. Small blood vessels are often also included as the hippocampal sulcus forms, folds, and fuses.

Clinical Issues

HCSRs are incidental findings of no clinical significance. They do not cause seizures and are not related to trauma.

Imaging

HCSRs are seen in 10-15% of normal high-resolution MR scans. They appear as a "string of beads" with multiple small round or ovoid cysts curving along the hippocampus between the dentate gyrus and subiculum, just medial to the temporal horn of the lateral ventricle. HCSRs follow CSF in signal intensity on all sequences. They suppress completely on FLAIR **(28-41)**, do not enhance, and do not restrict on DWI.

Differential Diagnosis

The major differential diagnosis HCSRs is **enlarged perivascular spaces**. When they occur in the temporal lobe, enlarged perivascular spaces are found in the subcortical white matter of the insula and anterior tip of the temporal lobe, not medial to the temporal horn of the lateral ventricle.

Neuroglial Cyst

Terminology

Neuroglial cysts (NGCs) are sometimes called **glioependymal cysts** or **neuroepithelial cysts**. They are benign fluid-containing cavities buried within the cerebral white matter.

Pathology

Location. Although NGCs occur throughout the neuraxis, they are usually supratentorial. The frontal lobe is the most common site. They often lie adjacent to—but do not communicate directly with—the cerebral ventricles.

Size and Number. Most NGCs are solitary unilocular cysts. They vary in size from a few millimeters up to several centimeters in diameter.

Gross Pathology. NGCs are rounded, smooth, unilocular cysts that contain clear CSF-like fluid.

Microscopic Features. Most NGCs are lined with a simple, nonstratified, low columnar/cuboidal epithelium **(28-42)**. The epithelium usually sits directly on deep cerebral WM without an intervening capsule or basement membrane.

Clinical Issues

Epidemiology. Parenchymal NGCs are uncommon, representing less than 1% of all intracranial cysts.

Demographics. NGCs occur in all age groups but are generally more common in adults. There is no sex predilection.

Presentation. NGCs are often asymptomatic and found incidentally at imaging or autopsy. The most common presenting symptom, if any, is headache.

Natural History. Many—if not most—NGCs remain stable over many years.

Treatment Options. Serial observation with imaging studies is the usual course. Large NGCs have been fenestrated or drained.

Imaging

General Features. NGCs are smooth, round or ovoid, fluid-containing cysts.

CT Findings. NGCs are fluid density, typically resemble CSF, do not contain calcifications, and do not hemorrhage.

MR Findings. Signal intensity varies with cyst content. Most NGCs are iso- or slightly hyperintense to CSF. They usually suppress on FLAIR, do not restrict, and do not enhance **(28-43)**. The parenchyma surrounding an NGC is usually normal or may show minimal gliosis.

Differential Diagnosis

The diagnosis of NGC is mostly a process of elimination, excluding other, sometimes more ominous possibilities.

The major differential diagnosis of NGC is an **enlarged perivascular space**. Most enlarged PVSs are multiple (not solitary) and occur as clusters of variably sized cysts. A **porencephalic cyst** is a result of an insult to the brain parenchyma. Porencephalic cysts communicate with the ventricle and are lined by gliotic or spongiotic white matter.

Arachnoid cysts are extraaxial, not intraaxial, and are lined with flattened arachnoid cells. **Epidermoid cysts** are almost always extraaxial, do not

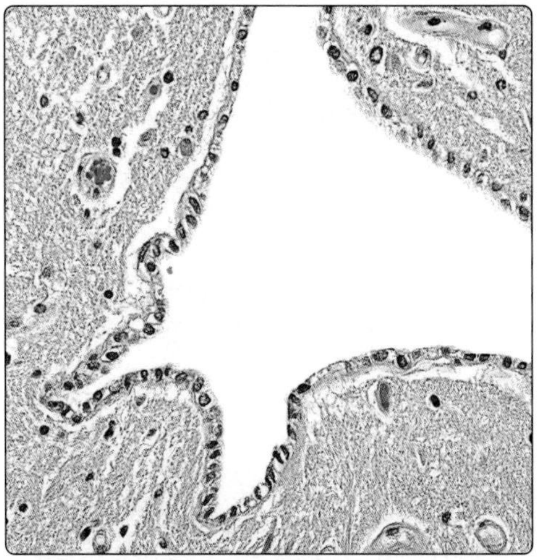

(28-42) Neuroglial cysts are lined by a single layer of cuboidal/low columnar epithelium. Cilia are rare. (Courtesy P. Burger, MD.)

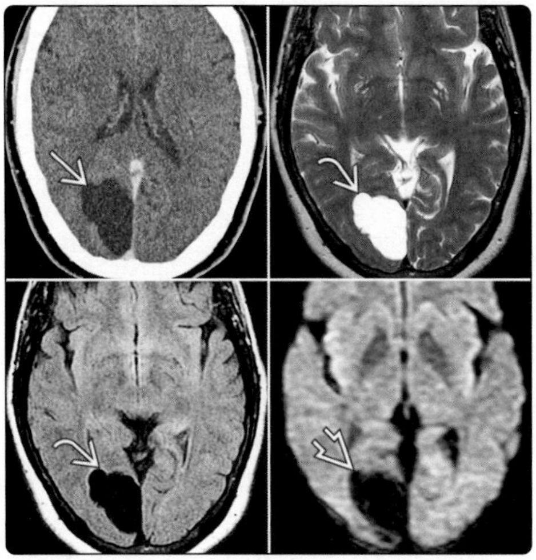

(28-43) Proven neuroglial cyst in the right occipital lobe does not enhance on CECT, follows CSF on T2/FLAIR, does not restrict.

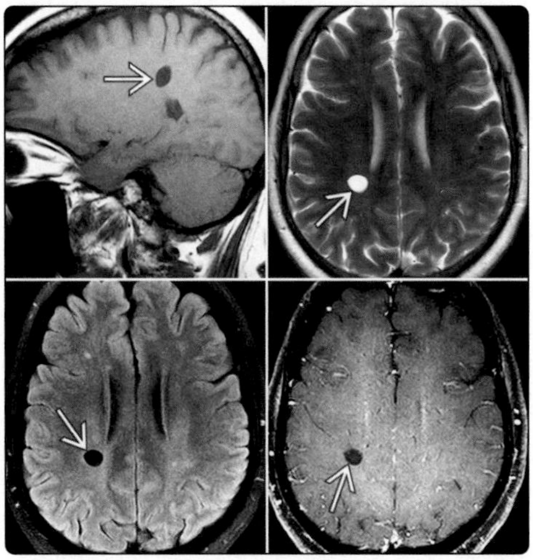

(28-44) MR shows a small presumed right parietal neuroglial cyst. The cyst follows CSF on all sequences and has been stable for 9 years.

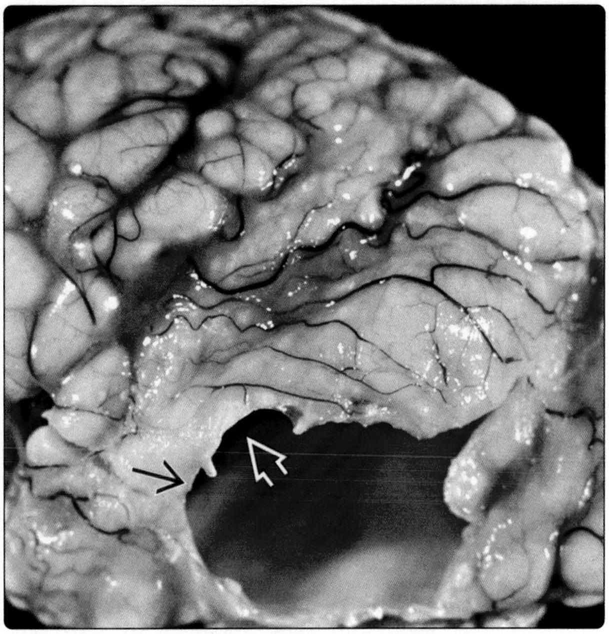

(28-45) Autopsy specimen shows a typical porencephalic cyst as a CSF-filled cavity that extends from the brain surface ⮕ to the ventricular ependyma ⮕. (Courtesy J. Townsend, MD.)

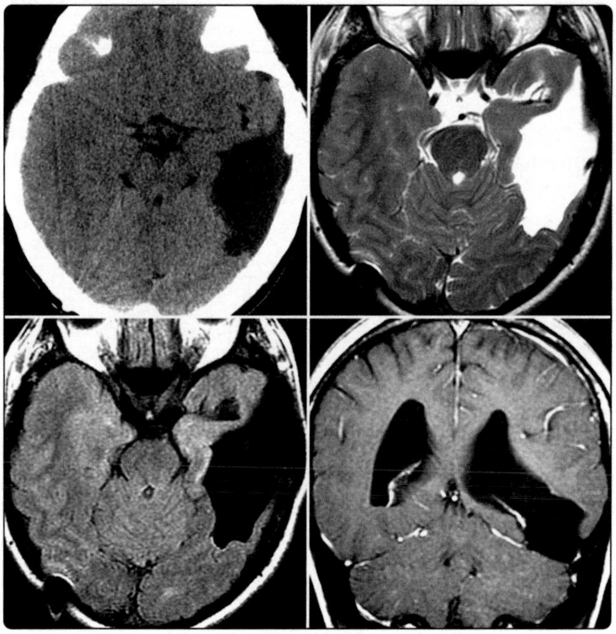

(28-46) NECT, MR scans show a posttraumatic porencephalic cyst extending from the surface of the temporal lobe to the temporal horn of the lateral ventricle. The cyst contains CSF.

suppress on FLAIR, and restrict on DWI. **Ependymal cysts** are intraventricular.

Neoplastic and **inflammatory cysts** generally do not follow CSF, often demonstrate wall enhancement or calcification, and are frequently surrounded by edema.

A variety of miscellaneous periventricular cysts occur in newborns or children. Some may persist into adulthood. These include connatal cysts, germinolytic cysts, and cystic periventricular leukomalacia (PVL). **Connatal cysts** are cystic ependyma-lined areas adjacent to the superolateral margins of the body and frontal horns of the lateral ventricles. They are relatively common and generally innocuous lesions caused by coarctation or coaptation of the walls of the frontal horns.

Germinolytic cysts are glia-lined cysts that lie along the caudothalamic groove. They are associated with inherited metabolic disorders (e.g., Zellweger) and congenital infections (e.g., CMV), often contain septations or hemosiderin, and do not enhance. **Cystic PVL** most frequently occurs in premature infants and is located dorsolaterally to the bodies of the lateral ventricles.

Porencephalic Cyst

Terminology

"Porencephaly" literally means a hole in the brain. Porencephalic cysts are congenital or acquired CSF-filled parenchymal cavities that usually—but not invariably—communicate with the ventricular system. These cysts or cavities also often communicate via a "pore" with the subarachnoid space.

Etiology

Porencephalic cysts are encephaloclastic lesions, the end result of a destructive process (e.g., trauma, infection, vascular insult, surgery) that compromises brain parenchyma.

Most porencephalic cysts are sporadic. A few inherited syndromes (e.g., autosomal-dominant familial porencephaly) have been reported.

Pathology

Porencephalic cysts range in size from a few centimeters to cysts that involve virtually an entire cerebral hemisphere.

Porencephalic cysts are deep, uni- or bilateral, smooth-walled cavities or excavations within the brain parenchyma. They are often "full-thickness" lesions, extending from the ventricle to the glia limitans of the cortex **(28-45)**. Occasionally, a thin rim of ependyma or subependymal white matter may separate the cyst from the ventricle.

Clinical Issues

Epidemiology. Porencephalic cysts are relatively common, especially in children, in whom they represent 2.5% of congenital brain lesions.

Presentation. Spastic hemiplegia, medically refractory epilepsy, and psychomotor retardation are the most common symptoms.

Natural History. Most porencephalic cysts remain stable for many years. Occasionally a porencephalic cyst will continue to sequester fluid and expand, causing mass effect.

Imaging

CT Findings. Porencephalic cysts are sharply marginated, smooth-walled, CSF-filled cavities that usually communicate directly with an adjacent ventricle **(28-46)**. The ipsilateral ventricle is often enlarged secondary to volume loss in the adjacent parenchyma.

Calcification is rare. Bone CT may show skull thinning and remodeling caused by chronic CSF pulsations.

A porencephalic cyst does not enhance.

MR Findings. Porencephalic cysts follow CSF signal intensity on all sequences **(28-46)**. Large cysts may show internal inhomogeneities secondary to spin dephasing. These cysts suppress completely on FLAIR although there is often a rim of hyperintense gliotic or spongiotic white matter around the cyst. No restriction on DWI is present.

Differential Diagnosis

The major differential diagnosis is **cystic encephalomalacia**. An encephalomalacic cavity is often more irregular and does not communicate with the adjacent ventricle.

Porencephalic cysts are lined by reactive gliosis (glial "scar"), which occurs when histologically benign astrocytes proliferate in and around damaged brain parenchyma. A porencephalic cyst with surrounding **reactive gliosis** must be distinguished from **spongiosis**, a process that represents tissue loss (not astrocytic proliferation) with formation of empty (spongiform) areas ("holes") in the brain. Gliosis is a low to medium cellularity lesion that is hyperintense on T2WI and does not suppress on FLAIR. Spongiosis is T2 hyperintense but suppresses on FLAIR.

An **arachnoid cyst** is extraaxial and does not communicate with the ventricle. **Schizencephaly** (literally "split brain") is a congenital lesion that can be either "open" or "closed lip." An "open lip" schizencephalic cleft can look very much like a porencephalic cyst but is lined with dysplastic gray matter, not gliotic white matter.

Hydranencephaly ("water on the brain") is a congenital lesion in which most of the supratentorial developing brain has been destroyed by arterial occlusion. Here the brain looks like a bag of water with little or no remnant cortex. Hydranencephaly is bilateral and symmetric, whereas most porencephalic cysts are unilateral or bilateral but asymmetric.

Intraventricular Cysts

Intraventricular cysts include choroid plexus cysts, colloid cysts, and ependymal cysts.

Choroid Plexus Cysts

Choroid plexus cysts (CPCs) are one of the most common types of intracranial cyst. Most are small and unremarkable. Occasionally, large cysts may appear somewhat atypical and cause diagnostic concern.

Terminology

A CPC is also often called a choroid plexus xanthogranuloma. CPCs are nonneoplastic noninflammatory cysts of the choroid plexus.

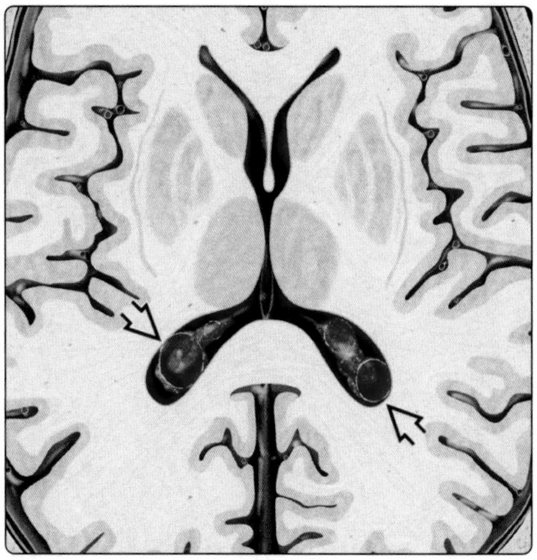

***(28-47)** Multiple cystic masses are in choroid plexus glomi ⇒; in adults, it increases with age. Most are degenerative xanthogranulomas.*

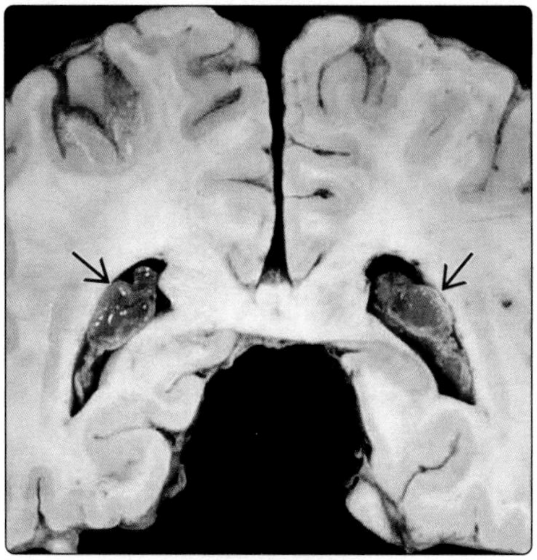

***(28-48)** Autopsy specimen shows multiple cysts in the choroid plexus glomi of both lateral ventricles ⇒. (Courtesy N. Nakase, MD.)*

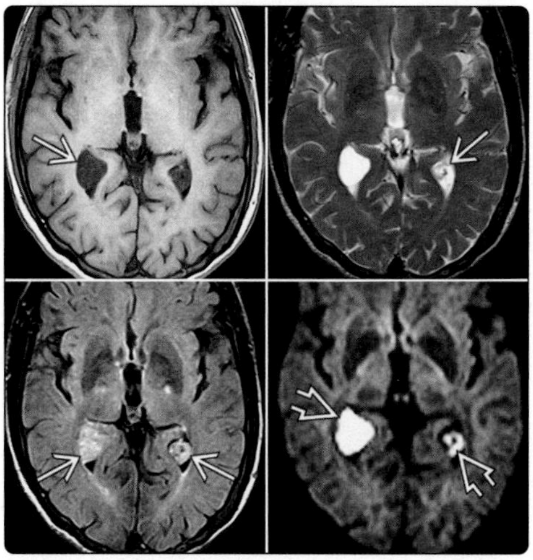

***(28-49)** Choroid plexus cysts are usually bilateral and hyperintense compared with CSF ⇒ and are often very bright on DWI ⇒.*

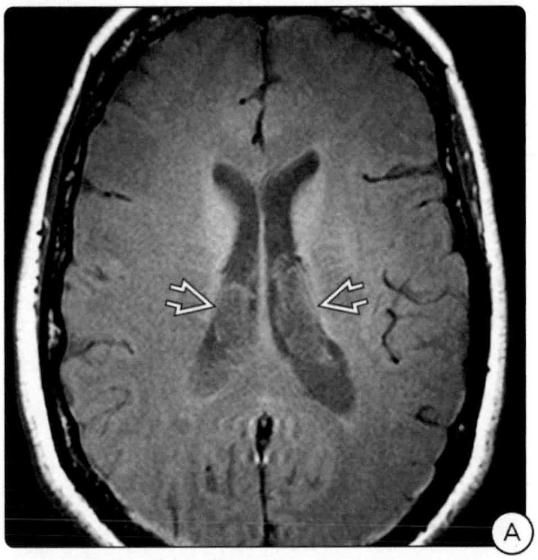

(28-50A) Variant choroid plexus cysts are in the body of the lateral ventricle. Cyst contents ➡ are slightly hyperintense compared with CSF.

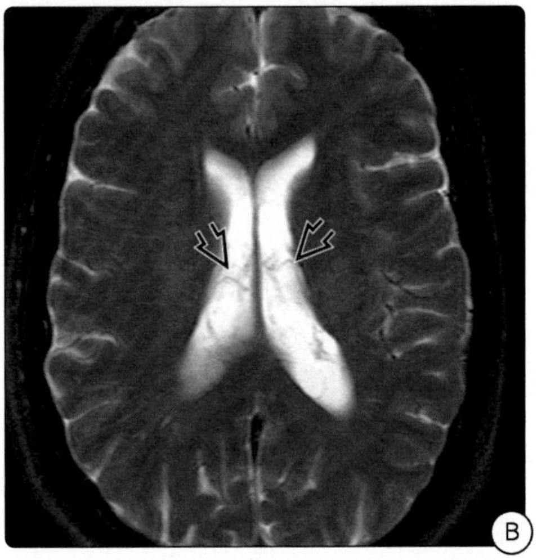

(28-50B) The cysts are so hyperintense on T2WI that the thin cyst walls are barely visible ➡.

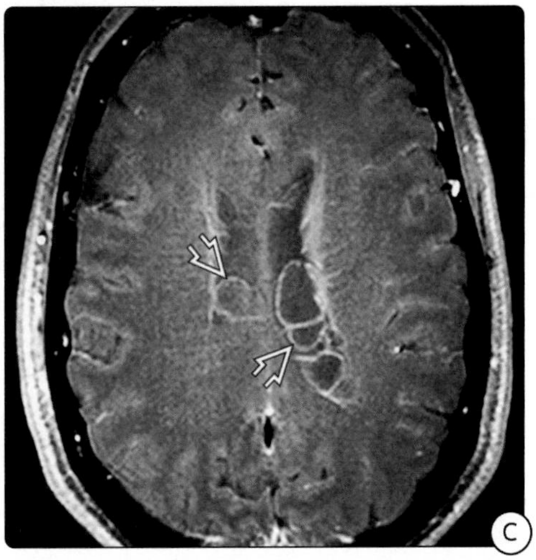

(28-50C) T1 C+ FS shows that the thin walls of these multiloculated choroid plexus cysts enhance moderately ➡.

Etiology

General Concepts. CPCs can be either congenital or acquired. Acquired lesions are much more common; lipid that accumulates from desquamating, degenerating choroid plexus epithelium coalesces into macrocysts and provokes a xanthomatous response.

Genetics. Large (> 10 mm), congenital CPCs can be associated with aneuploidy, particularly trisomy 18. CPCs, together with choroid plexus papillomas, also occur as part of Aicardi syndrome.

Pathology

Location. Most CPCs are found in the atrium of the lateral ventricle, within the choroid plexus glomus **(28-47)**.

Size and Number. CPCs are mostly small, ranging from a few millimeters up to 1 cm although occasionally larger cysts exceed 2 cm in diameter. Multiple bilateral lesions are significantly more common than solitary unilateral CPCs.

Gross Pathology. CPCs are nodular, partly cystic, yellowish-gray masses that are most often found in the choroid plexus glomus **(28-48)**. They are highly proteinaceous and often gelatinous. Gross hemorrhage is rare.

CHOROID PLEXUS CYSTS: ETIOLOGY, PATHOLOGY, AND CLINICAL ISSUES

Etiology
- Congenital
  - Aicardi syndrome
  - Trisomy 18
- Acquired
  - Desquamated, degenerated epithelium
  - Xanthomatous response

Pathology
- Bilateral, usually multiloculated
- Most common in glomi of choroid plexus
- Proteinaceous, gelatinous contents

Clinical Issues
- Most common intracranial cyst
- Most found incidentally
- Most common in fetus/infants, older adults

Clinical Issues

Demographics. CPCs are the most common of all intracranial cysts, occurring in up to 50% of autopsies. CPCs are found at both ends of the age spectrum. In adults, their prevalence increases with age, whereas fetal CPCs decrease with gestational age. There is no sex predilection.

Presentation and Natural History. Most adult CPCs are found incidentally and are asymptomatic, remaining stable for many years. Congenital CPCs are detected on prenatal ultrasound in 1% of fetuses during the second trimester and generally resolve during the third trimester. When detected postnatally, CPCs are of no clinical significance in otherwise normal neonates.

Imaging

CT Findings. CPCs are iso- to slightly hyperdense compared with intraventricular CSF. Irregular clumps of calcification around the margins are

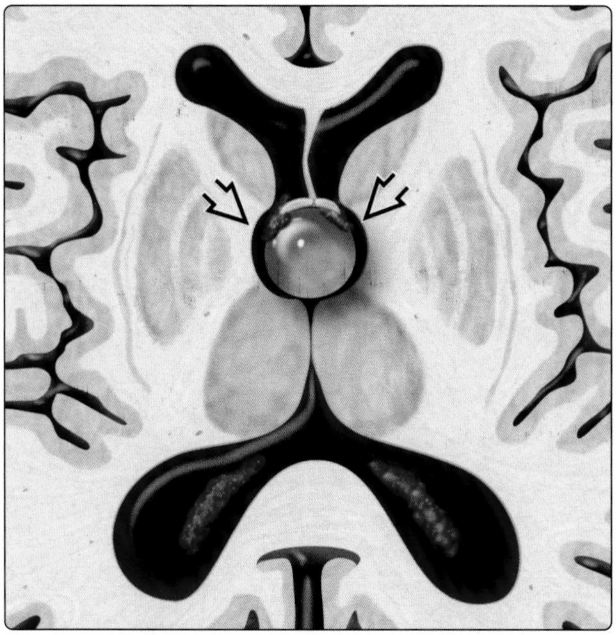

***(28-51)** Axial graphic shows a classic colloid cyst at the foramen of Monro causing mild/moderate obstructive hydrocephalus. Note that the fornices and choroid plexus are elevated and stretched over the cyst ⇨.*

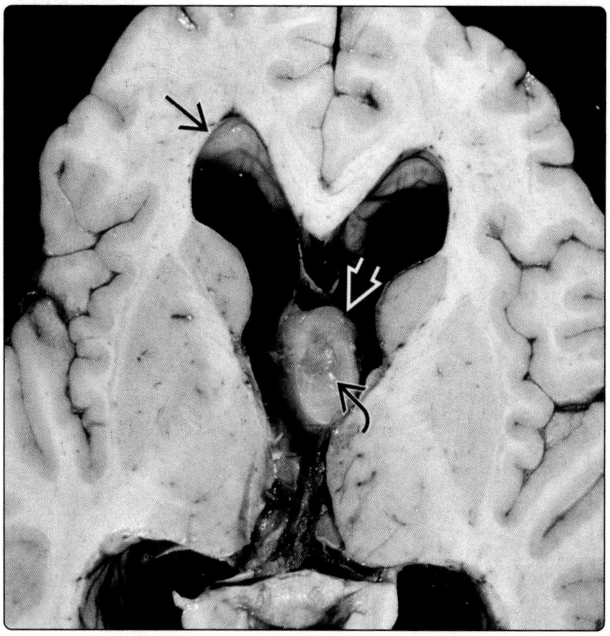

***(28-52)** Autopsy specimen demonstrates obstructive hydrocephalus ⇨ and a large gelatinous-appearing colloid cyst ➡ with a densely fibrotic inspissated center ⇨. Lesion is located within the foramen of Monro. (Courtesy R. Hewlett, MD.)*

common findings. Enhancement varies from none to a complete rim surrounding each cyst.

MR Findings. CPCs do not precisely follow CSF signal intensity. They are iso- to slightly hyperintense compared with CSF on T1WI and are hyperintense on PD and T2WI. FLAIR signal is variable **(28-49)**.

Enhancement following contrast administration varies from none to striking. Solid, ring, and nodular patterns occur **(28-50)**.

Between 60-80% of CPCs appear quite bright on DWI but often remain isointense with parenchyma on ADC. This may therefore represent pseudorestriction rather than true restricted diffusion.

Ultrasound. Fetal ultrasound may show multiple cysts of variable sizes.

Differential Diagnosis

The major differential diagnosis of a CPC is an **ependymal cyst**. Ependymal cysts generally displace and compress the choroid plexus rather than arise from it. Ependymal cysts usually behave much more like CSF than CPCs do. Intraventricular parasitic cysts, specifically those of **neurocysticercosis**, are relatively uncommon. They are not associated with the choroid plexus. A scolex is often present. Intraventricular **epidermoid cysts** occur but are rare in the lateral ventricles.

CHOROID PLEXUS CYST: IMAGING AND DDx

CT
- Iso-/mildly hyperdense
- Ca++ common

MR
- Iso-/mildly hyperintense to CSF on T1WI
- Hyperintense on PD/T2WI, FLAIR variable
- Variable enhancement (usually thin rim)
- Bright on DWI but isointense on ADC

Differential Diagnosis
- Most common = ependymal cyst
- Uncommon/rare
  - Epidermoid cyst (rarely intraventricular)
  - Cystic metastasis

Choroid plexus papilloma of the lateral ventricle is a tumor of children younger than 5 years old and enhances intensely. An enhancing, enlarged choroid plexus without frank cyst formation can also be seen with **Sturge-Weber malformation, collateral venous drainage,** and **diffuse villous hyperplasia**. Sturge-Weber and collateral venous drainage usually cause unilateral choroid plexus enlargement. The entire choroid plexus is enlarged in diffuse villous hyperplasia.

Colloid Cyst

Terminology

Colloid cysts (CCs) are also called paraphyseal cysts. They are unilocular, mucin-containing cysts that are almost always

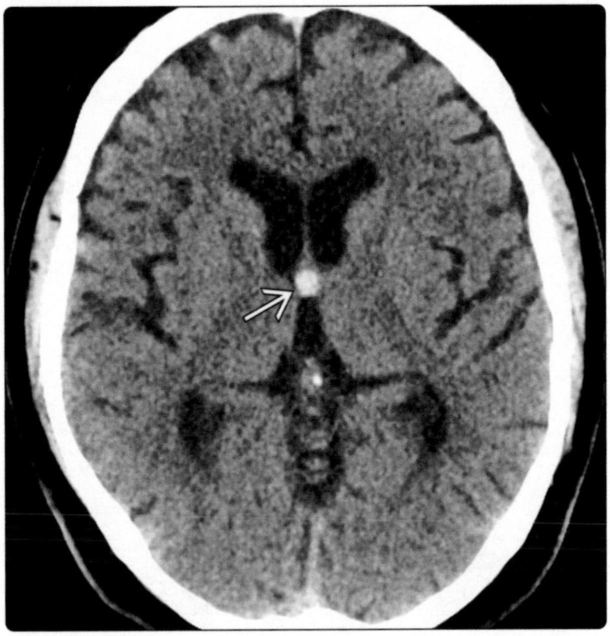

(28-53) *NECT scan reveals a classic colloid cyst as a well-circumscribed hyperdense mass* ➡ *in the foramen of Monro.*

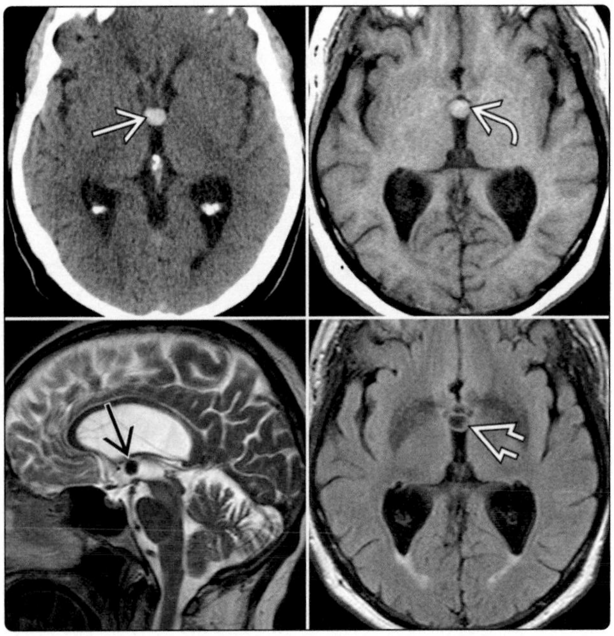

(28-54) *NECT scan shows hyperdense colloid cyst* ➡ *that is hyperintense on T1WI* ➡*, hypointense on T2WI* ➡*, with mixed signal intensity on FLAIR* ➡*.*

found wedged into the top of the third ventricle at the foramen of Monro **(28-51)**.

Etiology

General Concepts. CCs are endodermal—rather than neuroectodermal—cysts. They are similar to the other intracranial foregut-derived cysts, i.e., Rathke cleft and neurenteric cysts. Although their precise etiology is unknown, they are presumed to arise from ectopic endodermal elements that migrate into the embryonic diencephalic roof.

Genetics. No specific gene mutations have been identified. A few rare familial CCs have been described that appear to have an autosomal-recessive pattern of inheritance with variable penetrance.

Pathology

Location. More than 99% of CCs are wedged into the foramen of Monro, attached to the anterosuperior roof of the third ventricle. The posterior aspects of the frontal horns of the lateral ventricle are splayed laterally around the cyst, and the pillars of the fornix "straddle" the CC.

Size and Number. CCs are virtually always solitary lesions. Size varies from tiny (a few millimeters) up to 3 cm. Mean diameter is 1.5 cm.

Gross Pathology. CCs are smooth-walled, well-demarcated, spherical or ovoid cysts that have a gelatinous center of variable viscosity **(28-52)**. Gross hemorrhage is very rare.

Microscopic Features. The wall of a CC consists of a thin fibrous capsule that is lined with simple or pseudostratified columnar epithelium. Some ciliated and mucin-secreting goblet cells are interspersed throughout the cyst lining. Like other endodermal cysts, CCs are cytokeratin and EMA positive on immunohistochemistry.

Clinical Issues

Epidemiology. CCs account for about 1% of all intracranial tumors but cause 15-20% of all intraventricular tumors.

Demographics. Most symptomatic CCs present between the third and fifth decades. The peak age is 40 years. Pediatric CCs are rare; less than 8% of all patients are younger than 15 years at the time of initial diagnosis. There is no sex predilection.

Presentation. The clinical presentation of CCs is diverse, ranging from asymptomatic, incidentally discovered cysts (nearly half of all patients) to acute deterioration, coma, and death. CCs cause symptoms when they obstruct CSF flow at the foramina of Monro. Headache is the presenting symptom in 50-60% of symptomatic patients.

Natural History. Over 90% of CCs—especially small cysts found in older patients—are stable and do not enlarge. The roughly 10% that *do* enlarge tend to be larger lesions, often causing hydrocephalus, and found in younger patients. Incidental lesions rarely cause acute obstructive hydrocephalus or sudden neurological deterioration.

Cyst "apoplexy" with intracystic hemorrhage and sudden enlargement occurs but is rare.

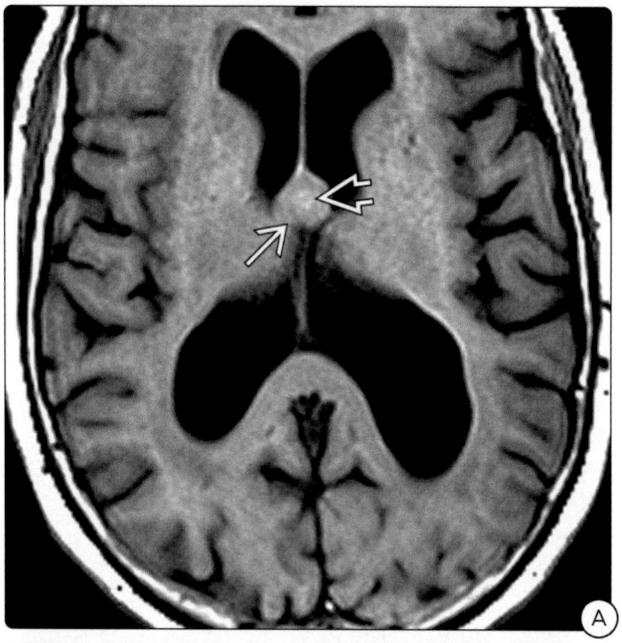

(28-55A) Axial T1WI in a 78y woman with headaches shows moderately enlarged lateral ventricles and isointense mass at the foramen of Monro ➡. Faint hyperintensity in the middle of the mass ➡ suggests inspissated mucous in a colloid cyst.

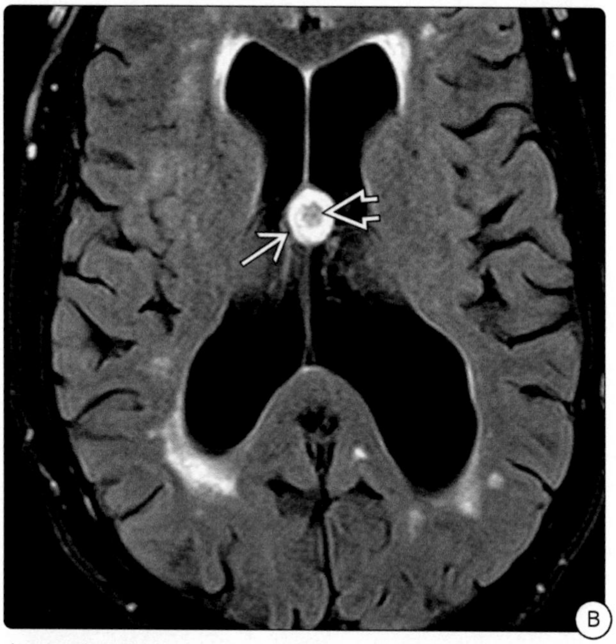

(28-55B) FLAIR in the same case shows that most of the cyst is hyperintense ➡. The center of the cyst appears isointense with brain ➡. Colloid cyst with inspissated mucous was removed at surgery.

COLLOID CYST: PATHOETIOLOGY AND CLINICAL ISSUES

Etiology
- Endodermal cyst
- Probably derived from ectopic elements in diencephalic roof

Pathology
- Foramen of Monro (> 99%)
- Size varies from a few millimeters up to 3 cm
- Fibrous capsule
- Cyst lining
  - Columnar epithelium
  - Mucin-secreting goblet cells
- Gelatinous center (variable viscosity)

Clinical Issues
- Epidemiology
  - 1% of all intracranial tumors
  - 15-20% of intraventricular masses
- Peak age = 40 years (rare in children)
- Asymptomatic, found incidentally (50%)
- Headache most common symptom
- Sudden obstruction can cause coma, death
- Stable, do not enlarge (90%)

Treatment Options. Small asymptomatic CCs that are discovered incidentally and followed with serial imaging rarely grow or cause obstructive hydrocephalus. However, their treatment is debated. Neuroendoscopic management has emerged as a safe, effective alternative to microsurgery with either a transcortical-transventricular or a transcallosal approach.

Imaging

General Features. CCs are well-delineated round or ovoid masses. Imaging appearance depends on their viscosity and/or cholesterol content. The relative amounts of mucous material, cholesterol, protein, and water content all affect density/signal intensity. Desiccated, inspissated cysts appear very different from water-rich lesions.

CT Findings. Density on NECT correlates directly with the hydration state of the cyst contents. Nearly two-thirds of all CCs are hyperdense compared with brain **(28-53)**, whereas one-third are iso- to hypodense **(28-56A)**. Hydrocephalus is variable. Intracystic hemorrhage and calcification are very rare.

Most CCs show no enhancement. Occasionally, a thin enhancing rim surrounds the cyst. Solid or nodular enhancement almost never occurs.

CTA/CTV demonstrates that the internal cerebral veins are displaced posterolaterally around the CC.

MR Findings. Signal intensity varies with cyst content.

Signal intensity on T1WI reflects cholesterol concentration. Most CCs are hyperintense compared with brain **(28-54)**, but one-third are isointense. Small isointense CCs may be very difficult to identify on T1WI.

Signal on PD and T2WI is more variable, as it is more reflective of water content. Most CCs are minimally hyperintense to brain on PD and usually isointense on T2WI **(28-54)**. A few CCs with inspissated contents are hypointense. Approximately 25% demonstrate mixed hypo- and hyperintensity (the "black hole" effect). Fluid-fluid levels are rare.

CCs do not suppress on FLAIR **(28-55)**, nor do they restrict on DWI.

CCs generally do not enhance. A thin peripheral rim of enhancement can be seen in some cases **(28-56)**.

Differential Diagnosis

A well-delineated focal hyperdense lesion at the foramen of Monro on NECT scan is virtually pathognomonic of a CC. Occasionally, extreme **ectasia of an artery**—usually the basilar artery—can mimic a CC although serial sections easily demonstrate the tubular nature of the ectatic vessel.

On MR, the most common "lesion" that mimics a CC is artifact caused by **pulsatile CSF flow**. Phase artifact propagated across the image is helpful in establishing the etiology. Multiplanar imaging and other pulse sequences are also helpful.

Neoplasms such as **metastasis** and **subependymoma** (usually in the frontal horn or foramen of Monro, not anterosuperior third ventricle) can be hyperdense on NECT scans. Large **craniopharyngiomas** and pituitary **macroadenomas** occasionally extend superiorly almost to the foramen of Monro. Multiplanar MR shows that the origin of these tumors is inferior to the third ventricle.

Rarely, an **astrocytoma** or **lymphoma** can infiltrate and thicken the fornices and thus mimic a CC. Most all of these neoplasms are diffusely infiltrating, nonfocal lesions that often show moderate to marked enhancement following contrast administration.

Other third ventricle/foramen of Monro **choroid plexus masses** such as papilloma, xanthogranuloma, and choroid plexus cysts are rare.

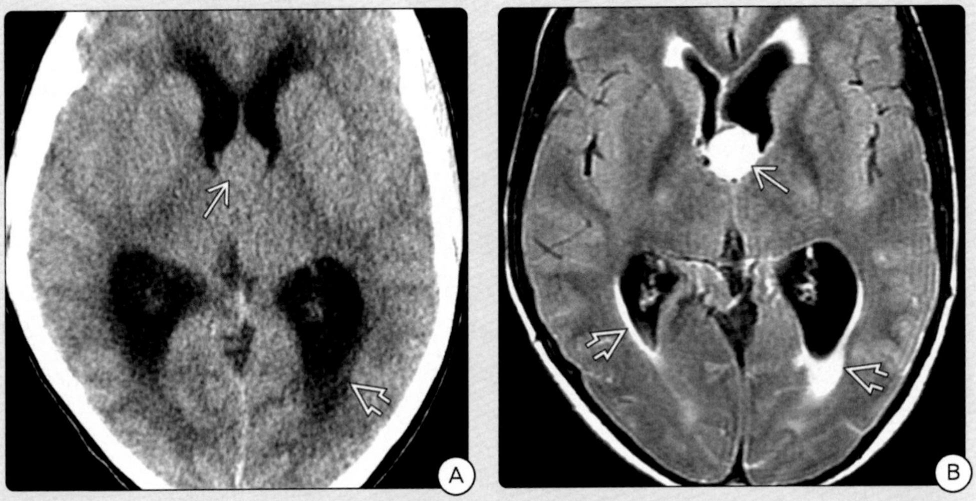

***(28-56A)** Patient had sudden-onset severe headache before he became comatose. Emergency NECT scan shows an isodense mass at the foramen of Monro → with enlarged ventricles. Note the "blurred" ventricular margins ⇨. **(28-56B)** FLAIR shows that the cyst is hyperintense →. The "halo" of fluid ⇨ around the lateral ventricles is secondary to obstructed drainage of interstitial fluid in the deep cerebral WM.*

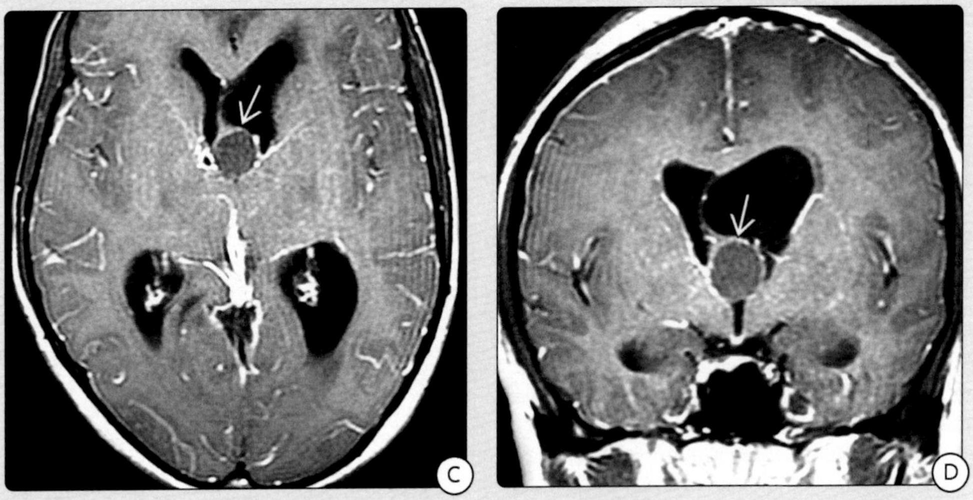

***(28-56C)** T1 C+ FS demonstrates a rim of enhancement around the cyst →. **(28-56D)** Coronal T1 C+ also shows the enhancing rim →. This is a variant colloid cyst.*

COLLOID CYST: IMAGING AND DDx

Imaging
- CT
  - 2/3 hyperdense
  - 1/3 iso- to hypodense
  - Usually do not enhance
- MR
  - Signal intensity varies with sequence, cyst contents
  - Typical: T1 hyper-, T2 hypointense
  - Inspissated: T2 hypointense
  - "Black hole" effect (25%)
  - Do not suppress on FLAIR
  - Generally do not enhance
  - Thin peripheral rim enhancement may occur
  - No restriction on DWI

Differential Diagnosis
- Most common
  - Ectatic basilar artery (NECT)
  - CSF flow artifact (MR)
- Less common
  - Metastasis
  - Subependymoma
  - Pituitary macroadenoma
  - Craniopharyngioma
- Rare but important
  - Low-grade astrocytoma
  - Lymphoma
  - Choroid plexus papilloma
  - Choroid plexus cyst
  - Xanthogranuloma

Ependymal Cyst

Terminology

Ependymal cysts are also called glioependymal cysts. Some authors consider ependymal cysts a subtype of neuroepithelial cyst.

Pathology

Ependymal cysts are solitary lesions that are most often found in the atrium of the lateral ventricles, where they may cause significant ventricular asymmetry **(28-57)**. Less commonly they occur in the brain parenchyma.

Ependymal cysts are rare lesions, accounting for less than 1% of all nonneoplastic intracranial cysts. Their precise pathogenesis is unknown.

Ependymal cysts are usually unilocular, thin walled, and filled with clear CSF-like liquid. They are lined by a layer of simple columnar or cuboidal cells that are similar to the normal endoventricular lining.

Clinical Issues

Ependymal cysts are typically asymptomatic and discovered incidentally at imaging or autopsy. Most patients present as young adults (under 40 years of age). Nonspecific symptoms such as headache and cognitive dysfunction are common. Large ependymal cysts occasionally cause obstructive hydrocephalus and increased intracranial pressure.

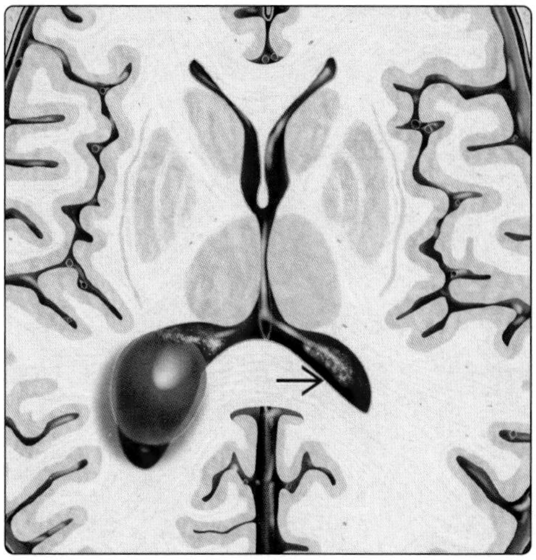

***(28-57)** Graphic depicts ependymal cyst of the lateral ventricle → as a CSF-containing simple cyst that displaces the choroid plexus around it.*

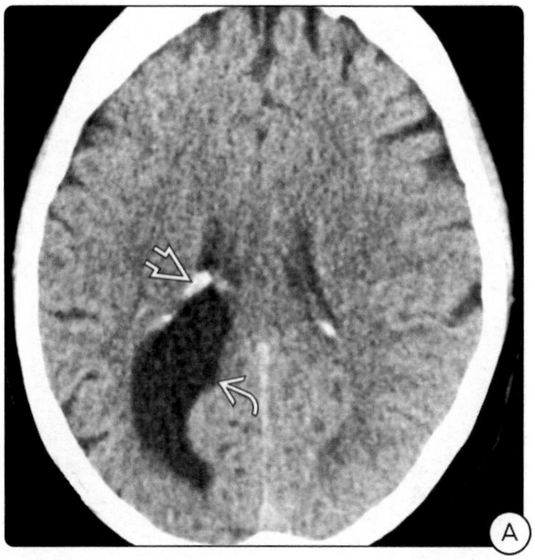

***(28-58A)** Axial NECT of ependymal cyst shows a CSF-containing mass → displacing the calcified choroid plexus around it →.*

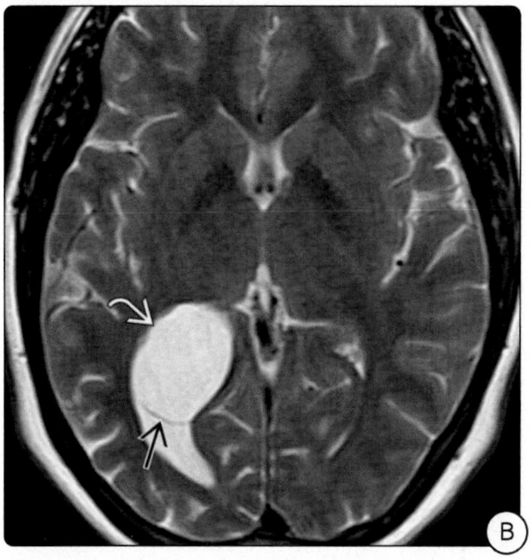

***(28-58B)** T2WI in the same case shows that the unilocular ependymal cyst → is exactly like CSF. Note distinct cyst wall →.*

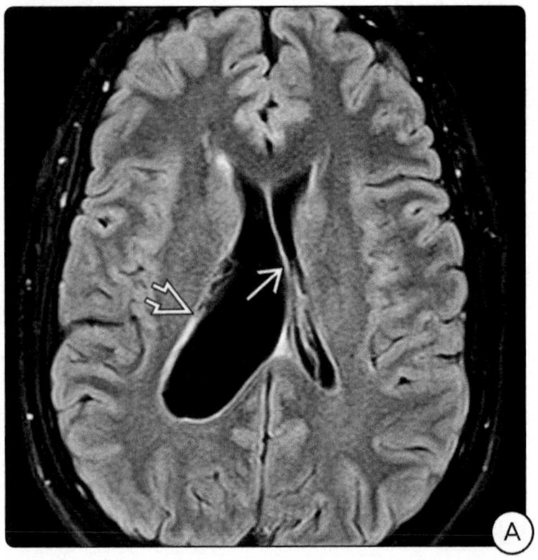

(28-59A) FLAIR, 27y man with severe headaches, shows enlarged body of right lateral ventricle ⇨, displaced septum pellucidum, fornices ➡.

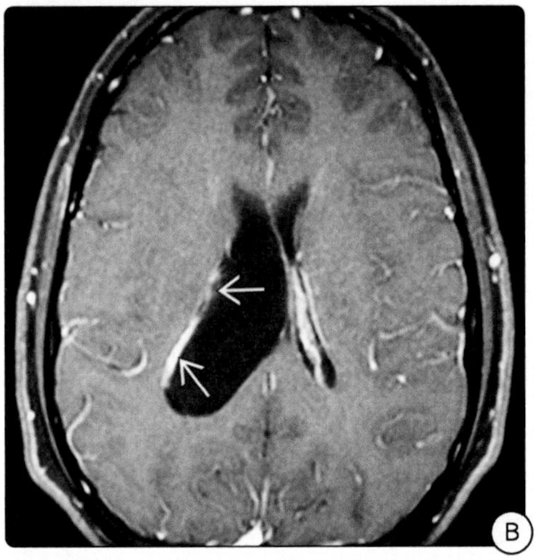

(28-59B) T1 C+ FS shows that the choroid plexus is displaced laterally ➡, but no intraventricular mass can be identified.

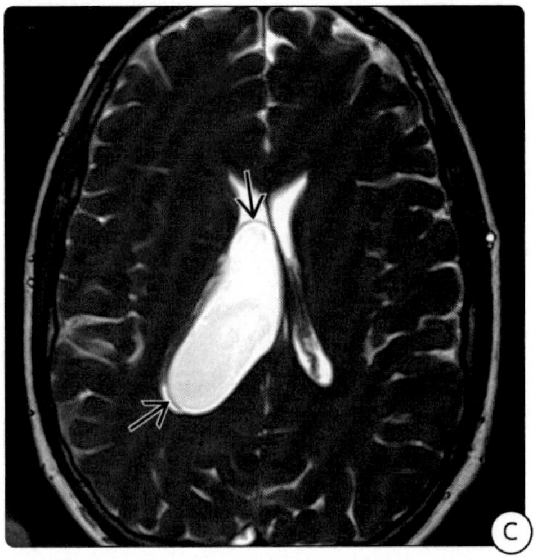

(28-59C) Constructive interference in steady state (CISS) clearly shows wall of an ependymal cyst ⇨ causing the ventricular dilatation.

Imaging

Ependymal cysts parallel CSF in density/signal intensity **(28-58)**. They suppress completely on FLAIR, do not enhance, and do not demonstrate diffusion restriction. Thin-section heavily T2-weighted sequences such as constructive interference in a steady state (CISS) may be necessary to delineate the cyst wall **(28-59)**.

Differential Diagnosis

Except for location, ependymal cysts may be indistinguishable on imaging from other benign intracranial cysts such as neuroglial cysts.

The major intraventricular mass that can mimic ependymal cyst is a **choroid plexus cyst**. Choroid plexus cysts are typically bilateral, often multilocular, and located within the choroid plexus glomi. Ependymal cysts arise *outside* the choroid plexus and usually displace it superolaterally.

Epidermoid cysts are rare in the lateral ventricle. They do not suppress completely on FLAIR and demonstrate diffusion restriction on DWI. **Arachnoid cysts** are identical to ependymal cysts in density and signal intensity but are rarely intraventricular. **Cystic metastases** to the choroid plexus are rare; nodular or irregular rim enhancement is typical.

EPENDYMAL CYST

Terminology
- Also called glioependymal or neuroepithelial cyst

Pathology
- 1% of intracranial cysts
- Solitary, usually unilocular
- Lined by columnar epithelium
- Contain CSF

Clinical Issues
- Most asymptomatic, discovered incidentally
- All ages, but usually < 40 years

Imaging
- Density, signal intensity = CSF
- No enhancement, no restriction

Differential Diagnosis
- Most common
  - Choroid plexus cyst
- Uncommon/rare
  - Epidermoid cyst
  - Arachnoid cyst
  - Cystic metastasis

Selected References

Extraaxial Cysts

Ajtai B et al: Imaging of intracranial cysts. Continuum (Minneap Minn). 22(5, Neuroimaging):1553-1573, 2016

Osborn AG, Preece MT. Intracranial cysts: radiologic-pathologic correlation and imaging approach. Radiology. 239(3):650-64, 2006

Arachnoid Cyst

Lee CH et al: Comparative analysis of bleeding risk by the location and shape of arachnoid cysts: a finite element model analysis. Childs Nerv Syst. 33(1):125-134, 2017

Nikolić I et al: The association of arachnoid cysts and focal epilepsy: hospital based case control study. Clin Neurol Neurosurg. 159:39-41, 2017

Chen Y et al: Treatment of middle cranial fossa arachnoid cysts: a systematic review and meta-analysis. World Neurosurg. 92:480-490.e2, 2016

Hall A et al: Spontaneous subdural haemorrhage from an arachnoid cyst: a case report and literature review. Br J Neurosurg. 1-4, 2016

Rabiei K et al: Prevalence and symptoms of intracranial arachnoid cysts: a population-based study. J Neurol. 263(4):689-94, 2016

Choroid Fissure Cyst

Tubbs RS et al: Progressive symptomatic increase in the size of choroidal fissure cysts. J Neurosurg Pediatr. 10(4):306-9, 2012

Epidermoid Cyst

Ravindran K et al: Intracranial white epidermoid cyst with dystrophic calcification - a case report and literature review. J Clin Neurosci. 42:43-47, 2017

Pikis S et al: Malignant transformation of a residual cerebellopontine angle epidermoid cyst. J Clin Neurosci. 33:59-62, 2016

Dermoid Cyst

Jin H et al: Intracranial dermoid cyst rupture-related brain ischemia: case report and hemodynamic study. Medicine (Baltimore). 96(4):e5631, 2017

McArdle DJ et al: Ruptured intracranial dermoid cyst. Pract Neurol. 16(6):478-479, 2016

Neurenteric Cyst

Singh P et al: Neurenteric cyst: magnetic resonance imaging findings in an adolescent. J Pediatr Neurosci. 12(1):29-31, 2017

Chakraborty S et al: Supratentorial neurenteric cysts: case series and review of pathology, imaging, and clinical management. World Neurosurg. 85:143-52, 2016

Chen CT et al: Neurenteric cyst or neuroendodermal cyst? Immunohistochemical study and pathogenesis. World Neurosurg. 96:85-90, 2016

Prasad GL et al: Ventral foramen magnum neurenteric cysts: a case series and review of literature. Neurosurg Rev. 39(4):535-44, 2016

Preece MT, Osborn AG, Chin SS, Smirniotopoulos JG. Intracranial neurenteric cysts: imaging and pathology spectrum. AJNR Am J Neuroradiol. 27(6):1211-6, 2006.

Pineal Cyst

Evans RW: Incidental findings and normal anatomical variants on MRI of the brain in adults for primary headaches. Headache. 57(5):780-791, 2017

Májovský M et al: Conservative and surgical treatment of patients with pineal cysts: a prospective case series of 110 patients. World Neurosurg. ePub, 2017

Starke RM et al: Pineal cysts and other pineal region malignancies: determining factors predictive of hydrocephalus and malignancy. J Neurosurg. 1-6, 2016

Parenchymal Cysts

Enlarged Perivascular Spaces

Sung J et al: Linear sign in cystic brain lesions ≥5 mm: a suggestive feature of perivascular space. Eur Radiol. ePub, 2017

Bakker EN et al: Lymphatic clearance of the brain: perivascular, paravascular and significance for neurodegenerative diseases. Cell Mol Neurobiol. 36(2):181-94, 2016

Ramirez J et al: Imaging the perivascular space as a potential biomarker of neurovascular and neurodegenerative diseases. Cell Mol Neurobiol. 36(2):289-99, 2016

Zhang X et al: Brain atrophy correlates with severe enlarged perivascular spaces in basal ganglia among lacunar stroke patients. PLoS One. 11(2):e0149593, 2016

Neuroglial Cyst

Ajtai B et al: Imaging of intracranial cysts. Continuum (Minneap Minn). 22(5, Neuroimaging):1553-1573, 2016

Porencephalic Cyst

Abergel A et al: Expanding porencephalic cysts: prenatal imaging and differential diagnosis. Fetal Diagn Ther. 41(3):226-233, 2017

Intraventricular Cysts

Colloid Cyst

Brostigen CS et al: Surgical management of colloid cyst of the third ventricle. Acta Neurol Scand. 135(4):484-487, 2017

Hamidi H et al: CT and MRI features of pediatric-aged colloid cysts: report of two cases. Case Rep Radiol. 2017:2467085, 2017

Beaumont TL et al: Natural history of colloid cysts of the third ventricle. J Neurosurg. 1-11, 2016

Byard RW: Variable presentations of lethal colloid cysts. J Forensic Sci. 61(6):1538-1540, 2016

Cox M et al: The isodense colloid cyst: an easily overlooked cause of intermittent acute obstructive hydrocephalus. Intern Emerg Med. ePub, 2016

Ependymal Cyst

El Damaty A et al: Neuroendoscopic approach to intracranial ependymal cysts. World Neurosurg. 97:383-389, 2017

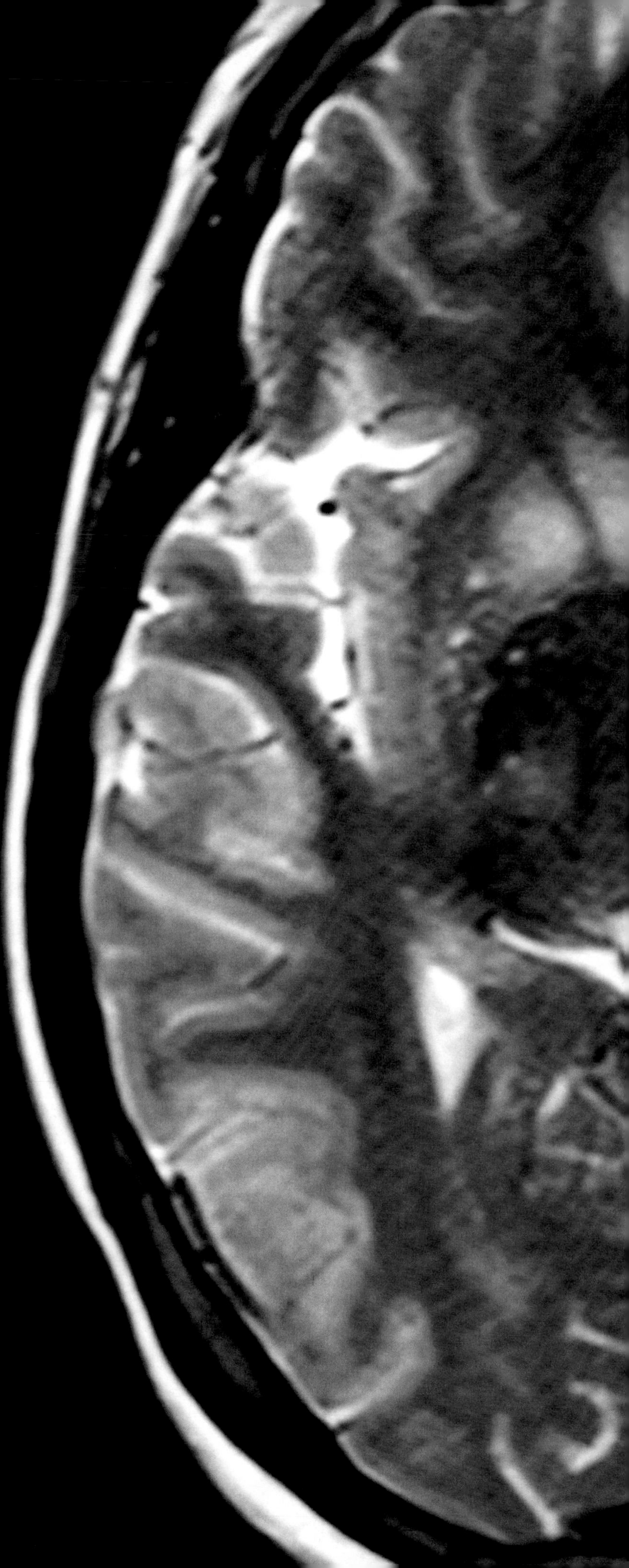

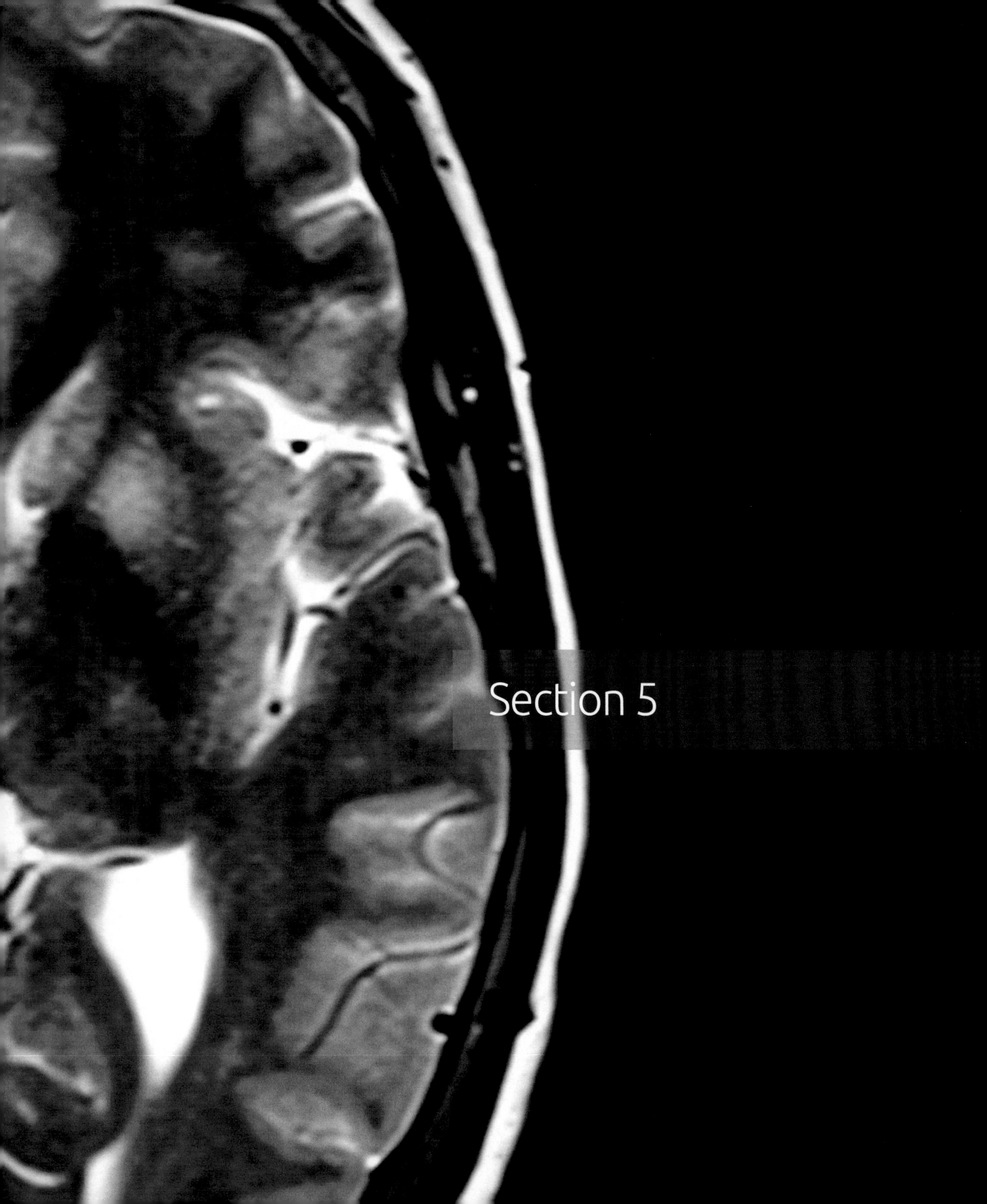

Section 5

Section 5

Toxic, Metabolic, Degenerative, and CSF Disorders

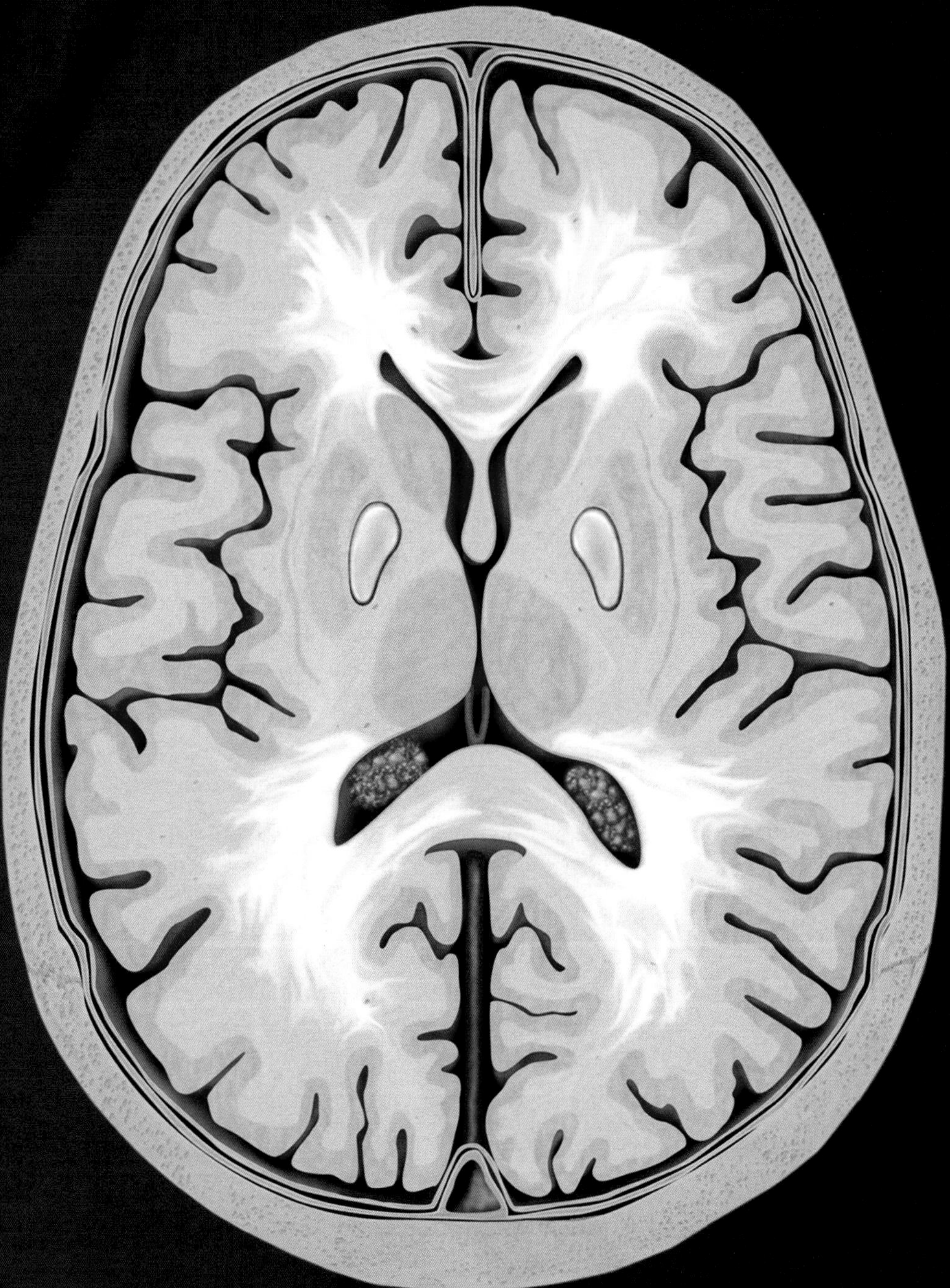

Approach to Toxic, Metabolic, Degenerative, and CSF Disorders

This part, devoted to toxic, metabolic, degenerative, and CSF disorders, addresses some of the most difficult and challenging issues in neuroimaging. In contrast to many other brain diseases, here the CNS effects are often secondary to systemic disorders. Patients who present acutely with encephalopathy may have unknown or undiagnosed metabolic derangements.

Metabolic disorders are relatively uncommon but important diseases in which imaging can play a key role in early diagnosis and appropriate patient management. Drug and alcohol abuse are increasing around the world, and the list of environmental toxins that can affect the CNS continues to increase. Recognizing toxic and metabolic-induced encephalopathies has become a clinical and imaging imperative. The two etiologies are often linked because many toxins induce metabolic derangements and some systemic metabolic diseases have a direct toxic effect on the brain.

With rapidly increasing numbers of aging people, the prevalence of dementia and brain degeneration is also becoming a global concern. Brain scans in elderly patients with mental status changes are now some of the most frequently requested imaging examinations.

Advanced MR techniques such as morphometric-volumetric analyses, diffusion tensor imaging, tractography, and iron content-sensitive imaging are now being used to obtain quantitative parameters that may increase diagnostic accuracy.

Because inherited and acquired toxic, metabolic, and degenerative brain disorders often affect the deep gray nuclei in a bilaterally symmetric pattern, we begin this section by considering the normal physiology, gross anatomy, and imaging of the basal ganglia and dopaminergic striatonigral system.

We then present an anatomy-based approach to the differential diagnosis of toxic, metabolic, and degenerative disorders. Shaded text boxes and representative cases illustrate this approach to—and some supplemental considerations for—imaging diagnosis.

Lastly, we briefly discuss normal age-related changes in the CNS, which lays the foundation for an imaging approach to dementia, brain degeneration, and CSF disorders.

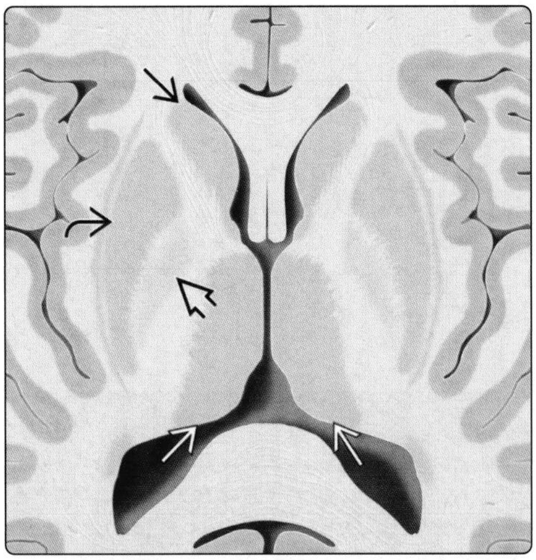

***(29-1)** Graphic depicts basal ganglia, caudate nucleus ➡, putamen ➡, globus pallidus (GP) ➡. Thalami ➡ form borders of the third ventricle.*

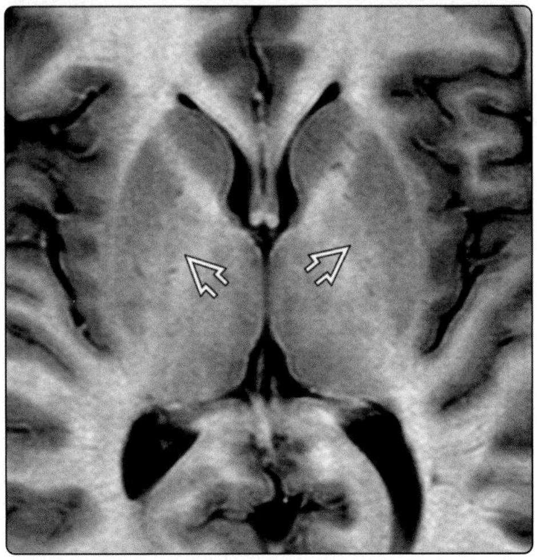

***(29-2)** Axial T1WI shows basal ganglia, thalami as isointense with gray matter. GP ➡ are slightly hyperintense to the caudate and putamen.*

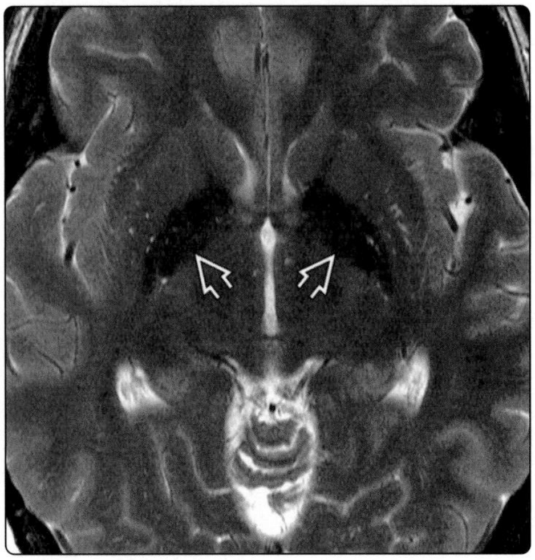

***(29-3)** On T2WI, the GP ➡ are more hypointense than putamen, caudate. Putamen reaches same hypointensity in 7th or 8th decade.*

Anatomy and Physiology of the Basal Ganglia and Thalami

Physiologic Considerations

Basal Ganglia Metabolism

By weight and volume, the brain is a small structure. However, relative to its size, the brain is one of the most metabolically active of all organs. It normally receives about 15% of total cardiac output, consumes about 20% of blood oxygen, and metabolizes up to 20% of blood glucose.

Because of its high intrinsic metabolic demands, the brain is exquisitely sensitive to processes that decrease delivery or utilization of blood, oxygen, and glucose. A variety of toxic substances do exactly that.

Two areas of the brain are especially susceptible to toxic and metabolic damage: the deep gray nuclei and the cerebral white matter (WM). The basal ganglia (BG) are highly vascular, rich in mitochondria, and loaded with neurotransmitters. The BG—especially the putamen and globus pallidus (GP)—are particularly susceptible to hypoxia or anoxia and are also commonly affected by toxins and metabolic derangements. The cerebral WM is particularly vulnerable to lipophilic toxic substances.

Dopaminergic Striatonigral System

The substantia nigra pars compacta (SNPc) contains most of the dopaminergic neuron population of the midbrain. Mesencephalic dopaminergic neurons help regulate voluntary movement. Degeneration of dopaminergic neurons in the SNPc reduces dopaminergic input to the striatum and results in movement disorders such as Parkinson disease. The dopaminergic striatonigral system is discussed in greater detail in Chapter 33.

Normal Gross Anatomy

The **BG** are symmetric paired subcortical (deep gray matter) nuclei that form the core of the extrapyramidal system and control motor activity. The BG consist of (1) the caudate nucleus (CNuc), (2) the putamen, and (3) the GP.

The caudate nucleus and putamen form the **corpus striatum**. Two other structures—the substantia nigra and subthalamic nuclei—are functionally related to the striatum. Together these structures form the striatonigral system.

Because of their triangular or lens shape, the putamen and GP together are also called the **lentiform nuclei (29-1)**.

The lentiform nuclei lie just deep to the insular cortex and are separated from it (from medial to lateral) by the WM of the external capsule, the gray matter of the claustrum, and the thin WM layer of the extreme capsule. Medially, the lentiform nuclei are separated from the caudate nucleus and thalamus by the anterior and posterior limbs of the internal capsule **(29-4)**.

The substantia nigra and subthalamic nuclei are considered next, as they are an integral part of the striatonigral system.

The thalami are the largest and most prominent of the deep gray matter nuclei but are generally not included in the term "basal ganglia." The thalami are also considered separately below.

Caudate Nucleus

The CNuc is a C-shaped structure with a large head, tapered body, and down-curving tail. The CNuc parallels the lateral ventricle body, forming part of its floor and lateral wall. The tail follows the curve of the temporal horn, lying along its roof. Anteriorly, the tail expands and becomes continuous with the posteroinferior aspect of the putamen. The most anterior aspect of the tail abuts—but remains separate from—the amygdala.

A deep groove called the sulcus terminalis separates the CNuc from the thalamus and covers a band of fibers called the stria terminalis. The ST runs all the way around the lateral ventricle from the amygdala to the hypothalamus.

The CNuc together with the putamen receives input from the cerebral cortex and is connected to the substantia nigra and GP.

Putamen

The putamen is the outermost part of the BG. Medially, the putamen is separated from the GP by a thin layer of WM fibers, the lateral (external) medullary lamina.

Globus Pallidus

The GP consists of two segments. The lateral (external) segment is separated from the medial segment by a thin layer of myelinated axons, the internal medullary lamina.

Thalamus

The thalami are symmetric, obliquely oriented ovoid masses of gray matter that lie posteromedial to the lentiform nuclei. The two thalami form the lateral walls of the third ventricle **(29-7)**. The anterior aspect of each thalamus abuts the foramen of Monro. The posterior thalamus bulges into the lateral ventricle atrium, whereas the dorsal surface forms part of the lateral ventricle floor. The stria terminalis demarcates the border between the thalamus and the body of the CNuc. The fornix curves above the thalamus and is separated from it by the choroid fissure.

Laterally, the thalami are separated from the GP by the posterior limb of the internal capsule. The thalami act as sensory and motor relay stations to the cortex.

Each thalamus is subdivided into several groups of nuclei (anterior, medial, and lateral thalamic). The lateral geniculate nuclei (part of the visual system) and medial geniculate nuclei (part of the auditory system) are also considered part of the thalamus. The pulvinar is the most posterior aspect of the thalamus and is nestled within the curve of the lateral ventricle, just in front of the atrium.

Substantia Nigra

The substantia nigra is located in the midbrain (mesencephalon). The substantia nigra appears black on gross anatomical sections because of high melanin levels in dopaminergic neurons. The substantia nigra is composed of two parts, a deep cell-rich pars compacta (SNPc) and a larger but less cellular segment, the pars reticulata.

Subthalamic Nucleus

The subthalamic nucleus (STN) is a small lens-shaped nucleus that lies in the upper midbrain, inferomedial to the thalamus and internal capsule and

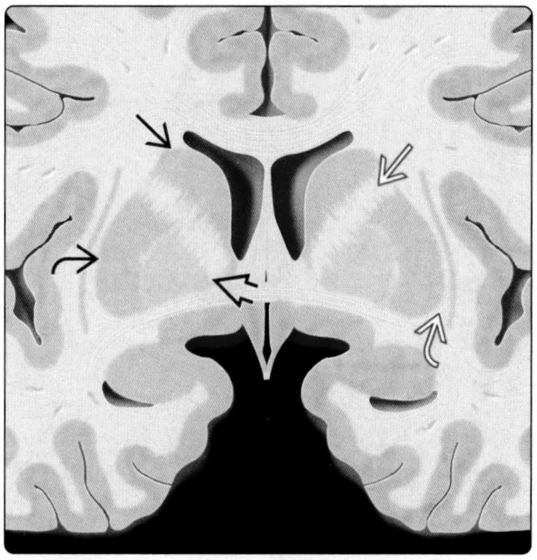

***(29-4)** Coronal graphic through frontal horns shows caudate nucleus ➙, putamen ➙, GP ➙, external capsule ➙, and internal capsule ➙.*

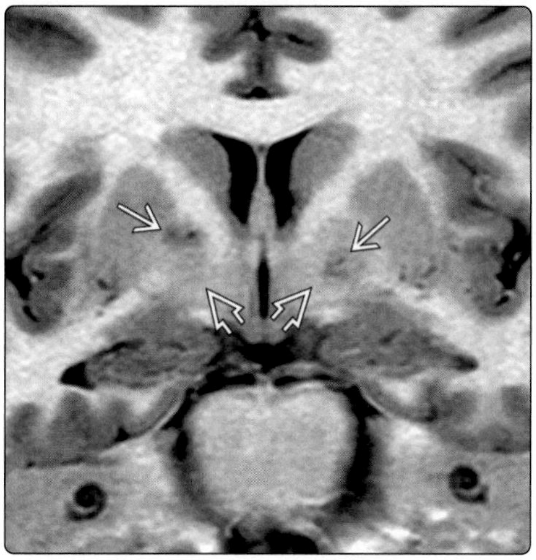

***(29-5)** On coronal T1WI, the GP ➙ are slightly hyperintense to the putamina except for punctate hypointensities caused by Ca++ ➙.*

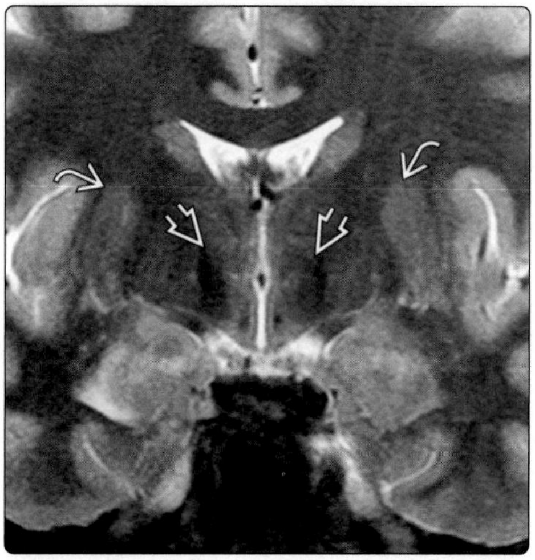

***(29-6)** Coronal T2WI shows that medial GP ➙ are the most hypointense of the basal ganglia. Putamina ➙ are isointense with cortex.*

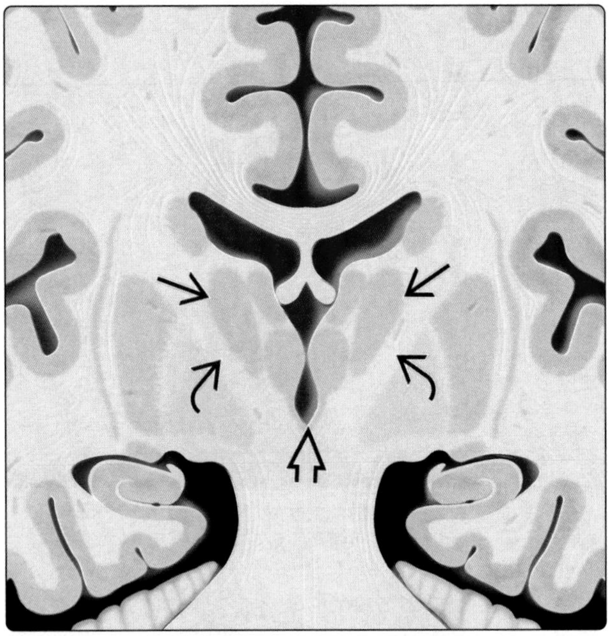

(29-7) Coronal graphic depicts the major thalamic subnuclei and their relationship to the third ventricle and internal capsules.

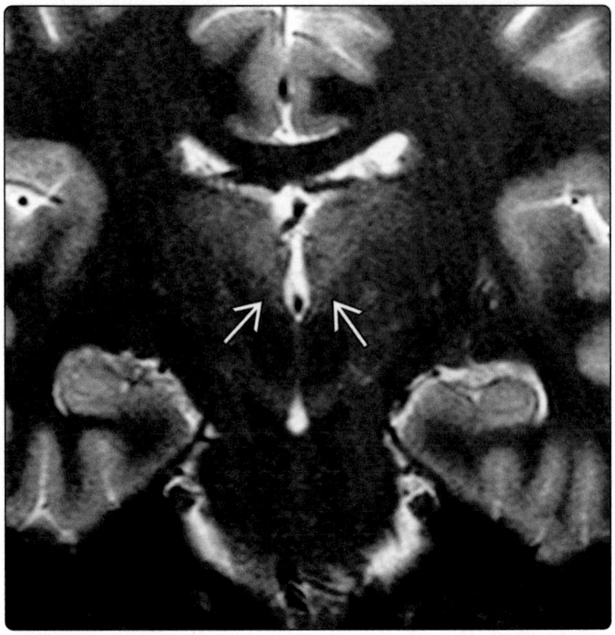

(29-8) Coronal T2WI through the posterior third ventricle shows that thalami are mostly isointense with the cortex.

superolateral to the red nucleus. The STN is wrapped by fibers of the substantia nigra but receives its main input from the GP.

Normal Imaging Anatomy

Although the lentiform nuclei, CNuc, thalami, and internal/external capsules can be identified on CT scans, their anatomy is best detailed on MR.

T1WI

The CNuc, putamina, and thalami are isointense with cortex on T1 scans. The globi pallidi are less cell-rich than either the putamen or caudate **(29-2)**. As the site of both physiologic calcification and age-related iron deposition, the GP segments vary in signal intensity **(29-5)**.

Calcification may cause T1 shortening and mild hyperintensity in the medial segment. The fully myelinated, compact WM in the internal and external capsules appears hyperintense relative to the BG.

T2WI

The CNuc, putamina, and thalami are isointense with cortical gray matter on T2 scans **(29-8)**. The myelin content in the GP is higher relative to the putamen **(29-3)** **(29-6)**, so it appears relatively more hypointense on T2WI. Increasing iron deposition occurs with aging, and the putamen becomes progressively more hypointense. A "dark" putamen is normal by the seventh or eighth decade of life.

T2*

The GP is hypointense relative to cortex on GRE or SWI imaging. By the seventh or eighth decade of life, iron deposition in the putamen "blooms," and the lateral putamen appears hypointense relative to the thalami but not as intensely hypointense as the GP. The age-associated changes of brain iron deposition are discussed in greater detail in Chapter 33.

Quantitative susceptibility mapping (QSM) is a new advanced MR technique that depicts and quantifies sources of magnetic susceptibility. Mapping iron—the dominant susceptibility source in the brain—has many important clinical applications, and QSM may assist in the early diagnosis of disorders such as amyotrophic lateral sclerosis and Parkinson disease.

Toxic and Metabolic Disorders

Many toxic, metabolic, systemic, and degenerative diseases affect the basal ganglia (BG) and thalami in a strikingly symmetric fashion.

When imaging discloses bilateral lesions that involve all the deep gray nuclei, the lesions are most often secondary to diffuse systemic or metabolic derangements.

Patchy, discrete, focal, and asymmetric lesions are more commonly infectious, postinfectious, traumatic, or neoplastic in origin.

Bilateral BG lesions have many potential causes. Diseases that specifically affect the putamen or globi pallidi in a bilaterally symmetric pattern have a somewhat different pathoetiologic spectrum.

Additional information such as patient age and specific imaging characteristics can also help establish a reasonable differential diagnosis.

In the subsequent chapters in this part, we consider toxic and metabolic disorders by diagnosis (e.g., chronic hepatic disease, acute hepatic encephalopathy, and hypoxic-ischemic encephalopathy).

Here we address the differential diagnosis of BG lesions first by general location (i.e., bilateral BG lesions) and then by sublocation. Entities within each differential diagnosis are categorized as common, less common, and rare but important.

Differential Diagnoses of Bilateral Basal Ganglia Lesions

The most common bilateral BG lesions are normal variants, such as physiologic calcification and prominent perivascular spaces. Vascular disease, hypoxic-ischemic insults, and common metabolic disorders, such as chronic liver failure, are the most frequent causes of abnormality.

Infection, toxins and drug abuse, or metabolic disorders, such as osmotic demyelination and Wernicke encephalopathy, are less common causes of bilateral BG lesions.

Careful evaluation of imaging findings outside the BG such as cortical or white matter (WM) involvement—together with clinical correlation and laboratory data—is essential to differentiate among the many disorders that cause bilateral BG abnormalities **(29-9) (29-10) (29-11) (29-12) (29-13) (29-14) (29-15) (29-16) (29-17) (29-18)**.

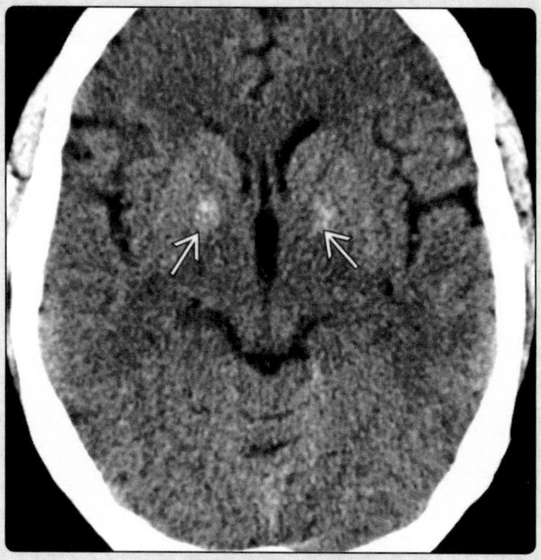

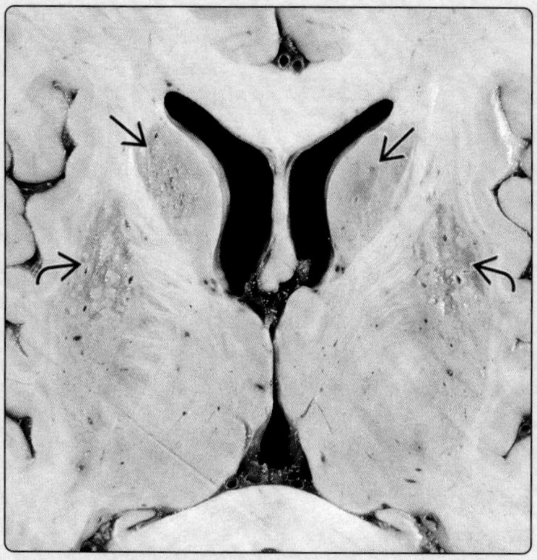

***(29-9)** Axial NECT scan in a 34y woman with headaches and normal neurologic examination shows normal bilateral symmetric physiologic calcifications in the medial GP ➡. **(29-10)** Autopsy case of hypoxia with acute striatal necrosis shows bilateral caudate nuclei ➡ and putamina ↪ lesions. The GP and thalami are spared. (Courtesy R. Hewlett, MD.)*

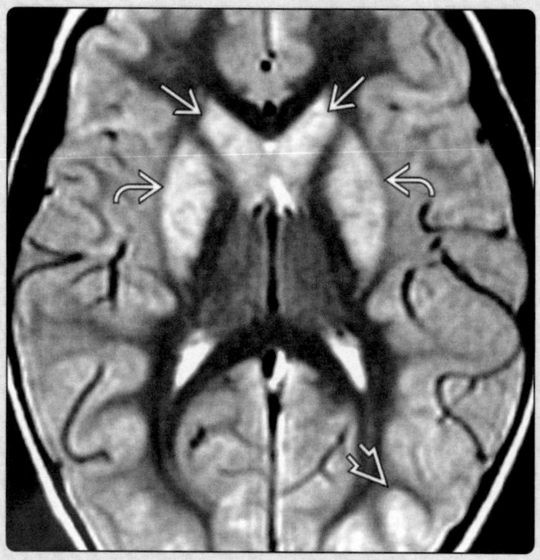

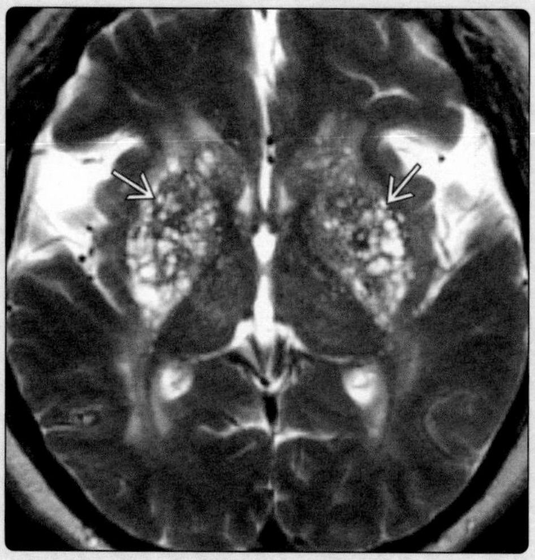

***(29-11)** Axial T2WI in a patient with anoxia, basal ganglia necrosis shows bilateral hyperintensity in caudate nuclei ➡, putamina, GP ↪, cortex ➡. The thalamus is relatively spared. **(29-12)** Axial T2WI shows innumerable variably sized CSF-like cysts in the caudate nuclei, putamina, and GP ➡ with relative sparing of the thalamus. These are unusually prominent enlarged perivascular spaces (sometimes called "état criblé" or "cribriform state").*

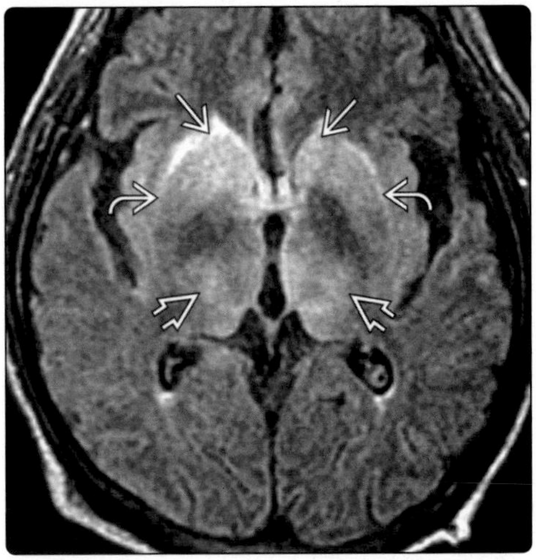

(29-13) FLAIR shows bilateral CNuc, putamina, thalamic hyperintensity; West Nile encephalitis. (Courtesy M. Colombo, MD.)

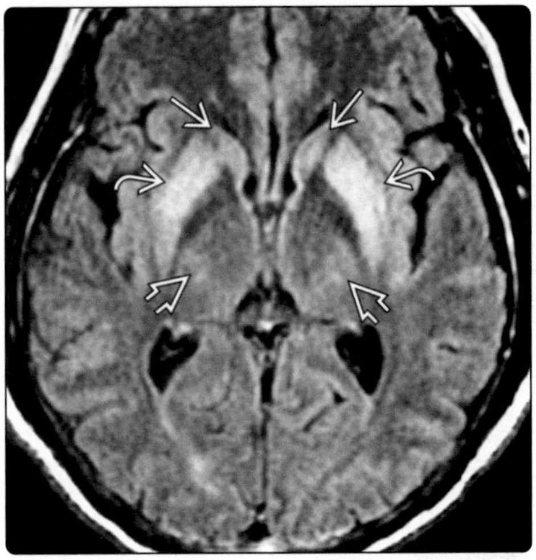

(29-14) Axial FLAIR shows CNuc, putamina, thalamic symmetric hyperintensity. This is extrapontine osmotic myelinolysis.

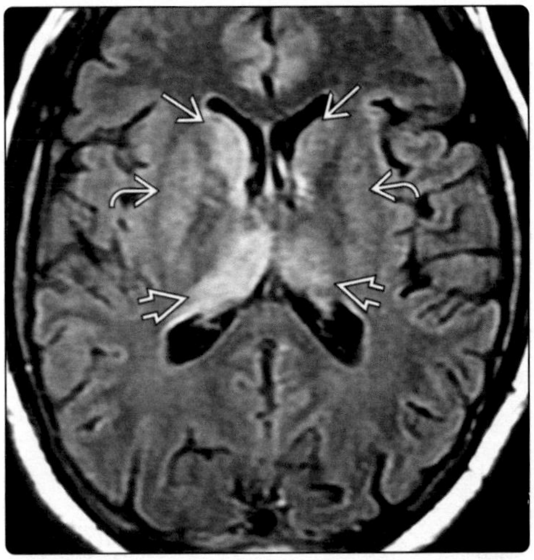

(29-15) Axial FLAIR shows bilateral but asymmetric CNuc, putamen, thalamic hyperintensity. This is deep vein occlusion.

COMMON BILATERAL BASAL GANGLIA LESIONS

Normal Variants
- Physiologic mineralization
  - Medial globus pallidus (GP) > > caudate, putamen
- Prominent perivascular spaces
  - Follow CSF, suppress on FLAIR

Vascular Disease
- Lacunar infarcts
  - Multiple bilateral, scattered, asymmetric
- Diffuse axonal/vascular injury
  - Hemorrhage, other lesions

Hypoxic-Ischemic Injury
- Hypoxic-ischemic encephalopathy (HIE)
  - BG ± cortex/watershed, hippocampi, thalami

Metabolic Disorders
- Chronic liver disease
  - GP, substantia nigra hyperintensity

LESS COMMON BILATERAL BASAL GANGLIA LESIONS

Infection/Postinfection
- Viral
  - Especially flaviviral encephalitides (West Nile virus, Japanese encephalitis, etc.)
- Postvirus, postvaccination
  - Acute disseminated encephalomyelitis (ADEM): patchy > confluent; WM, thalami, cord often involved
  - Acute striatal necrosis

Toxic Poisoning and Drug Abuse
- Carbon monoxide
  - GP (WM may show delayed involvement)
- Heroin
  - BG, WM ("chasing the dragon")
- Methanol
  - Putamen, WM
- Cyanide
  - Putamen (often hemorrhagic)
- Nitroimidazole
  - Dentate nuclei, inferior colliculi, splenium, BG

Metabolic Disorders
- Osmotic ("extrapontine") demyelination
  - BG, ± pons, WM
- Wernicke encephalopathy
  - Medial thalami, midbrain (periaqueductal), mammillary bodies

Vascular Disease
- Internal cerebral vein/vein of Galen/straight sinus thrombosis
  - BG, deep WM
- Artery of Percheron infarct
  - Bilateral thalami, midbrain ("V" sign)

Neoplasm
- Primary CNS lymphoma
  - Periventricular (WM, BG)
- Astrocytoma
  - Bithalamic "glioma"

RARE BUT IMPORTANT BILATERAL BASAL GANGLIA LESIONS

Metabolic Disorders
- Acute diabetic uremia
  - GP, putamen, caudate
- Acute hyperammonemia
  - Acute liver failure
  - Ornithine transcarbamylase deficiency, etc.
- Acute hyperglycemia
  - GP, caudate
- Severe hypoglycemia
  - Occipital cortex, hippocampi, ± WM

Infection and Inflammation
- Toxoplasmosis
  - Often HIV-positive, other ring-enhancing lesions
- Behçet disease
  - Midbrain often involved
  - Orogenital aphthous ulcers
- Chronic longstanding multiple sclerosis (MS)
  - BG become very hypointense
  - Putamina, thalami > GP, caudate nucleus (CNuc)
  - Extensive WM disease, volume loss
- Creutzfeldt-Jakob disease (CJD)
  - Anterior BG (caudate, putamen)
  - Posteromedial thalami (T2/FLAIR hyperintense "hockey stick" sign)
  - Variable cortical (occipital = Heidenhain variant)

Inherited Disorders
- Neurofibromatosis type 1 (NF1)
  - GP T1 hyperintensity, T2 hyperintense foci
- Mitochondrial encephalopathies
  - Mitochondrial encephalopathy with lactic acidosis and stroke-like episodes (MELAS), myoclonic epilepsy with ragged red fibers (MERRF)
  - Leigh disease (putamen, periaqueductal region, cerebral peduncles)
- Wilson disease
  - Putamina, CNuc, ventrolateral thalami
- Pantothenate kinase-associated neurodegeneration (PKAN)
  - GP ("eye of the tiger")
- Huntington disease
  - Atrophic CNuc, putamina
- Fahr disease
  - Dense symmetric BG, thalami, dentate nuclei, subcortical WM Ca++
- Iron storage disorders
  - Symmetric BG "blooming" hypointensity

Putamen Lesions

In general, the putamina are less commonly affected than either the globi pallidi or thalami. The most common lesion to affect the putamen is hypertensive hemorrhage. Acute hypertensive bleeds are usually unilateral although T2* scans often disclose evidence of prior hemorrhages.

Bilateral symmetric putamen lesions usually occur with more generalized BG involvement. However, there are some lesions that predominantly or almost exclusively involve the putamina.

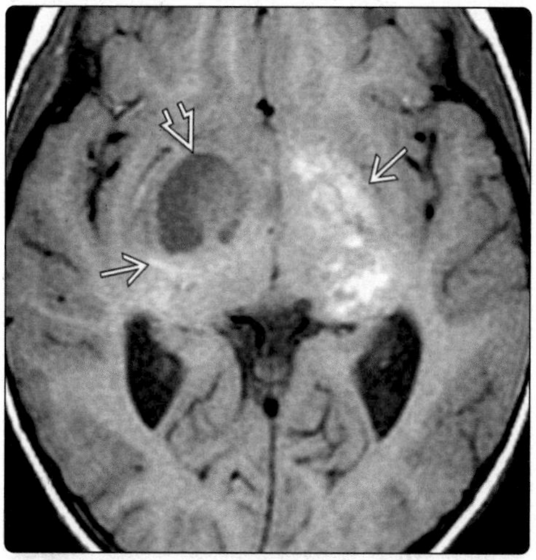

(29-16) Axial T1WI in a patient with NF1 shows multifocal basal ganglia (BG) hyperintensities ➡, large hypointensity ➡ from myelin vacuolization.

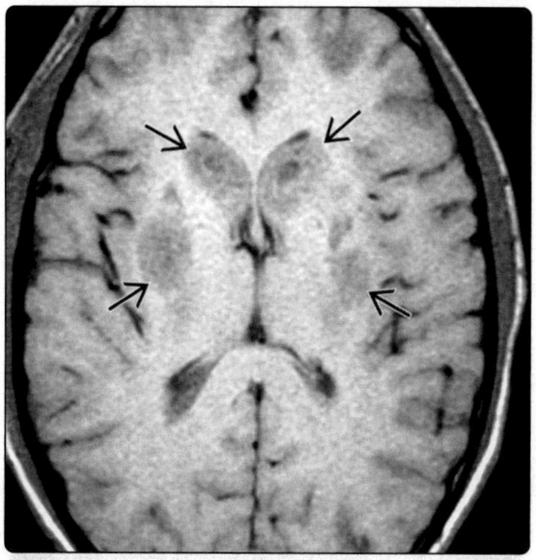

(29-17) Axial T1WI in a patient with mitochondrial encephalopathy (MERRF) shows multifocal hypointensities in the BG ➡.

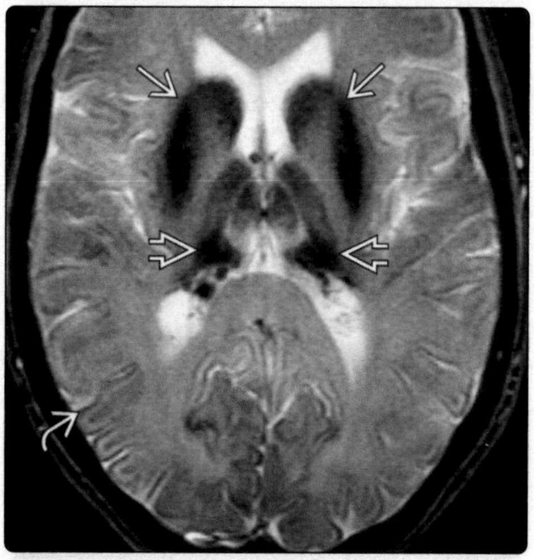

(29-18) T2 GRE in a patient with aceruloplasminemia shows symmetric "blooming" hypointensities in BG ➡, thalami ➡, cortex ➡.*

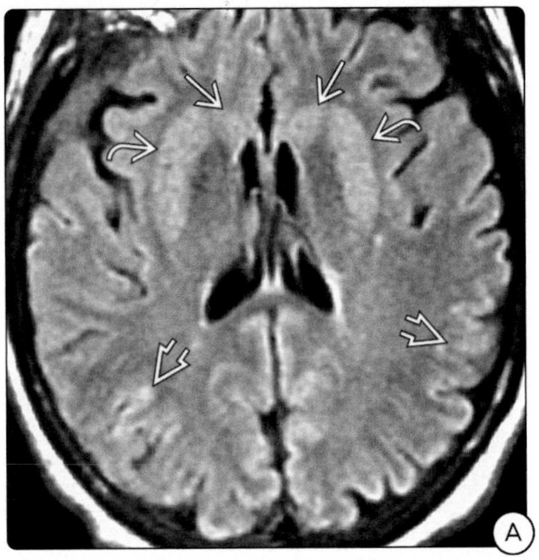

(29-19A) *FLAIR scan in a patient with anoxia shows bilateral putamina ➡, caudate nuclei ➡, and cortical ➡ hyperintensity.*

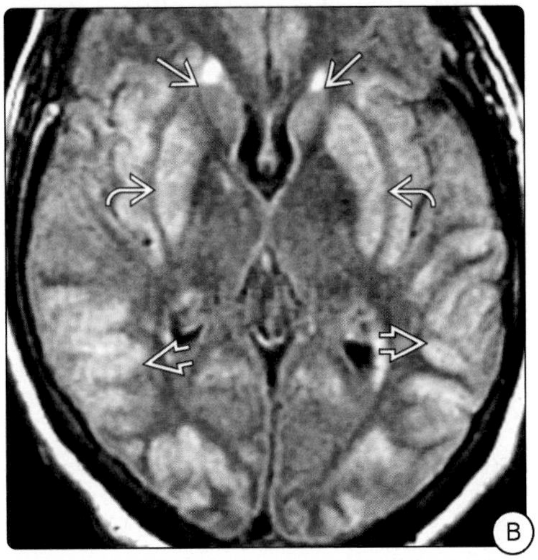

(29-19B) *FLAIR shows symmetric hyperintensity in the CNuc ➡, putamina ➡, cortex ➡. This is severe hypoglycemia. (Courtesy M. Castillo, MD.)*

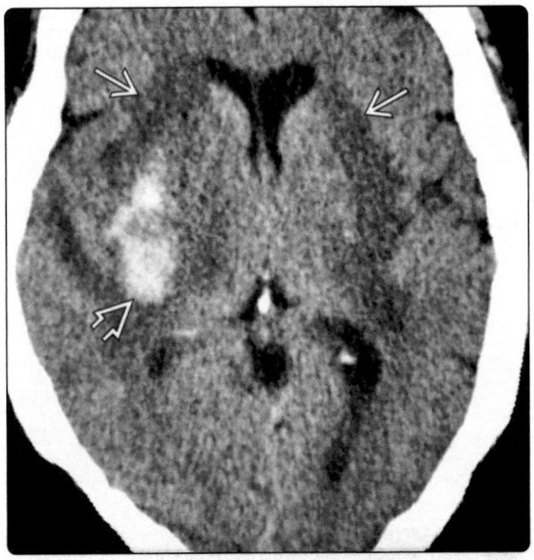

(29-20) *NECT shows symmetric hypointense putaminal lesions ➡, hemorrhage ➡; acute methanol toxicity. (Courtesy B. Hart, MD.)*

Toxic, metabolic, and hypoxic-ischemic events and degenerative disorders account for the vast majority of symmetric putamen lesions **(29-19A)** **(29-19B)** **(29-20)**.

COMMON PUTAMEN LESIONS

Metabolic Disorders
- Hypertensive hemorrhage
  - Lateral putamen/external capsule

Hypoxic-Ischemic Encephalopathy
- HIE in term infants
- Hypotensive infarction

LESS COMMON PUTAMEN LESIONS

Toxic Disorders
- Methanol toxicity*
  - Often hemorrhagic
  - ± Subcortical WM
- Osmotic demyelination
  - Extrapontine myelinolysis

Inherited Disorders
- Leigh disease
- Neuroferritinopathy
  - Putamina, GP, dentate

** Predominantly or almost exclusively involves the putamina*

RARE BUT IMPORTANT PUTAMEN LESIONS

Degenerative Diseases
- Huntington disease
  - CNuc, putamina
- Parkinson disease
  - Putamen hypointensity
- Multiple system atrophy
  - Parkinsonian type* (hyperintense putaminal rim)

Miscellaneous
- Creutzfeldt-Jakob disease*
  - Anterior putamina, CNuc
  - Posteromedial thalami
  - Variable cortex (± predominant or exclusive involvement)

** Predominantly or almost exclusively involves the putamina*

Globus Pallidus Lesions

The globus pallidus (GP) is the part of the BG that is most sensitive to hypoxia. The vast majority of symmetric GP lesions are secondary to hypoxic, toxic, or metabolic processes. Most cause bilateral symmetric abnormalities on imaging studies **(29-21)** **(29-22)** **(29-23)**.

The differential diagnosis of GP lesions can be approached by prevalence (common, less common, rare but important), etiology, age, imaging appearance, or a combination of these factors.

COMMON GLOBUS PALLIDUS LESIONS

Normal Variant
- Physiologic calcification
  - Medial GP

Hypoxic-Ischemic Encephalopathy
- Anoxia, hypoxia (near-drowning, cerebral hypoperfusion)
- Neonatal HIE (profound acute)

Toxic/Metabolic Disorders
- Chronic liver disease
  - T1 hyperintensity, T2* hypointensity
- Carbon monoxide
  - T2 hyperintense medial GP

LESS COMMON GLOBUS PALLIDUS LESIONS

Toxic/Metabolic Disorders
- Postopioid toxic encephalopathy
  - Often combined with HIE
- Hyperalimentation
  - Manganese deposition, short T1
- Chronic hypothyroidism
  - Punctate calcification
  - T1 hyperintensity, T2 hypointensity

Inherited Disorders
- NF1
- Leigh disease

RARE BUT IMPORTANT GLOBUS PALLIDUS LESIONS

Toxic/Metabolic Disorders
- Kernicterus
  - T1 shortening
- Cyanide poisoning
  - Hemorrhagic GP, laminar cortical necrosis

Inherited Disorders
- Fahr disease
  - Dense symmetric confluent calcification
- Wilson disease
  - T2 hyperintensity in GP, putamen
  - "Face of giant panda" sign in midbrain
- PKAN
  - "Eye of the tiger" (central T2 hyperintensity, peripheral hypointensity)
  - Not always present!
- Neurodegeneration with brain iron accumulation (NBIA)
  - GP, substantia nigra hypointensity ± putamen
- Maple syrup urine disease (MSUD)
  - Edema (GP, brainstem, thalami, cerebellar WM)
- Methylmalonic acidemia (MMA)
  - Symmetric GP T2 hyperintensity ± WM

Degenerative Diseases
- Hepatocerebral degeneration
  - 1% of patients with cirrhosis, portosystemic shunts
  - T1 shortening
- Progressive supranuclear palsy
  - Also affects subthalamic nucleus, substantia nigra

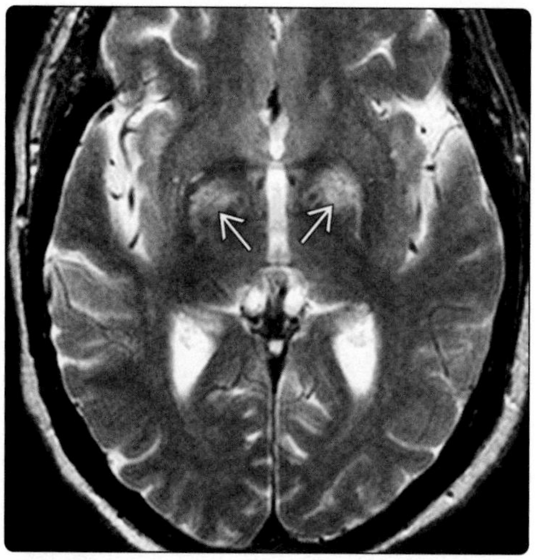

***(29-21)** T2WI in a patient with hypotensive infarct following narcotic overdose shows bilateral GP hyperintensities ➡.*

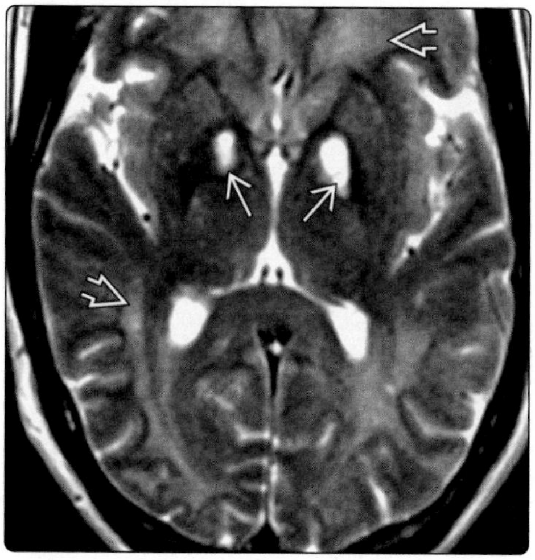

***(29-22)** T2WI shows bilateral medial GP hyperintensities ➡, confluent WM hyperintensity ➡; this is carbon monoxide poisoning.*

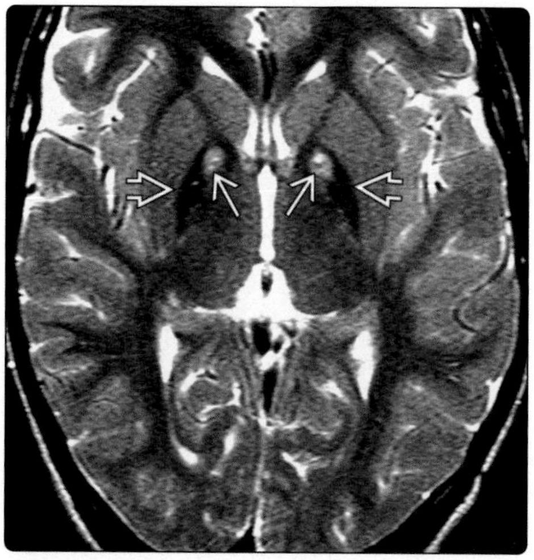

***(29-23)** T2WI shows classic "eye of the tiger" with medial GP hyperintensities ➡ surrounded by well-defined hypointensity ➡. This is PKAN.*

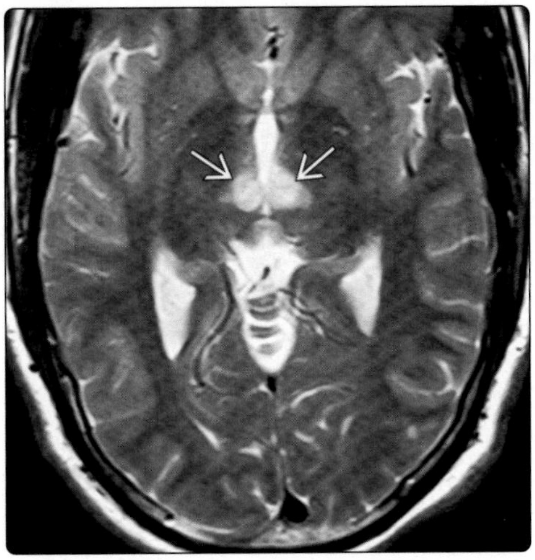

(29-24) *Axial T2WI shows bilateral medial thalamic infarcts ➡ caused by artery of Percheron occlusion.*

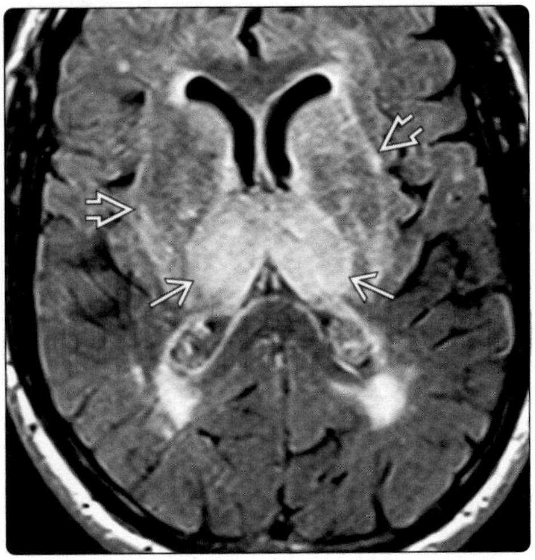

(29-25) *Axial FLAIR shows bithalamic lesions ➡ with less extensive involvement of putamina ➡ and GP. This is internal cerebral vein occlusion.*

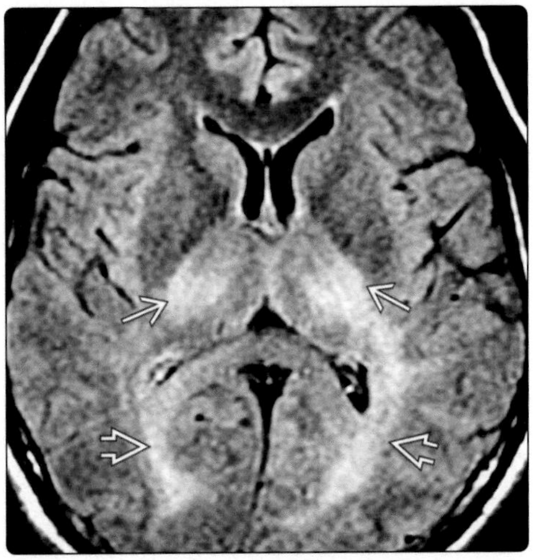

(29-26) *FLAIR scan in a patient with Epstein-Barr virus encephalitis shows bithalamic ➡ and occipital WM involvement ➡.*

Globus Pallidus Lesions by Age

Some GP lesions are common in adults but rare in children; others are seen primarily in the pediatric age group.

GLOBUS PALLIDUS LESIONS BY AGE

GP Lesions of Adulthood
- Hypoxia/anoxia
- Drug abuse
- Carbon monoxide poisoning
- Hepatic encephalopathy
- Hyperalimentation
- Hypothyroidism
- Wilson disease
- NBIA

GP Lesions of Childhood
- HIE
- NF1
- Leigh disease
- Wilson disease
- Kernicterus
- NBIA, PKAN
- MSUD
- MMA

Globus Pallidus Lesions by Appearance

Some GP lesions can be distinguished by their typical attenuation on CT or signal intensity on MR.

GLOBUS PALLIDUS LESIONS BY CHARACTERISTIC APPEARANCE

NECT Hypodensity
- HIE
- Carbon monoxide poisoning

NECT Hyperdensity
- Physiologic Ca++
- Hypothyroidism
- Fahr disease

T1 Hyperintensity
- Chronic hepatic encephalopathy
- Hyperalimentation (manganese deposition)
- NF1
- Hypothyroidism
- Kernicterus (acute)
- Wilson disease

T2 Hyperintensity
- HIE
- Drug abuse
- Carbon monoxide poisoning
- NF1
- Leigh disease
- Kernicterus (chronic)
- Wilson disease
- PKAN, MSUD, MMA

Thalamic Lesions

Because lacunar infarcts and hypertensive bleeds are so common, *unilateral* thalamic lesions are much more common than bilateral symmetric abnormalities.

UNILATERAL THALAMIC LESIONS

Common
- Lacunar infarction
- Hypertensive intracranial hemorrhage

Less Common
- NF1
- Diffuse astrocytoma (low-grade fibrillary)
- Glioblastoma multiforme
- Anaplastic astrocytoma
- ADEM

Rare But Important
- MS
- Unilateral internal cerebral vein thrombosis
- Germinoma

In contrast, *bilateral* symmetric thalamic lesions are relatively uncommon and have a somewhat limited differential diagnosis. As with the symmetric basal ganglia lesions discussed previously, bilateral thalamic lesions tend to be toxic, metabolic, vascular, infectious, or hypoxic-ischemic **(29-24)** **(29-25)** **(29-26)** **(29-27)** **(29-28)** **(29-29)**.

Bithalamic Lesions by Age

As with GP lesions, some symmetric bithalamic lesions—such as those caused by inherited metabolic disorders—are more common in infants and children. Others are seen primarily in adults. Some (e.g., acquired metabolic disorders, deep venous occlusion, ADEM) occur in all ages.

The most common and rare but important causes of bithalamic lesions in children and adults are shown in the boxes on the next page.

BITHALAMIC LESIONS BY AGE

Childhood Bithalamic Lesions
- Hypoxic-ischemic encephalopathy
- ADEM
- Bithalamic astrocytoma
- Inherited metabolic disorder
- Acquired metabolic disorders
- Toxic encephalopathy
- Deep venous occlusion
- Acute necrotizing encephalitis

Adult Bithalamic Lesions
- Deep venous occlusion
- Artery of Percheron, "top of the basilar" occlusion
- Profound hypoperfusion
- ADEM
- Wernicke encephalopathy
- Osmotic demyelination
- Vasculitis
- CJD

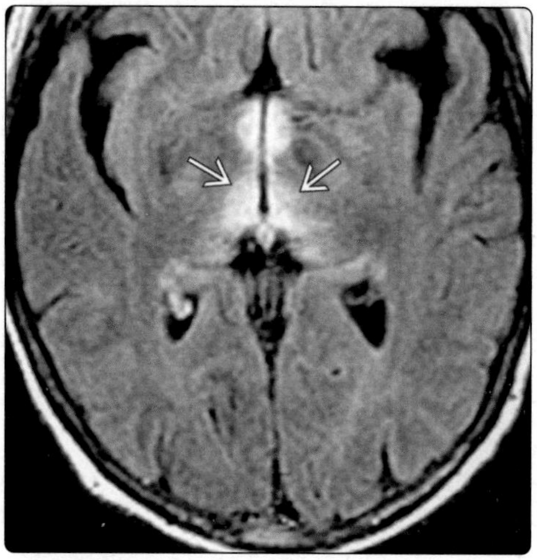

***(29-27)** FLAIR in a patient with Wernicke encephalopathy shows symmetric lesions in both medial thalami ➡.*

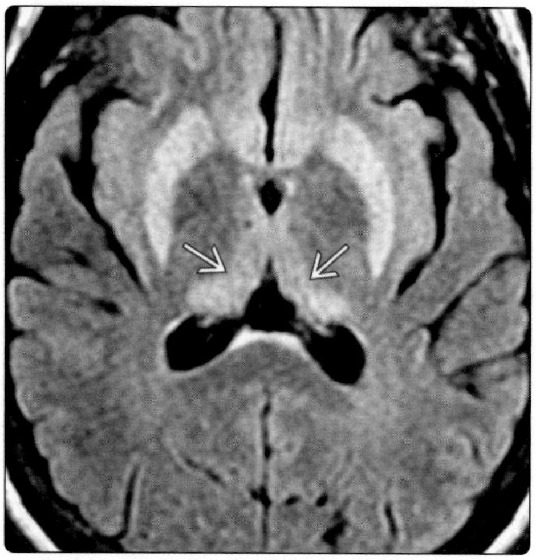

***(29-28)** FLAIR scan in a patient with CJD shows classic "hockey stick" sign ➡ as well as anterior caudate and putamen hyperintensity.*

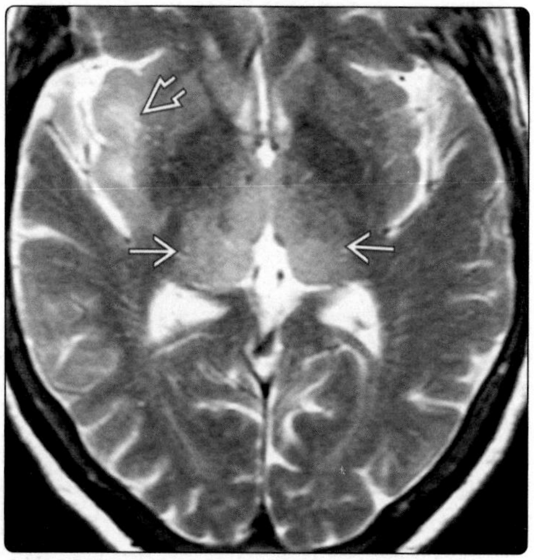

***(29-29)** T2WI shows bithalamic ➡ and right insular ➡ hyperintensity in a patient with gliomatosis cerebri, WHO grade II astrocytoma.*

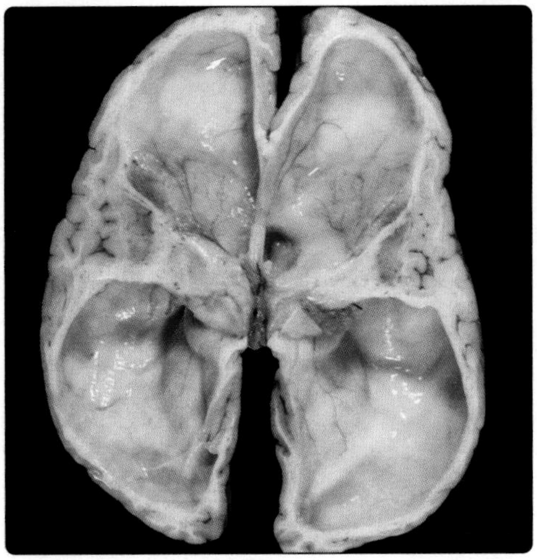

(29-30) Autopsy of severe obstructive hydrocephalus shows symmetrically enlarged lateral ventricles. (Courtesy R. Hewlett, MD.)

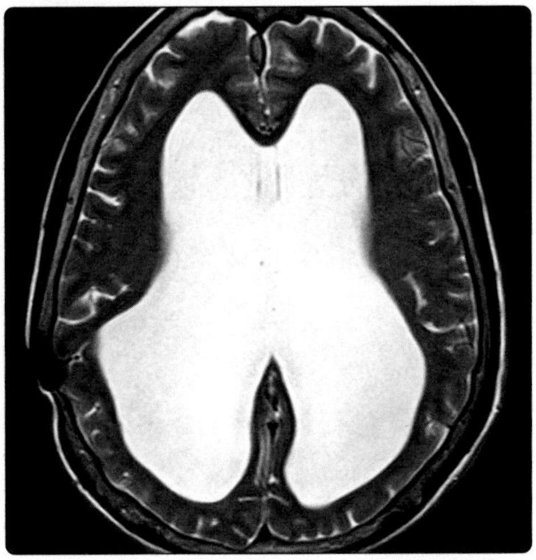

(29-31) T2WI in longstanding compensated shunted hydrocephalus shows symmetrical enlargement of both lateral ventricles.

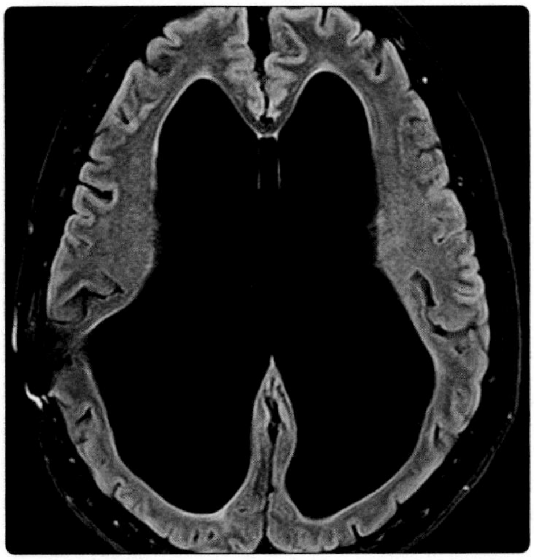

(29-32) FLAIR in the same case shows no evidence for periventricular fluid accumulation in this case of longstanding shunted hydrocephalus.

COMMON BITHALAMIC LESIONS

Vascular Lesions
- Deep venous occlusion
  - Thalami > GP, putamina
  - CNuc ± deep WM
- Arterial ischemia
  - Artery of Percheron infarct
  - "Top of the basilar" thrombosis
- Vasculitis

Hypoxic-Ischemic Encephalopathy
- Profound hypoperfusion
  - BG, hippocampi, cortex
- Usually occurs in full-term neonates

LESS COMMON BITHALAMIC LESIONS

Infection/Postinfection/Inflammatory Disorders
- ADEM
  - Usually with WM lesions
- Viral encephalitis
  - *Many* agents affect thalami
  - Epstein-Barr virus, West Nile virus, Japanese encephalitis, etc.
- CJD
  - "Hockey stick" sign
  - Pulvinar, medial thalami

Toxic/Metabolic Disorders
- Osmotic myelinolysis
  - Extrapontine involvement variable
  - Thalami
  - External capsules, putamina, CNuc
- Wernicke encephalopathy
  - Medial thalami (around 3rd ventricle)
  - Pulvinar
  - Midbrain (periaqueductal)
  - Mammillary bodies
  - Cortex variable
- Solvent inhalation
  - Toluene
  - Glue
  - Ethylene glycol
- Acute hypertensive encephalopathy (PRES)
  - Occipital lobes, watershed zones
  - "Atypical" PRES may involve BG, thalami
- Status epilepticus
  - Pulvinar
  - Corpus callosum splenium (usually transient excitotoxic)
  - Often hippocampi ± cortex

Neoplasms
- Bithalamic low-grade astrocytoma
- Germinoma
- Lymphoma

RARE BUT IMPORTANT BITHALAMIC LESIONS

Infection/Postinfection/Inflammatory Disorders

- MS (severe, chronic)
  - Hypointense BG on T2*
- Acute necrotizing encephalopathy of childhood
- Flavivirus encephalitis
- Neuro-Behçet

Inherited Disorders

- Mitochondrial disorders
- Krabbe disease
  - Hyperdense on CT, hypointense on T2
- Wilson disease
  - Putamina, CNuc > thalami
- Fahr disease
  - GP > thalami
- Fabry disease
  - T1 hyperintense posterior thalamus ("pulvinar")
  - M > > F
  - Strokes (territorial, lacunar)
  - Renal, cardiac disease

Neoplasm

- Glioblastoma
- Anaplastic astrocytoma

Paraneoplastic Syndromes

- Paraneoplastic can mimic prion disease (variant Creutzfeldt-Jakob disease)
- Limbic involvement not always present

Degenerative and CSF Disorders

Age-Related Changes

Normal age-related changes in the brain occur throughout life. Understanding the different stages of brain formation and normal progression of myelination is essential to diagnosing inherited metabolic disorders.

At the opposite end of the age spectrum, volume is normally lost in some parts of the brain, while other areas remain relatively intact. Abnormal mineral deposition in the basal ganglia can be a clue to degenerative and metabolic disorders. Understanding what is normal heavy metal deposition in different decades is a prerequisite to diagnosing these abnormalities on imaging studies.

Dementia and Brain Degeneration

Once an understanding of the normal aging brain is established, we discuss the pathology and imaging manifestations of dementia. Although identifying a "lobar predominant" pattern of volume loss on CT and standard MR can be accomplished in many cases, these are usually late-stage manifestations. The early diagnosis of dementing disorders increasingly relies on functional MR and PET studies. CNS degenerations from Parkinson disease to wallerian and hypertrophic olivary degeneration are considered. The anatomy and physiology of the brain dopaminergic system are briefly reviewed, as is the anatomy essential to evaluating pre- and postoperative deep brain stimulation.

Hydrocephalus and CSF Disorders

Because abnormalities of the brain CSF spaces are a common manifestation of brain degeneration in the elderly as well as a potentially treatable cause of encephalopathy, we devote the last chapter in this part to hydrocephalus and CSF disorders.

We first address the normal anatomy of the ventricles and CSF spaces as well as imaging variants that can be mistaken for disease.

Hydrocephalus, disorders of CSF production/circulation/absorption, and the newly described syndrome of inappropriately low-pressure acute hydrocephalus are then discussed. Lastly, we consider CSF leaks and sequelae including intracranial hypotension—conditions in which imaging plays an essential role in both diagnosis and patient management.

ABNORMALITIES OF VENTRICULAR SIZE

Large Ventricles

- Common
  - Aging brain (brain parenchyma volume loss)
  - Generalized encephalomalacia (posttrauma/infection, etc.)
  - Extraventricular obstructive hydrocephalus (meningitis, subarachnoid hemorrhage, etc.)
  - Dementias (Alzheimer, frontotemporal dementia, etc.)
- Less common
  - Intraventricular obstructive hydrocephalus
  - Colpocephaly (occipital horns)
  - Normal pressure hydrocephalus
  - Shunt failure
- Rare but important
  - Choroid plexus papilloma (CSF overproduction)
  - Megalencephaly syndromes
  - Huntington disease (frontal horns)

Small Ventricles

- Common
  - Normal (children, young adults)
  - Shunt failure ("slit ventricle" syndrome)
  - Increased intracranial pressure
- Less common
  - Diffuse cerebral edema
  - Intracranial hypotension
  - Idiopathic intracranial hypertension
- Rare but important
  - Brain death

Selected References

Anatomy and Physiology of the Basal Ganglia and Thalami

Avecillas-Chasin JM et al: Tractographical model of the cortico-basal ganglia and corticothalamic connections: improving our understanding of deep brain stimulation. Clin Anat. 29(4):481-92, 2016

Bonnier G et al: A new approach for deep gray matter analysis using partial-volume estimation. PLoS One. 11(2):e0148631, 2016

Daugherty AM et al: Accumulation of iron in the putamen predicts its shrinkage in healthy older adults: a multi-occasion longitudinal study. Neuroimage. 128:11-20, 2016

Guadalupe T et al: Human subcortical brain asymmetries in 15,847 people worldwide reveal effects of age and sex. Brain Imaging Behav. ePub, 2016

Sussman D et al: Developing human brain: age-related changes in cortical, subcortical, and cerebellar anatomy. Brain Behav. 6(4):e00457, 2016

Lopez WO et al: Optical coherence tomography imaging of the basal ganglia: feasibility and brief review. Braz J Med Biol Res. 48(12):1156-9, 2015

Toxic and Metabolic Disorders

Eskreis-Winkler S et al: The clinical utility of QSM: disease diagnosis, medical management, and surgical planning. NMR Biomed. 30(4), 2017

Barbagallo G et al: Multimodal MRI assessment of nigro-striatal pathway in multiple system atrophy and Parkinson disease. Mov Disord. 31(3):325-34, 2016

Eichler F et al: Inherited or acquired metabolic disorders. Handb Clin Neurol. 135:603-36, 2016

Hopes L et al: Magnetic resonance imaging features of the nigrostriatal system: biomarkers of Parkinson's disease stages? PLoS One. 11(4):e0147947, 2016

Rizzo G et al: Brain MR contribution to the differential diagnosis of Parkinsonian syndromes: an update. Parkinsons Dis. 2016:2983638, 2016

Salomão RP et al: A diagnostic approach for neurodegeneration with brain iron accumulation: clinical features, genetics and brain imaging. Arq Neuropsiquiatr. 74(7):587-96, 2016

Differential Diagnoses of Bilateral Basal Ganglia Lesions

Zaitout Z et al: A review of pathologies associated with high T1W signal intensity in the basal ganglia on magnetic resonance imaging. Pol J Radiol. 79:126-30, 2014

Bekiesinska-Figatowska M et al: Basal ganglia lesions in children and adults. Eur J Radiol. 82(5):837-49, 2013

Hegde AN et al: Differential diagnosis for bilateral abnormalities of the basal ganglia and thalamus. Radiographics. 31(1):5-30, 2011

Thalamic Lesions

Renard D et al: Thalamic lesions: a radiological review. Behav Neurol. 2014:154631, 2014

Smith AB et al: Bilateral thalamic lesions. AJR Am J Roentgenol. 192(2):W53-62, 2009

Toxic Encephalopathy

The list of toxins and poisons that affect the CNS is long and continues to grow. Some agents are deliberately injected, inhaled, or ingested, whereas others are accidentally encountered or administered in a controlled medical setting. Some toxins accumulate slowly, so their clinical manifestations are subtle and onset insidious. Others cause profound, virtually immediate CNS toxicity with rapid onset of coma and death. Still others—such as ethanol—have both acute and chronic effects.

Many illicit "street" drugs and synthetic "designer" CNS stimulants with innocent-sounding names such as "pink" and "bath salts" can have serious adverse impacts on the CNS. Dosage is highly variable and notoriously unreliable. Adulterated drugs are common, and contaminants may have additional adverse effects on their own.

A more recent development is the growth of so-called "legal high" drugs. Use of painkillers, "pep pills," and other legitimate pharmaceuticals for illicit or recreational purposes is becoming an epidemic, and overdoses (ODs) are increasingly common. An accurate history is often difficult to obtain in patients with suspected OD and clinical symptoms are frequently nonspecific. Presentation may also be confounded by "polydrug" abuse and secondary effects such as hypoxia that mask the underlying pathology. Acute effects on chronic underlying disease in abusers also contributes to the difficulty in sorting out which clinical and imaging findings can be attributed to specific drugs.

The vast majority of toxins with CNS manifestations cause bilateral, relatively symmetric lesions. Abnormalities in the deep gray nuclei (basal ganglia, thalamus) with varying white matter involvement are suggestive of toxic-metabolic causes.

In this chapter, we first focus on the most common types of toxic encephalopathies, beginning with the acute and long-term effects of alcohol on the brain followed by a discussion of drug abuse. Inhaled toxins (such as carbon monoxide and cyanide) and heavy metal poisoning are then considered. We conclude with treatment-related disorders.

Alcohol and Related Disorders

Alcohol [ethanol (EtOH)] is one of the most commonly abused substances in the world. EtOH has multiorgan effects, resulting in a wide range of diseases and disorders. EtOH causes different effects on different organs. Although the gastrointestinal system is exposed to higher concentrations of alcohol

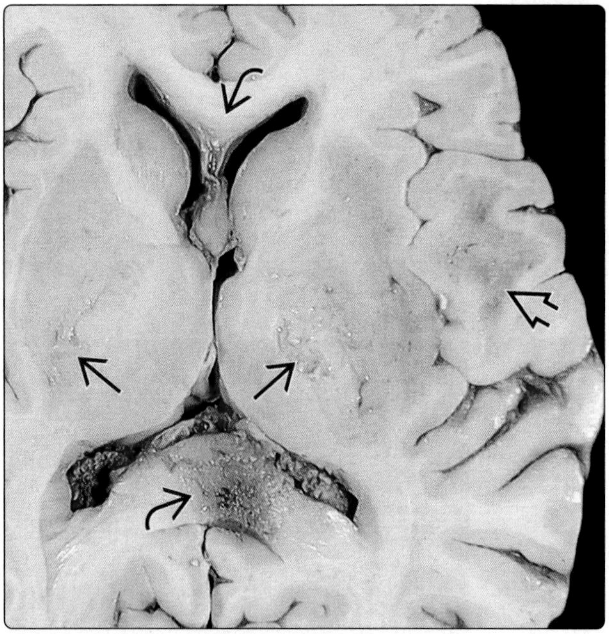

(30-1) Autopsy of acute EtOH poisoning shows brain swelling with necrosis in subcortical/deep white matter ➡, especially marked in the corpus callosum ➡. Basal ganglia/thalami are swollen, pale, infarcted ➡. (Courtesy R. Hewlett, MD.)

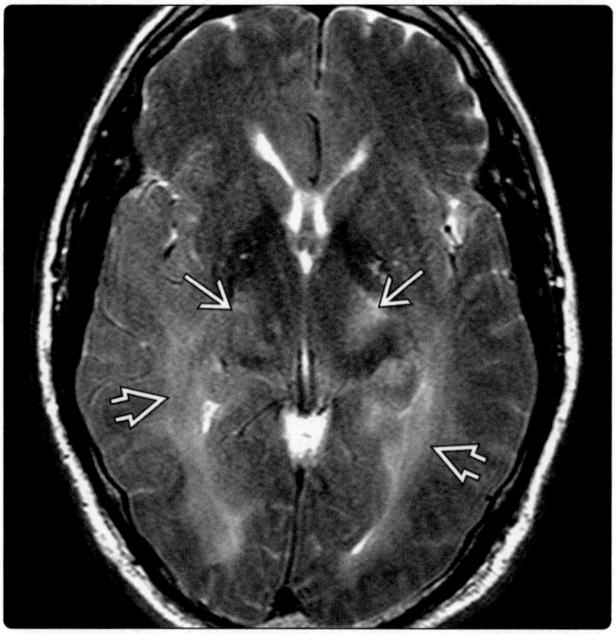

(30-2) T2WI in a comatose patient who drank 1 gallon of vodka or whisky daily for a full week shows diffuse brain swelling, hyperintense white matter ➡, bithalamic lesions ➡. This is acute alcohol poisoning.

than any other tissue, ethanol easily crosses the blood-brain barrier and is a potent neurotoxin. Both its short- and long-term effects on the central nervous system are profound.

Excessive alcohol consumption can result in chronic brain changes as well as acute, life-threatening neurologic disorders. Comorbid diseases such as malnutrition with vitamin deficiencies may lead to Wernicke encephalopathy. Altered serum osmolarity associated with alcohol abuse can cause acute demyelinating disorders.

We begin our discussion of alcohol and the brain by briefly considering the acute effects of alcohol poisoning. We then consider chronic alcoholic encephalopathy before turning to other complications of alcohol abuse, including alcohol-induced demyelination syndromes and Wernicke encephalopathy. We close the section with two less common forms of related abuse, i.e., methanol intoxication and ethylene glycol (antifreeze) ingestion.

Acute Alcohol Poisoning

Etiology

The acute effects of binge drinking are striking. EtOH inhibits Na^+/K^+ activity. Cellular swelling, life-threatening cytotoxic cerebral edema, and nonconvulsive status epilepticus may ensue **(30-1)**. A blood alcohol concentration of 0.40% typically results in unconsciousness, and a level exceeding 0.50% is usually lethal.

Acute alcohol poisoning is a complication of binge drinking and is most common in adolescents and young adults. The adolescent brain is also undergoing structural maturation and has a unique sensitivity to alcohol. Adolescent binge drinking reduces adult neurotransmitter gene expression, reduces basal forebrain function, and decreases the density of cholinergic neurons.

Binge drinkers are especially vulnerable to alcohol neurotoxicity. Binge drinkers represent a model for endophenotypic risk factors for alcohol misuse and early exposure to repeated binge cycles.

Imaging

Imaging findings in patients with acute alcohol poisoning include diffuse brain swelling and confluent hyperintensity in the supratentorial subcortical and deep white matter on T2/FLAIR **(30-2)**. Seizure-induced changes in the cortex, with gyral hyperintensity and diffusion restriction, may also be associated. DTI can detect brain changes after acute alcohol consumption that are not visible on conventional MR.

Chronic Alcoholic Encephalopathy

The long-term adverse effects of ethanol on the brain are much more common than those of acute alcohol poisoning. The effects are even more pronounced in immature brains. Recent fMR studies on alcohol use disorders (AUDs) have shown that even moderate repeated alcohol consumption can adversely affect the intrinsic functional architecture of adolescent brains.

Chronic alcohol-related brain damage can be divided into primary and secondary effects. We begin our discussion with the effects of EtOH itself on the brain and then consider secondary effects, which are mostly related to the sequelae of liver disease, malnutrition, malabsorption, and electrolyte disturbances.

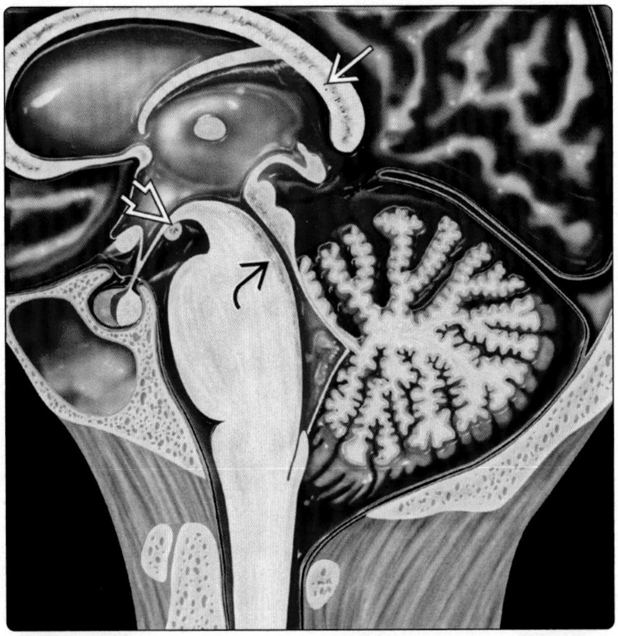

***(30-3)** Sagittal graphic shows generalized and superior vermian atrophy and corpus callosum necrosis ➡ related to alcoholic toxicity. Mammillary body ➡ and periaqueductal gray necrosis ⇗ is seen with Wernicke encephalopathy.*

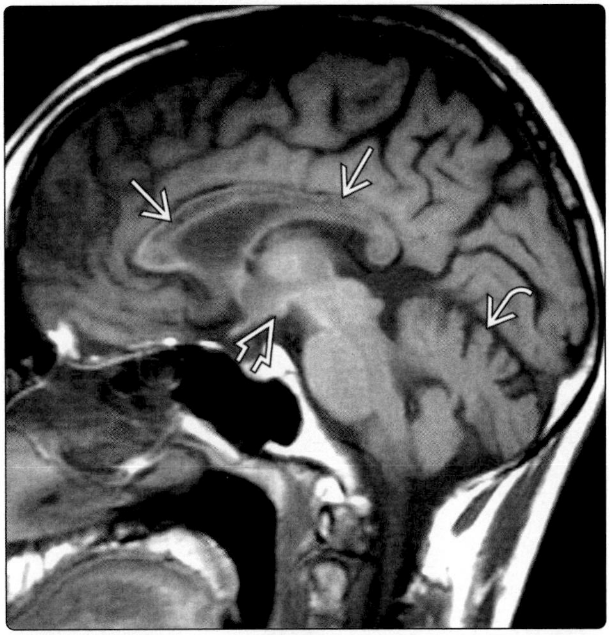

***(30-4)** Sagittal T1WI in chronic alcoholic encephalopathy and Marchiafava-Bignami disease shows hypointensity in the entire middle corpus callosum ➡. Mammillary bodies ➡ and superior vermis ➡ are atrophic. (Courtesy A. Datir, MD.)*

Etiology

Alcohol is readily absorbed through the gastric and small intestinal mucosae. A normally functioning liver breaks down nearly 90% of alcohol.

Chronic or harmful alchohol use leads to neurochemical, structural, and morphologic neuroplastic changes. EtOH readily crosses the blood-brain barrier, causing both direct and indirect neurotoxicity.

Direct brain toxicity is caused by upregulation of NMDA receptors, resulting in increased susceptibility to glutamate-mediated excitotoxicity. Other direct effects include the toxicity of acetaldehyde and related lipid peroxidation products, which can bind to brain tissue and initiate upregulation and expression of inflammatory factors. The resultant membrane injury, neuronal loss, and reduction of white matter volume reflect the indirect effects of alcohol neurotoxicity.

Repeated binge drinking damages the cortical and subcortical microstructure of the brain. Disturbed dendritic complexity occurs in areas of the prefrontal and parietal regions that mediate reward-related motivation.

Chronic EtOH abuse also dysregulates synaptic connectivity, causes increased apoptosis, and decreases expression of myelin protein-encoding genes in the frontal cortex, hippocampus, and cerebellum.

Pathology

Gross Pathology. The brain reflects the gross long-term effects of cumulative EtOH consumption **(30-3)**. Cerebral atrophy is evidenced by enlarged ventricles and sulci, particularly in the frontal lobes, and is due predominantly to reduced white matter volume.

Alcohol-induced cerebellar degeneration is also common. The folia of the rostral vermis and anterosuperior aspects of the cerebellar hemispheres are atrophic, separated by widened interfolial sulci.

Microscopic Features. Histologic changes in the cerebral hemispheres are nonspecific. Purkinje cell loss in the cerebellum, together with patchy loss of granular cells and molecular layer atrophy, reflects the alcohol-induced cerebellar degeneration.

Clinical Issues

The mechanisms that underlie alcohol's rewarding effects, the neuroadaptations from chronic exposure that contribute to tolerance and withdrawal, and the changes in fronto-striatal circuits that lead to loss of control and enhanced motivation to drink are complex and interdependent. Significant alterations in dopamine and serotonin-mediated neurotransmission also contribute to compulsive alcohol taking, dysphoria/depression, and other AUD-related disorders.

Imaging

General Features. A characteristic pattern of progressive brain volume loss is seen with chronic alcoholic encephalopathy. Initially, the superior vermis atrophies and the cerebellar fissures become prominent **(30-4)** **(30-5)** **(30-6)**. In later stages, the frontal white matter becomes involved, reflected by widened sulci and enlarged lateral ventricles. In the final stages, global volume loss is present **(30-7)**.

CT Findings. NECT scans show generalized ventricular and sulcal enlargement. The cerebral white matter is often abnormally hypodense and reduced in volume. The great horizontal fissure of the cerebellum and the superior vermian folia are unusually prominent relative to the patient's age.

MR Findings. Brain volume loss, especially in the prefrontal cortex, is common as is more focal atrophy of the superior vermis. Focal and confluent cerebral white matter hyperintensities on T2/FLAIR sequences are frequently present.

Chronic liver failure secondary to cirrhosis may cause basal ganglia hyperintensity on T1WI, probably secondary to manganese accumulation. Increased iron deposition in the basal ganglia and dentate nuclei may occur.

ACUTE/CHRONIC ALCOHOLIC ENCEPHALOPATHY

Acute Alcohol Poisoning
- Rare; caused by binge drinking
- Imaging
  - Diffuse cerebral edema
  - Acute demyelination

Chronic Alcoholic Encephalopathy
- Primary toxic effect on neurons
- Secondary effects related to liver, GI disease
  - Hepatic encephalopathy
  - Malnutrition, malabsorption, electrolyte imbalance
- Imaging
  - Atrophy (superior vermis, cerebellum, generalized)
  - White matter myelinolysis

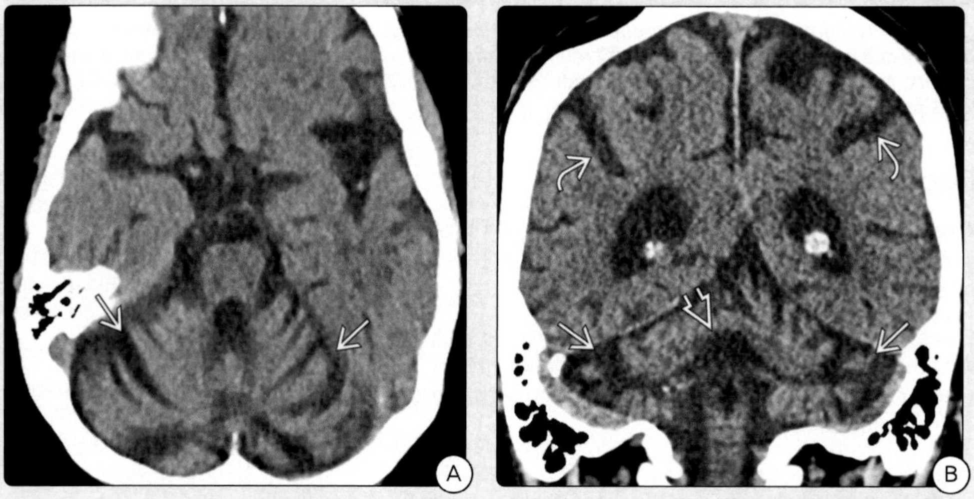

(30-5A) NECT in a 56y woman with chronic alcoholism and multiple falls shows severe cerebellar atrophy with grossly enlarged sulci ➡. (30-5B) Coronal NECT in the same case shows the striking cerebellar volume loss ➡. Note enlarged fourth ventricle ➡. The cerebral hemispheres also appear moderately atrophic with prominent superficial sulci ➡.

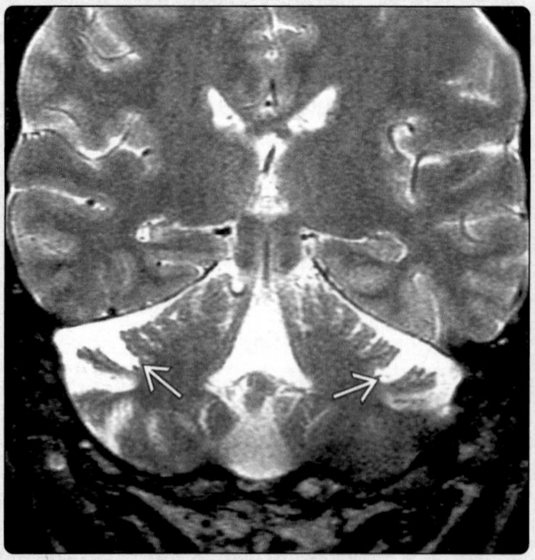

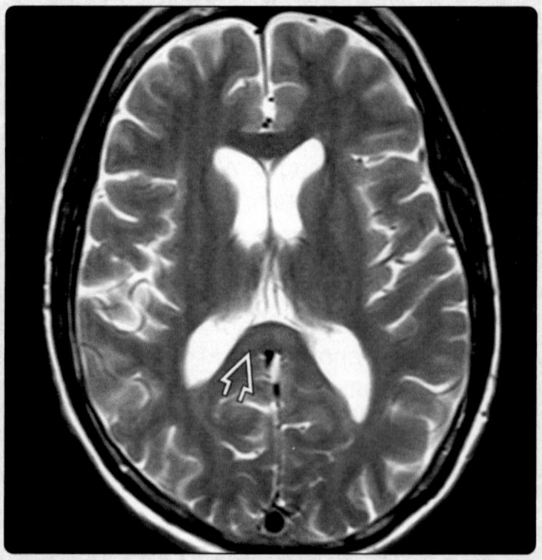

(30-6) Coronal T2WI in a 41y chronically alcoholic man shows marked atrophy of the superior cerebellum with striking widening of the horizontal fissures ➡. The supratentorial brain is relatively spared. (30-7) T2WI in a 30y chronically alcoholic patient with acute deterioration shows generalized volume loss. Note corpus callosum splenium lesion ➡; it restricted on DWI (not shown). This was alcohol-induced atrophy with acute toxic demyelination.

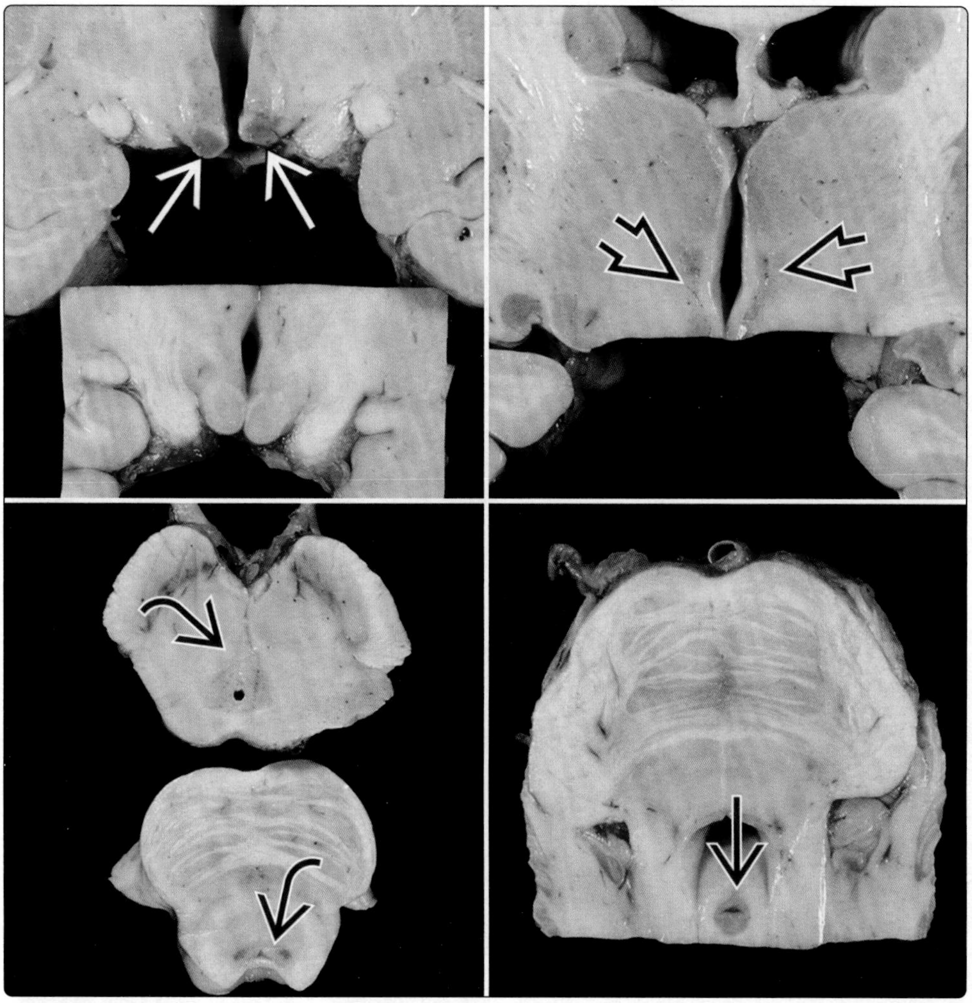

(30-8) Autopsy specimens are from a patient with Wernicke encephalopathy. (Upper left) Coronal section through the mammillary bodies shows hemorrhagic mammillary body necrosis ➡. The inset below the pathologic section shows normal mammillary bodies for comparison. (Upper right) Section through the third ventricle shows bithalamic necrosis around walls of the third ventricle ➡. (Lower left and right) Sections through the midbrain and upper pons show necrosis in periaqueductal gray matter ➡ and the bottom of the tectum ➡. (Courtesy R. Hewlett, MD.)

Wernicke Encephalopathy

Terminology

Wernicke encephalopathy (WE) is also known as Wernicke-Korsakoff syndrome. Both alcohol-related and non-alcohol-related Wernicke encephalopathy can occur.

Etiology

General Concepts. Common sequelae of chronic AUD include nutritional deficiencies, most notably thiamine (B1) deficiency. Thiamine is required to maintain membrane integrity and osmotic gradients across cell membranes. Inadequate thiamine results in lactic acidosis with intra- and extracellular edema.

Wernicke encephalopathy is caused by thiamine deficiency. Self-neglect and poor diet together with repeated vomiting may accompany alcoholism. Malnutrition with inadequate thiamine intake, decreased gastrointestinal absorption, and poor intracellular thiamine utilization may all contribute to the onset of alcoholic WE.

The underlying pathophysiology of *nonalcoholic* WE is identical to that of alcoholic WE, but the etiology is different. Malnutrition secondary to hyperemesis gravidarum (pregnancy-related vomiting), eating disorders, or bariatric surgery with drastically reduced thiamine intake is typical. Hyperemesis (e.g., pregnancy, chemotherapy) and prolonged hyperalimentation are other common causes of nonalcoholic WE.

A WE-like encephalopathy has also been reported with some drugs including antineoplastic agents such as ifosfamide. Toxicity is likely mediated through its metabolite chloroacetaldehyde, which may impair thiamine function.

Pathology

Location. The mammillary bodies, hypothalamus, medial thalamic nuclei (adjacent to the third ventricle), tectal plate, and periaqueductal gray matter are most commonly affected **(30-8)**. Less commonly involved areas include the cerebellum (especially the dentate nuclei), red nuclei, corpus callosum splenium, and cerebral cortex.

Gross Pathology. If WE occurs in the setting of chronic alcoholism, generalized brain atrophy (especially of the cerebellar vermis and frontal lobes) is present. Demyelination and petechial hemorrhages are common in the acute stage of

(30-9A) FLAIR scan in a patient with acute Wernicke encephalopathy shows hyperintensity in the periaqueductal gray matter and tectum . (30-9B) More cephalad FLAIR scan again shows the periaqueductal gray matter hyperintensity . Both mammillary bodies are also hyperintense .

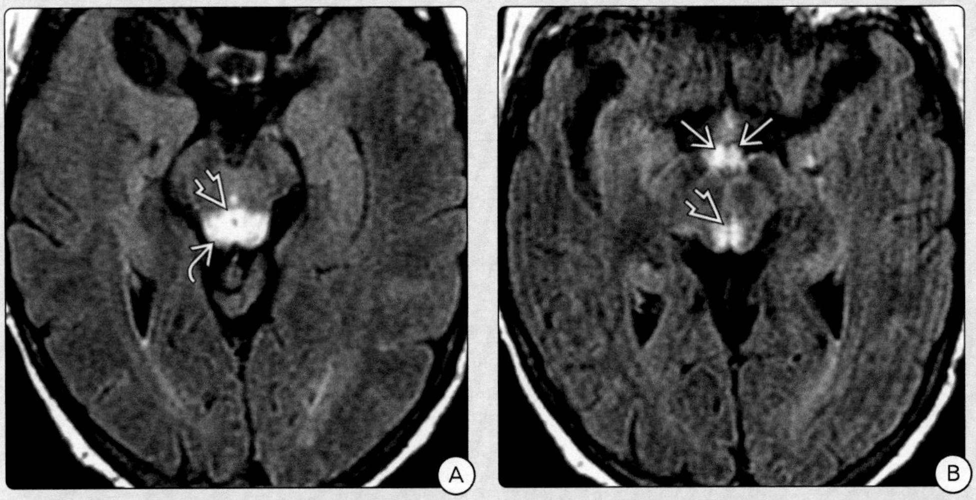

(30-9C) FLAIR scan shows hyperintensity in the medial thalami around the walls of the third ventricle . The hypothalamus is also involved. (30-9D) FLAIR scan through the cerebral convexities shows bilateral, relatively symmetric cortical hyperintensities .

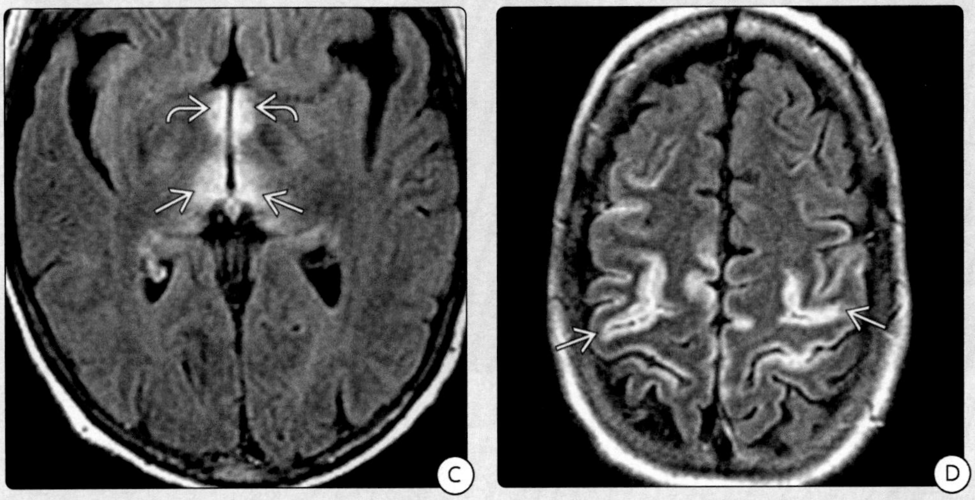

(30-9E) DWI in the same patient shows restricted diffusion in the mammillary bodies . The periaqueductal gray matter does not restrict, suggesting that the midbrain lesions seen on FLAIR may be somewhat less acute. (30-9F) Coronal T1 C+ demonstrates enhancement in the inferior colliculi .

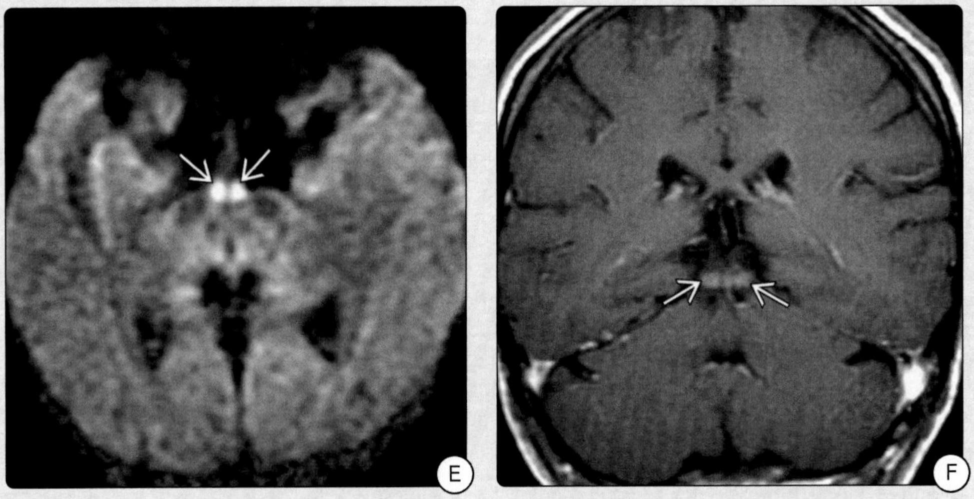

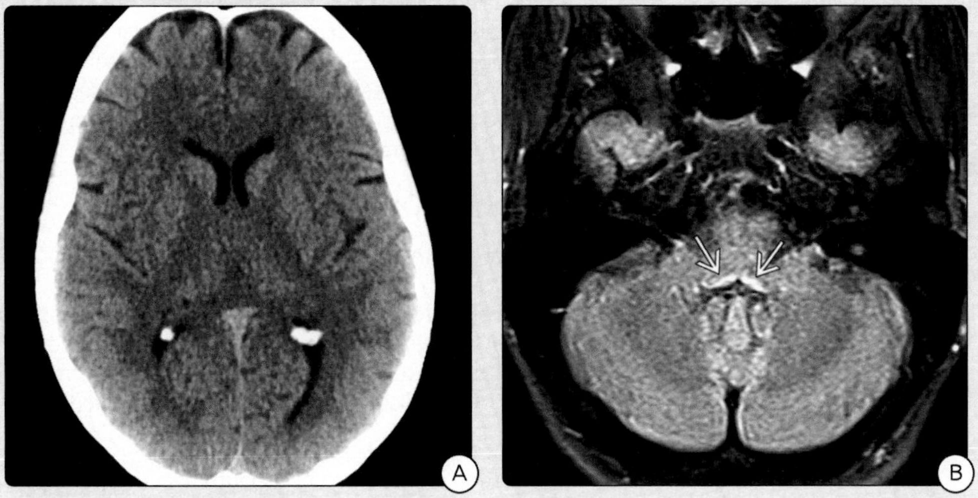

(30-10A) Axial NECT in a 28y woman with anorexia who experienced nystagmus after vomiting for several days appears grossly normal. (30-10B) Axial FLAIR in the same case shows symmetric hyperintensities in the dorsal medulla ➡.

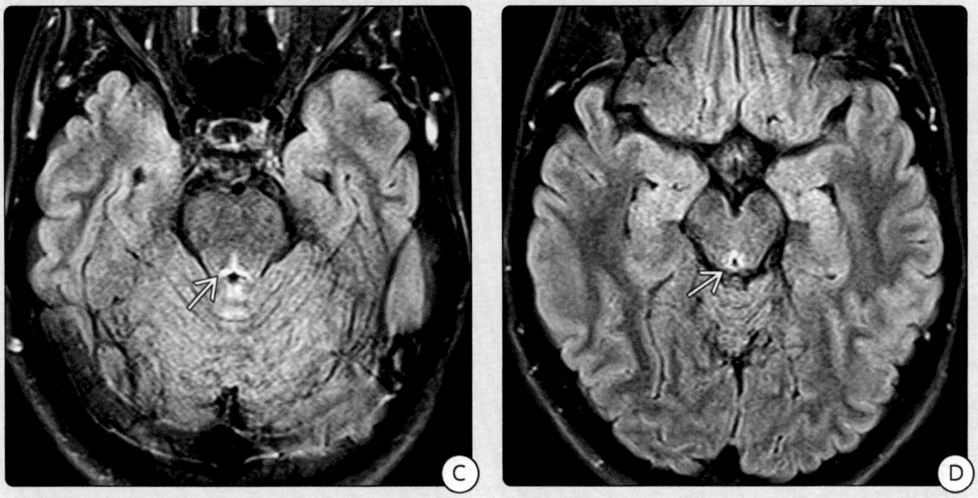

(30-10C) More cephalad FLAIR in the same case shows hyperintensity in the upper dorsal pons ➡. (30-10D) FLAIR through the midbrain and cerebral aqueduct in the same case shows symmetric hyperintensity surrounding the aqueduct ➡.

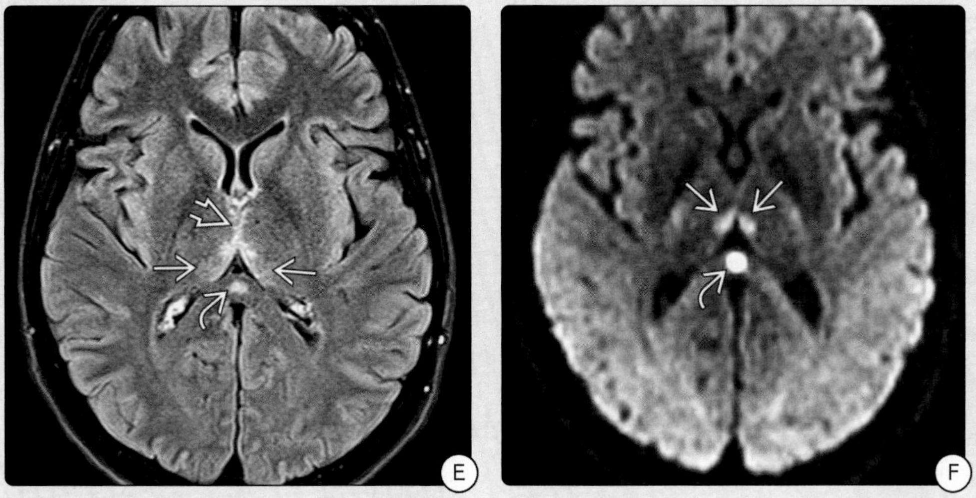

(30-10E) FLAIR through the basal ganglia shows symmetric hyperintensity in the putamina of both thalami ➡. Note hyperintensity along the walls of the third ventricle ➡, focal hyperintensity in the corpus callosum splenium ➡. (30-10F) DWI shows symmetric foci of restricted diffusion in the medial thalami ➡. Note focus in the corpus callosum splenium ➡. Nonalcoholic Wernicke encephalopathy was caused by malnutrition, intractable vomiting.

WE. Callosal necrosis, white matter rarefaction, and mammillary body atrophy can be seen in chronic WE.

Clinical Issues

Demographics. Alcohol dependence occurs in all countries and all socioeconomic groups. In the developed world, AUD is the most common cause of WE. Alcohol-related WE is dose dependent and occurs without sex or ethnicity predilection.

Almost half of all WE cases occur in nonalcoholics. Although WE is generally more common in adults, it *can and does occur in children!*

Presentation. Only 30% of patients demonstrate the classic WE clinical triad of (1) ocular dysfunction (e.g., nystagmus, conjugate gaze palsies, ophthalmoplegia), (2) ataxia, and (3) altered mental status (confusion). The majority of patients have polyneuropathy.

Natural History. Mortality of untreated WE is high. Rapid intravenous thiamine replacement is imperative to prevent the most severe sequelae of WE. Some survivors develop Korsakoff psychosis with severe retrograde amnesia, memory loss, and confabulation.

Imaging

Imaging—especially MR—is playing an increasingly important role in the early diagnosis of WE.

CT Findings. CT has a low sensitivity for the detection of WE and is generally unhelpful. NECT scans in acute WE are often normal. Subtle findings may include bilateral hypodensities around the third ventricle and midbrain. CECT may show subtle enhancement in the affected areas.

MR Findings. MR is much more sensitive than CT and is the procedure of choice in evaluating patients with possible WE. T1WI may show hypointensity around the third ventricle and cerebral aqueduct. In severe cases, petechial hemorrhages are present and may cause T1 hyperintensities in the medial thalami and mammillary bodies. T2* SWI sequences may be helpful in detecting microhemorrhages in the affected areas.

During the acute phase, T2/FLAIR hyperintensity can be seen in the affected areas **(30-9)**. Bilateral symmetric lesions in the putamina and medial thalami around the third ventricle are present in 85% of cases. The tectal plate and periaqueductal gray matter are involved in nearly two-thirds of cases. T2/FLAIR hyperintensity in the mammillary bodies is seen in 50-60% of cases.

Less commonly, the dorsal medulla is affected **(30-10)**. Cerebellar and symmetric cranial nerve involvement have been reported. Bilateral but asymmetric cortical hyperintensities can be present, and some cases show an isolated focus in the corpus callosum splenium **(30-10E)**.

DWI shows corresponding restricted diffusion in the affected areas **(30-9E)**. Some cases show an isolated focus of diffusion restriction in the corpus callosum splenium **(30-10F)**.

In about half of all alcoholic WE cases, postcontrast scans demonstrate enhancement of the periventricular and periaqueductal lesions. Strong uniform enhancement of the mammillary bodies is seen in up to 80% of acute cases and is considered pathognomonic of WE **(30-9F)**. With chronic WE, mammillary body atrophy ensues.

Differential Diagnosis

The medial thalami and midbrain can be symmetrically involved in **artery of Percheron (AOP) infarct** and **deep cerebral vein thrombosis (CVT)**. **Viral infections** such as influenza A and West Nile virus meningoencephalitis cause symmetric medial thalamic and midbrain lesions that may mimic WE. Mammillary bodies are usually not involved.

A rare but reported imaging differential diagnosis is demyelination in the spectrum of **neuromyelitis optica (NMO)**. Therefore, measurement of aquaporin 4 antibodies should be considered if no obvious cause for thiamine deficiency is present.

WERNICKE ENCEPHALOPATHY

Etiology
- Thiamine (vitamin B1) deficiency
- Alcohol related (50%), nonalcoholic (50%)

Pathology
- Acute = petechial hemorrhages (especially mammillary bodies), demyelination
- Chronic = callosal necrosis, mammillary atrophy

Clinical Issues
- Classic triad = ocular dysfunction, ataxia, altered mental status
- Can occur in children!
- Intravenous thiamine imperative

Imaging
- MR > > CT (usually unhelpful)
- T2/FLAIR hyperintensity, DWI restriction
    - Common = medial thalami (85%), periaqueductal gray matter (65%), mammillary bodies (60%), tectum (30%)
    - Less common = dorsal medulla (8%), cerebellum/cranial nerve nuclei (1%), corpus callosum splenium
- SWI may show microhemorrhages
- Enhancement varies
    - More common in alcoholic WE
    - Mammillary body enhancement pathognomonic

Differential Diagnosis
- Artery of Percheron infarct, deep cerebral vein thrombosis
- Viral infection (e.g., influenza A, West Nile virus)
- Neuromyelitis optica

Marchiafava-Bignami Disease

Marchiafava-Bignami disease (MBD) is a rare disorder characterized by osmotic demyelination—and later necrosis—of the corpus callosum.

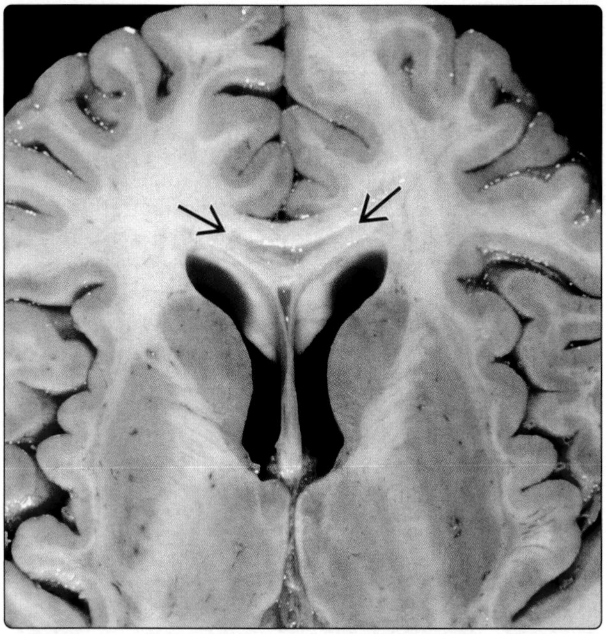

(30-11) *Autopsy specimen from a patient with Marchiafava-Bignami disease shows necrosis in the middle layers of the corpus callosum ➡, the classic pathology in this disorder. (Courtesy R. Hewlett, MD.)*

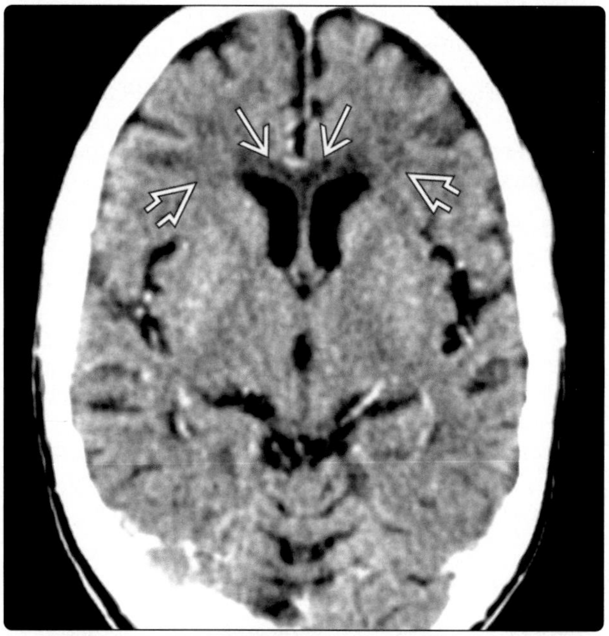

(30-12) *CECT scan in an alcoholic patient with Marchiafava-Bignami disease shows generalized cerebral atrophy and striking hypodensity in the corpus callosum genu ➡ and the adjacent white matter ➡. (Courtesy A. Datir, MD.)*

Terminology

MBD is also (incorrectly) known as "red wine drinkers' encephalopathy."

Etiology

MBD is primarily associated with chronic EtOH abuse. There is an anecdotal (but unproven) association with red wine. Rare cases of MBD in nonalcoholic patients have been reported. Most investigators attribute MBD to vitamin B complex deficiency (i.e., all eight B vitamins, in contrast to the more specific B1 deficiency of WE).

Pathology

Location. The imaging diagnosis of MBD is based on the presence of callosal lesions. Selective involvement of the middle layers along the entire length of the corpus callosum is highly suggestive of MBD **(30-11)**.

Extracallosal lesions do occur with MBD. Extension into the hemispheric white matter as well as internal capsule and middle cerebellar peduncle lesions have been reported. In addition, a specific type of cerebral cortical lesion, known as **Morel laminar sclerosis**, can be seen in the frontolateral cortex.

Gross Pathology. Corpus callosum degeneration is the hallmark of MBD and varies from demyelination to frank cystic necrosis with cavitation of the middle layers.

Clinical Issues

Epidemiology. MBD is rare. Most cases are found in middle-aged men.

Presentation. The clinical diagnosis of MBD is difficult and often confused with WE. Some investigators report that both diseases often occur together.

MBD presents in two major clinical forms. In acute MBD, rapid decline with impaired consciousness, seizures, muscular rigidity, and death within several days is typical. In the chronic form, interhemispheric disconnection syndrome (e.g., apraxia, hemialexia, dementia) can be seen and lasts from months to several years.

Natural History. Most patients who survive MBD have severe neurologic sequelae although a few cases with favorable outcome have been reported.

Treatment Options. If instituted quickly, intravenous vitamin B complex and methylprednisolone therapy may reverse the course of acute MBD.

Imaging

General Features. Selective involvement of the middle layers of the corpus callosum is typical. As with other alcohol-related disorders, MBD can also be accompanied by other alcohol-related pathologies. Chronic alcoholic encephalopathy with generalized brain volume loss is common. Electrolyte disturbances may cause osmotic demyelination.

CT Findings. CT may be normal in the acute stage of MBD. Chronic MBD shows linear hypodensity in the corpus callosum genu that, in the setting of chronic alcohol abuse, is highly suggestive of the diagnosis **(30-12)**.

MR Findings. The initial changes of *acute* MBD are best seen on sagittal FLAIR. Hyperintensity in the corpus callosum genu and frontoparietal cortex appears first, followed by splenial lesions. During the acute phase, the entire corpus callosum may appear swollen and hyperintense.

DWI is initially negative, suggesting that the FLAIR changes probably reflect intramyelinic vasogenic (not cytotoxic) edema. Restriction subsequently develops in the corpus callosum splenium.

Acute white matter lesions may also enhance **(30-13)**. Both peripheral (rim) or solid confluent patterns have been reported.

Chronic MBD with frank callosal necrosis is seen as thinning of the corpus callosum on sagittal T1WI with linear hypointensities in the middle layers **(30-4)**. In patients with chronic MBD, T2* susceptibility-weighted imaging may demonstrate multiple microbleeds in the cortical-subcortical regions and corpus callosum. Other changes associated with chronic alcohol abuse, such as cortical, cerebellar, and mammillary body atrophy, are common.

For inpatients with chronic MBD, DTI with fiber tracking discloses a substantial decrease in fibers crossing through the splenium.

Differential Diagnosis

In the setting of EtOH abuse, callosal lesions are highly suggestive of MBD. Other diseases that may affect the corpus callosum include **multiple sclerosis, axonal stretch injuries**, and **lacunar infarction**. All have patchy discontinuous lesions that rarely involve the entire length of the corpus callosum.

Methanol Intoxication

Methanol (MtOH) is a strong CNS depressant. Patients are often comatose, and an accurate history may be impossible to obtain. Moreover, few hospitals include methanol in their standard toxicology screens. Therefore, delayed diagnosis is common, and morbidity and mortality remain high. Imaging

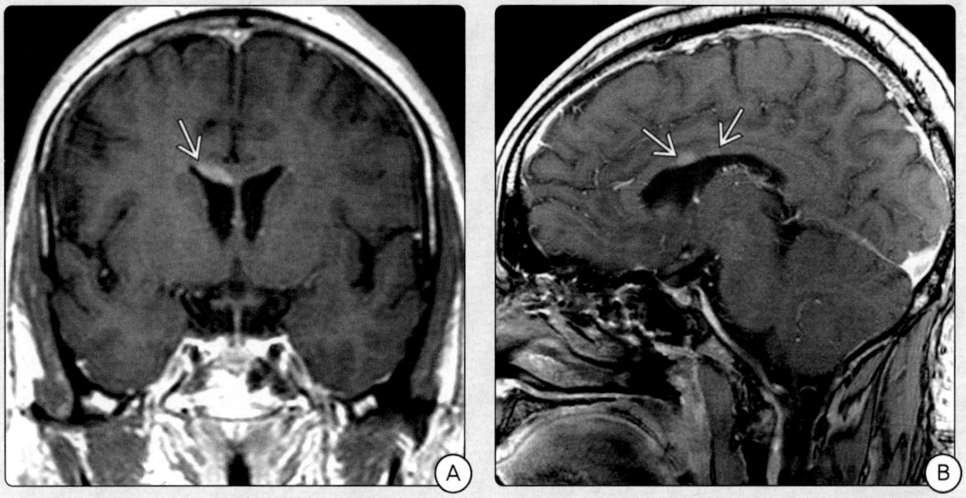

***(30-13A)** Coronal T1 C+ in a patient who "drinks like a fish" shows enhancement in the corpus callosum ➡. **(30-13B)** Sagittal T1 C+ FS scan shows enhancing lesions in the corpus callosum ➡.*

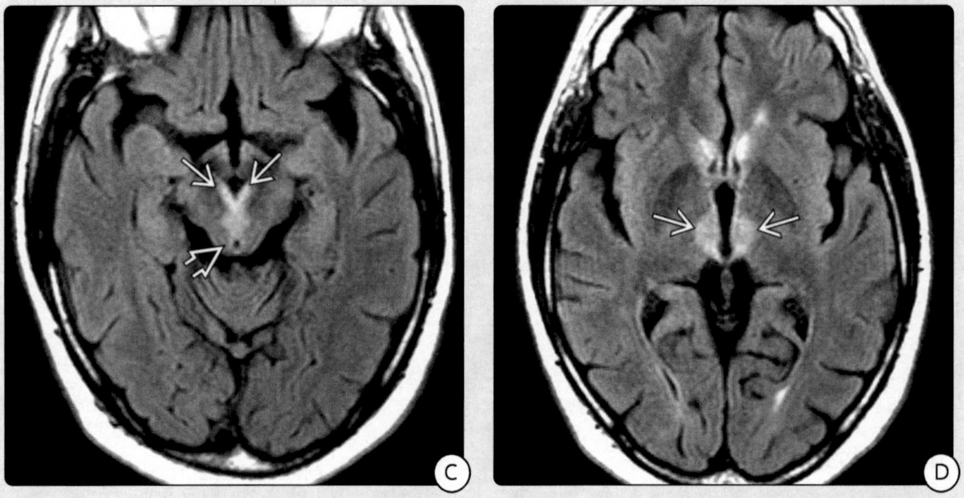

***(30-13C)** Axial FLAIR scan in the same patient shows symmetric hyperintensity in the midbrain ➡ and periaqueductal gray matter ➡. **(30-13D)** More cephalad scan shows hyperintensity in the medial thalami ➡, along the walls of the third ventricle. Acute Marchiafava-Bignami disease is shown with imaging findings of both acute demyelination and Wernicke encephalopathy. (Courtesy S. van der Westhuizen, MD.)*

may provide important clues to the diagnosis of possible MtOH toxicity.

Terminology

MtOH intoxication or poisoning is also known as methanol encephalopathy.

Etiology

MtOH is a common component of solvents, varnishes, perfumes, paint removers, antifreeze, and gasoline mixtures. It can be accidentally or intentionally ingested, inhaled, or absorbed transdermally. Some cases of MtOH poisoning result from the intake of illicit spirits ("moonshine").

MtOH is metabolized to formic and lactic acid, causing severe metabolic acidosis with arterial pHs ranging from 6.8 to 7.1. Increased anion and osmolar gaps are important laboratory clues to the presence of MtOH toxicity.

Pathology

Location. Bilateral basal ganglia necrosis is the most characteristic imaging feature of MtOH poisoning. Selective putamina involvement with relative sparing of the globi pallidi is common. Diffuse necrosis of the subinsular and subcortical white matter occurs in severe cases **(30-14)**.

There is no consistent relationship between clinical outcome and the extent of imaging abnormalities.

Clinical Issues

Epidemiology. Compared with ethanol-induced encephalopathy, MtOH poisoning is rare.

Demographics. Patients are overwhelmingly male. Peak age is between the third and fourth decades.

Presentation. A peculiarity of MtOH poisoning is the latent period between ingestion and the appearance of clinical

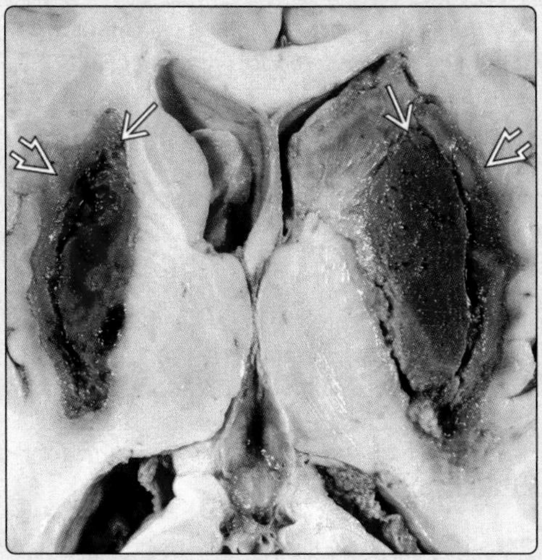

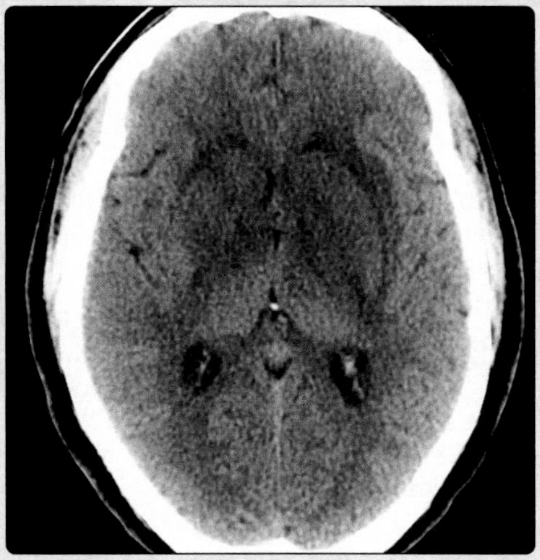

***(30-14)** Autopsy specimen from a patient with fatal methanol toxicity shows hemorrhagic necrosis in both putamina ➡ and subinsular white matter ➡. (Courtesy R. Hewlett, MD.) **(30-15)** Axial NECT in acute methanol poisoning shows confluent, symmetric hypointensities in the basal ganglia and internal capsules.*

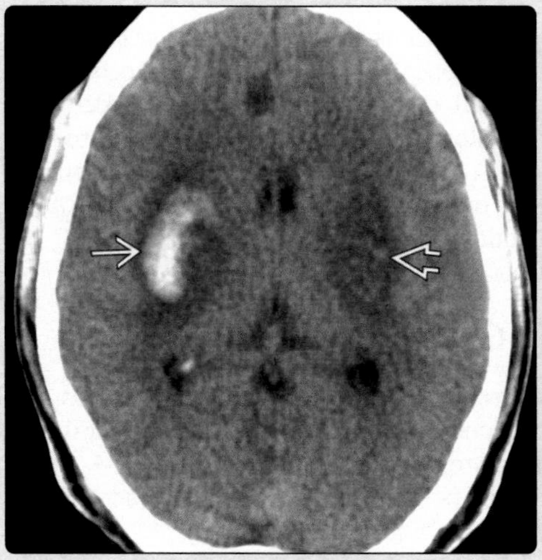

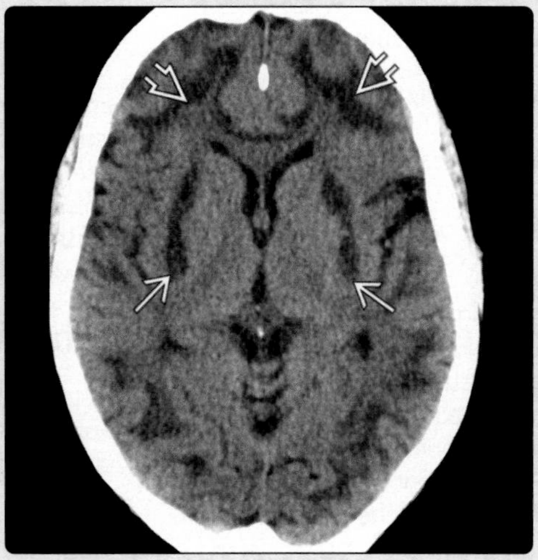

***(30-16)** NECT scan in a patient with subacute methanol poisoning shows confluent ➡ and patchy ➡ hemorrhagic putaminal necrosis. (Courtesy R. Ramakantan, MD.) **(30-17)** NECT scan in a patient who survived acute methanol poisoning shows shrunken, hypodense putamina ➡ and bilateral symmetric hypodensities in the subcortical white matter ➡.*

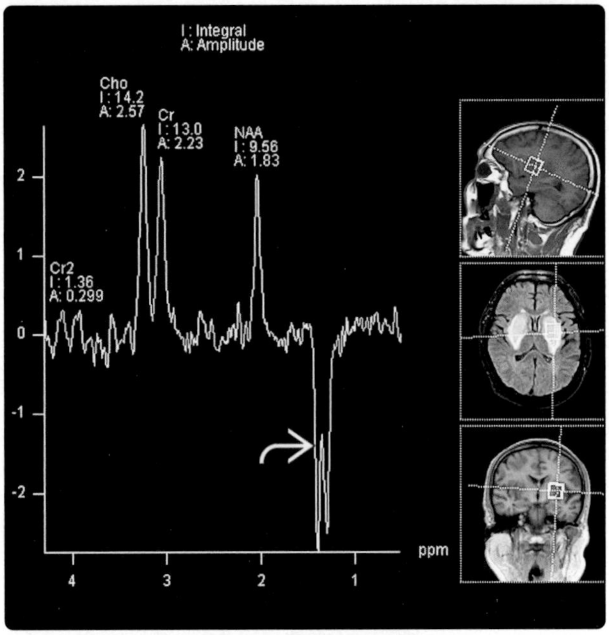

(30-18) Single-voxel MRS through the basal ganglia in a patient with methanol-induced putaminal necrosis shows reduced NAA and a huge lactate doublet ➔.

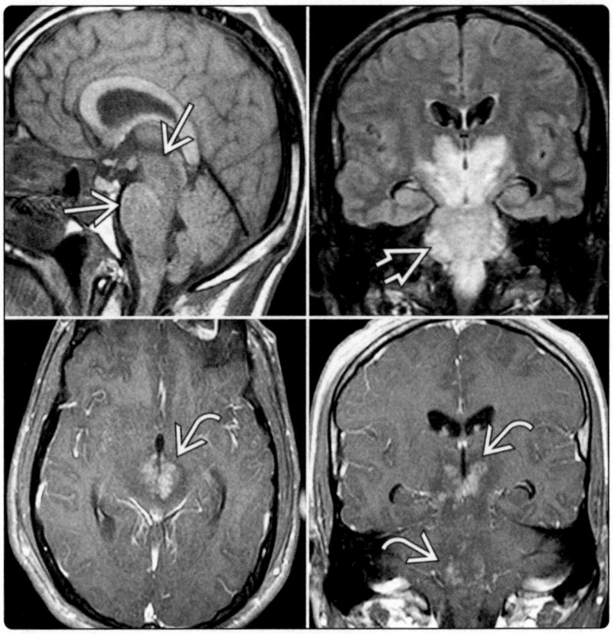

(30-19) Sagittal T1WI shows pons and midbrain hypointensity ➔, which is better seen as hyperintensity on coronal FLAIR ➔. Patchy enhancement is seen on T1 C+ ➔.

symptoms. Symptom onset is variable and often delayed, especially if ethanol is ingested simultaneously, as this slows MtOH metabolism. Between 85-90% of patients present with visual disturbances. Three-quarters of all patients have nonspecific gastrointestinal symptoms such as nausea and vomiting. Approximately 25% are comatose on admission.

Natural History. Ingestion of 30 mL of pure MtOH usually results in death. As little as 4 mL can result in blindness. Blood MtOH levels above 200 mg/L are considered toxic, and levels above 1,500 mg/L are potentially fatal.

Although the latency in symptom onset is variable, symptom progression may be rapid. Respiratory arrest and death can occur within a few hours.

Putaminal hemorrhage and insular subcortical white matter necrosis are associated with poor clinical outcome.

Treatment Options. MtOH is effectively treated with alkali to combat acidosis, antidotes (ethanol or fomepizole) to block production of formic acid, and hemodialysis to remove MtOH and formate.

Imaging

CT Findings. Initial NECT scan is normal in many patients with MtOH poisoning. Most patients who survive for more than 24 hours demonstrate bilateral symmetric hypodense lesions in the putamina, globi pallidi, and sometimes the deep cerebral white matter **(30-15)**. Hemorrhagic putaminal necrosis is seen in 15-25% of cases **(30-16)**. Enhancement is variable, ranging from none to peripheral enhancement of the putaminal lesions.

If the patient survives, cystic cavities form within the putamina, representing the chronic sequelae of MtOH poisoning **(30-17)**.

MR Findings. Bilateral putaminal and basal ganglia necrosis with variable white matter involvement is present. T2/FLAIR hyperintensity is seen with 25% exhibiting "blooming" foci on T2*. DWI shows restricted diffusion in the acute stage of methanol poisoning. MRS shows reduced NAA and markedly elevated lactate **(30-18)**.

Surviving patients have symmetric T2/FLAIR hyperintense lesions in the putamina with variable involvement of the subcortical white matter.

Differential Diagnosis

Bilateral symmetric putaminal lesions are not specific for MtOH and can be seen in **Wilson disease** and **mitochondrial encephalopathies** (e.g., Kearns-Sayre, Leigh). **Hypoxic-ischemic encephalopathy** involves the caudate and other deep gray nuclei in addition to the putamina. Acute **cyanide poisoning** is rare but can resemble MtOH encephalopathy. **Carbon monoxide poisoning** generally affects the globi pallidi rather than the putamina.

Ethylene Glycol Poisoning

Recent reports from the American Association of Poison Control Centers indicate that ethylene glycol is the third most common chemical responsible for deaths by nonpharmaceutical poisoning (following ethanol and carbon monoxide).

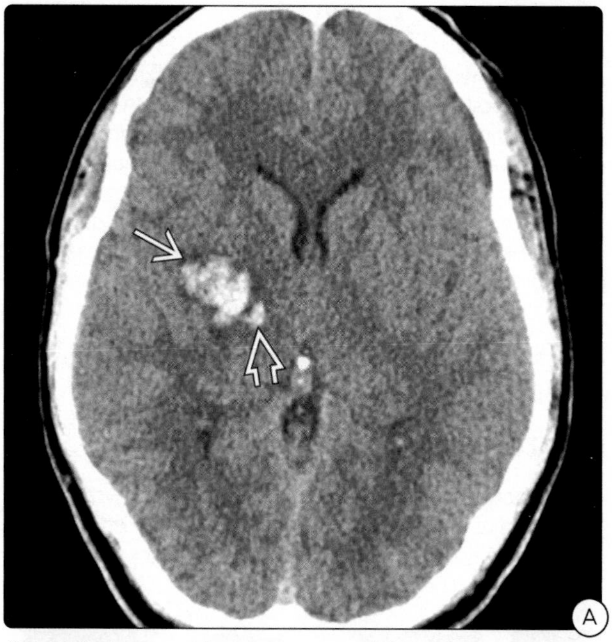

(30-20A) NECT scan shows a 32y man with amphetamine abuse, energy drink bingeing who presented with left hemiparesis and facial droop. Note focal acute hemorrhage in the right basal ganglia ➡ and posterior limb of the internal capsule ➡.

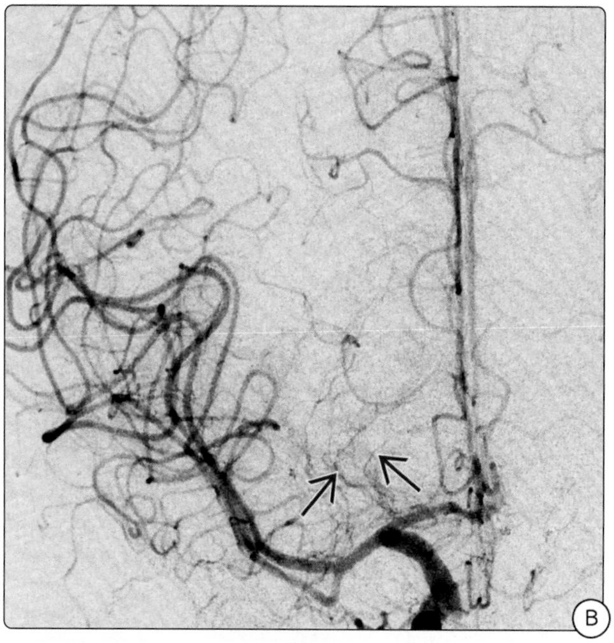

(30-20B) AP DSA in the same case obtained 24 hours later shows striking irregularity and beading of the medial and lateral lenticulostriate arteries ➡. This was drug-induced vasculitis.

Ethylene glycol is a colorless, odorless, sweet-tasting, but poisonous form of alcohol that is a common component found in many household products such as antifreeze, deicing solutions, and windshield wiper fluids. It may be ingested by alcoholics or, because of its sweet taste and the ease of access, it is often accidentally ingested by children and animals. Intake of even a small volume can prove lethal.

When ingested, ethylene glycol causes metabolic acidosis and can damage the brain, liver, kidneys, and lungs. The toxicity of ethylene glycol is mediated by its metabolites, mainly glycolic acid and oxalate. Glycolic acid is responsible for the metabolic acidosis. Glycolate is then metabolized to oxalate, which precipitates with calcium as calcium oxalate and is deposited in various tissues. The high anion gap of metabolic acidosis and osmolar gap resolve within 24 to 72 hours.

Early treatment with bicarbonate and ethanol or the alcohol dehydrogenase inhibitor 4-methylpyrazole (4MP, fomepizole) is very effective. Emergent hemodialysis is appropriate if the ethylene glycol level is more than 50 mg/dL and can be life saving.

Imaging findings of acute ethylene glycol toxicity include edema in the basal ganglia, thalami, midbrain, and upper pons **(30-19)**. Hemorrhagic putaminal necrosis, similar to that observed in methanol intoxication, can be seen in subacute and chronic cases.

Amphetamines and Derivatives

The "hedonic" and addictive properties of drugs of abuse—particularly amphetamines and cocaine—are at least in part related to increased dopamine levels in the synapses of monoaminergic neurons although multiple other neurotransmitter systems (e.g., serotonergic, GABAergic and glutamatergic circuits) are clearly involved in stimulant pharmacology.

CNS stimulants include cocaine, amphetamine, methamphetamine, methylenedioxymethamphetamine (MDMA), and methylphenidate. Although not a classic CNS stimulant, nicotine is a prototypic drug that is avidly self-administered and has some stimulating properties. All these drugs have a high human abuse liability.

Most addictive drugs are excitotoxic and cause two major types of pathologies: vascular events (e.g., ischemia, hemorrhage) and leukoencephalopathy.

Functional neuroimaging studies have also demonstrated that drugs of abuse are associated with dysfunctions in a range of overlapping brain regions. Working memory, inhibitory control, attention, and decision-making are all negatively impacted, the degree of which correlates with the severity and chronicity of abuse. In addition, CNS mitosis, migration, and cell survival in the fetus of a pregnant, substance-abusing woman are adversely affected.

Methamphetamine

Methamphetamine (MA or "meth") is a highly addictive psychostimulant drug. "Crystal" methamphetamine abuse has been steadily increasing over the past decade. Even a single acute exposure to MA can result in profound changes in cerebral blood flow. Both hemorrhagic and ischemic strokes occur **(30-20)** **(30-21)** **(30-22)**.

MR in chronic adult MA users demonstrates lower gray matter volumes on T1WI, especially in the frontal lobes, and more white matter hyperintensities on T2/FLAIR scans than are appropriate for the patient's age. MRS shows increased choline and myoinositol levels in the frontal lobes. DTI shows lower fractional anisotropy in the frontal lobes and higher ADC values in the basal ganglia.

MDMA ("Ecstasy")

3-,4-Methylenedioxymethamphetamine is also known as **MDMA** or **ecstasy**. Popular as a party drug, MDMA induces euphoria and sensory disturbances secondary to rapid release of potent vasoconstrictors from serotonergic synapses. MDMA can cause arterial constriction, vasculitis, or prolonged vasospasm with acute ischemic infarcts. MDMA-induced ischemia is most pronounced in serotonin-rich brain areas such as the globus pallidus and occipital cortex, which are especially vulnerable **(30-23)**.

Acute hippocampal necrosis with subsequent atrophy has been reported in chronic ecstasy users.

Benzodiazepines

Benzodiazepines, sometimes called "**benzo**," are psychoactive drugs used to treat anxiety, insomnia, seizures, muscle spasms, and alcohol withdrawal. Benzodiazepines such as

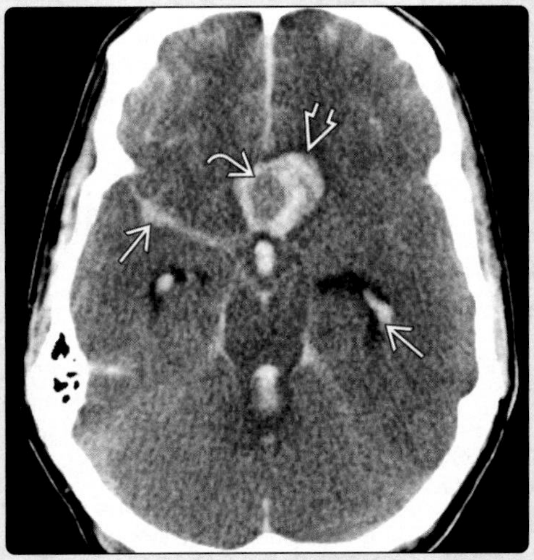

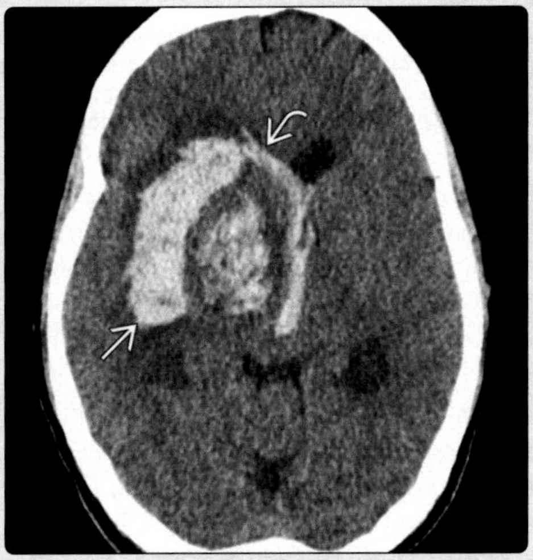

***(30-21)** A 32y female methamphetamine abuser had sudden severe headache and coma. NECT shows diffuse subarachnoid, intraventricular hemorrhage ➡ and focal interhemispheric hematoma ➡ surrounding an ACoA aneurysm ➡. **(30-22)** Axial NECT in a 35y female methamphetamine abuser shows a large basal ganglionic hemorrhage ➡ that has dissected into the lateral ventricle ➡.*

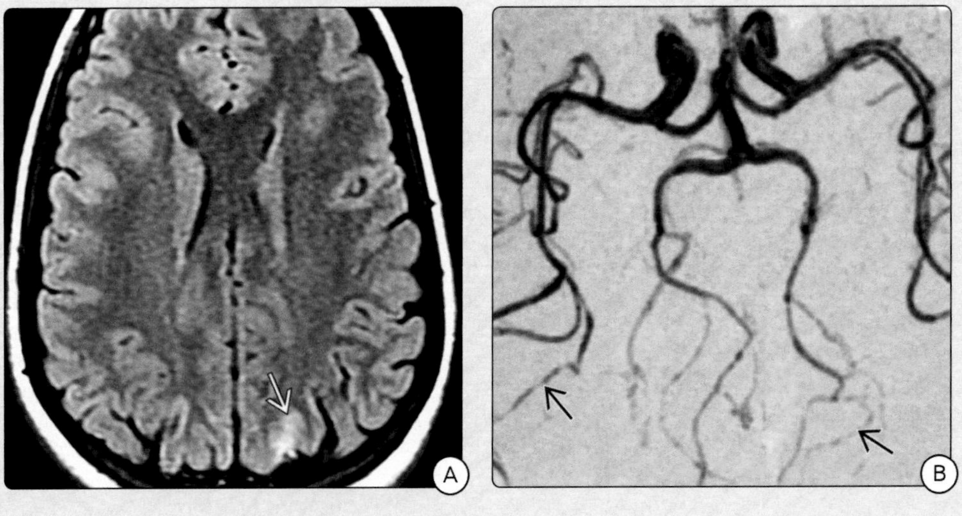

***(30-23A)** Axial FLAIR scan in a teenager who used MDMA ("ecstasy") at a "rave" party shows focal left occipital lobe hyperintensity ➡. (Courtesy P. Hildenbrand, MD.) **(30-23B)** MRA in the same patient shows alternating areas of narrowing and dilatation ➡ in the occipital, posterior parietal arteries, consistent with drug-induced vasculitis. (Courtesy P. Hildenbrand, MD.)*

temazepam and midazolam act selectively on GABA-A receptors in the brain, inhibiting or reducing the activity of neurons.

Benzodiazepine overdose has been associated with hypoxic-ischemic encephalopathy **(30-24)**, hemorrhagic ischemic strokes **(30-25)**, and delayed toxic leukoencephalopathy.

Cocaine

Cocaine can be sniffed/snorted, smoked, or injected. In its most common form (cocaine hydrochloride), it is ingested via the nasal mucosa. "Crack," the alkaloidal freebase form of cocaine hydrochloride, can also be smoked.

Etiology

Regardless of the route of administration, the adverse impact of cocaine on the brain is largely related to its vascular effects. Systemic hypertension can be extreme, causing spontaneous hemorrhagic strokes.

Rupture of a preexisting aneurysm or underlying vascular malformation accounts for nearly half of all cocaine-related hemorrhagic strokes **(30-28)**. Cocaine also facilitates platelet aggregation and may lead to thrombotic vascular occlusion.

Acute cerebral vasoconstriction and/or cocaine-induced vasculopathy may lead to ischemic strokes. Snorted cocaine causes severe vasoconstriction in the vascular plexus of the nasal septal mucosa (Kiesselbach plexus). Chronic abuse may lead to septal necrosis and perforation.

Pathology

Macroscopic hemorrhages, particularly in the putamen and external capsule, are the most common gross pathologic findings and are twice as common as ischemic strokes.

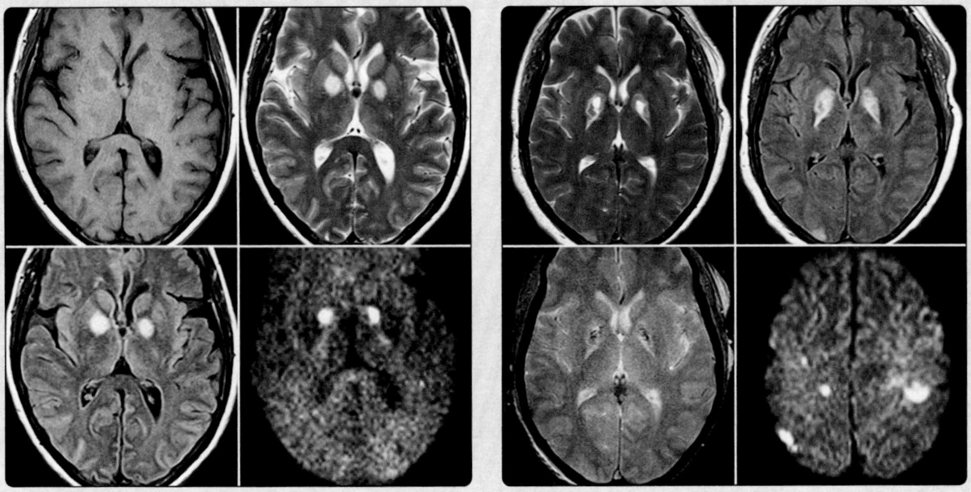

***(30-24)** A 60y depressed woman was found unconscious after overdose with benzodiazepines and opioids. Imaging shows bilateral symmetric globi pallidi lesions. **(30-25)** MR scans in a 45y bipolar woman with toxicology positive for opiates and benzodiazepines show globi pallidi and cortical infarcts. She also had symmetric hemorrhagic cerebellar infarcts (not shown).*

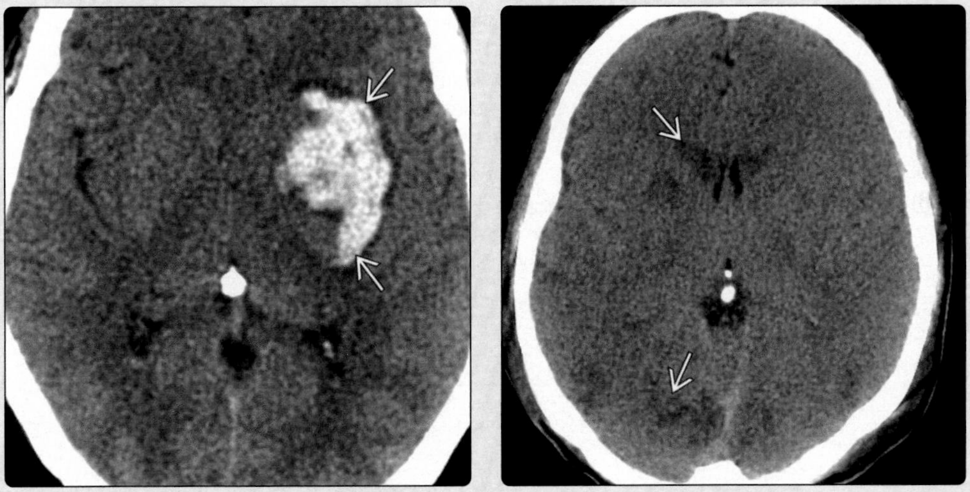

***(30-26)** NECT shows acute hypertensive hemorrhage with putamen/external capsule hemorrhage ➡ in a patient who abused cocaine. **(30-27)** NECT scan in a patient with cocaine abuse shows diffuse brain swelling and multifocal ischemic infarcts ➡.*

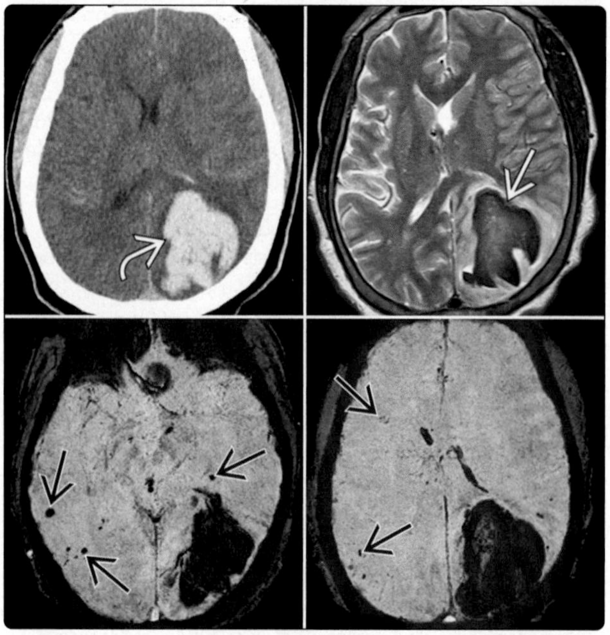

(30-28) (Upper L) NECT in polydrug abuse shows occipital hematoma ➡. (Upper R) T2WI 3 days later shows early subacute hematoma ➡. (Lower L, R) SWIs show multiple microbleeds ⇨. Unmasking of multiple cavernous malformations is shown.

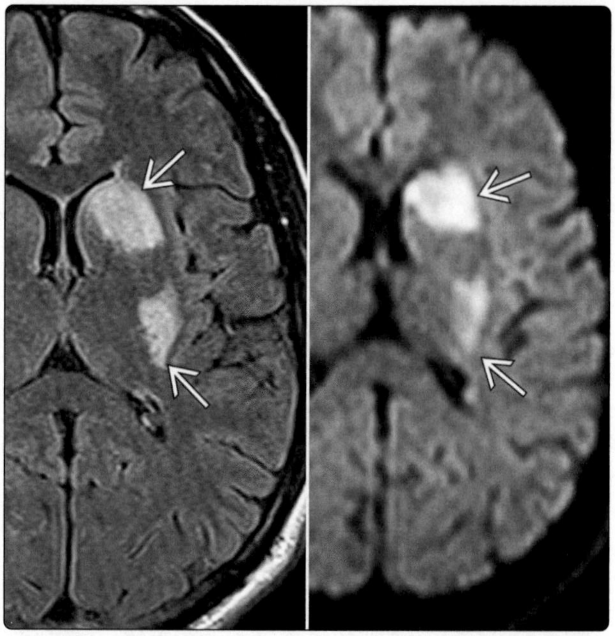

(30-29) Axial FLAIR scan (L) and DWI (R) in a 35y male cocaine abuser show ischemic infarcts in the left basal ganglia ➡.

Microscopically, cocaine arteriopathy is characterized by inflammatory changes and necrosis.

Clinical Issues

Epidemiology. Nearly one-third of strokes in patients younger than 45 years old are drug related, with 80-90% occurring in the fourth and fifth decades. Stroke risk is highest within the first 6 hours after drug use.

Presentation. Headache, seizure, and focal neurologic deficits are the most common symptoms.

Natural History. The onset of cocaine-related stroke may be immediate if hypertensive or subarachnoid hemorrhage occurs. Cocaine-induced vasculopathy with ischemic infarcts may occur up to a week after use.

Imaging

Strokes—both ischemic and hemorrhagic—are the major manifestations of cocaine-induced brain damage **(30-26)**. The hemorrhages can be parenchymal (secondary to hypertension or vascular malformation) **(30-28)** or subarachnoid (aneurysm rupture). Hypertensive bleeds are usually centered in the external capsule/putamen or in the thalamus.

Ischemic strokes can be caused by vasospasm, cocaine-induced vasoconstriction, vasculitis, or thrombosis **(30-27)**. Bilateral globus pallidus infarction has also been reported as a stroke subtype in cocaine abuse.

Acute cocaine-induced strokes are positive on DWI **(30-29)**. MRA, CTA, or DSA may show focal areas of arterial narrowing and irregularity.

Acute hypertensive encephalopathy with posterior reversible encephalopathy (PRES-like syndrome) can also occur. Vasogenic edema in the occipital lobes is the most common finding.

Differential Diagnosis

Unexplained parenchymal hemorrhage in young and middle-aged adults should prompt evaluation for possible drug abuse. **Embolic infarcts** as well as **vasculitis** may appear identical to cocaine vasculopathy.

COCAINE AND AMPHETAMINE EFFECTS ON THE BRAIN

Amphetamines

- Methamphetamine
  - Hemorrhagic, ischemic strokes
- MDMA ("ecstasy")
  - Vasospasm, infarcts
  - Location: occipital cortex, globus pallidus
- Benzodiazepines
  - Delayed toxic leukoencephalopathy

Cocaine

- Intracranial hemorrhage
  - Hypertensive intracranial hemorrhage (50%)
  - "Unmasked" aneurysm or arteriovenous malformation (50%)
- Ischemic stroke
  - Vasospasm, vasculitis
- Acute hypertensive encephalopathy
  - Posterior reversible encephalopathy syndrome (PRES)
  - Vasogenic edema (typically bioccipital)

Opioids and Derivatives

The ten drugs most frequently involved in overdose deaths include several opioids: **heroin, oxycodone, methadone, morphine, hydrocodone,** and **fentanyl**. Of these, heroin is the most commonly abused opioid.

In addition to the direct effects of opioids on the brain, impurities and additives may produce systemic pathology. Hypotension and anoxia may also complicate the clinical and imaging appearance of opioid toxicity.

Heroin

Heroin use has a direct and damaging effect on certain brain functions that are associated with impulsive and unhealthy decision making.

Heroin is usually injected intravenously. The most common acute complication of injected heroin is stroke. Globus pallidus ischemia, very similar to that seen in carbon monoxide poisoning, is common.

The most dramatic acute effects occur with inhaled heroin. The freebase form is heated over aluminum foil and the vapors inhaled (**"chasing the dragon"**). Heroin vapor inhalation causes a striking toxic leukoencephalopathy.

The most frequent secondary complication of heroin abuse is infection. Endocarditis is common and may result in septic emboli, brain abscesses, and vasculitis with mycotic aneurysm formation.

Etiology

Heroin causes both acute and chronic effects such as vasculopathy, leukoencephalopathy, and generalized brain volume loss. Stimulation of opioid receptors in vascular smooth muscle may cause reversible vasospasm. Immune-mediated response to additives in injected heroin may cause ischemia or vasculitis.

Pathology

Autopsied brains of patients with heroin-associated encephalopathy show a sponge-like appearance of the cerebral white matter. Microscopy demonstrates demyelination and white matter vacuolization. Because the cerebellum has a high density of opioid receptors, similar changes can be seen in its white matter.

Imaging

CT Findings. Acute CNS toxicity from inhaled heroin ("chasing the dragon") is characterized by symmetric hypodensities in the cerebellar white matter, sometimes described as a "butterfly wing" pattern **(30-30)**. The posterior cerebral white matter, posterior limb of the internal capsule, and globi pallidi are also commonly affected. The anterior limb of the internal capsule is typically spared.

MR Findings. T2 and FLAIR scans in patients with early heroin-related leukoencephalopathy show symmetric hyperintensity in the cerebellar white matter with relative sparing of the dentate nuclei. There is often selective symmetric involvement of the posterior limb of the internal capsule, the corticospinal tract, the medial lemniscus, and the tractus solitarius **(30-30)**.

Confluent hyperintensity in the cerebral white matter, including the corpus callosum, is common in severe cases of heroin vapor encephalopathy **(30-31)**. DWI shows acute diffusion restriction in the affected areas; MRS shows a lactate peak in the cerebral white matter.

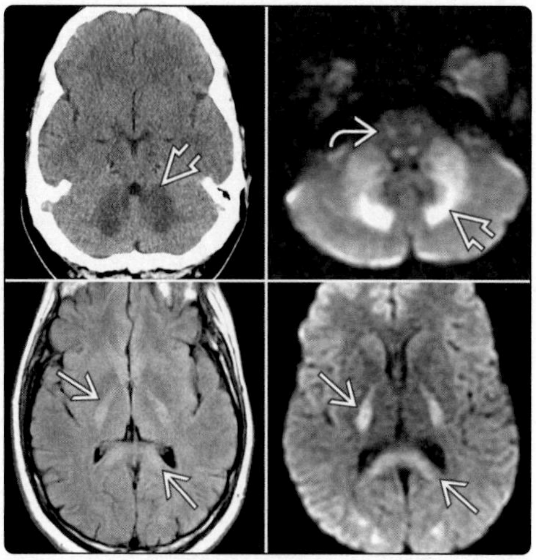

***(30-30)** Inhaled heroin results in abnormalities in pons ➡, cerebellum ➡, corpus callosum, and internal capsules ➡. (Courtesy K. Nelson, MD.)*

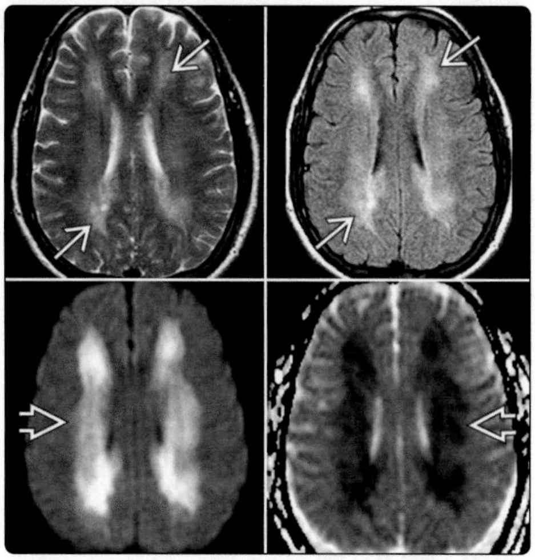

***(30-31)** "Chasing the dragon" shows hyperintensity ➡ and restricted diffusion ➡ in periventricular WM. (Courtesy M. Michel, MD.)*

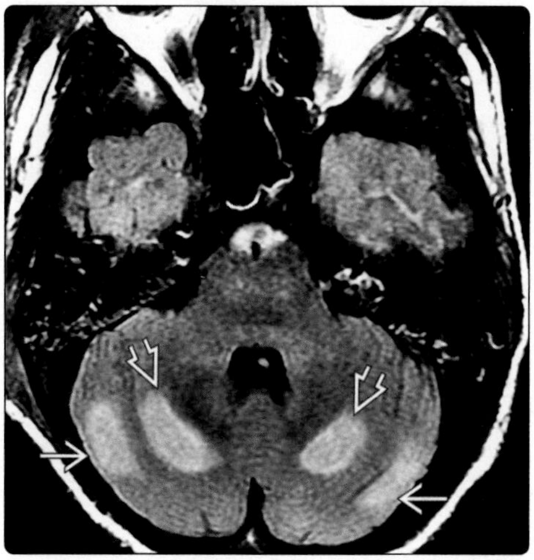

***(30-32)** FLAIR shows symmetric cerebellar ➡ and white matter lesions ➡ in oxycodone overdose.*

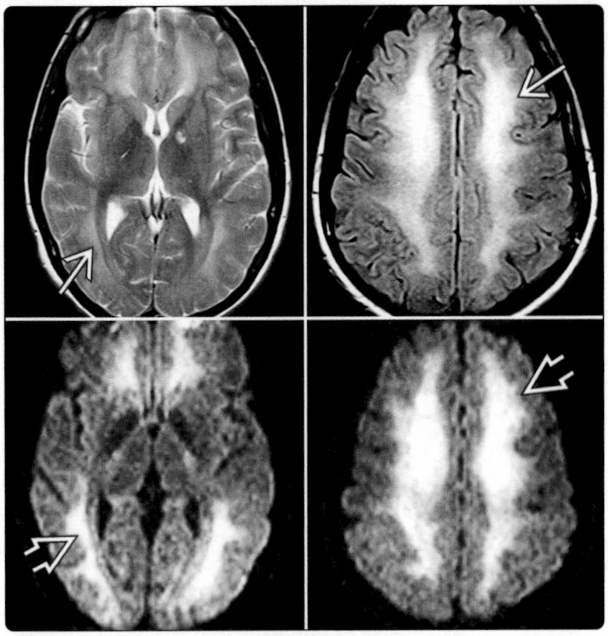

(30-33) MRs in a 33y woman who overdosed on methadone show striking symmetric confluent hyperintensity (leukoencephalopathy) on FLAIR and restricted diffusion on DWI .

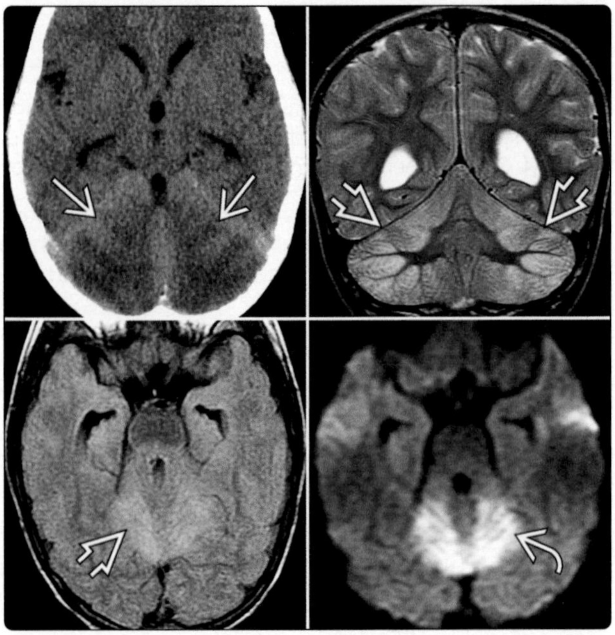

(30-34) Accidental methadone poisoning in a child shows bilateral cerebellar hypodensity on NECT , T2/FLAIR hyperintensity , and restricted diffusion .

Chronic heroin abuse can cause microvascular disease. Scattered multifocal hyperintensities in the subcortical or periventricular white matter are common but neither as prevalent nor as severe as seen with cocaine vasculopathy.

Longer duration of heroin use is also associated with more damaging effects on brain functions. fMR has demonstrated that heroin-induced brain changes may last long after abstinence.

Methadone

So-called substitute drugs such as the synthetic opioid methadone are used in the medication-assisted therapy for drug abuse/dependence as well as in the management of intractable pain. With increasing use and availability, methadone overdose is likewise growing.

A postopioid delayed toxic leukoencephalopathy similar to that caused by inhaled heroin has been reported with methadone. Diffuse, symmetric, confluent hyperintensity in the cerebral white matter on T2/FLAIR is seen **(30-33)**. Sparing of the subcortical U-fibers is typical. In contrast to heroin toxicity, cerebellar and brainstem changes are subtle or absent in adults. MRS shows elevated choline, decreased NAA, and increased lactate.

Accidental ingestion of methadone has been reported to cause severe cerebellar edema with acute obstructive hydrocephalus in children **(30-34)**.

Oxycodone

Imaging in the few reported cases of oxycodone and OxyContin overdose shows restricted diffusion in the cerebellar hemispheres and globi pallidi **(30-32)**.

OPIOID DRUGS

Heroin
- Injected
  - Most common = ischemic strokes
  - Globi pallidi, white matter (resembles carbon monoxide poisoning)
- Inhaled
  - "Chasing the dragon"
  - Most common = leukoencephalopathy
  - Cerebellum, cerebral white matter

Methadone
- Adults
  - Toxic leukoencephalopathy
- Children
  - Usually accidental ingestion
  - Cerebellar edema

Oxycodone
- Cerebellar, globus pallidus ischemia
- Less common = toxic leukoencephalopathy

Inhaled Gases and Toxins

Some drugs of abuse such as heroin have multiple potential routes of administration. Others are solely gases and therefore exclusively inhaled. Examples include toxins such as carbon monoxide and drugs of abuse such as nitrous oxide. Some toxins such as cyanide can be inhaled, ingested, or absorbed transdermally. Cyanides may also cause—or contribute to—deaths from smoke inhalation.

Inhaled vapors from volatile, intrinsically liquid agents include amyl nitrite ("poppers") and industrial solvents (e.g., toluene). Studies have shown that petrol sniffing is often the earliest inhaled drug used and increases both the likelihood and earlier use of other drugs.

Carbon Monoxide Poisoning

Terminology

Carbon monoxide (CO) is a colorless, odorless, tasteless gas that is produced by the incomplete combustion of various fuels. CO poisoning is caused by deliberate or accidental inhalation.

Etiology

The toxic effects of CO result mostly from impaired oxygen transport. CO combines reversibly with hemoglobin (Hgb) with over 200 times higher the affinity than that of oxygen. If carboxyhemoglobin (CO-Hgb) levels exceed 20%, brain and cardiac damage are common.

CO-Hgb impairs erythrocyte oxygen transport, reducing cellular oxygen and causing hypoxia. In addition, lipid peroxidation leads to oxidative injury. Peroxynitrites damage the vascular endothelium.

Pathology

Location. Because the globi pallidi are exquisitely sensitive to hypoxia, the hallmark of acute CO poisoning is symmetric globus pallidi necrosis **(30-35)** **(30-36)**. The cerebral white matter is the second most commonly affected and often

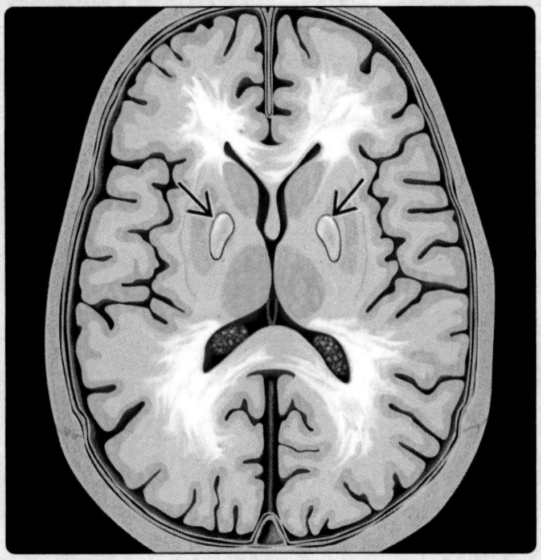

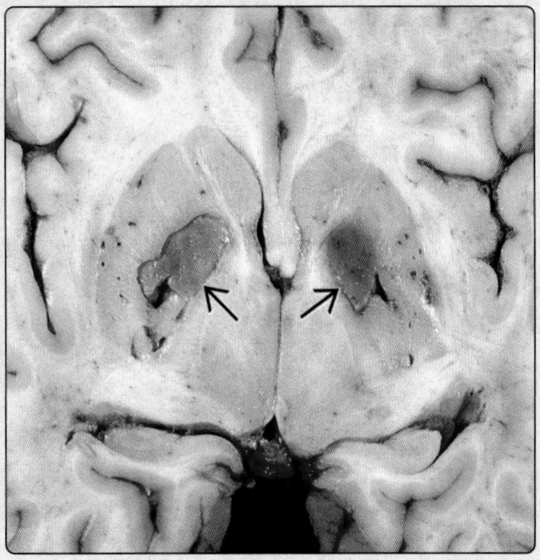

***(30-35)** Axial graphic shows the typical involvement of the brain by CO poisoning. The globi pallidi (GP) → are most affected, followed by the cerebral white matter. Pathologically, there is necrosis of the GP with variable areas of necrosis and demyelination in the white matter.* ***(30-36)** Autopsy of carbon monoxide poisoning shows symmetric coagulative (nonhemorrhagic) necrosis of both medial GP →. (Courtesy R. Hewlett, MD).*

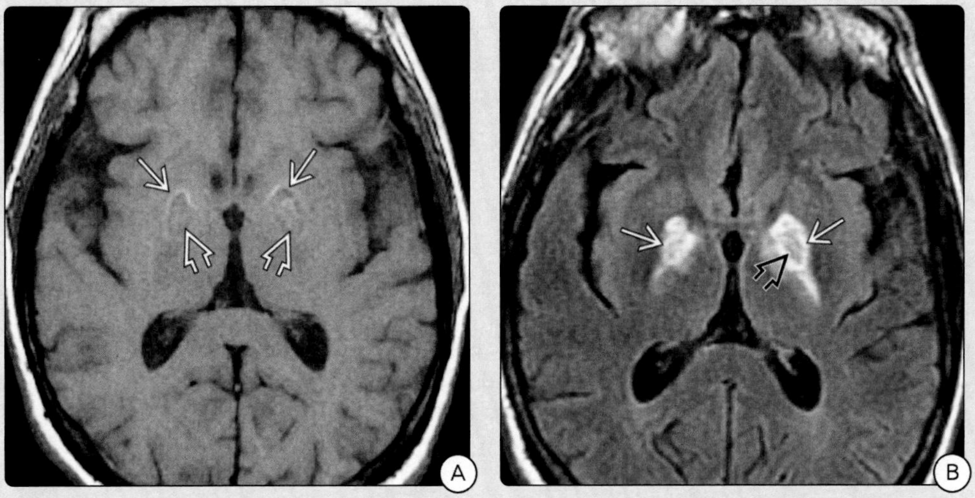

***(30-37A)** T1WI in a 49y man with CO poisoning shows symmetric lesions in both medial GP. Note faint hyperintense rim →, thin hypointense underlying rim, and central coagulative necrosis seen as mildly hyperintense lesions →.* ***(30-37B)** FLAIR scan in the same patient shows that the lesion is mostly hyperintense → with central isointense core →. The isointense parts of the lesions enhanced on T1 C+ (not shown).*

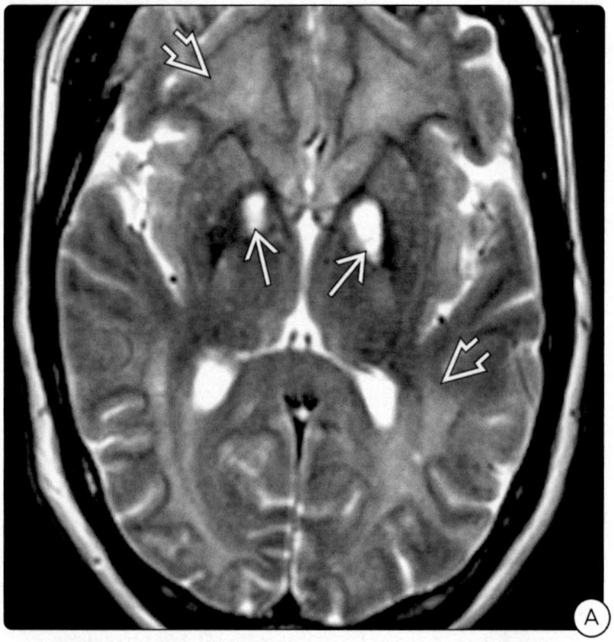

(30-38A) Axial T2WI in a patient with CO poisoning 2 weeks prior shows characteristic bilateral hyperintensities in globi pallidi ➡. Confluent hyperintensity now involves virtually all of the cerebral WM ➡, except the subcortical U-fibers.

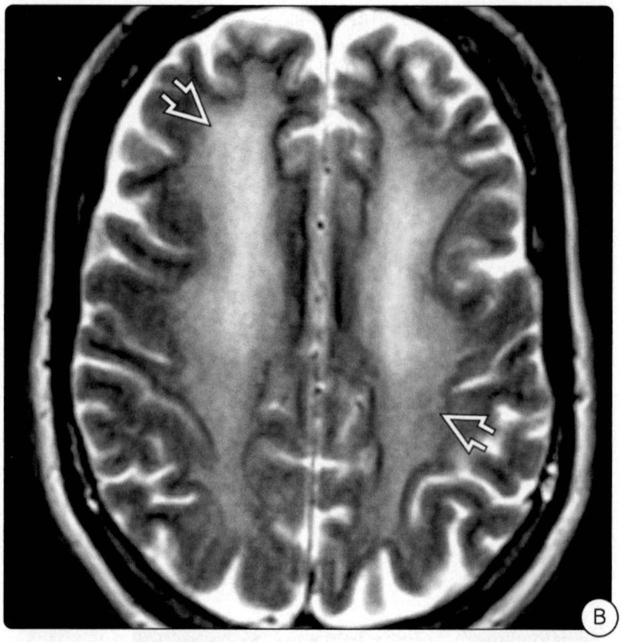

(30-38B) More cephalad T2WI shows that the hyperintensity involves most of the corona radiata ➡, mostly spares subcortical WM. This was "interval" (subacute) form of CO poisoning with toxic demyelination.

shows delayed demyelination and necrosis that may appear several weeks after the initial insult.

In addition to bilateral globi pallidi and cerebral white matter, various sites such as the cerebral cortex, cerebellum, hippocampus, amygdala, corpus callosum splenium, and insula are often involved.

Clinical Issues

Presentation and Natural History. Acute CO poisoning initially causes nausea, vomiting, headache, and impaired consciousness. Outcome depends on both duration and intensity of exposure. Seizures, coma, and death may ensue.

Patients who survive CO poisoning often develop delayed encephalopathy. Parkinson-like symptoms, memory deficits, and cognitive disturbances are common.

Treatment Options. Although there is some early success in therapies that target the downstream inflammatory and oxidative effects of CO poisoning, to date there is no available antidotal therapy. Hyperbaric oxygen significantly reduces the permanent neurologic and affective effects of CO poisoning. Early administration of 100% inspired oxygen may help mitigate long-term neuropsychiatric sequelae.

Imaging

CT Findings. Early NECT scans may be normal. Symmetric hypodensity in both globi pallidi develops within a few hours. Gross hemorrhage is rare. Variable diffuse hypodensity in the hemispheric white matter can be seen in severe cases.

MR Findings. Multiplanar MR (e.g., FLAIR, T2WI, and DWI) is the most sensitive technique for early detection of changes caused by CO poisoning. T1WI shows subtle hypointensity in the globi pallidi. A faint rim of hyperintensity caused by hemorrhage or coagulative necrosis may be present **(30-37A)**.

T2/FLAIR shows bilateral hyperintensities in the medial globi pallidi **(30-37B)**, with the putamina and caudate nuclei less commonly affected. A thin hypointense rim around the lesion may be present.

In addition to the hyperintense areas seen on T2WI, FLAIR imaging may disclose subtle involvement of the caudate nuclei, thalami, hippocampi, corpus callosum, fornices, and cerebral cortex.

DWI/ADC maps show restricted diffusion in the affected areas. Bilateral globi pallidi hyperintensities as well as foci of restricted diffusion in the subcortical white matter are typical. ADC in the cerebral white matter increases significantly, reflecting extensive microstructural tissue damage. DTI shows fractional anisotropy decline in associated cortical areas.

T2* GRE or SWI may show hypointensity in the globi pallidi suggestive of petechial hemorrhage.

Within a week after exposure, MRS shows elevated Cho/Cr and lowered NAA/Cr ratios, indicating increased membrane metabolism and decreased neuroaxonal viability.

Up to one-third of CO patients develop a **delayed leukoencephalopathy** with progressive white matter demyelination, the "interval" (subacute) form of CO poisoning. Extensive bilateral symmetric confluent areas of hyperintensity on T2/FLAIR are characteristic findings **(30-38)**.

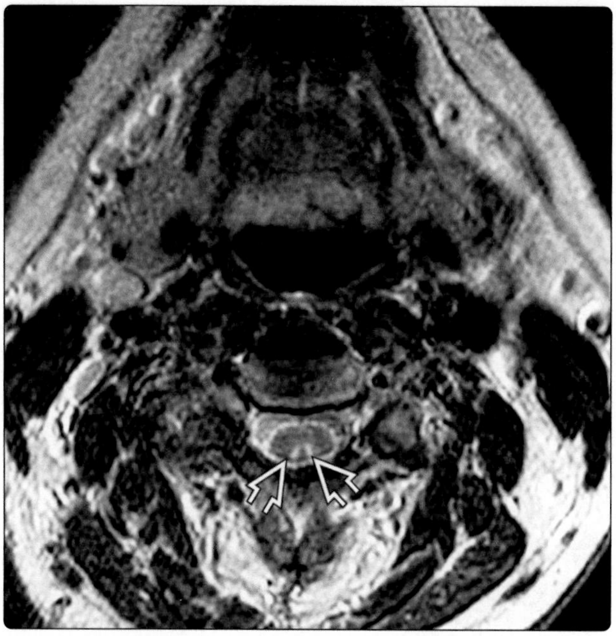

(30-39) Axial T2WI in a patient with nitrous oxide abuse shows selective symmetric demyelination of the posterior columns ➲, characteristic of subacute combined degeneration. (Courtesy C. Glastonbury, MBBS.)

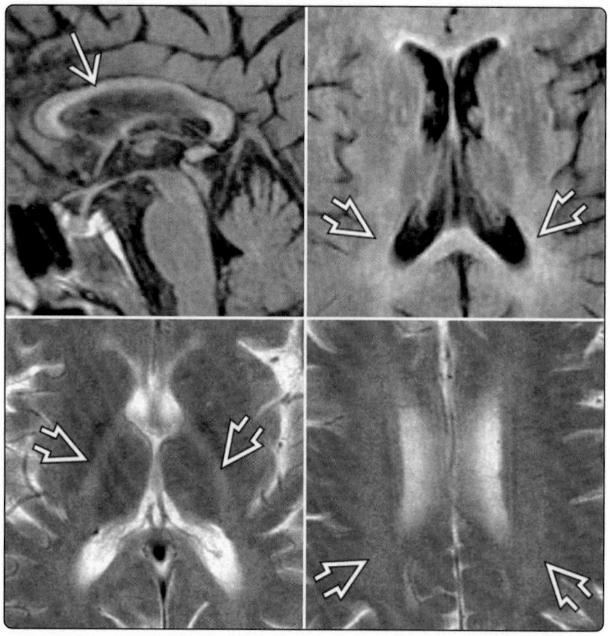

(30-40) Sagittal T1WI shows thinned corpus callosum ➲, and T2/FLAIR demonstrates confluent white matter hyperintensity ➲. This was toluene toxicity due to chronic glue sniffing. (Courtesy S. Lincoff, MD.)

Differential Diagnosis

The major differential diagnoses of CO poisoning are **hypoxic-ischemic encephalopathy** (HIE) and **drug abuse**. As they share some common pathophysiology, imaging findings often overlap. HIE generally affects the entire basal ganglia and hippocampi, less often the white matter or only the globi pallidi. **Organophosphate poisoning** (accidental or suicidal exposure) can cause bilateral hemorrhagic pallidal necrosis.

Wilson disease involves the basal ganglia, mesencephalon, pons, and dentate nuclei.

Mitochondrial encephalopathies, especially **Leigh disease**, generally affect younger patients. Brainstem and putamen lesions are more common than globi pallidi involvement.

Some **viral encephalitides**, such as Japanese encephalitis, preferentially affect the basal ganglia and thalami. **Creutzfeldt-Jakob disease** (CJD) is rapidly progressive and affects the caudate nuclei, anterior basal ganglia, and cortex. Posteromedial thalamic involvement (pulvinar) is common in CJD and rare in CO poisoning.

Nitrous Oxide

Nitrous oxide (N_2O), commonly known as "laughing gas," is an inhaled anesthetic supplement commonly used in dentistry and oral surgery. N_2O is extremely soluble in fatty compounds and is used as an aerosol spray propellant (e.g., whipped cream canisters and cooking sprays). Anesthetic gases, including N_2O, are sometimes inhaled for the putative euphoria.

Excess N_2O irreversibly oxidizes the cobalt ion of vitamin B12, which is necessary for methylation of myelin sheath phospholipids. Long-term nitrous oxide abuse causes progressive myelopathy and a peripheral polyneuropathy. The end result is **subacute combined degeneration of the spinal cord**. The dorsal columns and corticospinal tracts are preferentially affected **(30-39)**. Brain lesions are rare.

Toluene Abuse

The most important component of industrial solvents is toluene, so we focus our discussion on this particular solvent. Toluene, a colorless liquid found in glues, paint thinners, inks, and other industrial products, is lipid-soluble and rapidly absorbed by the CNS. Prolonged exposure through occupation or purposeful inhalation causes multifocal neurologic defects and optic neuropathy.

Terminology

Toluene, also called methylbenzene, is an aromatic hydrocarbon. Toluene poisoning results in **chronic solvent encephalopathy**.

Etiology

The common methods of solvent abuse are "sniffing" (direct inhalation from a container), "huffing" (inhalation from a soaked rag held over the nose and mouth), and "bagging" (inhalation from a plastic bag).

Pathology

Toluene preferentially affects the cerebral white matter and optic nerves, causing demyelination and gliosis. Iron deposition in the thalami and basal ganglia due to demyelination and axonal loss is also common.

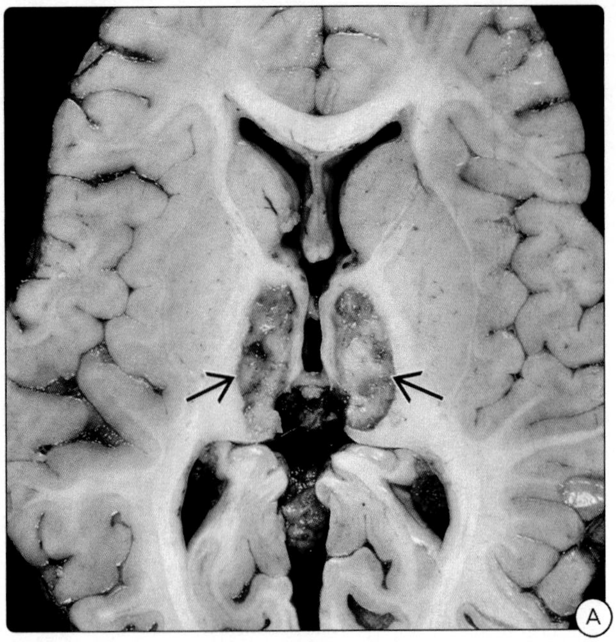

***(30-41A)** Autopsy specimen is from a patient with smoke inhalation, possibly from burning trash with vaporized cyanide. Note bilateral thalamic necrosis ➡. (Courtesy R. Hewlett, MD.)*

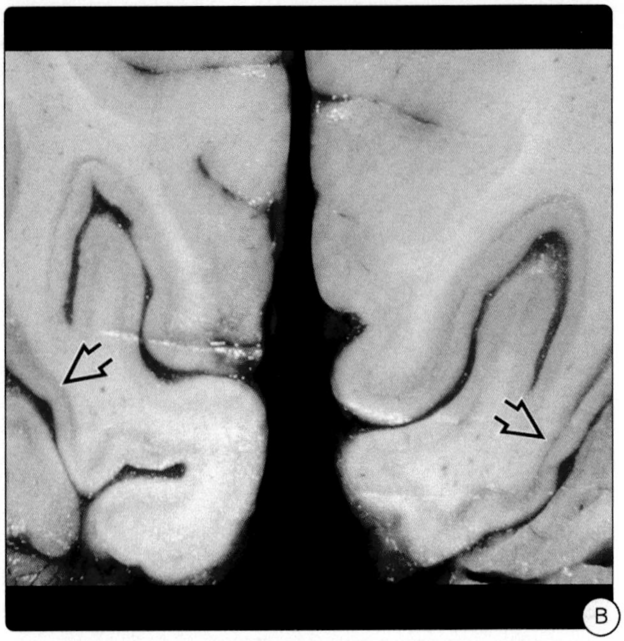

***(30-41B)** Coronal section through the occipital lobes of the same patient shows cortical laminar necrosis ➡. (Courtesy R. Hewlett, MD.)*

Clinical Issues

Solvent abuse is particularly prevalent among adolescents and young adults. Low cost and ease of access have led to increased prevalence in many countries. Regular long-term toluene abuse causes severe and irreversible cognitive impairment.

Imaging

Imaging in patients with acute toluene abuse is usually normal. Abnormalities are typically seen only after several years of chronic inhalant abuse. Diffuse white matter lesions are seen in nearly half of all patients, initially seen as T2/FLAIR hyperintensity in the deep periventricular white matter with subsequent spread into the centrum semiovale and subcortical areas. The internal capsule, cerebellum, and pons are often affected **(30-40)**.

Chronic prolonged toluene exposure also causes generalized atrophy with ventricular dilatation and enlarged subarachnoid spaces. White matter volume loss is seen as thinning of the corpus callosum. The extent of volume loss directly correlates with abuse duration.

Organophosphate Poisoning

Organophosphates (OPs) are common ingredients in pesticides. Because of their widespread agricultural use, ready availability, and easy accessibility, OPs are potential sources of accidental or suicidal exposure.

"Street pesticides" (illegal, unlabeled, and decanted agricultural pesticides used predominantly for urban household purposes) pose an increasing risk for significant pesticide exposures and poisonings in emerging nations.

The anticholinesterase effect of OPs causes three potential discrete neurologic syndromes. The initial acute effect is a life-threatening acute cholinergic crisis due to excessive stimulation of muscarinic receptors. The intermediate syndrome is characterized by cranial nerve palsies, proximal muscle weakness, delayed polyneuropathy, and Parkinson-like extrapyramidal symptoms.

Chronic or low-dose occupational exposure may result in neurobehavioral and neuropsychiatric disorders. There is increasing evidence that some cases of acquired amyotrophic lateral sclerosis (ALS) are linked to OP exposure.

Acute OP poisoning causes hemorrhagic basal ganglia necrosis with the "eye of the tiger" sign. On T2WI, a ring of marked hypointensity caused by excess iron accumulation surrounds a central hyperintense focus in the medial globus pallidus.

The differential diagnosis of OP poisoning includes other drug-induced causes of pallidal necrosis such as carbon monoxide poisoning. HIE and metabolic encephalopathies such as Leigh and Wilson diseases also affect the basal ganglia.

Cyanide Poisoning

Terminology

Cyanide (CN) is one of the most potent and deadly of all poisons. Cyanogenic compounds may be found in household or workplace substances and deliberately or accidentally ingested.

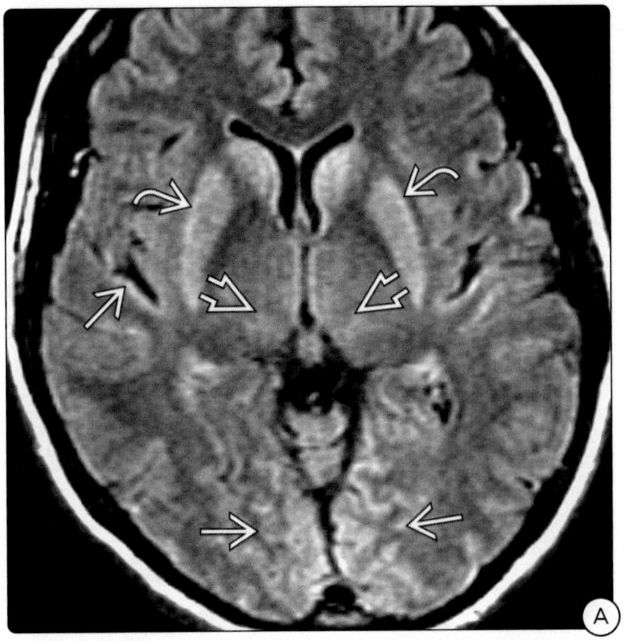

(30-42A) FLAIR scan in smoke inhalation with CN poisoning from burning plastic shows symmetric hyperintensity in caudate nuclei and putamina ➔, more subtle lesions in posteromedial thalami ➔, and curvilinear cortical hyperintensities ➔.

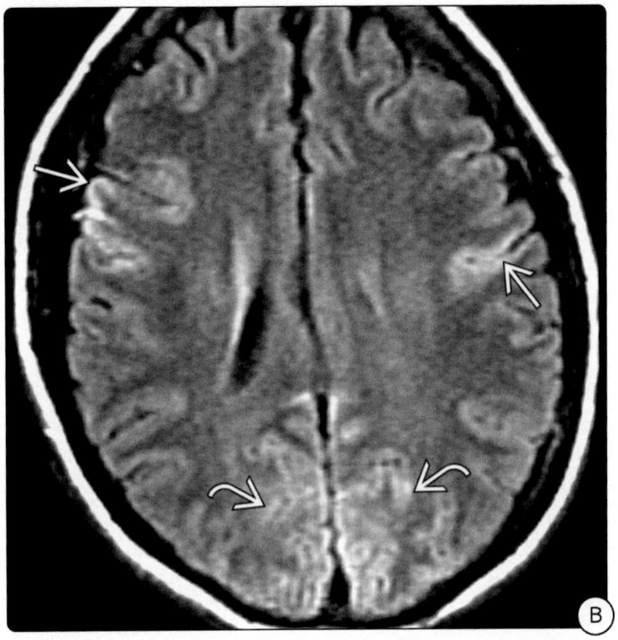

(30-42B) More cephalad scan in the same patient shows the cortical hyperintensities ➔, which are especially prominent in both occipital lobes ➔.

Acute CN intoxication is also called CN poisoning and is often the result of attempted suicide or smoke inhalation. Chronic CN toxicity is usually caused by occupational exposure to substances that contain cyanogenic compounds. Chronic CN exposure results in cyanide encephalopathy.

Etiology

CN exists in gas, solid, and liquid form. CN poisoning can occur by inhalation, ingestion, or transdermal absorption. Combustion of many common materials such as some fabrics and plastics may release CN and cyanogenic compounds. Cyanogenic compounds are also found in some foods, including almonds, the pits of stone fruits, Lima beans, and cassava root.

CN inactivates cytochrome oxidase, a key enzyme in the mitochondrial respiratory chain. Therefore, acute CN poisoning typically affects structures with high metabolic requirements. The basal ganglia and cortex are most commonly involved. Cerebral hypoxia may occur as part of the acute intoxication process, complicating both the diagnosis and treatment of CN poisoning.

Pathology

Hemorrhagic basal ganglia necrosis and laminar cortical necrosis are the pathologic hallmarks of CN poisoning **(30-41)**.

Clinical Issues

Patients with acute CN poisoning typically present with unresponsiveness, hemodynamic instability, and severe lactic acidosis. Because administered doses are usually high, acute CN poisoning is fatal in 95% of cases with death often occurring in minutes. Survivors may develop pseudo-parkinsonism with extrapyramidal symptoms.

INHALED GASES AND TOXINS

Carbon Monoxide Poisoning
- Acute: symmetric globi pallidi necrosis
- Subacute ("interval"): confluent leukoencephalopathy

Nitrous Oxide Abuse
- Brain lesions rare
- Subacute combined degeneration of the spinal cord
  - Hyperintensity in dorsal columns

Toluene (Solvent) Abuse
- Chronic, repeated use
  - Atrophy
  - White matter lesions
  - Thalami, substantia nigra, red nuclei, dentate lesions

Organophosphate (Pesticide) Poisoning
- Basal ganglia hemorrhage, necrosis
- "Eye of the tiger" sign

Cyanide Poisoning
- Suicide, smoke inhalation
- Basal ganglia hemorrhage, necrosis
- Laminar cortical necrosis

Imaging

MR is the modality of choice to depict lesion extent. Patients who survive the initial insult show symmetric hyperintensity in the basal ganglia and linear cortical hyperintensity on T2WI

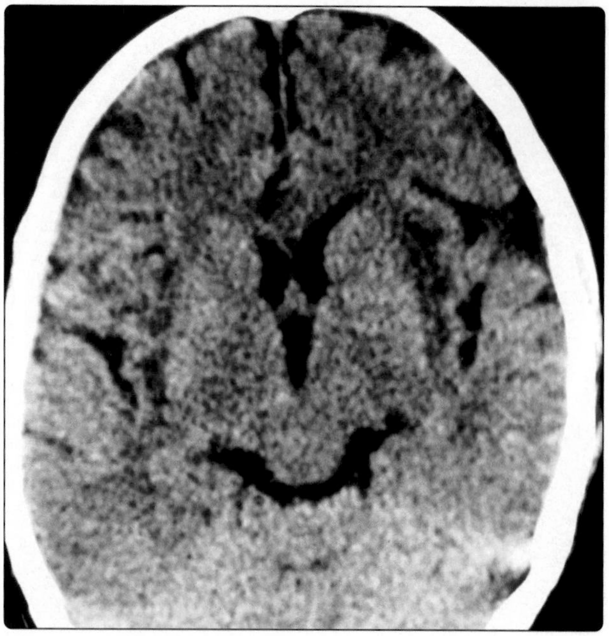

(30-43) NECT scan demonstrates volume loss in the frontal and temporal lobes attributable to lead poisoning. (Courtesy R. Ramakantan, MD.)

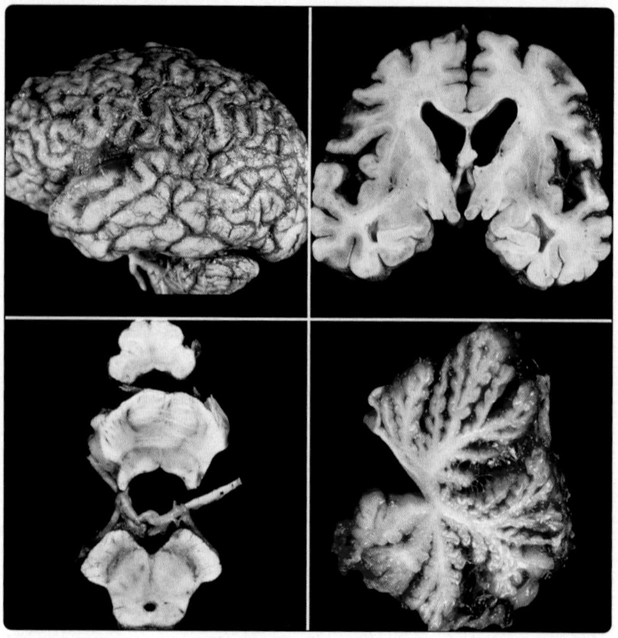

(30-44) Autopsy case of chronic mercury poisoning shows diffuse cortical, cerebellar volume loss. The medulla, pons, and midbrain also appear shrunken. (Courtesy R. Hewlett, MD.)

and FLAIR **(30-42)**. CN poisoning usually spares the hippocampi. T1 C+ scans typically show intense enhancement in the affected areas.

In the subacute and chronic stages, hemorrhagic necrosis causes T1 hyperintensity in the basal ganglia. Laminar necrosis results in serpentine linear hyperintensity in the cortex.

Differential Diagnosis

The most important differential diagnosis of CN poisoning is **hypoxic-ischemic encephalopathy**. It may complicate CN poisoning, and their features often overlap because the basal ganglia are affected in both disorders.

Metal Poisoning and Toxicity

A variety of metals can cause serious neurologic dysfunction when deposited in excess amounts in the CNS. **Manganese** accumulation is more common in the setting of chronic liver failure (see Chapter 32) but also occurs with occupational exposure. Other environmental toxins such as **lead** and **mercury** can cause significant neurotoxicity.

Lead Poisoning

Lead (Pb) is a potent and pervasive environmental neurotoxicant that is especially harmful during childhood development. Chronic Pb poisoning occurs in three forms: (1) a **gastrointestinal form** (anorexia, vomiting, lead "colic," etc.), (2) a **neuromuscular form** (muscle weakness, myalgias, peripheral neuritis, etc.), and (3) a **cerebral** or **neuropsychiatric form** (irritability, headache, encephalopathy, seizure, etc.). The cerebral form is common in children, whereas neuromuscular manifestations are more common in adults. The gastrointestinal form occurs in both age groups.

Lead-containing cooking utensils and indigenous medications are common sources of Pb poisoning in developing nations. Chronic lead exposure is associated with a significant and persistent impact on white matter microstructure.

Patients with moderate to severe lead encephalopathy usually have blood lead levels that exceed 70 µg/dL. In such cases, CT or MR may reveal volume loss, especially in the frontal cortex and subcortical WM **(30-43)**.

In less severe cases, DTI may reveal subtle changes such as decreased fractional anisotropy and diffusivity in the corona radiata and corpus callosum.

Mercury Poisoning

Mercury (Hg) occurs naturally in three forms: elemental Hg, mercury vapor, and organic/inorganic. Elemental mercury ("quicksilver") is liquid at room temperature. Liquid Hg is not absorbed through the skin and, if swallowed, passes through the GI tract without being absorbed. Mercury vaporizes easily, is highly diffusible, lipid soluble. Hg vapor is very toxic and easily absorbed.

Although occupational exposures to Hg still occasionally occur in manufacturing and mining, most current cases are caused by dermal absorption from illegal skin-lightening cosmetic products or bioconcentration of inorganic methylmercury in the food chain. Seafood (fish, marine mammals) is especially susceptible to contamination. Organic mercury poisoning is known as **Minamata disease**.

Gross pathology shows widespread cortical atrophy, white matter shrinkage, and thinning of the corpus callosum **(30-44)**. Severe spongiosis and gliosis with neuronal loss are seen on microscopic examination.

Imaging findings of Minamata disease include atrophy of the calcarine (visual) cortex, cerebellar vermis and hemispheres, and the postcentral cortex. Decreased regional blood flow in the cerebellum can be demonstrated even in the absence of cerebellar atrophy.

Treatment-Related Disorders

A comprehensive treatment of all iatrogenic abnormalities in the brain is far beyond the scope of this text. Here we discuss the most common disorders with a focus on treatment effects that must be recognized on imaging studies, namely radiation, chemotherapy, and surgery.

Radiation Injury

In the United States, approximately 100,000 primary and metastatic brain tumor patients each year survive long enough (more than 6 months) to develop some degree of radiation-induced injury (RII) to the brain.

CNS response to stressors and injuries such as ionizing radiation are modulated by responses of the brain's innate immune effector cells, the microglia. Exposure to high doses of ionizing radiation leads to the expression and release of proinflammatory cytokines and reactive oxygen species, leading to the tissue destruction that occurs with RII.

Many investigators divide RII into three phases: acute injury, early delayed injury, and late delayed injury. However, the pathophysiology and natural course of radiation therapy (XRT)-induced CNS injury are not well understood. Pathologically, radiation injury varies from mild transient vasogenic edema to frank necrosis. The damage that results from XRT depends on a number of variables including total dose, field size, number/frequency/fractionation of doses, whether chemotherapy is used in conjunction with XRT, and patient age.

Several different CNS tissues are affected by XRT. Vascular endothelial cells, oligodendrocytes, astrocytes, microglia, and neurons probably all interact in the brain's response to radiation injury.

Oligodendrocytes are especially sensitive. Vascular injury occurs in both early and late delayed injury. Once considered relatively radioresistant, neurons are now known to respond negatively to radiation and probably play a significant but as-yet-unidentified role in late radiation-induced cognitive impairment.

Acute Radiation Injury

Acute RII occurs days to weeks after irradiation and is very rarely encountered with modern XRT regimens. The major clinical manifestations of acute RII include headache and drowsiness.

Standard imaging studies are usually normal, although MRS, DTI, and fMR may detect changes before neurocognitive symptoms or anatomic alterations emerge. Occasionally, transient white matter edema secondary to changes in capillary permeability can be seen on T2/FLAIR sequences.

Biomarkers of pathology such as the mitochondrial translocator protein 18 kDa (TSPO) have facilitated in vivo characterization of microglial activation. In the future, microglial PET imaging may be a potential biomarker of early neuroinflammation from radiation-induced brain injury.

Early Delayed Radiation Injury

In early delayed RII, imaging abnormalities can be detected as early as 1 to 6 months after XRT is completed. Early delayed RII is characterized pathologically by transient demyelination and clinically by somnolence, attention deficits, and short-term memory loss. Patients may have significant cognitive impairments even in the absence of detectable anatomic abnormalities.

Confluent hypodense areas on NECT and periventricular white matter hyperintensity on T2/FLAIR are typical abnormalities. At this stage, RII changes are generally mild and reversible, often resolving spontaneously.

Late Delayed Radiation Injury

Late delayed RII is usually not observed until at least 6 months post irradiation. These late delayed injuries are viewed as progressive and largely irreversible, resulting from loss of glial and vascular endothelial cells.

Pathologically, coagulative necrosis in a "mosaic" pattern with coalescing foci produces a necrotizing leukoencephalopathy in the deep cerebral white matter. The subcortical association or U-fibers and corpus callosum are typically spared **(30-45)**. Vascular changes include fibrinoid necrosis, hyalinization, and sclerosis with thrombosis. Late delayed radiation necrosis is initially expansile and mass-like, with necrosis largely confined to white matter.

Initially, late delayed RII shows mass effect and variable enhancement on imaging studies. Later, volume loss, white matter spongiosis with confluent hyperintensity, and calcifications can be seen **(30-46)**.

Long-Term Sequelae of Radiation Injury

In addition to **necrotizing leukoencephalopathy**, long-term complications of XRT include vasculopathy, mineralizing microangiopathy, microvascular glomeruloid proliferation with telangiectasis (XRT-induced vascular malformations), and the development of radiation-induced neoplasms.

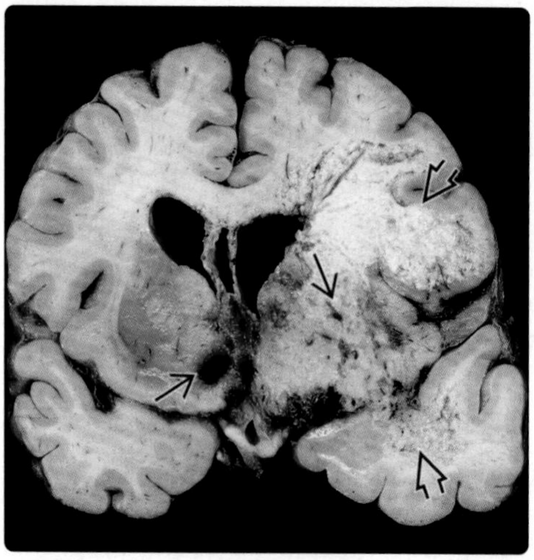

(30-45) Autopsy shows XRT-induced necrotizing leukoencephalopathy ⇒, hemorrhagic vascular malformations →. (Courtesy R. Hewlett, MD.)

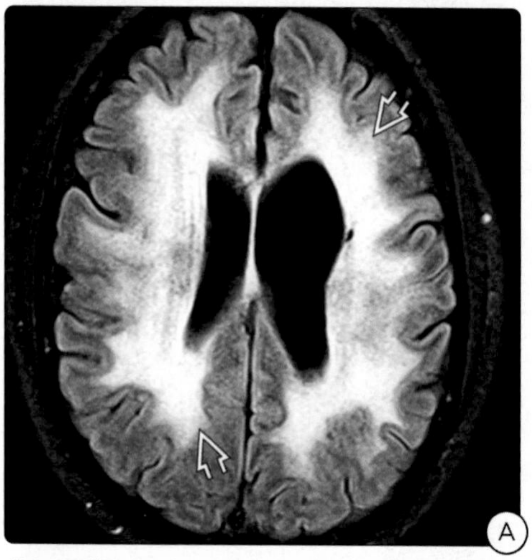

(30-46A) FLAIR in a patient with cognitive decline 3 years after whole-brain XRT for leukemia shows confluent WM hyperintensity ⇒.

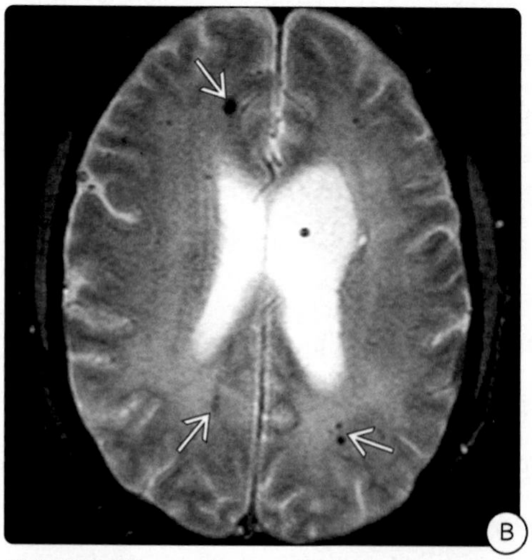

(30-46B) T2* scan shows multiple foci of gradient blooming →, necrotizing leukoencephalopathy with XRT-induced vascular malformations.

Radiation-induced vasculopathy with endothelial hyperplasia results in diffusely narrowed large and medium-sized arteries. Ischemic strokes and moyamoya-like disease may result **(30-47)**.

Mineralizing microangiopathy is usually seen in patients treated with combination XRT and chemotherapy. Mineralizing microangiopathy generally does not appear until at least 2 years following treatment; it is then seen as calcifications in the basal ganglia and subcortical white matter **(30-48)**.

Radiation-induced vascular malformations (RIVMs) are primarily capillary telangiectasias or cavernous malformations, most commonly seen in children who have received whole-brain radiotherapy for acute lymphoblastic leukemia. T2* (GRE, SWI) sequences demonstrate "blooming" microhemorrhages in the majority of patients **(30-49)**. It is uncommon to develop RIVMs less than 3 years following XRT. Children under 10 years of age at the time of irradiation are at higher risk.

Radiation-induced neoplasms are rare but often devastating. XRT is the single most important risk factor for developing a new primary CNS neoplasm. Approximately 70% are meningiomas, 20% malignant astrocytomas or medulloblastomas, and 10% sarcomas. Meningiomas occur an average of 17-20 years after treatment, whereas gliomas occur at a mean of 9 years. Sarcomas have a mean latency of 7 or 8 years following XRT.

RADIATION-INDUCED BRAIN INJURY

Pathology
- Microglial activation
- Proinflammatory cytokines

Three Phases of RII
- Acute radiation injury
  - Rare
  - T2/FLAIR may show white matter edema
  - TSPO-PET may show neuroinflammation
- Early delayed injury (at least 6 months)
  - Necrotizing leukoencephalopathy
  - Confluent hyperintensity
- Long-term sequelae
  - Necrotizing leukoencephalopathy
  - Vasculopathy, mineralizing microangiopathy
  - Vascular malformations (T2* "black dots")
  - Radiation-induced neoplasms

Chemotherapy Effects

Currently, the most common chemotherapy agents implicated in CNS toxicity are methotrexate, cytarabine, vincristine, asparaginase, and corticosteroids.

Unlike radiation injury, chemotherapy-associated acute toxic CNS injury is common. The two most frequent abnormalities are posterior reversible encephalopathy syndrome and treatment-induced leukoencephalopathy.

Posterior reversible encephalopathy syndrome (PRES) is addressed in detail in Chapter 32. In chemotherapy-related PRES, imaging findings are often atypical. The occipital lobes are frequently spared whereas the cerebellum, brainstem, and basal ganglia are frequently involved. Hemorrhage, contrast enhancement, and diffusion restriction—all relatively rare in "typical" PRES—are common.

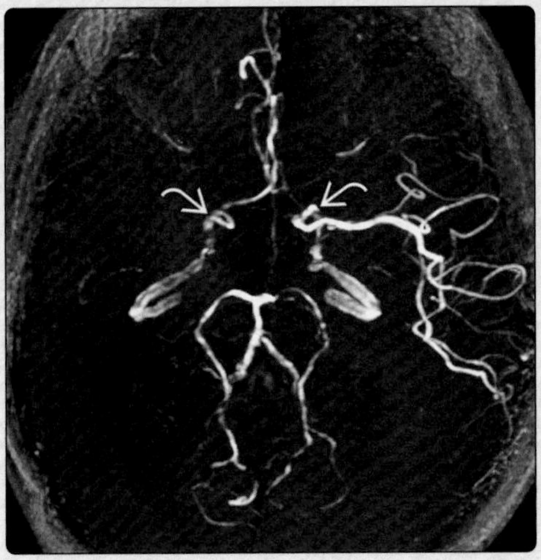

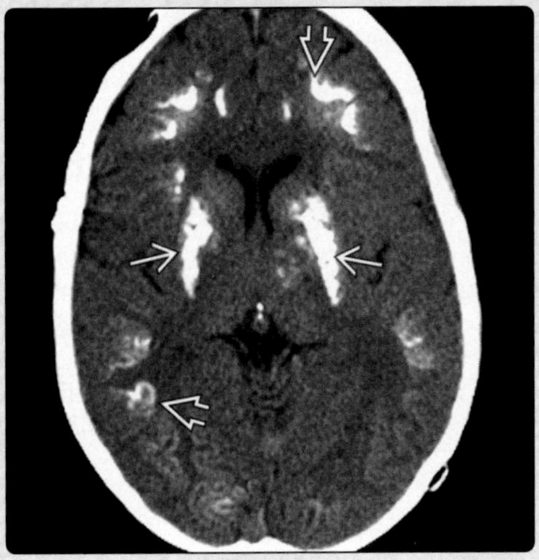

***(30-47)** MRA in a case with right MCA stroke years after XRT shows moyamoya and postradiation vasculopathy. Stenosis of both supraclinoid ICAs ➔ is present; right MCA is occluded. (Courtesy P. Hildenbrand, MD.) **(30-48)** NECT shows 20y man with XRT and chemo at age 8 for medulloblastoma. BG ➔, subcortical WM calcifications ➔ are characteristic of mineralizing microangiopathy. (Courtesy P. Chapman, MD.)*

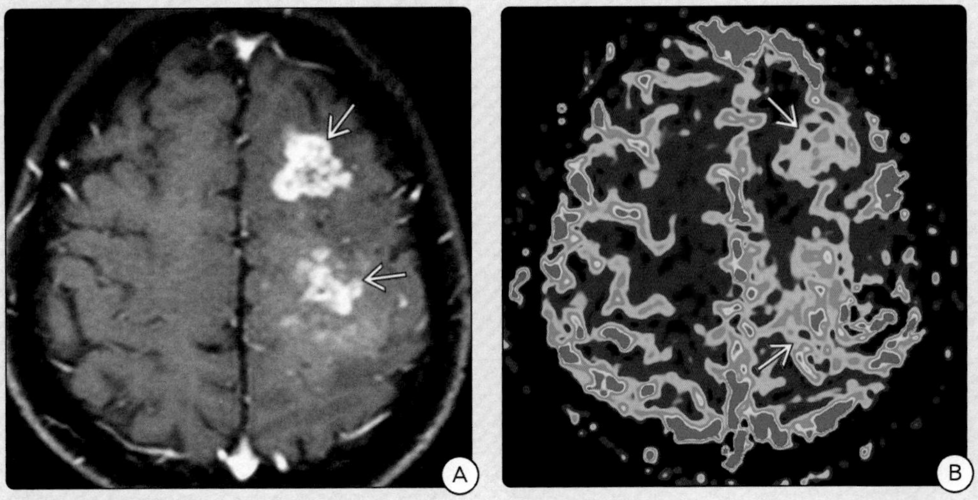

***(30-49A)** Patient with whole-brain radiation, chemo for anaplastic oligodendroglioma presented with seizure 5 years after treatment. T1 C+ FS shows multiple enhancing foci in left hemispheric WM ➔; delayed radiation necrosis vs. tumor recurrence. **(30-49B)** pMR shows elevated rCBV in the enhancing areas ➔, suggesting the enhancing foci represent recurrent tumor rather than necrotizing leukoencephalopathy.*

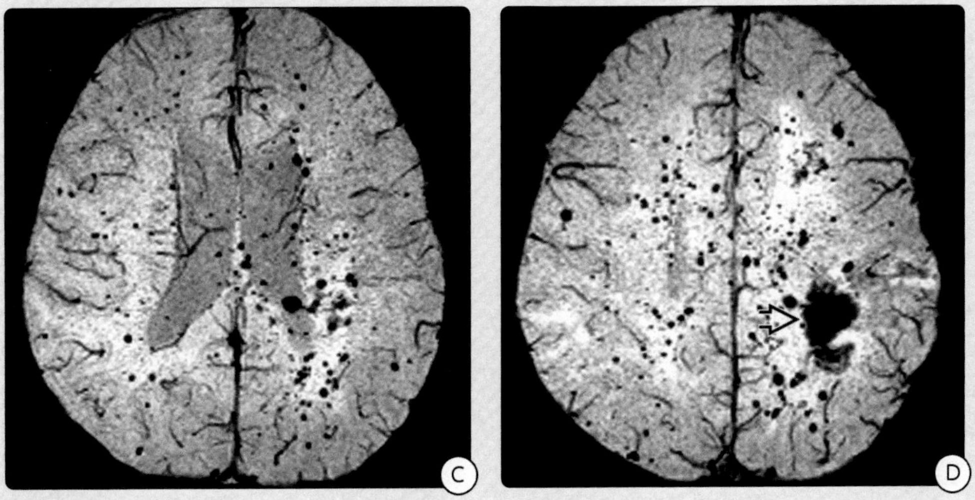

***(30-49C)** T2* SWI scan shows innumerable "blooming" hypointense foci in the WM, consistent with radiation-induced vascular malformations. **(30-49D)** More cephalad T2* SWI scan in the same patient shows additional small lesions and a larger focus ➔, consistent with hemorrhage into the recurrent neoplasm. Biopsy confirmed recurrence of anaplastic oligodendroglioma (WHO grade III), capillary telangiectases.*

CHEMOTHERAPY EFFECTS ON THE BRAIN

Clinical Issues

- Acute effects common
- Often reversible

Imaging

- PRES common
  - Atypical > typical imaging findings
  - Occipital lobes often spared
  - Hemorrhage, enhancement, restricted diffusion common
- Acute leukoencephalopathy
  - Reflects acute neurotoxicity
  - Transient T2/FLAIR periventricular hyperintensity

Treatment-induced leukoencephalopathy is especially common in patients treated with methotrexate. Acute neurotoxicity occurs in 5-18% of children treated for acute lymphoblastic leukemia. Bilateral, relatively symmetric, confluent areas of T2/FLAIR hyperintensity in the periventricular white matter are typical **(30-50)**. Imaging abnormalities typically resolve after treatment.

Effects of Surgery

Interpreting imaging findings in the postoperative brain can be challenging. Expected findings include pneumocephalus, focal hemorrhage, retraction edema, small subdural CSF collections (hygromas), etc. We focus on just two abnormalities that are important to recognize on imaging studies: retained surgical material ("textiloma") and sinking skin flap syndrome.

Textiloma

Textiloma—also known as muslinoma or gauzoma—is a foreign body reaction to retained surgical elements. The term has traditionally referred to reactions to surgical elements

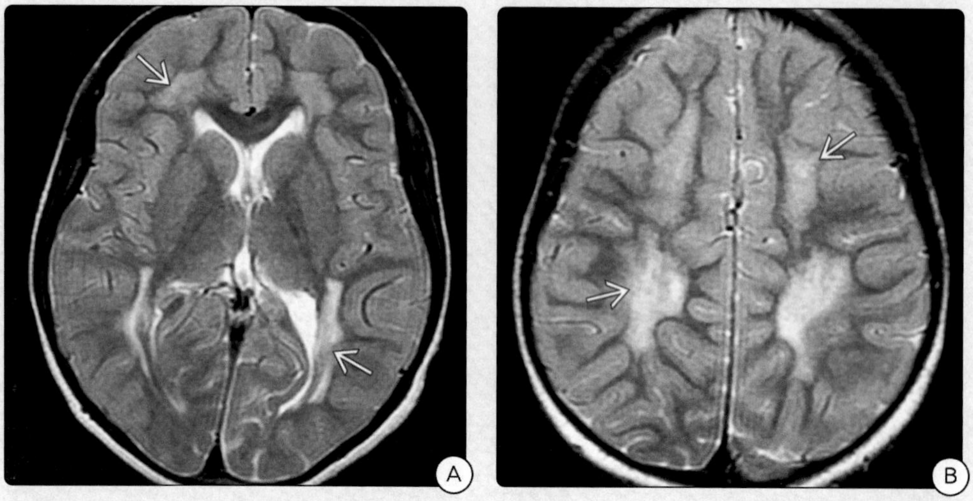

***(30-50A)** T2WI in a 5y child with acute deterioration following intrathecal methotrexate for ALL shows symmetric confluent hyperintensity in the deep periventricular WM. Note sparing of subcortical U-fibers. **(30-50B)** More cephalad scan in the same patient shows the confluent WM hyperintensity and spared subcortical WM. This is methotrexate-induced leukoencephalopathy.*

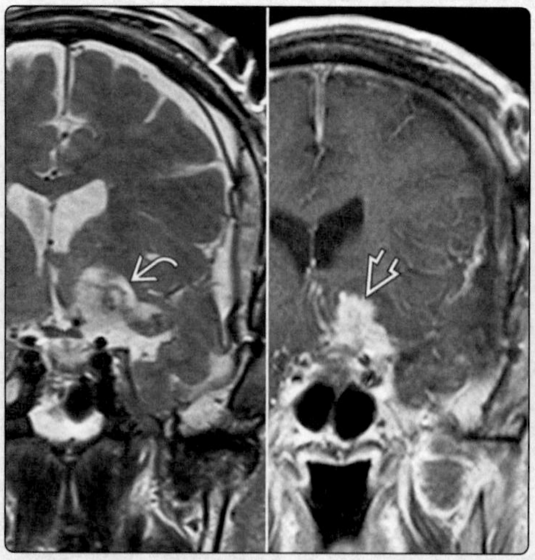

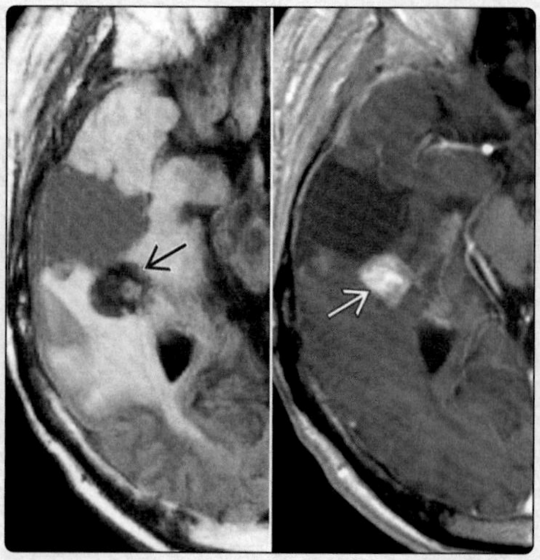

***(30-51)** T2WI (L), T1 C+ (R) after meningioma resection show that a mixed signal mass enhances strongly and uniformly; this is textiloma. **(30-52)** (L) Retained cotton ball after surgery is round and hypointense on FLAIR. (R) T1 C+ shows that the retained material enhances strongly but heterogeneously. This is textiloma. (Courtesy B. K. Kleinschmidt-DeMasters, MD.)*

inadvertently left in the operative bed but has recently been expanded to include reactions to intentionally placed surgical elements.

Intracranial textilomas are rare. Both resorbable and nonresorbable hemostatic agents may be placed in the surgical bed to provide persistent hemostasis after closure.

When they occur, textilomas can be mistaken for recurrent tumor or abscesses on imaging studies. Most surgically placed materials [e.g., cotton hemostats, muslin, or polytetrafluoroethylene (Teflon)] do not have signal abnormalities on MR and are visualized only when a foreign body reaction develops, forming a textiloma.

Nearly 40% of textilomas are hypointense on T2WI and FLAIR **(30-51)**. Many "bloom" on T2* (GRE, SWI) sequences. Restriction on DWI is variable. Most enhance; both solid and ring patterns occur **(30-52)**.

Sinking Skin Flap Syndrome

Sinking skin flap syndrome (SSFS)—also referred to as "syndrome of the trephined"—is an unusual cause of neurologic deterioration in patients who have undergone large decompressive craniectomy for uncontrollable brain swelling (usually following trauma or "malignant" hemispheric infarction).

The mechanism of SSFS has not been fully elucidated. Some authors suggest that the large cranial defect allows external (atmospheric) pressure to act on the brain, causing altered CSF dynamics. Significantly smaller CSF volumes have been measured in patients with SSFS. CSF leakage or ventriculo-peritoneal shunt overdrainage can exacerbate intracranial hypovolemia and result in clinical deterioration.

SSFS occurs in 20-25% of patients who survive decompressive surgery and in whom restorative cranioplasty is delayed. It typically presents weeks to months after craniectomy but most commonly occurs during the second postoperative month.

Presenting signs and symptoms vary, but the overwhelming majority of patients exhibit a visibly sunken skin flap. In severe cases, decreased consciousness and hemiparesis can occur. SSFS can become life-threatening, especially if exacerbated by CSF leak. Symptoms typically improve after cranioplasty.

Imaging shows skin flap depression below the level of the calvarium, often with an S-shaped configuration. Mass effect on the cortex, evidenced by sulcal effacement and buckling of the gray-white matter interface under the skin flap, is seen in nearly all cases.

Paradoxical deviation of midline structures away from the craniectomy site is typical. Midline shift of the interhemispheric fissure and/or septi pellucidi away from the sunken skin flap is seen in 75% of cases **(30-53)**.

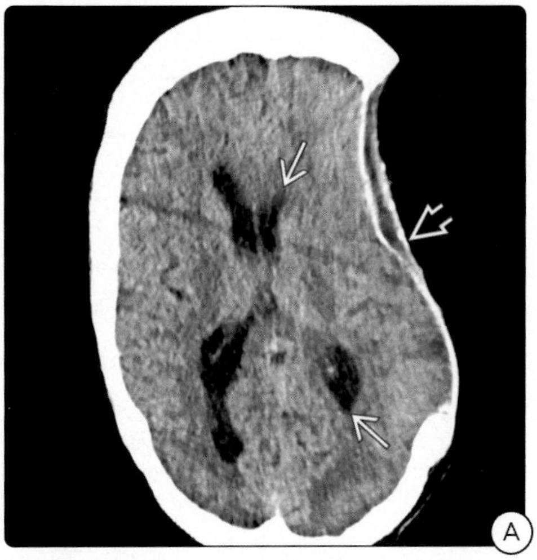

***(30-53A)** SSFS is 5 weeks after decompressive craniectomy. Duraplasty is sunken with S-shaped configuration ➡, mass effect on ventricles ➡.*

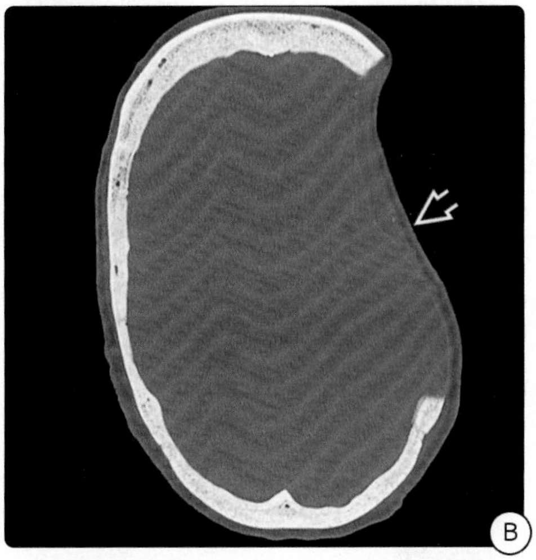

***(30-53B)** Bone CT shows the craniectomy defect and S-shape configuration of the sunken skin flap ➡.*

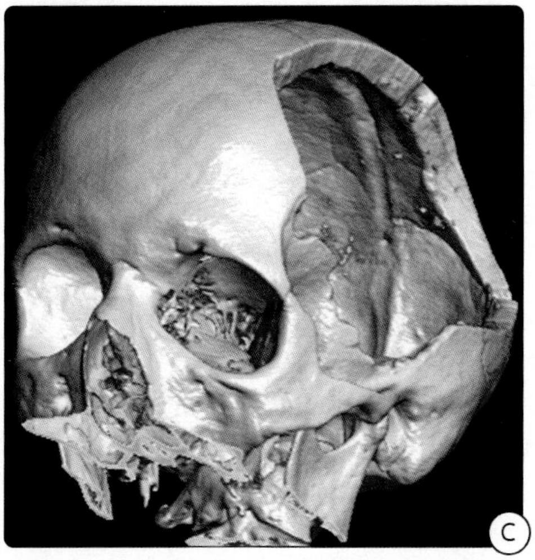

***(30-53C)** Bone CT with 3D SSD shows the extent to which the brain and duraplasty have sunken inward below the level of the craniectomy defect.*

Selected References

Alcohol and Related Disorders

Juhás M et al: Deep grey matter iron accumulation in alcohol use disorder. Neuroimage. 148:115-122, 2017

Volkow ND et al: Neurochemical and metabolic effects of acute and chronic alcohol in the human brain: studies with positron emission tomography. Neuropharmacology. 122:175-188, 2017

Logan C et al: Neuroimaging of chronic alcohol misuse. J Med Imaging Radiat Oncol. ePub, 2016

Wernicke Encephalopathy

Chamorro AJ et al: Differences between alcoholic and nonalcoholic patients with Wernicke encephalopathy: a multicenter observational study. Mayo Clin Proc. 92(6):899-907, 2017

Ashraf VV et al: Wernicke's encephalopathy due to hyperemesis gravidarum: clinical and magnetic resonance imaging characteristics. J Postgrad Med. 62(4):260-263, 2016

Hattingen E et al: Wernicke encephalopathy: SWI detects petechial hemorrhages in mammillary bodies in vivo. Neurology. 87(18):1956-1957, 2016

Liong CC et al: Nonalcoholic Wernicke encephalopathy: an entity not to be missed! Can J Neurol Sci. 43(5):719-20, 2016

Methanol Intoxication

Zakharov S et al: Acute methanol poisoning: prevalence and predisposing factors of haemorrhagic and non-haemorrhagic brain lesions. Basic Clin Pharmacol Toxicol. 119(2):228-38, 2016

Vaneckova M et al: Imaging findings after methanol intoxication (cohort of 46 patients). Neuro Endocrinol Lett. 36(8):737-44, 2015

Amphetamines and Derivatives

Montoya-Filardi A et al: The addicted brain: imaging neurological complications of recreational drug abuse. Radiologia. 59(1):17-30, 2017

Methamphetamine

Kish SJ et al: Brain dopamine neurone 'damage': methamphetamine users vs. Parkinson's disease - a critical assessment of the evidence. Eur J Neurosci. 45(1):58-66, 2017

Prakash MD et al: Methamphetamine: effects on the brain, gut and immune system. Pharmacol Res. 120:60-67, 2017

Wang TY et al: Pattern and related factors of cognitive impairment among chronic methamphetamine users. Am J Addict. 26(2):145-151, 2017

London ED et al: Chronic methamphetamine abuse and corticostriatal deficits revealed by neuroimaging. Brain Res. 1628(Pt A):174-85, 2015

MDMA ("Ecstasy")

Mueller F et al: Neuroimaging in moderate MDMA use: a systematic review. Neurosci Biobehav Rev. 62:21-34, 2016

Cocaine

Shrot S et al: Acute brain injury following illicit drug abuse in adolescent and young adult patients: spectrum of neuroimaging findings. Neuroradiol J. 30(2):144-150, 2017

Opioids and Derivatives

Morgan DJ et al: 2016 Update on medical overuse: a systematic review. JAMA Intern Med. 176(11):1687-1692, 2016

Warner M et al: Drugs most frequently involved in drug overdose deaths: United States, 2010-2014. Natl Vital Stat Rep. 65(10):1-15, 2016

Heroin

Lefaucheur R et al: Leucoencephalopathy following abuse of sniffed heroin. J Clin Neurosci. 35:70-72, 2017

Inhaled Gases and Toxins

Carbon Monoxide Poisoning

Kim DM et al: Acute carbon monoxide poisoning: MR imaging findings with clinical correlation. Diagn Interv Imaging. 98(4):299-30, 2017

Rose JJ et al: Carbon monoxide poisoning: pathogenesis, management and future directions of therapy. Am J Respir Crit Care Med. 195(5):596-606, 2017

Tsai PH et al: Early white matter injuries in patients with acute carbon monoxide intoxication: a tract-specific diffusion kurtosis imaging study and STROBE compliant article. Medicine (Baltimore). 96(5):e5982, 2017

Nitrous Oxide

Sellers WF: Misuse of anaesthetic gases. Anaesthesia. 71(10):1140-3, 2016

Toluene Abuse

Jayanth SH et al: Glue sniffing. Med Leg J. 85(1):38-42, 2017

Treatment-Related Disorders

Radiation Injury

Lumniczky K et al: Ionizing radiation-induced immune and inflammatory reactions in the brain. Front Immunol. 8:517, 2017

Balentova S et al: Molecular, cellular and functional effects of radiation-induced brain injury: a review. Int J Mol Sci. 16(11):27796-815, 2015

Chemotherapy Effects

Rossi Espagnet MC et al: Magnetic resonance imaging patterns of treatment-related toxicity in the pediatric brain: an update and review of the literature. Pediatr Radiol. 47(6):633-648, 2017

Effects of Surgery

Ashayeri K et al: Syndrome of the trephined: a systematic review. Neurosurgery. 79(4):525-34, 2016

Kleinschmidt-DeMasters BK: Textiloma (Muslinoma, Gauzoma, Gossypiboma). In: Diagnostic Pathology: Neuropathology, 2e, edited by Burger P et al. Salt Lake City, UT: Elsevier, 2016, pp 716-721

Vasung L et al: Radiological signs of the syndrome of the trephined. Neuroradiology. 58(6):557-68, 2016

Inherited Metabolic Disorders

Inherited metabolic disorders (IMDs)*—also known as* ***inborn errors of metabolism****—represent conditions in which a genetic defect leads to a deficiency of a protein (e.g., enzyme or non-enzyme protein) that subsequently affects mechanisms of synthesis, degradation, transport, and/or storage of molecules in the body. IMDs are relatively uncommon diseases that pose diagnostic dilemmas for clinicians and radiologists alike. IMDs can present at virtually any age from infancy well into the fifth and sixth decades, although infantile and childhood presentation is most common.*

Symptoms vary among the various disorders and within the degree of severity in patients with the same disorder. As radiologists, in the process of constructing an ordered, differential diagnosis, keeping the category of IMD in mind will serve our patients well. IMDs may mimic hypoxic ischemic injury (HII), sepsis, and CNS abnormalities attributed to underlying vascular (e.g., stroke) and congenital heart diseases. The most immediate impact on patient well-being of making a timely diagnosis of IMD is that many of these conditions can be treated effectively. Rapid therapeutic intervention can avoid irreversible brain injury. Additionally, if the IMD diagnosis is associated with a defined pattern of inheritance, this information is essential to parents who may be considering having other children. Our focus here will be on disorders most often presenting in the newborn, infant, and child.

Family history often provides clues to the diagnosis of IMDs. These clues include (1) families that are known to have members with IMD, (2) neonatal deaths that have occurred without cause, and (3) unexplained severe and progressive illness in childhood. When history is strongly suggestive of IMD in advance of childbirth, a rapid diagnostic and treatment plan can be established prior to parturition.

In utero, the placenta serves the function of an effective *dialysis unit,* removing toxic metabolites. Therefore, the newborn and young infant with some inherited metabolic disorders may initially appear clinically sound. The specific metabolic disorder will dictate, in large part, the pace of clinical presentation. The expression of this dysfunction may range between sudden neonatal death in the first few weeks of life to gradual deterioration after a symptom-free intmoyaerval of months to years. Interestingly, IMDs are rarely associated with premature birth.

The neonatal and young infant repertoire of physiologic responses to severe illness is limited. Respiratory distress, lethargy, weak suck, poor feeding, weight loss, vomiting, diarrhea, and dehydration are individually and in aggregate nonspecific symptoms and signs that may herald an underlying

Selected Myelination Milestones

Age	T1 Hyperintensity	T2 Hypointensity
Birth		
	Dorsal brainstem	Dorsal brainstem
	Posterior limb IC	Partial posterior limb IC
	Perirolandic gyri	Perirolandic gyri
	Corticospinal tracts	Corticospinal tracts
3-4 Months		
	Ventral brainstem	Posterior limb IC
	Anterior limb IC	
	CC splenium	
	Central, posterior corona radiata	
6 Months		
	Cerebellar WM	Ventral brainstem
	CC genu	Anterior limb IC
	Parietal, occipital WM	CC splenium, genu by 8-9 months
	Frontal WM by 9 months	
12 Months		
	Posterior fossa (≈ adult)	Most of corona radiata
	Most of corona radiata	Posterior subcortical WM
	Posterior subcortical WM	Occipital WM
18 Months		
	All WM except temporal, frontal U-fibers	All WM except temporal, frontal U-fibers, occipital radiations
24 Months		
	Anterior temporal, frontal U-fibers	Anterior temporal, orbital frontal U-fibers

(Table 31-1) *CC = corpus callosum; IC = internal capsule; WM = white matter. WM maturation is seen earlier on T1WI.*

IMD. Older affected children and adolescents may exhibit seizures, movement disorders, hypotonia, ataxia, autism, or delayed achievement of developmental milestones. Some IMDs will present with developmental delay including features of autism. Thus, there is a broad range of phenotypes among those affected.

In conceptualizing IMDs, consider these broad categories: (1) disorders that give rise to intoxication symptoms—accumulation of toxic compounds (e.g., maple syrup urine disease); (2) disorders involving energy metabolism—symptoms arising from a deficiency in energy production or utilization (e.g., mitochondrial defects, creatine deficiency states); (3) disorders involving large or complex molecules—abnormalities arising from disordered synthesis and/or catabolism of molecules that accumulate in cellular organelles (e.g., *lysosomal*—Gaucher disease or *peroxisomal*—Zellweger disease); (4) disorders involving neurotransmitters (e.g., glycine, serine, and pterin metabolism); and (5) other inherited disorders.

Neuroimaging has great potential to improve diagnostic accuracy (e.g., in some cases clinching the diagnosis—MRS and creatine deficiency states), follow therapeutic interventions, and monitor disease progression in patients afflicted with IMDs. The informed radiologist can merge his or her understanding of the pathogenetic and pathomorphologic underpinnings of the various IMDs with imaging observations. Specifically, we observe *what part of the brain is involved* (e.g., GM vs. WM), *what kind of involvement is present* (e.g., cortex, basal ganglia, white matter—subcortical, deep, or periventricular), and *what locations are most affected* (e.g., frontal lobes). Additional information such as the presence of cysts, calcifications, diffusion restriction, and pathologic enhancement aids in crystallizing the imaging differential diagnosis.

MR is routinely obtained in newborns, infants, and children with delayed neurologic development and when they present with neurologic disorders. Familiarization with the normal progression of white matter myelination is a prerequisite for detecting and understanding IMDs, as many of the metabolic derangements to be discussed exhibit early disturbance in the anticipated progression of myelination. We therefore begin this chapter with a review of how normal myelination progresses from birth through 2 years of life. DWI/DTI and MRS have become important adjunctive MR sequences to the comprehensive MR examination.

Once we have reviewed the patterns of normal myelination as assessed with MR, we continue with an overview and introduction of the IMDs. A discussion of classification systems is a recommended and practical approach to analyzing imaging. Selected discussion of the leukodystrophies and nonleukodystrophic white matter disorders focuses on abnormal myelin development, myelin degeneration, and hypomyelination. Those IMDs most often clinically encountered will be emphasized.

Normal Myelination and White Matter Development

General Considerations

Myelination

Myelination is an orderly, highly regulated, multistep process that begins during the fifth fetal month and is largely complete by 18-24 postnatal months. Some structures (e.g., cranial nerves) myelinate relatively early in fetal development, whereas others (e.g., optic radiations and fibers to/from association areas) often do not completely myelinate until the third or even the fourth decade of life. CNS myelin is produced by oligodendrocytes. The myelin sheath consists of multiple double membranes wrapped radially around axons. Myelin is rich in lipids, including cholesterol, glycolipids, and phospholipids.

Importantly, because white matter abnormalities form a constant part of many if not most **inborn metabolic diseases**, it is imperative that the radiologist have a firm grasp on normal patterns of myelination.

Brain myelination is an event involving more than oligodendrocytes; it is an interaction between oligodendrocytes, axons, astrocytes, and many soluble factors. Normal myelination follows a typical topographical pattern, progressing from **inferior to superior, central to peripheral,** and **posterior to anterior**. For example, the brainstem myelinates before the peripheral cerebellar hemispheres, the posterior limbs of the internal capsules myelinate before the anterior limbs, and the deep periventricular white matter (WM) myelinates before the subcortical U-fibers. The dorsal brainstem myelinates before the anterior brainstem, and—with the exception of the parietooccipital association tracts—occipital WM myelinates earlier than WM in the anterior temporal and frontal lobes.

CT

The hemispheres of normal term infants at birth appear well formed. The gyral pattern is mature with distinctly defined cortex and surface sulci. The lateral cerebral (sylvian) fissures may be slightly prominent but generally resemble those seen in older children. The frontal subarachnoid spaces and basal cisterns often appear prominent up to 1 year of age.

At birth, the WM is largely unmyelinated, so it appears quite hypoattenuating compared with regional gray matter due to the comparatively high water content of WM. There is a symmetry to the peripheral, deep, and periventricular pattern of normal neonatal and early infantile unmyelinated WM.

MR

MR allows visualization of the process of myelination. The appearance of WM maturation varies with two important factors, i.e., **patient age** and the **imaging sequence** employed. MR remains the imaging gold standard when it comes to in vivo assessment of brain formation, organization, and myelin maturation.

Unmyelinated WM is hypointense relative to gray matter on T1WI and hyperintense to gray matter on T2WI. As the WM matures, it becomes more hyperintense (T1 shortening) on T1WI. T1 shortening is related to water molecules within the myelin sheath that are tightly bound to macromolecules and the high myelin content of cholesterol and galactocerebroside. In fact, there are several properties of maturing WM that can be studied on clinical MR scanners and used in the clinical care arena. The normal progressive T2 shortening (hypointensity) that occurs in the first 2 years of life is due mainly to decreasing proton density within maturing myelin.

Consider these normal WM MR findings within the first 2 years of life: T1 and T2 shortening, decreasing mean diffusivity, decreased radial diffusivity, increased fractional anisotropy (FA), increased magnetization transfer, and increased bound water fraction of WM. In aggregate, during the *normal myelin maturational period*, the increasingly complex intracellular and extracellular structures that transiently bind water molecules exhibit dynamic T1/T2 relaxivity and diffusivity characteristics that affect T1 and T2 prolongation. Simply put, normal myelin maturation results in progressively reduced water content with MR demonstrating T1 hyperintensity and T2 hypointensity.

During the first 6-8 months of life, T1 shortening occurs earlier and is more conspicuous than T2 shortening. Therefore,T1-weighted sequences are best both to evaluate WM maturation and brain morphology. Partially myelinated structures will have high signal on T1 and T2 sequences (T1 and T2 shortening). Heavily weighted T2 sequences are sensitive to follow WM maturation between 6 and 18 months and to help characterize cortical organization and to assess other gray matter structures.

Therefore, fully myelinated WM has high T1 signal and low T2 signal. Normal myelin maturation results in progressively reduced WM water content with concomitant T2 hypointensity. The radiologist makes a mental note when interpreting MR examinations in the first 6 months of life that T1 shortening normally occurs before T2 shortening and is more prominent and that normal myelin T1 and T2 signal intensities vary during the process of myelination.

In the clinical neuroimaging arena, at a minimum, accurate evaluation of myelination status requires both T1 and T2 sequences with orthogonal planes advised. More advanced

__(31-1A)__ Axial T1WI in a normal 4m infant shows the medulla to be completely myelinated. Hyperintensity now extends into the medial cerebellar hemispheres, but the more peripheral WM remains unmyelinated and appears hypointense. __(31-1B)__ Axial ADC map shows hypointensity (mature myelin) in the dorsal brainstem, cranial nerve nuclei, as well as the middle cerebellar peduncles.

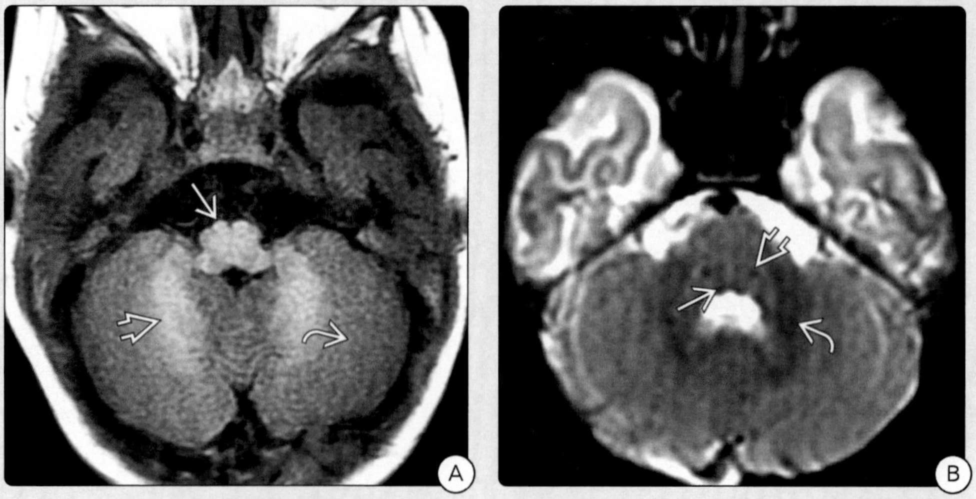

__(31-1C)__ Axial T1WI in the same patient shows normal T1 shortening in the PLIC and the subtle hyperintensity (normal myelination) in the ALIC. The optic radiation WM is beginning to myelinate. __(31-1D)__ Axial T2WI reveals hypointensity in the PLIC. The anterior limbs are beginning to myelinate and are not well seen between the hypointensity of the caudate and putamen.

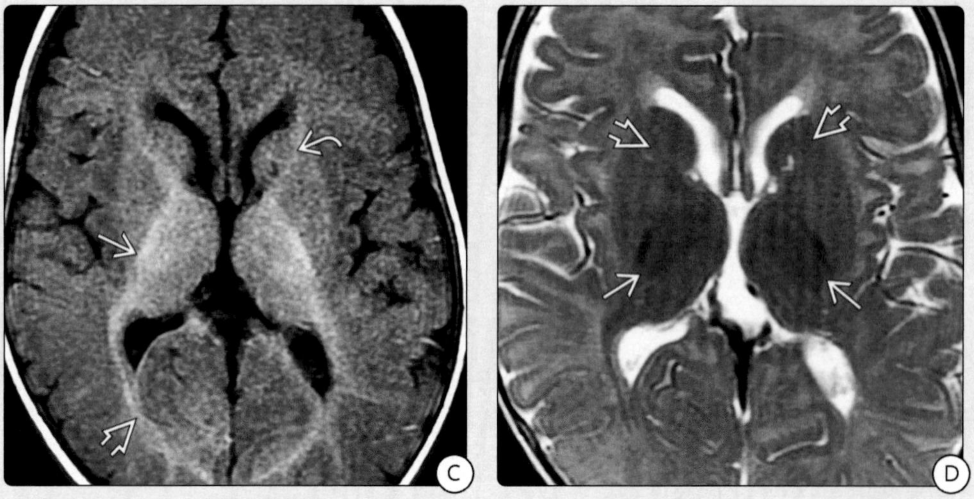

__(31-1E)__ Axial T1WI shows that WM in the corona radiata remains mostly unmyelinated at 4 months, although some myelination in WM of the perirolandic regions is present. __(31-1F)__ Axial T2WI shows the same patient. Except for the "smudgy" areas deep to the central sulci, WM in the corona radiata remains hyperintense and unmyelinated.

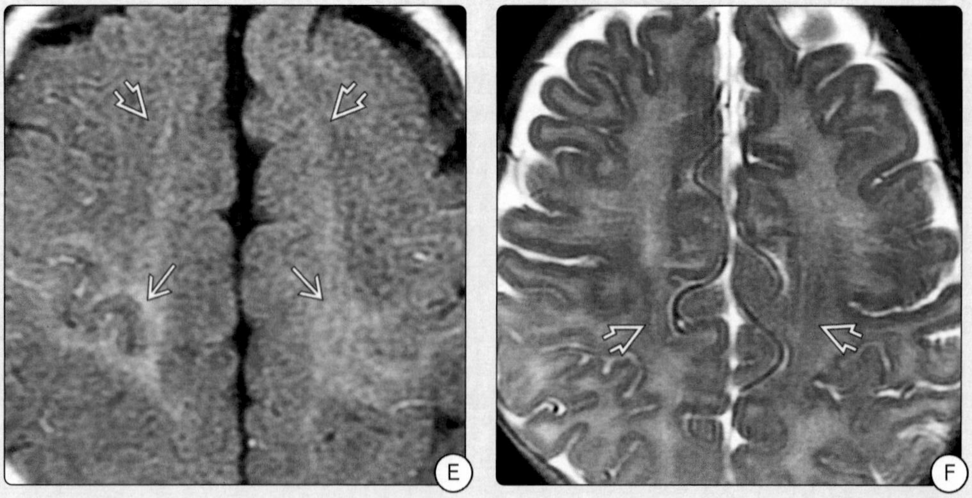

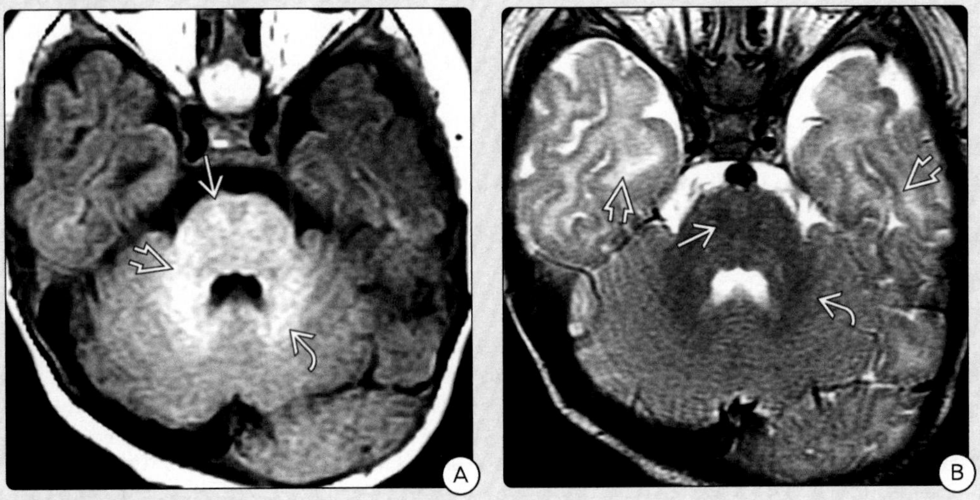

***(31-2A)** Axial T1WI at 6 months shows that the pons → and middle cerebellar peduncles → are completely myelinated and that normal hyperintense myelin now extends further into the cerebellar hemispheres →. **(31-2B)** Axial T2WI in the same patient shows striking contrast between the hypointense (myelinated) pons → and medial cerebellar WM → compared with the unmyelinated hyperintense WM in the temporal lobes →.*

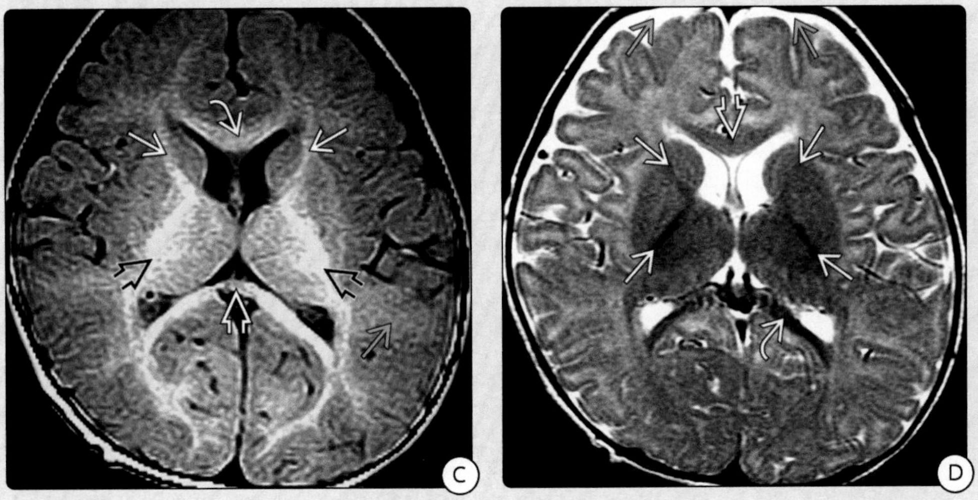

***(31-2C)** Axial T1WI at 6 months shows normal WM in the PLIC →, ALIC →, the corpus callosum splenium →, and genu →. The subcortical WM is unmyelinated → (isointense to cortex). **(31-2D)** Axial T2WI shows that both limbs → of the internal capsules are myelinated and hypointense (PLIC > ALIC). The splenium → is more hypointense than the genu →. Prominent frontal subarachnoid spaces → are normal at 6 months.*

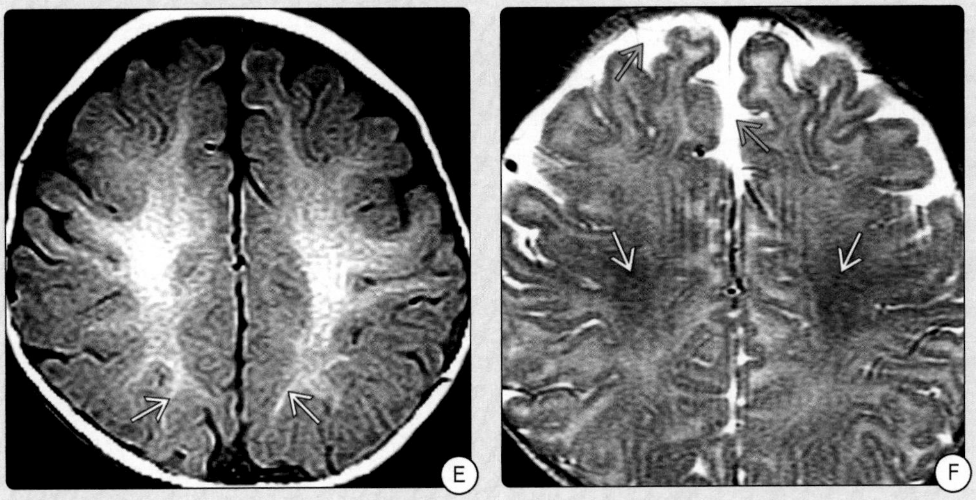

***(31-2E)** Axial T1WI shows normal myelin at 6 months extends into the peripheral subcortical WM, especially in parietal and occipital lobes →. **(31-2F)** Axial T2WI shows hypointensity in the corona radiata → is not as striking as hyperintensity on previous T1WI. Myelination on T2WI lags behind that seen on T1WI. Note the normal prominence of the frontal and interhemispheric subarachnoid spaces →.*

techniques such as DTI, magnetization transfer imaging (MTI), and T1/T2 relaxometry may provide additional information but do not supplant the utility of spin magnitude imaging. *When in doubt* about the pediatric patient's myelination status, particularly if a pathologic state of myelination is suspected, repeat MR in 6 months, and make sure that at least one of the MR examinations has been performed at or after the first year of life.

DWI/DTI. DWI/DTI is an important MR adjunct. Acute demyelination is often associated with restricted diffusion. Certain diffusion patterns are strongly suggestive of specific inborn errors of metabolism [e.g., crenulated ribbon of restricted diffusion at the depth of cerebral hemispheric sulci in urea cycle disorders, juxta-ventricular diffusion restriction in phenylketonuria (PKU), cerebellar WM and four bright dots of pontine diffusion restriction in maple syrup urine disease, and "worst case ever of hypoxic-ischemic encephalopathy-like DWI abnormalities" in isolated sulfite oxidase deficiency].

Magnetic Resonance Spectroscopy. A lactate doublet at 1.3 ppm is a nonspecific indicator of disturbed oxidative metabolism and may be seen in several inherited metabolic disorders. A prominent resonant peak at 3.55 ppm on long TE proton spectroscopy aquisitions is characteristic of nonketotic hyperglycinemia (myoinositol at 3.6 ppm is seen only at short TES). The PKU peak at 7.4 ppm is out of range of the standard clinical *x*-axis display.

Imaging of Normal Myelination

Selected major milestones of normal myelination on T1- and T2-weighted images are summarized earlier in the chapter **(Table 31-1)** and discussed in greater detail here. The radiologist who has committed these normal MR milestones to memory will be well suited to detect early pathologic states of myelination. Although a nonspecific finding, disordered myelination is common among many inborn metabolic errors or inborn errors of metabolism.

Birth to Three Months

T1WI. Compared with the timing of neuronal migration and sulcation, normal myelination lags in the fetus. However, during the early third trimester, the dorsal brainstem myelination is advancing.

On T1-weighted sequences, the brain of a full-term newborn resembles an adult's on T2WI, i.e., most of the cerebral WM has lower signal than gray matter. The dorsal brainstem (medial longitudinal fasciculus, medial and lateral lemnisci), decussation of the superior cerebellar peduncles, central cerebellar WM, posterior limb of the internal capsule (PLIC), ventrolateral thalami, corticospinal tracts, and the deep corona radiata adjacent to the lateral ventricles exhibit T1 hyperintensity (myelinated) in the normal term newborn. In the newborn posterior fossa, look for T1 hyperintensity within the brachium of the inferior colliculus and within the inferior and superior cerebellar peduncles.

At birth and throughout the first month of life, there is progressive hyperintensity within the central cerebellar hemispheres. This normal myelination proceeds peripherally throughout the third month of life. The entire PLIC becomes hyperintense by the end of the second month and the entire anterior limb of internal capsule by the third month of life. As an aside, the presence of the normal T1 hyperintense myelin marker in the PLIC in the newborn is an important marker when profound hypoxic ischemic injury (HII) to the deep nuclei is suspected.

T2WI. On T2WI, the WM of a term newborn infant resembles that of a T1 image in an adult, i.e. it has higher signal relative to gray matter. Hypointensity can be seen in corticospinal tract and dorsal brainstem, PLIC, and ventrolateral thalamus. The dentate nuclei of the cerebellum consist of gray matter and thus also appear hypointense. Normal T2 hypointensity is seen at birth within the brainstem cranial nerve nuclei and within the inferior and superior cerebellar peduncles. Always check for the presence of the normal newborn linear T2 hypointensity (myelin marker) within the PLIC when profound HII is suspected.

At birth, the rolandic and perirolandic gyri of the cortex appear quite hypointense. This corresponds to known early myelination of the WM within these gyri. An ill-defined "smudgy" hypointensity in the WM underlying the rolandic/perirolandic gyri is a normal finding shortly after birth.

Three to Six Months

T1WI. The anterior limb of the internal capsule and the proximal, most central WM of the cerebellar folia become hyperintense by three postnatal months **(31-1)**. High signal appears in the splenium of the corpus callosum (CC) by 4 months and can be identified in the genu at 6 months **(31-2)**. Remember, the CC myelinates from back to front.

T2WI. Focal linear low signal appears in the PLIC at the location of the corticospinal tracts normally at birth and represents an important landmark in assessing neonatal health. The entire PLIC and splenium of the CC show hypointensity at 6 months.

The last normal regions of T2 hypointensity are the orbital region of the frontal lobes and the most anterior temporal lobes. This normal progression of T2 hypointensity may not be complete until 28-30 months. WM in the deep corona radiata extending from the motor cortex toward the lateral ventricle body myelinates early, appearing "smudgy" and slightly hypointense **(31-2)**.

Potential diagnostic pitfall: normal tiny foci of T2 hypointensity may be seen immediately anterior to the frontal horn tips in preterm and term newborns. These represent small aggregates of germinal matrix and typically vanish by 44 postconceptual weeks. These should not be misdiagnosed as gray matter heterotopia.

Six Months to One Year

T1WI. The WM assumes a near-adult appearance by 8 months with hyperintensity extending throughout most of the cerebellum and hemispheric WM. The corona radiata is almost completely hyperintense except for its most anterior and peripheral fibers.

Continued normal progression of T1 hyperintensity within the subcortical white matter is seen through the seventh month of life in the occipital white matter and through 8-11 months in the frontal and temporal white matter. Only minimal T1 hyperintensity changes are normally seen after 11 months. By 11-12 months, the WM resembles that of an adult with hyperintensity extending into most of the subcortical U-fibers. Only the anterior temporal and most peripheral frontal lobe WM remain unmyelinated, appearing isointense with the overlying cortex **(31-3)**.

T2WI. Hypointensity appears throughout the CC genu by 8 months and in the anterior limb of the internal capsule by 11 months. The basal ganglia demonstrate diminishing T2 signal compared with subcortical WM by 5-7 months of life. Most of the deep WM tracts of the cerebral hemispheres show progressive hypointensity between 6 and 12 months of life. The subcortical WM with the exception of the perirolandic and calcarine regions (which demonstrate early T2 hypointensity) continues (from posterior to anterior) to demonstrate T2 hypointensity. Within the cerebral hemispheric WM, occipital hypointensity is seen by 12 months, and frontal subcortical WM hypointensity is seen by 20 months.

Historically, it has been said that subcortical WM myelination (T2 hypointensity) was complete by 24 months of life. However, with improvements in MR hardware and software, we know that peripheral myelin T2 hypointensity is complete closer to 30 months, at which time the WM assumes a near-adult appearance. The caveat or pitfall is the persistence of T2 hyperintensity that is seen in the normal **terminal zones** (see below).

Two Years to Adulthood

T1WI. Although little discernible T1 hyperintensity change is appreciated by most radiologists after 11 months of patient age, the anterior temporal lobe WM does not become completely hyperintense on T1 scans until 24-30 months. Although WM myelination is visually complete at this age, functional MR studies demonstrate that some active myelination continues well into adolescence.

T2WI. It is common to see symmetric *brush-border-like* high signal intensity regions in the WM, both lateral and dorsal to the atria of the lateral ventricles. These parietal and parietal occipital regions of association fibers (*terminal zones*) of incompletely myelinated WM are considered a normal finding. *Terminal zones* are isointense to surrounding WM on proton density, show an interposed zone or collar of normally myelinated WM between the ventricular ependyma and the terminal zones, and are not affiliated with signs of volume loss. Terminal zones may remain hyperintense on T2WI well into the second or even third decade **(31-3D)** **(31-3F)** **(31-4D)**.

The term *terminal zones* was coined due to the fact that some axons in these association regions may not stain for myelin until the fourth decade of life.

Scattered punctate and linear T2 hyperintense WM foci that suppress completely on FLAIR are also common. These are normal perivascular (Virchow-Robin) spaces and occur at all ages.

Classification of Inherited Metabolic Disorders

Overview

The sheer number and variety of inherited metabolic disorders (IMDs) are overwhelming. New entities together with their MR findings are constantly added to the ever-growing list of these disorders. Moreover, identifying one of these elusive diseases is a multidisciplinary endeavor requiring, not only correct interpretation of imaging features, but also appreciation at times of the subtle and nonspecific clinical derangements, pathogenetics, and biochemical defect(s) of IMDs. In some cases, brain, skin, or muscle biopsy may be necessary to establish a definitive diagnosis. Adding to these diagnostic challenges for clinician and radiologist alike are the facts that these disorders are rare and that the accumulated individual experience that a physician has in diagnosing and treating IMDs throughout a lifetime practice is often limited.

An exhaustive discussion of IMDs is far beyond the scope of this book. The interested reader is referred to the superb definitive texts by A. James Barkovich. In this chapter, we consider the major and some of the less common but important inherited neurometabolic diseases, summarizing the pathoetiology, genetics, demographics, clinical presentation, and key imaging findings of each.

CLASSIFICATION OF IMDs RESULTING FROM ACCUMULATION OR DEFICIENCY OF SPECIFIC METABOLITES

- Disorders of intermediary metabolism
- Amino acid metabolism
- Fatty acid oxidation and ketogenesis
- Carbohydrate metabolism
- Vitamin-related disorders
- Mitochondrial energy metabolism
- Mineral and peptide metabolism
- Disorders of biosynthesis and breakdown of complex molecules
- Peroxisomes
- Lysosomes
- Purine and pyrimidine metabolism
- Glycosylation
- Lipoprotein metabolism
- Bile acid and Heme metabolism
- Disorders of neurotransmitter metabolism
- Glycine and serine metabolism
- Pterin and biogenic amine metabolism
- γ-Aminobutyrate metabolism

We begin by considering several approaches to classifying these unusual but fascinating disorders. There are several strategies that can be used to conceptually frame IMDs. One way is to divide IMDs according to which cellular organelle

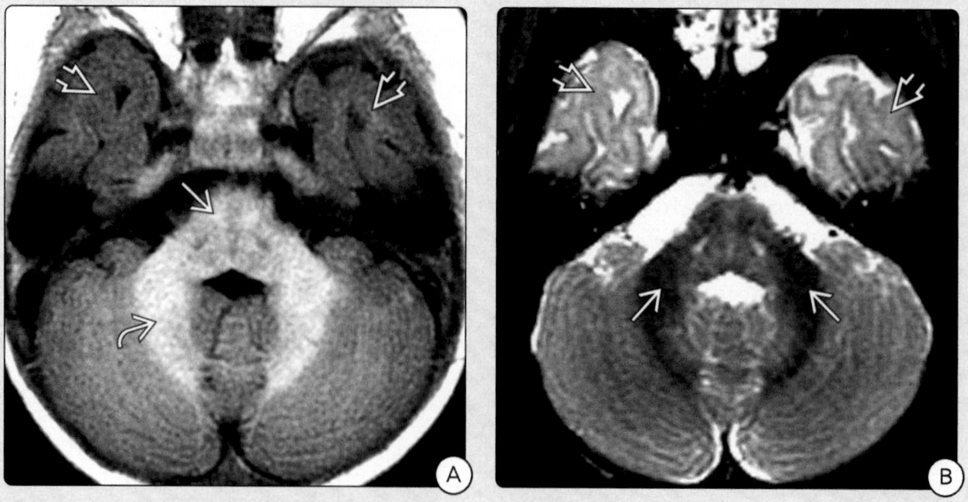

(31-3A) *Axial T1WI in a normal 12m infant shows the pons and cerebellum have a near-adult hyperintense appearance. The pons ➡ and middle cerebellar peduncles ➡ are completely myelinated. WM in anterior temporal lobe ➡ remains largely unmyelinated.* ***(31-3B)*** *Axial T2WI at 12 months shows hypointense (myelinated) cerebellar WM ➡ in contrast to the subcortical WM in both temporal lobes ➡, which is hyperintense.*

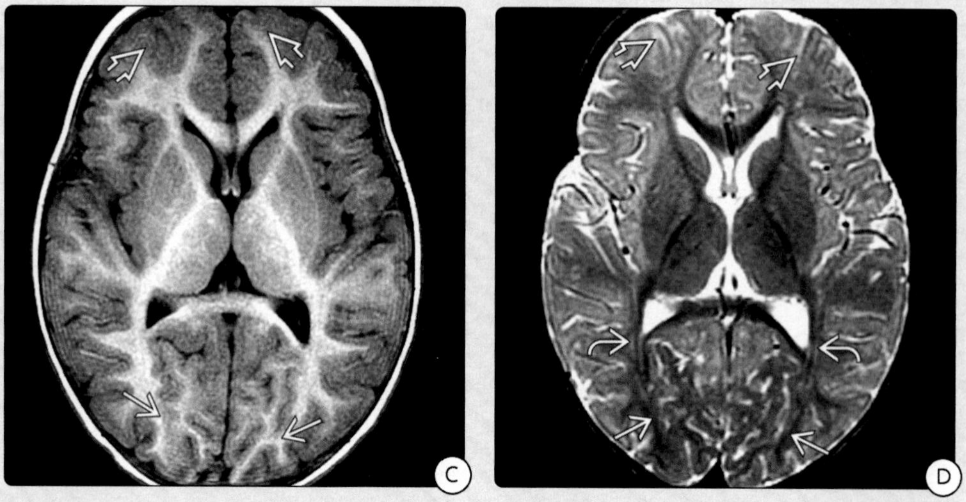

(31-3C) *Axial T1WI at 12 months shows "adult-like" myelination. Hyperintensity extends into the subcortical U-fibers in the occipital ➡ and parietal lobes to the undersurface of the cortex. Anterior frontal lobe U-fibers remain unmyelinated ➡.* ***(31-3D)*** *Axial T2WI shows hypointense subcortical U-fibers in occipital ➡ and parietal lobes but not in temporal or frontal lobes ➡. Some hyperintensity lateral to the trigones, occipital horns ➡ is normal.*

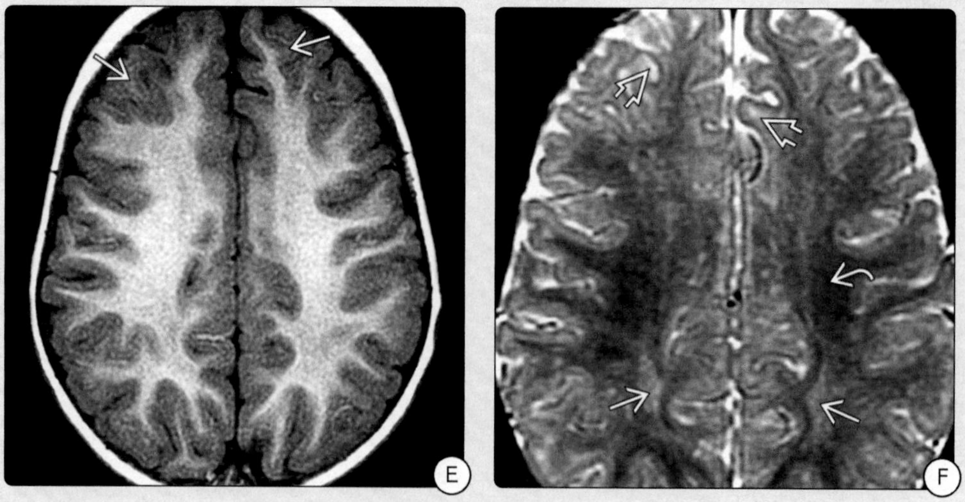

(31-3E) *Axial T2WI at 12 months shows myelination of corona radiata and that most U-fibers are mature (hyperintense). Some anterior U-fibers ➡ are unmyelinated.* ***(31-3F)*** *Axial T2WI shows that parietal and occipital U-fibers together with central corona radiata ➡ appear hypointense. The frontal and most superior U-fibers ➡ remain unmyelinated. Patchy hyperintense foci posterosuperior to the lateral ventricles ➡ are age appropriate.*

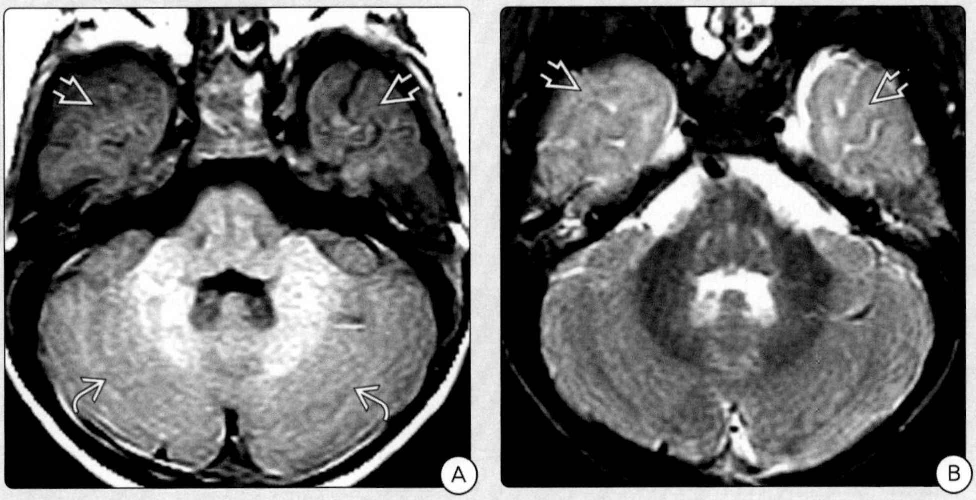

(31-4A) *Axial normal T1WI at 18 months shows the cerebellum looking adult-like hyperintense. WM of the cerebellar folia ➔ indicates that myelination is near complete. WM in the anterior temporal lobes ➔ remains unmyelinated.* ***(31-4B)*** *Axial T2WI shows a normal 18m child. The cerebellum is nearly completely myelinated. WM in the anterior temporal lobes remains hyperintense (unmyelinated) ➔.*

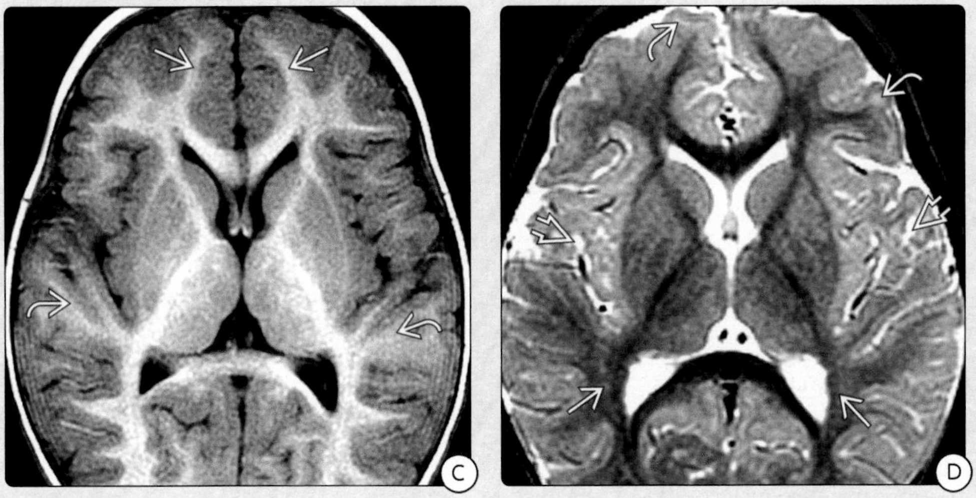

(31-4C) *At 18 months, axial T1WI shows that the normal anterior frontal ➔ and superior ➔ temporal U-fibers are completely myelinated at 18 months.* ***(31-4D)*** *Axial T2WI shows that in the same patient some temporal ➔ and frontal subcortical ➔ U-fibers remain hyperintense and unmyelinated. Persistent hyperintensity in the peritrigonal zones ➔ typically myelinates by 5 years.*

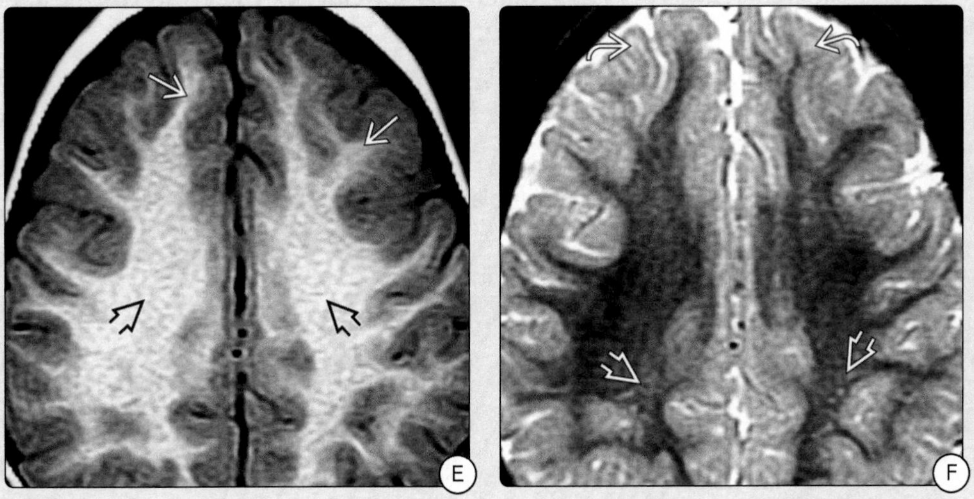

(31-4E) *At 18 months, axial T1WI shows WM of the corona radiata to be homogeneously hyperintense ➔. Normal myelin T1 shortening extends into the U-fibers ➔.* ***(31-4F)*** *Axial T2WI shows that, aside from some frontal subcortical U-fibers ➔, myelination in the corona radiata is complete. Patchy hyperintensities in the parietal association WM ➔ are perivascular spaces, which are normal at 3.0 T in children.*

(e.g., mitochondria, lysosomes) is predominantly affected. Another characterizes them by defects in a specific metabolic pathway (e.g., disorders of carbohydrate metabolism). Although intellectually sound, these methods lack the kind of pragmatic approach needed by the radiologist to be a contributing member of the clinical care team. To this end, we will emphasize—and advocate the use of—an approach to imaging analysis pioneered by A. James Barkovich that is primarily based on anatomic location and specific imaging features with an emphasis on MR—the **imaging-based approach.**

Organelle-Based Approach

Three cellular organelles are primarily affected in IMDs, i.e., the lysosomes, peroxisomes, and mitochondria. Classifying IMDs according to the affected organelle has the benefit of conceptual simplicity. However, many IMDs do not arise from disordered organelle formation or function, making this classification scheme less than comprehensive.

Lysosomal Diseases

Lysosomal disorders are characterized by abnormal lysosomes and disordered carbohydrate metabolism. The frequency of lysosomal disorders varies widely with geographic distribution. Some are far more frequent in certain locations because of the high prevalence of founder mutations.

The mucopolysaccharidoses are the classic lysosomal storage disorders. They result from deficiencies of enzymes involved in the degradation of mucopolysaccharides (glycosaminoglycans). Incompletely degraded mucopolysaccharides accumulate in the lysosomes, which often become enlarged and vacuolated. Prototypical mucopolysaccharidoses include **Hurler, Hunter, Sanfilippo,** and **Morquio** syndromes.

The gangliosidoses are rare lysosomal storage disorders characterized by deficient β-galactosidase. Abnormal oligosaccharides accumulate in the brain and viscera. Typical disorders are **GM1** and **GM2 gangliosidoses** (Tay-Sachs and Sandhoff diseases, respectively).

Peroxisomal Disorders

Peroxisomes contain multiple enzymes essential for normal growth and development. Inherited peroxisomal disorders can result in lack of organelle development or normally formed peroxisomes that nonetheless have disordered or deficient function of a single enzyme.

Deficiencies in peroxisomal formation result in syndromes such as **Zellweger syndrome, neonatal adrenoleukodystrophy,** and **infantile Refsum disease**. Disorders in which the peroxisomes are formed but function improperly include **X-linked adrenoleukodystrophy** and **classic Refsum disease**.

Mitochondrial Disorders

Mitochondrial disorders, also called respiratory chain disorders, are characterized by abnormal mitochondrial function. The result is impaired ATP (energy) production in affected cells.

Some mitochondrial disorders predominantly or exclusively affect striated muscle and therefore are not discussed in this text. Important mitochondrial encephalopathies include **Leigh syndrome, m**itochondrial **e**ncephalopathy with **l**actic **a**cidosis and **s**troke-like episodes (**MELAS**), **m**yoclonic **e**pilepsy with **r**agged **r**ed **f**ibers (**MERRF**), **Kearns-Sayre syndrome** (KSS), and **glutaric aciduria types 1 and 2**.

ORGANELLE-BASED CLASSIFICATION OF IMDs

Lysosomal Disorders
- Mucopolysaccharidoses
- Gangliosidoses
- Metachromatic leukodystrophy
- Krabbe disease
- Fabry disease

Peroxisomal Disorders
- Abnormal peroxisomal formation
  - Zellweger syndrome
  - Neonatal adrenoleukodystrophy
  - Infantile Refsum disease
- Abnormal peroxisomal function
  - X-linked adrenoleukodystrophy
  - Classic Refsum disease

Mitochondrial Disorders
- Leigh syndrome
- MELAS
- MERRF
- Kearns-Sayre
- Glutaric aciduria types 1 and 2

Metabolic Approach

Many IMDs result in accumulation of one or more abnormal metabolites such as ammonia, copper, or iron degradation products. These IMDs are summarized below and discussed in more detail later in the chapter.

Organic/Aminoacidopathies and Urea Cycle Disorders

The aminoacidopathies and urea cycle disorders result from disrupted nitrogen elimination and are characterized by hyperammonemia and elevated glutamine levels. Typical urea cycle disorders include **maple syrup urine disease, methylmalonic acidemia, ornithine transcarbamylase deficiency,** and **citrullinemia**.

Canavan disease is characterized by *N*-acetyl-L-aspartate (NAA) aciduria and NAA accumulation in the brain, which causes striking spongy degeneration.

Alexander disease results from mutations in the gene that encodes glial fibrillary acidic protein. Massive accumulation of Rosenthal fibers in astrocytes results in macrocephaly and a paucity of myelin in the frontal white matter.

Disorders of Copper Metabolism

Copper is an essential trace element required by all living organisms. However, excessive amounts of copper damage cells. Disruptions to normal copper homeostasis are the hallmarks of three genetic disorders: **Wilson disease, Menkes disease,** and **occipital horn disease**.

Brain Iron Accumulation Disorders

Iron accumulates within the basal ganglia and dentate nuclei during normal aging. A group of genetic disorders termed **n**eurodegeneration with **b**rain **i**ron **a**ccumulation (**NBIA**) are characterized by brain iron deposition in abnormal amounts and in abnormal locations. Neuronal death results.

SELECTED DISORDERS OF INTERMEDIARY METABOLISM

- Amino acid disorders
- Phenylketonuria
- Maple syrup urine disease
- Homocystinuria
- Galactosemia
- Tyrosinemia
- Disorders of glycogenesis (glycogen storage diseases, GSD)
- Glucose-6-phosphatase deficiency (GSD1, von Gierke disease)
- Lysosomal acid maltase deficiency (GSD2, Pompe disease)
- Disorders of gluconeogenesis
- Pyruvate carboxylase deficiency
- Pyruvate dehydrogenase deficiency
- Fatty acid oxidation disorders
- Organic acidurias (propionic, methylmalonic, isovaleric)
- Very-long-chain acyl-coenzyme A dehydrogenase deficiency
- Selected mitochondrial disorders
- Glutaric acidemia type 1
- Leigh syndrome
- Mitochondrial encephalopathy lactic acidosis and stroke (MELAS)
- Myoclonic epilepsy, ragged red fiber disease (MERRF)
- Kearns-Sayre

Imaging-Based Approach

Barkovich et al. have elaborated a practical imaging-based approach to the diagnosis of IMDs derived from the seminal work of van der Knaap and Valk. This approach is based on determining whether the disease involves primarily or exclusively (1) WM, (2) mostly GM, or (3) both. Furthermore, a heightened awareness of the region of the brain most heavily involved (e.g., periventricular WM vs. subcortical white matter or frontal lobe vs. parietal occipital lobes) and the presence of miscellaneous findings (e.g., cysts and/or calcifications) leads to greater specificity in the radiologist's differential diagnosis. In some cases, the aggregate of imaging findings leads to a specific unequivocal diagnosis (e.g., the MR and MRS findings in creatine transporter deficiency states).

In this text, we follow the **imaging-based approach**, the clinically practical classification based on the three above-mentioned categories of predominant imaging features (e.g., WM, GM, or both being involved). General findings for each individual category are delineated at the beginning of each section. We then discuss the major diagnostic entities in each imaging-based group. It is important to recognize that early imaging assessment with any IMD is of paramount importance, as the end-stage MR findings of these disorders may significantly overlap.

IMDs Predominantly Affecting White Matter

Historically, nearly all abnormalities of the white matter (WM) have been described as "leukodystrophies." The term leukodystrophy unfortunately is often loosely applied to all heritable disorders with WM changes on MR. *"Leukodystrophies"* have been further divided into three categories: (1) *dys*myelinating disorders (i.e., normal myelination does not occur), (2) *de*myelinating disease (i.e., myelin forms normally, is deposited around axons, but later breaks down or is destroyed), and (3) *hypo*myelinating diseases (i.e., here the WM may partially myelinate but never myelinates completely). Hypomyelinating leukoencephalopathies represent an important yet uncommon group of genetic disorders that cause delayed myelin maturation or undermyelination.

Updating our understanding and usage of terminology leads to greater understanding of the pathomorphology, genetics, and imaging characteristics of many disorders affecting WM, often becoming clinically evident in infants and children. **Leukodystrophies** are inherited disorders caused by an inborn metabolic defect. Leukodystrophies are characterized histopathologically by *demyelination* and clinically by *progressive neurologic deterioration, often leading to death.* Well-recognized leukodystrophies include metachromatic leukodystrophy, globoid cell leukodystrophy (Krabbe disease), and X-linked adrenoleukodystrophy. **Key leukodystrophy elements** include heritable inborn metabolic error and demyelination and inexorable clinical progression.

Of equal importance in the discussion of inherited WM abnormalities is the category of **nonleukodystrophic white matter changes (NLWMC).** Here, the histopathology may show arrested or highly delayed myelination, abnormal and irregular myelination, gliosis, spongiosis of the WM without demyelination, small WM infarctions, or enlarged Virchow-Robin spaces. Unlike many leukodystrophies, *NLWMCs demonstrate a more indolent clinical picture* and greater variability in the spectrum of MR abnormalities. **Key NLWMC elements** include disorders that are typically inherited, varied histopathology (i.e., demyelination not principle), and more indolent clinical progression.

From an imaging perspective, it can be difficult to determine whether a disorder is *dys*myelinating, *de*myelinating, or *hypo*myelinating. In structuring a differential diagnosis, it is

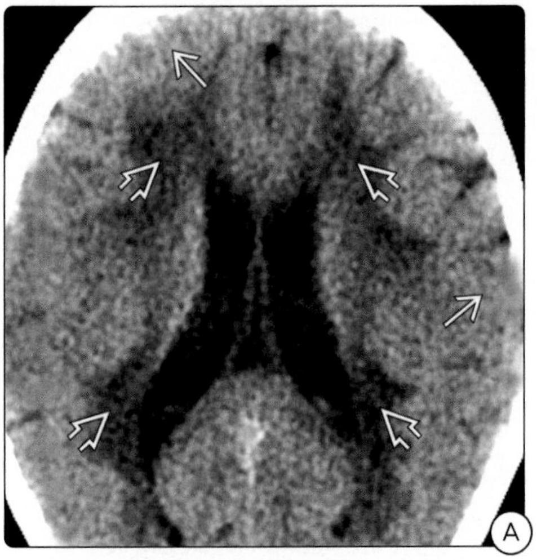

(31-5A) *Axial NECT in 6y boy with MLD shows periventricular WM hypoattenuation . The subcortical U-fibers are spared .*

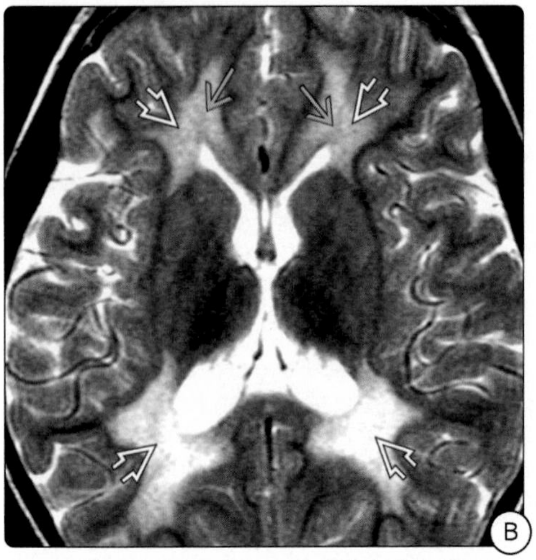

(31-5B) *Axial T2WI shows WM demyelination (hyperintensity) . Note "granular" hypointense frontal perivenular myelin sparing .*

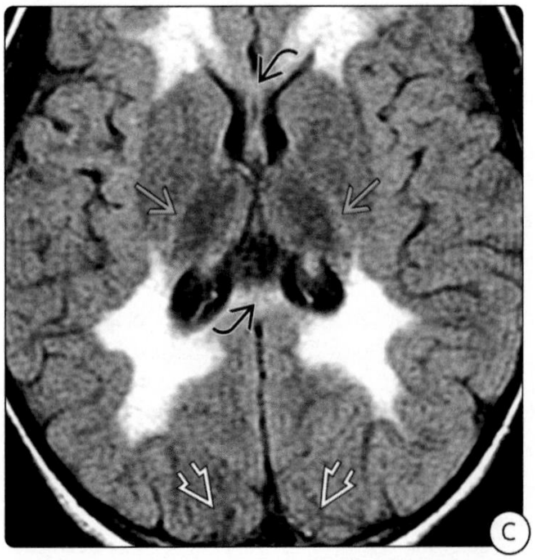

(31-5C) *Axial FLAIR shows the "butterfly" pattern of MLD. U-fibers appear normal . CC and PLIC are involved.*

important to determine whether the disorder primarily affects *deep* (periventricular) WM or the *subcortical* short association WM fibers (U-fibers). In a few diseases, both the deep and peripheral WM are affected.

Examples of leukodystrophies that exhibit early *deep* WM predominance include metachromatic leukodystrophy and X-linked adrenoleukodystrophy. Leukodystrophies that involve the *subcortical* U-fibers early in the disease course include megaloencephalic leukoencephalopathy with cysts and infantile Alexander disease. The latter two diagnoses also present with a large head.

Diseases in which virtually *all* the WM (both periventricular *and* subcortical) remains unmyelinated are rare. The imaging appearance in these disorders resembles that of a normal newborn brain with immature, almost completely unmyelinated WM. Here the entire WM—including the subcortical U-fibers—appears uniformly hyperintense on T2WI.

A good imaging rule of thumb, when interpretation of the MR in a newborn or infant *suggests a disorder of the WM*, is to repeat the MR in 6 months. Ideally, one of the MR examinations should follow the child's first birthday. This is particularly helpful in the hypomyelinating disorders in which there will be no discernible interval improvement in myelin milestones as assessed by MR.

Periventricular White Matter Predominance

The prototypical disorder that typically begins with symmetric deep WM involvement and spares the subcortical U-fibers until late in the disease course is metachromatic leukodystrophy (MLD). Others with a similar pattern of periventricular predominance include Krabbe disease (globoid cell leukodystrophy), X-linked adrenoleukodystrophy, and vanishing WM disease (VWMD).

MAJOR IMDs WITH PERIVENTRICULAR WM PREDOMINANCE

Common
- Metachromatic leukodystrophy
- Classic X-linked adrenoleukodystrophy

Less Common
- Globoid cell leukodystrophy (Krabbe disease)
- Vanishing WM disease

Rare But Important
- Phenylketonuria
- Maple syrup urine disease
- Merosin-deficient congenital muscular dystrophy

Metachromatic Leukodystrophy

Terminology. MLD, also known as sulfatide lipoidosis, is a devastating lysosomal storage disease caused by a reduction in or complete absence of arylsulfatase A (ARSA), resulting in the intralysosomal accumulation of sphingolipid sulfatide in tissues including the CNS and peripheral nervous system (PNS).

Etiology. MLD is caused by reduction of or complete absence of ARSA with failure of myelin breakdown and reutilization. It affects the CNS, PNS, and other tissues. Reduced or absent ARSA leads to increased lysosomal storage of sulfatide and eventually lethal demyelination. The late stage of disease is associated with progressive demyelination and diffuse cerebral atrophy.

ARSA gene is located at 22q13.31-qter. Over 110 mutations have been reported. Earlier onset is associated with greater reduction in *ARSA*.

Pathology. Grossly, a brain affected by MLD may be normal or demonstrate mild volume loss. Initially, the periventricular WM shows a grayish discoloration (e.g., "tigroid" or "leopard " pattern) with relatively normal-appearing subcortical U-fibers.

Demyelination is the main histopathologic feature and affects both the CNS and PNS. Characteristic PAS + material, reflecting brownish metachromasia (for which the disorder is named), is seen with acidic cresyl violet stain and represents intracellular deposits of cholesterol, phospholipids, and sulfatides. Deposition occurs within glial cells, plasma membranes, inner layer of myelin sheath, neurons, Schwann cells, and macrophages. Tissue assays for ARSA are positive. There is a distinctive lack of inflammation in the regions that demonstrate demyelination.

Clinical Issues. MLD is one of the most common of all inherited WM disorders with a prevalence of 1:100,000 live births. MLD is more common among Habbani Jews and Navajo American Indians. Prognosis is variable based on the clinical form of disease. The initial signs of MLD may appear at any age.

Three distinct clinical forms are currently recognized, late infantile (onset earlier than 3 years), juvenile (onset earlier than 16 years), and adult MLD. The *late infantile form* is the most common and typically presents in the second year of life with visuomotor impairment, gait disorder, and abdominal pain. Progressive decline and death within 4 years are expected. The *juvenile form* presents between 5-10 years, often with deteriorating school performance. Survival beyond 20 years is rare. The *adult form* may present with early-onset dementia, MS-like symptoms, and progressive cerebellar signs.

Established treatment options include hematopoietic stem cell transplantation. Therapies such as enzyme replacement and gene therapy with oligodendroglial or neural progenitor cells are still experimental.

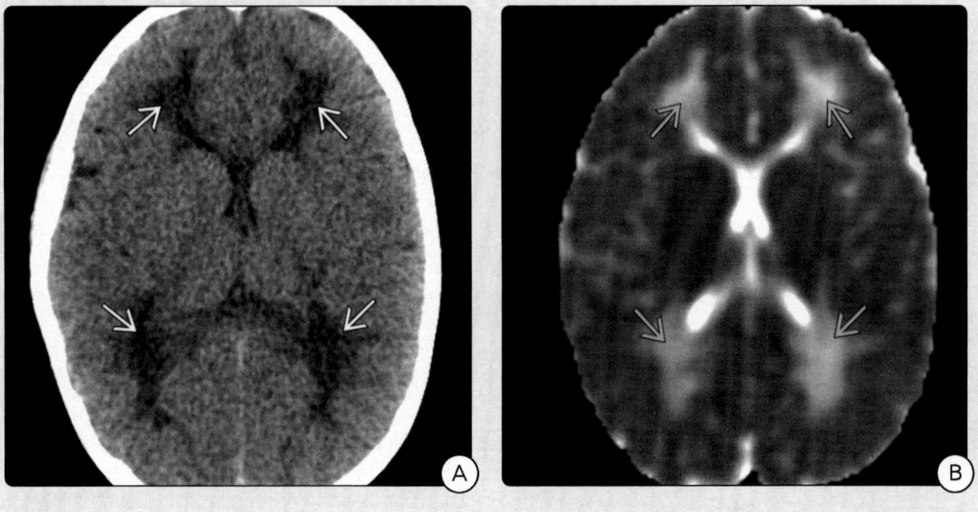

***(31-6A)** Axial NECT in a 4y boy with MLD shows symmetric periventricular diminished WM attenuation ➡. **(31-6B)** Axial ADC map in the same patient shows increased diffusivity (hyperintensity) within zones of "aging" demyelination →.*

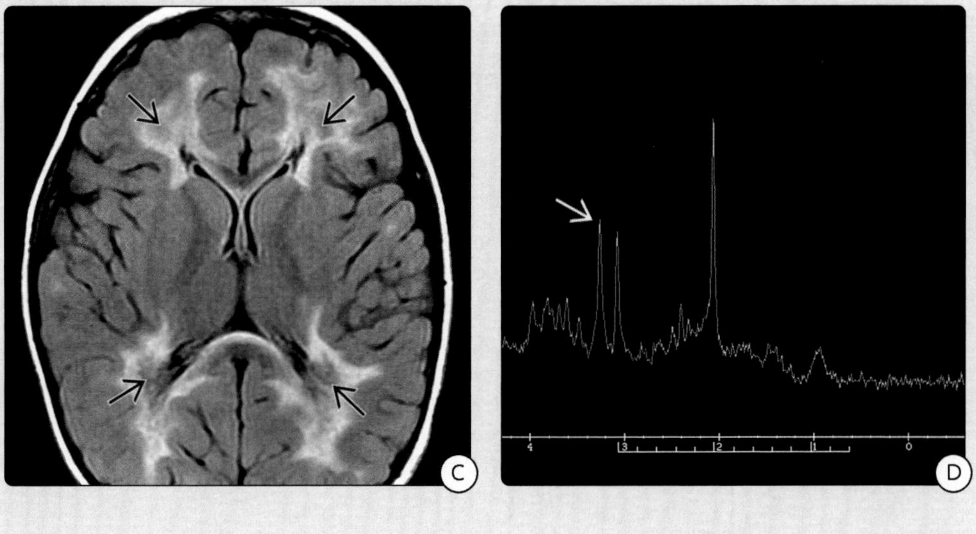

***(31-6C)** Axial FLAIR image in the same patient shows hyperintense zones of periventricular demyelination with inner granular or tigroid hypointensities → representing perivenular myelin sparing. **(31-6D)** MRS of the same patient shows that short TE (35 ms) proton spectroscopy of the left peritrigonal WM shows mild elevation of choline ➡, indicating cell membrane (myelin) turnover.*

Imaging. The early imaging hallmark of MLD is a confluent butterfly-shaped pattern of deep cerebral hemispheric altered CT attenuation and MR signal intensity. Depending on the clinical form of disease, the imaging changes may be rapidly progressive.

CT Findings. Early NECT shows symmetric diminished attenuation involving the central cerebral hemispheric white matter **(31-6)**. CECT shows no enhancement, and CT perfusion demonstrates reduced perfusion to the hemispheric WM. Cerebral atrophy is an expected nonspecific late finding.

MR Findings. The typical MR features of early MLD are confluent, symmetric, butterfly-shaped hyperintensities (i.e., T2/FLAIR) involving the periventricular WM. The subcortical U-fibers and cerebellum are typically spared until late in the disease. Serial MR shows a centrifugal spread of confluent T2/FLAIR hyperintensity. With disease progression, demyelination involves the corpus callosum (i.e., splenium), parietooccipital WM, and the frontal and then the temporal WM. Eventually, the progressive subcortical demyelination involves the subcortical U-fibers. Additional sites of late involvement include the corpus callosum, pyramidal tracts, and internal capsules. Islands of normal myelin around medullary veins in the WM may produce a striking "tiger," "tigroid," or "leopard" pattern with linear hypointensities in a sea of confluent hyperintensity **(31-7)**. This tigroid pattern reflects early sparing of perivenular myelin. No enhancement is seen on T1 C+. A few cases of MLD have been reported with enlarged, enhancing cranial nerves and/or cauda equina nerve roots.

DWI/DTI. Reduction of diffusivity in zones of active demyelination is seen. Regions of "burnt-out," aging, or chronic demyelination demonstrate increased diffusivity.

MRS. Nonspecific elevation of choline and myoinositol may be seen in early and active disease **(31-6)** **(31-8)**.

Differential Diagnosis. The major differential diagnosis of MLD includes other IMDs that primarily affect the periventricular WM. Globoid cell leukoencephalopathy (**Krabbe disease**) shows bithalamic hyperattenuation on NECT, involves the cerebellum early, and often demonstrates enlarged optic nerves and optic chiasm.

Pelizaeus-Merzbacher disease usually presents in neonates and shows almost total lack of myelination that does not show interval improvement on serial MRs. The cerebellum may be markedly atrophic.

Periventricular white matter injury (PVL) is associated with a history of low birthweight/preterm deliveries and clinical static spastic di- or quadriparesis and shows nonprogressive periventricular volume loss and T2/FLAIR hyperintensity.

Pseudo-TORCH demonstrates progressive cerebral and cerebellar demyelination and Ca++ involving brainstem, basal ganglia, and cerebral parenchyma. If the severity of WM involvement appears at first blush to represent the "worst case ever of MLD," consider pseudo-TORCH. The presence of elevated CSF neurotransmitters is noteworthy in pseudo-TORCH.

METACHROMATIC LEUKODYSTROPHY (MLD)

Etiology and Pathology
- Lysosomal storage disorder
- Decreased ARSA → sphingolipid accumulation
- Periventricular demyelination

Clinical Issues
- Most common inherited leukodystrophy
- Three forms
  - Late infantile (most common)
  - Juvenile
  - Adult (late onset)

Imaging
- Centrifugal spread of demyelination
  - Starts in corpus callosum splenium, deep parietooccipital WM
  - Frontal, temporal WM affected later
  - Spares subcortical U-fibers, cerebellum
- Classic = butterfly pattern
  - Symmetric hyperintensities around frontal horns, atria
- Tiger pattern
  - "Stripes" of perivenular myelin sparing in WM

Differential Diagnosis
- Other disorders that predominantly affect periventricular WM
  - Globoid cell leukodystrophy (Krabbe disease)
  - Pelizaeus-Merzbacher disease
  - Vanishing white matter disease
- Destructive disorders
  - Periventricular leukomalacia

TORCH including Zika virus infection is nonprogressive and often associated with micrencephaly and polymicrogyria. Variable WM changes (representing gliosis and demyelination) and varied patterns of Ca++ may be present.

Vanishing white matter disease (VWMD) begins in the periventricular WM but eventually involves all the hemispheric white matter. VWMD often cavitates and does not enhance.

Megalencephaly with leukoencephalopathy and cysts represents a slowly progressive disorder, associated with macrocephaly, spared cognition, demyelination with "swollen" WM, and eventual development of subcortical cysts (frontal, parietal, and temporal).

Sneddon syndrome also known as ARSA pseudodeficiency represents demyelination that may be triggered by a hypoxic event. The diagnosis can be confirmed by skin biopsy.

Ischemic white matter disease [e.g., moyamoya syndrome, as seen in Down syndrome, sickle cell disease, neurofibromatosis type 1 (NF1), and *ACTA2* gene mutation **(31-8)**] is a differential diagnosis of MLD. (Moyamoya disease is more common among children in Japan.) Deep white matter gliosis and demyelination, diminished size of circle of Willis, lateral cerebral fissure "candelabra" vessels, and hypertrophy of lenticulostriate vessels are seen **(31-8)**.

SELECTED WELL-KNOWN LEUKODYSTROPHIES

- Metachromatic leukodystrophy
- Globoid cell leukodystrophy (Krabbe disease)
- X-linked adrenoleukodystrophy
- Adrenomyeloneuropathy
- Canavan disease
- Alexander disease
- Refsum disease
- Cerebrotendinous xanthomatosis

SELECTED INHERITED DISEASES WITH NONLEUKODYSTROPHIC WM CHANGES

Arrested or Highly Delayed Myelination
- Pelizaeus-Merzbacher disease
- Infantile-onset neuronal degenerative disorders
  - Infantile GM1 and GM2 gangliosidosis
  - Infantile neuronal ceroid lipofuscinosis
  - Alpers disease
  - Menkes disease

Abnormal and Irregular Myelination
- Amino organic acidopathies
  - Phenylketonuria
  - Propionic acidemia
  - Maple syrup urine disease
  - Nonketotic hyperglycemia
- Chromosomal abnormalities (e.g., 18q syndrome)

Widespread White Matter Gliosis
- Lowe syndrome and galactosemia

Large Virchow-Robin Spaces
- Mucopolysaccharidoses

Small White Matter Infarctions
- Fabry disease and hyperhomocysteinemia

Status Spongiosis of Cerebral White Matter

Megalencephaly With Leukoencephalopathy and Cysts

X-Linked Adrenoleukodystrophy

Terminology. X-linked adrenoleukodystrophy (X-ALD) is also known as *childhood cerebral X-ALD* (CCALD). It was historically known as "bronze" Schilder disease and "melanodermic type leukodystrophy" before its adrenal involvement was recognized. At least five variants other than CCALD have been described, including presymptomatic X-ALD, adolescent (AdolCALD), adult (ACALD), adrenomyeloneuropathy (AMN), and Addison-only symptomatic female carriers.

Etiology. ALD is an inherited disorder of peroxisomal metabolism. Peroxisomes are ubiquitous organelles involved in catabolic pathways. Altered peroxisome metabolism in ALD results from absent or deficient acyl-CoA synthetase leading to impaired β-oxidation of very-long-chain fatty acids (VLCFAs). VLCFAs accumulate in the WM, causing a severe inflammatory demyelination ("brittle" myelin). Axonal degeneration in the posterior fossa and spinal cord are also typical of the disease.

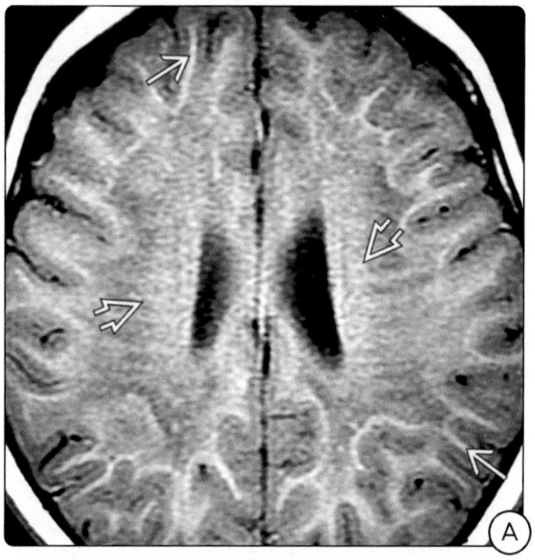

***(31-7A)** Axial T1MR shows MLD in a 2y boy with sparing of U-fibers, preserved striate myelin surrounding venules (tigroid pattern).*

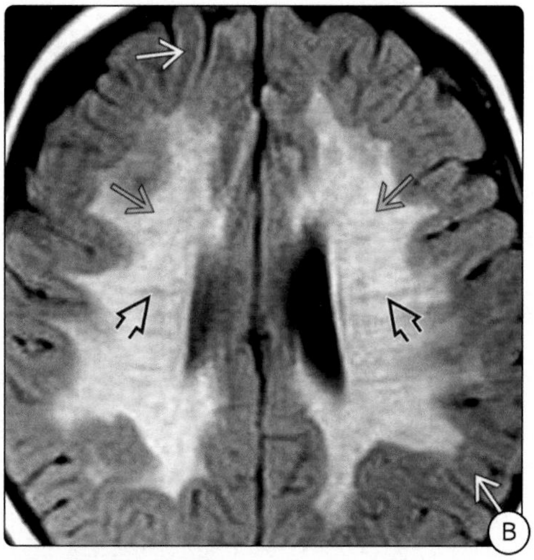

***(31-7B)** Axial FLAIR shows hyperintense demyelination, preserved perivenule myelin (tigroid pattern), sparing of U-fibers.*

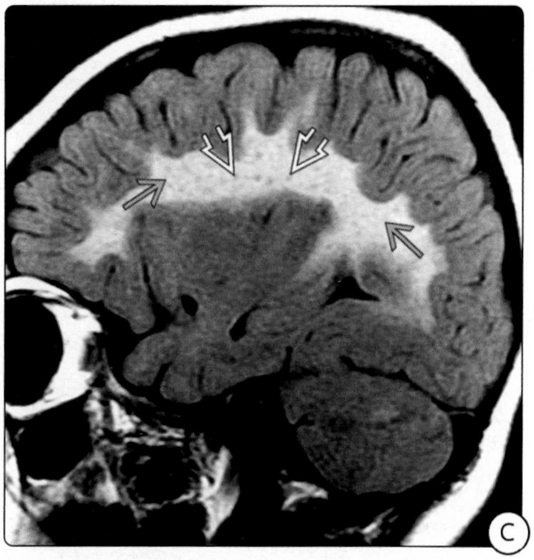

***(31-7C)** Sagittal FLAIR shows hypointense dots (leopard pattern) of preserved myelin within demyelinated WM sparing U-fibers.*

Genetics. ALD is an X-linked recessive disorder caused by mutations of the gene *ABCD1, which has been mapped to Xq28*. More than 500 mutations of the *ABCD1* gene have been described. The Xq28 chromosome normally codes for a peroxisomal membrane protein also known as an ATPase transporter protein, "traffic" ATPase.

Pathology. There are two distinctive active pathophysiologic processes in ALD. The first is axonal degeneration that predominates in the posterior fossa and spinal cord, and the second is a severe inflammatory demyelination.

Three distinct zones of myelin loss are seen in ALD **(31-11)**. The *innermost zone* consists of a necrotic core of demyelination with astrogliosis, ± Ca++. An *intermediate zone* of active demyelination and perivascular inflammation lies just outside the necrotic, "burned out" core of the lesion. The most *peripheral zone* consists of ongoing demyelination without inflammatory changes **(31-12)**.

Clinical Issues. X-ALD is the most common single protein or enzyme deficiency disease to present in childhood. The incidence is 1:20,000-50,000.

Several clinical forms of ALD and related disorders have been described. Phenotypes are unpredictable (even intrafamilial ALD). **Classic X-linked ALD** is the most common form (45%) and is seen almost exclusively in boys 5-12 years of age. Behavioral difficulties and deteriorating school performance are common. Hearing loss and skin bronzing may be seen. Approximately 10% of affected patients present acutely with seizures, adrenal crisis, acute encephalopathy, or coma.

Adrenomyeloneuropathy (AMN) is the second most common type (35%). It is another X-linked disorder that occurs primarily in male patients. It presents between 14 and 60 years, thus presenting later than classic X-ALD. AMN is characterized by axonal degeneration in the spinal cord more than the brain and peripheral nerves.

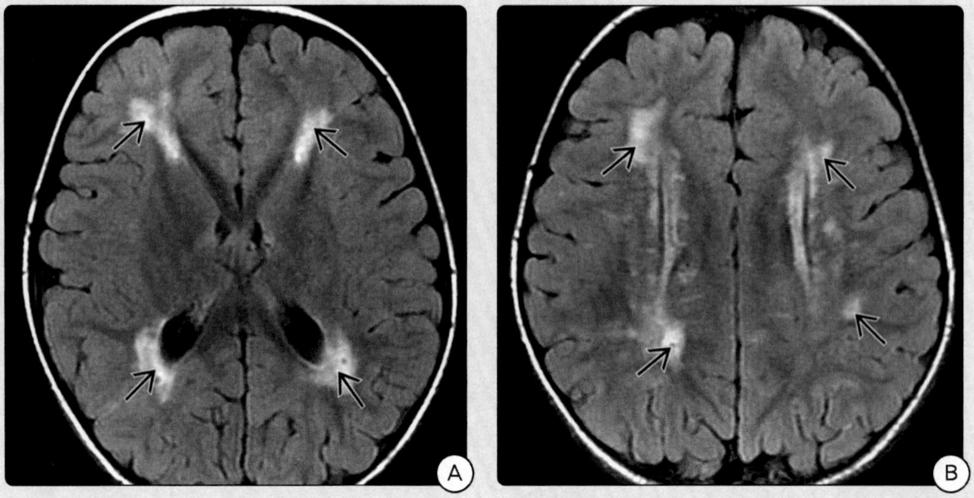

(31-8A) Axial FLAIR image in a 3y boy with ACTA2 gene mutation and stroke-like episodes shows central periventricular hyperintensities (gliosis and demyelination) ➙. Note the sparing of subcortical U-fibers. (31-8B) Axial FLAIR image in the same patient through cerebral convexities shows patchy WM hyperintensities ➙.

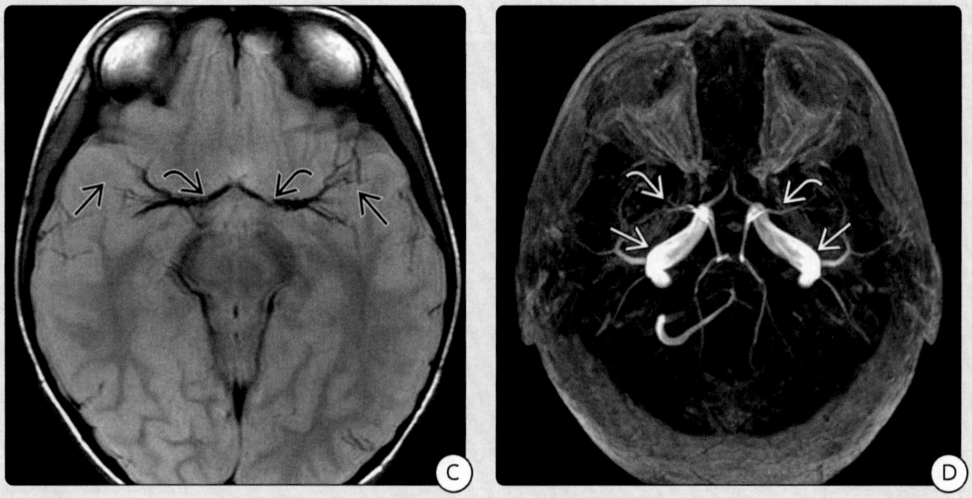

(31-8C) Axial PD MRI in the same patient shows diminished caliber of circle of Willis vasculature ➙ and conspicuous absence of vessels in the lateral cerebral fissures ➙, representing early moyamoya syndrome. (31-8D) Axial TOF MRA in the same patient with ACTA2 mutation shows striking diminished caliber of M1 and M2 segments of the middle cerebral arteries ➙. Note aneurysmal petrous carotids ➙.

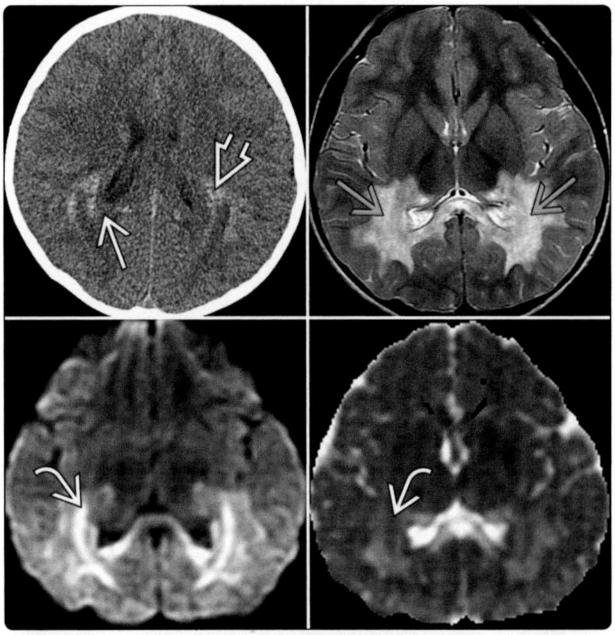

(31-9) Classic X-ALD shows periatrial WM hypoattenuation ➡ and calcifications ➡ on NECT. There is periatrial T2 hyperintensity ➡ and diffusion restriction ➡ in the actively demyelinating, inflammatory regions.

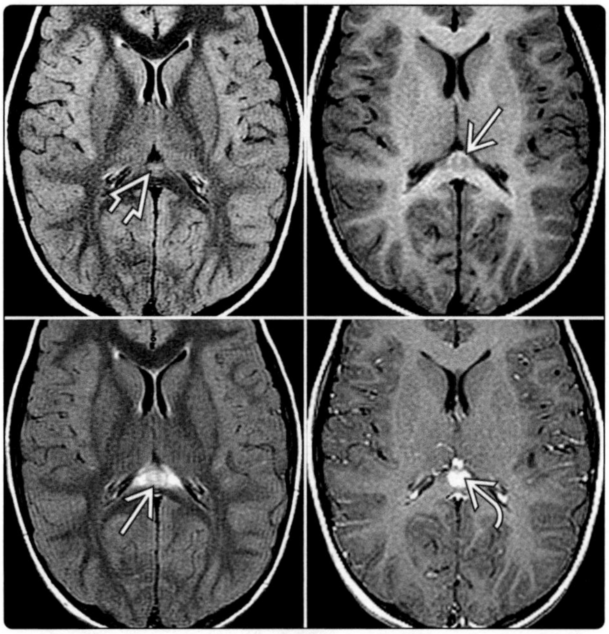

(31-10) FLAIR (upper left) in a 5y boy with early ALD shows a small hyperintense focus in the splenium ➡. Six months later, T1WI (upper right), FLAIR (lower left) show the increasing size of the lesion ➡. T1 C+ (lower right) shows enhancement ➡.

ADRENOLEUKODYSTROPHY (ALD): ETIOLOGY, PATHOLOGY, AND CLINICAL ISSUES

Etiology

- Peroxisomal disorder
- Impaired oxidation of VLCFAs

Pathology

- Severe inflammatory demyelination
- Three zones
  - Necrotic "burned out" core
  - Intermediate zone of active demyelination + inflammation
  - Peripheral demyelination without inflammation

Clinical Issues

- Classic X-linked ALD
  - Most common form (45%)
  - Preteen boys
  - Deteriorating cognition, school performance
- Adrenomyeloneuropathy (AMN)
  - Second most common form (35%)
  - Most common in male patients
- Addison disease without CNS involvement (20%)

Approximately 20% of X-ALD patients exhibit isolated adrenal insufficiency (**Addison disease**). Neurologic involvement is absent. Other less common forms of ALD include adolescent and adult-onset ALD and mild symptomatic disease in female carriers.

Untreated X-ALD carries a dismal prognosis. Relentless progression with spastic quadriparesis, blindness, deafness, and vegetative state is typical. Dietary intake of Lorenzo oil (a mixture of triolein and trierucin) has helped mitigate symptoms in some patients. Early bone marrow transplantation or hematopoietic stem cell gene therapy has improved clinical outcome for others.

Imaging. The definitive diagnosis of X-ALD is established by tissue assays for increased amounts of VLCFAs. When typical, imaging findings can be strongly suggestive of the diagnosis. Although CT scans are sometimes obtained as an initial screening study in children with encephalopathy of unknown origin, MR without and with IV contrast is the procedure of choice.

ALD: IMAGING AND DIFFERENTIAL DIAGNOSIS

Imaging

- X-linked ALD posterior predominance in 80%
  - Earliest finding: corpus callosum splenium hyperintensity
  - Spreads posterior to anterior, center to periphery
  - Intermediate zone often enhances, restricts
- Variant patterns
  - X-linked ALD with anterior predominance (10-15%)
  - AMN involves corticospinal tracts, cerebellum, cord more than hemispheric WM

Differential Diagnosis

- X-linked ALD pathognomonic if sex, age, imaging findings classic

CT Findings. NECT scans demonstrate hypoattenuation involving the corpus callosum splenium and WM around the atria and occipital horns. Calcification in the affected WM may be seen **(31-9)**. CECT typically shows enhancement around the central hypoattenuating WM.

MR Findings. A *posterior-predominant* pattern is seen in 80% of patients with X-ALD **(31-13)**. The earliest spin magnitude finding is T2/FLAIR hyperintensity in the middle of the corpus callosum splenium **(31-10)**. As the disease progresses, hyperintensity spreads from posterior to anterior and from the center to the periphery. The peritrigonal WM, corticospinal tracts, fornix, commissural fibers, plus the visual and auditory pathways can all eventually become involved.

The leading edge of demyelination appears hyperintense on T1WI but does not enhance **(31-14)**. The intermediate zone of active inflammatory demyelination typically enhances T1 C+. Thus, always include T1 C+ when imaging suspected leukodystrophy.

The *Loes MR scoring system* is a severity score based on the location, extent of disease, and atrophy. It divides the brain into nine regions with 23 subregions. Each region is scored for the presence (1) or absence (0) of atrophy, and every subregion is assessed as normal (0), unilateral abnormality (0.5), or bilateral abnormalities (1) in signal intensity.

Variant imaging patterns of X-ALDs are common. Approximately 10-15% of all patients with classic X-ALD have an *anterior predominant* demyelination; T2WI/FLAIR hyperintensity initially appears in the corpus callosum genu (not the splenium) and spreads into the frontal lobe WM **(31-15)**. Other atypical reported patterns include unilateral disease, disease with both bioccipital and bifrontal WM abnormality. Another variant involves only the internal capsules. In summary, X-ALD may present at an atypical age, demonstrate atypical sites of involvement, and lack enhancement. X-ALD may present with "mild" peritrigonal T2/FLAIR signal changes **(31-17)**. Rarely, the patient with X-ALD presents with Guillain-Barré-like acute demyelinating radiculopathy of the cauda equina nerve roots.

Imaging findings in patients with adrenomyeloneuropathy vary from those of patients with classic X-ALD. The cerebral

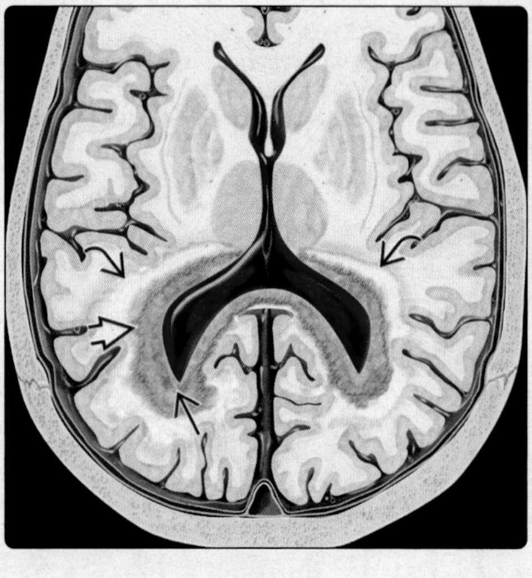

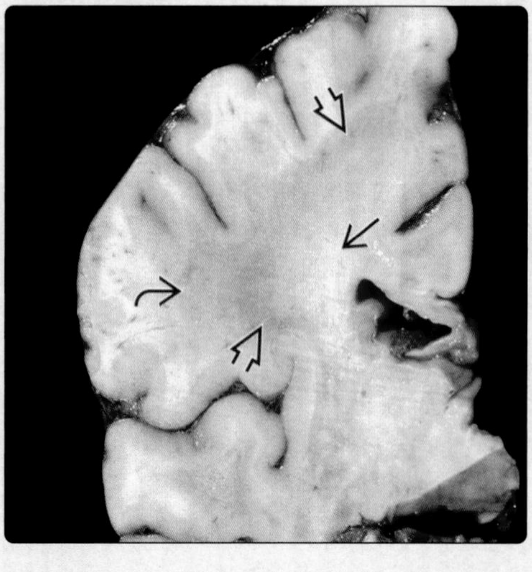

(31-11) Axial graphic of classic X-ALD shows deep zone of demyelination is burned out ➡; the intermediate zone ➡ shows active demyelination, inflammation, and advancing edge ➡ display ongoing demyelination. (31-12) Coronal autopsy section of X-ALD shows the three zones of myelin loss: "burned out" core ➡, intermediate zone (grayish region ➡), advancing edge (yellowish discoloration ➡). (AFIP Archives.)

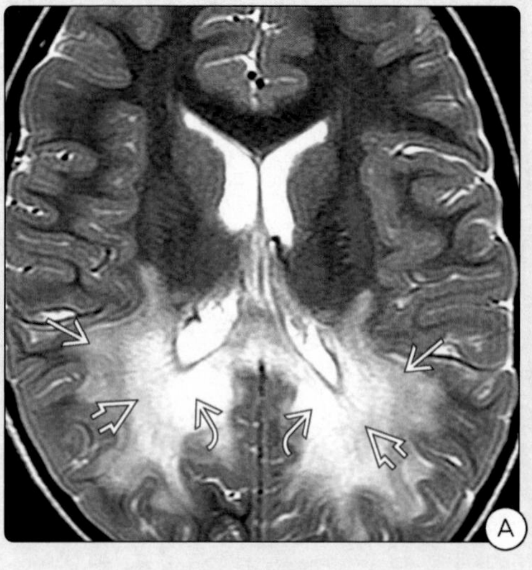

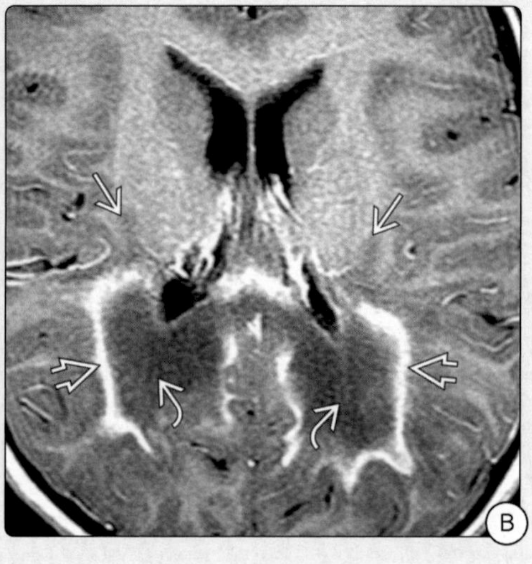

(31-13A) Axial T2WI in classic X-ALD shows periatrial hyperintense burned out WM ➡. Active demyelination, inflammation surrounding core is less hyperintense ➡. Most peripheral, leading edge zone ➡ shows ongoing demyelination without inflammatory changes. (31-13B) Axial T1 C+ FS in X-ALD shows intermediate zone of active demyelination enhances ➡, while leading edge ➡ and central burnt out cores ➡ do not.

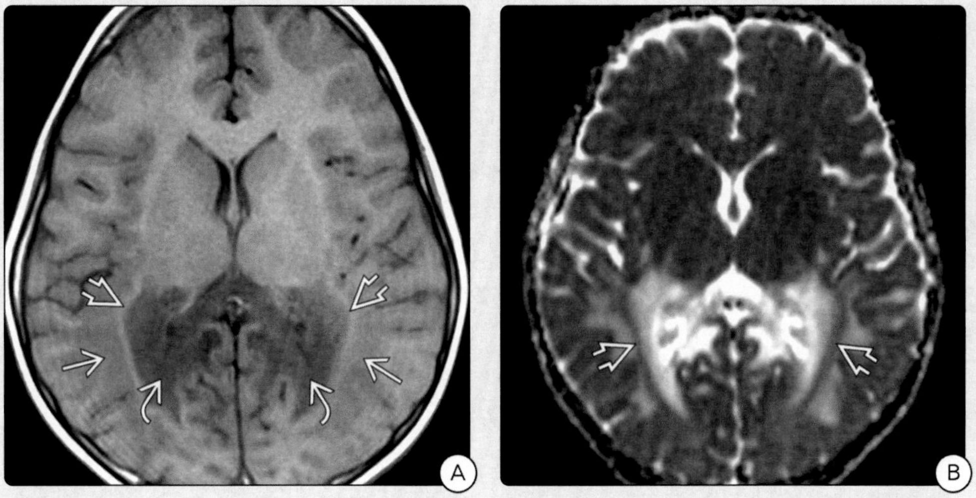

(31-14A) *Axial T1WI in classic X-ALD shows hypointense inner → burnt out core and outer → perimeter of demyelination. Note the T1 hyperintensity of the intermediate zone →.* ***(31-14B)*** *Axial ADC map in the same patient shows diffusion restriction (low ADC values) within the intermediate zone →. The inner core and outer perimeter of disease show increased diffusivity (hyperintensity).*

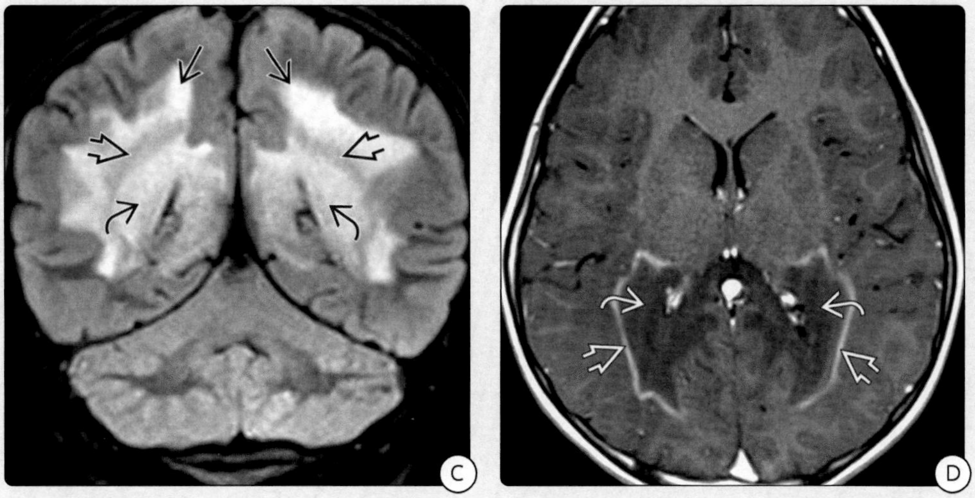

(31-14C) *Coronal FLAIR image in the same patient shows hyperintense inner ⟳ and outer zones → of demyelination and relatively hypointense intermediate zones →.* ***(31-14D)*** *Axial T1WI C+ in classic X-ALD shows enhancement of the intermediate zone of demyelination and inflammation →. Note the hypointensity of the "burned out " core ⟳.*

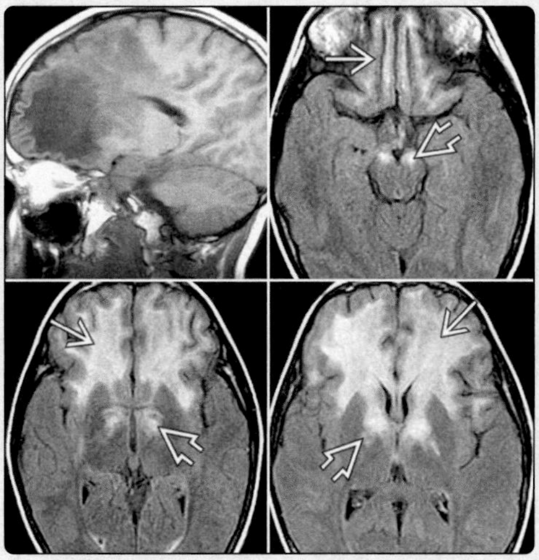

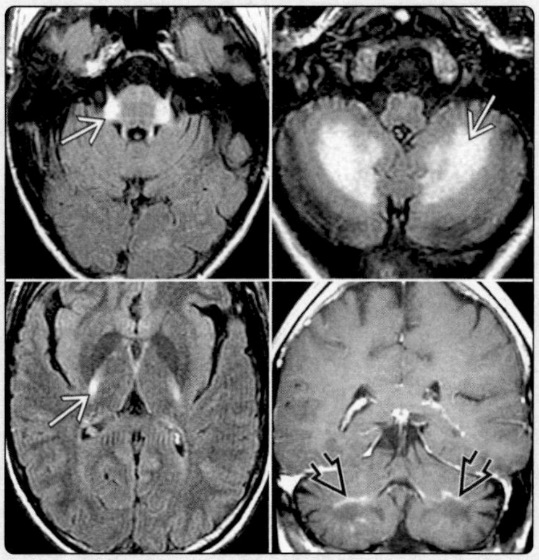

(31-15) *MR multiplanar images of an atypical variant of ALD show symmetric confluent frontal lesions → with sparing of parietooccipital WM. Note the involvement of internal capsules and cerebral peduncles →.* ***(31-16)*** *MRs in adrenomyeloneuropathy show a 33y woman with symmetric lesions in the cerebellar WM, lateral pons, CN V, superior cerebellar peduncles, and internal capsules →. Note the enhancement of the cerebellar lesions →.*

hemispheres are relatively spared with predominant involvement of the cerebellum, corticospinal tracts, and spinal cord **(31-16)**. Enhancement is typically absent.

DWI/DTI shows reduced diffusivity in active zones of demyelination and increased diffusivity in regions of "burnt-out" demyelination. DTI shows reduced connectivity (i.e., loss of fractional anisotropy) in WM that MR demonstrates as abnormal and in "normal" WM **(31-14)**.

MRS shows, at TE of 35 ms, peaks at 0.8-1.4 (i.e., cytosolic amino acids and VLCFA macromolecules). Reduced NAA may be detected prior to observed MR abnormality and predicts progression. Increased myoinositol, CHO, and lactate doublet are typical findings.

Differential Diagnosis. When X-ALD presents in patients of classic age and sex (i.e., 5- to 12-year-old boys) and with typical posterior predominance on imaging studies, the differential diagnosis is very limited.

Leukoencephalopathy with brainstem/spinal cord involvement and high lactate may resemble ALD but has a different clinical presentation and is caused by homozygous mutation in the *DARS2* gene. **Hypoglycemia** in neonates and young infants may involve the parietal and occipital WM and GM, CC splenium, calcar avis, peritrigonal WM with T2WI/FLAIR hyperintensity, and restricted diffusion. There is a lack of WM enhancement. **Alexander disease** is associated with macrocephaly and involves frontal WM (not peritrigonal as in typical X-ALD). WM enhances. **Metachromatic leukodystrophy** demonstrates symmetric nonenhancing periventricular T2/FLAIR hyperintensity.

Globoid Cell Leukodystrophy (Krabbe Disease)

Terminology. Globoid cell leukodystrophy (GLD) is also commonly known as Krabbe disease. GLD is characterized by the presence of unique "globoid" cells in the demyelinating

(31-17A) Axial T2WI shows an 8y boy with X-ALD with worsening behavioral problems. There are subtle asymmetric peritrigonal hyperintensities ➲. (31-17B) Axial FLAIR image in the same patient demonstrates hyperintensities ➲.

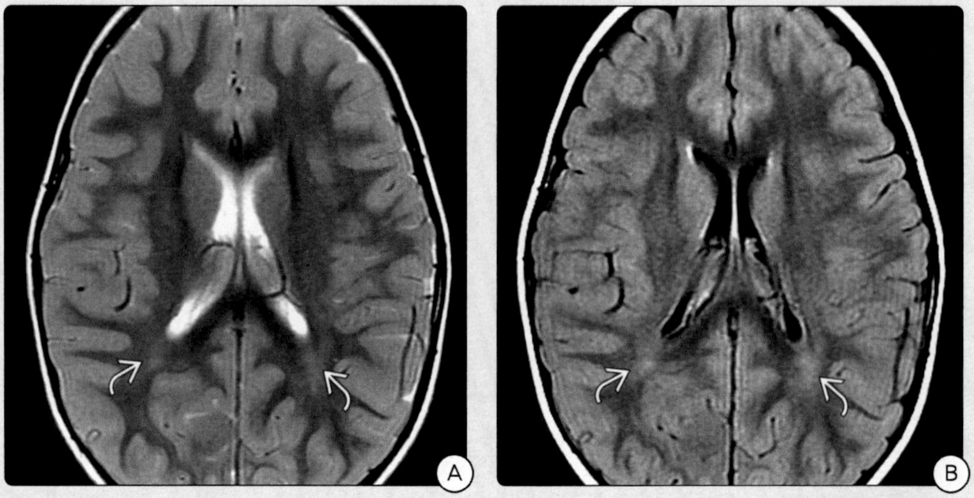

(31-17C) Axial DWI in the same patient shows very subtle qualitative diffusivity asymmetry in the peritrigonal regions ➲, showing relative diminished diffusivity. (31-17D) Axial T1WI C+ in the same patient shows "very subtle" patchy peritrigonal T1 shortening ➲ relative to other regions of peripheral WM.

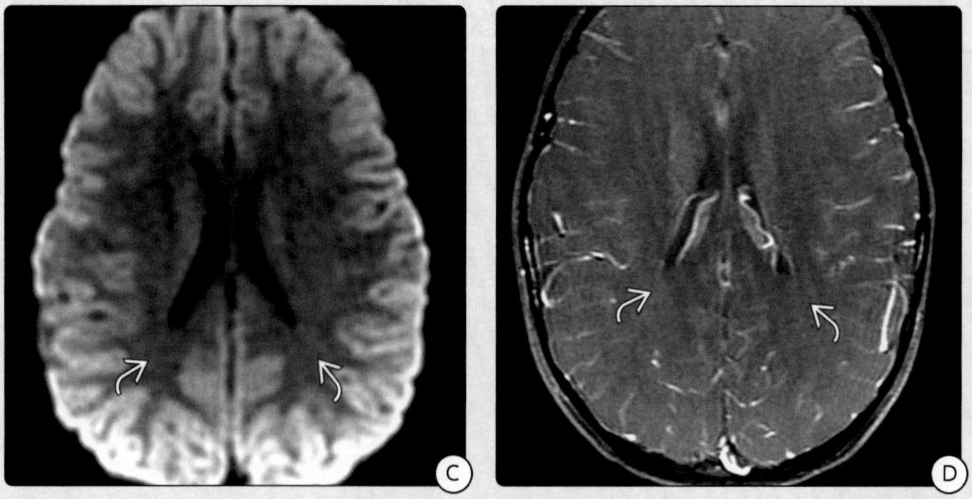

lesions. It is a progressive degenerative leukodystrophy of the CNS and peripheral nervous system.

Etiology and Pathology. GLD is an autosomal-recessive lysosomal storage disease caused by deficiency of the enzyme galactocerebroside β-galactosidase. Faulty galactose cleavage results in progressive psychosine accumulation in large ("globoid") multinucleated epithelioid cells. Psychosine (accumulations to ~ 100 times normal in Krabbe disease) is especially toxic to oligodendrocytes; the result is severe oligodendrocyte destruction with resultant demyelination. Psychosine upregulates AP-1 (a proapoptotic pathway) and downregulates NF-κB (antiapoptotic).

The brain demonstrates progressive volume loss with WM thinning, dilated ventricles, and enlarged sulci. The periventricular WM shows "grayish" discoloration. The subcortical U-fibers are typically spared. The optic and peripheral nerves can appear enlarged and fibrotic.

Typical histopathologic findings are extensive WM demyelination and gliosis with numerous conspicuous PAS-positive multinucleated macrophages ("globoid" cells). Electron microscopy shows dense crystalloid inclusions of galactocerebroside.

GLOBOID CELL LEUKODYSTROPHY (KRABBE DISEASE)

Etiology and Pathology
- Lysosomal storage disease
- Galactocerebroside β-galactosidase deficiency
- Psychosine accumulation in "globoid" cells
- Highly toxic to oligodendrocytes

Clinical Issues
- Female (80%)
- Three forms
  - Infantile (majority)
  - Juvenile
  - Adult (rare)

Imaging
- NECT: basal ganglia, thalamic Ca++
- MR
  - Periventricular WM, corticospinal hyperintensity
  - Subcortical U-fibers spared
  - Alternating "halos" around dentate nuclei
  - Optic nerve/chiasm enlarged ± other cranial nerves

Differential Diagnosis
- Other disorders with periventricular WM predominance
  - Metachromatic leukodystrophy
  - Vanishing WM disease
- Other lysosomal storage diseases
  - Neuronal ceroid lipofuscinosis
  - GM2 gangliosidosis

Genetics. GLD is an an autosomal-recessive lysosomal disorder. Gene mapping to Ch 14 (14q24.3 to 14q32.1) is needed to confirm the diagnosis.

Clinical Issues. GLD is a panethnic disease with an 80% female prevalence. Infantile, juvenile, and adult forms are recognized. The infantile form is the most common, typically presenting between 3 and 6 months with extreme irritability and feeding difficulties. Neonatal GLD is rapidly progressive and almost invariably fatal.

Hematopoietic stem cell transplantation halts progression in mild cases. Clinical and imaging manifestations may mitigate or reverse the disease.

Imaging

NECT Findings. Scans can be helpful in the diagnosis of GLD, unlike most other leukodystrophies. Bilaterally symmetric increased attenuation (i.e., globoid accumulation + calcification) in the thalami, basal ganglia, internal capsule, corticospinal tracts, and dentate nuclei of the cerebellum can sometimes be identified even prior to the development of visible abnormalities on standard MR sequences. Deep periventricular hypoattenuation is seen, and atrophy becomes apparent as CNS degeneration progresses.

MR Findings. Classic MR findings in GLD are corticospinal tract hyperintensity on T2/FLAIR with confluent symmetric demyelination in the deep periventricular WM. The subcortical U-fibers are typically spared. Bithalamic hypointensity on T2WI is common. The presence of globoid and Ca++ accumulation in the thalami and basal ganglia may lead to T1 shortening or hyperintensity.

Krabbe disease is one of the few leukodystrophies in which cerebellar findings appear early in the disease course. Alternating "halo" or ring-like hypointensities on T1WI and hyperintensities on T2WI can be identified in the cerebellar WM surrounding the dentate nuclei **(31-19)**.

Another distinctive feature of GLD is enlargement of the intracranial optic nerves and chiasm **(31-20C)**. Diffusely enlarged, enhancing cranial nerves and cauda equina nerve roots have also been reported in GLD.

Diffusion tensor imaging (DTI) may demonstrate reduced fractional anisotropy in the corticospinal tracts before other abnormalities appear. Relative anisotropy (RA) differences in thalami, basal ganglia, middle cerebellar peduncles, internal capsule, corpus callosum, and periventricular WM are seen. RA values can be followed after stem cell transplant (RA of untreated patients less than treated cohort).

MRS. Findings vary with age, including increased choline, myoinositol, and lactate and reduced NAA in affected areas; these are common yet nonspecific.

Differential Diagnosis. Although the histopathology of GLD is unique and virtually pathognomonic of the disease, the imaging differential diagnosis of GLD includes other leukodystrophies with periventricular WM predominance. The WM changes in **metachromatic leukodystrophy** and **vanishing white matter disease** may initially appear quite similar, but these disorders lack the basal ganglia/thalamic deposits typical of GLD.

Other lysosomal storage disorders that can mimic GLD include neuronal ceroid lipofuscinosis and the GM2 gangliosidoses. **Neuronal ceroid lipofuscinosis** (i.e., Batten disease) can have

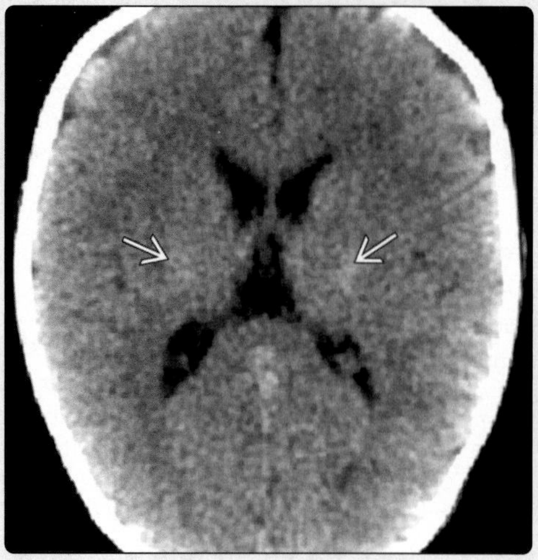

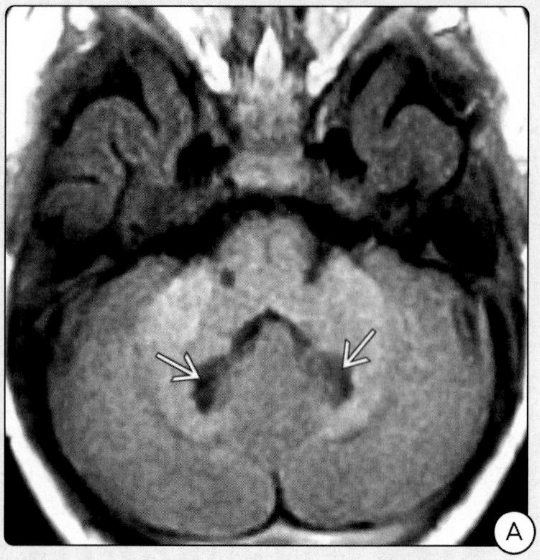

(31-18) *Axial NECT in an 18m girl with infantile GLD (Krabbe disease) shows symmetric hyperattenuation in both thalami ➡.* ***(31-19A)*** *Axial T1WI in a 6m infant with GLD shows striking hypointensity in the dentate nuclei ➡.*

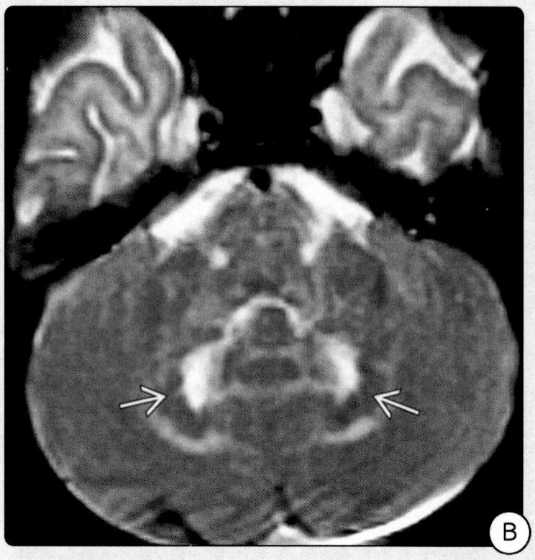

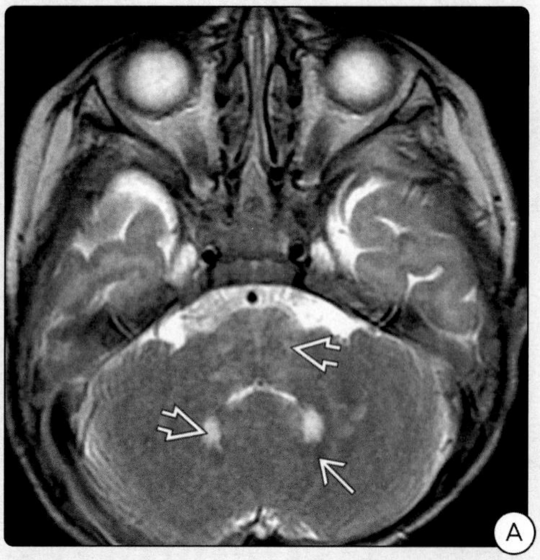

(31-19B) *Axial T2WI in the same patient shows "halos" of alternating hyper-/hypointensities ➡ characteristic of Krabbe disease (GLD).* ***(31-20A)*** *Axial T2WI of 4y boy with Krabbe disease shows patchy central cerebellar and brainstem hyper- ➡ and hypointensities ➡.*

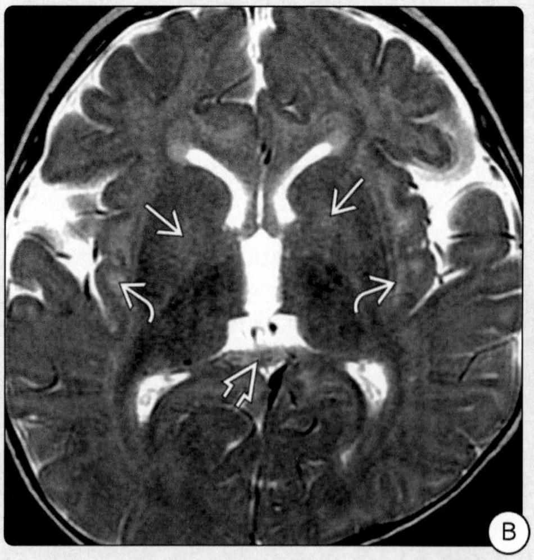

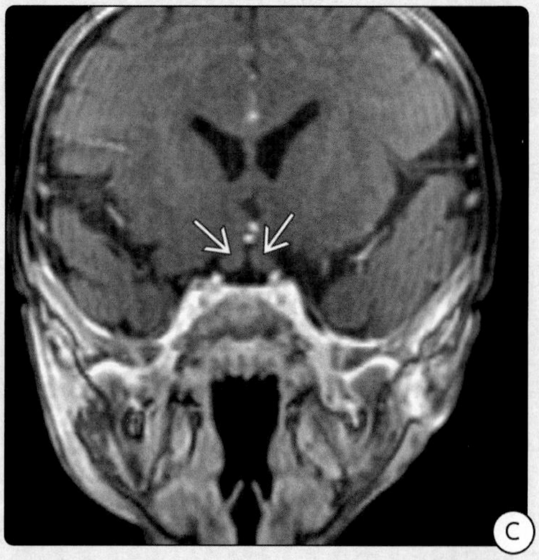

(31-20B) *Axial T2WI in the same patient shows T2 hyperintensity in GP ➡, splenium ➡, and subinsular WM ➡.* ***(31-20C)*** *Coronal T1WI C+ in the same GLD patient shows nonenhancing large optic nerves ➡, characteristic of Krabbe disease.*

hyperattenuating thalami on NECT. "Classic" infantile **GM2 gangliosidosis** (i.e., Tay-Sachs disease) shows similar thalamic hypointensity on T2WI. Late-onset GM2 shows progressive cerebellar atrophy. **NF1** demonstrates optic nerve enlargement in 15% of patients (i.e., optic nerve glioma) and shows characteristic T2WI/FLAIR hyperintensities in zones of myelin vacuolization or focal areas of signal intensity (FASI). Distinctive cutaneous phenotypic features are present.

Vanishing White Matter Disease

Terminology. Vanishing white matter disease (VWMD) has become recognized as one of the most prevalent inherited leukoencephalopathies. VWMD, formerly termed childhood ataxia with CNS hypomyelination, is an unusual leukoencephalopathy characterized by diffusely abnormal cerebral WM that literally "vanishes" over time. Cree leukoencephalopathy (i.e., a rare and severely progressive form of VWMD)—once considered a separate entity—is now considered an early-onset, especially severe form of VWMD. Other terms for VWMD that have been used include vanishing WM leukodystrophy and ovarian failure.

Etiology

Genetics. VWMD is an autosomal-recessive disorder caused by point mutation of genes responsible for encoding any of the five subunits of the eukaryotic translation inhibiting factor 2B (*EIF2B*). Mutation plays an essential role in the faulty initiation of mRNA translation to protein, particularly following exposure to physiologic stressors (e.g., heat, trauma, infection). This results in deficient protein recycling and intracellular accumulation of denatured proteins. This represents a fatal disorder.

Pathology. VWMD is also previously described as an orthochromatic sudanophilic leukodystrophy. This slowly progressive eventually cavitating WM disease involves the deep frontoparietal regions most severely affected with lesser involvement of the temporal lobes **(31-21)**. The basal ganglia, corpus callosum, anterior commissure, and internal capsules are characteristically spared. The gross appearance of the affected WM varies from grayish gelatinous discoloration to areas of cystic degeneration with frank cavitation. The cortex appears spared.

VWMD predominantly affects oligodendrocytes and astrocytes with relative sparing of neurons. Microscopic findings include myelin pallor, thinned myelin sheaths, vacuolation, a limited number of reactive astrocytes with atypical features, and cystic changes. There is no inflammatory component of the leukodystrophy. Paradoxical increase in oligodendrocytes can be seen in some areas with marked loss in others. The cerebellar WM is usually affected, and atrophy evolves. The cortex and gray matter structures appear normal. At autopsy, a cystic leukoencephalopathy is observed with both axons and myelin sheaths absent.

Clinical Issues. Classic VWMD presents in children 2-5 years of age. Development is initially normal, but progressive motor and cognitive impairment with cerebellar and pyramidal signs follows. Episodic deterioration is often associated with systemic illness, trauma, or emotional stress. Progression is typically slow. Death by adolescence is typical.

Cree leukoencephalopathy is an especially severe, rapidly progressive form of VWMD that affects infants between the ages of 3 and 9 months and is invariably fatal by 21 months of age **(31-22)**.

Approximately 15% of VWMD cases occur in adolescents and adults. Mean age of late-onset VWMD is 30 years. Learning disabilities with insidious, protracted cognitive impairment are typical. Stress-induced rapid neurologic deterioration with death is common.

Imaging

NECT Findings. Involved areas exhibit hypoattenuation. Calcifications are not typical. Eventually profound WM volume loss is seen.

MR Findings. Extensive confluent WM T1 hypointensity with T2/FLAIR hyperintensity is typical. The disease is initially periventricular but later spreads to involve the subcortical arcuate fibers. Over time, the affected WM undergoes rarefaction. Cavitary foci of CSF-like signal intensity develop **(31-21)**. Diffuse volume loss with enlarged ventricles and sulci is seen on serial studies. VWMD does not enhance.

DWI/DTI. Early reduced diffusivity in normal-appearing WM reflects brain degeneration. Anisotropy progressively decreases as disease progresses.

MRS. In time, reduced NAA, Cho, and Cr with normal myoinositol are seen on MRS and reflect early WM degeneration without reactive gliosis. Lactate may be present as disease progresses.

Differential Diagnosis. VWMD is not the only leukoencephalopathy that causes "melting away" or "vanishing" of the cerebral WM. Alexander disease and mitochondrial encephalopathies can be associated with WM rarefaction and cystic degeneration. **Alexander disease** presents with macrocephaly and is not associated with the episodic neurologic deterioration characteristic of VWMD; it demonstrates a frontoparietal gradient of disease. Frontal WM cysts can occur in end-stage disease. Approximately 10% of **mitochondrial encephalopathies** predominantly affect the WM and may form cavitations.

Globoid cell leukodystrophy (or **Krabbe disease**) may resemble severe VWMD clinically, but the imaging findings of basal ganglia/thalamic globoid material and calcifications and cerebellar "halos" help distinguish GLD from VWMD.

Phenylketonuria

Phenylketonuria (PKU) is the most common inborn error of amino acid metabolism, caused by mutations in the phenylalanine (Phe) hydroxylase (*PAH*) gene, which is mapped to chromosome 12q24.1. Elevated levels of Phe are toxic to the developing brain.

Neonates are often asymptomatic. Fair skin and blue eyes (reflecting difficulty in forming melanin) are common

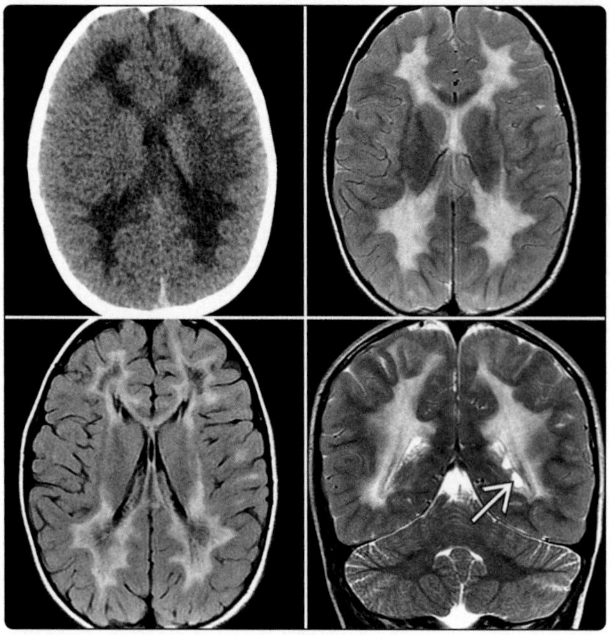

(31-21) Images show vanishing white matter disease in a 5y boy, originally diagnosed with MLD. Note the symmetric periventricular disease, spared U-fibers, and early cyst formation ➡. (Courtesy S. Harder, MD.)

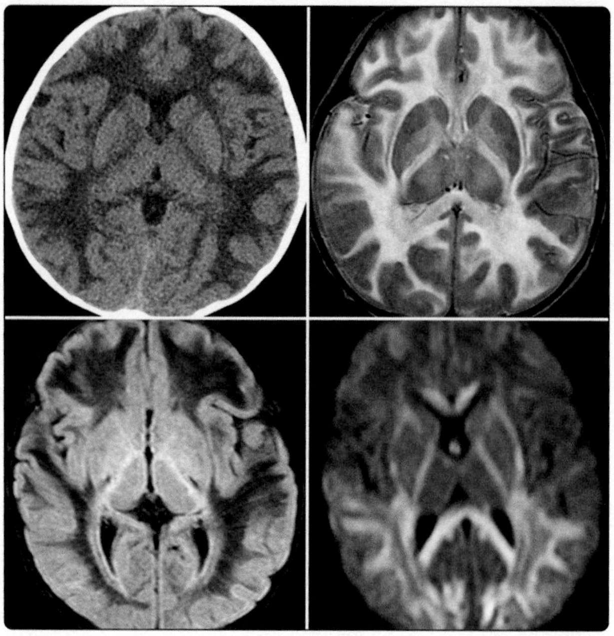

(31-22) Cree leukoencephalopathy (now recognized as a severe variant of vanishing white matter disease) in an 8m infant shows nearly complete lack of myelination.

phenotypes. Nonspecific signs and symptoms including eczema, developmental delay, seizures, and hyperactivity may herald the disease. Severe mental retardation and profound global developmental delay result if the disease remains untreated or if dietary protein restriction is not followed.

In the past, PKU was diagnosed by the presence of hyperphenylalaninemia and "musty-smelling" urine. Most PKU cases are now diagnosed through state health department-sponsored newborn metabolic disease-screening programs. With adherence to dietary protein restriction, mitigation of the ravages of this disease occurs. Early treatment is key to minimizing cognitive impairment.

Imaging. The MR in PKU can appear normal! When abnormality is detected, T2/FLAIR imaging shows hyperintensity in the periventricular WM, particularly frontal and peritrigonal regions **(31-23)** **(31-24)**. The subcortical arcuate fibers are spared. There is no enhancement following contrast administration **(31-24)**. Diffusion can be present and, when followed serially, may reflect a progression of disease or poor dietary control **(31-23)**. A *centrifugal* progression of PKU eventually leads to end-stage disease. MRS shows a Phe peak resonating at 7.37 ppm (which is missed on routine clinical MRS that only displays to 4 ppm).

Differential Diagnosis. Periventricular WM injury (PVL) (at-risk population of low birth weight, premature neonates who, when affected, eventually manifest signs and symptoms of cerebral palsy, a nonprogressive neurologic disorder), **metachromatic leukodystrophy** (demonstrating more confluent zones of deep WM T2/FLAIR hyperintensity), and **Krabbe disease** (optic and cranial nerve enlargement, thalamic hyperattenuation on NECT, MR showing T2/FLAIR hyperintensity in corticospinal tracts, deep cerebral WM, and early cerebellar involvement) are differential diagnoses for PKU.

Maple Syrup Urine Disease

Maple syrup urine disease (MSUD), also known as leucine encephalopathy, is an autosomal-recessive disorder of branched-chain amino acid (leucine, isoleucine, valine) metabolism. More than 50 different gene mutations governing enzyme components of *BCKDK* have been identified. Decreased activity of the branched chain α-keto acid dehydrogenase complex disrupts the Krebs cycle and results in elevated brain levels of leucine and other leukotoxic metabolites. In turn, these induce cytotoxic or intramyelinic edema and spongiform degeneration.

The overall prevalence is 1:850,000 live births with a greater frequency among Mennonites, people of Middle Eastern descent, and Ashkenazi Jews.

Infants with classic MSUD are initially normal. Breastfeeding delays onset of symptoms. Within days after birth, poor feeding, lethargy, vomiting, seizures, and encephalopathy may occur. In severe cases, the urine smells of maple syrup or burnt sugar. If the family history is positive for MSUD, immediate postparturition testing is necessary, and, if positive, start therapy within hours to assure excellent outcome.

Imaging. Transcranial US during the acute stage of MSUD edema shows hyperechogenicity reflecting edema within the thalami and basal ganglia, periventricular WM, brainstem, and cerebellum. In fact, unexplained cerebral hemispheric, basal ganglia, thalamic, brainstem, and cerebellar edema in the newborn should provoke a consideration of MSUD in the differential diagnosis.

NECT scans show profound hypoattenuation within the myelinated WM as well as within the dorsal brainstem, cerebellum, cerebral peduncles, and posterior limb of the internal capsule **(31-25)**.

MR shows striking T2/FLAIR hyperintensity involving the cerebellar WM, dorsal brainstem, cerebral peduncles, thalami, globi pallidi, posterior limbs of internal capsule, internal medullary lamina, and pyramidal and tegmental tracts **(31-26)**. Margins of parenchymal hyperintensity tend to become sharp during the subacute phase of disease. Imaging abnormalities are much more conspicuous infratentorially than supratentorially.

DWI/DTI shows restricted diffusion (e.g., low ADC values) in the T2/FLAIR hyperintense regions; look for *four-dot* brainstem sign **(31-26D)**!

MRS shows a peak at 0.9 ppm caused by accumulation of branched-chain α-keto amino acids **(31-26F)**. This peak is present at short (35 ms), intermediate (144 ms), and long (288 ms) PRESS MRS aquisitions, distinguishing them from the broad cytosolic amino acid peaks that only resonate at a short TE (35 ms).

Differential Diagnosis. Sepsis (brain MR expected to be normal), **Alexander disease** (T2 hyperintensity of the frontal WM and enhancement), **hypoxic ischemic injury** (with history of periparturitional distress, no significant symptom-free period), and **mitochondrial cytopathy** (episodic stroke-like clinical events of varied severity depending on the genotype of the disorder) should all be considered.

Nonketotic Hyperglycinemia

Nonketotic hyperglycinemia (NKH) is an autosomal-recessive disorder in glycine metabolism. It is the second most common inherited disorder of amino acid metabolism, PKU being first. Glycine is normally metabolized to the final end-products of ammonia and carbon dioxide. The estimated incidence is

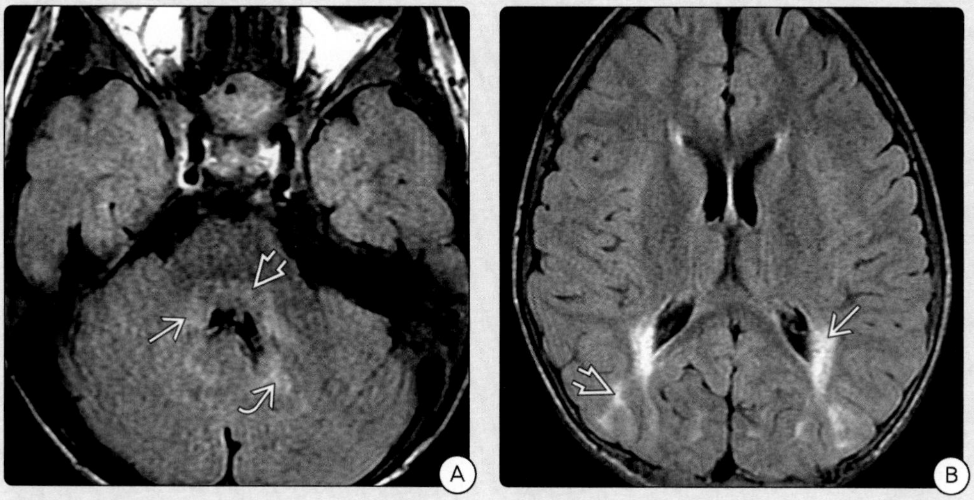

(31-23A) Axial FLAIR image in a 7y child with PKU shows patchy dorsal pontine ➡, central cerebellar ➡, and brachium pontis ➡ hyperintensities. (31-23B) Axial FLAIR image in the same patient shows confluent peritrigonal ➡ and subcortical ➡ hyperintensities.

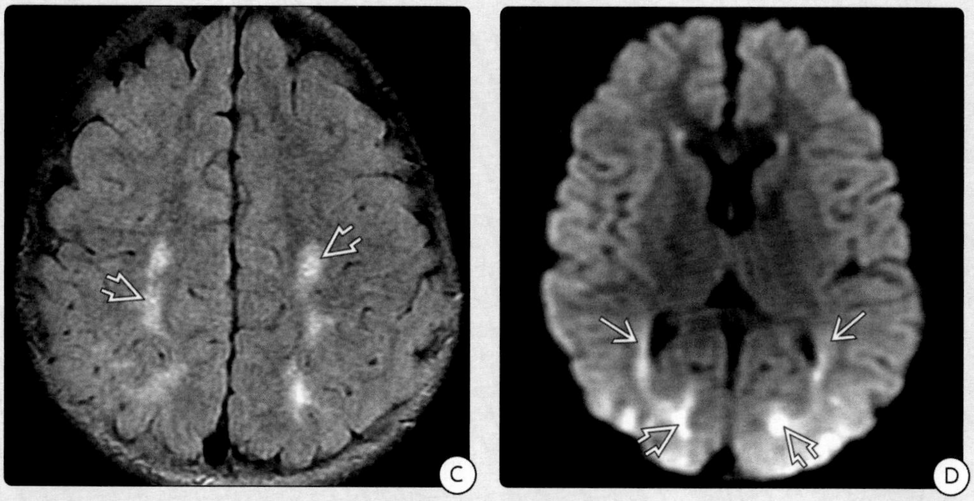

(31-23C) Axial FLAIR image through the convexities shows bilateral subcortical hyperintensities ➡ (WM vacuolization). (31-23D) Axial DWI in the same patient shows peritrigonal ➡ and parietal occipital ➡ WM diffusion hyperintensities, confirmed on ADC maps to represent "true" diffusion restriction.

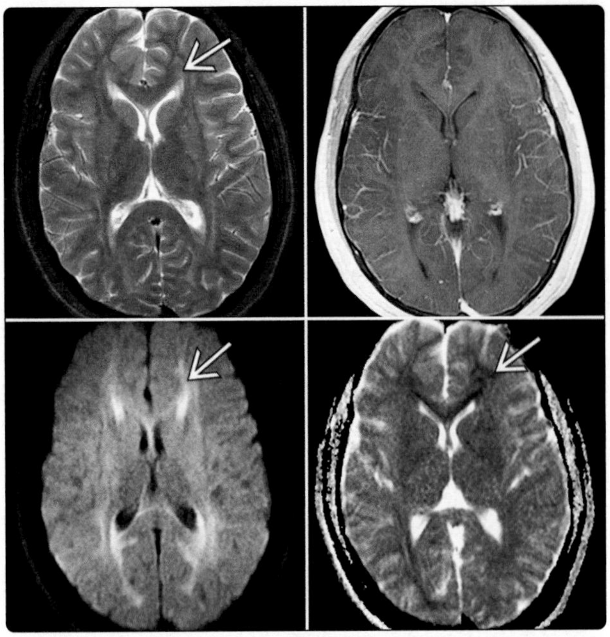

(31-24) Axial MRs show a 13y girl with PKU and mild cognitive impairment. Findings are subtle with periventricular WM hyperintensity ➡ (top L) showing no enhancement (top R) and restricting on DWI (bottom L and R).

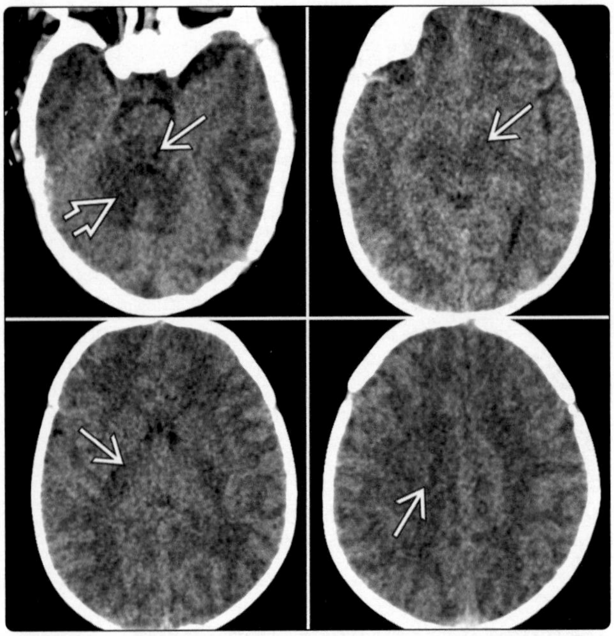

(31-25) Axial NECT in a 13d boy with MSUD shows edema (low attenuation) ➡ in the dorsal midbrain and central cerebellar WM ⇨, cerebral peduncles (upper R), internal capsules (lower L), and centrum semiovale.

1:60,000 live births. Eighty percent of affected newborns exhibit mutation of the *GLDC* gene, and 10% exhibit mutation of the *AMT* gene.

The affected newborn with NKH presents with lethargy, hypotonia, apnea, seizures, and often myoclonic jerks. When the diagnosis of NKH has been made, the oral administration of sodium benzoate has been shown to lower plasma levels of glycine although the CSF levels remain high. Such treatment may mitigate the severity of neurologic deterioration.

Imaging. Restricted diffusion and T2/FLAIR hyperintensity within the corticospinal tracts and flocculus of the cerebellum are common. One may appreciate a lack of expected normal myelin signal in the PLIC (T1WI hyper- and T2WI hypointensity) **(31-27A)**. Importantly, in the neonate with NKH, who presents with seizure, the initial MR may appear normal. MRS with glycine peak at 3.55 ppm on short and long TE proton spectroscopy **(31-27)** is characteristic. Normal myoinositol resonance at 3.6 ppm is detected on short, not long, TE MRS acquisitions **(31-27C)**. The initial MR may appear completely normal; thus, adjunctive MRS in the evaluation of newborn seizures is critical.

Differential Diagnosis. Hypoxic ischemic injury has a relevant health history and characteristic striatal, thalamic, and corticospinal tract involvement.

Hyperhomocysteinemia

Hyperhomocysteinemia (HHcy)—formerly known as homocystinuria—is a heterogeneous group of IMDs exhibiting autosomal-recessive inheritance that affects methionine metabolism, resulting in elevated plasma homocysteine.

HHcy patients are normal at birth but develop multisystem abnormalities involving the eye, skeleton, spinal dural dysplasia, vascular system, and CNS. Upward dislocation of the lens develops early and affects the majority of patients. Osteoporosis and kyphoscoliosis are common. Endothelial damage and hypercoagulability result in a high incidence of both arterial and venous occlusions, which occur at all ages.

Imaging. The major imaging manifestations of HHcy in the brain are vascular. Stenoocclusive disease in both the arterial and venous systems is typical. Microangiopathy from premature atherosclerosis, thrombolic arterial strokes, lacunar infarcts, sinovenous occlusion, and generalized volume loss are common. An increased number of T2/FLAIR WM hyperintensities is seen in patients with even mildly elevated plasma homocysteine levels **(31-28)**.

Differential Diagnosis. Mitochondrial disorders (episodic stroke events, lack of systemic HHcy phenotype) and **moyamoya disease** (obliterative vasculopathy in circle of Willis and other manifestations, like NF1) should be considered.

Congenital Muscular Dystrophy

The congenital muscular dystrophies (CMDs) have varied clinical manifestations. They are a heterogeneous group of myopathies of broad phenotypes and genotypes. They are autosomal-recessively inherited. Some infants and children present with hypotonia (i.e., *floppy newborn*) and muscle weakness without CNS symptoms. Others present with developmental delay, seizures, and blindness. Their MRs often show WM T2/FLAIR hyperintensities (e.g., *watery WM*). See Chapter 37 for discussion of CMDs and *cobblestone* abnormalities.

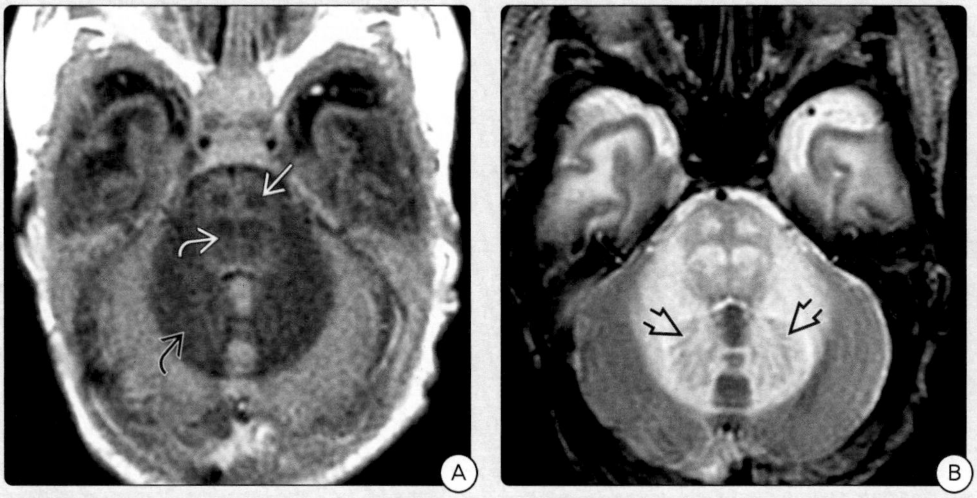

(31-26A) Axial T1WI shows an infant with MSUD who was normal at birth but developed seizures at 28 days. T1 hypointensity in the cerebellar WM, dorsal pons, and paired pyramidal/tegmental tracts is seen. **(31-26B)** Axial T2WI in the same patient shows well-delineated hyperintensity in the swollen cerebellar WM and pontine tracts with sparing of the dentate nuclei gray matter.

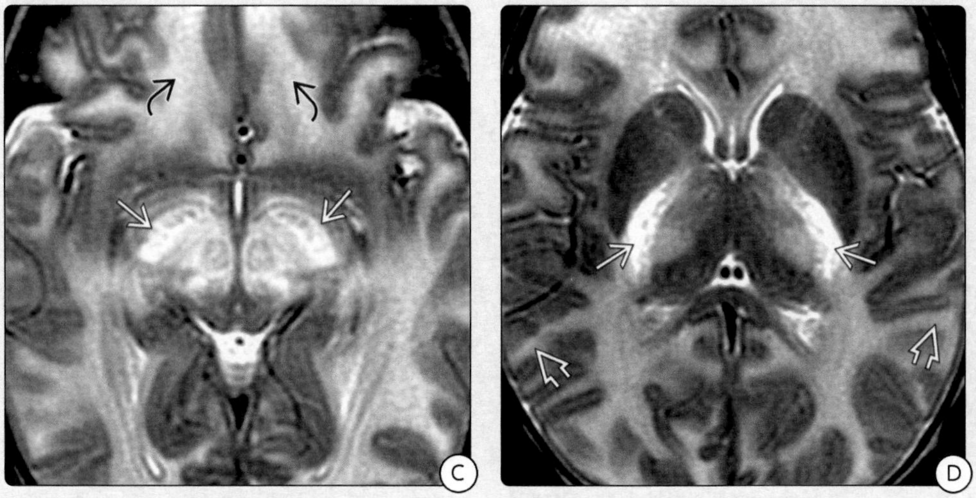

(31-26C) Axial T2WI in MSUD demonstrates striking midbrain edema extending into the cerebral peduncles. Note the relatively normal signal intensity of the unmyelinated cerebral hemispheric WM. **(31-26D)** Axial T2WI shows MSUD hyperintense edema in the myelinated posterior limbs of the internal capsules clearly and easily differentiated from the less hyperintense normal unmyelinated hemispheric WM.

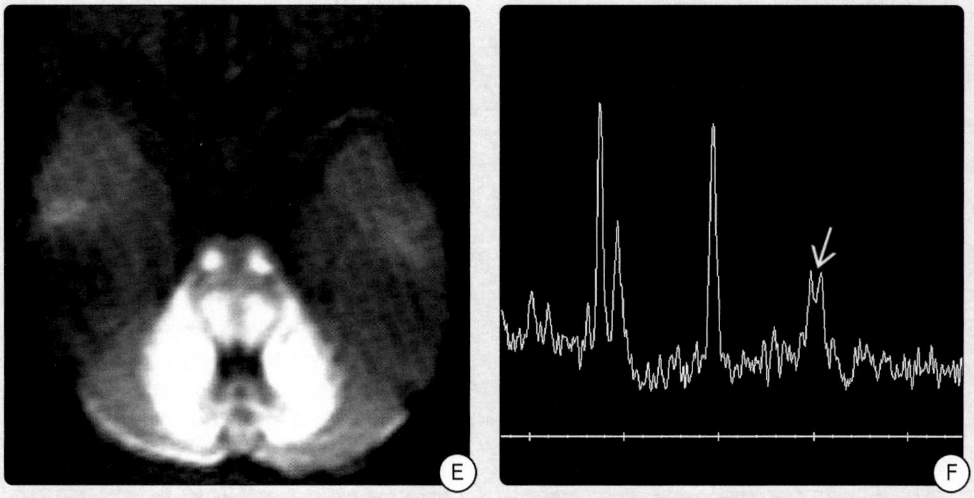

(31-26E) Axial DWI shows striking diffusion hyperintensity in the cerebellar WM and the segmental and pyramidal tracts. ADC maps confirmed true diffusion restriction. **(31-26F)** MRS at TE of 144 ms shows a peak at 0.9-1.0 ppm, representing branched chain a-keto acids, typically seen during acute metabolic decompensation in MSUD. At this TE, a lactate doublet would invert (J-coupling) at 1.33 ppm.

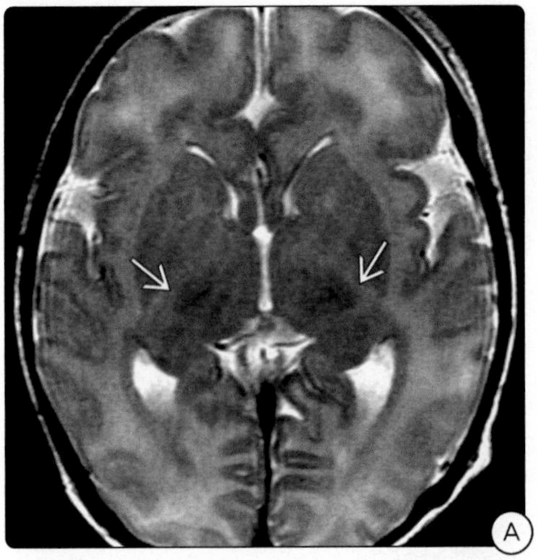

(31-27A) Axial T2WI shows a term newborn with nonketotic hyperglycinemia, seizures. Note lack of expected myelin hypointensity in the PLICs ➡.

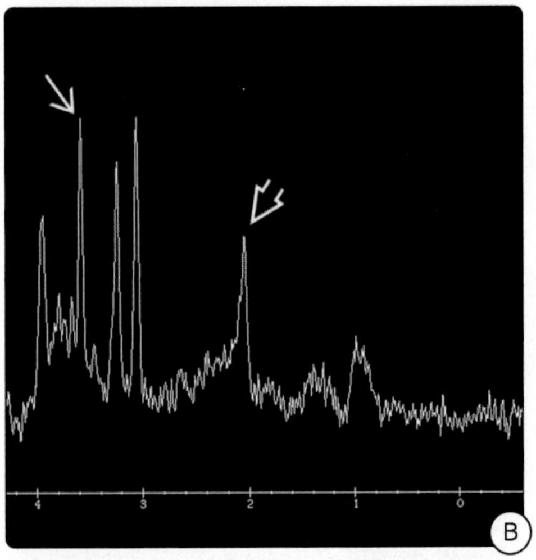

(31-27B) MRS short TE (35 ms) shows glycine peak at 3.55 ppm ➡. There is diminished NAA ➡. Glycine is not a normal MRS resonance!

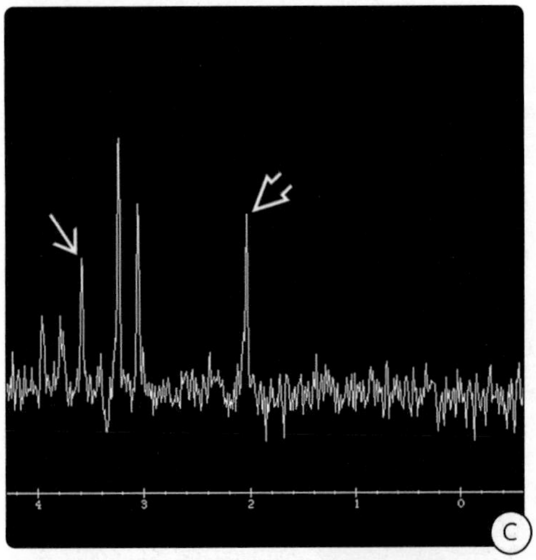

(31-27C) MRS long TE (288 ms) shows glycine peak (3.55 ppm) ➡, ↓ NAA ➡. Normal myoinositol (3.6 ppm) won't resonate at long TEs.

Most of the CMDs characterized by abnormal myelination are merosin-deficient CMDs. Muscle biopsy shows dystrophic changes with negative expression of merosin (laminin α2).

Imaging. These patients are usually hypotonic at birth ("floppy infant") and exhibit severely delayed motor milestones. MR shows diffuse confluent T2/FLAIR hyperintensity in the periventricular WM. The corpus callosum, internal capsule, and subcortical U-fibers are typically spared **(31-29)**.

Differential Diagnosis. States of hypomyelination (i.e., 4H, PMD in which myelination never progresses vs. CMD, with progressive neurologic decline), **MLD** (central cerebral hemispheric butterfly pattern of WM hyperintensity and *tigroid pattern* on T2/FLAIR), and **VWMD** (begins in the periventricular WM, relentlessly progresses, and may cavitate) should be considered.

Subcortical White Matter Predominance

IMDs that initially or predominantly affect the subcortical WM are much less common than those that begin with deep periventricular involvement. The most striking IMD with preferential involvement of the subcortical WM is megaloencephalic leukoencephaly with subcortical cysts (MLC), formally known as van der Knapp disease or van der Knapp leukoencephalopathy.

Megaloencephalic Leukodystrophy With Subcortical Cysts

Terminology. MLC is also known as vacuolating megaloencephalic leukoencephalopathy, formally called van der Knaap disease or vacuolating megaloencephalic leukoencephalopathy with benign slowly progressive course. MLC is a rare autosomal-recessive disorder with characteristic MR features and a variable but mild clinical course.

Etiology. MLC is a genetically heterogeneous disorder. Approximately 75% of cases are caused by mutations in the *MLC1* gene located on Chr. 22q(tel). MLC1 is an oligomeric membrane protein located in astrocyte-astrocyte junctions. A newly described mutation in the *HEPACAM* gene that encodes for the GlialCAM protein, an IgG-like hepatic and glial cell adhesion molecule, may account for the remaining cases. Both defects lead to abnormal cell junction trafficking with associated disturbed water homeostasis and osmotic balance and functional disturbance in volume-regulated anion channels (i.e., impaired osmoregulation). Patients with *HEPACAM* mutations develop a spectrum of abnormalities ranging from benign familial macrocephaly to MLC that is indistinguishable from that caused by *MLC1* mutation.

Pathology. Gross pathology shows a swollen cerebral hemispheric WM, relative occipital sparing, variable involvement of the subcortical arcuate fibers, frequent involvement of the external capsules, and sparing of the internal capsules with multiple variably sized subcortical cysts often initially involving the temporal lobes **(31-31)** **(31-32)**. The basal ganglia are spared. In the few reported cases of MLC with histopathology, extensive vacuolation is seen in the outer layers of myelin sheaths, accounting for the characteristic swollen appearance of the WM on MR.

Clinical Issues. MLC is distinguished clinically from other leukoencephalopathies by its remarkably slow course of neurologic deterioration. Infantile-onset macrocephaly is characteristic, but neurologic deterioration is often delayed. Age at symptom onset varies widely, ranging from birth to 25 years; median age of onset of prominent clinical symptoms is 6 months.

Pyramidal and cerebellar signs are common. Therefore, early motor developmental delay, gait ataxia, and hypotonia may be observed.

Eventually, progression to spastic tetraparesis occurs. Seizures are variable. Intellectual skills are typically preserved early in the disease, but slow cognitive decline is observed as the disease progresses. Although the geographical distribution of MLC is global, increased population isolates of MLC have been reported among Libyan Jewish, Turkish, and Agrawal Indian communities.

Imaging. Cranial US in symptomatic infants shows unexplained hyperechogenicity of affected WM. NECT will demonstrate hypoattenuation of the cerebral hemispheric WM.

The diagnosis of MLC is typically established by MR. Commonly, the magnitude of MR abnormalities appears much worse than the clinical appearance of the child. Macrocephaly with diffuse confluent WM T2/FLAIR hyperintensity in the subcortical WM is typical. The affected subcortical WM appears "watery" and swollen. The overlying gyri seemingly stretch over the swollen WM. The optic radiations, occipital subcortical WM, and basal ganglia are typically spared. The corpus callosum and internal capsule are usually normal. Variable involvement of the cerebellar WM is generally normal or only mildly affected. Characteristic CSF-like subcortical cysts develop in the anterior temporal lobes followed in frequency by fronto-parietal cysts. Unlike the "watery" WM, which exhibits T2/FLAIR hyperintensity, the cysts approximate the signal intensity of CSF on FLAIR. The number and size of the cysts may increase over time. The abnormal WM and cysts do not enhance on T1 C+.

On DWI/DTI, the increased water content within the interstitial spaces leads to reduced anisotropy and increased ADC values.

MRS shows mild to moderate reduced NAA and NAA:Cr ratio. Myoinositol is normal, with or without lactate. Cystic regions show reduction of all neurometabolites.

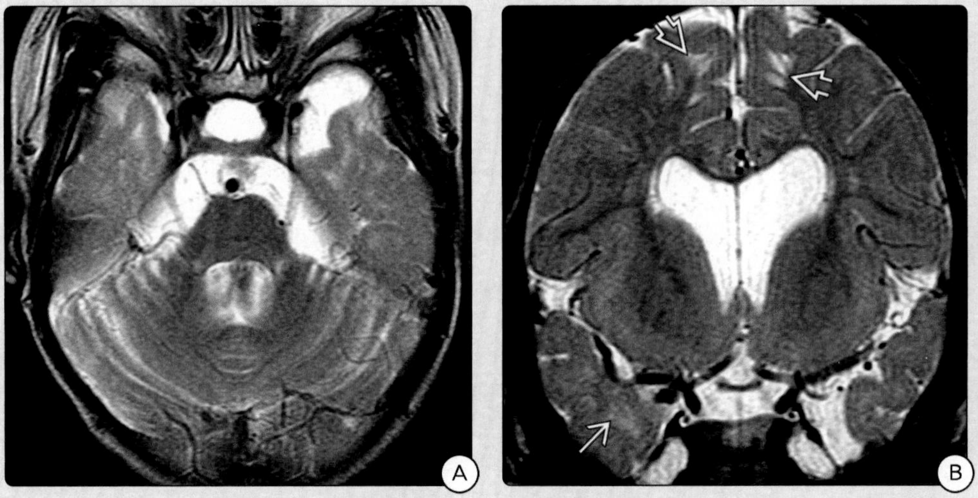

***(31-28A)** Axial T2WI in a 4y boy with hyperhomocysteinemia and a history of sinovenous occlusion as an infant shows generalized cerebellar atrophy. **(31-28B)** Coronal T2WI in the same patient shows cerebral atrophy, ventriculomegaly, patchy WM hyperintensity in the temporal lobe ➡, and frontal lobe perivascular demyelinating foci ➡.*

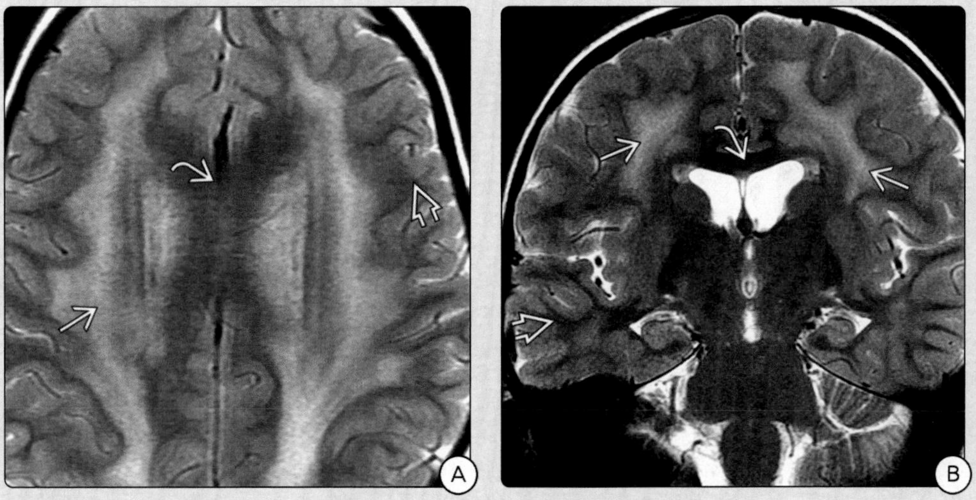

***(31-29A)** Axial T2WI in a 10y boy with merosin-deficient congenital muscular dystrophy shows confluent hyperintensity in the periventricular WM ➡. The subcortical arcuate fibers are spared ➡, as is the corpus callosum ➡. **(31-29B)** Coronal thin-section T2WI in the same patient shows the confluent hyperintensity in the deep WM ➡. The corpus callosum ➡ and subcortical WM ➡ are spared. No cortical malformations are seen.*

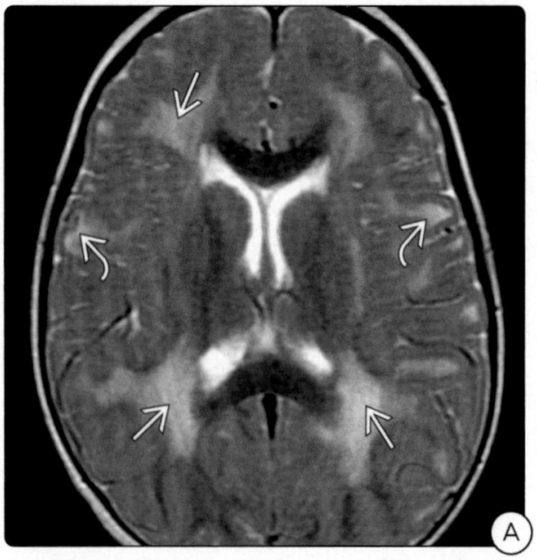

(31-30A) Axial T2WI in a 4y boy with merosin-deficient muscular dystrophy shows central ➡ and peripheral ➡ hyperintensities.

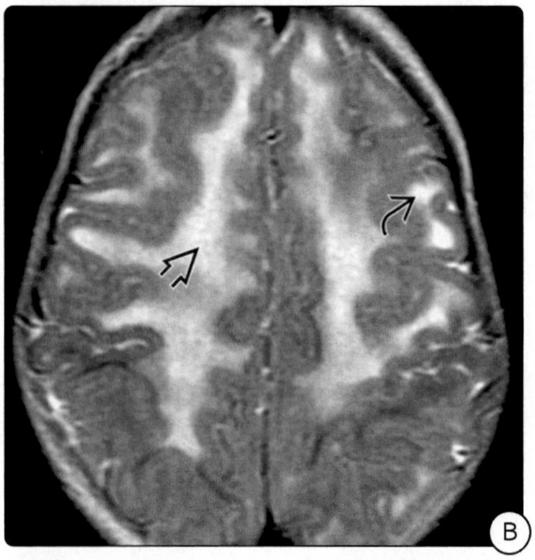

(31-30B) Axial T2WI in same patient shows confluent subcortical ➡ and centrum semiovale ➡ WM T2 hyperintensity.

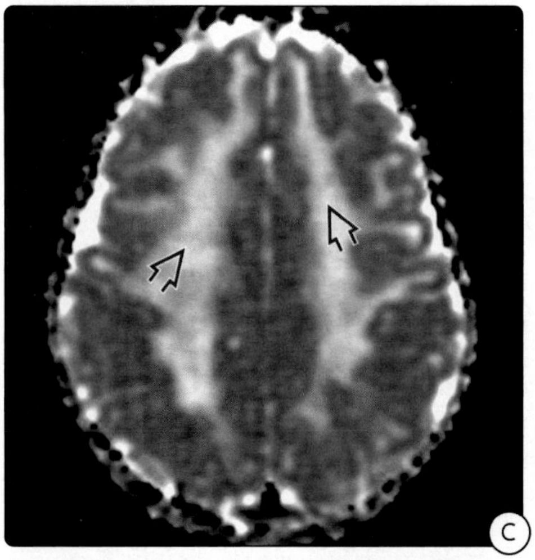

(31-30C) Axial ADC map through the cerebral convexities in the same patient shows WM increased diffusivity (ADC hyperintensity) ➡.

Differential Diagnosis. MLC must be distinguished from other IMDs with macrocrania. The two major considerations are **Canavan disease** and **Alexander disease**, both of which are characterized by much greater clinical disability.

Canavan disease almost always involves the basal ganglia, lacks the development of subcortical cysts, and demonstrates a large NAA peak on MRS. Canavan disease also shows very early involvement of the subcortical U-fibers, which may appear uninvolved in the early presentation of MLC.

Alexander disease demonstrates a *frontal* WM gradient, involves the basal ganglia, and often enhances following contrast administration.

Hypomyelinating Disorders

Hypomyelination refers to a permanent, substantial deficit in myelin deposition within the brain. *Hypomyelinating leukoencephalopathies* have been observed in the context of a number of genetic disorders that may share some clinical characteristics. These heterogeneous disorders exhibit reduced or absent myelination. *Hypomyelination* often reflects a deficiency of mature oligodendrocytes. Immature oligodendrocytes do not produce myelin; myelin is essential to axonal nourishment. Hypomyelination may be a primary hypomyelination syndrome or may be secondary to other pathologies. *Hypomyelinating* disorders differ from other WM diseases that are characterized by abnormal myelin formation (*dys*myelinating diseases) or myelin destruction (*de*myelinating diseases).

Some hypomyelinating disorders may be differentiated by their MR characteristics. These include **4H syndrome** (hypomyelination with hypogonadotropic hypogonadism and hypodontia), **Pelizaeus-Merzbacher disease** (PMD), **Pelizaeus-Merzbacher-like disease** (PMLD), **hypomyelination with atrophy of the BG and cerebellum** (HABC), **hypomyelination with congenital cataract** (HCC), and PMD-like diseases (GM1, GM2, Salla disease, and fucosidosis). These represent only a small number of hypomyelinating disorders that have been described.

HYPOMYELINATING DISORDERS

Most Common
- Hypomyelination of unknown cause
- 4H syndrome
- Pelizaeus-Merzbacher disease
- Pelizaeus-Merzbacher-like disease

Less Common
- Hypomyelination with congenital cataract
- GM2 gangliosidosis
- Salla disease (sialuria)
- Fucosidosis
- Cockayne syndrome
- GM1 gangliosidosis
- Hypomyelination with atrophy of the basal ganglia and cerebellum

Rare
- 18q-syndrome
- Cockayne syndrome
- Trichothiodystrophies (brittle, sulfur-deficient hair)

Most of the hypomyelinating leukoencephalopathies are lysosomal storage diseases. Although some have been identified and characterized, hypomyelinating disorders of unknown origin constitute the largest single category of these leukoencephalopathies.

The generally accepted imaging criterion for the diagnosis of hypomyelination is an unchanged pattern of deficient myelination on two successive MR scans obtained at least 6 months apart, with one of these MR studies being performed after 12 months of age **(31-35)**. For the interpreting radiologist, it is very helpful in the interpretation to assess and estimate the maturity pattern of myelination prior to reviewing the chronological age of the patient. Doing so will avoid predetermination bias. The most common MR finding is *mild* T2 hyperintensity in much or most of the cerebral hemispheric WM. In some cases, signal intensity on T1WI can appear deceptively normal. *Remember* to always adjust chronological age for degree of prematurity when interpreting infant brain MRs.

After hypomyelination of unknown etiology, the next most commonly diagnosed inherited hypomyelinating disorder is **4H syndrome**. The best-known hypomyelination syndrome is **Pelizaeus-Merzbacher disease**. 4H syndrome, PMD, and spastic paraplegia type 2 (SPG2) are caused by a mutation in the gene that encodes myelin proteolipid protein 1 (*PLP1*). 18q-syndrome (another hypomyelinating disorder) causes a hemizygous deletion (one copy of gene missing) of the *MBP* gene. Some experts consider PMD and 18q-syndrome to represent the prototypes of hypomyelination.

4H Syndrome

The diagnosis of 4H syndrome is based on the combination of hypomyelination on MR, hypogonadotropic hypogonadism, and hypodontia. The hypomyelination in 4H syndrome is distinctive. T2 *hypo*intensity of the optic radiations, pyramidal tracts in the posterior limb of the internal capsule, and anterolateral thalami together with cerebellar atrophy and mild cerebellar WM hyperintensity are characteristic **(31-34)**.

Pelizaeus-Merzbacher Disease

Terminology and Etiology. PMD is an X-linked disorder that results in nearly complete lack of myelination. Some (10-30%) of PMD patients exhibit defects in the *PLP1* gene located at Xq21-q22. The PMD brain looks like a *much less mature brain* than expected for the patient's chronological age.

PMD is a hypomyelinating disorder caused by variations in *PLP1*. Two forms of PMD are recognized: type 1 (classic) and type 2 (connatal). Classic PMD is an X-linked recessive disorder, whereas patients with the connatal form show either autosomal or X-linked recessive inheritance.

Most patients with PMD have homogeneous hyperintensity of the entire cerebral WM. The hyperintense WM in PMD is more *muted* than the striking T2 prolongation (hyperintensity) of the WM in demyelinating disorders. Cerebellar atrophy is common in PMD and *very* common in 4H syndrome.

Pathology. With advanced disease, the brain appears atrophic with normal cortex and shrunken, grayish, or gelatinous-appearing WM. Both the central and subcortical WM are affected. The cerebellar WM, brainstem, and spinal cord are also shrunken and gray. The optic nerves (which are brain tracts) are usually involved, but other cranial nerves (which are ensheathed with a different myelin protein called PMP 22) are normally myelinated.

Histopathology shows markedly reduced or absent oligodendrocytes with variable myelin staining. Cases of connatal PMD show almost complete lack of myelin staining, whereas more slowly progressive cases demonstrate preservation of myelin islets around blood vessels in a classic "tiger" or discontinuous pattern. Absent or deficient myelin sheaths contribute to what the pathologist describes as redundant myelin balls.

Clinical Issues. Although it is one of the most common hypomyelinating disorders, PMD causes only 5-7% of all the inherited leukodystrophies.

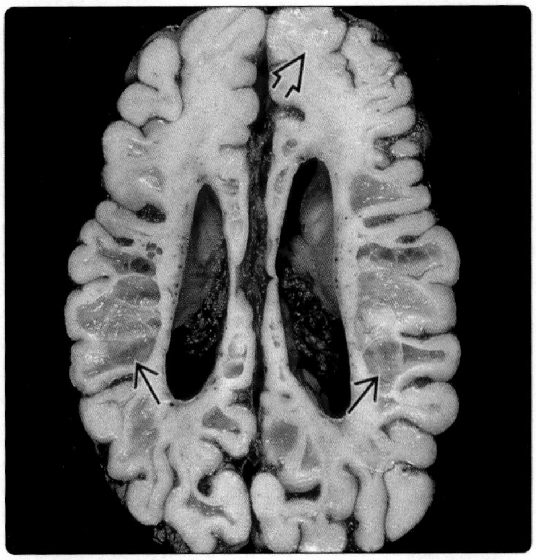

***(31-31)** MLC autopsy shows multiple subcortical cysts and WM rarefaction in frontal subcortical WM. (Courtesy R. Hewlett, MD.)*

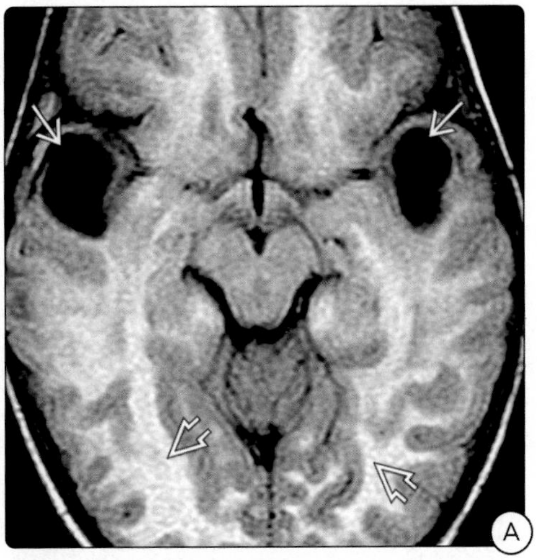

***(31-32A)** Axial FLAIR in a 22m child with MLC shows swollen, hyperintense, "watery" WM and CSF-like temporal subcortical cysts.*

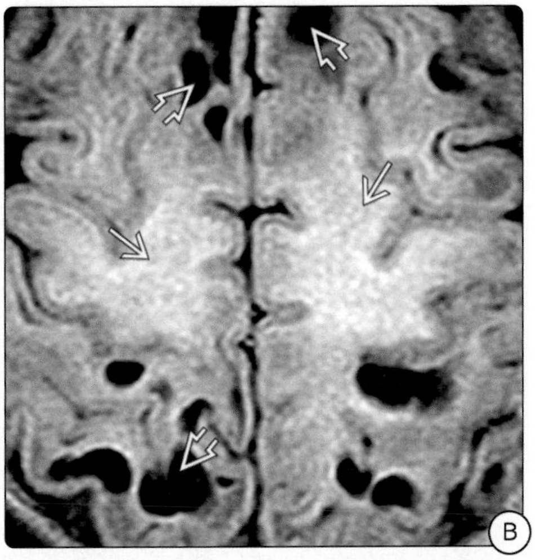

***(31-32B)** Axial FLAIR scan in a 2y child with MLC shows swollen, hyperintense subcortical WM. Note fluid-filled subcortical hypointense cysts.*

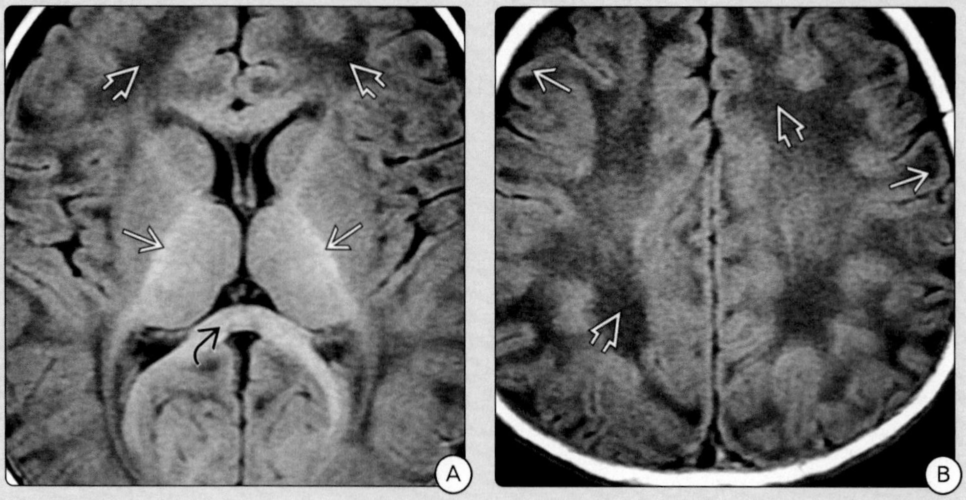

(31-33A) *Axial T1WI of a 6m boy with macrocephaly shows early findings of MLC. Normal myelination in the corpus callosum ➡ and internal capsules ➡ is seen, but the hemispheric WM is very hypointense and immature for age ➡.* ***(31-33B)*** *Axial T1WI in the same patient through the upper corona radiata shows striking lack of myelination ➡. Some of the gyri appear swollen ➡ although no frank subcortical cysts are yet identified.*

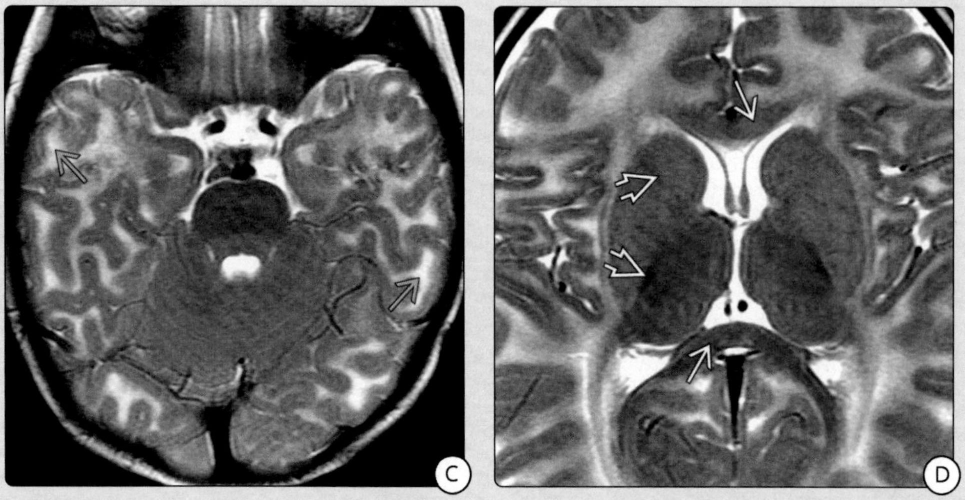

(31-33C) *Axial T2WI in the same patient shows hyperintensity throughout the WM of both temporal lobes, including the subcortical U-fibers ➡. The overlying cortex appears normal.* ***(31-33D)*** *Axial T2WI in the same patient shows normal for age myelination in the corpus callosum ➡ and delayed myelination of the internal capsules ➡. The remainder of the hemispheric WM appears abnormally "watery" and hyperintense.*

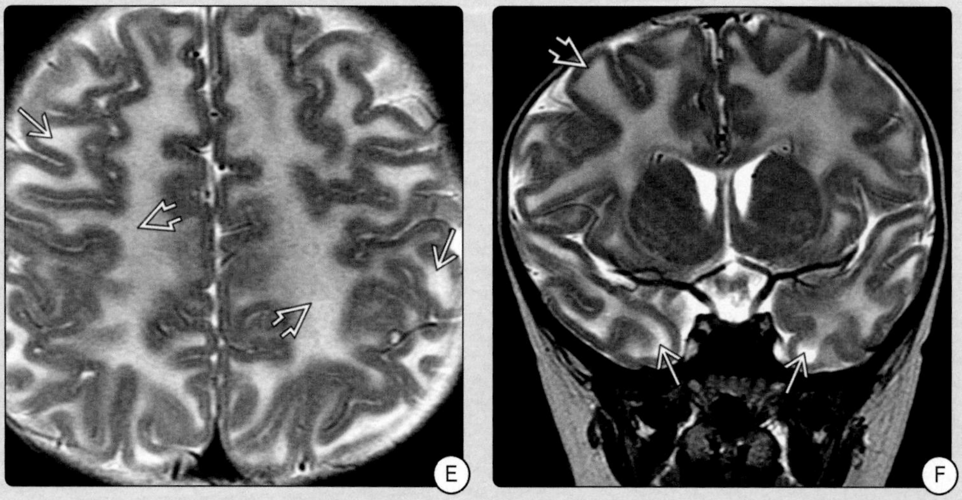

(31-33E) *Axial T2WI through the centrum semiovale in the same patient shows the subcortical WM ➡ to be more hyperintense than the central WM ➡, possibly indicating early cystic degeneration.* ***(31-33F)*** *Coronal T2WI shows the most hyperintense WM to be the medial temporal lobes ➡ compared with the swollen convexity gyri ➡. This probably represents the earliest development of the characteristic cysts seen in MLC.*

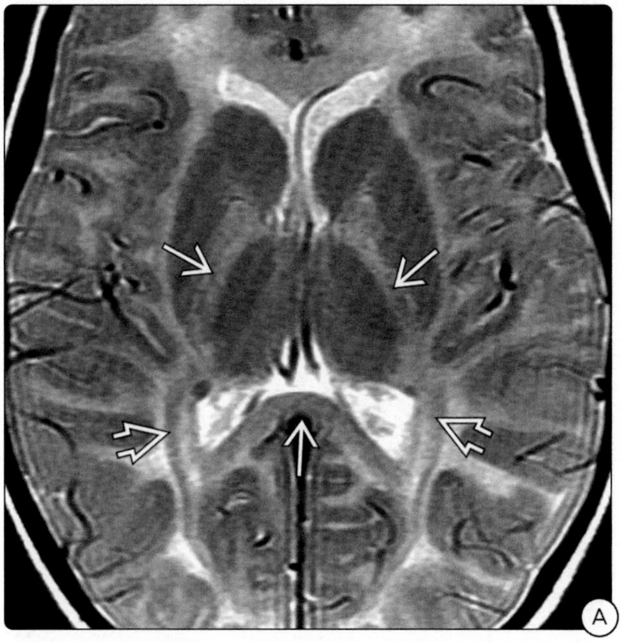

(31-34A) Axial T2WI in a 3y girl with 4H syndrome shows that most of the hemispheric WM is hyperintense. The T2 hypointensity in the optic tracts ➡ and posterior limb of the internal capsules ➡ are characteristic.

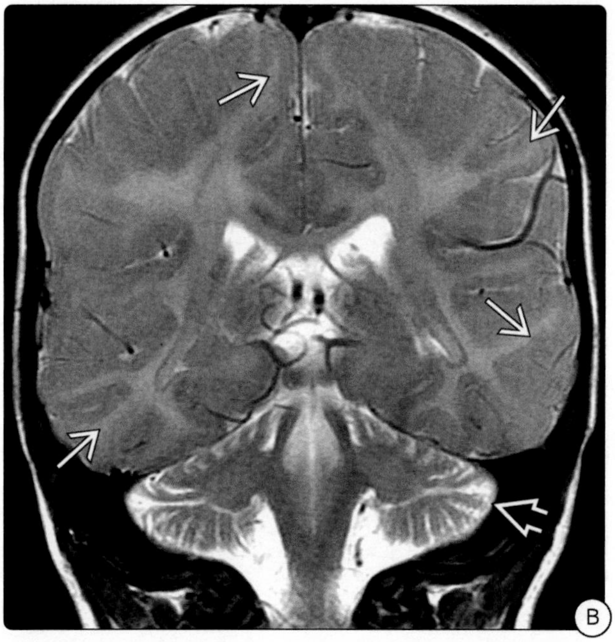

(31-34B) Coronal T2WI in the same patient shows that the absent myelination also involves the subcortical U-fibers ➡. The striking early cerebellar atrophy ➡ is characteristic of 4H syndrome.

Nearly 100% of classic PMD cases occur in male patients. Connatal PMD can affect either sex.

Mean age at diagnosis is helpful when interpreting MR studies and ordering the DDx in hypomyelinating disorders. PMD exhibits a broad age range of presentation (i.e., 1-30 years and a mean age of initial MR diagnosis of 4.7 years). Therefore, the diagnosis of PMD is often entertained in the mid-first decade. Common clinical features include hypotonia, developmental delay, inability to sit, and head titubation, with progression, nystagmus, and spasticity. The long-term prognosis is poor, and death often occurs in early childhood.

Imaging

MR Findings. The typical imaging appearance of PMD is nearly complete lack of myelination. The entire cerebral WM appears diffusely and homogeneously hyperintense on T2WI (yet not as hyperintense as demyelinating leukodystrophies). In some cases, preserved myelin around perivascular spaces gives the WM a "tigroid" pattern. Hyperintensity of the pyramidal tracts or entire pons is typically present. Progressive WM and cerebellar volume loss are common. Cavitary WM changes are typically absent.

DTI/DWI. ADC values predate T1- and T2-weighted signal changes. ADC values and radial diffusivity decrease with myelin maturation **(31-36A)**.

MRS. Relative increases in myoinositol, choline, and cytosolic (lipid) resonances with hypomyelination are common yet nonspecific. Choline is normally reduced with normal myelination **(31-36C)**.

Differential Diagnosis. The major differential diagnosis of PMD is **other hypomyelinating disorders**. Pyramidal tract and pontine hyperintensity are helpful distinguishing features. Patients with **4H syndrome** and **PMD-like disease** typically present clinically a bit later than **PMD** (i.e., in the late first decade). The MR in **4H syndrome** shows early cerebellar atrophy, relative T2 hypointensity within the anterior lateral thalami, and pyramidal tracts at the level of the PLICs. MR in **PMLD** patients shows T2 hyperintensity either within pontine pyramidal tracts alone or T2 hyperintensity throughout the pons. Patients with **fucosidosis** show T2 hypointensity of the globus pallidus and substantia nigra. Patients with **GM1/GM2** gangliosidosis show early T2 hyperintensity within the basal ganglia. Also consider **mucopolysaccharidoses** and **mitochondrial encephalopathies** in the differential diagnosis.

IMDs Predominantly Affecting Gray Matter

Inherited metabolic disorders (IMDs) that involve the gray matter (GM) without affecting the white matter (WM) are also known as poliodystrophies. They can be subdivided into those that involve the cortex and those that mostly affect the deep gray nuclei. Inherited GM disorders that involve the deep gray nuclei are significantly more common than those that primarily affect the cortex.

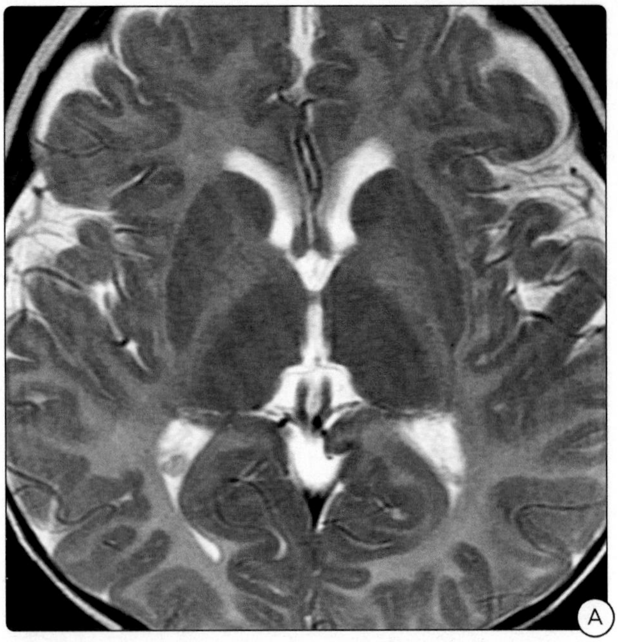

(31-35A) Axial T2WI in a 6m boy with PMD, delayed motor development, and normal head circumference shows almost complete absence of myelination, including the subcortical U-fibers. At this age, the internal capsules should be myelinated.

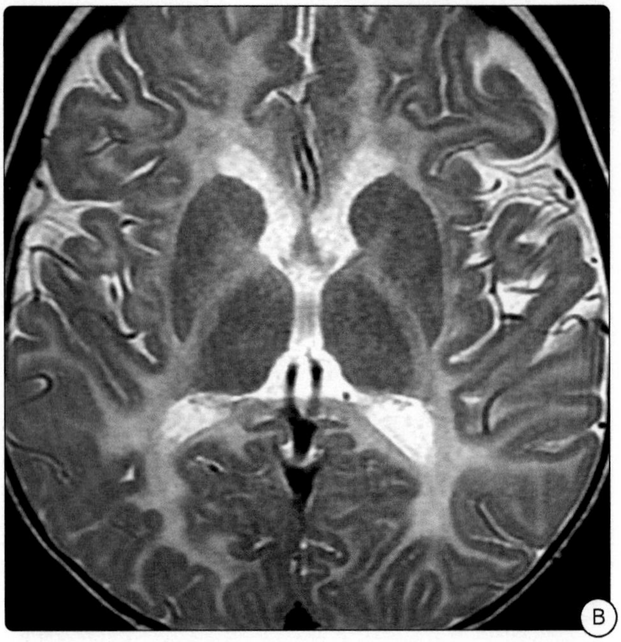

(31-35B) Axial T2WI in the same patient at age 3 years shows no interval progression of myelination. Genetic analysis showed PLP1 mutation, diagnostic for PMD. Serial MR is warranted when hypomyelination is suspected.

IMDs Primarily Affecting Deep Gray Nuclei

A number of inherited disorders affect mostly the basal ganglia and thalami. Three inborn errors of metabolism with specific predilection for the deep gray nuclei include (1) *pantothenate kinase-associated neurodegeneration* (PKAN), (2) *creatine deficiency syndromes*, and (3) a cytosine-adenine-guanine (CAG) repeat disorder called *Huntington disease*.

We begin this section with an overview of brain iron accumulation disorders before turning our attention specifically to PKAN, creatine deficiency syndromes, and Huntington disease. We close the section with a discussion of two inherited disorders with abnormal copper metabolism, **Wilson disease** and **Menkes disease**.

Brain Iron Accumulation Disorders

Some iron accumulation within the basal ganglia and dentate nuclei occurs as part of normal aging (see Chapter 33). Neurodegeneration with brain iron accumulation (NBIA) represents a clinically and genetically heterogeneous group of conditions characterized by progressive neurodegeneration and abnormally elevated brain iron.

Four major NBIA subtypes have been defined at the molecular genetic level: (1) PKAN (or NBIA type 1), (2) neuroferritinopathy (NBIA type 2), (3) infantile neuroaxonal dystrophy, and (4) aceruloplasminemia.

We focus our discussion on PKAN, the most common type of NBIA. We then briefly discuss the other three types.

PKAN

Terminology. PKAN was formerly known as Hallervorden-Spatz disease.

Etiology. PKAN is a rare familial autosomal-recessive disorder characterized by excessive iron deposition in the globus pallidus (GP) and substantia nigra (SN). It is caused by mutations in the pantothenate kinase gene (*PANK2*) localized to chromosome 20p12.2-13p13. More than 100 individual *PANK2* mutations have been described. It is estimated that approximately 50% of the cases occur sporadically.

Pathology. Grossly, PKAN is characterized by shrinkage and rust-brown discoloration of the medial GP, the reticular zone of the SN **(31-41)**, and sometimes the dentate nuclei. The red nuclei are generally spared. Granular pigment consisting of iron, lipofuscin, and neuromelanin accumulates in axonal "spheroids" (swollen distended axons), neurons, astrocytes, and microglia, which in turn causes neuronal loss and gliosis. Immunostaining for hyperphosphorylated tau reveals numerous neurofibrillary tangles. Microscopically, increased iron content is found in the GP interna and pars reticulata SN. Iron deposition is found within astrocytes, microglial cells, neurons, and around vessels. The "eye of the tiger" corresponds to regions of reactive astrocytes, dystrophic axons, and vacuoles in the anteromedial GP.

Clinical Issues. PKAN or NBIA type 1 can develop at any age. Four clinical forms are recognized: infantile (onset in the first year of life), late-infantile (onset between 2 and 5 years), juvenile or "classic" (onset between 7 and 15 years), and adult-onset NBIA type 1.

Most cases are diagnosed late in the first decade or during early adolescence. The disorder classically begins with slowly progressive gait disturbances and delayed psychomotor development. Choreoathetosis, dysarthria, and dystonia are observed. Hyperkinesia occurs in about 50% of cases. Progressive mental deterioration finally leads to dementia. In the later stages of the disease, the dyskinesias are replaced by rigid stiffness. An atypical clinical presentation is behavioral and psychiatric disorders, speech delay, and pyramidal and extrapyramidal disturbance.

PANK2 mutations are associated with younger age at onset, more rapid progression, and higher frequency of dystonia, dysarthria, intellectual impairment, and gait disturbances. Parkinsonism is seen predominantly in patients with adult-onset disease.

Imaging. Imaging findings reflect the anatomic distribution of the excessive iron accumulation. T2WI demonstrates marked hypointensity in the GP and SN. A small focus of central hyperintensity in the medial aspect of the very hypointense GP (the classic "eye of the tiger" sign) is caused by tissue gliosis and vacuolization **(31-37)**.

It is important to note that *not all cases of PKAN demonstrate the "eye of the tiger"* **(31-38)**. Additionally, detection of the T2/FLAIR hyperintense eye of the tiger may antedate the T2 hypointense border. T1WI may show GP T1 shortening reflecting the presence of ferritin-bound iron. T2WI shows diffuse pallidal hypointensity with a medial focus of T2 hyperintensity (*eye of the tiger*). In time, as the disease progresses, the "eye of the tiger" T2 hyperintensity "shrinks" and becomes less conspicuous. Striking, severe T2 shortening in the GP with hypointense "blooming" on T2* (GRE, SWI) **(31-39)** in a child or young adult should strongly suggest the diagnosis of an NBIA—either PKAN or infantile neuroaxonal dystrophy—even in the absence of an "eye of the tiger" sign **(31-38)**.

NECT shows variable features with pallidus showing either hypoattenuation, hyperattenuation, or normalcy.

PKAN does not enhance on T1 C+, nor does it demonstrate restricted diffusion although DTI demonstrates significantly increased fractional anisotropy in both the GP and SN. MRS shows decreased NAA peak and reduced NAA:Cr ratio consistent with neuraxonal loss. Increased myoinositol peak (at 3.6 ppm) and increased mI:Cr ratio at short TE are present, suggesting reactive glial proliferation.

Differential Diagnosis. Abnormal iron deposition in the basal ganglia occurs with PKAN as well as other NBIAs. **Aceruloplasminemia** and **neuroferritinopathy** are both adult-onset disorders. Both involve the cortex, which is spared in PKAN.

Disorders with increased T2 signal within the GP can be grouped within *metabolic* derangements and *toxic/ischemic* insults. These entities lack pallidal GRE and SWI "blooming."

Inherited metabolic disorders to consider in the differential diagnosis of BG T2 hyperintensity include **methylmalonic acidemia** (increased T2 signal in GP + WM T2 prolongation), **Canavan disease** (GP and other deep nuclei showing increased T2 signal, subcortical WM T2 hyperintensity, and significantly increased NAA:Cr), **guanidinoacetate methyltransferase deficiency** (GAMT) (with or without GP T2 hyperintensity, absent or severely reduced Cr on MRS), **neuroferritinopathy** (variable GP T2 hyperintensity), **Wilson disease, Leigh syndrome, infantile bilateral striatal necrosis**, and **mitochondrial encephalopathies**, which show striatal hyperintensity (not hypointensity or blooming). Additionally, they also predominantly involve the caudate and putamen, not the medial GP. **Toxic/ischemic insults include hypoxic ischemic injury** (positive health history, T2 hyperintensity involving striatum, GP, thalami, corticospinal tracts, with or without cortical involvement), *CO poisoning* (increased T2 signal involving GP, other deep

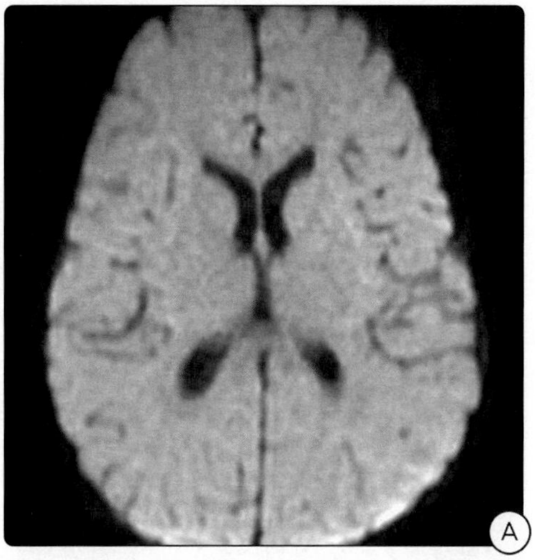

(31-36A) Axial DWI in a 3y hypotonic boy with PMD shows similar diffusivity of cortical GM and hemispheric WM.

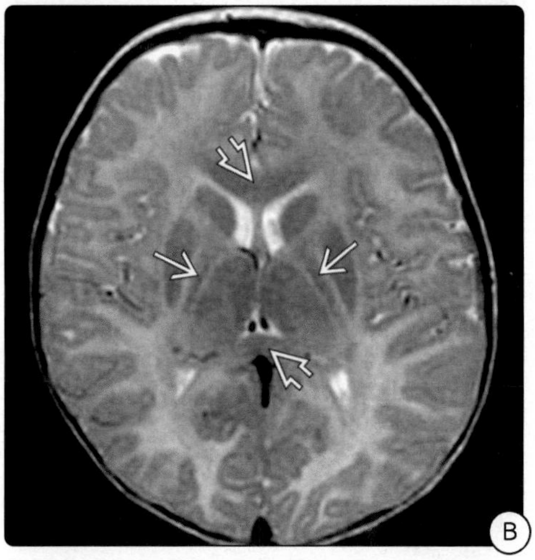

(31-36B) Axial T2WI in the same patient shows a lack of normal hypointense myelinated WM aside from the PLICs ➡ and corpus callosum ➡.

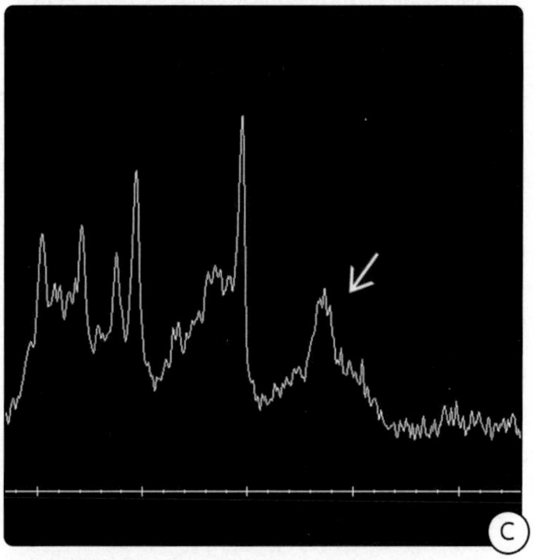

(31-36C) MRS short TE (35 ms) in the same patient elevated cytosolic amino acids in the 0.8- to 1.4-ppm range ➡.

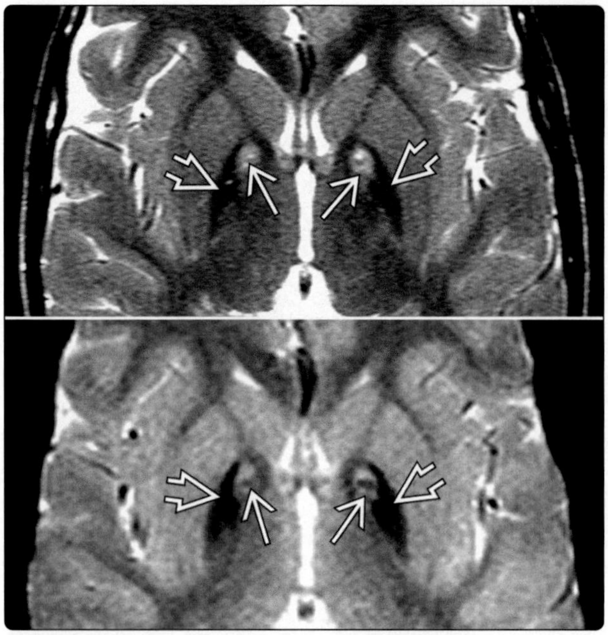

(31-37) T2WI (top), GRE (bottom) in a patient with PKAN show classic "eye of the tiger" sign with bilateral hyperintense central foci in the medial globi pallidi surrounded by striking hypointensity.

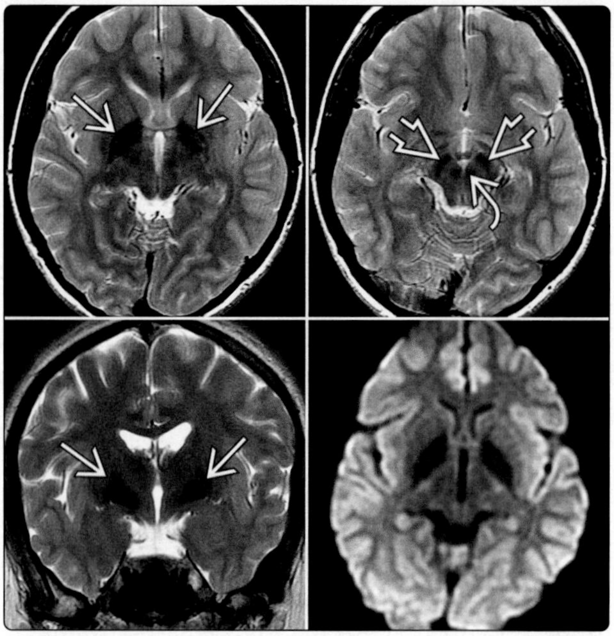

(31-38) Multiplanar MR shows a 19y woman with documented PKAN. Note the profound hypointensity in the GP, SN, red nuclei, and the lack of an "eye of the tiger" sign. DWI is normal (bottom right).

nuclei, cortex, and WM), **cyanide toxicity** (T2 increased within basal ganglia with or without hemorrhagic necrosis), and **kernicterus** (neonate) (increased T1/T2 GP).

Neuroferritinopathy. Mutations in the carboxy terminus of the ferritin light chain gene (*FTL*) interfere with the transport of iron. Redox active iron is deposited in neurons, causing oxidative stress with neuronal loss and gliosis. The result is **neuroferritinopathy**, an adult autosomal-dominant disorder, mean age of 39 years at onset.

The predominant clinical neuroferritinopathy phenotype is an extrapyramidal disorder with choreiform movements and focal dystonia. Early cognitive and psychiatric disturbances are absent, thus distinguishing neuroferritinopathy from Huntington disease.

Imaging. The earliest detectable imaging findings in neuroferritinopathy are T2* GRE and SWI hypointensity ("blooming") in the GP and SN. T2 hypointensity in the GP and SN, red nuclei, caudate, putamen, thalamus, and cerebral cortex typically follow. In later stages, gliosis and cystic degeneration in the medial GP may produce foci of T2 hyperintensity that causes an "eye of the tiger" appearance similar to that seen in PKAN (see above).

Infantile Neuroaxonal Dystrophy. Mutations in phospholipase A2 (*PLA2G6*) cause **infantile neuroaxonal dystrophy** (INAD), a severe psychomotor disorder showing progressive hypotonia, hyperreflexia, and tetraparesis. Median age at onset is 14 months. Rapid progression with a mean age of death of 9 years is typical.

Imaging. Children with INAD show striking cerebellar atrophy in over 95% of cases. T2/FLAIR hyperintensity in the cerebellum secondary to demyelination and gliosis is also common. Almost 50% of cases demonstrate abnormal iron deposition with T2 hypointensity in the GP and SN.

NBIA T2* HYPOINTENSITY

PKAN
- GP, SN, dentate nuclei
- "Eye of tiger" sign variable
- *Spares* cortex

Infantile Neuroaxonal Dystrophy
- Cerebellar atrophy (95%)
- T2* hypointensity in GP, SN (50%)
- *Spares* cortex

Neuroferritinopathy
- T2* hypointensity in GP, SN
- Then dentate/caudate nuclei, thalami
- *Affects* cortex

Aceruloplasminemia
- GP, caudate nuclei, putamen, thalamus
- Red nucleus, SN, dentate nuclei
- *Affects* cerebral, cerebellar cortices

Aceruloplasminemia. Homozygous mutations in the ceruloplasmin gene cause **aceruloplasminemia**, also known as hereditary ceruloplasmin deficiency. Ceruloplasmin carries over 95% of all plasma copper and acts as a ferroxidase, thus playing an important role in mobilizing tissue iron.

Aceruloplasminemia is a disease of middle-aged adults characterized by the clinical triad of diabetes, retinopathy, and neurologic symptoms (primarily dementia, craniofacial dyskinesia, and cerebellar ataxia). T2 and T2* (GRE, SWI) demonstrate striking hypointensity in the cerebral and cerebellar cortex, GP, caudate nucleus, putamen, thalamus, red nucleus, SN, and dentate nuclei **(31-40)**.

Imaging. MR is especially useful in diagnosing NBIAs. All feature iron deposition in the GP but differ in other associated findings. The distribution of T2 or T2* hypointensity can help distinguish between the different NBIA subtypes (see box below).

Creatine Deficiency Syndromes

Creatine (*kreas* in Greek) is required for the utilization of ATP-derived energy at sites of high energy utilization (i.e., muscle, brain, and heart). Specifically, creatine and creatine phosphate are essential for the storage and transmission of phosphate-bound energy in both muscle and brain. About half of our bodies' needs come from our diet, and the remainder is synthesized in the kidney and liver. Brain creatine deficiency syndromes are a group of rare disorders that include *guanidinoacetate methyltransferase (GAMT) deficiency*, *arginine:glycine amidinotransferase (AGAT) deficiency*, and *creatine transporter defect* (*SLC6A8*) (CRTR). The first two are inherited in an autosomal-recessive pattern, and the third is an X-linked recessive disorder. Dietary supplementation can partially or completely reverse the symptoms and imaging abnormalities, so making the diagnosis is crucial to patient management.

Imaging. MR may show variably conspicuous bilaterally symmetric T2/FLAIR hyperintensity and/or restricted diffusion within the globi pallidi **(31-42)**. MRS is often key to making this challenging diagnosis, showing a diminished or absent creatine peak on short and long TE studies at 2.0 ppm **(31-42)** **(31-43)**. Also, in GAMT deficiency, a guanidinoacetate peak will be detected at 3.8 ppm. MRS may be abnormal when MR appears normal **(31-43)**. This emphasizes the importance of always supplementing MR with MRS in infants and children with unexplained hypotonia and/or unexplained basal ganglia DWI and/or T2/FLAIR hyperintensity.

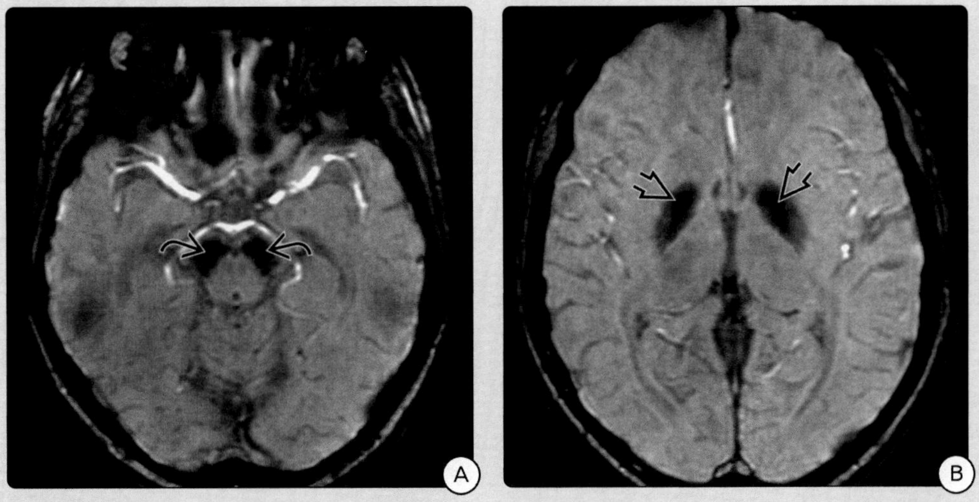

(31-39A) Axial SWI in a 9y boy with PKAN shows substantia nigra hypointensity. SWI is approximately six times more sensitive in detecting paramagnetic and diamagnetic effects in the brain than T2* GRE. (31-39B) Axial SWI in the same patient with PKAN shows GP hypointensity.

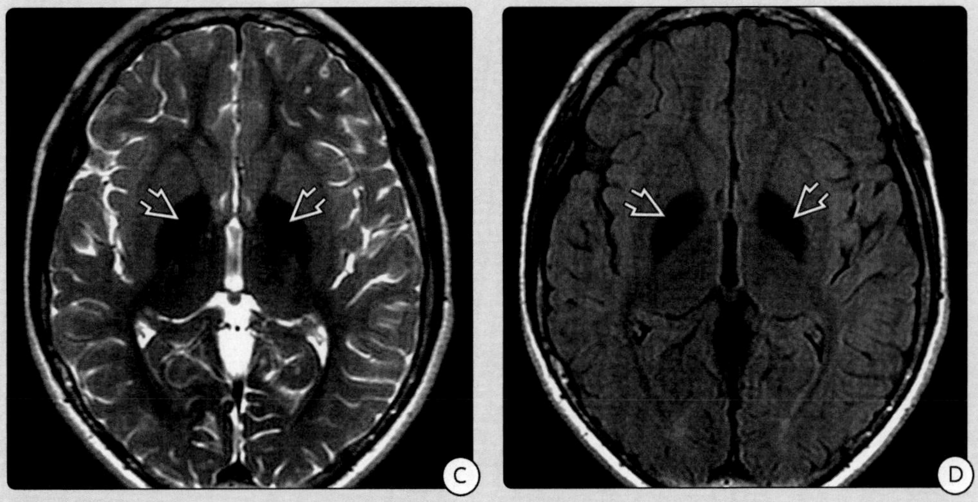

(31-39C) Axial T2WI in the same patient shows GP hypointensity. The central bright T2 eye of the tiger may either not be seen or become less apparent in time. (31-39D) Axial FLAIR in the same patient shows GP FLAIR hypointensity.

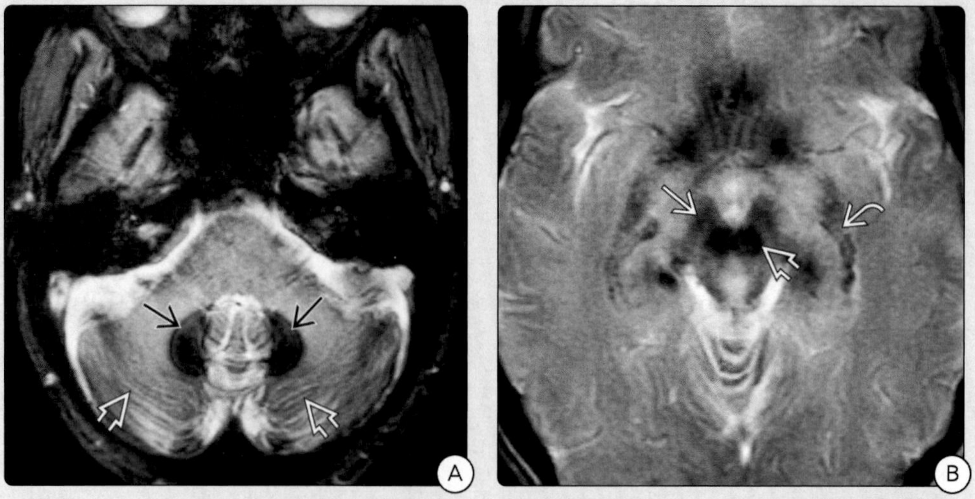

***(31-40A)** Axial T2* GRE scan in a 66y woman with aceruloplasminemia shows striking hypointensity in the dentate nuclei with subtle but definite linear "blooming" in the cerebellar cortex. **(31-40B)** Axial T2* GRE scan in the same patient shows symmetric "blooming" hypointensities in the substantia nigra, red nuclei, and inferior putamina.*

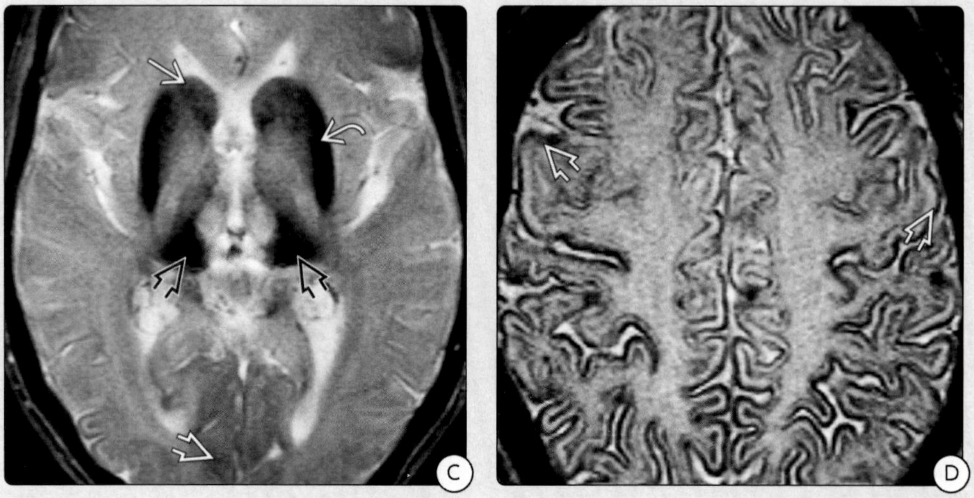

***(31-40C)** Axial T2* GRE, more cephalad shows profound symmetric hypointensity in the caudate nuclei, putamina, and both thalami. Note the subtle "blooming" hypointensity in the cortex as well. **(31-40D)** Axial T2* SWI scan in the same patient through the corona radiata demonstrates striking curvilinear hypointensity "etching" the entire cortex of both hemispheres.*

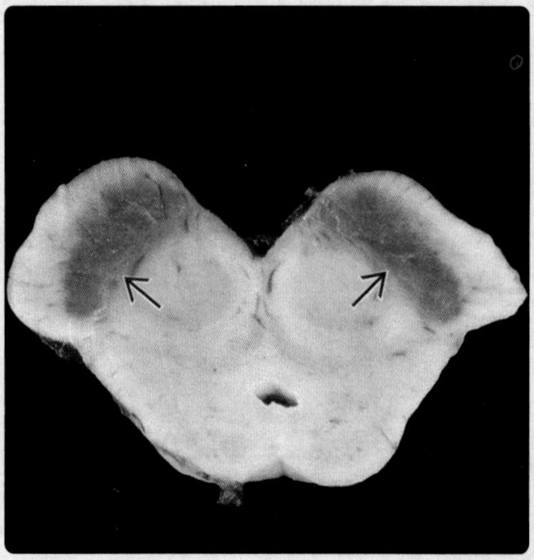

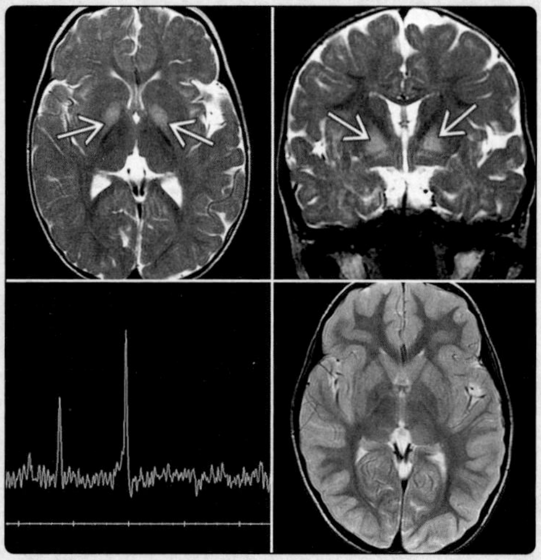

***(31-41)** Autopsy case of PKAN shows characteristic brownish discoloration caused by iron deposition in the substantia nigra (SN). (Courtesy E. T. Hedley-Whyte, MD.) **(31-42)** MR in an 11m infant with creatine deficiency shows hyperintensity in the globi pallidi. Long TE MRS shows absent Cr peak (2.0 ppm). With dietary supplementation, 3 years later MR is normal (bottom right).*

Differential Diagnosis. Differential diagnoses include **other disorders with increased T2/FLAIR signal within the GP**. This includes **metabolic disorders** such as **methylmalonic acidemia** (increased GP T2 signal and WM T2 hyperintensity), **neuroferritinopathy** (eye of the tiger and SWI GP blooming), **Canavan disease** (macrocephaly, subcortical WM T2 hyperintensity, GP increased T2 signal). **Toxic/ischemic insults** include **HII** (health history, striatal and thalamic DWI hyperintensity, with or without watershed ischemia), **CO poisoning** (increased GP, other deep nuclei, and WM T2/FLAIR hyperintensities), and **cyanide poisoning** (hemorrhagic necrosis and basal ganglia increased T2 signal).

Huntington Disease

Until recently, Huntington disease (HD) was thought to be regionally selective, affecting only GM (most specifically the caudate nuclei and putamina). Although advanced imaging techniques such as DTI have demonstrated that WM is also affected, the dominant imaging features are abnormalities of the deep gray nuclei. Therefore, we include HD in this section with the other IMDs that preferentially involve the striatum, manifesting with profound caudate nucleus atrophy.

Terminology and Etiology. HD is also known as Huntington chorea. HD is an autosomal-dominant chronic hereditary neurodegenerative disorder with complete penetrance. The responsible genetic defect occurs on the short arm of chromosome 4 (4p16.3) and codes for the protein huntingtin. The huntingtin gene includes a repeating CAG trinucleotide segment of variable length. It is more common in a paternally transmitted mutated allele. The presence of more than 38 repeats confirms the diagnosis of HD. There is a progressive increase in the length of the CAG repeat sequences with successive generations.

Pathology. Aggregates of huntingtin protein accumulate in axonal terminals, which eventually leads to the death of medium spiny neurons. Autopsy shows generalized cerebral atrophy with an average of 30% reduction in brain weight. Both the cortex and hemispheric WM are affected. The most characteristic gross abnormality is volume loss with rarefaction of the caudate nucleus, putamen, and globus pallidus **(31-44)** **(31-45)**.

Microscopically, HD features neuronal loss with huntingtin nuclear inclusions, astrocytic gliosis, and iron accumulation. The changes are most severe in the basal ganglia but can also be seen in other regions of the brain, including the cerebellum (which is less commonly involved in the adult).

Clinical Issues. The incidence of HD is 4-7:100,000 in most populations. Mean age at symptom onset is 35-45 years. Only 5-10% of patients present before the age of 20 years (juvenile-onset HD). In the juvenile-onset form, look for cerebellar atrophy in addition to caudate atrophy There is no sex predilection.

CAG repeat length and age influence both the expression and the progression of HD. Adult-onset HD is characterized by progressive loss of normal motor function, development of stereotypic choreiform movements, and deteriorating cognition. Once symptoms appear, the disease progresses relentlessly and results in death within 10-20 years.

Juvenile-onset HD is initially characterized by rigidity and dystonia, much more than by chorea. Cerebellar signs are also common.

Imaging. Standard imaging studies (CT, MR) are normal early in the disease course. As symptoms develop and progress, NECT scans show caudate atrophy with enlarged, outwardly convex frontal horns and variable generalized diffuse atrophy **(31-46)** with or without cerebellar atrophy.

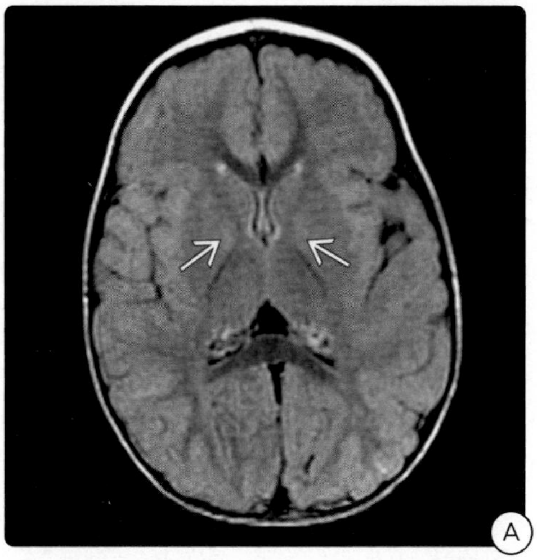

***(31-43A)** Axial FLAIR in a 10m hypotonic girl with creatine deficiency (GAMT deficiency) shows subtle GP hyperintensity ➡.*

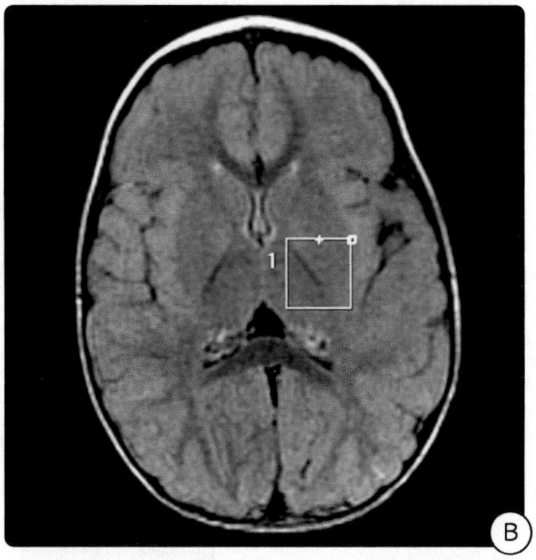

***(31-43B)** Axial FLAIR in the same patient shows BG MRS voxel placement.*

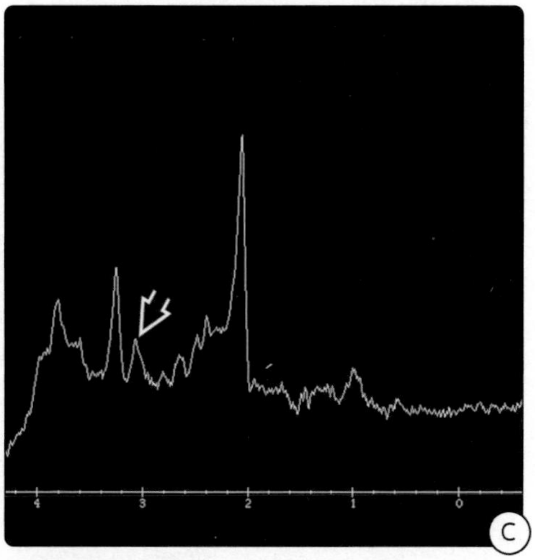

***(31-43C)** MRS short TE (35 ppm) shows diminished creatine peak at 2.0 ppm ➡.*

MR shows diffuse cerebral volume loss with T2/FLAIR hyperintensity in shrunken caudate heads. Putaminal hyperintensity is also common **(31-47)**. The pattern of cerebral volume loss may show predilection for the frontal lobes. There is no enhancement of involved structures.

MR volumetric studies can demonstrate decreased basal ganglia volumes years before the onset of motor disturbances. Voxel-based morphometry, DTI, and PET have also demonstrated abnormalities in the hemispheric WM and cortex of both asymptomatic carriers and patients with "premanifest" HD.

Magnetization transfer imaging (MTI) demonstrates peak height reduction proportionate to CAG repeat length in normal-appearing GM and WM. Disturbances in MTI are apparent in early HD and are homogeneous across both GM and WM.

Differential Diagnosis. Some acquired neurodegenerative disorders can mimic *adult* HD. These include **multiple system atrophy** (MSA), **corticobasal degeneration**, and **frontotemporal lobar dementia**. All these acquired disorders are often accompanied by basal ganglia atrophy, although, unlike in HD, the caudate nuclei are not disproportionately affected.

The differential diagnosis of *juvenile* HD includes **Leigh syndrome** (DWI hyperintensity and increased T2/FLAIR in the putamen, caudate, and tegmentum), late-stage **Wilson disease** (caudate and brainstem atrophy, increased symmetric signal in the caudate nucleus, putamen, midbrain, and pons and regions of caudate and putaminal irregular T2 hypointensities), and **PKAN** with choreoathetosis and dementia, which can mimic the symptoms of HD. The "eye of the tiger" sign in the medial GP distinguishes PKAN from HD.

(31-44) Axial graphic shows shrunken, atrophic caudate nuclei ➔ with the outwardly convex frontal horns ➔ that are typical of Huntington disease (HD). (31-45) Coronal autopsy of HD shows outwardly convex frontal horns ➔, severely shrunken caudate nuclei ➔, and atrophic putamina ➔. (Courtesy R. Hewlett, MD.)

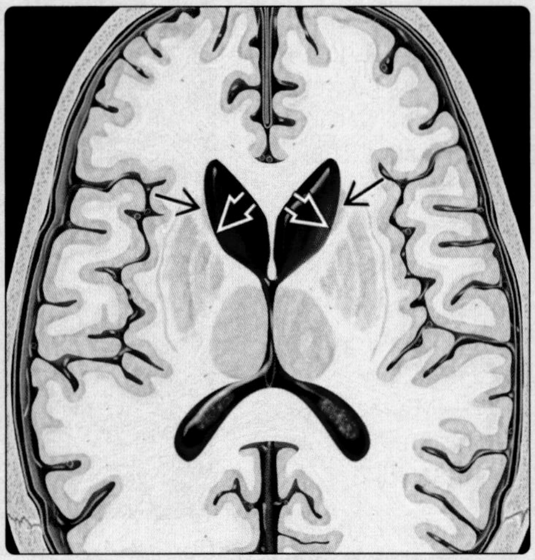

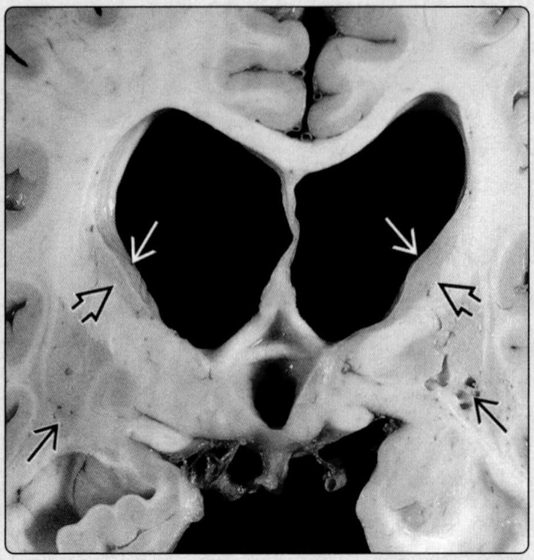

(31-46) Axial NECT of a patient with HD shows moderate generalized, severe caudate atrophy seen as outwardly convex frontal horns ➔. (Courtesy M. Huckman, MD.) (31-47) Axial FLAIR in a patient with HD shows almost nonexistent caudate heads ➔, basal ganglia atrophy, and thinned atrophic hyperintense putamina ➔.

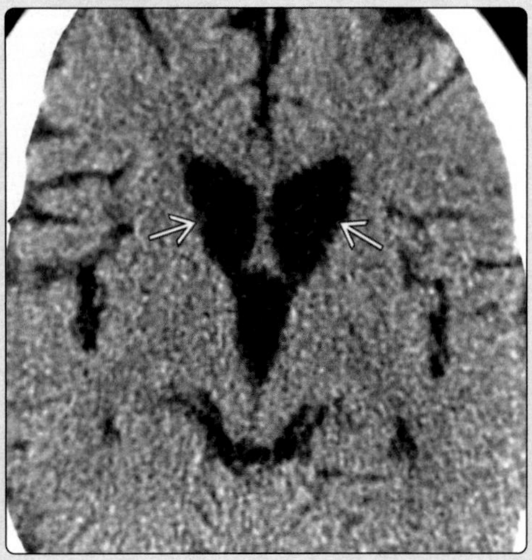

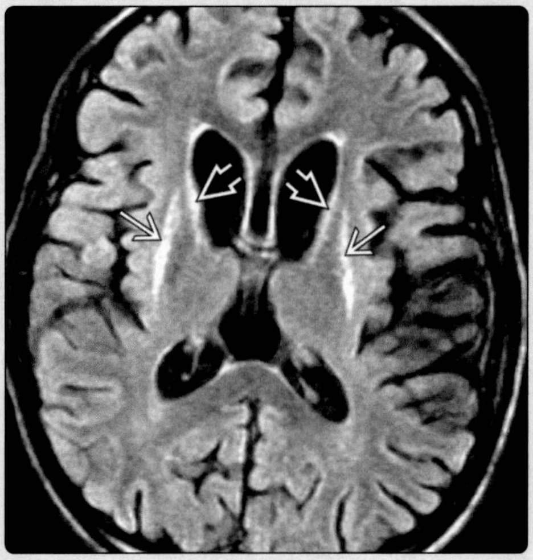

HUNTINGTON DISEASE

Etiology
- Autosomal-dominant, complete penetrance
- CAG trinucleotide repeat disorder

Pathology
- Caudate nuclei, putamina, GP
  - Huntingtin protein nuclear inclusions
  - Neuronal loss, gliosis, iron accumulation

Clinical
- Adult onset (35-45 years) = 90%
- Juvenile onset HD (< 20 years) = 10%

Imaging
- Caudate nuclei, putamina T2/FLAIR hyperintense
- Frontal horns outwardly convex

Disorders of Copper Metabolism

Copper is essential for normal brain development. Copper-containing proteins are a critical element in a number of enzymatic systems, including iron homeostasis. Copper homeostasis is a delicate balance that requires both adequate dietary intake and proper excretion. Excess copper is neurotoxic. Two disorders of copper metabolism—Wilson disease (WD) and Menkes disease—have striking CNS manifestations.

The major manifestations of WD are found in the basal ganglia, midbrain, and dentate nucleus of the cerebellum. Therefore, WD is discussed in this section with IMDs that predominantly affect the gray matter. A brief consideration of Menkes disease follows.

Wilson Disease

Etiology. WD is an uncommon autosomal-recessive disorder of copper trafficking caused by mutations in the *ATP7B* gene, which is found on chromosome 13q14.3q21.1. The mutation causes defective incorporation of cooper into ceruloplasmin and impaired biliary copper excretion. There is excessive accumulation of Cu in hepatocytes, which later spills into the circulation. Copper deposition in Golgi complexes and the mitochondria results in oxidative damage primarily to the liver, brain, kidney, skeletal system, and eye.

Pathology. Selective vulnerability of the corpus striatum to mitochondrial dysfunction accounts for the predominant basal ganglia volume loss seen in WD **(31-49)**. Gross pathologic features are nonspecific, with ventricular enlargement and widened sulci seen at autopsy in severe cases. Microscopic features include edema, necrosis, and spongiform changes in the basal ganglia. Variable gliosis and demyelination are present in the cerebral and cerebellar WM.

Clinical Issues. WD most commonly affects children and young adults. The reported incidence of symptomatic WD is 1:30,000-40,000, but the frequency of asymptomatic carriers is 1:90. There is no sex predilection.

Symptoms of early-onset WD (8-16 years of age) are usually related to liver failure. Later-onset WD symptoms are primarily neurologic and are generally recognized in the second or third decade. Dysarthria, dystonia, tremors, ataxia, Parkinson-like symptoms, and behavioral disturbances are common. Copper deposition in the cornea causes the characteristic greenish yellow Kayser-Fleischer rings seen on slit-lamp examination **(31-48)**.

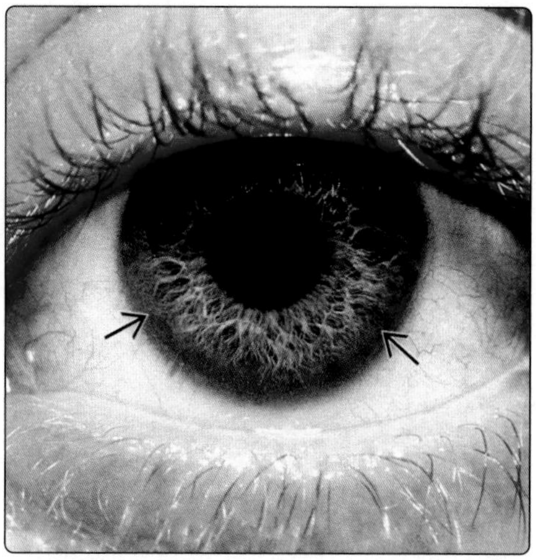

***(31-48)** Wilson disease (WD) is shown with classic peripheral greenish-yellow Kayser-Fleischer ring. (Courtesy AFIP Archives.)*

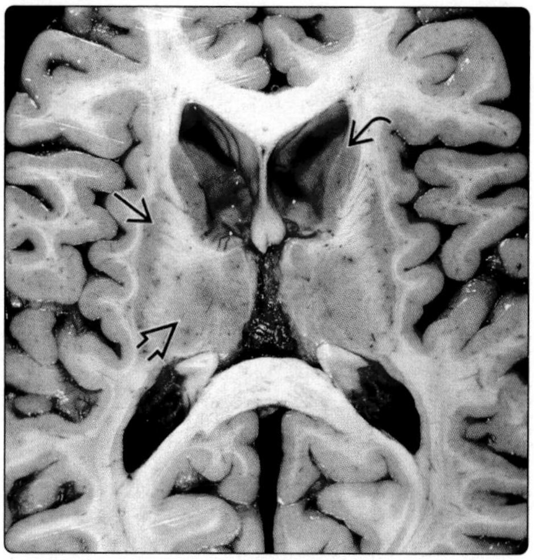

***(31-49)** Autopsy in WD shows atrophic putamina, caudate, and basal ganglia characteristic of WD. (Courtesy R. Hewlett, MD.)*

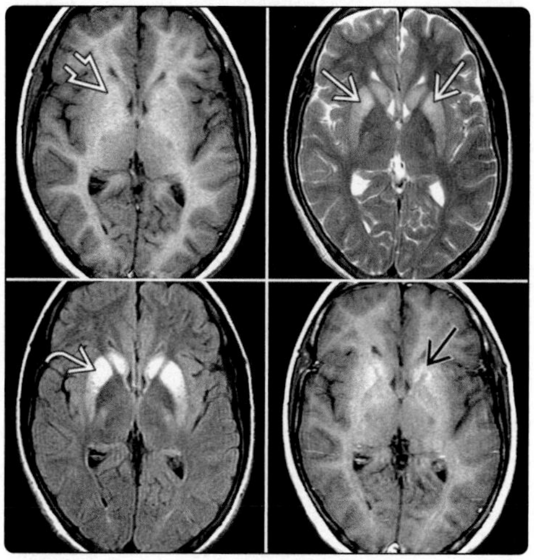

***(31-50)** Acute WD shows hyperintensity on T1 and T2WI, DWI restriction, and no enhancement. (Courtesy M. Ayadi, MD.)*

Clinical symptoms generally improve, and signal abnormalities on MR may diminish with appropriate treatment. Treatments include restriction of foods rich in Cu (i.e., nuts, mushrooms, chocolate), chelating drugs (i.e., Trientene), and liver transplantation. Untreated WD is always fatal.

WILSON DISEASE

Etiology
- Abnormal copper metabolism
- Autosomal recessive
- *ATP7B* gene mutations

Pathology
- Copper accumulates in hepatocytes, brain, eye
- Mitochondrial dysfunction damages basal ganglia

Clinical Issues
- Childhood WD: liver disease
- Young adults: Parkinson-like
- Kayser-Fleischer rings

Imaging
- T2/FLAIR hyperintensity
  - Putamina, caudate, thalami, midbrain
- T2* "blooming"

Differential Diagnosis
- Leigh syndrome
- PKAN

Imaging. NECT scans may be normal, especially early in the disease course. CT grossly underestimates WD pathology. Diffuse brain atrophy, widening of the frontal horns of the lateral ventricles, and striatal or thalamic hypoattenuation may be seen in advanced cases.

Signal intensity on T1WI is variable. Some cases demonstrate subtle hypointensity in the affected areas, whereas others show T1 shortening similar to that seen in chronic hepatic encephalopathy (see Chapter 32). BG T2 signal reflects paramagnetic effects of Cu.

The most common imaging finding of WD on MR is bilaterally symmetric T2/FLAIR hyperintensity (sometimes heterogeneous) in the putamina (70%), caudate nuclei (60%), ventrolateral thalami (55-60%), and midbrain (50%) **(31-50)**. Initially, *swelling* of the basal ganglia then atrophy are seen. Hyperintensity can sometimes be seen in the pons (20%), medulla (10-15%), and cerebellum (10%). The cerebral (25%) and cerebellar WM (10%) can show focal or diffuse confluent hyperintensities.

In 10-12% of cases, diffuse tegmental (midbrain) hyperintensity with sparing of the red nuclei gives an appearance that has been termed the **"face of a giant panda."**

T2* (GRE, SWI) sequences show blooming in the putamina, caudate nuclei, ventrolateral thalami, and often the dentate nuclei. Contrast enhancement is typically absent although mild enhancement can occur in the acute stages.

Restricted diffusion in the corpus striatum can be seen in the early stages of WD. Elevated ADC values consistent with necrosis and spongiform degeneration are seen in chronic longstanding WD. MRS shows reduced NAA and Cho and reduced myoinositol:creatine ratio in affected areas. PET shows markedly reduced glucose metabolism and diminished dopa-decarboxylase activity indicative of striatonigral dopaminergic pathway dysfunction.

Differential Diagnosis. The differential diagnoses of WD includes other inherited metabolic disorders that affect the basal ganglia, such as Leigh syndrome, NBIAs, the organic acidurias, and Japanese encephalitis (JE). **Leigh syndrome** (subacute necrotizing encephalomyelopathy) shows bilateral, symmetric, spongiform, and hyperintense lesions particularly in the *putamen* and brainstem. The WM is often affected in Leigh syndrome, whereas the caudate and thalamus are less commonly involved. MRS demonstrates elevated lactate levels in the basal ganglia. **Organic aciduria** (widened CSF spaces, symmetric WM T2/FLAIR hyperintensities, basal ganglial increased T2 signal) and **JE** (mosquito-borne illness showing characteristic homogeneous T2/FLAIR hyperintensities in the basal ganglia and posteromedial thalami) should be considered.

Likewise, **PKAN** can resemble WD. WD predominantly affects the putamina and caudate nuclei rather than the medial GP and lacks the "eye of the tiger" sign often seen in PKAN.

Menkes Disease. Menkes disease—also known as kinky hair syndrome—is an X-linked, multisystemic, lethal disorder of copper metabolism caused by *ATP7A* gene mutations. Severe classic Menkes disease is characterized by progressive neurodegeneration, connective tissue abnormalities, pili torti ("kinky" hair), and death in early childhood. It accounts for 90-95% of cases. A milder phenotype, **occipital horn syndrome**, also called Ehlers-Danlos type 9, is characterized by skeletal abnormalities and longer survival.

Imaging. Menkes disease shows severe brain atrophy with subdural fluid collections and excessive tortuosity and prominence of the intracranial arteries (remember: "kinky hair, kinky vessels") **(31-51A)** **(31-51B)**. Wormian bones, although nonspecific, are also seen **(31-51C)**. With progression in neurodegeneration and brain atrophy, development of subdural hemorrhage is common.

Differential Diagnosis. Differential diagnoses include **glutaric aciduria type I** (widened lateral cerebral fissures, GP increased DWI and T2/FLAIR signal), **hypoxic ischemic encephalopathy (HII)** (positive health history, nonprogressive neurologic features), **urea cycle defects** (initial diffuse cerebral edema, looks like "worst case ever" of HII), **TORCH infections** (microcephaly, Ca++, nonprogressive), and **Loeys-Dietz syndrome** (characterized by aneurysms of the aorta and other vessels, including intracranial, similar to Marfan syndrome).

IMDs Primarily Affecting Cortex

Compared with IMDs that affect the deep gray nuclei, disorders that exclusively or primarily affect the cortical GM are rare. Two prototypical IMDs that involve the cortex are briefly discussed here. These are **neuronal ceroid lipofuscinoses (NCLs)** and **Rett syndrome (RTT)**.

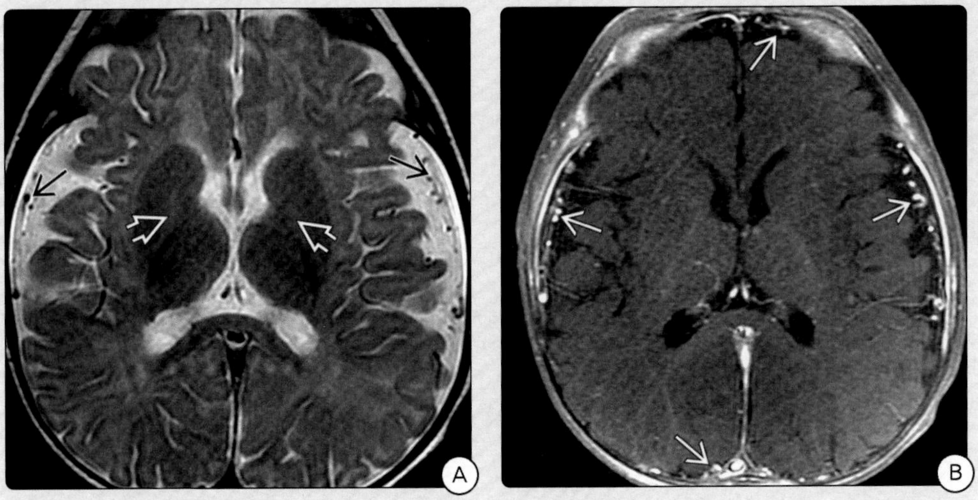

(31-51A) *Axial T2WI in a 5y child with Menkes shows widened sylvian fissures, T2 hyperintensity within the GP ➡, and prominent flow voids ⇨.* **(31-51B)** *Axial T1WI C+ in the same patient shows numerous tortuous LM enhancing vessels ➡.*

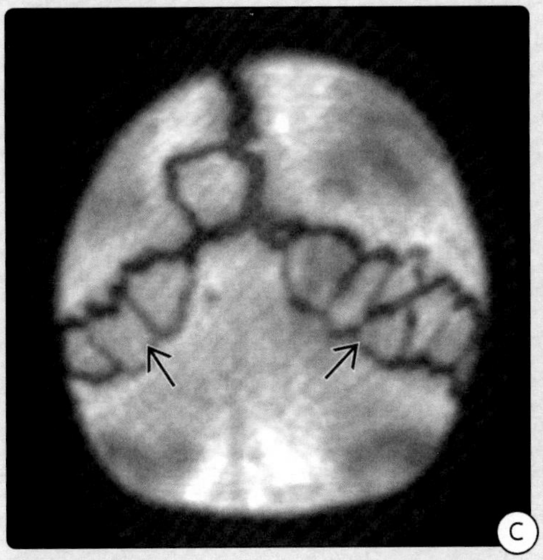

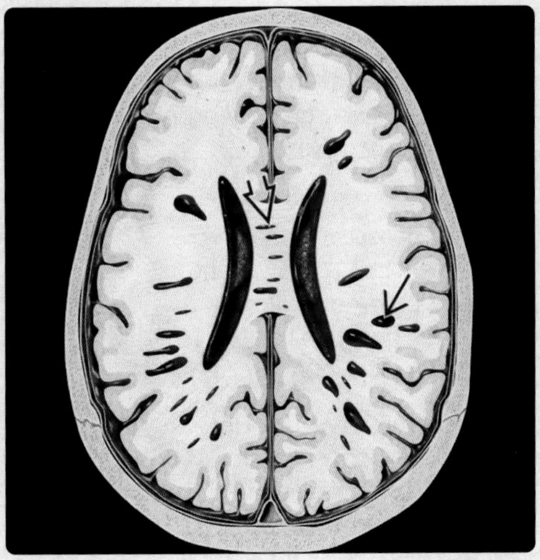

(31-51C) *Coronal NECT in the same Menkes patient through the lambdoid sutures shows numerous Wormian bones ⇨. More than six are too many.* **(31-52)** *MPS with dilated PVSs ⇨ is radially oriented in the WM. Posterior predominance and involvement of the corpus callosum ⇨ are seen.*

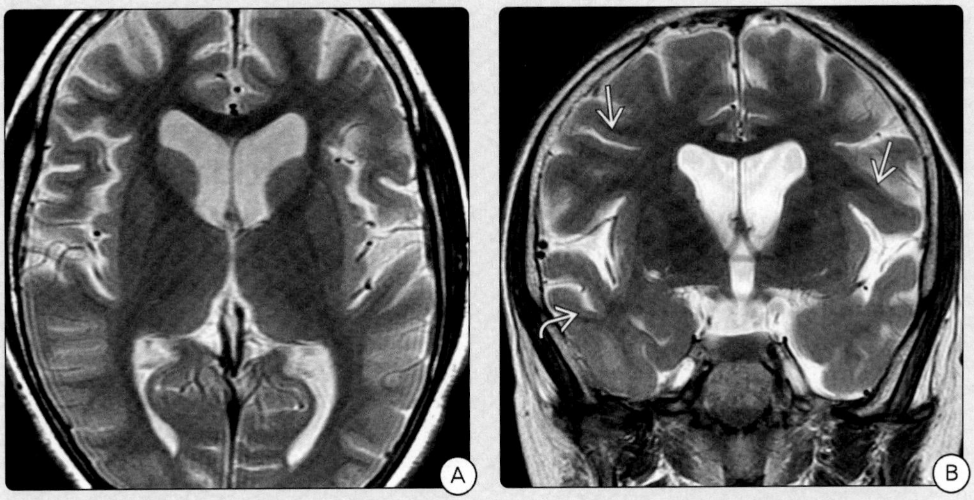

(31-53A) *Axial T2WI in a 7y girl with Rett syndrome shows enlarged frontal horns and striking frontotemporal sulcal enlargement due to predominant volume loss. The hemispheric WM appears normal.* **(31-53B)** *Coronal T2WI in the same patient shows thinned cortex in the posterior frontal ➡ and temporal ↪ lobes. Moderate volume loss with enlarged suprasellar cistern, sylvian fissures, and frontal SASs is present.*

Neuronal Ceroid Lipofuscinosis

The NCLs are a heterogeneous family of inherited neurodegenerative disorders characterized by accumulation of ceroid-lipopigment inclusions in neurons. A number of different types have been described. Previously, the NCLs were classified according to age at onset with infantile, late-infantile, juvenile (i.e., Batten disease), and adult forms (e.g., Kufs disease). The specific gene mutations that cause most forms have been identified, and the NCLs are now classified according to the eight affected genes (*CLN1-8*).

NCL is predominantly a childhood disease with an estimated incidence of 1:12,500. The diagnosis is established through clinicopathologic findings, enzymatic assay, and molecular genetic testing. Ultrastructural studies—usually from skin biopsy specimens—are used to confirm the presence and nature of lysosomal storage material (i.e., specific lipopigments).

Gross pathologic findings in the childhood NCLs are striking global atrophy with no specific lobar predominance. All NCLs demonstrate similar histopathologic features, i.e., abnormal accumulation of PAS- and Sudan black-positive inclusions in ballooned neurons. Cortical layers III, V, and VI are most severely affected. Progressive and selective neuronal loss and gliosis with secondary WM degeneration are universally present.

Imaging. The NCLs share common but nonspecific imaging features. Thalami and GP are hyperattenuating on NECT and hypointense on T2WI. Serial MR shows progressive atrophy with thinned cortex, enlarged ventricles, periventricular T2/FLAIR hyperintense rims, and prominent sulci.

Differential Diagnosis. Differential diagnoses include **HII-status marmoratus** (positive health history of perinatal hypoxic ischemic insult, nonprogressive hyperattenuating GP and thalami, striatal increased T2 signal, perirolandic atrophy), **Krabbe disease** (hyperattenuating on NECT thalami, caudate, and dentate nuclei, increased T2 signal cerebral WM), and **juvenile GM1 gangliosidoses** (hyperattenuating thalami on NECT, T2 hypointensity of ventral thalami, hypointense dorsal thalami).

Rett Syndrome

RTT is a progressive neurodevelopmental disorder that almost always affects girls. The majority of cases are sporadic, and no risk factors have been identified. A mutation in the methyl-CpG-binding protein-2 gene (*MECP2*) is identified in 80% of cases.

RTT occurs in 1:20,000 girls. Affected individuals are usually normal at birth with no obvious abnormalities. Head growth gradually decelerates after the first few months, and severe psychomotor retardation develops. Intellectual impairment, mood and behavioral changes, speech difficulty, truncal apraxia, and stereotypical hand waving develop.

Imaging. Imaging shows microcephaly with mild but diffuse reduction in both cortical and hemispheric WM volume **(31-53)**. The most prominent loss is seen in the frontal and anterior temporal cortex **(31-53)**. DTI shows reduced fractional anisotropy (FA) in the corpus callosum, internal capsule, frontal WM, and anterior cingulate gyrus with preservation or increased FA in the posterior corona radiata. MRS shows decreased NAA.

Differential Diagnosis. The clinical differential diagnosis of RTT includes NCL and autism. Cortical thinning in **NCL** is generalized and does not exhibit the frontotemporal pattern seen in RTT. **Autism** is excluded if the patient is *MECP2* mutation positive. Hypoxic ischemic encephalopathy to include watershed infarction is nonprogressive and associated with positive health history.

Disorders Affecting Both Gray and White Matter

In the last section of this chapter, we discuss inherited metabolic disorders (IMDs) that affect *both* gray and white matter. The pathoetiologies are quite variable and range from abnormal organelles to specific enzymatic dysfunctions.

Selected for discussion are the mucopolysaccharidoses (MPSs), Canavan disease, Alexander disease, peroxisomal spectrum disorders, and mitochondrial disorders.

Mucopolysaccharidoses

Terminology and Etiology

The MPSs are lysosomal storage disorders characterized by incomplete degradation and progressive accumulation of toxic glycosaminoglycan (GAG) in various organs. In the brain, this accumulation includes GAG deposits in the Virchow-Robin spaces, leptomeninges, and craniocervical junction ligamentous structures. GAG represents a CNS toxin. The MPSs were once grouped into a single entity and termed "gargoylism" for their supposedly characteristic facies.

The MPSs have a classification of 1-9. Each has a specific enzyme deficiency and gene defect that leads to the inability to break down GAG.

MPS 1H (Hurler) and MPS 1HS (Hurler-Scheie disease) have deficiency of α-L-iduronidase (4p16.3). MPS 2 (Hunter disease) is characterized by iduronate 2-sulfatase deficiency (Xq28). Other MPSs include MPS 3A (Sanfilippo disease), a deficiency of heparin N-sulfatase (17q25.3), MPS 4A (Morquio disease), a deficiency in galactose 6-sulfatase (16q24.3), and MPS 6 (Maroteaux-Lamy disease) associated with a deficiency in arylsulfatase B (5q11-q13).

Pathology

Autophagy is a highly regulated process in the lysosomal pathway that degrades proteins and damaged cellular organelles. Abnormal autophagy combined with the incomplete degradation and progressive accumulation of GAGs is the pathology that underlies the MPSs.

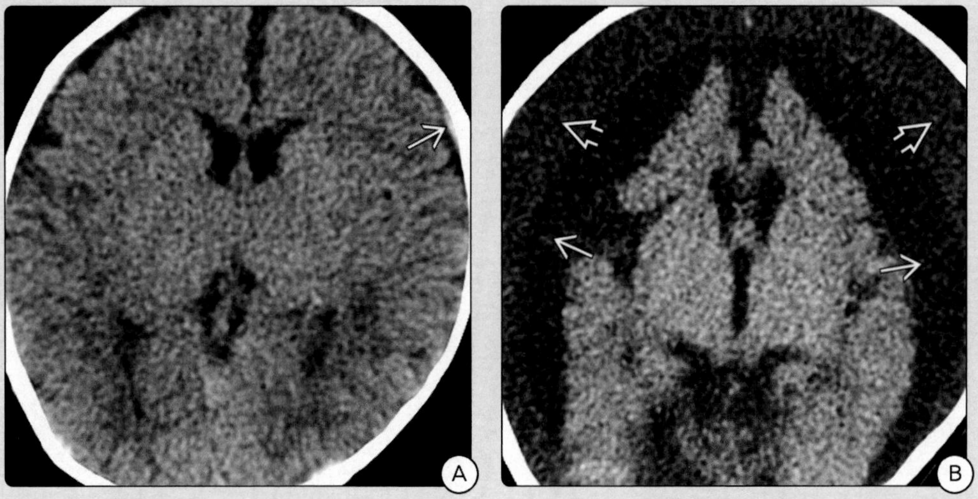

***(31-54A)** Initial axial NECT in a 7m infant with Menkes disease who initially presented with failure to thrive shows a thin-film left frontal subdural hematoma. **(31-54B)** Axial T1WI 9 months later shows large compressive chronic subdural hematomas. The brain is atrophic. The overlying subarachnoid spaces are grossly enlarged.*

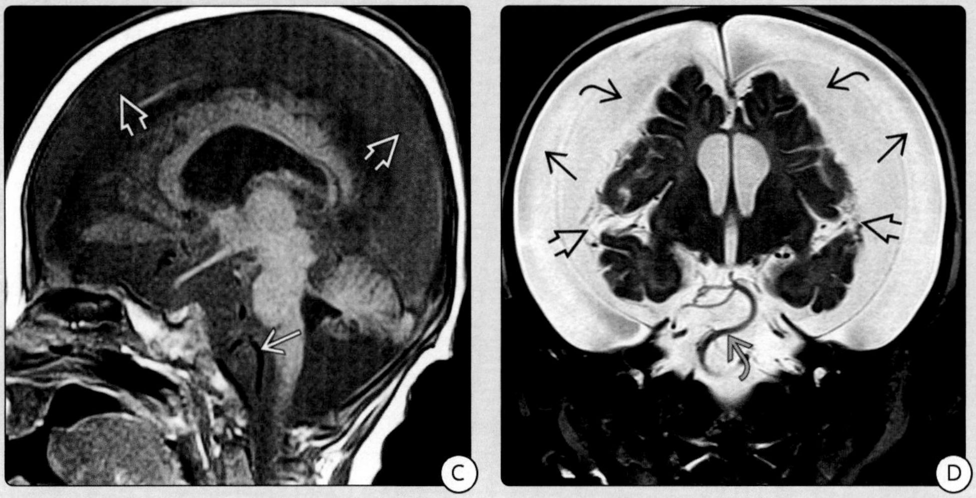

***(31-54C)** Sagittal T1WI in the same patient shows an atrophic brain and large chronic SDHs (cSDH). Note the tortuous "flow void" of the basilar artery within the enlarged premedullary cistern. **(31-54D)** Coronal T2WI in the same patient shows large cSDHs. Note the tortuous basilar artery and numerous cortical vessels in enlarged sylvian fissures. Profound brain atrophy and large SASs are seen.*

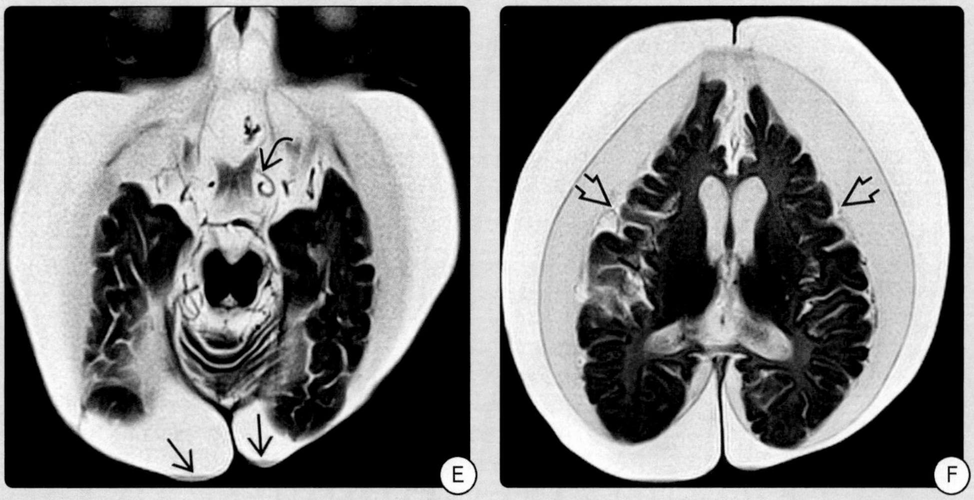

***(31-54E)** Axial T2WI of Menkes shows tortuous vessels. Marked brain atrophy and small dependent hematohygromas are seen. **(31-54F)** Axial T2WI shows the extremely atrophic brain, membrane containing cSDHs, inwardly displaced arachnoid. This is Menkes disease ("kinky hair, kinky vessels"). The severe brain atrophy, subdural fluid collections are typical, as is the excessive tortuosity of the intracranial arteries.*

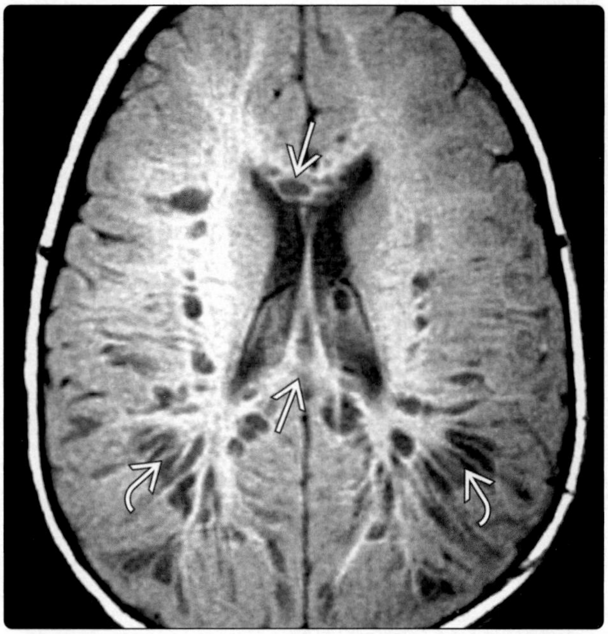

(31-55) T1WI in a toddler with MPS 1H (Hurler disease) shows markedly enlarged WM PVSs, including the corpus callosum .

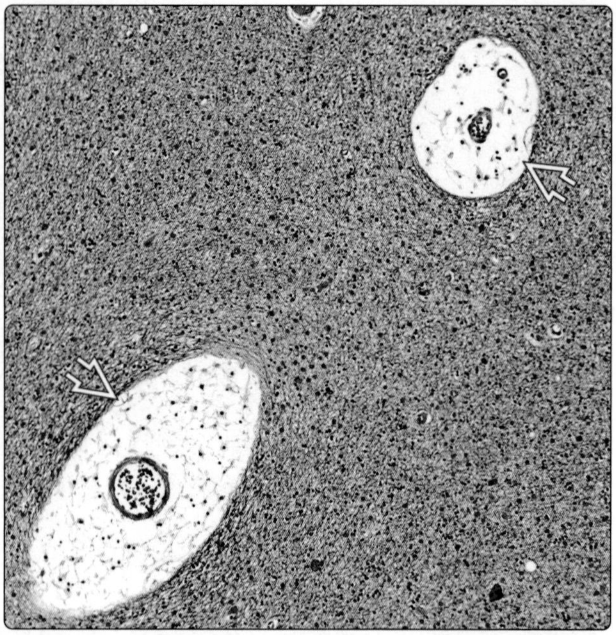

(31-56) MPS 1HS (Hurler-Scheie) myelin stain shows large PVSs packed with undegraded mucopolysaccharides. (Courtesy P. Shannon, MD.)

The two distinctive gross features of the MPSs are thickened meninges and dilated perivascular spaces (PVSs). The enlarged PVSs give a cribriform appearance to the brain on both pathology and imaging **(31-52)** **(31-55)**.

Microscopically, the MPSs are characterized by dilated PVSs packed with undegraded GAG **(31-56)**. GAG infiltrates the leptomeninges and ligaments as well.

Clinical Issues

Each MPS subtype has different clinical phenotypes. Clinical observations include macrocrania, coarse facies, bushy eyebrows, macroglossia, flat nasal bridge, hepatosplenomegaly, and skeletal dysostoses. Age at presentation varies, as do sex predilection and prognosis based on the inherited MPS type.

Hurler (MPS 1H) and Hunter (MPS 2) diseases are two of the most common "prototypical" MPSs. Hurler patients appear normal at birth but soon develop CNS symptoms, including delayed development and mental retardation. Untreated Hurler disease typically results in death by age 10.

MPS 2 (Hunter disease) is an X-linked disorder and is seen only in male patients. Hunter disease is characterized by progressive multisystem involvement in the CNS, joints, bones, heart, skin, liver, eyes, and other organs. Patients often survive into their mid teens but usually expire from cardiac disease.

Therapy for MPS includes bone marrow transplant and IV recombinant enzyme replacement therapies (i.e., α-L-iduronidase for MPS 1H).

Imaging

The prototypical imaging findings in MPSs are illustrated by Hurler (MPS 1H) and Hunter (MPS 2) diseases. The major features of these disorders are macrocephaly, frontal calvarial bossing, J-shaped sella, enlarged PVSs, WM abnormalities, pachymeningopathy, rosette formation of impacted teeth, broad ribs, dysostosis multiplex, and trident hands.

Macrocephaly. NECT and MR scans show an enlarged head, often with metopic "beaking" and scaphocephalic configuration **(31-57)**. Reduced attenuation of WM, progressive hydrocephalus, and atrophy of Virchow-Robin spaces are rarely seen on NECT. Sagittal MR scans also demonstrate a large head with craniofacial disproportion. Pannus of ligaments at craniocervical junction can be seen.

Enlarged Perivascular Spaces and WM Abnormalities. A striking sieve-like cribriform appearance in the posterior cerebral WM and corpus callosum is characteristic and is caused by numerous dilated PVSs **(31-55)** **(31-57)** **(31-58)** **(31-59)** **(31-61)**. Although sometimes called "Hurler holes," these enlarged PVSs are typical of both Hurler and Hunter diseases. They are much less common in the other MPSs.

NECT scans *may show* decreased attenuation with multifocal CSF-like regions in the WM and basal ganglia **(31-57)**.

T2 scans show CSF-like hyperintensity in the enlarged PVSs. The surrounding WM may show patchy or confluent hyperintensity. The PVSs themselves suppress completely on FLAIR **(31-58)** **(31-59C)**. A faint "halo" of hyperintensity often surrounds the lesions. Some MPS types (MPS 3A) demonstrate subtle enlargement of the PVSs.

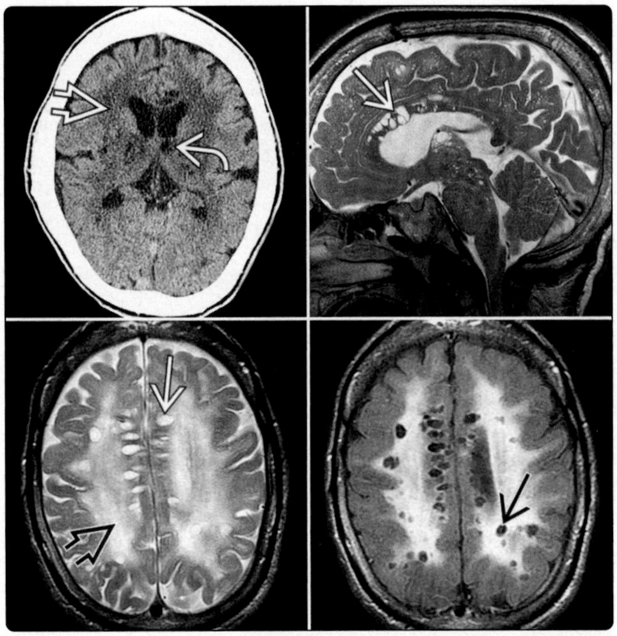

(31-57) NECT of Hunter disease shows WM ➡ and focal BG hypoattenuating lesions ➡. T2WI shows enlarged PVSs in corpus callosum ➡ and confluent WM disease ⇨. PVSs suppress on FLAIR ⇨; the WM disease remains hyperintense. This is MPS 2.

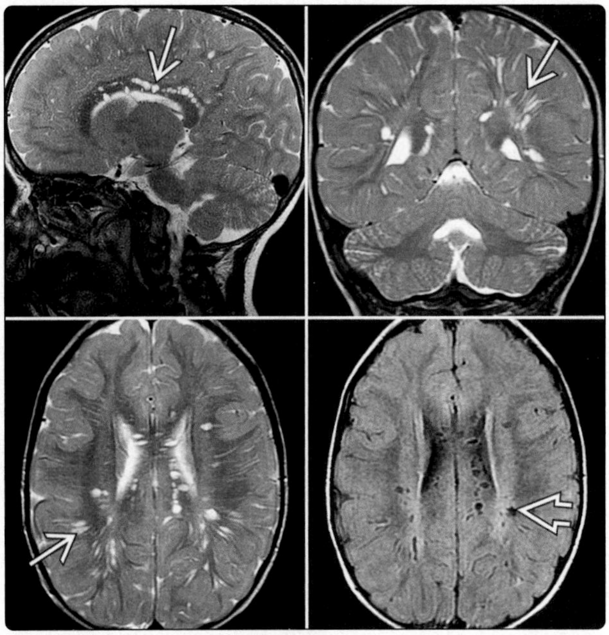

(31-58) Sagittal, coronal, axial T2 scans in a 2y boy with Hunter disease show multiple enlarged PVSs ➡. Note the posterior predominance and corpus callosum involvement. The lesions suppress on FLAIR ➡. This is MPS 2.

The enlarged PVSs do not "bloom" on T2* and do not enhance following contrast administration. These may be subtle in MPS 3A **(31-59)** **(31-61)**.

There is a linear correlation between the severity of WM abnormality and the cognitive impairment and developmental delay.

Pachymeningopathy. The meninges, especially around the craniovertebral junction, are often thickened and appear very hypointense on T2-weighted images **(31-60)**. In severe cases, the thickened meninges can compress the medulla or upper cervical cord. Odontoid dysplasia and a short C1 posterior arch—common in the MPSs—can exacerbate the craniovertebral junction stenosis, causing progressive myelopathy. A lumbar gibbus with a "beaked" L1 vertebral body is common in Hurler disease. The practical consideration here is to always assess the craniocervical junction for level and degree of compression and to image infants under an anesthesiologist's supervision to avoid sudden death.

Differential Diagnosis

The differential diagnosis of MPS is limited. **Prominent PVSs** can be normal findings in patients of any age. Although they can be seen in children and even infants, prominent PVSs are more common in middle-aged and older patients. No macrocephaly is present with this normal variant.

Dilated PVSs with a frontal predominance are a feature of **velocardiofacial syndrome**. Deviated carotid arteries in the pharynx are present, a finding not associated with the MPSs. **Hypomelanosis of Ito** may show dilated PVSs. Cutaneous hypopigmented zones with irregular borders are seen; seizures usually develop in the first year of life.

Canavan Disease

Canavan disease (CD) is a fatal autosomal-recessive neurodegenerative disorder for which there is currently no effective treatment. CD is the only identified genetic disorder caused by a defect in a metabolite—*N*-acetyl-L-aspartate (NAA)—that is produced exclusively in the brain.

Terminology

CD is also known as spongiform leukodystrophy, spongy degeneration of the CNS, aspartoacylase deficiency, aminoacylase 2 deficiency, and Canavan-van Bogaert-Bertrand disease.

Etiology

NAA is the second most abundant amino acid in the mammalian brain. NAA levels in the brain are normally maintained within a tightly regulated range. Aspartoacylase—the enzyme responsible for metabolizing NAA—is a signature marker of mature oligodendrocytes. Mutations in the *ASPA* gene, located on the long arm of chromosome 17, cause abnormal NAA accumulation in the brain and result in CD.

The how and why of excessive NAA, causing intramyelinic edema and myelin damage associated with CD, are unknown.

Pathology

The brain in CD appears grossly swollen. Microscopic analysis shows spongiform WM degeneration with swollen astrocytes in the globi pallidi and thalami.

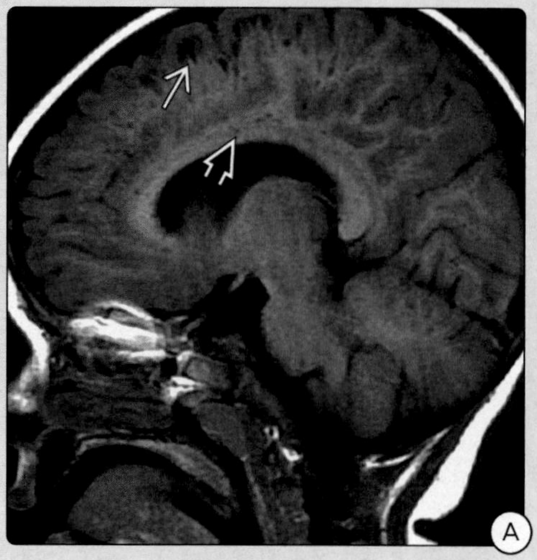

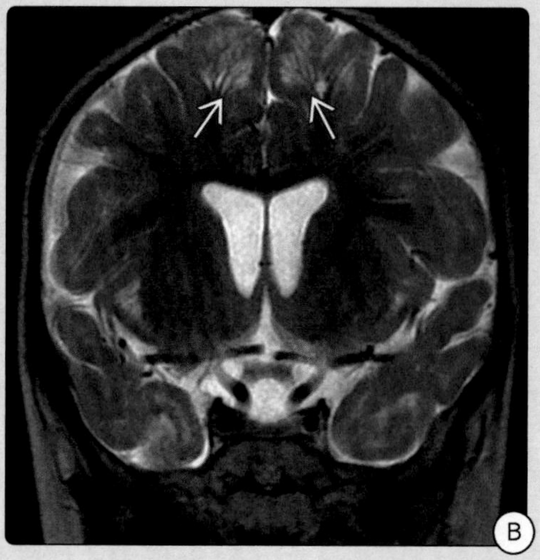

(31-59A) *Sagittal T1WI shows a 2y boy with MPS 3A with course facies, frontal bossing, and large subcortical* ➡ *and corpus callosum* ➡ *PVSs.* ***(31-59B)*** *Coronal T2WI in the same patient shows subtle frontal subcortical enlarged PVSs* ➡*. MPS 3A may have subtle MR findings.*

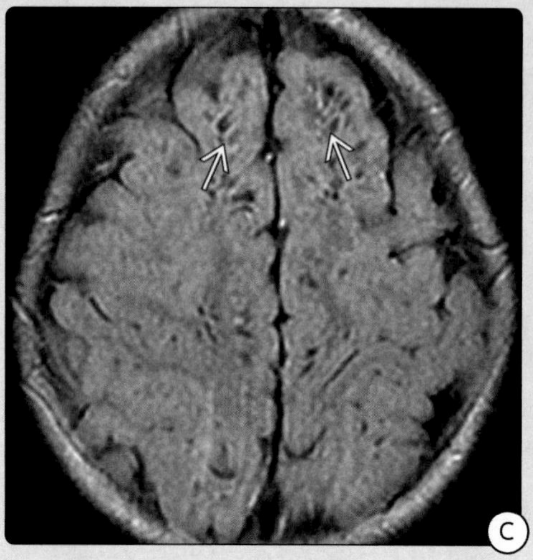

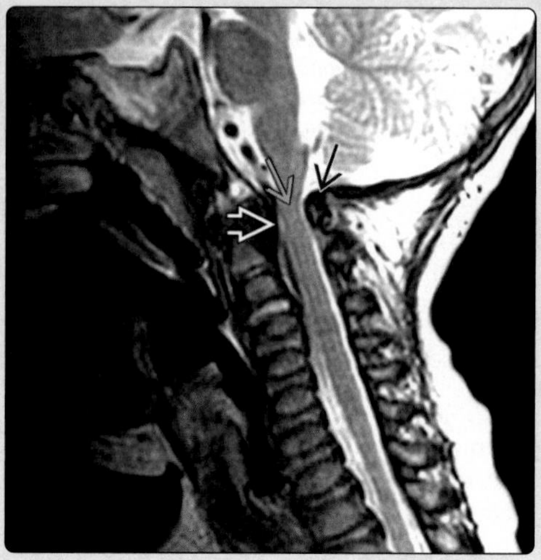

(31-59C) *Axial FLAIR in the same MPS 3A patient shows numerous enlarged hypointense PVSs* ➡*.* ***(31-60)*** *Sagittal T2WI in a patient with MPS 1H shows foramen magnum narrowing and cord compression* ⇨*. The CVJ narrowing is caused by a combination of a short posterior C1 arch* ⇨*, odontoid dysplasia, and thickened ligaments* ➡*.*

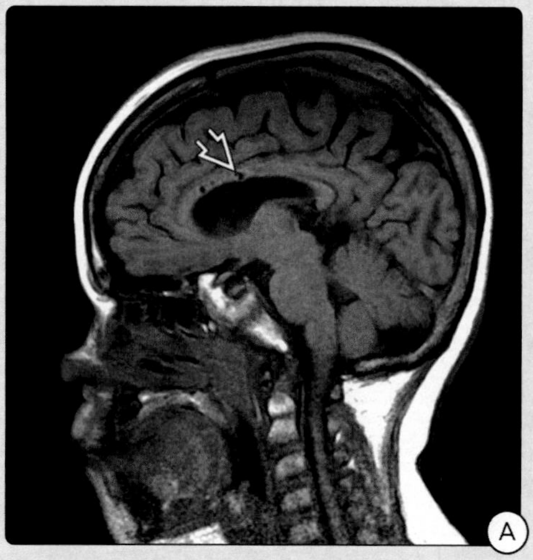

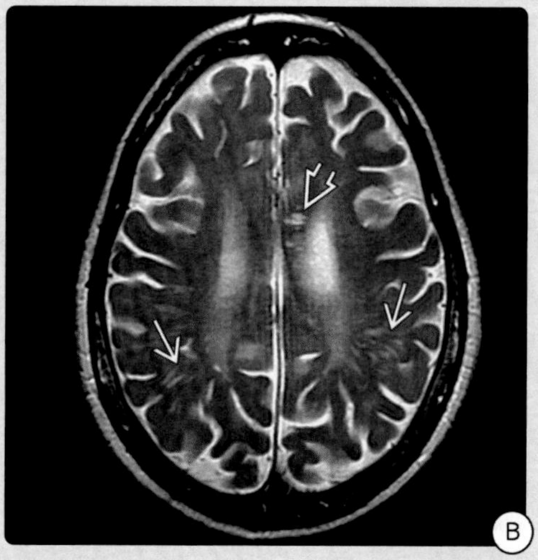

(31-61A) *Sagittal T1WI in a 4y child with MPS 3A (Sanfillipo) shows enlarged PVSs within the anterior body of the corpus callosum* ➡*.* ***(31-61B)*** *Axial T2WI in the same patient shows hyperintense enlarged PVSs in the corpus callosum* ➡ *and parietal WM* ➡*. Note the convexity sulcal prominence due to volume loss.*

Clinical Issues

CD is most common in Ashkenazi Jews and rare in other non-Jewish populations. One in 40 Ashkenazi Jews carries the mutated *ASPA* gene. There is no sex predilection.

Three clinical variants of CD are recognized. The *congenital form* presents within the first few days of life and leads to profound hypotonia with poor head control. Death rapidly ensues. The most common form by far is *infantile CD.* Infantile CD presents between 3 and 6 months and is characterized by hypotonia, macrocephaly, and seizures. Death between 1 and 2 years is typical. *Juvenile-onset CD* begins between 4 and 5 years of age and is the most slowly progressive form.

Imaging

NECT shows a large head with diffuse WM hypoattenuation in the cerebral hemispheres and cerebellum. The globi pallidi also appear hypoattenuating. CD does not enhance.

MR eventually shows virtually complete absence of myelination with confluent T2/FLAIR hyperintensity throughout the WM and globi pallidi. These involved regions show T1 prolongation. Early in the disease course, the subcortical arcuate fibers are initially affected, and the gyri may appear swollen **(31-62)**. Early occipital WM T2/FLAIR hyperintensity is observed. As the disease progresses, diffuse volume loss with ventricular and sulcal enlargement ensues. The hemispheric and cerebellar WM, basal ganglia, and cortex are all extensively affected. DWI reveals bright DWI signal with normal to reduced ADC values in the involved areas.

MRS is the key to the definitive imaging diagnosis of CD. Markedly elevated NAA is seen in virtually all cases **(31-63)**. Cr is reduced. An elevated myoinositol peak is sometimes present. The choline/creatine (Ch/Cr) ratio is reduced.

Differential Diagnosis

The major differential diagnosis of CD is **Alexander disease**. Both CD and Alexander disease cause macrocephaly, but an elevated NAA peak on MRS distinguishes the two disorders. Furthermore, Alexander disease exhibits a frontal WM predilection and enhancement; CD does neither.

Megalencephaly with leukoencephalopathy and cysts involves the subcortical arcuate fibers, as does CD; however, the basal ganglia are not affected. **Pelizaeus-Merzbacher disease** demonstrates virtually complete lack of myelination but does not cause macrocephaly and does not affect the basal ganglia. ADC values are increased. **Merosin-deficient congenital muscular dystrophy** spares involvement of the GP and thalami and demonstrates increased ADC values.

Alexander Disease

Terminology

Alexander disease (AxD) is also known as fibrinoid leukodystrophy, a misnomer given that it involves both white and gray matter.

Etiology

AxD patients have de novo heterozygous dominant mutations in the *GFAP* gene (17q21) in more than 95% of cases. *GFAP* encodes for glial fibrillary acidic protein, an intermediate filament protein that is expressed only in astrocytes. The parents of patients with infantile- or childhood-onset AxD are neurologically normal.

GFAP mutations cause precipitation and accumulation of mutant GFAP aggregates, which begins during fetal development.

Pathology

The brains of infants with AxD have markedly increased astrocytic density and are grossly enlarged. Dramatic myelin loss in the hemispheres, brainstem, cerebellum, and spinal cord makes the WM—especially in the frontal lobes—appear very pale. In severe cases, the WM appears partially or almost entirely cystic. The subcortical arcuate fibers are relatively spared. Cortical thinning with basal ganglia and thalamic atrophy is common.

The hallmark histopathologic feature of AxD is the presence of enormous numbers of Rosenthal fibers (RFs) in astrocytes. RFs are ovoid or rod-shaped eosinophilic cytoplasmic inclusion bodies. The striking lack of nearly all myelin in AxD is considered a secondary phenomenon that arises from severely disrupted astrocyte-derived myelination signaling.

Clinical Issues

AxD is rare, accounting for just 1-2% of childhood inherited leukodystrophies.

Three clinical forms are recognized: infantile, juvenile, and adult. In the infantile form, which is the most common, patients younger than 2 years present with megalencephaly, progressive psychomotor retardation, and seizures. Spasticity and eventually quadriplegia often develop. All forms eventually lead to death. Care is supportive.

Juvenile AxD presents between ages 2-12 years and is characterized by bulbar and cerebellar signs. Patients over the age of 12 years present with a variety of signs and symptoms, including ataxia, bulbar signs, and cognitive decline. Palatal myoclonus occurs in 40% of adult AxD cases.

Disease progression is variable. Patients with adult-onset AxD have a slower, more protracted course. Although imaging findings can be suggestive of the disease, the diagnosis of AxD is confirmed by increased GFAP CSF levels or *GFAP* gene analysis.

Imaging

NECT scans of infants with AxD show a large head with symmetric WM hypoattenuation in the frontal lobes that extends posteriorly into the caudate nuclei and internal/external capsules **(31-64A)**. AxD is one of the few IMDs that demonstrates enhancement following contrast. The other is X-ALD. Intense bifrontal periventricular enhancement can be seen on CECT scans early in the disease course.

MR shows macrocephaly, T1 hypointensity, and T2/FLAIR hyperintensity involving the frontal WM, caudate nuclei, and anterior putamina. Although infantile AxD involves the subcortical U-fibers early in the disease course, the periventricular WM is more severely affected in the juvenile and adults forms. A classic finding is a T1 hypointense, T2 hyperintense rim around the frontal horns. FLAIR scans may demonstrate cystic encephalomalacia in the frontal WM in more severe, protracted cases **(31-64)**.

A unique finding in AxD is enlargement of the caudate heads and fornices, which appear swollen and hyperintense. The thalami, globi pallidi, brainstem, and cerebellum are less commonly affected **(31-64B)**.

Unlike most IMDs, AxD can demonstrate moderate to striking enhancement on T1 C+. Rims of intense enhancement can be seen around the surfaces of the swollen caudate nuclei and affected frontal lobe WM **(31-64A)**. In the juvenile and adult forms, brainstem and cerebellar involvement can be striking and may even mimic a neoplasm.

MRS shows decreased NAA, elevated myoinositol, with variable choline and lactate. DWI shows normal to increased diffusivity in the affected WM.

Differential Diagnosis

The major differential diagnoses of AxD are other inherited leukodystrophies with macrocephaly. These primarily include **Canavan disease** and the **mucopolysaccharidoses**. Although both AxD and Canavan disease show almost complete lack of myelination with T2/FLAIR WM hyperintensity, the predilection of AxD for the frontal lobes, caudate heads, and enhancement helps distinguish it from Canavan disease.

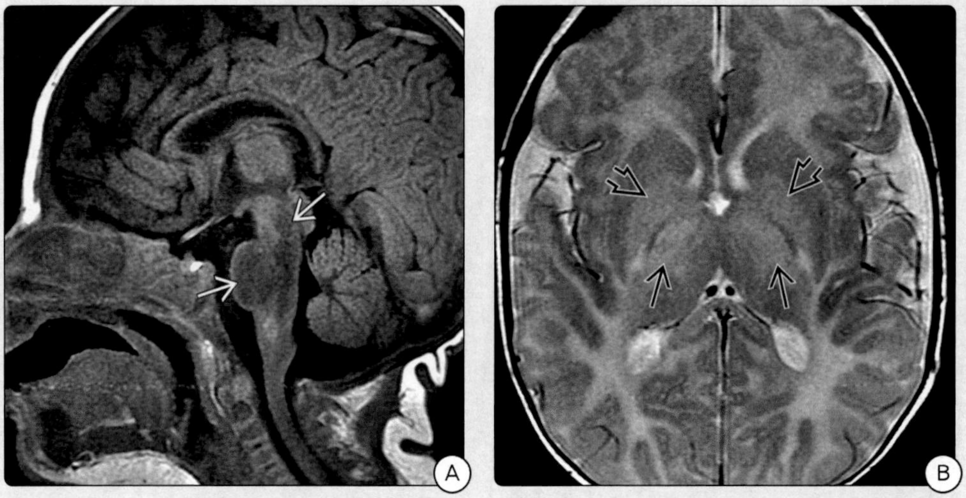

***(31-62A)** Sagittal T1WI in a 6y boy with Canavan disease shows hypointense "swollen" brainstem ➡ (i.e., spongiform degeneration). **(31-62B)** Axial T2WI in the same patient shows diffuse hyperintensity throughout the WM. Note the hyperintense globi pallidi ⇨ and thalami ⇨, representing involved WM tracts.*

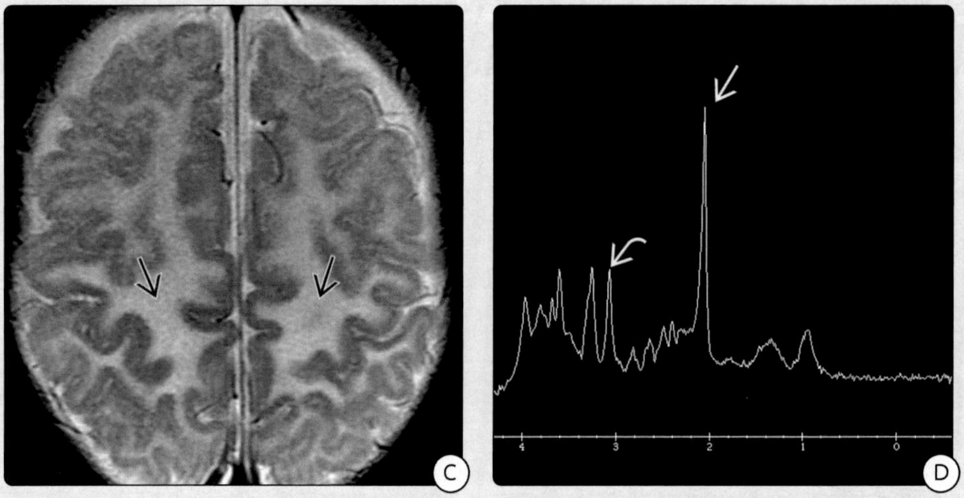

***(31-62C)** Axial T2WI in the same patient shows completely absent myelination and diffuse WM hyperintensity ⇨. **(31-62D)** Long TE MRS (i.e., 288 ms) shows an amplified NAA resonance at 2.0 ppm ➡. There is a reduction in the creatine peak ➡.*

DIFFERENTIAL DIAGNOSIS: CHILD WITH A LARGE HEAD

Common
- Normal variant
- Benign familial macrocrania
- Benign macrocrania of infancy

Less Common
- Nonaccidental trauma with subdural hematomas

Rare But Important
- Inherited metabolic disorder
  - Canavan disease
  - Alexander disease
  - Mucopolysaccharidoses
  - Megalencephaly with leukoencephalopathy and cysts
  - Glutaric aciduria type 1

The mucopolysaccharidoses, especially Hurler and Hunter diseases, display a striking "cribriform" appearance of the WM and corpus callosum caused by enlarged perivascular spaces. Deep gray involvement is absent, and the lesions do not enhance. Some of the MPSs—especially MPS-1—cause dural thickening, which is absent in AxD.

Megalencephaly with leukoencephalopathy and cysts has striking subcortical arcuate involvement early in the disease course, does not involve the basal ganglia, and does not enhance. **Glutaric aciduria type 1** shows characteristic widening of the lateral cerebral fissures, symmetric BG involvement, no enhancement, and periventricular WM involvement in severe cases.

Peroxisomal Biogenesis Disorders

Peroxisomes are small single-membrane-bound organelles that contain over 50 enzymes required for normal growth, development, and cellular metabolism. Biosynthesis of

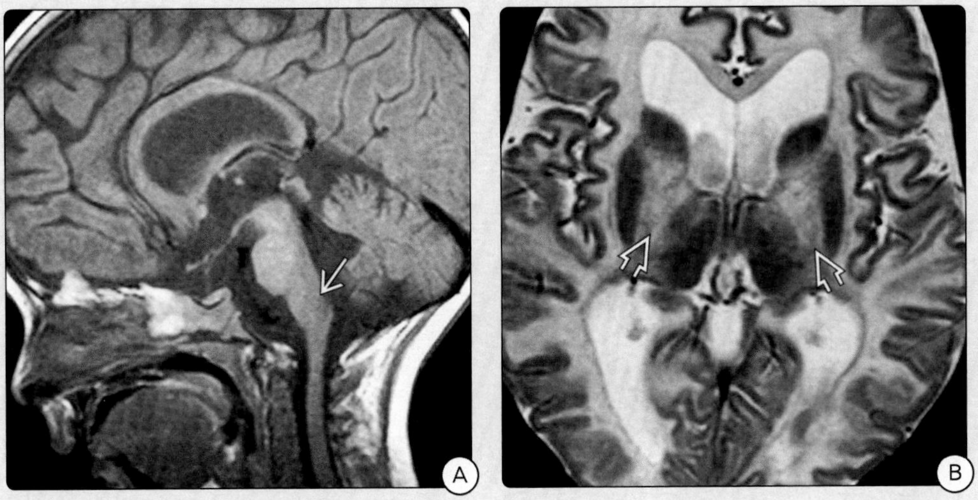

***(31-63A)** Sagittal T1WI in a 2y boy with Canavan disease shows macrocephaly. Volume loss involves the cerebral hemispheres and cerebellum. Note the swollen lower brainstem →. **(31-63B)** Axial T2WI shows diffuse WM hyperintensity throughout the WM, indicating complete absence of myelination. The globi pallidi → are hyperintense and shrunken.*

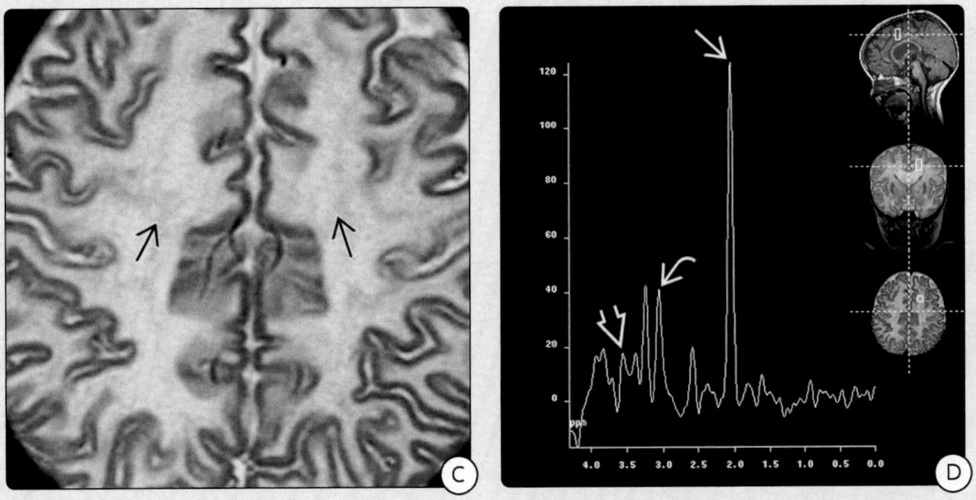

***(31-63C)** T2WI through the corona radiata in the same patient shows the virtually complete absence of myelination (hyperintense WM) →. The cortex appears thinned, and the sulci are enlarged. **(31-63D)** Multivoxel MRS of the WM with TE = 135 ms shows a markedly elevated NAA peak resonating at 2.0 ppm →. Cr → is significantly reduced. A small myoinositol peak → is present.*

(31-64A) Axial NECT in a 6m boy with macrocephaly and AxD shows anterior more than posterior WM hypoattenuation. (31-64B) Axial T1 C+ scan shows striking differentiation between the exceptionally hypointense frontal WM and the more normal-appearing parietooccipital WM. The hypointensity extends into the external capsules. Note the characteristic enhancing rims around the frontal horns.

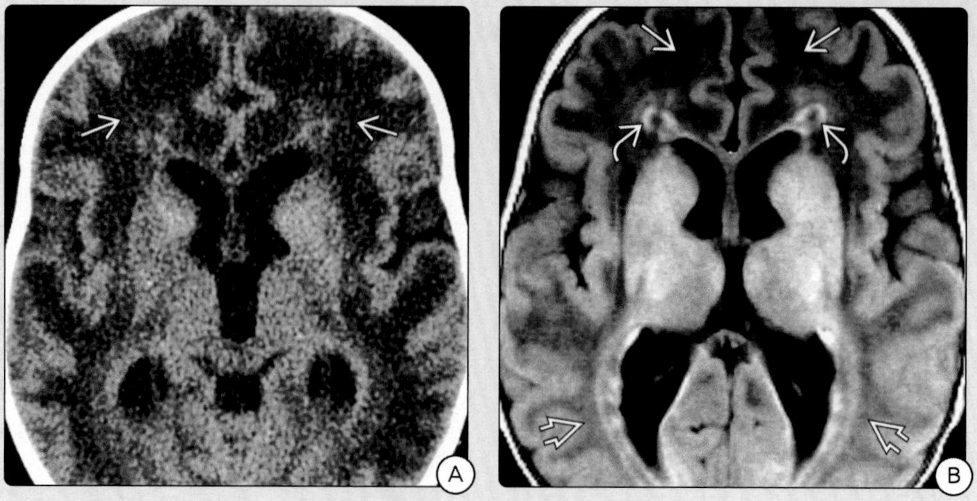

(31-64C) Axial T2WI shows hyperintense frontal WM; the parietooccipital WM is less involved on T2WI. Note external capsule involvement. The internal capsules are partially myelinated and thus appear less hyperintense than the frontal WM. The hypointense rim around the frontal horns is characteristic. (31-64D) Axial T1 C+ shows enhancement in the periventricular WM and basal ganglia.

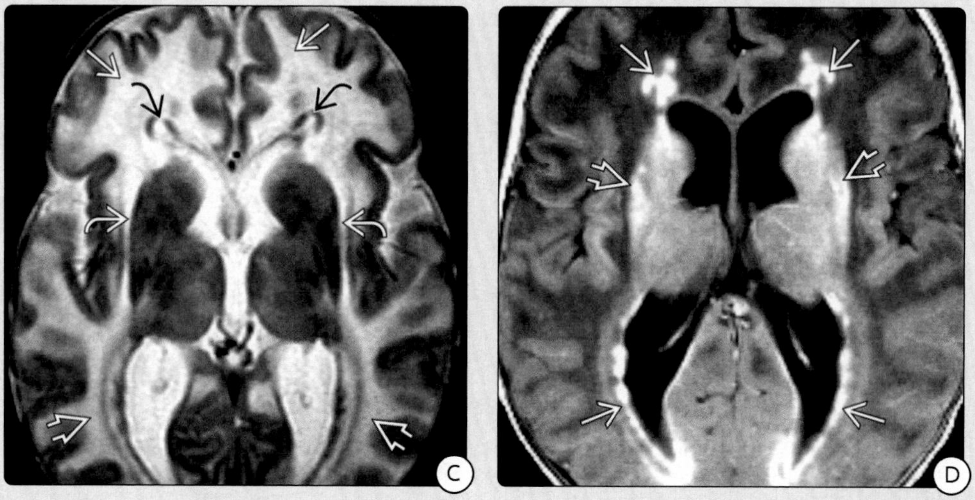

(31-64E) Coronal T1 C+ scan shows striking enhancement of the deep periventricular WM and basal ganglia. (31-64F) Sagittal T1 C+ scan displays enhancement of virtually all the deep periventricular WM and striking hypointensity of the frontal and anterior parietal WM with relative sparing of the occipital lobe.

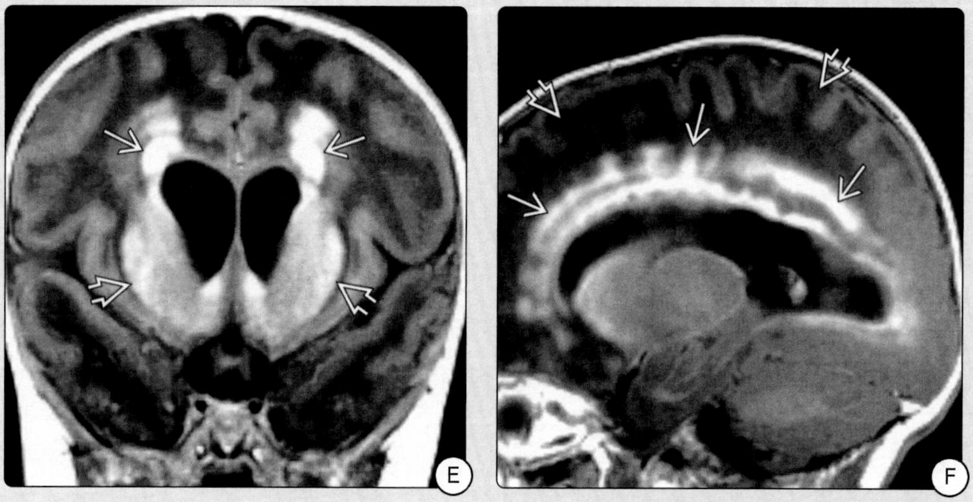

plasmalogens and β-oxidation of very-long-chain fatty acids (VLCFAs) are among the essential functions of peroxisomes. Genetic defects that affect either peroxisomal formation or enzymatic function cause a group of diseases called peroxisomal disorders.

Terminology

Synonyms are cerebrohepatorenal syndrome and Zellweger syndrome spectrum (ZSS). There are two main types of peroxisomal disorders. The most common type is caused by *single protein deficiencies within intact (morphologically normal) peroxisomes.* This group includes, among others, X-linked adrenoleukodystrophy (ALD), adrenomyeloneuropathy (AMN), and classic (adult) Refsum disease. ALD and AMN affect periventricular WM and were discussed earlier in the chapter.

The second less common group of peroxisomal disorders caused by *abnormal formation of peroxisomes* is discussed below. Disorders in which the peroxisomal organelles themselves fail to form normally are called peroxisomal biogenesis disorders (PBDs). PBDs are typically characterized by multiple (not single) enzymatic defects.

Four major PBDs are recognized: **Zellweger syndrome** (ZS, also called cerebrohepatorenal syndrome), neonatal adrenoleukodystrophy, infantile Refsum disease, and classic rhizomelic chondrodysplasia punctata. The first three disorders are grouped together and referred to as **Zellweger syndrome spectrum** (ZSS).

Etiology

PBDs are autosomal-recessive disorders caused by mutations in one of 13 peroxisomal assembly (*PEX*) genes. The most severe form is ZSS, which accounts for 80% of all cases and is characterized by nearly complete absence of peroxisomes.

Pathology

PBDs are characterized pathologically by germinal matrix injury, subependymal germinolytic cysts, disordered neuronal migration, and hypomyelination.

The most common gross findings are cerebral neocortical and cerebellar abnormalities. Brain atrophy and abnormal gyration—most often pachygyria or polymicrogyria—are common in patients with severe ZSS **(31-65)**. Defective peroxisomes in oligodendroglial cells also cause abnormal WM formation and maintenance.

Clinical Issues

PBDs are less common than many other inherited metabolic disorders. The estimated incidence is 1:20,000-100,000 live births. In contrast to ALD, there is no sex predilection.

The PBDs are clinically diverse, but frequent features include dysmorphic facies with large fontanelle and sutures, high forehead, and broad nasal bridge. Hepatointestinal dysfunction, hypotonia ("floppy infant"), seizures, retinitis pigmentosa, and psychomotor retardation are common.

The disease course of different PBDs varies considerably. The most severely affected neonates with ZS typically die by 6 months of age, whereas those with milder forms of the disease may survive more than 20 years.

Imaging

Imaging in PBDs is variable, but the most common features are disordered neuronal migration and abnormal myelination. ZSS is known by microgyria and pachygyria, often with bilaterally symmetric parasylvian lesions. Hypomyelinated WM is seen as confluent T2/FLAIR WM hyperintensity. Subependymal (caudothalamic) germinolytic cysts are common findings **(31-66)**. Hyperbilirubinemia may cause increased T1 signal intensity in the globi pallidi of older patients. T1WI C+ may show enhancement within the corticospinal tracts of the brainstem. MRS demonstrates lipid peaks on short TE sequences (i.e., TE 35 ms) between 0.80 and 1.33 ppm, reduced NAA, and increased Cho.

Differential Diagnosis

The major differential diagnosis of ZSS is **congenital cytomegalovirus** (CMV). Both ZSS and congenital CMV exhibit hypomyelination and cortical malformations. Calcifications are a more prominent feature of CMV, particularly along the caudostriatal groove, and the periventricular cysts (particularly anterior temporal) are strongly suggestive of CMV. Isolated **neuronal migration disorders** (e.g., bilateral perisylvian polymicrogyria) occur without other clinical and imaging stigmata of ZSS. **Pseudo-TORCH** shows basal ganglia, brainstem, thalamic, and periventricular Ca++. In pseudo-TORCH, the clinical course is that of progressive neurologic deterioration.

Mitochondrial Diseases (Respiratory Chain Disorders)

The mitochondria are cellular organelles that are the "power plants" responsible for energy production. Five complexes are embedded in the inner mitochondrial membrane and are responsible for oxidative phosphorylation (OXPHOS); defects in any one result in defective OXPHOS and deficient ATP production.

Mitochondrial disorders are caused by mitochondrial DNA (mtDNA) mutations and are among the most common of all IMDs. Although virtually every organ or tissue of the body can be affected, the nervous system and skeletal muscle are especially vulnerable because of their high energy demands.

Four major encephalomyopathic syndromes have been described and are considered here: *Leigh syndrome, Kearns-Sayre syndrome, MELAS,* and *MERRF.* We then discuss glutaric aciduria types 1 and 2, also caused by mtDNA-mediated enzyme abnormalities. Other mitochondrial disorders—including Alpers syndrome, infantile mitochondrial myopathy, and Leber hereditary optic neuropathy (LHON)—are very rare and not examined further in this text.

Mitochondrial disorders have significant clinical and imaging overlap and are challenging to distinguish from each other.

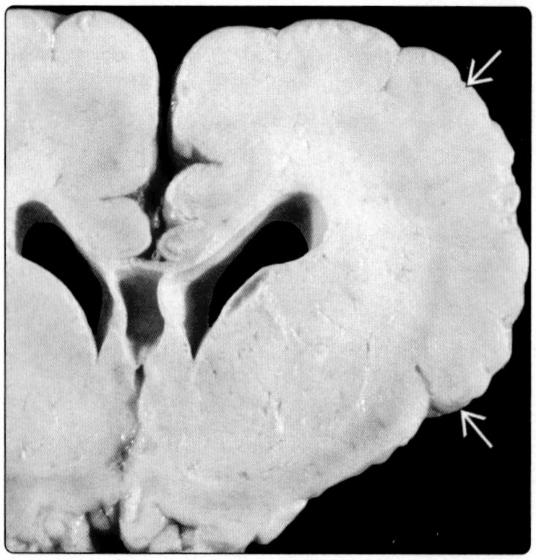

(31-65) Coronal autopsy specimen of ZSS shows abnormal gyration with pachy-, polymicrogyria ➡, poor sulcation. (Courtesy AFIP Archives.)

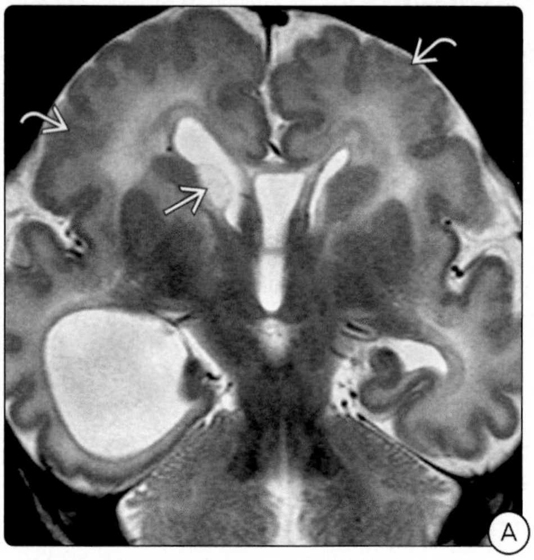

(31-66A) Coronal T2WI in newborn with ZSS shows a germinolytic cyst ➡ and several areas of polymicrogyria ➡.

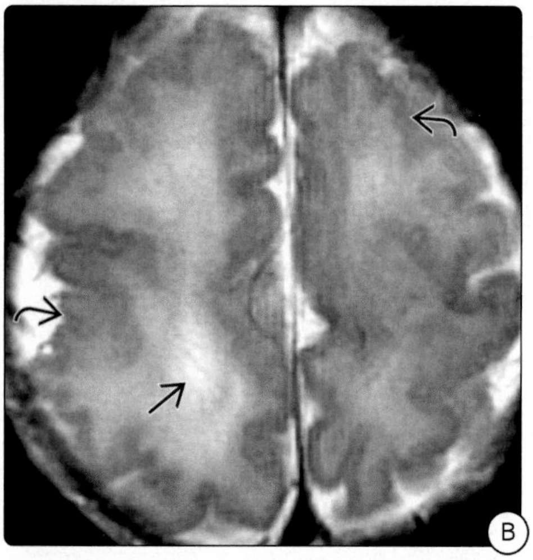

(31-66B) Axial T2WI in the same patient shows diffuse microgyria ➡ and foci of abnormal WM hyperintensity ➡.

Leigh Syndrome

Terminology and Etiology. Leigh syndrome (LS) is also known as subacute necrotizing encephalopathy. LS is caused by mutations that encode for OXPHOS enzymes, a group of disorders caused by defective terminal oxidative metabolism.

Pathology. LS demonstrates brownish gray gelatinous or cavitary foci within the basal ganglia, brainstem, dentate nuclei, thalami, and spinal cord with variable WM spongiform degeneration and demyelination.

Clinical Issues. Clinical manifestations of LS are variable. Most patients with LS present in infancy or childhood with failure to thrive, central hypotonia, developmental regression, ataxia, bulbar dysfunction, and ophthalmoplegia. Serum and/or CSF lactate levels are increased.

Imaging. MR in LS shows bilaterally symmetric areas of T2/FLAIR hyperintensity (often *speckled)* in the basal ganglia **(31-67)**. The putamina (especially the posterior segments) are consistently affected, as are the caudate heads. The dorsomedial thalami can also be involved, whereas the globi pallidi are less commonly affected. Acute lesions show swelling of the basal ganglia.

Mid and lower brainstem (pons/medulla) lesions are typical in LS and in a few cases can be the *only* finding. Symmetric lesions in the cerebral peduncles are common, and the periaqueductal gray matter is frequently affected. Brainstem lesions are especially common in cytochrome-C oxidase deficiency.

Acute lesions restrict on DWI but do not enhance. MRS of the brain and CSF typically shows a lactate doublet at 1.3 ppm. Lactate resonates above baseline at short (35 ms) and long (288 ms) TEs and inverts at an intermediate TE (144 ms).

Differential Diagnosis. As their imaging findings often overlap, the differential diagnosis of LS includes the other mitochondrial encephalomyopathies. **MELAS** typically shows stroke-like abnormalities in the cortical gray matter in a nonvascular distribution in the hemispheres, peripheral in location and often crossing vascular territories and sparing underlying white matter.

Metabolic and hypoxic-ischemic disease can mimic some findings of LS. **Wilson disease** (WD) shows T2/FLAIR hyperintensity in the putamina, midbrain, and thalami. The globi pallidi in WD often show T1 shortening secondary to hepatic failure. **Perinatal asphyxia (HII)** can affect the basal ganglia and mimic LS, and the corticospinal tracts and perirolandic cortex are commonly affected.

MELAS

Terminology and Etiology. Mitochondrial **e**ncephalomyopathy with **l**actic **a**cidosis and **s**troke-like episodes (MELAS) is caused by several different point mutations. A mitochondrial tRNA mutation at nucleotide 3.243 is found in most patients with MELAS.

Clinical Issues. The clinical triad of lactic acidosis, seizures, and stroke-like episodes is the classic presentation, but other common symptoms include progressive sensorineural hearing loss, migraines, episodic vomiting, alternating hemiplegia, and progressive brain injury. Cardiac abnormalities, renal dysfunction, GI motility disorders, and generalized muscle weakness are also common. The diagnosis of MELAS should always be considered when encountering an atypical stroke and encephalitis of seizure presentation with diffusion and DWI.

Abnormal mitochondria have been found in the arterial walls of MELAS patients, implicating a vasculogenic etiology. MELAS is an uncommon but important cause of childhood stroke. The prevalence is approximately 1.2-13.0 cases/100,000 live births. Mean age at symptom onset is 15 years, although some patients may not become symptomatic until 40-50 years of age.

Imaging. Imaging findings vary with disease acuity **(31-68)**. *Acute* MELAS often shows swollen T2/FLAIR hyperintense gyri. The underlying WM is normal, and the cortical abnormalities cross vascular distribution territories, distinguishing MELAS from acute cerebral infarction **(31-69)**. The parietal and occipital lobes are most commonly affected **(31-70C)**. The appearance of *strokes of differing ages* is often a clue to the diagnosis of MELAS. Gyral enhancement on T1 C+ is typical. Abnormal cortical vein T2/FLAIR signal hyperintensity has been reported in MELAS patients, perhaps representing vessel wall thickening and/or sluggish flow. MRA in MELAS shows no evidence of major vessel occlusion.

Chronic MELAS shows multifocal lacunar-type infarcts, symmetric basal ganglia calcifications, WM volume loss, and progressive atrophy of the parietooccipital cortex.

MRS is extremely helpful in the diagnosis of most mitochondrial encephalopathies. Nearly two-thirds of cases with MELAS show a prominent lactate "doublet" at 1.3 ppm in otherwise normal-appearing brain **(31-70D)**. **Caution**: one-third of cases show no evidence for elevated lactate levels in the brain parenchyma but may demonstrate a lactate peak in the ventricular CSF.

Differential Diagnosis. The differential diagnosis of MELAS includes major territorial **cerebral infarction**. MELAS spares the subcortical and deep WM and *crosses vascular territories* (often the middle and posterior cerebral distributions). **Prolonged seizures** can cause gyral swelling, hyperintensity,

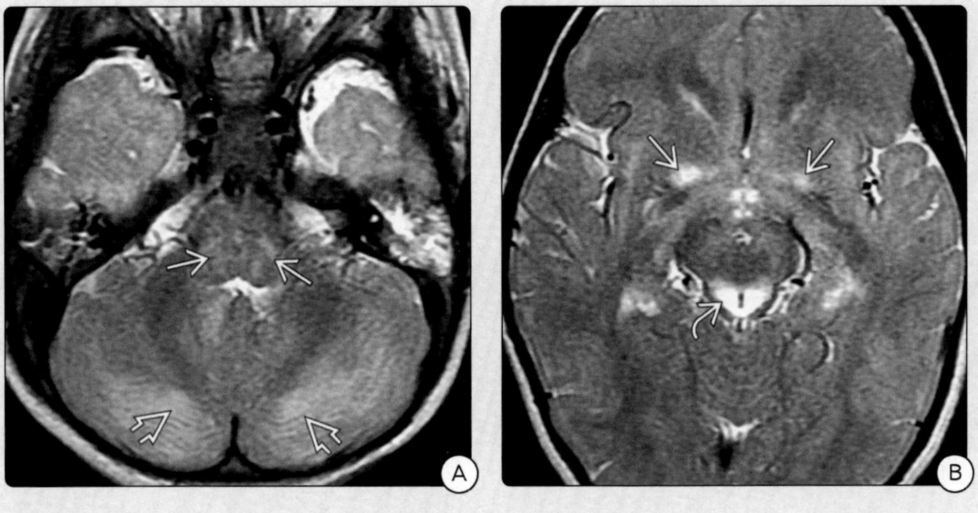

***(31-67A)** Axial T2WI in a 19y woman with Leigh syndrome shows bilaterally symmetric hyperintensities in the white matter of both cerebellar hemispheres ➡ and medulla ➡. **(31-67B)** Axial T2WI, more cephalad, in the same patient shows striking hyperintensity in the periaqueductal gray matter ➡. Note the globi pallidi hyperintensities ➡.*

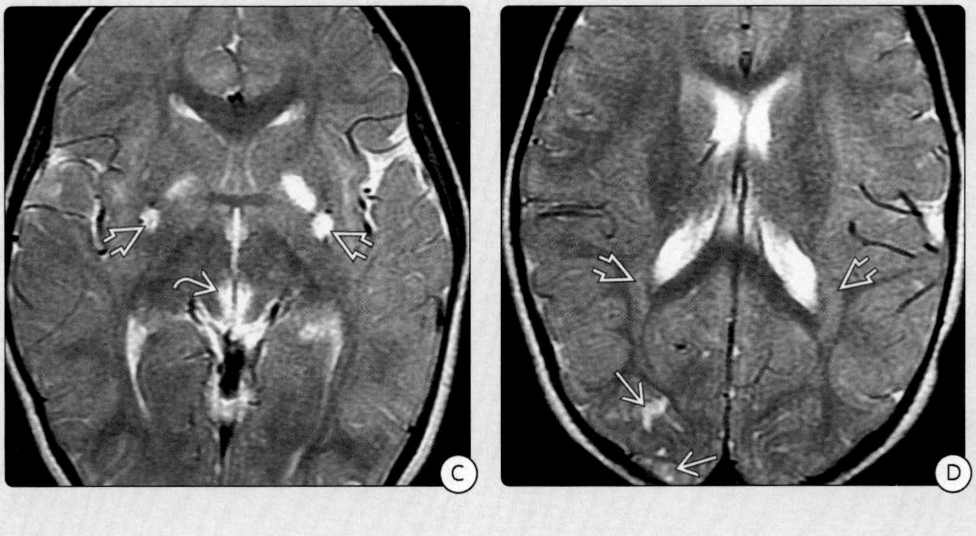

***(31-67C)** Axial T2WI in the same patient shows symmetric hyperintensity in the upper midbrain ➡ and basal ganglia ➡. **(31-67D)** Axial T2WI through the lateral ventricles shows focal hyperintensities in the right occipital cortex and subcortical WM ➡ consistent with infarction. Symmetric mild hyperintensity of peritrigonal WM ➡ represents normal terminal zones of late myelination in parietooccipital association fibers.*

and enhancement that appears identical to MELAS. MRS shows no evidence of elevated lactate levels in the CSF and normal-appearing brain.

LS often involves the brainstem, which is less commonly involved in MELAS. **MERRF** shows a propensity to involve the basal ganglia, caudate nuclei, and vascular watershed zones. Certain vitamin deficiencies **(congenital folate deficiency)** may simulate LS **(31-72)**.

Kearns-Sayre Syndrome

Terminology and Etiology. Kearns-Sayre syndrome (KSS), also known as Kearns-Sayre ophthalmoplegic syndrome, is another mtDNA disorder. A number of different gene deletions have been identified in KSS patients.

Pathology. The most typical and consistent pathologic finding of KSS is spongiform WM vacuolation. The cerebral hemispheres and midbrain are most commonly affected. The cerebellum, brainstem, and spinal cord are also frequently involved, whereas the corpus callosum and internal capsules are usually spared.

Clinical Issues. KSS typically presents in older children or young adults and is characterized by short stature, progressive external ophthalmoplegia, retinitis pigmentosa, sensorineural hearing loss, and ataxia.

Other organs are frequently involved in KSS. Heart block and proximal muscle weakness are common. Ragged red fibers are present on muscle biopsy.

Imaging. CT scans show variable symmetric basal ganglia calcifications. Mild cortical and cerebellar volume loss is common.

MR shows increased signal intensity in the basal ganglia, WM, and cerebellum on T2/FLAIR. The subcortical arcuate fibers, corticospinal tracts, cerebellum, and posterior brainstem are

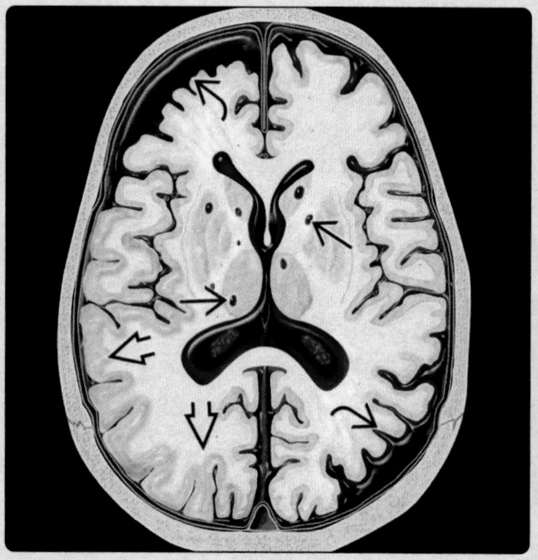

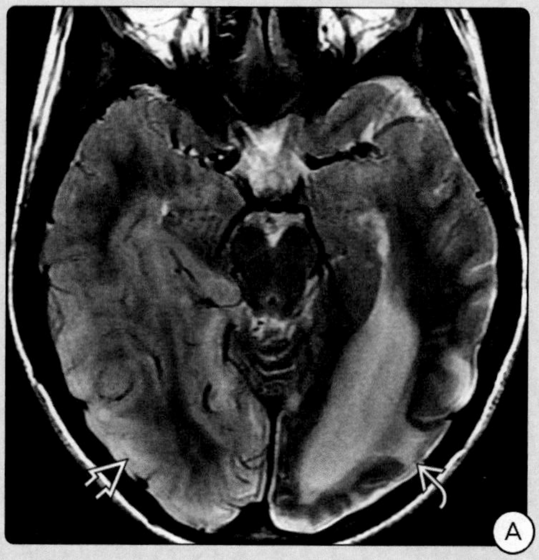

***(31-68)** Axial graphic depicts changes of MELAS with both acute and chronic lesions (lacunar infarcts ➡, cortical atrophy ➡). Acute manifestation is gyral edema that crosses vascular territories ➡, spares the underlying WM, and favors the posterior hemispheres. **(31-69A)** Axial T2WI in a 10y girl with MELAS shows residua of remote left parietooccipital infarct ➡ and acute right temporoparietal gyral swelling ➡ that spares the underlying WM.*

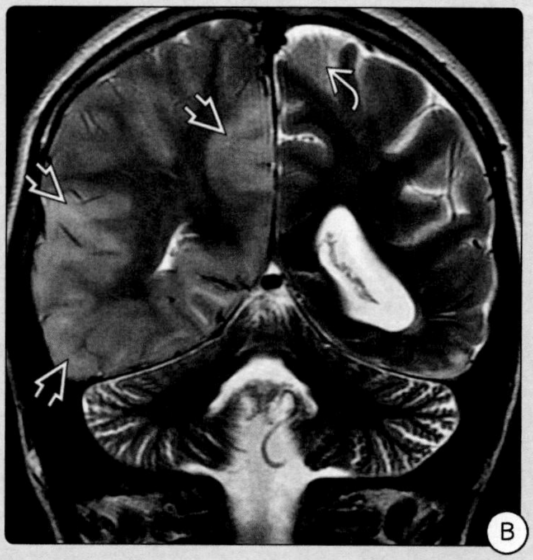

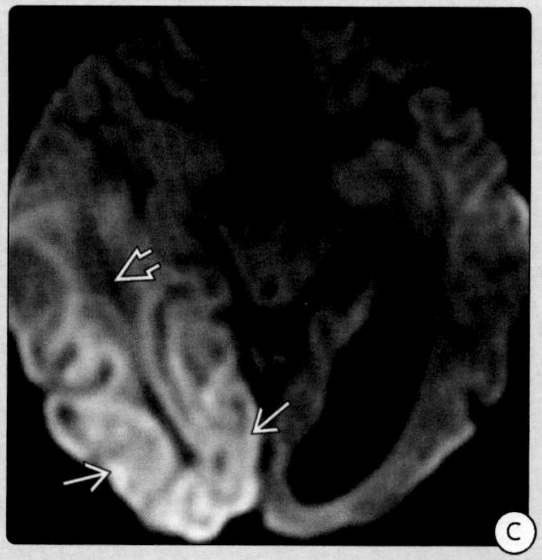

***(31-69B)** Coronal T2WI shows an enlarged left lateral ventricle and cortical atrophy ➡ with acute right gyral edema ➡, the "shifting spread" characteristic of MELAS. **(31-69C)** Axial DWI shows diffusion restriction ➡ in the acutely swollen edematous cortex with sparing of the underlying WM ➡. MRS (not shown) demonstrated a lactate doublet at 1.3 ppm in the normal-appearing brain.*

involved early in the disease course, whereas the periventricular WM remains relatively spared **(31-71)**.

DWI shows reduced diffusivity in the brainstem and subcortical WM. MRS demonstrates elevated lactate.

Differential Diagnosis. There is significant overlap between imaging findings in KSS and other mitochondrial disorders such as **MELAS**. Early involvement of the cortex in a nonvascular distribution—particularly the parietal and occipital lobes—is characteristic of MELAS but uncommon in KSS.

MERRF

Myoclonus **e**pilepsy with **r**agged **r**ed **f**ibers (MERRF) is another syndrome with mtDNA mutations that result in defective mitochondrial OXPHOS. MERRF is a multisystem disorder characterized by myoclonus (often the first symptom) followed by epilepsy, ataxia, weakness, cardiomyopathy, and dementia. Childhood onset is typical.

MERRF is typified pathologically by systemic degeneration involving the globus pallidus, substantia nigra, red nuclei, dentate nuclei, inferior olivary nuclei, cortex, and spinocerebellar tracts.

Imaging studies show watershed and basal ganglia infarcts. The major imaging differential diagnosis of MERRF is **MELAS**; the two disorders often overlap. Pathologically, the major differential diagnosis is **KSS**, as both can demonstrate the presence of ragged red fibers on muscle biopsy.

Glutaric Aciduria Type 1

Terminology. Glutaric aciduria type 1 (GA1), glutaric acidemia type 1, and mitochondrial glutaryl-coenzyme A dehydrogenase (*GCDH*) deficiency are synonyms.

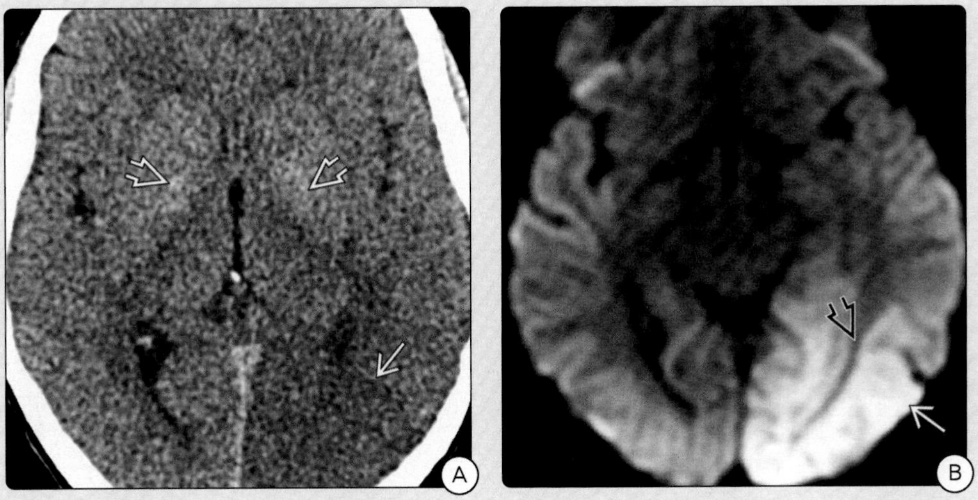

***(31-70A)** Axial NECT in a 7y child with MELAS shows parietal occipital swelling and increased attenuation within the globi pallidi. **(31-70B)** Axial DWI in the same patient shows restricted diffusion in the affected cortex with sparing of the underlying white matter. Initial diagnosis was ictal-related diffusion hyperintensity.*

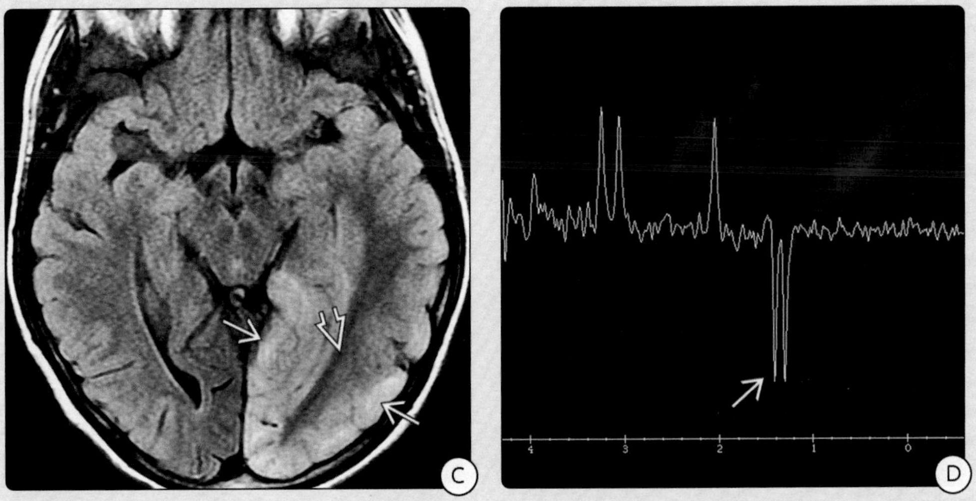

***(31-70C)** Axial FLAIR in the same patient shows hyperintensity of the involved cortex and sparing of the adjacent WM. **(31-70D)** MRS at intermediate TE (144 ms) shows inversion of the lactate doublet at 1.3 ppm. This demonstrates lactate J-coupling at intermediate TE.*

Etiology. GA1 is an autosomal-recessive IMD caused by deficiency of the mitochondrial enzyme *GCDH*. *GCDH* missense mutations (Chr 19p13.2) result in amino acid substitutions. *GCDH* is required for metabolism of lysine, hydroxylysine, and tryptophan. *GCDH* deficiency induces imbalances in neurotransmission. The accumulation of glutaric acid impedes operculization during the third trimester and postnatally leads to globi pallidi, dentate nuclei, and WM degeneration.

Pathology. Excess glutaric acid is neurotoxic. Cells in the basal ganglia and WM are especially vulnerable. Spongiform changes with neuronal loss, myelin splitting and vacuolation, and intramyelinic fluid accumulation are typical microscopic features of GA1.

Clinical Issues. The prevalence of GA1 is approximately 1:100,000 live births. There is a higher case rate among the old order Amish. The majority of infants with GA1 exhibit macrocephaly at birth. Most GA1 patients (85%) present during the first year of life, usually around the time of their first birthday with acute encephalopathy, seizures, dystonia, choreoathetosis, vomiting, and/or opisthotonus. These episodic crises are often triggered by febrile illness, immunization, or surgery. Approximately 25% present insidiously with dystonia without crisis. Disease progression is characterized by permanent motor and mental disability.

Patients may develop an acute Reye-like encephalopathy with ketoacidosis and vomiting. Hypoglycemia accompanied by elevated urinary organic acids is typical. Serum and urine metabolites may be completely normal between metabolic crises.

Therapy for GA1 requires limitation of lysine and tryptophan and administration or oral carnitine.

Imaging. The three "signature" imaging findings of classic GA1 are (1) macrocrania, (2) bilateral widened ("open") lateral cerebral or sylvian fissures (i.e., widened operculum), and (3)

(31-71A) Axial T2WI in a teenager with Kearns-Sayre syndrome demonstrates bilaterally symmetric hyperintensities in the pons ➡ and middle cerebellar peduncles ➡. (31-71B) T2WI through the basal ganglia shows abnormal signal intensities within the globi pallidi ➡ and posterior limbs of the internal capsules ➡.

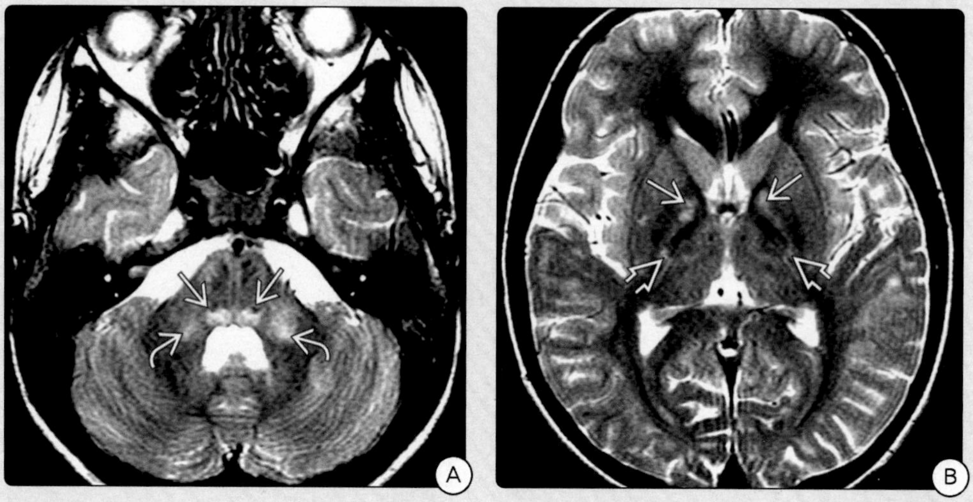

(31-71C) Axial T2WI through the lateral ventricles shows multifocal stripe-like hyperintensities in the periventricular ➡ and subcortical WM ➡. (31-71D) Coronal FLAIR in the same patient with KSS shows the involvement of the subcortical U-fibers ➡, corticospinal tracts/internal capsules ➡, and medial thalami ➡.

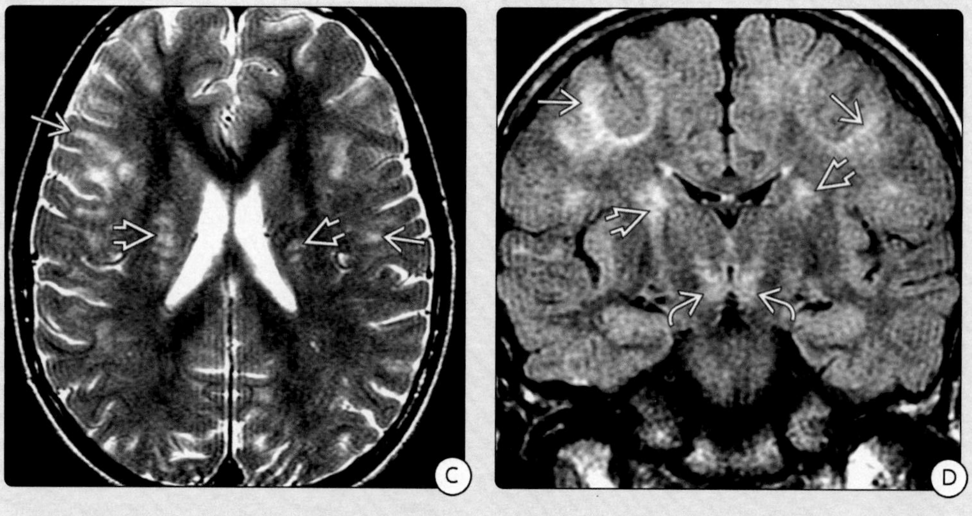

bilaterally symmetric basal ganglia lesions **(31-73)**. Severe GA1 may also cause diffuse hemispheric WM abnormalities (i.e., central and periventricular) **(31-75)** **(31-76A)**. Cerebellar dentate nuclei T2/FLAIR hyperintensity is common. T2/FLAIR hyperintensity may also involve the corpus striatum, substantia nigra, thalamus, and dentate nuclei.

GA1 infants in metabolic crisis often present with acute striatal necrosis. Bilateral diffusely swollen basal ganglia that are T2/FLAIR hyperintense and that restrict on DWI are typical **(31-74)** **(31-75)**. In between crises, GP and dentate findings "normalize" **(31-76)**.

Chronic GA1 causes enlarged CSF spaces and cerebral atrophy **(31-75)**. Volume loss leads to tearing of cortical dural bridging veins that cross from the brain surface to the superior sagittal venous sinus, resulting in recurrent subdural hematomas **(31-77)**.

GA1 does not enhance on T1 C+ scans. DWI in the acute phase or during crises shows restricted diffusion within the globi pallidi. MRS is nonspecific with reduced NAA, increased lipids, increased Cho:Cr ratio, and (during crisis) elevated lactate level **(31-76D)**.

Differential Diagnosis. The major differential diagnosis of GA1 is **subdural hemorrhage** occurring in the setting of **abusive head trauma**. However, GA1 is not associated with fractures, and the subdural hematomas associated with GA1 do not occur in the absence of enlarged CSF spaces and characteristic globi pallidi and other parenchymal T2/FLAIR and/or DWI changes.

Other causes of macrocephaly and conditions with middle cranial fossa cyst-like spaces in infants and children should be considered in the differential diagnosis. These include **hydrocephalus, benign expansion of the subarachnoid spaces (BESS)** of infancy (enlarged subarachnoid spaces) in the first year of life, **benign familial macrocephaly** (a normal variant), **middle cranial fossa arachnoid cysts** (i.e., usually unilateral), and other IMDs, such as the **mucopolysaccharidoses** (CSF-like mucopolysaccharide pachymeningeal deposition in all but Morquio type 4 MPS), **Canavan disease**, and **Alexander disease**.

Glutaric Aciduria Type 2

Glutaric aciduria type 2 (GA2) results from a defect in the mitochondrial electron transport chain at coenzyme Q.

Clinical Issues. Three phenotypes are reported, including neonatal onset with multiple associated congenital anomalies, neonatal onset without anomalies, and late-onset form. The neonatal onset form presents with overwhelming illness, including metastatic acidosis and severe hypoglycemia. The late-onset form presents with vomiting, hypoglycemia, and unexplained acidosis.

Imaging Findings. MR demonstrates symmetric T2/FLAIR hyperintensity involving the corpus striatum, caudate nucleus, putamen, middle cerebral peduncles, splenium of the corpus callosum, and hemispheric WM. The "open" sylvian fissures characteristic of GA1 are absent in GA2.

Differential Diagnosis. Diabetic ketoacidosis can be a clinical and imaging mimic of GA2; MR may show central herniation with resultant diencephalic ischemia and infarction. **Profound hypoxic ischemic injury (HII)** targets the striatum and thalami. A positive health history is typically present.

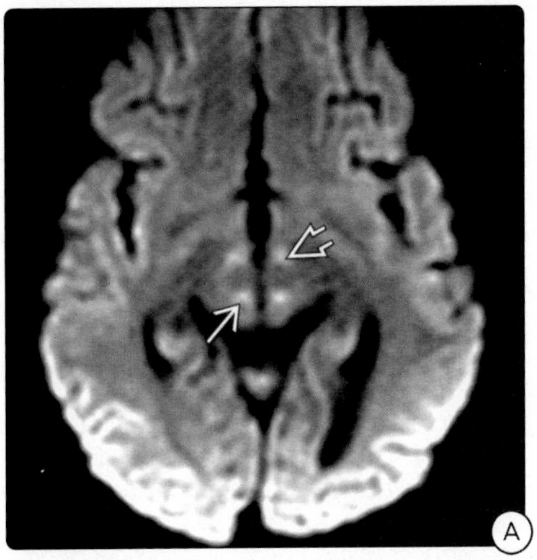

***(31-72A)** Axial DWI in a newborn with congenital folate deficiency shows midbrain ➡ and epithalamus ➡ restriction, confirmed on ADC.*

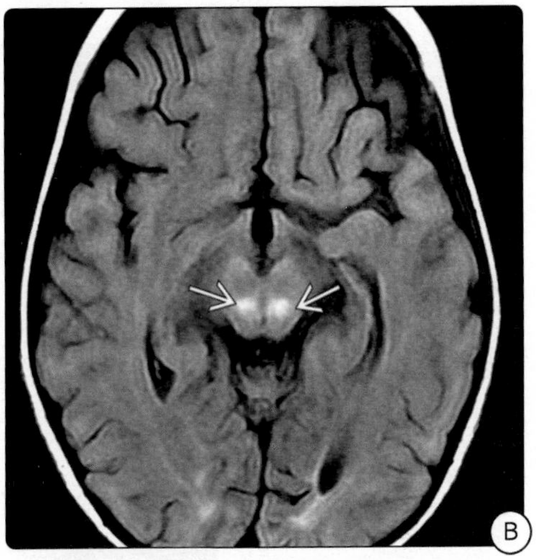

***(31-72B)** Axial FLAIR shows red nucleus hyperintensity ➡. Mild diffuse volume loss is noted.*

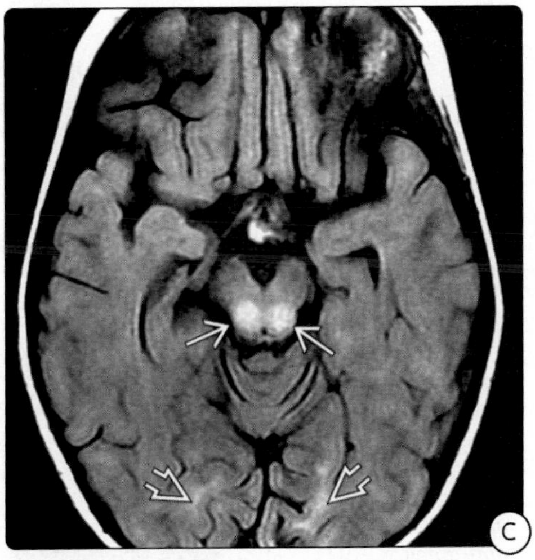

***(31-72C)** Axial FLAIR in the same patient shows swollen midbrain ➡ and occipital WM hyperintensities ➡.*

Urea Cycle/Ammonia Disorders

Ammonia is an important source of nitrogen and is required for amino acid synthesis as well as normal acid-base balance. When present in high concentrations, ammonia is toxic.

The urea cycle normally prevents excess accumulation of toxic nitrogen products by incorporating nitrogen into urea, which is then excreted in the urine. Interruption of the urea cycle results in elevated serum ammonia, which readily crosses the blood-brain barrier and causes diffuse cerebral edema. In chronic disease, atrophy with resultant ulegyria is seen.

Six disorders of the urea cycle have clinical importance. These include *ornithine transcarbamylase deficiency (OTCD), carbamoyl phosphate synthetase 1 deficiency, citrullinemia or argininosuccinate synthetase deficiency, argininosuccinate aciduria or argininosuccinate lyase deficiency, argininemia or arginase deficiency (AD), and N-acetylglutamate synthase deficiency.* The two classic and most common disorders are **OTCD** and **citrullinemia**. Both are characterized by diffuse brain swelling (which does not spare the basal ganglia) on NECT and MR scans.

Imaging

MR shows basal ganglia and cortical swelling with T2/FLAIR hyperintensity **(31-78)**. The peri-insular cortex is usually affected first (i.e., linear T2 prolongation and restricted diffusion between the globi pallidi and putamina), with involvement then extending into the frontal, parietal, temporal, and (finally) the occipital lobes **(31-78) (31-79)**. The globi pallidi, putamina, and thalami are affected with prolonged hyperammonemia and may show restricted diffusion **(31-78D) (31-78E)**. A characteristic pattern of "crenulated" subcortical diffusion restriction and T2 prolongation strongly suggests urea cycle disorder **(31-78E)**. MRS demonstrates increased lactate and glutamine-glutamate and eventually reduced NAA **(31-78)**.

(31-73) Axial graphic depicts typical findings of glutaric aciduria type 1. Note the symmetrically enlarged basal ganglia and the bilateral "open" sylvian or lateral cerebral fissures. The thalami appear normal. (31-74) Axial DWI in an infant in acute metabolic crisis with acute striatal necrosis shows restricted diffusion in the basal ganglia. Note the "open" sylvian fissures and sparing of the thalami.

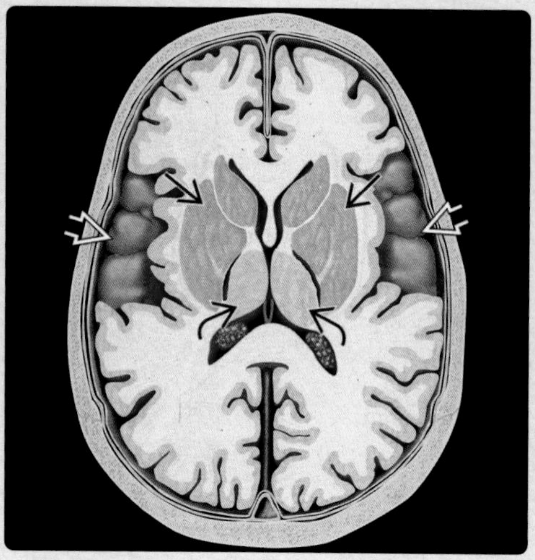

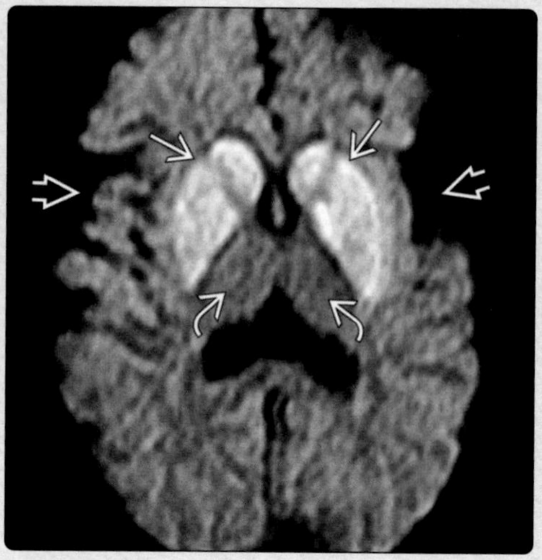

(31-75A) Axial T2WI in a 7m child with GA1 shows enlarged, hyperintense caudate nuclei, putamina, and globi pallidi with thalamic sparing. The sylvian fissures are enlarged. The hemispheric WM myelination is grossly delayed. (31-75B) Coronal T2WI in the same patient shows generalized brain volume loss, swollen basal ganglia, and delayed myelination. The sylvian fissures appear underoperculized and "open."

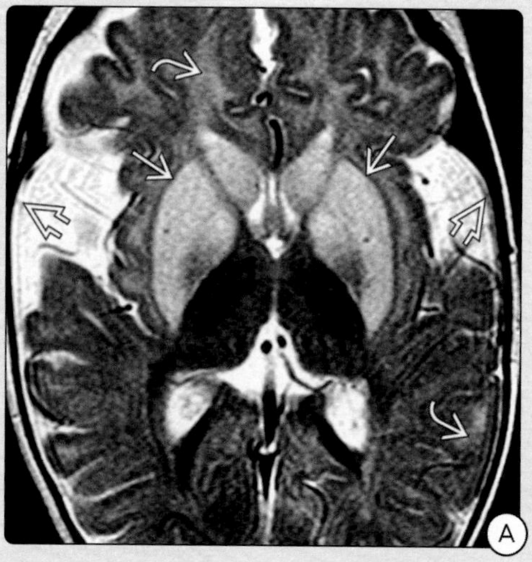

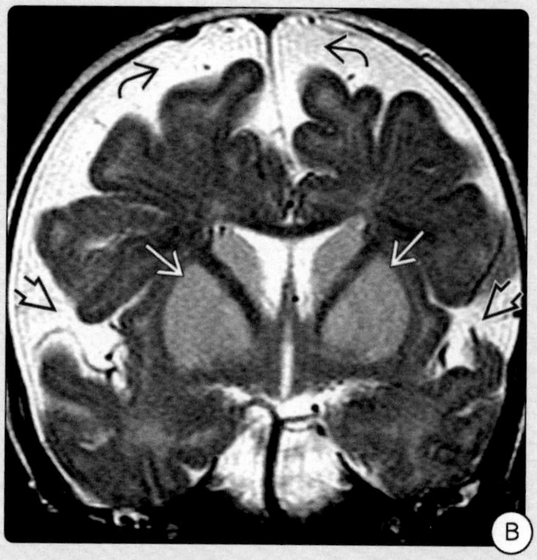

Differential Diagnosis

The major imaging differential diagnosis of acute hyperammonemia caused by urea cycle disorders is **hypoxic-ischemic encephalopathy** (HIE). Infants with HIE typically have more thalamic and perirolandic cortical abnormalities. **Neonatal herpes simplex encephalitis** (i.e., usually HSV type 2) is often associated with hepatitis and diffuse pulmonary involvement. HSV2 is nonpatterned and may present with diffuse edema.

Methylmalonic and Propionic Acidemias

Both **methylmalonic acidemia (MMA)** and **propionic acidemia (PPA)** are autosomal-recessive disorders that both present early in life with episodic ketoacidosis, lethargy, tachypnea, nausea, vomiting, progressive hypotonia, and seizures, eventually progressing to coma and death. Survivors show microcephaly, movement and psychomotor disorders, mental retardation, and ketoacidosis. Central hypotonia with pyramidal tract signs and symptoms at the time of clinical crisis is seen. Dystonia and choreoathetosis are common sequelae of basal ganglia involvement. Respective acids (methylmalonic/propionic) are detected in the urine. **Methylmalonic acidemia** is caused by mutation of the *MUT* gene located at 6p21, which encodes methylmalonic CoA mutase. **Propionic acidemia** is caused by mutations in the gene encoding propionyl-CoA carboxylase, *PCCA*.

Imaging

MR findings in both disorders are nonspecific yet reflective of increased water within involved tissues (therefore, reduced attenuation on NECT and T1 and T2 prolongation on MR). Neuroimaging findings vary based on the *specific acidemia* and the stage of brain maturation at the time of presentation. Ventricular enlargement, cortical atrophy, cerebellar volume

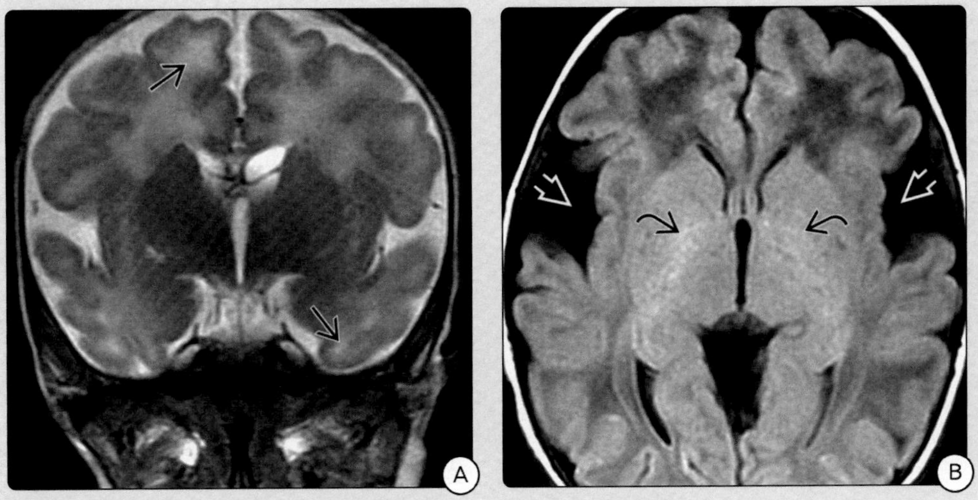

***(31-76A)** Coronal T2WI in a 14m girl with GA1 "between crises" shows diffuse delay in WM maturation →. Note the normal appearance of the BG. **(31-76B)** Axial T1WI in the same patient demonstrates open lateral cerebral (sylvian) fissures → and subtle T1 shortening within the globi pallidi (GP) →.*

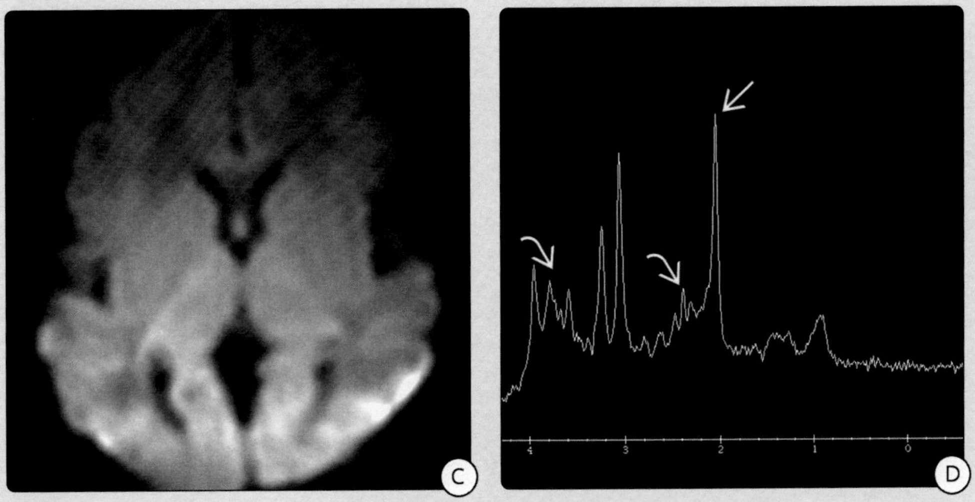

***(31-76C)** Axial DWI "in between crises" shows normal diffusivity of the basal ganglia. **(31-76D)** Short TE (35 ms) MRS in the same patient (in between crises) shows minimal decline of NAA → and elevation of excitatory neurotransmitters →.*

(31-77A) Axial NECT shows classic findings of GA1 in a 7m infant with a large head and delayed development. Note the "open" sylvian (lateral cerebral) fissures ➡ and large bifrontal hypoattenuating chronic subdural hematomas (cSDH) ➡. (31-77B) Axial NECT in the same patient demonstrates the holocranial compressive cSDHs ➡. The fluid attenuation of the cSDH is greater than sulcal SAS fluid ➡.

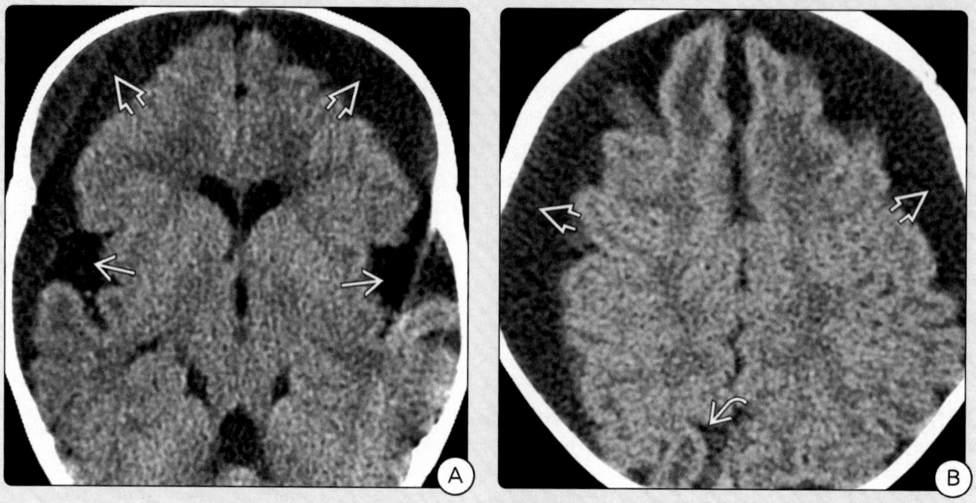

(31-77C) Axial FLAIR image shows the "open" sylvian fissures ➡ and the peripheral chronic SDHs ➡. (31-77D) Axial T2WI in the same patient shows the "open" sylvian fissures ➡, membrane-bound subdural fluid collections ➡, and significantly delayed myelination for a child 7 months of age. GP shows T2 hyperintensity ➡.

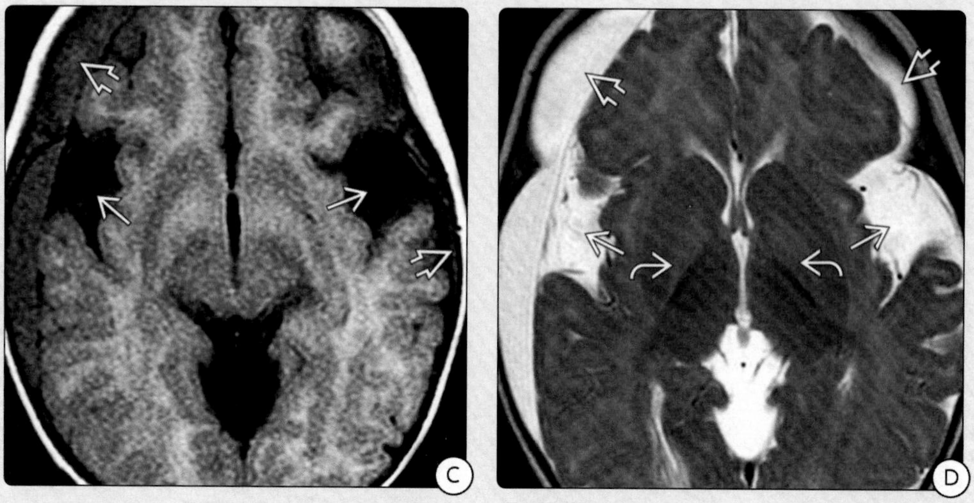

(31-77E) Axial DWI shows mild hyperintensity in the frontal WM ➡ and GP ➡. DWI abnormalities are more commonly seen during metabolic crises. (31-77F) Axial NECT scan 10 months later shows near complete resolution of the SDHs. A small residual cSDH is present over the right frontal and temporal lobes ➡. The sylvian fissures remain widened, typical of GA1.

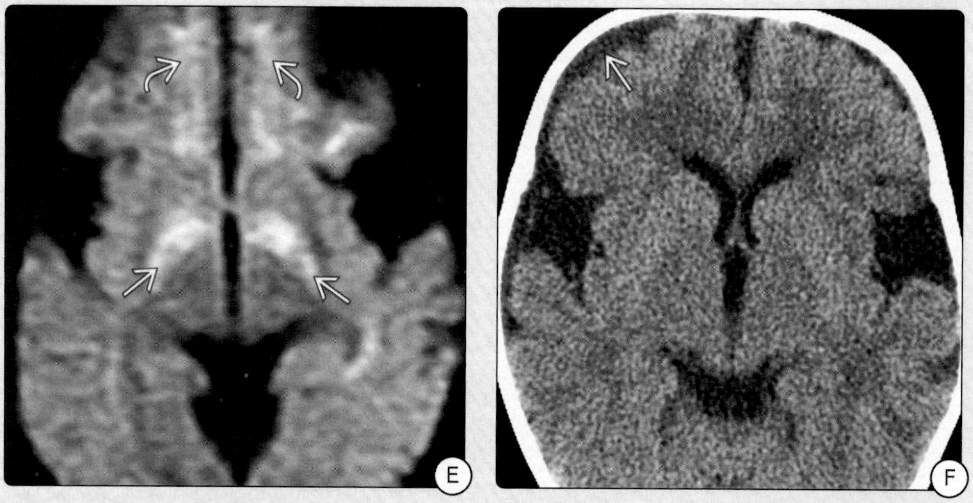

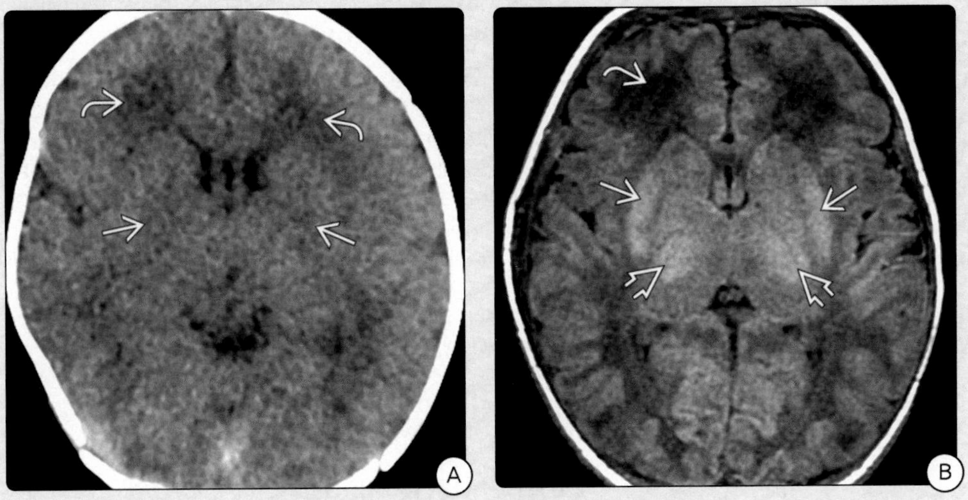

***(31-78A)** Axial NECT in a newborn boy with UCD (OTCD) shows reduced attenuation of basal ganglia and hemispheric WM. There was no history of HII.* ***(31-78B)** Axial T1WI in the same neonate shows basal ganglia and thalamic T1 hyperintensity. Note the hypointense frontal WM.*

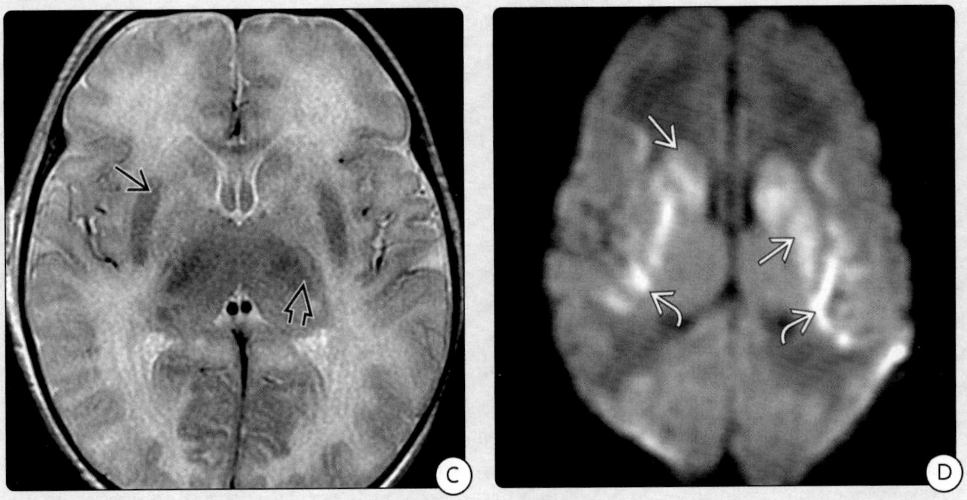

***(31-78C)** Axial T2WI in the same patient shows diffuse WM hyperintensity. Putaminal and thalamic hypointensity is demonstrated. Manganese, Ca++, and myelin breakdown products may contribute to reduced T2 signal.* ***(31-78D)** Axial DWI in the same newborn shows basal ganglia and subinsular diffusion hyperintensity.*

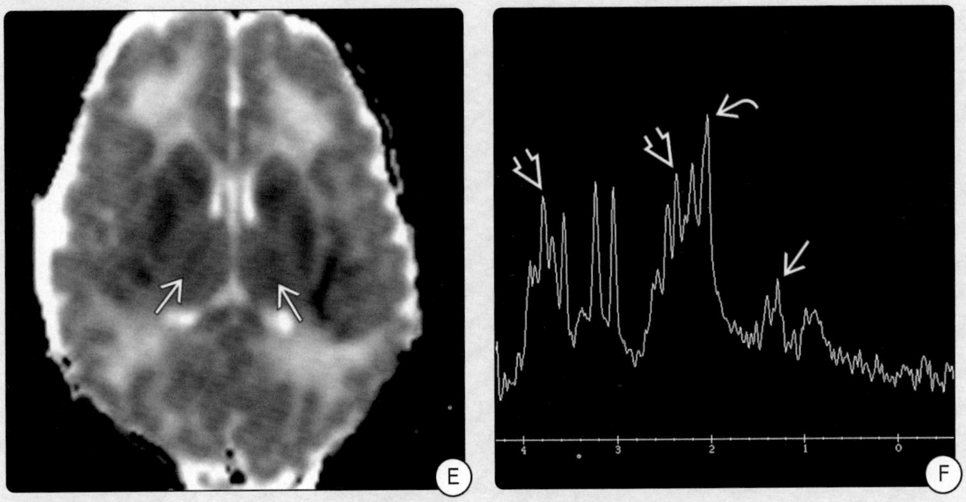

***(31-78E)** Axial ADC map in the same neonate shows restricted diffusion within the basal ganglia, subinsular regions, and thalami. OCDs may appear as "worst case ever HII," without HII history.* ***(31-78F)** MRS short TE (35 ms) of the left basal ganglion shows lactate doublet, increased excitatory neurotransmitters, and reduced NAA.*

loss, and T2/FLAIR hyperintensity involving the periventricular WM and globi pallidi are the most common abnormalities in **MMA**. Bilateral basal ganglia calcifications are present in 5-10% of cases of MMA. **PPA** involves the putamina and caudate nuclei and causes reduced myelination in the hemispheric WM **(31-80)**. MRS can not distinguish MMA from PPA. Both show reduced NAA and myoinositol and increased glutamate/glutamine.

Differential Diagnosis

Hypoxic ischemic injury (HII) of the profound type involves striatum and thalami as well as corticospinal tracts and hippocampi. **Carbon monoxide poisoning** targets the BG and is associated with often deep GM structures showing T2 prolongation.

Gangliosidoses

Clinically important forms of gangliosidoses include GM1 and GM2 [Tay-Sachs (TS), Sandhoff disease (SD), and GM2 variant AB]. They are biochemically distinct but clinically indistinguishable.

GM1 is a rare lysosomal storage disease. Deficiency of the lysosomal enzyme β-galactosidase results in accumulation of GM1 ganglioside in the brain (especially the basal ganglia) and oligosaccharide in the abdominal viscera. Three forms of the disease have been described, all being the result of mutations of the *GLB1* gene located on chromosome 3p21.33.

GM2 is an autosomal-recessive disorder of sphingolipid storage caused by a deficiency of hexosaminidase. Deficiency of isoenzyme A, coded by the *HEXA* gene at Chr 15q23-24, causes **TS**. β-Subunit deficiencies of both isoenzymes A and B coded by the *HEXB* gene at Chr 5q13 cause **SD**. The **GM2 AB variant** is caused by deficiency of the GM2 activator protein. All three forms are associated with an abnormal accumulation of GM2 ganglioside in the cytoplasm of neurons. This results in extensive neuronal loss and WM degeneration, leading to atrophy. Atrophy may be more cerebellar than cerebral.

GM1 and GM2, as well as GM2 AB variant (rare), exist in infantile, juvenile, and adult forms. Patients with infantile **GM1** present between birth and 6 months with coarse facial features, skeletal dysostosis, and hepatosplenomegaly. There is clinical overlap with Morquio type B disease. Juvenile-onset **GM1** presents with psychomotor retardation. Adult-onset disease is characterized by slowly progressive dystonia and ataxia, as well as extrapyramidal signs. The three forms of GM2 disease (TS, SD, and GM2 AB variant) share similar clinical and imaging features. In the most common infantile form, initial psychomotor retardation and hypotonia are followed by neurologic deterioration. Progressive weakness, choreiform movements, dystonia, and ataxia occur.

Imaging

In both GM1 and GM2, imaging findings are quite similar. Patients with infantile-onset gangliosidoses show preferential involvement of the thalami, small and hyperattenuating on NECT scans. The basal ganglia (striatum) and sometimes the cerebral and cerebellar WM are hypoattenuating on NECT. Patients with juvenile- or adult-onset disease may show only cerebellar atrophy.

MR scans in infantile-onset gangliosidosis may demonstrate T1 hyper- and hypointensity of the thalami. Variable T1 signal of the striatum and hypointense cerebral WM may be seen **(31-80)**. With disease progression, the globi pallidi and ventral thalami often appear profoundly shrunken and hypointense on T2WI. In **TS**, on T2WI, the ventral thalami are hypointense, and the dorsal thalami are hyperintense. In **SD**, the thalami are diffusely hypointense on T2WI **(31-80B)**. With the exception of the corpus callosum (which is often spared), the WM appears variably T2/FLAIR hyperintense. There is no enhancement, and DWI shows variable reduced diffusivity in the ventral thalami (TS). MRS shows reduced NAA and increased choline and myoinositol.

Differential Diagnosis

HII (status marmoratus) demonstrates atrophic hyperattenuating thalami, atrophic striatum, and perirolandic cortex. Nonprogressive neurologic deficits and positive health history are common. **Krabbe disease** demonstrates hyperattenuating thalami, caudate, and dentate nuclei. T2 prolongation involves the cerebral and cerebellar WM.

Fabry Disease

Fabry disease causes 1.5-5.0% of unexplained strokes in young patients and is present in 4-5% of men with unexplained left ventricular hypertrophy or cryptogenic stroke. As enzyme replacement therapy is now widely available, it is key to find Fabry disease before irreversible organ damage occurs.

Etiology and Pathology

Fabry disease is an X-linked lysosomal storage disorder of glycosphingolipid metabolism. Mutation in α-galactosidase leads to abnormal accumulation of glycosphingolipids in various tissues, especially in the vascular endothelium and smooth muscle cells. Impaired endothelial function results in progressive multisystem vasculopathy. The renal, cardiac, and cerebral vessels are severely affected. Cardiac emboli, large vessel arteriopathy, and microvascular disease all occur.

Clinical Issues

Infants with Fabry disease typically present with diffuse angiokeratomas, but late-onset Fabry disease is much more difficult to diagnose. Fabry-induced stroke often occurs before the definitive diagnosis has been established. Although mean onset of first stroke is 39 years in men and 45 years in women, nearly 22% of patients are younger than 30 years at initial presentation. Over 85% of strokes in Fabry disease are ischemic strokes. Hemorrhagic strokes are less common and usually occur secondary to renovascular hypertension.

Imaging

NECT scans show bilateral, often symmetric calcifications in the basal ganglia and thalami. Multifocal deep WM hypodensities consistent with lacunar infarcts can be

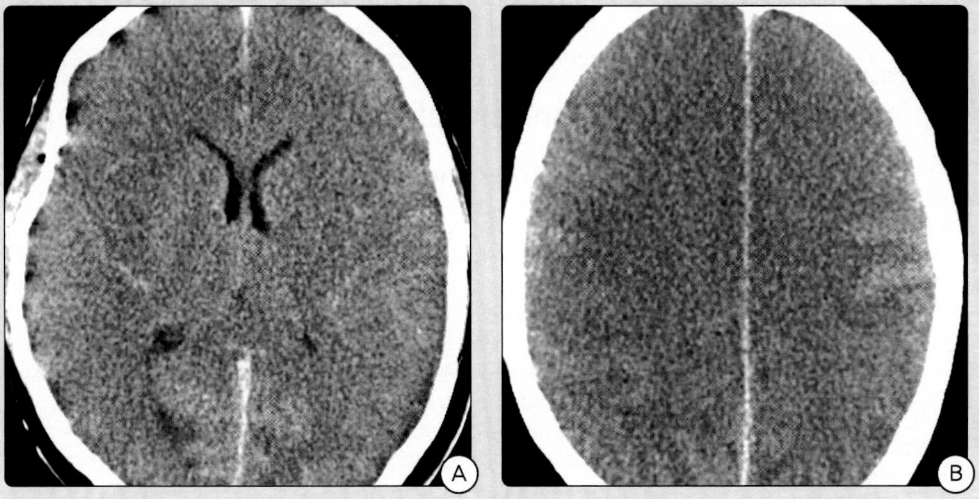

***(31-79A)** Axial NECT shows a 51y woman with ornithine transcarbamylase deficiency (OCTD), in acute metabolic crisis. Diffuse cerebral edema is seen. The cortex, basal ganglia, and thalami are of the same attenuation as the underlying WM. **(31-79B)** Axial NECT through the cerebral convexities shows swollen, hypoattenuating gyri and WM with complete effacement of all sulci.*

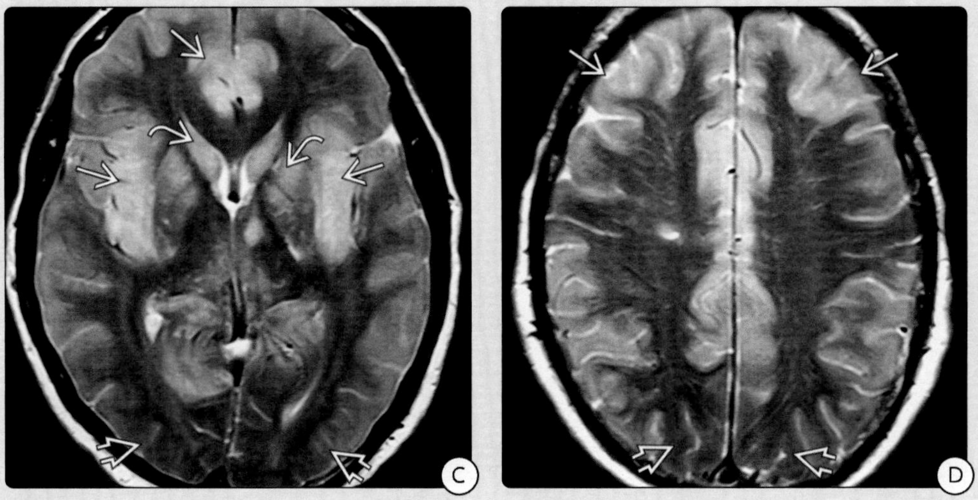

***(31-79C)** Axial T2WI in the same patient shows basal ganglia ➡ and cortical hyperintensity, most striking in the peri-insular and frontal cortices ➡. The occipital lobes ➡ are relatively spared. **(31-79D)** Axial T2WI in the same patient shows diffusely swollen cortex ➡. Again, the occipital lobes ➡ are relatively spared, a characteristic pattern in hyperammonemia caused by OTCD.*

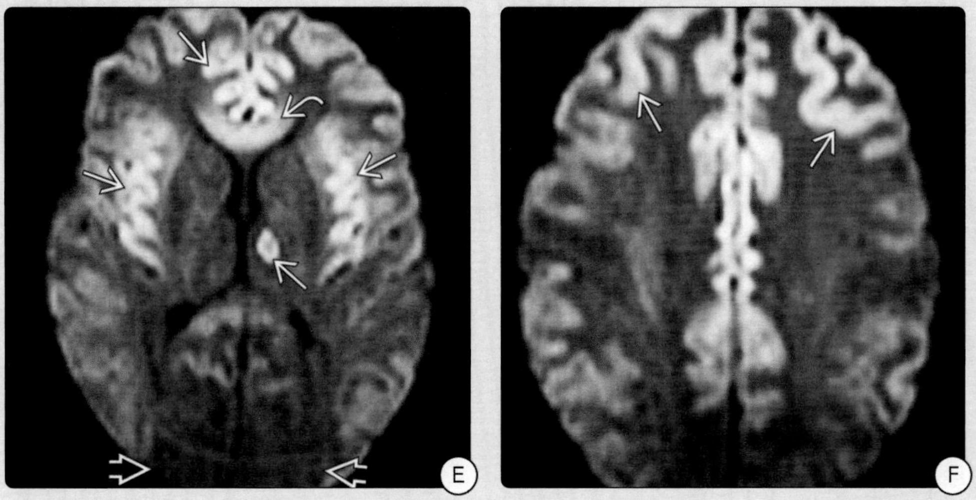

***(31-79E)** Axial DWI in the same patient shows diffusion hyperintensity in the peri-insular and frontal cortices ➡ and left thalamus with less striking involvement of the corpus callosum ➡. The occipital lobes ➡ show no evidence of restricted diffusion. **(31-79F)** Axial DWI more cephalad shows diffusion restriction ➡ (confirmed on ADC maps) involving the cortex and sparing the underlying WM of the corona radiata.*

identified in some cases. Patients with long-standing Fabry disease show volume loss with enlarged ventricles and sulci.

MR may show T1 shortening in the basal ganglia and thalami. The "pulvinar" sign (T1 hyperintensity in the posterior thalamus) is highly suggestive of Fabry disease. Between 45 and 50% of adult patients with Fabry disease have patchy multifocal T2/FLAIR hyperintensities in the basal ganglia, thalami, and cerebral WM. With time, the lesions increase in number and may become coalescent. Ten percent of patients demonstrate "blooming" hypointensities on T2* (GRE, SWI) due to microbleeds. Dolichoectasias is less common.

Differential Diagnosis

Look for other disorders marked by BG calcifications. **Fahr disease** causes bilateral, dense, thick calcifications in the BG and thalami. The cerebellum and GM-WM interfaces are frequently affected but generally not involved in Fabry disease. **Endocrinologic disorders** like hyperparathyroidism, hypoparathyroidism, pseudohypoparathyroidism, and hypothyroidism may have similar calcifications but lack the multifocal infarcts typical of Fabry disease.

Congenital Glycosylation Disorders

Etiology and Pathology

Carbohydrate-deficient glycoprotein (CDG) syndrome is a disorder in glycosylation of *N*-linked oligosaccharides. Genetically heterogeneous, autosomal recessive in inheritance, CDG1a is caused by mutation in the gene encoding *PMM2* (most common). Asparagine-*N*-linked oligosaccharide transfer deficiency is suspected. At autopsy, marked atrophy of the cerebellum is seen, especially the anterior vermis, pontine nuclei, and inferior olive. There are a complete loss of Purkinje cells and subtotal loss of cerebellar granular cells.

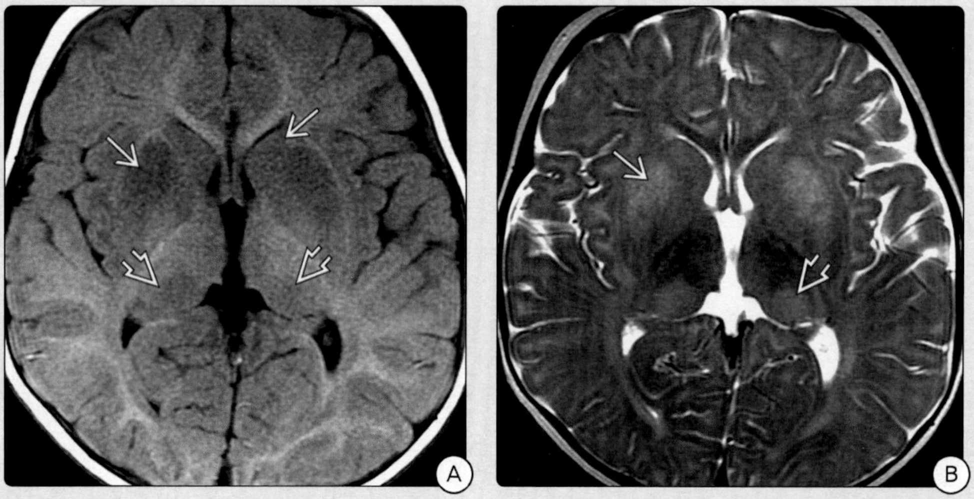

***(31-80A)** Axial T1WI shows an 11m boy with Tay-Sachs (TS) (GM2) with developmental regression. There are T1 hypointensity and swelling in the basal ganglia → and thalami →. **(31-80B)** Axial T2WI in the same infant shows basal ganglia → and thalamic → increased T2 signal. Note the peripheral enlarged SASs due to global volume loss.*

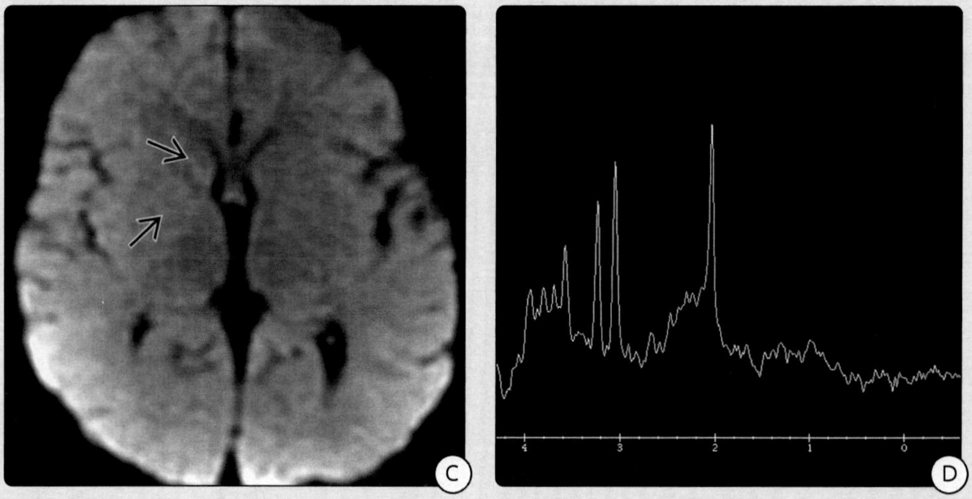

***(31-80C)** Axial DWI in the same patient shows subtle hyperintensity within the right basal ganglion →. **(31-80D)** MRS short TE (35 ms) shows minimal reduction of NAA and increase of myoinositol. No lactate was identified at 1.33 ppm.*

Clinical Issues

CDG ranges from severe infantile multisystem involvement to mild late-onset forms, with hypotonia, developmental delay, failure to thrive, stroke-like episodes, strabismus, ataxia, abnormal subcutaneous fat distribution, and nipple retraction.

Imaging

Sagittal imaging shows shrunken vermis with folial volume loss, fissural enlargement, and flattening of the inferior vermis. The ventral pons is small. DWI/ADC shows increased diffusivity within the affected cerebellum. There is cerebellar T2/FLAIR hyperintensity. MRS shows severely reduced NAA, reduced Cho, and increased myoinositol.

Differential Diagnosis

Differential diagnoses include isolated cerebellar atrophy in **ataxia-telangiectasia** with oculomucocutaneous telangiectasias, scattered WM foci of T2 hyperintensity and SWI hypointensity, **GM2 gangliosidosis** showing characteristic T1WI and T2WI findings of the thalami, and **Wilson disease** showing tortuous intracranial vessels (corkscrew) and cerebral and cerebellar atrophy and wormian bones.

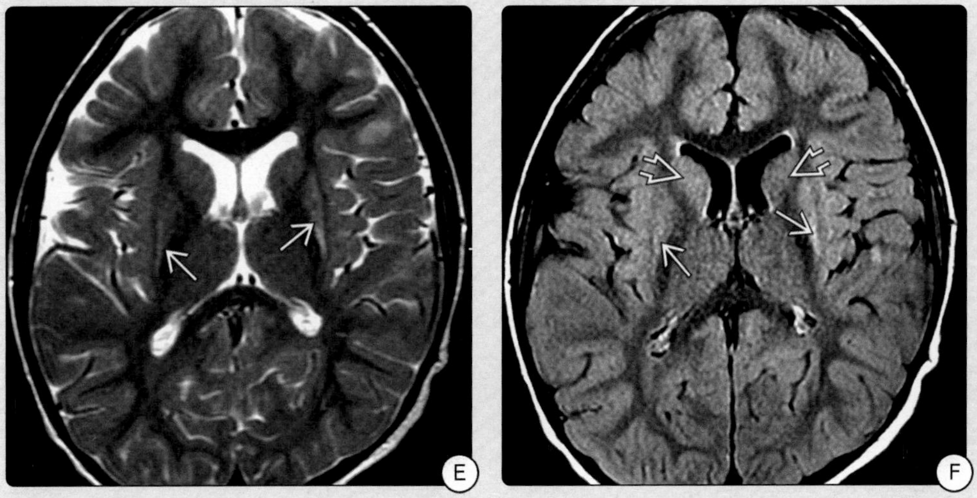

***(31-80E)** Axial T2WI in a 3y boy with propionic acidemia shows shrunken putamen ➡ with increased signal. Prominent SASs reflect atrophy. **(31-80F)** Axial FLAIR in the same patient shows hyperintense atrophic putamen ➡ and edematous caudate nuclei ➡. HII typically involves bilateral thalami.*

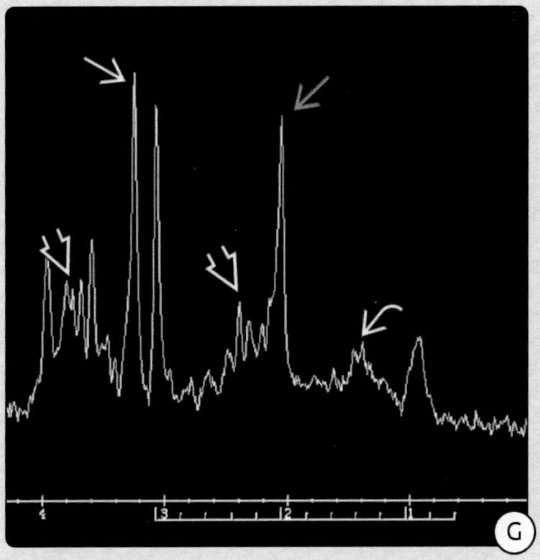

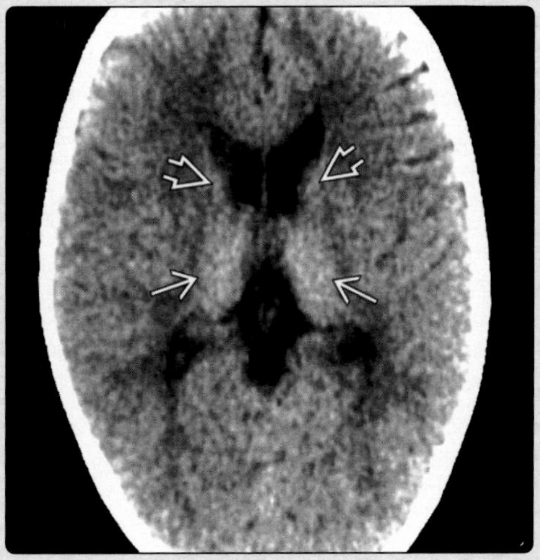

***(31-80G)** MRS, short TE (35 ms), shows increased choline ➡ and excitatory neurotransmitters ➡. A small lactate doublet ➡ and reduced NAA ➡ are seen. **(31-81)** NECT scan in a developmentally delayed 1y infant with infantile Tay-Sachs (TS) disease shows shrunken basal ganglia ➡ and hyperattenuating thalami ➡.*

Selected References

Normal Myelination and White Matter Development

Merrow C et al (eds): Diagnostic Imaging: Pediatrics, 3e. Salt Lake City, UT: Elsevier, 2017

Fogel BL et al: Clinical exome sequencing in neurogenetic and neuropsychiatric disorders. Ann N Y Acad Sci. 1366(1):49-60, 2016

Barkovich AJ, Koch BL, Moore KR (eds): Pediatric Neuroradiology, 2e. Salt Lake City, UT: Elsevier, 2015

Yang Y et al: Clinical whole-exome sequencing for the diagnosis of mendelian disorders. N Engl J Med. 369(16):1502-11, 2013

Classification of Inherited Metabolic Disorders

Saudubray JM et al (eds): Inborn Metabolic Diseases: Diagnosis and Treatment. Berlin, Germany: Springer, 2016

Longo MG et al: Brain imaging and genetic risk in the pediatric population, part 1: inherited metabolic diseases. Neuroimaging Clin N Am. 25(1):31-51, 2015

Saudubray JM: Neurometabolic disorders. J Inherit Metab Dis. 32(5):595-6, 2009

Overview

Barkovich AJ: Approach to normal myelination and metabolic disease. In: Diagnostic Imaging: Pediatric Neuroradiology, 2e, edited by Barkovich AJ, Koch BL, Moore KR. Salt Lake City, UT: Elsevier, 2015, pp. I-1-38-43

Barkovich AJ, Patay Z: Metabolic, toxic, and inflammatory brain disorders. In: Pediatric Neuroimaging, 5e, edited by Barkovich AJ, Raybaud C. Philadelphia, PA: Lippincott Williams & Wilkins, 2012, pp. 81-239

Metabolic Approach

Salmi H et al: Patients with organic acidaemias have an altered thiol status. Acta Paediatr. 101(11):e505-8, 2012

Leonard JV: Recent advances in amino acid and organic acid metabolism. J Inherit Metab Dis. 30(2):134-8, 2007

IMDs Predominantly Affecting White Matter

van Der Knaap MS and Valk J. Magnetic Resonance of Myelination and Myelin Disorders, 3e. New York, NY: Springer, 2005

van der Knaap MS et al. Non-leukodystrophic white matter changes in inherited disorders. Int J Neuroradiol. 1(1): 56–66, 1995

Periventricular White Matter Predominance

Butler CJ et al: Distinctive magnetic resonance imaging findings in neonatal nonketotic hyperglycinemia. Pediatr Neurol. 72:90-91, 2017

Zubarioglu T et al: Neonatal nonketotic hyperglycinemia: diffusion-weighted magnetic resonance imaging and diagnostic clues. Acta Neurol Belg. 116(4):671-673, 2016

Pinto WB et al: Brain MRI features in late-onset nonketotic hyperglycinemia. Arq Neuropsiquiatr. 73(10):891, 2015

Kanekar S et al: Characteristic MRI findings in neonatal nonketotic hyperglycinemia due to sequence changes in GLDC gene encoding the enzyme glycine decarboxylase. Metab Brain Dis. 28(4):717-20, 2013

Hypomyelinating Disorders

Steenweg ME et al: Magnetic resonance imaging pattern recognition in hypomyelinating disorders. Brain. 133(10):2971-82, 2010

IMDs Predominantly Affecting Gray Matter

Jones BV: Metabolic brain disease. In: Diagnostic Imaging: Pediatrics, 3e, edited by Carl Merrow et al. Salt Lake City, UT: Elsevier, 2017, pp 1090-1095

Barkovich AJ, Koch BL, Moore KR (eds): Pediatric Neuroradiology, 2e. Salt Lake City, UT: Elsevier, 2015

IMDs Primarily Affecting Deep Gray Nuclei

Viau KS et al: Evidence-based treatment of guanidinoacetate methyltransferase (GAMT) deficiency. Mol Genet Metab. 110(3):255-62, 2013

Longo N et al: Disorders of creatine transport and metabolism. Am J Med Genet C Semin Med Genet. 157C(1):72-8, 2011

Disorders Affecting Both Gray and White Matter

Mucopolysaccharidoses

Xing M et al: Radiological and clinical characterization of the lysosomal storage disorders: non-lipid disorders. Br J Radiol. 87(1033):20130467, 2014

Zafeiriou DI et al: Brain and spinal MR imaging findings in mucopolysaccharidoses: a review. AJNR Am J Neuroradiol. 34(1):5-13, 2013

Rasalkar DD et al: Pictorial review of mucopolysaccharidosis with emphasis on MRI features of brain and spine. Br J Radiol. 84(1001):469-77, 2011

Mitochondrial Diseases (Respiratory Chain Disorders)

Kurtcan S et al: MRS features during encephalopathic crisis period in 11 years old case with GA-1. Brain Dev. 37(5):546-51, 2015

Mohammad SA et al: Glutaric aciduria type 1: neuroimaging features with clinical correlation. Pediatr Radiol. 45(11):1696-705, 2015

Kölker S et al: Diagnosis and management of glutaric aciduria type I--revised recommendations. J Inherit Metab Dis. 34(3):677-94, 2011

Urea Cycle/Ammonia Disorders

Enns GM: Neurologic damage and neurocognitive dysfunction in urea cycle disorders. Semin Pediatr Neurol. 15(3):132-9, 2008

Gropman AL et al: Neurological implications of urea cycle disorders. J Inherit Metab Dis. 30(6):865-79, 2007

Methylmalonic and Propionic Acidemias

Fowler B et al: Causes of and diagnostic approach to methylmalonic acidurias. J Inherit Metab Dis. 31(3):350-60, 2008

Congenital Glycosylation Disorders

Feraco P et al: The shrunken, bright cerebellum: a characteristic MRI finding in congenital disorders of glycosylation type 1a. AJNR Am J Neuroradiol. 33(11):2062-7, 2012

Akaboshi S et al: Transient extreme spindles in a case of subacute Mycoplasma pneumoniae encephalitis. Acta Paediatr Jpn. 40(5):479-82, 1998

Acquired Metabolic and Systemic Disorders

The brain is highly susceptible to a number of acquired metabolic derangements. As occurs with inherited metabolic disorders and the toxic encephalopathies, the basal ganglia and cortex are especially vulnerable. Whereas the hemispheric white matter is less often affected, some acquired diseases such as osmotic demyelination may largely spare the gray matter and present with striking WM abnormalities.

In this chapter, we focus on acquired metabolic and systemic disorders that involve the CNS. We begin with the most common—hypertension—before turning our attention to abnormalities of glucose metabolism and thyroid/parathyroid function.

We then discuss seizure disorders, as sustained ictal activity with hypermetabolism can have profound effects on the brain. We begin with a brief delineation of normal temporal lobe and limbic anatomy as a prelude to the challenging topic of epilepsy. We finish the section by exploring the puzzling phenomena of the transient corpus callosum splenium lesion and transient global amnesia.

Finally, we consider a potpourri of acquired metabolic diseases, such as hepatic encephalopathy (both acute and chronic) and the osmotic demyelination syndromes.

Hypertensive Encephalopathies

If not recognized and treated, the effects of both acutely elevated blood pressure and chronic hypertension (HTN) on the brain can be devastating. We begin this section with a discussion of acute hypertensive encephalopathy, then delve into the CNS damage caused by HTN.

Acute Hypertensive Encephalopathy, Posterior Reversible Encephalopathy Syndrome

Terminology

The most common manifestation of acute hypertensive encephalopathy is **p**osterior **r**eversible **e**ncephalopathy **s**yndrome (PRES), also known as reversible posterior leukoencephalopathy syndrome (RPLS). Despite the syndrome's names, lesions are rarely limited to the "posterior"

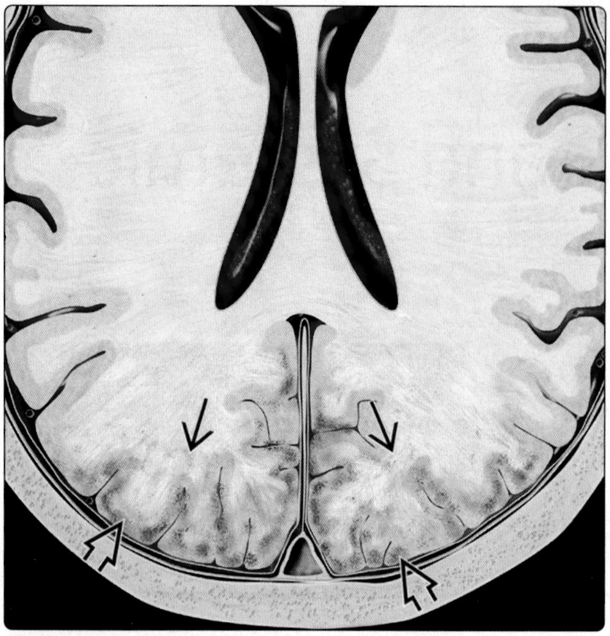

***(32-1)** Axial graphic shows cortical/subcortical vasogenic edema → in the posterior circulation, characteristic of PRES. Petechial hemorrhage ⇨ occurs in some cases but is unusual.*

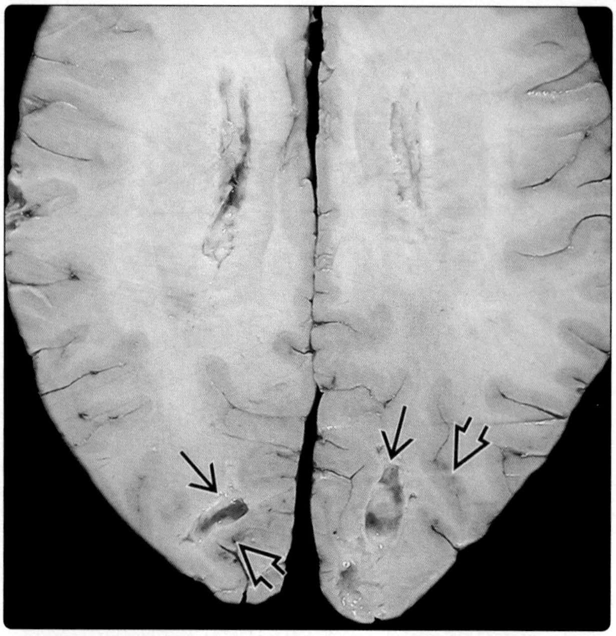

***(32-2)** Gross pathology of complicated PRES demonstrates diffuse cerebral edema with swollen gyri. Petechial hemorrhages ⇨ and foci of encephalomalacia secondary to infarction → are present. (Courtesy R. Hewlett, MD.)*

(parietooccipital) aspects of the brain (see below), and atypical is more common than "classical" PRES.

Etiology

General Concepts. The pathogenesis of PRES is not yet completely understood. The most common explanation is that severe HTN leads to failed cerebral autoregulation and breakthrough hyperperfusion with *vasodilatation*.

Excessive circulating cytokines may contribute to injury of the microvascular endothelium, increasing vascular permeability. Hydrostatic leakage and extravasation or transudation of fluid and macromolecules through damaged arteriolar walls into the adjacent brain interstitium result in vasogenic (not cytotoxic) edema **(32-1)**. However, between 15-20% of patients with PRES are normotensive or even hypotensive, whereas less than half have a mean arterial pressure above 140-150 mm Hg.

Alternative theories for the development of PRES invoke vasculopathy with vascular endothelial injury and dysfunction. Possible mechanisms for drug-induced PRES include direct toxic effects on vascular endothelial cells with release of endothelin, prostacyclin, and thromboxane A2.

Associated Conditions. PRES is associated with a multitude of diverse clinical entities, the most common of which are **eclampsia, HTN**, and **immunosuppressive treatment**.

Other conditions associated with PRES include renal failure with hemolytic-uremic syndrome (HUS), thrombotic thrombocytopenic purpura (TTP), autoimmune disorders (e.g., lupus nephropathy and acute glomerulonephritis), shock/sepsis syndrome, postcarotid endarterectomy with reperfusion syndrome, endocrine disorders, and stimulant drugs, such as ephedrine and pseudoephedrine.

Less common etiologies of PRES include ingestion of food products (such as licorice) containing substances that cause mineralocorticoid excess. The triad of HTN, hypokalemia, and metabolic alkalosis is typical. Patients with excess mineralocorticoids also have impaired endothelium-dependent vascular reactivity, which may contribute to the development of PRES.

Rarely, PRES is associated with the so-called SMART syndrome (**s**troke-like **m**igraine **a**ttacks after **r**adiation **t**herapy).

Pathology

The pathology of PRES is largely undefined, as PRES is rarely fatal and biopsied only in exceptional circumstances. Autopsied brains from patients with complicated PRES show diffuse cerebral edema. Intracranial hemorrhage complicates 15-25% of PRES cases. The most common finding is multiple bilateral petechial microhemorrhages in the occipital lobes **(32-2)**.

Microscopic features in PRES resemble those reported in malignant hypertensive encephalopathy. The occipital cortex, subcortical white matter (WM), and cerebellum demonstrate a range of microvascular pathology, including fibrinoid arteriolar necrosis with petechial hemorrhages, proteinaceous exudates, and macrophage infiltration along the perivascular spaces.

Pathologic evidence of partial irreversible damage has been documented in PRES despite radiographic resolution of abnormalities. Scattered microinfarcts, WM rarefaction with subpial gliosis, and hemosiderin deposition—especially in the posterior cerebrum—have been reported.

PRES: TERMINOLOGY, ETIOLOGY, AND CLINICAL ISSUES

Terminology

- **P**osterior **r**eversible **e**ncephalopathy **s**yndrome (PRES)
- *Lesions often not* just *posterior, not always reversible!*

Etiology

- HTN-induced dysautoregulation vs. vasospasm, ↓ perfusion
- ↑ ↑ BP → failed autoregulation → hyperperfusion
  - Vasogenic (not cytotoxic) edema
  - Endothelial dysfunction ± excessive circulating cytokines →"leaky" blood-brain barrier
  - Fluid, macromolecules ± blood extravasate
- Causes (HTN typical but not invariable)
  - Preeclampsia/eclampsia
  - Chemotherapy, immunosuppressive drugs
  - Thrombotic microangiopathies (e.g., HUS/TTP)
  - Renal failure
  - Shock/sepsis
  - Tumor lysis syndrome
  - Food/drug-induced mineralocorticoid excess

Clinical Issues

- All ages (peak = 20-40 years)
- F >> M
- BP usually ↑ ↑ *but*
  - < 50% have *mean* arterial pressure > 140-50 mm Hg
  - 15-20% normotensive or hypotensive
- Usually resolves completely with BP normalization

Clinical Issues

Epidemiology and Demographics. Although the peak age of onset is 20-40 years, PRES can affect patients of all ages from infants to the elderly. There is a moderate female predominance, largely because of the strong association of PRES and preeclampsia.

Preeclampsia is the most common overall cause of PRES. This pregnancy-specific disorder is characterized by HTN (blood pressure exceeding 140/90 mm Hg) and proteinuria occurring after 20 weeks of gestation in a previously normotensive patient. Preeclampsia and its variants affect approximately 5% of pregnancies and remain leading causes of both maternal and fetal morbidity.

Progression from preeclampsia to **eclampsia** occurs in 0.5% of patients with mild and 2-3% of patients with severe preeclampsia. Eclampsia is characterized by a peak systolic pressure of 160 mm Hg or greater, diastolic BO of 100 mg or greater, impaired renal function, thrombocytopenia, and/or evidence of microangiopathic hemolytic anemia, hepatocellular injury, pulmonary edema, and neurologic disturbances (primarily seizures).

Presentation. Although 92% of patients with PRES have acutely elevated blood pressure, *PRES can also occur in the absence of hypertension.* There is also no statistically significant association of blood pressure with imaging severity, hemorrhage, and cytotoxic edema.

The most common clinical symptoms and signs in patients with PRES are encephalopathy (50-80%), seizure (60-75%), headache (50%), visual disturbances (33%), and focal neurological deficit (10-15%).

PRES-associated seizures are typically single, short, uncomplicated grand mal type that terminate spontaneously during the first 24 hours. Serial or recurrent seizures as well as status epilepticus are uncommon.

Common comorbidities reported in recent series include steroids or immunosuppressants (40%), systemic lupus erythematosus (30%), kidney disease (20-30%), eclampsia (20%), and miscellaneous disorders such as vasculitis.

Natural History and Treatment Options. Reversibility is a typical feature of PRES and is associated with good prognosis. If the inciting substances or precipitating conditions are eliminated and any existing HTN is promptly treated, PRES often resolves with minimal or no residual abnormalities.

Extensive vasogenic edema, hemorrhage, and restricted diffusion on initial imaging are associated with worse clinical outcomes.

Severe PRES can be life-threatening. In rare cases, lesions are irreversible and permanent damage occurs, typically hemorrhagic cortical/subcortical or basal ganglionic infarcts.

Imaging

General Features. Three distinct imaging patterns of PRES have been described. The most common is a dominant **parietal-occipital pattern** (classic or typical PRES). Two less common (atypical) patterns are a **superior frontal sulcus pattern** (involvement of the mid and posterior aspects of the superior frontal sulcus) and a **holohemispheric watershed pattern** (involvement of the frontal, parietal, and occipital lobes along the internal watershed zones). Combinations of these three patterns as well as involvement of other anatomic areas (see below) are also common.

The parietooccipital lobes are involved in over 90% of PRES cases. These areas are considered particularly vulnerable because the comparatively sparse sympathetic innervation of the posterior circulation results in less protection against the effects of severe systemic HTN.

The frontal lobes are involved in 75-77% of cases, with the temporal lobes (65%) and cerebellum (50-55%) also commonly affected. Other atypical distributions include the basal ganglia and thalami, deep white matter, corpus callosum splenium, brainstem, and cervical spinal cord **(32-3)**.

As many PRES patients present with encephalopathy, seizure, severe headache, or visual disturbances, NECT scans are commonly obtained as an initial screening study. It is therefore extremely important to identify even subtle abnormalities that may be suggestive of PRES. **If the screening NECT is normal and PRES is suspected on clinical grounds, an MR**

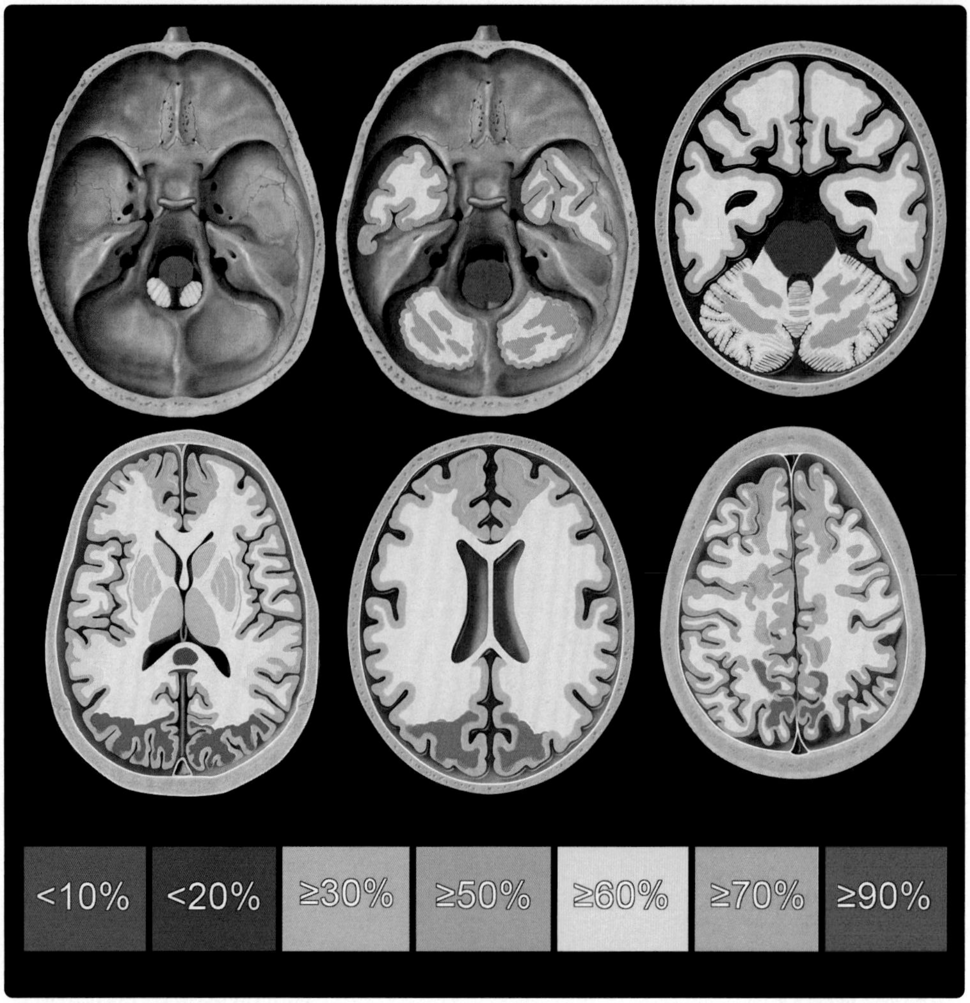

***(32-3)** Diagrammatic axial images show location and relative frequency of lesions in PRES. Although > 90% of PRES cases have lesions in the parietooccipital subcortical WM (classic PRES, shown in red), note multifocality is the rule, not the exception. Most cases of PRES also have lesions in areas other than the classic parietooccipital location. Both classic PRES (red) and the superior frontal sulcus pattern (orange) are frequently combined with additional lesions distributed along the hemispheric cortical (superficial) watershed zones (depicted in the lower right image). The cerebellum is affected in nearly half of PRES cases, whereas about one-third have basal ganglionic lesions (light blue). The pons, medulla, cervical spinal cord, and corpus callosum splenium are less common sites involved by PRES although in some cases ONLY the posterior fossa is affected. Remember: atypical PRES is actually more common than the classic isolated parieto-occipital involvement! (Adapted from Ollivier et al.)*

scan with DWI and T2* in addition to the routine sequences (T1 and T2/FLAIR) should be obtained.

CT Findings. Screening NECTs are normal in approximately one-quarter of all PRES cases **(32-5)**. Subtle patchy cortical/subcortical hypodensities—usually in the parietooccipital lobes, watershed zones, and/or cerebellum—may be the only visible abnormalities on NECT **(32-4)**.

PRES-associated intracranial hemorrhage is uncommon, seen in only 5-15% of cases. Three different patterns of PRES-associated intracranial hemorrhage occur and are found in almost equal proportions: focal parenchymal hematoma, multifocal hemorrhages (usually less than 5 mm), and convexity subarachnoid hemorrhage.

CECT is usually negative although severe cases may show patchy, nonconfluent cortical/subcortical enhancing foci.

MR Findings. PRES has both classic and atypical (i.e., variant) MR features. Keep in mind that (1) atypical PRES is actually more common than classic (i.e., purely parietal-occipital) PRES; (2) PRES is rarely *just* posterior; and (3) PRES is *not always reversible.*

Classic PRES demonstrates bilateral parietooccipital cortical/subcortical hypointensities that are hypointense on T1WI and hyperintense on T2/FLAIR **(32-5)**. T2* (GRE or SWI) sequences may demonstrate hemorrhagic foci **(32-7)**.

"Leaky" arterioles with loss of blood-brain barrier integrity may cause patchy cortical-subcortical enhancement on T1 C+ sequences.

Imaging findings in *atypical* PRES include involvement of the frontal lobes, watershed zones, basal ganglia and/or thalami, brainstem, cerebellum, and even the spinal cord **(32-6)**. Findings of both classic and atypical PRES very commonly occur together.

In unusual cases, brainstem and/or cerebellar lesions may be the *only* abnormality present. The spinal cord has been reported as a rare site of isolated PRES involvement.

Frank infarction is quite rare in PRES. Because most cases of PRES are caused by vasogenic—not cytotoxic—edema, DWI is usually negative. However, PRES with restricted diffusion occurs in 15-30% of cases and is usually seen as small foci of restricted diffusion within larger regions of nonrestricting vasogenic edema.

MR and CT perfusion studies have demonstrated both increased AND decreased perfusion in PRES. The most striking reported findings are in the occipital regions and cortical watershed zones.

Following blood pressure normalization, imaging findings in most cases of PRES resolve completely. Irreversible lesions are relatively uncommon, occurring in approximately 15% of cases. Imaging features associated with poor prognosis include lesions with low initial ADC, brainstem involvement, and the presence of hemorrhage on initial imaging studies.

Angiography. Vasculopathy is a common finding on CTA, MRA, or DSA in patients with PRES. Diffuse vessel constriction or narrowing, focal irregularity, and beaded appearance are typical but nonspecific angiographic findings in PRES. Whether these abnormalities reflect transient reversible vasoconstriction or vasculitis/vasculopathy is unclear.

Differential Diagnosis

The major differential diagnoses of PRES includes acute cerebral ischemia-infarction, vasculitis, hypoglycemia, status epilepticus, sinovenous thrombosis, reversible cerebral vasoconstriction syndrome, and the thrombotic microangiopathies.

PRES rarely involves *just* the posterior circulation, so **acute cerebral ischemia-infarction** is often easily distinguished. Bilateral PCA distribution infarcts are rare in the absence of "top of the basilar" thrombosis, which typically affects other areas such as the thalami, midbrain, and superior cerebellum.

Vasculitis can resemble PRES-induced vasculopathy at angiography. The distribution of lesions in vasculitis is much more random and less symmetric, usually does not demonstrate the parietooccipital predominance seen in PRES, and more often enhances following contrast administration.

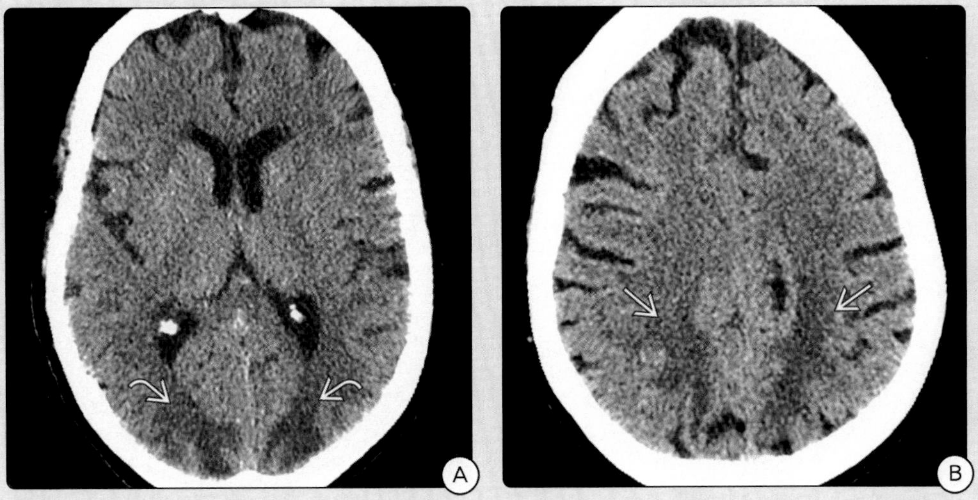

***(32-4A)** NECT in a 63y woman with severe hypertension and headache followed by seizure shows bioccipital hypodensities in the subcortical white matter ➡. **(32-4B)** More cephalad NECT in the same case shows symmetric hypodensity in the posterior parietal and high occipital white matter ➡.*

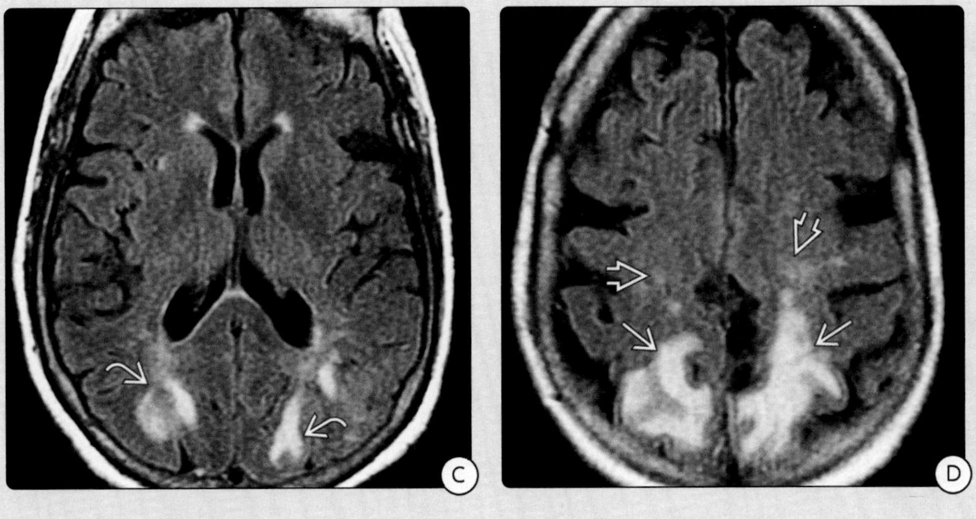

***(32-4C)** FLAIR in the same case shows patchy hyperintensity in the occipital white matter ➡ that mostly spares the cortex. **(32-4D)** More cephalad FLAIR shows confluent WM hyperintensity ➡ with sparing of the overlying cortex. Note extension into the adjacent watershed zones ➡. T2* GRE showed no hemorrhage, and DWI was negative. This is classic PRES.*

In contrast to vasculitis, high-resolution vessel wall imaging is usually negative in PRES.

Hypoglycemia typically affects the parietooccipital cortex and subcortical WM, so the clinical laboratory findings (i.e., low serum glucose, lack of systemic HTN) are important differentiating features. **Status epilepticus** can cause transient gyral edema but is rarely bilateral and can affect any part of the cortex.

Less common entities that can mimic PRES include **sinovenous thrombosis** and reversible cerebral vasoconstriction syndrome. Thrombosis of the posterior (descending) aspect of the superior sagittal sinus can cause patchy bilateral parietooccipital cortical/subcortical edema. Hemorrhage is common (rare in PRES), and CTV easily demonstrates the occluded sinus. **Reversible cerebral vasoconstriction syndrome** shares some features (e.g., convexal subarachnoid hemorrhage) with PRES but is typically limited to a solitary sulcus or just a few adjacent sulci.

Thrombotic microangiopathies (TMAs) can be difficult to differentiate from PRES solely on the basis of imaging features. Primary TMAs include ADAMTS13-mediated TMA (also known as thrombotic thrombocytopenic purpura, TTP) and Shiga toxin-mediated TMA (hemolytic-uremic syndrome, HUS).

Secondary TMAs are caused by an underlying disease process and include malignant HTN (mHTN), HELLP syndrome, autoimmune disorders, and disseminated intravascular coagulopathy (DIC).

PRES is a common manifestation in all the thrombotic microangiopathies, although the distinction between PRES and mHTN may be largely academic. The presence of diffuse cerebral edema and multifocal microhemorrhages is more typical of mHTN. Atypical location (brainstem, cerebellum, basal ganglia), restricted diffusion, and generalized cerebral edema are all more common in mHTN but also occur in PRES.

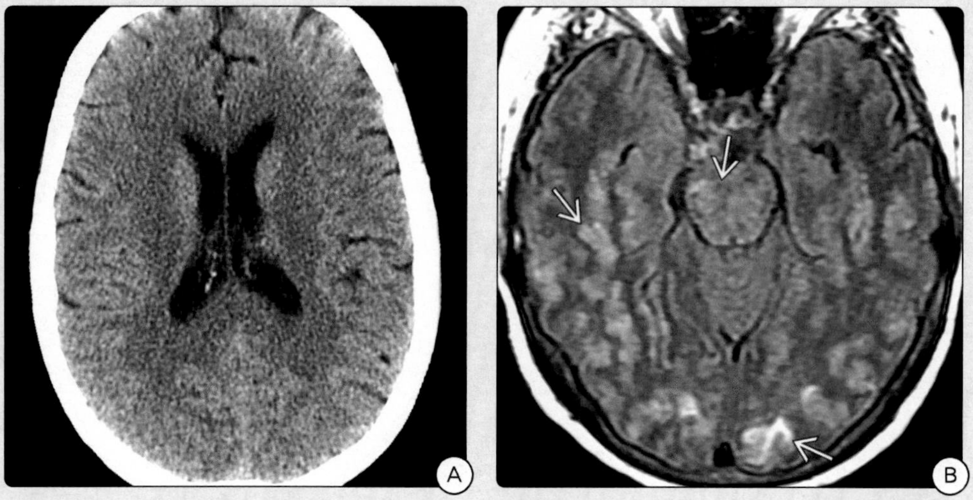

***(32-5A)** A 63y woman with end-stage renal disease had a seizure, then fell. Blood pressure on admission was 220/140. NECT scan performed to evaluate for intracranial hemorrhage shows normal findings. **(32-5B)** MR was obtained because of suspected PRES. FLAIR scan obtained 1 hour after the NECT shows multifocal patchy hyperintensities in the midbrain, posteroinferior temporal lobes, and parietooccipital cortex ➡.*

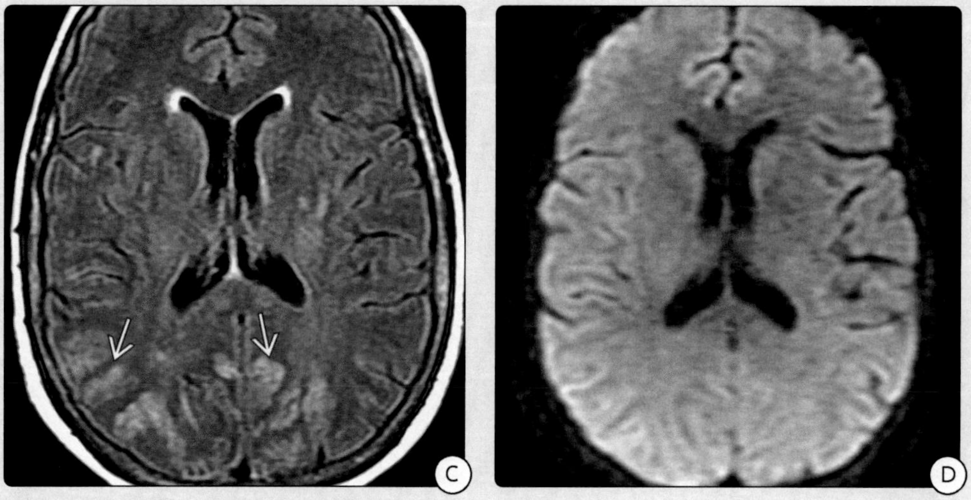

***(32-5C)** FLAIR image through the lateral ventricles shows bilateral, relatively symmetric lesions in the parietooccipital cortex ➡. **(32-5D)** DWI scan in the same patient shows no evidence for diffusion restriction. DWI scans are usually (although not invariably) normal in PRES because the edema is mostly vasogenic, not cytotoxic.*

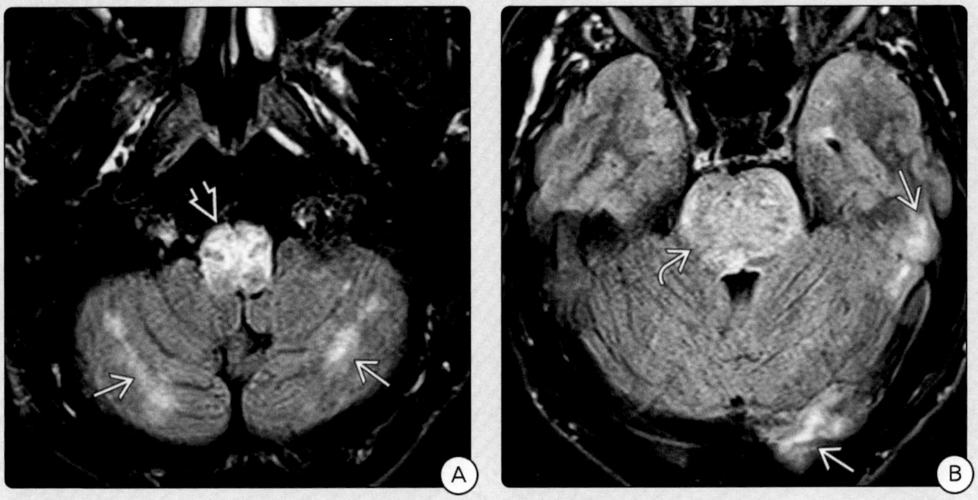

(32-6A) *Axial FLAIR in a 50y man with severe hypertension (BP = 200/120) shows confluent hyperintensity involving the entire medulla ➡. Note patchy hyperintensities in the white matter of both cerebellar hemispheres ➡.* **(32-6B)** *More cephalad FLAIR in the same case shows involvement of the pons ➡, occipital, and temporal subcortical white matter ➡.*

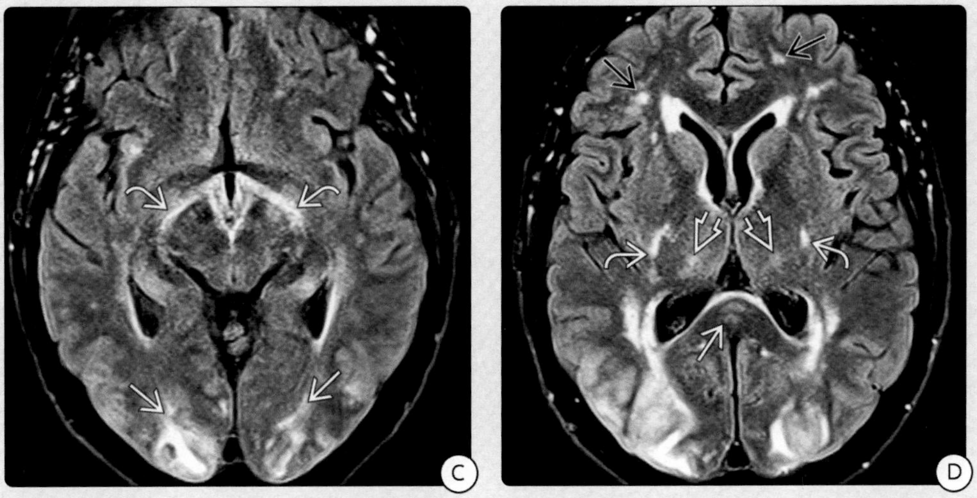

(32-6C) *More cephalad FLAIR in the same case shows hyperintensity in the optic tracts ➡ and occipital subcortical WM ➡.* **(32-6D)** *Additional lesions are present in the thalami ➡, internal capsules ➡, corpus callosum splenium ➡, and frontal WM ➡.*

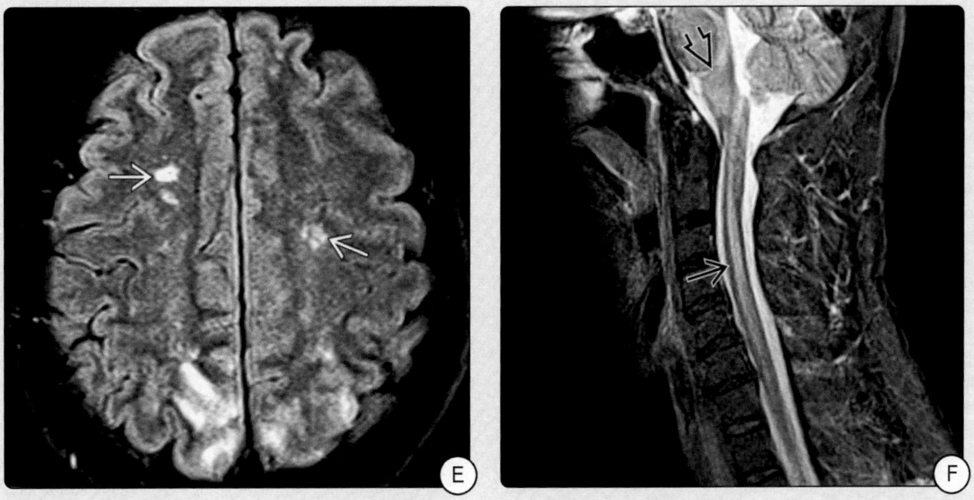

(32-6E) *More cephalad FLAIR shows lesions along the watershed zones ➡.* **(32-6F)** *Sagittal STIR of the cervical spine shows confluent hyperintensity extending from the medulla ➡ inferiorly throughout the entire cervical spinal cord ➡. This is atypical PRES.*

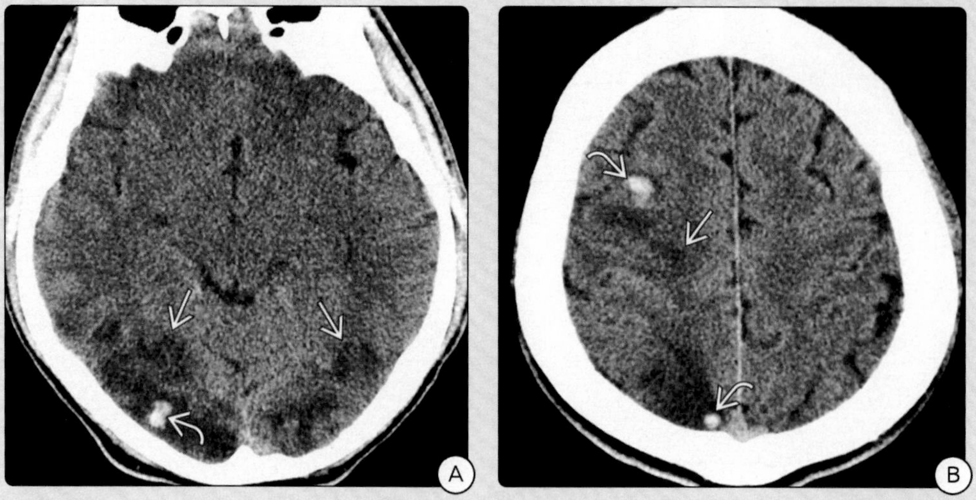

***(32-7A)** NECT in a 39y male methamphetamine abuser with headache, altered mental status, and vision loss shows bilateral parietal-occipital hypodense lesions with patchy hemorrhagic foci . **(32-7B)** NECT in the same case shows confluent hypodensities in the right hemispheric white matter . Note two additional hemorrhagic foci . This was read outside the hospital with the imaging diagnosis of hemorrhagic metastases.*

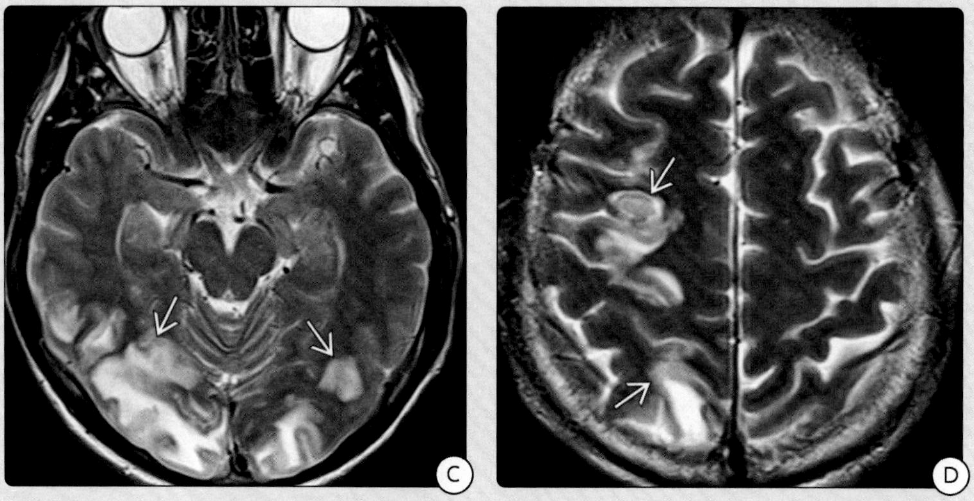

***(32-7C)** MR was obtained on admission. T2WI in the same case shows patchy and confluent parieto-occipital hyperintense lesions predominately in the subcortical WM. **(32-7D)** More cephalad T2WI shows lesions in the right hemisphere watershed zone.*

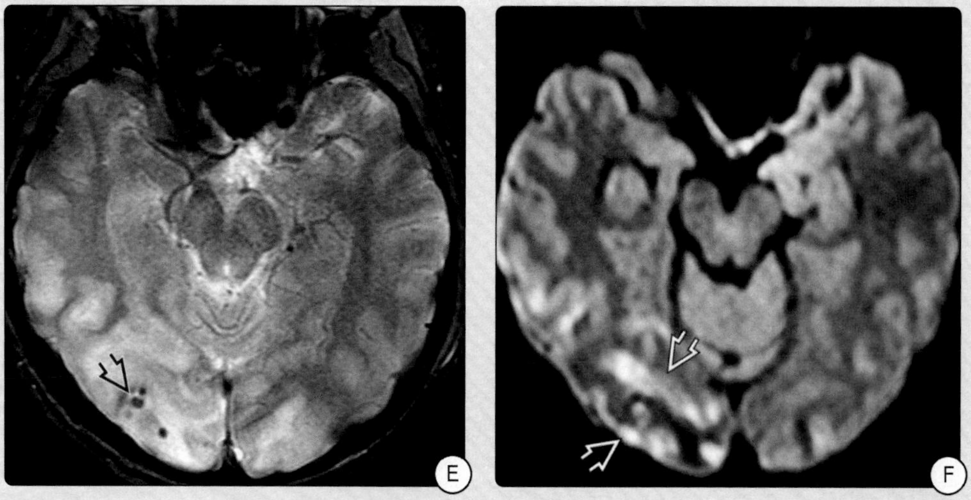

***(32-7E)** T2* GRE shows several "blooming" hemorrhagic foci . **(32-7F)** DWI shows patchy foci of restricted diffusion in the larger, more confluent areas of WM edema seen on the T2WIs. Blood pressure was 152/73. This was methamphetamine-induced PRES.*

PRES: IMAGING AND DDx

Three Anatomic Patterns

- Classic PRES
  - **Parietooccipital pattern** (> 90%)
- Variant PRES
  - **Superior frontal sulcus pattern** (70%)
  - **Holohemispheric watershed pattern** (50%)
  - Other: cerebellum (50%), basal ganglia (30%), brainstem (20%), spinal cord (< 10%)
- Combinations *very* common (> 90%)

CT

- Can be normal or only subtly abnormal
  - If PRES suspected and CT normal, get MR!
- Posterior cortical/subcortical hypodensities
- Gross hemorrhage rare (parenchymal > cSAH)

MR

- T2/FLAIR hyperintensity (parietooccipital most common)
- T2* (GRE/SWI) shows hemorrhage in 15-25%
- DWI usually but not invariably negative
- Enhancement none/mild (unless severe PRES)

Differential Diagnosis

- Posterior circulation ischemia-infarction
  - Top of the basilar syndrome
- Vasculitis
- Status epilepticus
- Hypoglycemia
- Thrombotic microangiopathy
  - Primary (ADAMTS13-mediated TMA/TTP, Shiga toxin-mediated HUS)
  - Secondary (mHTN, HELLP syndrome, autoimmune disorders, DIC)
- Sinovenous thrombosis
  - Internal cerebral veins, vein of Galen/straight sinus
- Reversible cerebral vasoconstriction syndrome

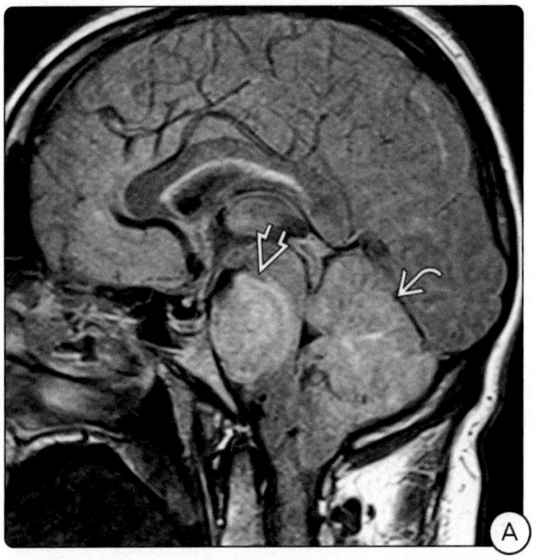

***(32-8A)** FLAIR in an encephalopathic 34y patient with severe headache, BP 240/120 shows swollen, hyperintense pons ⇨, cerebellum ↷.*

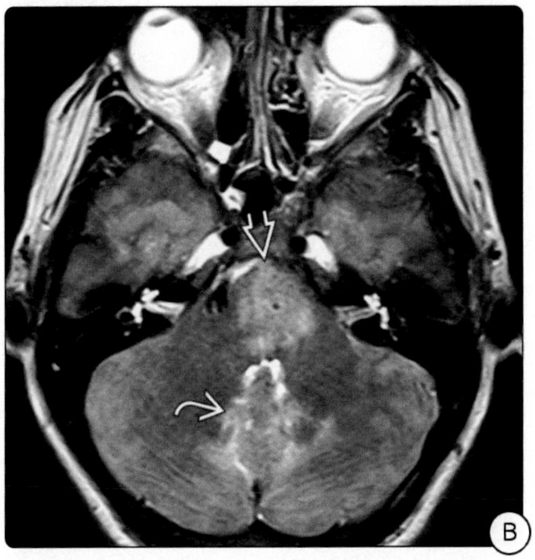

***(32-8B)** T2WI in the same case with mHTN shows pontine ⇨ and cerebellar ↷ confluent hyperintensity and mass effect.*

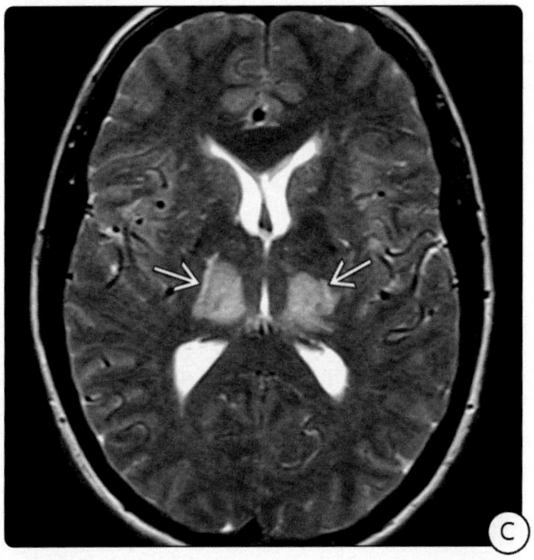

***(32-8C)** Symmetric thalamic hyperintensities ➔ are present. DWI (not shown) was negative. Findings resolved with aggressive BP treatment.*

Acute Hypertensive Encephalopathy and Malignant Hypertension

Terminology

Hypertensive encephalopathy occurs when elevated mean arterial pressure overcomes cerebral autoregulation. With the resulting loss of control of cerebral perfusion, cerebral blood flow (CBF) rises, the brain is hyperperfused, and vasogenic edema develops.

Malignant hypertension (mHTN), sometimes termed acute hypertensive crisis, is characterized clinically by extreme blood pressure elevation and papilledema. **Accelerated HTN** is identified by the presence of severe retinopathy (exudates, hemorrhages, arteriolar narrowing, spasm, etc.) without papilledema. Both forms of HTN are associated with severe vascular injury to the kidneys and other end-organs.

Etiology

Any form of hypertensive disorder, regardless of etiology, can precipitate a hypertensive crisis. **The abruptness of blood pressure elevation seems to be more important than the absolute level of either systolic or mean arterial blood pressure.**

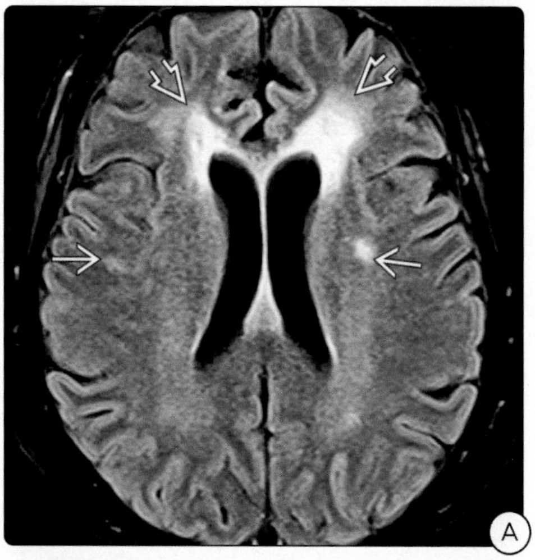

***(32-9A)** FLAIR in 54y woman with chronic renal failure, TTP, confusion shows bifrontal confluent ➡ and scattered WM ➡ hyperintensities.*

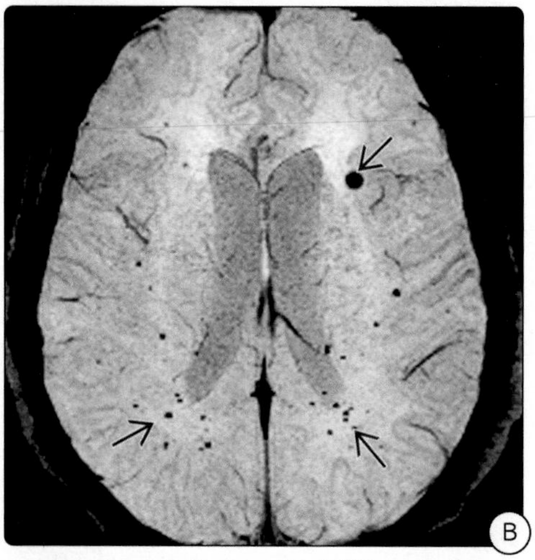

***(32-9B)** T2* SWI shows multiple "blooming" foci ➡ throughout the white matter. The cortex is spared.*

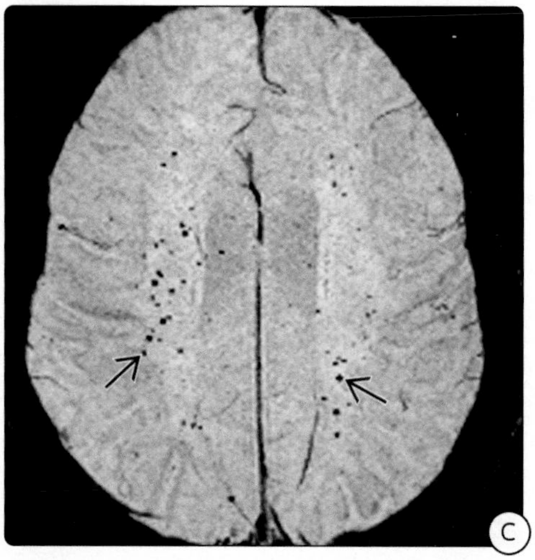

***(32-9C)** More cephalad T2* SWI demonstrates more blooming WM hypointensities ➡.*

mHTN in the setting of chronic hypertension is actually rare, occurring in less than 1% of all patients. Nevertheless, because the prevalence of HTN in the general population is so high, so-called *essential hypertension* (i.e., chronic HTN without an identifiable underlying cause) is still the most common overall condition predisposing to mHTN.

mHTN also occurs in previously normotensive individuals. Sudden onset of severe HTN can occur in children with acute glomerulonephritis and renal failure, pregnant women with eclampsia, and patients of all ages with substance abuse (e.g., cocaine). Less common causes of mHTN include pheochromocytoma crisis, clonidine withdrawal syndrome, drug interactions (e.g., monoamine oxidase inhibitor + tyramine), and autonomic overactivity in patients with spinal cord disorders.

Pathology

Macroscopically, the brain appears swollen and edematous. Gross parenchymal hematomas and perivascular petechial microhemorrhages may be present. Acute microinfarcts, especially in the basal ganglia and pons, are common.

Microscopic features of mHTN include arteriolar fibrinoid necrosis with fragmentation and loss of nuclear staining in the affected vessel walls. In HTN-associated thrombotic microangiopathy, some arterioles contain intraluminal platelet/fibrin thrombi, whereas others are surrounded by proteinaceous exudates or admixed fibrin and hemorrhage. Edema in the adjacent white matter is a typical associated finding.

Clinical Issues

Blood pressure in mHTN is severely elevated, with diastolic levels often exceeding 130-140 mm Hg. Headache with or without coexisting encephalopathy is the most frequent symptom and is often accompanied by visual disturbances, nausea, vomiting, and altered mental status. Congestive heart failure, deteriorating renal function, and anemia are common.

The complications of acute hypertensive crisis are generally reversible if the condition is diagnosed properly and appropriate therapy instituted quickly. Rapid blood pressure reduction typically results in prompt, dramatic improvement in hypertensive encephalopathy.

Imaging

Imaging findings in mHTN range from classic PRES-like features with parietooccipital predominance to "atypical" features. "Atypical" features are more common in mHTN compared with PRES. Brainstem-dominant hypertensive encephalopathy and basal ganglia and/or watershed lesions are common cerebral manifestations of mHTN **(32-8)**. Diffuse cerebral edema may be present in especially severe cases.

Lobar and/or multifocal parenchymal microhemorrhages in the cortex, basal ganglia, pons, and cerebellum are common in mHTN and are best seen as "blooming" foci on T2* sequences (GRE, SWI) **(32-9)**. Convexal subarachnoid hemorrhage with multiple foci of short-segment arterial stenoses resembling reversible cerebral vasoconstriction syndrome (RCVS) has been reported in a few cases of mHTN.

mHTN can cause widespread blood-brain barrier disruption with striking multifocal patchy enhancement following contrast administration **(32-10)**. Restricted diffusion with decreased ADC values on DWI is more common in mHTN compared with classic PRES.

Differential Diagnosis

The major differential diagnosis of mHTN is **PRES**. **TTP** with brain ischemia and microhemorrhages **(32-9)** can appear identical on imaging studies, and the distinction is established by clinical laboratory features, not imaging findings.

ACUTE HYPERTENSIVE ENCEPHALOPATHY

Terminology
- Also known as malignant hypertension, hypertensive crisis

Etiology
- Abrupt rise in BP > absolute value of BP
- Many causes
  - Idiopathic ("essential") HTN
  - Eclampsia
  - Drug abuse (cocaine, methamphetamine)
  - Immunosuppressant neurotoxicity
  - Renal (acute glomerulonephritis, HUS)
  - Other thrombotic microangiopathies
  - High altitude exposure
  - Collagen-vascular disease (e.g., scleroderma, lupus)
  - Pheochromocytoma crisis
  - Autonomic instability

Imaging
- Brainstem, basal ganglia > > cortex, watershed
- Microbleeds on T2* (GRE, SWI) common

Differential Diagnosis
- Major differential diagnosis is PRES (can, often does overlap)

Chronic Hypertensive Encephalopathy

Although the clinical and imaging manifestations of posterior reversible encephalopathy syndrome (PRES) and malignant hypertension (mHTN) can be dramatic and life-threatening, the effects of longstanding untreated or poorly treated HTN on end-organ function can be equally devastating.

Pathology

The most consistent histopathologic feature of chronic hypertensive encephalopathy (CHtnE) is a microvasculopathy characterized by arteriolosclerosis and lipohyalinosis (see Chapter 10). Stenosis and occlusion of small arteries and arterioles from layers of hyaline collagen deposition cause decreased oligodendrocyte density, myelin pallor, gliosis, and spongiform WM volume loss. Multiple lacunar infarcts are common.

Clinical Issues

CHtnE is most common in middle-aged and elderly patients. CHtnE affects men more often than women and is especially prevalent in African Americans. In addition to age and chronically elevated blood pressure, smoking is an independent risk factor for CHtnE. Metabolic syndrome (impaired glucose metabolism, elevated blood pressure, central obesity, and dyslipidemia) is increasingly common and contributes significantly to the worldwide burden of CHtnE.

The most common symptom of CHtnE is nonspecific headache. Stepwise or gradual progression of cognitive dysfunction is also common and may develop into frank vascular dementia.

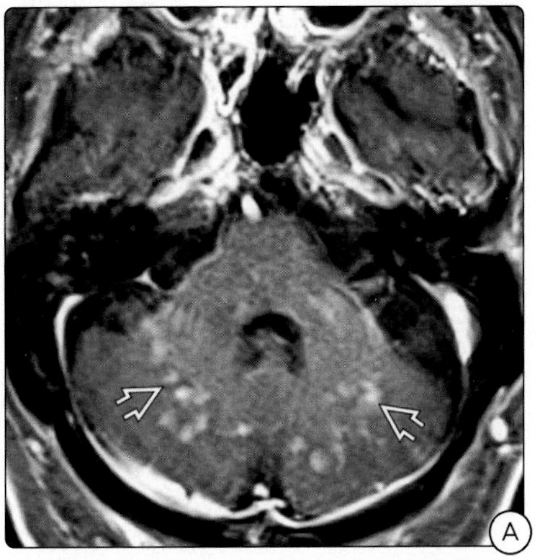

***(32-10A)** T1 C+ FS in a patient with mHTN shows multiple patchy foci of enhancement ➡ in the cerebellar white matter.*

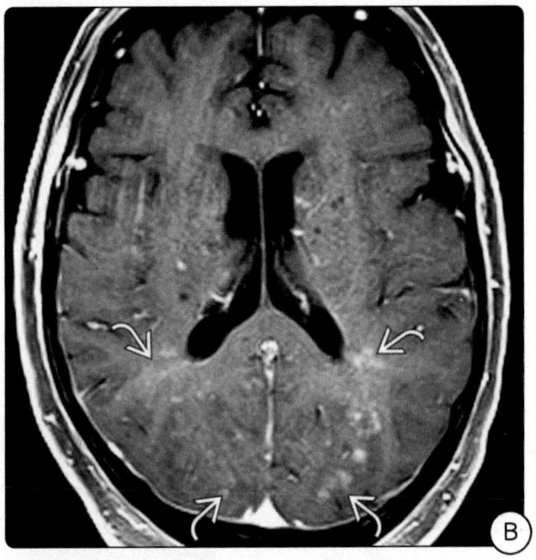

***(32-10B)** More cephalad T1 C+ FS shows multifocal patchy enhancement ➡ in the parieto-occipital lobes of both hemispheres.*

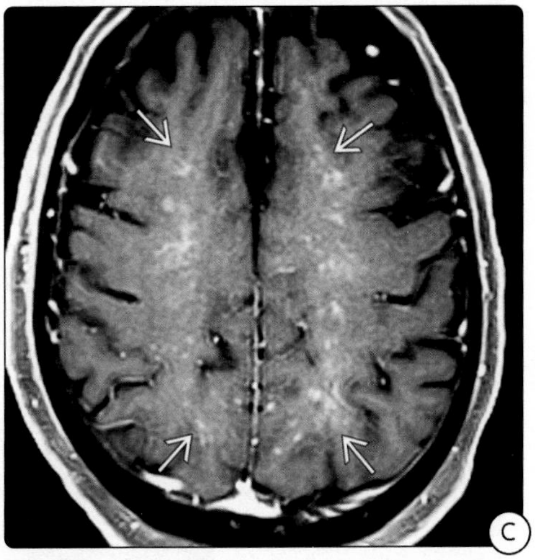

***(32-10C)** T1 C+ FS through the corona radiata shows extensive patchy enhancement ➡ in the subcortical white matter of both hemispheres.*

Approximately 1-2% of patients with chronic HTN develop an acute hypertensive emergency. In these "acute-on-chronic" hypertensive cases, blood pressure rises substantially and causes end-organ dysfunction. The brain is affected in approximately 15% of cases. Headache, seizure, focal neurological signs, or depressed consciousness are common symptoms. These patients have a 5% 1-year cumulative risk of subsequent ischemic stroke or intracranial hemorrhage.

Imaging

The two cardinal imaging features of CHtnE are (1) diffuse patchy and/or confluent WM lesions and (2) multifocal microbleeds. The WM lesions are concentrated in the corona radiata and deep periventricular WM—especially around the atria of the lateral ventricles. The damaged WM appears hypodense on NECT scans and hyperintense on T2/FLAIR imaging.

Multiple petechial bleeds ("microhemorrhages") are the second most common manifestation of CHtnE. These are not usually identifiable on NECT and may be invisible on standard MR sequences (FSE T2WI and FLAIR). T2* (GRE, SWI) scans show multiple "blooming" hypointensities ("black dots") that tend to be concentrated in the basal ganglia and cerebellum **(32-11)**.

Imaging findings in CHtnE can also reflect "acute-on-chronic" disease. T2* scans in the majority of patients with classic basal ganglia or lobar hypertensive hemorrhages demonstrate petechial microhemorrhages. Occasionally, patients with chronic longstanding HTN develop an acute hypertensive crisis and can demonstrate features of PRES superimposed on longstanding, chronic-appearing WM disease.

Differential Diagnosis

The major differential diagnosis of CHtnE is **cerebral amyloid angiopathy** (CAA). The WM lesions in both diseases often

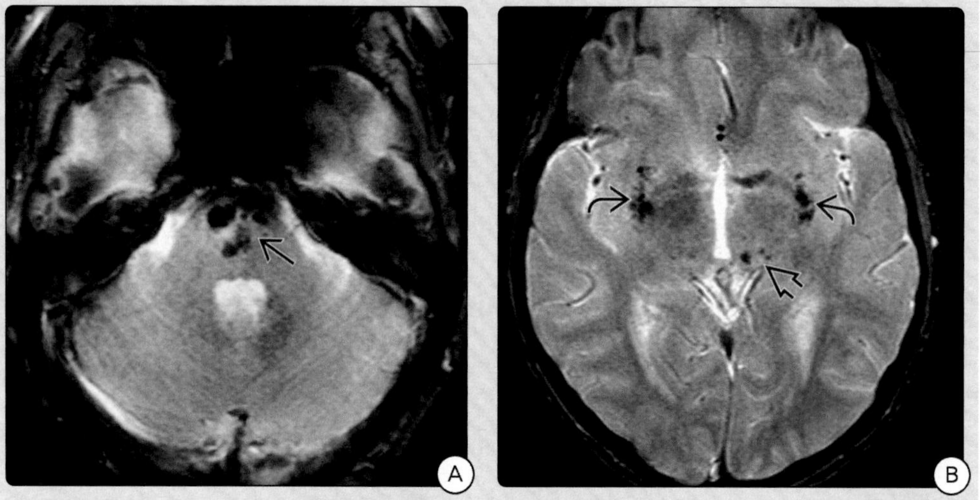

***(32-11A)** T2*GRE in a 37y woman with longstanding poorly treated hypertensions shows multiple "blooming" foci in the pons →. **(32-11B)** More cephalad T2* GRE in the same case shows multiple foci of blooming hypointensity in both external capsules/putamina → as well as in the thalami →.*

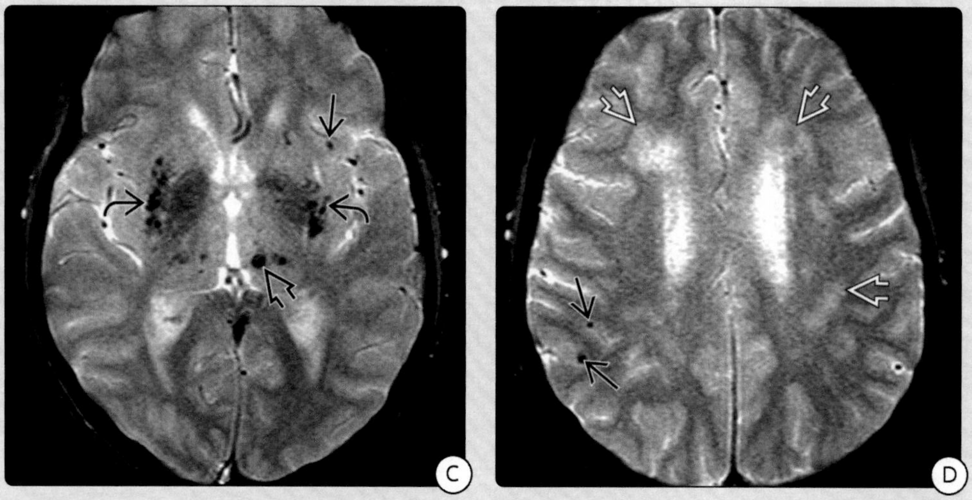

***(32-11C)** More cephalad T2* GRE shows innumerable hypointensities in the basal ganglia → and thalami →. A single focus of susceptibility is seen in the left insular cortex →. **(32-11D)** More cephalad T2* GRE shows additional foci of gradient susceptibility in the cortex →. Note extensive periventricular WM hyperintensities →. This is chronic hypertensive encephalopathy.*

appear similar, and both disorders can cause hemorrhagic microangiopathy. The microbleeds of CAA are more often peripheral (e.g., cortex, leptomeninges) and rarely affect the brainstem or cerebellum. Hypertensive microhemorrhages are most common in the basal ganglia and frequently can be identified in the pons and cerebellar hemispheres.

CHRONIC HYPERTENSIVE ENCEPHALOPATHY

Pathology
- Microvasculopathy
  - Arteriolosclerosis, lipohyalinosis
  - Myelin pallor, lacunar infarcts
  - Microbleeds (cerebellum, basal ganglia/thalami > cortex)

Clinical Issues
- Metabolic syndrome, headaches
- Can have "acute-on-chronic" HTN with encephalopathy

Imaging
- Diffuse patchy and/or confluent WM lesions
- Microbleeds on T2* (basal ganglia, cerebellum)

Differential Diagnosis
- Amyloid angiopathy (cortex > basal ganglia, cerebellum)
- CADASIL (younger patients, anterior temporal/external capsule WM lesions)

Cerebral autosomal-dominant arteriopathy without subcortical infarcts and leukoencephalopathy (CADASIL) can also mimic CHtnE. CADASIL typically presents in younger patients and causes multiple subcortical lacunar infarcts. Lesions in the anterior temporal lobes and external capsules are classic imaging findings of CADASIL.

Glucose Disorders

The brain is a glucose glutton, consuming more than half the body's total glucose. Because the brain does not store excess energy as glycogen, CNS function is highly dependent on a steady, continuous supply of blood glucose (see box below).

Blood glucose levels are tightly regulated and are normally maintained within a narrow physiologic range. Disorders of glucose metabolism—both *hypo*glycemia and *hyper*glycemia—can injure the CNS.

The neurologic manifestations of deranged glucose metabolism range from mild, reversible focal deficits to status epilepticus, coma, and death. Because the clinical and imaging manifestations differ in neonates from those of older children and adults, hypoglycemia in these two age groups is discussed separately.

The vast majority of hypoglycemia cases are acquired. A few inherited syndromes present with infantile hyperinsulinemic hypoglycemia as a secondary manifestation of systemic disease. The effects of hypoglycemia on the infant brain are identical, regardless of etiology, so they are discussed in this chapter.

Following the discussion of *hypo*glycemia, we turn our attention to *hyper*glycemia-associated disorders that affect the CNS.

GLUCOSE AND THE BRAIN

Normal Physiology
- Brain is a "glucose glutton"
  - Utilizes 100-150 g/day
- Glucose must be actively transported across blood-brain barrier
  - Glucose transport protein (GLUT-1)
- Glucose metabolism
  - Aerobic oxidation (20% of total body O_2 consumption)
  - Intracellular glucose converted to pyruvate
  - Then metabolized to ATP, phosphocreatine
- Glucose utilization linearly related to CBF
  - GM ≈ 5x WM
  - Mostly used for active ion transport, maintenance of membrane potentials
- Glucose homeostasis
  - Blood glucose concentration dynamic, tightly regulated
  - Brain monitors, "conducts" gut-CNS-endocrine axis
  - Complex interactions maintain normal glycemia

Abnormal Physiology
- Too much or too little glucose both injure brain
- Hyperglycemic > > hypoglycemic disorders

Pediatric/Adult Hypoglycemic Encephalopathy

Terminology

Hypoglycemia literally means low blood sugar and is caused by an imbalance between glucose supply and glucose utilization. Acute hypoglycemic brain injury is called hypoglycemic encephalopathy.

Etiology

Childhood hypoglycemic encephalopathy is most commonly associated with type 1 diabetes mellitus. Rarely, hypoglycemia occurs as an inherited disorder (see below) or secondary to insulin-secreting tumors.

In its most common adult setting—advanced type 2 diabetes—hypoglycemia typically results from the interplay between absolute or relative insulin excess and compromised glucose counterregulation; insulin in and of itself is not neurotoxic. Most cases of adult hypoglycemia occur as a side effect of diabetes treatment with insulin and sulfonylureas.

Factors other than absolute blood glucose levels also affect the presence and extent of hypoglycemic brain injury, including the duration and severity of hypoglycemia, presence

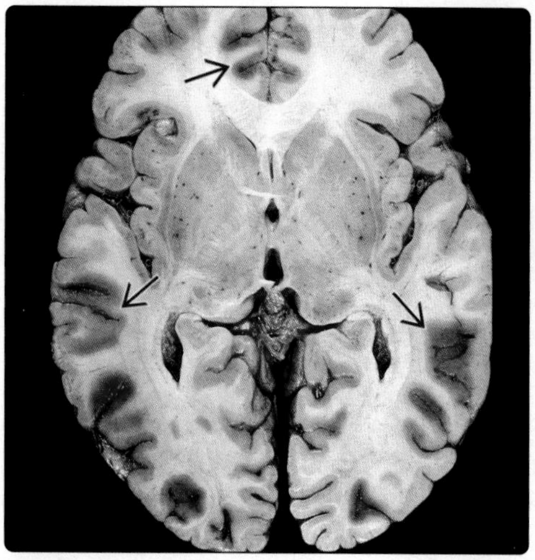

(32-12) Autopsy of severe hypoglycemia shows bilateral symmetric parietooccipital, frontal cortical necrosis →. (Courtesy R. Hewlett, MD.)

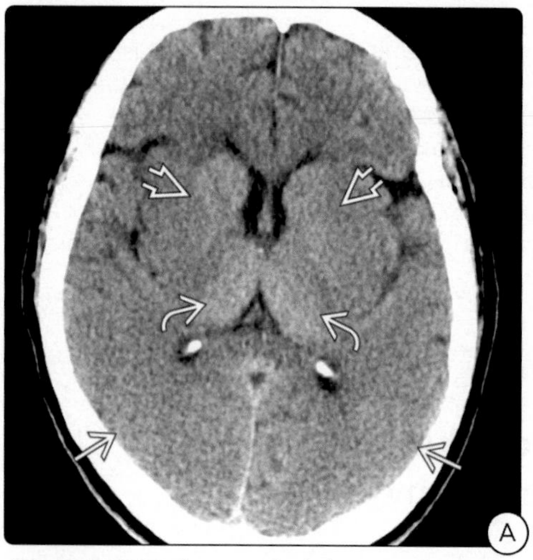

(32-13A) NECT shows typical changes of hypoglycemia with parietooccipital gyral swelling →, putamen hypodensity →, spared thalami ↷.

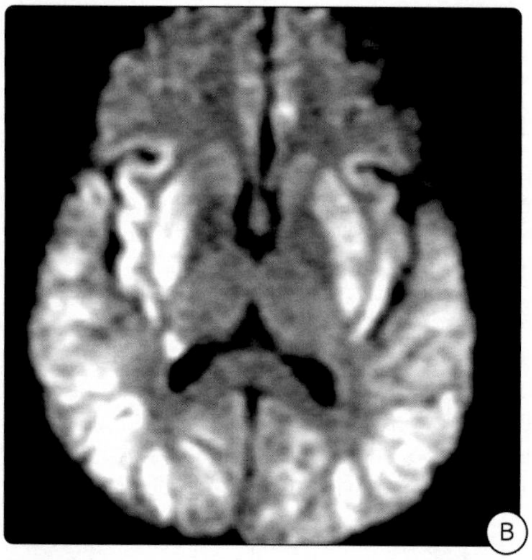

(32-13B) DWI in the same case of typical AHE shows restricted diffusion in parietooccipital cortex, putamina with thalamic and WM sparing.

and degree of hypoxia or other metabolic disturbances, cerebral blood flow, and CNS/cardiovascular metabolic requirements.

Pathology

Hypoglycemia has both direct and indirect effects on the brain, which is exquisitely sensitive to glucose insufficiency. Glucose insufficiency results in impaired oxygen utilization and compromised intracellular energy production. In addition, sustained glucose deprivation sensitizes microglial release of inflammatory mediators and may contribute to a number of comorbidities in diabetes and/or metabolic disorders.

Indirect effects of hypoglycemia occur secondary to the accumulation and release of excitatory neurotransmitters, which in turn accentuates the degree of hypoglycemic brain injury.

Cortical necrosis is the most common gross finding in hypoglycemic encephalopathy. Although the entire cortical ribbon can be affected, the parietooccipital regions are usually the most severely involved **(32-12)**. Other especially vulnerable areas include the basal ganglia, hippocampi, and amygdalae. The thalami, white matter, brainstem, and cerebellum are typically spared.

Clinical Issues

The typical hypoglycemic patient is an elderly diabetic on insulin replacement therapy with altered dietary glucose intake. Deliberate or accidental insulin overdose is more common in children and young or middle-aged adults.

Seizures, mental status changes, and coma are common symptoms of hypoglycemic encephalopathy. Prognosis varies with the extent of brain injury. If the basal ganglia are involved, the outcome is generally poor. If basal ganglia injury is minimal or absent, residual neurologic deficits are correlated with the severity of cortical injury.

Because of sympathoadrenergic effects, myocardial infarction and severe arrhythmias are common indirect effects of hypoglycemia and may account for the "dead in bed" syndrome.

Imaging

CT Findings. NECT scans typically show symmetrically hypodense parietal and occipital lobes. The putamina frequently appear hypodense, whereas the thalami are spared **(32-13)**. In severe cases, diffuse cerebral edema with near-total sulcal effacement and blurred gray-white matter interfaces can be seen.

MR Findings. T1 scans in patients with acute hypoglycemic encephalopathy can appear normal or demonstrate only gyral swelling and sulcal effacement. In the subacute and chronic stages, curvilinear gyral hyperintensity secondary to laminar necrosis may be present.

T2/FLAIR hyperintensity in the parietooccipital cortex and basal ganglia is typical of acute hypoglycemic encephalopathy **(32-14)**. The thalami, subcortical/deep WM, and cerebellum are generally spared. T2* scans generally show minimal or no "blooming" to suggest hemorrhage. Enhancement on T1 C+ is variable and, when present, usually mild.

DWI scans show restricted diffusion in the affected areas, predominately the posterior parietal and occipital cortex **(32-14)**. Cytotoxic corpus callosum splenium lesions with restricted diffusion have also been reported in association with hypoglycemia.

MRS demonstrates reduced NAA with or without a prominent lactate peak.

Differential Diagnosis

The most important differential diagnosis of hypoglycemic encephalopathy is **hypoxic-ischemic encephalopathy** (HIE). HIE typically occurs following cardiac arrest or global hypoperfusion. In contrast to hypoglycemic encephalopathy, the thalami and cerebellum are often affected in HIE. **Acute cerebral ischemia-infarction** is wedge-shaped, involving both the cortex and underlying WM.

Acute hypertensive encephalopathy (PRES) typically affects the parietooccipital cortex but spares most of the underlying WM and rarely restricts on DWI. PRES patients present with uncontrolled hypertension, not hypoglycemia.

Neonatal/Infantile Hypoglycemia

The immature brain is relatively resistant to hypoglycemia. Unlike older children and adults, neonates have lower absolute glucose demands and can utilize other substrates such as lactate to produce energy. Nevertheless, prolonged and/or severe hypoglycemia can result in devastating brain injury in newborn infants.

Terminology

The precise clinical/laboratory definition of neonatal/infantile hypoglycemia is controversial. Between 5 and 15% of normal term infants have initial plasma glucose values as low as 40-45 mg/dL. Currently accepted definitions of significant hypoglycemia in the newborn are glucose levels below 30-35 mg/dL in the first 24 hours after birth and 40-45 mg/dL thereafter.

Etiology

Congenital hyperinsulinism (HI) is the most common, most severe cause of *persistent* hypoglycemia in neonates and children. Mutations in 11 different genes cause congenital HI. The most common are inactivating mutations in the genes that encode the **pancreatic β-cell ATP-sensitive potassium (KATP) channel.**

Neonatal/infantile hypoglycemic encephalopathy is most often caused by maternal diabetes with poor glycemic control. Uncontrolled maternal diabetes leads to chronic fetal hyperglycemia in utero. This results in transient neonatal hyperinsulinemia and hypoglycemia of varying severity.

Neonatal hypoglycemia may also occur in the setting of **Beckwith-Wiedemann syndrome** (BWS), an inherited disorder with macrosomia, macroglossia, visceromegaly, omphalocele, embryonal tumors, adrenocortical cytomegaly, and renal abnormalities. Hypoglycemia due to HI occurs in approximately 50% of BWS cases. In most cases, BWS-associated hypoglycemia is mild and transient but can persist and—if undetected and untreated—pose significant risk for developmental sequelae.

Pathology

Transient, mild hypoglycemia generally does not injure the neonatal brain. Prolonged, severe hypoglycemia causes coagulative necrosis in the middle layers of the parietooccipital cortex and underlying WM.

Clinical Issues

Neonatal/infantile hypoglycemic encephalopathy typically presents in the first 3 days of life, usually within the first 24 hours. Large for gestation age babies have an increased risk of hypoglycemia even when they are not the product of diabetic pregnancies.

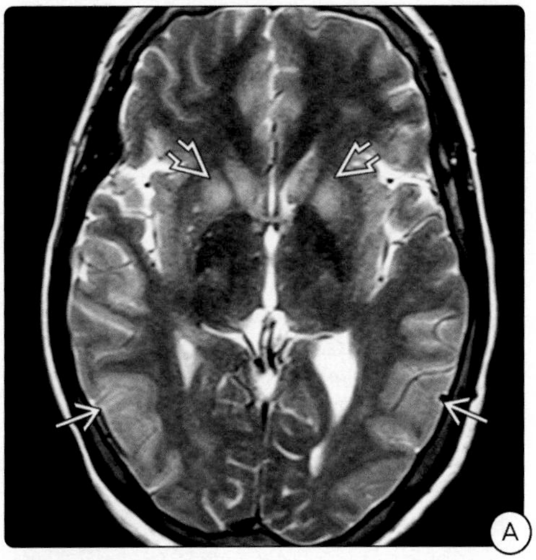

***(32-14A)** T2WI in a 21y diabetic patient "found down" shows bilateral parietooccipital cortical ➡ and basal ganglia hyperintensity ⇨.*

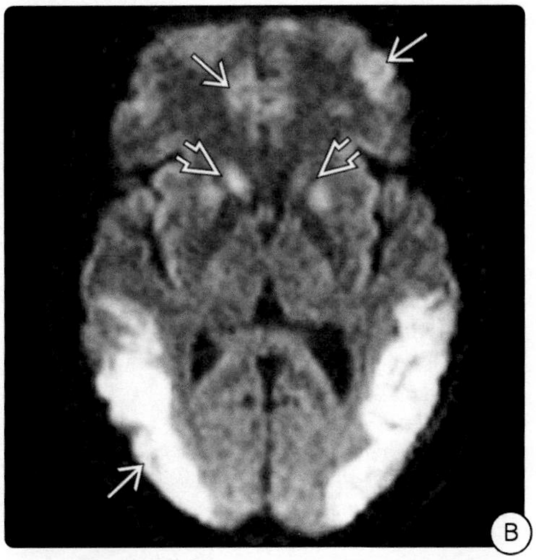

***(32-14B)** DWI in the same patient shows diffusion restriction in the cortex ➡ and basal ganglia ⇨. The thalami and WM are spared.*

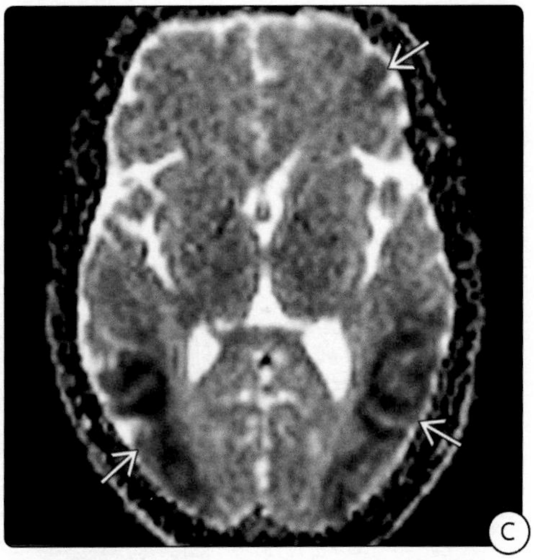

***(32-14C)** ADC map confirms restriction in the cortex ➡.*

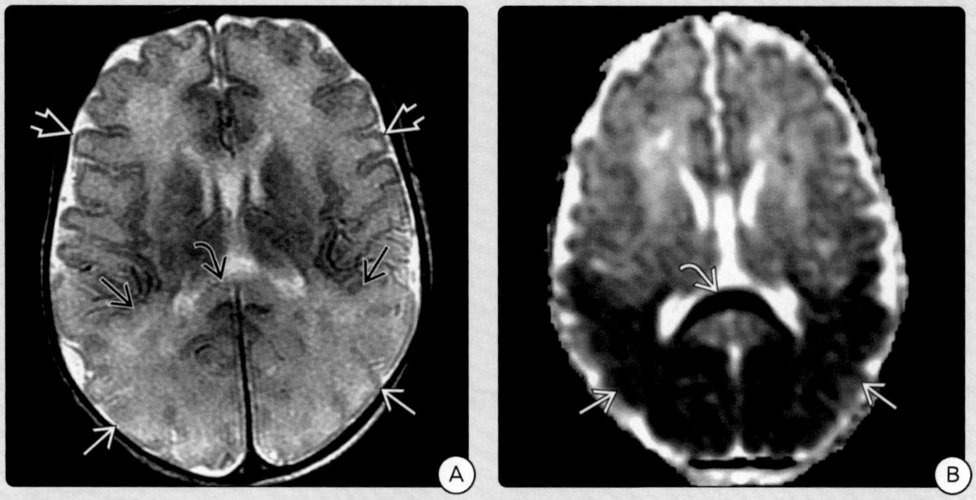

(32-15A) *Axial T2WI in a 5d infant with hypoglycemia shows effaced GM-WM interfaces in the parietooccipital lobes ➡ compared with the normal frontal lobes ➡. The cortex, underlying WM ➡, and corpus callosum splenium ➡ are swollen and hyperintense.* ***(32-15B)*** *ADC map in the same patient shows profound restricted diffusion in the parietal and occipital lobes ➡ and corpus callosum splenium ➡.*

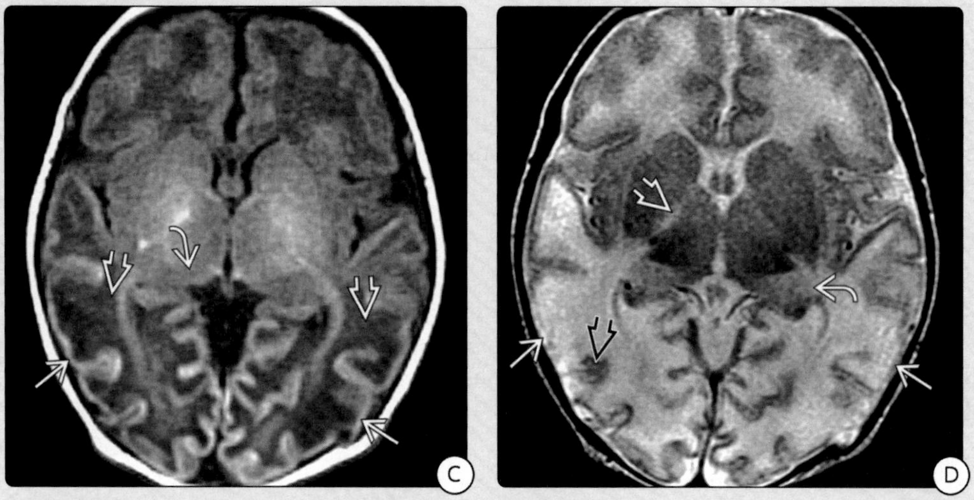

(32-15C) *T1WI in the same patient at 7 days shows swollen, markedly hypointense WM in the parietal and occipital lobes ➡, hyperintense, thinned cortex ➡, and hypointense pulvinars of the thalami ➡.* ***(32-15D)*** *T2WI at the same time shows thinned swollen cortex with patchy increased ➡ and decreased ➡ signal intensity, hyperintense pulvinars ➡, and abnormally hyperintense internal capsules ➡.*

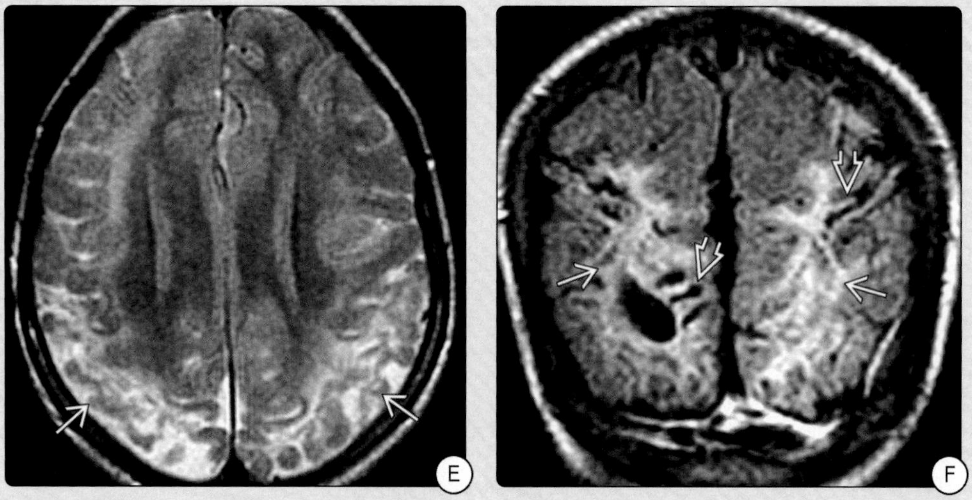

(32-15E) *Axial T2WI in the same infant at 1 year of age shows shrunken, hyperintense parietooccipital lobes with profound cortical loss, ulegyria, and encephalomalacic-appearing WM ➡.* ***(32-15F)*** *Coronal FLAIR scan, also performed at 1 year of age, shows extensive WM hyperintensity ➡ and thinned, shrunken gyri with focally enlarged sulci ➡.*

The precise level of hypoglycemia that requires treatment is controversial. Some experts recommend treating only symptomatic neonates with glucose concentrations below 45-50 mg/dL. The response to glucose therapy is typically prompt if the degree and duration of hypoglycemia are mild to moderate.

Hypoglycemia remains an important cause of brain injury in children with HI. Up to 50% suffer from neurodevelopmental disabilities.

HYPOGLYCEMIA

General Concepts
- Imbalance between glucose supply, utilization → hypoglycemia
- Can be mild, transient, asymptomatic
- Extent of brain injury depends on
  - Degree, duration of hypoglycemia
  - CBF, glucose utilization
  - Availability/utilization of alternative energy sources (e.g., lactate)
  - Exacerbating factors (e.g., hypoxia)
  - Recognition, prompt/appropriate treatment

Pediatric/Adult Hypoglycemia
- Etiology
  - Usually associated with diabetes
  - Absolute/relative insulin excess or glucose insufficiency
  - Energy production/O_2 utilization ↓, excitotoxic neurotransmitters ↑
- Pathology
  - Cortical necrosis
- Imaging
  - Hypodense/hyperintense parietooccipital cortex, basal ganglia
  - WM, thalami, cerebellum generally spared
  - Restricted diffusion common
  - May cause reversible corpus callosum splenium lesion

Neonatal/Infantile Hypoglycemia
- Etiology
  - Most common cause of transient hypoglycemia = maternal diabetes
  - Fetal hyperglycemia → neonatal hyperinsulinemia → hypoglycemia
  - Most common cause of severe, persistent hypoglycemia = congenital hyperinsulinemia (KATP mutation in 60%)
- Clinical issues
  - Usually presents in first 3 postnatal days
  - Glucose levels variable
- Imaging
  - Often similar to adult (posterior predominance)
  - Different: subcortical WM, thalami often involved
- Differential diagnosis
  - Term hypoxic-ischemic encephalopathy
  - Mitochondrial encephalopathy (MELAS)

Imaging

Some imaging findings in neonatal/infantile hypoglycemia resemble those of older children and adults, i.e., predominant involvement of the parietooccipital cortex and basal ganglia. However, white matter, thalamic, and cerebellar involvement are all relatively more common in neonates compared with hypoglycemic encephalopathy in older children and adults.

NECT scans in neonates with acute hypoglycemic encephalopathy show posterior brain hypodensity with effaced gray-white matter interfaces. In especially severe cases, the brain appears diffusely swollen and hypodense.

MR scans in the acute stages of neonatal hypoglycemic encephalopathy show T2/FLAIR hyperintensity and restricted diffusion in the parietooccipital cortex, subcortical WM, and corpus callosum splenium **(32-15A)** **(32-15B)**.

In the late acute/early subacute phase, the affected areas are swollen and edematous **(32-15C)** **(32-15D)**.

Cystic encephalomalacia may ensue. In chronic hypoglycemic encephalopathy, the parietooccipital cortices become atrophic, shrunken, and encephalomalacic **(32-15E)** **(32-15F)**.

Differential Diagnosis

As with older children and adults, the major differential diagnosis of neonatal hypoglycemic encephalopathy is **term hypoxic-ischemic injury** (HII). Hypoglycemic encephalopathy and HII often coexist, potentiating the extent of brain injury. Imaging findings in the two disorders may be indistinguishable.

Inherited mitochondrial disorders such as **mitochondrial encephalopathy with lactic acidosis and stroke-like episodes** (MELAS) may present with cortical swelling that spares the underlying WM. MELAS is rarely bilaterally symmetric and demonstrates much more markedly elevated lactate on MRS.

Hyperglycemia-Associated Disorders

There are three serious complications of diabetes mellitus (DM) that require prompt recognition, diagnosis, and treatment: (1) hypoglycemia (see above), (2) diabetic ketoacidosis (DKA), and (3) hyperglycemic hyperosmolar state (HHS).

In the past, there has been relatively little concern about the influence of hyperglycemia on the CNS. The accepted clinical axiom has been that, in diabetics, it is better to err on the side of having high blood glucose because of the greater risk of brain and physical injury associated with severe hypoglycemia. After all, the conventional thinking went the brain is protected from high glucose exposure by the blood-brain barrier, which reduces brain exposure to two-thirds that of the peripheral blood level.

Accumulating evidence now shows that hyperglycemia is toxic for the brain at any and all stages of life. In this section, we briefly discuss DM itself before turning our attention specifically to hyperglycemia-induced brain injury. We first

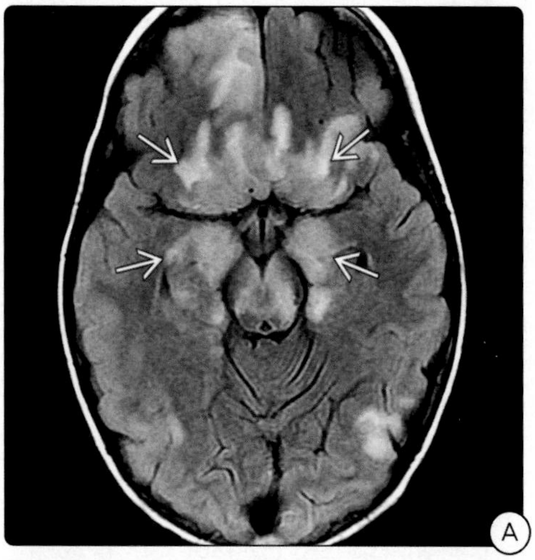

(32-16A) FLAIR in a child treated for DKA-associated cerebral edema shows hyperintensity ➡ from descending transtentorial herniation.

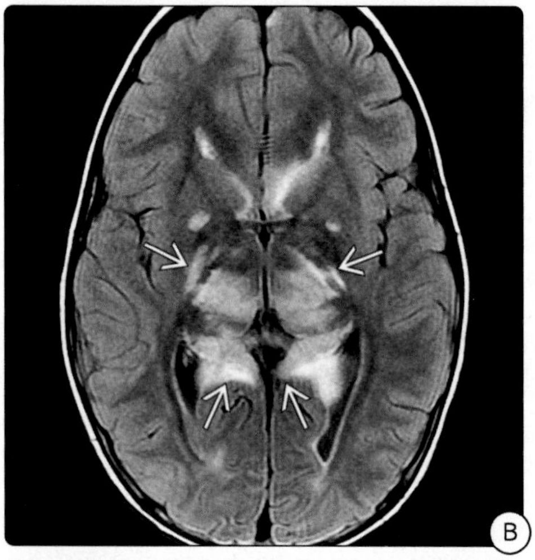

(32-16B) More cephalad FLAIR shows additional central hyperintensity ➡.

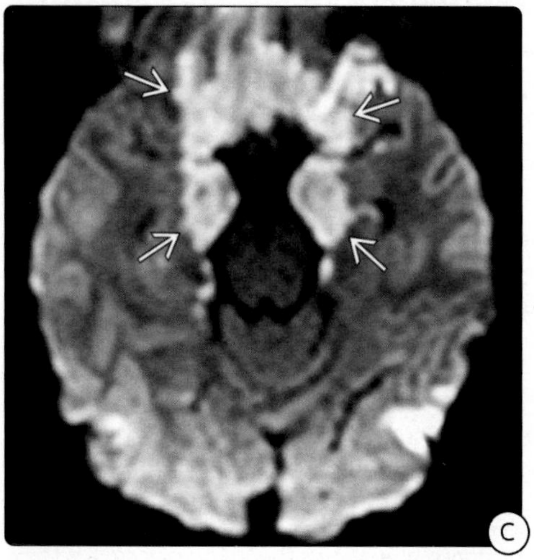

(32-16C) DWI shows restricted diffusion ➡ from bilateral central descending transtentorial herniation. Compare with Figure 3-10.

discuss the effects of *chronic* hyperglycemia on the brain, primarily seen as accelerated small vessel (microvascular) disease. We then consider two less common conditions associated with *acute* hyperglycemic changes in the CNS: DKA and HHS.

Diabetes

In **type 1 diabetes** (DM1), previously known as "juvenile diabetes," a lack of insulin results from the destruction of insulin-producing β cells in the pancreas, presumably secondary to an autoimmune-mediated process. DM1 accounts for only 5-10% of all patients with DM. Children with DM1 have slower growth of gray and white matter during the period of rapid brain maturation. Metaanalytic reviews have also documented subtle but real neurocognitive deficits in both children and adults with DM1.

The vast majority of patients with diabetes have **type 2 diabetes** (DM2), previously termed "adult-onset diabetes." DM2 is also known as non-insulin-dependent diabetes and is caused by relative insulin deficiency or cellular insulin resistance. DM2 occurs in both children and adults. Risk factors include low activity level, poor diet, and excess body weight.

Chronic Hyperglycemic Brain Injury

Hyperglycemia-induced brain injury can be chronic or acute. With the worldwide rise in obesity and the soaring prevalence of DM2, the effects of chronic hyperglycemia on the brain are increasingly recognized. Patients with DM2 have accelerated arteriolosclerosis and lipohyalinosis with silent infarcts, brain volume loss, and decreased cognitive functioning.

MR shows increased numbers of T2/FLAIR subcortical and periventricular hyperintensities, especially in the frontal WM, pons, and cerebellum. DTI demonstrates loss of microstructural integrity with decreased FA. Elevated myoinositol on MRS reflects gliosis, an indicator of brain injury.

Acute Hyperglycemic Brain Injury

Although acute brain injury in hyperglycemia is less common than in hypoglycemia, hyperglycemia can also cause major morbidity and significant mortality. Two acute conditions are associated with hyperglycemia: **DKA** and **HHS**. These two diseases can be considered the endpoints of a clinical laboratory continuum from DKA with minimal symptoms and normal osmolality to HHS with minimal or no ketosis and coma.

DKA and HHS are both caused by reduction in the net effective action of circulating insulin. Intracellular starvation stimulates the release of the counterregulatory hormones, glucagon, catecholamines, cortisol, and growth hormones. This leads to accelerated hepatic and renal glucose production and impaired glucose utilization in insulin-dependent peripheral tissues (e.g., muscle, liver, and adipose). The result is hyperglycemia, lipolysis (with release of free fatty acids into the circulation), and hepatic fatty acid oxidation (to ketone bodies).

DKA and HHS are also associated with glycosuria, which can cause osmotic diuresis with subsequent loss of water, sodium, potassium, and other electrolytes. In severe cases, secondary changes of acute osmotic demyelination can complicate the imaging findings of both disorders.

Diabetic Ketoacidosis. Although DKA can occur in patients with both DM1 and DM2, it is quite uncommon in DM2. DKA is defined as acidosis with a venous pH less than 7.3 or serum bicarbonate concentration less than 15 mmol/L in the presence of serum glucose concentration more than 11 mmol/L. DKA is characterized by glucosuria, ketonuria, and ketonemia.

DKA is often a recurrent disease. Mortality for each episode is relatively small (0.15-0.30%). Idiopathic cerebral edema accounts for at least two-thirds of fatal cases.

Imaging in patients with acute DKA is nonspecific, with vasogenic cerebral edema the most common abnormality. Younger age, severe acidosis, hypocapnia, and dehydration have all been cited as risk factors for DKA-related cerebral edema. If severe cerebral edema develops and is aggressively treated, survivors may show imaging evidence for bilateral (central) descending transtentorial herniation **(32-16)**.

Hyperglycemic Hyperosmolar State. HHS occurs almost exclusively in patients with DM2. Once considered a relatively rare condition seen only in the elderly population, the emergence of childhood DM2 means HHS now occurs in patients of all ages and is becoming significantly more common.

The clinical laboratory criteria for HHS include plasma glucose concentration > 33.3 mmol/L, serum bicarbonate concentration > 15 mmol/L, absent or minimal ketonuria and ketonemia, effective serum osmolality > 320 mOsm/kg, *and* the presence of stupor or coma. Unlike DKA, seizures are common. Glycosuria and hypernatremia from dehydration can lead to cerebral edema, osmotic demyelination, seizure, and cardiac arrest.

Imaging in HHS is uncommon. T2/FLAIR *hypo*intensity in the parietooccipital WM and transient lesions of the corpus callosum splenium have been reported. Patients treated for HHS with rapid correction of the hyperosmolar state may also develop osmotic demyelination with typical findings of central pontine myelinolysis (see below).

HYPERGLYCEMIA

General Concepts
- Spontaneous (rare) or diabetes-associated (common)
- Acute (rare) or chronic (common)

Hyperglycemia
- *Chronic* diabetes-associated brain injury
  - Accelerated arteriolosclerosis, impaired cognition
  - MR: decreased brain volume, increased WM hyperintensities
- *Acute* hypoglycemic brain injury
  - Diabetic ketoacidosis (DKA)
  - Hyperglycemic hyperosmolar state (HHS)
  - Hyperglycemia-induced hemichorea-hemiballismus (HIHH)
- Imaging
  - DKA: vasogenic cerebral edema ± osmotic demyelination
  - HHS: subcortical WM hypointensity
  - HIHH: unilateral T1 shortening in basal ganglia

Hyperglycemia-Induced Hemichorea-Hemiballismus

Also called delayed-onset diabetic striatopathy, the syndrome of hyperglycemia-induced hemichorea-hemiballismus (HIHH) is characterized by nonpatterned and involuntary unilateral movements. HIHH is a rare but potentially reversible complication of nonketotic hyperglycemia.

HIHH usually occurs in elderly patients, more often affects female patients, and may be the first ("unmasking") symptom of DM2. It can present as an acute, life-threatening manifestation of DM or develop 1-4 weeks after the hyperglycemic event when blood sugar has been controlled. Symptoms may resolve over days or persist for years.

MR findings are virtually pathognomonic of HIHH. T1 shortening in the basal ganglia contralateral to the hemichorea-hemiballism with sparing of the

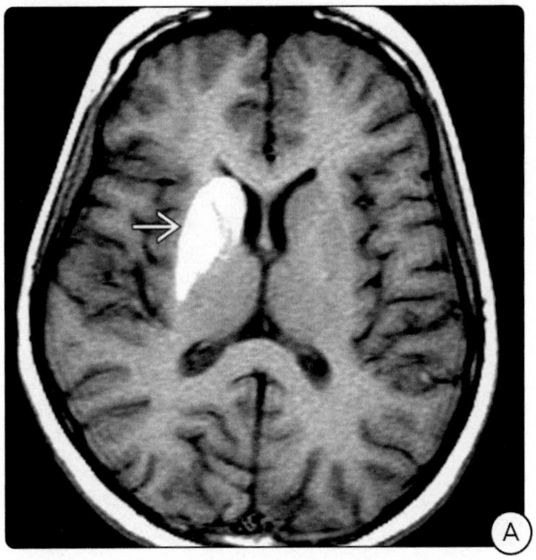

(32-17A) T1WI in hyperglycemia-induced hemichorea-hemiballismus (HIHH) shows uniformly hyperintense right basal ganglia ➡.

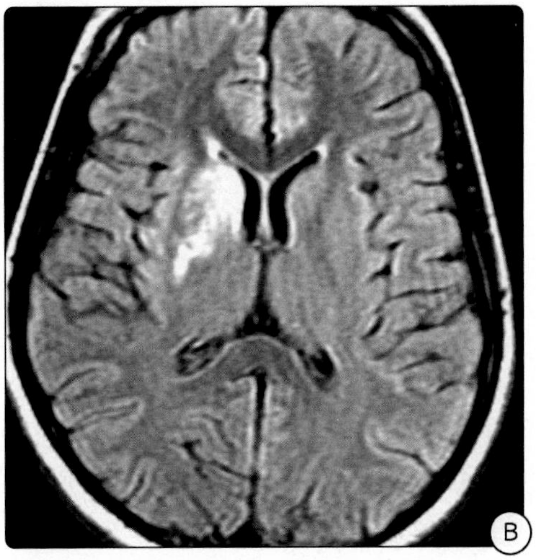

(32-17B) FLAIR in the same patient shows patchy hyperintensity in the right basal ganglia. The remainder of the brain appears normal.

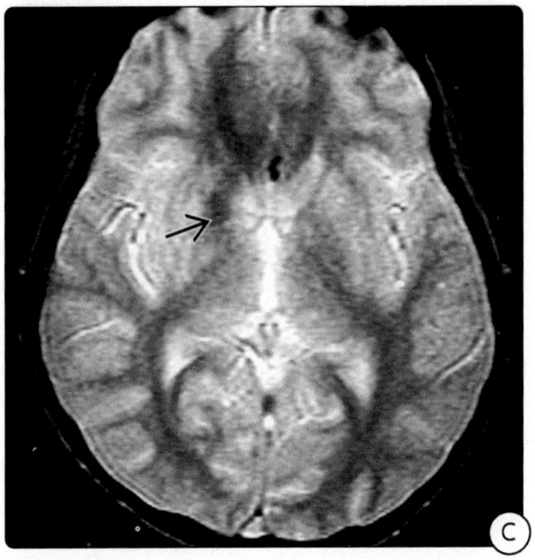

(32-17C) T2 GRE demonstrates minimal hypointensity in the globus pallidus ➡. (Courtesy K. K. Oguz, MD.)*

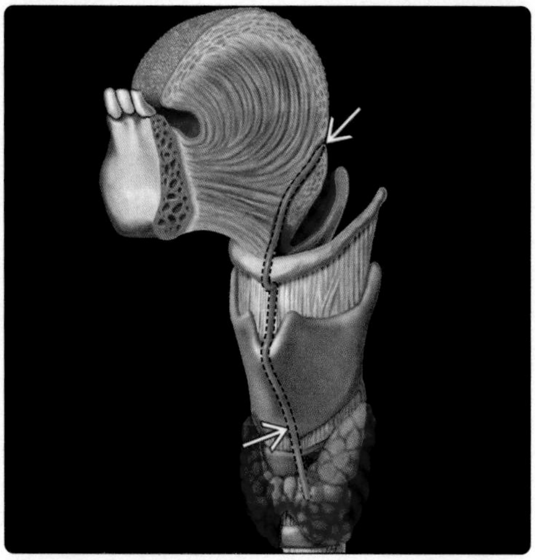

(32-18) Embryonic thyroid migrates inferiorly from the tongue to the neck. Ectopic thyroid can occur anywhere along the thyroglossal duct ➡.

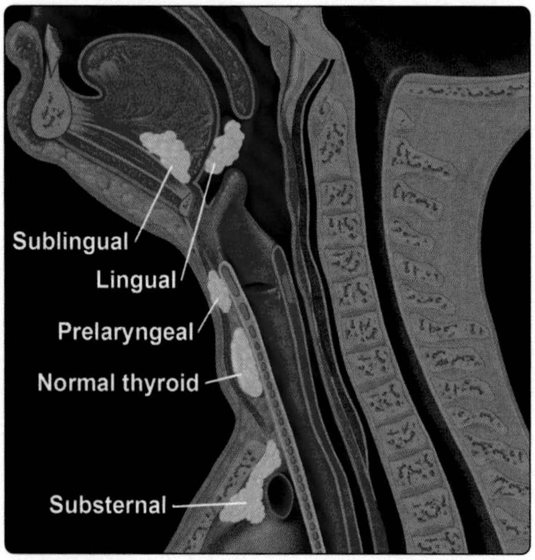

(32-19) Graphic depicts possible sites of ectopic thyroid along the thyroglossal duct, but they may also occur elsewhere (e.g., substernal).

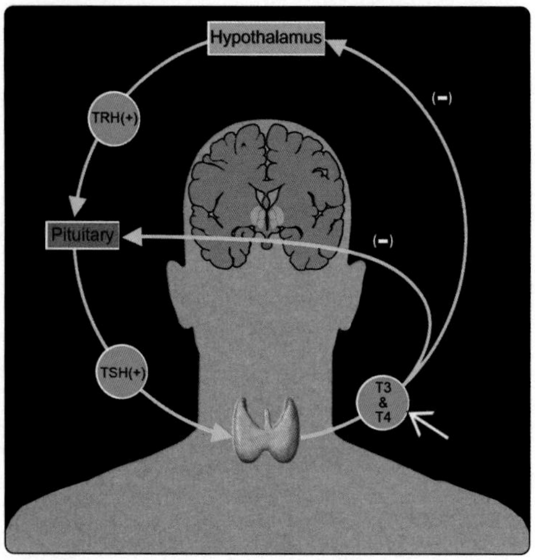

(32-20) Graphic depicts hypothalamic-pituitary-thyroid axis. T3 and T4 ➡ inhibit hypothalamic and pituitary stimulation of thyroid.

thalamus is characteristic **(32-17)**. In two-thirds of HIHH cases, T2* GRE or SWI demonstrates hypointense signal within the affected striatum. The signal abnormality probably represents manganese or zinc deposition, not calcium or hemorrhage.

Thyroid Disorders

Thyroid disorders are relatively common metabolic disturbances that are usually mild and rarely affect brain function. However, several imaging findings—some of them striking—have been associated with thyroid disease. Some can be mistaken for more serious disease (e.g., hypothyroid-induced pituitary hyperplasia mimicking pituitary adenoma), and a few (e.g., Hashimoto encephalopathy) can be life-threatening.

Hypothyroidism can be congenital or acquired. We begin our discussion of thyroid disease with congenital hypothyroidism before turning our attention to acquired hypothyroid disease and its imaging manifestations. We close the section with a brief consideration of hyperthyroid disease and its effects on the CNS.

Congenital Hypothyroidism

Hypothyroidism is one of the most frequent congenital endocrine disorders. Congenital hypothyroidism (CH) occurs in 1:2,000-4,000 newborns and is one of the most common preventable causes of mental retardation. If the diagnosis is made and treatment begun within a few weeks of birth, neurodevelopmental outcome is generally normal.

Newborns with CH normally have some initial residual thyroid function because maternal T4 crosses the placenta to the fetus. With a half-life of 6 days, however, maternal T4 will be almost completely metabolized and excreted by 3-4 weeks of age.

In developed countries with newborn screening programs, most infants with CH are diagnosed soon after birth. Serum TSH is elevated (typically more than 20-30 mU/L). In less developed countries, CH is often diagnosed later in childhood when suspicious clinical features lead to serum thyroid function testing or imaging studies. The most visible clinical feature is a facies suggestive of "cretinism," a term no longer used because of its pejorative implications.

Etiology and Presentation

CH can be caused by thyroid dysgenesis, dyshormonogenesis, or central hypothyroidism. Iodine deficiency and maternal thyroid disease can also cause hypothyroidism in neonates.

Maternal Factors. Transient CH can occur in preterm infants born in areas with endemic iodine deficiency or to families with a history of goiter.

In maternal autoimmune thyroiditis, IgG antibodies cross the placenta and may block fetal thyroid production. Medication or I-131 therapy for maternal hyperthyroidism or cancer can also act adversely on the fetus.

Thyroid Dysgenesis. Thyroid dysgenesis is the most common cause of CH, accounting for 70-75% of cases. Failure of normal thyroid gland development includes both abnormal gland formation and aberrant thyroid descent.

Ectopic thyroid tissue accounts for 25-50% of cases with thyroid dysgenesis. Ectopia can occur anywhere along the embryonic thyroglossal duct **(32-18)**, the path that the developing thyroid follows as it descends from the tongue base to the neck **(32-19)**. Hormone production in ectopic thyroids is low (despite the presence of functioning tissue) but not completely absent. In some cases, hormone production may be enough to delay clinical symptoms until adolescence.

Thyroid agenesis or **hypoplasia** accounts for 20-50% of CH cases and typically causes severe hypothyroidism with markedly depressed T4, elevated TSH, and undetectable levels of thyroglobulin.

Dyshormonogenesis. Inborn errors of thyroid hormone biosynthesis (dyshormonogenesis) account for 5-15% of CH cases. Here, defects occur in the biosynthesis, secretion, or utilization of thyroid hormone. These include enzymatic abnormalities, deficient iodide trapping due to sodium-iodide symporter defects, TSH resistance with abnormal TSH receptors on the follicular cell membranes, and peripheral thyroid hormone resistance with T3 receptor defects in peripheral cell nuclei.

Central (Secondary) Hypothyroidism. Pituitary or hypothalamic dysfunction causes 10-15% of CH cases. The gland is formed normally, but the hypothalamic-pituitary-thyroid axis is disrupted **(32-20)**. Most cases of secondary hypothyroidism are caused by decreased pituitary TSH and often occur in the setting of combined pituitary hormone deficiency. So-called tertiary hypothyroidism from low hypothalamic TSH is rare in children.

Imaging

Imaging studies of the face and neck demonstrate an ectopic thyroid in up to half of all CH cases. Nearly 90% occur at the tongue base, where they are seen as a well-delineated, round or ovoid, hyperdense midline mass on NECT and a T1 iso-/T2 hyperintense mass on MR. Avid uniform enhancement following contrast administration is typical.

Complete absence of the thyroid and thyroid hypoplasia accounts for most of the remaining cases. Although high-resolution ultrasound is considered the "gold standard" for measuring thyroid dimensions, it lacks sensitivity for detecting small ectopic glands and is often combined with scintigraphy—considered the "gold standard"—for the work-up of CH.

Nuclear medicine studies (Tc-99m pertechnetate or I-123 scans) are typically used to diagnose thyroid agenesis and demonstrate absent uptake (no activity in any of the expected sites) **(32-21)**. Inborn errors of thyroid hormone metabolism often appear as a small bilobed thyroid in the expected location **(32-22)**.

Brain MR in children with CH may show mild generalized atrophy with reduced WM volume and poor differentiation of cortical layers, enlarged sylvian fissures, and T2 hypointensity in the globi pallidi and substantia nigra.

Differential Diagnosis

As the central tongue base is the most common location for an ectopic thyroid **(32-24)**, the most important differential diagnoses are venous malformation or hemangioma, prominent/asymmetric lingual tonsil, and neoplasm (non-Hodgkin lymphoma). A lingual thyroid may expand dramatically during puberty. *In 75% of cases, a lingual thyroid is the only functioning thyroid tissue; it must not be mistaken for tumor and removed* **(32-25) (32-26)**!

Venous malformation exhibits prominent T2 hyperintensity. An upper airway **infantile hemangioma** is usually subglottic and asymmetric. A transglottic hemangioma involves multiple structures, not just the tongue base. **Prominent/asymmetric tonsillar tissue** has the same density/signal intensity as other lymphoid structures.

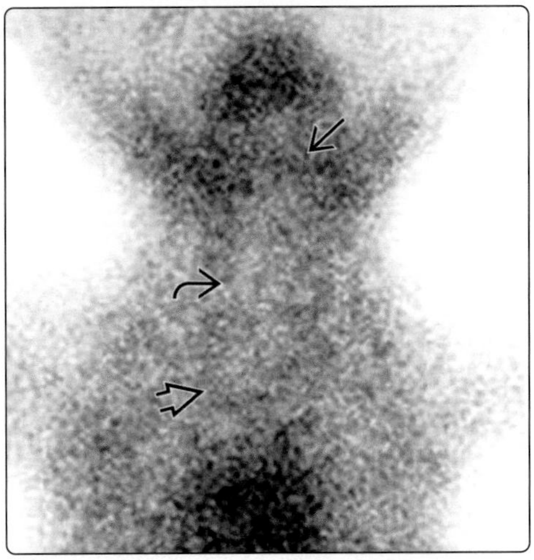

***(32-21)** Tc-99m in congenital hypothyroidism shows no uptake in oropharynx, tongue base →, neck →, mediastinum →. (J. P. O'Malley, MD.)*

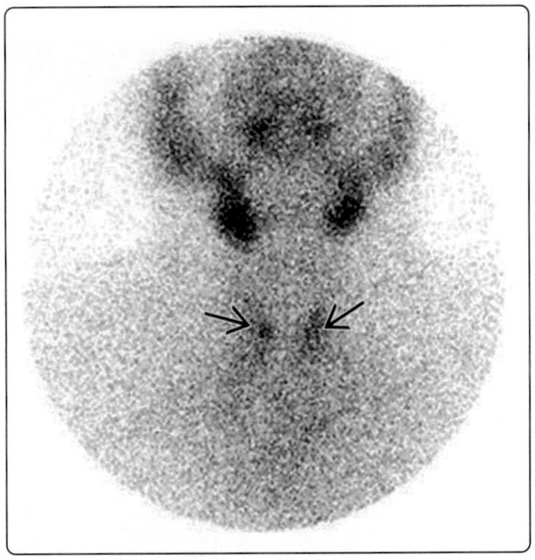

***(32-22)** Hypothyroidism secondary to organification defect with bilobed thyroid shows very low uptake →. (J. P. O'Malley, MD.)*

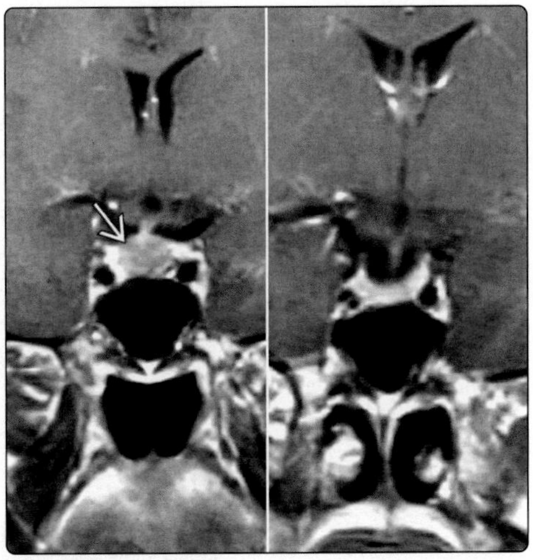

***(32-23)** (L) T1 C+ shows 8y boy with hyperplasia → initially called pituitary macroadenoma. (R) After PTH, pituitary is normal.*

Acquired Hypothyroid Disorders

Acquired hypothyroidism is much more common than the congenital variety, affecting eight to nine million Americans and many more patients worldwide. Acquired hypothyroidism has two important imaging manifestations: pituitary hyperplasia and Hashimoto thyroiditis/encephalopathy.

Pituitary Hyperplasia

Enlarged pituitary glands are common in young menstruating female patients and pregnant/lactating female patients. *Non*physiologic increase in pituitary volume—pathologic pituitary enlargement—is much less common and typically occurs in response to end-organ failure.

Hypothyroidism can result in secondary TSH cell hyperplasia, symmetrically enlarging the pituitary gland and mimicking a pituitary adenoma on imaging studies. Both physiologic and nonphysiologic pituitary hyperplasia are discussed in detail in Chapter 25. Most cases of hypothyroid-induced pituitary hyperplasia reverse with thyroid hormone replacement therapy **(32-23)**. Caution: Any prepubescent male patient thought to harbor a "pituitary macroadenoma" on imaging studies should undergo comprehensive endocrine evaluation, as macroadenomas are exceptionally rare in this age group!

Hashimoto Encephalopathy

Terminology and Etiology. Hashimoto encephalopathy is a rare but treatable condition typically associated with Hashimoto thyroiditis and characterized by high levels of anti-thyroid antibodies. Hashimoto encephalitis is also called "steroid-responsive encephalopathy with autoimmune thyroiditis." It is a well-recognized neurologic complication of autoimmune thyroid disease and is the most common cause of acquired hypothyroidism.

Occasionally, Hashimoto encephalopathy occurs with severe "iatrogenic" hypothyroidism, typically with inadequate

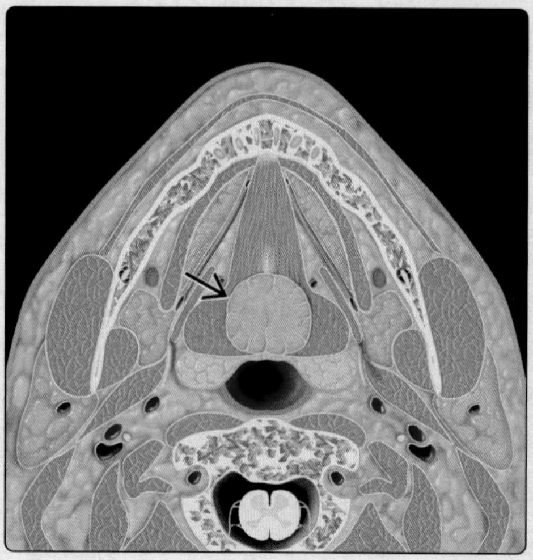

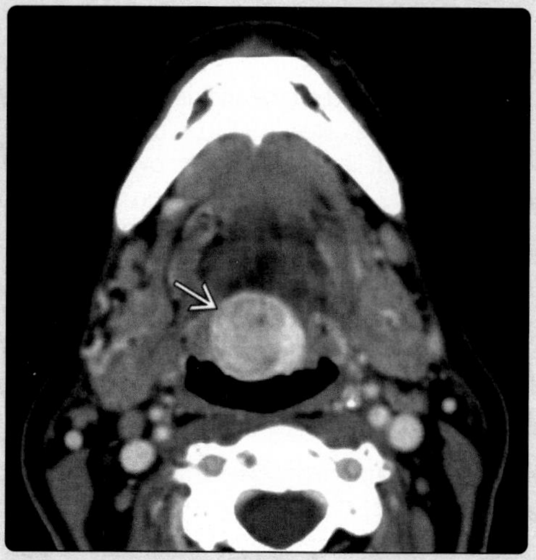

***(32-24)** Axial graphic depicts lingual thyroid → in the posterior midline of the tongue, deep to the foramen cecum. Sharply defined contour and midline location at the tongue base or floor of the mouth are typical of lingual thyroid. **(32-25)** CECT scan shows classic lingual thyroid →, seen as a uniformly enhancing midline mass in the base of the tongue.*

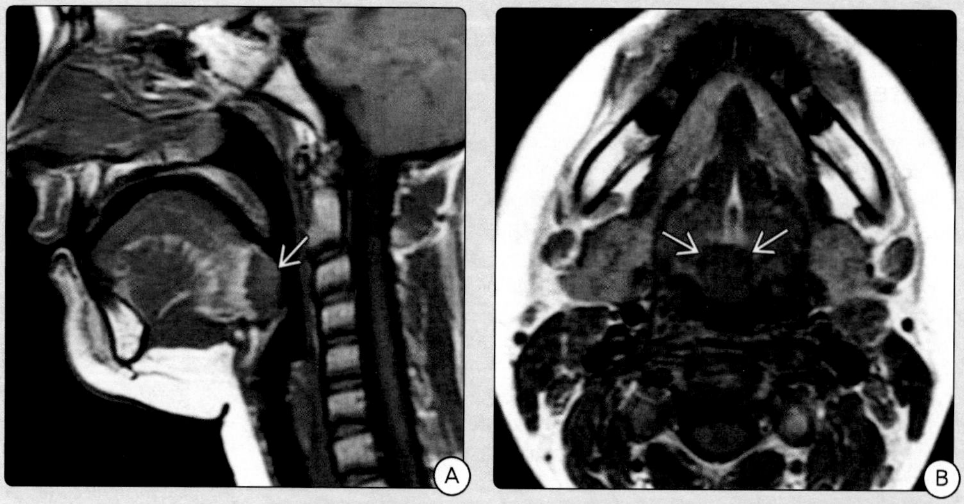

***(32-26A)** Sagittal T1WI in a 13y hypothyroid girl shows a well-delineated mass → at the tongue base. The mass is isointense with the intrinsic musculature of the tongue. **(32-26B)** Axial T1WI in the same patient shows that the mass → is midline and sharply demarcated. This is classic lingual thyroid.*

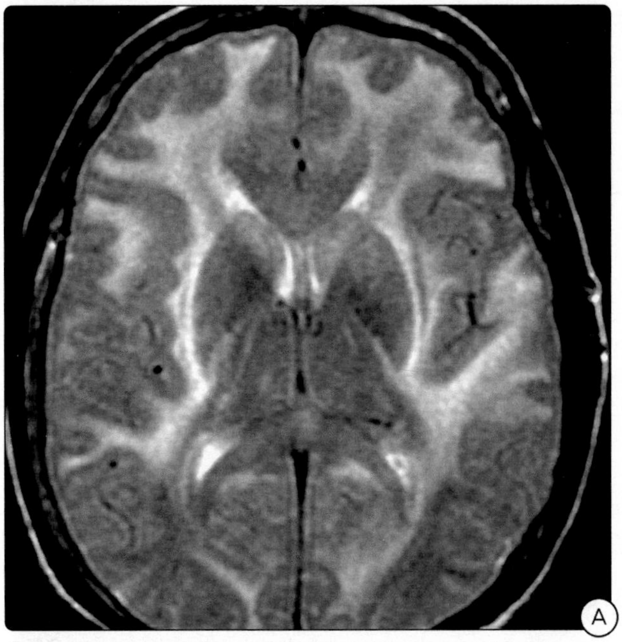

(32-27A) *Axial T2WI in a 58y woman with acute Hashimoto encephalopathy shows confluent, symmetric hyperintensity in the subcortical, deep WM.*

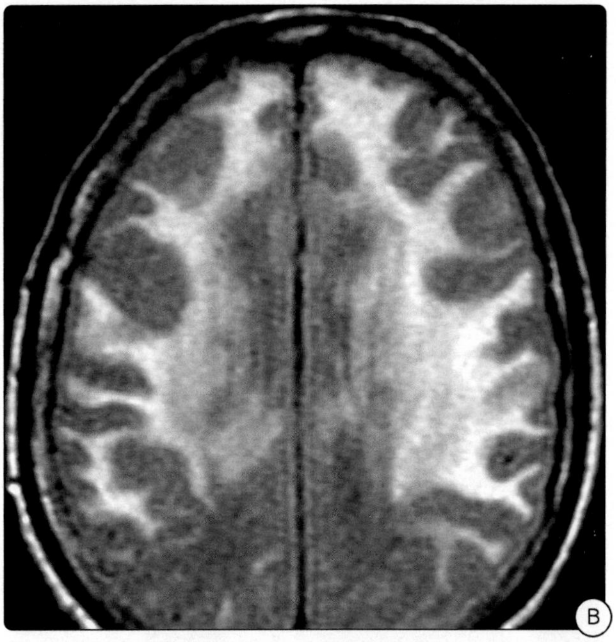

(32-27B) *FLAIR scan in the same patient shows involvement of the frontal subcortical WM with marked sparing of the occipital lobes.*

hormone replacement following thyroidectomy or radioactive I-131 treatment.

Clinical Issues. Hashimoto encephalopathy occurs in both children and adults. There is a moderate female predominance.

Most patients present with acute encephalopathy or severe neuropsychiatric disturbances (sometimes termed "myxedema madness"). Other common symptoms include seizures (66%), myoclonus (38%), and stroke (27%). Occasionally, patients present with more gradual cognitive decline and personality changes. These patients may be initially misdiagnosed as having "presenile" dementia.

Imaging. Approximately half of all patients with Hashimoto encephalopathy demonstrate imaging abnormalities. The most typical MR findings are diffuse confluent or focal T2/FLAIR hyperintensities in the subcortical and deep periventricular white matter. The occipital lobes are relatively spared **(32-27)**. Hashimoto encephalopathy typically does not enhance following contrast administration.

Hyperthyroidism

The most common manifestation of hyperthyroidism in the head and neck is thyroid ophthalmopathy (Graves disease). Brain involvement in hyperthyroidism occurs but is very rare.

Thyrotropin-secreting pituitary macroadenomas cause hyperthyroidism due to the syndrome of inappropriate TSH secretion. Hypocortisolemic states (e.g., Sheehan syndrome with peri- or postpartum pituitary necrosis) can also precipitate hyperimmunity and autoimmune hyperthyroidism.

There is an increased prevalence of psychiatric and behavioral disturbances in patients with hyperthyroidism, including apathetic hyperthyroidism and hyperthyroid dementia. Thyrotoxicosis can also cause disturbances of consciousness. Seizures, usually the generalized tonic-clonic type, occur in less than 1% of cases.

Brain imaging in hyperthyroidism is uncommon. A few cases of **acute idiopathic intracranial hypertension** ("pseudotumor cerebri") associated with hyperthyroidism have been reported.

THYROID DISORDERS

Congenital Hypothyroid Disorders
- Etiology
  - Thyroid dysgenesis, dyshormonogenesis, central hypothyroidism
- Imaging
  - Ectopic thyroid in 50% (90% at base of tongue)
  - Do not mistake for neoplasm!

Acquired Hypothyroid Disorders
- Pituitary hyperplasia
  - Prepubescent male patient with "fat" pituitary
- Hashimoto encephalopathy
  - WM edema (spares occipital lobes)

Hyperthyroidism
- Thyroid ophthalmopathy (Graves disease)
- Brain rarely imaged

Because of its effect on factor VIII activity, hyperthyroidism has also been reported as an independent risk factor for **dural venous sinus thrombosis**. Graves disease has been reported as a rare cause of **transient corpus callosum splenium**

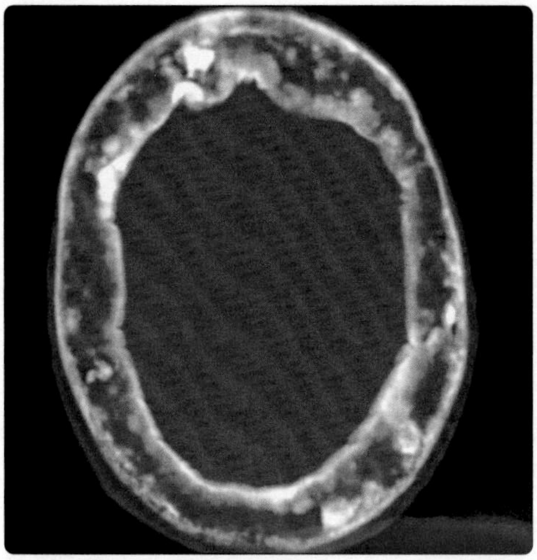

(32-28) NECT scan of the skull in a patient with HPTH shows the characteristic alternating "salt and pepper" foci of resorption and sclerosis.

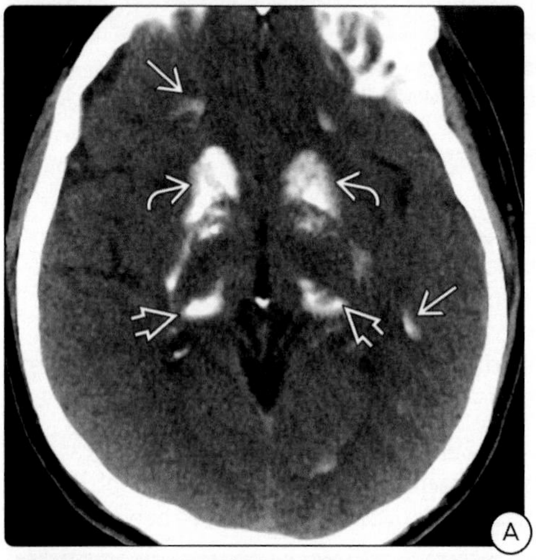

(32-29A) NECT in a 54y man with hyperparathyroidism shows extensive symmetric Ca++ in basal ganglia ➡, thalami ➡, cortex ➡.

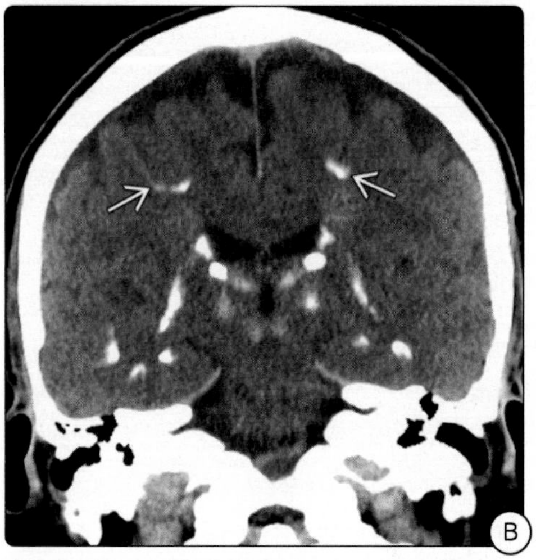

(32-29B) Coronal NECT in the same case shows how symmetric the basal Ca++ is. Note GM-WM interface calcifications ➡.

hyperintensity and an **MS-like multiphasic demyelinating autoimmune syndrome**.

Parathyroid and Related Disorders

The parathyroid glands lie in the visceral space of the neck. They are normally the size and shape of kidney beans and are closely adherent to the posterior surfaces of the thyroid lobes. Ectopic parathyroid glands are found in 2% of cases, typically just below the inferior thyroid pole, although they can be found from the upper neck to the mediastinum. Most patients have four parathyroid glands, 10% have five or more, and 3% have three or fewer glands.

Metabolic abnormalities related to parathyroid hormone dysfunction include primary and secondary hyperparathyroidism as well as hypoparathyroidism, pseudohypoparathyroidism, and pseudo-pseudohypoparathyroidism.

Hyperparathyroidism

The parathyroid glands control calcium metabolism by producing parathyroid hormone (PTH). Hyperparathyroidism (HPTH) is the classic disease of bone resorption, so imaging abnormalities may be seen in both the skull and brain.

HPTH can be an acquired (common) or inherited disorder (rare). Both conditions are briefly discussed in this chapter. HPTH can also be primary, secondary, or even tertiary. Because of the increasing number of patients on dialysis, the most common type is now secondary HPTH.

Primary Hyperparathyroidism

Etiology. In primary HPTH (1° HPTH), excessive levels of PTH result in unneeded bone resorption. The most common cause of 1° HPTH is **parathyroid adenoma**, responsible for 75-85% of cases. The second most common etiology is nonneoplastic parathyroid hyperplasia (10-20%). Parathyroid carcinoma is rare, accounting for just 1-5% of cases.

Sporadic 1° HPTH is much more common than hereditary HPTH. The most important inherited syndromes associated with 1° HPTH are multiple endocrine neoplasia (MEN) type 1, MEN type 2A, and familial isolated HPTH. Major features in patients with **MEN1** include parathyroid tumor (95%), pancreatic neuroendocrine tumor (40%), and pituitary neoplasm (30%). **MEN2A** is characterized by medullary thyroid carcinoma (99%), pheochromocytoma (50%), and parathyroid tumors (20-30%).

Clinical Issues. 1° HPTH is most common in middle-aged to older adults and relatively rare in children. There is a striking female predominance. 1° HPTH is characterized by hypercalcemia and hypophosphatemia (serum calcium is elevated; serum phosphorus is normal or decreased). HPTH is usually asymptomatic. General signs of symptomatic HPTH have been characterized as "stones, bones, abdominal groans, and psychic moans."

A recently described (and controversial) entity is called "normocalcemic primary hyperparathyroidism." Patients have elevated PTH levels but normal serum calcium and vitamin D levels.

Imaging. Standard two-phase contrast-enhanced CT has an overall pooled sensitivity of 73% and PPV of 81% for localization of the pathologic parathyroid gland to the correct quadrant. 4D-CT performs comparably well to US and sestamibi scans, with an overall sensitivity of 80-90%.

Bone CT demonstrates diffuse patchy **"salt and pepper" lesions** in the skull. These are caused by foci of bone resorption interspersed with variable patchy sclerosis **(32-28)**. Bilateral symmetric resorption of the lamina dura of the teeth may be present.

The most common findings in the brain are **basal ganglia calcifications** on NECT. Bilateral symmetric deposits in the globi pallidi, putamen, and caudate nuclei are typical. The thalami, subcortical WM, and dentate nuclei may also be affected **(32-29)**.

MR shows symmetric T1 shortening and T2 hypointensity in the basal ganglia. Mild to moderate "blooming" on T2* (GRE, SWI) sequences is typical. **"Brown tumors"**—solitary or multiple nonneoplastic lesions in the skull—are common (see below).

Secondary Hyperparathyroidism

Etiology. Secondary HPTH (2° HPTH) is characterized by PTH hypersecretion and parathyroid gland hyperplasia.

The most common cause of 2° HPTH is chronic renal disease (CRD). The majority of dialysis patients eventually develop 2° HPTH. Other etiologies of 2° HPTH include dietary calcium deficiency, vitamin D disorders, disrupted phosphate metabolism, and hypomagnesemia.

Clinical Issues. Most patients with 2° HPTH are older than 40 years at the time of initial diagnosis. There is no sex predilection. Serum calcium is normal or low, serum phosphorus is increased, and calcium-phosphate product is elevated. Vitamin D is low, almost always secondary to renal disease rather than dietary deficiency.

A common manifestation of CRD is renal osteodystrophy. Massive thickening of the calvaria and skull base narrows neural and vascular channels. Progressive cranial nerve involvement—most commonly compressive optic neuropathy—and carotid stenosis with ischemic symptoms are typical.

Imaging. 2° HPTH primarily affects the skull and dura; the brain parenchyma itself is usually normal. NECT scans show markedly thickened skull and facial bones, a condition sometimes referred to as **"uremic leontiasis ossea"** or "big head disease" **(32-30)**.

"Brown tumors" can be seen in both 1° HPTH and 2° HPTH. "Brown tumors" represent a reactive—not neoplastic—process caused by osteoclastic bone resorption. Fibrous replacement, hemorrhage, and necrosis lead to formation of brownish-appearing cysts. Solitary or multiple "brown tumors" are seen on bone CT as focal expansile lytic lesions with nonsclerotic margins. Signal intensity on MR is highly variable, reflecting the age and amount of hemorrhage as well as the presence of fibrous tissue and cyst formation **(32-32)**.

The classic intracranial finding in 2° HPTH is unusually extensive, **plaque-like dural thickening (32-31)**. Longstanding CRD can also result in extensive **"pipestem" calcifications** in the internal and external carotid arteries.

Tertiary Hyperparathyroidism

Tertiary HPTH (3° HPTH) results from longstanding 2° HPTH. Full-blown tertiary HPTH is rarely seen. The parathyroid gland becomes hyperplastic and does not respond appropriately to serum calcium levels (i.e., functions "autonomously"). Imaging findings are similar to those of 2° HPTH.

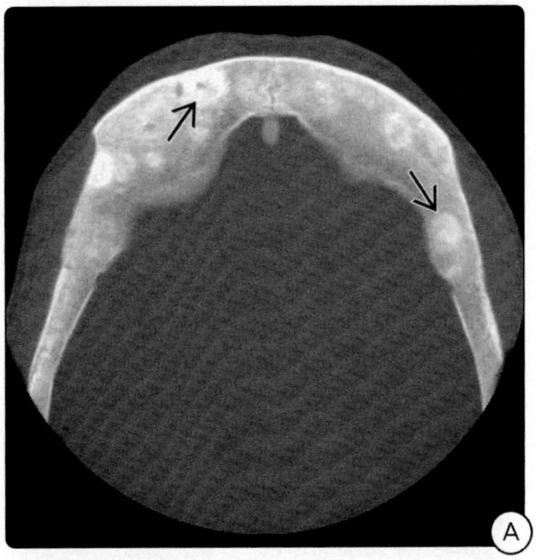

***(32-30A)** Axial bone CT in a patient with 2° HPTH shows leontiasis ossea with marked calvarial thickening, focal sclerotic "brown tumors" ⇒.*

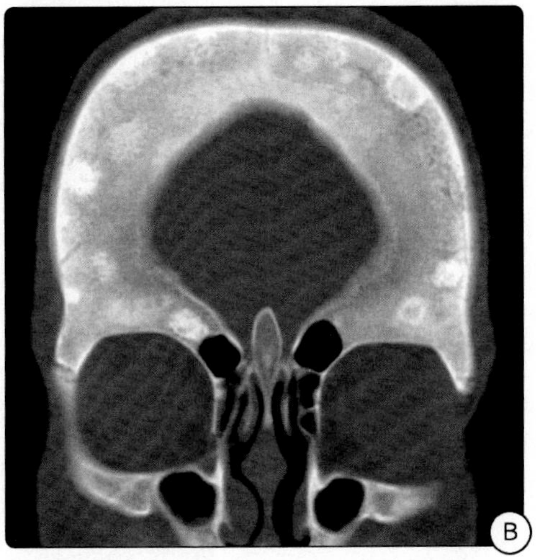

***(32-30B)** Coronal bone CT in the same patient demonstrates the striking calvarial thickening.*

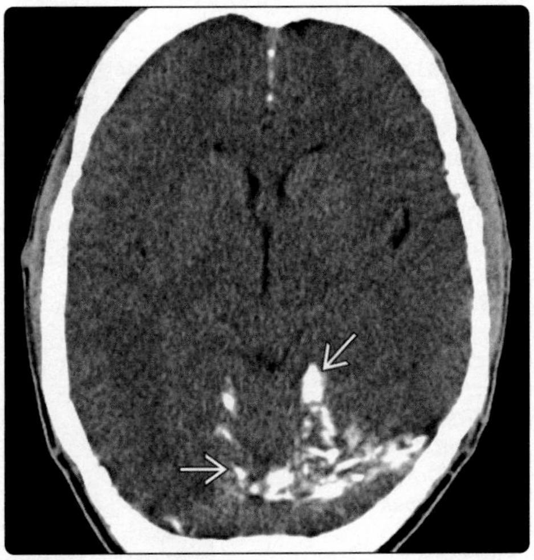

***(32-31)** NECT scan in a 31y man with ESRD shows markedly thickened, plaque-like deposits along the tentorium ➡.*

(32-32A) Sagittal T1WI shows a 34y man with 25-y history of renal failure on dialysis, known 2° HPTH, and "big head disease." He developed decreasing vision, swollen optic discs. Note markedly thickened skull ➡ with multiple "brown tumors" ➡, thickened calcified pannus around the odontoid ➡. (32-32B) Sagittal T1WI in same patient shows thickening of orbital wall ➡ and calvaria. Note well-delineated "brown tumors" of varying SI ➡.

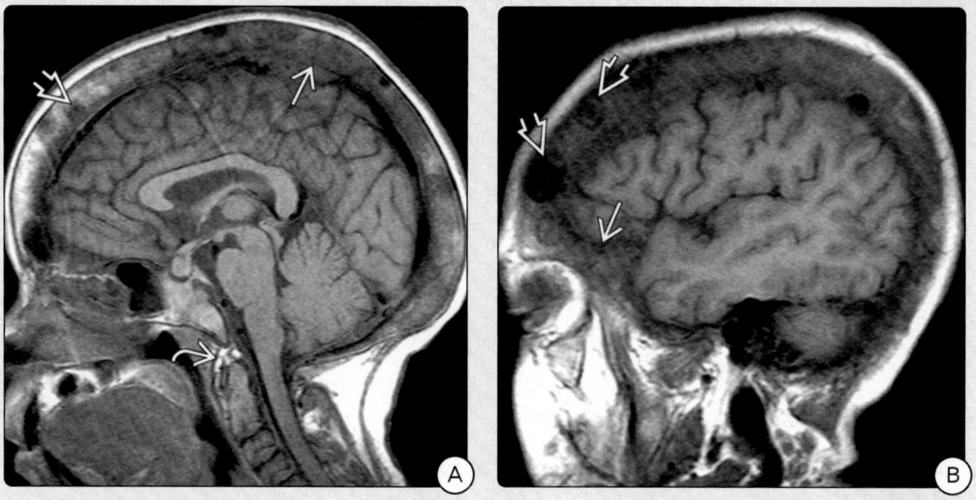

(32-32C) Axial T1WI shows the markedly thickened calvaria and focal lesions. (32-32D) T2WI shows thick calvaria ➡, multiple "brown tumors" of varying signal intensity ➡. Note that some of the more hyperintense lesions ➡ are virtually invisible on the T1WI to the left.

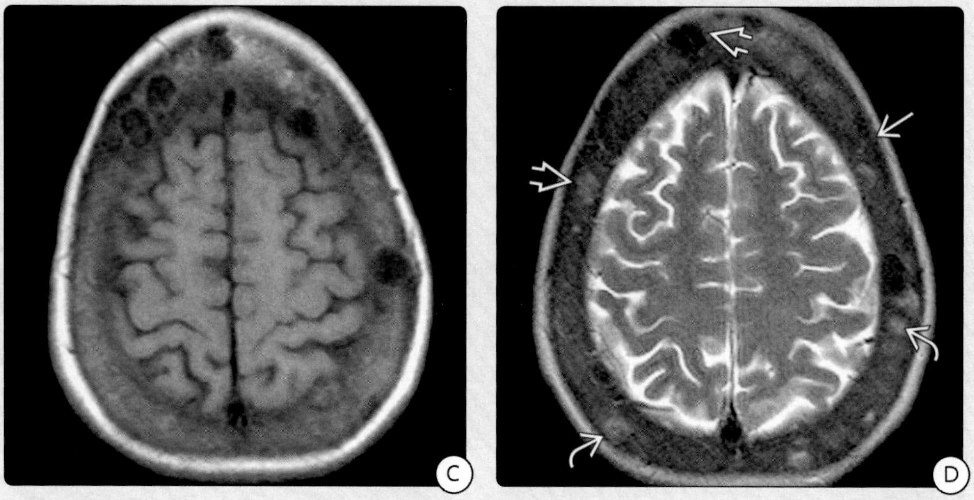

(32-32E) FLAIR scan shows the thick skull, multifocal "brown tumors." The underlying brain appears normal. (32-32F) Coronal T1 C+ FS shows that one of the "brown tumors" enhances ➡. Note thick dura ➡. The thickened bone causes significantly decreased volume of the orbits with compression of the optic nerve sheaths ➡ at the orbital apex. (All six images courtesy S. Chung, MD.)

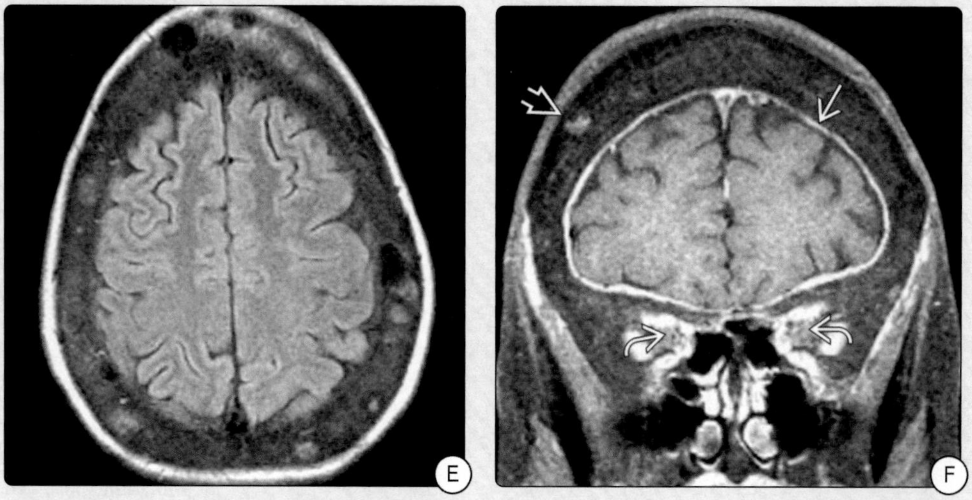

Hypoparathyroid Disorders

Three types of hypoparathyroidism are recognized: hypoparathyroidism, pseudohypoparathyroidism, and pseudo-pseudohypoparathyroidism. All three disorders share common features on brain imaging although their clinical presentation and laboratory findings vary.

Hypoparathyroidism

Childhood hypoparathyroidism (HP) usually presents around age five. It is probably an autoimmune-mediated disease with *decreased* parathyroid hormone (PTH) production. HP is characterized by hypocalcemia and hyperphosphatemia. Carpal-pedal spasm, tetany, seizures, and hyperreflexia are common presentations.

Ectopic calcification in brain tissue is one of the characteristic typical findings in HP on NECT scans **(32-33)**. The basal ganglia and thalami are the most common sites, followed by the cerebrum and cerebellum. Subcutaneous soft tissue calcifications are common in the extremities but rare in the head and neck.

The most striking extracranial imaging findings are related to osteosclerosis. Spinal ligament calcification/ossification, osteophyte formation, and enthesopathy (especially around the pelvis) are typical.

Adult HP is rare. The most common causes in adults are parathyroid gland injury and inadvertent removal during neck dissection in thyroid cancer, which carries a 37% risk of permanent HP.

Complications of chronic hypocalcemia in adults include renal dysfunction, nephrocalcinosis, kidney stones, basal ganglia calcifications, and posterior subcapsular cataracts, as well as low bone turnover and increased bone density.

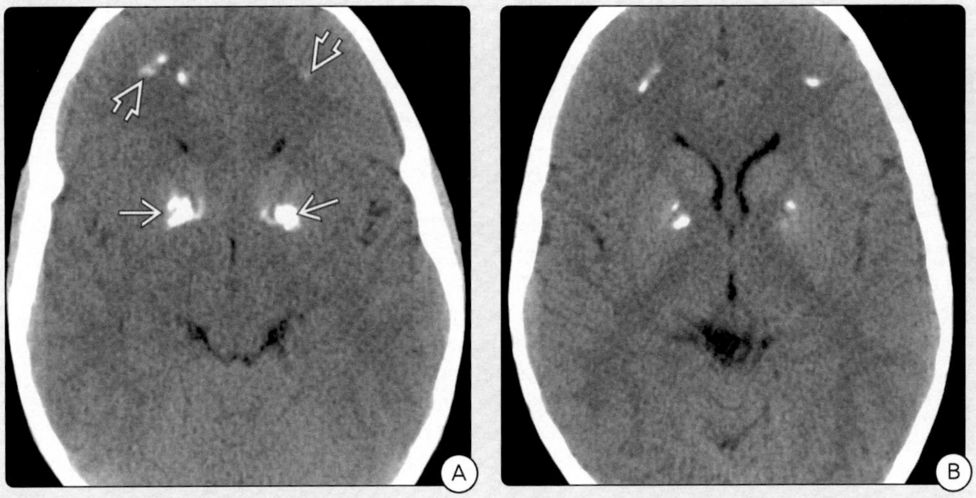

(32-33A) Axial NECT scan in a 7y patient with new onset of seizures and documented hypoparathyroidism shows symmetric calcifications in the globi pallidi ➡ with smaller calcific foci at the GM-WM interfaces ➡. (32-33B) Slightly more cephalad scan shows additional calcifications.

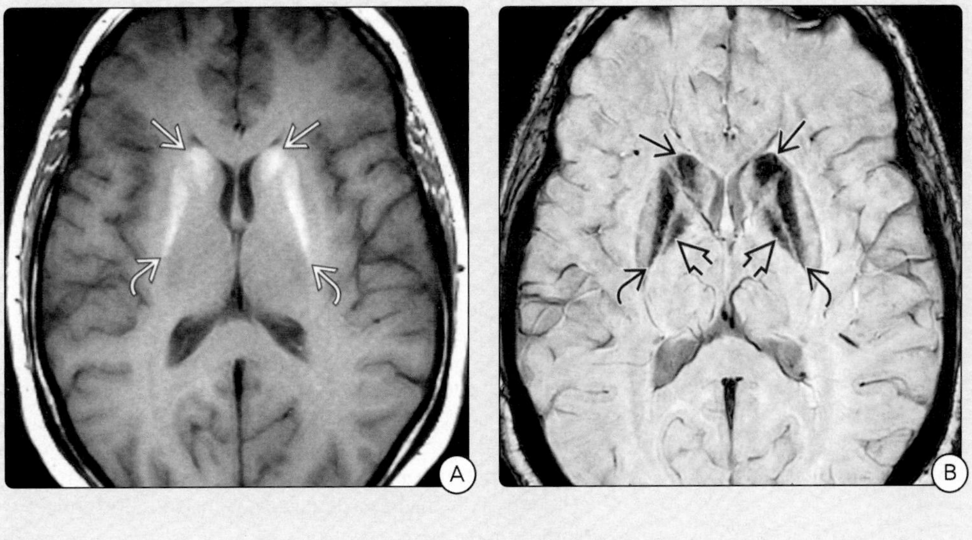

(32-34A) Axial T1WI in a 34y woman with PPHP on calcitriol shows symmetric T1 shortening in both caudate nuclei ➡ and putamina ➡. (32-34B) T2* SWI in the same case shows symmetric hypointensity in both caudate nuclei ➡, putamina ➡, and the globi pallidi ➡. (Courtesy P. Hildenbrand, MD.)

Pseudohypoparathyroidism and Pseudo-Pseudohypoparathyroidism

Both pseudohypoparathyroidism (PHP) and pseudo-pseudohypoparathyroidism (PPHP) are caused by mutations in *GNAS* and *STX16*, which confer resistance to PTH. In both disorders, the parathyroid glands produce PTH.

PHP is characterized by *elevated* PTH levels and PTH-resistant hypocalcemia and hyperphosphatemia. Obesity, round face, and mental retardation are the key clinical features. Albright hereditary osteodystrophy is a specific phenotype seen in autosomal-dominant PHP and is characterized by short fourth and fifth metacarpals and short stature.

PPHP is characterized by incomplete expression of PHP (hence the term "pseudo-pseudo"). PPHP typically shows no laboratory abnormalities, so calcium and phosphate levels are normal.

Bilateral symmetric calcifications in the basal ganglia and thalami, cerebellar hemispheres, subcortical WM, and occasionally the cerebral cortex are typical findings in both PHP and PPHP **(32-34)**.

PARATHYROID DISORDERS

Hyperparathyroidism
- 1° hyperparathyroidism (parathyroid adenomas)
  - "Salt and pepper" skull, "brown tumors"
  - Basal ganglia Ca++
- 2° (chronic renal failure)
  - Thick skull, face ("big head" disease) ± brown tumors
  - Plaque-like dural thickening, Ca++

Hypoparathyroid Disorders
- 3 types (distinguished by clinical, laboratory findings)
  - Hypoparathyroidism
  - Pseudohypoparathyroidism
  - Pseudo-pseudohypoparathyroidism
- All have Ca++ in basal ganglia > cerebrum, cerebellum

Primary Familial Brain Calcification (Fahr Disease)

Primary familial brain calcification (PFBC) is an inherited disorder that results in striking brain calcifications. Once thought to be idiopathic, it is included in this chapter (rather than Chapter 31 on inherited metabolic disorders), as its imaging findings closely resemble those seen in pseudohypoparathyroidism and pseudo-pseudohypoparathyroidism.

Terminology

PFBC, formerly termed Fahr disease, has also been termed idiopathic basal ganglia calcification and bilateral striopallidodentate calcinosis. PFBC is characterized by basal ganglia and extraganglionic calcifications, parkinsonism, and neuropsychiatric symptoms.

Etiology

PFBC is caused by mutations in four genes, namely *SLC20A2*, *PDGFB*, *PDGFRB*, and *XPR1*.

Pathology

Autopsies of the few described cases of PFBC disclose severe brain calcification in the basal ganglia, thalami, cerebral WM, cerebellar WM, and dentate nuclei. Severe cases show rows of small calcospherites along capillaries. In some cases, diffuse neurofibrillary tangles with Fahr-type calcification have been identified in patients with early-onset Alzheimer dementia.

Clinical Issues

Fahr disease is typically asymptomatic in the first and second decades. There is no sex predilection. Calcium-phosphorus metabolism and PTH levels are normal.

Deposition of calcium, along with other minerals, typically begins in the third decade, but symptoms develop one or two decades later, usually between ages 30 and 60 years. Clinical findings follow a bimodal distribution; schizophrenic-like psychosis typically presents in early adulthood with extrapyramidal symptoms, and subcortical dementia predominates in patients over the age of 50.

Imaging

CT Findings. NECT discloses extensive bilateral, relatively symmetric basal ganglia calcification in virtually all cases of PFBC. The lateral globus pallidus (GP) is the most severely affected with relative sparing of the medial GP. The putamen, caudate, thalami, dentate nuclei of the cerebellum, and both the cerebral and cerebellar WM (including the internal capsule) are commonly affected **(32-35)**. Thalamic and dentate nucleus calcification is most frequently associated with *SLC20A2* mutation.

PFBC does not enhance on CECT.

MR Findings. MRs in PFBC can be confusing. Signal intensity varies according to disease stage and the amount of calcification and heavy metal deposition. Calcification is typically hyperintense on T1WI but can be quite variable on T2WI **(32-35G)** **(32-35H)**.

T2/FLAIR scans may appear normal or mildly abnormal. They may also show extensive foci of T2 prolongation in the cerebral WM that can be so striking as to mimic toxic/metabolic demyelination **(32-36)**. The pattern of WM cysts with leukodystrophy seems to be a marker for *PDGFB* mutation.

T2* (GRE, SWI) scans show profound susceptibility changes with "blooming" hypointensity secondary to iron deposition **(32-35I)** **(32-35J)**. Fahr disease does not enhance on T1 C+ sequences.

Ultrasound. Transcranial sonography performed through the temporal bone acoustic windows demonstrates increased echogenicity in the basal ganglia, thalami, and substantia nigra.

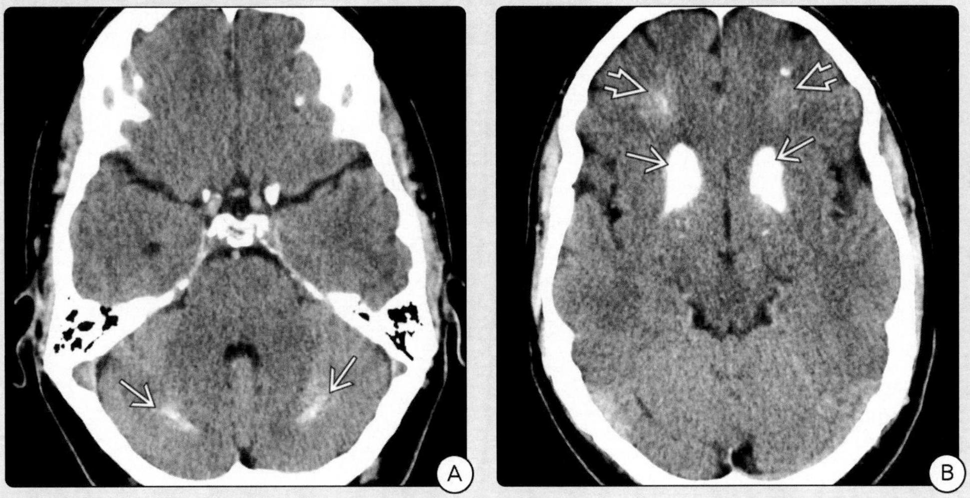

***(32-35A)** Series of axial NECT scans in a 51y man with Fahr disease shows bilaterally symmetric calcifications in the cerebellar white matter ➡. **(32-35B)** NECT scan shows very dense calcifications in both caudate nuclei and globi pallidi ➡, as well as more faint calcification in the frontal white matter ➡.*

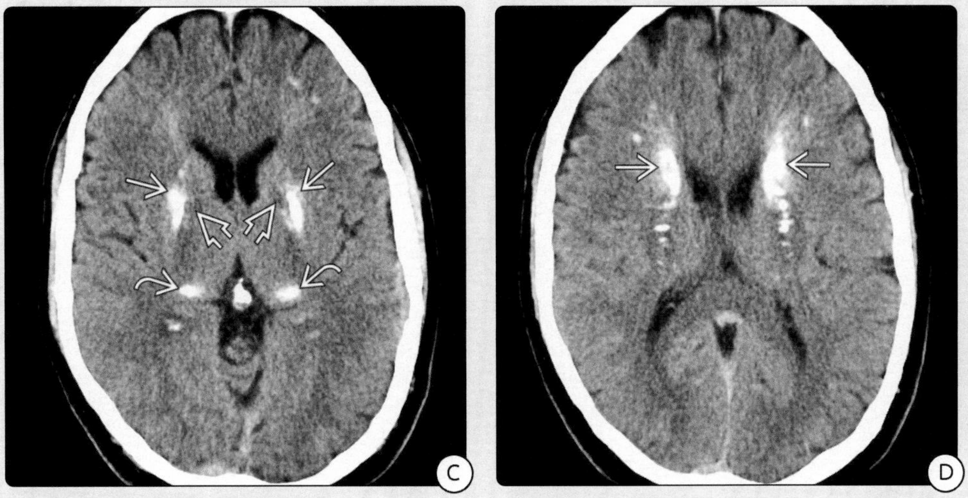

***(32-35C)** More cephalad NECT scan in the same patient shows calcification in the putamina and lateral globi pallidi ➡, with relative sparing of the most medial GP ➡. Calcification is present in the pulvinars of both thalami ➡. Punctate calcification is seen in the cerebral WM. **(32-35D)** More extensive calcification is present in the caudate heads ➡ and bodies.*

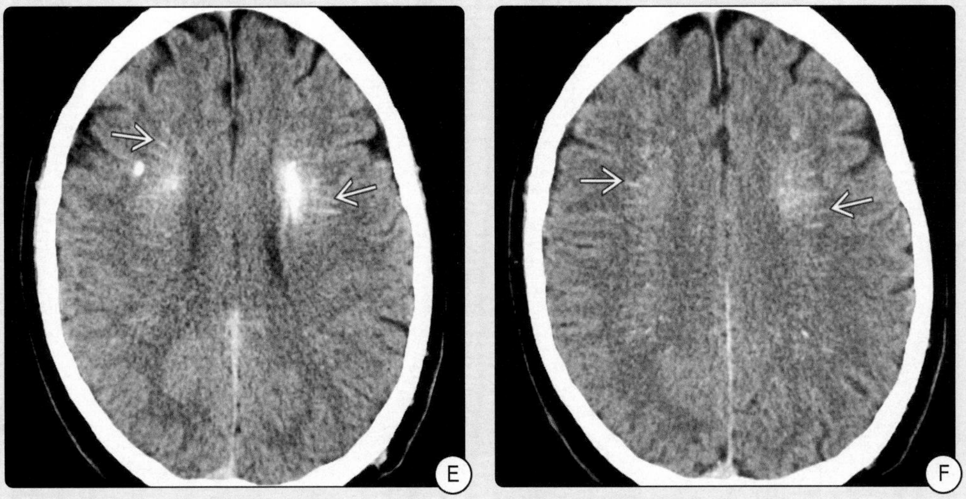

***(32-35E)** NECT scan shows linear calcification extending perpendicularly from the caudate nuclei into the cerebral white matter ➡. **(32-35F)** NECT scan through the corona radiata shows innumerable faint linear calcifications extending throughout the deep cerebral WM ➡.*

Nuclear Medicine. SPECT scans have demonstrated increased uptake in the temporal lobes with decreased basal ganglia uptake. This may reflect hyperactivation with disruption of the cortical-subcortical neural circuits responsible for the psychotic episodes often associated with Fahr disease.

Differential Diagnosis

Basal ganglia calcification is nonspecific and can be physiologic or the end result of a variety of toxic, metabolic, inflammatory, and infectious insults. Specific sublocation of the calcification can be very helpful in determining its underlying etiology.

The major differential diagnosis of PFBC is normal **physiologic calcification of the basal ganglia**. Age-related ("senescent") calcification in the basal ganglia is common, typically localized in the *medial* GP, relatively minor, and of no clinical significance. PFBC has much heavier, far more extensive calcification.

PRIMARY FAMILIAL BRAIN CALCIFICATION

Pathoetiology, Clinical Features

- Also known as Fahr disease
- Caused by 4 gene mutations (*SLC20A2* most common)
- Usually presents between 30 and 60 years
  - Extrapyramidal symptoms, dementia

Imaging Findings

- NECT
  - Extensive bilateral BG Ca++
  - Putamen, caudate, thalami, dentate nuclei
  - WM of hemispheres, cerebellum
- MR
  - T1 shortening in areas of calcification
  - ± T2/FLAIR WM hyperintensity, cysts
  - Extensive "blooming" on T2* (GRE/SWI)
  - DDx = physiological Ca++, PHP/PPHP

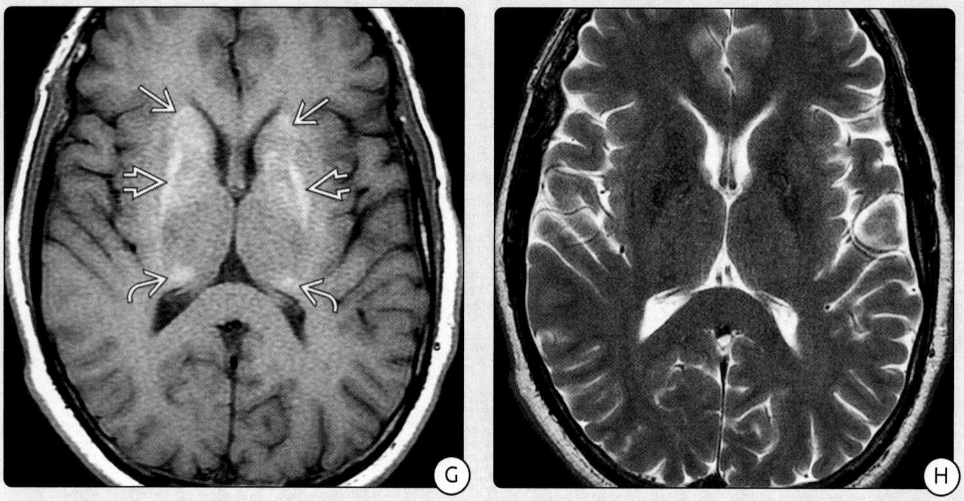

***(32-35G)** Axial T1WI in the same patient as shown on the previous page shows relatively symmetric hyperintensity in the caudate heads, lateral globi pallidi, and pulvinars of both thalami. **(32-35H)** T2WI in the same patient shows no visible abnormalities.*

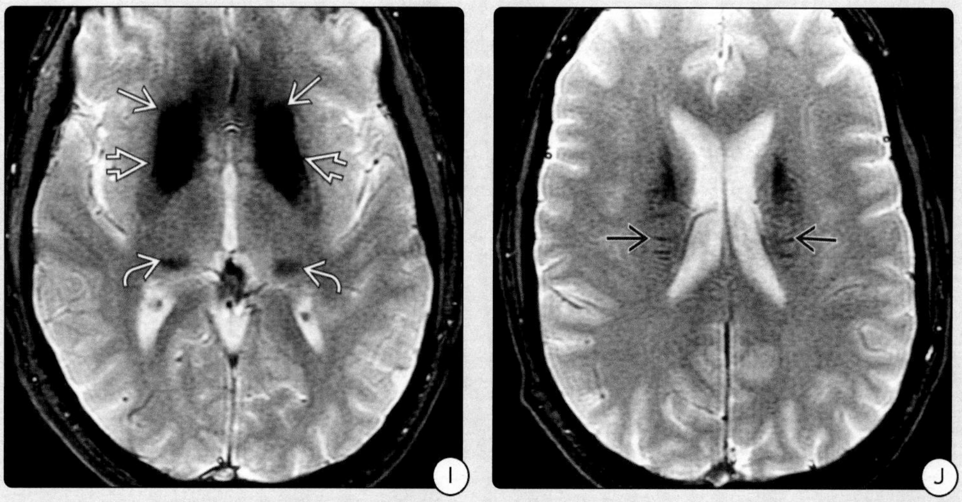

***(32-35I)** T2* GRE scan shows striking "blooming" in the same areas (caudate heads, globi pallidi, and thalamic pulvinars) as the calcifications on NECT scans and corresponding hyperintensities on the T1WI above. **(32-35J)** T2* GRE scan shows linear "blooming" foci extending perpendicularly from the caudate nuclei into the deep periventricular white matter.*

PFBC also demonstrates calcification in other locations, such as the thalami, dentate nuclei, and cerebral and cerebellar WM.

Parathyroid disorders (i.e., hyperparathyroidism, hypoparathyroidism, pseudohypoparathyroidism, and pseudo-pseudohypoparathyroidism) can all have calcification in a distribution similar to that of PFBC. In cases with severe hypocalcemia, acquired dystrophic brain calcifications can be so extensive that they mimic the appearance and distribution seen in PFBC. Serum calcium, phosphorus, and PTH levels are normal in PFBC and pseudo-pseudohypoparathyroidism.

Mineralizing microangiopathy is a late complication of radiation-induced brain injury. Some cases exhibit extensive symmetric cerebral calcifications with striopallidodentate, occipital, cerebellar, and U-fiber involvement that mimic PFBC.

Seizures and Related Disorders

Seizures can be precipitated by many infective, metabolic, toxic, developmental, neoplastic, or degenerative conditions and can affect numerous different areas of the brain. Because the temporal lobe is the most commonly affected site, we begin this section with a brief review of its normal gross and imaging anatomy. Special attention is given to the hippocampus as the site involved in mesial temporal sclerosis, an important imaging diagnosis.

We next consider the imaging manifestations of seizure activity. Two classic disorders represent the effects of chronic repeated seizures (mesial temporal sclerosis) and prolonged acute seizure activity (status epilepticus) on the brain.

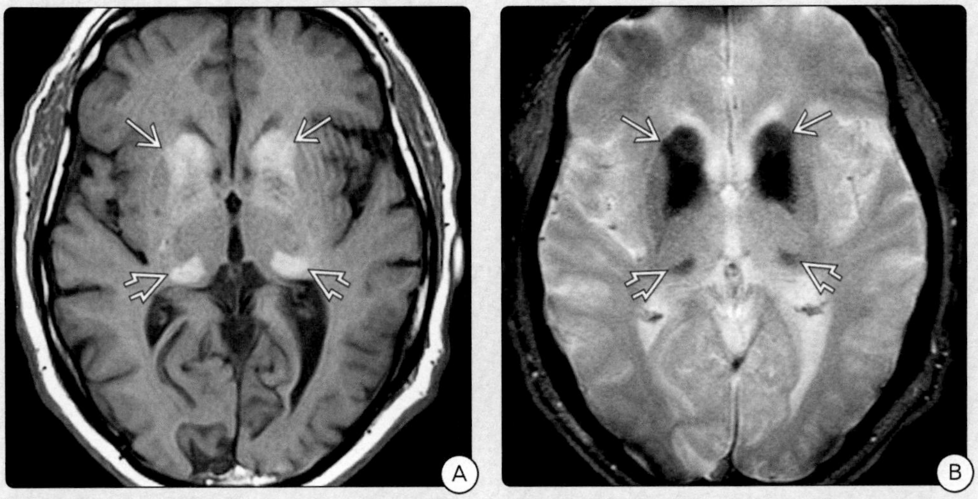

(32-36A) *Axial T1WI in a 67y man with epilepsy and known Fahr disease shows symmetric T1 shortening in the basal ganglia ➡ and pulvinars ➡ of both thalami.* ***(32-36B)*** *T2* GRE in the same case shows dense susceptibility "blooming" in the basal ganglia ➡ and thalami ➡ corresponding to the areas of T1 shortening.*

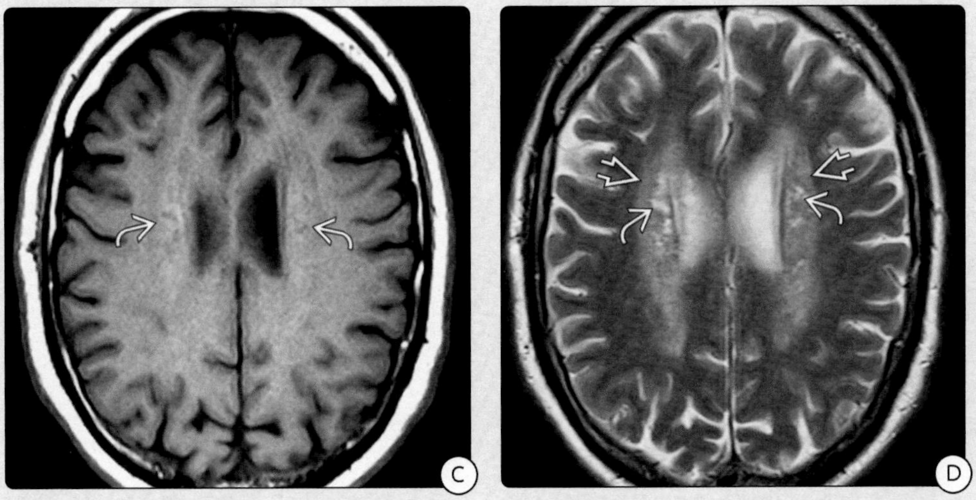

(32-36C) *More cephalad T1WI in the same case shows mixed foci of T1 shortening and hypointensity in the caudate nuclei and deep periventricular white matter ➡.* ***(32-36D)*** *T2WI in the same case shows extensive confluent areas of T2 hyperintensity in the deep WM ➡ intermixed with areas of cystic degeneration ➡ and hypointense foci. This pattern of WM cysts with leukodystrophy is characteristic for PDGFB mutation.*

We then discuss a newly described abnormality that can be seen with seizures (as well as a variety of other disorders), the "transient lesion of the corpus callosum splenium." The section concludes with a consideration of imaging findings in transient global amnesia, which specifically affects the hippocampus.

Normal Anatomy of the Temporal Lobe

Here, we briefly review general anatomy of the temporal lobe before focusing in greater detail on the hippocampus.

Gross Anatomy

Temporal Lobe. The temporal lobe lies inferior to the sylvian fissure. Its lateral surface presents three gyri: the superior temporal gyrus (contains the primary auditory cortex), the middle temporal gyrus (connects with auditory, somatosensory, visual association pathways), and the inferior temporal gyrus (contains the higher visual association area).

The temporal lobe also contains major subdivisions of the limbic system **(32-37)**. The parahippocampal gyrus lies on the medial surface of the temporal lobe and merges into the uncus **(32-38)**.

Hippocampus. The human hippocampus is a phylogenetically older part of the brain that plays a key role in memory. It can be affected by many common neurologic disorders, including acute ischemic stroke, transient global amnesia, epilepsy, and encephalitis.

The hippocampus is part of the limbic system, three nested C-shaped arches that surround the diencephalon and basal ganglia **(32-37)**. The hippocampus proper is part of the middle arch, which extends from the temporal to the frontal lobes.

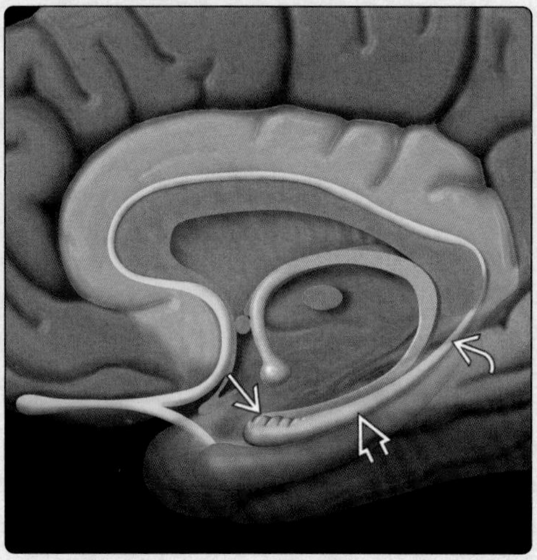

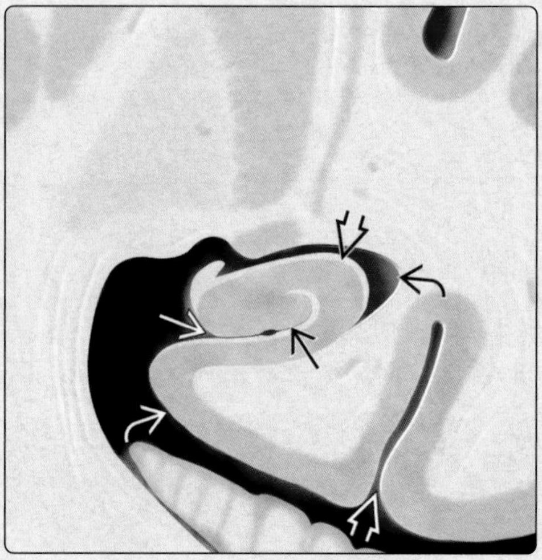

***(32-37)** Sagittal graphic shows 3 nested C-shaped arches of the limbic system. Hippocampus, indusium griseum are shown in yellow. Digitated anterior head, body, tail of the hippocampus lie along the floor of the temporal horn of the lateral ventricle. **(32-38)** Coronal graphic shows dentate gyrus, Ammon horn, parahippocampal gyrus, hippocampal sulcus, collateral sulcus, temporal horn of lateral ventricle.*

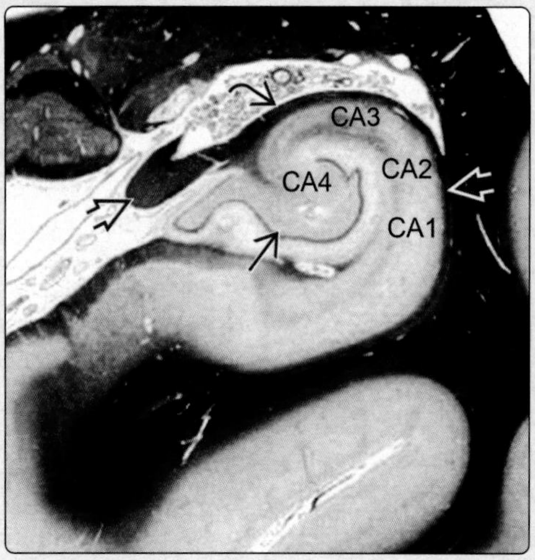

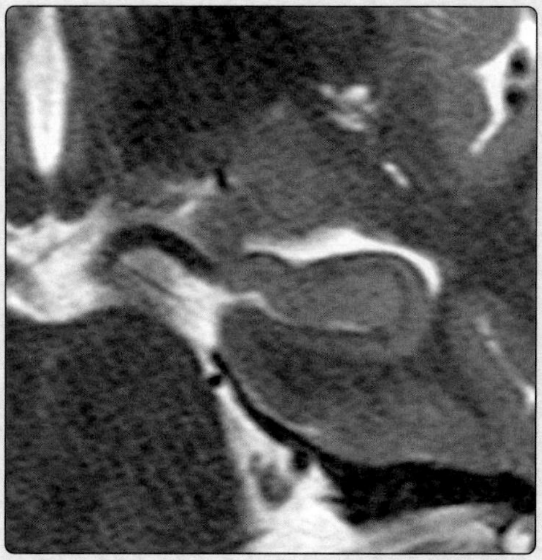

***(32-39)** Coronal histology shows CA1-4 zones of Ammon horn. The two U-shaped interlocking layers of gray matter formed by the dentate gyrus inside and Ammon horn outside comprise the hippocampus and are nicely seen. WM (stained purple) of the alveus and fimbria is external to the GM of the Ammon horn. **(32-40)** High-resolution coronal T2WI shows normal hippocampus with distinct layers of white and gray matter.*

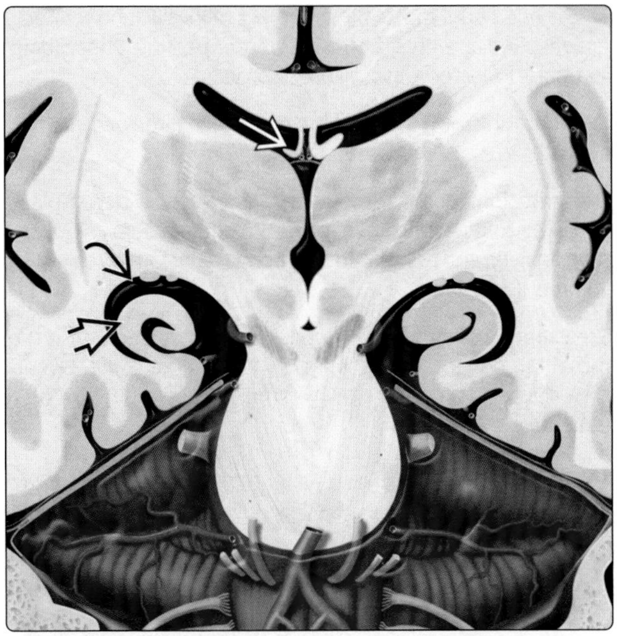

(32-41) Coronal graphic depicts typical mesial temporal sclerosis. The right hippocampus ⇨ is atrophied and sclerotic with loss of normal internal architecture. The right temporal horn ⇨ is enlarged, and the ipsilateral fornix ➡ is small.

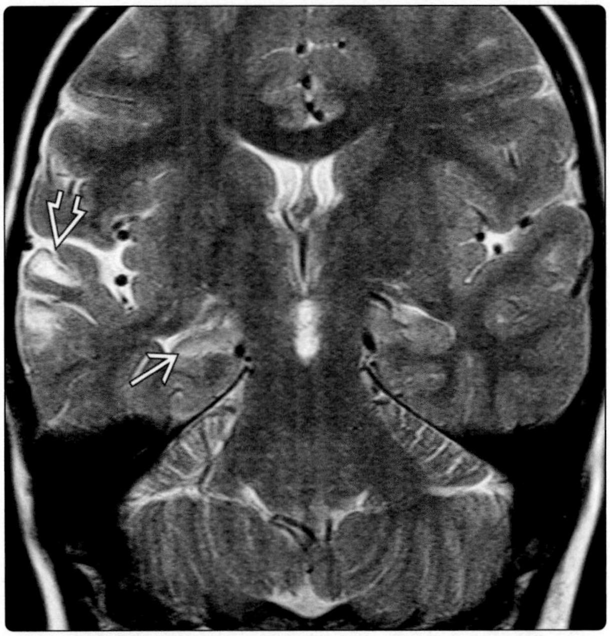

(32-42) Coronal T2WI in a 27y man with history of intractable epilepsy and remote closed head trauma shows temporal lobe encephalomalacia ⇨. The shrunken, hyperintense right hippocampus ➡ is consistent with MTS.

The hippocampus lies on the medial aspect of the temporal horn and bulges into its floor. The hippocampus has three anatomic segments: the head (pes hippocampus, the digitated anterior part), the body (cylindrical), and a posterior tail that narrows and curves around the corpus callosum splenium **(32-37)**.

On coronal sections through the body, the hippocampus is composed of two interlocking U-shaped layers of gray matter: the Ammon horn and the dentate gyrus. The Ammon horn—the hippocampus proper—forms the more superolateral, upside-down "U," while the dentate gyrus forms the inferomedial "U" **(32-39)**.

The Ammon horn is subdivided into four zones based on width, cell size, and cell density. These zones are designated as CA1, CA2, CA3, and CA4. CA1 (also known as the Sommer sector) is the lateral, outermost zone and consists of small pyramidal cells that are especially vulnerable to anoxia. CA2 curves superomedially from CA1 and consists of a narrow band of cells that are relatively resistant to anoxia. CA3 is a wide loose band that merges into CA4, the innermost zone. CA4 is enveloped by the dentate gyrus.

Imaging Anatomy

The superior, middle, and inferior temporal gyri are best seen on sagittal MR scans.

The hippocampus is best depicted on coronal MR scans performed perpendicular to the long axis of the hippocampus. Thin-section true IR (or 3D T1 SPGR), high-resolution T2WI, and coronal whole-brain FLAIR scans are recommended.

Coronal scans show the hippocampus as a seahorse-shaped structure immediately below the choroid fissure and temporal horn of the lateral ventricle **(32-40)**. The parahippocampal gyrus is separated from the dentate gyrus by the hippocampal sulcus. The collateral sulcus is an important landmark that lies just inferolateral to the parahippocampal gyrus.

Mesial Temporal (Hippocampal) Sclerosis

Temporal lobe epilepsy (TLE) is the most common form of partial complex epilepsy and can occur with or without mesial temporal sclerosis.

Terminology

Mesial temporal sclerosis (MTS), also known as hippocampal sclerosis (HS) is the most common overall localization-related form of epilepsy **(32-41)**. Its most common manifestation is complex partial seizures.

Etiology

A variety of events such as trauma or infection may precipitate intractable complex partial seizures **(32-42)**. The end result is MTS. Although the precise pathophysiology of how and why MTS develops is unclear, inflammatory processes or prolonged seizures with hippocampal hypoxic-ischemic injury are considered the most likely candidates.

Pathology

MTS is characterized grossly by atrophy of the hippocampus and adjacent structures **(32-41)**. The hippocampal body (85-90%) is the most commonly affected site, followed by the tail (60%) and head (50%). Approximately 15-20% of cases are bilateral but usually asymmetric.

The CA1 and CA4 areas are the most susceptible to hypoxic-ischemic damage, but all regions of the hippocampus can be affected. Neuronal loss with chronic astrogliosis is the typical histologic finding.

Clinical Issues

Epidemiology. Nearly 10% of all individuals experience a seizure in their lifetime. Two-thirds of these are nonrecurrent febrile/nonfebrile seizures. Peak prevalence is bimodal (< 1 year and > 55 years of age). One-third of patients develop repeated seizures ("epilepsy").

Approximately 20% of patients with epilepsy have complex partial seizures. Of these, 35-50% are pharmacoresistant and are refractory to anticonvulsant therapy. Current estimates based on a USA population of 325 million indicate that as many as 143,000-191,000 patients suffer from drug-resistant HS-TLE.

MTS is one of the most common types of localization-related epilepsy and accounts for the majority of patients undergoing temporal lobectomy for seizure disorder.

Demographics. MTS is a disease of older children and young adults. There is no sex predominance.

Presentation. Most patients with MTS present with complex partial seizures lasting 1-2 minutes. Preceding "auras" with fear, anxiety, and associated autonomic symptoms are common.

Treatment Options. Anteromedial temporal lobectomy is the most common treatment for MTS with drug-resistant TLE and is successful in reducing or eliminating seizures in 70-90% of patients.

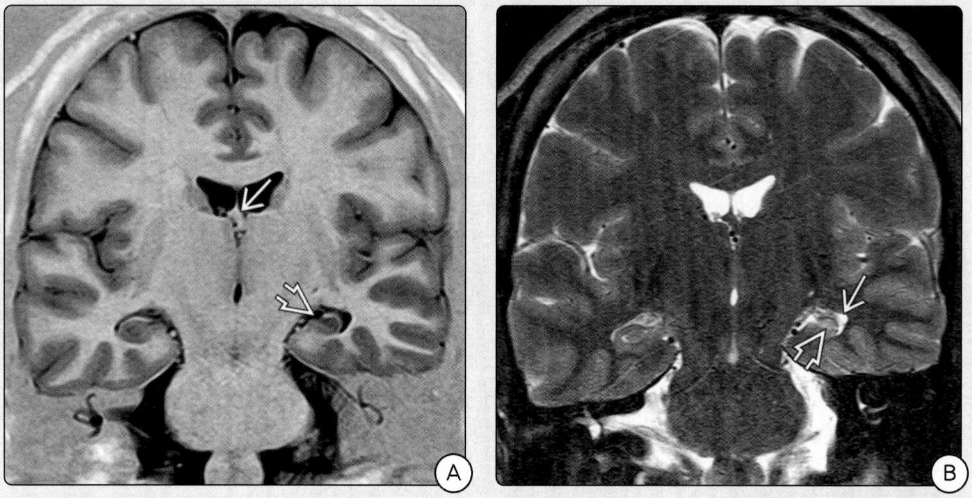

***(32-43A)** Coronal true inversion recovery scan in a 37y woman with temporal lobe epilepsy shows shrunken left hippocampus ➡. The ipsilateral fornix ➡ is small. **(32-43B)** Coronal thin-section T2WI in the same patient shows that the shrunken left hippocampus is hyperintense ➡. The temporal horn ➡ is mildly enlarged compared with the right side.*

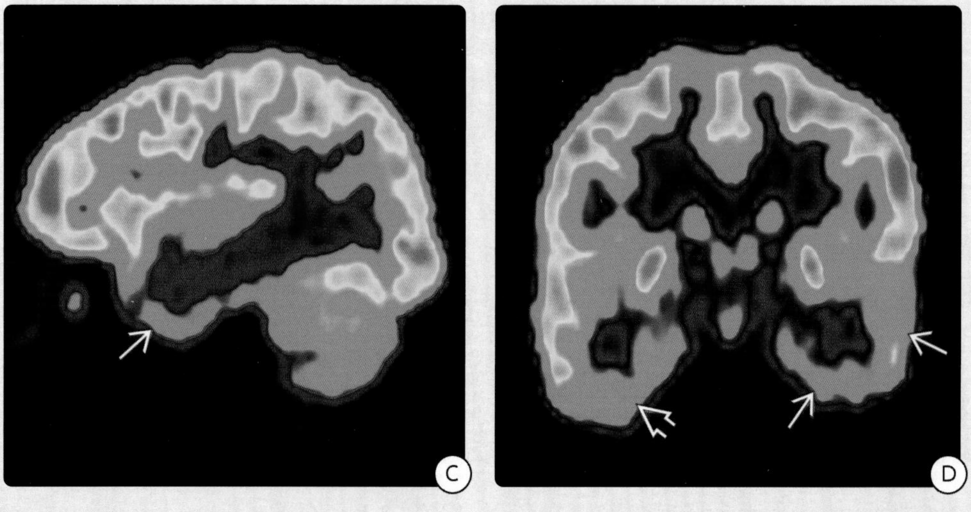

***(32-43C)** Sagittal FDG PET shows marked hypometabolism in the affected temporal lobe ➡. **(32-43D)** Coronal FDG PET scan in the same patient shows that the entire left temporal lobe ➡ is markedly hypometabolic. Note reduced metabolism in the right temporal lobe ➡, possibly reflecting chronic subclinical mirroring seizures.*

Imaging

MR Findings. Imaging markers of MTS are found in 60-70% of patients with TLE. True coronal IR or 3D SPGR sequences show a shrunken hippocampus with atrophy of the ipsilateral fornix and widening of the adjacent temporal horn and/or choroid fissure **(32-43)**. Abnormal T2/FLAIR hyperintensity with obscuration of the internal hippocampal architecture is typical **(32-42)**. MTS typically does not enhance following contrast administration.

DWI shows increased diffusivity on ADC and hyperintensity on DWI (T2 "shine-through"). The spectroscopic hallmark of TLE is reduced NAA in the epileptogenic focus, presumably secondary to neuronal loss. Cho and Cr are typically unchanged. In MTS, NAA is reduced—and not just in the hippocampus.

Widespread alterations in extrahippocampal and even extratemporal regions can be demonstrated in MTS. High-resolution DTI shows evidence of diffusion abnormalities of the ipsilateral fimbria-fornix, parahippocampal WM bundle, and the uncinate fasciculus and is helpful in predicting postoperative seizure outcome. Resting-state fMR demonstrates that the inferior cingulum bundle undergoes degeneration in tandem with ipsilateral hippocampal volume loss.

Nuclear Medicine Findings. FDG PET is one of the most sensitive imaging procedures for diagnosing MTS. Temporal lobe hypometabolism is the typical finding **(32-43)**. SPECT shows hyperperfusion in the epileptogenic zone during seizure activity; hypoperfusion in the interictal period is common.

Angiography. In the past, most patients with intractable TLE who were candidates for temporal lobe resection underwent a Wada test (intracarotid amobarbital test) to evaluate language lateralization and assess risk for postoperative memory disorders. With new noninvasive techniques such as resting fMR mapping, the utilization of Wada testing is declining precipitously. It is no longer used in many epilepsy centers.

Differential Diagnosis

The major differential diagnosis of MTS is status epilepticus. **Status epilepticus** can be subclinical and may cause transient gyral edema with T2/FLAIR hyperintensity and/or enhancement in the affected cortex as well as the hippocampus.

A **low-grade glioma** (WHO grade II astrocytoma, oligodendroglioma, or oligoastrocytoma) in the temporal lobe can cause drug-resistant TLE. Gliomas are usually T2/FLAIR hyperintense and cause mass effect, not volume loss. Cortically based neoplasms associated with TLE include **dysembryoplastic neuroepithelial tumor (DNET)**. DNET typically is a well-demarcated, "bubbly" mass that is often associated with adjacent cortical dysplasia. **Cortical dysplasia** is isointense with GM but frequently causes T2 hyperintensity in the underlying temporal lobe WM.

Cystic-appearing lesions in the temporal lobe that are hyperintense on T2WI include **prominent perivascular spaces, hippocampal sulcus remnants**, and **choroid fissure cysts**. These "leave me alone" lesions all behave like CSF and suppress on FLAIR.

Status Epilepticus

Terminology

Status epilepticus (SE) is a prolonged (more than 30 minutes), continuously active seizure with EEG-demonstrated seizure activity. Two or more seizures without full recovery between the events is also considered SE. SE can be focal or generalized; generalized convulsive SE is potentially life-threatening if not controlled.

Etiology

Prolonged ictal activity induces hypermetabolism with increased glucose utilization. Perfusion increases but is still insufficient to match glucose demand. The result is compromised cellular energy production, cytotoxic cell swelling, and vasogenic edema. With prolonged severe seizure activity, the blood-brain barrier may become permeable, permitting leakage of fluid and macromolecules into the extracellular spaces.

Pathology

Transient vasogenic and/or cytotoxic edema causes cortical swelling that typically spares the underlying WM.

Imaging

General Features. Imaging findings in SE vary with acuity and severity. Most acute periictal abnormalities are reversible and normalize within a few days. Irreversible changes do occur, especially with generalized convulsive SE.

CT Findings. Initial NECT scans may be normal or show gyral swelling with sulcal effacement and parenchymal hypodensity. CECT may demonstrate gyral enhancement in a nonvascular distribution.

MR Findings. Periictal MR shows T2/FLAIR hyperintensity with gyral swelling **(32-44)**. The subcortical and deep WM is relatively spared. Crossed cerebellar diaschisis, ipsilateral thalamic involvement, and basal ganglia lesions are seen in some cases.

Gyriform enhancement on T1 C+ varies from none to striking. Diffusion restriction with uni- or bilateral hippocampal, thalamic, and cortical lesions is common **(32-45) (32-46)**. Ictal DWI and pMR demonstrating hyperperfusion can be especially useful in the diagnosis of nonconvulsive SE.

Scans performed a week to several months following SE may show permanent abnormalities, including focal brain atrophy, cortical laminar necrosis, and mesial temporal sclerosis.

Differential Diagnosis

The major differential diagnosis of periictal brain swelling is **acute cerebral ischemia-infarction**. Acute cerebral ischemia occurs in a typical vascular territorial distribution, is wedge-shaped (involving both GM and WM), and is positive on DWI *before* T2/FLAIR hyperintensity develops. In ongoing SE, DWI and T2 signal changes typically occur simultaneously.

Cerebritis may cause a T2/FLAIR hyperintense mass that restricts on DWI. Cerebritis typically involves the subcortical WM as well as the cortex. **Herpes encephalitis** is typically preceded by a viral prodrome, affects the limbic system, is frequently bilateral but asymmetric, and often demonstrates petechial hemorrhage.

Acute onset **of mitochondrial encephalopathy with lactic acidosis and stroke-like episodes** (MELAS) may affect the cortex in a nonvascular distribution. MRS in the noninvolved brain usually demonstrates a lactate peak. **Transient global amnesia** causes tiny dot-like foci of restricted diffusion in the lateral hippocampus.

IMAGING IN SEIZURE DISORDERS

Mesial Temporal Sclerosis
- Hippocampal ± fornix volume loss
  - 80-85% unilateral
- Loss of internal architecture
  - T2/FLAIR hyperintensity
  - FDG PET hypometabolic

Status Epilepticus
- Gyriform T2/FLAIR hyperintensity, spares WM
- Nonvascular distribution
- May restrict on DWI, exhibit hyperperfusion
- Subacute/chronic effects
  - Atrophy, cortical laminar necrosis
  - Mesial temporal sclerosis

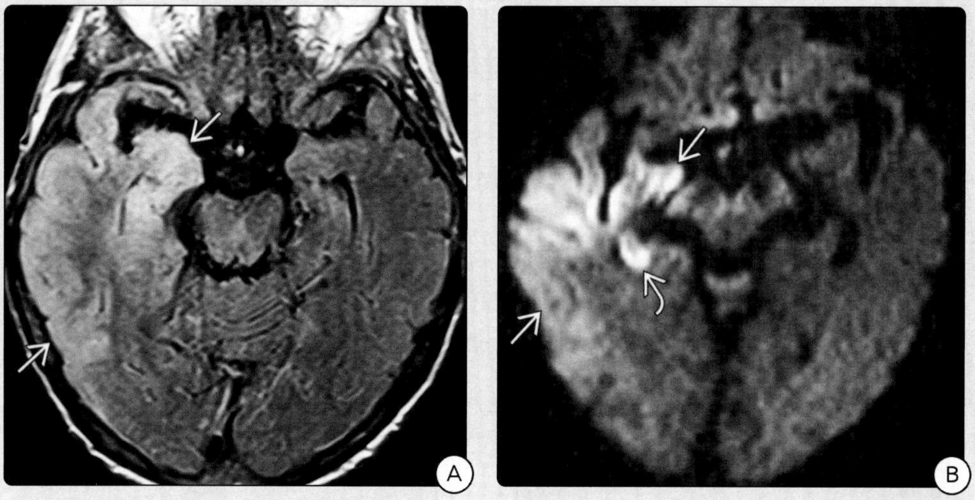

***(32-44A)** Axial FLAIR in a 79y man with prolonged seizure shows gyral swelling and hyperintensity in a nonvascular distribution involving the temporal and parietal cortex. The underlying WM is spared. **(32-44B)** DWI in the same case shows restricted diffusion in the edematous cortex of the temporal and parietal lobes. Note restriction in the ipsilateral hippocampus .*

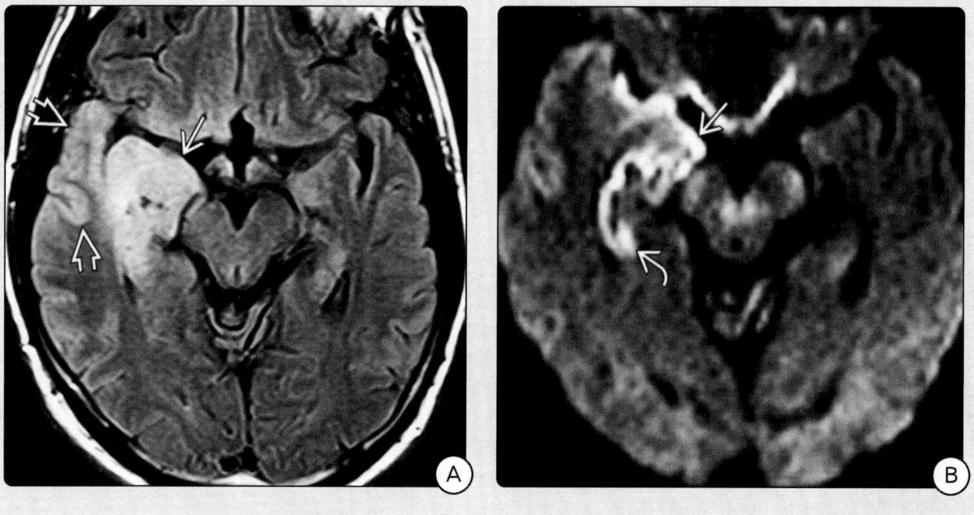

***(32-45A)** Axial FLAIR in a 58y man with new onset of drug-refractory seizures shows mass-like hyperintensity in the right medial temporal lobe . Note hyperintensity of the lateral temporal lobe cortex . **(32-45B)** DWI shows restricted diffusion in the uncus and hippocampus of the right temporal lobe. EEG confirmed temporal lobe epilepsy. Biopsy and resection revealed diffusely infiltrating astrocytoma.*

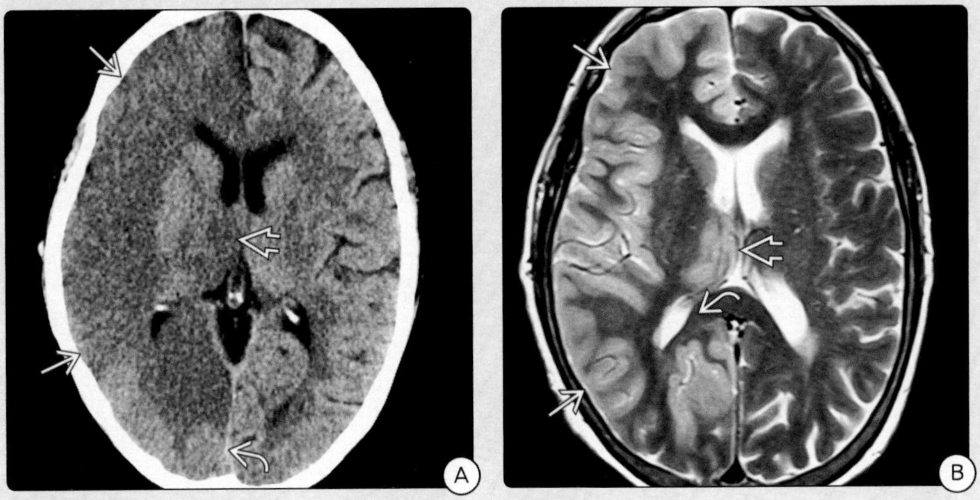

(32-46A) *NECT in a 52y woman in status epilepticus for 24 hours shows diffuse hypodensity in the right hemisphere that involves both the gray and white matter ➡. Patchy hypodensity is present in the right thalamus ➡. The right occipital cortex ➡ and left hemisphere are spared.* ***(32-46B)*** *T2WI in the same case shows diffuse gyral ➡ and right thalamic ➡ swelling and hyperintensity. The WM in the parietal lobe and corpus callosum ➡ is subtly abnormal.*

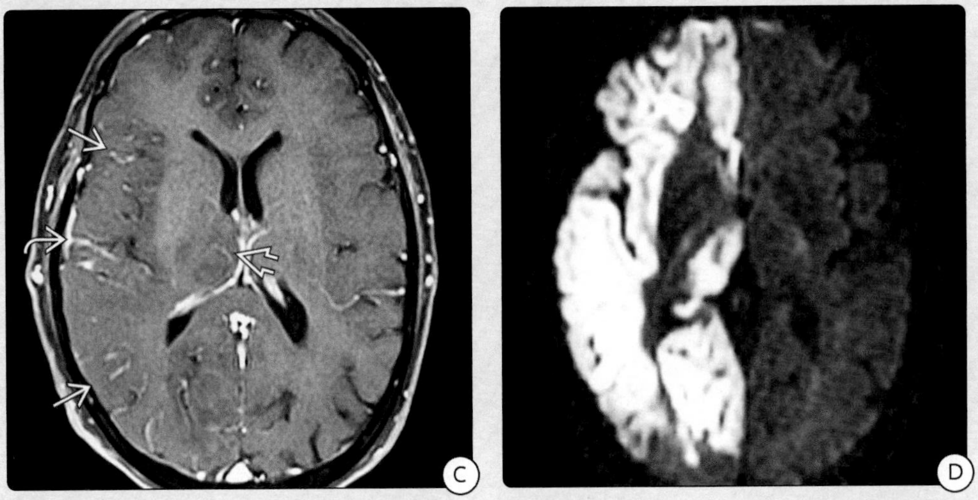

(32-46C) *T1 C+ FS shows corresponding cortical, thalamic ➡ hypointensity. Note engorgement of right cortical vessels ➡ and draining veins ➡ compared with the normal left side.* ***(32-46D)*** *DWI shows markedly restricted diffusion in the right hemisphere cortex, subcortical WM, and thalamus.*

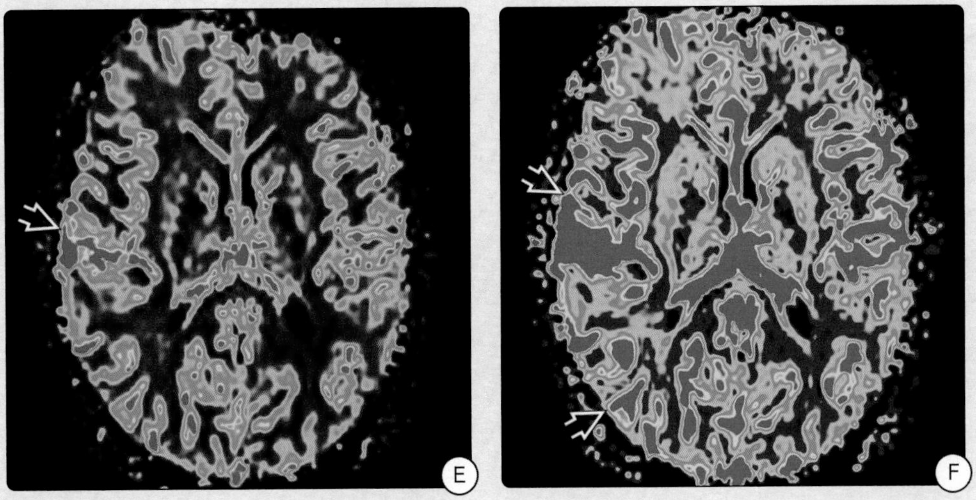

(32-46E) *MR perfusion with cerebral blood flow shows modestly elevated rCBF ➡.* ***(32-46F)*** *The rCBV map shows increased blood volume throughout the right hemisphere ➡ compared with the left.*

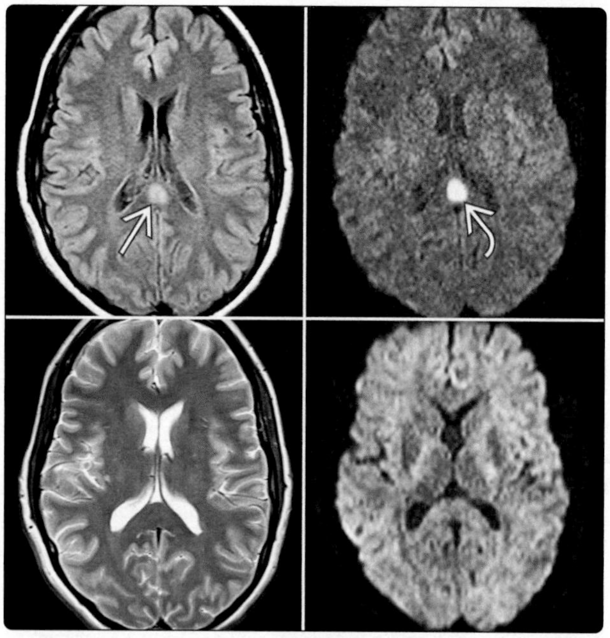

***(32-47)** A patient taken off antiseizure medications 3 weeks prior to imaging shows round FLAIR hyperintense lesion → in CC splenium (top L) that restricts on DWI ↪ (top R). Repeat scan 2 weeks later shows that the lesions have resolved. This is CLCC.*

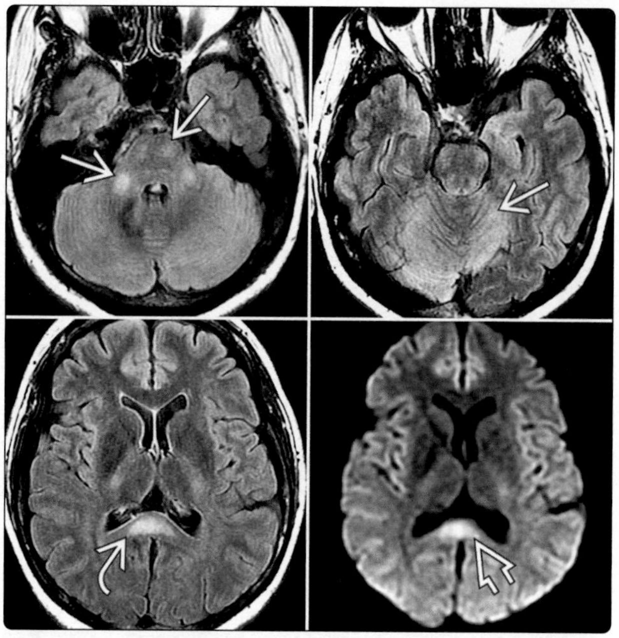

***(32-48)** Series of FLAIR scans in viral encephalitis shows lesions → in pons, peduncles, and cerebellar hemisphere. Corpus callosum splenium lesion ↪ restricts on DWI ⇨. This is virus-associated CLCC.*

Cytotoxic Lesions of the Corpus Callosum

Terminology

Cytotoxic lesions of the corpus callosum (CLCCs) are acquired lesions that have been associated with a number of different entities. Because they are (1) often reversible and (2) most common in the corpus callosum splenium, they have also been called transient or reversible splenial lesions.

Pathoetiology

Precisely how and why CLCCs appear and then disappear is unknown. Most investigators believe CLCCs are a cytokinopathy with secondary excitotoxic glutaminergic-associated intracellular edema. The corpus callosum—especially the splenium—has a high density of excitatory amino acid, toxin, and drug receptors and is hence more vulnerable to the development of cytotoxic edema.

Associated Conditions

CLCCs were first identified in patients with epilepsy and were initially considered a seizure- and/or drug-related reversible abnormality. The use and subsequent withdrawal of antiepileptic drugs is the most commonly associated condition. CLCCs typically appear between 24 hours and 3 weeks after antiepileptic therapy is discontinued.

The second most common cause of CLCC is infection, usually a viral encephalitis that may also cause a mild febrile encephalopathy (sometimes termed MERS, or mild encephalopathy with reversible splenial lesion). Influenza virus, rotavirus, measles, human herpesvirus-6, West Nile virus, Epstein-Barr virus, varicella-zoster virus, mumps, and adenoviruses have all been reported with CLCCs as have bacterial meningoencephalitis and malaria.

Metabolic derangements such as hypoglycemia and hypernatremia, acute alcohol poisoning, malnutrition, and vitamin B12 deficiency are the third most common group of CLCC-associated disorders. Eclampsia and hemolytic-uremic syndrome have been reported as rare possible causes.

Miscellaneous reported associations include migraine headache, trauma, high-altitude cerebral edema, systemic lupus erythematosus, internal cerebral vein occlusion, Charcot-Marie-Tooth disease, and neoplasms.

Clinical Issues

CLCCs themselves are usually asymptomatic and discovered incidentally on imaging studies. Variable degrees of encephalopathy reported with CLCCs may be caused by the inciting pathology, not the lesion itself.

Most CLCCs resolve spontaneously and disappear although not all lesions are completely reversible.

Imaging

On imaging studies, typical CLCCs are round to ovoid homogeneous, nonhemorrhagic lesions centered in the corpus callosum splenium. They are mildly hypointense on T1WI, hyperintense on T2/FLAIR, do not enhance, and demonstrate restricted diffusion **(32-47)** **(32-48)**. A variant type of CLCC that involves the entire corpus callosum splenium and extending into the forceps major has been termed the "boomerang" sign. Rarely, CLCCs extend anteriorly from the splenium into the corpus callosum body.

CLCCs typically resolve completely within a few days or weeks, and follow-up imaging studies are normal.

CYTOTOXIC LESIONS OF THE CORPUS CALLOSUM

Terminology
- Also called reversible or transient splenial lesions

Pathoetiology
- Cytokinopathy with glutamate-induced intracellular edema
- Associated with
  - Seizures
  - Drugs (antiepileptic, metronidazole, etc.)
  - Infections (often but not invariably viral)
  - Metabolic disorders (alcohol, Wernicke, osmotic)
  - Neoplasms, chemotherapy
  - Trauma

Clinical Features
- Usually asymptomatic, incidental
- Typically (but not invariably) resolves spontaneously

Imaging Findings
- Round, ovoid or "boomerang-shaped" lesion
- Splenium > > > body, central > > eccentric
- T2/FLAIR hyperintense
- Restricts on DWI
- Does not enhance

Transient Global Amnesia

Terminology

Transient global amnesia (TGA) is a unique neurologic disorder characterized by (1) sudden memory loss without other signs of cognitive or neurologic impairment and (2) complete clinical recovery within 24 hours.

As a clinical syndrome, TGA is easily recognized. The patient has isolated transient amnesia with normal consciousness and no other neurologic or cognitive disturbances.

Etiology

The underlying etiology of TGA is unknown. Paroxysmal neuronal discharges or epileptic phenomena (e.g., spreading cortical depression, seizure with delayed neuronal injury), migraine with aura, ischemic stroke or hypoxia, local nonischemic energy failures, and venous congestion have all been proposed as possible pathologic mechanisms.

Clinical Issues

Most TGA patients are between 50 and 70 years; TGA is rare under the age of 40. There is no sex predilection. A typical scenario is a middle-aged patient who suddenly starts forgetting conversations within minutes and tends to repeat the same questions. Isolated anterograde amnesia with preserved alertness, attention, and personal identity are consistent features. EEGs are normal in 80-90% of cases with the remainder showing minor nonepileptiform activity. Symptoms resolve in 24 hours or less.

Recurrences are relatively rare (5-10% per year). Population-based studies have demonstrated that having a TGA episode does not increase the risk of

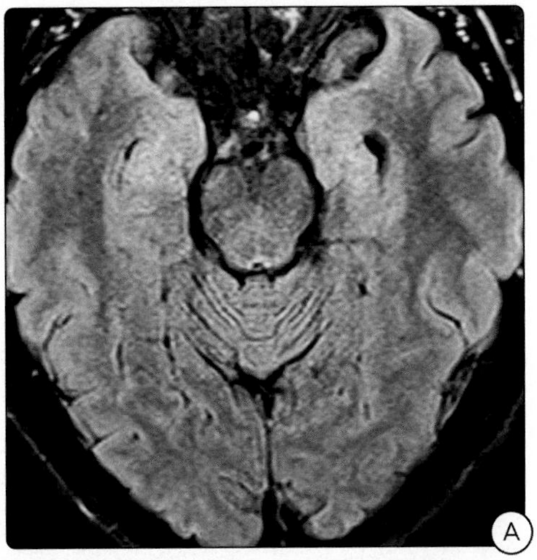

***(32-49A)** Axial FLAIR in a 70y woman with sudden onset of confusion and amnesia is normal.*

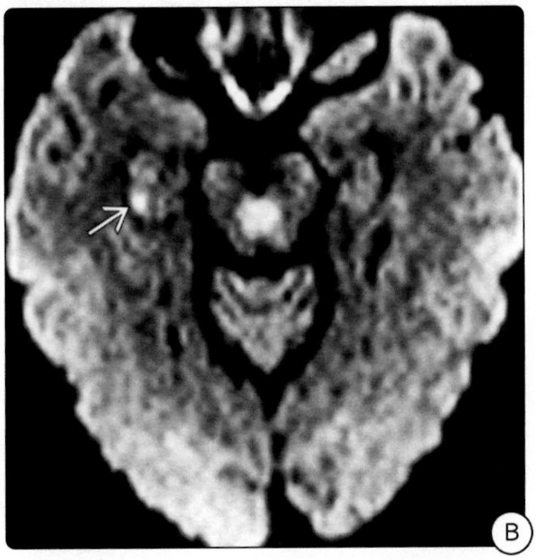

***(32-49B)** DWI shows small focus of restricted diffusion in right hippocampus ➡. Symptoms resolved; follow-up scan was normal. This is TGA.*

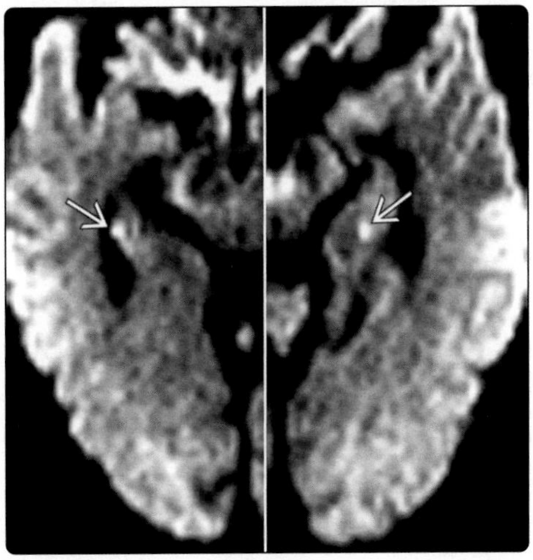

***(32-50)** DWI in 65y man with sudden anterograde memory loss shows foci of restricted diffusion in both hippocampi ➡. This is TGA.*

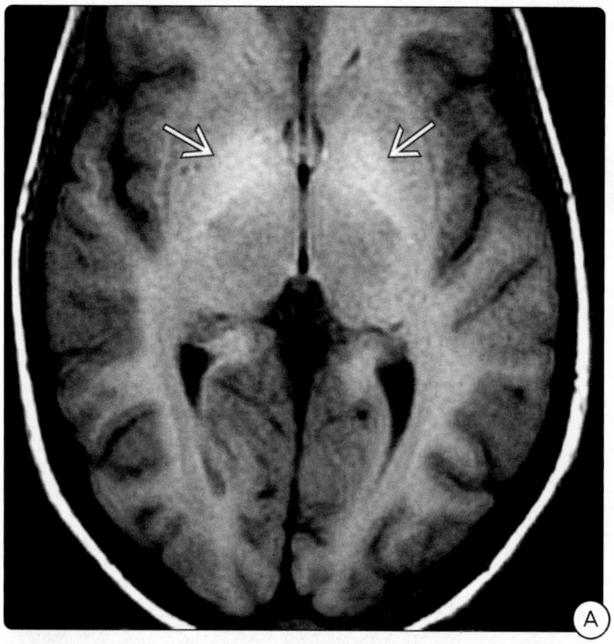

(32-51A) *Axial T1WI in a 31y patient with chronic liver failure demonstrates symmetric T1 shortening in the globi pallidi ➡.*

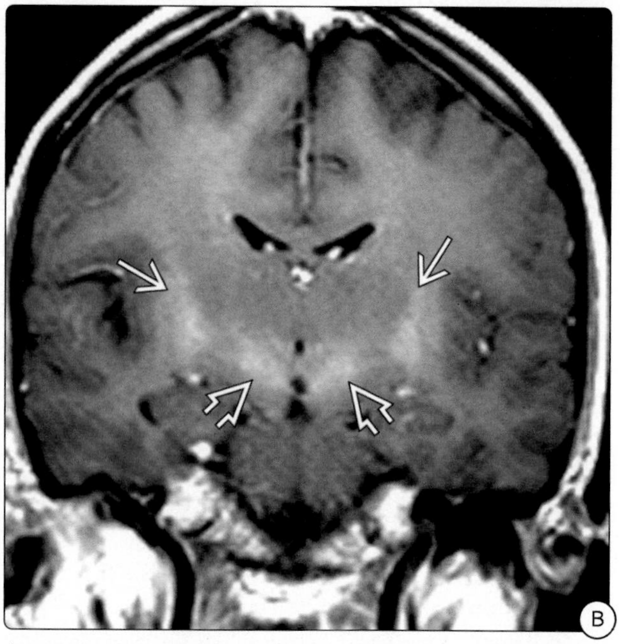

(32-51B) *Coronal T1 C+ scan shows the symmetric basal ganglia hyperintensity ➡ as well as hyperintensity in both cerebral peduncles and substantia nigra ⇨. Findings are classic for chronic hepatic encephalopathy.*

subsequent cerebrovascular events, seizures, or cognitive impairment.

Imaging

CT scans are invariably normal, and standard MR sequences (T2/FLAIR) typically show no abnormalities.

Nearly 80% of patients with TGA develop focal hippocampal abnormalities on DWI **(32-49)**. Thin sections (3 mm) obtained at high b-values (at least 2,000) and higher field strength magnets increase sensitivity.

The typical findings of TGA are 1-2 mm of punctate or dot-like foci of restricted diffusion in the CA1 area of the hippocampus. These appear as hyperintensities along the lateral aspect of the hippocampus, just medial to the temporal horn. Lesions can be single (55%) or multiple (45%), unilateral (50-55%) or bilateral (45-50%) **(32-50)**. The body of the hippocampus is most commonly involved, followed by the head.

DWI abnormalities in TGA increase significantly with time following symptom onset. Between 0-6 hours, 34% show foci of restricted diffusion. This increases to 62% in patients imaged between 6 and 12 hours and to 67% of patients between 12 and 24 hours. By day three, 75% of patients demonstrate abnormalities. Follow-up scans typically show complete resolution by day 10.

A few reported cases have demonstrated both hypoperfusion and hypometabolism in the hippocampus on PET or SPECT.

Differential Diagnosis

The two major differential diagnoses of TGA are stroke and seizure. A strategic embolic stroke isolated to the mesial temporal area, thalamus, or fornix can produce isolated amnestic syndromes and mimic TGA clinically. TGA lesions are often multiple. Their exclusive location in the hippocampus mitigates against typical embolic infarcts. However, acute **isolated punctate hippocampal infarction** can be indistinguishable from TGA based on imaging studies alone.

Seizures can cause transient diffusion restriction but typically involve moderate to large areas of the cortex. The dot-like lesions in TGA are distinctly different from the cortical gyriform ribbons of restricted diffusion seen in **status epilepticus** and the posterior-predominant lesions seen in **hypoglycemic seizures**.

Thiamine deficiency with acute **Wernicke encephalopathy** can present as a fulminant disorder with relative preservation of consciousness. Lesions are found in the medial thalami, mammillary bodies, periaqueductal region, and tectal plate. The hippocampi are spared.

Miscellaneous Disorders

Hepatic Encephalopathy

Hepatic encephalopathy (HE) is an important cause of morbidity and mortality in patients with severe liver disease. HE is classified into three main groups: minimal HE (also known as latent or subclinical HE), chronic HE, and acute HE.

Although the precise mechanisms responsible for HE remain elusive, elevated blood and brain ammonia levels have been strongly implicated in the pathogenesis of hepatic encephalopathy.

Ammonia is metabolized primarily in the liver via the urea cycle. When the metabolic capacity of the liver is severely diminished, ammonia detoxification is compromised. Nitrogenous wastes accumulate and easily cross the blood-brain barrier. Ammonia and its principal metabolite, glutamine, interfere with brain mitochondrial metabolism and energy production. Increased osmolarity in the astrocytes causes swelling and loss of autoregulation and results in cerebral edema.

We first discuss chronic HE, then focus on the acute manifestations of liver failure and its most fulminant manifestation, hyperammonemic encephalopathy.

Chronic Hepatic Encephalopathy

Chronic hepatic encephalopathy is a potentially reversible clinical syndrome that occurs in the setting of chronic severe liver dysfunction. Both children and adults are affected. Most patients have a longstanding history of cirrhosis, often accompanied by portal hypertension and portosystemic shunting.

NECT scans typically are normal or show mild volume loss. In the vast majority of cases, MR scans show bilateral symmetric hyperintensity in the globi pallidi and substantia nigra on T1WI, probably secondary to manganese deposition **(32-51)**. T1 hyperintensity has also been reported in the pituitary gland and hypothalamus but is less common. The T1 hyperintensity in the striatopallidal system may decrease or even disappear completely after liver transplantation.

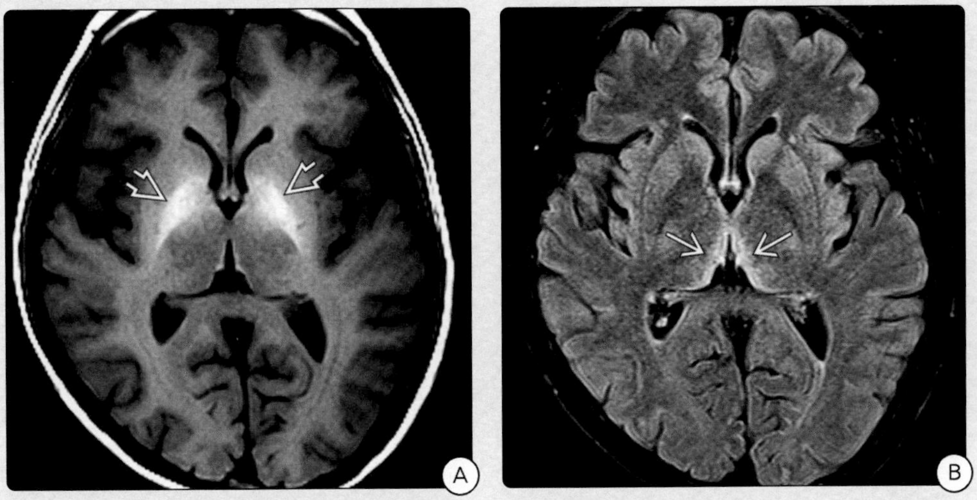

***(32-52A)** A patient with chronic liver failure on total parenteral nutrition developed symptoms of acute encephalopathy with confusion and disorientation. Axial T1WI shows striking, symmetric T1 shortening in the globi pallidi ➡. **(32-52B)** Axial FLAIR in the same case shows symmetric hyperintensity ➡ in the medial thalami around the third ventricle.*

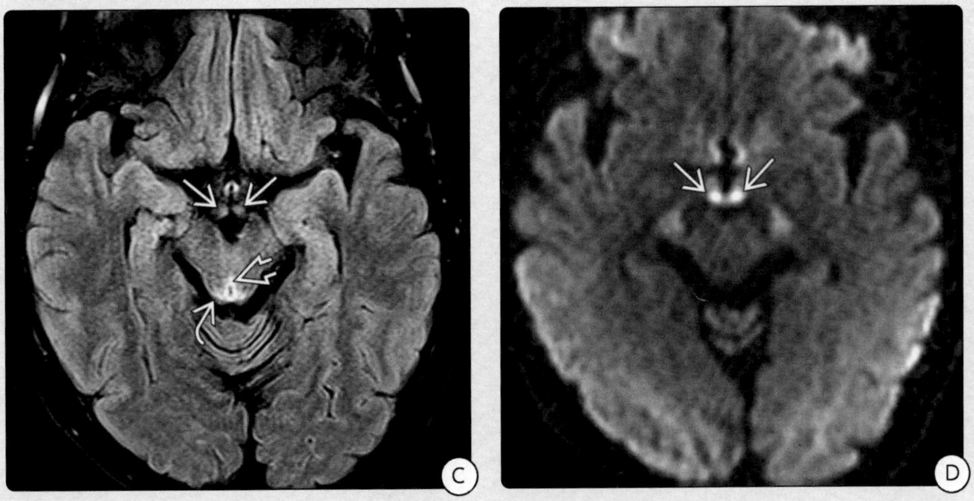

***(32-52C)** Axial FLAIR through the midbrain shows hyperintensity around the periaqueductal gray matter ➡ and tectal plate ➡. Note subtle hyperintensity in both mammillary bodies ➡. **(32-52D)** DWI in the same case shows restricted diffusion in the mammillary bodies ➡. Imaging changes are consistent with acute-on-chronic liver failure manifested as nonalcoholic Wernicke encephalopathy.*

Acute-On-Chronic Liver Failure

Acute-on-chronic liver failure (ACLF) is acute deterioration in liver function in an individual with preexisting chronic liver disease, commonly cirrhosis. Hepatic and extrahepatic organ failure—often renal dysfunction—is common in ACLF and is associated with substantial short-term mortality. Precipitating factors include bacterial and viral infections, alcoholic hepatitis, and surgery. In more than 40% of cases, no precipitating event is identified.

Changes in consciousness as a result of acute hepatic encephalopathy are common and range from mild confusion to coma. Imaging reflects a combination of chronic liver disease (see above) and superimposed changes of acute liver dysfunction, such as hyperammonemia with cortical edema (see below) or Wernicke encephalopathy **(32-52)**.

Acute Hepatic Encephalopathy and Hyperammonemia

Terminology. Acute hepatic encephalopathy (AHE) is caused by hyperammonemia, which can be both hepatic *and* nonhepatic. Hyperammonemia, systemic inflammation (including sepsis, bacterial translocation, and insulin resistance), and oxidative stress are key factors mediating clinical deterioration.

Etiology. Although acute hepatic decompensation is the most common cause of hyperammonemia in adults, drug toxicity is also an important consideration. Valproate, asparaginase, acetaminophen, and chemotherapy have all been implicated in the development of hyperammonemic encephalopathy. Other important nonhepatic causes of hyperammonemia include hematologic disease, parenteral nutrition, bone marrow transplantation, urinary tract infection, and fulminant viral hepatitis.

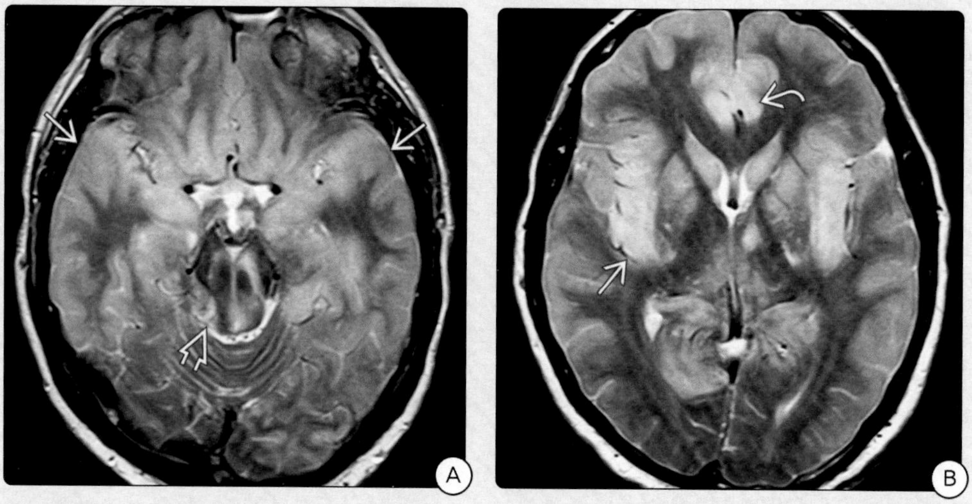

***(32-53A)** T2WI in a 51y woman with acute, fulminant liver failure and severe hyperammonemia shows diffuse cortical swelling ➡ that largely spares the underlying WM. Note central herniation with the midbrain compressed by the herniating temporal lobes ➡. **(32-53B)** More cephalad T2WI shows cortical swelling; hyperintensity is most pronounced in the insular cortex ➡, cingulate gyri ➡, and basal ganglia/thalami with posterior cortical sparing.*

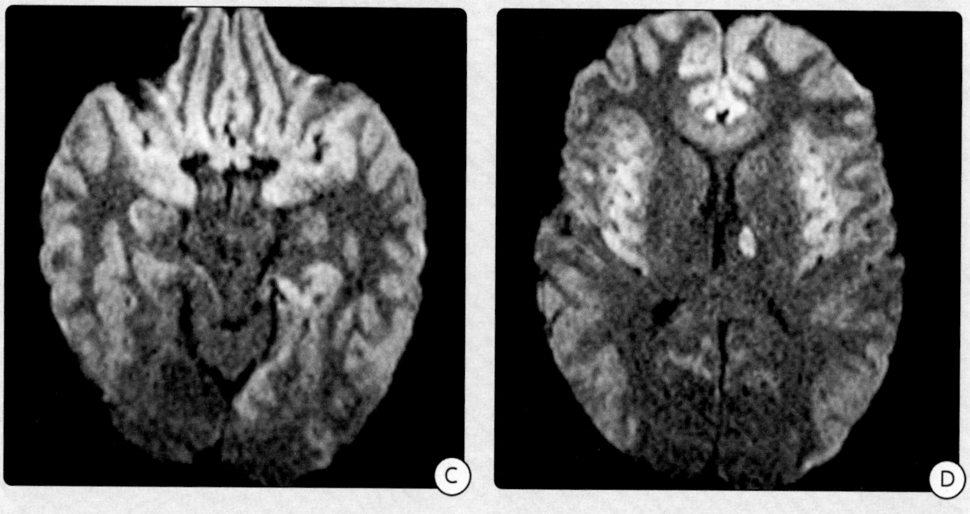

***(32-53C)** DWI shows restricted diffusion in the frontal, temporal, and parietal cortex with relative sparing of the posterior occipital lobes. **(32-53D)** More cephalad DWI shows striking symmetrical restriction in the cortex with sparing of the underlying WM and posterior occipital lobes. This is classic acute hepatic encephalopathy.*

Inherited urea cycle abnormalities or organic acidemias such as citrullinemia and ornithine transcarbamylase deficiency are other potential causes of acute hyperammonemic encephalopathy (see Chapter 31).

Many patients with AHE have multiple systemic and metabolic abnormalities. Hypoxic injury, seizures, and hypoglycemia all exacerbate the acute toxic effects of ammonia on the brain.

Pathology. AHE is characterized grossly by laminar necrosis of the cerebral cortex. Severe cytotoxic edema in astrocytes with anoxic neuronal damage is the typical histologic appearance of AHE.

Clinical Issues. Early clinical manifestations of hyperammonemia can be seen with plasma ammonia levels of 55-60 μmol/L. Irritability, lethargy, vomiting, and somnolence are typical. Progressively decreasing consciousness, seizures, and coma are the principal manifestations of severe AHE and are usually seen when ammonia levels are at least four times the normal range.

AHE is a life-threatening disorder with high morbidity and mortality. There is a significant positive correlation between arterial ammonia and the presence of brain herniation.

Recognition and aggressive treatment of AHE are critical to patient outcome. Therapeutic strategies fall into one of three categories, ammonia-lowering strategies, treatment aimed at modulation of neurotransmitter action, and strategies aimed at modulating inflammation.

Imaging. In the early stages of AHE, NECT scans may show only minimal cerebral edema with mild sulcal effacement. As the brain swelling increases, the gray-white matter interfaces are "blurred," the hemispheres become diffusely hypodense, and complete central brain descending herniation ensues **(32-53A)**.

On T1WI, the gyri appear swollen and hypointense. The CSF spaces are compressed. Bilaterally symmetric T2/FLAIR hyperintensity in the insular cortex, cingulate gyri, and basal ganglia is typical, as is relative sparing of the perirolandic and occipital regions **(32-53B)**. More diffuse cortical injury with involvement of the thalami and brainstem is also common. The hemispheric white matter is typically spared.

AHE restricts strongly on DWI **(32-53C)** **(32-53D)**. MRS may show a glutamate-glutamine peak at short echo times.

Differential Diagnosis. The major differential diagnoses of AHE/hyperammonemia are hypoglycemia, hypoxic-ischemic encephalopathy, status epilepticus, and Wernicke encephalopathy. **Hypoglycemia** is a common comorbidity in patients with chronic HE. Acute hypoglycemia typically affects the parietooccipital gray matter, whereas early AHE may spare the posterior cortex. Serum glucose is low, and ammonia is normal.

Hypoxic-ischemic encephalopathy may be difficult to distinguish from AHE on imaging alone. Nevertheless, symmetric involvement of the insular cortex and cingulate gyri should suggest AHE. **Status epilepticus** is usually unilateral, and, although the thalamus is often involved, the basal ganglia are generally spared. **Wernicke encephalopathy** affects the medial thalami, mammillary bodies, tectal plate, and periaqueductal gray matter. The cerebral cortex and basal ganglia are less commonly involved.

ACUTE vs. CHRONIC HEPATIC ENCEPHALOPATHY

Chronic Hepatic Encephalopathy
- More common
- Etiology
  - Chronic severe liver disease (cirrhosis)
- Imaging
  - T1 hyperintense globi pallidi, substantia nigra
  - Probably due to manganese deposition

Acute Hepatic Encephalopathy
- Rare
- Etiology
  - Usually associated with hyperammonemia
  - Acute liver decompensation (viral hepatitis, etc.)
  - Drug toxicity (acetaminophen, valproate, etc.)
  - Parenteral nutrition, infection
- Imaging findings = those of hyperammonemia
  - Bilateral swollen T2/FLAIR hyperintense gyri
  - Most severe: insular cortex, cingulate gyri
  - ± Basal ganglia, thalami
  - DWI 4+
  - MRS may show glutamate-glutamine peak

Bilirubin Encephalopathy

Terminology

Bilirubin encephalopathy (BRE), also known as kernicterus, is caused by hyperbilirubinemia. A milder form of chronic BRE is termed bilirubin-induced neurologic dysfunction (BIND).

Etiology

In kernicterus, the liver is basically unable to conjugate insoluble bilirubin into water-soluble bilirubin diglucuronide.

It is unclear how bilirubin gets into the brain. Neonatal hyperbilirubinemia results in unconjugated bilirubin passing across an immature or compromised blood-brain barrier.

Hyperbilirubinemia is associated with a number of predisposing conditions, including prematurity, hemolytic disorders (especially blood group incompatibility), breast feeding, significant loss of birth weight, polycythemia, and dehydration. Inherited or acquired defects of bilirubin conjugation, glucose metabolism, GI transit disorders, and drugs that compete with bilirubin for albumin binding are other factors that increase the risk of BRE.

Pathology

The cardinal gross pathologic feature is yellow discoloration of the globi pallidi, mammillary bodies, substantia nigra, subthalamic nuclei, hippocampi, dentate nuclei, and spinal cord **(32-54)**. The major histologic feature of acute BRE is

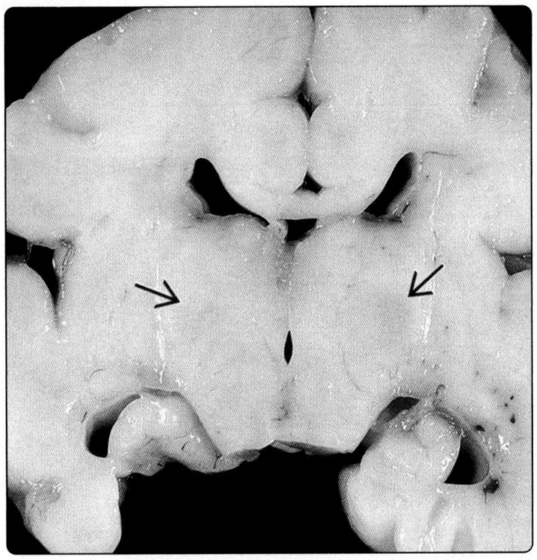

(32-54) Coronal autopsy specimen of bilirubin encephalopathy shows obvious yellow staining of the globi pallidi ➡. (Courtesy R. Hewlett, MD.)

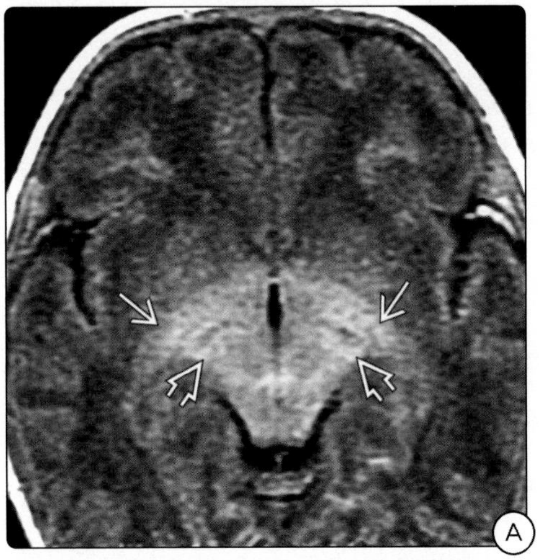

(32-55A) Axial T1WI in a 5d girl with bilirubin encephalopathy shows hyperintensity in the subthalamic nuclei ➡ and substantia nigra ➡.

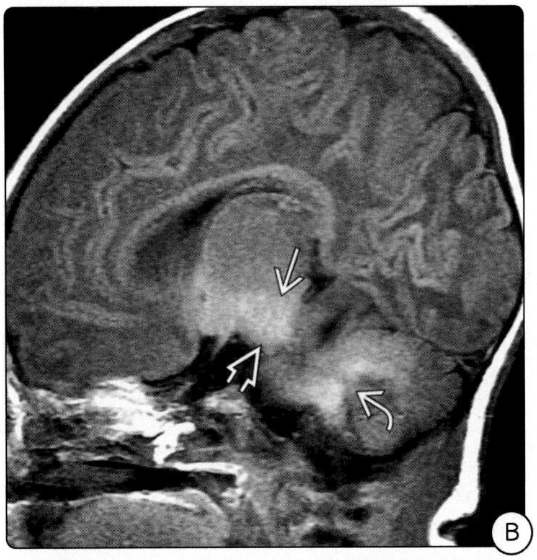

(32-55B) Sagittal T1WI in the same patient shows the hyperintensity in the subthalamic nuclei ➡, midbrain ➡, and dentate nuclei ➡.

neuronal necrosis with little or no inflammatory reaction. Demonstration of bilirubin pigment within the neurons is uncommon.

Clinical Issues

Although neonatal jaundice is common, kernicterus is rare in developed countries. The estimated incidence in the United States is approximately five cases per year.

Not all infants with kernicterus exhibit symptoms. Neonates with overt hyperbilirubinemia present in the first few days of life. Jaundice, stupor, hypotonia, and poor sucking are followed by opisthotonus and hyperreflexia.

Findings in children with classic chronic kernicterus vary in severity. Most show some type of movement disorder, most commonly athetosis. Other abnormalities include auditory disturbances, oculomotor impairments (particularly upward gaze), and teeth with dysplastic enamel. Frank mental retardation is relatively uncommon.

Patients with BIND may show subtle neurodevelopmental disabilities without the classic clinical findings of kernicterus.

Imaging

MR is the procedure of choice, as CT is almost always normal. T1 scans during the *acute* stages of BRE show bilaterally symmetric hyperintensities in the globi pallidi (GP), subthalamic nuclei, substantia nigra, hippocampi, and dentate nuclei **(32-55)**. The thalami and cortex are typically spared. T2 scans are typically normal in the acute stage.

Chronic BRE may show T2/FLAIR hyperintensity in the typical areas. Bilateral hippocampal sclerosis with volume loss and T2 hyperintensity is common.

DWI is normal in both acute and chronic BRE. MRS shows decreased NAA:Cho and NAA:Cr ratios. Preterm infants with BRE may demonstrate increased glutamate-glutamine.

Differential Diagnosis

The major imaging differential diagnoses of BRE are the other disorders that cause GP abnormalities. The GP is an area of especially high metabolic activity with significant glucose and oxygen demands, which is thus vulnerable to a number of metabolic and systemic diseases.

In term neonates with suspected BRE, the major differential diagnosis is acute **hypoxic-ischemic injury** (HII). In term HII, the putamen is the most commonly affected site. T2/FLAIR hyperintensity and restricted diffusion are typical in HII but absent in BRE.

Bilaterally symmetric T1 hyperintense GP are seen in **chronic liver failure, hyperalimentation**, and **nonketotic hyperglycemia**. **Neurofibromatosis type 1** can also cause mild T1 shortening in the GP. Late sequelae of **carbon monoxide poisoning** can cause T1 shortening and T2 hyperintensity in the medial GP.

Uremic Encephalopathy

Uremic encephalopathy (UE) is a well-known complication in patients with renal failure and is characterized by a brain syndrome with various neurologic symptoms. UE can occur with any uremia, including glomerulonephritis, hemolytic-uremic syndrome, and thrombotic thrombocytopenic purpura.

Presentation and imaging findings depend on the site and extent of CNS involvement. Three general patterns have been described.

The most common type of UE is characterized by *cortical involvement*. Patients present with confusion, visual impairment, and headaches. Imaging findings are usually those of typical PRES (see above), and the edema is vasogenic. In especially severe cases, the cortex is diffusely affected **(32-56)**. Imaging abnormalities usually reverse when uremic toxins are removed by dialysis and metabolic acidosis is corrected.

In the *basal ganglia* type of UE, the patients are usually chronic diabetics who present with acute onset of encephalopathy. Movement disorders are common, and bilateral symmetrical T2/FLAIR hyperintensity in the basal ganglia and internal and external or extreme capsules are typical MR findings. Lesions may exhibit restricted diffusion. Hemorrhage is rare, and findings usually regress after dialysis.

Less commonly, nondiabetic, nonhypertensive dialysis-naive patients with uremia present with an atypical, predominately *white matter* pattern of involvement. Bilateral, symmetric T2/FLAIR hyperintensities and restricted diffusion in the centrum semiovale are present **(32-57)**.

Hyperthermic Encephalopathy

Acute heat-related illness is a spectrum of disorders that ranges from minor heat cramps and heat exhaustion to life-threatening heat stroke. Heat stroke is defined clinically as a core body temperature exceeding 40°C. It can cause delirium, seizures, and coma. Morbidity and mortality in patients suffering from heat stroke range between 10 and 50%.

Heat stroke can be exertional (exercise-induced) and nonexertional (classic) heat stroke. Classic heat stroke risk factors include high ambient temperature and humidity, dehydration, alcohol abuse, and some medications (antihypertensive or psychiatric). Both ends of the age spectrum—infants and the very old—are especially susceptible.

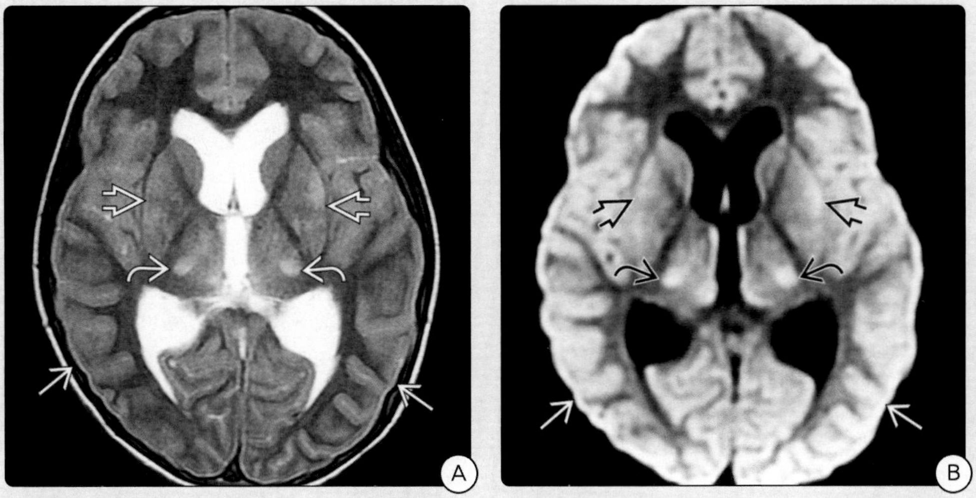

***(32-56A)** T2WI in an encephalopathic 8y girl with HUS and acute renal failure shows diffuse swelling with hyperintensity of the basal ganglia, thalami, and cortex. **(32-56B)** DWI shows marked, symmetric restricted diffusion throughout the entire cortex, basal ganglia, and thalami. Uremic encephalopathy with combined cortical and basal ganglia involvement is shown.*

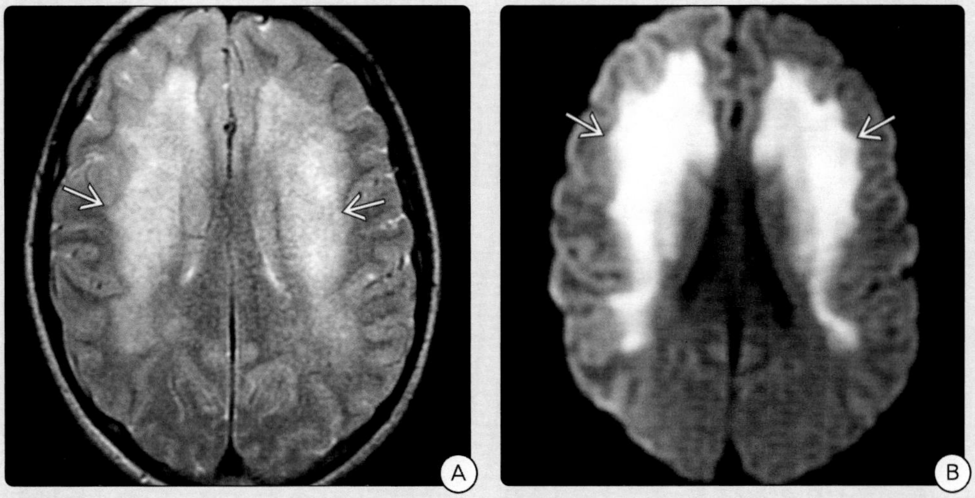

***(32-57A)** T2WI in 13y girl with uremia and metabolic acidosis shows symmetric, confluent hyperintensity in the corona radiata. **(32-57B)** DWI and ADC (not shown) demonstrate restricted diffusion in the WM of both hemispheres. This is acute uremic encephalopathy.*

Because the Purkinje cells in the cerebellum are especially susceptible to thermic injury, typical NECT findings include diffuse cerebellar edema **(32-58A)**. The cerebral cortex and subcortical white matter can also appear diffusely hypodense **(32-58B)**.

MR may demonstrate T2/FLAIR hyperintensity in the cerebellum, basal ganglia/thalami, hippocampus, and cerebral cortex **(32-58)**. Restricted diffusion in the affected areas is common.

Osmotic Encephalopathy

Acute electrolyte and osmolality disorders can cause alarming alterations in mental status. Extreme hyperosmolality is rare; hypoosmolar states are much more common. The most common hypoosmolar state is hyponatremia, and the most common osmotic encephalopathy is **osmotic demyelination syndrome** (ODS).

Terminology

ODS was formerly called **central pontine myelinolysis** (when it affected only the pons) or, if it involved both the pons and **extrapontine myelinolysis**, osmotic myelinolysis. ODS is now the preferred term.

Etiology

ODS occurs with osmotic stress, classically occurring when wide fluxes in serum sodium levels are induced by too-rapid correction of hyponatremia. ODS also occurs in many other disorders, such as AIDS, organ transplantation (particularly liver), hemodialysis, correction of hypoglycemia or hypernatremia, and hematologic malignancies (i.e., leukemia and lymphoma).

Serum hypotonicity triggers cells to lose inorganic and organic osmolytes to prevent catastrophic swelling. If the rise of serum tonicity surpasses the point of intracellular organic

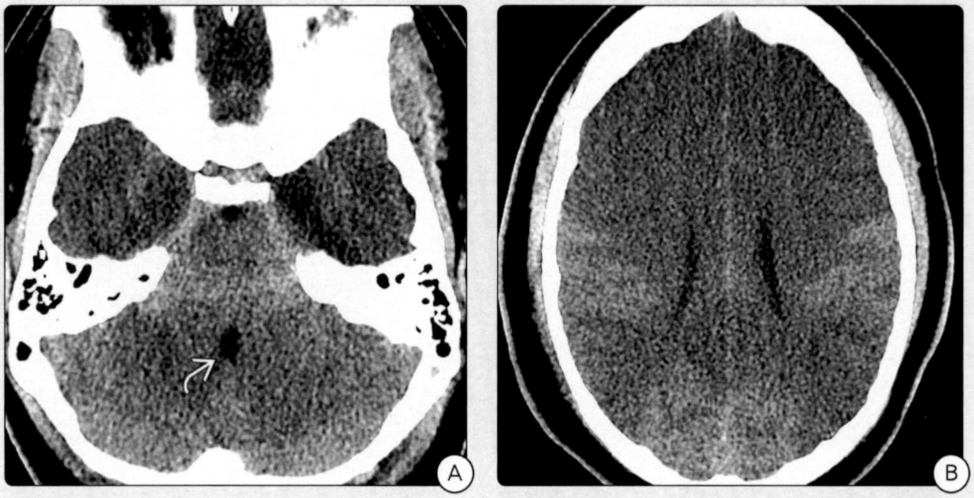

***(32-58A)** A teenage athlete became confused and disoriented during high-intensity exercise in a hot, humid climate then lapsed into coma. NECT 6 days after admission shows diffusely swollen cerebellum, temporal lobes with compressed 4th ventricle ➲. **(32-58B)** More cephalad NECT shows diffuse hemisphere swelling and obliterated GM-WM interfaces.*

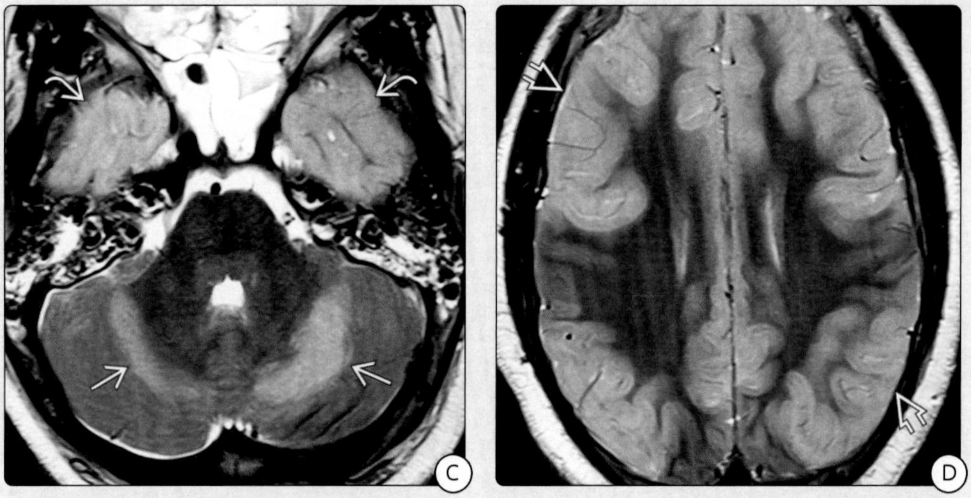

***(32-58C)** T2WI shows diffuse swelling and hyperintensity of both temporal lobes ➲. The cerebellar white matter is also hyperintense ➲. **(32-58D)** More cephalad T2WI shows diffuse cortical hyperintensity ➲. This is heat stroke. (Courtesy P. Hudgins, MD.)*

osmole generation, the cells shrink, injuring oligodendroglial cells and separating myelin from axons. Oligodendrocytes, which form the myelin sheaths, are particularly vulnerable to osmotic changes. Myelin sheaths can rupture and split when osmotic stress on oligodendrocytes is severe.

Pathology

Location. ODS is traditionally considered primarily a pontine lesion **(32-59) (32-62)**. However, multifocal involvement is common and typical. Only 50% of ODS cases have isolated pontine lesions. In 30% of cases, myelinolytic foci occur both outside and inside the pons. The basal ganglia and hemispheric WM are common sites. WM demyelination is exclusively extrapontine in 20-25% of cases.

Other parts of the CNS that can be involved in ODS include the cerebellum (especially the middle cerebellar peduncles), basal ganglia, thalami, lateral geniculate body, and hemispheric WM. Some ODS cases involve the cortex.

Gross Pathology. Grossly, the central pons is abnormally soft and exhibits a rhomboid or trident-shaped area of grayish tan discoloration. The peripheral pons is spared. Laminar cortical necrosis can occur in ODS, either primarily or in association with hypoxia or anoxia. In such cases, the affected cortex appears soft and pale.

Microscopic Features. Microscopically, ODS is characterized by myelin loss with relative sparing of axons and neurons. Active demyelination without evidence of significant inflammation is typical. The presence of reactive astrocytes and abundant foamy, lipid-laden macrophages is characteristic.

Clinical Issues

Epidemiology and Demographics. ODS is a rare disorder, and its exact prevalence is unknown. It can occur at any age but is most common in middle-aged patients (peak = 30-60 years).

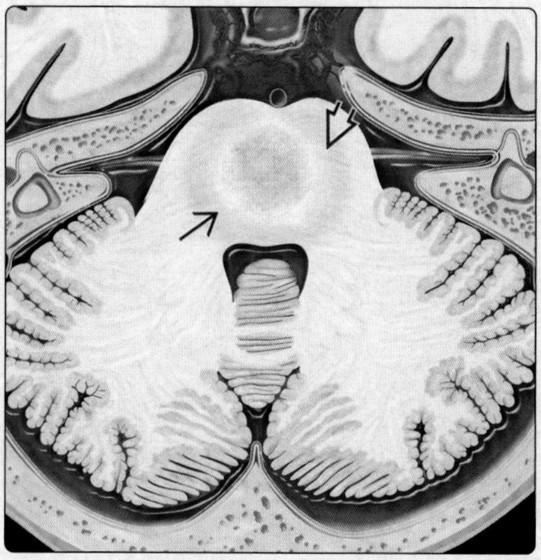

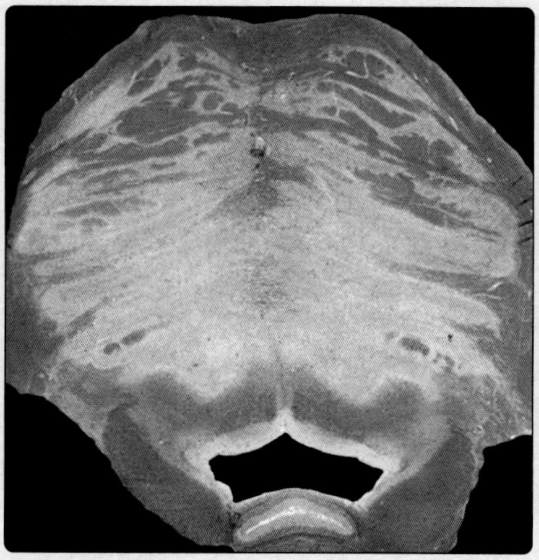

***(32-59)** Graphic shows acute osmotic central pontine demyelination. Note sparing of peripheral WM, traversing corticospinal tracts.* ***(32-60)** Low-power photomicrograph shows acute CPM with Luxol fast blue (myelin) stain. Note that demyelination (pink) largely spares the periphery of the pons and crossing transverse pontine WM tracts (blue). (From Agamanolis DP, Neuropathology, 2e, 2012.)*

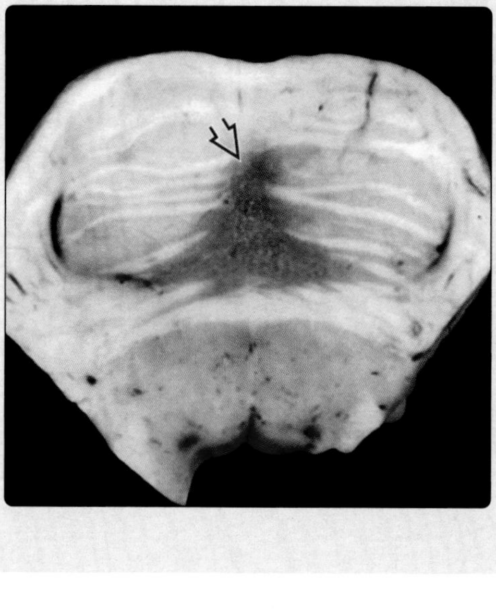

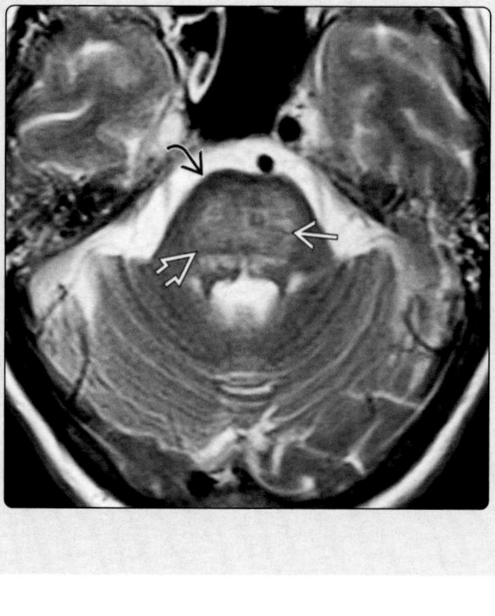

***(32-61)** Gross pathology of remote CPM shows triangular shape of brown discolored demyelination in the central pons. (From Agamanolis DP, op cit.)* ***(32-62)** T2WI shows classic acute osmotic demyelination in CPM. The peripheral pons is spared as are the corticospinal tracts and transverse pontine fibers.*

There is a moderate male predominance. Pediatric patients with ODS typically have diabetes or anorexia.

The most common causes of ODS are rapid correction of hyponatremia, alcoholism, liver transplantation, and malnutrition.

Comorbid conditions that predispose patients to developing ODS include renal, adrenal, pituitary, and paraneoplastic disease. Prolonged vomiting (e.g., hyperemesis gravidarum), severe burns, transplants, and prolonged diuretic use may all contribute to the development of ODS.

In hyponatremic patients, the initial step is to differentiate hypotonic from nonhypotonic hyponatremia. The former is further differentiated on the basis of urine osmolality, urine sodium level, and volume status. Recently identified parameters including fractional uric acid excretion and plasma copeptin concentration improve diagnostic accuracy.

Presentation. The most common presenting symptoms of ODS are altered mental status and seizures. A biphasic clinical course is common. As normonatremia is restored, mental status improves but can then rapidly deteriorate. Other findings include pseudobulbar palsy, dysarthria, and dysphagia. Movement disorders are common when myelinolysis involves the basal ganglia.

Natural History. The outcome of ODS varies significantly, ranging from complete recovery to coma and death. Some patients survive with minimal or no residual deficits. In severe cases, the patient may become quadriparetic and "locked in."

Treatment Options. Initial serum sodium in ODS is usually under 115-120 mmol/L and serum osmolality less than 275 mOsm/kg. Although there is no consensus regarding the optimal correction rates for hyponatremia, correction of more than 12 mmol/L/day seems to increase the risk of ODS.

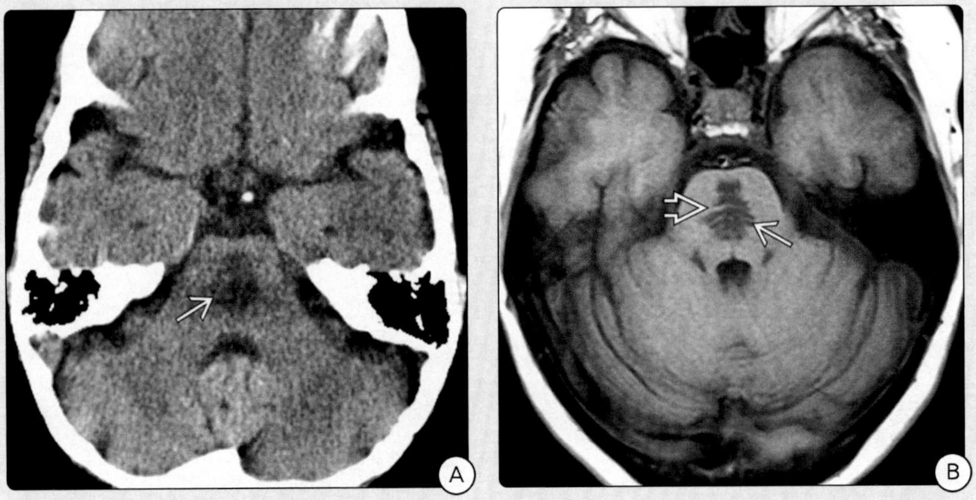

***(32-63A)** NECT scan in a 37y woman with osmotic demyelination syndrome shows a triangular central pontine hypodensity ➡. **(32-63B)** T1WI in the same patient shows that the lesion is hypointense ➡. The transverse pontine fibers are spared and are seen here as lines of preserved brain ➡ passing from one side to the other.*

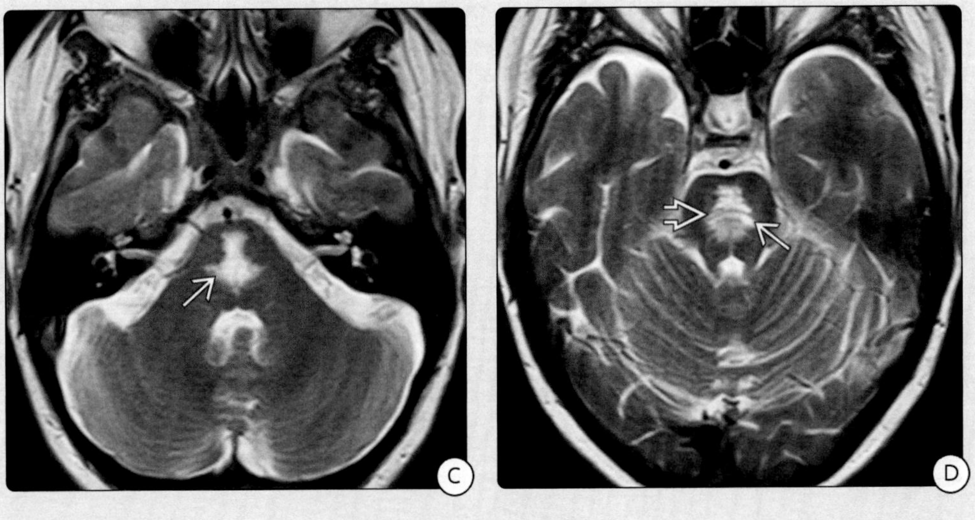

***(32-63C)** T2WI shows the symmetric "trident" or "bat wing" shape of pontine myelinolysis ➡. The peripheral pons is spared. **(32-63D)** More cephalad T2WI through the upper pons shows the lesion ➡ with "stripes" of preserved myelinated transverse pontine tracts ➡ seen crossing the lesion.*

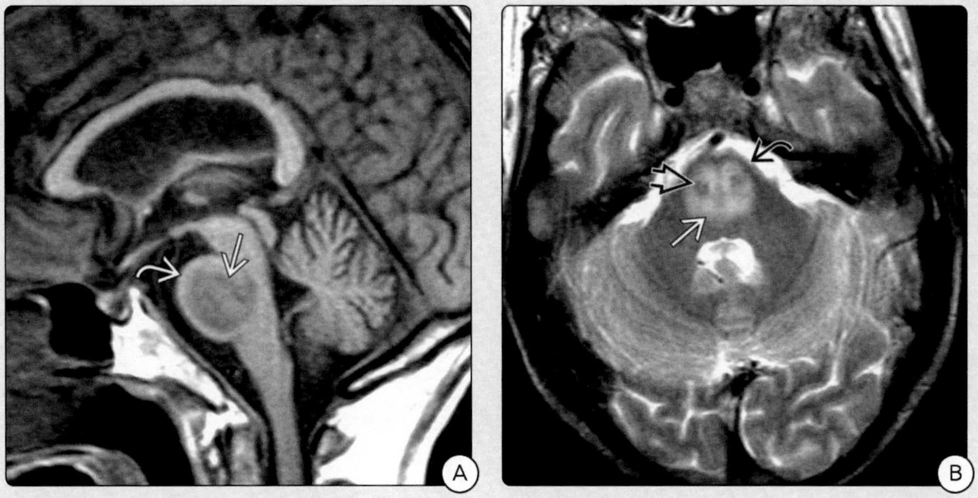

***(32-64A)** Sagittal T1WI shows a 44y alcoholic man with vomiting, seizures, and acutely altered mental status. The central pons is slightly swollen and hypointense →, whereas the peripheral pons → is spared. **(32-64B)** T2WI in the same patient shows symmetric central hyperintensity → with sparing of the peripheral pons → and corticospinal tracts →.*

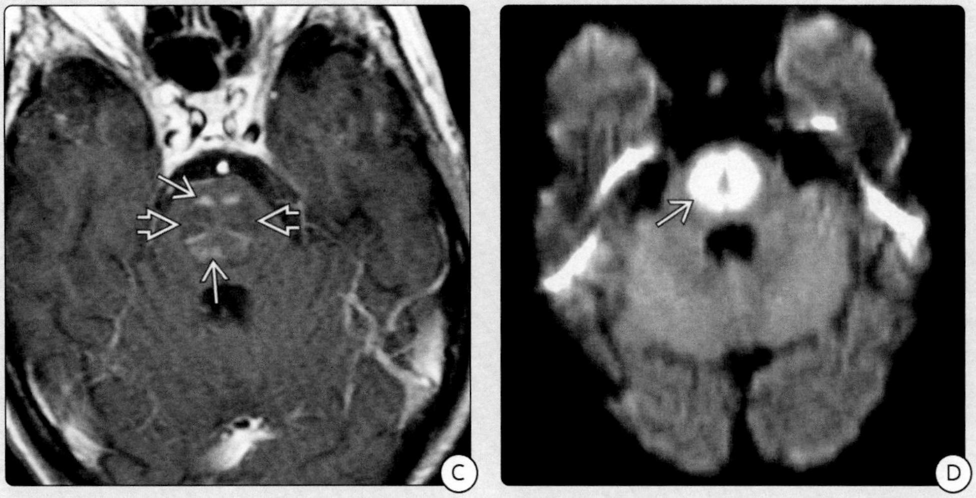

***(32-64C)** Axial T1 C+ scan in the same patient shows patchy but symmetric enhancement in the affected WM → with sparing of the corticospinal tracts →. **(32-64D)** DWI in the same patient shows acutely restricted diffusion →. ODS with acute demyelination can both enhance and restrict.*

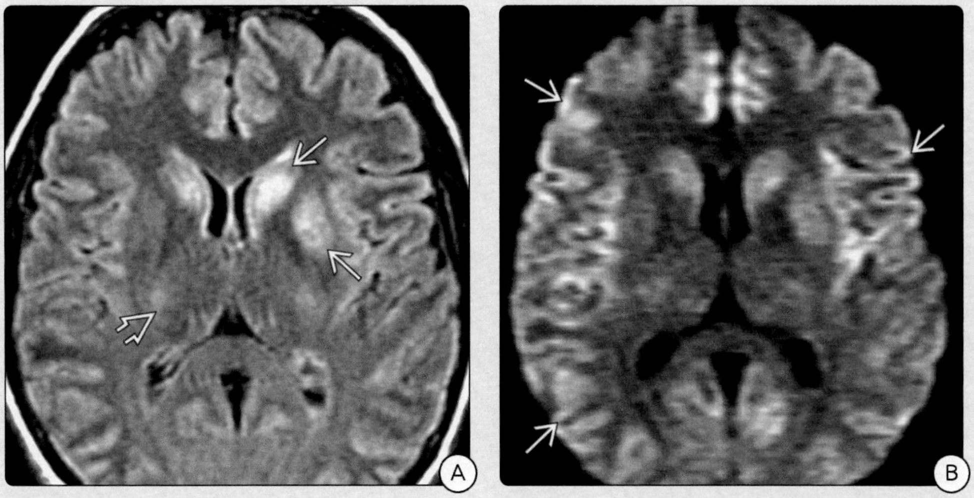

***(32-65A)** A variant case of ODS is illustrated by this axial FLAIR scan in a 56y man with confusion after rapid correction of hyponatremia. Note hyperintensity in the basal ganglia → and both thalami →. **(32-65B)** DWI shows that the cortex is also diffusely but somewhat asymmetrically affected →. Cortical laminar necrosis can sometimes be seen in ODS.*

***(32-66A)** Variant ODS with both pontine and extrapontine myelinolysis is illustrated by this case of a 46y alcoholic man who became severely hyponatremic following surgery, then was rapidly corrected. Sagittal T1WI shows a band of hypointensity in the central pons ➡ with peripheral sparing. **(32-66B)** T2WI shows central pontine hyperintensity ➡ with symmetric lesions in both major cerebellar peduncles ⇨.*

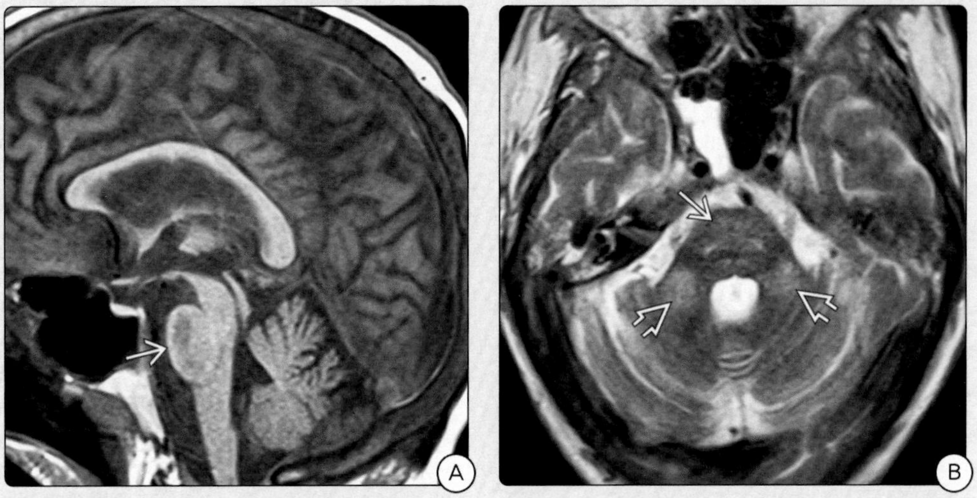

***(32-66C)** DTI with b = 3,000 shows a cruciform area of restricted diffusion in the central pons ➡ together with large ovoid areas of restricted diffusion in both major cerebellar peduncles ⇨. **(32-66D)** More cephalad DTI shows restricted diffusion in both lateral geniculate bodies ➡ and the subthalamic nuclei ⇨.*

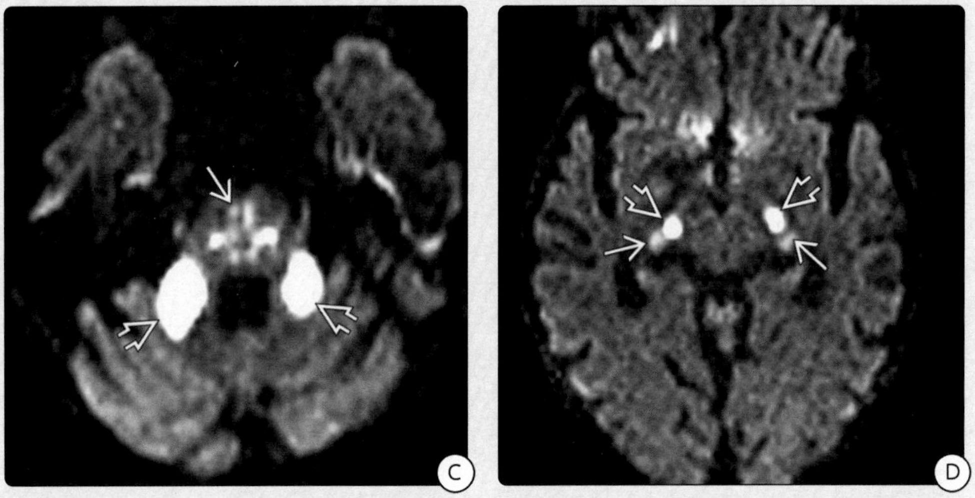

***(32-66E)** DTI through the lateral ventricles shows symmetric restriction in the posterior limbs of both internal capsules ➡ and thalami ⇨. **(32-66F)** Color DTI map shows preserved peripheral pontine fibers in green ➡ with disruption of the central pontine WM ⇨. The transverse pontine tracts (in red) are preserved ↪.*

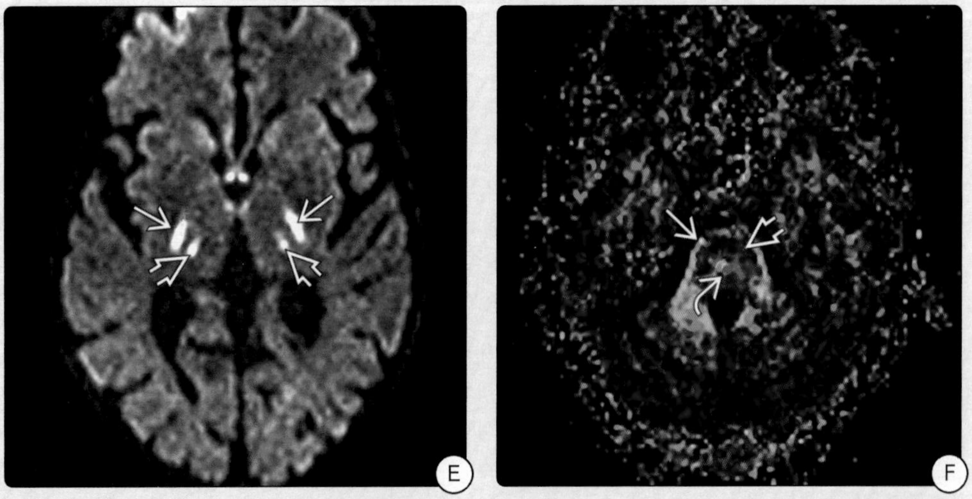

ODS may also occur (1) in normonatremic patients and (2) independent of changes in serum sodium!

Imaging

General Features. Imaging findings in ODS typically lag 1 or 2 weeks behind clinical symptoms.

CT Findings. NECT scans can be normal or show hypodensity in the affected areas, particularly the central pons **(32-63A)**.

MR Findings. Standard MR sequences may be normal in the first several days. Eventually, ODS becomes hypointense on T1WI and hyperintense on T2/FLAIR. The lesions are typically well demarcated and symmetric. Pontine ODS is often round or sometimes "trident"-shaped **(32-61)** **(32-63C)**. The peripheral pons, corticospinal tracts, and transverse pontine fibers are spared **(32-62)**. Involvement of the basal ganglia and hemispheric WM is seen in at least half of all cases ("extrapontine myelinolysis").

T2* (GRE, SWI) shows no evidence of hemorrhage.

In approximately 20% of acute ODS cases, enhancement in the midline and rim of the affected region may form a distinct "trident-shaped" lesion. Late acute or subacute ODS lesions may demonstrate moderate confluent enhancement on T1 C+ **(32-64)**. Enhancement typically resolves within a few weeks after onset.

DWI is the most sensitive sequence for acute ODS and can demonstrate restricted diffusion when other sequences are normal **(32-64D)** **(32-65)**. DTI shows disruption of central pontine WM with sparing of peripheral, transverse tracts **(32-66)**.

Differential Diagnosis

The major differential diagnosis of "central" ODS is pontine ischemia-infarction. **Basilar perforating artery infarcts** involve the surface of the pons and are usually asymmetric.

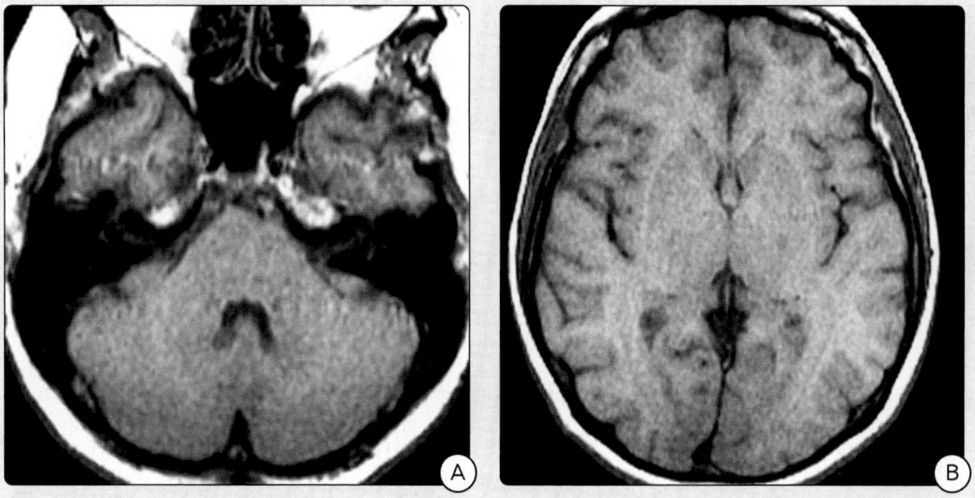

***(32-67A)** T1WI of the posterior fossa in a patient with newly diagnosed multiple sclerosis shows no abnormalities. **(32-67B)** More cephalad scan through the basal ganglia shows no abnormalities. Signal intensity in the globi pallidi is normal.*

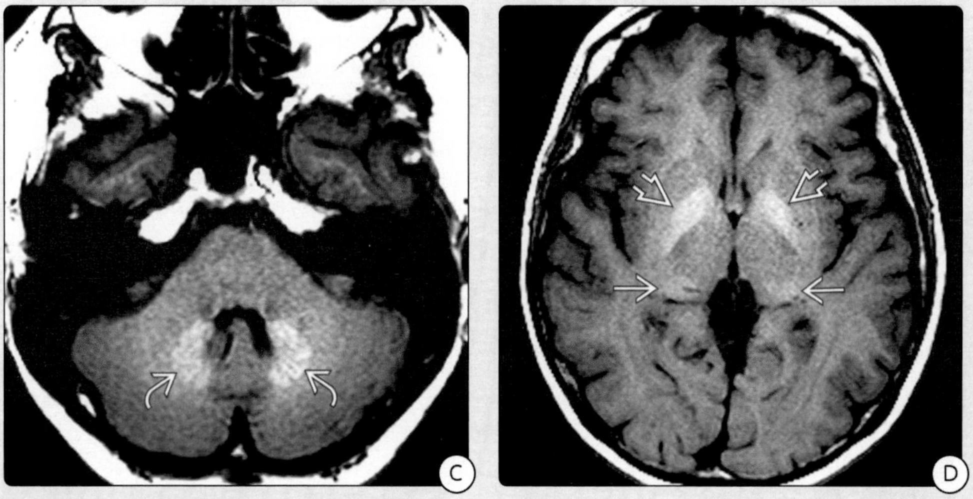

***(32-67C)** Axial T1WI in the same case 12 years later after multiple scans with GBCA were administered to assess disease course and treatment response shows distinct hyperintensity in both dentate nuclei ➡. **(32-67D)** More cephalad T1WI shows interval development of T1 shortening in both globi pallidi ➡. Note less striking but definite hyperintensity in the pulvinars of both thalami ➡. This is presumed gadolinium deposition.*

Demyelinating disease can involve the pons but is rarely symmetric. Sagittal FLAIR scans usually demonstrate lesions elsewhere, especially along the callososeptal interface.

Neoplasm rarely mimics ODS. Pontine gliomas can expand the pons and appear hyperintense on T2/FLAIR scans. They are neoplasms of children and young adults. Metastatic disease in the posterior fossa is typically in the cerebellum, not the pons.

The major differential diagnosis of extrapontine ODS with basal ganglia and/or cortical involvement is metabolic disease. **Hypertensive encephalopathy** (PRES) can involve the pons but does not spare the peripheral WM tracts. The basal ganglia are affected in **Wilson disease** and **mitochondrial disorders**, but the pons is less commonly involved.

OSMOTIC DEMYELINATION SYNDROMES

Terminology, Etiology
- ODS (formerly pontine, extrapontine myelinolysis)
- Serum hypotonicity → cells lose osmoles, shrink
- Oligodendrocytes especially vulnerable to osmotic stress
- Note: can occur without serum sodium disturbances!

Location
- 50% pons (spares periphery, transverse pontine tracts)
- 30% pons + extrapontine (BG, thalami, WM)
- 20-25% exclusively extrapontine
- ± Cortical laminar necrosis

Imaging
- Hypointense on T1, hyperintense on T2
    - "Trident" sign on T2WI, T1 C+ in acute ODS
- May restrict on DWI

Heavy Metal Deposition Disorders

Various metals are essential nutrients in humans; concentration abnormalities may cause metal deposition in the brain. Many metals affect the signal intensity of brain structures on MR. A few of these are discussed in this closing section. Gadolinium deposition from repeated MR contrast administration causes high signal intensity in the dentate nucleus, globus pallidus, and pulvinar.

Brain iron deposition occurs as a part of normal aging. However, excessive iron is neurotoxic. Ferritin, a protein that contains iron nanoparticles, induces reactive oxygen species formation and inhibits glutamate uptake from synaptic junctions, potentially leading to neurodegeneration.

Manganese Deposition

Manganese overload causes high signal intensity in the globi pallidi on T1WI and is commonly identified in patients with chronic liver disease **(32-51)** **(32-52)**.

Gadolinium Deposition

Gadolinium-based contrast agents (GBCAs) have been widely used in MR for almost 30 years. Initially, the use of GBCAs was felt to carry minimal risk. In 2006, nephrogenic systemic fibrosis (NSF) was linked to GBCA administration in patients with advanced renal disease, and the FDA has subsequently mandated a "black box" warning on all patients with eGFRs less than 30 mL/min/1.72-m^2.

GBCA-related toxicities arise from the deposition of gadolinium ions in various tissues, which also varies among the different GBCAs. All GBCAs consist of a gadolinium ion (GD^3+) complexed with a chelating ligand. In general, macrocyclic and ionic agents have higher stability than linear and nonionic agents, respectively. Immediate adverse reactions to GBCAs are uncommon, and serious ones are exceedingly rare.

A number of studies have reported a significant correlation between the degree of hyperintensity in the dentate nucleus and globus pallidus on T1WIs and the number of previous GBCA administrations. Increased signal intensity of these structures on unenhanced T1WIs can be a possible consequence of multiple applications of GBCAs even in the absence of renal impairment **(32-67)**.

Although some authors have used the term *gadolinium deposition disease* and linked it to various clinical symptoms, to date there are no well-controlled, independently validated studies that support such an association.

Iron Overload Disorders

Iron overload disorders encompass a broad spectrum of both inherited and acquired etiologies. Elevated brain iron in myelinated structures has been demonstrated in hemochromatosis and inherited neurodegeneration with brain iron accumulation. Inherited disorders of iron metabolism are discussed in Chapter 31. Acquired iron overload disorders are briefly addressed here.

Acquired brain iron overload is called **siderosis**. When iron deposition occurs along cranial nerves or the pial surface of the brain, it is termed **superficial siderosis. Hemochromatosis** is the pathologic accumulation of intracellular iron in parenchymal tissues.

In the brain, superficial siderosis is more common than iron accumulation within the cortex itself (i.e., hemochromatosis). Superficial siderosis is usually caused by trauma, tumor, prior surgery, or repeated subarachnoid hemorrhage from an arteriovenous malformation or aneurysm. Amyloid angiopathy is a common cause of siderosis in elderly patients.

The **pituitary gland**, especially the anterior lobe, is very sensitive to early toxic effects from iron overload. Progressive iron deposition causes pituitary hypointensity on T2WI.

Iron deposition in the **choroid plexus** occurs in the setting of hematologic dyscrasias such as sickle cell disease. NECT scans are typically normal, but T2* (GRE, SWI) MR shows symmetric "blooming" hypointensity in the choroid plexus. Superficial siderosis along the **brain surfaces** and **cranial nerves** is usually linked with repeated subarachnoid hemorrhages. T2* scans show "blooming" along the pial surfaces.

Selected References

Hypertensive Encephalopathies

Acute Hypertensive Encephalopathy, Posterior Reversible Encephalopathy Syndrome

Fischer M et al: Posterior reversible encephalopathy syndrome. J Neurol. ePub, 2017

Hiremath SB et al: Susceptibility-weighted angiography and diffusion-weighted imaging in posterior reversible encephalopathy syndrome - is there an association between hemorrhage, cytotoxic edema, blood pressure and imaging severity? J Neuroradiol. ePub, 2017

Ollivier M et al: Neuroimaging features in posterior reversible encephalopathy syndrome: A pictorial review. J Neurol Sci. 373:188-200, 2017

Schweitzer AD et al: Imaging characteristics associated with clinical outcomes in posterior reversible encephalopathy syndrome. Neuroradiology. 59(4):379-386, 2017

Shankar J et al: Posterior reversible encephalopathy syndrome: a review. Can Assoc Radiol J. 68(2):147-153, 2017

Acute Hypertensive Encephalopathy and Malignant Hypertension

Thind G et al: Malignant hypertension as a rare cause of thrombotic microangiopathy. BMJ Case Rep. 2017, 2017

Timmermans SA et al: Patients with hypertension-associated thrombotic microangiopathy may present with complement abnormalities. Kidney Int. 91(6):1420-1425, 2017

Mitaka H et al: Malignant hypertension with thrombotic microangiopathy. Intern Med. 55(16):2277-80, 2016

Shi L: ED 08-4 Diagnosis and treatment of hypertensive emergency in children. J Hypertens. 34 Suppl 1 - ISH 2016 Abstract Book:e373-e374, 2016

Glucose Disorders

Pediatric/Adult Hypoglycemic Encephalopathy

Shah P et al: Hyperinsulinaemic hypoglycaemia in children and adults. Lancet Diabetes Endocrinol. ePub, 2016

Neonatal/Infantile Hypoglycemia

De Leon DD et al: Congenital hypoglycemia disorders: new aspects of etiology, diagnosis, treatment and outcomes: highlights of the Proceedings of the Congenital Hypoglycemia Disorders Symposium, Philadelphia April 2016. Pediatr Diabetes. 18(1):3-9, 2017

Ferriero DM: The vulnerable newborn brain: imaging patterns of acquired perinatal injury. Neonatology. 109(4):345-51, 2016

Hyperglycemia-Associated Disorders

Siwakoti K et al: Cerebral edema among adults with diabetic ketoacidosis and hyperglycemic hyperosmolar syndrome: incidence, characteristics, and outcomes. J Diabetes. 9(2):208-209, 2017

Soto-Rivera CL et al: Suspected cerebral edema in diabetic ketoacidosis: is there still a role for head CT in treatment decisions? Pediatr Crit Care Med. 18(3):207-212, 2017

Yu F et al: T2*-based MR imaging of hyperglycemia-induced hemichorea-hemiballism. J Neuroradiol. 44(1):24-30, 2017

Barrot A et al: Neuroimaging findings in acute pediatric diabetic ketoacidosis. Neuroradiol J. 29(5):317-22, 2016

Malone JI: Diabetic central neuropathy: CNS damage related to hyperglycemia. Diabetes. 65(2):355-7, 2016

Umpierrez G et al: Diabetic emergencies - ketoacidosis, hyperglycaemic hyperosmolar state and hypoglycaemia. Nat Rev Endocrinol. 12(4):222-32, 2016

Thyroid Disorders

Keller-Petrot I et al: Congenital hypothyroidism: role of nuclear medicine. Semin Nucl Med. 47(2):135-142, 2017

Kocova M et al: Diagnostic approach in children with unusual symptoms of acquired hypothyroidism. When to look for pituitary hyperplasia? J Pediatr Endocrinol Metab. 29(3):297-303, 2016

Parathyroid and Related Disorders

Hyperparathyroidism

Sharata A et al: Management of primary hyperparathyroidism: can we do better? Am Surg. 83(1):64-70, 2017

Hypoparathyroid Disorders

Abate EG et al: Review of hypoparathyroidism. Front Endocrinol (Lausanne). 7:172, 2017

Tafaj O et al: Pseudohypoparathyroidism: one gene, several syndromes. J Endocrinol Invest. 40(4):347-356, 2017

Simpson C et al: Pseudopseudohypoparathyroidism. Lancet. 385(9973):1123, 2015

Primary Familial Brain Calcification (Fahr Disease)

Batla A et al: Deconstructing Fahr's disease/syndrome of brain calcification in the era of new genes. Parkinsonism Relat Disord. 37:1-10, 2017

Hascalovici JR et al: Diffuse symmetric cerebral calcifications: an emerging clinical pivot. Can J Neurol Sci. 44(2):190-191, 2017

Seizures and Related Disorders

Normal Anatomy of the Temporal Lobe

Dekeyzer S et al: "Unforgettable" - a pictorial essay on anatomy and pathology of the hippocampus. Insights Imaging. 8(2):199-212, 2017

Mesial Temporal (Hippocampal) Sclerosis

Asadi-Pooya AA et al: Prevalence and incidence of drug-resistant mesial temporal lobe epilepsy in the United States. World Neurosurg. 99:662-666, 2017

Stefanits H et al: Seven-Tesla MRI of hippocampal sclerosis: an in vivo feasibility study with histological correlations. Invest Radiol. ePub, 2017

Shih YC et al: Hippocampal atrophy is associated with altered hippocampus-posterior cingulate cortex connectivity in mesial temporal lobe epilepsy with hippocampal sclerosis. AJNR Am J Neuroradiol. 38(3):626-632, 2017

AlQassmi A et al: Benign mesial temporal lobe epilepsy: a clinical cohort and literature review. Epilepsy Behav. 65:60-64, 2016

Status Epilepticus

Cabrera Kang CM et al: Survey of the diagnostic and therapeutic approach to new-onset refractory status epilepticus. Seizure. 46:24-30, 2017

Shimogawa T et al: The initial use of arterial spin labeling perfusion and diffusion-weighted magnetic resonance images in the diagnosis of nonconvulsive partial status epileptics. Epilepsy Res. 129:162-173, 2017

Cytotoxic Lesions of the Corpus Callosum

Fong CY et al: Mild encephalitis/encephalopathy with reversible splenial lesion (MERS) due to dengue virus. J Clin Neurosci. 36:73-75, 2017

Starkey J et al: Cytotoxic lesions of the corpus callosum that show restricted diffusion: mechanisms, causes, and manifestations. Radiographics. 37(2):562-576, 2017

Bajaj BK et al: "Boomerang sign": an ominous-looking finding in reversible maladies. Neurol India. 64(2):330-1, 2016

Ka A et al: Mild encephalopathy with reversible splenial lesion: an important differential of encephalitis. Eur J Paediatr Neurol. 19(3):377-82, 2015

Malhotra HS et al: Boomerang sign: clinical significance of transient lesion in splenium of corpus callosum. Ann Indian Acad Neurol. 15(2):151-7, 2012

Transient Global Amnesia

Förster A et al: Isolated punctuate hippocampal infarction and transient global amnesia are indistinguishable by means of MRI. Int J Stroke. 12(3):292-296, 2017

Miscellaneous Disorders

Hepatic Encephalopathy

Hanquinet S et al: Globus pallidus MR signal abnormalities in children with chronic liver disease and/or porto-systemic shunting. Eur Radiol. ePub, 2017

Ishii N et al: Parkinsonism and high-intensity midbrain lesions on T2-weighted imaging in hepatic encephalopathy: a case report. Neurol Sci. ePub, 2017

Bernal W et al: Acute-on-chronic liver failure. Lancet. 386(10003):1576-87, 2015

Butterworth RF: Pathogenesis of hepatic encephalopathy and brain edema in acute liver failure. J Clin Exp Hepatol. 5(Suppl 1):S96-S103, 2015

Bilirubin Encephalopathy

Chang PW et al: Update on predicting severe hyperbilirubinemia and bilirubin neurotoxicity risks in neonates. Curr Pediatr Rev. ePub, 2017

Ribeiro BN et al: Chronic kernicterus: magnetic resonance imaging findings. Radiol Bras. 49(6):407-408, 2016

Uremic Encephalopathy

Kim DM et al: Uremic encephalopathy: MR imaging findings and clinical correlation. AJNR Am J Neuroradiol. 37(9):1604-9, 2016

Camara-Lemarroy CR et al: Bilateral cytotoxic edema of the centrum semiovale in uremic encephalopathy. J Neurol Sci. 345(1-2):260-1, 2014

Hyperthermic Encephalopathy

Kalaiselvan MS et al: A retrospective study of clinical profile and outcomes of critically ill patients with heat-related illness. Indian J Anaesth. 59(11):715-20, 2015

Li J et al: Heat stroke: typical MRI and (1)H-MRS features. Clin Imaging. 39(3):504-5, 2015

Osmotic Encephalopathy

Beh SC: Temporal evolution of the trident and piglet signs of osmotic demyelination syndrome. J Neurol Sci. 373:268-273, 2017

Diringer M: Neurologic manifestations of major electrolyte abnormalities. Handb Clin Neurol. 141:705-713, 2017

Heavy Metal Deposition Disorders

Conte G et al: Signal intensity change on unenhanced T1-weighted images in dentate nucleus and globus pallidus after multiple administrations of gadoxetate disodium: an intraindividual comparative study. Eur Radiol. ePub, 2017

Fraum TJ et al: Gadolinium-based contrast agents: a comprehensive risk assessment. J Magn Reson Imaging. ePub, 2017

Hoggard N et al: T1 hyperintensity on brain imaging subsequent to gadolinium-based contrast agent administration: what do we know about intracranial gadolinium deposition? Br J Radiol. 90(1069):20160590, 2017

Dementias and Brain Degenerations

Worldwide public health efforts to improve living conditions, prevent disease, and enhance medical treatment have resulted in a 30-year increase in life expectancy over the past century. Individuals over 65 years of age now represent 13% of the population, and people aged 85 years and older are the fastest growing segment of the population.

One in three adults over 85 years suffers from Alzheimer disease or other forms of dementia. Despite the global increase in both the incidence and prevalence of Alzheimer disease, it is the only leading cause of death that we are currently unable to prevent or cure. New treatments to slow disease progression are being developed; most rely on early identification of at-risk individuals before clinical symptoms emerge.

Innovative technologies, such as tau imaging and novel MR sequences for connectivity analyses, represent new, exciting frontiers in the early identification of dementing disorders. A detailed discussion of these experimental techniques is beyond the scope of this book. While some illustrative case examples are included here, the overall purpose of this chapter is to discuss normal and abnormal brain aging changes on imaging modalities that are generally available to practicing neuroradiologists.

Understanding the biology and imaging of normal aging is a prerequisite to understanding the pathobiology of degenerative brain diseases. Therefore, we first delineate normal age-related changes in brain structure and function.

We then turn our attention to dementias and brain degenerative disorders. **Dementia** is a loss of brain function that affects memory, thinking, language, judgment, and behavior. Dementia has many causes but most often occurs secondary to degenerative processes in the brain.

Neurodegeneration occurs when neurons in specific parts of the brain, spinal cord, or peripheral nerves die. Although dementia always involves brain degeneration, not all neurodegenerative disorders are dementing illnesses. Some neurodegenerative disorders (e.g., Parkinson disease) can have associated dementia, but most do not.

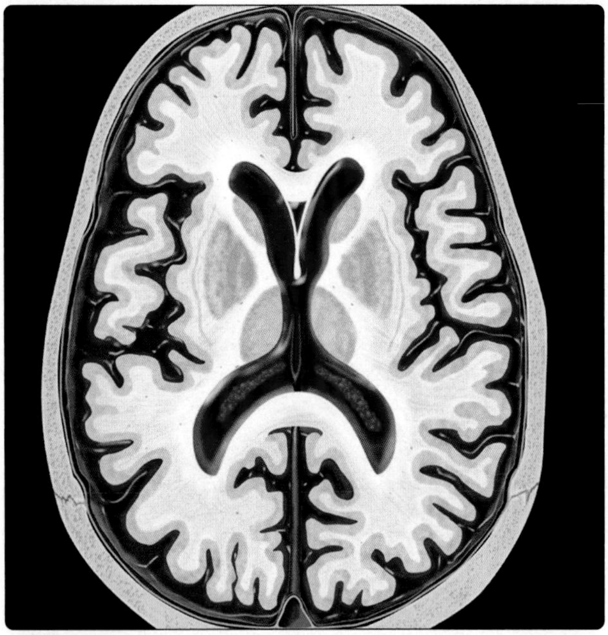

(33-1) Axial graphic depicts a normally aging brain in an 80y patient. Note the widening of sulci and ventricles in the absence of any parenchymal abnormalities.

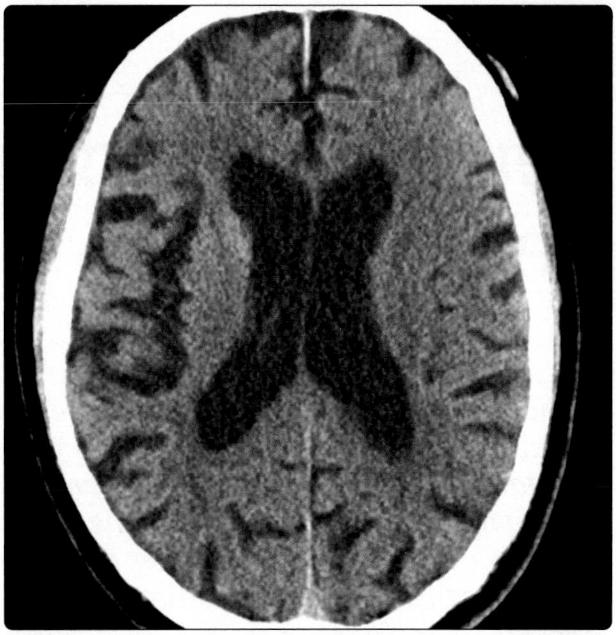

(33-2) NECT scan in a 100y, independent, cognitively normal man who had a ground-level fall shows mildly enlarged ventricles and sulci with no evidence of white matter lesions.

The Normal Aging Brain

Introduction to the Normal Aging Brain

Terminology

Age-related changes take place in virtually all parts of the brain and occur at all ages. The term **"normal aging brain"** as used in this chapter refers to the spectrum of normal age-related neuroimaging findings as delineated by the Rotterdam Scan Study (RSS). The RSS is a continuing population-based longitudinal study that began in the 1990s and includes advanced MR sequences. The population includes persons 45 years and older who are scanned every 3-4 years.

The term **"successfully aging brain"** previously referred to patients whose *anatomic* imaging studies do not demonstrate markers of small vessel ("microvascular") disease, such as white matter (WM) hyperintensities with arteriolosclerosis and lipohyalinosis, silent lacunar infarcts, and microbleeds.

Recent studies of *functional* connectivity have demonstrated that the brain's intrinsic networks undergo progressive disgregation (i.e., separation and parting) from clinically normal aging across progressive states of cognitive impairment to full-blown Alzheimer disease (AD). *Functional* imaging definitions of successful brain aging therefore include older individuals whose brain connectivity maps are considered normal.

Various methods to determine *cognitive* status in the elderly include the designation of "clinically normal (CN)" on the Alzheimer Disease Cooperative Study Preclinical Alzheimer Cognitive Composite (ADCS-PACC). The ADCS-PACC combines tests that assess episodic memory, timed executive function, and global cognition.

Genetics

Genetic factors affect brain aging and contribute to age-related cognitive decline. Apolipoprotein E (specifically *APOE-*ε4) and six novel risk-associated single-nucleotide polymorphisms (SNPs) on chromosome 17q25 are genetic variants that are robustly associated with brain pathology on MR.

Epigenetic dysregulation has also been identified as a pivotal player in aging as well as age-related cognitive decline and degenerative disorders. Major epigenetic mechanisms including DNA methylation and demethylation, chromatin remodeling, and noncoding RNAs are involved in normal aging and in the pathophysiology of the most common neurodegenerative diseases.

Biomarkers

The National Institute on Aging-Alzheimer's Association (NIA-AA) criteria for normal aging vs. preclinical AD use five biomarkers to classify individuals as either amyloid-β-positive or amyloid-β-negative and as neurodegeneration-positive or neurodegeneration-negative. Biomarkers of fibrillary β-amyloid deposition are high ligand retention on amyloid PET and low levels of amyloid-β42 in the CSF.

The biomarkers of AD-related neurodegeneration are high levels of tau in CSF, brain hypometabolism as assessed by 18F FDG PET, and atrophy as determined by anatomic MR.

Pathology

Gross Pathology. Overall brain volume decreases with advancing age and is indicated by a relative increase in the size of the CSF spaces. Widened sulci with proportionate enlargement of the ventricles are common **(33-1)**. Although minor thinning of the cortical mantle occurs with aging, the predominant neuroanatomic changes occur in the subcortical WM.

Microscopic Features. Physiologic brain aging is accompanied by ubiquitous degeneration of neurons and oligodendrocytes. Neuronal dysfunction—rather than frank neuronal loss—seems to predominate with a reduction in cell size (rather than number). Dendritic pruning and loss of synapses occur in selected areas (e.g., the hippocampus) but not globally.

The subcortical WM demonstrates decreased numbers of myelinated fibers, increased extracellular space, and gliosis. Perivascular (Virchow-Robin) spaces in the subcortical WM and basal ganglia enlarge.

Three histologic markers are associated with dementias: **senile plaques (SPs), neurofibrillary tangles (NFTs)**, and **Lewy bodies**. All can be identified to some extent in normal aging brains, so the border between normal and "preclinical" dementia is unclear. Decades may elapse between initial cortical accumulations of NFTs and SPs and the development of overt cognitive changes.

SPs are extracellular amyloid deposits that accumulate in cerebral gray matter. Nearly half of cognitively intact older individuals demonstrate moderate or frequent SP density.

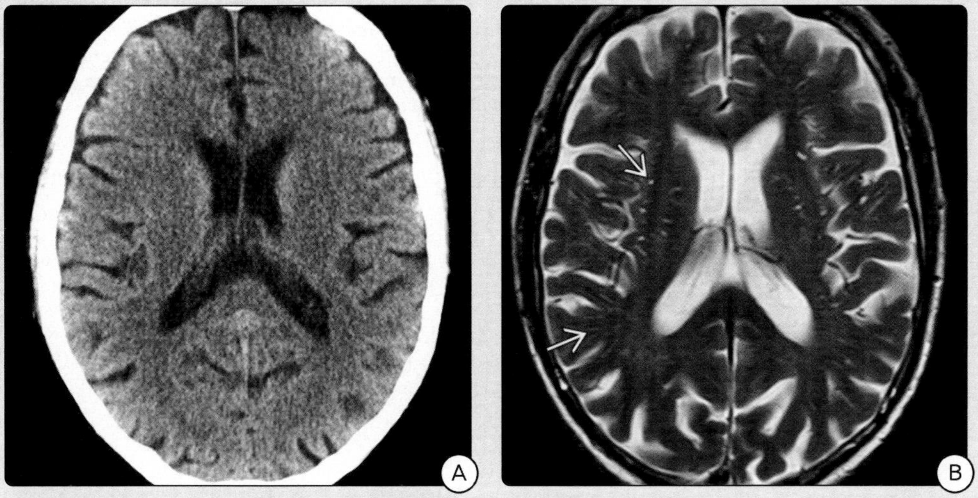

***(33-3A)** NECT scan in a 71y, neurologically normal man with a squamous cell carcinoma of the pinna shows mildly enlarged ventricles and sulci with normal-appearing white matter. **(33-3B)** T2WI in the same patient shows multifocal round and linear hyperintensities ➡ that probably represent prominent but normal perivascular spaces.*

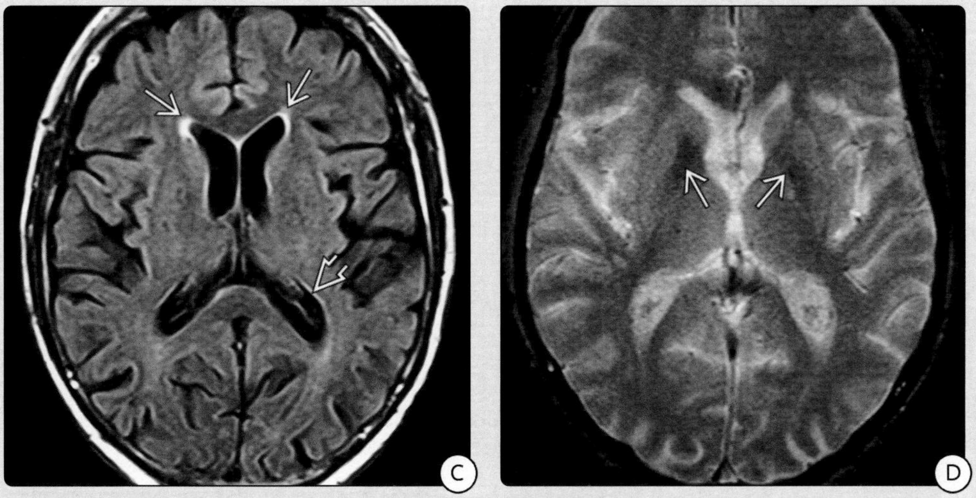

***(33-3C)** FLAIR scan in the same patient shows frontal periventricular "caps" ➡ and a thin hyperintense rim around the lateral ventricles ⇨. **(33-3D)** T2* GRE scan in the same patient shows hypointensity in the globi pallidi ➡ but not in the putamina or thalami. No microbleeds are present. This is a normal "successfully" aging brain.*

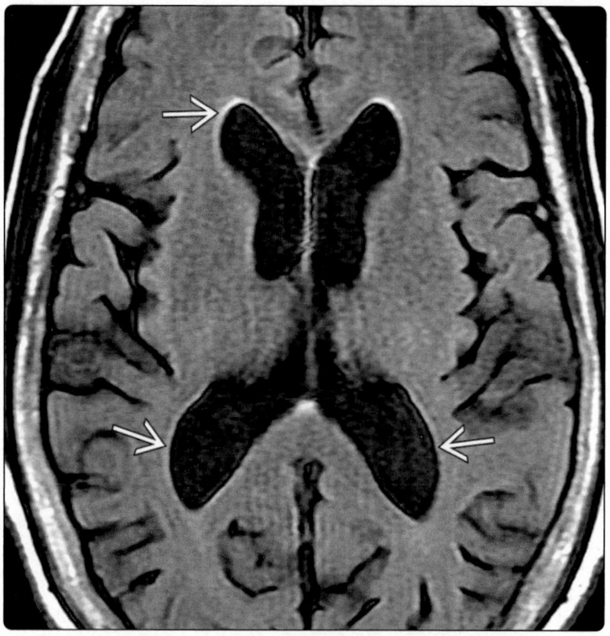

(33-4) FLAIR in a normal 79y man shows enlargement of ventricles, sulci due to age-related volume loss. Smooth, thin periventricular hyperintense rim around lateral ventricles ➡ is normal. Note lack of lacunar infarcts, WM hyperintensities.

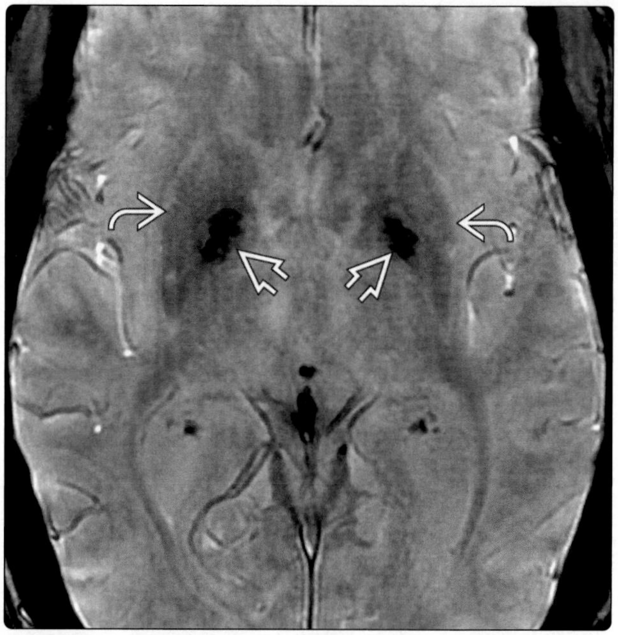

(33-5) T2* SWI in a 67y normal woman shows striking hypointensity in the globi pallidi ➡ and less prominent hypointensity in the putamina ➡ from iron deposition. (Both cases from Imaging in Neurology.)

NFTs are caused by tau aggregations within neurons. The Braak pathoanatomic staging divides AD into six distinct stages based on the topographical distribution of NFTs. Braak stage 5 or 6 NFTs are found in 6% of cognitively normal cases.

Lewy bodies are intraneuronal clumps of α-synuclein and ubiquitin proteins. They are found in 5-10% of cognitively intact individuals.

Clinical Issues

Epidemiology and Demographics. Brain maturation continues well into the third decade of life, after which brain aging predominates. Although the incidence of dementias increases dramatically with aging, nearly two-thirds of patients over 85 years of age remain neurologically intact and cognitively normal.

Presentation. Most older people with memory loss *do not* have dementia. As we age, we all experience memory deficits. As Dr. Gary Small, director of the UCLA Longevity Center put it, "To forget where you placed your keys, that's normal. If you forget how to use your keys, that's a problem."

Imaging the Normal Aging Brain

Because age-associated brain pathology begins long before clinical symptoms develop, imaging plays an increasingly central role in evaluating older patients for early signs of dementia. Just as imaging findings reflect the dramatic changes in brain morphology that occur with fetal and postnatal development, others mirror normal alterations in the aging brain.

CT Findings

The normal aging brain demonstrates mildly enlarged ventricles and widened sulci on NECT scans **(33-2)**. Punctate calcifications in the medial basal ganglia are physiologic.

Curvilinear calcifications in the cavernous carotid arteries and vertebrobasilar system are common. The significance of macrovascular calcification as a marker of microvascular disease is debated.

A few scattered patchy WM hypodensities are common, but confluent subcortical hypointensities, especially around the atria of the lateral ventricles, are a marker of arteriolosclerosis.

CECT scans demonstrate no foci of parenchymal enhancement in normal aging brains.

MR Findings

T1WI. T1-weighted images show mild but symmetric ventricular enlargement and proportionate prominence of the subarachnoid spaces. The corpus callosum may appear mildly thinned on sagittal T1 scans. Prominent perivascular spaces are a normal finding. They are filled with interstitial fluid (not CSF) but behave like CSF on all imaging sequences.

T2/FLAIR. White matter hyperintensities (WMHs) and lacunar infarcts on T2/FLAIR scans are highly prevalent in the elderly. They are associated with cardiovascular risk factors such as diabetes and hyperlipidemia. "Successfully" aging brains may demonstrate a few scattered nonconfluent WMHs (a reasonable number is one WMH per decade).

Perivascular spaces increase in prevalence and size with aging and are seen on T2WI as well-delineated round, ovoid, or linear CSF-like collections in the basal ganglia, subcortical WM, midbrain, etc. (see Chapter 28) **(33-3)**. PVSs suppress completely on FLAIR. Between 25 and 30% may display a thin, smooth, hyperintense rim. Lacunar infarcts typically demonstrate an irregular hyperintense rim around the lesions.

FLAIR scans in normal older patients demonstrate a smooth, thin, periventricular hyperintense rim around the lateral ventricles that probably represents increased extracellular interstitial fluid in the subependymal WM **(33-4)**. A "cap" of hyperintensity around the frontal horns is common and normal.

T2* (GRE, SWI). Brain iron is not present at birth but gradually accumulates as part of normal development. Iron accumulation is greatest in the pars reticulata of the substantia nigra (SN), followed by the globus pallidus (GP), where iron deposition progresses from medial to lateral. The red nucleus and putamen are other common sites where ferritin normally accumulates. Iron deposition in the GP and SN plateaus in early adulthood, but iron storage in the putamen continues well past 80 years of age.

Ferric iron deposition is best demonstrated on T2* sequences. Susceptibility-weighted images (SWI) are more sensitive than gradient-refocused (GRE) images. As field heterogeneity and magnetic susceptibility effects are proportional to field strength, hypointensity increases on 3.0-T images.

Hypointensity on T2* scans is normal in the medial GP **(33-5)**. Putaminal hypointensity is typically less prominent until the eighth decade. The caudate nucleus shows a scarce iron load at any age. The thalamus does not normally exhibit any hypointensity on T2* sequences.

Microbleeds on T2* scans are common in the aging brain. GRE and SWI sequences demonstrate cerebral microbleeds in 20% of patients over age 60 years and one-third of patients aged 80 years and older. Although common and therefore *statistically* "normal," microbleeds are not characteristic of *successful* brain aging. Basal ganglia and cerebellar microbleeds are usually indicative of chronic hypertensive encephalopathy. Lobar and cortical microbleeds are typical of amyloid angiopathy and are associated with worse cognitive performance.

DTI. The deleterious effect of WM changes on cognition depends on lesion burden, volume loss, and characteristics such as WM integrity that may not be apparent on standard imaging sequences. Even "normal-appearing white matter" may demonstrate loss of fractional anisotropy on DTI.

MRS. MRS shows a gradual decrease in NAA in the cortex, cerebral WM, and temporal lobes with concomitant increases in both Cho and Cr.

FDG PET/pMR

FDG PET studies show a gradual decrease in rCBF with aging, particularly in the frontal lobes. Patients with low total brain perfusion on pMR studies have more WMHs, but the precise relationship to cognitive performance is unclear.

Differential Diagnosis

The correlation between cognitive performance and brain imaging is complex and difficult to determine. Therefore, the major differential diagnosis of a normal aging brain is **mild cognitive impairment** and early "preclinical" **AD**. WMHs are markers of microvascular disease, so there is considerable overlap between normal brains and those with **subcortical arteriosclerotic encephalopathy**.

Dementias

Dementia is an acquired impairment in intellectual abilities that affects multiple cognitive domains including memory, language, and visuospatial skills. Emotional ability changes, behavioral alterations, and deteriorating ability to execute the activities of daily living are common. Dementia is one of the greatest fears people have about aging.

The three most common dementias are **Alzheimer disease, dementia with Lewy bodies**, and **vascular dementia (VaD)**. Together they account for the vast majority of all dementia cases. Less frequent causes include **frontotemporal lobar degeneration** (formerly known as Pick disease) and **corticobasal degeneration**. It can be difficult to distinguish between the various dementia syndromes because clinical features frequently overlap and so-called mixed dementias are common.

As new disease-modifying agents enter clinical practice, correctly diagnosing dementia type is becoming increasingly important. Assessment of patients with a potential dementing illness requires a detailed clinical history and careful physical examination as well as evaluation of cognition, behavior, and functional and social capacity.

Currently there is no single *behavioral* marker that can reliably discriminate Alzheimer disease—by far the most common dementing disorder—from other major dementia syndromes. As imaging plays a growing role in the diagnosis of dementias, we discuss each major type. Where possible, we point out features and new advanced imaging modalities that help distinguish the different types from potentially reversible nondementing disorders.

Alzheimer Disease

Alzheimer disease (AD) remains the only leading cause of death for which no disease-modifying treatment exists and age is by far the greatest risk factor. At least one-third of older individuals in the USA will die with dementia, largely due to AD.

Three ongoing longitudinal studies, namely the Alzheimer's Disease Neuroimaging Initiative (ADNI), the Australian Imaging, Biomarkers and Lifestyle (AIBL) study, and the ADCS Prevention Initiation, have recently been joined by a new study, the Harvard Aging Brain Study (HABS). These and other important initiatives aim to predict the emergence of clinical symptoms and elucidate the molecular, functional, and structural imaging markers that signal the transition from

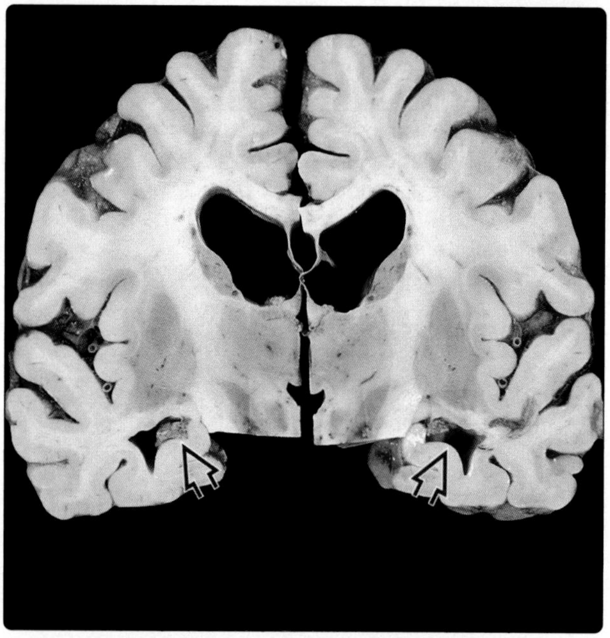

(33-6) Autopsy specimen from a patient with histologically proven early Alzheimer disease shows enlarged lateral ventricles. Temporal horns are proportionally enlarged, and hippocampi ➲ appear mildly atrophic. (R. Hewlett, MD.)

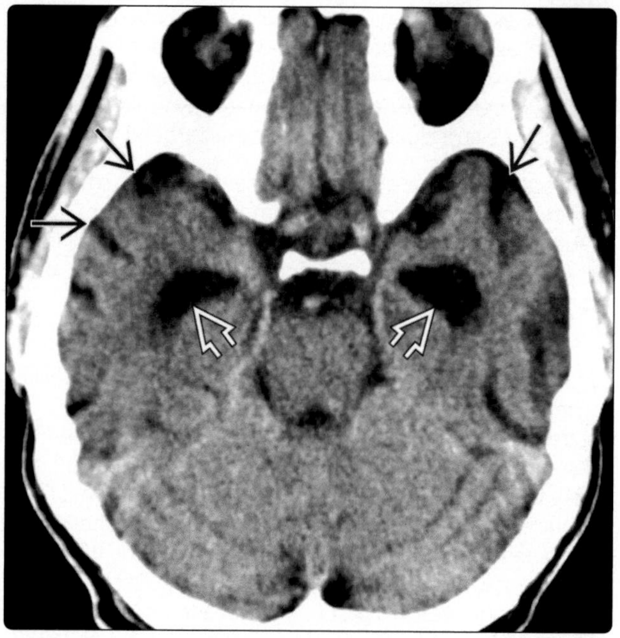

(33-7) Axial NECT scan in a 54y woman with severe early-onset Alzheimer disease shows markedly enlarged temporal horns ➲ and sulci ➔.

normal cognition to preclinical AD that characterizes the earliest stages along the trajectory of this devastating disorder.

Terminology

AD is a progressive neurodegenerative condition that leads to cognitive decline, impaired ability to perform the activities of daily living, and a range of behavioral and psychologic conditions.

AD is also known as senile dementia of Alzheimer type. There is increasing evidence that AD is not a single, all-encompassing disorder but instead a continuum of severity. The pathogenic process of AD is prolonged and may extend over several decades. A prodromal **preclinical/asymptomatic disease** (i.e., pathology is present, but cognition remains intact) may exist for years before evidence of **mild cognitive impairment** (MCI) develops.

Etiology

General Concepts. AD is characterized by an "amyloid cascade." Amyloidosis is one of the earliest events in the neuropathologic cascade leading to AD. Reduced clearance of the protein aggregate amyloid-β (Aβ) results in its aggregation in neurons. The **Aβ**42 residue is both insoluble and highly neurotoxic. Aβ42 clumps form **senile plaques** in the cortical gray matter. Aβ42 deposits also thicken the walls of cortical and leptomeningeal arterioles, causing **amyloid angiopathy**.

The majority of Aβ accumulation occurs before the progressive structural neurodegeneration and cognitive decline occur. One-third of *clinically normal* patients with elevated Aβ are in the preclinical stage of AD.

Another key feature of AD is **tauopathy**. Abnormal phosphorylation of a microtubule-associated protein known as "tau" eventually leads to the development of **neurofibrillary tangles** and **neuronal death**. CSF tau levels are almost tripled in patients with AD.

Genetics. The ε4 allele is the ancestral form of apolipoprotein E (*APOE*) and is associated with both higher absorption of cholesterol at the intestinal level and higher plasma cholesterol levels in carriers. Both the ε4 and *MTHFR* polymorphisms are known risk factors for late-onset AD (the most common type) and cerebrovascular disease (including VaD, see below).

Approximately 10% of AD cases have a strong family history of the disorder. Three autosomal-dominant gene mutations are associated with early-onset AD: amyloid precursor protein (*APP*) and presenilin 1 and 2 (*PSEN1 and PSEN2*).

Pathology

Gross Pathology. Brains affected by AD show generalized (whole-brain) atrophy with shrunken gyri, widened sulci, and ventricular expansion (especially the temporal horns). Changes are most marked in the medial temporal and parietal lobes **(33-6)**. The frontal lobes are commonly involved, whereas the occipital lobes and motor cortex are relatively spared.

The hippocampus is severely affected in 75% of cases. Relative hippocampal sparing is seen in 10%, and limbic-predominance accounts for 15% of AD cases.

Microscopic Features. The three characteristic histologic hallmarks of AD are senile plaques, neurofibrillary tangles, and

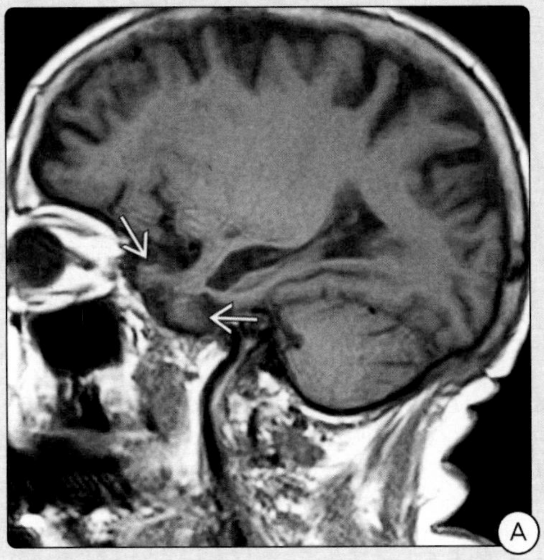

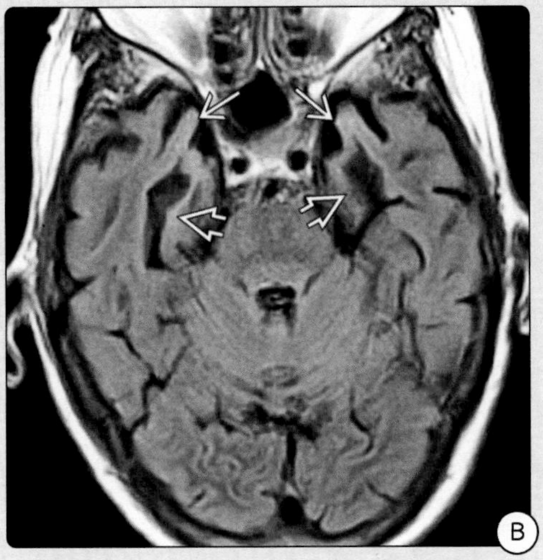

(33-8A) *Sagittal T1WI in a 67y woman with clinically definite AD shows markedly atrophic temporal lobe.* ***(33-8B)*** *Axial FLAIR in the same patient shows severely shrunken, hyperintense hippocampi and medial temporal lobes.*

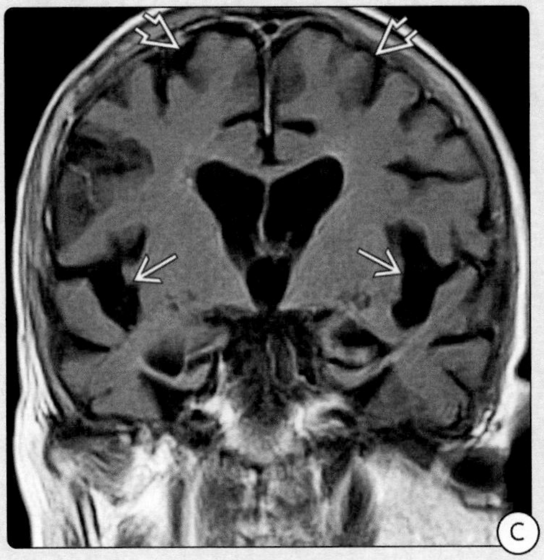

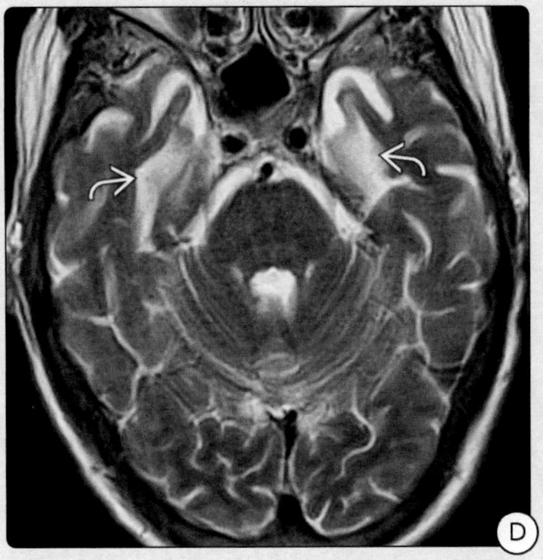

(33-8C) *Coronal FLAIR shows the striking temporal lobe atrophy with enlarged sylvian fissures and relative preservation of frontal lobe volume.* ***(33-8D)*** *T2WI shows that the temporal horns of the lateral ventricles are markedly enlarged.*

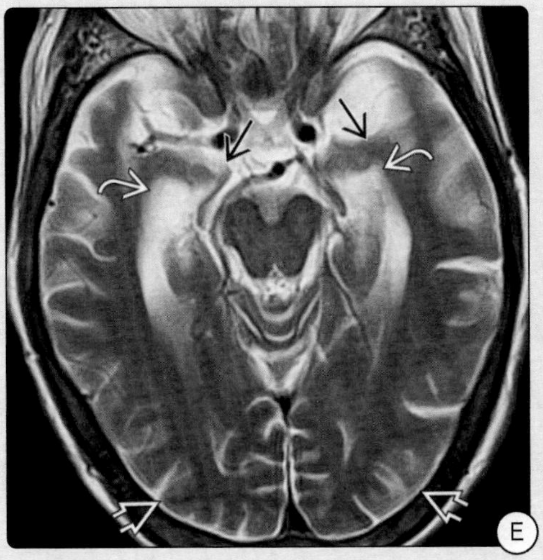

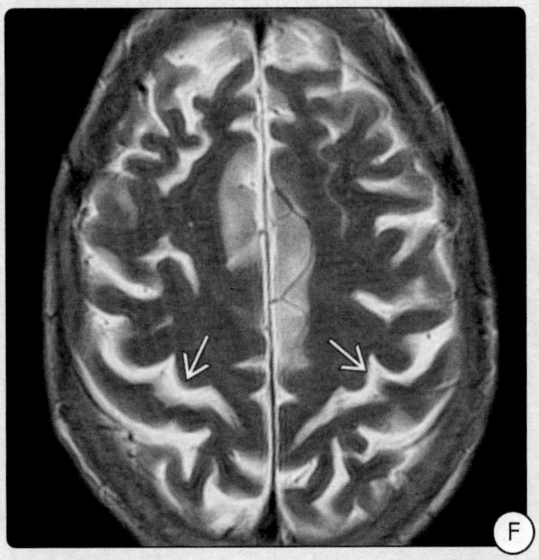

(33-8E) *More cephalad T2WI in the same patient shows enlarged temporal horns and disproportionate volume loss in the temporal lobes compared with the normal-appearing occipital lobes.* ***(33-8F)*** *Scan through the upper cerebral hemispheres shows symmetric parietal lobe atrophy.*

exaggerated neuronal loss. All are characteristic of—but none is specific for—AD.

AD also often coexists with other pathologies, such as vascular disease or Lewy bodies. Variable amounts of amyloid deposition in arterioles of the cortex and leptomeninges (amyloid angiopathy) are present in over 90% of AD cases. Vascular and AD pathology are additive; patients with both have clinically more severe dementia.

Staging, Grading, and Classification. There are several scales for the histologic staging of Alzheimer pathology. One of the most widely used—the Braak and Braak system—is based on the topographic distribution of neurofibrillary tangles and neuropil threads, with grades from 1 to 6. The Consortium to Establish a Registry for Alzheimer Disease (CERAD) scale is based on the quantity of neocortical neuritic plaques in relation to age.

A third system (the Poly Pathology AD Assessment 9 or PPAD9) is based not just on neurofibrillary tangles and neuritic plaques, but also a combination of other factors, including the extent of neuronal degeneration, microvacuolization, cytoarchitectural disorder, and gliosis. Each finding is calculated for nine different regions of the brain.

To date, correlation between these major staging systems is suboptimal. Choice of staging system affects the evaluation of AD pathology and therefore the final diagnosis.

Clinical Issues

Epidemiology and Demographics. AD is the most common cause of dementia, accounting for approximately 50-60% of all cases and affecting more than 35 million people worldwide. The World Alzheimer Report predicts that this number will almost double by 2030 and will exceed 100 million by 2050.

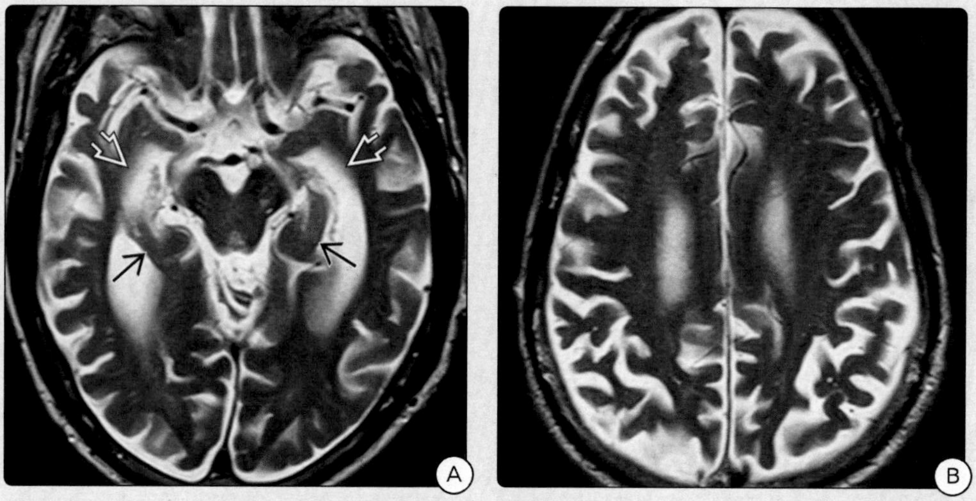

***(33-9A)** Axial T2WI in a 74y man with cognitive decline shows generalized volume loss. Both temporal horns ➡ are prominent, and the hippocampi → appear atrophic. **(33-9B)** More cephalad T2WI in the same case shows generalized volume loss without an obvious lobar predominant pattern.*

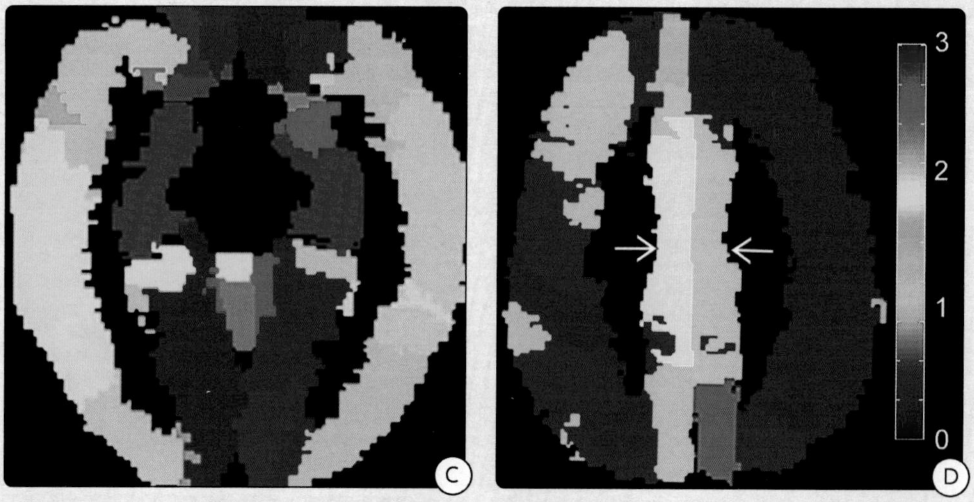

***(33-9C)** Thin-section MP-RAGE images in the same case were used to create a difference map with age-matched controls. The hippocampus volumes are 3 standard deviations below normal, whereas the right temporal lobe is 2 SDs below normal (see color graph on next panel). **(33-9D)** More cephalad image compared with age-matched controls shows that the right and left posterior cingulate gyri ➡ are nearly 2 SDs below normal. This is Alzheimer disease.*

Age is the biggest risk factor for developing AD. The prevalence of AD is 1-2% at age 65 and increases by 15-25% each decade. In the "oldest-old" patients (more than 90 years), with mixed pathologies—typically AD plus VaD—predominate.

Diagnosis. AD represents a disease spectrum that ranges from cognitively normal individuals with elevated Aβ through those who exhibit the very first, minimal signs of cognitive impairment (MCI) on the ADCS-PACC to frank AD.

Historically, the *definitive* diagnosis of AD was made only by biopsy or autopsy. The *clinical* diagnosis of AD using the National Institute of Neurological Disorders and Stroke-Alzheimer Disease and Related Disorders (NINDS-ADRA) criteria defines three levels of certainty: possible, probable, and definite AD. The diagnosis of definite AD currently requires the clinical diagnosis of probable AD *plus* neuropathologic confirmation.

The Alzheimer Disease Neuroimaging Initiative (ADNI) is an ongoing longitudinal, multicenter study designed to identify clinical, imaging, genetic, and biochemical biomarkers for the early detection and tracking of AD. The ADNI standardized datasets are currently the most commonly used references for the computer-aided diagnosis of dementia.

Presentation. Minimal cognitive impairment causes a slight but noticeable (and measurable) decline in cognitive abilities. The mildest MCI is a single cognitive domain (amnestic) form that is characterized by memory loss beyond that expected for age and education. Here global cognitive function is maintained, and the capacity to perform activities of daily living is preserved.

Individuals with MCI do not meet the diagnostic guidelines for dementia but are nevertheless at increased risk of eventually developing AD or another type of dementia.

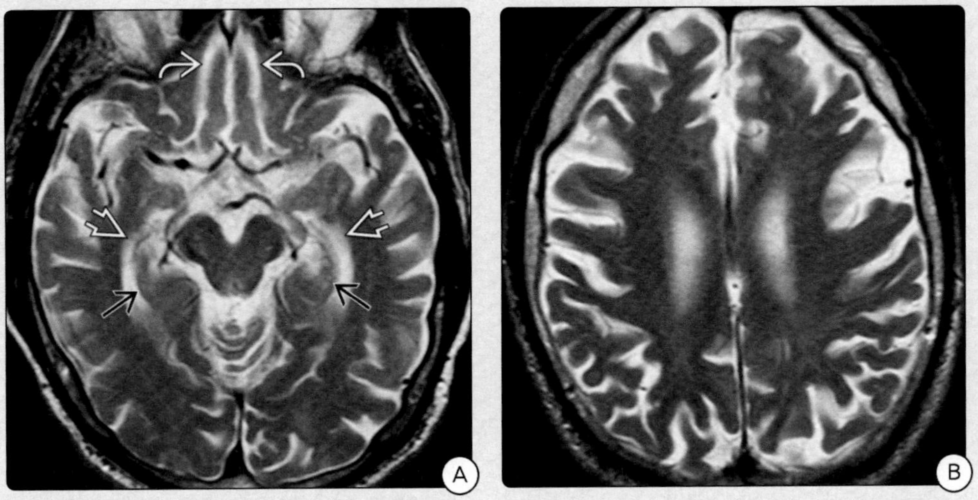

***(33-10A)** Axial T2WI in a 74y man with mild cognitive impairment shows generalized volume loss with mildly increased size of the temporal horns and decreased size of the hippocampi. The inferior frontal lobes appear shrunken, and the adjacent sulci are enlarged. **(33-10B)** More cephalad T2WI in the same case shows generalized sulcal enlargement without obvious lobar predominance.*

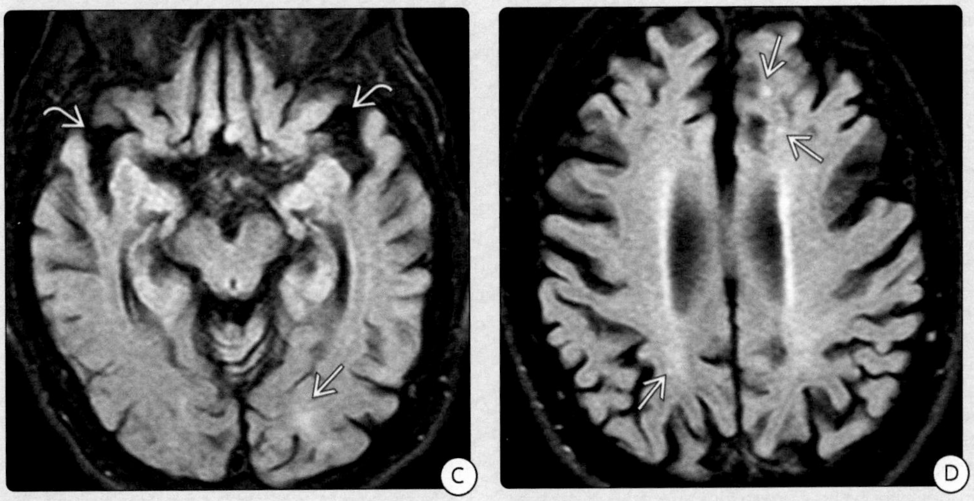

***(33-10C)** FLAIR MR in the same case shows that the sylvian fissures are moderately enlarged. The visualized white matter appears normal for the patient's age with only scattered ill-defined hyperintensities. **(33-10D)** More cephalad FLAIR shows generalized volume loss with slight frontal predominance. Only a few white matter hyperintensities are identified. The clinical diagnosis was probable Alzheimer disease.*

(33-11) NeuroQuant® morphometry obtained using thin-section MP-RAGE and age-matched controls shows a hippocampal occupancy score (HOC) of 0.58. The hippocampal volumes are at the 4th percentile, and the inferior lateral ventricle volumes are at the 96th percentile for age. The mesial temporal lobes are more than 2 SDs below normal.

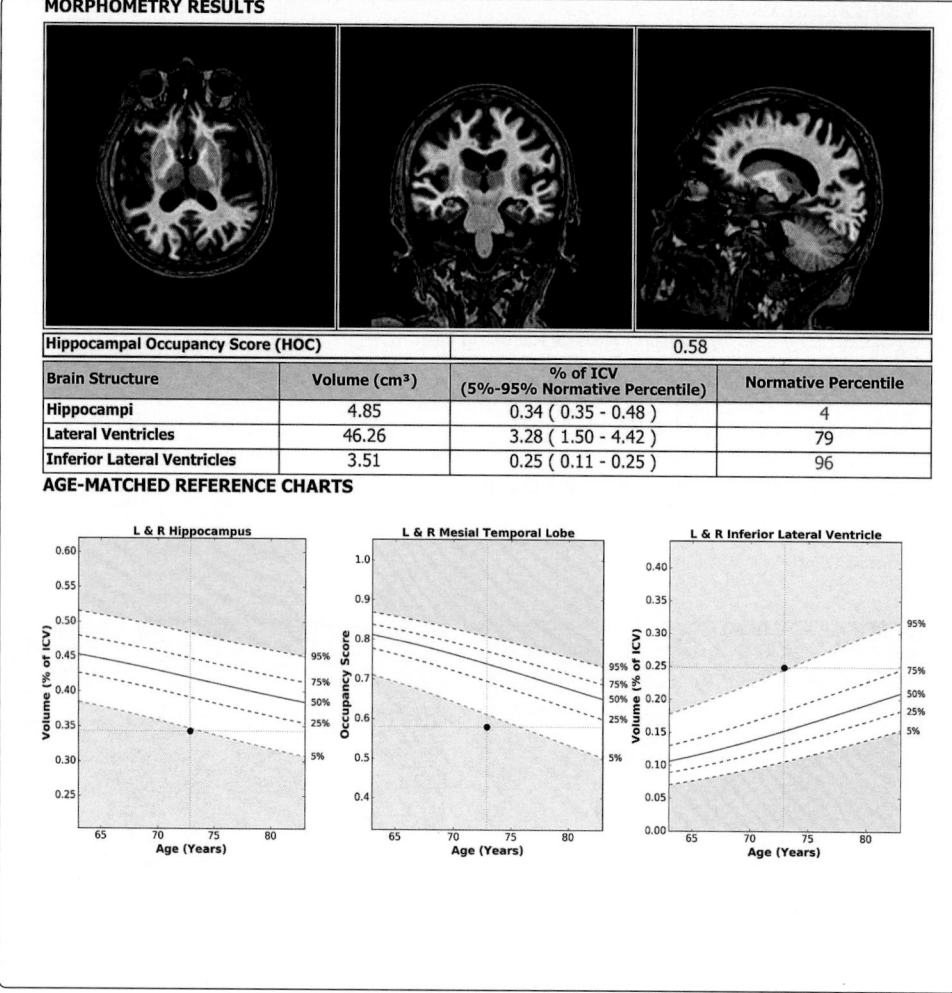

MORPHOMETRY RESULTS

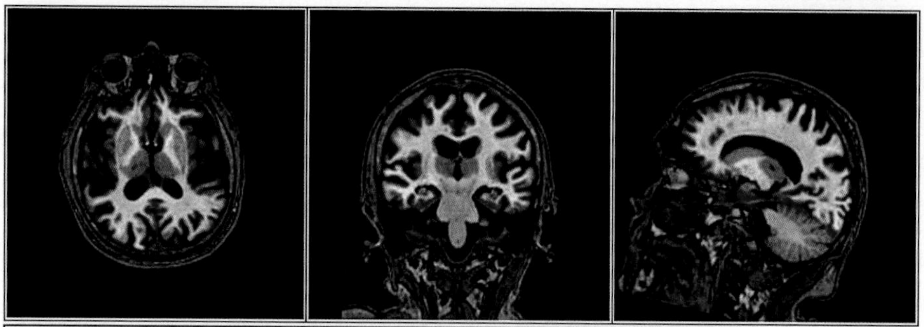

Hippocampal Occupancy Score (HOC)	0.58

Brain Structure	Volume (cm³)	% of ICV (5%-95% Normative Percentile)	Normative Percentile
Hippocampi	4.85	0.34 (0.35 - 0.48)	4
Lateral Ventricles	46.26	3.28 (1.50 - 4.42)	79
Inferior Lateral Ventricles	3.51	0.25 (0.11 - 0.25)	96

AGE-MATCHED REFERENCE CHARTS

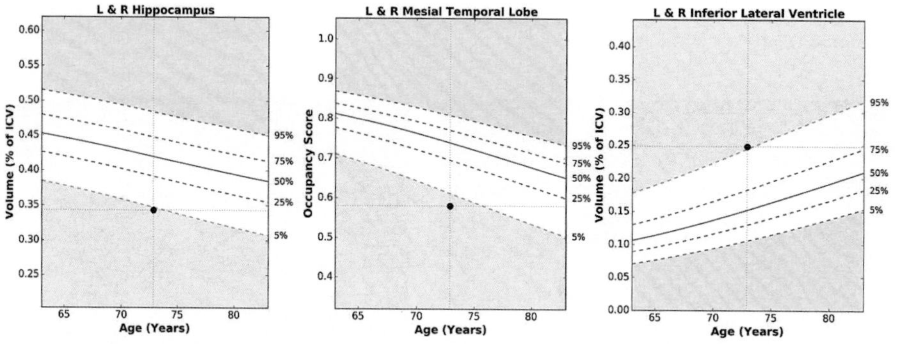

Patients with very early AD show impaired short-term memory. As the disease progresses, memory deficits increase and are associated with neuropsychiatric changes, difficulties in finding words and spatial cognition, and reduced executive functioning. Motor, sensory, and gait disturbances are uncommon until relatively late in the disease.

Natural History and Treatment Options. AD is a chronic disease. Progression is gradual, and patients live an average of 8-10 years after diagnosis. Between 5 and 10% of patients with MCI progress to probable AD each year.

There are no established treatments to prevent or reverse AD. Many current disease-modifying drugs focus on reducing Aβ amyloidosis. Treating MCI patients with cholinesterase inhibitors or NMDA receptor antagonists may transiently improve cognitive functioning but does not delay conversion from MCI to AD.

Imaging

General Features. One of the most important goals of routine CT and MR is to identify specific abnormalities that could support the clinical diagnosis of AD. The other major role is to exclude alternative etiologies that can mimic AD clinically, i.e., "causes of reversible dementia" (see below).

The introduction of radiotracers for the noninvasive in vivo quantification of Aβ burden in the brain has revolutionized the approach to the imaging evaluation of AD.

CT Findings. NECT is a helpful screening procedure that may exclude potentially reversible or treatable causes of dementia, such as subdural hematoma and normal pressure hydrocephalus. Otherwise, CT scans are generally uninformative, especially in the early stages of AD.

Medial temporal lobe atrophy is generally the earliest identifiable finding on CT **(33-7)**. Late findings include generalized cortical atrophy.

MR Findings. The current role of conventional 1.5- and 3.0-T MR in the evaluation of patients with dementing disorders is to (1) exclude other causes of dementia, (2) identify region-specific patterns of brain volume loss (e.g., "lobar-predominant" atrophy), and (3) identify imaging markers of comorbid vascular disease, such as amyloid angiopathy.

The most common morphologic changes on standard MR are thinned gyri, widened sulci, and enlarged lateral ventricles. The medial temporal lobe—particularly the hippocampus and entorhinal cortex—are often disproportionately affected **(33-8)** **(33-10)** as are the posterior cingulate gyri **(33-9)**.

MORPHOMETRY RESULTS

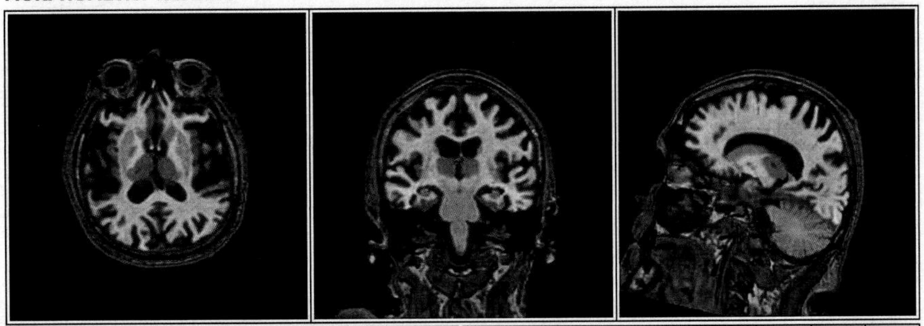

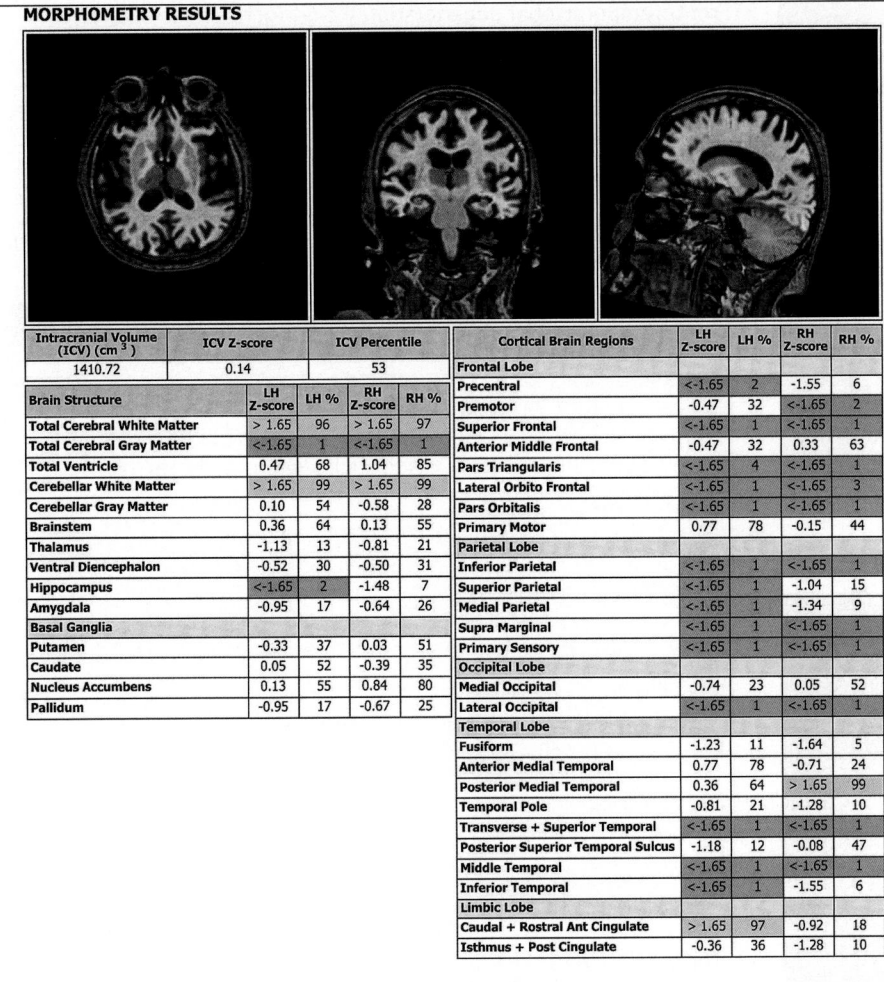

Intracranial Volume (ICV) (cm ^{3})	ICV Z-score	ICV Percentile
1410.72	0.14	53

Brain Structure	LH Z-score	LH %	RH Z-score	RH %
Total Cerebral White Matter	> 1.65	96	> 1.65	97
Total Cerebral Gray Matter	<-1.65	1	<-1.65	1
Total Ventricle	0.47	68	1.04	85
Cerebellar White Matter	> 1.65	99	> 1.65	99
Cerebellar Gray Matter	0.10	54	-0.58	28
Brainstem	0.36	64	0.13	55
Thalamus	-1.13	13	-0.81	21
Ventral Diencephalon	-0.52	30	-0.50	31
Hippocampus	<-1.65	2	-1.48	7
Amygdala	-0.95	17	-0.64	26
Basal Ganglia				
Putamen	-0.33	37	0.03	51
Caudate	0.05	52	-0.39	35
Nucleus Accumbens	0.13	55	0.84	80
Pallidum	-0.95	17	-0.67	25

Cortical Brain Regions	LH Z-score	LH %	RH Z-score	RH %
Frontal Lobe				
Precentral	<-1.65	2	-1.55	6
Premotor	-0.47	32	<-1.65	2
Superior Frontal	<-1.65	1	<-1.65	1
Anterior Middle Frontal	-0.47	32	0.33	63
Pars Triangularis	<-1.65	4	<-1.65	1
Lateral Orbito Frontal	<-1.65	1	<-1.65	3
Pars Orbitalis	<-1.65	1	<-1.65	1
Primary Motor	0.77	78	-0.15	44
Parietal Lobe				
Inferior Parietal	<-1.65	1	<-1.65	1
Superior Parietal	<-1.65	1	-1.04	15
Medial Parietal	<-1.65	1	-1.34	9
Supra Marginal	<-1.65	1	<-1.65	1
Primary Sensory	<-1.65	1	<-1.65	1
Occipital Lobe				
Medial Occipital	-0.74	23	0.05	52
Lateral Occipital	<-1.65	1	<-1.65	1
Temporal Lobe				
Fusiform	-1.23	11	-1.64	5
Anterior Medial Temporal	0.77	78	-0.71	24
Posterior Medial Temporal	0.36	64	> 1.65	99
Temporal Pole	-0.81	21	-1.28	10
Transverse + Superior Temporal	<-1.65	1	<-1.65	1
Posterior Superior Temporal Sulcus	-1.18	12	-0.08	47
Middle Temporal	<-1.65	1	<-1.65	1
Inferior Temporal	<-1.65	1	-1.55	6
Limbic Lobe				
Caudal + Rostral Ant Cingulate	> 1.65	97	-0.92	18
Isthmus + Post Cingulate	-0.36	36	-1.28	10

***(33-12)** NeuroQuant® morphometry results are the same case illustrated on the previous page. Detailed analyses of total cerebral gray matter, hippocampi, and several cortical brain regions (frontal, parietal, temporal) are grossly abnormal, highlighted in red.*

T1-weighted MP-RAGE data can be used to quantify regional brain atrophy using open-source (i.e., FreeSurfer), proprietary, or commercial (i.e., NeuroQuant®) automated volumetric analyses **(33-11)**. 7-T MR can identify abnormalities in the hippocampal subfields. The most consistent finding is reduction in CA1 volume (specifically CA1-SRLM) **(33-12)**.

T2* (GRE, SWI) sequences are much more sensitive than standard FSE in detecting cortical microhemorrhages that may suggest comorbid amyloid angiopathy.

MRS shows decreased NAA and increased myoinositol in patients with AD, even during the early stages of the disease **(33-13)**. The NAA:myoinositol ratio is relatively sensitive and highly specific in differentiating AD patients from the normal elderly. NAA:Cr ratio in the posterior cingulate gyri and left occipital cortex predicts conversion from MCI to probable AD with relatively high sensitivity and good specificity.

DTI in patients with AD shows decreased FA in multiple regions, especially the superior longitudinal fasciculus and corpus callosum splenium. Reduced FA reflects early microstructural WM changes.

Functional Neuroimaging. fMR shows decrease in intensity and/or extent of activation in the frontal and temporal regions in cognitive tasks. pMR may demonstrate subtly reduced rCBV in the temporal and parietal lobes in MCI patients.

Nuclear Medicine. 18F FDG PET demonstrates areas of regional hypometabolism **(33-14)** and helps distinguish AD from other lobar-predominant dementias (e.g., frontotemporal lobar degeneration).

PET using amyloid-binding radiotracers such as 11[C] PiB (Pittsburgh compound B) has emerged as one of the best techniques for early AD diagnosis. Aβ deposition occurs well before symptom onset and likely represents preclinical AD in asymptomatic individuals and prodromal AD in patients with MCI.

Differential Diagnosis

The most difficult distinction is differentiating **normal age-related degenerative processes** and early "preclinical" AD.

"Mixed dementias" are common, especially in patients over the age of 90 years. **VaD** is the most common dementia associated with AD. Lacunar and cortical infarcts are typical findings in VaD. **Cerebral amyloid angiopathy** often coexists with AD. **Lewy bodies** are sometimes found in AD patients ("Lewy body variant of AD").

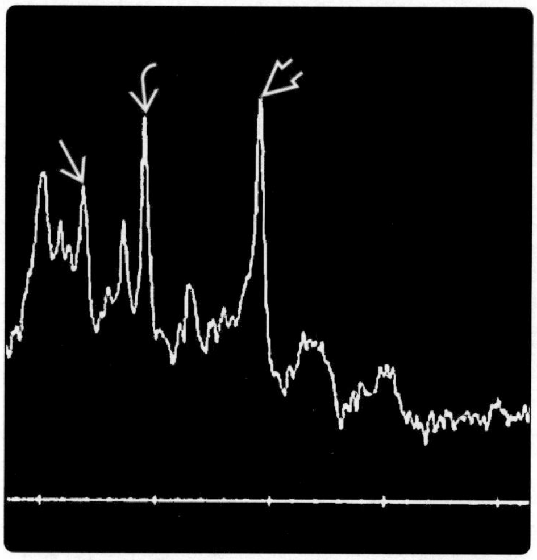

***(33-13)** MRS in AD shows elevated myoinositol (mI) peak. The NAA-to-mI ratio is decreased; creatine (Cr) peak is decreased.*

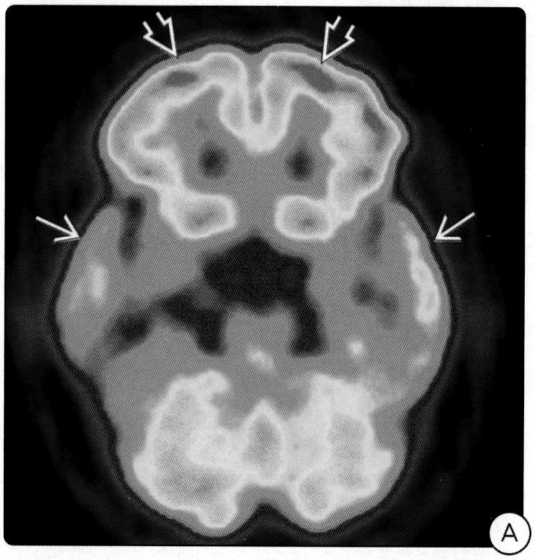

***(33-14A)** 18F FDG PET in AD shows markedly reduced metabolism in both temporal lobes with comparatively normal frontal lobes.*

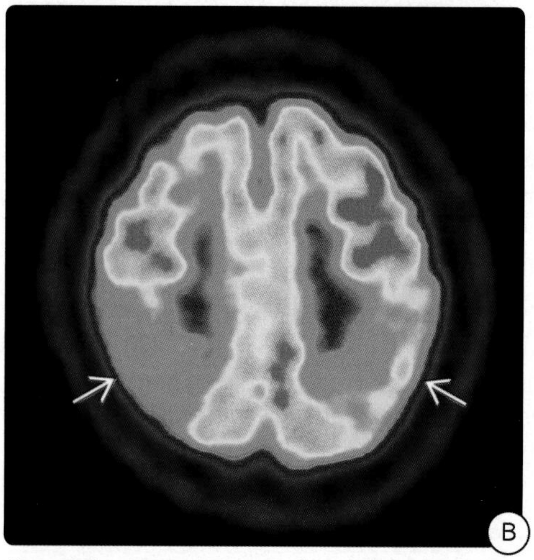

***(33-14B)** Parietal hypometabolism on cephalad PET shows temporal/parietal hypometabolism; preserved frontal activity common.*

Frontotemporal lobar degeneration shows frontal and/or anterior temporal atrophy and hypometabolism; the parietal lobes are generally spared. **Dementia with Lewy bodies** typically demonstrates generalized, nonfocal hypometabolism. Patients with **corticobasal degeneration** have prominent extrapyramidal symptoms.

Causes of reversible dementia that can be identified on imaging studies include mass lesions, such as chronic subdural hematoma or neoplasm, vitamin deficiencies (thiamine, B12), endocrinopathy (e.g., hypothyroidism), and normal pressure hydrocephalus.

ALZHEIMER DISEASE

Pathoetiology
- Neurotoxic "amyloid cascade"
  - Aβ42 accumulation → senile plaques, amyloid angiopathy
- Tauopathy → neurofibrillary tangles, neuronal death

Clinical Issues
- Most common dementia (50-60% of all cases)
- Prevalence increases 15-25% per decade after 65 years
- Pathology begins *at least* a decade before clinical symptoms emerge
  - "Clinically normal" on preclinical Alzheimer cognitive composite
  - Aβ in clinically normal predicts significant longitudinal decline

Imaging
- Frontoparietal dominant lobar atrophy
  - Hippocampus, entorhinal cortex
  - FDG PET shows hypometabolism
  - Amyloid-binding markers, such as 11[C] PiB
- Amyloid angiopathy
  - Present in > 95% of cases
  - T2* cortical "blooming black dots""
  - With or without cortical siderosis

Differential Diagnosis
- Exclude reversible dementias!
  - Subdural hematoma
  - Normal pressure hydrocephalus
- DDx
  - Normal aging
  - Vascular dementia
  - Frontotemporal lobar degeneration
  - AD often mixed with other dementias (especially vascular)

Vascular Dementia

Cerebrovascular disease is a common cause of cognitive decline. The burden of "silent" microvascular disease and its long-term deleterious effect on cognition is becoming increasingly well recognized, as is its link with AD as a significant comorbidity.

Terminology

Vascular dementia (VaD) is sometimes also called multiinfarct dementia, vascular cognitive disorder, vascular cognitive impairment, subcortical ischemic vascular dementia, and poststroke dementia. All are broadly encompassing terms for cognitive dysfunction associated with—and presumed to be caused by—vascular brain damage.

Etiology

Inherited Vascular Dementias. Monogenic disorders are estimated to cause approximately 5% of all strokes and 10% of vascular dementias.

Known monogenic disorders that can cause VaD are (1) **c**erebral **a**utosomal-**d**ominant **a**rteriopathy with **s**ubcortical **i**nfarcts and **l**eukoencephalopathy (CADASIL, caused by *NOTCH3* mutations on chromosome 19) and **c**erebral **a**utosomal-**r**ecessive **a**rteriopathy with **s**ubcortical **i**nfarcts and **l**eukoencephalopathy (CARASIL, caused by mutations in the *HTRA1* gene); (2) Fabry disease (an X-linked lysosomal disease caused by a mutation of the *GLA* gene); (3) **p**ontine **a**utosomal-**d**ominant **m**icroangiopathy **a**nd **l**eukoencephalopathy (PADMAL, i.e., *COL4A1*-A2 gene-related arteriopathies); (4) **r**etinal **v**asculopathy with **c**erebral **l**eukodystrophy (RCVL, associated with *TREX1* mutation); and (5) the recently-described Forkhead Box C1 mutations (*FOXC1*).

Sporadic Vascular Dementias. Most cases of VaD are sporadic and are caused by the cumulative burden of cerebrovascular lesions. Risk factors for VaD include hypertension, dyslipidemia, and smoking. Mutations in the *MTHFR* gene correlate with elevated levels of plasma homocysteine and are associated both with AD and vasculogenic cognitive impairment.

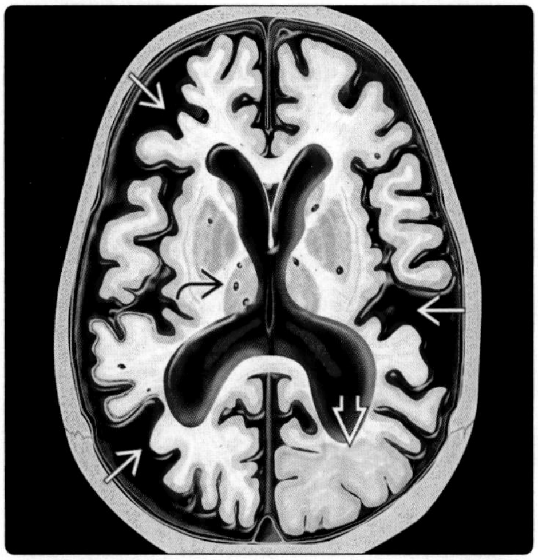

(33-15) Graphic of VaD shows multiple chronic infarcts ➡, acute left occipital lobe infarct ➡, and small basal ganglia lacunar infarcts ↗.

VASCULAR DEMENTIA: ETIOLOGY

Inherited (≈ 10%)
- CADASIL
  - Most common inherited cerebral small vessel disease
  - Autosomal-dominant; *NOTCH3* mutation
  - MR after 35 years of age always abnormal!
  - WM lesions, lacunae
  - Especially anterior temporal, external capsule; corpus callosum
- CARASIL
  - Autosomal-recessive; *HTRA1* mutation
- Fabry disease
  - X-linked recessive; α-GAL A (*GLA*) mutation
  - WM lesions, lacunae; T1 hyperintense pulvinar

Sporadic or Mixed (≈ 90%)
- VaD = 2nd most common dementia
- Multiple etiologies
  - Systemic hyperlipidemia, cardiovascular risk factors
  - *MTHFR* mutations (increased plasma homocysteine)
  - Amyloid angiopathy

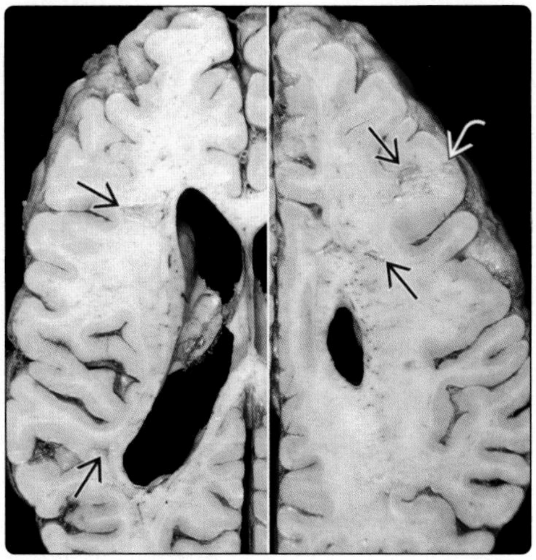

(33-16) VaD shows multiple WM ➡, cortical ➡ lacunae at the level of the lateral ventricle (L), corona radiata (R). (Courtesy R. Hewlett, MD.)

Pathology

Gross Pathology. The most common readily identifiable gross finding in VaD is multiple infarcts with focal atrophy **(33-15)** **(33-17)**. Multiple subcortical lacunar infarcts **(33-16)** and/or widespread white matter ischemia are more common than cortical branch occlusions or large territorial infarcts **(33-17)**.

Microscopic Features. Vessel wall modifications are the most common and presumably the earliest identifiable changes associated with VaD. **Arteriolosclerosis** and **amyloid angiopathy** are the major underlying pathologies in small vessel vascular disease. Myelin loss and modifications in perivascular spaces are the next most common vascular findings in dementia.

So-called **microinfarcts**—minute foci of neuronal loss, gliosis, pallor, or frank cystic degeneration—and other cerebrovascular lesions are seen at autopsy in nearly two-thirds of patients with VaD and more than half of all cases with other dementing disorders (e.g., AD, dementia with Lewy bodies). Lesions are found in all brain regions and are especially common in the cortex, subcortical WM, and basal ganglia.

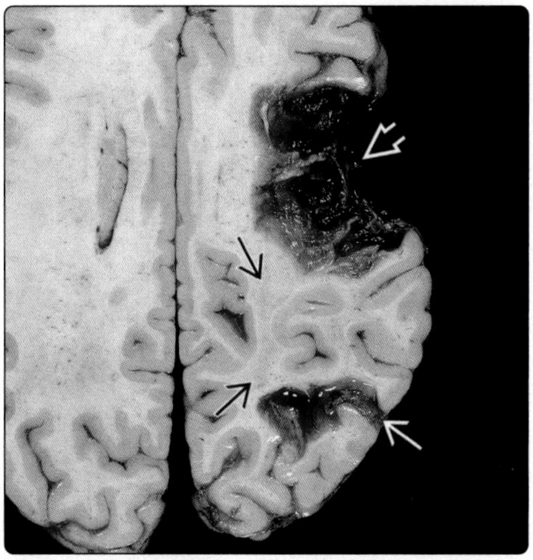

(33-17) Autopsied multiinfarct dementia shows territorial ➡, cortical ➡ infarcts, WM lesions ➡ in the left hemisphere. (Courtesy R. Hewlett, MD.)

Clinical Issues

Epidemiology and Demographics. VaD is the second most common cause of dementia (after AD) and accounts for approximately 10% of all dementia cases in developed countries. VaD is a common component of "mixed" dementias and is especially prevalent in patients with AD.

The incidence of VaD increases with age. Risk factors include hypertension, diabetes, dyslipidemia, and smoking. There is a moderate male predominance.

Recently proposed definitions of major VaD subtypes include (1) poststroke dementia, (2) mixed dementias (i.e., with AD, diffuse Lewy disease), (3) subcortical ischemic VaD (mostly small vessel disease with lacunar infarcts and subcortical ischemic white matter lesions) that incorporates the overlapping clinical entities of Binswanger disease and lacunar state, and (4) multiinfarct dementia (multiple large cortical infarcts).

VASCULAR DEMENTIA: PATHOLOGY AND CLINICAL ISSUES

Pathology
- Small > large vessel
- Atherosclerosis, arteriolosclerosis, amyloid angiopathy

Clinical Issues
- 2nd most common dementia (10%)
- Multiple strokes; episodic step-like deterioration
- Subtypes
  - Poststroke dementia
  - Mixed dementias
  - Subcortical ischemic VaD
  - Multiinfarct dementia

Presentation. A history of multiple stroke-like episodes with focal neurologic deficits is characteristic of patients with VaD.

(33-18A) Axial FLAIR in an 82y woman with vascular dementia (VaD) shows a small lacunar infarct ➡, a focal cortical infarct ⇨, and subcortical WM hyperintensities ➡. (33-18B) More cephalad FLAIR scan in the same patient shows additional WM hyperintensities ➡.

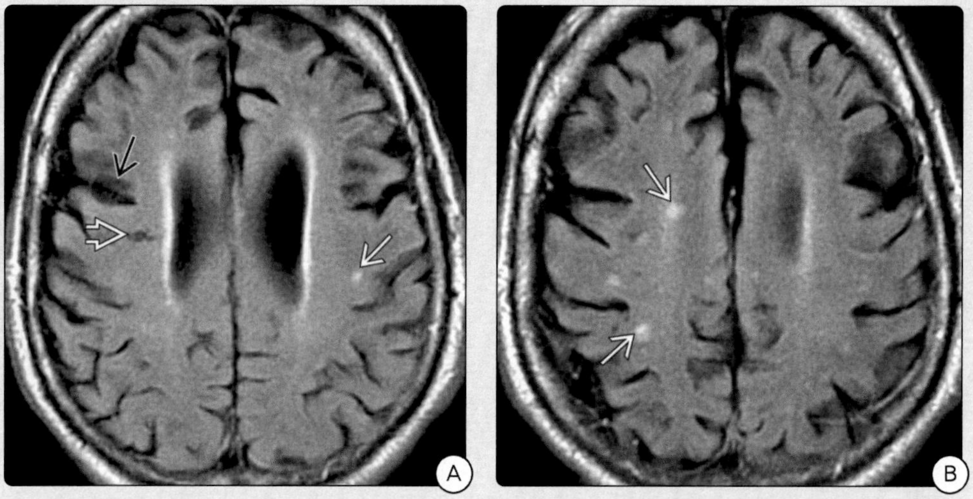

(33-18C) T2 GRE sequence in the same patient shows the lacunar ⇨ and cortical ⇨ infarcts but no "blooming" hypointensities, suggestive of amyloid angiopathy. (33-18D) PET scan shows normal age-matched controls (second row) and the patient's scan (third row). Note multifocal cortical areas of decreased glucose metabolism ➡. Z-score map (bottom) shows severely affected areas in green. (Courtesy N. Foster, MD.)*

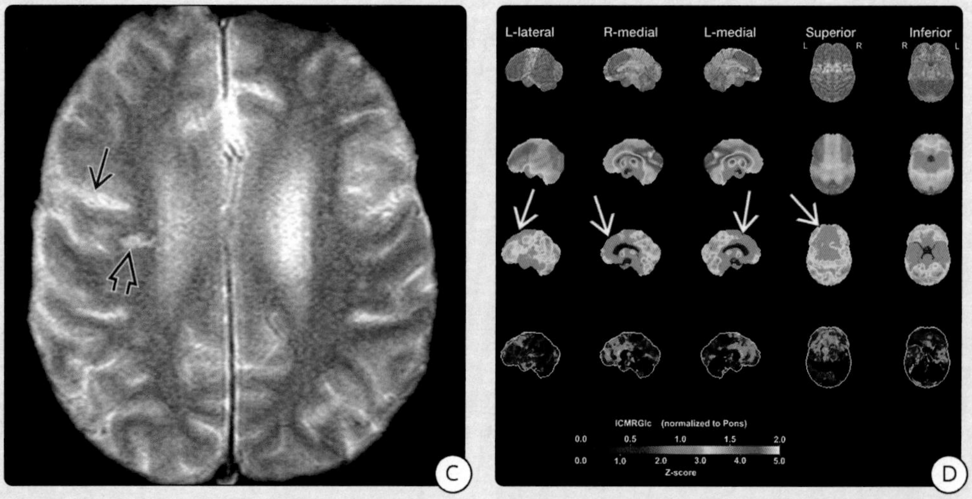

Mood and behavioral changes are more typical than memory loss.

Natural History. Progressive, episodic, stepwise neurologic deterioration interspersed with intervals of relative clinical stabilization is the typical pattern of VaD.

Imaging

General Features. The general imaging features of VaD are those of multifocal infarcts and WM ischemia.

CT Findings. NECT scans often show generalized volume loss with multiple cortical, subcortical, and basal ganglia infarcts. Patchy or confluent hypodensities in the subcortical and deep periventricular WM, especially around the atria of the lateral ventricles, are typical.

MR Findings. T1WI often shows greater than expected generalized volume loss. Multiple hypointensities in the basal ganglia and deep WM are typical. Focal cortical and large territorial infarcts with encephalomalacia can be identified in many cases.

T2/FLAIR scans show multifocal diffuse and confluent hyperintensities in the basal ganglia and cerebral WM. The cortex and subcortical WM are commonly affected **(33-18)**. T2* sequences may demonstrate multiple "blooming" hypointensities in the cortex and along the pial surface of the hemispheres **(33-19)** **(33-20)**.

DTI may demonstrate decreased FA and increased ADC values in otherwise normal-appearing or minimally abnormal WM. Multiple regions are affected, especially the inferior-frontal-occipital fascicles, corpus callosum, and superior longitudinal fasciculus.

Nuclear Medicine. FDG PET shows multiple diffusely distributed areas of hypometabolism, generally without specific lobar predominance **(33-18D)** **(33-19D)**.

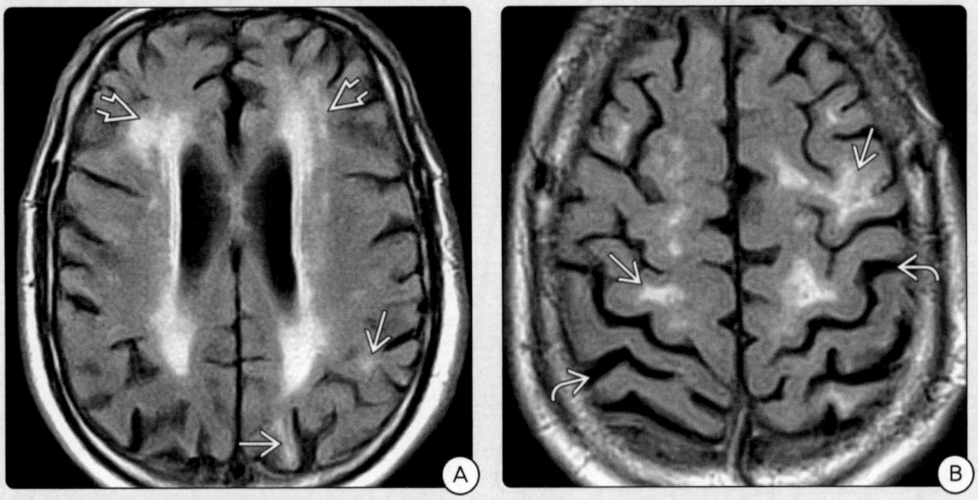

***(33-19A)** FLAIR scan in a 76y normotensive demented man shows multifocal confluent hyperintensities in the subcortical ➡, deep periventricular WM ➡. **(33-19B)** More cephalad FLAIR scan in the same patient shows significant lesion burden in the subcortical WM ➡. Note enlarged parietal sulci ➡.*

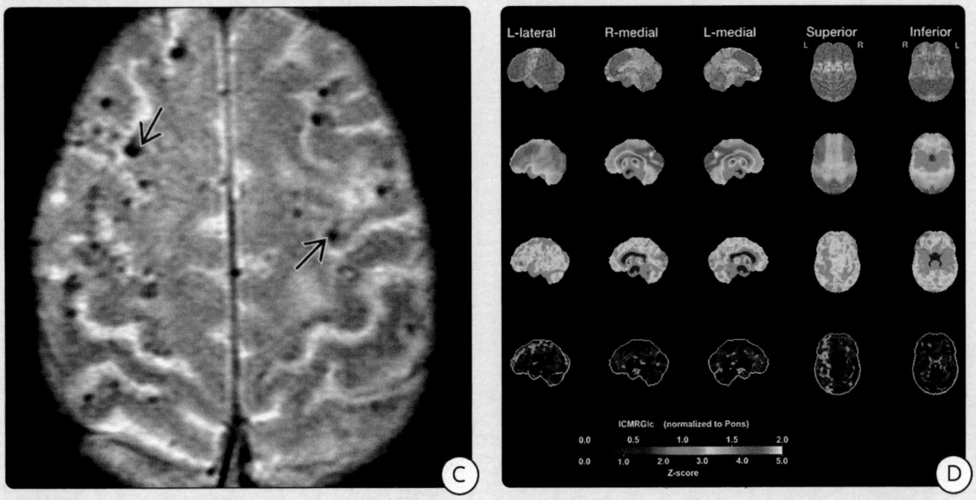

***(33-19C)** T2* GRE scan in the same patient shows multifocal cortical "blooming" hypointensities ➡ characteristic of cerebral amyloid angiopathy. **(33-19D)** PET scan in the same patient shows multifocal areas of decreased glucose metabolism (third row) compared with age-matched normal controls (second row). Z-score map (bottom row) shows the diffuse nature of the lesions seen in VaD. (Courtesy N. Foster, MD.)*

Differential Diagnosis

The major differential diagnosis of VaD is **Alzheimer disease**. The two disorders overlap and often coexist. AD typically shows striking and selective volume loss in the temporal lobes, especially the hippocampi. The basal ganglia are typically spared in AD, whereas they are often affected in VaD.

CADASIL is the most common *inherited* cause of VaD. Onset is typically earlier than in *sporadic* VaD. Anterior temporal and external capsule lesions are highly suggestive of CADASIL.

Frontotemporal lobar degeneration (FTLD) is characterized by early onset of behavior changes, whereas visuospatial skills remain relatively unaffected. Frontotemporal atrophy with knife-like gyri is typical.

VASCULAR DEMENTIA: IMAGING AND DIFFERENTIAL DIAGNOSIS

Imaging
- Varies with subtype
  - Often mixed
- General features
  - Multifocal infarcts (lacunae, cortical > large territorial)
  - WM ischemia (patchy and/or confluent T2/FLAIR hyperintensities)
  - T2* "blooming black dots" (amyloid or HTN)

Differential Diagnosis
- Alzheimer disease
- CADASIL (most common *inherited* VaD)
- FTLD
- Lewy body disease
- Cerebral amyloid angiopathy 7

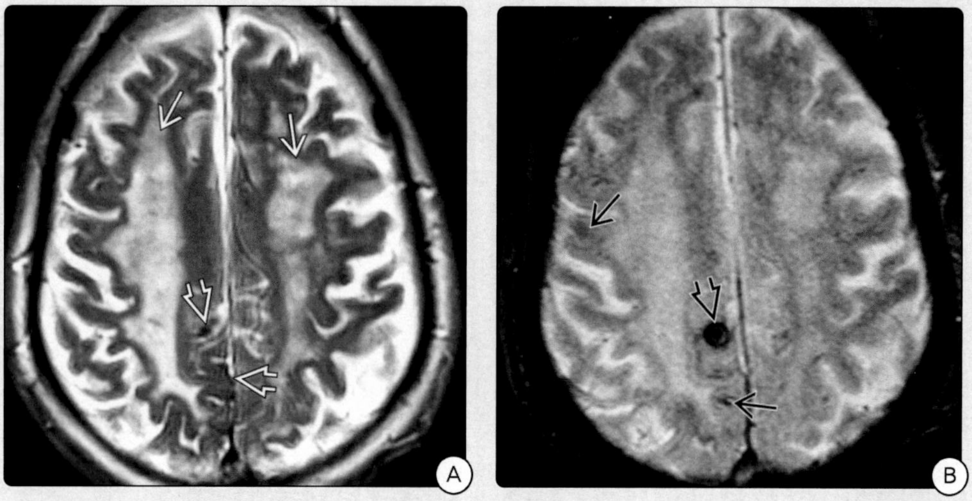

***(33-20A)** Axial T2WI in a 76y woman with a history of multiple strokes and clinical diagnosis of VaD shows generalized volume loss with confluent subcortical WM hyperintensity →. Insensitivity of FSE scans to hemorrhage is demonstrated by this case; only faint hypointensities → can be identified. **(33-20B)** T2* GRE shows a round, focal "blooming" lesion → with several faint linear hypointensities →.*

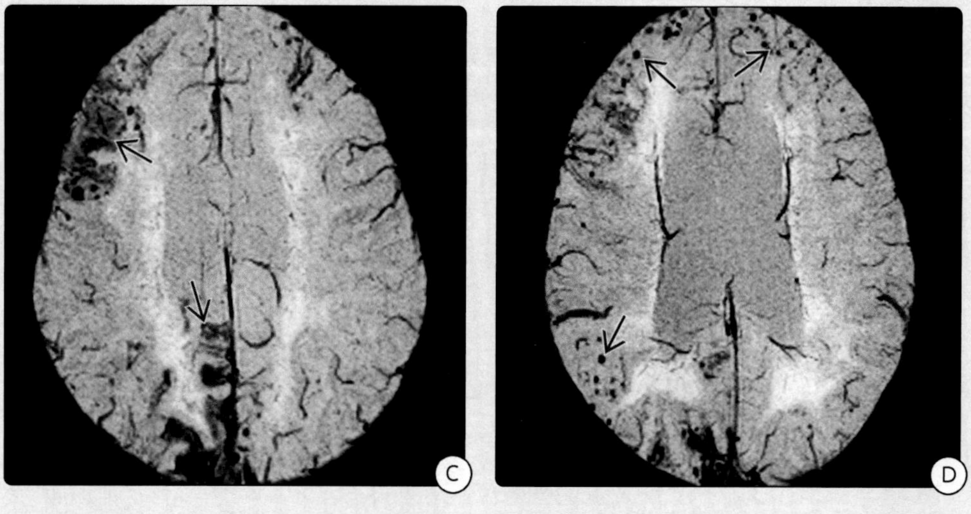

***(33-20C)** T2* SWI sequence in the same patient shows much more extensive confluent cortical and pial hypointensities →. **(33-20D)** Lower T2* SWI scan shows multiple tiny cortical "black dots" → characteristic of amyloid angiopathy, the underlying cause of this patient's vascular dementia. T2* sequences should be an integral part of all MR protocols in patients with dementia.*

Dementia with Lewy bodies (DLB) may be difficult to distinguish from VaD without biopsy. The entire brain is hypometabolic, and atrophy is generally minimal or absent. DLB typically occurs without infarcts.

Cerebral amyloid angiopathy commonly coexists with both AD and VaD and may be indistinguishable without biopsy.

Frontotemporal Lobar Degeneration

Terminology

Frontotemporal lobar degeneration (FTLD) is a clinically, pathologically, and genetically heterogeneous group of disorders—sometimes called frontotemporal dementias (FTDs)—that principally affect the frontal and temporal lobes.

FTLD is a "disorder of threes." There are three main genetic mutations, three principal histologies, and three major associated clinical syndromes. All three can exist separately or in combination with amyotrophic lateral sclerosis (ALS, see below). The FTLD spectrum also includes Parkinson disease with dementia.

Etiology

Genetics. Mutations in three major genes, *MAPT*, *GRN*, and *C9orf72*, along with several other less common gene mutations account for most cases of FTLD. Approximately 10% of cases are caused by mutations in the microtubule-associated protein tau gene (*MAPT*), whereas another 10% have mutations in the progranulin gene (*GRN*).

Tau protein—the product of *MAPT*—is responsible for the assembly/disassembly of microtubules, vital for intracellular transport. Mutations in *MAPT* drive FTLD-tau pathology. These mutations lead to abnormal tau accumulations in neurons and/or glia known as Pick bodies.

FTLD-TDP pathology is associated with either mutations in *GRN* or expansions in *C9orf72*. The semantic dementia variant of FTLD and ALS are both TDP-43 proteinopathies. A key characteristic of both is the presence of TDP-43 or the protein fused in sarcoma (FUS) immunoreactive cytoplasmic inclusions in neuronal and glial cells. TDP-43 and FUS are nuclear carrier proteins involved in the regulation of reactive nitrogen species metabolism.

Pathology

Gross Pathology. FTLDs are characterized by severe frontotemporal atrophy with neuronal loss, gliosis, and spongiosis of the superficial cortical layers **(33-21)**. The affected gyri are thinned and narrowed, causing the typical appearance of knife-like gyri. The posterior brain regions, especially the occipital poles, are relatively spared until very late in the disease process **(33-22)**.

Microscopic Features. The three principal FTLD histologies are characterized by abnormal neuronal (and sometimes glial) accumulations of aggregated proteins. These are (1) tau, (2) TDP-43, and (3) FUS proteins.

In approximately 45% of cases, the neuronal intracytoplasmic inclusions are composed of the microtubule-associated protein, tau, and termed **FTLD-tau**. In most cases the neuronal tau occurs as either Pick bodies (round or oval silver-staining inclusions) or neurofibrillary tangle-like structures. Pick bodies are most commonly found in the dentate gyrus, amygdala, and frontal and temporal neocortex.

In about 50% of FTLD cases, the RNA- and DNA-binding protein TDP-43 is present in dystrophic neurites. These cases are termed **FTLD-TDP**.

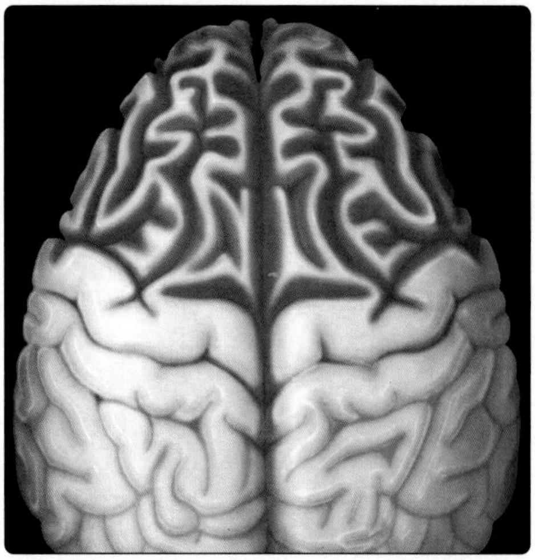

***(33-21)** Graphic shows frontal atrophy in late-stage FTLD with "knife-like" gyri. Parietooccipital lobes are spared.*

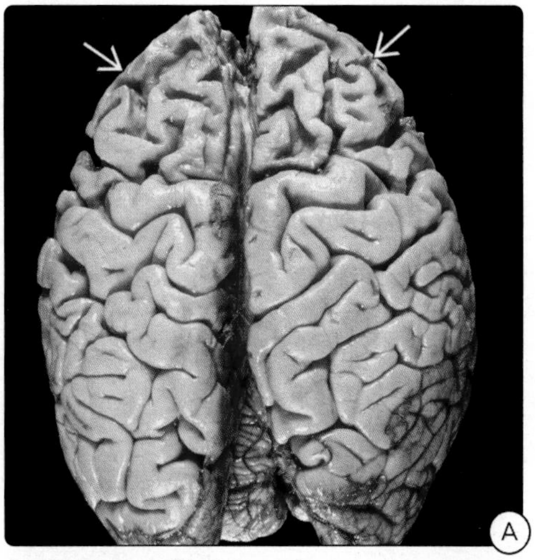

***(33-22A)** Autopsy of FTLD shows striking atrophy of the frontal gyri ➡ and normal-appearing parietal and occipital lobes.*

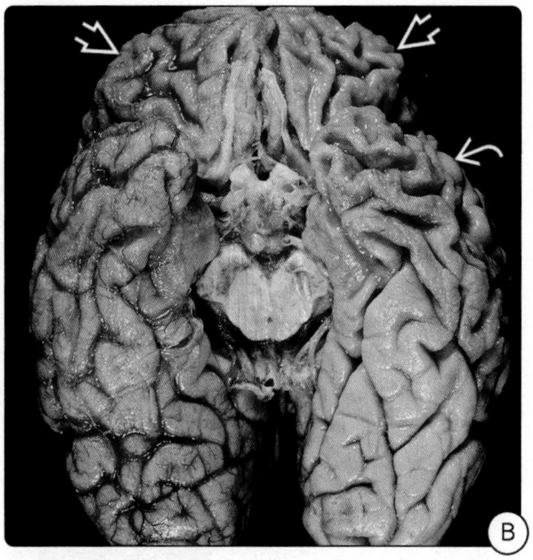

***(33-22B)** Submentovertex view in the same case shows striking frontal ➡ and temporal lobe atrophy ➡. (Courtesy R. Hewlett, MD.)*

The remaining 5% of cases show inclusions composed of the protein FUS. These cases are described as **FTLD-FUS**. In a very small minority of cases no inclusions are seen.

Clinical Issues

Epidemiology and Demographics. FTLD is the second most common cause of "presenile dementia," accounting for 20% of all cases in patients under the age of 65 years. FTLD occurs between the third and ninth decades, but the average age at disease onset is typically around 60 years, younger than seen in AD and other neurodegenerative disorders.

Excluding alcoholic encephalopathy, FTLD is the third most common overall cause of dementia (after AD and VaD), constituting 10-25% of all dementia cases. The estimated prevalence varies between 5 and 15 cases/100,000. Up to 40% of patients have a history of a similar disorder within their families. An autosomal-dominant pattern of inheritance is seen in 10% of cases.

Presentation. Three different *clinical* subtypes of FTLD are recognized. The most common is **behavioral-variant frontotemporal dementia** (bvFTD), which accounts for more than half of all cases. Core behavioral features of bvFTD are personality changes and social disinhibition. In contrast to AD, visuospatial functions are initially well preserved.

A second, less common syndrome is **semantic dementia** (SD), a disorder of conceptual knowledge. Patients with SD exhibit behavioral changes and difficulties with language comprehension while speech itself remains relatively fluent.

The third clinical syndrome is termed **progressive nonfluent aphasia** (PNFA). PNFA is a disorder of expressive language associated with asymmetric atrophy of the left hemisphere.

There is a clinical overlap between bvFTD and progressive supranuclear palsy and corticobasal syndrome.

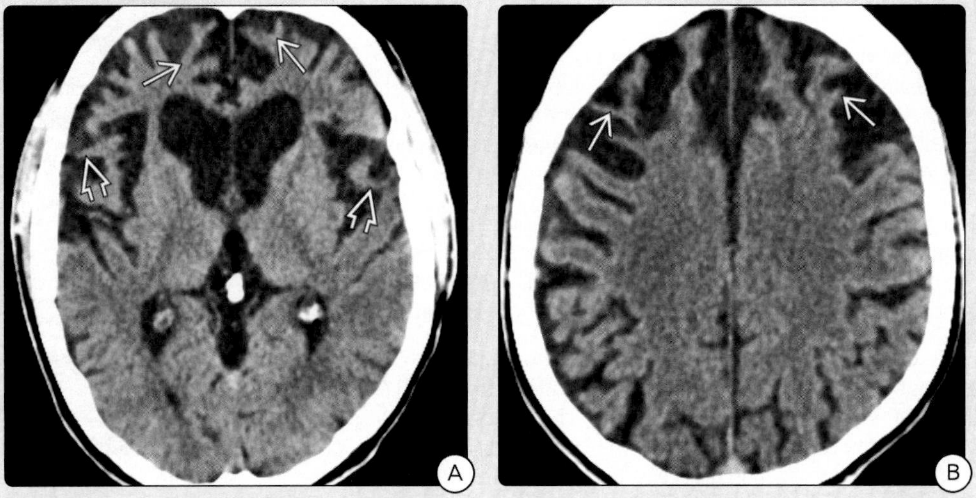

***(33-23A)** NECT scan in a 59y man with FTLD shows striking frontal atrophy with knife-like gyri ➡. Note temporal lobe atrophy ➡ with markedly enlarged sylvian fissures. The parietal and occipital lobes appear normal. **(33-23B)** More cephalad scan in the same patient shows the frontal-predominant atrophy ➡ especially well. The parietal sulci are also moderately prominent for a patient of this age.*

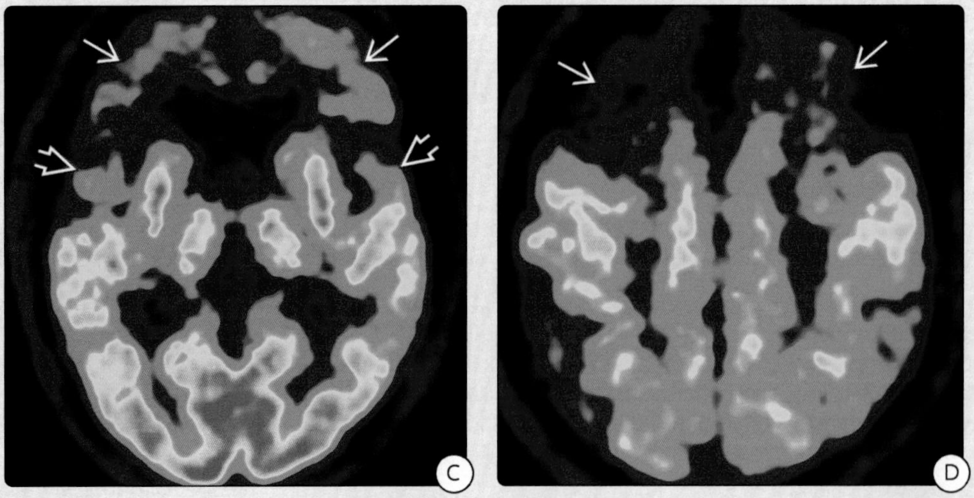

***(33-23C)** FDG PET in the same patient shows markedly decreased glucose metabolism in both frontal lobes ➡. The temporal lobes ➡ are somewhat less severely affected. The occipital lobes both appear normal. **(33-23D)** More cephalad scan in the same patient shows striking frontal hypometabolism ➡, but the parietal lobes also show moderately reduced glucose utilization.*

The correlation between histopathology and clinical syndromes varies. bvFTD is histopathologically heterogeneous, whereas SD is usually associated with TDP pathology and PNFA with tau pathology.

Natural History. Median survival for patients with FTLD is 6-11 years following symptom onset.

Imaging

General Features. Neuroimaging features of the FTDs should be assessed according to whether they produce focal temporal or extratemporal (e.g., frontal) atrophy, whether the pattern is relatively symmetric or strongly asymmetric, and which side (left versus right) is most severely affected.

CT Findings. Abnormalities on CT represent late-stage FTLD. Severe symmetric atrophy of the frontal lobes with lesser volume loss in the temporal lobes is the most common finding **(33-23)**.

MR Findings. Whereas standard T1 scans may show generalized frontotemporal volume loss, voxel-based morphometry can discriminate between various *pathologic* subtypes. FTLD-tau is associated with strongly asymmetric atrophy involving the temporal and/or extratemporal (i.e., frontal) regions. FTLD-TDP disease shows asymmetric, relatively localized temporal lobe atrophy.

Clinical FTLD subtypes also correlate with frontal-versus-temporal and left-versus-right atrophy predominance. The SD subtype shows bilateral temporal volume loss but little or no frontal atrophy **(33-24)**. bvFTD and PNFA both demonstrate bilateral frontal and temporal volume loss, but the right hemisphere is most affected in bvFTD, whereas left-sided volume loss dominates in PNFA.

WM damage also occurs in FTLD and is probably secondary to damage in the overlying cortex. DWI shows elevated mean diffusivity in the superior frontal gyri, orbitofrontal gyri, and anterior temporal lobes.

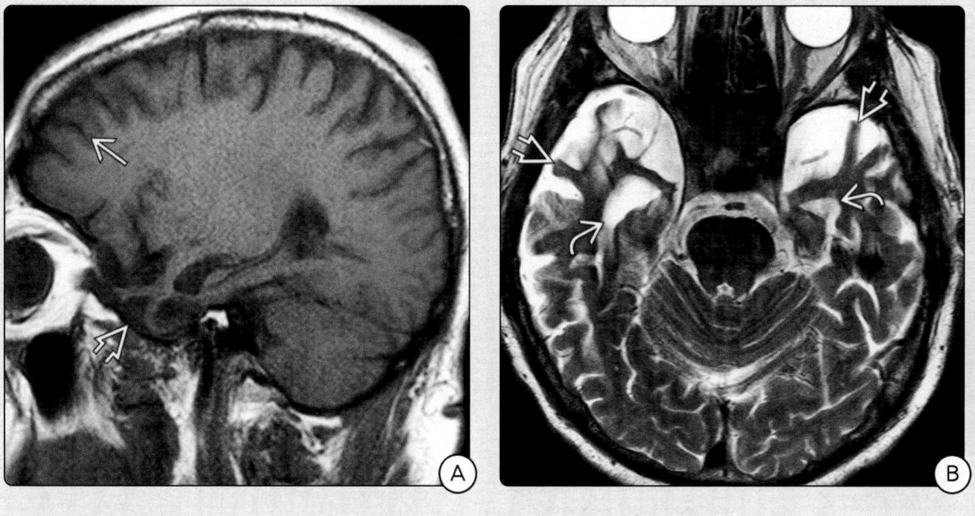

***(33-24A)** Series of images in a 63y man with FTLD shows the utility of detailing cerebral atrophy patterns. Note striking temporal lobe volume loss ➡ with relatively well-preserved frontal gyri ➡. **(33-24B)** Axial T2WI in the same patient shows striking, relatively symmetric temporal lobe atrophy with knife-like gyri ➡ and markedly enlarged temporal horns of the lateral ventricles ➡.*

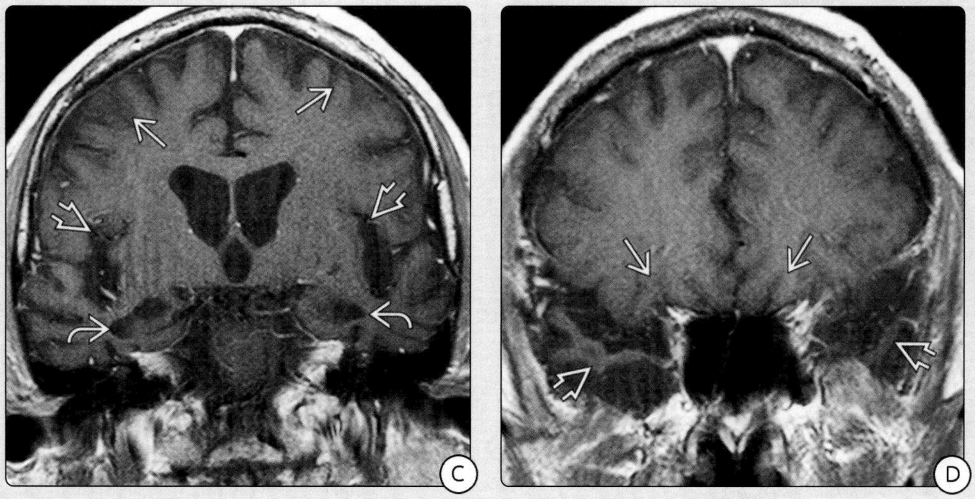

***(33-24C)** Coronal T1 C+ scan in the same patient shows symmetrically enlarged sylvian fissures ➡ and temporal horns ➡, indicating temporal lobe volume loss. The posterior frontal gyri ➡ appear normal. **(33-24D)** More anterior coronal scan shows shrunken, knife-like temporal lobe gyri ➡ and normal frontal gyri ➡. The relatively symmetric, predominantly temporal lobe atrophy is most consistent with the SD FTLD subtype.*

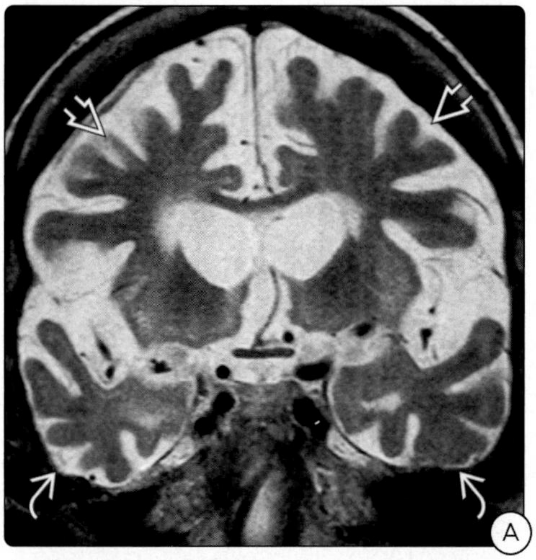

(33-25A) *Coronal T2WI in a 64y woman with FTLD shows severe volume loss, especially in the frontal and temporal lobes.*

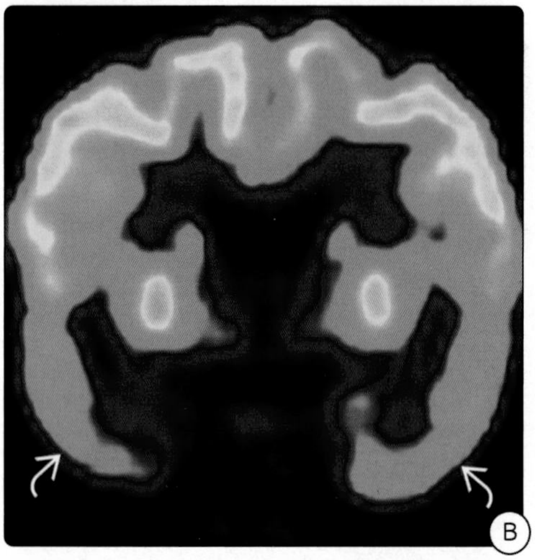

(33-25B) *Coronal FDG PET-CT shows severe hypometabolism in both temporal lobes.*

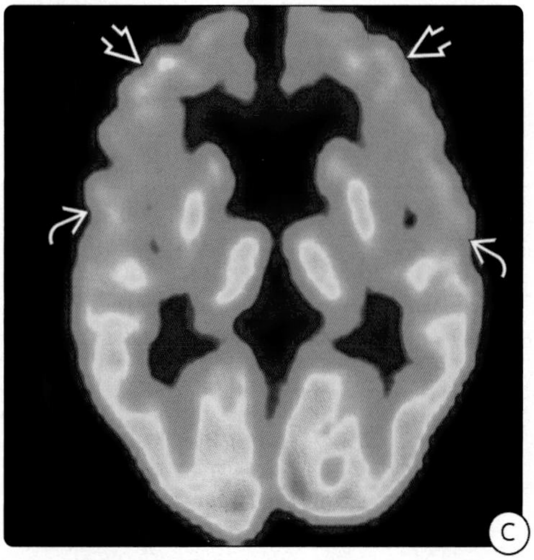

(33-25C) *Axial FDG PET-CT shows hypometabolism in both frontal and temporal lobes characteristic of FTLD.*

DTI with reduced FA in the superior longitudinal fasciculus is common in bvFTD and correlates with behavior disturbances, whereas the inferior longitudinal fasciculus is more affected in the SD variant. MRS shows decreased NAA and elevated myoinositol in the frontal lobes.

Nuclear Medicine Findings. FDG PET scans show hypoperfusion and hypometabolism in the frontal and temporal lobes **(33-25)**.

Differential Diagnosis. The major differential diagnoses of FTLD are AD (parietal lobe, hippocampi more than frontal) and VaD (WM, basal ganglia lacunae).

FRONTOTEMPORAL LOBAR DEGENERATION

Etiology
- Three major mutations
  - *MAPT*
  - *GRN*
  - *C9orf72*

Pathology
- Three major types
  - FTLD-tau (45%)
  - FTLD-TDP (50%)
  - FTLD-FUS (5%)

Clinical Issues
- Second most common cause of "presenile" dementia
- Accounts for 20% of all cases < 65 years of age
- Three major subtypes
  - Behavioral variant (bvFTD)
  - Semantic dementia (SD)
  - Progressive nonfluent aphasia (PNFA)

Imaging
- Classify atrophy (volumetric MR best)
  - Temporal vs. extratemporal (frontal) predominance
  - Symmetric or asymmetric
- 18F FDG PET
  - Frontotemporal hypometabolism

Differential Diagnosis
- Alzheimer disease
  - Parietal, temporal > frontotemporal
- Vascular dementia
  - Multifocal infarcts
  - WM ischemic changes

Lewy Body Dementias

Lewy body dementias include **dementia with Lewy bodies** (DLB), **Parkinson disease dementia** (PDD), and the **Lewy body variant** (LBV) **of Alzheimer disease** (LBAD). All three diseases have significant clinicopathologic overlap.

Terminology

Lewy body dementias are characterized by the presence of Lewy bodies (see below).

Etiology

Lewy bodies are spherical intraneuronal protein aggregates that consist primarily of α-synuclein (α-syn), a presynaptic microtubule-associated misfolded protein similar to tau. DLB is therefore considered a **synucleinopathy** and belongs to a group of disorders with α-synuclein gene mutations that also includes Parkinson disease, PDD, multisystem atrophy, pure autonomic failure, and REM sleep behavior disorder.

Pathology

Gross Pathology. The gross appearance of DLB resembles early AD. Frontotemporal and parietal atrophy is generally mild to moderate, whereas the hippocampi and occipital lobes are typically spared **(33-26)**. There is marked depigmentation of the substantia nigra and locus ceruleus.

Microscopic Features. The histopathologic hallmark of DLB is the presence of Lewy body inclusions in the cortex and brainstem, especially the substantia nigra and dorsal mesopontine GM. Loss of tegmental dopamine and basal forebrain cholinergic cell populations is typical.

Some pathologic hallmarks of AD, namely amyloid plaques and neurofibrillary tangles, can be found in many patients with DLB. In turn, Lewy body inclusions have also been identified in some Alzheimer patients (LBAD).

Clinical Issues

Epidemiology and Demographics. DLB is now recognized as the second most common neurodegenerative dementia, accounting for approximately 15-20% of all cases.

Presentation and Diagnosis. Because DLB symptoms can resemble other more commonly recognized dementias (AD, PDD), it is widely underrecognized as a cause of progressive cognitive decline and is often diagnosed only at autopsy.

Three core diagnostic features of DLB have been defined: (1) recurrent visual hallucinations and visuospatial disturbances, (2) spontaneous parkinsonism, and (3) fluctuating cognition with variations in attention, executive function, and alertness. The presence of two of these three features is considered evidence of probable DLB.

Natural History. Patients with pure DLB have annual rates of atrophy and ventricular enlargement that are comparable to those of age-matched controls and less marked than those of patients with AD.

Imaging

General Features. The most commonly used neuroimaging technique for the diagnosis of LBD is dopaminergic imaging of the basal ganglia with a sensitivity of 87% and specificity of 94% for differentiating between LBD and other dementia types such as PDD.

Despite the prominent visual symptoms that often characterize DLB, major occipital volume loss is not a typical finding. Standard anatomic imaging studies are often normal or show only mild generalized volume loss.

MR Findings. T1 scans show only mild generalized atrophy without lobar predominance **(33-27)**. T2/FLAIR may demonstrate nonspecific WM hyperintensities that are similar to those found in cognitively normal aging patients.

Manual and automated volumetric studies generally show relatively little cortical atrophy. Reduced volume in the hypothalamus, basal forebrain, and midbrain may be seen in some severe cases. There is usually more putaminal and relatively less medial temporal lobe atrophy in DLB compared with AD.

DTI demonstrates increased mean diffusivity in the amygdala and decreased FA in the inferior longitudinal and inferior occipitofrontal fasciculi. MRS shows relatively normal NAA:Cr ratios.

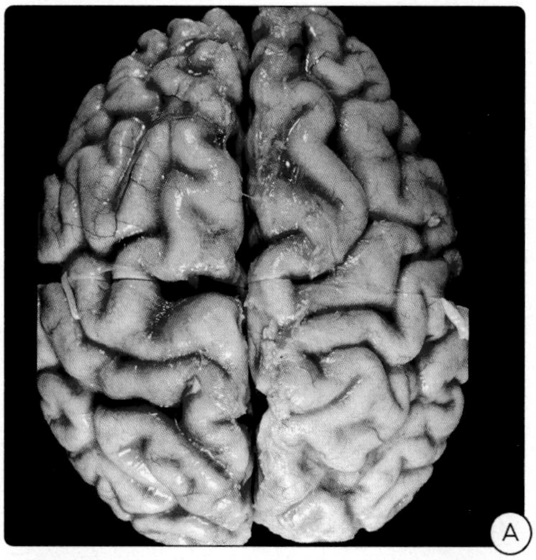

***(33-26A)** Autopsy case of dementia with diffuse Lewy bodies shows mild generalized volume loss without specific lobar predominance.*

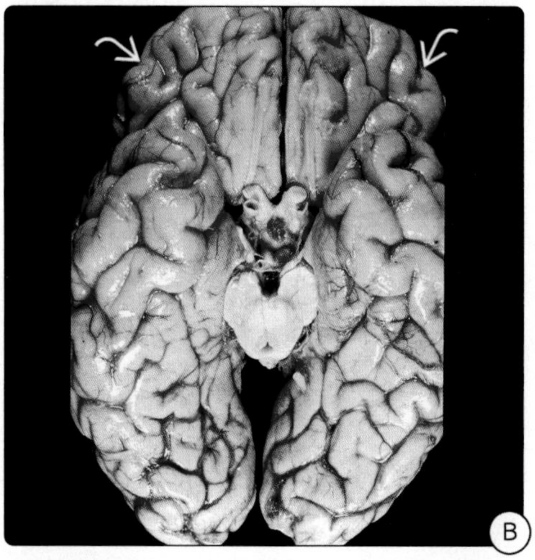

***(33-26B)** Submentovertex view in the same case shows mild frontal volume loss ➘. The temporal lobes appear normal.*

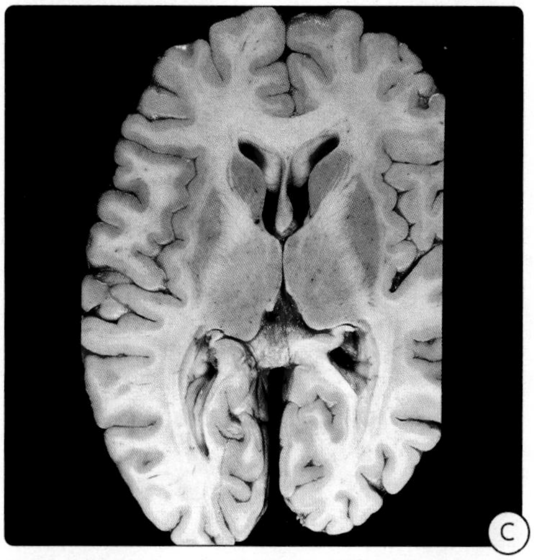

***(33-26C)** Axial section shows mildly enlarged lateral ventricles, normal occipital lobes; diffuse Lewy body disease. (Courtesy R. Hewlett, MD.)*

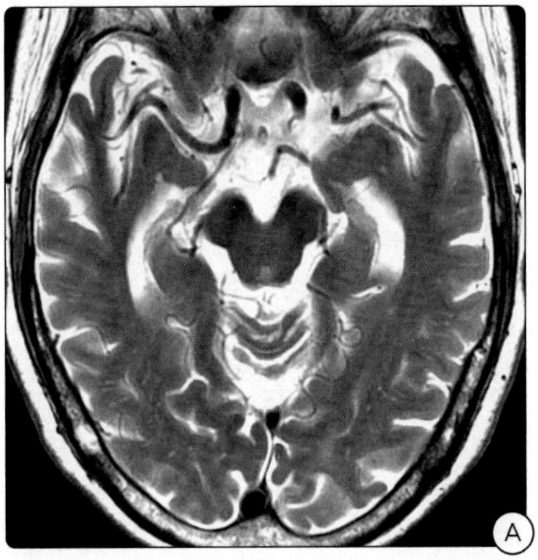

***(33-27A)** T2WI in a patient with cognitive decline and visual hallucinations shows mild diffuse atrophy. Occipital lobes appear relatively normal.*

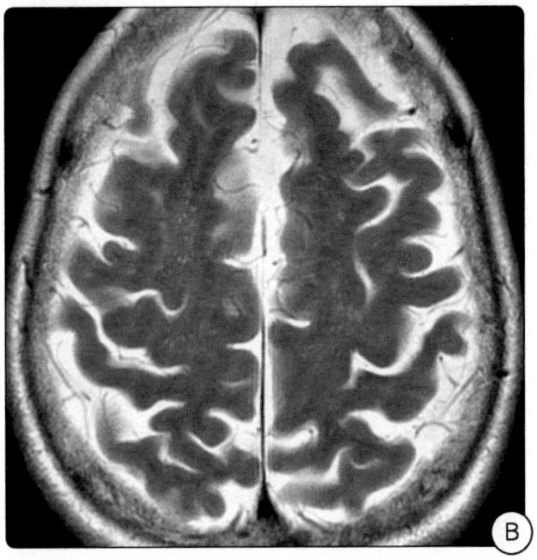

***(33-27B)** More cephalad scan in the same patient shows mild symmetric and diffuse volume loss. Clinical diagnosis was probable DLB.*

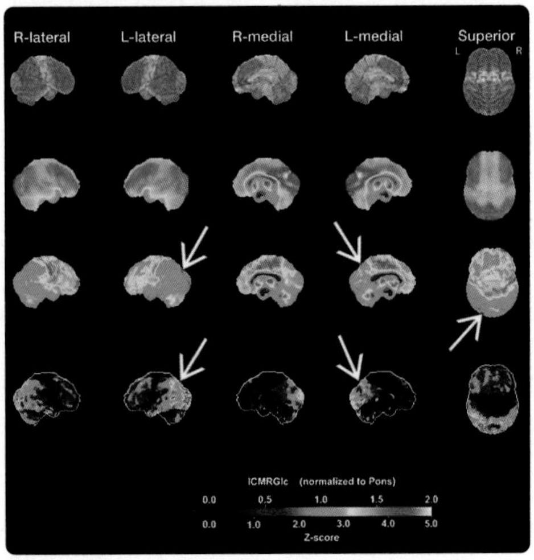

***(33-28)** FDG PET scan in another patient with DLB shows occipital hypometabolism ➡. (Courtesy N. Foster, MD.)*

Nuclear Medicine. Occipital hypometabolism on FDG PET and reduced cerebral blood flow on SPECT-HMPAO or pMR are typical of DLB **(33-28)**. The primary visual cortex is especially affected.

Presynaptic dopamine transporter (DaT) imaging with the FP-CIT ligand shows almost absent uptake in the putamen and markedly reduced uptake in the caudate. Cholinergic radioligands may help identify the profound cholinergic neuronal loss that occurs in DLB and PDD.

Differential Diagnosis

The major differential diagnosis of DLB is **Parkinson disease with dementia (PDD)**. The second most important differential diagnosis is **Alzheimer disease (AD)**. Hippocampal hypometabolism and volume loss are more common in AD. **Multiple system atrophy** and the parkinsonian tauopathies **progressive supranuclear palsy** and **corticobasal degeneration** can be difficult to distinguish from DLB. **Posterior cortical atrophy** (see below) can mimic DLB clinically but generally occurs in younger patients.

LEWY BODY DEMENTIAS

Etiology

- α-synuclein mutation
- Others = Parkinson disease dementia, AD (variant with Lewy bodies), multisystem atrophy

Pathology

- Lewy bodies with α-synuclein inclusions
- Striatonigral degeneration
- Tegmental dopamine, basal forebrain cholinergic cells seriously reduced
  - Substantia nigra depigmented

Clinical Issues

- 2nd most common neurodegenerative dementia
- Visual symptoms, spontaneous parkinsonism, cognition reduced

Imaging

- MR nonspecific (mild generalized atrophy)
- SPECT dopaminergic imaging best
  - DaT scan shows sharply reduced uptake putamen, caudate

Differential Diagnosis

- Other dementias with parkinsonism (e.g., PDD, multisystem atrophy)
- Alzheimer disease (Lewy body variant)

Miscellaneous Dementias

Creutzfeldt-Jakob Disease

Transmissible spongiform encephalopathies (TSEs), also known as **prion diseases**, are a group of neurodegenerative disorders that includes **Creutzfeldt-Jakob disease** (CJD), **kuru**, **Gerstmann-Sträussler-Schenker** syndrome, and **fatal familial insomnia**. Animal TSEs include scrapie (from sheep and goats), chronic wasting disease (from mule deer and elk), bovine spongiform encephalopathy ("mad cow disease"), and feline encephalopathy (from domestic cats).

Kuru was the first recognized human TSE, occurring in the Fore population of Papua New Guinea. Kuru is a uniformly fatal cerebellar ataxic syndrome; it has now almost disappeared with the discontinuation of cannibalism, the only source of human-to-human transmission.

CJD is the most common human TSE and has a worldwide distribution. CJD is unique, as it is both an infectious and neurogenetic dementing disorder. CJD is the archetypal human TSE and is detailed in the following discussion.

Etiology. CJD is a rapidly progressive neurodegenerative disorder caused by proteinaceous infectious particles ("prions") that are devoid of DNA and RNA. The abnormal prion protein, PrP(Sc), is a misfolded isoform (a β-pleated sheet) of the normal host prion protein, PrP(C). The abnormal form propagates itself by recruiting the normal isoform and imposing its conformation on the homologous host cell protein. *The conformational conversion of PrP(C) to PrP(Sc) is the fundamental event underlying all prion diseases.*

Four types of CJD are recognized: **sporadic** (sCJD), **familial** or **genetic** (gCJD), **iatrogenic** (iCJD), and **variant** (vCJD). sCJD is the most common type. gCJD is caused by diverse mutations in the *PRNP* gene. iCJD is caused by prion-contaminated materials (e.g., surgical instruments, dura mater grafts, cadaveric corneal transplants, and pituitary-derived human growth hormone). vCJD typically results from the transmission of bovine spongiform encephalopathy from cattle to humans. vCJD is also known as "new variant" CJD.

Pathology. Gross pathology shows ventricular enlargement, caudate atrophy, and cortical volume loss that varies from minimal to striking **(33-29)**. The white matter is relatively spared.

The classic triad of histopathologic findings in CJD is marked neuronal loss, spongiform change, and striking astrogliosis. The cerebral and cerebellar cortex are often most severely affected although the basal ganglia and thalami are also frequently involved. Amyloid plaques can be identified in 10% of cases.

Various deposits of PrP(Sc) are present, and PrP(Sc) immunoreactivity is the gold standard for the neuropathologic diagnosis of human prion diseases.

HUMAN PRION DISEASES

Sporadic (Idiopathic) Prion Diseases (85%)
- sCJD
- Sporadic fatal insomnia, variably protease-sensitive prionopathy

Acquired (Infectious) Prion Diseases (2-5%)
- iCJD (due to medical interventions)
- Kuru
- vCJD

Familial (Inherited/Genetic) Prion Diseases (5-15%)
- iCJD
- Gerstmann-Sträussler-Scheinker syndrome
- Fatal familial insomnia

Epidemiology and Demographics. CJD now accounts for more than 90% of all human prion diseases. Approximately 85% of CJD cases are sporadic (sCJD) with an annual worldwide incidence of one to two cases per million. Peak age of onset is 55-75 years. There is no sex predilection. gCJD causes most of the remaining cases (5-15%). vCJD and iCJD together now account for less than 5%.

vCJD typically presents in younger patients between 15 and 40 years. Psychiatric symptoms predominate. Approximately 220 vCJD cases have been reported with most—but not all—occurring in the United Kingdom. The incidence of vCJD has declined in recent years, but small numbers of new cases are still identified.

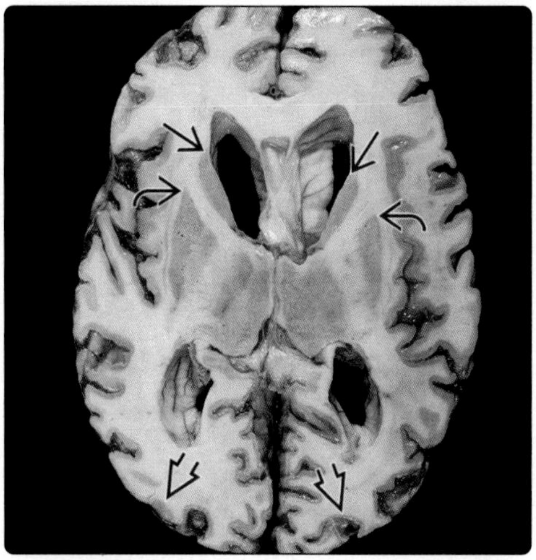

***(33-29)** sCJD shows caudate ➙, anterior basal ganglia atrophy ➙, cortical thinning especially in the occipital lobes ➙. (Courtesy R. Hewlett, MD.)*

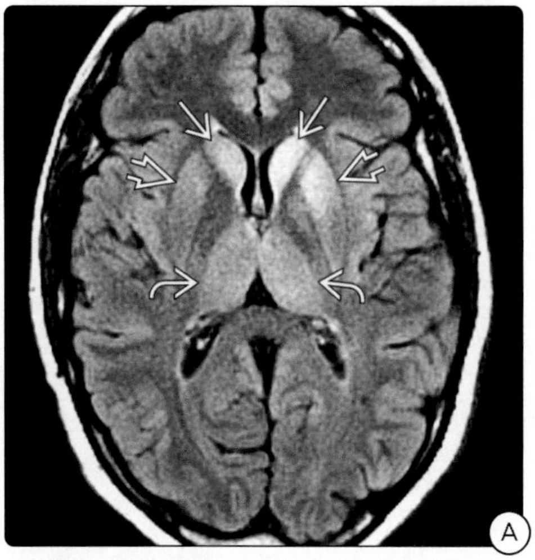

***(33-30A)** Axial FLAIR shows classic findings of sCJD with hyperintense caudate nuclei ➙, anterior putamina ➙, and thalami ➙.*

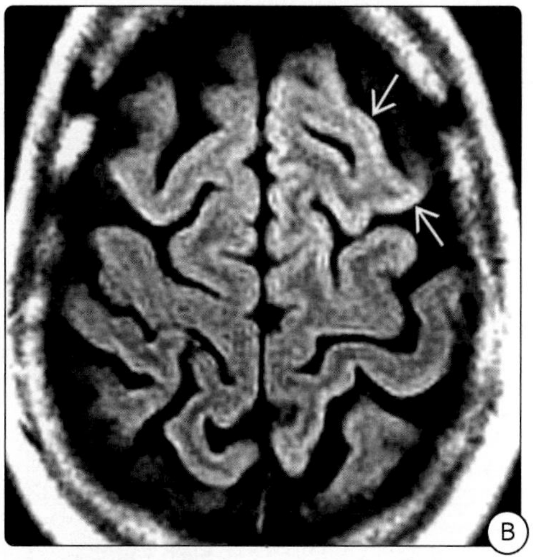

***(33-30B)** More cephalad FLAIR shows subtle hyperintensity in the left frontal cortex ➙. This is autopsy-proven sCJD.*

Clinical Issues. CJD is a progressive, fatal illness. Over 90% of patients progress from normal function to death in under a year. Median survival is approximately 4 months, although vCJD progresses more slowly.

The diagnosis of CJD is complex and is often based on the exclusion of other, more frequent causes of rapidly progressive dementia. The definitive diagnosis of sCJD requires autopsy or brain biopsy.

The current WHO guidelines for the antemortem diagnosis of sCJD use a combination of clinical manifestations, EEG, and a laboratory measure of CSF 14-3-3. More recent criteria such as the European MRI-CJD Consortium include imaging manifestations in the diagnosis of probable CJD.

Five clinicopathologic subtypes of sCJD have been identified. Three subtypes prominently affect cognitive functions, and the other two impair cerebellar motor activities. In the most common subtype, rapidly worsening dementia is followed by myoclonic jerks and akinetic mutism. In two-thirds of sCJD cases, EEG shows a characteristic pattern of periodic bi- or triphasic complexes.

Two less common but important presentations of sCJD are the so-called **Brownell-Oppenheimer variant** (a pure cerebellar syndrome) and the **Heidenhain variant** (pure visual impairment leading to cortical blindness).

Imaging. CJD primarily involves the gray matter structures of the brain. The cerebral cortex, hippocampus, basal ganglia, thalami, and the cerebellum are the most frequently affected areas. WM disease is much less common and is usually a late finding.

CT scans are typically normal although serial studies may show progressive ventricular dilatation and sulcal enlargement.

MR with DWI is the imaging procedure of choice. T1 scans are often normal but may show faint hyperintensities in the

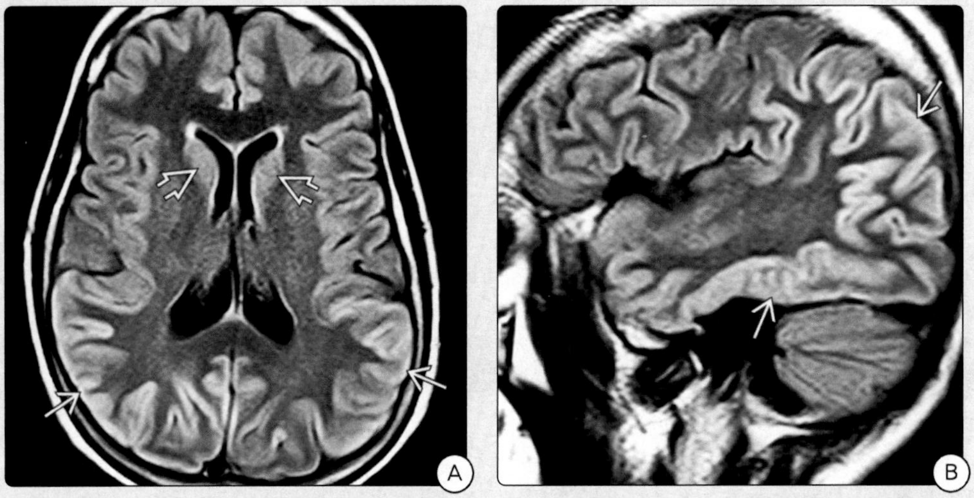

***(33-31A)** Series of images demonstrates classic findings of the Heidenhain variant of sCJD. Axial FLAIR scan shows bilateral cortical hyperintensity in both occipital lobes ➡. Although the anterior caudate nuclei ➡ appear mildly hyperintense, the basal ganglia are generally spared. **(33-31B)** Sagittal FLAIR scan demonstrates occipital, posterior temporal hyperintensity ➡. The frontal and anterior parietal lobes are spared.*

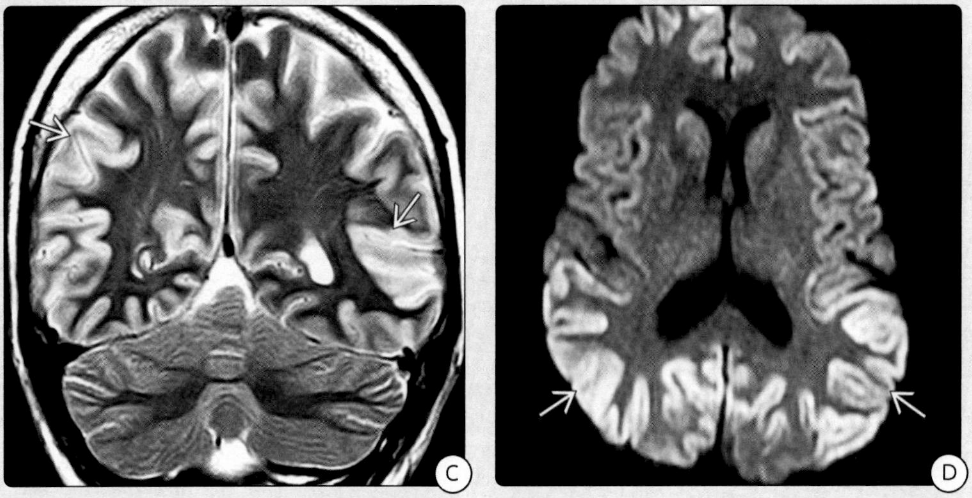

***(33-31C)** Coronal T2WI in the same patient shows striking hyperintensity in both occipital cortices ➡. **(33-31D)** DWI shows striking diffusion restriction in the cortex ("cortical ribboning") of both occipital lobes ➡. The underlying WM is spared. This is sCJD.*

posterior thalami **(33-33)**. FLAIR hyperintensity or restricted diffusion in the caudate nucleus and putamen or in at least two cortical regions (temporal-parietal-occipital "cortical ribboning") are considered highly sensitive and specific (96% and 93%, respectively) for the diagnosis of sCJD **(33-30)**. Occipital lobe involvement predominates in the Heidenhain variant **(33-31)**, whereas the cerebellum is primarily affected in the Brownell-Oppenheimer variant.

T2/FLAIR hyperintensity in the posterior thalamus ("pulvinar" sign) or posteromedial thalamus ("hockey stick" sign) is seen in 90% of vCJD cases but can also occur in sCJD **(33-32)**. CJD does not enhance on T1 C+.

Differential Diagnosis. CJD must be distinguished from other causes of rapidly progressive dementia, such as **viral encephalitis, paraneoplastic limbic encephalitis**, and the recently characterized **autoimmune-mediated inflammatory disorders,** such as voltage-gated K-channel, NMDAR, or GABA encephalopathies. These CJD "mimics" can usually be excluded with appropriate serologic examination.

Common disorders with rare presentations that can mimic CJD include **hypoxic-ischemic encephalopathy**, liver failure with **hepatic encephalopathy, Wernicke encephalopathy, hypoglycemia**, and thyroid dysfunction (**Hashimoto encephalopathy**).

Other dementias such as **Alzheimer disease** and **frontotemporal lobar degeneration** are more insidiously progressive. The basal ganglia involvement in CJD is a helpful differentiating feature. Unlike most dementing diseases, CJD also shows striking diffusion restriction.

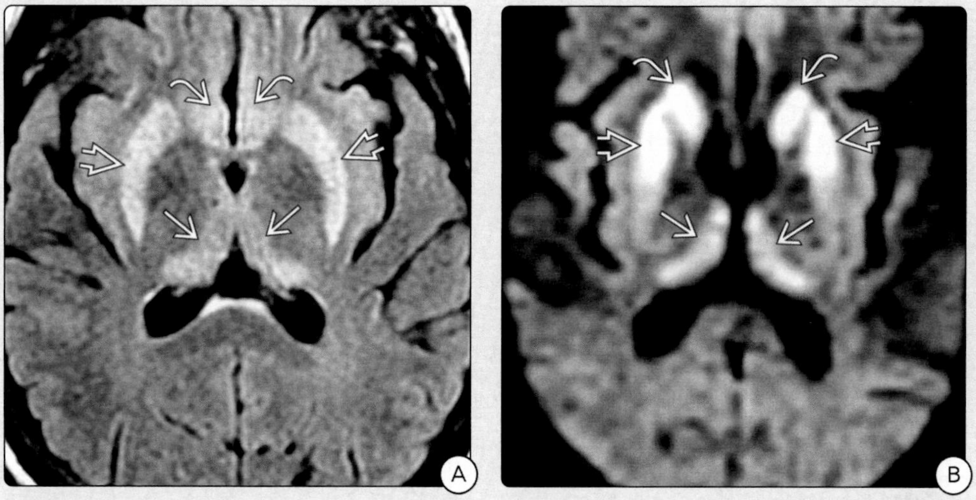

(33-32A) Axial FLAIR in a patient with sCJD shows the classic "hockey stick" sign in the posteromedial thalami ➡. The anterior caudate nuclei ➡ and both putamina ➡ are also involved. (33-32B) DWI in the same patient with sCJD shows corresponding strong diffusion restriction in the posteromedial thalami ➡, caudate nuclei ➡, and putamina ➡.

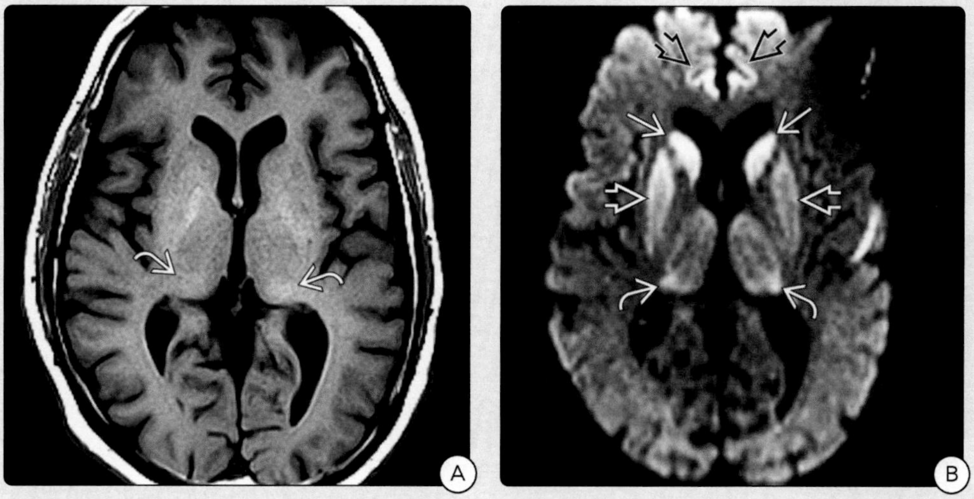

(33-33A) Axial T1WI in a 64y man with biopsy-proven sCJF shows faint hyperintensities ➡ in the pulvinars of both thalami. (33-33B) DWI in the same case shows symmetric, strongly restricted diffusion in the thalami ➡, putamina ➡, caudate nuclei ➡, and frontal lobe cortex ➡.

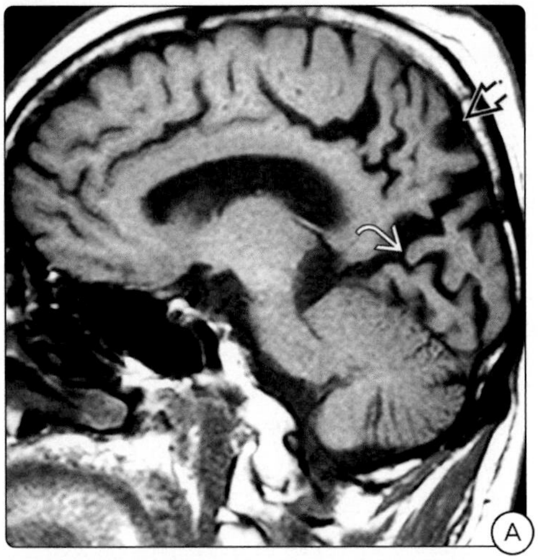

(33-34A) Sagittal T1WI in a 64y woman with visual agnosia, left cortical blindness shows striking atrophy of parietal , occipital lobes.

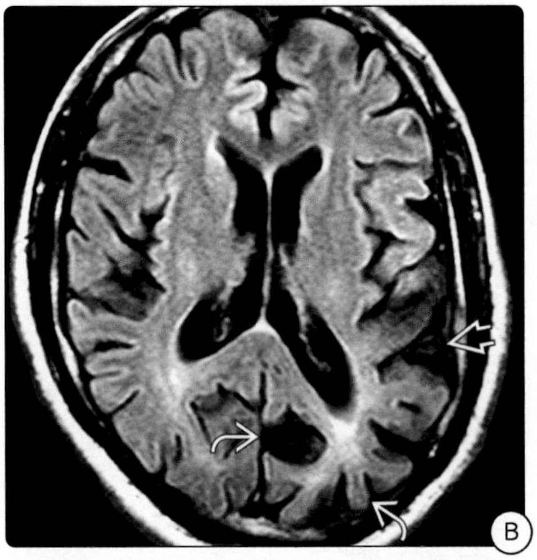

(33-34B) Axial FLAIR shows normal frontal lobes, atrophic left parietal , occipital lobes characteristic of posterior cortical atrophy.

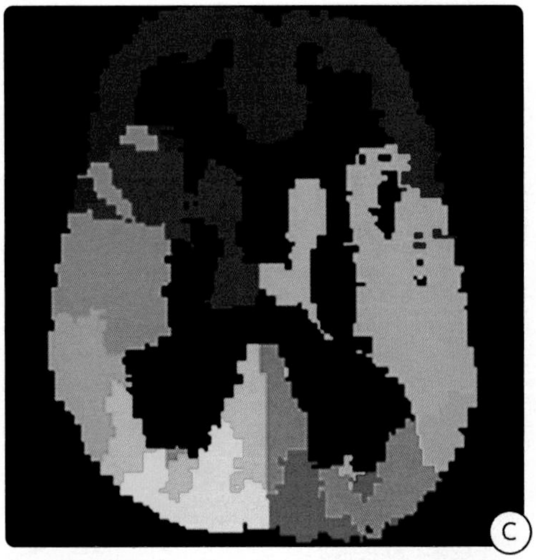

(33-34C) Compared with age-matched control, the patient shows abnormal left parietal (green) and occipital lobes (red/orange, yellow).

CREUTZFELDT-JAKOB DISEASE

Pathology and Etiology

- Most common human transmissible spongiform encephalopathy
- CJD is a prion disease
  - Proteinaceous particles without DNA, RNA
  - Misfolded isoform PrP(Sc) of normal host PrP(C)
  - Propagated by conformational conversion of PrP(C) to PrP(Sc)
- 4 CJD types recognized
  - Sporadic (sCJD) (85%)
  - Genetic/familial (gCJD) (5-15%)
  - Iatrogenic (iCJD) (2-5%)
  - Variant ("mad cow" disease, vCJD) (< 1%)

Clinical Issues

- Peak age = 55-75 years
- Rapidly progressive dementia, death in sCJD within 4 months

Imaging

- T2/FLAIR hyperintensity
  - Basal ganglia, thalami, cortex
  - "Pulvinar" sign: posterior thalami
  - "Hockey stick" sign: posteromedial thalami
  - Occipital cortex in Heidenhain variant
- Restricted diffusion

Posterior Cortical Atrophy

Posterior cortical atrophy (PCA) is a rare neurodegenerative syndrome characterized by insidious onset and selective, gradual decline in visuospatial and visioperceptual skills with relative sparing of other cognitive domains such as memory and language.

Some investigators consider PCA an atypical ("visual variant") form of AD, whereas others define it a separate neurodegenerative syndrome. In contrast to AD, neuropathologic studies of PCA report that the highest density of neurofibrillary tangles and senile plaques is in the parietooccipital regions, while the frontal lobes are relatively less involved. Mixed, multiple (e.g., PCA-AD), or variant pathologies are common.

PCA typically presents in the mid-50s or early 60s and primarily affects the parietal, occipital, and occipitotemporal cortex with relative sparing of the frontal and inferomedial temporal lobes. Biparietal (dorsal), occipitotemporal (ventral), and primary visual (caudal) variants have been described within the PCA spectrum of disease.

Occipito-parietal or occipito-temporal atrophy on MR is typical **(33-34)** *although not all patients with PCA demonstrate discernible volume loss.* Asymmetric involvement is common. FDG PET/SPECT shows hypometabolism in the parietooccipital lobes and both frontal eye fields.

The major imaging differential diagnosis of PCA is the **occipital (Heidenhain) variant of CJD**. Although the clinical and histopathologic features of both diseases overlap, PCA demonstrates greater right parietal with less left medial temporal and hippocampal atrophy. Other clinical considerations include **Alzheimer disease, dementia with Lewy bodies**, and **corticobasal degeneration**.

Degenerative Disorders

In this section, we consider a range of brain degenerations. Although some (such as Parkinson disease, PD) can be associated with dementia, most are not. Because PD occurs more often as a movement disorder than a dementing illness, it is discussed with other degenerative diseases.

The use of deep brain stimulators (DBSs) in treating patients with disabling akinetic-rigid PD is increasingly common, so a brief review of the dopaminergic striatonigral system and its relevant anatomy will be helpful before we discuss PD.

Basal Ganglia

The basal ganglia are part of the complex neuronal circuits that play a key role in the integration and execution of motor, cognitive, and emotional function. The subthalamic nucleus (STN) and globus pallidus interna (GPi)—both targets in DBS—are components of a large segregated cortical-subcortical network of white matter fibers.

Advanced diffusion imaging techniques enable detection of multiple fiber orientations in complex neuroanatomical regions that can be used to map white matter connectivity between the STN and the GP. As PD is increasingly being viewed as a circuit disorder, visualizing the inhibitory pallido-subthalamic fibers that project from the GP pars externa (GPe) to the STN and excitatory subthalamo-pallidal fibers that project from the STN to the GPi and the GPe may become clinically relevant in DBS placement.

Dopaminergic Striatonigral System

Dopaminergic neurons are found throughout the brain, but by far the largest collections lie in the midbrain. Here dopaminergic neurons are located in three specific areas: the ventral tegmental area (VTA), the pars compacta of the substantia nigra (SNPc), and the retrobulbar field. Neurons in the VTA project to the frontal cortex and ventral striatum, whereas SNPc neurons project to the putamen and caudate nuclei. Mesencephalic dopaminergic neurons help regulate voluntary movement and influence reward behavior.

Dopamine transporter (DaT) scans are used to differentiate essential tremor from the presynaptic dopaminergic degeneration in PD. Striatal loss of dopamine transporters occurs in the various parkinsonian syndromes and cannot be used to differentiate between PD and other disorders such as multiple system atrophy (MSA), dementia with Lewy bodies (DLB), corticobasal degeneration (CBD), and progressive supranuclear palsy (PSP).

Relevant Gross Anatomy

The striatonigral system consists of the **basal ganglia** (caudate nucleus, putamen, and globus pallidus), the **substantia nigra (SN)**, and the **subthalamic nucleus (STN)**. The gross and imaging anatomy of the basal ganglia is discussed in Chapter 32.

The **SN** lies in the midbrain tegmentum between the cerebral peduncles and red nuclei (RN). The SN consists of pigmented gray matter that extends through the midbrain from the pons to the subthalamic region. The SN has two parts: the **pars compacta** (which contains *dopaminergic* cells) and the **pars reticularis** (which contains *GABAergic* cells). The **RN** is a round gray matter formation that lies medial to the SN and serves as a relay station between the cerebellum, globus pallidus, and cortex **(33-35)**.

The **STN** is a small lens-shaped structure that measures approximately 100-125 mm³ in total volume. The SN envelopes the anterior and inferior borders of the STN **(33-36)**. The STN lies just inside the internal capsule, 1-2 mm from the anterolateral edge of the RN.

The *superior* border of the STN is formed by the lenticular fasciculus while the *lateral* aspect of the STN abuts the internal capsule. The *medial* border of

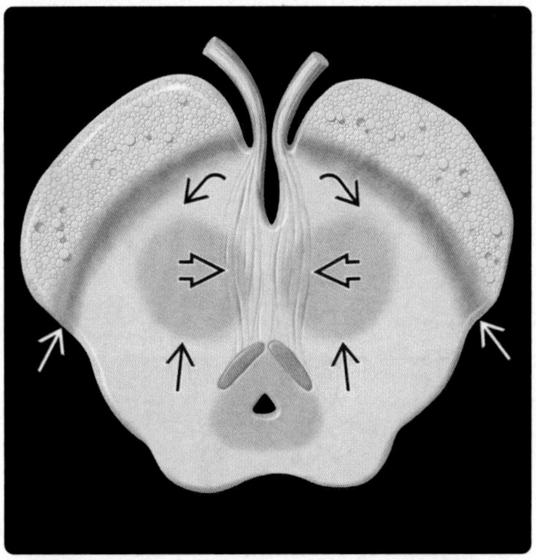

***(33-35)** Graphic of midbrain depicts substantia nigra ➡, red nuclei ⇨, pars compacta ⇗, and CN3 nuclei and tracts ⇨.*

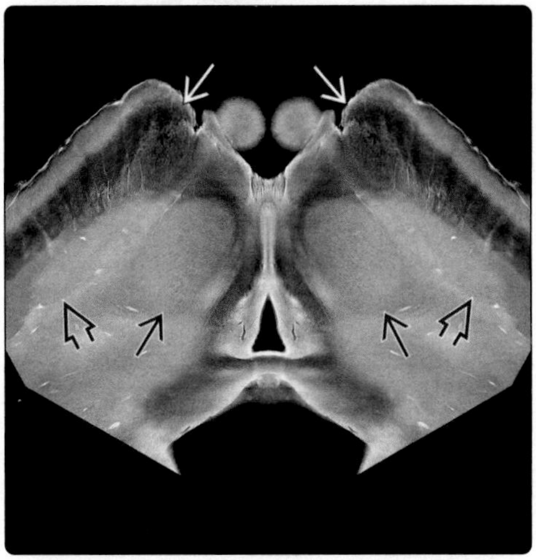

***(33-36)** 9-T MR shows subthalamic nuclei ⇨ between red nuclei ⇨, substantia nigra ➡. (Courtesy T. P. Naidich, MD, B. N. Delman, MD.)*

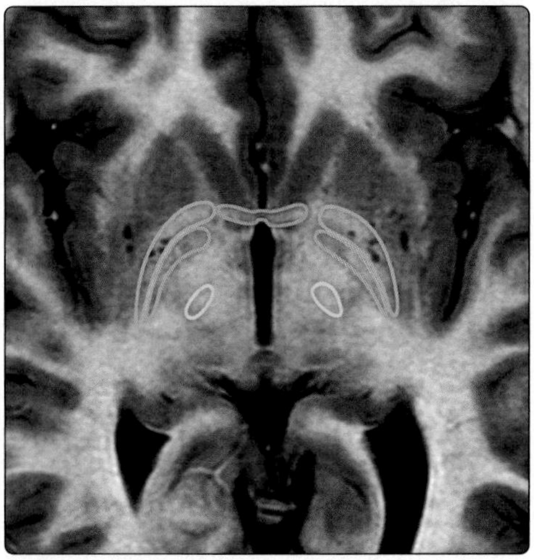

***(33-37)** Axial 3-T T1WI in a normal patient shows approximate locations of GPe (green), GPi (red), and STN (orange).*

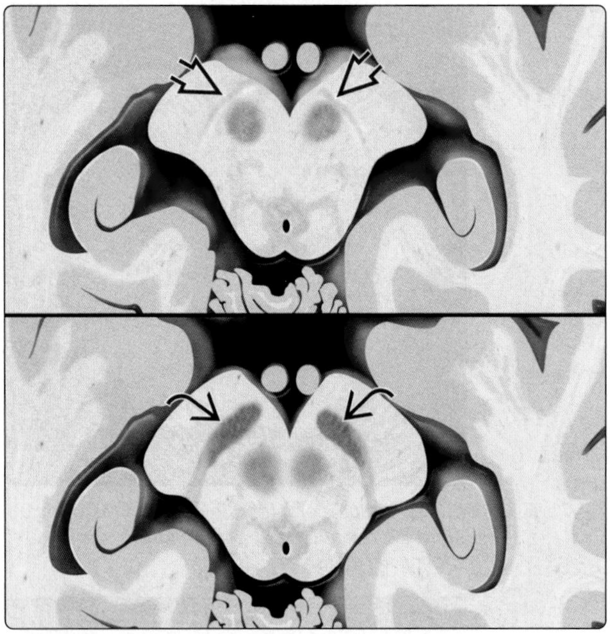

***(33-38)** Axial diagram shows midbrain atrophy with narrowing and depigmentation of the substantia nigra (SN) in Parkinson disease (top) relative to normal anatomy (bottom, STN). Note narrowing of pars compacta between red nuclei, SN.*

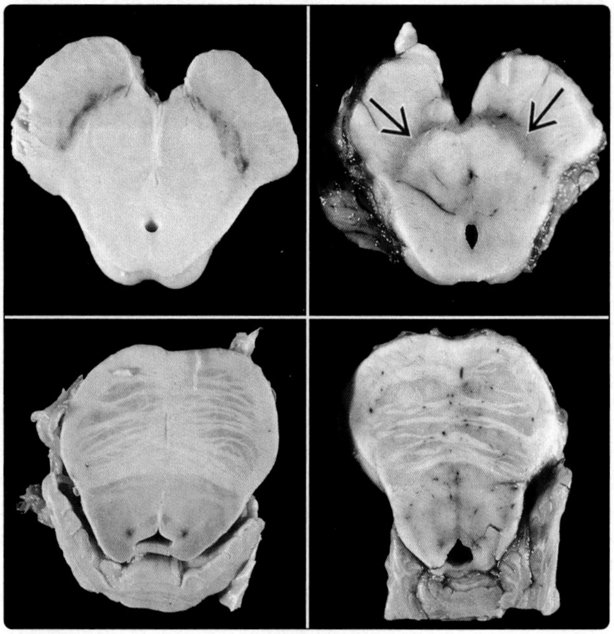

***(33-39)** Autopsied sections compare normal midbrain (L) to one affected by Parkinson disease (R). Note midbrain volume loss in PD, abnormal pallor of the substantia nigra . (Courtesy R. Hewlett, MD.)*

the STN is formed by a band of subthalamic white matter—the zona incerta (ZI)—that lies between it and the RN **(33-38)**.

The STN is currently the preferred target for both direct (imaging-based) and indirect (atlas-based) stereotactic DBS electrode placement in the treatment of movement disorders. Recent studies have demonstrated that both STN volumes and neuron numbers decrease with age, which might influence the efficacy of DBS in a geriatric population.

Imaging Anatomy

On thin-section 1.5- or 3.0-T T2-weighted MR scans, the STNs are seen as hypointense almond-shaped structures that are obliquely oriented in all three standard planes. In the axial plane, the STN lies between the SN anterosuperiorly and the RN posteromedially. The hypointensity of the STN blends imperceptibly into that of the SN, but medially the white matter of the ZI separates the STN from the RN.

The midpoint of the STN lies between 9.7-9.9 mm lateral to the midline. Its position (and the correct location of the tip of a DBS) can thus be estimated on CT scans by finding the upper cerebral peduncles and measuring 9-10 mm from the midline.

Parkinson Disease

Terminology

Parkinson disease (PD) is a multisystem neurodegenerative disorder that affects diverse neural pathways and several neurotransmitter circuits. The constellation of resting tremor, bradykinesia, and rigidity is often termed **parkinsonism**. PD accounts for approximately 75% of all cases of parkinsonism.

When PD is accompanied by dementia, it is referred to as **Parkinson disease dementia** (PDD). When PD is combined with other clinical signs, it is called "**Parkinson plus**," an overarching term that includes **multiple system atrophy** and **progressive supranuclear palsy** (see below).

PD is classified *clinically* as a neurodegenerative disorder, *histopathologically* as a **Lewy body disease**, and *immunohistochemically* as a **synucleinopathy**.

Etiology

General Concepts. Although a number of environmental factors have been implicated, aging is the most significant known risk factor for PD.

In PD, degeneration of dopaminergic neurons in the SNPc reduces dopaminergic input to the striatum. Neuronal degeneration is relatively advanced histopathologically before it becomes apparent clinically. By the time clinical symptoms develop, over 60% of dopaminergic neurons are lost and 80% of striatal dopamine is already depleted.

The death of dopaminergic neurons in PD is regional and very selective with neuronal loss centered mainly in the SNPc. The precise mechanisms underlying the susceptibility of dopaminergic neurons and regional propensity for cell death in the SNPc are poorly understood.

Genetics. The vast majority of PD cases are genetically complex. Nearly two decades ago, mutation in the α-synuclein locus was the first gene identified in PD. To date, genome-wide association studies have identified 26 PD risk loci. Approximately 5-10% of patients have a monogenic form of PD, with autosomal-dominant mutations in *SNCA*, *LRRK2*, and *VPS35* and autosomal-recessive mutations in *PINK1*, *PARK7*,

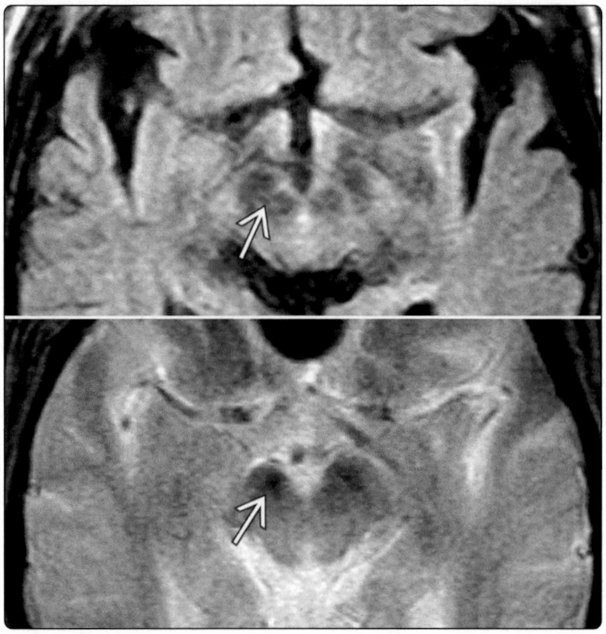

***(33-40)** Axial FLAIR (top) and T2* GRE (bottom) in a 61y man show mild midbrain volume loss with narrowed SNPc, especially on the right side ➡, where it is difficult to delineate the border between the substantia nigra and red nucleus.*

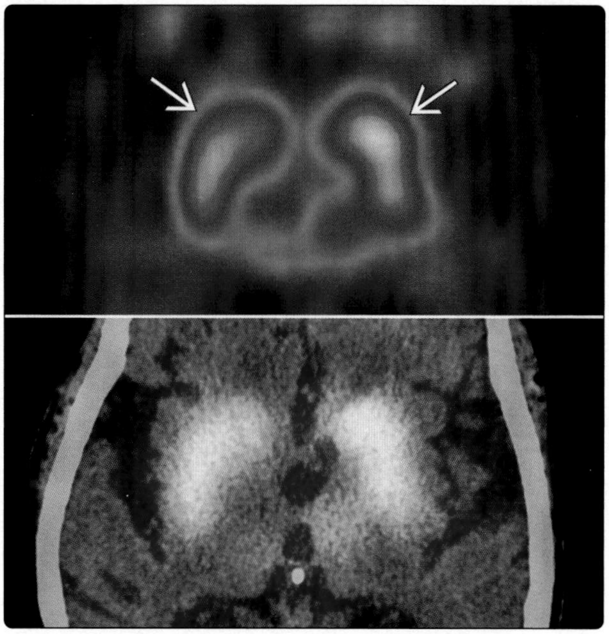

***(33-41)** DaT scan (top) shows normal uptake in caudate, putamen in an 83y man with tremor. The double "comma-shaped" configuration ➡ is a classic normal finding. (Bottom) Fused PET CT in the same case is negative for Parkinson disease.*

and Parkin, cause the disease to manifest with high penetrance. Between 10-20% cases of PD are familial, but most are sporadic.

Pathology

Gross Pathology. The midbrain may appear mildly atrophic with a splayed or "butterfly" configuration of the cerebral peduncles **(33-38)**. Depigmentation of the substantia nigra is a common pathologic feature of PD and is related to loss of neuromelanin **(33-39)**.

Microscopic Features. The most devastating effects of PD are seen in the dopaminergic striatonigral system. The two histopathologic hallmarks of PD are (1) severe depletion of dopaminergic neurons in the SNPc and (2) the presence of Lewy bodies (LBs) in the surviving neurons. Immunohistochemistry shows that the LBs stain positively for ubiquitin and α-synuclein.

Staging, Grading, and Classification. PD is divided into six (Braak) stages, which correlate clinical symptoms with the distribution of LBs. LBs begin to accumulate well before diagnosis. The disease process in the brainstem generally pursues an ascending course.

Stages 1 and 2 are preclinical. In stage 1, the LBs are confined to the medulla and the olfactory system. As the disease progresses, LBs spread into the upper brainstem and forebrain. At Braak stage 3, numerous LBs are present in the SN, loss of dopaminergic neurons is evident, the forebrain cholinergic system is involved, and the first clinical symptoms begin to emerge.

In Braak stage 4, the limbic system becomes involved. In the most advanced stages (Braak stages 5 and 6), LBs are distributed throughout the entire neocortex.

Clinical Issues

Epidemiology and Demographics. PD is both the most common movement disorder and the most common of the Lewy body diseases. Its distribution is worldwide, and the estimated overall prevalence is 150-200:100,000. There is a slight male predominance.

Peak age at onset is 60 years; PD onset under 40 years is uncommon. Rarely, PD occurs as a juvenile-onset autosomal-dominant dystonia.

Presentation. PD diagnosis depends on a constellation of symptoms. The three cardinal clinical features of PD are (1) resting tremor, (2) rigidity, and (3) bradykinesia (slowness in executing movements). An expressionless face, sometimes termed "masked" or "stone" face, is a common manifestation of bradykinesia.

Other classic symptoms are "pill-rolling" tremor, "cogwheel" or "lead pipe" rigidity, and postural instability with shuffling gait. Rigidity occurs in both agonist and antagonist muscles, affects movements in both directions, and can be elicited at very low speeds of passive movement.

Dementia eventually develops in 40% of PD patients. Other less common features of PD include autonomic dysfunction, behavioral abnormalities, depression, and sleep disturbances.

Natural History. PD typically follows a slowly progressive course with an overall mean duration of 13 years. Falls and "gait freezing" eventually become a major cause of disability.

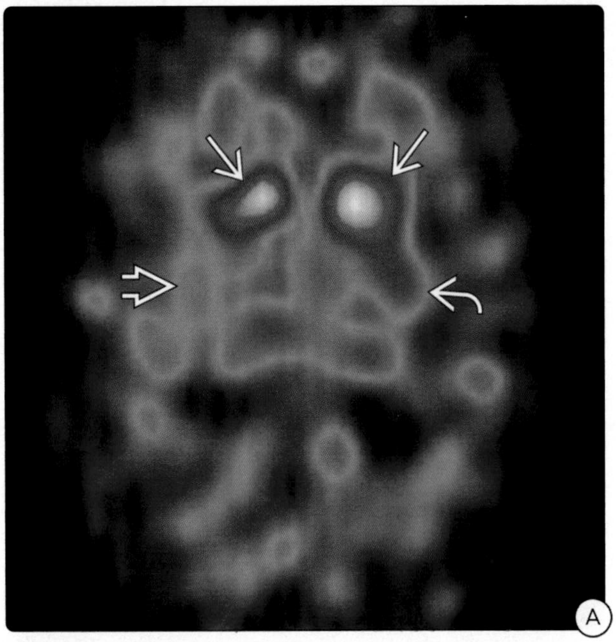

(33-42A) DaT scan in a 78y man with clinical diagnosis of Parkinson disease shows normal uptake in the heads of both caudate nuclei, absence of uptake in the right putamen, and markedly reduced uptake in the left putamen.

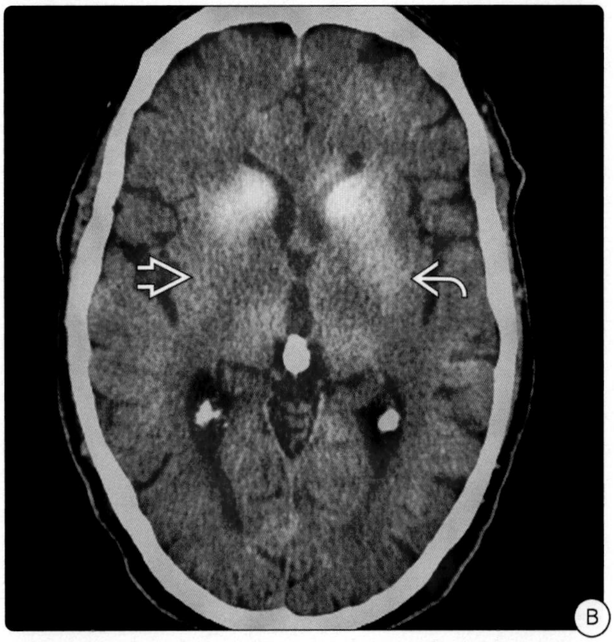

(33-42B) PET CT with fused DaT scan, NECT in the same case shows absence of uptake in the right putamen and greatly reduced uptake in the left consistent with the clinical diagnosis of Parkinson disease.

Treatment Options

Medical Treatment. A number of medications are available to control PD symptoms. Levodopa was introduced more than 40 years ago and remains the most efficacious treatment, especially in young patients. As SNPc dopamine-secreting neurons are lost, striatal dopamine levels become increasingly dependent on peripherally administered levodopa. Motor complications of levodopa such as "wearing off," dyskinesias, and "on-off" phenomena are common.

Emerging disease-modifying therapies such as adenosine A2A antagonists, MAO-b inhibitors, and dopamine agonists are under consideration, as is gene therapy to enhance in vivo dopamine production.

Surgical Options. High-frequency stimulation of deep brain structures is now preferred to ablative/lesional therapy. Deep brain stimulation (DBS) has become the preferred technique for treating a gamut of advanced PD-related symptoms.

The STN is considered one of the most optimal DBS targets. Electrodes are inserted via burr holes 25-30 mm lateral to the sagittal sutures, 20-30 mm anterior to the coronal sutures, and angled approximately 60% from the horizontal plane of the anterior-posterior commissure line. Electrode positions are determined from preoperative MR or by using standard computerized atlases.

The distance of the STN from the midline varies somewhat from individual to individual. As the STN is often difficult to identify on standard MR, many neurosurgeons identify the red nucleus and position the DBSs slightly anterolateral to it. Recent studies indicate that some patients—those with a so-called dominant STN—may do as well with one DBS as with bilateral electrodes.

Imaging

CT Findings. CT is used primarily following DBS placement to evaluate electrode position **(33-43)** and to check for surgical complications. Correct positioning in the STN is seen when the tips of the electrodes are approximately 9 mm from the midline and located just inside the upper margin of the cerebral peduncles **(33-43)**. Complications include ischemia **(33-44)**. Transient inflammatory changes may develop around the electrodes **(33-45)**. These typically appear within a few weeks and then gradually resolve.

MR Findings. Conventional MR alone is not sufficiently sensitive in diagnosing and differentiating neurodegenerative parkinsonian syndromes. Mild midbrain volume loss with a "butterfly" configuration can be seen at 1.5 T in some *late*-stage cases of PD. Findings that may support the diagnosis of PD include thinning of the pars compacta (with "touching" RNs and "smudging" of the SNs) and loss of normal SN hyperintensity on T1WI **(33-40)**.

The STNs are difficult to identify on standard 1.5- and 3.0-T MR scans, as their hypointensity blends in with the hypointensity of the SN. At 7.0 T, the shapes and boundaries of the SN on susceptibility-weighted sequences, which normally appear smooth and arch-like, may become irregular ("serrated" or "lumpy-bumpy") and blurred in PD patients.

Nuclear Medicine. The most sensitive imaging techniques for an *early* diagnosis of parkinsonian syndromes are SPECT and PET. DaT-SPECT is used to assess integrity of presynaptic dopaminergic nerve cells in patients with movement disorders **(33-41)**. Decreased uptake of I-123 FP-CIT is considered highly suggestive of PD **(33-42)**, but is also seen in other parkinsonian degenerations.

Differential Diagnosis

DaT-SPECT imaging enables differentiation of neurodegenerative causes of parkinsonism from other movement or tremor disorders in which the study is typically normal.

When dementia is present, the major differential diagnosis of PDD is **dementia with Lewy bodies**. The clinical features overlap and are distinguished by whether parkinsonism precedes dementia by more than a year. If so, the diagnosis is PDD rather than LBD.

PARKINSON DISEASE

Etiology and Pathology

- Degeneration of dopaminergic neurons in SNPc
  - Reduced dopaminergic input to striatum
  - 60% of SNPc neurons lost, 80% striatal dopamine depleted before clinical PD develops
- Substantia nigra (SN) becomes depigmented
- Pars compacta thins
- Lewy bodies develop
  - PD is most common Lewy body disease

Clinical Issues

- Peak age = 60 years
- 3 cardinal features
  - Resting tremor
  - Rigidity
  - Bradykinesia

Treatment Options

- Medical
  - Levodopa (L-dopa), other drugs
- Surgical
  - Deep brain stimulation (DBS)
  - Electrodes implanted into subthalamic nuclei

Imaging

- Difficult to diagnose on standard MR
  - ± Midbrain atrophy
  - ± Thinned, irregular SN
  - ± "Touching" SN, red nuclei
- Dopamine transporter (DaT) imaging
  - PET or SPECT can show decreased uptake

Multiple System Atrophy

Terminology

Multiple system atrophy (MSA) is an adult-onset sporadic neurodegenerative disorder that is one of the more common **Parkinson-plus** syndromes. Parkinson-plus syndromes exhibit the classic dyskinetic features of PD plus additional deficits that are not present in simple idiopathic PD. Parkinson-plus syndromes include MSA, progressive supranuclear palsy (PSP), and corticobasal degeneration (CBD). Each will be discussed in turn.

MSA includes three disorders that were previously regarded as separate entities: striatonigral degeneration, olivopontocerebellar atrophy, and Shy-Drager syndrome. These disorders are all now recognized as clinical MSA subtypes.

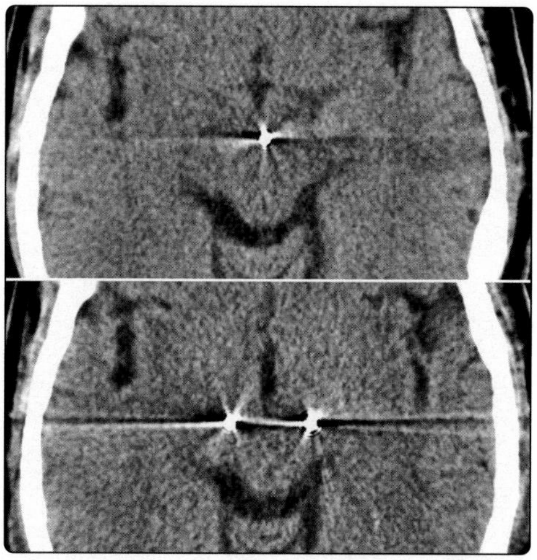

***(33-43)** Incorrect placement of left DBS (top) superomedial to STN is before repositioned left DBS, new right DBS (bottom) in correct position.*

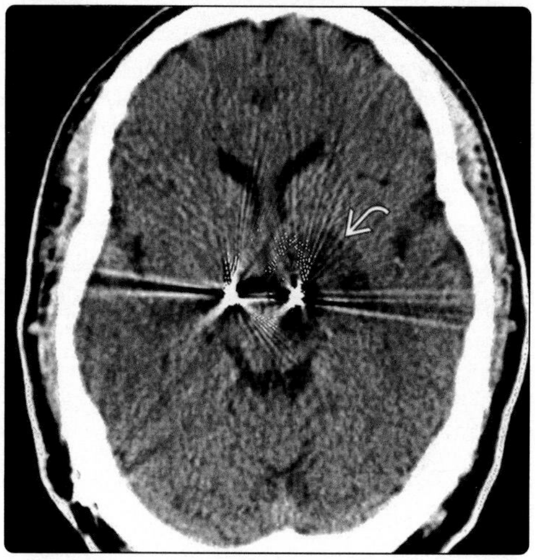

***(33-44)** NECT shows bilateral DBS placement with complication of midbrain, basal ganglia subacute infarction ➢.*

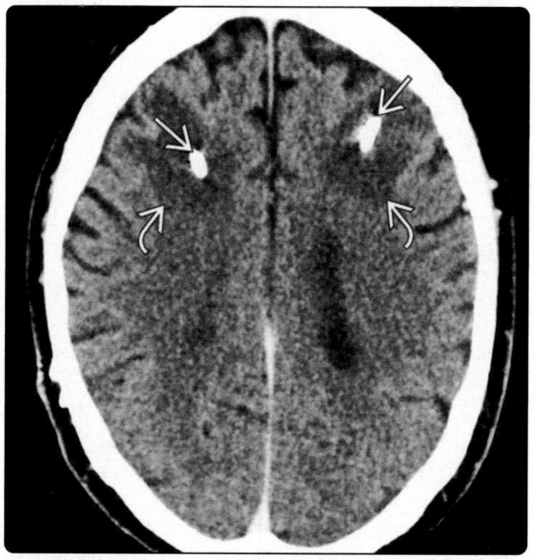

***(33-45)** NECT 4 wks after bilateral DBS shows leads ➡ surrounded by hypodensity ➢. This is transient inflammatory reaction, not infection.*

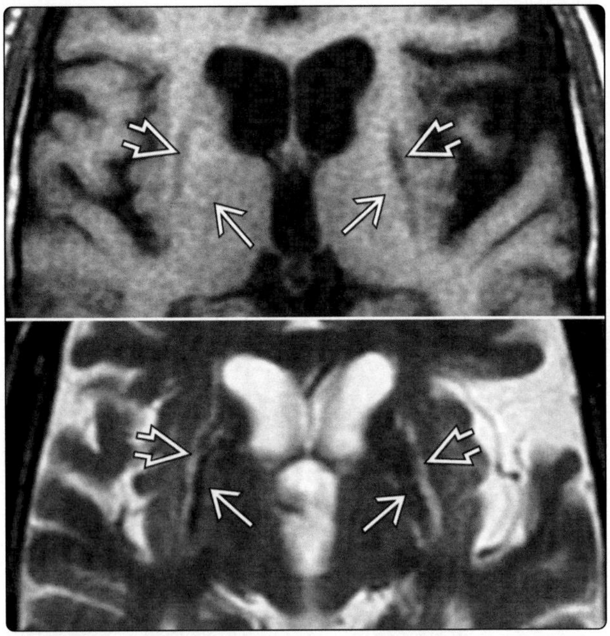

***(33-46)** Axial T1WI (top) and T2WI (bottom) show changes of MSA-P. Note large ventricles/sulci and thinned, atrophic putamina ➡ with an irregular lateral rim of hypo- and hyperintensity ➡.*

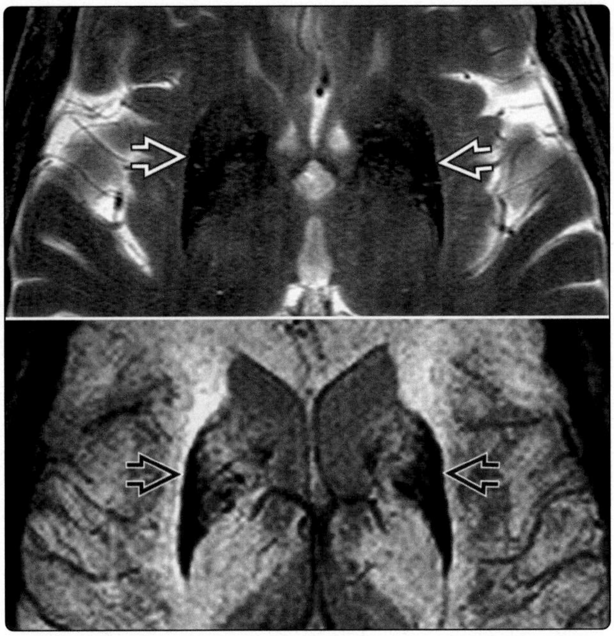

***(33-47)** (Top) Axial T2WI in a 62y patient with MSA-P shows abnormal putaminal hypointensity ➡. (Bottom) MIP SWI shows shrunken, hypointense putamina with irregular lateral margins ➡. (Images reformatted from Imaging in Neurology.)*

MULTIPLE SYSTEM ATROPHY: TERMINOLOGY, PATHOLOGY, AND CLINICAL ISSUES

Terminology

- Parkinson-plus syndrome
- 3 disorders now considered part of MSA
  - Striatonigral degeneration
  - Olivopontocerebellar atrophy
  - Shy-Drager syndrome

Pathology

- MSA-P (parkinsonian)
  - Substantia nigra depigmented
  - Putamen atrophic, grayish discoloration
- MSA-C (cerebellar)
  - "Flat" atrophic pons
  - "Beaked" appearance
  - Cerebellar peduncles/hemispheres atrophic
- Microscopic features
  - Glial (not neuronal!) cytoplasmic inclusions
  - Immunohistochemistry (+) for synuclein, ubiquitin

Clinical Issues

- Divided into subtypes by dominant symptoms
  - Parkinsonian → MSA-P
  - Cerebellar → MSA-C
  - Autonomic → MSA-A
- Parkinsonian features in 85-90% of all MSA patients
- Mean onset = 58 years, duration = 5.8 years

MSA subtypes are identified by dominant symptomatology. When parkinsonian (i.e., extrapyramidal) symptoms predominate, the disease is designated **MSA-P**. If cerebellar symptoms such as ataxia predominate, the disorder is designated **MSA-C**. When signs of autonomic failure such as orthostatic hypotension, global anhidrosis, or urogenital dysfunction predominate, the condition is designated **MSA-A.**

Etiology and Pathology

The etiology of MSA is unknown.

Gross pathology shows two distinct atrophy patterns. MSA-P shows depigmentation and pallor of the substantia nigra. The putamen may be atrophic and show a grayish discoloration secondary to lipofuscin pigment accumulation. In MSA-C, marked volume loss in the cerebellum, pons, middle cerebellar peduncles (MCPs), and medulla gives the pons a "beaked" appearance **(33-48)**. MSA-A may demonstrate a combination of these patterns.

Microscopically, MSA is characterized by glial cytoplasmic inclusions that are immunopositive for α-synuclein and ubiquitin.

Clinical Issues

Mean age of onset is 58 years; mean disease duration is 5.8 years.

Parkinson-like features are present in 85-90% of all MSA patients, regardless of subtype. Other symptoms such as dysautonomia, cerebellar ataxia, and pyramidal signs can occur in any combination. Nearly two-thirds of MSA cases are classified as parkinsonian type (MSA-P) and 32% as MSA-C. Some degree of symptomatic dysautonomia is present in almost all patients but is rarely the dominant feature. Less than 5% of MSA patients have MSA-A.

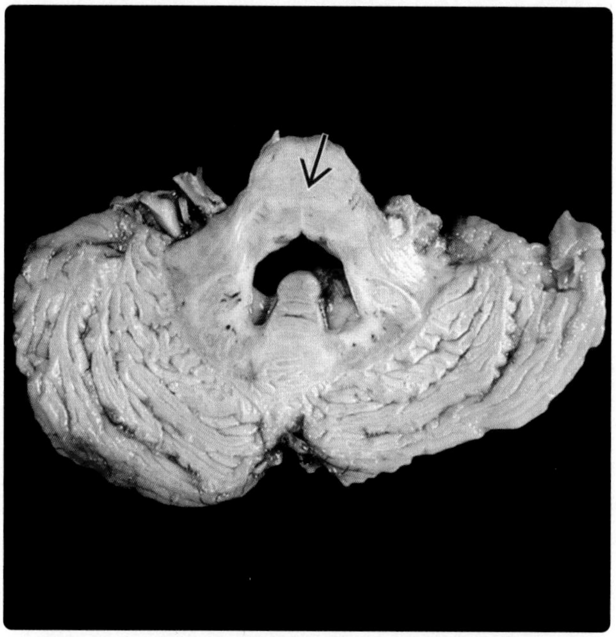

(33-48) MSA-C shows cerebellar atrophy, shrunken middle cerebellar peduncles, and small pons with "hot cross bun" sign ⇒. (Courtesy J. Townsend, MD.)

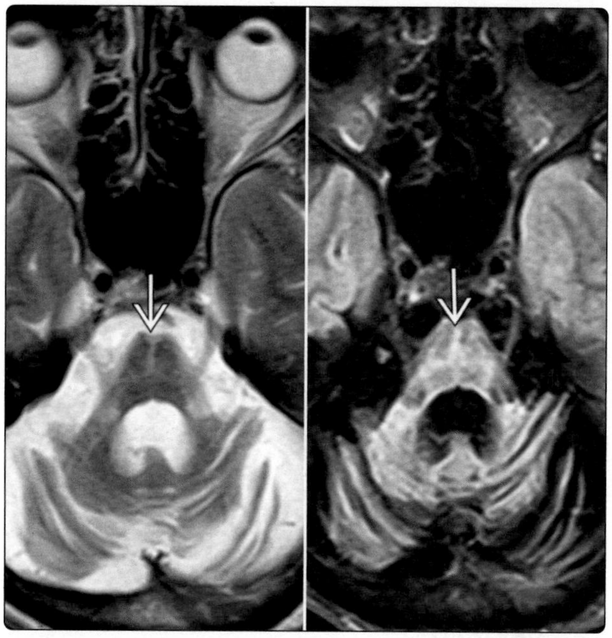

(33-49) (L) T2WI and (R) FLAIR in MSA-C show severe pontine, cerebellar atrophy with distinct hyperintense "hot cross bun" sign ⇒.

Imaging

General Features. Although there can be some overlap, the imaging findings for the two most common MSA subtypes (MSA-C and MSA-P) are somewhat different.

CT Findings. NECT scans in MSA-C show cerebellar atrophy with the hemispheres more severely affected than the vermis. A small flattened pons and an enlarged fourth ventricle are common associated findings. Cortical atrophy—especially involving the frontal and parietal lobes—may be present. Findings in MSA-P are less obvious; NECT may demonstrate shrunken putamina with flattened lateral margins.

MR Findings

MSA-P. In patients with MSA-P, the putamina appear small and hypointense on T2WI and often have a somewhat irregular high signal intensity rim along their lateral borders on 1.5-T scans (**"hyperintense putaminal rim"** sign) **(33-46)**. This finding is nonspecific, as it can be seen in some cases of CBD as well as in over one-third of normal patients.

T2* (GRE, SWI) scans show significantly higher iron deposition in the putamen compared with both age-matched controls and patients with PD **(33-47)**. DTI shows decreased FA in the pons and middle cerebellar peduncle.

MSA-C. T1 scans in MSA-C show a shrunken pons and medulla, symmetric cerebellar atrophy, small concave-appearing MCPs, and an enlarged fourth ventricle.

T2/FLAIR scans demonstrate a cruciform hyperintensity in the pons termed the **"hot cross bun"** sign **(33-49)**. The "hot cross bun" sign results from selective loss of myelinated transverse pontocerebellar fibers and neurons in the pontine raphe.

DWI shows elevated ADC in the pons, middle cerebellar peduncles, cerebellar WM, and dentate nuclei.

DTI demonstrates decreased volume of fiber bundles and reduced FA in the degenerated transverse pontocerebellar fibers. Corticospinal tract involvement is often inapparent on standard T2WI but can be demonstrated clearly with DTI.

Nuclear Medicine. 123I-Ioflupane SPECT (DaT) scans are usually normal in MSA.

MULTIPLE SYSTEM ATROPHY: IMAGING AND DDx

Imaging
- MSA-P
  - Small shrunken, hypointense putamina on T2/FLAIR
  - ± T2/FLAIR hyperintense lateral rim
  - Increased putaminal iron deposition on T2*
- MSA-C
  - Cerebellar atrophy
  - Small, concave middle cerebellar peduncles
  - Shrunken "beaked" pons, "hot cross bun" sign
  - Reduced FA in transverse pontocerebellar, corticospinal tracts
- MSA-A
  - No distinctive imaging findings

Differential Diagnosis
- Parkinson disease
- Atypical parkinsonian syndromes (progressive supranuclear palsy, corticobasal degeneration)
- Spinocerebellar ataxia
- Hypoglycemia (transient MCP hyperintensity)

Differential Diagnosis

The major differential diagnosis of MSA is **Parkinson disease**. Clinical findings often overlap. Imaging shows that the width of the middle cerebellar peduncles is diminished in MSA-C but not PD. Putaminal iron deposition appears earlier and is more prominent in MSA-P compared with PD. DTI also shows decreased FA in the middle cerebral peduncles in MSA-P.

Atypical parkinsonian syndromes (e.g., **progressive supranuclear palsy** and **corticobasal degeneration**) can also be difficult to distinguish clinically from MSA, but regional ADC values and MCP widths are normal.

Spinocerebellar ataxia can look identical to MSA-C, demonstrating atrophic, hyperintense middle cerebellar peduncles and a "hot cross bun" sign. **Hypoglycemia** can cause transient hyperintensity and acutely restricted diffusion in the MCPs and pyramidal tracts.

Progressive Supranuclear Palsy

Terminology

Progressive supranuclear palsy (PSP)—also known as Steele-Richardson-Olszewski syndrome—is a neurodegenerative disease characterized by supranuclear gaze palsy, postural instability, and mild dementia.

Etiology and Pathology

Unlike Lewy body disease, Parkinson disease (PD), and multiple system atrophy (MSA) (which are synucleinopathies), PSP is a **tauopathy**. When tau protein is fibrilized, it becomes less soluble, and its microtubule-stabilizing properties are reduced. PSP shares many clinical, pathologic, and genetic features with other tau-related diseases, such as corticobasal degeneration (CBD) and tau-positive frontotemporal lobar degeneration (FTLD).

The major gross pathologic findings are substantia nigra and locus ceruleus depigmentation with midbrain atrophy. Variable atrophy of the pallidum, thalamus, and subthalamic nucleus together with mild symmetric frontal volume loss may also be present **(33-50)** **(33-51)**.

Pathologic heterogeneity is common in PSP. Histologic findings consistent with other coexisting neurodegenerative diseases, such as Alzheimer disease or diffuse Lewy body disease, are present in the majority of cases.

PSP is characterized histopathologically by neuronal loss and astrocytic gliosis. Tau-immunoreactive cellular inclusions accumulate within both neurons and glia (in "tufted" or star-shaped astrocytes). The distribution of tau inclusions is predominantly subcortical with the globus pallidus, STN, substantia nigra, and brainstem most severely affected. Cortical involvement is common.

Clinical Issues

Epidemiology and Demographics. PSP is the second most common form of parkinsonism (after idiopathic PD) and is the most common of the so-called Parkinson-plus syndromes.

The prevalence of PSP is age dependent and estimated at 6-10% that of PD.

Presentation and Natural History. PSP symptom onset is insidious, typically beginning in the sixth or seventh decade. Peak onset is 63 years, and no cases have been reported in patients under the age of 40.

Two PSP phenotypes are recognized: Richardson syndrome (PSP-RS) and parkinsonian-type PSP (PSP-P). PSP-RS is the classic, more common presentation with lurching gait, axial dystonia, and early ocular symptoms. Vertical supranuclear gaze palsy is the definitive diagnostic feature but typically develops years after disease onset.

One-third of patients exhibit the PSP-P phenotype. Parkinsonism dominates the early clinical picture with bradykinesia, rigidity, normal eye movements, and transient response to levodopa.

Although disease course is variable, PSP is a progressive neurodegenerative process. Neuropsychiatric symptoms develop in over half the patients within two years of disease onset. In 15-30% of cases, cognitive decline and behavioral changes are the presenting complaints and can remain the only clinical feature throughout the disease course.

Imaging

CT Findings. NECT scans show variable midbrain volume loss with prominent interpeduncular and ambient cisterns. Mild to moderate ventricular enlargement is common.

MR Findings. Sagittal T1- and T2-weighted images show midbrain atrophy with a concave upper surface (the **"penguin"** or **"hummingbird" sign**) **(33-52)**. Volumetric calculations show that the sagittal midbrain is less than 70 mm^3 and that the midbrain:pons ratio is less than 0.15, only half that of normal controls.

Axial scans show a widened interpeduncular angle and abnormal concavity of the midbrain tegmentum. However, PSP, CBD, MSA, and Lewy body disease may all exhibit increased cerebral peduncle angle.

In addition to a small midbrain, enlarged third ventricle, and prominent perimesencephalic cisterns, the quadrigeminal plate is often thinned. Cerebellar atrophy is common, and the *superior* cerebellar peduncles also frequently appear atrophic.

DTI indices (FA, mean diffusivity, etc.) demonstrate widespread WM abnormalities that are often mild or inapparent on T2/FLAIR. WM changes are more severe in PSP-RS.

Nuclear Medicine. FDG PET shows glucose hypometabolism in the midbrain and along medial frontal regions. Dopamine transporter (DaT) radioligands show uniformly decreased dopamine nerve terminals in both the caudate nuclei and putamen. Tau-PET accumulation is markedly distinct compared with that of amyloid burden in aging and Alzheimer disease.

Differential Diagnosis

The major differential diagnosis includes **other tauopathies**, such as **CBD** and some forms of **FTLD**. All share common molecular mechanisms and are therefore probably part of the same disease spectrum. **Alzheimer disease**, **PD**, and **MSA-P** usually do not exhibit severe atrophy of the superior colliculi that is seen with PSP.

PROGRESSIVE SUPRANUCLEAR PALSY

Etiology and Pathology
- Abnormal tau protein ("tauopathy")
- Substantia nigra depigmented
- Prominent midbrain atrophy

Clinical Issues
- Second most common cause of parkinsonism
- Insidious onset (sixth, seventh decades)
- Neuropsychiatric symptoms develop in 50%

Imaging
- Midbrain volume loss
  - "Penguin" or "hummingbird" sign on sagittal T1WI
  - Quadrigeminal plate thinned (especially superior colliculi)
  - Adjacent cisterns increased
- Midbrain, medial frontal hypometabolism

Differential Diagnosis
- Other tauopathies
  - Corticobasal degeneration
  - Some forms of FTLD
- Alzheimer, PD, MSA-P
  - No disproportionate atrophy of midbrain, superior colliculi

Corticobasal Degeneration

Terminology

Corticobasal degeneration (CBD) is an uncommon sporadic neurodegenerative and dementing disorder whose characterization continues to evolve. Once thought to represent a distinct clinicopathologic entity, CBD has multiple clinical phenotypes and different associated syndromes. The umbrella terms **corticobasal syndrome** (CBS) and CBS/CBD have been used to acknowledge the clinicopathologic heterogeneity of CBD.

Etiology

CBD, PSP, and the FTD-tau subset of frontotemporal dementia are all characterized by tau inclusions in neurons and glia. These tauopathies have overlapping mutations, largely through the *MAPT* clade.

Pathology

The most common gross features of CBD are asymmetric frontoparietal atrophy, especially in the motor and sensory areas. The temporal and occipital cortex are relatively spared. Striatonigral degeneration is seen with striking atrophy and discoloration of the substantia nigra. The putamen, pallidum, thalamus, and hypothalamus are affected to a lesser degree.

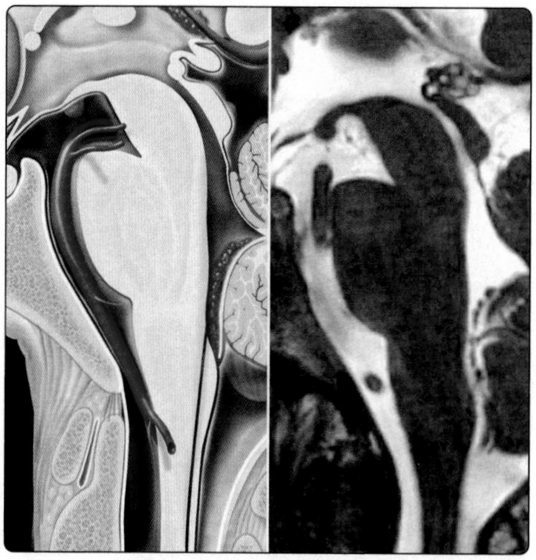

***(33-50)** Sagittal graphic (L) and high-resolution T2WI (R) together show normal midbrain and pons.*

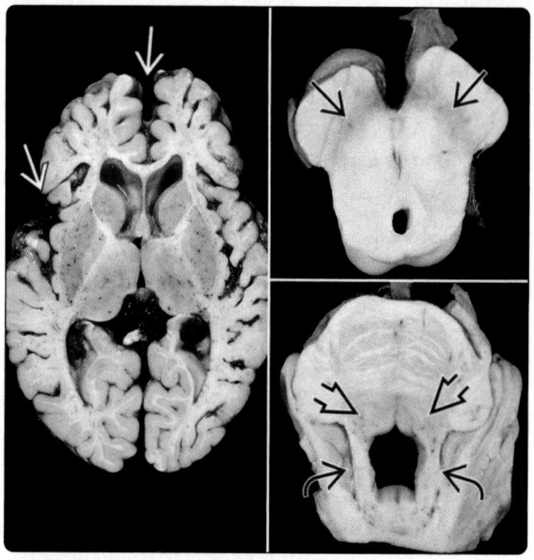

***(33-51)** PSP with frontotemporal atrophy ➡, depigmented SN ➡, locus ceruleus ➡, small superior cerebellar peduncles ➡ (R. Hewlett).*

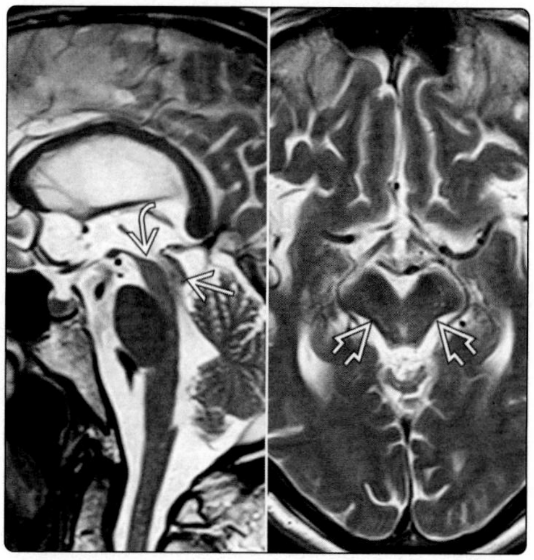

***(33-52)** PSP shows small midbrain with upper concavity and "penguin" or "hummingbird" sign ➡, tectal atrophy ➡, and concave midbrain ➡.*

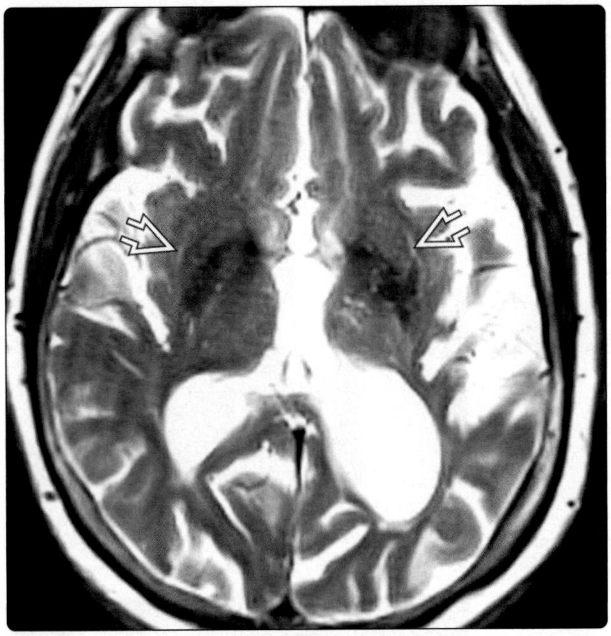

***(33-53)** Axial T2WI in a 72y woman with corticobasal degeneration (CBD) shows the hyperintense putaminal rim ➲ characteristic of CBD. This finding can also be seen in some cases of MSA-P and in 35-40% of normal patients.*

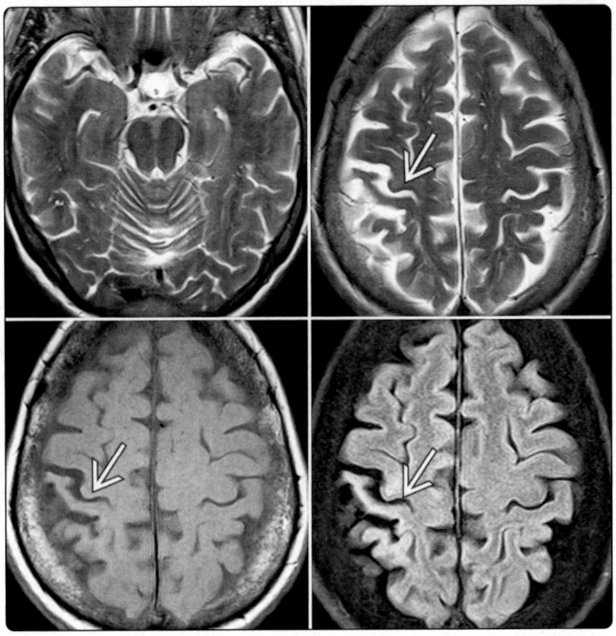

***(33-54)** CBD is in a 66y woman with spastic left arm. The temporal and occipital lobes appear normal. Note asymmetric atrophy, thin cortex, and hyperintense WM in the right perirolandic region ➲.*

Microscopically, CBD is characterized by neuronal achromasia (pale ballooned neurons) and tau-positive cytoplasmic inclusions in astrocytes within the atrophic cortex.

Clinical Issues

CBD typically affects patients 50-70 years of age. Its onset is both insidious and progressive. CBD can be associated with a broad variety of motor, sensory, behavioral, and cognitive disturbances. Levodopa-resistant, asymmetric, akinetic-rigid parkinsonism and limb dystonia (usually affecting an arm) are classic findings. Rigidity is followed by bradykinesia, gait disorder, and tremor. "Alien limb phenomenon" occurs in 50% of cases.

Variable cortical features of CBD include cognitive decline with impaired language production (nonfluent aphasia) and symptoms such as visuospatial dysfunction that mimic posterior cortical atrophy. Learning and memory are relatively preserved.

Imaging

Conventional imaging studies show moderate but asymmetric frontoparietal atrophy, contralateral to the side that is more severely affected clinically. The dorsal prefrontal and perirolandic cortex, striatum **(33-53)**, and midbrain tegmentum are the most severely involved regions. FLAIR scans may show patchy or confluent hyperintensity in the rolandic subcortical WM **(33-54)**.

SPECT and PET demonstrate asymmetric frontoparietal and basal ganglia/thalamic hypometabolism. Studies using striatal dopamine transporter imaging are sometimes helpful in differentiating CBD from other neurodegenerative disorders such as Parkinson disease.

Differential Diagnosis

CBD is a member of the parkinsonian group of disorders. The clinical differential diagnosis of CBD therefore includes **Parkinson disease, progressive supranuclear palsy**, and **multiple system atrophy**. In patients with cognitive dysfunction, symptoms can also mimic **dementia with Lewy bodies** or one of the **frontotemporal lobar degeneration syndromes**.

Amyotrophic Lateral Sclerosis

Terminology

Amyotrophic lateral sclerosis (ALS) is also known as motor neuron disease (ALS/MND) or Lou Gehrig disease.

Etiology

General Concepts. Upper motor neurons (UMNs) in the primary motor cortex send axons inferiorly along the corticospinal tract (CST) to pass through the brainstem, decussate at the cervicomedullary junction, and travel into the spinal cord. There, they synapse with anterior horn cells [lower motor neurons (LMNs)].

ALS is characterized by progressive degeneration of motor neurons in both the brain and spinal cord. Whether the degeneration is a neuronopathy (i.e., begins in the cell body and proceeds in an anterograde fashion) or an axonopathy with retrograde degeneration is unknown.

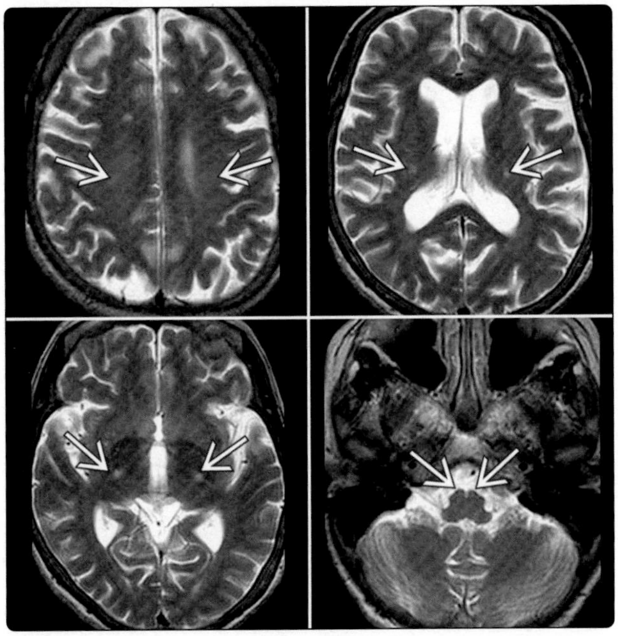

(33-55) Axial T2WI in a patient with ALS shows prominent hyperintensity along the course of the CSTs ➡. Remember that the CSTs are typically slightly hyperintense on T2WI, especially at 3 T. (From Imaging in Neurology.)

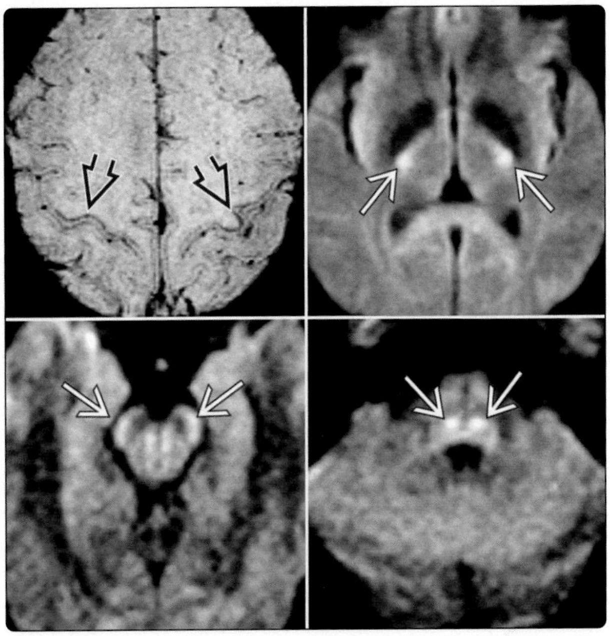

(33-56) SWI in a patient with ALS shows blooming hypointensity ("motor band sign") ⇨ in both precentral gyri. DWI shows symmetric hyperintensities ➡ in the posterior limbs of the internal capsules, cerebral peduncles, and medulla.

As is the case with many other neurodegenerations, it is now recognized that ALS is a heterogeneous condition associated with more than one pathogenic mechanism and with different clinical manifestations and trajectories.

Genetics. Mutations in several genes appear to be associated with familial ALS: *C9orf72*, *SOD1*, *TARDBP*, and *FUS*.

Pathology

Gross Pathology. Evidence of widespread muscle atrophy affecting limb and intercostal muscles and the diaphragm is typical at autopsy. Macroscopically, the brain is generally unremarkable, but mild focal atrophy of the precentral gyrus can be seen in some cases.

Microscopic Features. The major histopathologic change in ALS is loss of motor neurons in the motor cortex, brainstem, and anterior horns of the spinal cord. Demyelination, axonal degeneration, and astrocytosis are typical features.

An RNA-mediated proteinopathy with mutated *TARDBP* and *FUS* occurs in both FTLD and ALS. Immunohistochemistry demonstrates the presence of TDP-43 ubiquitinated cytoplasmic inclusion bodies in motor neurons. Extramotor pathology is also commonly found in the frontal cortex and CA4 neurons of the hippocampus.

Clinical Issues

Epidemiology and Demographics. ALS has an incidence of 1-2 per 100,000 per year and is the most common motor neuron disease, representing approximately 85% of all cases.

ALS is mostly sporadic; 10-15% of cases are familial. The average age of onset in familial ALS is 10 years earlier than in sporadic ALS.

Presentation. Signs of *both* UMN and LMN disease are generally required for the clinical diagnosis of ALS. Evidence of UMN degeneration includes hypertonicity, hyperreflexia, and pathologic reflexes. LMN disease results in muscle fasciculations, atrophy, and weakness.

Although ALS shares the same genetic spectrum with FTLD, muscle weakness is its dominant feature, and dementia rarely—if ever—occurs. Disease onset is typically insidious, as at least 30% of anterior horn cells are lost before weakness becomes clinically apparent.

Natural History. Although median survival from diagnosis to death is between 3 and 4 years, 10% of patients survive beyond 10 years. Death is generally from respiratory failure due to diaphragm weakness.

ALS: PATHOLOGY AND CLINICAL ISSUES

Terminology and Etiology
- Lou Gehrig disease
- Progressive motor neuron atrophy in brain, spinal cord

Pathology
- Brain macroscopically normal
- Loss of motor neurons

Clinical Issues
- Sporadic > familial ALS
- Insidious onset
- Both upper and lower motor neuron symptoms
- Death from respiratory failure

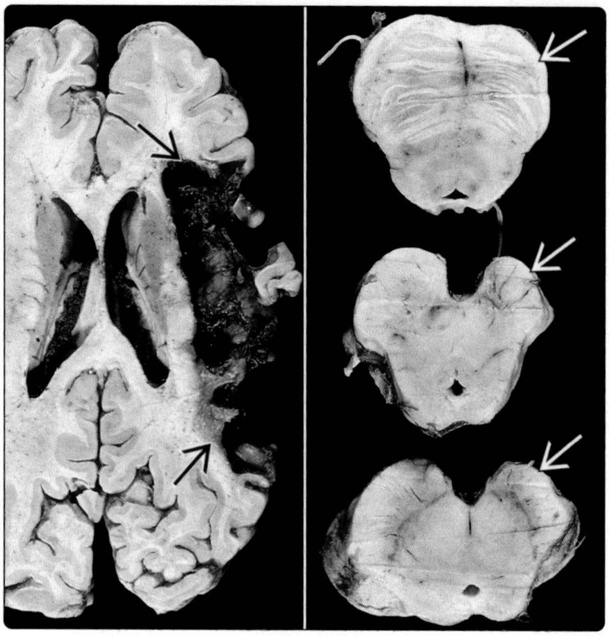

(33-57) ***Autopsy specimen from a patient with chronic WaD following large left MCA infarct ⮕ shows volume loss in the left cerebral peduncle and upper pons ➡. (Courtesy R. Hewlett, MD.)***

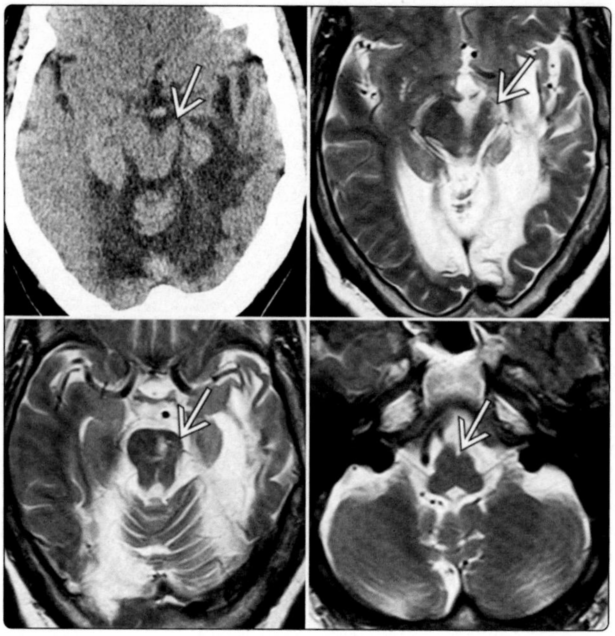

(33-58) ***NECT (upper left) and a series of T2 scans demonstrate changes of chronic WaD following major territorial infarction. Note atrophy of the left cerebral peduncle, upper pons, and midbrain ➡.***

Imaging

MR Findings. Standard MR in many—perhaps even the majority of—ALS patients is normal. Macroscopic atrophy on T1WI is uncommon in ALS. Voxel-based morphometry may demonstrate subtle gray matter atrophy in the precentral gyri.

T2/FLAIR hyperintensity is unusual but can occur anywhere from the subcortical WM through the posterior limb of the internal capsule, cerebral peduncles, pons to the medullary pyramids, and spinal cord. Changes are usually most prominent in the posterior limbs of the internal capsules and cerebral peduncles **(33-55)**. As the CST is normally slightly hyperintense, this finding lacks both sensitivity and specificity as an imaging "biomarker" for ALS.

T2* SWI may demonstrate hypointensity in the precentral cortex, the so-called "motor band sign" **(33-56)**. DWI may show increased diffusivity and reduced FA in the CSTs. Tractography may demonstrate subcortical truncation or pruning of the CST fibers.

Differential Diagnosis

The major differential diagnosis of ALS is the **normal hyperintensity of compact, fully myelinated WM tracts**. The CST is typically slightly hyperintense on T2 scans, especially at 3.0 T.

Another diagnostic consideration is **primary lateral sclerosis** (PLS). PLS is a juvenile-onset autosomal-recessive motor neuron disease that affects only upper motor neurons. **Wallerian degeneration** can cause T2/FLAIR hyperintensity along the CST but is unilateral.

Other disorders that may demonstrate T2 hyperintensity along the CSTs include **demyelinating** and **inflammatory diseases**, metabolic disorders such as **acute hypoglycemic coma**, and **infiltrating neoplasms** (most commonly high-grade astrocytomas).

ALS: IMAGING AND DIFFERENTIAL DIAGNOSIS

Imaging
- T2/FLAIR often normal
  - CST hyperintensity occurs but uncommon
  - Posterior limb internal capsules (ICs), cerebral peduncles
- DTI shows reduced FA
  - Tractography shows thinning of one or both subcortical CSTs
- T2* SWI
  - "Motor band sign" (hypointensity in motor cortex)

Differential Diagnosis
- Most common: normal!
  - CST normally slightly hyperintense
  - Especially in posterior limb of IC, peduncles
- Less common
  - Wallerian degeneration (unilateral)
  - Primary lateral sclerosis
  - Demyelinating disease
  - Tumor infiltration

Wallerian Degeneration

Axonal degeneration can occur via several mechanisms, the most common being *anterograde* (or wallerian) and *retrograde* ("dying back") degeneration. In diseases such as multiple

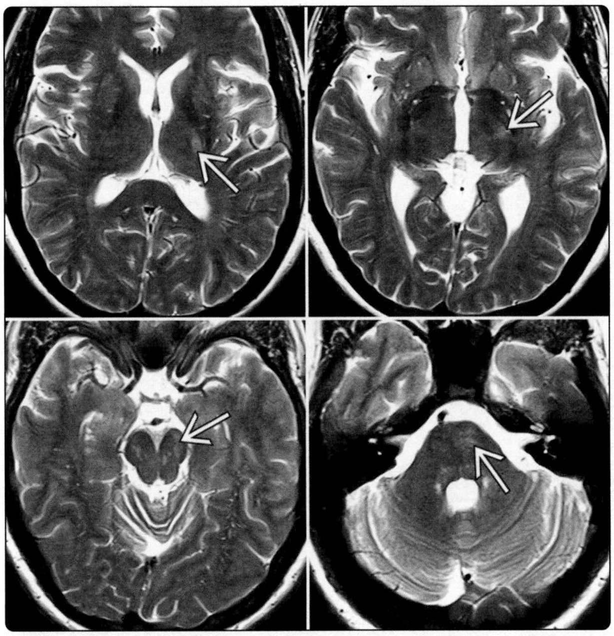

(33-59) A patient with acute WaD was imaged 3 weeks following left hemisphere tumor resection. MR scans show CST hyperintensity ➡ without volume loss.

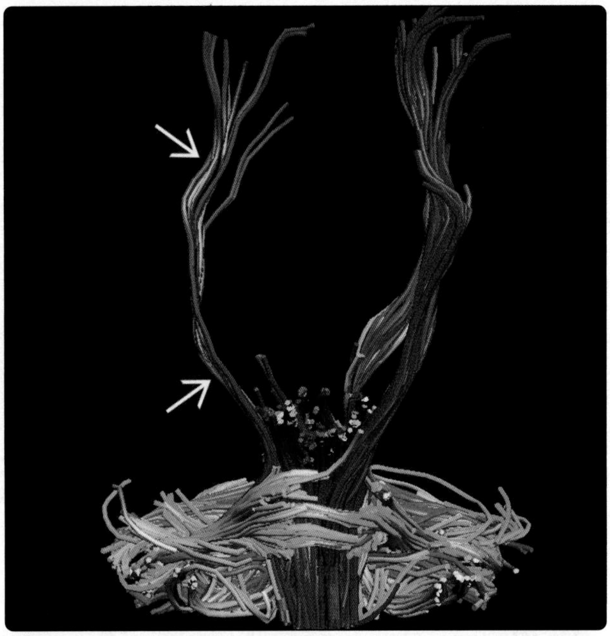

(33-60) DTI in a patient with chronic WaD after a right basal ganglionic-internal capsule infarct shows marked diminution in the right CST ➡. (Courtesy N. Agarwal, MD.)

sclerosis, inflammation-associated axonal transport disturbances—so-called "focal axonal degeneration"—may precede axonal transection and the ensuing axonal self-destruction by wallerian degeneration (WaD).

Terminology

WaD is an intrinsic anterograde degeneration of distal axons and their myelin sheaths caused by detachment from—or injury to—their proximal axons or cell bodies.

Etiology

In the brain, WaD most often occurs after trauma, infarction, demyelinating disease, or surgical resection. Descending WM tracts ipsilateral to the injured neurons degenerate—but not immediately. Axons may stay morphologically stable for the first 24-72 hours. The distal part of the axon then undergoes progressive fragmentation that proceeds directionally along the axon stump.

Most forms of acute axonal degeneration involve a stepwise "cascade" of events. After the initial insult, the myelin sheath first retracts from its axon at the nodes of Ranvier, followed by axonal degeneration. The myelin sheath itself then degenerates with breakdown of its protein components and degradation of the lipids. The final result is granular disintegration of the axonal cytoskeleton and volume loss in the affected WM tracts or nerves.

Pathology

Virtually any WM tract or nerve in the brain, spinal cord, or peripheral nervous system can exhibit changes of WaD. The caudally directed motor fiber pathways of the descending corticospinal tract (CST) are the most common sites of visible brain involvement. Other affected locations include the corpus callosum, optic radiations, fornices, and cerebellar peduncles.

In chronic WaD, midbrain and pons volume loss ipsilateral to a destructive lesion (e.g., a large territorial infarct) are grossly visible **(33-57)**. Microscopic findings include early changes of myelin disintegration and axon breakdown.

Clinical Issues

Imaging abnormalities in WaD (see below) seem to correlate with motor deficits and poor outcome.

Imaging

CT Findings. NECT scans are insensitive in the acute-subacute stages of WaD. Atrophy of the ipsilateral cerebral peduncle is the most common finding in chronic WaD **(33-58)**.

MR Findings. The development of visible WaD following stroke, trauma, or surgery is unpredictable. Fewer than half of all patients with motor deficits following acute cerebral infarction demonstrate T2/FLAIR hyperintensities or diffusion restriction in the CST that might herald WaD **(33-59)**.

When it does develop, T2/FLAIR hyperintensity along the CST ipsilateral to the damaged cortex may occur as early as 3 days after major stroke onset ("pre-wallerian degeneration") but more typically becomes visible between 3 and 4 weeks later. The hyperintensity may be transient or permanent.

Chronic changes of WaD include foci of frank encephalomalacia with volume loss of the ipsilateral peduncle, rostral pons, and medullary pyramid. Chronic WaD does not

(33-61A) Axial T2WI in a patient with biopsy-proven acute WaD shows a mass-like hyperintense lesion in the deep left cerebral white matter ➡. (33-61B) Hyperintensity in continuity with the hemispheric WM lesion is seen in the left corticospinal tract ➡. Compare with mild, normal hyperintensity in the right cerebral peduncle ➡.

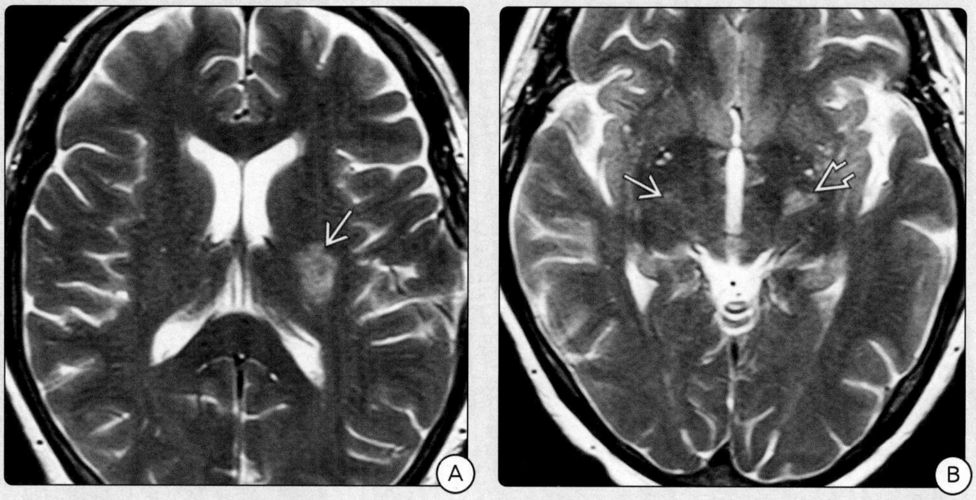

(33-61C) Coronal T2WI shows hyperintensity in continuity from the deep WM lesion ➡ all the way along the internal capsule ➡, through the pons ➡, and down into the medulla ➡. (33-61D) Coronal T1 C+ FS shows enhancement along the cephalad internal capsule ➡.

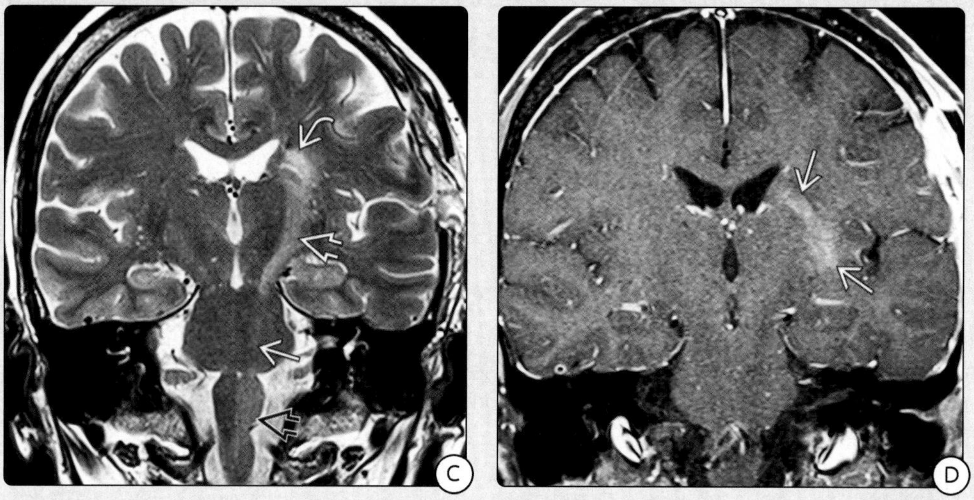

(33-61E) Coronal DWI shows diffusion restriction in the left corticospinal tract ➡. (33-61F) Color DTI shows some reduction in the blue (superior to inferior) fiber tracts in the left internal capsule ➡.

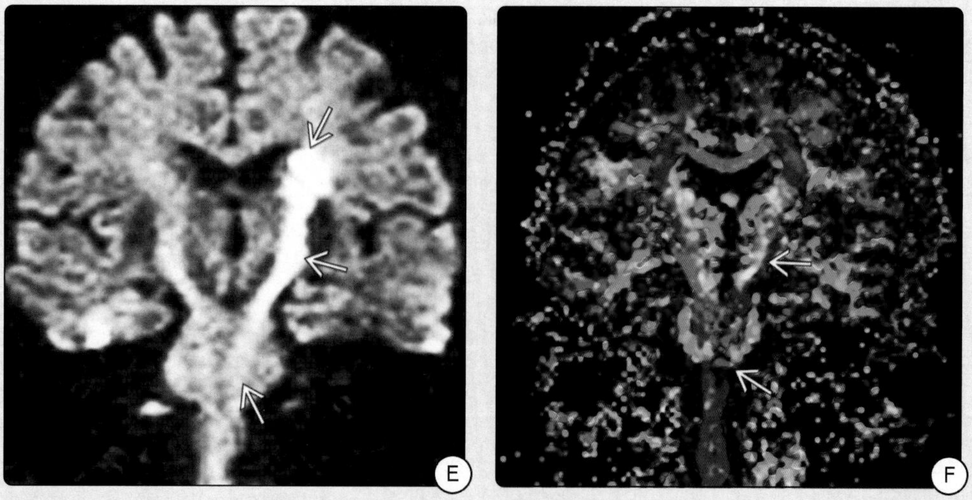

enhance on T1 C+, but acute degeneration may show transient mild enhancement (33-61).

Transient restricted diffusion in the CST may develop in acute ischemic stroke within 48-72 hours. Recent studies show that restricted diffusion can occur beyond the CST. The most commonly reported area is the corpus callosum (primarily the splenium), which should not be mistaken for acute ischemia, as it most likely reflects the early phase of secondary neuronal degeneration.

Other WM tracts can undergo WaD with an insult to their neuronal cell bodies. These include the corticopontocerebellar tract, dentate-rubro-olivary pathway (Guillain-Mollaret triangle), posterior column of the spinal cord, limbic circuit, and optic pathway.

Microstructural changes in WM tracts are especially well demonstrated with DTI **(33-60)**. Chronic hemispheric infarction shows decreased mean diffusivity (MD) and fractional anisotropy (FA) with absence of color in the CST **(33-61)**.

Differential Diagnosis

The major differential diagnosis of WaD is primary neurodegenerative disease. The T2/FLAIR hyperintensity sometimes seen in **amyotrophic lateral sclerosis** is bilateral and extends from the subcortical WM adjacent to the motor cortex into the brainstem. High-grade infiltrating primary brain tumors (typically **anaplastic astrocytoma** or **glioblastoma multiforme**) infiltrate along compact WM tracts but cause expansion, not atrophy.

Hypertrophic Olivary Degeneration

In order to understand the imaging findings in hypertrophic olivary degeneration (HOD), it is necessary first to understand the underlying anatomy of the medulla and the functional connections between the olives, red nuclei, and cerebellum.

Anatomy of the Medulla and Guillain-Mollaret Triangle

Two prominent ventral bulges are present on the anterior surface of the medulla: the pyramids and olives. The **pyramids** are paired structures, separated in the midline by the ventral median fissure of the medulla. The pyramids contain the ipsilateral corticospinal tracts above their decussation.

The **olives** are a crenulated complex of gray nuclei that are lateral to the pyramids and separated from them by the ventrolateral (preolivary) sulcus **(33-62)**.

The **Guillain-Mollaret triangle** consists of the **ipsilateral inferior olivary nucleus** (ION), **contralateral dentate nucleus** (DN), and **ipsilateral red nucleus** (RN) together with their three connecting neural pathways, i.e., the **olivocerebellar tract, dentatorubral tract,** and **central tegmental tract**.

Olivocerebellar fibers from the ipsilateral ION cross the midline through the inferior cerebellar peduncle, connecting it with the contralateral DN and cerebellar cortex.

Dentatorubral fibers then enter the superior cerebellar peduncle (brachium conjunctivum) and decussate in the midbrain to connect to the opposite RN. The ipsilateral central tegmental tract then descends from the RN to the ipsilateral ION, completing the Guillain-Mollaret triangle **(33-63)**.

Terminology

HOD is a secondary degeneration of the ION caused by injury to the dentato-rubro-olivary pathway. Interruption of the dentato-rubro-olivary pathway at any point can cause HOD.

Etiology

Unlike other degenerations, in hypertrophic olivary degeneration, the degenerating structure (the olive) becomes hypertrophic rather than atrophic. Cerebellar symptoms and olivary hypertrophy typically develop many months after the inciting event. Understanding the clinical and pathologic underpinnings of HOD as well as its imaging manifestations will help avoid potential misinterpretation of this unusual lesion as an ischemic event, neoplasm, or focus of tumefactive demyelination.

HOD is a transsynaptic degeneration caused by lesions in the Guillain-Mollaret triangle. Lesions in the dentatorubral or central tegmental (rubro-olivary) tracts functionally deafferent the olive and cause HOD more often than lesions located in the olivocerebellar pathway.

The primary causative lesion in developing HOD is often **hemorrhage**, either from hypertension, surgery, vascular malformation, or trauma. **Pontomesencephalic stroke** also occasionally causes HOD. **Postoperative pediatric cerebellar mutism** (POPCMS) is a well-recognized complication that affects children undergoing posterior fossa brain tumor resection. Interruption of the dentato-thalamo-cortical pathway is recognized as its anatomic substrate. The proximal structures of the DTC pathway also form a segment of the Guillain-Mollaret triangle, so bilateral HOD is common in patients with POPCMS.

Some cases of mitochondrial disorders with *POLG* and *SURF1* mutations have been described as causing HOD. Occasionally, no inciting lesion can be identified.

Pathology

Location. Three distinct patterns develop, all related to the location of the inciting lesion. In **ipsilateral HOD**, the primary lesion is limited to the central tegmental tract of the brainstem. In **contralateral HOD**, the primary lesion is located within the cerebellum (either the DN or the superior cerebellar peduncle). In **bilateral HOD**, the lesion involves both the central tegmental tract and the superior cerebellar peduncle.

Approximately 75% of HOD cases are unilateral and 25% bilateral.

Gross Pathology. Olivary hypertrophy is seen grossly as asymmetric enlargement of the anterior medulla. The contralateral RN often appears pale. In chronic HOD, the

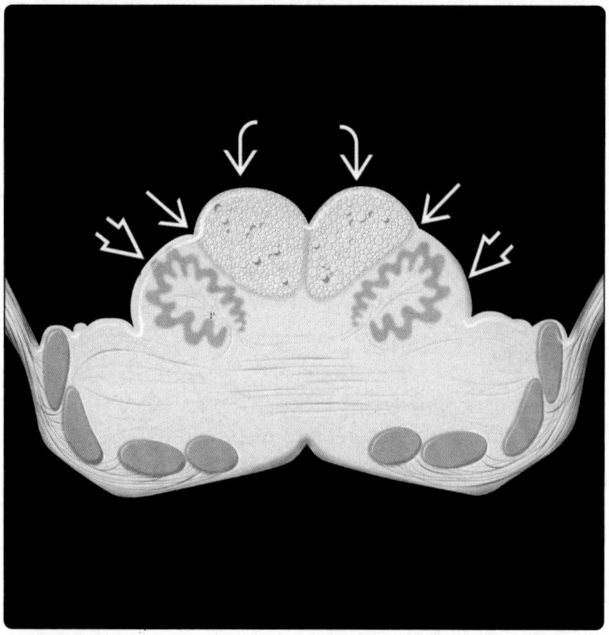

(33-62) Axial graphic of the upper medulla shows the medullary pyramids ➪ on each side of the ventral median fissure. The olives ➪ lie just posterior to the preolivary sulci ➪.

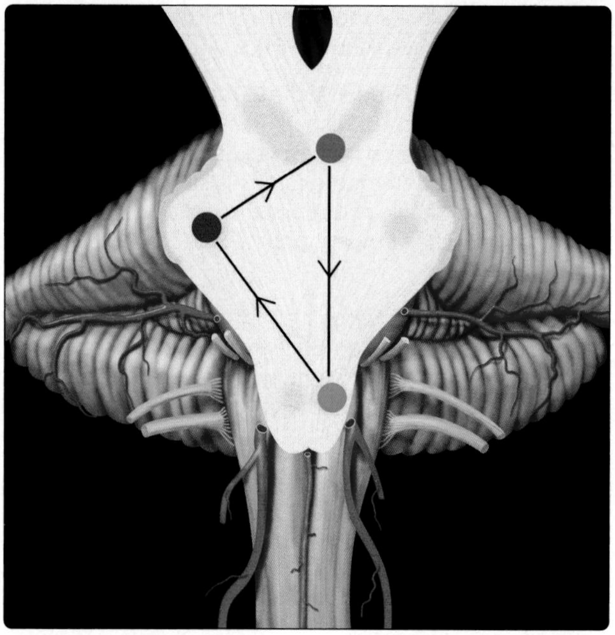

(33-63) Coronal graphic depicts the Guillain-Mollaret triangle. The triangle is composed of the ipsilateral inferior olivary nucleus (green), the dentate nucleus (blue) of the contralateral cerebellum, and the ipsilateral red nucleus (red).

ipsilateral ION and contralateral cerebellar cortex may be shrunken and atrophic.

Microscopic Features. Interruption of the Guillain-Mollaret triangle functionally deafferents the olive. The result is vacuolar cytoplasmic degeneration, neuronal enlargement, and proliferation of gemistocytic astrocytes. The enlarged neurons and proliferating astrocytes cause the initial hypertrophy. Over time, the affected olive atrophies.

HYPERTROPHIC OLIVARY DEGENERATION

Etiology
- Interruption of Guillain-Mollaret triangle
- Usually secondary to midbrain lesion
- Also postoperative pediatric cerebellar mutism

Pathology
- Inferior olives hypertrophy
  - Can be uni- or bilateral
  - Ipsi- or contralateral to primary lesion

Clinical Issues
- Rare; can occur at any age
- Delayed onset
  - Usually occurs 4-12 months after insult
- Palatal myoclonus, dentatorubral tumor

Clinical Issues

Epidemiology and Demographics. HOD is rare. It has been reported in patients of all ages, from young children to the elderly. There is no sex predilection.

Presentation and Natural History. The classic clinical presentation of HOD is palatal myoclonus, typically developing 4-12 months following the brain insult.

Imaging

General Features. The development of HOD is a delayed process. Although changes can sometimes be detected within 3 or 4 weeks after the initial insult, maximum hypertrophy occurs between 5 and 15 months. The hypertrophy typically resolves in 1-3 years, and the ION eventually becomes atrophic.

CT Findings. Although NECT scans may demonstrate the primary inciting lesion (e.g., hemorrhage), the HOD is generally not depicted.

MR Findings. T1 scans are usually normal or show mild enlargement of the ION. T2/FLAIR hyperintensity without enlargement of the ION occurs in 4-6 months but may be detectable as early as 3 weeks after the initial insult. Between 6 months and several years later, the ION appears both hyperintense and hypertrophied **(33-64)** **(33-65)**. Although the hypertrophy typically resolves and atrophy eventually ensues, the hyperintensity may persist indefinitely.

HOD does not enhance on T1 C+.

T2* SWI imaging may detect degeneration of the RN, seen as loss of the normal RN hypointensity; the signal should be similar to that of the substantia nigra.

Nuclear Medicine. PET shows increased metabolic activity in the early stages of HOD, whereas SPECT may demonstrate hyperperfusion.

HOD: IMAGING AND DIFFERENTIAL DIAGNOSIS

Imaging
- Maximum hypertrophy at 5-15 months
  - Usually resolves in 1-3 years
  - Then ION atrophies
- ION T2/FLAIR hyperintensity
- Does not enhance

Differential Diagnosis
- Common
  - MS, neoplasm
  - Perforating artery infarct
- Rare but important
  - Metronidazole neurotoxicity

Differential Diagnosis

Other lesions with T2/FLAIR hyperintensity in the anterior medulla include **demyelinating disease, neoplasm**, and **perforating artery infarction. Metronidazole neurotoxicity** exhibits bilateral, symmetric T2/FLAIR hyperintense lesions in the corpus callosum splenium and RN as well as the caudate, lentiform, olivary, and dentate nuclei.

Spinocerebellar Ataxias

Spinocerebellar ataxias (SCAs), also known as spinocerebellar atrophy/degeneration or inherited olivopontocerebellar atrophy, represent a clinically and genetically heterogeneous group of disorders. An ever-growing number of SCAs have been reported with more than 60 types identified to date.

Most SCAs are inherited and are progressive neurodegenerative disorders. SCAs are grouped into two

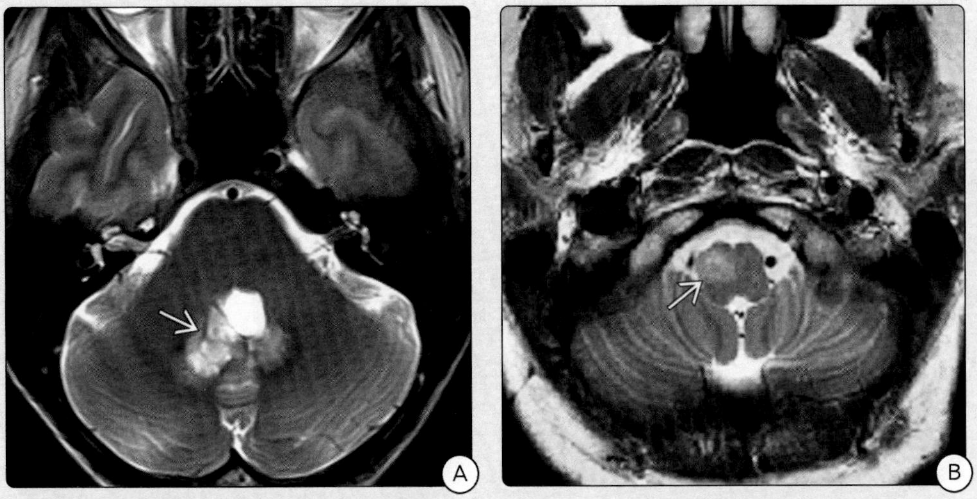

***(33-64A)** Axial T2WI in a patient who developed palatal myoclonus 6 months after medulloblastoma resection shows surgical changes in the right dentate nucleus ➡. **(33-64B)** Axial T2WI through the medulla in the same patient shows unilateral hypertrophic olivary degeneration ➡.*

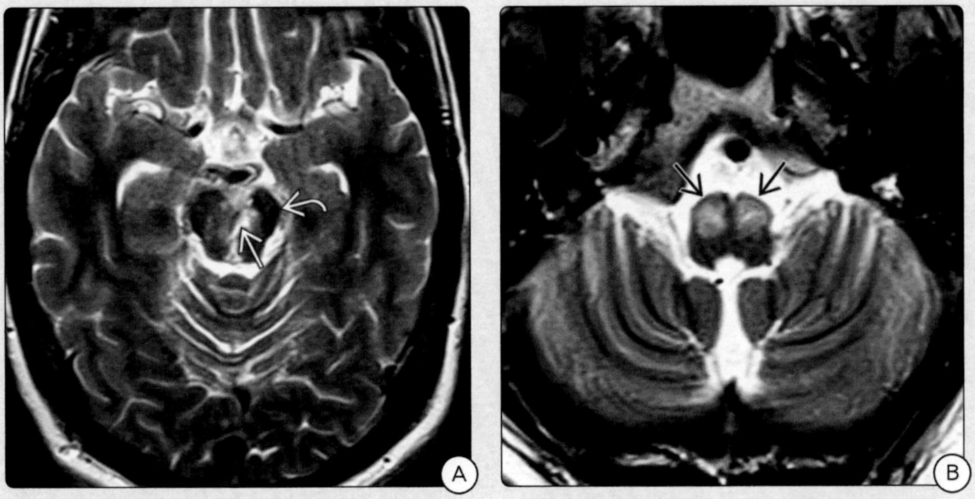

***(33-65A)** A 24y man developed palatal myoclonus 3 months after midbrain infarction. Axial T2WI shows the infarct ➡ and some volume loss in the left side of the midbrain ↶. **(33-65B)** T2WI through the medulla shows expansion, hyperintensity of both olives ➡. This is acute hypertrophic olivary degeneration. Follow-up scans (not shown) disclosed olivary atrophy.*

subtypes by pattern of inheritance, autosomal-dominant and autosomal-recessive types.

Autosomal-Recessive SCAs

Friedreich ataxia is the most common autosomal-recessive SCA. Autosomal-recessive SCAs typically become symptomatic before the age of 20 years **(33-66)** **(33-68)**. Extra-CNS involvement is frequent, and peripheral sensorimotor neuropathy is a common feature. Despite early onset, the clinical course is slowly progressive. Imaging typically shows a normal cerebellum with spinal cord and/or brainstem volume loss.

Autosomal-Dominant SCAs

The autosomal-dominant ataxias usually present at an older age with mean onset between the third and fourth decades of life. Gait disorders, abnormal eye movements, and macular degeneration are common. The course is relentlessly progressive and usually fatal.

Imaging findings in the autosomal-dominant SCAs vary with type **(33-67)**. Brainstem volume loss is generally more prominent than cerebellar atrophy, which often affects the vermis without involving the hemispheres. The pons is atrophic in SCA1, whereas the entire brainstem is small in SCA3. The cerebellum is atrophic in SCA6.

Cerebral Hemiatrophy (Dyke-Davidoff-Masson)

Terminology and Etiology

Dyke-Davidoff-Masson syndrome (DDMS), also known as cerebral hemiatrophy, is typically caused by an in utero or early childhood cerebral insult, such as an infarct, trauma, or (less commonly) infection.

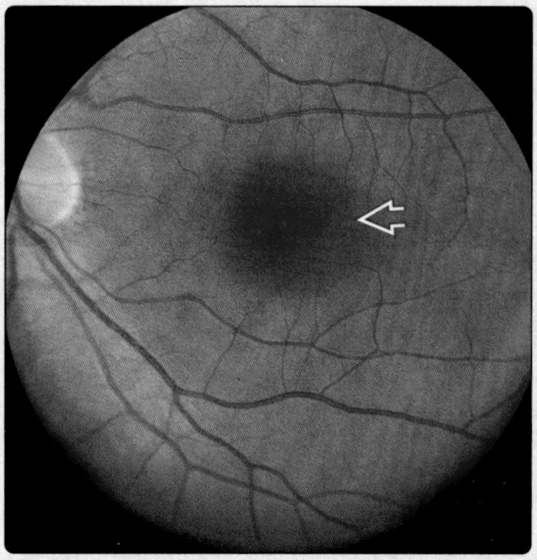

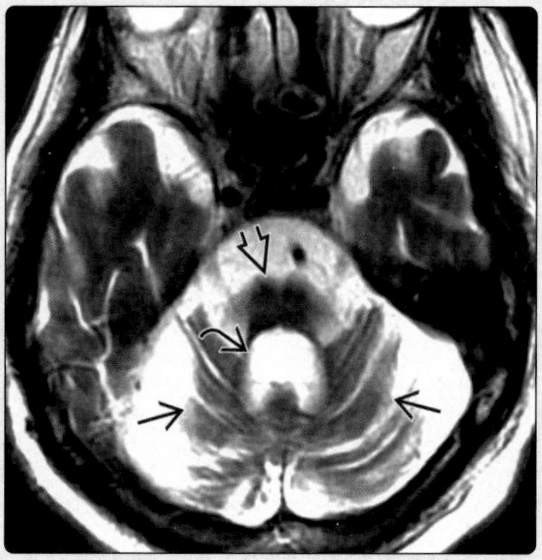

***(33-66)** Funduscopic examination in a patient with SCA7 shows striking pigmented maculopathy ➡. The patient presented with changes in visual acuity and color vision. (Courtesy K. Digre, MD, Imaging in Neurology.) **(33-67)** Axial T2WI in a patient with SCA2 shows a shrunken pons ➡, markedly atrophic cerebellar hemispheres ➡, and an enlarged 4th ventricle ➡.*

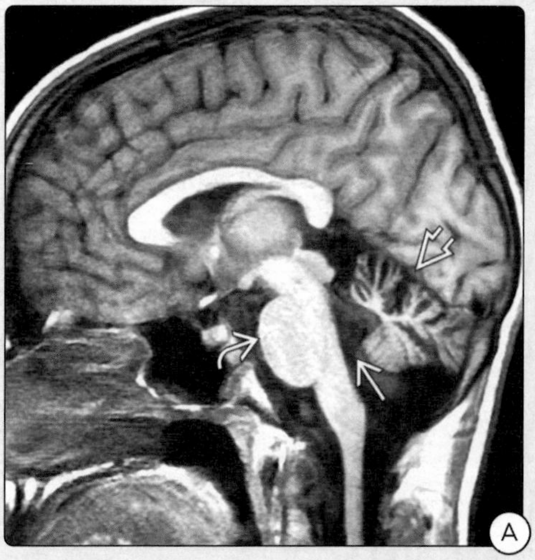

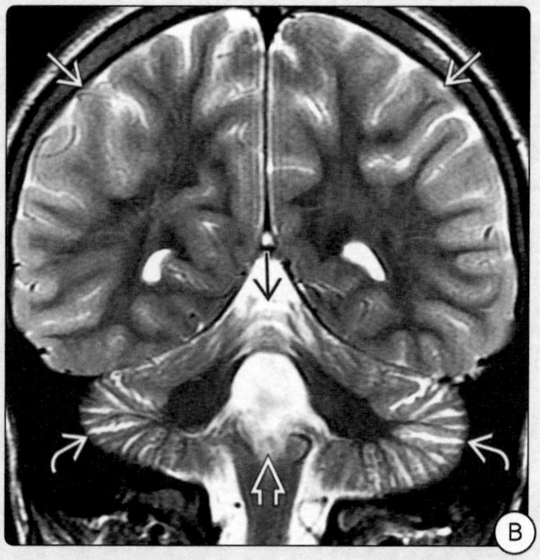

***(33-68A)** Sagittal T1WI in a 13y boy with autosomal-recessive spastic ataxia of Charlevoix-Saguenay shows normal cerebral hemispheres, pons ➡. Vermis ➡ is grossly atrophic; 4th ventricle ➡ is markedly enlarged. **(33-68B)** Coronal T2WI shows the normal cerebral hemispheres ➡. 4th ventricle ➡ is markedly enlarged, and cerebellar fissures ➡ appear prominent because folia are thinned. Vermis ➡ is markedly atrophic. (From Imaging in Neurology.)*

Lack of ipsilateral brain growth causes the calvaria and diploic space to thicken, whereas the paranasal sinuses and mastoids become enlarged and hyperaerated **(33-69)**.

Clinical Issues

Patients typically present with contralateral hemiplegia or hemiparesis. Seizures, facial asymmetry, and mental retardation are common.

Imaging

General Features. The affected hemisphere demonstrates diffuse volume loss with encephalomalacia and gliosis. Left-sided hemiatrophy is more common (70%) than right-sided hemiatrophy.

CT Findings. NECT scans show an atrophic hemisphere with enlarged sulci and dilatation of the ipsilateral ventricle. The superior sagittal sinus and interhemispheric fissure are often displaced across the midline **(33-70)**.

Bone CT shows variable degrees of calvarial thickening, elevation of the sphenoid wing and petrous temporal bone, and expanded sinuses and mastoids.

MR Findings. T1WI shows hemispheric volume loss with prominent sulci and cisterns. T2/FLAIR scans demonstrate encephalomalacia with shrunken hyperintense gyri and subcortical WM **(33-71)**. The ipsilateral cerebral peduncle is usually small. Atrophy of the contralateral cerebellum is common, secondary to crossed cerebellar diaschisis.

DDMS neither enhances on T1 C+ nor demonstrates restricted diffusion.

Differential Diagnosis

The major differential diagnosis is **Sturge-Weber syndrome** (SWS). DDMS lacks the enhancing pial angioma, enlarged choroid plexus, and typical dystrophic cortical calcifications of SWS. **Rasmussen encephalitis** lacks the calvarial changes typical of DDMS and demonstrates more focal encephalomalacia, typically in the medial temporal lobe and around the sylvian fissure.

In **hemimegalencephaly**, the abnormal hemisphere is enlarged (not small as in DDMS) and has dysplastic-appearing features caused by hamartomatous overgrowth. **Large territorial MCA infarcts** that occur after the age of 2 or 3 years do not cause the calvarial changes that typify DDMS.

CEREBRAL HEMIATROPHY

Terminology and Etiology
- Also known as Dyke-Davidoff-Masson syndrome
  - Others = cerebral hemihypoplasia, unilateral cerebral hypoplasia
- Can be congenital (infantile) or acquired (early childhood)
- In utero, early childhood insult to developing brain
  - Infarction (e.g., unilateral ICA or MCA occlusion, aortic coarctation)
  - Less commonly, infection, perinatal insult
- Trauma (1st 2 years of life)
- One hemisphere fails to develop or involutes
  - Calvarium thickens
  - Falx/tentorium, superior sagittal sinus insert off-midline

Clinical Issues
- Contralateral hemiparesis
- With or without facial asymmetry
- Seizures, variable mental retardation

Imaging Findings
- Small, atrophic hemisphere
  - Encephalomalacia, gliosis
  - Ipsilateral ventricle, sulci enlarged
  - Ipsilateral cerebral peduncle usually small
  - Contralateral cerebellar hemisphere often atrophic
- Ipsilateral calvarial thickened
  - Paranasal sinuses prominent
  - Greater sphenoid wing elevated
  - Petrous temporal bone often enlarged, overpneumatized
- Falx inserts off-midline

Differential Diagnosis
- Sturge-Weber syndrome
- Rasmussen encephalitis

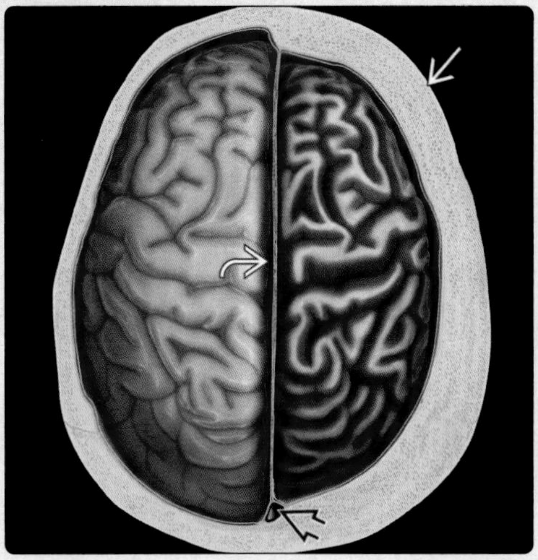

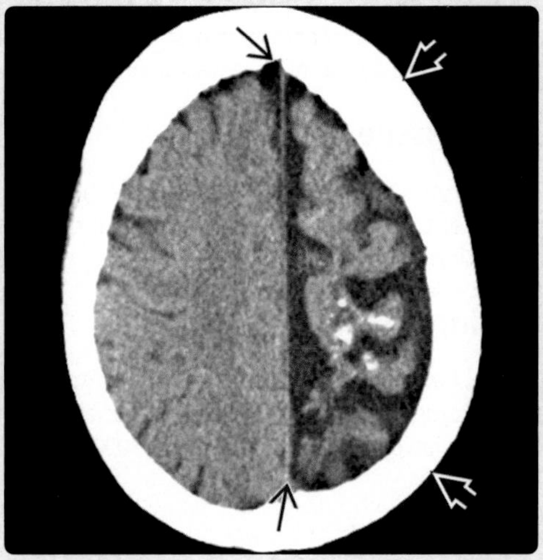

***(33-69)** Axial graphic depicts Dyke-Davidoff-Masson syndrome with shrunken, atrophic left hemisphere, thickened calvaria, off-midline insertion of the falx, and superior sagittal sinus. **(33-70)** NECT scan shows the typical findings of Dyke-Davidoff-Masson with significant atrophy and dystrophic calcification in the left hemisphere. The falx inserts off the midline, and the overlying calvaria is thickened.*

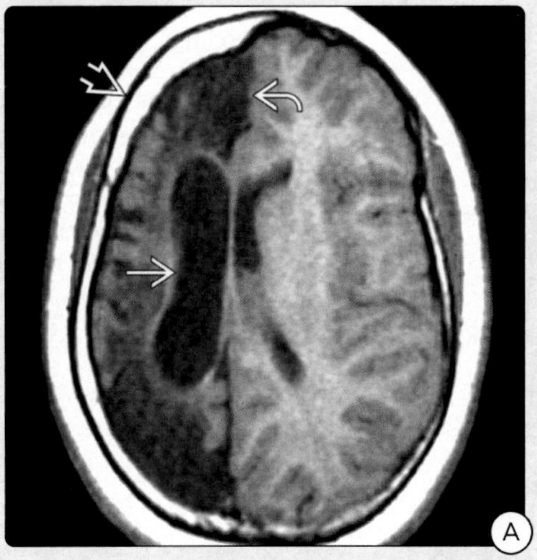

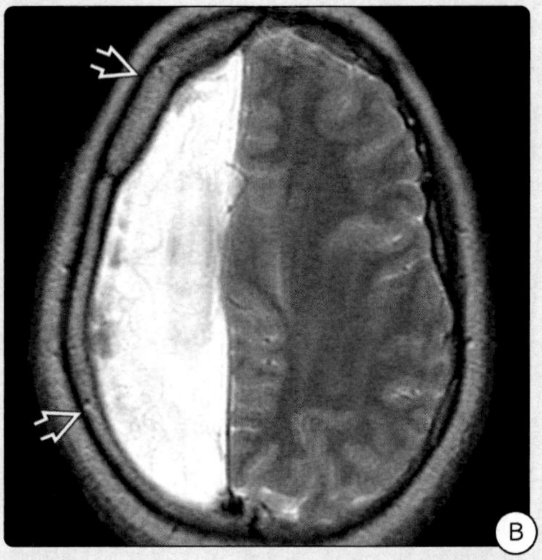

***(33-71A)** Axial T1WI in a 13y patient with longstanding seizures and left hemiparesis shows striking right cerebral hemiatrophy with enlarged lateral ventricle, off-midline falx and interhemispheric fissure, and thickened calvaria. **(33-71B)** More cephalad T2WI in the same patient shows that CSF fills the space above the atrophic right hemisphere. Compare the thickened calvaria with the normal-appearing left side.*

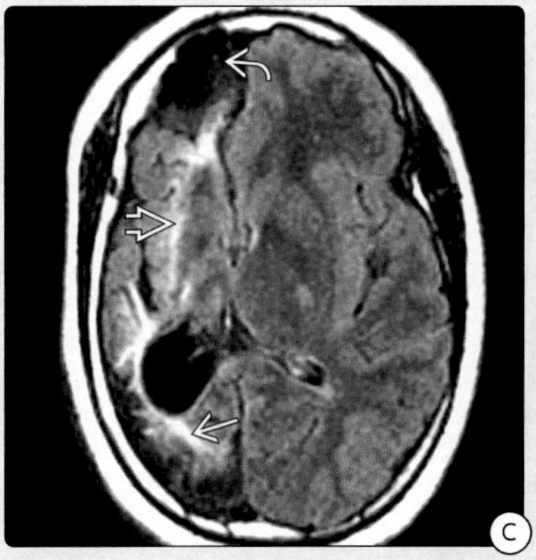

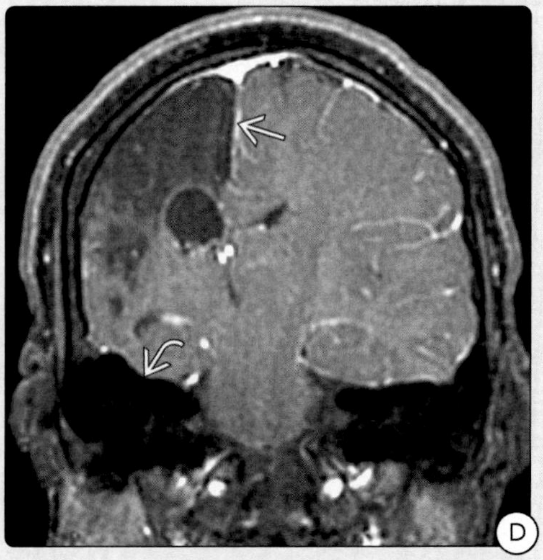

***(33-71C)** FLAIR scan in the same patient shows cortical atrophy with extensive WM gliosis, shrunken basal ganglia, and prominent right frontal sinus. **(33-71D)** Coronal T1 C+ FS scan in the same patient shows elevation, hyperaeration of the right temporal bone, and off-midline insertion of the falx and superior sagittal sinus. (Courtesy M. Edwards-Brown, MD.)*

Selected References

The Normal Aging Brain

Danka Mohammed CP et al: MicroRNAs in brain aging. Mech Ageing Dev. ePub, 2017

Dekeyzer S et al: "Unforgettable" - a pictorial essay on anatomy and pathology of the hippocampus. Insights Imaging. 8(2):199-212, 2017

Di Benedetto S et al: Contribution of neuroinflammation and immunity to brain aging and the mitigating effects of physical and cognitive interventions. Neurosci Biobehav Rev. 75:114-128, 2017

Hullinger R et al: Molecular and cellular aspects of age-related cognitive decline and Alzheimer's disease. Behav Brain Res. 322(Pt B):191-205, 2017

Lardenoije R et al: The epigenetics of aging and neurodegeneration. Prog Neurobiol. 131:21-64, 2015

Imaging the Normal Aging Brain

Spiegel AM et al: Epigenetic contributions to cognitive aging: disentangling mindspan and lifespan. Learn Mem. 21(10):569-74, 2014

Dementias

Alzheimer Disease

Buckley RF et al: Functional network integrity presages cognitive decline in preclinical Alzheimer disease. Neurology. ePub, 2017

Dallaire-Théroux C et al: Radiological-pathological correlation in Alzheimer's disease: systematic review of antemortem magnetic resonance imaging findings. J Alzheimers Dis. 57(2):575-601, 2017

Dickie DA et al: Whole brain magnetic resonance image atlases: a systematic review of existing atlases and caveats for use in population imaging. Front Neuroinform. 11:1, 2017

Donohue MC et al: Association between elevated brain amyloid and subsequent cognitive decline among cognitively normal persons. JAMA. 317(22):2305-2316, 2017

Masdeu JC: Future directions in imaging neurodegeneration. Curr Neurol Neurosci Rep. 17(1):9, 2017

McKiernan EF et al: 7T MRI for neurodegenerative dementias in vivo: a systematic review of the literature. J Neurol Neurosurg Psychiatry. ePub, 2017

Pagani MM et al: Progressive disgregation of brain networking from normal aging to Alzhimer's disease. Independent component analysis on FDG-PET data. J Nucl Med. ePub, 2017

Sørensen L et al: Differential diagnosis of mild cognitive impairment and Alzheimer's disease using structural MRI cortical thickness, hippocampal shape, hippocampal texture, and volumetry. Neuroimage Clin. 13:470-482, 2016

Lardenoije R et al: The epigenetics of aging and neurodegeneration. Prog Neurobiol. 131:21-64, 2015

Tabatabaei-Jafari H et al: Cerebral atrophy in mild cognitive impairment: a systematic review with meta-analysis. Alzheimers Dement (Amst). 1(4):487-504, 2015

Vascular Dementia

Di Donato I et al: Cerebral autosomal dominant arteriopathy with subcortical infarcts and leukoencephalopathy (CADASIL) as a model of small vessel disease: update on clinical, diagnostic, and management aspects. BMC Med. 15(1):41, 2017

Ikram MA et al: Genetics of vascular dementia - review from the ICVD working group. BMC Med. 15(1):48, 2017

Quinn TJ et al: Diagnosis in vascular dementia, applying 'Cochrane diagnosis rules' to 'dementia diagnostic tools'. Clin Sci (Lond). 131(8):729-732, 2017

Roseborough A et al: Associations between amyloid β and white matter hyperintensities: A systematic review. Alzheimers Dement. ePub, 2017

Santos CY et al: Pathophysiologic relationship between Alzheimer's disease, cerebrovascular disease, and cardiovascular risk: a review and synthesis. Alzheimers Dement (Amst). 7:69-87, 2017

Smith EE: Clinical presentations and epidemiology of vascular dementia. Clin Sci (Lond). 131(11):1059-1068, 2017

Søndergaard CB et al: Hereditary cerebral small vessel disease and stroke. Clin Neurol Neurosurg. 155:45-57, 2017

Frontotemporal Lobar Degeneration

Mann DM et al: Frontotemporal lobar degeneration: pathogenesis, pathology and pathways to phenotype. Brain Pathol. ePub, 2017

Olney NT et al: Frontotemporal dementia. Neurol Clin. 35(2):339-374, 2017

Prpar Mihevc S et al: Nuclear trafficking in amyotrophic lateral sclerosis and frontotemporal lobar degeneration. Brain. 140(Pt 1):13-26, 2017

Li YQ et al: Frontotemporal lobar degeneration: mechanisms and therapeutic strategies. Mol Neurobiol. 53(9):6091-6105, 2016

Lewy Body Dementias

Agosta F et al: Advanced magnetic resonance imaging of neurodegenerative diseases. Neurol Sci. 38(1):41-51, 2017

Galasko D: Lewy body disorders. Neurol Clin. 35(2):325-338, 2017

McAleese KE et al: TDP-43 pathology in Alzheimer's disease, dementia with Lewy bodies and ageing. Brain Pathol. 27(4):472-479, 2017

Nag S et al: TDP-43 pathology and memory impairment in elders without pathologic diagnoses of AD or FTLD. Neurology. 88(7):653-660, 2017

Gomperts SN: Lewy body dementias: dementia with Lewy bodies and Parkinson disease dementia. Continuum (Minneap Minn). 22(2 Dementia):435-63, 2016

Hogan DB et al: The prevalence and incidence of dementia with Lewy bodies: a systematic review. Can J Neurol Sci. 43 Suppl 1:S83-95, 2016

Ingelsson M: Alpha-synuclein oligomers-neurotoxic molecules in Parkinson's disease and other Lewy body disorders. Front Neurosci. 10:408, 2016

Walker Z et al: Lewy body dementias. Lancet. 386(10004):1683-97, 2015

Miscellaneous Dementias

Crutch SJ et al: Consensus classification of posterior cortical atrophy. Alzheimers Dement. ePub, 2017

Gaudino S et al: Neuroradiology of human prion diseases, diagnosis and differential diagnosis. Radiol Med. 122(5):369-385, 2017

Iwasaki Y: Creutzfeldt-Jakob disease. Neuropathology. 37(2):174-188, 2017

Mead S et al: CJD mimics and chameleons. Pract Neurol. 17(2):113-121, 2017

Degenerative Disorders

Pujol S et al: In vivo exploration of the connectivity between the subthalamic nucleus and the globus pallidus in the human brain using multi-fiber tractography. Front Neuroanat. 10:119, 2017

Zwirner J et al: Subthalamic nucleus volumes are highly consistent but decrease age-dependently-a combined magnetic resonance imaging and stereology approach in humans. Hum Brain Mapp. 38(2):909-922, 2017

Plantinga BR et al: Ultra-high field MRI post mortem structural connectivity of the human subthalamic nucleus, substantia nigra, and globus pallidus. Front Neuroanat. 10:66, 2016

Parkinson Disease

Braak H et al: Neuropathological staging of brain pathology in sporadic Parkinson's disease: separating the wheat from the chaff. J Parkinsons Dis. 7(s1):S73-S87, 2017

Frey KA: Molecular imaging of extrapyramidal movement disorders. Semin Nucl Med. 47(1):18-30, 2017

Graebner AK et al: Clinical impact of 123I-Ioflupane SPECT (DaTscan) in a movement disorder center. Neurodegener Dis. 17(1):38-43, 2017

Lill CM: Genetics of Parkinson's disease. Mol Cell Probes. 30(6):386-396, 2016

Sako W et al: Imaging-based differential diagnosis between multiple system atrophy and Parkinson's disease. J Neurol Sci. 368:104-8, 2016

Booth TC et al: The role of functional dopamine-transporter SPECT imaging in parkinsonian syndromes, part 1. AJNR Am J Neuroradiol. 36(2):229-35, 2015

Multiple System Atrophy

Chen B et al: Usefulness of diffusion-tensor MRI in the diagnosis of Parkinson variant of multiple system atrophy and Parkinson's disease: a valuable tool to differentiate between them? Clin Radiol. 72(7):610.e9-610.e15, 2017

Wang N et al: Using 'swallow-tail' sign and putaminal hypointensity as biomarkers to distinguish multiple system atrophy from idiopathic Parkinson's disease: a susceptibility-weighted imaging study. Eur Radiol. 27(8):3174-3180, 2017

Progressive Supranuclear Palsy

Hall B et al: in vivo tau PET imaging in dementia: pathophysiology, radiotracer quantification, and a systematic review of clinical findings. Ageing Res Rev. 36:50-63, 2017

Lee Y et al: Volumetric analysis of the cerebellum in patients with progressive supranuclear palsy. Eur J Neurol. 24(1):212-218, 2017

Yokoyama JS et al: Shared genetic risk between corticobasal degeneration, progressive supranuclear palsy, and frontotemporal dementia. Acta Neuropathol. 133(5):825-837, 2017

Tipton PW et al: Cerebral peduncle angle: unreliable in differentiating progressive supranuclear palsy from other neurodegenerative diseases. Parkinsonism Relat Disord. 32:31-35, 2016

Corticobasal Degeneration

Yokoyama JS et al: Shared genetic risk between corticobasal degeneration, progressive supranuclear palsy, and frontotemporal dementia. Acta Neuropathol. 133(5):825-837, 2017

Amyotrophic Lateral Sclerosis

Hardiman O et al: The changing picture of amyotrophic lateral sclerosis: lessons from European registers. J Neurol Neurosurg Psychiatry. ePub, 2017

van Es MA et al: Amyotrophic lateral sclerosis. Lancet. ePub, 2017

Vajda A et al: Genetic testing in ALS: a survey of current practices. Neurology. 88(10):991-999, 2017

Chakraborty S et al: The "motor band sign:" susceptibility-weighted imaging in amyotrophic lateral sclerosis. Can J Neurol Sci. 42(4):260-3, 2015

Wallerian Degeneration

Bekiesinska-Figatowska M et al: Diffusion restriction in the corticospinal tracts and the corpus callosum in neonates after cerebral insult. Brain Dev. 39(3):203-210, 2017

Chen YJ et al: Wallerian degeneration beyond the corticospinal tracts: conventional and advanced MRI findings. J Neuroimaging. 27(3):272-280, 2017

Singh S et al: Relationship of acute axonal damage, Wallerian degeneration, and clinical disability in multiple sclerosis. J Neuroinflammation. 14(1):57, 2017

Tricaud N et al: Wallerian demyelination: chronicle of a cellular cataclysm. Cell Mol Life Sci. ePub, 2017

Hypertrophic Olivary Degeneration

Smets G et al: The dentato-rubro-olivary pathway revisited: new MR imaging observations regarding hypertrophic olivary degeneration. Clin Anat. 30(4):543-549, 2017

Avula S et al: Post-operative pediatric cerebellar mutism syndrome and its association with hypertrophic olivary degeneration. Quant Imaging Med Surg. 6(5):535-544, 2016

Spinocerebellar Ataxias

Beaudin M et al: Systematic review of autosomal recessive ataxias and proposal for a classification. Cerebellum Ataxias. 4:3, 2017

Cerebral Hemiatrophy (Dyke-Davidoff-Masson)

Gökçe E et al: Radiological imaging findings of Dyke-Davidoff-Masson syndrome. Acta Neurol Belg. ePub, 2017

Thakkar PA et al: Dyke-Davidoff-Masson syndrome: a rare cause of cerebral hemiatrophy in children. J Pediatr Neurosci. 11(3):252-254, 2016

Hydrocephalus and CSF Disorders

The brain CSF spaces include the ventricular system—a series of interconnected, CSF-filled cavities—and the subarachnoid space. Understanding the normal anatomy of these CSF spaces and their variants is a prerequisite to deciphering their pathology. We therefore begin this chapter with a brief discussion of the normal development of the ventricles and CSF spaces, then delineate their normal gross and imaging anatomy.

We next describe normal variants, which should not be mistaken for disease, then turn our attention to hydrocephalus and the manifestations of elevated CSF pressure, including idiopathic intracranial hypertension ("pseudotumor cerebri"). We close the chapter with a discussion of CSF leaks and intracranial hypotension.

Normal Development of the Ventricles and Cisterns

Ventricles

The embryonic ventricular system is a series of interconnected fluid-filled chambers that arise as expansions from the central cavity of the embryonic neural tube. As the developing brain bends and expands, it forms forebrain, midbrain, and hindbrain vesicles. The forebrain cavity divides into two lateral ventricles, which develop as outpouchings from the rostral third ventricle and are connected to it by the interventricular foramen (foramen of Monro) **(34-1)**.

The cerebral aqueduct develops from the midbrain vesicle. The fourth ventricle develops from the hindbrain cavity and merges proximally with the aqueduct and caudally with the central canal of the spinal cord. In the coronal plane, the developing lateral and third ventricles form a central H-shaped monoventricle that continues inferiorly into the aqueduct and then connects to the fourth ventricle.

At the eleventh or twelfth gestational week, the inferomedial aspect of the fourth ventricular roof thins and opens, creating the foramen of Magendie. The foramina of Luschka open shortly thereafter, establishing communication between the developing ventricular system and subarachnoid space.

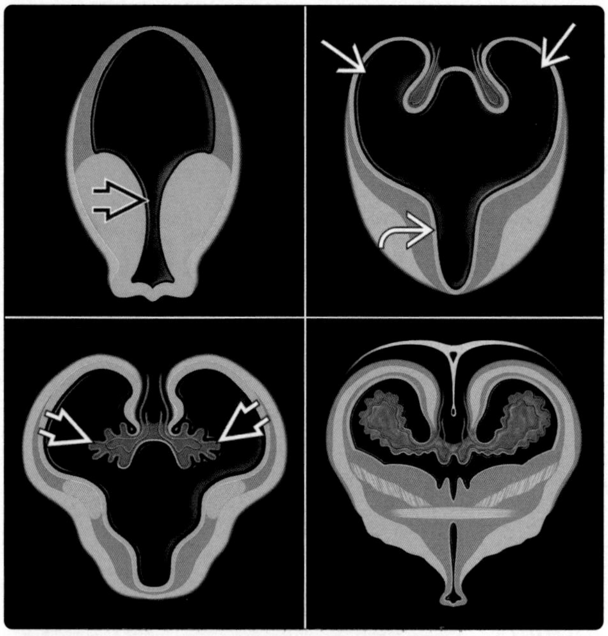

(34-1) Embryology of forebrain, ventricles, choroid plexus shows central cavity of neural tube ⇒ develops outpouchings ⇒ from rostral 3rd ventricle ⇒, forming H-shaped monoventricle. Choroid plexus ⇒ develops along choroid fissure.

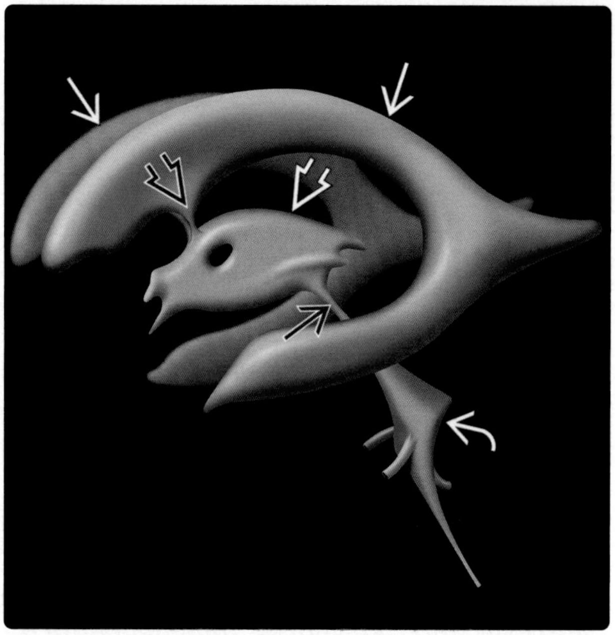

(34-2) Graphic depicts the paired lateral ventricles ⇒, foramen of Monro ⇒, third ventricle ⇒, aqueduct ⇒, fourth ventricle ⇒ with its three-outlet foramina, and inferiorly directed obex.

Choroid Plexus

The embryonic choroid plexus forms where infolded meningeal mesenchyme—the tela choroidea—contacts the ependymal lining of the ventricles. The invagination occurs along the entire choroidal fissure, a narrow cleft that lies in the medial lateral ventricle between the fornix and the thalamus. Initially, the fetal choroid plexus is large relative to the size of the lateral ventricles, occupying nearly three-quarters of the ventricular lumen. As the brain and ventricular system grow, the choroid plexus gradually diminishes in relative volume.

Subarachnoid Spaces

The leptomeninges are derived from a gelatinous layer of paraxial mesoderm—the primary meninx or "meninx primitiva"—that envelops the neural tube. At gestational day 32, the innermost zone of the primary meninx systematically degenerates, forming irregular spaces on the ventral aspect of the rhombencephalon. These spaces then extend caudally and dorsally, eventually coalescing to form the fluid-filled leptomeninges.

Normal Anatomy of the Ventricles and Cisterns

Ventricular System

The ventricular system is composed of four interconnected ependyma-lined cavities that lie deep within the brain **(34-2)**. The paired lateral ventricles communicate with the third ventricle via the Y-shaped foramen of Monro. The third ventricle communicates with the fourth ventricle via the cerebral aqueduct (of Sylvius). In turn, the fourth ventricle communicates with the subarachnoid space.

Lateral Ventricles

Each lateral ventricle is a C-shaped structure with a body, atrium, and three projections ("horns"). We consider each part of the lateral ventricle from front to back.

The **body** of the lateral ventricle passes posteriorly under the corpus callosum. Its floor is formed by the dorsal thalamus, and its medial wall is bordered by the fornix. Laterally, it curves around the body and tail of the caudate nucleus.

The **atrium** contains the choroid plexus glomus and is formed by the convergence of the body with the temporal and occipital horns. The **temporal horn** extends anteroinferiorly from the atrium and is bordered on its floor and medial wall by the hippocampus. The **occipital horn** is surrounded entirely by white matter tracts, principally the geniculocalcarine tract and the forceps major of the corpus callosum.

The **frontal horn** is the most anterior segment of the lateral ventricle. Its roof is formed by the corpus callosum genu, and it is bordered inferolaterally by the head of the caudate nucleus. The septi pellucidi are thin bilayered membranes that extend from the corpus callosum to the foramen of Monro, forming the medial borders of both frontal horns.

Foramen of Monro

The foramen of Monro (interventricular foramen) is a Y-shaped structure with two long arms extending toward each lateral ventricle and a short inferior common stem that

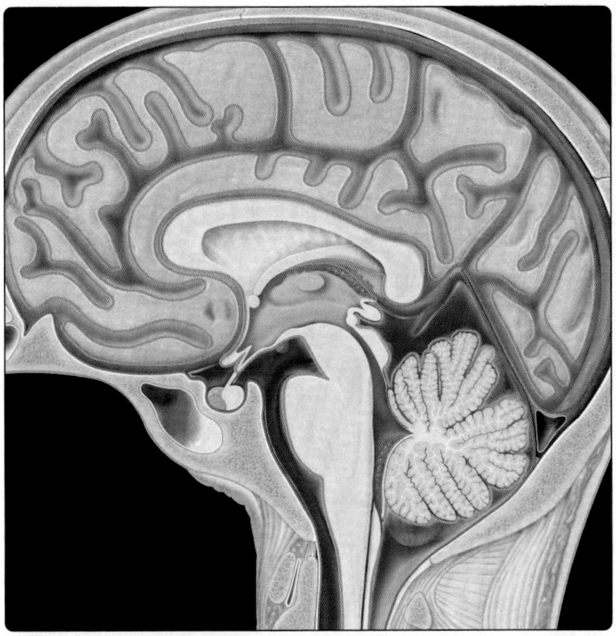

(34-3) Sagittal graphic depicts subarachnoid spaces with CSF (blue) between arachnoid (purple) and pia (orange). The pia is closely adherent to the brain, while the arachnoid loosely adheres to the dura.

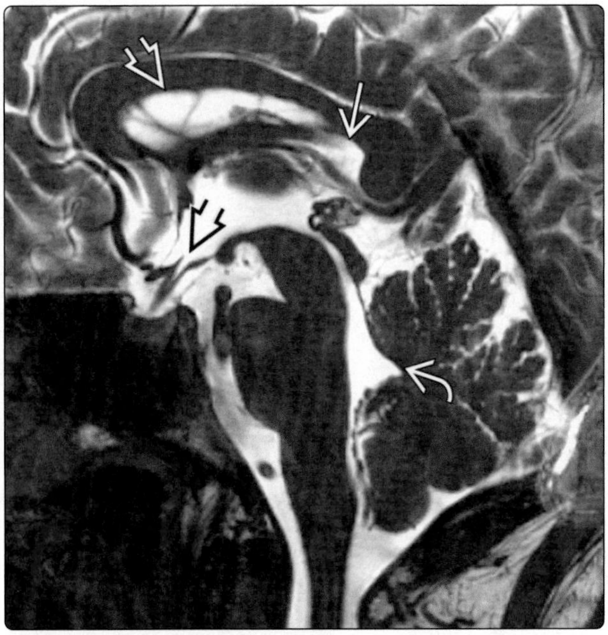

(34-4) Sagittal T2WI shows lateral ventricle ➡, velum interpositum ➡, "pointed" recesses of the anterior third ventricle ➡, and fastigium of the fourth ventricle ➡.

connects with the roof of the third ventricle. The anterior borders of the foramen on Monro are formed by the pillars (bodies) of the fornices. The posterior border is formed by the choroid plexus.

Third Ventricle

The third ventricle is a single, slit-like, midline, vertically oriented cavity that lies between the thalami. Its roof is formed by the tela choroidea, a double layer of invaginated pia. The anterior commissure lies along the anterior border of the third ventricle. The floor of the third ventricle is formed by the optic chiasm, hypothalamus, mammillary bodies, and roof of the midbrain tegmentum.

The third ventricle has two inferiorly located projections, the slightly rounded **optic recess** and the more pointed **infundibular recess**. Two small recesses, the **suprapineal** and **pineal recesses**, form the posterior border of the third ventricle. A variably sized interthalamic adhesion (the massa intermedia) lies between the lateral walls of the third ventricle.

Cerebral Aqueduct

The cerebral aqueduct is an elongated tubular conduit that lies between the midbrain tegmentum and the quadrigeminal plate. It connects the third ventricle with the fourth ventricle.

Fourth Ventricle

The fourth ventricle—sometimes called the rhomboid fossa—is a diamond-shaped cavity that lies between the dorsal pons and the vermis **(34-3)** **(34-4)**. The fourth ventricle has five distinct recesses. The **fastigium** is a prominent triangular dorsal midline outpouching that points toward the vermis. The **posterior superior recesses** are paired, slender, CSF-filled pouches that curve over the cerebellar tonsils. The **lateral recesses** curve anterolaterally from the fourth ventricle, passing under the major cerebellar peduncles into the lower cerebellopontine angle cisterns **(34-5)**.

The fourth ventricle gradually narrows as it courses inferiorly, forming the **obex**. Near the cervicomedullary junction, the obex becomes continuous with the central canal of the spinal cord. The junction between the obex and central canal is demarcated by a prominent dorsal "bump" formed by the nucleus gracilis.

Choroid Plexus, CSF, and Brain Interstitial Fluid

The CSF space is a dynamic pressure system with a hydrostatic balance between CSF production and absorption. CSF pressure determines intracranial pressure. With lumbar puncture, the CSF should appear clear with opening pressure ranging from 3-4 mm Hg before 1 year of age to 10-15 mm Hg (100-180 mm H_2O) in adults.

Anatomy

The choroid plexus (CP) is composed of numerous highly vascular papillary or frond-like excrescences. These papillae consist of a central connective tissue core covered by ependyma-derived secretory epithelium.

CP is present in all parts of the ventricular system except for the cerebral aqueduct and the frontal and occipital horns of the lateral ventricles.

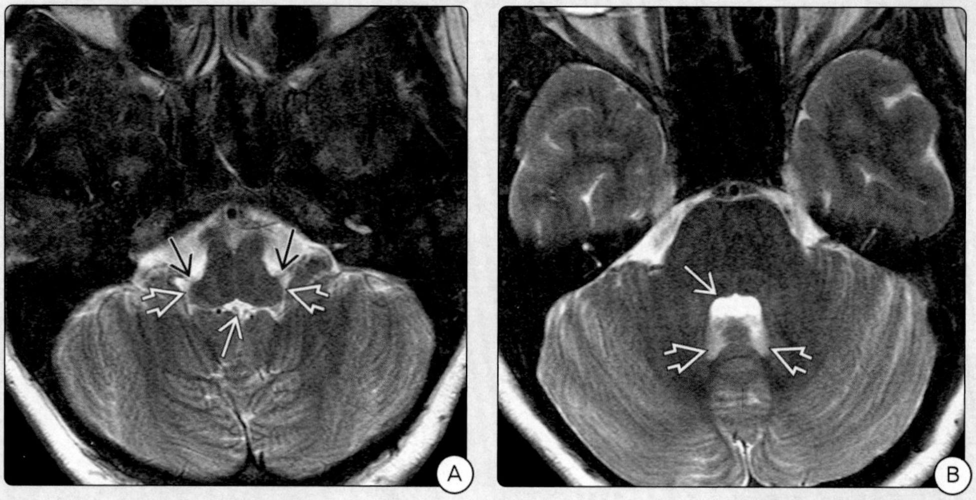

(34-5A) *These 3.0-T T2 scans demonstrate normal ventricular anatomy. Inferior fourth ventricle ➡ contains small "dots" of choroid plexus. The posterolateral recesses ➡ and foramina of Luschka ➡ are indicated.* ***(34-5B)*** *The body of the fourth ventricle resembles a kidney bean on its side. Note indentations caused by the facial colliculi ➡. The posterior superior recesses ➡ cap the cerebellar tonsils.*

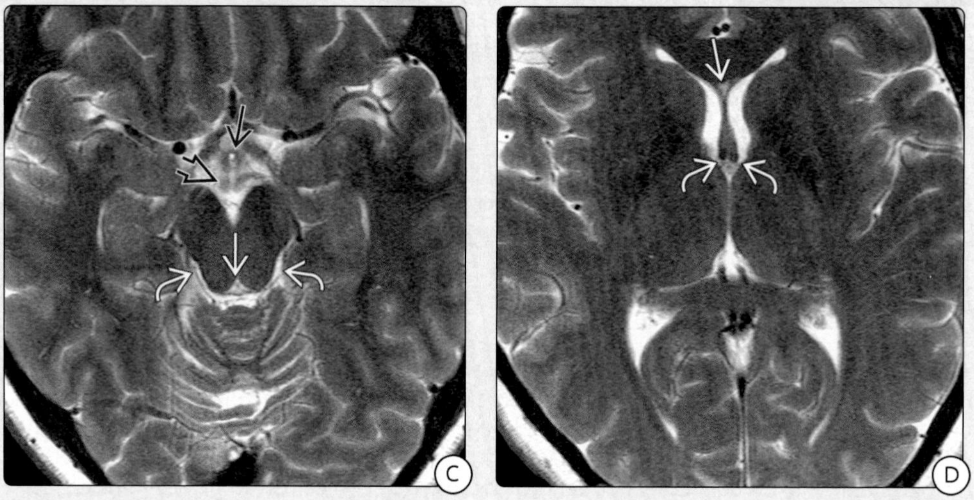

(34-5C) *Suprasellar cistern with the hypothalamus and infundibular recess of 3rd ventricle ➡, mammillary bodies ➡ are clearly seen. Cerebral aqueduct is small and triangular ➡. Quadrigeminal cisterns ➡ contain choroidal arteries, basal vein of Rosenthal, and the trochlear nerves.* ***(34-5D)*** *Frontal horns of the lateral ventricles are separated by the septi pellucidi. A tiny CSP is present ➡. Note foramen of Monro with its two connections ➡.*

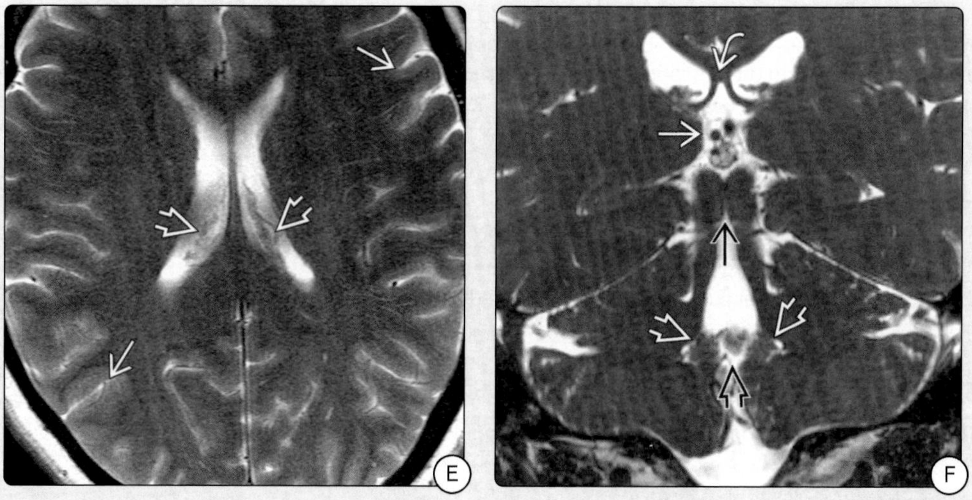

(34-5E) *Choroid plexus ➡, vessels course anteromedially toward the foramen of Monro (seen on lower section). Surface sulci ➡ are small but well delineated in this normal scan.* ***(34-5F)*** *Coronal scan shows velum interpositum ➡ lying below fornices ➡. The rhomboid 4th ventricle joins the aqueduct above ➡. Midline foramen of Magendie ➡, posterosuperior recesses ➡ capping cerebellar tonsils are shown.*

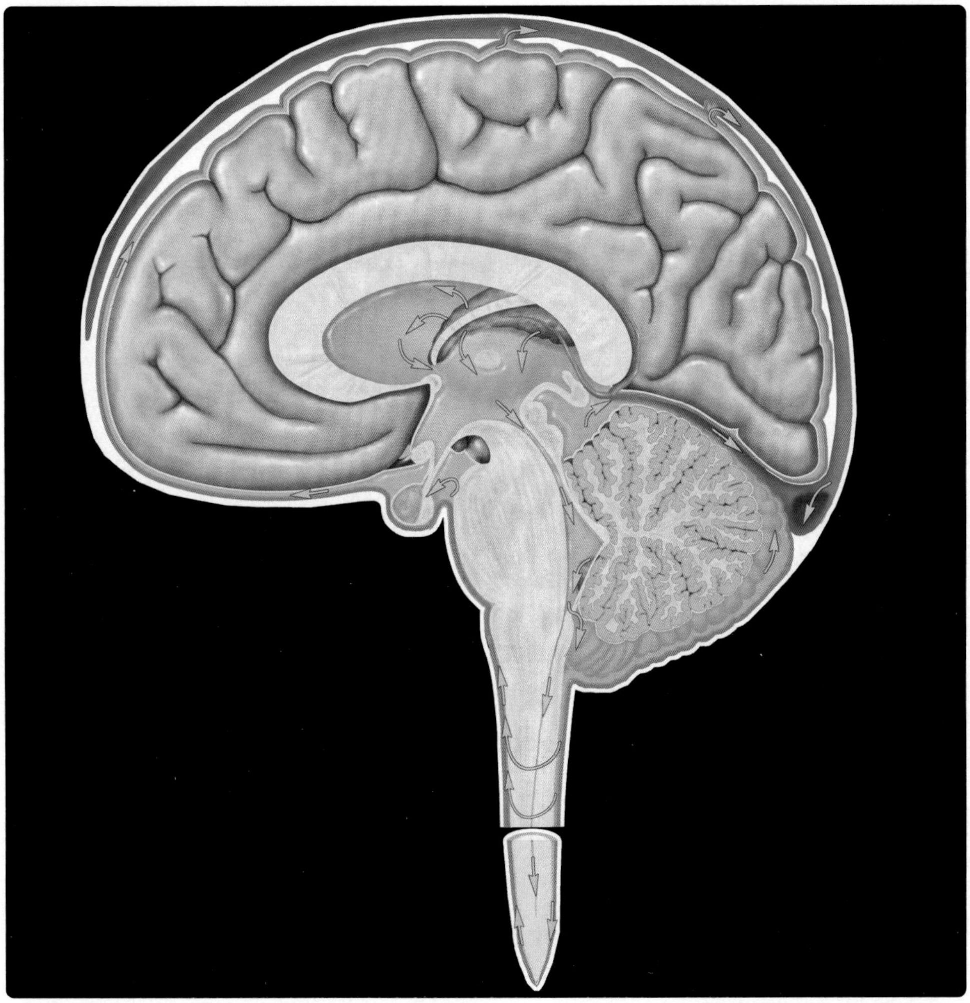

(34-6) Sagittal graphic depicts classic model of normal CSF circulation. In this model, CSF is mostly produced by the lateral ventricular choroid plexus and flows in a unidirectional manner from the lateral ventricles through the short Y-shaped foramen of Monro into the third ventricle. From there, CSF passes through the long, narrow cerebral aqueduct into the fourth ventricle. The fourth ventricle has three outlet foramina, the midline foramen of Magendie and the two lateral foramina of Luschka. When CSF exits the fourth ventricle into the cisterna magna, it circulates throughout the subarachnoid cisterns, including those in the spinal canal. CSF is eventually resorbed primarily through the arachnoid granulations into the dural venous sinuses. In newer models of brain CSF-interstitial fluid (ISF) homeostasis, some CSF is probably absorbed into the brain and passes via the paravascular spaces through the cribriform plate into the cervical lymphatics.

The largest mass of CP is the **glomus**, located in the atrium of the lateral ventricles. The CP extends anterosuperiorly from the glomus along the floor of the lateral ventricle, lying between the fornix and the thalamus. It also extends anteroinferiorly from the glomus into the temporal horn, where it fills the choroidal fissure and lies superomedial to the hippocampus.

The CP of the lateral ventricles passes into and through the foramen of Monro, curving posteriorly along the roof of the third ventricle and terminating near the suprapineal recess. The third ventricle CP is often hypoplastic and inapparent on imaging studies.

The CP of the fourth ventricle extends from the midline, protruding laterally through the foramen of Luschka into the cerebellopontine angle cisterns. These tufts of choroid plexus are located anterior to the flocculus, inferolateral to the CN VII/VIII complex, and posterosuperior to the CN IX, X, and XI complex.

Function

The CP has two major functions: CSF production and maintenance of the blood-CSF barrier. In adult humans, the CP epithelium forms CSF at the rate of about 0.4 mL per minute or about 500-600 mL every 24 hours. CSF is turned over about four times a day, allowing for the removal of waste products.

The CP is not the only source of CSF. Brain interstitial fluid (ISF) is a significant extrachoroidal source of CSF. Smaller potential sources of CSF production include the ventricular ependyma and brain capillaries.

In adult humans, there are 280 mL of ISF and 140 mL of CSF, of which 30 mL are in the ventricles, 80 mL in the cerebral subarachnoid space (SAS), and 30 mL in the spinal SAS.

The CP maintains the blood-CSF barrier via tight junctions between epithelial cells. The exchange of substances between the brain extracellular fluid and the CSF across the blood-CSF barrier is highly regulated. Specialized subpopulations of CP epithelial cells are responsible for the transfer of plasma proteins from blood to the CSF via the albumin-binding protein SPARC.

CSF Circulation and Homeostasis

Traditional Model of CSF Homeostasis. The longstanding, classic model of CSF homeostasis was based on the *circulation theory* in which the majority of CSF is produced by the CP, then circulates from the ventricles into the SASs. In this model, CSF flow in the ventricular cavities is unidirectional and rostrocaudal. CSF exits the fourth ventricle into the SASs through the medial foramen (of Magendie) and the two lateral foramina (of Luschka), which form the only natural communications between the ventricles and the SAS **(34-6)**.

In the classic model, CSF resorption was thought to occur mostly via *bulk flow*, driven by the hydrostatic pressure difference between the CSF and cerebral veins. Flow-sensitive MR has now demonstrated that CSF motion is actually *pulsatile* and is driven by pressure waves from intracranial blood vessels generated during the cardiac cycle. This results in a relatively small net flow from the ventricles toward the SAS.

Updated Model of CSF and ISF Homeostasis. New evidence suggests that the traditional model of CSF production, circulation, and function is too simplistic and much more complex than previously thought. It is now recognized that CSF plays an essential role in the maintenance of brain ISF homeostasis and that the two are intimately interrelated in maintaining normal brain function. The main sources of ISF are the blood and CSF.

In the updated CSF-ISF model, the brain perivascular spaces (PVSs) (Virchow-Robin) and paravascular spaces play a critical role in CSF homeostasis. The PVSs form a key component of the brain's "protolymphatic" or *"glymphatic" system*. The PVSs are lined with leptomeningeal (pial) cells that coat the PVSs as well as arteries and veins in the SAS, thus separating CSF in the SAS from the brain parenchyma and PVSs.

Human brain capillaries are formed by an endothelium that separates them from the extracellular space (ECS). Fibrous astrocytes form end-feet that completely surround the capillaries. A basement membrane separates the astrocyte end-feet from the capillary endothelium. The capillary endothelial basement membrane is fused with the layer of basement membrane adjacent to the astrocyte end-feet and is also shared with contractile pericytes. The endothelial cells, astrocytes, and pericytes are all involved in the regulation of blood-brain barrier permeability.

ISF diffuses through the ECS and then drains via bulk flow along the basement membranes of cerebral capillaries. ISF circulation likely occurs through the water-selective aquaporin (AQP) channels of the glymphatic system, key factors in regulating ECS water homeostasis. AQP4 is highly expressed in astrocytic end-feet and also appears to be crucial for fluid exchange between the CSF and ISF.

A substantial amount of ISF exits the brain via connections between the perivascular spaces and leptomeningeal arteries. Tracer experiments show that both CSF and ISF drain through the cribriform plate to lymphatics of the head and neck.

Estimates are that CSF drainage is approximately one-third via arachnoid granulations (and possibly lymphatics) in the cranial dura mater, one-third via paravascular spaces adjacent to intracerebral arteries and around leptomeningeal arteries passing through the cribriform plate to the cervical lymphatics/deep cervical lymph nodes, and one-third via spinal vessels.

Finally, in this model of CSF and ISF homeostasis, drainage of extracellular fluids in the CNS and integrity of the brain glymphatic system is important for not only volume regulation, but also clearance of waste products such as amyloid-β (Aβ) from the brain parenchyma.

Subarachnoid Spaces/Cisterns

The **subarachnoid spaces** (SASs) lie between the pia and arachnoid **(34-3)**. The **sulci** are small, thin SASs that are interposed between the gyral folds. Focal expansions of the SASs form the brain CSF cisterns. Numerous pial-covered septa cross the SASs from the brain to the arachnoid, which is loosely attached to the inner layer of the dura.

The major cisterns are found at the base of the brain above the sella turcica, around the brainstem, at the tentorial apex, adjacent to the cerebellopontine angles, and above/below the foramen magnum. All SASs normally communicate freely with each other and the ventricular system, providing natural pathways for disease dissemination **(34-5)**.

Normal Variants

Age-Related Changes

Morphometrical age- and sex-related studies using three-dimensional volume rendering derived from standard 3-T MR scans show that an increase in lateral ventricular volume is a constant, linear function of age throughout life.

Asymmetric Lateral Ventricles

Asymmetric lateral ventricles can be identified on imaging studies in approximately 5-10% of normal patients. The asymmetry is typically mild to moderate **(34-7)**. Bowing, deviation, or displacement of the septi pellucidi across the midline is common; by itself, it neither indicates pathology nor implicates an etiology for nonspecific headache.

Severe degrees of asymmetry, diffuse nonfocal ventricular enlargement, or evidence of transependymal CSF migration should prompt a search for possible accompanying disorders.

The major differential diagnosis for asymmetric lateral ventricles is **unilateral obstructive hydrocephalus**. Unilateral obstructive hydrocephalus is rare, occurring when only one arm of the foramen of Monro becomes occluded **(34-8)**. Membranous obstruction of the foramen of Monro can be overlooked and is best differentiated from benign ventricular asymmetry using special MR techniques (see below).

Cavum Septi Pellucidi and Vergae

Terminology

A **cavum septi pellucidi** (CSP) is a fluid-filled cavity that lies between the frontal horns of the lateral ventricles **(34-9)**. A **cavum vergae** (CV) is an elongated finger-like posterior extension from the CSP that lies between the fornices **(34-10)**.

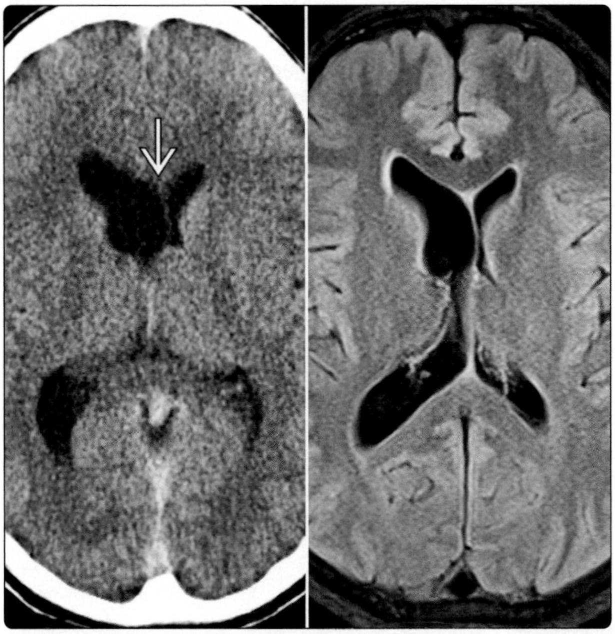

(34-7) (L) NECT shows that the right lateral ventricle is larger than the left, septum pellucidum is displaced across the midline. (R) FLAIR shows that the ventricular asymmetry is normal without evidence for obstruction.

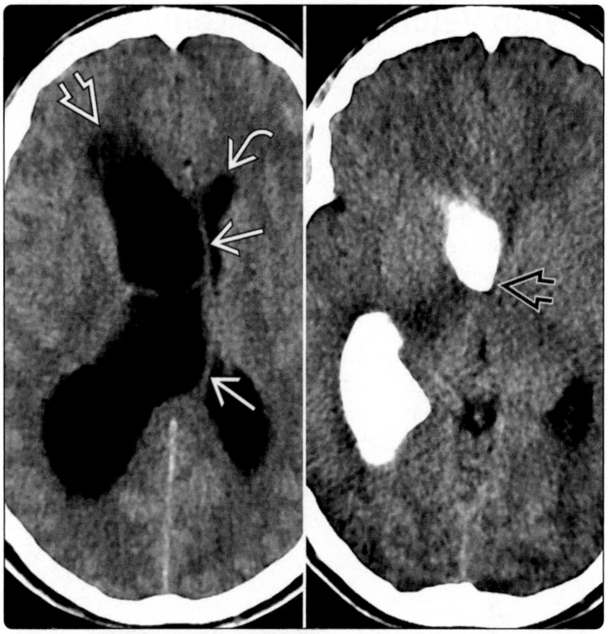

(34-8) (L) NECT shows enlarged, blurred right lateral ventricle , normal left , displaced septum pellucidum, and fornix . (R) Contrast ventriculogram shows obstruction is at right limb of the foramen of Monro ; unilateral obstructive hydrocephalus.

A CSP may occur in isolation, but a CV occurs only in combination with a CSP. When the two occur together, the correct Latin terminology is "cavum septi pellucidi et vergae." In common usage, the combination is often referred to simply as a CSP.

Etiology

The septum pellucidum consists of two paired glial membranes ("leaflets") that develop at about 12 weeks of gestation. These embryonic leaflets are initially unfused, and the cavity between them is filled with CSF. Normally the two leaflets eventually fuse, and the cavity between them is obliterated. The fused membranes then become the **septum pellucidum**.

If the two leaflets fail to fuse, the persisting cavity between them has two different names. Anterior to the foramen of Monro it is called a **CSP**. Its posterior continuation between the fornices is designated the **CV**.

Clinical Issues

CSP prevalence decreases with increasing age. By 3-6 months of age, the CSP is closed in 80-85% of infants. The reported prevalence of CSP and CV in adults ranges from 1-5%. A CSP is usually asymptomatic and is typically a "leave-me-alone" lesion found incidentally on imaging studies.

Imaging

CT and MR. The appearance of CSPs and CVs on CT and MR varies from an almost inapparent, slit-like cavity to a prominent collection measuring several millimeters in diameter. A CSP is isodense with CSF on NECT and follows CSF signal intensity exactly on MR. It suppresses completely on FLAIR.

In rare cases, an unusually large CSP/CV creates significant mass effect, splaying the fornices and leaves of the septi pellucidi laterally.

Ultrasound. A CSP is present in 100% of fetuses and is therefore always identified during obstetric sonography. The CSP increases in size between 19-27 gestational weeks, plateaus at 28 weeks, and then gradually closes from back to front. By term, the posterior part is usually fused, and, in 85% of cases, the CSP is completely closed by 3-6 postnatal months. A CSP may persist into adulthood as a normal variant.

Differential Diagnosis

The location and appearance of a CSP with or without a CV is virtually pathognomonic and should not be confused with a **cavum velum interpositum** (CVI). A CVI is a thin, triangular CSF space that overlies the thalami and third ventricle. A CVI typically occurs *without* a CSP.

An **absent septum pellucidum** lacks septal leaves, and the frontal horns appear as a single squared-off or "box-like" CSF cavity. An **asymmetric lateral ventricle** has a fused septi pellucidi that may be displaced across the midline. **Ependymal cysts** in the frontal horn are rare. When present, they focally displace the septi pellucidi rather than splaying its leaves apart.

Cavum Velum Interpositum

Terminology

The velum interpositum (VI) is a thin translucent membrane formed by two infolded layers of pia-arachnoid. The VI is adherent to the undersurface of the fornices and extends laterally over the thalami to become continuous with the choroid plexus of the lateral ventricles. Together with the fornices, the VI forms the roof of the third ventricle (see Chapter 20).

The VI is often CSF-filled and open posteriorly, communicating directly with the quadrigeminal cistern. In such cases, it is called a cavum velum interpositum (CVI) **(34-11)**. A CVI is considered a normal anatomic variant.

Clinical Issues

CVIs can be found at any age. They are usually asymptomatic and discovered incidentally on imaging studies. Mild nonspecific and nonfocal headache is the most common reported symptom.

Imaging

On imaging studies, a CVI appears as a triangular CSF space that curves over the thalami between the lateral ventricles. Its apex points toward the foramen of Monro **(34-12)**.

CVI size varies from an almost inapparent slit-like cavity to a round or ovoid cyst-like mass that elevates and splays the fornices superiorly while flattening and displacing the internal cerebral veins inferiorly **(34-12)**.

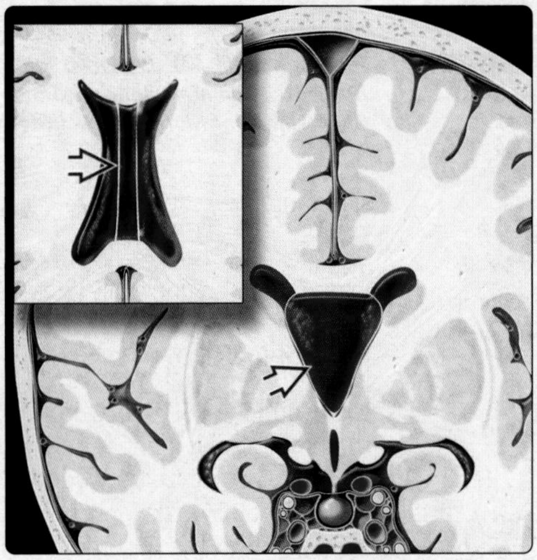

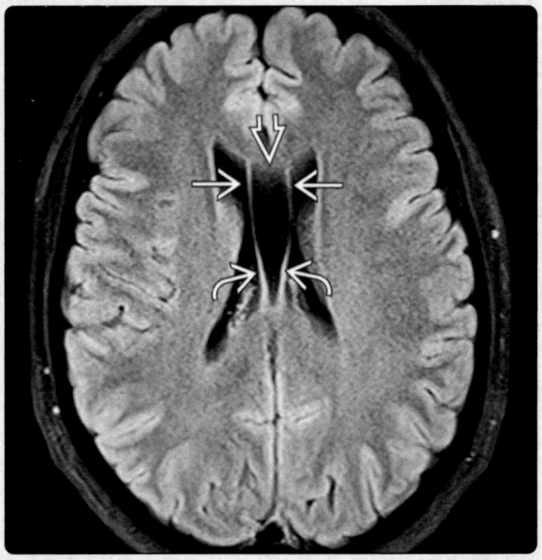

***(34-9)** Coronal graphic with axial inset shows classic cavum septi pellucidi (CSP) with cavum vergae (CV) ➾. The CSP appears triangular on the coronal image but finger-like on the axial view. **(34-10)** Axial FLAIR shows a CSP with CV. The leaves of the septum pellucidum ➙ and bodies of the fornices ➙ are splayed apart by a contiguous CSF-containing cavity ➙ that lies between them. This is a normal variant.*

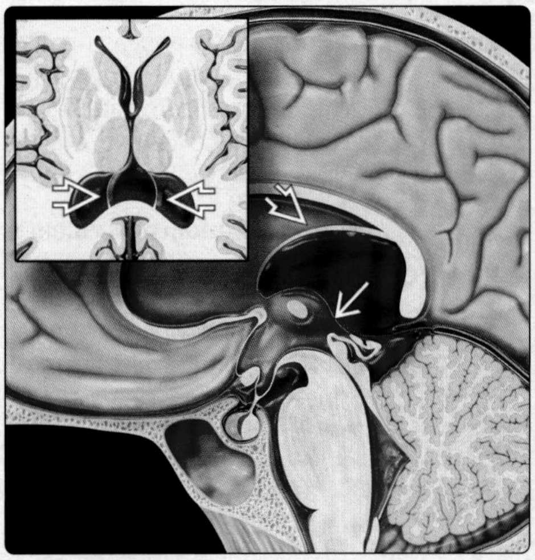

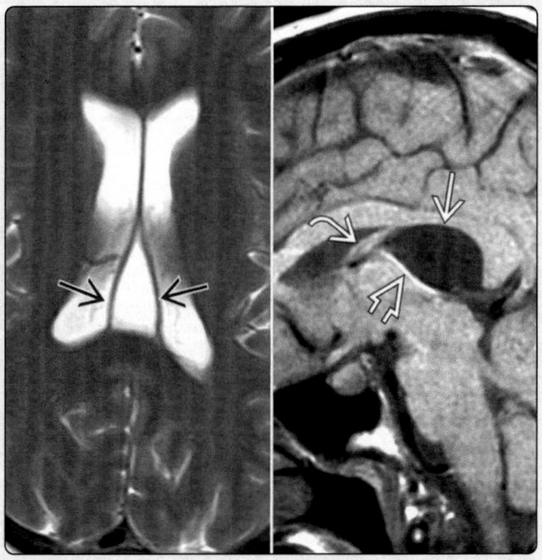

***(34-11)** Sagittal graphic with axial inset shows a cavum vellum interpositum (CVI). Note the elevation and splaying of the fornices ➙. Also noted is the inferior displacement of the internal cerebral veins and third ventricle ➙. **(34-12)** On axial T2WI (L) a CVI is triangular and separates the fornices ➾. On the sagittal image (R), CVI ➙ flattens the internal cerebral vein inferiorly ➙ but elevates and displaces the fornix superiorly ➙.*

A CVI is isodense with CSF on NECT and isointense on all MR sequences. It suppresses completely on FLAIR, does not enhance, and does not restrict on DWI.

Differential Diagnosis

The major differential diagnosis of CVI is epidermoid cyst. An **epidermoid cyst** of the VI can occur but is rare. An epidermoid cyst shows some diffusion restriction and does not suppress completely on FLAIR. A large CVI may be impossible to distinguish from an **arachnoid cyst** in the VI on the basis of imaging studies alone. A **CSP with CV** is elongated and finger-shaped, not triangular.

Enlarged Subarachnoid Spaces

Enlarged subarachnoid spaces (SASs) occur in three conditions: communicating hydrocephalus, brain atrophy, and benign enlargement of the SASs. Communicating hydrocephalus (both the intra- and extraventricular types) is discussed below. Brain atrophy—sometimes inappropriately called "hydrocephalus ex vacuo"—is discussed in Chapter 33 as a manifestation of aging and brain degeneration. In this section, we discuss benign physiologic enlargement of the SAS.

Terminology

Idiopathic enlargement of the SASs with normal to slightly increased ventricular size is common in infants. Large CSF spaces in developmentally and neurologically normal children with or without macrocephaly may be called benign SAS enlargement, benign idiopathic external hydrocephalus, benign external hydrocephalus, and benign extracerebral fluid collections of infancy. The preferred term is **benign enlargement of the SASs (BESS)**.

Etiology

The precise etiology of benign enlarged SASs in infants is unknown but probably related to immature CSF drainage pathways. Pacchionian granulations do not fully mature until 12-18 postnatal months, by which time the benign SAS enlargement generally resolves.

There is no known genetic predisposition, although 80% of infants with benign enlarged SASs have a family history of macrocephaly.

Pathology

Grossly, the SASs appear deep and unusually prominent but otherwise normal **(34-13)**. There are no subdural membranes present that would suggest chronic subdural hematomas or effusions.

Clinical Issues

Epidemiology and Demographics. The incidence of benign enlargement of the SASs is difficult to ascertain. It is reported on 2-65% of imaging studies for macrocrania in children under 1 year of age.

Benign enlarged SASs typically present between 3 and 8 months. There is a 4:1 M:F predominance.

Presentation. Occipitofrontal head circumference (OFC) tends to be in the high-normal range at birth and increases rapidly within the first few months. Macrocrania with OFC above the 95th percentile is typical at presentation.

There are no findings indicative of elevated intracranial pressure or nonaccidental trauma. Mildly delayed development is present in about half of all cases, but normal milestones are eventually reached.

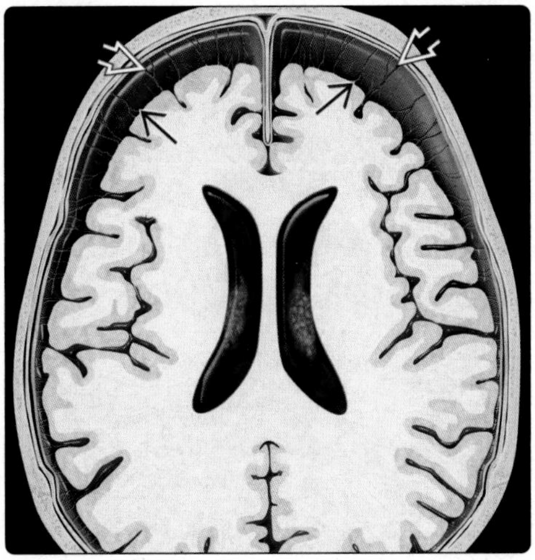

***(34-13)** Graphic depicts benign enlarged frontal SASs ⇒. Posterior SASs are normal. Note cortical veins crossing the prominent SASs ➡.*

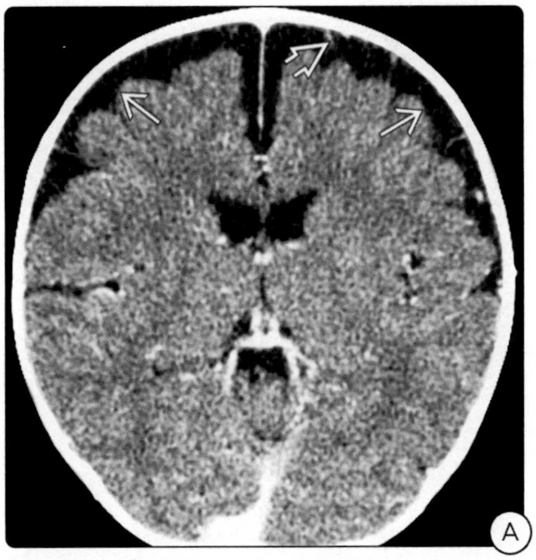

***(34-14A)** CECT scan in a 7m infant shows prominent bifrontal, interhemispheric subarachnoid spaces ➡ and bridging veins ➡.*

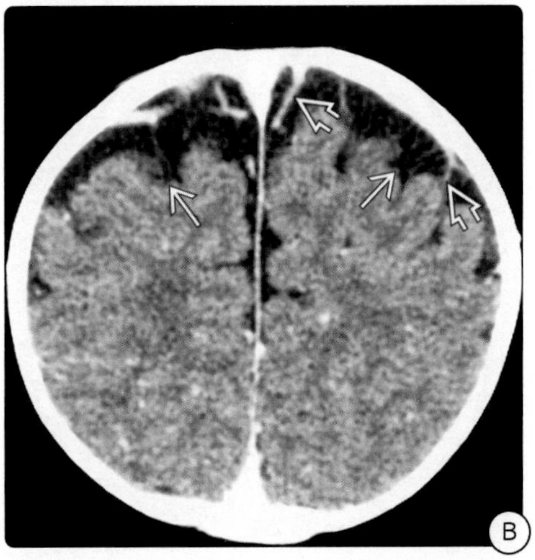

***(34-14B)** More cephalad CECT in the same patient shows fluid collections ➡, bridging veins ➡. These are benign enlarged SASs of infancy.*

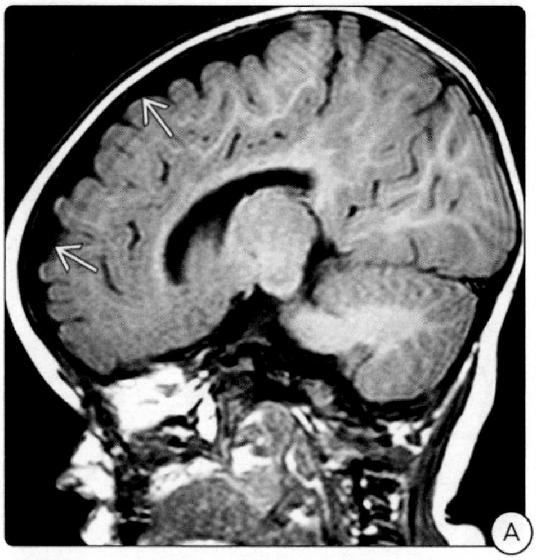

(34-15A) Sagittal T1WI in a normal 7m infant with a large head shows macrocrania and enlarged frontal subarachnoid spaces ➡.

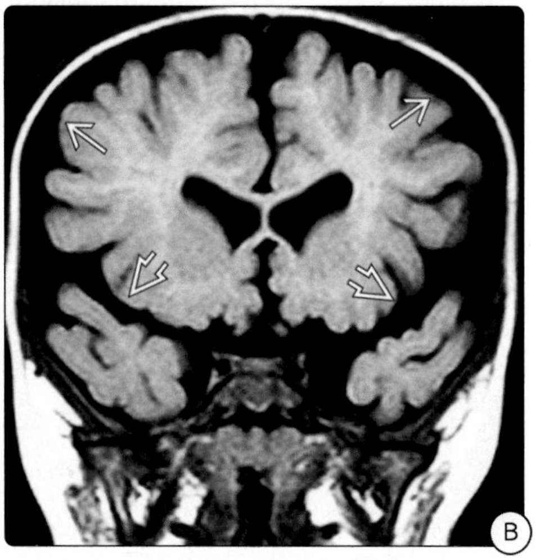

(34-15B) Coronal T1WI in the same patient demonstrates prominent SASs ➡ and sylvian fissures ⇨.

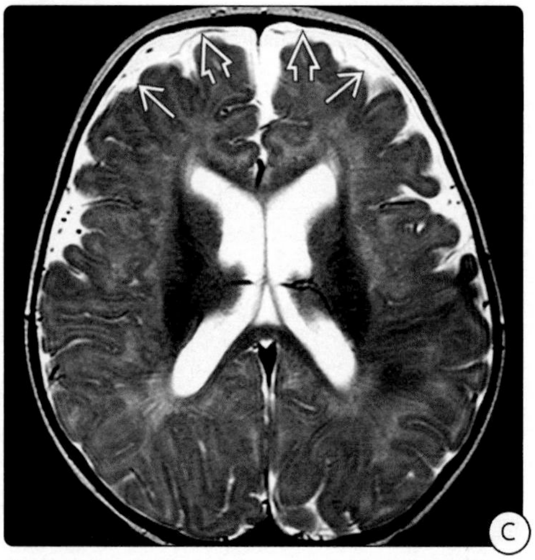

(34-15C) Axial T2WI shows prominent frontal, interhemispheric subarachnoid spaces ➡ and bridging veins ⇨.

Natural History. Benign enlarged SASs are a self-limited phenomenon that typically resolve by 12-24 months without intervention. The associated macrocephaly may resolve by 2 years, but it often levels off, remaining at the 98th percentile. Some authors report a greater prevalence of incidental subdural collections in children with increasing degrees of BESS and caution that this finding is not necessarily indicative of abusive head injury.

Treatment Options. No treatment is generally required.

Imaging

The frontal SASs in infants can normally appear somewhat prominent, reaching maximum size at about 7 months. The presence of prominent SASs in and of itself does not establish the diagnosis of benign enlarged SASs; head circumference should be at or above the 95th percentile.

CT Findings. Typical NECT findings in infants with benign enlarged SASs are prominent bifrontal and anterior interhemispheric SASs larger than 5 mm in diameter, enlarged suprasellar/chiasmatic cisterns, prominent sylvian fissures, and mildly enlarged lateral and third ventricles. The posterior and convexity sulci appear normal.

CECT scans demonstrate bridging veins traversing the SAS **(34-14)**. There is *no* evidence of thickened enhancing membranes to suggest subdural hematoma or hygroma.

MR Findings. Fluid in the enlarged frontal SASs exactly parallels CSF because it *is* CSF **(34-15)**. The fluid suppresses completely on FLAIR, and there is no evidence of "blooming" on T2* (GRE, SWI). Enhancing veins can be seen traversing the SASs on T1 C+. DWI is normal.

Ultrasound. Ultrasound shows increased craniocortical width with linear echogenic foci caused by bridging veins that can be seen coursing directly into the superior sagittal sinus. Color Doppler demonstrates venous structures traversing the prominent SASs.

Differential Diagnosis

The major differential diagnoses of benign enlarged SASs are atrophy, extraventricular obstructive hydrocephalus, and nonaccidental trauma. In **atrophy**, the OFC is normal to small. In **extraventricular obstructive hydrocephalus** secondary to infection or trauma, the fourth ventricle is frequently enlarged, and the CSF in the extraaxial spaces does not parallel that of CSF in density or signal intensity.

Occasionally, infants with benign enlarged SASs have minor superimposed hemorrhagic subdural collections, similar to those sometimes observed with arachnoid cysts. In such infants, **abusive head trauma** must be a consideration until careful screening discloses no substantiating evidence of inflicted injury.

CSF Flow Artifacts

Normal CSF has long T1 and T2 relaxation times, causing the familiar dark and bright signal, respectively. CSF-related artifacts in the brain and spine are common on MR scans, primarily due to the to-and-fro pulsatile nature of CSF motion. Although a complete discussion of CSF flow-related phenomena is beyond the scope of this text, we briefly describe three examples of major CSF artifacts that can mimic pathology on MR.

CSF flow-related phenomena are caused by time-of-flight (TOF) effects, turbulent flow, and patient motion.

Time-of-Flight Effects

TOF effects can result in **signal loss** (dark CSF signal) or flow-related enhancement, which produces bright CSF signal. TOF signal loss is directly related to CSF velocity and most prominent where flow is accelerated through narrow confines. Typical locations for TOF signal loss are around the foramen of Monro and in the third and fourth ventricles **(34-17)**.

Incomplete CSF nulling on FLAIR scans causes sulcal-cisternal CSF to appear spuriously bright, mimicking subarachnoid hemorrhage, infection, or metastatic disease **(34-18)**.

Entry-slice phenomena are most striking on T1 scans. Bright signal is caused by inflow of unsaturated spins that have full longitudinal magnetization. The first slices of the imaging volume show the most prominent flow-related enhancement effects, which are most pronounced in the lower posterior fossa on axial sequences and around the foramen of Monro on coronal images. These entry-slice phenomena create artifacts that can mimic masses.

Turbulent Flow

Turbulent flow causes varied flow velocities and different directions with signal loss secondary to intravoxel spin dephasing. In the brain, turbulent flow with signal loss is common in the cerebral aqueduct, the fourth ventricle, and around pulsating vessels. This effect is especially pronounced around the basilar artery, where it can mimic aneurysmal dilatation.

Motion Artifacts

The most problematic artifact on MR is voluntary patient motion. Voluntary patient motion can be minimized with verbal reminders or mild sedation. Some patient motion is both intrinsic and involuntary, caused by pulsating arteries or CSF.

Pulsation artifacts along the phase-encoding direction cause propagation of "ghosting" artifacts in a straight linear band across the entire imaged plane. Phase-encoding artifacts are often seen as alternating foci of bright and dark signal **(34-16)**.

Hydrocephalus

The term "hydrocephalus" literally means "water head." The term "ventriculomegaly" means enlargement of the ventricular system. Remember: the terms **"hydrocephalus" and "ventriculomegaly" are descriptive findings, not a diagnosis!** The role of imaging is to **find the etiology of the ventricular enlargement**.

Hydrocephalus has traditionally been regarded as an abnormality in the formation, flow, or resorption of CSF. If normal CSF flow is impeded by a blockage within the ventricular system, CSF production continues and the ventricles enlarge. In the classic model, hydrocephalus can also result from an imbalance between CSF production and absorption. When CSF absorption through the arachnoid granulations is compromised, the ventricles enlarge, and hydrocephalus results. Absorption can be blocked at any level within the subarachnoid cisterns, e.g., within the cisterna magna, at the basilar cisterns, or along the cerebral convexities.

In the newest attempt to understand the development of hydrocephalus, aquaporin (AQP)-mediated brain water homeostasis and/or clearance of both CSF and ISF into the PVSs and blood are compromised. The molecular mechanisms that drive AQP4 modifications in hydrocephalus that fail to facilitate removal of excess water are still relatively unknown.

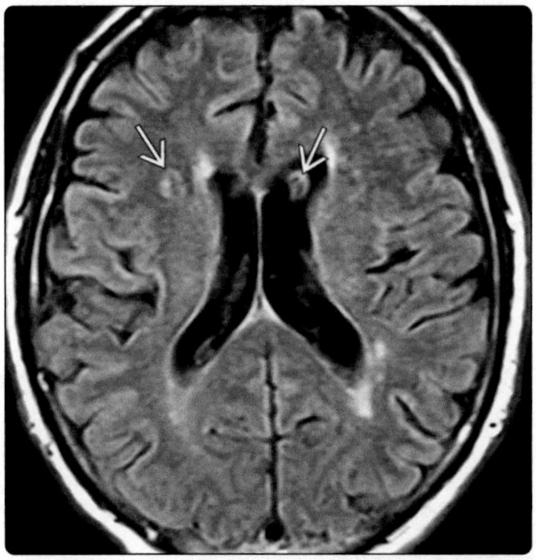

***(34-16)** Phase-encoding artifact propagates horizontally across ventricles and parenchyma →.*

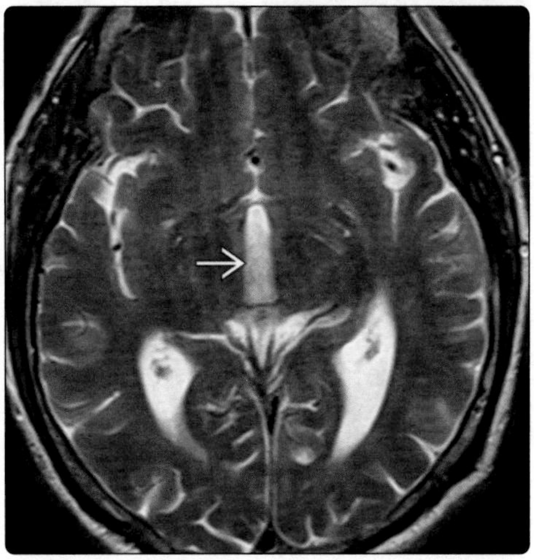

***(34-17)** Axial T2WI shows hypointense CSF in the upper third ventricle → caused by pulsatile CSF flow through the foramen of Monro.*

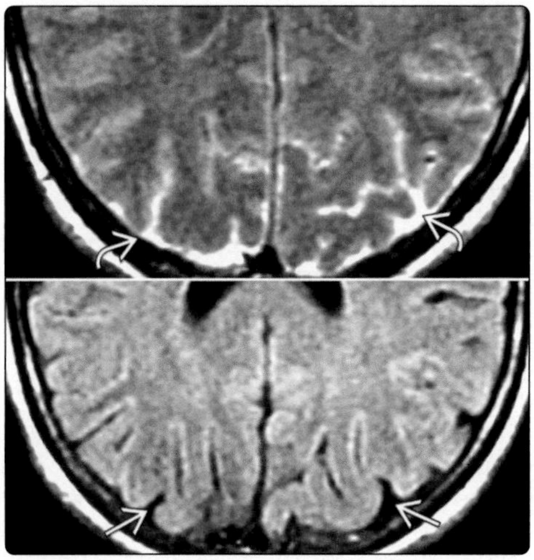

***(34-18)** (Top) FLAIR with incomplete fluid suppression, CSF in sulci → appears hyperintense. (Bottom) Corrected suppression → looks normal.*

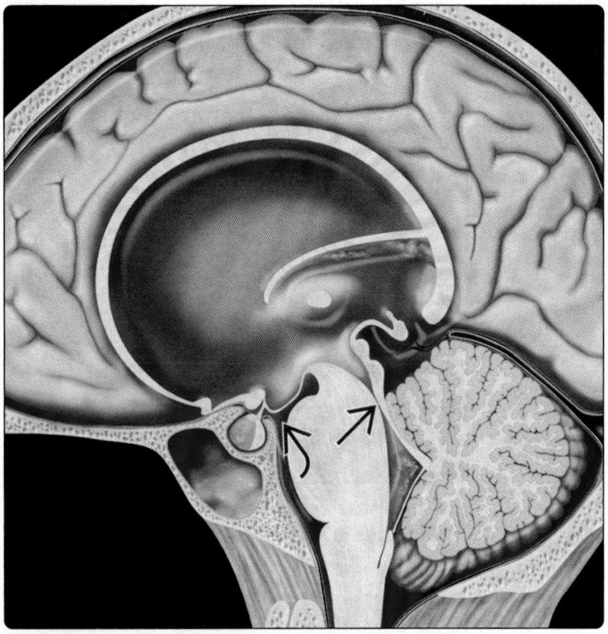

(34-19) Triventricular IVOH shows markedly enlarged lateral, third ventricles, stretched corpus callosum, funnel-shaped cerebral aqueduct with distal obstruction. Note normal size of fourth ventricle and bulging floor of third ventricle .

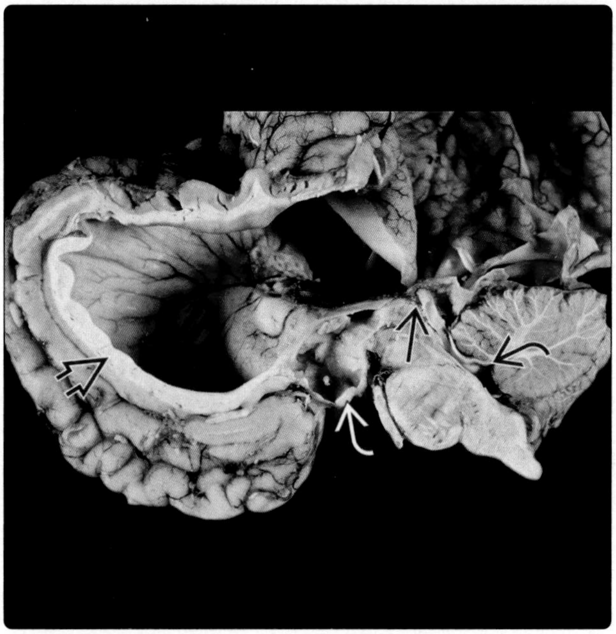

(34-20) Sagittal autopsy case shows aqueduct stenosis , massively enlarged lateral ventricle , ballooned third ventricle , and normal fourth ventricle . (Courtesy Rubinstein Collection, AFIP Archives.)

Hydrocephalus is the most common disorder requiring neurosurgical intervention in children. Its treatment consumes a disproportionate share of healthcare dollars, approaching nearly a billion dollars a year in the United States alone. Once considered predominantly a disease of childhood, hydrocephalus is now increasingly recognized as a less common but still important cause of neurologic disability in adults.

Terminology

A rigorous definition of hydrocephalus is surprisingly difficult. Its terminology and classification are a matter of continuing debate. We follow the common approach of subclassifying hydrocephalus by the presumed site of CSF obstruction, i.e., inside [**intraventricular obstructive hydrocephalus** (VOH)] or outside the ventricles [**extraventricular obstructive hydrocephalus** (EVOH)]. The distinction is important, as treatment for IVOH (CSF diversion) differs from that of EVOH (membrane fenestration).

The outdated term "ex vacuo hydrocephalus" referring to ventricular and cisternal enlargement caused by parenchymal volume loss is no longer used.

Etiology

When abnormally large cerebral ventricles are identified on imaging studies, the diagnostic imperative is to find the cause of the hydrocephalus. The presence of enlarged ventricles with elevated intracranial pressure is only one presentation along a spectrum that ranges from idiopathic intracranial hypertension ("pseudotumor cerebri") to the recently recognized, enigmatic syndrome of low-pressure hydrocephalus.

In the pediatric age group, a majority of cases are caused by congenital defects of the CSF pathway. Adult-onset hydrocephalus is usually secondary to different pathologies that encompass a heterogeneous group of disorders. The most common is intracranial hemorrhage (45%, most often caused by aneurysmal subarachnoid hemorrhage) followed by neoplasm (30%) and head injury or infection (5% each). Normal pressure hydrocephalus (11%) and idiopathic intracranial hypotension (4%) together account for 15% of cases.

Intraventricular Obstructive Hydrocephalus

Terminology

IVOH is used to designate physical obstruction at or proximal to the fourth ventricular outlet foramina. The term "noncommunicating hydrocephalus" is no longer used.

Etiology

General Concepts. IVOH can be **congenital** or **acquired**, **acute** (aIVOH) or **chronic** (cIVOH). Congenital IVOH occurs with disorders such as aqueductal stenosis.

Although aIVOH can occur suddenly (e.g., foramen of Monro obstruction by a colloid cyst), it usually develops over a period of weeks or even months. Any gradually expanding intraventricular mass (such as a neoplasm or cyst) can cause IVOH, as can an extraventricular mass of sufficient size to occlude a critical structure (e.g., the cerebral aqueduct).

When the ventricles become obstructed, CSF outflow is impeded. As CSF production continues, the ventricles expand.

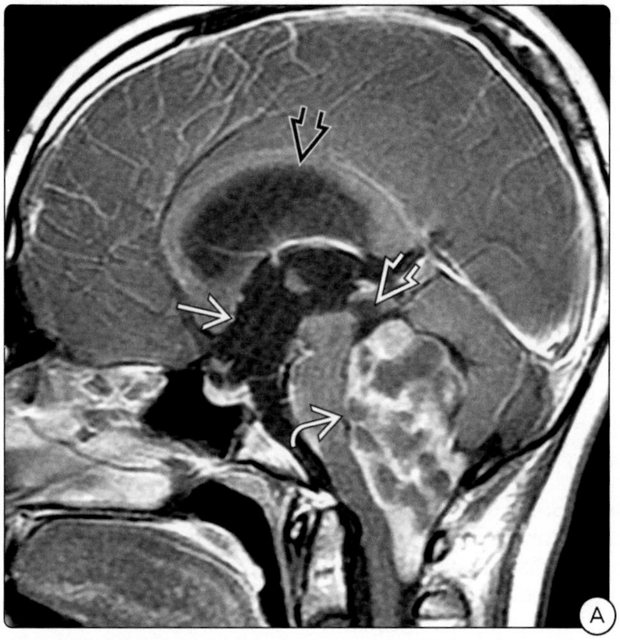

(34-21A) Sagittal T1 C+ shows a heterogeneously enhancing mass expanding the 4th ventricle. The upper 4th ventricle and cerebral aqueduct are enlarged as are the third and lateral ventricles.

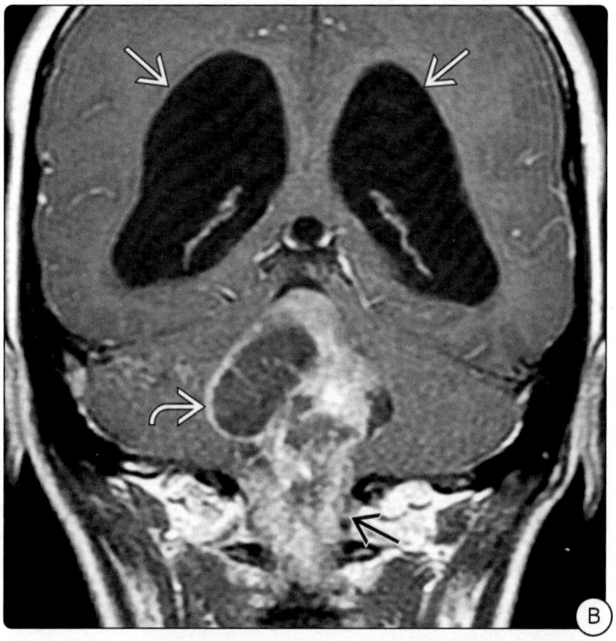

(34-21B) Coronal T1 C+ in the same case shows 4th ventricular mass extrudes inferiorly through the cisterna magna into the upper cervical canal. Note symmetrically enlarged lateral ventricles. Ependymoma was found at surgery.

As the ventricles expand, increased pressure is exerted on the adjacent brain parenchyma. Increased intraparenchymal pressure compromises cerebral blood flow, reducing brain perfusion. The increased pressure also compresses the subependymal veins, which reduces absorption of brain interstitial fluid via the deep medullary veins and perivascular spaces. The result is **periventricular interstitial edema**. Whether the edema results from CSF extruding across the ventricular ependyma (**"transependymal CSF flow"**) or accumulation of brain extracellular fluid is unknown.

In chronic "compensated" IVOH, the ventricles expand slowly enough that CSF homeostasis is relatively maintained. Periventricular interstitial edema is minimal or absent.

Pathoetiology. The general causes of obstructive hydrocephalus range from developmental/genetic abnormalities to trauma, infection, intracranial hemorrhage, neoplasms, and cysts.

The most common cause of acquired IVOH is intraventricular inflammatory or posthemorrhagic membranous obstruction. The most common sites of obstructing membranes are, in order, the foramina of Luschka, the cerebral aqueduct, and the foramen of Magendie. The foramen of Monro is a relatively rare location.

Intraventricular masses are the next most common cause of acquired IVOH. The prevalence of specific pathologies varies with location. Colloid cyst is the most common mass found at the foramen of Monro, followed by tuberous sclerosis (subependymal nodules and giant cell astrocytoma). After benign (membranous) obstruction, the most common lesions to obstruct the aqueduct of Sylvius are tectal plate glioma and pineal region neoplasms.

The fourth ventricle is a common site for neoplasms that can cause obstructive hydrocephalus. In children, medulloblastoma is the most common tumor that causes IVOH, followed by ependymoma, pilocytic astrocytoma, diffusely infiltrating astrocytoma, and atypical teratoid/rhabdoid tumor (AT/RT).

In adults, metastases, hemangioblastoma, epidermoid cyst, and choroid plexus papilloma are fourth ventricular lesions that may cause hydrocephalus. Inflammatory cysts (e.g., neurocysticercosis) occur throughout the ventricular system and in patients of all ages.

Genetics. Congenital hydrocephalus can be syndromic or nonsyndromic. To date, only one gene—the neural cell adhesion molecule L1 (*L1CAM*)—has been recognized as a cause of congenital hydrocephalus. X-linked hydrocephalus (hereditary aqueduct stenosis) is caused by mutation in the *L1CAM* gene.

Pathology

Grossly, the ventricles proximal to the obstruction appear ballooned **(34-19)** **(34-20)**. The ependyma is thinned and may be focally disrupted or even absent. The corpus callosum (CC) is thinned and displaced superiorly against the rigid, unyielding falx cerebri. Focal encephalomalacic changes are common in the CC body.

Microscopic examination shows that the ependymal lining is discontinuous or inapparent. The periventricular extracellular space is increased, and the surrounding WM is rarefied and stains pale. The cortex is relatively well preserved.

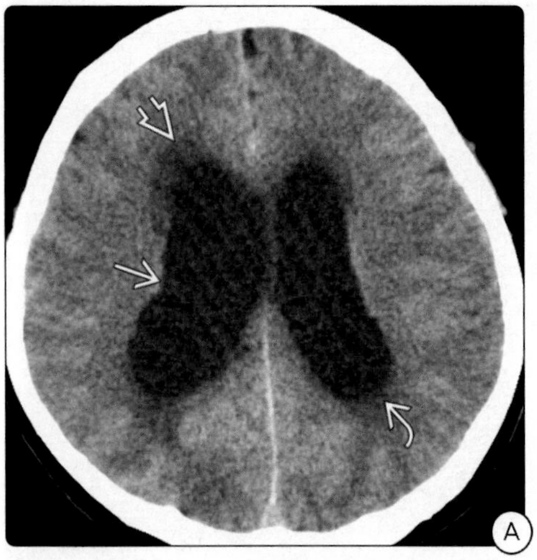

(34-22A) NECT in a 52y woman shows "tight" brain, large lateral ventricles, "blurred" margins, periventricular hypodense "halo.

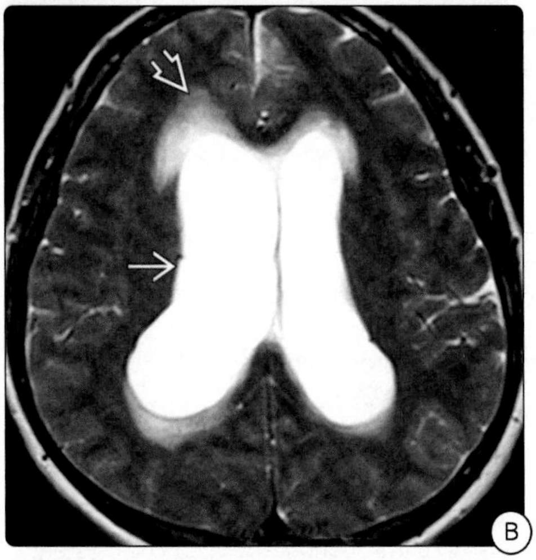

(34-22B) Axial T2WI in same patient, who had headaches, shows large lateral ventricles with extensive periventricular fluid accumulation.

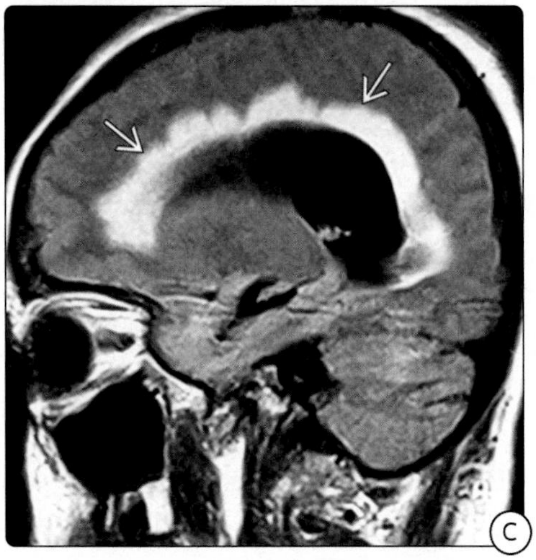

(34-22C) Sagittal FLAIR shows hyperintense "fingers" extending along the entire margin of the lateral ventricle, acute IVOH (GBM of fornix).

Clinical Issues

Epidemiology and Demographics. IVOH can affect people at any age, from the fetus (in utero congenital hydrocephalus) to the elderly. There is no sex predilection except for primary congenital hydrocephalus, in which the M:F ratio is 2.6:1.0.

Presentation. The presentation of IVOH varies with acuity and severity. Headache is the most common overall symptom, and papilledema is the most common sign. Nausea, vomiting, and CN VI palsy are also common with aIVOH.

Natural History. The natural history of IVOH varies. Most cases are typically progressive unless treated. Untreated severe aIVOH can result in brain herniation with coma and even death. Some patients with slowly developing compensated IVOH may not present until late in adult life (e.g., the recently recognized syndrome of late-onset aqueductal stenosis).

Treatment Options. CSF diversion (shunt, ventriculostomy, endoscopic fenestration of the third ventricle floor) is common, often performed as a first step before definitive treatment of the obstruction (e.g., removal of a colloid cyst or resection of an intraventricular neoplasm).

Imaging

General Features. A number of measurements have been devised to quantify hydrocephalus. These include indices such as diameter of the frontal horns in relation to the inner table of the skull (ventricular or Evans index), frontal horn radius, and ventricular angle. The utility of such two-dimensional measurements versus visual judgment is uncertain. Computer-generated volume measurements have been proposed as providing better normative standards but are time-consuming and difficult to obtain.

Despite its acknowledged inaccuracies, subjective neuroradiologic evaluation remains the most common method of assessing ventricular size. Hydrocephalus is usually diagnosed when the ventricles appear disproportionately enlarged relative to the subarachnoid spaces.

Although NECT scans are often used as an emergent screening procedure in patients with headache and signs of increased intracranial pressure, MR is the procedure of choice. Multiplanar MR best delineates the hydrocephalus and often permits identification of its etiology.

On axial studies, helpful general imaging findings include enlarged temporal horns of the lateral ventricles (out of proportion to the basal subarachnoid spaces). The frontal horns assume a "rounded" appearance. The third ventricle—which usually appears slit-like on axial views—expands, losing its normal tapered appearance. The walls first become parallel, then expand outward so that the third ventricle appears oblong or ovoid. As the ventricles continue to enlarge, the subarachnoid cisterns and convexity sulci may become compressed, and gyri appear flattened against the calvaria.

Sagittal views show that the CC is thinned, stretched, bowed upward, and, in severe cases, even impacted against the falx cerebri. The anterior recesses of the third ventricle enlarge, losing their normal "pointed" appearance **(34-21)**.

In cases of cIVOH, pulsating CSF in the third ventricle pounds the central skull base relentlessly. The bony sella turcica gradually enlarges and assumes an "open" configuration. In severe cases, the anterior third ventricle may protrude into the sella itself.

If both lateral and third ventricles are enlarged but the fourth ventricle remains normal (e.g., as occurs with aqueductal stenosis), the condition is termed **triventricular hydrocephalus**. If all four chambers of the ventricular system are enlarged, it is called **quadriventricular hydrocephalus**. Quadriventricular hydrocephalus is caused by a mass in the fourth ventricle or obstruction of the outlet foramina (typically infection or subarachnoid hemorrhage).

In approximately 0.5-1.0% of IVOH cases, just one lateral ventricle is enlarged (**"unilateral hydrocephalus"**). Most cases are acquired and associated with intraventricular neurocysticercosis or the presence of a membranous web at the junction of the inferior frontal horn with the foramen of Monro.

CT Findings. Imaging findings vary with acuity and severity. NECT scans in aIVOH demonstrate enlarged lateral and third ventricles, whereas the size of the fourth ventricle varies. The temporal horns are prominent, the frontal horns are "rounded," and the margins of the ventricles appear indistinct or "blurred." Periventricular fluid—whether from compromised drainage of interstitial fluid or transependymal CSF migration—causes a "halo" of low density in the adjacent WM **(34-22A)**. The sulci and basal cisterns appear compressed or indistinct.

MR Findings. Axial T1WI shows that both lateral ventricles are symmetrically enlarged. On sagittal views, the CC appears thinned and stretched superiorly, whereas the fornices and internal cerebral veins are displaced inferiorly.

In aIVOH, T2 scans may demonstrate "fingers" of CSF-like hyperintensity extending outward from the lateral ventricles into the surrounding WM **(34-22B)**. Fluid in the periventricular "halo" does not suppress on FLAIR **(34-22C)**. In longstanding chronic "compensated" hydrocephalus, the ventricles appear enlarged and the WM attenuated but without a thick periventricular "halo" **(34-23)**.

High-resolution thin-section T2WI, FIESTA, or CISS sequences exquisitely delineate the CSF spaces and may demonstrate subtle abnormalities not detected on standard sequences. 2D cine-phase contrast imaging is helpful to depict CSF dynamics in the aqueduct and around the foramen magnum.

Complications of Hydrocephalus. In severe cases of IVOH, the CC becomes compressed against the free inferior margin of the falx **(34-24)** **(34-25)**. This can cause pressure necrosis and loss of callosal axons, the so-called **corpus callosum impingement syndrome** (CCIS). In acute CCIS, the CC may initially appear swollen and hyperintense on T2WI and FLAIR. Subacute and chronic changes are seen as encephalomalacic foci in a shrunken, atrophic-appearing CC. In 15% of treated IVOH cases, the CC shows T2/FLAIR hyperintensity after decompression. In rare cases, the hyperintensity extends beyond the CC itself into the periventricular WM **(34-26)**.

Massive ventricular enlargement may weaken the medial wall of the lateral ventricle enough that a pulsion-type diverticulum of CSF extrudes through the inferomedial wall of the atrium **(34-27)**. Such **medial atrial diverticula** may cause significant mass effect on the posterior third ventricle, tectal plate, and aqueduct. Large atrial diverticula can herniate inferiorly through the tentorial incisura into the posterior fossa, compressing the vermis and fourth ventricle **(34-28)**.

In rare cases, the ependyma may actually rupture and spill CSF into the adjacent WM (**"ventricular disruption"**), creating a fluid-filled cleft in the hemisphere.

Differential Diagnosis

The major differential diagnosis of IVOH is **extraventricular obstructive hydrocephalus** (see below). Patients often have a history of aneurysmal

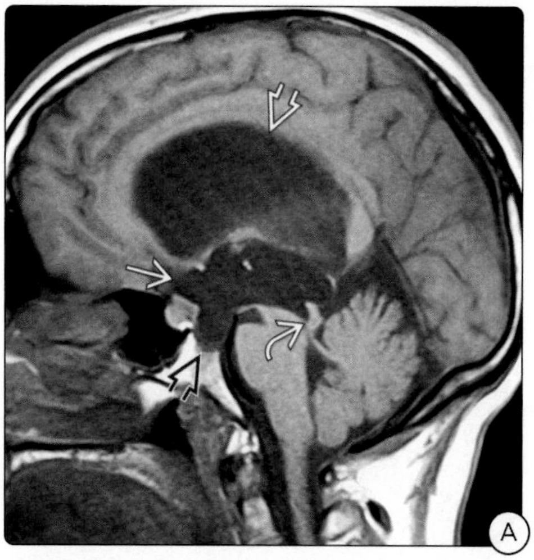

***(34-23A)** T1WI in a 22y woman with longstanding aqueductal stenosis ➡ shows enlarged lateral ➡, third ventricles ➡ with remodeled clivus ➡.*

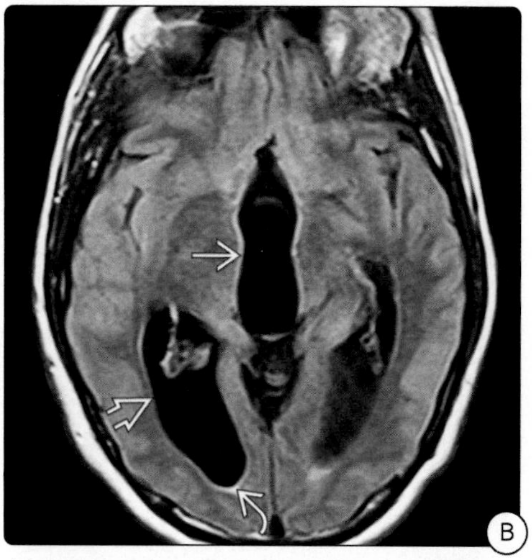

***(34-23B)** Axial FLAIR shows enlarged third ➡, lateral ➡ ventricles with minimal hyperintense rim ➡.*

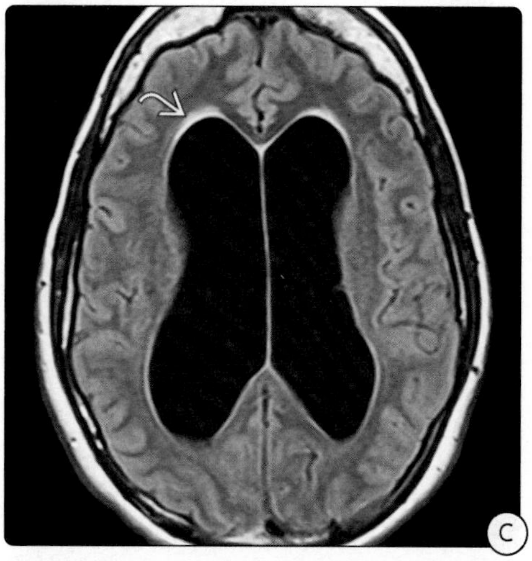

***(34-23C)** More cephalad FLAIR shows marked symmetrically enlarged ventricles, thin fluid rim ➡. This is chronic compensated IVOH.*

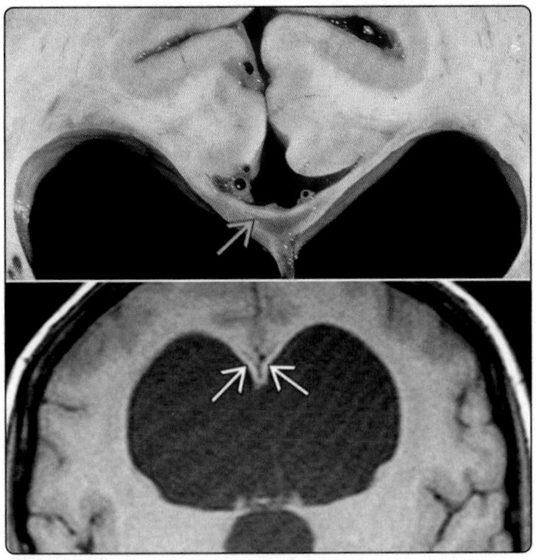

(34-24) (Top) IVOH, encephalomalacic CC are caused by falx impingement. (Bottom) T1WI shows CC impingement.

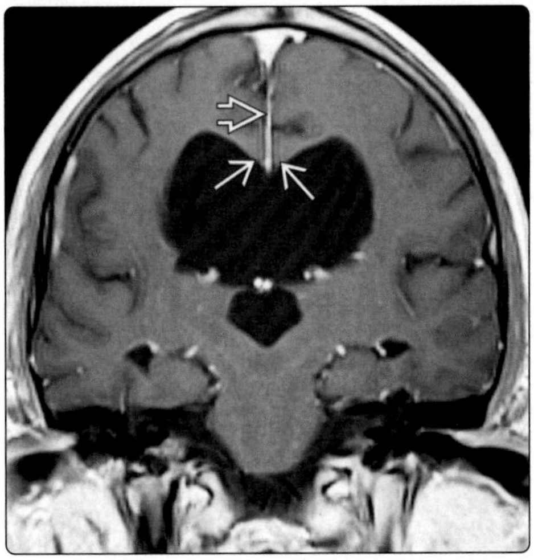

(34-25) Coronal T1 C+ of longstanding IVOH shows the lateral ventricles, corpus callosum are forced upward against the falx cerebri.

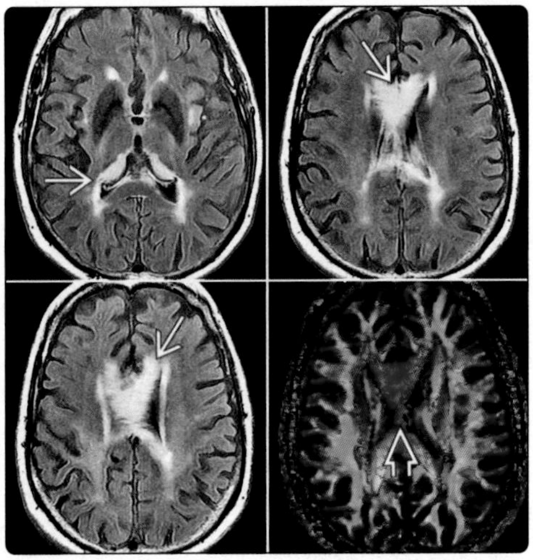

(34-26) CCIS with decompression, postshunt FLAIR shows hyperintensity in CC, periventricular WM, disrupted fibers on DTI.

subarachnoid hemorrhage or meningitis. The lateral, third, and fourth ventricles are symmetrically and proportionately enlarged.

Parenchymal volume loss causes secondary dilatation of the ventricles (ventriculomegaly) with proportional enlargement of the surface sulci and cisterns. In infants with large ventricles, measuring head size is a critical component of the total evaluation. The finding of large ventricles in a large head favors hydrocephalus; seeing large ventricles with a normal to small head is more common with congenital anomalies or volume loss (atrophy).

A helpful feature to distinguish obstructive hydrocephalus from atrophy is the appearance of the temporal horns. In obstructive hydrocephalus, they appear rounded and moderately to strikingly enlarged. If the IVOH is acute, a periventricular "halo" is often present.

Even with relatively severe volume loss, the temporal horns retain their normal kidney bean shape and are only minimally to moderately enlarged. The lateral ventricle margins remain sharply defined. Periventricular hypodensity appears patchy and is caused by chronic microvascular ischemia, not interstitial edema or transependymal CSF migration.

Normal pressure hydrocephalus is typically a disorder of older adults and is typified clinically by progressive dementia, gait disturbance, and incontinence (see below). The ventricles often appear disproportionately enlarged relative to the sulci and cisterns.

Overproduction hydrocephalus is rare, associated with choroid plexus papilloma and the even rarer villous hyperplasia. The choroid plexus glomus is enlarged and avidly enhancing.

INTRAVENTRICULAR OBSTRUCTIVE HYDROCEPHALUS

Terminology, Etiology
- Proximal to 4th ventricle outlet foramina
- Can be congenital or acquired, acute or chronic
  - Postinflammation/posthemorrhage
  - Obstructing intraventricular mass

Acute Obstructive Hydrocephalus
- Ventricles proximal to obstruction are ballooned
- "Blurred" margins of ventricles
- Periventricular fluid accumulation (CSF, ISF, or both)
  - "Halo" ± "fingers" of fluid around ventricles
  - T2 hyperintense, does not suppress on FLAIR

Chronic Compensated Obstructive Hydrocephalus
- Large ventricles, no periventricular "halo"
- ± Callosal impingement, atrial diverticula

Extraventricular Obstructive Hydrocephalus

Terminology

In extraventricular obstructive hydrocephalus (EVOH), the obstruction is located outside the ventricular system.

Etiology

The obstruction causing EVOH can be located at any level from the fourth ventricular outlet foramina to the arachnoid granulations. Subarachnoid hemorrhage—whether traumatic or aneurysmal—is the most frequent cause. Other common etiologies include purulent meningitis, granulomatous meningitis, and disseminated CSF metastases.

EXTRAVENTRICULAR OBSTRUCTIVE HYDROCEPHALUS

Terminology
- Formerly called "communicating" hydrocephalus
- Obstruction outside ventricular system
  - Any site from 4th ventricle foramina to arachnoid granulations

Etiology
- Most common
  - Subarachnoid hemorrhage (aneurysm > trauma)
- Less common
  - Meningitis (bacterial, granulomatous)
  - Metastases

Imaging
- > 50% show no discernible etiology
- Use CISS to look for obstructing membranes

Pathology

Gross pathology demonstrates generalized ventricular dilatation **(34-30)**. The basal cisterns and convexity sulci may be filled with acute or chronic exudates **(34-29)**, meningeal fibrosis, or arachnoid adhesions.

Clinical Issues

As with IVOH, the presentation of EVOH varies with acuity and severity. The most common symptom is headache followed by signs of increased intracranial pressure such as papilledema, nausea, vomiting, and diplopia.

Imaging

CT Findings. The classic appearance of EVOH on NECT scans is that of symmetric, proportionally enlarged lateral, third, and fourth ventricles. The basal subarachnoid spaces are hyperdense in acute subarachnoid hemorrhage and may

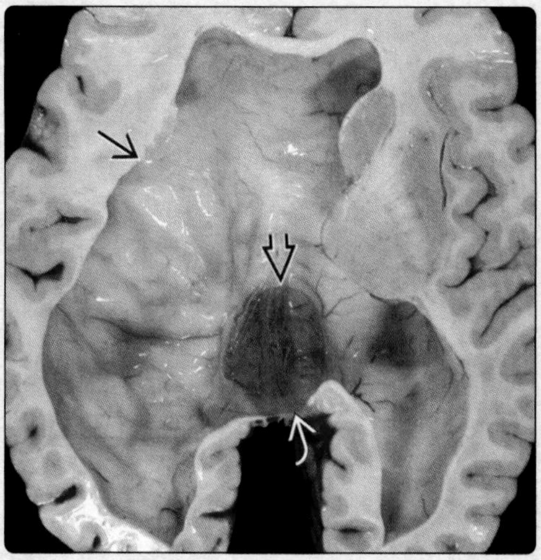

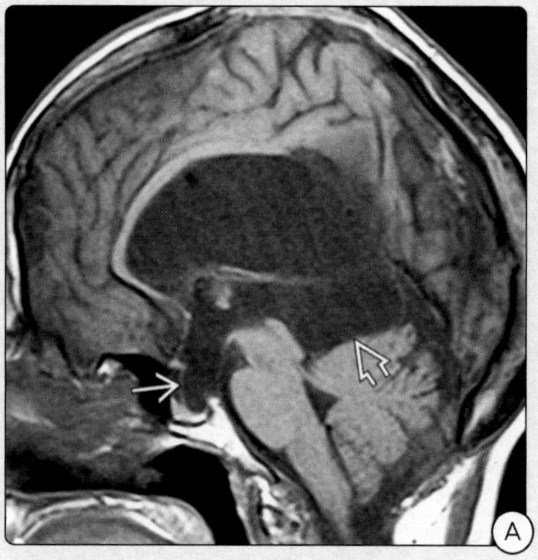

***(34-27)** Autopsy of longstanding obstructive hydrocephalus with markedly enlarged lateral ventricles shows the pouch of an atrial diverticulum extending medially, inferiorly through the tentorial incisura. (Courtesy R. Hewlett, MD.) **(34-28A)** Triventricular hydrocephalus is shown with intrasellar herniation of the third ventricle, CSF collection compressing/displacing the vermis.*

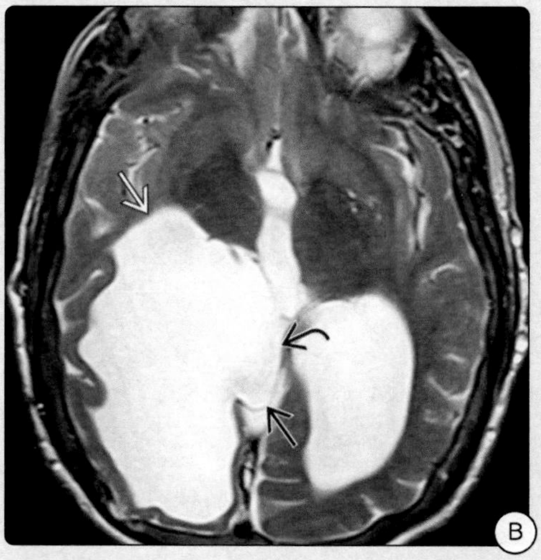

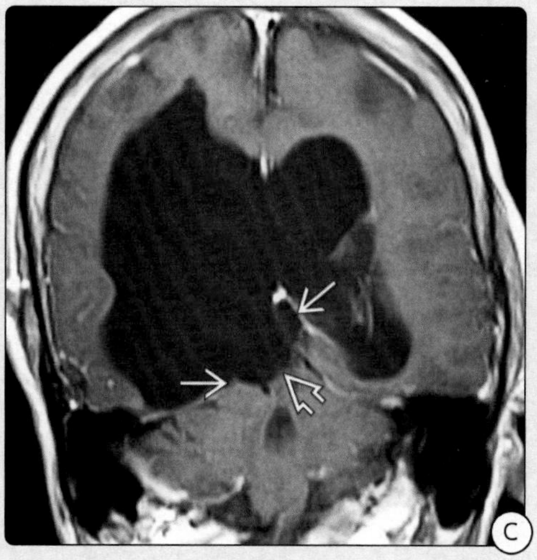

***(34-28B)** T2WI in the same patient shows enlarged lateral ventricles with a right medial atrial diverticulum and thinned but intact ventricular wall. **(34-28C)** Coronal T1 C+ nicely shows the medial atrial diverticulum herniating through the tentorial incisura, compressing the vermis.*

appear isodense and effaced in pyogenic or neoplastic meningitis. CECT scans may demonstrate enhancement in cases of EVOH secondary to infection or neoplasm.

MR Findings. The same imaging sequences used in IVOH apply to the evaluation of EVOH **(34-31)**. If the hydrocephalus is caused by acute subarachnoid hemorrhage or meningitis, the CSF appears "dirty" on T1WI and hyperintense on FLAIR. T1 C+ scans may demonstrate sulcal-cisternal enhancement.

In contrast to IVOH, more than half the cases of EVOH have no discernible cause for the obstruction on standard MR sequences. In such cases, it is especially important to identify subtle thin membranes that may be causing the extraventricular obstruction.

The CSF cisterns, ventricles, and outlet foramina are best demonstrated by special pulse sequences such as 3D constructive interference in the steady state (3D-CISS).

With the use of high-resolution 3D-CISS, thin membranous obstruction can be demonstrated in nearly 20% of patients with unexplained hydrocephalus. Even if the membrane is not visualized directly, differences in CSF signal intensity proximal and distal to the culprit membrane are helpful in localizing the obstruction.

Differential Diagnosis

The major differential diagnosis of EVOH is **IVOH**. In some cases—even with special sequences such 3D-CISS—it may be difficult, if not impossible, to localize the level of the obstruction.

Overproduction Hydrocephalus

Overproduction hydrocephalus is uncommon and results from excessive CSF formation. The choroid plexus epithelium is extremely efficient, having the highest rate of ion and water transport of any epithelium in the human body.

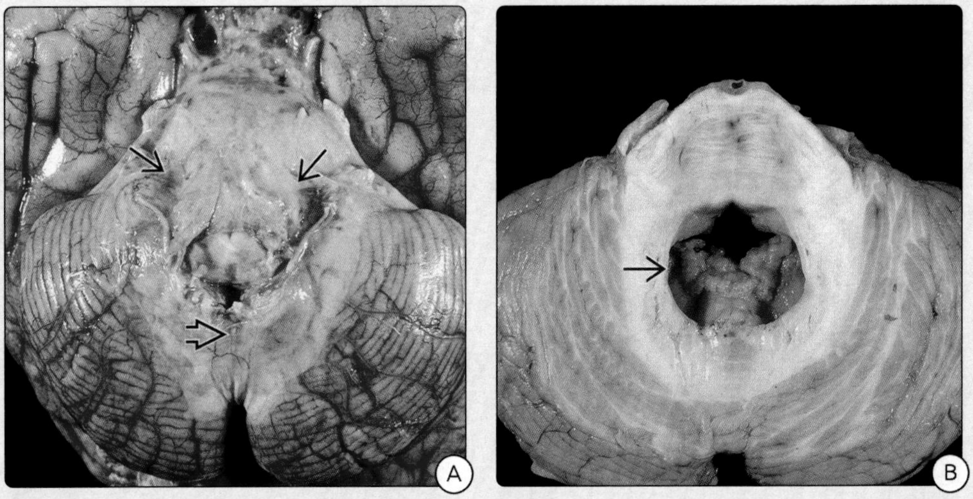

***(34-29A)** Extensive tuberculous meningitis with thick exudate in the basal cisterns occludes the foramina of Magendie ⇨ and Luschka →. **(34-29B)** Axial section through the cerebellum shows that the fourth ventricle → is markedly enlarged and rounded ("ballooned").*

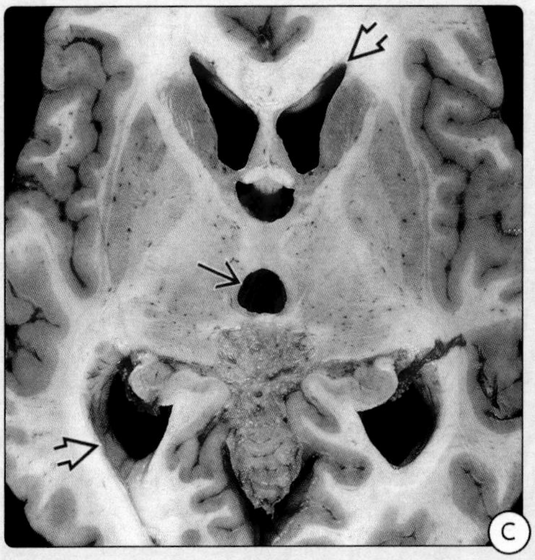

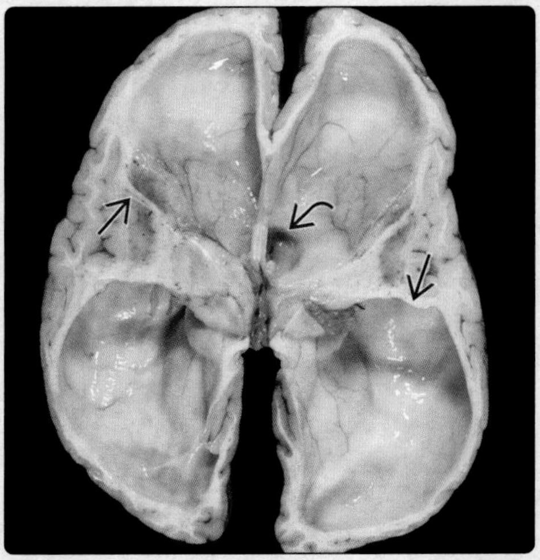

***(34-29C)** Third → and both lateral ventricles ⇨ are enlarged. This is extraventricular "communicating" hydrocephalus. (All three images courtesy R. Hewlett, MD.) **(34-30)** Axial gross pathology in another case of chronic EVOH secondary to tuberculous meningitis shows massively enlarged lateral ventricles →. Note enlarged foramen of Monro ↩. (Courtesy R. Hewlett, MD.)*

Approximately 80% of CSF is produced by the choroid plexus, but at least 20% is generated from the brain ISF. The flow of brain ISF is not unidirectional and can contribute to both net CSF production and reabsorption.

Some investigators believe that—at least in children—CSF overproduction is an underrecognized cause of hydrocephalus **(34-32)**. Panventricular enlargement is the most common imaging finding but is not invariably present.

Choroid plexus papillomas (CPPs) are the most common cause of overproduction hydrocephalus (see Figure 18-39). CPPs account for 2-4% of childhood neoplasms and typically occur in children younger than 5 years. Some CPPs produce enormous amounts of CSF, overwhelming the capacity of the arachnoid villi and other structures to absorb the excess fluid. **Choroid plexus carcinomas** (CPCas) can also cause overproduction hydrocephalus but are only a tenth as common as CPPs. Imaging findings of both CPP and CPCa are delineated in Chapter 18.

Diffuse villous hyperplasia of the choroid plexus (DVHCP) is a rare cause of overproduction hydrocephalus. CSF production in DVHCP can exceed 3 L per day. DVHCP is histologically normal with little to no pleomorphism or hyperchromasia. Imaging studies in DVHCP show severe hydrocephalus with massive enlargement of the entire choroid plexus. The diffusely enlarged choroid plexus enhances strongly and often contains multiple nonenhancing cysts of varying sizes. DVHCP can be difficult to distinguish from rare bilateral CPPs, which typically cause focal—not diffuse—enlargement of the choroid plexus.

Benign, nonneoplastic **choroid plexus cysts** have also been reported as another rare cause of overproduction and triventricular obstructive hydrocephalus in children.

Normal Pressure Hydrocephalus

There are no currently accepted evidence-based guidelines for either the diagnosis or treatment of normal pressure

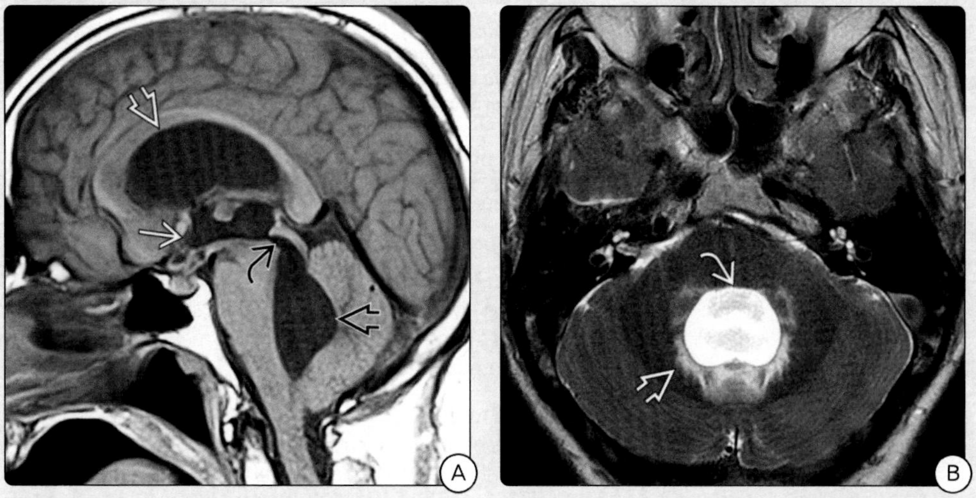

(34-31A) Sagittal T1WI in a patient with headache and history of meningitis shows markedly enlarged fourth ventricle ⇨ and aqueduct ↗. The third ➡ and lateral ➡ ventricles are also enlarged. (34-31B) Axial T2WI in the same case shows the markedly enlarged 4th ventricle ➡ with edema in the adjacent cerebellum ⇨.

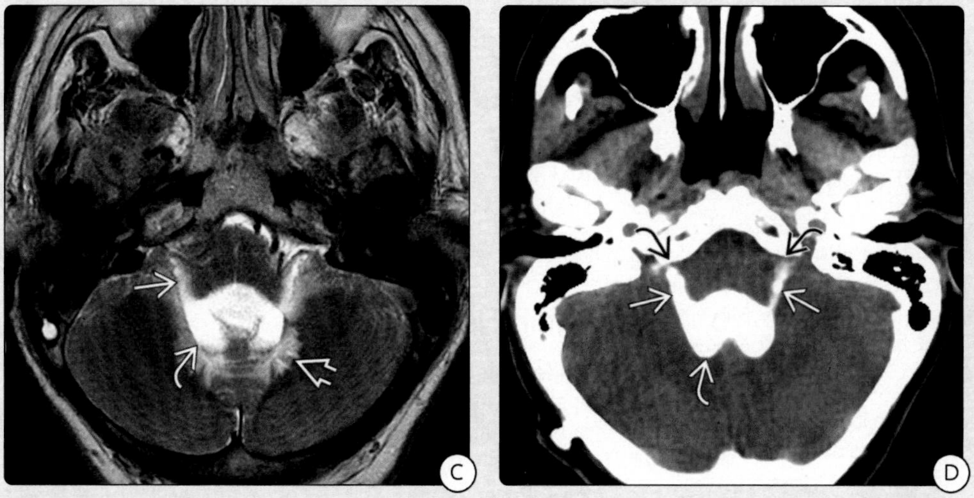

(34-31C) T2WI shows marked enlargement of the posterosuperior ➡ and lateral ➡ recesses of the fourth ventricle and CSF migration into the adjacent cerebellum ⇨. (34-31D) Contrast was injected through a ventriculostomy in the lateral ventricle. Axial NECT shows that contrast fills the fourth ventricle ➡ and lateral recesses ➡ but is obstructed at the outlet foramina ↗. EVOH is secondary to meningitis.

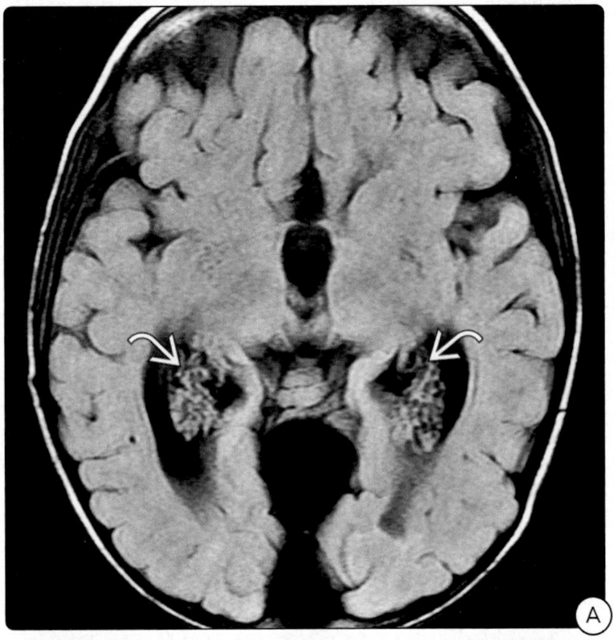

***(34-32A)** Axial FLAIR in a 3y boy with progressively increasing head size shows enlarged third and lateral ventricles with unusually prominent choroid plexus glomi ➡ in the atria of the lateral ventricles.*

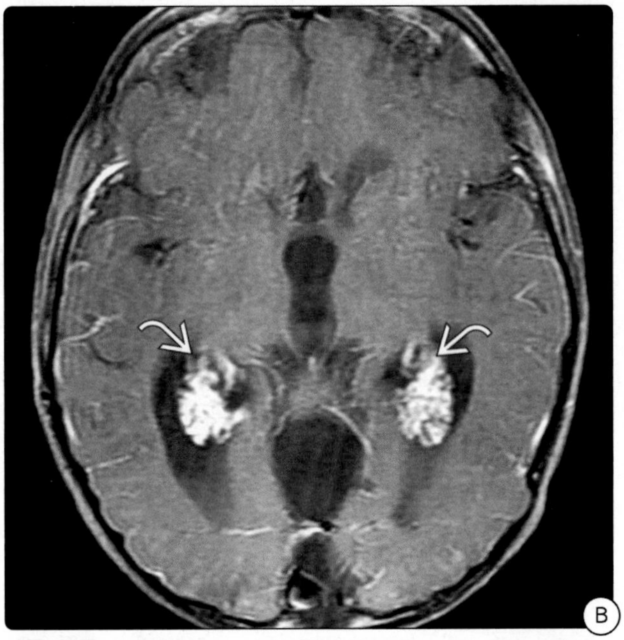

***(34-32B)** T1 C+ FS in the same case shows the enlarged, intensely enhancing choroid plexi ➡. This is choroid plexus hyperplasia with overproduction hydrocephalus. Duplication of the short arm of chromosome 9 was found on genetic analysis.*

hydrocephalus (NPH). In this section, we briefly review the syndrome and summarize the spectrum of imaging findings that—in conjunction with clinical history and neurologic examination—may suggest the diagnosis.

Terminology

NPH was first described by Hakim and Addams as "symptomatic occult hydrocephalus with 'normal' CSF pressure." NPH is characterized by ventriculomegaly with normal CSF pressure but altered CSF hydrodynamics.

NPH has also been called idiopathic adult hydrocephalus syndrome. **Primary** or **idiopathic NPH** (iNPH) is distinguished from **secondary NPH** (sNPH), in which there is a known antecedent such as subarachnoid hemorrhage, traumatic brain injury, or meningitis.

Etiology

The pathogenesis of NPH is poorly understood and remains controversial. Whether NPH reflects abnormal brain structure, disturbed blood flow, or altered CSF circulation (or a combination of all three) is unclear.

Animal studies have demonstrated that disruption of the periventricular matrix integrity could result in pressure gradients that favor progressive ventriculomegaly. Movement of CSF into the parenchyma in the form of interstitial edema may result.

Recent studies of NPH also suggest that CSF and ISF stasis with excess fluid in the interstitial spaces disrupts the balance between hydrostatic and osmotic pressures, reversing ISF flow. In turn, this could result in impaired or failed removal of neurotoxic compounds such as β-amyloid and tau from the brain parenchyma.

PET and SPECT studies all indicate widespread cortical and subcortical hypometabolism in NPH. Decreased global and regional cerebral blood flow and accelerated microvascular disease also contribute to the parenchymal degeneration that often accompanies NPH.

Other proposed etiologies invoke altered viscoelastic properties of the ventricular walls and adjacent parenchyma with a resultant "water hammer" effect of CSF pulsations. In this model, elevated arterial pulsations cannot be transmitted to the cortical veins and perivascular spaces due to reduced compliance. Intermittent high pressure "B" waves together with altered compliance of the venous system and craniospinal subarachnoid space have also been posited as potential etiologies for NPH.

Pathology

The ventricles appear grossly enlarged. The periventricular WM often appears abnormal with or without frank lacunar infarction. Neurofibrillary tangles and other microscopic changes typically found in Alzheimer disease are seen in 20% of cases.

Clinical Issues

Epidemiology and Demographics. NPH accounts for approximately 5-6% of all dementias. The reported prevalence of NPH is 0.5-3.0% in the elderly population. Although it is most common in patients older than 60 years, NPH also occasionally occurs in children following intraventricular hemorrhage or meningitis. There is a moderate male predominance.

NPH is designated as "possible" or "probable" based on the combination of clinical findings, imaging studies, and response to high volume lumbar tap.

Presentation. The nature and severity of symptoms as well as the disease course vary in NPH. Impaired gait and balance are the typical initial symptoms. The classic triad of dementia, gait disturbance, and urinary incontinence is present in a minority of patients and typically represents advanced disease. While gait disturbances are seen in most cases, not all patients exhibit impaired cognition.

Natural History. The natural history of NPH has not been well characterized, nor is the tempo of progression uniform. Many patients experience continuing cognitive and motor decline.

Treatment Options. Some patients initially respond dramatically to ventricular shunting ("shunt-responsive" NPH). The favorable response to shunting varies from about 35-40% in patients with clinically "possible" NPH to 65% in patients diagnosed with "probable" NPH.

Long-term outcome is more problematic. Although early gait improvement is common, only one-third of patients experience continued improvement 3 years after shunting. Cognition and urinary incontinence are even less responsive.

Imaging

General Features. Imaging studies in suspected NPH are necessary but insufficient to establish the definitive diagnosis of NPH. The goal of identifying patients who are likely to improve following ventriculoperitoneal shunting likewise remains elusive.

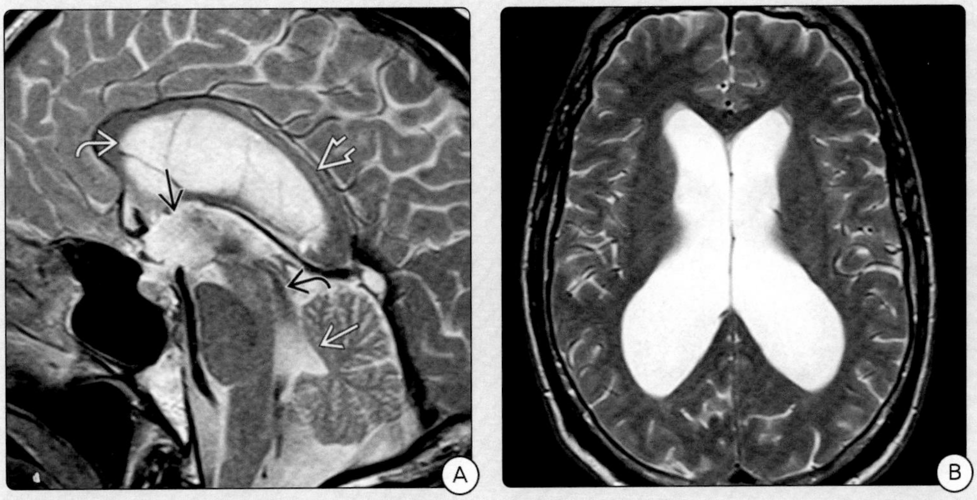

***(34-33A)** Sagittal T2WI in a 74y man shows proportionately enlarged lateral, third, and fourth ventricles with an exaggerated aqueductal "flow void". Note abnormal signal in thinned corpus callosum. **(34-33B)** Axial T2WI shows symmetrically enlarged lateral ventricles with normal sulci and normal white matter.*

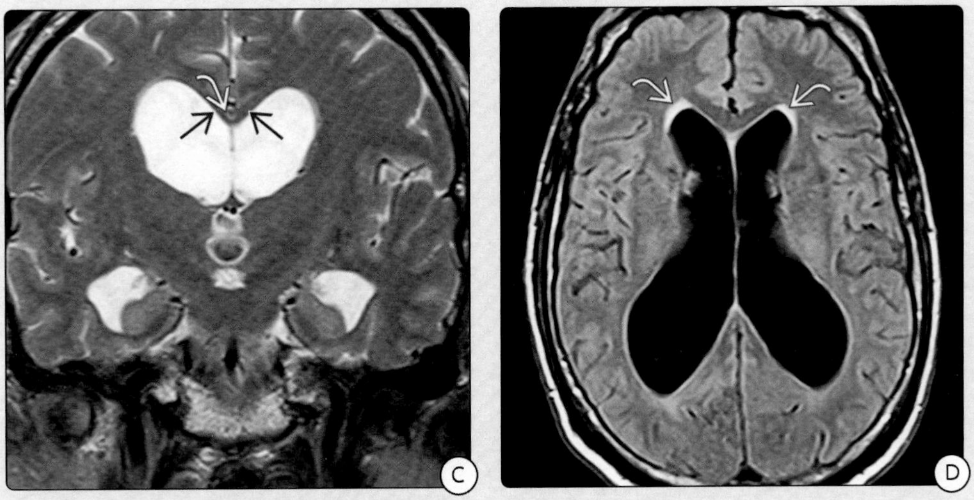

***(34-33C)** Coronal T2WI shows the enlarged lateral ventricles pushing the corpus callosum against the falx cerebri with thin area of encephalomalacia (compare with Figure 34-24). **(34-33D)** Axial FLAIR shows thin rim of periventricular fluid accumulation, best seen around the frontal horns of the lateral ventricles. Aqueductal stroke volume was 72 µL. This was normal pressure hydrocephalus.*

The most common general imaging feature of NPH is a degree of ventriculomegaly (Evans index of at least 0.3) that appears out of proportion to sulcal enlargement ("ventriculosulcal disproportion").

CT Findings. NECT scans show enlarged lateral ventricles with rounded frontal horns. The third ventricle is moderately enlarged, whereas the fourth ventricle appears relatively normal.

The basal cisterns and sylvian fissures may be somewhat prominent, but, compared with the degree of ventriculomegaly, generalized sulcal enlargement is mild. Periventricular hypodensity is common and often represents a combination of increased interstitial fluid and WM rarefaction secondary to microvascular disease.

MR Findings. T1 scans show large lateral ventricles. The convexity and medial subarachnoid spaces may appear decreased or "tight," whereas the basal cisterns and sylvian fissures are often enlarged. The corpus callosum is usually thinned. Most patients have a mild to moderate periventricular "halo" on T2/FLAIR **(34-34)**. A prominent, exaggerated "hyperdynamic" aqueductal "flow void" may be present **(34-33)**.

CSF flow studies are generally accepted as a supplementary tool for the assessment of shunt-responsive NPH. Either 2D or 3D phase-contrast studies may show hypermotile flow and markedly elevated aqueductal stroke volume. An aqueductal stroke volume greater than 42 µL has been associated with shunt responsiveness although a significant percentage of patients with lower stroke volumes also may respond to shunt surgery.

Recent studies show NPH patients have hyperdynamic CSF flow with increased velocity and volume in *both* systole and diastole. The inflow during diastole exceeds that of systole, so the net flow direction is caudo-cranial, the reverse of normal.

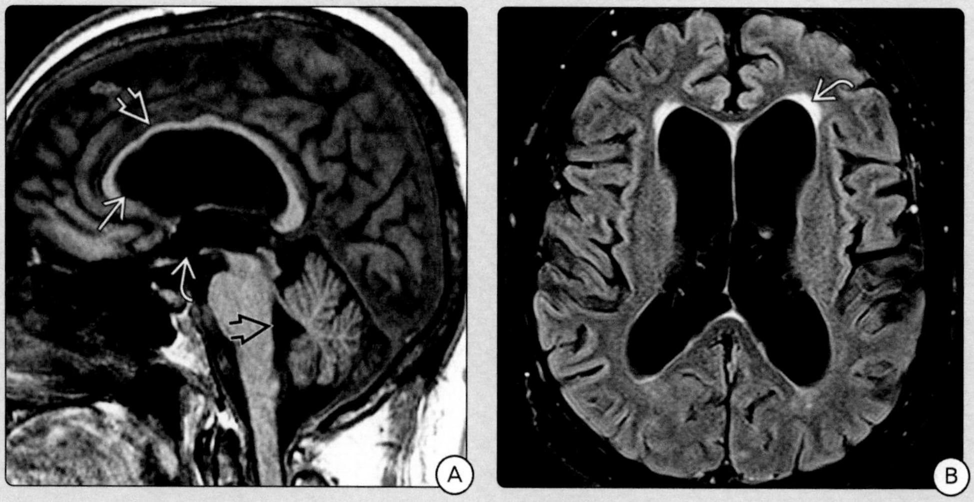

(34-34A) Sagittal MP-RAGE in a 72y man with progressive confusion and gait apraxia shows large lateral, third, and fourth ventricles with normal-appearing sulci. The corpus callosum appears stretched and thinned. (34-34B) Axial FLAIR shows striking symmetric enlargement of both lateral ventricles. The sulci and white matter appear normal. The hyperintense rim surrounding the ventricles is more prominent than normal.

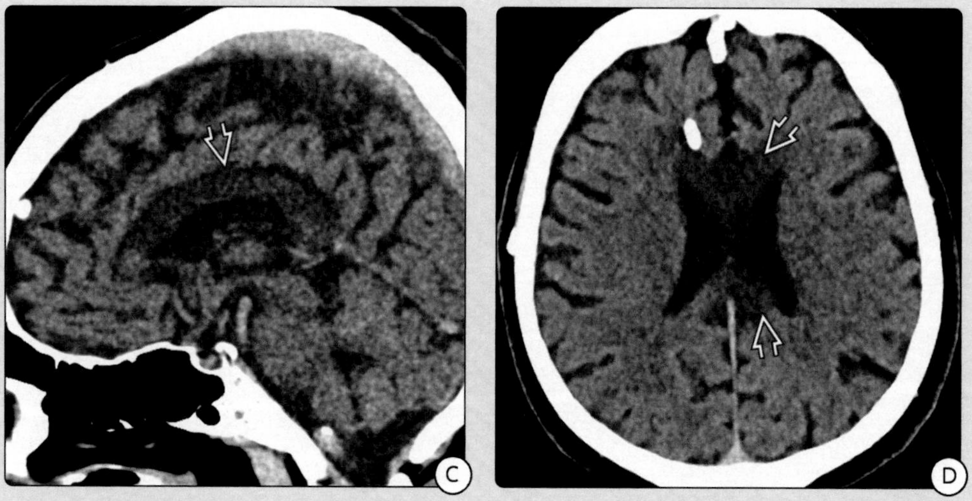

(34-34C) Normal pressure hydrocephalus was diagnosed, and the patient was shunted. NECT 3 months later shows normal thickness of the corpus callosum, but it appears unusually hypodense. (34-34D) Axial NECT shows the hypodense corpus callosum. This is shunted NPH with callosal impingement syndrome following decompression.

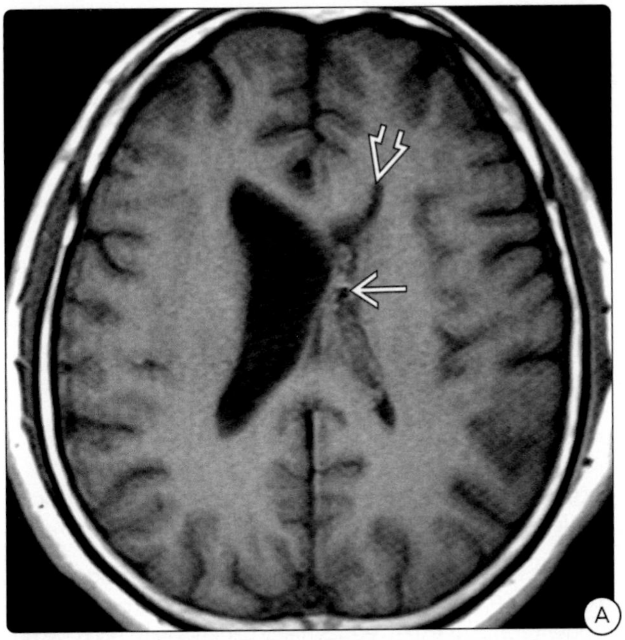

***(34-35A)** Axial T1WI in a patient with ventriculoperitoneal shunt and headache shows shunt catheter ➡ in a collapsed, slit-like left lateral ventricle ➡. The right lateral ventricle is moderately enlarged; the sulci appear normal.*

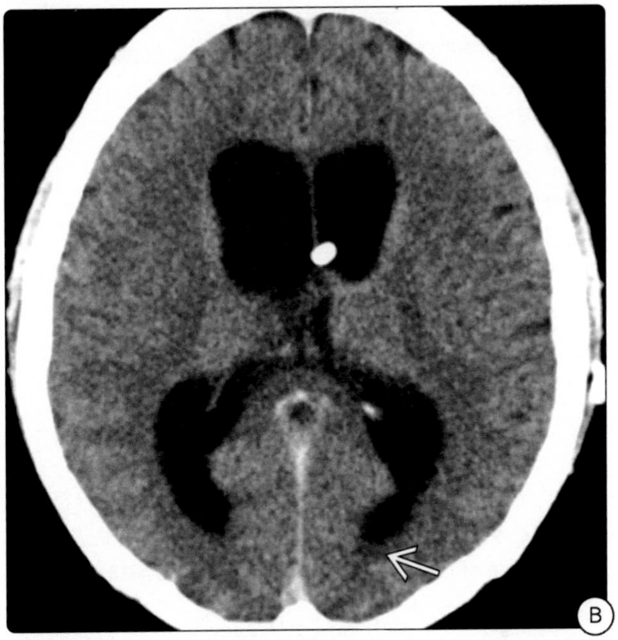

***(34-35B)** The shunt was replaced. The patient had acute neurologic deterioration 10 days later. NECT shows "ballooned" ventricles, periventricular edema ➡, small sulci. EVD showed unexpectedly low pressure, consistent with SILPAH.*

This hyperdynamic flow reversal may play a key role in the development of ventriculomegaly in NPH patients.

DTI is a good marker of WM pathology and shows increased FA in the posterior limb of the internal capsule. Increased diffusivity in the same tract can be seen as early as 2 weeks following shunting.

Nuclear Medicine. Prominent ventricular activity at 24 hours on In-111 DTPA cisternography is considered a relatively good indicator of NPH. 18F FDG PET shows decreased regional cerebral metabolism.

Differential Diagnosis

The major difficulty in diagnosing iNPH is distinguishing it from other neurodegenerative disorders. Up to 75% of patients with NPH have another neurodegenerative disorder, most commonly **Alzheimer disease** and **vascular dementia**. In **age-related atrophy**, both the ventricles and the subarachnoid spaces are proportionately enlarged.

Syndrome of Inappropriately Low-Pressure Acute Hydrocephalus

Most patients with acute obstructive hydrocephalus have ventriculomegaly and elevated intracranial pressure (ICP). However, a small subset of patients with acute obstructive hydrocephalus have ventriculomegaly with inappropriately *low* ICP.

Terminology

The syndrome of inappropriately low-pressure acute hydrocephalus (SILPAH) has sometimes been called "negative-pressure hydrocephalus." As opening pressures are not always "negative" (i.e., subzero), the terms SILPAH or "very low-pressure hydrocephalus" are more accurate.

Etiology

Once thought to occur only in patients with a preexisting ventriculoperitoneal shunt, SILPAH is now known to occur in other patients, too. The common factor is isolation of the ventricular system from a subarachnoid space that leaks (or is drained of) CSF, resulting in low brain turgor and decreased ICP. CSF production continues, builds up, and expands the ventricles.

Clinical Issues

SILPAH is both uncommon and—because of its enigmatic and counterintuitive nature—often unrecognized.

Patients with SILPAH present with progressive neurologic deterioration, *acute* progressive ventriculomegaly, and ICP that is inappropriately low when an external ventricular drain (EVD) is inserted **(34-35)**. SILPAH affects patients of all ages; 20% are children.

Shunted patients with SILPAH typically have opening pressures less than 0 mm H_2O. Patients without a shunt typically have much lower than expected pressures that rapidly become even lower. In both scenarios, ICP is too low to allow CSF drainage with normal EVD protocols.

Treatment by neck wrapping with a tensor bandage and/or lowering the EVD to negative levels typically results in clinical improvement and resolution of the ventriculomegaly. Reestablishing communication between the ventricular system and the SAS may be required to correct ICP dynamics.

OTHER HYDROCEPHALUS

Overproduction Hydrocephalus
- Rare
- Results from CSF overproduction
  - Choroid plexus tumor > > hyperplasia
- Imaging shows panventricular enlargement

Normal Pressure Hydrocephalus
- Ventriculomegaly with normal CSF pressure, altered fluid dynamics
- Accounts for ≈ 5% of dementias
- Dementia, gait apraxia, incontinence (minority)
- Imaging diagnosis difficult
  - Disproportionately enlarged ventricles vs. sulci
  - MR may show exaggerated aqueductal "flow void," elevated stroke volume
  - In-111 DTPA cisternography, intraventricular tracer at 24 hours

Syndrome of Inappropriately Low-Pressure Acute Hydrocephalus
- Progressive neurologic deterioration
  - Acute progressive obstructive hydrocephalus
  - CSF opening pressure very low or negative
- Imaging
  - Like acute obstructive hydrocephalus with elevated ICP
  - Quadriventricular enlargement
  - Small/inapparent sulci common
- Differential diagnosis
  - Acute obstructive hydrocephalus with elevated ICP
  - Idiopathic intracranial hypotension
  - Critical postcraniotomy CSF hypovolemia

Arrested Hydrocephalus
- No/minimal overt symptoms
  - No stigmata of elevated ICP
  - Ventriculomegaly often incidental, unexpected MR finding
  - May be stable for years
- May cause subtle neurologic deterioration
  - Rare = sudden, fatal decompensation

Imaging

Imaging findings are identical to those of acute severe obstructive hydrocephalus. "Quadriventricular" enlargement, "halos" of periventricular interstitial edema, and small—sometimes almost inapparent—subarachnoid spaces are present **(34-35)**.

Differential Diagnosis

The major differential diagnosis of SILPAH is the much more common syndrome of **acute obstructive hydrocephalus** with elevated ICPs. Imaging findings are identical, so the definitive diagnosis is established only when EVD discloses unexpectedly low ICP.

SILPAH must be differentiated from **idiopathic intracranial hypotension**, a disorder also characterized by low ICP (see below). Intracranial hypotension is characterized by downward displacement of the central core brain structures, midbrain sagging, tonsillar descent, and dural thickening/enhancement.

Critical postcraniotomy CSF hypovolemia can cause marked cerebral hypotension with dramatic downward migration of intracranial structures. In both idiopathic intracranial hypotension and postcraniotomy CSF hypovolemia, the ventricles are usually small, not large.

Arrested Hydrocephalus

Arrested hydrocephalus (AH) has also been called asymptomatic hydrocephalus, occult hydrocephalus, compensated hydrocephalus, long-standing overt ventriculomegaly of adulthood, and late-onset idiopathic aqueductal stenosis. Moderate to severe triventricular enlargement without evidence for periventricular fluid accumulation is present on imaging studies and may remain stable for years **(34-36)** **(34-37)**.

Patients with AH rarely present with symptoms or stigmata of elevated ICP, and the diagnosis of hydrocephalus is often incidental and unexpected. As many patients with AH have no overt symptoms or evidence of neurologic deterioration, some clinicians have advocated a conservative approach with serial imaging and "watchful waiting."

Whether AH patients benefit from ventriculo-peritoneal shunt or third ventriculostomy remains unresolved with limited data to guide clinical decision making. Improvement in headaches and neuropsychiatric outcomes has been reported in some cases following CSF diversion. Despite clinical and imaging stability, some investigators believe longstanding ventriculomegaly is not benign and may be associated with cognitive decline and even sudden, fatal decompensation.

Idiopathic Intracranial Hypertension

Terminology

Idiopathic intracranial hypertension (IIH), also known as **benign intracranial hypertension**, is preferred to the term **pseudotumor cerebri**. IIH is characterized by unexplained elevation of ICP not related to an intracranial mass lesion, a meningeal process, or cerebral venous thrombosis. Patients with elevated ICP secondary to certain medications or transverse dural venous sinus stenosis are nonetheless still classified as having IIH.

Etiology and Pathology

The precise etiology of IIH is unknown. An obese phenotype with elevated body mass index is common. Disturbed CSF-ISF drainage through the "glymphatic pathway" has been invoked by some investigators.

It is unclear whether the dural venous sinus stenosis found in the vast majority of IIH patients is a cause (from venous outflow obstruction) or an effect (from extrinsic compression) of elevated ICP, or both.

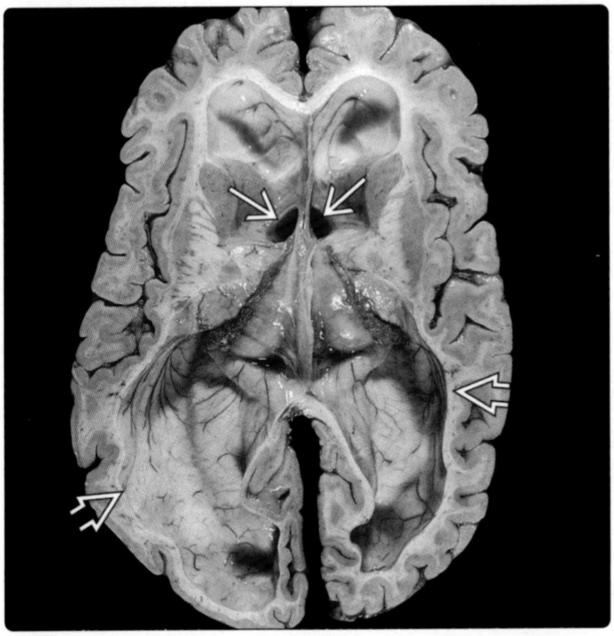

(34-36) Longstanding "compensated" IVOH from aqueductal stenosis shows symmetrically enlarged lateral ventricles and dilated foramen of Monro ➡. WM ➡ is severely reduced in volume, but cortex appears normal. (Courtesy R. Hewlett, MD.)

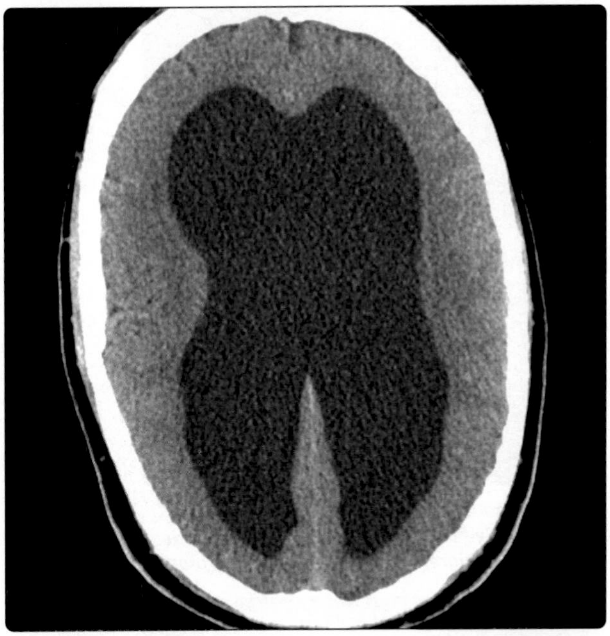

(34-37) NECT in a cognitively normal 73y man with headaches, normal neurological examination shows markedly enlarged lateral ventricles without periventricular fluid accumulation. Serial examinations showed no change; arrested hydrocephalus.

Clinical Issues

Epidemiology and Demographics. IIH is rare, but the incidence is rising with the worldwide obesity epidemic in industrialized nations. A recent epidemiology study reported an incidence of 23/100,000/year when stratified for reproductive age, female sex, and weight.

Presentation. Classically, IIH presents in overweight women who are 20-45 years of age although recent studies have confirmed a rising incidence in obese children, especially girls.

Headache is the most constant symptom (90-95%) followed by tinnitus and visual disturbances. Papilledema is the most common sign on neurologic examination. Cranial nerve deficits, usually limited to CN VI, are common.

Comorbidities are common and include—among others—polycystic ovarian syndrome, metabolic syndrome, obstructive sleep apnea, and hypervitaminosis A.

The definitive diagnosis of IIH is established by lumbar puncture, which demonstrates elevated ICP (>200 mm H_2O in adults or 280 mm H_2O in children) with normal CSF composition.

Natural History. Visual loss is the major morbidity in IIH. In fulminant IIH, visual loss can progress rapidly and become irreversible **(34-38)**.

Treatment Options. A 2015 Cochrane review concluded that there is no current consensus on the best management strategy for IIH. The two key approaches are to preserve visual function and reduce long-term headache disability.

Serial CSF removal (10-20 mL at initial LP) often temporarily ameliorates IIH-associated headache. Weight reduction and pharmacologic intervention can be effective in some patients. Acetazolamide is the mainstay of medical therapy for IIH, lowering ICP by its effects on choroid plexus CSF secretion.

Most recently, venous sinus stenting in patients who have transverse sinus stenosis has been successful in improving symptoms and reducing papilledema. Occasionally, spontaneous resolution of the stenosis occurs in obese patients with nonsurgical weight loss or following bariatric surgery.

Imaging

Neuroimaging is used to (1) exclude identifiable causes of increased ICP (e.g., neoplasm or obstructive hydrocephalus) and (2) detect findings associated with IIH.

The most significant imaging findings of IIH include **flattening of the posterior globes, distension of the perioptic subarachnoid space with or without a tortuous optic nerve, intraocular optic nerve protrusion, partial empty sella**, and **transverse venous sinus stenosis (34-39) (34-41)**. The presence of one or a combination of these signs—especially transverse sinus stenosis—significantly increases the odds of IIH, but their absence does not rule out IIH. *Prepubescent children have significantly lower frequencies of these findings compared with adults and adolescents!*

MR Findings. Sagittal scans show a partial empty sella. Here the pituitary gland occupies less than 50% of the pituitary fossa, and its superior surface appears concave. Dilated optic nerve sheaths are common, often appearing kinked and tortuous. The posterior globe is flattened or concave, and

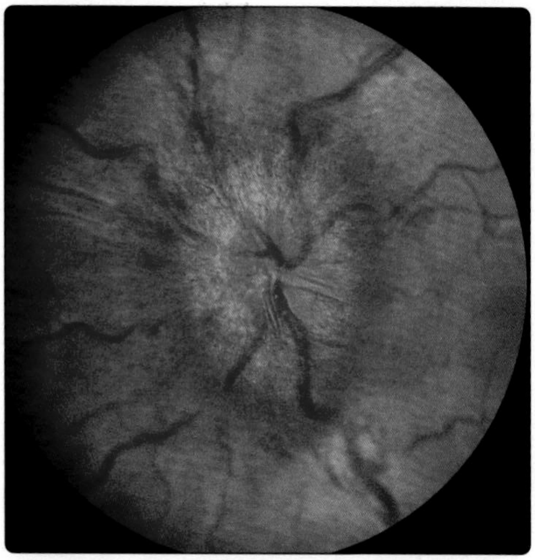

(34-38) Funduscopic image shows findings of severe papilledema with elevated, blurred optic disc (From K. Digre, MD, in Imaging in Neurology.)

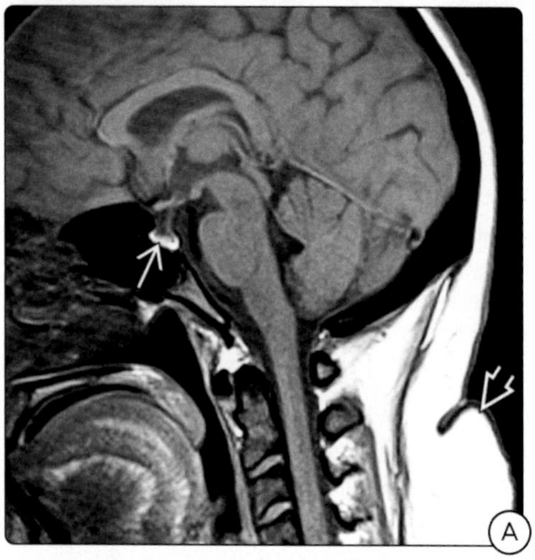

(34-39A) Sagittal T1WI in a 33y obese woman shows excessive subcutaneous fat ➡ and a partial empty sella ➡.

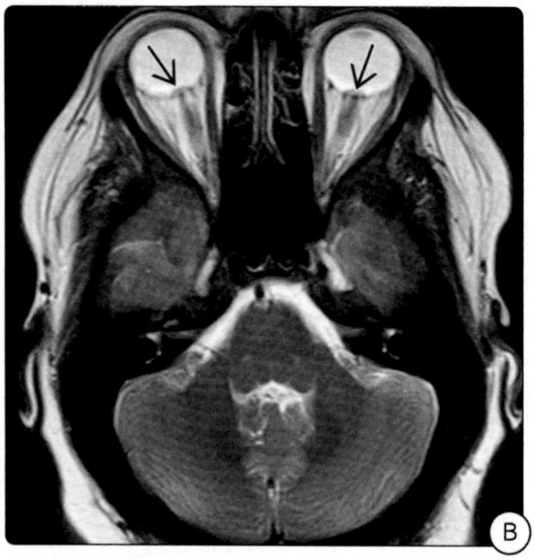

(34-39B) T2WI shows flattening of the globes, intraocular protrusion of optic nerve heads ➡. At LP the OP was 440 mm H_2O. This was IIH.

intraocular protrusion of the optic nerve may be visible **(34-40)**. In some patients, the optic nerve head enhances on T1 C+ FS sequences.

The prevalence of other reported findings such as slit-like or "pinched" ventricles (10%), "tight" subarachnoid spaces (small sulci and cisterns), and inferiorly displaced tonsils may be present. Cerebellar tonsillar ectopia may be present and sometimes even "peg-like" in configuration, mimicking Chiari I malformation.

Meningoceles or cephaloceles protruding through osseous defects in the skull base are common, especially in extremely obese patients. CSF leaks are common **(34-43)**, and CT or gadolinium MR cisternography may identify which of several bony defects is leaking.

CTV/MRV. The single most sensitive finding in IIH is a thinned, narrowed transverse-sigmoid sinus. Contrast-enhanced MRV has a pooled sensitivity of 97% in discriminating IIH patients and is helpful in differentiating a hypoplastic sinus segment from thrombosis (which is rare in IIH).

CT Findings. Solitary or multiple skull base osseous-dural defects are common. These appear as thinned, deossified, and/or dehisced bone with "sagging" of meninges through the bony defect. "Pits" around the margins of the temporal bones are also frequent.

Differential Diagnosis

The most important differential diagnosis in patients with suspected IIH is **secondary intracranial hypertension** (i.e., increased ICP with an identifiable cause). Although dilated optic nerve sheaths ("hydrops") and flattened posterior globes indicate elevated ICP, they can be seen in both secondary and idiopathic intracranial hypertension. Ventriculomegaly is more common in secondary intracranial hypertension, whereas the ventricles are usually normal to small in IIH.

Dural sinus thrombosis is another important consideration. T2* (GRE, SWI) shows "blooming" thrombus in the affected sinuses. MRV and CTV demonstrate a cigar-shaped, long-segment clot.

IDIOPATHIC INTRACRANIAL HYPERTENSION

Terminology and Etiology
- Also known as benign intracranial hypertension
- Often no cause identified (idiopathic)

Clinical Issues
- F > M; obesity = definite risk
- Peak 20-45 years
- Headache, tinnitus, vision loss, LP > 200 mm H_2O

Imaging
- Dilated optic nerve sheaths
- Intraoptic disc protrusion
- Flat posterior globe
- Partial empty sella
- "Tight" brain, ± tonsillar herniation
- ± Dural sinus thrombosis, stenosis

CSF Shunts and Complications

Although endoscopic third ventriculostomy is gaining acceptance, the standard treatment for all types of obstructive hydrocephalus remains placement of a shunt for CSF diversion.

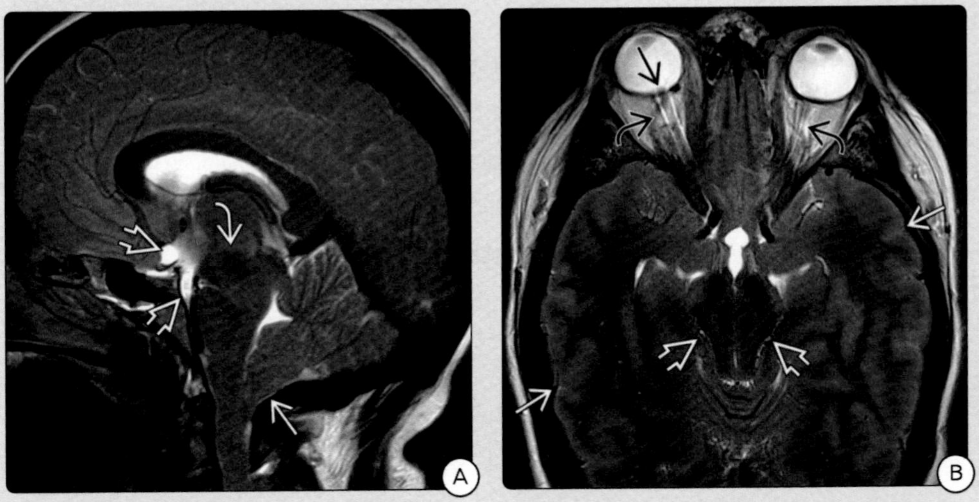

(34-40A) T2WI in 30y woman with headache, papilledema shows midbrain sagging →, tonsillar displacement →, distended anterior 3rd ventricle recesses →. (34-40B) Axial T2WI shows distended optic nerve sheaths →, intraoptic protrusion of nerve head →, brain swelling with midbrain herniation →. Note sulcal obliteration → with "tight" appearance to brain. Lumbar puncture OP was 600 mm. This was severe IIH.

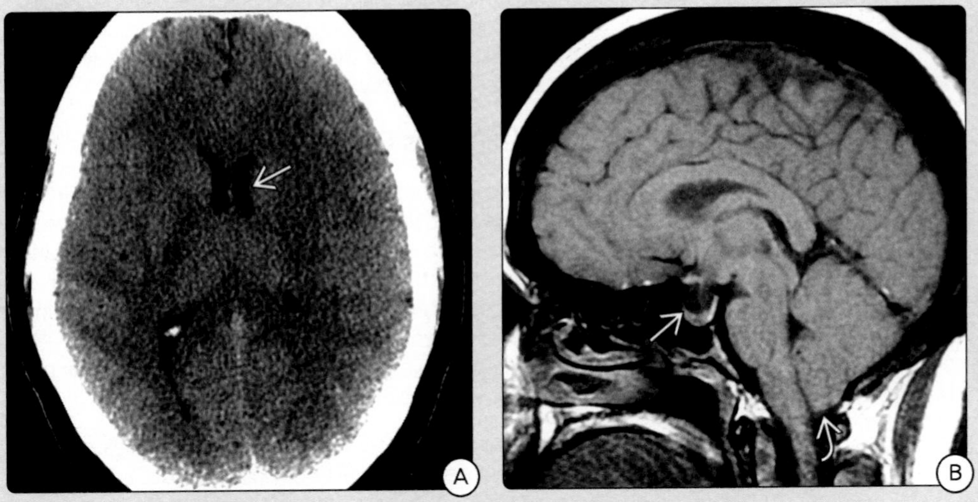

(34-41A) Axial NECT scan in a 29y woman with severe intractable headaches shows small lateral ventricles → and almost inapparent sulci over the surfaces of the hemispheres. (34-41B) Sagittal T1WI in the same patient shows partially empty sella → and mild tonsillar descent → without significant midbrain "slumping" or dural engorgement.

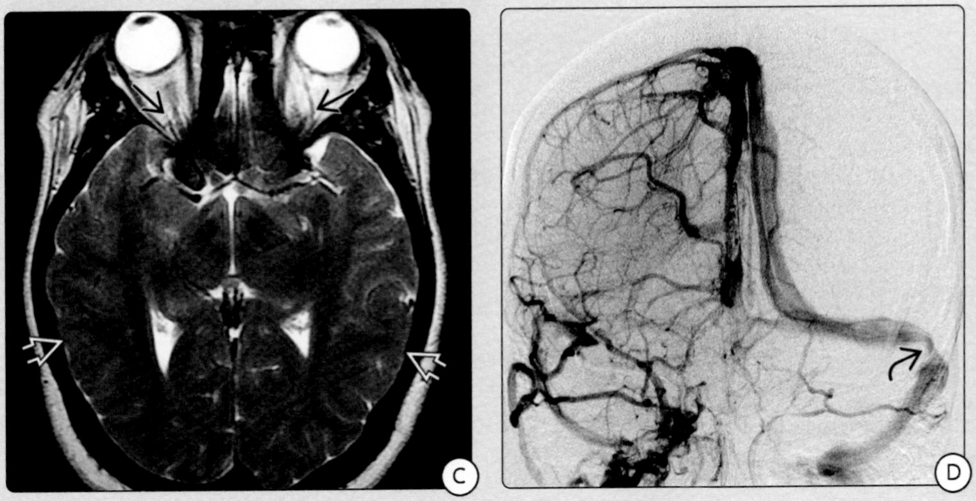

(34-41C) T2WI shows subtle dilatation of optic nerve sheaths → and relative lack of CSF-filled sulci over brain surfaces →. The globes appear normal. (34-41D) AP DSA shows left transverse sinus stenosis → with 10 mm Hg gradient. A stent was placed across the stenosis with resolution of the patient's headaches. Venous sinus stenosis or web causing intracranial hypertension is an uncommon but potentially remediable cause of IIH.

Placement of ventricular shunts are one of the most common of all neurosurgical procedures. Multiple surgeries are the rule, not the exception; approximately 50% of ventricular shunts in children fail in the first 2 years, and the vast majority have failed by 10 years after insertion.

The costs and lifelong morbidity associated with shunt placement to treat both childhood and adult hydrocephalus are substantial. More than half of all pediatric and adult patients require shunt revision. Almost 55% of children have four or more shunt revisions, and nearly 10% experience three or more shunt infections. Direct treatment-related costs for patients of all ages with hydrocephalus exceed $1 billion annually in the USA alone.

Imaging is a key component in evaluating patients with CSF diversions. Shunt failure can result in either enlarging or collapsing ventricles. The most common imaging manifestation of shunt failure is enlarging ventricles. CT is generally the preferred technique to assess patients with intracranial shunt catheters. Alternative modalities include transfontanelle ultrasound and new rapid MR techniques such as fast steady-state gradient-recalled-echo (SS-GRE) sequences.

We now briefly examine some of the most common causes of shunt malfunction.

Mechanical Failure

Mechanical failures represent nearly 75% of shunt malfunctions. Disconnection or fracture account for another 15% or so.

Most ventriculoperitoneal shunts have several components. The commonly used systems consist of three pieces: (1) a ventricular catheter connected to (2) an inline valve and (3) a distal peritoneal catheter. Shunt discontinuity can occur at any site, but disconnection is most common at the junctions of the various components.

The most common imaging modality to assess mechanical failure is a shunt series. Although some evidence suggests only a small number (less than 1%) of shunt series help in surgical decision making, shunt series are still frequently requested studies.

Standard shunt series are composed of skull (two views), neck, chest, and abdomen/pelvis radiographs to track shunt trajectory and integrity. Accurate diagnosis of shunt fractures and disconnections is complicated by three factors: (1) the wide variety of systems used, (2) the accumulation of residual "abandoned" catheter fragments in patients who have undergone multiple shunt revisions, and (3) nonradiopaque shunt segments. Careful comparison of current and prior studies is essential to determine whether the "active" shunt system is intact.

Programmable Valve Failures

Many neurosurgeons now use a programmable rather than a fixed-pressure valve for the treatment of hydrocephalus. Such devices allow noninvasive adjustment of valve pressure settings. (In up to 50% of cases, the opening pressure of an implanted valve has to be changed, sometimes months or even years later.)

Imaging is often performed to assess valve settings. Interested readers are referred to the comprehensive guide to valves and their radiographic appearances by Lollis et al. 2010.

Slit Ventricle Syndrome

Some shunted hydrocephalus patients exhibit clinical signs of shunt failure without evidence of ventricular enlargement, a condition called slit ventricle syndrome (SVS) **(34-42)**.

The etiology of SVS is controversial. Some patients have scarred ventricular walls with decreased compliance and reduced tolerance for the normal fluctuations in intracranial pressure. Others may have low pressure with collapsed ventricles secondary to overdrainage or CSF leak. Intermittent or partial shunt obstruction may be a contributory factor.

Comparison to prior imaging studies is essential. NECT scans show that one or both lateral ventricles are small or slit-like. Functional studies show that the shunt may fill slowly but still functions, although flow is often reduced.

Miscellaneous Complications

Decompression of longstanding hydrocephalus and CSF overdrainage both increase the risk of **subdural hematoma**. Intraventricular scarring and adhesions can block CSF flow from one compartment to another, causing an **encysted "trapped" (isolated) ventricle**. Continued CSF production can result in massive enlargement of the affected ventricle. Infection is a relatively uncommon complication but can result in meningitis, ventriculitis, and pyocephalus.

Abdominal complications from ventriculoperitoneal shunts include loculated CSF collections ("pseudocysts"), ascites, and bowel perforations. Distal shunt obstruction can cause shunt failure and hydrocephalus.

COMMON CSF SHUNT COMPLICATIONS

Mechanical
- Shunt discontinuity, fracture

Programmable Valve
- Valve setting too high, low

Miscellaneous
- Overdrainage (slit ventricle syndrome)
- Ventricles trapped, encysted

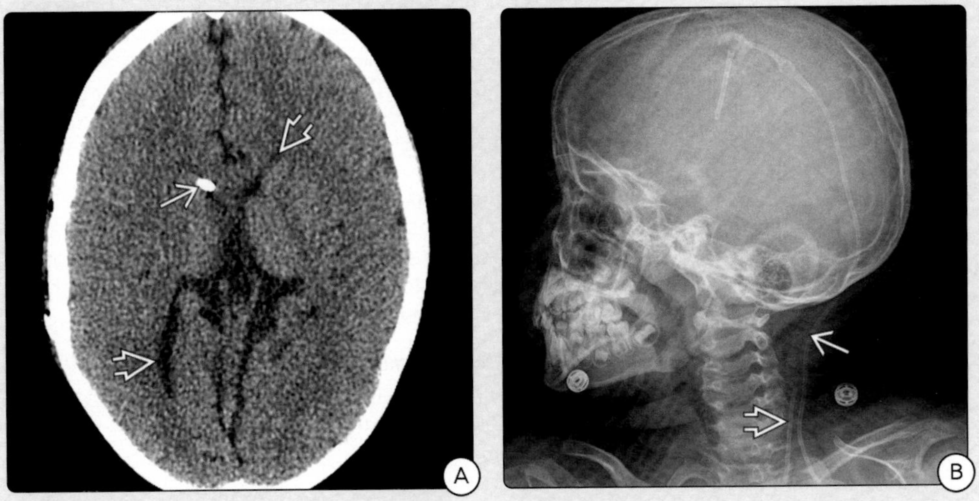

(34-42A) *NECT scan in an infant with shunted hydrocephalus shows shunt →, slit-like lateral ventricles →. Despite the shunt failure, the patient was asymptomatic.* ***(34-42B)*** *Skull radiograph obtained at the same time shows contiguity of the active shunt →. An abandoned shunt fragment in the neck is present →.*

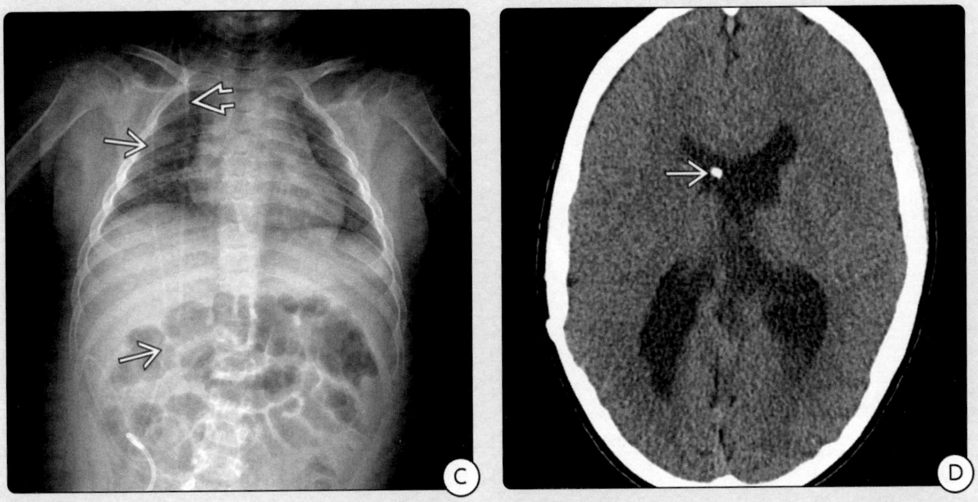

(34-42C) *Chest radiograph obtained as part of shunt series confirms contiguity of the actively functioning shunt → and shows distal aspect of the abandoned shunt fragment →.* ***(34-42D)*** *Several years later, the child developed severe headaches. NECT scan shows the ventricular catheter segment → has not changed in position. However, the lateral ventricles now appear moderately enlarged compared with the prior baseline examination.*

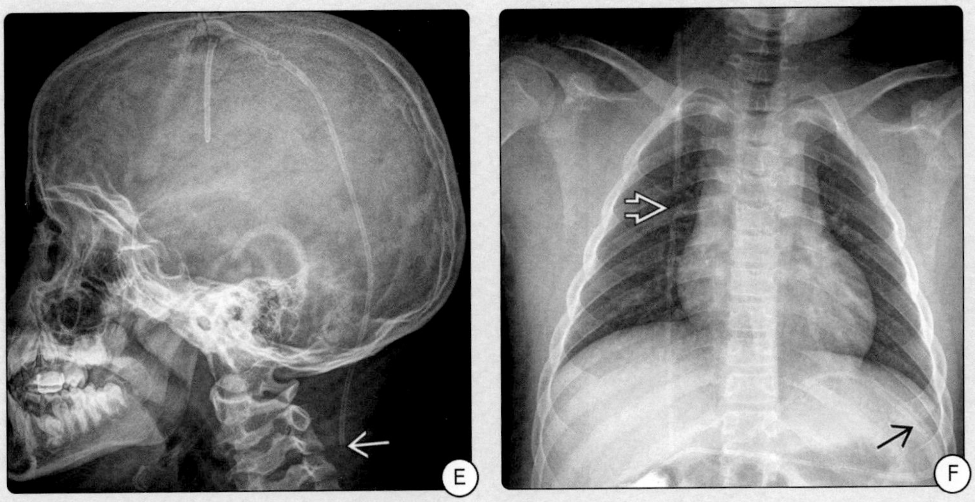

(34-42E) *Compared with the lateral skull radiograph from the prior shunt series (Figure 34-42B), the active catheter now abruptly terminates in the neck →.* ***(34-42F)*** *Chest radiograph shows a second discontinuity in the catheter →. The distal segment is coiled in the left upper quadrant →, a suboptimal position. (All six images courtesy K. Moore, MD.)*

CSF Leaks and Sequelae

CSF Leaks

Terminology

CSF anywhere outside the subarachnoid space of the brain and spine is abnormal. CSF leaks are named by location, e.g., CSF rhinorrhea (nasopharynx), CSF otorrhea (temporal bone).

Etiology

CSF leaks can be congenital or acquired. Congenital CSF leaks can occur with a cephalocele, persistent craniopharyngeal canal, or cribriform plate defect.

Acquired CSF leaks can be spontaneous, posttraumatic, or iatrogenic. Spontaneous intracranial CSF leaks are most commonly associated with arachnoid granulations in the lateral sphenoid sinus. Posttraumatic CSF leaks typically occur with fractures of the sphenoid sinus, cribriform plate, or ethmoid roof. Iatrogenic CSF leaks are seen with skull base surgery or following functional endoscopic sinus surgery.

Clinical Issues

Epidemiology and Demographics. CSF leaks can occur in patients of all ages. Trauma, prior skull base operation, and sinonasal surgery are common antecedents. Spontaneous CSF leaks usually develop in middle-aged obese women with idiopathic intracranial hypertension.

Presentation. The most common symptoms are CSF rhinorrhea, especially if the nasal discharge increases with Valsalva or head-down maneuvers.

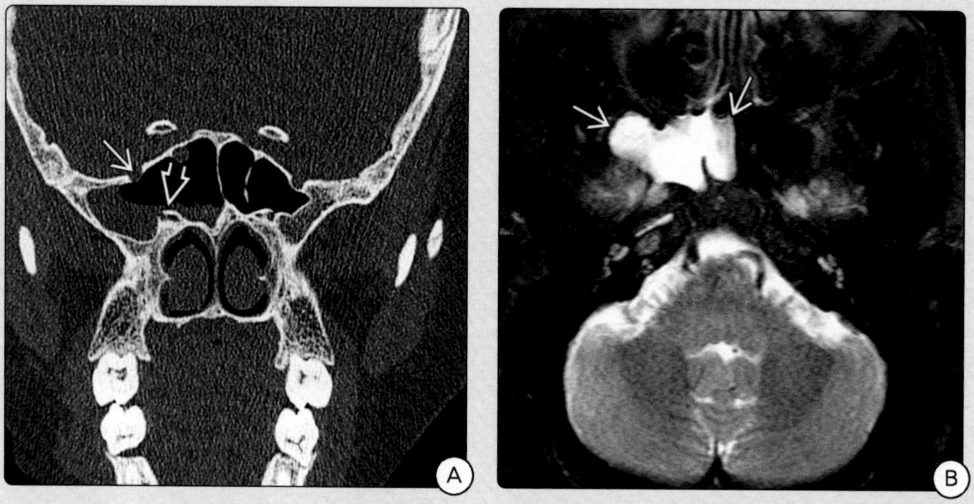

***(34-43A)** Bone CT in a patient with a spontaneous CSF leak shows a defect in the right sphenoid wing → and sphenoid sinus air-fluid level ⇒. **(34-43B)** T2 FS scan in the same patient shows fluid filling the right sphenoid sinus ⇒. The left sphenoid is normally aerated. In-111 DTPA cisternogram (not shown) demonstrated activity in nose and sphenoid sinus, confirming CSF leak. (Courtesy H. R. Harnsberger, MD.)*

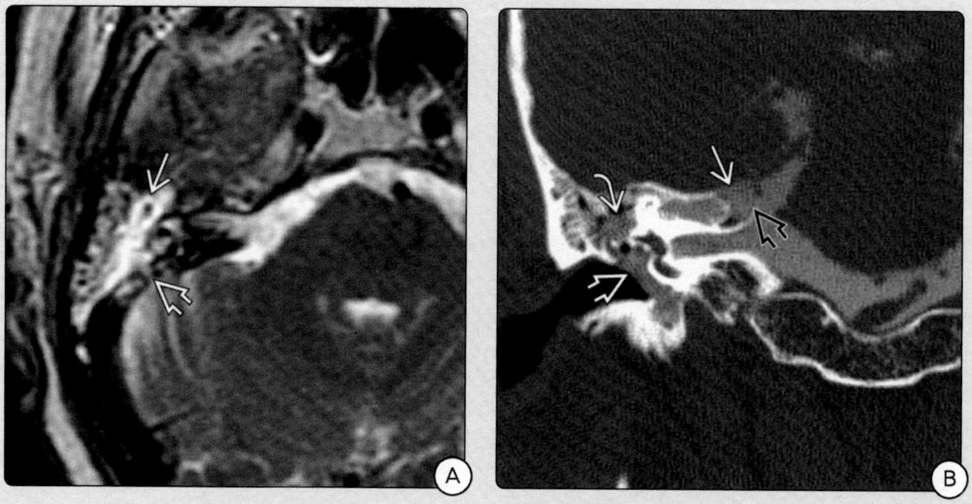

***(34-44A)** Axial T2WI in a patient with severe headaches and recurrent meningitis shows fluid filling the right mastoid → and filling defect in temporal bone ⇒. **(34-44B)** Coronal CT cisternogram in the same patient shows contrast in the CPA cistern entering the petrous temporal bone → through a defect caused by a giant arachnoid granulation ⇒, then filling the mastoid ↷ and middle ear ⇒. (Courtesy H. R. Harnsberger, MD.)*

Imaging

CT Findings. Bone CT with multiplanar reformations is the procedure of choice and may obviate the need for invasive CT cisternography. A bone defect, with or without an air-fluid level in the adjacent sinus, is the typical finding **(34-43)**. Defects under 3 or 4 mm may be difficult to detect, especially in areas where the bone is normally very thin.

CT cisternography is indicated if standard bone CT is negative or shows more than one potential leakage site **(34-44)**.

MR Findings. MR is generally used only if CT is negative or the presence of brain parenchyma within a cephalocele is suspected. T2 scans disclose an osseous defect with fluid in the adjacent sinus cavity.

Nuclear Medicine. In isotope cisternography, CSF is labeled with intrathecal Tc-99m or In-111 DTPA, and the activity over the head and spine is scanned. Pledgets can be packed into the nose or ear and then counted, usually 1-2 hours after tracer injection. Pledget counts should be at least 1.5 times the serum count.

Differential Diagnosis

The major differential diagnosis of a cranial CSF leak is a **skull base defect without CSF leak**. Some areas of the skull base—such as the cribriform plate, olfactory recesses, and petrous ridges—are often very thin.

Intracranial Hypotension

Intracranial hypotension is a poorly understood, frequently misdiagnosed entity that can present with a wide variety of symptoms. Imaging is key to the diagnosis, sometimes providing the first insight into the cause of often puzzling symptoms.

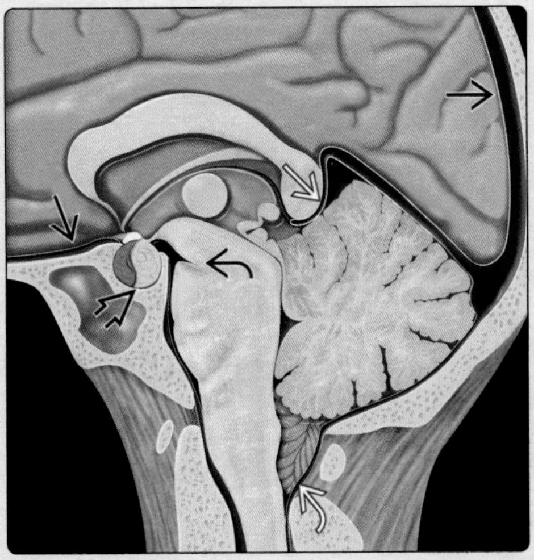

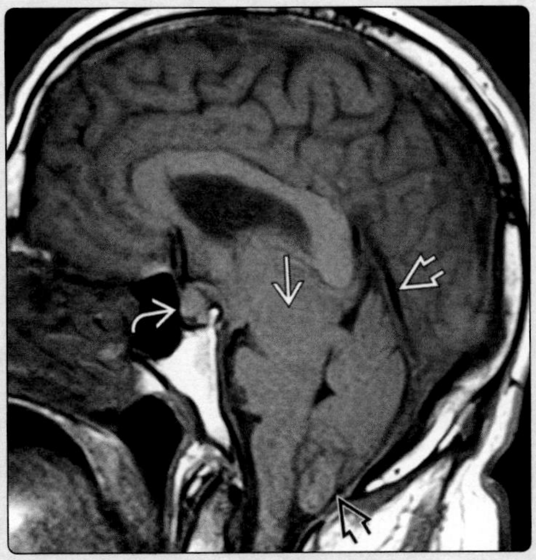

***(34-45)** Intracranial hypotension (ICH) is shown with distended dural sinuses , enlarged pituitary , and herniated tonsils . Central brain descent causes midbrain "slumping," inferiorly displaced pons, "closed" pons-midbrain angle , splenium depressing ICV/V of G junction . **(34-46)** Sagittal T1WI in patient with severe ICH shows severe midbrain, pons sagging , fat pituitary , low-lying tonsils , and prominent venous sinuses .*

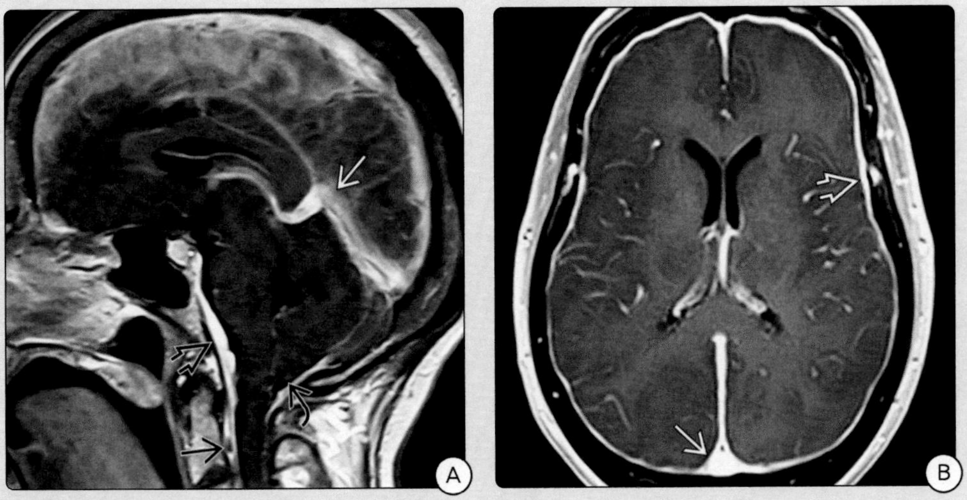

***(34-47A)** Sagittal T1 C+ in a 58y woman with postural headaches shows extensive dura-arachnoid thickening, enhancement that extends into the upper cervical spine . Midbrain slumping and tonsillar herniation are minimal. Venous sinuses are engorged . **(34-47B)** Axial T1 C+ shows venous engorgement , diffuse dura-arachnoid thickening, and enhancement . ICH is secondary to spinal CSF leak (not shown).*

Terminology

Intracranial hypotension is also known as **CSF hypovolemia syndrome**.

Etiology

Intracranial hypotension can be spontaneous (SIH) or acquired. Common antecedent causes include lumbar puncture, spinal surgery, and trauma. Patients with Marfan and Ehlers-Danlos syndromes have abnormal connective tissue and an increased risk of CSF rupture through the congenitally weakened dura.

Spinal meningeal diverticula can rupture suddenly and may be responsible for many cases of "spontaneous" intracranial hypotension. Occasionally, CSF leaks occur through a dural tear caused by a cervical or lumbar disc-osteophyte complex. In contrast to idiopathic intracranial hypertension, skull base CSF leaks rarely cause SIH.

Pathology

CSF hypovolemia and hypotension (lumbar OP < 60 mm H_2O) result in venous and dural interstitial engorgement with brain descent ("sagging") **(34-45)**. The dura itself typically appears normal without evidence of neoplasia or inflammation. Longstanding cases of SIH may have dura-arachnoid fibrosis with nests of prominent meningothelial cells that should not be mistaken for meningioma.

Clinical Issues

Epidemiology and Demographics. The true incidence of SIH is unknown. Estimated prevalence is 1:50,000 per year. Although SIH can occur at any age, peak prevalence is in the third and fourth decades. There is a moderate female predominance.

Presentation. Symptoms range widely, from mild headache to coma. The classic presentation of SIH is a severe orthostatic

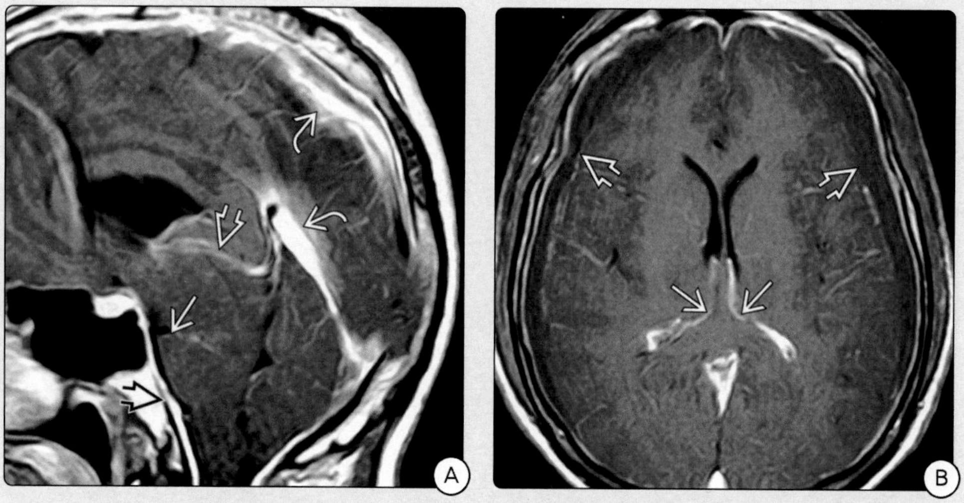

***(34-48A)** Downward herniation can become severe; large subdural hematomas (SDHs) may develop, as happened in this case. Sagittal T1 C+ scan shows severe midbrain "slumping" and downward compression of the pons ➡, flattened internal cerebral veins ➡, thick dural enhancement ➡, and venous sinus distension ➡. **(34-48B)** T1 C+ FS scan demonstrates medially displaced ICVs and ventricles ➡ and bilateral SDHs ➡.*

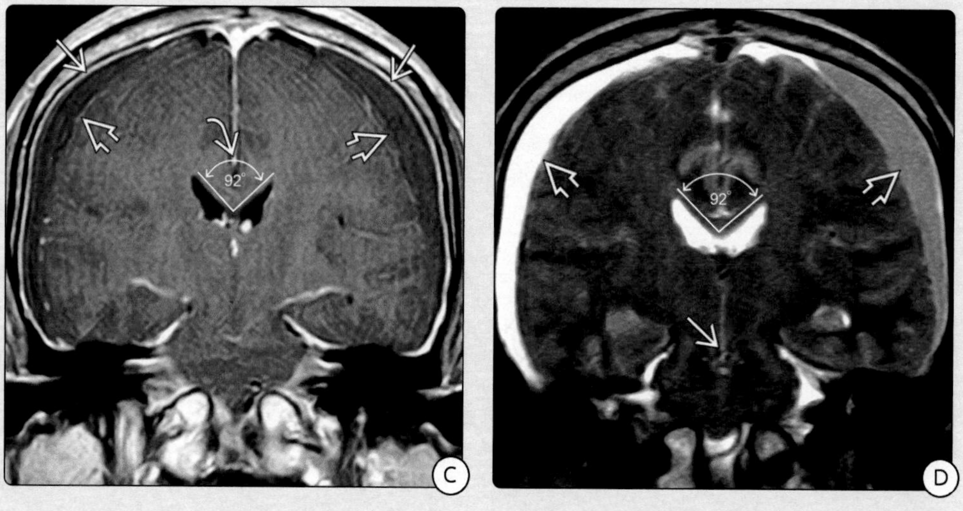

***(34-48C)** Coronal T1 C+ shows the SDHs ➡, diffuse dural enhancement ➡, and markedly decreased ("closed") ventricular angle ➡ from downward traction on the central core structures of the brain. **(34-48D)** Coronal T2WI in the same patient shows downward displacement of the slit-like third ventricle ➡ through the tentorial incisura, SDHs of different ages ➡, and "closed" ventricular angle.*

headache that is relieved by lying down. (Loss of approximately 10% of the total CSF volume is required to induce orthostatic headache.)

Nonorthostatic headache, nuchal rigidity, and visual disturbances are less common. Severe cases may present with progressive encephalopathy. Orthostatic or postural headache can have posterior neck pain or stiffness,vomiting, or photophobia. Hyperprolactinemia with stalk effect caused by the infundibular compression may be present.

Natural History. Most cases of SIH resolve spontaneously. In rare cases, severe unrelieved brain descent can result in coma or even death.

Treatment Options. Treatment is aimed at restoring CSF volume. Fluid replacement and bed rest can be sufficient in many cases. In others, epidural blood patch or surgical repair may be required. Emergent intrathecal saline infusion may be lifesaving in obtunded, severely encephalopathic patients.

Epidural blood patch is often performed on the basis of clinical and brain imaging findings alone. If low- and high-volume patches are unsuccessful, further studies may be necessary to localize precisely the level of the CSF leak.

INTRACRANIAL HYPOTENSION

Etiology and Pathology

- CSF hypovolemia leads to brain "sags," dural/venous sinuses increase
- Can be spontaneous (idiopathic) or acquired

Clinical Issues

- Most common symptom = headache
    - ± Orthostatic
- Severe intracranial hypotension can cause coma, even death

MR Findings

- Common
    - Midbrain "sags" down
    - Angle between midbrain, pons decreases (< 50°)
    - Pontomammillary distance < 5.5 mm
    - Optic chiasm/hypothalamus draped over prominent pituitary
    - Diffusely thickened enhancing dura (reduced with time)
    - "Fat" pituitary
- Less common
    - Pons, midbrain may appear "fat"
    - ± Tonsils displaced downward
    - Effaced cisterns/sulci
    - Small lateral ventricles ± atria "tugged" inferomedially
    - ± Subdural collections (hygromas > frank hematomas)
    - Enlarged dural sinuses with outwardly bulging (convex) margins
- Rare but important
    - Ventricular angle on coronal imaging decreases
    - Torn bridging cortical veins
    - Subarachnoid hemorrhage, superficial siderosis

Imaging

Although CT is often obtained as an initial screening study in patients with severe or intractable headache, MR of the brain and spine is the procedure of choice to evaluate possible SIH. A spectrum of findings occurs with SIH; only rarely are *all* imaging signs present in the same patient! Almost 20% of patients with clinically apparent intracranial hypotension have NO abnormal brain MR findings!

CT Findings. CT scans in SIH are often normal. The most obvious findings are subdural fluid collections. Subtle CT clues to the presence of SIH include effacement of the basal cisterns (especially the suprasellar subarachnoid space), medial herniation of the temporal lobes into the tentorial incisura, small ventricles with medial deviation of the atria of the lateral ventricles, and a "fat" pons.

MR Findings. Between 90-95% of SIH patients have one or more key findings on standard MR scans.

T1WI. Sagittal T1 scans show brain descent in approximately half of all cases **(34-46)**. Midbrain "sagging" with the midbrain displaced below the level of the dorsum sellae, decreased angle between the peduncles and pons below 50°, shortened pontomammillary distance below 5.5 mm, and flattening of the pons against the clivus are typical findings **(34-47)**. Caudal displacement of the tonsils is common but not invariably present.

The optic chiasm and hypothalamus are often draped over the sella, effacing the suprasellar cistern. The pituitary gland appears enlarged in at least 50% of all cases **(34-46)** **(34-50C)**.

Axial scans show that the basal cisterns are effaced. The pons often appears elongated and "fat" **(34-49B)**. Midbrain anatomy is distorted with decreased width and increased anteroposterior diameter **(34-49C)**. The temporal lobes are displaced medially over the tentorium into the incisura. The lateral ventricles are usually small and distorted, as they are pulled medially and inferiorly by the brain "sagging" **(34-48)**.

In cases with severe brain descent, coronal scans may show that the angle between the roof of the lateral ventricles progressively decreases (< 120°) as brain sagging increases **(34-48)** **(34-50)**.

The dural sinuses often appear distended with outwardly convex margins and exaggerated "flow voids" **(34-49E)**. Between 15-50% of cases have subdural fluid collections (hygromas > hematomas) **(34-48)**.

T2/FLAIR. The slit-like third ventricle is displaced downward and on axial scans appears almost superimposed on the midbrain and hypothalamus **(34-49C)**.

T1 C+. One of the most consistent findings in SIH, seen in 80-85% of cases, is diffuse dural thickening with intense enhancement. Linear dural thickening may extend into the internal auditory canals, down the clivus, and through the foramen magnum into the upper cervical canal **(34-47)**. On axial imaging the engorged enhancing cervical venous plexuses may appear like a "draped curtain," narrowing the canal and even mimicking sarcoid or metastatic disease.

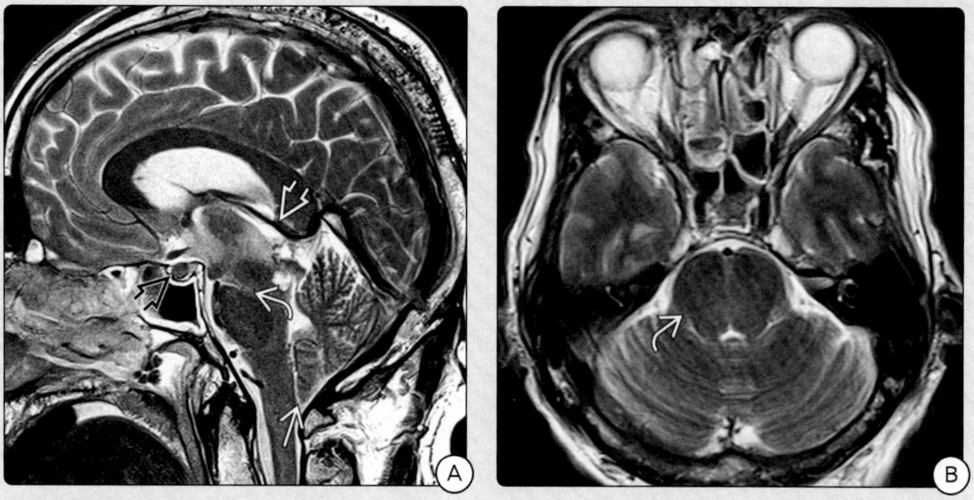

***(34-49A)** Sagittal T2WI in a 57y man with headaches and acute encephalopathy shows severe midbrain slumping, tonsillar descent, fat pituitary gland, and flattening of the internal cerebral vein/vein of Galen angle. **(34-49B)** Axial T2WI in the same case shows a "fat"-appearing pons.*

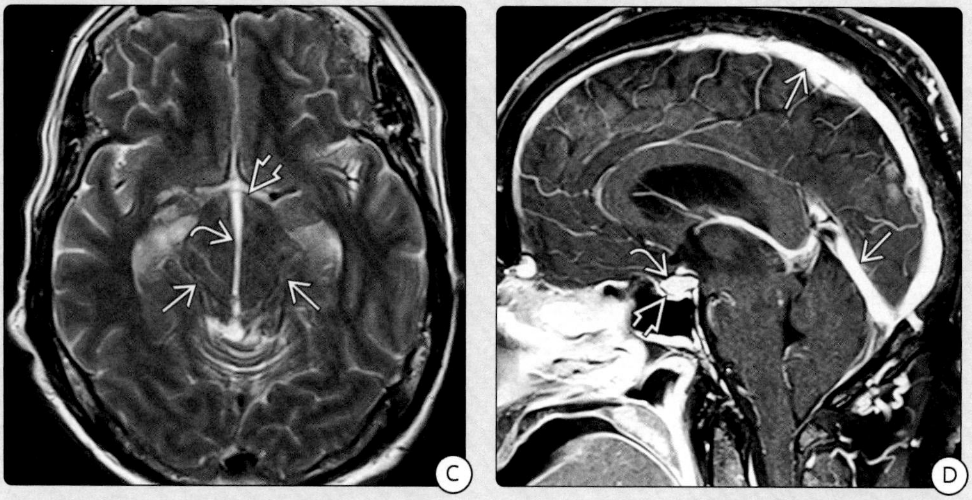

***(34-49C)** More cephalad T2WI in the same case shows a "fat," elongated midbrain with a low-lying third ventricle seen in the same plane as the midbrain and hypothalamus. **(34-49D)** Sagittal T1 C+ shows engorged dural venous sinuses, a prominent, enhancing pituitary gland, and enlarged inferior intercavernous sinus.*

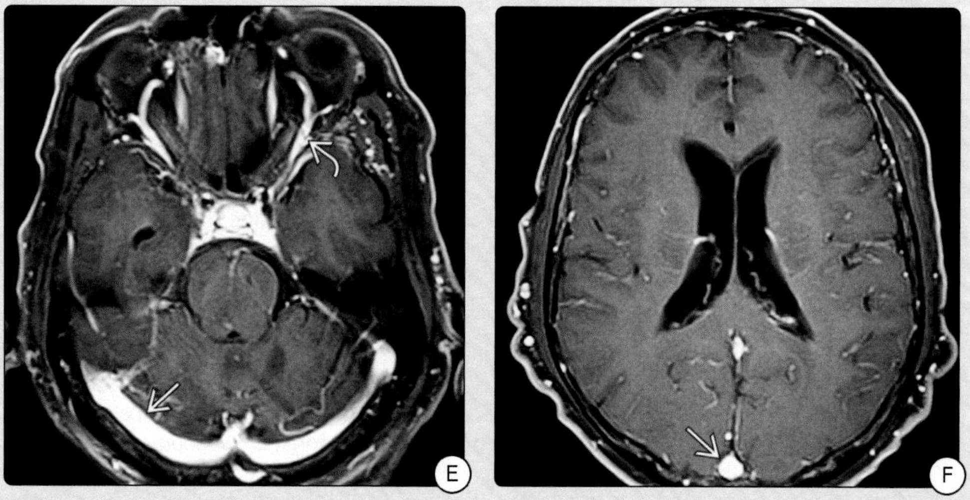

***(34-49E)** Axial T1 C+ FS shows prominent dural venous sinuses and superior ophthalmic veins. **(34-49F)** More cephalad T1 C+ FS shows enlarged, rounded enhancing superior sagittal sinus but no dura-arachnoid enhancement. Severe intracranial hypotension often has minimal or no abnormal dura-arachnoid thickening and enhancement.*

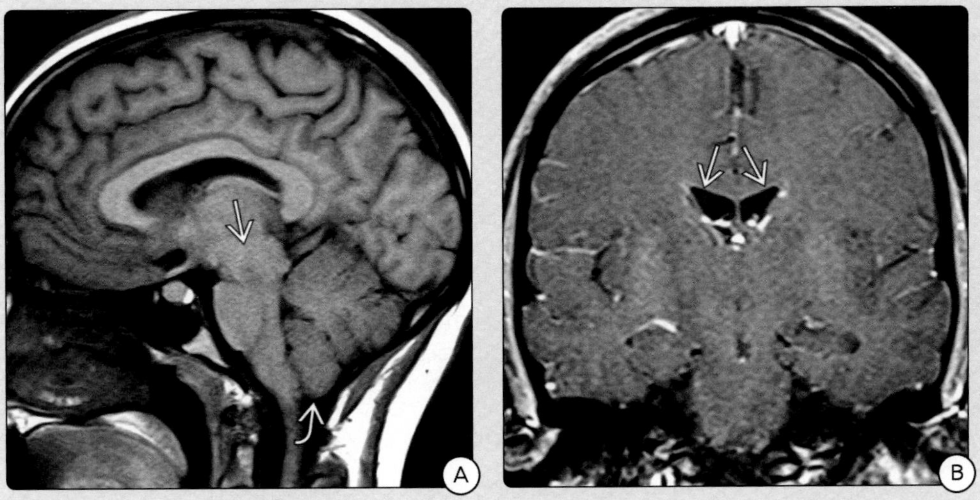

(34-50A) *Sagittal T1WI in a 25y woman with headaches shows mild midbrain slumping . The cerebellar tonsils measured 7 mm below the foramen magnum but are normally shaped. This was called Chiari 1 malformation.* ***(34-50B)*** *Coronal T1 C+ in the same case shows normal callosoventricular angle and no evidence for abnormal dura-arachnoid enhancement.*

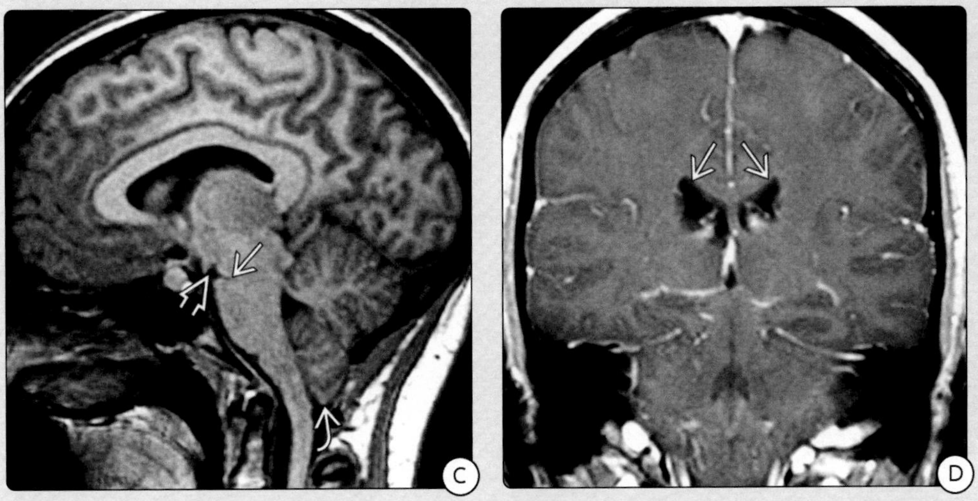

(34-50C) *The patient's headaches worsened. One year later, sagittal MP-RAGE shows more severe midbrain slumping with decreased mesencephalon-pontine angle that measures less than 45°. Tonsillar descent has increased. The mamillopontine distance was 4 mm.* ***(34-50D)*** *Coronal T1 C+ shows decreased callosal-ventricular angle compared with the prior scan.*

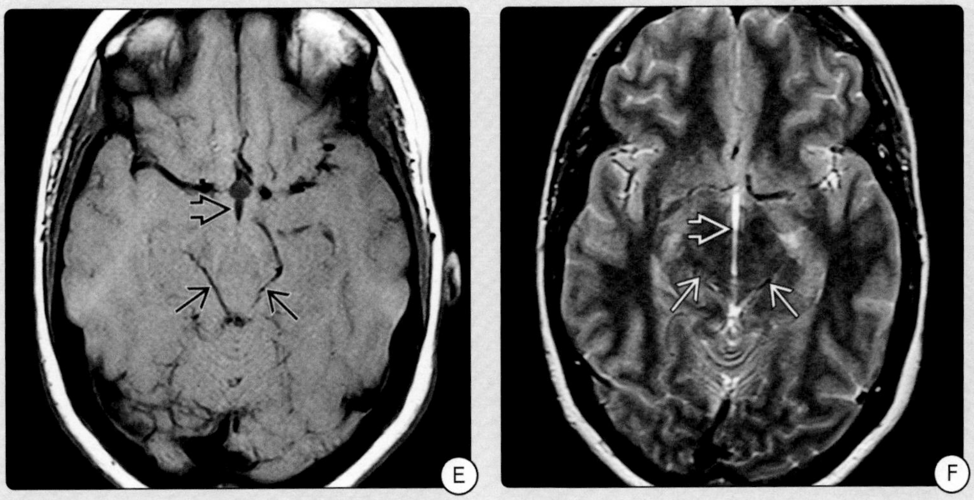

(34-50E) *Axial T1WI shows decreased CSF spaces with a "tight brain" appearance. The midbrain is elongated and concave laterally . The third ventricle is inferiorly displaced over the hypothalamus.* ***(34-50F)*** *Axial T2WI shows elongated midbrain and elongated and inferiorly displaced 3rd ventricle . No abnormal dura-arachnoid enhancement was seen on T1 C+. ICH was initially misdiagnosed as Chiari 1 malformation.*

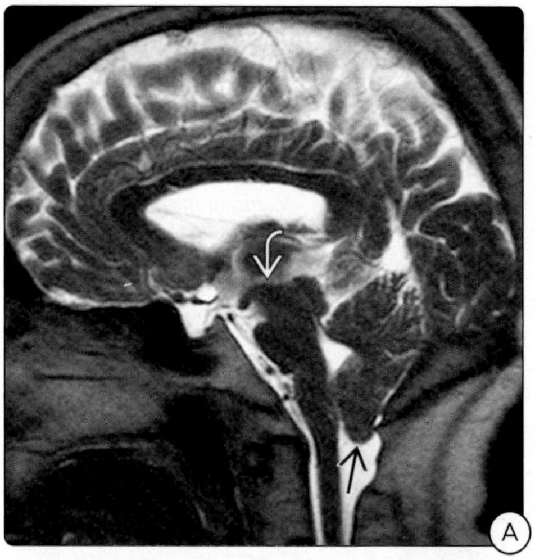

***(34-51A)** T2WI in 48y woman (severe HA) shows inferiorly displaced tonsils, slumping midbrain; called Chiari 1, decompressed surgically.*

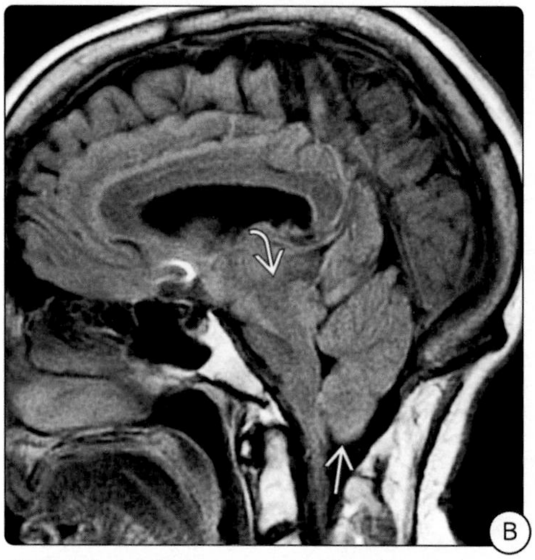

***(34-51B)** Headaches worsened over 2 years. FLAIR shows severe midbrain slumping, vermis displaced posteroinferiorly.*

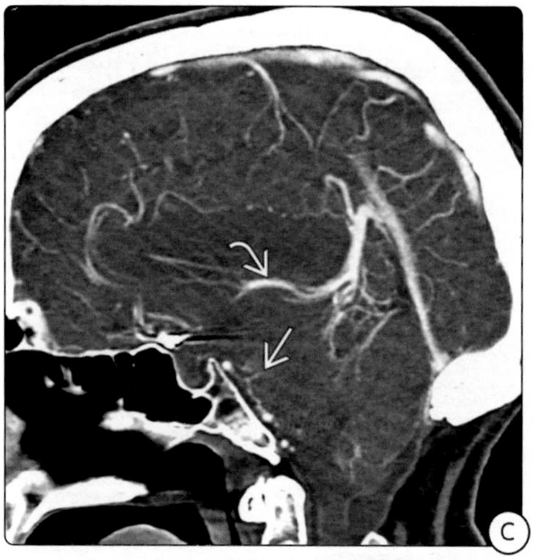

***(34-51C)** CTA shows flattened ICV, pons displaced downward. Severe intracranial hypotension was misdiagnosed as Chiari 1.*

Dural enhancement is time dependent and gradually decreases over time. Patients with chronic SIH may have no dural enhancement despite ongoing CSF leakage detectable on CT myelography.

T2* (GRE, SWI). Tearing of bridging veins caused by brain sagging can result in subarachnoid hemorrhage and superficial siderosis.

Spine Imaging. CT myelography (CTM) with immediate and delayed imaging is considered the gold standard for finding a CSF leak. MR of the entire spine with heavily T2-weighted sequences ("MR myelogram") can be helpful in identifying meningeal diverticula with pericyst extraarachnoid CSF.

Nuclear Medicine. In-111 DTPA, intrathecal radionuclide cisternography can detect extradural egress of tracer. SPECT/CT fusion imaging is very helpful to determine the precise spinal level responsible for the CSF leak.

Differential Diagnosis

The major differential diagnosis of intracranial hypotension is **Chiari 1 malformation**. In rare SIH cases, prolapse of the cerebellar tonsils can be mistaken for a Chiari I malformation **(34-51)**. However, in Chiari I the only intracranial abnormality is displaced tonsils, which appear peg-like with vertically oriented folia. Other findings of SIH are absent. *Mistaking SIH for Chiari 1 on imaging studies can lead to decompressive surgery, worsening CSF hypovolemia, and clinical deterioration!*

Selected References

Normal Anatomy of the Ventricles and Cisterns

Stratchko L et al: The ventricular system of the brain: anatomy and normal variations. Semin Ultrasound CT MR. 37(2):72-83, 2016

Choroid Plexus, CSF, and Brain Interstitial Fluid

Bakker EN et al: Lymphatic clearance of the brain: perivascular, paravascular and significance for neurodegenerative diseases. Cell Mol Neurobiol. 36(2):181-94, 2016

Cherian I et al: Exploring the Virchow-Robin spaces function: a unified theory of brain diseases. Surg Neurol Int. 7(Suppl 26):S711-S714, 2016

Normal Variants

Asymmetric Lateral Ventricles

Barzilay E et al: Fetal brain anomalies associated with ventriculomegaly or asymmetry: an MRI-based study. AJNR Am J Neuroradiol. 38(2):371-375, 2017

Nigri F et al: Hydrocephalus caused by unilateral foramen of Monro obstruction: a review on terminology. Surg Neurol Int. 7(Suppl 12):S307-13, 2016

Cavum Septi Pellucidi and Vergae

Saba L et al: MR and CT of brain's cava. J Neuroimaging. 23(3):326-35, 2013

Cavum Velum Interpositum

Tubbs RS et al: Cavum velum interpositum, cavum septum pellucidum, and cavum vergae: a review. Childs Nerv Syst. 27(11):1927-30, 2011

Enlarged Subarachnoid Spaces

Fingarson AK et al: Enlarged subarachnoid spaces and intracranial hemorrhage in children with accidental head trauma. J Neurosurg Pediatr. 19(2):254-258, 2017

Tucker J et al: Macrocephaly in infancy: benign enlargement of the subarachnoid spaces and subdural collections. J Neurosurg Pediatr. 1-5, 2016

Hydrocephalus

Intraventricular Obstructive Hydrocephalus

Langner S et al: Diagnosis and differential diagnosis of hydrocephalus in adults. Rofo. ePub, 2017

Bir SC et al: Epidemiology of adult-onset hydrocephalus: institutional experience with 2001 patients. Neurosurg Focus. 41(3):E5, 2016

Desai B et al: Hydrocephalus: the role of cerebral aquaporin-4 channels and computational modeling considerations of cerebrospinal fluid. Neurosurg Focus. 41(3):E8, 2016

Kestle JR et al: Introduction: Pediatric hydrocephalus: a continuing evolution in our understanding and management. Neurosurg Focus. 41(5):E1, 2016

Extraventricular Obstructive Hydrocephalus

Bir SC et al: Epidemiology of adult-onset hydrocephalus: institutional experience with 2001 patients. Neurosurg Focus. 41(3):E5, 2016

Hong J et al: Surgical management of arrested hydrocephalus: case report, literature review, and 18-month follow-up. Clin Neurol Neurosurg. 151:79-85, 2016

Overproduction Hydrocephalus

Cox JT et al: Choroid plexus hyperplasia: a possible cause of hydrocephalus in adults. Neurology. 87(19):2058-2060, 2016

Karimy JK et al: Cerebrospinal fluid hypersecretion in pediatric hydrocephalus. Neurosurg Focus. 41(5):E10, 2016

Spennato P et al: Acute triventricular hydrocephalus caused by choroid plexus cysts: a diagnostic and neurosurgical challenge. Neurosurg Focus. 41(5):E9, 2016

Normal Pressure Hydrocephalus

Yin LK et al: Reversed aqueductal cerebrospinal fluid net flow in idiopathic normal pressure hydrocephalus. Acta Neurol Scand. ePub, 2017

Daou B et al: Revisiting secondary normal pressure hydrocephalus: does it exist? A review. Neurosurg Focus. 41(3):E6, 2016

Keong NC et al: Imaging normal pressure hydrocephalus: theories, techniques, and challenges. Neurosurg Focus. 41(3):E11, 2016

Syndrome of Inappropriately Low-Pressure Acute Hydrocephalus

Barami K et al: The cerebral venous system and the postural regulation of intracranial pressure: implications in the management of patients with cerebrospinal fluid diversion. Childs Nerv Syst. 32(4):599-607, 2016

Hamilton MG et al: Syndrome of inappropriately low-pressure acute hydrocephalus (SILPAH). Acta Neurochir Suppl. 113:155-9, 2012

Idiopathic Intracranial Hypertension

Chan JW: Current concepts and strategies in the diagnosis and management of idiopathic intracranial hypertension in adults. J Neurol. ePub, 2017

Hartmann AJ et al: Imaging features of idiopathic intracranial hypertension in children. J Child Neurol. 32(1):120-126, 2017

Matloob SA et al: Effect of venous stenting on intracranial pressure in idiopathic intracranial hypertension. Acta Neurochir (Wien). ePub, 2017

Raper DMS et al: Effect of body mass index on venous sinus pressures in idiopathic intracranial hypertension patients before and after endovascular stenting. Neurosurgery. ePub, 2017

CSF Shunts and Complications

Lollis SS et al: Programmable CSF shunt valves: radiographic identification and interpretation. AJNR Am J Neuroradiol. 31(7):1343-6, 2010

CSF Leaks and Sequelae

Intracranial Hypotension

Holbrook J et al: Imaging of intracranial pressure disorders. Neurosurgery. 80(3):341-354, 2017

Capizzano AA et al: Atypical presentations of intracranial hypotension: comparison with classic spontaneous intracranial hypotension. AJNR Am J Neuroradiol. 37(7):1256-61, 2016

Kranz PG et al: Time-dependent changes in dural enhancement associated with spontaneous intracranial hypotension. AJR Am J Roentgenol. 207(6):1283-1287, 2016

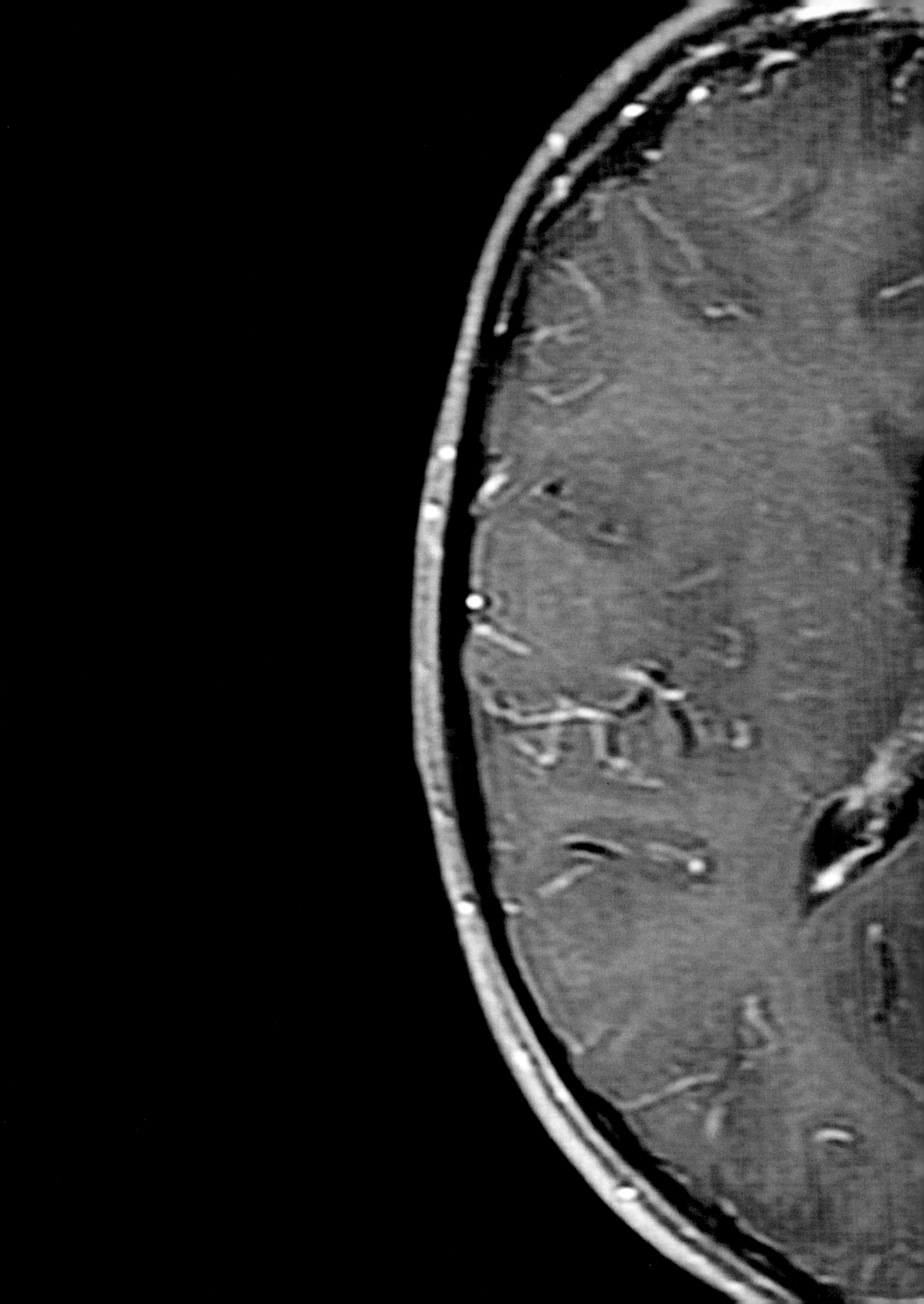

Section 6

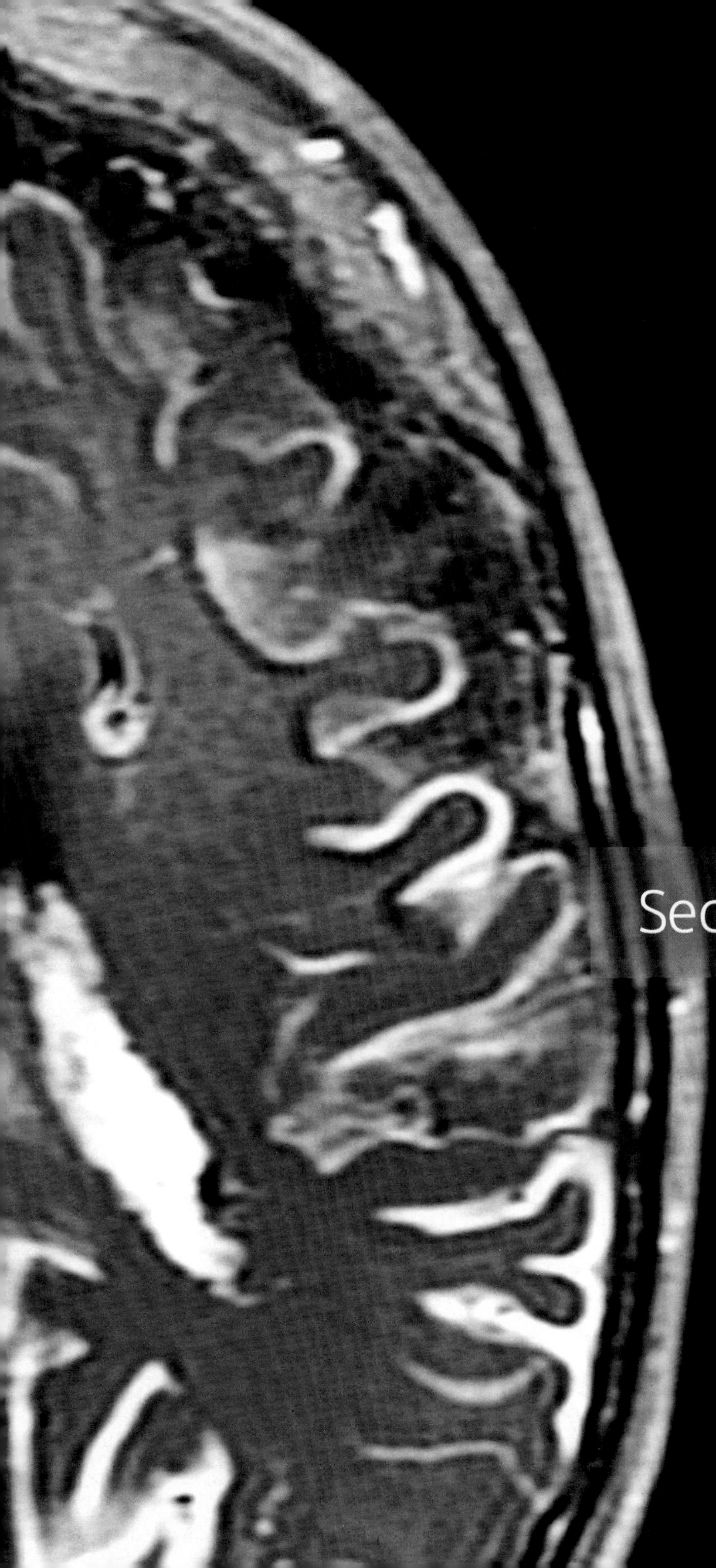

Section 6

Congenital Malformations of the Skull and Brain

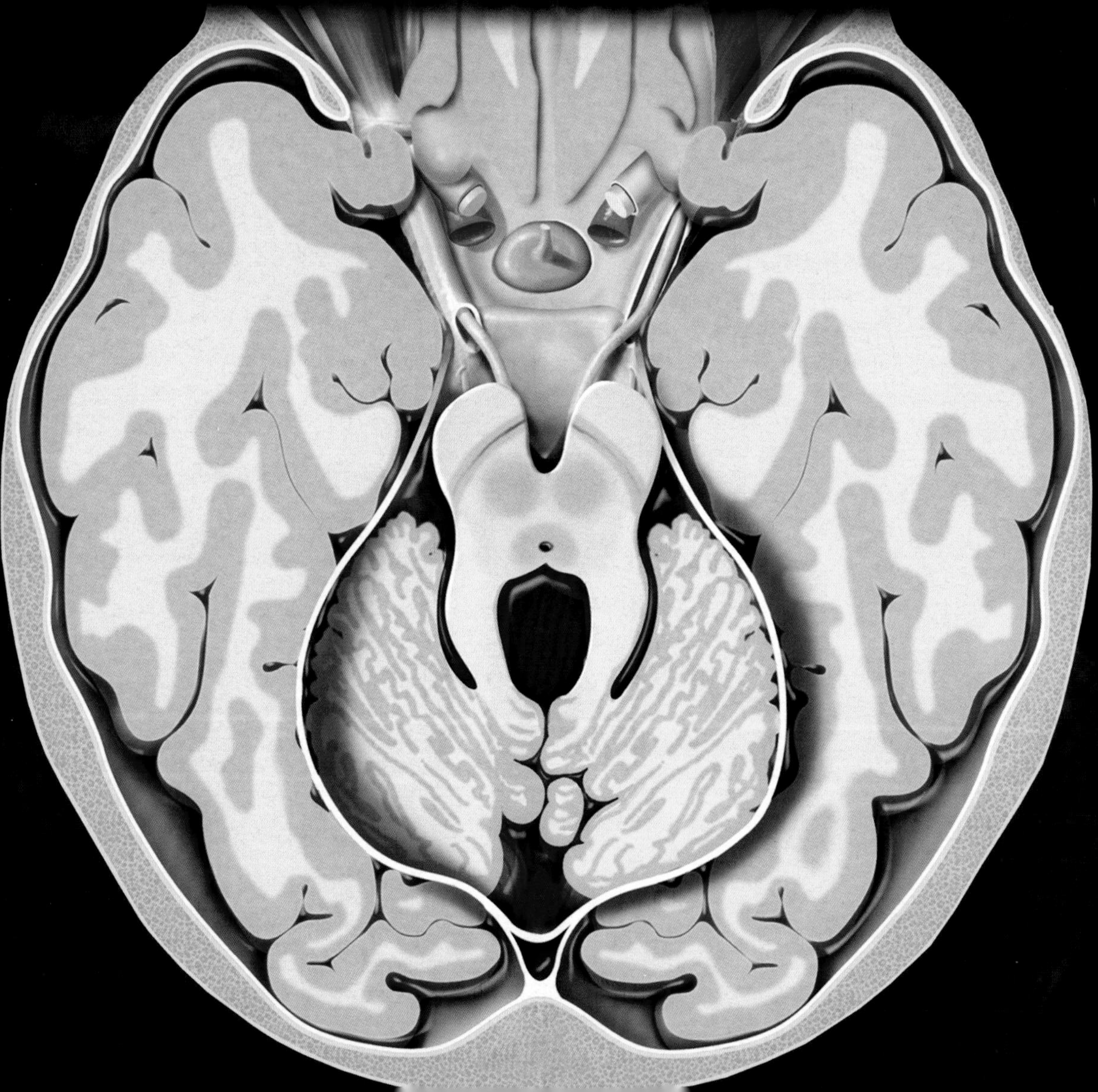

Embryology and Approach to Congenital Malformations

A basic knowledge of normal brain development and maturation provides the essential foundation for understanding congenital malformations, the subject of the final part of this book.

This text approaches embryology step by step, discussing different aspects of CNS development with their relevant pathology. Some concepts have already been elucidated in previous chapters. Myelination maturation from birth to age three was discussed in Chapter 31 with inherited metabolic disorders, and development of the ventricles and choroid plexus was presented in conjunction with the discussion of hydrocephalus and CSF disorders in Chapter 34.

Here, we briefly consider normal development of the cerebral hemispheres and cerebellum. We first focus on the basics of neurulation and neural tube closure, then turn our attention to how the neural tube flexes, bends, and evolves into the forebrain, midbrain, and hindbrain. Developmental errors and the resulting malformations that may occur at each stage are briefly summarized. (They are discussed in detail in subsequent chapters.)

Growth of the cerebral hemispheres with their elaboration into lobes, the development of sulci and gyri, patterns of gray matter migration, and layering of the neocortex are all succinctly delineated. Development of the three major brain commissures (corpus callosum, anterior commissure, and hippocampal commissure) is detailed in Chapter 37 as a prelude to our consideration of callosal anomalies.

We then touch lightly on the complex choreography required for proper development of the midbrain and hindbrain structures (pons, cerebellum, and medulla). We include a brief discussion of how the midbrain and cerebellum develop. The final section of this chapter suggests an approach to analyzing brain malformations.

Cerebral Hemisphere Formation

The major embryologic events in brain development begin with neurulation, neuronal proliferation, and neuronal migration. The processes of operculization, gyral and sulcal development, and the earliest steps in myelination all take place later, between gestational weeks 11 and birth.

Neurulation

Neural Tube and Brain Vesicles

The earliest step in brain development occurs during the third fetal week when the three layers of the trilaminar germ disc emerge. The **neural plate**

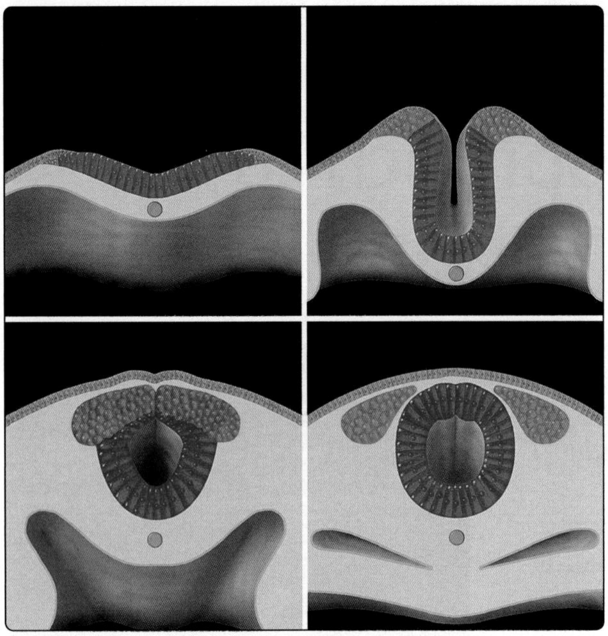

(35-1) Graphic shows the formation and closure of the neural tube. The neural plate (red) forms, folds, and fuses in the midline. The neural and cutaneous ectoderm then separate. Notochord (green) and neural crest (blue) are shown.

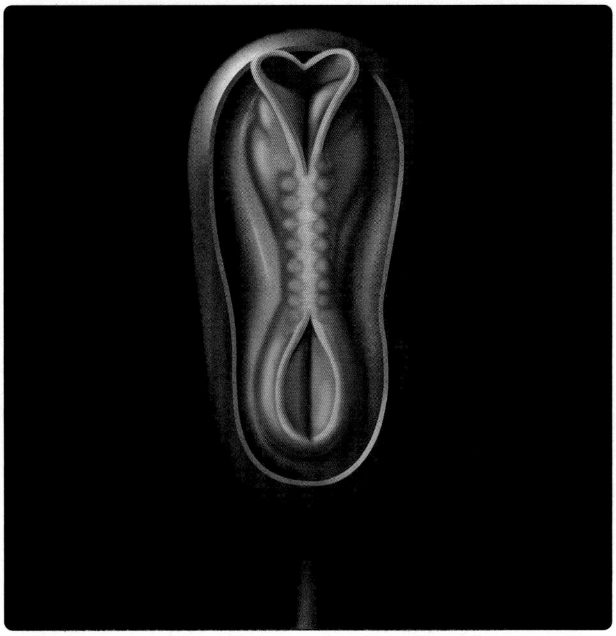

(35-2) The neural tube closes in a bidirectional zipper-like manner, starting in the middle and proceeding toward both ends.

develops at the cranial end of the embryo as a thickening of ectoderm on either side of the midline.

During the fourth fetal week, the neural plate indents and thickens laterally, forming the **neural folds**. The neural folds bend upward, meet in the midline, and then fuse to form the **neural tube**. The primitive **notochord** lies ventral to the neural tube, and the **neural crest** cells are extruded and migrate laterally. The neural tube forms the brain and spinal cord, whereas the neural crest gives rise to peripheral nerves, roots, and ganglia of the autonomic nervous system **(35-1)**.

As the neural tube closes, the neuroectoderm (which will form the CNS) separates from the cutaneous ectoderm in a process known as disjunction. Upon completion of disjunction, the cutaneous ectoderm fuses in the midline, dorsal to the closed neural tube.

Neural tube closure probably begins at two or three levels in the middle of the embryo **(35-2)**. Closure proceeds bidirectionally in a zipper-like fashion along the length of embryo. The cephalic and caudal ends of the neural tube (the so-called anterior and posterior neuropores) do not fuse until the twenty-fifth and twenty-seventh gestational days, respectively.

Three primary brain vesicles—the **prosencephalon** (forebrain), **mesencephalon** (midbrain), and **rhombencephalon** (hindbrain)—also form during the fourth week. The embryonic brain grows rapidly and begins to bend, forming several flexures **(35-3)**.

During the fifth week, the forebrain further divides into two vesicles, forming the **telencephalon** and the **diencephalon**. The hindbrain divides into the **metencephalon** and **myelencephalon**. Together with the mesencephalon, the brain now has five definitive or "secondary" vesicles **(35-4)**.

Neurulation Errors

Errors in neurulation result in a spectrum of congenital anomalies. The most severe is **anencephaly**—essentially complete absence of the cerebral hemispheres—which is caused by failure of the anterior neuropore to close (see Chapter 38). Various types of **cephaloceles** also result from abnormalities of neurulation.

Incomplete closure of the posterior neuropore results in **spina bifida**. If the neuroectoderm fails to separate completely from the cutaneous ectoderm, **myelomeningocele** results. Abnormal neurulation of the hindbrain leads to a **Chiari 2 malformation** (see Chapter 36).

Neuronal Proliferation

Embryonic Stem Cells

*Pluri*potent embryonic stem cells are derived from the inner cell mass of the 4- to 5-day blastocyst. These cells are able to proliferate and differentiate into all three germ layers (ectoderm, mesoderm, endoderm). MicroRNAs seem to play an important role as genetic regulators of stem cell development, differentiation, growth, and neurogenesis.

Histogenesis of Neurons and Glia

As the cerebral vesicles develop and expand, layers of stem cells arise around the primitive ventricular ependyma, forming the germinal matrix. These neural stem cells (NSCs) are *multi*potent cells that generate the main CNS phenotypes, i.e.,

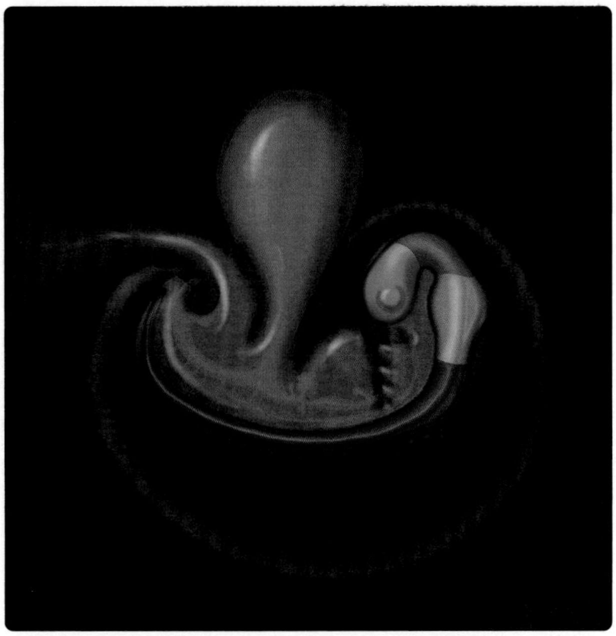

(35-3) Development of primary vesicles is depicted. The prosencephalon (green) gives rise to the forebrain, the mesencephalon (purple) to the midbrain, and the rhombencephalon (light blue) to the hindbrain.

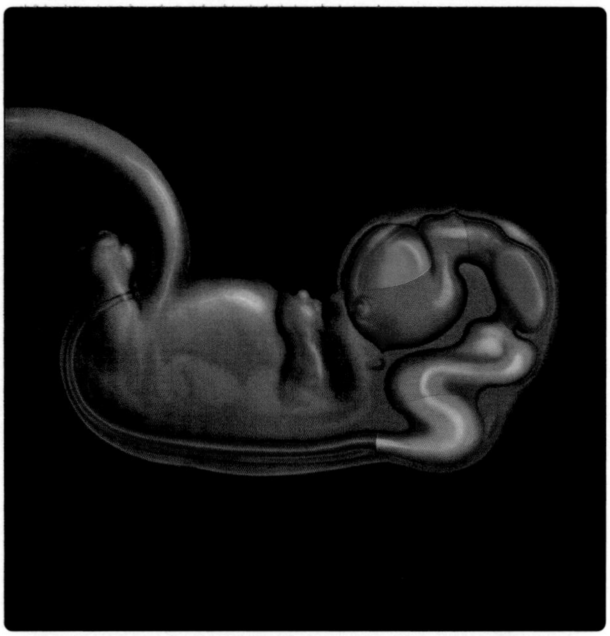

(35-4) The brain develops flexures as prosencephalon gives rise to telencephalon (green) and diencephalon (red). Mesencephalon (purple) elongates while rhombencephalon gives rise to metencephalon (yellow) and myelencephalon (light blue).

neurons, astrocytes, and oligodendrocytes. NSCs are found primarily in the germinal zones (see Chapter 16).

*Pluri*potent NSCs in the specialized subventricular zone of the germinal matrix give rise to neuroblasts ("primitive" or "young" **neurons**) that migrate through the developing telencephalon to form the cortical mantle zone, the precursor of the definitive cortex. Axons from the migrating neurons form an intermediate zone between the germinal matrix and cortical mantle that will eventually become the cerebral white matter.

Some NSCs become specialized **radial glial cells** (RGCs) that will eventually span the entire hemisphere from the ventricular ependyma to the pia. RGCs are also stem cells and can give rise to both neurons and glia. Elongated cell bodies of the RGCs serve as a "rope ladder" that guides migrating neurons from the germinal matrix to the cortex.

Astrocytes arise from two sources: glial progenitor cells in the ventricular zone and RGCs in the intermediate zone. **Oligodendrocytes** arise from oligodendrocyte precursor cells in the ventricular and subventricular zones. Before differentiating into myelinating oligodendrocytes, these precursor cells proliferate, migrate, and then spread throughout the CNS.

Errors in Histogenesis

Errors in histogenesis and differentiation result in a number of embryonal neoplasms, including medulloblastoma and primitive neuroectodermal tumors. Problems with NSC proliferation and differentiation also contribute to malformations of cortical development (see below).

Neuronal Migration

As a result of steadily improving imaging techniques, malformations of cerebral cortical development (MCDs) are now being identified with greater frequency. Understanding how neurons are formed, migrate, organize, and then connect is essential to recognizing and understanding MCDs.

Genesis of Cortical Neurons

Neurogenesis occurs in a predictable manner with sequential generation of specific neural subtypes from designated areas in the germinal matrix. For example, glutamatergic cerebral cortical neurons arise in dorsal ventricular zones, whereas GABAergic neurons destined for the striatum originate in the more ventral zones.

Once the "young" neurons have been generated in the germinal matrix and dorsal ventricular zones, they must leave their "home" to reach their final destination (the cortex). The definitive cerebral cortex develops through a highly ordered process of neuronal proliferation, migration, and differentiation. The neocortex of the cerebral hemispheres has six cell layers, each with its own distinctive pattern of organization and connections.

Neuronal Migration

Migration of newly proliferated neurons occurs along scaffolding provided by the RGCs. Neurons travel from the germinal zone to the cortical mantle in a generally "inside-out" sequence. Cells initially form the deepest layer of the cortex with each successive migration ascending farther outward and progressively forming more superficial layers. Each migrating

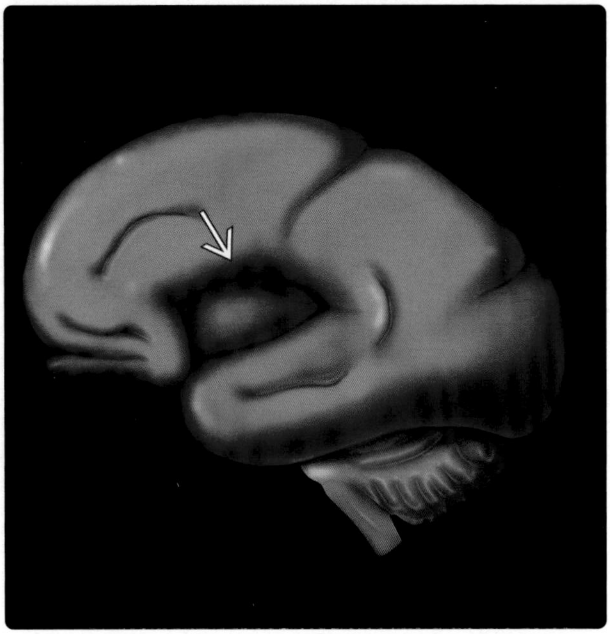

***(35-5)** Embryonic brain at 22 weeks is mostly agyric with shallow lateral cerebral (sylvian) fissures ➡. Prosencephalon (green), metencephalon (yellow), myelencephalon (light blue) are shown. Mesencephalic and midbrain structures are not visible.*

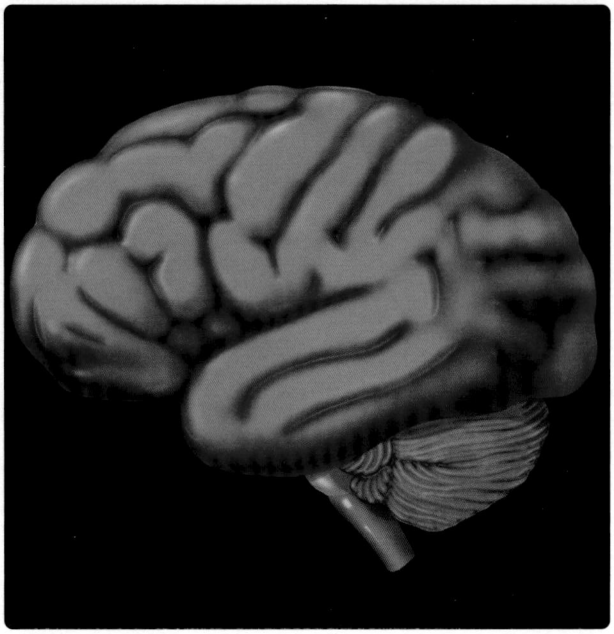

***(35-6)** With advancing gestational age, multiple secondary and tertiary gyri develop, and the number and complexity of the cerebellar folia increase.*

group passes through layers already laid down by the earlier-arriving cells.

Peak neuronal migration occurs between 11-15 fetal weeks although migration continues up to 35 weeks.

Errors in Neuronal Migration and Cortical Organization

The primary result of errors at these stages are **malformations of cortical development**. Problems with NSC proliferation or differentiation, migration, and cortical organization can all result in developmental anomalies of the neocortex. Examples include **microcephaly, megalencephaly, heterotopias, cortical dysplasias**, and **lissencephaly**.

Operculization, Sulcation, and Gyration

Lobulation and Operculization

The cerebral hemispheres first appear as outpouchings of the embryonic telencephalon. The hemispheres are initially almost featureless; the cortex is thin and smooth. The fetal cerebral vasculature covers the brain surface in a basket-like network of thin-walled, undifferentiated vessels.

The cerebral hemispheres expand, first covering the diencephalon and then the midbrain and hindbrain. The roofs of the hemispheres grow more rapidly than the floors. As the hemispheres elongate and rotate, they assume a "C" shape with the caudal ends turning ventrally to form the temporal lobes.

Sulcation and Gyration

Sulcation and gyration—the **progressive folding** of the telencephalon into a complex pattern of lobes and gyri—occurs relatively late in embryonic development. Shallow triangular surface indentations along the sides of the hemisphere—the beginnings of the lateral cerebral (sylvian) fissures—first appear between the fourth and fifth fetal months **(35-5)**.

As the forebrain enlarges, the emerging frontal, parietal, and temporal lobes begin to overhang the lateral fissures, forming the opercula. As the opercula develop and the lateral indentations deepen, cortex that was once on the brain surface becomes completely covered **(35-6)**. This tissue—now buried in the depths of the lateral cerebral (sylvian) fissures—forms the insula ("island of Reil"). The sylvian fissures gradually lose their "open" fetal configuration and assume their narrow slit-like adult configuration.

The definitive middle cerebral arteries follow the indented surfaces of the insulae, first dipping into and then out of the sylvian fissures to ramify over the lateral surfaces of the frontal, parietal, and temporal lobes.

After the sylvian fissures form **(35-7)**, the next groups of surface indentations to appear are the calcarine and parietooccipital sulci **(35-8)**, followed by the central sulci **(35-9)**. Gyral development occurs most rapidly around the sensorimotor and visual pathways.

Anomalies in Sulcation and Gyration

Developmental errors in operculization, sulcation, and gyration are relatively uncommon. **Microcephaly** with

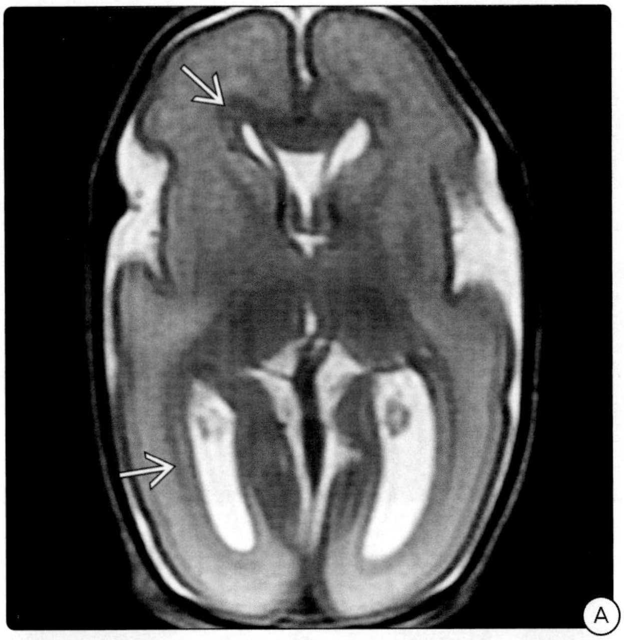

(35-7A) *Axial T2WI shows a 26-week, 5-day premature infant. The lateral cerebral (sylvian) fissures are just beginning to form. The hypointensity around the ventricles ➡ is mostly in the germinal matrix.*

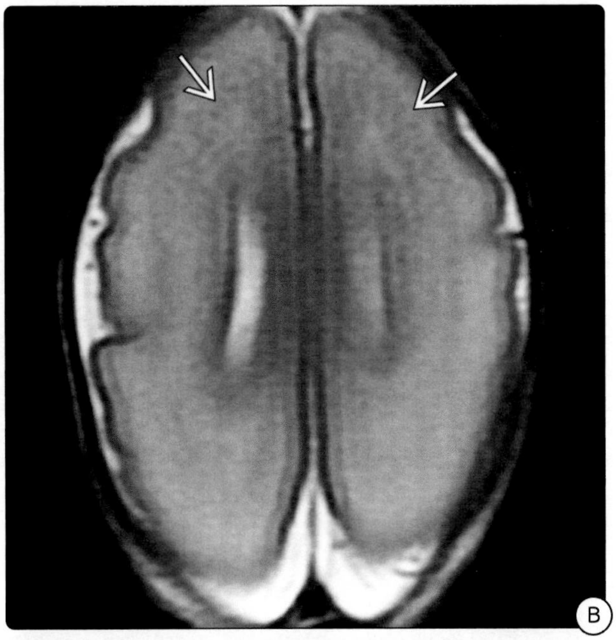

(35-7B) *Image through the corona radiata shows that the brain is almost completely smooth with only a few shallow sulci. Waves of hypointense migrating neurons ➡ give the WM a layered and "smudgy" appearance.*

simplified gyral pattern and **microlissencephaly** are representative anomalies that have too few gyri and abnormally shallow sulci.

Myelination

Myelination occurs in an orderly, predictable manner and can be detected as early as 20 fetal weeks. Normal brain myelination patterns as well as abnormalities in myelin formation and maintenance are discussed in greater detail in Chapter 31. In general, myelination proceeds from **inferior to superior**, from **back to front**, and from **central to peripheral**.

Midbrain and Hindbrain Development

We now summarize the major embryologic events involved in forming the midbrain and hindbrain. A description of the consequences of errors in their development follows.

Major Embryologic Events

The mesencephalon gives rise to the brainstem, and the rhombencephalon elaborates into the medulla, pons, and cerebellum. Each is "patterned" along both the rostral-caudal and dorsal-ventral axes. The mesencephalon is divided into ventral (tegmentum) and dorsal (tectum) regions. Likewise, the metencephalon is divided into ventral (pons) and dorsal (cerebellum) regions.

The pons is formed by a proliferation of cells and fiber tracts along the ventral metencephalon. The alar plates of the rhombencephalon ("rhombencephalic lips") thicken to form cerebellar plates, which in turn proliferate and eventually form the two cerebellar hemispheres and midline vermis. Embryologically, the cerebellum is an extension of the midline and thus part of the dorsal pons.

The rhombencephalic lips fuse, forming the cerebellar commissures in the roof of the fourth ventricle. Each hemisphere subsequently fuses and fissures in a cranial-to-caudal direction.

Formation of the fourth ventricle is a complex process. A ridge of developing choroid plexus divides the emerging fourth ventricle into anterior and posterior membranous areas. Normally, the anterior membrane is incorporated into the developing choroid plexus, whereas the posterior membranous area persists and eventually cavitates, forming the midline foramen of Magendie. Precisely how and when the lateral foramina open is unknown.

Midbrain-Hindbrain Anomalies

A number of different classifications of midbrain and hindbrain malformations have been proposed. Barkovich et al. use an approach that categorizes lesions according to developmental and genetic considerations. Such a system makes consummate sense and certainly aids understanding the pathogenesis of these fascinating anomalies. However, the more traditional morphologic-based approach in which malformations are grouped according to imaging findings is the simplest for radiologists to follow. The interested reader is referred to the publications cited at the end of Chapter 36.

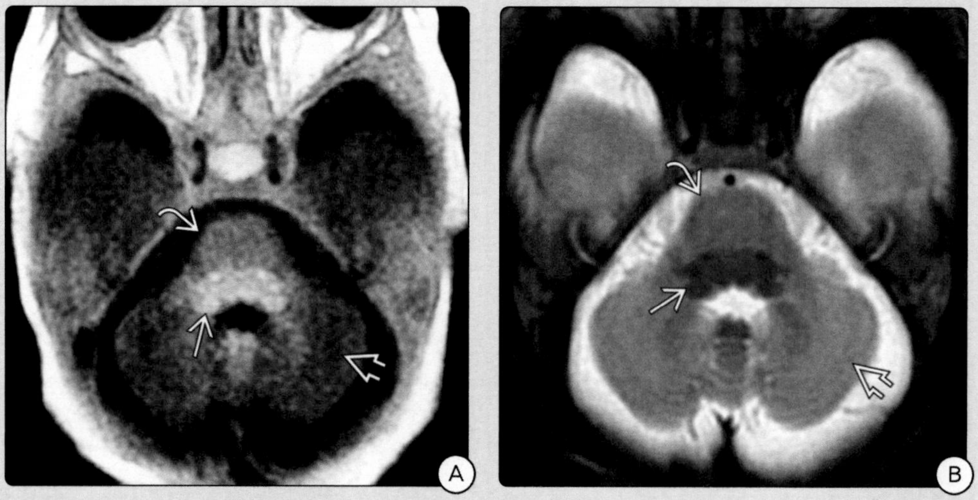

***(35-8A)** Axial T2WI in a normal 30-week premature infant shows hyperintensity (myelination) in the dorsal brainstem →. The ventral brainstem → and cerebellar WM → are hypointense and unmyelinated. **(35-8B)** T2WI in the same patient shows the dorsal brainstem → is myelinated and appears hypointense compared with the hyperintense (unmyelinated) ventral pons → and cerebellar WM →.*

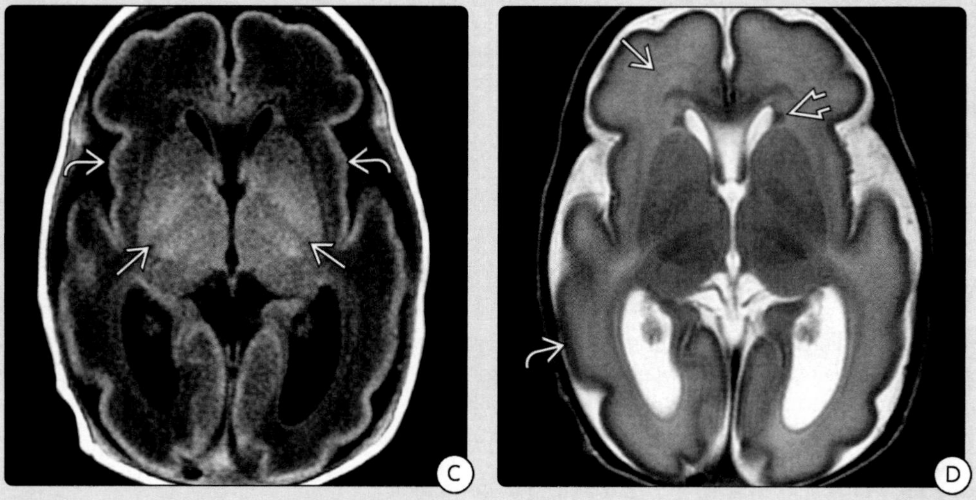

***(35-8C)** T1WI shows that the posterior limbs of the internal capsules → are unmyelinated. Cerebral WM is completely unmyelinated and shows relative lack of gyration and sulci. Note shallow, open-appearing lateral cerebral (sylvian) fissures →. **(35-8D)** T2WI shows layers of hypointensity → that represent migrating neurons and germinal matrix residua →. Thin cortex → and shallow, incompletely formed sulci are normal for such a premature infant.*

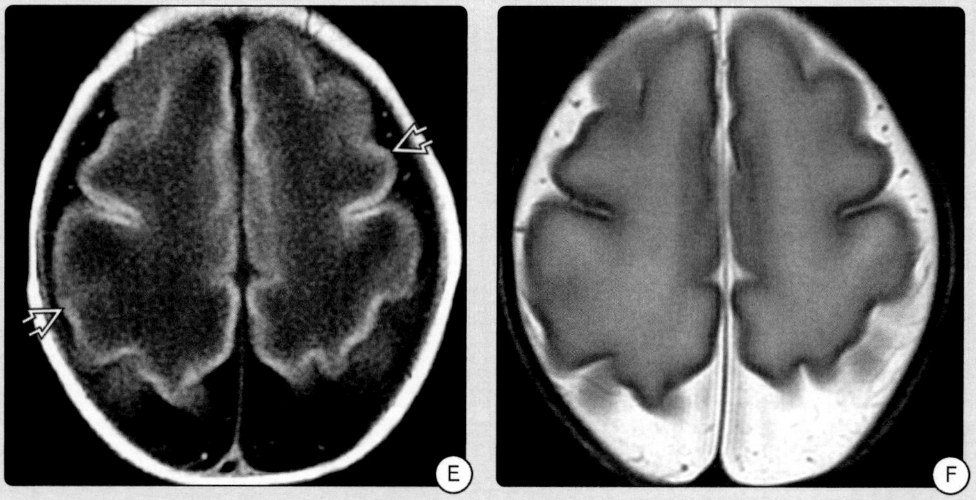

***(35-8E)** T1WI through the corona radiata shows that the WM is hypointense and completely unmyelinated. The sulci are primitive appearing and very shallow, related to immaturity. The cortical GM is thin →. **(35-8F)** T2WI shows the WM is hyperintense compared with hypointensity of the thin but normal cerebral cortex. This early in development, the brain looks like a "water bag" of unmyelinated WM covered by a thin, incomplete shell of GM.*

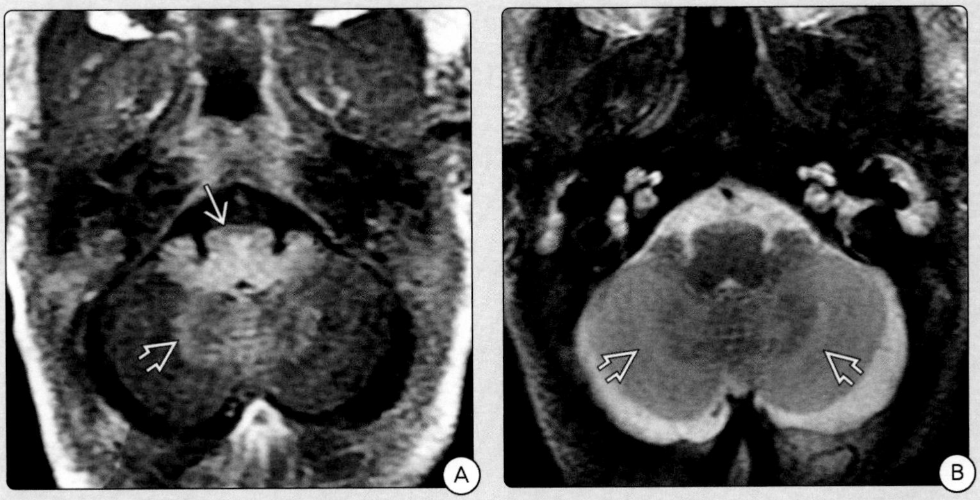

(35-9A) Axial T1WI shows a normal 33-week, 3-day gestation premature infant. The medulla → has myelinated and increased in signal intensity, as have the flocculi and dentate nuclei ⇨. (35-9B) Axial T2WI shows that the medulla, flocculi, and dentate nuclei are hypointense, but the cerebellar hemisphere WM ⇨ remains unmyelinated and hyperintense.

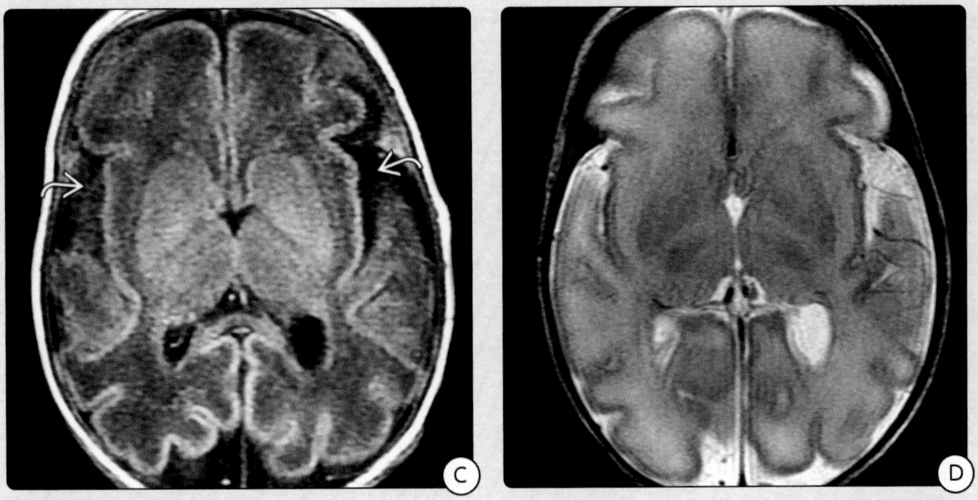

(35-9C) As the opercula continue developing, the lateral cerebral (sylvian) fissures ↷ appear progressively less prominent. (35-9D) T2WI shows that the WM of the cerebral hemispheres remains unmyelinated and hyperintense.

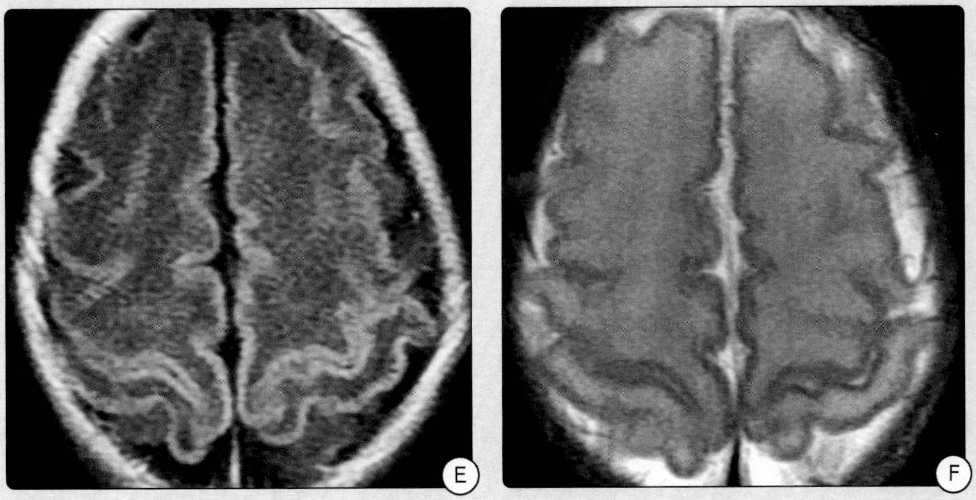

(35-9E) More surface sulci and gyri are now apparent, especially in the parietal and occipital lobes. The cortex appears thicker. Compare to scans of the 30-week premature infant on Figure 35-8. The increased sulcation and gyration of both hemispheres are quite striking. (35-9F) At 33 weeks, the WM of the corona radiate is completely unmyelinated.

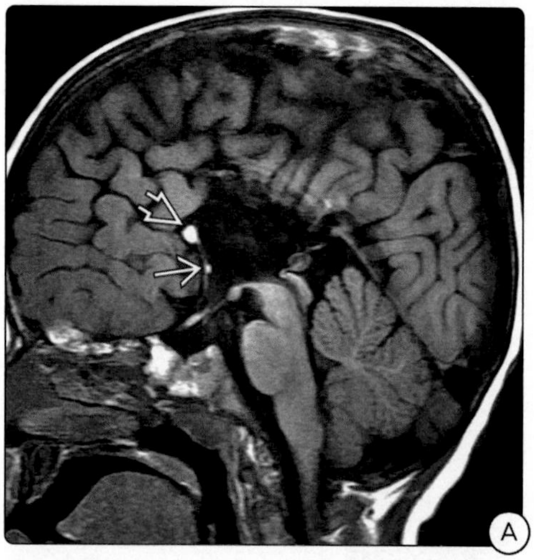

(35-10A) Sagittal midline T1WI shows classic callosal agenesis. The anterior commissure is present, as is a tiny remnant of the genu .

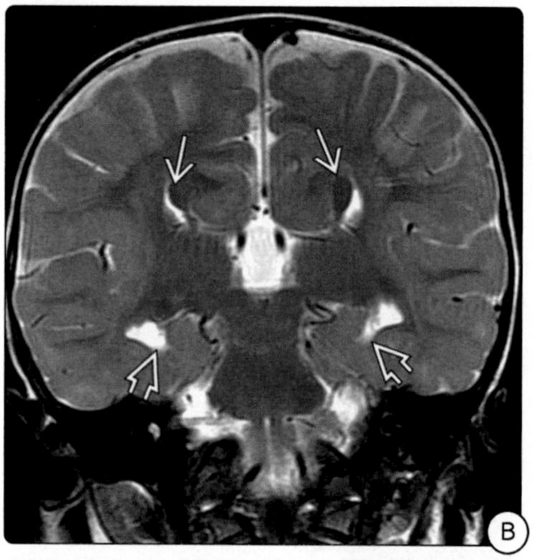

(35-10B) Coronal T2WI shows Probst bundles indenting the lateral ventricles. Note vertically oriented hippocampi .

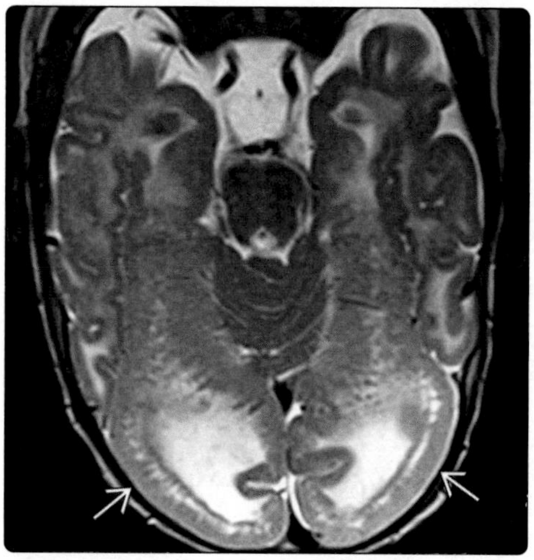

(35-11) Axial T2WI shows "cobblestone" lissencephaly in both occipital poles . (Courtesy M. Warmuth-Metz, MD.)

Imaging Approach to Brain Malformations

Technical Considerations

CT

Clinicians sometimes order NECT scans as an initial screening procedure in a patient with seizures or suspected brain malformation. Although parenchymal calcifications, ventricular size/configuration, and major abnormalities can be identified, subtle abnormalities such as cortical dysplasia are difficult to detect and easy to overlook.

Bone CT is helpful in depicting midline facial defects, synostoses, and anomalies of endochondral bone.

MR

MR is the procedure of choice. The two most important factors are gray-white matter differentiation and high spatial resolution. Many pediatric neuroradiologists recommend a sagittal T1 or T1 FLAIR sequence, volumetric T1 sequences (e.g., MP-RAGE), and sagittal and coronal heavily T2-weighted sequences with very long TR/TEs. 3D imaging acquisitions allow isotropic orthogonal reformations.

A T2* sequence (GRE, SWI) can be a helpful addition if abnormal mineralization or vascular anomaly is suspected. DTI tractography is valuable when commissural anomalies are identified on initial sequences.

Contrast-enhanced T1 and FLAIR sequences are generally optional, as they add little useful information in most congenital malformations. However, they can be very helpful in delineating associated vascular anomalies. DWI and MRS are useful in evaluating mass lesions and inborn errors of metabolism.

Image Analysis

The following approach to analyzing imaging studies is modified and adapted from A. James Barkovich's guidelines on imaging evaluation of the pediatric brain (see reference cited in Chapter 36).

Sagittal Images

Begin with the midline section, and examine the craniofacial proportion. At birth, the ratio of calvaria to face should be 5:1 or 6:1. At 2 years, it should be 2.5:1. In adults and children over the age of 10 years, it should be approximately 1.5:1. Assess myelination of midline structures such as the corpus callosum and brainstem.

The most common of all brain malformations are anomalies of the cerebral commissures (especially the corpus callosum), which can be readily identified on sagittal T1 scans **(35-10A)**. Commissural anomalies are also the most common malformation associated with other anomalies and syndromes, so, if you see one, keep looking! Look for abnormalities of the pituitary gland and hypothalamus. Evaluate the size and shape of the third ventricle, especially its anterior recesses.

Look for other lesions such as lipomas and cysts. These are often midline or paramidline and can be readily identified. The midline sagittal scan also permits a very nice evaluation of the posterior fossa structures. Does the fourth ventricle appear normal? Can you find its dorsally pointing fastigium?

Evaluate the position of the tonsils and the craniovertebral junction for anomalies.

If the lateral and third ventricles are large and the fourth ventricle appears normal, look for a funnel-shaped aqueduct indicating aqueductal stenosis. If you see aqueductal stenosis, look at the quadrigeminal plate carefully to see whether the cause might be a low-grade tectal glioma.

Sagittal images are also especially useful in evaluating the cerebral cortex. Is the cortex too thick? Too thin? Irregular? "Lumpy-bumpy"? Anomalies of cortical development such as pachygyria and cortical dysplasia associated with brain clefting ("schizencephaly") are often most easily identified on sagittal images. Finally, note position and size of the vein of Galen, straight sinus, and torcular Herophili.

Coronal Images

Cortical dysplasias are often bilateral and most frequently cluster around the sylvian fissure. Coronal scans make side-to-side comparison relatively easy. Follow the interhemispheric fissure (IHF) all the way from front to back. If the hemispheres are in contiguity across the midline, holoprosencephaly is present. If the IHF appears irregular and the gyri "interdigitate" across the midline, the patient almost certainly has a Chiari 2 malformation.

Evaluate the size, shape, and position of the ventricles. If the third ventricle appears "high riding" and the frontal horns of the lateral ventricles look like a "Viking helmet," corpus callosum dysgenesis is present **(35-10B)**.

If the frontal horns appear squared-off or box-like, look carefully for an absent cavum septi pellucidi. Absent cavum septi pellucidi is seen in septooptic dysplasia (SOD) and often occurs with callosal dysplasia or schizencephaly. If absent septi pellucidi is noted, look for fusion of the anterior columns of the fornix

Carefully evaluate the temporal horns and hippocampi to make sure that they are normally folded and oriented horizontally (not vertically, as often occurs with holoprosencephaly, lissencephaly, callosal anomalies, and malformations of cortical development).

Axial Images

The combination of a true T1WI together with a long TR/TE T2WI is necessary in evaluating all cases of delayed development to assess myelin maturation. The thickness and configuration of the cortical mantle are well seen **(35-11)**. The size, shape, and configuration of the ventricles is easily evaluated on these sequences.

After 6-8 months of age, FLAIR sequences are especially useful in evaluating abnormalities such as focal or Taylor cortical dysplasia and the flame-shaped subcortical WM hyperintensities seen in tuberous sclerosis complex **(35-12)**.

Don't forget the posterior fossa! The fourth ventricle in axial plane is normally shaped like a kidney bean on its side. If the vermis is absent and the cerebellar hemispheres appear continuous from side to side, rhombencephalosynapsis is present **(35-13)**. If the fourth ventricle and superior cerebellar peduncles resemble a molar tooth, then a molar tooth malformation is present **(35-14)**.

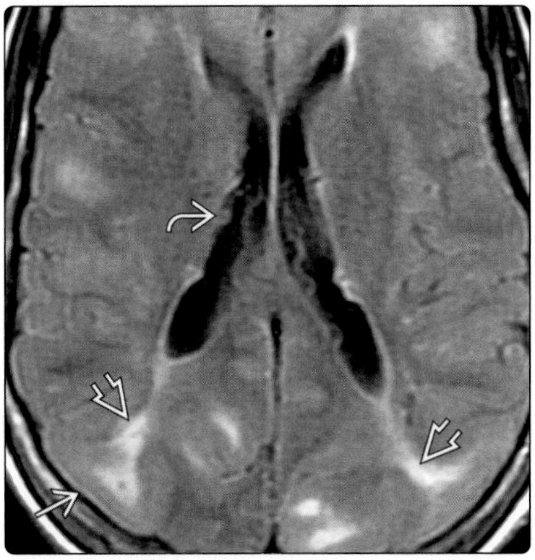

(35-12) FLAIR shows subependymal nodules ➡ and cortical tubers ➡ with subcortical hyperintensities ➡ of tuberous sclerosis.

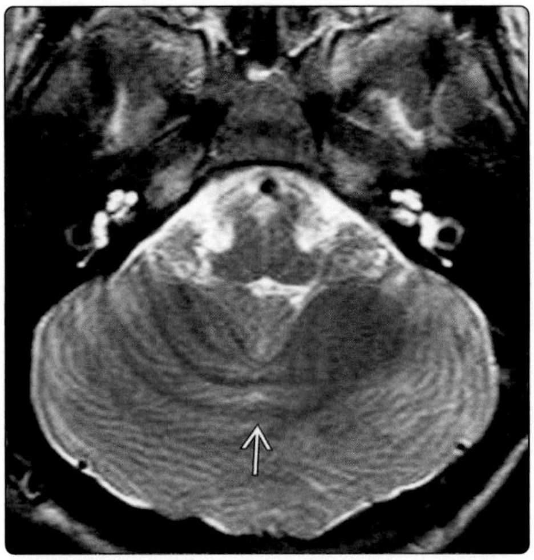

(35-13) T2WI of rhombencephalosynapsis shows continuity of cerebellar hemispheres across the midline ➡. (Courtesy M. Warmuth-Metz, MD.)

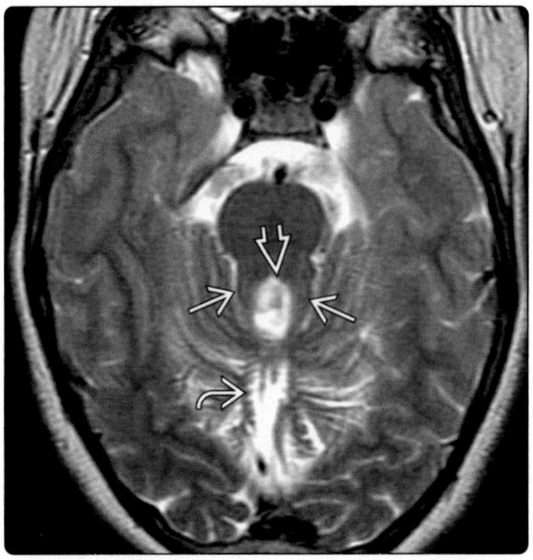

(35-14) T2WI shows "molar tooth" anomaly, elongated upper 4th ventricle ➡, thick superior cerebellar peduncles ➡, and "split" vermis ➡.

Posterior Fossa Malformations

The cerebellum is one of the earliest cerebral structures to develop. Its development is also unusually protracted as cellular proliferation, migration, and maturation extend into the first few postnatal months. It is therefore particularly vulnerable to development mishaps.

Neural structures in the posterior fossa are derived from the embryonic hindbrain (rhombencephalon), whereas the mesencephalon gives rise to midbrain structures. Mesodermal elements give rise to the meninges and bone that surround and protect the neural structures. Developmental errors in either give rise to the spectrum of midbrain and hindbrain malformations that we will discuss in this chapter. A summary of the imaging findings of these malformations is presented at the end of this chapter **(Table 36-1)**.

We begin our discussion of posterior fossa malformations with the anomalies known as Chiari malformations. Moving to the hindbrain, we consider the Dandy-Walker spectrum and a group of miscellaneous malformations.

We review the normal posterior fossa anatomy as the foundation for understanding these lesions. Some structures (e.g., the fourth ventricle, arteries, dural venous sinuses, cranial nerves) have been discussed in detail in previous chapters. Here, we summarize the major anatomic features specifically as they relate to the posterior fossa itself.

Posterior Fossa Anatomy

Gross Anatomy

The posterior fossa (PF) is the largest and deepest of all the cranial fossae. It is a bowl-shaped, relatively protected space that lies below the tentorium. The PF contains the *hindbrain* with the brainstem (pons, medulla) anteriorly, the vermis, and the cerebellar hemispheres posterolaterally.

The *midbrain* lies within the tentorial incisura. The midbrain represents the transition between the cerebral hemispheres above and the pons and cerebellar hemispheres below the tentorium.

PF CSF-containing spaces include part of the cerebral aqueduct, the fourth ventricle, and CSF cisterns that surround the brainstem and cerebellum.

Bone and Dura

The dorsum sellae of the sphenoid body and **clivus** of the basioccipital bone form the anterior wall of the PF. Laterally, the PF is bordered by the petrous temporal bone. The occipital squamae form most of its concave floor, and

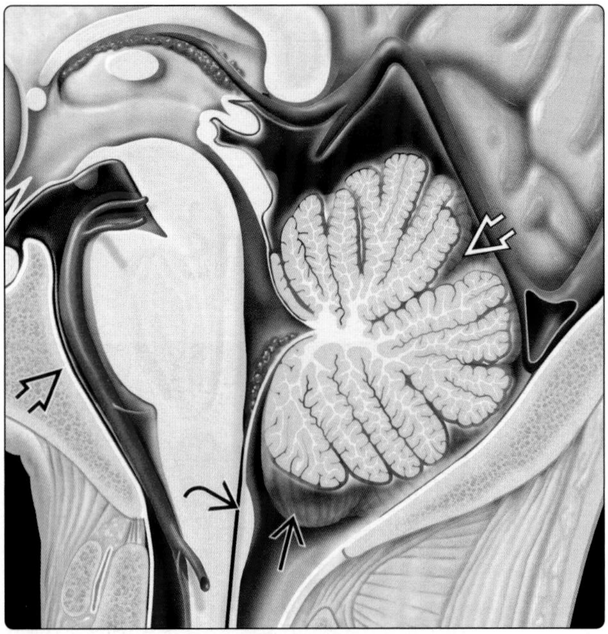

***(36-1)** Graphic shows anterior PF bordered by clivus ⇨. Note rounded tonsil ⇨. Nucleus gracilis ⇨, junction between 4th ventricle obex, and central canal lie above foramen magnum. Primary fissure of vermis ⇨ lies along tentorial surface.*

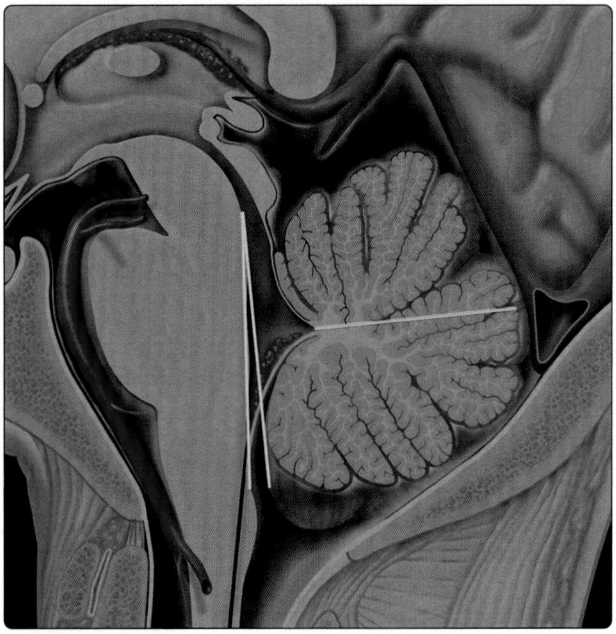

***(36-2)** Graphic shows that normal tegmento-vermian angle (yellow) should be ≤ 18°. The fastigium-declive line (blue) extends from the fastigium of the 4th ventricle to the declive. Approximately 50% of the vermis should lie below this line.*

the tent-shaped tentorium cerebelli covers the PF superiorly. The PF communicates superiorly with the supratentorial compartment through the U-shaped **tentorial incisura** and inferiorly with the cervical subarachnoid space through the ovoid **foramen magnum**.

A layer of dura with a loosely adherent arachnoid membrane lines the bony part of the PF. The cranial dura has two layers, an inner (meningeal) and an outer (endosteal) layer, that are fused together except where they separate to enclose the dural venous sinuses.

The meningeal layer of the dura covers the PF with two prominent crescentic infoldings, the leaves of the **tentorium cerebelli**, that separate the infra- from the supratentorial compartments. A large U-shaped central opening, the **tentorial incisura**, contains the midbrain. Variable amounts of the upper cerebellar hemispheres and vermis project into the tentorial hiatus behind the midbrain.

The convex outer margins of the dura split posteriorly along the occipital squamae to contain the sinus confluence (torcular herophili) and transverse sinuses, attaching laterally to the temporal bones and posteriorly to the occipital bone. The **falx cerebelli** consists of one or more small crescentic folds of dura that project into the cisterna magna and attach superiorly to the undersurface of the tentorium.

The dura divides into two distinct layers as it passes inferiorly through the foramen magnum into the upper cervical canal. The endosteal layer becomes the periosteum of the vertebral canal, and the meningeal layer becomes the dura of the thecal sac. In the spine, the two layers are separated by fat, the epidural venous plexus, and loose connective tissue.

Brainstem

The brainstem has three anatomic divisions: the midbrain, pons, and medulla. The **midbrain** (mesencephalon) lies partly above and partly below the tentorium. It courses through the tentorial incisura, connecting the pons and cerebellum with the basal forebrain structures and cerebral hemispheres.

The bulb-shaped **pons** nestles into the gentle curve of the clivus **(36-1)**. Its ventral aspect contains both transverse pontine fibers and the large descending white matter (WM) tracts that are continuous with the cerebral peduncles superiorly and the medullary pyramids inferiorly. Its dorsal part—the tegmentum—is common to all three brainstem structures (midbrain, pons, medulla) and contains the reticular formation and multiple cranial nerve nuclei.

The **medulla** is the most caudal brainstem segment and represents the transition from the brain to the spinal cord. Its ventral (anterior) segment contains the olives and pyramidal tracts. An important imaging landmark is the prominent "bump" along the dorsal medulla created by the nucleus gracilis. This demarcates the junction between the fourth ventricle (obex) and central canal of the spinal cord. The nucleus gracilis normally lies above the foramen magnum.

Cerebellum

The cerebellum is a bilobed structure located posterior to the brainstem and fourth ventricle. It consists of two hemispheres and the midline vermis.

Each cerebellar hemisphere has three surfaces: superior (tentorial), inferior (suboccipital), and anterior (petrosal). The superior surface abuts the undersurface of the tentorium. The

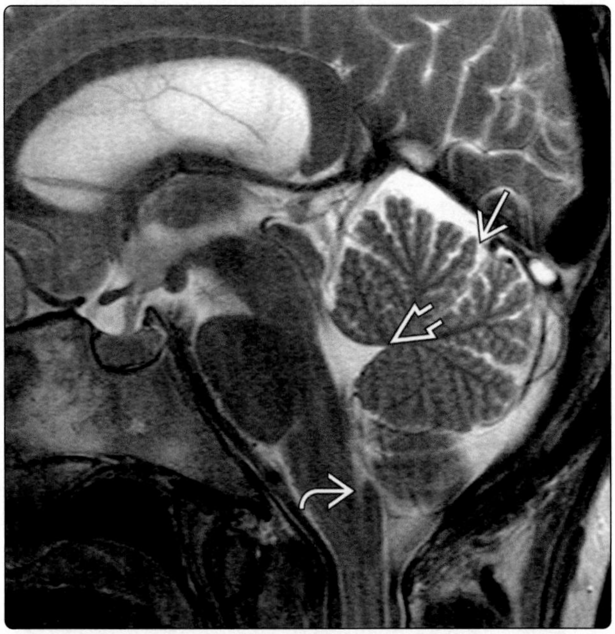

(36-3) Sagittal T2WI shows normal PF imaging landmarks: nucleus gracilis with junction of the 4th ventricle and central canal of the spinal cord, fastigium of the 4th ventricle, and primary fissure of the vermis.

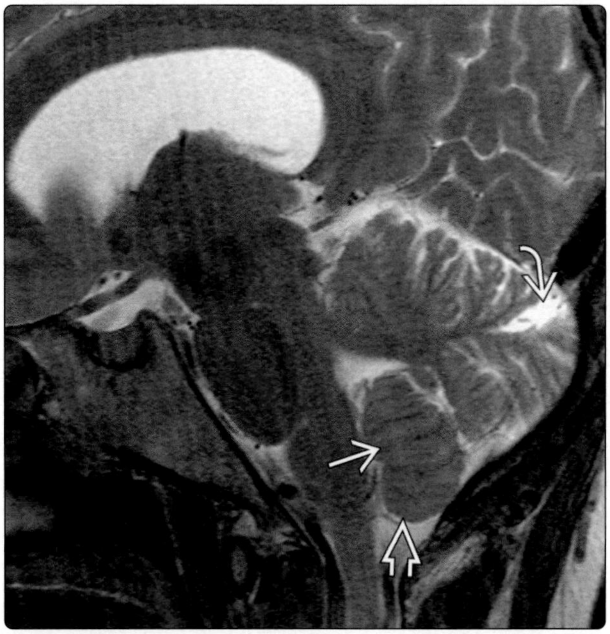

(36-4) Slightly more lateral scan reveals the horizontally oriented folia, rounded bottom of the tonsil, and the horizontal fissure.

inferior surface is mostly bordered by the occipital squamae, and the anterior surface lies along the posterior wall of the petrous temporal bone.

Fissures divide the cerebellum into lobes and lobules. The most prominent is the large **horizontal fissure**. This deep cleft wraps around the cerebellum and separates its superior from the inferior surfaces. The obliquely oriented **primary fissure** divides the cerebellum into anterior and posterior lobes. Smaller fissures subdivide the lobes into lobules.

Prominent superficial landmarks of the cerebellar hemispheres include the cerebellar **tonsils**, which extend inferomedially from the biventral lobules **(36-1)**. A small nubbin of tissue, the **flocculus**, lies below each middle cerebellar peduncle and projects anteriorly into the cerebellopontine angle cistern.

Three paired peduncles attach the cerebellar hemispheres to the brainstem. The **superior cerebellar peduncles** (brachium conjunctivum) connect the cerebellum to the cerebral hemispheres via the midbrain. The superior cerebellar peduncles contain efferents to the red nucleus and thalamus.

The **middle cerebellar peduncles** (brachium pontis) connect the cerebellum to the pons and represent the continuation of the corticopontine tracts. The **inferior cerebellar peduncles** (also known as the restiform bodies) connect the cerebellum to the medulla and contain spinocerebellar tracts and tracts to the vestibular nuclei.

The **vermis** lies between both cerebellar hemispheres, behind the fourth ventricle. Its lobules are (moving clockwise from the fourth ventricle roof) the lingula, central lobule, culmen, declive, folium, tuber, pyramid, uvula, and nodulus. The prominent **primary fissure** continues across the vermis from the cerebellar hemispheres and separates the culmen from the declive. With the exception of the lingula, each vermian lobule is also in direct contiguity with an adjoining lobule of the cerebellar hemisphere.

The cerebellar cortex is a continuous sheet of tissue that is folded in accordion-like fashion to form a series of prominent ridges. The cortex has three main layers. The **molecular layer** is the most superficial and is a relatively neuron-sparse layer. The **Purkinje cell layer** primarily contains Purkinje cells, which are arranged in a single row between the more superficial molecular layer and the deeper granular layer. The **granular layer** is the most complex and most cellular, containing the bodies and axons of granular neurons.

Fourth Ventricle and Cisterns

Anatomy of the fourth ventricle is delineated in more detail in Chapter 34.

The **fourth ventricle** is a complex diamond-shaped space that runs along the dorsal pons and upper medulla. Important anatomic landmarks are the dorsally pointed **fastigium**, the midline **foramen of Magendie** (the outlet from the fourth ventricle into the cisterna magna), and the paired **lateral recesses** that empty into the cerebellopontine angle (CPA) cisterns via the **foramina of Luschka**. Choroid plexus extends from the 4th ventricle through its lateral recesses, protruding into the adjacent CPA cisterns. Bulbous tufts of choroid plexus in the CPA cistern are eponymously named "Bochdalek's flower basket" and are a normal finding on imaging studies.

The **posterior superior recesses** are thin, blind-ending, ear-like outpouchings that curve over the tops of the cerebellar tonsils. The **obex** is the inferior extension of the fourth ventricle and communicates directly with the central canal of the cervical spinal cord.

The major PF cisterns are the prepontine cistern, the cerebellopontine angle cistern, and the variably sized cisterna magna. Part of the cisterna magna (the **vallecula**) extends superiorly between the two cerebellar tonsils and is connected to the fourth ventricle via the foramen of Magendie.

Arteries, Veins, and Dural Sinuses

The arteries of the PF are detailed in Chapter 8; the veins and dural venous sinuses are discussed in Chapter 9.

Cranial Nerves

The cranial nerves—together with the cisterns through which they course and the bony foramina through which they enter or leave the cranial cavity—are discussed in detail in Chapter 23.

Imaging Anatomy

Sagittal Plane

Midline images show the smooth floor of the fourth ventricle extending from the cerebral aqueduct above to the obex below. The junction of the obex and central canal is marked by a dorsal bump, the nucleus gracilis **(36-3)**. The nucleus gracilis normally lies above a line drawn between the tip of the clivus anteriorly and the rim of the foramen magnum posteriorly ("basion-opisthion line").

The sharply pointed fastigium forms a triangle of CSF whose apex points toward the vermis. The primary fissure of the vermis faces the tentorium, dividing the culmen from the declive. Approximately 50% of the vermis should lie below a line from the fastigium to the declive **(36-2)**.

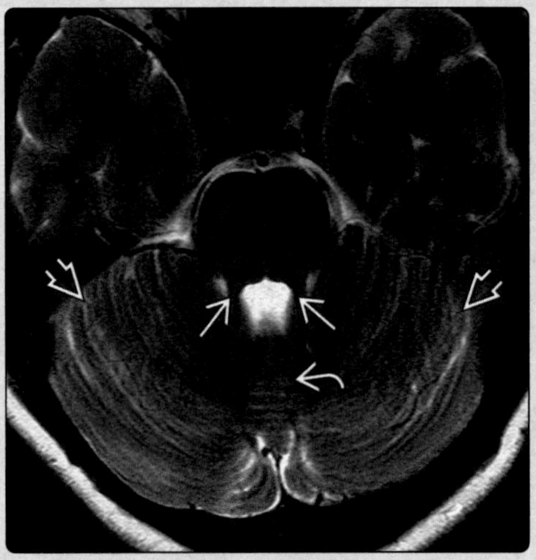

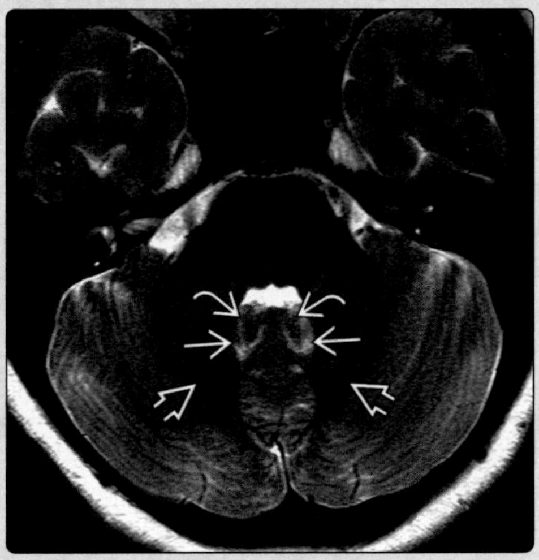

***(36-5)** Axial T2WI shows normal superior cerebellar peduncles, vermis, and horizontal fissures of the cerebellum. **(36-6)** Axial scan through the body of the fourth ventricle shows CSF-filled posterior superior recesses capping the tops of the cerebellar tonsils. Dentate nuclei are mineralized and hypointense.*

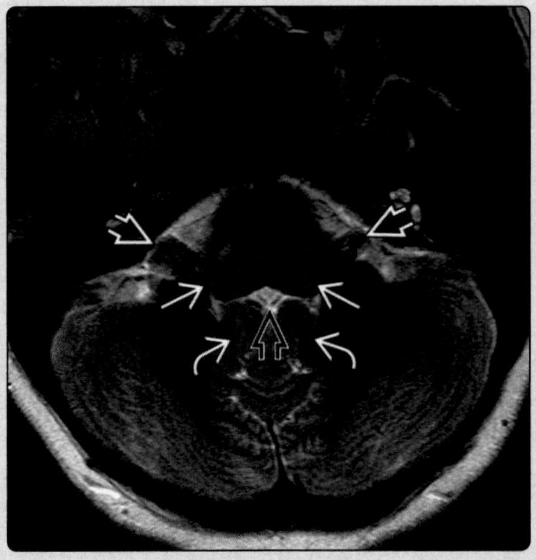

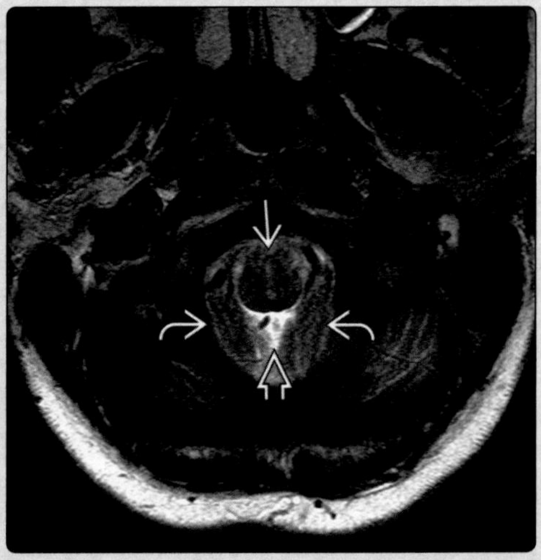

***(36-7)** More inferior scan through the bottom of the fourth ventricle shows the midline foramen of Magendie, lateral recesses, tonsils, and floccular lobes of the cerebellum projecting into cerebellopontine angle cisterns. **(36-8)** T2WI through the foramen magnum shows the medulla, cerebellar tonsils, and vallecula lying between the tonsils at the bottom of the cisterna magna.*

Just slightly lateral to the midline, the cerebellar tonsils can be identified as ovoid structures lying between the vermis and inferior fourth ventricle. Normal tonsils display horizontally oriented folia and a gently rounded bottom **(36-4)**. More lateral sections through the hemispheres show the dentate nuclei, the brachium pontis, and the primary fissure of the cerebellum.

Axial Plane

Images through the upper PF show the vermis and superior surfaces of the cerebellar hemispheres lying behind the pons and midbrain, just inside the tentorial incisura. Slightly farther down, the superior cerebellar peduncles are seen as thin white matter bands lying along either side of the upper fourth ventricle **(36-5)**.

At the level of the middle cerebellar peduncles, the body of the fourth ventricle resembles a kidney bean on its side. The two bumps along its anterior aspect are the facial colliculi, and the midline posterior bump is the nodulus of the vermis. Sometimes, the thin posterior superior recesses can be seen capping the tops of the cerebellar tonsils **(36-6)**. Anterolaterally, a flocculus projects from each hemisphere into the cerebellopontine angle cistern.

Moving inferiorly, the lateral recesses of the fourth ventricle pass anterolaterally under the middle cerebellar peduncles **(36-7)**. Tufts of choroid plexus pass through the lateral recesses and the foramina of Luschka into the inferior cerebellopontine angle cisterns just medial to the flocculi.

The cerebellar tonsils can be identified just above or at the foramen magnum. The vallecula—part of the cisterna magna that receives the midline foramen of Magendie—is the CSF space that lies between the tonsils **(36-8)**. The medulla lies just in front of (and medial to) the cerebellar tonsils. The anterior medulla is marked by paired "bumps" of tissue: the pyramids and the olives.

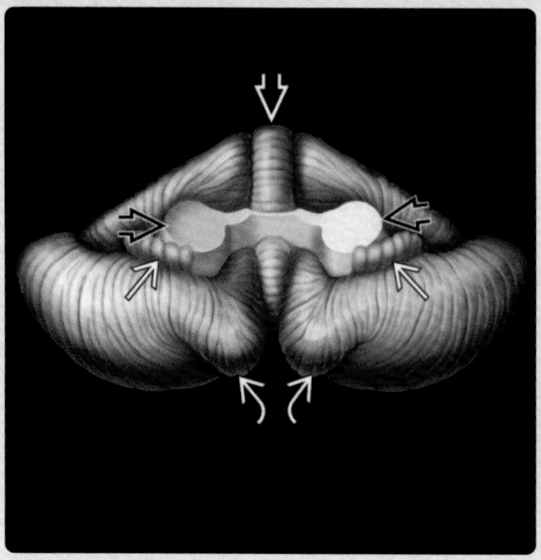
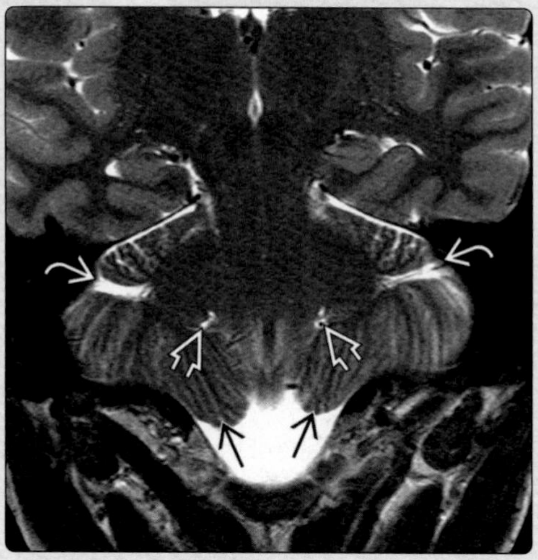

***(36-9)** Coronal graphic shows brachium pontis (middle cerebellar peduncles), vermis, flocculi, and tonsils projecting inferiorly from the biventral lobules. **(36-10)** Coronal T2WI shows tonsils, foramina of Luschka, and horizontal fissures.*

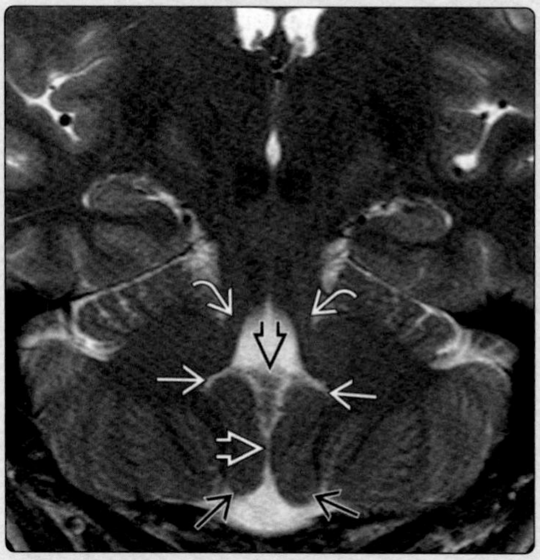
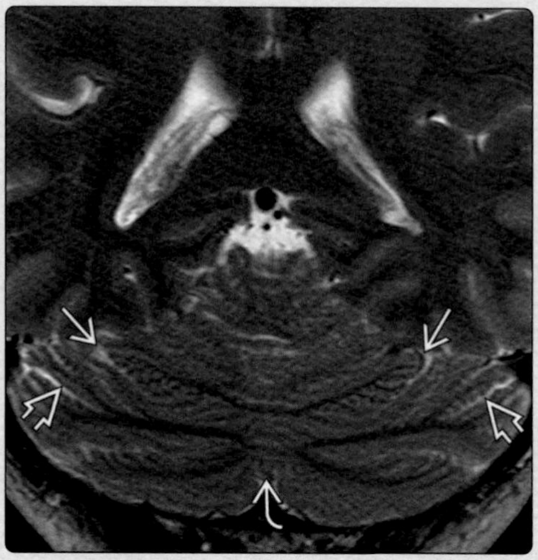

***(36-11)** More posterior coronal image shows foramen of Magendie, vermis, superior cerebellar peduncles, and posterior superior recesses capping tonsils. **(36-12)** More posterior T2WI shows the primary fissures, horizontal fissures, and midline vermis.*

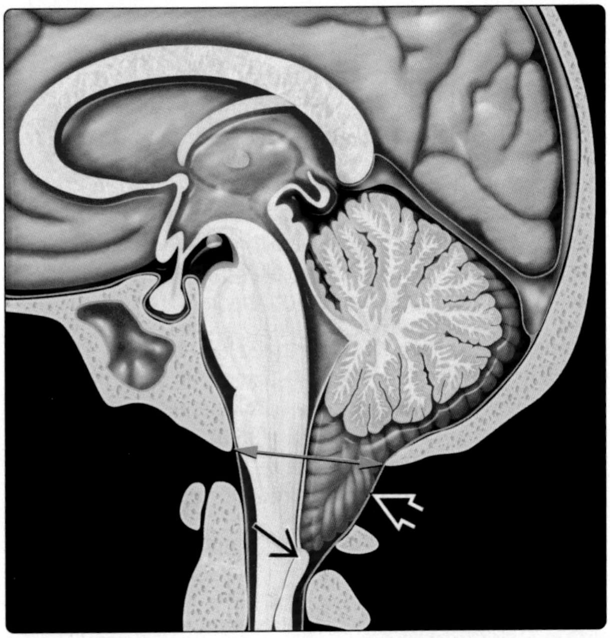

(36-13) Chiari 1 malformation shows the basion-opisthion line shown in green. Note the low-lying, pointed tonsil with vertically oriented folia ➡. The nucleus gracilis ➡ is inferiorly displaced.

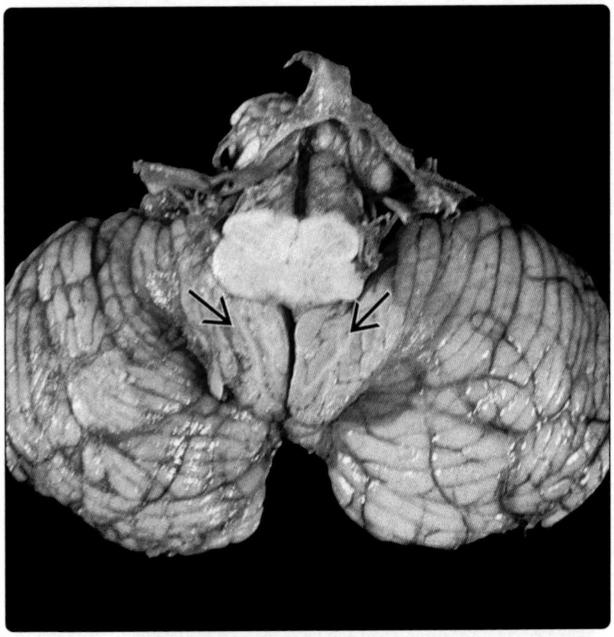

(36-14) Semiaxial view of autopsy case shows Chiari 1 malformation. Note inferiorly displaced tonsils with vertically oriented folia ➡. (Courtesy E. T. Hedley-Whyte, MD.)

Coronal Plane

Images through the anterior "belly" of the pons show the large biventral lobules of the inferior cerebellar hemispheres with the cerebellar tonsils projecting inferomedially **(36-9)** **(36-10)**. The flocculi lie just in front of the horizontal fissure **(36-9)**.

Moving posteriorly, the rhomboid or diamond shape of the fourth ventricle can be appreciated. Thin caps of CSF, the posterior superior recesses, cover the tops of the cerebellar tonsils **(36-11)**. Inferiorly, the fourth ventricle opens into the cisterna magna via the foramen of Magendie. The large middle cerebellar peduncles are seen along the sides of the fourth ventricle. More posteriorly, the vermis can be seen lying between the two hemispheres **(36-12)**.

Chiari Malformations

Introduction to Chiari Malformations

Chiari malformations were first described in the late nineteenth century by the Austrian pathologist Hans Chiari. He described what seemed to be a related group of hindbrain malformations associated with hydrocephalus and divided them into three types: Chiari 1-3.

Chiari 1 and 2 are pathogenetically distinct disorders. **Chiari 1** involves inferior dislocation of the cerebellar tonsils **(36-13)**; **Chiari 2** is always associated with myelodysplasia and involves herniation of the medulla and vermis. **Chiari 3** is classically characterized as herniation of posterior fossa contents through a low occipitocervical bony defect.

"Chiari 4 malformation" was originally used to designate what is now recognized as primary cerebellar agenesis, not a hindbrain herniation. The term has been abandoned.

Some authors have expanded the Chiari spectrum to include variants such as **Chiari 0** (syrinx without frank tonsillar herniation), **Chiari 1.5** (caudal protrusion of brainstem in addition to the tonsils), and **Chiari 5** (Chiari 2 plus occipital or high cervical myelomeningocele). These variants are controversial and are briefly discussed at the end of this section.

Chiari 1

Overview

Type 1 Chiari malformation (CM1) is defined as caudal cerebellar tonsillar ectopia. However, the precise distance of the tonsils below the foramen magnum (FM) required to diagnose CM1 is not agreed upon. Some investigators consider tonsillar ectopia measuring 5 mm or more as sufficient to establish the diagnosis of CM1. However, other investigators insist additional abnormalities such as tonsillar deformity, obliterated retrotonsillar CSF spaces, or altered CSF flow dynamics should also be present.

Abnormalities of the cervical spinal cord are common in CM1. A complex CSF-filled cavity with multiple septations of spongy glial tissue is typical. *Glia*-lined cord cavitations are generally referred to as **syringomyelia**. The term **hydromyelia** refers to an *ependyma*-lined expansion of the central canal. In CM1, extensive areas of ependymal denuding and astrocytic scarring make it difficult to distinguish between hydro- and syringomyelia even on histologic examination. Therefore, these nonneoplastic, septated, paracentral, fluid-containing

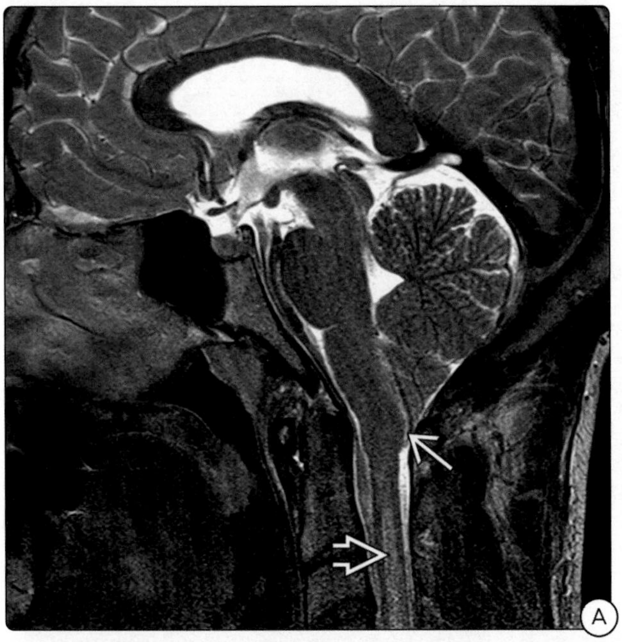

(36-15A) Sagittal T2WI in a 23y man with classic Chiari 1 malformation shows a low-lying, pointed tonsil ➡ and normal-sized posterior fossa. Cord T2 hyperintensity ➡ represents "pre-syrinx" state.

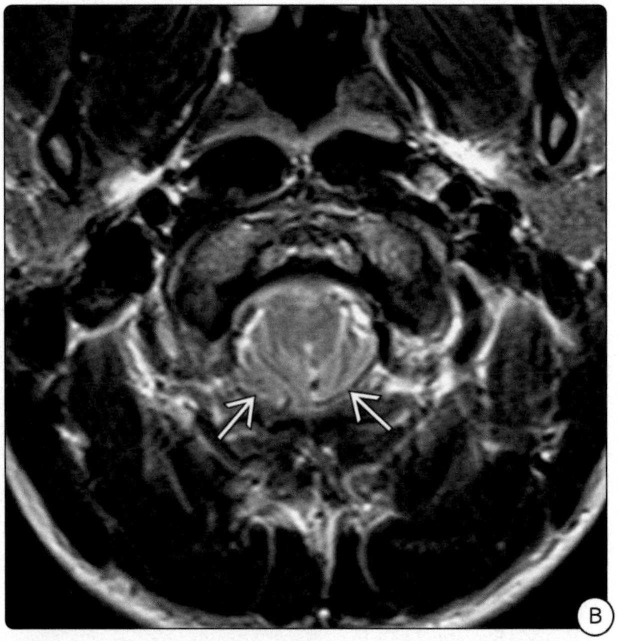

(36-15B) Axial T2WI in the same patient shows "crowded" foramen magnum with obliterated retrotonsillar CSF spaces ➡.

cavitations are often referred to as **hydrosyringomyelia** or simply syrinx.

Etiology

General Concepts. The pathogenesis of CM1 is incompletely understood and remains controversial. Genetic, nongenetic, and epigenetic factors have all been proposed.

Primary paraxial mesodermal insufficiency with underdeveloped occipital somites has also been invoked to explain the development of CM1. Other theories suggest that disorders of neural crest-derived elements could lead to hyper- or hypoossification of the basi-chondro-cranium, resulting in morphometric changes in the posterior fossa.

A combination of altered bony anatomy and abnormal CSF hydrodynamics is the most widely accepted concept.

Abnormal Posterior Fossa. Many—but by no means all—patients with CM1 demonstrate abnormal geometry of the bony posterior fossa (*"normal-sized hindbrain housed in a too-small bony envelope"*). Various combinations of congenitally reduced clival length, shortened basiocciput, and craniovertebral junction (CVJ) fusion anomalies may all result in diminished posterior cranial fossa depth and/or an abnormally small posterior fossa volume.

Altered CSF Dynamics. Syringomyelia is present in 40-80% of individuals with symptomatic CM1. Its etiology is also a controversial subject. Tonsillar impaction and posterior arachnoid adhesions cause increased resistance to CSF flow between the intracranial and spinal subarachnoid spaces. Systolic piston-like descent of the impacted tonsils may create abnormal intraspinal CSF pressure waves, which in turn could result in the development of hydrosyringomyelia in the upper cervical cord.

Altered CSF hydrodynamics with accelerated flow velocity and increased pressure gradients may also cause or contribute to the displacement of brain tissue out of the cranium and into the upper cervical canal.

Genetics. Familial aggregation studies, twin studies, the cosegregation of CM1 with known genetic conditions such as achondroplasia and Klippel-Feil syndrome, and recent genome-wide analyses all provide strong evidence for a genetic component of CM1.

Although the specific genetic causes of CM1 are not yet fully elucidated, chromosomes 9q21 and 15q21 (also the site of the fibrillin-1 gene, the major cause of Marfan syndrome) have been implicated in some studies. Researchers have identified five regions of the X chromosome linked to FG syndrome, which is also associated with increased prevalence of CM1.

Pathology

Grossly, the herniated tonsils in CM1 are inferiorly displaced and grooved by impaction against the opisthion **(36-14)**. They often appear firm and sclerotic. Arachnoid thickening and adhesions around the CVJ are common. Microscopically, degenerative changes with Purkinje and granular cell loss may be present.

Clinical Issues

Epidemiology and Demographics. CM1 is the most common of the Chiari malformations and can be identified in patients of all ages. Its estimated prevalence in the general population is 0.6-1.0%, but recent studies have found a Chiari 1

(36-16A) Sagittal T1WI shows "crowded" foramen magnum and tonsillar ectopia with the "pointed" appearance that is typical of Chiari 1. Note syrinx in the upper cervical cord. (36-16B) Sagittal T2WI shows "pointed" tonsil and obliquely oriented tonsillar folia. Multiple septations in the syrinx cavity are clearly seen. The inferior fourth ventricle is somewhat elongated, and the nucleus gracilis is slightly low-lying.

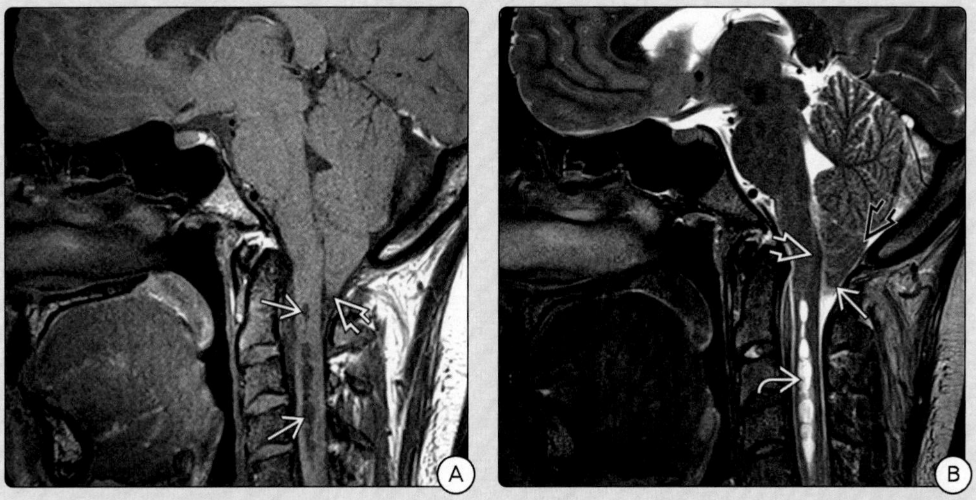

(36-16C) Sagittal T1 C+ FS shows that the syrinx does not enhance. (36-16D) Axial T2WI shows a well-demarcated CSF cavity in the middle of the central cervical spinal cord. It is not possible by imaging to distinguish between ependyma-lined dilatation of the central canal (hydromyelia) and glia-lined paracentral cord cavitations (syringomyelia), so the term hydrosyringomyelia is generally used to designate this CM1-associated finding.

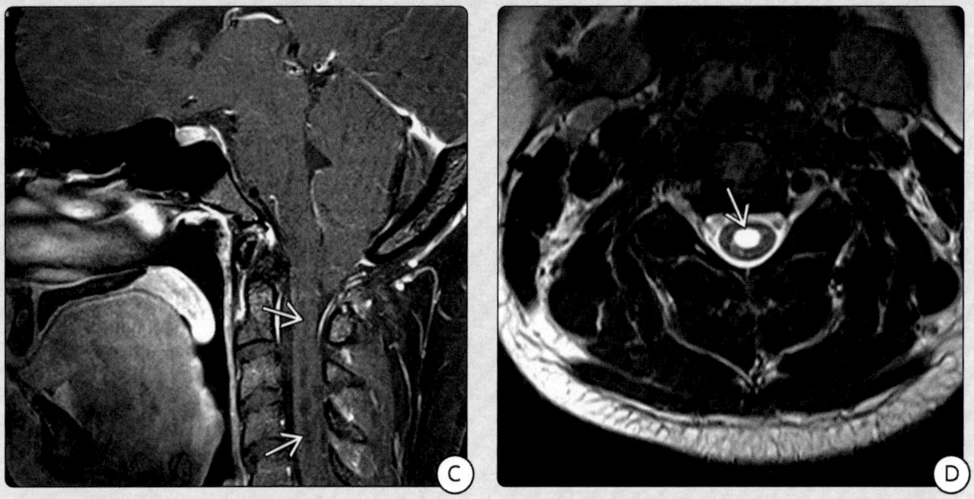

(36-16E) T2WI in the same patient shows tonsils and a compressed and slightly deformed medulla, giving the appearance of the "crowded" foramen magnum typical of CM1. (36-16F) Sagittal phase-contrast CSF flow study in systole (L) and diastole (R) shows normal CSF flow in front of the cervicomedullary junction and no posterior flow in the foramen magnum. Tonsillar "crowding" and adhesions prevent normal CSF circulation.

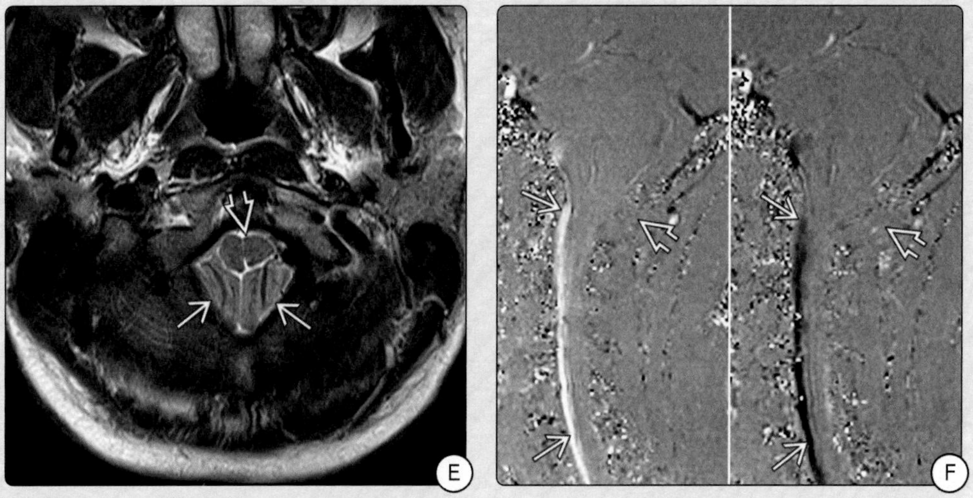

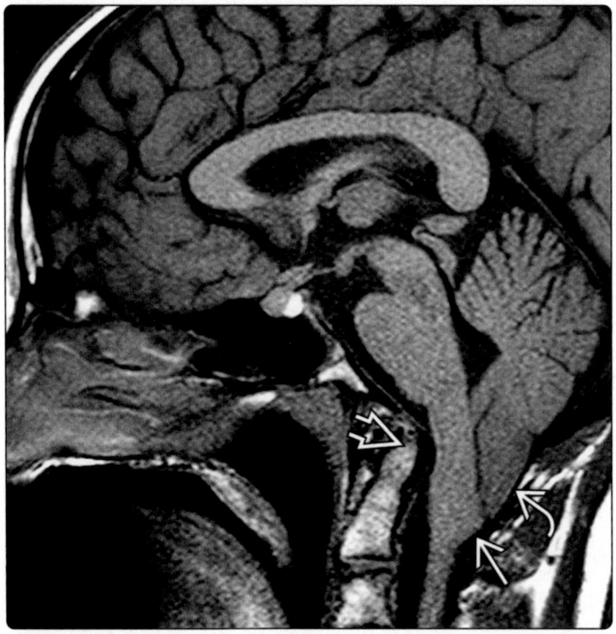

***(36-17)** Sagittal T1WI shows severe Chiari I malformation. The tonsils are pointed inferiorly ➡, lying 15 mm below the crowded foramen magnum. The obex and nucleus gracilis are kinked and displaced inferiorly ➡. The odontoid is retroflexed ➡.*

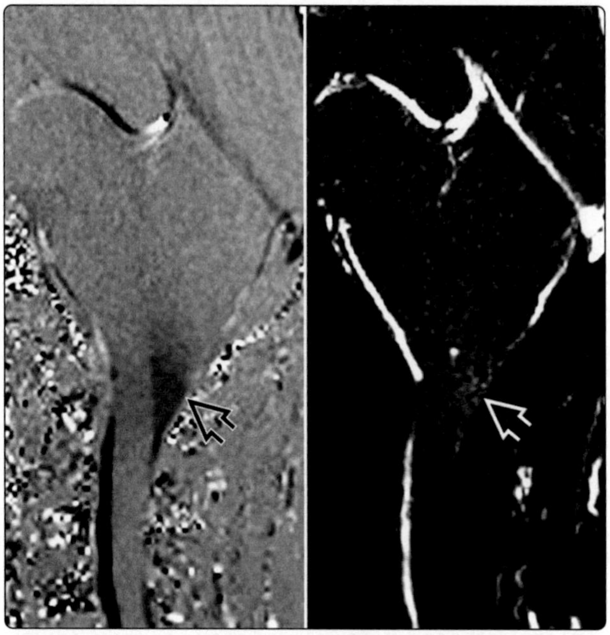

***(36-18)** 2D phase-contrast cine CSF flow study in Chiari I shows change in signal from dark ➡ to bright ➡ behind the cervical spinal cord, consistent with "pistoning" tonsillar pulsations.*

malformation in 3.6% of children undergoing routine brain or cervical spine MR. There is no sex predilection.

A CM1-associated syrinx is rare in infants under 1 year, but the incidence rises with age. This age-related increase is most pronounced in the first 5 years of life.

Presentation. One-third to half of all patients with CM1 on imaging are asymptomatic at the time of diagnosis.

Presentation of symptomatic CM1 differs with age. Children who are 2 years and younger most commonly present with oropharyngeal dysfunction (nearly 80%). Those between 3 and 5 years present with headache (57%) or scoliosis (38%). Children with holocord syringohydromyelia demonstrate altered pain, temperature, and vibratory sensation.

Uncommon presentations include hypersomnolence and sleep apnea. Valsalva-induced suboccipital headache (i.e., with coughing or sneezing), neck pain, and syncope are common in adults.

Natural History. The natural history of CM1 varies. Many patients remain asymptomatic. Some investigators believe that the degree of tonsillar ectopia in CM1 gradually increases with time and is associated with a greater likelihood of becoming symptomatic.

Outcomes of CM1-associated syringomyelia are likewise uncertain. Longitudinal studies show that a syrinx remains stable or decreases in size in nearly 90% of pediatric patients who have minimal neurologic symptoms. Others develop progressive scoliosis, spinal cord symptoms, or bulbar deficits. Such deficits are sometimes precipitated or exacerbated by relatively minor head or neck injury.

Treatment Options. Like almost everything else about CM1, management is controversial. Asymptomatic tonsillar ectopia in the absence of an associated syrinx or scoliosis is usually not treated. Periodic surveillance of patients with documented hydrosyringomyelia is generally recommended, as 12% of syringes show increase in size and may require craniocervical decompression if symptoms worsen.

Treatment of symptomatic CM1 attempts to restore normal CSF fluid dynamics at the FM. Craniospinal CSF stroke volume, maximal cord displacement during the cardiac cycle, and evidence for collateralization of venous drainage around the FM correlate with favorable outcome following surgical decompression.

Imaging

General Features. The basion-opisthion line (BOL) is a line drawn from the tip of the clivus to the posterior rim of the FM **(36-13)**. Measuring the distance from this line to the inferior margin of the cerebellar tonsils on sagittal MR defines tonsillar position.

Midline tonsillar descent 5 mm or more below the BOL—often considered diagnostic of Chiari 1—is by itself a poor criterion for definitive diagnosis. Tonsils 6 mm below the FM are common during the first decade of life. Almost 15% of normal patients have tonsils that lie 1-4 mm below the FM, and 0.5-1.0% have tonsils that project 5 mm into the upper cervical canal.

Great caution should be exercised in establishing a diagnosis of CM1, especially on the basis of borderline tonsillar ectopia alone. Unless (1) the tonsils appear compressed and pointed (peg-like) instead of gently rounded **(36-15A)**, (2) the tonsillar folia are angled obliquely or inferiorly (instead of horizontally), and (3) the retrocerebellar CSF spaces at the FM/C1 level are effaced **(36-15B)**, the diagnosis may not be warranted. Low-lying tonsils that retain their rounded shapes and are surrounded by normal-appearing CSF spaces are usually asymptomatic and of no diagnostic significance.

CT Findings. NECT scans may reveal a "crowded" FM and effaced retrotonsillar CSF space. Bone CT often demonstrates a combination of undersized, shallow posterior cranial fossa, short clivus, and CVJ assimilation anomalies. Look carefully for calvarial anomalies, as nearly 10% of patients with nonsyndromic single-suture craniosynostosis have CM1.

MR Findings. Sagittal T1 and T2 scans show "pointed" tonsils with more vertically oriented folia, obliterated retrocerebellar and premedullary subarachnoid spaces, and a "crowded" FM. The posterior fossa may appear normal or somewhat small with a short clivus and steeply angled straight sinus. In contrast to Chiari 2, the 4th ventricle usually displays a normal fastigium (dorsal point). In some cases, the inferior fourth ventricle is mildly elongated, and the nucleus gracilis—which demarcates the end of the obex and beginning of the central canal—can appear slightly low-lying **(36-16)**.

The proximal cervical spinal cord should be carefully examined for the presence of hydrosyringomyelia. T2/FLAIR parenchymal hyperintensity without frank cyst formation may indicate a "pre-syrinx" state **(36-15A)**.

The diameter of the central canal relative to the cord normally decreases significantly during the first few years of life. A CSF-like central cord cavity 3 mm or larger on axial scans is abnormal in older children and adults and should be considered a syrinx. Mean syrinx size in a large series of CM1 patients was nearly 8 mm in width and averaged nine vertebral levels in length.

Sagittal phase-contrast CSF flow studies show diminished or absent alternating bright (systolic) and dark (diastolic) signals behind the cervicomedullary junction. Any change in signal intensity of the cerebellar tonsils in cine mode suggests tonsillar pulsations **(36-18)**.

Associated Abnormalities. Complete imaging evaluation in CM1 includes the brain, CVJ, and entire spine. Mild to moderate hydrocephalus is present in 10% of patients with CM1. Callosal dysgenesis is seen in 3.0% and absent septi pellucidi in 2.4% of cases. Other supratentorial anomalies are uncommon.

Hydrosyringomyelia is present in 10-20% of asymptomatic patients and 40-80% of symptomatic CM1 patients. Associated skeletal anomalies include a retroverted dens, clival-C2 body angle < 122°, hypoplastic C1 ring, Klippel-Feil anomaly, basilar invagination, platybasia, CVJ fusion anomalies, kyphosis, and/or scoliosis.

Differential Diagnosis

Congenital tonsillar descent (CM1) must be distinguished from **normal variants** (mild uncomplicated tonsillar ectopia). The most important pathologic differential diagnosis is *acquired* tonsillar herniation caused by increased intracranial pressure **or** intracranial hypotension.

Increased intracranial pressure due to supratentorial mass effect with transmission of the pressure cone through the tentorial incisura can be easily distinguished from CM1. Signs of descending transtentorial herniation are present along with downward midbrain displacement. Tonsillar herniation in such cases is a secondary effect and should *not* be termed "acquired Chiari 1."

Intracranial hypotension shows a constellation of other findings besides inferiorly displaced tonsils. "Slumping" midbrain, enlarged pituitary gland, draping of the optic chiasm and hypothalamus over the dorsum sellae, subdural hematoma, engorged venous sinuses, and dura-arachnoid thickening and enhancement are typical abnormalities. *Mistaking intracranial hypotension for CM1 can have disastrous consequences, as surgical decompression may exacerbate brainstem "slumping."*

Approximately 20% of patients with **idiopathic intracranial hypertension** exhibit cerebellar tonsillar ectopia ≥ 5 mm. Half have a peg-like tonsil configuration, and many have a low-lying obex. Looking for other signs of idiopathic intracranial hypertension (e.g., optic nerve head protrusion into the globe) is essential to avoid misdiagnosis as Chiari 1.

Other conditions that reduce posterior cranial fossa volume can also displace the tonsils below the foramen. Such causes of **cranial constriction** include craniosynostosis, achondroplasia, acromegaly, and Paget disease. Cranial "settling" from rheumatoid arthritis, osteogenesis imperfecta, hereditary connective tissue disorders, and occipitoatlantoaxial joint instability can also force the tonsils below the FM.

CHIARI 1 MALFORMATION

Clinical Issues
- Most common Chiari malformation
- Found in 3-4% of children on routine brain imaging
- Up to 50% asymptomatic
- Valsalva-induced suboccipital headache, neck pain
- Holocord hydrosyringomyelia
  - Progressive scoliosis ± lower extremity pain
  - Abnormalities of temperature, vibratory sensation

Imaging Findings
- General features
  - Caudal tonsillar ectopia (≥ 5 mm below foramen magnum, FM)
  - Pointed, peg-like tonsils with angled folia
  - "Crowded" FM with effaced CSF spaces
  - Diminished/absent CSF flow at posterior FM
  - Syrinx in 10-20% asymptomatic, 40-80% symptomatic patients
- Differential diagnosis
  - Normal "low-lying" tonsils (rounded, no disturbed CSF flow)
  - Acquired herniation (elevated ICP, intracranial hypotension)

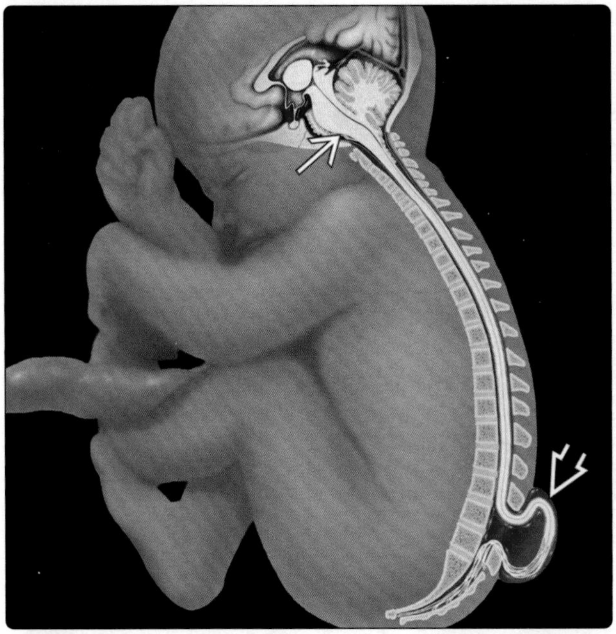

(36-19) Graphic depicts a fetus with Chiari 2 malformation with the spinal cord tethered into a myelomeningocele.

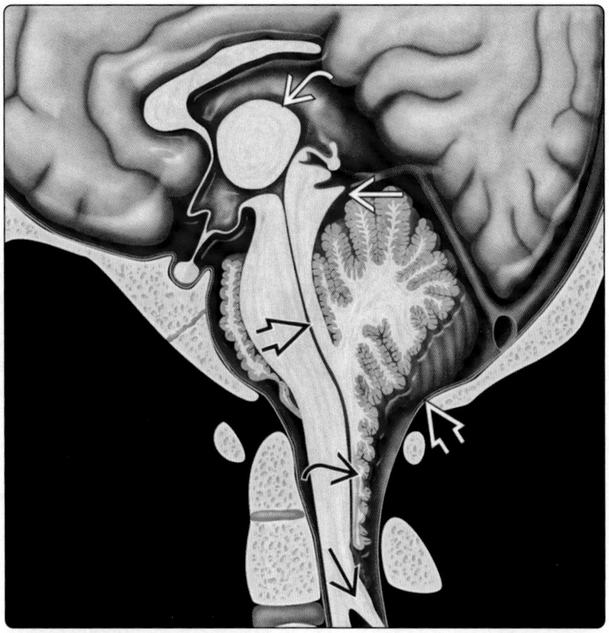

(36-20) Graphic shows CM2 with small posterior fossa, large massa intermedia, "beaked" tectum, callosal dysgenesis, elongated fourth ventricle with "cascade" of inferiorly displaced nodulus and choroid plexus, and medullary spur.

Chiari 2

Terminology and Definition

Chiari 2 malformation (CM2) is a complex hindbrain malformation that is almost always associated with myelodysplasia (myelomeningocele) **(36-19)**.

Etiology

General Concepts. CM2 is a disorder of neural tube closure but also involves paraxial mesodermal abnormalities of the skull and spine. A number of steps are required for proper neural tube closure and formation of the focal expansions that subsequently form the cerebral vesicles and ventricles. Skeletal elements of both the skull and vertebral column become "modeled" around the neural tube.

Only if the posterior neuropore closes will the developing ventricles expand sufficiently for a normal-sized posterior fossa to form around the hindbrain. If this does not happen, the cerebellum develops in a small posterior fossa with abnormally low tentorial attachments. The growing cerebellum is squeezed cephalad through the tentorial incisura and stretched inferiorly through the foramen magnum (FM).

Genetics. Nearly half of all neural tube closure anomalies have mutations on the methylene-tetra-hydrofolate reductase gene (*MTHFR*). Maternal folate deficiency and teratogens such as anticonvulsants have been linked to increased risk of CM2.

Pathology

Grossly, a broad spectrum of findings can be present in CM2. Myelomeningocele and a small posterior fossa with concave clivus and petrous pyramids are virtually always present **(36-20)**. The cerebellar vermis (typically the nodulus) is displaced inferiorly along the dorsal aspect of the cervical spinal cord. The fourth ventricle, pons, and medulla are elongated and partially dislocated into the cervical spinal canal. The lower medulla may be kinked.

Unlike Chiari 1, supratentorial abnormalities are the rule in CM2, not the exception. Hydrocephalus is present in the majority of cases, and aqueductal stenosis is common. Corpus callosum dysgenesis and gray matter anomalies such as polymicrogyria and heterotopias are frequent **(36-21)** **(36-22)** **(36-23)** **(36-24)** **(36-25)** **(36-26)**.

Clinical Issues

Epidemiology and Demographics. The overall prevalence of CM2 is 0.44 in 1,000 live births but has been decreasing with prophylactic maternal folate therapy. A dose of 4 mg per day reduces the risk of CM2 by at least 70%.

Presentation. CM2 is identified in utero with ultrasound or fetal screening for elevated α-fetoprotein. At birth, coexistent myelomeningocele and hydrocephalus are dominant clinical features in over 90% of cases. Lower cranial nerve deficits, apneic spells, and bulbar signs may be present. Lower extremity paralysis, sphincter dysfunction, and spasticity often develop later.

Treatment Options. Fetal repair of myelomeningocele is increasingly common and may reduce subsequent symptoms.

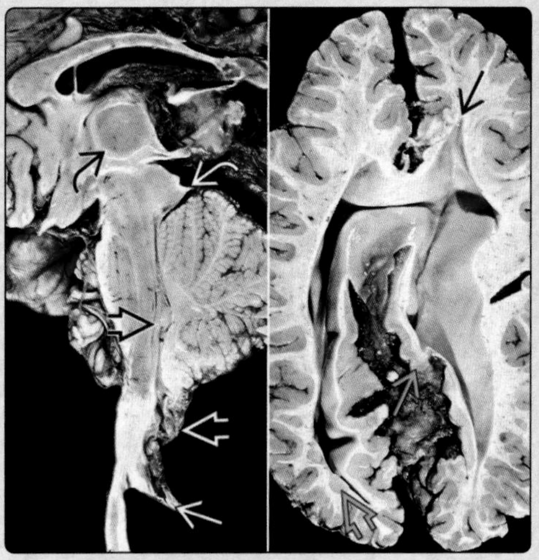

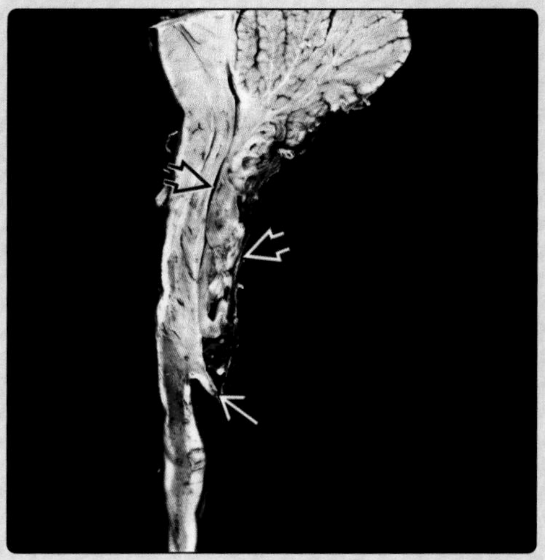

(36-21) (L) CM2 shows medullary spur, "cascade" of nodulus, CP behind medulla, elongated "soda straw" 4th ventricle, "beaked" tectum, large massa intermedia. (T. P. Naidich, MD.) (R) CM2 has stenogyria, heterotopic GM, "pointed" lateral ventricles. (E. T. Hedley-Whyte, MD.) (36-22) CM2 shows medullary spur, "cascade" of nodulus, choroid plexus, elongated "straw-like" 4th ventricle. (R. Hewlett, MD.)

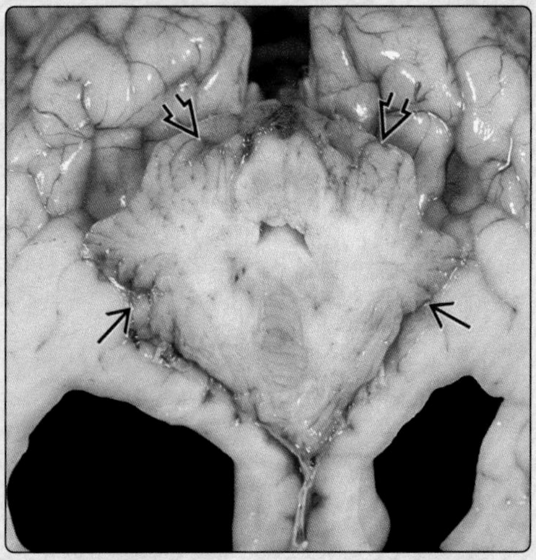

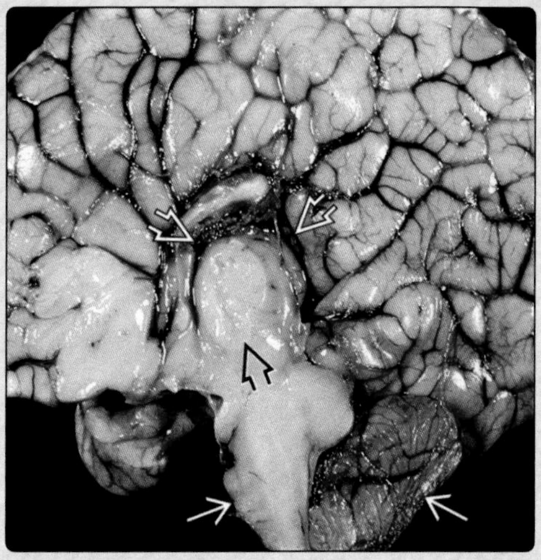

(36-23) Autopsy of CM2 shows a very small posterior fossa, cerebellar hemispheres "creeping" anteriorly around the medulla. (Courtesy R. Hewlett, MD.) (36-24) Autopsy of CM2 shows a very small posterior fossa, huge massa intermedia, corpus callosum dysgenesis with radiating gyri converging on a "high-riding" third ventricle that is open dorsally to the interhemispheric fissure. (Courtesy R. Hewlett, MD.)

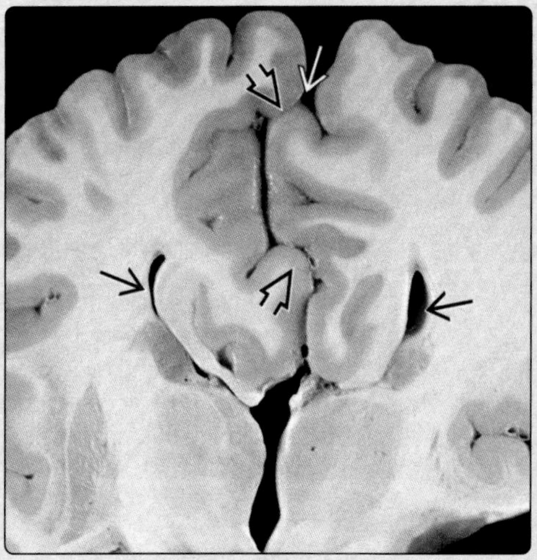

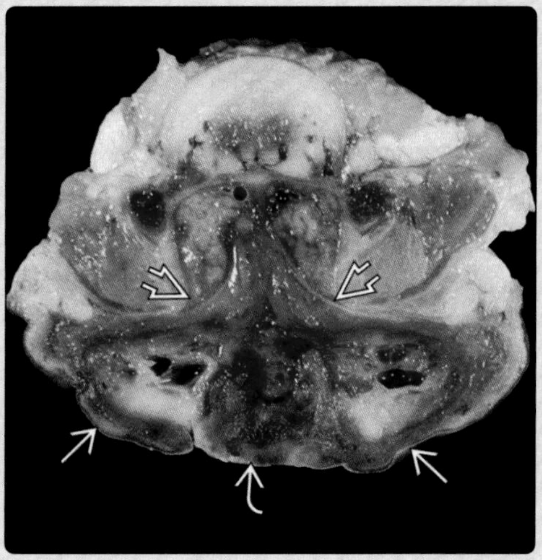

(36-25) Coronal autopsy of CM2 shows corpus callosum agenesis with "Viking helmet" or "moose head" appearance to third, lateral ventricles. Note interdigitating gyri creating an irregular, "serrated" appearance to the interhemispheric fissure. (J. Townsend, MD.) (36-26) Axial view shows autopsied spine from CM2. Note wide dorsal dysraphism and myelomeningocele with exposed neural placode. (R. Hewlett, MD.)

Surgical repair within 72 hours following delivery reduces mortality and morbidity from the open dysraphism.

Imaging

CM2 affects many regions of the skull, brain, and spine, so a variety of imaging abnormalities may be seen.

Skull and Dura. The calvarial vault forms from membranous bone. With failure of neural tube closure and absence of fetal brain distension, normal induction of the calvarial membranous plates does not occur. Disorganized collections of collagen fibers and deficient radial growth of the developing calvaria ensue, resulting in **lacunar skull** (i.e., Lückenschädel) **(36-27)**. The skull defects ("craniofenestra") are caused by the mesenchymal abnormality and are *not* a consequence of increased intracranial pressure.

Focal calvarial thinning and a "scooped-out" appearance are typical imaging findings of lacunar skull. The calvaria appears thinned with numerous circular or oval lucent defects and shallow depressions. The craniofenestra diminish with age and typically resolve by 6 months, although some scalloping of the inner table often persists into adulthood.

A **small, shallow, bony posterior fossa** with low-lying transverse sinuses is almost always present in CM2. A **large, "gaping" FM** is common. **Concave petrous temporal bones** and a **short concave clivus** are often present **(36-28)**.

Dural abnormalities are common. A widened, open, **heart-shaped tentorial incisura** and **thinned, hypoplastic**, or **fenestrated falx** are frequent findings. The fenestrated falx allows gyri to cross the midline. Interdigitating gyri and the deficient falx result in the appearance of an **irregular interhemispheric fissure** on imaging studies **(36-28C) (36-29C)**.

Midbrain, Hindbrain, and Cerebellum. Hindbrain and cerebellum anomalies are a constant in CM2. The medulla and

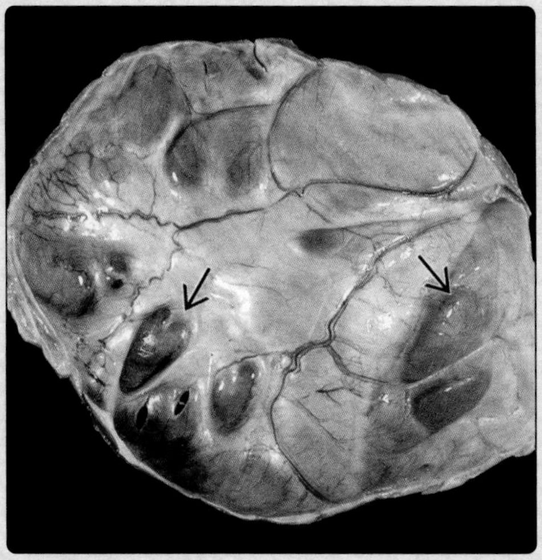

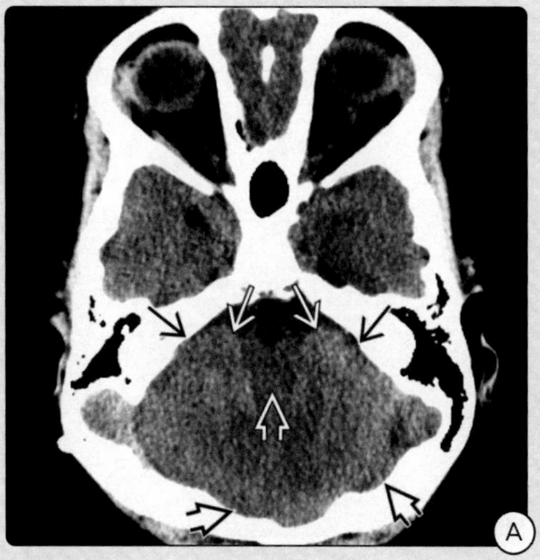

A

***(36-27)** Autopsy case of lacunar (Lückenschädel) skull in CM2 shows multiple "scooped" out foci of thinned, almost translucent bone ➙. (Courtesy R. Hewlett, MD.) **(36-28A)** NECT scan of a patient with CM2 shows a small posterior fossa with concave petrous ridges ➙, scalloped inner table ➙, no visible fourth ventricle, and "creeping" cerebellar hemispheres ➙ almost enveloping an elongated, inferiorly stretched medulla ➙.*

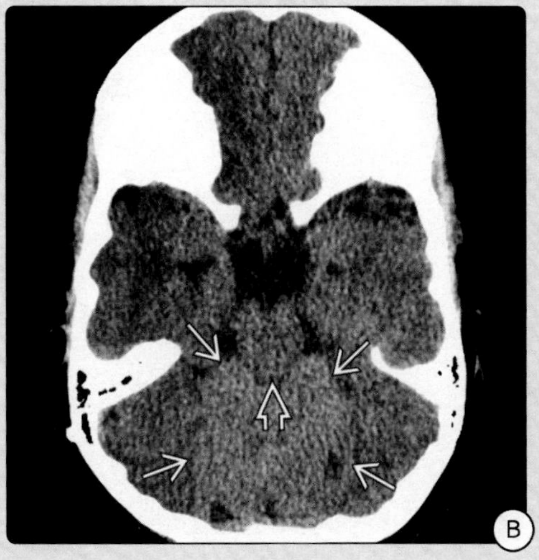

B

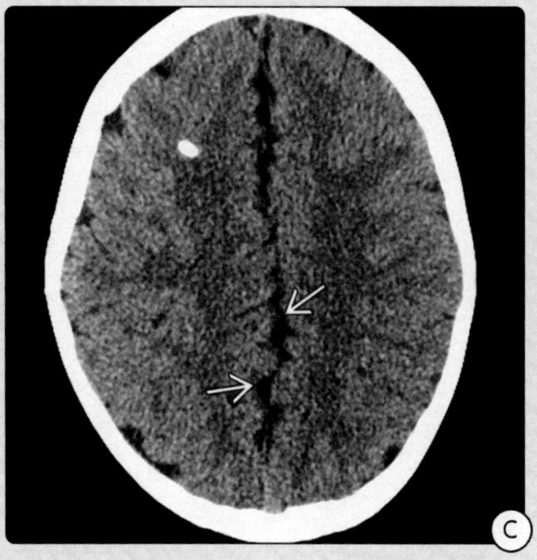

C

***(36-28B)** NECT scan in the same patient shows widely gaping, heart-shaped incisura with "towering" cerebellum protruding superiorly ➙ and mild "beaking" of the tectum ➙. **(36-28C)** More cephalad scan in the same patient shows the typical "serrated" appearance of the interhemispheric fissure ➙ due to the interdigitating gyri typically seen in CM2.*

cerebellar vermis (*not* the tonsils!) are displaced downward into the upper cervical canal for a variable distance. The **inferiorly displaced cerebellar tissue** is typically the **nodulus**, with variable contributions from the uvula and pyramid. A **cervicomedullary "kink"** with a **"medullary spur"** is common in the upper cervical canal but may lie as low as T1-4 in severe cases.

On sagittal T1 and T2 scans, the inferiorly displaced vermis, medulla, and choroid plexus form a **"cascade" of tissue** that protrudes downward through the gaping FM to lie behind the spinal cord. The superiorly herniated cerebellum may compress and deform the quadrigeminal plate, giving the appearance of a **"beaked" tectum (36-29A) (36-29B)**.

In addition to the cephalocaudal displacement of posterior fossa contents, the cerebellar hemispheres often curve anteromedially around the brainstem. In severe cases, the pons and medulla appear nearly engulfed by the "creeping" cerebellum on axial imaging studies.

The cerebellar hemispheres and vermis are pushed upward through the incisura, giving the appearance of a **"towering" cerebellum** on coronal T1 and T2 scans **(36-29D)**.

Ventricles. Abnormalities of the ventricles are present in over 90% of CM2 patients. The fourth ventricle is caudally displaced, typically lacks a fastigium (dorsal point), and appears thin and elongated (**"soda straw" fourth ventricle**). The third ventricle is often large and has a very **prominent massa intermedia (36-29A)**.

The lateral ventricles vary in size and configuration. Hydrocephalus is almost always present at birth. The atria and occipital horns are often disproportionately enlarged (**"colpocephaly"**), suggesting the presence of callosal and forceps major dysgenesis.

Following shunting, the lateral ventricles frequently retain a **serrated** or **scalloped appearance**. A large CSF space between the occipital lobes often persists.

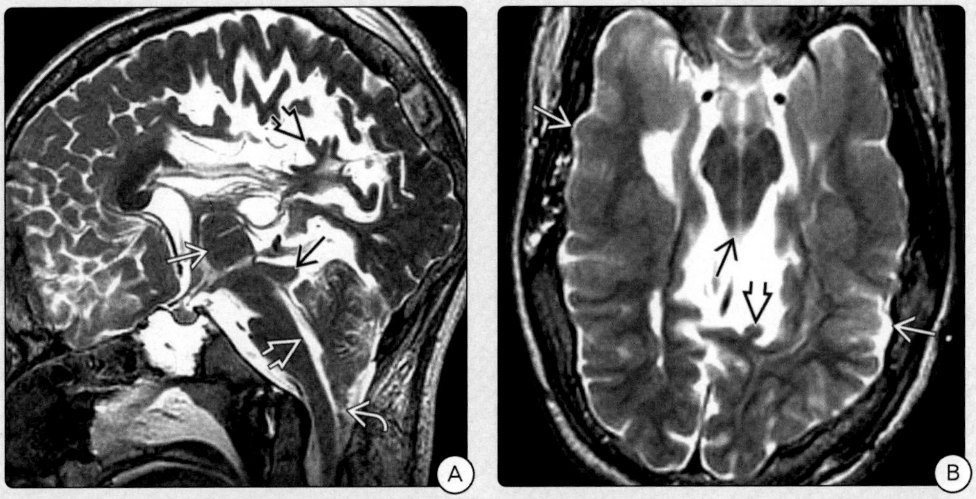

***(36-29A)** Sagittal image in a 13y patient demonstrates many features of Chiari 2, including small posterior fossa, elongated "soda straw" fourth ventricle, "cascade" of vermis/choroid plexus behind the medulla, "beaked" tectum, large massa intermedia, and multiple gyral malformations ("stenogyria"). **(36-29B)** Axial T2WI shows "beaked" tectum, stenogyria, and scalloped calvaria.*

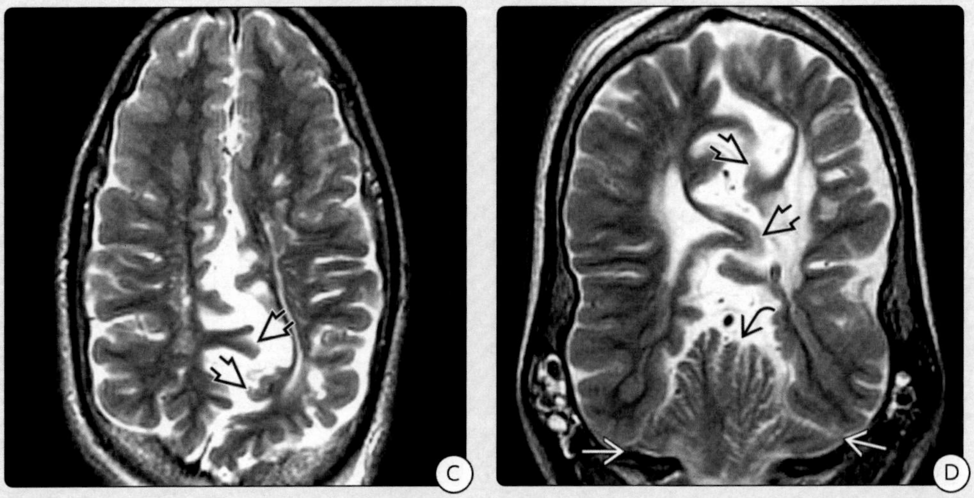

***(36-29C)** Axial T2WI shows fenestrated falx with shortened interdigitating gyri, irregular "serrated" appearance to interhemispheric fissure. **(36-29D)** Coronal T2WI shows low-lying transverse sinuses with a very small posterior fossa, "towering" cerebellum that protrudes upward through the tentorial incisura, and interdigitating gyri, giving a "serrated" appearance to the interhemispheric fissure.*

Cerebral Hemispheres. Malformations of cortical development, such as **polymicrogyria**, contracted narrow gyri (**"stenogyria"**) **(36-29B)**, and **heterotopic gray matter**, are frequent associated findings.

Callosal dysgenesis is found in nearly two-thirds of all cases, and **abnormalities of the fornices** are also common.

Spine and Spinal Cord. Open spinal dysraphism with **myelomeningocele** is present in almost all cases of CM2. **Hydrosyringomyelia** is seen in 50%.

Differential Diagnosis

The major differential diagnosis of CM2 is other Chiari malformations.

In **Chiari 1**, it is the tonsils (not the vermis) that are herniated inferiorly. Myelomeningocele is absent, and, other than being somewhat small, the posterior fossa and its contents appear relatively normal.

If findings of CM2 plus a low occipital or high cervical cephalocele are present, the diagnosis is **Chiari 3**.

A few cases of posteriorly angled odontoid, brainstem descent, and tonsillar ectopia without myelodysplasia have been described and are considered by some investigators as **Chiari 1.5** (see below).

Severe chronic shunted congenital hydrocephalus may cause cerebellar herniation upward through the tentorial incisura, but brainstem descent and myelomeningocele are absent.

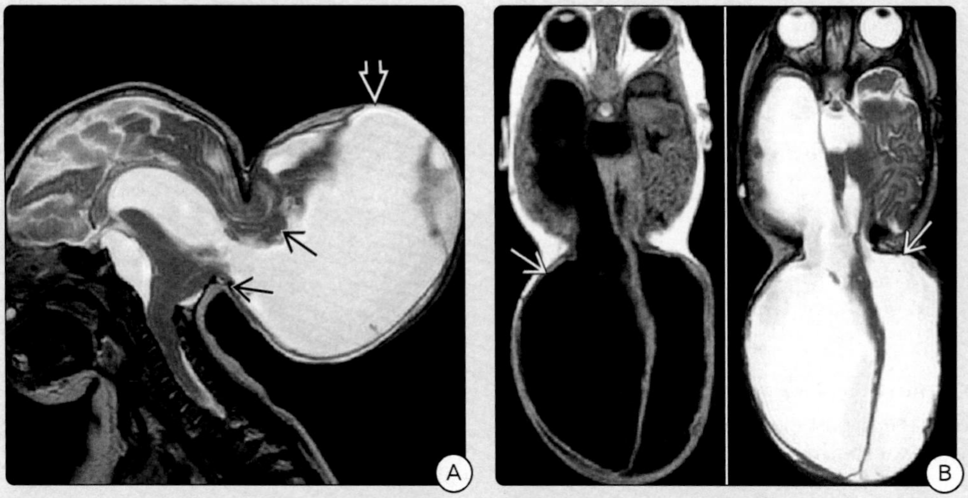

***(36-30A)** Sagittal T2WI in a 3d infant shows Chiari 3 with a cephalocele that contains herniated dysplastic brain and CSF in continuity with a lateral ventricle. **(36-30B)** Axial T1WI (L), T2WI (R) in the same patient show extension of the lateral ventricles into the cephalocele. (Courtesy G. Hedlund, DO.)*

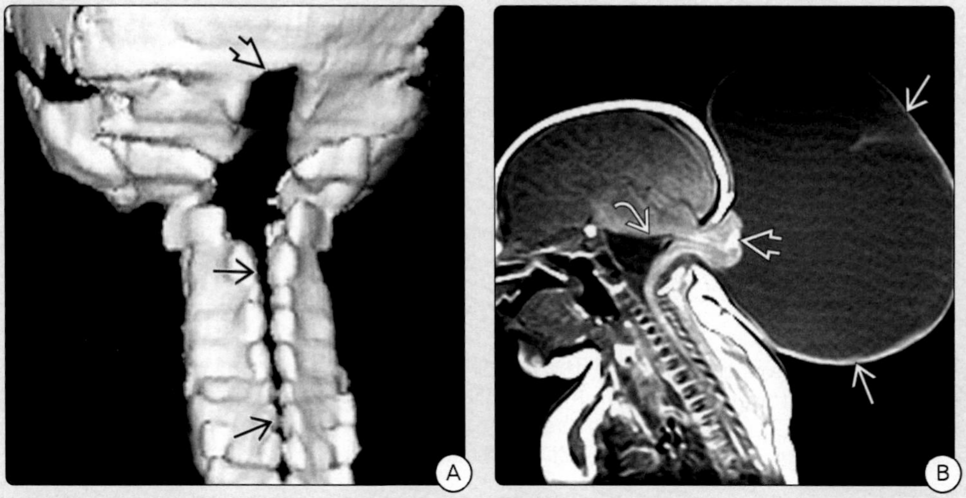

***(36-31A)** Chiari 3 is shown with extensive cranium bifidum extending from the occipital bone through the entire cervical spine. **(36-31B)** Sagittal T1WI in the same patient with cranium bifidum and Chiari 3 shows an enormous meningocele sac with herniated, dysplastic-appearing brain. The fourth ventricle is enlarged, elongated, and "tugged" toward the cephalocele. (Courtesy A. Illner, MD.)*

CHIARI 2 MALFORMATION

Pathoetiology
- Complex hindbrain malformation with myelomeningocele
  - Posterior neuropore closure disorder
  - Developing vesicles fail to expand
  - Paraxial mesodermal abnormalities (skull, spine)
- Result = "too small" bony posterior fossa

Clinical Issues
- Prevalence reduced with maternal folate
- Myelomeningocele, hydrocephalus dominate clinical picture at birth

Imaging Findings
- Myelomeningocele (almost always)
- Lacunar skull
- Small posterior fossa
- Abnormal dura (gaping FM, heart-shaped incisura, fenestrated falx)
- Inferiorly displaced medulla, vermis lead to "cascade" of tissue
- Cervicomedullary "kink," medullary "spur"
- "Towering" and "creeping" cerebellum
- "Soda straw" fourth ventricle
- Prominent massa intermedia
- Hydrocephalus, shunted ventricles appear scalloped
- Callosal dysgenesis
- Stenogyria, gray matter heterotopias

Chiari 3

Terminology

Chiari 3 malformation (CM3) is the rarest of the Chiari malformations. CM3 consists of a small posterior fossa with a caudally displaced brainstem and variable herniation of meninges/posterior fossa contents through a low occipital or upper cervical bony defect.

Pathology

The cephalocele contains meninges together with variable amounts of brain tissue, vessels, and CSF spaces. The brain is often featureless, dysplastic-appearing, and disorganized with extensive gliosis and gray matter heterotopias.

Clinical Issues

The cephalocele in CM3 generally appears as a large skin-covered, sac-like suboccipital mass protruding posteroinferiorly from the craniovertebral junction. Microcephaly is common, and, in extreme cases, the cephalocele exceeds the cranium in size **(36-30)**.

Some cases are diagnosed with antenatal ultrasound. Other patients present at birth with bulbar and long tract signs, seizures, and developmental delay. Surgical mortality is high, and prognosis is generally poor because survivors usually have severe residual neurologic deficits.

Imaging

NECT scans show bony features similar to those seen in CM2, i.e., a small posterior cranial fossa, short scalloped clivus, lacunar skull, a defect in the ventral chondral portion of the supraoccipital bone, and low cranium bifidum that may extend inferiorly to involve much of the cervical spine **(36-31)**.

MR best delineates sac contents, which often include dysplastic-appearing cerebellum and/or brainstem, as well as distorted CSF spaces and vessels. A deformed fourth and sometimes third ventricle can be partially found within the mass of herniated brain and meninges. Veins, dural sinuses, and even the basilar artery are sometimes "pulled" into the defect.

Differential Diagnosis

The differential diagnosis of CM3 includes isolated occipital cephalocele, iniencephaly, and syndromic occipital cephaloceles. **Isolated occipital cephalocele** lacks the typical intracranial features of CM2 and is not associated with cervical dysraphism.

Iniencephaly is an occipital cephalocele with extensive spinal dysraphism and fixed retroflexion of the neck ("stargazer" fetus). **Syndromic occipital cephalocele** occurs with other specific features (e.g., in Meckel-Gruber and Goldenhar-Gorlin syndromes).

CHIARI 3 MALFORMATION

Pathology
- Small posterior fossa
- Caudally displaced brainstem
- Low occipital or upper cervical bony defect
- Cephalocele with herniation of meninges, dysplastic brain, ventricles

Sac May Contain
- Meninges
- Dysplastic brain
- Deformed ventricle(s)
- Blood vessels (venous sinuses, arteries)

Chiari Variants

Some additions to the original Chiari classification have been proposed by neurosurgeons to account for hindbrain herniations that do not conform to the classic Chiari 1-3 definitions. Although these concepts are controversial and have not been universally adopted, radiologists should at least be familiar with them.

Chiari 0 Malformation

This variant consists of hydrosyringomyelia and foramen magnum (FM) "crowding." Chiari 0 differs from Chiari 1, as *the cerebellar tonsils are normally positioned* (i.e., either above or less than 3 mm below the FM) **(36-32)**.

Chiari 0 patients are typically symptomatic (usually because of the syrinx). A smaller than normal posterior fossa (particularly

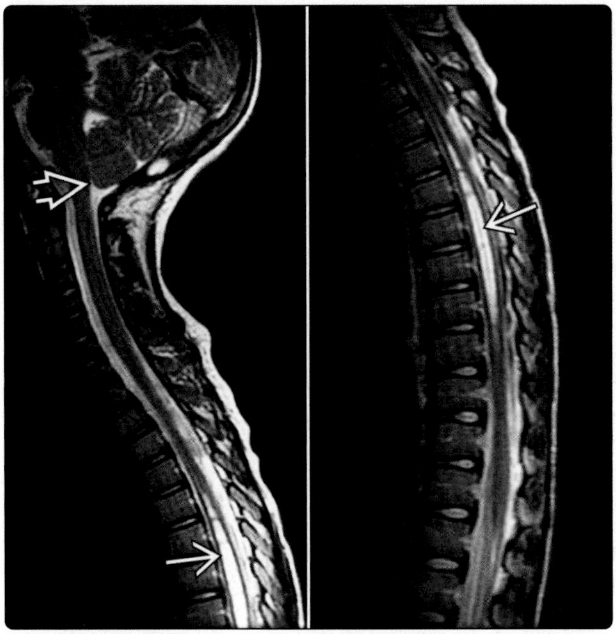

(36-32) Sagittal T2 scans show Chiari 0 malformation with thoracic syrinx ➡. The cerebellar tonsil ➡ is rounded and in normal position, but the FM appears "crowded" posteriorly.

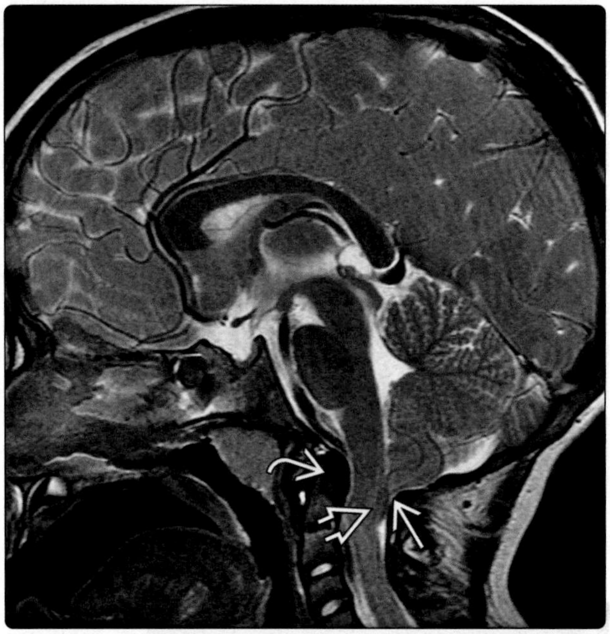

(36-33) Sagittal T2WI in a 6y girl with Chiari 1.5 malformation shows retroflexed odontoid ➡, tonsillar herniation ➡, crowded FM, and low-lying nucleus gracilis ➡. The clival-C2 body angle is normal (i.e., > 122°).

with a short clivus) and the presence of embryonic membranes at the foramen magnum may accentuate the craniovertebral junction obstruction.

Chiari 1.5 Malformation

Terminology. The term Chiari 1.5 malformation (CM1.5) has been coined by neurosurgeons to designate a "complex Chiari" malformation in which cerebellar tonsillar herniation is complicated by other abnormalities (e.g., caudally displaced brainstem and fourth ventricle and/or cervicomedullary "kink"). CM1.5 differs from classic CM1 in that *caudal descent of the brainstem is present, and tonsillar herniation is typically more severe.* CM1.5 differs from CM2, as *myelomeningocele is absent.*

Clinical Issues. Recent large series show that cases fulfilling the imaging criteria for CM1.5 represent approximately 22% of all patients 16 years or younger referred for surgical management of Chiari-related malformations.

Age at diagnosis is usually younger compared with CM1 although no single sign or symptom is peculiar to CM1.5. The most frequent symptom is headache (often Valsalva induced). Progressive scoliosis and syrinx-related symptoms such as extremity paresthesias are common.

Symptomatic patients with "classic" CM1 often require only suboccipital decompression (with or without duraplasty), whereas patients with "complex" CM1.5 abnormalities may require other additional interventions, such as transoral odontoid resection and occipitocervical fusion. Outcomes are similar, suggesting that CM1.5 is just a more severe subtype of CM1 rather than a unique type of Chiari malformation.

Imaging. In addition to tonsillar ectopia (see above), patients with CM1.5 demonstrate several other significant imaging abnormalities. The major finding that differentiates CM1.5 from CM1 is the presence of brainstem herniation through the FM (hence the term "Chiari 1.5 malformation"). Elongation/caudal displacement of the brainstem and fourth ventricle and displacement of the obex below the FM are common **(36-33)**. FM "crowding" with a medullary "kink" or "bulb" is often present in addition to the inferiorly displaced tonsils.

Bony abnormalities are common in CM1.5. These include a "retroflexed" odontoid, abnormal clival-cervical angle, occipitalization of the atlas, basilar invagination with odontoid compression of the brainstem, and scoliosis. Syringomyelia is present in 50% of cases, but spina bifida and myelodysplasia are absent.

Differential Diagnosis. The major differential diagnosis of CM1.5 is **CM1**. As management strategies differ, the distinction is important. Although both CM1.5 and CM1 share common features, such as tonsillar descent and bony anomalies, caudal brainstem descent distinguishes the two malformations.

Chiari 4 Malformation

The terms "primary cerebellar agenesis" or "severe cerebellar hypoplasia" should be used instead of "Chiari 4 malformation." The posterior fossa is normal in size and mostly filled with CSF. The pons is small and appears flat. There is no myelomeningocele, and the intracranial features of Chiari 2 are absent.

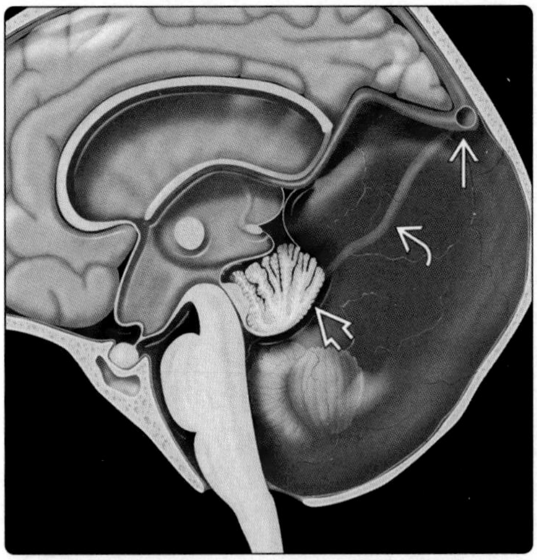

(36-34) Elevated torcular, steeply angled TS, superiorly rotated hypoplastic cerebellar vermis, and hydrocephalus reveal DWM.

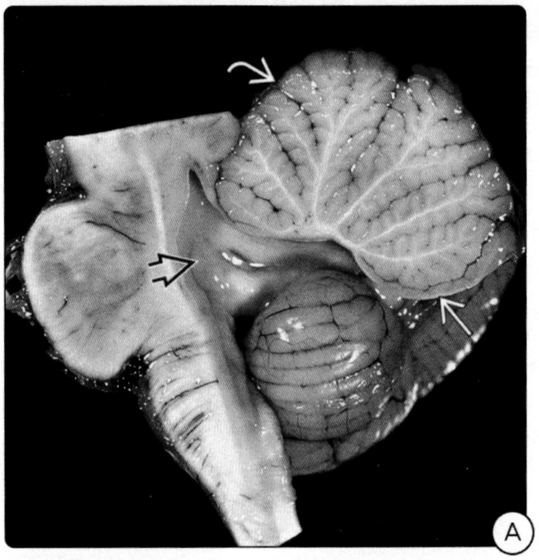

(36-35A) Autopsy of DWC shows mildly hypoplastic, superiorly rotated vermis, 4th ventricle open dorsally to a large CSF cyst.

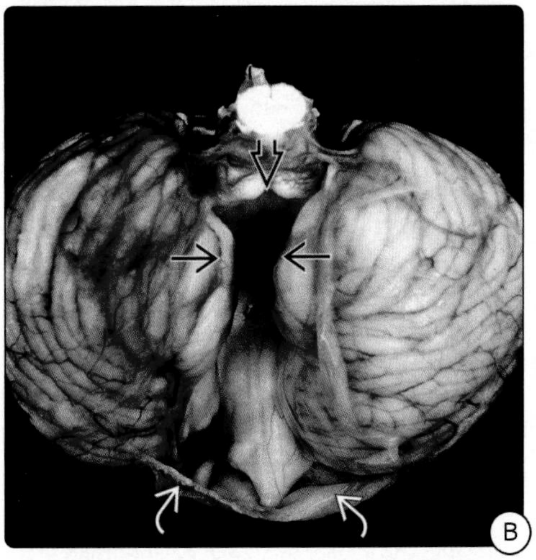

(36-35B) DWC shows normal 4th ventricle floor opening through widened vallecula into a dorsal cyst. (Courtesy R. Hewlett, MD.)

Hindbrain Malformations

Cystic Posterior Fossa Anomalies and the Dandy-Walker Continuum

Terminology

The Dandy-Walker continuum (DWC) is a spectrum of anomalies that includes **Dandy-Walker malformation (DWM), vermian hypoplasia (VH), Blake pouch cyst (BPC)**, and **mega cisterna magna (MCM)**. Two measurements are important in distinguishing these entities: (1) the *tegmento-vermian angle* (the angle formed by lines along the anterior surface of the vermis and the dorsal surface of the brainstem, normally < 18°) and (2) the *fastigium-declive line* (a line drawn from the fastigium—the dorsal "point" of the 4th ventricle on sagittal images—and the dorsal most point of the vermis) **(36-2)**.

Dandy-Walker malformation (DWM) is a generalized disorder of mesenchymal development that affects both the cerebellum and overlying meninges. It consists of a large PF with a high-inserting venous sinus confluence, large PF pia-ependyma-lined cyst extending dorsally from the fourth ventricle, and varying degrees of vermian and cerebellar hemispheric hypoplasia **(36-34)**. The fourth ventricle choroid plexus is absent.

Vermian hypoplasia (VH) is part of the DWC spectrum. There is superior rotation of the vermis, increased tegmento-vermian angle (18-45°), and variable cerebellar hypoplasia (diminished vermian volume below the fastigium-declive line). The overall posterior fossa volume is normal in VH.

Blake pouch cyst (BPC) is an ependyma-lined protrusion of the fourth ventricle through the foramen of Magendie into the retrovermian cistern. The fourth ventricle choroid plexus is present but displaced into the superior cyst wall. The tegmento-vermian angle is increased, but the *vermis is normal* in size and configuration. The fourth ventricle has a "key hole" appearance.

Mega cisterna magna (MCM) is an enlarged retrocerebellar CSF collection (> 10 mm). There is no mass effect on the cerebellar hemispheres or vermis. The vermis is normal as is the tegmento-vermian angle (< 18°). Cerebellar veins and elements of the falx cerebelli can be seen crossing through the MCS.

Etiology

Embryology. If (1) the anterior membranous area of the embryonic fourth ventricle fails to incorporate properly into the choroid plexus or (2) there is delayed opening of the foramen of Magendie, CSF pulsations cause the nonintegrated anterior membranous area to balloon posteriorly within the PF. This large CSF-filled cyst does not communicate with the subarachnoid space.

Etiology and Genetics. Three main DWM causative genes have been identified: *FOXC1* on chromosome 3q24 and the linked *ZIC1* and *ZIC4* genes on chromosome 6q25.3. Each member of the ZIC gene family encodes a highly related zinc-finger transcription factor that is broadly expressed throughout cerebellar development. Both *ZIC1* and *ZIC4* have key roles in the regulation of both cerebellar size and normal cerebellar foliation. Zic proteins compete or interact with Gli proteins to regulate Shh signaling, which is crucial for normal cerebellar development.

DWM is accompanied by more than 18 types of chromosomal abnormality and co-occurs with more than 40 genetic syndromes. In addition, DWM can arise as a result of maternal diabetes, use of warfarin, or fetal infection by cytomegalovirus, rubella, or Zika virus.

Known clinical associations with DWM include PHACES, neurocutaneous melanosis (Figure 39-67), midline anomalies, and trisomy 18.

Pathology

Gross Pathology. The most striking gross findings in DWM are (1) an enlarged PF with (2) upward displacement of the tentorium and accompanying venous sinuses and (3) cystic dilatation of the fourth ventricle. Vermian abnormalities range from complete absence to varying degrees of hypoplasia. In DWM, the 4th ventricle choroid plexus is absent.

DWM is frequently associated with other CNS anomalies. Almost two-thirds of patients have gyral abnormalities (e.g., pachy- or polymicrogyria and heterotopic GM). Callosal dysgenesis is common. Craniofacial, cardiac, and urinary tract anomalies are frequent.

Microscopic Features. The PF cyst in DWM is typically lined by two layers: an outer layer of pia-arachnoid and an inner layer of ependyma. Occasionally, microscopic remnants of cerebellar tissue are present in the cyst wall.

Clinical Issues

Epidemiology and Demographics. DWM is the most common congenital cerebellar malformation with an estimated prevalence of 1:5,000 live births. There is a slight female predominance (F:M = 1.5-2:1).

Presentation. The most common presentation of DWM is increased intracranial pressure secondary to hydrocephalus. Despite the extensive cerebellar abnormalities, cerebellar signs are relatively uncommon.

Natural History. Early death is common in classic DWM. If DWM is relatively mild and uncomplicated by other CNS anomalies, intelligence can be normal and neurologic deficits minimal.

Treatment Options. CSF diversion, usually ventriculoperitoneal shunting with or without cyst shunting or marsupialization, is the standard treatment for DWM-related hydrocephalus.

Imaging

The spectrum of imaging abnormalities in DWM is broad, affecting—to varying degrees—the skull and dura, ventricles and CSF spaces, and brain.

Skull and Dura, Venous Sinuses. In contrast to CM2, in which the PF is abnormally small, the PF in DWM is strikingly enlarged. The straight sinus, sinus confluence, and tentorial apex are elevated above the lambdoid suture ("lambdoid-torcular inversion"). The transverse sinuses descend at a steep angle from the torcular herophili toward the sigmoid sinuses **(36-36)**.

The occipital bone may appear scalloped, focally thinned, and remodeled with *all* posterior fossa cysts. Retrocerebellar CSF cysts (formerly termed "mega cisterna magna") often demonstrates partially infolded dura-arachnoid (falx cerebelli) on axial T2 scans. The falx cerebelli is usually absent in DWM.

Ventricles and Cisterns. The floor of the fourth ventricle is present and appears normal in DWM. The anterior medullary velum and fastigium are absent. The choroid plexus is absent, and the fourth ventricle opens dorsally to a variably sized CSF-containing cyst that balloons posteriorly behind and between the cerebellar hemisphere remnants.

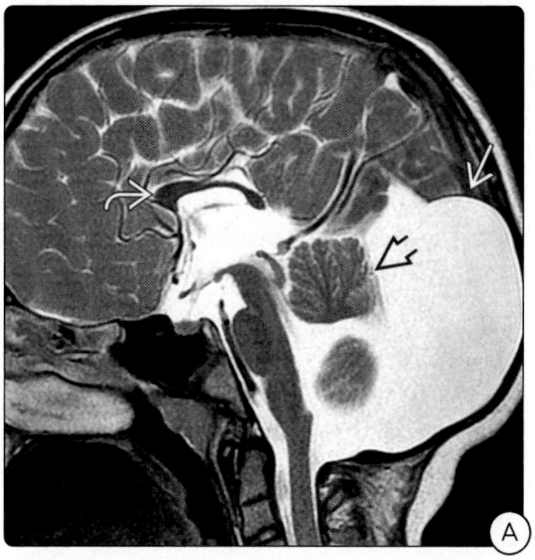

***(36-36A)** DWM shows large PF cyst elevating torcular →, superiorly rotated vermian remnant →, small pons, dysgenetic corpus callosum →.*

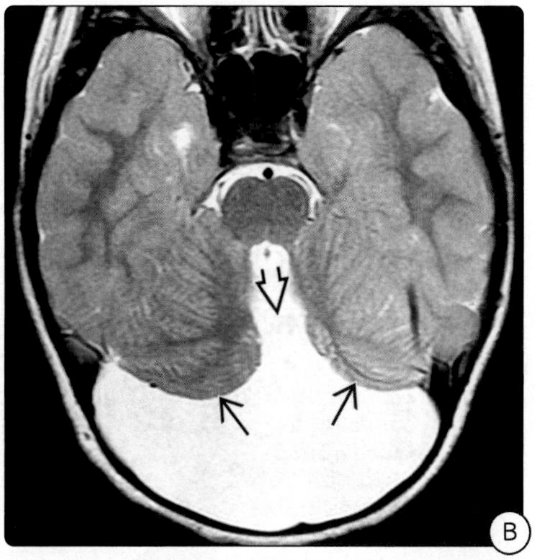

***(36-36B)** Axial T2WI in DWM shows 4th ventricle open dorsally → to the large PF cyst. Cerebellar hemispheres are small, "winged" anteriorly →.*

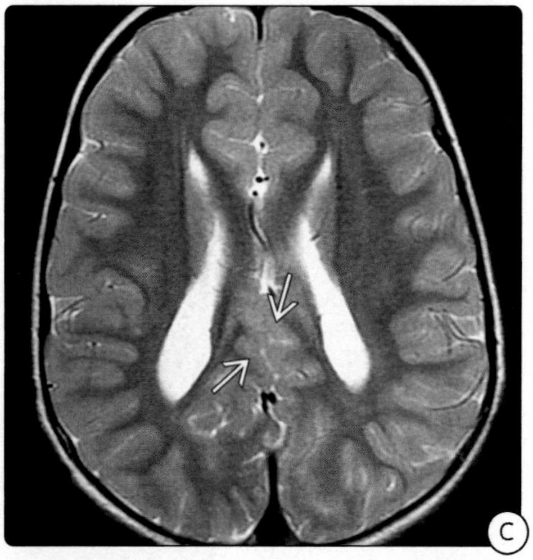

***(36-36C)** Axial T2WI in the same case shows callosal dysgenesis with polymicrogyria →.*

Generalized obstructive hydrocephalus is present in over 80% of neonates with DWM at birth. If callosal dysgenesis is present, the lateral ventricles are widely separated and may have unusually prominent occipital horns (colpocephaly).

In DWC (previously called Dandy Walker "variant"), the fourth ventricle has a "keyhole" configuration on axial imaging caused by a widely patent vallecula that communicates with a prominent cisterna magna **(36-37)** **(36-38)**.

BPC is an ependyma-lined protrusion from the fourth ventricle. The vermis is normal in size and morphology but is elevated and superiorly rotated with increased tegmento-vermian angle (18-45°). The posterior fossa is normal in size.

The fourth ventricle is normal in retrocerebellar arachnoid cysts and shows a normal fastigium (dorsal point) on sagittal MR scans.

Brainstem, Cerebellum, and Vermis. The brainstem appears normal in mild forms of DWM but often appears somewhat small in moderate to more severe DWM.

The vermis is normal in BPC and retrocerebellar arachnoid cysts. Varying degrees of vermian hypoplasia are seen in DWM **(36-39)** **(36-40)**. The inferior lobules are often hypoplastic in mild DWC. In classic DWM, the vermian remnant is rotated and elevated above the large PF cyst.

The cerebellar hemispheres appear normal in VH and BPCs but are hypoplastic in DWM. In severe cases of DWM, the cerebellar remnants appear "winged" outward and displaced anterolaterally.

Retrocerebellar arachnoid cysts exert mass effect on the cerebellar hemispheres, which otherwise appear normal in morphology.

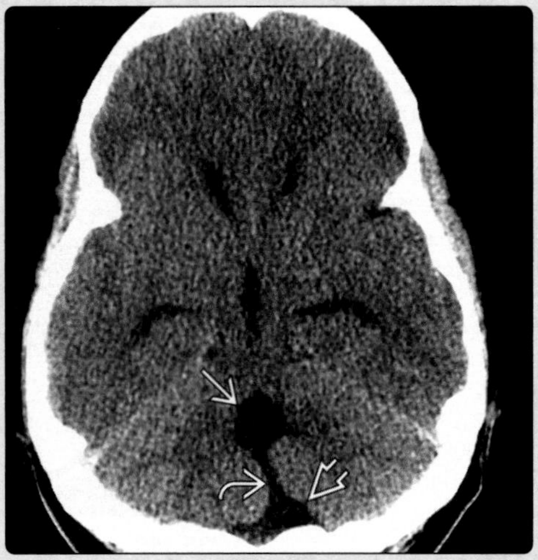

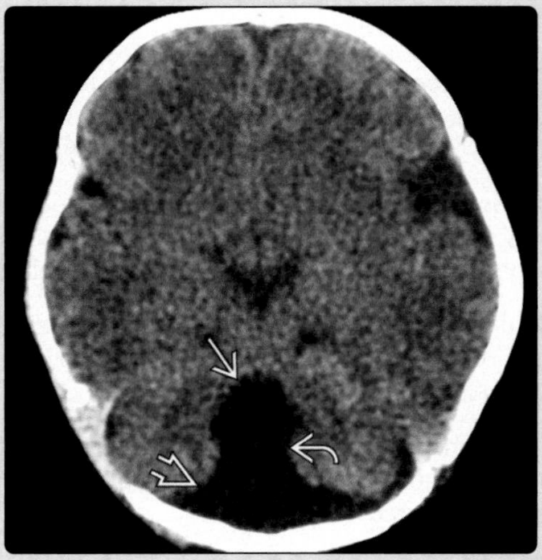

***(36-37)** NECT scan in an 11y girl with mild DWC-VH shows the "keyhole" appearance of the fourth ventricle opening into the prominent foramen magnum via an enlarged foramen of Magendie. **(36-38)** Axial NECT scan in a 10d infant shows a more pronounced "keyhole" deformity of mild DWC-VH with inferior vermian hypoplasia and a large fourth ventricle opening into the cisterna magna via a gaping foramen of Magendie.*

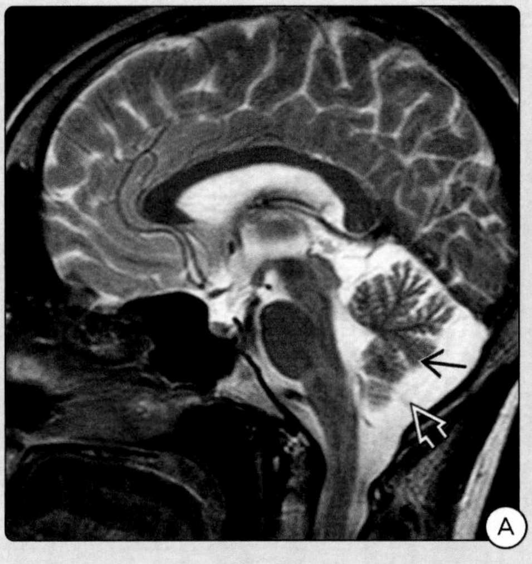

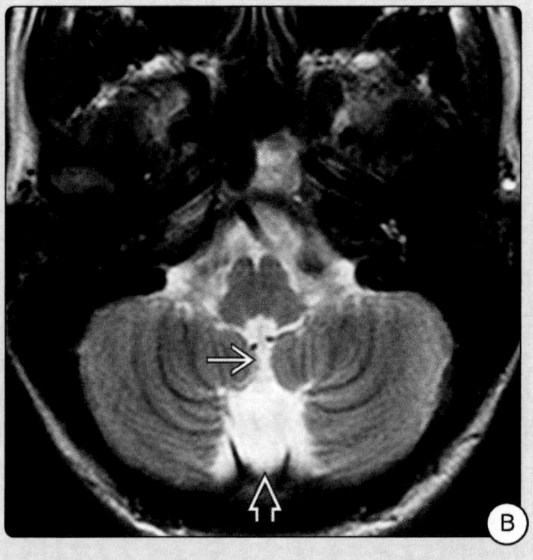

***(36-39A)** Sagittal T2WI in an asymptomatic 30y woman shows a very prominent cisterna magna, somewhat hypoplastic-appearing inferior vermis. **(36-39B)** Axial T2WI in the same patient shows the mild inferior vermian hypoplasia (VH), prominent cisterna magna, and wide foramen of Magendie. This is mild DWC with mega cisterna magna (MCM).*

Associated Abnormalities. Other CNS abnormalities are present in 70% of DWM. The most common finding is callosal agenesis or dysgenesis. A dorsal interhemispheric cyst may be present. Gray matter abnormalities (e.g., heterotopias, clefts, and pachy- and polymicrogyria) are common associated abnormalities.

DANDY-WALKER CONTINUUM (DWC): DIFFERENTIAL DIAGNOSIS

Dandy-Walker Malformation (DWM)
- Large posterior fossa (PF)
- Cyst extending posteriorly from fourth ventricle
- Vermian agenesis or hypogenesis
  - Seriously increased tegmento-vermian angle (> 45°)
- Torcular-lambdoid inversion

Vermian Hypoplasia (VH)
- Old term = Dandy-Walker variant
- Reduced vermian tissue below fastigium-declive line
- Superior rotation of vermis
  - Increased tegmento-vermian angle (18-45°)
- PF normal size

Blake Pouch Cyst (BPC)
- Ependyma-lined protrusion from fourth ventricle
- Normal size and morphology of vermis
- Elevated vermis
  - Increased tegmentovermian angle (18-45°)

Mega Cisterna Magna (MCM)
- Enlarged retrocerebellar CSF (> 10 mm)
- No mass effect on vermis or cerebellum
- Normal vermis
  - Tegmento-vermian angle < 18°
- Fluid crossed by veins, falx cerebelli
- May scallop, remodel occiput**
  - ** All categories in DWC may "scallop" inner occipital bone

Arachnoid Cyst
- Not truly in the Dandy-Walker Continuum
  - Cerebellopontine angle > retrovermian
- No communication with 4th ventricle
- No crossing veins or falx cerebelli
- Causes mass effect

Differential Diagnosis

Thin-section sagittal and coronal MRs are crucial in differentiating posterior fossa fluid collections. They often appear similar and without knowledge of cyst wall histopathology can be difficult to distinguish from each other. The best approach is to describe the cyst by location, assess vermian development including measurement of the tegmento-vermian angle and the fastigium-declive line, and determine the mass effects—if any—on surrounding structures.

Because Dandy-Walker really is a spectrum, there are many "in between" cases. From a clinical perspective, it is most important for the radiologist to specifically describe vermian, cerebellar, and any coexisting supratentorial anomalies (see shaded box above).

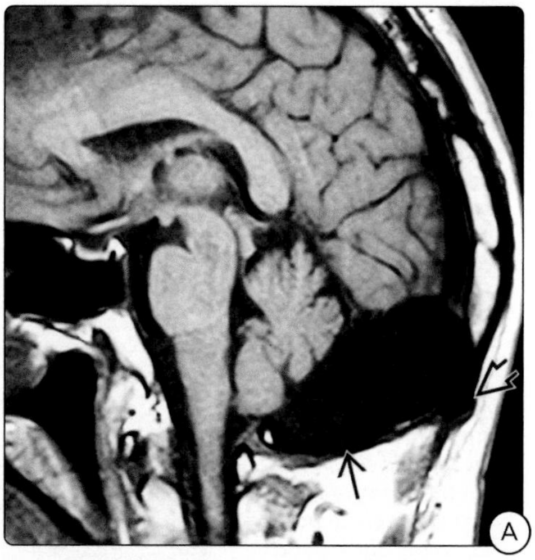

***(36-40A)** Sagittal T1WI shows mild DWC (MCM). Note thinned, scalloped occipital bone. Pons, vermis, 4th ventricle are normal.*

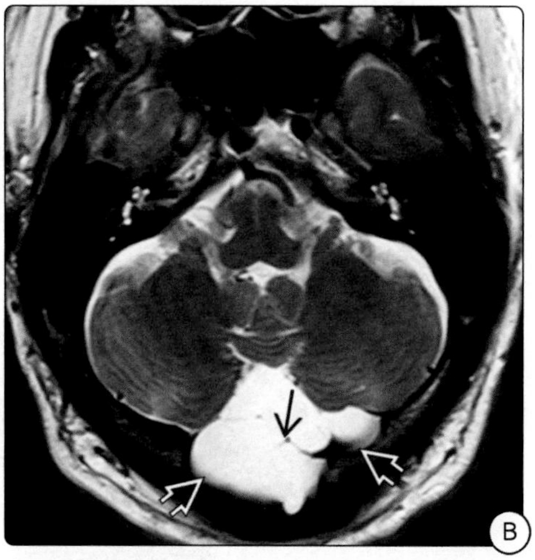

***(36-40B)** Axial T2WI in the same patient shows bone "scalloping" and partially infolded dura-arachnoid of falx cerebelli.*

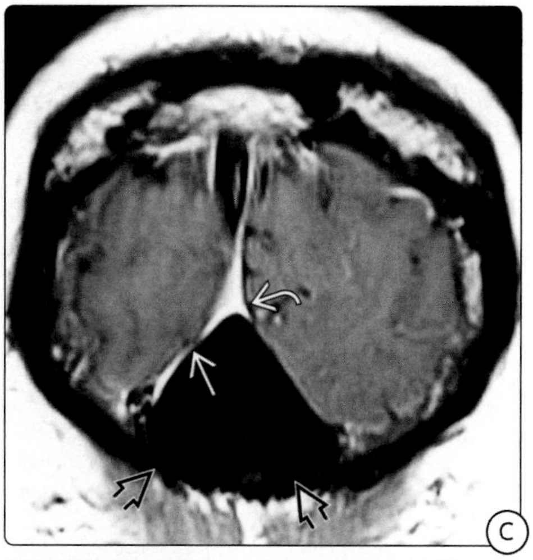

***(36-40C)** Coronal T1 C+ shows that MCM can elevate the posterior tentorium and torcular herophili.*

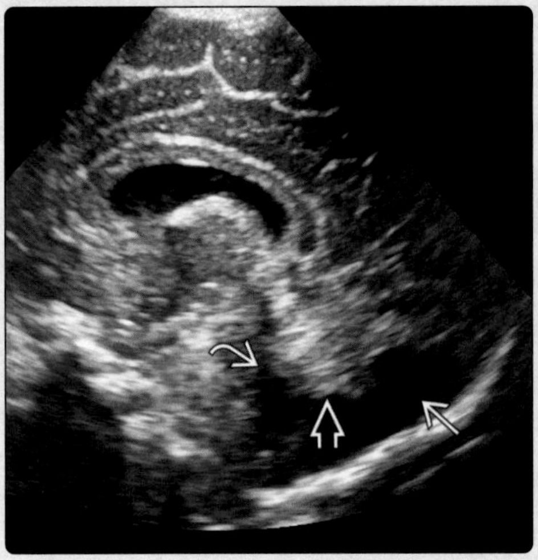

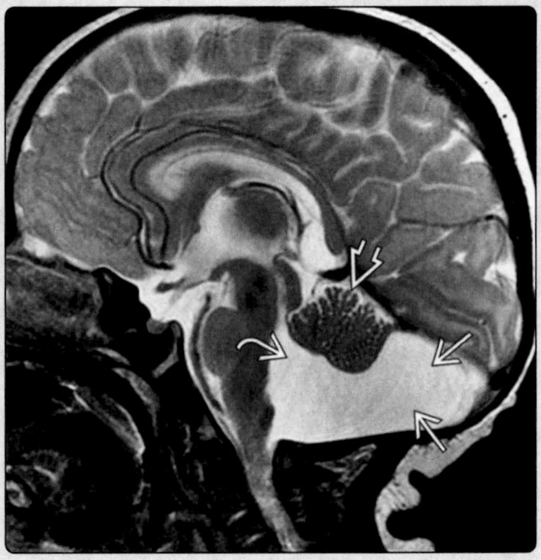

***(36-41)** Sagittal ultrasound in a newborn infant shows a cystic posterior fossa fluid collection →. The tegmento-vermian angle is increased →, and the vermis → appears rotated superiorly. **(36-42)** Sagittal T2WI at 17 weeks of age shows the rim → of a fluid-filled cyst that has extruded posteriorly from the 4th ventricle. The vermis → is intact but rotated superiorly, and the tegmento-vermian angle is increased →. This is Blake pouch cyst.*

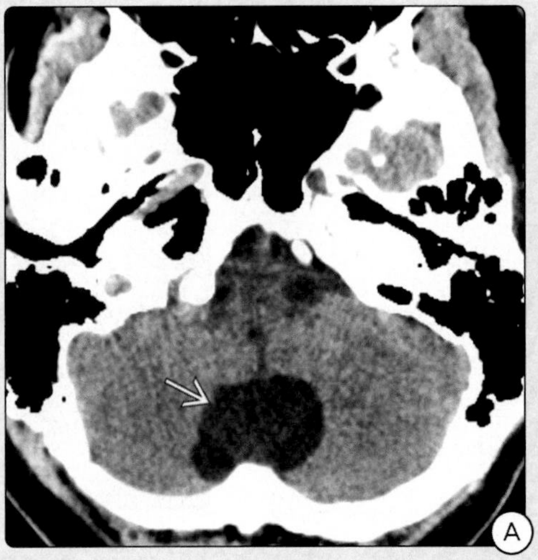

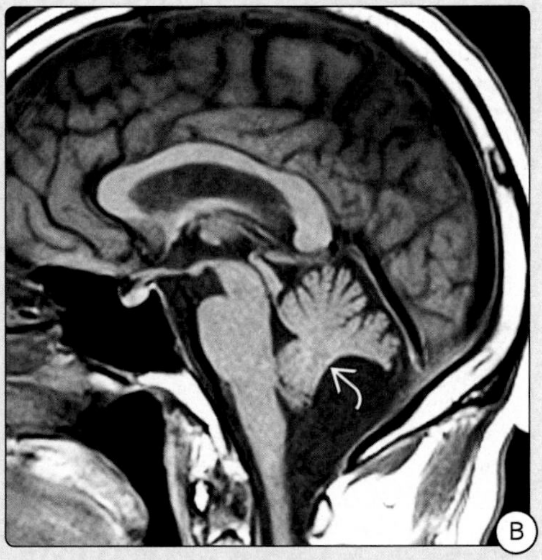

***(36-43A)** NECT in a 58y man with TIAs shows a well-delineated rounded retrocerebellar CSF-like fluid collection →. **(36-43B)** Sagittal T1W shows that the fluid collection is isointense with CSF and exerts mass effect on the inferior vermis →.*

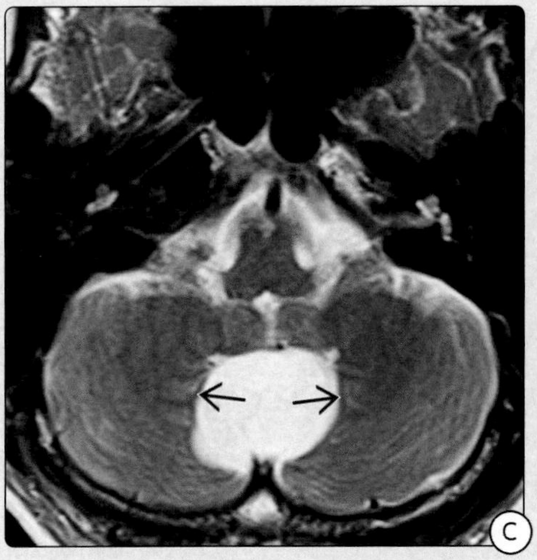

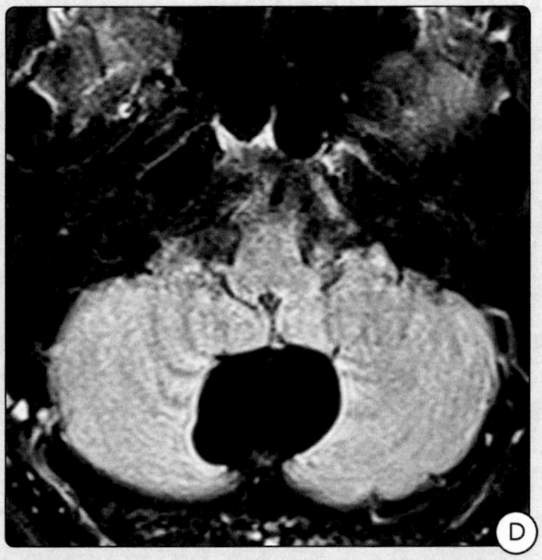

***(36-43C)** Axial T2WI shows that the fluid collection is well delineated and displaces adjacent cerebellum laterally →. No veins or falx cerebelli cross the collection, which is isointense with CSF. **(36-43D)** Axial FLAIR shows that the fluid collection suppresses completely. This is retrocerebellar arachnoid cyst.*

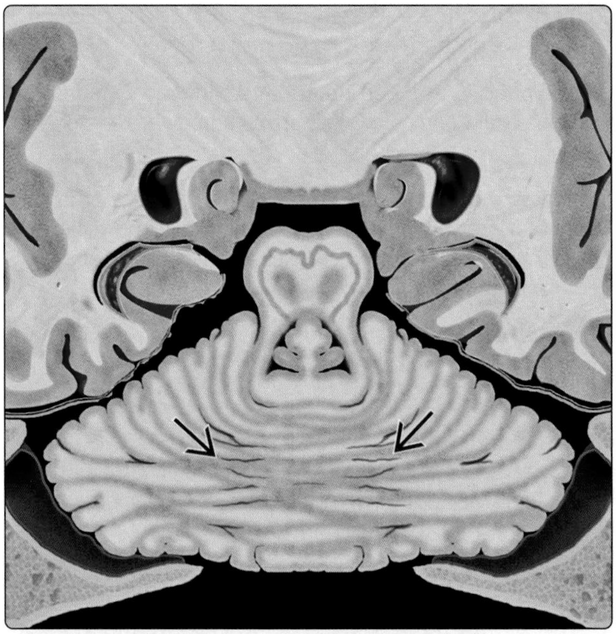

(36-44) Coronal graphic of rhombencephalosynapsis shows that no vermis is present in the midline of the cerebellum. Instead, the folia, interfoliate sulci, and cerebellar white matter ⇨ are continuous across the cerebellar midline.

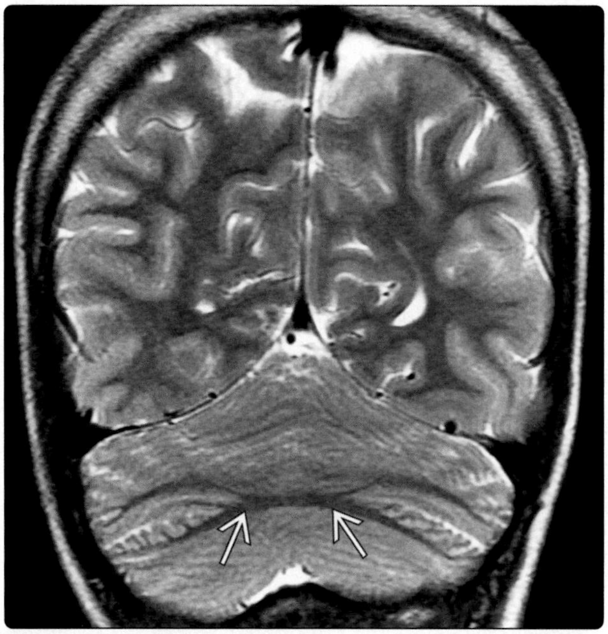

(36-45) Coronal T2WI shows classic rhombencephalosynapsis. Note absent vermis, transversely oriented folia, continuity of cerebellar white matter across the midline ➡.

A **retrocerebellar arachnoid cyst** is not part of DWC. It is a midline arachnoid-lined cyst located behind the vermis and fourth ventricle that does not communicate with the latter. Although there may be mass effect on the cerebellum, there is no associated hydrocephalus and no communication with the 4th ventricle. The cerebellum otherwise appears normal. Veins and a falx cerebelli do not traverse the CSF collection.

In the absence of other findings, a prominent **retrocerebellar CSF collection** > 10 mm with crossing vessels and a traversing falx cerebelli is most often a mega cisterna magna (MCM), a normal variant that is of no clinical significance.

Miscellaneous Malformations

A number of less common PF malformations occur. We now discuss several of those in which the abnormalities are largely defined by imaging features: rhombencephalosynapsis, Joubert syndrome, cerebellar hypoplasias, and unclassified dysplasias.

Rhombencephalosynapsis

Terminology. Rhombencephalosynapsis is a midline brain malformation characterized by (1) a "missing" cerebellar vermis and (2) apparent fusion of the cerebellar hemispheres **(36-44)**.

Pathology. Severity ranges from mild (partial absence of the nodulus and anterior and posterior vermis) to complete (the entire vermis, including the nodulus, is absent). Dorsal midline continuity of the cerebellar hemispheres is characteristic. The tonsils, dentate nuclei, and superior cerebellar peduncles are usually fused.

Clinical Issues. Rhombencephalosynapsis can be seen in patients with **VACTERL** (**v**ertebral anomalies, **a**nal atresia, **c**ardiovascular anomalies, **t**racheo**e**sophageal fistulas, **r**enal anomalies, and **l**imb defects).

Imaging. Sagittal MR scans show an upwardly rounded fastigial recess of the fourth ventricle and lack of the normal midline foliar pattern of the vermis. Coronal and axial images show transverse folia and continuity of the cerebellar white matter across the midline **(36-45)**. Images through the rostral fourth ventricle may demonstrate a diamond or pointed shape.

Aqueductal stenosis and hydrocephalus are common. Absent cavum septi pellucidi is seen in half of all cases. The thalami, fornices, and tectum may be partially or completely fused. Other forebrain anomalies include absent olfactory bulbs and corpus callosum dysgenesis.

Joubert Syndrome and Related Disorders

Terminology and Classification. Joubert syndrome (JS) and related disorders (JSRD) are a group of syndromes in which the obligatory hallmark is the "molar tooth" sign, a complex mid- and hindbrain malformation that resembles a molar tooth on axial MR scans.

Anomalies of the kidneys, eyes, extremities, liver, and bile ducts are common in the JSRD spectrum. Six major JSRD phenotypic subgroups are recognized: pure JS, JS with ocular defect, JS with renal defect, JS with oculo-renal defects, JS with hepatic defect, and JS with oro-facio-digital defects.

Classic JS is the "pure" syndrome. The oculo-renal form is termed CORS (**c**erebello-**o**culo-**r**enal **s**yndrome). JS with preaxial or mesoaxial polydactyly and orofacial defects is known as type 6 **o**ro-**f**acial-**d**igital syndrome (OFD-6). COACH syndrome consists of **c**erebellar vermis hypoplasia, **o**ligophrenia, **a**taxia, **o**cular **c**oloboma, and **h**epatic fibrosis.

Etiology. With the exception of rare X-linked recessive cases, JSRD follows autosomal-recessive inheritance. Mutations in at least 10 affected genes that help regulate normal axon growth and decussation have been identified in JS and JSRD.

JSRD is genetically heterogeneous. Molar tooth disorders are, at least in part, "ciliopathies" with mutations of ciliary/centrosomal proteins that affect cell migration.

Pathology. JSRD is characterized grossly by a dysmorphic vermis with sagittal clefting, nondecussating enlarged superior cerebellar peduncles, and an elongated rounded fastigium of the fourth ventricle **(36-46)** **(36-47)**. The anteroposterior diameter of the midbrain is reduced. Microscopically, dysplasias and heterotopias of the cerebellar nuclei are common.

Clinical Issues. The estimated incidence of JSRD is 1:80,000-100,000 live births. There is no sex predilection.

JSRD typically presents in infancy and childhood. Coloboma, encephalocele, and polydactyly are commonly associated with JSRD.

The classic clinical presentation is a child with developmental delay, ataxia, and oculomotor and respiratory abnormalities. Nystagmus, alternating hyperapnea and hyperpnea, and seizures are common.

Imaging. Axial NECT scans demonstrate vermian clefting and an oddly shaped fourth ventricle with a "bat wing" configuration.

MR is the cornerstone in establishing a diagnosis of JSRD. Midline sagittal scans show a small dysmorphic vermis. The fourth ventricle appears deformed with a thin upwardly

(36-46) Axial graphic shows Joubert malformation. Thickened superior cerebellar peduncles → around an elongated 4th ventricle form the classic "molar tooth" sign. Note cleft cerebellar vermis →. (36-47) Autopsy specimen of JSRD shows foreshortened midbrain with narrowed isthmus →, thick superior cerebellar peduncles →, "bat wing" 4th ventricle →, and clefted superior vermis ➡. (Courtesy R. Hewlett, MD.)

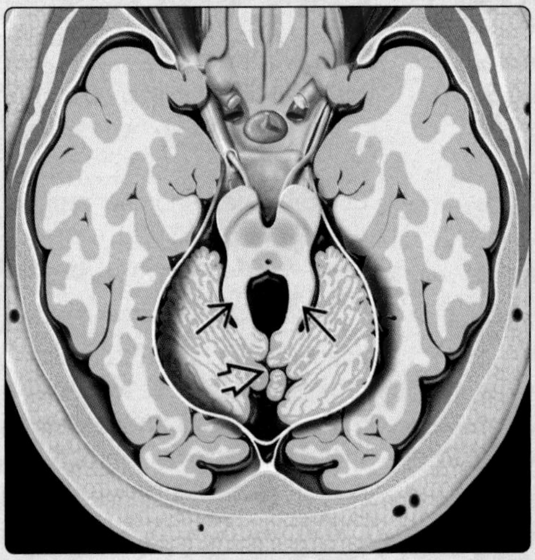

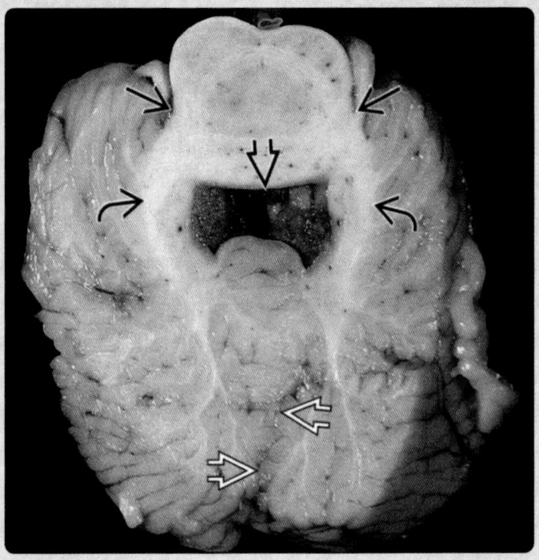

(36-48A) Sagittal T2WI in a patient with classic Joubert shows small misshapen vermis ➡, upwardly convex superior fourth ventricle →, and rounded enlarged fastigial point ➡. (36-48B) Axial scan in the same patient shows "molar tooth" sign, foreshortened midbrain with narrow isthmus ➡, thick superior cerebellar peduncles ➡ surrounding an elongated fourth ventricle, and disorganized cleft vermis ➡.

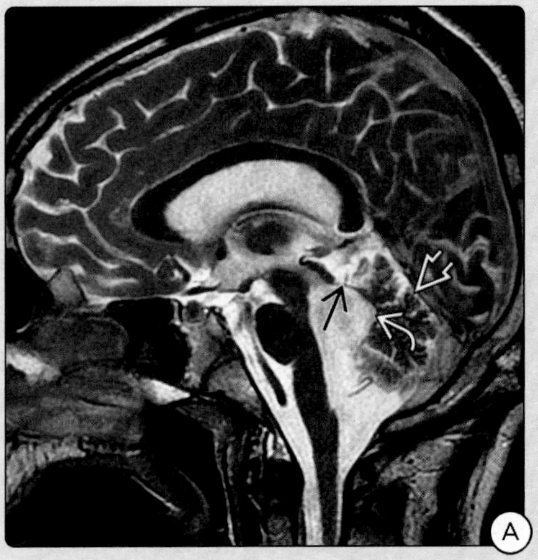

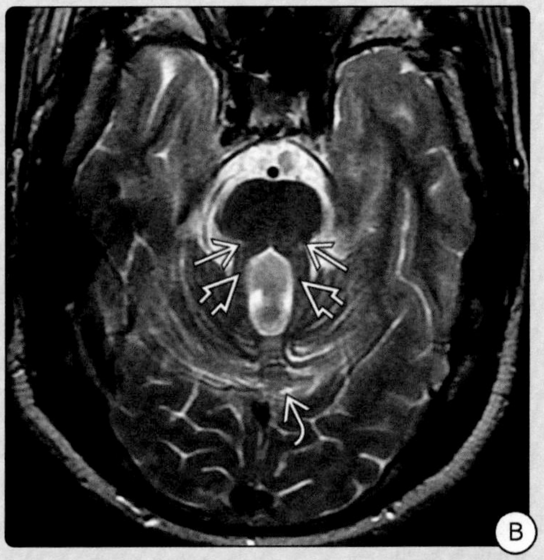

convex roof and loss of the normal pointed fastigium **(36-48A)**.

Axial scans demonstrate the classic "molar tooth" appearance with foreshortened midbrain, narrow isthmus, deep interpeduncular fossa, and thickened superior cerebellar peduncles surrounding an oblong or diamond-shaped fourth ventricle. The superior vermis is clefted, and the cisterna magna may appear enlarged **(36-48B)**.

DTI shows that fibers of the superior cerebellar peduncles do not decussate in the mesencephalon and that the corticospinal tracts fail to cross in the caudal medulla.

Differential Diagnosis. The major imaging differential diagnosis of JSRD is **vermian and pontocerebellar hypoplasia**, in which the vermis is small but is not clefted. In **rhombencephalosynapsis**, the cerebellar hemispheres and dentate nuclei are fused across the midline, not split.

Multiple syndromes exhibit "molar tooth" posterior fossa malformations. Genetic analysis may be required to distinguish among different JSRD subtypes.

Cerebellar Hypoplasia and Unclassified Dysplasias

In severe cases of cerebellar hypoplasia, the cerebellar hemispheres and vermis are almost completely absent, and the pons is hypoplastic **(36-49)**.

Unclassified cerebellar dysplasias are not associated with other known malformations or syndromes such as molar tooth malformation or Dandy-Walker continuum. A variety of findings including enlarged, vertically oriented fissures or clefts **(36-50)**, disordered or primitive foliation, lack of normal white matter arborization, gray matter heterotopias, and small cyst-like cavities in the subcortical white matter are some of the many abnormalities seen in such cases **(36-51)**.

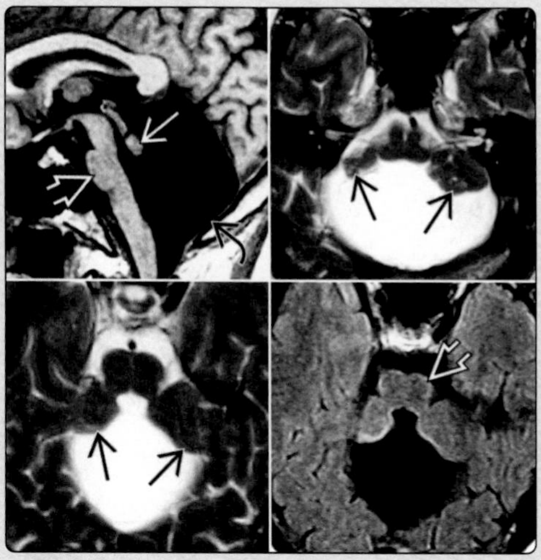

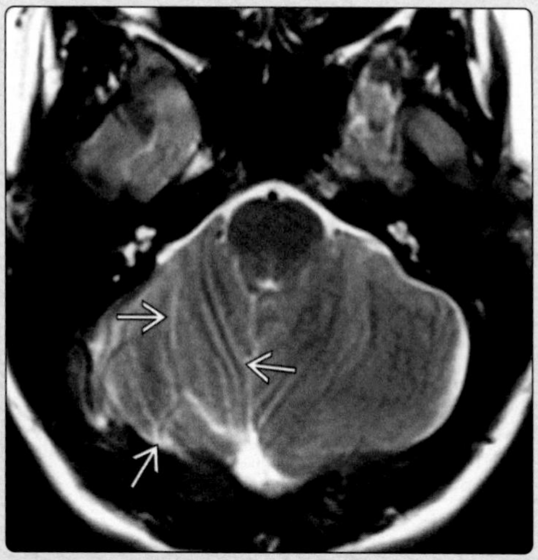

***(36-49)** Extreme cerebellar hypoplasia is seen with small brainstem ➡, nearly "empty" appearing but normal-sized PF ➡, tiny nubbins of vermian ➡, and cerebellar remnants ➡. **(36-50)** Axial T2WI of a patient with unclassified cerebellar dysplasia shows several clefts ➡ with abnormal-appearing and misaligned folia.*

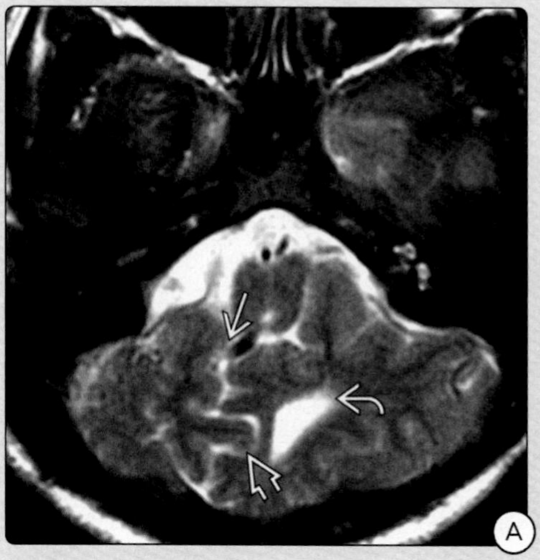

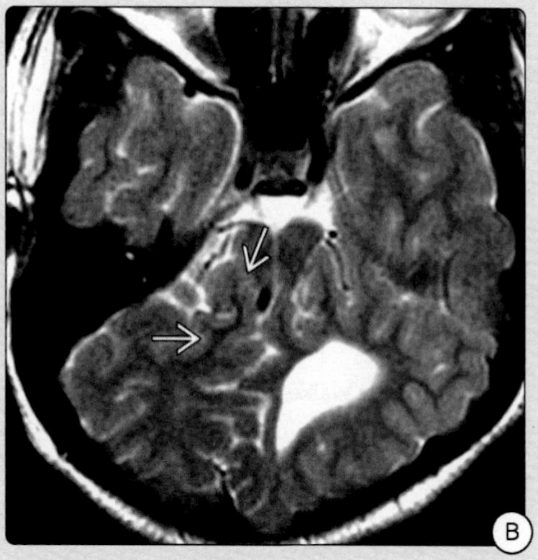

***(36-51A)** Unclassified cerebellar dysplasia is seen with cleft ➡, interdigitating dysplastic folia ➡, and hemispheric cyst ➡. **(36-51B)** More cephalad scan in the same patient shows the cyst, cleft, and appearance of polymicrogyria ➡ in the grossly abnormal folia.*

Hindbrain Malformations: Imaging

	Vermis Position	Vermis Size	Torcular Position	Cerebellar Hemispheres	Fourth Ventricle
Mega cisterna magna	N	N	N	N	N
Blake pouch cyst	Rotated	N	N	N	Enlarged; communicates with posterior fossa via valleculae
Arachnoid cyst	May be displaced	N or compressed	N	N or compressed	N or compressed
Vermian dysgenesis	May be rotated	Small or absent	N	N	Abnormal shape; lacks normal fastigial point
Dandy-Walker malformation	Rotated	Small or absent	Elevated	Often small	Dilated, enlarged; lacks normal fastigial point
Cerebellar hypoplasia	N	Small	N	Small	N or small
Pontocerebellar hypoplasia	N	Small	N	Small	Pontine bulge missing
Cerebellar disruption	N	N or small	N	Asymmetric; one smaller, abnormal structure	Variable depending on part of cerebellum disrupted
Rhombencephalosynapsis	N/A	Absent	N	Fused with continuous horizontal folia	Small; lacks normal fastigial point
Joubert syndrome	N	Small or absent, clefted	N	Small	Large (associated with elongated superior cerebellar peduncles and "molar tooth" sign)

(Table 36-1) *N = normal.*

Selected References

Chiari Malformations

Chiari 1

Abu-Arafeh I et al: Headache, Chiari malformation type 1 and treatment options. Arch Dis Child. 102(3):210-211, 2017

Alperin N et al: Magnetic resonance imaging-based measures predictive of short-term surgical outcome in patients with Chiari malformation type I: a pilot study. J Neurosurg Spine. 26(1):28-38, 2017

Wang J et al: Acquired Chiari malformation and syringomyelia secondary to space-occupying lesions: a systematic review. World Neurosurg. 98:800-808.e2, 2017

Poretti A et al: Chiari type 1 deformity in children: pathogenetic, clinical, neuroimaging, and management aspects. Neuropediatrics. 47(5):293-307, 2016

Chiari Variants

Moore HE et al: Magnetic resonance imaging features of complex Chiari malformation variant of Chiari 1 malformation. Pediatr Radiol. 44(11):1403-11, 2014

Hindbrain Malformations

Cystic Posterior Fossa Anomalies and the Dandy-Walker Continuum

Abdel Razek AA et al: Magnetic resonance imaging of malformations of midbrain-hindbrain. J Comput Assist Tomogr. 40(1):14-25, 2016

Boltshauser E et al: Cerebellar cysts in children: a pattern recognition approach. Cerebellum. 14(3):308-16, 2015

Cotes C et al: Congenital basis of posterior fossa anomalies. Neuroradiol J. 28(3):238-53, 2015

Nelson MD Jr et al: A different approach to cysts of the posterior fossa. Pediatr Radiol. 34(9):720-32, 2004

Miscellaneous Malformations

Poretti A et al: Joubert syndrome: neuroimaging findings in 110 patients in correlation with cognitive function and genetic cause. J Med Genet. ePub, 2017

Abdel Razek AA et al: Magnetic resonance imaging of malformations of midbrain-hindbrain. J Comput Assist Tomogr. 40(1):14-25, 2016

Poretti A et al: Cerebellar and brainstem malformations. Neuroimaging Clin N Am. 26(3):341-57, 2016

Poretti A et al: Pre- and postnatal neuroimaging of congenital cerebellar abnormalities. Cerebellum. 15(1):5-9, 2016

Poretti A et al: Prenatal cerebellar disruptions: neuroimaging spectrum of findings in correlation with likely mechanisms and etiologies of injury. Neuroimaging Clin N Am. 26(3):359-72, 2016

Poretti A et al: The pediatric cerebellum. Neuroimaging Clin N Am. 26(3):xiii-xiv, 2016

Poretti A et al: Fetal diagnosis of rhombencephalosynapsis. Neuropediatrics. 46(6):357-8, 2015

Poretti A et al: Cerebellar hypoplasia: differential diagnosis and diagnostic approach. Am J Med Genet C Semin Med Genet. 166(2):211-26, 2014

Commissural and Cortical Maldevelopment

Corpus callosum dysgenesis and malformations of cortical development (MCDs) are two of the most important congenital brain anomalies. Anomalies of the cerebral commissures are the most common of all congenital brain malformations, and corpus callosum dysgenesis is the single most common malformation that accompanies other developmental brain anomalies.

Although they affect very different parts of the forebrain, commissural and cortical malformations share a very important feature: they arise when migrating precursor cells fail to reach their target destinations.

We begin this chapter with a brief consideration of normal development and anatomy of the cerebral commissures, then focus on callosal dysgenesis as the most important anomaly that affects these white matter tracts.

We devote the second half of the chapter to MCDs, which are intrinsically epileptogenic and may be responsible for 25-40% of all medically refractory childhood epilepsies. Prior to the development of high-resolution MR techniques, many complex partial epilepsies were considered cryptogenic. Their imaging detection, localization, and characterization have become increasingly important in patient management.

Normal Development and Anatomy of the Cerebral Commissures

In this section, we briefly review normal development of the commissures and then delineate their gross and imaging anatomy.

Normal Development

The telencephalon has three major commissural tracts: the corpus callosum (CC), which is the largest and most prominent, the anterior commissure (AC), and the hippocampal (posterior) commissure (HC). Coordinated transfer of information between the cerebral hemispheres is essential for normal brain function and occurs via these three axonal commissures.

Commissural development is a carefully choreographed process in which axons from cortical neurons are actively guided across the midline to reach their targets in the contralateral hemisphere. The axon-guidance receptor *DCC* **gene** (deleted in colorectal carcinoma) is a master regulator of midline

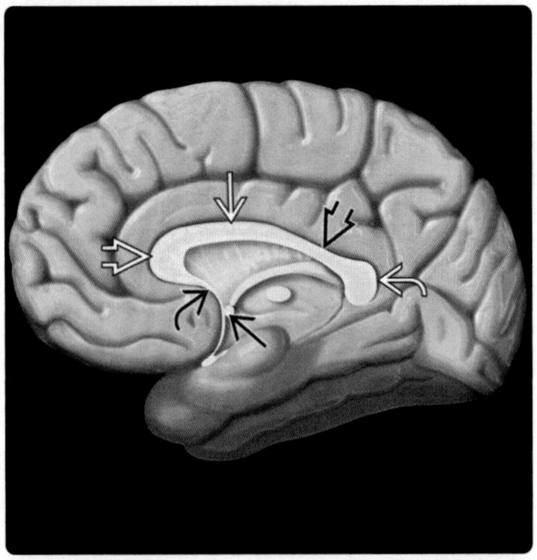

***(37-1)** Graphic shows anterior commissure and corpus callosum segments: rostrum, genu, body, isthmus, and splenium.*

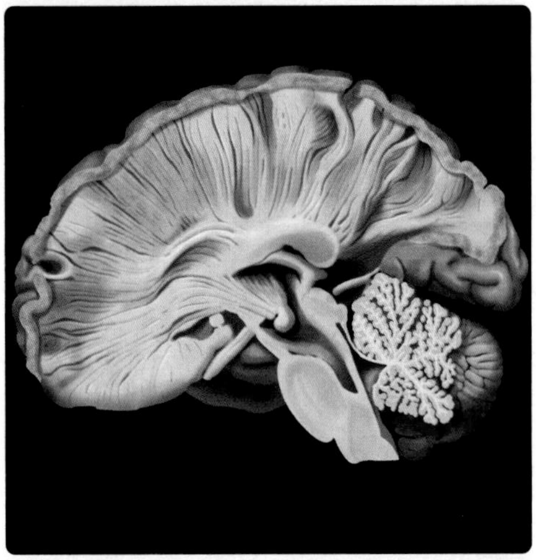

***(37-2)** Sagittal graphic shows white matter tracts of corona radiata converging to form corpus callosum.*

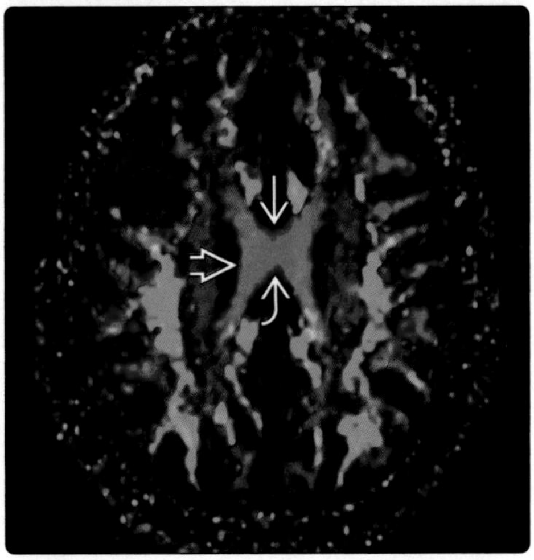

***(37-3)** DTI shows normal red X-shaped corpus callosum formed by the genu with forceps minor, body, splenium with forceps major.*

crossing and normal development of white-matter projections throughout the human CNS.

The AC is the first forebrain commissure to develop (eighth fetal week). The hippocampal commissure (HC) forms posteriorly around week 11 and is followed by axons that eventually become the posterior body and splenium of the CC.

The CC forms in two separate segments. Between 13 and 14 fetal weeks, anterior axons cross a guiding structure called the glial sling, while others follow the HC posteriorly. The genu, rostrum, and body appear in rapid succession; the splenium does not form until 18-19 weeks. Fiber bundles in the anterior and posterior callosum eventually unite to form a single continuous structure, the definitive corpus callosum.

At birth, the CC is very thin and relatively flat in gross appearance. It continues to grow for several postnatal months. As myelination proceeds, the genu and splenium thicken noticeably. Both the length and thickness of the CC also increase. By 10 months of age, the overall appearance resembles that of a normal adult.

Normal Gross and Imaging Anatomy

Corpus Callosum

The CC is the largest and most important of the forebrain commissures. It is composed of five parts. From front to back, these are the rostrum, genu, body, isthmus, and splenium. The **rostrum** is the smallest segment and connects the orbital surfaces of the frontal lobes. A prominent anterior "knee"—the **genu**—connects the lateral and medial frontal lobes **(37-1)**. White matter fibers curve anterolaterally from the genu into the frontal lobes as the forceps minor.

The longest CC segment is the **body** (also called the truncus or trunk). Its fibers pass laterally and intersect with projection fibers of the corona radiata. The body connects broad regions of each hemispheric cortex together and forms a red *X* on axial DTI scans **(37-3)**.

The **isthmus** is a shorter, slightly narrower area that lies between the posterior body and splenium. The isthmus connects the pre- and postcentral gyri and auditory cortex with their counterparts in the contralateral hemisphere. The **splenium** is the expanded, rounded termination of the CC. Most of its fibers curve posterolaterally into the occipital lobes **(37-2)** as the **forceps major.**

Sagittal T1 and T2 scans demonstrate the rostrum as a thin WM tract that curves posteroinferiorly from the genu. The dorsal CC surface is typically not straight but has a slightly "wavy" appearance with a distinct posterior narrowing—the isthmus—just before the CC widens again into the splenium **(37-4)**.

Coronal scans show the CC curving from side to side across the midline. Anteriorly, the genu is seen as a continuous band of WM connecting the frontal lobes. More posteriorly, the CC lies above the fornices. Bands of WM fibers fan outward from the splenium into the forceps major.

Anterior Commissure

The AC is a transversely oriented bundle of compact, heavily myelinated fibers that crosses the midline anterior to the fornix. It is much smaller than the CC but is a crucial anatomic landmark for stereotactic neurosurgery.

The AC lies in the anterior wall of the third ventricle **(37-5)**. From the midline, it curves laterally in the basal forebrain and splits into two fascicles.

The smaller more anterior bundle courses toward the orbitofrontal cortex and olfactory tract. The much larger posterior bundle splays out into the temporal lobe. The AC connects the anterior parts of the temporal lobes **(37-6)** and lies anterosuperior to the temporal horn of the lateral ventricle.

On sagittal T1 scans, the AC is seen as a hyperintense ovoid structure lying midway up the anterior wall of the third ventricle. On axial T2 scans, the AC can be identified as a compact well-defined hypointense band of tissue lying just in front of the third ventricle. As it courses laterally, both sides of the AC curve slightly anteriorly to resemble an archer's bow on axial MR scans.

Hippocampal Commissure

The HC is the smallest of the three major commissures. It is a transversely oriented fiber bundle that crosses the midline in the posterior pineal lamina.

In contrast to the CC and AC, the HC is less easily distinguished on MR scans. In the midline sagittal plane, its myelinated fibers blend imperceptibly with those of the inferomedial WM in the CC splenium. On coronal scans through the lateral ventricle atria, the HC can be seen lying below the CC, where its fibers blend in with those of the fornices.

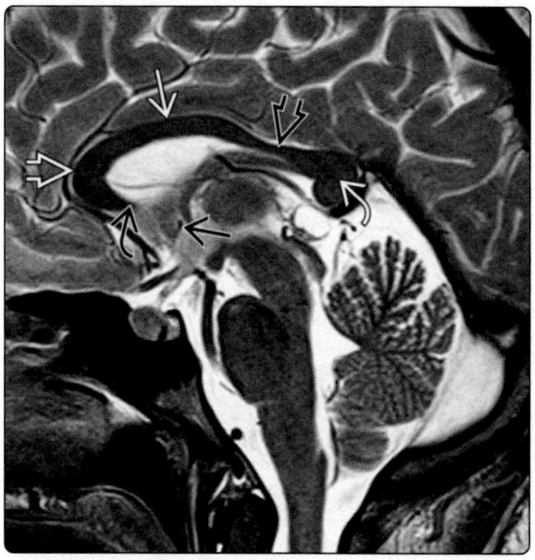

***(37-4)** Sagittal T2WI shows anterior commissure (AC) ➡, rostrum ➡, genu ➡, body ➡, isthmus ➡, and splenium ➡ of CC.*

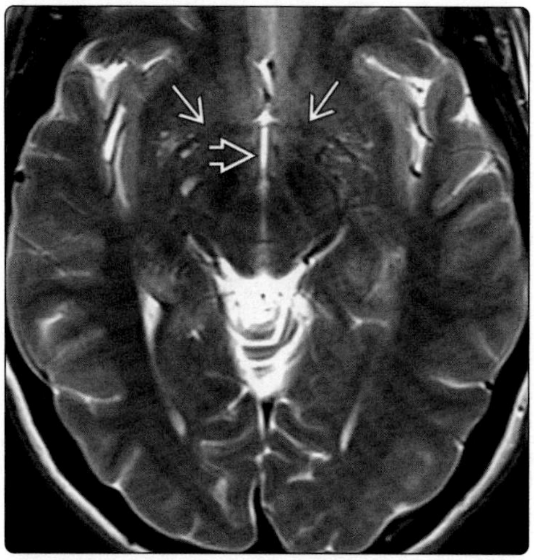

***(37-5)** Axial T2WI shows the compact, hypointense, bow-shaped AC ➡ passing in front of the third ventricle ➡.*

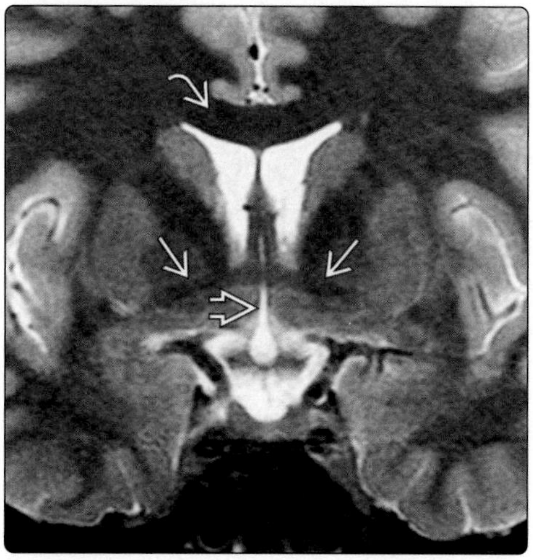

***(37-6)** Coronal T2WI shows the AC ➡, third ventricle ➡, and body of the corpus callosum ➡.*

Commissural Anomalies

Any one of or combination of the three forebrain commissures can be affected by developmental failures. Recognizing the surprisingly broad spectrum of commissural malformations and delineating any associated abnormalities is essential for accurate and complete diagnosis.

We now discuss corpus callosum malformations together with some representative syndromes and associated lesions.

Callosal Dysgenesis Spectrum

Terminology

The corpus callosum (CC) can be completely absent (agenesis) **(37-7)** **(37-8)** or partially formed (hypogenesis). **Complete CC agenesis** is almost always accompanied by the absence of the hippocampal commissure (HC). The anterior commissure (AC), which forms 3 weeks earlier than the CC, is usually present and normal. If the CC is hypogenetic, the posterior segments and the inferior genu and rostrum are usually absent.

Pathology

In *complete* CC agenesis, all five segments are missing. The **cingulate gyrus** is absent on sagittal sections, whereas the hemispheres demonstrate a radiating **"spoke-wheel" gyral pattern** extending perpendicularly to the roof of the third ventricle **(37-9)**.

On coronal sections, the **"high-riding" third ventricle** looks as if it opens directly into the interhemispheric fissure. It is actually covered by a thin membranous roof that bulges into the interhemispheric fissure, displacing the fornices laterally. The lateral ventricles have upturned, pointed corners **(37-8)**.

A prominent longitudinal WM tract called the **Probst bundle** is situated just inside the apex of each ventricle **(37-7)**. These bundles consist of the misdirected commissural fibers, which should have crossed the midline but instead course from front to back, indenting the medial walls of the lateral ventricles.

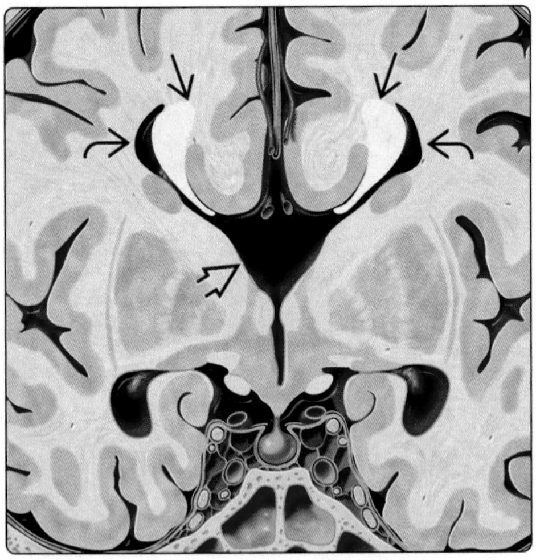

(37-7) Agenesis of CC (ACC) shows "Viking helmet," "high-riding" 3rd ventricle ➡, pointed lateral ventricles ➡, and Probst bundles ➡.

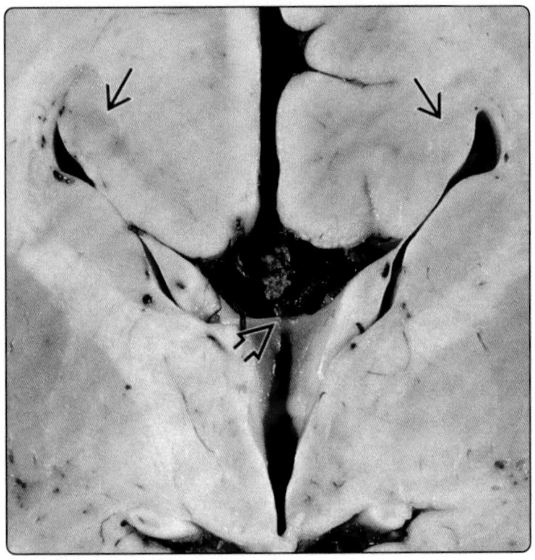

(37-8) Coronal autopsy of coronal agenesis shows thin third ventricle roof ➡, Probst bundles ➡. (Courtesy J. Townsend, MD.)

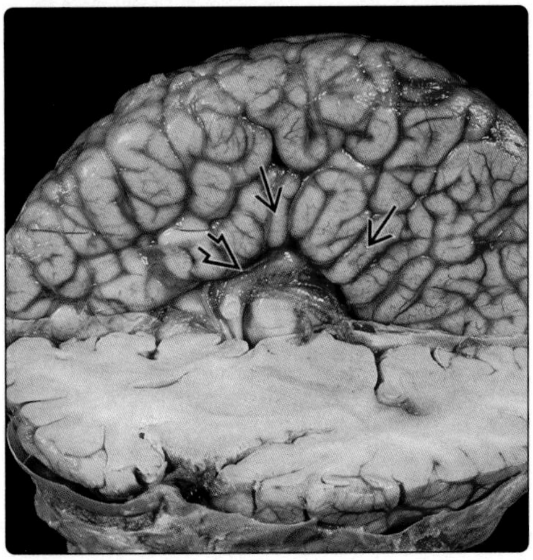

(37-9) ACC in Aicardi syndrome shows "radiating" gyri ➡ converging on "high-riding" third ventricle ➡. (Courtesy R. Hewlett, MD.)

The septi pellucidi often appear absent but actually have widely separated leaves that course laterally—not vertically—from the fornices to the Probst bundles.

Axial sections show that the lateral ventricles are parallel and nonconverging. The occipital horns are often disproportionately dilated, a condition termed colpocephaly.

The gross pathology of CC *hypogenesis* varies according to which segments are missing. The splenium is usually small or absent.

Clinical Issues

Epidemiology and Demographics. CC dysgenesis is the most common CNS malformation and is found in 3-5% of individuals with neurodevelopmental disorders. It has a prevalence of at least 1:4,000 live births. Nonsyndromic CC dysgenesis is found in patients of all ages.

Presentation. Minor CC dysgenesis/hypogenesis is often discovered incidentally on imaging studies or at autopsy. Major commissural malformations are associated with seizures, developmental delay, and symptoms secondary to disruptions of the hypothalamic-pituitary axis.

CALLOSAL DYSGENESIS: PATHOETIOLOGY AND CLINICAL ISSUES

Terminology
- Complete absence of corpus callosum (CC) = agenesis
  - Hippocampal commissure (HC) absent
  - Anterior commissure (AC) often present
  - All 3 absent = tricommissural agenesis
- Hypogenetic, dysgenetic CC
  - Rostrum, splenium often absent in partial agenesis
  - Partial posterior agenesis = HC, splenium, ± posterior body

Etiology and Pathology
- Embryonic guiding mechanisms fail
  - Axons may fail to form
  - Molecular guidance fails
  - Glial sling and/or HC fail to develop normally
  - Failure to guide axons across midline
- Multiple genes implicated

Clinical Issues
- Most common CNS malformation
- Found in 3-5% of neurodevelopmental disorders

Imaging

CT Findings. Axial NECT scans show parallel, nonconverging, widely separated lateral ventricles. Disproportionate enlargement of the occipital horns is common.

MR Findings. Sagittal T1 and T2 scans best demonstrate complete CC absence or partial dysgenesis.

Complete Corpus Callosum Agenesis. With complete agenesis, the third ventricle appears continuous with the interhemispheric fissure and is surrounded dorsally by fingers of radiating gyri that "point" toward the third ventricle **(37-10)**.

A midline interhemispheric cyst may be present above the third ventricle. Such cysts can be ventricular outpouchings or separate structures that do not communicate with the ventricular system.

An azygous anterior cerebral artery (ACA) can be seen "wandering" upward in the interhemispheric fissure. Look for associated malformations of the eyes, hindbrain, and hypothalamic-pituitary axis.

Axial scans demonstrate the parallel lateral ventricles especially well. The prominent myelinated tracts of the Probst bundles can appear quite prominent **(37-14)**.

Coronal scans show a "Viking helmet" or "moose head" appearance caused by the curved, upwardly pointed lateral ventricles and "high-riding" third ventricle that expands into the interhemispheric fissure. The Probst bundles are seen as densely myelinated tracts lying just inside the lateral ventricle bodies. The hippocampi appear abnormally rounded and vertically oriented. Moderately enlarged temporal horns are common. Look for malformations such as heterotopic gray matter **(37-13)**.

DTI is especially helpful in depicting CC agenesis. The normal red (right-to-left encoded) color of the corpus callosum is absent. Instead, prominent front-to-back (green) tracts of the Probst bundles are seen **(37-15)**.

Corpus Callosum Hypogenesis. In partial agenesis, the rostrum and splenium are usually absent **(37-11)**, and the remaining genu and body often have a "blocky," thickened appearance **(37-12)**. The hippocampal commissure is typically absent, but the AC is generally preserved and often appears quite normal or even larger than usual.

Angiography. In complete CC agenesis, CTA, DSA, and MRA demonstrate an azygous ACA that courses directly upward within the interhemispheric fissure **(37-16B)**.

Differential Diagnosis

The major differential diagnosis of CC dysgenesis is destruction caused by **trauma, surgery (callosotomy)**, or **ischemia**. Occasionally, if the **hippocampal commissure** forms but the CC is absent, the HC may mimic a remnant portion of the CC on sagittal images. Coronal views show that the HC connects the fornices, not the hemispheres.

CALLOSAL DYSGENESIS: IMAGING AND DDx

Sagittal
- Partial or complete CC agenesis
- Third ventricle appears "open" to interhemispheric fissure
- Cingulate gyrus absent → gyri "radiate" outward from third ventricle

Axial
- Lateral ventricles parallel, nonconverging, widely separated
- Probst bundles = WM along medial margins of lateral ventricles

Coronal
- "Viking helmet" or "moose head" appearance
- "High-riding" third ventricle
- Pointed, upcurving lateral ventricles
- Probst bundles

Differential Diagnosis
- Corpus callosum present but damaged
    - Trauma
    - Surgery (callosotomy)
    - Ischemia (rare)

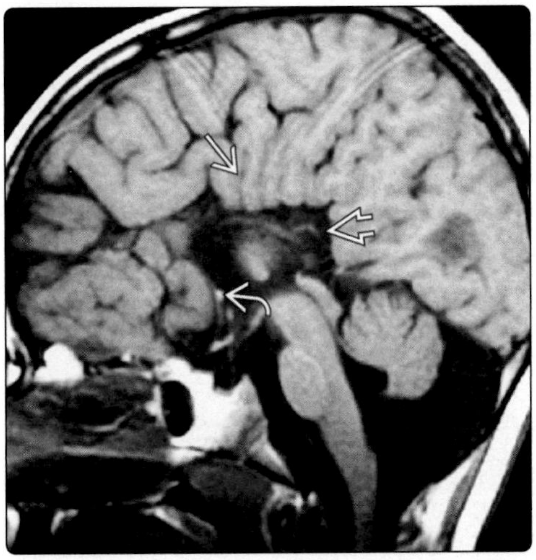

***(37-10)** "Spoke-wheel" gyri ➡ converge on third ventricle ➡. Anterior commissure is normal ➡. Hippocampal commissure is absent. This is ACC.*

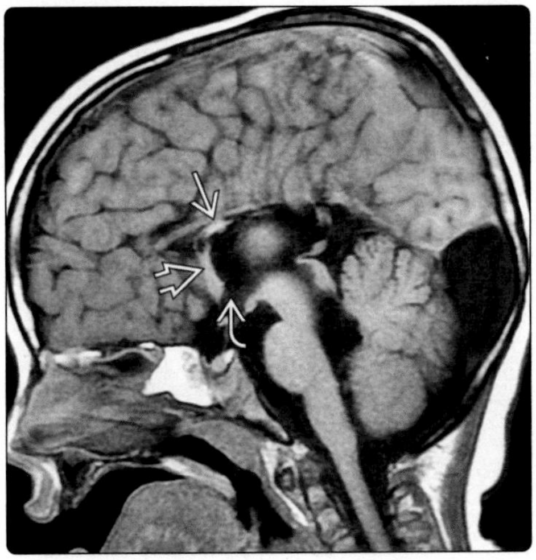

***(37-11)** Genu ➡, remnant of body ➡ are present. Rostrum ➡, splenium are absent. This is CC hypogenesis.*

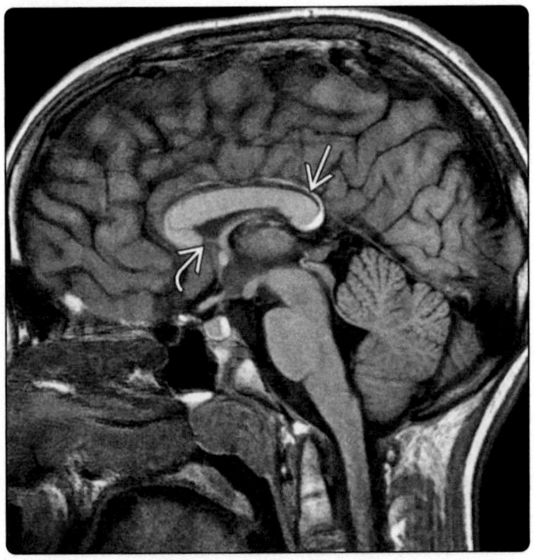

***(37-12)** CC appears short and "blocky" with absent rostrum ➡, tapered splenium with curvilinear lipoma ➡; mild callosal hypogenesis.*

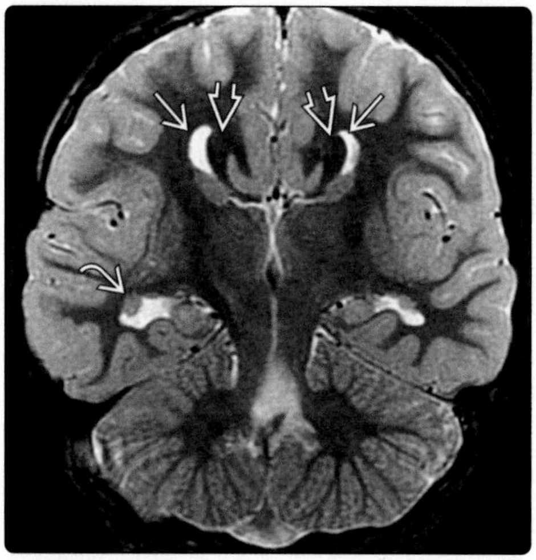

(37-13) Coronal T2WI shows "Viking helmet" of ACC with curving, upturned lateral ventricles, Probst bundles, and heterotopic GM.

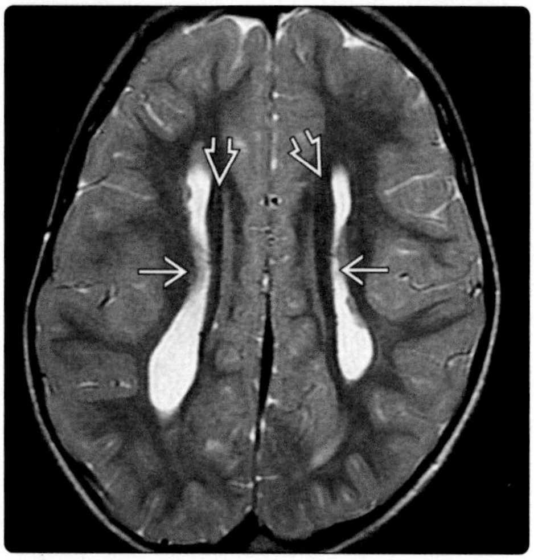

(37-14) Axial scan shows parallel, "nonconverging" lateral ventricles and Probst bundles.

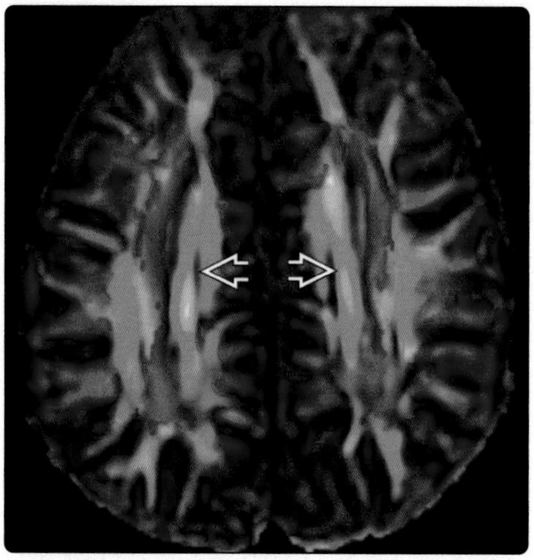

(37-15) Axial DTI shows absence of normal red X-shaped corpus callosum. Probst bundles are green, indicating anterior-to-posterior course.

Associated Anomalies and Syndromes

The corpus callosum (CC) forms at the same time the cerebral hemispheres and cerebellum are undergoing rapid changes. Neuronal migration also peaks during the same period. Although CC dysgenesis can occur as an isolated phenomenon, it is not surprising that—of all the malformations—CC anomalies are the single most common malformation associated with other CNS anomalies and syndromes.

Malformations Associated With Callosal Dysgenesis

Chiari 2 malformation, Dandy-Walker spectrum, frontonasal dysplasia, median cleft face syndromes, syndromic **craniosynostoses, hypothalamic-pituitary** anomalies, **cerebellar hypoplasia/dysplasia**, and **malformations of cortical development** all have an increased prevalence of CC anomalies. CC agenesis and regional increases in cortical thickness are the most common brain morphologic defects in **fetal alcohol syndrome**.

Genetic Conditions With Callosal Involvement

Anomalies of the cerebral commissures have been described in nearly 200 different syndromes! A few of the more striking examples are included here.

Aicardi Syndrome. Aicardi syndrome is an X-linked neurodevelopmental disorder associated with severe cognitive and motor impairment. It occurs almost exclusively in female patients and is defined by the diagnostic triad of CC dysgenesis, chorioretinal lacunae, and infantile spasms. Other common associated abnormalities are polymicrogyria, periventricular and subcortical heterotopic gray matter, and choroid plexus papillomas.

Callosal agenesis or hypogenesis—often with interhemispheric cysts—is the most common anatomic abnormality in Aicardi syndrome **(37-16)**. DTI in patients with Aicardi syndrome shows gross deficits in white matter organization, with absence of multiple major corticocortical association WM tracts such as the left arcuate fasciculus.

Apert Syndrome. Apert syndrome is also called acrocephalosyndactylia type 1. Apert syndrome is characterized by craniostenosis, mid-face hypoplasia, and symmetric syndactylia of the hands and feet. Associated CNS malformations are frequent; the most common are CC or septi pellucidi hypoplasias.

CRASH Syndrome. CRASH syndrome—also known as **X-linked hydrocephalus** and hereditary stenosis of the aqueduct of Sylvius—is a rare inherited disorder characterized by **c**orpus callosum hypoplasia, mental **r**etardation, **a**dducted thumbs, **s**pastic paraplegia, and **h**ydrocephalus. CRASH is caused by mutation in the gene (*L1CAM*) that regulates the L1 cell adhesion molecule, which plays an essential role in normal development of the CNS.

L1CAM mutations cause neurological alterations, including severe intellectual disabilities summarized as **L1 syndrome**.

22q11.2 Deletion Syndrome. The 22q11.2 deletion syndrome (22qDS) is also known as **DiGeorge syndrome**. Atypical facial morphometry, obsessive-compulsive disorder, autistic spectrum disorder, and other psychological disturbances are common in patients with 22qDS. Many patients have an abnormally large, misshapen CC.

Williams Syndrome. Williams syndrome (WS) is caused by a microdeletion of genes on locus 7q11.23, which is crucial for neuronal migration and maturation. Overall brain size is reduced, and some degree of CC dysgenesis is typical. The CC in WS is smaller or shorter than normal with a less concave shape.

Fragile X Syndrome. Fragile X syndrome is an X-linked disorder caused by the expansion of a single trinucleotide gene sequence (CGG) on the X chromosome and the most common inherited cause of mental retardation in boys. The CC is generally thinned but present.

Morning Glory Syndrome. Morning glory syndrome is a rare optic disc anomaly named for its characteristic appearance on funduscopic examination. A wide funnel-shaped excavation of the optic disc **(37-17)** with whitish central gliosis is surrounded by retinal vessels that emerge from the disc periphery. CNS findings include retinal coloboma **(37-18)**, scleral staphyloma, optic nerve cyst, and midline disorders such as CC dysgenesis, basal encephalocele, and frontonasal dysplasia.

MALFORMATIONS AND SYNDROMES ASSOCIATED WITH CALLOSAL DYSGENESIS

Malformations
- Chiari 2
- Dandy-Walker
- Frontonasal dysplasia, clefts
- Cerebellar hypoplasia/dysplasia
- Hypothalamic-pituitary axis malformations
- Malformations of cortical development
- Malformations

Inherited Syndromes (> 200)
- Aicardi syndrome
- Apert syndrome
- CRASH syndrome
- 22q11.2 deletion syndrome (DiGeorge)
- Morning glory syndrome

Thick Corpus Callosum

An congenitally thick corpus callosum ("mega" corpus callosum) is an extremely rare condition. Only a few genetic disorders are associated with mega corpus callosum **(37-19)**. Reported syndromes include neurofibromatosis type 1 (NF1), FG syndrome, and Cohen syndrome. A constellation of findings designated megalencephaly-polymicrogyria-mega-corpus callosum syndrome is recognized as an Online Mendelian Inheritance in Man disorder (OMIM 603387).

Malformations of Cortical Development Overview

Three Stages of Malformations

The umbrella term malformations of cortical development (MCD) is used to denote a heterogeneous group of focal or diffuse lesions that develop during cortical ontogenesis.

The three major stages of cortical development are **proliferation, neuronal migration**, and **postmigrational development**. These stages have some overlap; proliferation continues after neuronal migration starts, and postmigrational development (e.g., process of cortical organization) begins before neuronal migration ends. In addition, cells resulting from abnormal proliferation often neither migrate nor organize properly.

Barkovich et al. suggest classifying MCDs according to which of the three development stages is primarily affected. Group I consists of **abnormalities**

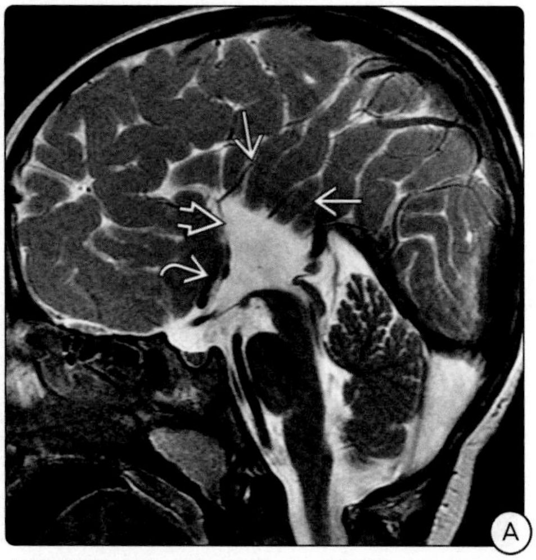

(37-16A) Sagittal T2WI in Aicardi shows ACC with absent cingulate gyrus, "high-riding" third ventricle ➡, radiating gyri ➡, azygous ACA ➡.

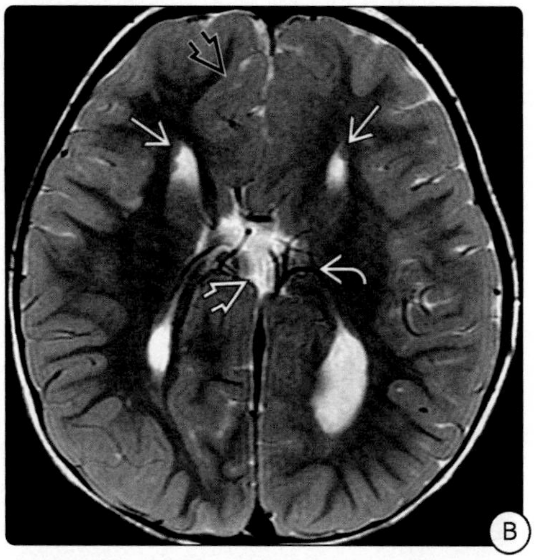

(37-16B) Axial T2WI shows interhemispheric cyst ➡, azygous ACA ➡, parallel lateral ventricles, heterotopic GM ➡, and pachygyria ➡.

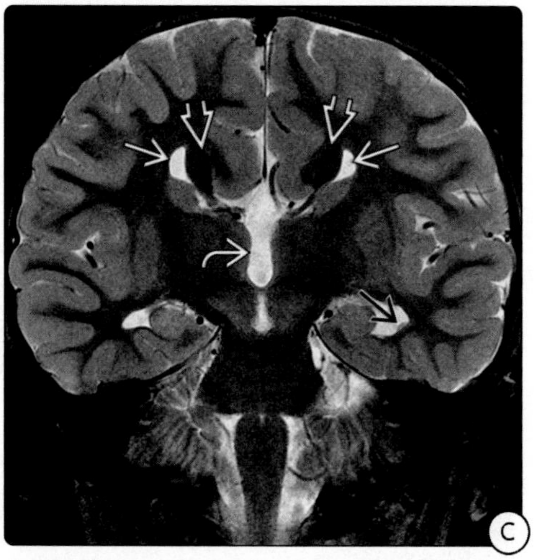

(37-16C) Coronal T2WI has "moose head," high-riding 3rd ventricle ➡, pointed lateral ventricles ➡, Probst bundles ➡, and heterotopic GM ➡.

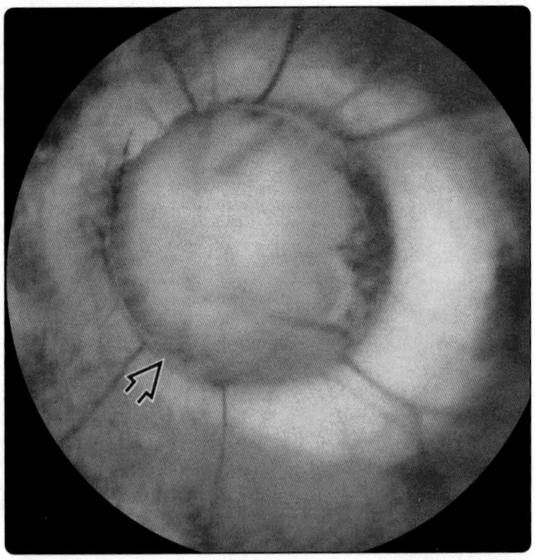

(37-17) Funduscopic photograph shows morning glory syndrome with enlarged, cup-shaped optic disc ⇒. (From Diagnostic Ophthalmology.)

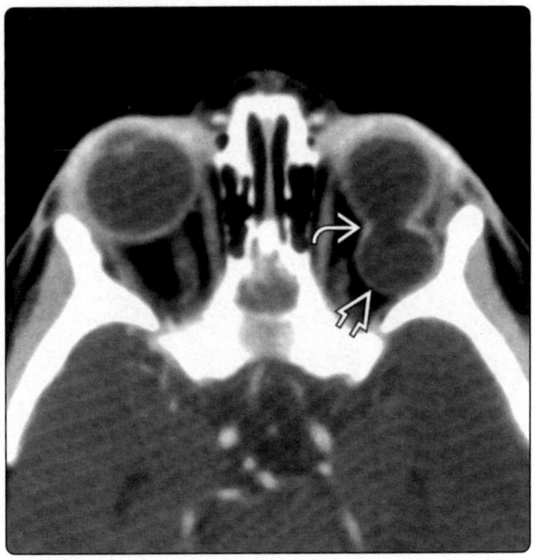

(37-18) CECT shows coloboma ➡ with dehiscence of posterior globe through large optic disc ➡. (From Diagnostic Ophthalmology.)

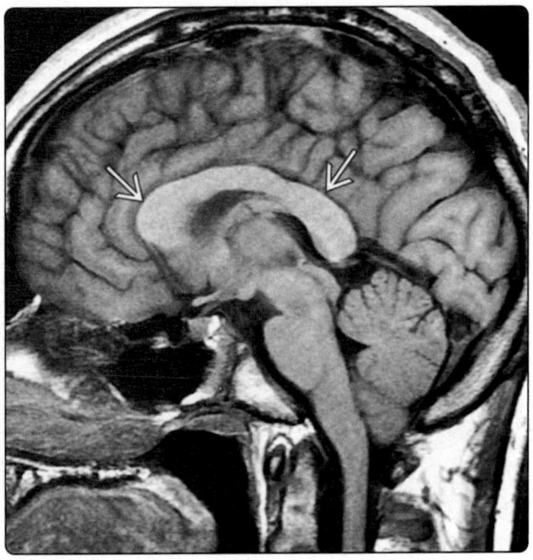

(37-19) Sagittal T1WI shows thickened corpus callosum ➡ in FG syndrome, an X-linked disorder with hypotonia and intellectual disabilities.

of neuronal and glial proliferation or apoptosis (resulting in either too many or too few cells). Three subcategories reflect malformations due to (A) reduced proliferation or accelerated apoptosis (congenital microcephalies), (B) increased proliferation or decreased apoptosis (megalencephalies), and (C) abnormal proliferation (focal and diffuse dysgenesis and dysplasia).

Group II represents **abnormalities of neuronal migration** and has been divided into four subgroups: (A) abnormalities in the neuroependyma during initiation of migration cause periventricular nodular heterotopia; (B) lissencephalies are caused by *generalized* abnormalities of transmantle migration; (C) *localized* abnormalities of transmantle migration result in subcortical heterotopia; and (D) terminal migration anomalies and defects in the pial limiting membranes result in cobblestone malformations.

MALFORMATIONS OF CORTICAL DEVELOPMENT

I. Malformations Secondary to Glial/Neuronal Proliferation or Apoptosis

- A. Microcephaly
- B. Megalencephaly
    - Polymicrogyria and megalencephaly
- C. Cortical dysgeneses with abnormal cell proliferation
    - Cortical tubers
    - Focal cortical dysplasia (FCD IIb, Taylor type)
    - Hemimegalencephaly

II. Malformations Secondary to Abnormalities of Neuronal Migration

- A. Heterotopia
    - Periventricular nodular heterotopia
- B. Lissencephaly spectrum
    - Agyria
    - Pachygyria
    - Subcortical band heterotopia
- C. Subcortical heterotopia and sublobar dysplasia
    - Large focal collections of neurons in deep WM
- D. Cobblestone malformations
    - Congenital muscular dystrophies

III. Abnormalities of Postmigrational Development

- A. Polymicrogyria
- B. Schizencephaly
- C. Focal cortical dysplasia (types I and III)
- D. Postmigrational microcephaly

Abnormalities of **postmigrational development** comprise group III. These result from injury to the cortex during later stages and are associated with prenatal and perinatal insults.

Malformations With Abnormal Cell Numbers/Types

Microcephalies

Microcephaly (MCPH), which literally means "small head," can be primary (genetic) or secondary (nongenetic).

Primary MCPH is a congenital malformation caused by a defect in brain development. Secondary MCPH is an *acquired* disorder resulting from an insult that affects fetal, neonatal, or infantile brain growth. Ischemia, infection, maternal diabetes, and trauma are the most common causes. A few examples of MCPH microcephaly induced by intrauterine infection are illustrated in Chapter 12. In this section, we focus on primary (congenital) microcephaly.

Terminology and Classification

Microcephaly is defined as a head circumference more than three standard deviations below the mean for age and sex. In primary MCPH, there is no evidence of other causes of small brain such as craniostenosis, perinatal infection, or trauma.

Barkovich et al. classify primary MCPH on the basis of morphologic characteristics such as gyral patterns, cortical thickness, the presence of heterotopias or other malformations, and normal versus delayed myelination. The gyral pattern can be normal, "simplified," microgyric, or pachygyric.

Three types of primary microcephaly are recognized. **Microcephaly with simplified gyral pattern** (MSG) is the most common and the mildest form **(37-20)**. Simplified gyri and abnormally shallow sulci are the hallmarks of MSG. The cortex is normal or thinned, not thickened. The gyri are also reduced in number and demonstrate a "simplified" pattern. Various MSG subtypes are described with normal or delayed myelination, heterotopias, and arachnoid cysts.

Microlissencephaly is characterized by severe microcephaly and abnormal sulcation. The brain is extremely small, and the sulcation pattern appears greatly simplified or almost completely smooth **(37-22)**. The cortex is thickened, usually measuring more than 3 mm. In **microcephaly with extensive polymicrogyria**, the brain is small, and polymicrogyria is the predominant gyral pattern **(37-21)**.

Etiology and Pathology

Glioneuronal proliferation and apoptosis both play key roles in determining brain size, so abnormalities in either can result in microcephaly. Familial primary microcephaly is an autosomal-recessive disorder with a single clinical phenotype and genetic heterogeneity.

Several chromosomal syndromes are characterized by mental retardation and microcephaly. These include trisomy 21 (Down), trisomy 18 (Edward), cri-du-chat ("cat cry," 5p syndrome), Cornelia de Lange, and Rubinstein-Taybi syndromes.

Clinical Issues

Epidemiology and Demographics. The incidence of primary MCPH ranges from 1:10,000-30,000. Most cases of primary (genetic) microcephaly are detected in utero or shortly after birth.

Presentation and Natural History. Mental retardation, developmental delay, and seizures are the most common clinical symptoms. Prognosis is variable.

Imaging

General Features. The craniofacial ratio is decreased (usually ≤ 1.5:1). The forehead is often slanted, and the calvarial sutures may appear overriding.

CT Findings. Bone CT shows a small cranial vault, often with closely apposed and overlapping sutures. In older children, the skull is thickened, and the sinuses appear overpneumatized.

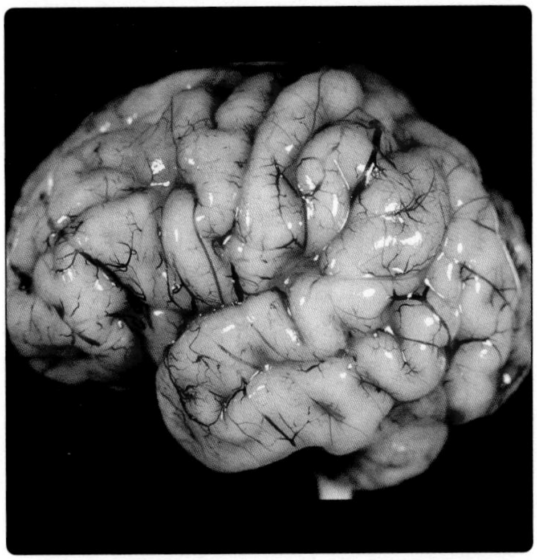

***(37-20)** Autopsy shows microcephaly, simplified gyral pattern. The gyri appear less convoluted than normal. (Courtesy R. Hewlett, MD.)*

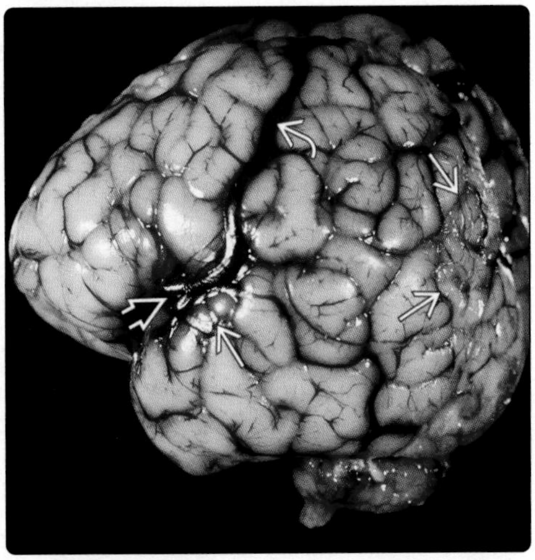

***(37-21)** Microcephaly also shows polymicrogyria, abnormal veins in sylvian fissure, large vein of Trolard. (Courtesy R. Hewlett, MD.)*

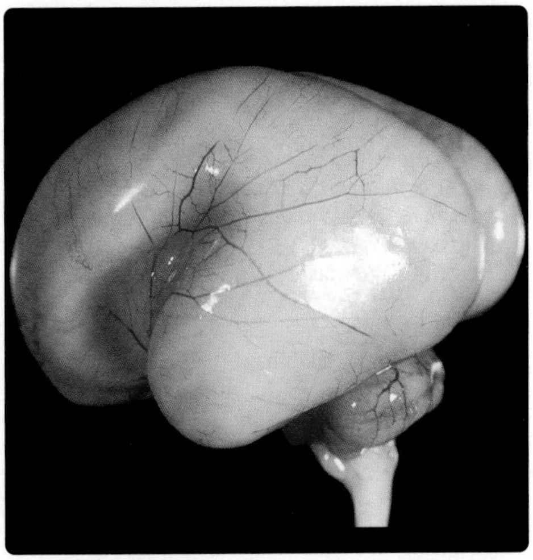

***(37-22)** Microcephaly with LIS looks like that of a 24-week fetus with smooth surface, shallow sylvian fissure. (Courtesy R. Hewlett, MD.)*

The cortical surface can be normal, simplified, microlissencephalic, or polymicrogyric. The ventricles may appear normal or moderately enlarged.

MR Findings. Sagittal T1WI demonstrates slanted frontal bones and a marked decrease in cranial-to-facial proportions **(37-23)**. The brain can appear small but relatively normal, small with simplified gyral pattern, or microlissencephalic.

In microcephaly with simplified gyral pattern, the gyri are fewer in number and appear simplified. The sulci are shallow (25-50% of normal depth). Delayed myelin milestones may be present. Associated anomalies such as callosal dysgenesis and cephaloceles are common.

T2* (GRE, SWI) sequences are helpful to delineate secondary insults with hemorrhagic residua.

Differential Diagnosis

The major diagnostic dilemma is differentiating primary from **secondary microcephaly**. Calcifications, cysts, gliosis, and encephalomalacia are more common in microcephaly secondary to TORCH, Zika virus infection, trauma, or ischemic encephalopathy.

Focal Cortical Dysplasias

The distinctive histological features of focal cortical dysplasia (FCD) were first characterized by Taylor et al. (1971). It is now recognized that FCD is a common cause of medically refractory epilepsy in both children and adults. Surgical resection is an increasingly important treatment option, so recognition and accurate delineation of FCD on imaging studies are key to successful patient management.

(37-23A) Sagittal T1WI in a patient with primary microcephaly shows craniofacial disproportion with a 1.5:1 ratio, sloping forehead ➡. Note the thin dysplastic corpus callosum ➡ and simplified gyral pattern ➡. (37-23B) T2WI in the same patient shows the simplified gyral pattern with too few gyri and shallow-appearing sulci. The eyes are disproportionately large.

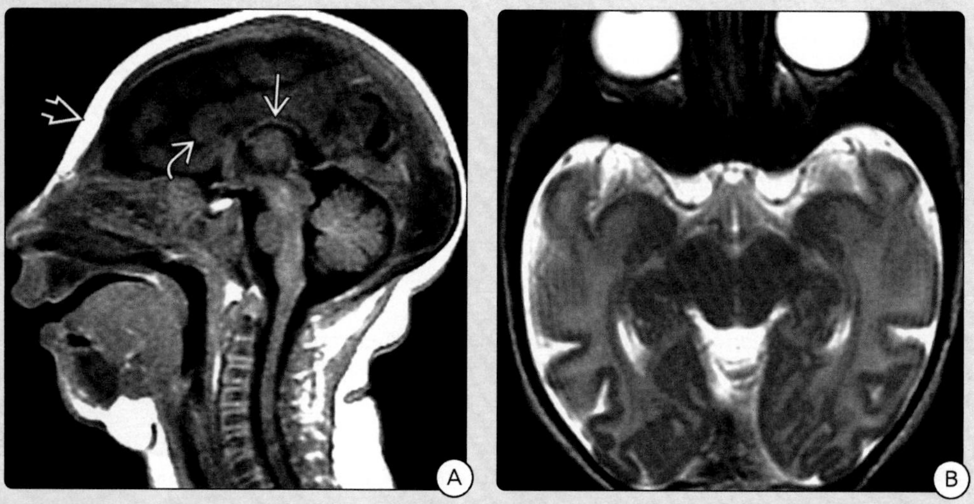

(37-23C) T2WI through the ventricles shows the simplified gyral pattern with numerous shallow sulci. Cortical thickness appears normal, but myelination is delayed. (37-23D) T2WI in the same patient again shows the simplified gyral pattern. Compare Figure 37-20.

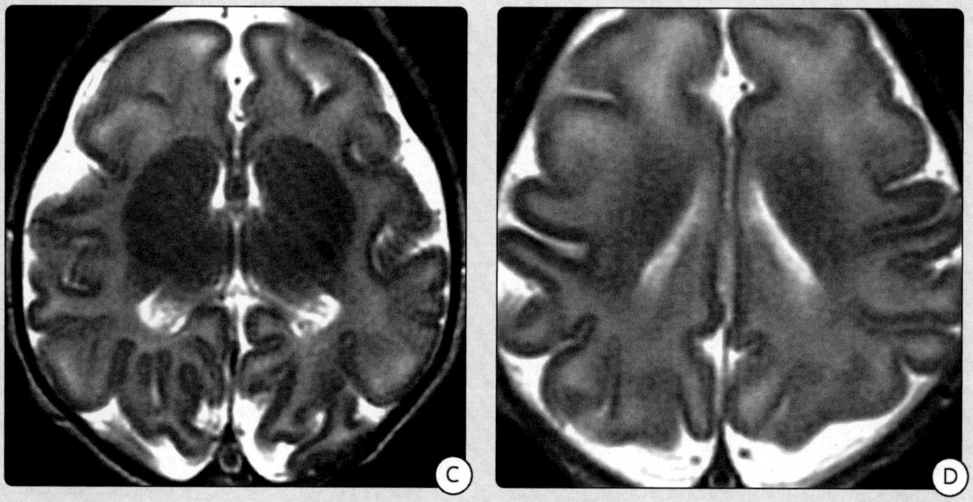

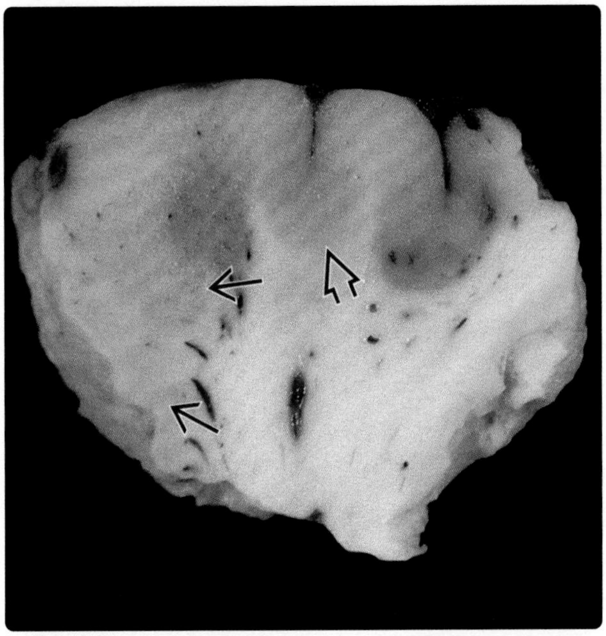

***(37-24)** Resected surgical specimen from a patient with intractable epilepsy shows a classic "funnel-shaped" area of thickened cortex, blurred gray-white interface ➲. Contrast with adjacent normal sulcus and gyrus ➲. (Courtesy R. Hewlett, MD.)*

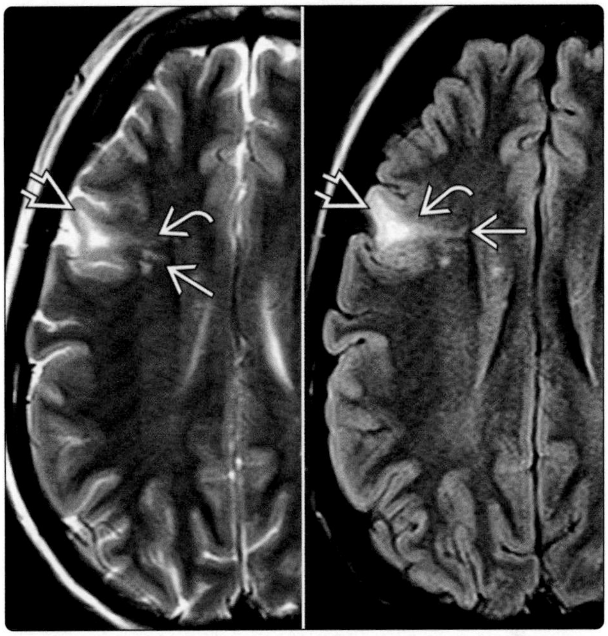

***(37-25)** T2WI (L), FLAIR (R) show pathologically proven FCDIIb. Note funnel-shaped malformation ➲ with indistinct gray-white matter interface ➲ and curvilinear hyperintense foci ➲ extending toward the lateral ventricle.*

Terminology and Classification

FCDs—sometimes called **Taylor cortical dysplasia**—are localized regions of nonneoplastic malformed gray matter.

The International League Against Epilepsy (ILAE) has established a three-tiered classification of FCD based on clinical, imaging, and neuropathologic findings (e.g., lamination disturbances or cytoarchitectural/cellular dysplasia).

FCD type I is an isolated malformation with abnormal cortical layering that demonstrates either vertical (radial) persistence of developmental microcolumns (FCD type Ia) or loss of the horizontal hexalaminar structure (FCD type Ib) in one or multiple lobes. FCD type Ic is characterized by both patterns of abnormal cortical layering.

FCD type II is an isolated lesion characterized by altered cortical layering and dysmorphic neurons either without (type IIa) or with **balloon** (type IIb) **cells**. Type II is the most common type of FCD.

The third type of FCD, **FCD type III** is a postmigrational disorder associated with principal pathologies such as ischemia, infection, trauma, etc. In such cases, cytoarchitectural abnormalities occur together with hippocampal sclerosis (FCD type IIIa), epilepsy-associated tumors (FCD type IIIb), vascular malformations (FCD type IIIc), or—in the case of FCD type IIId—other epileptogenic lesions acquired in early life.

Etiology

The molecular pathology and genetics of FCD are intensely investigated but incompletely understood. Decreased expression of BMP-4 and increased expression of double cortin-like protein that is critically involved in neuronal division and radial migration have been found in both FCDIIb and cortical tubers.

The most convincing data implicate mammalian target of rapamycin (mTOR) cascade abnormalities as the cause of FCD. FCD type IIb specimens typically have sequence alterations in the *TSC1* (hamartin) gene and resemble the cortical tubers in tuberous sclerosis complex (TSC).

Extensive cortical malformations can be caused by prenatal infections (e.g., TORCH). HPV-16 infection and oncoprotein expression have also been found in a large series of resected FCDIIb specimens.

Pathology

Gross Pathology. Surgical specimens often appear grossly normal. A funnel-shaped configuration of mildly thickened, slightly firm cortex with poor demarcation from the underlying white matter is characteristic **(37-24)**.

Microscopic Features. The histopathologic hallmarks of FCD are disorganized cytoarchitecture and neurons with abnormal shape, size, and orientation.

FCD type II has pronounced cytoarchitectural disturbances. Dysmorphic neurons with increased diameter of their cell bodies and nuclei are found in both types IIa and IIb. Cortical thickness is increased, and the gray-white matter interface is blurred in both subtypes.

Prominent balloon cells together with lack of myelin and oligodendrocytes are typical of type IIb. These balloon cells are

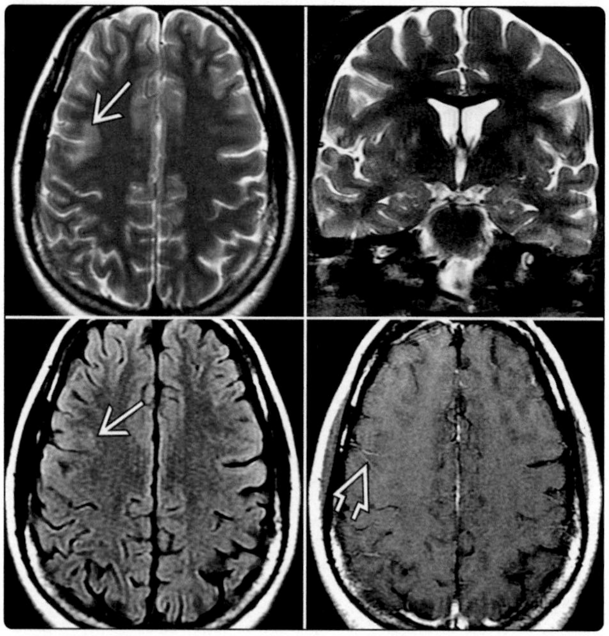

***(37-26)** Images show subtle findings of FCD ➡. Signal intensity is similar to GM on both T2/FLAIR. T1 C+ shows enhancement of "primitive" cortical veins ⇨ over the focal dysplasia. (Courtesy P. Hildenbrand, MD.)*

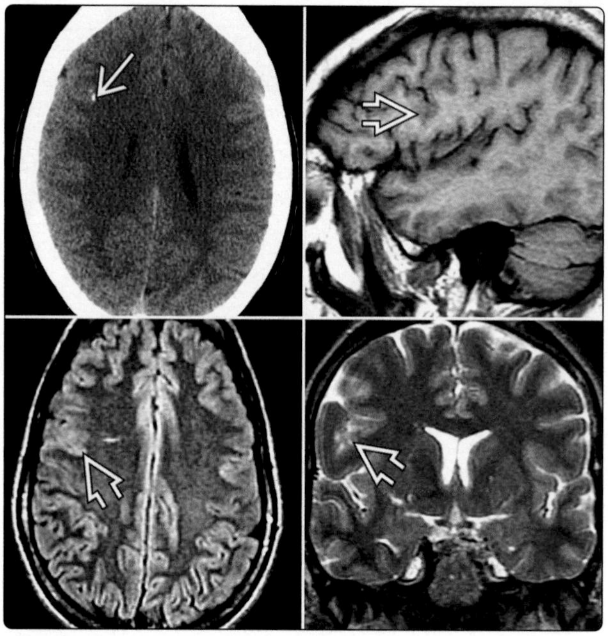

***(37-27)** Images in a different patient show very subtle findings of FCD ⇨, including a tiny focus of calcification ➡ on NECT. This is biopsy-proven FCD. (Courtesy P. Hildenbrand, MD.)*

histologically identical to giant cells in the tubers from TSC patients.

Clinical Issues

Epidemiology and Demographics. As a group, FCDs are the single most common cause of severe early-onset drug-resistant epilepsy in children and young adults. FCD type II is found in 15-20% of patients undergoing epilepsy surgery. There is no sex predilection.

Presentation and Natural History. FCD-associated seizures usually begin in the first decade but can present in adolescence or even adulthood. Patients with FCD type Ia are typically young with early seizure onset and severe psychomotor retardation.

Treatment Options. Medically resistant chronic epilepsy secondary to FCD may be treated by surgical resection. Outcome varies with FCD subtype; excellent seizure control is reported in 70-100% of patients with FCD type IIb.

Imaging

General Features. Imaging findings of FCD are often subtle. Most foci are smaller than 2 cm in diameter and can be difficult to detect, especially on standard imaging studies. Larger lesions can mimic neoplasm or focal demyelination.

CT Findings. CT scans are usually normal unless the lesion is unusually large. A few patients with calcified FCD type IIb lesions have been reported **(37-27)**.

MR Findings. MR findings in FCD depend on lesion size and type. For example, FCD type Ia causes only mild hemispheric hypoplasia without other visible lesions.

FCD type IIb shows a localized area of increased cortical thickness and a funnel-shaped area of blurred gray-white interface at the bottom of a sulcus, the **"transmantle MR" sign (37-25)**. Signal intensity varies with age. In neonates and infants, FCD type IIb appears hyperintense on T1WI and mildly hypointense on T2WI. In older patients, FCD appears as a wedge-shaped area of T2/FLAIR hyperintensity extending from the bottom of a sulcus into the subcortical and deep WM **(37-26)**.

A subcortical linear or curvilinear focus of T2/FLAIR hyperintensity sometimes extends toward the superolateral margin of the lateral ventricle **(37-25)**.

FCD type IIb does not enhance on T1 C+. It shows increased diffusivity and decreased FA on DWI. MRS shows decreased NAA:Cr and elevated myoinositol. Perfusion MR shows normal or reduced rCBV.

The recently defined FCD type III is primarily encountered in patients with hippocampal sclerosis (FCD IIIa). Anterior temporal lobe volume loss with abnormal WM hyperintensity on T2/FLAIR with otherwise normal-appearing cortex is characteristic.

Voxel-based morphometry, statistical parametrical mapping, and texture analysis are advanced techniques that may increase detection of epileptogenic lesions in patients with negative standard MR scans.

Functional Imaging. Ictal SPECT, PET, and magnetoencephalography (MEG) can be beneficial tools in patients with normal MRs who are suspected of harboring FCD. Fused images have been used to guide intraoperative lesionectomy. Functional imaging has also been used in

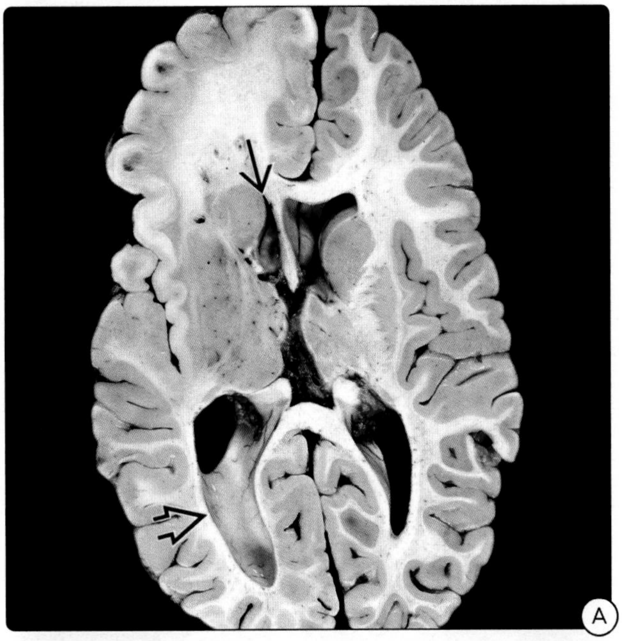

(37-28A) Hemimegalencephaly shows enlarged right hemisphere with "overgrown" WM. Note pointed frontal horn ➡ and enlarged occipital horn ➡.

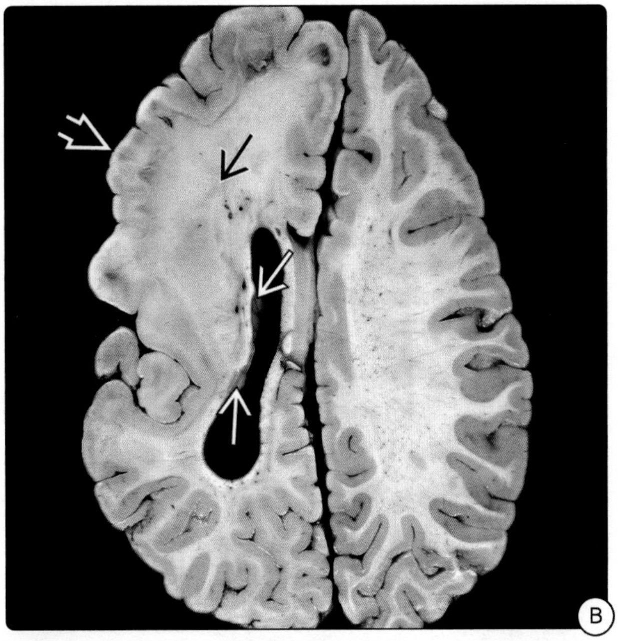

(37-28B) More cephalad image shows large hemisphere/ventricle with subependymal heterotopic GM ➡, polymicrogyria ➡, and "overgrown" WM with abnormal myelination ➡. (Courtesy B. Horten, MD.)

conjunction with subdural and depth electrodes to localize the ictal zone.

FOCAL CORTICAL DYSPLASIA

ILAE Classification

- FCD I: Cortical dyslamination
- FCD II: Cortical dyslamination with dysmorphic neurons
  - FCD IIA = without balloon cells
  - FCD IIb = with balloon cells (most common)
- FCD III: Cortical lamination abnormalities + additional pathology in adjoining area

Pathology and Clinical Issues

- Mass-like with thickened cortex, indistinct GM-WM junction
- Most common cause of refractory epilepsy

Imaging

- Focal/wedge-shaped mass, blurred GM-WM interface
- Subcortical T2/FLAIR hyperintensity

Differential Diagnosis

The major differential diagnosis of FCD (especially type IIb) includes neoplasm, tuberous sclerosis, and demyelinating disease. The most common **cortically based neoplasms** associated with longstanding epilepsy include dysembryoplastic neuroepithelial tumor (DNET), ganglioglioma, oligodendroglioma, and low-grade diffusely infiltrating astrocytoma (WHO grade II). It may be difficult (if not impossible) to distinguish between FCD and neoplasm on the basis of imaging findings alone.

The cortical lesions in **tuberous sclerosis complex** can look very similar to FCD type IIb. Both can calcify; both are funnel- or flame-shaped and involve the cortex and subcortical WM. TSC usually demonstrates other imaging stigmata such as subependymal nodules.

A solitary **demyelinating lesion** can mimic FCD. The myelin and oligodendrocyte loss in FCD results in similar signal intensity changes, i.e., T2/FLAIR hyperintensity. "Tumefactive" demyelination often has an incomplete enhancing rim, whereas FCD does not enhance. Serial MRs may be helpful in distinguishing FCD from demyelinating disease.

Hemimegalencephaly

Terminology

Hemimegalencephaly (HMEG)—also called unilateral megalencephaly—is a rare malformation characterized by enlargement and cytoarchitectural abnormalities of all or part of one cerebral hemisphere.

Etiology

The precise etiology of HMEG is unknown. Some investigators believe HMEG and FCD represent a single disease spectrum with phenotypic variability. In this view, HMEG represents a hemispheric FCD with aberrant PI3K/AKT/mTOR signaling playing the key role in developing malformations of cortical development ("TORopathies").

HMEG can occur as an isolated malformation, but approximately 30% of cases are syndromic. Associations with Proteus, Klippel-Weber-Trenaunay, and epidermal nevus syndromes, neurofibromatosis type 1, and hypomelanosis of Ito have been reported.

Pathology

Gross Pathology. The affected hemisphere appears enlarged and grossly dysplastic. Abnormal gyral pattern, cortical dysgenesis, enlarged lateral ventricle, and white matter hypertrophy are common. Areas of dysplastic hamartomatous overgrowth are present, and the gray-white matter junction is often indistinct **(37-28)**.

Microscopic Features. Severe cortical dyslamination, hypertrophic and dysmorphic neurons, and parenchymal and leptomeningeal glioneuronal heterotopias are typical histologic features of HMEG. Balloon cells are identified in half of all cases.

The white matter is often grossly abnormal and poorly myelinated. Gray matter heterotopias and clusters of hypertrophic astrocytes are frequent findings. Gliosis, WM vacuolation, and cystic changes are common.

Clinical Issues

Epidemiology and Demographics. HMEG is rare, representing less than 5% of MCDs diagnosed on imaging studies.

Presentation, Natural History, and Treatment Options. HMEG usually presents in infancy and is characterized by macrocrania, developmental delay, and seizures. Extracranial hemihypertrophy of part or all of the ipsilateral body may be present.

Prognosis is poor because seizures are usually intractable and developmental delay is severe. HMEG-associated seizures are usually resistant to anticonvulsants. Anatomic or functional hemispherectomy has had variable success, as *abnormalities in*

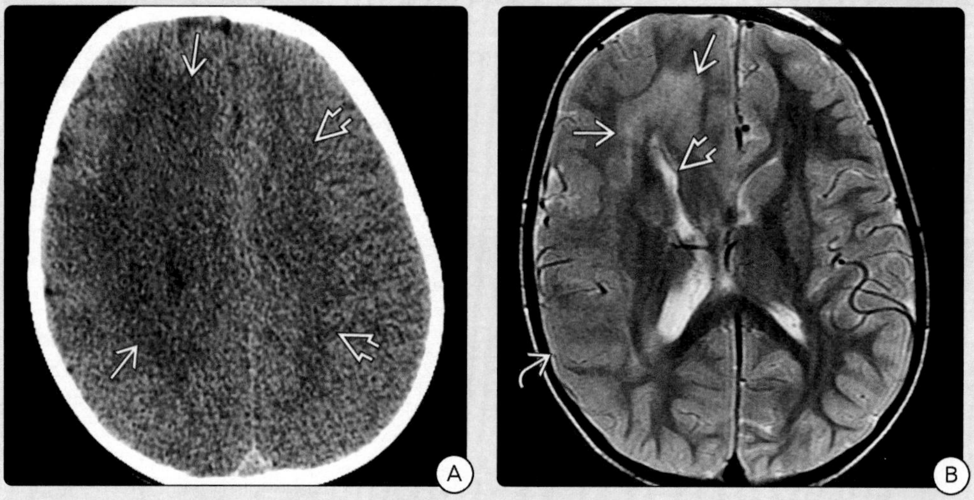

***(37-29A)** NECT in a 4y girl with hemimegalencephaly, intractable seizures shows enlarged right hemisphere, hemicranium with enlarged WM in the corona radiata ➡. Compare this to the normal-appearing WM of the left hemisphere ➡. **(37-29B)** T2WI in the same patient shows enlarged hemisphere, hyperintense WM ➡, enlarged deformed lateral ventricle ➡, thickened dysplastic cortex ➡. Again compare to the normal left side.*

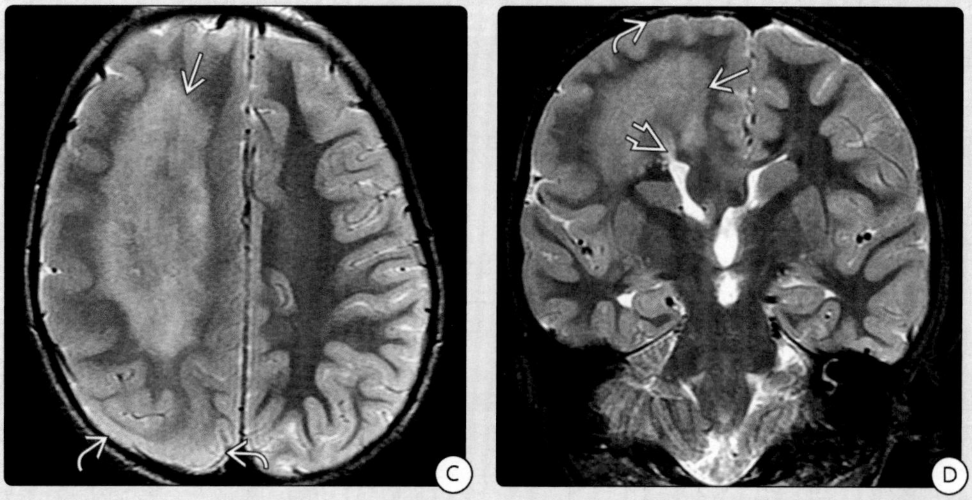

***(37-29C)** T2WI through the corona radiata in the same patient shows hypertrophied heterogeneously hyperintense WM ➡ and pachygyria ➡. **(37-29D)** Coronal T2WI in the same patient shows the hyperplastic, hyperintense WM ➡, deformed pointed lateral ventricle ➡, and polymicrogyria ➡.*

the contralateral "normal" hemisphere are common and so should be carefully searched for as part of surgical planning.

Imaging

General Features. HMEG is characterized by an enlarged, dysplastic-appearing hemisphere with abnormal gyration, thickened cortex, and white matter abnormalities. The lateral ventricle usually appears enlarged and deformed. In rare cases, the dysplastic changes involve only part of one hemisphere ("focal," "localized," or "lobar" hemimegalencephaly).

CT Findings. NECT shows an enlarged hemisphere and hemicranium. The posterior falx often appears displaced across the midline **(37-29)**. Abnormal white matter myelination may increase in attenuation, making the contralateral "normal" WM appear unusually hypodense. Dystrophic calcifications are common.

CECT may disclose abnormal, "uncondensed," primitive-appearing superficial veins over regions of severely dysplastic cortex.

HEMIMEGALENCEPHALY

Pathology
- Enlarged hemisphere
- Thick cortex + focal subcortical masses of dysplastic GM
- WM abnormally myelinated

Imaging
- Large, dysplastic-appearing hemisphere
- Ipsilateral ventricle large, malformed
- Falx inserts off midline
- Focal mass(es) of heterotopic GM can mimic neoplasm
- DDx = FCD, TSC, neoplasm (gangliocytoma)

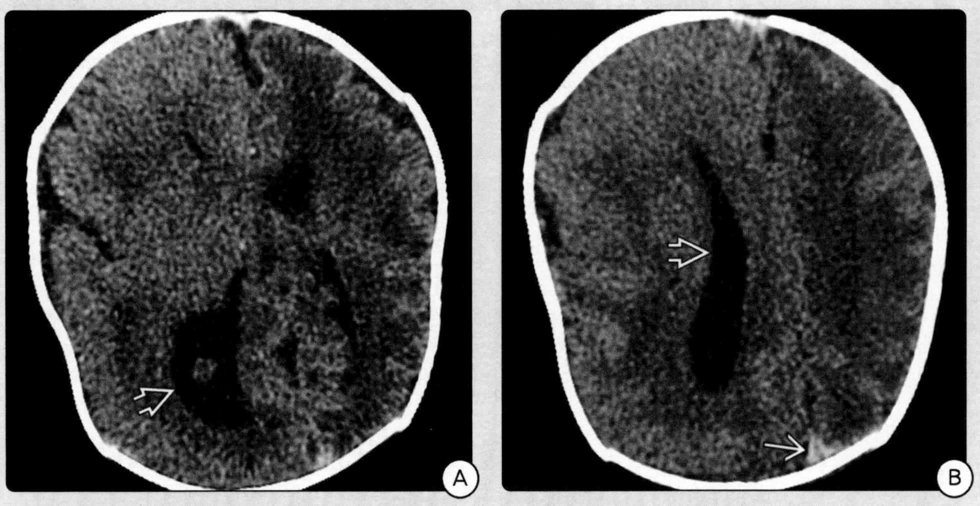

(37-30A) NECT scan in a 35w premature infant shows enlarged right hemisphere, lateral ventricle ➡. The right hemispheric WM appears less hypodense than the left. (37-30B) More cephalad scan in the same patient shows the enlarged right hemisphere, lateral ventricle ➡, and off-midline insertion of the falx ➡. Initial diagnosis was left MCA stroke.

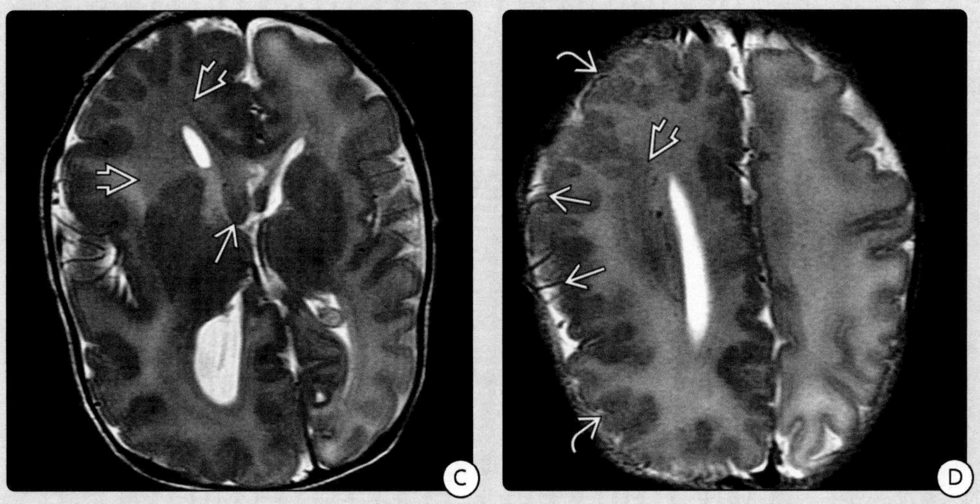

(37-30C) T2WI in the same patient shows expanded right hemispheric WM that appears "dirty" ➡ (i.e., less hyperintense than the unmyelinated left WM). Note the markedly enlarged fornices ➡. (37-30D) More cephalad T2WI shows that corona radiata WM is less hyperintense than normal ➡, and there is extensive cortical thickening with polymicrogyria ➡. Note the prominent, primitive-appearing veins ➡.

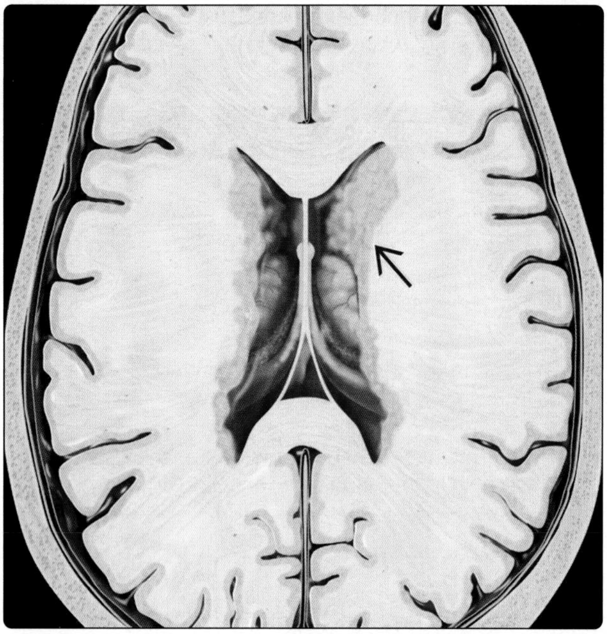

(37-31) Axial graphic shows extensive bilateral subependymal heterotopia ➡ lining the lateral ventricles. The gray matter cortical ribbon is thin, and the sulci are shallow.

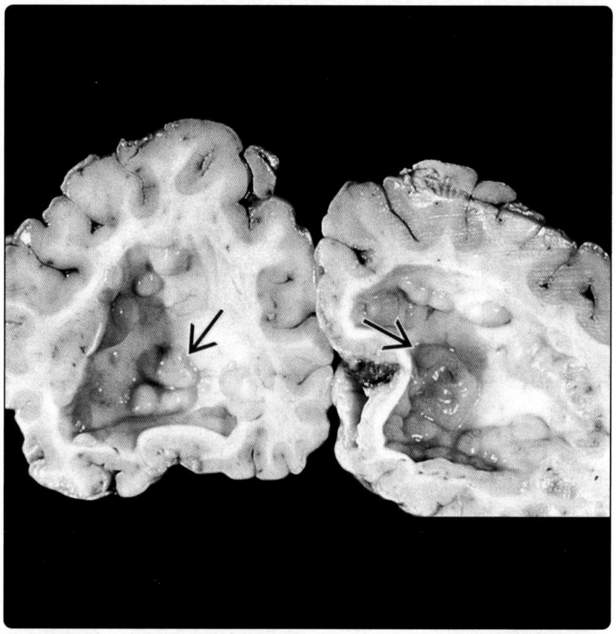

(37-32) Autopsy specimen shows nodules of subependymal heterotopic gray matter ➡. Ventricles are enlarged, and the overlying cortex is thin. (Courtesy J. Ardyn, MD.)

MR Findings. The cortex often appears thickened and "lumpy-bumpy" on T1 scans. Myelination is disordered and accelerated with shortened T1. Neuronal heterotopias are common. The ipsilateral ventricle is usually enlarged and deformed. In severe cases, almost no normal hemispheric architecture can be discerned.

T2 scans show areas of pachy- and polymicrogyria with indistinct borders between gray and white matter **(37-30)**. White matter signal intensity on T2/FLAIR is often heterogeneous with cysts and gliosis-like hyperintensity **(37-29)**.

Differential Diagnosis

The major differential diagnosis of HMEG is a **focal malformation of cortical development**. Although the entire hemisphere is usually involved in HMEG, cases of "focal" or "lobar" megalencephaly are difficult to distinguish. They show identical histologic features. The presence of associated extracerebral abnormalities (e.g., limb hemihypertrophy) may be a helpful differentiating feature.

Tuberous sclerosis complex with widespread cortical dysplasia does not enlarge the hemisphere and exhibits other imaging stigmata, such as subependymal nodules, cortical/subcortical tubers, and radial glial bands.

Cases of severe HMEG with almost no identifiable normal anatomic landmarks can be mistaken for neoplasm, typically **gangliocytoma**. Other than dysplastic cerebellar gangliocytoma (Lhermitte-Duclos disease), tumors consisting only of neoplastic neurons (often with dysplastic features) are exceptionally rare. The newly described multinodular and vacuolating neuronal tumor of the cerebrum has a distinct imaging appearance, i.e., a focal cluster of T2/FLAIR hyperintense "bubbles" on the undersurface of the cortex, and does not have the dysmorphic appearance of HMEG.

In all of the differential diagnostic considerations listed above, color FA maps are helpful in delineating the GM-WM junction and demonstrating the WM hypertrophy or hypermyelination so characteristic of HMEG.

Abnormalities of Neuronal Migration

Abnormalities of neuronal migration are divided into four main subgroups as discussed above. We begin with the heterotopias and then turn to lissencephaly spectrum disorders. The section concludes with a brief discussion of subcortical heterotopias, sublobar dysplasias, and cobblestone complex.

Heterotopias

Arrest of normal neuronal migration along the radial glial cells can result in grossly visible masses of "heterotopic" gray matter. These collections come in many shapes and sizes and can be found virtually anywhere between the ventricles and the pia. They can be solitary or multifocal and exist either as an isolated phenomenon or in association with other malformations.

Periventricular Nodular Heterotopia

Periventricular nodular heterotopia (PVNH) is the most common form of cortical malformation in adults. Here one or more subependymal nodules of gray matter (GM) line the lateral walls of the ventricles **(37-31)** **(37-32)**. PVNH can be unilateral focal, unilateral diffuse, bilateral focal, and bilateral diffuse. Nodules of PVNH follow GM in density/signal intensity and do not enhance following contrast administration **(37-33)**.

PVNH commonly occurs with other abnormalities. The most common is ventriculomegaly followed by agenesis of the corpus callosum and cortical dysplasia. *FLNA* mutations, when present in the X-linked dominant form, cause bilateral ectopic GM nodules, which are perinatal lethal in male patients.

Less commonly, PVNH lines most or even all of the lateral ventricular walls. Collections of round or ovoid nodules indent the lateral walls of the ventricles, giving them a distinctive "lumpy-bumpy" appearance. They follow GM on all sequences, do not enhance, and—unlike the subependymal nodules of tuberous sclerosis—do not calcify. The overlying cortex often appears thinned, but sulcation and gyration are typically normal.

The major differential diagnosis of PVNH is the subependymal nodules of **tuberous sclerosis**.

Subcortical Heterotopias

Subcortical heterotopias are malformations in which large, focal, mass-like collections of neurons are found in the deep cerebral white matter anywhere from the ependyma to the cortex **(37-34)**. The involved portion of the affected hemisphere is abnormally small, and the overlying cortex appears thin and sometimes dysplastic **(37-35)**.

In other forms of heterotopia, focal masses of ectopic GM occur in linear or swirling curved columns of neurons that extend through normal-appearing white matter from the ependyma to the pia. The overlying cortex is thin, and the underlying ventricle often appears distorted **(37-36)**. The

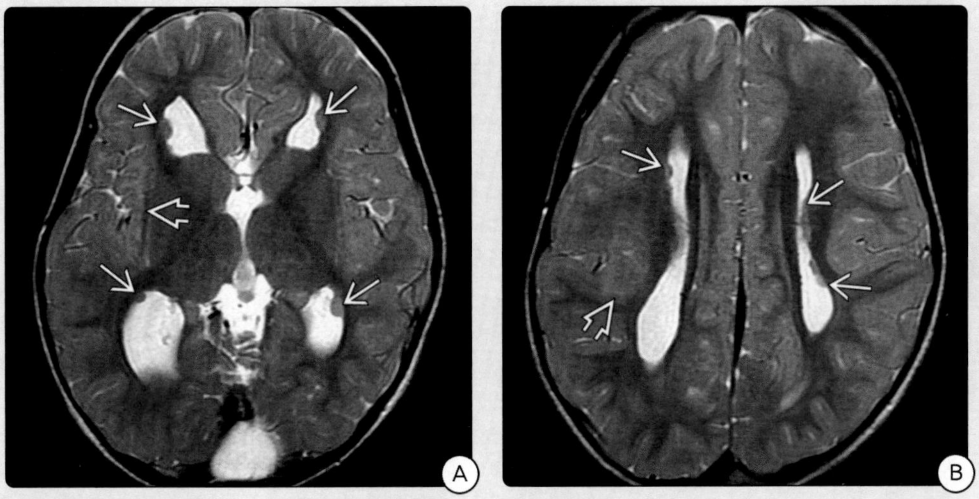

***(37-33A)** Axial T2WI in a patient with corpus callosum agenesis shows multiple nodules of subependymal heterotopic gray matter ➡. Cortex shows perisylvian areas of pachy- and polymicrogyria ➡. **(37-33B)** More cephalad image in the same patient shows additional foci of subependymal heterotopic GM ➡ and cortical dysplasia ➡.*

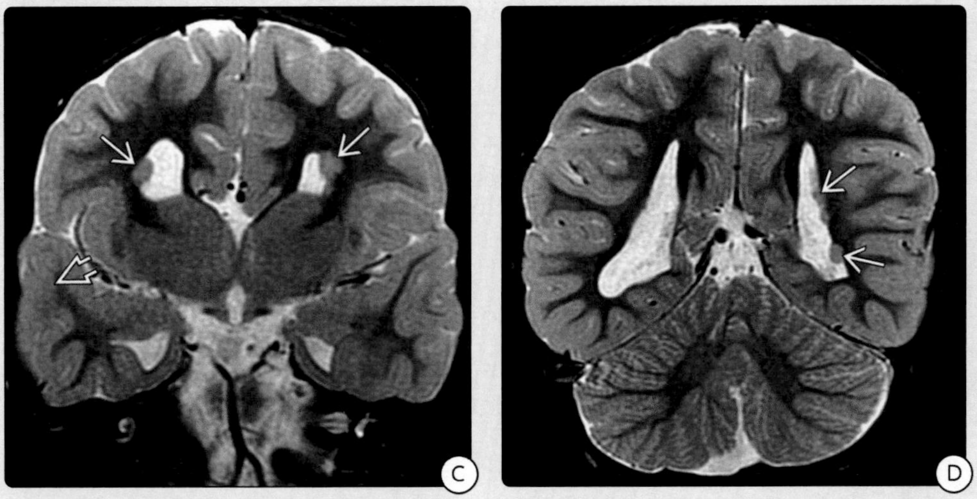

***(37-33C)** Coronal T2WI in the same patient nicely demonstrates the subependymal heterotopias ➡ and pachy- and polymicrogyria ➡. **(37-33D)** T2WI through the atria of the lateral ventricles shows the subependymal heterotopias ➡. The heterotopias followed gray matter signal intensity on all sequences.*

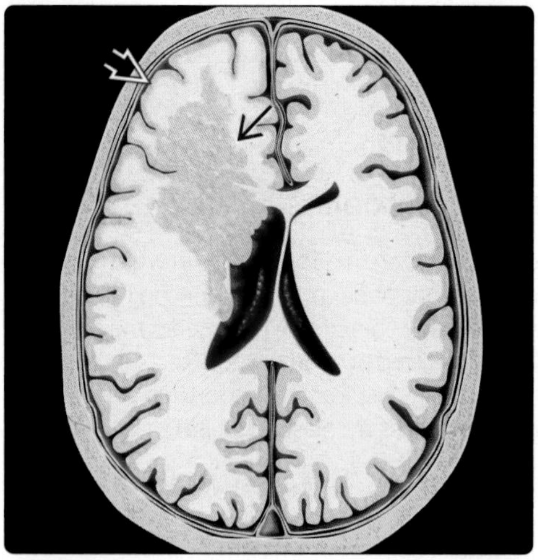

(37-34) Graphic depicts subcortical heterotopia. The large, focal, mass-like collection of gray matter ⇒, thin overlying cortex ➡ are typical.

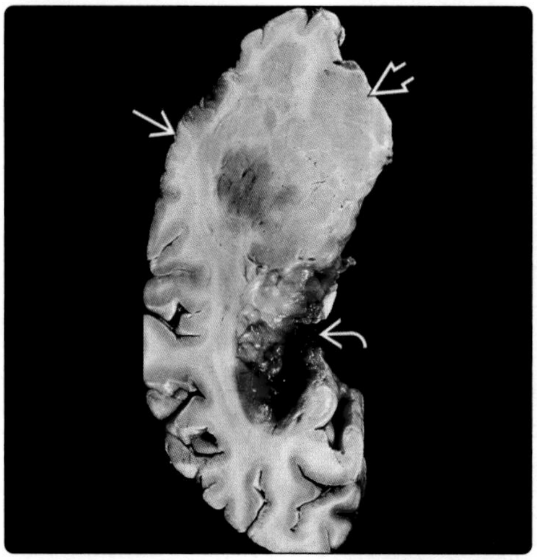

(37-35) Autopsy shows dysplastic lateral ventricle ➡, mass-like GM heterotopias ➡ under thin, polymicrogyric cortex ➡. (AFIP Archives.)

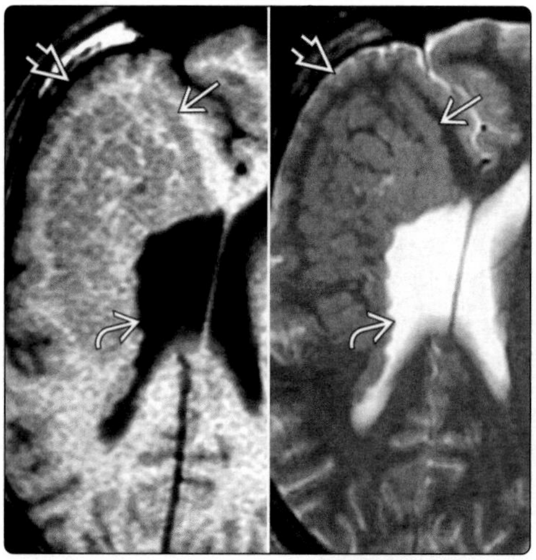

(37-36) T1 (L), T2 (R) show mass of heterotopic GM ➡, thin overlying cortex ➡, deformed underlying ventricle ➡ mimicking neoplasm.

masses follow GM on all sequences, do not demonstrate edema, and do not enhance.

Occasionally ribbon-like bands of heterotopic GM (**subcortical band heterotopia**) form partway between the lateral ventricles and cortex **(37-37)**. Although these have been described with megalencephaly and polymicrogyria, most are probably part of the "double cortex" form of lissencephaly (see below).

The major differential diagnosis of subcortical heterotopia is neoplasm, most specifically **gangliocytoma**. Because the histologic features of GM heterotopia are so similar to those of gangliocytoma, recognizing that the imaging findings are characteristic of a PVNH is essential to avoid misdiagnosis.

Lissencephaly Spectrum

Malformations due to widespread abnormal transmantle migration include **agyria, pachygyria**, and **band heterotopia**. All are part of the **lissencephaly spectrum**.

Terminology

The term lissencephaly (LIS) literally means "smooth brain." The spectrum of LISs ranges from severe (agyria) to milder forms, including abnormally broad folds (pachygyria) or a heterotopic layer of gray matter embedded in the white matter below the cortex (subcortical band heterotopia).

In classic LIS (cLIS), the brain surface lacks normal sulcation and gyration. **cLIS** is also called **type 1 lissencephaly** or **four-layer lissencephaly** to differentiate it from cobblestone cortical malformation. Agyria is defined as a thick cortex with absence of surface gyri (**"complete" lissencephaly**).

True agyria with complete loss of all gyri is relatively uncommon. Most cases of cLIS show parietooccipital agyria with some areas of broad, flat gyri ("pachygyria") and shallow sulci along the inferior frontal and temporal lobes (**"incomplete" LIS**).

Some rare forms of LIS are associated with a disproportionately small cerebellum and are referred to as **lissencephaly with cerebellar hypoplasia**.

Variant LIS (vLIS) consists of thick cortex and reduced sulcation without a cell-sparse zone. Examples include X-linked LIS with callosal agenesis and ambiguous genitalia and LIS with *RELN* signaling pathway mutations.

Subcortical band heterotopia is also called **"double cortex" syndrome** and is the mildest form of cLIS **(37-37)**.

Etiology

Genetics. Between 5 and 22 gestational weeks, primitive neurons (neuroblasts) are generated from mitotic neural stem cells in the ventricular zone (VZ), a region close to the lateral ventricles. Guided by radial glial fibers, postmitotic neuroblasts migrate outward from the VZ to populate the cortical plate.

cLIS is caused by mutation in three genes that regulate the outward migration of neuroblasts: *PAFAH1B1* (often called it alias LIS1), *DCX* (double cortex gene) and *TUBA1A*. The majority of patients with cLIS have LIS1 defects. Another 10-15% have *DCX* mutations, whereas *TUBA1A* accounts for 1-4% of cLIS cases.

LIS1 is deleted in all patients with Miller-Dieker syndrome. *DCX* mutations can cause cLIS (typically in male patients) but are also common in female patients with subcortical band heterotopia (SBH). Almost all cases of familial

SBH are due to *DCX* mutations. *TUBA1A*-related LIS typically demonstrates a posterior to anterior gradient of severity and can also be associated with cerebellar hypoplasia, dysmorphic basal ganglia, callosal dysgenesis, and congenital microcephaly.

Pathology

Gross Pathology. In cLIS, the external surface of the brain shows a marked lack of gyri and sulci. In the most severe forms, the cerebral hemispheres are smooth with poor operculization and underdeveloped sylvian fissures. Coronal sections demonstrate a markedly thickened cerebral cortex with broad gyri and reduced volume of the underlying white matter **(37-38)**.

Microscopic Features. In cLIS, the normal six-layer cortex is replaced by a thick four-layer cortex. From the outermost to the innermost, these layers are (1) a thin subpial molecular layer, (2) a thin outer cortex composed of disorganized large pyramidal neurons, (3) a "cell-sparse" zone that consists mostly of axons (myelinated after the age of 2 years), and (4) a broad inner band of disorganized neurons. The white matter is severely reduced in volume and often contains foci of heterotopic neurons.

Clinical Issues

Epidemiology and Demographics. LIS occurs in 1-4:100,000 live births. Patients with band heterotopia are almost always female.

Presentation. Patients with cLIS typically exhibit moderate to severe developmental delay, impaired neuromotor functions, variable mental retardation, and seizures. Microcephaly and mildly dysmorphic facies are frequent. Patients with band heterotopia typically present with developmental delay and a milder seizure disorder.

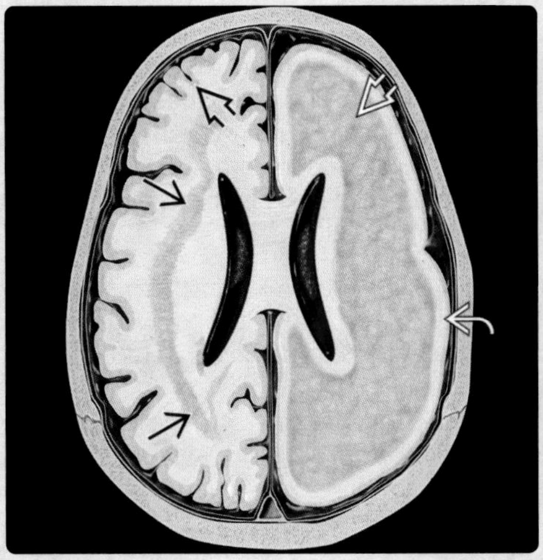

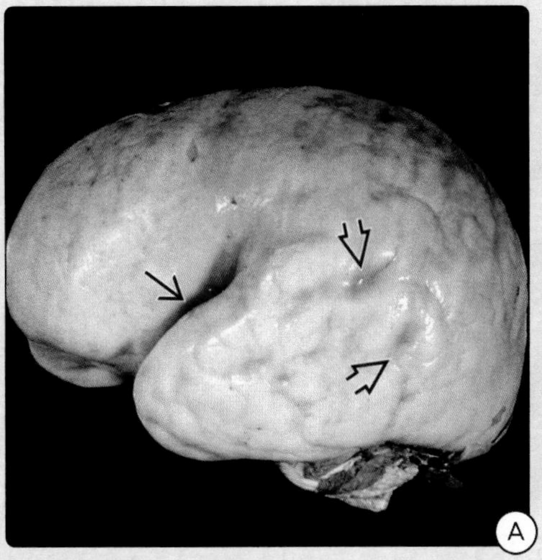

(37-37) Axial graphic shows classic lissencephaly in the left hemisphere with thick subcortical gray matter band ➡, thin cortex, and "cell-sparse" zone ➡. The right hemisphere demonstrates milder lissencephaly with band heterotopia ("double cortex" syndrome) ➡ and thin outer cortex ➡. (37-38A) Lissencephaly shows shallow sylvian fissure ➡, near-complete lack of sulcation. A few shallow surface indentations ➡ are present.

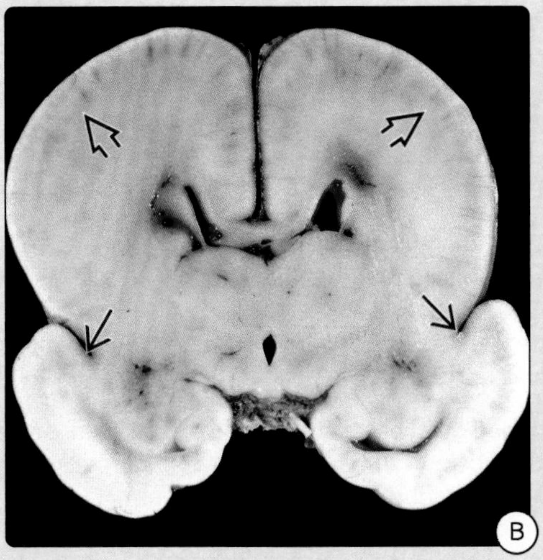

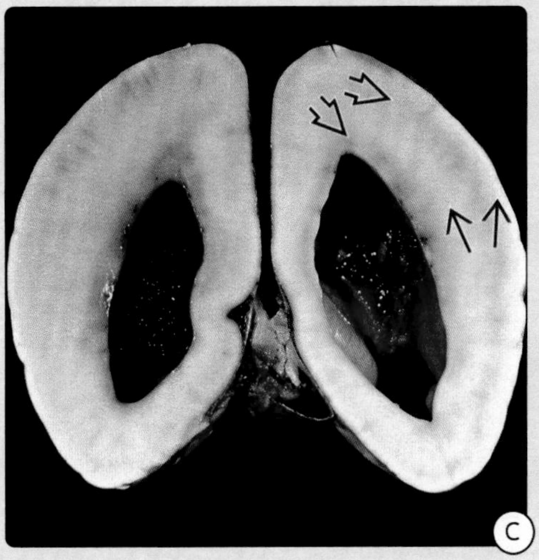

(37-38B) Coronal section shows "hourglass" configuration with shallow sylvian fissures ➡, absent sulci, and thick incompletely layered cortex ➡. (37-38C) Posterior coronal section shows occipital horn dilatation ("colpocephaly") and alternating bands of GM ➡ and WM ➡. (Courtesy R. Hewlett, MD.)

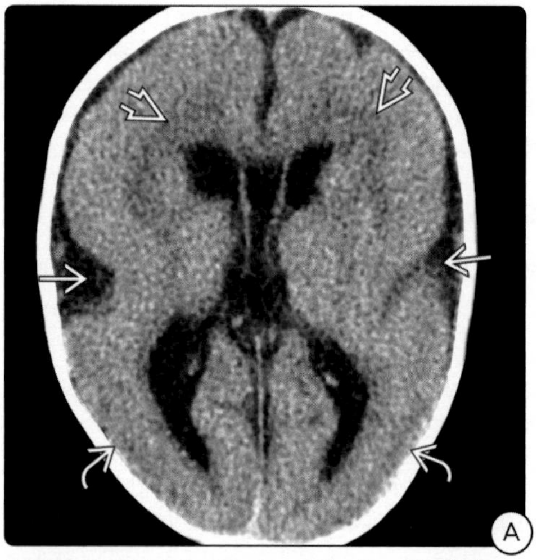

(37-39A) NECT shows smooth brain with shallow sylvian fissures ⇒, thick cortex ⇒, and reduced WM ⇒. The ventricles are moderately enlarged.

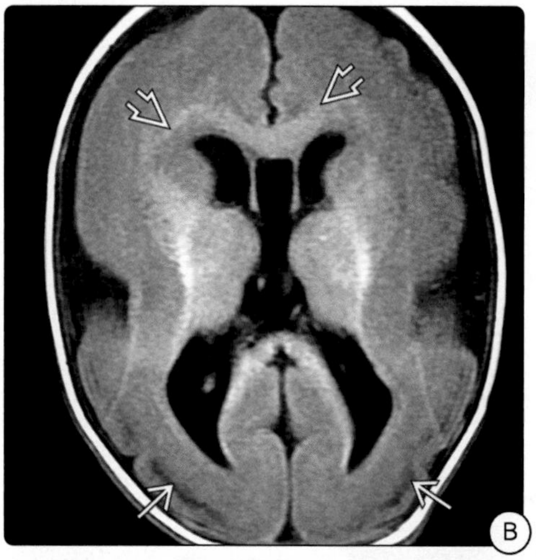

(37-39B) T1WI shows flat gyri, thin outer, thick inner layers of GM separated by a hypointense "cell-sparse" layer ⇒. WM volume ⇒ is reduced.

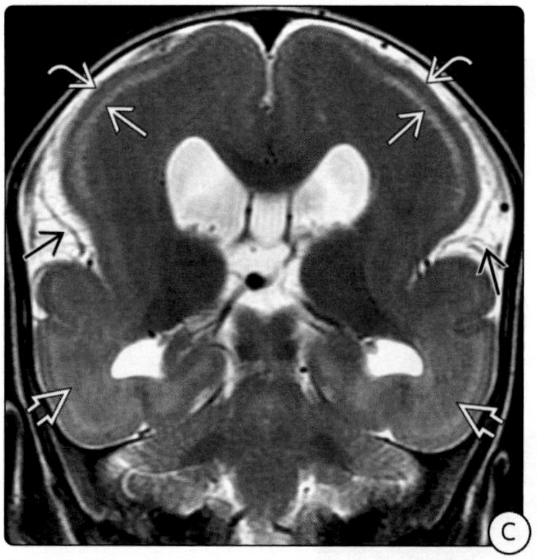

(37-39C) Coronal T2WI shows thin cortex ⇒, hyperintense "cell-sparse" layer ⇒, thickened inner band of GM ⇒ and primitive veins ⇒.

Patients with cLIS and severe facial deformities are diagnosed with **Miller-Dieker syndrome** (MDS). Frontal bossing, hypertelorism, upturned nose, small jaw, and prominent upper lip with thin vermilion border are characteristic features of MDS.

Imaging

General Features. Imaging in patients with complete cLIS (agyria) shows a smooth, featureless brain surface with shallow sylvian fissures and large ventricles. The cortex is thickened, and the WM is diminished in volume. The normal finger-like interdigitations between the cortical GM and subcortical WM are absent. In some cases, the cerebellum appears hypoplastic.

CT Findings. Axial NECT scans in cLIS show an "hourglass" or "figure-eight" appearance caused by the flat brain surface and shallow, wide sylvian fissures. A thick band of relatively well-delineated dense cortex surrounds a thinner, smooth band of white matter **(37-39A)**.

CECT scans show prominent "primitive-appearing" veins running in the shallow sylvian fissures and coursing over the thickened cortices.

MR Findings

Classic Lissencephaly. In **cLIS**, T1 scans show a smooth cortical surface, a thick band of deep GM that is sharply demarcated from the underlying WM, and large ventricles. T2 sequences are best to distinguish the separate cortical layers. A thin outer cellular layer that is isointense with GM covers a hyperintense "cell-sparse" layer. The WM layer is smooth and reduced in volume. A deeper, thick layer of arrested migrating neurons is common and may mimic band heterotopia **(37-39B)** **(37-39C)**.

Callosal anomalies are common in cLIS. The predominant abnormality is callosal hypogenesis. The corpus callosum has a thin flat body with a more vertically oriented splenium. DTI shows marked "pruning," rarefaction, and disorganization of subcortical association fibers (U-fibers). FA and axial diffusivity are decreased, and radial diffusivity is increased. The main WM tracts also appear aberrant and heterotopic.

Variant Lissencephaly. In **vLIS**, sulcation is reduced, and the cortex appears thick (although not as thick as in cLIS). There is no "cell-sparse" layer.

Band Heterotopia or "Double Cortex" Syndrome. In **band heterotopia**, a band of smooth GM is separated from a relatively thicker, more gyriform cortex by a layer of normal-appearing white matter.

MR scans show a more normal gyral pattern with relatively thicker cortex. The distinguishing feature of band heterotopia is its "double cortex," a homogeneous layer of gray matter separated from the ventricles and cerebral cortex by layers of normal-appearing WM **(37-40)**.

Differential Diagnosis

Extremely premature brain is smooth at 24-26 gestational weeks and normally has a "lissencephalic" appearance (see Chapter 35). Although in utero MR can identify fetal lissencephaly between 20 and 24 weeks, false positives are common in the second trimester. Full sulcation and gyration do not develop completely until approximately 40 weeks.

In **microcephaly with simplified gyral pattern**, the head circumference is at least three standard deviations below normal. Too few gyri, abnormally shallow sulci, and a normal or thin (not thick) cortex are present.

cLIS should also be distinguished from the so-called **cobblestone lissencephalies** (type 2 lissencephaly or LIS2). Here the brain surface appears "pebbly" instead of smooth. LIS2 is typically associated with congenital muscular dystrophies (see below).

Pachygyria histologically resembles cLIS but is more localized, often multifocal, and usually asymmetric. In contrast to cLIS, the gray-white matter junction along the thickened cortex is indistinct.

Cytomegalovirus-associated LIS may demonstrate periventricular calcifications as well as germinal zone and anterior temporal cysts.

LISSENCEPHALY SPECTRUM

Classic Lissencephaly (cLIS)
- Pathology: thick, 4-layer cortex
  - Thin subpial layer
  - Thin outer cortex
  - "Cell-sparse" zone
  - Broad inner band of disorganized neurons
- Clinical issues
  - cLIS + severe facial anomalies = Miller-Dieker
- Imaging
  - Smooth, "hourglass" brain
  - Flat surface, shallow "open" sylvian fissures

Band Heterotopia ("Double Cortex")
- Clinical issues
  - Almost always in female patients
- Imaging: looks like "double cortex"
  - Thin, gyriform cortex
  - Normal-appearing WM under cortex
  - Smooth inner band of GM
  - Normal-appearing periventricular WM

Differential Diagnosis
- Extremely premature brain
  - cLIS looks like 20- to 24-week fetal brain
- Microcephaly with simplified gyral pattern
  - Brain size ≥ 3 standard deviations below normal
- Cobblestone lissencephalies (type 2 LIS)
  - Associated with congenital muscular dystrophies
  - "Pebbly" (cobblestone) surface, not smooth
- Pachygyria
  - More localized, often multifocal
  - GM-WM interface indistinct
- Congenital CMV
  - Often microcephalic
  - Smooth brain, periventricular Ca++

Cobblestone Lissencephaly

Cobblestone lissencephaly is also known as type 2 lissencephaly and is genetically, embryologically, pathologically, and radiologically distinct from type 1 ("classic") lissencephaly.

Terminology

Cobblestone lissencephaly is also called **cobblestone cortical malformation** (CCM) and is characterized by an uneven, nodular, "pebbly" brain surface that resembles a cobblestone street. Almost all cases of cobblestone lissencephaly are associated with ocular anomalies and occur as a part of a congenital muscular dystrophy (CMD) syndrome.

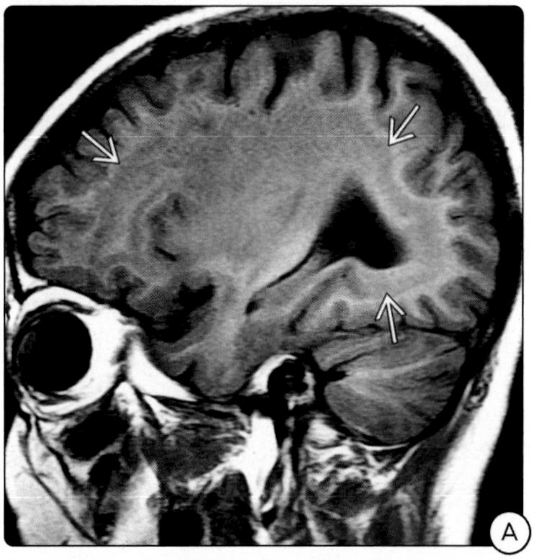

(37-40A) Sagittal T1WI shows band heterotopia with thin outer cortex, myelinated WM, band of GM ➡, periventricular WM ("double cortex").

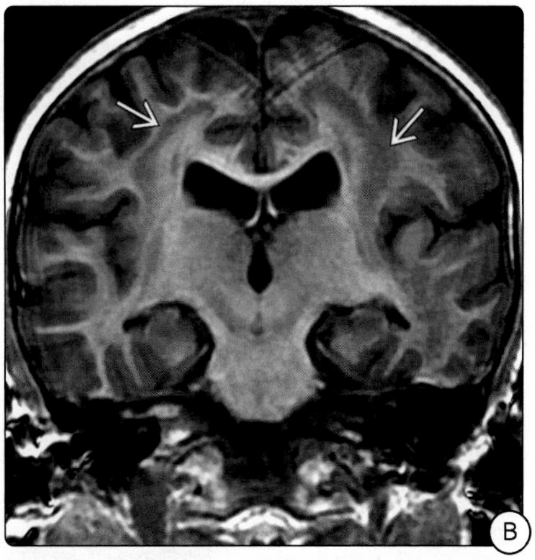

(37-40B) Coronal SPGR in the same patient nicely demonstrates bilateral homogeneous-appearing bands of subcortical heterotopic gray matter ➡.

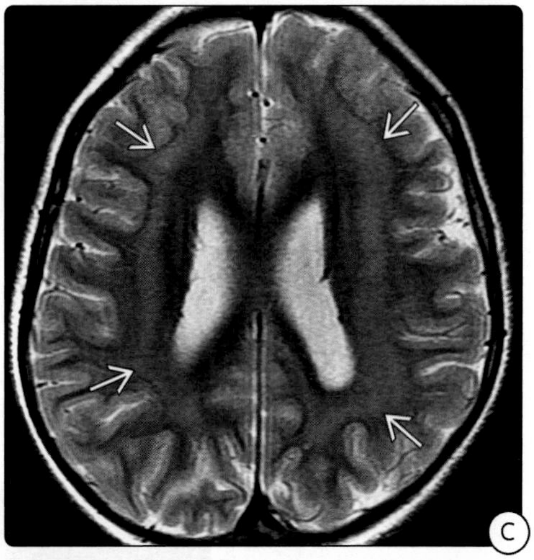

(37-40C) Axial T2WI in the same patient shows that the subcortical bands ➡ follow GM signal intensity. The overlying cortex is thin.

Three major CMD phenotypes are associated with CCM: **Walker-Warburg syndrome** (WWS), **muscle-eye-brain disease** (MEB), and **Fukuyama congenital muscular dystrophy** (FCMD).

Etiology

Cobblestone cortex results from abnormalities caused by defects in the limiting pial basement membrane. Overmigration of neuroblasts through these breaches results in an extracortical layer of aberrant gray matter nodules—the "cobblestones"—on the brain surfaces.

CCM is genetically heterogeneous but is mostly due to autosomal-recessive defects in α-dystroglycan-*O*-glycosylation and is therefore termed a **dystroglycanopathy**.

Pathology

Gross Pathology. Grossly, the brain is usually small. Broadened gyri and loss of sulci give the brain its lissencephalic appearance. The affected areas exhibit a "lumpy-bumpy" appearance **(37-41)**. In WWS, the entire brain is often involved, whereas patients with MEB and FCMD show variable amounts of affected cortex, usually the posterolateral parietal and occipital lobes.

The cerebral WM volume is reduced, and the cortex appears irregularly thickened. The GM-WM junction can have an irregular and nodular appearance.

The brainstem is almost always small. The cerebellum is often small, and its folia are frequently fused and disorganized. From 15-20% of patients with WWS also have a Dandy-Walker malformation.

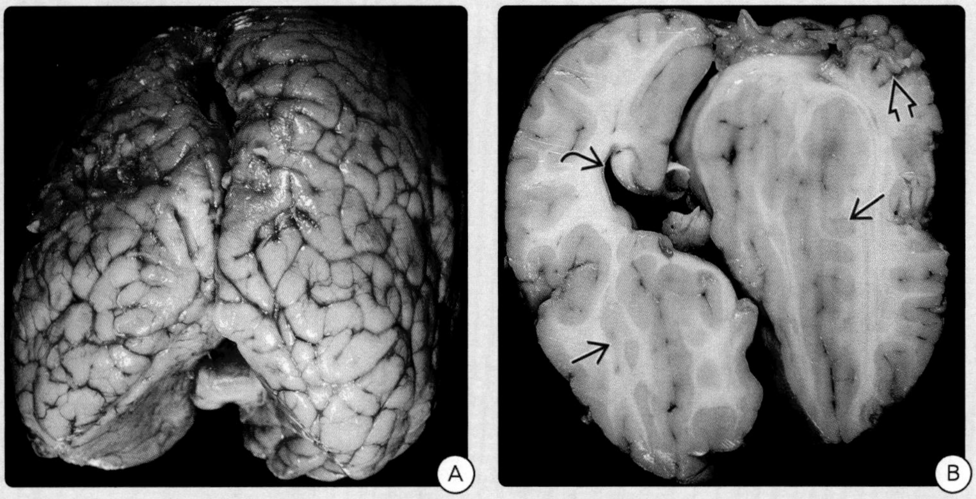

***(37-41A)** Cobblestone lissencephaly is named for the nodular, "pebbly" appearance of the brain surface, which resembles the surface of a cobblestone street. **(37-41B)** Coronal section shows cobblestone cortex ⇨, multiple lines, columns, swirls, and nodules of subcortical heterotopic gray matter ⇨. The right lateral ventricle ⇨ is grossly malformed with nodules of subependymal heterotopic GM.*

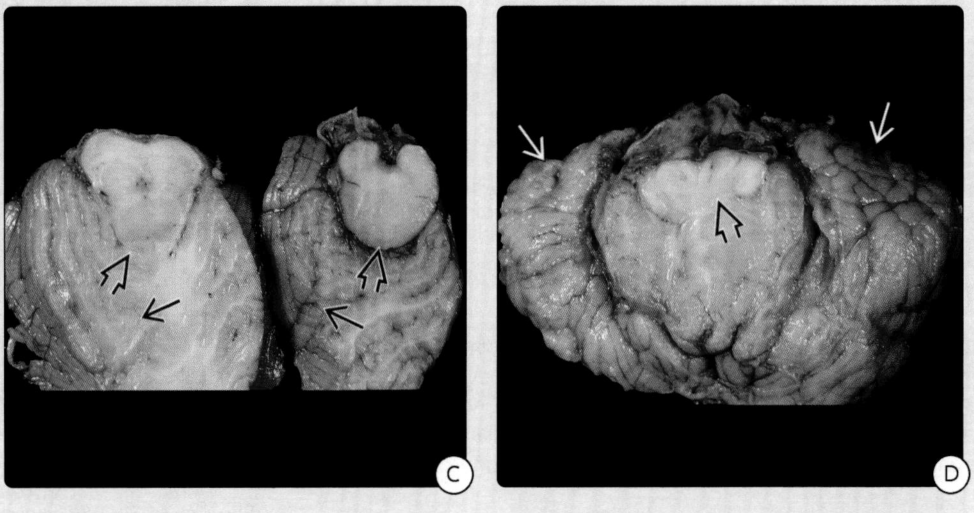

***(37-41C)** Sections through the midbrain and cerebellum show thick fused colliculi ⇨ and bizarre dysplastic cerebellar folia ⇨. **(37-41D)** More inferior section shows a small medulla ⇨ and distinct "pebbly" appearance to the cerebellar hemispheres and vermis ➡. (All four images courtesy R. Hewlett, MD.)*

Microscopic Features. The histopathology of type 2 lissencephaly shares many features with polymicrogyria. The cortex is unlayered and highly disorganized. Unlike type 1 ("classic") lissencephaly, no recognizable laminations are identified. There are numerous areas in which a breach in the pial-glial limitans has occurred, possibly providing a migratory route for aberrant neurons.

Histopathology of skeletal muscle shows classic features of CMD, i.e., degenerating and regenerating muscle fibers with marked fibrosis.

Clinical Issues

Epidemiology and Demographics. All the CMDs are rare. WWS is the most severe form and is found worldwide. MEB is intermediate in severity and is found primarily in Finland. FCMD—the mildest form—occurs almost exclusively in Japan and in patients of Japanese descent.

Presentation and Natural History. The hallmark of all type 2 lissencephalies is the combination of CMD with CNS involvement. Most patients present during the first year of life, but the relative degree of weakness varies.

WWS is characterized by the triad of CMD, brain anomalies (primarily cobblestone cortex), and ocular abnormalities. Infants with WWS have profound hypotonia ("floppy baby"), ocular abnormalities (such as colobomas and persistent hypoplastic primary vitreous), severe developmental delay, and seizures. Most affected individuals do not survive beyond 1 or 2 years.

MEB patients are hypotonic and have impaired vision, seizures, and mental retardation. The eye findings are usually present at birth, and motor retardation often presents earlier than symptoms caused by brain involvement.

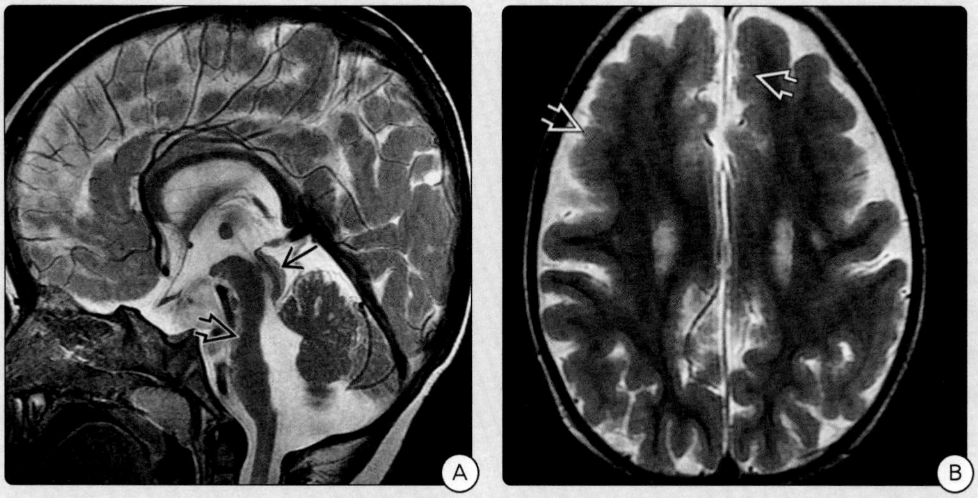

***(37-42A)** Sagittal T2WI shows a patient with cobblestone lissencephaly associated with muscle-eye-brain disease. Note enlarged, fused collicular plate →, small pons ⇨ with "kinked" appearance to the midbrain, and the thin upwardly arched corpus callosum. **(37-42B)** Axial T2WI in the same patient shows frontal-predominant cobblestone lissencephaly ⇨.*

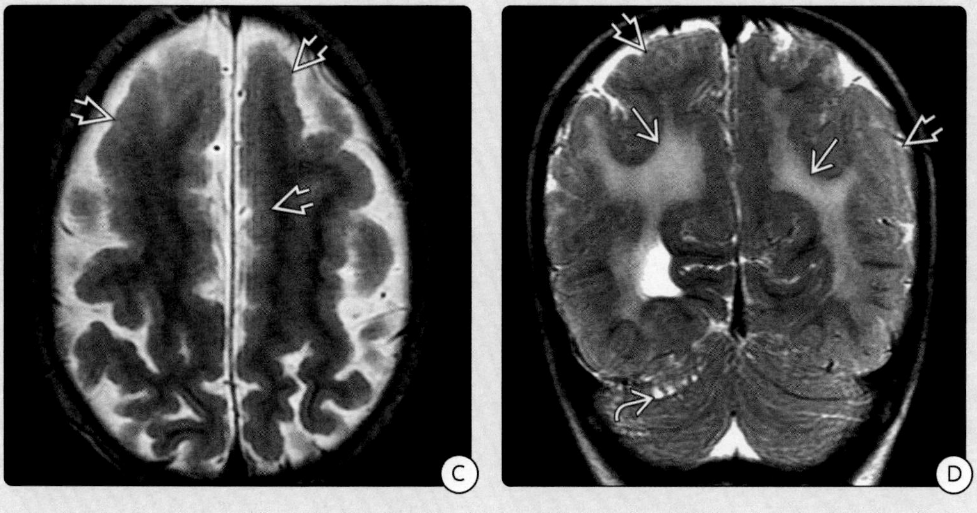

***(37-42C)** More cephalad scan in the same patient nicely demonstrates the distinctive cobblestone appearance of the thickened frontal gyri ⇨. **(37-42D)** Coronal T2WI in the same patient shows delayed myelination ⇨, cobblestone cortex ⇨, and cerebellar cysts ⇨.*

Infants with FCMD present with hypotonia, developmental delay, and seizures. The eye abnormalities are less severe than those of WWS or MEB.

Imaging

Walker-Warburg Syndrome. WWS has a distinctive appearance on MR. Part or all of the cortex is grossly thickened with nodules of disorganized neurons on the surface (accounting for the cobblestone appearance) and linear bundles of GM that project into the underlying WM. Hydrocephalus is common. The brainstem is usually hypoplastic and appears "kinked", the tectum is enlarged, and the cerebellum appears small and dysmorphic with abnormal foliation.

Multiple tiny cerebellar cysts are typical of WWS. They are best demonstrated on thin-section, high-resolution T2WI and suppress completely with FLAIR.

Muscle-Eye-Brain Disease. Retinal detachment with microphthalmia is typical with MEB. Cortical dysplasia, polymicrogyria, and hypoplasia of the inferior vermis are typical **(37-42)** although the cortical dysplasia may not be apparent on MR until several postnatal months.

Fukuyama Congenital Muscular Dystrophy. Patients with FCMD have temporooccipital cobblestone cortex. The brainstem is small, and the collicular plate appears enlarged and fused. The cerebellum is grossly dysmorphic with disorganized folia and subcortical T2/FLAIR hyperintense cysts.

Differential Diagnosis

The major differential diagnosis of type 2 lissencephaly with CMD includes type 1 ("classic") lissencephaly and polymicrogyria. CMD is not a feature of **type 1 lissencephaly**. In **polymicrogyria**, the absence of eye anomalies and muscle weakness are helpful distinguishing features.

__(37-43)__ Coronal oblique graphic shows the thickened "pebbly" gyri of polymicrogyria involving the frontal ⇒ and temporal ⇒ opercula. Note abnormal sulcation and the irregular cortical-white matter interface ⇒ in the affected regions. __(37-44)__ Autopsy shows pachy- and polymicrogyria. Note several foci of tiny nodules ("gyri piled on top of gyri") ⇒, giving brain surface irregular "pebbly" appearance. (R. Hewlett, MD.)

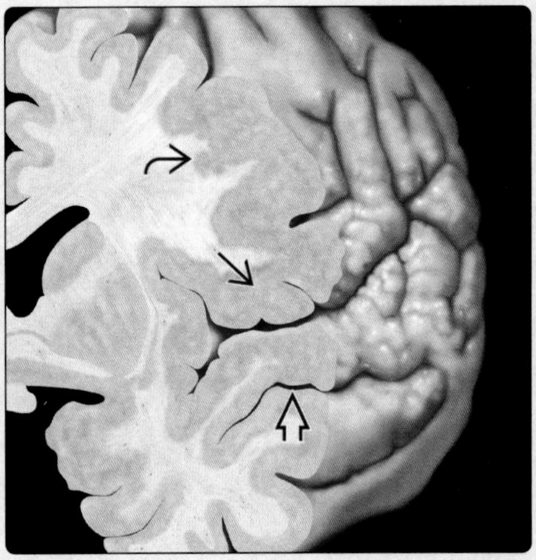

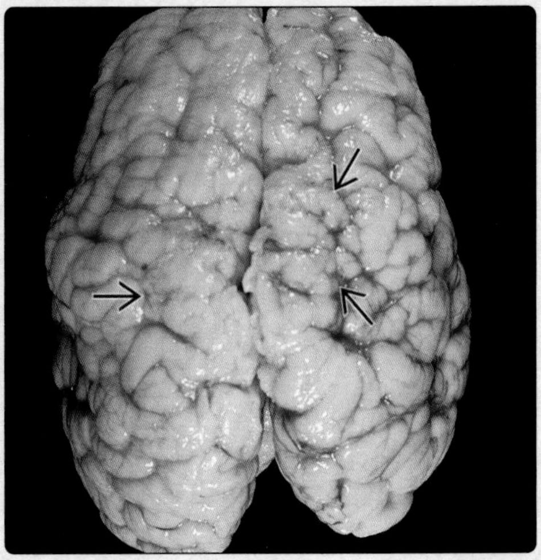

__(37-45A)__ Axial T2WI in a 2w infant with seizures shows multiple foci of polymicrogyria ⇒. The left hemisphere is much more severely affected than the right. __(37-45B)__ Coronal T2WI in the same patient also shows the polymicrogyria ⇒. The appearance of multiple tiny nodules of gray matter piled on top of gyri is characteristic.

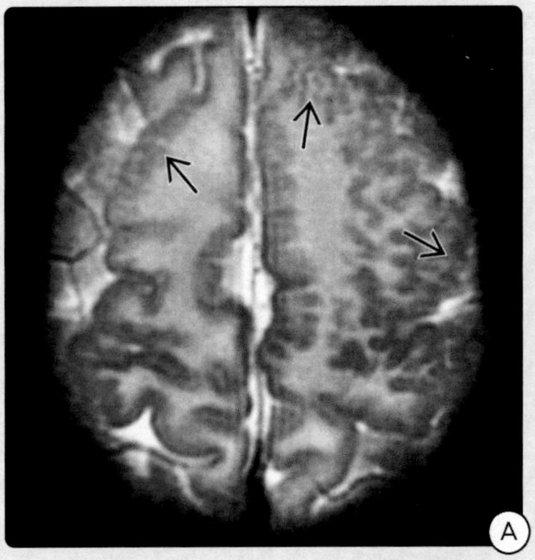

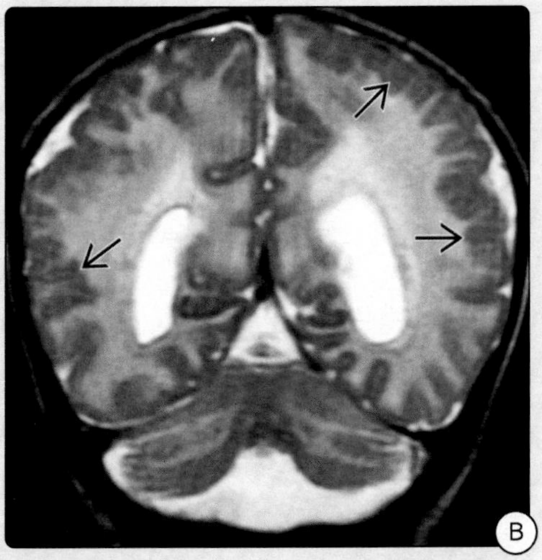

Malformations Secondary to Abnormal Postmigrational Development

According to Barkovich et al., the third group of cortical malformations is secondary to abnormal postmigrational development and typically reflects infectious or ischemic insults. This group was formerly designated "abnormalities of cortical organization." It is currently divided into four subtypes of polymicrogyria (PMG) according to whether clefts (schizencephaly) are present and whether they occur as part of a recognized multiple malformation syndrome or an inherited metabolic disorder.

Polymicrogyria

Terminology and Etiology

The signature feature of PMG is an irregular cortex with numerous small convolutions and shallow or obliterated sulci. The appearance is that of tiny miniature gyri piled on top of other disorganized gyri **(37-43)**.

Mutations in the tubulin genes are common. The phenotypic spectrum of *TUBA1A* mutations includes bilateral perisylvian PMG with dysmorphic basal ganglia, cerebellar vermis dysplasia, and pontine hypoplasia.

Encephaloclastic insults such as infection (e.g., TORCH, Zika virus infection), intrauterine vascular accident (e.g., middle cerebral artery occlusion), trauma, and metabolic disorders have also been implicated in the development of PMG.

Pathology

Location. Bilateral perisylvian PMG is the most common location (61% of cases). Generalized (13%), frontal (5%), and parasagittal parietooccipital (3%) sites are less common. Associated periventricular GM heterotopias are found in 11% of cases, and other anomalies such as schizencephaly are common.

Gross Pathology. The gross findings of PMG vary widely. PMG can involve a single gyrus or most of an entire cerebral hemisphere. It can be uni- or bilateral, symmetric or asymmetric, and focal or diffuse.

Part or all of the brain surface is covered by innumerable heaped up and fused tiny gyri, giving it a "lumpy-bumpy" appearance that has been likened to the look and feel of Morocco leather **(37-44)**. Bilateral disease—especially in the perisylvian regions—is present in the majority of cases. Abnormal lateral ventricle configuration and dysmorphic basal ganglia are common in PMG-associated tubulinopathies **(37-46)**.

Microscopic Features. Microscopically, the cortical ribbon appears thin and excessively folded. Two main histological types of PMG—unlayered and four-layered forms—occur. In the unlayered form, a continuous molecular layer is present without any discernible laminar organization. In four-layered PMG, the cortex shows complex folding, fusion, and branching. A laminar structure composed of a molecular layer, outer neuronal layer, nerve fiber layer, and inner neuronal layer is present.

Clinical Issues

PMG can present at any age. PMG is the most common imaging abnormality seen in infants with congenital cytomegalovirus infection. Some types of

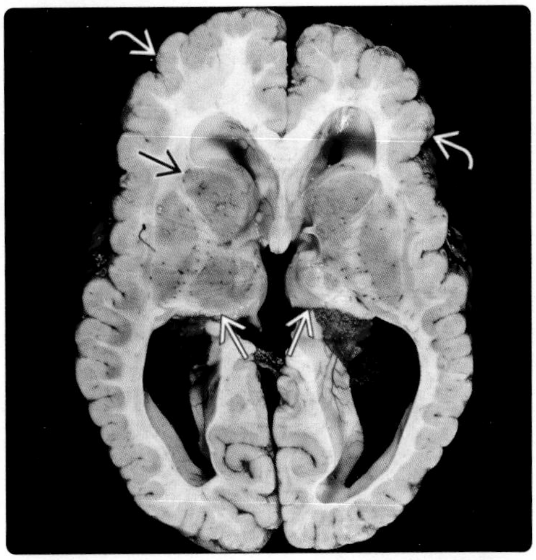

***(37-46)** Tubulinopathy shows PMG, grossly enlarged caudate heads, dysplastic-appearing putamina, small thalami. (R. Hewlett, MD.)*

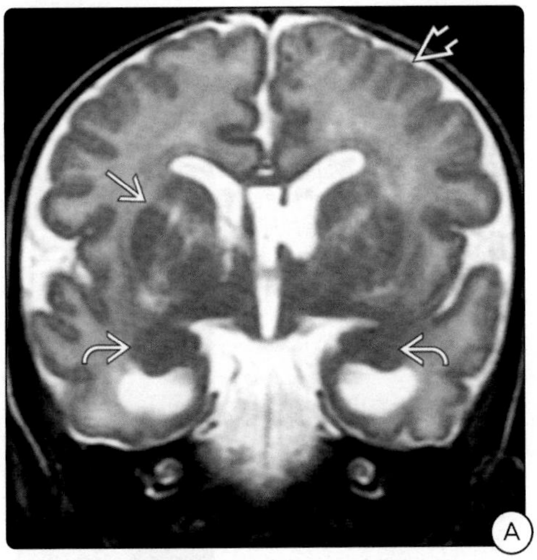

***(37-47A)** Coronal T2WI shows PMG with dysmorphic-appearing basal ganglia and large amygdalae.*

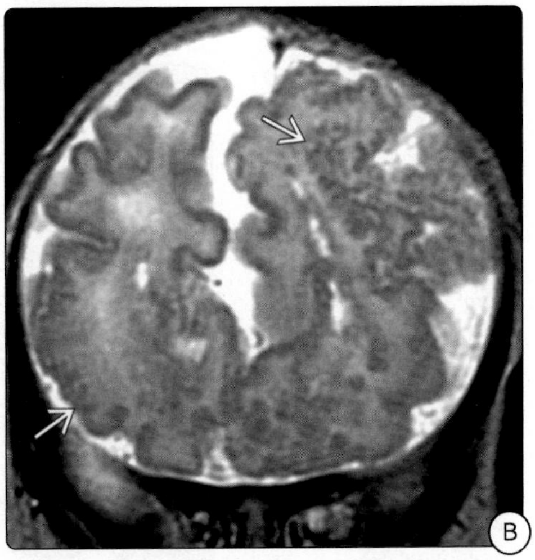

***(37-47B)** More anterior coronal T2WI shows PMG as innumerable small nodular gray matter foci studding the surfaces of both hemispheres.*

PMG are more common in male patients, suggesting the involvement of X-linked genes.

Symptoms depend on the location and extent of PMG, ranging from global developmental delay to focal neurologic deficit(s) and seizures. Perisylvian PMG is a known congenital cause of bilateral opercular syndrome (Foix-Chauvany-Marie syndrome), which is characterized by paralysis of the facial, tongue, pharynx, and masticatory muscles.

Imaging

Multiplanar MR with high-resolution thin sections is required for complete delineation and detection of subtle lesions. Thickened or overfolded cortex with nodular surfaces and irregular "stippled" gray-white matter interfaces are the most characteristic findings **(37-45)**. The basal ganglia often appear dysmorphic **(37-47)**.

Diffusion-weighted imaging often demonstrates increased ADC values in the white matter underlying the PMG, the ipsilateral deep gray nuclei, and the corpus callosum.

Differential Diagnosis

The major differential diagnosis of polymicrogyria is **type 2 lissencephaly** (cobblestone malformation). The absence of congenital muscular dystrophy and "Z-shaped" brainstem is a helpful clinical distinction.

Sometimes **pachygyria** can be confused with PMG. The cortex in PMG is thin, nodular, and excessively folded. In **focal cortical dysplasia**, the gray matter is thickened, and the GM-WM interface is blurred.

In **schizencephaly**, the dysplastic cortex lining the cleft may appear "pebbled," but the cleft distinguishes it from PMG.

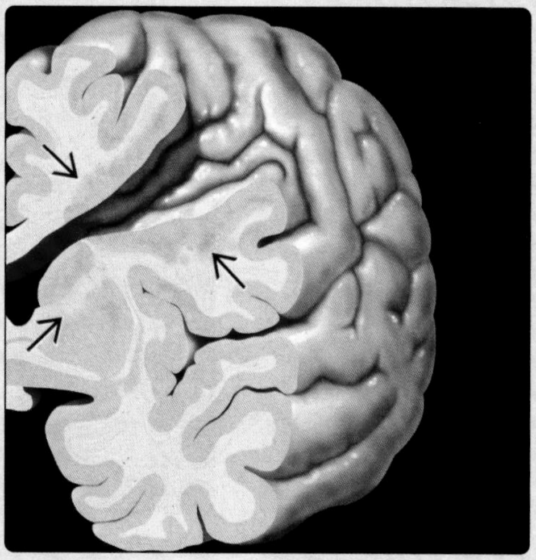

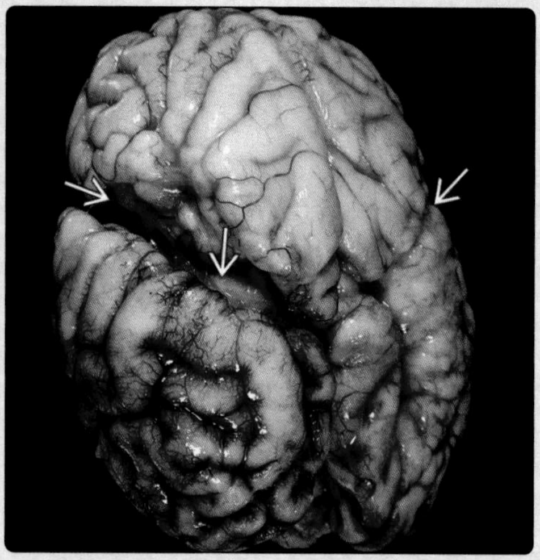

***(37-48)** Coronal oblique graphic shows an "open lip" schizencephaly in the frontal lobe. Note irregular gray-white matter interface of the cortex lining the cleft, indicating its dysplastic nature. **(37-49)** Autopsy shows bilateral schizencephalic clefts. Note that the thick, abnormal cortex curves over the "lips" of the clefts and follows them all the way medially to the ventricular ependyma. (Courtesy R. Hewlett, MD.)*

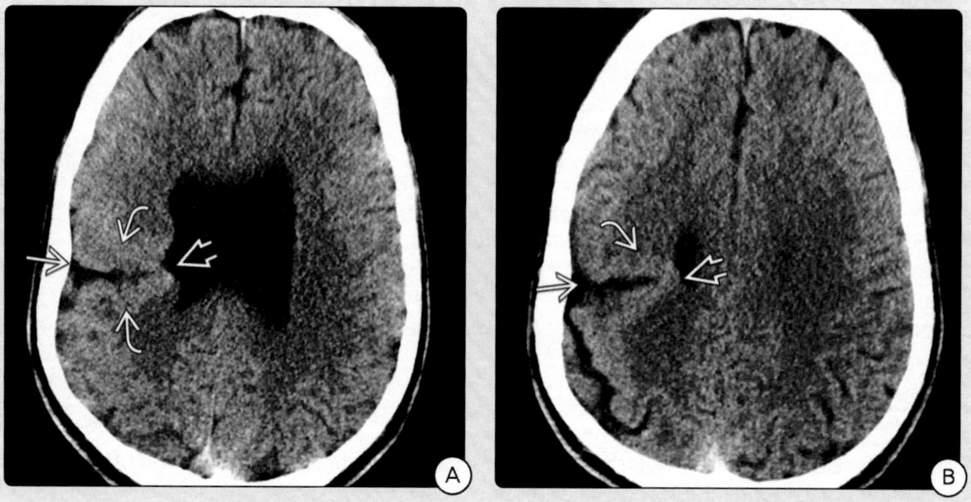

***(37-50A)** NECT in a 19y man following minor head trauma shows the classic findings of unilateral schizencephaly. A nipple-like outpouching of CSF from the lateral ventricle is continuous with a thin "seam" of CSF that extends to the surface of the hemisphere. The cleft is lined with dysplastic-appearing GM. **(37-50B)** More cephalad scan shows cleft and dysplastic GM extending to ventricular ependyma.*

Schizencephaly

Terminology

Schizencephaly (literally meaning "split brain") is a gray-matter-lined cleft that extends from the ventricular ependyma to the pial surface of the cortex. The cleft spans the full thickness of the affected hemisphere **(37-48)**.

Etiology

Once thought to represent an early malformation of cortical development, schizencephaly is now regarded as a disorder with heterogeneous causes. Destructive vascular lesions (e.g., middle cerebral artery occlusion) and infections (e.g., TORCH) occurring before 28 fetal weeks are considered likely etiologies. Focal destruction of radial glial fibers with impaired neuronal migration has been invoked as the potential consequence of these early vascular or infectious insults.

COL4A1 mutation can cause schizencephaly and periventricular calcifications closely resembling congenital TORCH infection. *COL4A1* encodes type IV collagen, which is expressed in all human tissues, especially the vasculature. Up to one-third of schizencephaly cases have an associated non-CNS abnormality secondary to vascular disruption (e.g., amniotic band syndrome or gastroschisis).

Pathology

Grossly, the brain exhibits a deep cleft that extends from its surface to the ventricle. The cleft is surrounded and lined by disorganized, dysmorphic-appearing cortex **(37-49)**. The "lips" of the cleft can be fused or closely apposed ("closed lip" schizencephaly) or appear widely separated ("open lip" schizencephaly). Clefts may be associated with a range of other macroscopic abnormalities involving the septi pellucidi, corpus callosum, optic chiasm, and hippocampus.

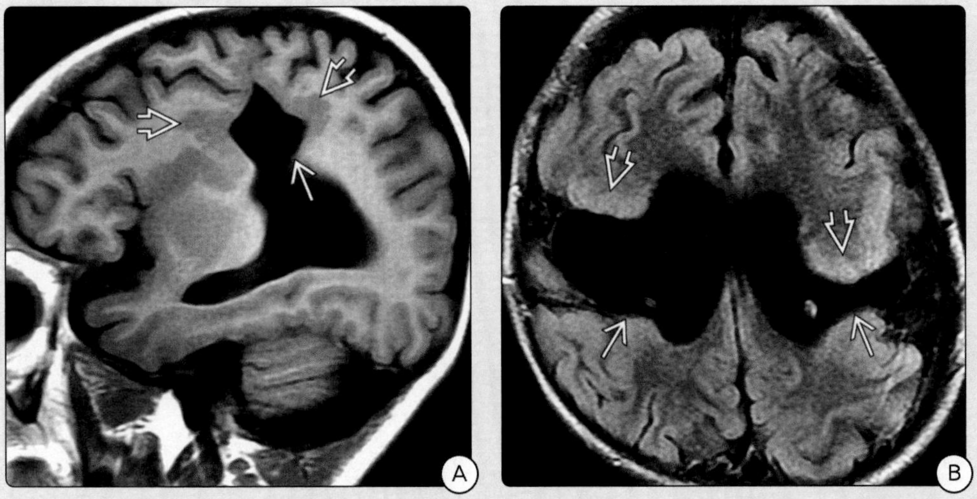

***(37-51A)** Sagittal T1WI shows a large CSF-filled cleft ➡ extending superiorly from the lateral ventricle. The cleft is lined with dysplastic-appearing gray matter ➡. **(37-51B)** FLAIR scan in the same patient shows bilateral schizencephalic clefts ➡ that are lined by dysplastic GM ➡. The clefts suppress completely.*

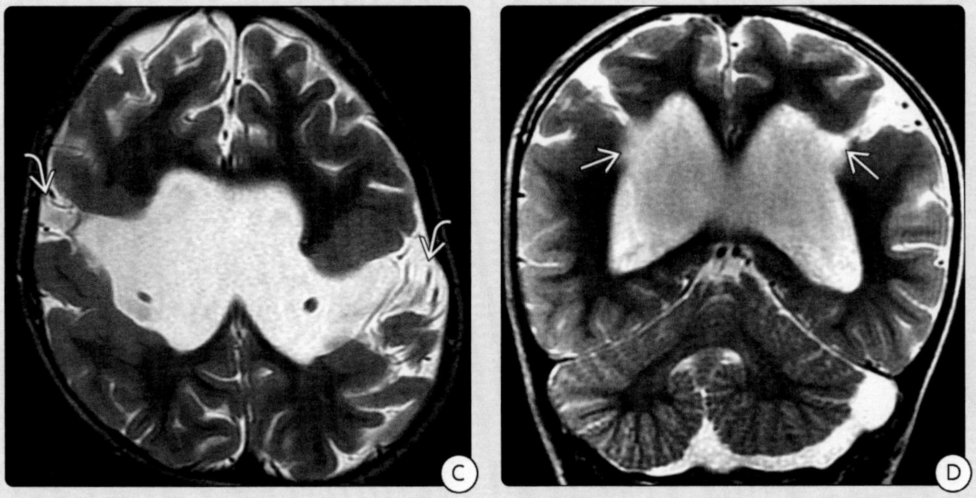

***(37-51C)** Axial T2WI shows that the open "lips" of both clefts contain prominent "flow voids" ➡ consistent with the primitive, "uncondensed" cortical veins that commonly accompany schizencephaly. **(37-51D)** Coronal T2WI shows the pointed "nipples" ➡ of CSF that extend outward from the ventricles into the schizencephalic clefts.*

Microscopically, the gray matter that lines the cleft is disorganized and does not exhibit normal cortical layers.

Clinical Issues

Schizencephaly is rare. There is no sex predilection. The most common clinical manifestations are drug-resistant epilepsy, developmental delay, and motor impairment. The severity of the motor and mental deficits correlates with the extent of the anatomic defect. "Open lip" clefts usually result in the most significant impairment. A unilateral "closed lip" cleft may cause only seizures. A few cases are discovered incidentally.

Imaging

The key imaging features of schizencephaly are (1) a CSF-filled defect extending from the ventricle wall to the pial surface and (2) dysplastic gray matter lining the cleft.

NECT scans typically show a focal V-shaped outpouching or "dimple" of CSF extending outward from the lateral ventricle **(37-50)**. The clefts can be uni- (60%) or bilateral (40%) with prominent ("open lip") **(37-52)** or barely visible ("closed lip") **(37-53)**. The cortex lining the cleft is hyperdense relative to white matter and interrupts the relatively uniform appearance of the corona radiata.

Common associated abnormalities are absent septi pellucidi (70% of cases) and a focally thinned or dysgenetic corpus callosum.

MR is more sensitive than CT, especially in delineating associated abnormalities, such as cortical dysplasia (polymicrogyria, pachygyria) and heterotopic gray matter. The cleft follows CSF signal intensity on all sequences **(37-51)** **(37-52)** **(37-53)**.

DSA or CTA/MRA have demonstrated occlusion or absence of the middle cerebral artery in some cases.

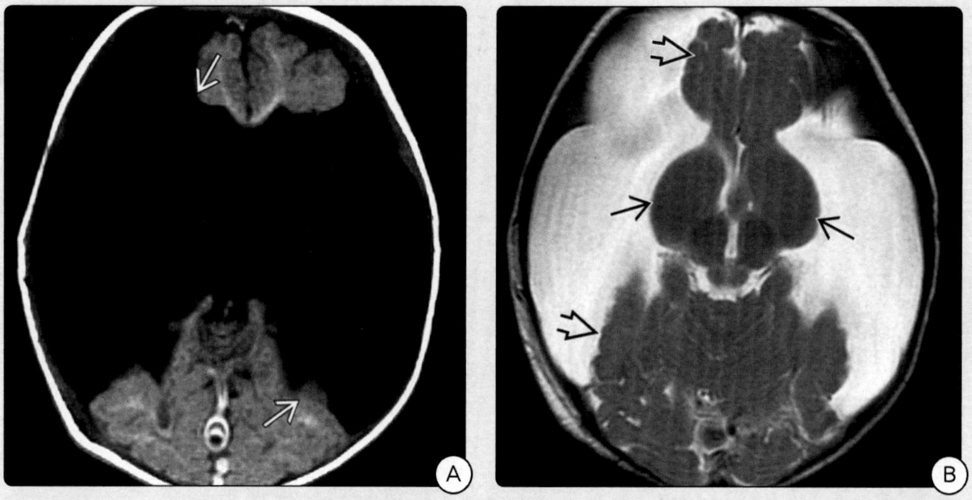

***(37-52A)** Axial T1WI shows severe "open lip" schizencephalic clefts ➡ in both hemispheres. **(37-52B)** T2WI shows the thalami ⇨ and some brain remnants ⇨ in the frontal and occipital poles.*

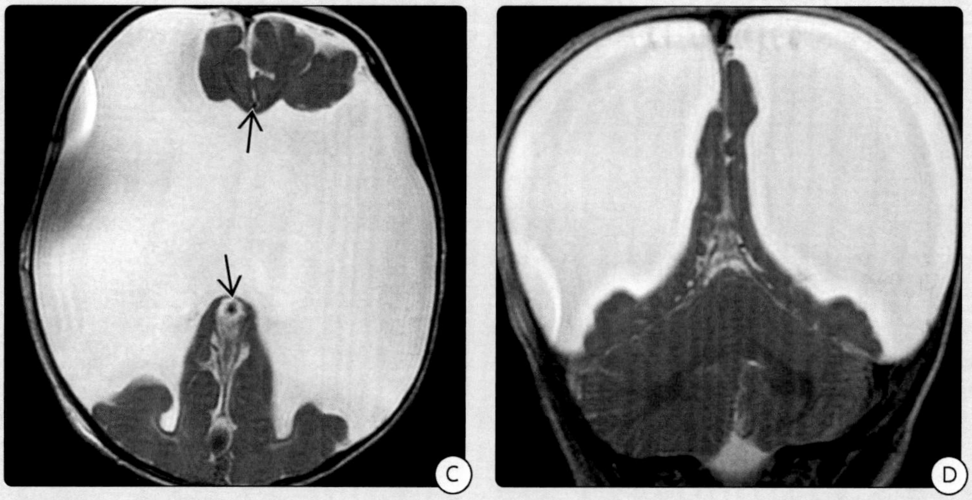

***(37-52C)** More cephalad scan shows presence of a falx and interhemispheric fissure ⇨ distinguishing this extreme case of schizencephaly from holoprosencephaly. The remnant anterior, posterior "nubbins" of brain are different from the thin rim of cortex around the maximally enlarged lateral ventricles in severe hydrocephalus. **(37-52D)** Coronal T2WI shows no cortex external to the huge "open" schizencephalic clefts.*

Differential Diagnosis

The differential diagnosis of CSF-filled brain defects includes both developmental and destructive lesions. The major differential diagnosis of schizencephaly is **porencephaly**. In porencephaly, the cleft is lined by gliotic white matter, not dysplastic gray matter.

A large **arachnoid cyst** can mimic "open lip" schizencephaly. An arachnoid cyst displaces the adjacent cortex, which is otherwise normal in appearance. Occasionally, malformations in focal cortical development are seen with an arachnoid cyst.

Transmantle **heterotopia** or deeply infolded **polymicrogyria** may be difficult to distinguish from schizencephaly with closed, nearly fused "lips." Multiple imaging planes with high-resolution T2WI or thin-section T1-weighted sequences with 3D reformatting and shaded surface displays are helpful in differentiating these entities.

SCHIZENCEPHALY

Etiology
- In utero encephaloclastic lesion (vascular, infection)?
- *COL4A1* mutation (can mimic TORCH)

Pathology
- Cleft ("seam") from ependyma to pia
  - Can be closed or open, uni- or bilateral
  - Lined by dysplastic gray matter

Imaging
- NECT
  - Outpouching ("nipple") from lateral ventricle
  - CSF-filled cleft lined with dysplastic GM
- MR
  - Cleft lining follows cortex signal on all sequences
  - Corpus callosum dysgenesis, other abnormalities common

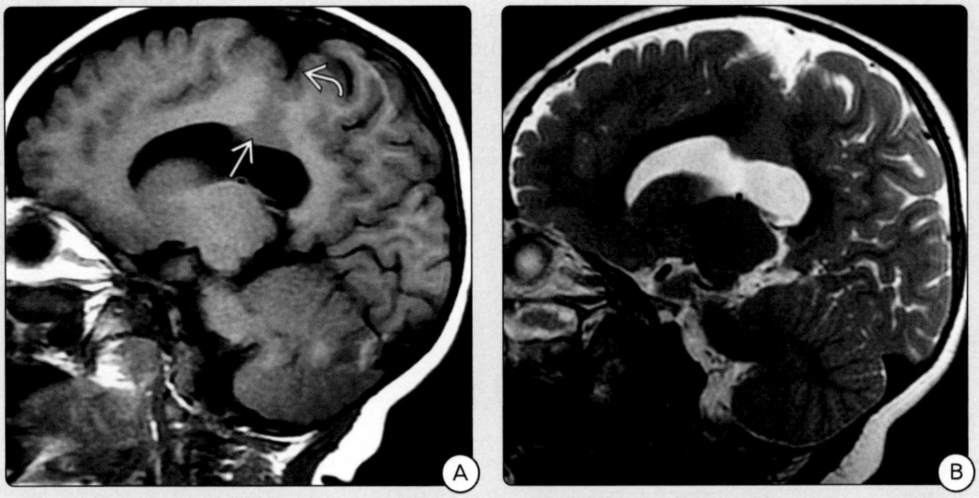

(37-53A) Unilateral "closed lip" schizencephaly is illustrated by this case. Note gray matter extending from the ventricle ➡ to the pial surface of the brain ➡. (37-53B) Sagittal T2WI shows that the GM lining the cleft is the same signal intensity as the cortex.

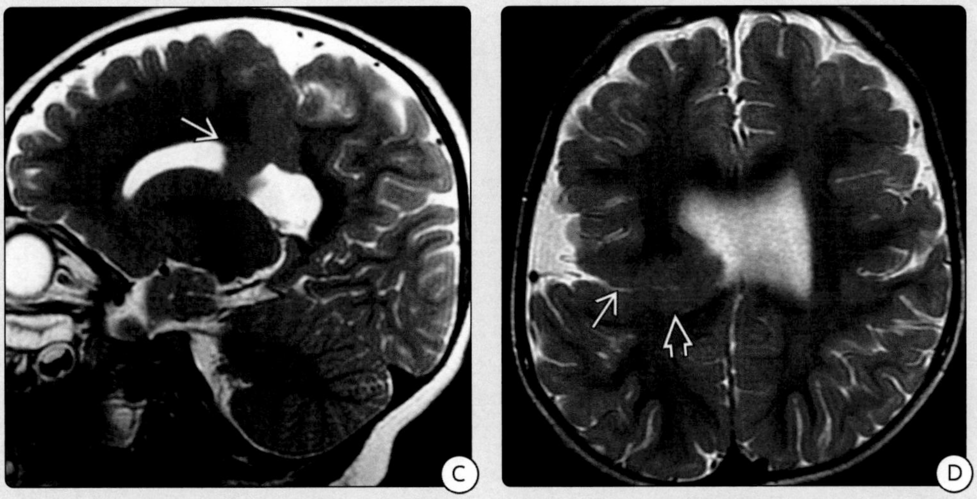

(37-53C) Sagittal T2WI shows that the heterotopic GM around the cleft bulges into the lateral ventricle body ➡. (37-53D) Axial T2WI shows the heterotopic GM ➡ surrounding the cleft ➡, which is difficult to discern, as it is so thin.

Selected References

Normal Development and Anatomy of the Cerebral Commissures

Normal Development

Jamuar SS et al: Biallelic mutations in human DCC cause developmental split-brain syndrome. Nat Genet. 49(4):606-612, 2017

Scola E et al: Fetal development of the corpus callosum: insights from a 3T DTI and tractography study in a patient with segmental callosal agenesis. Neuroradiol J. 29(5):323-5, 2016

Normal Gross and Imaging Anatomy

Vannucci RC et al: Development of the corpus callosum: an MRI study. Dev Neurosci. ePub, 2016

Andronikou S et al: Corpus callosum thickness in children: an MR pattern-recognition approach on the midsagittal image. Pediatr Radiol. 45(2):258-72, 2015

Di Ieva A et al: The indusium griseum and the longitudinal striae of the corpus callosum. Cortex. 62:34-40, 2015

Commissural Anomalies

Callosal Dysgenesis Spectrum

Unterberger I et al: Corpus callosum and epilepsies. Seizure. 37:55-60, 2016

Filippi CG et al: Lesions of the corpus callosum and other commissural fibers: diffusion tensor studies. Semin Ultrasound CT MR. 35(5):445-58, 2014

Thick Corpus Callosum

Nguyen LS et al: A nonsense variant in HERC1 is associated with intellectual disability, megalencephaly, thick corpus callosum and cerebellar atrophy. Eur J Hum Genet. 24(3):455-8, 2016

Budai C et al: Polymicrogyria, large corpus callosum and psychomotor retardation in four-year-old girl: potential association based on MR findings. A case report and literature review. Neuroradiol J. 27(5):590-4, 2014

Malformations of Cortical Development Overview

Barkovich AJ et al: Pediatric Neuroimaging, 5th ed. Philadelphia, PA: Lippincott, Williams & Wilkins, 2012

Malformations With Abnormal Cell Numbers/Types

Focal Cortical Dysplasias

Knerlich-Lukoschus F et al: Clinical, imaging, and immunohistochemical characteristics of focal cortical dysplasia Type II extratemporal epilepsies in children: analyses of an institutional case series. J Neurosurg Pediatr. 19(2):182-195, 2017

Siedlecka M et al: Focal cortical dysplasia: molecular disturbances and clinicopathological classification (Review). Int J Mol Med. 38(5):1327-1337, 2016

Crino PB: Focal cortical dysplasia. Semin Neurol. 35(3):201-8, 2015

Taylor DC et al: Focal dysplasia of the cerebral cortex in epilepsy. J Neurol Neurosurg Psychiatry. 34(4):369-87, 1971

Hemimegalencephaly

Crino PB: The enlarging spectrum of focal cortical dysplasias. Brain. 138(Pt 6):1446-8, 2015

Oikawa T et al: Utility of diffusion tensor imaging parameters for diagnosis of hemimegalencephaly. Neuroradiol J. 28(6):628-33, 2015

Abnormalities of Neuronal Migration

Heterotopias

Seniaray N et al: PET MRI coregistration in intractable epilepsy and gray matter heterotopia. Clin Nucl Med. 42(3):e171-e172, 2017

Hung PC et al: Clinical and neuroimaging findings in children with gray matter heterotopias: a single institution experience of 36 patients. Eur J Paediatr Neurol. 20(5):732-7, 2016

Kobayashi Y et al: Megalencephaly, polymicrogyria and ribbon-like band heterotopia: a new cortical malformation. Brain Dev. 38(10):950-953, 2016

Jamuar SS et al: Somatic mutations in cerebral cortical malformations. N Engl J Med. 371(8):733-43, 2014

Lissencephaly Spectrum

Fry AE et al: The genetics of lissencephaly. Am J Med Genet C Semin Med Genet. 166C(2):198-210, 2014

Malformations Secondary to Abnormal Postmigrational Development

Polymicrogyria

Bahi-Buisson N et al: The wide spectrum of tubulinopathies: what are the key features for the diagnosis? Brain. 137(Pt 6):1676-700, 2014

Holoprosencephalies, Related Disorders, and Mimics

In this chapter, we discuss the holoprosencephalies and related disorders. Holoprosencephalies and variants such as syntelencephaly are classified as anomalies of ventral prosencephalon development. Other anomalies of the ventral prosencephalon include septooptic dysplasia (with or without anomalies of the hypothalamic-pituitary axis) and arrhinencephaly, both of which are discussed in this chapter.

We also consider two midline facial anomalies—solitary median maxillary central incisor syndrome and congenital pyriform aperture stenosis/choanal atresia spectrum—that are often present in holoprosencephaly or arrhinencephaly.

Finally, we conclude the chapter with a brief discussion of hydranencephaly, an in utero acquired destruction of the cerebral hemispheres that can sometimes be confused with alobar holoprosencephaly or severe "open lip" schizencephaly.

Anencephaly

Anencephaly (literally meaning "no brain") occurs when the cephalic end of the neural tube fails to close, resulting in absence of the forebrain, skull, and scalp. The remaining brain—usually only the brainstem—is not covered by bone or skin. Most anencephalic fetuses are aborted or die shortly after birth **(38-1)**.

Two rare lethal malformations—**aprosencephaly** and **atelencephaly** (AP/AT)—are intermediate in the continuum between anencephaly and holoprosencephaly. AP/AT is now considered the most severe end of the holoprosencephaly spectrum. These three extreme malformations are usually diagnosed at fetal MR, sonography, or postmortem examination **(38-2)**.

Holoprosencephaly

Holoprosencephaly (HPE) spans a continuum from alobar to lobar forms. Although each is delineated separately, keep in mind that the HPEs are really a spectrum with no clear boundaries that reliably distinguish one type from another.

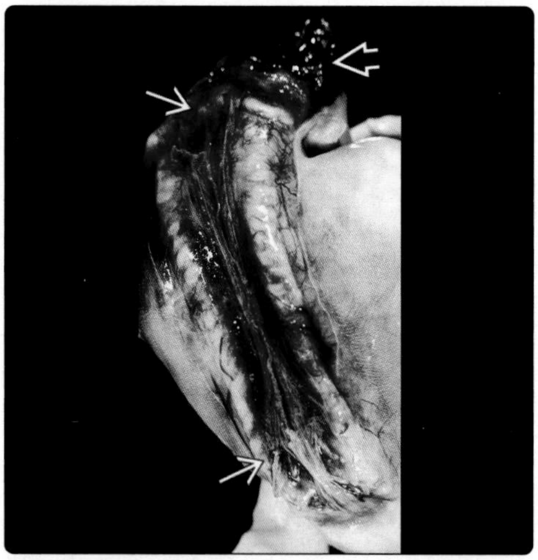

(38-1) *Autopsy shows total failure of neural tube closure with complete spine dysraphism* ➡ *and anencephaly* ➡. *(Courtesy R. Hewlett, MD.)*

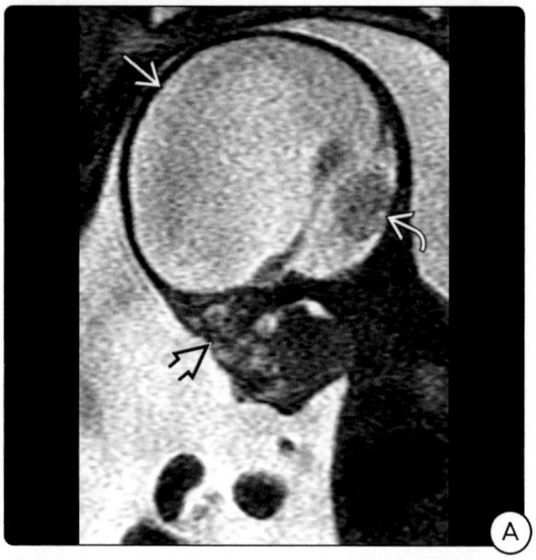

(38-2A) *Fetal sagittal T2WI in aprosencephaly shows no supratentorial brain* ➡, *absent nose* ⇨, *and small remnant of cerebellum* ➡.

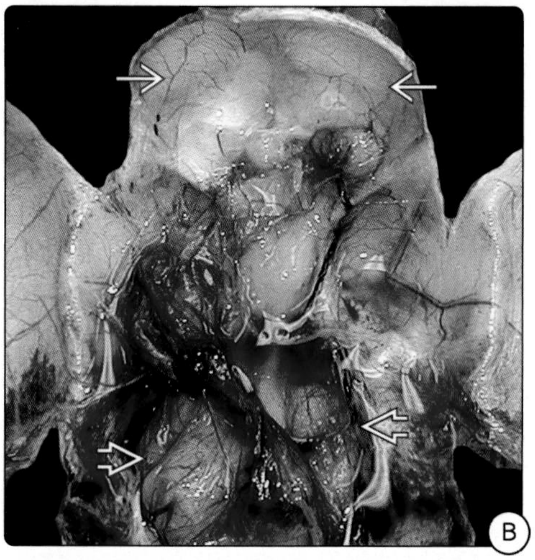

(38-2B) *Autopsy of same case, seen from above, shows no supratentorial tissue* ➡. *Only cerebellum is present* ➡ *(T. Winters, MD).*

Overview

In HPE, the fetal forebrain fails to bifurcate into two hemispheres. "Holoprosencephaly" literally means a single ("holo") ventricle involving the embryonic prosencephalon ("pros") of the brain ("encephaly"). As ventral induction is closely related to facial development, HPE is also associated with a number of characteristic facial anomalies.

Although the phenotype of HPE is quite variable, it can be grouped into two major classes, namely **classic HPE** and an HPE variant known as **middle interhemispheric variant of holoprosencephaly** (MIH HPE) or syntelencephaly.

Classic HPE as described by DeMyer (1977) can be further subdivided into three subtypes based on severity although HPE is a continuum that ranges from the most severe type (**alobar** HPE) to milder **lobar** forms. In the most severe forms, a central monoventricle is present, whereas diencephalic-derived structures such as the basal ganglia remain fused in the midline.

An intermediate type, **semilobar** HPE, is more severe than alobar HPE but not nearly as well differentiated as the lobar variety. The distinction between these three forms is based primarily on the presence or absence of a midline fissure separating the hemispheres.

Etiology

Embryology. The fetal forebrain starts as a featureless, fluid-filled frontal sac. In the earliest stages, bilateral outpouchings from the neural tube initially form a single central fluid-filled cavity ("monoventricle"). A key group of specialized cells called the roof plate is involved in the division of this single forebrain vesicle into the two cerebral hemispheres. Failure of this process leads to some forms of holoprosencephaly.

General Concepts. Between one-quarter and one-half of HPE patients have a recognized syndrome (e.g., Pallister-Hall) or a single gene defect. Nonsyndromic HPE has previously been associated with a number of environmental teratogens (e.g., retinoic acid and alcohol) and maternal factors such as prepregnancy diabetes, smoking, and substance abuse. However, recent studies have cast doubt on these assertions.

Genetics. Genetically determined proteins are involved in normal forebrain roof plate function. Among the most prominent are members of the fibroblast growth factor (Fgf), Bmp, and Wnt proteins as well as Shh, Zic2, Neurogenin2, Six3, and TGIF.

Studies have shown that mutations in any of at least nine genes involved in the *Shh* signaling pathway can cause HPE in humans although this pathway accounts for only 17% of familial HPE. Variations in the homeobox protein Six3 have been shown to result in different forms of HPE.

Clinical Issues

Epidemiology and Demographics. HPE is the most common human forebrain malformation. The overall incidence of HPE varies from 1:250 aborted conceptuses to 1:10,000-20,000 live births.

Presentation. Presentation and prognosis in HPE both vary widely. Craniofacial malformations such as cyclopia or single proboscis, hypotelorism, nasal anomalies, and facial clefts occur in approximately 75-80% of cases. The statement "the face predicts the brain" means that the most severe facial defects generally (although not invariably) are found with the most severe intracranial anomalies **(38-3)**.

Nearly three-quarters of HPE patients have endocrinopathies; severity generally correlates with the degree of hypothalamic nonseparation. An association between HPE and hypothalamic hamartoma also exists.

Natural History. Fetuses with severe alobar HPE are often spontaneously aborted, and severely affected children frequently die as neonates. Surviving individuals usually exhibit variable mental retardation and seizures. Pituitary insufficiency and congenital anosmia with absent CN I ("arrhinencephaly") are other common clinical features of HPE.

Imaging

Imaging findings range from a pancake-like holosphere with central monoventricle (alobar HPE) to well-differentiated, almost completely separated hemispheres with minimal abnormalities (lobar HPE). The septum pellucidum is absent in all cases of HPE.

Alobar Holoprosencephaly

Terminology and Pathology

Alobar holoprosencephaly (aHPE) is the most severe form of HPE. No midline fissure divides the brain into two separate cerebral hemispheres, and no identifiable lobes are seen. The basal ganglia are usually present but fused. The falx and sagittal sinus are absent, as are the olfactory bulbs and tracts. The optic nerves can be normal, fused, or absent.

The brain itself is often smaller than normal. Its configuration varies from flat ("pancake") to cup- or ball-shaped. The sylvian fissures are unformed, and the brain surface often appears completely agyric **(38-3B)** or minimally sulcated with shallow sulci and flat, disordered gyri.

Cut sections demonstrate a single crescent-shaped monoventricle that opens dorsally into a large CSF-filled dorsal cyst **(38-4)**.

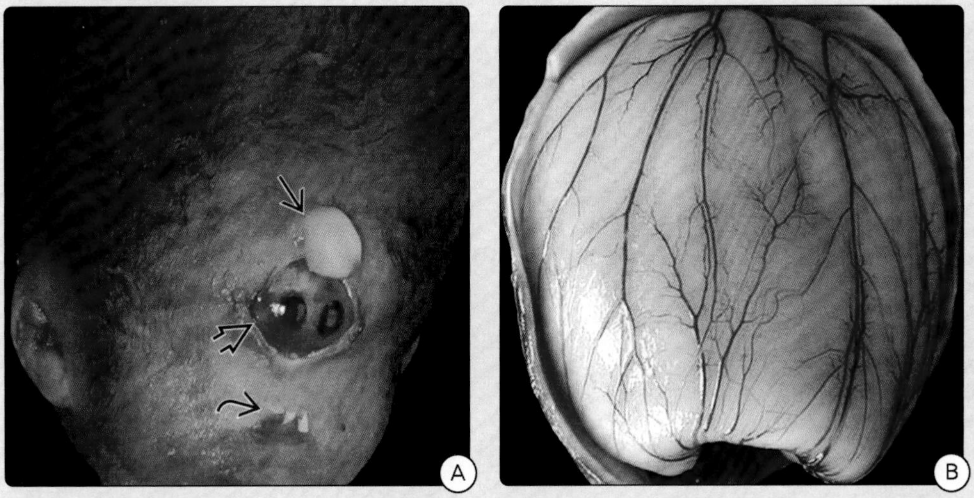

***(38-3A)** Clinical photograph of aborted fetus with alobar holoprosencephaly shows extreme facial anomalies with central proboscis, cyclops, and slit-like oral cavity. **(38-3B)** View of autopsied brain in the same case shows completely smooth, featureless brain with no evidence of sulcation, gyration, or midline structures such as the falx or interhemispheric fissure. (Courtesy R. Hewlett, MD.)*

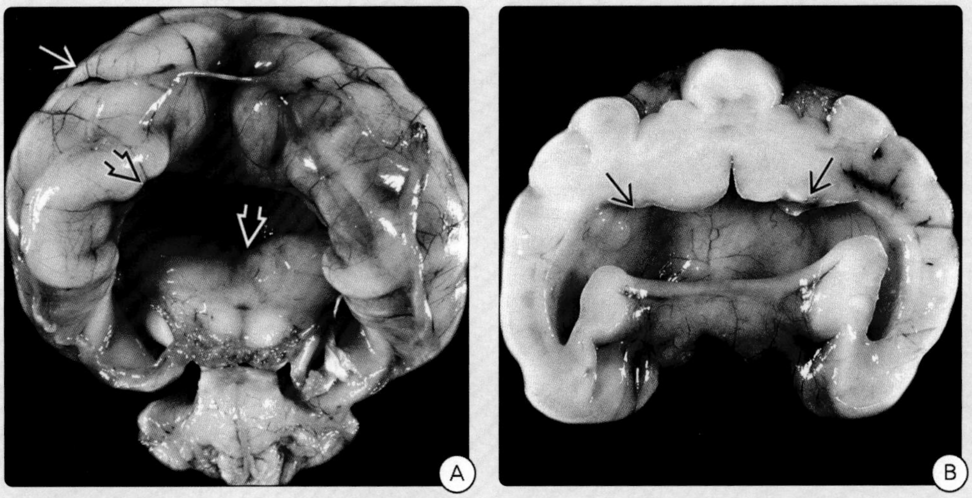

***(38-4A)** Autopsy of alobar holoprosencephaly shows large dorsal cyst, fused thalami, and rudimentary hemispheres with minimal sulcation and gyration. **(38-4B)** Coronal cut section in the same case demonstrates no evidence of midline fissure with fusion of the rudimentary hemispheres across the midline. The central monoventricle has a "horseshoe" shape. (Courtesy J. Townsend, MD.)*

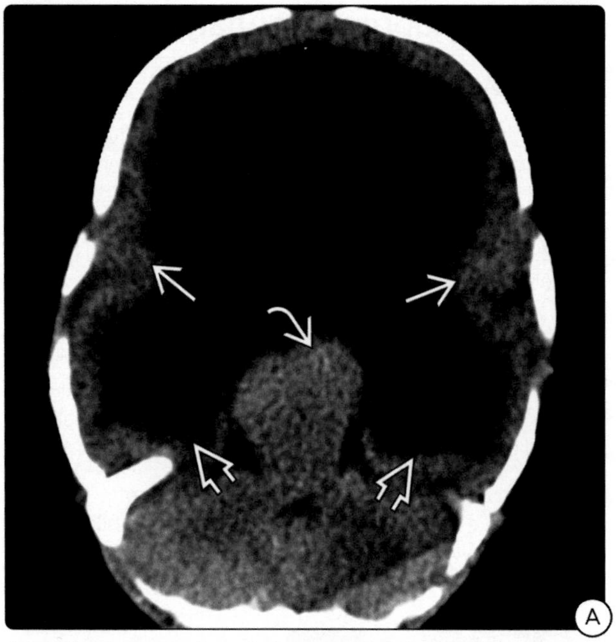

(38-5A) NECT scan shows holoprosencephaly. Small rim of cortex surrounds "horseshoe" central monoventricle. Thalami are fused.

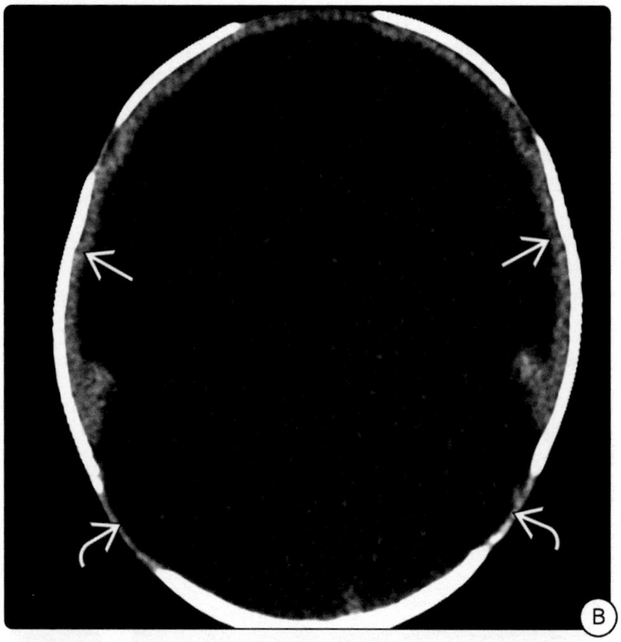

(38-5B) More cephalad scan in the same patient shows a large dorsal cyst and central monoventricle with thin rim of surrounding brain. No falx or interhemispheric fissure is present.

Clinical Issues

aHPE has a high intrauterine lethality and stillbirth rate. It is found in 1:250 terminated pregnancies and approximately 1:15,000 live births. In utero demise and stillbirths are common.

With severe facial deformities such as cyclopia and proboscis, survival is often less than 1 week. Prognosis in surviving infants is poor. At least half of all patients with aHPE die in less than 5 months, and 80% die before 1 year of age.

Imaging

No normal ventricles can be identified. NECT scans show a CSF-filled horseshoe-shaped cavity that is usually continuous posteriorly with a large dorsal cyst **(38-5)**.

Sagittal T1 scans show a thin anteroinferior pancake of tissue with poor gyration and no discernible midline fissure. Most of the calvaria appears CSF-filled and virtually featureless. In contrast, the brainstem and cerebellum often seem relatively normal.

Coronal scans best demonstrate the central monoventricle. The septi pellucidi and third ventricle are absent, as are the falx cerebri and interhemispheric fissure. The cerebral mantle is fused across the midline anteriorly. The brain appears thin and almost agyric, although a few shallow sulci may be present. The basal ganglia are small and fused across the midline. There are no discernible commissures.

Axial scans show that the brain is completely fused across the midline without evidence of an anterior interhemispheric fissure. The monoventricle opens dorsally into a large CSF-filled cyst.

Vascular anomalies associated with aHPE include a rete of vessels and azygous anterior cerebral artery.

Differential Diagnosis

The major differential diagnosis of aHPE is **hydranencephaly**. In hydranencephaly, the face is normal. A falx is present, but most of the cerebral tissue has been destroyed, usually by an intrauterine vascular accident or infection.

Semilobar Holoprosencephaly

Terminology and Pathology

Semilobar holoprosencephaly (sHPE) is intermediate in severity between alobar HPE and lobar HPE. A gradation of findings is present. The most severe sHPE shows a rudimentary interhemispheric fissure and incomplete falx **(38-6)**. The temporal horns of the lateral ventricle may be partially formed, but the septi pellucidi are absent. A dorsal cyst is often present.

Imaging

With progressively better-differentiated sHPE, more of the interhemispheric fissure appears formed **(38-7)**. The deep nuclei exhibit various degrees of separation. If a rudimentary third ventricle is present, the thalami may be partially separated. The basal ganglia and hypothalami are still largely fused. The caudate heads are continuous across the midline **(38-8)**.

A corpus callosum splenium is present, but the body and genu are absent. Barkovich points out that (1) holoprosencephaly is the only malformation in which the posterior corpus callosum

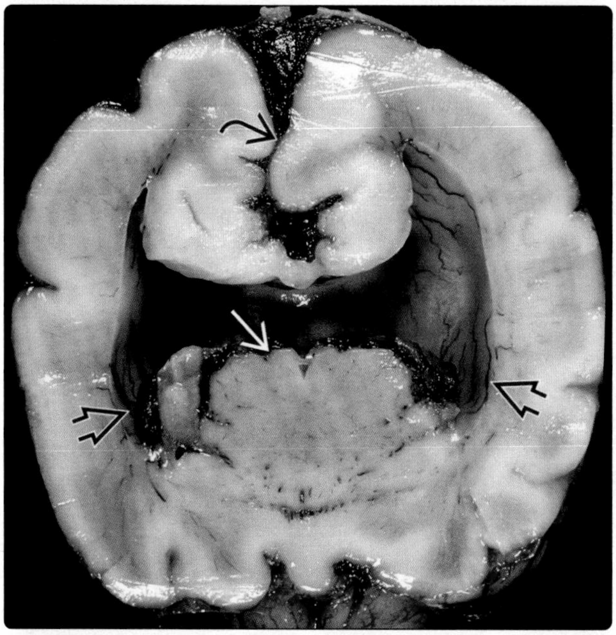

(38-6) Coronal autopsy case of severe semilobar HPE shows H-shaped central ventricle with primitive-appearing temporal horns, fused basal ganglia, and rudimentary interhemispheric fissure. (Courtesy R. Hewlett, MD.)

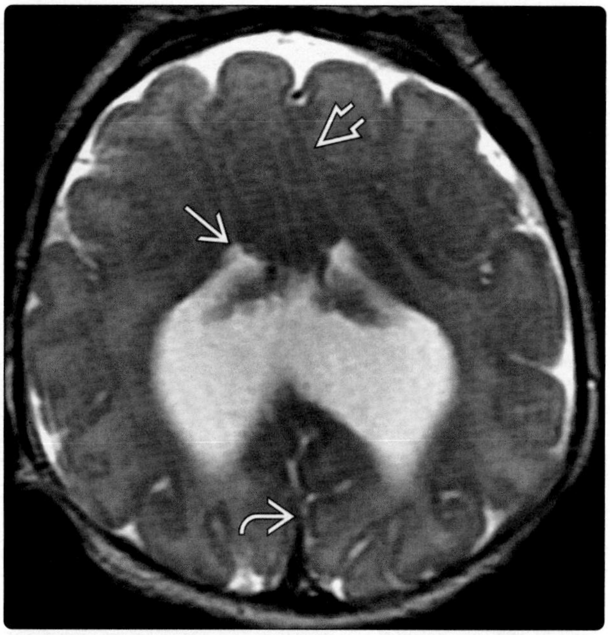

(38-7) Axial T2WI shows severe sHPE with rudimentary posterior interhemispheric fissure, primitive ventricular horns, and anterior midline fusion. Diffuse frontal migration arrest with subcortical heterotopic GM is also present.

forms while the anterior aspects are absent and (2) the farther anteriorly the corpus forms, the better the brain is developed.

Associated abnormalities include a dorsal cyst (present in one-third of cases) and vascular anomalies, such as azygous anterior cerebral artery and rudimentary deep veins.

Differential Diagnosis

The major differential diagnoses of sHPE are **alobar HPE and lobar HPE**, depending on the severity of the sHPE.

Lobar Holoprosencephaly

Terminology and Pathology

Lobar HPE is the best differentiated of the HPEs. The interhemispheric fissure and falx are clearly developed, although their most anterior aspects are often somewhat shallow and dysplastic-appearing.

The third ventricle and lateral ventricular horns are generally well formed, although the septi pellucidi are absent and the frontal horns almost always appear dysmorphic. The hippocampi are present but often more vertically oriented than normal.

Clinical Issues

Patients with lobar HPE are less severely affected compared with individuals with sHPE. Mild developmental delay, hypothalamic-pituitary dysfunction, and visual disturbances are the most common symptoms.

Imaging

In lobar HPE, the cerebral hemispheres—including the thalami and most of the basal ganglia—are mostly separated. At least some of the most rostral and ventral portions of the frontal lobes are continuous across the midline **(38-9)**. The anterior columns of the fornix are fused. The thalami and basal ganglia are separated, although the caudate heads may remain fused.

The frontal horns of the lateral ventricles are present but dysplastic-appearing. The temporal and occipital horns are better defined, and the third ventricle generally appears normal. There are no septi pellucidi.

The corpus callosum is present and can be normal, incomplete, or hypoplastic. The splenium and most of the body can usually be identified, although the genu and rostrum are often absent. In contrast to isolated or syndromic corpus callosum dysgenesis, there are no Probst bundles in any of the HPEs.

The walls of the hypothalamus remain unseparated, and the optic chiasm is often smaller than normal. The olfactory bulbs are present in well-differentiated lobar HPE. The pituitary gland can be flattened, hypoplastic, or ectopic.

Associated vascular anomalies include an azygous anterior cerebral artery.

Differential Diagnosis

The major differential diagnosis of lobar HPE is **septooptic dysplasia** (SOD). Some authors consider SOD the best differentiated of the HPE spectrum. In contrast to lobar HPE,

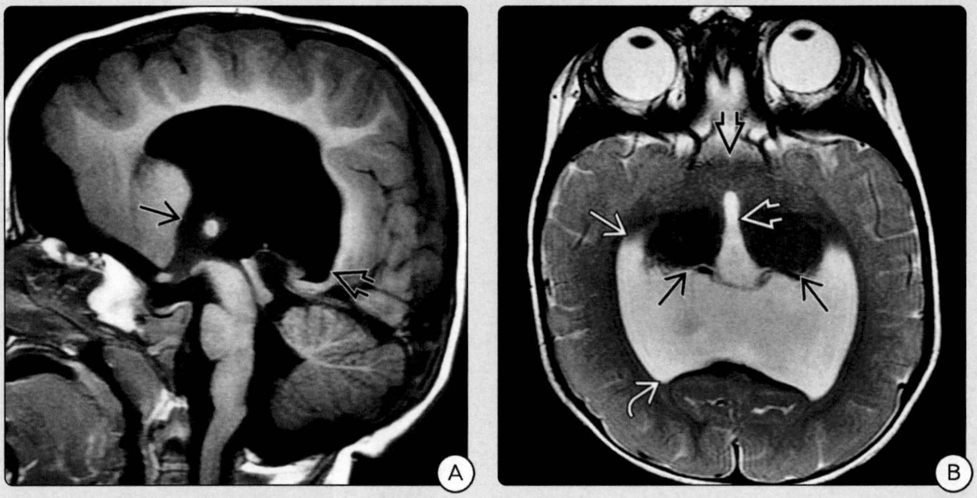

***(38-8A)** Sagittal T1WI shows sHPE with partial differentiation of third ventricle, occipital horns. The midbrain, pons, and cerebellum are comparatively normal. **(38-8B)** Axial T2WI in the same patient shows mild hypotelorism with no other midface anomalies. Rudimentary temporal and occipital horns are present. The third ventricle is partially formed. The thalami are separated, but the hypothalamus remains fused.*

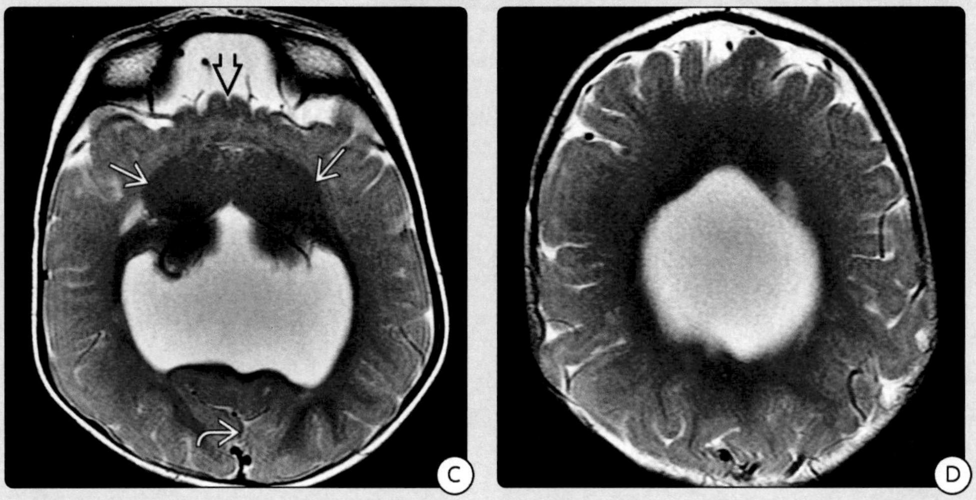

***(38-8C)** More cephalad T2WI in the same patient shows fused basal ganglia, rudimentary posterior interhemispheric fissure, and absence of anterior interhemispheric fissure with the brain fused across the midline. **(38-8D)** More cephalad scan shows the upper aspect of a poorly differentiated central monoventricle. The corpus callosum and all normal midline structures are absent.*

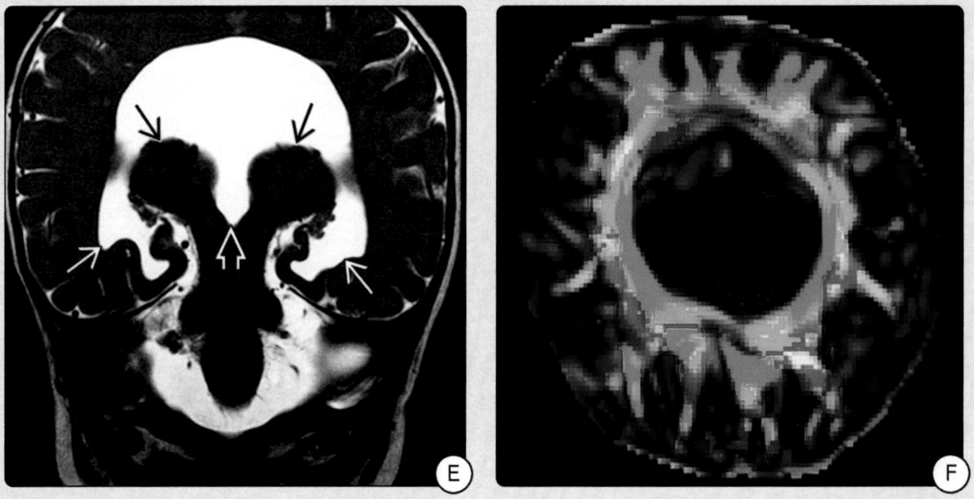

***(38-8E)** Coronal T2WI shows the monoventricle with rudimentary temporal horns. A partially formed third ventricle separates the thalami. The interhemispheric fissure is absent. **(38-8F)** Color DTI shows the central monoventricle surrounded by unindentifiable disorganized, chaotic white matter tracts.*

the frontal horns are well formed in SOD. **Arrhinencephaly** may resemble lobar HPE, but the olfactory bulbs are usually present in lobar HPE.

In the **middle interhemispheric variant of HPE** (syntelencephaly), the corpus callosum genu and splenium are formed; however, the body is missing, and the posterior frontal lobes are continuous across the midline.

HOLOPROSENCEPHALIES (BASED ON DEMYER'S THREE DEGREES OF SEVERITY)

Classic Holoprosencephaly

- Alobar holoprosencephaly
  - Most severe; high intrauterine lethality
  - "Pancake" brain with central monoventricle
  - Basal ganglia fused; no falx, no interhemispheric fissure (IHF)
- Semilobar holoprosencephaly
  - Rudimentary falx, posterior IHF
  - Primitive ventricular horns, third ventricle
  - Thalami often separated, but basal ganglia fused
- Lobar holoprosencephaly
  - Best-differentiated form of classic HPE
  - Basal ganglia separated, falx/IHF present except anteroinferiorly
  - Ventral frontal lobes remain fused across midline

Variant Holoprosencephaly

- Midline (middle) interhemispheric holoprosencephaly
- Septopreoptic holoprosencephaly

Holoprosencephaly Variants

Several holoprosencephaly (HPE) variants have been identified, including syntelencephaly and septopreoptic HPEs. Arrhinencephaly, which some authors consider a variant of HPE, is considered together with septooptic dysplasia later in the chapter.

Middle Interhemispheric Variant of Holoprosencephaly

The middle interhemispheric variant of HPE (MIH) is also known as **syntelencephaly**. Here the anterior and posterior hemispheres are separated by the falx and interhemispheric fissure, but their midsections are fused across the midline **(38-10)**. In contrast to classic HPE, the ventral aspects of the basal forebrain are largely spared, so the basal ganglia and olfactory sulci appear normal.

Imaging findings in MIH are diagnostic. Sagittal T1 and T2 scans show that the corpus callosum splenium and genu are present but that the body is absent. The posterior frontal lobes are continuous across the midline on coronal images. The lateral ventricle bodies appear narrow and fused.

Axial scans show the anterior and posterior parts of the interhemispheric fissure and the absence of the midsection. The falx also narrows and disappears in both the posterior frontal and anterior parietal regions. In 85% of cases, the sylvian fissures course superiorly and meet in a coronally oriented, cortically lined fissure that is continuous across the midline **(38-11A) (38-11B) (38-11D)**.

On coronal imaging, a single common ventricle lacking a septum pellucidum is present. A nodule of gray matter is perched along the dorsal aspect of the fused lateral ventricles, forming a characteristic central ventricular "notch" **(38-11C)**. The third ventricle is well formed.

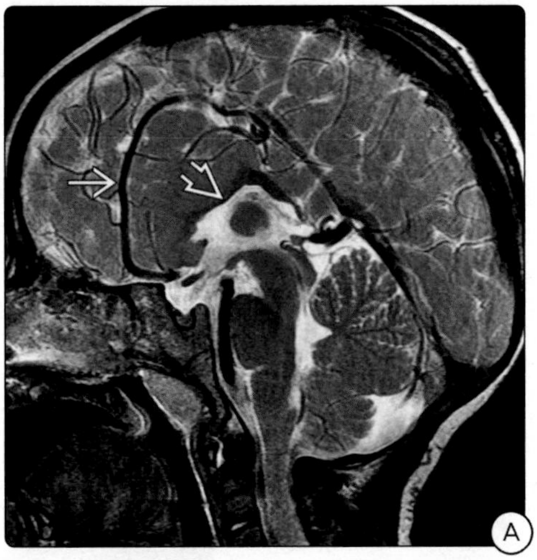

(38-9A) Sagittal T2WI of lobar HPE shows well-differentiated brain, nearly normal-appearing third ventricle, and azygous ACA.

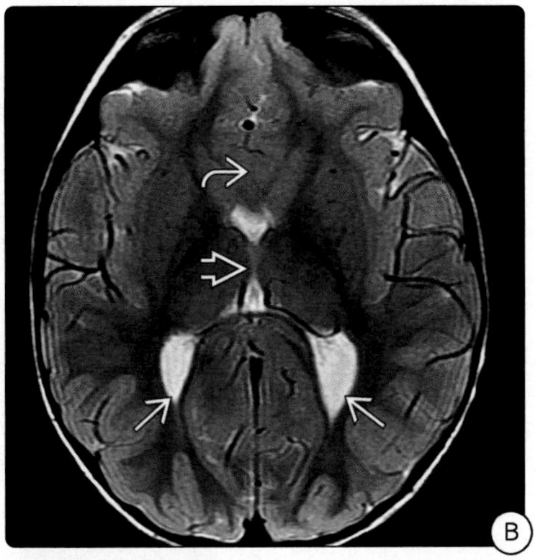

(38-9B) Axial T2WI shows well-developed occipital horns, third ventricle, and minimal anterior midline fusion.

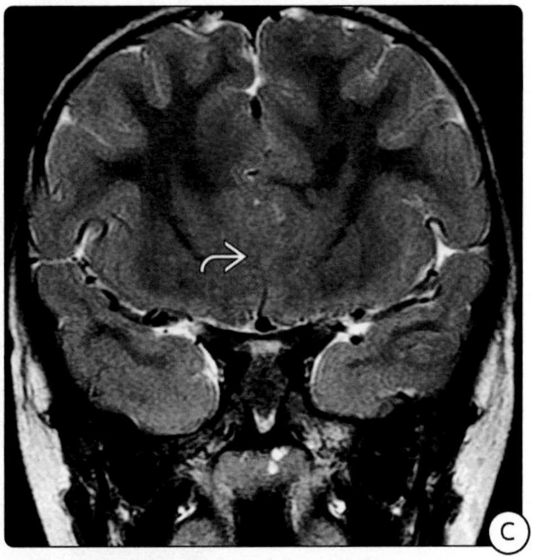

(38-9C) Coronal T2WI shows that the anteroinferior frontal cortex is fused across the midline.

(38-10) Axial graphic depicts syntelencephaly with absent midsection of the interhemispheric fissure, upward extension of an anomalous sylvian fissure across the midline, and foci of both gray and white matter that bridge the hemispheres. (38-11A) Axial NECT scan in a patient with syntelencephaly shows that the midportions of the hemispheres appear fused across the midline with bridges of both white and gray matter.

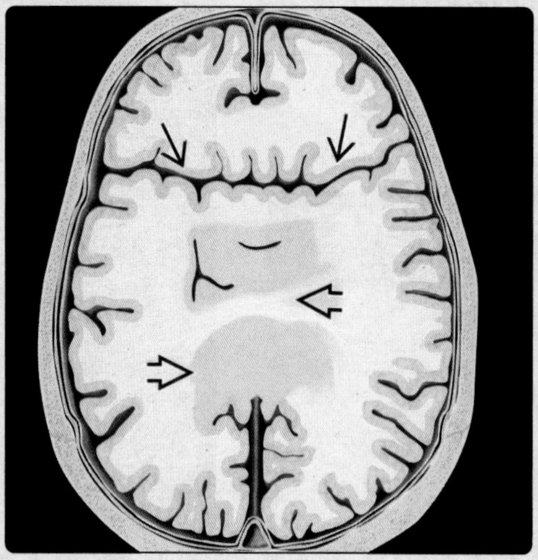

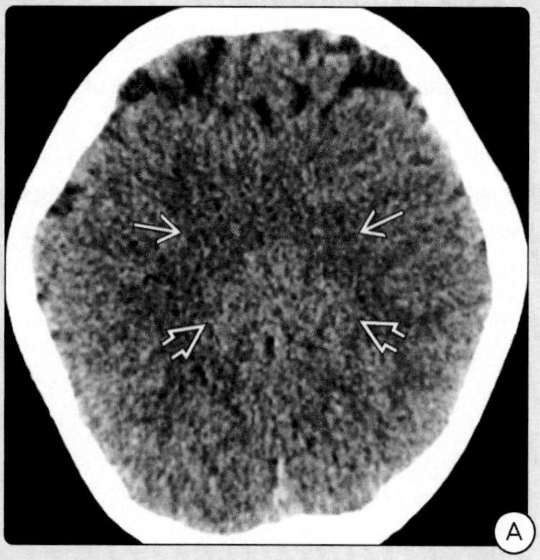

(38-11B) Sagittal T1WI shows classic findings of MIH. Corpus callosum genu and splenium are present without an intervening body. Note dysplastic gray matter deforming the lateral ventricle. (38-11C) Coronal T2 shows fused, "notched" lateral ventricles with a nodule of gray matter perched on top of the fused lateral ventricle. The posterior frontal lobes are continuous across the midline without an interhemispheric fissure.

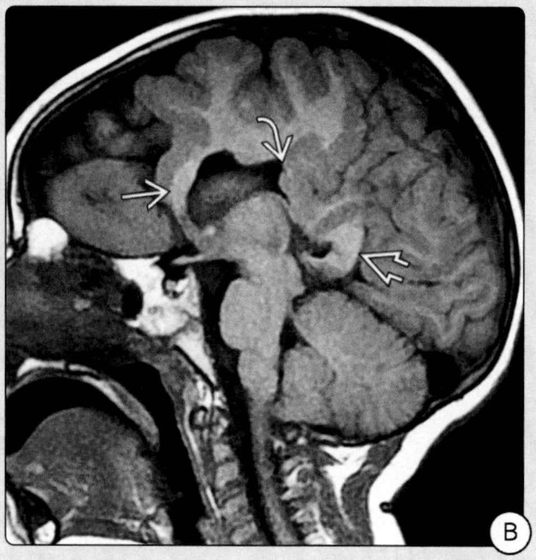

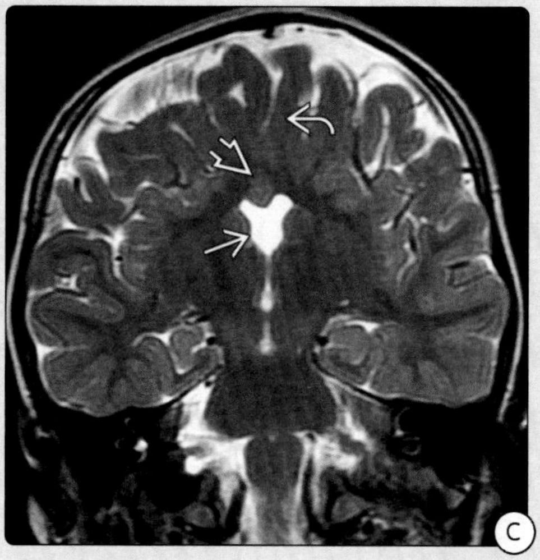

(38-11D) Axial T2WI shows that abnormal sylvian fissures continue superiorly, meeting over the cerebral convexities and crossing the midline. (38-11E) Axial DTI in the same patient shows WM tracts in the posterosuperior frontal lobes meeting and crossing in the midline.

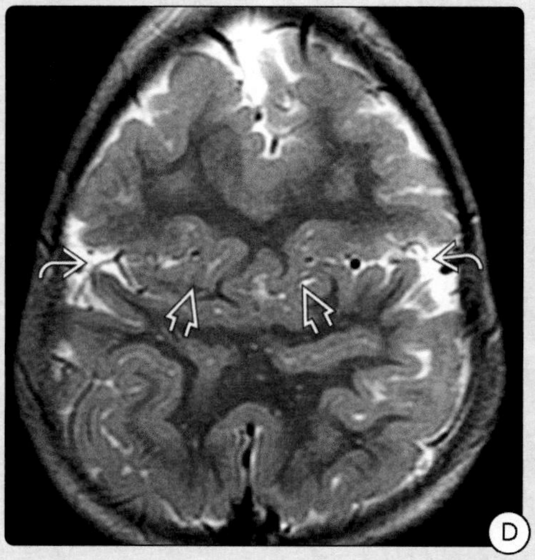

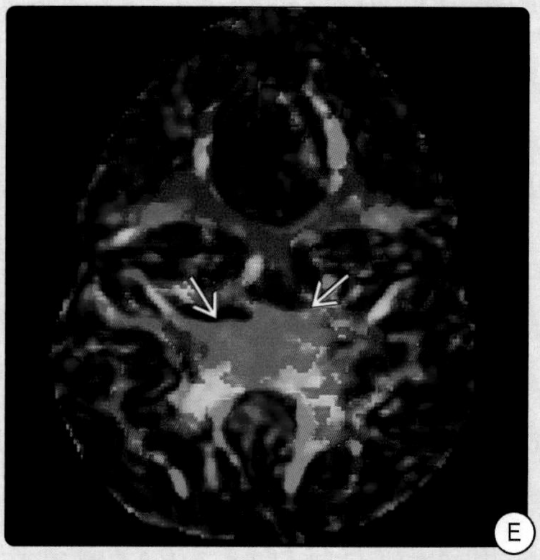

DTI shows that the callosal body and central cingulum fibers are absent, but all other major WM tracts have a normal course, thickness, and integrity. The horizontal white matter tracts cross the midline just under the fused cortex **(38-11E)**.

Septopreoptic Holoprosencephaly

Several very mild forms of HPE have been described in which the failure of hemispheric separation is restricted to the septal (subcallosal) and/or preoptic regions or both. Patients with these types of HPE—termed septopreoptic holoprosencephaly—often present with mild midline craniofacial malformations. These variants include **solitary median maxillary central incisor** (SMMCI) and **congenital nasal pyriform aperture stenosis** (CNPAS). Both are briefly discussed here.

Solitary Median Maxillary Central Incisor Syndrome

SMMCI syndrome is a rare malformation that consists of multiple (mainly midline) defects. Most authors suggest that SMMCI is an HPE variant, although others consider it a distinct entity.

Neonates with SMMCI often present with breathing difficulties secondary to nasal obstruction. Neurodevelopmental delay and endocrine abnormalities such as short stature and precocious puberty are common associated findings.

Imaging findings in SMMCI range from isolated dental abnormalities with a single maxillary incisor and V-shaped palate to more complex abnormalities that involve the brain **(38-12)**. Anomalies of the fornix, septi pellucidi, and anterior

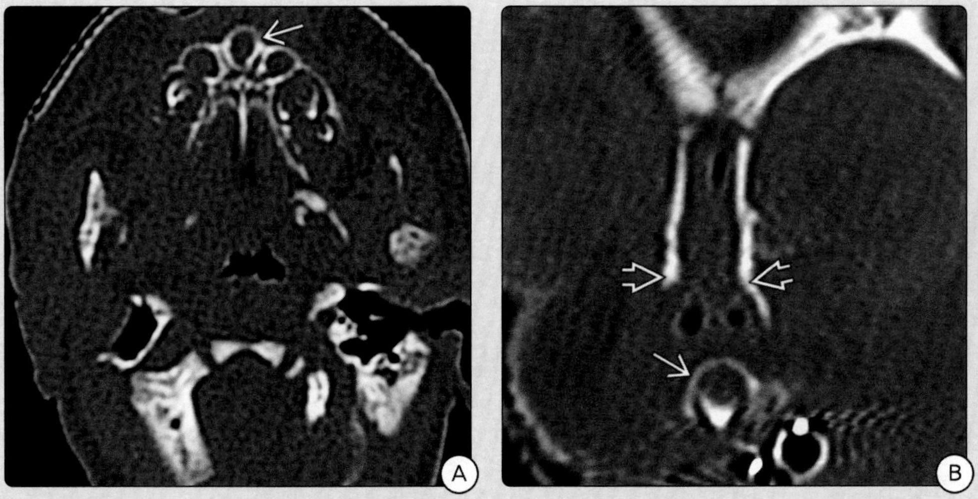

***(38-12A)** Axial bone CT in a 3d infant with breathing difficulty shows a single midline maxillary incisor ➡. **(38-12B)** Coronal bone CT in the same patient shows the central incisor ➡ and narrowed pyriform aperture stenosis ➡. In the term newborn, the normal aperture width should be > 8 mm.*

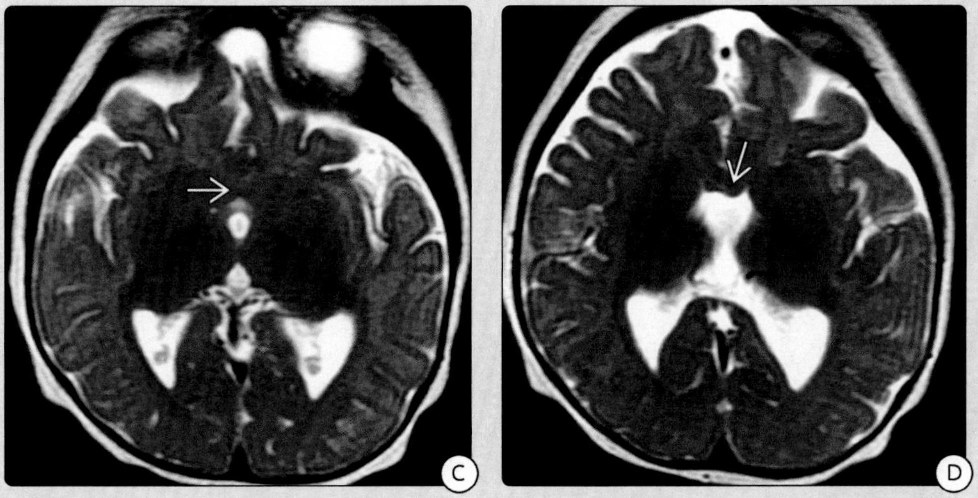

***(38-12C)** Axial T2WI in the same patient at age 7 months shows lobar HPE with mild hypotelorism and fusion across the ventral frontal lobes ➡. **(38-12D)** More cephalad scan shows absent septi pellucidi and thickened dysplastic-appearing fused fornices ➡.*

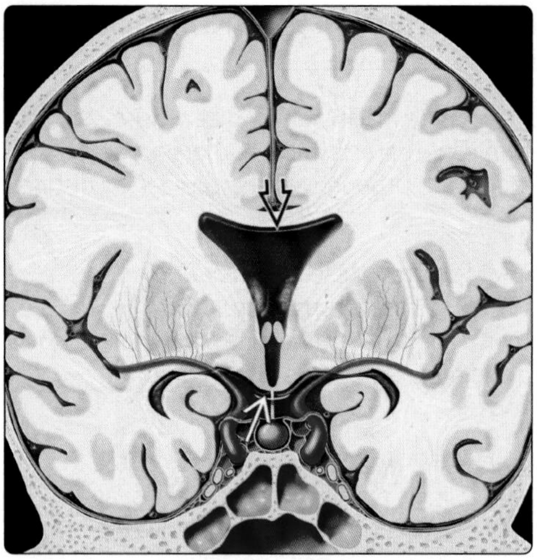

(38-13) Coronal graphic shows SOD with absent cavum septi pellucidi with flat-roofed anterior horns and small optic chiasm.

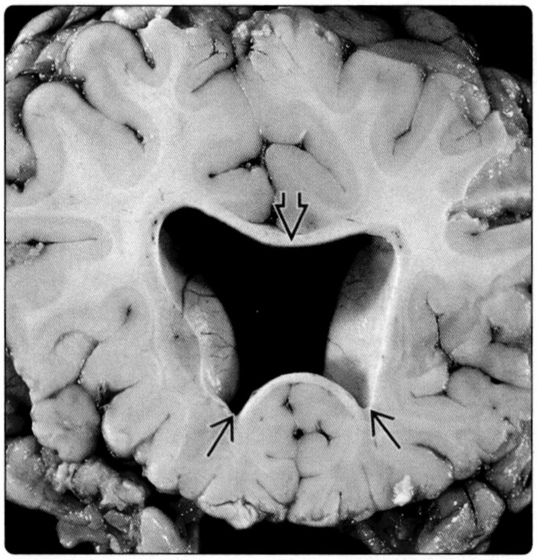

(38-14) Cavum septi pellucidi are absent; box-like lateral ventricles with inferiorly pointed frontal horns are seen. (J. Townsend, MD.)

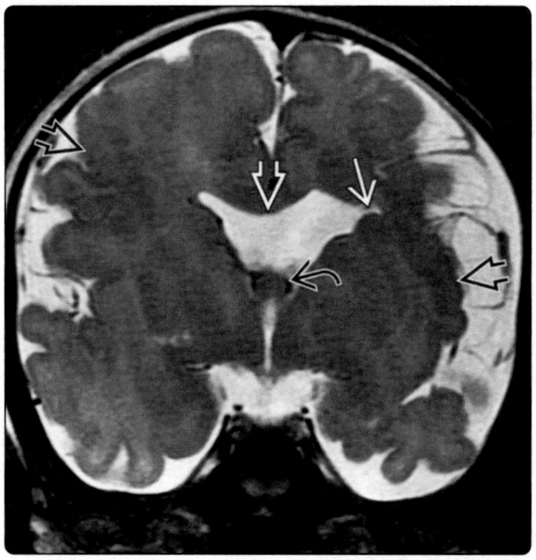

(38-15) Coronal T2WI in newborn shows absent cavum septi pellucidi, schizencephaly, extensive polymicrogyria, fused fornices.

corpus callosum are often present. An azygous anterior cerebral artery is common. Pituitary stalk hypoplasia occurs in some cases.

Congenital Nasal Pyriform Aperture Stenosis

CNPAS can exist as an isolated abnormality with choanal atresia, midnasal stenosis, or pyriform aperture stenosis. CNPAS may also coexist with SMMCI. CNPAS is associated with a high incidence of hypothalamic-pituitary-adrenal axis dysfunction, cleft palate, and inner ear anomalies.

VARIANT HOLOPROSENCEPHALY

Middle Interhemispheric Variant Holoprosencephaly

- Also known as syntelencephaly
- Corpus callosum genu, splenium present; middle absent
  - Only brain malformation with that morphology
- Midsections of falx, interhemispheric fissure absent
- Posterior frontal gray/white matter fused across midline

Septopreoptic Holoprosencephaly

- Solitary median maxillary central incisor syndrome (SMMCI)
  - Single midline incisor
  - Often coexists with nasal anomalies
  - Brain anomalies of fornix, septi pellucidi, corpus callosum common
- Congenital nasal pyriform aperture stenosis (CNPAS)
  - Choanal atresia, midnasal stenosis, pyriform aperture stenosis
  - Often coexists with SMMCI
  - Hypothalamic-pituitary-adrenal axis dysfunction common

Related Midline Disorders

Septooptic Dysplasia

Some authors consider septooptic dysplasia (SOD) simply a very well-differentiated form of lobar holoprosencephaly (HPE). However, the lack of ventral midline fusion and the heterogeneous nature of the disorder are more consistent with a separate but related midline malformation.

Terminology and Pathology

SOD is also known as de Morsier syndrome. Two cardinal pathologic features define SOD: (1) absence of the septum pellucidum and (2) optic nerve hypoplasia **(38-13)** **(38-14)**.

When SOD occurs with other anomalies such as schizencephaly or callosal dysgenesis, the syndrome is sometimes called SOD plus **(38-15)**.

Etiology and Genetics

Most SOD cases are sporadic. Some are autosomal-dominant or -recessive cases. Mutation of the homeobox gene *HESX1* has been identified in a few cases.

Clinical Issues

The most common clinical feature of SOD is visual impairment. Nearly two-thirds of SOD patients also develop endocrine abnormalities from hypothalamic-pituitary insufficiency (e.g., hypoglycemic seizures).

SEPTOOPTIC DYSPLASIA: PATHOLOGY AND CLINICAL FEATURES

Pathology

- Cardinal pathologic features
  - Absent septi pellucidi
  - Optic nerve/chiasm hypoplasia

Clinical Features

- Hormonal dysfunction in nearly two-thirds
  - Pituitary insufficiency
  - Growth hormone deficiency, hypothyroid most common
  - Rare = precocious puberty
- Neurodevelopmental delay common

Imaging

Imaging findings in SOD are diagnostic. Three orthogonal planes are crucial to identifying all the findings. Thin-section coronal T1- and T2-weighted images show absent or hypoplastic septi pellucidi. The frontal horns appear "squared-off" or box-like with distinct inferior pointing. The optic chiasm and one or both optic nerves appear small in most cases **(38-16)**.

Sagittal images show that the septi pellucidi are absent and the fornices are low-lying, giving the lateral ventricles an "empty" appearance **(38-17A)**.

Isolated absence of the septi pellucidi is relatively rare, so look carefully for other anomalies. The majority of patients with SOD have malformations of cortical development (e.g., heterotopias, schizencephaly **(38-17B)**, and polymicrogyria) in addition to optic nerve hypoplasia. Others exhibit a small pituitary gland with thin or absent stalk and an ectopic

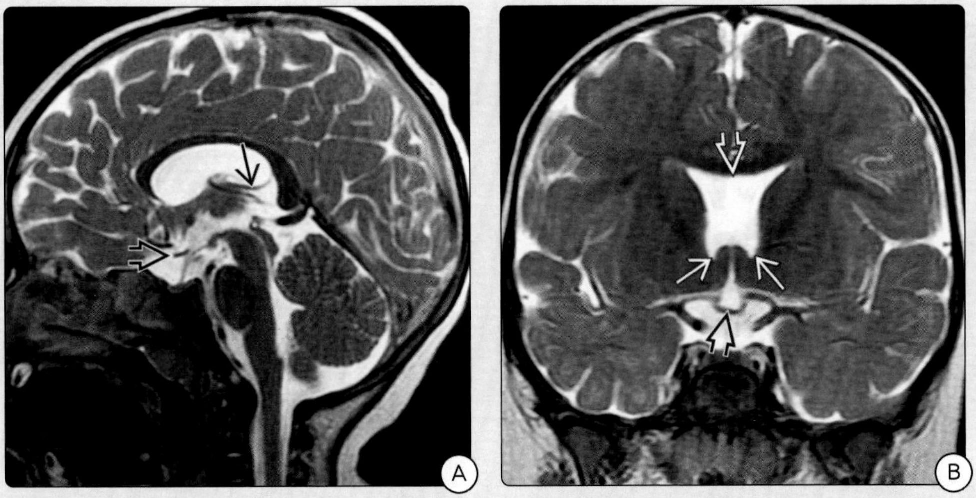

***(38-16A)** Sagittal T2WI in a 13m boy with septooptic dysplasia (SOD) shows an empty-appearing lateral ventricle with low-lying fornix ⇨. The optic chiasm ⇨ appears small. **(38-16B)** Coronal T2WI shows the hypoplastic optic chiasm ⇨, absent septi pellucidi ➡, and the peculiar box-like or "squared-off" appearance of the frontal horns. The inferior pointing ➡ of both frontal horns is also characteristic of SOD.*

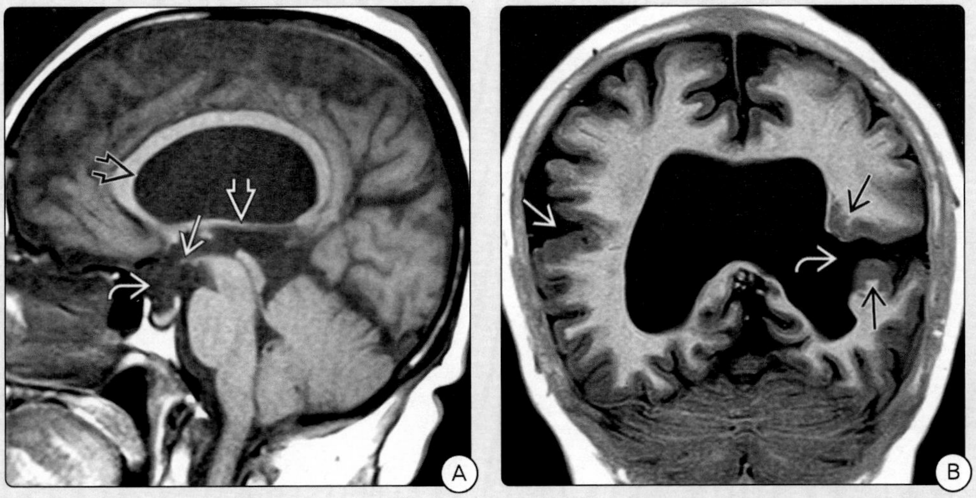

***(38-17A)** Sagittal T1WI in a 26y woman with SOD shows extreme hypoplasia of the optic chiasm ➡, small pituitary gland with inapparent stalk ➡, and low-lying fornices ➡ that give a striking "empty" appearance to the lateral ventricle ⇨. **(38-17B)** Coronal IR in the same case shows unilateral schizencephaly with dysplastic gray matter ⇨ lining the cleft ➡. Note contralateral polymicrogyria ➡.*

neurohypophysis. Olfactory tract/bulb hypoplasia and incomplete hippocampal rotation are common.

SEPTOOPTIC DYSPLASIA: IMAGING

Imaging Findings
- Absent septum pellucidum
  - "Squared-off" frontal horns, pointed inferiorly on coronal T2WI
- Hypoplastic optic nerves, chiasm
- Look for
  - Malformations of cortical development
  - Thin stalk, small gland, ectopic posterior pituitary

Differential Diagnosis

The major differential diagnosis of SOD is well-differentiated **lobar HPE**. The olfactory bulbs are present in lobar HPE but are frequently absent in SOD. The cerebral hemispheres and basal ganglia are completely separated in SOD.

Arrhinencephaly

Arrhinencephaly (ARR) is a congenital malformation in which the olfactory bulb and tracts are absent **(38-18) (38-19) (38-20) (38-21)**. Although ARR can exist in isolation, most cases occur with multiple other midline facial anomalies such as cleft palate, cleft lip, and nasal and/or ocular malformations.

Common associated intracranial abnormalities include abnormalities of the hypothalamic-pituitary axis, callosal dysgenesis, and alobar and semilobar HPE.

When olfactory aplasia/hypoplasia occurs with hypogonadotropic hypogonadism, it is termed **Kallmann syndrome**. Olfactory agenesis occurs in approximately 25% of patients with **CHARGE** (**c**oloboma, **h**eart malformations,

(38-18) Submentovertex graphic depicts the normal olfactory bulbs →, trigones →, and lateral olfactory stria → passing into the temporal lobes. (38-19) Coronal T2WI in a normal newborn shows olfactory bulbs → and normal olfactory sulci →.

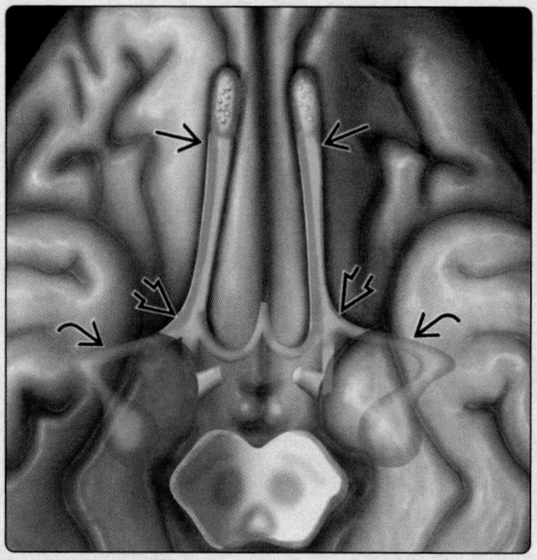

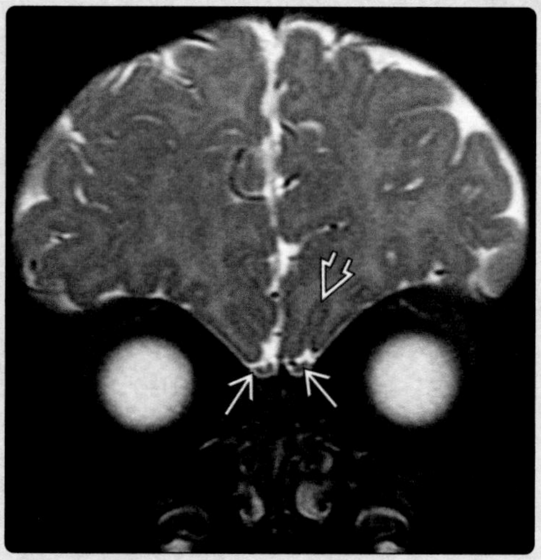

(38-20) Autopsy case of arrhinencephaly shows absent olfactory bulbs and shallow, deformed olfactory sulci →. (Courtesy R. Hewlett, MD.) (38-21) Coronal T2WI in a newborn with multiple congenital anomalies demonstrates arrhinencephaly with absent olfactory bulbs → and no olfactory sulci →. (Courtesy S. Blaser, MD.)

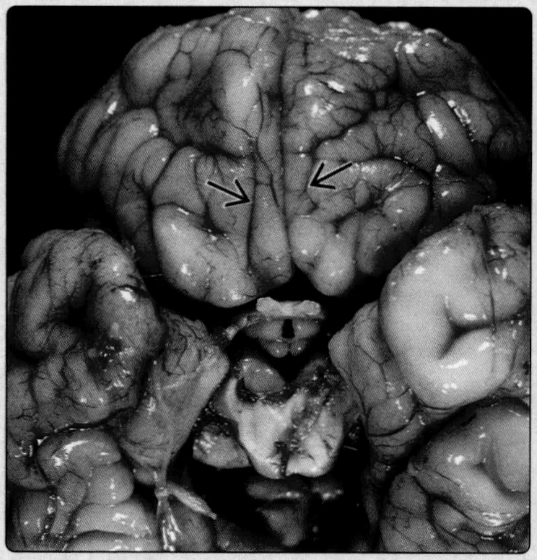

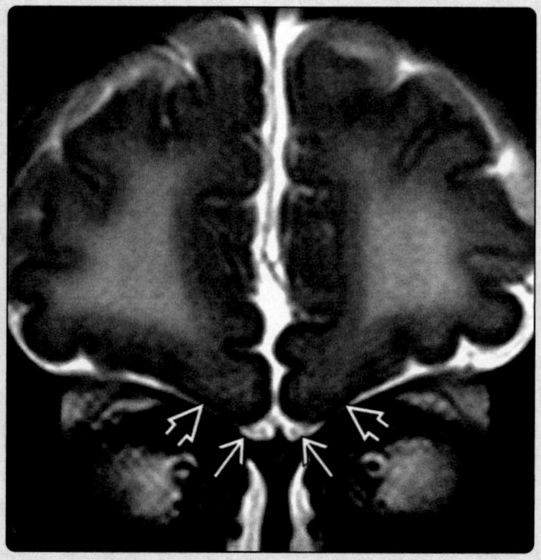

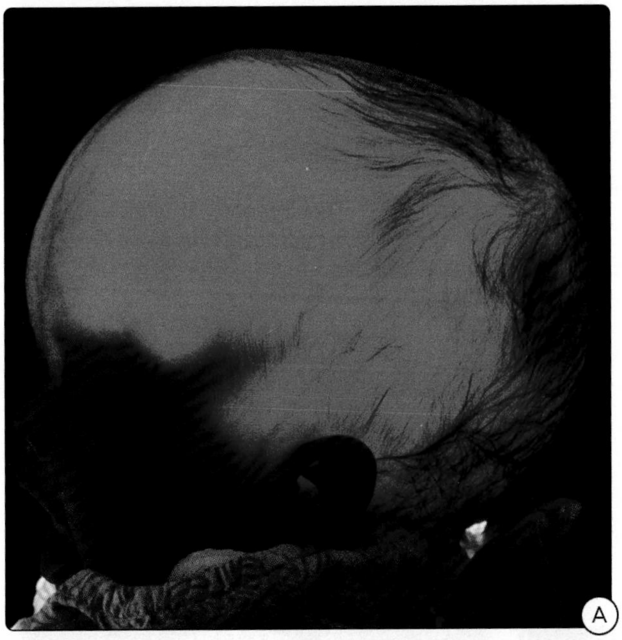

(38-22A) *Autopsy case of hydranencephaly demonstrates a large head with striking transillumination indicating that most of the cranium is water-filled.*

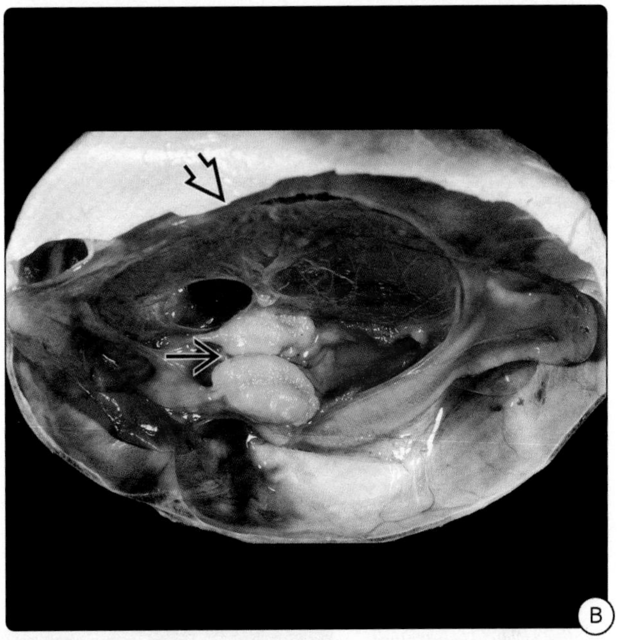

(38-22B) *The thinned calvarium ➩ has been partially removed to show the fluid-filled cavity. The hemispheres are absent ("water-bag brain"), and only the basal ganglia are present. Note separation ➩. (Courtesy R. Hewlett, MD.)*

choanal **a**tresia, developmental **r**etardation, **g**enital anomalies, **e**ar anomalies) syndrome.

Holoprosencephaly Mimics

Hydranencephaly

Although some authors consider hydranencephaly a congenital malformation, it is actually the consequence of severe brain destruction in utero. We discuss it here, as it is important to recognize and distinguish hydranencephaly from other disorders such as alobar holoprosencephaly or maximal hydrocephalus.

Terminology

The term hydranencephaly is a contraction of "hydroanencéphalie" and literally means water without the brain. In hydranencephaly, the cerebral hemispheres are completely or almost completely missing. Instead, a membranous sac filled with CSF, glial tissue, and ependyma is present. In rare instances, only one hemisphere is destroyed. This condition is termed **hemihydranencephaly**.

Etiology and Pathology

The precise etiology of hydranencephaly is unknown, but most investigators believe compromise of the internal carotid artery circulation before 16 gestational weeks followed by diffuse liquefactive necrosis of the cerebral mantle is responsible. Maternal trauma, toxins, twin-twin transfusion syndrome, massive hemorrhage, and infection have all been cited as possible contributory factors. *COL4A1* mutations with large prenatal hemorrhages have been implicated in some cases.

In hydranencephaly, most of the cerebral hemispheres have been destroyed and are totally or partially replaced by translucent thin-walled sacs of CSF that fill most of the supratentorial space **(38-22)** **(38-23)**. The outer layer consists of leptomeninges, and the inner layer is glial tissue without demonstrable ependymal elements.

The falx is intact. Cortical loss is massive but seldom complete. The medial temporal lobes, brainstem, cerebellum, and parts of the thalami—all supplied by the posterior circulation—are often relatively preserved. As some of the choroid plexus is also supplied by the posterior circulation, CSF continues to be elaborated but not normally resorbed. This distends the fluid-filled sacs that are the dominant pathologic feature of hydranencephaly.

Hydranencephaly usually occurs sporadically without other associated malformations. Fowler syndrome is a rare autosomal-recessive disorder in which hydranencephaly is accompanied by glomeruloid vasculopathy of the CNS vessels and neurogenic muscular atrophy.

Clinical Issues

Hydranencephaly occurs in 1-2 per 10,000 live births and represents 0.6% of CNS malformations in perinatal/neonatal autopsy series.

Prognosis is poor. Half of liveborn infants with hydranencephaly die within the first postnatal month, and 85% die by the end of the first year. Occasional long-term survivors have been reported. The major management problem is controlling the macrocephaly that usually accompanies hydranencephaly. Patients with hemihydranencephaly have a better prognosis and may experience long-term survival.

Imaging

General Features. A normal or large head with fluid-filled cranial vault ("water bag" brain) and small nubbins of remnant brain with a normal falx cerebri and posterior fossa are the typical findings **(38-22)** **(38-23)**.

CT Findings. NECT scans show that CSF almost completely fills the supratentorial space. The falx cerebri is generally intact and appears to "float" in the water-filled cranial vault **(38-24)**. The basal ganglia are present and separated but may appear moderately atrophic. Small remnants of the medial frontal and parietooccipital lobes can be present.

MR Findings. MR demonstrates a largely absent cerebral mantle. The falx is easily identified **(38-25)**. The fluid-filled spaces follow CSF on all sequences, although some signal heterogeneity is often present secondary to CSF pulsations. In hemihydranencephaly, one hemisphere appears absent, and the CSF-filled space often displaces the falx across the midline.

Differential Diagnosis

The most important differential diagnosis of hydranencephaly **(38-25)** is severe **obstructive hydrocephalus** (OH). In severe OH (e.g., secondary to aqueductal stenosis), a thin cortex can be seen compressed against the dura and inner table of the calvaria **(38-26)**.

In **alobar holoprosencephaly**, the falx and interhemispheric fissure are absent. The basal ganglia are fused **(38-27)**. Severe **bilateral "open lip" schizencephaly** has large transmantle CSF clefts that are lined with dysplastic-appearing cortex **(38-28)**. Severe **cystic encephalomalacia** shows large ventricles with multiple parenchymal CSF-filled cavities.

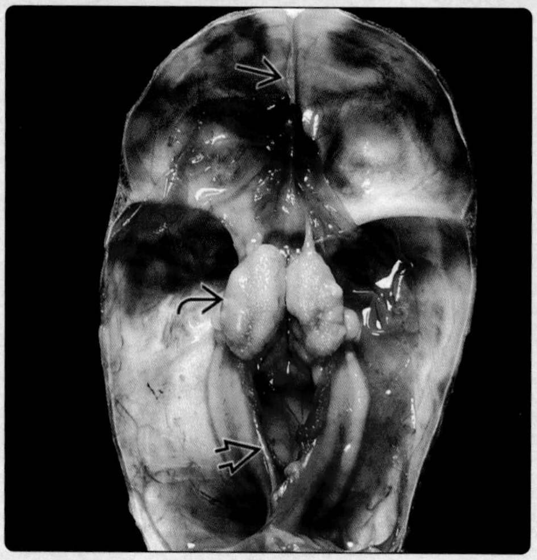

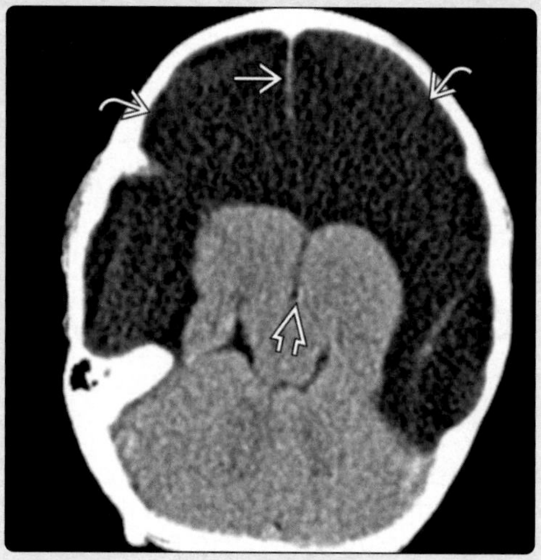

***(38-23)** This is the same case as Figure 38-22, seen from above. A falx cerebri ➡ and tentorium ➡ are present, as are the separated basal ganglia ➡. The hemispheres are absent. (Courtesy R. Hewlett, MD.) **(38-24)** NECT shows hydranencephaly. Both hemispheres are replaced by CSF. BG/thalami are separated ➡, falx is present ➡. No brain is visible over CSF-filled cavities ➡.*

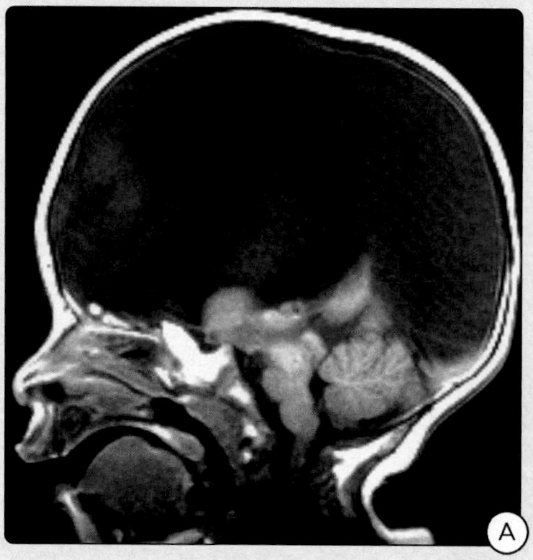

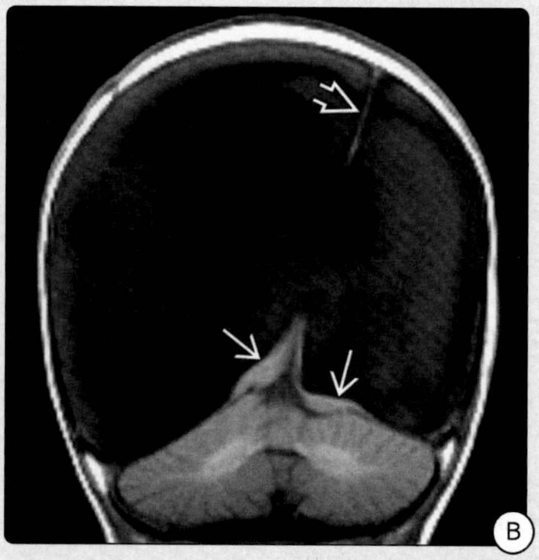

***(38-25A)** Sagittal T1WI shows hydranencephaly with macrocephaly; CSF fills virtually all of the supratentorial spaces. Brainstem and cerebellum are normal. **(38-25B)** Coronal T1WI in the same case shows expanded, CSF-filled cranial vault, only tiny remnants of brain ➡. A falx is present ➡. (Courtesy A. Illner, MD.)*

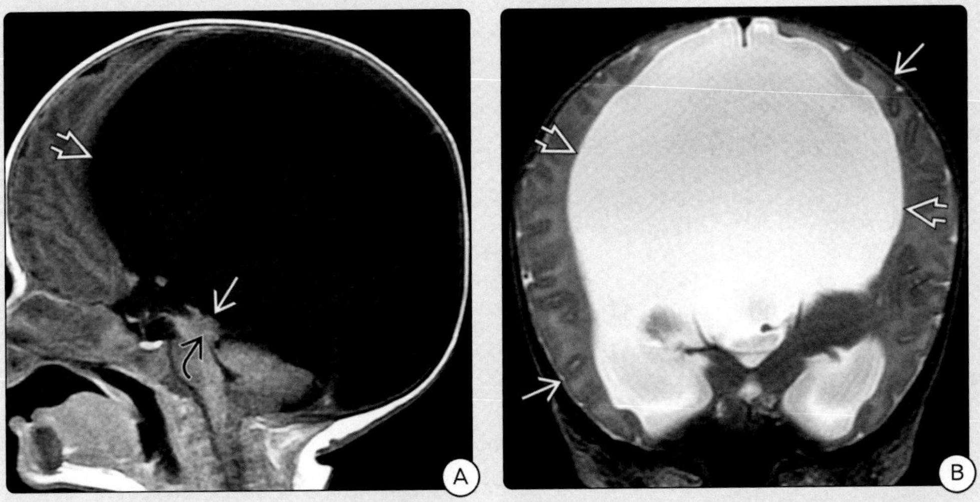

***(38-26A)** Sagittal T1WI in a 4-week infant with macrocrania shows massively enlarged lateral ventricles and tectal dysplasia causing aqueductal stenosis. **(38-26B)** Coronal T2WI shows the massively enlarged lateral ventricles. There is a thin rim of compressed but normally formed cortex and subcortical WM lying under the calvarium. This is maximal hydrocephalus.*

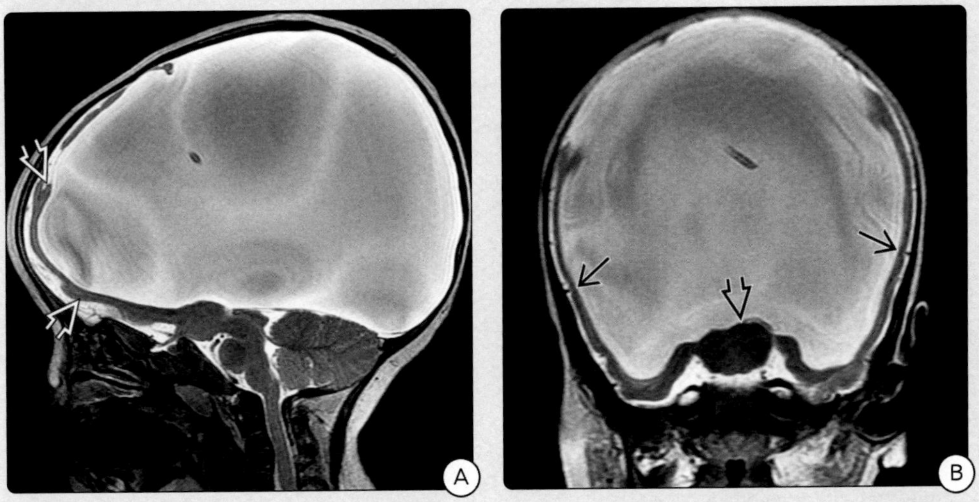

***(38-27A)** This is alobar holoprosencephaly. Sagittal T2WI shows enlarged head with relatively normal-appearing posterior fossa. Almost the entire calvarium is occupied by the CSF-filled monoventricle covered by a very thin rim of featureless brain. **(38-27B)** Coronal T2WI shows a horseshoe-shaped monoventricle. The basal ganglia are fused. Note absent falx, thin rim of smooth dysplastic-appearing brain.*

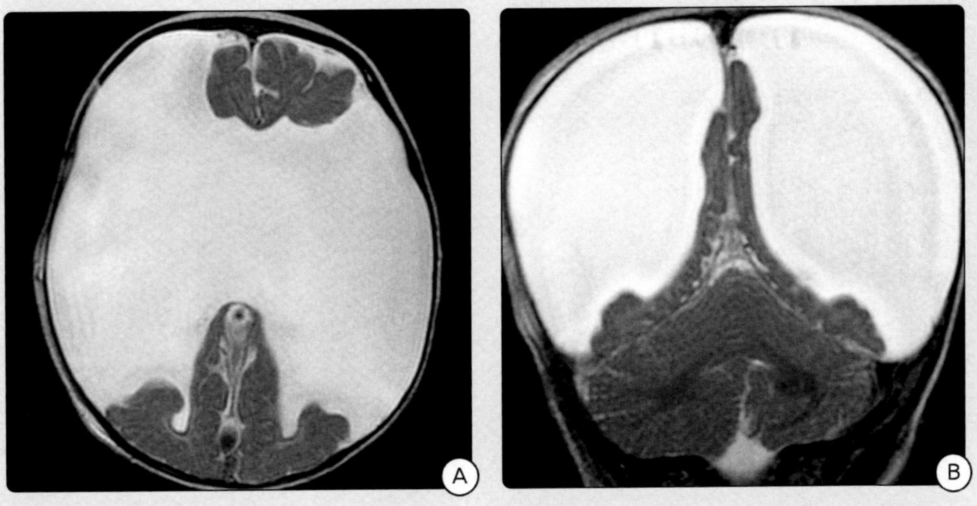

***(38-28A)** Axial T2WI shows severe "open lip" schizencephaly, another cause of "water-bag brain" appearance. **(38-28B)** Coronal T2WI in the same case shows that the falx and tentorium are normal. The massive "open lip" schizencephalic clefts are lined by dysplastic-appearing gray matter.*

Selected References

Holoprosencephaly

Yang E et al: A practical approach to supratentorial brain malformations: what radiologists should know. Radiol Clin North Am. 55(4):609-627, 2017

Dubourg C et al: Mutational spectrum in holoprosencephaly shows that FGF is a new major signaling pathway. Hum Mutat. 37(12):1329-1339, 2016

Gupta S et al: Roof plate mediated morphogenesis of the forebrain: new players join the game. Dev Biol. 413(2):145-52, 2016

Kaliaperumal C et al: Holoprosencephaly: antenatal and postnatal diagnosis and outcome. Childs Nerv Syst. 32(5):801-9, 2016

DeMyer W: Holoprosencephaly. In: Handbook of Clinical Neurology, Vol. 30, edited by Vinker PI, Bruyn JW. Amsterdam, The Netherlands: North Holland Publishing, 1977, pp 431-478

Alobar Holoprosencephaly

Pucciarelli V et al: Facial evaluation in holoprosencephaly. J Craniofac Surg. 28(1):e22-e28, 2017

Rosa RFM et al: Trisomy 18 and holoprosencephaly. Am J Med Genet A. ePub, 2017

Semilobar Holoprosencephaly

Pucciarelli V et al: Facial evaluation in holoprosencephaly. J Craniofac Surg. 28(1):e22-e28, 2017

Barkovich AJ et al: Pediatric Neuroimaging, 5e. Philadelphia, PA: Lippincott Williams & Wilkins, 2012

Lobar Holoprosencephaly

Pucciarelli V et al: Facial evaluation in holoprosencephaly. J Craniofac Surg. 28(1):e22-e28, 2017

Holoprosencephaly Variants

Middle Interhemispheric Variant of Holoprosencephaly

Bulakbasi N et al: The middle interhemispheric variant of holoprosencephaly: magnetic resonance and diffusion tensor imaging findings. Br J Radiol. 89(1063):20160115, 2016

Virta M et al: Adult with middle interhemispheric variant of holoprosencephaly: neuropsychological, clinical, and radiological findings. Arch Clin Neuropsychol. 31(5):472-9, 2016

Yahyavi-Firouz-Abadi N et al: Case 236: middle interhemispheric variant of holoprosencephaly. Radiology. 281(3):969-974, 2016

Septopreoptic Holoprosencephaly

Esen E et al: Pyriform aperture enlargement in all aspects. J Laryngol Otol. 1-4, 2017

de Boutray M et al: Median cleft of the upper lip: a new classification to guide treatment decisions. J Craniomaxillofac Surg. 44(6):664-71, 2016

Yang S et al: Congenital nasal pyriform aperture stenosis in association with solitary median maxillary central incisor: unique radiologic features. Radiol Case Rep. 11(3):178-81, 2016

Ginat DT et al: CT and MRI of congenital nasal lesions in syndromic conditions. Pediatr Radiol. 45(7):1056-65, 2015

Poelmans S et al: Genotypic and phenotypic variation in six patients with solitary median maxillary central incisor syndrome. Am J Med Genet A. 167A(10):2451-8, 2015

Related Midline Disorders

Septooptic Dysplasia

Alt C et al: Clinical and radiologic spectrum of septo-optic dysplasia: review of 17 cases. J Child Neurol. ePub, 2017

Koizumi M et al: Endocrine status of patients with septo-optic dysplasia: fourteen Japanese cases. Clin Pediatr Endocrinol. 26(2):89-98, 2017

Ryabets-Lienhard A et al: The optic nerve hypoplasia spectrum: review of the literature and clinical guidelines. Adv Pediatr. 63(1):127-46, 2016

Arrhinencephaly

de Boutray M et al: Median cleft of the upper lip: a new classification to guide treatment decisions. J Craniomaxillofac Surg. 44(6):664-71, 2016

Kaliaperumal C et al: Holoprosencephaly: antenatal and postnatal diagnosis and outcome. Childs Nerv Syst. 32(5):801-9, 2016

Holoprosencephaly Mimics

Hydranencephaly

Adhikari EH et al: Infant outcomes among women with Zika virus infection during pregnancy: results of a large prenatal Zika screening program. Am J Obstet Gynecol. 216(3):292.e1-292.e8, 2017

Pavone P et al: Hydranencephaly: cerebral spinal fluid instead of cerebral mantles. Ital J Pediatr. 40(1):79, 2014

Familial Cancer Predisposition Syndromes

***The term* cancer predisposition syndrome *is used to describe familial cancers in which a clear mode of inheritance can be established. The 2016 WHO classifies these as* familial tumor syndromes.**

The term **neurocutaneous syndromes** denotes a group of CNS disorders that are characterized by brain malformations or neoplasms and skin/eye lesions. These disorders have also been called **phakomatoses**. The term is derived from the Greek root *phako*, which refers to the lens; phakomatosis thus means a tumor-like condition of the eye (lens).

Most—but not all—neurocutaneous syndromes are inherited. Most—but not all—are associated with a distinct predilection to develop CNS neoplasms; these have also been called **inherited cancer syndromes**. Most—but again not all—of these also have characteristic cutaneous lesions. Many—but not all—also have prominent visceral and connective tissue abnormalities.

Cancer predisposition syndromes are typically uncommon, monogenic, high-penetrance disorders. Next-generation sequencing can identify patients who possess the germline genetic variants that underlie these disorders. Despite the availability of accurate genetic testing, many individuals are diagnosed on purely clinical grounds. In others, characteristic imaging features provide the first suggestion that a patient may have an inherited cancer syndrome.

In this chapter, we consider familial tumor syndromes that involve the nervous system, beginning with the neurofibromatoses and schwannomatosis. Major attention is also directed to tuberous sclerosis, von Hippel-Lindau disease, and Li-Fraumeni syndrome. We close with a brief discussion of rare familial tumor syndromes including Cowden and Turcot syndromes.

Neurofibromatosis and Schwannomatosis

Neurofibromatosis is not a single entity but a group of genetically and clinically distinct disorders with few overlapping features. Although they are the most common CNS tumor predisposition syndromes, neurofibromatoses are multisystem disorders with both neoplastic and nonneoplastic manifestations.

Two types of neurofibromatosis are widely recognized: neurofibromatosis type 1 (NF1) and neurofibromatosis type 2 (NF2).

A third related disorder—schwannomatosis—is a rare non-NF1/NF2 syndrome characterized by multiple nonvestibular schwannomas. Together,

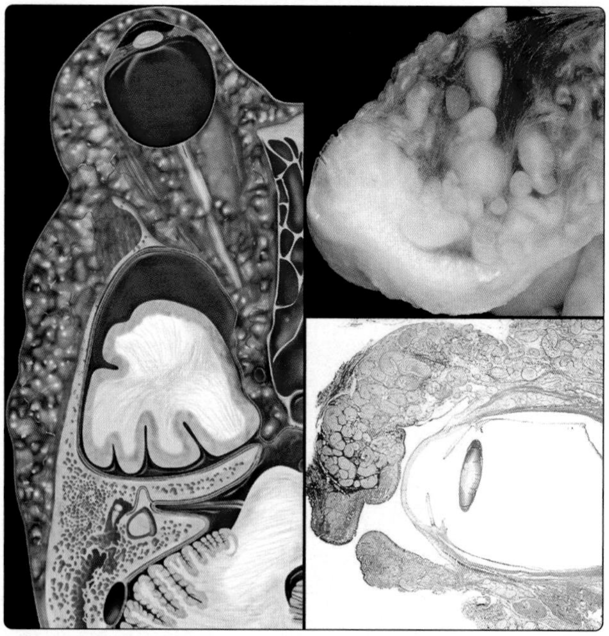

(39-1) Graphic (L) and surgical specimens (AFIP Archives) (R) depict neurofibromatosis type 1 (NF1) with typical plexiform neurofibroma of orbit, eyelid, and scalp.

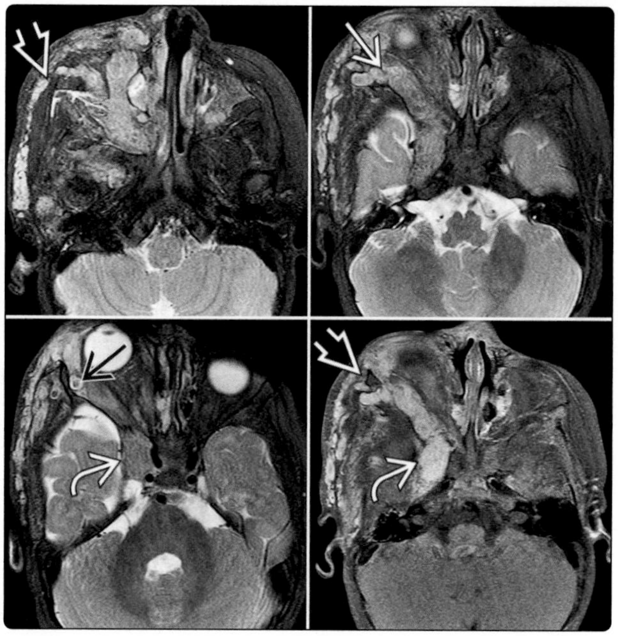

(39-2) Series of three T2WIs, one T1 C+ FS shows enhancing plexiform neurofibroma infiltrating orbit, masticator space, and cavernous sinus. Lesion is hyperintense with typical target appearance.

these three inherited disorders affect approximately 100,000 persons in the United States alone.

Neurofibromatosis Type 1

Terminology

Neurofibromatosis type 1 (NF1) was formerly known as **von Recklinghausen disease** or "peripheral neurofibromatosis." Because NF1 often has central lesions, the term "peripheral neurofibromatosis" should not be used. When extreme, NF1 can be highly disfiguring and is sometimes dubbed "elephantiasis neuromatosa" or "elephant man disease."

NF1 is one of the most common of all genetic syndromes with a prevalence of 1:3,000. An uncommon form, **segmental NF1** (formerly called neurofibromatosis type 5), affects one region of the body (e.g., a limb) or sometimes just a single dermatome. Segmental NF1 is a mosaicism in which localized disease results from a postzygotic *NF1* gene mutation.

An even more uncommon NF1 type is **localized NF1**. Localized NF1 is isolated to a small area and is caused by a sporadic *somatic* (not germline) mutation.

Etiology

General Concepts. NF1 is an autosomal-dominant disorder with variable expression, a high rate of new mutations, and virtually 100% penetrance by age 20.

Genetics. NF1 is caused by mutation of the *NF1* gene on chromosome 17q11.2. This large gene has one of the highest rates of spontaneous mutation in the entire human genome. Mutations vary from complete gene deletions to insertions, stop and splicing mutations, as well as amino acid substitutions and chromosomal rearrangements.

Mutations inactivate the gene that encodes the protein product **neurofibromin**. Neurofibromin is a cytoplasmic protein that functions as a tumor suppressor protein through negative regulation of the RAS oncogene. Unopposed Ras activation leads to enhanced activation of the downstream RAF/MEK/ERK, PI3K/AKT/mTOR, and cAMP signaling pathways, which are critical for control of cellular growth and differentiation. NF1 is therefore considered a **"Ras-opathy."**

Neurofibromin also acts as a regulator of neural stem cell proliferation and differentiation; it is required for normal glial and neuronal development. The oligodendrocyte myelin glycoprotein—a major myelin protein—is also embedded in the *NF1* gene and is often also mutated.

Neurofibromin is expressed at low levels in all cells with higher levels expressed in the CNS (astrocytes and oligodendrocytes as well as neurons, Schwann cells) and skin (melanocytes).

Approximately half of all NF1 cases are familial. Nearly 50% are sporadic ("de novo") and represent new mutations. NF1 patients already harboring a heterozygous germline *NF1* mutation develop neurofibromas upon somatic mutation of the second (wild-type) *NF1* allele. About 10% of NF1 patients display somatic mosaicism.

Pathology

CNS lesions are found in 15-20% of patients. A variety of nonneoplastic lesions as well as benign and malignant tumors are associated with NF1. An increased risk of non-CNS malignancies also occurs in NF1 patients.

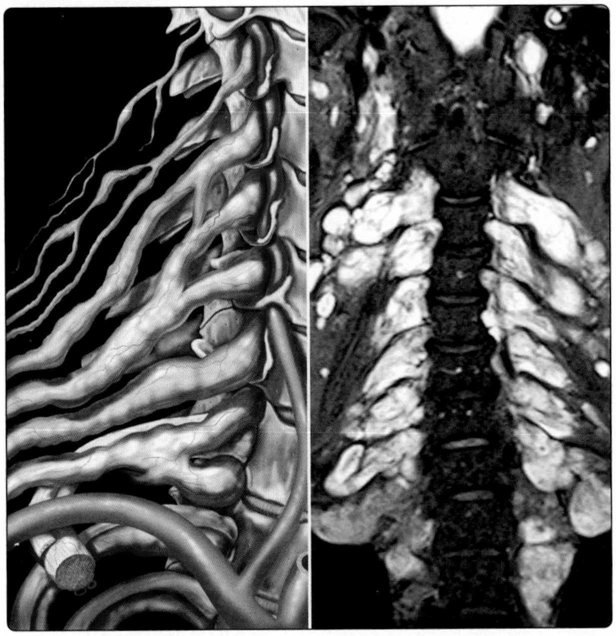

(39-3) Plexiform neurofibroma involving cervical nerve roots is depicted in the graphic (L) and on a coronal STIR scan (R).

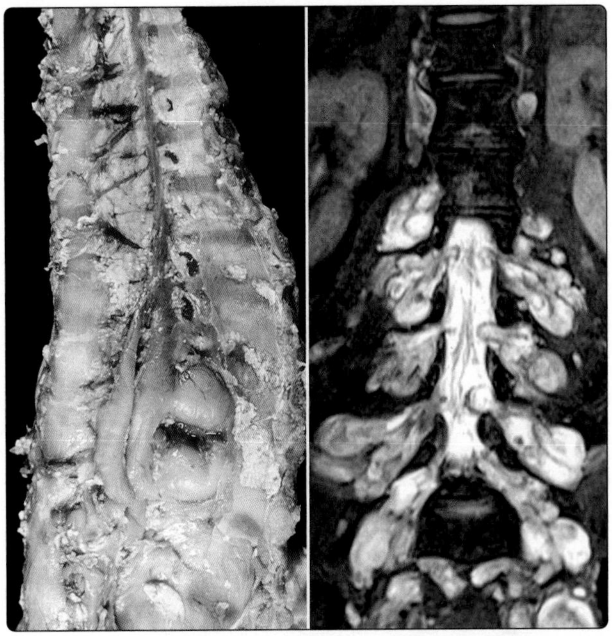

(39-4) Coronal autopsy specimen (L) and coronal STIR (R) show plexiform neurofibroma of thoracolumbar nerve roots. (Autopsy courtesy R. Hewlett, MD.)

Nonneoplastic CNS Lesions. Multiple waxing and waning **dysplastic white matter lesions** on T2/FLAIR are commonly identified in patients with NF1 (see below). Histopathologically, these lesions represent zones of myelin vacuolization and dysgenesis, not hamartomas. These lesions follow a benign course with regression by 20 years.

Uncommon nonneoplastic CNS lesions include macrocephaly and subependymal glial nodules. Hydrocephalus occurs in 10-15% of cases. **Dural ectasia** may cause dilatation of the optic nerve sheaths, Meckel cave, or internal auditory canals.

Arteriopathy occurs in at least 6% of cases. The most common manifestation is progressive intimal fibrosis of the supraclinoid internal carotid arteries, resulting in moyamoya. Both intra- and extracranial aneurysms and arteriovenous fistulas occur in NF1 but are relatively rare. The vertebral arteries are more commonly affected than the carotid arteries.

CNS Neoplasms. CNS tumors occur in approximately 20% of individuals with NF1. A variety of both benign and malignant tumors occur. All involve tumorigenesis of neural crest-derived cells and can be found in both the central and peripheral nervous systems. Benign NF1-related neoplasms include neurofibromas and schwannomas. Malignant tumors include malignant peripheral nerve sheath tumors and gliomas.

Neurofibromas. A spectrum of NF1-associated neurofibromas occurs. Tumors derived from skin sensory nerves are designated cutaneous or **dermal neurofibromas**. The prevalence of dermal neurofibromas increases with age, so more than 95% of adults with NF1 have at least one lesion.

Dermal neurofibromas are benign tumors that are composed of Schwann cells, fibroblasts, mast cells, and perineural cells. These tumors arise from a single fascicle within a peripheral nerve and appear as soft, well-circumscribed pedunculated or sessile lesions that range in size from 1 mm to 2 cm. Most patients develop more tumors as they age, and some have literally thousands of dermal neurofibromas.

Less commonly, a tumor within a larger subcutaneous nerve appears as a more diffuse mass within the dermis (**"diffuse" subcutaneous neurofibroma**). Neither dermal nor subcutaneous neurofibromas undergo malignant transformation.

Plexiform neurofibromas (PNFs) are distinct from dermal neurofibromas and are virtually pathognomonic of NF1. PNFs develop in 30-50% of individuals with NF1, typically manifesting at birth and growing most rapidly during the first decade of life.

PNFs are generally large bulky tumors usually associated with major nerve trunks and plexuses. PNFs are rope-like, diffusely infiltrating, noncircumscribed transspatial lesions that resemble a bag of worms **(39-1)**.

The scalp and orbit are common sites for PNFs **(39-2)** **(39-5)** **(39-6)**. Spinal neurofibromas and PNFs are found in approximately 40% of patients with NF1 **(39-3)** **(39-4)**.

Malignant Peripheral Nerve Sheath Tumors. Although most PNFs remain benign, 10-15% become malignant. Deep-seated PNFs are at particular risk for development into malignant peripheral nerve sheath tumors (**MPNSTs**). Individuals with NF1 have an 8-13% cumulative lifetime risk of developing an MPNST. MPNST is an aggressive, deadly tumor with a high rate of metastases and poor overall prognosis.

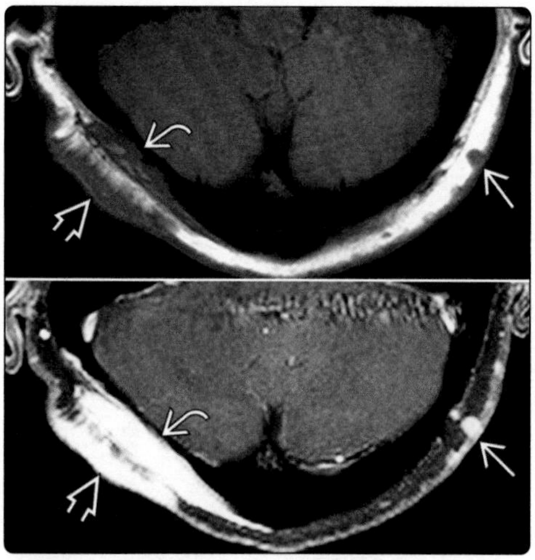

(39-5) NF1 shows discrete, enhancing dermal neurofibromas, infiltrating plexiform neurofibroma, and eroding skull.

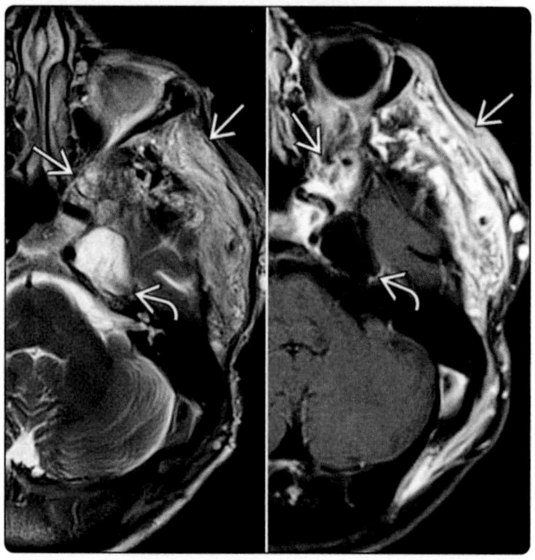

(39-6) (L) T2WI, (R) T1 C+ show scalp/orbit neurofibroma and dural dysplasia with enlarged Meckel cave.

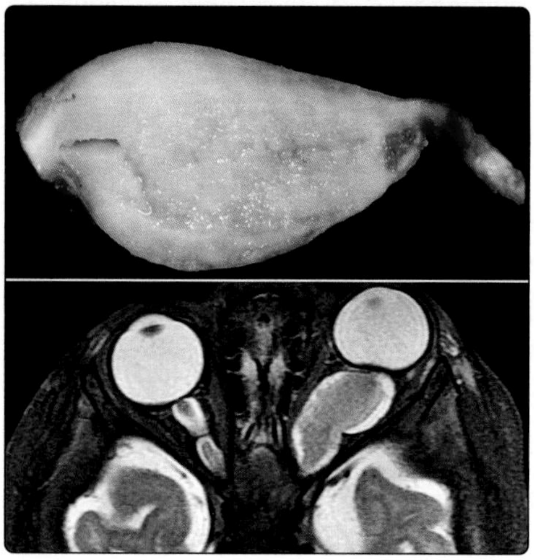

(39-7) Optic nerve glioma in NF1 (top), axial T2WI (bottom) show fusiform enlargement of optic nerve. Nerve sheaths are partly patulous.

MPNSTs may also include rhabdomyoblastic and other heterologous elements. These histologically mixed neoplasms—referred to as **malignant Triton tumors**—are very characteristic of NF1.

Gliomas. The overwhelming majority of CNS neoplasms in NF1 are grade I **pilocytic astrocytomas** (PAs). Approximately 80% of NF1 PAs arise in the optic pathway, 15% occur in the brainstem, and 5% occur in other regions.

Optic pathway gliomas (OPGs) occur in 15-20% of patients with NF1 and can be uni- or bilateral **(39-7)**. Any part of the optic pathway can be involved. Some OPGs affect just the optic nerve, whereas others involve the optic chiasm and optic tracts.

NF1-associated gliomas of the medulla, tectum, and pons are typically indolent neoplasms. Approximately 20% are malignant (WHO grades II-IV). These include **diffusely infiltrating ("low-grade") fibrillary astrocytoma, anaplastic astrocytoma**, and **glioblastoma**.

Non-CNS Neoplasms. NF1 is associated with an increased risk of leukemia (especially juvenile myelomonocytic leukemia and myelodysplastic syndromes), gastrointestinal stromal tumors (6%), and adrenal or extraadrenal pheochromocytoma (0.1-5.0%).

Rare NF1-associated systemic neoplasms include rhabdomyosarcoma, juvenile xanthogranuloma, melanoma, thyroid medullary carcinoma, and glomus tumors.

NF1-ASSOCIATED NEOPLASMS

Common
- Dermal neurofibromas (95% of adults)
- Plexiform neurofibromas (PNFs) (30-50%)
- Spinal neurofibromas

Less Common
- Pilocytic astrocytoma (80% of gliomas)
  - 80% in optic pathway (15-20% of NF1 patients)
  - 15% brainstem
  - 5% other locations (cerebellum, cerebral hemispheres)
- Other astrocytomas (20%)
  - Diffusely infiltrating fibrillary astrocytoma (WHO grade II)
  - Anaplastic astrocytoma (WHO grade III)
  - Glioblastoma (WHO grade IV)

Rare But Important
- Malignant peripheral nerve sheath tumor
  - Develops in 8-13% of PNFs
- Juvenile chronic myeloid leukemia
- Gastrointestinal stromal tumor
- Pheochromocytoma
- Rhabdomyosarcoma
- Juvenile xanthogranuloma
- Melanoma
- Thyroid medullary carcinoma
- Glomus tumors

Clinical Issues

Epidemiology and Demographics. NF1 is one of the most common CNS single-gene disorders, affecting 1:3,000 live births. There is no sex predilection.

Presentation. The clinical manifestations of NF1 are quite heterogeneous, and intrafamilial variation is common. Although absence of visible stigmata does not exclude the diagnosis of NF1, most patients exhibit characteristic cutaneous lesions **(39-8)**. Most are diagnosed as children or young adults.

Characteristic features include cutaneous neurofibromas (present in almost all adults with NF1), hyperpigmentary skin abnormalities with café au lait macules (95%) **(39-9)**, inguinal/axillary freckling (65-85%), and iris hamartomas or Lisch nodules **(39-10)**. Funduscopic examination using near-infrared reflectance demonstrates bright patchy choroidal nodules in 70% of pediatric patients and 80% of adults.

Other less common NF1-associated features include distinctive skeletal abnormalities such as sphenoid dysplasia (3-11%), long bone deformities (1-4%), pseudarthroses, and progressive kyphoscoliosis.

Cardiovascular anomalies occur in approximately 25% of individuals with NF1. Conotruncal cardiac defects, pulmonary valvular stenosis, and arterial hyperplasia are typical anomalies. NF1-related vasculopathy may present as renovascular hypertension, abdominal aortic coarctation, and strokes.

Cognitive impairment is common in NF1 and manifests primarily as learning difficulties and attention deficit disorder.

General surveillance recommendations in children with NF1 include annual physical examination (including ophthalmologic examination up to age 5 years), developmental assessment, and regular blood pressure monitoring. Additional specialist evaluations depend on associated CNS, skeletal, or cardiovascular manifestations.

Clinical Diagnosis. Molecular diagnostic testing distinguishes NF1 from other disorders that share similar phenotypic features. With the exception of PNF, most clinical stigmata of NF1 also occur in other disorders (e.g., multiple café au lait macules in McCune-Albright syndrome). Consensus criteria for the clinical diagnosis of NF1 are summarized in the box below.

NF1: DIAGNOSTIC CLINICAL FEATURES (AT LEAST TWO REQUIRED)

Cutaneous Lesions

- ≥ 6 café au lait spots (earliest manifestation)
  - Prepubertal: ≥ 0.5 cm
  - Postpubertal: ≥ 1.5 cm
- Freckling of armpits or groin
- ≥ 2 neurofibromas (any type)
- 1 plexiform neurofibroma

Eye Abnormalities

- ≥ 2 Lisch nodules (pigmented iris hamartomas)
- Optic pathway pilocytic astrocytoma

Distinctive Bone Lesion

- Sphenoid dysplasia/absence
- Long bone cortex dysplasia/thinning

Family History

- First-degree relative with NF1

Natural History. Prognosis in NF1 is variable and relates to its specific manifestations. Median age at death for all NF1 patients is 59 years. Increased mortality is related to MPNST, glioma, cardiovascular disease, and organ compression by neurofibromas.

The foci of myelin vacuolization **(39-18)** increase in number and size over the first decade, then regress, and eventually disappear. They are rarely identified in adults, and their relationship to intellectual impairment is uncertain.

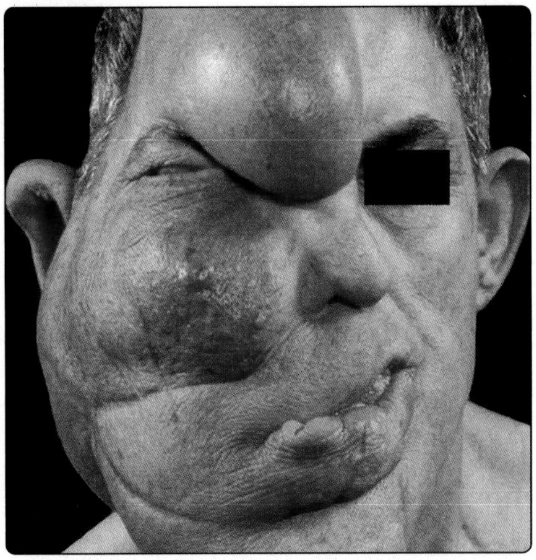

***(39-8)** Clinical photo reveals extensive facial plexiform neurofibroma. (Courtesy A. Ersen, MD.)*

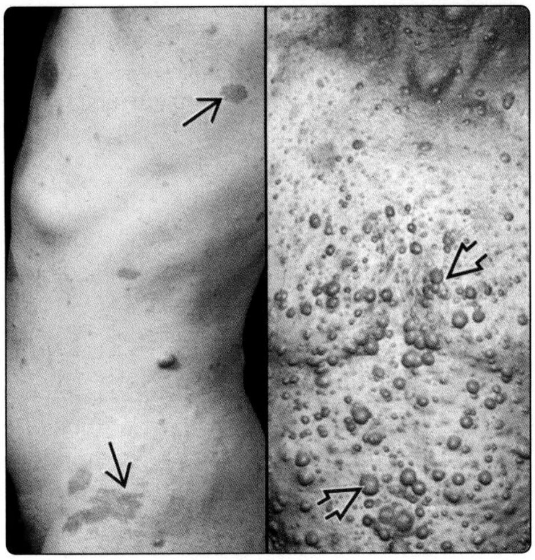

***(39-9)** Photographs show multiple café au lait spots (L) ⇨ and cutaneous neurofibromas ⇨ (R) in NF1. (Courtesy A. Ersen, MD.)*

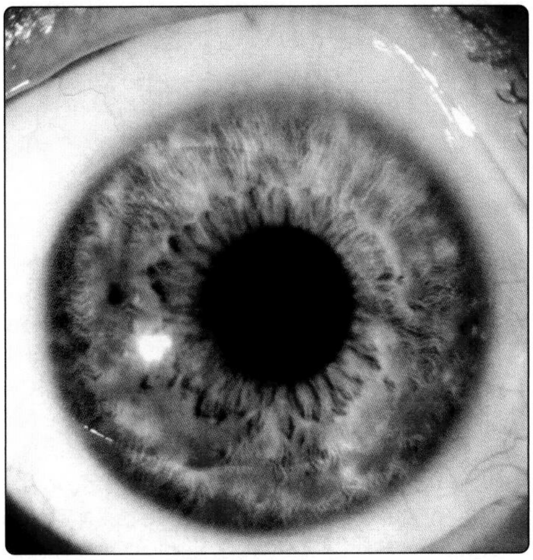

***(39-10)** Clinical photo shows multiple Lisch nodules in a patient with NF1. (Courtesy A. Ersen, MD.)*

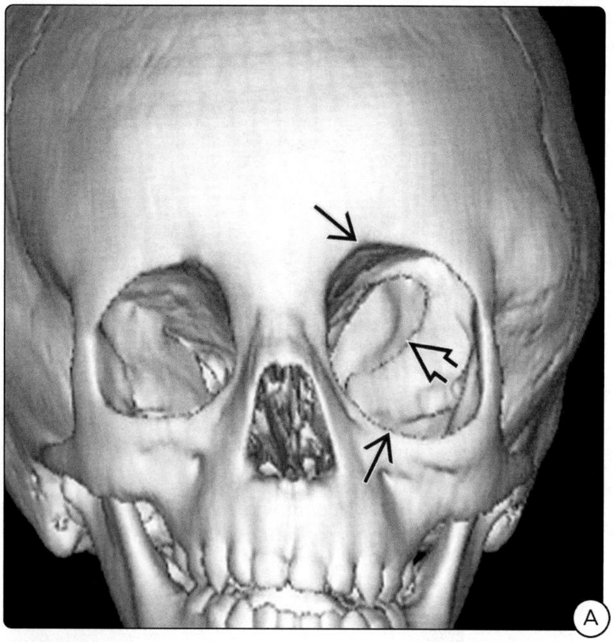

(39-11A) 3D bone CT in a patient with NF1 and sphenoid dysplasia shows enlarged left orbit → and widened superior orbital fissure ⇨.

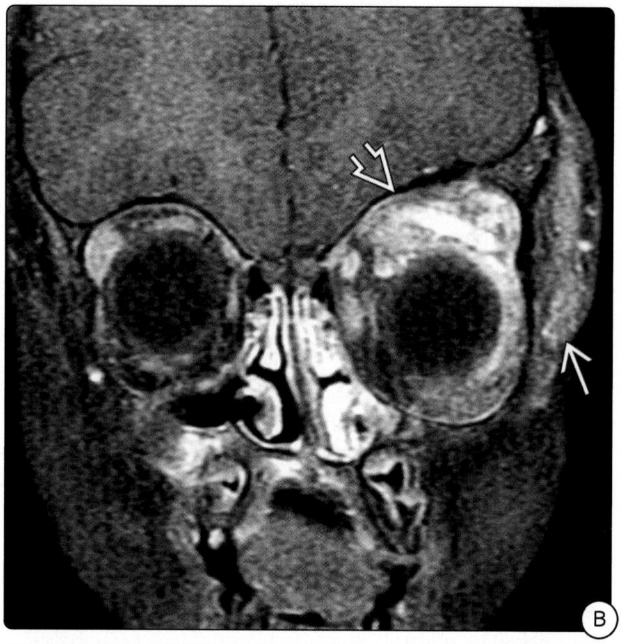

(39-11B) Coronal T1 C+ FS scan in the same patient shows enhancing plexiform neurofibroma infiltrating the orbit ⇨ and high deep masticator space →.

Treatment Options. Foci of myelin vacuolization do not undergo neoplastic transformation and do not require treatment.

Imaging

Imaging features vary with the specific type of NF1-related abnormalities. The use of whole-body short tau inversion recovery (STIR) sequences for both identifying tumors and assessing overall tumor burden in clinical trials is becoming more widespread although standard CNS-focused sequences are illustrated here.

Nonneoplastic CNS Lesions. Bone dysplasias occur in the skull, spine, and long bones (e.g., pseudarthroses). NECT scans may demonstrate a hypoplastic sphenoid wing **(39-11A)** and enlarged middle cranial fossa, with or without an associated arachnoid cyst. Protrusion of the anterior temporal lobe may result in ipsilateral proptosis. The globe is frequently enlarged ("buphthalmos"), and a plexiform neurofibroma is often present **(39-11B)**.

Dural dysplasia with patulous spinal dura **(39-12)** as well as enlarged optic nerve sheaths, internal auditory canals, and Meckel caves can occur **(39-13)**.

Dysplastic white matter lesions are seen as multifocal hyperintensities on T2/FLAIR imaging. These foci represent zones of myelin vacuolization (ZMVs) and are seen in 70% of children with NF1. They generally increase in size and number until approximately 10 years of age but then wane and disappear **(39-19)**. ZMVs are rarely seen in adults.

The most common sites are the globi pallidi (GP), centrum semiovale, cerebellar WM, dentate nuclei, thalamus, and brainstem **(39-18)**. Most are smaller than 2 cm in diameter **(39-19)**. They generally exhibit little or no mass effect although the corpus callosum may appear thickened in severe cases. Confluent midbrain, tectum, brainstem, and hypothalamic lesions with unusually extensive myelin vacuolization can occasionally cause mass effect and even obstructive hydrocephalus.

Most ZMVs are iso- or minimally hypointense on T1WI although GP lesions are often mildly hyperintense. ZMVs do not enhance following contrast administration and demonstrate increased ADC values on DWI.

Most NF1-associated **vascular lesions** are extracranial and range from renal artery stenosis to aortic coarctation and aneurysmal dilatations of the great vessels.

Relentless endothelial hyperplasia can cause progressive stenosis of the intracranial internal carotid arteries, resulting in a moyamoya pattern. Careful scrutiny of the intracranial vasculature demonstrates attenuation of the middle cerebral artery "flow voids" **(39-14)**.

CNS Neoplasms

Neurofibromas. Patients with **cutaneous neurofibromas** often demonstrate solitary or multifocal discrete round or ovoid scalp lesions that are hypointense to brain on T1WI and hyperintense on T2WI. A target sign with a hyperintense rim and relatively hypointense center is common. Strong but heterogeneous enhancement following contrast administration is typical.

PNFs are most common in the orbit, where they are seen as poorly marginated serpentine masses that infiltrate the orbit, extraocular muscles, and eyelids **(39-11B)**. They often extend inferiorly into the pterygopalatine fossa and buccal spaces as well as superiorly into the adjacent scalp and masticator spaces. Transspatial extension into the neck is common. PNFs enhance strongly and resemble a "bag of worms."

Malignant Peripheral Nerve Sheath Tumors. **MPNSTs** arising within a PNF can be difficult to detect and to differentiate from the parent tumor. MPNSTs tend to be more heterogeneous in signal intensity, often exhibiting intratumoral cysts, perilesional edema, and peripheral enhancement. Whole-body F-18 FDG PET/CT may be helpful in distinguishing benign tumors from MPNSTs.

Gliomas. The most common glioma in NF1 is **pilocytic astrocytoma**. Optic pathway glioma (OPG) is the most common lesion and is seen as a diffuse, fusiform, or bulbous enlargement of one or both optic nerves **(39-7)**. Tumor may extend posteriorly into the optic chiasm, superiorly into the hypothalamus, fornices, and cavum septi pellucidi, laterally into the temporal lobes, posteriorly into the optic tracts and lateral geniculate bodies, and posteroinferiorly into the cerebral peduncles and brainstem **(39-15)**.

Signal intensity is variable. Most OPGs are isointense with brain on T1WI and iso- to moderately hyperintense on T2WI. Enhancement on T1 C+ FS scans varies from none to striking.

MRS is generally not helpful, as pilocytic astrocytomas often demonstrate a malignant-appearing spectrum with elevated choline and increased Cho:Cr ratio. Neither extent of signal intensity nor enhancement indicates malignancy, so interval surveillance is necessary. NF1-associated OPGs can be stable for many years or involute spontaneously.

NF1-associated **low-grade fibrillary astrocytomas** can be difficult to distinguish from FASIs. They are usually moderately hypointense on T1WI and hyperintense on T2WI and show progression on follow-up imaging.

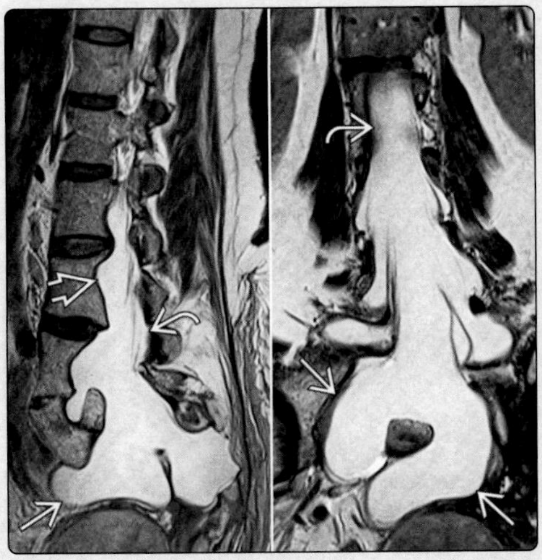

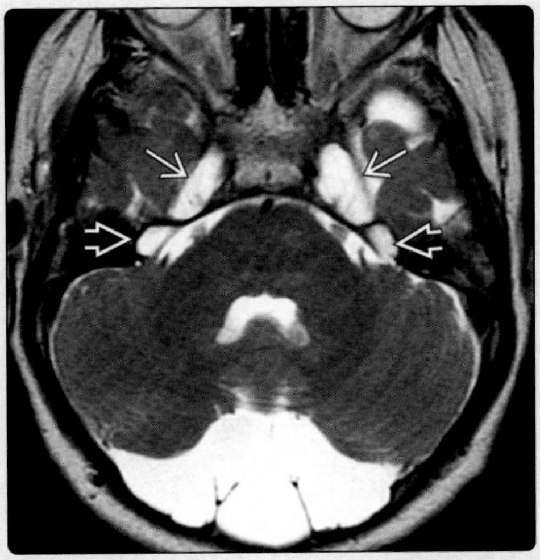

***(39-12)** Sagittal (L) and coronal (R) T2WIs show NF1 with extreme dural ectasia ➡ causing posterior vertebral scalloping ➡ and extensive meningoceles ➡. **(39-13)** T2WI in NF1 shows CSF-filled patulous Meckel caves ➡ and internal auditory canals ➡.*

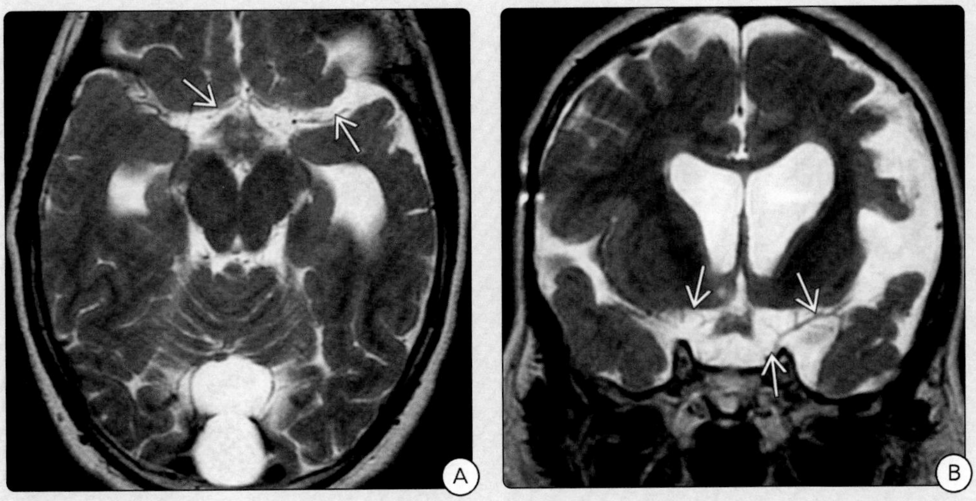

***(39-14A)** Axial T2WI in a teenager with NF1 shows extremely attenuated anterior and middle cerebral arteries ➡, a vascular manifestation of NF1. **(39-14B)** Coronal T2WI in the same patient shows the typical appearance of moyamoya in NF1 with markedly attenuated supraclinoid internal carotid, anterior cerebral, and middle cerebral arteries ➡.*

(39-15A) Axial T2WI in a patient with NF1 shows an enlarged hyperintense left optic nerve ➡, a prosthetic globe ➡, and a hyperintense mass ➡ in the pons. (39-15B) More cephalad T2WI shows enlarged optic chiasm ➡, mass extending into right midbrain ➡, and foci of abnormal signal intensity in both medial temporal lobes and the left midbrain ➡.

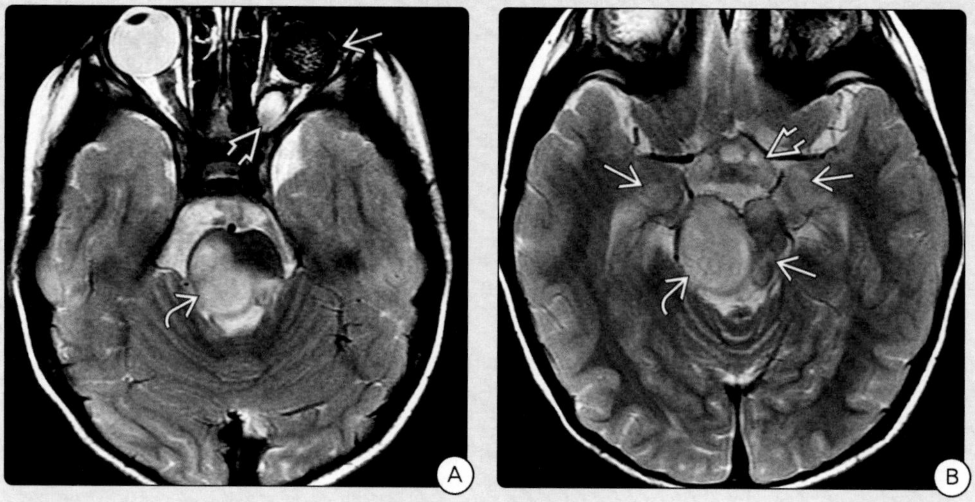

(39-15C) T1 C+ FS scan shows intense enhancement in the enlarged optic chiasm ➡, medial temporal lobes ➡, and midbrain ➡. (39-15D) More cephalad scan shows that the enhancement extends posteriorly along both optic radiations ➡. Biopsy demonstrated pilocytic astrocytoma (WHO grade I) without evidence of malignant degeneration.

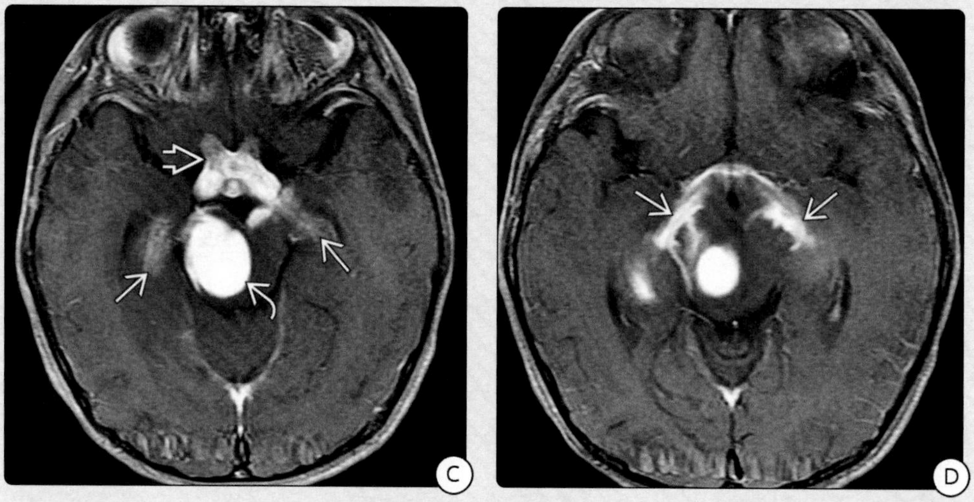

(39-16) Precontrast (L) and postcontrast (R) T1WIs in an 18y man with NF1 shows a circumscribed cyst ➡ with enhancing nodule ➡. This is hemispheric pilocytic astrocytoma, WHO grade I. (39-17) (L) T1 C+ FS in a 30y woman with NF1, headaches shows a tiny enhancing focus ➡ in the left parieto-occipital lobe. The patient was lost to follow-up but returned 12 years later. The mass ➡ is very large, abuts the dura ➡. This is gliosarcoma, WHO IV.

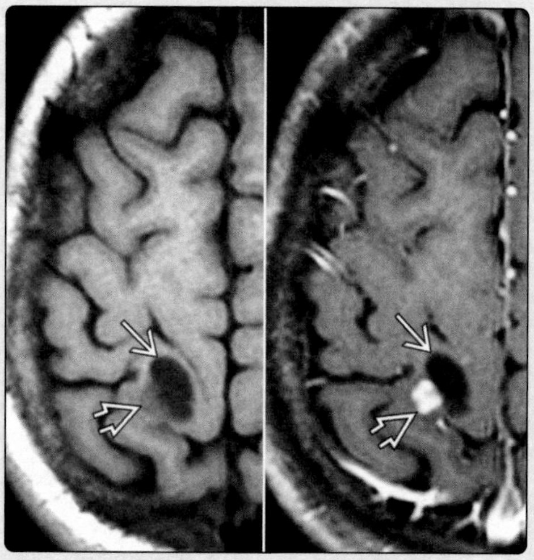

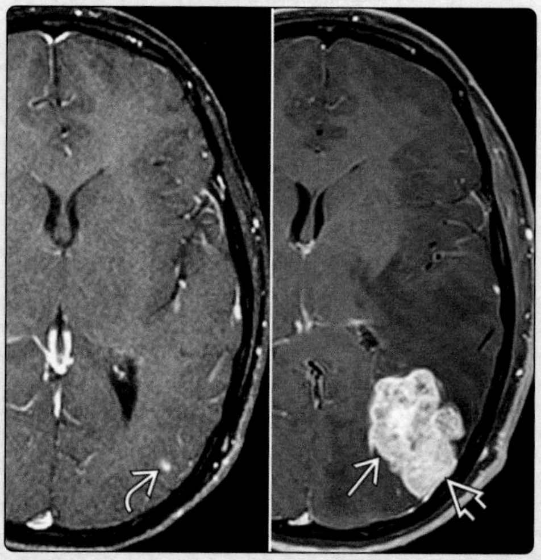

Anaplastic astrocytoma and **glioblastoma multiforme** are more aggressive, more heterogeneous tumors that demonstrate relentless progression. A progressively enlarging mass that enhances following contrast administration in a child with NF1 should raise suspicion of malignant neoplasm.

NF1: IMAGING

Scalp/Skull, Meninges, and Orbit

- Dermal neurofibromas
  - Solitary/multifocal scalp nodules
  - Increases with age
  - Localized, well-circumscribed
- Plexiform neurofibroma
  - Pathognomonic of NF1 (30-50% of cases)
  - Large, bulky infiltrative transspatial lesions
  - Scalp, face/neck, spine
  - Orbit lesions may extend into cavernous sinus
- Sphenoid wing dysplasia
  - Hypoplasia → enlarged orbital fissure
  - Enlarged middle fossa ± arachnoid cyst
  - Temporal lobe may protrude into orbit
- Dural ectasia
  - Tortuous optic nerve sheath
  - Patulous Meckel caves
  - Enlarged IACs

Brain

- Hyperintense T2/FLAIR WM foci
  - Wax in first decade, then wane
  - Rare in adults
- Astrocytomas
  - Most common: pilocytic
  - Optic pathway, hypothalamus > brainstem
  - Malignant astrocytoma (anaplastic astrocytoma, glioblastoma multiforme) less common

Arteries

- Progressive ICA stenosis → moyamoya
- Fusiform ectasias, arteriovenous fistulas
  - Vertebral > carotid

Differential Diagnosis

In combination with appropriate clinical findings (see above), the presence of ZMVs on MR with or without OPG is diagnostic of NF1. In and of themselves, multifocal T2/FLAIR hyperintensities are nonspecific and can be seen in a variety of nonneoplastic disorders, including **demyelinating disease** and **viral encephalitis**. Unlike NF1, viral encephalitis has an acute clinical course and is usually associated with encephalopathy.

Unusually extensive, confluent FASIs can mimic **neoplasm** (i.e., pilocytic astrocytoma, diffusely infiltrating low-grade astrocytoma, anaplastic astrocytoma, glioblastoma multiforme, or gliomatosis cerebri). Both FASIs and gliomas are part of the NF1 spectrum, so follow-up imaging may be necessary.

A recently described disorder parallels NF1 in some ways—multiple café au lait macules, axillary freckling, and macrocephaly—but the causative gene (*SPRED1*) is different. This disorder has been termed **NF1-like syndrome**. Patients lack cutaneous neurofibromas or PNFs, typical NF1 bone lesions, and optic pathway gliomas.

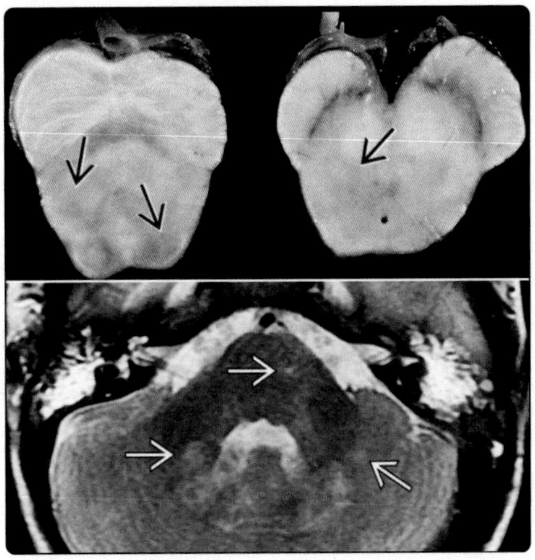

***(39-18)** Autopsied NF1 (top) shows foci of discolored WM ⇨ (AFIP). T2WI (bottom) shows hyperintense lesions ➡ in pons, cerebellum.*

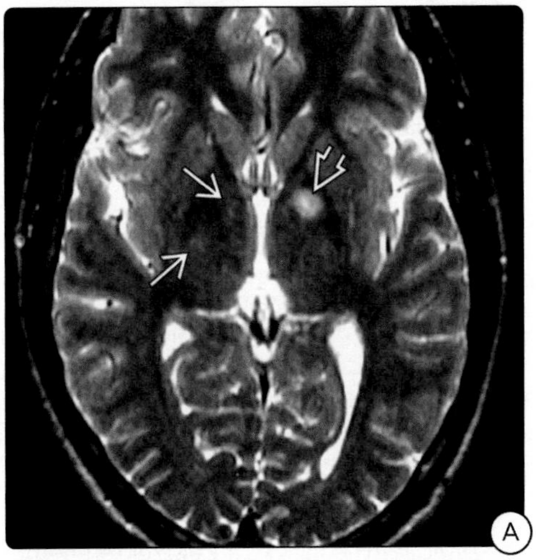

***(39-19A)** T2WI in a child with NF1 shows zones of myelin vacuolization (ZMVs) in right ➡ and left basal ganglia ⮚.*

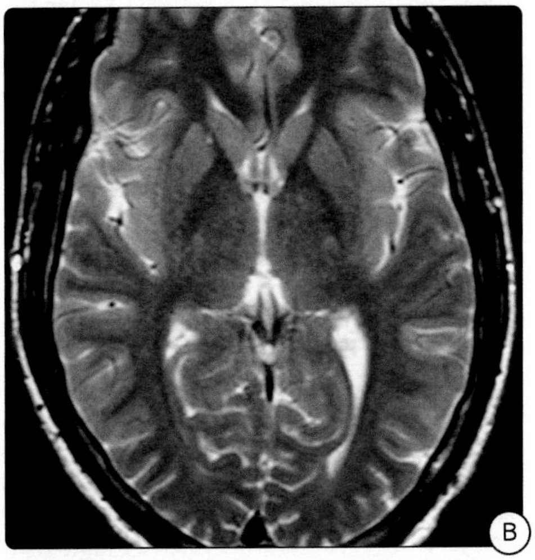

***(39-19B)** Six years later, the ZMVs have resolved completely without residual abnormality.*

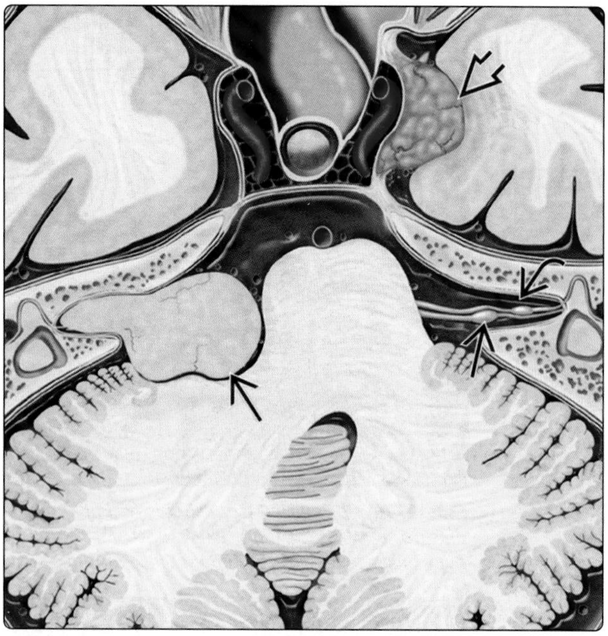

(39-20) Graphic depicts classic NF2 with bilateral vestibular schwannomas ➡, facial schwannoma ➡, and cavernous sinus meningioma ➡.

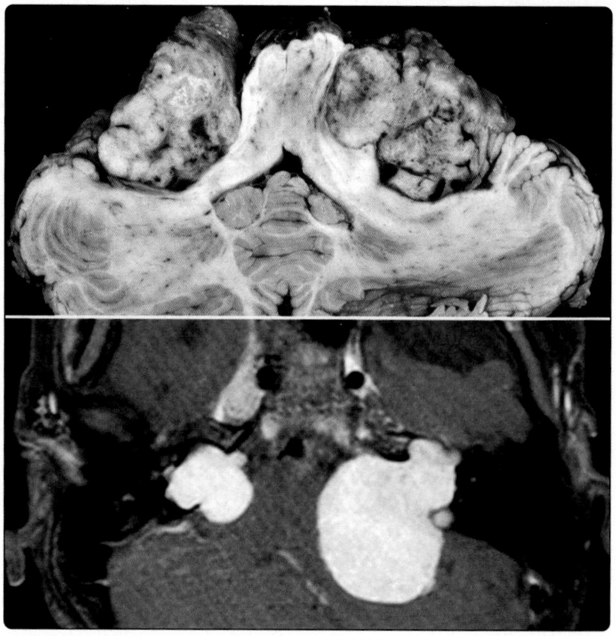

(39-21) Autopsy (top) shows bilateral vestibular schwannomas in NF2. (A. Ersen, MD.) Typical T1 C+ scan (bottom) shows bilateral vestibular and facial schwannomas and right cavernous sinus trigeminal schwannoma.

Neurofibromatosis Type 2

Although historically grouped with NF1, neurofibromatosis type 2 (NF2) is a distinct syndrome with totally different mutations, clinical features, and imaging findings. Neurofibromas characterize NF1 and are composed of Schwann cells plus fibroblasts. Schwannomas (especially bilateral vestibular schwannomas) are the major feature of NF2 and contain only Schwann cells.

The associated neoplasms are also different from those in NF1. Astrocytomas are found in NF1, whereas ependymomas and meningiomas are the predominant tumors in NF2.

There is only one similarity between NF1 and NF2: they both predispose affected individuals to develop benign Schwann cell tumors.

Terminology

NF2 is also known as neurofibromatosis with bilateral vestibular ("acoustic") schwannomas. Historically, NF2 was termed central neurofibromatosis (to distinguish it from so-called peripheral neurofibromatosis, i.e., NF1). The term von Recklinghausen neurofibromatosis is associated only with NF1 and should not be used for NF2.

Etiology

General Concepts. Like NF1, NF2 is an autosomal-dominant disorder. About half of all cases occur in individuals with no family history of NF2 and are caused by newly acquired germline mutations. Approximately 30% of these patients have mosaic genetic alterations.

Genetics. NF2 is caused by mutations of the *NF2* gene on chromosome 22q12. The *NF2* gene encodes the protein Merlin (**m**oesin-**e**rzin-**r**adixin-**l**ike prote**in**), which is also known as schwannomin. Merlin is implicated in the regulation of membrane organization and cytoskeleton-based cellular processes, such as adhesion, migration, cell-cell contact, and signaling.

Merlin functions as a growth inhibitor and tumor suppressor and regulates antiangiogenic factors. Inactivating mutations of the *NF2* gene result in loss of contact-dependent inhibition of proliferation and cause predominantly benign neoplasms (schwannomas and meningiomas). Biallelic *NF2* inactivation is detected in the majority of sporadic meningiomas and nearly all schwannomas.

Pathology

Location. CNS lesions are present in virtually all patients with NF2.

The most common NF2-related schwannomas are vestibular schwannomas (VSs) **(39-20)**. Approximately 50% of patients have nonvestibular schwannomas (NVSs). The most common locations for NVSs are the trigeminal and oculomotor nerves. NF2-associated schwannomas of the trochlear and lower cranial nerves occur but are relatively rare.

Meningiomas occur in approximately half of all patients with NF2 and can be found anywhere in the skull and spine. The most frequent sites are along the falx and cerebral convexities.

Intracranial ependymomas are rare in NF2. Most are found in the spinal cord, especially within the cervical cord or at the cervicomedullary junction.

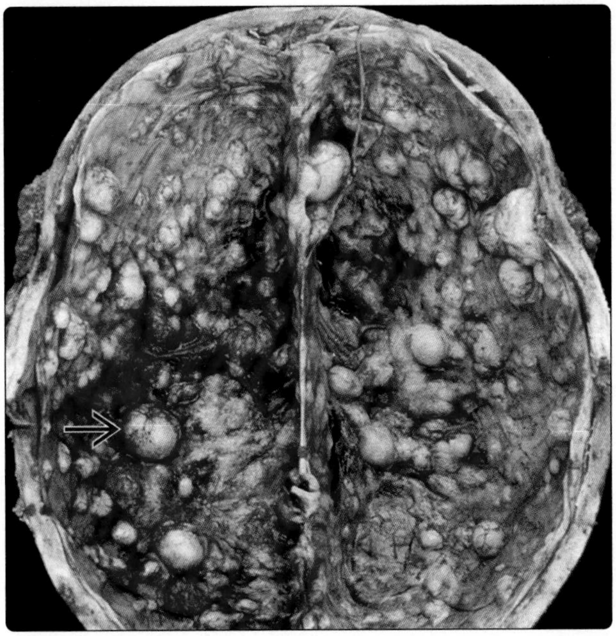

(39-22) Autopsy specimen demonstrates innumerable small meningiomas ⇒, a common finding in NF2. (From DP: Neuropathology, 2e.)

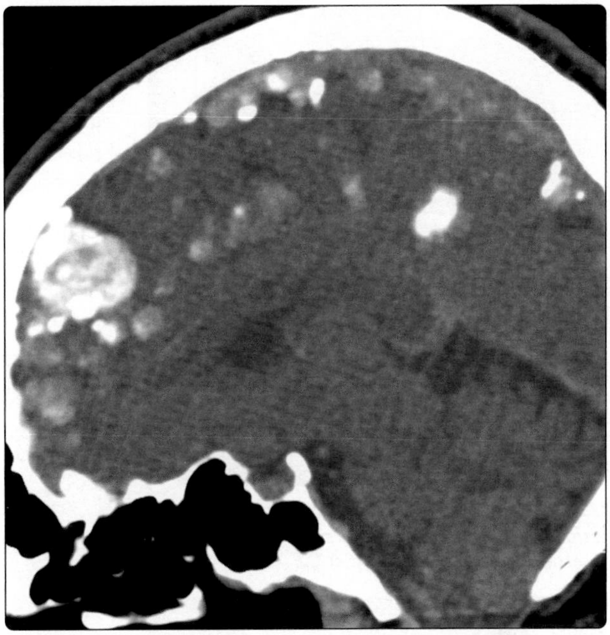

(39-23) Sagittal NECT in a 31y woman with NF2, multiple intracranial and spinal schwannomas shows innumerable hyperdense calcified masses that abut the dura and falx characteristic of NF2-associated meningiomatosis.

Size and Number. NF2-related schwannomas, meningiomas, and ependymomas are often multiple. The presence of bilateral VSs is pathognomonic of NF2; adult patients with NF2 have an average of three meningiomas.

Size varies from tiny to several centimeters. Innumerable tiny schwannomas ("tumorlets") throughout the cauda equina are seen in the majority of patients. Intramedullary ependymomas are often small; multiple tumors are present in nearly 60% of patients.

Gross Pathology. NF2 is characterized by multiple schwannomas, meningiomas, and ependymomas. Virtually all patients have bilateral VSs, considered the hallmark of NF2 **(39-21)**. Most schwannomas are well-delineated round or ovoid encapsulated masses that are attached to—but do not infiltrate—their parent nerves.

Multiple meningiomas are the second pathologic hallmark of NF2 **(39-22)**. They are found in approximately 50% of patients and may be the presenting feature (especially in children). Meningiomas appear as unencapsulated but sharply demarcated masses.

Microscopic Features. Schwannomas are composed of neoplastic Schwann cells. Areas of alternating high and low cellularity (Antoni A pattern) are admixed with foci that exhibit microcysts and myxoid changes (Antoni B pattern). Schwann cells are strongly immunoreactive for S100 and usually do not express Merlin.

Benign nerve sheath tumors, especially of the peripheral nerves, can occasionally exhibit hybrid features of both neurofibroma AND schwannoma.

Staging, Grading, and Classification. Although NF2-associated schwannomas often have higher proliferative activity than sporadic tumors, they are not necessarily more aggressive. They are considered WHO grade I tumors.

Most NF2-associated meningiomas are WHO grade I neoplasms. Among symptomatic resected meningiomas, grades II and III tumors are found in 29% and 6% of cases, respectively. NF2-associated ependymomas—especially those in the spinal cord—are generally indolent and carry a favorable prognosis.

Clinical Issues

Epidemiology and Demographics. NF2 is much less common than NF1, with an estimated prevalence of 1:25,000 births. There is no geographic, ethnic, or sex predilection.

Presentation. Unlike NF1 patients, individuals with NF2 generally do not become symptomatic until the second to fourth decades; symptoms often precede definitive diagnosis by 5-8 years. Average age at initial diagnosis is 17-24 years; less than 20% of patients with NF2 present under the age of 15.

Unlike NF1, most of the clinical features of NF2 involve the nervous system. Cutaneous schwannomas and/or juvenile subcapsular opacities may be the first visible manifestations of NF2. Café au lait spots are seen in only one-quarter of patients and are both less prominent and fewer in number than in individuals with NF1.

Most adult patients exhibit CN VIII dysfunction with progressive sensorineural hearing loss, tinnitus, and difficulties with balance. Other common symptoms include facial pain and/or paralysis, vertigo, and seizures. Hearing loss is relatively

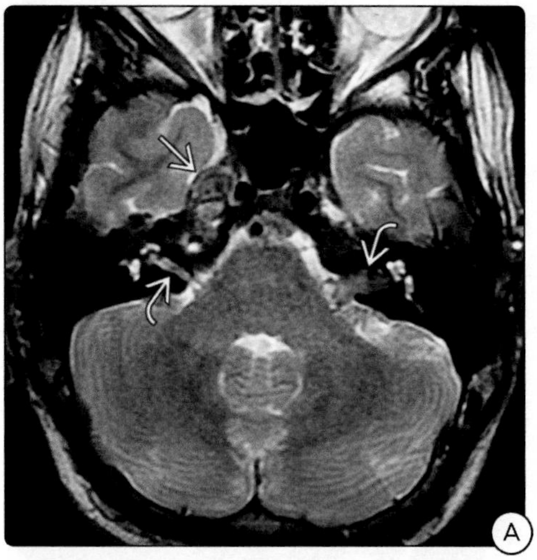

(39-24A) T2WI in a 14y boy with NF2 reveals lesions in the right cavernous sinus and both internal auditory canals (IACs).

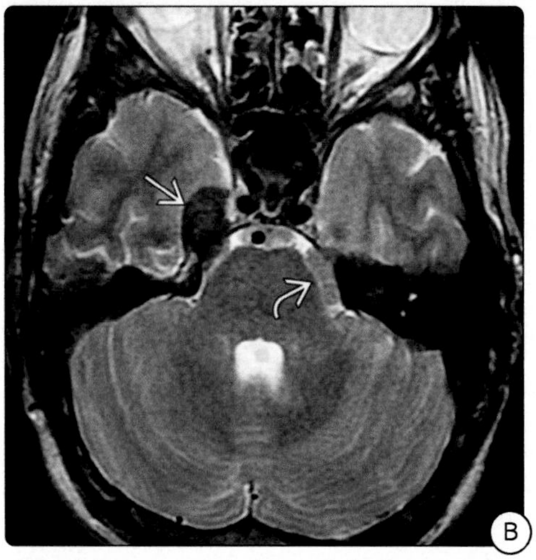

(39-24B) More cephalad T2WI in in the same case shows a hypodense mass in the right cavernous sinus and lesions in the left CPA cistern.

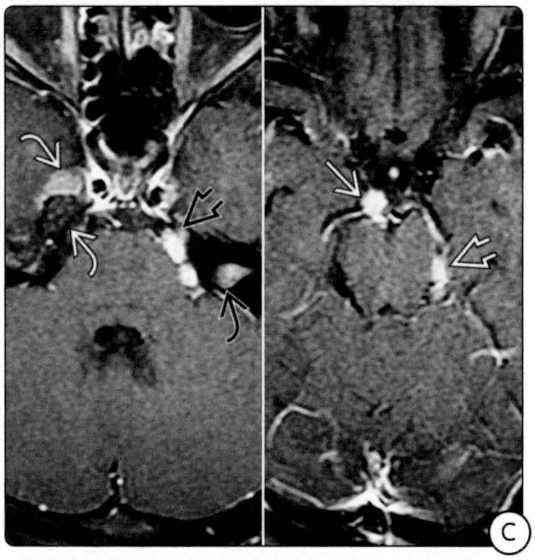

(39-24C) T1 C+ FS scans show right cavernous sinus meningioma, CN III, and left CNs IV, V, and VIII schwannomas.

uncommon in children. Subcapsular cataracts, seizures, facial nerve palsy, and other cranial neuropathies are common.

Many NF2-related meningiomas are asymptomatic and discovered incidentally on imaging studies; if symptoms appear, seizures or focal neurologic deficits are the most common. Spinal cord ependymomas are asymptomatic in 75% of patients.

Clinical Diagnosis. The definitive diagnosis of NF2 is established genetically. Similar to NF1, consensus criteria have been developed for the clinical diagnosis and are summarized in the box below. Findings are divided into those of "definite" and "probable" NF2.

NF2: DIAGNOSTIC CLINICAL FEATURES

Definite NF2
- Bilateral vestibular schwannomas (VSs)
- First-degree relative with NF2 *and* unilateral VS diagnosed before 30 years of age
- *Or* first-degree relative with NF2 *and* 2 of the following
  - Meningioma
  - Glioma
  - Schwannoma
  - Juvenile posterior subcapsular lenticular opacities or cataracts

Probable NF2
- Unilateral VS diagnosed < 30 years of age *and* 1 of the following
  - Meningioma
  - Glioma
  - Schwannoma
  - Juvenile posterior subcapsular lenticular opacities or cataracts
- ≥ 2 meningiomas *and* 1 of the following
  - 1 VS diagnosed < 30 years of age
  - 1 meningioma, glioma, schwannoma, or lens opacity

Natural History. Actuarial survival for NF2 patients after diagnosis is 85% at 5 years, 67% at 10 years, and 38% at 20 years. Although NF2-associated meningiomas have a mean annual growth rate of 1.5 mm, de novo meningiomas with brain edema may require active treatment.

NF2-associated intracranial neoplasms often demonstrate a "saltatory" growth pattern characterized by alternating periods of growth and quiescence.

As new tumors can develop and radiographic progression and symptom development are unpredictable, continued surveillance is necessary.

Treatment Options. Treatment is increasingly conservative with the use of stereotaxic radiosurgery and drugs like bevacizumab, a monoclonal antibody against VEGF. Current recommended MR surveillance includes imaging at 1, 5, and 10 years postoperatively.

Imaging

General Features. The cardinal imaging feature of NF2 is bilateral vestibular schwannomas.

CT Findings. NECT scans typically demonstrate a mass in one or both cerebellopontine angle (CPA) cisterns. Both schwannomas and meningiomas are typically iso- to slightly hyperdense on NECT **(39-23)** and exhibit strong enhancement following contrast administration.

Nonneoplastic choroid plexus calcifications in atypical locations (e.g., temporal horn) are a rare manifestation of NF2 but can be striking. Bone CT typically shows that one or both internal auditory canals are widened, whereas schwannomas of other cranial nerves may demonstrate enlargement and remodeling of their exit foramina.

MR Findings. MR findings of NF2-related schwannomas and meningiomas are similar to those of their sporadic counterparts. If NF2 is suspected on the basis of brain imaging, the entire spine and spinal cord should be screened. High-resolution T2WI and contrast-enhanced sequences disclose asymptomatic tiny schwannomas **(39-24)** **(39-27)** and intramedullary ependymomas **(39-25)** in at least half of all individuals with NF2 **(39-26)**.

Dural enhancement at the porus acusticus is present in approximately 10% of extracanalicular VSs. Although it may represent dural reaction, hypervascularity, or neoplastic infiltration, it portends increased tumor adherence and greater likelihood of subtotal resection and should be considered in surgical planning.

Differential Diagnosis

The major differential diagnosis of NF2 is **schwannomatosis**. Schwannomatosis is characterized by multiple NVSs. Meningiomas are less common in schwannomatosis. **Multiple meningiomatosis** is characterized by multifocal meningiomas without schwannomas.

NF1 vs. NF2 vs. SCHWANNOMATOSIS

Neurofibromatosis Type 1
- Common (90% of all neurofibromatosis cases)
- Chromosome 17 mutations
- Almost always diagnosed by age 10
- Cutaneous/eye lesions common (> 95%)
  - Café au lait spots
  - Lisch nodules
  - Cutaneous neurofibromas (often multiple)
  - Plexiform neurofibromas (pathognomonic)
- CNS lesions less common (15-20%)
  - T2/FLAIR hyperintensities (myelin vacuolization; lesions wax, then wane)
  - Astrocytomas (optic pathway gliomas—usually pilocytic—other gliomas)
  - Sphenoid wing, dural dysplasias
  - Moyamoya
  - Neurofibromas of spinal nerve roots

Neurofibromatosis Type 2
- Much less common (10% of all neurofibromatosis cases)
- Chromosome 22 mutations
- Usually diagnosed in second to fourth decades
- Cutaneous, eye lesions less prominent
  - Mild/few café au lait spots
  - Juvenile subcapsular opacities
- CNS lesions in 100%
  - Bilateral vestibular schwannomas (almost all)
  - Nonvestibular schwannomas (50%)
  - Meningiomas (50%)
  - Cord ependymomas (often multiple)
  - Schwannomas of spinal nerve roots

Schwannomatosis
- Very rare; usually de novo mutation
- Multiple *nonvestibular* schwannomas ± meningioma
- *SMARCB1* (INI1) and *LZTR1* mutations

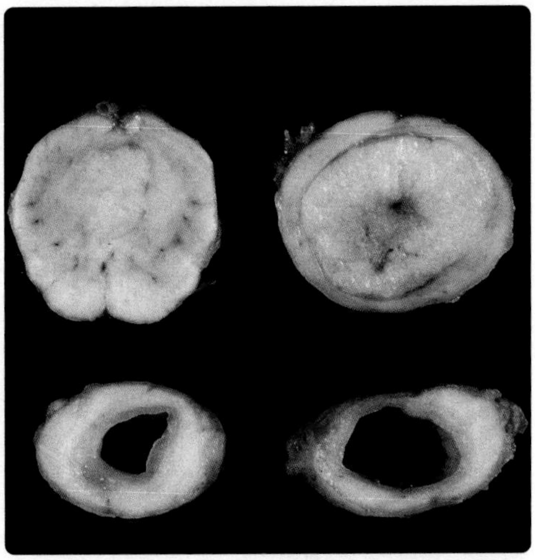

(39-25) Axial gross pathology in NF2 shows intramedullary ependymoma with cyst expanding cervical cord. (Courtesy R. Hewlett, MD.)

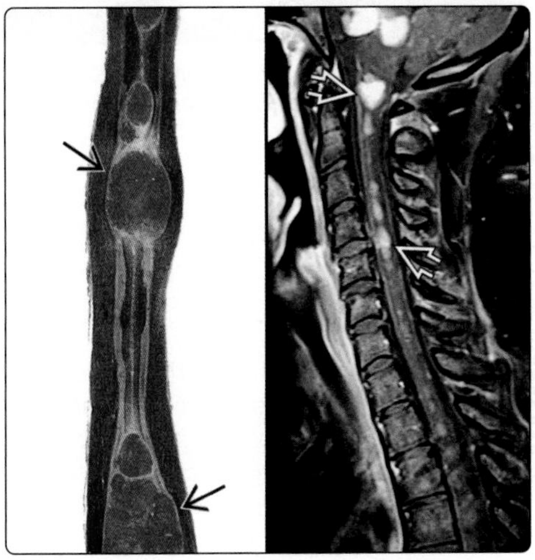

(39-26) Autopsy (L) shows intramedullary ependymomas. (Courtesy A. Ersen, MD.) (R) T1 C+ shows multiple cord ependymomas in NF2.

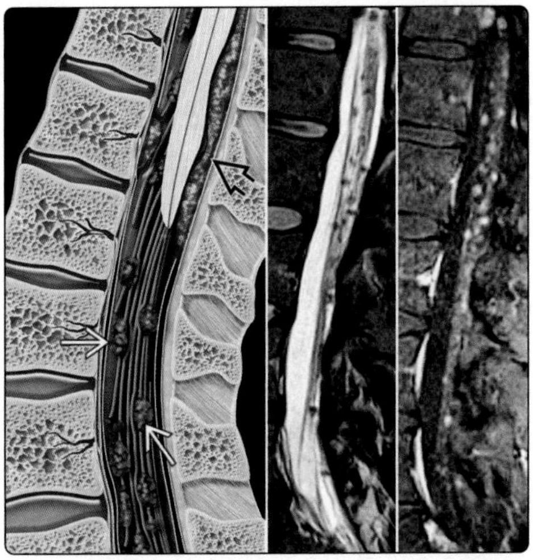

(39-27) NF2 graphic (L) depicts spinal "tumorlets", meningioma. T2WI (middle), T1 C+ (R) show cauda equina schwannomas.

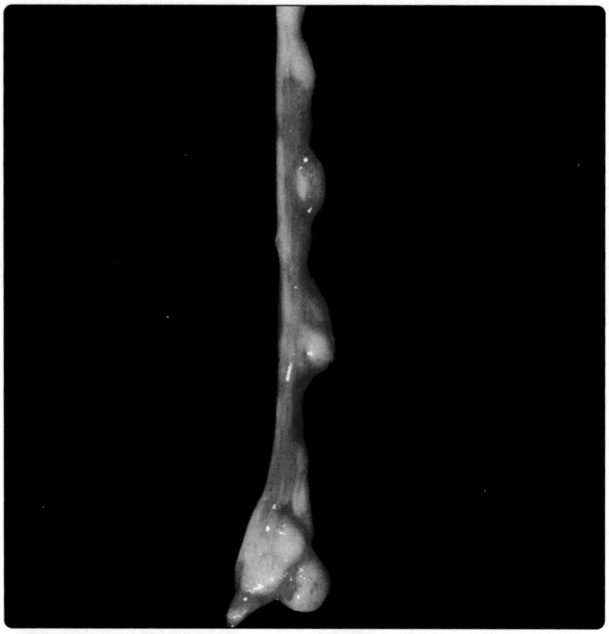

(39-28) Gross pathology of schwannomatosis shows multiple eccentric, expanded foci along this peripheral nerve. (From DP: Neuropathology, 2e.)

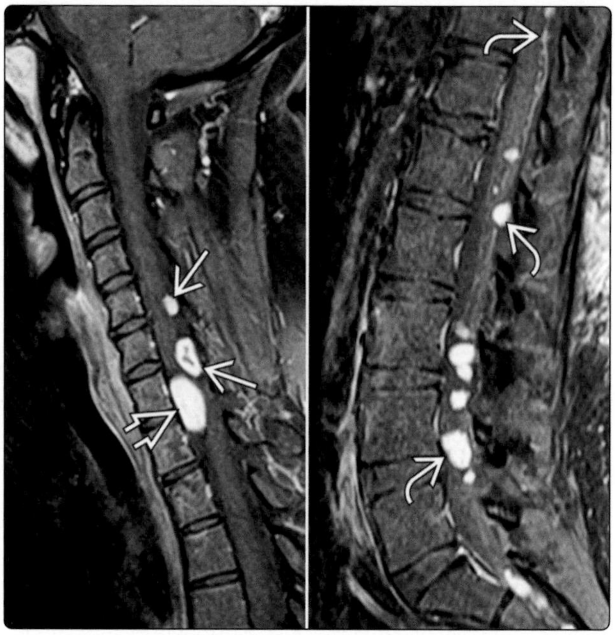

(39-29) T1 C+ FS of (L) cervical, (R) lumbar spine in a 32y woman with arm pain, numbness show cervical meningioma ➡, schwannomas ➡ plus innumerable cauda equina schwannomas ➡. Intracranial scan was negative; this is schwannomatosis.

Schwannomatosis

Terminology

Schwannomatosis, which is the third major form of neurofibromatosis, is a rare hereditary cancer syndrome in which patients develop multiple **nonvestibular schwannomas**. Schwannomatosis is a paradigm for a tumor predisposition syndrome caused by the concomitant mutational inactivation of two or more tumor suppressor genes.

Unlike NF1 and NF2, most cases of schwannomatosis arise de novo. Less than 15% appear to be familial. The rate of transmission to offspring is low, likely due to the high rate of genetic mosaicism in founder mutations.

Etiology and Pathology

Despite the clinical overlap with NF2, schwannomatosis is not caused by germline NF2 mutations. Instead, germline mutations of either the *SMARCB1* or *LZTR1* tumor suppressor genes occur in 85% of familial and 40% of sporadic schwannomatosis patients. Large parts of chromosome 22q harboring, not only *SMARCB1* and *LZTR1*, but also *NF2* are affected.

Multiple schwannomas of the spine (75%), subcutaneous tissues (15%), and nonvestibular cranial nerves (10%) are characteristic **(39-28)**. Schwannomas vary from multiple discrete nodules to plexiform lesions. Histologic features are those of typical schwannoma.

Recent evidence indicates that schwannomatosis patients with *SMARCB1* mutations are at risk to develop multiple cranial meningiomas. Nearly two-thirds of meningiomas in patients with this tumor predisposition syndrome are located at the falx cerebri.

Clinical Issues

Schwannomatosis is the rarest of the neurofibromatoses, affecting 1:40,000 births. Symptoms vary, but pain is the most common presentation. Multiple painful progressive swellings in the body without the characteristic features of NF1 and NF2 should raise the suspicion of schwannomatosis. Prognosis is excellent, as anaplastic transformation is very rare.

Imaging and Differential Diagnosis

Cranial nonvestibular schwannomas are common and resemble both sporadic and NF2-associated schwannomas. Multiple enhancing nodules occur along the cauda equina and peripheral nerves. Meningiomas occur but are uncommon compared with NF2.

The major differential diagnosis of schwannomatosis is **NF2**. By definition, schwannomatosis lacks the bilateral VSs characteristic of NF2.

Other Common Familial Tumor Syndromes

Tuberous Sclerosis Complex

Tuberous sclerosis complex (TSC) is a neurocutaneous syndrome characterized by the formation of nonmalignant hamartomas and neoplastic lesions in the brain, heart, skin, kidney, lung, and other organs. It is associated with autism, seizures, and neurocognitive and behavioral disabilities. Because its clinical manifestations vary widely, establishing the diagnosis of TSC was particularly challenging prior to the advent of modern neuroimaging and genetic phenotyping.

Terminology

TSC has also been called Bourneville or Bourneville-Pringle disease. The classic clinical triad of TSC consists of facial lesions ("adenomata sebaceum"), seizures, and mental retardation.

Etiology

General Concepts. Approximately 50% of TSC cases are inherited and follow an autosomal-dominant pattern. The other half represents de novo mutations and germline mosaicism.

Genetics. Two separate genes are mutated or deleted in TSC: *TSC1* and *TSC2*. *TSC2* mutations are approximately five times as frequent as those affecting *TSC1*.

The *TSC1* gene is located on chromosome 9q34 and encodes a protein called **hamartin**. The *TSC2* gene is localized to chromosome 16p13.3 and encodes the **tuberin** protein. Mutations in either gene are identified in 75-85% of patients with TSC.

The TSC1/TSC2 protein dimer complex functions as a tumor suppressor. Hamartin/tuberin inhibits the complex signaling pathway called mammalian target of rapamycin (mTOR). The mTOR protein product is a component of two complexes, mTORC1 and mTORC2. Activation of either mTORC regulates protein synthesis and cell growth. Mutations that lead to increased mTOR activation promote cellular disorganization, overgrowth, and abnormal differentiation that may result in tumorigenesis.

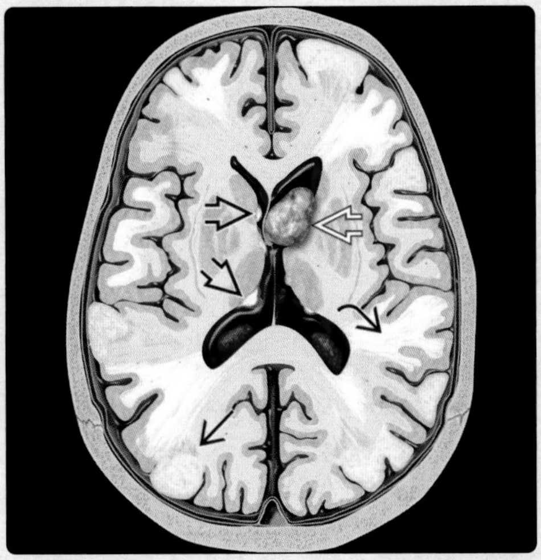

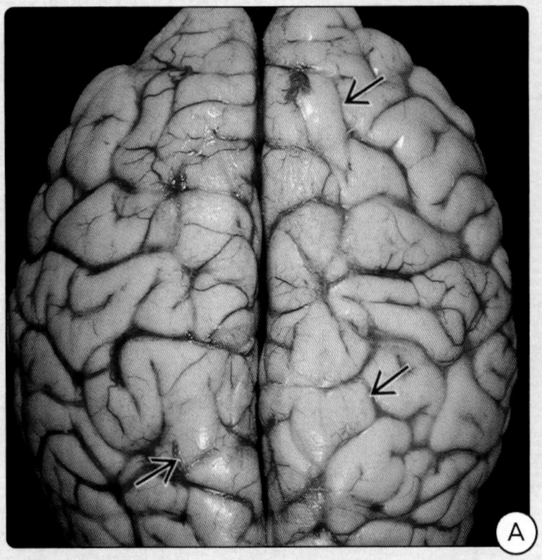

***(39-30)** Axial graphic of typical brain involvement in tuberous sclerosis complex (TSC) shows a giant cell astrocytoma in the left foramen of Monro, subependymal nodules, radial migration lines, and cortical/subcortical tubers. **(39-31A)** Autopsy specimen from a patient with TSC shows multiple expanded gyri with the potato-like appearance characteristic of cortical tubers.*

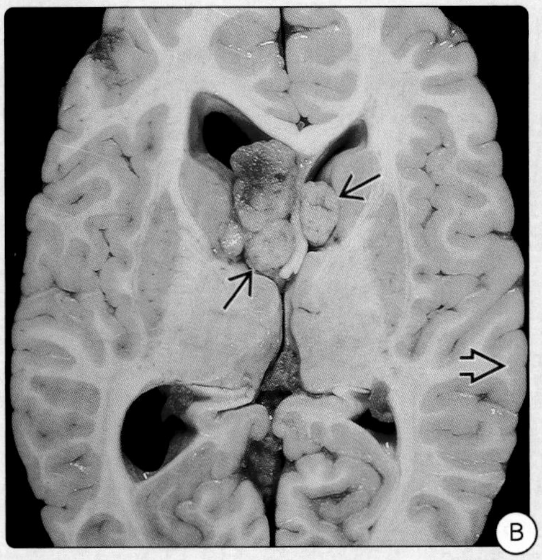

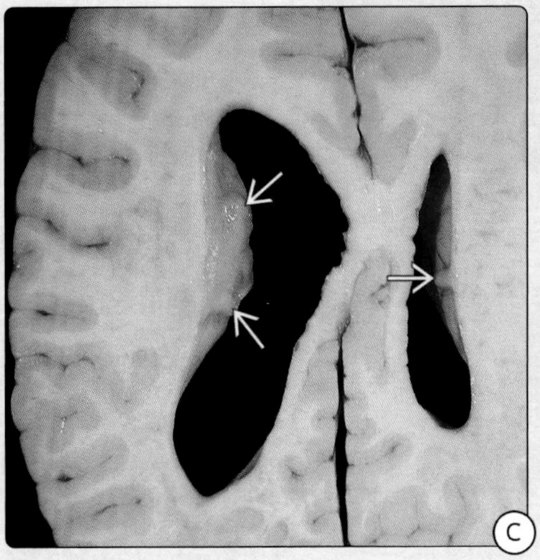

***(39-31B)** Axial cut section from the same case shows bilateral subependymal giant cell astrocytomas and cortical tubers. **(39-31C)** Axial section from the same case through the lateral ventricles shows the "heaped-up" appearance of subependymal nodules along the striothalamic groove. (All three images courtesy R. Hewlett, MD.)*

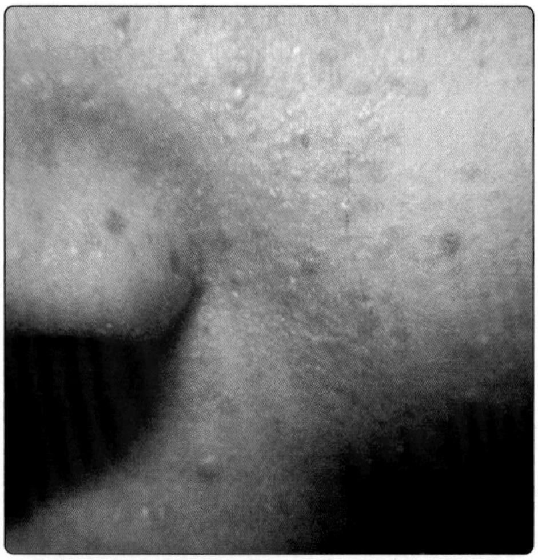

***(39-32)** Clinical photo shows the typical facial "adenomata sebaceum" seen in tuberous sclerosis complex. (Courtesy B. Krafchik, MD.)*

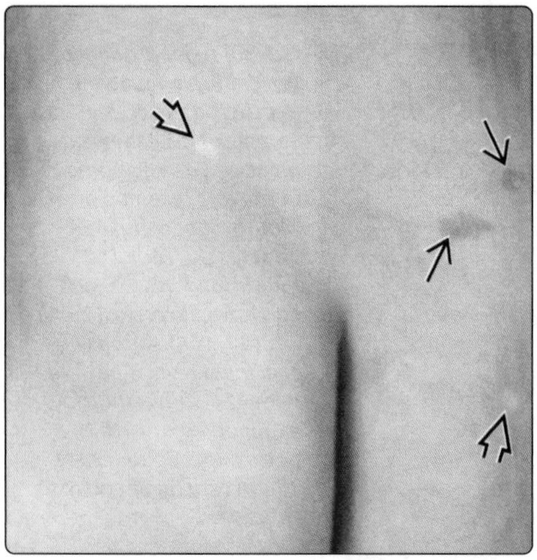

***(39-33)** TSC is shown with "ash leaf" spots ➲. Other macules show areas of hyperpigmentation ➲. (Courtesy B. Krafchik, MD.)*

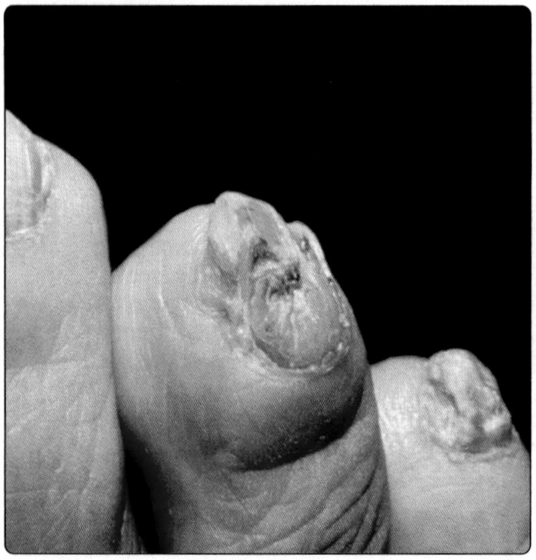

***(39-34)** Periungual fibromas are common in the toes and fingernails in patients with TSC. (Courtesy B. Krafchik, MD.)*

Multiple genotype-phenotype studies have demonstrated that *TSC2* mutations are associated with a more severe disease phenotype with more and larger tubers, more radial migration lines, and more subependymal nodules (SENs) compared with *TSC1*.

Pathology

The four major pathologic features of TSC in the brain are **cortical tubers, SENs, white matter (WM) lesions**, and **subependymal giant cell astrocytoma (39-30) (39-31)**.

Cortical Tubers. Cortical tubers are glioneuronal hamartomas. They are found in over 90% of TS patients and appear as firm, whitish, pyramid-shaped, elevated areas of smooth gyral thickening, with or without central depressions. Cortical tubers grossly resemble potatoes ("tubers").

Microscopically, cortical tubers consist of giant cells and dysmorphic neurons with foci of gliosis, disrupted lamination, and disordered myelin. Balloon cells similar to those seen in Taylor-type focal cortical dysplasia (FCD IIb) are also commonly found in tubers. Tubers do not undergo malignant transformation.

Subependymal Nodules. SENs are located immediately beneath the ependymal lining of the lateral ventricles, along the course of the caudate nucleus.

SENs appear as elevated, rounded, hamartomatous lesions that grossly resemble candle guttering or drippings. They often calcify with increasing age. SENs along the caudothalamic groove adjacent to the foramen of Monro may undergo neoplastic transformation into subependymal giant cell astrocytoma (SEGA).

White Matter Lesions. WM lesions are almost universal in patients with TSC. They appear as foci of bizarre dysmorphic neurons and balloon cells in the subcortical WM and/or fine radial lines extending outward from the ependymal ventricular surface toward the cortex. These radial migration lines often terminate in a tuber.

Subependymal Giant Cell Astrocytoma. SEGA is seen almost exclusively in the setting of TSC, occurring in 6-9% of patients. Grossly, SEGAs appear as well-circumscribed solid intraventricular masses located near the foramen of Monro. SEGAs are WHO grade I tumors that often cause obstructive hydrocephalus but do not invade adjacent brain. Although most SEGAs are unilateral, bilateral tumors occur in 10-15% of cases.

Typical microscopic features are large (not truly giant), plump cells that resemble astrocytes and/or ganglion cells in a fibrillar background. Tumor cell GFAP positivity varies, but most SEGAs are positive for neurofilament protein, neuron-specific enolase, and synaptophysin on immunohistochemistry.

Intratumoral calcifications are relatively common, but necrosis is rare. Mitoses are few, and the MIB-1 index is generally low.

Clinical Issues

Epidemiology and Demographics. TSC is the second most common inherited tumor syndrome (after NF1) with a prevalence of approximately 1:6,000 live births. Almost 80% of cases are diagnosed before the age of 10 years. Between 20 and 30% are diagnosed during the first year of life when infantile spasms are observed in the patients with a positive family history. Patients with *TSC2* mutations are diagnosed an average of 9 years earlier than patients with a *TSC1* mutation.

Presentation. TSC patients generally present within the first two decades of life. The most common skin lesions are hypomelanotic macules, which are ovoid depigmented areas with irregular margins that are best visualized by ultraviolet light (Woods lamp). These "ash leaf" spots are seen in over 90% of cases and may be the first visible manifestation of TSC **(39-33)**. Other common cutaneous findings such as forehead plaques, shagreen patches, facial angiofibromas ("adenoma sebaceum") **(39-32)**, and periungual fibromas **(39-34)** usually do not appear until after puberty.

Clinical Diagnosis. The clinical diagnosis of TSC is problematic because all cutaneous features are age-dependent and may not become apparent until later in childhood. The classic triad of facial "adenomata sebaceum" **(39-32)**, seizures, and mental retardation is seen in only 30% of patients.

The various clinical features of TSC are designated as either major or minor features. Based on these features, the diagnosis is divided into definite, probable, and possible TSC (see box below). Although DNA testing is useful for diagnosis and determining the causative mutation, approximately 30% of patients with definite TSC have negative results for *TSC1* and *TSC2* mutations.

TSC: DIAGNOSTIC CLINICAL FEATURES

Diagnosis
- Definite TSC
  - 2 major features *or* 1 major + 2 minor
- Probable TSC
  - 1 major + 1 minor feature
- Possible TSC
  - 1 major *or* ≥ 2 minor features

Major Features
- Identified clinically
  - ≥ 3 hypomelanotic ("ash leaf") macules (97%)
  - Facial angiofibromas (75%) or forehead plaque (15-20%)
  - Shagreen patch (45-50%)
  - Ungual/periungual fibroma (15%)
  - Multiple retinal hamartomas (15%)
- Identified on imaging
  - Subependymal nodules (98%)
  - Cortical tubers (95%)
  - Cardiac rhabdomyoma (50%)
  - Renal angiomyolipoma (50%)
  - Subependymal giant cell astrocytoma (15%)
  - Lymphangioleiomyomatosis (1-3%)

Minor Features
- Identified clinically
  - Gingival fibromas (70%)
  - Affected first-degree relative (50%)
  - Pitting of dental enamel (30%)
  - Retinal achromic patch (35%)
  - Confetti-like skin macules (2-3%)
- Identified on imaging
  - WM hamartomas, radial migration lines (100%)
  - Hamartomatous rectal polyps (70-80%)
  - Nonrenal hamartomas (40-50%)
  - Bone cysts (40%)
  - Renal cysts (10-20%)

Natural History. TSC is characterized by wide phenotypic variation in disease severity and natural course. Neurologic manifestations—primarily intractable seizures from brain hamartomas and obstructive hydrocephalus

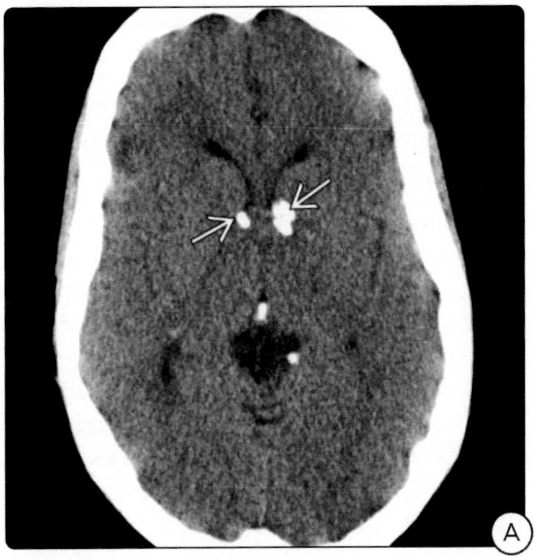

***(39-35A)** NECT in a 22y woman with TSC demonstrates typical calcifications ➡ seen in subependymal nodules.*

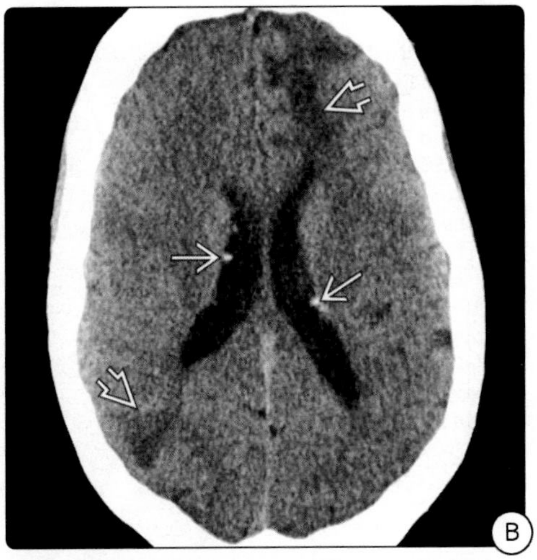

***(39-35B)** NECT scan shows additional calcified SENs ➡, wedge-shaped hypodensities ➡ characteristic of the WM lesions in TSC.*

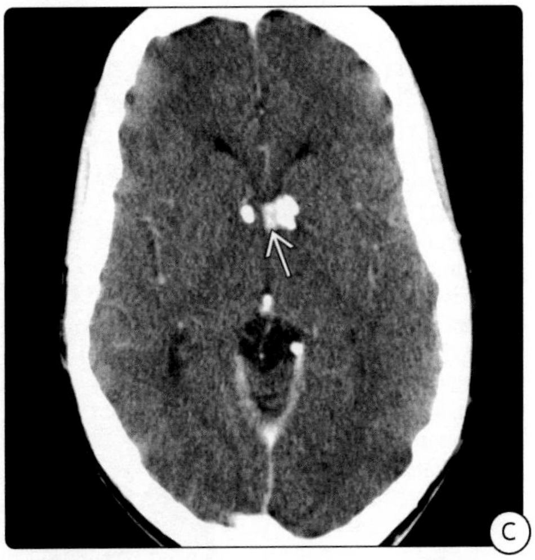

***(39-35C)** CECT scan shows enhancement ➡ adjacent to the foramen of Monro, suspicious for subependymal giant cell astrocytoma (SEGA).*

secondary to SEGA—are the leading cause of morbidity and mortality.

SEGAs are benign and usually slow-growing neoplasms. Although they can develop at any age, they are most frequent in patients between 5-19 years of age.

Treatment Options. Until recently, few treatment options other than surgery for SEGA existed. Rapamycin inhibitors such as everolimus and sirolimus have been approved for the treatment of TSC-associated SEGAs in patients with TSC. When growing cells are treated with rapamycin, both mTORC1 and mTORC2 are depleted. Downregulation of general protein synthesis, upregulation of macroautophagy, and activation of stress-responsive anabolic proteins occur.

Imaging

General Features. Imaging studies in TSC are abnormal in over 98% of all patients.

CT Findings

Cortical Tubers. Neonatal and infantile cortical tubers are initially seen as hypodense cortical/subcortical masses within broadened and expanded gyri **(39-35B)**. The lucency decreases with age; tubers in older children and adults are mostly isodense with cortex.

Calcifications in cortical tubers progressively increase with age. By 10 years, 50% of affected children demonstrate one or more globular or gyriform cortical calcifications. Between 15 and 25% of all TSC patients demonstrate focal cerebellar calcifications.

Subependymal Nodules. SENs are a near-universal finding in TSC. Most are found along the caudothalamic groove. The walls of the atria and temporal horns of the lateral ventricles are less common sites.

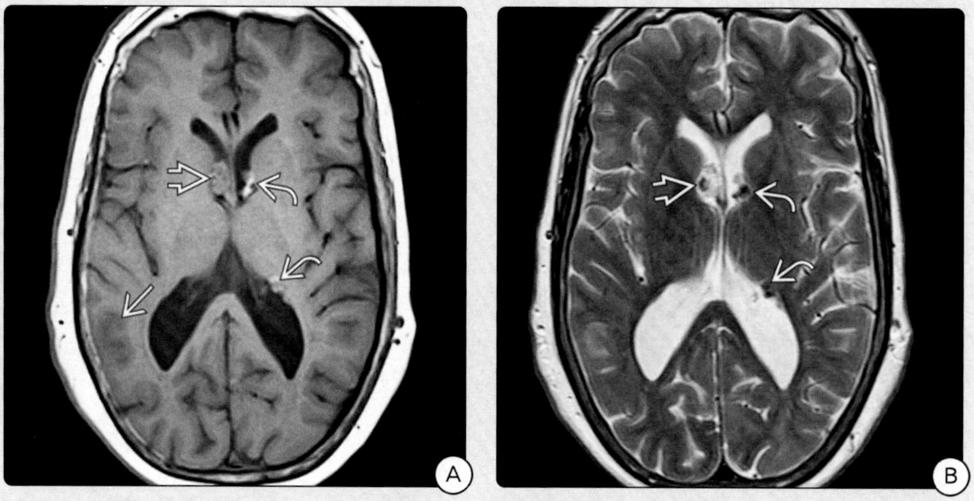

(39-36A) T1WI in a 42y man with TSC shows multiple hyperintense calcified SENs and SEGA in the right frontal horn. Note poorly defined gray-white matter junctions of typical cortical tubers. (39-36B) T2WI in the same case shows the hypointense calcified SENs and mixed signal intensity SEGA .

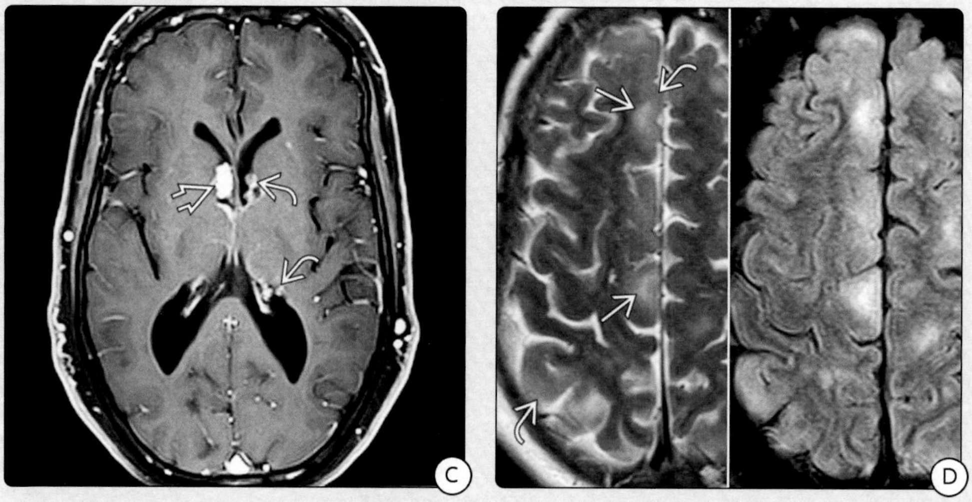

(39-36C) T1 C+ FS shows that the SEGA enhances intensely. The SENs also enhance moderately. (39-36D) T2WI (L), FLAIR (R) show cortical tubers as expanded, hyperintense gyri with poor gray-white matter differentiation , and "flame-shaped" subcortical hyperintensities . The tubers are easier to appreciate on the FLAIR image.

SENs are rarely calcified in the first year of life. Calcification in SENs increases with age. Eventually, 50% demonstrate some degree of globular calcification **(39-35A)**. SENs typically do not enhance on CECT scans. An enhancing or enlarging SEN—especially if located near the foramen of Monro—is suspicious for SEGA **(39-35C)**.

White matter lesions. Most WM lesions are relatively small and difficult to detect on CT scans.

Subependymal giant cell astrocytoma. SEGAs show mixed density on NECT scans and frequently demonstrate focal calcification. Frank hemorrhage is rare. Moderate enhancement on CECT is typical.

MR Findings. In general, MR is much more sensitive than CT in depicting parenchymal abnormalities in TSC. Findings vary with lesion histopathology, patient age, and imaging sequence.

Cortical tubers. In infants, tubers appear as thickened hyperintense cortex compared to the underlying unmyelinated WM on T1WI and become moderately hypointense on T2WI. "Streaky" linear or wedge-shaped T2/FLAIR hyperintense bands may extend from the tuber all the way through the WM to the ventricular ependyma **(39-37)**.

Signal intensity changes after myelin maturation. Tubers gradually become more isointense relative to cortex on T1WI (unless calcification is present and causes T1 shortening). Occasionally the outer margin of a tuber is mildly hyperintense to GM, while the subcortical component appears hypointense relative to WM **(39-39)**.

Tubers in older children and adults demonstrate mixed signal intensity on T2/FLAIR. The periphery of the expanded gyrus is isointense with cortex while the deeper component is strikingly hyperintense. Between 3-5% of cortical tubers show mild enhancement on T1 C+ imaging.

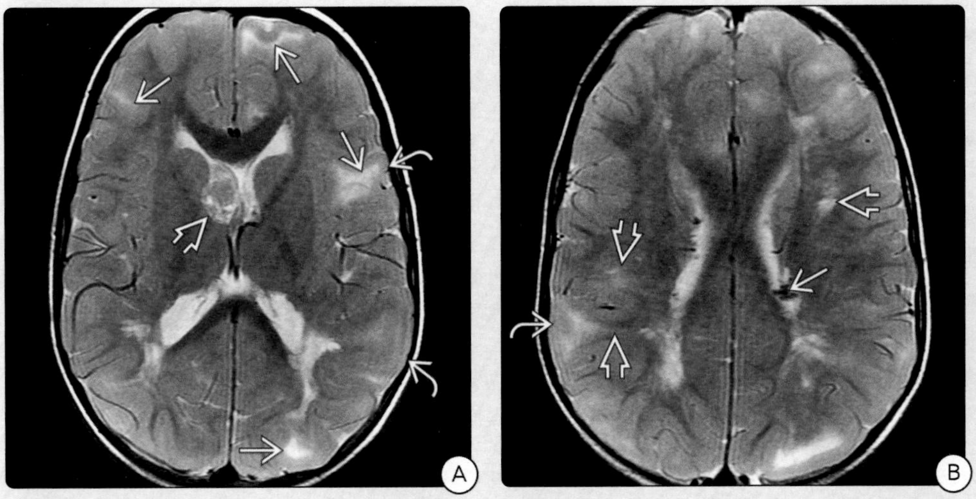

(39-37A) T2WI in a 3y child with TSC shows linear/flame-shaped WM hyperintensities under cortical tubers. A SEGA in right frontal horn does not invade the adjacent parenchyma. (39-37B) More cephalad scan demonstrates cortical tubers and multiple radial hyperintensities extending outward from the ventricles through the corona radiata toward cortical tubers. Calcified SENs appear hypointense relative to brain.

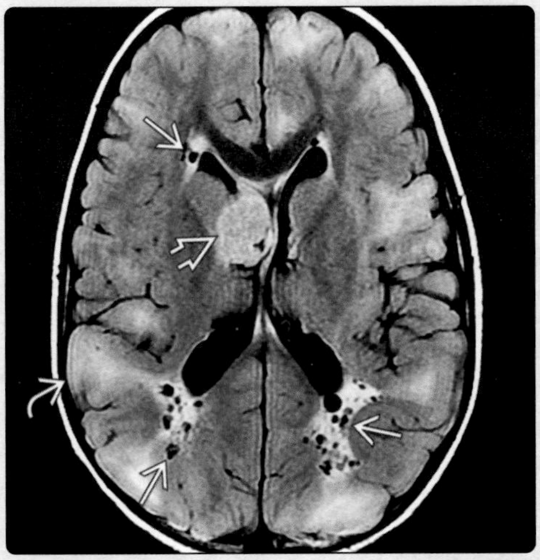

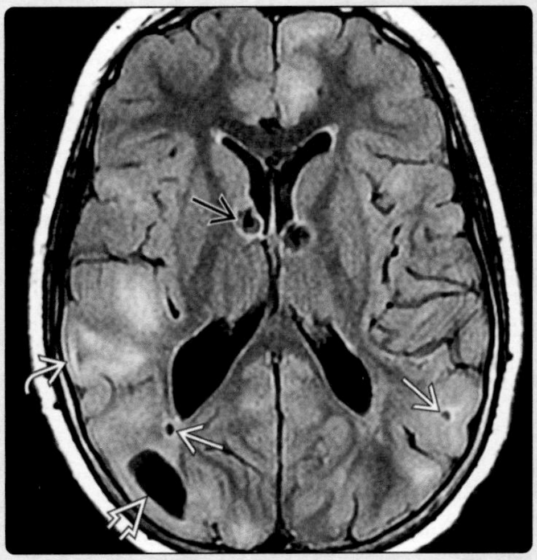

(39-38) Axial FLAIR in a 5y boy with TSC shows a SEGA, multiple cortical tubers, and numerous CSF-like cysts in the deep periventricular white matter. (39-39) Axial FLAIR in an 11y boy with TSC shows SENs, cortical tubers, one large subcortical component, and several small deep WM CSF-like cysts.

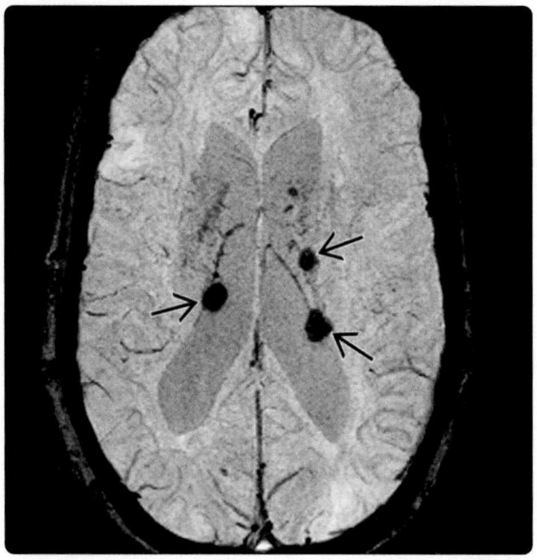

(39-40) Axial MIP of an SWI in a patient with TSC shows that calcified SENs ➡ "bloom" on T2* sequences.

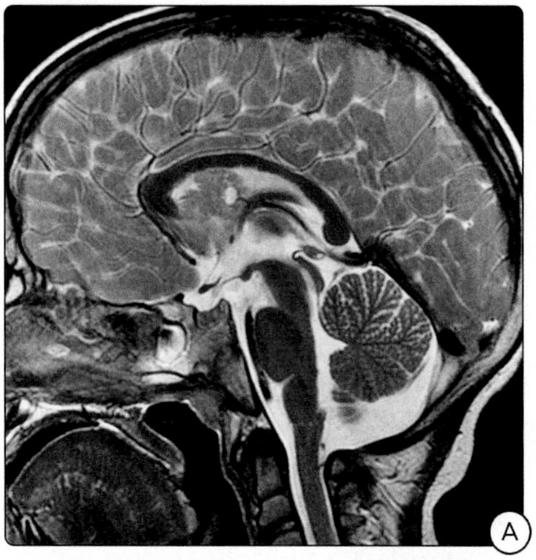

(39-41A) Sagittal T2WI shows that a SEGA in the frontal horn is wedged into the foramen of Monro.

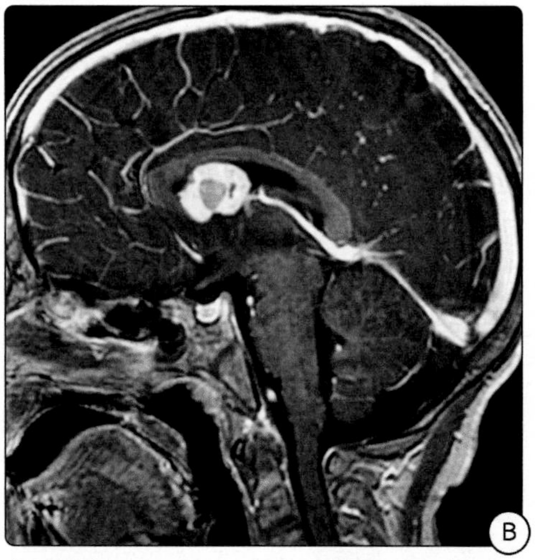

(39-41B) Sagittal postcontrast MP-RAGE shows that the SEGA enhances intensely but heterogeneously.

Subependymal nodules. SENs are seen as small (generally < 1.3 cm) nodular "bumps" or "candle gutterings" that protrude from the walls of the lateral ventricles **(39-36)**. In the unmyelinated brain, SENs appear hyperintense on T1WI and hypointense on T2WI. With progressive myelination, the SENs gradually become isointense with WM.

Calcified SENs appear variably hypointense on T2WI or FLAIR **(39-39)** and are easily identified on T2* sequences (GRE, SWI) **(39-40)**. They can be distinguished from blood products on the SWI phase map, as Ca++ is diamagnetic and appears bright, whereas paramagnetic substances (blood products) are hypointense.

Enhancement of SENs following contrast administration is variable. About half of all SENs show moderate or even striking enhancement, which—in contrast to enhancement on CECT—does not indicate malignancy.

SENs are stable lesions. However, as SENs near the foramen of Monro may become malignant, close interval follow-up is essential. It is the interval change in size seen on serial examinations—not the degree of enhancement—that is significant. Some investigators suggest an increase of greater than 20% demonstrated on two consecutive MR scans as defining a SEGA.

White Matter Lesions. WM lesions are seen in 100% of cases. Even though they are considered a "minor" criterion for TSC, their appearance is highly characteristic of the disease. Streaky linear or wedge-shaped lesions extend along radial bands from the ventricles to the undersurfaces of cortical tubers **(39-37)**. In the unmyelinated brain, these linear foci (radial migration lines) appear mildly hyperintense to WM on T1WI. In older children and adults, they are hyperintense on T2/FLAIR sequences.

Small round cyst-like parenchymal lesions are seen in nearly 50% of TS cases. They are typically located in the deep periventricular white matter **(39-38)**. They are often multiple and resemble CSF, i.e., they suppress on FLAIR and do not enhance.

Subependymal Giant Cell Astrocytoma. Although SEGAs can occur anywhere along the ventricular ependyma, the vast majority are found near the foramen of Monro. SEGAs are mixed signal intensity on both T1- and T2WI **(39-41)**. Virtually all enhance moderately strongly on T1 C+ scans **(39-36C)**.

SEGAs become symptomatic when they obstruct the foramen of Monro and cause hydrocephalus. Even large SEGAs rarely invade brain.

Miscellaneous CNS Lesions. Cerebellar tubers can be identified in 10-40% of cases and are always associated with supratentorial lesions. Other uncommon abnormalities include hemimegalencephaly, cerebellar malformations, and linear, clump-like, or gyriform parenchymal calcifications. Aneurysms (mostly fusiform aortic and intracranial) are seen in 1% of TSC.

Differential Diagnosis

Brain somatic mutations in *TSC1* and *TSC2* can cause **focal cortical dysplasia (FCD)**. Although FCD can appear identical on imaging studies and histopathology, lesions are typically solitary, whereas cortical tubers are almost always multiple. Foci of **subependymal heterotopic gray matter** can resemble SENs, but most SENs calcify and often enhance on T1 C+ sequences.

SEGAs can resemble other frontal horn/septum pellucidum lesions such as **subependymoma**. Subependymomas are tumors of middle-aged and older individuals, and other TSC stigmata such as cortical tubers and SENs are absent.

The WM T2/FLAIR hyperintense streaks of radial glial lines extend from the subventricular zone to cortical tubers. **Medullary veins** follow the same general course but appear hypointense on T2* SWI and enhance following contrast administration. The CSF-like white matter cysts can resemble **enlarged perivascular spaces** but are typically embedded within abnormal-appearing WM.

TSC: IMAGING

Cortical Tubers
- Broad, expanded gyrus
- CT: initially hypodense; Ca++ increases with age
  - 50% of patients eventually develop ≥ 1 calcified tuber(s)
- MR: periphery isointense, subcortical portion T2/FLAIR hyperintense

Subependymal Nodules
- CT: Ca++ rare in first year, increases with age
  - 50% eventually calcify; don't enhance
- MR: T1 hyper-, T2 hypointense; 50% enhance

White Matter Lesions
- T2/FLAIR hyperintense radial lines/wedges
- CSF-like cysts in deep periventricular WM

Subependymal Giant Cell Astrocytoma
- CT: mixed-density mass at foramen of Monro, moderate enhancement
- MR: heterogeneous signal, strong enhancement

Miscellaneous Lesions
- Vascular (usually fusiform aneurysms), seen in 1% of cases
- Parenchymal calcifications

von Hippel-Lindau Disease

Terminology

von Hippel-Lindau disease (VHL) is also known as von Hippel-Lindau syndrome and familial cerebello-retinal angiomatosis. VHL is characterized by retinal and CNS hemangioblastomas (HBs) **(39-42)**, endolymphatic sac tumors (ELSTs) **(39-43)**, abdominal neoplasms (adrenal pheochromocytomas, clear cell renal carcinomas), and pancreatic and renal cysts **(39-44)**.

Etiology

General Concepts. VHL is an autosomal-dominant familial tumor syndrome with marked phenotypic variability and age-dependent penetrance.

Genetics. Mutations in the *VHL* tumor suppressor gene on chromosome 3p25.3 cause inactivation of the VHL protein (pVHL) and increased expression of factors such as PDGF and VEGF, which in turn leads to angiogenesis and tumorigenesis. Approximately 20% of tumors in patients with VHL result from de novo germline mutations.

Two VHL phenotypes are recognized, distinguished by the presence or absence of associated pheochromocytoma. Type 1 has a *low risk* of pheochromocytoma and is caused by truncating mutations of the *VHL* gene. Type 2 is caused by missense mutations and has a *high risk* of developing pheochromocytoma. Type 2 VHL is subdivided into type 2A [low risk of renal cell carcinoma (RCC), 2B (high risk of RCC), and 2C (familial pheochromocytoma without either hemangioblastoma or RCC)].

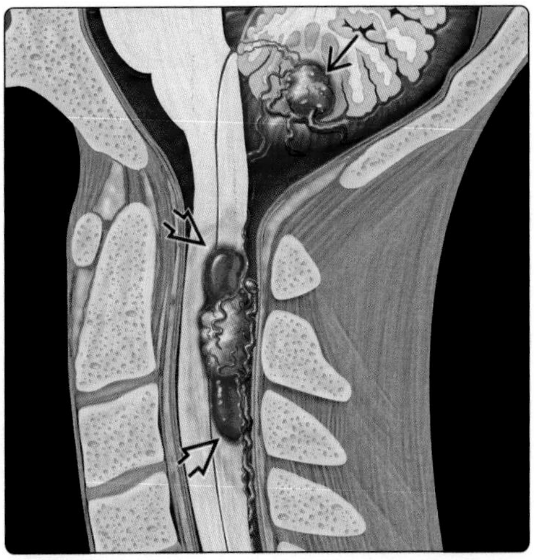

***(39-42)** Two HBs in VHL show spinal cord tumor has associated cyst ➡, causing myelopathy. Small cerebellar HB ➡ would be asymptomatic.*

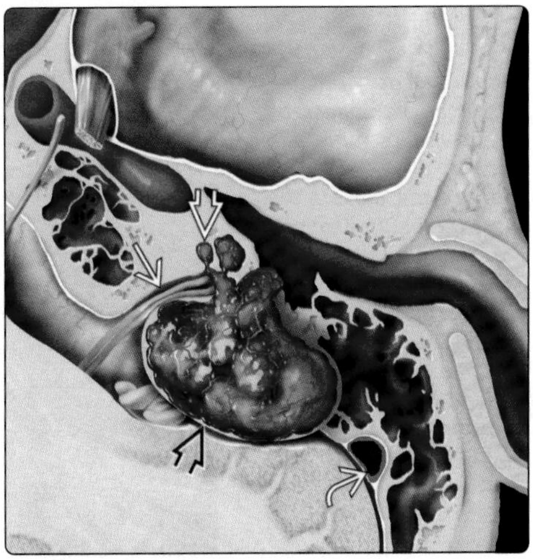

***(39-43)** ELST ➡ is a lytic, vascular, hemorrhagic mass between IAC ➡ and sigmoid sinus ➡. Note tendency to fistulize inner ear ➡.*

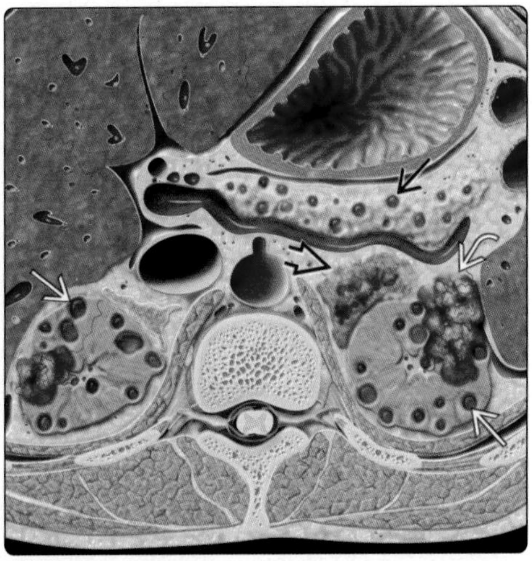

***(39-44)** Abdominal VHL lesions include bilateral renal cysts ➡, carcinomas ➡, pancreatic cysts ➡, and adrenal pheochromocytoma ➡.*

VHL: GENETICS

Type 1 VHL
- Genotype = truncating mutations
- Phenotype
  - *Low* risk for pheochromocytoma (PCC)
  - Retinal angioma, CNS hemangioblastomas (HBs)
  - Renal cell carcinoma (RCC), pancreatic cysts, neuroendocrine tumors

Type 2 VHL
- Genotype = missense mutation
- Phenotypes
  - *All have high risk* of PCC
  - Type 2A (low risk of RCC); retinal angiomas, CNS HBs
  - Type 2B (high risk of RCC); retinal angioma, CNS HBs, pancreatic cysts, neuroendocrine tumor
  - Type 2C (risk for PCC only); no HB or RCC

Pathology

Many of these de novo mutations result in mosaicism. Here patients have clinical signs of the disease, but genetic testing may be negative because not all tissues carry the mutation.

The great majority of VHL patients harbor significant CNS disease. The two most common VHL-related CNS neoplasms are craniospinal **HBs** (found in 60-80% of all VHL cases) and **ELSTs** (seen in 10-15% of patients).

Hemangioblastomas. HBs are well-circumscribed red or yellowish masses that usually abut a pial surface. The vast majority of intracranial HBs are infratentorial; the dorsal half of the cerebellum is the most common site, followed by the medulla.

Approximately 10% are supratentorial; the most common site is the pituitary stalk (30% of all supratentorial HBs and 3% of those in patients with VHL). Most are asymptomatic and do

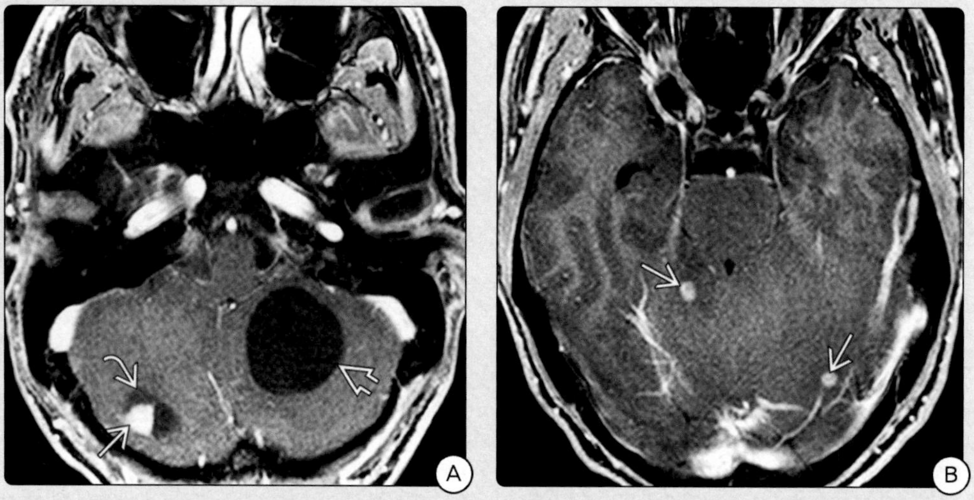

***(39-45A)** Axial T1 C+ FS scan in an asymptomatic 26y man with pancreatic cysts and a strong family history of VHL shows a large cystic mass in the left cerebellar hemisphere → and a smaller cyst → with enhancing nodule → in the right hemisphere. **(39-45B)** More cephalad scan in the same case shows two tiny enhancing nodules →.*

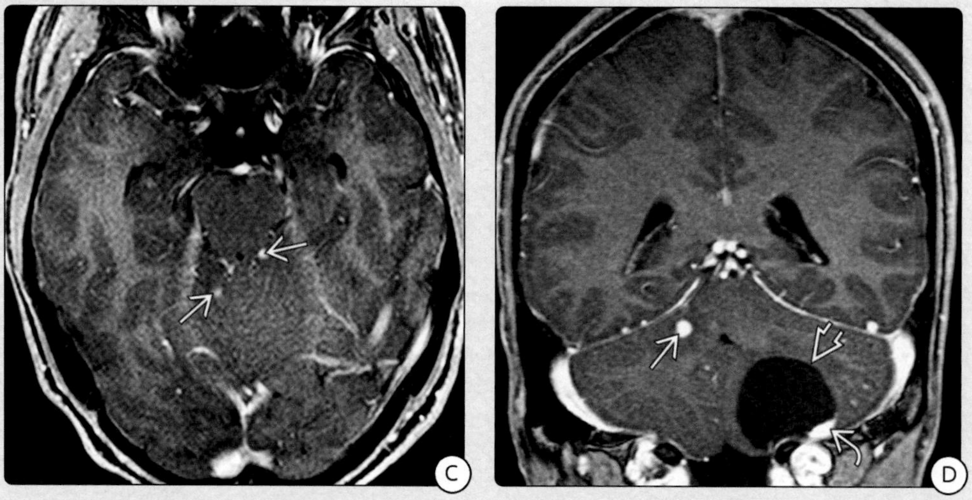

***(39-45C)** Even more cephalad scan in the same patient shows another two tiny enhancing nodules in the upper cerebellum →. **(39-45D)** Coronal T1 C+ shows the enhancing nodule → associated with the large left cerebellar cyst. The nodule abuts a pial surface; the cyst wall → consists of compressed, gliotic brain and does not enhance. Note separate enhancing nodule → in the right hemisphere. This is classic VHL-associated hemangioblastoma.*

not require treatment. Less common locations are along the optic pathways and in the cerebral hemispheres.

Nearly half of all VHL-associated HBs occur in the spinal cord. Intraspinal HBs are often multiple and are frequently associated with a syrinx.

Between one-quarter and one-third of HBs are solid; two-thirds are at least partially cystic and contain amber-colored fluid. One or more cysts together with a variably sized mural tumor nodule is the typical appearance. HBs are highly vascular with large arteries and prominent draining veins.

Two microscopic features dominate HBs and are identical in both sporadic and VHL-associated cases: a rich capillary network and large, vacuolated, variably lipid-laden stromal cells with clear cytoplasm. The cyst wall is nonneoplastic compressed brain with prominent piloid gliosis and Rosenthal fibers.

HBs often demonstrate nuclear pleomorphism and hyperchromasia with scattered large, dark nuclei. Mitoses are absent or few, and MIB-1 is generally low. HBs are designated as WHO grade I neoplasms.

Retinal Hemangioblastomas ("Angiomas"). Retinal capillary angiomas are the typical ocular lesions of VHL and are seen in half of all cases. Retinal angiomas are small but often multifocal, and almost 50% are bilateral. They are identical in histopathology to CNS HBs; the differing terminology reflects ophthalmologic tradition, not histopathologic diagnosis.

Endolymphatic Sac Tumors. ELSTs are slow-growing, benign but locally aggressive papillary cystadenomatous tumors of the endolymphatic sac. Sporadic ELSTs are more common than VHL-associated tumors. Approximately 10-15% of VHL patients develop an ELST; of these, 30% are bilateral.

Grossly, ELSTs appear as vascular "heaped up" tumors along the posterior aspect of the petrous temporal bone.

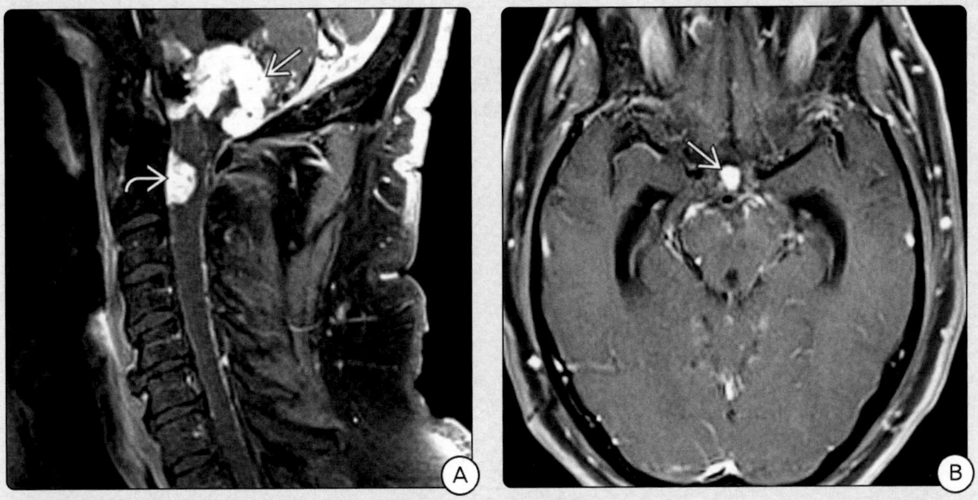

(39-46A) Sagittal T1 C+ scan in a 38y man with VHL shows multiple HBs in the cerebellum ➡ and cervical spinal cord ➡. (39-46B) Axial T1 C+ FS scan in the same patient demonstrates an enlarged enhancing pituitary stalk ➡.

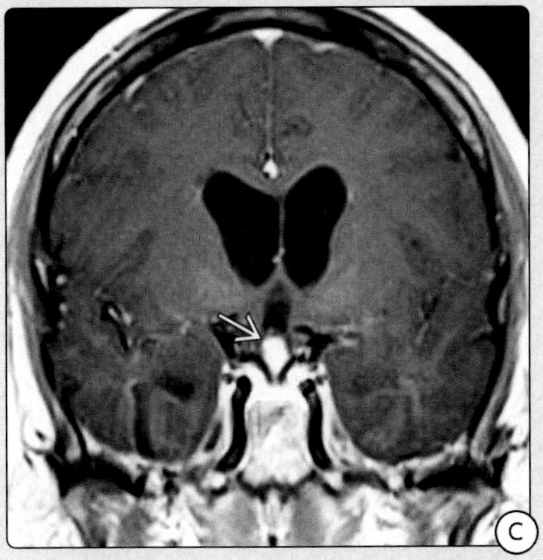

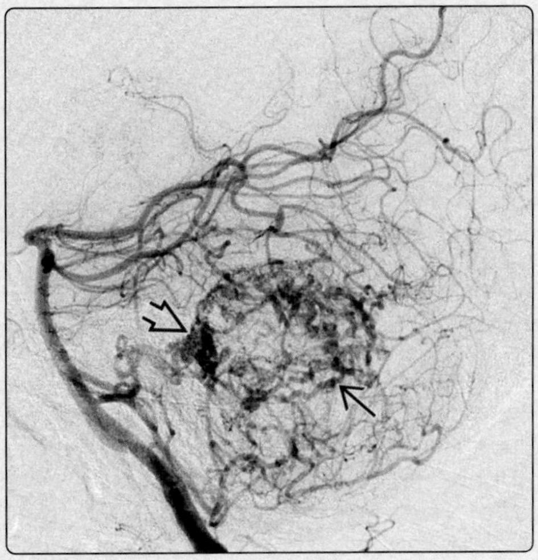

(39-46C) Coronal T1 C+ scan shows that the pituitary stalk is enlarged and enhances intensely ➡. The patient's endocrine status was normal. The pituitary infundibulum is the most common site for supratentorial HBs in VHL. (39-47) Lateral DSA shows typical angiographic findings in HBs. The lesions exhibit mass effect, intense vascular "stain" ➡, and striking neovascularity with tortuous, irregular-appearing vessels ➡.

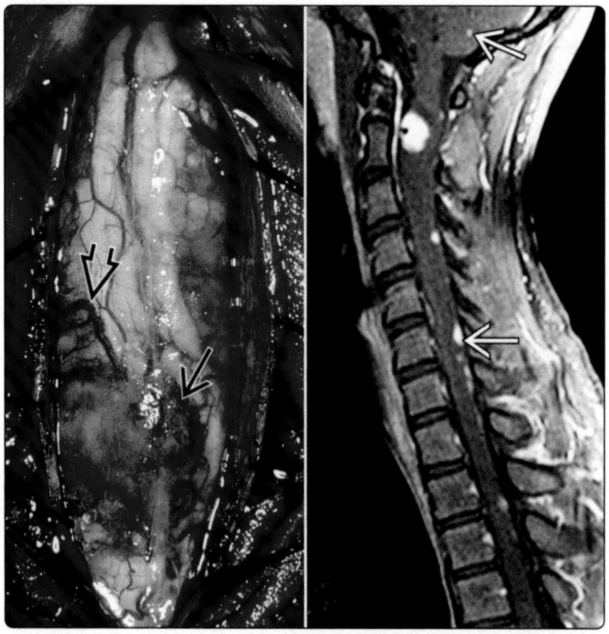

(39-48) (L) Intraoperative photograph shows typical dorsal subpial location of HB nodule and prominent vessels. (R) Sagittal T1 C+ shows multiple HBs.

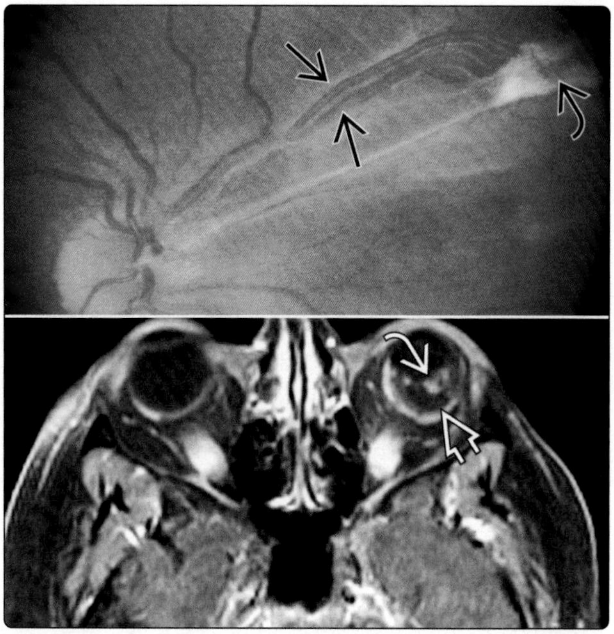

(39-49) (Top) Funduscopic examination in VHL shows peripheral retinal angioma supplied by prominent arteries. (From Imaging in Neurology.) (Bottom) T1 C+ FS shows enhancing angioma with retinal detachment in VHL.

Microscopically, ELSTs demonstrate interdigitating papillary processes embedded in sheets of dense fibrous tissue. Cystic foci and evidence of old and recent hemorrhage are common.

VHL: PATHOLOGY

CNS Neoplasms
- HBs (60-80%)
  - Retinal HBs ("angiomas") (50%)
- Endolymphatic sac tumors (10-15%)

Visceral Lesions
- Renal lesions (2/3 of all VHL patients)
  - Cysts (50-75%)
  - Clear cell renal carcinomas (25-45%)
- Adrenal pheochromocytoma (10-20%)
  - Hallmark of type 2 VHL
- Pancreatic cysts (35-70%), nonsecretory islet cell tumors (5-10%)
- Epididymal cysts, cystadenomas (60% of male patients, often bilateral)
- Broad ligament cystadenomas (female patients, rare)

Clinical Issues

Epidemiology and Demographics. VHL is uncommon; estimated incidence is 1:35,000-50,000 live births.

Presentation and Clinical Diagnosis. Because all VHL-associated lesions can also occur as sporadic (i.e., nonfamilial) events, a clinical diagnosis of VHL disease in a patient without a positive family history requires the presence of at least two tumors (see box below).

Age at diagnosis varies. Although VHL can present in children and even infants, most patients become symptomatic as young adults. Painless visual loss from retinal angioma-induced hemorrhage is often the first symptom (mean: 25 years).

Tumors are the presenting feature in approximately 40% of cases. HBs, pheochromocytomas, and endolymphatic tumors typically become symptomatic in the 30s, whereas RCCs tend to present somewhat later. Mean age at diagnosis of symptomatic RCCs is 40 years, but asymptomatic tumors are frequently detected earlier on screening abdominal CT.

VHL: DIAGNOSTIC CLINICAL FEATURES

No Family History of VHL
- ≥ 2 CNS HBs *or*
- 1 CNS HB + visceral tumor

Positive Family History of VHL
- 1 CNS HB *or*
- Pheochromocytoma *or*
- Clear cell renal carcinoma

Natural History. VHL-associated HBs demonstrate a "saltatory" growth pattern characterized by quiescent periods (averaging slightly over 2 years) interspersed with periods of growth. Nearly half of all patients develop de novo lesions after the initial diagnosis of VHL.

The two major causes of death in VHL patients are RCC (50%) and HBs. Overall median life expectancy is 49 years.

Surveillance Recommendations. Imaging is crucial in the identification and surveillance of extra-CNS lesions.

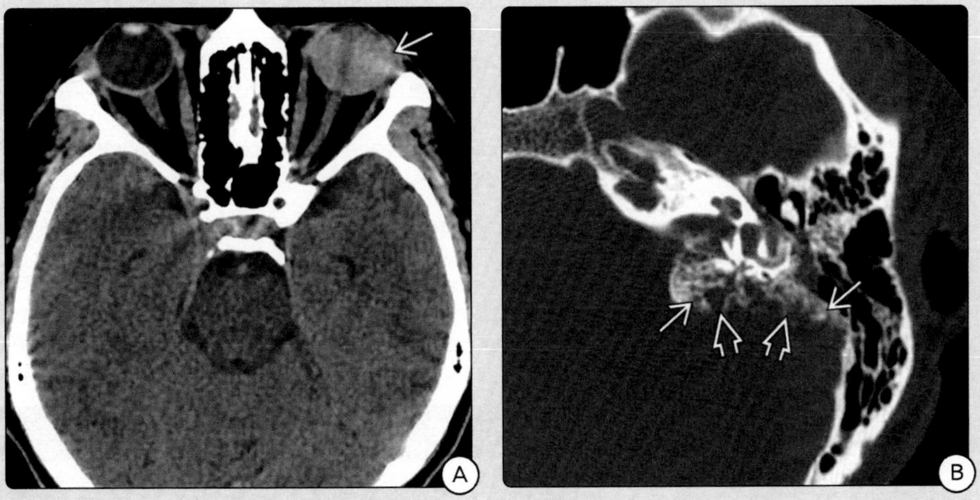

(39-50A) *NECT in a 51y patient with known VHL, sensorineural hearing loss shows classic feature of VHL: hyperdense V-shaped hemorrhagic retinal detachment caused by underlying "angioma" (retinal HB).* ***(39-50B)*** *Temporal bone CT in same patient shows a lytic infiltrative lesion along left posterior petrous temporal bone. Note preserved "spicules" of bone within lesion. Location between the IAC, sigmoid sinus is characteristic for ELST.*

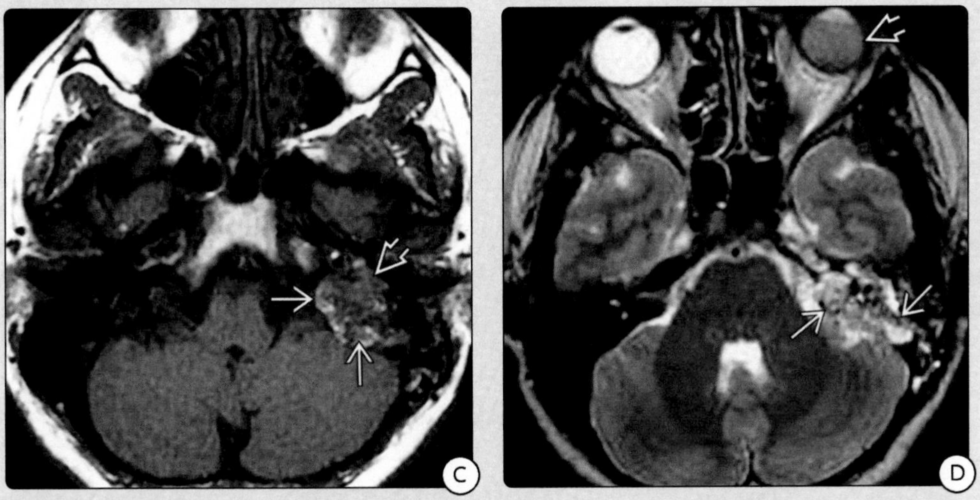

(39-50C) *Axial T1WI in the same patient shows that the lesion is mixed iso- and hyperintense relative to brain.* ***(39-50D)*** *The lesion is heterogeneously hyperintense on T2WI. Note that the left vitreous body is hypointense compared with the normal right side.*

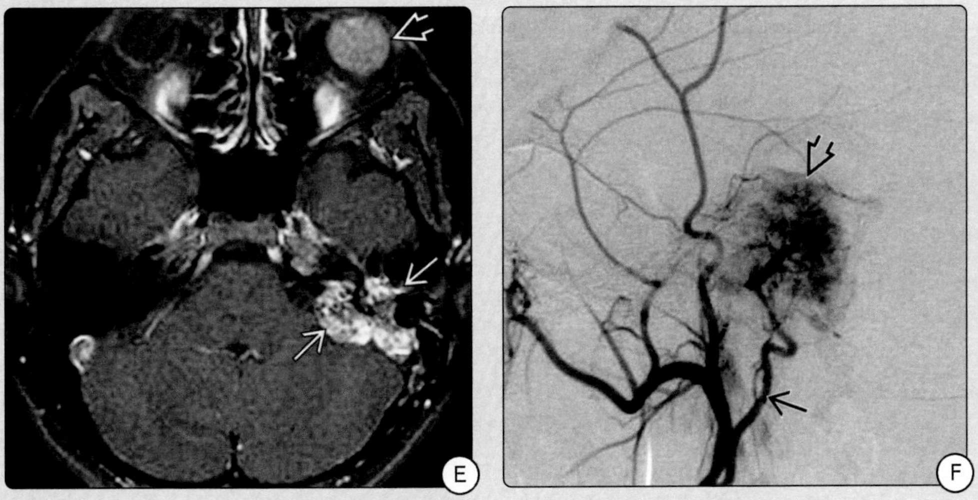

(39-50E) *Axial T1 C+ FS scan in the same patient shows that the lesion enhances intensely but heterogeneously. Note hyperintense retinal hemorrhage.* ***(39-50F)*** *Lateral selective external carotid angiogram shows that the enlarged posterior auricular artery supplies the highly vascular tumor. This is classic endolymphatic sac tumor in VHL. (All six images courtesy D. Shatzkes, MD.)*

Identification of RCC is especially important because it is the major malignant neoplasm of VHL and one of the leading causes of mortality.

Patients with a family history of VHL should undergo annual screening (ophthalmoscopy, physical/neurologic examination) beginning in infancy or early childhood. Brain MRs are recommended every 1-3 years starting in adolescence. Abdominal MR or ultrasound screening for RCC and pancreatic tumors is recommended annually, beginning at age 16.

Methods for pheochromocytoma screening vary. Blood pressure should be monitored and 24-hour urine catecholamines obtained annually. More intense surveillance beginning at age 8 years should be considered in families at high-risk for pheochromocytoma (i.e., type 2 VHL).

Treatment Options. Laser treatment for angioma-induced retinal hemorrhages is common. Surgical resection of HBs is generally based on symptoms, not evidence of radiologic progression.

Imaging

General Features. The best imaging clue for VHL is the presence of two or more CNS HBs **(39-45)** or one HB plus a visceral lesion or concomitant presence of retinal hemorrhage (highly suggestive of intraocular HB).

Hemangioblastomas. HB-associated peritumoral cysts are common and often underlie neurologic morbidity and mortality. Approximately two-thirds of HBs are cystic; one-third are solid or mixed solid/cystic lesions. NECT scans typically demonstrate a hypodense cyst with isodense mural nodule that abuts the pial surface of the cerebellum. The tumor nodule enhances intensely on CECT.

MR shows that the cyst is slightly to moderately hyperintense to CSF on T1WI and iso- to hyperintense on T2/FLAIR. Signal intensity of the nodule is variable; large lesions may show prominent "flow voids." Hemorrhage is common, and peritumoral edema varies.

Tumor nodules enhance strongly on T1 C+ **(39-46)**. Enhanced scans often demonstrate several tiny nodules in the cerebellum and/or spinal cord **(39-48)**. Less commonly, HBs are identified in the pituitary stalk (the most common supratentorial site) **(39-46B)** **(39-46C)**, optic tracts, or cerebral hemispheres. An uncommon manifestation of recurrent VHL-associated HB, disseminated leptomeningeal hemangioblastomatosis, is seen as multiple tumor nodules with diffuse pial enhancement of the spinal cord and/or brain.

DSA demonstrates one or more intensely vascular masses with prolonged tumor "blush" and variable arteriovenous shunting **(39-47)**.

Retinal Hemangioblastomas ("Angiomas"). Retinal angiomas (actually small capillary HBs) are usually visualized as hemorrhagic retinal detachments that are hyperdense compared with normal vitreous on NECT. Tiny enhancing nodules can sometimes be identified on T1 C+ MR **(39-49)**.

Endolymphatic Sac Tumors. ELSTs are located along the posterior petrous temporal bone between the internal auditory canal and the sigmoid sinus. The imaging hallmark of ELST is that of a retrolabyrinthine mass associated with osseous erosion. Bone CT shows an infiltrative, poorly circumscribed, lytic lesion with central intratumoral bone spicules **(39-50)**.

MR demonstrates T1 hyperintense foci in 80% of cases. Signal intensity is mixed hyper- and hypointense on T2WI. Heterogeneous enhancement is seen following contrast administration. ELSTs are vascular lesions that may demonstrate prominent "flow voids" on MR and prolonged tumor "blush" on DSA **(39-50F)**.

VHL: IMAGING

Multiple Hemangioblastomas
- Diagnostic of VHL
- 2/3 cystic, 1/3 solid
- Nodule abuts pia
- 50% in cord (dorsal > ventral surface)
  - Multiple tiny "tumorlets" along cord common
  - Disseminated leptomeningeal hemangioblastomatosis

Retinal "Angiomas"
- Hemorrhagic retinal detachment
  - V-shaped hyperdense posterior globe
  - Plus other HB = highly suggestive of VHL
- With or without enhancing "dots" (tiny HBs)

Uni- or Bilateral Endolymphatic Sac Tumors
- Dorsal T-bone
  - Between IAC, sigmoid sinus
- Infiltrative, lytic, intratumoral bone spicules
- T1 iso-/hyperintense; T2 hyperintense
- Strong enhancement

Differential Diagnosis

The major differential diagnosis of VHL in the brain is **sporadic non-VHL-associated hemangioblastoma**. Between 60-80% of HBs are sporadic tumors *not* associated with VHL. Multiple HBs and/or supratentorial lesions are highly suggestive of VHL.

A **pilocytic astrocytoma** with cyst and mural tumor nodule can resemble a solitary HB. Pilocytic astrocytomas are solitary tumors of children, whereas HBs are rarely seen in patients younger than 15 years. In contrast to HB, the tumor nodule in pilocytic astrocytoma typically does not abut a pial surface.

Vascular metastases can mimic multiple HBs but are rarely isolated to the cerebellum and/or spinal cord.

Rare Familial Cancer Syndromes

A number of other neurocutaneous syndromes have been identified in recent years.

As with the more common inherited cancer syndromes discussed above, the neoplasms associated with these disorders do not differ much—if at all—from their sporadic counterparts. They are histopathologically identical and often feature the same genetic mutations. What sets them apart is the *constellation* of clinical features—often skin lesions—combined with systemic and CNS neoplasms.

We close the chapter with a brief consideration of these interesting syndromes.

Li-Fraumeni Syndrome

Terminology

Li-Fraumeni syndrome (LFS) is also known as the sarcoma family syndrome of Li and Fraumeni. LFS is an autosomal-dominant familial tumor syndrome characterized by a lifelong increased risk of developing multiple malignant tumors in a variety of organ systems, including the brain.

Etiology

Nearly three-quarters of all patients have loss-of-function germline mutations in the tumor suppressor gene *TP53* (sometimes termed the "guardian of the genome"). Two newly discovered exons of the gene, 9β and 9γ, are the targets of inactivating mutation events in breast, liver, and head and neck tumors.

Pathology

CNS Tumors. Nearly half of all CNS neoplasms in LFS are astrocytomas, primarily the diffusely infiltrating fibrillary type (WHO grades II-IV) and gliosarcoma **(39-51)** **(39-52)**.

Choroid plexus tumors (15%) **(39-53)** and medulloblastoma/primitive neuroectodermal tumor (PNET) (10-12%) are the next most common types. Ependymoma, oligodendroglioma, and meningioma together account for less than 5% of LFS-associated neoplasms. Histologically, LFS-

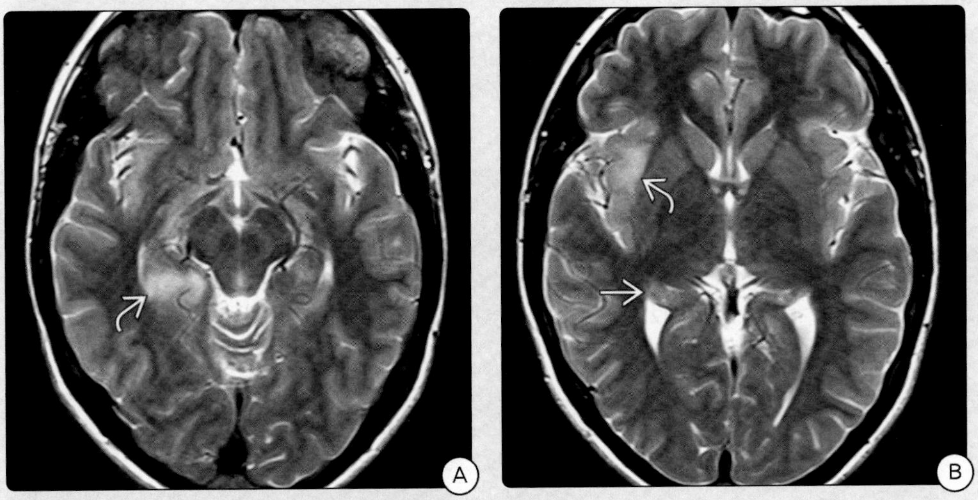

(39-51A) T2WI from a surveillance MR in a 16y girl with Li-Fraumeni and proven TP53 mutation shows an infiltrating hyperintense mass ➡ in the right hippocampus and posteromedial temporal lobe. (39-51B) More cephalad T2WI shows an infiltrating hyperintense mass ➡ in the right insula, hippocampus ➡. The mass did not enhance on T1 C+. Biopsy disclosed diffusely infiltrating astrocytoma, WHO grade II.

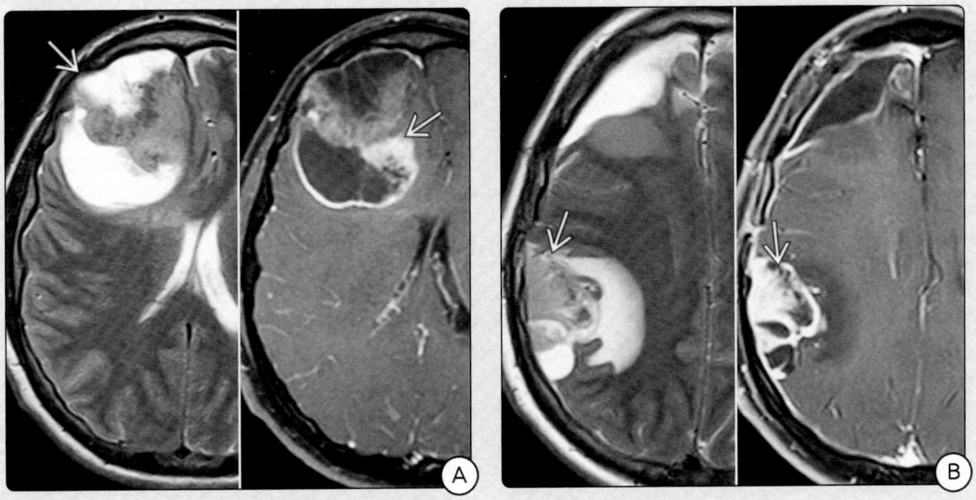

(39-52A) (L) Axial T2WI and (R) T1 C+ scans in a 22y man with Li-Fraumeni show surgically proven glioblastoma ➡. (39-52B) Six months following resection, a new dura-based lesion ➡—a gliosarcoma—has developed.

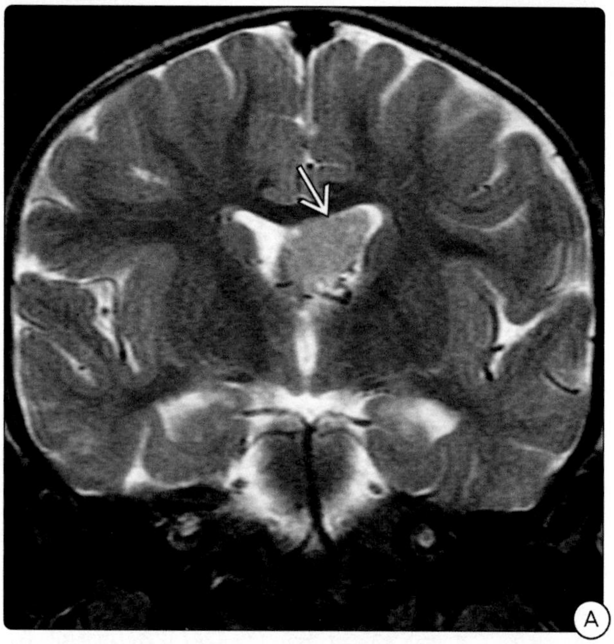

(39-53A) Coronal T2WI in a child with Li-Fraumeni syndrome shows a mass ➡ filling and slightly expanding the body of the left lateral ventricle.

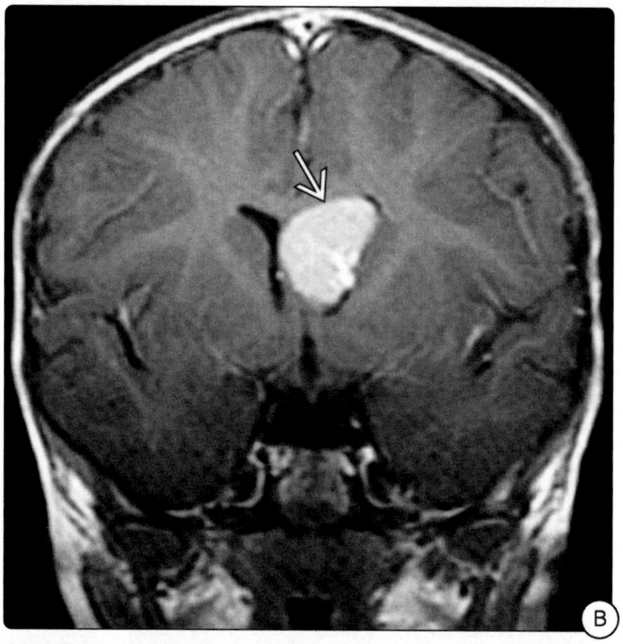

(39-53B) Coronal T1 C+ scan in the same patient shows that the mass ➡ enhances intensely and quite uniformly. Final histopathologic diagnosis was choroid plexus carcinoma.

associated neoplasms are indistinguishable from their sporadic counterparts.

Extraneural Manifestations. Together with brain tumors, breast cancer and sarcomas (osteosarcomas and soft tissue tumors) account for almost 75% of LFS-associated neoplasms. Other reported LFS-associated neoplasms with *TP53* mutations include hematopoietic and lymphoid tumors, lung cancer, skin cancers, stomach cancer, and ovarian cancer.

Clinical Issues

The revised diagnostic clinical criteria for LFS are shown in the accompanying box.

Prognosis is poor; almost half of all patients develop an invasive cancer by age 30 and have a lifelong increased risk of osteosarcoma, soft tissue sarcoma, leukemia, breast cancer, brain tumors, melanoma, and adrenal cortical tumors. Age at tumor onset in LFS patients is significantly younger compared with their sporadic counterparts.

Individuals with LFS have a 50% chance of developing cancer by age 40. Lifetime risk approaches 75% in male patients and almost 100% in female patients, as breast cancer is the most common LFS-associated malignancy. Adrenocortical carcinoma associated with *TP53* germline mutation develops almost exclusively in children.

LI-FRAUMENI SYNDROME: DIAGNOSTIC CLINICAL FEATURES

Patient With
- Sarcoma diagnosed < 45 years of age *and*
- First- or second-degree relative with
  - Any cancer diagnosed < 45 years *or*
  - Any sarcoma at any age

Or With
- Multiple tumors (exception = breast)
  - 2 of which are known LFS-associated neoplasms *and*
  - The first of which occurred < age 45 years *or*
  - Adrenocortical carcinoma or choroid plexus tumor

Imaging

Brain imaging in LFS patients with CNS symptoms varies with tumor type. Imaging findings and differential diagnoses in LFS-associated CNS neoplasms are similar to those of their sporadic counterparts.

Differential Diagnosis

The differential diagnosis of LFS is sporadic neoplasms. Imaging findings are similar, so definitive diagnosis requires clinical correlation and genetic analysis.

Cowden Syndrome

Terminology

Cowden syndrome (CS) is also known as **multiple hamartoma-neoplasia syndrome** and phosphate and tensin homolog **(PTEN) hamartoma tumor syndrome**.

CS involves hamartomatous overgrowth of tissues of all three embryonic origins. The characteristic hamartomas of CS are noncancerous lesions of the skin, mucous membranes, and gastrointestinal tract. The classic brain hamartoma is dysplastic gangliocytoma of the cerebellum, also known as **Lhermitte-Duclos disease** (LDD). If CS and LDD occur together, the disorder is known as **COLD** (**Co**wden-**L**hermitte-**D**uclos syndrome).

CS is a multisystem disease that carries an increased lifetime risk of developing certain cancers as well as benign neoplasms. Breast, thyroid, endometrial, colorectal, and renal cancers are the major systemic carcinomas associated with CS.

Etiology

CS is an autosomal-dominant disorder with variable expression and age-related penetrance. Over 80% of patients have germline mutation of the *PTEN* tumor suppressor gene with downstream abnormalities in the mTOR signaling pathways involved in cell proliferation, cell cycle progression, and apoptosis.

Pathology

The most common brain imaging finding is nonspecific macrocephaly, with or without foci of heterotopic GM **(39-54)** **(39-55)**.

The most characteristic associated lesion is dysplastic cerebellar gangliocytoma **(39-56)** (see Chapter 19). Grossly, marked enlargement of the cerebellar hemisphere/vermis is present. The folia are enlarged and distorted but not obliterated. Macrocephaly with heterotopic GM foci is common. Microscopic features include accumulation of abnormal ganglion cells in the inner granule cell layer, loss of Purkinje cells in the middle layer, and thickening with hypermyelination of the outer (molecular) layer.

CS patients are also at increased risk of meningiomas and glial tumors, including glioblastoma and gliosarcoma.

Clinical Issues

Epidemiology and Demographics. CS is uncommon; its estimated incidence is 1:200,000-250,000. Age at onset is variable. Most cases have been identified in adults, but LDD can occur in infants.

Presentation. In addition to multiple tumors and hamartomas, CS patients may also have megalencephaly, heterotopic GM, hydrocephalus, mental retardation, and seizures. Other features include gastrointestinal polyps as well as various benign breast, thyroid, and uterine lesions.

Characteristic mucocutaneous lesions (trichilemmomas, acral keratoses, papillomatous lesions) are present in 99% of CS patients by the third decade of life.

Clinical Diagnosis. CS is diagnosed clinically by the presence of pathognomonic lesions or a combination of major and minor criteria (see box below). The pathognomonic criteria are those features most likely to be associated with CS, whereas the major and minor criteria are not as specific.

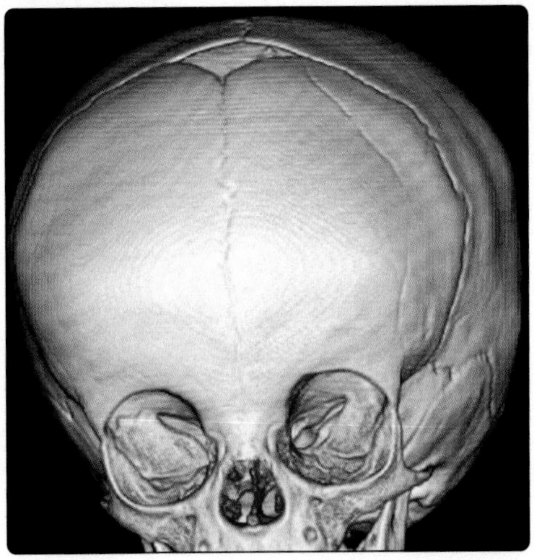

***(39-54)** 3D CT in a 16m boy with skin lesions characteristic of Cowden syndrome (CS) and PTEN mutation shows gross macrocephaly.*

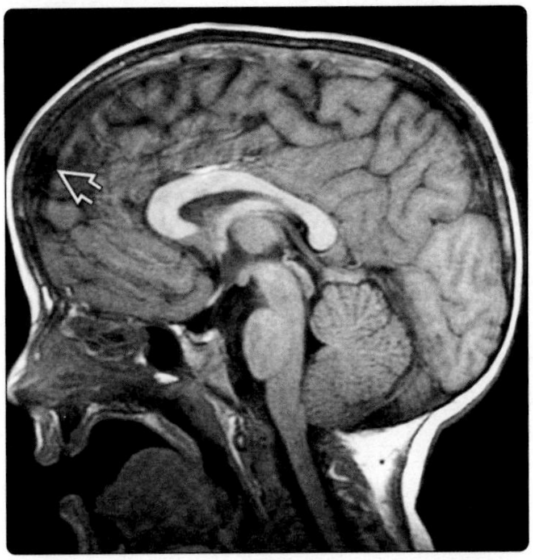

***(39-55)** Sagittal T1WI in a 6y boy with CS and macrocephaly shows increased craniofacial proportion and prominent frontal bossing ➲.*

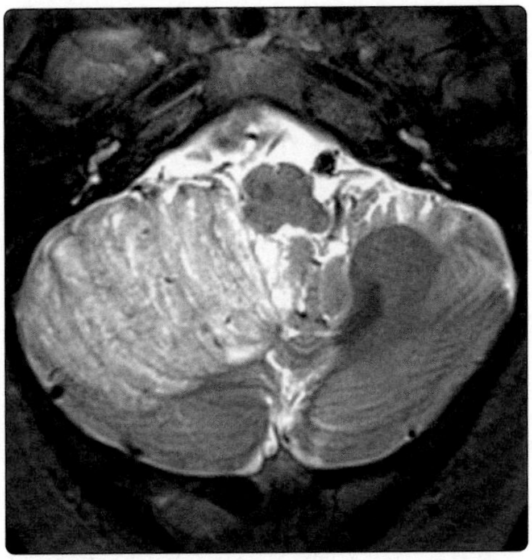

***(39-56)** Axial T2WI shows dysplastic cerebellar gangliocytoma (Lhermitte-Duclos disease) with thickened, striated cerebellar folia.*

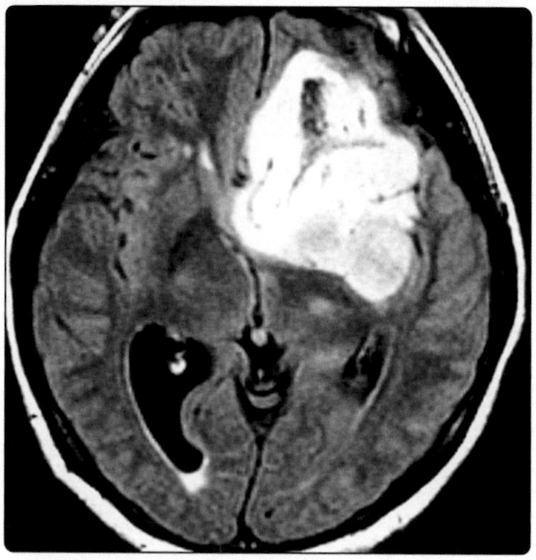

(39-57) FLAIR scan in type 1 Turcot shows heterogeneously hyperintense left frontal mass, anaplastic astrocytoma. (Courtesy T. Tihan, MD.)

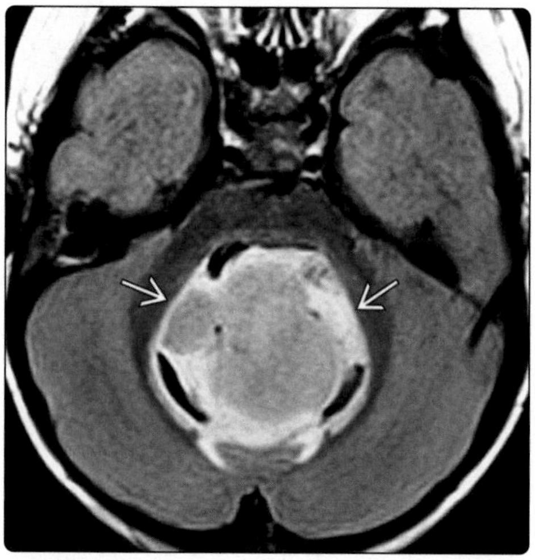

(39-58) FLAIR scan in type 2 Turcot shows typical appearance of medulloblastoma ➡. (Courtesy T. Tihan, MD.)

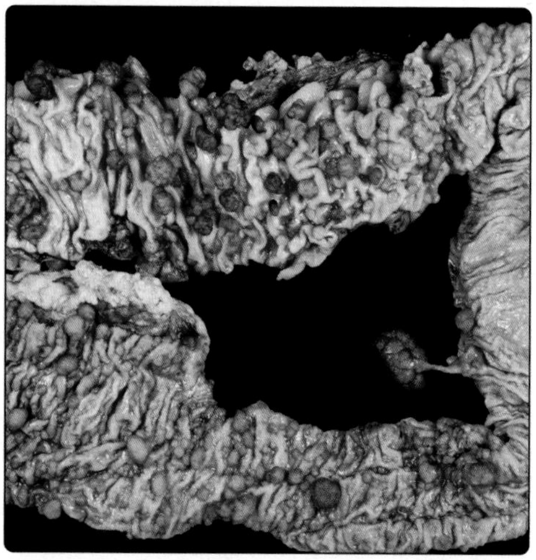

(39-59) Surgical colon specimen from a patient with type 2 Turcot shows innumerable small polyps. (Courtesy T. Tihan, MD.)

COWDEN SYNDROME: DIAGNOSTIC CLINICAL FEATURES

Pathognomonic Criteria
- Dysplastic cerebellar gangliocytoma (Lhermitte-Duclos disease) *and*
- Characteristic mucocutaneous lesions
  - Papillomatous lesions
  - Facial trichilemmomas
  - Acral keratoses

Major Criteria
- Breast cancer
- Thyroid cancer (especially follicular)
- Endometrial cancer
- Macrocephaly
  - Occipitofrontal circumference > 97th percentile

Minor Criteria
- Other thyroid lesions
- Mental retardation
- GI polyps
- Fibrocystic breast disease
- Lipomas
- Fibromas
- Genitourinary tumors (especially renal cell carcinoma)
- Genitourinary structural malformations
- Uterine fibroids

Natural History. CS carries a significantly increased lifetime risk of developing malignancies. Women with CS have a 50% lifetime risk of developing breast cancer, 10% risk for follicular thyroid cancer, and 5-10% risk of developing endometrial cancer. The risk is even higher for patients with germline *PTEN* mutations and includes renal and colorectal cancers as well as melanoma.

Imaging

Imaging findings of dysplastic cerebellar gangliocytoma in the setting of CS/PTEN hamartoma tumor syndrome are identical to those of LDD. An enlarged cerebellar hemisphere with thickened folia in a "corduroy" or "tiger-striped" appearance is typical.

Differential Diagnosis

LDD plus CS is diagnostic of COLD. Patients with LDD should be screened for CS and vice versa. A dysplastic cerebellar gangliocytoma without a characteristic mucocutaneous lesion or other criteria (e.g., breast cancer, thyroid lesions) is simply **Lhermitte-Duclos disease**.

Turcot Syndrome

Terminology

Turcot syndrome (TS) is a rare autosomal-dominant disorder characterized by primary CNS neoplasms and two different forms of colorectal polyps.

In type 1 Turcot (TS1) (**hereditary nonpolyposis colorectal cancer, HNPCC**, also known as Lynch syndrome), colorectal, endometrial, gastric, pancreaticobiliary, and genitourinary tumors occur together with malignant astrocytomas.

In type 2 Turcot, colorectal tumors (**familial adenomatous polyposis, FAP**) and skin lesions (such as epidermoid cysts) occur together with medulloblastoma and craniofacial exostosis **(39-57)** **(39-58)** **(39-59)**.

Etiology

TS1 (HNPCC) is associated with biallelic DNA mismatch repair mutations. In type 2 Turcot, mutations in the *APC* gene are present. APC is a large protein complex in the WNT signaling pathway controlling cell proliferation and differentiation. CNS tumors in FAP patients are typically the WNT-subtype medulloblastoma.

Pathology

Three CNS neoplasms—medulloblastoma, anaplastic astrocytoma, and glioblastoma—account for 95% of all Turcot-associated brain tumors. The histologic features of these tumors are indistinguishable from those of their sporadic counterparts.

Clinical Issues

Patients with type 1 Turcot-associated anaplastic astrocytoma or glioblastoma present *earlier* than those with nonsyndromic tumors. Median age at onset is 18 years. Family history of polyposis is absent.

Patients with type 2 Turcot-associated medulloblastoma present *later* than patients in the general embryonal tumor population. Median age is 15 years. Patients with type 2 Turcot frequently have a family history of polyposis.

Imaging

Imaging findings in Turcot-related CNS neoplasms are identical to those of their nonsyndromic counterparts.

Nevoid Basal Cell Carcinoma Syndrome

Terminology

Nevoid basal cell carcinoma syndrome (NBCCS) is also known as Gorlin or Gorlin-Goltz syndrome. Patients with NBCCS exhibit a broad spectrum of neurodevelopmental disorders and are predisposed to develop multiorgan benign and malignant neoplasms.

Etiology

NBCCS is an autosomal-dominant disease with full penetrance but variable clinical phenotypes. NBCCS is caused by germline mutations of the *PTCH1* gene on chromosome 9q22. This gene encodes a glycoprotein that is a binding site for the *SHH* gene.

Pathology

The CNS neoplasm most commonly associated with NBCCS is **medulloblastoma.** Most are desmoplastic medulloblastomas, SHH subtype.

Systemic NBCCS-associated lesions include **basal cell carcinomas** and **epidermal cysts, multiple keratocystic odontogenic tumors** (KOTs) **(39-60)**, and **skeletal anomalies** (e.g., bifid ribs).

Clinical Issues

Epidemiology and Demographics. NBCCS has a prevalence of 1:57,000 in population-based studies.

Presentation. Patients are usually diagnosed by age 5-10 years. Basal cell carcinomas are the most common initial presentation and may appear as early as 2 years of age. Multiple enlarging jaw masses are frequent and can be asymptomatic or painful.

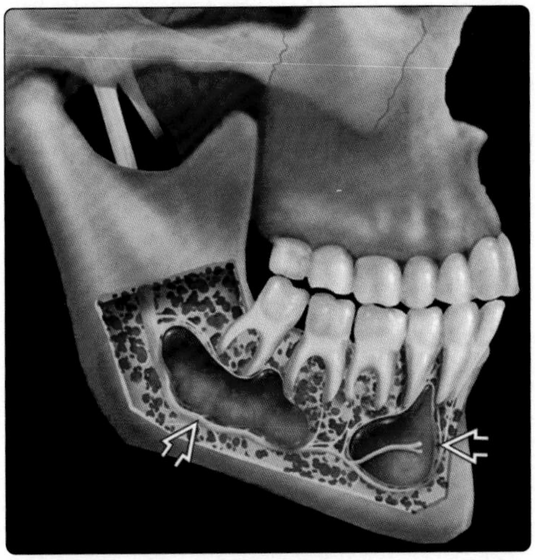

(39-60) NBCCS graphic shows classic appearance of multiple odontogenic keratocysts. Lesions splay teeth roots and displace nerves.

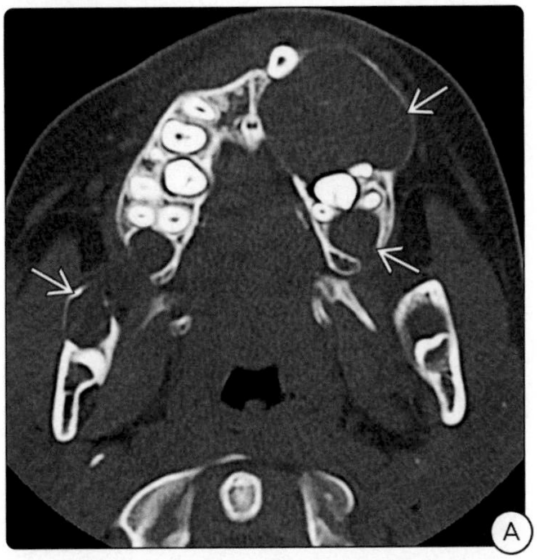

(39-61A) Bone CT in a 9y boy with NBCCS shows multiple lytic lesions in the maxilla and mandible. These are typical odontogenic keratocysts.

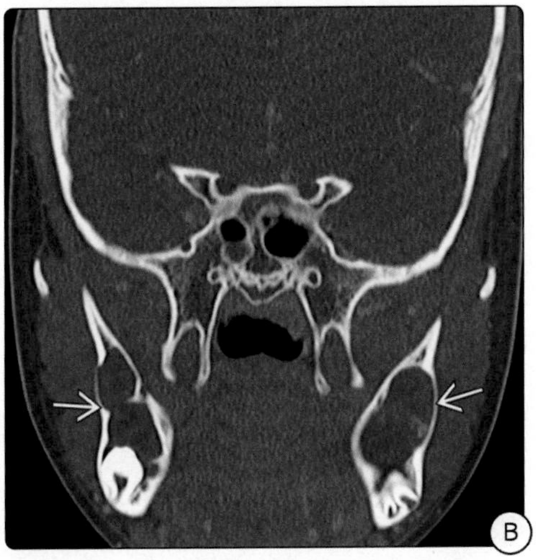

(39-61B) Coronal bone CT in the same patient nicely demonstrates the expansile, lobulated nature of the cysts.

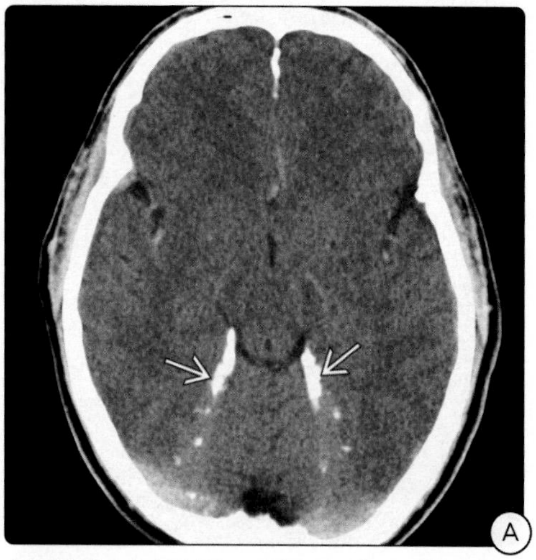

(39-62A) Axial NECT scan in a patient with NBCCS demonstrates dense lamellar calcifications ➡ along the tentorium cerebelli.

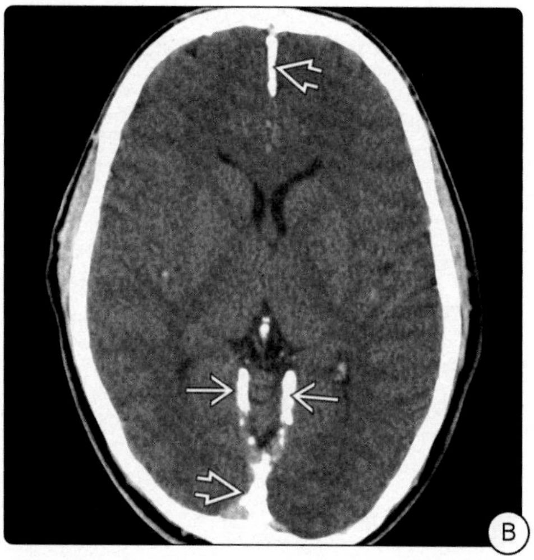

(39-62B) More cephalad NECT in the same patient shows dense calcification at the tentorial apex ➡ and along the falx cerebri ➡.

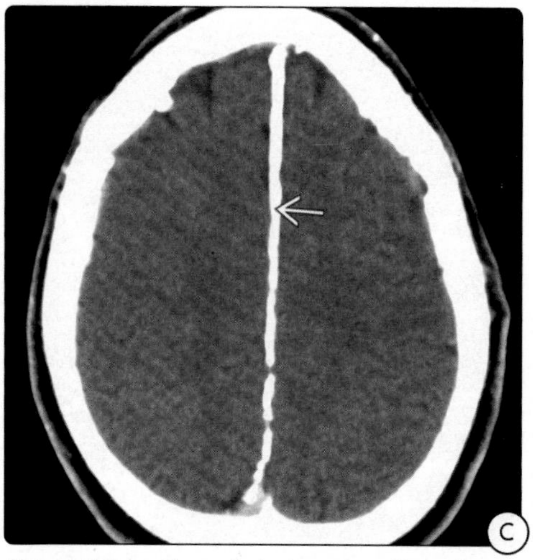

(39-62C) Scan through the corona radiata shows that the falx is thickly and densely calcified ➡.

Medulloblastomas develop in 4-20% of patients and present within the first 2 years of life, typically with symptoms of obstructive hydrocephalus.

Natural History. The major morbidity and mortality in NBCCS is caused by its associated neoplasms. Basal carcinomas often become more aggressive after puberty and may exhibit distant metastases. KOTs eventually develop in 80% of patients and have a high recurrence rate.

Imaging

Typical brain/head and neck abnormalities seen in NBCCS are multiple jaw cysts, macrocephaly, dense lamellar dural calcifications, and medulloblastoma.

Keratocystic Odontogenic Tumors. KOTs are seen as multiple expansile, well-corticated cysts in the mandible and maxilla on bone CT. They can be uni- or multilocular and often exhibit scalloped borders **(39-61)**. They typically do not enhance on CECT scans.

KOTs exhibit low to intermediate signal intensity on T1WI and appear heterogeneously hyperintense on T2WI.

Dural Calcifications. Abnormal dural calcification eventually develops in 80% of patients older than 20 years **(39-62)**. Subtle flecks of calcium deposition along the falx can occur in very young children and—together with the unusually early appearance of medulloblastoma—should suggest the diagnosis of NBCCS.

Thick, slightly irregular lamellar calcifications along the falx, tentorium, petroclinoid ligaments, and diaphragma sellae are typical findings in teenagers and adults with NBCCS.

Medulloblastoma. The imaging appearance of NBCCS-associated medulloblastoma is identical to that of nonsyndromic tumors. Although SHH-subtype desmoplastic MBs can occur anywhere in the posterior fossa, the lateral cerebellum is the most characteristic location.

Differential Diagnosis

The major differential diagnosis of the abnormal calcifications in NBCCS is **physiologic** or **metabolic-related dural calcifications** (e.g., as occurs with secondary hyperparathyroidism). Physiologic calcification is much less striking and is rarely seen in young children. Thick dural calcifications can be seen in patients with chronic renal failure and long-term hemodialysis.

The differential diagnosis of KOTs includes **periapical (radicular) cysts**—usually unilocular and associated with dental caries—and **dentigerous (follicular) cysts**. Dentigerous cysts are seen as a single unilocular cyst surrounding the crown of an unerupted tooth.

The differential diagnoses of NBCCS-related medulloblastoma are **sporadic (nonsyndromic) medulloblastoma** and **atypical teratoid/rhabdoid tumor**. As imaging findings of the tumors are identical, look for other differentiating features, such as atypical dural calcifications and jaw cysts.

Rhabdoid Tumor Predisposition Syndrome

Rhabdoid tumor predisposition syndrome (RTPS) is characterized by markedly increased risk of developing malignant rhabdoid tumors. Most cases are caused by biallelic germline mutations with inactivation of the *SMARCB1* (INI1/SNF5) tumor suppressor gene on chromosome 22q11.

The most common CNS tumor in RTPS is **atypical teratoid/rhabdoid tumor** (AT/RT). AT/RT is composed of poorly differentiated neuroectodermal and mesenchymal elements. The rhabdoid component can be subtle, making the diagnosis difficult.

Approximately 60% of AT/RTs are found in the posterior fossa. Tumors tend to be large bulky masses with mixed cystic and solid components that demonstrate variable enhancement following contrast administration **(39-63)**. Dissemination at the time of initial diagnosis is common.

Other familial CNS tumors associated with RTPS include **choroid plexus carcinoma**, which has the same *SMARCB1* inactivating mutation.

The most common non-CNS neoplasm in RTPS is malignant rhabdoid tumor (MRT) of the kidney. Prognosis is poor; MRTs are highly aggressive cancers that occur in young children and are generally lethal within months or a few years.

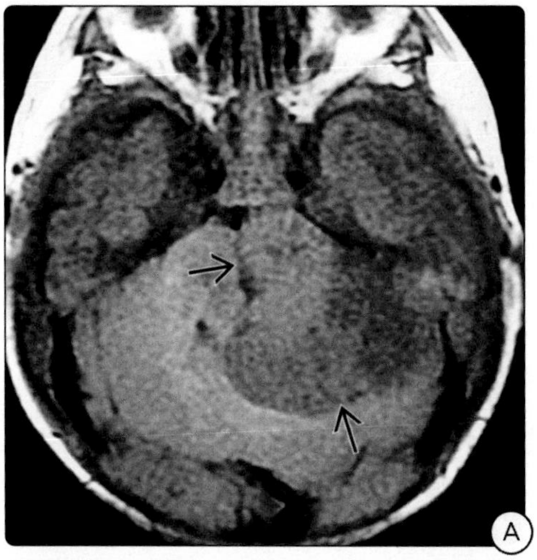

(39-63A) T1WI in a 4m infant with vomiting and bulging fontanelle shows a large, heterogeneous posterior fossa mass ⇨.

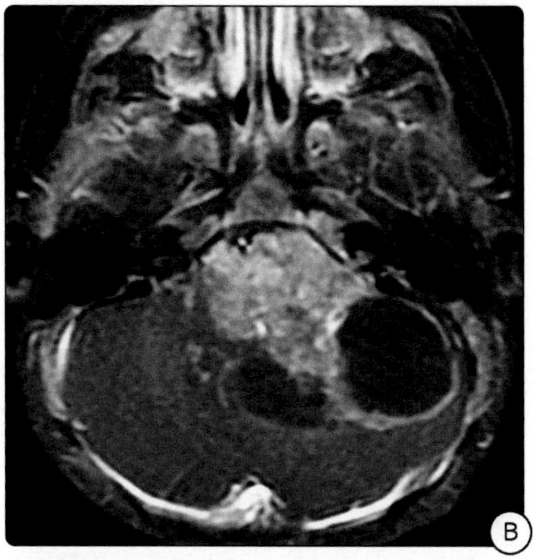

(39-63B) The mass enhances strongly but heterogeneously and has large necrotic-appearing nonenhancing components.

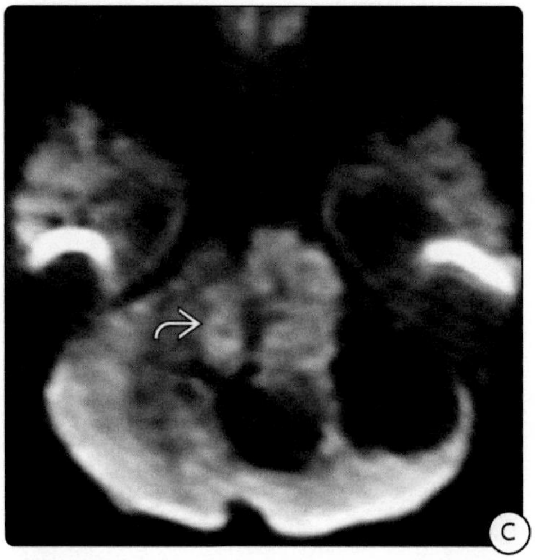

(39-63C) The solid, enhancing portion of the mass shows moderate diffusion restriction ⇨. This is AT/RT.

Meningioangiomatosis

Terminology

Meningioangiomatosis (MA) is a rare neurocutaneous syndrome characterized by a focal hamartomatous lesion that involves the pia and underlying cerebral cortex.

Etiology and Pathology

Although its precise etiology is unknown, MA is a benign, slow-growing lesion of presumed hamartomatous or developmental origin. MA can occur as a solitary or multifocal lesion.

Grossly, MA appears as a reddish gyriform mass that infiltrates the pia and underlying brain. MA can occur without or with an accompanying neoplasm (most commonly meningioma).

Microscopic features are those of a plaque-like intracortical and leptomeningeal proliferation consisting of small blood vessels, meningothelial cells, and fibroblasts. The adjacent cortex may show dense gliosis and neurofibrillary tangles. MIB-1 index is low.

Clinical Issues

MA can occur sporadically or as a *forme fruste* of neurofibromatosis type 2 (NF2). Sporadic MA usually occurs as a single lesion in a child or young adult who presents with seizures or persistent headaches.

Imaging

NECT scans typically demonstrate an iso- to slightly hyperdense cortically based lesion with nodular, linear, or gyriform calcification. The frontal or temporal lobes are the most common sites. Mass effect is minimal or absent. Little or no enhancement is seen on CECT.

MA is iso- to hypointense on T1WI. Although signal intensity on T2WI varies, most MAs are moderately hypointense to adjacent brain with variable amounts of associated edema or gliosis.

T1 C+ shows mild to moderate serpentine enhancement extending over the surface of adjacent gyri and into adjacent sulci. In some cases, cortical infiltration along the penetrating perivascular spaces thickens the cortex and obliterates the normal gray-white matter interface.

A few cases of MA with associated focal cortical dysplasia have been reported.

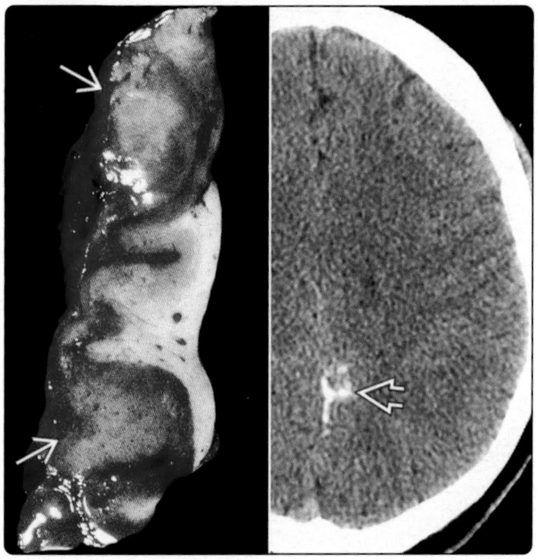

(39-64) *(L) MA shows thickened cortex invaded by vascular-appearing tissue ➡. (AFIP Archives.) (R) NECT shows Ca++ ➡ in MA (different case).*

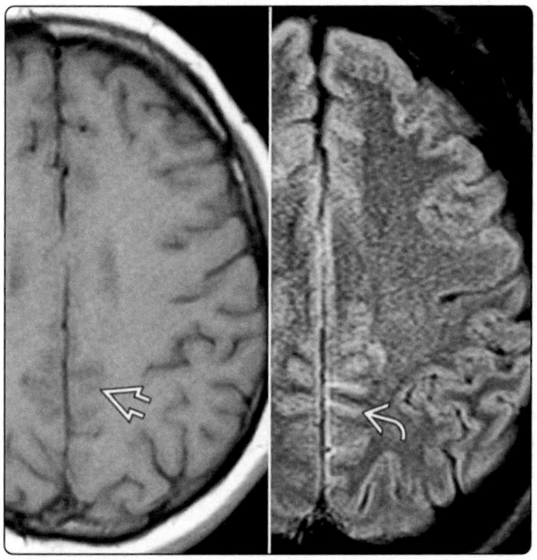

(39-65) *(L) T1WI (same case as above CT) shows subtle effacement of posterior medial sulci ➡ with hyperintensity on FLAIR ➡ (R).*

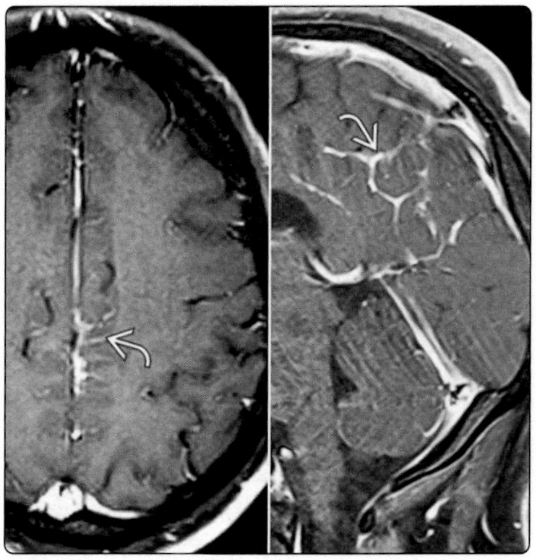

(39-66) *Axial (L), sagittal (R) T1 C+ FS scans in the same case show sulcal enhancement ➡. This is presumed meningioangiomatosis.*

Differential Diagnosis

The most important differential diagnosis of MA is **neoplasm**. Imaging findings are not pathognomonic, so the definitive diagnosis is generally a pathologic one. *It is extremely important that the neuropathologist does not mistake MA for an invasive atypical or malignant meningioma!* MA does not recur after complete resection and does not require radiation or adjuvant chemotherapy.

MENINGIOANGIOMATOSIS

Pathology
- Benign mass of proliferating meningothelial cells, small vessels
- Curvilinear plaque-like lesion
- May show focal brain invasion

Clinical Issues
- *Forme fruste* of NF2

Imaging
- Iso-/hypointense on T1WI; usually hypointense on T2WI
- Serpentine enhancement ± perivascular space invasion

Differential Diagnosis
- Invasive neoplasm

Neurocutaneous Melanosis

Terminology

Neurocutaneous melanosis (NCM) is a rare nonfamilial syndrome characterized by a single giant and/or multiple congenital melanocytic nevi, excessive proliferation of melanin-containing cells in the leptomeninges, and benign and malignant tumors of the CNS **(39-67)**.

Etiology

Scattered melanocytes are normally present in the pia over the convexities and around the base of the brain, ventral brainstem, and parts of the spinal cord. Focal or diffuse proliferation of these melanin-producing cells in the skin and meninges results in NCM.

Melanocytes are derived from neural crest cells (NCCs). Around 8-10 weeks of gestation, NCC-derived pluripotent precursors migrate to the fetal epidermis via the paraspinal ganglia and peripheral nerve sheath, ultimately generating differentiated melanocytes.

NCM is thought to be a neurocristopathy caused by neural crest aberration during early embryonic development. Some abnormalities in neural tube-derived cells also occur, possibly resulting in NCM-associated brain malformation (e.g., Dandy-Walker malformation) **(39-69)**.

Pathology

CNS disease can be parenchymal or leptomeningeal, benign or malignant. **Melanosis** consists of focal collections of histologically benign melanotic cells. A malignant **melanoma** consists of proliferating anaplastic melanotic cells. The estimated prevalence of malignant melanoma in the setting of NCM is 40-60%.

Grossly, leptomeningeal melanosis appears as superficial dark gray or black pigmentation in the pia **(39-69)**. The most common locations for parenchymal melanotic deposits are the amygdala and cerebellum, followed by the pons, thalami, and inferior frontal lobes.

Clinical Issues

Between 60-70% of patients with NCM develop symptoms, usually before 5 years of age. Seizures and signs of elevated intracranial pressure can occur both with leptomeningeal melanosis and malignant melanoma. The prognosis in symptomatic NCM is extremely poor.

Imaging

Uni- or bilateral round or ovoid T1 hyperintensities in the anterior temporal lobes are the most characteristic findings. Focal or diffuse T1 shortening in the leptomeninges with serpentine enhancement on T1 C+ scans is much less common and is generally seen only in cases in which melanotic deposits have undergone malignant transformation **(39-68)**.

Hydrocephalus is common. Cortical invasion along the penetrating perivascular spaces may cause significant mass effect and edema.

Between 8 and 10% of patients with NCM harbor an associated Dandy-Walker malformation.

NEUROCUTANEOUS MELANOSIS

Pathology
- Black or grayish deposits
- Leptomeninges, amygdala, cerebellum
- Benign or malignant melanotic cells

Imaging
- T1 hyperintensities
  - Round/ovoid deposits in amygdala
  - Uni- or bilateral
- Serpentine pial lesions, perivascular space invasion in malignant
- Variable enhancement
- 8-10% Dandy-Walker malformation

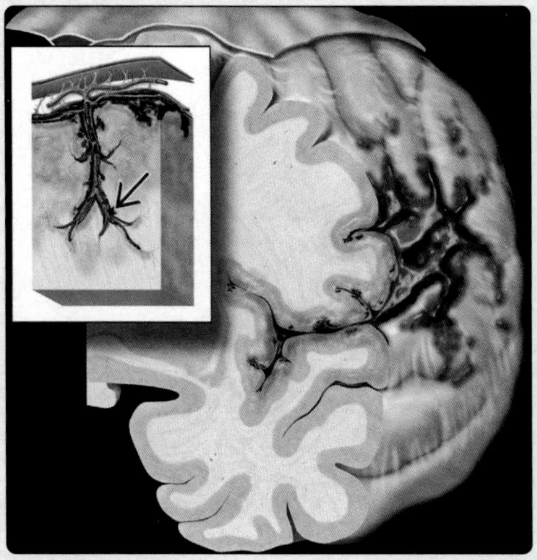
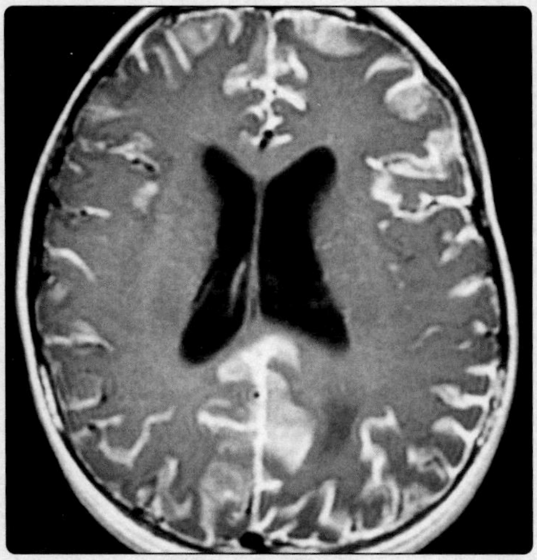

***(39-67)** Graphic shows localized dark (melanotic) pigmentation of the leptomeninges. Inset demonstrates extension of melanosis into the brain substance along the Virchow-Robin spaces. **(39-68)** Axial T1 C+ MR in a patient with extensive neurocutaneous melanosis shows diffuse pia-subarachnoid space enhancement. (Courtesy M. Martin, MD.)*

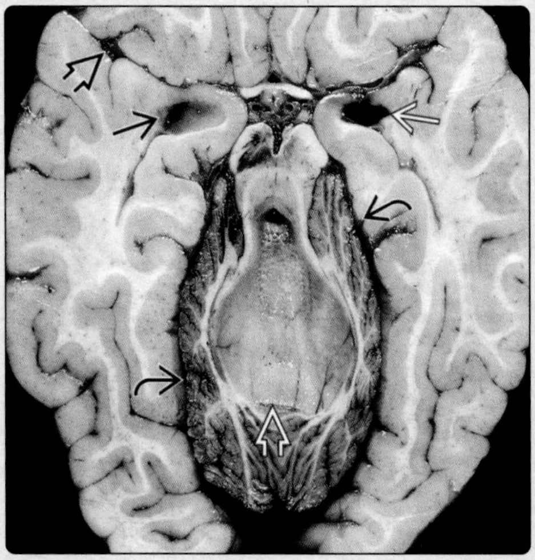
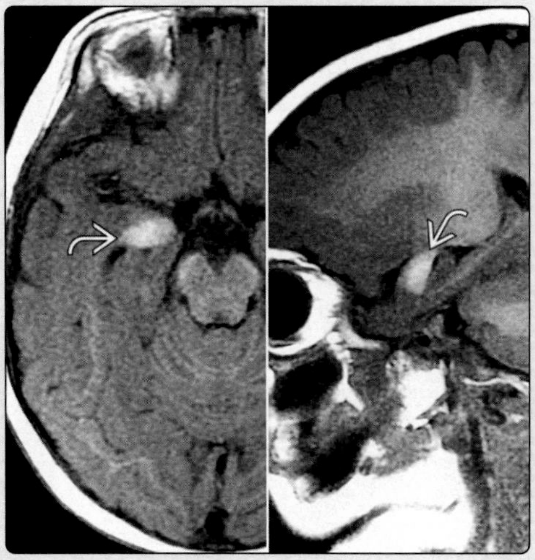

***(39-69)** Autopsy of NCM shows ovoid melanotic deposits in right, left amygdalae. Black discoloration in sylvian fissures and over the cerebellum represents diffuse leptomeningeal melanin deposits. Note Dandy-Walker malformation seen in 8-10% of NCM. (Courtesy R. Hewlett, MD.) **(39-70)** Axial (L), sagittal (R) T1WIs in a child with NCM show the characteristic ovoid T1 hyperintense melanotic deposit in the amygdala.*

Encephalocraniocutaneous Lipomatosis

Encephalocraniocutaneous lipomatosis (ECCL), also known as Haberland or Fishman syndrome, is a rare congenital neurocutaneous disorder whose hallmark CNS lesions are benign lipomas of the brain and spinal cord. All reported cases of ECCL are sporadic. A nonhereditary, autosomal mutation that may survive only in a mosaic state may be the cause of the clinical manifestations of ECCL.

ECCL is characterized clinically by ocular choristomas (typically lipodermoids), a smooth hairless scalp lipoma called a nevus psiloliparus **(39-71)**, and subcutaneous cervicofacial fatty soft tissue masses. Approximately one-half of all patients have seizures, and one-third demonstrate mild or moderate mental retardation.

Most patients with ECCL have one or more CNS lipomas. ECCL-associated lipomas have a predilection for the posterior fossa and spine. They are generally stable but may increase with age **(39-72)**, becoming moderately large and extending over multiple spinal segments. Other congenital anomalies of the meninges such as arachnoid cysts and meningioangiomatosis are common.

Epidermal Nevus Syndrome

Epidermal nevus syndrome consists of an epidermal nevus (EN)—a benign congenital skin hamartoma—with developmental abnormalities of the skin, eyes, and CNS with variable involvement of the musculoskeletal, cardiovascular, and urogenital systems **(39-73)**.

Several different types of nevi are included as part of epidermal nevus syndrome. The main component can be keratinocytic, sebaceous, follicular, apocrine, or eccrine. Pigmented hairy nevi, nevus comedonicus, inflammatory

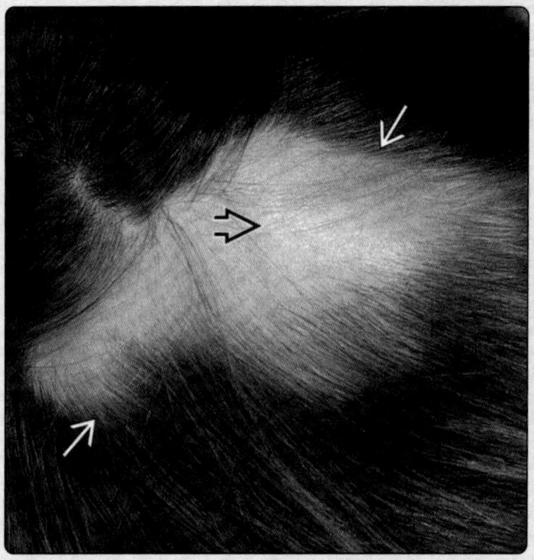

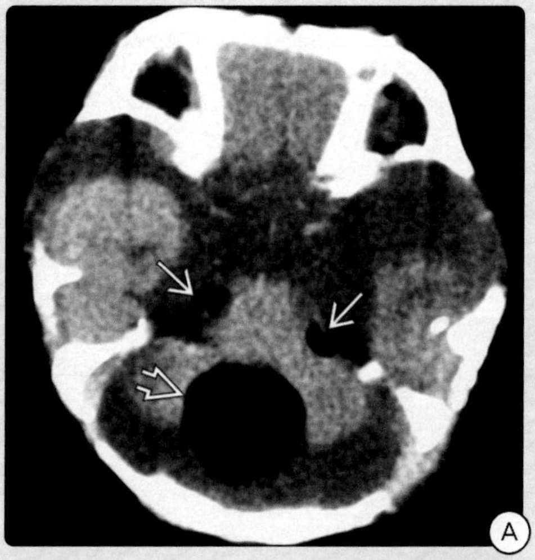

***(39-71)** Clinical photograph demonstrates a nevus psiloliparus, the dermatologic token of ECCL. A focal area of alopecia ➡ (hair loss) covers an underlying scalp lipoma ⇨, seen here as a rubbery, slightly elevated mass. (Courtesy A. Illner, MD.) **(39-72A)** NECT scan in a 2y child with ECCL shows focal lipomas in both cerebellopontine angle (CPA) cisterns ➡ and the cisterna magna ⇨.*

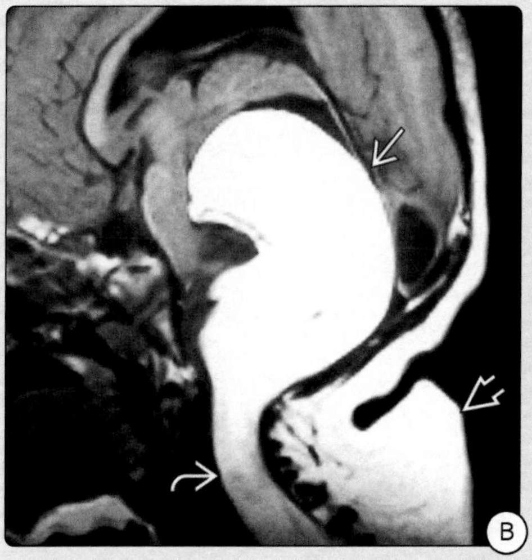

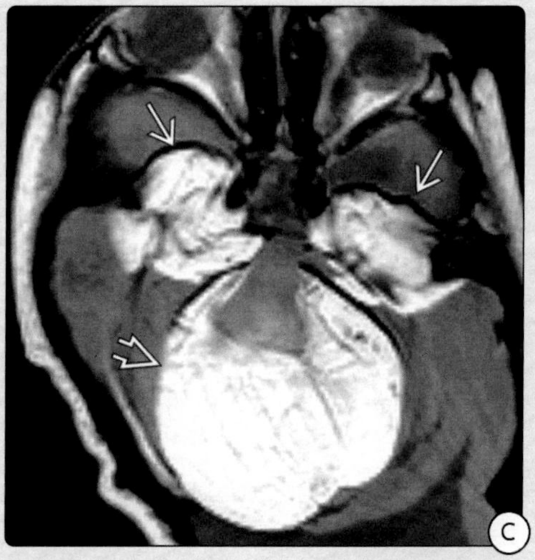

***(39-72B)** Three years later, sagittal T1WI shows a very large suboccipital lipoma ➡. The cisterna magna lipoma has massively increased in size. It now occupies almost the entire posterior fossa ⇨ and extends inferiorly into the upper cervical spinal canal ↪. **(39-72C)** Axial PD shows the large posterior fossa lipoma ⇨. The CPA lipomas have also increased in size, now extending into both Meckel caves ➡.*

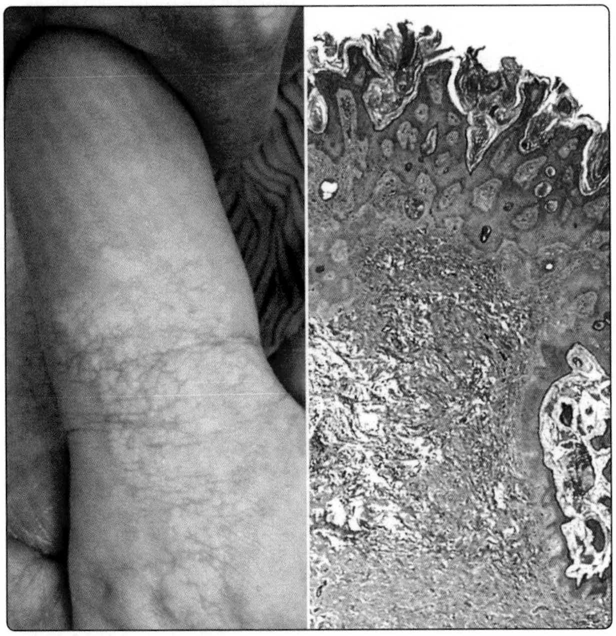

(39-73) (L) Epidermal nevus (EN) is a warty band of hypopigmented growth. (Courtesy University of Utah Department of Dermatology.) (R) EN shows hyperkeratosis, papillomatosis, and acanthosis. (Courtesy J. Comstock, MD.)

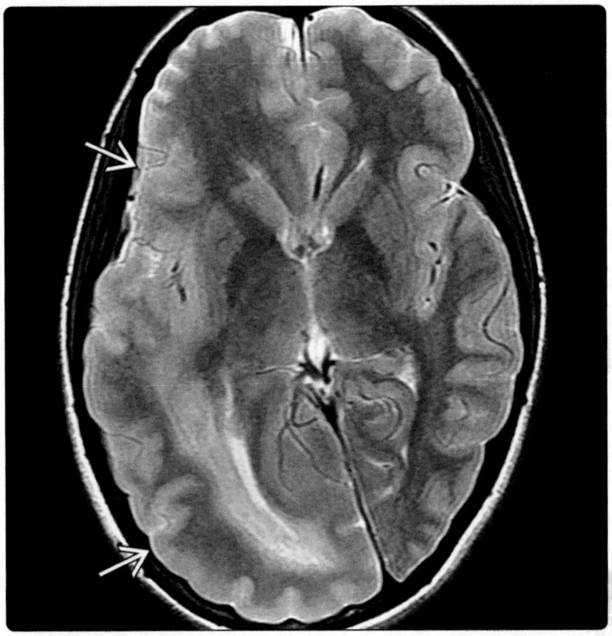

(39-74) Axial T2WI shows right hemisphere hemimegalencephaly ➡, the most common CNS malformation seen in epidermal nevus syndrome.

linear verrucous epidermal nevus, and linear sebaceous nevi are common manifestations.

ENs are caused by genetic mosaicism (represented by two or more different but coexisting clones of the same cell line). Embryonic epidermal cells appear early in fetal development. They proliferate and then migrate from their origin in neural crest to their destinations along so-called Blaschko lines. Mutated cells are phenotypically manifested along this pathway, resulting in the characteristic distribution of ENs.

ENs are present at birth or develop during the first few years of life. Clinically, an epidermal nevus is seen as a linear or zosteriform warty plaque that may exhibit scaly discoloration. Most are found on the neck, trunk, and extremities.

CNS malformations are present in the majority of patients with EN syndrome. The most common are malformations of cortical development (hemimegalencephaly, pachygyria-polymicrogyria) **(39-74)**. Eye lesions are present in 40-70% of patients and include ocular colobomas, choristomas (epibulbar dermoids and lipodermoids), and optic nerve dysplasia.

Proteus Syndrome

Proteus syndrome (PS) is a rare hamartomatous disorder with multiple and diverse somatic manifestations. Mosaicism for activating mutations in *AKT1* causes PS. AKT is part of the mTORC1 signaling pathway, so PS shares some genetic features with other disorders such as PTEN hamartoma tumor syndrome, TSC1/TSC2, and **PIK3CA-related overgrowth spectrum**.

PS is characterized by localized, progressive, postnatal limb overgrowth with bony distortion, dysregulated adipose tissue, epidermal nevi, and CNS malformations. Hemimegalencephaly, pachygyria-polymicrogyria, and heterotopic gray matter are common associated abnormalities.

CNS TUMORS IN RARE FAMILIAL CANCER SYNDROMES

Li-Fraumeni Syndrome
- Most have *TP53* mutations
  - *TP53* = "guardian of the genome"
- Astrocytoma, choroid plexus neoplasms, medulloblastoma

Cowden (MHAM) Syndrome
- *PTEN* mutations
- With Lhermitte-Duclos = COLD syndrome

Turcot Syndrome
- Type 1 = HNPCC (Lynch syndrome); type 2 = FAP
- Type 1 = AA, GBM; type 2 = WNT medulloblastoma

Nevoid Basal Cell Carcinoma (Gorlin) Syndrome
- *PTCH1* mutations
- Medulloblastoma (usually SHH-subtype)

Rhabdoid Tumor Predisposition Syndrome
- *SMARCB1*/INI1/SNFS mutations
- AT/RT

Neurocutaneous Melanosis
- Leptomeningeal melanoma

Selected References

Neurofibromatosis and Schwannomatosis

Vijapura C et al: Genetic syndromes associated with central nervous system tumors. Radiographics. 37(1):258-280, 2017

Kresak JL et al: Neurofibromatosis: a review of NF1, NF2, and schwannomatosis. J Pediatr Genet. 5(2):98-104, 2016

Neurofibromatosis Type 1

Evans DGR et al: Cancer and central nervous system tumor surveillance in pediatric neurofibromatosis 1. Clin Cancer Res. 23(12):e46-e53, 2017

Karmakar S et al: The role of the immune system in neurofibromatosis type 1-associated nervous system tumors. CNS Oncol. 6(1):45-60, 2017

Ahlawat S et al: Current whole-body MRI applications in the neurofibromatoses: NF1, NF2, and schwannomatosis. Neurology. 87(7 Suppl 1):S31-9, 2016

Neurofibromatosis Type 2

Evans DGR et al: Cancer and central nervous system tumor surveillance in pediatric neurofibromatosis 2 and related disorders. Clin Cancer Res. 23(12):e54-e61, 2017

Lloyd SK et al: Hearing optimization in neurofibromatosis type 2: a systematic review. Clin Otolaryngol. ePub, 2017

Miller ME et al: Long-term MRI surveillance after microsurgery for vestibular schwannoma. Laryngoscope. ePub, 2017

Schwannomatosis

Kehrer-Sawatzki H et al: The molecular pathogenesis of schwannomatosis, a paradigm for the co-involvement of multiple tumour suppressor genes in tumorigenesis. Hum Genet. 136(2):129-148, 2017

Other Common Familial Tumor Syndromes

Tuberous Sclerosis Complex

Cardis MA et al: Cutaneous manifestations of tuberous sclerosis complex and the paediatrician's role. Arch Dis Child. ePub, 2017

Gokare P et al: The tuberous sclerosis complex gets fatter. Oncotarget. 8(26):41780-41781, 2017

Ji S et al: Combined targeting of mTOR and Akt using rapamycin and MK-2206 in the treatment of tuberous sclerosis complex. J Cancer. 8(4):555-562, 2017

von Hippel-Lindau Disease

Huntoon K et al: Biological and clinical impact of hemangioblastoma-associated peritumoral cysts in von Hippel-Lindau disease. J Neurosurg. 124(4):971-6, 2016

Shanbhogue KP et al: von Hippel-Lindau disease: review of genetics and imaging. Radiol Clin North Am. 54(3):409-22, 2016

Rare Familial Cancer Syndromes

Kennedy RA et al: An overview of autosomal dominant tumour syndromes with prominent features in the oral and maxillofacial region. Head Neck Pathol. ePub, 2017

Vijapura C et al: Genetic syndromes associated with central nervous system tumors. Radiographics. 37(1):258-280, 2017

Li-Fraumeni Syndrome

Guha T et al: Inherited TP53 mutations and the Li-Fraumeni syndrome. Cold Spring Harb Perspect Med. 7(4):a026187, 2017

Kratz CP et al: Cancer screening recommendations for individuals with Li-Fraumeni syndrome. Clin Cancer Res. 23(11):e38-e45, 2017

Cowden Syndrome

Heaney RM et al: Cowden syndrome: serendipitous diagnosis in patients with significant breast disease. Case series and literature review. Breast J. 23(1):90-94, 2017

Ngeow J et al: Clinical implications for germline PTEN spectrum disorders. Endocrinol Metab Clin North Am. 46(2):503-517, 2017

Turcot Syndrome

Waller A et al: Familial adenomatous polyposis. J Pediatr Genet. 5(2):78-83, 2016

Nevoid Basal Cell Carcinoma Syndrome

Kennedy RA et al: An overview of autosomal dominant tumour syndromes with prominent features in the oral and maxillofacial region. Head Neck Pathol. ePub, 2017

Shiohama T et al: Brain morphology in children with nevoid basal cell carcinoma syndrome. Am J Med Genet A. 173(4):946-952, 2017

Rhabdoid Tumor Predisposition Syndrome

Foulkes WD et al: Cancer surveillance in Gorlin syndrome and rhabdoid tumor predisposition syndrome. Clin Cancer Res. 23(12):e62-e67, 2017

Johansson G et al: Recent developments in brain tumor predisposing syndromes. Acta Oncol. 55(4):401-11, 2016

Meningioangiomatosis

Nascimento FA et al: Meningioangiomatosis: a disease with many radiological faces. Can J Neurol Sci. 43(6):847-849, 2016

Neurocutaneous Melanosis

Kolin DL et al: CSF cytology diagnosis of NRAS-mutated primary leptomeningeal melanomatosis with neurocutaneous melanosis. Cytopathology. 28(3):235-238, 2017

Levy R et al: Melanocytic nevi in children: a review. Pediatr Ann. 45(8):e293-8, 2016

Encephalocraniocutaneous Lipomatosis

Kocak O et al: Encephalocraniocutaneous lipomatosis, a rare neurocutaneous disorder: report of additional three cases. Childs Nerv Syst. 32(3):559-62, 2016

Epidermal Nevus Syndrome

Israni A et al: Cutaneous and brain malformations of epidermal nevus syndrome: a classical image. J Pediatr Neurosci. 11(3):285-286, 2016

Proteus Syndrome

Nathan N et al: Mosaic disorders of the PI3K/PTEN/AKT/TSC/mTORC1 signaling pathway. Dermatol Clin. 35(1):51-60, 2017

Sachdeva P et al: Proteus syndrome with neurological manifestations: a rare presentation. J Pediatr Neurosci. 12(1):109-111, 2017

Vascular Neurocutaneous Syndromes

A number of syndromes with prominent cutaneous manifestations occur without associated neoplasms. Many of these are disorders in which both cutaneous and intracranial vascular lesions are the predominant features. These ***vascular phakomatoses*** *may be segmental, involve a large region, or occur as a localized vascular lesion.*

Some vascular phakomatoses, such as Sturge-Weber syndrome, are present at birth (i.e., congenital) but are *not* inherited. Others, including hereditary hemorrhagic telangiectasia, have specific gene mutations and known inheritance patterns. We delineate these and other pertinent features of the major vascular neurocutaneous syndromes here.

Capillary Malformation Syndromes

In the updated classification scheme adopted by the International Society for the Study of Vascular Anomalies, port-wine stains and associated syndromes [e.g., Sturge-Weber syndrome (SWS) and others] are grouped under the heading of capillary malformations.

In this section on capillary malformation syndromes, we discuss SWS, capillary-lymphatic-venous malformation (often called Klippel-Trenaunay syndrome), and capillary malformation-arteriovenous malformation.

Sturge-Weber Syndrome

SWS is noteworthy among neurocutaneous syndromes; it is one of the very few syndromes that is sporadic, i.e., not familial and not inherited. It is also one of the most disfiguring syndromes, as a prominent nevus flammeus ("port-wine birthmark," PWB) is seen in the vast majority of cases. Neurological problems such as epilepsy, focal deficits, and mental retardation are common.

Imaging has always played a central role in the diagnosis and management of SWS. With the advent of functional imaging, we are gaining new insights into the clinical manifestations and pathophysiology of this disorder.

Terminology

SWS is also known as **encephalo-trigeminal angiomatosis**. Its hallmarks are variable combinations of (1) a dermal capillary-venular malformation (the PWB) in the sensory distribution of the trigeminal nerve, (2) retinal choroidal

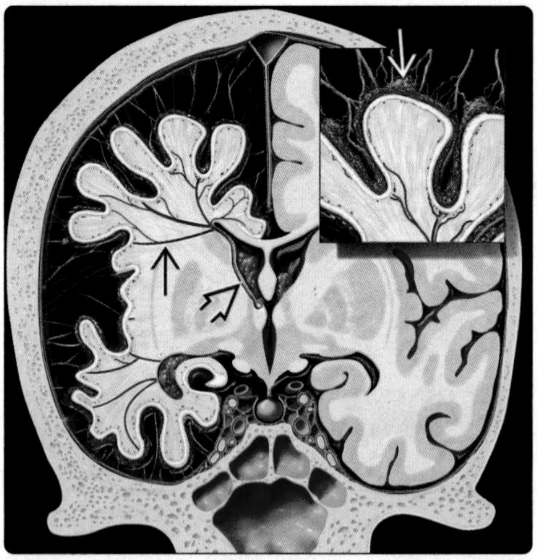

(40-1) ***SWS shows pial angiomatosis ➡, deep medullary collaterals ⇨, enlarged choroid plexus ⇨, and atrophy of the right cerebral hemisphere.***

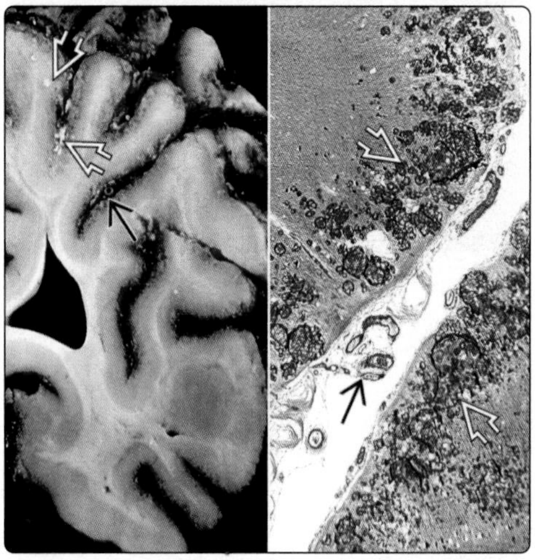

(40-2) ***Gross image (L), photomicrograph (R) of SWS show cortical atrophy, calcifications ➡, and pial angioma ⇨ within sulci. (AFIP Archives.)***

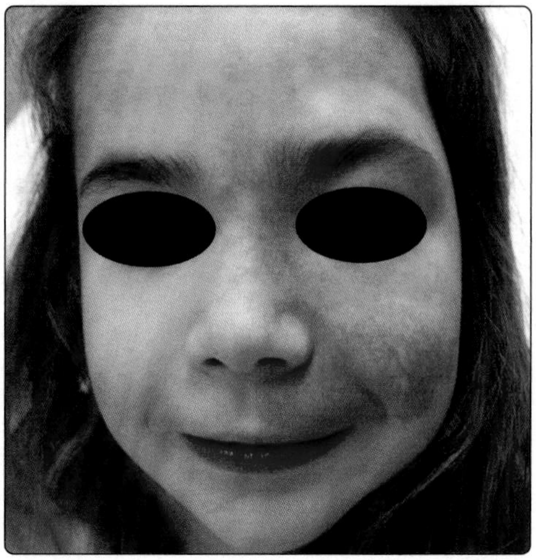

(40-3) ***Photograph shows the classic CN V_1-V_2 nevus flammeus characteristic of SWS.***

angioma (either with or without glaucoma), and (3) a cerebral capillary-venous leptomeningeal angioma.

Etiology

Once considered an enigma, the pathoetiology of SWS is now demystified. In 2013, postzygotic somatic activating mutations in *GNAQ* were identified in both SWS and nonsyndromic PWB-type capillary malformations (so-called SWS type II, i.e. PWB without a vascular pial malformation).

Endothelial cells in SWS skin and brain lesions strongly express somatic R183Q *GNAQ* mutation. The mutation results in hyperactivation of several downstream pathways including RAS-MEK-ERK and (indirectly) mTOR.

GNAQ mutations cause an overlapping phenotypic spectrum of vascular and melanocytic birthmarks. Depending on when they occur, they can lead to differing dermal phenotypes, either vascular alone (SWS), pigmentary alone (extensive dermal melanocytosis), or both (phakomatosis pigmentovascularis).

Pathology

A tangle of thin-walled vessels—multiple enlarged capillaries and venous channels—forms the characteristic leptomeningeal (pial) angioma. The angioma covers the brain surface, dipping into the enlarged sulci between shrunken apposing gyri **(40-1)**.

The most common location is the parietooccipital region, followed by the frontal and temporal lobes. Part or all of one hemisphere can be affected. SWS is unilateral in 80% of cases and is typically ipsilateral to the facial angioma. Bilateral involvement is seen in 20% of cases. Infratentorial lesions are seen in 11% of cases.

Dystrophic laminar cortical calcifications are typical **(40-2)**. Frank hemorrhage and large territorial infarcts are rare.

Clinical Issues

Demographics. SWS is rare with an estimated prevalence of 1:40,000-50,000 live births. There is no sex predilection.

Presentation. The vast majority of SWS patients exhibit a nevus flammeus—formerly termed a facial "angioma" or "port-wine stain"—that is plainly visible at birth. It can be uni- (63%) or bilateral (31%) and is distributed over the skin innervated by one or more sensory branches of the trigeminal nerve. CN V_1 (forehead and/or eyelid) or a combination of CN V_1-V_2 (plus cheek) are the most common sites **(40-3)**. All three trigeminal divisions are involved in 13% of cases. Approximately one-third of patients have ocular or orbital abnormalities such as a diffuse choroidal hemangioma ("tomato catsup fundus") **(40-5A)**, congenital glaucoma with an enlarged globe (buphthalmos), and optic disc colobomas.

Occasionally the facial vascular malformation involves the midline and may even extend to the chest, trunk, and limbs. *No facial nevus flammeus is present in 5% of cases,* so lack of a visible port-wine nevus does not rule out SWS!

Similarly, presence of a PWB is *not* sufficient in and of itself for the definitive diagnosis of SWS. Patients with PWBs in the CN V_1 distribution have only a 10-20% risk of SWS although the risk increases with size, extent, and bilaterality of the nevus flammeus.

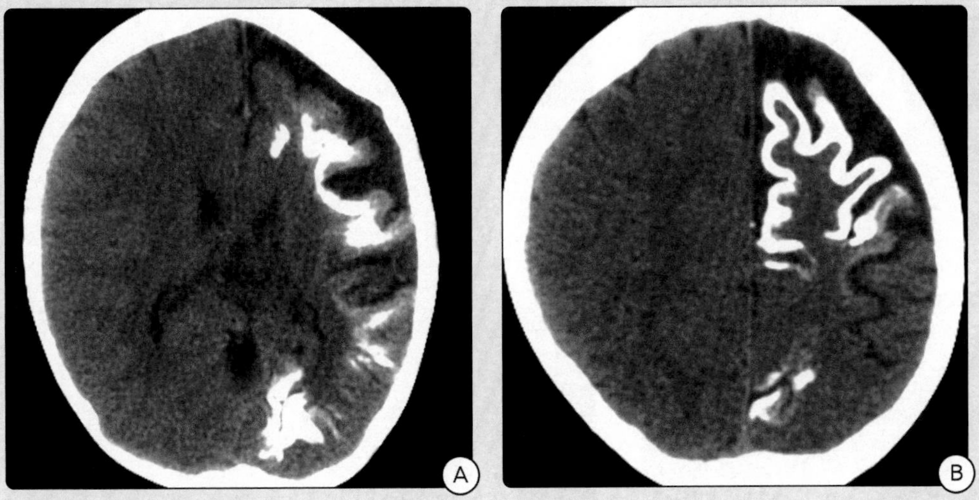

***(40-4A)** NECT in an 8y girl with SWS shows striking cortical atrophy and extensive calcifications in the cortex and subcortical WM throughout most of the left cerebral hemisphere. **(40-4B)** More cephalad NECT in the same patient shows the typical serpentine gyral calcifications together with significant volume loss.*

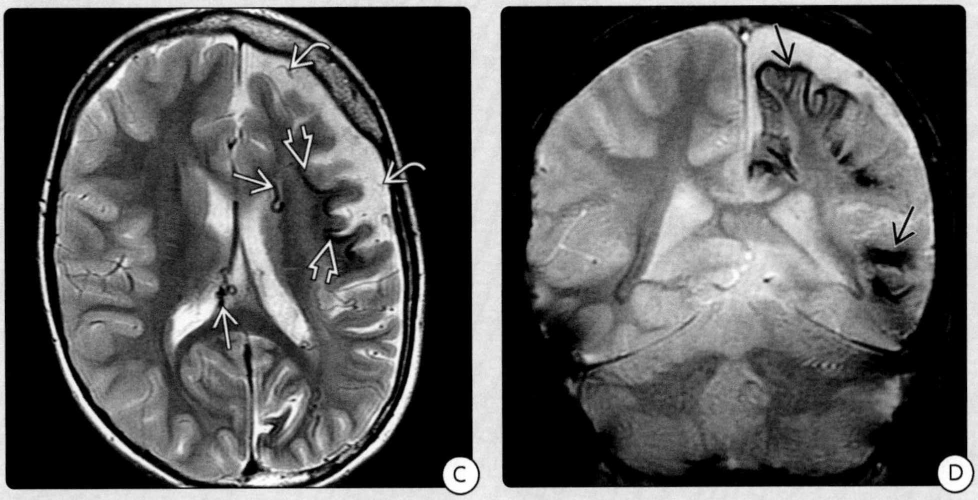

***(40-4C)** T2WI in the same patient shows atrophy with thinned cortex, extensive curvilinear hypointensity in the GM-WM interface ➯. Note the prominent "flow voids" in the subependymal veins ➔. The CSF in the enlarged subarachnoid space appears somewhat "dirty" with enlarged traversing trabeculae and veins ➱. **(40-4D)** Coronal T2* GRE scan shows "blooming" of the extensive cortical/subcortical calcifications →.*

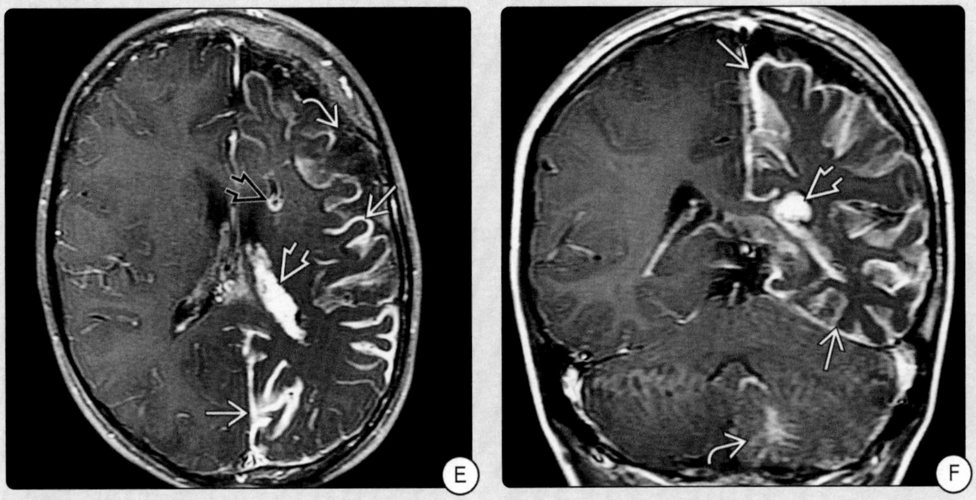

***(40-4E)** T1 C+ FS shows serpentine enhancement covering gyri, filling sulci ➔ with grayish "dirty" CSF ➱. Note enlargement, enhancement of ipsilateral choroid plexus ➯ and draining subependymal vein ➾. **(40-4F)** Coronal T1 C+ shows pial angioma ➔ and enlarged choroid plexus ➯. Developmental venous anomaly is seen in left cerebellar hemisphere ➱.*

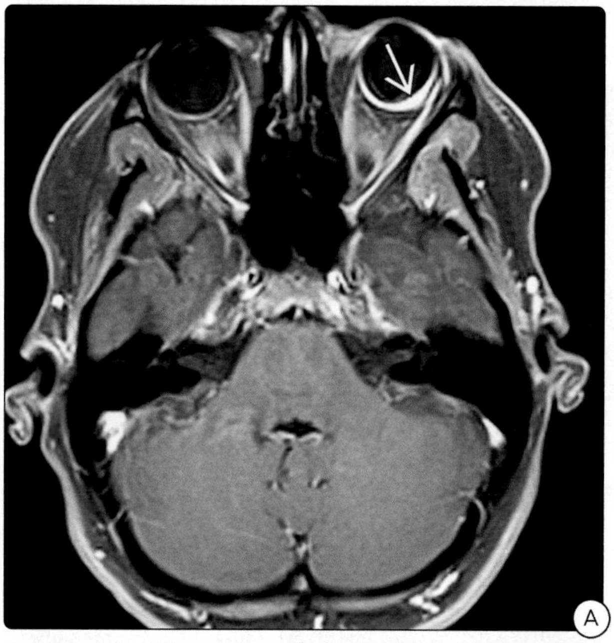

***(40-5A)** T1 C+ FS in a patient with SWS and left vision loss shows a diffuse choroidal angioma, seen here as a thick crescent of contrast enhancement around the posterior segment of the globe.*

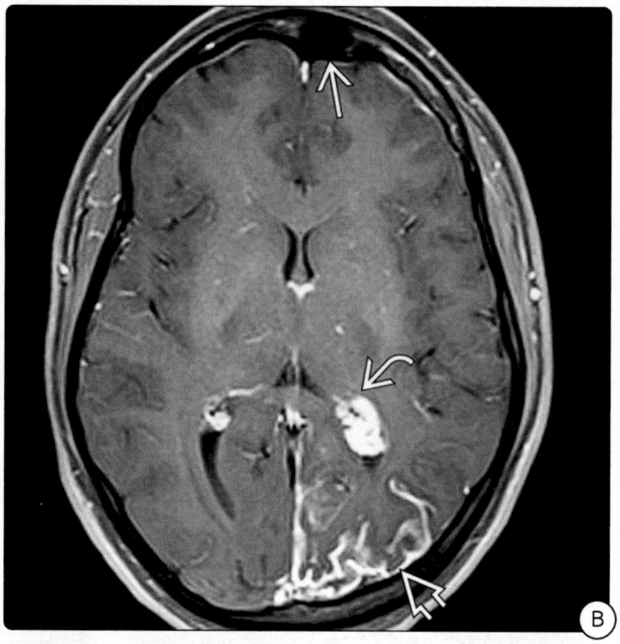

***(40-5B)** T1 C+ FS in the same case shows left occipital pial enhancement with enlarged, enhancing ipsilateral choroid plexus . The left hemisphere is slightly atrophic, and the left frontal sinus is enlarged .*

Seizures developing in the first year of life (75-90%), glaucoma (70%), hemiparesis (30-65%), and migraine-like headaches are other common manifestations of SWS.

Occasionally, children with SWS also have extensive cutaneous capillary malformations, limb hypertrophy, and vascular and/or lymphatic malformations. These children are diagnosed as having **Klippel-Trenaunay syndrome** (KTS), which is also known as angioosteohypertrophy or hemangiectatic hypertrophy. SWS and KTS most likely represent phenotypic variations within the same spectrum.

Endocrine disorders are a newly recognized aspect of SWS. Patients with SWS have a significantly increased risk of growth hormone deficiency and central hypothyroidism.

Natural History. SWS-related seizures are often medically refractory and worsen with time. Progressive hemiparesis and stroke-like episodes with focal neurologic deficits are common. Most patients are mentally retarded.

Treatment Options. Despite adequate treatment with antiepileptic drugs, seizure control is achieved in less than half of all cases. Early lobectomy or hemispherectomy in infants with drug-resistant epilepsy and widespread hemispheric angioma may be an option in severe cases.

Imaging

General Features. Neuroimaging is used to identify the intracranial pial angioma and the sequelae of longstanding venous ischemia. This enables the radiologist to (1) establish or confirm the diagnosis of SWS and (2) evaluate the extent and severity of intracranial involvement.

Sequential examinations of SWS patients show progressive cerebral cortical-subcortical atrophy, especially during the first years of life. *Findings may be minimal or absent in newborn infants, so serial imaging is necessary in suspected cases.*

CT Findings. NECT is especially useful to depict the dystrophic cortical/subcortical calcifications that are one of the imaging hallmarks of SWS **(40-4B)**. (Note that the calcifications are in the underlying brain, not the pial angioma). Cortical calcification, atrophy, and enlargement of the ipsilateral choroid plexus are typical findings in older children and adults with SWS.

Heavily calcified cortex correlates with decreased perfusion in the underlying WM and is also associated with more severe epilepsy.

Bone CT shows thickening of the diploë and enlargement with hyperpneumatization of the ipsilateral frontal sinuses secondary to longstanding volume loss in the underlying brain. Dense cortical calcifications may obscure enhancement of the pial angioma on CECT, but an enlarged enhancing choroid plexus can usually be identified.

MR Findings. T1 and T2 scans show volume loss in the affected cortex with enlargement of the adjacent subarachnoid spaces **(40-4C)** **(40-7)**. Myelination is usually normal or even accelerated, and malformations of cortical development may be present. White matter ischemic damage with subcortical T2/FLAIR hyperintensities in the affected hemisphere is common in older patients.

Prominent trabeculae and enlarged veins often cross the subarachnoid space, making the CSF appear somewhat grayish or "dirty" **(40-4E)**.

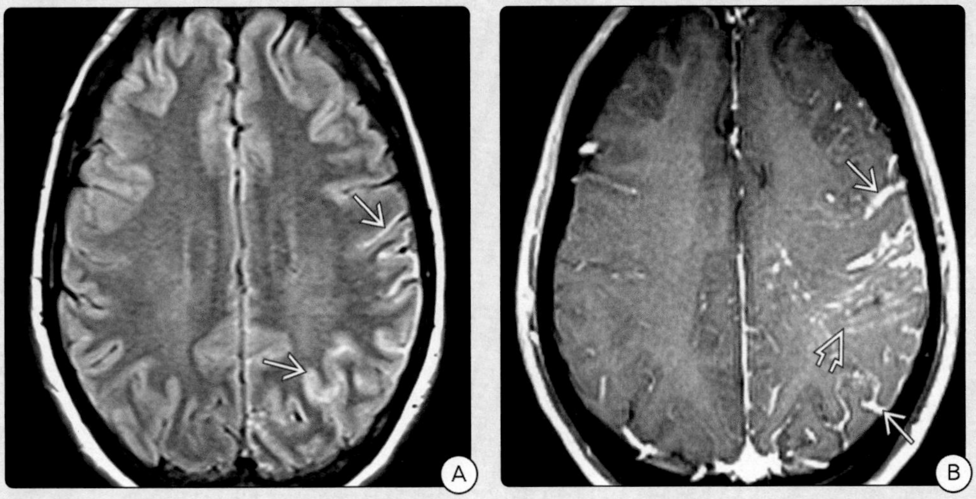

***(40-6A)** Axial FLAIR scan in a 25y woman with seizures and SWS shows left parietooccipital sulcal hyperintensity ("ivy" sign) →. **(40-6B)** T1 C+ FS scan in the same patient shows that the enhancing pial angioma fills the affected sulci →. Note the linear enhancing foci caused by enlarged medullary veins → that provide collateral venous drainage into the subependymal veins and galenic system.*

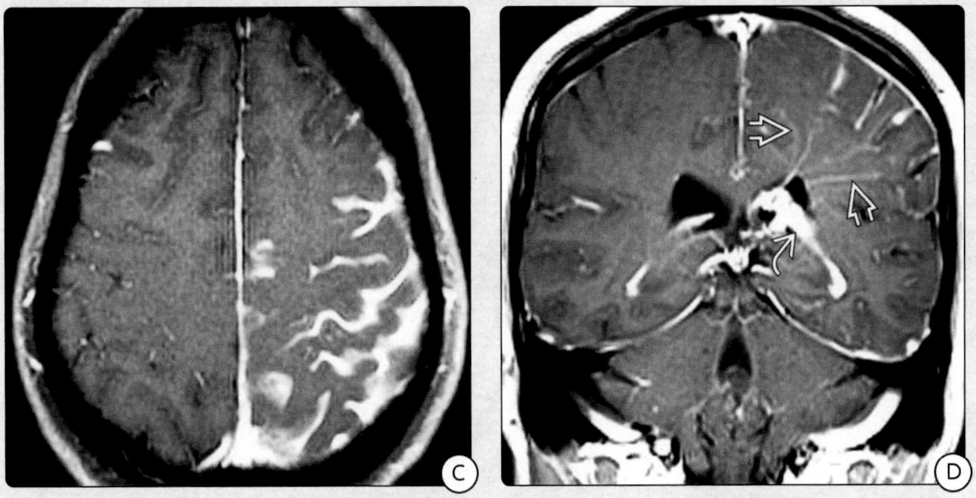

***(40-6C)** More cephalad T1 C+ scan in the same patient shows that the sulci and subarachnoid spaces are enlarged, completely filled by the enhancing pial angioma. **(40-6D)** Coronal T1 C+ scan nicely demonstrates the prominent enhancing medullary veins → as they drain through the hemispheric white matter to converge on the subependymal veins that line the lateral ventricles. The ipsilateral choroid plexus → is markedly enlarged.*

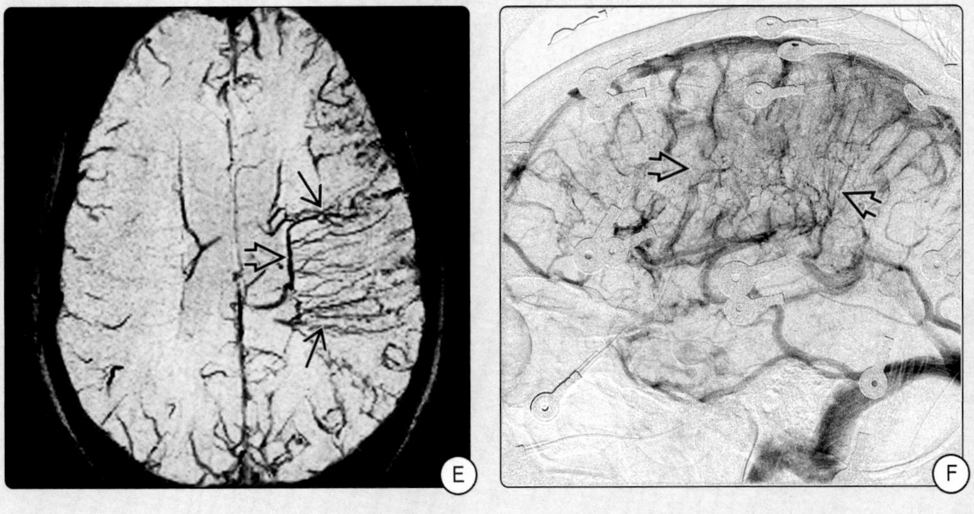

***(40-6E)** Axial T2* susceptibility-weighted image (SWI) demonstrates deoxyhemoglobin in the enlarged, tortuous medullary veins → that are slowly draining into enlarged subependymal veins →. **(40-6F)** Venous-phase DSA in the same patient performed as part of a Wada test for language localization shows a paucity of normal cortical veins with a prolonged vascular "blush" caused by contrast stasis in multiple enlarged medullary veins →.*

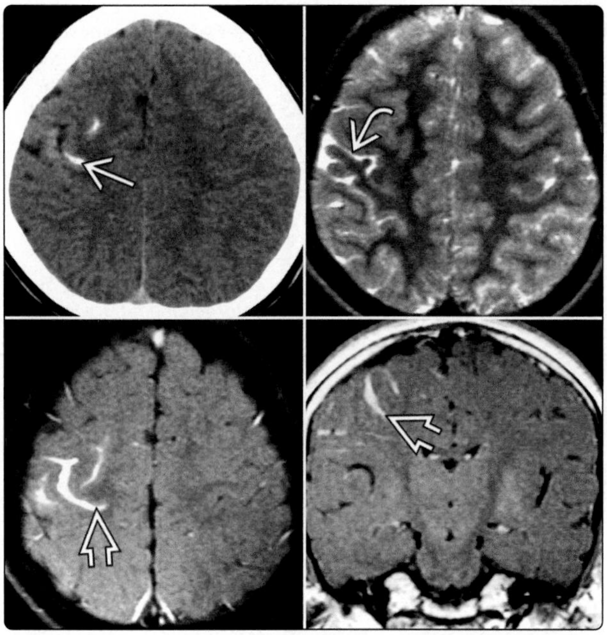

(40-7) Variant SWS case shows focal Ca++, atrophy, and a very localized enhancing pial angioma that fills just a few adjacent sulci.

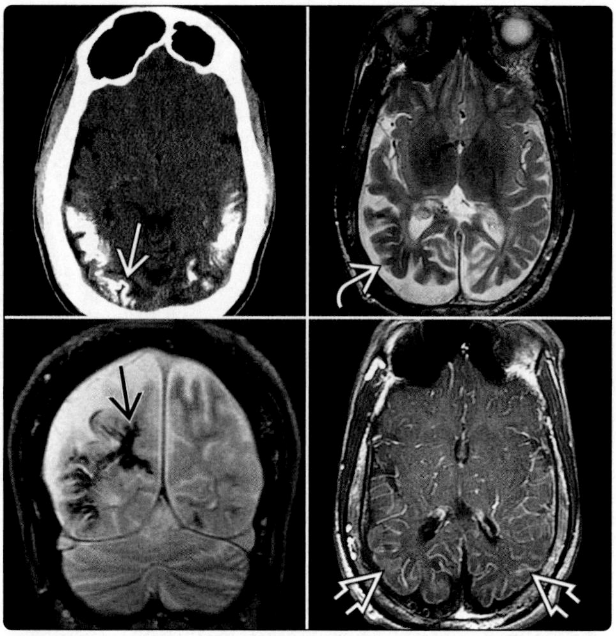

(40-8) Images from a 17y boy with KTS show bilateral gyriform parenchymal calcifications that "bloom" on T2, parietal occipital atrophy, and extensive bilateral enhancing pial angiomata.*

Dystrophic cortical/subcortical calcifications are seen as linear hypointensities on T2WI that "bloom" on T2* (GRE, SWI) **(40-4D)**. SWI scans often demonstrate linear susceptibility in enlarged medullary veins **(40-6E)**.

FLAIR scans may demonstrate serpentine hyperintensities in the sulci, the "ivy" sign **(40-6A)**. DWI is usually negative unless acute ischemia is present.

Postcontrast T1WI or FLAIR sequences best demonstrate the pial angioma. Serpentine enhancement covers the underlying gyri, extending deep into the sulci and sometimes almost filling the subarachnoid space **(40-6C)**. Enlarged medullary veins—sources of compensatory collateral venous drainage—can sometimes be identified as linear enhancing foci extending deep into the hemispheric white matter **(40-6D)**. The ipsilateral choroid plexus is almost always enlarged and enhances intensely **(40-5B)**.

T1 C+ is particularly helpful in the newborn, infant, or young child with dark skin pigmentation and SWS who presents with seizures and has not yet exhibited focal brain atrophy.

Angiography. DSA typically demonstrates a lack of superficial cortical veins with corresponding dilatation of deep medullary and subependymal veins **(40-6F)**. The arterial phase is normal.

Differential Diagnosis

The major differential diagnoses of SWS are other vascular neurocutaneous syndromes. Patients with **meningioangiomatosis** (MA) typically lack the PWB seen in SWS. The meningeal angioma of MA often extends into the adjacent brain along the perivascular spaces. Cutaneous or ophthalmoscopic findings help differentiate other vascular neurocutaneous syndromes, such as **blue rubber bleb nevus syndrome** and **Wyburn-Mason syndrome** from SWS.

STURGE-WEBER SYNDROME

Etiology
- Congenital but sporadic, not inherited
- Postzygotic (i.e., somatic) mutation in *GNAQ*
  - Causes both SWS, nonsyndromic "port-wine birthmarks" (PWBs)

Pathology
- Pial (leptomeningeal) angioma
- Cortical venous ischemia, atrophy
- Parietooccipital > frontal

Clinical Issues
- Unilateral facial nevus flammeus
  - Also known as PWB
- Usual cutaneous distribution = CN $V1_1$, $V_2 > V_3$
  - Can be bilateral or even absent

Imaging
- CT
  - Atrophic cortex
  - Ipsilateral calvaria thick, sinuses enlarged
  - Cortical Ca++ (*not* in angioma!) increases with age
- MR
  - Cortical/subcortical hypointensity on T2
  - Ca++ "blooms" on T2*
  - Angioma enhances (unilateral 80%, bilateral 20%)
  - Ipsilateral choroid plexus enlarged
  - Enlarged medullary veins

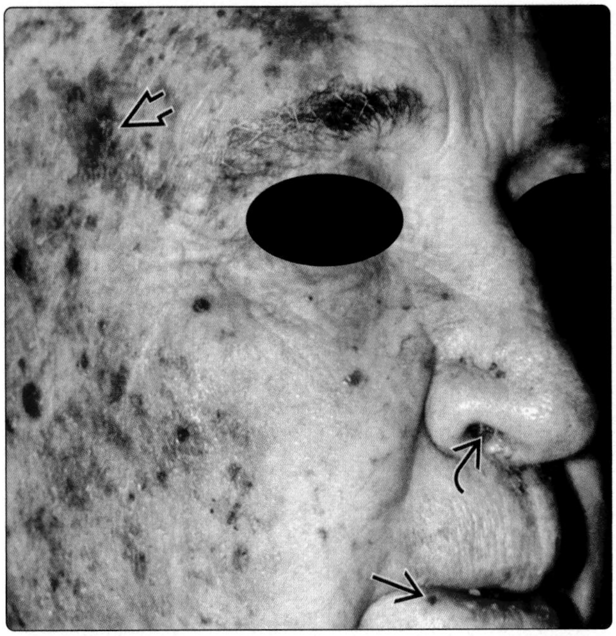

(40-9) Clinical photograph of a patient with HHT and multiple episodes of severe epistaxis shows multiple mucocutaneous telangiectasias of the scalp, nose, and lips.

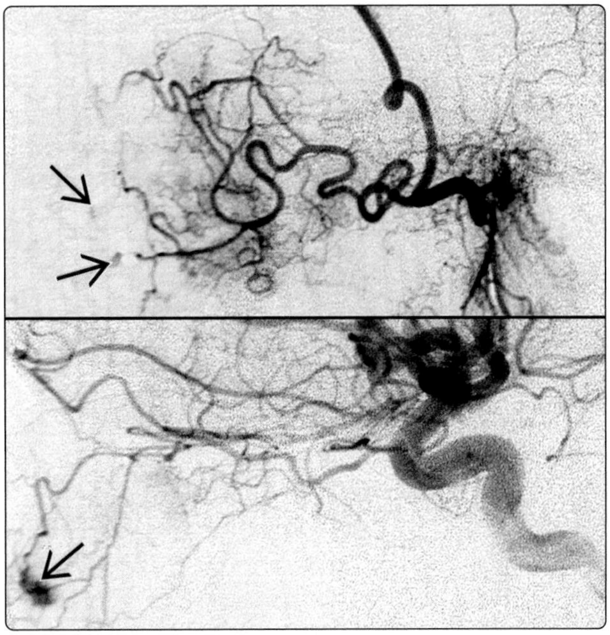

(40-10) ECA (top), ICA (bottom) angiograms in a patient with HHT and epistaxis show tiny capillary telangiectases in the nasal and orbital mucosa.

Klippel-Trenaunay Syndrome

Klippel-Trenaunay syndrome (KTS)—also called Klippel-Trenaunay-Weber syndrome—is characterized by capillary-lymphatic-venous malformations anywhere in the body. The classic clinical triad of KTS includes (1) capillary malformation, seen in 98% of patients either as cutaneous hemangiomas or port-wine stains, (2) limb overgrowth, which may include the underlying bones and soft tissues, and (3) venous varicosities.

KTS shares overlapping features with SWS. Intracranial lesions, i.e., pial angiomas, are rare. When present, they are often bilateral **(40-8)**.

Capillary Malformation-Arteriovenous Malformation

Capillary malformation-arteriovenous malformation (CM-AVM) is characterized by small multifocal capillary malformations that may occur anywhere on the body, typically on the face and limbs. CM-AVM syndrome is a **RASA1 disorder.** About 30% of affected individuals also have associated AVMs or arteriovenous fistulas (AVFs) in the skin, muscle, bone, spine, or brain.

Some patients with a *RASA1* pathogenic variant have the clinical diagnosis of **Parkes-Weber syndrome (PWS).** PWS patients have capillary malformations and limb overgrowth but also have AVFs. Here multiple micro-AVFs are associated with a cutaneous capillary stain and overgrowth of an affected limb. In contrast to PWS and KTS, patients with CM-AVM do not exhibit limb overgrowth.

Cutaneous and/or mucosal capillary malformations can also occur with microcephaly (**capillary malformation-microcephaly syndrome**) or megalencephaly (**megalencephaly-capillary malformation syndrome**).

Other Vascular Phakomatoses

Hereditary Hemorrhagic Telangiectasia

Terminology

Hereditary hemorrhagic telangiectasia (HHT) is also known as **Osler-Weber-Rendu** or Rendu-Osler-Weber syndrome. HHT is an autosomal-dominant monogenetic disorder with considerable intrafamilial variability and is characterized pathologically by widely distributed, multisystem angiodysplastic lesions.

Etiology

Mutations in three genes (*ENG, ACVRL1*/ALK1, and *SMAD4*) cause approximately 85-95% of HHT cases by affecting the TGF-β signaling pathway, leading to downstream changes in vascular cell proliferation. These changes ultimately result in the formation of telangiectasias and AVMs in multiple organ systems, including the brain.

ENG (endoglin) gene mutations cause **type 1 HHT** and are associated with mucocutaneous telangiectases, early onset of epistaxis, pulmonary arteriovenous fistulas (AVFs), and brain arteriovenous malformations (AVMs). *ACVRL1*/ALK1 mutation causes **type 2 HHT**, is associated with lower penetrance and milder disease, and presents primarily as GI bleeds and pulmonary arterial hypertension. *SMAD4* mutations cause **HHT/juvenile polyposis combined syndrome**.

HEREDITARY HEMORRHAGIC TELANGIECTASIA: ETIOLOGY AND PATHOLOGY

Etiology

- Type 1 HHT
  - Endoglin (*ENG*) mutation
  - Mucocutaneous telangiectases, epistaxis, pulmonary AVFs/brain AVMs
- Type 2 HHT
  - *ACVRL1*/ALK1 mutation
  - Milder; predominantly GI bleeds

Pathology

- Neurovascular malformations 10-20%
  - > 50% multiple
- Two main types
  - Approximately 50:50
  - "Nidal" brain AVMs
  - Capillary vascular malformations
- Other intracranial vascular malformations
  - Developmental venous anomaly 12%
  - Cavernous malformations 2-4%
  - Capillary telangiectases (mucocutaneous common; rare in brain 1-3%)
  - Pial AVF < 1%

Pathology

Between 10-20% of patients with a diagnosis of definite HHT have brain vascular malformations. Two main types are common: (1) nidus-type AVMs and (2) capillary vascular malformations. AVFs—common in the lung—are rare in the brain. Nonshunting lesions in HHT include developmental venous anomalies, capillary telangiectasias, and cavernous malformations.

"Nidal" brain AVMs account for slightly less than half of all HHT neurovascular manifestations and are found in 10% of all patients. Nearly 60% are solitary, whereas multiple lesions are present in 40%; approximately 80% are supratentorial, whereas 20% are infratentorial.

Capillary vascular malformations account for slightly over half of all neurovascular manifestations of HHT. They are typically supratentorial (86%), are often peripherally located in the brain, and are almost always < 1 cm.

Capillary telangiectasias are distinct from capillary vascular malformations and consist of numerous thin-walled ectatic capillaries interspersed in normal brain parenchyma. Feeding arteries are absent although sometimes a draining vein can be identified. Brain capillary telangiectasias are relatively rare in HHT (2-4%). They are typically found in the pons or medulla and are occult on DSA.

Other manifestations of HHT include pial AVFs and nonshunting lesions, such as **developmental venous anomalies** (12%) and **cavernous malformations** (3-4%). **Pial AVFs** are rare, accounting for just 1% of all HHT-related brain vascular malformations. **Malformations of cortical development**—usually perisylvian polymicrogyria—are found in 12% of HHT cases.

Clinical Issues

Epidemiology and Demographics. HHT is a rare but probably underdiagnosed disease, with a prevalence of 1-2:10,000. There is no sex predilection.

Presentation. The most common features of HHT are nosebleeds and telangiectases on the lips, hands, and oral mucosa **(40-9)**. Epistaxis typically begins by age 10, and 80-90% have nosebleeds by age 21 **(40-10)**. The onset of visible telangiectases is generally 5-30 years later than for epistaxis. Almost 95% of affected individuals eventually develop mucocutaneous telangiectases.

The diagnosis of HHT is considered "confirmed" in an individual with three or more of the following: (1) nosebleeds, (2) mucocutaneous telangiectases, (3) visceral AVM, and (4) a first-degree relative in whom HHT has been diagnosed. Identification of a heterozygous pathogenic variant in one of the causative genes can establish the diagnosis if clinical features are inconclusive.

Most experts agree that patients with HHT should be screened for cerebral vascular malformations at least once during their clinical evaluation. Repeat screening is low-yield, as the rate of de novo formation of brain AVMs in this population is exceedingly low.

Natural History. HHT displays age-related penetrance with increasing manifestations developing over a lifetime; penetrance approaches 100% by age 40. Epistaxis increases in frequency and severity and, in some cases, can require multiple transfusions or even become life-threatening.

Although most HHT-associated brain AVMs are small and have a low Spetzler-Martin grade, 20% present with rupture, and nearly 50% are symptomatic.

Approximately 50% of adults with HHT eventually develop gastrointestinal bleeding, usually after the age of 50 years. Iron deficiency anemia is more common than acute GI hemorrhage.

Shunting of air, thrombi, and bacteria through pulmonary AVMs can cause TIAs, strokes, and cerebral abscesses.

Treatment Options. Laser coagulation of mucosal telangiectases can be effective. Cerebral AVMs greater than 1.0 cm in diameter are usually treated with surgery, embolotherapy, and/or stereotactic radiosurgery.

Imaging

Brain MR without and with contrast enhancement is the recommended screening procedure for patients diagnosed with HHT and, when possible, should be obtained within the first six months of life. Molecular diagnostics may obviate further imaging. In adults, if no AVMs are detected on initial MR scans, further screening for cerebral AVMs is unnecessary.

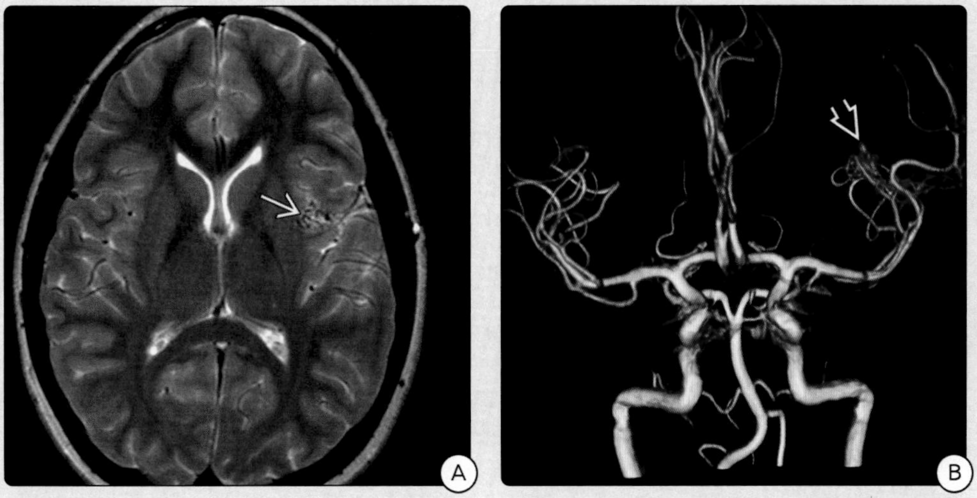

***(40-11A)** Axial T2WI from a screening MR in an 18y patient with nosebleeds and a parent with a pulmonary AVM shows an abnormal cluster of flow voids → along the left insular cortex. **(40-11B)** 3D TOF MRA in the same case shows a corresponding tangle of vessels → in the left sylvian fissure.*

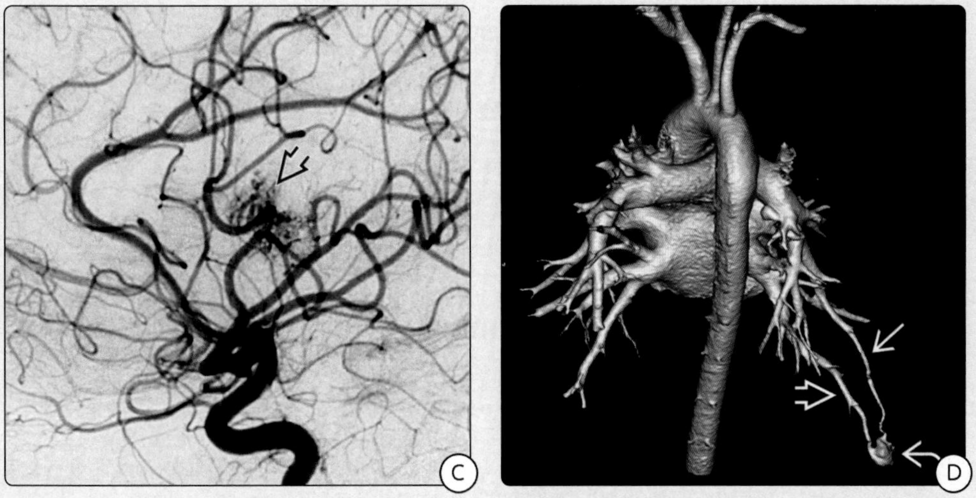

***(40-11C)** Lateral DSA of the left internal carotid artery, arterial phase, shows a 2-cm AVM →. This is Spetzler grade 2. **(40-11D)** Posterior 3D chest CTA in the same case shows a pulmonary AVM → with its feeding artery → and draining vein →. (All four images courtesy C. Merrow, MD.)*

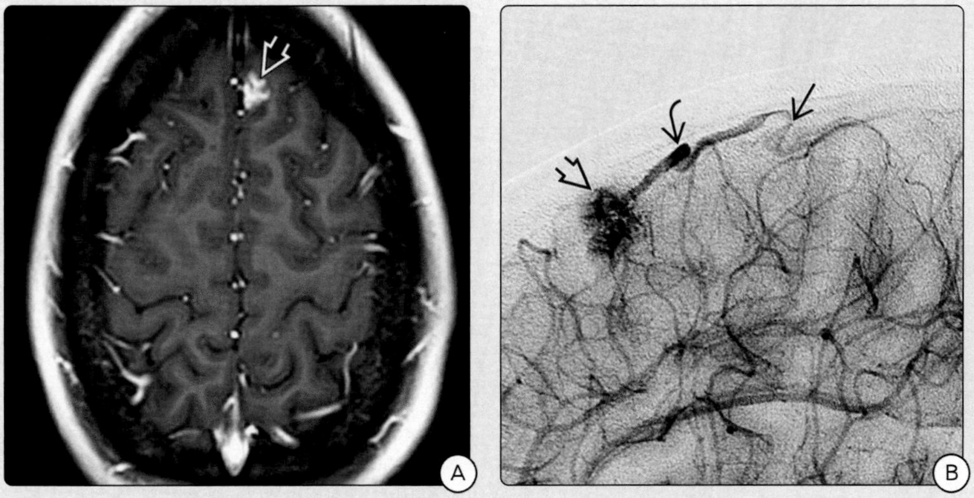

***(40-12A)** Screening T1 C+ MR in an 18y man with a family history of HHT shows an irregularly shaped focus of intense contrast accumulation →. **(40-12B)** Magnified view of the DSA in the same case shows that a tangle of vessels → appears to contain little or no normal brain. The early opacifying vein → is seen emptying into the superior sagittal sinus →. This is typical small nidus-type AVM in HHT. The lesion has been stable for 8 years.*

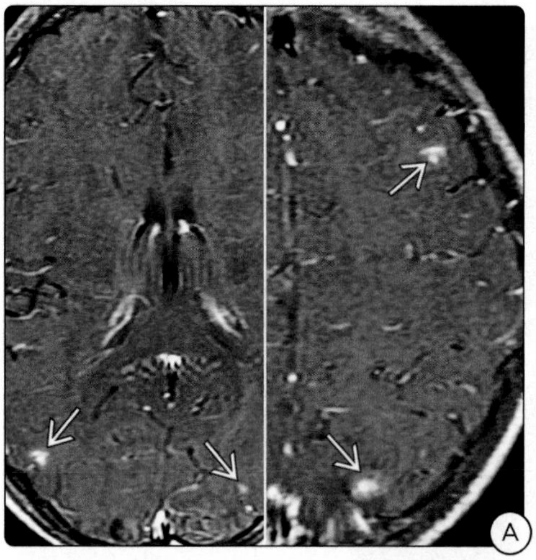

(40-13A) ***Axial T1 C+ FS scans in an 11y girl with HHT show multiple foci of fluffy "stain-like" enhancement →.***

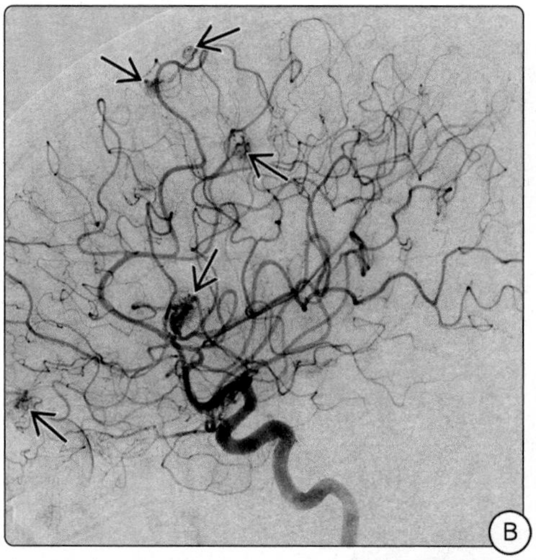

(40-13B) ***Lateral DSA in a 54y woman with HHT shows five small capillary vascular malformations → in the left cerebral hemisphere.***

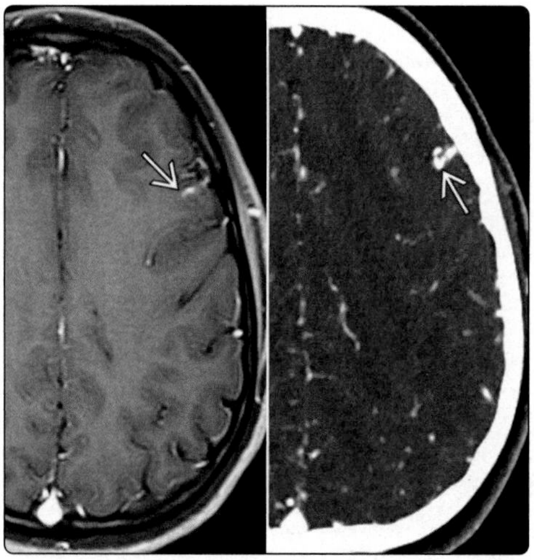

(40-14) ***(L) T1 C+ FS, (R) CTA in an asymptomatic 16y girl with HHT show focus of tubular enhancement →. This is a dural AVF.***

Although some HHT-associated **AVMs** are large, nearly 90% are small (Spetzler-Martin 2 or less). Large lesions can demonstrate prominent "flow voids" on T2WI **(40-11A)**; smaller lesions are seen as "speckled" enhancing foci on T1 C+ studies **(40-12A)**.

Capillary vascular malformations do not show "flow voids" on MR and are defined by a "blush" of abnormal vessels on the late arterial/capillary phase on DSA or an area of fluffy "stain-like" enhancement on T1 C+ MR **(40-13A)**. A dilated feeding artery that empties directly into a draining vein is typical of an **AVF** **(40-14)**.

Capillary telangiectasias are most common in the pons and are usually invisible on T2/FLAIR. A faint "brush-like" area of enhancement is seen on T1 C+, whereas T2* sequences show decreased signal intensity.

HEREDITARY HEMORRHAGIC TELANGIECTASIA: IMAGING

Capillary Vascular Malformations
- Slightly > 50% of HHT vascular malformations
- No "flow voids" on MR
- "Blush" of fluffy, "stain-like" enhancement on T1 C+

AVMs
- Slightly < 50%
- Most are Spetzler grades ≤ 2
  - Multiple AVMs 40%
- Large lesions rare
  - "Flow voids" on T2WI
- Small lesions show "speckled" enhancement on T1 C+
- Feeding artery, nidus, draining vein on DSA
- Other vascular malformations less common
- Perisylvian polymicrogyria 12%

PHACE Syndrome

Children with CNS vascular malformations often have associated broader vascular conditions, such as HHT (considered above), PHACES, and the *RASA1* mutation-related disorder capillary malformation-arteriovenous malformation syndrome. We close this chapter with a discussion of these uncommon but important phakomatoses.

Terminology

PHACE syndrome is an acronym for **p**osterior fossa malformations, **h**emangioma, **a**rterial cerebrovascular anomalies, **c**oarctation of the aorta and cardiac defects, and **e**ye abnormalities (sometimes called PHACES with the addition of the less common **s**ternal clefting or **s**upraumbilical raphe).

PHACE is characterized clinically by a large infantile hemangioma (IH) that is associated with developmental defects. A definitive diagnosis of PHACE is determined when a **craniofacial hemangioma** is present together with one or more characteristic extracutaneous anomalies (see below).

Etiology

The precise etiology of PHACE is unknown, and genetic studies of PHACE syndrome are ongoing. A germ-line mutation has been ruled out, as there are no known familial cases.

The infantile hemangioma and cerebral vasculopathy appear to be linked by common *in utero* morphogenic event(s) with the insult occurring early in embryogenesis, probably during the fifth fetal week or even earlier.

Developmental errors in the neural plate, neural crest, and adjacent cephalic mesoderm have been implicated in the PHACE structural anomalies. Segmental neural crest cell disturbances could result in the formation of facial and intracranial hemangiomas in the same embryonic metamere. Neural crest cells also contribute to formation of the optic vesicles, possibly explaining the eye malformations that often occur as part of the syndrome.

Pathology

Hemangiomas are—by definition—found in 100% of PHACE patients. Hemangiomas are true vascular neoplasms and are the most common benign tumor of infancy, occurring in 2-3% of neonates and 10-12% of children under 1 year of age. The majority are sporadic, nonsyndromic lesions; only 20% meet the diagnostic criteria for PHACE.

Cutaneous Hemangiomas. The topographic distribution of PHACE-associated hemangiomas is significant. Patients with lesions in the upper half of the face typically have structural brain, cerebrovascular, and ocular abnormalities **(40-15)**, whereas hemangiomas in a mandibular ("beard-like") distribution are associated with ventral developmental defects, such as sternal abnormalities and supraumbilical raphe.

The hemangiomas in PHACE can be single (70%) or multiple (30%). Trans- and multispatial lesions are common.

Extracutaneous Hemangiomas. Extracutaneous hemangiomas occur in 20-25% of patients. The subglottis is the most common site and can cause potentially life-threatening airway obstruction.

Ophthalmologic findings are present in 30% of cases. Choroidal hemangiomas, colobomas, microphthalmos, and optic atrophy are common eye lesions in PHACE.

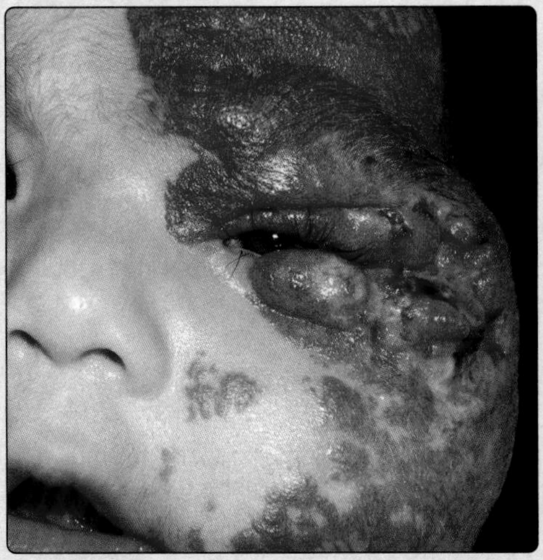

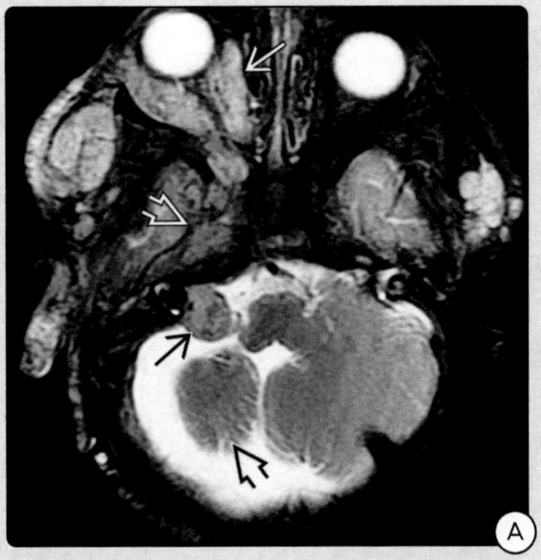

__(40-15)__ Clinical photograph of a patient with PHACES shows a typical facial infantile hemangioma. (Courtesy S. Yashar, MD.) __(40-16A)__ T2WI in an infant with PHACES shows a hemangioma filling the right orbit ➡, extending posteriorly into the cavernous sinus ➡ and cerebellopontine angle ➡. Note hypoplasia of the ipsilateral cerebellar hemisphere ➡.

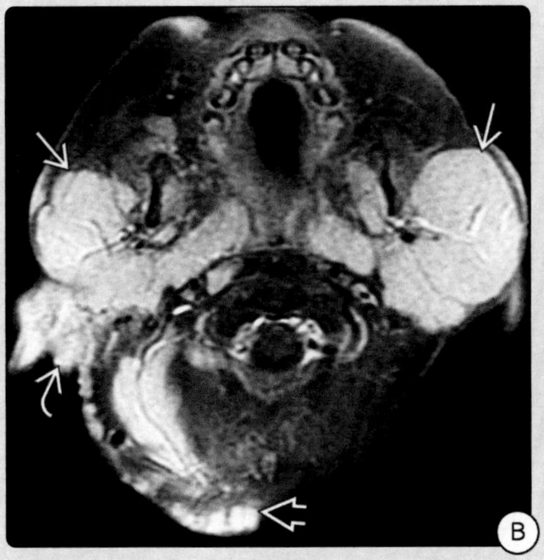

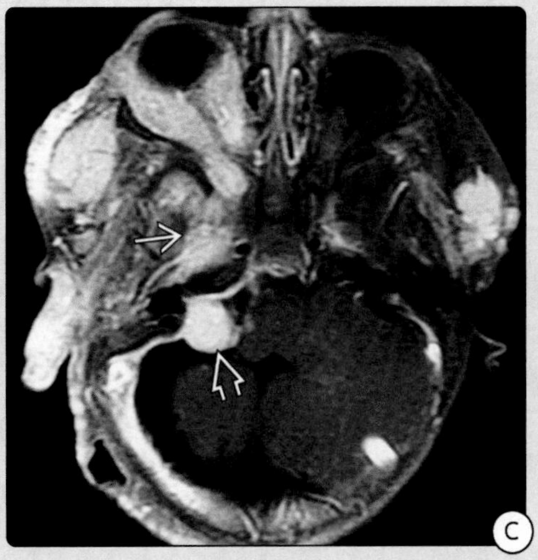

__(40-16B)__ Axial T1 C+ FS in the same patient shows intensely enhancing hemangiomas in massively enlarged parotid glands ➡ and the right ear ➡. Hemangioma also infiltrates the scalp ➡ and posterior cervical space. __(40-16C)__ More cephalad T1 C+ FS scan shows the intracranial extension of the hemangioma into the cavernous sinus ➡ and cerebellopontine angle cistern ➡.

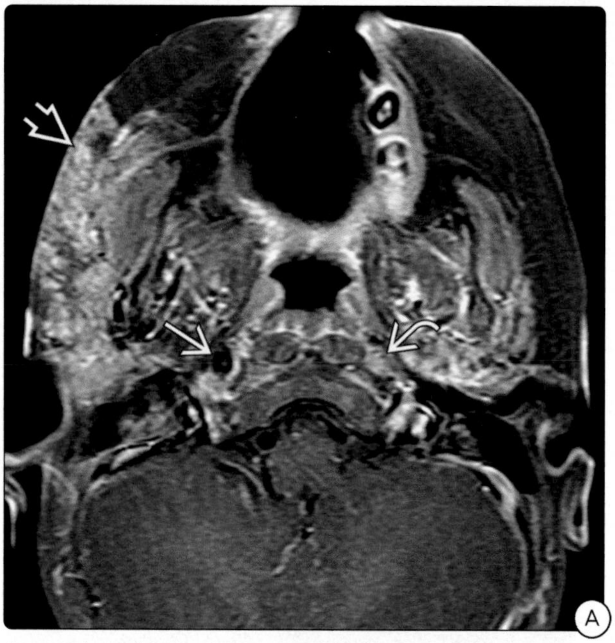

(40-17A) Axial T1 C+ FS in a patient with PHACE(S) shows an enhancing facial angioma ➔. There is no left ICA flow void ➔ as a result of ICA atresia. Contrast with normal right ICA flow void ➔.

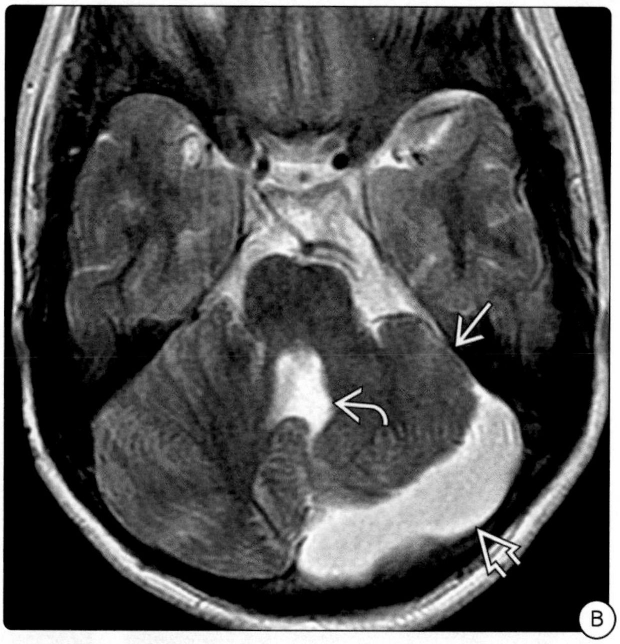

(40-17B) T2WI in the same case shows cerebellar hypoplasia and cortical malformation ➔ with a prominent retrocerebellar CSF space ➔. The fourth ventricle also appears malformed ➔. (From DI: Head and Neck, 3e.)

Although not included in the acronym PHACE, otologic abnormalities are also common. These include middle ear atelectasis, tympanic membrane hemangiomas with conductive hearing loss, skin and cartilage ulcerations, and dysphagia.

Intracranial Hemangiomas. Intracranial hemangiomas are relatively uncommon. When present, they exhibit a predilection for the cavernous sinus and cerebellopontine angle cistern and are generally ipsilateral to the facial hemangioma.

Other Intracranial Malformations. Nonvascular intracranial malformations are present in 30-80% of all PHACE patients. Posterior fossa malformations are identified in 50-75% of these cases and range from focal regions of cerebellar dysplasia or hypoplasia to various cystic malformations, including Dandy-Walker spectrum. Other associated anomalies include corpus callosum dysgenesis, septi pellucidi anomalies, polymicrogyria, gray matter heterotopias, and arachnoid cysts.

Noncutaneous Systemic Manifestations. Over 90% of PHACE patients have more than one extracutaneous finding. Ventral developmental defects such as sternal clefting and supraumbilical raphe are common. Two-thirds of all patients have vasculopathy or exhibit cardiac anomalies.

PHACE-Associated Arteriopathy. PHACE-related vasculopathy includes a number of congenital and progressive large vessel lesions. Arterial anomalies of the craniocervical vasculature are seen in over 75% of patients. Aortic coarctation (35%), arterial occlusions (21%), progressive stenoses (18%), and saccular aneurysms (13%) are the most common potentially symptomatic anomalies. Persistent embryonic arteries (most often a persistent trigeminal artery) are seen in 17% of cases. Aberrant course or origin, extreme dolichoectasia, and dysgenesis/agenesis of the internal carotid and/or vertebral arteries and circle of Willis are also frequent anomalies.

Clinical Issues

A large segmental IH of the face or scalp should prompt screening for PHACE syndrome. Smaller IHs with other characteristic/major anomalies (e.g., midline ventral defects, aortic coarctation, etc.) should also undergo complete evaluation for PHACE.

Epidemiology and Demographics. PHACES is a rare syndrome, but the exact incidence is unknown. The F:M ratio is 9:1.

Presentation. The cutaneous hemangiomas in PHACE are typically bulky, plaque-like geographic lesions **(40-15)**. Unlike the port-wine birthmark of Sturge-Weber syndrome, PHACE-related hemangiomas are not always confined to a specific dermatome and are often transspatial.

Natural History. The prognosis in PHACE typically depends on the type and severity of the associated anomalies, not the hemangioma itself. Hemangiomas generally proliferate during the first year of life and then involute spontaneously over the next 5-7 years (or more). Most remain asymptomatic and are managed by close observation. Occasionally hemangiomas behave more aggressively, causing visual impairment, skeletal deformities, airway obstruction, high-output cardiac failure, bleeding, or ulceration.

Treatment Options. Treatment options for symptomatic hemangiomas include steroids or propranolol and pulsed dye laser. Saccular aneurysms can be treated by coiling or clipping, whereas progressive stenoocclusive disease is sometimes treated with neurosurgical revascularization.

Imaging

CT Findings. NECT may demonstrate soft tissue masses in the orbit, face, and neck as well as cerebellar hypoplasia. CECT depicts hemangiomas as lobulated or plaque-like, intensely enhancing, infiltrating masses. Bone CT may show a small or absent carotid canal.

MR Findings. MR is the best technique to evaluate the presence and extent of craniofacial hemangiomas and to delineate coexisting intracranial malformations **(40-16)**.

T1 scans depict callosal dysgenesis and cerebellar anomalies. Gray matter heterotopias are best seen on T2WI. Proliferating hemangiomas appear hyperintense on T2WI **(40-16A)** and may exhibit prominent internal "flow voids." Intense homogeneous enhancement following contrast administration is typical **(40-16)** **(40-17)**.

Angiography. The prevalence of congenital heart disease in PHACE ranges from 40-67% with aortic coarctation in 20-30%. Aortic arch anomalies are common and unusually complex. The arch obstruction is most often long segment rather than the discrete juxtaductal narrowing seen in nonsyndromic coarctation.

Various anomalies of the craniofacial vasculature also occur in PHACE. These include hypoplasia or aplasia of the internal carotid or vertebral arteries, aberrant origin and/or course of cranial arteries, persistent embryonic vascular anastomoses (typically persistent trigeminal artery), kinking and/or ectasia of major arteries, saccular aneurysms, and progressive arterial stenoses **(40-18)**.

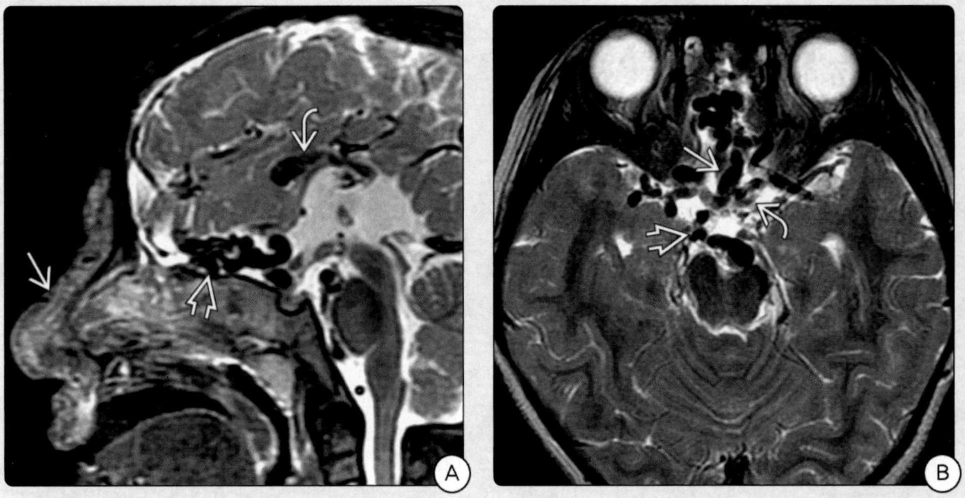

***(40-18A)** Sagittal T2WI in a 2y patient with a sternal anomaly shows an involuting facial hemangioma. Note corpus callosum hypogenesis and serpentine flow voids from an ectatic, tortuous azygous ACA. **(40-18B)** Axial T2 FS in the same case at age 4 shows marked tortuosity and ectasia of the azygous ACA and the right posterior communicating artery. The left ICA is hypoplastic.*

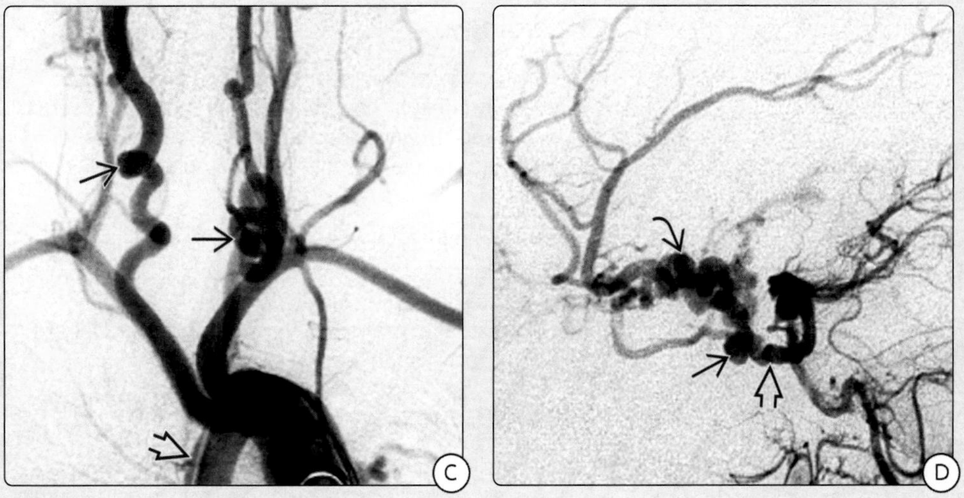

***(40-18C)** Anteroposterior DSA in the same case demonstrates extracranial vasculopathy with right aortic arch and tortuous, ectatic common carotid arteries. **(40-18D)** Lateral DSA in the same case via a right vertebral artery injection shows absent internal carotid artery, persistent trigeminal artery with saccular aneurysm, and tortuous, ectatic azygous ACA. (Courtesy C. Robson, MBChB.)*

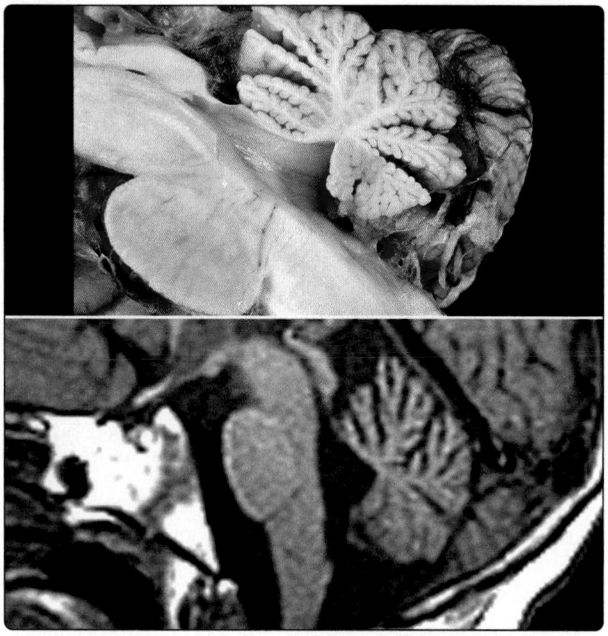

(40-19) (Top) Sagittal autopsy in ataxia-telangiectasia shows severe atrophy of vermis and cerebellum. (Bottom) 4y child with ataxia-telangiectasia shows striking vermian atrophy. (Courtesy S. Blaser, MD.)

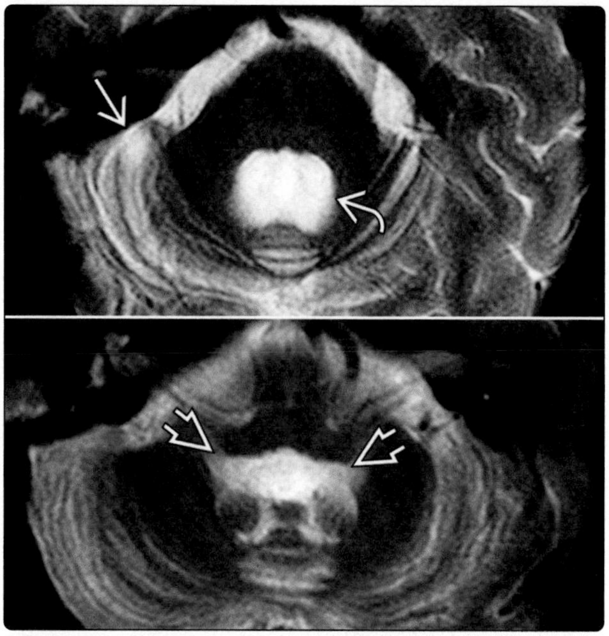

(40-20) (Top) T2WI in a 19y man with ataxia-telangiectasia shows marked cerebellar atrophy ➔, large fourth ventricle ↪. (Bottom) Note severe atrophy, enlarged lateral recesses of the 4th ventricle ⇨. The supratentorial brain was entirely normal.

PHACE(S) SYNDROME

Terminology
- **P**osterior fossa malformations
- **H**emangioma
- **A**rterial cerebrovascular anomalies
- **C**oarctation of the aorta and cardiac defects
- **E**ye abnormalities
- ± **S**ternal clefting or supraumbilical raphe

Pathology
- Hemangiomas (vascular neoplasm, not malformation)
- Ipsilateral cerebellar hypoplasia
- Posterior fossa cystic lesions (e.g., Dandy-Walker) common
- Arterial stenoses/occlusions, saccular aneurysms, aberrant vessels

Clinical Issues
- Hemangiomas proliferate, then involute

Imaging
- T1 C+ FS MR to delineate hemangiomas
- CTA/MRA to evaluate for vascular anomalies

Differential Diagnosis

The major differential diagnosis of PHACE is **Sturge-Weber syndrome** (SWS). The facial hemangioma can be (and often is) mistaken for the port-wine stain (nevus flammeus) of SWS. Patients with SWS lack the noncutaneous systemic manifestations of PHACE. The leptomeningeal angioma of SWS appears relatively thin and serpentine, covering the pial surface of the underlying dystrophic cortex, which is shrunken and contains linear calcifications. The intracranial hemangioma of PHACE usually involves the cavernous sinus and/or cerebellopontine angle, appearing more focal and mass-like.

Ataxia-Telangiectasia

Terminology and Etiology

Ataxia-telangiectasia (AT), also known as Louis-Bar syndrome, is a genetically based multisystem disorder. AT is a rare autosomal-recessive disorder characterized by progressive cerebellar atrophy and ataxia, oculocutaneous telangiectasias, immunodeficiency, radiosensitivity, and predisposition to malignancies. AT is caused by a mutation in the ataxia telangiectasia mutated gene, *ATM*. *ATM* mutations cause cells to be driven to oxidative stress and carcinogenesis.

Pathology

The major neuropathologic findings of AT occur in the cerebellum **(40-19)**. The cerebellar hemispheres and vermis show marked atrophy, reflecting the pronounced loss of Purkinje and granule cells that is the pathologic marker of this disease.

At least one-third of all AT patients develop malignancies. The most common cancers in younger patients are lymphomas and lymphoid leukemias. Nonlymphoid epithelial tumors, mainly breast and gastric carcinomas, represent 15-25% of AT-related neoplasms and develop primarily in adults.

Clinical Issues

AT patients demonstrate heterogeneous clinical manifestations. Mucocutaneous telangiectasis usually begin to appear in early childhood but may be minimal or absent.

Neurologic findings include hyperkinesia, progressive truncal and cerebellar ataxia, dysarthria, oculomotor apraxia, choreoathetosis, and progressive neurodegeneration.

Imaging and Differential Diagnosis

Diagnostic tests involving ionizing radiation should be avoided when possible to minimize the risk of mutations and subsequent tumor development, so MR is the procedure of choice for evaluating the intracranial manifestations of AT.

Initial MR in early childhood is typically normal. By the age of 10 years, cerebellar atrophy is the most consistent finding. The atrophy is initially evident in the vermis and eventually progresses to the cerebellar peduncles and hemispheres **(40-20)**.

Multiple capillary telangiectasias in the cerebral hemispheres, cerebellum, and brainstem can be seen as faint brush-like enhancing foci on T1 C+ scans or multifocal "blooming black dots" on T2* (GRE, SWI) sequences. MRS may show increased Cho in the cerebellum.

The major *clinical* differential diagnosis of AT is **cerebral palsy**. Cerebral palsy rarely involves the cerebellum. Serum α-fetoprotein (AFP) is markedly elevated in AT and helps distinguish the disorder.

Unless imaging evidence for multiple cutaneous and/or brain capillary telangiectasias is present, the cerebellar atrophy can be indistinguishable from an ever-growing number of recessive **inherited spinocerebellar degenerations with progressive ataxia**. In Freidreich ataxia—the most common—the cerebellum is generally normal, whereas the spinal cord and brainstem are atrophic. The pons is typically normal in AT. Elevated Cho on MRS may also help distinguish early AT from other forms of ataxia.

Blue Rubber Bleb Nevus Syndrome

Blue rubber bleb nevus syndrome (BRBNS) is a rare disorder characterized by multiple venous malformations. BRBNS is caused by a somatic mutation in the receptor tyrosine kinase or *TEK*, the gene encoding TIE2. *TEK* is a controller of endothelial cell assembling and remodeling that organizes the vascular network and recruits the perivascular cells necessary for stabilizing vessel walls. The same mutation also occurs in sporadic multifocal venous malformations.

BRBNS usually affects the skin, oral cavity, and gastrointestinal tract. Small raised bluish, compressible rubber- or "bleb-like" nevi are the clinical hallmarks of this disorder **(40-21)**.The most common presentation is iron deficiency anemia caused by intestinal bleeding.

CNS lesions occur in 15-20% of cases. Reported imaging manifestations include an extensive network of developmental venous anomalies with or without sinus pericranii **(40-22)** **(40-23)**.

Wyburn-Mason Syndrome

Wyburn-Mason syndrome, also known as congenital unilateral retinocephalic vascular malformation syndrome, is a rare nonhereditary neurocutaneous syndrome that presents with unilateral AVMs of the brain, orbit, and face. Craniofacial vascular malformations can involve the eyelids and orbits as well as the retina and optic nerve **(40-24)** **(40-25)**. Lesions range from barely visible to large tangles of dilated, tortuous vessels. Patients with extensive retinal AVMs are at high risk for visual loss, whereas patients with brain AVMs are at risk for parenchymal hemorrhage **(40-26)**.

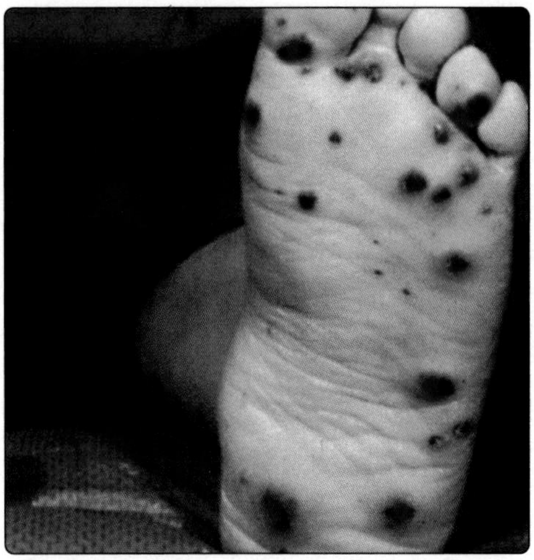

***(40-21)** Photo of a patient with BRBNS shows multiple elevated and bluish skin "blebs" on the foot. (Courtesy AFIP Archives.)*

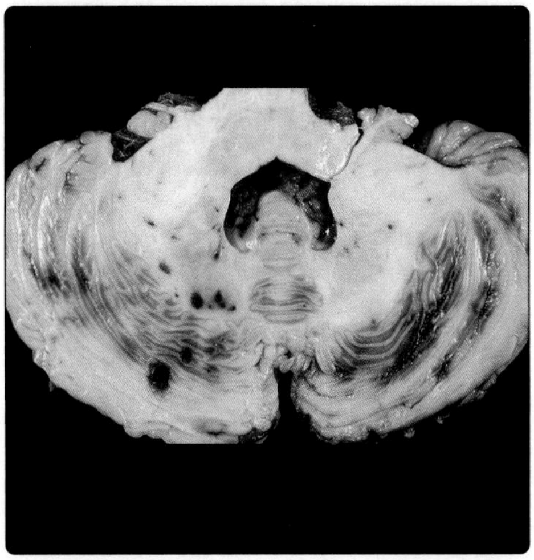

***(40-22)** Axial cut section through the cerebellum shows multiple developmental venous anomalies (DVAs) characteristic of BRBNS. (R. Hewlett, MD.)*

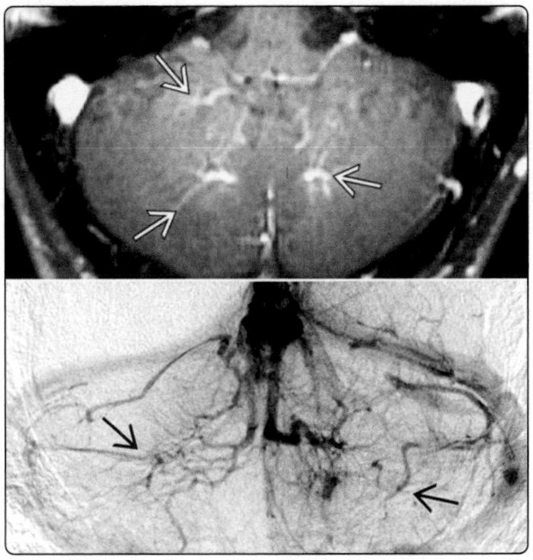

***(40-23)** (Top) T1 C+ FS scan in a patient with probable BRBNS shows bilateral enhancing DVAs ➡. (Bottom) AP DSA shows bilateral DVAs ⇨.*

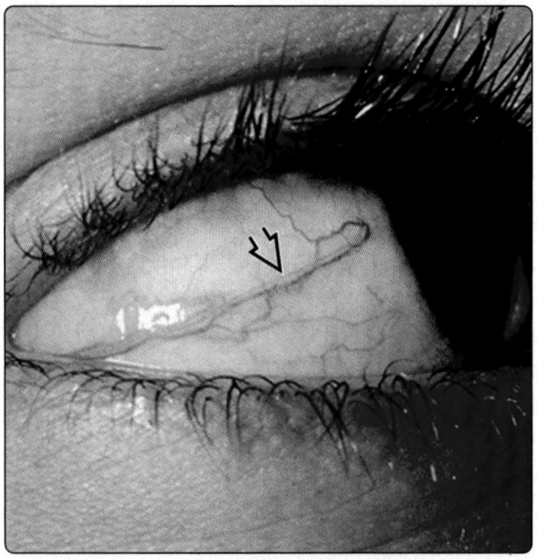

***(40-24)** Clinical photograph in a patient with Wyburn-Mason syndrome shows dilated scleral vessels ➲. (Courtesy T. P. Naidich, MD.)*

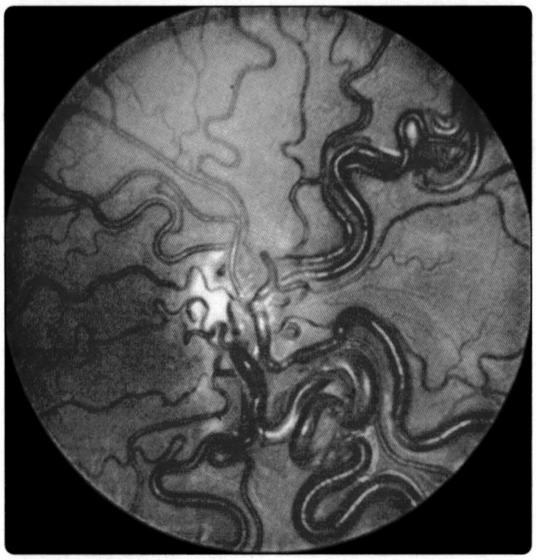

***(40-25)** Funduscopy in Wyburn-Mason syndrome shows markedly enlarged arteries, veins from retinal AVM. (Courtesy T. P. Naidich, MD.)*

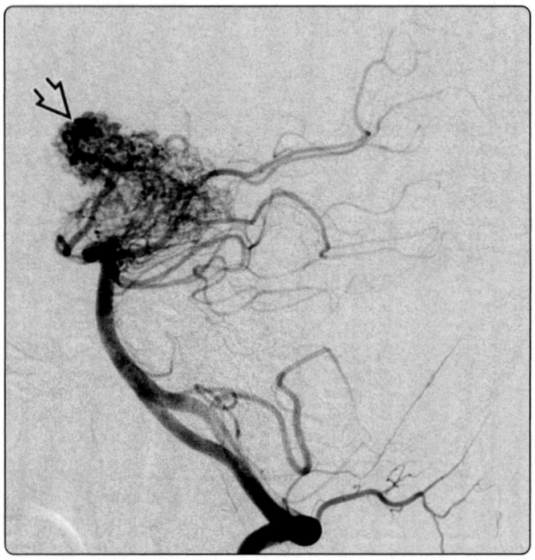

***(40-26)** DSA in probable Wyburn-Mason syndrome shows a large midbrain AVM ➲. The lesion was treated with stereotaxic radiosurgery.*

Selected References

Capillary Malformation Syndromes

Kirkorian AY et al: Genetic basis for vascular anomalies. Semin Cutan Med Surg. 35(3):128-36, 2016

Sturge-Weber Syndrome

Huang L et al: Somatic GNAQ mutation is enriched in brain endothelial cells in Sturge-Weber syndrome. Pediatr Neurol. 67:59-63, 2017

Pilli VK et al: Clinical and metabolic correlates of cerebral calcifications in Sturge-Weber syndrome. Dev Med Child Neurol. ePub, 2017

Pilli VK et al: Enlargement of deep medullary veins during the early clinical course of Sturge-Weber syndrome. Neurology. 88(1):103-105, 2017

Wetzel-Strong SE et al: The pathobiology of vascular malformations: insights from human and model organism genetics. J Pathol. 241(2):281-293, 2017

Comi AM et al: Leveraging a Sturge-Weber gene discovery: an agenda for future research. Pediatr Neurol. 58:12-24, 2016

Kirkorian AY et al: Genetic basis for vascular anomalies. Semin Cutan Med Surg. 35(3):128-36, 2016

Capillary Malformation-Arteriovenous Malformation

Banzic I et al: Parkes Weber syndrome-diagnostic and management paradigms: a systematic review. Phlebology. 32(6):371-383, 2017

Wetzel-Strong SE et al: The pathobiology of vascular malformations: insights from human and model organism genetics. J Pathol. 241(2):281-293, 2017

Other Vascular Phakomatoses

Hereditary Hemorrhagic Telangiectasia

Palagallo GJ et al: The prevalence of malformations of cortical development in a pediatric hereditary hemorrhagic telangiectasia population. AJNR Am J Neuroradiol. 38(2):383-386, 2017

Wetzel-Strong SE et al: The pathobiology of vascular malformations: insights from human and model organism genetics. J Pathol. 241(2):281-293, 2017

Brinjikji W et al: Neurovascular manifestations of hereditary hemorrhagic telangiectasia: a consecutive series of 376 patients during 15 years. AJNR Am J Neuroradiol. 37(8):1479-86, 2016

PHACE Syndrome

Mamlouk MD et al: PHACE syndrome and cerebral cavernous malformations: association or simply microhemorrhages? Childs Nerv Syst. ePub, 2017

Garzon MC et al: PHACE syndrome: consensus-derived diagnosis and care recommendations. J Pediatr. 178:24-33.e2, 2016

Winter PR et al: PHACE syndrome--clinical features, aetiology and management. Acta Paediatr. 105(2):145-53, 2016

Ataxia-Telangiectasia

Vijapura C et al: Genetic syndromes associated with central nervous system tumors. Radiographics. 37(1):258-280, 2017

Blue Rubber Bleb Nevus Syndrome

Soblet J et al: Blue rubber bleb nevus (BRBN) syndrome is caused by somatic TEK (TIE2) mutations. J Invest Dermatol. 137(1):207-216, 2017

Kirkorian AY et al: Genetic basis for vascular anomalies. Semin Cutan Med Surg. 35(3):128-36, 2016

Anomalies of the Skull and Meninges

Anomalies of the skull and meninges represent maldevelopment of the embryonic mesenchyme. These include cephaloceles, other skull base defects such as nasal gliomas or dermoids, congenital calvarial defects, and other meningeal malformations, including lipomas.

We previously discussed how the brain itself develops in Chapter 35. This final chapter of the book focuses on anomalies of the brain coverings, the skull, and meninges. We begin with skull base embryology, which is key to understanding the malformations discussed.

Normal Development and Anatomy of the Skull Base

Embryology

The skull base (SB) arises primarily from cartilaginous precursors that ossify in an orderly manner from posterior to anterior and from lateral to medial. More than 100 separate ossification centers participate in developing the definitive SB **(41-1)**.

Forehead and Nose

Prior to the eighth week of gestation, two transient but important spaces are present in the developing forehead and nose: the fonticulus frontalis and prenasal space. The **fonticulus frontalis** lies between the partially ossified frontal bone above and the nasal bones below. The **prenasal space** is a transient dura-filled structure that lies between the nasal bones and the unossified chondrocranium **(41-2A)**.

As the chondrocranium begins to ossify, it leaves some cartilage in front that later becomes the nasal capsule. By this stage, the fonticulus frontalis has closed. The prenasal space then involutes, leaving a small dural diverticulum anterior to the crista galli called the **foramen cecum**. The foramen cecum continues anteroinferiorly as a transient dura-lined channel called the **anterior neuropore**.

The foramen cecum and anterior neuropore establish a temporary connection between the anterior cranial fossa and the nose **(41-2B)**. The anterior neuropore normally regresses completely, leaving a small remnant of the foramen cecum **(41-2C)**. The foramen cecum is approximately 4 mm in diameter at birth and is normally completely ossified by 2 years of age.

Skull Base

At birth, the *anterior* skull base is composed mostly of cartilage with relatively limited ossification. Ossification of the crista galli and cribriform plate begins at 2 months and is nearly complete by 2 years of age. The foramen cecum ossifies last.

The *central* skull base forms from approximately 24 ossification centers. Major named centers include the presphenoid (planum sphenoidale), postsphenoid (basisphenoid with the posterior half of the sella, dorsum sellae, and upper clivus), alisphenoid (greater sphenoid wing), and orbitosphenoid (lesser sphenoid wing). The **intersphenoidal synchondrosis** lies between the presphenoid and the postsphenoid (basisphenoid).

The **sphenooccipital synchondrosis** lies between the basisphenoid and basiocciput. It is one of the last sutures to fuse (not completed until age 15-20 years). The embryonic **craniopharyngeal canal**—a Rathke pouch remnant—is a transient tract from the nasopharynx to the pituitary fossa that passes between chondrification centers for the developing pre- and postsphenoid bones. The craniopharyngeal canal is typically obliterated by the twelfth gestational week. It is replaced by the transient **intersphenoidal synchondrosis**, which normally closes around three postnatal months.

The *posterior* skull base consists primarily of the occipital bone, which has four major ossification centers located around the foramen magnum. In contrast to the anterior and central skull base segments, the posterior skull base is almost completely ossified by birth. However, the sutures remain unfused until the second decade. The petrooccipital and occipitomastoid sutures are among the last of all the cranial sutures to close (15-17 years).

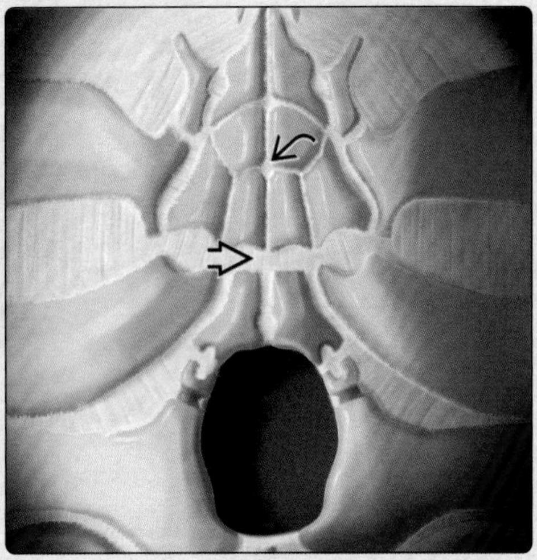

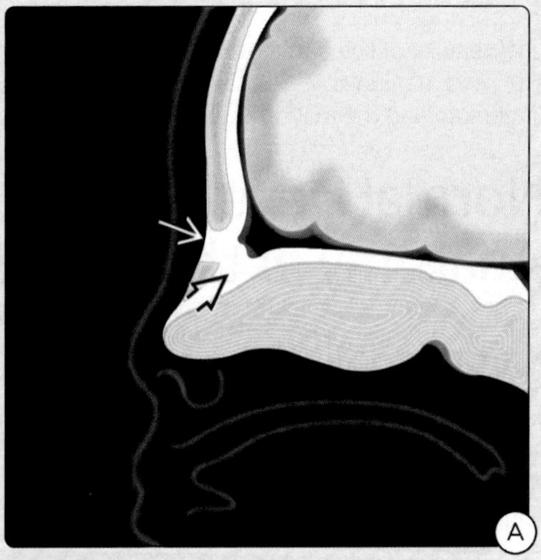

***(41-1)** Skull base ossification centers show sphenooccipital synchondrosis (between postsphenoid and basiocciput) and craniopharyngeal canal (in intersphenoidal synchondrosis, between pre- and postsphenoid). **(41-2A)** Developing dura is white; unossified chondrocranium is blue. Fonticulus frontalis lies between partially ossified frontal and nasal bones. Prenasal space is in dura, between nasal bones/cartilage.*

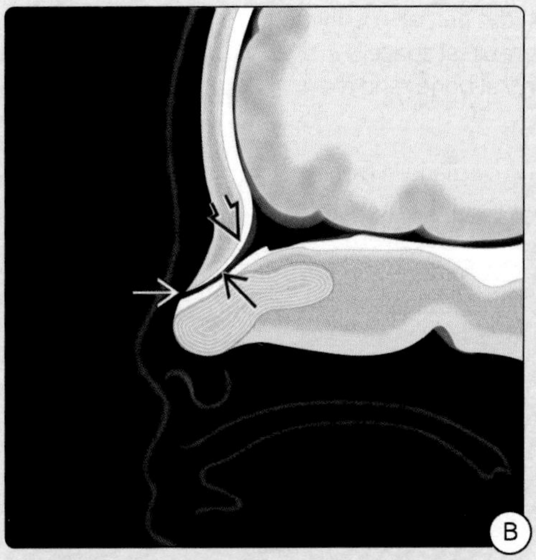

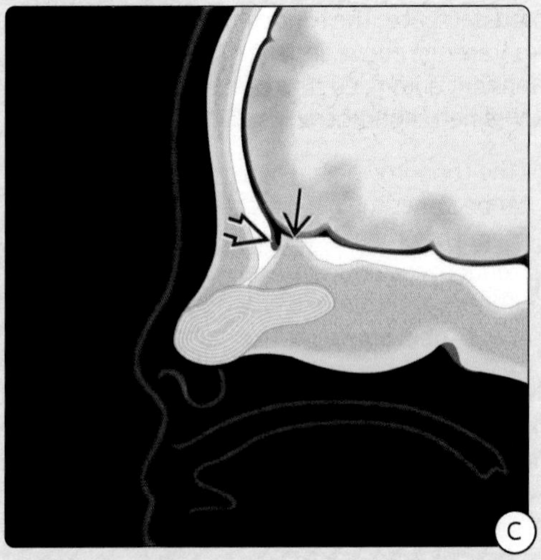

***(41-2B)** Over time, fonticulus frontalis closes. Chondrocranium is now mostly ossified. Cartilage of developing nasal capsule is blue. Prenasal space, now encased in bone and lined with dura, becomes foramen cecum. Dura-lined channel (anterior neuropore) is open at dorsum of nose. **(41-2C)** Graphic depicts a later stage of development, by which point anterior neuropore has regressed. Foramen cecum remnant and crista galli are shown.*

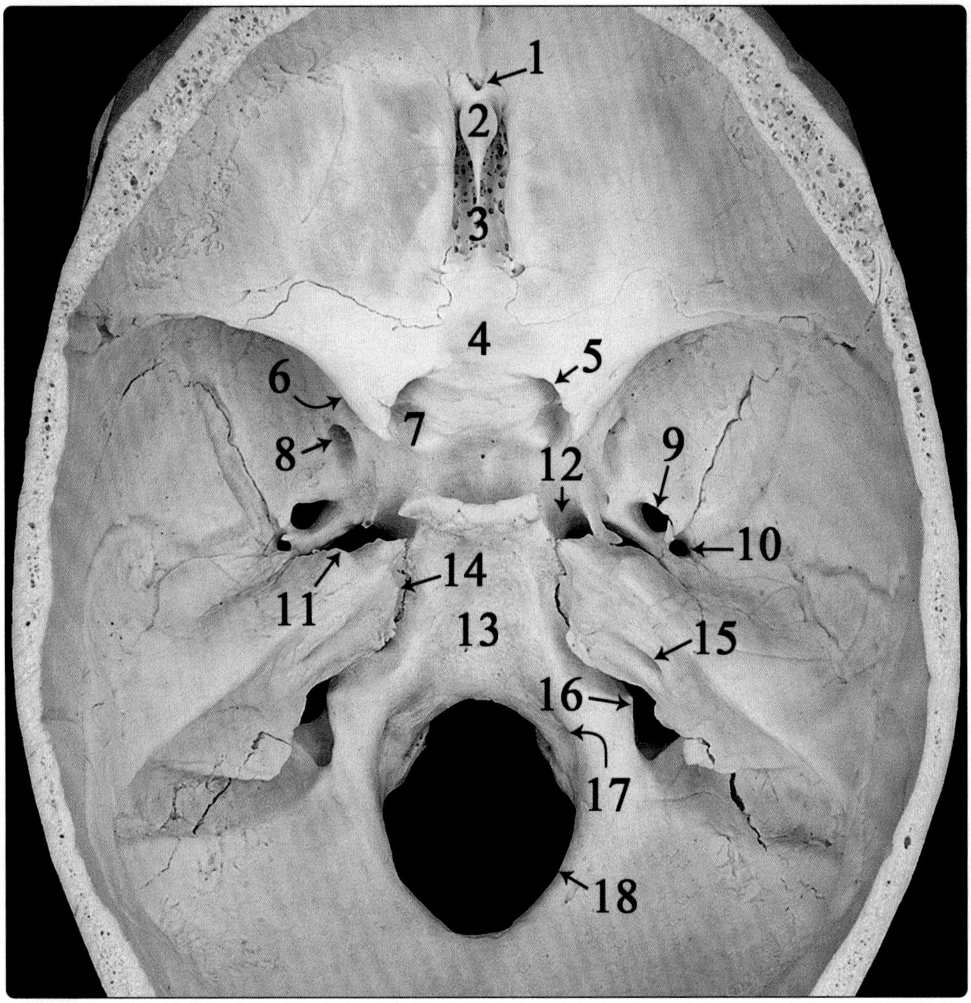

***(41-3)** Endocranial view of the adult skull shows the following: foramen cecum (1), crista galli (2), cribriform plate (3), planum sphenoidale (4), lesser sphenoid wing and optic canal (5), superior orbital fissure (6), endocranial openings of carotid canal (7, 12), foramen rotundum (8), foramen ovale (9), foramen spinosum (10), foramen lacerum (11), clivus (13), petrooccipital fissure (14), internal auditory canal (15), jugular foramen (16), jugular tubercle overlying hypoglossal canal (17), and the foramen magnum (18). (Courtesy M. Nielsen, MS.)*

Relevant Gross Anatomy

Here we briefly delineate the important aspects of the anterior and central segments of the skull base. A detailed description of cranial nerves—their origins, courses, and imaging appearances—is included in Chapter 23.

Anterior Skull Base

The *endocranial* surface of the anterior skull base (ASB) forms the floor of the anterior cranial fossae. The endocranial surface is composed of the orbital plates of the frontal bones, the ethmoid bone with its cribriform plate and sinus roof, and the lesser sphenoid wing. The *exocranial* surface of the ASB forms the orbital roofs and abuts the nose.

Important bony landmarks of the endocranial ASB are shown **(41-3)**. In this specimen, the foramen cecum (1) persists as a small bony midline pit immediately in front of the crista galli (2). The olfactory recesses with the sieve-like cribriform plate (3) lie on either side of the crista galli. A flat bony surface, the planum sphenoidale (4), extends posteriorly from the cribriform plate of the ethmoid bone to the sella turcica.

The lesser wings of the sphenoid bone overhang the optic canals (5), superior orbital fissures (6), and endocranial openings for the internal carotid arteries (7). The optic nerves and ophthalmic arteries pass through the optic canals. The superior orbital fissures transmit the superior orbital veins and oculomotor (CN III) and trochlear (CN IV) nerves, as well as ophthalmic divisions of the trigeminal nerves (CN V_1) and the abducens nerves (CN VI).

Central Skull Base

The endocranial surface of the central skull base (CSB) forms the sella turcica and medial floors of the middle cranial fossae. It is composed of the greater sphenoid wing, the basisphenoid, and the temporal bone anterior to the petrous ridge. A central depression, the sella turcica, is bordered anteriorly by the tuberculum sellae and anterior clinoid processes. The posterior border of the sella is formed by the dorsum sellae, a prominent bony projection that lies anteromedial to the petrous apices.

Important CSB foramina include the foramen rotundum (8), which transmits the maxillary division of the trigeminal nerve CN V_2, and the foramen ovale (9), which transmits the mandibular nerve CN V_3. The foramen spinosum (10) lies posterolateral to the foramen ovale. The middle meningeal artery enters the cranial cavity through the foramen spinosum.

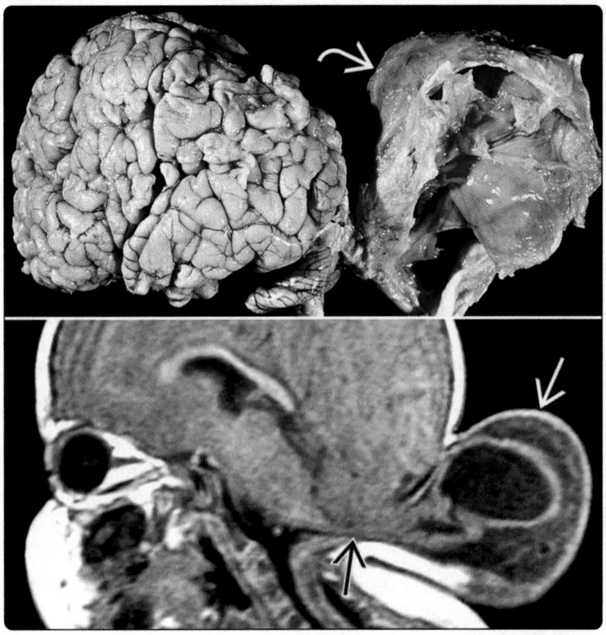

(41-4) (Top) Autopsy shows occipital cephalocele ➡, brain with pachy-/polymicrogyria. (E. T. Hedley-Whyte, MD.) (Bottom) Sagittal T1WI shows occipitocervical meningoencephalocele ➡ with traction of cervicomedullary junction ➡.

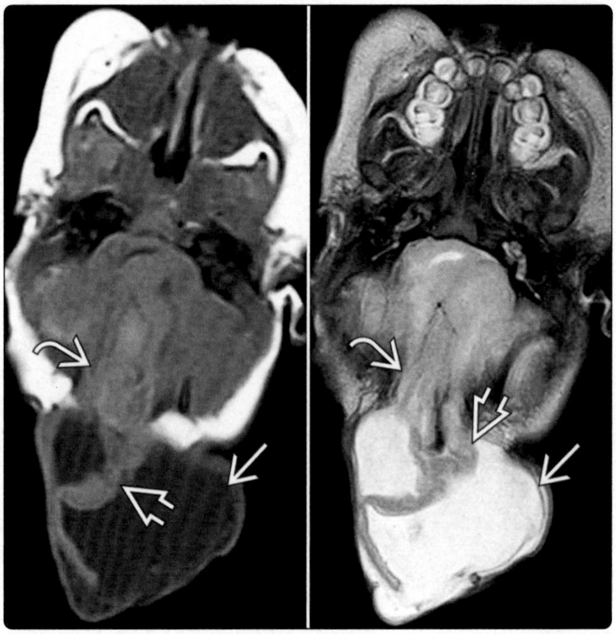

(41-5) (L) T1WI, (R) T2WI show an occipital cephalocele that contains meninges and CSF ➡ and dysplastic brain ➡. Note traction and distortion of the cerebellum ➡.

The foramen lacerum (11) is an irregular cartilage-filled aperture that lies between the sphenoid bone and petrous apex. The internal carotid arteries exit the petrous temporal bone at the endocranial carotid canal (12). The dorsum sellae continues posteroinferiorly as the upper part of a smooth concavity, the clivus (13).

Posterior Skull Base

The posterior skull base (PSB) is formed by the temporal bones posterior to the petrous ridges and the occipital bone. The petrooccipital fissure (14) lies between the petrous apex and the occipital bone.

The internal acoustic meatus (15) lies along the posterior aspect of the petrous temporal bone and transmits the facial (CN VII) and vestibulocochlear nerves (CN VIII) as well as the labyrinthine artery, which is a small branch of the anterior inferior cerebellar artery.

The jugular foramen (16) lies below the internal acoustic meatus. The jugular foramen transmits CNs IX-XI, the jugular bulb, and the inferior petrosal sinus. The hypoglossal canal (17) transmits CN XII. The foramen magnum (18) contains the medulla, both vertebral arteries, and the spinal segment of CN XI.

Cephaloceles

"Cephalocele" is a generic term for the protrusion of intracranial contents through a calvarial or skull base defect. Cephaloceles that contain herniations of brain tissue, meninges, and CSF are called **meningoencephaloceles**. If the meninges and accompanying CSF are herniated *without* brain tissue, the lesion is termed a **meningocele**.

An **atretic cephalocele** is a small defect that contains just dura, fibrous tissue, and degenerated brain tissue. Atretic cephaloceles most commonly occur at the obelion (along the sagittal suture on a level with the parietal foramina). A **gliocele** is a glia-lined pouch that contains only CSF.

Cephaloceles can be congenital or acquired lesions. They are generally classified by location and are named according to the roof and floor of the bone(s) through which they herniate. They can be open or skin-covered. Most congenital cephaloceles have coexisting intracranial abnormalities of varying severity. Cephalocele prevalence and type vary significantly with geographic location and ethnicity.

Cephalocele imaging has four goals: (1) depict the osseous defect, (2) delineate the sac and define its contents, (3) map the course of adjacent arteries and determine the integrity of the dural venous sinuses, and (4) identify any coexisting anomalies.

CT should be avoided when investigating frontonasal masses or suspected sphenoethmoidal cephaloceles in the central skull base during the first 18 months of life. This helps reduce both false positive and false negative examinations during a time of active ossification. The imaging modality of choice is MR with a small FOV (10 or 12 cm).

We now discuss four of the most common forms of cephalocele: occipital, frontoethmoidal, parietal, and skull base cephaloceles.

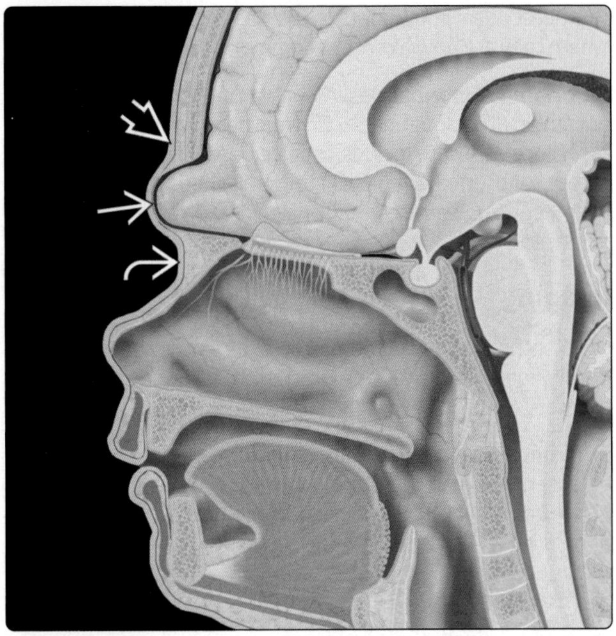

***(41-6)** Graphic depicts frontonasal cephalocele with brain herniating ➡ through a patent fonticulus frontalis between the frontal bone above ➡ and nasal bone ➡ below.*

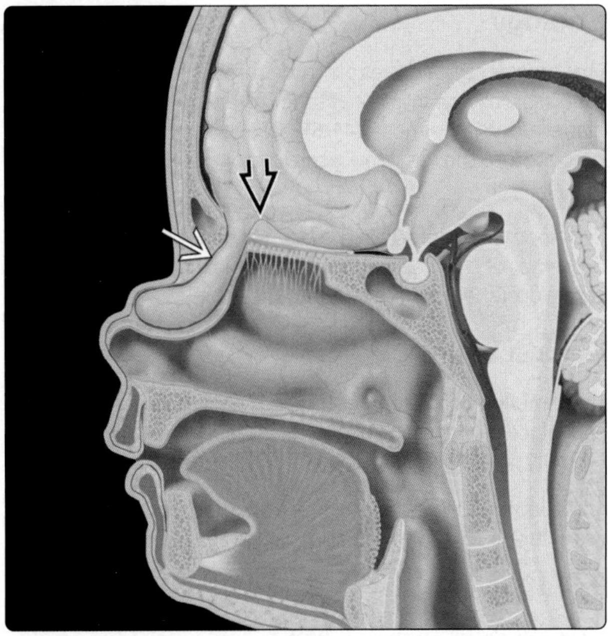

***(41-7)** Graphic demonstrates nasoethmoidal cephalocele with brain ➡ herniating into the nose through a patent foramen cecum in front of the crista galli ➡.*

Occipital Cephaloceles

Terminology and Classification

Three subtypes of occipital cephalocele are recognized and identified according to the involved bone(s). From most to least extensive, they are **occipitocervical** (involving the occipital bone, foramen magnum, and neural arches of the upper cervical spine) **(41-4)**, **low occipital** (involving the occipital bone and foramen magnum), and **high occipital** (involving the occipital bone only).

Clinical Issues

Occipital cephaloceles account for 75% of cephaloceles in European and North American Caucasians. There is a 2.4:1 male predominance.

Occipital cephaloceles are almost always recognized at birth as a variably sized occipital or suboccipital soft tissue mass. The affected infant is often microcephalic with visible craniofacial disproportion. Neurodevelopmental outcome is related to cephalocele size and contents as well as the presence and type of associated abnormalities.

Imaging

Bone CT with 3D reconstruction delineates the osseous defect well, and multiplanar MR best depicts the sac and its contents. The herniated brain—which can derive from both supra- and infratentorial structures—is always abnormal, appearing dysmorphic, disorganized, and dysplastic **(41-5)**. Depending on the size of the cephalocele, severe traction and distortion of the brainstem and supratentorial structures can be present. Dura and CSF-filled structures (including the fourth ventricle and sometimes part of the lateral ventricles) are often contained within the sac. In addition to delineating the sac and its contents, identifying the course and integrity of the dural venous sinuses is essential for preoperative planning.

At least half of all patients with occipital cephaloceles have associated abnormalities such as callosal dysgenesis, cerebellar malformations (including Chiari 2 and Dandy-Walker spectrum disorders), and gray matter heterotopias.

Frontoethmoidal Cephaloceles

Terminology and Classification

Frontoethmoidal cephaloceles are also called **sincipital cephaloceles**. In frontoethmoidal cephaloceles, brain parenchyma herniates through a persisting dural projection into the midface, typically the forehead, dorsum of the nose, or orbit.

There are three subtypes of frontoethmoidal cephaloceles. The **frontonasal** subtype is most common, representing 40-60% of frontoethmoidal cephaloceles.

In the **nasoethmoidal** subtype (30%), the sac herniates through a midline foramen cecum defect into the prenasal space.

The least common subtype is **nasoorbital** (10%). Here the cephalocele herniates through the maxilla and lacrimal bone into the inferomedial orbit.

Etiology

Frontonasal cephaloceles protrude through an unobliterated *fonticulus frontalis* into the anterior forehead at the glabella/dorsum of nose **(41-6)**. Nasoethmoidal cephaloceles herniate into the nasal cavity through a *patent foramen cecum* **(41-7)**.

Developmental defects in the lacrimal bones and frontal processes of the maxillary bones result in a nasoorbital cephalocele, which herniates into the orbit.

Clinical Issues

Epidemiology and Demographics. Frontoethmoidal cephaloceles represent 10-15% of all cephaloceles and are typically present at birth. There is no sex predilection.

Frontoethmoidal cephaloceles are the most common type of cephalocele seen in southeast Asia and among ethnic southeast Asian immigrants to the United States and Europe, where they are now almost as common as the occipital type.

Associated Abnormalities. Associated abnormalities are present in 80% of patients with frontoethmoidal cephaloceles. These include hypertelorism and eye anomalies, corpus callosum dysgenesis, interhemispheric lipomas, hydrocephalus, seizures, neuronal migration anomalies, and microcephaly.

Imaging

NECT scans show a well-demarcated, heterogeneous, mixed-density mass that extends extracranially through a bony defect.

In a **frontonasal cephalocele**, brain herniates into the forehead between the frontal bones above and the nasal bones below **(41-8)**. In the **nasoethmoidal** type, the nasal bone is bowed anteriorly by the cephalocele, and the crista

***(41-8A)** 3D CT soft tissue reconstruction in a newborn with a frontonasal encephalocele shows a large mass → protruding anteriorly between the eyes. **(41-8B)** 3D reformatted bone CT shows a well-delineated frontonasal bony defect → just above the bridge of the nose.*

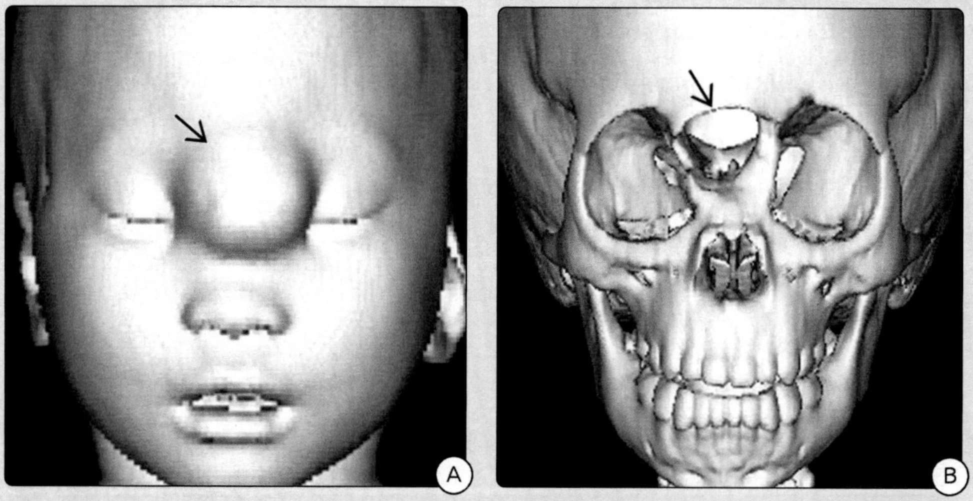

***(41-8C)** Sagittal T1WI in same patient shows the skin-covered soft tissue mass → protrudes through a patent fonticulus frontalis →. Note absence of corpus callosum with "high-riding" third ventricle, azygous anterior cerebral artery →. Chiari 1 malformation with tonsillar herniation → is also present. **(41-8D)** T2WI shows cephalocele is mostly dysplastic brain →. Note arachnoid cyst →, polymicrogyria →. (Courtesy M. Michel, MD.)*

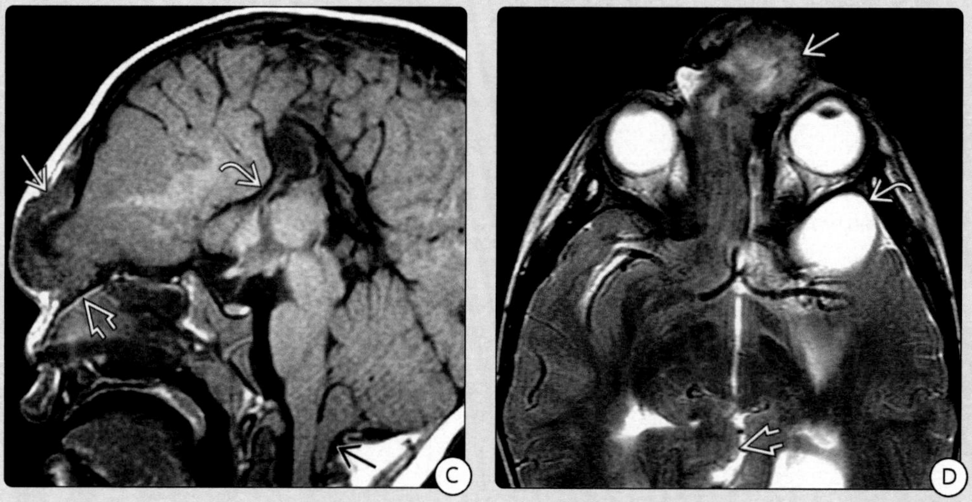

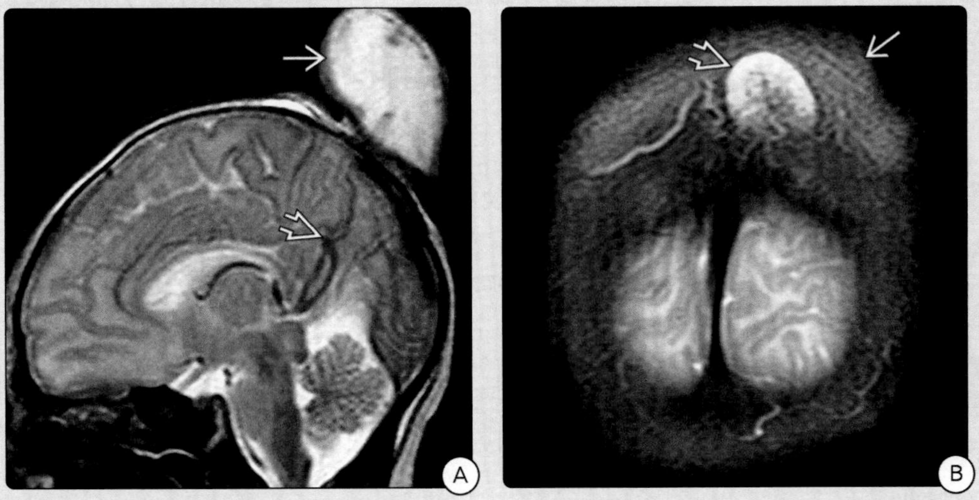

***(41-9A)** Sagittal T2WI shows classic parietal cephalocele ➡ in the midline over the posterior vertex. The cephalocele is associated with a falcine sinus ➡. (Courtesy G. Hedlund, DO.) **(41-9B)** Coronal T2WI in another case shows a scalp mass ➡ with underlying parietal cephalocele ➡. (Courtesy K. Moore, MD.)*

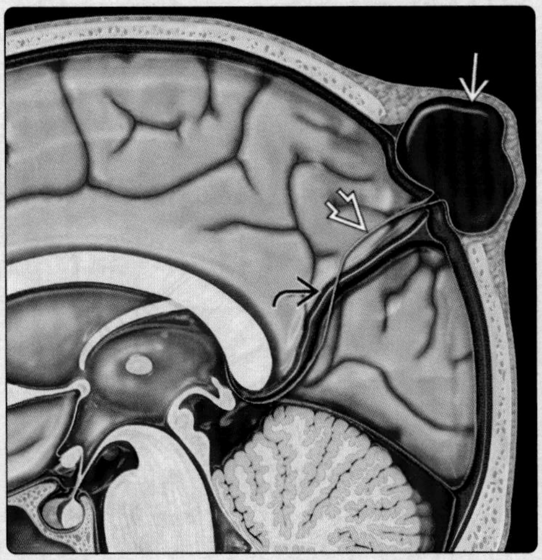

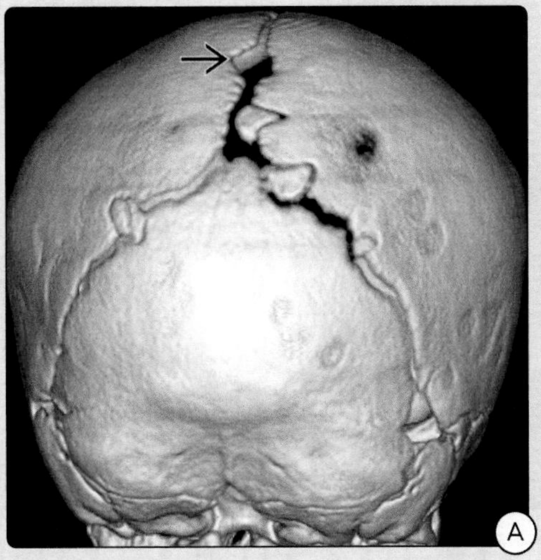

***(41-10)** Sagittal graphic demonstrates a skin-covered atretic parietal cephalocele ➡ associated with a dura-lined sinus tract ➡ and a persistent falcine sinus ➡. **(41-11A)** 3D rendered bone CT in a child with an atretic parietal cephalocele demonstrates a small, well-demarcated midline skull defect ➡.*

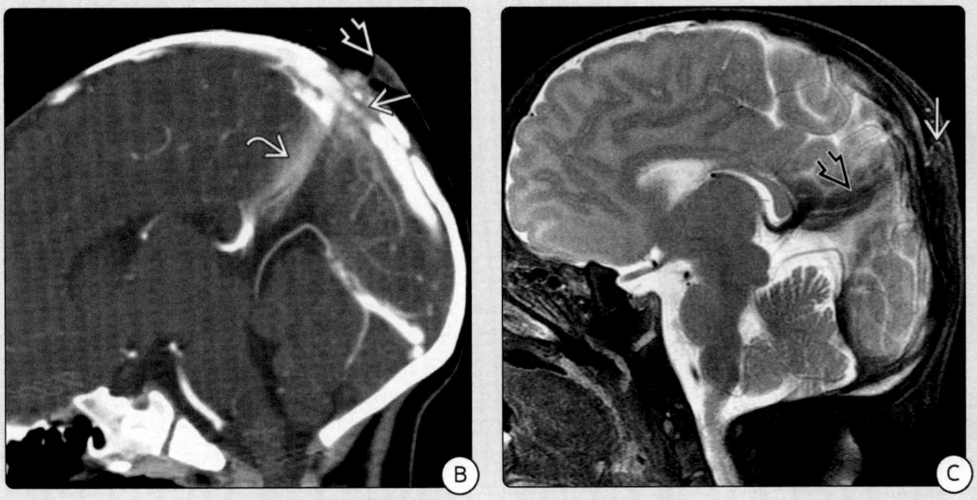

***(41-11B)** CTA in the same patient shows persistent falcine sinus ➡ and atretic cephalocele ➡ passing between the split superior sagittal sinus ➡. **(41-11C)** Sagittal T2WI in the same patient demonstrates the persistent falcine sinus ➡ and a tiny atretic cephalocele ➡. (All three images courtesy K. Moore, MD.)*

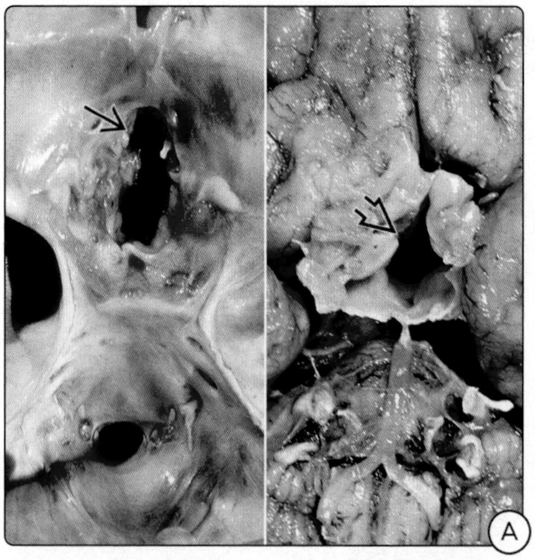

(41-12A) Autopsy of sphenoethmoidal cephalocele shows central skull base defect ⇒. Basal view of brain shows the cephalocele sac ⇒.

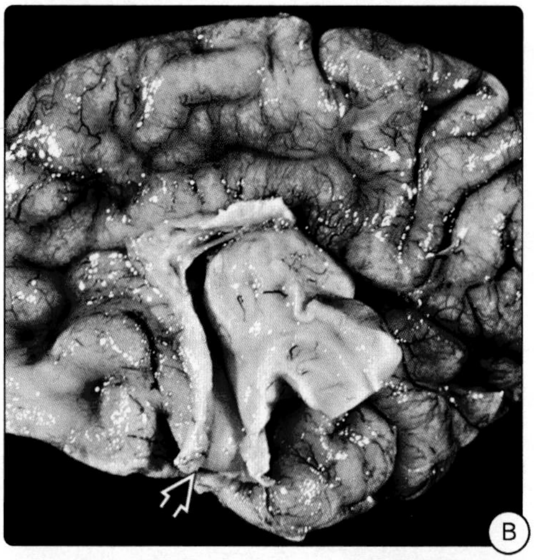

(41-12B) Sagittal view shows the cephalocele ⇒, pachygyria, and corpus callosum dysplasia. (Courtesy E. T. Hedley-Whyte, MD.)

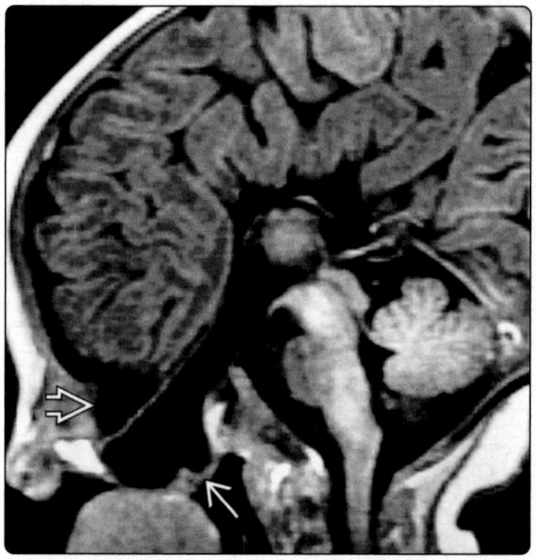

(41-13) Sagittal T1WI shows sphenoethmoidal cephalocele ⇒. Hypothalamus and anterior third ventricle ➡ are retracted into the sac.

galli is posterior to the defect. The cribriform plate is deficient or absent; the crista galli may be absent or bifid. A **nasoorbital cephalocele** protrudes inferomedially into the orbit through a defect in the lacrimal/frontal process of the maxillary bone.

MR shows a soft tissue mass in direct contiguity with the intracranial parenchyma. The mass is usually heterogeneous in signal intensity but mostly appears isointense with cortex. It does not enhance following contrast administration.

Differential Diagnosis

The major differential diagnoses of a frontoethmoidal cephalocele are nasal dermal sinus with or without associated dermoids/epidermoids and nasal cerebral heterotopia (nasal "glioma"). All three lesions present clinically as midline nasal masses. All three have similar embryologic origin (i.e., the dura that normally extends through the embryonic foramen cecum between the developing nasal bone and nasal cartilage fails to regress).

A **nasal dermal sinus** is seen clinically as a small dimple or pit on the nose. It is the opening of a dermal-lined sinus tract that extends intracranially for a variable distance. A dermoid or epidermoid cyst can develop anywhere along the tract. Nasal dermal sinuses have an epithelial lining and do not contain brain parenchyma.

A **nasal glioma** is a congenital nonneoplastic heterotopia that consists of dysplastic glial tissue. Most nasal gliomas are extranasal (60%), located along the dorsum of the nose. Approximately one-third are intranasal, lying under the nasal bones. MR scans show no connection between the mass and intracranial contents.

Parietal Cephaloceles

Parietal cephaloceles comprise just 5-10% of all cephaloceles. Most have significant underlying brain and vascular anomalies, such as a persistent falcine sinus, sinus pericranii, and/or partial absence of the straight sinus.

MR without and with contrast enhancement is best to delineate parietal cephalocele contents **(41-9)**. Because of the proximity to the superior sagittal sinus, it is important to delineate the position of all dural sinuses and adjacent cortical draining veins with MRV, CTV, or DSA prior to surgery.

A number of parietal cephaloceles are termed **atretic cephaloceles** (APCs), small lesions that typically present as midline scalp masses near the posterior vertex **(41-10)**. They have been associated with maternal folate deficiency and valproic acid use. APCs have limited defects in the skull that are best visualized on 3D bone CT. They are often associated with a persistent falcine sinus and frequently split the superior sagittal sinus **(41-11)**.

Skull Base Cephaloceles

Skull base cephaloceles account for 10% of all cephaloceles. They result from developmental failure of proper skull base ossification, which in turn allows migration of neural crest cells and their derivatives through the bony defect.

Skull base cephaloceles can be midline or off-midline (lateral) and are subtyped according to which bony component(s) they involve. There are three types of midline skull base cephaloceles. **Sphenopharyngeal** cephaloceles involve just the sphenoid body, whereas **sphenoethmoidal** lesions affect both the sphenoid and ethmoid bones **(41-12)**. **Transethmoidal** cephaloceles herniate through the cribriform plate.

Lateral basal cephaloceles can be **sphenomaxillary** (orbital fissure plus maxillary sinus with herniation into the pterygopalatine fossa) or **sphenoorbital** (through the sphenoid bone into the orbit).

Occasionally, **middle cranial fossa arachnoid granulations** are seen as multiple focal outpouchings (arachnoid "pits") in the greater sphenoid ala. These skull base defects can be associated with CSF leak or skull base cephalocele.

Imaging of skull base cephaloceles is essential to delineate the sac contents completely. The pituitary gland, optic nerves and chiasm, hypothalamus, and third ventricle can all be displaced inferiorly into the cephalocele **(41-13)**.

Intracranial anomalies are frequent findings in association with skull base cephaloceles. Midline anomalies such as corpus callosum dysgenesis and an azygous anterior cerebral artery are common.

Persistent Craniopharyngeal Canal

Terminology

Persistent craniopharyngeal canal (PCPC) is also known as persistent hypophyseal or basipharyngeal canal.

Etiology and Clinical Issues

PCPC is a rare developmental anomaly with a persistent tract in the intersphenoidal synchondrosis **(41-14)** that extends from the nasopharynx to the bottom of the pituitary fossa. It is usually small, uncomplicated, and noted incidentally on imaging studies or at autopsy. However, occasionally PCPCs can present as large complex skull base lesions with cysts, cephaloceles, midline craniofacial malformations, or pituitary anomalies. Some cases have been linked to genetic defects in *SOX3,* an early developmental transcription factor involved in pituitary development.

Imaging

High-resolution bone CT with 3D reformatted images best delineates the skull base abnormality. Most PCPCs are small, typically less than 1.5 mm in diameter. A larger lesion appears as a smoothly marginated cylindrical or ovoid midline bony "canal" extending obliquely downward from the sellar floor to the nasopharynx.

MR findings depend on the contents within the canal. Small, uncomplicated PCPCs may be difficult to identify. Larger lesions show variable signal intensity within the canal itself. Coronal images sometimes show the adenohypophysis sitting on the top of the PCPC, resembling a "golf ball on a tee."

Associated anomalies of the midface (e.g., hypertelorism, cleft palate, and sphenopharyngeal cephaloceles) or pituitary gland/stalk (e.g., duplicated gland, ectopic adenoma, and hypothalamic hamartoma) are common.

Differential Diagnosis

The major differential diagnosis of PCPC is a **sphenooccipital synchondrosis**, a linear developmental cleft between the basisphenoid and basiocciput. The sphenooccipital synchondrosis gradually decreases in size with increasing age and usually disappears by adulthood. It lies *behind* the dorsum sellae; a PCPC lies *in front of* the dorsum **(41-16)**.

A **persistent medial basal canal** is a developmental variant of the lower clivus and occurs posteroinferior to the sphenooccipital synchondrosis **(41-15)**.

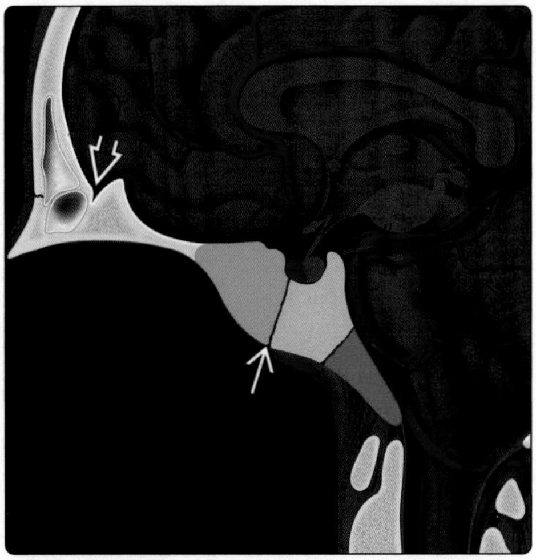

***(41-14)** Presphenoid (green), postsphenoid with basisphenoid (yellow), basiocciput (red), foramen cecum, and intersphenoid synchondrosis.*

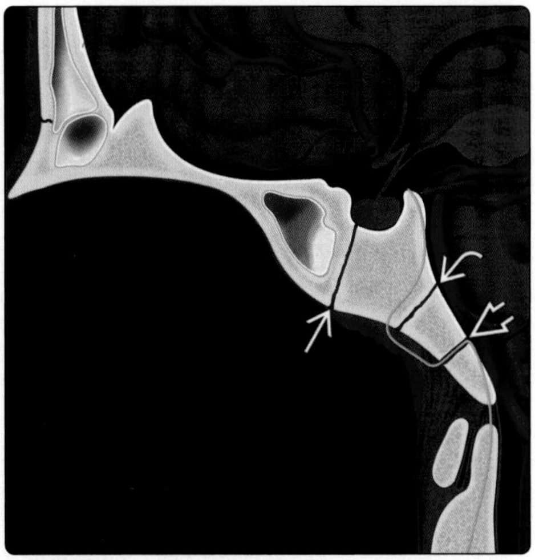

***(41-15)** Intersphenoid and sphenooccipital synchondroses and notochord migration path (green) forming medial basal canal are shown.*

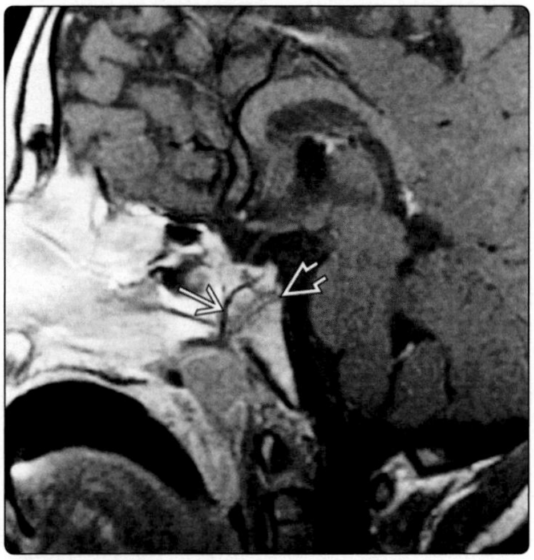

***(41-16)** Sagittal T1WI shows persistent craniopharyngeal canal and sphenooccipital synchondrosis posterior to the PCPC.*

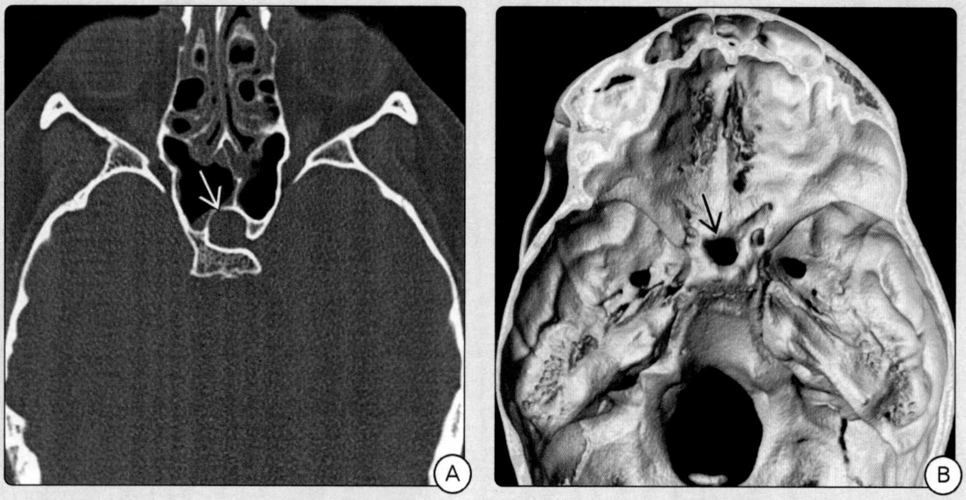

***(41-17A)** Axial bone CT in a 22y woman with chronic diabetes insipidus and headaches demonstrates a persistent craniopharyngeal canal (PCPC), seen here as a smoothly marginated, well-demarcated defect in the central basisphenoid ➡. **(41-17B)** 3D reformatted image nicely shows the PCPC ➡ and its relationship to other structures in the central skull base.*

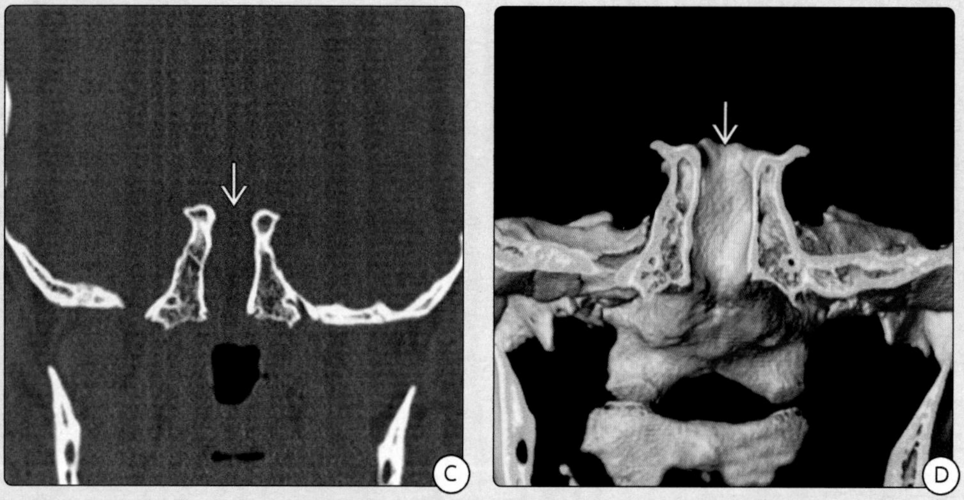

***(41-17C)** Coronal bone CT shows the enlarged PCPC appearing as an elongated tube ➡ that connects the sella with the nasopharynx. **(41-17D)** Coronal 3D bone CT elegantly demonstrates the cylindrical shape of the PCPC ➡.*

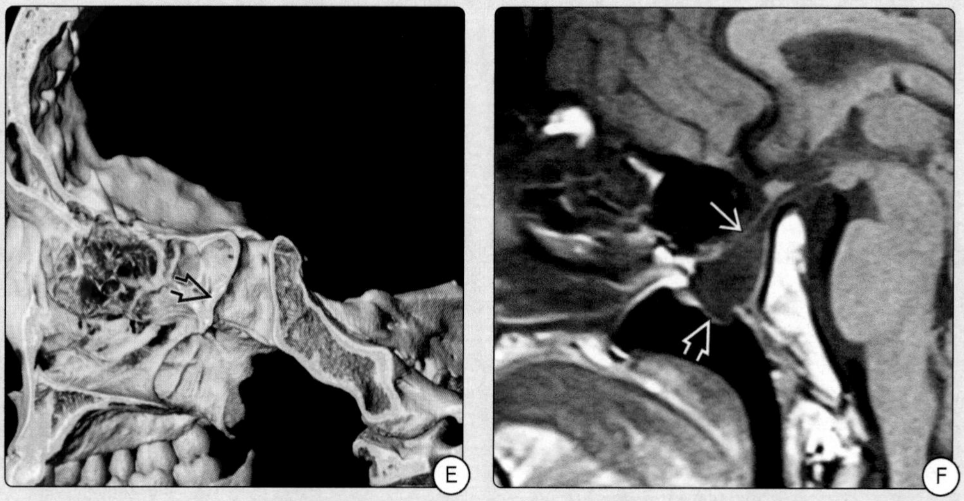

***(41-17E)** Sagittal 3D rendering of the bone CT shows that the PCPC appears to widen slightly ➡ as it approaches the upper aerodigestive tract. **(41-17F)** Sagittal T1-weighted MR shows a sphenoidal cephalocele ➡ traversing the PCPC and bulging into the roof of the nasopharynx ➡. (All six images courtesy P. Chapman, MD.)*

CEPHALOCELES

Occipital Cephaloceles
- Most common in European/North American Caucasians
- 75% of cephaloceles, M:F = 2.4:1
- Typically contains dysplastic brain

Frontoethmoidal Cephaloceles
- 10-15% of cephaloceles
- Southeast Asian predominance
- Frontonasal (40-60%)
  - Through fonticulus frontalis into forehead
- Nasoethmoidal (30%)
  - Through patent foramen cecum into nose
- Nasoorbital (10%)
  - Through lacrimal bone/maxilla into orbit

Parietal Cephaloceles
- 5-10% of cephaloceles
- Most are atretic
  - Associated with falcine sinus, sinus pericranii

Skull Base Cephaloceles
- 10% of cephaloceles
- Brain anomalies common (e.g., callosal dysgenesis)

Persistent Craniopharyngeal Canal
- Less than 1%, usually incidental finding
- Large complex lesions rare
  - Associated with pituitary anomalies
  - May have sphenoidal cephalocele

Craniosynostoses

Craniosynostosis Overview

Terminology

Craniosynostosis is also known as **craniostenosis, sutural synostosis**, and **cranial dysostosis**. The craniosynostoses are a heterogeneous group of disorders characterized by abnormal head shape. Craniosynostosis can be nonsyndromic (70-75% of cases) or syndromic.

Etiology

The calvaria normally expands during infancy and early childhood to accommodate the growing brain. This mostly occurs at narrow seams of undifferentiated mesenchyme—the cranial sutures—that lie between adjacent bones. Compared with most major embryonic structures such as the brain and cardiovascular systems, the cranial sutures form relatively late (at around 16 weeks of gestation).

Normal sutures permit skull growth perpendicular to their long axis. As long as the brain grows rapidly, the calvaria expands. As brain growth slows, the sutures close.

The normal order of closure is metopic first, followed by the coronal and then the lambdoid sutures. The sagittal suture normally closes last. Craniostenosis occurs when osseous obliteration of one or more sutures occurs prematurely.

Skull distortion occurs from a combination of (1) restriction of skull growth perpendicular to the prematurely fused suture and (2) compensatory overgrowth at the nonfused sutures.

Clinical Issues

Craniosynostosis can be associated with neurological and/or vascular compromise. Severe deformities can be cosmetically disfiguring and socially stigmatizing. Precisely when the anatomical and functional anomalies become clinically relevant varies from patient to patient and thus requires a tailored approach to treatment.

Imaging

Imaging plays an essential role in recognition of craniosynostoses, identification of coexisting brain anomalies, preoperative treatment planning, and postoperative follow-up.

Craniosynostoses can be nonsyndromic or syndromic and may affect a single suture or multiple sutures. In this section, we discuss representative examples of each type.

Nonsyndromic Craniosynostosis

Terminology and Etiology

Nonsyndromic craniosynostoses (NCSs) are genetically determined lesions that occur in the absence of a recognizable syndrome.

The genetic component is believed to be suture specific. For example, genome-wide association studies have identified strong and reproducible associations between sagittal NCS and *BMP2* and *BBS9,* whereas gene mutations are relatively rare in metopic NCS.

Coronal NCS has a stronger genetic component compared with other forms. Several diverse genes include *FGFR3*, *TWIST1*, *EFNB1*, and *TCF12* (which are also associated with syndromic forms of craniosynostosis). The genetic basis of lambdoid NCS—the rarest type—is unknown.

Pathology

Location. Approximately 60% of all single-suture craniosynostosis cases involve premature fusion of the sagittal suture, followed in frequency by those that involve the coronal (22%) and metopic (15%) sutures. Lambdoid craniosynostosis is very rare, causing just 2% of all cases.

Classification. Craniosynostosis is generally classified by head shape as **scaphocephaly** or dolichocephaly (long and narrow) **(41-18)**, **brachycephaly** (broad and flattened) **(41-21)**, **trigonocephaly** (triangular at the front) **(41-19)**, or **plagiocephaly** (skewed) **(41-20)**.

Gross Pathology. Gross examination shows fibrous or bony sutural "bridging." Focal synostosis or diffuse bony "beaking" along the affected suture are typical findings.

CRANIOSYNOSTOSIS: ETIOLOGY AND PATHOLOGY

Normal Suture Development
- Late (16 weeks' gestation)
- Metopic closes first, then coronal, then lambdoid
- Sagittal closes last

Pathology
- Location
  - Sagittal (60%, most common single suture)
  - Coronal (22%)
  - Metopic (15%)
  - Lambdoid (2%)
  - Multiple (5%)
- Gross pathology
  - Suture obliterated by diffuse or focal bony "beaking"

Clinical Issues

Epidemiology. The overall prevalence of craniosynostosis is estimated at 1:2,000-2,500 live births.

Sporadic (nonsyndromic) craniosynostoses are more common than syndrome-associated cases, accounting for 75% of all craniosynostoses. Between 85-90% of these involve only a single suture, whereas 5-15% are multisuture synostoses.

Demographics. Sex varies with craniostenosis type. Both scaphocephaly and trigonocephaly have a moderate male predominance (M:F = 3.1:1 and M:F = 2:1, respectively).

Presentation. Most craniosynostoses—even syndromic ones—are not detected during pregnancy. Affected infants generally present during the first year of life. The most common presentation is unusual head shape with craniofacial asymmetry.

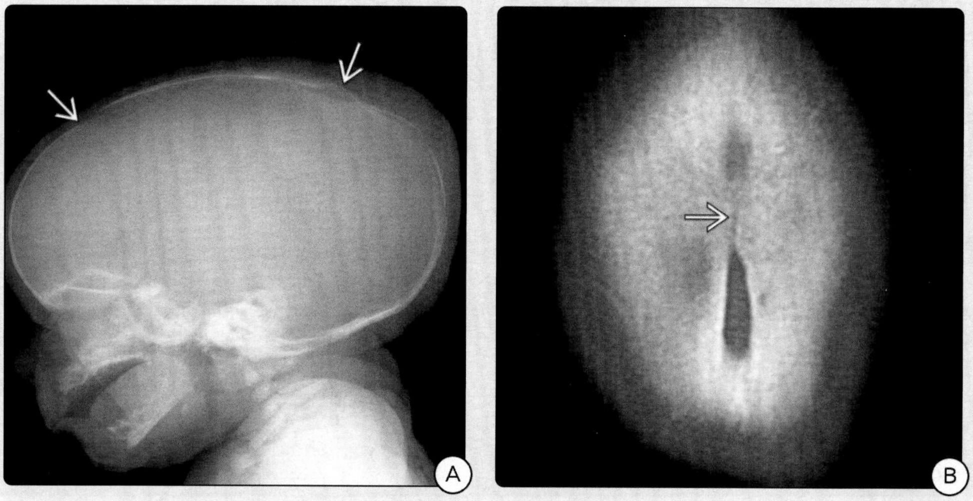

***(41-18A)** Lateral radiograph of a newborn shows pronounced scaphocephaly with unusually severe elongation of the calvaria in the anteroposterior plane →. **(41-18B)** Bone CT in the same patient shows the elongated configuration of the skull. Note severe narrowing with almost complete obliteration of the superior sagittal suture →.*

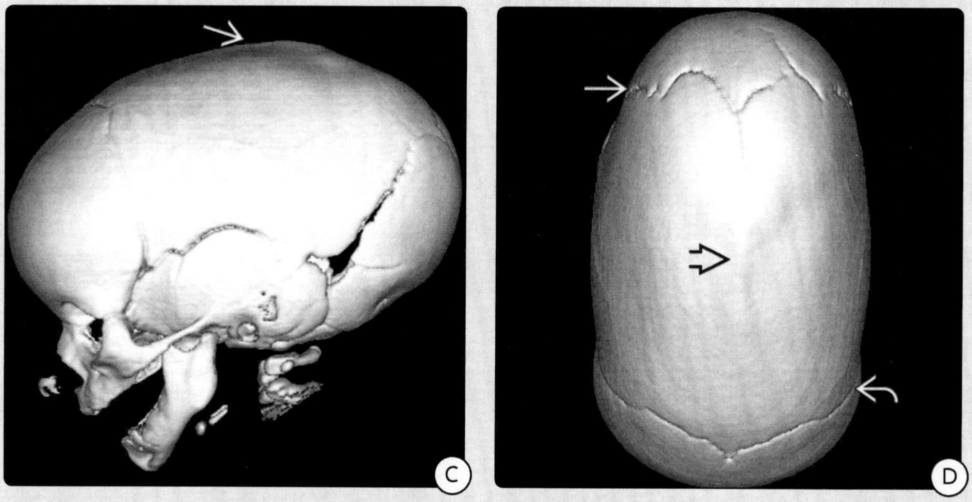

***(41-18C)** Bone CT with 3D shaded surface display (SSD) in the same patient shows pronounced elongation of the skull. Note ridge of bone along the vertex → that resembles the keel of a ship. **(41-18D)** Coronal 3D SSD in the same patient shows normal-appearing coronal → and lambdoid ↩ sutures. The sagittal suture is completely fused and demonstrates the elevated midline ridge of bone ⇨, characteristic of scaphocephaly. (Courtesy K. Moore, MD.)*

Natural History. Severe deformities may lead to hydrocephalus, elevated intracranial pressure, compromised cerebral blood flow, and airway obstruction.

Treatment Options. Mild deformities are sometimes treated with physiotherapy and head repositioning or orthotic helmet. Severe skull deformities may require one or more surgeries to remodel the cranial vault.

Imaging

General Features. Digital radiographs are sufficient to identify simple single-suture craniosynostoses. However, in addition to identifying the deformity and affected suture, preoperative planning requires careful imaging assessment of calvarial and dural venous sinus anatomy. Delineating associated intra- and extracranial abnormalities is especially important in evaluating patients with multiple or syndromic synostoses.

CT Findings. Although the diagnosis of cranial synostosis can be made clinically or on plain film radiographs, thin-section CT scans with multiplanar reconstruction and 3D shaded surface display (SSD) are invaluable for detailed evaluation and preoperative planning. However, the radiologist should always rely heavily on "CT source data" rather than surface-rendered images to avoid false positive diagnoses!

Head shape generally predicts which suture(s) will be abnormal, but CT is required to determine whether part or all of the affected suture(s) is fused.

Scaphocephaly. Scaphocephaly, also known as dolichocephaly, is caused by sagittal suture synostosis. Patients with scaphocephaly demonstrate an elongated skull with decreased transverse and increased AP measurements. Forehead bossing is common. In severe cases, the sagittal suture is elevated, and the elongated ridge of bone resembles the keel of a ship **(41-18)**.

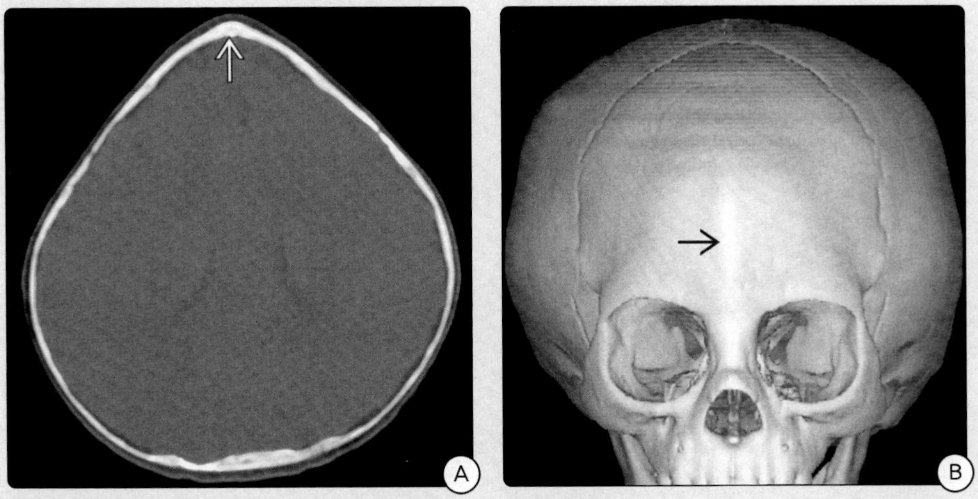

***(41-19A)** Axial NECT in an 18m child with trigonocephaly shows triangular anterior pointing of the skull ➡. The calvaria appears widened in the transverse plane. **(41-19B)** Anteroposterior projection of the 3D SSD in the same patient shows premature metopic suture synostosis with a distinct vertical ridge of bone ⇨.*

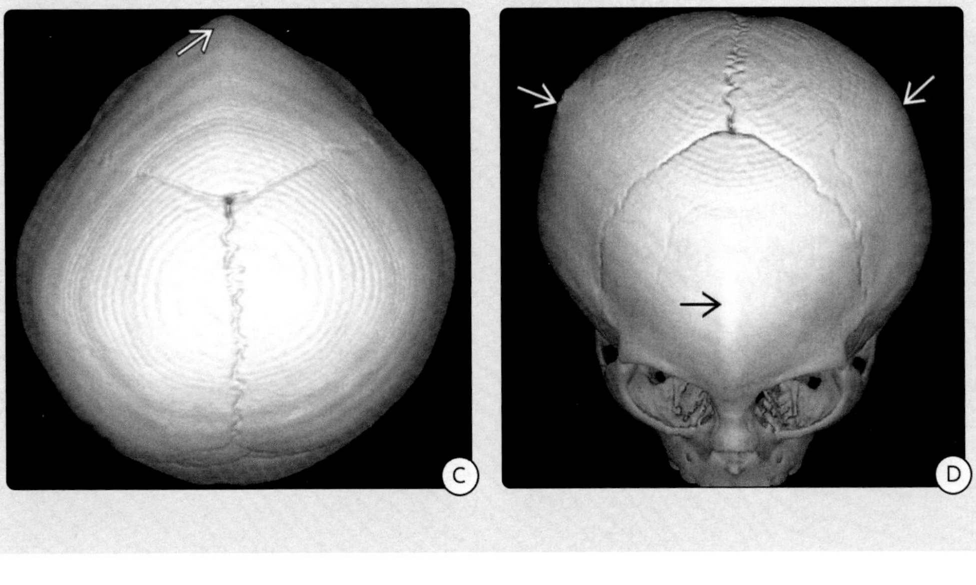

***(41-19C)** Vertex view of the SSD demonstrates the distinct triangular shape of the forehead ➡, characteristic of trigonocephaly secondary to metopic suture synostosis. **(41-19D)** Angled view shows the widened transverse diameter of the calvaria ➡ and the midline elevated bony ridge along the obliterated metopic suture ⇨. (Courtesy K. Moore, MD.)*

Brachycephaly. Brachycephaly is caused by bicoronal or bilambdoid synostosis. In such cases, the skull appears widened in the transverse dimension while shortened from front to back **(41-21A)**. Craniofacial deformities such as bilateral "harlequin" orbits—peculiar bony deformities seen as elevation/elongation of the superolateral orbit walls—are common.

Trigonocephaly. Trigonocephaly is caused by synostosis of the metopic suture. The forehead appears wedge-shaped or triangular **(41-19)**. Hypotelorism is common.

Plagiocephaly. In plagiocephaly, the calvaria is very asymmetric. Unilateral single or asymmetric multiple sutural fusions can produce this appearance. In unilateral coronal synostosis, the hemicalvaria is shortened and pointed; it may be associated with a unilateral "harlequin" eye **(41-21B)**. If the lambdoid suture is fused, the skull assumes a more trapezoid appearance with occipital flattening and posterior ear displacement **(41-20)**.

Turricephaly. Turricephaly or "towering" skull is a more extreme deformity caused by bicoronal or bilambdoid synostosis.

Oxycephaly. The coronal, sagittal, and lambdoid sutures are all fused in oxycephaly.

Kleeblattschädel. Kleeblattschädel is also known as "cloverleaf" skull. Bicoronal and bilambdoid synostoses cause an unusual pattern of bulging temporal bones, towering skull, and shallow orbits **(41-22)**.

MR Findings. MR is helpful to rule out coexisting anomalies. Hydrocephalus, corpus callosum dysgenesis, and gray matter abnormalities may be present but are more common in syndromic craniosynostoses. MRA or CTA is useful to delineate venous sinus drainage prior to surgical intervention.

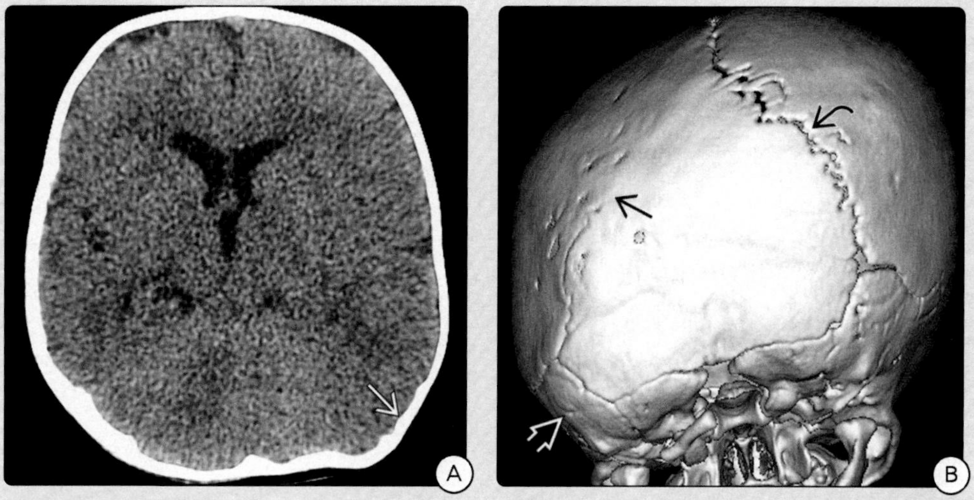

(41-20A) NECT scan in a 6m boy with plagiocephaly shows an asymmetric, flattened posterior skull bulging in the left posterior parietooccipital area ➡. (41-20B) 3D shaded surface display in the same patient shows synostosis of the left lambdoid suture ⇨ with posterior bulging of the calvaria ➡. The right lambdoid suture ⇨ appears normal. (Courtesy K. Moore, MD.)

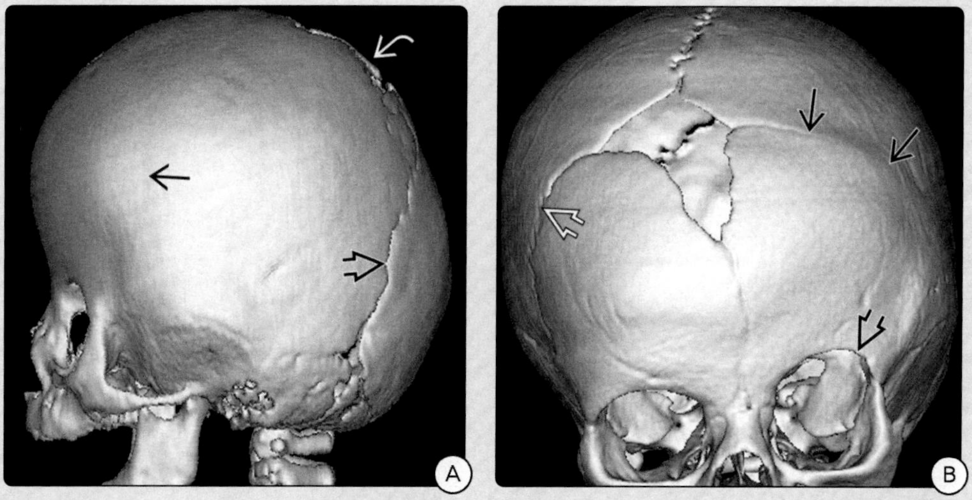

(41-21A) Newborn infant is shown with brachycephaly caused by bicoronal synostosis. Coronal suture is completely fused ⇨, while the lambdoid ⇨ and sagittal ➡ sutures are open. (41-21B) The right coronal suture ➡ appears normal. The left ⇨ is ridged and fused. Note characteristic "uplifting" of the superolateral orbital rim ⇨, giving the classic "harlequin" appearance of unilateral coronal craniosynostosis. (Courtesy K. Moore, MD.)

CRANIOSYNOSTOSIS: IMAGING

Scaphocephaly
- Most common type: sagittal suture synostosis
- Elongated skull with midline bony ridge

Brachycephaly
- Bicoronal or bilambdoid synostosis
- Coronal → widened transverse dimension ± "harlequin" orbit
- Lambdoid → flattened occiput

Trigonocephaly
- Metopic suture synostosis, "quizzical eye"

Plagiocephaly
- Unilateral coronal or multiple sutures

"Cloverleaf" Skull
- Bicoronal + bilambdoid synostoses

Syndromic Craniosynostoses

Syndromic craniosynostoses account for just 25-30% of all cranial synostoses. In syndromic disease, the craniosynostosis presents as one feature of a genetic syndrome due to chromosomal defects or mutations in genes within interconnected signaling pathways.

Compared with their sporadic, nonsyndromic counterparts, syndromic craniosynostoses are much more likely to be associated with additional craniofacial or skeletal anomalies, such as limb abnormalities, dysmorphic facial features, and skull deformity. In addition, brain malformations are common, and developmental delay is more frequent. In contrast to nonsyndromic craniosynostoses (in which the sagittal suture is most often affected), bilateral coronal synostosis is the most common pattern in these patients.

Nearly 200 inherited syndromes have been described in conjunction with craniosynostosis. More than 60 different

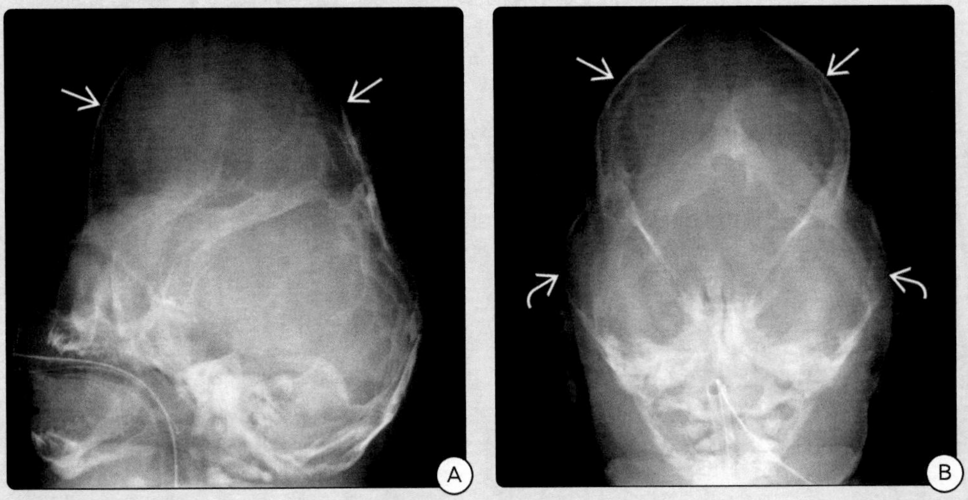

***(41-22A)** Syndromic craniosynostosis is demonstrated by this lateral radiograph in a newborn with Pfeiffer syndrome. Note the unusual "towering" configuration ➡ of the calvaria. **(41-22B)** AP radiograph shows the "towering" skull ➡ especially well. Also note the symmetrically protruding temporal fossae ➡, which create the classic "cloverleaf" appearance of Kleeblattschädel skull.*

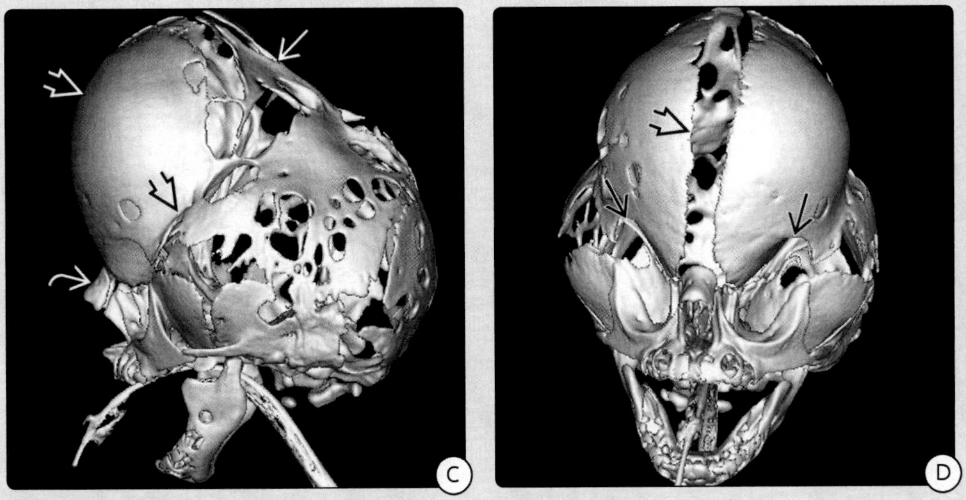

***(41-22C)** Sagittal 3D SSD shows abnormal head shape with "towering" skull ➡, frontal bossing ➡, mandibular and facial hypoplasia ➡, protruding temporal fossae ➡. Premature closure of the squamosal, coronal, lambdoid, and sagittal sutures is present. Multiple "holes" are foci of thinned calvaria. **(41-22D)** Frontal SSD shows widened metopic suture ➡ and "harlequin" orbits with superolaterally pointed rims ➡. (K. Moore, MD.)*

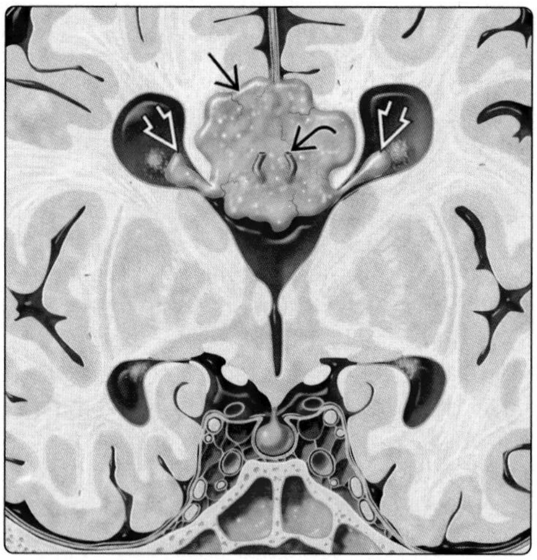

(41-23) *CC agenesis with interhemispheric lipoma ➡ encases ACAs ➡ and extends through choroidal fissure into both lateral ventricles ➡.*

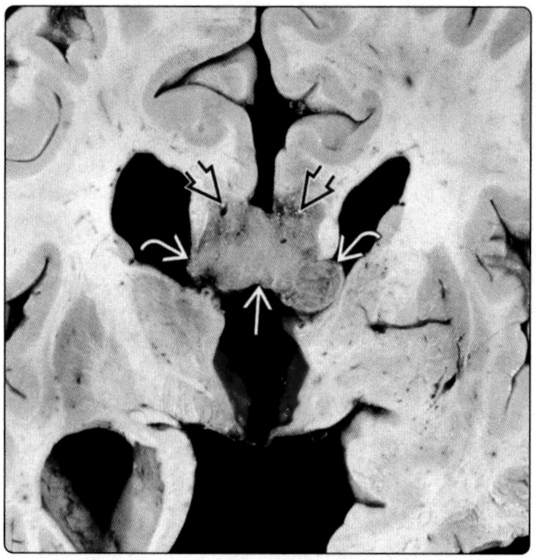

(41-24) *Autopsy shows interhemispheric lipoma ➡ encasing both ACAs ➡ and extending into lateral ventricles ➡. (Courtesy AFIP Archives.)*

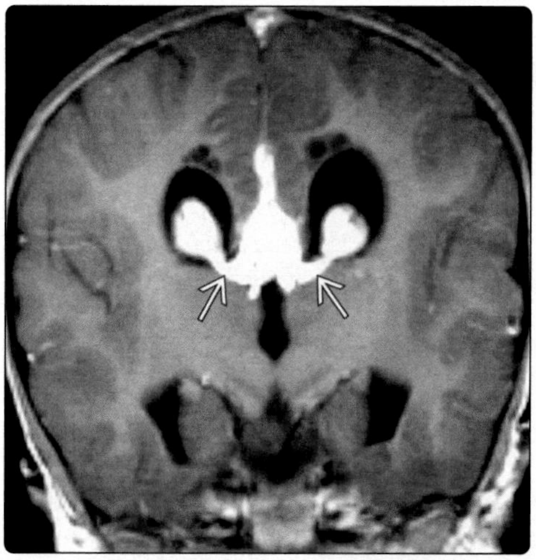

(41-25) *Coronal T1WI shows lipoma with extension through choroidal fissures into both lateral ventricles ➡ and the choroid plexi.*

mutations have been identified, reflecting the extreme genetic heterogeneity of this disorder. Mutations in the *FGFR2* gene account for several of the most severe syndromic craniosynostoses, including Apert, Pfeiffer, and Crouzon syndromes.

We first discuss acrocephalosyndactyly types 1-5, using the eponyms by which these syndromes are most commonly known. We then mention some of the rare acrocephalopolysyndactylies.

Apert Syndrome

Apert syndrome is also known as **acrocephalosyndactyly type 1**. Craniosynostosis with hypertelorism, midface hypoplasia, and cervical spine anomalies is common. Severe symmetric hand and foot syndactyly is present in most patients. Bilateral coronal synostosis is the most common calvarial anomaly.

Of all the syndromic craniosynostoses, patients with Apert syndrome are most severely affected in terms of intellectual disability, developmental delay, CNS malformations, hearing loss, and limb anomalies.

Intracranial anomalies occur in more than half of all Apert cases and include hydrocephalus, callosal dysgenesis, and abnormalities of the septi pellucidi (25-30% each). Cavum vergae and arachnoid cysts are seen in 10-12% of cases. Venous anomalies and Chiari 1 malformation are less common associations.

Acrocephalosyndactyly type2, also known as Apert-Crouzon or Crouzon syndrome, shows many of the same features seen in Apert syndrome. However, affected individuals more commonly have multiple suture calvarial involvement. Hypertelorism and exophthalmos are prominent features. Both types 1 and 2 acrocephalosyndactyly are associated with *FGFR2* mutations.

Saethre-Chotzen Syndrome

Saethre-Chotzen syndrome is also known as **acrocephalosyndactyly type 3**. A specific mutation in *TWIST1* has been associated with this disorder. Duplicated distal phalanges, cone-shaped hallux epiphysis, and syndactyly of the second and third digits are characteristic findings in the extremities.

Waardenburg Syndrome

Waardenburg syndrome (WS) is also known as **acrocephalosyndactyly type 4**. WS is characterized by pigmentation abnormalities and sensorineural hearing loss. Depigmented patches of skin and hair and vivid blue eyes or heterochromia irides are common.

At least six genes are involved in WS, including *SOX10*; mutations in these genes affect myelination. Central myelin deficiency with cerebral and cerebellar hypoplasia is common in the neurological variant of WS. Peripheral demyelinating neuropathy can result in Hirschsprung disease.

Pfeiffer Syndrome

Pfeiffer syndrome is formally known as **acrocephalosyndactyly type 5**. Multiple sutures are typically affected, and severe deformities such as a "cloverleaf" skull are common **(41-22)**.

Carpenter Syndrome

Carpenter syndrome is an autosomal-recessive **acrocephalopolysyndactyly** caused by biallelic mutations in *RAB23*. Craniosynostosis is a consistent and severe component. As the name implies, both polydactyly and syndactyly are often present. Umbilical hernia, malformed ears, mental retardation, and hypogenitalism in male patients are all common associations.

Greig Syndrome

Greig **cephalopolysyndactyly** syndrome (GCPS) is characterized by multiple limb and craniofacial anomalies. GCPS is an autosomal-dominant inherited disorder caused by heterozygous mutation or deletion of *GLI3*.

Trigonocephaly with metopic or sagittal synostosis is a distinctive presenting feature of GCPS. Pre- and postaxial polydactyly and cutaneous syndactyly of hands and feet are common. Corpus callosal dysgenesis and mild cerebral ventriculomegaly are recognized associations.

Meningeal Anomalies

Anomalies of the cranial meninges commonly accompany other congenital malformations such as Chiari 2 malformation. **Lipomas** and **arachnoid cysts** are two important intracranial abnormalities with meningeal origin. Arachnoid cysts were considered in detail in Chapter 28. We therefore conclude our discussion of congenital anomalies by focusing on lipomas.

Lipomas

The 2016 WHO places intracranial lipomas in the mesenchymal, nonmeningothelial CNS neoplasms under "Other Mesenchymal Tumours," but also notes that "whether these various lesions (i.e., lipomas and complex lipomatous lesions) are neoplasms or malformative overgrowths is yet to be determined."

We include lipomas in this chapter rather than in the discussion of intracranial neoplasms because of their frequent association with other congenital malformations.

Fat—adipose tissue—is not normally found inside the arachnoid. Therefore, any fatty tissue inside the skull or spine is abnormal. Because fat deposits commonly accompany congenital malformations such as callosal dysgenesis **(41-23)** or tethered spinal cord, imaging studies should be closely scrutinized for the presence of additional abnormalities.

Terminology

So-called ordinary lipoma is the most common of all soft tissue tumors and is composed of mature adipose tissue. "Complex lipomatous lesions" may contain other mesenchymal tissues such as striated muscle and have sometimes been referred to as choristomas.

Etiology

Intracranial lipomas are uncommon lesions whose etiology remains poorly understood. Two explanations have been offered.

Lipomas were once thought to be congenital anomalies. This theory postulates that lipomas arise as malformations of the **embryonic meninx primitiva** (the undifferentiated mesenchyme). The primitive meninx normally differentiates into the cranial meninges, invaginating along the choroid fissure of the lateral ventricle. Maldifferentiation and persistence of the meninx was thought to result in deposits of mature adipose tissue, i.e., fat, along the subpial surface of the brain and spinal cord and within the lateral ventricles.

Recent fluorescence in situ hybridization (FISH) and comparative genomic hybridization (CGH) studies have identified clonal cytogenetic aberrations in

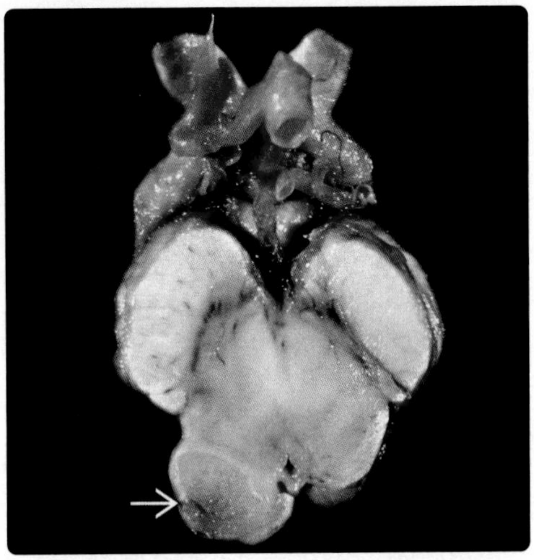

***(41-26)** Autopsy case demonstrates subpial lipoma ➡ attached to quadrigeminal plate. (Courtesy E. T. Hedley-Whyte, MD.)*

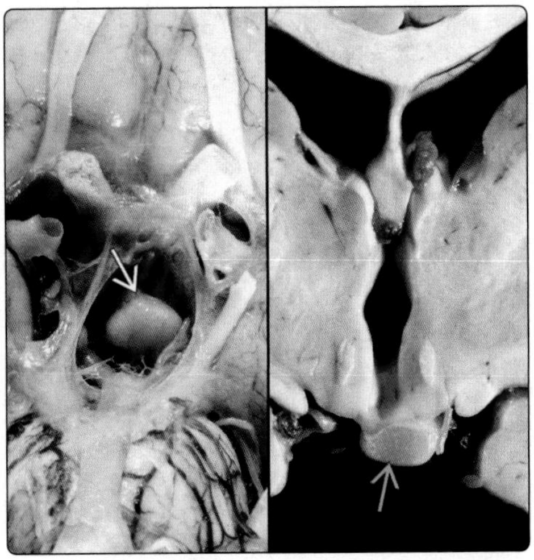

***(41-27)** (L) Autopsy shows suprasellar lipoma ➡. (R) Coronal section shows lipoma ➡ attached to hypothalamus. (J. Townsend, MD.)*

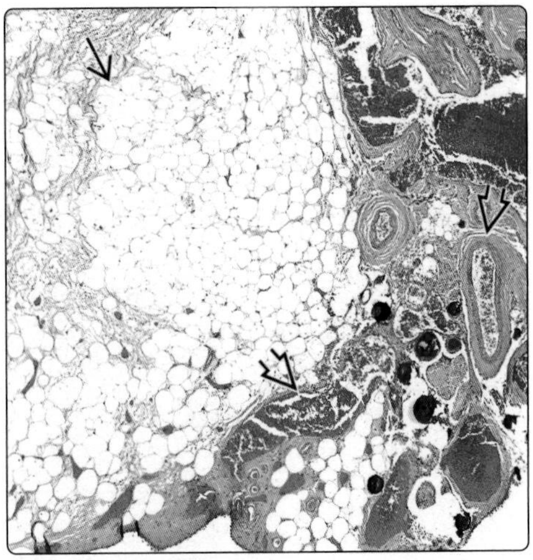

***(41-28)** Low-power photomicrograph shows normal fat cells ➡. Prominent vessels ➡ course through lesion. (Courtesy E. Rushing, MD.)*

nearly 60% of ordinary systemic lipomas. The 12q13-15 region is the most commonly involved site.

Pathology

Location. Nonsyndromic lipomas are usually solitary lesions that can be found in virtually any location in the body, including the CNS. Nearly 80% of intracranial lipomas are supratentorial, and most occur in or near the midline. The interhemispheric fissure is the most common overall site (40-50%) **(41-24)**. Lipomas curve over the dorsal corpus callosum, often extending through the choroidal fissures into the lateral ventricles or choroid plexus **(41-25)**.

Between 15-25% are located in the quadrigeminal region, usually attached to the inferior colliculi or superior vermis **(41-26)**. Approximately 15% are suprasellar, attached to the undersurface of the hypothalamus or infundibular stalk **(41-27)**. About 5% of lipomas are found in the sylvian fissure.

Approximately 20% of lipomas are infratentorial. The cerebellopontine angle cistern is the most common posterior fossa site (10%).

Size and Number. Lipomas are generally solitary lesions that vary from tiny, barely perceptible fatty collections to huge bulky masses. Most are less than 5 cm in diameter.

Gross Pathology. Lipomas appear as bright yellow, lobulated soft masses. They usually adhere to the pia and underlying parenchyma. At least one-third encase adjacent vessels and/or cranial nerves **(41-24)**.

Microscopic Features. Lipomas are composed of mature, nonneoplastic-appearing adipose tissue with relatively uniform fat cells **(41-28)**. Patchy hyalinization and calcification can be present.

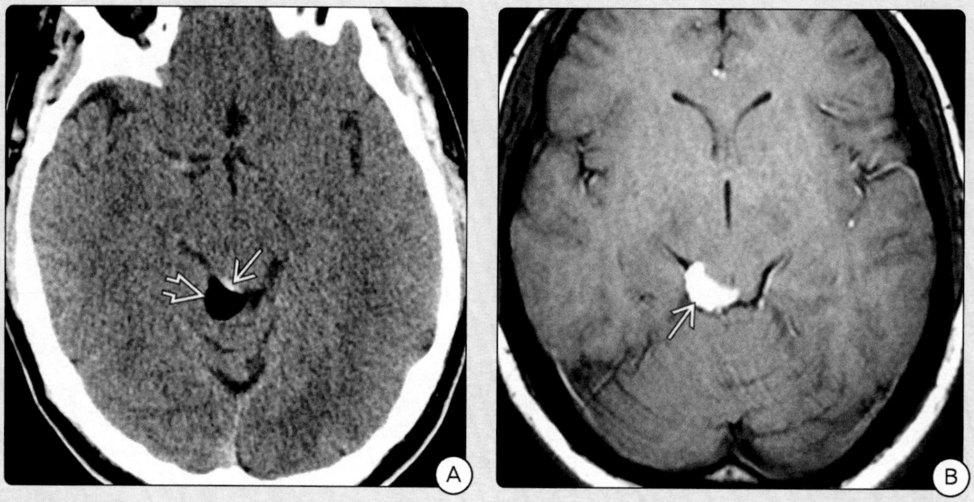

***(41-29A)** Axial NECT scan shows well-delineated, hypodense (-75 HU) lipoma ➡ attached to the quadrigeminal plate. Some calcification is present ➡. **(41-29B)** Axial T1WI shows that the hyperintense lipoma ➡ is attached to the quadrigeminal plate without a distinct medial border.*

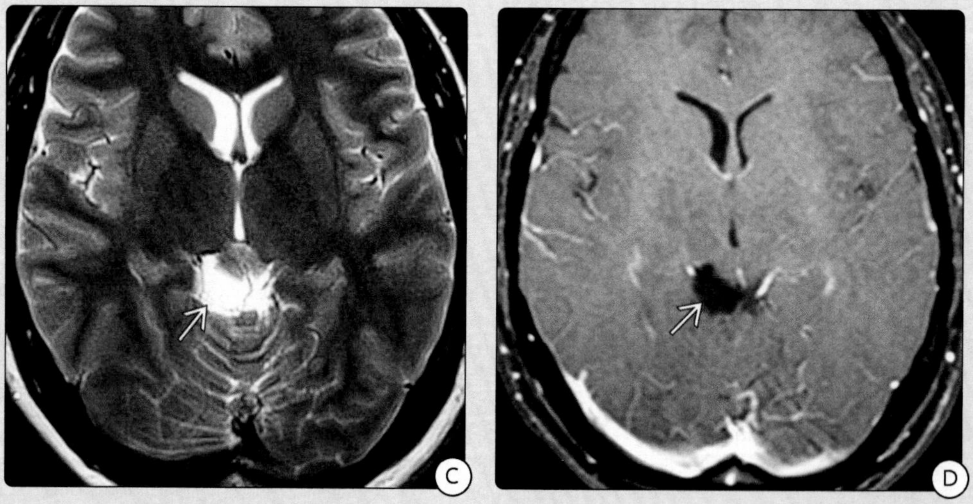

***(41-29C)** FSE T2WI shows that the lipoma ➡ remains hyperintense (because of J-coupling) and cannot be distinguished from the adjacent CSF in the quadrigeminal cistern. **(41-29D)** T1 C+ FS demonstrates that the lipoma ➡ suppresses completely and does not enhance.*

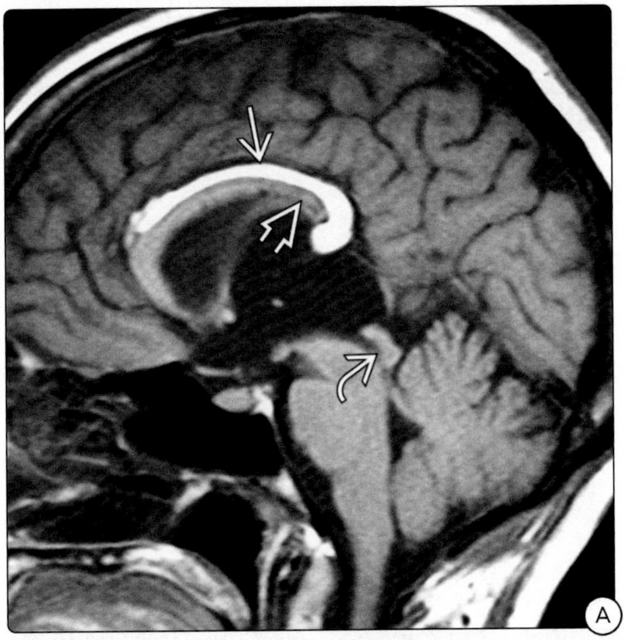

(41-30A) Sagittal T1WI shows aqueductal stenosis ➡, curvilinear lipoma ➡ with thin posterior body, and absent splenium of corpus callosum ➡.

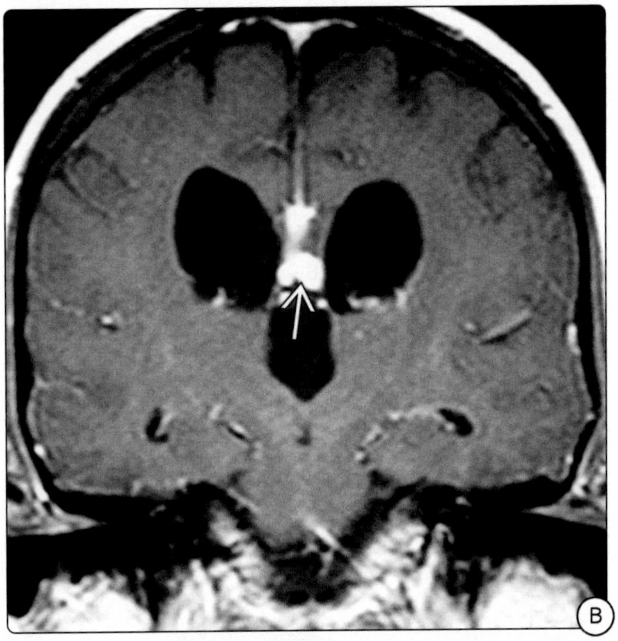

(41-30B) Coronal T1 C+ scan demonstrates the interhemispheric lipoma ➡. (Courtesy A. Maydell, MD.)

INTRACRANIAL LIPOMAS: ETIOLOGY AND PATHOLOGY

Etiology

- Two theories
  - Maldifferentiation of embryonic meninx primitiva
  - Genetic aberration

Pathology

- Usually solitary
- Supratentorial (80%)
  - Interhemispheric fissure (40-50%)
  - Quadrigeminal (15-25%)
  - Suprasellar (15%)
- Infratentorial (20%)
- Gross appearance: lobulated, yellow
- Microscopic: mature, nonneoplastic adipose tissue

Clinical Issues

Epidemiology and Demographics. Lipomas are relatively rare, accounting for less than 0.5% of intracranial masses. They can be found in patients of all ages. There is a slight female predominance.

Presentation. Lipomas are rarely symptomatic and are usually incidental findings on imaging studies. Headache, seizure, hypothalamic disturbances, and cranial nerve deficits have been reported in a few cases.

Syndromic intracranial lipomas occur in encephalocraniocutaneous lipomatosis (see Chapter 39) and Pai syndrome (cutaneous lipomas and facial clefts).

Natural History. Lipomas are benign lesions that remain stable in size. Some may expand with corticosteroid use.

Treatment Options. Lipomas are generally considered "leave me alone" lesions. Because they encase vessels and nerves, surgery has high morbidity and mortality.

Imaging

General Features. Lipomas are seen as well-delineated, somewhat lobulated extraaxial masses that exhibit fat density/signal intensity.

Two morphologic configurations of interhemispheric fissure lipomas are recognized on imaging studies: a **curvilinear** type (a thin, pencil-like mass that curves around the corpus callosum body and splenium) and a **tubulonodular** type (a large, bulky interhemispheric fatty mass). Dystrophic calcification occurs in both types but is more common in tubulonodular lesions.

CT Findings. NECT scans show a hypodense mass that measures -50 to -100 HU. Calcification varies from extensive—nearly two-thirds of bulky tubulonodular interhemispheric lipomas are partially calcified—to none, generally seen in small lesions in other locations **(41-29A)** **(41-31A)**. Lipomas do not enhance on CECT scans.

MR Findings. Lipomas follow fat signal on all imaging sequences. They appear homogeneously hyperintense on T1WI and become hypointense with fat suppression **(41-29)**. Lipomas exhibit chemical-shift artifact in the frequency-encoding direction.

Signal on T2WI varies. Fat becomes hypointense on standard T2WI but remains moderately hyperintense on fast spin-echo studies because of J-coupling. Fat is hypointense on STIR and appears hyperintense on FLAIR. No enhancement is seen following contrast administration.

On SWI, lipomas show hyperintensity surrounded by a low-signal intensity band along the fat-water interface that is more prominent than seen on T2* GRE sequences.

Other CNS malformations are common. The most frequent are corpus callosum anomalies. These range from mild dysgenesis (usually with curvilinear lipomas) **(41-30)** to agenesis (with bulky tubulonodular lipomas) **(41-25)** **(41-31)**.

Differential Diagnosis

Although fat does not appear inside the normal CNS, it *can* be found within the dura and cavernous sinus. **Metaplastic falx ossification** is a normal variant that can resemble an interhemispheric lipoma. Dense cortical bone surrounding T1 hyperintense, fatty marrow is the typical finding.

The major differential diagnosis of an intracranial lipoma is an unruptured **dermoid cyst**. Dermoids generally measure 20-40 HU, often calcify, and demonstrate more heterogeneous signal intensity on MR.

INTRACRANIAL LIPOMAS

Clinical Issues
- Less than 0.5% of intracranial masses
- Usually found incidentally, "leave me alone" lesions

Imaging
- NECT: -50 to -100 HU
  - Ca++ rare except in tubulonodular lesions
- MR: "just like fat"
  - Other intracranial malformations common
  - Often surrounds, encases vessels/nerves

Differential Diagnosis
- Dermoid cyst
- Falx ossification

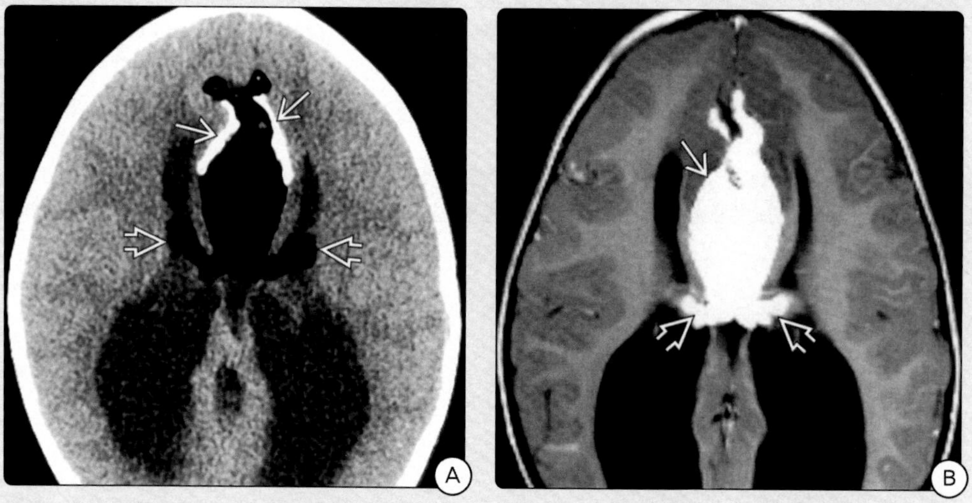

***(41-31A)** Axial NECT scan shows corpus callosum agenesis with parallel, nonconverging lateral ventricles. Large, partially calcified tubulonodular interhemispheric lipoma extends into both lateral ventricles through choroidal fissures. **(41-31B)** Axial T1WI shows hyperintense lipoma between the nonconverging lateral ventricles. Extension into the lateral ventricles through the choroid fissures is especially well demonstrated.*

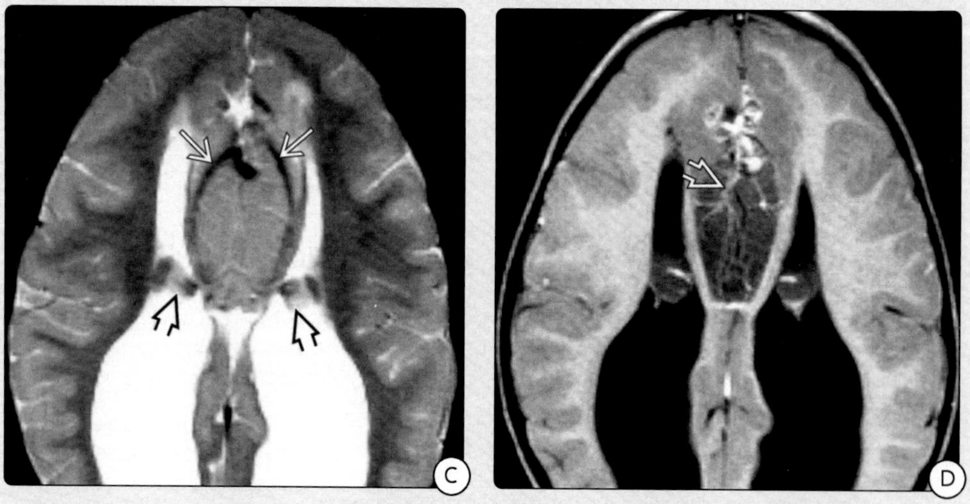

***(41-31C)** Standard T2WI shows that the lipoma is hypointense; the calcifications show as curvilinear hypointensities. Note extension into lateral ventricles. **(41-31D)** Axial T1 C+ FS scan shows that the lipoma becomes profoundly hypointense. Note enhancing vessels coursing through the lipoma.*

Selected References

Normal Development and Anatomy of the Skull Base

Conley LM et al: Imaging of the central skull base. Radiol Clin North Am. 55(1):53-67, 2017

Bernard S et al: The human occipital bone: review and update on its embryology and molecular development. Childs Nerv Syst. 31(12):2217-23, 2015

Blaser SI et al: Skull base development and craniosynostosis. Pediatr Radiol. 45 Suppl 3:S485-96, 2015

Rijken BF et al: The formation of the foramen magnum and its role in developing ventriculomegaly and Chiari I malformation in children with craniosynostosis syndromes. J Craniomaxillofac Surg. 43(7):1042-8, 2015

Zhang Q et al: Morphological and morphometric study on sphenoid and basioccipital ossification in normal human fetuses. Congenit Anom (Kyoto). 51(3):138-48, 2011

Cephaloceles

Yucetas SC et al: A retrospective analysis of neonatal encephalocele predisposing factors and outcomes. Pediatr Neurosurg. 52(2):73-76, 2017

Ramdurg SR et al: Pediatric encephaloceles: a series of 20 cases over a period of 3 years. J Pediatr Neurosci. 10(4):317-20, 2015

Occipital Cephaloceles

Ivashchuk G et al: Chiari III malformation: a comprehensive review of this enigmatic anomaly. Childs Nerv Syst. 31(11):2035-40, 2015

Frontoethmoidal Cephaloceles

Zabsonre DS et al: Frontoethmoidal cephalocele: our experience of eleven cases managed surgically. Pediatr Neurosurg. 50(1):7-11, 2015

Tirumandas M et al: Nasal encephaloceles: a review of etiology, pathophysiology, clinical presentations, diagnosis, treatment, and complications. Childs Nerv Syst. 29(5):739-44, 2013

Parietal Cephaloceles

Mazzucchi E et al: Parietal intradiploic encephalocele in an adult: a delayed complication of pediatric head injury? Childs Nerv Syst. 33(2):217-219, 2017

Shi C et al: Symptomatic parietal intradiploic encephalocele-a case report and literature review. J Neurol Surg Rep. 78(1):e43-e48, 2017

Demir MK et al: Atretic cephaloceles: a comprehensive analysis of historical cohort. Childs Nerv Syst. 32(12):2327-2337, 2016

Santos SF et al: Atretic parietal encephalocoele. BMJ Case Rep. 2016, 2016

Skull Base Cephaloceles

Ogiwara H et al: Surgical treatment of transsphenoidal encephaloceles: transpalatal versus combined transpalatal and transcranial approach. J Neurosurg Pediatr. 11(5):505-10, 2013

Persistent Craniopharyngeal Canal

Sajisevi M et al: Nasopharyngeal masses arising from embryologic remnants of the clivus: a case series. J Neurol Surg Rep. 76(2):e253-e257, 2015

Alatzoglou KS et al: SOX3 deletion in mouse and human is associated with persistence of the craniopharyngeal canal. J Clin Endocrinol Metab. 99(12):E2702-8, 2014

Craniosynostoses

Craniosynostosis Overview

Lattanzi W et al: Genetic advances in craniosynostosis. Am J Med Genet A. 173(5):1406-1429, 2017

Nonsyndromic Craniosynostosis

Lee BS et al: Management options of non-syndromic sagittal craniosynostosis. J Clin Neurosci. 39:28-34, 2017

Syndromic Craniosynostoses

Lee BS et al: Management options of non-syndromic sagittal craniosynostosis. J Clin Neurosci. 39:28-34, 2017

Fernandes MB et al: Apert and Crouzon syndromes-cognitive development, brain abnormalities, and molecular aspects. Am J Med Genet A. 170(6):1532-7, 2016

Hwang SK et al: Update of diagnostic evaluation of craniosynostosis with a focus on pediatric systematic evaluation and genetic studies. J Korean Neurosurg Soc. 59(3):214-8, 2016

Saal HM: Genetic evaluation for craniofacial conditions. Facial Plast Surg Clin North Am. 24(4):405-425, 2016

Wang JC et al: Syndromic craniosynostosis. Facial Plast Surg Clin North Am. 24(4):531-543, 2016

Meningeal Anomalies

Lipomas

Atallah A et al: Limitations and pitfalls in prenatal diagnosis of pericallosal curvilinear lipoma based on a specific imaging pattern. Ultrasound Obstet Gynecol. ePub, 2017

Agostini A et al: Molecular characterization of the t(4;12)(q27~28;q14~15) chromosomal rearrangement in lipoma. Oncol Lett. 12(3):1701-1704, 2016

Niwa T et al: Interhemispheric lipoma, callosal anomaly, and malformations of cortical development: a case series. Neuropediatrics. 47(2):115-8, 2016

Yilmaz MB et al: Pericallosal lipomas: a series of 10 cases with clinical and radiological features. Turk Neurosurg. 26(3):364-8, 2016

Yilmaz MB et al: Lipoma of the quadrigeminal cistern: report of 12 cases with clinical and radiological features. Turk Neurosurg. 25(1):16-20, 2015

Erol FS et al: How innocent is corpus callosum dysgenesis? Pediatr Neurosurg. 49(1):24-8, 2013

Mehemed TM et al: Fat-water interface on susceptibility-weighted imaging and gradient-echo imaging: comparison of phantoms to intracranial lipomas. AJR Am J Roentgenol. 201(4):902-7, 2013

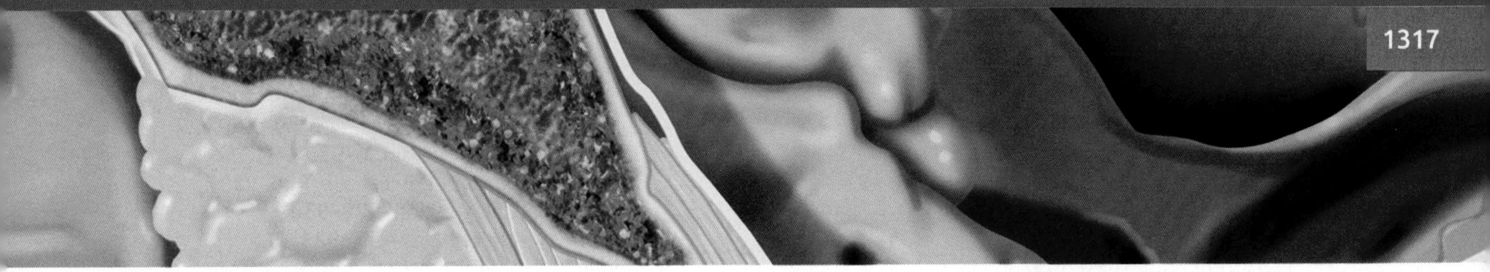

Index

Index

B

Index

Index

E

Index

G

H

I

J

K

L

N

Index

P

Index

Q

R

S

T

U

V

W

X

Y

Z